T0393302

Wintrobe's
CLINICAL
HEMATOLOGY

FIFTEENTH EDITION

VOLUME 1

Wintrobe's CLINICAL HEMATOLOGY

FIFTEENTH EDITION

Editors

Robert T. Means, Jr., MD, MACP
Professor of Internal Medicine
Clinical Professor of Pathology
James H. Quillen College of Medicine
East Tennessee State University
Johnson City, Tennessee

George M. Rodgers, MD, PhD
Professor of Medicine
Department of Medicine/Hematology
University of Utah Health Sciences Center
Salt Lake City, Utah

Bertil Glader, MD, PhD
Stanford Medicine Professor of Pediatric
 Hematology/Oncology
Professor of Pathology (by courtesy)
Medical Director, RBC Special Studies Lab
Stanford University School of Medicine
Stanford, California

Daniel A. Arber, MD
Donald West and Mary Elizabeth King Professor
 and Chair
Department of Pathology
University of Chicago
Chicago, Illinois

Frederick R. Appelbaum, MD
Deputy Director
Fred Hutchinson Cancer Research Center
Professor
University of Washington School of Medicine
Seattle, Washington

Angela Dispenzieri, MD
Serene and Francis C. Durling Professor of Medicine
Division of Hematology and Division of Clinical Chemistry
Departments of Internal Medicine and Laboratory Medicine
Mayo Clinic
Rochester, Minnesota

Todd A. Fehniger, MD, PhD
Professor of Medicine
Division of Oncology
Department of Medicine
Washington University School of Medicine
Saint Louis, Missouri

Laura C. Michaelis, MD
Armand J. Quick Professor of Medicine
Chief, Division of Hematology/Oncology
Medical College of Wisconsin
Milwaukee, Wisconsin

John P. Leonard, MD
Senior Associate Dean for Innovation and Initiatives
Richard T. Silver Distinguished Professor of Hematology
 and Medical Oncology
Weill Department of Medicine
Weill Cornell Medicine
New York Presbyterian Hospital
New York, New York

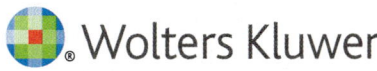
. Wolters Kluwer

Philadelphia • Baltimore • New York • London
Buenos Aires • Hong Kong • Sydney • Tokyo

Acquisitions Editor: Joe Cho
Associate Director of Content Development: Anne Malcolm
Development Editor: Eric McDermott
Editorial Coordinator: Remington Fernando
Editorial Assistant: Kristen Kardoley
Marketing Manager: Kirsten Watrud
Production Project Manager: Frances Gunning
Manager, Graphic Arts & Design: Stephen Druding
Manufacturing Coordinator: Lisa Bowling
Prepress Vendor: TNQ Technologies

Fifteenth edition

9 8 7 6 5 4 3 2 1

Printed in Mexico.

Library of Congress Cataloging-in-Publication Data

ISBN-13: 978-1-975184-69-8

Cataloging in Publication data available on request from publisher.

---

shop.lww.com

QUADM0623

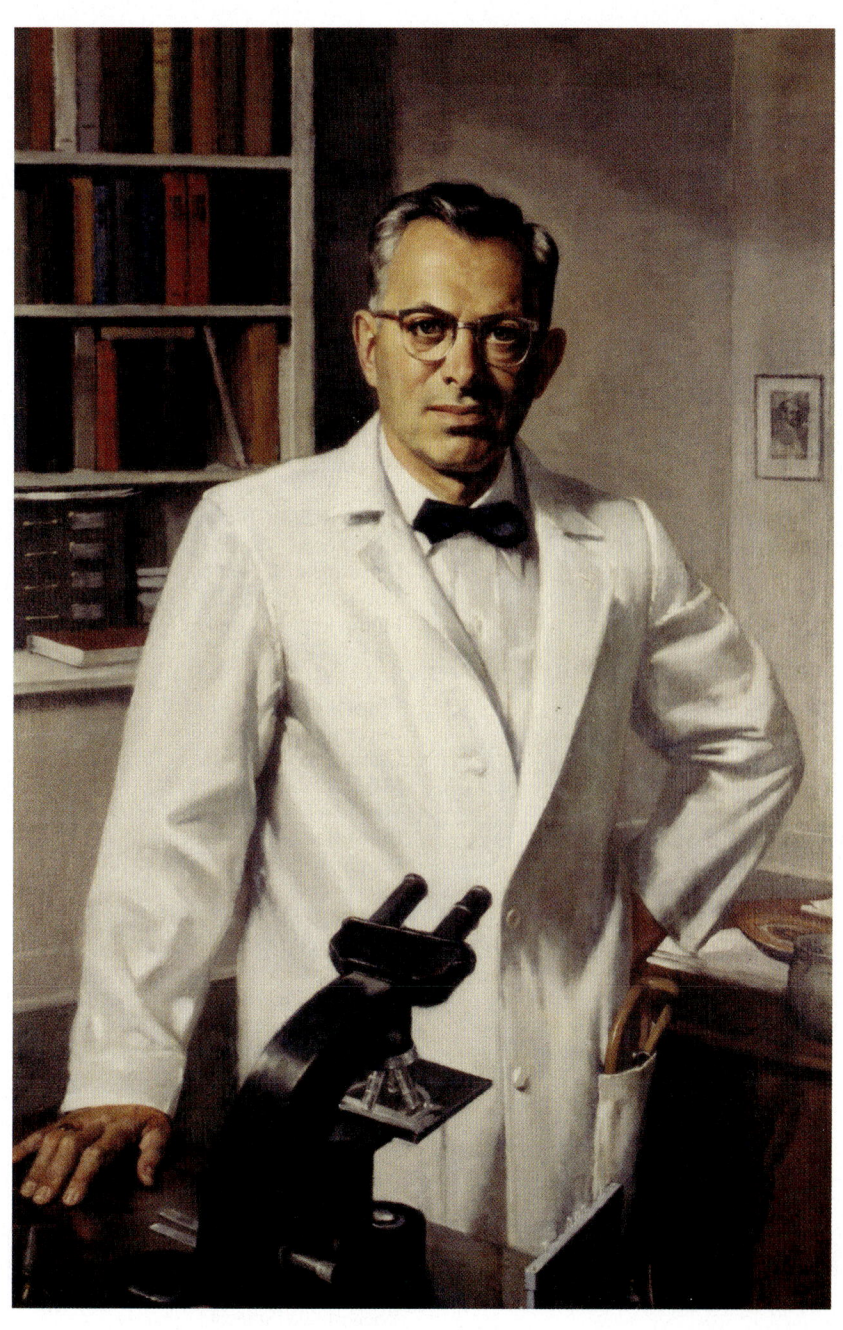

Contributors

Yasmin M. Abaza, MD
Assistant Professor of Medicine
Division of Hematology and Oncology, Leukemia Program
Robert H. Lurie Comprehensive Cancer Center
Northwestern University Feinberg School of Medicine
Chicago, Illinois

Archana M. Agarwal, MD
Professor
Department of Pathology
University of Utah Health Sciences
Salt Lake City, Utah

Jessica K. Altman, MD
Professor of Medicine
Director, Leukemia Program
Division of Hematology and Oncology
Robert H. Lurie Comprehensive Cancer Center
Northwestern University Feinberg School of Medicine
Chicago, Illinois

Richard F. Ambinder, MD, PhD
Professor
Department of Oncology
Johns Hopkins School of Medicine
Baltimore, Maryland

Claudio Anasetti, MD
Emeritus Member
Department of Blood & Marrow Transplantation and Cellular
    Immunotherapy
Moffitt Cancer Center
Tampa, Florida

Jennifer Andrews, MD
Associate Professor
Departments of Pathology, Microbiology & Immunology (Division
    of Transfusion Medicine) and Pediatrics (Division of Hematology/
    Oncology)
Vanderbilt University Medical Center
Nashville, Tennessee

Stephen M. Ansell, MD, PhD
Professor of Medicine
Division of Hematology
Mayo Clinic
Rochester, Minnesota

Frederick R. Appelbaum, MD
Deputy Director
Fred Hutchinson Cancer Research Center
Professor
University of Washington School of Medicine
Seattle, Washington

Daniel A. Arber, MD
Donald West and Mary Elizabeth King Professor and Chair
Department of Pathology
University of Chicago,
Chicago, Illinois

Yan Asmann, PhD
Associate Professor of Biomedical Informatics
Mayo Clinic
Jacksonville, Florida

Ehab Atallah, MD
Professor of Medicine
Department of Medicine
Medical College of Wisconsin
Milwuakee, Wisconsin

Maria R. Baer, MD
Professor
Department of Medicine
University of Maryland School of Medicine
Baltimore, Maryland

James C. Barton, MD
Clinical Professor of Medicine
Department of Medicine
University of Alabama at Birmingham
Medical Director
Southern Iron Disorders Center
Brookwood Medical Center
Birmingham, Alabama

Elisabeth M. Battinelli, MD, PhD
Associate Professor
Division of Hematology
Associate Chief of Research Hematology Division
Associate Director Special Coagulation Laboratory
Brigham and Women's Hospital
Harvard Medical School
Harvard Institute of Medicine
Boston, Massachusetts

Linda B. Baughn, PhD, FACMG
Associate Professor
Department of Laboratory Medicine and Pathology
Division of Hematopathology
Mayo Clinic
Rochester, Minnesota

Jeffrey J. Bednarski II, MD, PhD
Assistant Professor
Pediatrics
Washington University in St. Louis School of Medicine
St. Louis, Missouri

A. Dean Befus, BSc, MSc, PhD
Professor Emeritus
Department of Medicine
University of Alberta
Edmonton, Alberta, Canada

Trisha R. Berger, PhD
Department of Cancer Center
Massachusetts General Hospital
Charlestown, Massachusetts

Peter Leif Bergsagel, MD
Consultant
Department of Medicine
Mayo Clinic Arizona
Scottsdale, Arizona

Nancy Berliner, MD
Chief, Division of Hematology
Department of Medicine
Prigham and Women's Hospital
Boston, Massachusetts

Brian C. Betts, MD
Associate Professor of Medicine
Division of Hematology, Oncology, and Transplantation
Program Co-Leader, Transplantation and Cellular Therapy, Masonic
    Cancer Center
Minneapolis, Minnesota

Venetia Bigley, MB, BChir, PhD
MRC Senior Clinical Fellow, Honorary Consultant Hematologist
Translational and Clinical Research Institute
Newcastle University
Newcastle upon Tyne, United Kingdom

Daniel K. Borger, MS
MD/PhD Candidate
Ruth L. and David S. Gottesman Institute for Stem Cell Biology and
    Regenerative Medicine
Albert Einstein College of Medicine
Bronx, New York

Justin C. Boucher, PhD
Postdoc Fellow
Department of Clinical Science
Moffitt Cancer Center
Tampa, Florida

Evan M. Braunstein, MD, PhD
Assistant Professor
Department of Medicine
Johns Hopkins School of Medicine
Baltimore, Maryland

Robert A. Brodsky, MD
Professor of Medicine and Oncology
Division of Hematology, Department of Medicine
Johns Hopkins University
Baltimore, Maryland

Kathleen E. Brummel-Ziedins, PhD
Professor
Department of Biochemistry, Retired
University of Vermont
Colchester, Vermont

Francis K. Buadi, MB, ChB
Associate Professor
Division of Hematology
Department of Medicine
Mayo Clinic
Rochester, Minnesota

Loredana Bury, PhD
Department of Medicine and Surgery
Section of Internal and Cardiovascular Medicine
University of Perugia
Perugia, Italy

Carrie L. Butler, PhD
Assistant Professor
Department of Pathology & Laboratory Medicine
David Geffen School of Medicine
University of California Los Angeles
Los Angeles, California

David C. Calverley, MD
Clinical Associate Professor of Medicine
Department of Medicine
University of British Columbia
Vancouver, British Columbia, Canada

Paul A. Carpenter, MBBS, BSc(Med)
Medical Director Long Term Follow-Up
Fred Hutchinson Cancer Center
Professor of Pediatrics
University of Washington
Seattle, Washington

J. Michael Cecka, PhD
Professor Emeritus
Department of Pathology and Laboratory Medicine
University of California at Los Angeles
Los Angeles, California

Devon S. Chabot-Richards, MD
Associate Professor
Department of Hematopathology and Molecular Genetic Pathology
University of New Mexico
Albuquerque, New Mexico

Namrata S. Chandhok, MD
Assistant Professor of Clinical Medicine
Department of Hematology
University of Miami
Sylvester Comprehensive Cancer Center
Miami, Florida

William C. Chapman, MD
Professor
Department of Surgery
Washington University in St Louis
St Louis, Missouri

William C. Chapman, Jr., MD
Resident Physician
Department of Surgery
Washington University in St Louis
St Louis, Missouri

Robert D. Christensen, MD
Professor
Department of Pediatrics
University of Utah Health
Salt Lake City, Utah

Matthew Collin, BM, BCh, MA, DPhil
Professor of Hematology
Newcastle University
Newcastle upon Tyne, United Kingdom

Utpal P. Davé, MD
Co-director Hematopoiesis and Hematologic Malignancies Program
   at the Indiana University Melvin and Bren Simon Comprehensive
   Cancer Center and R.L. Roudebush VA Medical Center
Associate Professor of Medicine
Associate Professor of Microbiology and Immunology
Division of Hematology/Oncology
Department of Medicine
Indiana University School of Medicine
Indianapolis, Indiana

Marco L. Davila, MD, PhD
Senior Member
Department of Blood and Marrow Transplantation-Cellular
   Immunotherapy
H. Lee Moffitt Cancer Center and Research Institute
Tampa, Florida

Najet Debili, PhD
UMR (unité mixte de recherche) 1287
INSERM (Institut nationale de la Santé et de la recherche)
Université Paris Saclay
Gustave Roussy
Villejuif, France

Michael W. Deininger, MD, PhD
Executive Vice President and Chief Scientific Officer, Versiti
Director and Senior Investigator, Versiti Blood Research Institute
Cathy and Mike White Chair of Hematology
Professor, Division of Hematology and Oncology, Department of
   Medicine
Milwaukee, Wisconsin

Judah A. Denburg, MD, FRCP(C)
William J. Walsh Chair in Medicine
Michael G. DeGroote School of Medicine
Professor of Medicine
Faculty of Health Sciences
McMaster University
Hamilton, Ontario, Canada

Pinkal Desai, MD, MPH
Assistant Professor of Medicine
Weill Cornell Medical College
Charles, Lillian, and Betty Neuwirth Clinical Scholar in
   Oncology
Clinical Director EIPM Molecular Aging Institute
Leukemia Program
New York-Presbyterian Hospital
New York, New York

Robert J. Desnick, MD, PhD
Dean for Genetics and Genomic Medicine
Department of Genetics and Genomic Sciences
Icahn School of Medicine at Mount Sinai/ Mount Sinai Health
   System
New York, New York

Amy E. DeZern, MD, MHS
Associate Professor of Oncology and Medicine
Division of Hematologic Malignancies
Sidney Kimmel Comprehensive Cancer Center
The Johns Hopkins University School of Medicine
Baltimore, Maryland

Bhagirathbhai Dholaria, MBBS
Assistant Professor
Department of Hematology Oncology
Vanderbilt University Medical Center
Nashville, Tennessee

David Dingli, MD, PhD
Professor of Medicine
Department of Hematology and Internal Medicine
Mayo Clinic College of Science and Medicine
Rochester, Minnesota

Angela Dispenzieri, MD
Serene and Francis C. Durling Professor of Medicine
Division of Hematology and Division of Clinical Chemistry
Departments of Internal Medicine and Laboratory Medicine
Mayo Clinic
Rochester, Minnesota

Alexander Drelick, MD
Assistant Professor
Department of Medicine, Division of Infectious Diseases-
   Transplantation-Oncology Program
Weill Cornell Medical College
New York, New York

Ashkan Emadi, MD, PhD
Professor of Medicine and Pharmacology
Associate Director for Clinical Research
Marlene & Stewart Greenebaum Comprehensive Cancer Center
Director, Translational Genomics Laboratory
University of Maryland School of Medicine
Baltimore, Maryland

Jeremie E. Estepp, MD
Director of Global Hematology
Departments of Global Pediatric Medicine and Hematology
St. Jude Children's Research Hospital
Memphis, Tennessee

Stephen J. Everse, PhD
Associate Professor
Department of Biochemistry
Larner College of Medicine
University of Vermont
Burlington, Vermont

Emanuela Falcinelli, PhD
Department of Medicine and Surgery, Section of Internal and
   Cardiovascular Medicine
University of Perugia
Perugia, Italy

Min Fang, MD, PhD, FACMG
Professor, Clinical Research Division, Fred Hutchinson Cancer
   Center
Professor of Laboratory Medicine and Pathology
University of Washington Medical Center
Director of Cytogenetics
Seattle, Washington

Rawan G. Faramand, MD
Assistant Professor
Blood and Marrow Transplant and Cellular Immunotherapy
H. Lee Moffitt Cancer Center
Tampa, Florida

Todd A. Fehniger, MD, PhD
Professor of Medicine
Division of Oncology
Department of Medicine
Washington University School of Medicine
Saint Louis, Missouri

Andrew L. Feldman, MD
Professor
Department of Laboratory Medicine and Pathology
Mayo Clinic College of Medicine
Rochester, Minnesota

Mark D. Fleming, MD, DPhil
Pathologist-in-Chief
Department of Pathology
Boston Children's Hospital
Boston, Massachusetts

Rafael Fonseca, MD
Chief Innovation Officer
Getz Family Professor of Cancer, Distinguished Mayo Investigator
Division of Hematology and Oncology
Mayo Clinic Arizona
Phoenix, Arizona

Francine Foss, MD
Professor of Medicine
Departments of Hematology and Stem Cell Therapies
Yale University School of Medicine
New Haven, Connecticut

Aharon G. Freud, MD, PhD
Associate Professor
Department of Pathology
The Ohio State University
Columbus, Ohio

Richard C. Friedberg, MD, PhD, FCAP
President
8064 Associates
Longmeadow, Massachusetts

Debra L. Friedman, MD, MS
Professor of Pediatrics, Division Director
Department of Pediatric Hematology and Oncology
Vanderbilt University Medical Center
Nashville, Tennessee

Patrick G. Gallagher, MD
Professor
Departments of Pediatrics, Pathology, and Genetics
Yale University School of Medicine
New Haven, Connecticut

Varsha Gandhi, PhD
Professor and Chair ad interim
Department of Experimental Therapeutics
The University of Texas MD Anderson Cancer Center
Houston, Texas

Eric A. Gehrie, MD
Executive Physician Director of Direct Patient Care and Emerging
    Cell and Gene Therapy Solutions
American Red Cross
Washington, DC

Tracy I. George, MD
Professor of Pathology
Spencer Fox Eccles School of Medicine at the University of Utah
President and Chief Scientific Officer
ARUP Laboratories
Salt Lake City, Utah

Morie A. Gertz, MD
Consultant
Department of Hematology
Mayo Clinic
Rochester, Minnesota

Florent Ginhoux, PhD
Directeur de Laboratoire
Gustave Roussy Cancer Campus, Villejuif, France
Institut National de la Santé et de la Recherche
    Médicale (INSERM) U1015
Equipe Labellisée – Ligue Nationale contre le Cancer, Villejuif,
    France
Singapore Immunology Network (SIgN), Agency fora Science,
    Technology, and Research (A*STAR), Singapore
Shanghai Institute of Immunology
Shanghai Jiao Tong University School of Medicine, Shanghai, China
Translational Immunology Institute
SingHealth Duke-NUS Academic Medical Centre, Singapore

Bertil Glader, MD, PhD
Stanford Medicine Professor of Pediatric Hematology/Oncology
Professor of Pathology (by courtesy)
Medical Director, RBC Special Studies Lab
Stanford University School of Medicine
Stanford, California

Ronald S. Go, MD
Hematologist
Department of Medicine
Mayo Clinic
Rochester, Minnesota

Wilson I. Gonsalves, MD
Consultant, Associate Professor of Medicine
Department of Hematology
Mayo Clinic
Rochester, Minnesota

Lawrence T. Goodnough, MD
Professor of Pathology and Hematology
Department of Pathology
Stanford University School of Medicine
Stanford, California

Jason Gotlib, MD, MS
Professor of Medicine (Hematology)
Stanford Cancer Institute / Stanford University School of Medicine
Stanford, California

Rachael F. Grace, MD, MMSc
Associate Professor, Harvard Medical School
Department of Pediatric Hematology/Oncology
Boston Children's Hospital, Dana-Farber/Boston Children's Cancer
    and Blood Disorders Center
Boston, Massachusetts

John P. Greer, MD
Professor, Emeritus
Departments of Medicine and Pediatrics
Vanderbilt University Medical Center
Nashville, Tennessee

Patricia T. Greipp, DO
Consultant, Division of Hematopathology
Department of Laboratory Medicine and Pathology
Mayo Clinic
Rochester, Minnesota

Paolo Gresele, MD, PhD
Full Professor of Internal Medicine
Department of Medicine and Surgery, Section of Internal and
    Cardiovascular Medicine
University of Perugia
Perugia, Italy

Michael R. Grever, MD
Professor Emeritus
Department of Internal Medicine
The Ohio State University
Columbus, Ohio

Nitya Gulati, MBBS, FAAP
Assistant Professor, Pediatric Hematology/Oncology
Department of Pediatrics
Baylor College of Medicine/Texas Children's Hospital
Houston, Texas

Roy M. Gulick, MD, MPH
Chief, Division of Infectious Diseases
Rochelle Belfer Professor in Medicine
Department of Medicine
Weill Cornell Medicine
New York, New York

Jane Silva Hankins, MD, MS
Member
Department of Pediatric Global Medicine
St Jude Children's Research Hospital
Memphis, Tennessee

Michael M. Henry, MD
Director, Histiocytosis Program
Center for Cancer and Blood Disorders
Phoenix Children's Hospital
Phoenix, Arizona

Michelle Hickey, PhD, D(ABHI)
Associate Director, UCLA Immunogenetics Center
Associate Professor, UCLA Department of Pathology and Laboratory
    Medicine
UCLA Immunogenetics Center
UCLA David Geffen School of Medicine
Los Angeles, California

Marie Hollenhorst, MD, PhD
Clinical Instructor, Research Scientist
Brigham and Women's Hospital, Division of Hematology
Harvard Medical School
Boston, Massachusetts

Pedro Horna, MD
Associate Professor
Division of Hematopathology
Mayo Clinic
Rochester, Minnesota

Stephen P. Hunger, MD
Chief, Division of Oncology
Department of Pediatrics
Children's Hospital of Philadelphia
Philadelphia, Pennsylvania

Nitin Jain, MD
Associate Professor
Department of Leukemia
The University of Texas MD Anderson Cancer Center
Houston, Texas

Nathalie Javidi-Sharifi, MD, PhD
Clinical Fellow
Department of Medical Oncology
Dana Farber Cancer Institute
Boston, Massachusetts

Dragan Jevremovic, MD, PhD
Professor of Pathology
Department of Laboratory Medicine and Pathology
Mayo Clinic
Rochester, Minnesota

Stacy A. Johnson, MD, MSCI
Professor of Medicine
Division of General Internal Medicine
University of Utah School of Medicine
Salt Lake City, Utah

James B. Johnston, MB, BCh, FRCP(C)
Professor
Department of Internal Medicine, Section of Medical Oncology &
    Hematology
University of Manitoba
Winnipeg, Manitoba, Canada

Ridas Juskevicius, MD
Hematopathologist
PathGroup
Nashville, Tennessee

Theodosia A. Kalfa, MD, PhD
Professor of Pediatrics
Department of Hematology
Cancer and Blood Diseases Institute
Cincinnati Children's Hospital Medical Center
Department of Pediatrics
University of Cincinnati College of Medicine
Cincinnati, Ohio

Jennifer L. Kamens, MD
Instructor
Department of Pediatric Hematology/Oncology
Stanford University
Palo Alto, California

Prashant Kapoor, MD, FACP
Associate Professor of Medicine
Consultant
Division of Hematology
Mayo Clinic
Rochester, Minnesota

Neil E. Kay, MD
Consultant
Department of Medicine/Division of Hematology
Mayo Clinic
Rochester, Minnesota

Saad S. Kenderian, MD
Hematologist, Assistant Professor of Medicine, Oncology, and
    Immunology
Division of Hematology and Department of Molecular Medicine
Mayo Clinic
Rochester, Minnesota

Eugene Khandros, MD, PhD
Assistant Professor of Pediatrics
Division of Hematology
The Children's Hospital of Philadelphia
Perelman School of Medicine at the University of Pennsylvania
Philadelphia, Pennsylvania

Annette S. Kim, MD, PhD
Associate Professor
Department of Pathology
Brigham and Women's Hospital, Harvard Medical School
Boston, Massachusetts

Rebecca L. King, MD
Professor
Division of Hematopathology
Mayo Clinic
Rochester, Minnesota

Matthew M. Klairmont, MD
Fellow
Department of Pathology
New York University School of Medicine
New York, New York

Rami Komrokji, MD
Section Head Leukemia & MDS; Vice Chair
Department of Malignant Hematology
Moffitt Cancer Center
Tampa, Florida

Shalin Kothari, MD
Assistant Professor of Medicine (Hematology)
Department of Internal Medicine/Hematology
Yale University
New Haven, Connecticut

Taxiarchis Kourelis, MD
Associate Professor of Medicine
Department of Hematology
Mayo Clinic
Rochester, Minnesota

Marianna Kulka, PhD
Team Lead and Senior Researcher
National Research Council Canada
Adjunct Professor
Department of Medical Microbiology and Immunology
University of Alberta
Edmonton, Alberta, Canada

Shaji K. Kumar, MD
Mark and Judy Mullins Professor of Hematological Malignancies
Consultant, Division of Hematology
Professor of Medicine
Mayo Clinic
Rochester, Minnesota

Gary Kupfer, MD
Professor
Departments of Oncology, Pediatrics, and Medicine
Georgetown University
Washington, DC

Andrew T. Kuykendall, MD
Assistant Member
Department of Malignant Hematology
Moffitt Cancer Center
Tampa, Florida

Janet L. Kwiatkowski, MD, MSCE
Director, Thalassemia Program
Division of Hematology
Children's Hospital of Philadelphia
Professor of Pediatrics
Department of Pediatrics
Perelman School of Medicine at the University of Pennsylvania
Philadelphia, Pennsylvania

Robert A. Kyle, MD
Professor of Medicine
Division of Hematology
Mayo Clinic
Rochester, Minnesota

Ann LaCasce, MD, MMSc
Associate Professor of Medicine
Department of Medical Oncology
Dana Farber Cancer Institute
Boston, Massachusetts

Norman Lacayo, MD
Associate Professor of Pediatrics
Department of Pediatrics/Division of Hematology-Oncology, SCT
    and RM
Stanford University
Palo Alto, California

Paige Lacy, PhD
Professor
Department of Medicine
University of Alberta
Edmonton, Alberta

Nahal Rose Lalefar, MD
Associated Professor of Pediatrics
Pediatric Hematology/Oncology and Bone Marrow Transplantation
UCSF Benioff Children's Hospital Oakland
Oakland, California

Andre Larochelle, MD, PhD
Principal Investigator
Cellular and Molecular Therapeutics Branch
National Heart, Lung and Blood Institute
National Institutes of Health
Bethesda, Maryland

John P. Leonard, MD
Senior Associate Dean for Innovation and Initiatives
Richard T. Silver Distinguished Professor of Hematology and
    Medical Oncology
Weill Department of Medicine
Weill Cornell Medicine
New York Presbyterian Hospital
New York, New York

Ming Y. Lim, MBBChir, MSCR
Associate Professor
Division of Hematology and Hematologic Malignancies
Department of Internal Medicine
University of Utah
Salt Lake City, Utah

Daniel C. Link, MD
Professor
Department of Medicine
Washington University
St. Louis, Missouri

Jeffrey M. Lipton, MD, PhD
Frances and Thomas Gambino Professor of Hematology/Oncology
Professor of Pediatrics and Molecular Medicine
Zucker School of Medicine at Hofstra/Northwell
Hempstead, New York

Clara Lo, BS, MD
Clinical Associate Professor
Department of Pediatric Hematology
Stanford University School of Medicine
Palo Alto, California

Frederick L. Locke, MD
Chair
Department of Blood and Marrow Transplant and Cellular
    Immunotherapy
Moffitt Cancer Center
Tampa, Florida

Matthew R. Lordo, BSc
MD/PhD Student
Department of Pathology
The Ohio State University
Columbus, Ohio

Scott B. Lovitch, MD, PhD
Assistant Professor
Department of Pathology
Brigham and Women's Hospital
Boston, Massachusetts

Jonathan J. Lyons, MD
Lasker Scholar
Chief, Translational Allergic Immunopathology Unit
Laboratory of Allergic Diseases
NIAID/NIH
Bethesda, Maryland

Kenneth G. Mann, PhD
Professor Emeritus
Department of Biochemistry and Medicine
University of Vermont
Burlington, Vermont

Jennifer Marvin-Peek, MD
Department of Internal Medicine
Vanderbilt University Medical Center
Nashville, Tennessee

Katie Maurer, MD, PhD
Fellow
Department of Oncology/Hematology
Dana-Farber Cancer Institute
Boston, Massachusetts

Marcela V. Maus, MD, PhD
Director of Cellular Immunotherapy
Associate Professor
Cancer Center, Department of Medicine
Massachusetts General Hospital, Harvard Medical School
Charlestown, Massachusetts

Margaret M. McGovern, MD, PhD
Professor of Genetics
Yale University School of Medicine
New Haven, Connecticut

Christopher McKinney, MD
Assistant Professor of Pediatrics
Center for Cancer and Blood Disorders
Children's Hospital Colorado
University of Colorado
Aurora, Colorado

Kelly M. McNagny, PhD
Professor of Biomedical Engineering and Medical Genetics
The University of British Columbia
Vancouver, British Columbia, Canada

Robert T. Means, Jr., MD, MACP
Professor of Internal Medicine
Clinical Professor of Pathology
James H. Quillen College of Medicine
East Tennessee State University
Johnson City, Tennessee

Reid W. Merryman, MD
Instructor of Medicine
Department of Medical Oncology
Dana-Farber Cancer Institute
Boston, Massachusetts

Dean D. Metcalfe, MD
Chief, Mast Cell Biology Section
Laboratory of Allergic Diseases
National Institute of Allergy and Infectious Diseases
Bethesda, Maryland

Laura C. Michaelis, MD
Armand J. Quick Professor of Medicine
Chief, Division of Hematology/Oncology
Medical College of Wisconsin
Milwaukee, Wisconsin

Eli Muchtar, MD
Associate Consultant
Division of Hematology
Mayo Clinic
Rochester, Minnesota

Manali Mukherjee, MSc, PhD
Assistant Professor
Division of Respirology
Department of Medicine, McMaster University
Hamilton, Ontario, Canada

Erin Mulvey, MD
Assistant Professor of Medicine
Division of Hematology and Medical Oncology
Weill Cornell Medicine
New York, New York

Bethany L. Mundy-Bosse, PhD
Assistant Professor
Department of Internal Medicine, Division of Hematology
The Ohio State University
Columbus, Ohio

Mark A. Murakami, MD
Assistant Professor
Department of Medicine
Harvard Medical School
Boston, Massachusetts

Parameswaran Nair, MD, PhD, FRCP, FRCPC
Frederick E. Hargreave Teva Innovation Chair in Airway Diseases
Professor of Medicine, McMaster University
Staff Respirologist, St. Joseph's Healthcare Hamilton
Hamilton, Ontario, Canada

Anupama Narla, MD
Assistant Professor
Department of Pediatrics, Division of Hematology/Oncology
Stanford University
Stanford, California

Elizabeta Nemeth, PhD
Professor
Department of Medicine
UCLA David Geffen School of Medicine
Los Angeles, California

Paul M. Ness, MD
Senior Director, Transfusion Medicine
Department of Pathology
Johns Hopkins Medical Institutions
Baltimore, Maryland

Eva Niklinska, MD
Resident
Department of Dermatology
Vanderbilt University Medical Center
Nashville, Tennessee

Ariela Noy, MD
Member and Attending Physician Department
Department of Medicine/Lymphoma Service
Memorial Sloan Kettering Cancer Center
Professor
Department of Medicine
Weill Cornell Medical College
New York, New York

Maureen M. O'Brien, MD, MS
Professor of Clinical Pediatrics
Department of Pediatrics
Cincinnati Children's Hospital Medical Center
University of Cincinnati College of Medicine
Cincinnati, Ohio

Kristen O'Dwyer, MD
Associate Professor
Department of Medicine
University of Rochester Medical Center
Rochester, New York

Robin K. Ohls, MD
August L. "Larry" Young Presidential Professor of Pediatrics
Chief, Division of Neonatology
University of Utah
Salt Lake City, Utah

Attilio Orazi, MD, FRCPath
Professor of Pathology
Chair, Department of Pathology
Paul L. Foster School of Medicine
Texas Tech University Health Sciences Center
El Paso, Texas

Thomas Orfeo, PhD
Assistant Professor
Department of Biochemistry
Larner College of Medicine
University of Vermont
Burlington, Vermont

Eric Padron, MD
Associate Member and Scientific Director
Department of Malignant Hematology
Moffitt Cancer Center
Tampa, Florida

Suchitra Pandey, MD
Clinical Associate Professor
Department of Pathology
Stanford University School of Medicine
Stanford, California

Sameer A. Parikh, MBBS
Consultant
Department of Hematology
Mayo Clinic
Rochester, Minnesota

Christopher Y. Park, MD, PhD
Professor
Department of Pathology
NYU Grossman School of Medicine
New York, New York

Charles J. Parker, MD
Professor of Medicine
Department of Medicine
University of Utah School of Medicine
Salt Lake City, Utah

Mrinal M. Patnaik, MD
Professor of Internal Medicine
Division of Hematology and Department of Internal Medicine
Mayo Clinic College of Medicine
Rochester, Minnesota

Shilpa Paul, PharmD, BCOP
Clinical Pharmacy Specialist
Department of Pharmacy
The University of Texas MD Anderson Cancer Center
Houston, Texas

Naveen Pemmaraju, MD
Associate Professor
Department of Leukemia
The University of Texas MD Anderson Cancer Center
Houston, Texas

Jess F. Peterson, MD
Consultant
Laboratory Medicine and Pathology
Mayo Clinic
Rochester, Minnesota

John D. Phillips, PhD
Professor
Department of Medicine, Division of Hematology
University of Utah School of Medicine
Salt Lake City, Utah

Joseph Pidala, MD, PhD
Senior Member
Blood and Marrow Transplantation and Cellular Immunotherapy
H. Lee Moffitt Cancer Center and Research Institute
Tampa, Florida

Markus Plate, MD
Assistant Professor of Clinical Medicine
Department of Medicine, Division of Infectious Diseases-
    Transplantation-Oncology Program
Weill Cornell Medicine
New York, New York

Anna Porwit, MD, PhD
Professor
Department of Clinical Sciences, Oncology and Pathology
Lund University, Faculty of Medicine
Lund, Sweden

Graeme R. Quest, MD, MSc, FRCPC
Assistant Professor
Department of Pathology and Molecular Medicine
Queen's University
Kingston, Ontario, Canada

John G. Quigley, MB, FRCPC
Professor
Department of Medicine
Division of Hematology/Oncology
University of Illinois at Chicago
Chicago, Illinois

Parul Rai, MD
Assistant member
Department of Hematology
St Jude Children's Research Hospital
Memphis, Tennessee

Amit Rajaram, DO
Physician
Department of Hematology/Oncology
Phoenix Children's Hospital
Phoenix, Arizona

S. Vincent Rajkumar, MD
Professor of Medicine
Division of Hematology
Mayo Clinic
Rochester, Minnesota

Hana Raslova, PhD
Research Director
UMR (unité mixte de recherche) 1287
INSERM (Institut nationale de la Santé et de la recherche)
Gustave Roussy
Villejuif, France

Elaine F. Reed, BS, MS, PhD
Professor
UCLA Immunogenetics Center
Department of Pathology and Laboratory Medicine
David Geffen School of Medicine
University of California, Los Angeles
Los Angeles, California

George M. Rodgers, MD, PhD
Professor of Medicine
Department of Medicine/Hematology
University of Utah Health Sciences Center
Salt Lake City, Utah

Maxim Rosario, MB, BCh, BAO, DPhil
Assistant Professor
Department of Pathology
Johns Hopkins University
Baltimore, Maryland

Lisa Giulino Roth, MD
Associate Professor
Department of Pediatrics
Weill Cornell Medical College
New York, New York

Rachel B. Salit, MD
Associate Professor
Fred Hutchinson Cancer Center
Associate Professor
University of Washington Medical Center
Seattle, Washington

Michael J. Satlin, MD
Associate Professor
Department of Medicine, Pathology and Laboratory Medicine
Weill Cornell Medicine
New York, New York

Bipin N. Savani, MD
Professor of Medicine
Department of Medicine
Vanderbilt University Medical Center
Nashville, Tennessee

Laura G. Schuettpelz, MD, PhD
Associate Professor
Department of Pediatrics
Washington University
St. Louis, Missouri

Adam C. Seegmiller, MD, PhD
Professor
Department of Pathology, Microbiology, and Immunology
Vanderbilt University Medical Center
Nashville, Tennessee

Alix E. Seif, MD, MPH
Associate professor
Center for Childhood Cancer Research
Children's Hospital of Philadelphia
Department of Pediatrics
Perelman School of Medicine
of the University of Pennsylvania
Philadelphia, Pennsylvania

Mikkael A. Sekeres, MD, MS
Professor of Medicine
Chief, Division of Hematology
Sylvester Cancer Center, University of Miami
Miami, Florida

Tarsheen K. Sethi, MD, MSCI
Assistant Professor of Medicine
Department of Hematology
Yale University School of Medicine
New Haven, Connecticut

Aaron C. Shaver, MD, PhD
Associate Professor
Department of Pathology, Microbiology, and Immunology
Vanderbilt University
Nashville, Tennessee

Akiko Shimamura, MD, PhD
Professor of Pediatrics
Department of Pediatric Hematology-Oncology
Boston Children's Hospital, Harvard Medical School
Boston, Massachusetts

Danielle Shin, MD, PhD
Adjunct Clinical Instructor
Department of Pediatric Hematology/Oncology
Stanford University
Palo Alto, California

Heather M. Smetana, MLS(ASCP), SBB
Laboratory Supervisor
Department of Pathology and Transfusion Medicine
Johns Hopkins Medical Institutions
Baltimore, Maryland

Christine Moore Smith, MD
Assistant Professor of Clinical Pediatrics
Division of Pediatric Hematology/Oncology
Vanderbilt University Medical Center/Vanderbilt-Ingram Cancer
    Center
Nashville, Tennessee

Kristi J. Smock, MD
Professor
Department of Pathology
University of Utah Health Sciences Center
Medical Director, Hemostasis/Thrombosis Laboratory
ARUP Laboratories
Salt Lake City, Utah

Nwe Nwe Soe, MBBS, PhD, F(ACHI)
Director, AdventHealth Tissue Typing Laboratory
Central Florida Pathology Associates PA
Orlando, Florida

Rebecca A. Sosa, PhD
Assistant Professor of Pathology and Laboratory Medicine, UCLA
Assistant Director of UCLA Immunogenetics Center
Department of Pathology and Laboratory Medicine
UCLA
Los Angeles, California

Sally P. Stabler, MD
Professor
Department of Medicine, Division of Hematology
University of Colorado School of Medicine, Anschutz Medical
    Campus
Aurora, Colorado

Martin H. Steinberg, MD
Professor of Medicine, Pediatrics, Pathology, and Laboratory
    Medicine
Boston University Chobanian and Avedisian School of Medicine
Boston, Massachusetts

Martin S. Tallman, MD
Professor of Medicine
Division of Hematology and Oncology, Leukemia Program
Robert H. Lurie Comprehensive Cancer Center
Northwestern University Feinberg School of Medicine
Chicago, Illinois

Tsewang Tashi, MD
Assistant Professor
Division of Hematology and Hematologic Malignancies
Huntsman Cancer Institute, University of Utah
Salt Lake City, Utah

Christiane D. Thienelt, MD
Associate Professor of Medicine/Hematology
RMR VAMC/University of Colorado
Aurora, Colorado

Mary Ann Thompson, MD, PhD
Associate Professor
Department of Pathology, Microbiology, and Immunology
Vanderbilt University Medical Center
Nashville, Tennessee

Troy R. Torgerson, MD, PhD
Director, Experimental Immunology
Allen Institute for Immunology
Seattle, Washington

Han-Mou Tsai, MD
Visiting Professor of Medicine
State University of New York Downstate Medical Center
Brooklyn, New York

William Vainchenker, MD, PhD
Director of Research
UMR (unité mixte de recherche) 1287
INSERM (Institut nationale de la Santé et de la recherche)
Université Paris Saclay
Gustave Roussy
Villejuif, France

Madeleine Verhovsek, BSc, MD, FRCPC
Associate Professor
Department of Medicine and Pathology & Molecular Medicine
McMaster University
Hamilton, Ontario, Canada

Srdan Verstovsek, MD, PhD
United Energy Resources, Inc. Professor of Medicine
Director, Hanns A. Pielenz Clinical Research Center
for Myeloproliferative Neoplasms
Department of Leukemia
MD Anderson Cancer Center
Houston, Texas

Mrigender Singh Virk, MD
Clinical Assistant Professor
Department of Pathology
Stanford University School of Medicine
Stanford, California

Laura F. Walsh, MD
Osler Housestaff
Department of Internal Medicine
Johns Hopkins Hospital
Baltimore, Maryland

Mark C. Walters, MD
Jordan Family Director
Blood & Marrow Transplant, UCSF Benioff Children's Hospital
Professor and Chief, Hematology Division
UCSF Department of Pediatrics
Oakland, California

Russell E. Ware, MD, PhD
Director, Division of Hematology
Department of Pediatrics
Cincinnati Children's Hospital
Cincinnati, Ohio

Rahma Warsame, MD
Associate Professor of Medicine & Oncology
Department of Hematology
Mayo Clinic
Rochester, Minnesota

Nina Weichert-Leahey, MD
Physician
Department of Pediatric Oncology/Hematology
Dana-Farber Cancer Institute
Bosto, Massachusetts

Makiko Yasuda, MD, PhD
Associate Professor
Department of Genetics and Genomic Sciences
Icahn School of Medicine at Mount Sinai
New York, New York

Ji Yuan, MD, PhD
Associate Professor
Department of Laboratory Medicine and Pathology
Mayo Clinic
Rochester, Minnesota

James L. Zehnder, MD
Professor of Pathology and Medicine (Hematology)
Director of Clinical Pathology, Department of Pathology
Stanford University School of Medicine
Stanford, California

Bing Melody Zhang, MD, MS
Department of Pathology
Stanford University, School of Medicine
Palo Alto, California

Qiuheng Jennifer Zhang, PhD
Professor
University of California, Los Angeles
Los Angeles, California

John A. Zic, MD, MMHC
Professor of Dermatology
Vice Chair for Clinic Affairs
Executive Medical Director Dermatology Clinic
Director, VU Cutaneous Lymphoma Clinic
Department of Dermatology
Vanderbilt University Medical Center
Nashville, Tennessee

Jeff P. Zwerner, MD, PhD
Assistant Professor
Department of Dermatology
Vanderbilt University
Nashville, Tennessee

Preface

The red blood cell indices (mean corpuscular volume [MCV], mean corpuscular hemoglobin [MCH], and mean corpuscular hemoglobin concentration [MCHC]) have become so ingrained in the way clinicians think about anemia that it is difficult to realize that somebody actually derived their formulas and established a classification of anemia based upon them. This was in fact done by Maxwell Wintrobe, a young faculty member at Tulane, in publications that appeared in 1929 and 1930.[1-3] It was not his only major contribution as a clinical scientist although it was one of his earliest. However, almost four decades after his death in 1986, Dr. Wintrobe is best remembered as the eponymous founding author of the *Wintrobe's Clinical Hematology* textbook.

As the 15th edition of *Wintrobe's Clinical Hematology* is being assembled in the fall of 2022, it has been 80 years since the publication of the first edition in 1942, a single-author textbook called *Clinical Hematology*. Dr. George Rodgers, the longest-serving of the current *Wintrobe* editors, and Drs. John H. Ward and Paul F. Bray, two of Dr. Wintrobe's trainees and colleagues, recently celebrated this in a publication that displayed the first 14 editions (*Figure*).[4] The 1942 edition was not Dr. Wintrobe's first venture into hematology textbook writing. In the late 1920s, he and his department chair John Musser wrote a 157-page section on diseases of the blood for *Tice's Practice of Medicine*, a serialized multivolume textbook. This experience led directly to his decision to undertake authorship of a comprehensive textbook of hematology some dozen years later.[5]

The first six editions of *Clinical Hematology* were written by Wintrobe himself as a sole author. For the 7th and 8th editions, former fellows were recruited as coauthors: John Athens, Thomas Bithell, Dane Boggs, John Foerster, Richard Lee, and John Lukens. With the 9th edition, the first to appear after Dr. Wintrobe's death, the title was changed to *Wintrobe's Clinical Hematology*, and the book became a multicontributor edited work. Drs Athens, Bithell, Foerster (9th-11th editions), Lee (9th and 10th editions), and Lukens (9th-11th editions) were the initial editors. Over the years, there have been transitions in the editorial team: John Greer (10th-14th editions), Frixos Paraskevas (10th-13th editions), George Rodgers (10th edition to the present), Bertil Glader (11th edition to the present), Daniel Arber (12th edition to the present), Robert Means (12th edition to the present), Alan List (13th and 14th editions), Frederick Appelbaum (14th edition to the present), Angela Dispenzieri (14th edition to the present), and Todd Fehniger (14th edition to the present). John Leonard and Laura Michaelis have joined as of this edition, covering the areas formerly overseen by Drs. Greer and List.

A textbook like this, however, is not solely the product of its editors. *Wintrobe's Clinical Hematology* continues to benefit from the generous efforts of physicians and scientists around the world who have accepted the editors' invitations to share their expertise through their chapters. The editors are profoundly grateful to them for their contributions which make this the definitive textbook that it is.

Wintrobe's Clinical Hematology continues to evolve. The chapters on hematopoietic cell transplantation now include newer aspects of cellular therapy. A new chapter on clonal hematopoiesis has been added. Therapeutic and diagnostic algorithms have been revised to accommodate new guidelines and new scientific developments.

The audience for *Wintrobe's Clinical Hematology* encompasses the entire spectrum of health care providers, including medical students, nurses, residents, nurse practitioners, physician assistants, clinicians, and scientists. The book reviews the science, the methods of diagnosis, and the evidence for the basis of therapeutic decisions. The artwork has been redrawn for color, and numerous photomicrographs have been provided that illustrate the role of hematopathology in diagnosis.

The book is divided into eight parts: (1) Laboratory Hematology; (2) The Normal Hematologic System; (3) Transfusion Medicine; (4) Disorders of Red Blood Cells; (5) Disorders of Hemostasis and Coagulation; (6) Disorders of Leukocytes, Immunodeficiency, and the Spleen; (7) Hematologic Malignancies; and (8) Hematopoietic Cellular Therapy (previously Hematopoietic Cell Transplantation). Emphasis continues to be placed on four components of diagnosis: the morphology of the peripheral smear, bone marrow, lymph nodes, and other tissues; flow cytometry; cytogenetics; and molecular markers and mutations. Therapeutic principles are discussed on the basis of pathogenesis and an accurate diagnosis.

There were many people at Wolters Kluwer who supported the book, particularly Anne Malcolm, Nicole Dernoski, Sean McGuire, Thomas Celona, Eric McDermott, Oliver Raj, Remington Fernando, Frances Gunning, and Kirsten Watrud. We are appreciative of all the production efforts of Kiruthiga Sowndararajan and TNQ Technologies.

The Wintrobe tradition in hematology textbooks began in the late 1920s. The editors are honored to continue that tradition into its second century.

ROBERT T. MEANS, JR.

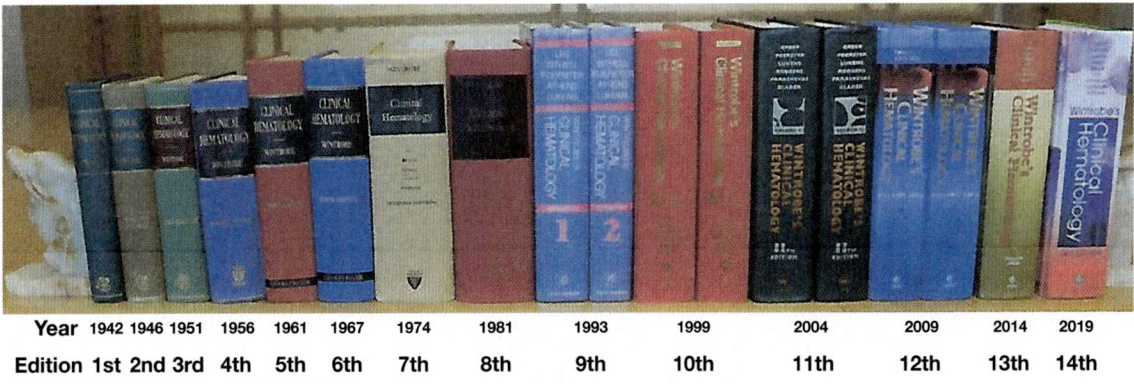

Year	1942	1946	1951	1956	1961	1967	1974	1981	1993	1999	2004	2009	2014	2019
Edition	1st	2nd	3rd	4th	5th	6th	7th	8th	9th	10th	11th	12th	13th	14th

FIGURE (Reproduced from Rodgers GM, Ward JH, Bray PF. 80 years of *Clinical Hematology. Br J Haematol.* 2022;198(5):802, with permission.)

References

1. Wintrobe MM. The erythrocyte in man. *Medicine*. 1930;9(2):195.
2. Wintrobe MM. The volume and hemoglobin content of the red blood corpuscle. *Am J Med Sci*. 1929;177:513-523.
3. Wintrobe MM. A simple and accurate hematocrit. *J Lab Clin Med*. 1929;15:287-289.
4. Rodgers GM, Ward JH, Bray PF. 80 years of *Clinical Hematology*. *Br J Haematol*. 2022;198(5):802.
5. Wintrobe MM. *Hematology, The Blossoming of a Science: A Story of Inspiration and Effort*. Lea & Febiger; 1985:1-563.

Acknowledgments

I wish to thank my wife, Stacey, and our children, Casey, Robert, and Patrick, for their support and tolerance during the preparation of this book; the many teachers and colleagues who have guided me as mentors and examples in science and medicine, particularly Shu-Yung Chen, Joachim Pfitzner, James B. Walker, Robert D. Collins, Roger M. DesPrez, Richard Borreson, Mark Udden, Richard Vilter, Herbert Flessa, Makio Ogawa, Frederick C. de Beer, John Flexner, and Sanford B. Krantz; and, above all, my late parents, Ann and Bob Means, who were my first and best teachers.

ROBERT T. MEANS, JR.

I acknowledge Ayleah Hansen for expert word processing and my numerous contributors for their outstanding chapters. This is the sixth edition of this textbook I have been involved with; it has been a pleasure working with my coeditors and contributors on this edition.

GEORGE M. RODGERS

I wish to acknowledge the many outstanding colleagues, both chapter authors and fellow editors, whom I have had the privilege to work with in the development of this new edition. I also want to acknowledge my students, residents, and fellows who continue to make the teaching of clinical hematology so meaningful. Lastly, but most of all, I want to recognize the understanding and support of my wonderful wife, Lou Ann, my children, and their families.

BERTIL GLADER

I wish to thank my wife, Carol Park, for her constant support, and our children, James and William, who make every day a joy. I also thank my current and past trainees, colleagues, and mentors, all of whom are continuous sources of knowledge.

DANIEL A. ARBER

I would like to thank the chapter authors and the editorial staff of Wolters Kluwer for creating an outstanding text and making my job easy.

FREDERICK R. APPELBAUM

Thanks to my husband, Greg, for his understanding and support and to my extraordinary colleagues and mentors at the Mayo Clinic, most notably Morie A. Gertz, Robert A. Kyle, and Ayalew Tefferi.

ANGELA DISPENZIERI

I deeply thank all of the authors who worked diligently to write chapters of the very highest quality for this edition. I would also like to acknowledge the Hematology/Oncology trainees and my laboratory members for providing feedback on this text, as well as my mentors and colleagues who helped introduce me to Hematology: Michael Caligiuri, Stuart Kornfeld, Timothy Ley, Nancy Bartlett, and John DiPersio. Most of all I thank my wife, Megan Cooper, and my children, Max and Eleanor, for their ever-present support and understanding.

TODD A. FEHNIGER

Thanks to my family, friends, and professional colleagues for their continued support, inspiration, and encouragement. I want to specifically acknowledge Robert Means for his mentorship and staunch and kind support. Finally, I would like to express my deep gratitude for this edition's numerous contributors for their outstanding chapters. It has been a pleasure and privilege to be part of producing this endeavor. I am humbled and honored to be part of the team.

LAURA C. MICHAELIS

I want to thank my fellow editors and the many chapter authors for their extensive effort, knowledge, and time in developing this new edition. It is truly a labor of love, and a reflection of collaboration and commitment in furthering the education and training of hematologists, supporting colleagues and most importantly helping patients. I appreciate all of the wisdom, compassion, and interaction I have been fortunate to receive from those who have trained me in this field as well as those who I continue to learn from on a regular basis. Hematology is truly a wonderful community of which to be a member. Most importantly, I appreciate all of the understanding and support I have received over many years from my family—including my wife Leah and our children Maddie, Abbie, and Zach.

JOHN P. LEONARD

Contents

VOLUME 2

Part 7   HEMATOLOGIC MALIGNANCIES

Part **8**   HEMATOPOIETIC CELLULAR THERAPY

The Wintrobe Legacy

In 2007, the late Dr. Herbert L. Fred, Professor Emeritus of Medicine at the University of Texas McGovern Medical School in Houston, published a reminiscence that chronicled the life and contributions of Dr. Max Wintrobe.[1] Beginning in 1954, Dr. Fred, spent five years working with Max, four as his house officer (including one as chief resident) and one as a member of his staff. Dr. John Greer invited Dr. Fred to contribute a discussion of the Wintrobe legacy in hematology and medicine to the 14th edition. Here is Dr. Fred's response:

> I am honored by this invitation and grateful for the opportunity to recount my mentor's outstanding career. As the story unfolds, I share my views of Wintrobe, the man, and emphasize with love and respect his monumental contributions to the fields of hematology, medical education, and patient care.

Dr. Fred passed away not long after the 14th edition went to press. It is our pleasure to include his contribution.

THE EARLY YEARS (1901-1927)

Max was born in Sanok, Poland, on October 27, 1901, to Herman and Ethel Weintraub. The village of Sanok was part of the Austrian Empire at the time, but became part of Poland after World War I. Because of religious persecution in his homeland, Max and his Jewish parents fled in 1906 to Halifax, Nova Scotia, where four brothers of his mother lived.

An only child (*Figure 1*), Max characterized his father as an honest man with no great ambition for himself or for his son. On the other hand, Max was very close to his mother, whom he described as a

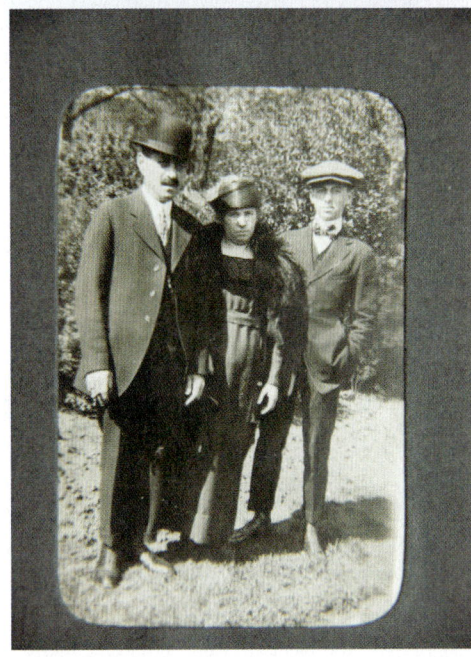

FIGURE 2 Max with his parents, ca. 1917. (Courtesy of Susan Wintrobe Walker.)

caring, liberal, and unprejudiced person. He credited her for teaching him the values of a good education and hard work.

In 1912, Max moved with his parents to Winnipeg, Manitoba, where he later attended St. John's High School. According to officials at that school, Max Weintraub was a student there in 1915 and 1916. Furthermore, his high school art box bears the inscription "Max" on its top.

At the age of 15 years and 10 months, Max entered the University of Manitoba, where he spent four years getting a general education (*Figure 2*). Authorities at the University confirm that Max's last name on entry there was Weintraub; however, on his diploma, it was Wintrobe. Thus, sometime during those four years, Max's name changed from Weintraub to Wintrobe. The questions how and why the change occurred remain unanswered.

He began medical school at the University of Manitoba in 1921 and graduated first in his class in 1925.[2] He divided his time there between work and play, never working to the point of extreme fatigue or late into the night—a habit similar to that of his idol and role model, William Osler.

During his sophomore year, he learned about the Johns Hopkins University School of Medicine and wanted to transfer there, but he could not afford the tuition or the added expenses of travel and living away from home. So he gave up the idea of going there but not the desire—a desire that strengthened when, as an intern, he read Harvey Cushing's *The Life of Sir William Osler*.

One other aspect of Max's sophomore year is noteworthy. To ease his financial constraints, he took a job in the hospital's blood bank. He later told me that working in that blood bank was the spark that ignited his passion for hematology.

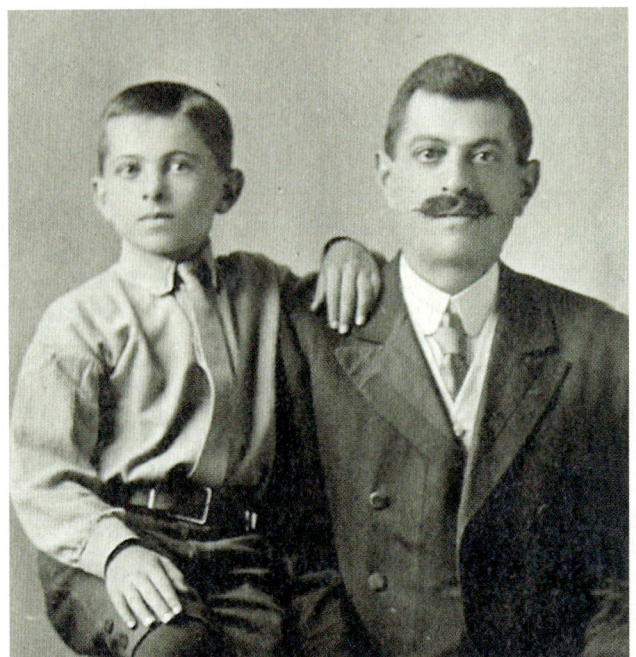

FIGURE 1 Max with his father, 1907. (Courtesy of Susan Wintrobe Walker.)

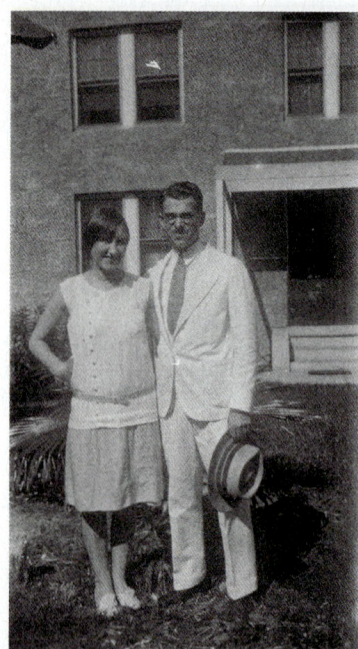

FIGURE 3 **Max and Becky—newlyweds in New Orleans, 1928.** (Courtesy of the Special Collections Department, J. Willard Marriott Library, University of Utah.)

CREATING A SUBSPECIALTY: TULANE (1927-1930)

In September of 1927, Max accepted a job in New Orleans as assistant in medicine at Tulane University. At that time, there was no such discipline as hematology, but Max would change that. Years later, he considered the move to New Orleans as the most fortunate decision of his life.[3]

With a salary of $1800 per year, Max could now marry his sweetheart, Rebecca (Becky) Zanphir, whom he had met when she was a freshman in college and he a freshman in medical school. They were married in Winnipeg on January 1, 1928, and returned to New Orleans (*Figure 3*) to live in a small, one-room apartment with secondhand furniture.

His work at Tulane—enhanced by superb clinical material at Charity Hospital—produced monumental results. Among the most memorable was his invention of the famous Wintrobe hematocrit (*Figure 4*),[4] which would allow for accurate determination of the volume of packed red blood cells after centrifugation. It could also measure the erythrocyte sedimentation rate,[5] the volume of packed white blood cells and platelets, and changes in appearance of the plasma.[6] Because there were no reliable normal blood values at the time,[7] Max made careful observations of various populations, including Tulane medical students and women from Sophie Newcomb College.[8] An integral part of that effort was Max's derivation of the red blood cell indices,[9,10] from which he classified anemias into three basic forms: microcytic, normocytic, and macrocytic.[11] That classification has been the standard ever since, and determining the red blood cell indices is still done daily in laboratories throughout the world.

In 1929, Max earned a PhD at Tulane. His thesis was a monograph titled "The Erythrocyte in Man,"[12] which he submitted for publication in the journal *Medicine*. The editor of that journal, Alan Chesney, was also Dean of the Johns Hopkins University School of Medicine. Impressed by the monograph, Chesney invited Max to join the Hopkins staff as an instructor in Clinical Microscopy. Max happily accepted.

ESTABLISHING A LEGACY: JOHNS HOPKINS (1930-1943)

Arriving in Baltimore in 1930, Max and Becky encountered blatant anti-Semitism. Otherwise, Max found Hopkins to be everything he had hoped for. And it was there that his reputation as a clinical investigator,

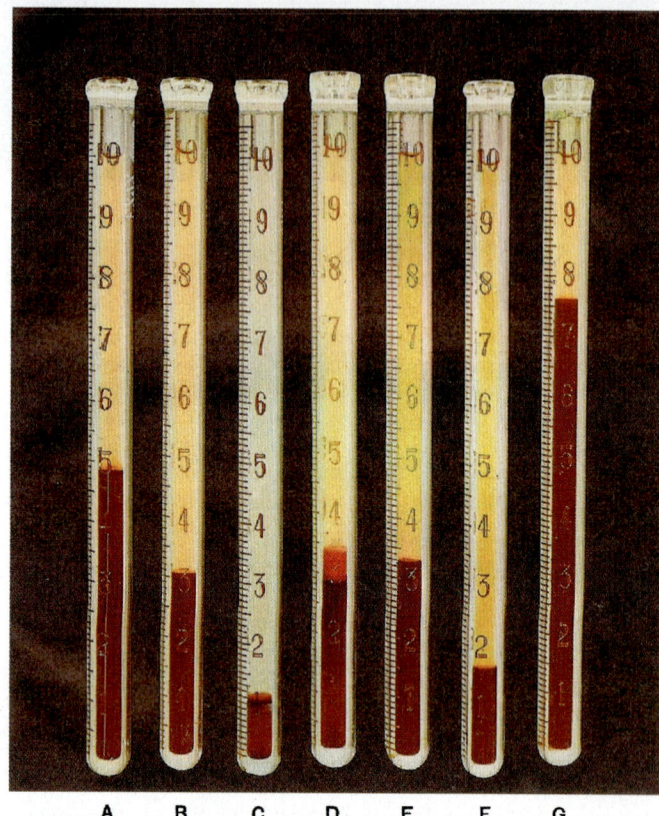

FIGURE 4 **Wintrobe hematocrit tube.** The appearance of blood in various conditions. A, Normal blood. B, Anemia with chronic infection. C, Iron deficiency anemia with pale blood plasma. D, Chronic myeloid leukemia with distinct layers of white cells and platelets above the red cells. E, Posthepatic jaundice with moderate anemia. The coloring of the blood plasma results from biliary obstruction. F, Pernicious anemia with a small amount of red cells, a narrow layer of white cells and platelets, and icteric plasma consequent to hyperbilirubinemia. G, Polycythemia.

teacher, and hematologist blossomed. After three years at Hopkins, Max became Chief of the Clinic for Nutritional, Gastrointestinal, and Hematological Disorders. Two years later, he was promoted to associate in medicine.

In 1937, Becky gave birth to their daughter, Susan. And after six more years at Hopkins, Max accepted an offer to become the first Chair of Medicine at the newly formed four-year medical school at the University of Utah in Salt Lake City.

CEMENTING THE LEGACY: UTAH (1943-1986)

Max's goal in Utah was to establish a first-rate medical school where teaching, research, and the best possible medical care would receive equal dedication. He not only achieved his goal, but he also became the guiding spirit of that school.

On January 7, 1944, four months into his new job, Max took pride in the birth of his son, Paul. For the next eight and one-half years, the Wintrobes were a happy, handsome group. Then, on August 14, 1952, disaster struck. The four of them were riding in a small convertible on a slippery mountain road in Wyoming, when the brakes failed, forcing their vehicle into the path of an oncoming car. The ensuing crash killed Paul. Susan suffered serious head wounds and fractures of the spine and pelvis. Max and Becky escaped with minor injuries.

The loss of his son devastated Max. As a result, he dedicated subsequent editions of his textbook not only to his wife, as he had done before the accident, but also to the memory of their son, Paul.

One of Max's early achievements was to obtain the school's first research grant ever—$100,000 to study muscular dystrophy and other hereditary and metabolic disorders. It was also the first research grant ever awarded by the National Institutes of Health and was renewed annually for 23 years.

While at the helm, Max and his associate, George Cartwright, built a hematology training program second to none. It graduated approximately 110 fellows, 85% of whom became associated with medical schools or research institutes around the world.[13]

Accounts of Max's scientific and academic achievements are available elsewhere.[1,2,8] A few highlights, however, are worth mentioning here:

- Devised his hematocrit[4] and derived the red blood cell indices[9,10];
- Gave the first account of a cryoglobulin in the blood[14];
- Offered the first description of Fabry disease in an American patient[15];
- Provided the first evidence that Cooley anemia (thalassemia major) is a homozygous disorder[16];
- Emphasized the role of nutritional factors, particularly the B vitamins, in hemopoiesis[17];
- Pioneered in studying the effects of nitrogen mustard, folate antagonists, and adrenocorticosteroids on the hemopoietic system[18-21];
- Called attention to the potential of chloramphenicol to produce aplastic anemia[22];
- Led the drive to recognize and publicize adverse reactions to drugs.[23-25]

He wrote three books and more than 400 medical articles. His textbook, *Clinical Hematology*, appeared in 1942 as a single-author, exhaustively and meticulously referenced, 792-page tome. He remained the sole author for the first six editions. For the seventh edition, which comprised 1896 pages, he appointed five of his former fellows as coeditors.

Max coedited *Harrison's Principles of Internal Medicine* from 1951 through 1966 and was its editor-in-chief for the sixth and seventh editions in 1970 and 1974, respectively.

He edited and partly wrote his second book, *Blood, Pure and Eloquent: A Story of Discovery, of People, and of Ideas*.[26] It offers a history of scientific discovery in hematology and contains written accounts from some of the scientists responsible for those discoveries. This work won the 1980 American Medical Writers Association book award for physicians.

His third book, *Hematology, the Blossoming of a Science: A Story of Inspiration, and Effort*,[3] was published in 1985, a year before he died. It is his autobiography, together with a history of hematology, brilliantly unfolded in the context of the lives of the men and women who contributed to the development of the discipline.

Max lectured in numerous countries, received myriad awards for his research and teaching, headed many prestigious organizations and committees, and trained hundreds of house officers and scores of hematologists. He served as President of the Association of American Physicians (1956-1957), the Association of Professors of Medicine (1965-1966), and the American Society of Hematology (1971-1972). In 1973, he was elected to the National Academy of Sciences.

He was the Chair at Utah for 24 years, stepping down in 1967. Three years later, the University named him Distinguished Professor of Internal Medicine, its highest academic rank.

PASSING THE TORCH

Max demanded much of those around him, but never more than he demanded of himself. He abhorred excuses, expected top effort, and praised only those whose performance was exceptional. He was firm but fair. He played no favorites and complemented or condemned trainees and colleagues just as rapidly and convincingly as he did the custodial staff or hospital administrator. He had the rare ability to criticize someone's work without making the individual feel personally attacked. He listened perceptively and spoke authoritatively, never leaving his audience in doubt as to where he and they stood, and why.

He rarely seemed satisfied. "No matter how good a job we do, we can always do a better one," he would say. Indeed, had I discovered the

cure for leukemia, his response surely would have been, "That's fine, Herb, but why didn't you do that *last* year?"

Two other statements of his have stuck with me through the years. "If I do my job well," he said, "I'll never win a popularity contest." In that regard, he often added, "I'd rather be respected than loved."

Although he never wasted a moment at work, Max knew when to relax and how to play. He was an avid skier, appreciated the fine arts—especially the symphony—and enjoyed travel. He was all business in the hospital but charming in his home. He and Becky loved to entertain and were incomparably gracious, whether hosting one couple such as my wife and me, or giving their annual lawn party for the faculty, house staff, fellows, newcomers, and other friends.

With trainees always high on his priority list, Max instituted a policy whereby students, house officers, and fellows were the first to examine all patients, whether private or nonpaying. Later, this policy was widely emulated.

As a teacher, Max used the Socratic method, asking many questions but giving few answers. He strongly believed that one could learn much from *any* patient, regardless of how routine the case appeared.

He invariably discovered something in the medical history or physical examination that others had missed or inappropriately ignored. He taught best, however, by setting examples—particularly the examples of hard work, self-discipline, self-education, clear thinking, intellectual honesty, and intellectual curiosity. And his unwavering commitment to excellence made him intolerant of mediocrity.

SUMMING IT UP

In the 20th century, Maxwell Myer Wintrobe (*Figure 5*) was a giant among physician-scientists. His death from heart failure on December 9, 1986, at the age of 85, ended six decades of outstanding clinical research and teaching.

What he accomplished is truly amazing, considering that he had no mentors and no formal hematologic training. Yet his work established hematology as a distinct subspecialty. His textbook, *Clinical Hematology*, was the most authoritative in its field. And his model fellowship training program produced scores of academic and practicing hematologists around the world. No wonder this man, by his own

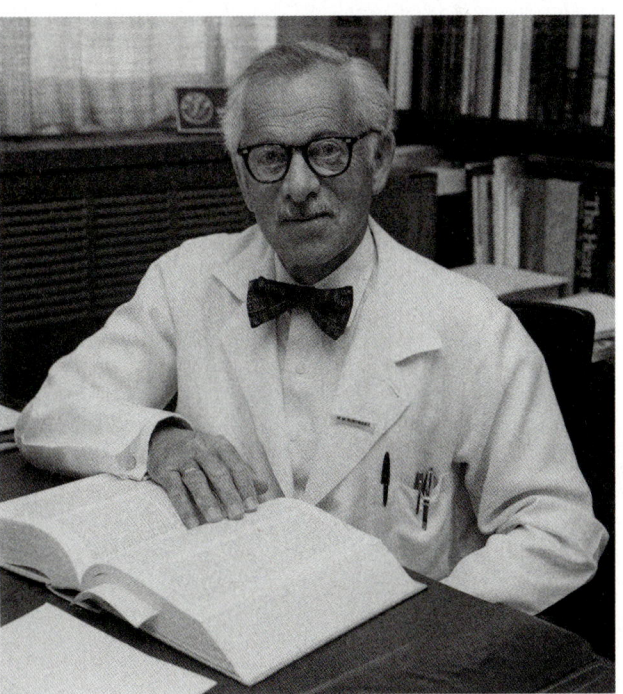

FIGURE 5 **Max at the pinnacle of his career, ca. 1980.** (Courtesy of the Special Collections Department, J. Willard Marriott Library, University of Utah.)

efforts, achieved lasting international renown and earned a front-row seat in the pantheon of world-class figures.

Even more powerful was Max's impact on those around him. He favorably and profoundly influenced countless medical students, house officers, and fellows, giving their lives new impetus and direction. To me, that was, and is, his finest and most durable contribution.

References

1. Fred HL. Maxwell Myer Wintrobe: new history and a new appreciation. *Tex Heart Inst J.* 2007;34:328-335.
2. Spivak JL. Maxwell Wintrobe, in his own words. *Br J Haematol.* 2003;121:224-232.
3. Wintrobe MM. *Hematology, the Blossoming of a Science: A Story of Inspiration and Effort.* Lea & Febiger; 1985.
4. Wintrobe MM. A simple and accurate hematocrit. *J Lab Clin Med.* 1929;15:287-289.
5. Wintrobe MM, Landsberg JW, A standardized technique for the blood sedimentation test. *Am J Med Sci.* 1935;189:102-115.
6. Wintrobe MM. Macroscopic examination of the blood: discussion of its value and description of the use of a single instrument for the determination of sedimentation rate, volume of packed red cells, leukocytes and platelets, and of icterus index. *Am J Med Sci.* 1933;185:58-71.
7. Weisse AB. *Chapter 5: Maxwell M. Wintrobe, M.D., Ph.D. (1901-).* In: *Conversations in Medicine: The Story of Twentieth-Century American Medicine in the Words of Those Who Created It.* New York University Press; 1984;75-92.
8. Valentine WN. *Maxwell Myer Wintrobe: October 27, 1901-December 9, 1986.* In: *Biographical Memoirs.* Vol 59. National Academy Press; 1990;446-472.
9. Wintrobe MM. The volume and hemoglobin content of the red blood corpuscle: simple method of calculation, normal findings, and value of such calculations in the anemias. *Am J Med Sci.* 1929;177:513-523.
10. Wintrobe MM. Classification of the anemias on the basis of differences in the size and hemoglobin content of the red corpuscles. *Proc Soc Exp Biol Med.* 1930;27:1071-1073.
11. Wintrobe MM. Anemia: classification and treatment on the basis of differences in the average volume and hemoglobin content of the red corpuscles. *Arch Intern Med.* 1934;54:256-258.
12. Wintrobe MM. The erythrocyte in man. *Medicine (Baltimore).* 1930;9:195-251.
13. Boggs DR, Maxwell M, Wintrobe. *Blood.* 1973;41:1-5.
14. Wintrobe MM, Buell MV, Hyperproteinemia associated with multiple myeloma. *Bull Johns Hopkins Hosp.* 1933;52:156-165.
15. Fessas P, Wintrobe MM, Cartwright GE. Angiokeratoma corporis diffusum universale (Fabry); first American report of a rare disorder. *AMA Arch Intern Med.* 1955;95:469-481.
16. Wintrobe MM, Matthews E, Pollack R, Dobyns BM. A familial hemopoietic disorder in Italian adolescents and adults: resembling Mediterranean disease (thalassemia). *JAMA.* 1940;114:1530-1538.
17. Wintrobe MM. The search for an experimental counterpart of pernicious anemia. *AMA Arch Intern Med.* 1957;100:862-869.
18. Goodman LS, Wintrobe MM, Dameshek W, Goodman MJ, Gilman A, McLennan MT. Nitrogen mustard therapy. Use of methyl-bis (beta-chloroethyl) amine hydrochloride and tris (beta-chloroethyl) amine hydrochloride for Hodgkin's disease, lymphosarcoma, leukemia and certain allied and miscellaneous disorders. *J Am Med Assoc.* 1946;132:126-132. [Reproduced in *JAMA.* 1984;251:2255-2261.]
19. Wintrobe MM, Huguley CM Jr., McLennan MT, Lima LP. Nitrogen mustard as a therapeutic agent for Hodgkin's disease, lymphosarcoma and leukemia. *Ann Intern Med.* 1947;27:529-540.
20. Wintrobe MM, Huguley CM Jr., Nitrogen mustard therapy for Hodgkin's disease, lymphosarcoma, the leukemias, and other disorders. *Cancer.* 1948;1:357-382.
21. Wintrobe MM, Cartwright GE, Palmer JG, Kuhns WJ, Samuels LT. Effect of corticotrophin and cortisone on the blood in various disorders in man. *AMA Arch Intern Med.* 1951;88:310-336.
22. Smiley RK, Cartwright GE, Wintrobe MM. Fatal aplastic anemia following chloramphenicol (chloromycetin®) administration. *J Am Med Assoc.* 1952;149:914-918.
23. Wintrobe MM. The therapeutic millennium and its price: adverse reactions to drugs. In: Talalay P, Murnaghan JH, eds. *Drugs in our Society.* The Johns Hopkins Press; 1964;107-114.
24. Cartwright GE, Wintrobe MM, Blood disorders caused by drug sensitivity. *AMA Arch Intern Med.* 1956;98:559-566.
25. Wintrobe MM. The problems of drug toxicity in man—a view from the hematopoietic system. *Ann N Y Acad Sci.* 1965;123:316-325.
26. Wintrobe MM. *Blood, Pure and Eloquent: A Story of Discovery, of People, and of Ideas.* McGraw-Hill Book Company; 1980.

Part 1

LABORATORY HEMATOLOGY

Chapter 1 ■ Examination of the Blood and Bone Marrow

KRISTI J. SMOCK

INTRODUCTION

Since the advent of microscopy several hundred years ago, there have been continual advances in our ability to identify and quantify the components of blood and bone marrow. One important advance was the invention of the Coulter counter in the 1950s, which allowed accurate automated counting of large numbers of cells. In the present time, evaluation of blood and bone marrow counts and morphology, along with important ancillary studies, is essential for accurate diagnosis of hematologic disorders and for monitoring disease progression and response to therapy. This chapter introduces the fundamental concepts and limitations that underlie laboratory evaluation of the blood and bone marrow and introduces additional testing that may aid in evaluating hematologic disorders.

Blood elements include erythrocytes (red blood cells [RBCs]), leukocytes (white blood cells [WBCs]), and platelets. RBCs are the most numerous cells in the blood and are required for tissue respiration. RBCs lack nuclei and contain hemoglobin (Hg), an iron-containing protein that transports oxygen and carbon dioxide. WBCs include a variety of cell types that have specific immune functions and characteristic morphologic appearances. WBCs are nucleated and include neutrophils, lymphocytes, monocytes, eosinophils, and basophils. Platelets are cytoplasmic fragments derived from bone marrow megakaryocytes that function in hemostasis.

Blood evaluation requires quantification of the cellular elements by either manual or automated methods. Automated methods are more commonly used, are more precise than manual procedures, and provide additional data regarding cellular characteristics. Automated methods also require less technical time and minimize the possibility of human error. However, the automated measurements describe average cellular characteristics but do not adequately describe the variability of individual values. For example, a bimodal population of small (microcytic) and large (macrocytic) RBCs might be reported as average normal cell size. Therefore, a thorough blood examination also requires microscopic evaluation of a stained blood film to complement hematology analyzer data.

SPECIMEN COLLECTION

Proper specimen collection is essential for acquisition of accurate laboratory data for hematologic specimens. Before a specimen is obtained, careful thought as to what studies are needed will aid in optimal collection of samples. Communication with laboratory personnel is helpful in ensuring proper handling and test performance.

Several preanalytical factors may affect hematologic measurements, and specimens should be collected in a standardized manner to reduce data variability. For example, patient activity, level of hydration, medications, gender, age, race, smoking, and anxiety level may significantly affect hematologic parameters.[1-3] Similarly, the age and storage conditions of the specimen may affect the quality of the data collected.[4-6] Thus, data such as patient age, gender, and time of specimen collection as well as pertinent correlative clinical information should be noted.

Most often, blood is collected by venipuncture into vacuum collection tubes containing an anticoagulant.[7] The three most commonly used anticoagulants are tripotassium or trisodium salts of ethylenediaminetetraacetic acid (EDTA), trisodium citrate, and heparin. EDTA is the preferred anticoagulant for blood counts because it produces complete anticoagulation with minimal morphologic and physical effects on cells. Heparin causes a bluish coloration of the background when a blood smear is stained with Wright-Giemsa but does not affect cell size or shape. Heparin is often used for red cell testing and functional or immunologic analysis of leukocytes. Trisodium citrate is the preferred anticoagulant for platelet and coagulation studies. Anticoagulated blood may be stored at 4°C for a 24-hour period without significantly altering cell counts or cellular morphology.[4] However, it is preferable to perform hematologic analysis as soon as possible after the blood is obtained.

RELIABILITY OF TESTS

In addition to proper acquisition of specimens, data reliability requires accurate and precise testing methods. Both manual and automated testing of hematologic specimens must be interpreted considering expected test accuracy and precision (reproducibility), particularly when evaluating the significance of small changes. Accuracy is the difference between the measured value and the true value, which implies that a true value is known. Clearly, this may present difficulties when dealing with biologic specimens. The Clinical and Laboratory Standards Institute (CLSI), formerly the National Committee for Clinical Laboratory Standards, has developed standards to assess the performance characteristics of automated blood cell analyzers.[8] Automated instrumentation requires careful calibration and regular quality control and quality assurance procedures to reach expected performance goals for accuracy and reproducibility.

CELL COUNTS

As previously mentioned, cell counts are obtained manually or by automated hematology analyzers. Because blood contains large numbers of cells, sample dilution is required for accurate analysis. The type of diluent depends on the cell type to be enumerated. RBC counts require dilution with an isotonic medium, whereas for WBC or platelet counts, a diluent that lyses the more numerous RBCs is used to simplify counting and avoid errors. The highest degree of precision occurs when many cells are evaluated. Clearly, automated methods are superior to manual methods for counting large numbers of cells and minimizing statistical error. Recent comparisons of hematology analyzers showed good between-instrument concordance for basic blood count parameters, but with less agreement for measurements such as reticulocyte counts, nucleated RBCs, WBC differentials, indicating that manual review remains a valuable tool.[9-11]

Manual RBC, WBC, and platelet counts are performed using a microscope after dilution of the sample in a hemocytometer, a specially constructed counting chamber that contains a specific blood volume. This process is time-consuming, requires a great deal of technical expertise, and has largely been replaced by automated methods. There are a variety of automated hematology analyzers available from manufacturers, such as Abbott, Beckman Coulter, Siemens, Sysmex, Horiba, and others. Analyzer selection depends on the volume of samples to be tested and the specific needs of the laboratory and health care system. The analyzers range in price and workload capacity from those that would be appropriate for an individual physician's office or point-of-care facility to those needed in a busy high-volume reference laboratory.

Automated hematology analyzers sample directly from phlebotomy tubes and use volumes as small as 150 μL for a full complete blood count (CBC) analysis.[9] They perform a variety of hematologic measurements in addition to basic cell counting, such as Hb concentration, red cell size, and leukocyte differentials. They may also perform more specialized testing, such as reticulocyte and nucleated RBC counts, and flagging of blasts, left shift, and variant lymphocytes.[9,12,13] Current analyzers utilize combinations of techniques to detect and differentiate specific cell types, including electrical impedance, radiofrequency conductivity, laser light scattering, flow cytometry, fluorescence detection, cytochemistry, and monoclonal antibodies (*Figures 1.1* and *1.2*).[9,12,13] Using flow-cytometric technologies, some analyzers detect specific blood cell populations by antigen expression, such as detection of CD34-positive peripheral blood stem cells or leukemic blasts.[9,14,15] Integration of data from various sources of information has improved the accuracy of the five-part differential and decreased the numbers of unidentifiable cells requiring manual review for identification, although analyzers do still frequently generate flags for abnormalities that require further investigation.[16-18] The

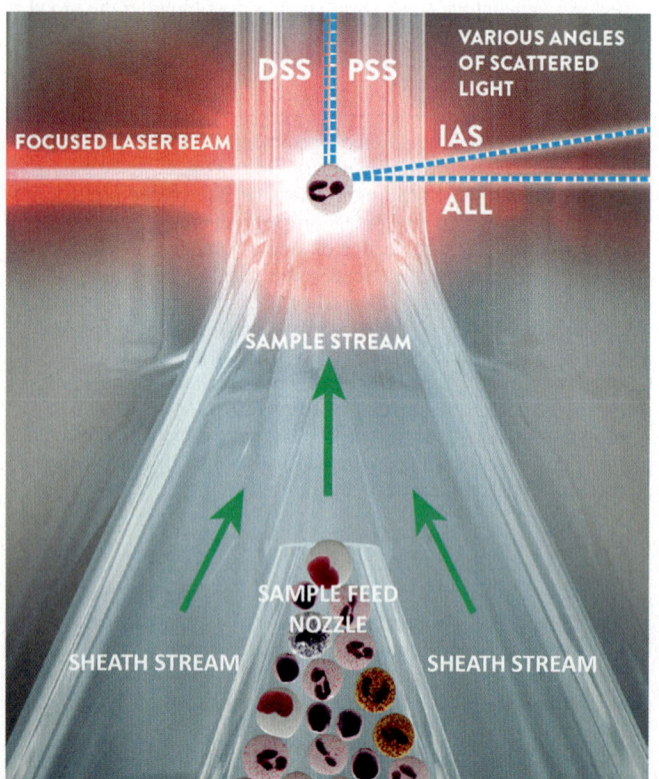

FIGURE 1.1 Optical flow-cytometric technology used in automated hematology analyzers. A suspension of cells is passed through a flow chamber and focused into a single-cell sample stream. The cells pass through a chamber and interact with a laser light beam. The scatter of the laser light beam at different angles is recorded, generating signals that are converted to electronic information about cell size, structure, internal structure, and granularity. (Cell-Dyn is a trademark of Abbott or its related companies. Reproduced with permission of Abbott, © 2022. All rights reserved.)

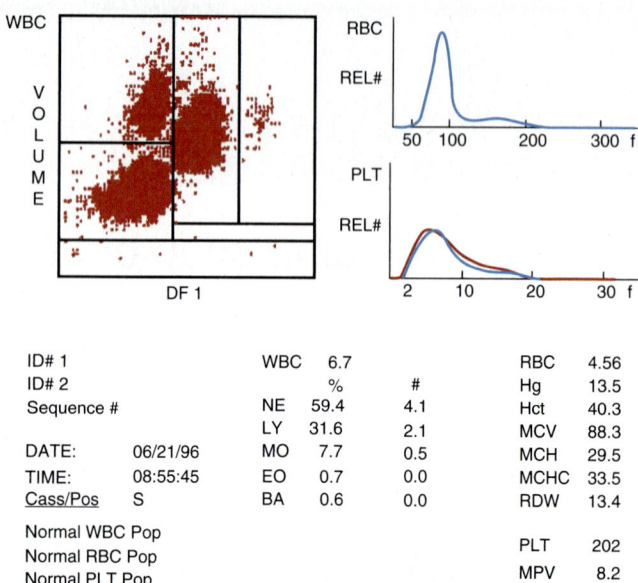

ID# 1		WBC	6.7		RBC	4.56
ID# 2			%	#	Hg	13.5
Sequence #		NE	59.4	4.1	Hct	40.3
		LY	31.6	2.1	MCV	88.3
DATE:	06/21/96	MO	7.7	0.5	MCH	29.5
TIME:	08:55:45	EO	0.7	0.0	MCHC	33.5
Cass/Pos	S	BA	0.6	0.0	RDW	13.4
Normal WBC Pop						
Normal RBC Pop					PLT	202
Normal PLT Pop					MPV	8.2

FIGURE 1.2 Histograms and printout generated by the Coulter automated hematology analyzer utilizing light scatter and electrical impedance. BA, basophil; DF 1, differential; EO, eosinophil; Hct, hematocrit; Hg, hemoglobin; LY, lymphocyte; MCH, mean corpuscular hemoglobin; MCHC, mean corpuscular hemoglobin concentration; MCV, mean corpuscular volume; MO, monocyte; MPV, mean platelet volume; NE, neutrophil; PLT, platelet; RBC, red blood cell; RDW, red cell distribution width; REL, relative; WBC, white blood cell.

International Consensus Group for Hematology Review has suggested criteria that should lead to manual review of a specimen after automated analysis and differential counting.[15,16]

RED BLOOD CELL PARAMETERS

RBCs are defined by three quantitative values: the volume of packed red cells or hematocrit (Hct), the amount of Hb, and the red cell number per unit volume (RBC). Three additional indices describing average qualitative characteristics of the red cell population are also collected. These are mean corpuscular volume (MCV), mean corpuscular hemoglobin (MCH), and mean corpuscular hemoglobin concentration (MCHC). All these values are routinely determined by hematology analyzers.

Volume of Packed Red Cells (Hematocrit)

The Hct is the proportion of the volume of a blood sample that is occupied by red cells. Hct may be determined manually by centrifugation of blood at a given speed and time in a standardized glass tube with a uniform bore, as was originally described by Wintrobe.[19] The height of the column of red cells after centrifugation compared with total blood sample volume yields the Hct. Macromethods (using 3-mm test tubes) with low-speed centrifugation or micromethods using capillary tubes and high-speed centrifugation may be used.

Manual methods of measuring Hct are simple and accurate means of assessing red cell status. They are easily performed with little specialized equipment, allowing adaptation for situations in which automated cell analysis is not readily available or for office use. However, several sources of error are inherent in the technique. The spun Hct measures the red cell volume, not red cell mass. Therefore, patients in shock or with volume depletion may have normal or high Hct measurements because of hemoconcentration despite a decreased red cell mass. Technical sources of error in manual Hct determinations usually arise from inappropriate concentrations of anticoagulants, poor mixing of samples, or insufficient centrifugation.[19] Another inherent error in manual Hct determinations arises from trapping of plasma in the red cell column. This may account for 1% to 3% of the volume in microcapillary tube methods, with macrotube methods trapping relatively more plasma.[20,21] It should be noted that abnormal red cells (e.g., sickle cells, microcytic cells, macrocytic cells, or spherocytes) often trap higher volumes of plasma because of increased cellular rigidity, possibly accounting for up to 6% of the red cell volume.[21] Very high Hcts, as in polycythemia, may also have excess plasma trapping. Manual Hct methods have a coefficient of variation (CV) of approximately 2%.[20]

Automated analyzers do not depend on centrifugation techniques to determine Hct, but instead calculate Hct using direct measurements of red cell number and red cell volume as follows: Hct = red cell number × mean red cell volume. Alternatively, some analyzers measure Hct directly by comparing the sum of all RBC size measurements to the volume of the specimen. Automated Hct values closely parallel manually obtained measurements, and the manual Hct is used as the reference method for hematology analyzers (with correction for the error induced by plasma trapping). Errors of automated Hct calculation are more common in patients with polycythemia[22] or abnormal plasma osmotic pressures.[23] Manual methods of Hct determination may be preferable in these cases. The CV of most automated Hcts is <1.5%.[24,25]

Hemoglobin Concentration

Hb is an intensely colored protein, allowing its measurement by spectrophotometric techniques. Hb is found in the blood in a variety of forms, including oxyhemoglobin, carboxyhemoglobin, methemoglobin, and other minor components. These may be converted to a single stable compound, cyanmethemoglobin, by mixing blood with Drabkin solution (contains potassium ferricyanide and potassium cyanide).[26] Sulfhemoglobin is not converted but is rarely present in significant amounts. The absorbance of the cyanmethemoglobin is measured in a spectrophotometer at 540 nm to determine Hb. This technique is used both in manual determinations and in most automated hematology analyzers, although cyanide-free methods are used by some. Hb is reported in grams per deciliter (g/dL) of whole blood. The main errors in measurement arise from dilution errors or increased sample turbidity caused by improperly lysed red cells, leukocytosis, or increased levels of lipid or protein in the plasma.[27-29] Older analyzers reported spurious increases in Hb levels when white cell counts exceeded 30×10^9/L because of increased turbidity, but this is decreased with newer flow systems so that Hb levels remain extremely accurate in the face of WBC counts as high as 100×10^9/L.[24] With automated methods, the precision for Hb determination is <1% (CV).[24,25]

Red Cell Count

Manual methods for counting red cells have proven to be very inaccurate, and automated counters provide a much more accurate reflection of red cell numbers.[30] Both erythrocytes and leukocytes are counted after whole blood dilution in an isotonic solution. Because the number of red cells (expressed as 10^{12} cells/L) greatly exceeds the number of white cells (by a factor of 500 or more), the error introduced by counting both cell types is negligible. However, when marked leukocytosis is present, red cell counts and volume determinations may be erroneous, unless corrected for white cells. The observed precision for RBC counts using automated hematology analyzers is approximately 1% (CV)[24,25] compared with a minimum estimated value of 11% with manual methods.[30]

Mean Corpuscular Volume

The average volume of the RBC is a useful parameter that is used to classify anemias and may provide insights into the pathophysiology of red cell disorders.[31] The MCV is measured in femtoliters (fL or 10^{-15} L) and is usually measured directly in automated analyzers by dividing the sum of the individual RBC volumes by the RBC count but may also be calculated from the RBC count and the Hct using the following formula[19]:

$$MCV = Hct(L/L) \times 1000/\text{red cell count}(10^{12}/L)$$

The CV in most automated systems is approximately 1%,[24,25] compared with 10% for manual methods.[20] Agglutination of cells, as with cold agglutinin disease or paraproteinemia, may result in a falsely elevated MCV.[32] Most automated analyzers gate out MCV values above 360 fL, thereby excluding most red cell clumps, although this may falsely lower calculated Hct determinations. In addition, severe hyperglycemia (glucose > 600 mg/dL) may cause osmotic swelling of the red cells, leading to a falsely elevated MCV, which could also lead to a falsely high Hct and falsely decreased MCHC.[23,33] Leukocytosis may also spuriously elevate MCV values.[27]

Mean Corpuscular Hemoglobin

MCH is a measure of the average Hb content per RBC. It may be calculated manually or by automated methods using the following formula[19]:

$$MCH = \text{hemoglobin}(g/L)/\text{red cell count}(10^{12}/L)$$

MCH is expressed in picograms (pg, or 10^{-12} g). In anemias secondary to impaired Hb synthesis, such as iron deficiency anemia, Hb mass per red cell decreases, resulting in a lower MCH value. MCH measurements may be falsely elevated by hyperlipidemia[29] because increased plasma turbidity will erroneously elevate Hb measurement. The CV for automated analysis of MCH is 1% to 2% in most modern analyzers, compared with approximately 10% for manual methods.[20,25]

Mean Corpuscular Hemoglobin Concentration

The average concentration of Hb in a given red cell volume, or MCHC, may be calculated by the following formula[19]:

$$MCHC = \text{hemoglobin}(g/dL)/Hct(L/L)$$

The MCHC is expressed in grams of Hb per deciliter of packed RBCs, representing the ratio of Hb mass and the volume of red cells. Except for hereditary spherocytosis and some cases of homozygous sickle cell or hemoglobin C disease, MCHC values will not exceed 37 g/dL. This level is close to the solubility value for Hb, and further increases in Hb may lead to crystallization. The accuracy of the MCHC determination is affected by factors that have an impact on measurement of either Hct (plasma trapping or the presence of abnormal red cells) or Hb (hyperlipidemia and leukocytosis), which is methodology specific.[27] The CV for MCHC for automated methods ranges between 1.0% and 1.5%.[24]

As noted earlier, the MCV, MCH, and MCHC reflect average values and may not adequately describe blood samples when mixed populations of red cells are present. For example, in sideroblastic anemias, a dimorphic red cell population of both microcytic hypochromic and normocytic normochromic cells may be present, yet the indices may be normochromic and normocytic. It is important to examine the blood smear as well as instrument red cell histograms to detect such dimorphic populations.[16] The MCV is an extremely useful value in classification of anemias,[24,31,34] but the MCH and MCHC often do not add significant, clinically relevant information.

Red Cell Distribution Width

The red cell distribution width (RDW) is a red cell measurement that quantitates cellular volume heterogeneity, reflecting the range of red cell sizes within a sample.[35] RDW has been proposed to be useful in early classification of anemia because it becomes abnormal earlier in nutritional deficiency anemias than other red cell parameters, especially in cases of iron deficiency anemia.[36] RDW is particularly useful in characterizing microcytic anemia, allowing discrimination between uncomplicated iron deficiency anemia (high RDW and normal-to-low MCV) and uncomplicated heterozygous thalassemia (normal RDW and low MCV),[36] although other tests are usually required to confirm the diagnosis. RDW is also useful in identifying red cell fragmentation, agglutination, or dimorphic cell populations (including patients who have had transfusions, have sideroblastic anemias, or have been recently treated for a nutritional deficiency).[36,37] RDW is increased in common conditions such as cardiovascular disease, diabetes, cancer, and infections, and increased RDW has been found to predict mortality in certain settings.[38]

Reticulocyte Counts

Determination of the numbers of reticulocytes or immature, non-nucleated RBCs that still contain RNA provides useful information about the capacity of the bone marrow to synthesize and release red cells in response to anemia and helps to distinguish between decreased RBC production and enhanced peripheral destruction. Corrected reticulocyte counts or the reticulocyte production index (RPI) can be used to compare the magnitude of reticulocytosis with the magnitude of anemia to determine whether the bone marrow response is adequate. In the past, reticulocyte counts were performed manually using supravital staining with methylene blue, which stains precipitated RNA as a dark-blue meshwork or granules (at least two per cell).[39] Normal values for reticulocytes in adults are 0.5% to 1.5%, although they may be 2.5% to 6.5% in newborns (falling to adult levels by the second week of life). Because there are relatively low numbers of reticulocytes, the CV for manual reticulocyte counting is relatively large (10%-20% or higher).[40,41]

To increase the accuracy of reticulocyte counting, automated detection methods using fluorescent dyes that bind to RNA allow for many more cells to be analyzed, thereby increasing the accuracy and precision of counts.[42,43] Most hematology analyzers offer automated reticulocyte counting and can report reticulocyte numbers with routine CBC parameters. CVs of 10% or less can be achieved using automated analyzers.[24,25,44] Differences in reticulocyte counts obtained from different analyzers have been observed, which are likely related to instrument-specific technologies.[9] Current instruments also have the capability to report novel reticulocyte parameters such as immature reticulocyte fraction (IRF) and reticulocyte cellular indices such as cell volume and Hb content. The IRF quantitates younger reticulocytes identified by more intense staining with RNA stains. However, the clinical utility of these novel parameters is still being investigated and differences between instruments have been reported.[45] Potential clinical uses for IRF include as an indicator of early marrow recovery in bone marrow transplant, an indicator of response to treatment with erythropoietic stimulating agents, and as an alternative to the manually calculated RPI.[43]

Nucleated Red Blood Cell Counts

Circulating nucleated red blood cells (NRBCs) are abnormal in adults and are seen in conditions such as acute hemolysis and hypoxic stress, reflecting an increase in marrow erythropoietic activity, and can also be seen with bone marrow involvement by hematologic or other malignancies. NRBCs are also normally seen in newborns, particularly premature newborns, and young infants. Modern hematology analyzers provide enumeration of circulating NRBCs, with results expressed as number of NRBCs per volume of blood and as a percentage per 100 WBCs. Automated counts have been historically challenging because these cells have a size and nucleus similar to mature lymphocytes and misclassification as lymphocytes can lead to errors in the total leukocyte count and differential. Correction of WBC counts may be necessary in the presence of high numbers of NRBCs. Although analyzers have become more sophisticated in the identification of NRBCs, a study of five common hematology analyzers demonstrated poor concordance of NRBC counts between instruments and between automated and manual counts, likely representing differences in instrument technologies.[9]

LEUKOCYTE ANALYSIS

White Blood Cell Counts

Leukocytes (WBCs) may also be enumerated by either manual methods or automated hematology analyzers. WBCs are counted after dilution of blood in a diluent that lyses the RBCs (usually acid or detergent). The much lower numbers of leukocytes present require less dilution of the blood than is needed for RBC counts. As with red cell counts, manual leukocyte counts have more inherent error, with CVs ranging from 6.5% in cases with normal or increased white cell counts to 15% in cases with decreased white cell counts.[46] Automated methods characteristically yield CVs in the 1% to 3% range for normal or elevated counts but also with increased CVs (approximately 6%) for low WBC counts.[24,25] Automated leukocyte counts may be falsely elevated, with inaccurate differentials, in the presence of cryoglobulins or cryofibrinogen,[47] giant platelets or platelet clumps,[48] and nucleated RBCs, or when there is incomplete lysis of red cells, possibly requiring manual counting. Falsely low neutrophil counts have also been reported because of granulocyte agglutination secondary to surface immunoglobulin interactions.[49]

Leukocyte Differentials

WBCs are analyzed to find the relative percentage of each cell type in a differential leukocyte count. This information can be used to determine absolute counts for each cell type by multiplying the percentage by the total WBC count. Uniform standards for performing manual differential leukocyte counts on blood smears have been proposed by the CLSI[50] to ensure reproducibility of results between laboratories. It is important to scan the entire blood smear at low power to ensure that all atypical cells and cellular distribution patterns are recognized. In wedge-pushed smears, leukocytes tend to aggregate in the feathered edge and side of the blood smear rather than in the center of the slide. Larger cells in particular (blasts and monocytes) tend to aggregate at the edges of the blood smear.[51] The use of coverslip preparations and spinner systems tends to minimize this artifact of cell distribution. For wedge-pushed smears, it is recommended that a battlement pattern of smear scanning be used in which one counts fields in one direction, then changes direction and counts an equal number of fields before changing direction again to minimize distributional errors.[50]

In manual leukocyte counts, three main sources of error are found: distribution of cells on the slide, cell recognition errors, and statistical sampling errors. Poor blood smear preparation and staining are major contributors to cell recognition and cell distribution errors. Statistical errors are the main source of error inherent in manual counts because of the small sample size in counts of 100 or 200 cells. The CV in manual counts is between 5% and 10% and is also highly dependent on the skill of the technician performing the differential. Accuracy may be improved by increasing the numbers of cells counted, but for practical purposes, most laboratories will do a differential on 100 white cells.[13,52]

Automated leukocyte differentials markedly decrease the time and cost of performing routine examinations as well as improving precision with CVs of approximately 3% for normal neutrophil and lymphocyte counts.[25,52,53] However, automated analysis is incapable of accurately identifying and classifying all types of cells and is particularly insensitive to abnormal or immature cells, especially in small numbers. There have been some improvements in the ability of instrument to identify immature granulocytes, including blasts.[13] However, a comparison of five analyzers demonstrated that samples containing blasts may be missed, in particular with low WBC counts, and that blasts may sometimes be misclassified as other cell types, such as variant lymphocytes. Instrument blast flags may also be generated in samples where circulating blasts are not subsequently confirmed by microscopy.[9,54] For these reasons, instrument flags for possible abnormal white cell populations indicate the need for examination by a skilled morphologist.[16,53]

Hematology analyzers identify cells based on the combinations of cellular size, cell complexity, and staining characteristics, allowing for generation of a five-part differential count that enumerates neutrophils, monocytes, lymphocytes, eosinophils, and basophils.[24] Most analyzers use flow-cytometric techniques where the cells are suspended in diluent and passed through an optical flow cell in a continuous stream so that single cells are analyzed (*Figure 1.1*). The differential data are plotted as a histogram (*Figure 1.2*), which displays and classifies cell populations based on their characteristics. Lymphocytes are characterized as small unstained cells (no myeloperoxidase staining). Atypical/reactive lymphocytes, some blasts, circulating plasma cells, or other abnormal cells are larger than mature lymphocytes with low internal complexity and no myeloperoxidase activity and are classified as large unstained cells. Neutrophils have higher internal complexity (because of the segmented nucleus and granules) and appear as larger cells. Eosinophils appear smaller than neutrophils because they tend to absorb some of their own light scatter. Monocytes have lower levels of complexity, are usually found between neutrophils and lymphocytes, and can be challenging to accurately classify.[13] To enumerate basophils, which are few in number and lack specific staining characteristics, a basophil-nuclear lobularity channel may be utilized. For this determination, RBCs and WBCs are differentially lysed, leaving bare leukocyte nuclei, except for basophils, which are resistant to lysis, and can then be counted based on relatively large cell size because of the retained cytoplasm. Analysis using this technique examines thousands of cells per sample, increasing statistical accuracy, although the accuracy of automated basophil counts is still recognized as a challenge for all analyzers.[13,24,55]

Hematology analyzers may have settings that allow for evaluation of red cell and white cell populations in very hypocellular specimens, such as body fluids. Because higher numbers of cells are evaluated, the accuracy of cell counts and differential counting is improved over manual counting methods.[56-59] However, manual techniques are still commonly used for cerebrospinal fluid and body fluid specimens.[13]

Automated digital image analysis is now used by some hematology analyzers. For instance, CellaVision has an automated image analyzer that captures digital images of cells in a stained smear and classifies them to provide a differential that includes mature and immature WBCs and other cells, such as variant lymphocytes and plasma cells.[55] The images are reviewed by trained technologists to further refine the classifications if needed. RBC and platelet counts and morphology can also be analyzed.[60] The systems have the capacity to store images and are useful in training technologists as well as providing an easily accessible means, whereby smears obtained at different times from a single patient may be compared morphologically.[61] These systems perform well in normal blood specimens but have limitations in their ability to identify morphologically abnormal cells, so specimens with dysplastic changes, unusual morphologic variants, or significant artifacts may not be evaluable or may provide false data.[13,55,62-65] Often, these systems will designate a certain percentage of cells as unclassifiable, requiring review by a technologist for definitive identification of the cell type and completion of the differential.

PLATELET ANALYSIS

Platelets are anucleate cytoplasmic fragments that are 2 to 4 μm in diameter. As with the other blood components, they may be counted by either manual or automated methods. Manual methods involve dilution of blood samples and enumeration in a counting chamber or hemocytometer using phase-contrast microscopy. Sources of error are similar to other manual counting techniques and include dilution errors and low numbers of events counted. The CV of manual methods, especially in patients with thrombocytopenia, may be >15%.[66] Platelets are counted in automated hematology analyzers after removal of red cells by sedimentation or centrifugation or using whole blood. Platelets are identified by light scatter, impedance characteristics, and/or platelet antigen– or platelet-specific cytoplasmic staining.[24,60] These give reliable platelet counts with a CV of approximately 3% in the normal range. However, achieving accurate counts in patients with thrombocytopenia remains a challenge, and CVs in thrombocytopenic samples are closer to 5%.[25] Falsely low platelet counts may be caused

by the presence of large platelets, platelet clumps/agglutinins,[48] or adsorption of platelets to leukocytes.[67] Fragments of RBCs or WBCs may falsely elevate the automated platelet count, but this usually gives rise to an abnormal histogram that identifies the spurious result.[68,69]

Automated hematology analyzers also determine mean platelet volume (MPV), which has been correlated with several disease states.[70] In general, MPV has an inverse relationship with platelet count, with larger platelet volumes (secondary to new platelet production) seen in thrombocytopenic patients in whom platelets are decreased because of peripheral destruction (as in immune thrombocytopenia).[70-73] MPV may also be increased in myeloproliferative disorders. However, it should be noted that platelets tend to swell during the first 2 hours in EDTA anticoagulant, shrinking again with longer storage.[73,74] Decreased MPV has been associated with megakaryocytic hypoplasia and cytotoxic drug therapy.[75]

Other platelet parameters may also be reported, depending on the analyzer. The immature platelet fraction, or reticulated platelets, represents newly released platelets that retain residual RNA, analogous to red cell reticulocytes.[60] Reticulated platelet counts are determined using RNA staining dyes, give an estimate of thrombopoiesis, and may be useful in distinguishing platelet destruction syndromes from hypoplastic platelet production in bone marrow failure conditions.[60,76,77] Normal values vary between 3% and 20%, and 2.5- to 4.5-fold increases in reticulated platelet counts are seen in the clinical setting of immune thrombocytopenia.[77] Increased reticulated platelets may herald the return of platelet production after chemotherapy.[78] However, differences between methods for identifying immature platelets limit comparisons between clinical studies that use different analytical methods.[77]

ADVANTAGES AND SOURCES OF ERROR WITH AUTOMATED HEMATOLOGY

Clearly, the use of automated hematology analyzers has reduced laboratory costs and turnaround time while also improving the accuracy and reproducibility of blood counts. Thorough verification of hematology analyzers prior to clinical use and adequate technical and quality control procedures are essential.[8,25,79] Despite the high level of accuracy and precision, automated hematology analyzers may generate a warning flag in 10% to 25% of samples, requiring manual examination of the blood smear.[2,4,16-18,80] Blood smear examination still plays an important role in characterizing these samples. Some cell types are only identified morphologically, such as Sézary cells, and red cell morphology is best analyzed by direct smear examination.[34] While there have been recent advances allowing increased automation of blood smear morphologic analysis with analyzers that use artificial intelligence algorithms and digital image analysis, there is a lack of standardization between methods, and improvements are still needed in accuracy of cell classifications.[81]

Certain disease states are associated with spuriously high or low results from analyzers, although some of these are specific to a particular type of instrumentation (summarized in *Table 1.1*). Therefore, values obtained from the automated hematology analyzer must be interpreted in the context of clinical findings. As previously mentioned, careful examination of the stained blood film often imparts additional information that may not be reflected in the average values reported by the automated CBC.

MORPHOLOGIC ANALYSIS OF BLOOD CELLS

Careful evaluation of a well-prepared blood smear is an important part of the evaluation of hematologic disease. Although a specific diagnosis may be suggested by the data obtained from an automated hematology analyzer, many diseases may have normal blood counts but abnormal cellular morphology. Examples of abnormal red cells that may be seen in the peripheral blood smear examination and that are associated with specific disease states are found in *Table 1.2*. Morphologic analysis may be greatly hampered by poorly prepared or stained blood smears.

Table 1.1. Disorders and Conditions That May Reduce the Accuracy of Blood Cell Counting

Component	Disorder/Condition	Effect on Cell Count	Rationale
Red cells	Microcytosis or schistocytes	May underestimate RBC	Lower threshold of RBC counting window is greater than microcyte size
	Howell-Jolly bodies	May spuriously elevate platelet count (in whole blood platelet counters only)	Howell-Jolly bodies are similar in size to platelets
	Polycythemia	May underestimate RBC	Increased coincidence counting
White cells	Leukocytosis	Overestimate RBC	Increased coincidence counting
	Acute leukemia and chronic lympho-cytic leukemia, viral infections	May spuriously lower WBC	Increased fragility of leukocytes, including immature forms
	Chemotherapy of acute leukemia	May artifactually increase platelet count	Leukemic cell nuclear or cytoplasmic fragments identified as platelets
Platelets	Platelet agglutinins	May underestimate platelet count, sometimes with spurious increase in WBC	Platelet clumping Aggregates may be identified as leukocytes
Plasma	Cold agglutinins	May underestimate RBC with spurious macrocytosis	Red cell doublets, triplets, etc. have increased volume
	Cryoglobulins, cryofibrinogens	Variation in platelet count	Protein precipitates may be identified as platelets

Some of these examples affect counts only when certain instruments are used. The effects depend on methodology, dilution, solutions used, and specimen temperatures.
Abbreviations: RBC, red blood cell count; WBC, white blood cell count.
Adapted from Koepke JA. *Laboratory Hematology.* Churchill Livingstone; 1984. Copyright © 1984 Elsevier. With permission.

Preparation of Blood Smears

Blood films may be prepared on either glass slides or coverslips. Each method has specific advantages and disadvantages.[82] Blood smears are often prepared from samples of anticoagulated blood remaining after automated hematologic analysis. However, artifacts in cell appearance and staining may be induced by anticoagulant.[7] Optimal morphology and staining are obtained from nonanticoagulated blood, most often from a finger-stick procedure. Mechanical dragging of the cells across the glass of the slide or coverslip and uneven distribution of blood may also distort the cells; however, these artifacts are minimized with proper technique.

Coverslip smears (*Figure 1.3A*) are prepared using a good grade of flat, no. 1, 0.5-in square (or 22 × 22 mm) coverslips that are free of lint, dust, and grease. Such coverslips allow optimal spreading of the blood over the surface and minimal artifact. Usually, high-quality coverslips do not require additional cleaning, although there may be some deterioration with age. Plastic "nonwettable" coverslips are not satisfactory for these preparations. The smear is prepared by holding the coverslip by two adjacent corners between the thumb and index finger. A small drop of fresh or anticoagulated blood is placed in the center of the coverslip. The size of the drop of blood is critical. If the drop is too large, a thick smear results. If the drop of blood is too small, a very thin smear is obtained. A second coverslip is then grasped in a similar manner with the other hand, placed across the first coverslip, and rotated 45° with a steady, rapid, and gentle motion. The two coverslips are then immediately pulled apart and allowed to air-dry. If done properly, this procedure produces two coverslips with even dispersion of blood without holes or excessively thick areas.[83]

Blood smears may also be prepared on clean glass slides by the wedge method (*Figure 1.3B*). This often leads to irregular distribution of cells on the slide, a distinct disadvantage over the coverslip procedure. However, glass slides are less fragile, are easier to handle, and may be labeled more easily than coverslips. To prepare a slide blood smear, a drop of blood is placed in the middle of the slide approximately 1 to 2 cm from one end. A second spreader slide is placed at a 30° to 45° angle and moved backward to contact the blood drop. The blood drop will spread along the slide edge and then the spreader slide is moved rapidly forward. This technique creates a film of blood that is 3 to 4 cm long. Artifacts may be introduced by irregular edges in the spreader and by the speed at which the spreader is moved. Glass slide preparations have increased incidence of accumulation of the larger white cells at the edges of the film, introducing cellular distribution errors. Fast movement of the spreader results in a more uniformly distributed population of cells.[83,84]

Automated techniques for blood smear preparation have also been developed, and some instruments have integrated automated blood smear preparation technology, thus allowing smear preparation directly from the CBC tube. Two major types of approaches are used: centrifugation and mechanical spreaders. Centrifugation techniques are often most useful when a small number of cells must be concentrated in a small area, as in preparing smears of cells in fluids such as cerebrospinal fluid.[85] Mechanical spreaders mimic the manual technique and are useful when large numbers of blood smears are prepared.[86] In general, smears made by automated techniques are inferior to those made by an experienced technician.

Routine Staining of Blood Smears

Blood smears are usually stained with either Wright or May-Grünwald-Giemsa stains. Both stains are modifications of the Romanowsky procedure.[84] The stain may be purchased commercially or made in the laboratory. The basic stain is formulated from methylene blue and eosin. Giemsa stains use known quantities of acid bichromate to form the converted azure compounds. The Wright stain formulation uses sodium bicarbonate to convert methylene blue to methylene azure, which stains the cell. All types of Romanowsky stains are water insoluble but can be dissolved in methyl alcohol. The stain must be free of water to avoid RBC artifacts. This may be avoided by fixation of slides or coverslips in anhydrous methanol before staining.[87]

Optimal staining conditions must be established for each new batch of stain. The methylene blue conversion to azure compounds continues to occur while the stain is in the bottle, so staining conditions may change over time. Methyl azures are basic dyes that impart a violet-blue coloration when binding to the acidic components of the cell, such as nucleic acids and proteins. The eosin reacts with the basic cellular elements, imparting a reddish hue to cytoplasmic components and Hb. A properly stained slide has a pink tint. The red cells will have an orange-to-pink coloration, and leukocytes have purplish-blue nuclei. The Romanowsky stains differentially stain leukocyte granules, which aids in morphologic analysis of the cells. Thus, neutrophil granules are slightly basic and stain weakly with the azurophilic component. The eosinophils contain a strongly basic spermine derivative and stain strongly with eosin. In contrast, basophil granules contain

Table 1.2. Pathologic Red Cells in Blood Smears

Red Cell Type	Description	Underlying Change	Disease State Associations
Acanthocyte (spur cell)	Irregularly spiculated red cells with projections of varying length and dense center	Altered cell membrane lipids	Abetalipoproteinemia, parenchymal liver disease, post splenectomy
Basophilic stippling	Punctuate basophilic inclusions	Precipitated ribosomes (RNA)	Coarse stippling: Lead intoxication, thalassemia Fine stippling: A variety of anemias
Bite cell (degmacyte)	Smooth semicircle taken from one edge	Heinz body pitting by spleen	Glucose-6-phosphate dehydrogenase deficiency, drug-induced oxidant hemolysis
Burr cell (echinocyte) or crenated red cell	Red cells with short, evenly spaced spicules and preserved central pallor	May be associated with altered membrane lipids	Usually artifactual; seen in uremia, bleeding ulcers, gastric carcinoma
Cabot rings	Circular, blue, threadlike inclusion with dots	Nuclear remnant	Post splenectomy, hemolytic anemia, megaloblastic anemia
Ovalocyte (elliptocyte)	Elliptically shaped cell	Abnormal cytoskeletal proteins	Hereditary elliptocytosis
Howell-Jolly bodies	Small, discrete, basophilic, dense inclusions; usually single	Nuclear remnant (DNA)	Post splenectomy, hemolytic anemia, megaloblastic anemia
Hypochromic red cell	Prominent central pallor	Diminished hemoglobin synthesis	Iron deficiency anemia, thalassemia, sideroblastic anemia
Macrocyte	Red cells larger than normal (>8.5 μm), well filled with hemoglobin	Young red cells, abnormal red cell maturation	Increased erythropoiesis; oval macrocytes in megaloblastic anemia; round macrocytes in liver disease
Microcyte	Red cells smaller than normal (<7.0 μm)	Diminished hemoglobin	Hypochromic red cell
Pappenheimer bodies	Small, dense, basophilic granules	Iron-containing siderosome or mitochondrial remnant	Sideroblastic anemia, post splenectomy
Polychromatophilia	Grayish or blue hue often seen in macrocytes	Ribosomal material	Reticulocytosis, premature marrow release of red cells
Rouleaux	Red cell aggregates resembling stack of coins	Red cell clumping by circulating paraprotein	Paraproteinemia
Schistocyte (helmet cell)	Distorted, fragmented cell; two or three pointed ends	Mechanical distortion in microvasculature by fibrin strands, disruption by prosthetic heart valve	Microangiopathic hemolytic anemia (disseminated intravascular coagulation, thrombotic thrombocytopenic purpura, hemolytic uremic syndrome, prosthetic heart valves, severe burns)
Sickle cell (drepanocyte)	Bipolar, spiculated forms, sickle-shaped, pointed at both ends	Molecular aggregation of HbS	Sickle-cell disorders, not including S trait
Spherocyte	Spherical cell with dense appearance and absent central pallor, usually decreased diameter	Decreased membrane surface area	Hereditary spherocytosis, immune hemolytic anemia
Stomatocyte	Mouth or cuplike deformity	Membrane defect with abnormal cation permeability	Hereditary stomatocytosis, immune hemolytic anemia
Target cell (codocyte)	Targetlike appearance, often hypochromic	Increased redundancy of cell membrane	Liver disease, post splenectomy, thalassemia, hemoglobin C disease
Teardrop cell (dacrocyte)	Distorted, drop-shaped cell	Altered bone marrow architecture	Myelofibrosis, myelophthisic anemia

Adapted from Kjeldsberg C, Perkins SL, eds. *Practical Diagnosis of Hematologic Disorders.* 5th ed. ASCP Press; 2010. Copyright © 2010 by American Society for Clinical Pathologists.

predominately acidic proteins and stain a deep blue-violet. No precipitate should overlie the cells because this indicates the use of slides or coverslips that were not cleaned properly. Dust on slides may also induce artifacts. Staining solutions should be filtered or replaced weekly, if used heavily, to avoid precipitation.[84]

Occasionally, an excessive blue coloration of the cells is seen. This may be caused by excessive staining times, improperly prepared or aged buffer that is too alkaline, old blood smears, or blood smears that are too thick. The quality of the staining may be improved by quick and vigorous rinsing with distilled water. If the areas of the slide between cells are staining, it usually indicates inadequate washing of the slide, heparin anticoagulation, or possible paraproteinemia. When the staining appears too pink or red, the usual problem is the buffer that is too acidic. This results in pale-stained leukocyte nuclei, excessively orange RBCs, and bright red eosinophil granules. Other causes

of excessive red or pink coloration include inadequate staining times or excessive washing of the slide. Most often, problems with staining are caused by problems with the pH of the solutions, and the use of new buffer solutions often corrects the problem.[87]

Examination of the Blood Smear

The blood smear should be initially examined under an intermediate power (×10 to ×20 objective) to assess the adequacy of cellular distribution and staining. An estimate of the WBC count may also be made at this power, and scanning for abnormal cellular elements, such as blasts or nucleated RBCs, can be performed. It is important to scan the entire blood smear to ensure that abnormal populations, which may be concentrated at the edges of the smear, are not missed. The use of an oil-immersion lens (×50 or ×100) or high-power dry lens (×40 or ×60) is usually sufficient for performing leukocyte differential counts,

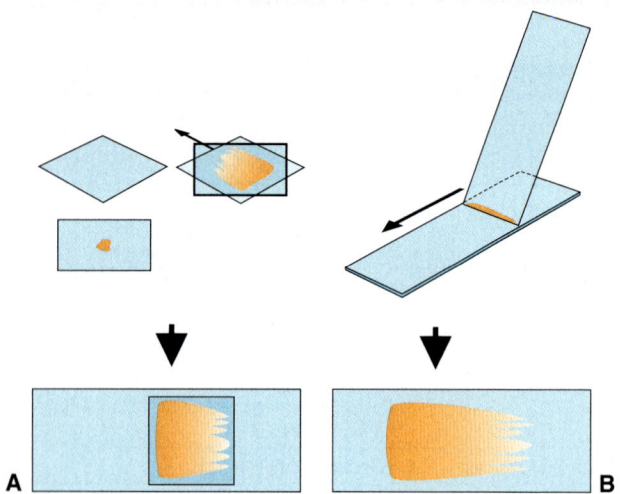

FIGURE 1.3 Preparation of blood smears. Blood smears may be prepared by the coverslip (A) or slide wedge method (B). Coverslip smears are prepared by placing a drop of blood in the center of a coverslip and spreading the blood by rotating a second coverslip over it. Wedge smears are prepared by placing a drop of blood on a slide and using a second slide to push the blood out along the length of the slide. (Adapted and redrawn from Bauer J. *Clinical Laboratory Methods.* 9th ed. C.V. Mosby; 1982.)

although a ×100 oil lens may be necessary for identification of cellular inclusions or abnormal cytoplasmic granules. Systematic evaluation of the blood smear is essential so that all cell types are examined and characterized. Each cell type should be evaluated for both quantitative and qualitative abnormalities.[88,89]

It is difficult to evaluate quantitative abnormalities of red cells on a blood smear; however, the RBCs should be evaluated for variations in size, shape, Hb content and distribution, and the presence of cellular inclusions. The red cells are usually unevenly distributed throughout the blood film. Optimal red cell morphology is seen in an area of the smear where the red cells are close together but do not overlap. Areas where the red cells are spread too thinly or thickly have increased artifacts. In some blood smears, the red cells appear to stick together, forming what appear to be stacks of RBCs, termed rouleaux. This finding may be mimicked in normal patients in areas of the smear where the red cells are too closely packed. However, if rouleaux are seen even in thinner areas of the blood film, it suggests the presence of a paraprotein coating the red cells and causing agglutination because of loss of normal electrostatic repulsion between red cells. Areas of the blood smear that are too thin will have loss of red cell central pallor, mimicking spherocytes.[88]

Red cells should be uniform in size and shape, with an average diameter of 7.2 to 7.9 µm. This may be evaluated by use of a micrometer or by comparison with the diameter of a small lymphocyte nucleus, which is approximately the same size or slightly smaller. Variation in red cell size is called anisocytosis. Cells that are larger than 9 µm and well hemoglobinized are considered macrocytes. Less mature erythrocytes are macrocytic and have a bluish tint to the Hb (polychromatophilia) or have fine basophilic stippling of the cell because of remnant RNA and ribosomes. Microcytes are cells with a diameter of <6 µm.[88,89]

Normal erythroid cells are round. Variations in red cell shape are called poikilocytosis. The red cell should have a pale central area (central pallor) with a rim of red-to-orange Hb. Hypochromia reflects poor hemoglobinization and results in a very thin rim of Hb or an increased area of central pallor. Abnormal distribution of Hb may result in the formation of a cell with a central spot of Hb surrounded by an area of pallor, called a target cell. Abnormal Hbs may also form crystals. Spherocytes and macrocytes lack an area of central pallor because of increased thickness of the cell. Red cells may also contain inclusions, such as remnants of nuclear material (Howell-Jolly bodies), remnants of mitochondria or siderosomes (Pappenheimer bodies),[89]

or infectious agents (malarial parasites, babesiosis).[90,91] In addition, red cell fragments, or schistocytes, suggestive of red cell mechanical destruction are more easily detected by blood smear examination, and underestimation of schistocyte numbers has been reported when using automated methods on hematology analyzers.[92-94] Observer bias in blood smear examination can be reduced by following standardized guidelines for schistocyte identification and quantification.[94]

Platelet counts and morphology are evaluated next. Platelets appear as small blue cytoplasmic fragments with red-to-purple granules. Platelets are usually 1 to 2 µm in diameter with wide variation in shape. Platelet counts may be estimated from the blood film. Normal platelet counts should have several (5-15) platelets per oil-immersion field or approximately 1 platelet for 10 to 20 RBCs.[95] It should be noted that platelets may aggregate if blood is not anticoagulated, properly, or a finger-stick preparation is used, and this may cause the spurious impression of a low platelet count.[96]

Finally, leukocyte morphology and distribution are analyzed. The number of leukocytes may be estimated by scanning the blood film at an intermediate power. Mechanical effects leading to abnormal distribution of larger cells should be excluded by examination of the edges of the blood film in particular.[88] White cells at the edges of the blood smear may appear artifactually smaller (because of cellular shrinkage and poor spreading of the cell) or larger (because of cell disruption and excessive spreading). Care must be taken when making the smear because cells, particularly neoplastic cells, may be more easily disrupted by excessive mechanical pressure than normal leukocytes. Optimal morphology of the leukocytes requires that those blood smears be made promptly. Significant artifacts begin to be observed in blood that has been held for several hours and include cytoplasmic vacuolation, nuclear karyorrhexis, and cytoplasmic disruption.[7]

The WBCs normally seen in the blood smear include neutrophils, eosinophils, basophils, lymphocytes, and monocytes. The presence of immature myeloid cells (myelocytes, metamyelocytes, promyelocytes, and blasts) is distinctly abnormal.[89] At least 100 cells should be identified and counted to yield a manual WBC differential.[88,89] In addition to identifying relative populations of white cells by performing a differential count, the cells should be closely examined for morphologic abnormalities of the cytoplasm and nucleus. For example, infection or growth factor therapy often leads to increased prominence of the primary (azurophilic) granules in neutrophils, termed toxic granulation.[95,97] In contrast, many myelodysplastic disorders are characterized by hypogranularity of neutrophils in addition to abnormal nuclear segmentation.[98] Cytoplasmic inclusions may be seen in some storage disorders or infections.[89,91,99]

Other Means of Examining Blood

Occasionally, it is necessary to examine fresh blood as a wet mount. Wet preparations are made by placing a drop of blood on a slide, covering the drop with a coverslip, and surrounding the coverslip with petroleum jelly or paraffin wax to seal the edges. If needed, the blood may be diluted with isotonic saline, or in some cases, it may be fixed with buffered glutaraldehyde for later examination. The blood may then be viewed with light or phase-contrast microscopy. Some organisms, such as spirochetes and trypanosomes, may be detected by movement in wet mount preparations, although more definitive testing, such as serology or molecular organism detection, is more frequently used.

Supravital staining is performed on living motile cells and helps avoid artifacts induced by smear preparation, fixation, and staining.[100] However, such preparations are not permanent, a distinct disadvantage. Supravital stains are often used to detect red cell inclusions. These include crystal violet staining that detects Heinz bodies or denatured Hb inclusions that appear as irregularly shaped purple bodies within the red cell. Brilliant cresyl blue may be used to precipitate and stain unstable Hbs, such as hemoglobin Zurich and hemoglobin H.[101] The most commonly used supravital stain is new methylene blue or brilliant cresyl blue, used for manual reticulocyte determinations,[42] although the use of automated methods of reticulocyte determination by CBC analyzers has largely replaced manual methods. Reticulocytes are not identified positively on Wright-stained blood smears, although their presence is suggested by polychromatophilia of RBCs. Automated reticulocyte counts may have increased errors in the presence of Heinz bodies[102] or Howell-Jolly bodies[103] in the red cells. Normal reference values for reticulocytes are influenced by patient age, sex, and physical activity level.[104]

BONE MARROW EXAMINATION

Diagnosis and management of many hematologic diseases depends on the evaluation of the bone marrow. Bone marrow examination usually involves two separate but interrelated specimens. The first is a cytologic preparation of bone marrow cells obtained by aspiration of the marrow and preparing a smear of the cells, allowing excellent visualization of cell morphology and detailed enumeration of the marrow cellular elements. The second specimen is a needle core biopsy of the bone and associated marrow, allowing optimal evaluation of bone marrow cellularity, fibrosis, infections, or infiltrative diseases.

Indications for bone marrow examination include further workup of hematologic abnormalities observed in the peripheral blood smear; evaluation of primary bone marrow tumors; staging for bone marrow involvement by metastatic tumors; assessment of infectious disease processes, including fever of unknown origin; and evaluation of storage diseases. Before a bone marrow examination is performed, clear diagnostic goals about the information to be obtained from the procedure should be defined, and decisions made about whether any special studies are needed, to ensure that all necessary specimens may be collected and handled correctly.

Several sites may be used for bone marrow aspiration and biopsy.[105,106] In part, the site chosen reflects the normal distribution of bone marrow and the age of the patient. At birth, hematopoietic marrow is found in all bones of the body. However, by early childhood, fat cells begin to replace the bone marrow hematopoietic cells in the extremities so that adults have hematopoiesis limited to the axial skeleton and proximal portions of the extremities.[105] Thus, younger children may have marrow examinations from the anteromedial tibial area, whereas adult marrow is best sampled from the sternum at the second intercostal space or from either the anterior or posterior iliac crests. Sternal marrows do not allow a biopsy to be performed, and several possible complications, including hemorrhage and pericardial tamponade, may occur if the inner table of the sternum is penetrated by the needle at areas other than the second intercostal space. The sternal marrow space in an adult is only approximately 1 cm thick at the second intercostal space, so care must be taken to avoid penetrating the chest cavity, although sternal bone marrow needles have guards to prevent penetration of the needle beyond the sternal plate. In contrast, little morbidity is associated with iliac crest aspiration and biopsy, and the posterior iliac crest is the most common site for bone marrow sampling.[107] The anterior iliac crest may be used if previous radiation, surgery, or discomfort does not allow a posterior approach.

Bone Marrow Aspiration and Biopsy

Bone marrow is a semifluid and is easily aspirated through a needle. Many types of needles have been used for performing marrow aspiration. Most are 14 to 18 gauge, and many have a removable obturator, which prevents plugging of the needle before aspiration, and a stylet that may be used to express the bone marrow biopsy sample (*Figure 1.4*). Some models, primarily used for sternal bone marrow aspiration procedures, have adjustable guards that limit the extent of needle penetration and reduce morbidity.[107] Most bone marrow needles are disposed of after one use, and specific longer needles that may be used for obese patients and mechanical drills to aid in bone penetration are available commercially.

In most cases, marrow aspiration and biopsy may be carried out with little risk of patient discomfort, provided adequate local anesthesia is used. Apprehensive patients may be sedated before the procedure. The procedure is performed under sterile conditions. The skin at the site of the biopsy is shaved, if necessary, and cleaned with a disinfectant solution. The skin, subcutaneous tissue, and periosteum in the area of the biopsy are anesthetized with a local anesthetic, such

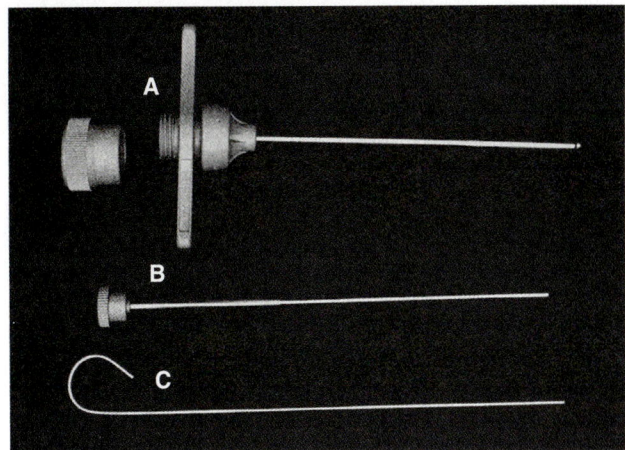

FIGURE 1.4 Jamshidi bone marrow aspiration and biopsy needle. This type of hollow needle with a beveled tip (A) is satisfactory for percutaneous biopsy of the bone marrow. The needle is inserted with the obturator (B) in place. The biopsy is expressed from the needle using the stylet (C).

as 1% lidocaine, using a 25-gauge needle. Care must be taken to fully anesthetize the periosteum, where most of the bone pain fibers are located. After the anesthetic has taken effect, a small cut is made in the skin overlying the biopsy site, and the marrow aspiration needle is inserted through the skin, subcutaneous tissues, and bone cortex with a slight rotating motion. Entrance of the needle into the bone marrow cavity should be sensed as a slight give or as an increase in the speed of needle advancement. The needle obturator is removed, and the needle is attached to a 10- or 20-mL syringe. Aspiration of the marrow is achieved by rapid suctioning with the syringe so that 0.2 to 2.0 mL of bloody fluid is obtained. Aspiration may cause a very brief, sharp pain. If no pain is noted and no marrow is obtained, the needle may be rotated, and suction applied again. If no marrow is obtained, relocation to another sampling site may be required.[106,108]

The aspirated material is given to a technical assistant, who makes smears of the material (*Figure 1.5*) and assesses the quality of the material by noting the presence of marrow spicules. The smears must be made quickly to avoid clotting in a manner like that described for blood smears using either coverslips or slides to spread the marrow (*Figure 1.3*). After smears are made, the aspirate may be allowed to clot to form a histologic clot section for processing. In some cases, where immediate slide preparation is not available, the bone marrow may be aspirated into a tube containing a small amount of anticoagulant to impede clotting. The aspirate may later be filtered and submitted for histologic processing into a particle clot section. EDTA is the best anticoagulant to use because it introduces the least amount of morphologic artifact to the specimen.[108] If additional material is needed for flow cytometry, cytogenetics, culture, or other special studies, additional aspirations may be performed by withdrawing the needle and repositioning it in a new site and drawing marrow into appropriate tubes. Morphologic examination requires the best sample, and the aspirations for ancillary studies should be performed after the initial aspiration. Occasionally, a portion of an anticoagulated marrow aspirate is spun down to obtain a buffy coat, thereby concentrating the cellular elements. In some instances, no marrow can be aspirated (dry tap). In these cases, it is essential to make smears from material at the tip of the needle and to make touch preparations from the biopsy, as outlined here, to allow cytologic examination of the bone marrow elements.[106,108]

The bone marrow core biopsy (*Figure 1.6*) may be performed using the same skin incision if the aspirate has been performed in the iliac crest area. A separate biopsy needle that is slightly larger than the needle used for aspiration may be used, or the same needle that was used for the bone marrow aspiration may be reused. Care must be taken to reposition the needle biopsy site away from the area where the aspiration was performed to avoid collection of a specimen

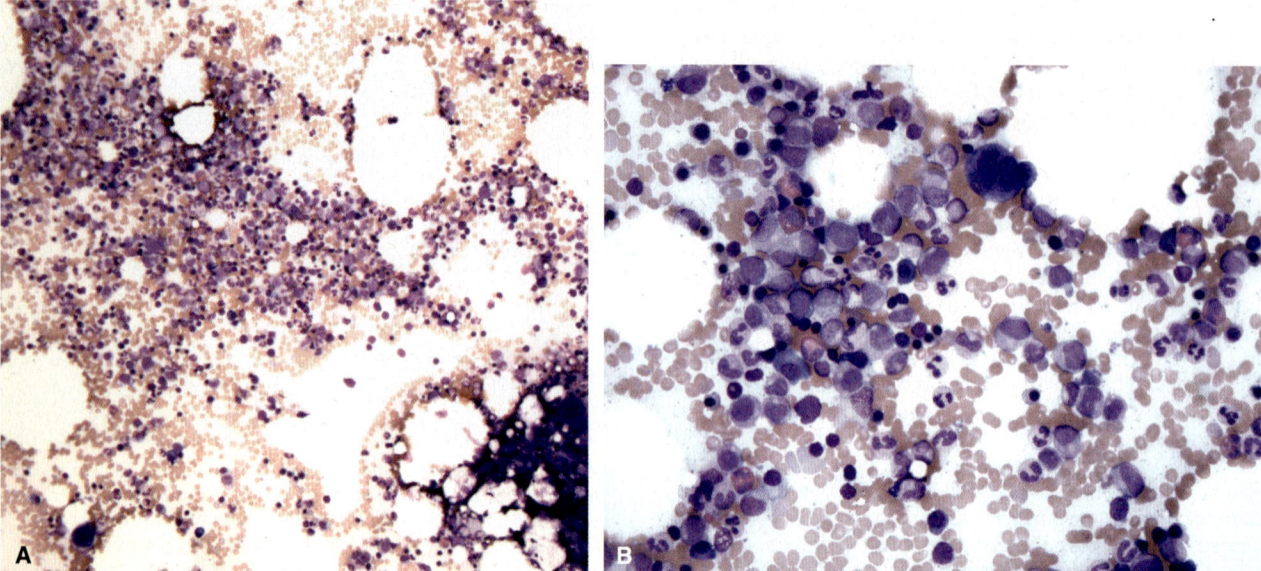

FIGURE 1.5 Bone marrow aspirate smear stained with Wright-Giemsa stain. The bone marrow aspirate shows a central spicule with dispersion of hematopoietic precursor cells around the spicule. The preparation allows for optimal evaluation of cytologic features of the bone marrow precursor cells. Panel A (low power) demonstrating distribution of hematopoietic cells near the darkly staining bone marrow spicule in a bone marrow aspirate. Panel B (high power) demonstrating cytologic features of bone marrow aspirate hematopoietic cells.

with extensive artifact induced by the aspiration procedure.[109] The use of a biopsy needle may require more pressure to enter the bone because of the larger bore size. Once the needle is in place in the bone, the stylet may be inserted to give an approximation of the size of the bone core within the needle. The biopsy needle is rotated and gently rocked to free the biopsy from the surrounding bone and then advanced slightly farther. The biopsy is then removed from the bone by withdrawing the needle, and slight positive pressure may be applied using a syringe. The biopsy is expressed from the needle by the stylet. Touch preparations of the bone biopsy should be made, particularly if no aspirate has been obtained, to allow cytologic examination of the bone marrow elements. The bony core is then fixed, decalcified, and processed for histologic examination.[110,111] Ancillary testing can often be performed on additional bone marrow cores when no material can be aspirated, so collection of more than one core biopsy may be necessary.

Once the biopsy is completed, manual pressure is applied to the site for several minutes to achieve hemostasis. The site is then bandaged, and the patient is instructed to remain recumbent to apply further pressure for approximately 30 to 60 minutes. If a patient is thrombocytopenic, pressure bandages should be applied and the site checked frequently for prolonged bleeding.

Staining and Evaluation of Bone Marrow Aspirates and Touch Preparations

The bone marrow aspirate or touch preparation slides are stained with either Wright or May-Grünwald-Giemsa stains, like blood smears. These stains allow excellent morphologic detail and allow differential counts to be performed. Unstained smears should be retained for possible special stains, if indicated.[106,108]

Evaluation of bone marrow aspirates gives little information about the total cellularity of the bone marrow because of fluctuations in cell

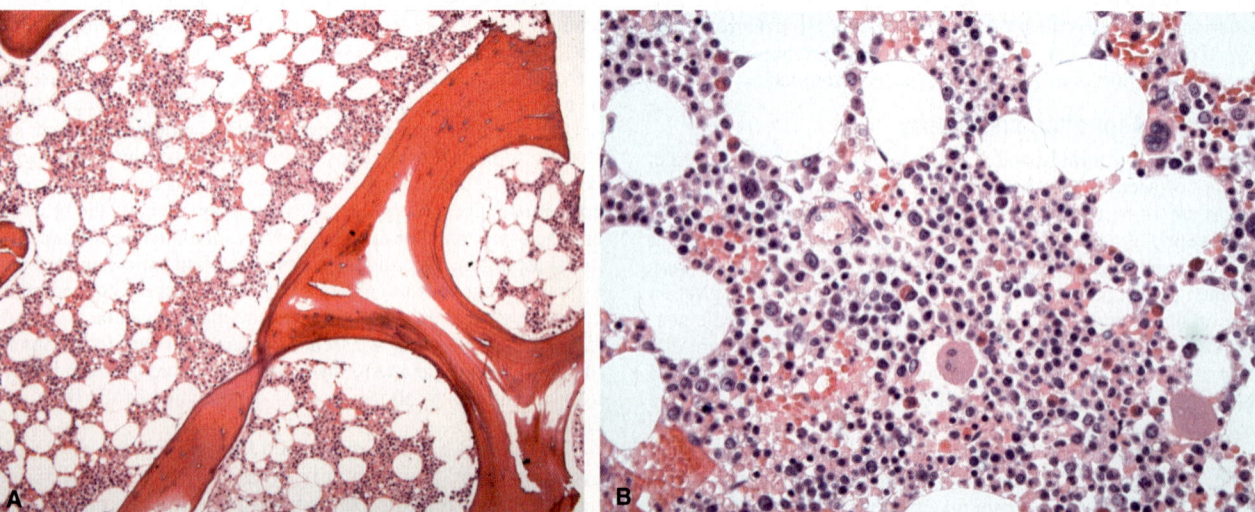

FIGURE 1.6 Bone marrow core biopsy. Histologic preparation of the bone marrow core biopsy following fixation and decalcification. The biopsy is stained with hematoxylin and eosin. This preparation allows for optimal evaluation of bone marrow cellularity and interaction of bone marrow cells with bony trabeculae and is helpful in evaluating extrinsic features, such as metastatic tumor or fibrosis in the marrow. Panel A (low power) showing bony spicules and marrow in section of bone marrow core biopsy. Panel B (high power) showing morphologic detail of hematopoietic tissue within the section.

Table 1.3. Differential Counts of Bone Marrow Aspirates From 12 Healthy Men

	Mean (%)	Observed Range (%)	95% Confidence (%)
Neutrophilic series (total)	53.6	49.2-65.0	33.6-73.6
Myeloblast	0.9	0.2-1.5	0.1-1.7
Promyelocyte	3.3	2.1-4.1	1.9-4.7
Myelocyte	12.7	8.2-15.7	8.5-16.9
Metamyelocyte	15.9	9.6-24.6	7.1-24.7
Band	12.4	9.5-15.3	9.4-15.4
Segmented	7.4	6.0-12.0	3.8-11.0
Eosinophilic series (total)	3.1	1.2-5.3	1.1-5.2
Myelocyte	0.8	0.2-1.3	0.2-1.4
Metamyelocyte	1.2	0.4-2.2	0.2-2.2
Band	0.9	0.2-2.4	0-2.7
Segmented	0.5	0-1.3	0-1.1
Basophilic and mast cells	<0.1	0-0.2	–
Erythrocytic series (total)	25.6	18.4-33.8	15.0-36.2
Pronormoblasts	0.6	0.2-1.3	0.1-1.1
Basophilic	1.4	0.5-2.4	0.4-2.4
Polychromatophilic	21.6	17.9-29.2	13.1-30.1
Orthochromatic	2.0	0.4-4.6	0.3-3.7
Lymphocytes	16.2	11.1-23.2	8.6-23.8
Plasma cells	1.3	0.4-3.9	0-3.5
Monocytes	0.3	0-0.8	0-0.6
Megakaryocytes	<0.1	0-0.4	–
Reticulum cells	0.3	0-0.9	0-0.8
Myeloid-to-erythroid ratio	2.3	1.5-3.3	1.1-3.5

Laboratory Hematology

counts induced by peripheral blood contamination of the bone marrow specimen and preparation artifacts. An overall impression of the cellularity may be given (i.e., cellular or paucicellular). More accurate evaluation of bone marrow cellularity requires examination of the bone marrow biopsy or particle clot section, although the biopsy represents a tiny fraction of the total marrow and may also be subject to sampling error.[106,110] The stained aspirate smear will have a central zone of dark marrow particles and stroma surrounded by a thinner area of dispersed bone marrow cells and red cells (*Figure 1.5*). Low-power examination allows evaluation of the adequacy of cellularity and of the presence of megakaryocytes. Infiltrating tumor cells or granulomas may also be seen by scanning the aspirate smear at low power.[108]

The aspirate smear allows cytologic examination of the bone marrow cells. A minimum of 500 nucleated cells should be evaluated under oil-immersion magnification in most marrows. Only intact cells are evaluated; all bare nuclei are excluded. Counting is performed in an area where few bare nuclei are present and the cells are not overlapping, found in clusters, or artifactually distorted because of the spreading artifact. This is usually in the dispersed cell zone adjacent to the spicule. It should be noted that spicules may be absent in pediatric marrows where marrow cells will be uniformly dispersed. Reference ranges for the percentage of bone marrow cell types vary widely between laboratories and are used only as guides for what is to be expected in normal bone marrow samples[108] (for example of reference ranges, see *Table 1.3*). The proportions of each cell type and progression of the maturational sequence for myeloid and erythroid elements are determined from the differential. In addition, the myeloid-to-erythroid ratio may be calculated.

Differences in cell differential results among infants, children, and adults exist (*Table 1.4*).[106,108,110,112] In general, lymphocytes are more commonly seen in the marrow of children, especially those younger than 4 years, where they may compose up to 40% of the marrow cellularity.[113] Plasma cells are rare in the marrow of infants and children. Lymphocytes are much less numerous in adult marrows, usually making up <20% of adult marrow cellularity. Lymphocyte and plasma cell counts in adults tend to be quite variable, perhaps reflecting the tendency of these cells to be unevenly distributed in the bone marrow of adults. Often, lymphoid cells are found in nodular aggregates in older adults, and plasma cells tend to be associated with blood vessels.[114]

During the first month of life, bone marrow erythroid cells are prominent because of high levels of erythropoietin[115]; thereafter, the erythroid cells make up 10% to 40% of the marrow cells. Relatively few early erythroid precursors (normoblasts) are usually seen, and more mature forms predominate. Erythroid cells should be examined for abnormalities in morphology as well as iron content because these features are often deranged in pathologic states. Myeloid cells are usually the predominant bone marrow element, and more mature cells predominate over immature myeloblasts. Children tend to have higher numbers of eosinophils and eosinophilic precursor cells than do adults, although many medications, allergies, or infections may increase the bone marrow eosinophil count. Megakaryocytes constitute the least abundant cell type seen in the bone marrow, usually making up <1% of the cells.[106]

In addition to the hematopoietic cells, a variety of other cells may be seen in bone marrow aspirates in varying proportions, including macrophages, mast cells, stromal cells, and fat cells. In children, osteoblasts and osteoclasts may be seen, although these cells are rare in adults, and their presence may indicate metabolic bone disease.[106,108,110] Normally, these other cells make up <1% of the total

Table 1.4. Changes in Differential Counts of Bone Marrow With Age

		Birth	1 mo-1 y	1-4 y	4-12 y	Adult
Neutrophilic series	Mean (%)	60	33	50	52	57
	95% limits	42-78	17-47	32-68	35-69	39-79
Eosinophilic series	Mean (%)	3	3	6	3	3
	95% limits	1-5	1-5	2-10	1-5	1-5
Lymphocytes	Mean (%)	14	47	22	18	17
	95% limits	3-25	34-63	8-36	12-28	10-24
Erythrocytic	Mean (%)	14	8	19	21	22
	95% limits	2-28	2-16	11-27	11-31	10-30
Myeloid-to-erythroid ratio	Mean	4.3	4.0	2.6	2.5	2.6

The means and 95% confidence limits were calculated by combining data published in Osgood EE, Seaman AJ. The cellular composition of bone marrow as obtained by sternal puncture. *Physiol Rev.* 1939;24:105–114, with the data in *Table 1.3*.

marrow cellularity; however, they may be increased in a variety of reactive and pathologic processes. Aspirate smears are excellent for the evaluation of macrophage hemophagocytosis[116] or storage disorders.[108]

Examination of Bone Marrow Histologic Sections

Bone marrow core biopsies and the clot section obtained from the aspiration procedure are usually fixed in formalin or in a coagulative fixative, such as B5 or zinc formalin. The bony core will require decalcification before histologic processing. The fixed materials are processed and embedded in paraffin or plastic, and sections are made for examination. The bone marrow biopsy and clot sections are stained with either hematoxylin and eosin or Giemsa stains for morphologic examination[106,110] (*Figure 1.6*).

Bone marrow biopsies are useful in the evaluation of bone marrow cellularity. Several caveats must be kept in mind when assessing cellularity. Studies show variations in cellularity even within the same biopsy site[112] as well as between different anatomic sites. However, comparisons of the relative proportions of myeloid, erythroid, and megakaryocytic cells appear to be constant even in widely separated biopsy sites.[106,112] In older patients, the subcortical area is often hypocellular, and care must be taken to obtain a large enough biopsy to allow adequate evaluation of the marrow away from this area.[112] The bone marrow biopsy section provides the best representation of the bone marrow and its anatomic relationships, such as normal localization of immature myeloid cells adjacent to bony trabeculae. Evaluation of nonhematopoietic elements, such as bony trabeculae, blood vessels, and stroma, requires a biopsy specimen.

The clot section, which is prepared from the bone marrow aspirate material, has a degree of inherent artifact because the bone marrow is removed from its normal relationships with bone, blood vessels, and other stromal elements. Cellularity estimations may be falsely elevated secondary to collapse of the normal stromal network in a clot section.[106]

In addition to providing information about the anatomic distribution and relationships of hematopoietic cells, the bone marrow biopsy is useful for the evaluation of infiltrative processes, such as carcinoma, lymphoma, other tumors, granulomatous inflammation, and fibrosis.[106] Occasionally, the marrow is so involved with an infiltrative process that no aspiration can be obtained (dry tap), and the biopsy provides the only diagnostic material.[117,118]

SPECIAL STAINS

Several special stains may be performed on peripheral blood smears, bone marrow aspirate smears, bone marrow touch preparations, and bone marrow biopsy materials, and will provide additional information about the cell lineage beyond what is obtained by standard staining with Giemsa or hematoxylin and eosin stains. Special stains generally fall into two categories: cytochemical stains that use cellular enzymatic reactions to impart staining and immunocytochemical stains that identify cell-specific antigen epitopes. These stains are particularly useful in characterization of primary hematologic or metastatic malignancies.

Cytochemical Stains

Cytochemical stains are useful in the diagnosis and classification of acute leukemias, although this utility has been lessened by identification of lineage-specific markers by flow cytometry. They allow identification of myeloid and lymphoid acute leukemias, as well as providing one basis for subclassification of the acute myeloid leukemias. These stains were widely used in morphologic subclassifications, such as the French-American-British system,[119] but their use has decreased because of wide availability of flow-cytometric and other ancillary tests.[120] Cytochemical stains are usually performed on peripheral blood films, bone marrow aspirates, or touch preparations made from bone marrow biopsies. Best results are obtained using freshly obtained materials; however, some reactions may be carried out on materials that are several years old.[121]

Myeloperoxidase

Primary granules of neutrophils and secondary granules of eosinophils contain myeloperoxidase. Monocytic lysosomal granules are faintly positive. Lymphocytes and nucleated RBCs lack the enzyme.[120,122] Staining is caused by oxidation of 3-amino-9-ethylcarbazole or 4-chloro-1-naphthol substrates by myeloperoxidase in the cell to form a brown-colored precipitate.

The myeloperoxidase enzyme is sensitive to light, and smears should be stained immediately or sheltered from light. Enzymatic activity in cells may diminish over time, so the stain should not be performed in blood or marrow aspirate smears older than 3 weeks. Permount coverslip mounting medium (Fisher Scientific, Pittsburgh, PA) may cause fading of the stain. Myeloperoxidase is also sensitive to heat and methanol treatment. Erythroid cells may stain for peroxidase after methanol treatment because of a nonenzymatic interaction between the staining reagents and Hb (pseudoperoxidase or Lepehne reaction). Antibodies to myeloperoxidase are available for both flow-cytometric analysis and immunohistochemical staining in fixed tissue sections.[123]

Sudan Black B

Sudan black B stains intracellular lipid and phospholipids. The pattern of staining closely parallels the myeloperoxidase reaction, with positive staining of granulocytic cells and eosinophils, weak monocytic staining, and no staining of lymphocytes, although some positivity may be seen in azurophilic granules of lymphoblasts.[120] Sudan black

B has an advantage over myeloperoxidase in that it may be used to stain older blood or bone marrow smears, and there is little fading of the stain over time.[122]

Specific (Naphthol AS-D Chloroacetate) Esterase

The specific (naphthol AS-D chloroacetate) esterase stain, also called the Leder stain, is used to identify cells of the granulocytic series.[120,122] It does not stain lymphocytes and monocytes. Because of enzymatic stability in formalin-fixed, paraffin-embedded tissues, this stain is extremely useful for identifying granulocytes and mast cells in tissue sections and is particularly helpful in the diagnosis of extramedullary myeloid tumors (granulocytic sarcoma and chloroma) of blasts found in tissues.[121] The cellular esterase enzyme hydrolyzes the naphthol AS-D chloroacetate substrate.[122] This reaction product is then coupled to a diazo salt to form a bright red-pink reaction product at the site of enzymatic activity. The enzyme activity is inhibited by the presence of mercury, acid solutions, heat, and iodine which may give rise to false-negative staining results.

Nonspecific (α-Naphthyl Butyrate or α-Naphthyl Acetate) Esterases

Nonspecific (α-naphthyl butyrate or α-naphthyl acetate) esterase stains are used to identify monocytic cells but do not stain granulocytes or eosinophils.[120,122,124] Mature T-lymphocytes stain with a characteristic focal, dotlike pattern. The stain also reacts with macrophages, histiocytes, megakaryocytes, and some carcinomas. The α-naphthyl butyrate stain is considered to be more specific, although slightly less sensitive, than the α-naphthyl acetate stain.[122] Differential staining with the different esterases is seen in megakaryoblasts, which do not stain with the α-naphthyl butyrate, but stain with the α-naphthyl acetate substrate.[121]

Terminal Deoxynucleotidyl Transferase

Terminal deoxynucleotidyl transferase (TdT) is an intranuclear enzyme that catalyzes the addition of deoxynucleotide triphosphates to the 3′-hydroxyl ends of oligonucleotides or polydeoxynucleotides without the need for a template strand.[125] TdT is found normally in the nucleus of thymocytes and immature lymphoid cells within the bone marrow but is not found in mature lymphocytes, and it is a useful marker in identifying acute lymphoblastic leukemias and lymphomas. TdT activity is found in approximately 90% of acute lymphoblastic leukemias as well as in a small subset of acute myeloid leukemias.[126,127] TdT levels may be measured biochemically, by cytochemical staining with an immunofluorescent detection technique, by flow cytometry after permeabilization of freshly collected cells, or by immunohistochemical methods.[120,128,129] Indirect immunofluorescent staining is very sensitive and may be applied to air-dried samples several weeks after collection, although it is not often used because of the widespread use of flow cytometry. Immunohistochemical methods of TdT detection are useful in paraffin-embedded tissue sections and can be used on touch preps.[126]

Leukocyte Alkaline Phosphatase

Alkaline phosphatase activity is found in the cytoplasm of neutrophils, osteoblasts, vascular endothelial cells, and some lymphocytes. The alkaline phosphatase level of peripheral blood neutrophils is quantitated by the leukocyte alkaline phosphatase (LAP) score and is useful as a screening test to differentiate chronic myeloid leukemia from leukemoid reactions and other myeloproliferative disorders.[130] The LAP score is usually performed using the Kaplow procedure.[131] This method uses a naphthol AS-BI phosphate as the substrate, which is coupled to fast violet B salt by the enzyme to produce a bright red reaction product that is visualized over neutrophils. The LAP score is determined by evaluation of the staining intensity (ranging from 0 to 4+) of 100 counted neutrophils or bands. Normal LAP scores range from 15 to 130, but there may be variation in these ranges between laboratories. Many different disease states may cause elevation or depression of the LAP score. Patients with chronic myeloid leukemia have low LAP scores (usually between 0 and 13). Paroxysmal nocturnal hemoglobinuria and some myelodysplastic syndromes may also be characterized by low LAP scores. Leukemoid reactions in response to infection and other myeloproliferative neoplasms (primary myelofibrosis and polycythemia vera) often have an elevated LAP score.[130] There is rapid loss of alkaline phosphatase activity in samples drawn in EDTA anticoagulant.[131] The test is optimally performed on fresh capillary blood finger-stick smears or on blood anticoagulated with heparin and should be performed within 48 hours after collection of the sample. The blood smears may be held in the freezer for 2 to 3 weeks with little loss of activity.

Acid Phosphatase

Acid phosphatase is found in all hematopoietic cells, but the highest levels are found in macrophages and osteoclasts. A localized dotlike pattern is seen in many T-lymphoblasts, but this staining pattern is not reliable. The tartrate-resistant acid phosphatase (TRAP) is an isoenzyme of acid phosphatase that is found in high levels in the cells of hairy cell leukemia and osteoclasts.[132] Several methods of measuring TRAP activity have been described, but one using naphthol AS-BI phosphoric acid coupled to fast garnet GBC is reliable and reproducible.[133] Not all cases of hairy cell leukemia stain for TRAP, and staining intensity may be variable. Positive TRAP staining may also be seen in some activated T-lymphocytes, macrophages, some histiocytes (such as Gaucher cells), mast cells, and some marginal zone lymphomas.[134] TRAP staining may also be detected by immunohistochemical methods in fixed tissue sections.[135]

Periodic Acid-Schiff

The periodic acid-Schiff (PAS) stain detects intracellular glycogen and neutral mucopolysaccharides, which are found in variable quantities in most hematopoietic cells.[122,136] PAS staining is seen in blasts of both acute lymphoblastic and acute myeloid leukemias, although there is great variability between cases.[136] Erythroleukemias demonstrate an intense diffuse cytoplasmic positivity with PAS, which may be helpful in diagnosis.[137] In addition, PAS staining is very useful in demonstrating the abnormal glucocerebrosidase accumulation in Gaucher disease.[138]

Iron

Cellular iron is found as either ferritin or hemosiderin. It is identified in cells by the Perls or Prussian blue reaction, in which ionic iron reacts with acid ferrocyanide to impart a blue color.[122,136,139] The stain is used to identify iron in nucleated RBCs (sideroblastic iron) and histiocytes (reticuloendothelial iron) or to identify Pappenheimer bodies in erythrocytes. Normally, red cell precursors contain one or more small (<1 μm in diameter) blue granules in 20% to 50% of the cells. When increased numbers of these granules surround at least two-thirds of the nucleus of the red cell precursor, the cell is called a ringed sideroblast.[140] The stain is best used on bone marrow aspirate smears but can also be used on blood films and aspirate clot tissue sections. Decalcification of the bone marrow core biopsy may lead to loss of iron from the cells, leading to a false impression of low iron.

Toluidine Blue

Toluidine blue specifically marks basophils and mast cells by reacting with the acid mucopolysaccharides in the cell granules to form metachromatic complexes. Malignant mast cells or basophils may have low levels of acid mucopolysaccharides and may not react with this stain.[141] Specific immunohistochemical markers, such as those staining for mast cell tryptase, may be more specific in identification of mast cells than toluidine blue staining.[142,143]

Immunocytochemical Stains

Immunocytochemical staining is based on the use of an antibody that recognizes a specific antigenic epitope on a cell. There is a high level of specificity. In general, these stains may be applied to blood smears, bone marrow aspirates, cellular suspensions, or tissue sections. Not all antibody preparations are equally effective on all types of specimens, and staining procedures may vary depending on the specimen type. A wide variety of antibodies specific to hematopoietic cellular antigens is available commercially. Some of the newer antibodies have replaced classical cytochemical stains and may be useful on older or fixed specimens.

Immunocytochemical staining of fresh blood or bone marrow cell suspensions or cell suspensions from tissues and analysis by flow cytometry is a common ancillary testing modality that is employed when a hematologic malignancy is suspected.[144,145] The flow cytometer detects both light scatter data and the presence of specific fluorochrome-labeled antibodies that have bound to the cell surface. The use of different fluorochromes can allow more than one antibody to be studied simultaneously on the same cell by means of different excitation wavelengths. The study of these cell surface markers allows rapid and accurate analysis of lymphomas and leukemias, enumeration of T-cell subsets, and identification of tumor cells. In addition, recent advances have allowed detection of intracytoplasmic or nuclear antigens, such as myeloperoxidase and TdT, by flow-cytometric analysis.[144] In many cases, particularly in the acute leukemias, the flow-cytometric analysis of an acute leukemia provides important prognostic information that is not available through cytochemical staining and is useful in detection of minimal residual disease.[126,144,146,147]

Immunohistochemical staining is the use of specific antibody probes on tissue sections or smears of blood and bone marrow. This allows the localization of a specific antigenic epitope to the cell surface, cytoplasm, or nucleus. The antigen binding may then be detected by immunofluorescence, which requires a special fluorescence microscope, or by enzymatic formation of a colored reaction product linked to the antigen-antibody complex. Immunoenzymatic staining techniques include immunoperoxidase, immunoalkaline phosphatase, and avidin-biotin techniques.[148,149] These procedures allow study of the specimen with standard light microscopy and provide a permanent record of staining that may be reexamined. In the past, the repertoire of antibodies available for use on paraffin-embedded tissues was limited, and many antibodies required frozen sections of fresh tissues to be used. Over time, however, there has been a large increase in the number of antibodies that can be used on fixed and processed tissues.[150,151] Automated immunostaining instruments have become available that allow highly reproducible results and require less technician time and expertise.

OTHER LABORATORY STUDIES

Cytogenetic Analysis

Many hematologic malignancies and premalignant conditions are associated with specific cytogenetic changes.[137,152-154] These include distinctive changes in chromosome number, translocations, and inversions of genetic material. These chromosomal changes are often associated with activation or increased transcription of oncogenes and may contribute to acquisition of a malignant phenotype.[155] Cytogenetic analysis is an important element in diagnosing hematologic disorders, identifying specific prognostic subgroups, and monitoring for progression of disease or residual disease after therapy, and is integral to the most current classification of hematologic malignancies, such as the World Health Organization classification.[137,156-161] Both standard chromosomal preparations and fluorescent-labeled in situ hybridization techniques may be used for cytogenetic analysis of chromosomal changes.

Molecular Genetics

In addition to standard morphologic analysis and cytogenetics, analysis of molecular changes in hematologic malignancies has become commonplace.[154,156,158,160,162-164] Using Southern blot, polymerase chain reaction (PCR), and sequencing techniques, hematopoietic proliferations may be studied for genetic alterations associated with the development of malignancy. Molecular genetic analysis was initially used to identify monoclonality in lymphoid neoplasms by

identifying either immunoglobulin (B-cell) or T-cell receptor gene rearrangements.[165] This finding is extremely useful in classification of lymphoproliferative disorders that may be difficult to diagnose on morphologic grounds alone or that lack specific phenotypic markers.[166] In the past few years, there has been an explosion in the use of molecular techniques to detect abnormalities that previously had been detected only by conventional cytogenetics or had gone undetected. Common tests include the *BCR-ABL1* translocations seen in chronic myeloid leukemia and acute leukemia and are used to monitor efficacy of treatment,[167] *BCL2* translocations characteristic of follicular lymphomas,[168] the t(15;17) associated with acute promyelocytic leukemia,[169,170] *JAK2* mutations associated with myeloproliferative neoplasms,[171,172] and *NPM1*, *FLT3*, *CEBPA*, *IDH1*, and *IDH2* mutations, which are prognostic factors, and sometimes therapeutic targets, in acute myeloid leukemia.[161,173-175] In chronic myeloid leukemia, *BCR-ABL1* kinase domain mutation analysis can be performed to detect mutations that lead to imatinib resistance.[176,177] It should be anticipated that more clinically useful genetic tests will be developed as technology advances. Molecular studies have an advantage over conventional morphologic and cytogenetic analyses in that they may detect very small populations of malignant cells (as few as 1%-5% of the cells in a sample), may allow for quantification of low levels of transcripts to allow monitoring of disease status, and can lead to more rapid test completion (especially with PCR-based testing). Molecular tests are most useful when guided by clinical and morphologic findings or in monitoring residual disease after therapy because they do not provide effective screening capability for additional genetic alterations that may affect prognosis, which is a utility of conventional cytogenetic analysis.[178,179]

The high degree of sensitivity makes molecular testing very attractive for the purpose of monitoring for disease persistence or recurrence after therapy. Previously, molecular genetic studies required collection of fresh or frozen diagnostic material; however, many of the newer assays can make use of formalin-fixed materials with sensitivity like that of fresh or frozen materials. This allows analysis to be performed on a wider range of cases, including archival materials. The topic of molecular genetics is covered in further detail in Chapter 4.

Electron Microscopy

The electron microscope allows examination of ultrastructural details of a cell. In the past, electron microscopy was used as a research tool and, occasionally, as a diagnostic tool for difficult hematologic diagnoses. However, with the advent of increasing numbers of specific immunocytochemical stains, the use of the electron microscope as a diagnostic tool for hematopathologic processes has been largely discontinued.

References

1. Cheng CK, Chan J, Cembrowski GS, et al. Complete blood count reference interval diagrams derived from NHANES III: stratification by age, sex, and race. *Lab Hematol.* 2004;10(1):42-53.
2. Schwartz J, Weiss ST. Cigarette smoking and peripheral blood leukocyte differentials. *Ann Epidemiol.* 1994;4(3):236-242.
3. Lim EM, Cembrowski G, Cembrowski M, et al. Race-specific WBC and neutrophil count reference intervals. *Int J Lab Hematol.* 2010;32(6 pt 2):590-597.
4. Wood BL, Andrews J, Miller S, et al. Refrigerated storage improves the stability of the complete blood cell count and automated differential. *Am J Clin Pathol.* 1999;112(5):687-695.
5. Song KS, Song JW. Changes of platelet parameters determined by the Bayer ADVIA 120 with EDTA sample age. *Platelets.* 2005;16(3-4):223-224.
6. Daves M, Zagler EM, Cemin R, et al. Sample stability for complete blood cell count using the Sysmex XN haematological analyser. *Blood Transfus.* 2015;13(4):576-582.
7. CLSI. *Tubes and Additives for Venous and Capillary Blood Specimen Collection; Approved Standard*, 6th ed. CLSI document GP39-A6. Clinical and Laboratory Standards Institute; 2010.
8. CLSI. *Validation, Verification, and Quality Assurance of Automated Hematology Analyzers; Approved Standard*, 2nd ed. CLSI document H26-A2. Clinical and Laboratory Standards Institute; 2010.
9. Bruegel M, Nagel D, Funk M, et al. Comparison of five automated hematology analyzers in a university hospital setting: Abbott cell-dyn Sapphire, Beckman Coulter DxH 800, Siemens Advia 2120i, Sysmex XE-5000, and Sysmex XN-2000. *Clin Chem Lab Med.* 2015;53(7):1057-1071.
10. Malecka M, Ciepiela O. A comparison of Sysmex-XN 2000 and Yumizen H2500 automated hematology analyzers. *Pract Lab Med.* 2020;22:e00186.

11. Genc S, Dervisoglu E, Erdem S, et al. Comparison of performance and abnormal cell flagging of two automated hematology analyzers: Sysmex XN 3000 and Beckman Coulter DxH 800. *Int J Lab Hematol.* 2017;39(6):633-640.

12. Becker PH, Fenneteau O, Da Costa L. Performance evaluation of the Sysmex XN-1000 hematology analyzer in assessment of the white blood cell count differential in pediatric specimens. *Int J Lab Hematol.* 2016;38(1):54-63.

13. Chabot-Richards DS, George TI. White blood cell counts: reference methodology. *Clin Lab Med.* 2015;35(1):11-24.

14. Shelat SG, Canfield W, Shibutani S. Differences in detecting blasts between ADVIA 2120 and Beckman-Coulter LH750 hematology analyzers. *Int J Lab Hematol.* 2010;32(1 pt 2):113-116.

15. Barnes PW, Eby CS, Shimer G. Blast flagging with the UniCel DxH 800 Coulter cellular analysis system. *Lab Hematol.* 2010;16(2):23-25.

16. Barnes PW, McFadden SL, Machin SJ, et al. The International Consensus Group for hematology review: suggested criteria for action following automated CBC and WBC differential analysis. *Lab Hematol.* 2005;11(2):83-90.

17. Depoorter M, Goletti S, Latinne D, et al. Optimal flagging combinations for best performance of five blood cell analyzers. *Int J Lab Hematol.* 2015;37(1):63-70.

18. Novis DA, Walsh M, Wilkinson D, et al. Laboratory productivity and the rate of manual peripheral blood smear review: a College of American Pathologists Q-Probes study of 95,141 complete blood count determinations performed in 263 institutions. *Arch Pathol Lab Med.* 2006;130(5):596-601.

19. Wintrobe M. A simple and accurate hematocrit. *J Lab Clin Med.* 1929;15:287-289.

20. Fairbanks VF. Nonequivalence of automated and manual hematocrit and erythrocytic indices. *Am J Clin Pathol.* 1980;73(1):55-62.

21. Pearson TC, Guthrie DL. Trapped plasma in the microhematocrit. *Am J Clin Pathol.* 1982;78(5):770-772.

22. Guthrie DL, Pearson TC. PCV measurement in the management of polycythaemic patients. *Clin Lab Haematol.* 1982;4(3):257-265.

23. Beautyman W, Bills T. Letter: osmotic error in measurements of red-cell volume. *Lancet.* 1974;2(7885):905-906.

24. Bourner G, Dhaliwal J, Sumner J. Performance evaluation of the latest fully automated hematology analyzers in a large, commercial laboratory setting: a 4-way, side-by-side study. *Lab Hematol.* 2005;11(4):285-297.

25. Vis JY, Huisman A. Verification and quality control of routine hematology analyzers. *Int J Lab Hematol.* 2016;38(suppl 1):100-109.

26. CLSI. *Reference and Selected Procedures for the Quantitative Determination of Hemoglobin in Blood: Approved Standard-*3rd ed. CLSI document H15-A3. Clinical and Laboratory Standards Institute; 2000.

27. Cornbleet J. Spurious results from automated hematology cell analyzers. *Lab Med.* 1983;14:509-514.

28. Linz LJ. Elevation of hemoglobin, MCH, and MCHC by paraprotein: how to recognize and correct the interference. *Clin Lab Sci.* 1994;7(4):211-212.

29. Campbell NR, Edwards AL, Brant R, et al. Effect on lipid, complete blood count and blood proteins of a standardized preparation for drawing blood: a randomized controlled trial. *Clin Invest Med.* 2000;23(6):350-354.

30. ICSH. Reference method for the enumeration of erythrocytes and leucocytes. International Council for standardization in haematology; prepared by the expert panel on cytometry. *Clin Lab Haematol.* 1994;16(2):131-138.

31. Hermiston ML, Mentzer WC. A practical approach to the evaluation of the anemic child. *Pediatr Clin.* 2002;49(5):877-891.

32. Bessman JD, Banks D. Spurious macrocytosis, a common clue to erythrocyte cold agglutinins. *Am J Clin Pathol.* 1980;74(6):797-800.

33. Savage RA, Hoffman GC. Clinical significance of osmotic matrix errors in automated hematology: the frequency of hyperglycemic osmotic matrix errors producing spurious macrocytosis. *Am J Clin Pathol.* 1983;80(6):861-865.

34. Tefferi A, Hanson CA, Inwards DJ. How to interpret and pursue an abnormal complete blood cell count in adults. *Mayo Clin Proc.* 2005;80(7):923-936.

35. ICSH. ICSH recommendations for the analysis of red cell, white cell and platelet size distribution curves. Methods for fitting a single reference distribution and assessing its goodness of fit. International Committee for Standardization in Haematology. ICSH Expert Panel on Cytometry. *Clin Lab Haematol.* 1990;12(4):417-431.

36. Aslan D, Gumruk F, Gurgey A, et al. Importance of RDW value in differential diagnosis of hypochromic anemias. *Am J Hematol.* 2002;69(1):31-33.

37. Roberts GT, El Badawi SB. Red blood cell distribution width index in some hematologic diseases. *Am J Clin Pathol.* 1985;83(2):222-226.

38. Lippi G, Mattiuzzi C, Cervellin G. Learning more and spending less with neglected laboratory parameters: the paradigmatic case of red blood cell distribution width. *Acta Biomed.* 2016;87(3):323-328.

39. ICSH. Proposed reference method for reticulocyte counting based on the determination of the reticulocyte to red cell ratio. The Expert Panel on Cytometry of the International Council for Standardization in Haematology. *Clin Lab Haematol.* 1998;20(2):77-79.

40. Davis BH, Bigelow NC, Koepke JA, et al. Flow cytometric reticulocyte analysis. Multiinstitutional interlaboratory correlation study. *Am J Clin Pathol.* 1994;102(4):468-477.

41. Higgins JM. Red blood cell population dynamics. *Clin Lab Med.* 2015;35(1):43-57.

42. Riley RS, Ben-Ezra JM, Tidwell A, et al. Reticulocyte analysis by flow cytometry and other techniques. *Hematol Oncol Clin North Am.* 2002;16(2):373-420.

43. Piva E, Brugnara C, Spolaore F, et al. Clinical utility of reticulocyte parameters. *Clin Lab Med.* 2015;35(1):133-163.

44. Siekmeier R, Bierlich A, Jaross W. Determination of reticulocytes: three methods compared. *Clin Chem Lab Med.* 2000;38(3):245-249.

45. Buttarello M. Laboratory diagnosis of anemia: are the old and new red cell parameters useful in classification and treatment, how? *Int J Lab Hematol.* 2016;38(suppl 1):123-132.

46. Bentley SA, Johnson A, Bishop CA. A parallel evaluation of four automated hematology analyzers. *Am J Clin Pathol.* 1993;100(6):626-632.

47. Fohlen-Walter A, Jacob C, Lecompte T, et al. Laboratory identification of cryoglobulinemia from automated blood cell counts, fresh blood samples, and blood films. *Am J Clin Pathol.* 2002;117(4):606-614.

48. Lombarts AJ, de Kieviet W. Recognition and prevention of pseudothrombocytopenia and concomitant pseudoleukocytosis. *Am J Clin Pathol.* 1988;89(5):634-639.

49. Berliner S, Fusman R, Rotstein R, et al. Electronic counter-related pseudoleukopenia: more than a rare occurrence. *Haematologica.* 2001;86(2):210-211.

50. CLSI. *Reference Leukocyte (WBC) Differential Count (Proportional) and Evaluation of Instrumental Methods*; Approved Standard-2nd ed. CLSI document H20-A2; 2007.

51. Benattar L, Flandrin G. Comparison of the classical manual pushed wedge films, with an improved automated method for making blood smears. *Hematol Cell Ther.* 1999;41(5):211-215.

52. Rumke C. *The Statistically Expected Variability in Differential Counting.* College of American Pathologists; 1978.

53. Hyun BH, Gulati GL, Ashton JK. Differential leukocyte count: manual or automated, what should it be? *Yonsei Med J.* 1991;32(4):283-291.

54. Petrone J, Jackups R, Jr, Eby CS, et al. Blast flagging of the Sysmex XN-10 hematology analyzer with supervised cell image analysis: impact on quality parameters. *Int J Lab Hematol.* 2019;41(5):601-606.

55. Da Costa L. Digital image analysis of blood cells. *Clin Lab Med.* 2015;35(1):105-122.

56. Harris N, Kunicka J, Kratz A. The ADVIA 2120 hematology system: flow cytometry-based analysis of blood and body fluids in the routine hematology laboratory. *Lab Hematol.* 2005;11(1):47-61.

57. Aulesa C, Mainar I, Prieto M, et al. Use of the Advia 120 hematology analyzer in the differential cytologic analysis of biological fluids (cerebrospinal, peritoneal, pleural, pericardial, synovial, and others). *Lab Hematol.* 2003;9(4):214-224.

58. Paris A, Nhan T, Cornet E, et al. Performance evaluation of the body fluid mode on the platform Sysmex XE-5000 series automated hematology analyzer. *Int J Lab Hematol.* 2010;32(5):539-547.

59. de Jonge R, Brouwer R, van Rijn M, et al. Automated analysis of pleural fluid total and differential leukocyte counts with the Sysmex XE-2100. *Clin Chem Lab Med.* 2006;44(11):1367-1371.

60. D'Souza C, Briggs C, Machin SJ. Platelets: the few, the young, and the active. *Clin Lab Med.* 2015;35(1):123-131.

61. Horiuchi Y, Tabe Y, Idei M, et al. The use of CellaVision competency software for external quality assessment and continuing professional development. *J Clin Pathol.* 2011;64(7):610-617.

62. Cornet E, Perol JP, Troussard X. Performance evaluation and relevance of the CellaVision DM96 system in routine analysis and in patients with malignant hematological diseases. *Int J Lab Hematol.* 2008;30(6):536-542.

63. Briggs C, Longair I, Slavik M, et al. Can automated blood film analysis replace the manual differential? An evaluation of the CellaVision DM96 automated image analysis system. *Int J Lab Hematol.* 2009;31(1):48-60.

64. Ceelie H, Dinkelaar RB, van Gelder W. Examination of peripheral blood films using automated microscopy; evaluation of Diffmaster Octavia and Cellavision DM96. *J Clin Pathol.* 2007;60(1):72-79.

65. Kratz A, Bengtsson HI, Casey JE, et al. Performance evaluation of the CellaVision DM96 system: WBC differentials by automated digital image analysis supported by an artificial neural network. *Am J Clin Pathol.* 2005;124(5):770-781.

66. Lawrence JB, Yomtovian RA, Dillman C, et al. Reliability of automated platelet counts: comparison with manual method and utility for prediction of clinical bleeding. *Am J Hematol.* 1995;48(4):244-250.

67. Dale N, Shumacher H. Platelet satellitism-new results with automated instruments. *Lab Med.* 1982;13:300-304.

68. Akwari AM, Ross DW, Stass SA. Spuriously elevated platelet counts due to microspherocytosis. *Am J Clin Pathol.* 1982;77(2):220-221.

69. Hammerstrom J. Spurious platelet counts in acute leukaemia with DIC due to cell fragmentation. *Clin Lab Haematol.* 1992;14(3):239-243.

70. Noris P, Klersy C, Zecca M, et al. Platelet size distinguishes between inherited macrothrombocytopenias and immune thrombocytopenia. *J Thromb Haemostasis.* 2009;7(12):2131-2136.

71. Niethammer AG, Forman EN. Use of the platelet histogram maximum in evaluating thrombocytopenia. *Am J Hematol.* 1999;60(1):19-23.

72. Diquattro M, Gagliano F, Calabro GM, et al. Relationships between platelet counts, platelet volumes and reticulated platelets in patients with ITP: evidence for significant platelet count inaccuracies with conventional instrument methods. *Int J Lab Hematol.* 2009;31(2):199-206.

73. Eicher JD, Lettre G, Johnson AD. The genetics of platelet count and volume in humans. *Platelets.* 2018;29(2):125-130.

74. McShine RL, Sibinga S, Brozovic B. Differences between the effects of EDTA and citrate anticoagulants on platelet count and mean platelet volume. *Clin Lab Haematol.* 1990;12(3):277-285.

75. Bessman JD, Gilmer PR, Gardner FH. Use of mean platelet volume improves detection of platelet disorders. *Blood Cell.* 1985;11(1):127-135.

76. Pons I, Monteagudo M, Lucchetti G, et al. Correlation between immature platelet fraction and reticulated platelets. Usefulness in the etiology diagnosis of thrombocytopenia. *Eur J Haematol.* 2010;85(2):158-163.

77. Buttarello M, Mezzapelle G, Freguglia F, et al. Reticulated platelets and immature platelet fraction: clinical applications and method limitations. *Int J Lab Hematol.* 2020;42(4):363-370.

78. Ryningen A, Apelseth T, Hausken T, et al. Reticulated platelets are increased in chronic myeloproliferative disorders, pure erythrocytosis, reactive thrombocytosis and prior to hematopoietic reconstitution after intensive chemotherapy. *Platelets.* 2006;17(5):296-302.

Laboratory Hematology

79. Verbrugge SE, Huisman A. Verification and standardization of blood cell counters for routine clinical laboratory tests. *Clin Lab Med.* 2015;35(1):183-196.

80. Sireci A, Schlaberg R, Kratz A. A method for optimizing and validating institution-specific flagging criteria for automated cell counters. *Arch Pathol Lab Med.* 2010;134(10):1528-1533.

81. Kratz A, Lee SH, Zini G, et al. Digital morphology analyzers in hematology: ICSH review and recommendations. *Int J Lab Hematol.* 2019;41(4):437-447.

82. Vives Corrons JL, Van Blerk M, Albarede S, et al. Guidelines for setting up an external quality assessment scheme for blood smear interpretation. Part II: survey preparation, statistical evaluation and reporting. *Clin Chem Lab Med.* 2006;44(8):1039-1043.

83. Wenk RE. Comparison of five methods for preparing blood smears. *Am J Med Technol.* 1976;42(3):71-78.

84. Houwen B. Blood film preparation and staining procedures. *Clin Lab Med.* 2002;22(1):1-14.

85. McGoogan E, Colgan TJ, Ramzy I, et al. Cell preparation methods and criteria for sample adequacy. International Academy of cytology task force summary. Diagnostic cytology towards the 21st Century: an International expert Conference and tutorial. *Acta Cytol.* 1998;42(1):25-32.

86. Adler SL, Groner W, Ornstein L. Fully automated preparation of high-quality stained blood films. *Anal Quant Cytol.* 1981;3(3):216-224.

87. Dunning K, Safo AO. The ultimate Wright-Giemsa stain: 60 years in the making. *Biotech Histochem.* 2011;86(2):69-75.

88. Barth D. Approach to peripheral blood film assessment for pathologists. *Semin Diagn Pathol.* 2012;29(1):31-48.

89. Jenkins C, Hewamana S. The blood film as a diagnostic tool. *Br J Hosp Med (Lond).* 2008;69(9):M144-M147.

90. Prokocimer M, Potasman I. The added value of peripheral blood cell morphology in the diagnosis and management of infectious diseases—part 1: basic concepts. *Postgrad Med J.* 2008;84(997):579-585.

91. Blevins SM, Greenfield RA, Bronze MS. Blood smear analysis in babesiosis, ehrlichiosis, relapsing fever, malaria, and Chagas disease. *Cleve Clin J Med.* 2008;75(7):521-530.

92. Tefferi A, Elliott MA. Schistocytes on the peripheral blood smear. *Mayo Clin Proc.* 2004;79(6):809.

93. Schapkaitz E, Mezgebe MH. The clinical significance of schistocytes: a prospective evaluation of the International Council for standardization in hematology schistocyte guidelines. *Turk J Haematol.* 2017;34(1):59-63.

94. Zini G, d'Onofrio G, Briggs C, et al. ICSH recommendations for identification, diagnostic value, and quantitation of schistocytes. *Int J Lab Hematol.* 2012;34(2):107-116.

95. Kabutomori O, Kanakura Y, Watani YI. Induction of toxic granulation in neutrophils by granulocyte colony-stimulating factor. *Eur J Haematol.* 2002;69(3):187-188.

96. Moreno A, Menke D. Assessment of platelet numbers and morphology in the peripheral blood smear. *Clin Lab Med.* 2002;22(1):193-213.

97. Al-Gwaiz LA, Babay HH. The diagnostic value of absolute neutrophil count, band count and morphologic changes of neutrophils in predicting bacterial infections. *Med Princ Pract.* 2007;16(5):344-347.

98. Widell S, Hellstrom-Lindberg E, Kock Y, et al. Peripheral blood neutrophil morphology reflects bone marrow dysplasia in myelodysplastic syndromes. *Am J Hematol.* 1995;49(2):115-120.

99. Kaplan J, De Domenico I, Ward DM. Chediak-Higashi syndrome. *Curr Opin Hematol.* 2008;15(1):22-29.

100. Schwind JL. The supravital method in the study of the cytology of blood and marrow cells. *Blood.* 1950;5(7):597-622.

101. Williamson D. The unstable haemoglobins. *Blood Rev.* 1993;7(3):146-163.

102. Espanol I, Pedro C, Remacha AF. Heinz bodies interfere with automated reticulocyte counts. *Haematologica.* 1999;84(4):373-374.

103. Lofsness KG, Kohnke ML, Geier NA. Evaluation of automated reticulocyte counts and their reliability in the presence of Howell-Jolly bodies. *Am J Clin Pathol.* 1994;101(1):85-90.

104. Banfi G, Mauri C, Morelli B, et al. Reticulocyte count, mean reticulocyte volume, immature reticulocyte fraction, and mean sphered cell volume in elite athletes: reference values and comparison with the general population. *Clin Chem Lab Med.* 2006;44(5):616-622.

105. Hyun BH, Stevenson AJ, Hanau CA. Fundamentals of bone marrow examination. *Hematol Oncol Clin N Am.* 1994;8(4):651-663.

106. Riley RS, Hogan TF, Pavot DR, et al. A pathologist's perspective on bone marrow aspiration and biopsy: I. Performing a bone marrow examination. *J Clin Lab Anal.* 2004;18(2):70-90.

107. Bain BJ. Bone marrow biopsy morbidity and mortality. *Br J Haematol.* 2003;121(6):949-951.

108. Bain BJ, Bailey K. Pitfalls in obtaining and interpreting bone marrow aspirates: to err is human. *J Clin Pathol.* 2011;64(5):373-379.

109. Islam A. Bone marrow aspiration before bone marrow core biopsy using the same bone marrow biopsy needle: a good or bad practice? *J Clin Pathol.* 2007;60(2):212-215.

110. Hyun BH, Gulati GL, Ashton JK. Bone marrow examination: techniques and interpretation. *Hematol Oncol Clin N Am.* 1988;2(4):513-523.

111. Wilkins BS, Clark DM. Making the most of bone marrow trephine biopsy. *Histopathology.* 2009;55(6):631-640.

112. Hartsock RJ, Smith EB, Petty CS. Normal variations with aging of the amount of hematopoietic tissue in bone marrow from the anterior iliac crest. A study made from 177 cases of sudden death examined by necropsy. *Am J Clin Pathol.* 1965;43:326-331.

113. Rosse C, Kraemer MJ, Dillon TL, et al. Bone marrow cell populations of normal infants; the predominance of lymphocytes. *J Lab Clin Med.* 1977;89(6):1225-1240.

114. Hasserjian RP. Reactive versus neoplastic bone marrow: problems and pitfalls. *Arch Pathol Lab Med.* 2008;132(4):587-594.

115. Kling PJ, Schmidt RL, Roberts RA, et al. Serum erythropoietin levels during infancy: associations with erythropoiesis. *J Pediatr.* 1996;128(6):791-796.

116. Gupta A, Tyrrell P, Valani R, et al. The role of the initial bone marrow aspirate in the diagnosis of hemophagocytic lymphohistiocytosis. *Pediatr Blood Cancer.* 2008;51(3):402-404.

117. Humphries JE. Dry tap bone marrow aspiration: clinical significance. *Am J Hematol.* 1990;35(4):247-250.

118. Novotny JR, Schmucker U, Staats B, et al. Failed or inadequate bone marrow aspiration: a fast, simple and cost-effective method to produce a cell suspension from a core biopsy specimen. *Clin Lab Haematol.* 2005;27(1):33-40.

119. Bennett JM, Catovsky D, Daniel MT, et al. Proposed revised criteria for the classification of acute myeloid leukemia. A report of the French-American-British Cooperative Group. *Ann Intern Med.* 1985;103(4):620-625.

120. Paessler ME, Helfrich M, Wertheim GBW. Cytochemical staining. *Methods Mol Biol.* 2017;1633:19-32.

121. Klobusicka M. Reliability and limitations of cytochemistry in diagnosis of acute myeloid leukemia. Minireview. *Neoplasma.* 2000;47(6):329-334.

122. Hayhoe FG. Cytochemistry of the acute leukaemias. *Histochem J.* 1984;16(10):1051-1059.

123. Saravanan L, Juneja S. Immunohistochemistry is a more sensitive marker for the detection of myeloperoxidase in acute myeloid leukemia compared with flow cytometry and cytochemistry. *Int J Lab Hematol.* 2010;32(1 pt 1):e132-136.

124. Strober W. Wright-Giemsa and nonspecific esterase staining of cells. *Curr Protoc Cytom.* 2001. Appendix 3:Appendix 3D.

125. Thai TH, Kearney JF. Isoforms of terminal deoxynucleotidyltransferase: developmental aspects and function. *Adv Immunol.* 2005;86:113-116.

126. McGregor S, McNeer J, Gurbuxani S. Beyond the 2008 World Health Organization classification: the role of the hematopathology laboratory in the diagnosis and management of acute lymphoblastic leukemia. *Semin Diagn Pathol.* 2012;29(1):2-11.

127. Drexler HG, Sperling C, Ludwig WD. Terminal deoxynucleotidyl transferase (TdT) expression in acute myeloid leukemia. *Leukemia.* 1993;7(8):1142-1150.

128. Al Gwaiz LA, Bassioni W. Immunophenotyping of acute lymphoblastic leukemia using immunohistochemistry in bone marrow biopsy specimens. *Histol Histopathol.* 2008;23(10):1223-1228.

129. Roma AO, Kutok JL, Shaheen G, et al. A novel, rapid, multiparametric approach for flow cytometric analysis of intranuclear terminal deoxynucleotidyl transferase. *Am J Clin Pathol.* 1999;112(3):343-348.

130. Li CY. The role of morphology, cytochemistry and immunohistochemistry in the diagnosis of chronic myeloproliferative diseases. *Int J Hematol.* 2002;76(suppl 2):6-8.

131. Kaplow LS. Leukocyte alkaline phosphatase in disease. *CRC Crit Rev Clin Lab Sci.* 1971;2(2):243-278.

132. Moss DW, Raymond FD, Wile DB. Clinical and biological aspects of acid phosphatase. *Crit Rev Clin Lab Sci.* 1995;32(4):431-467.

133. Lamp EC, Drexler HG. Biology of tartrate-resistant acid phosphatase. *Leuk Lymphoma.* 2000;39(5-6):477-484.

134. Dunphy CH. Reaction patterns of TRAP and DBA.44 in hairy cell leukemia, hairy cell variant, and nodal and extranodal marginal zone B-cell lymphomas. *Appl Immunohistochem Mol Morphol.* 2008;16(2):135-139.

135. Sherman MJ, Hanson CA, Hoyer JD. An assessment of the usefulness of immunohistochemical stains in the diagnosis of hairy cell leukemia. *Am J Clin Pathol.* 2011;136(3):390-399.

136. Crook L, Liu PI, Cannon A, et al. Histochemistry of bone marrow aspirations. *Ann Clin Lab Sci.* 1980;10(4):290-304.

137. WHO. *World Health Organization Classification of Tumours of Haematopoietic and Lymphoid Tissues.* 4th ed. IARC Press; 2008.

138. Chen M, Wang J. Gaucher disease: review of the literature. *Arch Pathol Lab Med.* 2008;132(5):851-853.

139. Gomori G. Microtechnical demonstration of iron: a Criticism of its methods. *Am J Pathol.* 1936;12(5):655-664.

140. Tham KT, Cousar JB. Combined silver Perls's stain for differential staining of ringed sideroblasts and marrow iron. *J Clin Pathol.* 1993;46(8):766-768.

141. Klatt EC, Lukes RJ, Meyer PR. Benign and malignant mast cell proliferations. Diagnosis and separation using a pH-dependent toluidine blue stain in tissue section. *Cancer.* 1983;51(6):1119-1124.

142. Johnson MR, Verstovsek S, Jorgensen JL, et al. Utility of the World Heath Organization classification criteria for the diagnosis of systemic mastocytosis in bone marrow. *Mod Pathol.* 2009;22(1):50-57.

143. Ribatti D. The staining of mast cells: a historical overview. *Int Arch Allergy Immunol.* 2018;176(1):55-60.

144. Davis BH, Holden JT, Bene MC, et al. Bethesda International Consensus recommendations on the flow cytometric immunophenotypic analysis of hematolymphoid neoplasia: medical indications. *Cytometry B Clin Cytom.* 2007;72(suppl 1):S5-S13.

145. Weir EG, Borowitz MJ. Flow cytometry in the diagnosis of acute leukemia. *Semin Hematol.* 2001;38(2):124-138.

146. Gaipa G, Buracchi C, Biondi A. Flow cytometry for minimal residual disease testing in acute leukemia: opportunities and challenges. *Expert Rev Mol Diagn.* 2018;18(9):775-787.

147. Wood BL. Principles of minimal residual disease detection for hematopoietic neoplasms by flow cytometry. *Cytometry B Clin Cytom.* 2016;90(1):47-53.

148. Leong TY, Cooper K, Leong AS. Immunohistology—past, present, and future. *Adv Anat Pathol.* 2010;17(6):404-418.

149. Scanziani E. Immunohistochemical staining of fixed tissues. *Methods Mol Biol.* 1998;104:133-140.

150. Lu J, Chang KL. Practical immunohistochemistry in hematopathology: a review of useful antibodies for diagnosis. *Adv Anat Pathol.* 2011;18(2):133-151.

151. Garcia CF, Swerdlow SH. Best practices in contemporary diagnostic immunohistochemistry: panel approach to hematolymphoid proliferations. *Arch Pathol Lab Med.* 2009;133(5):756-765.

152. Morrissette JJ, Bagg A. Acute myeloid leukemia: conventional cytogenetics, FISH, and moleculocentric methodologies. *Clin Lab Med.* 2011;31(4):659-686.

153. Tiu RV, Visconte V, Traina F, et al. Updates in cytogenetics and molecular markers in MDS. *Curr Hematol Malig Rep.* 2011;6(2):126-135.

154. Sever C, Abbott CL, de Baca ME, et al. Bone marrow Synoptic reporting for hematologic neoplasms: guideline from the College of American pathologists pathology and laboratory quality center. *Arch Pathol Lab Med.* 2016;140(9):932-949.

155. Rowley JD. The critical role of chromosome translocations in human leukemias. *Annu Rev Genet.* 1998;32:495-519.

156. Kolialexi A, Tsangaris GT, Kitsiou S, et al. Impact of cytogenetic and molecular cytogenetic studies on hematologic malignancies. *Anticancer Res.* 2005;25(4):2979-2983.

157. Arber DA, Stein AS, Carter NH, et al. Prognostic impact of acute myeloid leukemia classification. Importance of detection of recurring cytogenetic abnormalities and multilineage dysplasia on survival. *Am J Clin Pathol.* 2003;119(5):672-680.

158. Swerdlow SH, Campo E, Pileri SA, et al. The 2016 revision of the World Health Organization classification of lymphoid neoplasms. *Blood.* 2016;127(20): 2375-2390.

159. Bennett JM. Changes in the updated 2016: WHO classification of the myelodysplastic syndromes and related myeloid neoplasms. *Clin Lymphoma Myeloma Leuk.* 2016;16(11):607-609.

160. Arber DA, Orazi A, Hasserjian R, et al. The 2016 revision to the World Health Organization classification of myeloid neoplasms and acute leukemia. *Blood.* 2016;127(20):2391-2405.

161. WHO. *World Health Organization Classification of Tumours of Haematopoietic and Lymphoid Tissues.* Revised 4th ed. IARC Press; 2017.

162. Yeung DT, Parker WT, Branford S. Molecular methods in diagnosis and monitoring of haematological malignancies. *Pathology (Phila).* 2011;43(6):566-579.

163. Ramchandren R, Jazaerly T, Bluth MH, et al. Molecular diagnosis of hematopoietic neoplasms: 2018 update. *Clin Lab Med.* 2018;38(2):293-310.

164. Bacher U, Shumilov E, Flach J, et al. Challenges in the introduction of next-generation sequencing (NGS) for diagnostics of myeloid malignancies into clinical routine use. *Blood Cancer J.* 2018;8(11):113.

165. Sen F, Vega F, Medeiros LJ. Molecular genetic methods in the diagnosis of hematologic neoplasms. *Semin Diagn Pathol.* 2002;19(2):72-93.

166. Wang HW, Raffeld M. Molecular assessment of clonality in lymphoid neoplasms. *Semin Hematol.* 2019;56(1):37-45.

167. Hughes T, Branford S. Molecular monitoring of BCR-ABL as a guide to clinical management in chronic myeloid leukaemia. *Blood Rev.* 2006;20(1):29-41.

168. Wrench D, Montoto S, Fitzgibbon J. Molecular signatures in the diagnosis and management of follicular lymphoma. *Curr Opin Hematol.* 2010;17(4):333-340.

169. Randolph TR. Acute promyelocytic leukemia (AML-M3)—Part 2: molecular defect, DNA diagnosis, and proposed models of leukemogenesis and differentiation therapy. *Clin Lab Sci.* 2000;13(2):106-116.

170. Hasan SK, Lo-Coco F. Utilization of molecular phenotypes to detect relapse and optimize the management of acute promyelocytic leukemia. *Clin Lymphoma Myeloma Leuk.* 2010;10(suppl 3):S139-S143.

171. Anastasi J. The myeloproliferative neoplasms including the eosinophilia-related myeloproliferations associated with tyrosine kinase mutations: changes and issues in classification and diagnosis criteria. *Semin Diagn Pathol.* 2011;28(4):304-313.

172. Smith CA, Fan G. The saga of JAK2 mutations and translocations in hematologic disorders: pathogenesis, diagnostic and therapeutic prospects, and revised World Health Organization diagnostic criteria for myeloproliferative neoplasms. *Hum Pathol.* 2008;39(6):795-810.

173. Gale RE, Green C, Allen C, et al. The impact of FLT3 internal tandem duplication mutant level, number, size, and interaction with NPM1 mutations in a large cohort of young adult patients with acute myeloid leukemia. *Blood.* 2008;111(5): 2776-2784.

174. Schlenk RF, Dohner K, Krauter J, et al. Mutations and treatment outcome in cytogenetically normal acute myeloid leukemia. *N Engl J Med.* 2008;358(18):1909-1918.

175. Schnittger S, Schoch C, Kern W, et al. Nucleophosmin gene mutations are predictors of favorable prognosis in acute myelogenous leukemia with a normal karyotype. *Blood.* 2005;106(12):3733-3739.

176. La Rosee P, Hochhaus A. Molecular pathogenesis of tyrosine kinase resistance in chronic myeloid leukemia. *Curr Opin Hematol.* 2010;17(2):91-96.

177. Weisberg E, Manley PW, Cowan-Jacob SW, et al. Second generation inhibitors of BCR-ABL for the treatment of imatinib-resistant chronic myeloid leukaemia. *Nat Rev Cancer.* 2007;7(5):345-356.

178. Swansbury J. Cytogenetic studies in hematologic malignancies: an overview. *Methods Mol Biol.* 2003;220:9-22.

179. Bain BJ. Overview. Cytogenetic analysis in haematology. *Best Pract Res Clin Haematol.* 2001;14(3):463-477.

Laboratory Hematology

Chapter 2 ■ Clinical Flow Cytometry

ANNA PORWIT

DEFINITION

One of the meanings of the word *flow* is "to move with a continual shifting of the component particles." The term *cytometry* refers to counting (*metry*) cells (*cyto*). Thus, flow cytometry (FCM) is a method that employs a fluid stream to carry cells through a counter. FCM evaluates multiple parameters of individual cells (or other particles) by measuring the characteristics of light they scatter or the photons they emit as they stream through a light source. The strength of this technology lies in its high throughput (measurement of high numbers of cells in a short time) and in its ability to capture many parameters per cell, assessing them individually. Currently, the principal applications of FCM in the clinical practice are routine cell counters and immunophenotyping. This chapter focuses on clinical application of FCM in hematology, mainly in diagnosis of hematologic malignancies. However, some functional assays (e.g., phosphorylation, cytokine secretion, and apoptotic) that are being introduced into clinical practice are also briefly discussed.

HISTORICAL BACKGROUND

FCM dates back to the work done in Stockholm by Caspersson and coworkers, who in the 1930s demonstrated that DNA content, measured by ultraviolet and visible light absorption in unstained cells, doubled during the cell cycle.[1,2] In 1950, Coons and Kaplan reported on the detection of antigens in tissues using fluorescein-conjugated antibody methods, which prompted widespread use of fluorescence microscopes.[3] In 1953, W. H. Coulter patented the so-called Coulter principle and built the first FCM machine, in which blood cells in saline suspensions passed one by one through a small orifice and were detected by changes of electrical impedance at the orifice. The Coulter principle started to be applied for cell counting in clinical hematology.[4] After the first paper in *Science* by Fulwyler,[5] the era of standard use of FCM for cell sorting started beginning with publications from the L. A. Herzenberg Laboratory at Stanford University, California, the United States, in the early 1970s.[6] Soon after, the first flow cytometers became commercially available from Becton Dickinson (now BD Biosciences), followed by other companies. FCM came into clinical use in the late 1980s, at first only in specialized laboratories. In the 1990s and early 2000s, three- and four-color analyses became a standard diagnostic method for immunophenotyping of hematologic samples. Many clinical solutions and standardization efforts were initialized by Orfao and coworkers, from the University of Salamanca, Spain.[7] In the 2010s, 8- and 10-color FCM became a standard clinical method.[8-10] In research settings, applications using 19-parameter FCM combining 17 fluorescence channels with forward scatter (FS) and side scatter (SS) have been reported.[11]

PRINCIPLES OF FLOW CYTOMETRY

For reliable analysis, the specimen must be in a monodisperse suspension. In a flow cytometer, isotonic fluid is forced under pressure into a tube that delivers it to the flow cell, where a fluid column with laminar flow and a high flow rate is generated (the so-called sheath fluid). The sample is introduced into the flow cell by a computer-driven syringe in the center of the sheath fluid, creating a coaxial stream within a stream (the so-called sample core stream). The pressure of the sheath stream hydrodynamically aligns the cells or particles so that they are presented to the light beam one at a time. FCM measures the amount of light emitted by fluorochromes associated with individual cells or particles (*Figure 2.1*). New flow cytometers have three to six lasers. For application in FCM, antibodies are conjugated with fluorochromes, dyes that absorb the light from the laser and emit light at longer wavelengths.[12] A list of fluorochromes commonly used in clinical FCM is given in *Table 2.1*. The emitted light is focused by a lens onto fiber-optic cables and transmitted to octagonal detectors (*Figure 2.1*). Filters in front of each of a series of detectors restrict the light that reaches the detector to only a small range of wavelengths (referred to as channels). The sensors convert the photons to electrical impulses that are proportional to the number of photons received and to the number of fluorochrome molecules bound to the cell. The fluorescent emissions are of low intensity and are amplified by photomultiplier tubes (PMTs). PMTs count the specific photons, and the remaining light is reflected to the next filter, where the process is repeated. Thus, most of the cell-associated fluorescence detected in a given channel is emitted by fluorochrome-coupled antibodies or other fluorescent reagents of interest. Electrical impulses from photoelectrons collected by PMTs are converted to digital signals. Acquired FCM data are electronically stored in so-called list-mode files that are a part of the medical record of the patient.[13]

A pair of light scatter channels provides an approximate measure of cell size (FS) and granularity (SS). FS and SS are used to set the threshold for separating debris, erythrocytes, and platelets from viable nucleated cells. Live cells scatter more light than dead and apoptotic cells and therefore have higher FS. SS signals are collected with fluorescent light at right angles to the beam and are dependent on light reflected from internal structures of the cell. Cells with high granularity or vacuoles, such as granulocytes or monocytes, will have higher SS than ones with no granules, such as lymphocytes or immature precursor (blast) cells.

Most cells have low numbers of native fluorescent molecules that define their background fluorescence. Some of the light may come from spillover fluorescence emitted by a reagent measured in a different channel. The interference is corrected by applying fluorescence

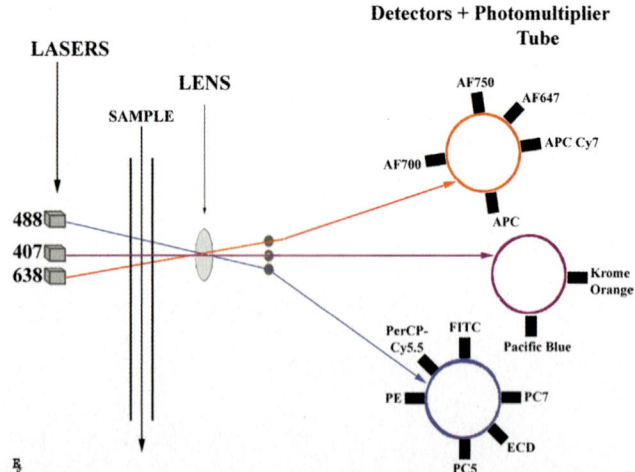

FIGURE 2.1 Principles of multicolor flow cytometry. A single-cell suspension is hydrodynamically focused with sheath fluid to intersect lasers (three-laser system is shown). Fluorescence signals are collected by multiple fluorescence emission detectors, separate for every laser. Examples of fluorochromes detected by different lasers are given according to *Table 2.1*. Detected signals are amplified by photomultiplier tubes and converted to digital form for analysis.

compensation based on data from single-stained samples. This is usually done using cells or beads before or during the data acquisition phase.[14] However, modern FCM data analysis software also allows collection of uncompensated data and applying compensation during analysis. Before data acquisition, standard reference particles (fluorescent microspheres) should be used to adjust the PMT voltage settings so that the beads fall in approximately the same location or the same "target channels," predetermined for each fluorochrome.[15]

Cell Sorting

Some flow cytometers are capable of physically separating the cells (fluorescence-activated cell sorter) based on differences in any measurable parameters.[16] Sorting is achieved by formation of droplets. The basic components of any sorter are as follows:

- A droplet generator
- A droplet-charging and deflecting system

Table 2.1. Fluorochromes Commonly Used in Clinical Flow Cytometry

Probe	Ex (nm)	Em (nm)	Acronym/Comments
AmCyan	405	489	
Vio Bright V423	405	420	
Pacific Blue	405	455	PcB
Brilliant Violet 421	405	421	BV421
BD Horizon V450	405	455	
Alexa Fluor 405	405	421	
BD Horizon V500	405	500	
Krome Orange	405	428	
Pacific Orange	405	551	
R-Phycoerythrin	480; 565	578	PE
Red 613	480; 565	613	PE-Texas Red
PE-Cy5 conjugates	480; 565; 650	670	Cy-Chrome, Tri-Color, Quantum Red
PE-Cy7 conjugates	480; 565; 743	767	PE-Cy7
Peridinin chlorophyll protein	490	675	PerCP
TruRed	490,675	695	PerCP-Cy5.5
Fluorescein isothiocyanate	495	519	FITC
Rhodamine isothiocyanate	547	572	TRITC
X-Rhodamine	570	576	XRITC
Texas Red	589	615	TR
PE-TR-X	595	620	ECD
Allophycocyanin	650	660	APC
APC-H7	627-640	782	APC-H7
APC-Cy7 conjugates	650; 755	767	APC-CY7
Alexa Fluor 647	650	668	
Alexa Fluor 700	696	719	
Alexa Fluor 750	752	779	
Cyanine 5	(625); 650	670	Cy5
Cyanine 5.5	675	694	Cy5.5
Cyanine 7	743	767	Cy7
Nucleic Acid Probes			
4',6-Diamidino-2-phenylindole	345	455	DAPI, AT-selective
SYTOX Blue	431	480	DNA
SYTOX Green	504	523	DNA
Ethidium bromide	493	620	
7-Aminoactinomycin D	546	647	7-AAD, CG-selective
Acridine Orange	503	530/640	DNA/RNA
Thiazole Orange	510	530	TO (RNA)
Propidium iodide	536	617	PI
DRAQ5	633	660	
DRAQ7	633	670	

Abbreviations: Em, peak emission wavelength; Ex, peak excitation wavelength.

Laboratory Hematology

- A collection component
- The electronic circuitry for coordinating the timing and generation of droplet-charging pulses

The flow chamber is attached to a piezoelectric crystal, which vibrates at a certain frequency so that when the fluid carrying the cells passes through the nozzle, forming a jet in air with a velocity of 15 m/s, the vibration causes the jet to break up in precisely uniform droplets, approximately 30,000 to 40,000/s. Each droplet, when separated from the jet, can be charged, and deflected by a steady electric field and is collected in a receptacle. Almost every cell is isolated in a separate droplet. When the cell is analyzed, a sorting decision is made, and until the proper electrical charge pulse is applied to the droplet containing the cell, there is a transit time determined by several factors, such as flow velocity, droplet separation, and the cell preparation. If two cells cannot be separated, the sorting is aborted.

Monoclonal Antibodies

Advances of FCM would not be possible without the development of monoclonal antibodies (MAbs). By the Nobel Prize–winning hybridoma technology developed in 1975 by Köhler and Milstein,[17] lymphocytes from the spleen of an immunized mouse can be immortalized by fusion to myeloma cells that have lost the ability to make their own immunoglobulins (Igs) but are capable of unlimited mitotic divisions. Through limited dilutions, individual cell lines (hybridomas) that produce an antibody of unique specificity, avidity, and isotype can be established. In the early days of the application of MAbs to immunology, many laboratories immunized mice with leukocytes. The obtained hybridomas produced many antibodies that reacted with leukocytes, but the identities of the molecular targets were not known. The reactivity spectrum of the antibody could be described by staining multiple different cell types, and in most cases, the target antigen could be isolated by immunoprecipitation or Western blotting and its molecular weight and other structural characteristics determined.

The first round of multilaboratory, blind, comparative analyses of antibodies was performed during the first human leukocyte differentiation antigen (HLDA) workshop held in 1982 in Paris, France.[18] Statistical analysis of data from several laboratories revealed "clusters of differentiation," named for the statistical procedure of cluster analysis and for the focus on leukocyte differentiation. Antibodies thought to be detecting the same molecule, and the molecule itself, were given a "CD" designation.[19] An organization called the HLDA Council was established, and 10 subsequent HLDA workshops have characterized more than 370 CD antigens. The HLDA Council reviewed and modified the objectives of HLDA in 2004 and changed the name of the organization to human cell differentiation molecules (HCDM). The reasoning behind the name change to HCDM was to break with tradition while retaining the letters "CD" to maintain emphasis on molecules of human origin, to extend focus from leukocytes to other cell types interacting with leukocytes such as endothelial cell or stromal cell molecules, and to broaden the scope from cell-surface molecules to any molecule whose expression reflects differentiation, recognizing the growing values of intracellular molecules. The HCDM Council keeps a comprehensive database of CD molecules (www.hcdm.org). CD antigens, which are most often applied in hematologic immunophenotyping, are listed in *Table 2.2*.

Table 2.2. List of CD Antigens Most Commonly Used in Flow Cytometry Immunophenotyping of Hematologic Samples

CD	Expression in Normal Hematopoietic Cell Types	MW (kDa)	Function
CD1a	Cortical thymocytes, Langerhans cells, dendritic cells	49	Antigen presentation, w/β2m
CD2	Thymocytes, T cells, NK cells	50	CD58 ligand, adhesion, T-cell activation
CD3	T cells, thymocyte subset		w/TCR, TCR surface expression/signal transduction
CD4	Thymocyte subset, T-cell subset, monocytes, macrophages	55	MHC class II coreceptor, HIV receptor, T-cell differentiation/activation
CD5	Thymocytes, T-cell, B-cell subset	67	CD72 receptor, TCR or BCR signaling, TB interaction
CD7	Thymocytes, T cells, NK cells, small subset of hematopoietic progenitors	40	T costimulation
CD8	Thymocyte subset, T-cell subset, NK subset	32-34	MHC class I coreceptor, receptor for some mutated HIV-1, T-cell differentiation/activation
CD9	Eosinophils, basophils, platelets, activated T cells	22-27	Cellular adhesion and migration
CD10	B-cell precursors, germinal center B cells, thymocyte subset, neutrophils	100	Zinc-binding metalloproteinase, B-cell development
CD11a	Lymphocyte subsets, granulocytes, monocytes, macrophages	180	CD11a/CD18 receptor for ICAM-1, -2, -3; intercellular adhesion; T-cell costimulation
CD11b	Granulopoietic cells, NK cells	170	Binds CD54, ECM, and iC3b
CD11c	Dendritic cells, granulopoietic cells, NK cells, and B-cell and T-cell subsets	150	Binds CD54, fibrinogen, and iC3b
CD13	Granulopoietic cells, monocytes	150-170	Zinc-binding metalloproteinase, antigen processing, receptor for coronavirus strains
CD14	Monocytes, macrophages, Langerhans cells	53-55	Receptor for LPS/LBP, LPS recognition
CD15	Neutrophils, eosinophils, monocytes		Adhesion
CD16	Neutrophils, macrophages, NK cells	50-65	Component of low-affinity Fc receptor, phagocytosis, and ADCC
CD19	B cells, plasma cells	95	Complex w/CD21 and CD81, BCR coreceptor, B-cell activation/differentiation
CD20	B cells	33-37	B-cell activation

(Continued)

Table 2.2. List of CD Antigens Most Commonly Used in Flow Cytometry Immunophenotyping of Hematologic Samples (Continued)

CD	Expression in Normal Hematopoietic Cell Types	MW (kDa)	Function
CD21	B-cell and T-cell subsets	145, 110	Complement C3d and EBV receptor, complex w/CD19 and CD81, BCR coreceptor
CD22	B cells	150	Adhesion, B-mono, BT interactions
CD23	B cells, eosinophils, platelets	45	CD19-CD21-CD81 receptor, IgE low-affinity receptor, signal transduction
CD24	Thymocytes, erythrocytes, lymphocytes, myeloid cells	35-45	Binds P-selectin
CD25	Activated B cells and T cells	55	IL-2Rα, w/IL-2Rβ, and γ to form high-affinity complex
CD30	Reed-Sternberg cells, T-cell lymphomas	110	Treatment with anti-CD30 MAb
CD33	Granulopoietic cells, monocytes, dendritic cells	67	Adhesion
CD34	Hematopoietic precursors	105-120	Stem cell marker, adhesion, CD62L receptor
CD36	Platelets, monocytes, erythropoietic precursors	88	A scavenger and thrombospondin receptor, adhesion, phagocytosis
CD38	High expression on B-cell precursors, plasma cells, and activated T cells; low on granulopoietic cells	45	Ecto-ADP-ribosyl cyclase, cell activation
CD41	Platelets, megakaryocytes	125/22	w/CD61 forms GPIIb, binds fibrinogen, fibronectin, vWF, thrombospondin, platelet activation and aggregation
CD42a	Platelets, megakaryocytes	22	Complex w/CD42b, c, and d; receptor for vWF and thrombin; platelet adhesion to subendothelial matrices
CD45	Hematopoietic cells, multiple isoforms from alternative splicing	180-240	Tyrosine phosphatase, enhanced TCR and BCR signals
CD55	Ubiquitous		Decay accelerating factor, GPI anchored
CD56	NK subset, T-cell subset	175-185	Neural cell adhesion molecule
CD57	NK subset, T-cell subset	110	HNK-1
CD58	T-cell and B-cell subsets, macrophages	40-70	Ligand of the T-lymphocyte CD2 glycoprotein
CD59	Ubiquitous	18-20	Complement regulatory protein, GPI anchored
CD61	Platelets, megakaryocytes	105	Integrin β_3, adhesion, CD41/CD61, or CD51/CD61 mediate adhesion to ECM
CD62L	B-cell subsets, T-cell subsets, monocytes, granulocytes, NK cells, thymocytes	74, 95	CD34, GlyCAM, and MAdCAM-1 receptor; leukocyte homing; tethering; rolling
CD64	Monocytes, neutrophils	72	FCγRI, increases on neutrophils in sepsis
CD65	Granulopoietic cells		Phagocytosis
CD66	Neutrophils	90	Cell adhesion
CD68	Monocytes, neutrophils, basophils, mast cells	110	Macrosialin
CD71	Proliferating cells, erythroid precursors, reticulocytes	95	Transferrin receptor, iron uptake
CD79	B cells, plasma cells	33-37	Component of BCR, BCR surface expression and signal transduction
CD103	B-cell and T-cell subsets	150, 25	w/Integrin β_7, binds E-cadherin, lymph homing/retention
CD117	Hematopoietic progenitors, mast cells	145	Stem cell factor receptor, hematopoietic progenitor development/differentiation
CD123	Basophils, dendritic cell subset, hematopoietic progenitors	70	IL-3Rα, w/CDw131
CD133	Hematopoietic stem cells subset	120	
CD158 A-K	KIR molecules		Killer cell immunoglobulin-like receptors
CD159c	NK	40	w/MHC class I HLA-E molecules, forms heterodimer with CD94
CD200	Thymocytes, T-cell and B-cell subsets	43	
CD207	Langerin		
CD247	CD3-zeta		
CD235a	Erythropoietic precursors	36	Glycophorin A
CD271	PDCD-1		Programmed cell death receptor 1
CD326	EpCAM		Epithelial cell adhesion molecule

For a comprehensive list and characteristics, please see www.hcdm.org.

Abbreviations: ECM, extracellular matrix; GP, glycoprotein; GPI, glycosylphosphatidylinositol; HLA, human leukocyte antigen; MHC, major histocompatibility complex; MW, molecular weight; NK, natural killer; vWF, von Willebrand factor.

Laboratory Hematology

Sample Preparation

Appropriate samples for clinical FCM include peripheral blood (PB), bone marrow (BM) aspirate, disaggregated tissues including lymph node (LN) and other soft-tissue biopsies as well as fine-needle aspirations (FNAs) and BM core biopsies, cerebrospinal fluid (CSF), other body fluids including effusions and lavage fluids, and nuclei from paraffin-embedded tissue for DNA ploidy assays. All unfixed clinical FCM specimens should be considered biohazardous and labeled as such in accordance with national or regional safety standards. A test requisition form, whether printed or electronic, should accompany all specimens. This form should include unique patient identifiers, age, sex, diagnosis (if previously established) or suspect condition under consideration, name of the physician submitting the specimen, pertinent medication, or recent treatment (including dates of chemotherapy or radiation), date and time of specimen collection, and source of the specimen (such as BM aspirate, CSF). The requested test should appear on the specimen label or on the requisition accompanying the specimen. Complete blood count should be provided for PB and BM samples. For PB, ethylenediaminetetraacetic acid (EDTA), sodium heparin, or acid citrate dextrose may be used. For BM aspirates, sodium heparin is the preferred anticoagulant and is required if cytogenetic testing is to be performed on the same specimen. All tissue biopsies intended for FCM evaluation, including LN or other tissue biopsies, should be transported in an adequate volume of an appropriate transport medium in a sterile container to optimize cell viability.[20] CSF samples should be stabilized or analyzed immediately owing to potential toxic effects on cell viability.[21]

All clinical samples should be analyzed as soon as possible. Twenty-four hours is preferred, but 48 hours is considered the longest acceptable time frame for analysis of nonstabilized samples. If transport time is longer, a viability report is mandatory, and the results should be interpreted cautiously. Room temperature (18°-25°C) is recommended for storage and transport. For specimens that are not highly degenerated, nonviable cells can be excluded from the analysis by meticulous FS vs SS gating. Dead cells trap fluorochrome-conjugated antibodies and increase background fluorescence. Fluorescent, DNA-binding dyes (*Table 2.1*) that are excluded from viable cells with intact plasma membranes, and thus positive in nonviable cells, can also be applied.

Whole-PB/BM analysis with erythrocyte lysis is recommended for clinical leukocyte immunophenotyping. Immunophenotyping of density gradient (Ficoll)-separated mononuclear cells should not be used because of selective cell loss. Samples to be stained for surface immunoglobulin (sIg) should be thoroughly washed before incubation with MAbs to avoid false-negative results owing to the presence of serum Igs.[20] For surface staining, the "stain-lyse-wash" or "bulk-lyse-stain-wash" methods provide the best signal discrimination. Erythrocytes are either lysed after staining in individual tubes or before staining and then samples are divided into individual tubes for staining (recommended for minimal residual disease [MRD] studies). Several commercial lysis reagents are available. Some of the lysis reagents also contain a fixative. If erythropoietic compartment is to be evaluated, lysis is not recommended, and nucleated cells can be acquired using the fluorescent DNA-binding dye and the so-called live gate method to exclude erythrocytes.[22]

For staining, cells are incubated with appropriate amounts of titrated MAbs and then cells are washed before acquisition. Evaluation of intracellular epitopes, including proteins, epigenetic protein modifications (such as protein phosphorylation and methylation), DNA, or RNA, generally requires that the target cell population be fixed and permeabilized to allow antibodies or target-binding dyes to cross the cytoplasmic (cyt.) and nuclear membranes. Commercial fixation and permeabilization kits, with recommended protocols, are available from several manufacturers.[23] For newly developed tests, it is useful to check whether the obtained intracellular staining is associated with an expected localization, using fluorescence microscopy. The specificity of the applied I antibody should also be ensured. For cytoplasmic or nuclear staining, it is important to use antibody conjugates that are free of unconjugated fluorochrome molecules that can stick to intracellular proteins nonspecifically. When simultaneous detection of surface and intracellular epitopes is necessary, the surface staining is performed first, then cells are fixed and permeabilized, and finally intracellular epitopes are stained.

Fluorochromes and Panels

Panel selection should be based on specimen type with consideration of information provided by clinical history, medical indication, and morphology.[24] Several guidelines and consensus papers proposing choice of antigens for diagnosis of various hematologic malignancies have been published.[25] Selecting which antibody combinations best delineate, distinguish, and measure key differences within the target populations of interest and the number of simultaneously measured antibodies is a critical step of FCM assays. Serial dilution antibody titrations against both positive and negative cellular targets are necessary for antibody optimization. The choice of fluorochrome conjugate can affect background, specificity, and dynamic range of measurement. Typically, one would choose a fluorochrome with the best quantum efficiency/yield as the antibody conjugate to identify the lowest antigen density to obtain the best possible signal-to-noise ratio possible. It is of high importance to reliably distinguish between antigen-positive and antigen-negative cell populations to accurately measure the population of positive cells. This can be a challenge in populations of cells weakly expressing antigens. Fluorescence-minus-one controls give the maximum fluorescence expected for a specific population in a channel when the reagent used in that channel is omitted.[26] These controls include both autofluorescence of the cells and the spillover that may be present even after compensation corrections; therefore, such controls are best suited to determine boundaries between positive and negative cells for each subset.

Often, the same anchor gating antibodies are used in every tube, thereby allowing consistent population gating strategies across all tubes of a panel. In immunophenotyping of lymphocyte subsets and in the diagnosis of leukemia/lymphoma, CD45 anchor gating has been shown to provide differential population identification correlated to morphologic microscopic differentials (*Figure 2.2*)[25,27,28]:

- Mature lymphocytes are characterized by low SS and strong CD45 expression (lymph region, *Figure 2.2B*).
- Monocytes have higher SS and strong CD45 expression (monocyte region, *Figure 2.2B*).
- Erythropoietic precursors are CD45 negative and have low SS (CD45− ery region, *Figure 2.2B*).
- Granulopoietic precursors and granulocytes are weakly CD45 positive and have high SS (CD45dim, gran region, *Figure 2.2B*).
- Early hematopoietic precursors of various lineages, including CD34+ stem cells, are characterized by low CD45 expression and low SS (blast region, *Figure 2.2B*).

The localization of these subpopulations on the CD45/SS plot can be confirmed by multicolor staining of various lineage-associated antigens together with CD45 (*Figure 2.2C-K*) and visualization of cell clusters positive for given antigen combinations on the CD45/SSC plot (*Figure 2.2B*) by the so-called back-gating using color-coding.[28]

In multicolor FCM, lineage-associated antigens that are broadly expressed through maturation of investigated cell lineage can be used for gating in conjunction with SSC and CD45 (such as CD19 for B cells, CD3 for T cells; *Figures 2.2-2.4*). Both 8- and 10-color panels for immunophenotyping of hematologic malignancies have been published.[8,25,29]

Examples of 10-color panels for leukemia and lymphoma, currently used at the Flow Cytometry Laboratory, Department of Pathology, Lund University Hospital, Stockholm, Sweden, are given in *Table 2.3*.

Data Analysis and Reporting

Fluorescence data may be presented using either linear or logarithmic amplification. In linear amplification, fluorescence differences are directly proportional to differences of fluorochrome concentration between cells. Logarithmic amplification compresses a wide input range, which may cause difficulties in resolving populations with

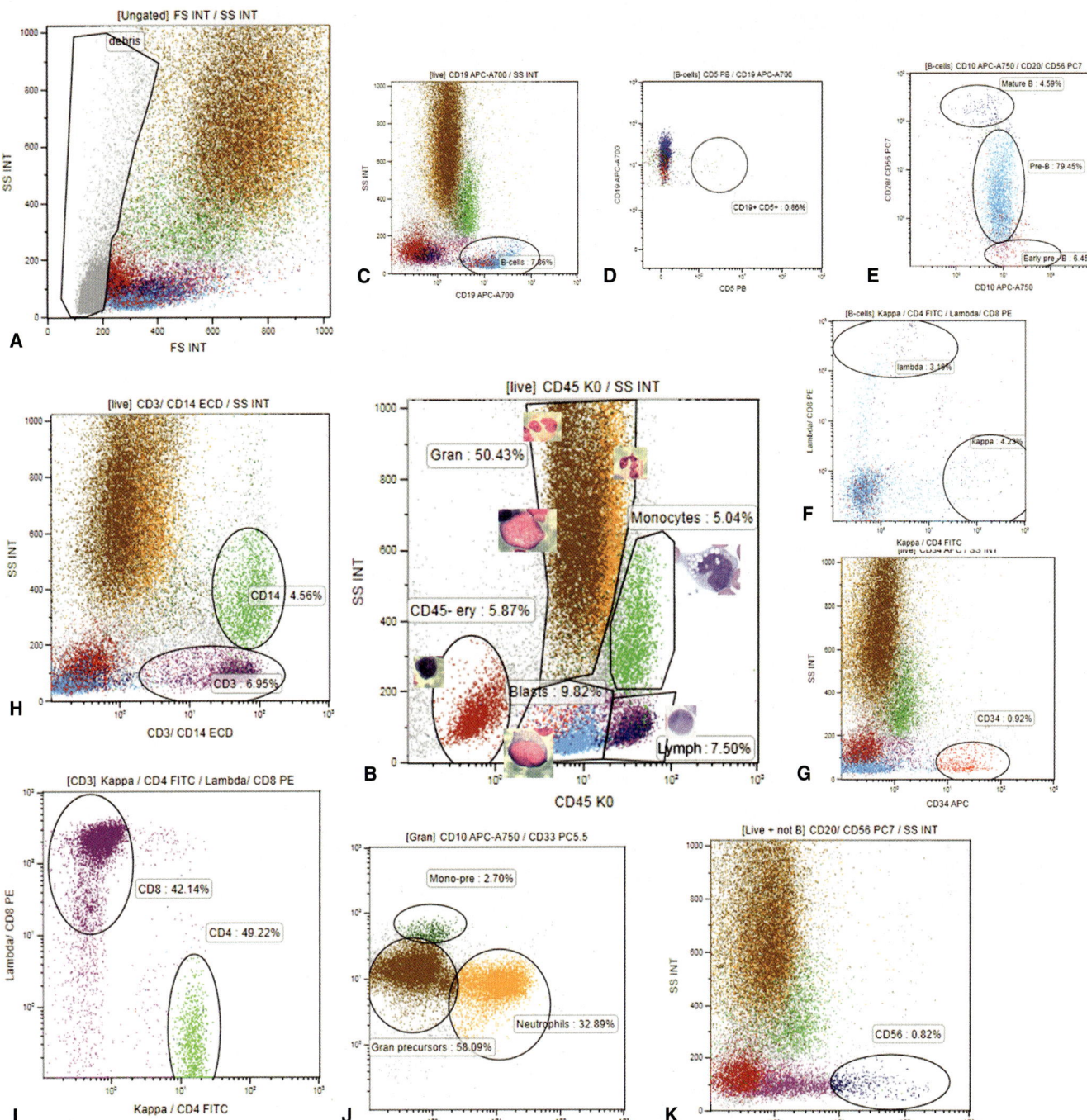

FIGURE 2.2 Bone marrow (BM) mapping with polychromatic flow cytometry. Reactive bone marrow sample from a young patient was analyzed with a screening 10-color 14 MAb panel[30] on a Navios flow cytometer and Kaluza software (Beckman Coulter). The screening BM panel (*Table 2.3*, row 1) was used. The analysis starts with the creating of the "live cells" gate by removal of dead cells, erythrocyte, and platelet aggregates on FS/SS plot (A). A CD45/SS plot is created within the live cell gate (B). Regions for lymphocytes (CD45^{bright}/SS^{low}), monocytes (CD45^{bright}/SS^{high}), granulopoietic cells (CD45^{dim}/SS^{high}), CD45^{dim}/SS^{low} blasts, and CD45^{-}/SS^{low} erythropoietic cells are determined. The B-cell gate is created from the live cell gate on the CD19/SC plot (C). The presence of CD5 positive B cells is investigated using a CD5/CD19 plot (D). The presence of CD10^{+} B cells is looked for by analysis of CD20 and CD10 expression within the B-cell gate (E). In this patient, no CD5^{+} B cells were detected, but a significant fraction of B cells showed a B-cell precursor immunophenotype with a normal maturation pattern (E). If a CD5^{+} or CD10^{+} B-cell population is present, a new gate can be created within plot (D) or (E). B-cell clonality is analyzed within the B-cell gate (F). In this patient, most B cells are negative for light-chain expression, consistent with B-cell precursors. Note that most of CD10^{+}/CD20^{dim} B-cell precursors (cyan dots) fall into the blast gate in the CD45/SS plot (B). κ- and λ-positive B cells have normal κ to λ ratio. If CD5 and/or aberrant CD10^{+} B cells were present, clonality of B cells would be analyzed within the specific CD5^{+}/CD19^{+} or CD10^{+}/CD19^{+} gate. The fraction of CD34^{+} cells (red dots) is estimated within the live cell gate on the CD34/SS plot (G). If increased numbers of CD34^{+} cells are found, they are further analyzed for CD33, CD19, and CD10 expression. CD3^{+} T-cell and CD14^{+} monocyte gates are created on the CD45/CD3^{+}CD14 plot within the live cell gate (H). Fractions of CD4^{+} (violet dots) and CD8^{+} T cells (light green dots) are esti-mated within the CD3^{+} gate (I). CD4-to-CD8 ratio was normal (1.16). Granulopoietic cells are analyzed on CD33/CD10 plot within the "Gran" gate, and fractions of mature neutrophils (CD33^{+}CD10^{+}, orange dots) and granulopoietic precursors (CD33^{+} CD10^{-}, brown dots) are estimated (J). CD14^{-}CD33 bright monocytic precursors can also be enumerated (green dots). Finally, the fraction of CD56^{+} NK cells (dark blue dots) can be evaluated on a CD20^{+}56/SS plot using the Boolean gate of live cells AND non-B cells to exclude CD20^{+} B cell from analysis (K). Various cell populations are back-gated and visualized on both FS/SS and CD45/SS plots (A and B). FS, forward scatter; NK, natural killer; SS, side scatter.

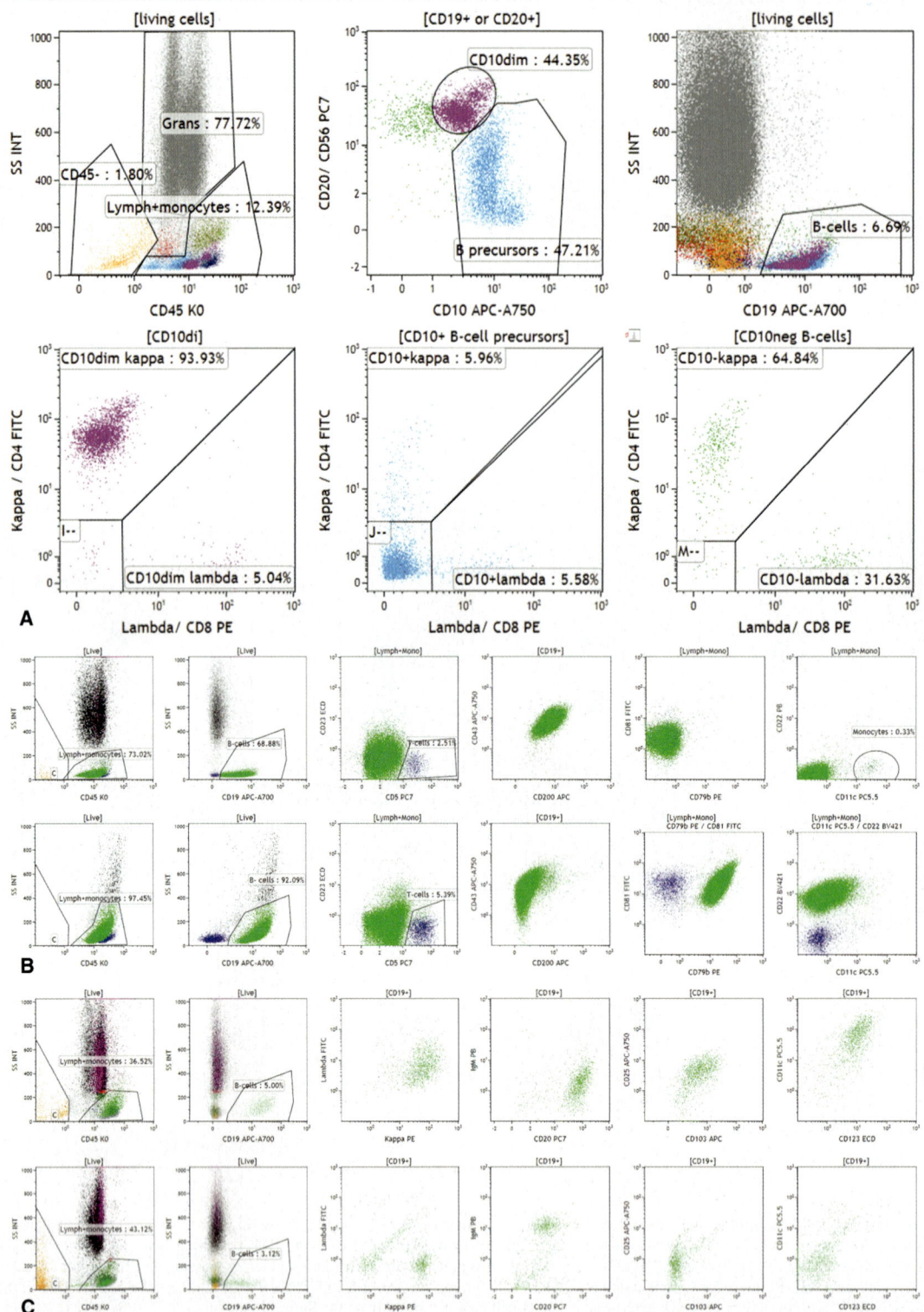

FIGURE 2.3 Examples of analysis of B-cell lymphoma using Navios flow cytometer and Kaluza software (Beckman Coulter). A, Screening panel for bone marrow[30] (*Table 2.3*, row 1). The "live" gate is created by excluding debris and doublets. Fractions of lymphocytes, granulocytes, and monocytes are evaluated as shown in *Figure 2.2*. The B-cell gate is created on a CD19/SS plot. Expression of CD10 is analyzed within the B-cell population. In this sample, a CD10+/CD20$^{neg/dim}$ population of B-cell precursors (cyan dots) and aberrant CD20+CD10^{dim} lymphoma cells population (violet dots) as well as a minor population of CD20+/CD10− mature normal B cells (green dot) were noted. The analysis of κ and λ light-chain expression shows monotypic expression of κ in lymphoma cells, whereas normal cells were polytypic and B-cell precursors negative for sIg. Correlation with bone marrow biopsy revealed follicular lymphoma infiltrates. B, The CLL vs MCL panel (*Table 2.3*, row 3) was applied. The upper panel exemplifies a case of B-CLL with low CD23 expression. A population of B cells (green dots) with weak κ positivity, weak CD20 expression, and CD5 expression was found on screening (not shown). The analysis shows a CD200+, CD43+, CD81$^{neg/dim}$, CD79b−, CD22−, CD11c− immunophenotype. Th lower panel exemplifies findings in a fine-needle aspirate from a lymph node MCL. A population of B cells (green dots) with strong κ positivity, strong CD20 expression, and CD5 expression was found on screening (not shown). The analysis shows a CD200−, CD43+, CD81+, CD79b+, CD22+, CD11c$^{−/dim}$ immunophenotype. MCL diagnosis was confirmed by morphology and FISH for t(11;14). C, The HCL panel (*Table 2.3*, row 4) was applied. The upper panel exemplifies a bone marrow sample with a small population of B cells with a hairy cell leukemia phenotype. Screening showed κ+ CD5−CD10− B cells (5%) (not shown). The analysis with HCL panel confirmed a κ+ B-cell population positive for CD20^{bright}, IgM, CD103, CD25, CD11c, and CD123. Bone marrow biopsy confirmed HCL infiltrates. The lower panel exemplifies a small population of monoclonal B cells in a bone marrow sample from a patient with Waldenström macroglobulinemia. Screening showed κ+ CD5−CD10− B cells (3%) (not shown). Analysis with HCL panel confirmed a κ+ B-cell population positive for CD20^{dim} and IgM but negative for CD103, CD25, CD11c, and CD123. CLL, chronic lymphocytic leukemia; FISH, fluorescence in situ hybridization; HCL, hairy cell leukemia; IgM, immunoglobulin M; MAb, monoclonal antibody; MCL, mantle cell lymphoma; sIg, surface immunoglobulin.

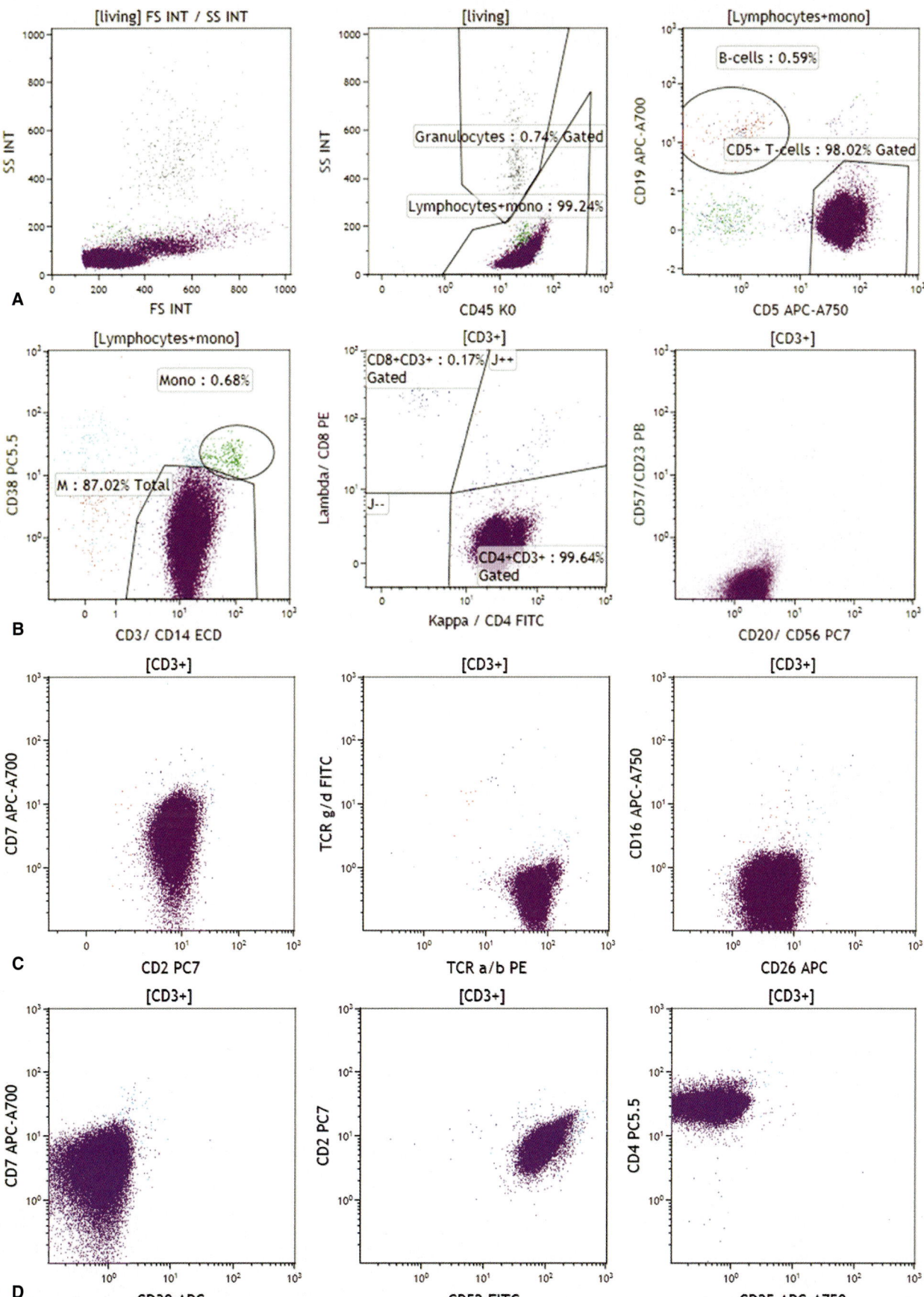

FIGURE 2.4 Example of aberrant T-cell population detected in peripheral blood of a patient with lymphocytosis (WBC 80 × 10⁹/L). Ten-color MAb panels and Navios flow cytometer (Beckman Coulter) were used. Screening analysis showed that 98% of blood cells were CD5⁺CD3⁺ lymphocytes. Further analysis with additional panels[31] showed that majority of CD3⁺ cells were CD4⁺, CD56⁻, CD57⁻, CD7⁺/dim, CD2⁺, TCRα/β⁺, CD16⁻, CD30⁻, CD52⁺⁺, and CD25⁻. Antibody TCRBC1[100] showed that all CD4+ cells were positive, suggesting a monoclonal T-cell population. Clonal TCR rearrangement was later confirmed by PCR. Extra panels showed that TdT and myeloid markers were negative. In combination with cytology that showed medium-sized lymphoid cells with nucleoli, a final diagnosis of T-cell prolymphocytic leukemia was rendered. TdT, terminal deoxynucleotidyl transferase; MAb, monoclonal antibody; TCR, T-cell receptor.

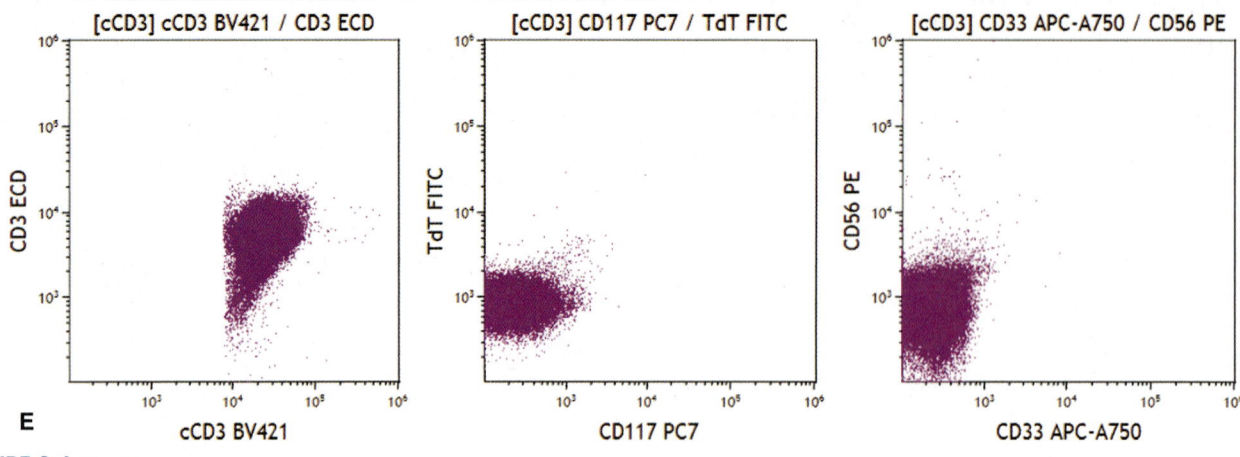

FIGURE 2.4 Cont'd

Table 2.3. Examples of 10-Color Flow Cytometry Panels in Immunophenotyping of Leukemia and Lymphoma

Panel	FITC[a]	PE	ECD	PC5.5	PC7	APC	APC-AF700	APC-AF750	PB/BV421	KO
Screening BM[30]	κ/CD4	λ/CD8	CD3/CD14	CD33	CD20/CD56	CD34	CD19	CD10	CD5	CD45
Screening PB/tissue[31]	κ/CD8	λ/CD4	CD3/CD14	CD38	CD20/CD56	CD10	CD19	CD5	CD57/CD23	CD45
CLL vs MCL	CD81	CD79b	CD23	CD11c	CD5	CD200	CD19	CD43	CD22	CD45
HCL vs SMZL vs LPL	Λ	κ	CD123	CD11c	CD20	CD103	CD19	CD25	IgM	CD45
AML/MDS-granulo	CD56	CD13	CD14	CD10	CD117	CD11b	CD34	CD33	CD16	CD45
AML/MDS-mono	CD36	CD7	CD64	HLA-DR	CD117	CD123	CD34	CD33	CD38	CD45
MDS-ery	CD71	CD13	CD117		CD105	DRAQ5[b]			CD36	CD45
ALL-B	CD66	CD58	CD20	CD38	CD19	CD123	CD34	CD10	CD22	CD45
ALL-T	CD99	CD1a	CD3	CD4	CD5	CD7	CD2	CD10	CD8	CD45
MPAL	TdT	MPO	CD2	HLA-DR	CD19	cytCD79	CD34	CD33	cytCD3	CD45

These panels are in current (December 2017) clinical use at the Flow Cytometry Lab, Department of Pathology, Lund University Hospital, Lund, Sweden.
Abbreviations: ALL, acute lymphoblastic leukemia; AML, acute myeloid leukemia; BM, bone marrow; CLL, chronic lymphocytic leukemia; HCL, hairy cell leukemia; LPL, lymphoplasmacytic lymphoma; MCL, mantle cell lymphoma; MDS, myelodysplastic syndrome; MPAL, mixed phenotype acute leukemia; PB, peripheral blood; SMZL, splenic marginal zone lymphoma.
[a]Characteristics of fluorochromes are given in *Table 2.1.*
[b]Nuclear dye.

similar fluorescence intensities. "Logicle" (or "biexponential") displays have recently been designed for the display of FCM data so that they not only incorporate the useful features of logarithmic displays but also provide accurate visualization of populations with low or background fluorescence.[23] During analysis, data are presented in the form of:

- Histograms (for one parameter), where relative fluorescence or scatter is on the *x*-axis and the number of events with given characteristics on the *y*-axis
- Two-parameter dot plots, where each signal is visualized by one dot and given a parameter on the *x*- and *y*-axis; various cell populations can be then "painted" with different colors
- Density plots, where hot spots indicate large numbers of events resulting from discrete populations of cells and colors can give the graph a three-dimensional feel
- Contour diagrams, where joined lines represent similar numbers of cells

New software applications where multiparameter data can be analyzed using principal component analysis and unsupervised artificial intelligence–based methodology are also available.[32,33]

Analysis is usually focused on identifying and quantifying subsets of cells. A successful analysis will depend on correct marker selection and panel design. Cell counts and percentages are typically reported. The choice of gating strategy depends on the panel used and specific populations of interest. In immunophenotyping of PB and BM, the analysis can be focused on lymphocytes (CD45^{bright} gate)—B lymphocytes, immature precursor/blast gate (CD45^{dim}), T lymphocytes, and natural killer (NK) cells—and on monocytes, or include all living cells in the sample (debris excluded). In tissue samples (LNs, FNA, and body fluids), a broad lymphocyte gate is usually applied. The parent population should be clearly identified when percentages are reported: a fraction may represent a percentage of all living cells in the sample (debris excluded), a percentage of lymphocytes, a percentage of B cells, a percentage of T cells, or a percentage of blasts.

In hematology, assays are usually designed to characterize abnormal cell populations or stages of cell development. In these tests, marker intensities are used to identify the immunophenotype of the cells at various stages of differentiation. Therefore, markers with good dynamic range and proper spillover compensation are critical. Intensity results are typically compared to beads or internal control populations, such as normal mature cells. If fluorescence intensity is comparable to that in normal mature cells, it is reported as "normal": positive, "dim" if it is weaker than in a normal cell population, or "bright" if it is stronger than in normal cells.

Most currently used analysis software allows cross-platform application for analysis and makes it possible to create analysis templates, which are a useful tool for assuring that the analysis is always performed in the same way.[25] Templates help to include all critical elements, and they can serve as an example of how the analysis should be performed. Owing to the highly complex nature of multiparameter analysis, it is recommended that experienced interpreters with knowledge of instrumentation, software, and data analysis produce the templates and supervise the reporting. The final report should contain[24,34]:

1. Demographic identification of the patient
2. Identification of the hospital or division sending the sample
3. Type of specimen (BM aspirate, PB, and other biologic fluids)
4. Timing of observation (first diagnosis or follow-up)
5. Diagnostic hypothesis made by the sender
6. A list of antigens and the type of immunofluorescence analysis carried out
7. Absolute number of cells in the sample
8. Quality of the sample, in terms of viability
9. General description of the gating procedure
10. Immunophenotype of abnormal cells present in the sample
11. Description of other (normal) cells
12. Diagnostic conclusions
13. Comments and/or recommendations for further testing

Validation of Assays and Quality Assurance

In clinical settings, the results obtained in FCM must be interpreted in relation to the clinical information and to the results of other techniques applied in the diagnostic workup (morphology, cytogenetics, molecular genetics, and fluorescence in situ hybridization [FISH]), which can also be used to validate the information provided by FCM. Newly established panels should be validated by comparison to reference methodology, interlaboratory comparison, or verification with specimens obtained from patients with a confirmed diagnosis. A minimum of 20 samples (10 normal and 10 abnormal) is recommended for accuracy assessment. The acceptance criteria will also be variable depending on the required degree of accuracy for the intended use; nevertheless, they should be clearly defined for each assay. Ninety percent or greater agreement between methods is generally required for accuracy.[20,23,35]

All instruments should follow daily quality checks according to manufacturers' recommendations. Participation in a suitable external quality assurance (EQA) program should be undertaken. Many proficiency testing programs are in existence operating at local, national, or international levels. The more common uses of FCM should be subjected to EQA, and many of the larger international programs, such as those operated by UK NEQAS (United Kingdom National External Quality Assessment Service) for Leukocyte Immunophenotyping[35] and the College of American Pathologists, offer FCM EQA programs for leukemia and lymphoma diagnosis, lymphocyte subset monitoring, paroxysmal nocturnal hemoglobinuria (PNH), and CD34+ stem cell enumeration. Many of these programs use stabilized material, enabling samples to be transported long distances such that data from large international cohorts can be examined to search for any instrument or reagent bias. The frequency of the samples issued by such programs is recommended to be at least four times per year to ensure continued performance monitoring.

NORMAL HEMATOPOIESIS

Knowledge of levels and expression patterns of various antigens in normal hematopoietic cells at different stages of development provides a frame of reference for recognition of abnormal differentiation patterns. Following reports by Terstappen et al, several groups provided descriptions of clearly delineated differentiation stages of various hematopoietic cell lineages.[36-42] A detailed review of all available data is beyond the scope of this chapter; a summary of the most important and well-established issues is provided in the subsequent section.

Immature Cells of Normal Bone Marrow

CD34+ hematopoietic progenitor and precursor cells (HPCs) that constitute most cells of the CD45^{dim} (blast) region are a heterogeneous cell population. A small fraction of pluripotent stem cells with long-term repopulating cell activity has been associated with the Lineage (Lin) marker–negative (CD2−, CD3−, CD14−, CD16−, CD19−, CD24−, CD56−, CD66b−, CD235− [Lin−])/CD34+/CD38− phenotype. These cells are very rare in normal BM (usually <0.1%) but may increase in regenerating BM and in myelodysplastic syndromes (MDSs).[43] CD34+/CD45^{dim} cells also include a major fraction of HPC already committed to different hematopoietic lineages (erythroid, neutrophil, monocytic, dendritic cell [DC], basophil, mast cell [MC], eosinophil, and megakaryocytic) and variable numbers of CD34+ B-cell precursors.[44,45] Human stem cells are defined by expression of CD90 and CD49f, and are CD45RA negative. Early myeloid progenitors are isolated based on the expression of interleukin (IL)-3 receptor, α chain (CD123) or FLT3 (CD135), and CD45RA. Myeloid, but not erythroid, progenitors express CD123 and CD135, and the transition from common myeloid to granulocyte-macrophage progenitor is marked by acquisition of CD45RA.[46]

Granulocytic Differentiation

Several antigens change their expression intensity during maturation of granulopoiesis. Characteristic normal patterns for various antigen combinations have been identified using multicolor analysis.[25,28,40,41] Continuous variation in the expression of CD13, CD11b, and CD16 that occurs as the blasts/promyelocytes mature to neutrophils makes the combinations of these antigens very useful in delineating granulocyte maturation (*Figure 2.5*).[47] CD13 is expressed at high levels on CD34+ HPCs and CD117+ precursors (mainly promyelocytes). CD13 is then downregulated and dimly expressed on intermediate precursors (myelocytes) and is gradually upregulated again as the granulocytic cells develop into segmented neutrophils. CD11b and CD16 are initially expressed at low levels, but their expression increases during maturation (*Figure 2.6*).

Expression of CD33 is particularly useful if followed together with expression of human leukocyte antigen-D related (HLA-DR). CD34+ cells are HLA-DR positive and become weakly positive for CD33. With maturation, CD34 disappears, and CD33 expression is upregulated, followed by downregulation of HLA-DR and slight downregulation of CD33 in most mature forms.[41] CD15 and CD65 appear when cells are restricted to neutrophil differentiation. CD66, CD16, and CD10 are the markers of mature, band, and segmented neutrophil granulocytes, respectively, and can be applied to evaluate blood contamination of aspirates.[48] The sequence of marker expression during neutrophil differentiation is summarized in *Table 2.4*. It has been confirmed by cell-culture studies and sorting experiments.[49]

Monocytic Differentiation

CD14, CD36, and CD64 are considered as monocyte-associated markers, with CD14 being the most specific. During maturation toward promonocytes, progenitors downregulate CD34 and CD117 and gain the expression of CD64, CD33, HLA-DR, CD36, and CD15, with an initial mild decrease in CD13 and an increase in CD45. Maturation toward mature monocytes leads to a progressive increase in CD14, CD11b, CD13, CD36, CD300e, and CD45, with a mild decrease in HLA-DR and CD15. Classic mature monocytes show expression of bright CD14, bright CD33, variably bright CD13, bright CD36 and CD64, and low CD15 and CD16.[50]

Blood monocytes can be separated into three major subsets according to their expression of CD14 and CD16 (*Figure 2.4*): CD14++CD16− classical monocytes (cMo), CD14++CD16+ intermediate monocytes (iMo), and CD14−/lowCD16+ nonclassical (ncMo).[51]

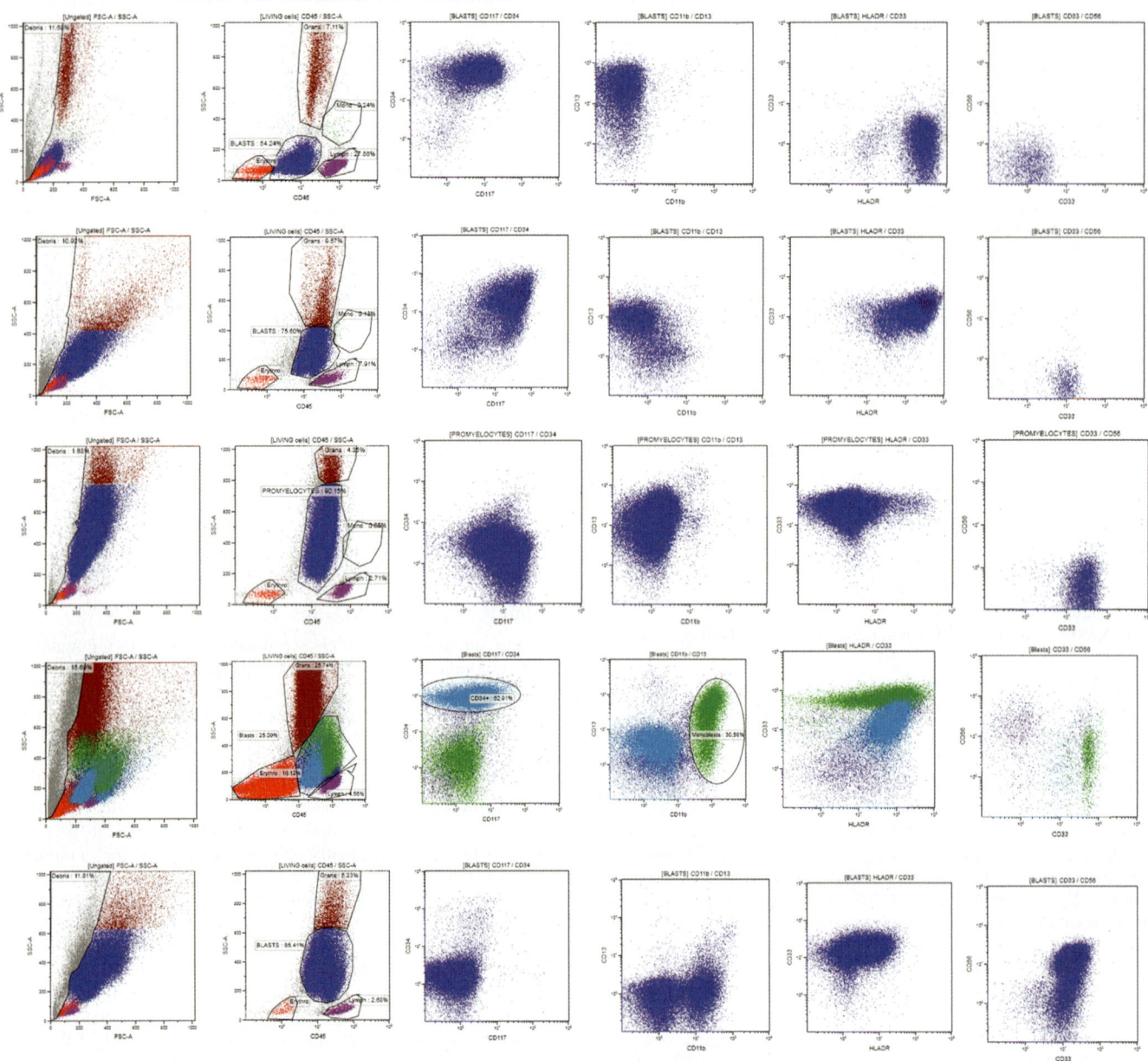

FIGURE 2.5 Examples of various scatter characteristics of CD45^{dim} blast population and patterns of antigen expression in AML. Bone marrow samples were stained with an eight-color MAb panel and acquired on a FACS-CANTOII flow cytometer (BD Biosciences). The panel consisted of CD56FITC/CD13PE/CD34 PerCPCy5.5/CD117PECy7/CD33APC/CD11b APCCy7/HLADR PBlue/CD45 AmCyan. Analysis was performed using Kaluza software (Beckman Coulter). After removal of dead cells and debris, blasts, lymphocytes, monocytes, and granulopoietic precursors/granulocytes were gated on the CD45/SS plot. Further analysis of antigen expression was performed within the blast population (dark blue dots) except for myelomonocytic leukemia (fourth row) where the monocyte gate was added (green dots). The upper row of plots shows an example of AML without differentiation showing agranular blasts, positive for CD34, CD117, CD13, and HLA-DR but negative for CD33 and CD56. The second row shows an example of AML with granulocytic differentiation as demonstrated by partial expression of CD11b and SS characteristics. Blasts are strongly positive for CD34, CD117, CD13, CD33, and HLA-DR but negative for CD56. The third row shows an example of APL with characteristic high SS and negative CD34, HLA-DR, CD11b, heterogeneous CD13, strong CD33, and no expression of CD56. The fourth row shows an example of myelomonocytic AML where a population of blasts (dark blue) and a population of aberrant monocytes were detected. Blasts were positive for CD34, CD33, CD11b, and HLA-DR but negative for CD117 and CD13. Both blasts and monocytes showed aberrant expression of CD56. The fifth row shows an example of monoblastic leukemia, which was negative for CD34, CD117, and CD13 but showed strong expression of CD33 and CD56, dim HLA-DR, and partial expression of CD11b. AML, acute myeloid leukemia; APL, acute promyelocytic leukemia; HLA, human leukocyte antigen; MAb, monoclonal antibody; SS, side scatter.

Erythropoietic Differentiation

Early erythropoietic precursors are found in the blast area and can be identified by very bright CD44, bright CD71, intermediate CD36, positivity for HLA-DR, and expression of CD117 with "dim" CD45. Glycophorin A (CD235a) is expressed at a low level at this stage. Maturation to the basophilic erythroblast is accompanied by a decrease in CD44, appearance of CD105, disappearance of CD45, and acquisition of bright CD235a expression. At transition to the polychromatophilic/orthochromatophilic stage, erythroblasts show loss of HLA-DR, CD105, followed by decrease in CD44 and a mild decrease in CD36.[22,25,52]

Lymphocyte Differentiation

The average reported relative frequencies of major lymphoid subsets in various types of tissues are given in *Table 2.5*. Each laboratory should establish its own ranges.

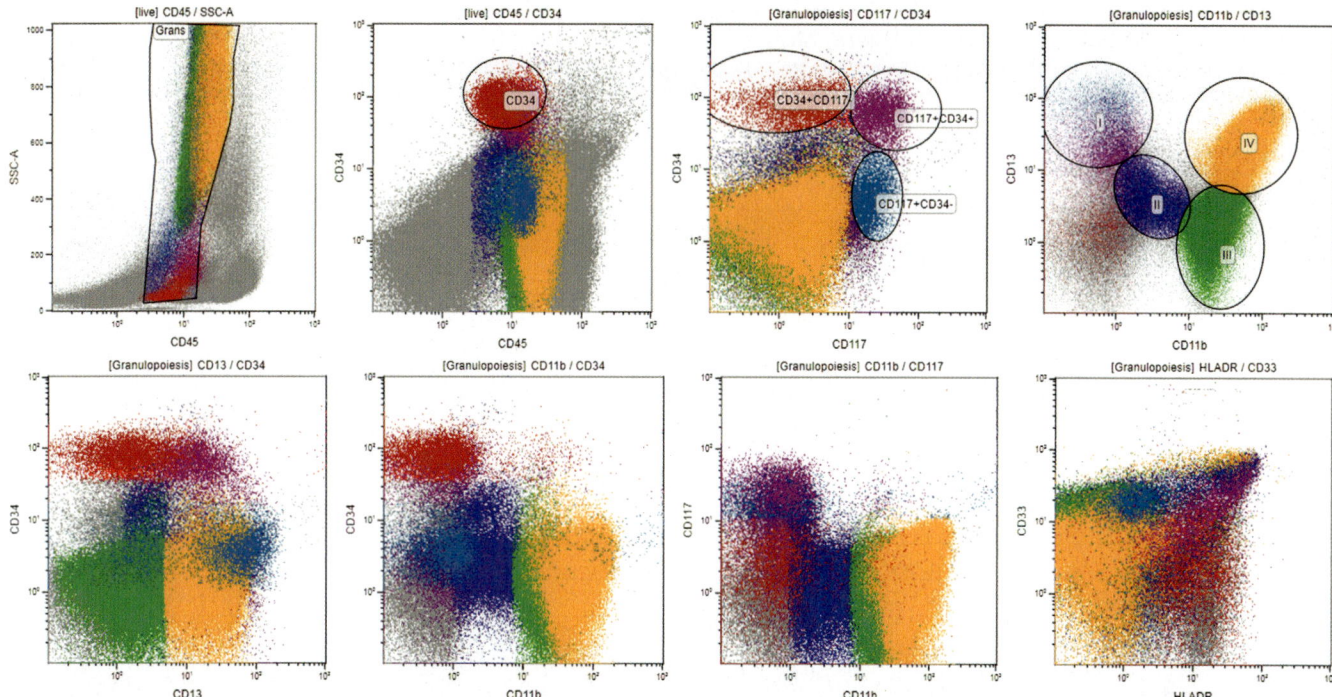

FIGURE 2.6 Flow cytometry analysis of maturation in granulopoiesis. Reactive bone marrow samples were stained with an eight-color MAb panel and acquired on a FACS-CANTOII flow cytometer (BD Bioscience). The panel consisted of CD56FITC/CD13PE/CD34 PerCPCy5.5/CD117PECy7/CD33APC/CD11b APCCy7/HLADR PBlue/CD45 AmCyan. Analysis was performed using Kaluza software (Beckman Coulter). Granulopoietic cells and blasts were gated on CD45/SS plot within a live cell gate (upper left). CD34+ cells were gated in a live cell gate, and a Boolean gate was created by adding both gates (called granulopoiesis). Expression of CD34 and CD117 showed three populations: CD34+/CD117−, CD34+/CD117+, and CD117+/CD34−. The right upper plot shows maturation in granulopoiesis corresponding to promyelocytes (I: CD13++/+ CD11b−), myelocytes (II: CD13+/dim, CD11bdim), metamyelocytes/bands (III: CD13dim, CD11bright), and mature neutrophils (IV: CD13bright, CD11bbright). The lower row of plots illustrates the position of these various subsets in other antigen expression plots. All granulopoietic cells were negative for CD56 (not shown). MAb, monoclonal antibody.

B Cells

B-cell differentiation in the normal human BM has been extensively studied by several groups that described characteristic patterns of antigen expression on consecutive stages of B-cell precursors (*Table 2.6* and *Figure 2.7*).[38,53] The changes in antigen expression in B-lineage committed cells can be summarized as follows[25,54]:

- CD34+CD10+ terminal deoxynucleotidyl transferase (TdT)+CD79a+CD19− common lymphoid progenitor: early B stage.
- CD34+CD19+CD10+TdT+CD20−cyt.IgM− pro B-cell stage.
- After downregulation of CD34 and TdT, they become CD34−CD19+CD10+CD20 heterogeneous pre-B that can be further subdivided into I and II subsets.
- CD34−CD19+CD20+CD10dim/−IgM+ immature B cells.
- After expression of light chains, cells become CD10−CD19+CD20+IgM+IgD+ mature B cells.

Pre-B and immature B cells constitute the most B cells in BM of children, whereas mature B cells are most frequent in adult BM.[38]

In children with BM regeneration after infection or chemotherapy and in transient hyperplasia of B-cell progenitors, subpopulations of immature and mature B cells coexpressing CD5 have been identified. CD5+ B cells are the major population of B cells in fetal life, and their percentage decreases with age.[55] Knowledge of antigen expression patterns of B-cell subsets in normal BM is essential for follow-up studies of MRD in patients treated for B-cell acute lymphoblastic leukemia (B-ALL).[38,56]

T Cells

T-cell production is maintained throughout life by thymic seeding of BM-derived progenitors. Rare (<0.1%) T-cell restricted precursors, which express pre-Tα protein on the cell surface and are CD34+CD7+CD45RA+, are identified in human BM. It has been suggested that CD34+CD10+CD24− progenitors present in both BM and thymus constitute a thymus-seeding population and may replace CD34+CD7+CD45RA+ cells in the postnatal period.[57] However, the frequency of these cells in normal BM is lower than 1×10^{-4}.[39] No TdT-positive T cells expressing cyt.CD3 are found in normal BM.[39] Most mature T cells in the BM coexpress CD7, CD5, CD2, and membrane CD3 and are either CD4 or CD8 positive. However, minor subsets of CD7+ cells lacking other "pan-T" antigens, small subsets with coexpression of CD4 and CD8, and a subset lacking CD4 and CD8 have been identified. A small population of CD7− T cells (<10% of T cells) can also be seen in normal and reactive conditions.[58]

Minor Bone Marrow Cell Subsets

In healthy donors, *eosinophils* represent 2% to 3% of blood leukocytes. Numbers of eosinophilic precursors may vary considerably in reactive BM. Eosinophilic myelocytes can be identified by high SS, intermediate CD45 (at a level slightly higher than neutrophilic myelocytes), low-to-intermediate CD11b, intermediate CD13, and low CD33, with bright CD66b and no CD16 expression. Mature eosinophils show increased levels of CD45 and CD11b, with a decrease in CD33, and are negative for CD16.[59]

Basophils are the least common granulocyte subset (0.5% of total blood leukocytes and about 0.3% of nucleated BM cells in healthy individuals). Basophils are positive for CD9, CD13, CD22 (dimmer than mature B lymphocytes), CD25dim, CD33, CD38bright, CD45 (dimmer than lymphocytes and brighter than myeloblasts), and CD123bright, and are negative for CD3, CD4, CD19, CD34, CD15, CD64, CD117, and HLA-DR.[60] In some individuals, basophils are positive for CD11b.

Bone marrow mast cells (BMMCs) are present in normal BM at a very low frequency (0.021% ± 0.0025% of the nucleated cells).[61] BMMCs are clearly identifiable on the basis of their light scatter properties and strong CD117 expression. Normal BMMCs are virtually always positive for CD9, CD11c, CD29, CD33, CD43, CD44, CD45,

Table 2.4. Surface Marker Expression During Maturation of Granulopoietic Precursors in the Bone Marrow

Antigen	Blasts	Promyelocytes	Myelocytes	Metamyelocytes	Bands	Segmented Neutrophils
CD10	–	–	–	–	–	+
CD11a	D	d	d	+	+	+
CD11b	–	–	d	+	+	b
CD11c	–	–	d	D	D	d
CD13	D	+	+	D	d/+	b
CD15	–/+	d/+	+	+	+	+
CD16	–	–	–	D	+	b
CD18	+	+	b	+	+	+
CD24	–	–	+	+	+	+
CD33	–/d/+	b	+	D	D	D
CD34	d/+	–	–	–	–	–
CD35	–	–	–	–	D	D
CD44	B	+	d	D	+	B
CD45RA	D	d	–	–	–	–
CD45RO	–	–	–	D	+	B
CD54	+	+	–/d	–/d	–/d	–/d
CD55	B	+	+	B	B	B
CD59	B	b	b	B	B	B
CD62L	+	+	+	+	+	+
CD64	D	d	+	+	–	–
CD65	–/+	d	+	+	B	B
CD66a	–	–	+	+	+	+
CD66b	–	b	b	+	+	+
CD66c	–	b	b	+	+	+
CD117	D	+	–	–	–	–
CD133	D	–	–	–	–	–

Abbreviations: –, negative; +, positive; –/+ or (d), partially positive (or dim); b, bright, strongly positive; d, dim, weakly positive.

Table 2.5. Average Relative Frequency of Major Lymphoid Cell Subsets in Normal Tissues

Subset	Peripheral Blood[a] Children (%)		Peripheral Blood[a] Adults (%)	Bone marrow[b] (%)		Lymph Nodes[a] (%)	Tonsils[a] (%)	Spleen[a] (%)
	2-5 y	5-15 y		Children	Adults			
CD19+ B cells	24	17	12	10	3	41	51	55
CD3+ T cells	64	68	72	6	12	56	49	31
CD4+ CD3+ T-helper	37	38	44	3.2	6.5	48	42	17
CD4+CD8+ T-cytotoxic	24	26	24	2.6	4.2	10	6	14
Natural killer (all NK subsets)	10	13	13	2	4	1	<1	15

[a]Percentage of cells in the lymphocyte region (CD45 bright).
[b]Percentage of total bone marrow cells.

CD49d, CD49e, CD51, CD54, CD71, and FcεRI antigens. Other markers such as CD11b, CD13, CD18, CD22, CD35, CD40, and CD61 display a variable expression in normal individuals. BMMCs are negative for CD34, CD38, and CD138 antigens.[62]

DCs comprise two main subpopulations: conventional DCs (cDCs) and interferon-producing plasmacytoid (pDCs). Human cDCs are Lin⁻HLA-DR⁺ cells that express high levels of CD11c and consist of a blood DC antigen (BDCA)3⁺ (CD141⁺) and a CD141⁻/CD1c⁺ population.[63] Human Lin⁻HLA-DR⁺ pDCs are defined by the absence of CD11c expression and by high levels of CD123 (the IL-3Rα chain) and BDCA2.[64] The CD11c⁺HLA-DR⁺BDCA3⁻ population can be further subdivided into CD16⁺

Table 2.6. Immunophenotypic Changes Detected by Flow Cytometry During B-Cell Development in Normal Bone Marrow

	CLP	Early B	Pro-B	Pre-B I	Large Pre-B II	Small Pre-B II	Immature B	Mature B	Plasma Cells
CD34	+	+	+	−	−	−	−	−	−
CD10	+	+	+	+	+	+	+/dim	−	−
CD19	−	−	+	+	+	+	+	+	+
cyt.CD79a	−	+	+	+	+	+	+	+	+
cyt.CD22	−	+	+	+	+	+	+	+	+
TdT	−	−	+	−	−	−	−	−	−
mCD22	−	Dim	dim	+	+	+	+	+	−
CD20	−	−	+	+	+	+	+	+	−
sIgM	−	−	−	−	−	−	+	+	−
sIgD	−	−	−	−	−	−	−	+	−
sIg κ or λ	−	−	−	−	−	−	−	+	−
cyt.Ig κ or λ	−	−	−	−	−	−	−	+	+

Abbreviations: CLP, common lymphoid precursor; cyt. cytoplasmic; Ig, immunoglobulin; s, surface; TdT, terminal deoxynucleotidyl transferase.

and CD16⁻ populations. cDCs in lymphoid tissues arise from a distinct population of committed cDC precursors (pre-cDCs) that originate in BM and migrate via blood. Spleen cDCs arise from a distinct population of Lin⁻CD11c⁺ major histocompatibility complex (MHC) class II neg immediate pre-cDCs. Pre-cDCs originate from BM Lin⁻CD117^int FLT3⁺CD115⁺ common DC progenitors. The direct progenitor of pDCs is contained within the CD34 low compartment of cord blood, fetal liver, and BM. These progenitors (pro-pDCs) coexpress CD45RA, CD4, and high levels of CD123.[54]

NK cells are positive for CD2 and CD7 but negative for CD3 and CD5. In humans, there are two major subsets of NK cells: one expressing high levels of CD56 and low or no CD16 (CD56^bright CD16^+/−), and the other that is CD56⁺CD16^bright. CD56^bright CD16^+/− cells display relatively lower cytolytic activity and produce more cytokines than the CD56⁺CD16^bright cells and are considered as less mature precursors of CD56^dim cells.[65,66] A putative-committed NK-cell precursor population has been found within CD34^low CD45RA⁺α4β7^high CD7^+/− CD10⁻ BM population, and these cells give rise to CD56^high CD16⁻ NK cells in vitro. The immature NK cells developing from committed NK-cell precursors are defined by expression of CD161 (NKR-P1). These cells do not express CD56 or CD16. Immature NK cells can be induced to express these markers as well as the activating and inhibitory receptors, CD94 (NKG2A) and killer inhibitory receptors (KIR, CD158), upon culture with stromal cells and cytokines such as IL-15 or FLT3-L.[54] NK-cell development is accompanied by early expression of stimulatory coreceptor CD244, and NK-cell developmental intermediates have also been detected in LNs and tonsils.[67] A total of 30% to 60% of CD56^dim CD16^bright NK cells in healthy adults express CD57, which is not expressed on immature CD56^bright NK cells. CD57⁺ NK cells express a repertoire of NK-cell receptors, suggestive of a more mature phenotype, and proliferate less when stimulated with target cells and/or cytokines.[68]

MULTICOLOR ANALYSIS OF HEMATOLOGIC MALIGNANCIES

Detailed immunophenotypic information necessary for diagnosis and prognosis of various hematologic diseases, based on both FCM and immunohistochemistry, is provided in their respective chapters. The FCM findings important for diagnosis of most common entities are summarized in the subsequent section.

Immunophenotyping of B-Cell Lymphoproliferative Disorders

Normal/reactive B-cell populations in blood, BM, and lymphatic tissue are polyclonal, with an average Igκ-to-Igλ ratio of 1.5 (range 0.9-3) (*Figure 2.2*).[69,70] An increase in polyclonal B cells in blood, called persistent polyclonal B-cell lymphocytosis (PPBL), is characterized by a chronic, stable, persistent, and polyclonal increase in B cells (median 5×10^9/L), the presence of binucleated lymphocytes in the PB, and a polyclonal increase in serum IgM. Most patients are asymptomatic, but isochromosome 3q with a common minimally amplified genomic region in the *MECOM* gene has been described in some cases.[71] Development of malignant lymphoma and monoclonal gammopathy of undetermined significance has been reported in PPBL patients.

B-cell malignancies are clonal expansions of B cells that express only one type of Ig light chain (κ or λ). Analysis of light-chain expression in the total B-cell population and in CD5/CD19- or CD10/CD19-positive cells forms the basis for B-cell lymphoma diagnosis (*Figure 2.3A*). Typical immunophenotypes found in various mature B-cell lymphoma subtypes are summarized in *Table 2.6*. An issue that may cause diagnostic problems is the demonstration of small monoclonal B-cell populations in the BM samples taken during investigations for staging of diffuse large B-cell lymphoma (DLBCL). As FCM sensitivity increases, it becomes more likely that small abnormal populations are detected; how these relate to the neoplastic cells found in other organs is not clear. In some cases, a clonal relationship to the diagnostic lymphoma sample has been demonstrated.[72] However, if the histopathologic signs of lymphoma involvement are missing, these cells may represent the so-called monoclonal B-cell lymphocytosis (MBL; see "Monoclonal B-Cell Lymphocytosis"). Therefore, interpretation of FCM results in BM samples should be always integrated with clinical findings and BM biopsy analysis.

B-Cell Chronic Lymphocytic Leukemia

The characteristic immunophenotype of chronic lymphocytic leukemia (CLL) includes positivity for CD19, CD5, CD23, CD43, and CD200, often expression of IgM with or without IgD, weak expression of CD20, CD22, and Ig light chains, and negative or "dim" CD79b and CD81 (*Figure 2.3B*).[73] FMC7 (an antibody recognizing one of the CD20 epitopes) is negative or only partially expressed in most cases. CD11c, CD25, and other markers that recognize adhesion molecules are variably positive in CLL. Levels of marker expression have been

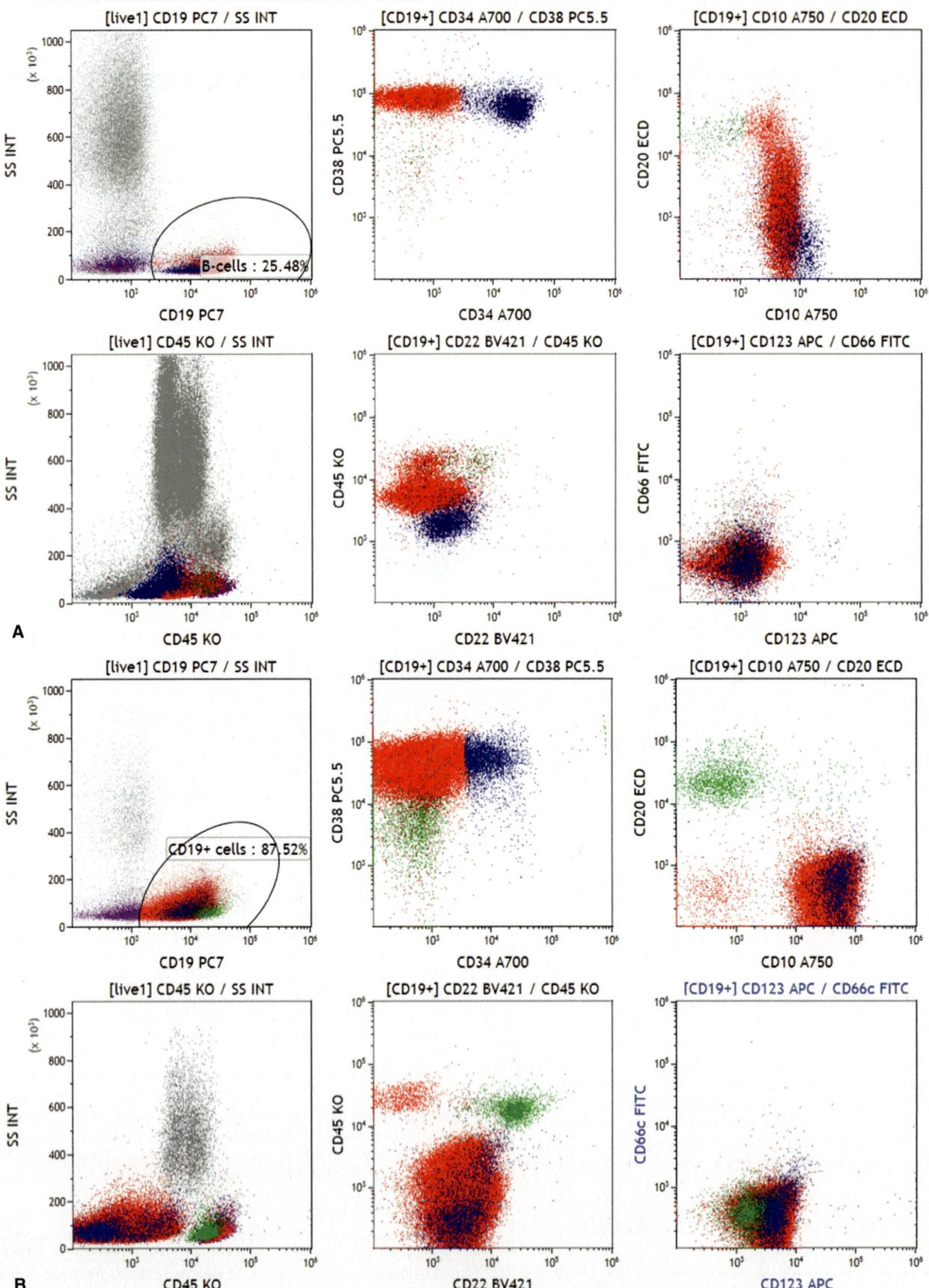

FIGURE 2.7 Example of antigen expression in a case of B-cell precursor lymphoblastic leukemia/lymphoma in comparison to normal bone marrow B cells in a child. Bone marrow samples were analyzed with B-ALL panel (*Table 2.3*). To acquire sufficient numbers of B cells, 500,000 events were analyzed on a normal bone marrow sample, and 50 000 cells were acquired on the B-ALL sample. CD19$^+$ B cells were gated on the CD19/SS plot. Normal antigen expression patterns are shown in (A), and corresponding plots for a B-ALL case are shown in (B). Leukemic cells show aberrant immunophenotype CD45$^{neg/dim}$CD20−CD10^{++}CD34$^-$. B-ALL, B-cell acute lymphoblastic leukemia; MAb, monoclonal antibody; SS, side scatter.

shown to associate with genetic/molecular changes: trisomy 12 cases showed increased CD38 expression, and higher CD38 was observed in IGHV-unmutated (U) vs IGHV-mutated (M) cases. CD20 expression intensity was increased in IGHV-U vs IGHV-M. Del13q cases demonstrated lower CD22 expression intensity. Cases without cytogenetic abnormality exhibited higher CD19 and CD22 expression. Del17p cases demonstrated lower CD25. High and very-high CLL-IPI risk groups were associated with high CD38 expression and low CD25.[74] Most CLL cases express the wingless-type family member 5a (Wnt5a) receptor ROR1 (tyrosine kinase-like orphan receptor). High levels of expression (ROR1[high]) have been associated with shorter treatment-free survival.[75] According to the World Health Organization (WHO) 2016 update, the level of abnormal B cells in blood has to reach 5×10^9/L for a CLL diagnosis to be established.[76]

Monoclonal B-Cell Lymphocytosis

Monoclonal B-cell lymphocytosis (MBL) is an asymptomatic hematologic condition defined by the presence of monoclonal B lymphocytes detected in the PB of persons who do not have CLL, other B-lymphoproliferative disorders, or underlying conditions such as infectious and/or autoimmune diseases. Initial criteria have been based on detection of a monoclonal B-cell population in the PB with an overall κ-to-λ ratio >3:1 or 0.3:1, or >25% of B cells lacking or expressing low-level surface Ig in conjunction with a specific phenotype.[77] Three different types of MBL have been described, defined on the basis of CD19 positivity, CD5 presence or absence, and CD20 intensity. The most common MBL type is the CLL-like MBL that coexpresses CD19 and CD5, and CD23 with dim expression of CD20. The second type is similar to CLL but shows bright CD20 expression. B cells in the third type of MBL do not express CD5; these are classified as CD5[−] MBL or non–CLL-like MBL.[78] The reported prevalence depends on the sensitivity of applied FCM methodology. Studies performed using four-color FCM with a sensitivity of detection commonly used for detection of MRD in patients with CLL (1 clonal cell per 1×10^5 events) showed a 5% prevalence of CLL-like MBL in adults aged over 60. Another study, using a much higher sensitivity of FCM, analyzed 5×10^6 PB cells per individual and identified CLL-like MBL in 12% of all tested subjects and in 20% of adults over 60 years.[79] The level of abnormal B cells at 0.5×10^9/L has been used as a cutoff for low-level and higher-level MBL.[77] Finding of peripheral MBL should always be correlated with clinical data and interpreted in the absence of peripheral lymphadenopathy, splenomegaly, and extensive lymphoid BM infiltrates.

Mantle Cell Lymphoma

Mantle cell lymphoma (MCL) typically expresses bright CD20, CD5, FMC7, and bright-to-moderate sIg but lacks CD23 and CD200 (*Table 2.7* and *Figure 2.3B*).[80] However, MCL cases positive for CD23 and

negative for FMC7 as well as rare CD5[−] cases have been found.[81] Therefore, confirmation of MCL diagnosis by FISH for t(11;14) is recommended. Cyclin D1 expression can also be detected by FCM,[82] but this method is not routinely applied in most diagnostic laboratories.

Lymphoplasmacytic Lymphoma and Marginal Zone Lymphoma

These two entities are difficult to differentiate by FCM. The typical immunophenotype findings include the strong expression of sIg and cyt.Ig (IgM in Waldenström macroglobulinemia [WM], IgG, or IgA in lymphoplasmacytic lymphoma [LPL]). The characteristic antigen expression pattern is sIgD[+/−] CD19[+]CD20[+]CD22[+]CD79a[+]FMC7[+]CD38[+]CD103[−]CD5[−]CD10[−]CD23[−]CD25[−]CD11c[+/−]CD43[+/−]CD27[+/−] (*Figure 2.3C*).[83] Detection of somatic mutations in *MYD88* and/or *CXCR4* may confirm a WM diagnosis.[84] A minority of splenic marginal zone lymphoma (SMZL) cases express CD5, which often correlates with higher WBC. However, leukemic presentation of MCL should be excluded. Some SMZL cases are CD23 positive. In LPL, a monotypic plasma cell (PC) population that is strongly CD38/CD138 positive and positive for CD19 and CD45 can often be found.[85] Splenic diffuse red pulp small B-cell lymphoma cells in blood and BM are characterized by a similar phenotype, as given earlier, but are usually CD11c positive.[86]

Hairy Cell Leukemia and Hairy Cell Leukemia Variant

Both hairy cell leukemia (HCL) and hairy cell leukemia variant (HCLv) strongly express CD103, CD11c, CD20, CD22, and CD19 and are negative for CD5, CD23, and, in most cases, CD38 (*Figure 2.3C*). HCL cells are often large (can be found in the monocyte region) and are positive for CD25 and CD123 in contrast to HCLv cells that are smaller and CD25 negative.[87]

Follicular Lymphoma

The follicular lymphoma (FL) cells usually express sIg, more frequently IgM[+]/IgD[+/−] than IgG or rarely IgA, together with B-cell-associated antigens (CD19, CD20, CD22, CD79a, and CD79b), and, in most cases, CD10 (*Figure 2.3A*). Expression of CD19 and CD22 is often weaker than in normal B cells.[88] FL cells are usually CD5[−], CD43[−], and CD23[−/+], CD11c[−/+]. The weaker expression of CD38 helps to differentiate between FL cells and CD10-positive B-cell precursors.[89] Cytoplasmic BCL2 detection in CD10[+] cells can be useful to detect FL cells in cases with partial involvement.[70]

Burkitt Lymphoma

Burkitt lymphoma (BL) cells often display a similar phenotype to FL cells (CD19[+], CD20[+], and CD10[+]) but have a bright CD38 expression. The CD23[−]/FMC7[+] immunophenotype has been reported as

Table 2.7. Flow Cytometry Immunophenotypic Features of Major B-Lineage Lymphoproliferative Disorders

WHO 2016 Category	CD19	CD20	CD22	CD23	CD10	CD5	CD11c	CD103	CD25	CD123	sIg
CLL	+#	+d/−	d/−	+	−	+	±	−	±	−	d
HCL	+	+b	+	−	−/(+)	−	+	+	+	+	b
HCLv	+	+	+	−	−/(+)	−	±	+/(−)	−	−(+)	b
SMZL	+	+−	+	−	−	−	+	−/(+)	±	−	+
MCL	+	+b	+	−/(+d)	−	+	−	−	−	−	b
FL	+	+	+	±	+	−	−	−	−	−	+
DLBCL	+	+/(−)	+	±	±	±	±	−/(+)	−	−	±
BL	+	+	+	−	+	−	−	−	−	−	+/(−)

Abbreviations: BL, Burkitt lymphoma; CLL, chronic lymphocytic leukemia; DLBCL, diffuse large B-cell lymphoma; FL, follicular lymphoma; HCL, hairy cell leukemia; HCLv, HCL variant; MCL, mantle cell lymphoma; SMZL/SLVL, splenic marginal zone lymphoma, splenic lymphoma with villous lymphocytes; WHO, World Health Organization; +#, most cases positive; −, most cases negative; ±, can be positive or negative; +/(−), usually positive, rarely negative; −/(+), usually negative, rarely positive; b, bright; d, dim.

significantly associated with *MYC* rearrangement.[90] BL cells usually lack CD44 and CD54, which are often expressed in CD10-positive DLBCLs.[91] Moreover, BL usually shows negative or dim CD39 and CD95, whereas CD43 and CD81 are brightly expressed.[92] A combination of CD38% > 90, CD10% > 80, CD10 MFI > 10 with high KI67 and low BCL2 expression has been found particularly useful in differentiating BL from other high-grade lymphomas.[93]

High-Grade Lymphomas

High-grade lymphomas with two or three translocations, including *MYC* (e.g., t[8;14]) and *BCL2* (t[14;18]) or *BCL6* (involving chromosome 3q27), the so-called double-hit or triple-hit lymphomas, which can present in the leukemic phase, have been shown to display a common phenotype including a marked decrease in expression of CD20 ranging from dim to absent as compared to normal follicle center B cells. Other common features of this immunophenotype include positivity for CD10, variably decreased expression of CD45; and variably increased expression of CD38. In addition, Ig light-chain restriction with decreased intensity or complete absence of light-chain expression was noted in these cases.[93-95] The latter cases have to be tested for nuclear TdT expression, and, when present, the differential diagnosis of B-ALL should be considered. However, some double-hit lymphoma cases with TdT expression have been described.[96]

Diffuse Large B-Cell Lymphoma

Diffuse large B-cell lymphoma (DLBCL) is a heterogeneous group of lymphomas with variable immunophenotype. Pathologic findings in DLBCL may include high-scatter, low/negative expression of sIg, CD20, and CD45 (*Table 2.7*). FCM may be of use in differentiating between two major subgroups of DLBCL (germinal center type, usually CD10[+], and activated B-cell type, usually CD10[-]).[97] CD5-positive DLBCL cases have been reported and may have a worse prognosis.[98] It has been suggested that FCM may improve the prognostic value of BM staging procedures.[99] However, small populations of pathologic large cells that are easily seen in BM biopsies may, in some cases, be difficult to delineate by FCM against a background of reactive BM cells. In staging of DLBCL, it is important to analyze high numbers of BM cells to be able to evaluate B-cell light-chain sIg expression, even in cases where B cells represent only a minor portion of the BM cell population.

Immunophenotyping of T-Cell Lymphoproliferative Disorders

FCM detection of aberrant T-cell populations requires good understanding of T-cell biology and knowledge of normal T-cell subsets. Reactive conditions may cause a predominance of some T-cell subpopulations, which can be interpreted as immunophenotypic "aberrancy." Also, reactive T-cell populations, particularly in the setting of chronic stimulation, may comprise a limited number of clonotypes (i.e., are oligoclonal) and therefore are prone to producing clonal TCR (T-cell receptor) rearrangement results. A single antibody (anti-TRBC1; JOVI-1 antibody clone) against one of the two mutually exclusive T-cell receptor β-chain constant domains was identified as a useful marker to assess Tαβ-cell clonality (*Figure 2.4*). In 96% of samples containing clonal Tαβ-cells in which the approach was validated, monotypic expression of TRBC1 was confirmed.[100]

A characteristic dynamic of CD8[+] immune response, including CD8[+] lymphocytosis with an increase in CD38 and HLA-DR expression in the acute phase and expansion of CD57[+]CD8[+] subset in the chronic phase, was described in viral infections, such as that of Epstein-Barr virus and human immunodeficiency virus (HIV).[101] Chronic activation of the immune system may lead to an increase in CD8[+]CD57[+] T cells.[102] Application of TRBC1 antibody is of help to determine whether molecular clonality studies should be performed.

An integrated approach combining morphology, immunophenotyping, and molecular analysis is necessary to differentiate between reactive and malignant T-cell lymphoproliferations. Immunophenotypic findings in the most common T-cell lymphoproliferative disorders are summarized in *Table 2.8*.[25]

T-Cell Prolymphocytic Leukemia

Leukemic cells are usually positive for CD7, CD2, CD5, and CD3, although about 20% do not express membrane CD3 but are cyt. CD3 positive. CD7- and/or CD45-negative cases have been reported. T-cell prolymphocytic leukemia (T-PLL) cells are usually CD4 positive and CD8 negative (60%), but in a fraction of cases, T-PLL cells may express both CD4 and CD8 or are CD4 negative and CD8 positive or negative for both CD4 and CD8. CD25 and NK-cell markers (CD56, CD57, and CD16) as well as T-cell-precursor–related markers CD1a and TdT are negative. T-PLL cells are usually CD52[bright] (*Figure 2.4*).[103,104]

Adult T-Cell Leukemia/Lymphoma

In most patients, adult T-cell leukemia/lymphoma (ATLL) cells express CD2, CD4, CD5, CD25, CD45RO, CD29, T-cell receptor αβ, CCR4, and HLA-DR (the phenotype of activated CD4[+] memory T cells). The frequency of CD4[+]CCR4[+]CD26[-] correlated with HTLV-1 virus load in infected subjects. ATLL cells usually lack CD7 and CD26, and exhibit lower CD3 expression than normal T cells. Expression of CCR7 and CD127 indicated a more aggressive ATLL, whereas in patients with the more indolent form, leukemic cells were CCD7[-] and CD127[-].[105]

Sézary Syndrome

The typical immunophenotype of Sézary syndrome cells in blood includes positivity for CD2, CD3, CD4, and CD5. CD7 is expressed in only 50% of patients. Loss of CD3, CD2, and unusually bright CD5 expression has been reported. CD8, CD25, and CD26 are usually negative. Sézary cells have an immunophenotype characteristic for T-central memory cells (CD4[+]CD27[+]CD26[-]CD45RA[-]). By comparison, CD4[+] cells in patients with inflammatory erythroderma are CD27 negative.

According to the international guidelines, a flow-cytometric assay for SS and MF should include the following six antibodies: CD3, CD4, CD7, CD8, CD26, and CD45. Gating strategies to identify abnormal T cells should be based on the identification of subsets with distinctly homogeneous immunophenotypic properties that are different from those expected for normal T cells. The blood concentration of abnormal cells, based on any immunophenotypic abnormalities indicative of MF or SS, should be calculated by either direct enumeration or a dual-platform method, and reported.[106]

Angioimmunoblastic T-Cell Lymphoma

A predominant T-cell population is usually positive for CD2, CD4, CD5, CD7, and CD45 but negative for CD8, CD19, CD20, CD30, CD38, and CD56. Lack of one or more of the "pan-T" cell markers in a subset of T cells may be found. Aberrant expression of CD10 in at least a fraction of CD4[+] T-cell population is a characteristic feature.[107]

T-Cell Large Granular Lymphocyte Leukemia

Most cases of T-cell large granular lymphocyte (T-LGL) leukemia are characterized by an expansion of CD3[+]CD8[+] TCRαβ T cells. Rarely, CD3[+]CD4[+]CD8[+] TCRαβ or CD4[-]CD8[-] TCRγδ T cells may be found. It has been shown that leukemic T-LGLs have CD3[+]CD8[+]CD45RA[+]CD62L[-] immunophenotype consistent with effector/memory CD45RA T cells. Leukemic T-LGLs often express CD57. Loss of CD5 and/or CD7 may occur. Correlation of the flow-cytometric and molecular genetic results with the other clinical and laboratory findings is critical before the final diagnosis of T-LGL leukemia is established. The level of aberrant T-cell population ≥2 × 10⁹/L is the suggested level for diagnosis of T-LGL leukemia. However, in appropriate clinical settings, lower counts (>0.4 × 10⁹/L) may be compatible with the diagnosis.[108]

Chronic NK-Cell Proliferations

Chronic NK-cell proliferations are characterized by CD3[-]CD56[+] and/or CD16[+] cells. Further information can be obtained by investigation of expression pattern of killer cell Ig-like receptors (KIRa, CD158)

Table 2.8. Flow Cytometry Immunophenotypic Findings in Major Categories of Mature T/NK-Cell Non-Hodgkin Leukemia/Lymphoma

WHO Category[a]	mCD3	Cyt CD3	CD4	CD8	CD2	CD5	CD7	CD10	HLA-DR	CD25	CD56	CD57	CD16
T-PLL	+/−	+	+/−	− (+)	+	+	+ (−)	−	− (+)	−	−	−	−
ATLL	+	+	+	−	+	+	−/d	−	+	+	−	−	−
SS	+/d	+	+	−	+ (−)	+	− (+)	−	+/−	− (+)	−	−	−
AITL	+/−	+	+	−	+/d	+/d	+/d	+	+/−	−	−	−	−
ALC	+/−	+/−	+/−	− (+)	+/−	−	−	−	+/−	−	+	+	−
LGL	+	+ (−)	−	+	+	−/+	−/+	−	+	−	− (+)	+	+/−
ANKL	−	−	−	−/+	+	−	−	−	−/+	−	+b	−/−	+
HSTCL	+/−	+	−	−/d/+	+	− (+)	+ (−)	−	+	−	−/+	− (+)	−/+
PTCL	+/−	−	+/−	+/−	+	−/+	+/−	−	+/−	− (+)	− (+)	−	−

[a]*Diagnostic* categories of WHO 2016 classification.
Abbreviations: (+) or (−) some cases positive or negative; AITL, angioimmunoblastic T-cell lymphoma; ALC, anaplastic large-cell lymphoma; ANKL, aggressive natural killer-cell leukemia; ATLL, adult T-cell leukemia/lymphoma; b (bright) strong positive staining; d (dim), weak positive staining; HSTCL, hepatosplenic T-cell lymphoma; LGL; large granular lymphocyte leukemia; PTCL, peripheral T-cell lymphoma; SS, Sézary syndrome; T-PLL, T-cell prolymphocytic leukemia.

on these cells. These receptors are encoded by at least two distinct families of genes and gene products, which are members of the Ig gene superfamily. In NK-LGL, approximately one-third of cases exhibit restricted expression of a single (or multiple) KIR isoform. The remaining NK-LGL cases lack detectable expression of the three ubiquitously expressed KIRs, CD158a, CD158b, and CD158e. The uniform absence of these KIRs on NK cells is aberrant because in normal NK-cell populations, there are subsets positive for each. In contrast to normal NK cells that show variable staining intensity, NK lymphoproliferations also often show uniform bright expression of CD94 exclusively paired with NKG2A to form an inhibitory receptor complex. Abnormal loss of CD161 expression is also frequent in NK-LGL.[109]

Aggressive NK-Cell Leukemia

The typical immunophenotype in aggressive NK-cell leukemia is CD2[+], CD16[+], and CD56[+], with loss of CD7 in some cases and variable expression of CD8 and CD57. Blasts are negative for membrane CD3, myeloid markers, and CD123.[110]

Hepatosplenic T-Cell Lymphoma

The most common immunophenotype is CD2[+], CD3[+], CD4[−], CD5[−], CD7[+], CD8[−], γδ TCR[+], but CD8-positive cases do occur. Decreased expression of CD3 and/or CD7 has also been reported. Usually, some NK-cell markers (CD56 and/or CD16) are present. The normal T-cell counterpart for hepatosplenic T-cell lymphoma is thought to be a functionally immature cytotoxic γδ T cell of the splenic pool with *Vδ1* gene usage. A "variant form" showing αβ TCR[+] and similar clinical features has been described.[111,112]

Immunophenotyping of Plasma Cell Myeloma

Consensus guidelines on FCM in multiple myeloma (MM) and other clonal PC-related disorders recommend simultaneous assessment of the expression of CD38 and CD138 with acquisition of at least 100 000 "events" at diagnosis and to ensure that at least 3000 "events" with broad gated CD38[bright]/CD138+ characteristics and at least 100 PCs are analyzed. Clonality of PCs should be evaluated by analysis of cytoplasmic Ig expression.

The most common aberrant features of PCs in myeloma in comparison to normal PCs are as follows:

- Decreased or absent expression of CD19, CD27, CD38, CD81, and CD45
- Overexpression of CD28, CD33, and CD56
- Asynchronous expression of CD20, CD117, and sIg[113]

Because almost all MM cases show aberrant immunophenotypic features, FCM has been used in several studies to assess MRD in MM, and if enough cells are acquired, it may reach a sensitivity of 10^{-5}.[25,114,115]

Immunophenotyping of Acute Leukemia

The use of CD45/SS gating is widely used for the identification of pathologic cells in acute leukemia because blasts usually appear in a position of progenitor cells on the SS/CD45 dot plots of normal BM (*Figures 2.2* and *2.5*).[116] However, leukemic cell populations may be found in the granulocyte gate in acute promyelocytic leukemia or monocyte gate in acute myeloid leukemia (AML) with monocytic differentiation. In rare cases, CD45 is not suitable for gating purposes because of the marked heterogeneity of the leukemic population or the limited number of blasts present in the hemodiluted sample. In such cases, other markers such as CD34, CD117, CD13, or CD33 may be of help. A good correlation between frequencies of blasts determined by FCM and by morphology has been reported. Lower blast counts by FCM in comparison to percentages of cells with blast morphology in BM smears may be because of enrichment of blasts in BM fragments (spicules). A possible bias can also be introduced by hematopathologists who choose "representative" areas of the smear for blast counting or by a relative hemodilution of samples submitted for FCM analysis.[48] Immunophenotyping provides information needed for lineage assignment, analysis of the degree of heterogeneity of the abnormal cell population either because of the existence of different pathologic clones or because of the presence of cells in different stages of maturation, and further characterization of aberrant phenotypes for MRD follow-up.

Lineage Assignment and Mixed Phenotype Acute Leukemias

FCM is essential for diagnosis of mixed phenotype acute leukemias (MPALs) that belong within the acute leukemia of ambiguous origin category and are characterized by coexpression of the markers of different lineages.[117] In cases of biclonal/bilineal proliferations, two different blast populations can be detected. In other cases, transitional patterns with only part of the blast population being biphenotypic together with two separate populations can be seen and rarely one population of biphenotypic blasts is present. For the myeloid lineage, cytoplasmic myeloperoxidase (MPO) detected by cytochemistry or immunohistochemistry or by FCM with an anti-MPO antibody is considered as the most significant marker. FCM allows for the detection of MPO even in some cases of minimally differentiated AML that are negative by cytochemistry. MPO positivity per se is not required for myeloid lineage assignment in leukemias that are not MPAL that lack B- and T-lineage associated markers.[117] Also, a population that would otherwise fulfill immunophenotypic criteria for MPO-negative AML can be accepted as a myeloid part of MPAL. Moreover, cases of otherwise clear-cut B-ALL with weak MPO expression have been described.[118] To establish differentiation toward monocytic lineage, which may lack MPO, the presence of nonspecific esterase by cytochemistry or the detection of surface CD14, CD11c, CD36, CD64, or intracytoplasmic lysozyme can be used. B-lineage assignment is based on CD19 expression. If the CD19 labeling is bright, the presence of another B-lymphocyte marker is considered enough to establish B lineage. If CD19 expression is of low intensity, the presence of two other B-lineage-associated markers will be necessary. Cytoplasmic CD79a, cytoplasmic CD22, cytoplasmic CD24, cytoplasmic CD10, intracytoplasmic μ chains, or (less frequently expressed in MPAL) CD20 or CD21 can be applied. The strongest marker indicating T lineage is the strong cytoplasmic expression of CD3. The presence of other T-cell-associated markers, such as CD2, CD5, or CD7, can add to the diagnosis of MPAL, although some of these markers can be seen on myeloid cells in AML and MDS.[25]

Acute Myeloid Leukemia

The utility of individual myeloid-associated markers for AML diagnosis is limited because of aberrant expression of these markers in many cases of ALL. Immunologic diagnosis of AML is established by expression of at least two myeloid-associated markers in the absence of criteria for diagnosis of B-ALL, T-cell acute lymphoblastic leukemia/lymphoma (T-ALL), and MPAL.[119] Immunophenotyping by FCM is especially useful in the differential diagnosis between ALL and minimally differentiated AML[120] and in the diagnosis of leukemic presentation of pDC neoplasms that are characterized by coexpression of bright CD123, bright HLA-DR, CD4, CD56, CD36, and the absence of other lineage-associated markers (MPO⁻, cytoplasmic CD3⁻, and CD19⁻).[121]

Characteristic antigen expression patterns have been associated with AML with recurrent chromosomal abnormalities (*Table 2.9*).[122] These patterns may help in planning directed FISH or molecular studies in cases with limited material.

Several attempts at immunologic classification of AML, though showing limited clinical utility, have been published. Most prognostic implications may be because of immunophenotypes reflecting

Table 2.9. Immunophenotypic Patterns Associated With Recurrent Specific Cytogenetic Abnormalities in Leukemia

	Cytogenetic Abnormality	Characteristic Flow Cytometry Findings
AML	t(8;21)(q22;q22.1), *RUNX1-RUNX1T1*	At least a fraction of blasts with CD34^{bright}, often coexpressing CD19 and TdT but not CD10 Granulocytic differentiation (CD13, CD33, MPO, and CD15), aberrant expression of CD56 common No monocytic differentiation
AML	inv(16)(p13.1q22) or t(16;16)(p13.1;q22) *CBF-MYH11*	Distinct populations of blasts, granulocytic, and monocytic (CD14, CD4, CD64) precursors Coexpression of CD34 and CD64 common Eosinophils can be delineated by high SS and low FS than neutrophils and CD16 negative Often CD2 on blasts and precursors
AML	t(9;11)(p21.3;q23.3) *KMT2A-MLLT3*	MAb 7.1 positivity Monocytic differentiation (HLA-DR, CD4^{dim}, CD11b, CD13, CD15, CD36, CD33, and CD64)
AML	*NPM1* mutated	Most often blasts CD34⁻, often HLA-DR⁻, CD117⁺, CD123⁺, CD33^{bright}, CD110⁺ Show granulocytic differentiation (CD15⁺) Monocytic differentiation in 30% of cases Some cases only CD33^{bright} and MPO^{bright} with no differentiation
AML	inv(3)(q21.3;q26.2) or t(3;3)(q21.3;q26.2) *GATA2, MECOM*	Positive for CD34, CD117, CD13, CD33, HLA-DR, and MPO
AML	t(6;9)(p23;q34.1) *DEK-NUP214*	CD9⁺, CD13⁺, CD33⁺, CD117⁺, and HLA-DR⁺ May be CD34⁻ at presentation but CD34⁺ at relapse Basophils are often increased (CD123⁺⁺, HLA-DR⁻)
AMkL	t(1;22)(p13.3;q13.1) *RBM15-MKL1*	Megakaryocytic differentiation CD41⁺, CD61⁺ often together with CD34, HLA-DR
APL	t(15;17)(q24.1;q21.2) *PML-RARA*	Hypergranular: most cases CD34⁻, HLA-DR⁻, CD11b⁻, CD11c⁻, CD117⁺, MPO⁺, CD33^{bright}, CD13 heterogeneous, CD15$^{-/dim}$ Hypogranular: often CD2⁺, subsets positive for CD34 and/or HLA-DR present
ALL (B)	t(4;11)(q21.3-q22.1;q23.3) *AFF1-KMT2A*	CD34⁺, CD19⁺, CD10⁻, CD20⁻, CD13, and/or CD33 may be positive, often CD15 and/or CD65⁺, 7.1⁺, cyt.IgM⁻
ALL (B)	t(9;22)(q34.1;q11.2) *BCR-ABL1*	CD34⁺⁺, CD19⁺, CD10⁺, CD20$^{-/+}$, CD25⁺, CD13, CD33, CD66c often positive, CD15⁻, CD65⁻, 7.1⁻, cyt.IgM⁻
ALL (B)	IGH-*CLRF* fusion	CLRF overexpression
ALL (B)	t(12;21)(p13.2;q22.1) *ETV6-RUNX1*	CD34$^{+/-}$, CD19⁺, CD10⁺, CD20$^{-/+}$, CD13, and/or CD33 often positive, CD66c⁻, CD15⁻, CD65⁻, 7.1⁻, cyt.IgM⁻
ALL (B)	Hyperdiploid	CD34⁺ or subset, CD19⁺, CD10⁺⁺⁺, CD123⁺⁺, CD20$^{-/+}$, CD13⁻, CD33⁻, CD66c$^{-/+}$, CD15⁻, CD65⁻, 7.1⁻, cyt.IgM⁻
ALL (B)	t(1;19)(q23;p13.3) *TCF3-PBX1*	CD34⁻ or subset, CD19⁺, CD10⁻ or subset, CD20⁺, CD13⁻, CD33⁻ CD66c$^{-/+}$, CD15⁻, CD65⁻, 7.1⁻, cyt.IgM⁺
ALL (T)	*FLT3* activating mutation	Expression of CD117 and CD135

Abbreviations: AML, acute myeloid leukemia; ALL, acute lymphoblastic leukemia; APL, acute promyelocytic leukemia; cyt., cytoplasmic; FS, forward scatter; HLA-DR, human leukocyte antigen-D related; Ig, immunoglobulin; MPO, myeloperoxidase; SS, side scatter.

underlying genetic aberrancies. However, owing to the genetic complexity of AML, clear-cut correlations are difficult to establish.[123]

In general, immunophenotypic patterns of AML (*Figure 2.5*) can be described as less differentiated (purely blastic) or as showing signs of maturation toward one or several lineages. Consequently, AML can show a single or two or more populations of malignant cells. AML showing maturation toward granulocytic lineage usually displays (at least on a fraction of cells) markers associated with myeloid immaturity (CD34 and CD117) combined with variable expression of other myeloid lineage (CD13 and/or CD33) and at least some positivity for markers associated with granulocytic maturation, such as CD15 and/or CD65. AMLs with myelomonocytic differentiation also display a population of cells demonstrating expression of CD14; coexpression of CD36 and CD64; or bright expression of CD33, CD4, CD11b, and/or CD11c. By contrast, acute monoblastic and monocytic leukemias usually show a single population of aberrant cells with evidence of monocytic differentiation (bright CD36, CD64, CD14, and/or CD4), which are usually CD34 and/or CD117 positive. Positivity for megakaryocytic (CD41a, CD42b, and CD61) or erythroid lineage involvement (glycophorin A, CD36, CD71[++]) must be interpreted cautiously because the possible adherence of platelets or red cell membrane fragments to the blast cells may lead to unspecific positivity and misclassification. Correlation with morphologic and immunohistochemical findings is necessary. The rare cases of acute basophilic leukemia reported have shown expression of common myeloid antigens such as CD13 and CD33, as well as CD9, CD11b, CD22, and CD123.[25,124]

Using FCM, aberrant phenotypes (also called leukemia-associated immunophenotype) can be detected in >90% of patients with AML. For correct interpretation of follow-up samples and detection of MRD, the immunophenotypic pattern of the diagnostic sample and a thorough knowledge of the immunophenotype of various cell populations in normal and regenerating BM are necessary. New 8- to 10-color approaches rely on common comprehensive panels applied at both diagnosis and follow-up, allowing detection of aberrant cells in most patients using a sequential gating strategy.[25,125-127]

Acute Lymphoblastic Leukemia

Leukemic cells in ALL clearly disclose their belonging to a B-cell or T-cell lineage. As in AML, specific immunophenotypes in ALL have been associated with major groups of chromosomal aberrations[122] (*Table 2.9*).

B-ALL is characterized by expression of CD19, HLA-DR, and TdT together with several B-cell markers such as membrane and/or cytoplasmic CD22 and cytoplasmic CD79a. In many cases, CD45 is negative. Five immunologic subtypes, roughly corresponding to sequential stages of B-cell differentiation, have been recognized. However, the existence of CD10-negative normal early B-cell progenitors is controversial. B-ALL can be immunologically classified into[119] the following:

- B I/pro-B/early B: CD10[−], CD20[−], cytoplasmic IgM[−], sIg[−]
- B II/common/early B: CD10[+], CD20[+/−], cytoplasmic IgM[−], sIg[−]
- B III/pre-B: CD10[+], CD20[+/−], cytoplasmic IgM[+], sIg[−]
- B IV/mature B: Tdt[+/−], CD10[+/−], CD20[+], cytoplasmic IgM[−], sIg[+] (κ or λ)

T-cell lineage in *T-ALL* is established by expression of cytoplasmic CD3, cytoplasmicTdT, and cytoplasmic CD7, which are found in most cases.[39] Other T-cell-associated markers are variably expressed. In some cases, weak expression of cytoplasmic CD79a has been reported.[128] The European Group for the Immunologic Classification of Leukemia proposed the following classification[119]:

- Pro-T (or T-I) positive for only CD7
- Pre-T (or T-II) positive for CD2 and/or CD5 and/or CD8
- Cortical T (or T-III) positive for CD1a (irrespective of other markers)
- Mature T (T-IV) positive for surface CD3 and negative for CD1a (irrespective of other markers)

An early T-cell precursor (ETP) subtype, characterized by an aggressive clinical course and carrying an immunophenotype associated with ETPs, has been identified. ETPs are a subset of thymocytes that recently migrated from the BM to the thymus; they retain multilineage differentiation potential, suggesting their direct derivation from hematopoietic stem cells. The immunophenotype of the ETP subtype of T-ALL includes a lack of CD1a and CD8, very weak or negative CD5, and expression of one or more early precursor or myeloid-associated markers, such as CD117, CD34, HLA-DR, CD13, CD33, CD11b, and/or CD65.[129]

In >95% of both B-ALL and T-ALL cases, leukemic blasts display aberrant immunophenotypes, allowing us to distinguish them from normal B-cell precursors (*Figure 2.7*) and normal BM T cells.[38,39] MRD detection by FCM is well established and already included in some clinical trials.[130] Characteristic immunophenotypes must be identified at diagnosis for each patient by comparing the cell marker profile of leukemic blasts to that of normal and regenerating BM samples. Transient changes in immunophenotypes of residual leukemic cells have been reported, but some aberrant features are usually retained.[131] Sensitivity of MRD detection at 0.01% can be achieved, provided that sufficient numbers of cells are analyzed (1×10^6) in each antibody combination.

Myelodysplastic Syndromes and Chronic Myelomonocytic Leukemia

Several groups described various aberrant immunophenotypic features in the BM of patients with MDS, and FCM has been recommended by European LeukemiaNet as one of the ancillary diagnostic procedures.[132] The WHO 2016 update acknowledged that FCM may provide useful information when integrated with morphology and cytogenetics.[133] Standardization efforts concerning FCM diagnostics in MDS resulted in several publications by the International/European LeukemiaNet Working Group for Flow Cytometry.[134-137] For screening purposes, a four-parameter score (the so-called Ogata score) can be applied. The score includes evaluation of the CD34[+] myeloid blast fraction (normal <2% BM cells), the fraction of B-cell precursors within the CD34[+] cell population (normal > 5%), the SS ratio between granulocytes and lymphocytes (normal > 6) and the CD45 expression ratio between lymphocytes and CD34[+] cells (normal between 4 and 7.5), and values >2 have been significantly associated with MDS and MDS/MPN.[30,138]

A detailed knowledge of normal immunophenotypes of BM cells is necessary for full evaluation of aberrant features suggestive of MDS.[134] Findings in chronic myelomonocytic leukemia (CMML) are similar to those described in MDS, with the high numbers of monocytes and monocytic precursors being the main difference. Some of most important immunophenotypic characteristics of dysplasia are summarized in the subsequent section.

Progenitor Cells

Both lymphoid and myeloid progenitor cells are found in the CD45[dim]/SS[low] region (*Figure 2.2*). A large study by Kern et al found a good correlation between numbers of blasts counted by morphology and FCM in MDS patients.[139] Several reports consider 2% CD34[+] myeloid blasts as a limit for a significantly increased blast number in the BM.[140] Regardless of the numbers, aberrant phenotypes of blasts give very important diagnostic and prognostic information and may even be used in evaluation of response to therapy. The most common aberrancies are abnormal expression of CD45, CD33, CD38, CD117, and HLA-DR and overexpression of CD5, CD7, CD11b, CD15, and CD56.[134,141,142]

Maturing Myeloid Compartment

The most consistently reported aberration of the maturing myeloid cell compartment is the lower SS that is due to lower-than-normal granularity seen also by morphology in BM smears. The aberrant maturation patterns detected using CD13 and CD16 and/or CD13 and CD11b MAb combinations; altered expression of CD45, CD33; asynchronous expression of CD34; and expression of lineage infidelity markers such as CD2, CD7, and CD56 are the frequently reported changes.[140,141] However, it has to be pointed out that various aberrant features observed in MDS patients can occasionally be found in patients with nonclonal cytopenias. Some authors suggest that aberrant FCM findings in the immature precursor population are more specific for MDS than those in maturing granulopoietic cells.[143]

Monocytes

The numbers of monocytes in BM and PB of MDS patients are usually not increased, but this population may show aberrant features in approximately 25% of MDS patients.[139] The finding of two or more aberrant features is very rare in reactive monocytes.[144] Aberrant features described in MDS are similar to those found in CMML. Increased expression of CD56 is most frequently reported. However, this feature is not specific for MDS and could be found in patients with infections and after growth factor treatment. Findings that were only rarely found in monocytes from patients with reactive monocytosis are decreased expression of CD13, CD11b, CD43, and/or HLA-DR and aberrant expression of CD2. Moreover, CMML patients show a characteristic increase (>94%) in the CD14+/CD16− classic monocyte fraction in blood, whereas intermediate CD14+/CD16+ and nonclassic CD14−/CD16+ fractions are relatively decreased.[145]

Erythropoietic Cells

The erythropoietic fraction is often increased in MDS patients. Evaluation of the erythropoietic fraction is more reliable on nonlysed BM.[22] Aberrant expression of CD71 and CD36 markers is the most common aberrant finding.[51,146] However, FCM signs of erythropoietic dysplasia may also be seen in some patients with hemolytic anemia and aplastic anemia.[42]

Lymphoid Cells

B-cell lymphoid progenitors (CD19+/CD10+/CD34+/−) are usually markedly diminished or absent in MDS BMs.[138] Analysis of the mature B-cell compartment should be carried out to exclude underlying B-cell lymphoma.[30]

Myeloproliferative Neoplasms

In CML, reported abnormalities include aberrant expression of CD56 on precursors and differentiating myeloid cells,[147] decreased CD16 on granulocytes,[148] and decreased L-selectin (CD62L) and P-selectin (CD62P) expression on CD34+ cells.[149] Aberrant expression of lymphoid antigens, such as CD2, CD5, and CD7, may be seen on the myeloid blasts in CML blast crisis. An increasing population with a B-lymphoid precursor phenotype may indicate the possibility of lymphoblastic transformation.

In non-CML myeloproliferative neoplasm (MPN), the most common changes were aberrant findings in the CD34+ cell compartment or aberrant expression of CD13, CD33, HLA-DR, and/or CD16 on maturing granulopoietic precursors. BM eosinophils, identified by expression of relatively bright CD11b, CD13, CD15, and CD45, without CD16, are expanded markedly in the patients with putative chronic eosinophilic leukemia. A higher rate of basophils with an abnormal immunophenotype was also detected in different MPNs. Increased CD56 expression and small size of granulocytes as measured by FS were described in primary myelofibrosis.[41,150] Increase in cells in the blast gate and emerging aberrant phenotypes in the blast population herald transformation to AML.

OTHER APPLICATIONS OF FLOW CYTOMETRY IN HEMATOLOGY

Paroxysmal Nocturnal Hemoglobinuria

FCM is a standard method for diagnosis of PNH. In PNH, the somatic mutation of the X-linked phosphatidylinositol glycan complementation class A (*PIGA*) gene causes a partial or absolute inability to make glycosylphosphatidylinositol (GPI)-anchored proteins. Antigens such as CD55, CD58, CD59, CD14, CD16, and CD24 are affected. The channel-forming toxin aerolysin and the preform pro-aerolysin bind selectively and with high affinity to GPI anchor. An inactive aerolysin variant conjugated with Alexa Fluor 488 (FLAER-A) is now widely used to detect GPI-anchored protein deficient (*Figure 2.8*).[151] Current guidelines include a combination of CD235a-FITC and CD59-PE for detection of GPI-deficient RBC, FLAER-A/CD24-PE/CD15-PECy5/CD45-PECy7 for detection of GPI-deficient granulocytes, and FLAER-A/CD14-PE/CD64-PECy5/CD45-PECy7 for GPI-deficient monocytes[152] (*Figure 2.8*). High-resolution assays allow detection of GPI-deficient RBC at the sensitivity level 10^{-5} and GPI-deficient WBC at 10^{-4}, which has also been noted in patients with aplastic anemia and MDS.[153]

Red Blood Cell Analysis

Clinical application of FCM to study erythropoiesis and nonclonal RBC disorders has been reviewed in Chesney et al.[154] Enumeration of reticulocytes and detection of hemoglobin F (HbF)-positive erythrocytes are briefly summarized in the subsequent section.

Reticulocyte Enumeration

Several RNA dyes may be applied in hematology analyzers and FCMs to enumerate reticulocytes (e.g., Oxazine 750, CD4K 530, New Methylene Blue, Auramine O, and Thiazole Orange [TO]). Dyes show differing sensitivities to stain the RNA of reticulocytes. Various analyzers use different technologies to identify positive cells (fluorescence, light scattering, and absorbance) and a software program that is more or less capable of separating reticulocytes from erythrocytes (because there is a physiologic continuum between these populations) and from other cells, such as platelets or nucleated RBCs.[155,156] Fluorescence intensity will depend on the RNA content and is correlated to reticulocyte maturity. The immature reticulocyte fraction (the sum of reticulocyte fractions with medium and high fluorescence) provides information on activity of erythropoiesis. TO can also be applied together with CD59-PE for detection of GPI-deficient reticulocytes, which may be of advantage in transfused PNH patients.

Hemoglobin F (Fetal Maternal Hemorrhage and Sickle Cell Anemia)

Fetal maternal hemorrhage from a Rhesus factor–positive (Rh+) fetus to an Rh− mother may lead to immunization of the mother against fetal alloantigens. Therefore, standard clinical practice is to administer Rh immune globulin to all Rh− women at 28 weeks of gestation and within 72 hours of delivery of an Rh+ infant. Measurement of the amount of HbF in the maternal circulation helps to determine the amount of Rh immune globulin to administer. FCM method for fetal-maternal hemorrhage detection uses a fluorochrome-conjugated anti-HbF MAb to detect HbF inside permeabilized RBCs.[157] Weakly positive red cells (termed F cells) may be found in genetic disorders, such as hereditary persistence of fetal hemoglobin, sickle cell anemia, and thalassemia major.[158] In patients with sickle cell anemia treated with hydroxyurea, monitoring the percentages of F cells can be applied to determine treatment efficacy.

Fetal cells can be distinguished from F cells by much higher fluorescence intensity. Adequate gating is necessary to determine the percentage of fetal cells in the mother's RBCs, where only the "bright" cluster is considered as fetal cells. To determine the quantity of fetal hemorrhage (in milliliters of fetal blood), the percentage of fetal RBC is multiplied by a factor of 50 (assuming that maternal blood volume is 5.0 L).

Analysis of Platelets

FCM analysis of platelets is usually performed on whole blood drawn into 3.2% to 3.8% citrate anticoagulant. Other anticoagulants can also be applied for platelet enumeration, but EDTA and heparin are not recommended for analysis of platelet activation or activity due to interference with glycoprotein (GP) IIb-IIIa complex. Blood samples should not be subjected to cold and should be processed within 15 minutes of drawing. Platelets can be differentiated from other blood cells by their FS and SS properties and/or expression of platelet-specific antigens (e.g., CD41, CD42, or CD61). FCM analysis of platelets can help to establish a diagnosis of specific platelet disorders[159] such as:

- Bernard-Soulier syndrome, inherited deficiency of the GPIb-IX-V complex, where decreased expression of GPIb (CD42b), GPIX (CD42a), and GPV (CD42d) is noted

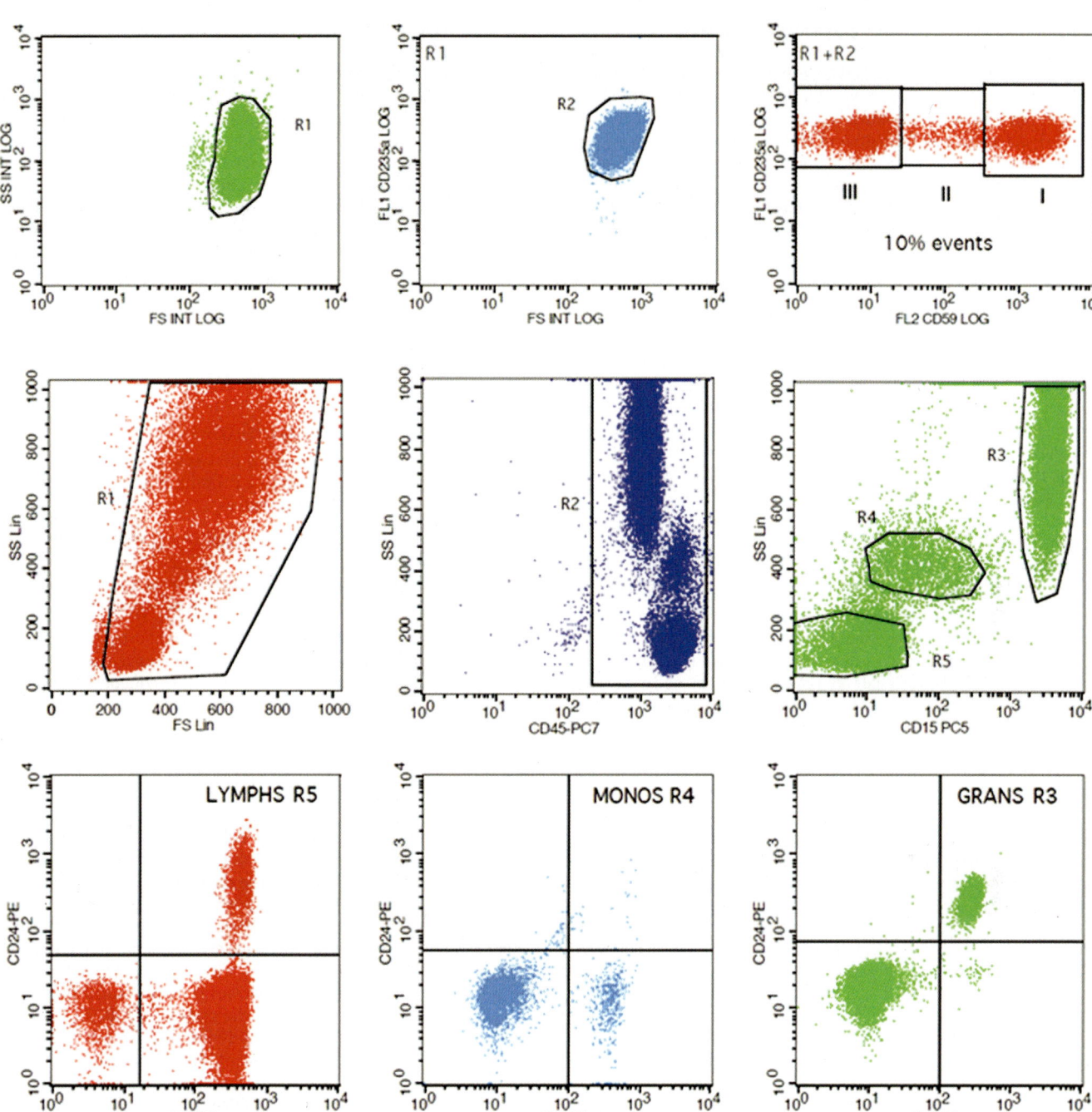

FIGURE 2.8 Enumeration of blood for markers associated with paroxysmal nocturnal hemoglobinuria (PNH). Upper row: the red blood cell (RBC) assay using CD23a⁻FITC/CD59-PE staining. RBCs are gated on FS and SS (R1, upper left plot) and displayed on FS vs CD235a FITC plot (upper middle). CD235a-positive RBCs are gated (R2). RBCs from regions R1 + R2 are analyzed for CD59 expression (right upper plot). Normal RBCs (CD59 bright) are in region I. RBCs with PNH-related phenotypes (i.e., with CD59^{dim} expression or CD59 negative) are in regions II and III, respectively. Middle and lower rows: white blood cell (WBC assay) using staining with FLAER, CD24PE, CD15PECy5, and CD45PECy7. Light scatter voltages were established so that all nucleated cells were visible above the FS threshold (middle left) and debris was excluded with a combination of light scatter and CD45 gating (middle plot). CD45⁺ events were displayed on CD15 vs SS plot (middle right plot) and granulocytes (bright CD15, high SS), monocytes (dim CD15 and intermediate SS) and lymphocytes (CD15-negative, low SS) were gated. Each of these populations was displayed on a FLAER vs CD24 plot (bottom row). PNH granulocytes (FLAER negative and CD24 negative) were enumerated in the bottom right plot (lower left quadrant). Normal granulocytes were enumerated in the upper right quadrant. Gated monocytes were similarly displayed (bottom row middle) and the PNH monocytes (FLAER negative and CD24 negative) were enumerated in the lower left quadrant. Gated lymphocytes (bottom row left) were assessed for PNH phenotypes in the lower left quadrant. Normal T lymphocytes (FLAER⁺ and CD24⁻) are visible in the lower right quadrant, and normal B lymphocytes (FLAER⁺ and CD24⁺) are visible in the upper right quadrant. FS, forward scatter; SS, side scatter. (Courtesy of Dr D. Robert Sutherland, Laboratory Medicine Program, University Health Network, Toronto General Hospital, Toronto, Ontario, Canada.)

- Glanzmann thrombasthenia, inherited deficiency of integrin $\alpha_{IIb}\beta_3$, where aberrant expression of CD41 (GPIIb) and CD61 (GPIIIa) is found
- Dense granule storage pool deficiency can be detected by studying uptake and release of mepacrine as fluorescent marker together with CD63 expression[160]

- von Willebrand disease, where the new FCM method microfluidic FCM method has been introduced[161]

Immature platelets (also called reticulated platelets) may be identified using TO dye.[162] This method can be applied to differentiate regenerative vs nonregenerative thrombocytopenia and assess regeneration after BM transplant.

Several antibodies bind to activated but not to resting platelets (activation-dependent antibodies). Markers of platelet activation include PAC1 (that detects conformational changes in integrin $\alpha_{IIb}\beta_3$), CD62P (P-selectin), and formation of platelet-derived microparticles (PMPs). Measurements of platelet activation by FCM may assist in diagnosis and treatment of acute coronary syndromes, acute cerebrovascular ischemia, and several other conditions. Studies of platelet activation have also been widely employed in monitoring of specific antiplatelet therapies.[163]

Heparin-Induced Thrombocytopenia

Heparin-induced thrombocytopenia (HIT) is a rare but potentially serious complication of heparin use. Prompt diagnosis is crucial and requires the integration of clinical assessment and laboratory testing. Primary screening to exclude HIT is performed by the immunologic detection of antibodies against PF4-heparin complex, but FCM functional tests are needed for positive diagnosis and prediction of thrombotic complications. Heparin-dependent activation of donor platelets by patient plasma can be detected using increased binding of annexin-V to platelets and elevated number of PMPs.[164,165]

STEM CELL TRANSPLANTATION

CD34+ Cell Enumeration

Enumeration of CD34+ cells is an essential tool for peripheral blood stem cell (PBSC) harvest, providing a rapid assessment of graft adequacy. Most transplant centers determine graft adequacy based on the number of CD34+ cells per kilogram of patient body weight. Mobilization of PBSC is typically done using granulocyte colony-stimulating factor alone or in combination with chemotherapy. PB CD34+ counts have been shown to correlate with PB CD34 apheresis collections and have been utilized to decide when apheresis should start. Mobilization success is influenced by several factors, such as prior therapy, mobilization strategy, and underlying disease. Clinical guidelines for CD34+ cell quantitation in PB and PBSC for the International Society for Hematotherapy and Graft Engineering based CD34+ cell enumeration on four parameters: FS, SS, CD45, and CD34 staining intensity (*Figure 2.9*).[166] A viability dye 7-aminoactinomycin D (7-AAD) and fluorescent-counting beads were subsequently added to create a single-platform assay (*Figure 2.9*) and to avoid potential calculation errors from using FCM and hematology analyzer.[167] UK NEQUAS surveys showed that the methodology is still in need of standardization and that several laboratories did not perform the gating correctly.[168] New flow cytometers allowing direct volumetric cell analyses (CD34+ cells per microliter) and quantitation without the need of the beads have been introduced and shown to give comparable results as the standard single-platform protocol.[169]

Human Leukocyte Antigen Antibody Detection

The primary goal of HLA antibody testing for transplant patients is to assess potential risk for graft rejection. The selection of a matched donor and appropriate posttransplant treatment is determined by patient HLA antibody status. Posttransplant formation of antibodies against HLA class I and II antigens heralds graft rejection. FCM cross-match (FCXM), introduced in the 1980s, involves incubation of purified donor mononuclear cells with the patient's serum and subsequent detection of cell-bound antibodies by fluorochrome-conjugated antihuman Ig serum. By varying the type of secondary antibody, the isotype of antibody (IgG, IgM, or IgA) can be determined, and by adding MAbs to B- and T-lineage-associated markers, reactivity in B lymphocytes and T lymphocytes can be evaluated separately.

Solid-phase immunobinding assays utilized purified HLA proteins as targets. Beads that can be identified by a unique level of fluorescence are coated with HLA class I or II proteins to create a screening pool of HLA antigens. By using multiple different phenotypes distributed over several arrays, patient-specific HLA specificities can be determined.

However, these assays are very cumbersome and require up to 15 tubes per patient. The Luminex platform (Luminex Corp, Austin, TX, USA) allows up to 100 individual beads to be evaluated in a single multiplexed assay. Each bead has a unique fluorescent signature and is coated by a different antigen. A PE-conjugated antihuman IgG is used to detect the binding of patient serum to the beads. However, a fraction of patients have very broadly reactive HLA antibodies, making all beads positive. Introduction of recombinant technology and coating the beads with single HLA antigens make it possible to clearly delineate the antibody reactivity of each patient. Combination of the highly sensitive antibody assessment with FCXM contributes to better selection of donor-recipient pairs and better transplant outcomes.[170-172]

SOME APPLICATIONS OF FLOW CYTOMETRY IN IMMUNODEFICIENCY, AUTOIMMUNE, AND INFECTIOUS DISEASES

Primary Immunodeficiency Diseases

Over 350 primary immunodeficiency diseases (PIDs) have been clinically identified.[173] The majority of PIDs have an abnormality that could be detected by FCM assay, such as:

- Mutations in genes that affect the relative representation of a specific cell subset
- Mutations in genes that affect the expression of a specific antigen
- Mutations in genes that affect a particular cell function

Routine immunophenotyping of blood lymphocyte subsets, detection of CD154 upregulation, and oxidative burst assay for the screening diagnosis of granulomatous diseases are the commonly employed FCM assays in PID diagnosis. FCM findings in the most common PID categories are summarized in *Table 2.10*.[174]

Flow Cytometry Detection of HLA-B27

HLA-B27, an MHC class I molecule, is related to a major risk factor for a group of diseases now called spondyloarthritis, which consists of psoriatic arthritis, reactive arthritis, arthritis related to inflammatory bowel disease, a subgroup of juvenile idiopathic arthritis, and ankylosing spondylitis. This association is present in many genetically diverse populations and across all major HLA-B27 subtypes.[175]

The presence of HLA-B27 in 80% to 90% of patients with ankylosing spondylitis and the spontaneous spondyloarthritis-like disease in HLA-B27 transgenic rats suggests a direct and dominant effect of the gene encoding this molecule. However, only a small proportion of people in the general population who harbor HLA-B27 (5%-6% in Caucasians) develop ankylosing spondylitis, and HLA-B27 explains only 20% to 40% of the genetic susceptibility to ankylosing spondylitis, suggesting the contribution of additional genes. Genomewide association studies have allowed the identification of several of these additional genes. HLA-B27 typing using MAbs and FCM analysis of their reactivity in a gated T-cell population is used extensively. However, the cross-reactivity of anti-"B27" murine MAbs, particularly with the common HLA-B7 antigen, has been a problem. A one-tube test, employing two "B27" MAb reagents, has been developed.[176] This test securely detects the HLA-B*27 allele product B*2705, B*2702, and B*2708, and reacts with many of the other rare B*27 allele products tested. In addition, other HLA-B antigens, notably HLA-B7, do not interfere with accurate HLA-B27 assignment. However, even when using the recommended dual anti-B27 typing reagents, patients reacting with one antibody only should be retested using a DNA-based technique. In general, the FCM method is consistent with genetic testing in 99% of patients.[177]

Human Immunodeficiency Virus Infection

FCM studies provide important clinical information that helps predict disease outcome and guide treatment decisions in HIV-positive patients. CD4+ T-cell counts, together with viral load, are the strongest predictors of disease progression. CD4 depletion is also one of

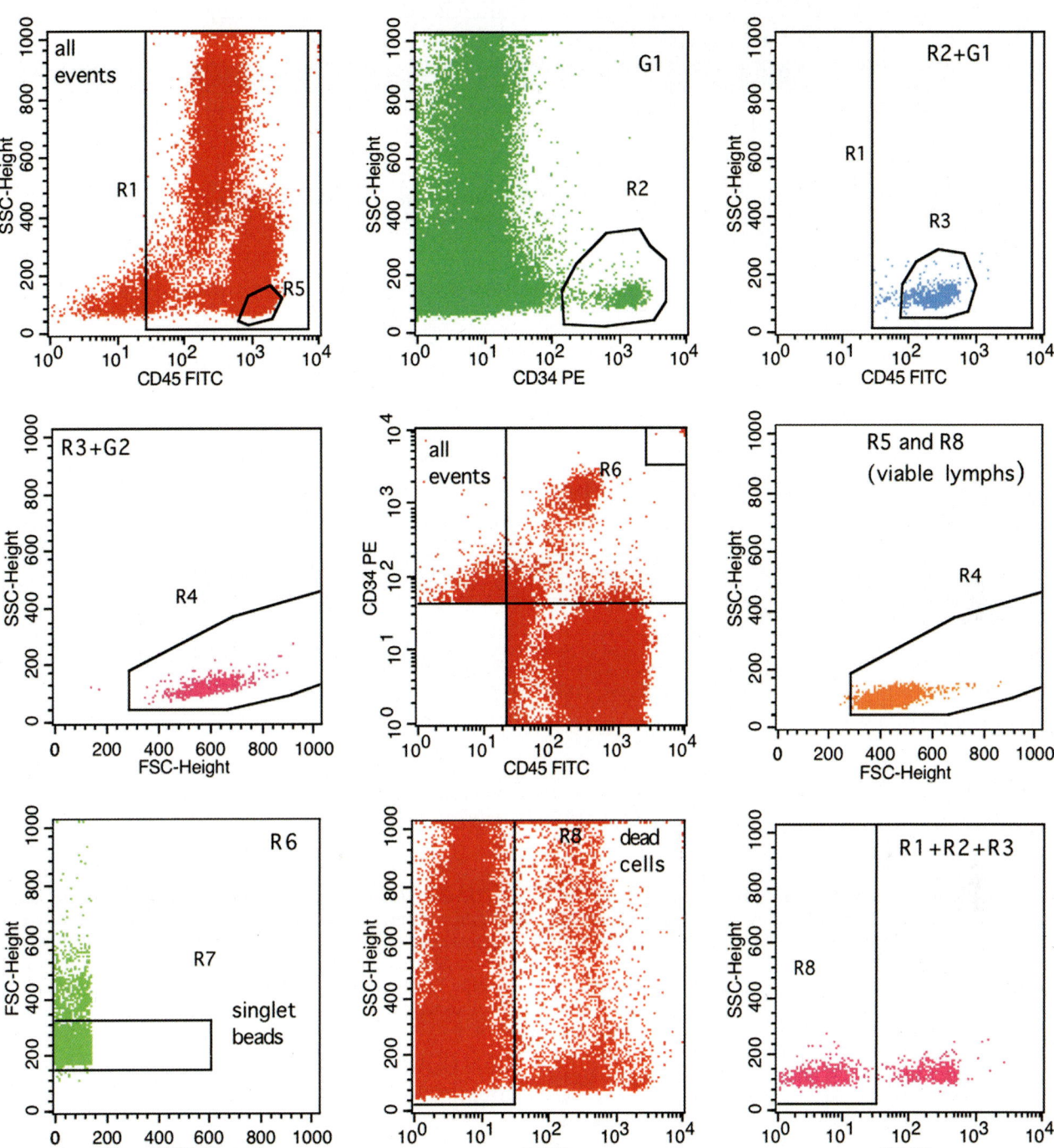

FIGURE 2.9 Enumeration of viable CD34+ cells according to ISHAGE protocol. An apheresis sample that had been stored overnight at room temperature was stained with the Stem-Kit reagent set and analyzed on a BD Biosciences FACSCalibur cytometer equipped with CellQuest. Viable CD34+ cells were identified using Boolean gating and regions R1 through R4 (all upper plots and left middle row plots), including only viable (7-AAD−) cells from region R8 (right lower row plot). Viable lymphocytes from region R5 (left upper plot) and R8 are displayed on the left middle plot, and the duplicate blast-lymphocyte region R4 adjusted to include the smallest viable lymphocytes. Duplicate gating region R4 on plot 4 self-adjusts accordingly. Middle plot shows the position of a "live" gate in the bottom left corner, which excludes debris resulting from lyse-no-wash sample processing of PB, CB, and BM sample types. The number of CD34+ cells in region R4 is compared with the total number of singlet beads counted during the same acquisition and present in the same list-mode file. In the example shown, total beads are gated in region R6 in the middle plot and displayed in the left lower plot (time vs forward scatter). Singlet beads are then delineated and enumerated in gating region R7. Sample analysis was performed using CellQuest Pro software using semiautomated Expression Editors. For earlier versions of CellQuest, the absolute number of

viable CD34+ cells per microliter is calculated as follows: $\dfrac{\text{\#CD34}^+\text{ cells} \times \text{bead concentration} \times \text{DF}}{\text{\#single beads}}$ where #CD34+ cells are determined from logic gate G4

(vCD34 in gate stats = R1 + R2 + R3 + R4 + R8), the bead concentration is specified by the manufacturer, DF is the sample dilution factor, and the singlet bead count is determined from plot 7 (singlet beads in gate stats = R6 + R7). The right lower plot shows the total CD34+ cells (viable and nonviable) from gating regions R1 + R2 + R3 only and shows viable cells on-scale in about the first decade of fluorescence. This plot is useful when samples with poor viability are to be analyzed because it is easier to set region R8 in this plot vs the middle lower plot. Additionally, it shows that the fluorescence compensation between PMT 2 (CD34PE) and PMT 3 (7-AAD) is optimally set. BM, bone marrow; CB, complete blood; ISHAGE, International Society for Hematotherapy and Graft Engineering; PB, peripheral blood; PMT, photomultiplier tube; 7-AAD, 7-aminoactinomycin D. (Courtesy of Dr D. Robert Sutherland, Laboratory Medicine Program, University Health Network, Toronto General Hospital, Toronto, Ontario, Canada.)

Table 2.10. Flow Cytometry in the Diagnosis of Major Primary Immune Deficiency

Primary Immune Deficiency Type	Main Findings
Congenital agammaglobulinemia X-linked (XLA)	Absence (or very low numbers) of CD20$^+$ and/or CD19$^+$ B lymphocytes Absence of intracellular Bruton tyrosine kinase (BTK) in monocytes and platelets
Common variable immunodeficiency (CVID)	Expansion of CD21^{low} B cells Absence of memory switched B cells Lack of inducible costimulator (ICOS) upregulation on T cells following activation CD19 deficiency (in the presence of CD20) B-cell activating factor-receptor (BAFF-R) deficiency
Severe combined immunodeficiency (SCID)	Wide range of defects: Adenosine deaminase deficiency: lack of T cells, B cells, and NK cells Janus kinase 3 deficiency: lack of T cells and NK cells RAG1/2 deficiency: lack of T cells and B cells CD3δ, ε, or ζ deficiency: lack of T cells
Hyper-IgM syndromes	Decrease in CD40 and/or CD40 ligand (CD154) expression on activated CD4$^+$ cells
Wiskott-Aldrich syndrome (WAS)	Decrease in CD8$^+$ cells and increase in NK cells Decreased expression of WAS protein
Defects in the interleukin-12/23-Interferon-γ circuit	Aberrant expression of IL-12 receptor β1 and interferon (IFN)-γ receptor 1
Toll-like receptor pathway defects	Absence of shedding of CD62L from the surface of granulocytes
Chronic granulomatous disease	Low results of nicotinamide adenine dinucleotide phosphate (NADPH) oxidase activity assay following granulocyte activation
Leukocyte adhesion deficiency type 1 (LAD1)	Decreased or absent CD11a, CD11b, CD11c, and CD18 on granulocytes
Immune dysregulation, polyendocrinopathy, enteropathy, X-linked inheritance syndrome	Decreased/absent factor forkhead box protein 3 (FOXP3) expression in T cells
Autoimmune lymphoproliferative syndrome	Elevated levels of CD4$^-$CD8$^-$ (double negative) T-cell receptor α/β–positive T cells Low memory B cells (CD20$^+$CD27$^+$)[en] Increased CD8$^+$CD57$^+$ T cells
X-linked lymphoproliferative syndrome	Very low numbers of NK T cells CD3$^+$CD16$^+$CD56$^+$Vα24$^+$Vβ11$^+$ Decreased/absent signaling lymphocyte activation molecule (SLAM)-associated protein (SAP) or X-linked inhibitor of apoptosis (XIAP) protein
Familial hemophagocytic lymphohistiocytosis	Defects in expression of perforin, syntaxin-11 Diminished expression of CD107 on NK cells

the signs of the acute retroviral syndrome that occurs in some patients soon after infection and is characterized by general symptoms, high viral burden, plasma tumor necrosis factor (TNF)-α, C-reactive protein, D-dimer, and adverse prognosis.[178]

Single-platform technology (SPT) is designed to enable determinations of both absolute and percentage lymphocyte subset values using a single tube. Previously, most absolute T-cell numbers were derived from three measurements determined with two different instruments, a hematology analyzer and an FCM (dual-platform technology). A gating strategy for identifying lymphocytes using CD45 fluorescence and side-scattering characteristics is now the preferred method for identifying lymphocytes. The obligatory panel includes CD45, CD3, CD4, and CD8. Commercial bead-counting reagents for SPT have resulted in decreased interlaboratory variability. A single-tube model can easily be employed even in countries with limited resources.[179] Point-of-care testing with small CD4 analyzers may facilitate linking to care in resource-limited settings.[180] However, in 2015, the WHO recommended antiviral treatment to be offered to all HIV-infected individuals, independent of CD4 counts.[181] This may diminish the role and frequency of CD4 testing in HIV patients in the future.

Analysis of Antigen-Specific T Cells

FCM detection of antigen-specific T cells became possible by the development of fluorochrome-labeled MHC peptide complex (the so-called tetramers) technology. MHC class I tetramers usually consist of four MHC class I Gps loaded with peptide and labeled with streptavidin bound to a fluorochrome. During incubation with the lymphocytes, the tetramer will bind to CD8$^+$ T cells that express a T-cell receptor capable of recognizing the specific peptide. MHC class II tetramers are more difficult to produce but have also been developed and applied to study CD4$^+$ cell responses.[182]

Tetramer technology is also used in functional assays to study proliferation of epitope-specific T cells or for analysis of T cells responding to viruses or vaccines. Tetramer-positive T-cell subset analysis is used to determine the quality of the T-cell response and to sort antigen-specific T cells. Another emerging use of tetramer technology is CAR-T-cell therapy.[183]

CELLULAR DNA CONTENT AND CELL CYCLE ANALYSIS

FCM methods for measuring DNA content rely on cells being labeled with a fluorochrome that is expected to stain DNA stoichiometrically and the intensity of DNA-associated fluorescence is obtained. Staining of live cells (the so-called supravital staining) is used mainly for cell sorting based on their DNA content. A variety of methods for FCM DNA analysis of fixed cells has been reported, differing in cell permeabilization, choice of fluorochrome, and applicability to different cell populations. In general, precipitating fixatives (alcohols and acetone) are preferred over cross-linking reagents (formaldehyde and glutaraldehyde). The most common fluorochromes are 4′,6-diamidino-2-phenylindole, propidium iodide (PI), and 7-AAD (Table 2.1). Staining with PI required preincubation with RNase to digest RNA; RNase should be free of DNase activity. The method of isolating nuclei from paraffin-embedded tissues can be applied to determine DNA ploidy and cell phase in archival materials.[184] The results of cellular DNA content are presented in the form of frequency histograms. The DNA analysis software allows estimation of the percentage of cells in the G$_1$, S, and G$_2$/M phases of the cell cycle as well as the frequency of apoptotic cells with fractional (sub-G$_1$) DNA content[184,185] (Figure 2.10). Before the DNA content is analyzed, cell

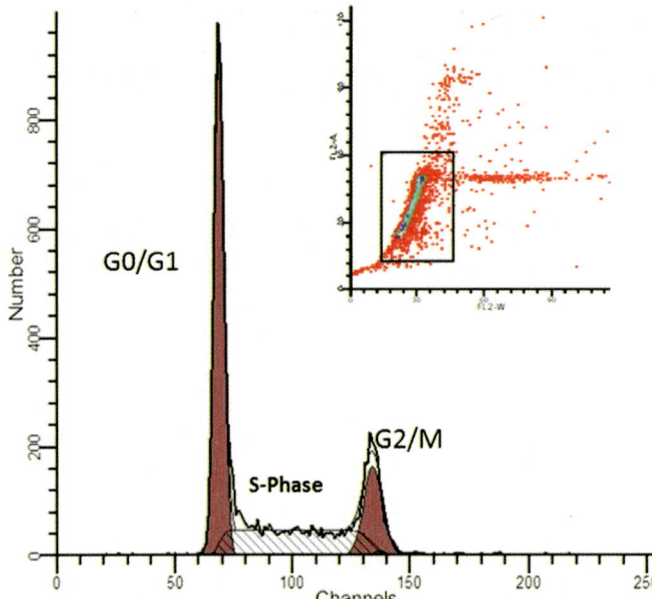

FIGURE 2.10 Schematic presentation of DNA analysis using DNA fluorochrome. Frequency of cells in $G_{0/1}$, S, and G_2/M phases can be determined. Inset shows gating of single cells using FL-W vs FL-A plot. A, area; FL, fluorescence; W, width.

aggregates have to be removed from the analysis window by gating single cells on FL-width vs FL-area plots.

DNA staining can be combined with immunophenotyping by labeling of live cells with a fluorochrome-conjugated MAb and supravital DNA staining or subsequent short fixation in 0.5% to 1% paraformaldehyde in phosphate buffer serum before DNA fluorochrome is applied.

In hematology, DNA ploidy studies by FCM have determined prognosis in B-ALL and PC myeloma. In ALL, a DNA index (DI) ≥ 1.16, the so-called hyperdiploidy, is of favorable significance, whereas hypodiploidy (<40 chromosomes, DI < 0.9) is related to poor prognosis. Near-haploid ALL with 24 to 30 chromosomes and low-hypodiploid ALL with 31 to 39 chromosomes have been defined as distinct ALL subgroups. DI analysis is especially useful in detection of cases with the so-called masked hypodiploidy, where the doubling of either a low-hypodiploid or a near-haploid clone results in an apparently high-hyperdiploid karyotype.[186] In myeloma, hyperdiploidy is related to a better response to bortezomib treatment,[187] whereas hyperhaploidy is related to a worse outcome.[188]

Analysis of DNA replication was at first performed using direct incorporation of ^{3}H- or ^{14}C-labeled thymidine, and ^{3}H-uridine incorporation was used for analysis of RNA content. Incorporation of 5-bromo-2-deoxyuridine (BrdU) was subsequently applied, based on quenching of the Hoechst 33358 fluorescence by BrdU. Distribution of BrdU-containing cells through the cell cycle was studied by combining Hoechst 33358 with BrdU-resistant dye such as ethidium bromide or with mithramycin. The so-called click chemistry approach allows measuring DNA synthesis and RNA replication simultaneously, by applying 5-ethyl-2′-deoxyuridine as a DNA precursor and 5-ethyluridine as an RNA precursor. These precursors can be detected with fluorochrome-tagged azides by means of a copper(I)-catalyzed [3 + 2] cycloaddition reaction.[189]

FUNCTIONAL ASSAYS

Monitoring of Cytokine Profiles

Current FCM technologies allow the simultaneous quantification of multiple cytokines with characterization of cytokine-producing cell subsets. Antibodies to studied cytokines can be combined with lineage markers such as CD4, CD8, and CD3 and/or memory/effector phenotype markers such as CCR7, CD57, CD27, or CD45RO.

Intracellular cytokine assays are usually performed after short-term stimulation required for induction of cellular activation and cytokine production. Cytokines can be detected after secretion inhibitors such as monensin or brefeldin are applied, and proteins are retained intracellularly. Intracellular staining is performed after fixation and permeabilization.[190] One of the clinical applications includes studies of cytokine secretion by T cells in aplastic anemia.[191]

Multiplex cytokine bead arrays are used to quantify soluble plasma cytokines (e.g., Luminex technology). Distinct cytokine profiles were detected, allowing differentiation between patients with aplastic anemia (characterized by high levels of thrombopoietin and granulocyte colony-stimulating factor) and hypoplastic MDS (characterized by high levels of TNF-α, IL-6, chemokine [C-C motif] ligand 3, IL-1 receptor antagonist, and hepatocyte growth factor).[192] Very high levels of several cytokines (such as IL-6, IL-2R, IL-10, TNF-RI, and macrophage inflammatory protein-1α) were detected with the Luminex methodology in children with anaplastic large cell lymphoma by comparison with other non-Hodgkin lymphoma subtypes.[193]

Protein Phosphorylation

The use of phospho-specific antibodies allows detection of the transient alterations induced by kinases and phosphatases involved in cell signaling. Phosphorylation refers to the addition of a phosphate to one of the amino acid side chains of a protein. Many of the proteins that are phosphorylated upon reception of a signal are protein kinases as well. This organization of kinases produces a phosphorylation cascade, in which one protein kinase is activated by phosphorylation upon reception of a signal; this kinase then phosphorylates the next kinase in the cascade. However, FCM methodology to detect phosphorylation is considered challenging.[194] Signaling responses have to be determined by comparing the basal level to the activated state of the enzyme. Often, multiple growth factors should be applied for studies of activation (e.g., SCF and FLT3 for the extracellular signal-regulated kinase [ERK] pathway), and inhibitors are used for appropriate controls (e.g., MEK inhibitor U0126 for the ERK pathway). Appropriate fixation and permeabilization protocols have to be applied, depending on the studied protein. Responses are usually transient, and the time point of measurement is crucial. A high level of consistency in experimental procedures is needed.

Phosphoflow method made it possible to detect activated NF-κB p65 and phosphorylated STAT1, STAT3, STAT5, and STAT6, together with the B-cell differentiation antigens CD19, CD27, and CD38. Applying these methods on in vitro-induced human B-cell differentiation cultures showed significantly different steady-state levels, and responses to stimulation, of phosphorylated signaling proteins in CD27-expressing B-cell and antibody-secreting populations.[195] By tracking differential phosphorylation states of specific proteins, phosphoflow gains importance as a screening tool to identify genes and drugs to turn intracellular signaling on and off in various diseases.[196]

Apoptosis

Apoptosis (or programmed cell death) plays an essential role in the survival of the organism and is considered as an imperative component of various processes, including normal cell turnover, proper development and functioning of the immune system, multiplication of mutated chromosomes, hormone-dependent atrophy, normal embryonic development, elimination of indisposed cells, and maintenance of cell homeostasis. The importance of apoptosis has prompted development of FCM assays capable of measuring this process. Examples of FCM methods employed in apoptosis research include[197]:

- Detection of scatter changes corresponding to cell shrinkage (lower FS and unchanged or increased SC in early phase, and low FS and SC in late phase)
- FCM detection of mitochondrial inner transmembrane potential ($\Delta\Pi_m$) loss using lipophilic cationic probes (e.g., Rh123 or $DiOC_6(3)$) that are readily taken up by live cells and accumulated in mitochondria

- FCM detection of caspase activation using fluorochrome-labeled inhibitors of caspases or detection of cleavage of poly-ADP-ribose polymerase using an antibody that recognized the 89-kDa product of cleavage
- FCM detection of changes in the plasma membrane during apoptosis using fluorochrome-labeled annexin-V that binds to exposed phosphatidylserine on the cell surface
- FCM detection of changes in plasma membrane permeability
- FCM detection of nuclear fragmentation using sub-G_0 fraction in DNA analysis or assessment of DNA strand breaks by TdT-mediated dUTP-biotin nick-end labeling
- Gradual decrease in cyanine SYTO staining in apoptotic cells

Because apoptosis is a rapid process, knowledge of the time-window when specific markers can be detected is crucial. Moreover, antigen loss often occurs at early stages of apoptosis, causing problems in immunophenotyping apoptotic cells. In hematology, increased apoptosis has been implicated as one of major pathophysiological mechanisms in development of MDSs.[198]

References

1. Caspersson TO. History of the development of cytophotometry from 1935 to the present. *Anal Quant Cytol Histol.* 1987;9(1):2-6.
2. Shapiro HM. The evolution of cytometers. *Cytometry A.* 2004;58(1):13-20.
3. Coons AH. The beginnings of immunofluorescence. *J Immunol.* 1961;87:499-503.
4. Blades AN, Flavell HC. Observations on the use of the Coulter model D electronic cell counter in clinical haematology. *J Clin Pathol.* 1963;16:158-163.
5. Fulwyler MJ. Electronic separation of biological cells by volume. *Science.* 1965;150(3698):910-911.
6. Hulett HR, Bonner WA, Barrett J, Herzenberg LA. Cell sorting: automated separation of mammalian cells as a function of intracellular fluorescence. *Science.* 1969;166(3906):747-749.
7. Orfao A, Ortuno F, De SM, Lopez A, San MJ. Immunophenotyping of acute leukemias and myelodysplastic syndromes. *Cytometry A.* 2004;58(1):62-71.
8. van Dongen JJ, Lhermitte L, Bottcher S, et al. EuroFlow antibody panels for standardized n-dimensional flow cytometric immunophenotyping of normal, reactive and malignant leukocytes. *Leukemia.* 2012;26(9):1908-1975.
9. Cherian S, Levin G, Lo WY, et al. Evaluation of an 8-color flow cytometric reference method for white blood cell differential enumeration. *Cytometry B Clin Cytom.* 2010;78(5):319-328.
10. Porwit A. Immunophenotyping of selected hematologic disorders focus on lymphoproliferative disorders with more than one malignant cell population. *Int J Lab Hematol.* 2013;35(3):275-282.
11. Chattopadhyay PK, Hogerkorp CM, Roederer M. A chromatic explosion: the development and future of multiparameter flow cytometry. *Immunology.* 2008;125(4):441-449.
12. Cunningham RE. Overview of flow cytometry and fluorescent probes for flow cytometry. *Methods Mol Biol.* 2010;588:319-326.
13. Davis BH, Holden JT, Bene MC, et al. 2006 Bethesda International Consensus recommendations on the flow cytometric immunophenotypic analysis of hematolymphoid neoplasia: medical indications. *Cytometry B Clin Cytom.* 2007;72(suppl 1):S5-S13.
14. Szaloki G, Goda K. Compensation in multicolor flow cytometry. *Cytometry A.* 2015;87(11):982-985.
15. Wang L, Hoffman RA. Standardization, calibration, and control in flow cytometry. *Curr Protoc Cytom.* 2017;79(1):3.1-1.3.27.
16. Ibrahim SF, van den Engh G. Flow cytometry and cell sorting. *Adv Biochem Eng Biotechnol.* 2007;106:19-39.
17. Köhler G, Milstein C. Continuous cultures of fused cells secreting antibody of predefined specificity. *Nature.* 1975;256(5517):495-497.
18. Bernard A, Boumsell L. The clusters of differentiation (CD) defined by the first international workshop on human leucocyte differentiation antigens. *Hum Immunol.* 1984;11(1):1-10.
19. Zola H, Swart B. The human leucocyte differentiation antigens (HLDA) workshops: the evolving role of antibodies in research, diagnosis and therapy. *Cell Res.* 2005;15(9):691-694.
20. Lambert C, Yanikkaya Demirel G, Keller T, et al. Flow cytometric analyses of lymphocyte markers in immune oncology: a comprehensive guidance for validation practice according to laws and standards. *Front Immunol.* 2020;11:2169.
21. de Jongste AH, Kraan J, van den Broek PD, et al. Use of TransFix cerebrospinal fluid storage tubes prevents cellular loss and enhances flow cytometric detection of malignant hematological cells after 18 hours of storage. *Cytometry B Clin Cytom.* 2014;86(4):272-279.
22. Violidaki D, Axler O, Jafari K, et al. Analysis of erythroid maturation in the nonlysed bone marrow with help of radar plots facilitates detection of flow cytometric aberrations in myelodysplastic syndromes. *Cytometry B Clin Cytom.* 2020;98(5):399-411.
23. Tanqri S, Vall H, Kaplan D, et al. Validation of cell-based fluorescence assays: practice guidelines from the ICSH and ICCS-part III-analytical issues. *Cytometry B Clin Cytom.* 2013;84(5):291-308.
24. Wood BL, Arroz M, Barnett D, et al. 2006 Bethesda International Consensus recommendations on the immunophenotypic analysis of hematolymphoid neoplasia by flow cytometry: optimal reagents and reporting for the flow cytometric diagnosis of hematopoietic neoplasia. *Cytometry B Clin Cytom.* 2007;72(suppl 1):S14-S22.
25. Porwit A, Béné MC, eds. *Multiparameter Flow Cytometry in the Diagnosis of Hematological Malignancies.* Cambridge University Press; 2018.
26. Roederer M. Spectral compensation for flow cytometry: visualization artifacts, limitations, and caveats. *Cytometry.* 2001;45(3):194-205.
27. Borowitz MJ, Guenther KL, Shults KE, Stelzer GT. Immunophenotyping of acute leukemia by flow cytometric analysis. Use of CD45 and right-angle light scatter to gate on leukemic blasts in three-color analysis. *Am J Clin Pathol.* 1993;100(5):534-540.
28. Arnoulet C, Bene MC, Durrieu F, et al. Four-and five-color flow cytometry analysis of leukocyte differentiation pathways in normal bone marrow: a reference document based on a systematic approach by the GTLLF and GEIL. *Cytometry B Clin Cytom.* 2010;78(1):4-10.
29. Porwit A, Rajab A. Flow cytometry immunophenotyping in integrated diagnostics of patients with newly diagnosed cytopenia: one tube 10-color 14-antibody screening panel and 3-tube extensive panel for detection of MDS-related features. *Int J Lab Hematol.* 2015;37(suppl 1):133-143.
30. Rajab A, Porwit A. Screening bone marrow samples for abnormal lymphoid populations and myelodysplasia-related features with one 10-color 14-antibody screening tube. *Cytometry B Clin Cytom.* 2015;88(4):253-260.
31. Rajab A, Axler O, Leung J, Wozniak M, Porwit A. Ten-color 15-antibody flow cytometry panel for immunophenotyping of lymphocyte population. *Int J Lab Hematol.* 2017;39(suppl 1):76-85.
32. Costa ES, Arroyo ME, Pedreira CE, et al. A new automated flow cytometry data analysis approach for the diagnostic screening of neoplastic B-cell disorders in peripheral blood samples with absolute lymphocytosis. *Leukemia.* 2006;20(7):1221-1230.
33. Béné MC, Lacombe F, Porwit A. Unsupervised flow cytometry analysis in hematological malignancies: a new paradigm. *Int J Lab Hematol.* 2021;43(suppl 1):54-64.
34. Del Vecchio L, Brando B, Lanza F, et al. Recommended reporting format for flow cytometry diagnosis of acute leukemia. *Haematologica.* 2004;89(5):594-598.
35. Du L, Grover A, Ramanan S, Litwin V. The evolution of guidelines for the validation of flow cytometric methods. *Int J Lab Hematol.* 2015;37(suppl 1):3-10.
36. Terstappen LW, Levin J. Bone marrow cell differential counts obtained by multidimensional flow cytometry. *Blood Cell.* 1992;18(2):311-330. discussion 331-332.
37. Macedo A, Orfao A, Ciudad J, et al. Phenotypic analysis of CD34 subpopulations in normal human bone marrow and its application for the detection of minimal residual disease. *Leukemia.* 1995;9(11):1896-1901.
38. Lucio P, Parreira A, van den Beemd MW, et al. Flow cytometric analysis of normal B cell differentiation: a frame of reference for the detection of minimal residual disease in precursor-B-ALL. *Leukemia.* 1999;13(3):419-427.
39. Porwit-MacDonald A, Bjorklund E, Lucio P, et al. BIOMED-1 concerted action report: flow cytometric characterization of CD7+ cell subsets in normal bone marrow as a basis for the diagnosis and follow-up of T cell acute lymphoblastic leukemia (T-ALL). *Leukemia.* 2000;14(5):816-825.
40. van Lochem EG, van der Velden VH, Wind HK, te Marvelde JG, Westerdaal NA, van Dongen JJ. Immunophenotypic differentiation patterns of normal hematopoiesis in human bone marrow: reference patterns for age-related changes and disease-induced shifts. *Cytometry B Clin Cytom.* 2004;60(1):1-13.
41. Kussick SJ, Wood BL. Using 4-color flow cytometry to identify abnormal myeloid populations. *Arch Pathol Lab Med.* 2003;127(9):1140-1147.
42. Della Porta MG, Malcovati L, Invernizzi R, et al. Flow cytometry evaluation of erythroid dysplasia in patients with myelodysplastic syndrome. *Leukemia.* 2006;20(4):549-555.
43. Goardon N, Nikolousis E, Sternberg A, et al. Reduced CD38 expression on CD34+ cells as a diagnostic test in myelodysplastic syndromes. *Haematologica.* 2009;94(8):1160-1163.
44. Matarraz S, Lopez A, Barrena S, et al. The immunophenotype of different immature, myeloid and B-cell lineage-committed CD34+ hematopoietic cells allows discrimination between normal/reactive and myelodysplastic syndrome precursors. *Leukemia.* 2008;22(6):1175-1183.
45. Jafari K, Tierens A, Rajab A, Musani R, Schuh A, Porwit A. Visualization of cell composition and maturation in the bone marrow using 10-color flow cytometry and radar plots. *Cytometry B Clin Cytom.* 2018;94(2):219-229.
46. Doulatov S, Notta F, Laurenti E, Dick JE. Hematopoiesis: a human perspective. *Cell Stem Cell.* 2012;10(2):120-136.
47. Stetler-Stevenson M, Arthur DC, Jabbour N, et al. Diagnostic utility of flow cytometric immunophenotyping in myelodysplastic syndrome. *Blood.* 2001;98(4):979-987.
48. Loken MR, Chu SC, Fritschle W, Kalnoski M, Wells DA. Normalization of bone marrow aspirates for hemodilution in flow cytometric analyses. *Cytometry B Clin Cytom.* 2009;76(1):27-36.
49. Edvardsson L, Dykes J, Olsson ML, Olofsson T. Clonogenicity, gene expression and phenotype during neutrophil versus erythroid differentiation of cytokine-stimulated CD34+ human marrow cells in vitro. *Br J Haematol.* 2004;127(4):451-463.
50. Matarraz S, Almeida J, Flores-Montero J, et al. Introduction to the diagnosis and classification of monocytic-lineage leukemias by flow cytometry. *Cytometry B Clin Cytom.* 2017;92(3):218-227.
51. Wong KL, Tai JJ, Wong WC, et al. Gene expression profiling reveals the defining features of the classical, intermediate, and nonclassical human monocyte subsets. *Blood.* 2011;118(5):e16-e31.
52. Eidenschink Brodersen L, Menssen AJ, Wangen JR, et al. Assessment of erythroid dysplasia by "difference from normal" in routine clinical flow cytometry workup. *Cytometry B Clin Cytom.* 2015;88(2):125-135.
53. McKenna RW, Washington LT, Aquino DB, Picker LJ, Kroft SH. Immunophenotypic analysis of hematogones (B-lymphocyte precursors) in 662 consecutive bone marrow specimens by 4-color flow cytometry. *Blood.* 2001;98(8):2498-2507.

54. Blom B, Spits H. Development of human lymphoid cells. *Annu Rev Immunol.* 2006;24:287-320.
55. Loken MR, Shah VO, Dattilio KL, Civin CI. Flow cytometric analysis of human bone marrow. II. Normal B lymphocyte development. *Blood.* 1987;70(5):1316-1324.
56. Seegmiller AC, Kroft SH, Karandikar NJ, McKenna RW. Characterization of immunophenotypic aberrancies in 200 cases of B acute lymphoblastic leukemia. *Am J Clin Pathol.* 2009;132(6):940-949.
57. Six EM, Bonhomme D, Monteiro M, et al. A human postnatal lymphoid progenitor capable of circulating and seeding the thymus. *J Exp Med.* 2007;204(13):3085-3093.
58. Reinhold U, Abken H, Kukel S, et al. CD7-T cells represent a subset of normal human blood lymphocytes. *J Immunol.* 1993;150(5):2081-2089.
59. Berdnikovs S. The twilight zone: plasticity and mixed ontogeny of neutrophil and eosinophil granulocyte subsets. *Sem Immunopath.* 2021;43(3):337-346.
60. Han X, Jorgensen JL, Brahmandam A, et al. Immunophenotypic study of basophils by multiparameter flow cytometry. *Arch Pathol Lab Med.* 2008;132(5):813-819.
61. Escribano L, Diaz-Agustin B, Bellas C, et al. Utility of flow cytometric analysis of mast cells in the diagnosis and classification of adult mastocytosis. *Leuk Res.* 2001;25(7):563-570.
62. Orfao A, Escribano L, Villarrubia J, et al. Flow cytometric analysis of mast cells from normal and pathological human bone marrow samples: identification and enumeration. *Am J Pathol.* 1996;149(5):1493-1499.
63. Yu CI, Becker C, Metang P, et al. Human CD141+ dendritic cells induce CD4+ T cells to produce type 2 cytokines. *J Immunol.* 2014;193(9):4335-4343.
64. Dzionek A, Fuchs A, Schmidt P, et al. BDCA-2, BDCA-3, and BDCA-4: three markers for distinct subsets of dendritic cells in human peripheral blood. *J Immunol.* 2000;165(11):6037-6046.
65. Cooper MA, Fehniger TA, Caligiuri MA. The biology of human natural killer-cell subsets. *Trends Immunol.* 2001;22(11):633-640.
66. Yu J, Freud AG, Caligiuri MA. Location and cellular stages of natural killer cell development. *Trends Immunol.* 2013;34(12):573-582.
67. Freud AG, Yu J, Caligiuri MA. Human natural killer cell development in secondary lymphoid tissues. *Semin Immunol.* 2014;26(2):132-137.
68. Angelo LS, Banerjee PP, Monaco-Shawver L, et al. Practical NK cell phenotyping and variability in healthy adults. *Immunol Res.* 2015;62(3):341-356.
69. Deneys V, Mazzon AM, Marques JL, Benoit H, De Bruyere M. Reference values for peripheral blood B-lymphocyte subpopulations: a basis for multiparametric immunophenotyping of abnormal lymphocytes. *J Immunol Methods.* 2001;253(1-2):23-36.
70. Laane E, Tani E, Bjorklund E, et al. Flow cytometric immunophenotyping including Bcl-2 detection on fine needle aspirates in the diagnosis of reactive lymphadenopathy and non-Hodgkin's lymphoma. *Cytometry B Clin Cytom.* 2005;64(1):34-42.
71. Cornet E, Mossafa H, Courel K, Lesesve JF, Troussard X. Persistent polyclonal binucleated B-cell lymphocytosis and MECOM gene amplification. *BMC Res Notes.* 2016;9:138.
72. Tierens AM, Holte H, Warsame A, et al. Low levels of monoclonal small B cells in the bone marrow of patients with diffuse large B-cell lymphoma of activated B-cell type but not of germinal center B-cell type. *Haematologica.* 2010;95(8):1334-1341.
73. Rawstron AC, Kreuzer KA, Soosapilla A, et al. Reproducible diagnosis of chronic lymphocytic leukemia by flow cytometry: an European Research Initiative on CLL (ERIC) & European Society for Clinical Cell Analysis (ESCCA) harmonisation project. *Cytometry B Clin Cytom.* 2018;94(1):121-128.
74. Balakrishna J, Basumallik N, Matulonis R, et al. Intensity of antigen expression reflects IGHV mutational status and Dohner-defined prognostic categories in chronic lymphocytic leukemia, monoclonal B-cell lymphocytosis, and small lymphocytic lymphoma. *Leuk Lymphoma.* 2021;62(8):1828-1839.
75. Cui B, Ghia EM, Chen L, et al. High-level ROR1 associates with accelerated disease progression in chronic lymphocytic leukemia. *Blood.* 2016;128(25):2931-2940.
76. Swerdlow SH, Campo E, Pileri SA, et al. The 2016 revision of the World Health Organization classification of lymphoid neoplasms. *Blood.* 2016;127(20):2375-2390.
77. Strati P, Shanafelt TD. Monoclonal B-cell lymphocytosis and early-stage chronic lymphocytic leukemia: diagnosis, natural history, and risk stratification. *Blood.* 2015;126(4):454-462.
78. Shim YK, Middleton DC, Caporaso NE, et al. Prevalence of monoclonal B-cell lymphocytosis: a systematic review. *Cytometry B Clin Cytom.* 2010;78(suppl 1):S10-S18.
79. Nieto WG, Almeida J, Romero A, et al. Increased frequency (12%) of circulating chronic lymphocytic leukemia-like B-cell clones in healthy subjects using a highly sensitive multicolor flow cytometry approach. *Blood.* 2009;114(1):33-37.
80. Challagundla P, Medeiros LJ, Kanagal-Shamanna R, Miranda RN, Jorgensen JL. Differential expression of CD200 in B-cell neoplasms by flow cytometry can assist in diagnosis, subclassification, and bone marrow staging. *Am J Clin Pathol.* 2014;142(6):837-844.
81. Gao J, Peterson L, Nelson B, Goolsby C, Chen YH. Immunophenotypic variations in mantle cell lymphoma. *Am J Clin Pathol.* 2009;132(5):699-706.
82. Jain P, Giustolisi GM, Atkinson S, et al. Detection of cyclin D1 in B cell lymphoproliferative disorders by flow cytometry. *J Clin Pathol.* 2002;55(12):940-945.
83. Berger F, Traverse-Glehen A, Felman P, et al. Clinicopathologic features of Waldenstrom's macroglobulinemia and marginal zone lymphoma: are they distinct or the same entity? *Clin Lymphoma.* 2005;5(4):220-224.
84. Treon SP, Cao Y, Xu L, Yang G, Liu X, Hunter ZR. Somatic mutations in MYD88 and CXCR4 are determinants of clinical presentation and overall survival in Waldenstrom macroglobulinemia. *Blood.* 2014;123(18):2791-2796.
85. Rosado FG, Morice WG, He R, Howard MT, Timm M, McPhail ED. Immunophenotypic features by multiparameter flow cytometry can help distinguish low grade B-cell lymphomas with plasmacytic differentiation from plasma cell proliferative disorders with an unrelated clonal B-cell process. *Br J Haematol.* 2015;169(3):368-376.
86. Kanellis G, Mollejo M, Montes-Moreno S, et al. Splenic diffuse red pulp small B-cell lymphoma: revision of a series of cases reveals characteristic clinico-pathological features. *Haematologica.* 2010;95(7):1122-1129.
87. Shao H, Calvo KR, Gronborg M, et al. Distinguishing hairy cell leukemia variant from hairy cell leukemia: development and validation of diagnostic criteria. *Leuk Res.* 2013;37(4):401-409.
88. Demurtas A, Stacchini A, Aliberti S, Chiusa L, Chiarle R, Novero D. Tissue flow cytometry immunophenotyping in the diagnosis and classification of non-Hodgkin's lymphomas: a retrospective evaluation of 1,792 cases. *Cytometry B Clin Cytom.* 2013;84(2):82-95.
89. Mantei K, Wood BL. Flow cytometric evaluation of CD38 expression assists in distinguishing follicular hyperplasia from follicular lymphoma. *Cytometry B Clin Cytom.* 2009;76(5):315-320.
90. Maleki A, Seegmiller AC, Uddin N, Karandikar NJ, Chen W. Bright CD38 expression is an indicator of MYC rearrangement. *Leuk Lymphoma.* 2009;50(6):1054-1057.
91. Schniederjan SD, Li S, Saxe DF, et al. A novel flow cytometric antibody panel for distinguishing Burkitt lymphoma from CD10+ diffuse large B-cell lymphoma. *Am J Clin Pathol.* 2010;133(5):718-726.
92. Cardoso CC, Auat M, Santos-Pirath IM, et al. The importance of CD39, CD43, CD81, and CD95 expression for differentiating B cell lymphoma by flow cytometry. *Cytometry B Clin Cytom.* 2018;94:451-458.
93. Tsagarakis NJ, Papadhimitriou SI, Pavlidis D, et al. Contribution of immunophenotype to the investigation and differential diagnosis of Burkitt lymphoma, double-hit high-grade B-cell lymphoma, and single-hit MYC-rearranged diffuse large B-cell lymphoma. *Cytometry B Clin Cytom.* 2020;98(5):412-420.
94. Wu D, Wood BL, Dorer R, Fromm JR. "Double-Hit" mature B-cell lymphomas show a common immunophenotype by flow cytometry that includes decreased CD20 expression. *Am J Clin Pathol.* 2010;134(2):258-265.
95. Roth CG, Gillespie-Twardy A, Marks S, et al. Flow cytometric evaluation of double/triple hit lymphoma. *Oncol Res.* 2016;23(3):137-146.
96. Geyer JT, Subramaniyam S, Jiang Y, et al. Lymphoblastic transformation of follicular lymphoma: a clinicopathologic and molecular analysis of 7 patients. *Hum Pathol.* 2015;46(2):260-271.
97. Hans CP, Weisenburger DD, Greiner TC, et al. Confirmation of the molecular classification of diffuse large B-cell lymphoma by immunohistochemistry using a tissue microarray. *Blood.* 2004;103(1):275-282.
98. Alinari L, Gru A, Quinion C, et al. De novo CD5+ diffuse large B-cell lymphoma: adverse outcomes with and without stem cell transplantation in a large, multicenter, rituximab treated cohort. *Am J Hematol.* 2016;91(4):395-399.
99. Okamoto H, Uoshima N, Muramatsu A, et al. For kyoto clinical hematology study group investigators. Combination of bone marrow biopsy and flow cytometric analysis: the prognostically relevant central approach for detecting bone marrow invasion in diffuse large B-cell lymphoma. *Diagnostics (Basel).* 2021;11(9):1724.
100. Muñoz-García N, Lima M, Villamor N, et al. Anti-TRBC1 antibody-based flow cytometric detection of T-cell clonality: standardization of sample preparation and diagnostic implementation. *Cancers (Basel).* 2021;13(17):4379.
101. Lynne JE, Schmid I, Matud JL, et al. Major expansions of select CD8+ subsets in acute Epstein-Barr virus infection: comparison with chronic human immunodeficiency virus disease. *J Infect Dis.* 1998;177(4):1083-1087.
102. Strioga M, Pasukoniene V, Characiejus D. CD8+ CD28-and CD8+ CD57+ T cells and their role in health and disease. *Immunology.* 2011;134(1):17-32.
103. Chen X, Cherian S. Immunophenotypic characterization of T-cell prolymphocytic leukemia. *Am J Clin Pathol.* 2013;140(5):727-735.
104. Sud A, Dearden C. T-cell prolymphocytic leukemia. *Hematol Oncol Clin North Am.* 2017;31(2):273-283.
105. Kagdi HH, Demontis MA, Fields PA, Ramos JC, Bangham CR, Taylor GP. Risk stratification of adult T-cell leukemia/lymphoma using immunophenotyping. *Cancer Med.* 2017;6(1):298-309.
106. Horna P, Wang SA, Wolniak KL, et al. Flow cytometric evaluation of peripheral blood for suspected Sézary syndrome or mycosis fungoides: international guidelines for assay characteristics. *Cytometry B Clin Cytom.* 2021;100(2):142-155.
107. Loghavi S, Wang SA, Jeffrey Medeiros L, et al. Immunophenotypic and diagnostic characterization of angioimmunoblastic T-cell lymphoma by advanced flow cytometric technology. *Leuk Lymphoma.* 2016;57(12):2804-2812.
108. Lamy T, Loughran TP, Jr. How I treat LGL leukemia. *Blood.* 2011;117(10):2764-2774.
109. Morice WG. The immunophenotypic attributes of NK cells and NK-cell lineage lymphoproliferative disorders. *Am J Clin Pathol.* 2007;127(6):881-886.
110. Ruskova A, Thula R, Chan G. Aggressive natural killer-cell leukemia: report of five cases and review of the literature. *Leuk Lymphoma.* 2004;45(12):2427-2438.
111. Shi Y, Wang E. Hepatosplenic T-cell lymphoma: a clinicopathologic review with an emphasis on diagnostic differentiation from other T-cell/natural killer-cell neoplasms. *Arch Pathol Lab Med.* 2015;139(9):1173-1180.
112. Yabe M, Medeiros LJ, Wang SA, et al. Distinguishing between hepatosplenic T-cell lymphoma and gammadelta T-cell large granular lymphocytic leukemia: a clinicopathologic, immunophenotypic, and molecular analysis. *Am J Surg Pathol.* 2017;41(1):82-93.
113. Flores-Montero J, de Tute R, Paiva B, et al. Immunophenotype of normal vs. myeloma plasma cells: toward antibody panel specifications for MRD detection in multiple myeloma. *Cytometry B Clin Cytom.* 2016;90(1):61-72.
114. Stetler-Stevenson M, Paiva B, Stoolman L, et al. Consensus guidelines for myeloma minimal residual disease sample staining and data acquisition. *Cytometry B Clin Cytom.* 2016;90(1):26-30.
115. Munshi NC, Avet-Loiseau H, Rawstron AC, et al. Association of minimal residual disease with superior survival outcomes in patients with multiple myeloma: a meta-analysis. *JAMA Oncol.* 2017;3(1):28-35.
116. Lacombe F, Durrieu F, Briais A, et al. Flow cytometry CD45 gating for immunophenotyping of acute myeloid leukemia. *Leukemia.* 1997;11(11):1878-1886.

117. Porwit A, Béné MC. Multiparameter flow cytometry applications in the diagnosis of mixed phenotype acute leukemia. *Cytometry B Clin Cytom.* 2019;96(3):183-194.

118. Borowitz MJ. Mixed phenotype acute leukemia. *Cytometry B Clin Cytom.* 2014;86(3):152-153.

119. Bene MC, Castoldi G, Knapp W, et al. Proposals for the immunological classification of acute leukemias. European group for the immunological characterization of leukemias (EGIL). *Leukemia.* 1995;9(10):1783-1786.

120. Bene MC, Bernier M, Casasnovas RO, et al. Acute myeloid leukaemia M0 – haematological, immunophenotypic and cytogenetic characteristics and their prognostic significance: an analysis in 241 patients. *Br J Haematol.* 2001;113(3):737-745.

121. Deotare U, Yee KW, Le LW, et al. Blastic plasmacytoid dendritic cell neoplasm with leukemic presentation: 10-Color flow cytometry diagnosis and HyperCVAD therapy. *Am J Hematol.* 2016;91(3):283-286.

122. Hrusak O, Porwit-MacDonald A. Antigen expression patterns reflecting genotype of acute leukemias. *Leukemia.* 2002;16(7):1233-1258.

123. van Solinge TS, Zeijlemaker W, Ossenkoppele GJ, Cloos J, Schuurhuis GJ. The interference of genetic associations in establishing the prognostic value of the immunophenotype in acute myeloid leukemia. *Cytometry B Clin Cytom.* 2018;94(1):151-158.

124. Peters JM, Ansari MQ. Multiparameter flow cytometry in the diagnosis and management of acute leukemia. *Arch Pathol Lab Med.* 2011;135(1):44-54.

125. Zhou Y, Wood BL. Methods of detection of measurable residual disease in AML. *Curr Hematol Malig Rep.* 2017;12(6):557-567.

126. Schuurhuis GJ, Heuser M, Freeman S, et al. Minimal/measurable residual disease in AML: a consensus document from the European LeukemiaNet MRD Working Party. *Blood.* 2018;131(12):1275-1291.

127. Chen X, Cherian S. Role of minimal residual disease testing in acute myeloid leukemia. *Clin Lab Med.* 2021;41(3):467-483.

128. Pilozzi E, Pulford K, Jones M, et al. Co-expression of CD79a (JCB117) and CD3 by lymphoblastic lymphoma. *J Pathol.* 1998;186(2):140-143.

129. Coustan-Smith E, Mullighan CG, Onciu M, et al. Early T-cell precursor leukaemia: a subtype of very high-risk acute lymphoblastic leukaemia. *Lancet Oncol.* 2009;10(2):147-156.

130. Campana D, Pui CH. Minimal residual disease-guided therapy in childhood acute lymphoblastic leukemia. *Blood.* 2017;129(14):1913-1918.

131. Gaipa G, Basso G, Aliprandi S, et al. Prednisone induces immunophenotypic modulation of CD10 and CD34 in nonapoptotic B-cell precursor acute lymphoblastic leukemia cells. *Cytometry B Clin Cytom.* 2008;74(3):150-155.

132. Malcovati L, Hellstrom-Lindberg E, Bowen D, et al. Diagnosis and treatment of primary myelodysplastic syndromes in adults: recommendations from the European LeukemiaNet. *Blood.* 2013;122(17):2943-2964.

133. Arber DA, Hasserjian RP. Reclassifying myelodysplastic syndromes: what's where in the new WHO and why. *Hematol Am Soc Hematol Educ Program.* 2015;2015:294-298.

134. Porwit A, van de Loosdrecht AA, Bettelheim P, et al. Revisiting guidelines for integration of flow cytometry results in the WHO classification of myelodysplastic syndromes-proposal from the International/European LeukemiaNet Working Group for Flow Cytometry in MDS. *Leukemia.* 2014;28(9):1793-1798.

135. van de Loosdrecht AA, Alhan C, Bene MC, et al. Standardization of flow cytometry in myelodysplastic syndromes: report from the first European LeukemiaNet working conference on flow cytometry in myelodysplastic syndromes. *Haematologica.* 2009;94(8):1124-1134.

136. van de Loosdrecht AA, Ireland R, Kern W, et al. Rationale for the clinical application of flow cytometry in patients with myelodysplastic syndromes: position paper of an International Consortium and the European LeukemiaNet Working Group. *Leuk Lymphoma.* 2013;54(3):472-475.

137. Westers TM, Ireland R, Kern W, et al. Standardization of flow cytometry in myelodysplastic syndromes: a report from an international consortium and the European LeukemiaNet Working Group. *Leukemia.* 2012;26(7):1730-1741.

138. Della Porta MG, Picone C, Pascutto C, et al. Multicenter validation of a reproducible flow cytometric score for the diagnosis of low-grade myelodysplastic syndromes: results of a European LeukemiaNET study. *Haematologica.* 2012;97(8):1209-1217.

139. Kern W, Haferlach C, Schnittger S, Haferlach T. Clinical utility of multiparameter flow cytometry in the diagnosis of 1013 patients with suspected myelodysplastic syndrome: correlation to cytomorphology, cytogenetics, and clinical data. *Cancer.* 2010;116(19):4549-4563.

140. Porwit A. Is there a role for flow cytometry in the evaluation of patients with myelodysplastic syndromes? *Curr Hematol Malig Rep.* 2015;10(3):309-317.

141. van de Loosdrecht AA, Westers TM. Cutting edge: flow cytometry in myelodysplastic syndromes. *J Natl Compr Cancer Netw.* 2013;11(7):892-902.

142. Alhan C, Westers TM, van der Helm LH, et al. Absence of aberrant myeloid progenitors by flow cytometry is associated with favorable response to azacitidine in higher risk myelodysplastic syndromes. *Cytometry B Clin Cytom.* 2014;86(3):207-215.

143. Truong F, Smith BR, Stachurski D, et al. The utility of flow cytometric immunophenotyping in cytopenic patients with a non-diagnostic bone marrow: a prospective study. *Leukemia Res.* 2009;33(8):1039-1046.

144. Xu Y, McKenna RW, Karandikar NJ, Pildain AJ, Kroft SH. Flow cytometric analysis of monocytes as a tool for distinguishing chronic myelomonocytic leukemia from reactive monocytosis. *Am J Clin Pathol.* 2005;124(5):799-806.

145. Selimoglu-Buet D, Wagner-Ballon O, Saada V, et al. Characteristic repartition of monocyte subsets as a diagnostic signature of chronic myelomonocytic leukemia. *Blood.* 2015;125(23):3618-3626.

146. Westers TM, Cremers EM, Oelschlaegel U, et al. Immunophenotypic analysis of erythroid dysplasia in myelodysplastic syndromes. A report from the IMDSFlow working group. *Haematologica.* 2017;102(2):308-319.

147. Lanza F, Bi S, Castoldi G, Goldman JM. Abnormal expression of N-CAM (CD56) adhesion molecule on myeloid and progenitor cells from chronic myeloid leukemia. *Leukemia.* 1993;7(10):1570-1575.

148. Carulli G, Gianfaldoni ML, Azzara A, et al. FcRIII (CD16) expression on neutrophils from chronic myeloid leukemia. A flow cytometric study. *Leuk Res.* 1992;16(12):1203-1209.

149. Martin-Henao GA, Quiroga R, Sureda A, Gonzalez JR, Moreno V, Garcia J. L-selectin expression is low on CD34+ cells from patients with chronic myeloid leukemia and interferon-a up-regulates this expression. *Haematologica.* 2000;85(2):139-146.

150. Ouyang J, Zheng W, Shen Q, et al. Flow cytometry immunophenotypic analysis of Philadelphia-negative myeloproliferative neoplasms: correlation with histopathologic features. *Cytometry B Clin Cytom.* 2015;88(4):236-243.

151. Sutherland DR, Kuek N, Davidson J, et al. Diagnosing PNH with FLAER and multiparameter flow cytometry. *Cytometry B Clin Cytom.* 2007;72(3):167-177.

152. Borowitz MJ, Craig FE, Digiuseppe JA, et al. Guidelines for the diagnosis and monitoring of paroxysmal nocturnal hemoglobinuria and related disorders by flow cytometry. *Cytometry B Clin Cytom.* 2010;78(4):211-230.

153. Sutherland DR, Illingworth A, Keeney M, Richards SJ. High-sensitivity detection of PNH red blood cells, red cell precursors, and white blood cells. *Curr Protoc Cytom.* 2015;72:6.37.1-6.37.30.

154. Chesney A, Good D, Reis M. Clinical utility of flow cytometry in the study of erythropoiesis and nonclonal red cell disorders. *Methods Cell Biol.* 2011;103:311-332.

155. Buttarello M. Laboratory diagnosis of anemia: are the old and new red cell parameters useful in classification and treatment, how?. *Int J Lab Hematol.* 2016;38(suppl 1):123-132.

156. Buttarello M, Rauli A, Mezzapelle G. Reticulocyte count and extended reticulocyte parameters by Mindray BC-6800: reference intervals and comparison with Sysmex XE-5000. *Int J Lab Hematol.* 2017;39(6):596-603.

157. Farias MG, Dal Bo S, Castro SM, et al. Flow cytometry in detection of fetal red blood cells and maternal f cells to identify fetomaternal hemorrhage. *Fetal Pediatr Pathol.* 2016;35(6):385-391.

158. Othman J, Orellana D, Chen LS, Russell M, Khoo TL. The presence of F cells with a fetal phenotype in adults with hemoglobinopathies limits the utility of flow cytometry for quantitation of fetomaternal hemorrhage. *Cytometry B Clin Cytom.* 2018;94(4):695-698.

159. Linden MD. Platelet flow cytometry. *Methods Mol Biol.* 2013;992:241-262.

160. Cai H, Mullier F, Frotscher B, et al. Usefulness of flow cytometric mepacrine uptake/release combined with CD63 assay in diagnosis of patients with suspected platelet dense granule disorder. *Semin Thromb Hemost.* 2016;42(3):282-291.

161. Lehmann M, Ashworth K, Manco-Johnson M, Di Paola J, Neeves KB, Ng CJ. Evaluation of a microfluidic flow assay to screen for von Willebrand disease and low von Willebrand factor levels. *J Thromb Haemost.* 2018;16(1):104-115.

162. Ibrahim H, Nadipalli S, Usmani S, DeLao T, Green L, Kleiman NS. Detection and quantification of circulating immature platelets: agreement between flow cytometric and automated detection. *J Thromb Thrombolysis.* 2016;42(1):77-83.

163. Busuttil-Crellin X, McCafferty C, Van Den Helm S, et al. Guidelines for panel design, optimization, and performance of whole blood multi-color flow cytometry of platelet surface markers. *Platelets.* 2020;31(7):845-852.

164. Favaloro EJ. Laboratory tests for identification or exclusion of heparin induced thrombocytopenia: HIT or miss? *Am J Hematol.* 2018;93(2):308-314.

165. Kerenyi A, Beke Debreceni I, Olah Z, et al. Evaluation of flow cytometric HIT assays in relation to an IgG-Specific immunoassay and clinical outcome. *Cytometry B Clin Cytom.* 2017;92(5):389-397.

166. Sutherland DR, Anderson L, Keeney M, Nayar R, Chin-Yee I. The ISHAGE guidelines for CD34+ cell determination by flow cytometry. International Society of Hematotherapy and Graft Engineering. *J Hematother.* 1996;5(3):213-226.

167. Sutherland DR, Nayyar R, Acton E, Giftakis A, Dean S, Mosiman VL. Comparison of two single-platform ISHAGE-based CD34 enumeration protocols on BD FACSCalibur and FACSCanto flow cytometers. *Cytotherapy.* 2009;11(5):595-605.

168. Whitby A, Whitby L, Fletcher M, et al. ISHAGE protocol: are we doing it correctly? *Cytometry B Clin Cytom.* 2012;82(1):9-17.

169. Mariani M, Colombo F, Assennato SM, et al. Evaluation of an easy and affordable flow cytometer for volumetric haematopoietic stem cell counting. *Blood Transfus.* 2014;12(3):416-420.

170. Bray RA, Tarsitani C, Gebel HM, Lee JH. Clinical cytometry and progress in HLA antibody detection. *Methods Cell Biol.* 2011;103:285-310.

171. Reed EF, Rao P, Zhang Z, et al. Comprehensive assessment and standardization of solid phase multiplex-bead arrays for the detection of antibodies to HLA-drilling down on key sources of variation. *Am J Transplant.* 2013;13(11):3050-3051.

172. Liwski RS, Greenshields AL, Conrad DM, et al. Rapid optimized flow cytometric crossmatch (FCXM) assays: the Halifax and Halifaster protocols. *Hum Immunol.* 2018;79(1):28-38.

173. Picard C, Al-Herz W, Bousfiha A, et al. Primary immunodeficiency diseases: an update on the classification from the international union of immunological societies expert committee for primary immunodeficiency 2015. *J Clin Immunol.* 2015;35(8):696-726.

174. O'Gorman MRG. Flow cytometry assays in primary immunodeficiency diseases. *Methods Mol Biol.* 2018;1678:321-345.

175. Garg N, van den Bosch F, Deodhar A. The concept of spondyloarthritis: where are we now? *Best Pract Res Clin Rheumatol.* 2014;28(5):663-672.

176. Darke C, Coates E. One-tube HLA-B27/B2708 typing by flow cytometry using two "Anti-HLA-B27" monoclonal antibody reagents. *Cytometry B Clin Cytom.* 2010;78(1):21-30.

177. Skalska U, Kozakiewicz A, Maslinski W, Jurkowska M. HLA-B27 detection-comparison of genetic sequence-based method and flow cytometry assay. *Reumatologia.* 2015;53(2):74-78.

178. Crowell TA, Colby DJ, Pinyakorn S, et al. Acute retroviral syndrome is associated with high viral burden, CD4 depletion, and immune activation in systemic and tissue compartments. *Clin Infect Dis.* 2018;66(10):1540-1549.

179. Kestens L, Mandy F. Thirty-five years of CD4 T-cell counting in HIV infection: from flow cytometry in the lab to point-of-care testing in the field. *Cytometry B Clin Cytom.* 2017;92(6):437-444.

180. Desai MA, Okal DO, Rose CE, et al. Effect of point-of-care CD4 cell count results on linkage to care and antiretroviral initiation during a home-based HIV testing campaign: a non-blinded, cluster-randomised trial. *Lancet HIV.* 2017;4(9):e393-e401.

181. *WHO Guidelines Approved by the Guidelines Review Committee. Consolidated Guidelines on the Use of Antiretroviral Drugs for Treating and Preventing HIV Infection: Recommendations for a Public Health Approach.* 2nd ed. World Health Organization; 2016.

182. Sims S, Willberg C, Klenerman P. MHC-peptide tetramers for the analysis of antigen-specific T cells. *Expert Rev Vaccines.* 2010;9(7):765-774.

183. Meeuwsen MH, Wouters AK, Jahn L, et al. A broad and systematic approach to identify B cell malignancy-targeting TCRs for multi-antigen-based T cell therapy. *Mol Ther.* 2021;S1525-0016(21):00404-4.

184. Darzynkiewicz Z, Halicka HD, Zhao H. Analysis of cellular DNA content by flow and laser scanning cytometry. *Adv Exp Med Biol.* 2010;676:137-147.

185. Darzynkiewicz Z, Huang X, Zhao H. Analysis of cellular DNA content by flow cytometry. *Curr Protoc Immunol.* 2017;119:5.7.1-5.7.20.

186. Safavi S, Paulsson K. Near-haploid and low-hypodiploid acute lymphoblastic leukemia: two distinct subtypes with consistently poor prognosis. *Blood.* 2017;129(4):420-423.

187. Mateos MV, Gutierrez NC, Martin-Ramos ML, et al. Outcome according to cytogenetic abnormalities and DNA ploidy in myeloma patients receiving short induction with weekly bortezomib followed by maintenance. *Blood.* 2011;118(17):4547-4553.

188. Sawyer JR, Tian E, Shaughnessy JD, Jr, et al. Hyperhaploidy is a novel high-risk cytogenetic subgroup in multiple myeloma. *Leukemia.* 2017;31(3):637-644.

189. Darzynkiewicz Z, Traganos F, Zhao H, Halicka HD, Li J. Cytometry of DNA replication and RNA synthesis: historical perspective and recent advances based on "click chemistry". *Cytometry A.* 2011;79(5):328-337.

190. Lovelace P, Maecker HT. Multiparameter intracellular cytokine staining. *Methods Mol Biol.* 2018;1678:151-166.

191. Kordasti S, Marsh J, Al-Khan S, et al. Functional characterization of CD4+ T cells in aplastic anemia. *Blood.* 2012;119(9):2033-2043.

192. Feng X, Scheinberg P, Wu CO, et al. Cytokine signature profiles in acquired aplastic anemia and myelodysplastic syndromes. *Haematologica.* 2011;96(4):602-606.

193. Mellgren K, Hedegaard CJ, Schmiegelow K, Muller K. Plasma cytokine profiles at diagnosis in pediatric patients with non-Hodgkin lymphoma. *J Pediatr Hematol Oncol.* 2012;34(4):271-275.

194. Hedley DW, Chow S, Shankey TV. Cytometry of intracellular signaling: from laboratory bench to clinical application. *Methods Cell Biol.* 2011;103:203-220.

195. Marsman C, Jorritsma T, Ten Brinke A, van Ham SM. Flow cytometric methods for the detection of intracellular signaling proteins and transcription factors reveal heterogeneity in differentiating human B cell subsets. *Cells.* 2020;9(12):2633.

196. Wu S, Jin L, Vence L, Radvanyi LG. Development and application of 'phosphoflow' as a tool for immunomonitoring. *Expert Rev Vaccines.* 2010;9(6):631-643.

197. Telford WG. Multiparametric analysis of apoptosis by flow cytometry. *Methods Mol Biol.* 2018;1678:167-202.

198. Karlic H, Herrmann H, Varga F, et al. The role of epigenetics in the regulation of apoptosis in myelodysplastic syndromes and acute myeloid leukemia. *Crit Rev Oncol Hematol.* 2014;90(1):1-16.

Laboratory Hematology

Chapter 3 ■ Cytogenetics

PATRICIA T. GREIPP • JESS F. PETERSON • LINDA B. BAUGHN • MIN FANG

INTRODUCTION

Cytogenetics is the study of chromosome structure and function. The field of cytogenetics has evolved significantly over the past 60 years. From conventional chromosome analysis by karyotype to fluorescence in situ hybridization (FISH), to chromosomal microarray analysis (CMA), each technique today plays a critical role in the diagnosis and prognostic risk stratification of hematologic malignancies. An increasing number of disease entities catalogued in the *World Health Organization Classification of Tumours of Haematopoietic and Lymphoid Tissues*[1-3] are defined by chromosomal abnormalities. Research into recurrent chromosomal abnormalities has been integral to the identification of genes important in malignant transformation, and extension of this investigation has yielded promise for targeted therapies.

This chapter focuses on the evolution and application of cytogenetic techniques as well as the nomenclature system utilized in the interpretation of cytogenetic testing. Recurrent cytogenetic rearrangements that occur in specific hematologic malignancies are detailed in corresponding chapters.

HISTORY

The association of mitotic aberrancies in the nucleus with malignancy was made in 1890 by von Hansemann.[4] The proposal that chromosomal abnormalities served as the basis for the change from normal cell division to malignant growth, driven by what is now known as a clonal population of cells, was made by Boveri in 1914 in the landmark publication "The Origin of Malignant Tumors."[5] Painter's analysis of testicular tissue in paraffin-embedded specimens in the early 1920s led to the description of the Y chromosome and a proposal that the number of chromosomes in human cells was 48.[6] Ultimately, Tjio and Levan in 1956 pioneered cell culturing techniques achieving mitotic arrest utilizing colchicine and utilizing hypotonic solution to improve spreading of metaphases which helped lead to the understanding that the human diploid chromosome number was actually 46.[7] Levan and Van Steenis went on in 1966 to describe nonrandom chromosome gains and losses in a series of human tumors, which became the basis for the important role of karyotyping in cancer genetics.[8,9] Emerging theories on the role of chromosome abnormalities in oncogenesis in the 1970s and 1980s included Knudson's two-hit mutational hypothesis leading to cancer[10] and the description by Sandberg[11] of chromosomal breakage leading to translocations, inversions, insertions, and deletions as the origin of cancer.[10] A model of carcinogenesis was described by Weinberg in 1989 as a series of oncogenic events leading to the malignant phenotype.[12]

The distinction for the etiology of chromosomal abnormalities as germline (constitutional), occurring in every cell of the body, or acquired (somatic), occurring only in a neoplastic clone, began with the description of constitutional trisomy 21 and its association with Down syndrome by Lejeune in 1959.[13] Nowell and Hungerford[14] in 1960, still utilizing unbanded chromosome analysis techniques, identified the first structural chromosomal abnormality, specific for a type of cancer, when they described the small "Philadelphia" chromosome (so-called Ph chromosome or Ph+) and its association with chronic myeloid leukemia (CML) (*Figure 3.1*). It wasn't until 1973 with the use of chromosome banding techniques that Janet Rowley[15] characterized the origin of the Philadelphia chromosome as a balanced reciprocal translocation between the long arms of chromosomes 9 and 22 (*Figure 3.2*). The breakpoint on chromosome 9 was determined to be 9q34 involving the *ABL1* locus, and the breakpoint on chromosome

22 is 22q11.2 involving the *BCR* locus which is now known to lead to the formation of a chimeric fusion protein (*Figure 3.3*). The resulting upregulation of tyrosine kinase activity leads to increased cell division in the clonal cell.[16] Targeted therapy directed against the increased tyrosine kinase activity by imatinib revolutionized the treatment of patients with CML[17] and has paved the way for ongoing discoveries in cytogenetics that are leading to other targeted approaches to treating cancer.

CYTOGENETIC METHODS FOR ANALYSIS OF HEMATOLOGIC MALIGNANCIES

Specimens

The ideal specimens for hematologic cytogenetic analysis are 2 to 3 mL of bone marrow aspirate or 5 to 10 mL of peripheral blood, which are typically collected in a sodium heparin tube and should be transferred to the laboratory in ambient temperature within 24 hours. However, upon receipt into the laboratory, specimens are commonly split to perform concurrent molecular testing, such as reverse transcription polymerase chain reaction, for which heparin is not ideal.

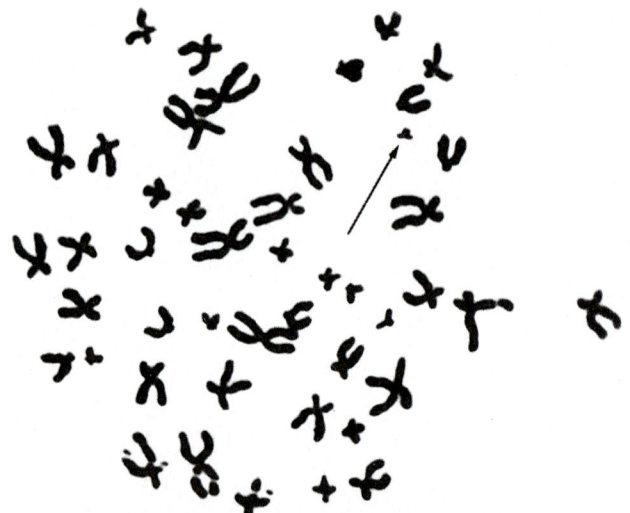

FIGURE 3.1 An unbanded metaphase spread from bone marrow cells of a patient with chronic myeloid leukemia depicting the Ph chromosome. Arrow indicates the Philadelphia chromosome (Ph chromosome).

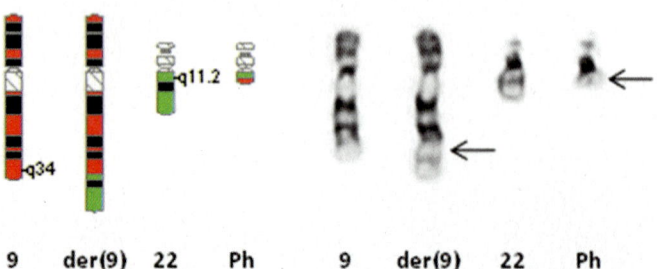

9   der(9)   22   Ph   9   der(9)   22   Ph

FIGURE 3.2 Illustration of t(9;22) observed in chronic myeloid leukemia and B-cell acute lymphoblastic leukemia/lymphoma. Ideogram of chromosomes 9 and 22 on left with partial karyogram on right. Arrows indicate breakpoints.

INTERPHASE FUSION FISH: *BCR::ABL1*

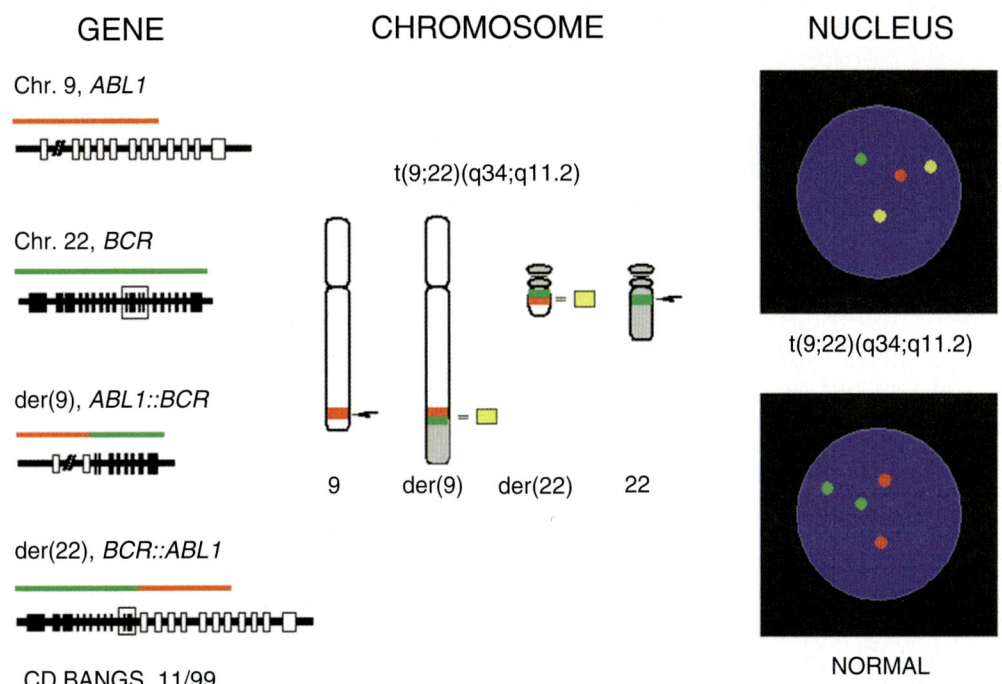

GENE   CHROMOSOME   NUCLEUS

Chr. 9, *ABL1*

Chr. 22, *BCR*

der(9), *ABL1::BCR*

der(22), *BCR::ABL1*

CD BANGS, 11/99

t(9;22)(q34;q11.2)

9   der(9)   der(22)   22

t(9;22)(q34;q11.2)

NORMAL

FIGURE 3.3 Fluorescence in situ hybridization (FISH) illustration of t(9;22) with red-labeled *ABL1* probe spanning the breakpoint at 9q24, and green-labeled *BCR* probe spanning the breakpoint at 22q11.2. At right, nuclei showing abnormal and normal signal pattern with yellow fusions indicating *BCR::ABL1*.

Therefore, tubes containing acid-citrate-dextrose are increasingly being utilized to collect specimens to meet the needs of both cytogenetic assays and molecular testing. Other specimens can also be analyzed by cytogenetic methods. With special preparation, mitotic cells can be cultured from bone core specimens. Lymph node tissue can be transported in normal saline-RPMI transport media or Ringer's solution with antibiotics and, upon arrival into the laboratory, can be minced to form a cell suspension.

The different cytogenetic analysis methods require different specimen preparation and are described in the corresponding sections of this chapter (*Table 3.1*). In general, once a specimen is accessioned into the laboratory, sample processing should not be delayed. Each of the hematologic specimens described here contains dividing cells that can be cultured (without mitogenic stimulation) to produce metaphase spreads for banded chromosome analysis (karyotype analysis) or analyzed by direct methods to analyze interphase nuclei by FISH or DNA can be extracted for CMA. If transportation is prolonged or processing is delayed, the viability of malignant cells (particularly B-lymphoblasts) can be compromised, and overgrowth of normal myeloid cells can hinder the detection of chromosomal abnormalities driving a hematologic malignancy.

Karyotype Analysis

Karyotype analysis can be performed on numerous types of dividing tissue and can help to render diagnoses for constitutional (germline) chromosome conditions (i.e., trisomy 21), as well as acquired (somatic) chromosomal abnormalities associated with different types of malignancies. Karyotype analysis is an essential part, particularly for the diagnostic workup of acute leukemia, per the joint guidelines developed by the College of American Pathologists and the American Society of Hematology and endorsed by the American Society of Clinical Oncology.[18,19] Chromosome analysis requires living, dividing cells that are arrested in metaphase using a substance that inhibits spindle fiber formation during mitosis (e.g., Colcemid, Velban). Typically, specimens from patients suspected with a hematologic malignancy are placed into short-term unstimulated cell suspension cultures (direct, 24-, 48-, or 72-hours). This process is distinct from the preparation of a specimen for constitutional analysis, which involves the stimulation of T-cells by a mitogen such as phytohemagglutinin (PHA). In each case, after arrest in metaphase is achieved, the cells are then "harvested" using a hypotonic solution (sodium chloride or sodium citrate) and fixed using a mixture of methanol and acetic acid. Slides are made by dropping the cell suspension on the slides and drying or "aging" them in optimal humidity and temperature conditions. The slides are aged and then banded using trypsin (or pepsin) and Giemsa (or Wright or Leishman) stain. This produces the G-banding (or reverse; R-banded) pattern, or the classic dark and light bands on the individual pairs of chromosomes, which can be analyzed comparatively for abnormalities under a microscope (*Figure 3.4*). Each of the autosomes (chromosome pairs 1-22) and sex chromosomes (X and Y) has classic banding patterns recognizable by specially trained personnel. Banded metaphases are identified and analyzed using a light microscope equipped with high-resolution objectives (typically ×10 oculars, with ×63 or ×100 objectives, enlarged up to 1000× their normal size). Images then are acquired using a charge-coupled device camera, and a computer software application is utilized by the technologist to create the karyogram, which represents the chromosomal content of an individual cell.

Karyotype analysis for hematologic neoplasia evaluation requires complete analysis of a minimum of 20 metaphase spreads from two or more primary cultures if possible with the production of a minimum of two karyograms, including one for each clone and subclone.[20] Technologists (or automated imaging systems) scan the slides looking for abnormal metaphases. Normal metaphases are typically present on the slide, and it is often the poorer-quality metaphases that contain cytogenetic abnormalities that represent the malignant clone. Chromosomes are counted to detect for numeric abnormalities (trisomies or monosomies) and chromosome pairs are analyzed: by matching band by band, assessing for structural abnormalities, such as translocations, deletions, and insertions. Clonal abnormalities are described and documented. Clonal anomalies are defined as two or

Table 3.1. Comparison of Cytogenetic Analysis Methods

Methodology	Detectable Abnormalities	Undetectable Abnormalities	Additional Notes
Karyotype analysis	1. Aneusomies, CNVs (>5 ~ 10 Mb) 2. Balanced and unbalanced rearrangements, 3. Primary clone(s) and/or subclones	1. CNVs (<5 Mb) 2. cnLOH 3. Cryptic gene rearrangements	Provides a low-resolution, whole-genome view of single metaphase(s). Typically performed on peripheral blood, bone marrow aspirates, and/or lymph node specimens. Requires living cells.
FISH	1. Aneusomies 2. CNVs (>30,000 kb) 3. Balanced and unbalanced chromosomal rearrangements 4. Cryptic gene rearrangements not visible by CCA	1. Chromosomal abnormalities not targeted by FISH probes 2. Elucidating some structural abnormalities by interphase-nuclei analysis 3. cnLOH	Provides a targeted evaluation for the detection of recurrent chromosomal abnormalities in hematologic neoplasms. Can perform on a variety of specimen types. Does NOT require living cells. Quick TAT.
Chromosomal microarray analysis	1. Aneusomies 2. CNVs (>5 ~ 10 kb) 3. Unbalanced chromosomal rearrangements 4. cnLOH	1. Balanced rearrangements 2. Elucidating some structural abnormalities 3. Low-level clones and/or subclones (<15% ~ 20% of neoplastic cells)	Provides a high-resolution, whole-genome view of the genome. Does NOT require living cells.
NGS (MPseq and OGM)	1. Aneusomies 2. CNVs (>5 ~ 10 kb) 3. Unbalanced chromosomal rearrangements 4. cnLOH	1. SNVs 2. Low-level clones and/or subclones (<15% ~ 20% of neoplastic cells)	
NGS (long-read or long-insert WGS)	1. Aneusomies 2. CNVs (>5 ~ 10 kb) 3. Unbalanced chromosomal rearrangements 4. cnLOH 5. SNVs	1. Low-level clones and/or subclones (<15% ~ 20% of neoplastic cells)	

Abbreviations: CCA, conventional chromosome analysis; cnLOH, copy-neutral loss of heterozygosity; CNV, copy number variant; FISH, fluorescence in situ hybridization; MPseq, mate pair sequencing; NGS, next-generation sequencing; OGM, optical genome mapping; SNV, single nucleotide variants; TAT, turnaround time; WGS, whole-genome sequencing.

more cells with the same structural abnormality or same additional chromosome (trisomy), whereas loss of a chromosome (monosomy) must be observed in three or more cells to be considered clonal.[21] Karyograms are then generated as both an analytical and a documentary tool, and the chromosome analysis interpretation is formulated and reported by the laboratory.

CYTOGENETIC NOMENCLATURE

It is important for the hematopathologist to have a basic understanding of cytogenetic nomenclature, because they often are asked to incorporate these data into an integrated or comprehensive report, including all clinical laboratory analytic data on individuals with hematologic malignancies (i.e., flow cytometry, molecular and cytogenetic analytic data). The International System for Human Cytogenomic Nomenclature (ISCN)[22] is the accepted method of describing the karyotype of an individual or tumor (*Table 3.2*). There are very specific rules for how this information is presented. This is the internationally accepted cytogenetic language that, using alpha/numeric/symbolic string text, allows one laboratory to describe what was observed in the karyotype and another laboratory to understand what that means. Every few years, this system of nomenclature is updated. The most recent update was in 2020. ISCN first came into existence in 1978; however, there were several conferences held from 1960 until then to codify the human karyotype, with banded ideograms first introduced in 1971. An ideogram is a scientific illustration of the light and dark bands, sub-bands, and sub-sub-bands observed by metaphase chromosome analysis. Each chromosome has its own particular set of recognized bands, which allows it to be identified as such (*Figure 3.5*). For instance, all human chromosome #1s look very similar to one another, having the same pattern of light and dark bands, with the exception of a known variant region near the centromere. Chromosomes are divided into short arm and long arm by the centromere or primary constriction, which mediates attachment to the spindle fiber apparatus in mitosis. Bands in the short arm are labeled "p," whereas bands in the long arm are labeled "q." Each chromosome arm has landmark bands, which demarcate the regions of the chromosome arm (this is the first number indicated after the p or q designation). These regions are then divided into bands, and possibly sub-bands or sub-sub-bands. Bands are numbered in an increasing order starting at the centromere and proceeding toward the end of the chromosome arm (or telomere). The total number of chromosomes observed is stated first, with the sex chromosome designation given following a comma. There are normally no spaces between the numbers, letters, and punctuations that make up the karyotype designation. As an example, a female patient with the Philadelphia chromosome would have a karyotype written as "46,XX,t(9;22)(q34;q11.2)[18]/46,XX[2]," meaning that she has the Ph or t(9;22) in 18 of her metaphases (18 in []), a slash designating a second normal cell line with 46,XX (or normal chromosomes) in two metaphases (2 in []). The breakpoint in chromosome #9 is at band 9q34 (long arm or q arm, region 3, band 4 or band three four, not thirty-four), and the breakpoint in chromosome #22 is at sub-band 22q11.2 (long arm or q arm, region 1, band 1, sub-band .2 or band one one point two, not eleven point two). There are rules as well for describing both interphase and metaphase FISH.

FLUORESCENCE IN SITU HYBRIDIZATION ANALYSIS

In situ hybridization was first described by Gall and Pardue in 1969[23] when they hybridized radioactively labeled probes to highly repetitive sequences in mouse and *Drosophila*. In 1981, Harper and Saunders[24] used a similar technique using tritiated (^{3}H) nucleotides to label probes and autoradiographic methods to map human genes. Also in 1981, Langer et al[25] introduced biotin-labeled probes for gene mapping purposes, which could be detected with streptavidin-conjugated antibodies that had been fluorescently tagged. In 1988, Pinkel et al[26] described chromosome painting probes, while Kallioniemi et al[27] in 1992 introduced comparative genome hybridization (CGH) using metaphase chromosomes as the interrogator.

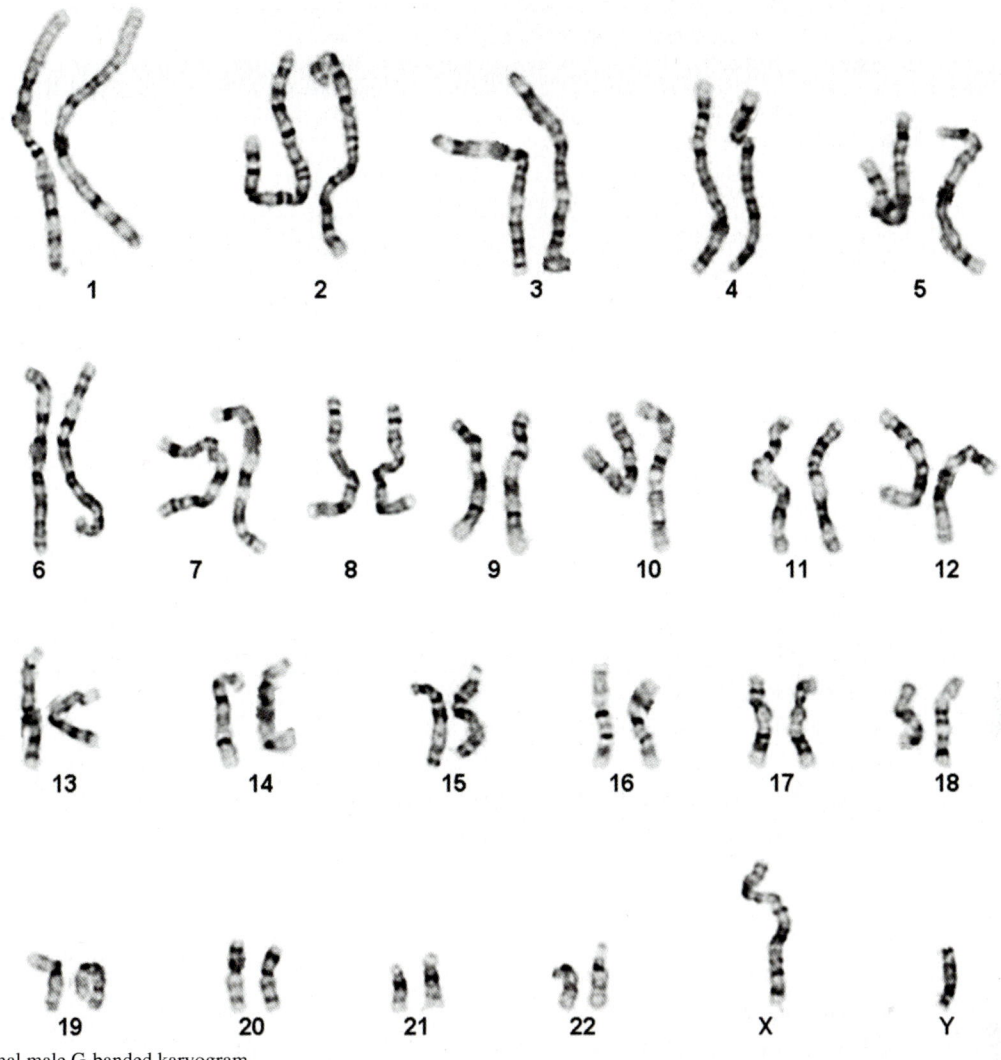

FIGURE 3.4 Normal male G-banded karyogram.

In situ hybridization takes advantage of the genetic code, the complementary strands of DNA, and their unique, as well as repetitive, sequences. Probes are designed with a particular DNA sequence in mind. These probes are labeled so that they can be detectable once they have hybridized to the DNA. Target DNA, in the form of metaphase chromosomes or interphase nuclei, is denatured, as is the DNA probe, using formamide, heat, and salt. The slide/DNA is then reannealed so that the DNA probe can hybridize to its complementary target DNA sequence. After hybridization is complete (from a few hours to overnight), the slides are washed and counterstained, and the hybridization is visualized. In this manner, questions of loss, gain, or juxtapositioning of target sequences can be answered.

Most DNA probes used for in situ hybridization are directly labeled with fluorochromes and visualized using a fluorescent microscope and the proper filter sets, once the hybridization has taken place. FISH probes can be single-copy probes, unique sequence probes, or repetitive probes. Whole-chromosome paint probes and spectral karyotyping are no longer used clinically. Single-copy probes can be used to determine copy number (gain or loss) of a single locus or specific chromosome or can be designed in combination to detect gene rearrangements (dual-color, dual-fusion probe sets to detect specific gene fusions, or break-apart probe sets to detect a specific gene rearrangements). Single-copy probes can also be used to detect amplification of a locus, such as the *RUNX1* gene region (intrachromosomal amplification of chromosome 21 or iAMP21) observed in B-cell acute lymphoblastic leukemia/lymphoma. Repetitive probes can also

be used primarily for chromosome enumeration. These are typically chromosome-specific alpha satellite repeats (e.g., DXZ1 and DYZ3 located at the centromeres of the X and Y chromosomes, respectively).

For hematologic neoplasms, FISH is commonly offered as disease-specific panels that are mainly performed on, but not limited to, bone marrow aspirates, peripheral bloods, and/or formalin-fixed paraffin-embedded (FFPE) tissue specimens. Unlike conventional chromosome studies, FISH can be performed on fresh or aged specimens (does not require living cells) and can provide clinicians with results within 24 hours of specimen receipt. In addition, FISH can achieve greater analytic sensitivity compared to karyotype analysis by evaluating significantly more cells (typically at least 100 nuclei for interphase FISH). Limitations of FISH analysis include the inability to detect chromosomal abnormalities not targeted by FISH probes (including loss of heterozygosity [LOH]), the inability to further characterize some structural abnormalities (when evaluating interphase nuclei), and artifacts introduced via sectioning through nuclei when evaluating fresh or FFPE tissue specimens.

FLUORESCENCE IN SITU HYBRIDIZATION NOMENCLATURE

FISH nomenclature has also been established by the ISCN.[22] FISH can be of either metaphase chromosomes or interphase nuclei. Both have different nomenclature rules. Metaphase FISH is always

Table 3.2. Frequently Used ISCN Symbols and Abbreviated Terms

Symbol/Term	Interpretation
add	Additional material of unknown origin. Unknown material that replaces a chromosome segment may result in increase or decrease in the length of the chromosome arm.
Approximate sign (~)	Denotes intervals and boundaries of a chromosome segment or number of chromosomes, fragments, or markers; also used to denote a range of number of copies of a chromosome region
arr	Chromosomal microarray, array
Brackets, angle (<>)	Surround the ploidy level
Brackets, square ([])	Surround the number of cells
c	Constitutional anomaly
chr	Chromosome
Comma (,)	Separates chromosome number, sex chromosomes, and chromosome abnormalities
con	Connected signals in interphase FISH
cp	Composite karyotype; cp[20]. Karyotype contains many heterogeneous clonal abnormalities among 20 metaphases analyzed. Chromosome number may be given as a range.
Cth	Chromothripsis
Decimal point (.)	Denotes sub-bands
del	Deletion
der	Derivative chromosome (from a translocation or other rearrangement)
dic	Dicentric chromosome (two centromeres)
dmin	Double minute (amplified material, acentric fragments)
dup	Duplication
hsr	Homogeneously staining region (amplified material within a chromosome)
i	Isochromosome (two long arms or two short arms without the other)
idem	Denotes the stemline karyotype in a subclone
inc	Incomplete karyotype (partially analyzable)
ins	Insertion
inv	Inversion
ish	In situ hybridization
mar	Marker chromosome (unidentified origin)
Minus sign (−)	Loss
Multiplication sign (×)	Multiple copies
nuc	Nuclear
p	Short arm of a chromosome
Parentheses ()	Surround structurally altered chromosomes and breakpoints
Period (.)	Separates various techniques
Plus sign (+)	Gain of additional hybridization signal in FISH (++ = gain of 2 signals)
q	Long arm of a chromosome
Question mark (?)	Questionable identification of a chromosome, chromosome structure, or breakpoint
r	Ring chromosome
sep	Separated signals (in FISH)
sl	Stemline. The most basic clone of a tumor population. It is listed first. Subclones (sidelines) are referred to as sdl1, sdl2, etc.
Slant line, single (/)	Separates clones
Slant line, double (//)	Separates chimeric clones (cross-sex transplant; host//donor)
t	Translocation

Abbreviations: FISH, fluorescence in situ hybridization; ISCN, International System for Human Cytogenomic Nomenclature.

prefaced by the term "ish," followed by the locus of the DNA probe used or the abnormality observed. The presence, absence, or appearance of the FISH probes is then described. As an example, an individual who has CML and is Ph chromosome positive might have metaphase FISH (using a dual-fusion FISH strategy), which would be written as:

$$46,XX,t(9;22)(q34;q11.2)[20].ish$$
$$t(9;22)(ABL1+,BCR+;BCR+,ABL1+)[3]$$

The semicolon separates one chromosome from the other descriptively and shows that although some of *ABL1* has remained at 9q34,

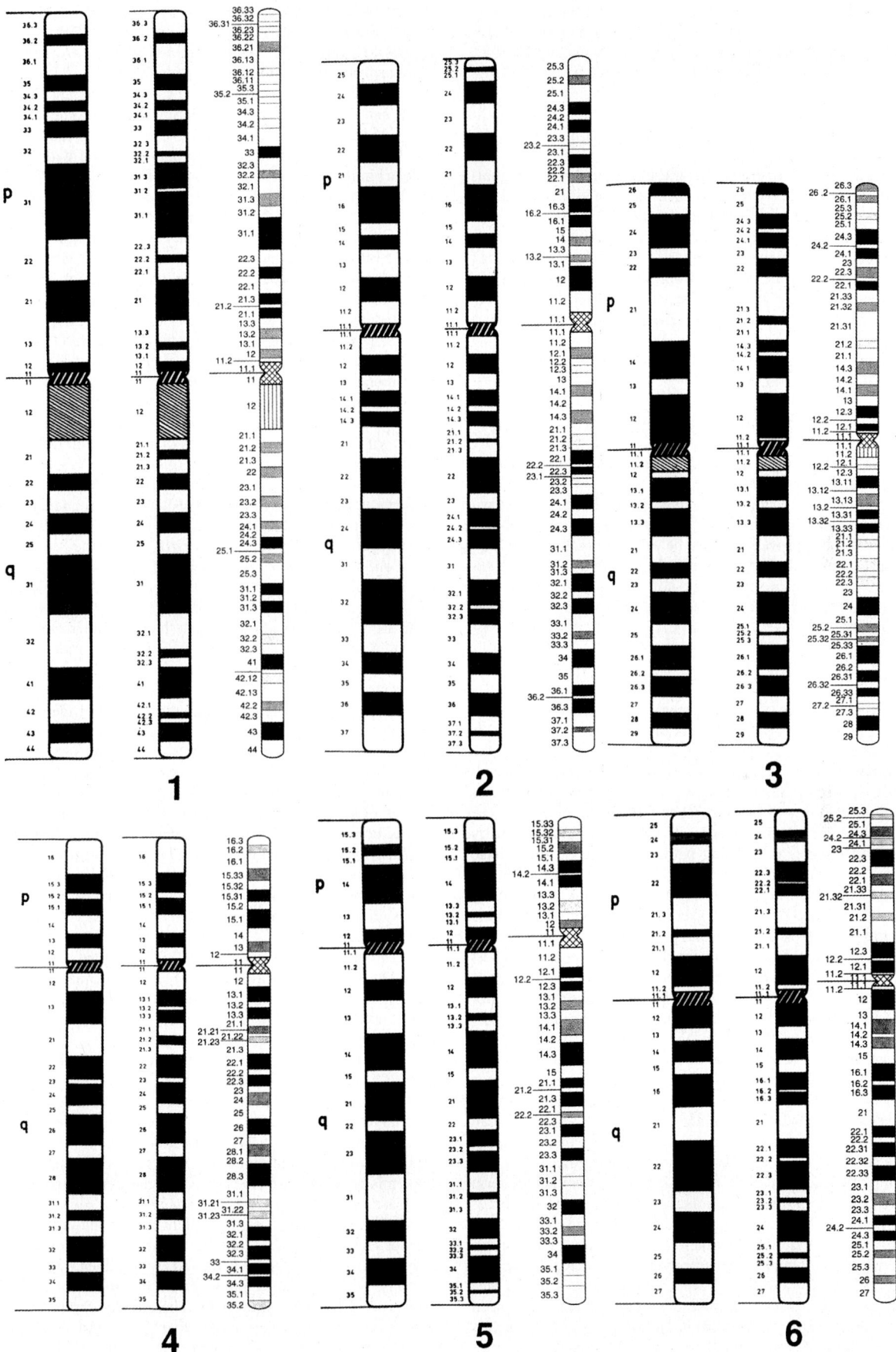

FIGURE 3.5 Ideogram of normal G-banded chromosomes 1-6 at 400, 550, and 850 band level of resolution.

some is now translocated to 22q11.2, next to *BCR*, and vice versa. Interphase FISH of this same individual would typically involve scoring 200 interphase nuclei for their signal patterns. This would be described by using the term "nuc ish," followed by the pattern that was observed. This can be expressed best as:

$$\text{nuc ish}(ABL1, BCR) \times 3(ABL1 \text{ con } BCR \times 2)[200]$$

The foregoing scenario shows that there are three *ABL1* signals and three *BCR* signals; however, two each of these signals are connected ("con") or fused, representing both the *BCR::ABL1* and the *ABL1::BCR* sequence fusions. The double colon (::) denotes the fusion of *ABL1* with *BCR*. This is the standardized method proposed in 2021 by the HUGO Gene Nomenclature Committee to designate gene fusions.[28] Previously, there was not a formal convention for depicting fusion of two genes and they could be separated by a hyphen (-) or a forward slash (/).

Alternatively, if the patient has a normal karyotype and no evidence of the *BCR::ABL1* translocation:

$$\text{nuc ish}(ABL1, BCR) \times 2[200] \text{ or nuc ish}(ABL1 \times 2, BCR \times 2)[200]$$

In other words, there are two distinct *ABL1* signals and two distinct *BCR* signals, with no fusion of the two.

It is important to note that although many of the FISH probes used for leukemias, lymphomas, and other solid tumors are US Food and Drug Administration approved, all must be validated in the laboratory. Such validation must determine the analytic sensitivity and specificity of each probe and establish normal cutoff values or thresholds for determining whether a FISH assay is positive or negative for the aberrant signal pattern.

CHROMOSOMAL MICROARRAY ANALYSIS

A comprehensive analysis of the cancer genome has become a standard research approach to identify new disease loci that may ultimately lead to new therapeutic strategies. One way of studying the genomes of malignancies is to use CMA, also known as chromosome genomic array testing (CGAT), to discern copy number changes or LOH or copy-neutral loss of heterozygosity (cnLOH).

While karyotype analysis relies on dividing cells and the ability to recognize differences in banding patterns visible on metaphase chromosomes by light microscopy, CMA/CGAT uses any number of known DNA sequences (single-nucleotide polymorphisms [SNPs], exons, introns, etc.) and determines their copy number and/or allele status. Karyotype analysis has a resolution of approximately 5 to 10 Mb (megabase pairs or million base pairs of DNA), even at its highest resolution, whereas CMA/CGAT can detect much smaller anomalies on the order of 50 to 100 kb pairs (a 100 times higher resolution). Karyotype analysis can detect structural rearrangements, whether balanced (two copies of every gene or DNA sequence, just not in the correct order) or unbalanced (one or three copies vs the normal two); however, CMA/CGAT cannot detect balanced rearrangements (i.e., balanced translocations or inversions). It can detect only copy number changes, often referred to as copy number variants (CNVs). CNVs can be benign, disease associated, or of unknown significance. Disease-associated CNVs are often called copy number aberrations.

When first introduced in 1992, Kallioniemi et al[27] coined the term comparative genomic hybridization using metaphase chromosomes as the interrogator. CGH arrays were made up of probes that were either bacterial artificial chromosomes (BACs) or oligonucleotides (typically 25-60 bp in length) that were synthesized, specific, unique DNA sequences. BAC CGH arrays were the first arrays used clinically for the detection of copy number changes.[29,30] This was seen as a way to do multiple FISH tests simultaneously. These arrays were initially "targeted" arrays that had about 800 probes specific for numerous microdeletion/microduplication syndromes, as well as other Mendelian disorders with associated disease loci. Over the years,

these have been replaced by the more robust oligonucleotide arrays. Oligo arrays typically have anywhere from 44,000 unique sequence probes to over a million. Most clinical laboratories that employed oligo arrays use ones that have between 60,000 and 180,000 probes to detect CNVs. This detection is performed by labeling patient or tumor DNA and control DNA with different fluorochromes (typically Cy3 and Cy5), denaturing the array DNA as well as the target and control DNAs, and hybridizing them together, along with Cot-1 DNA to reduce binding to repetitive sequences. The DNAs will find and hybridize to complementary array probe sequences. After washing, the array is read by a laser, which determines the color and intensity of each spot on the array. Using a proprietary software application, correcting for dye bias and other artifacts, copy number calls are made according to established parameters, typically the $\log_2$ ratios of the intensities of the different fluorochromes. In most cases, the imbalanced regions can be detected by as few as three to five consecutive oligonucleotide probes. However, these CGH arrays require control DNA for comparative hybridization and cannot detect allelic imbalances. They have now been replaced by newer generation of arrays that contain SNP probes, preferably in addition to oligo probes. SNP arrays were initially used for genome-wide association studies to find associations of particular SNPs with disease; however, it was discovered that they could also be used to determine copy number (*Figure 3.6*).[31,32] SNP array analysis is slightly different, in that it utilizes SNPs to determine copy number changes in comparison to the expected SNP frequencies, as control DNA is not used. SNPs vary from individual to individual. Individuals have different SNPs: one is arbitrarily called the "A allele" and the other one the "B allele." It is expected that everyone has two different SNP alleles at various loci (they are AA, AB, or BB). The copy number analysis of SNP array data generally uses two parameters, comparing the observed test sample fluorescence intensity values with expected reference values: the $\log_2$ R intensity ratio, and the allelic intensity ratio or "B allele frequency." The latter is used to determine stretches of homozygosity (copy-neutral changes where only one SNP allele is detected, presumably from either LOH or identity by descent/relatedness/consanguinity). Most SNP arrays now also include unique oligo sequences, other than the SNPs, because they enhance the ability of the SNP array to detect copy number changes. These new generation arrays contain about 1 million SNP probes and another 1 to 2 million oligo probes. They no longer require comparative hybridization of both target and control genomes. Instead, a reference genome database has been generated from thousands of normal individuals to serve as controls and used during the bioinformatic analysis of the data. Therefore, the term CGH is no longer appropriate. The technology is referred to as chromosomal microarray (CMA) or chromosome genomic array testing (CGAT) in current literature and clinical practice. The advantage of CMA/CGAT is its unique capability to detect clinically significant LOH, particularly in cancer analysis. Many clinical diagnostic laboratories have adopted CMA/CGAT because of their robustness and ease of use, particularly when compared with the original pure SNP arrays.

There is substantial evidence supporting the clinical utility of CMA/CGAT.[33-37] It has now become the "standard of care" in many academic centers and is widely performed by both academic and commercial laboratories. Recent National Comprehensive Cancer Network (NCCN) guidelines also included CMA/CGAT for the workup of several hematological malignancies, such as B-cell acute lymphoblastic leukemia (B-ALL), myelodysplastic syndrome or myeloproliferative neoplasm, and plasma cell neoplasm.

CMA/CGAT can detect smaller, cryptic anomalies and help to further characterize the genomic imbalance of a tumor better than karyotype or FISH (*Figure 3.7A and B*); however, there are some limitations.[38] Malignancies can often be heterogeneous, with multiple clones present in only a few cells. These underrepresented clones may well be missed, if they are in less than 15% of the cells. CMA/CGAT cannot detect balanced rearrangements, which are commonly observed in hematologic malignancies. Ploidy changes (pure triploidy or tetraploidy, etc) are not detectable either. Yet another issue is determining

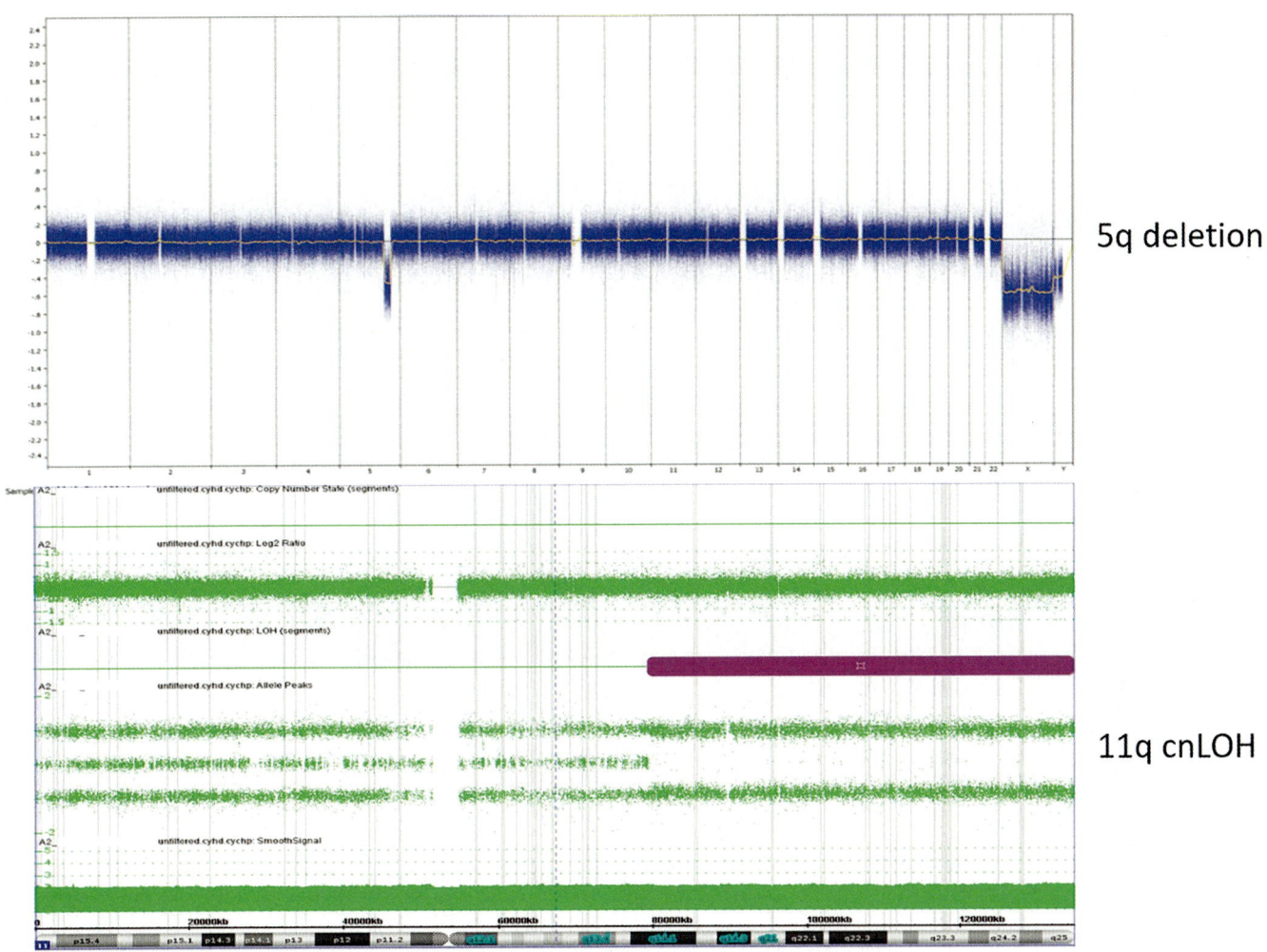

FIGURE 3.6 **Detection of 5q deletion and 11q copy-neutral loss of heterozygosity (cnLOH) by chromosomal microarray/chromosome genomic array testing (CMA/CGAT) in a patient with myelofibrosis.** The upper panel shows the $\log_2$ ratio of each chromosome arranged according to chromosome number from left to right with the X and Y sex chromosomes at the right end. Within each chromosome, the probe signals are aligned from the short arm on the left and long arm on the right, separated by the centromeric region without probe coverage. The copy number aberration (CNA) shown is consistent with the karyotype finding of 46,XY,del(5)(q31q33)[19]/46,XY[1]. The lower panel displays the chromosome 11 with a large segmental cnLOH that is only detectable by microarrays with single-nucleotide polymorphism (SNP) probes.

Laboratory Hematology

whether CNVs or regions of LOH observed in a tumor are constitutional (and not disease related) or acquired, because often normal control DNA from the patient is unavailable. This can be addressed by analyzing a subsequent remission sample or a germline tissue, such as skin fibroblasts or buccal swab. If a CNV or LOH remains detectable at the same level (close to 100%) in both the diagnostic sample and the remission sample (or the germline tissue), it is of constitutional origin. If a CNV or LOH is no longer detectable, or at a significantly lower level, in the remission sample, it is an acquired clonal aberration. Many databases of common variants from normal individuals are available for in silico analysis of the data to distinguish constitutional from acquired CNVs and regions of LOH.

CHROMOSOME GENOMIC ARRAY TESTING NOMENCLATURE

CMA/CGAT nomenclature has evolved significantly since its introduction in the ISCN (2005) edition. According to the most recent version ISCN (2020) under the section "Microarrays," results are described with the preface "arr," followed by the chromosome band and genomic coordinates of any copy number gain, loss, or cnLOH included in brackets (starting position ending position) and the

respective copy number of the specified genomic region.[22] Genome build is specified immediately after "arr" unless only aneuploidy or whole-chromosome-arm changes are seen. The estimated clone size (or level of mosaicism) is included in a bracket [ ] immediately following the abnormality. Each alteration is separated by a comma, ordered according to the chromosome number, with the sex chromosome abnormalities listed first, and from the end of the short arm (pter) to the end of the long arm (qter). For example, a female acute myeloid leukemia (AML) patient with 13q cnLOH in 80% of the cells along with a subclone of *CEBPA* deletion on 19q in 50% of the cells would have the CMA/CGAT results described as "arr[GRCh38] (13q)x2 hmz [0.8],19q13.11(33,329,934_33,355,534)x1[0.5]." Sex chromosome info is not listed in this case, indicating no sex chromosome abnormality was evident.

DIAGNOSTIC AND PROGNOSTIC IMPACT OF CHROMOSOMAL ABNORMALITIES

As stated earlier, the WHO system[1,2] has classified many leukemias and lymphomas according to their cytogenetic or molecular abnormalities. Many of these have not only diagnostic significance but prognostic significance as well. *Table 3.3* provides a sampling of

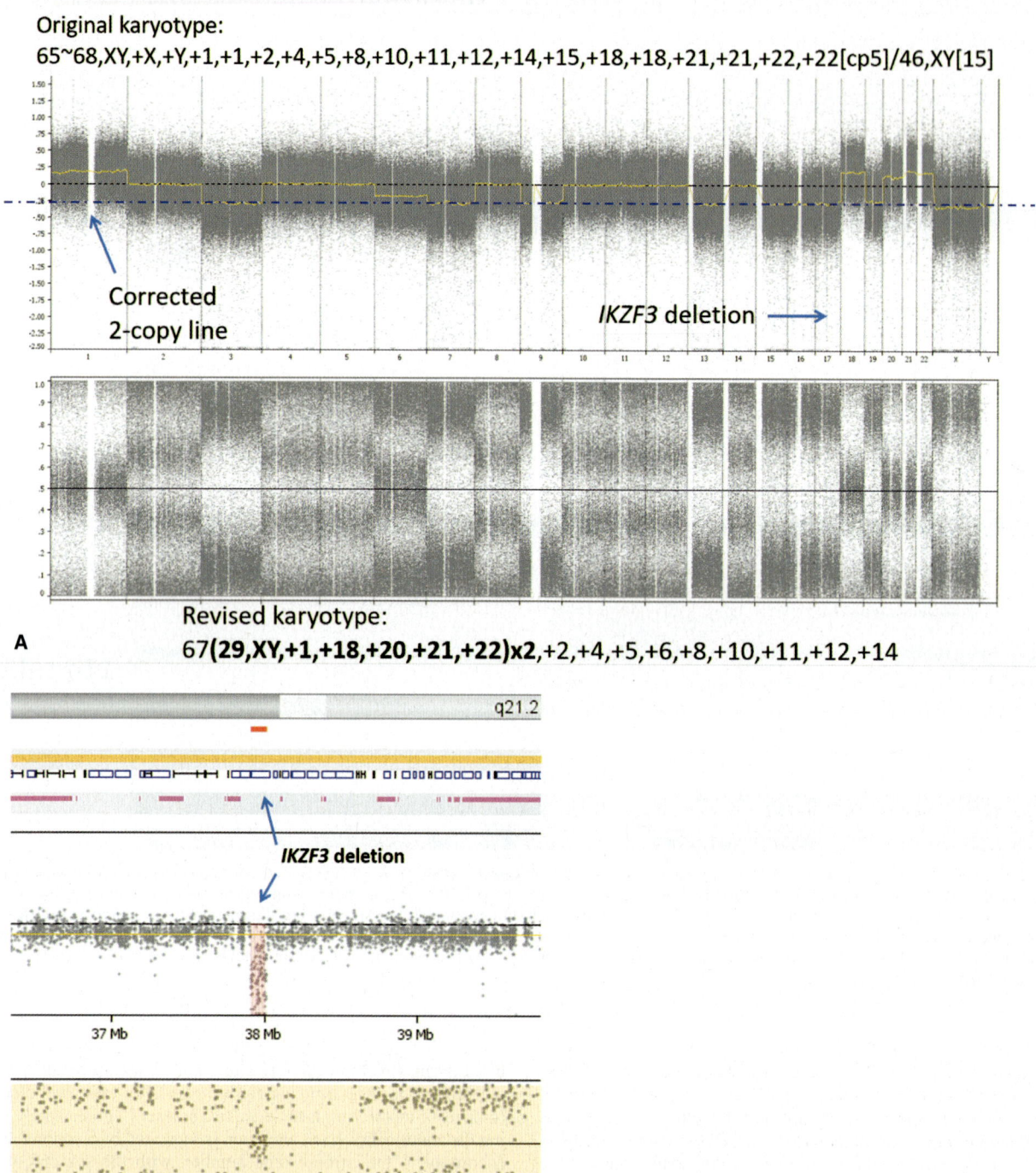

FIGURE 3.7 **A, Chromosome genomic array testing/chromosome microarray (CGAT/CMA) for a patient with B-cell acute lymphoblastic leukemia, with original karyotype written above the upper panel.** The upper panel represents the copy number abnormalities; the lower panel shows the B-allele frequency plot. Chromosome count: four copies of chromosomes 1, 18, 20, 21, and 22; three copies of chromosomes 2, 4, 5, 6, 8, 10, 11, 12, and 14; two copies of chromosomes X, Y, 3, 7, 9, 13, 15, 16, 17, and 19, each with copy-neutral loss of heterozygosity. Arrow depicts deletion of *IKZF3* gene on chromosome 17. A revised karyotype based on CGAT findings is written under the lower panel. A zoomed-in view of *IKZF* gene region is shown in panel (B). B, Regional view of *IKZF3* deletion at 17q12 against the background of copy-neutral loss of heterozygosity of chromosome 17. (Adopted from Fang M, Becker PS, Linenberger M, et al. Adult low-hypodiploid acute B-lymphoblastic leukemia with IKZF3 deletion and TP53 mutation: comparison with pediatric patients. *Am J Clin Pathol.* 2015;144:263-270. Reproduced by permission of American Society for Clinical Pathology.)

chromosomal rearrangements associated with hematologic malignancies. Although this table is by no means exhaustive, it does inform the reader as to the significance of a number of anomalies (*Table 3.3*). Comprehensive catalogs of chromosomal rearrangements are available online: "The Atlas of Genetics and Cytogenetics in Oncology and Haematology" (http://atlasgeneticsoncology.org) and the "Mitelman Database of Chromosome Aberrations in Cancer" (http://cgap.nci.nih.

gov/Chromosomes/Mitelman). Newer technologies, including CMA/CGAT, allow better risk stratification when combined with conventional cytogenetics, such as karyotype analysis and FISH. Two entities that benefit from this approach are AML and chronic lymphocytic leukemia (CLL). Please refer to disease-specific chapters in this book for more comprehensive descriptions of all clinically significant chromosome abnormalities.

Table 3.3. Selected Chromosome Abnormalities in Hematologic Malignancies and Diagnostic or Prognostic Value

Disease	Significance	References
ALCL	t(2p23) with *ALK* rearrangement is diagnostic; t(2;5) is the most common	3
AML	inv(3)/t(3;3) with *MECOM* rearrangement, –5/5q–, t(6;9), –7/7q–, t(11q23) with *KMT2A* rearrangement (except t(9;11)), 13q cnLOH, –17/17p (*TP53*), complex karyotype, and monosomal karyotype are unfavorable	37,39-41
	t(8;21), inv(16)/t(16;16), and t(15;17) are favorable	
B-ALL	t(9;22), t(4;11), iAMP21, and low hypodiploidy/near haploid (including masked), Ph-like ALL, are unfavorable	33
	t(12;21) and hyperdiploidy with +4 and +10 are favorable	
BL	t(8;14), t(14;22), and t(2;8) with *MYC* rearrangement are diagnostic	3
CLL	11q– (*ATM* deletion), –17/17p– (*TP53*), and complex abnormal (by karyotype or CMA/CGAT) are unfavorable	34,42
	trisomy 12 (+12) is common; 13q– is favorable	
CML	t(9;22) [*BCR::ABL1*] is diagnostic	3
	Additional abnormalities (extra Ph, +8, i(17q), etc) are associated with accelerated phase and/or blast crisis	
FL	t(14;18) and t(2;18) with *BCL2* rearrangement is diagnostic	3
MCL	t(11;14) [IGH::*CCND1*] is diagnostic	3
MDS	–5/5q–, –7/7q-, +8, and 20q– are most common	43,44
	inv(3)/t(3;3), –7, double including 7q–/–7, complex karyotype are unfavorable	
MDS/MPN	9p cnLOH is common	35
MPN	1q+, 9p– (*CDKN2A/B* deletion), and 20q– are common	35
MM	1p–/1q+, t(4;14), t(14;16), t(14;20), and –17/17p– are unfavorable	36,45,46
	Monosomy 13 by karyotype analysis is unfavorable	
	t(11;14) and –13/13q– are common by FISH	

Abbreviations: ALCL, anaplastic large-cell lymphoma; AML, acute myeloid leukemia; B-ALL, B-cell acute lymphoblastic leukemia/lymphoma; BL, Burkitt lymphoma; CGAT, chromosome genomic array testing; CLL, chronic lymphocytic leukemia; CMA, chromosome microarray; CML, chronic myeloid leukemia; FISH, Fluorescence in situ hybridization; FL, follicular lymphoma; MCL, mantle cell lymphoma; MDS, myelodysplastic syndrome; MM, multiple myeloma; MPN, myeloproliferative neoplasm.
This table shows a selected group of representative chromosome abnormalities and is not meant to be comprehensive or complete. Only favorable and unfavorable risk categories are specified. Please refer to disease-specific chapters in this book for more comprehensive descriptions of all clinically significant chromosome abnormalities.

Acute Myeloid Leukemia

According to the 2017 WHO classification,[1-3] there are certain entities of AML defined by their cytogenetic or molecular abnormalities (recurrent genetic abnormalities). The t(8;21) and the inv(16) and its variants, both core binding factor abnormalities, as well as the t(15;17), when observed by karyotype, FISH, or polymerase chain reaction, are considered distinct forms of AML, even if the percent blasts are below 20%. All of these have been associated with a good or favorable outcome.[40] The t(9;11)(p22;q23) is an entity with an intermediate risk, even though all other translocations involving 11q23 are of high risk.

Risk stratification tools for AML patients based on cytogenetics have been developed and refined over the past 20 years. The most widely utilized system is the 2017 European LeukemiaNet categorization strategy (ELN2017),[40] which incorporates mutation status into cytogenetic risk stratification. Patients in the favorable group show t(8;21), inv(16)/t(16;16), *NPM1* mutation, or biallelic *CEBPA* mutation, whereas those in the unfavorable group display monosomy 5 or 7, 5q deletion, inv(3)/t(3;3), t(6;9), 11q23 (or *KMT2A/MLL*) rearrangements except t(9;11), abnormalities of 17p, *RUNX1* mutation, complex karyotypes (CKs), with three or more abnormalities, or monosomal karyotype (MK), defined as either loss of at least two autosomes or loss of one autosome along with at least one well-defined structural abnormality. MK has been associated with a worse prognosis than even CK, although hematopoietic cell transplantation appears to mitigate the extremely poor outcome to some degree.[47-49] The ELN2017 is largely consistent with the UK Medical Research Council tool that was based on karyotype only and also included 7q deletion in the unfavorable group.[39] Recently, multiple retrospective studies suggested

poor prognostic impact of submicroscopic deletions of 4q24 (*TET2*) and 17q11.2 (*NF1*), amplification of 21q22 (*ERG*), and cnLOH of 13q (*FLT3*) based on CMA/CGAT.[37] The AML risk stratification tools continue to evolve as new genomic methods identify novel biomarkers.

Chronic Lymphocytic Leukemia

In CLL, karyotype analysis of blood or bone marrow was not very successful, in part because of the lack of neoplastic B cells that are actively dividing. Use of B-cell mitogens during in vitro culturing, such as CpG oligonucleotide DSP30, has significantly improved the diagnostic yield of karyotype analysis for CLL.[50-52] Investigators have also shown that approximately 80% of patients with CLL have clonal chromosomal abnormalities that can be detected in nondividing cells of the blood using interphase FISH by employing a number of DNA probes specific for the chromosomal abnormalities known to be associated with CLL. This group of probes is called a "FISH Panel." Döhner et al[53] reported a CLL risk stratification based on FISH abnormalities alone. They found that those patients with a FISH result of 13q deletion as a sole abnormality (13q–) had a good prognosis, whereas those with trisomy 12 or normal result were in the intermediate group. They also found that patients with 11q deletion showed rapid progression and shorter survival, and those with a *TP53* deletion (17p deletion) were in the worst prognostic group. Current NCCN Guidelines specify 11q– and 17p– as unfavorable, trisomy 12 as intermediate, and as a sole abnormality del(13q) is considered favorable.[54] For the past 20 years, this four-probe FISH panel has been widely used to stratify CLL patients. However, it does not detect genome-wide abnormalities as do karyotype analysis and CMA/CGAT. When complex genome-wide

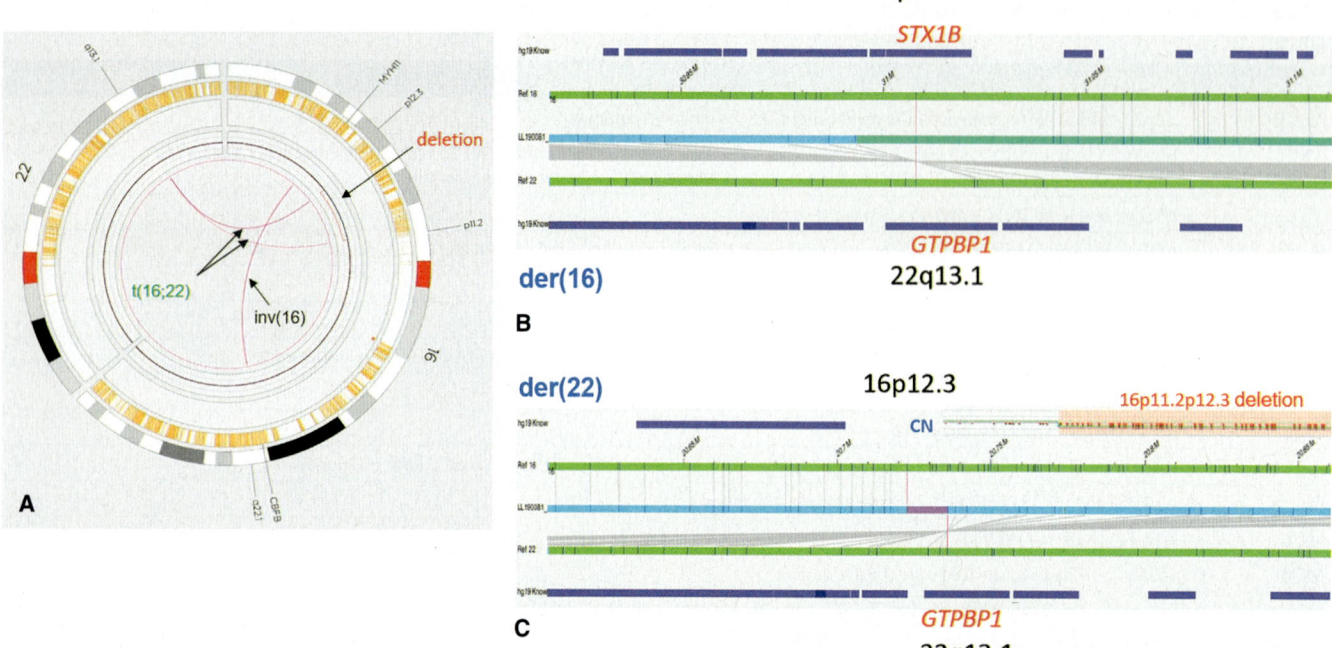

FIGURE 3.8 Optical genomic mapping (OGM) result for a patient with acute myeloid leukemia. The karyotype finding was 46,XX,inv(16)(p13.1q22),t(16;22) (p11.2;q13)[14]/46,XX[6]. OGM not only identified both inv(16) and t(16;22) but also detected a submicroscopic deletion of 16p11.2p12.3 at the translocation breakpoint. A, Circos plot displays the three structural abnormalities identified on chromosomes 16 and 22. The outermost circle demonstrates the cytogenetics ideogram of the involved chromosomes. The innermost circle shows translocations and rearrangements. The middle circles display copy number alterations (deletions or gains) and other structural variants. B, Derivative chromosome 16 [der(16)] showing the patient DNA sequence (gray tracks) mapped to both the chromosome 16 reference sequence and the chromosome 22 reference sequence (green tracks) with the breakpoints mapped to the *STX1B* gene on chromosome 16 and *GTPBP1* on chromosome 22 (blue tracks). C, Derivative chromosome 22 [der(22)] showing a deletion of 16p from the copy number track (inlet CN) in addition to the translocation.

clonal abnormalities are found in a CLL patient, they have been shown to impart a worse prognosis.[42,55] The European Research Initiative on CLL (ERIC) defined the CK by the presence of >3 chromosome abnormalities; but independent poor prognosis was more definitively associated with a CK with ≥5 chromosome aberrations.[55] Although genomic complexity has not been explicitly defined for abnormalities identified by CMA/CGAT, and it is not yet currently considered a surrogate for CK, increasing numbers of genomic lesions identified by CMA/CGAT have been associated with a worse outcome.[56-58] Nevertheless, CMA/CGAT has the advantage of detecting chromosome abnormalities in nondividing cells. For a good review of abnormalities detected by CMA analysis in CLL with extensive references, see Chun et al.[34]

NEXT-GENERATION SEQUENCING

New molecular technologies, such as next-generation sequencing and other novel techniques, can now be utilized to identify structural variants (SVs) and CNVs with improved sensitivity and specificity above traditional cytogenetic techniques. One of these techniques, mate-pair sequencing (MPseq), is a variation of whole-genome sequencing (WGS) that utilizes a specialized library preparation of long input DNA followed by circularization, fragmentation, and sequencing of smaller paired end fragments.[59,60] MPseq has been used to identify SVs and CNVs in the context of numerous malignancies including multiple myeloma, AML, lymphoma, B-ALL, and others.[61-66] Other alternative technologies include optical genome mapping (OGM) based on imaging of ultrahigh-molecular-weight DNA. OGM is an emerging technology that has the potential to also replace traditional cytogenetic methodologies in the analysis of various malignancies (*Figure 3.8*).[67-69] A limitation of MPseq and OGM is the inability

to identify single-nucleotide variants (SNVs) due to the relative low depth of sequencing for MPseq and no bona fide sequencing for OGM. This limitation has been overcome with the use of WGS involving long-read or long-insert DNA fragments that can provide all genomic variants (SNVs, SVs, and CNVs) within a single assay in an unbiased fashion. This approach has been utilized in the context of AML within the clinical setting and demonstrated the feasibility of utilizing WGS as a replacement technology to cytogenetic analysis in myeloid malignancies.[70]

ACKNOWLEDGMENT

The authors acknowledge Athena M. Cherry, PhD, and Charles D. Bangs who composed an earlier version of this chapter.

References

1. Arber DA, Orazi A, Hasserjian R, et al. The 2016 revision to the World Health Organization classification of myeloid neoplasms and acute leukemia. *Blood.* 2016;127(20):2391-2405.
2. Swerdlow SH, Campo E, Pileri SA, et al. The 2016 revision of the World Health Organization classification of lymphoid neoplasms. *Blood.* 2016;127(20):2375-2390.
3. Swerdlow SH, Campo E, Harris NL, et al. *WHO Classification of Tumours of Haematopoietic and Lymphoid Tissues.* 4th ed. IARC Press; 2017.
4. von Hansemann D. Ueber asymmetrische zelltheilung in epithelkrebsen und deren biologische bedeutung. *Virchow's Arch Path Anat.* 1890;119:299-326.
5. Boveri T. *Zur frage der entstehung maligner tumoren [The origin of malignant tumors].* Gustav Fischer; 1914.
6. Painter TS. Studies in mammalian spermatogenesis. II. The spermatogenesis of man. *J Exp Zool.* 1923;37:291-321.
7. Tijo HJ, Levan A. The chromosome numbers of man. *Hereditas.* 1956;42:1-6.
8. Levan A. Non-random representation of chromosome types in human tumor stemlines. *Hereditas.* 1966;55:28-38.
9. Van Steenis H. Chromosomes and cancer. *Nature.* 1966;209(5025):819-821.

10. Knudson AG, Jr. Mutation and cancer: statistical study of retinoblastoma. *Proc Natl Acad Sci U S A*. 1971;68(4):820-823.

11. Sandberg AA. A chromosomal hypothesis of oncogenesis. *Cancer Genet Cytogenet*. 1983;8(4):277-285.

12. Weinberg RA. Oncogenes, antioncogenes, and the molecular bases of multistep carcinogenesis. *Cancer Res*. 1989;49(14):3713-3721.

13. Lejeune J, Gautier M, Turpin R. Study of somatic chromosomes from 9 mongoloid children. [Article in French]. *C R Hebd Seances Acad Sci*. 1959;248(11):1721-1722.

14. Nowell PC, Hungerford DA. A minute chromosome in human chronic granulocytic leukemia. *Science*. 1960;132:1497-1501.

15. Rowley JD. Letter: a new consistent chromosomal abnormality in chronic myelogenous leukaemia identified by quinacrine fluorescence and Giemsa staining. *Nature*. 1973;243(5405):290-293.

16. Chissoe SL, Bodenteich A, Wang YF, et al. Sequence and analysis of the human ABL gene, the BCR gene, and regions involved in the Philadelphia chromosomal translocation. *Genomics*. 1995;27(1):67-82.

17. Deininger MW, Druker BJ. Specific targeted therapy of chronic myelogenous leukemia with imatinib. *Pharmacol Rev*. 2003;55(3):401-423.

18. Arber DA, Borowitz MJ, Cessna M, et al. Initial diagnostic workup of acute leukemia: guideline from the College of American Pathologists and the American Society of Hematology. *Arch Pathol Lab Med*. 2017;141(10):1342-1393.

19. de Haas V, Ismaila N, Advani A, et al. Initial diagnostic work-up of acute leukemia: ASCO clinical practice guideline endorsement of the College of American Pathologists and American Society of Hematology guideline. *J Clin Oncol*. 2019;37(3):239-253.

20. Mikhail FM, Biegel JA, Cooley LD, et al. Technical laboratory standards for interpretation and reporting of acquired copy-number abnormalities and copy-neutral loss of heterozygosity in neoplastic disorders: a joint consensus recommendation from the American College of Medical Genetics and Genomics (ACMG) and the Cancer Genomics Consortium (CGC). *Genet Med*. 2019;21(9):1903-1916.

21. Second international workshop on chromosomes in leukemia. General report. *Cancer Genet Cytogenet*. 1980:93-96.

22. McGowan-Jordan J, Hastings RJ, Moore S, eds. *ISCN 2020: An International System for Human Cytogenomic Nomenclature*. S. Karger; 2020.

23. Gall JG, Pardue ML. Formation and detection of RNA-DNA hybrid molecules in cytological preparations. *Proc Natl Acad Sci U S A*. 1969;63(2):378-383.

24. Harper ME, Saunders GF. Localization of single copy DNA sequences of G-banded human chromosomes by in situ hybridization. *Chromosoma*. 1981;83(3):431-439.

25. Langer PR, Waldrop AA, Ward DC. Enzymatic synthesis of biotin-labeled polynucleotides: novel nucleic acid affinity probes. *Proc Natl Acad Sci U S A*. 1981;78(11):6633-6637.

26. Pinkel D, Landegent J, Collins C, et al. Fluorescence in situ hybridization with human chromosome-specific libraries: detection of trisomy 21 and translocations of chromosome 4. *Proc Natl Acad Sci U S A*. 1988;85(23):9138-9142.

27. Kallioniemi A, Kallioniemi OP, Sudar D, et al. Comparative genomic hybridization for molecular cytogenetic analysis of solid tumors. *Science*. 1992;258(5083):818-821.

28. Bruford EA, Antonescu CR, Carroll AJ, et al. HUGO Gene Nomenclature Committee (HGNC) recommendations for the designation of gene fusions. *Leukemia*. 2021;35(11):3040-3043.

29. Shaffer LG, Kashork CD, Saleki R, et al. Targeted genomic microarray analysis for identification of chromosome abnormalities in 1500 consecutive clinical cases. *J Pediatr*. 2006;149(1):98-102.

30. Shaw-Smith C, Redon R, Rickman L, et al. Microarray based comparative genomic hybridisation (array-CGH) detects submicroscopic chromosomal deletions and duplications in patients with learning disability/mental retardation and dysmorphic features. *J Med Genet*. 2004;41(4):241-248.

31. Gunderson KL, Steemers FJ, Lee G, Mendoza LG, Chee MS. A genome-wide scalable SNP genotyping assay using microarray technology. *Nat Genet*. 2005;37(5):549-554.

32. Syvanen AC. Toward genome-wide SNP genotyping. *Nat Genet*. 2005;37(suppl):S5-S10.

33. Akkari YMN, Bruyere H, Hagelstrom RT, et al. Evidence-based review of genomic aberrations in B-lymphoblastic leukemia/lymphoma: report from the cancer genomics consortium working group for lymphoblastic leukemia. *Cancer Genet*. 2020;243:52-72.

34. Chun K, Wenger GD, Chaubey A, et al. Assessing copy number aberrations and copy-neutral loss-of-heterozygosity across the genome as best practice: an evidence-based review from the Cancer Genomics Consortium (CGC) working group for chronic lymphocytic leukemia. *Cancer Genet*. 2018;228-229:236-250.

35. Kanagal-Shamanna R, Hodge JC, Tucker T, et al. Assessing copy number aberrations and copy neutral loss of heterozygosity across the genome as best practice: an evidence based review of clinical utility from the cancer genomics consortium (CGC) working group for myelodysplastic syndrome, myelodysplastic/myeloproliferative and myeloproliferative neoplasms. *Cancer Genet*. 2018;228-229:197-217.

36. Pugh TJ, Fink JM, Lu X, et al. Assessing genome-wide copy number aberrations and copy-neutral loss-of-heterozygosity as best practice: an evidence-based review from the Cancer Genomics Consortium working group for plasma cell disorders. *Cancer Genet*. 2018;228-229:184-196.

37. Xu X, Bryke C, Sukhanova M, et al. Assessing copy number abnormalities and copy-neutral loss-of-heterozygosity across the genome as best practice in diagnostic

38. Shao L, Akkari Y, Cooley LD, et al. Chromosomal microarray analysis, including constitutional and neoplastic disease applications, 2021 revision: a technical standard of the American College of Medical Genetics and Genomics (ACMG). *Genet Med*. 2021;23(10):1818-1829.

39. Grimwade D, Hills RK, Moorman AV, et al. Refinement of cytogenetic classification in acute myeloid leukemia: determination of prognostic significance of rare recurring chromosomal abnormalities among 5876 younger adult patients treated in the United Kingdom Medical Research Council trials. *Blood*. 2010;116(3):354-365.

40. Dohner H, Estey E, Grimwade D, et al. Diagnosis and management of AML in adults: 2017 ELN recommendations from an international expert panel. *Blood*. 2017;129(4):424-447.

41. Gronseth CM, McElhone SE, Storer BE, et al. Prognostic significance of acquired copy-neutral loss of heterozygosity in acute myeloid leukemia. *Cancer*. 2015;121(17):2900-2908.

42. Chatzikonstantinou T, Demosthenous C, Baliakas P. Biology and treatment of high-risk CLL: significance of complex karyotype. *Front Oncol*. 2021;11:788761.

43. Greenberg PL, Tuechler H, Schanz J, et al. Revised international prognostic scoring system for myelodysplastic syndromes. *Blood*. 2012;120(12):2454-2465.

44. Deeg HJ, Scott BL, Fang M, et al. Five-group cytogenetic risk classification, monosomal karyotype, and outcome after hematopoietic cell transplantation for MDS or acute leukemia evolving from MDS. *Blood*. 2012;120(7):1398-1408.

45. Lussier T, Schoebe N, Mai S. Risk stratification and treatment in smoldering multiple myeloma. *Cells*. 2021;11(1):130.

46. Rajkumar SV. Multiple myeloma: 2012 update on diagnosis, risk-stratification, and management. *Am J Hematol*. 2012;87(1):78-88.

47. Breems DA, Van Putten WL, De Greef GE, et al. Monosomal karyotype in acute myeloid leukemia: a better indicator of poor prognosis than a complex karyotype. *J Clin Oncol*. 2008;26(29):4791-4797.

48. Fang M, Storer B, Estey E, et al. Outcome of patients with acute myeloid leukemia with monosomal karyotype who undergo hematopoietic cell transplantation. *Blood*. 2011;118(6):1490-1494.

49. Medeiros BC, Othus M, Fang M, Roulston D, Appelbaum FR. Prognostic impact of monosomal karyotype in young adult and elderly acute myeloid leukemia: the Southwest Oncology Group (SWOG) experience. *Blood*. 2010;116(13):2224-2228.

50. Muthusamy N, Breidenbach H, Andritsos L, et al. Enhanced detection of chromosomal abnormalities in chronic lymphocytic leukemia by conventional cytogenetics using CpG oligonucleotide in combination with pokeweed mitogen and phorbol myristate acetate. *Cancer Genet*. 2011;204(2):77-83.

51. Struski S, Gervais C, Helias C, Herbrecht R, Audhuy B, Mauvieux L. Stimulation of B-cell lymphoproliferations with CpG-oligonucleotide DSP30 plus IL-2 is more effective than with TPA to detect clonal abnormalities. *Leukemia*. 2009;23(3):617-619.

52. Rigolin GM, Cibien F, Martinelli S, et al. Chromosome aberrations detected by conventional karyotyping using novel mitogens in chronic lymphocytic leukemia with "normal" FISH: correlations with clinicobiologic parameters. *Blood*. 2012;119(10):2310-2313.

53. Dohner H, Stilgenbauer S, Benner A, et al. Genomic aberrations and survival in chronic lymphocytic leukemia. *N Engl J Med*. 2000;343(26):1910-1916.

54. *NCCN Clinical Practice Guidelines in Oncology: Chronic Lymphocytic Leukemia/Small Lymphocytic Lymphoma*. Version 2.2022. NCCN.org. Accessed March 8, 2022.

55. Baliakas P, Jeromin S, Iskas M, et al. Cytogenetic complexity in chronic lymphocytic leukemia: definitions, associations, and clinical impact. *Blood*. 2019;133(11):1205-1216.

56. Ouillette P, Collins R, Shakhan S, et al. Acquired genomic copy number aberrations and survival in chronic lymphocytic leukemia. *Blood*. 2011;118(11):3051-3061.

57. Kujawski L, Ouillette P, Erba H, et al. Genomic complexity identifies patients with aggressive chronic lymphocytic leukemia. *Blood*. 2008;112(5):1993-2003.

58. Bloehdorn J, Braun A, Taylor-Weiner A, et al. Multi-platform profiling characterizes molecular subgroups and resistance networks in chronic lymphocytic leukemia. *Nat Commun*. 2021;12(1):5395.

59. Johnson SH, Smadbeck JB, Smoley SA, et al. SVAtools for junction detection of genome-wide chromosomal rearrangements by mate-pair sequencing (MPseq). *Cancer Genet*. 2018;221:1-18.

60. Smadbeck JB, Johnson SH, Smoley SA, et al. Copy number variant analysis using genome-wide mate-pair sequencing. *Genes Chromosomes Cancer*. 2018;57(9):459-470.

61. Aypar U, Smoley SA, Pitel BA, et al. Mate pair sequencing improves detection of genomic abnormalities in acute myeloid leukemia. *Eur J Haematol*. 2019;102(1):87-96.

62. Peterson JF, Blackburn PR, Webley MR, et al. Identification of a novel ZBTB20-JAK2 fusion by mate-pair sequencing in a young adult with B-lymphoblastic leukemia/lymphoma. *Mayo Clin Proc*. 2019;94(7):1381-1384.

63. Schultz MJ, Blackburn PR, Cogbill CH, et al. Characterization of a cryptic PML-RARA fusion by mate-pair sequencing in a case of acute promyelocytic leukemia with a normal karyotype and negative RARA FISH studies. *Leuk Lymphoma*. 2020;61(4):975-978.

64. Smadbeck J, Peterson JF, Pearce KE, et al. Mate pair sequencing outperforms fluorescence in situ hybridization in the genomic characterization of multiple myeloma. *Blood Cancer J*. 2019;9(12):103.

Laboratory Hematology

65. Polonis K, Schultz MJ, Olteanu H, et al. Detection of cryptic CCND1 rearrangements in mantle cell lymphoma by next generation sequencing. *Ann Diagn Pathol.* 2020;46:151533.

66. Sharma N, Smadbeck JB, Abdallah N, et al. The prognostic role of MYC structural variants identified by NGS and FISH in multiple myeloma. *Clin Cancer Res.* 2021:27(19):5430-5439.

67. Lestringant V, Duployez N, Penther D, et al. Optical genome mapping, a promising alternative to gold standard cytogenetic approaches in a series of acute lymphoblastic leukemias. *Genes Chromosomes Cancer.* 2021;60(10):657-667.

68. Neveling K, Mantere T, Vermeulen S, et al. Next-generation cytogenetics: comprehensive assessment of 52 hematological malignancy genomes by optical genome mapping. *Am J Hum Genet.* 2021;108(8):1423-1435.

69. Luhmann JL, Stelter M, Wolter M, et al. The clinical utility of optical genome mapping for the assessment of genomic aberrations in acute lymphoblastic leukemia. *Cancers.* 2021;13(17):4388.

70. Duncavage EJ, Schroeder MC, O'Laughlin M, et al. Genome sequencing as an alternative to cytogenetic analysis in myeloid cancers. *N Engl J Med.* 2021;384(10):924-935.

Chapter 4 ■ Molecular Diagnosis in Hematology

BING MELODY ZHANG • JAMES L. ZEHNDER

INTRODUCTION

In the last several decades, the extensive genetic studies of hematologic disorders within the research realm have led to accelerated discovery of new disease-causing or disease-associated genetic abnormalities and significantly improved the understanding of disease etiology. Many genetic changes that provide important diagnostic, prognostic, or predictive values have been translated into routine clinical care. Testing for genetic changes has become an integral part of the laboratory workup for most hematologic malignancies and many nonmalignant hematologic disorders as well. The molecular testing methodologies have also evolved in breadth, resolution, and complexity to accommodate the increasing clinical needs. In this chapter, we will review the commonly used molecular diagnostic technologies for detection of genetic alterations and applications of molecular diagnosis in both malignant and nonmalignant hematologic disorders.

COMMONLY USED METHODOLOGIES IN MOLECULAR DIAGNOSTICS

Extraction of Nucleic Acids

Isolation of the appropriate type of nucleic acid for testing is the starting point for molecular assays. DNA is more stable than RNA in general with the exception that it is fragmented by acid treatment in decalcified bone marrow trephines and therefore unsuitable for downstream molecular testing. RNA is subject to quick degradation in blood, bone marrow, and other tissue specimens, so timely sample processing is key to a better preservation of RNA. It is more advantageous to use RNA than DNA as the analyte for fusion detection in hematologic neoplasms.[1]

Polymerase Chain Reaction

Polymerase chain reaction (PCR) is the basis and central technique for most molecular genetic assays. Through repeated cycles of denaturation, annealing, and extension, unique targeted DNA regions can be rapidly amplified exponentially with high specificity to generate an adequate amount of DNA fragments for subsequent genetic analysis. Both end-point PCR and real-time PCR are routinely used in molecular diagnostics. The amplification products of end-point PCR can be visualized with gel or capillary electrophoresis for fragment size–based analysis. These amplicons are also used as the input materials for Sanger sequencing or genotyping assays. Real-time PCR and digital PCR can be used for quantitative analysis of template nucleic acid[1,2] (*Figure 4.1*).

Amplification-Refractory Mutation System

Amplification-refractory mutation system (ARMS) is a modified PCR technique used to detect known point mutations. Besides the primers used to amplify an internal control, each of the two multiplex PCR reactions contains a primer matching the sequence of either wild-type or mutant target genomic sequence with the only nucleotide difference at the 3′ end of the primer. Resolving the amplicons from both reactions on a gel can inform both the presence and zygosity of mutations[3] (*Figure 4.2A*).

Multiplex Ligation-Dependent Probe Amplification

Multiplex ligation-dependent probe amplification (MLPA) is a modified multiplex PCR method used for DNA copy number quantification. Each probe is composed of two oligonucleotides matching adjacent DNA sequences. The hybridized oligonucleotides can be ligated and amplified with universal primers to generate amplicons of unique lengths, which can then be separated and identified by electrophoresis.[4,5] MLPA has been proven to be an accurate and reliable method

to detect relatively large deletions, duplications, and amplifications[6,7] (*Figure 4.2B*).

Restriction Enzyme Digestion

Restriction enzymes recognize specific short sequences and can cleave the DNA at the exact site. A gene mutation may create or obliterate a restriction enzyme site and therefore can be detected through restriction enzyme digestion of amplified DNA fragments. Although this conventional method is technically straightforward, it can at best be applied to a small fraction of known mutations that alter the restriction sites.[3]

SNaPshot Genotyping

SNaPshot is a multiplex primer base extension method coupled with capillary electrophoresis developed for the analysis of single-nucleotide variants (SNVs). First, a conventional multiplex PCR is performed using primers flanking the targeted SNV, followed by the SNaPshot reaction during which allele-specific primers anneal one base before the SNV of interest and extend with dideoxynucleotides (ddNTPs) labeled with fluorescence. Then, SNVs are detected with capillary electrophoresis. This technique allows the detection of one to multiple SNVs simultaneously in a single assay. SNaPshot assays are usually custom-designed to interrogate for known hotspot mutations.[8] It can reliably detect mutations present at 10% allele fraction and works well on paraffin-embedded tissue.[9] This method is not designed to detect mutations present at locations other than the SNVs of interest (*Figure 4.3*).

Sanger Sequencing

This dideoxy chain termination technique developed by Frederick Sanger has been the gold standard for determining DNA base composition.[10] A DNA sequence of interest is amplified in the presence of a primer and ddNTP chain terminators labeled with fluorescence. The different color signals corresponding to the four different nucleotides are then compiled by laser detection during capillary electrophoresis in an automated sequencer. This method can be used to precisely detect both unknown and known mutations. Its limitations include financial cost and analytical sensitivity (10% ~ 20%)[1] (*Figure 4.4A*).

Next-Generation Sequencing

Next-generation sequencing (NGS), also known as high-throughput sequencing, allows millions of sequencing reactions to happen in parallel and therefore achieves much higher throughput than the Sanger sequencing method. Different sequencing platforms use different approaches, such as creating microreactors and/or attaching DNA molecules to solid surfaces or beads, to generate quantifiable short reads[11] (*Figure 4.4B and C*). NGS has entered the realm of clinical diagnostics and is now widely used in molecular pathology laboratories for both somatic and germline mutation detection.[12] The DNA regions covered by NGS vary from single gene, to targeted multigene panels, to whole exome/transcriptome/genome.[13,14] NGS not only enables sensitive and comprehensive mutation profiling but also represents an alternative approach for translocation and copy number variation (CNV) detection in a genome-wide fashion.[15,16]

APPLICATIONS OF MOLECULAR GENETIC TESTING IN HEMATOLOGIC MALIGNANCIES

Cytogenetic and molecular features are increasingly incorporated into the World Health Organization (WHO) Classification of Hematologic and Lymphoid Neoplasms.[17] The diagnosis of specific myeloid and

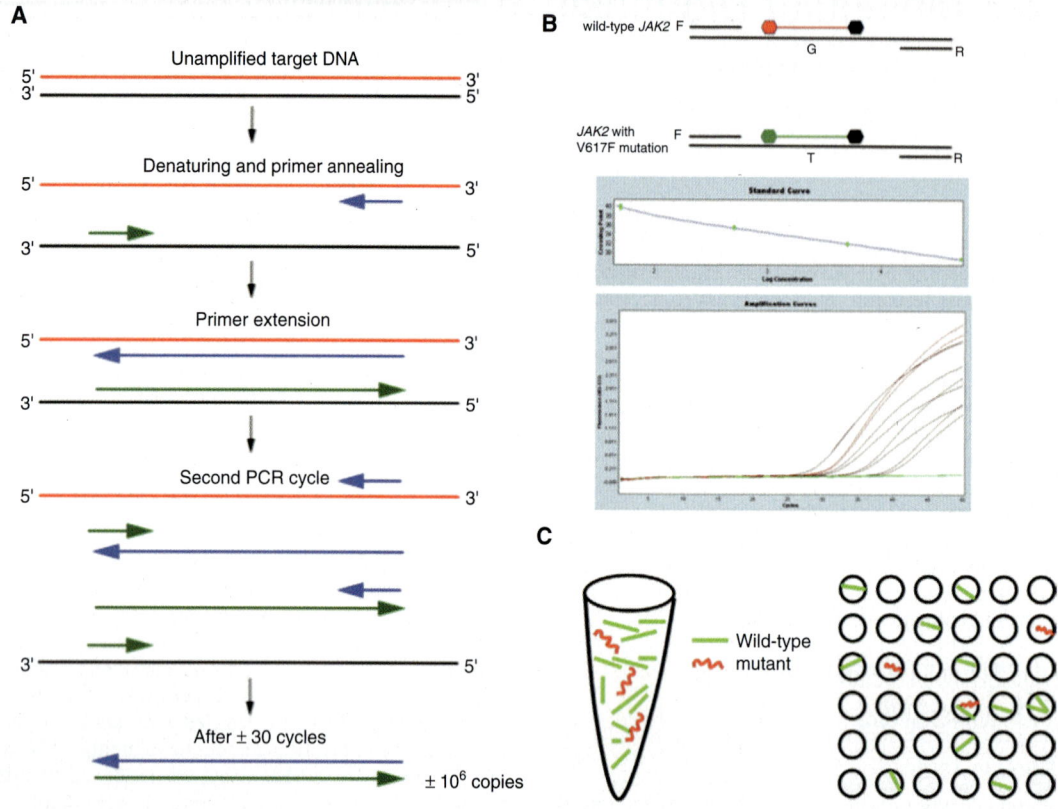

FIGURE 4.1 Polymerase chain reaction (PCR). A, End-point PCR. Unamplified double-strand template DNA is first denatured into two single strands by heating. Then, specific primers (green and blue arrows) anneal to the desired target sequences and the complementary strand is synthesized. The repeated PCR cycles of denaturing, primer annealing, and extension result in exponential amplification of the target sequence. B, Real-time PCR. The upper panel shows the design of a TaqMan qPCR assay for detection of the *JAK2* V617F mutation. The forward (F) and reverse (R) primers are identical, and the different fluorescent probes are used to detect the wild-type (red) and mutated (green) sequences. The 3′ moiety (black) on the probes represents the quencher dye. The middle panel shows an example of the standard curve generated by plotting the known absolute quantities of the standards versus the corresponding crossing points in PCR. The lower panel shows a representative example of *JAK2* TaqMan qPCR amplification curves of four standards and a V617F-positive patient sample (bright red color). The final result is reported as a relative quantity of the V617F *JAK2* derived by dividing the number of V617F mutant *JAK2* copies by the total number of *JAK2* copies (wild type and mutant). C, Digital PCR. Unlike conventional PCR (shown on the left) where mutant and wild-type alleles are mixed together in one reaction and rare mutants compete for reagents with usually more abundant wild-type DNA, digital PCR method dilutes the sample and compartmentalizes individual sequences so that ideally each reaction contains at most one copy of the DNA molecular of interest. Therefore, digital PCR can achieve increased sensitivity by giving mutant sequences equal access to reagents. The numbers of positive and negative reactions are used to calculate the quantity of DNA molecules of interest in the original sample based on Poisson statistics. (A, Reproduced with permission from Raby BA. Tools for genetics and genomics: Polymerase chain reaction. In: Post TW, ed. *UpToDate.* UpToDate. Accessed on November 1, 2021. Copyright © 2021 UpToDate, Inc. and its affiliates and/or licensors. All rights reserved. B, Image adapted from Jones D. Molecular Diagnosis in Hematology. *13e of Wintrobe's Clinical Hematology.* C, Reprinted from Sedlak RH, Jerome KR. Viral diagnostics in the era of digital polymerase chain reaction. *Diagn Microbiol Infect Dis.* 2013;75(1):1-4. Copyright © 2013 Elsevier. With permission.)

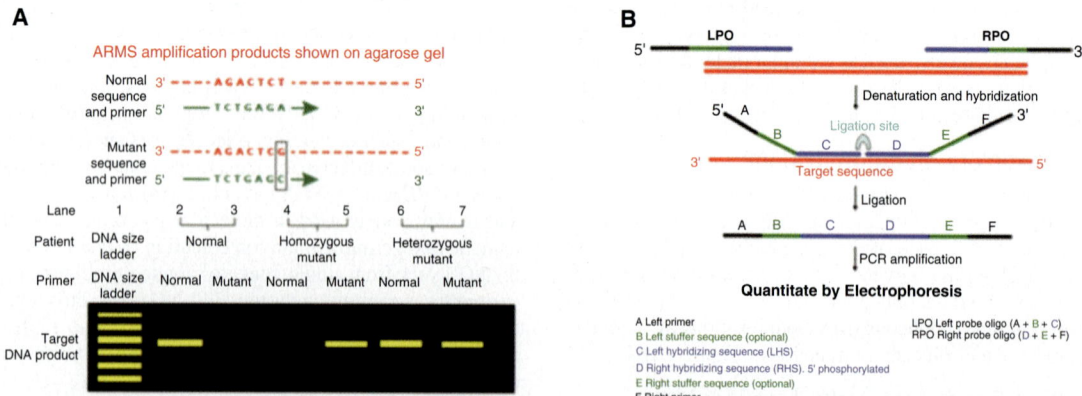

FIGURE 4.2 A, Amplification-refractory mutation system (ARMS). In this example, separate primers (green) are designed to match the normal or mutant gene sequences. The mutant base and the corresponding altered base on the mutant primer are indicated in the box. The polymerase chain reaction (PCR) products are resolved on an agarose gel with band patterns corresponding to the presence of the wild-type or mutant DNA sequence. Lanes 2 and 3: Individual homozygous wild-type; lanes 4 and 5: individual homozygous for the mutation; lanes 6 and 7: individual heterozygous for the mutation. B, Multiplex ligation-dependent probe amplification (MLPA). Two probes with flanking sequence tags are annealed adjacent to each other on the target sequence and then ligated using a DNA ligase. The ligated sequences are subsequently amplified using universal primers with fluorescent labels and quantified. The different size of stuffer sequence between hybridizing sequence and primer sequence, or extended length of the hybridizing sequences, renders a distinct size of each PCR product and allows for identification by electrophoresis. LPO, left probe oligonucleotide; RPO, right probe nucleotide. (A, Reproduced with permission from Schrijver I, Zehnder JL. Tools for genetics and genomics: cytogenetics and molecular genetics. In: Post TW, ed. *UpToDate.* UpToDate. Accessed on September 20, 2021. Copyright © 2021 UpToDate, Inc. and its affiliates and/or licensors. All rights reserved. B, From Zhi J, Hatchwell E. Human MLPA Probe Design (H-MAPD): a probe design tool for both electrophoresis-based and bead-coupled human multiplex ligation-dependent probe amplification assays. *BMC Genomics.* 2008;9:407. http://creativecommons.org/licenses/by/2.0)

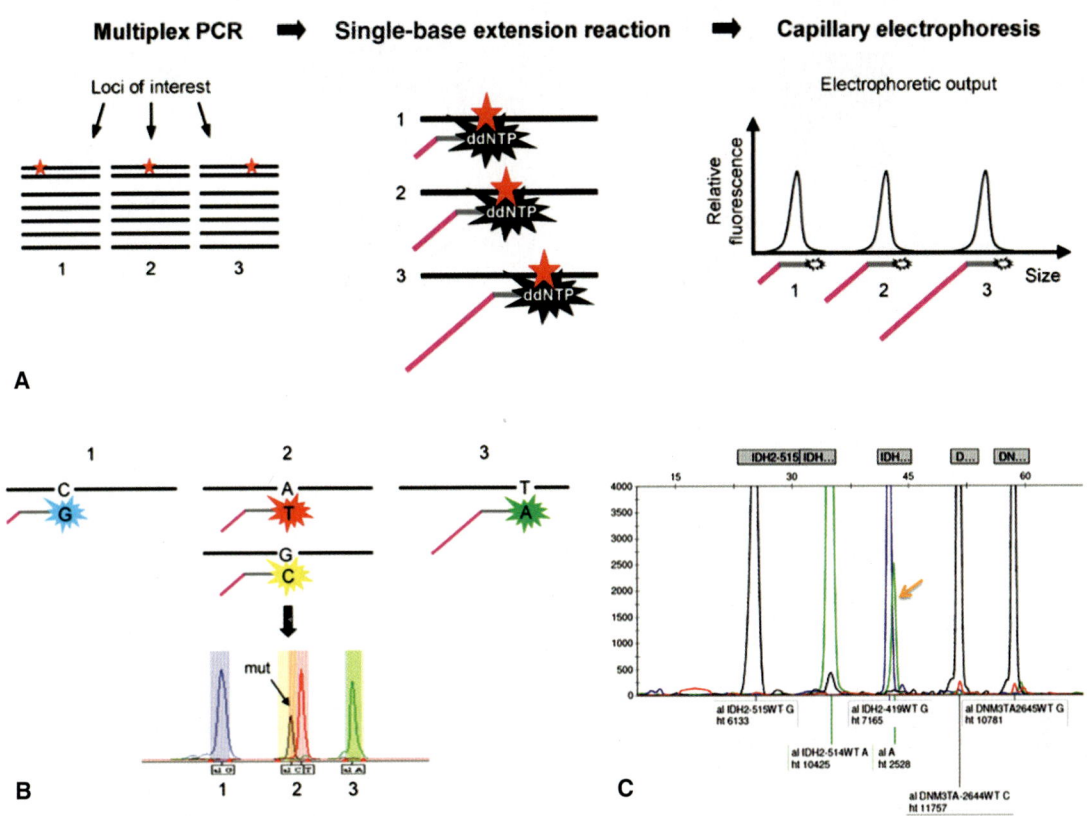

FIGURE 4.3 SNaPshot genotyping. A, This method starts with a multiplex polymerase chain reaction (PCR) and target sequences harboring loci of interest are amplified. Subsequently, in a single-base extension sequencing reaction, allele-specific probes fluorescently labeled with dideoxynucleotides (ddNTPs) and different in size are used to interrogate loci of interest. The products of this step are resolved by capillary electrophoresis and the identity of each locus is determined by the position of its corresponding fluorescent peak in the spectrum. **B,** The nucleotide at each locus is identified by the molecular weight and color of the fluorescently labeled ddNTPs. Therefore, mutant and wild-type alleles can be distinguished based on the slightly different positions and the color of the corresponding peaks. **C,** Example of IDH2 mutation by SNaPshot. A c.419G>A (p.R140Q) mutation (green peak, indicated by arrow) in the IDH2 gene is detected by SNaPshot. (A and B, From Dias-Santagata D, Akhavanfard S, David SS, et al. Rapid targeted mutational analysis of human tumours: a clinical platform to guide personalized cancer medicine. *EMBO Mol Med.* 2010;2(5):146-158. Copyright © 2010 EMBO Molecular Medicine. Reprinted by permission of John Wiley & Sons, Inc.)

lymphoid malignancies is discussed in other chapters of this book. In this chapter, we will focus on how molecular tests are used to assist with diagnosis and prognosis of diseases.

Somatic Single-Nucleotide Variant and Small Insertion/Deletion Detection

Many somatic genetic alterations have been identified in myeloid and lymphoid malignancies, and findings of new mutations are emerging almost every day. The diagnostic, prognostic, and predictive values of some of the mutations, especially in myeloid neoplasms, have been confirmed in prior studies. The pathogenic mutations in myeloproliferative neoplasms (MPNs) typically drive cell growth, whereas the pathogenic mutations in acute myeloid leukemia (AML) and myelodysplastic syndrome (MDS) often impair maturation.[1] A list of genes with recurrent mutations detected in myeloid neoplasm is shown by function groups in *Table 4.1.*[13]

The conventional testing strategy is to perform single gene assays targeting a particular genetic alteration using PCR or Sanger sequencing methods for genes with significance in the clinical management of patients (e.g., *FLT3*, *NPM1*, *KIT*, and *CEBPA*). Detection of *JAK2* p.V617F or *CALR* frameshift mutations in patients with suspected MPNs provides supporting evidence for the diagnosis.

With the elucidation of the mutational landscape in myeloid malignancies, the increasing access to NGS technology and decrease in sequencing costs, molecular pathology laboratories are rapidly adopting NGS-based multigene panels for myeloid mutation profiling. Instead of running multiple single-gene tests separately, this high-throughput and comprehensive approach can provide mutation information for all genes covered on the panel at the same time. The

method has been proven to be robust, provides a much broader scope of sequence information, and achieves superior sensitivity compared to Sanger sequencing. At the same time, however, NGS is also associated with higher cost, longer turnaround time, and requirements of setting up an infrastructure for bioinformatic analysis and gene variant curation. Some institutions have developed and started to use an integrated omics approach in the research setting—genome, exome, and transcriptome, in paired normal-tumor analysis.[14] The advantages of this approach include capturing genetic alterations on a genome-scale instead of being limited by the genomic regions covered by a panel, cross validation of findings of genetic alterations, distinguishing somatic versus germline variants, and identifying translocations, copy number variations in addition to SNVs and small insertions/deletions (indels). The applicability of such a comprehensive approach in the clinical setting remains to be established in the near future; however, RNA-based NGS analysis has demonstrated complementary clinical value, especially when used in combination with DNA-based NGS analysis.[18]

Molecular assessment of minimal/measurable residual disease (MRD) may be done by multiparameter flow cytometry (Chapter 2), chimerism evaluation following allogeneic hematopoietic stem cell transplantation, PCR methods targeting specific genetic variants (e.g., *NPM1*) or translocations (e.g., *PML::RARA*), and NGS methods. The utility of the qRT-PCR-based assessment of *NPM1* in *NPM1* mutation–positive AML has been demonstrated to have superior prognostic value compared with the baseline diagnostic molecular genetic markers.[19,20] NGS panel–based MRD assessments have emerged as sensitive and specific indicators of residual disease status.[21] The general approach to employing NGS methods is that there must be a prior

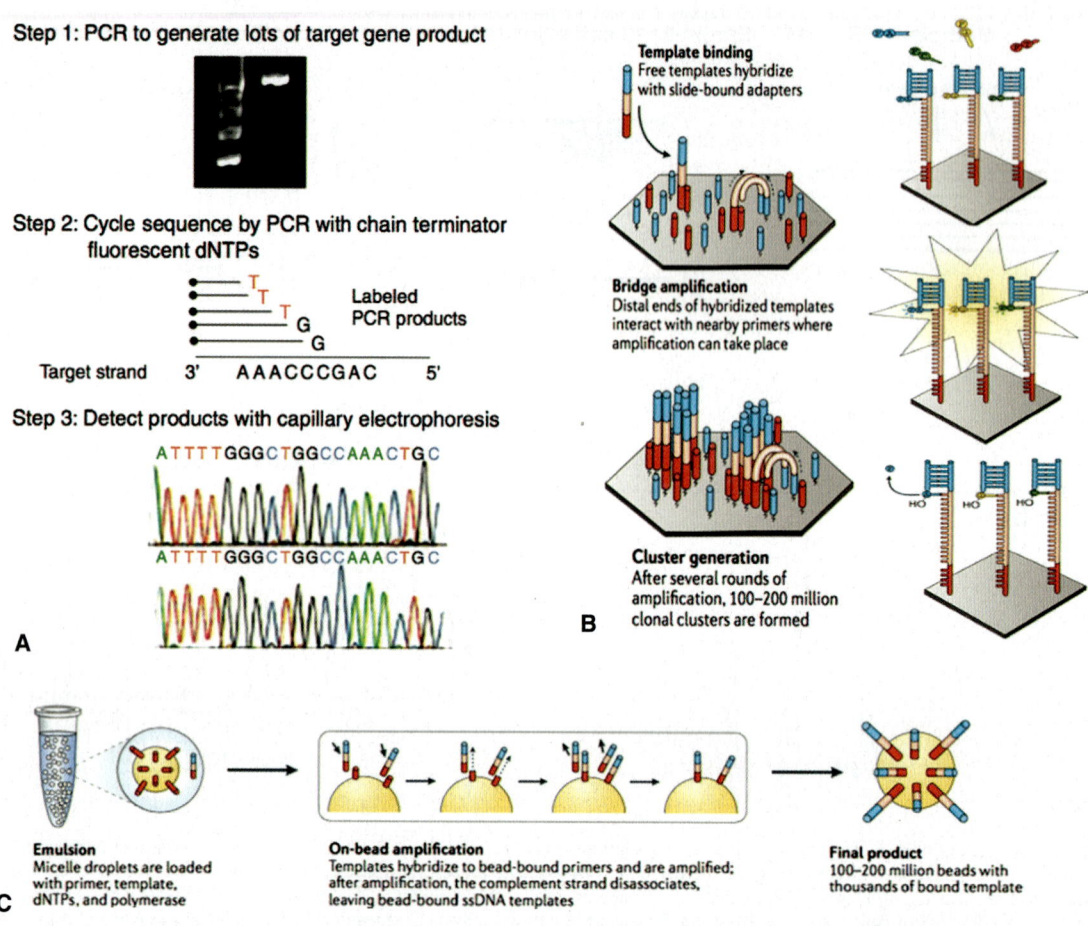

FIGURE 4.4 Sequencing methods. A, Steps of Sanger sequencing method. Amplicons of target gene regions are generated by polymerase chain reaction (PCR) and confirmed by electrophoresis. Then, unidirectional (asymmetric) PCR using the amplicons from the first step as template along with primer in a reaction containing normal nucleotides are mixed with chain terminating fluorescent deoxynucleotides (dNTPs). The products from the asymmetric PCR terminated at every possible base are separated by capillary electrophoresis followed by laser detection of the fluorochrome. A software application that normalizes the peak heights to produce the electropherogram is used for base-calling. B, Solid-phase bridge amplification–based next-generation sequencing. On the left, fragmented template DNA is ligated to adapter sequences and then bound to a primer immobilized on a solid support, such as a flow cell. The free end can interact with other primers to form a bridge structure. Subsequent PCR creates a second strand using the immobilized primers and generates large numbers of clonal clusters. On the right, the key steps of the Illumina sequencing-by-synthesis method—nucleotide addition, imaging, and cleavage—are shown. Fluorophore-labeled, terminally blocked nucleotides hybridize to complementary bases and are imaged with laser channels. Fluorophores are then cleaved and washed from the flow cell at the end of each cycle. C, Emulsion PCR–based next-generation sequencing. Fragmented template DNA is ligated to adapter sequences and captured in an aqueous droplet (micelle), along with a bead covered with complementary adapters, dNTPs, primers, and DNA polymerase. PCR is performed within the micelle and generating thousands of copies of the same DNA sequence on each bead. (A, Image copyright Jones D. Molecular diagnosis in hematology. *13e of Wintrobe's Clinical Hematology.* B and C, Adapted by permission from Nature: Goodwin S, McPherson JD, McCombie WR. Coming of age: ten years of next-generation sequencing technologies. *Nat Rev Genet.* 2016;17(6):333-351. Copyright © 2016 Springer Nature.)

Table 4.1. Genes With Recurrent Genetic Alterations Detected in Myeloid Neoplasms Grouped by Function[13]

Groups by Function	Genes
Signaling molecules	*JAK2, KIT, NRAS, FLT3, KRAS, PTPN11, CBL, JAK3, CSF3R, ABL1, BRAF, HRAS, CBLB, GNAS, CALR*
Regulators of DNA methylation	*IDH1, IDH2, TET2, DNMT3A*
Epigenetic regulators	*ASXL1, EZH2, SETBP1, KMT2A, BCOR, KDM6A, BCORL1*
Tumor suppressors	*TP53, WT1, PHF6, FBXW7, PTEN*
Myeloid transcription factors	*CEBPA, RUNX1, CBFB, NPM1, GATA1, GATA2, ETV6, IKZF1*
Splicing factors	*SF3B1, SRSF2, U2AF1, ZRSR2*
Cohesin complex	*STAG2, SMC1A, SMC3, RAD21*

baseline assessment of somatic variants at the time of diagnosis or active disease. Germline variants need to be excluded from MRD analysis. The bioinformatics challenge is to separate the signal of the previously identified variants from the background noise of the system. Excluding variants linked with clonal hematopoiesis (e.g., *DNMT3A, ASXL1, TET2,* also termed DAT) and focusing on pathogenic variants over variants of unknown significance also improve test specificity. Depending on the bioinformatic pipeline employed, the sensitivity of targeted NGS MRD assay is routinely <0.5% and can reach <0.1%. Emerging variants can also be detected at the standard sensitivity of the diagnostic NGS panel, generally 1% to 5%. Thus, NGS-based MRD testing is gaining popularity as a valuable tool in assessing disease status in AML patients following therapeutic interventions.

Clonality Analysis and Minimal Residual Disease Monitoring of Lymphoproliferative Disorders

It can be diagnostically challenging to distinguish clonal lymphoproliferations seen in lymphoid leukemias and lymphomas from benign lymphoid expansions. In addition to immunophenotyping by flow cytometry, PCR-based analysis of B-cell and T-cell receptor (TCR) rearrangements has been widely used as an important ancillary test.

Precursor B cells arise in the bone marrow and migrate into the peripheral blood as naïve forms. The further maturation of B cells is dependent on the recognition of an antigen that binds to the B-cell receptor, composed of two immunoglobulin heavy chains (IGH) and two immunoglobulin light chains (either IGK or IGL). Precursor T cells similarly arise in the bone marrow and then migrate to thymus.[1] Precursor T and B cells undergo rearrangements of their receptors during early development by recombining certain variable (V) and joining (J) gene segments, with or without diversity (D) segment. Random nucleotide insertions happen within the joining regions to further increase the sequence diversity.[22] All cells within a clonal B or T cell proliferation will have the same receptor sequence and identical PCR-amplified V(D)J fragment size. Due to the variation in rearranged Ig or TCR, the sizes of V(D)J amplicons of a polyclonal B- or T-cell population follow the Gaussian distribution. A monoclonal population, on the other hand, will demonstrate a distinct size peak on capillary electrophoresis representing the same receptor sequence (as assessed by amplicon size) shared by the clonal cells. The aforementioned differences form the foundation of multiplex PCR–based clonality analysis, which is currently widely used in clinical diagnostic laboratories.[21] While this methodology is fast and relatively inexpensive to perform, the lack of specific sequence information poses limitations. For example, two or more independent amplicons of the same size could be falsely interpreted as a single clone.

Historically, MRD monitoring for B-cell malignancies has been carried out using allele-specific oligonucleotide real-time PCR (ASO-PCR) with IGH used commonly as a target. The primer or probe is designed to anneal to the most variable CDR3 region specific to each patient's tumor clone. This method can achieve an analytical sensitivity of 10^{-5}, higher than the sensitivity of flow-cytometric method (10^{-4}) for clonal B-cell populations.[23] The limitations of this method include the following: (1) the patient's tumor clone sequence is necessary for the assay design; (2) the method is labor-intensive and expensive; (3) the method is unable to detect emerging new predominant clone or clonal evolution. For the foregoing reasons, ASO-PCR-based MRD assessment is usually restricted to the research setting.

The NGS-based clonality assays overcome the major limitations inherent to the conventional qualitative and quantitative PCR-based methods. It affords the capability to identify specific clonal sequences in both B- and T-cell populations and detect MRD following therapeutic interventions. These assays no longer rely on fragment size for clonality pattern recognition, but rather provide sequences along with the corresponding numbers of sequencing reads of all the clonotypes in the sampled antigen receptor repertoire. The results generated by this method are more sensitive and specific compared with those by the fragment size-based clonality analysis (*Figure 4.5*). The quantitative nature of NGS method also significantly reduces ambiguity and variation in interpretation of clonality patterns.[24-26]

The NGS-based T- and B-cell gene rearrangement assays with the capability of accurately identifying and quantifying individual clonotypes provide unique advantages in MRD monitoring and have become more widely utilized in the evaluation of lymphoid neoplasms in recent years. Both commercial in vitro diagnostic tests offered by reference laboratories and diagnostic tests established by institutional molecular pathology laboratories using standardized commercial reagents have been reported to achieve a sensitivity of 10^{-6}.[27,28]

Translocation/Fusion Detection

Besides SNVs and small indels, recurrent tumor-specific chromosomal translocations, which contribute directly to malignant transformation,

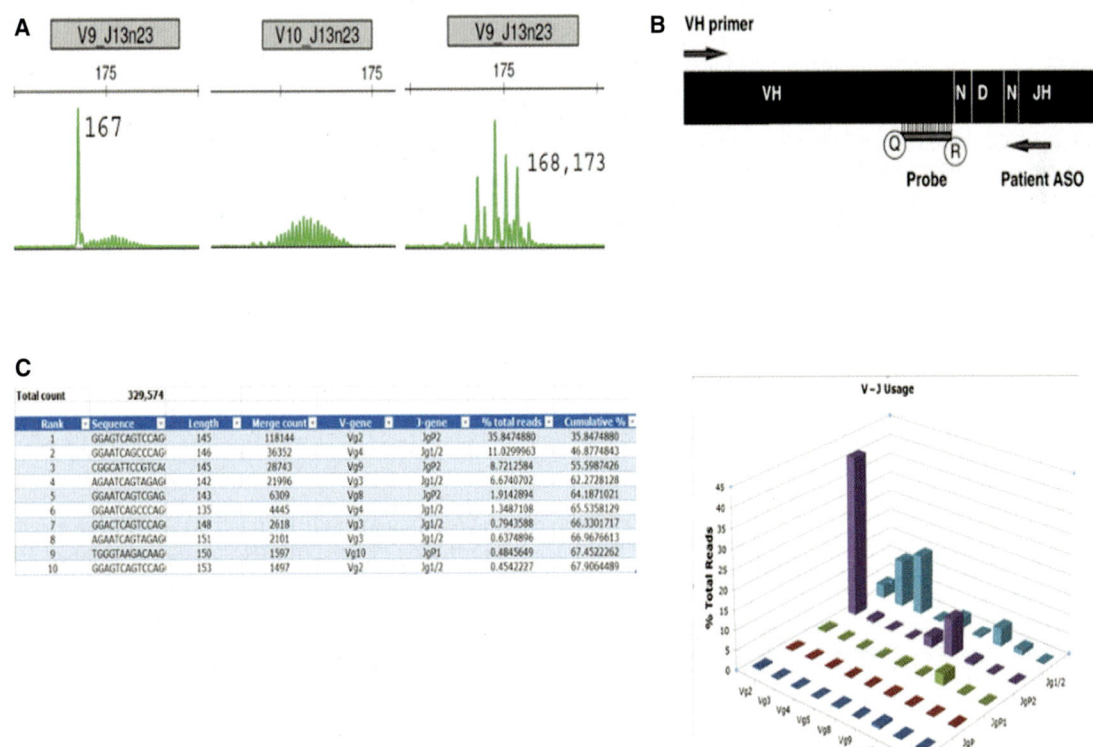

FIGURE 4.5 Clonality analysis and design of allele-specific oligonucleotide PCR (ASO-PCR) for minimal residual disease detection. A, Patterns by conventional capillary electrophoresis–based clonality analysis. From left to right, representative monoclonal, polyclonal, and oligoclonal patterns are shown. B, ASO-PCR assay design. In this example, the tumor-specific immunoglobulin heavy chain (IGH) sequence for each individual patient is used for the design of primers and TaqMan probe so that one primer and/or the probe anneals to the most variable sequence region to ensure highly specific amplification of the tumor clone. C, Next-generation sequencing (NGS)-based clonality analysis. With this approach, the individual clonotype sequences and counts within the sampled repertoire are obtained. The table on the left shows the rank, sequence, length, merge counts, V-gene, J-gene, % total reads, and cumulative% for the top 10 clonotypes of this patient with a clonal T-cell process. The graph on the right shows the V and J segment usage in the sampled T-cell receptor gamma (TRG) repertoire.

Laboratory Hematology

have been identified in many myeloid and lymphoid malignancies. Translocation, which involves recombination of chromosome segments, can result in the formation of a new fusion gene, or protein overexpression by juxtaposing positive regulatory elements from one gene to coding sequences of another.[1] Detection and quantitation of the fusion genes can provide important diagnostic and prognostic information.

One classical example of translocation in hematologic malignancies is the Philadelphia chromosome, a hallmark of chronic myeloid leukemia (CML) and also the first chromosome abnormality described in human malignancies. The reciprocal t(9;22)(q34;q11.2) leads to the creation of *BCR::ABL1*, a transcriptionally active fusion gene, which encodes a chimeric protein involved in leukemogenesis. Furthermore, *BCR::ABL1* is also central to the pathogenesis of 20% ~ 25% of adult and about 5% of pediatric B-cell acute lymphoblastic leukemias.[29] The two most commonly used molecular methods for detecting translocations are PCR and fluorescence in situ hybridization (FISH). There are pros and cons associated with each approach. FISH is rapid and technically straightforward. It enables the targeted detection of translocations without the need of knowing sequence-level details.[30] PCR method, on the other hand, requires the knowledge of sequence information, but has a higher analytical sensitivity. Qualitative and quantitative PCR methods have been used in standard clinical practice for diagnosis, treatment assessment, and MRD monitoring of CML and Ph+ ALL.

Another commonly used molecular test for fusion detection is *PML::RARA* as a result of the t(15;17)(q22;q21) which defines acute promyelocytic leukemia (APL). The major manifestation of the chimeric PML::RARA protein is a maturation block at the promyelocyte stage of myeloid differentiation, leading to the accumulation of neoplastic blasts and promyelocytes. With rare exceptions, both FISH and PCR methods can detect this fusion gene. PCR has the advantage of detecting the three major fusion transcripts and rare submicroscopic complex translocations. More importantly, we can use quantitative PCR to monitor MRD of APL following treatment.[31] The *PML::RARA* transcript level at the end of consolidation therapy is of high predictive value for relapse.[32]

In recent years, major advances have been made in the computational methods for NGS-based fusion detection. RNA sequencing (RNAseq) covers the transcribed genome (~2% of total genome) and can detect multiple splice variants from one translocation event.[33] Due to its relatively low cost and fast turnaround time, RNAseq is emerging as a reasonable choice for unbiased comprehensive fusion detection in molecular diagnostic laboratories.

Circulating Tumor DNA

Cell-free DNA (cfDNA), extracellular DNA molecules circulating in the bloodstream, was first described in 1948.[34] Since then, there have been significant advancements in elucidating the origin, characteristics as well as potential applications of cfDNA analysis. Circulating tumor DNA (ctDNA), also known as "liquid biopsy," is cfDNA originating from tumor cells. Due to the noninvasive nature of the associated procedure, ctDNA harboring specific genetic alterations has emerged as a promising diagnostic and prognostic biomarker in clinical oncology in recent years.[35] In the setting of hematological malignancies, clinical ctDNA assessment may add value to the cell-based testing, such as enabling characterization of the genetic landscape on a wider scale where the disease tissues contain low malignant cell fraction or the primary lesions are difficult to approach for technical reasons. Furthermore, the ctDNA analysis also holds promise for the monitoring of disease burden in non-Hodgkin lymphoma.[36-39]

APPLICATIONS OF MOLECULAR GENETIC TESTING IN NONMALIGNANT HEMATOLOGIC DISORDERS

In addition to malignant hematologic disorders, molecular testing also plays important roles in the diagnosis and stratification of patients with nonmalignant hematologic disorders. Several major disease categories are briefly discussed here.

Thalassemias

Thalassemias are quantitative defects that lead to reduced or absent levels of one type of globin chain, creating an imbalance in the ratio of alpha-like chains to non–alpha-like chains. The excess chains that fail to incorporate into hemoglobin form nonfunctional aggregates and precipitate within the red blood cells (RBCs), which lead to premature RBC destruction.[40]

At the genetic level, large deletions involving one or more alpha-globin genes account for the majority of alpha thalassemia cases, and other types of genetic alterations (SNVs, small indels in regions critical for alpha-globin gene expression) are less common. Although DNA-based testing is rarely used as a first-line test, it is useful for confirming the diagnosis in patients with suspected thalassemia, particularly in the setting of prenatal and newborn screening to provide the possibility of early diagnosis, genetic counseling, and early institution of appropriate treatment. The molecular testing method of choice depends on the type of suspected variants. For detection of gross deletions, GAP-PCR with primers flanking the deletion breakpoints, MLPA, and array comparative genomic hybridization can be used. For detection of SNVs and small indels, sequencing analysis can be performed.[41]

Beta-thalassemias are heterogeneous at the genetic level with more than 200 disease-causing mutations identified so far. In contrast to alpha-thalassemias, the majority of beta thalassemia cases are caused by SNVs or small indel variants leading to frameshifts in the *HBB* gene. Allele-specific PCR or microarray method can be used to detect the commonly occurring mutations, and sequencing analysis is the choice for unbiased mutation screening. The possibility of larger deletions can be investigated using MLPA.[42]

Bone Marrow Failure Syndromes

Bone marrow failure syndromes, a group of disorders with complex pathophysiology characterized by a common phenotype of peripheral cytopenia(s) and/or hypoplastic bone marrow,[43] can be acquired or inherited. The inherited forms of bone marrow failure syndromes (IBMFS) are phenotypically complex and genetically heterogeneous disorders associated with inadequate hematopoietic cell production, congenital anomalies, and a predisposition to malignancy.[44] More than 25% of pediatric patients and approximately 10% of young adults presenting with aplastic anemia have a genetic etiology.[45] The main recognized mechanisms include DNA repair defects (Fanconi anemia), ribosomopathies (Shwachman-Diamond and Diamond-Blackfan anemia), telomere defects (dyskeratosis congenita), and others.[46] Despite the relative rarity of IBMFS, they are associated with very high morbidity and mortality. Timely and accurate diagnosis of patients with underlying IBMFS allows appropriate clinical monitoring for clonal evolution so that hematopoietic stem cell transplantation can be initiated prior to MDS or leukemia development. The genetic diagnosis would also inform the selection of hematopoietic stem cell donors and identification of affected siblings. Moreover, genetic counseling of family members would also be possible.[47]

Molecular studies of these disorders can provide critical insight into hematopoietic cell biology. To date, over 50 disease-causing genes (*Table 4.2*[43]) for IBMFS have been identified and new discoveries keep emerging to further elucidate the pathophysiology of these disorders. Both single-gene Sanger sequencing tests and targeted multigene NGS panels are available to provide genetic evidence for IBMFS, which often impose diagnostic challenges clinically.[44]

Hemostatic Disorders

The delicate hemostatic balance is maintained by a complex interplay of coagulation cascade, natural antithrombotic systems, fibrinolytic mechanisms, and platelets. Genetic defects in certain factors can break the balance and lead to increased risk of thrombosis or bleeding. Inherited bleeding, thrombotic or platelet disorders affect ~300/million births.[48]

The most frequently ordered molecular tests for patients with thrombophilia are Factor V Leiden and Prothrombin 20210G > A. The p.R506Q mutation in the factor V gene occurs at one of the cleavage

Table 4.2. Known Disease-Causing Genes for Inherited Bone Marrow Failure Syndromes[31]

Inherited Bone Marrow Failure Syndromes	Known Disease-Causing Genes
Fanconi anemia	*FANCA, FANCB, FANCC, FANCD1, FANCD2, FANCE, FANCF, FANCG, FANCI, FANCL, FANCM*
Dyskeratosis congenita	*DKC1, TERT, TR, TINF2, RTEL1, NOP10, NHP2, WRAP53, NOP10, NHP2, WRAP53, C16orf57, CTC1*
Diamond-Blackfan anemia	*RPS24, RPS17, RPS7, RPS10, RPS19, RPS26, RPS27, RPS29, RPL5, RPL11, RPL26, RPL15, RPL27, RPL35*
Shwachman-Diamond syndrome	*SBDS*
Congenital amegakaryo-cytic thrombocytopenia	*MPL*
Severe congenital neutropenia	*ELA2, HAX1, AK2, GFI1, WASP, CSF3R, G6PC3, GATA1, JAGN1, VPS45*
Thrombocytopenia absent radii	*RBM8A*
Radioulnar synostosis with amegakaryocytic thrombocytopenia	*HOXA11*
Pearson syndrome	Contiguous gene deletion/duplication syndrome involving several mtDNA genes

sites by activated protein C and renders a less efficient degradation by protein C. The risk of thrombosis is increased 2- to 10-fold in heterozygotes and >10-fold in homozygotes for this mutation.[49,50] The prothrombin 20210G>A mutation in the 3′-untranslated region is associated with increased plasma prothrombin level and considered as an independent risk factor for thrombotic disease.[51,52] Genotyping assays, most commonly melting curve analysisbased method, have been widely used to accurately detect these two mutations.

Hemophilia (A and B) and von Willebrand disease (VWD) are the most common and well-known bleeding disorders. The value of molecular genetic testing for hemophilia lies in carrier status determination, prenatal diagnosis, prediction of inhibitor development, and possibly responsiveness to immune tolerance induction.[53] Genetic testing of VWD is more controversial due to the large size and highly polymorphic nature of the *VWF* gene, in addition to the challenge imposed by a pseudogene. It has been suggested that genetic testing should be limited only to specific situations, such as identifying large deletions in patients with VWD type 3 that would place them at higher risk of developing neutralizing antibodies and anaphylactic reactions upon treatment, or situations in which therapeutic options would be significantly different upon accurate diagnosis (e.g., type 2N and 2B VWD).[54,55]

Inherited platelet disorders (IPDs) with abnormalities in platelet number or function, in contrast to coagulation disorders, have high genetic heterogeneity. More than 50 IPD-causing genes are reported, although many of those genetic findings had not yet been translated into clinical molecular testing.[56,57] As NGS-based genetic testing for IPDs is becoming more available and more sequence variants are detected, it has become evident that variant curation and interpretation guidelines tailored for this heterogeneous group of disorders would be needed to minimize discrepancies among different clinical laboratories. For this reason, the Clinical Genome Resource (ClinGen) established an expert panel to perform American College of Medical Genetics and Genomics and the Association for Molecular Pathology (ACMG/AMP) rule specification and classification for IPD genetic variants.[58]

FUTURE DIRECTIONS

Hematology has been the discipline at the forefront of using molecular methods to understand disease etiology, diagnose disease, and stratify patients based on prognosis and response to therapies. In recent years, the revolutionary advancements in sequencing technologies offer exciting new opportunities not only in the research realm to improve understanding of disease mechanisms but also in the clinical molecular diagnostics of hematologic disorders. Various NGS-based multigene targeted panels are increasingly used in molecular pathology laboratories across the country, including panels for both malignant and nonmalignant hematologic disorders. Although these typically require a longer turnaround time, they serve as a great complementation and/or alternative to the conventional single-gene testing by providing comprehensive information on clinically significant biomarkers or actionable mutations, which forms the foundation for precision medicine in hematology. Some academic medical centers and reference laboratories have started offering whole-exome or whole-genome sequencing as a clinical test for suspected inherited disorders. Various computational tools have also been developed for better and more streamlined bioinformatic analysis.

In the coming years, it is foreseeable that integrated omics analysis, especially both DNA- and RNA-based, will likely gain further popularity and be utilized by more molecular diagnostic laboratories. Molecular and cytogenetic technologies will be increasingly converged into NGS-based platforms. The escalated speed of new discoveries of disease-causing genes and novel biomarkers in hematology facilitated by NGS technology would require a fast and flexible way of translating the findings with confirmed clinical utility into clinical testing to benefit the patients. As the cost of whole-exome/genome sequencing further decreases, more molecular diagnostic assays based on these platforms will be available. Single-cell-based genetic analysis, which can be very informative in elucidating clonal evolution of AML, is currently performed primarily in the research setting and may be more amenable to clinical use as the technology further matures and the cost decreases. The evolving knowledge of molecular pathogenesis of hematologic diseases also enables and drives the increasing incorporation of molecular evidence into disease classifications.

References

1. Jones D. Molecular diagnosis in hematology. *13e of Wintrobe's Clinical Hematology*. Wolters Kluwer; 2013:58-64.
2. Raby BA. *Tools for Genetics and Genomics: Polymerase Chain Reaction.* 2016 UpToDate. Updated August 9, 2016. Accessed January 23, 2018. https://www.uptodate.com/contents/tools-for-genetics-and-genomics-polymerase-chain-reaction
3. Schrijver I, Zehnder JL, Cherry AM. *Tools for Genetics and Genomics: Cytogenetics and Molecular Genetics.* 2016 UpToDate. Updated September 19, 2016. Accessed January 23, 2018. https://www.uptodate.com/contents/tools-for-genetics-and-genomics-cytogenetics-and-molecular-genetics
4. Schouten JP, McElgunn CJ, Waaijer R, et al. Relative quantification of 40 nucleic acid sequences by multiplex ligation-dependent probe amplification. *Nucleic Acids Res.* 2002;30(12):e57.
5. Zhi J, Hatchwell E. Human MLPA Probe Design (H-MAPD): a probe design tool for both electrophoresis-based and bead-coupled human multiplex ligation-dependent probe amplification assays. *BMC Genom.* 2008;9:407.
6. Yau SC, Bobrow M, Mathew CG, et al. Accurate diagnosis of carriers of deletions and duplications in Duchenne/Becker muscular dystrophy by fluorescent dosage analysis. *J Med Genet.* 1996;33(7):550-558.
7. Bunyan DJ, Eccles DM, Sillibourne J, et al. Dosage analysis of cancer predisposition genes by multiplex ligation-dependent probe amplification. *Br J Cancer.* 2004;91(6):1155-1159.
8. Paneto GG, Careta FP. Designing primers for SNaPshot technique, C. Basu (ed.), *Methods in Molecular Biology*, Vol 1275.
9. Fariña Sarasqueta A, Moerland E, de Bruyne H, et al. SNaPshot and StripAssay as valuable alternatives to direct sequencing for KRAS mutation detection in colon cancer routine diagnostics. *J Mol Diagn.* 2011;13(2):199-205.
10. Sanger F, Nicklen S, Coulson AR. DNA sequencing with chain-terminating inhibitors. *Proc Natl Acad Sci U S A.* 1977;74:5463-5467.
11. Goodwin S, McPherson JD, McCombie WR. Coming of age: ten years of next-generation sequencing technologies. *Nat Rev Genet.* 2016;17(6):333-351.
12. Black JS, Salto-Tellez M, Mills KI et al. The impact of next generation sequencing technologies on haematological research--A review. *Pathogenesis* 2015;2:9e16.
13. Kuo FC, Dong F. Next-generation sequencing-based panel testing for myeloid neoplasms. *Curr Hematol Malig Rep.* 2015;10(2):104-111.
14. Zhang J, Walsh MF, Wu G, et al. Germline mutations in predisposition genes in pediatric cancer. *N Engl J Med.* 2015;373(24):2336-2346.

Laboratory Hematology

15. Shen W, Szankasi P, Sederberg M, et al. Concurrent detection of targeted copy number variants and mutations using a myeloid malignancy next generation sequencing panel allows comprehensive genetic analysis using a single testing strategy. *Br J Haematol.* 2016;173(1):49-58.

16. Byron SA, Van Keuren-Jensen KR, Engelthaler DM, et al. Translating RNA sequencing into clinical diagnostics: opportunities and challenges. *Nat Rev Genet.* 2016;17(5):257-271.

17. Swerdlow SH, Campo E, Pileri SA, et al. The 2016 revision of the World Health Organization classification of lymphoid neoplasms. *Blood.* 2016;127(20):2375-2390.

18. He J, Abdel-Wahab O, Nahas MK, et al. Integrated genomic DNA/RNA profiling of hematologic malignancies in the clinical setting. *Blood.* 2016;127(24):3004-3014.

19. Schnittger S, Kern W, Tschulik C, et al. Minimal residual disease levels assessed by NPM1 mutation-specific RQ-PCR provide important prognostic information in AML. *Blood.* 2009;114(11):2220-2231.

20. Ivey A, Hills RK, Simpson MA, et al. Assessment of minimal residual disease in standard-risk AML. *N Engl J Med.* 2016;374(5):422-433.

21. Heuser M, Freeman SD, Ossenkoppele GJ, et al. Update on MRD in acute myeloid leukemia: a consensus document from the European LeukemiaNet MRD Working Party. *Blood.* 2021;138(26):2753-2767.

22. van Dongen JJM, Langerak AW, Brüggemann M, et al. Design and standardization of PCR primers and protocols for detection of clonal immunoglobulin and T-cell receptor gene recombinations in suspect lymphoproliferations: report of the BIOMED-2 Concerted Action BMH4-CT98-3936. *Leukemia (2003) 17,* 2257-2317.

23. Ritgen M, BöTtcher S, Dreger P, et al. Evaluation of minimal residual disease in chronic lymphocytic leukemia. *Haematologica Rep.* 2005;1(2):5-8.

24. van den Brand M, Rijntjes J, Möbs M, et al. Next-generation sequencing-based clonality assessment of Ig gene rearrangements: a multicenter validation study by EuroClonality-NGS. *J Mol Diagn.* 2021;23(9):1105-1115.

25. Scheijen B, Meijers RWJ, Rijntjes J, et al. Next-generation sequencing of immunoglobulin gene rearrangements for clonality assessment: a technical feasibility study by EuroClonality-NGS. *Leukemia.* 2019;33(9):2227-2240.

26. Ho CC, Tung JK, Zehnder JL, et al. Validation of a next-generation sequencing-based T-cell receptor gamma gene rearrangement diagnostic assay: transitioning from capillary electrophoresis to next-generation sequencing. *J Mol Diagn.* 2021;23(7):805-815.

27. Arcila ME, Yu W, Syed M, et al. Establishment of immunoglobulin heavy (IGH) chain clonality testing by next-generation sequencing for routine characterization of B-cell and plasma cell neoplasms. *J Mol Diagn.* 2019;21(2):330-342.

28. Ching T, Duncan ME, Newman-Eerkes T, et al. Analytical evaluation of the clonoSEQ Assay for establishing measurable (minimal) residual disease in acute lymphoblastic leukemia, chronic lymphocytic leukemia, and multiple myeloma. *BMC Cancer.* 2020;20(1):612.

29. Schrijver I, Zehnder JL, Cherry AM. *Genetic Abnormalities in Hematologic and Lymphoid Malignancies.* 2017 UpToDate. Updated February 8, 2016. Accessed January 23, 2018. https://www.uptodate.com/contents/genetic-abnormalities-in-hematologic-and-lymphoid-malignancies

30. Wolff DJ, Bagg A, Cooley LD, et al. Guidance for fluorescence in situ hybridization testing in hematologic disorders. *J Mol Diagn.* 2007;9(2):134-143.

31. Grimwade D, Lo Coco F. Acute promyelocytic leukemia: a model for the role of molecular diagnosis and residual disease monitoring in directing treatment approach in acute myeloid leukemia. *Leukemia.* 2002;16(10):1959-1973.

32. Santamaría C, Chillón MC, Fernández C, et al. Using quantification of the PML-RARalpha transcript to stratify the risk of relapse in patients with acute promyelocytic leukemia. *Haematologica.* 2007;92(3):315-322.

33. Wang Q, Xia J, Jia P, et al. Application of next generation sequencing to human gene fusion detection: computational tools, features and perspectives. *Brief Bioinform.* 2013;14(4):506-519.

34. Mandel P, Metais P. Les acides nucléiques du plasma sanguin chez l'homme [Nuclear Acids in Human Blood Plasma]. *C R Seances Soc Biol Fil.* 1948;142(3-4):241-243.

35. Peng Y, Mei W, Ma K, et al. Circulating tumor DNA and minimal residual disease (MRD) in solid tumors: current horizons and future perspectives. *Front Oncol.* 2021;11:763790.

36. Buedts L, Vandenberghe P. Circulating cell-free DNA in hematological malignancies. *Haematologica.* 2016;101(9):997-999.

37. Tan X, Yan H, Chen L, et al. Clinical value of ctDNA in hematological malignancies (lymphomas, multiple myeloma, myelodysplastic syndrome, and leukemia): a meta-analysis. *Front Oncol.* 2021;11:632910.

38. Ogawa M, Yokoyama K, Imoto S, et al. Role of circulating tumor DNA in hematological malignancy. *Cancers.* 2021;13(9):2078.

39. Roschewski M, Dunleavy K, Pittaluga S, et al. Circulating tumour DNA and CT monitoring in patients with untreated diffuse large B-cell lymphoma: a correlative biomarker study. *Lancet Oncol.* 2015;16(5):541-549.

40. Hoppe C. *Methods for Hemoglobin Analysis and Hemoglobinopathy Testing.* 2017 UpToDate. Updated January 9, 2018. Accessed January 23, 2018. https://www.uptodate.com/contents/methods-for-hemoglobin-analysis-and-hemoglobinopathy-testing

41. Galanello R, Cao A. Alpha-thalassemia. *Genet Med.* 2011;13(2):83-88.

42. Cao A, Galanello R. Beta-thalassemia. *Genet Med.* 2010;12(2):61-76.

43. Adam S, Sanchis DM, El-Kamah G, et al. Concise review: getting to the core of inherited bone marrow failures. *Stem Cell.* 2017;35(2):284-298.

44. Wilson DB, Link DC, Mason PJ, et al. Inherited bone marrow failure syndromes in adolescents and young adults. *Ann Med.* 2014;46(6):353-363.

45. Alter BP. Bone marrow failure: a child is not just a small adult (but an adult can have a childhood disease). *Hematology Am Soc Hematol Educ Program.* 2005;2005:96-103.

46. DeZern AE, Brodsky RA. Genetic panels in young patients with bone marrow failure: are they clinically relevant? *Haematologica.* 2016;101(11):1275-1276.

47. Zhang MY, Keel SB, Walsh T, et al. Genomic analysis of bone marrow failure and myelodysplastic syndromes reveals phenotypic and diagnostic complexity. *Haematologica.* 2015;100(1):42-48.

48. Simeoni I, Stephens JC, Hu F, et al. A high-throughput sequencing test for diagnosing inherited bleeding, thrombotic, and platelet disorders. *Blood.* 2016;127(23):2791-2803.

49. Bertina RM, Koeleman BPC, Koster T et al. Mutation in blood coagulation factor V associated with resistance to activated protein C. *Nature* 1994;369:64-67.

50. Dahlback B. New molecular insights into the genetics of thrombophilia: resistance to activated protein C caused by Arg506 to Gln mutation in Factor V as a pathogenic risk factor for venous thrombosis. *Thrombosis and Hemostasis.* 1995;74:139-148.

51. Poort SR, Rosendaal FR, Reitsma PH, et al. A common genetic variation in the 3' UTR of the prothrombin gene is associated with elevated plasma prothrombin levels and an increase in venous thrombosis. *Blood.* 1996;88:3698-3703.

52. Rosendaal FR, Siscovick DS, Schwartz SM, et al. A common prothrombin variant (20210 G>A) increases the risk of myocardial infarction in young women. *Blood.* 1997;90:1747-1750.

53. Swystun LL, James P. Using genetic diagnostics in hemophilia and von Willebrand disease. *Hematology Am Soc Hematol Educ Program.* 2015;2015:152-159.

54. Ng C, Motto DG, Di Paola J. Diagnostic approach to von Willebrand disease. *Blood.* 2015;125(13):2029-2037.

55. Branchford BR, Di Paola J. Making a diagnosis of VWD. *Hematology Am Soc Hematol Educ Program.* 2012;2012:161-167.

56. Westbury SK, Mumford AD. Genomics of platelet disorders. *Haemophilia.* 2016;22(suppl 5):20-24.

57. Lentaigne C, Freson K, Laffan MA, et al. Inherited platelet disorders: toward DNA-based diagnosis. *Blood.* 2016;127(23):2814-2823.

58. Ross JE, Zhang BM, Lee K, et al. Specifications of the variant curation guidelines for ITGA2B/ITGB3: ClinGen platelet disorder variant curation panel. *Blood Adv.* 2021;5(2):414-431.

Section 1 ■ HEMATOPOIESIS

Chapter 5 ■ Origin and Development of Blood Cells

DANIEL K. BORGER • ROBERT T. MEANS JR

BLOOD CELLS AND HEMATOPOIESIS

The cellular constituents of blood are divided into two lineages. The **myeloid** lineage consists of erythrocytes, megakaryocytes/platelets, granulocytes, and monocytes (although erythrocytes and megakaryocytes/platelets are often excluded from this classification). The **lymphoid** lineage consists of B cells, T cells, and the innate lymphoid cells. The structural and functional differences between these lineages, and between the cell types within each lineage, can be extreme. However, despite this diversity, all of these cells are the progeny of a single multipotent stem cell: the **hematopoietic stem cell** (**HSC**). HSCs reside within the bone marrow, where they are constantly giving rise to blood cells through a process called **hematopoiesis**. This process includes both maintenance of the HSC pool by tightly regulated HSC proliferation (i.e., **self-renewal**) and continuous replenishment of blood through gradual commitment of HSCs to single hematopoietic lineages and maturation into functional blood cells (i.e. **differentiation**). Along the path to differentiation, there are numerous intermediate cell types called **hematopoietic progenitor cells**, which exhibit varying levels of multipotency depending on the extent of differentiation, but which have lost the ability to self-renew long term (*Figure 5.1*).

The scale of hematopoiesis is massive and singular among human organ systems. It is estimated that 90% of the cells in the adult human body belong to the hematopoietic system[1] (albeit a much smaller proportion of the body's cells by weight, due to their relatively small size). It is also estimated that hematopoietic cells constitute a similar proportion of total cellular turnover in the body. Hundreds of billions of new hematopoietic cells are produced *each day*, dwarfing the turnover seen in the skin and intestinal epithelium.[2] But in spite of the scale of hematopoiesis, this process is exquisitely tuned to meet physiological needs. In a healthy individual, the numbers of the various cell types within the blood are kept in relatively constant ranges. Variations in erythrocyte numbers in particular are minimal, with values 30% above or below the norm having significant effects on health. To maintain this balance, and to respond to challenges like hemorrhage or infection, the regulation of hematopoiesis is complex. Some regulatory factors influence hematopoiesis by directly affecting HSCs and the most primitive progenitors. In contrast, some factors play key roles in fostering the production of a specific lineage. Such lineage-specific regulation is necessary because of the widely varying life spans and functions of the different mature blood cell types. Regulation can be local, mediated by cells that reside alongside HSCs and progenitors in the bone marrow. It can also be systemic, driven by factors from the liver or,

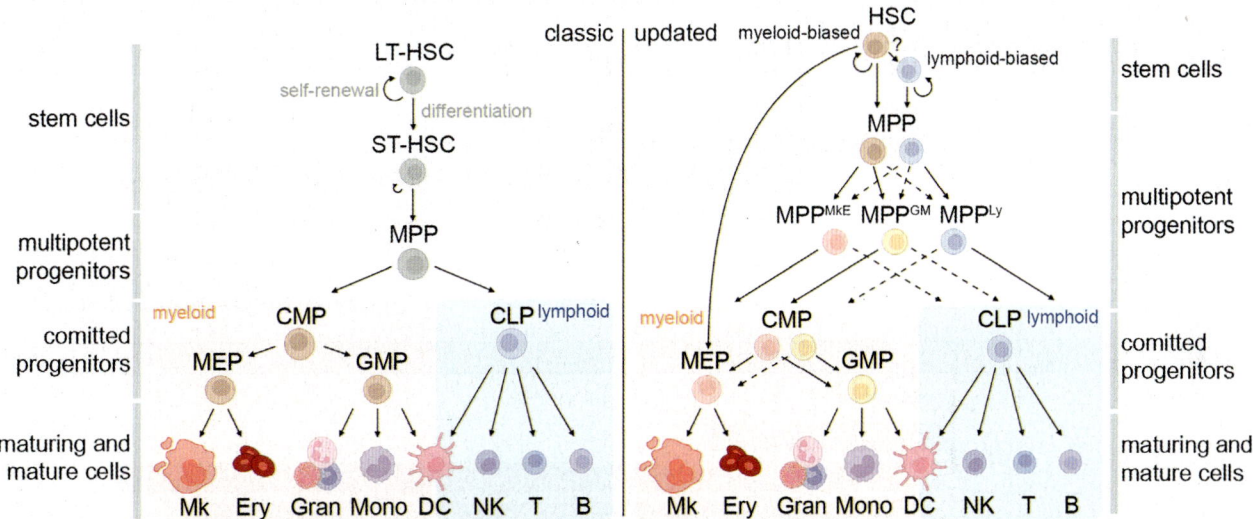

FIGURE 5.1 **The classical and updated schema of the hematopoietic hierarchy.** The updated view reflects the current appreciation that certain progenitors preferentially differentiate into certain cell types, a phenomenon termed "bias." CMP, common myeloid progenitor; DC, dendritic cell; Ery, erythrocyte; GMP, granulocyte-monocyte progenitor; Gran, granulocyte; LT-HSC, long-term HSC; MEP, megakaryocyte erythrocyte progenitor; Mk, megakaryocyte; Mono, monocyte; MPP, multipotent progenitor; MPP^{GM}, granulocyte/monocyte-biased MPP; MPP^{Ly}, lymphoid-biased MPP; MPP^{MkE}, Megakaryocyte/erythroid-biased MPP; NK, natural killer cell; ST-HSC, short-term HSC. (Created with BioRender.com.)

during inflammation, the immune system. In extreme conditions of stress, HSCs can even be driven to colonize other organs, such as the liver and spleen, in a process called **extramedullary hematopoiesis**.

This chapter presents an overview of the HSC and the process of hematopoiesis. Many conclusions presented here are based on experiments carried out in murine systems, although conclusions drawn from human research will be highlighted where it exists. As this is a vibrant field of research, experimental approaches to studying hematopoiesis in both humans and mice will also be discussed. All hematopoietic lineages are discussed, although more focused and detailed discussions of the differentiation of specific cell types can be found in later chapters.

ORIGINS AND DEVELOPMENT OF HEMATOPOIESIS

Extraembryonic Hematopoiesis

During prenatal development in mammals, the sites of hematopoiesis change several times, and hematopoietic cells themselves emerge in three major hematopoietic waves (*Figure 5.2*). The first two of these waves do not include HSCs and initiate within the extraembryonic yolk sack. They therefore constitute a phase known as extraembryonic hematopoiesis.

The first hematopoietic wave begins in the yolk sac around embryonic day (E) 7.5 in mice[3] and E16 in humans,[4] when hematopoietic progenitors emerge from mesodermal structures within the yolk sac known as **blood islands**. These progenitors rapidly mature to give rise to three cell types: macrophages, erythroid cells, and megakaryocytes. In addition to unipotent progenitors for these three lineages, there is evidence that this wave contains bipotential macrophage-erythroid progenitors[5] and megakaryocyte-erythroid progenitors[6,7] in both mice and humans.[8] However, no single common progenitor

has been identified. The erythroid progenitors of this first wave are distinct from those found later in fetal and adult life, when erythroid cells are continuously maturing and gradually entering circulation. Instead, this first erythropoietic wave occurs synchronously, providing the embryo proper with a wave of primitive erythroblasts when circulation is established between E8.5 to E10 in the mouse[9] and E21 in humans.[10] These cells are also distinct in that they continue maturing in the embryonic circulation, leaving the yolk sac as large nucleated erythroblasts, but eventually enucleating as they circulate.[11] Additionally, these cells undergo a process termed maturational globin switching, where expression of primitive β-globin (βH1 in mice, ε in humans) is replaced by expression of more mature chains (εγ globin in mice, γ in humans). α-globins undergo similar switching, with ζ chain expression being replaced by α1- and α2-globins.[12] The platelets derived from this first wave are released into the blood starting around E10.5 and, like the erythroblasts, exhibit immature features.[7] The primitive macrophages that arise from this wave gradually replace a population of maternal-derived macrophages which can be found in the yolk sac and embryo proper before the first wave emerges.[5] This initial hematopoietic wave is termed **primitive hematopoiesis**, due to both the absence of intermediate progenitors found in later hematopoiesis and the primitive features of the terminally differentiated cells that emerge from this wave.

This first wave is quickly followed by a second wave of progenitors emerging from the yolk sac beginning around E8.5 in mice, which consists mostly of erythroid-myeloid progenitors (EMPs).[13] Unlike the first wave of progenitors that arise in the yolk sac and rapidly mature in situ, EMPs mature outside of the yolk sac and ultimately give rise to fully differentiated cells without the primitive features seen in earlier hematopoietic cells. As this hematopoietic wave gives rise to phenotypically mature cells, and proceeds through the same intermediate progenitor populations that are seen in the adult, this wave is

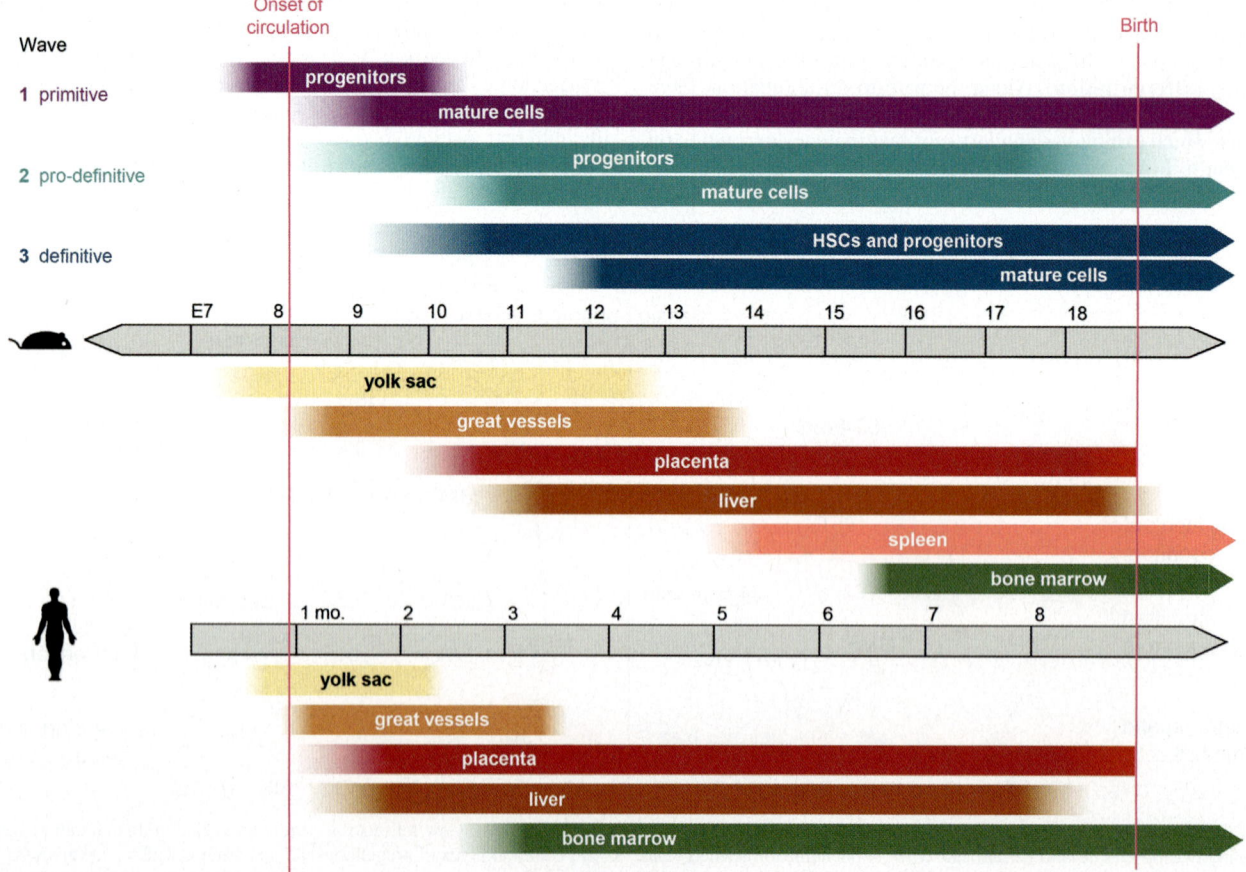

FIGURE 5.2 Sites of and timing of hematopoiesis. The time during which progenitors and mature cells of each hematopoietic wave can be identified in mice is shown, alongside the time during which hematopoiesis can be identified in each of the indicated organs in both mice and humans.

typically described as the onset of **definitive hematopoiesis**, although the absence of HSCs means it is occasionally called prodefinitive.[3] By E10.5 in the mouse, significant numbers of EMPs have left the yolk sac and migrated through the vitelline vein to the developing fetal liver.[6] By E11.5, they have established erythropoiesis in the fetal liver, with mature enucleated erythrocytes entering circulation.[14] Notably, when compared to HSC-derived erythroid progenitors found in the fetal liver later in development (see next section, *Genesis of HSCs*), EMP-derived erythroid progenitors have a much lower requirement for erythropoietin (EPO), a vital cytokine for erythroid differentiation. Since the fetal liver is relatively EPO restricted, yolk sac–derived EMPs therefore remain the dominant source of erythrocytes until birth.[15] Concurrent with this establishment of fetal liver erythropoiesis, EMPs in the fetal liver are also giving rise to megakaryocytes, granulocytes, and monocytes.[16] Beyond addressing the immediate hematopoietic needs of the embryo, these yolk sac–derived myeloid cells also give rise to tissue-resident macrophages and microglia, which persist after birth and throughout adulthood.[16,17] Additionally, and contrary to the earlier belief that adaptive immune cells did not develop until after the emergence of HSCs, *Rag1*-expressing lymphomyeloid-restricted (i.e., lacking erythrocytic or megakaryocytic potential) progenitors with B- and T-cell potential also emerge in the yolk sac during this second hematopoietic wave.[18-20] In contrast to the first hematopoietic wave, this second wave has not been conclusively identified in humans, although it appears that the developing human liver is seeded by erythroid and myeloid progenitors during embryonic week 4 (E28-35) of embryonic life, with definitive erythropoiesis arising during week 5 and enucleated erythrocytes entering fetal circulation by week 8.[21]

Genesis of HSCs

Because the first hematopoietic cells arise within the yolk sac, it was initially posited that the first HSCs also emerge there.[22,23] However, pioneering experiments in avian chimeras demonstrated that the yolk sac can only transiently contribute to hematopoiesis, and that hematopoietic cells present in later embryonic stages and after birth are derived from the intraembryonic compartment, suggesting that HSCs must arise from some intraembryonic tissue.[24-26] It had been known since the early 20th century that hematopoietic foci could be found in walls of major vessels early in embryonic development, but again, work in avian embryos was the first to establish experimentally that highly primitive hematopoietic precursors emerged at the walls of the developing aorta.[27,28] Subsequent studies in mice looking at the area encompassing the dorsal aorta—termed the para-aortic splanchnopleura (P-Sp) at E8, which evolves into the **aorta-gonad-mesonephros** (AGM) by E9—found that the precirculation E8 P-Sp contains hematopoietic progenitor activity[29,30] and that the E10.5 AGM could provide long-term multilineage reconstitution activity (LTR) in lethally irradiated adult mice, experimental confirmation of the presence of HSCs.[31]

Analogous to the AGM in mice, CD34+ cells on the ventral aspect of the dorsal aorta in human embryos at approximately 5 weeks of gestation are able to give rise to hematopoietic progenitors in culture.[32] Cell suspensions from the AGM region of embryos were capable of LTR in irradiated immunocompromised mice as early as 32 days of gestation, at least 5 days earlier than the yolk sac (see section *Hematopoietic Stem Cell Studies in Xenograft Models*).[33]

Around E11 in mice[34] and the fifth week of gestation in humans,[35] hematopoietic cells (both primitive and definitive) colonize the fetal liver. Dramatic expansion of HSCs occurs at this site (daily doubling in absolute numbers of HSC from E12.5-E14.5 in mice).[34] HSCs also circulate to the fetal spleen at approximately E13, but do not robustly expand there.[36] Because hematopoiesis shifts to the bone marrow prior to birth, fetal liver HSC numbers plateau then decline.[37] The first adult-repopulating HSCs are found in the murine fetal bone marrow at E16.5,[38] and the first evidence of hematopoietic activity in human fetal bone marrow is seen around 14 weeks of gestation.[39] In the mouse, the spleen continues to make a modest contribution to postnatal hematopoiesis. On the other hand, the bone marrow is the exclusive site of hematopoiesis under normal circumstances in humans.

The placenta represents a previously overlooked major site of hematopoiesis, where HSCs appear around E10.5 at the same time as they appear in the AGM.[40,41] Unlike the AGM, HSC numbers in the placenta rapidly expand, with 25-fold more HSCs in the placenta than in the AGM by E12.5. This is followed by a similarly rapid decline.[40] Because the placenta is directly upstream of fetal liver circulation and because the dramatic expansion of HSC in the fetal parallels that of the placenta, it has been suggested that the placenta acts as a temporary niche to expand HSCs in preparation for fetal liver colonization. It has also been proposed that the placenta is a site of de novo HSC emergence independent from the AGM. Indeed, explant and stromal coculture experiments of mesodermal tissue of the placenta prior to the establishment of circulation demonstrated erythroid and myeloid potential.[42,43] The concept of a de novo generated HSC was bolstered by in vitro culture of E8 to E9 placenta from Ncx1−/− animals, which lack a heartbeat and die by E10.5. Without circulatory contribution, the midgestation site had definitive hematopoietic cells with myelo-erythroid and lymphoid potential.[44] However, LTR HSC cannot be isolated from the placenta of Ncx1−/− animals because of developmental retardation. HSC activity is also found in the proximal vitelline and umbilical arteries, where clusters of endothelium-associated hematopoietic cells have also been identified.[45]

Vascular Origins of Hematopoiesis

Cells of vascular origin or potential are believed to be the cellular intermediates through which the mesoderm gives rise to hematopoietic cells. It was initially posited that hematopoietic cells emerged from bipotential **hemangioblasts** with both vascular and hematopoietic potential found in the posterior region of the primitive streak in the developing mouse at E7.[46] Other studies had suggested that a committed vascular cell was the precursor to HSCs. Supportive of an endothelial origin of HSCs is the presence of numerous endothelial cell markers on AGM HSCs, including CD31, VE-cadherin, and Tie-2.2. Furthermore, AGM HSCs and endothelial cells in the ventral wall of the E10 to E11 dorsal aorta both express Ly6A (Sca-1), c-Kit, CD34, Runx1, SCL, and GATA-2.1 Fate-mapping studies elegantly showed that VE-cadherin–expressing endothelia contribute to AGM and adult HSCs, whereas lineage tracing of subendothelial mesenchyme with myocardin-Cre animals did not result in labeling of HSCs.[47] Consistently, when *Runx1*, an essential gene in definitive hematopoiesis, was specifically deleted in VE-cadherin–expressing cells (endothelial and hematopoietic cells), but not Vav1-expressing cells (only hematopoietic cells), there was a severe disruption in hematopoietic development that was associated with 65% fetal lethality.[48] Others showed that expression of Runx1-binding partner core-binding factor-β in Ly6A-expressing hemogenic endothelium was sufficient for HSC formation.[49] Furthermore, novel imaging studies revealed de novo emergence of phenotypically defined HSCs directly from ventral aortic hemogenic endothelial cells.[50] Unifying the proposed hemangioblast and hemogenic endothelium origin, Lancrin and colleagues described that hemangioblasts generate hematopoietic cells through a hemogenic endothelium intermediate.[51] Altogether, these observations have supported the concept of blood cell development commencing with mesodermal cells that pass through vascular intermediates.

Common Critical Genes in Independent Origins of Hematopoiesis

Gene knockout experiments have provided significant insight into the critical regulators of embryonic hematopoiesis. Bone morphogenetic protein-4 (Bmp4), Flk1, Tal1/Scl, Lmo2, Gata-2, and Runx1 all play important roles for both primitive and definitive hematopoiesis.[52,53] Bmp4 is a critical signaling molecule to specify the dorsal-ventral axis in development. Although the posterior portion of the epiblast in development is fated to give rise to hematopoietic activity, the neurally fated anterior fragment can retain the ability to produce hematopoietic cells by addition of Bmp4.[54] Bmp4 is crucial for hematopoietic development because Bmp4-deficient embryos mostly die around the gastrulation stage, and those that do survive have less yolk sac mesoderm and less lateral plate mesoderm (from which the AGM will develop).[54,55] In definitive hematopoiesis, Bmp4 is expressed by endothelial cells in the ventral portion of the developing dorsal aorta and the subjacent mesoderm.[52] Using murine ES cells, it was shown that Bmp4 is necessary for mesodermal precursor expression of the receptor tyrosine kinase Flk1 and the basic helix-loop-helix transcription factor Tal1/Scl.[56]

The initiation of yolk sac hematopoiesis is dependent on the mesoderm and endoderm layers acting in concert because soluble factors from endoderm substantially bolster the production of endothelial and hematopoietic cells by murine yolk sac mesoderm explants.[57] One of the candidate soluble factor interactions is vascular endothelial growth factor (VEGF) derived from endoderm and its receptor Flk1 on the mesoderm.[58,59] Indeed, Flk1-deficient embryos do not develop vessels or yolk sac blood islands and die in utero between E8.5 and E9.5.[60] To overcome this early developmental mortality, Shalaby and colleagues performed complementation studies with chimeras of Flk1-heterozygous and Flk1-mutant ES cells and demonstrated convincingly that Flk1 is also required for the generation of definitive endothelial and hematopoietic cells.[61] It was later shown that Flk1 signaling appears to not be required intrinsically for endothelial and hematopoietic formation because Flk1-deficient embryonic stem (ES) cells are able to give rise to endothelial and hematopoietic lineages in vitro[62,63]; instead, Flk1 is likely required for the migration of mesoderm cells from the posterior primitive streak to the yolk sac.[61] In concordance with the importance of VEGF-Flk1 signaling axis, VEGF derived from the visceral endoderm, but interestingly not mesoderm, is sufficient for endothelial and hematopoietic differentiation.[64]

The transcription factor Tal1/Scl[65-67] and the transcriptional regulator Lmo2[68] are both expressed in the yolk sac mesoderm prior to the onset of primitive hematopoiesis and then subsequently expressed in both endothelial and hematopoietic cells. Gene knockout of *Tal1/Scl*[69,70] or *Lmo2*[71] results in decreased endothelial cells and abrogates yolk sac blood cell production. These genes are also critical for definitive hematopoiesis, as demonstrated by complementation studies with ES cell chimeras.[72-74] Tal1/Scl has numerous functions in the onset of hematopoiesis: it specifies lateral plate mesoderm to a hematopoietic fate, represses cardiomyogenesis in prospective hemogenic endothelium and endocardium, acts in concert with the VEGF-Flk1 axis to initiate primitive hematopoiesis, and acts in concert with Runx1 to promote endothelial to hematopoietic transition.[53,75]

Gata-2–deficient animals have severely impaired primitive hematopoiesis and die at E10.5.[76] *Gata-2*–haploinsufficient embryos have normal yolk sac hematopoiesis,[77] but have a reduction in AGM HSCs, which is consistent with its expression on aortic endothelium and its proposed role in the expansion of hemogenic endothelial progenitors.[78] Runx1 has also been demonstrated to be crucial in definitive hematopoiesis because *Runx1* invalidation abrogates definitive myeloid, lymphoid, and HSC accumulation in the yolk sac, AGM, and fetal liver.[79-81] Runx1 is thought to be crucial cell autonomously because complementation studies fail to demonstrate hematopoietic contribution by *Runx1*-null ES cells.[80] Although Runx1 was initially thought to be dispensable in murine primitive erythropoiesis, later studies have recently shown that the morphology and gene expression of erythrocytes are aberrant in Runx1-deficient animals.[82]

THE HEMATOPOIETIC STEM CELL

The modern definition of the HSC is a functional definition, consisting of two defining features. The first is the ability to differentiate into all hematopoietic cell types. The second is the ability to self-renew, producing more HSCs of similar differentiation and self-renewal capacity. These features together enable HSCs to power hematopoiesis in the long term, that is, for anywhere from months to decades.

Conception and Discovery of the HSC
The Age of Morphologists

By the end of the 19th century, it was relatively well established that the bone marrow represented the site of origin of blood cells,

and inquiry shifted to what processes gave rise to these cells. Paul Erlich, using new synthetic dyes and staining and cell fixation techniques which allowed for more precise morphologic characterization and classification of blood and marrow cells, was able to identify a primitive cell type which he postulated was the progenitor of all granulocytes. However, Erlich hypothesized that lymphocytes had a separate origin from myeloid cells and thus that there were two unrelated hematopoietic lineages. Later, using refined staining methods, Artur Pappenheim was able to observe various transitional cells and organize them into a relational scheme—a tree whose various branches when traced backward converged to a mononuclear cell that had none of the distinct features of the end-stage blood cells or the transitional cells. He posited that this cell was so morphologically primitive that it could be the common ancestor of *all* blood cells, both myeloid and lymphoid. Although by 1900 most morphologists accepted the idea of ancestral hematopoietic cells giving rise to progressively more mature cells, there was lasting debate between the so-called monophyleticists and dualists.[83,84]

The Advent of Transplantation

By the 1950s, a new tool had been adopted to study hematopoiesis: high-energy radiation. In 1951, it was discovered that mice and guinea pigs can be protected against otherwise lethal whole-body irradiation by injections of bone marrow from other animals of their species.[85] Several years later, using bone marrow from donor mice bearing an identifiable chromosomal marker, it was shown that hematopoiesis in the irradiated recipient mice was reconstituted by cells from the donor marrow—that is, the protected animals were hematopoietic chimeras.[86] These discoveries would revolutionize both the study of hematopoiesis and the treatment of hematological diseases.

Using this new transplantation approach, James Till and Ernest McCulloch were finally able to offer experimental proof of the existence of a single ancestral cell with multilineage potential. Looking in the spleens of mice 1 week after transplantation, they found macroscopic colonies containing cells of multiple hematopoietic lineages. These colonies were the progeny of individual transplanted cells, termed spleen colony-forming units (CFUs-S). Because the cells in these CFU-S colonies could, in turn, be injected into secondary, irradiated mice and again give rise to colonies, the CFU-S apparently replicated themselves in vivo.[87] While early studies could not demonstrate lymphoid cells in CFU-S colonies,[88,89] subsequent studies identified both lymphoid and myeloid progenitors within these colonies, indicating the CFU-S was multipotent.[90] However, although the CFU-S assay was able to demonstrate multilineage differentiation capacity and limited self-renewal via secondary transplantation, it could not demonstrate any long-term hematopoietic contribution from the CFU-S, since spleen colonies are eventually resorbed.

Definitive Evidence for HSCs

Animal reconstitution experiments with hematopoietic cells that were individually genetically marked have demonstrated the multipotent and self-renewing nature of HSCs.[91,92] In these marking experiments, hematopoietic cells were infected in vitro with a recombinant retrovirus that was able to integrate its DNA (provirus) into a cell but could not replicate and spread to other cells. The one-time, random integration of the provirus into the DNA of an individual cell provides a specific marker for the progeny of that cell that develops in an animal after transplantation. Random integration assures that each provirus has unique flanking sequences of DNA and thus has a high probability of yielding a DNA fragment of a distinguishable size after cutting with a restriction enzyme that does not cut the provirus. Several months after transplantation of the genetically marked cells and establishment of hematopoiesis, it is typically observed that all types of cells in the blood and lymphoid organs contain progeny of an individually marked cell, proving that it was multipotent. Often, these clones of marked cells continue to contribute to all of the hematopoietic lineages in the animal for an extended period. Also, when these primary recipient animals are subsequently used as donors for secondary recipient animals, frequently the same clones of HSCs are apparent in these secondary recipients. This persistence can even be demonstrated in tertiary recipients.[93,94] Demonstrating the ability of HSCs to self-renew over a long period, long-term reconstitution of the myeloid and lymphoid compartments can be achieved by transplantation of a single murine HSC,[95-97] indicating that a single HSC is the smallest repopulating unit. Dick and colleagues demonstrated that a single-cell transplant of human CD34+ CD38− CD45RA− CD90 (Thy1)+ Rho^lo CD49f+ cells into immunocompromised mice was able to provide multilineage reconstitution,[98] indicating that the HSC is also the smallest repopulating unit in humans.

Identification and Isolation of HSCs

The identification of relatively immature HSCs from more committed progenitor cells based on the various physical properties, functional attributes, and immunophenotypic markers has greatly advanced the field of hematopoiesis.[99] HSCs can be identified by their ability to efficiently efflux dyes. The most common methods utilize the dye Hoechst 33342, which when excited at two wavelengths yields a characteristic "side population" on flow cytometry[100] because of dye efflux. While this functional property enriches for HSCs, it precludes prospective isolation for further characterization or clinical application. Prospective isolation can be achieved through phenotypic identification with antibodies and gene-driven fluorescent proteins. In mice, the prospective isolation of HSC and progenitor populations derives from work by Weissman and colleagues, who initially proposed the combination of Sca-1 (Ly-6A/E)+, c-Kit+, Flk2−, CD90 (Thy-1)+, and negative for lineage markers (CD3, B220, Mac-1, Gr-1, and Ter119) as a highly purified population enriched for *in vivo* repopulating HSCs[101-104] (*Table 5.1*). The enrichment of long-term repopulating activity in the CD34^lo fraction was shown subsequently.[95] In 2005, Morrison developed a novel marker set to identify highly enriched HSCs and demonstrated that signaling lymphocyte and activation molecule (SLAM) markers were found to be differentially expressed on bone marrow lineage- Sca-1+ c-kit+ (LSK) populations such that CD150+ CD244− CD48− CD41− was the population enriched for murine HSC in vivo repopulating capacity.[105] Other studies have pointed to further enrichment in the endothelial protein C receptor-positive (EPCR and CD201), CD105-positive (endoglin), and CD229-negative[106-109] fractions of the HSC pool. This group also showed that α-catulin–expressing cells are enriched for HSCs with 1 in 3.1 α-catulin+ CD150+ CD48− LSK having long-term multipotent repopulating activity.[110] Additionally, the Weissman lab demonstrated that 78% of Hoxb5^hi CD150+ CD34^−/lo Flk2− LSK cells have long-term

Table 5.1. Flow Cytometric Definitions of HSCs, MPPs, and Single-Lineage Progenitors

Population	Phenotype
Hematopoietic stem cell (HSC)	Lin− Sca-1+ Kit+ Flk2− CD34− CD90 (Thy-1)+ CD150+ CD244− CD48− EPCR+ Hoechst 33342 Side Population+ CD105+ CD229− α-catulin+ HoxB5+ Pdzk1ip1+
Multipotent progenitors (MPPs)	Lin− Sca-1+ kit+ Thy1− Flk2+ CD150− CD105− CD229−
Common lymphoid progenitor	Lin− Sca-1^lo Kit^lo Thy1^lo IL-7R+
Common myeloid progenitor	Lin− Sca-1− Kit + FcγR^int CD34+
Granulocyte-macrophage progenitor (GMP)	Lin− Sca-1− Kit+ FcγR^hi CD34+
Megakaryocyte erythrocyte progenitor	Lin− Sca-1− Kit+ FcγR− CD34−
Macrophage dendritic cell progenitor	Lin− Sca-1− Kit^hi Flk2+ CX₃CR1+ CD115+

Abbreviations: CD, cluster of designation; Flk2, fms-like kinase-2; Lin−, lineage negative (Gr1− CD11b− CD3− B220− Ter119−); Sca-1, stem cell antigen 1.

multipotent repopulating activity,[111] and Sawai et al described that 36% of Pdzk1ip1+ CD45+ EPCR+ CD48− CD150+ cells were able to confer multilineage reconstitution in single-cell transplant experiments.[112]

In humans, CD34+ CD38− CD90+ CD45RA− Rho^lo CD49f+ cells that are negative for lineage markers (CD2, CD3, CD4, CD7, CD8, CD10, CD11b, CD14, CD19, CD20, CD56, CD235a) are considered highly enriched for in vivo repopulating HSCs.[98,113,114] The successes in mouse models have led to human phase I clinical trials that successfully demonstrated sustained hematopoiesis when HSCs purified by immunophenotyping were transplanted into irradiated patients.[115-117]

For example, the content of long-term repopulating HSCs within the same immunophenotyped LSK Thy1^lo fraction can change in aged mice, previously transplanted mice, and mobilized mice.[118] Reliability of CD34 in mice of various age groups has also been questioned.[119] Use of the CD150+ CD48-gating scheme, rather than Thy1 with LSK gating, retains the fidelity in frequency of long-term repopulating HSCs in aged, transplanted, and mobilized mice.[118] Nonetheless, it still is unknown if the SLAM markers retain fidelity in mutant mice. Moreover, other surface markers can also be modulated by environmental cues. This is illustrated by the Sca-1 upregulation that occurs in inflammatory settings likely secondary to type I interferon exposure,[120,121] which can erroneously lead to conclusions about HSCs based on a population of committed progenitors that artifactually acquired the Sca-1 antigen. Furthermore, not all mouse strains express the prospective HSC antigens, such as Thy1.1 or Sca-1.[122,123] Thus, conclusions drawn about HSCs in mouse or man need to be verified by functional assays in order to demonstrate multipotency and long-term repopulation.

Polyclonal Contribution of HSCs

It has been noted that not all HSC clones are long lived; some produce progeny for varying periods and then apparently become extinct. Also, marked clones have been observed to begin contributing to hematopoiesis after some period of posttransplantation latency, indicating that dormancy is possible. Thus, these studies have demonstrated that, after transplantation, some HSCs contribute continuously to hematopoiesis for a long time—in mice, apparently for the whole lifetime of the animal. Other HSCs contribute and then become extinct, and finally, some may remain dormant for some period and then contribute. Additional transplantation studies of marked HSCs in mice[124] have suggested that polyclonal hematopoiesis is more common and that long-term contribution by individual stem cells is more rare than the earlier studies indicated.[93,94] Newer technologies combining viral barcoding, high-throughput sequencing, and multicolor fate mapping of HSC have confirmed this polyclonal contribution of HSCs after transplantation.[125-127] In fact, fate-mapping studies with mathematical modeling in nonirradiated animals demonstrate that hematopoiesis is even more polyclonal than estimated by transplantation studies.[128-130] Studies using retroviral insertion-site analyses for larger animals, particularly nonhuman primates, have also provided some evidence of polyclonal hematopoiesis.[131-133] A recent remarkable study in four transplanted Wiskott-Aldrich syndrome patients utilized lentiviral transduction for clonal tracking of >89 000 cells.[134] Assessment of 15 lineages of blood and bone marrow cells up to 4 years after transplant revealed polyclonal hematopoiesis with a few thousand HSC/progenitor clones sustaining multilineage blood cell production.

HSC Quiescence

Compared to downstream CD34+ LSK murine multipotent progenitors (MPPs) (*Figure 5.3*) of which 90% are in cell cycle, <10% of CD34− CD48− CD150^hi LSK HSCs are cycling.[116] Even within this phenotypically identified HSC pool, investigators have used label-retaining tracking approaches to functionally distinguish the existence of two types of HSC: homeostatic (or hematopoietic stress activated) and dormant HSC, which represent 70% to 80% and 20% to 30% of the HSC pool, respectively.[116,117,135] Whereas homeostatic HSC divides every 28 to 36 days, dormant HSC divides only every 145 to 193 days, or about five times per lifetime.[116,120] Human HSCs have been estimated

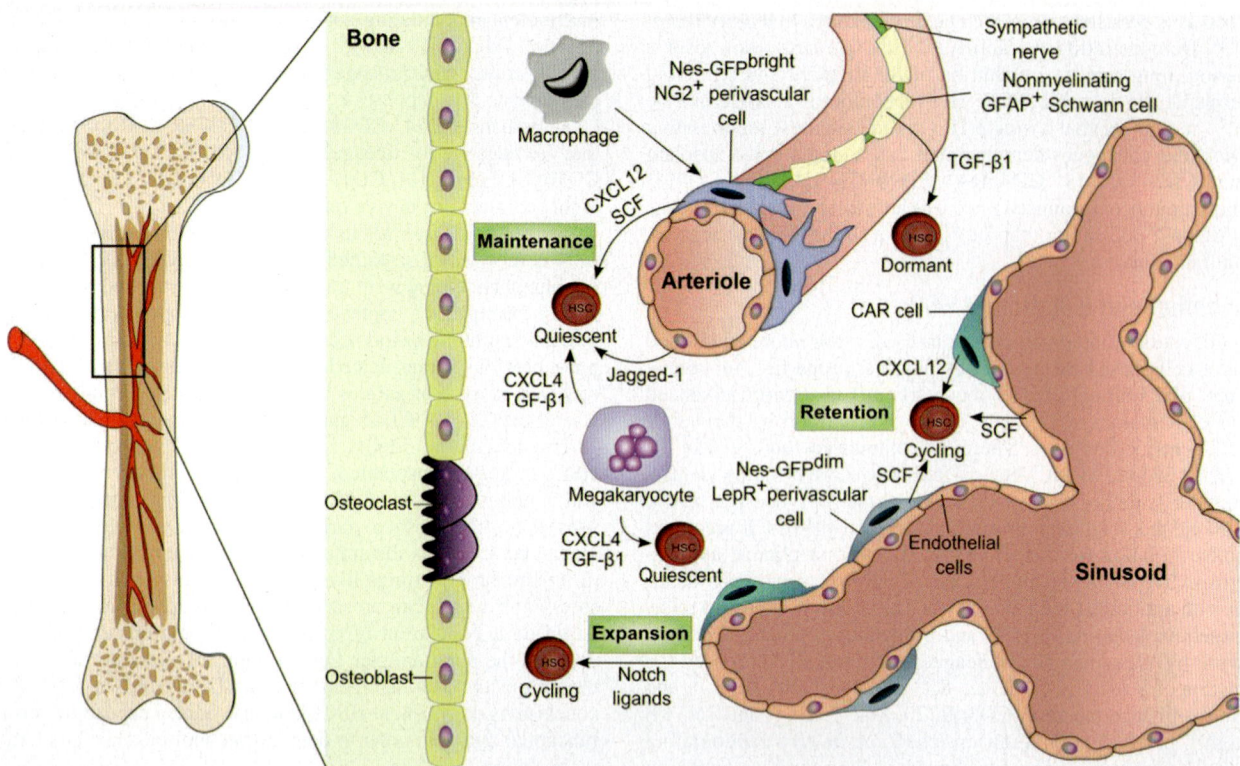

FIGURE 5.3 Hematopoietic stem cell niche. HSC behaviors (e.g., quiescence, dormancy, and cycling) are regulated through direct interactions with *Nestin*-GFP[bright] NG2[+] periarteriolar mesenchymal cells, *Nestin*-GFP[dim] LepR[+] perisinusoidal CXCL12-abundant reticular (CAR) mesenchymal cells, sinusoidal endothelial cells, and megakaryocytes. HSCs are also regulated indirectly by macrophages and sympathetic nerves. HSC, hematopoietic stem cell; SCF, stem cell factor; TGF-β, transforming growth factor-β. (Reprinted from Boulais PE, Frenette PS. Making sense of hematopoietic stem cell niches. *Blood.* 2015;125:2621-2629. Copyright © 2015 American Society of Hematology. With permission.)

to divide once every 40 weeks and compared to mice, cats, and baboons have an even higher percentage of quiescent to contributing HSCs.[136] This differential cycling has functional consequences. It has been described that exit from dormancy provokes physiologic DNA damage that accumulates over time and likely contributes to hematopoietic dysfunction with aging.[137] Although both homeostatic and dormant HSCs provide long-term repopulation in lethally irradiated recipients, only dormant HSC provides complete long-term repopulation in secondary transplants.[116,135]

HSCs in Culture

Repopulation studies in irradiated mice, as well as experience with bone marrow transplantation in humans, provide strong evidence that HSCs can replicate and expand extensively in vivo. Replicating the scale of this in vitro expansion of transplantable HSCs in culture represents a significant advance for clinical medicine and would be useful in a number of settings. Human umbilical cord blood (UCB) is an important alternative source of transplantable HSCs, but the limited number of HSCs present in a single unit of UCB poses a risk, as low cell dose of transplanted UCB units delays engraftment and increases the chances of treatment-related mortality.[138,139] Although double umbilical cord blood transplants (dUCBTs) have improved the rate of sustained engraftment, it is still associated with delayed engraftment and higher risk of engraftment failure when compared to bone marrow or mobilized peripheral blood transplant.[140] Similarly, autologous transplantation, which is used in certain malignancies, can be limited by the number of HSCs and progenitors, as some individuals do not respond to the drugs used to mobilize HSCs into peripheral blood.[141,142] Using culture to expand cell numbers and thereby accelerate engraftment would be valuable in these cases. The emergence of gene editing as an HSC therapy, which in some cases requires time in culture, means a culture setting that preserves HSC function could also benefit this new therapeutic modality. Thus, a successful ex

vivo expansion strategy would both preserve HSC function and permit HSC self-renewal in order to expand the number of transplantable HSCs during the culture period.

However, numbers of mouse and human HSCs generally decline relative to input numbers over time in culture[143-146] even though clonal analysis indicates that some HSC clones proliferate.[144] Also, for uncertain reasons, repopulating activity is lost when cultured HSCs enter the cell cycle to actively proliferate.[147] Cultured HSCs also exhibit reduced expression of a number of integrins, resulting in impaired homing.[148,149] Advances in culture components and techniques have gradually begun to improve culture, and clinical trials with UBC have played a large role in this. These clinical trials typically involve culturing one UCB unit (the "manipulated" unit) and coinfusing with a freshly thawed nonmanipulated UCB unit. Patients coinfused with these mixed units are compared to patients receiving a conventional dUCBT. Early ex vivo culture of human CD34[+] UCB cells with various combinations of cytokines for 10 to 14 days demonstrated moderate increases in progenitor cell numbers, but had no effects on clinically relevant outcomes, such as time to neutrophil recovery.[150] However, a number of newer factors have shown more promise, accelerating engraftment of cultured UCB units (summarized in *Table 5.2*). The studies all supplement the culture with the cytokines stem cell factor (SCF), thrombopoietin (TPO), and Flt3 ligand (Flt3l). Interleukin (IL)-3 and IL-6 are often included, as well.

As is shown in *Table 5.2*, the speed of neutrophil and platelet engraftment is of great interest in UCB transplantation, since neutropenia and thrombocytopenia are major sources of complications in the context of transplantation. However, rapid myeloid engraftment is likely driven by more committed progenitors.[163] Measuring relative engraftment of manipulated and unmanipulated units gives a better picture of what is happening at the level of stem cells. In the trial with the Notch ligand Delta 1, 2 out of 10 patients (20%) had persistence of the manipulated graft 180 days after transplantation. This is in spite

Table 5.2. Clinical Trials Assessing Strategies for ex vivo Expansion of UCB Units

Drug	Reference	Proposed Mechanism	Culture Period	CD34+ Expansion	Trial Type	Major Findings (vs Unmanipulated UCB)
Long-term culture						
SR-1	Wagner et al, 2016[151]	AhR antagonism inhibits differentiation	15 d	330-fold	Phase I/II	Accelerated neutrophil and platelet engraftment No effect on TRM or 1 y OS
UM171	Cohen et al, 2019[152]	Modulates proteasome activity preserves in vivo chromatin modifications[153]	7 d	35-fold	Phase I/II	No effect on neutrophil and platelet engraftment Some promise in improving TRM and 1 y OS
Nicotinamide	Horwitz et al, 2014[154]	SIRT1 deacetylase antagonist promotes self-renewal	21 ± 2 d	72-fold	Phase I	Accelerated neutrophil and platelet engraftment
	Horwitz et al, 2019[155]			33-fold	Phase I/II	Accelerated neutrophil and platelet engraftment No effect on 2 y OS
	Horwitz et al, 2021[156]			66-fold	Phase III	Accelerated neutrophil and platelet engraftment Lower rates of posttransplant infections No effect on 2 y OS
TEPA	de Lima et al, 2008[157]	Copper chelator inhibits differentiation	21 d	6-fold	Phase I/II	-
	Stiff et al, 2018[158]			90-fold	Phase II/III	Accelerated neutrophil and platelet engraftment Improved 100 d OS
Delta1	Delaney et al, 2010[159]	Notch agonist promotes self-renewal	17-21 d	164-fold	Phase I	Accelerated neutrophil engraftment
BM MSC coculture	De Lima et al, 2012[160]	Mimics in vivo niche	7 d coculture +14 d	30-fold		Accelerated neutrophil and platelet engraftment
Short-term (pretreatment)						
dmPGE$_2$	Cutler et al, 2013[161]	PTGER2 and PTGER4 agonist promotes expression of homing and self-renewal genes	2 h	-	Phase I	Accelerated neutrophil engraftment
FT-VI + GDP-fucose	Popat et al, 2015[162]	Forces fucosylation of P- and E-selectin, improving homing	30 min		Phase I	Accelerated neutrophil and platelet engraftment

Abbreviations: AhR, aryl hydrocarbon receptor; dmPGE$_2$, 16,16-Dimethyl prostaglandin E2; FT-VI, fucosyltransferase-VI; GDP-fucose, guanosine diphosphate fucose; MSC, mesenchymal stromal cell; OS, overall survival; SIRT1, sirtuin 1; SR-1, StemRegenin-1; TRM, transplant-related mortality; TEPA, tetraethylenepentamine; UCB, umbilical cord blood.

The Normal Hematologic System

of coinfusion with a nonmanipulated unit containing T cells capable of rejecting the manipulated unit.[159] With StemRegenin-1, 6 of the 17 patients (35%) exhibited high levels of myeloid and lymphoid donor chimerism from the manipulated unit out to 300 days. Five of the 17 patients (29%) exhibited myeloid engraftment that declined over time.[151] These results suggest the preservation of at least short-term self-renewing cells during ex vivo culture, although not to the degree of observed CD34+ cell expansion or expansion of severe combined immunodeficiency (SCID)-repopulating cells (a functional measure of human HSC activity in xenograft models, see section *Hematopoietic Stem Cell Studies in Xenograft Models*) as seen in prior murine studies of these molecules.[159,164] In the case of coculture with bone marrow mesenchymal stromal cells (MSCs), 6 months posttransplantation, blood cells derived from the manipulated cord blood graft were present in 13% of the patients, and long-term engraftment was largely derived from the unmanipulated graft.[157] This strategy to utilize MSCs to expand early progenitors therefore appears to come at the expense of long-term repopulating ability. Efforts have therefore been made to engineer both MSC[165] and endothelial cells[166,167] to better support hematopoietic cells in culture, or eschew coculture and mimic features of the in vivo extracellular matrix.[168] This remains an active field of research, with many discoveries with regard to culture systems and conditions that are yet to be applied to human studies.[169]

With the development of induced pluripotent stem cell (iPSC) technology, the derivation of HSCs from iPSCs has become an area of active investigation. Proof of concept that human iPSCs could differentiate into hematopoietic cells was initially established by coinjection of human iPSCs with the murine OP9 stromal cell line into immunocompromised mice.[170,171] The resulting teratomas yielded HSCs capable of serial transplantation. Because generation of blood cells in vivo under xenograft settings is not clinically feasible, ex vivo derivation protocols have been actively investigated. Although multilineage cells have been derived from iPSCs in vitro, conditions that generate cells robust long-term in vivo engraftment have yet to be identified.[172,173] Future strategies for successfully generating self-renewing multipotent HSCs from reprogrammed somatic cells include (1) optimization of transcription factor cocktails for derivation by following physiologic developmental principles, (2) selection of starting cells that are epigenetically related to HSCs (e.g., blood progenitors and endothelial cells), (3) augmentation of HSC expansion conditions (as stated earlier), and (4) maintenance of bone marrow homing molecules in culture.[172,173]

HEMATOPOIETIC PROGENITOR CELLS

Committed Hematopoietic Progenitor Cells

Committed hematopoietic progenitor cells are progeny of HSCs that have begun to differentiate and can no longer confer long-term reconstitution of all hematopoietic lineages in myeloablated animals. *Figure 5.1* depicts the HSC and downstream committed progenitors, and notably, only HSCs have the capacity to self-renew, as indicated by the reflexive arrows. This schematic is a working model that is constantly under revision with numerous nuances that preclude neat boundaries in differentiation potentials of progenitor cells.[174-176] Nonetheless, whichever branching scheme is utilized, each successive stage has a more restricted differentiation potential, and there is a succession of commitment steps. Similar to the manner in which molecular processes determining self-renewal vs commitment decisions for stem cells are not completely understood, neither are the molecular events that lead to subsequent commitment steps. Although phenotypic markers can largely, although not definitively, distinguish cells with stem cell (as opposed to just progenitor cell) potential, the unique contribution of progenitor cells (as opposed to progenitor cells that derive from transferred HSCs) is not well understood. It is known that although a single HSC can yield long-term, multilineage donor contribution, supporting total bone marrow or progenitor cells must be coinfused to allow short-term hematopoiesis; otherwise, survival is not possible. This demonstrates that in clinical transplantation or hematopoietic recovery from myeloablative regimens, progenitor cells are just as critical, if not more critical, than HSCs in the short term after conditioning. Clonal tracking of HSC/progenitors in humans suggests that the majority of blood production is derived from short-term rather than long-term HSC/progenitors.[134]

Multilineage Progenitors

The first committed progenitor without capacity to self-renew is the MPP. Although initially regarded as an HSC assay, the majority of CFU-S colonies cannot provide long-term reconstitution of ablated animals and are in fact MPP. Under culture conditions in semisolid medium with adequate supportive growth factors, these progenitor cells can form colonies of multiple cell lineages in vitro.[177,178] Similar multilineage colonies can also be demonstrated in vitro in human hematopoietic cell populations.[179] When the hematopoietic cells reach maturity, the lineage composition of the colonies can be determined by picking out the colonies and spreading the cells on microscope slides, followed by conventional staining techniques or by immunostaining using lineage marker antibodies. Not all multilineage colonies that appear in in vitro or in vivo assays contain all cell lineages. For example, some colonies contain granulocytes, erythrocytes, macrophages, and megakaryocytes (mixed colonies), other colonies contain GM colonies, and so forth. *Table 5.3* describes a variety of hematopoietic progenitor stages that are defined by in vitro assays.

The observation that colonies with various combinations of lineages occur has been interpreted in several ways (models) to explain how cells are committed to become a particular type of blood cell.[180] The data favor the idea that there are multiple commitment steps and that these steps lead to loss of specific lineage potential in a definite order. The first lineage commitment step separates lymphoid from myeloid potential, then GM potential is separated from erythroid/megakaryocyte potential, and so on, until finally, a descendant cell has only one lineage capability. This idea of successive commitment steps is embodied in *Figure 5.1*. Although this idea is probably generally correct, there are variant models that differ somewhat in their interpretation.[175] Also, it must be remembered that in vitro growth conditions may not be permissive for all possible lineages to appear in a colony. Thus, caution must be exercised in interpreting the exact lineage commitment pathways. For example, multilineage progenitors, CFU-S, and in vitro–derived multilineage colonies had been thought to be incapable of generating lymphoid cells. However, several studies have shown that lymphoid cells are produced by several such progenitors, but that they were not observed previously because growth factor support for colony development was not permissive for descendant lymphoid cells.[90,181,182]

By flow cytometry, these MPPs, first described by Morrison and Weissman,[101,183] have been characterized as Lin- Sca-1+ c-kit+ Thy1.1- Flk2+ (*Table 5.1*).[102] Further phenotypic enrichment of MPP[184] can be resolved in the VCAM1+ and CD150− CD105− populations.[107] In an elegant mouse model utilizing Flk2-Cre animals, fate mapping revealed that the vast majority of adult hematopoietic cells in the blood, bone marrow, and spleen arise from an Flk2-expressing cell in the steady state and hematopoietic stress, confirming the hub-role of MPPs that express Flk2.[185] An important caveat is that although clear-cut definitions, such as HSC vs MPP vs more committed progenitors, facilitate our understanding of hematopoiesis and are continuously refined, there is likely some fluidity to the cell type definitions and/or the model of stepwise loss of potential because lineage-biased HSC and MPP have been described.[109,173,176,186-189] Indeed, elegant studies with single human CD34+ cells suggest that adult bone marrow contains few oligopotent progenitors, and instead, unilineage progenitors and subsequent mature progeny descend directly from HSC or MPPs.[190]

Single-Lineage Progenitors

The descendants of the multilineage colony-forming cells are ultimately restricted to a single-lineage potential. The more mature, single-lineage-committed progenitor cells are assayed in vitro by their

Table 5.3. Colony-Forming Capacity of Hematopoietic Progenitors Assayed in Vitro

In vitro Progenitor Name	Progenitor Stage/Potential	Factors
CAFC (#)—"cobblestone area–forming cell"	Mouse CAFC (28-40), possible stem cells. Mouse CAFC (<28), multilineage.	Irradiated BM stromal layer with horse serum and hydrocortisone.
LTC-IC—"long-term culture-initiating cell"	Multilineage, possibly stem cells.	Irradiated BM stromal layer with horse serum and hydrocortisone.
CFU-GEMM—"CFU-granulocyte, erythrocyte, macrophage, megakaryocyte"	Multilineage.	Kit ligand, IL-11, GM-CSF, EPO
CFU-GM—"CFU-granulocyte macrophage"	Granulocytes and macrophages.	Kit ligand, GM-CSF
CFU-E—"CFU-erythrocyte"	Late-stage erythrocyte progenitor.	EPO and IGF-1
BFU-E—"burst-forming unit-erythrocyte"	Early-stage erythrocyte progenitor.	EPO, Kit ligand, IGF-1
CFU-G—"CFU-granulocyte"	Granulocytes.	G-CSF
CFU-M—"CFU-macrophage"	Macrophages.	CSF-1
CFU-Mk—"CFU-megakaryocyte"	Megakaryocytes.	TPO, IL-3, Kit ligand
CFU-preB—"CFU-preB lymphocytes"	B cells.	Kit ligand, IL-7
CFU-DL—"CFU dendritic/Langerhans cells"	Dendritic cells/Langerhans cells.	GM-CSF, TNF-α

Abbreviations: #, number of days of culture; BM, bone marrow; CFU, colony-forming unit; EPO, erythropoietin; G-CSF, granulocyte colony–stimulating factor; GM-CSF, granulocyte-macrophage colony-stimulating factor; IGF-1, insulin-like growth factor 1; IL, interleukin; TNF-α, tumor necrosis factor-α.

ability to form colonies. These progenitor cells include CFU-G, CFU-M, CFU-E, colony-forming unit megakaryocyte (CFU-MK),[191-193] CFU- preB,[194,195] and CFU-DL[196,197] for CFUs granulocyte, macrophage, erythrocyte, megakaryocyte, B lymphocyte, and dendritic/Langerhans cell, respectively (*Table 5.3*). In some lineages, it is possible to observe stages of maturity within the lineage-committed progenitors. For example, the single-lineage–producing burst-forming unit erythroid (BFU-E) is a more immature erythroid progenitor than the CFU-E, forming colonies of many more mature erythroid cells after a longer period of time than the CFU-E.

With the advent of flow cytometry, many of these populations now have phenotypic counterparts (*Table 5.1*). Flow cytometry allows for more precise separation of populations and assessment of the progenitor activity, even to the single-cell level. The MPP is thought to give rise to more committed oligopotent progenitors, specifically the common lymphoid progenitor (CLP)[198] and common myeloid progenitor (CMP).[199] CLPs give rise to B cells, T cells, and natural killer (NK) cells, whereas CMPs spawn the erythroid, megakaryocyte, and myeloid lineages. The CMP subsequently branches off to the more committed oligopotent MEP and granulocyte-macrophage progenitor (GMP). The GMP subdivides into granulocytes and macrophage dendritic cell progenitors,[200] which produce the respective eponymous lineages. A review of the surface markers for these populations can be found in *Table 5.1*. Recent single-cell analyses of progenitors isolated from fetal liver, as compared to bone marrow, demonstrated differences in oligopotentiality across development.[190] Whereas the human fetal liver contains numerous oligopotent cells (i.e., MEP, CMP, and GMP) with few unilineage progenitors, adult bone marrow hematopoiesis is dominated by committed unilineage progenitors that derive directly from HSCs or MPPs. Similarly, single-cell analyses of adult murine bone marrow suggest little contribution of oligopotent cells to steady-state hematopoiesis, even though cell fate plasticity can be seen in a stressed environment, such as after transplantation.[201]

Terminal Phases of Differentiation

Cells in the final stages of hematopoiesis are sufficiently differentiated that they can be identified by morphology using light microscopy. These cells are erythroblasts, myelocytes, monocytes, and megakaryocytes, and, because of the vastly amplifying cell divisions that occur by the time the final stages are reached, these cells are by far the most prevalent cells seen in hematopoietic tissues. They are only capable of a few cell divisions, on the order of one to four, yet they are undergoing dramatic specialized changes associated with terminal phases of differentiation/maturation. The erythroblasts rapidly accumulate hemoglobin and begin to assemble a unique membrane skeleton that later maintains the shape and deformation properties of the mature erythrocytes. The nucleus of the erythroblast becomes condensed and is extruded from the cell, leaving an irregular, organelle-containing reticulocyte. Subsequently, over the course of a few days, extensive remodeling occurs within the reticulocyte that eliminates the internal organelles and changes the membrane so that the biconcave erythrocyte is formed. This remodeling process involves extensive, selective proteolysis. In myeloid cells, granules that contain specific proteolytic enzymes are formed in the cytoplasm. The nuclei undergo a condensation process that ultimately results in a multilobular nucleus that is retained in the mature cell. Maturing monocyte precursors undergo similar changes. Terminal-stage megakaryocytes replicate their DNA and undergo several nuclear divisions without cytokinesis; thus, they become polyploid. Dense granules form in the cytoplasm, and the cytoplasm becomes highly compartmentalized by demarcation membranes. Platelets form as small portions of the demarcated megakaryocyte cytoplasm separate from the whole cell.

HEMATOPOIETIC STEM AND PROGENITOR CELL ASSAYS

While surface markers are useful as surrogate markers of HSCs, the definition of an HSC is ultimately a functional definition: a cell with the ability to give rise to all hematopoietic lineages in the long term.

Furthermore, under certain circumstances, HSC surface markers may change (see previous section *Enrichment of Hematopoietic Stem Cells*). Definitive studies of HSCs must therefore make use of functional assays. There are numerous such assays with differing levels of stringency, limitations, and appropriateness to the question being addressed.[202]

Colony-Forming Unit Assays
Long-Term In Vitro Assays

The various progenitors quantified by in vitro assays are shown in *Table 5.3*.

In humans and mice, two types of progenitor cells called long-term culture-initiating cells (LTC-ICs) and cobblestone area–forming cells (CAFCs) can be detected using LTC assays. Because these assays extend beyond 2 to 3 weeks when most committed progenitors proliferate and differentiate, these committed progenitors are lost from the cultures after 3 weeks. However, by 5 weeks or more of LTC, more immature progenitors that are dormant during the initial weeks but which possess extensive proliferating capacity have continued to proliferate. One type of LTC assay detects early-stage hematopoietic progenitors that are capable of initiating long-term hematopoiesis in culture after seeding them onto irradiated stromal cell monolayers (human[203,204] and mouse[205,206]). These LTC-ICs[203] sustain production of multilineage progenitors for 4 to 6 weeks. In some instances, these cultures have been extended for more than 10 to 12 weeks.[207,208] This continued production of hematopoietic progenitors of multiple lineages in individual cultures is measured after several weeks by harvesting the cultured cells and doing secondary assays for various types of lineage-committed progenitors. LTCs require a supporting stromal monolayer that is commonly generated from bone marrow–derived mesenchymal or fibroblast cells. The stromal layer supports the proliferation and differentiation of seeded hematopoietic progenitor cells, but at later times, it sloughs from the culture dish and fails to sustain continuation of the culture. In CAFC assays, islands or colonies of hematopoietic cells can be recognized morphologically in situ.[205] These cobblestone colonies integrate within the supporting stromal layer, forming clusters of flattened, optically dense, morphologically homogeneous appearing cells tightly adherent with the stromal layer.[209,210] CAFC assays are one-step cultures in contrast to LTC-IC assays, which require plating of fresh hematopoietic cells on established stromal layers. Using limiting dilution and Poisson statistics, the frequency of CAFC or LTC-IC in a test population or following culture can be determined.[204-206,208,211]

Assays of murine bone marrow cells for LTC-ICs and for day 28 CAFCs yield estimates of 1 to 4 LTC-ICs or CAFCs per 10^5 marrow mononuclear cells—a value comparable to that obtained for HSCs in repopulation assays.[212,213] A modification of the mouse LTC-IC assay[194,214] has led to a demonstration that some LTC-ICs form lymphoid as well as myeloid progenitors in vitro. However, LTC-ICs do not necessarily correspond in a 1:1 ratio to hematopoietic repopulating units. For example, several studies have shown that ex vivo expansion of hematopoietic cell populations with growth factors in culture leads to a loss of in vivo repopulating cells,[148,181] although measured LTC-ICs do not decrease in parallel. Despite these shortcomings, the LTC-IC assay is advantageous when an estimate of HSC frequency is required in scenarios in which the test population of HSCs has a defect in homing or engraftment capability, which would result in underestimation of the reduction in HSC activity when used in transplant assays (see in the subsequent section).

In Vivo Hematopoietic Assays

A large number of in vivo assays exist which can measure a broad of HSC functions, including homing, survival, proliferation, and differentiation. Homing and subsequent development of donor-derived blood cells is referred to as **hematopoietic engraftment**. To sustain lifelong hematopoiesis in the host, transplanted HSCs must self-renew and re-establish an HSC pool. Because in vivo assays can be monitored for a prolonged period for survival, proliferation, and differentiation of transplanted HSCs and, ultimately, the establishment of donor-derived hematopoiesis, they remain the gold standard for measuring the true functional potential of HSCs. It is worth noting that these assays can only confirm HSC activity within a transplanted cell population, and these methods cannot be used to prospectively isolate HSCs.

There are broadly three ways to assess long-term repopulating HSC activity in vivo: the competitive repopulation assay,[215] the limiting dilution assay,[212] and the serial transplantation assay.[216] The nomenclature of these assays is unfortunate, as both the competitive repopulation assay and the limiting dilution assay measure competitive repopulation, that is, the ability of a test sample to engraft alongside competitor bone marrow. Adding further confusion, limiting dilution assays are frequently called competitive repopulating unit assays, whereas competitive repopulation assays use the repopulating unit.

All three of these assays rely on the ability to discriminate between the sample of interest and host or competitor cells after transplantation. The first studies of engraftment used retrovirus to label and track engraftment, but the development of congenic mice strains with distinguishable surface markers has reduced the complexity of engraftment experiments. Congenic mice strains share the same genetic background, which differs at a single gene locus. This system uses two congenic lines expressing different alleles of CD45 (CD45.1 and CD45.2), which is broadly expressed by hematopoietic cells. Antibodies that specifically recognize one of the two CD45 alleles are widely available, allowing CD45.1- and CD45.2-expressing cells to be distinguished within a single mouse using flow cytometry. However, due to imperfect congenicity, hematopoietic cells from these two strains differ in their engraftment potential.[217] The development of a targeted CD45.1 knock-in point mutation in the CD45.2 mouse strain has solved this problem for experiments where equal engraftment potential is important.[218] Furthermore, this system cannot be used to evaluate erythroid or platelet engraftment, as these cells do not express CD45. Other systems, such as tracking hemoglobin variants or using a ubiquitously expressed green fluorescent protein (GFP) transgene, must be used to evaluate engraftment of these lineages.

In the competitive repopulation assay and limiting dilution assay, lethally irradiated animals are typically supplied with a standard, quantified competitor cell population to provide short-term hematopoietic reconstitution. These competitor "support" bone marrow cells limit the potential replicative stress on the small number of HSCs in the test sample following transplantation.[213] Competitive repopulation assays involve transplanting a test population with unknown HSC content—this can be whole bone marrow from an experimental model or a population of cells sorted based on immunophenotypic markers—along with a population of standard, although not necessarily definitively known, HSC content. The clonal contribution of HSCs is not a linear process and can display stochastic fluctuations in the short term after transplantation. It has been determined that individual oncoretroviral-marked HSCs gave stable contribution to hematopoiesis, starting at 6 months posttransplant.[93] Using a congenic system, it was demonstrated that this stability arises 16 weeks after transplantation, whereas more committed progenitors gradually lose reconstituting capacity by 16 weeks after transplant.[173] A minimum of 16 weeks and an optimal time frame of 6 months have been suggested as the interval to wait prior to assessment of donor contribution in transplantation-based HSC assays in mice.[202] The major drawback of the competitive repopulation assay is that it makes a statement regarding the relative number of HSCs, precluding definitive statement on the actual HSC content of a test sample.

In order to enumerate the actual number of HSCs in a test population, limiting dilution analysis is used instead.[212] In this assay, serial dilutions of a test cell population are transplanted into a group of animals. From the known dilutions of test cells given in the transplants and the percentage of mice without donor chimerism (defined as <0.1% or <1%, see in the subsequent section) yielded by each test cell dose, one can calculate the number of HSCs in a test sample by using limiting dilution analysis and Poisson statistic.[124,212] A variation of this assay uses limiting dilutions of genotypically distinct donor cells to transplant into stem cell–deficient W/Wv mice that can be used as hosts rather than lethally irradiated mice.[219] A second variation uses, as hosts, mice that have been transplanted previously and thus have a reduced or weakened endogenous stem cell competition

capacity. Although the limiting dilution assay is the gold standard to enumerate HSCs, it is time- and resource-intensive. In addition, other vagaries and considerations must be undertaken when designing limiting dilution experiments. When chimerism studies relied on Southern blot detection, <5% test-derived cells was considered as a mouse negative for engraftment. However, because flow cytometry and congenic markers have allowed for much enhanced sensitivity in detecting fine changes in engraftment, most studies utilize <1% as the threshold. Although some investigators propose a <0.1% threshold, it is controversial whether detecting such low levels of chimerism is accurate.[202] Caution should also be taken when enumerating HSC numbers in animals with mutation that affects proliferation kinetics of progenitors. If progenitors specifically have increased proliferative capacity, they may erroneously indicate enhanced HSC repopulating capacity, and likewise, decreased proliferative potential of progenitors might artifactually suggest reduced HSC repopulating activity.

The most stringent functional test (although not necessarily as sensitive or quantitative) is the serial transplantation assay, which involves successive rounds of transplantation, 16-week engraftment period, and retransplantation of recipient bone marrow into new recipients. This is the preferred method to demonstrate changes in HSC numbers when there is a perturbation in homing, engraftment, self-renewal, altered progenitor proliferative, or differentiation capacity.[202] Using serially diluted amounts of bone marrow in the primary transplant, the serial transplantation assay can be combined with the limiting dilution assay to add further stringency to this assay. However, this is rarely done because of the enormous resource requirements.

TRACKING HEMATOPOIETIC STEM CELLS AND THEIR PROGENY

Hematopoietic Stem Cell Studies in Xenograft Models

The need to study human hematopoiesis experimentally, and to assess novel therapeutic approaches in preclinical leukemia models, has generated a demand for xenogeneic transplant models using mice. The first of these humanized mouse models were generated in the late 1980s in an effort to establish models with which to study HIV infection. They were enabled by the chance discovery of mice with a spontaneously occurring *SCID* mutation,[220] which blocked B and T cell development, later identified to be a mutation in the gene encoding DNA-dependent protein kinase catalytic subunit (*Prkdc*), which is vital for repairing the double-stranded DNA breaks which occur during V(D)J recombination.[221,222] Transfer of human peripheral blood leukocytes[223] or fetal hematopoietic tissues[224] into these *SCID* mutation-bearing mice allowed for the establishment of human B and T cells, but not myeloid cells, without rejection by the host mice. Both myeloid and lymphoid engraftment was achieved in *SCID* mice by transplanting human bone marrow after sublethal irradiation of the mice.[225] Human hematopoietic cells with this ability to engraft long-term in a sublethally irradiated immunodeficient mouse are termed SCID-repopulating cells, the frequency of which can be determined by limiting dilution analyses (see previous section *In Vivo Hematopoietic Assays*). This assay remains perhaps the most common and definitive means of assessing functional human HSCs in an experimental setting.

However, the field advanced past the use of this initial *SCID* model. *SCID* mice were bred into the non–obese diabetic (NOD) background, and the resulting NOD-*SCID* mice demonstrated much improved engraftment of human cells compared to *SCID* mice.[88] In addition to its existing defects in innate immunity, the NOD background contains a mutation in the *Sirpa* gene that allows murine macrophages to recognize human CD47, a potent "don't eat me" signal, thereby reducing phagocytosis of transplanted human cells and boosting subsequent engraftment.[89] Derivatives of these NOD-*SCID* mice have become the most broadly used xenograft models, alongside derivatives of the RAG1[90] and RAG2[226] knockout mice that have similar deficiencies in adaptive immunity to *SCID* mice. In addition to the depletion of lymphocytes achieved in the NOD-*SCID* and RAG knockout lines, reduction or elimination of NK cell activity can further improve human hematopoietic engraftment. β2-Microglobulin, encoded by *B2m*, is an essential component of the major histocompatibility complex (MHC) class I molecule, and null alleles in the *B2m* gene lead to impairment of NK cells and other MHC class I–dependent cells.[91,92] As a result, NOD-*SCID β2M*[null] mice better support engraftment, proliferation, and differentiation of immature human hematopoietic progenitors.[93-96] Another approach to eliminating NK cells is targeting the IL-2 receptor, which is vital for NK cell maturation. This has been done either using antibodies against IL-2Rβ[227] or via a knockout of the common γ chain (IL-2rg[−/−]), which eliminates IL-2 signaling.[228] The NOD-*SCID IL-2rg*[−/−] (NSG) mouse is perhaps the most used strain for human xenotransplantation studies today, exhibiting 50-fold higher CD34[+] cell engraftment compared to NOD/SCID mice. NSG mice were utilized to demonstrate that 14% to 28% of single human Thy1[+] Rho[lo] CD49f[+] could give rise to multilineage reconstitution.[98]

Engraftment of certain lineages remains difficult in NSG mice. One of the main challenges for recapitulating human hematopoiesis in the mouse is the limited cross-reactivity of murine cytokines with human receptors. Whereas early efforts to supplement transplanted mice with exogenous human cytokines often resulted in supraphysio-logic levels of cytokines, recent advances, such as the generation of a mouse strain bearing simultaneous knock-in of human TPO, IL-3/granulocyte-macrophage colony-stimulating factor (GM-CSF), and CSF-1,[229,230] have allowed for enhanced reconstitution of the human myeloid and NK cell compartment. Additionally, an NSG mouse strain bearing the *Kit* loss-of-function allele *Kit*[W41] is able to achieve circulating human erythrocytes.[231] Although many challenges remain, innovations in the realm of xenograft hematopoietic transplantation are rapidly improving the modeling of human hematopoiesis in vivo, and these models have already granted insights into human hematopoiesis that could not be achieved by human studies alone.

Hematopoietic Stem Cell Studies in Large Animal Models

Important differences between the kinetics and behavior of HSCs in large animals and rodents have been identified.[232] The production of blood cells for the whole life span of a mouse is equivalent to blood cell production of a human in a single day. This limited replication demand as a result of the relatively short murine life span poses a significant challenge to determine the long-term repopulating activity of human hematopoietic cell populations transplanted into immunodeficient mice. Human cells have been found to persist for several years after in utero transplantation into fetal sheep.[233] Several large animal models are available for HSC studies, including feline, canine, ovine, and nonhuman primates,[234] but the genetic and biologic similarity between humans and nonhuman primates suggests that the nonhuman primate model is probably the best available model to study human hematopoiesis in vivo.[133,235] Another advantage of using nonhuman primates is that their relatively long life span (up to 30 years) compared to rodents (up to 3 years) allows long-term monitoring after transplantation, irradiation, cytokine therapy, chemotherapy, and other perturbations to the hematopoietic system. Simultaneous transplantation of genetically marked autologous cells in lethally irradiated nonhuman primates and immune-deficient mice demonstrated that the reconstituting cells in primates and in mice are distinct, suggesting a lack of overlap between these two cell populations.[236] The successful long-term repopulation potential of transplanted zinc finger nuclease–modified HSCs in irradiated nonhuman primate models has been demonstrated.[237] This, in addition to the use of CRISPR/Cas9 for deletion of CCR5 from human HSC/progenitor cells,[238] indicates the feasibility of a genome-editing technology for potential human cell transplantation.

TRAFFICKING OF HEMATOPOIETIC STEM AND PROGENITOR CELLS

Homing of Hematopoietic Stem Cells

Besides providing a source of growth factors for hematopoietic cells, the stroma of hematopoietic organs directs the trafficking of these cells. This trafficking occurs during embryonic development as the

primary organs of hematopoiesis change from the AGM to the fetal liver to the spleen and bone marrow. Additionally, some hematopoietic stem and progenitor cells (HSPCs) migrate continuously between the bone marrow and blood in normal adult animals.[239] Although not discussed further here, such trafficking to particular tissues is also critical for mature leukocytes to migrate specifically to areas of inflammation. Trafficking is composed of two parts: (1) egress from source tissue (typically the bone marrow), termed "mobilization" and (2) directed movement toward target tissue, termed "homing."

Homing is the process by which circulating HSPCs bind to the endothelium and extravasate, entering the bone marrow where they selectively interact with specific stromal cells and matrix proteins to initiate and sustain long-term hematopoiesis.[240] Homing occurs not only for HSPCs that are circulating under normal physiological conditions but is also essential for the successful engraftment of transplanted stem cells. Like the receptor-counterreceptor interactions that govern the inflammatory recruitment of mature leukocytes, the endothelial-progenitor cells interactions that govern homing are dependent on selectins, integrins, and chemokines.

The selectin family of cytoadhesion molecules are designated E-selectin, P-selectin, and L-selectin. HSPC tethering to the endothelial surface is dependent on endothelial P-selectin and E-selectin binding to fucosylated P-selectin glycoprotein ligand-1 on HSCs and progenitors.[241,242] Once bound to the endothelial surface, shear stress from blood flow allows for rolling of HSPCs along the endothelial surface, in a similar manner as leukocytes.

Integrins are heterodimeric, transmembrane proteins in which the α and β subunits are joined noncovalently. Both subunits have extracellular and intracellular domains. In all, 18 types of β subunits and 8 types of α subunits are known, although only a few of the possible heterodimer combinations have been found on hematopoietic or stromal cells and implicated in hematopoiesis. The definitive homing to and subsequent retention of HSC/progenitors in the extravascular space is dependent on integrins $\alpha_4\beta_1$,[241,243-249] $\alpha_4\beta_7$,[250] $\alpha_5\beta_1$,[247,251,252] $\beta6$,[253] and $\alpha_9\beta_1$[254]; CD44[255-257]; and VCAM-1[242-244,258].

The most critical chemokine receptor in HSPC homing is CXCR4, which recognizes the chemoattractant CXCL12.[259,260] CXCL12, secreted by bone marrow stroma, is the only known chemokine that elicits a directed chemotactic response in HSCs.[261,262] Mice lacking CXCL12 or CXCR4 have defective hematopoiesis in fetal bone marrow as a result of a decreased ability of HSCs to move from the fetal liver to the marrow cavity.[263,264] Antibodies against CXCR4 block engraftment of human CD34-enriched HSCs and progenitors when transplanted into SCID mice.[260,265] In addition, CXCL12 potentiates binding of circulating progenitors to the vascular endothelium by activating the integrins VLA-4, VLA-5, and lymphocyte function–associated antigen (LFA),[251,266,267] as well as CD44 and hyaluronic acid.[255] CXCL12 can thus help drive arrest of rolling HSPCs on the endothelium and subsequently guide extravasation into the bone marrow parenchyma in cooperation with $\alpha_4\beta_1$-, LFA-, CD44-, and Flt3-dependent interactions.[251,255,268]

Mobilization of Hematopoietic Stem Cells

In preclinical models, recruitment of circulating HSPCs has been implicated in toll-like receptor–mediated myeloid differentiation in tissues[269] and the development of repair-phenotype macrophages after liver injury,[270] but their in vivo steady-state relevance is still unclear. But enforced egress of HSPCs into circulation with pharmacologic agents, such as chemotherapy or hematopoietic growth factor administration, has been utilized in clinical medicine to procure HSPCs for transplantation, a process termed **stem cell mobilization**. Mobilized peripheral blood now represents the most common donor source for HSPC transplantations.[271] These mobilized grafts have several advantages over traditional bone marrow grafts for transplantation, including ease of harvesting, higher HSC yields, and faster hematopoietic engraftment following transplantation. G-CSF is the most commonly utilized mobilizing agent. Although early observations suggested that the mechanism of G-CSF mobilization depended on the enhanced levels of proteolytic enzymes in the marrow cavity to cleave adhesion

The Normal Hematologic System

factors tethering HSC/progenitors in the bone marrow, unperturbed levels of mobilization in animals deficient of virtually all serine protease activity have cast doubt on this as the primary mechanism.[272] More recent data indicate that reduced production of stem cell retention factors, of which the most important is CXCL12, rather than increased degradation, mediates mobilization.[273]

The sympathetic nervous system has been implicated in HSC/progenitor mobilization. β-Adrenergic signals from sympathetic nerve terminals in the bone marrow are critical for this abrogated stromal production of retention factors.[273,274] Consistently, the β2-agonist clenbuterol increases mobilization yields in mice.[274] Notably, neurotoxic chemotherapy, such as cisplatin and vincristine, or diabetes can cause a chronic sympathetic nervous system lesion that impairs HSC/progenitor mobilization.[275,276] Neuroprotection with glial-derived neural factor or 4-methylcatechol was able restore mobilization yield in the presence of neuropathy. Furthermore, there is a circadian time–dependent oscillation in HSC/progenitor trafficking,[277] which points to optimal times to harvest peripheral blood HSC/progenitors in mobilized mice and humans.[278]

Abrogation of bone marrow macrophage-derived retention signals is another mechanism of G-CSF–induced mobilization.[279-281] G-CSF-R expressed on CD68-expressing cells, presumably bone marrow macrophages, is sufficient for HSC/progenitor mobilization.[279] Bone marrow macrophages produce a protein factor, possibly oncostatin M, that promotes CXCL12 production by stromal cells.[281,282] This cross talk is downmodulated in response to G-CSF mobilization. It is likely that VCAM1 expressed at high levels on BM macrophages also directly adheres to HSCs and can be targeted to promote HSC mobilization.[283,284] A different α-smooth muscle actin- and cyclooxygenase 2–expressing macrophage population was also shown to induce CXCL12 expression on stromal cells.[285] Interestingly, bone marrow macrophage consumption of aged neutrophils appears to be a physiologic signal to downmodulate CXCL12 production in order to release HSC/progenitors to replenish the myeloid compartment.[286]

Another widely utilized agent for clinical HSC/progenitor mobilization is the CXCR4 antagonist AMD3100 (plerixafor). AMD3100 is capable of mobilizing HSCs within hours and synergizes with the mobilizing effects of G-CSF.[287] Because up to 30% of patients are "poor mobilizers" and thus do not mobilize a sufficient number of HSC/progenitors with standard clinical protocols, novel strategies to enhance mobilization efficiency are under active investigation.[288,289] Among the agents being investigated as adjuncts to G-CSF and AMD3100 include GM-CSF, SCF, TPO, human growth hormone, IL-8 analog, antibodies to VLA-4, retinoic acid receptor-α agonists, TPO receptor agonists, Flt3l, epithelial growth factor antagonists, and small molecule antagonists of α4 β1/α9β1.[290-293]

LINEAGE COMMITMENT

Branch Points of Hematopoiesis

Multiple lineage relationship models of hematopoiesis have been proposed over the years.[175] Discrepancies among multiple models can be partially explained by the differential predication of the models on differentiation potential vs physiologic production. Whereas certain progenitors may have particular differentiation potentials when cultured in vitro with the appropriate cytokines or in vivo in emergency scenarios, these potentials may not be evident under steady-state physiology. Where possible, assessment of lineage commitment by genetic lineage tracing is the most physiologic method to assess physiologic progenitor-progeny relationships in vivo.

Role of Particular Transcription Factors

Some specific transcription factors exhibit hematopoietic lineage–restricted expression and some are known to be essential for the complete differentiation of individual lineages. Two examples of transcription factors whose lineage associations are more fully understood are GATA-1, which is essential for terminal erythrocyte and megakaryocyte differentiation, and PU.1, which is essential for B

lymphocyte as well as macrophage development.[294,295] Specific factors not only play a direct role in the expression of lineage-specific genes but also, in some cases, appear to antagonize transcription factors important for other lineages; thus, they can repress the expression of genes characteristic of other lineages. For example, GATA-1 can suppress PU.1 activity, and PU.1 can suppress GATA-1 activity by direct protein interactions that block the function of each other.[295,296] PU.1 and GATA-1 play positive roles in the transcription of their own genes (autoregulatory loops).[297,298] Thus, hypothetically, an excess of GATA-1 over PU.1 could downregulate PU.1 expression at the level of transcription, and excess PU.1 could likewise downregulate GATA-1. In multipotent cells, it is known that there is expression at low levels of sets of genes characteristic of multiple hematopoietic lineages.[299] Thus, commitment appears to occur not only by upregulation of a single-lineage program of gene expression but also by the irreversible suppression of competing differentiation programs. Because of observations such as those described earlier for GATA-1 and PU.1 and because the forced overexpression of particular transcription factors can cause lineage switches in certain in vitro cell systems, some investigators have proposed that the transcription factor profile (stoichiometry relationships) of multipotent cells directs their lineage commitment decisions through cross-antagonism mechanisms.[295,300] A transcription factor network has been proposed in which combinations of specific lineage–instructive transcription factors at various stages of hematopoietic differentiation from HSCs to lineage-specific progenitor cells play roles in cell fate decisions.[301] Of note, recent high-resolution single-cell analyses of HSCs call into question this model of the deterministic role of stoichiometric ratios of transcription factors. An unexpected finding was that GATA-1 was never expressed on HSCs on their path to GM differentiation, PU.1 was inconsistently expressed on HSCs on their path to megakaryocytic-erythroid (MegE) differentiation, and they did not observe a reproducible PU.1-GATA-1 double-positive stage through which all differentiating HSCs pass.[302] These findings argue that although PU.1-GATA-1 interaction and antagonism can potentially serve as a reinforcing mechanism making terminal differentiation irreversible, it was not the primary determinant of MegE vs GM lineage fate. Subsequent studies in other cell lineage decisions will further clarify the contribution of transcription factor stoichiometry in differentiation decisions.

Role of Micro-RNAs

Micro-RNAs (miRNAs) are 18 to 24 nucleotide-noncoding RNAs that bind the 3′-untranslated region of target messenger RNA (mRNA), resulting in mRNA degradation or impaired translation efficiency.[303] miRNAs rise and fall as cells differentiate along the hematopoietic spectrum because these miRNAs fine-tune the expression of cytokines and transcription factors that are required for lineage commitment and differentiation. Because the role of miR-181 in B-lymphoid differentiation was first demonstrated in 2004,[304] there have been many reports on the role of various miRNAs in hematopoiesis.[305] Loss of function of all miRNAs can be studied broadly using gene knockdown models of Dicer, an RNAse that is critical for miRNA biosynthesis. For example, conditional knockout of Dicer in the B-cell[306] and T-cell[307] compartments impairs development of mature B lymphocytes and T lymphocytes, respectively, indicating a role of miRNAs in lymphocyte differentiation. More precisely, particular hematopoietic populations can be assessed for miRNAs that are expressed, and these candidate miRNAs can be specifically knocked down. For example, this has been used to show that miR-155 inhibits erythropoiesis and megakaryopoiesis,[308,309] but is critical in T-cell and B-cell function.[310-314] The influence of miRNAs is pervasive because they play essential roles in HSCs[315] and in the regulation of erythropoiesis,[316] megakaryopoiesis,[317] myelopoiesis,[318] and lymphopoiesis.[319]

Hematopoietic Cytokines

The purification of EPO from the urine of anemic patients in 1977 spurred investigation to find other comparable growth factors for other hematopoietic lineages.[320] Although taken for granted now because most of the discovered hematopoietic cytokines have thus far been made readily available in recombinant protein form and validated by genetic mouse models, there was substantial controversy in the hematopoietic growth factor field in the 1970s, 1980s, and 1990s. Most of the early work on these glycoprotein growth factors was derived from studies of "conditioned media," which were necessary and greatly stimulatory for hematopoietic cell colony growth. What particularly confounded researchers about the discovered CSFs was its polyfunctionality.[320] For example, until specialized utilization of different cytoplasmic domains downstream of the same receptor was described, it was unclear how G-CSF could promote the battery of cellular responses from survival, proliferation, differentiation commitment, maturation induction, and functional stimulation.[320,321] Another puzzling aspect of hematopoietic growth factors was the ability of one cytokine to act on many cell types and the ability of multiple cytokines to exert influence on a single-cell type. Exemplifying the latter, G-CSF, GM-CSF, IL-3, CSF-1, SCF, and IL-6 all expand granulocytic colonies.[320] This does not necessarily just reflect redundancy because there is synergistic activity among IL-3, G-CSF, GM-CSF, and CSF-1 in myeloid colony formation.[322] Based on certain structural and functional features of the receptors for hematopoietic growth factors, two families of ligands/receptors have been recognized: the cytokine receptor family and the tyrosine kinase receptor family (*Table 5.4*). Notably, synergy is most prominent when utilizing combinations of cytokines using both sets of receptors. *Table 5.4* presents a list of cytokines, their receptors, and expression patterns.

Factors That Act on Multilineage Progenitors

In vitro cultures of hematopoietic colony–forming cells have continued to be very useful in defining growth factor effects on various lineages of cells.[323-328] Many of the hematopoietic growth factors exhibit positive growth effects on HSCs or progenitors with multilineage potential, or both. These include KitL, GM-CSF, G-CSF, CSF-1, IL-3, IL-4, IL-6, IL-11, IL-12, fetal liver, leukemia-inhibitory factor, oncostatin M, and TPO.[329-332] In addition, some members of this same group can support differentiation of certain cell types to late stages or even to full maturity. For example, G-CSF, GM-CSF, CSF-1, IL-3, KitL, and IL-6

can all support formation of small neutrophilic granulocytic colonies, and CSF-1 and GM-CSF can also support macrophage colonies and mixed granulocyte/macrophage colonies.[329]

Potentiation of hematopoietic cell production in in vitro assays by combinations of growth factors can occur in two basic ways. First, a combination of growth factors may allow proliferation and differentiation of individual cells that would otherwise die or remain dormant in the presence of a single factor. Second, potentiation can occur by enhanced proliferation in the presence of the combined factors. The latter effect appears to apply to the examples of the combined effect of KitL with G-CSF, GM-CSF, IL-3, IL-6, or EPO on expansion of populations of progenitors.[333-335] The numbers of colonies formed in the presence of the combinations are not increased greatly, but there is a large increase in the size of the colonies. The proliferation of HSCs, however, appears to be an example of a requirement of a combination of factors for recruitment of dormant cells into proliferation and differentiation.[180,329,336-338]

When growth factors with effects on multilineage progenitors act alone or in combination, the result of early rounds of proliferation and differentiation is the generation of progeny that become committed individually to form different lineages of mature cells. For some lineages, the resultant single-lineage progenitors cannot complete differentiation and maturation without lineage-specific factors; thus, caution must be taken in interpreting negative results. For example, late committed erythroid progenitors (CFU-E) require EPO, or they die. Likewise, appearance of lymphoid cells requires IL-7, and maturation of megakaryocytes and formation of platelets are greatly enhanced by TPO. Thus, the full development of hematopoietic cells from stem cells or early-stage progenitors requires the action of growth factors (alone or in combination) that support the multilineage progenitors and, in addition, growth factors that support terminal differentiation of committed single-lineage progenitors.

Granulocyte Growth Factors

Granulocytes are composed of neutrophils, eosinophils, and basophils. Neutrophils are best known for their ability to rapidly arrive and exert effector responses at sites of tissue injury, whereas basophils and eosinophils are critical in responding to parasitic infections and also promoting allergic reactions. In vitro colony-forming assays have indicated the importance of G-CSF and IL-5 in the support of differentiation of neutrophils[122,262] and eosinophils,[339,340] respectively. This is substantiated by the neutropenia and increased bacterial susceptibility observed in mice deficient in G-CSFR[341] and impaired parasite–induced eosinophilia observed in IL-5–deficient animals[342] (*Table 5.5*). Nonetheless, the existence of neutrophils and eosinophils in the steady state indicates redundancy with other cytokines. IL-3 has been implicated in basophil differentiation. Although IL-3–deficient animals do not lack basophils, IL-3 is important in stimulating GMPs to differentiate into basophils in mice.[343,344]

GM-CSF has also been implicated in in vitro granulocyte colony formation[191,345]; however, no neutropenia is observed in GM-CSF–deficient animals.[346] Interestingly, mice deficient in G-CSF, GM-CSF, and CSF-1 still have neutrophils, suggesting extensive redundancy/collaboration among the hematopoietic cytokines.[347] G-CSF and GM-CSF not only support differentiation of late-stage progenitors but also can activate the resulting mature blood cells, stimulating functions such as phagocytosis.[348-350] Importantly, G-CSF (filgrastim) is used clinically to treat patients with neutropenia.

Mast Cell Growth Factors

Mast cell differentiation in vitro is supported by c-Kit.[339,350-354] The importance of c-Kit-KitL signaling in mast cell differentiation is validated in vivo by the absence of mast cells in animals deficient in KitL (Sl/Sld mice) or c-Kit (W/Wv)[355] (*Table 5.5*). KitL also activates mature mast cells, causing them to release histamine.[354]

Monocyte/Macrophage Growth Factors

In mice, monocytes consist of at least two subtypes: (1) the classic Gr1[hi] subset (CD14+ CD16− in humans, also known as "inflammatory

Table 5.4. Classification of Hematopoietic Factors Based on Their Receptor Types

	Receptors Consisting of:	Examples
Cytokine-type receptors	A single unique peptide chain	EPO, TPO, G-CSF
	Complexes containing GP130[a]	IL-6, IL-11, IL-12, LIF, OSM
	A ligand-specific common α subunit and/or common GP140 β_c subunits	IL-3, IL-5, GM-CSF
	A common γ_c subunit and ligand-specific α and/or β subunits	IL-2, IL-4, IL-7, IL-9, IL-15
	Two or more unique subunits	IFN-α, IFN-β, IFN-γ
RTK-type receptors	EGF family receptors (type I)	TGF-α
	Insulin family receptors (type II)	IGF-1
	PDGF subfamily with five Ig-like domains (type III)	Kit ligand, CSF-1, Flk-2 ligand
	PDGF subfamily with seven Ig-like domains (type V)	Flk-1 ligand

[a]GP130 serves as the signal transducer, plus an additional ligand-binding unit.
Abbreviations: CSF-1, colony-stimulating factor 1 (also known as macrophage colony–stimulating factor, or M-CSF); EGF, epidermal growth factor; EPO, erythropoietin; Flk-2 ligand, fms-like kinase 2 (also known as fms-like tyrosine kinase 3 ligand, or Flt3l); G-CSF, granulocyte colony–stimulating factor; GM-CSF, granulocyte-macrophage colony-stimulating factor; GP, glycoprotein; IFN, interferon; IGF, insulin growth factor; IL, interleukin; LIF, leukemia-inhibitory factor; OSM, oncostatin M; PDGF, platelet-derived growth factor; TGF, transforming growth factor; TPO, thrombopoietin.

monocytes") and (2) the nonclassic Gr1^{lo} (CD14$^{-/lo}$ CD16$^+$ in humans, also known as "resident monocytes") subset.[356] Monocytes are critical mediators of inflammation, whether beneficially in combating pathogens or detrimentally in contributing to atherosclerotic plaques and mediating inflammatory disorders. Although monocytes express high levels of the CSF-1R, they are still present in normal numbers in animals with defects in CSF-1 (Csf1op/op) or deficiency in CSF-1R (Csf1r$^{-/-}$)[357] (*Table 5.5*), indicating that other cytokines contribute or at least can compensate for defective CSF-1R signaling. Monocytes are also present at normal levels in GM-CSF–deficient animals.[346] Mice deficient in G-CSF, GM-CSF, and CSF-1 still have monocytes present, albeit at reduced numbers, again suggesting redundancy among cytokines for differentiation and maintenance of monocytes.[347]

Macrophage differentiation and survival in vitro can be supported by the CSF-1 cytokine.[358] Tissue-resident macrophages are severely reduced in Csf1op/op or deficiency in Csf1r$^{-/-}$ (*Table 5.5*).[357] Both of these deficient strains develop osteopetrosis owing to failure to develop osteoclasts. Although other macrophage populations are normal, lung macrophages are severely reduced in numbers in GM-CSF–deficient animals and develop a characteristic alveolar proteinosis.[346] Importantly, CSF-1 treatment in mice and patients after HSC transplantation protects from infections and improves survival.[359,360]

Megakaryocyte Growth Factors

In vitro colony-forming assays have been developed for quantifying megakaryocyte progenitor cells, termed CFUs-MK. As in the case for other early committed progenitors, the growth of such colonies is augmented by several of the CSFs with multilineage activity, such as IL-3, IL-6, GM-CSF, KitL, and IL-11.[193,361,362] Unlike granulocytes and monocytes, bone marrow production of platelets is regulated by the number of platelets in the blood. Reduction of platelet numbers in rodents by antiplatelet antibodies or by exchange transfusion of platelet-poor blood causes an increase in the number of

megakaryocytes in the hematopoietic tissues as well as an increase in their size and ploidy; conversely, platelet transfusion decreases these parameters.[193] Such manipulations did not affect CFU-MK numbers in the hematopoietic tissues,[363] leading to the speculation that megakaryocyte differentiation and platelet production are controlled by a thrombopoietic factor that is induced by thrombocytopenia.[193,364]

TPO is a growth factor that has been identified as the physiologic regulator of platelet production, exerts its effect through the activation of a cytokine receptor termed MPL.[365-367] MPL was identified earlier as the viral oncogene product of the mouse retrovirus, myeloproliferative leukemia virus.[368] Recombinant TPO increases megakaryocyte and platelet numbers in vivo and stimulates CFU-MK growth in vitro.[369,370] Mice bearing homozygous, nonfunctional alleles of MPL are viable with greatly diminished platelet numbers,[330] indicating that although TPO is not essential for platelet production, it is a strong in vivo regulator of the process. TPO production has been shown to be regulated by blood platelet numbers,[370] and platelet numbers regulate the mRNA for TPO in the marrow and spleen but not in the liver and kidney.[371] It is not yet clear whether the modulation of TPO mRNA in these organs is responsible for the regulation of overall TPO protein levels. Several studies indicate that TPO is constitutively synthesized in the liver and that its level in blood is determined by its removal from circulation by binding to MPL on platelets and bone marrow megakaryocytes.[365] Mice lacking TPO have approximately 10% of the normal number of platelets[330] (*Table 5.5*). Although early efforts to treat thrombocytopenia with recombinant TPO was complicated by the development of antibodies to endogenous TPO-causing thrombocytopenia, two FDA-approved drugs, including a TPO mimetic and TPO-R agonists, offer new hope to treat clinical thrombocytopenia.[372]

Erythroid Growth Factors

The physiologic regulator of erythrocyte production is EPO, and this regulation is very precise, keeping the red blood cell mass within very narrow limits.[373] EPO acts on committed erythroid progenitors to support the later phases of erythroid differentiation.[373] The regulation is achieved by EPO's action to modulate apoptosis of these progenitors. The production of EPO is regulated by the tissue O$_2$ tension in the vicinity of specialized EPO-producing cells in the kidney. These cells are peritubular cells, located in the renal cortex.[374-376] By sensing O$_2$ tension, they essentially measure the oxygen delivery capacity of the blood, and they adjust EPO production to achieve the number of erythrocytes needed for normal tissue O$_2$ tension. The liver also contains specialized cells that can produce EPO in an oxygen-dependent manner, although, in adult animals, the contribution of the liver to total EPO production is much less than that of the kidney. In specialized kidney and liver cells, the transcription of the EPO gene is controlled by an oxygen-dependent transcription factor, hypoxia-inducible factor (HIF), that interacts with DNA sequences corresponding to the 3′-untranslated sequence of the mRNA and also with sequences in the EPO promoter region.[377] HIF ubiquitination and subsequent proteasomal degradation are dependent on the hydroxylation of two specific prolines[378-380] and an asparagine of HIF[381,382] by nonheme, iron-containing hydroxylases that use molecular oxygen as a substrate for the reactions. With normoxia, HIF is rapidly hydroxylated and degraded. With hypoxia, HIF is not hydroxylated and degraded, but it forms part of a transcription complex that binds the 3′ enhancer sequence and induces EPO gene transcription. In addition, tissue specificity of expression in the kidney requires specific, cis-acting DNA sequences far upstream (between 6 and 14 kb pairs) of the coding sequence.[383,384] EPO is secreted rapidly into the circulation, and it binds in the bone marrow to EPO receptors on erythroid progenitor cells in the CFU-E through early erythroblast stages. The EPO-EPO receptor interaction not only triggers signal transduction but leads to endocytosis and degradation of both the EPO and EPO-R.[385] This erythroid progenitor–mediated consumption of EPO appears to be a major determinant of the metabolic fate of EPO both in vitro[386] and in vivo.[387] Loss of function of EPO or the EPO receptor in knockout mice leads to embryonic death at approximately day 13 of gestation owing to the failure of production of definitive erythrocytes[388,389]

Table 5.5. Phenotypes Caused by Nonfunctional Mutations in Genes for Hematopoietic Growth Factors or Their Receptors

Factor	Observed Effects
Kit ligand	No functional alleles: Embryonic death associated with no production of fetal hematopoietic cells and other developmental failures. Partially functional allele: Deficiency of hematopoiesis, mast cell deficiency, anemia, and also other defects in pigmentation and in gametogenesis
IL-3	Lack of function does not appear to affect hematopoiesis
GM-CSF	Alveolar proteinosis
CSF-1	Osteopetrosis, alveolar proteinosis, reduced macrophage, normal monocytes
G-CSF	Neutrophil deficiency; approximately 20% of normal numbers; impaired mobilization of neutrophils; demonstrated to be susceptible to some infections
IL-5	Eosinophil deficiency
TPO	Platelet deficiency, approximately 10% of normal numbers
EPO	Embryonic death; failure to produce fetal erythrocytes caused by apoptosis of the late progenitors in the fetal liver; production of some embryonic blood cells
Flt3 ligand	Deficiencies in immune system and in myeloid progenitors and CLP; more severe defects in the case of knockout of the ligand than knockout of the receptor (FLT3)
IL-7	Reduced thymic and peripheral lymphoid cellularity, including B-cell and T-cell development

Abbreviations: CLP, common lymphoid progenitor; CSF-1, colony-stimulating factor 1; EPO, erythropoietin; Flt3 ligand, fms-like tyrosine kinase 3 (also known as fms-like kinase 2 ligand, or Flk2 ligand); G-CSF, granulocyte colony–stimulating factor; GM-CSF, granulocyte-macrophage colony-stimulating factor; IL, interleukin; TPO, thrombopoietin.

(*Table 5.5*). Also, importantly, recombinant EPO has been used clinically to treat patients with anemia.

KitL is also required for erythroid cell development as shown by its requirement for growth of human BFU-E in vitro under serum-free conditions.[39] C-Kit is present on multilineage progenitors and on the BFU-E, and it persists on erythroid progenitors up to the proerythroblast stage. KitL thus has a stimulatory effect on erythroid progenitors throughout most early stages, including those of the CFU-E and proerythroblast, when EPO stimulation becomes essential for further development.

In addition, insulin-like growth factor 1 (IGF-1) appears to have a specific role in erythroid development because it appears necessary for proper erythroid differentiation in serum-free cultures.[391,392] Other multilineage growth factors, such as IL-3 and GM-CSF, have a stimulatory effect on BFU-E growth in vitro, although there does not appear to be a specific requirement for these factors.

Lymphocyte Growth Factors

Methods for culture of B lymphocytes and their progenitor cells were originally described by Whitlock and Witte.[393] Subsequently, a colony assay for B-cell progenitors, CFU-preB, was described, in which it was found that IL-7 is a very potent growth stimulatory factor for these progenitors.[195] The role of IL-7 in lymphoid cell development in vivo was demonstrated by generating mice in which the gene for the IL-7 receptor is nonfunctional. These mice have a profound reduction in thymic and peripheral lymphoid cellularity with defects in B-cell and T-cell development[394] (*Table 5.5*). Because of its importance in B-cell growth in vitro, IL-7 has been incorporated into culture media when examining the lineage potential of early multilineage progenitors.[182,194,214] Flt3l and SCF are also crucial in lymphoid commitment because the CLPs are severely reduced in deficient animals.[395]

Supportive vs Instructive Signals

There remains controversy over whether cytokines play a stochastic (supportive) or deterministic (instructive) role in determining cell fate because there are clear examples that accommodate both models. The idea that lineage differentiation is random and thus that cytokines merely play a role in proliferation or survival of the progeny after a differentiation decision has been made is supported by the persistence of myeloid cells in animals deficient in G-CSF, GM-CSF, and CSF-1.[347] Along the same lines, overexpression of antiapoptotic proteins can rescue erythroid and T-lymphocyte deficiencies caused by the absence of EPO[396] and IL-7R,[397,398] respectively, indicating that these cytokines are not critical for differentiation.

Still, even in the example of antiapoptotic rescue of IL-7R–deficient mice, B-cell development is not rescued.[397] In fact, IL-7 receptor signaling upregulates expression of the B-cell–specific transcription factor and its target genes; otherwise, B cells become arrested at the pre-proB-cell stage, indicating that IL-7 instructs B-cell differentiation.[399] Other examples of an instructive role of cytokines on committed progenitors include the demonstration that enforced GM-CSF signaling can redirect lymphoid progenitors to a myeloid fate,[400] G-CSF upregulates expression of C/EBPα, a critical transcription factor in neutrophil production, in bipotent GMPs,[401] and G-CSF and CSF-1 differentially instruct CMPs to adopt a granulocyte or macrophage fate, respectively.[402] Interestingly, when single HSCs were treated with CSF-1, the myeloid master regulator PU.1 was upregulated, promoting myelomonocytic commitment[403]; thus, CSF-1 could have an instructive role even on HSCs.

HEMATOPOIETIC MICROENVIRONMENTS

Stroma of Hematopoietic Organs

The stroma is composed of nonhematopoietic cells that provide structure and regulate hematopoietic cells in lymphoid tissues. These cells include mesenchymal lineage cells, such as MSC, pericytes, osteocytes, adipocytes, and also endothelia and nerves.[404] The stroma also contains an extracellular matrix that provides a structural network to which hematopoietic progenitors and stromal cells are anchored. This matrix is composed of various fibrous proteins, glycoproteins, and proteoglycans that are produced by the stromal cells, including collagens, fibronectin, laminin, tenascin, and proteoglycans.[405,406] The stroma is functionally important in hematopoiesis through its regulation of HSC/progenitor renewal, proliferation, differentiation, and trafficking. One example that illustrates stromal-hematopoietic interactions was discovered in studies of mice that have mutations in either of two particular genes[407]: the white spotting locus (nonfunctional allele W) and the steel locus (nonfunctional allele Sl). Each of these genes is essential for hematopoiesis. Mouse embryos that are homozygous for null alleles of either of these genes die at an early stage of embryogenesis without forming any blood cells. However, mice have been found and bred that bear mutant alleles of each of the two genes that retain partial function (Wv and Sld alleles). Heterozygous mice of the Sl/Sld or the W/Wv genotypes are phenotypically similar to one another, with a lack of cutaneous pigment, sterility, and congenital anemia.[407] Reciprocal bone marrow transplantation studies between normal, wild-type mice and heterozygous mice, Sl/Sld, and W/Wv revealed that W/Wv mice have defective HSCs but a functional microenvironment that can support transplants of normal HSCs. Conversely, the Sl/Sld mice have functional HSCs and can thus serve as donors for marrow transplants, but these mice have a defective microenvironment (stroma) for hematopoiesis; thus, their defect cannot be corrected by the receipt of HSCs from normal donor mice. The mechanism of impaired hematopoiesis caused by mutations in these two genes was understood after the cloning of the genes at the W and Sl loci. The W gene encodes the cell surface receptor protein c-Kit,[408,409] and the Sl gene encodes KitL protein.[410-412] C-Kit is a cell surface receptor on HSC/progenitors, and KitL is expressed by stromal cells. KitL is produced in two forms as a result of alternative splicing of the mRNA: a soluble form and a membrane-bound form.[413,414] Both the soluble form and the stromal cell membrane–bound form of KitL can stimulate HSCs, the former by free ligand receptor binding and the latter by cell-cell contact. Activation of c-Kit is essential for the survival and development of immature hematopoietic progenitors. KitL is just one of a large number of hematopoietic growth factors produced by stromal cells.

Hematopoietic Stem Cell Niches in Bone Marrow

The concept of the HSC niche as a microenvironment promoting the maintenance of HSCs was proposed by Schofield in 1978, but only over the past decade has the functional role of the niche been demonstrated in experimental animal models.[415] A comparison of niche cell candidates can be found in *Table 5.6*. Although osteoblasts were described as the initial putative HSC niche cell,[416-418] a number of observations have called into question the niche activity of osteoblasts: (1) organs with extramedullary hematopoiesis, such as the spleen and liver, do not have osteoblasts, suggesting that they are dispensable; (2) reductions in osteoblasts are not necessarily associated with reductions in HSC numbers in bone marrow[419-423]; (3) compared to nestin + mesenchymal cells, sorted osteoblasts from bone have low expression of CXCL2, KitL, and Vcam1, three microenvironmental factors implicated in the maintenance and retention of HSC[281]; (4) DT injection in Cxcl12-DTR-GFP mice did not reduce osteoblast numbers, suggesting that osteoblasts do not express high levels of CXCL12[424]; (5) although homotypic interactions between N-cadherin on osteoblasts and HSCs have been implicated as a critical niche interaction,[418] there have been conflicting data on the effect of N-cadherin loss of function on HSCs,[421,425-427] and N-cadherin is broadly expressed in mesenchymal cells, including MSCs; and (6) deletion of CXCL12 or KitL from osteoblasts had no effect on HSC content in the bone marrow.[423,428,429]

A "vascular zone" at the center of the marrow cavity consisting of a thin meshwork of fenestrated sinusoidal vessels has been suggested to be the site of a possible vascular niche.[430] However, the sinusoidal network is uniformly distributed throughout the bone marrow.[431] A role of the vasculature for supporting HSCs is suggested by the proximity of CD150+ CD48– Lin– HSC to sinusoidal endothelial cells in the bone marrow.[105] The Rafii group and others have demonstrated that

Table 5.6. Candidates for Cellular Identity of the Hematopoietic Stem and Progenitor Cell Niche

Cell Type	Phenotype	Niche Factors Produced
Osteoblasts	N-cadherin$^+$ CD45$^-$	N-cadherin
Endothelial cells ("Vascular niche")	VE-Cadherin$^+$ VEGFR2$^+$ VEGFR3$^+$ Tie2$^+$	Jagged1, Jagged2, KitL
Mesenchymal lineage pericytes	CD45$^-$ Ter119$^-$ CD31$^-$ Nestin$^+$ NG2$^+$ LeptinR$^+$ CD105$^+$ CD51$^+$ PDGFRα$^+$ PDGFRβ$^+$	CXCL12, Angpt1, KitL, VCAM1
Non–myelinating Schwann cells	GFAP$^+$	CXCL12, Angpt1, KitL, TPO, TGFβ
Megakaryocytes	CXCL4$^+$	CXCL4, TGFβ, FGF1, TPO, IGF-1/IGFBP3

Abbreviations: Angpt1, Angiopoietin 1; FGF1, fibroblast growth factor-1; IGF1, insulin growth factor-1; IGFBP3, insulin-like growth factor binding protein-3; KitL, Kit ligand; NQ, not quantified; TGFβ, transforming growth factor-β; TPO, thrombopoietin; VCAM1, vascular cell adhesion molecule 1.

endothelial cells are critical in vivo regulators of HSC self-renewal, differentiation, and recovery from hematopoietic stress.[432-434] Cxcl12 or KitL deletion with Tie2-Cre reduces HSC.[390,395,396] Of note, compared to mesenchymal lineage cells, endothelial cells produce much lower levels of the niche factors, such as Cxcl2, Angpt1, KitL, and Vcam1.[281]

Nakauchi and colleagues have asserted that latent transforming growth factor-β (TGF-β)-expressing, GFAP+ population of non–myelinating Schwann cells, are critical for HSC maintenance because celiac ganglionectomy rapidly led to the degeneration and loss of nonmyelin Schwann cells and reduced HSC content in the bone marrow.[435] Whether this population of cells expresses the appropriate HSC maintenance factors and whether more specific depletion of this population results in the same reduction in HSC content will further elucidate the relative contribution of this niche to HSC maintenance.

Another source of quiescence-promoting TGF-β could be megakaryocytes in the bone marrow.[436] Approximately 20% of phenotypic HSCs are found attached to megakaryocytes in the bone marrow.[436,437] Dovetailing well with the clinical observation that megakaryocyte dysplasia is frequently seen in myelodysplastic syndrome/acute myeloid leukemia, four recent reports found that megakaryocytes regulate HSCs.[436-439] These papers demonstrated a novel example of the progeny regulating its upstream stem cell precursor. Depending on the context, megakaryocytes maintained HSC quiescence through platelet factor-4,[437] TGF-β,[436] and TPO,[438] or promoted expansion of HSC and fibroblast growth factor-1,[436] IGF-1, and insulin-like factor–binding protein-3.[439] Although the function of megakaryocytes on the steady-state niche remains to be determined, these reports suggest that the megakaryocyte can regulate HSC proliferation.

The putative HSC niche cell with the most supporting evidence is the mesenchymal lineage pericyte, marked by high Cxcl12 expression,[424] nestin,[273,431] neural/glial antigen,[37,52] leptin receptor (lepR),[423,429] Prx1,[390,395] PDGFRα,[395,440] Sca-1,[395] and CD51.[440] These cells express high levels of Cxcl12, KitL, Angpt1, and Vcam1.[273,423,424,428,429,440] Importantly, Cxcl12 or KitL deletion from these pericytes reduced HSC.[390,395,396] Expression of the transcription factor Foxc1 from these mesenchymal lineage cells was also shown to be a critical regulator of the niche.[441] Furthermore, human CD146$^+$ MSCs/adventitial reticular cells express angiopoietin and are able to self-renew and form hematopoietic microenvironments in immunocompromised mice.[442] There appears to be at least two subsets of pericytes: nestinhi lepR-arteriolar and the more ubiquitous reticular nestinint lepR$^+$ sinusoidal types.[404,431] The most quiescent HSC resides near the arteriolar and megakaryocytic niches, and disruption of these niches results in HSC proliferation. Because pericytes are osteoprogenitors found in both the endosteum and bone marrow proper, this can reconcile previous findings supporting both an osteoblastic and vascular HSC niche.[443] *Figure 5.3* summarizes the cellular components and interactions within the HSC niche.

Adhesion Molecules in the Hematopoietic Niche

The adhesion molecules of all families are transmembrane proteins, and many can act as receptors that activate specific intracellular signaling pathways. These adhesion molecules/receptors, in turn, may be regulated by other intracellular signaling pathways.[444-446] Thus, the interactions of hematopoietic cells with stromal cells and matrix can be highly modulated by the adhesion receptors, both in transmitting signals from the microenvironment into the cell and in translating the state of intracellular signaling pathways into changes in the number and affinities of adhesion molecules. Activation of c-Kit by SCF modulates adhesion functions that are mediated by integrins α4 β1 (VLA-4) and α5β1 (VLA-5).[249,447,448]

Several of the adhesion molecules on hematopoietic cells specifically bind to sites on particular matrix macromolecules. For example, HSC/progenitors bind to fibronectin, primarily through interaction with the integrin receptors α4β1 and α5β1.[405,445,449-451] Another cytoadhesion molecule that interacts with several matrix macromolecules is CD44, which binds with glycosaminoglycans (hyaluronic acid being the major CD44 ligand).[452] The proteoglycans, proteins with extensive sulfation such as heparan sulfate and chondroitin sulfate, are extracellular matrix proteins that may contribute to adhesion between the stroma and the hematopoietic progenitor cells.[453-457] The proteoglycans can also concentrate soluble growth factors. For example, GM-CSF binds to heparan sulfate in the marrow matrix.[458,459]

Erythroid Niches in Bone Marrow

Before stromal niches for HSCs were proposed in 1978, the first nurse cell in the hematopoietic system was proposed 2 decades earlier, in 1958, to be macrophages promoting red blood cell development in erythroblastic islands.[460,461] Early reports showed that these macrophage-erythroblast interactions in vitro support the proliferation and viability of developing red cells, believed to be mediated by VCAM-1- VLA-4, CD51-ICAM4, and erythrocyte membrane protein homotypic interactions.[461] Recent data have shown that erythroblast islands indeed exist and have functional relevance in vivo.[284] Although depletion of macrophages has no steady-state effect on erythropoiesis because they are critical in both the production of young erythrocytes and consumption and aged erythrocytes, erythroid recovery was delayed in macrophage-depleted animals in murine models of acute blood loss, hemolytic anemia, total body irradiation, or chemotherapy. Furthermore, macrophages were found to support pathologic erythropoiesis in murine models of thalassemia and polycythemia vera, and importantly, macrophage depletion was able to restore effective erythropoiesis in these models.[284,462] Mechanistically, macrophages appear to promote proliferation of erythroid precursors in vitro.[422] Although macrophage depletion produced no deficit in erythroblast proliferation or apoptosis on a per cell basis in vivo, macrophage expression of VCAM1 in the bone marrow and BMP4 in the spleen allowed erythroblasts to remain in optimal anatomic locations for expansion under stress conditions.[284] Endothelial cell-selective adhesion molecule upregulation of macrophages has also been implicated in promoting stress erythropoiesis.[463] A recent study also showed that splenic classic dendritic cells can be stimulated to support stress erythropoiesis in response to the alarmin signaling via CD24 by increasing the production of KitL and EPO.[464] Besides hematopoietic cells, the aforementioned mesenchymal lineage cells that form the putative HSC niche also regulate young red blood cells because erythroblasts are reduced after depletion of CXCL12-expressing cells.[424]

Lymphoid Niches in Bone Marrow

The CXCR4-CXCL12 axis has been implicated in B-cell development because chimeric mice reconstituted with CXCR4-deficient fetal liver cells have reduced B-cell precursors.[465] As Nagasawa and colleagues investigated CXCL12-expressing niches for B cells in the bone marrow, they discovered that the earliest committed B-cell precursors, the pre-proB cells, localized around CXCL12-abundant reticular (CAR) cells, which did not express IL-7.[466] As they matured to proB cells, they migrated away from CAR cells to IL-7–expressing stromal cells. Then, after peripheral maturation, plasma cells home back to the bone marrow to reside near CAR cells. It is unclear how CAR cells that do not express IL-7 promote B-cell development. It is possible that CAR cells retain pre-proB cells and plasma cells so that a third cell type can exert regulation. Indeed, there is evidence that macrophage inhibitory factor derived from bone marrow–resident dendritic cells is able to promote survival B cells in the bone marrow.[467] Consistent with a critical role of CXCL12 production from CAR cells in maintaining early B cells, depletion of CAR cells reduced CLP and proB cells.[424] Similarly, *Cxcl12* and *Il-7* deletion from mesenchymal lineage pericytes reduced B-cell lymphoid progenitors.[423,428,468,469] In addition, *Cxcl12* or *Scf* deletion from IL-7–expressing cells reduced HSC and MPP, suggesting an overlapping niche for HSC, MPP, and B-cell lymphoid progenitors.

Prior work had implicated a supportive role for osteoblasts in B-lymphoid precursors.[417,420,423,469,470] Indeed, mice with *Cxcl12* deleted from mature osteoblasts had a small reduction in B-lymphoid progenitors that did not result in lymphopenia.[423] However, it was recently shown that mice with *Il-7* deleted from mature osteoblasts did not have a reduction in B-lymphoid progenitors.[468] While these results are compatible with a role for osteoblasts in CXCL12-mediated retention, but not IL-7–mediated differentiation, of B-lymphoid progenitors, it is also possible that the Col2.3 promoter used to target osteoblasts may have off-target expression in mesenchymal progenitors.

Scadden and colleagues demonstrated that the Notch ligand DLL4 expressed on bone marrow osteoblasts was required for the generation of T-cell precursors and mature T cells.[471] B-lymphoid progenitors and mature B cells were largely unaffected. Future work will be needed to clarify the niches allowing lymphoid commitment and differentiation.

PERSPECTIVES

The hematologic system is a tightly regulated organ system in which a host of different cell types with varied developmental potential and effector capacity work in concert to ensure efficient oxygen delivery, hemostasis, and immunosurveillance. They are regulated by each other and also by the nonhematopoietic stroma. In spite of all this complexity, most hematopoietic cells originate from HSCs in the bone marrow. This is critical in the context of bone marrow transplantation and other clinical scenarios in which a rebooted hematopoietic system is desired. The following chapters will discuss examples when the hematopoietic system becomes dysregulated.

ACKNOWLEDGMENTS

The authors wish to acknowledge the contributions of the late Dr. Paul Frenette, who was the lead author of this chapter in the 13th and 14th editions, and had agreed to revise it for the 15th edition. Daniel K. Borger, who had been recruited by Dr. Frenette as his coauthor for this edition, agreed to revise the chapter with Robert Means following Dr. Frenette's untimely death. Dr. Andrew Chow also contributed to earlier versions of this chapter.

References

1. Sender R, Fuchs S, Milo R. Revised estimates for the number of human and bacteria cells in the body. *PLoS Biol.* 2016;14(8):e1002533.
2. Sender R, Milo R. The distribution of cellular turnover in the human body. *Nat Med.* 2021;27(1):45-48.
3. Dzierzak E, Speck NA. Of lineage and legacy: the development of mammalian hematopoietic stem cells. *Nat Immunol.* 2008;9(2):129-136.
4. Ivanovs A, Rybtsov S, Ng ES, Stanley EG, Elefanty AG, Medvinsky A. Human haematopoietic stem cell development: from the embryo to the dish. *Development.* 2017;144(13):2323-2337.
5. Bertrand JY, Jalil A, Klaine M, Jung S, Cumano A, Godin I. Three pathways to mature macrophages in the early mouse yolk sac. *Blood.* 2005;106(9):3004-3011.
6. Palis J, Robertson S, Kennedy M, Wall C, Keller G. Development of erythroid and myeloid progenitors in the yolk sac and embryo proper of the mouse. *Development.* 1999;126(22):5073-5084.
7. Tober J, Koniski A, McGrath KE, et al. The megakaryocyte lineage originates from hemangioblast precursors and is an integral component both of primitive and of definitive hematopoiesis. *Blood.* 2007;109(4):1433-1441.
8. Klimchenko O, Mori M, Distefano A, et al. A common bipotent progenitor generates the erythroid and megakaryocyte lineages in embryonic stem cell-derived primitive hematopoiesis. *Blood.* 2009;114(8):1506-1517.
9. McGrath KE, Koniski AD, Malik J, Palis J. Circulation is established in a stepwise pattern in the mammalian embryo. *Blood.* 2003;101(5):1669-1676.
10. Palis J. Primitive and definitive erythropoiesis in mammals. *Front Physiol.* 2014;5:3.
11. Kingsley PD, Malik J, Fantauzzo KA, Palis J. Yolk sac-derived primitive erythroblasts enucleate during mammalian embryogenesis. *Blood.* 2004;104(1):19-25.
12. McGrath K, Palis J. Ontogeny of erythropoiesis in the mammalian embryo. *Curr Top Dev Biol.* 2008;82:1-22.
13. Frame JM, McGrath KE, Palis J. Erythro-myeloid progenitors: "definitive" hematopoiesis in the conceptus prior to the emergence of hematopoietic stem cells. *Blood Cells Mol Dis.* 2013;51(4):220-225.
14. McGrath KE, Frame JM, Fromm GJ, et al. A transient definitive erythroid lineage with unique regulation of the β-globin locus in the mammalian embryo. *Blood.* 2011;117(17):4600-4608.
15. Soares-da-Silva F, Freyer L, Elsaid R, et al. Yolk sac, but not hematopoietic stem cell-derived progenitors, sustain erythropoiesis throughout murine embryonic life. *J Exp Med.* 2021;218(4):e20201729.
16. Gomez Perdiguero E, Klapproth K, Schulz C, et al. Tissue-resident macrophages originate from yolk-sac-derived erythro-myeloid progenitors. *Nature.* 2015;518(7540):547-551.
17. Ginhoux F, Greter M, Leboeuf M, et al. Fate mapping analysis reveals that adult microglia derive from primitive macrophages. *Science.* 2010;330(6005):841-845.
18. Böiers C, Carrelha J, Lutteropp M, et al. Lymphomyeloid contribution of an immune-restricted progenitor emerging prior to definitive hematopoietic stem cells. *Cell Stem Cell.* 2013;13(5):535-548.
19. Yoshimoto M, Montecino-Rodriguez E, Ferkowicz MJ, et al. Embryonic day 9 yolk sac and intra-embryonic hemogenic endothelium independently generate a B-1 and marginal zone progenitor lacking B-2 potential. *Proc Natl Acad Sci U S A.* 2011;108(4):1468-1473.
20. Yoshimoto M, Porayette P, Glosson NL, et al. Autonomous murine T-cell progenitor production in the extra-embryonic yolk sac before HSC emergence. *Blood.* 2012;119(24):5706-5714.
21. Migliaccio G, Migliaccio AR, Petti S, et al. Human embryonic hemopoiesis. Kinetics of progenitors and precursors underlying the yolk sac----liver transition. *J Clin Invest.* 1986;78(1):51-60.
22. Moore MA, Metcalf D. Ontogeny of the haemopoietic system: yolk sac origin of in vivo and in vitro colony forming cells in the developing mouse embryo. *Br J Haematol.* 1970;18(3):279-296.
23. Weissman IL, Baird S, Gardner RL, Papaioannou VE, Raschke W. Normal and neoplastic maturation of T-lineage lymphocytes. *Cold Spring Harbor Symp Quant Biol.* 1977;41(pt 1):9-21.
24. Dieterlen-Lievre F. On the origin of haemopoietic stem cells in the avian embryo: an experimental approach. *J Embryol Exp Morphol.* 1975;33(3):607-619.
25. Dieterlen-Lièvre F, Beaupain D, Martin C. Origin of erythropoietic stem cells in avian development: shift from the yolk sac to an intraembryonic site. *Ann Immunol (Paris).* 1976;127(6):857-863.
26. Lassila O, Eskola J, Toivanen P, Martin C, Dieterlen-Lievre F. The origin of lymphoid stem cells studied in chick yold sac-embryo chimaeras. *Nature.* 1978;272(5651):353-354.
27. Dieterlen-Lièvre F, Martin C. Diffuse intraembryonic hemopoiesis in normal and chimeric avian development. *Dev Biol.* 1981;88(1):180-191.
28. Cormier F, Dieterlen-Lièvre F. The wall of the chick embryo aorta harbours M-CFC, G-CFC, GM-CFC and BFU-E. *Development.* 1988;102(2):279-285.
29. Godin IE, Garcia-Porrero JA, Coutinho A, Dieterlen-Lièvre F, Marcos MA. Para-aortic splanchnopleura from early mouse embryos contains B1a cell progenitors. *Nature.* 1993;364(6432):67-70.
30. Medvinsky AL, Samoylina NL, Müller AM, Dzierzak EA. An early pre-liver intraembryonic source of CFU-S in the developing mouse. *Nature.* 1993;364(6432):64-67.
31. Müller AM, Medvinsky A, Strouboulis J, Grosveld F, Dzierzak E. Development of hematopoietic stem cell activity in the mouse embryo. *Immunity.* 1994;1(4):291-301.
32. Tavian M, Coulombel L, Luton D, Clemente HS, Dieterlen-Lièvre F, Péault B. Aorta-associated CD34+ hematopoietic cells in the early human embryo. *Blood.* 1996;87(1):67-72.
33. Ivanovs A, Rybtsov S, Welch L, Anderson RA, Turner ML, Medvinsky A. Highly potent human hematopoietic stem cells first emerge in the intraembryonic aorta-gonad-mesonephros region. *J Exp Med.* 2011;208(12):2417-2427.
34. Morrison SJ, Hemmati HD, Wandycz AM, Weissman IL. The purification and characterization of fetal liver hematopoietic stem cells. *Proc Natl Acad Sci U S A.* 1995;92(22):10302-10306.
35. Abe J. Immunocytochemical characterization of lymphocyte development in human embryonic and fetal livers. *Clin Immunol Immunopathol.* 1989;51(1):13-21.
36. Bertrand JY, Desanti GE, Lo-Man R, Leclerc C, Cumano A, Golub R. Fetal spleen stroma drives macrophage commitment. *Development.* 2006;133(18):3619-3628.
37. Khan JA, Mendelson A, Kunisaki Y, et al. Fetal liver hematopoietic stem cell niches associate with portal vessels. *Science.* 2016;351(6269):176-180.

The Normal Hematologic System

38. Coşkun S, Chao H, Vasavada H, et al. Development of the fetal bone marrow niche and regulation of HSC quiescence and homing ability by emerging osteolineage cells. *Cell Rep*. 2014;9(2):581-590.

39. Charbord P, Tavian M, Humeau L, Péault B. Early ontogeny of the human marrow from long bones: an immunohistochemical study of hematopoiesis and its microenvironment. *Blood*. 1996;87(10):4109-4119.

40. Gekas C, Dieterlen-Lièvre F, Orkin SH, Mikkola HK. The placenta is a niche for hematopoietic stem cells. *Dev Cell*. 2005;8(3):365-375.

41. Ottersbach K, Dzierzak E. The murine placenta contains hematopoietic stem cells within the vascular labyrinth region. *Dev Cell*. 2005;8(3):377-387.

42. Corbel C, Salaün J, Belo-Diabangouaya P, Dieterlen-Lièvre F. Hematopoietic potential of the pre-fusion allantois. *Dev Biol*. 2007;301(2):478-488.

43. Zeigler BM, Sugiyama D, Chen M, Guo Y, Downs KM, Speck NA. The allantois and chorion, when isolated before circulation or chorio-allantoic fusion, have hematopoietic potential. *Development*. 2006;133(21):4183-4192.

44. Rhodes KE, Gekas C, Wang Y, et al. The emergence of hematopoietic stem cells is initiated in the placental vasculature in the absence of circulation. *Cell Stem Cell*. 2008;2(3):252-263.

45. Gordon-Keylock S, Sobiesiak M, Rybtsov S, Moore K, Medvinsky A. Mouse extra-embryonic arterial vessels harbor precursors capable of maturing into definitive HSCs. *Blood*. 2013;122(14):2338-2345.

46. Huber TL, Kouskoff V, Fehling HJ, Palis J, Keller G. Haemangioblast commitment is initiated in the primitive streak of the mouse embryo. *Nature*. 2004;432(7017):625-630.

47. Zovein AC, Hofmann JJ, Lynch M, et al. Fate tracing reveals the endothelial origin of hematopoietic stem cells. *Cell Stem Cell*. 2008;3(6):625-636.

48. Chen MJ, Yokomizo T, Zeigler BM, Dzierzak E, Speck NA. Runx1 is required for the endothelial to haematopoietic cell transition but not thereafter. *Nature*. 2009;457(7231):887-891.

49. Chen MJ, Li Y, De Obaldia ME, et al. Erythroid/myeloid progenitors and hematopoietic stem cells originate from distinct populations of endothelial cells. *Cell Stem Cell*. 2011;9(6):541-552.

50. Boisset JC, van Cappellen W, Andrieu-Soler C, Galjart N, Dzierzak E, Robin C. In vivo imaging of haematopoietic cells emerging from the mouse aortic endothelium. *Nature*. 2010;464(7285):116-120.

51. Lancrin C, Sroczynska P, Stephenson C, Allen T, Kouskoff V, Lacaud G. The haemangioblast generates haematopoietic cells through a haemogenic endothelium stage. *Nature*. 2009;457(7231):892-895.

52. Cumano A, Godin I. Ontogeny of the hematopoietic system. *Annu Rev Immunol*. 2007;25:745-785.

53. Hoang T, Lambert JA, Martin R. SCL/TAL1 in hematopoiesis and cellular reprogramming. *Curr Top Dev Biol*. 2016;118:163-204.

54. Johansson BM, Wiles MV. Evidence for involvement of activin A and bone morphogenetic protein 4 in mammalian mesoderm and hematopoietic development. *Mol Cell Biol*. 1995;15(1):141-151.

55. Winnier G, Blessing M, Labosky PA, Hogan BL. Bone morphogenetic protein-4 is required for mesoderm formation and patterning in the mouse. *Genes Dev*. 1995;9(17):2105-2116.

56. Park C, Afrikanova I, Chung YS, et al. A hierarchical order of factors in the generation of FLK1- and SCL-expressing hematopoietic and endothelial progenitors from embryonic stem cells. *Development*. 2004;131(11):2749-2762.

57. Belaoussoff M, Farrington SM, Baron MH. Hematopoietic induction and respecification of A-P identity by visceral endoderm signaling in the mouse embryo. *Development*. 1998;125(24):5009-5018.

58. Breier G, Clauss M, Risau W. Coordinate expression of vascular endothelial growth factor receptor-1 (flt-1) and its ligand suggests a paracrine regulation of murine vascular development. *Dev Dyn*. 1995;204(3):228-239.

59. Dumont DJ, Fong GH, Puri MC, Gradwohl G, Alitalo K, Breitman ML. Vascularization of the mouse embryo: a study of flk-1, tek, tie, and vascular endothelial growth factor expression during development. *Dev Dyn*. 1995;203(1):80-92.

60. Shalaby F, Rossant J, Yamaguchi TP, et al. Failure of blood-island formation and vasculogenesis in Flk-1-deficient mice. *Nature*. 1995;376(6535):62-66.

61. Shalaby F, Ho J, Stanford WL, et al. A requirement for Flk1 in primitive and definitive hematopoiesis and vasculogenesis. *Cell*. 1997;89(6):981-990.

62. Hidaka M, Stanford WL, Bernstein A. Conditional requirement for the Flk-1 receptor in the in vitro generation of early hematopoietic cells. *Proc Natl Acad Sci U S A*. 1999;96(13):7370-7375.

63. Schuh AC, Faloon P, Hu QL, Bhimani M, Choi K. In vitro hematopoietic and endothelial potential of flk-1(-/-) embryonic stem cells and embryos. *Proc Natl Acad Sci U S A*. 1999;96(5):2159-2164.

64. Damert A, Miquerol L, Gertsenstein M, Risau W, Nagy A. Insufficient VEGFA activity in yolk sac endoderm compromises haematopoietic and endothelial differentiation. *Development*. 2002;129(8):1881-1892.

65. Drake CJ, Brandt SJ, Trusk TC, Little CD. TAL1/SCL is expressed in endothelial progenitor cells/angioblasts and defines a dorsal-to-ventral gradient of vasculogenesis. *Dev Biol*. 1997;192(1):17-30.

66. Elefanty AG, Begley CG, Hartley L, Papaevangeliou B, Robb L. SCL expression in the mouse embryo detected with a targeted lacZ reporter gene demonstrates its localization to hematopoietic, vascular, and neural tissues. *Blood*. 1999;94(11):3754-3763.

67. Kallianpur AR, Jordan JE, Brandt SJ. The SCL/TAL-1 gene is expressed in progenitors of both the hematopoietic and vascular systems during embryogenesis. *Blood*. 1994;83(5):1200-1208.

68. Manaia A, Lemarchandel V, Klaine M, et al. Lmo2 and GATA-3 associated expression in intraembryonic hemogenic sites. *Development*. 2000;127(3):643-653.

69. Robb L, Lyons I, Li R, et al. Absence of yolk sac hematopoiesis from mice with a targeted disruption of the scl gene. *Proc Natl Acad Sci U S A*. 1995;92(15):7075-7079.

70. Shivdasani RA, Mayer EL, Orkin SH. Absence of blood formation in mice lacking the T-cell leukaemia oncoprotein tal-1/SCL. *Nature*. 1995;373(6513):432-434.

71. Warren AJ, Colledge WH, Carlton MB, Evans MJ, Smith AJ, Rabbitts TH. The oncogenic cysteine-rich LIM domain protein rbtn2 is essential for erythroid development. *Cell*. 1994;78(1):45-57.

72. Porcher C, Swat W, Rockwell K, Fujiwara Y, Alt FW, Orkin SH. The T cell leukemia oncoprotein SCL/tal-1 is essential for development of all hematopoietic lineages. *Cell*. 1996;86(1):47-57.

73. Robb L, Elwood NJ, Elefanty AG, et al. The scl gene product is required for the generation of all hematopoietic lineages in the adult mouse. *EMBO J*. 1996;15(16):4123-4129.

74. Yamada Y, Warren AJ, Dobson C, Forster A, Pannell R, Rabbitts TH. The T cell leukemia LIM protein Lmo2 is necessary for adult mouse hematopoiesis. *Proc Natl Acad Sci U S A*. 1998;95(7):3890-3895.

75. Van Handel B, Montel-Hagen A, Sasidharan R, et al. Scl represses cardiomyogenesis in prospective hemogenic endothelium and endocardium. *Cell*. 2012;150(3):590-605.

76. Tsai FY, Keller G, Kuo FC, et al. An early haematopoietic defect in mice lacking the transcription factor GATA-2. *Nature*. 1994;371(6494):221-226.

77. Ling KW, Ottersbach K, van Hamburg JP, et al. GATA-2 plays two functionally distinct roles during the ontogeny of hematopoietic stem cells. *J Exp Med*. 2004;200(7):871-882.

78. Minegishi N, Ohta J, Yamagiwa H, et al. The mouse GATA-2 gene is expressed in the para-aortic splanchnopleura and aorta-gonads and mesonephros region. *Blood*. 1999;93(12):4196-4207.

79. Cai Z, de Bruijn M, Ma X, et al. Haploinsufficiency of AML1 affects the temporal and spatial generation of hematopoietic stem cells in the mouse embryo. *Immunity*. 2000;13(4):423-431.

80. Okuda T, van Deursen J, Hiebert SW, Grosveld G, Downing JR. AML1, the target of multiple chromosomal translocations in human leukemia, is essential for normal fetal liver hematopoiesis. *Cell*. 1996;84(2):321-330.

81. Wang Q, Stacy T, Binder M, Marin-Padilla M, Sharpe AH, Speck NA. Disruption of the Cbfa2 gene causes necrosis and hemorrhaging in the central nervous system and blocks definitive hematopoiesis. *Proc Natl Acad Sci U S A*. 1996;93(8):3444-3449.

82. Yokomizo T, Hasegawa K, Ishitobi H, et al. Runx1 is involved in primitive erythropoiesis in the mouse. *Blood*. 2008;111(8):4075-4080.

83. Tavassoli M. Bone marrow: the seedbed of blood. In: Wintrobe M, ed. *Blood, Pure and Eloquent*; McGraw-Hill; 1980:57-79.

84. Lajtha LG. The common ancestral cell. In: Wintrobe M, ed. *Blood, Pure and Eloquent*. McGraw-Hill; 1980:80-95.

85. Lorenz E, Uphoff D, Reid TR, Shelton E. Modification of irradiation injury in mice and guinea pigs by bone marrow injections. *J Natl Cancer Inst*. 1951;12(1):197-201.

86. Ford CE, Hamerton JL, Barnes DW, Loutit JF. Cytological identification of radiation-chimaeras. *Nature*. 1956;177(4506):452-454.

87. Till JE, Mc CE. A direct measurement of the radiation sensitivity of normal mouse bone marrow cells. *Radiat Res*. 1961;14:213-222.

88. Siminovitch L, McCulloch EA, Till JE. The distribution of colony-forming cells among spleen colonies. *J Cell Comp Physiol*. 1963;62:327-336.

89. Wu AM, Till JE, Siminovitch L, McCulloch EA. A cytological study of the capacity for differentiation of normal hemopoietic colony-forming cells. *J Cell Physiol*. 1967;69(2):177-184.

90. Lepault F, Ezine S, Gagnerault MC. T- and B-lymphocyte differentiation potentials of spleen colony-forming cells. *Blood*. 1993;81(4):950-955.

91. Keller G, Paige C, Gilboa E, Wagner EF. Expression of a foreign gene in myeloid and lymphoid cells derived from multipotent haematopoietic precursors. *Nature*. 1985;318(6042):149-154.

92. Lemischka IR, Raulet DH, Mulligan RC. Developmental potential and dynamic behavior of hematopoietic stem cells. *Cell*. 1986;45(6):917-927.

93. Jordan CT, Lemischka IR. Clonal and systemic analysis of long-term hematopoiesis in the mouse. *Genes Dev*. 1990;4(2):220-232.

94. Capel B, Hawley RG, Mintz B. Long- and short-lived murine hematopoietic stem cell clones individually identified with retroviral integration markers. *Blood*. 1990;75(12):2267-2270.

95. Osawa M, Hanada K, Hamada H, Nakauchi H. Long-term lymphohematopoietic reconstitution by a single CD34-low/negative hematopoietic stem cell. *Science*. 1996;273(5272):242-245.

96. Smith LG, Weissman IL, Heimfeld S. Clonal analysis of hematopoietic stem-cell differentiation in vivo. *Proc Natl Acad Sci U S A*. 1991;88(7):2788-2792.

97. Matsuzaki Y, Kinjo K, Mulligan RC, Okano H. Unexpectedly efficient homing capacity of purified murine hematopoietic stem cells. *Immunity*. 2004;20(1):87-93.

98. Notta F, Doulatov S, Laurenti E, Poeppl A, Jurisica I, Dick JE. Isolation of single human hematopoietic stem cells capable of long-term multilineage engraftment. *Science*. 2011;333(6039):218-221.

99. Shizuru JA, Negrin RS, Weissman IL. Hematopoietic stem and progenitor cells: clinical and preclinical regeneration of the hematolymphoid system. *Annu Rev Med*. 2005;56:509-538.

100. Goodell MA, Brose K, Paradis G, Conner AS, Mulligan RC. Isolation and functional properties of murine hematopoietic stem cells that are replicating in vivo. *J Exp Med*. 1996;183(4):1797-1806.

101. Morrison SJ, Weissman IL. The long-term repopulating subset of hematopoietic stem cells is deterministic and isolatable by phenotype. *Immunity*. 1994;1(8):661-673.

102. Christensen JL, Weissman IL. Flk-2 is a marker in hematopoietic stem cell differentiation: a simple method to isolate long-term stem cells. *Proc Natl Acad Sci U S A*. 2001;98(25):14541-14546.

103. Spangrude GJ, Heimfeld S, Weissman IL. Purification and characterization of mouse hematopoietic stem cells. *Science*. 1988;241(4861):58-62.
104. Ikuta K, Weissman IL. Evidence that hematopoietic stem cells express mouse c-kit but do not depend on steel factor for their generation. *Proc Natl Acad Sci U S A*. 1992;89(4):1502-1506.
105. Kiel MJ, Yilmaz OH, Iwashita T, Yilmaz OH, Terhorst C, Morrison SJ. SLAM family receptors distinguish hematopoietic stem and progenitor cells and reveal endothelial niches for stem cells. *Cell*. 2005;121(7):1109-1121.
106. Chen CZ, Li M, de Graaf D, et al. Identification of endoglin as a functional marker that defines long-term repopulating hematopoietic stem cells. *Proc Natl Acad Sci U S A*. 2002;99(24):15468-15473.
107. Pronk CJ, Rossi DJ, Månsson R, et al. Elucidation of the phenotypic, functional, and molecular topography of a myeloerythroid progenitor cell hierarchy. *Cell Stem Cell*. 2007;1(4):428-442.
108. Balazs AB, Fabian AJ, Esmon CT, Mulligan RC. Endothelial protein C receptor (CD201) explicitly identifies hematopoietic stem cells in murine bone marrow. *Blood*. 2006;107(6):2317-2321.
109. Oguro H, Ding L, Morrison SJ. SLAM family markers resolve functionally distinct subpopulations of hematopoietic stem cells and multipotent progenitors. *Cell Stem Cell*. 2013;13(1):102-116.
110. Acar M, Kocherlakota KS, Murphy MM, et al. Deep imaging of bone marrow shows non-dividing stem cells are mainly perisinusoidal. *Nature*. 2015;526(7571):126-130.
111. Chen JY, Miyanishi M, Wang SK, et al. Hoxb5 marks long-term haematopoietic stem cells and reveals a homogenous perivascular niche. *Nature*. 2016;530(7589):223-227.
112. Sawai CM, Babovic S, Upadhaya S, et al. Hematopoietic stem cells are the major source of multilineage hematopoiesis in adult animals. *Immunity*. 2016;45(3):597-609.
113. Pang WW, Price EA, Sahoo D, et al. Human bone marrow hematopoietic stem cells are increased in frequency and myeloid-biased with age. *Proc Natl Acad Sci U S A*. 2011;108(50):20012-20017.
114. Czechowicz A, Weissman IL. Purified hematopoietic stem cell transplantation: the next generation of blood and immune replacement. *Immunol Allergy Clin*. 2010;30(2):159-171.
115. Michallet M, Philip T, Philip I, et al. Transplantation with selected autologous peripheral blood CD34+Thy1+ hematopoietic stem cells (HSCs) in multiple myeloma: impact of HSC dose on engraftment, safety, and immune reconstitution. *Exp Hematol*. 2000;28(7):858-870.
116. Wilson A, Laurenti E, Oser G, et al. Hematopoietic stem cells reversibly switch from dormancy to self-renewal during homeostasis and repair. *Cell*. 2008;135(6):1118-1129.
117. Trumpp A, Essers M, Wilson A. Awakening dormant haematopoietic stem cells. *Nat Rev Immunol*. 2010;10(3):201-209.
118. Yilmaz OH, Kiel MJ, Morrison SJ. SLAM family markers are conserved among hematopoietic stem cells from old and reconstituted mice and markedly increase their purity. *Blood*. 2006;107(3):924-930.
119. Matsuoka S, Ebihara Y, Xu M, et al. CD34 expression on long-term repopulating hematopoietic stem cells changes during developmental stages. *Blood*. 2001;97(2):419-425.
120. van der Wath RC, Wilson A, Laurenti E, Trumpp A, Liò P. Estimating dormant and active hematopoietic stem cell kinetics through extensive modeling of bromodeoxyuridine label-retaining cell dynamics. *PLoS One*. 2009;4(9):e6972.
121. Essers MA, Offner S, Blanco-Bose WE, et al. IFNalpha activates dormant haematopoietic stem cells in vivo. *Nature*. 2009;458(7240):904-908.
122. Spangrude GJ, Brooks DM. Mouse strain variability in the expression of the hematopoietic stem cell antigen Ly-6A/E by bone marrow cells. *Blood*. 1993;82(11):3327-3332.
123. Spangrude GJ, Brooks DM. Phenotypic analysis of mouse hematopoietic stem cells shows a Thy-1-negative subset. *Blood*. 1992;80(8):1957-1964.
124. Zhong RK, Astle CM, Harrison DE. Distinct developmental patterns of short-term and long-term functioning lymphoid and myeloid precursors defined by competitive limiting dilution analysis in vivo. *J Immunol*. 1996;157(1):138-145.
125. Lu R, Neff NF, Quake SR, Weissman IL. Tracking single hematopoietic stem cells in vivo using high-throughput sequencing in conjunction with viral genetic barcoding. *Nat Biotechnol*. 2011;29(10):928-933.
126. Yu VWC, Yusuf RZ, Oki T, et al. Epigenetic memory underlies cell-autonomous heterogeneous behavior of hematopoietic stem cells. *Cell*. 2016;167(5):1310-1322.e17.
127. Verovskaya E, Broekhuis MJ, Zwart E, et al. Asymmetry in skeletal distribution of mouse hematopoietic stem cell clones and their equilibration by mobilizing cytokines. *J Exp Med*. 2014;211(3):487-497.
128. Busch K, Klapproth K, Barile M, et al. Fundamental properties of unperturbed haematopoiesis from stem cells in vivo. *Nature*. 2015;518(7540):542-546.
129. Busch K, Rodewald HR. Unperturbed vs. post-transplantation hematopoiesis: both in vivo but different. *Curr Opin Hematol*. 2016;23(4):295-303.
130. Sun J, Ramos A, Chapman B, et al. Clonal dynamics of native haematopoiesis. *Nature*. 2014;514(7522):322-327.
131. Kim HJ, Tisdale JF, Wu T, et al. Many multipotential gene-marked progenitor or stem cell clones contribute to hematopoiesis in nonhuman primates. *Blood*. 2000;96(1):1-8.
132. Shi PA, Hematti P, von Kalle C, Dunbar CE. Genetic marking as an approach to studying in vivo hematopoiesis: progress in the non-human primate model. *Oncogene*. 2002;21(21):3274-3283.
133. Schmidt M, Zickler P, Hoffmann G, et al. Polyclonal long-term repopulating stem cell clones in a primate model. *Blood*. 2002;100(8):2737-2743.
134. Biasco L, Pellin D, Scala S, et al. In vivo tracking of human hematopoiesis reveals patterns of clonal dynamics during early and steady-state reconstitution phases. *Cell Stem Cell*. 2016;19(1):107-119.
135. Foudi A, Hochedlinger K, Van Buren D, et al. Analysis of histone 2B-GFP retention reveals slowly cycling hematopoietic stem cells. *Nat Biotechnol*. 2009;27(1):84-90.
136. Catlin SN, Busque L, Gale RE, Guttorp P, Abkowitz JL. The replication rate of human hematopoietic stem cells in vivo. *Blood*. 2011;117(17):4460-4466.
137. Walter D, Lier A, Geiselhart A, et al. Exit from dormancy provokes DNA-damage-induced attrition in haematopoietic stem cells. *Nature*. 2015;520(7548):549-552.
138. Rubinstein P, Carrier C, Scaradavou A, et al. Outcomes among 562 recipients of placental-blood transplants from unrelated donors. *N Engl J Med*. 1998;339(22):1565-1577.
139. Laughlin MJ, Barker J, Bambach B, et al. Hematopoietic engraftment and survival in adult recipients of umbilical-cord blood from unrelated donors. *N Engl J Med*. 2001;344(24):1815-1822.
140. Robinson SN, Simmons PJ, Yang H, Alousi AM, Marcos de Lima J, Shpall EJ. Mesenchymal stem cells in ex vivo cord blood expansion. *Best Pract Res Clin Haematol*. 2011;24(1):83-92.
141. Gertz MA, Wolf RC, Micallef IN, Gastineau DA. Clinical impact and resource utilization after stem cell mobilization failure in patients with multiple myeloma and lymphoma. *Bone Marrow Transplant*. 2010;45(9):1396-1403.
142. Giralt S, Costa L, Schriber J, et al. Optimizing autologous stem cell mobilization strategies to improve patient outcomes: consensus guidelines and recommendations. *Biol Blood Marrow Transplant*. 2014;20(3):295-308.
143. Rebel VI, Dragowska W, Eaves CJ, Humphries RK, Lansdorp PM. Amplification of Sca-1+ Lin- WGA+ cells in serum-free cultures containing steel factor, interleukin-6, and erythropoietin with maintenance of cells with long-term in vivo reconstituting potential. *Blood*. 1994;83(1):128-136.
144. Fraser CC, Szilvassy SJ, Eaves CJ, Humphries RK. Proliferation of totipotent hematopoietic stem cells in vitro with retention of long-term competitive in vivo reconstituting ability. *Proc Natl Acad Sci U S A*. 1992;89(5):1968-1972.
145. van der Sluijs JP, van den Bos C, Baert MR, van Beurden CA, Ploemacher RE. Loss of long-term repopulating ability in long-term bone marrow culture. *Leukemia*. 1993;7(5):725-732.
146. Verfaillie CM. Can human hematopoietic stem cells be cultured ex vivo? *Stem Cell*. 1994;12(5):466-476.
147. Glimm H, Eisterer W, Lee K, et al. Previously undetected human hematopoietic cell populations with short-term repopulating activity selectively engraft NOD/SCID-beta2 microglobulin-null mice. *J Clin Invest*. 2001;107(2):199-206.
148. Szilvassy SJ, Meyerrose TE, Ragland PL, Grimes B. Homing and engraftment defects in ex vivo expanded murine hematopoietic cells are associated with down-regulation of beta1 integrin. *Exp Hematol*. 2001;29(12):1494-1502.
149. Berrios VM, Dooner GJ, Nowakowski G, et al. The molecular basis for the cytokine-induced defect in homing and engraftment of hematopoietic stem cells. *Exp Hematol*. 2001;29(11):1326-1335.
150. Dahlberg A, Delaney C, Bernstein ID. Ex vivo expansion of human hematopoietic stem and progenitor cells. *Blood*. 2011;117(23):6083-6090.
151. Wagner JE, Jr, Brunstein CG, Boitano AE, et al. Phase I/II trial of StemRegenin-1 expanded umbilical cord blood hematopoietic stem cells supports testing as a stand-alone graft. *Cell Stem Cell*. 2016;18(1):144-155.
152. Cohen S, Roy J, Lachance S, et al. Hematopoietic stem cell transplantation using single UM171-expanded cord blood: a single-arm, phase 1-2 safety and feasibility study. *Lancet Haematol*. 2020;7(2):e134-e145.
153. Chagraoui J, Girard S, Spinella JF, et al. UM171 preserves epigenetic marks that are reduced in ex vivo culture of human HSCs via potentiation of the CLR3-KBTBD4 complex. *Cell Stem Cell*. 2021;28(1):48-62.e6.
154. Horwitz ME, Chao NJ, Rizzieri DA, et al. Umbilical cord blood expansion with nicotinamide provides long-term multilineage engraftment. *J Clin Invest*. 2014;124(7):3121-3128.
155. Horwitz ME, Wease S, Blackwell B, et al. Phase I/II study of stem-cell transplantation using a single cord blood unit expanded ex vivo with nicotinamide. *J Clin Oncol*. 2019;37(5):367-374.
156. Horwitz ME, Stiff PJ, Cutler C, et al. Omidubicel vs standard myeloablative umbilical cord blood transplantation: results of a phase 3 randomized study. *Blood*. 2021;138(16):1429-1440.
157. de Lima M, McMannis J, Gee A, et al. Transplantation of ex vivo expanded cord blood cells using the copper chelator tetraethylenepentamine: a phase I/II clinical trial. *Bone Marrow Transplant*. 2008;41(9):771-778.
158. Stiff PJ, Montesinos P, Peled T, et al. Cohort-controlled comparison of umbilical cord blood transplantation using carlecortemcel-L, a single progenitor-enriched cord blood, to double cord blood unit transplantation. *Biol Blood Marrow Transplant*. 2018;24(7):1463-1470.
159. Delaney C, Heimfeld S, Brashem-Stein C, Voorhies H, Manger RL, Bernstein ID. Notch-mediated expansion of human cord blood progenitor cells capable of rapid myeloid reconstitution. *Nat Med*. 2010;16(2):232-236.
160. de Lima M, McNiece I, Robinson SN, et al. Cord-blood engraftment with ex vivo mesenchymal-cell coculture. *N Engl J Med*. 2012;367(24):2305-2315.
161. Cutler C, Multani P, Robbins D, et al. Prostaglandin-modulated umbilical cord blood hematopoietic stem cell transplantation. *Blood*. 2013;122(17):3074-3081.
162. Popat U, Mehta RS, Rezvani K, et al. Enforced fucosylation of cord blood hematopoietic cells accelerates neutrophil and platelet engraftment after transplantation. *Blood*. 2015;125(19):2885-2892.
163. Theilgaard-Mönch K, Raaschou-Jensen K, Schjødt K, et al. Pluripotent and myeloid-committed CD34+ subsets in hematopoietic stem cell allografts. *Bone Marrow Transplant*. 2003;32(12):1125-1133.
164. Boitano AE, Wang J, Romeo R, et al. Aryl hydrocarbon receptor antagonists promote the expansion of human hematopoietic stem cells. *Science*. 2010;329(5997):1345-1348.
165. Nakahara F, Borger DK, Wei Q, et al. Engineering a haematopoietic stem cell niche by revitalizing mesenchymal stromal cells. *Nat Cell Biol*. 2019;21(5):560-567.

166. Seandel M, Butler JM, Kobayashi H, et al. Generation of a functional and durable vascular niche by the adenoviral E4ORF1 gene. *Proc Natl Acad Sci U S A.* 2008;105(49):19288-19293.

167. Butler JM, Gars EJ, James DJ, Nolan DJ, Scandura JM, Rafii S. Development of a vascular niche platform for expansion of repopulating human cord blood stem and progenitor cells. *Blood.* 2012;120(6):1344-1347.

168. Bai T, Li J, Sinclair A, et al. Expansion of primitive human hematopoietic stem cells by culture in a zwitterionic hydrogel. *Nat Med.* 2019;25(10):1566-1575.

169. Wilkinson AC, Igarashi KJ, Nakauchi H. Haematopoietic stem cell self-renewal in vivo and ex vivo. *Nat Rev Genet.* 2020;21(9):541-554.

170. Suzuki N, Yamazaki S, Yamaguchi T, et al. Generation of engraftable hematopoietic stem cells from induced pluripotent stem cells by way of teratoma formation. *Mol Ther.* 2013;21(7):1424-1431.

171. Amabile G, Welner RS, Nombela-Arrieta C, et al. In vivo generation of transplantable human hematopoietic cells from induced pluripotent stem cells. *Blood.* 2013;121(8):1255-1264.

172. Daniel MG, Pereira CF, Lemischka IR, Moore KA. Making a hematopoietic stem cell. *Trends Cell Biol.* 2016;26(3):202-214.

173. Dykstra B, Kent D, Bowie M, et al. Long-term propagation of distinct hematopoietic differentiation programs in vivo. *Cell Stem Cell.* 2007;1(2):218-229.

174. Ceredig R, Rolink AG, Brown G. Models of haematopoiesis: seeing the wood for the trees. *Nat Rev Immunol.* 2009;9(4):293-300.

175. Kawamoto H, Ikawa T, Masuda K, Wada H, Katsura Y. A map for lineage restriction of progenitors during hematopoiesis: the essence of the myeloid-based model. *Immunol Rev.* 2010;238(1):23-36.

176. Eaves CJ. Hematopoietic stem cells: concepts, definitions, and the new reality. *Blood.* 2015;125(17):2605-2613.

177. Johnson GR, Metcalf D. Pure and mixed erythroid colony formation in vitro stimulated by spleen conditioned medium with no detectable erythropoietin. *Proc Natl Acad Sci U S A.* 1977;74(9):3879-3882.

178. Nakahata T, Ogawa M. Identification in culture of a class of hematopoietic colony-forming units with extensive capability to self-renew and generate multipotential hemopoietic colonies. *Proc Natl Acad Sci U S A.* 1982;79:3843-3847.

179. Fauser AA, Messner HA. Proliferative state of human pluripotent hemopoietic progenitors (CFU-GEMM) in normal individuals and under regenerative conditions after bone marrow transplantation. *Blood.* 1979;54(5):1197-1200.

180. Ogawa M. Differentiation and proliferation of hematopoietic stem cells. *Blood.* 1993;81(11):2844-2853.

181. Brandt JE, Bartholomew AM, Fortman JD, et al. Ex vivo expansion of autologous bone marrow CD34(+) cells with porcine microvascular endothelial cells results in a graft capable of rescuing lethally irradiated baboons. *Blood.* 1999;94(1):106-113.

182. Ball TC, Hirayama F, Ogawa M. Lymphohematopoietic progenitors of normal mice. *Blood.* 1995;85(11):3086-3092.

183. Morrison SJ, Wandycz AM, Hemmati HD, Wright DE, Weissman IL. Identification of a lineage of multipotent hematopoietic progenitors. *Development.* 1997;124(10):1929-1939.

184. Lai AY, Lin SM, Kondo M. Heterogeneity of Flt3-expressing multipotent progenitors in mouse bone marrow. *J Immunol.* 2005;175(8):5016-5023.

185. Boyer SW, Schroeder AV, Smith-Berdan S, Forsberg EC. All hematopoietic cells develop from hematopoietic stem cells through Flk2/Flt3-positive progenitor cells. *Cell Stem Cell.* 2011;9(1):64-73.

186. Pietras EM, Reynaud D, Kang YA, et al. Functionally distinct subsets of lineage-biased multipotent progenitors control blood production in normal and regenerative conditions. *Cell Stem Cell.* 2015;17(1):35-46.

187. Woolthuis CM, Park CY. Hematopoietic stem/progenitor cell commitment to the megakaryocyte lineage. *Blood.* 2016;127(10):1242-1248.

188. Gekas C, Graf T. CD41 expression marks myeloid-biased adult hematopoietic stem cells and increases with age. *Blood.* 2013;121(22):4463-4472.

189. Sanjuan-Pla A, Macaulay IC, Jensen CT, et al. Platelet-biased stem cells reside at the apex of the haematopoietic stem-cell hierarchy. *Nature.* 2013;502(7470):232-236.

190. Notta F, Zandi S, Takayama N, et al. Distinct routes of lineage development reshape the human blood hierarchy across ontogeny. *Science.* 2016;351(6269):aab2116.

191. Metcalf D. Control of granulocytes and macrophages: molecular, cellular, and clinical aspects. *Science.* 1991;254(5031):529-533.

192. Eaves AC, Eaves CJ. Erythropoiesis in culture. *Clin Haematol.* 1984;13:371-391.

193. Hoffman R. Regulation of megakaryocytopoiesis. *Blood.* 1989;74(4):1196-1212.

194. Lemieux ME, Rebel VI, Lansdorp PM, Eaves CJ. Characterization and purification of a primitive hematopoietic cell type in adult mouse marrow capable of lymphomyeloid differentiation in long-term marrow "switch" cultures. *Blood.* 1995;86(4):1339-1347.

195. Suda T, Okada S, Suda J, et al. A stimulatory effect of recombinant murine interleukin-7 (IL-7) on B-cell colony formation and an inhibitory effect of IL-1 alpha. *Blood.* 1989;74(6):1936-1941.

196. Reid CD, Stackpoole A, Meager A, Tikerpae J. Interactions of tumor necrosis factor with granulocyte-macrophage colony-stimulating factor and other cytokines in the regulation of dendritic cell growth in vitro from early bipotent CD34+ progenitors in human bone marrow. *J Immunol.* 1992;149(8):2681-2688.

197. Szabolcs P, Avigan D, Gezelter S, et al. Dendritic cells and macrophages can mature independently from a human bone marrow-derived, post-colony-forming unit intermediate. *Blood.* 1996;87(11):4520-4530.

198. Kondo M, Weissman IL, Akashi K. Identification of clonogenic common lymphoid progenitors in mouse bone marrow. *Cell.* 1997;91(5):661-672.

199. Akashi K, Traver D, Miyamoto T, Weissman IL. A clonogenic common myeloid progenitor that gives rise to all myeloid lineages. *Nature.* 2000;404(6774):193-197.

200. Fogg DK, Sibon C, Miled C, et al. A clonogenic bone marrow progenitor specific for macrophages and dendritic cells. *Science.* 2006;311(5757):83-87.

201. Paul F, Arkin Y, Giladi A, et al. Transcriptional heterogeneity and lineage commitment in myeloid progenitors. *Cell.* 2015;163(7):1663-1677.

202. Purton LE, Scadden DT. Limiting factors in murine hematopoietic stem cell assays. *Cell Stem Cell.* 2007;1(3):263-270.

203. Sutherland HJ, Lansdorp PM, Henkelman DH, Eaves AC, Eaves CJ. Functional characterization of individual human hematopoietic stem cells cultured at limiting dilution on supportive marrow stromal layers. *Proc Natl Acad Sci U S A.* 1990;87(9):3584-3588.

204. Murray L, Chen B, Galy A, et al. Enrichment of human hematopoietic stem cell activity in the CD34+Thy-1+Lin-subpopulation from mobilized peripheral blood. *Blood.* 1995;85(2):368-378.

205. Ploemacher RE, van der Sluijs JP, van Beurden CA, Baert MR, Chan PL. Use of limiting-dilution type long-term marrow cultures in frequency analysis of marrow-repopulating and spleen colony-forming hematopoietic stem cells in the mouse. *Blood.* 1991;78(10):2527-2533.

206. Neben S, Anklesaria P, Greenberger J, Mauch P. Quantitation of murine hematopoietic stem cells in vitro by limiting dilution analysis of cobblestone area formation on a clonal stromal cell line. *Exp Hematol.* 1993;21(3):438-443.

207. Hao QL, Thiemann FT, Petersen D, Smogorzewska EM, Crooks GM. Extended long-term culture reveals a highly quiescent and primitive human hematopoietic progenitor population. *Blood.* 1996;88(9):3306-3313.

208. Kusadasi N, Oostendorp RA, Koevoet WJ, Dzierzak EA, Ploemacher RE. Stromal cells from murine embryonic aorta-gonad-mesonephros region, liver and gut mesentery expand human umbilical cord blood-derived CAFC(week6) in extended long-term cultures. *Leukemia.* 2002;16(9):1782-1790.

209. Ploemacher RE, van der Sluijs JP, Voerman JS, Brons NH. An in vitro limiting-dilution assay of long-term repopulating hematopoietic stem cells in the mouse. *Blood.* 1989;74(8):2755-2763.

210. Breems DA, Blokland EA, Neben S, Ploemacher RE. Frequency analysis of human primitive haematopoietic stem cell subsets using a cobblestone area forming cell assay. *Leukemia.* 1994;8(7):1095-1104.

211. Mahmud N, Patel H, Hoffman R. Growth factors mobilize CXCR4 low/negative primitive hematopoietic stem/progenitor cells from the bone marrow of nonhuman primates. *Biol Blood Marrow Transplant.* 2004;10(10):681-690.

212. Szilvassy SJ, Humphries RK, Lansdorp PM, Eaves AC, Eaves CJ. Quantitative assay for totipotent reconstituting hematopoietic stem cells by a competitive repopulation strategy. *Proc Natl Acad Sci U S A.* 1990;87(22):8736-8740.

213. Harrison DE, Jordan CT, Zhong RK, Astle CM. Primitive hemopoietic stem cells: direct assay of most productive populations by competitive repopulation with simple binomial, correlation and covariance calculations. *Exp Hematol.* 1993;21(2):206-219.

214. Lemieux ME, Eaves CJ. Identification of properties that can distinguish primitive populations of stromal-cell-responsive lymphomyeloid cells from cells that are stromal-cell-responsive but lymphoid-restricted and cells that have lympho-myeloid potential but are also capable of competitively repopulating myeloablated recipients. *Blood.* 1996;88(5):1639-1648.

215. Harrison DE. Competitive repopulation: a new assay for long-term stem cell functional capacity. *Blood.* 1980;55(1):77-81.

216. Rosendaal M, Hodgson GS, Bradley TR. Organization of haemopoietic stem cells: the generation-age hypothesis. *Cell Tissue Kinet.* 1979;12(1):17-29.

217. Waterstrat A, Liang Y, Swiderski CF, Shelton BJ, Van Zant G. Congenic interval of CD45/Ly-5 congenic mice contains multiple genes that may influence hematopoietic stem cell engraftment. *Blood.* 2010;115(2):408-417.

218. Mercier FE, Sykes DB, Scadden DT. Single targeted exon mutation creates a true congenic mouse for competitive hematopoietic stem cell transplantation: the C57BL/6-CD45.1(STEM) mouse. *Stem Cell Rep.* 2016;6(6):985-992.

219. Orlic D, Fischer R, Nishikawa S, Nienhuis AW, Bodine DM. Purification and characterization of heterogeneous pluripotent hematopoietic stem cell populations expressing high levels of c-kit receptor. *Blood.* 1993;82(3):762-770.

220. Bosma GC, Custer RP, Bosma MJ. A severe combined immunodeficiency mutation in the mouse. *Nature.* 1983;301(5900):527-530.

221. Jhappan C, Morse HC,IIIrd, Fleischmann RD, Gottesman MM, Merlino G. DNA-PKcs: a T-cell tumour suppressor encoded at the mouse scid locus. *Nat Genet.* 1997;17(4):483-486.

222. Morrison C, Smith GC, Stingl L, Jackson SP, Wagner EF, Wang ZQ. Genetic interaction between PARP and DNA-PK in V(D)J recombination and tumorigenesis. *Nat Genet.* 1997;17(4):479-482.

223. Mosier DE, Gulizia RJ, Baird SM, Wilson DB. Transfer of a functional human immune system to mice with severe combined immunodeficiency. *Nature.* 1988;335(6187):256-259.

224. McCune JM, Namikawa R, Kaneshima H, Shultz LD, Lieberman M, Weissman IL. The SCID-hu mouse: murine model for the analysis of human hematolymphoid differentiation and function. *Science.* 1988;241(4873):1632-1639.

225. Lapidot T, Pflumio F, Doedens M, Murdoch B, Williams DE, Dick JE. Cytokine stimulation of multilineage hematopoiesis from immature human cells engrafted in SCID mice. *Science.* 1992;255(5048):1137-1141.

226. Jones RJ, Wagner JE, Celano P, Zicha MS, Sharkis SJ. Separation of pluripotent haematopoietic stem cells from spleen colony-forming cells. *Nature.* 1990;347(6289):188-189.

227. Kerre TC, De Smet G, De Smedt M, et al. Adapted NOD/SCID model supports development of phenotypically and functionally mature T cells from human umbilical cord blood CD34(+) cells. *Blood.* 2002;99(5):1620-1626.

228. Hiramatsu H, Nishikomori R, Heike T, et al. Complete reconstitution of human lymphocytes from cord blood CD34+ cells using the NOD/SCID/gammacnull mice model. *Blood.* 2003;102(3):873-880.

229. Theocharides AP, Rongvaux A, Fritsch K, Flavell RA, Manz MG. Humanized hemato-lymphoid system mice. *Haematologica.* 2016;101(1):5-19.

230. Rongvaux A, Willinger T, Martinek J, et al. Development and function of human innate immune cells in a humanized mouse model. *Nat Biotechnol.* 2014;32(4):364-372.
231. Rahmig S, Kronstein-Wiedemann R, Fohgrub J, et al. Improved human erythropoiesis and platelet formation in humanized NSGW41 mice. *Stem Cell Rep.* 2016;7(4):591-601.
232. Abkowitz JL, Catlin SN, Guttorp P. Evidence that hematopoiesis may be a stochastic process in vivo. *Nat Med.* 1996;2(2):190-197.
233. Srour EF, Zanjani ED, Brandt JE, et al. Sustained human hematopoiesis in sheep transplanted in utero during early gestation with fractionated adult human bone marrow cells. *Blood.* 1992;79(6):1404-1412.
234. Wagner JL, Storb R. Preclinical large animal models for hematopoietic stem cell transplantation. *Curr Opin Hematol.* 1996;3(6):410-415.
235. Mahmud N, Devine SM, Weller KP, et al. The relative quiescence of hematopoietic stem cells in nonhuman primates. *Blood.* 2001;97(10):3061-3068.
236. Horn PA, Thomasson BM, Wood BL, Andrews RG, Morris JC, Kiem HP. Distinct hematopoietic stem/progenitor cell populations are responsible for repopulating NOD/SCID mice compared with nonhuman primates. *Blood.* 2003;102(13):4329-4335.
237. Peterson CW, Wang J, Norman KK, et al. Long-term multilineage engraftment of autologous genome-edited hematopoietic stem cells in nonhuman primates. *Blood.* 2016;127(20):2416-2426.
238. Mandal PK, Ferreira LM, Collins R, et al. Efficient ablation of genes in human hematopoietic stem and effector cells using CRISPR/Cas9. *Cell Stem Cell.* 2014;15(5):643-652.
239. Wright DE, Wagers AJ, Gulati AP, Johnson FL, Weissman IL. Physiological migration of hematopoietic stem and progenitor cells. *Science.* 2001;294(5548):1933-1936.
240. Perlin JR, Sporrij A, Zon LI. Blood on the tracks: hematopoietic stem cell-endothelial cell interactions in homing and engraftment. *J Mol Med (Berl).* 2017;95(8):809-819.
241. Frenette PS, Subbarao S, Mazo IB, von Andrian UH, Wagner DD. Endothelial selectins and vascular cell adhesion molecule-1 promote hematopoietic progenitor homing to bone marrow. *Proc Natl Acad Sci U S A.* 1998;95(24):14423-14428.
242. Hidalgo A, Frenette PS. Enforced fucosylation of neonatal CD34+ cells generates selectin ligands that enhance the initial interactions with microvessels but not homing to bone marrow. *Blood.* 2005;105(2):567-575.
243. Mazo IB, Gutierrez-Ramos JC, Frenette PS, Hynes RO, Wagner DD, von Andrian UH. Hematopoietic progenitor cell rolling in bone marrow microvessels: parallel contributions by endothelial selectins and vascular cell adhesion molecule 1. *J Exp Med.* 1998;188(3):465-474.
244. Papayannopoulou T, Craddock C, Nakamoto B, Priestley GV, Wolf NS. The VLA4/VCAM-1 adhesion pathway defines contrasting mechanisms of lodgement of transplanted murine hemopoietic progenitors between bone marrow and spleen. *Proc Natl Acad Sci U S A.* 1995;92(21):9647-9651.
245. Zanjani ED, Flake AW, Almeida-Porada G, Tran N, Papayannopoulou T. Homing of human cells in the fetal sheep model: modulation by antibodies activating or inhibiting very late activation antigen-4-dependent function. *Blood.* 1999;94(7):2515-2522.
246. Scott LM, Priestley GV, Papayannopoulou T. Deletion of alpha4 integrins from adult hematopoietic cells reveals roles in homeostasis, regeneration, and homing. *Mol Cell Biol.* 2003;23(24):9349-9360.
247. Potocnik AJ, Brakebusch C, Fässler R. Fetal and adult hematopoietic stem cells require beta1 integrin function for colonizing fetal liver, spleen, and bone marrow. *Immunity.* 2000;12(6):653-663.
248. Papayannopoulou T, Nakamoto B. Peripheralization of hemopoietic progenitors in primates treated with anti-VLA4 integrin. *Proc Natl Acad Sci U S A.* 1993;90(20):9374-9378.
249. Papayannopoulou T, Priestley GV, Nakamoto B. Anti-VLA4/VCAM-1-induced mobilization requires cooperative signaling through the kit/mkit ligand pathway. *Blood.* 1998;91(7):2231-2239.
250. Katayama Y, Hidalgo A, Peired A, Frenette PS. Integrin alpha4beta7 and its counter-receptor MAdCAM-1 contribute to hematopoietic progenitor recruitment into bone marrow following transplantation. *Blood.* 2004;104(7):2020-2026.
251. Peled A, Kollet O, Ponomaryov T, et al. The chemokine SDF-1 activates the integrins LFA-1, VLA-4, and VLA-5 on immature human CD34(+) cells: role in transendothelial/stromal migration and engraftment of NOD/SCID mice. *Blood.* 2000;95(11):3289-3296.
252. van der Loo JC, Xiao X, McMillin D, Hashino K, Kato I, Williams DA. VLA-5 is expressed by mouse and human long-term repopulating hematopoietic cells and mediates adhesion to extracellular matrix protein fibronectin. *J Clin Invest.* 1998;102(5):1051-1061.
253. Qian H, Tryggvason K, Jacobsen SE, Ekblom M. Contribution of alpha6 integrins to hematopoietic stem and progenitor cell homing to bone marrow and collaboration with alpha4 integrins. *Blood.* 2006;107(9):3503-3510.
254. Schreiber TD, Steinl C, Essl M, et al. The integrin alpha9beta1 on hematopoietic stem and progenitor cells: involvement in cell adhesion, proliferation and differentiation. *Haematologica.* 2009;94(11):1493-1501.
255. Avigdor A, Goichberg P, Shivtiel S, et al. CD44 and hyaluronic acid cooperate with SDF-1 in the trafficking of human CD34+ stem/progenitor cells to bone marrow. *Blood.* 2004;103(8):2981-2989.
256. Christ O, Kronenwett R, Haas R, Zöller M. Combining G-CSF with a blockade of adhesion strongly improves the reconstitutive capacity of mobilized hematopoietic progenitor cells. *Exp Hematol.* 2001;29(3):380-390.
257. Vermeulen M, Le Pesteur F, Gagnerault MC, Mary JY, Sainteny F, Lepault F. Role of adhesion molecules in the homing and mobilization of murine hematopoietic stem and progenitor cells. *Blood.* 1998;92(3):894-900.
258. Ulyanova T, Scott LM, Priestley GV, et al. VCAM-1 expression in adult hematopoietic and nonhematopoietic cells is controlled by tissue-inductive signals and reflects their developmental origin. *Blood.* 2005;106(1):86-94.
259. Kim CH, Broxmeyer HE. In vitro behavior of hematopoietic progenitor cells under the influence of chemoattractants: stromal cell-derived factor-1, steel factor, and the bone marrow environment. *Blood.* 1998;91(1):100-110.
260. Peled A, Petit I, Kollet O, et al. Dependence of human stem cell engraftment and repopulation of NOD/SCID mice on CXCR4. *Science.* 1999;283(5403):845-848.
261. Aiuti A, Webb IJ, Bleul C, Springer T, Gutierrez-Ramos JC. The chemokine SDF-1 is a chemoattractant for human CD34+ hematopoietic progenitor cells and provides a new mechanism to explain the mobilization of CD34+ progenitors to peripheral blood. *J Exp Med.* 1997;185(1):111-120.
262. Wright DE, Bowman EP, Wagers AJ, Butcher EC, Weissman IL. Hematopoietic stem cells are uniquely selective in their migratory response to chemokines. *J Exp Med.* 2002;195(9):1145-1154.
263. Nagasawa T, Hirota S, Tachibana K, et al. Defects of B-cell lymphopoiesis and bone-marrow myelopoiesis in mice lacking the CXC chemokine PBSF/SDF-1. *Nature.* 1996;382(6592):635-638.
264. Zou YR, Kottmann AH, Kuroda M, Taniuchi I, Littman DR. Function of the chemokine receptor CXCR4 in haematopoiesis and in cerebellar development. *Nature.* 1998;393(6685):595-599.
265. Kollet O, Spiegel A, Peled A, et al. Rapid and efficient homing of human CD34(+) CD38(-/low)CXCR4(+) stem and progenitor cells to the bone marrow and spleen of NOD/SCID and NOD/SCID/B2m(null) mice. *Blood.* 2001;97(10):3283-3291.
266. Imai K, Kobayashi M, Wang J, et al. Selective secretion of chemoattractants for haemopoietic progenitor cells by bone marrow endothelial cells: a possible role in homing of haemopoietic progenitor cells to bone marrow. *Br J Haematol.* 1999;106(4):905-911.
267. Peled A, Grabovsky V, Habler L, et al. The chemokine SDF-1 stimulates integrin-mediated arrest of CD34(+) cells on vascular endothelium under shear flow. *J Clin Invest.* 1999;104(9):1199-1211.
268. Fukuda S, Broxmeyer HE, Pelus LM. Flt3 ligand and the Flt3 receptor regulate hematopoietic cell migration by modulating the SDF-1alpha(CXCL12)/CXCR4 axis. *Blood.* 2005;105(8):3117-3126.
269. Massberg S, Schaerli P, Knezevic-Maramica I, et al. Immunosurveillance by hematopoietic progenitor cells trafficking through blood, lymph, and peripheral tissues. *Cell.* 2007;131(5):994-1008.
270. Si Y, Tsou CL, Croft K, Charo IF. CCR2 mediates hematopoietic stem and progenitor cell trafficking to sites of inflammation in mice. *J Clin Invest.* 2010;120(4):1192-1203.
271. van Rood JJ, Oudshoorn M. Eleven million donors in bone marrow donors worldwide! Time for reassessment? *Bone Marrow Transplant.* 2008;41(1):1-9.
272. Levesque JP, Liu F, Simmons PJ, et al. Characterization of hematopoietic progenitor mobilization in protease-deficient mice. *Blood.* 2004;104(1):65-72.
273. Méndez-Ferrer S, Michurina TV, Ferraro F, et al. Mesenchymal and haematopoietic stem cells form a unique bone marrow niche. *Nature.* 2010;466(7308):829-834.
274. Katayama Y, Battista M, Kao WM, et al. Signals from the sympathetic nervous system regulate hematopoietic stem cell egress from bone marrow. *Cell.* 2006;124(2):407-421.
275. Lucas D, Scheiermann C, Chow A, et al. Chemotherapy-induced bone marrow nerve injury impairs hematopoietic regeneration. *Nat Med.* 2013;19(6):695-703.
276. Ferraro F, Lymperi S, Méndez-Ferrer S, et al. Diabetes impairs hematopoietic stem cell mobilization by altering niche function. *Sci Transl Med.* 2011;3(104):104ra101.
277. Méndez-Ferrer S, Lucas D, Battista M, Frenette PS. Haematopoietic stem cell release is regulated by circadian oscillations. *Nature.* 2008;452(7186):442-447.
278. Lucas D, Battista M, Shi PA, Isola L, Frenette PS. Mobilized hematopoietic stem cell yield depends on species-specific circadian timing. *Cell Stem Cell.* 2008;3(4):364-366.
279. Christopher MJ, Rao M, Liu F, Woloszynek JR, Link DC. Expression of the G-CSF receptor in monocytic cells is sufficient to mediate hematopoietic progenitor mobilization by G-CSF in mice. *J Exp Med.* 2011;208(2):251-260.
280. Winkler IG, Sims NA, Pettit AR, et al. Bone marrow macrophages maintain hematopoietic stem cell (HSC) niches and their depletion mobilizes HSCs. *Blood.* 2010;116(23):4815-4828.
281. Chow A, Lucas D, Hidalgo A, et al. Bone marrow CD169+ macrophages promote the retention of hematopoietic stem and progenitor cells in the mesenchymal stem cell niche. *J Exp Med.* 2011;208(2):261-271.
282. Albiero M, Poncina N, Ciciliot S, et al. Bone marrow macrophages contribute to diabetic stem cell mobilopathy by producing oncostatin. M. *Diabetes.* 2015;64(8):2957-2968.
283. Haldar M, Kohyama M, So AY, et al. Heme-mediated SPI-C induction promotes monocyte differentiation into iron-recycling macrophages. *Cell.* 2014;156(6):1223-1234.
284. Chow A, Huggins M, Ahmed J, et al. CD169^{+} macrophages provide a niche promoting erythropoiesis under homeostasis and stress. *Nat Med.* 2013;19(4):429-436.
285. Ludin A, Itkin T, Gur-Cohen S, et al. Monocytes-macrophages that express α-smooth muscle actin preserve primitive hematopoietic cells in the bone marrow. *Nat Immunol.* 2012;13(11):1072-1082.
286. Casanova-Acebes M, Pitaval C, Weiss LA, et al. Rhythmic modulation of the hematopoietic niche through neutrophil clearance. *Cell.* 2013;153(5):1025-1035.
287. Broxmeyer HE, Orschell CM, Clapp DW, et al. Rapid mobilization of murine and human hematopoietic stem and progenitor cells with AMD3100, a CXCR4 antagonist. *J Exp Med.* 2005;201(8):1307-1318.
288. Bensinger W, DiPersio JF, McCarty JM. Improving stem cell mobilization strategies: future directions. *Bone Marrow Transplant.* 2009;43(3):181-195.
289. To LB, Levesque JP, Herbert KE. How I treat patients who mobilize hematopoietic stem cells poorly. *Blood.* 2011;118(17):4530-4540.
290. Bakanay ŞM, Demirer T. Novel agents and approaches for stem cell mobilization in normal donors and patients. *Bone Marrow Transplant.* 2012;47(9):1154-1163.

291. He S, Chu J, Vasu S, et al. FLT3L and plerixafor combination increases hematopoietic stem cell mobilization and leads to improved transplantation outcome. *Biol Blood Marrow Transplant*. 2014;20(3):309-313.

292. Ryan MA, Nattamai KJ, Xing E, et al. Pharmacological inhibition of EGFR signaling enhances G-CSF-induced hematopoietic stem cell mobilization. *Nat Med*. 2010;16(10):1141-1146.

293. Cao B, Zhang Z, Grassinger J, et al. Therapeutic targeting and rapid mobilization of endosteal HSC using a small molecule integrin antagonist. *Nat Commun*. 2016;7:11007.

294. Shivdasani RA, Orkin SH. The transcriptional control of hematopoiesis. *Blood*. 1996;87(10):4025-4039.

295. Graf T. Differentiation plasticity of hematopoietic cells. *Blood*. 2002;99(9):3089-3101.

296. Rekhtman N, Choe KS, Matushansky I, Murray S, Stopka T, Skoultchi AI. PU.1 and pRB interact and cooperate to repress GATA-1 and block erythroid differentiation. *Mol Cell Biol*. 2003;23(21):7460-7474.

297. Chen H, Ray-Gallet D, Zhang P, et al. PU.1 (Spi-1) autoregulates its expression in myeloid cells. *Oncogene*. 1995;11(8):1549-1560.

298. Tsai SF, Strauss E, Orkin SH. Functional analysis and in vivo footprinting implicate the erythroid transcription factor GATA-1 as a positive regulator of its own promoter. *Genes Dev*. 1991;5(6):919-931.

299. Hu M, Krause D, Greaves M, et al. Multilineage gene expression precedes commitment in the hemopoietic system. *Genes Dev*. 1997;11(6):774-785.

300. Nerlov C, Tenen DG, Graf T. Regulatory interactions between transcription factors and their role in hematopoietic lineage determination. In: Zon L, ed. *Hematopoiesis: A Developmental Approach*. Oxford University Press; 2001:363-367.

301. Laiosa CV, Stadtfeld M, Graf T. Determinants of lymphoid-myeloid lineage diversification. *Annu Rev Immunol*. 2006;24:705-738.

302. Hoppe PS, Schwarzfischer M, Loeffler D, et al. Early myeloid lineage choice is not initiated by random PU.1 to GATA1 protein ratios. *Nature*. 2016;535(7611):299-302.

303. Ambros V. The functions of animal microRNAs. *Nature*. 2004;431(7006):350-355.

304. Chen CZ, Li L, Lodish HF, Bartel DP. MicroRNAs modulate hematopoietic lineage differentiation. *Science*. 2004;303(5654):83-86.

305. Havelange V, Garzon R. MicroRNAs: emerging key regulators of hematopoiesis. *Am J Hematol*. 2010;85(12):935-942.

306. Koralov SB, Muljo SA, Galler GR, et al. Dicer ablation affects antibody diversity and cell survival in the B lymphocyte lineage. *Cell*. 2008;132(5):860-874.

307. Muljo SA, Ansel KM, Kanellopoulou C, Livingston DM, Rao A, Rajewsky K. Aberrant T cell differentiation in the absence of Dicer. *J Exp Med*. 2005;202(2):261-269.

308. Georgantas RW,IIIrd, Hildreth R, Morisot S, et al. CD34+ hematopoietic stem-progenitor cell microRNA expression and function: a circuit diagram of differentiation control. *Proc Natl Acad Sci U S A*. 2007;104(8):2750-2755.

309. Romania P, Lulli V, Pelosi E, Biffoni M, Peschle C, Marziali G. MicroRNA 155 modulates megakaryopoiesis at progenitor and precursor level by targeting Ets-1 and Meis1 transcription factors. *Br J Haematol*. 2008;143(4):570-580.

310. Rodriguez A, Vigorito E, Clare S, et al. Requirement of bic/microRNA-155 for normal immune function. *Science*. 2007;316(5824):608-611.

311. Thai TH, Calado DP, Casola S, et al. Regulation of the germinal center response by microRNA-155. *Science*. 2007;316(5824):604-608.

312. Vigorito E, Perks KL, Abreu-Goodger C, et al. microRNA-155 regulates the generation of immunoglobulin class-switched plasma cells. *Immunity*. 2007;27(6):847-859.

313. Teng G, Hakimpour P, Landgraf P, et al. MicroRNA-155 is a negative regulator of activation-induced cytidine deaminase. *Immunity*. 2008;28(5):621-629.

314. Dorsett Y, McBride KM, Jankovic M, et al. MicroRNA-155 suppresses activation-induced cytidine deaminase-mediated Myc-Igh translocation. *Immunity*. 2008;28(5):630-638.

315. Hong SH, Kim KS, Oh IH. Concise review: exploring miRNAs—toward a better understanding of hematopoiesis. *Stem Cell*. 2015;33(1):1-7.

316. Zhao G, Yu D, Weiss MJ. MicroRNAs in erythropoiesis. *Curr Opin Hematol*. 2010;17(3):155-162.

317. Li H, Zhao H, Wang D, Yang R. microRNA regulation in megakaryocytopoiesis. *Br J Haematol*. 2011;155(3):298-307.

318. O'Connell RM, Zhao JL, Rao DS. MicroRNA function in myeloid biology. *Blood*. 2011;118(11):2960-2969.

319. Belver L, Papavasiliou FN, Ramiro AR. MicroRNA control of lymphocyte differentiation and function. *Curr Opin Immunol*. 2011;23(3):368-373.

320. Metcalf D. Hematopoietic cytokines. *Blood*. 2008;111(2):485-491.

321. Santini V, Scappini B, Indik ZK, Gozzini A, Ferrini PR, Schreiber AD. The carboxy-terminal region of the granulocyte colony-stimulating factor receptor transduces a phagocytic signal. *Blood*. 2003;101(11):4615-4622.

322. Metcalf D, Nicola NA. The clonal proliferation of normal mouse hematopoietic cells: enhancement and suppression by colony-stimulating factor combinations. *Blood*. 1992;79(11):2861-2866.

323. Matsunaga T, Kato T, Miyazaki H, Ogawa M. Thrombopoietin promotes the survival of murine hematopoietic long-term reconstituting cells: comparison with the effects of FLT3/FLK-2 ligand and interleukin-6. *Blood*. 1998;92(2):452-461.

324. Matsunaga T, Hirayama F, Yonemura Y, Murray R, Ogawa M. Negative regulation by interleukin-3 (IL-3) of mouse early B-cell progenitors and stem cells in culture: transduction of the negative signals by betac and betaIL3 proteins of IL-3 receptor and absence of negative regulation by granulocyte-macrophage colony-stimulating factor. *Blood*. 1998;92(3):901-907.

325. Metcalf D. Lineage commitment and maturation in hematopoietic cells: the case for extrinsic regulation. *Blood*. 1998;92(2):345-347. discussion 352.

326. Yagi M, Ritchie KA, Sitnicka E, Storey C, Roth GJ, Bartelmez S. Sustained ex vivo expansion of hematopoietic stem cells mediated by thrombopoietin. *Proc Natl Acad Sci U S A*. 1999;96(14):8126-8131.

327. Zandstra PW, Lauffenburger DA, Eaves CJ. A ligand-receptor signaling threshold model of stem cell differentiation control: a biologically conserved mechanism applicable to hematopoiesis. *Blood*. 2000;96(4):1215-1222.

328. Gilliland DG, Griffin JD. The roles of FLT3 in hematopoiesis and leukemia. *Blood*. 2002;100(5):1532-1542.

329. Metcalf D. Hematopoietic regulators: redundancy or subtlety? *Blood*. 1993;82(12):3515-3523.

330. Alexander WS, Roberts AW, Nicola NA, Li R, Metcalf D. Deficiencies in progenitor cells of multiple hematopoietic lineages and defective megakaryocytopoiesis in mice lacking the thrombopoietic receptor c-Mpl. *Blood*. 1996;87(6):2162-2170.

331. Yonemura Y, Kawakita M, Fujimoto K, et al. Effects of short-term administration of recombinant human erythropoietin on rat megakaryopoiesis. *Int J Cell Clon*. 1992;10:18-27.

332. Young JC, Bruno E, Luens KM, Wu S, Backer M, Murray LJ. Thrombopoietin stimulates megakaryocytopoiesis, myelopoiesis, and expansion of CD34+ progenitor cells from single CD34+Thy-1+Lin- primitive progenitor cells. *Blood*. 1996;88(5):1619-1631.

333. McNeice IK, Langley KE, Zsebo KM. Recombinant human stem cell factor synergizes with GM-CSF, IL-2, and Epo to stimulate human progenitor cells of the myeloid and erythroid lineages. *Exp Hematol*. 1991;19:226-231.

334. Metcalf D, Nicola NA. Direct proliferative actions of stem cell factor on murine bone marrow cells in vitro: effects of combination with colony-stimulating factors. *Proc Natl Acad Sci U S A*. 1991;88(14):6239-6243.

335. Muta K, Krantz SB, Bondurant MC, Dai CH. Stem cell factor retards differentiation of normal human erythroid progenitor cells while stimulating proliferation. *Blood*. 1995;86(2):572-580.

336. Migliaccio G, Migliaccio AR, Valinsky J, et al. Stem cell factor induces proliferation and differentiation of highly enriched murine hematopoietic cells. *Proc Natl Acad Sci U S A*. 1991;88(16):7420-7424.

337. Leary AG, Zeng HQ, Clark SC, Ogawa M. Growth factor requirements for survival in G0 and entry into the cell cycle of primitive human hemopoietic progenitors. *Proc Natl Acad Sci U S A*. 1992;89(9):4013-4017.

338. Miura N, Okada S, Zsebo KM, Miura Y, Suda T. Rat stem cell factor and IL-6 preferentially support the proliferation of c-kit-positive murine hemopoietic cells rather than their differentiation. *Exp Hematol*. 1993;21(1):143-149.

339. Yamaguchi Y, Suda T, Suda J, et al. Purified interleukin 5 supports the terminal differentiation and proliferation of murine eosinophilic precursors. *J Exp Med*. 1988;167(1):43-56.

340. Dickason RR, Huston DP. Creation of a biologically active interleukin-5 monomer. *Nature*. 1996;379(6566):652-655.

341. Lieschke GJ, Grail D, Hodgson G, et al. Mice lacking granulocyte colony-stimulating factor have chronic neutropenia, granulocyte and macrophage progenitor cell deficiency, and impaired neutrophil mobilization. *Blood*. 1994;84(6):1737-1746.

342. Herbert DR, Lee JJ, Lee NA, Nolan TJ, Schad GA, Abraham D. Role of IL-5 in innate and adaptive immunity to larval Strongyloides stercoralis in mice. *J Immunol*. 2000;165(8):4544-4551.

343. Ohmori K, Luo Y, Jia Y, et al. IL-3 induces basophil expansion in vivo by directing granulocyte-monocyte progenitors to differentiate into basophil lineage-restricted progenitors in the bone marrow and by increasing the number of basophil/mast cell progenitors in the spleen. *J Immunol*. 2009;182(5):2835-2841.

344. Valent P, Dahinden CA. Role of interleukins in the regulation of basophil development and secretion. *Curr Opin Hematol*. 2010;17(1):60-66.

345. Metcalf D, Nicola NA. *The Hematopoietic Colony Stimulating Factors: From Biology to Clinical Applications*. Cambridge University Press; 1995.

346. Stanley E, Lieschke GJ, Grail D, et al. Granulocyte/macrophage colony-stimulating factor-deficient mice show no major perturbation of hematopoiesis but develop a characteristic pulmonary pathology. *Proc Natl Acad Sci U S A*. 1994;91(12):5592-5596.

347. Hibbs ML, Quilici C, Kountouri N, et al. Mice lacking three myeloid colony-stimulating factors (G-CSF, GM-CSF, and M-CSF) still produce macrophages and granulocytes and mount an inflammatory response in a sterile model of peritonitis. *J Immunol*. 2007;178(10):6435-6443.

348. Fleischmann J, Golde DW, Weisbart RH, Gasson JC. Granulocyte-macrophage colony-stimulating factor enhances phagocytosis of bacteria by human neutrophils. *Blood*. 1986;68(3):708-711.

349. Vadas MA, Nicola NA, Metcalf D. Activation of antibody-dependent cell-mediated cytotoxicity of human neutrophils and eosinophils by separate colony-stimulating factors. *J Immunol*. 1983;130(2):795-799.

350. Handman E, Burgess AW. Stimulation by granulocyte-macrophage colony-stimulating factor of Leishmania tropica killing by macrophages. *J Immunol*. 1979;122(3):1134-1137.

351. Wershil BK, Tsai M, Geissler EN, Zsebo KM, Galli SJ. The rat c-kit ligand, stem cell factor, induces c-kit receptor-dependent mouse mast cell activation in vivo. Evidence that signaling through the c-kit receptor can induce expression of cellular function. *J Exp Med*. 1992;175(1):245-255.

352. Valent P, Spanblöchl E, Sperr WR, et al. Induction of differentiation of human mast cells from bone marrow and peripheral blood mononuclear cells by recombinant human stem cell factor/kit-ligand in long-term culture. *Blood*. 1992;80(9):2237-2245.

353. Irani AM, Nilsson G, Miettinen U, et al. Recombinant human stem cell factor stimulates differentiation of mast cells from dispersed human fetal liver cells. *Blood*. 1992;80(12):3009-3021.

354. Lukacs NW, Kunkel SL, Strieter RM, et al. The role of stem cell factor (c-kit ligand) and inflammatory cytokines in pulmonary mast cell activation. *Blood*. 1996;87(6):2262-2268.

355. Galli SJ, Kitamura Y. Genetically mast-cell-deficient W/Wv and Sl/Sld mice. Their value for the analysis of the roles of mast cells in biologic responses in vivo. *Am J Pathol*. 1987;127(1):191-198.

356. Auffray C, Sieweke MH, Geissmann F. Blood monocytes: development, heterogeneity, and relationship with dendritic cells. *Annu Rev Immunol.* 2009;27:669-692.

357. Chitu V, Stanley ER. Colony-stimulating factor-1 in immunity and inflammation. *Curr Opin Immunol.* 2006;18(1):39-48.

358. Davies JQ, Gordon S. Isolation and culture of murine macrophages. *Methods Mol Biol.* 2005;290:91-103.

359. Nemunaitis J, Shannon-Dorcy K, Appelbaum FR, et al. Long-term follow-up of patients with invasive fungal disease who received adjunctive therapy with recombinant human macrophage colony-stimulating factor. *Blood.* 1993;82(5):1422-1427.

360. Kandalla PK, Sarrazin S, Molawi K, et al. M-CSF improves protection against bacterial and fungal infections after hematopoietic stem/progenitor cell transplantation. *J Exp Med.* 2016;213(11):2269-2279.

361. Broudy VC, Lin NL, Kaushansky K. Thrombopoietin (c-mpl ligand) acts synergistically with erythropoietin, stem cell factor, and interleukin-11 to enhance murine megakaryocyte colony growth and increases megakaryocyte ploidy in vitro. *Blood.* 1995;85(7):1719-1726.

362. Banu N, Wang JF, Deng B, Groopman JE, Avraham H. Modulation of megakaryocytopoiesis by thrombopoietin: the c-Mpl ligand. *Blood.* 1995;86(4):1331-1338.

363. Burstein SA, Adamson JW, Erb SK, Harker LA. Megakaryocytopoiesis in the mouse: response to varying platelet demand. *J Cell Physiol.* 1981;109(2):333-341.

364. Williams N, Eger RR, Jackson HM, Nelson DJ. Two-factor requirement for murine megakaryocyte colony formation. *J Cell Physiol.* 1982;110(1):101-104.

365. Kuter DJ, Begley CG. Recombinant human thrombopoietin: basic biology and evaluation of clinical studies. *Blood.* 2002;100(10):3457-3469.

366. Kaushansky K. Thrombopoietin: the primary regulator of platelet production. *Blood.* 1995;86(2):419-431.

367. Debili N, Wendling F, Cosman D, et al. The Mpl receptor is expressed in the megakaryocytic lineage from late progenitors to platelets. *Blood.* 1995;85(2):391-401.

368. Souyri M, Vigon I, Penciolelli JF, Heard JM, Tambourin P, Wendling F. A putative truncated cytokine receptor gene transduced by the myeloproliferative leukemia virus immortalizes hematopoietic progenitors. *Cell.* 1990;63(6):1137-1147.

369. Farese AM, Hunt P, Boone T, MacVittie TJ. Recombinant human megakaryocyte growth and development factor stimulates thrombocytopoiesis in normal nonhuman primates. *Blood.* 1995;86(1):54-59.

370. Wendling F, Maraskovsky E, Debili N, et al. cMpl ligand is a humoral regulator of megakaryocytopoiesis. *Nature.* 1994;369(6481):571-574.

371. McCarty JM, Sprugel KH, Fox NE, Sabath DE, Kaushansky K. Murine thrombopoietin mRNA levels are modulated by platelet count. *Blood.* 1995;86(10):3668-3675.

372. Kuter DJ. Biology and chemistry of thrombopoietic agents. *Semin Hematol.* 2010;47(3):243-248.

373. Koury MJ, Bondurant MC. The molecular mechanism of erythropoietin action. *Eur J Biochem.* 1992;210(3):649-663.

374. Koury ST, Bondurant MC, Koury MJ. Localization of erythropoietin synthesizing cells in murine kidneys by in situ hybridization. *Blood.* 1988;71:524-527.

375. Lacombe C, Da Silva JL, Bruneval P, et al. Peritubular cells are the site of erythropoietin synthesis in the murine hypoxic kidney. *J Clin Invest.* 1988;81(2):620-623.

376. Koury ST, Koury MJ, Bondurant MC, Caro J, Graber SE. Quantitation of erythropoietin-producing cells in kidneys of mice by in situ hybridization: correlation with hematocrit, renal erythropoietin mRNA, and serum erythropoietin concentration. *Blood.* 1989;74(2):645-651.

377. Wang GL, Jiang BH, Rue EA, Semenza GL. Hypoxia-inducible factor 1 is a basic-helix-loop-helix-PAS heterodimer regulated by cellular O2 tension. *Proc Natl Acad Sci U S A.* 1995;92(12):5510-5514.

378. Jaakkola P, Mole DR, Tian YM, et al. Targeting of HIF-alpha to the von Hippel-Lindau ubiquitylation complex by O2-regulated prolyl hydroxylation. *Science.* 2001;292(5516):468-472.

379. Ivan M, Kondo K, Yang H, et al. HIFalpha targeted for VHL-mediated destruction by proline hydroxylation: implications for O2 sensing. *Science.* 2001;292(5516):464-468.

380. Yu F, White SB, Zhao Q, Lee FS. HIF-1alpha binding to VHL is regulated by stimulus-sensitive proline hydroxylation. *Proc Natl Acad Sci U S A.* 2001;98(17):9630-9635.

381. Lando D, Peet DJ, Whelan DA, Gorman JJ, Whitelaw ML. Asparagine hydroxylation of the HIF transactivation domain a hypoxic switch. *Science.* 2002;295(5556):858-861.

382. Sang N, Fang J, Srinivas V, Leshchinsky I, Caro J. Carboxyl-terminal transactivation activity of hypoxia-inducible factor 1 alpha is governed by a von Hippel-Lindau protein-independent, hydroxylation-regulated association with p300/CBP. *Mol Cell Biol.* 2002;22(9):2984-2992.

383. Semenza GL, Koury ST, Nejfelt MK, Gearhart JD, Antonarakis SE. Cell-type-specific and hypoxia-inducible expression of the human erythropoietin gene in transgenic mice. *Proc Natl Acad Sci U S A.* 1991;88(19):8725-8729.

384. Koury ST, Bondurant MC, Semenza GL, Koury MJ. The use of in situ hybridization to study erythropoietin gene expression in murine kidney and liver. *Microsc Res Tech.* 1993;25(1):29-39.

385. Sawyer ST, Krantz SB, Goldwasser E. Binding and receptor-mediated endocytosis of erythropoietin in Friend virus-infected erythroid cells. *J Biol Chem.* 1987;262(12):5554-5562.

386. Gross AW, Lodish HF. Cellular trafficking and degradation of erythropoietin and novel erythropoiesis stimulating protein (NESP). *J Biol Chem.* 2006;281(4):2024-2032.

387. Chapel S, Veng-Pedersen P, Hohl RJ, Schmidt RL, McGuire EM, Widness JA. Changes in erythropoietin pharmacokinetics following busulfan-induced bone marrow ablation in sheep: evidence for bone marrow as a major erythropoietin elimination pathway. *J Pharmacol Exp Therapeut.* 2001;298(2):820-824.

388. Wu H, Liu X, Jaenisch R, Lodish HF. Generation of committed erythroid BFU-E and CFU-E progenitors does not require erythropoietin or the erythropoietin receptor. *Cell.* 1995;83(1):59-67.

389. Lin CS, Lim SK, D'Agati V, Constantini F. Differential effects of an erythropoietin receptor gene disruption on primitive and definitive erythropoiesis. *Genes Dev.* 1996;10(2):154-164.

390. Dai CH, Krantz SB, Zsebo KM. Human burst-forming units-erythroid need direct interaction with stem cell factor for further development. *Blood.* 1991;78:2493-2497.

391. Sawada K, Krantz SB, Dessypris EN, Koury ST, Sawyer ST. Human colony-forming units-erythroid do not require accessory cells, but do require direct interaction with insulin-like growth factor-I and/or insulin for erythroid development. *J Clin Invest.* 1989;83:1701-1708.

392. Muta K, Krantz SB, Bondurant MC, Wickrema A. Distinct roles of erythropoietin, insulin-like growth factor, and stem cell factor in the development of erythroid progenitor cells. *J Clin Invest.* 1994;94:34-43.

393. Whitlock CA, Witte ON. Long-term culture of B lymphocytes and their precursors from murine bone marrow. *Proc Natl Acad Sci U S A.* 1982;79(11):3608-3612.

394. Peschon JJ, Morrissey PJ, Grabstein KH, et al. Early lymphocyte expansion is severely impaired in interleukin 7 receptor-deficient mice. *J Exp Med.* 1994;180(5):1955-1960.

395. Nagasawa T. Microenvironmental niches in the bone marrow required for B-cell development. *Nat Rev Immunol.* 2006;6(2):107-116.

396. Dolznig H, Habermann B, Stangl K, et al. Apoptosis protection by the Epo target Bcl-X(L) allows factor-independent differentiation of primary erythroblasts. *Curr Biol.* 2002;12(13):1076-1085.

397. Kondo M, Akashi K, Domen J, Sugamura K, Weissman IL. Bcl-2 rescues T lymphopoiesis, but not B or NK cell development, in common gamma chain-deficient mice. *Immunity.* 1997;7(1):155-162.

398. Akashi K, Kondo M, Cheshier S, et al. Lymphoid development from stem cells and the common lymphocyte progenitors. *Cold Spring Harbor Symp Quant Biol.* 1999;64:1-12.

399. Kikuchi K, Lai AY, Hsu CL, Kondo M. IL-7 receptor signaling is necessary for stage transition in adult B cell development through up-regulation of EBF. *J Exp Med.* 2005;201(8):1197-1203.

400. Iwasaki-Arai J, Iwasaki H, Miyamoto T, Watanabe S, Akashi K. Enforced granulocyte/macrophage colony-stimulating factor signals do not support lymphopoiesis, but instruct lymphoid to myelomonocytic lineage conversion. *J Exp Med.* 2003;197(10):1311-1322.

401. Dahl R, Walsh JC, Lancki D, et al. Regulation of macrophage and neutrophil cell fates by the PU.1:C/EBPalpha ratio and granulocyte colony-stimulating factor. *Nat Immunol.* 2003;4(10):1029-1036.

402. Rieger MA, Hoppe PS, Smejkal BM, Eitelhuber AC, Schroeder T. Hematopoietic cytokines can instruct lineage choice. *Science.* 2009;325(5937):217-218.

403. Mossadegh-Keller N, Sarrazin S, Kandalla PK, et al. M-CSF instructs myeloid lineage fate in single haematopoietic stem cells. *Nature.* 2013;497(7448):239-243.

404. Birbrair A, Frenette PS. Niche heterogeneity in the bone marrow. *Ann N Y Acad Sci.* 2016;1370(1):82-96.

405. Yoder MC, Williams DA. Matrix molecule interactions with hematopoietic stem cells. *Exp Hematol.* 1995;23(9):961-967.

406. Gattazzo F, Urciuolo A, Bonaldo P. Extracellular matrix: a dynamic microenvironment for stem cell niche. *Biochim Biophys Acta.* 2014;1840(8):2506-2519.

407. Russell ES. Hereditary anemias of the mouse: a review for geneticists. *Adv Genet.* 1979;20:357-459.

408. Chabot B, Stephenson DA, Chapman VM, Besmer P, Bernstein A. The proto-oncogene c-kit encoding a transmembrane tyrosine kinase receptor maps to the mouse W locus. *Nature.* 1988;335(6185):88-89.

409. Geissler EN, Ryan MA, Housman DE. The dominant-white spotting (W) locus of the mouse encodes the c-kit proto-oncogene. *Cell.* 1988;55(1):185-192.

410. Copeland NG, Gilbert DJ, Cho BC, et al. Mast cell growth factor maps near the steel locus on mouse chromosome 10 and is deleted in a number of steel alleles. *Cell.* 1990;63(1):175-183.

411. Huang E, Nocka K, Beier DR, et al. The hematopoietic growth factor KL is encoded by the Sl locus and is the ligand of the c-kit receptor, the gene product of the W locus. *Cell.* 1990;63(1):225-233.

412. Zsebo KM, Williams DA, Geissler EN, et al. Stem cell factor is encoded at the Sl locus of the mouse and is the ligand for the c-kit tyrosine kinase receptor. *Cell.* 1990;63(1):213-224.

413. Anderson DM, Lyman SD, Baird A, et al. Molecular cloning of mast cell growth factor, a hematopoietin that is active in both membrane bound and soluble forms. *Cell.* 1990;63(1):235-243.

414. Flanagan JG, Chan DC, Leder P. Transmembrane form of the kit ligand growth factor is determined by alternative splicing and is missing in the Sld mutant. *Cell.* 1991;64(5):1025-1035.

415. Yin T, Li L. The stem cell niches in bone. *J Clin Invest.* 2006;116(5):1195-1201.

416. Calvi LM, Adams GB, Weibrecht KW, et al. Osteoblastic cells regulate the haematopoietic stem cell niche. *Nature.* 2003;425(6960):841-846.

417. Visnjic D, Kalajzic Z, Rowe DW, Katavic V, Lorenzo J, Aguila HL. Hematopoiesis is severely altered in mice with an induced osteoblast deficiency. *Blood.* 2004;103(9):3258-3264.

418. Zhang J, Niu C, Ye L, et al. Identification of the haematopoietic stem cell niche and control of the niche size. *Nature.* 2003;425(6960):836-841.

419. Wilson A, Trumpp A. Bone-marrow haematopoietic-stem-cell niches. *Nat Rev Immunol.* 2006;6(2):93-106.

420. Zhu J, Garrett R, Jung Y, et al. Osteoblasts support B-lymphocyte commitment and differentiation from hematopoietic stem cells. *Blood.* 2007;109(9):3706-3712.

421. Kiel MJ, Radice GL, Morrison SJ. Lack of evidence that hematopoietic stem cells depend on N-cadherin-mediated adhesion to osteoblasts for their maintenance. *Cell Stem Cell.* 2007;1(2):204-217.

The Normal Hematologic System

422. Bowers M, Zhang B, Ho Y, Agarwal P, Chen CC, Bhatia R. Osteoblast ablation reduces normal long-term hematopoietic stem cell self-renewal but accelerates leukemia development. *Blood.* 2015;125(17):2678-2688.

423. Ding L, Morrison SJ. Haematopoietic stem cells and early lymphoid progenitors occupy distinct bone marrow niches. *Nature.* 2013;495(7440):231-235.

424. Omatsu Y, Sugiyama T, Kohara H, et al. The essential functions of adipo-osteogenic progenitors as the hematopoietic stem and progenitor cell niche. *Immunity.* 2010;33(3):387-399.

425. Hosokawa K, Arai F, Yoshihara H, et al. Cadherin-based adhesion is a potential target for niche manipulation to protect hematopoietic stem cells in adult bone marrow. *Cell Stem Cell.* 2010;6(3):194-198.

426. Hosokawa K, Arai F, Yoshihara H, et al. Knockdown of N-cadherin suppresses the long-term engraftment of hematopoietic stem cells. *Blood.* 2010;116(4):554-563.

427. Kiel MJ, Acar M, Radice GL, Morrison SJ. Hematopoietic stem cells do not depend on N-cadherin to regulate their maintenance. *Cell Stem Cell.* 2009;4(2):170-179.

428. Greenbaum A, Hsu YM, Day RB, et al. CXCL12 in early mesenchymal progenitors is required for haematopoietic stem-cell maintenance. *Nature.* 2013;495(7440):227-230.

429. Ding L, Saunders TL, Enikolopov G, Morrison SJ. Endothelial and perivascular cells maintain haematopoietic stem cells. *Nature.* 2012;481(7382):457-462.

430. Kopp HG, Avecilla ST, Hooper AT, Rafii S. The bone marrow vascular niche: home of HSC differentiation and mobilization. *Physiology.* 2005;20:349-356.

431. Kunisaki Y, Bruns I, Scheiermann C, et al. Arteriolar niches maintain haematopoietic stem cell quiescence. *Nature.* 2013;502(7473):637-643.

432. Hooper AT, Butler JM, Nolan DJ, et al. Engraftment and reconstitution of hematopoiesis is dependent on VEGFR2-mediated regeneration of sinusoidal endothelial cells. *Cell Stem Cell.* 2009;4(3):263-274.

433. Butler JM, Nolan DJ, Vertes EL, et al. Endothelial cells are essential for the self-renewal and repopulation of Notch-dependent hematopoietic stem cells. *Cell Stem Cell.* 2010;6(3):251-264.

434. Kobayashi H, Butler JM, O'Donnell R, et al. Angiocrine factors from Akt-activated endothelial cells balance self-renewal and differentiation of haematopoietic stem cells. *Nat Cell Biol.* 2010;12(11):1046-1056.

435. Yamazaki S, Ema H, Karlsson G, et al. Nonmyelinating Schwann cells maintain hematopoietic stem cell hibernation in the bone marrow niche. *Cell.* 2011;147(5):1146-1158.

436. Zhao M, Perry JM, Marshall H, et al. Megakaryocytes maintain homeostatic quiescence and promote post-injury regeneration of hematopoietic stem cells. *Nat Med.* 2014;20(11):1321-1326.

437. Bruns I, Lucas D, Pinho S, et al. Megakaryocytes regulate hematopoietic stem cell quiescence through CXCL4 secretion. *Nat Med.* 2014;20(11):1315-1320.

438. Nakamura-Ishizu A, Takubo K, Fujioka M, Suda T. Megakaryocytes are essential for HSC quiescence through the production of thrombopoietin. *Biochem Biophys Res Commun.* 2014;454(2):353-357.

439. Heazlewood SY, Neaves RJ, Williams B, Haylock DN, Adams TE, Nilsson SK. Megakaryocytes co-localise with hemopoietic stem cells and release cytokines that up-regulate stem cell proliferation. *Stem Cell Res.* 2013;11(2):782-792.

440. Pinho S, Lacombe J, Hanoun M, et al. PDGFRα and CD51 mark human nestin+ sphere-forming mesenchymal stem cells capable of hematopoietic progenitor cell expansion. *J Exp Med.* 2013;210(7):1351-1367.

441. Omatsu Y, Seike M, Sugiyama T, Kume T, Nagasawa T. Foxc1 is a critical regulator of haematopoietic stem/progenitor cell niche formation. *Nature.* 2014;508(7497):536-540.

442. Sacchetti B, Funari A, Michienzi S, et al. Self-renewing osteoprogenitors in bone marrow sinusoids can organize a hematopoietic microenvironment. *Cell.* 2007;131(2):324-336.

443. Bianco P. Bone and the hematopoietic niche: a tale of two stem cells. *Blood.* 2011;117(20):5281-5288.

444. Giancotti FG, Ruoslahti E. Integrin signaling. *Science.* 1999;285(5430):1028-1032.

445. Lévesque JP, Simmons PJ. Cytoskeleton and integrin-mediated adhesion signaling in human CD34+ hemopoietic progenitor cells. *Exp Hematol.* 1999;27(4):579-586.

446. Liu S, Kiosses WB, Rose DM, et al. A fragment of paxillin binds the alpha 4 integrin cytoplasmic domain (tail) and selectively inhibits alpha 4-mediated cell migration. *J Biol Chem.* 2002;277(23):20887-20894.

447. Takahira H, Gotoh A, Ritchie A, Broxmeyer HE. Steel factor enhances integrin-mediated tyrosine phosphorylation of focal adhesion kinase (pp125FAK) and paxillin. *Blood.* 1997;89(5):1574-1584.

448. Kapur R, Cooper R, Zhang L, Williams DA. Cross-talk between alpha(4)beta(1)/alpha(5)beta(1) and c-Kit results in opposing effect on growth and survival of hematopoietic cells via the activation of focal adhesion kinase, mitogen-activated protein kinase, and Akt signaling pathways. *Blood.* 2001;97(7):1975-1981.

449. Verfaillie CM, Benis A, Iida J, McGlave PB, McCarthy JB. Adhesion of committed human hematopoietic progenitors to synthetic peptides from the C-terminal heparin-binding domain of fibronectin: cooperation between the integrin alpha 4 beta 1 and the CD44 adhesion receptor. *Blood.* 1994;84(6):1802-1811.

450. Yin Z, Giacomello E, Gabriele E, et al. Cooperative activity of alpha4beta1 and alpha4beta7 integrins in mediating human B-cell lymphoma adhesion and chemotaxis on fibronectin through recognition of multiple synergizing binding sites within the central cell-binding domain. *Blood.* 1999;93(4):1221-1230.

451. Chan JY, Watt SM. Adhesion receptors on haematopoietic progenitor cells. *Br J Haematol.* 2001;112(3):541-557.

452. Ghaffari S, Smadja-Joffe F, Oostendorp R, et al. CD44 isoforms in normal and leukemic hematopoiesis. *Exp Hematol.* 1999;27(6):978-993.

453. Wight TN, Kinsella MG, Keating A, Singer JW. Proteoglycans in human long-term bone marrow cultures: biochemical and ultrastructural analyses. *Blood.* 1986;67(5):1333-1343.

454. Siczkowski M, Clarke D, Gordon MY. Binding of primitive hematopoietic progenitor cells to marrow stromal cells involves heparan sulfate. *Blood.* 1992;80(4):912-919.

455. Minguell JJ, Hardy C, Tavassoli M. Membrane-associated chondroitin sulfate proteoglycan and fibronectin mediate the binding of hemopoietic progenitor cells to stromal cells. *Exp Cell Res.* 1992;201(1):200-207.

456. Uhlmann DL, Luikhart SD. The role of proteoglycans in the adhesion and differentiation of hematopoietic cells. In: Long MW, Wicha MS, eds. *The Hematopoietic Microenvironment.* Johns Hopkins University Press; 1993:232-245.

457. Bruno E, Luikart SD, Long MW, Hoffman R. Marrow-derived heparan sulfate proteoglycan mediates the adhesion of hematopoietic progenitor cells to cytokines. *Exp Hematol.* 1995;23:1212-1217.

458. Gordon MY, Riley GP, Watt SM, Greaves MF. Compartmentalization of a haematopoietic growth factor (GM-CSF) by glycosaminoglycans in the bone marrow microenvironment. *Nature.* 1987;326(6111):403-405.

459. Roberts R, Gallagher J, Spooncer E, Allen TD, Bloomfield F, Dexter TM. Heparan sulphate bound growth factors: a mechanism for stromal cell mediated haemopoiesis. *Nature.* 1988;332(6162):376-378.

460. Bessis M. Erythroblastic island, functional unity of bone marrow. *Rev Hematol.* 1958;13(1):8-11.

461. Chasis JA, Mohandas N. Erythroblastic islands: niches for erythropoiesis. *Blood.* 2008;112(3):470-478.

462. Ramos P, Casu C, Gardenghi S, et al. Macrophages support pathological erythropoiesis in polycythemia vera and β-thalassemia. *Nat Med.* 2013;19(4):437-445.

463. Sudo T, Yokota T, Okuzaki D, et al. Endothelial cell-selective adhesion molecule expression in hematopoietic stem/progenitor cells is essential for erythropoiesis recovery after bone marrow injury. *PLoS One.* 2016;11(4):e0154189.

464. Kim TS, Hanak M, Trampont PC, Braciale TJ. Stress-associated erythropoiesis initiation is regulated by type 1 conventional dendritic cells. *J Clin Invest.* 2015;125(10):3965-3980.

465. Egawa T, Kawabata K, Kawamoto H, et al. The earliest stages of B cell development require a chemokine stromal cell-derived factor/pre-B cell growth-stimulating factor. *Immunity.* 2001;15(2):323-334.

466. Tokoyoda K, Egawa T, Sugiyama T, Choi BI, Nagasawa T. Cellular niches controlling B lymphocyte behavior within bone marrow during development. *Immunity.* 2004;20(6):707-718.

467. Sapoznikov A, Pewzner-Jung Y, Kalchenko V, Krauthgamer R, Shachar I, Jung S. Perivascular clusters of dendritic cells provide critical survival signals to B cells in bone marrow niches. *Nat Immunol.* 2008;9(4):388-395.

468. Cordeiro Gomes A, Hara T, Lim VY, et al. Hematopoietic stem cell niches produce lineage-instructive signals to control multipotent progenitor differentiation. *Immunity.* 2016;45(6):1219-1231.

469. Terashima A, Okamoto K, Nakashima T, Akira S, Ikuta K, Takayanagi H. Sepsis-induced osteoblast ablation causes immunodeficiency. *Immunity.* 2016;44(6):1434-1443.

470. Wu JY, Purton LE, Rodda SJ, et al. Osteoblastic regulation of B lymphopoiesis is mediated by Gs{alpha}-dependent signaling pathways. *Proc Natl Acad Sci U S A.* 2008;105(44):16976-16981.

471. Yu VW, Saez B, Cook C, et al. Specific bone cells produce DLL4 to generate thymus-seeding progenitors from bone marrow. *J Exp Med.* 2015;212(5):759-774.

Chapter 6 ■ The Birth, Life, and Death of Red Blood Cells: Erythropoiesis, the Mature Red Blood Cell, and Cell Destruction

JOHN G. QUIGLEY • ROBERT T. MEANS JR • BERTIL GLADER

Our understanding of the birth, life, and death of the red blood cell (RBC) derives from a long history of findings generated by the techniques of classical biochemistry, microscopic anatomy, and physiology, and by recent insights at the molecular level. For many aspects of RBC biology, observations demonstrated throughout the 20th century continue to inform science and medical practice. For that reason, the authors believe it is appropriate that the references cited in this chapter span the years from 1929 to 2021.

ERYTHROPOIESIS

Concept of the Erythron

"There is, unfortunately, no name for this tissue (or organ), and it will save a good deal of paraphrasing and probably some confusion if we make one and call it *erythron*."[1]

Erythropoiesis is the process by which red cells are produced in the bone marrow. For descriptive purposes, the process can be divided into various stages, including the commitment of pluripotent stem cell progeny to erythroid differentiation, the erythropoietin (Epo)-independent or early phase of erythropoiesis, and the Epo-dependent late phase of erythropoiesis. Under normal conditions, erythropoiesis results in a red cell production rate of approximately 2.4 million RBCs per second,[2] by which the red cell mass in the body remains constant at approximately 25 trillion circulating RBCs at steady state. This indicates the presence of precise regulatory control mechanisms. The control mechanisms regulating the later phases of erythropoiesis are better understood than those regulating the early phases. The hormone Epo is established as the major factor governing red cell production.[3] Erythropoiesis involves a large number of cells at different stages of maturation, from stem cell progeny committed to erythroid differentiation to the mature circulating red cell (*Figure 6.1*). The whole mass of these erythroid cells has been termed the erythron,[1] a concept that emphasizes the functional unity of the red cells, their morphologically recognizable marrow precursors, and the functionally defined progenitors of these precursors. The concept of the erythron as a tissue has thus far contributed significantly to the understanding of the physiology and pathology of erythropoiesis.

ERYTHROID CELLS

Committed Erythroid Progenitors

The processes leading from the undifferentiated hematopoietic stem cell (HSC) to erythroid commitment are explored in Chapter 5. Recent studies indicate that the transcription factors GATA2, TAL1, and ERG form an integrated circuit that specifies stem cell-to-erythroid transition.[4] Erythroblasts in the bone marrow are generated from proliferation and differentiation of earlier, more immature erythroid cells termed erythroid progenitors. These progenitor cells are detectable functionally by their ability to form in vitro erythroid colonies.[5] The development of tissue culture techniques for cloning hematopoietic progenitor cells in semisolid culture media in vitro led to the recognition and assay in the human and murine bone marrow of at least two erythroid progenitors, the colony-forming unit-erythroid (CFU-E) and the burst-forming unit-erythroid (BFU-E). Under the influence of cytokines, these progenitors grow in semisolid culture media and give rise to colonies of well-hemoglobinized erythroblasts. The morphological

and functional phenotyping of committed erythroid progenitors have been improved by the identification of stage-specific cell-surface protein markers and, more recently, the description of their transcriptional landscapes using single cell RNA sequencing.[6]

Colony-Forming Unit-Erythroid

The CFU-E is an erythroid cell closely related to the proerythroblast.[7] Under the influence of Epo, it gives rise (in 2-3 days in murine, and in 5-8 days in human marrow) to colonies of 8 to 32 well-hemoglobinized cells.[7,8] The clonal origin of these colonies has been demonstrated, for example, by glucose-6-phosphate dehydrogenase (G6PD) isoenzyme analysis.[9] Morphologically, CFU-E purified from progenitor cell cultures appear as immature cells with fine nuclear chromatin; well-defined, large nucleoli; a high nuclear-cytoplasmic ratio; a perinuclear clear zone; and basophilic cytoplasm with pseudopods. On electron microscopy, they appear as primitive blasts with dispersed nuclear chromatin, prominent nucleoli, and an agranular cytoplasm containing clumps of mitochondria and frequent pinocytotic vesicles (of unknown function).[10] The number of CFU-E in the human marrow ranges from 50 to 400/10^5 light-density, nonadherent, mononuclear cells, varying significantly with the methods used for cell separation, and the culture conditions. The majority of CFU-E are actively synthesizing DNA as

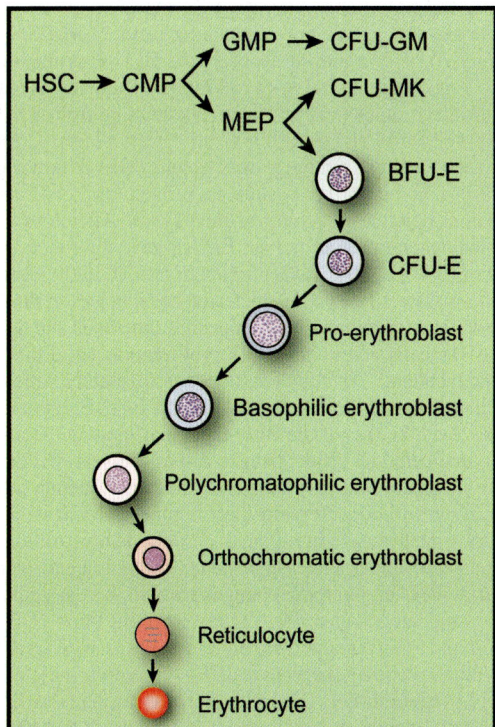

FIGURE 6.1 Schematic representation of the differentiation of erythroid cells from multipotent hematopoietic stem cells. CFU-E, colony-forming unit-erythroid; CFU-GM, colony-forming unit-granulocyte-monocyte; CFU-MK, colony-forming unit-megakaryocyte; CMP, common myeloid progenitor; FU-E, burst-forming unit-erythroid; GMP, granulocyte-monocyte progenitor; MEP, megakaryocyte-erythroid progenitor.

demonstrated by a 70% to 90% cell death after a short exposure to ³H-thymidine in vitro (³H-thymidine suicide assay), or cycle-specific chemotherapeutic agents in vivo.[11] In intact animals, the size of the CFU-E compartment depends on the levels of circulating Epo. Anemia associated with high Epo levels or with the administration of Epo leads to expansion of the CFU-E compartment, whereas transfusion-induced polycythemia leads to low Epo levels and a significant reduction of the CFU-E compartment.[12] The CFU-E is the most Epo-sensitive cell, carrying the highest density of Epo receptors (EpoRs) on its surface, and is absolutely dependent on Epo for survival. In the absence of Epo, CFU-E rapidly undergoes apoptosis (programmed cell death),[10,13] likely related to a lack of Epo-induced expression of the antiapoptotic protein Bcl-X(L).[14] However, while the first phase of CFU-E differentiation is Epo dependent, the later stages are not.[15]

Highly purified CFU-Es have been isolated from murine fetal liver cells. These cells express c-kit, the receptor for the cytokine stem cell factor (SCF), are negative for a number of lineage markers (Ter119, B220, Mac-1, CD3, Gr-1, CD32/16, Sca-1, and CD41) and have high cell surface expression of the transferrin receptor (TfR) (CD71) and of the heat stable antigen CD24.[16]

Burst-Forming Unit-Erythroid

The BFU-E is an erythroid progenitor that is less mature than the CFU-E and is more closely related to the multipotent HSC, with fewer than 25% of cells undergoing active DNA synthesis.[11,12] Unlike CFU-E, BFU-E have a (limited) capacity for self-renewal and are detectable in the peripheral blood at a concentration of 0.02% to 0.05% of light-density mononuclear blood cells.[17,18] Morphologically, the BFU-E is also smaller than CFU-E and appears as an immature blast cell with moderately basophilic cytoplasm, occasional pseudopods, very fine nuclear chromatin, and large nucleoli.[16,19] On electron microscopy, the cytoplasm contains polyribosomes that are less abundant than in CFU-E, while the nucleus contains small amounts of clumped heterochromatin and prominent nucleoli.[19]

In the presence of Epo and under the influence of cytokines that act on early hematopoietic cells, such as interleukin-3 (IL-3), IL-6, granulocyte-macrophage colony-stimulating factor (GM-CSF), thrombopoietin (Tpo), and, importantly, SCF, the BFU-E progenitor gives rise, in 5 to 7 days in mice and in 14 to 17 days in humans, to clusters of many erythroid colonies (a large "burst") containing from 500 to more than 30 to 40,000 well-hemoglobinized erythroblasts. Conversely, cytokines such as transforming growth factor (TGF)-β, tumor necrosis factor (TNF)-α, and interferon-γ suppress progenitor proliferation. The BFU-E is considered a progenitor of the CFU-E. After 6 to 8 days in culture, cells generated from human BFU-E have the functional characteristics of CFU-E.[10] The concentration of BFU-E in the human bone marrow varies from 10 to 50/10⁵ nucleated cells; however, this number fluctuates widely depending on cell separation methods and the culture conditions. The early stages of BFU-E proliferation and differentiation are Epo independent[12,19]; however, they are absolutely dependent on IL-3 for their survival.[19] Only 20% of blood BFU-E express detectable EpoR,[19] and the size of the BFU-E compartment in the marrow of animals is unaffected by acute changes in the levels of circulating Epo induced by anemia or transfusional polycythemia.[12] Anemia can induce BFU-E cycling without affecting their numbers,[20] and in vitro Epo induces DNA synthesis.[21] In humans, chronic administration of Epo is also associated with an increase in the concentration and cycling status of marrow BFU-E; but these changes are also seen in granulocytic-monocytic, and megakaryocytic colony-forming units (CFUs-GM, CFU-MK), and multilineage progenitors such as CFU-granulocye/erythroid/monocyte/megakaryocyte (CFU-GEMM), indicating that, at the early progenitor cell level, the marrow responds to Epo as an organ in a non–lineage-specific manner.[22] Therefore, the early stages of erythropoiesis at the BFU-E level appear to be Epo independent, with Epo dependence developing at a stage between BFU-E and CFU-E.[19] However, the distinction between early (BFU-E) and late (CFU-E) erythroid progenitors is by itself artificial. There are a variety of cells between BFU-E and CFU-E that form a continuum of erythroid progenitors at different stages of differentiation with properties between

those of BFU-E and those of CFU-E.[11] During erythroid development, early progenitors of high proliferative potential and a relatively low cycling status with absolute dependence on IL-3 and responsiveness to, but not dependence on Epo, differentiate progressively through various stages into later progenitors of low proliferative potential and a high cycling status that are IL-3 independent and completely Epo dependent.

Studies in mice and in humans allow for prospective identification of these broad progenitor populations using cell surface markers.[23] While both BFU-E and CFU-E express c-kit, murine BFU-Es are distinguished from CFU-E in that they have much lower cell surface expression of CD24 and CD71.[16] The type III TGF-β receptor (endoglin, CD105) has been identified as a cell surface marker that can distinguish "early" from "late" BFU-E.[24] It has been proposed that BFU-Es comprise the majority of the Lin⁻ CD34⁺ CD38⁺ IL-3Rα⁻/ᶫᵒ CD45RA⁻ CD71⁺ CD105⁻ cells in human bone marrow, while the Lin⁻ CD34⁺ CD38⁺ IL-3Rα⁻/ᶫᵒ CD45RA⁻ CD71ⁱⁿᵗ/⁺ CD105⁺ population contains CFU-E.[25]

Erythroid Precursors

The least mature recognizable erythrocyte precursor cell is known as the proerythroblast (or pronormoblast). The various stages of maturation, in order of increasing maturity, are proerythroblasts, basophilic erythroblasts, polychromatophilic erythroblasts, and orthochromatic erythroblasts. The morphologic characteristics of each stage, as seen with light microscopy after staining with Romanowsky dyes, are widely agreed upon. Cytoplasmic maturation is assessed by the change in staining characteristics, with the deep blue color derived from the high RNA content of immature cells giving way to the red color characteristic of hemoglobin. Nuclear maturation is evaluated by the disappearance of nucleoli and chromatin condensation as nuclear activity decreases. In addition, there is a gradual decrease in cell size and EpoR expression and terminally, exit from the cell cycle.

Stages of Erythroblastic Differentiation

The proerythroblast is a round or oval cell of moderate to large size (14-19 µm diameter) (*Figure 6.2A*). It possesses a relatively large nucleus, occupying perhaps 80% of the cell, and a rim of basophilic cytoplasm. Nucleoli may be prominent. Only small amounts

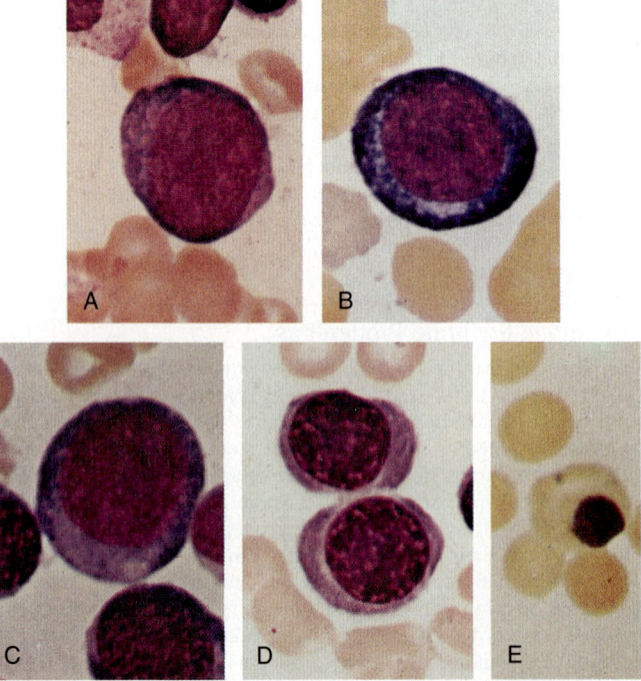

FIGURE 6.2 Erythroblasts. Proerythroblast (A); basophilic erythroblast (B); early (C) and late (D) polychromatophilic erythroblasts; orthochromatic erythroblast with stippling (E). Magnification × 1000; Wright stain.

of hemoglobin are present that cannot be detected by Giemsa stain. When compared to myeloblasts and lymphoblasts, the cytoplasm is more homogeneous and condensed and may appear granular. A small, pale area may be found in the cytoplasm, probably corresponding to the Golgi apparatus.[26]

The basophilic erythroblast is similar to the proerythroblast except that nucleoli are no longer visible and the cell is smaller (12-17 μm in diameter) (*Figure 6.2B*). Condensation of chromatin (formation of heterochromatin) begins and, on light microscopy, the chromatin may appear coarse and granular; thus, there is little resemblance to the myeloblast. Ribosomes reach their maximum number during this stage (reflecting protein synthesis rates), and thus the cytoplasm is deeply basophilic.

The first faint blush of hemoglobin, as indicated by one or more pink areas near the nucleus in dry fixed preparations, introduces the next stage, the polychromatophilic erythroblast (*Figure 6.2C* and *D*). Increasing chromatin condensation is seen and irregular masses of chromatin are formed. Nucleoli are not visible. The nucleus is smaller (7-9 μm) as is the cell as a whole (12-15 μm).

When the cytoplasm possesses almost its full complement of hemoglobin, the cell is termed an orthochromatic erythroblast (*Figure 6.2E*), the smallest of the nucleated erythrocyte precursors (8-12 μm in diameter). At this stage, the nucleus undergoes pyknotic degeneration, the chromatin becomes greatly condensed, and the nucleus shrinks. It may assume various bizarre forms such as buds, rosettes, or clover leaves prior to extrusion (*Figure 6.3*).

After the nucleus is extruded, the cell is known as a reticulocyte. These cells are larger than mature erythrocytes, perhaps 20% greater in volume.[27] They retain certain cytoplasmic organelles, such as residual ribosomes, mitochondria, and the Golgi complex (*Figure 6.3C* and *D*), and have special staining characteristics. Methyl alcohol or similar fixative agents used in staining cause precipitation of the ribosomal RNA. Such cells may thus appear uniformly blue or gray (diffuse basophilia), or basophilic shades may be intermingled with pink-staining areas (polychromatophilia or polychromasia). Certain supravital staining techniques (see Chapter 1) cause the ribosomal RNA to precipitate or aggregate into a network of strands or clumps termed reticulum, for example, cresyl blue agglutinates ribosomes. As the reticulocyte matures, the various organelles decrease in number. Usually, the mitochondria disappear first and the ribosomes last. "Autophagic vacuoles" (secondary lysosomes) containing degenerated organelles may be seen. The shape of the reticulocyte, as revealed by the scanning electron microscope, differs from that of the mature erythrocyte. Only in the late stages of maturation does the biconcave disc shape of the mature red cell appear.

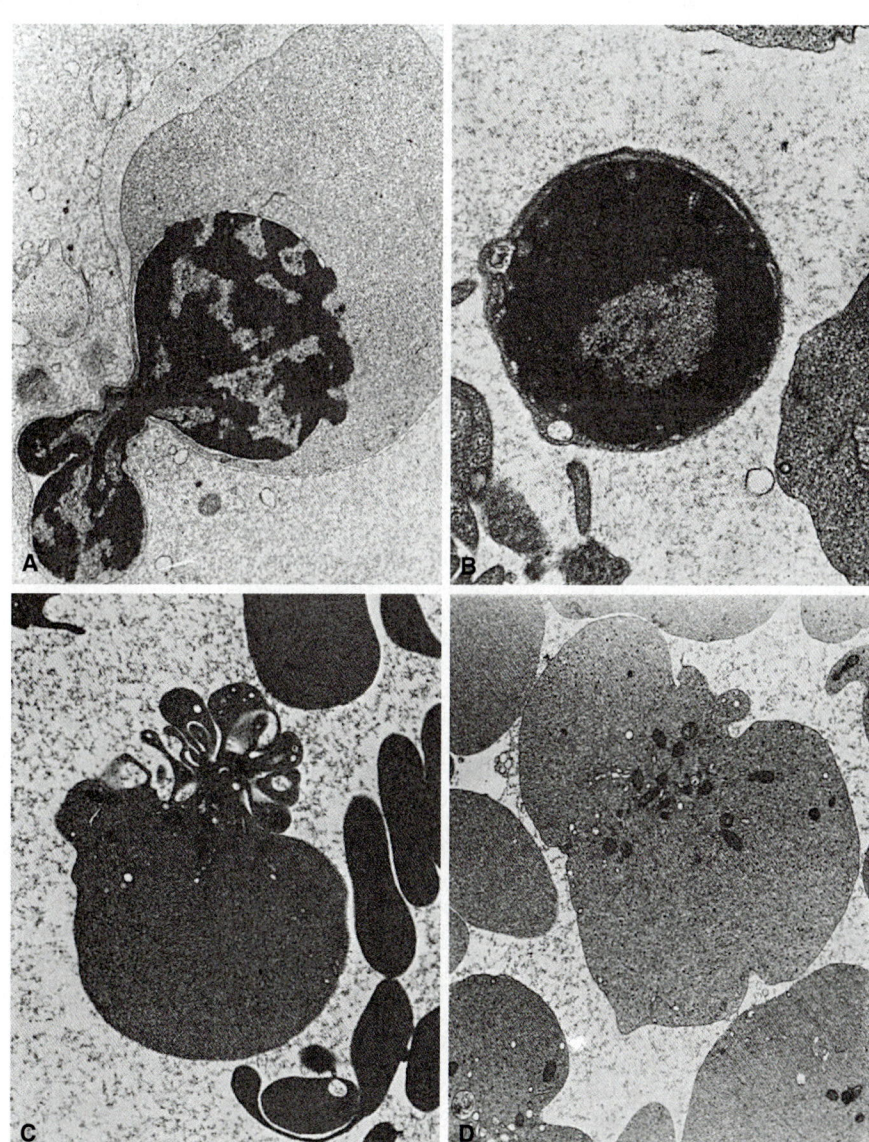

FIGURE 6.3 Formation of reticulocytes. A, Erythroblast expelling nucleus. B, Erythroblast nucleus after expulsion, with rim of cytoplasm. C, Reticulocyte immediately after expulsion of nucleus. D, Reticulocyte. (Courtesy of Dr Carl Kjeldsberg.)

Flow Cytometric Analysis of Erythroid Precursors

Populations of murine or human erythroid precursors may be distinguished broadly by cell surface antigens. Analyses of murine hematopoietic tissues (bone marrow, spleen,[28] or fetal liver[29]) demonstrate that the TfR (CD71) is expressed at very high levels by the early erythroid precursors, proerythroblasts and early basophilic erythroblasts (for iron uptake for high-level heme synthesis), and that CD71 expression then decreases with erythroid maturation (and decreasing heme synthesis). On the other hand Ter-119 (an antibody that recognizes an antigen associated with the predominant mature red cell membrane glycoprotein, glycophorin A [GPA]) is expressed at intermediate levels in proerythroblasts and subsequently at high levels in more differentiated precursors.[28] Thus, double immunostaining for these antigens (while excluding anucleate red cells) results in four cell populations, $CD71^{high}Ter119^{med}$, $CD71^{high}Ter119^{high}$, $CD71^{med}Ter119^{high}$, and $CD71^{low}Ter119^{high}$, corresponding broadly to proerythroblasts, basophilic, polychromatophilic, and orthochromatic murine erythroblasts, respectively, while gating by cell size and nuclear size can help in further refining these populations.[30] Similar immunostaining patterns have also been described during differentiation of human erythroid precursors; however, TfR expression appears to be more variable. Studies of human proerythroblast maturation indicate that the combination of CD36 (a high affinity scavenger receptor) and CD235a (GPA) or CD71 expression can be reliably used to discern basophilic, polychromatophilic and orthochromatic erythroblasts by flow cytometry.[24]

Proliferation and Maturation of the Erythron

Within the erythron, cellular maturation and proliferation proceed simultaneously. While BFU-E progenitors have some limited self-renewal capacity, CFU-E and the erythroid precursors are functionally destined to mature, and incapable of self-maintenance. In response to acute demands, such as hemorrhage or hemolysis, maintenance of the erythron occurs primarily through the action of Epo promoting both progenitor proliferation (in part through increasing the CFU-E pool by reducing apoptosis)[19] and accelerating terminal maturation. As discussed, a majority of CFU-E progenitors, however, are already in cycle and can undergo at most three to five divisions with maximal Epo stimulation, thus limiting the erythron response. With greater (or more chronic) demands, there appears to be an increase in BFU-E self-renewal divisions to further increase the size of the CFU-E pool.[31] Even greater requirements, for example, during recovery from bone marrow irradiation, necessitate input from the stem cell compartment (see Chapter 5). When severe anemia is present from birth, for example, in patients with the congenital hemolytic anemia thalassemia major (Chapter 35), there is, in addition to maximal expansion of the various erythroid progenitor and precursor compartments, expansion of the sites of erythropoiesis from the axial bones (vertebra, pelvis, clavicles, ribs, and sternum) to other sites, potentially including the femurs, humeri, skull, spleen, liver, and even thymus.

A scheme of the proliferation of the erythron and its various stages of development is presented in *Figure 6.1*. It takes approximately 2 weeks (14-17 days) for a cell at the BFU-E stage to mature into erythroblasts. Within 6 to 10 days, a BFU-E proliferates and differentiates into a CFU-E, which needs another 5 to 7 days to proliferate and develop into basophilic erythroblasts: a period during which the CFU-E undergoes three to five successive divisions. Three to five cell divisions also occur during the maturation of erythroid precursors.[32] Thus, 8 to 32 mature red cells are derived from each proerythroblast. Cell division ceases at the stage of polychromatophilic erythroblasts. Orthochromatic erythroblasts cannot synthesize DNA and, therefore, cannot divide. Two events may decrease the yield of cells: either death of erythrocytes before or shortly after release from the marrow (ineffective erythropoiesis) (Chapter 24), or a skipped cell division, a phenomenon that may occur with increased Epo stimulation and that results in a large hemoglobin-poor cell (Chapter 2). These events occur to a limited extent in normal subjects but occur more frequently under pathologic circumstances.

The biochemical events that occur in stem cell progeny during commitment to erythroid differentiation remain incompletely understood. The same holds true for the committed early erythroid progenitor BFU-E.

This cell is IL-3 dependent and expresses only small numbers of EpoR.[19] Within 72 hours in culture, it becomes fully dependent on Epo ("mature" BFU-E) and, in its presence, proliferates and differentiates into CFU-E progenitors.[10,19] With Epo stimulation, there is selective upregulation of transcription factors including GATA1[33] (related to demethylation),[34] KLF1 (also known as EKLF1),[35] and NFE2.[36] GATA1 interacts with SCL/Tal1 (complexed with LMO2, LDB1, and E2A), or with KLF1, and others, in multiprotein complexes that associate with, and activate (or, for example, with Gfi-1b, repress) erythroid genes.[31,37-39]

At this (CFU-E) stage, a number of differentiation events can be detected. Epo induces an increase in mRNA synthesis, closely followed by induction of murine globin gene transcription.[40] Other biochemical events associated with terminal erythroid differentiation include increased uptake of calcium, glucose, and amino acids; synthesis of TfRs; increased iron uptake; heme and globin synthesis; and the appearance of erythrocyte membrane proteins (e.g., anion exchanger-1 (AE1; also called band 3 and band 4.1)[41-43] There is a GATA1-dependent phase of differentiation, regulating EpoR, antiapoptotic genes (especially *BCL-X(L)*), and alpha (α-) globin gene expression that is then succeeded by a KLF1-dependent phase.[44] KLF1 appears to regulate expression of genes essential for many key aspects of terminal erythroid differentiation including those encoding for major cytoskeletal and cell membrane proteins (ankyrin, AE1, band 4.1, dematin, glycophorins A and C), iron transport proteins (TfR at the cell membrane and mitoferrin-1 in mitochondria[45]), heme synthesis enzymes, α- and beta (β-)globin chains, and α-hemoglobin stabilizing protein (AHSP, which stabilizes α-globin chains and increases their affinity for β-globin chains[35,46,47]).

Recent studies also demonstrate the importance of alterations in cell metabolism during erythroid differentiation. For example the protein complex mTORC1,[48] which couples protein translation to nutrient availability, appears critical for differentiation. Epo-EpoR–induced activation of the AKT pathway (see below) increases mTORC1 signaling during erythropoiesis, promoting, for example, translation of mRNAs encoding mitochondria-associated proteins. Mitochondrial biogenesis in response to mTORC1 stimulation during erythroid differentiation is essential to produce the adenosine triphosphate (ATP) needed to fuel the large amount of heme and globin production that occurs over 2 to 3 days in the developing erythrocyte[49]; additionally, mitochondria are the site of heme synthesis. Loss of mitochondrial proteins such as PHB2 or TFAM in developing murine red cells moderates the normal large increase in mitochondrial mass, is associated with decreased differentiation, proliferation, and survival, and results in anemia. The sensing of sufficient cytosolic levels of the branched chain amino acid leucine is a prime activator of mTORC1,[48] and deficiency or inhibition of LAT3, a leucine importer, also impacts hemoglobin production in murine RBCs, with decreased translation of globin-encoding transcripts.[50] Another amino acid, glutamine, is also essential both for erythroid lineage specification of HSC[51] and heme synthesis during late erythropoiesis.[52]

Not surprisingly, other regulators of mitochondrial capacity, energy metabolism, or function are also critical during erythropoiesis. The anemia of copper deficiency appears to be related to erythroid mitochondrial metabolic reprogramming,[53] while knockdown of transcriptional coactivators important for mitochondrial biogenesis, PGC-1α, and/or PGC-1β (haploinsufficient in myelodysplastic syndromes with chromosome 5q deletion (see Chapter 80)) impacts both Hb production and erythroid development.[54,55] Of clinical relevance, studies indicate that leucine supplementation may improve the defects in globin synthesis and the anemia observed in Diamond-Blackfan anemia (DBA), by activating mTOR,[56] while the use of mTORC1 inhibitors in cancer therapeutics is associated with development of anemia.[57]

Hemoglobin synthesis continues as the cell matures into a basophilic erythroblast, and, at the polychromatophilic erythroblast stage, enough hemoglobin has accumulated in the cytoplasm to give the cell the mild acidophilic reaction that is detected by Romanowsky stains. Hemoglobin synthesis continues through the orthochromatic stage and persists at a very low rate in the reticulocyte after enucleation. Mature red cells, lacking ribosomes, cannot synthesize hemoglobin. As previously noted, morphologic evidence of decreasing nuclear activity (heterochromatin formation) can be seen as early as the basophilic erythroblast stage. By the orthochromatic stage, the nucleus is completely inactive, unable to synthesize either

DNA or RNA. The factors leading to cessation of nuclear activity are not fully understood, but may be related to the intracellular hemoglobin concentration.[55] Hemoglobin is found within the nucleus, perhaps transported by biliverdin reductase (BVR) as heme (see Heme Oxygenase section below).[58-60] After reaching a critical concentration,[58] nuclear hemoglobin may then react with nucleohistones, bringing about chromosomal inactivation and nuclear condensation. According to this hypothesis, the number of cell divisions and the ultimate erythrocyte size are related to the rate of hemoglobin synthesis. For example, microcytic cells are produced in iron deficiency because it takes longer to reach the critical hemoglobin concentration and the generation time is unaffected; hence, more cell divisions occur before nuclear inactivation, and the resulting cell is small. In contrast, the macrocytes observed when erythropoiesis is stimulated may be related to an Epo-induced acceleration of hemoglobin synthesis, which in turn leads to an earlier onset of nuclear degeneration and fewer cell divisions. Consistent with this hypothesis is the observation that the mean corpuscular hemoglobin concentration is relatively constant in a variety of mammalian species, even though erythrocyte size varies greatly. Studies indicate that deacetylation of nucleohistones is critical for heterochromatin formation and nuclear condensation, and inhibition of deacetylation (by, for example, HDAC inhibition specifically inhibition of HDAC2[61] or ectopic expression of the histone acetyl transferase Gcn5) impedes chromatin condensation and enucleation during terminal erythroid differentiation.[62]

After the nucleus degenerates, it is extruded from the cell.[63] This process, as observed in living erythroblasts by phase contrast microscopy,[64] is completed in 5 to 60 minutes. The extruded nucleus or "pyrrenocyte" carries with it a rim of cytoplasm, including ribosomes, hemoglobin, and occasional mitochondria.

Enucleation resembles cytokinesis during asymmetric cell division and does not seem to require the presence of extracellular matrix proteins or accessory cells.[20] However, the rate of enucleation of murine erythroleukemia cells is increased when cultured in fibronectin-coated tissue culture dishes.[65] Among the various cytoskeletal proteins, filamentous actin plays an important role in the process of enucleation, accumulating between the extruding nucleus and the incipient reticulocyte, and forming a "cortical actin ring." Notably, cytochalasin D, an inhibitor of filamentous actin, causes complete inhibition of enucleation.[20,66] A Rac GTPase that activates mDia2, a formin involved in nucleation of actin filaments, is absolutely required for formation of the actin ring and enucleation.[67] Colchicine, which disrupts microtubule formation, also impairs enucleation.[68] Interestingly, none of the major erythroid cytoskeletal proteins are found in the region of the cell membrane where the nucleus is extruded, suggesting degradation at the site of extrusion. Nurse cells are macrophages at the center of an island of erythroblasts that appear to regulate terminal erythropoiesis, supplying developmental signals, iron (and possibly heme[69]) to adjacent erythroid cells.[70] Erythroblast macrophage protein (EMP), expressed on erythroblasts and macrophages, appears to be important for erythroblast island formation and erythroblast enucleation. However, like Rac GTPase-deficient cells, EMP-deficient erythroid cells have impaired differentiation that may decrease nuclear condensation and enucleation rates.[71]

MicroRNAs are small non–protein-coding RNAs that each downregulates multiple genes posttranscriptionally; and their importance in erythropoiesis is increasingly being recognized.[72] Studies suggest a role for miR-191 in erythroid enucleation. miR-191 is normally downregulated with erythroid differentiation; however, overexpression represses Mxi1 and Riok3, preventing the physiologic downregulation of Gcn5 expression, chromatin condensation, and enucleation.[73] Downregulation of a number of other factors also impacts terminal erythroid maturation including epigenetic factors (e.g., TET enzymes, Asxl1), cytoskeletal factors (e.g., dynein), and transcription factors (e.g., KLF1, Foxo3) among others.[74]

Within the marrow, enucleation sometimes may occur as the erythroblast traverses the endothelial cell layer that forms the sinus wall.[75] The erythroblast cytoplasm and small organelles (ribosomes and mitochondria) squeeze through endothelial cell cytoplasmic pores 1 to 4 μm in diameter, but the more rigid nucleus cannot conform to this pore size. The nucleus is thus "pitted" from the cell. Passage through the endothelial pores is not essential to enucleation, however, as it is observed in vitro.[20,64] Soon after enucleation, nuclei are engulfed by macrophages.

The enucleated cell may remain within the marrow as a reticulocyte for several days. After release from the marrow, the reticulocyte may be sequestered for 1 to 2 days in the spleen.[76] As the reticulocyte matures to an adult erythrocyte, it loses its ability to synthesize hemoglobin.[77] RNA is catabolized by a ribonuclease and the resulting oligonucleotides are further degraded by phosphodiesterases and phosphatases to nucleotides. A specific pyrimidine 5′-nucleotidase found in reticulocytes dephosphorylates pyrimidine nucleotides, and the free pyrimidine bases can then leak out of the cell. Of clinical note, the pyrimidine 5′-nucleotidase is lacking because of hereditary deficiency, or dysfunctional due to lead poisoning,[78] RNA degradation is retarded, and basophilic stippling due to retained RNA aggregates becomes prominent.

BIOSYNTHESIS OF HEMOGLOBIN

Because hemoglobin accounts for approximately 90% of the dry weight of the mature red cell, the biosynthesis of this protein is intimately related to erythropoiesis. To put hemoglobin biosynthesis in context, each red cell contains 270×10^6 molecules of hemoglobin, each with 4 globin chains and 4 heme moieties. When we consider that a normal adult makes 2.4 million red cells per second, this means our erythron synthesizes and coordinates 2.6 quadrillion (10^{15}) heme and 2.6 quadrillion globin molecules per second.

As detailed in the previous section, many of the morphologic criteria used in staging the maturation of erythrocyte precursors are related to hemoglobin production and content. Furthermore, the initial events associated with the differentiation of CFU-E into erythrocyte precursors include the activation of genes relating to hemoglobin synthesis.[40] Three complex metabolic pathways are required for hemoglobin synthesis, corresponding to the three structural components of hemoglobin: Protein (globin), protoporphyrin, and iron. The first two of these are discussed below. Iron metabolism is described in Chapter 25.

Globin Biosynthesis
Globin Genes and the Structure of Chromatin
Distinct structural genetic loci exist for each of the polypeptide chains in hemoglobin. Thus, there are α, β, γ, δ, and ε genes. In most human populations, the α genetic locus is duplicated, and there are four (two pairs of) identical α genes in normal subjects.[79] There are also at least two different pairs of γ genes, one (Gγ) coding for a γ-chain with glycine at position 136 and another (Aγ) coding for a γ-chain with alanine at the same position.[80] In contrast, only single gene pairs code for the β- and δ-chains, respectively.

The α-gene cluster (approximately 30 kb), located on the short arm of chromosome 16, also contains the locus encoding for the ζ-chain.[81] The β-gene cluster (approximately 50 kb), located on chromosome 11, also includes the genes for the Gγ-, Aγ-, δ-, and ε-globins.[81,82] A schematic representation is shown in *Figure 6.4*.

The globin genes are discussed in detail in Chapter 36.

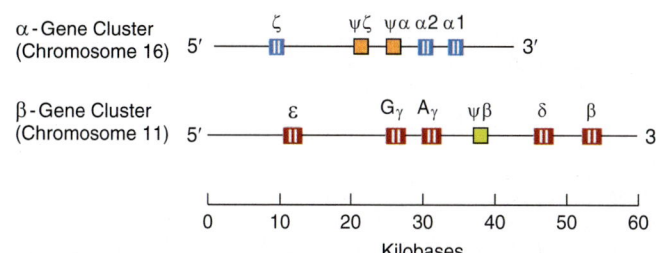

FIGURE 6.4 Organization of the human globin gene clusters on chromosomes 16 and 11. Solid areas within genes represent coding sequences; open areas represent intervening sequences. Each cluster includes pseudogenes ($\Psi\zeta$, $\Psi\alpha$, $\Psi\beta$), which have sequence homology to functional genes but include mutations that prevent their expression.

Regulation of Globin Synthesis

Heme is of particular importance in regulating the rate of globin synthesis.[83,84] It stimulates globin synthesis in intact reticulocytes and cell-free systems, and, in its absence, polyribosomes disaggregate.[85] The major effect of heme is exerted on the chain initiation step in translation. In the absence of heme, an inhibitor of globin synthesis accumulates.[86,87] This inhibitor, a heme-regulated eIF2α kinase (HRI), acts by phosphorylating the α-subunit of an initiation factor, eIF-2, that promotes binding of the initiator transfer RNA, tRNAMetf, to ribosomes, and by so doing shuts down protein synthesis (predominantly globin).[88,89] HRI, which has two heme binding sites (or heme regulatory motifs, HRMs) serves as a sensitive intracellular heme "sensor" that closely balances heme availability with globin chain production to prevent the accumulation of excessive unfolded globin proteins.[90] Studies of the *Hri* knockout mouse verify the importance of this protective mechanism during high-level hemoglobin synthesis, since in its absence steady state protein synthesis is considerably increased. HRI function is especially important in iron deficiency: in these circumstances the continued globin production in *hri*–/– mice results in cytotoxic globin protein precipitates, oxidative stress, and apoptosis of late erythroid precursors.[91] The red cells of iron-deficient *hri*–/– mice are normocytic/hyperchromic rather than microcytic/hypochromic and have globin chain inclusions, likely due to continued globin production. HRI also serves to ameliorate the phenotype of β-thalassemia in mice models, minimizing the production and accumulation of α-globin aggregates, apoptosis of erythroid precursors, and the ineffective erythropoiesis. Recent work indicates that HRI is also activated by oxidative stress (as occurs during erythropoiesis in β-thalassemia).[92] HRI-mediated inhibition of eIF2 activates the integrated stress response (ISR) and activating transcription factor 4 (ATF4) and through this (and other unknown mechanisms) also serves to regulate mTORC1 and its effects on protein translation.[93]

Notably, in addition to its effects on globin translation, heme also exerts positive effects on globin transcription, through nuclear binding to the globin gene transcriptional repressor Bach1 during erythroid differentiation.[94]

Heme Biosynthesis

Porphyrins are heterocyclic organic rings composed of four pyrrole subunits that are usually linked by methine bridges; their conjugation to diverse divalent metal ions such as Mg^{2+}, Co^{2+}, and Fe^{2+} gives rise to the "pigments of life," that is, chlorophyll, vitamin B_{12}, and heme, respectively. Heme, which is a complex of ferrous iron with the tetrapyrrole protoporphyrin IX, is ubiquitous in aerobic cells and essential for cellular oxidation-reduction reactions. It serves as a critical component of hemoproteins, including cytochromes (for mitochondrial respiratory chain electron transfer and drug metabolism), oxidases (e.g., NADPH oxidase) and peroxidases, catalases and synthases (e.g., nitric oxide synthase, NOS), in addition to the oxygen storage and transport molecules, myoglobin and hemoglobin.[95-102] The four pyrrole rings of protoporphyrin IX are designated A, B, C, and D. At the periphery of the tetrapyrrole are eight sites where side chains are located. In heme, the iron atom is inserted "like a gem"[101] into the center of the tetrapyrrole. Note that heme is the ferrous iron complex of protoporphyrin IX; however, the term *heme* is also used in the generic sense in the literature to indicate iron protoporphyrin IX without regard to the oxidation state (valence) of the iron.

Porphyrins are cyclically conjugated tetrapyrroles that have a number of common properties. They are very stable, essentially flat molecules and the macrocyclic ring itself has little or no affinity for water. All porphyrins are intensely colored and they have an extremely intense absorption band at approximately 400 nm, the so-called Soret band. All porphyrins fluoresce, but fluorescence is characteristically lost when metals are bound to form metalloporphyrins. Exceptions include Mg-porphyrins and Zn-porphyrins, which fluoresce despite their metal content (Chapter 28). Of the known porphyrins, five are of importance in humans: Uroporphyrin (two isomers), coproporphyrin (two isomers), and protoporphyrin (one isomer). Fully reduced

porphyrins are called porphyrinogens and comprise most of the tetrapyrroles that are intermediates in heme biosynthesis. Porphyrinogens are colorless, do not fluoresce, cannot bind metal ions, and are extremely unstable with regard to oxidation, which changes them to porphyrins. If uroporphyrinogen or coproporphyrinogen is oxidized to its corresponding porphyrins, they cannot function as substrates for the heme biosynthetic enzymes and must eventually be excreted in the urine (the porphyrins with many carboxyl groups—"uroporphyrins") and stool (porphyrins with few carboxyl groups—"coproporphyrins"). Uroporphyrinogen and coproporphyrinogen can occur in four isomeric forms. Of these, only two are known to occur naturally in mammalian tissues, namely, isomer forms I and III. Without exception, all biologically functional tetrapyrroles are derived from uroporphyrinogen III. Uroporphyrinogen I and coproporphyrinogen I are useless by-products of heme synthesis (see Chapter 28). Once formed, most uroporphyrinogen I is enzymatically decarboxylated to coproporphyrinogen I and excreted as the oxidized compound, coproporphyrin I.

The first of eight steps in the biosynthesis of heme (*Figure 6.5*) is the condensation of glycine and succinyl coenzyme A (CoA) to yield 5-aminolevulinic acid (ALA).[103,104] The formation of 10^9 molecules of heme/RBC implies high intracellular demand for glycine and succinyl-CoA during erythropoiesis. Extracellular glycine is primarily supplied by the transporter GlyT1, and gene knockout in mice[105] or, in a rat model, transport inhibition by a potent selective inhibitor, bitopertin results in a hypochromic microcytic anemia.[106] Expression of the glutamine transporter SLC38a5 is upregulated with nucleoside (SLC28a3) and other transporters by GATA1 during erythroid precursor differentiation[107] and recent studies indicate glutamine serves as the major source of succinyl-CoA for heme synthesis.[52] The condensation reaction occurs in the mitochondrial matrix and the enzyme catalyzing this reaction (ALA synthase [ALAS]) plays a key regulatory role in the biosynthesis of heme. Of clinical interest, ALAS requires pyridoxal phosphate as a cofactor,[108] and vitamin B6 has been used in the treatment of sideroblastic anemias for over 60 years (see Chapter 26). Subsequently, the reduced cyclic tetrapyrrole coproporphyrinogen III is formed in the cytosol from ALA in a series of 4 enzymatic reactions. Note that the product of step 2 is the monopyrrole porphobilinogen, the primary building block for all natural tetrapyrroles, including hemes, chlorophylls, and the vitamin B_{12} derivatives (cobalamins).

Coproporphyrinogen III is then transported back by across the outer mitochondrial membrane from the cytoplasm into the mitochondrial intermembrane space for the three subsequent reactions required to form heme. First, propionic acid side chains at positions 2 and 4 are oxidatively decarboxylated by the enzyme coproporphyrinogen oxidase, forming protoporphyrinogen IX, which is then oxidized by protoporphyrinogen IX oxidase to protoporphyrin IX. The enzymes protoporphyrinogen IX oxidase and ferrochelatase (FECH), catalyzing the penultimate and final steps of heme synthesis, are both localized at the mitochondrial inner membrane—protoporphyrinogen IX oxidase is an intermembrane space–facing protein, while FECH is exposed to the matrix—thus, a channeling of protoporphyrinogen IX and protoporphyrinogen IX through an enzyme complex formed by protoporphyrinogen IX oxidase and FECH within the inner membrane has been proposed, based on biochemical studies and the crystal structure of the two enzymes.[109,110] The final step, the addition of one atom of Fe^{2+} to protoporphyrin IX by FECH, which results in the formation of protoheme or heme *b*, occurs on the matrix side of the inner membrane, necessitating heme transfer, by as yet unidentified transporters (perhaps an isoform of feline leukemia virus subgroup C receptor (FLVCR1b[111]; see below), across both the inner and outer membranes again in order to reach the cytosol.

The biosynthesis of the specific porphyrins is discussed in detail in Chapter 28.

Biosynthesis of Heme

The insertion of ferrous iron into protoporphyrin IX to form heme is catalyzed by the enzyme FECH within the mitochondrial matrix. FECH (EC 4.99.1.1) is the best characterized of the heme biosynthesis enzymes.[112] The enzyme, which functions as a dimer appears to

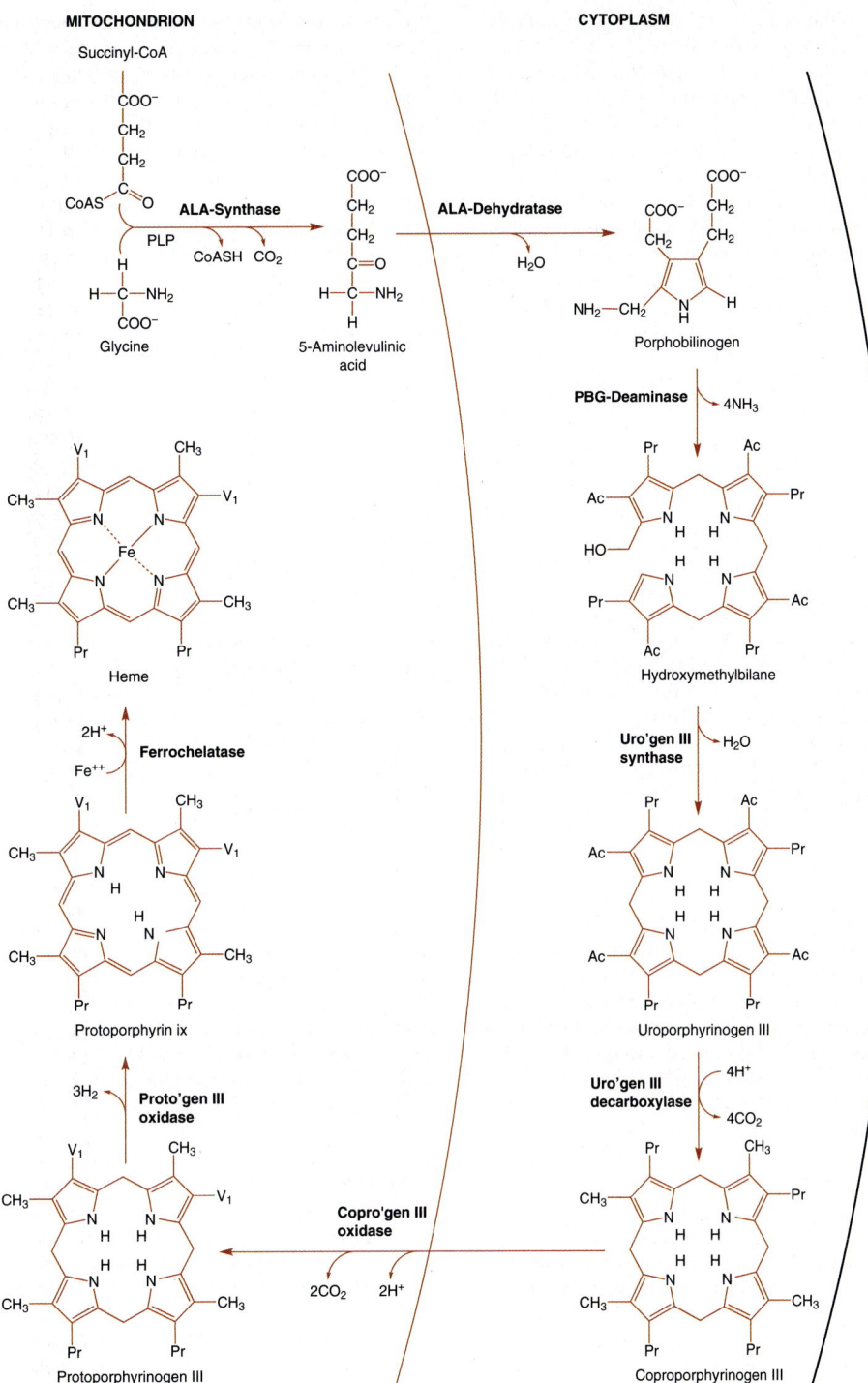

FIGURE 6.5 Heme biosynthetic pathway. Ac, acetate; ALA, δ-aminolevulinic acid; CoA, coenzyme A; CoAS, succinyl-CoA; CoASH, uncombined coenzyme A; COPRO'GEN, coproporphyrinogen; PBG, porphobilinogen; PLP, pyridoxal 5′-phosphate; Pr, propionate; PROTO'GEN, protoporphyrinogen IX (not III); URO'GEN, uroporphyrinogen; Vi, vinyl. (Modified from Bottomley SS, Muller-Eberhard U. Pathophysiology of heme synthesis. *Semin Hematol.* 1988;25(4):282-302. Copyright © 1988 Elsevier. With permission.)

be tightly bound to, or is an integral part of the inner mitochondrial membrane,[113] likely complexed with protoporphyrinogen IX oxidase dimers on the other side of the membrane.[114] Insertion of the iron appears to involve distortion of the planar porphyrin by FECH.[112] No cofactors are required for activity. While the in vivo substrates are ferrous iron and protoporphyrin, in vitro, the enzyme can also catalyze incorporation of iron, cobalt, or zinc into several dicarboxylic porphyrins (protoporphyrin, mesoporphyrin, and deuteroporphyrin).[96] Of clinical interest, an increase in zinc incorporation into protoporphyrin occurs in the context of iron deficiency and lead poisoning, but may

also occur when excess protoporphyrins are produced, for example, in X-linked protoporphyria due to gain-of-function mutations of ALAS2 (see Chapter 28).

Studies in cell lines demonstrate that FECH interacts with mitoferrin-1 (Mfrn1; Slc25a37)—a mitochondrial inner membrane importer of iron upregulated during erythroid differentiation.[115] In elegant studies, it has been shown that Mfrn1 is stabilized by an inner membrane ATP-binding cassette (ABC) transporter known as ABC-me or ABCB10,[116] allowing high efficiency iron uptake into mitochondria for optimal heme synthesis.[117] Further studies show that FECH,

Mfrn1, and ABCB10 are coinduced during MEL cell erythroid differentiation and that Mfrn1 and ABCB10 interact with FECH.[115] The gene encoding ABCB10 was originally identified in a screen of mouse genes upregulated by GATA1 and expression is regulated by heme.[116] Hematopoietic-specific deletion of ABCB10 in adult mice results in high levels of protoporphyrin IX, mitochondrial iron deposits, heme deficiency, and arrested erythropoiesis.[118] The potential substrate of the ABCB10 transporter has not been identified, but heme, which needs to be transferred from the matrix across two mitochondrial membranes into the cytosol, is a candidate. Apart from its use for heme synthesis, mitochondrial iron is also required for mitochondrial Fe-S cluster biogenesis. Fe-S clusters are modular protein cofactors consisting of iron and sulfur, usually linked by bonds joining the cysteine sulfur atoms of a polypeptide ("scaffold") protein to iron atoms of the cluster. They function, for example, as part of enzyme catalytic centers (e.g., aconitase, succinate dehydrogenase).[119] FECH contains a NO-sensitive Fe-S cluster that is attached at the C-terminus.[112] Although the cluster is not required for catalytic function or as a supply of ferrous iron, the enzyme is sensitive to the availability of Fe-S clusters. For example, when Fe-S cluster synthesis is impaired in MEL cells, due to deficiency of the scaffold proteins or iron required for Fe-S cluster biosynthesis, then apo-FECH is rapidly degraded in mitochondria, indicating a direct link between biosynthesis of Fe-S clusters and heme.[120] Recent studies indicate that a small hemoprotein, PGRMC1, functions as a heme chaperone or sensor for the off-loading of heme from FECH, and inhibition impacts erythroid differentiation in vitro.[121] In addition, Epo-activated protein kinase A phosphorylates and activates FECH to also regulate heme synthesis.[122]

The gene encoding FECH is comprised of 11 exons spread out across 45 kb on chromosome 18q21.3.[123] The promoter region has been examined in detail using in vitro and in vivo studies.[124,125] Sp1, NF-E2, and GATA1 elements are identified in the promoter region and a fragment of the promoter containing these binding sites allows expression in hematopoietic cells derived from transgenic embryonic mouse cells where a single copy of a reporter construct was inserted. In vivo erythroid specificity is mediated by NF-E2 elements between 300 and 1100 bp upstream of the transcriptional start site.[124] In vitro assays in K562 cells, the Kruppel-like transcription factor, KLF-13, activates the promoters for porphobilinogen deaminase, 5-aminolevulinate synthase, and ferrochelatase genes.[126] Mutations of the FECH gene are associated with erythropoietic porphyria. Of clinical interest, loss-of-function mutations of the FECH gene in humans are associated with an increase in erythrocyte metal-free protoporphyrins and the disease erythropoietic protoporphyria (Chapter 28).

Regulation of the Heme Biosynthetic Pathway

δ-ALA Synthase

The regulation of a biosynthetic pathway generally occurs at the first enzymatic reaction synthesizing a precursor compound committed to ultimate incorporation into the final product.[127] Frequently, such reactions are strongly exergonic and essentially irreversible. These generalizations hold true for the heme biosynthetic pathway. Control of the pathway is exerted primarily through the enzyme catalyzing the first committed and rate-limiting step, ALAS. However, regulation of the ubiquitous enzyme ALAS1 differs markedly from that of the erythroid-specific enzyme ALAS2.[101,128]

Non-erythroid ALAS1 Regulation

About 15% of the daily production of heme is generated in the liver by ALAS1 for cytochromes and enzymes. The amount of ALAS1 is regulated by induction and repression of enzyme synthesis,[129] and may increase by up to 300-fold.[130] The enzyme has a short half-life, allowing a rapid response to changes in the demand for heme and, thus, ALA.[131] The enzyme may be induced by a number of chemicals, drugs, and nonglucocorticoid steroids.[129] Negative feedback by the pathway end-product, heme, plays a critical central role in ALAS1 regulation, repressing transcription,[132] decreasing the half-life of the mRNA and, through binding to HRMs in the 5′ end of the protein, preventing translocation of the enzyme into the mitochondrial matrix,[133]

direct enzyme inhibition, and a Lon peptidase1–dependent breakdown.[108] When the amount of intracellular heme is high, ALAS1 synthesis is repressed, when the amount of heme is low, synthesis is induced. Agents that interfere with heme synthesis can induce ALAS1, and agents that induce the synthesis of hemoproteins (e.g., induction of cytochrome p450 enzymes by barbiturates), potentially depleting a putative pool of "free" or "uncommitted" heme, can produce a similar effect.[134,135] Agents that exert these effects on ALAS1 synthesis induction are clinically important, as they may precipitate acute attacks in patients with AIP and related disorders of porphyrin metabolism (see Chapter 28).

Early studies indicated that ALAS1 synthesis is induced during fasting, which can precipitate porphyria attacks, and that nutritional supplements (e.g., glucose loading) may ameliorate these acute episodes. Handschin et al have shown that this occurs because ALAS1 expression is induced by the concerted actions of peroxisome proliferator-activated receptor γ coactivator 1α (PGC-1α) and the transcription factors FOXO1 and nuclear respiratory factor-1 on the ALAS1 promoter.[136] PGC-1α, which coactivates nuclear receptors or transcription factors to regulate mitochondrial biogenesis and oxidative phosphorylation, is induced by low glucose levels or glucagon and repressed by high glucose or insulin.[137] Presumably, ALAS1-mediated heme synthesis is required for de novo mitochondrial respiratory chain cytochrome (hemoprotein) synthesis during mitochondrial biogenesis, as a response to decreased cellular ATP levels. Of interest, ALAS1 expression and thus hepatic cytochrome p450 enzyme synthesis is repressed in a liver-specific knockdown of the heme exporter FLVCR in mice, likely related to an increase in intracellular heme levels.[138] More recently, it has been demonstrated that in cancer cells, ALAS1 activity, and thus heme synthesis, is coordinated with heme export by FLVCR in order to suppress the tricyclic acid cycle—succinyl-CoA used for heme synthesis is an important TCA intermediate derived from glutamine metabolism—and thus oxidative phosphorylation, a mechanism important for cancer cell proliferation.[139]

Erythroid ALAS2 Regulation

In contrast to regulation of ALAS1, regulation of ALAS2 in erythroid cells is coordinated with heme synthesis, iron assimilation, and, importantly, globin synthesis. With erythroid differentiation there is coordination of cellular iron assimilation, heme, and globin synthesis to safely allow maximal hemoglobin synthesis within a short timespan without the buildup of individual, potentially cytotoxic components (see below). Regulation of erythroid heme involves the induction of the enzymes of the heme biosynthetic pathway and their regulation once induced,[101,128] regulation of iron uptake and its delivery to FECH in the mitochondria, and the regulated export of the newly formed heme from the mitochondria to the cytosol to bind to globin chains.

Initial studies suggested that the heme biosynthesis pathway enzymes were sequentially induced with erythroid differentiation (from ALAS2 to FECH[140]); however, subsequent studies in MEL cells[141] and maturing populations of human erythroblasts[142] indicate early upregulation of FECH with ALAS2, with synthesis of mRNAs for the terminal three pathway enzymes upregulated within 12 hours of erythroid induction of MEL cells with dimethylsulfoxide (DMSO). In contrast to the repressive effects of heme on ALAS1 in hepatocytes, in erythroid cells, intracellular heme appears necessary for induction of the biosynthetic pathway enzymes, perhaps through upregulation of the erythroid transcription factor NF-E2,[143] and/or inhibition of the transcriptional repressor Bach1.[94] For example, studies of ALAS2-deficient MEL cells following their "erythroid" induction with DMSO demonstrate a lack of erythroid differentiation (as assessed by a lack of upregulation of mRNAs for ALA dehydratase, porphobilinogen deaminase, FECH, and β-globin), that is, at least partially reversed by addition of heme to DMSO, in keeping with studies by others of ALAS2-deficient cell lines.[144]

As discussed, unlike *ALAS1*, there is an IRE in the 5′ UTR of the *ALAS2* gene. Therefore, depletion of cytosolic iron (believed to exist in a putative labile iron pool) in erythroid precursors should result in binding of IRP1 and IRP2 to the IRE of *ALAS* transcripts, preventing translation. Thus, it is the supply of iron to the erythroid precursor that ultimately controls heme synthesis. To allow maximal heme synthesis—which requires ~20 mg of iron for the 20 g of erythrocytes generated in adult humans every day—iron is delivered to the bone marrow in the form of ferric-transferrin (Fe-Tf) that is rapidly bound by TfR1 present in large numbers on the cell surface of erythroid precursors (up to 10^6 receptors per cell[145]). In addition, the mitochondrial iron importer, MFN1, becomes stabilized in a macrocomplex with FECH and ABCB10 following upregulation of ABCB10 with erythroid differentiation, thus facilitating the transfer of iron across the mitochondrial inner membrane to FECH. By necessity, there must also be upregulation of an unidentified heme transporter to export heme from the mitochondria into the cytosol (perhaps ABCB10, FLVCR1b,[111] or another mitochondrial transporter upregulated with heme synthesis).[146] As a feedback mechanism, "uncommitted" or "free" heme appears to inhibit either Fe-Tf-TfR endocytosis, or iron release from Tf to prevent unnecessary iron uptake.[101,147] Like ALAS1, ALAS2 also has HRMs located in the 5′ end of its targeting leader sequence and, in vitro, micromolar quantities of heme inhibit translocation of ALAS2 into isolated mitochondria; however, whether excess uncommitted heme also impedes ALAS2 translocation in erythroid precursors is unclear.[133,148]

Both ALAS1 and ALAS2 also appear to be regulated by the CLPX-CLPP system, a mitochondrial unfoldase and proteasome-like complex. Of clinical relevance, the importance of this system is demonstrated by the development of erythropoietic protoporphyria in a family related to a ClpX mutation that resulted in decreased ALAS2 degradation.[149]

ALAS2 and ferritin mRNAs contain an IRE in their 5′ UTR, and their translation is therefore susceptible to low cytosolic iron levels. Although TfR1 contains IRE modules in its 3′ UTR and its mRNA should be stabilized (predominantly by IRP2[150]) under these conditions, the standard posttranscriptional regulatory model by which cytosolic iron levels controls iron transport, utilization, and storage via the IRE/IRP system (see Chapter 25) appears to become uncoupled in differentiating erythroid cells. In erythroid cells, ALAS2 is translated, while ferritin translation is blocked, and high expression of TR1 persists despite high Fe-Tf delivery. Analyses of erythroid progenitors in culture indicate that, with differentiation, these cells behave as if a "low cytosolic iron" condition exists.[151] This is in keeping with a hypothesis of iron delivery by which iron released from Fe-Tf-fFR complexes in the endosome bypasses the cytosol to be delivered to the mitochondria by direct contact between these two organelles.[152] An alternative theory is that MFN1 functions as a highly efficient mitochondrial iron importer driving cytosolic iron transfer across inner mitochondrial membranes for heme or Fe/S synthesis. In addition, it is suggested that the presence of large numbers of ALAS2 transcripts overwhelms the IRE/IRP system.[151]

Critical Balance Between Iron Assimilation, Heme, and Globin Synthesis

There are a number of mechanisms that protect erythroid precursors from the results of any imbalance between iron assimilation, heme, and globin synthesis. While each component is essential for hemoglobin synthesis, individually they are all potentially cytotoxic and it is therefore crucial that α- and β-globin chains and heme are produced in the 2:2:4 ratio necessary to form the stable complex of $\alpha_2\beta_2$ and four heme molecules that comprise hemoglobin A. The toxicity of free iron is well known, related to its intrinsic ability to generate highly reactive hydroxyl radicals from hydrogen peroxide in the Fenton reaction, while "free" or uncommitted heme is lipophilic and toxic to cells, promoting lipid peroxidation and reactive oxygen species (ROS) production, causing membrane injury and ultimately cell apoptosis.[102,153,154] The cytotoxicity arising from an imbalance in the production of α-globin and β-globin chains is best illustrated by the pathophysiology of β-thalassemia (Chapter 35), where the relative excess in α-globin production and the resultant precipitation of these globin chains triggers oxidative stress and cytotoxicity.[155] Among the protective systems identified to date are as follows:

(i) Heme regulation
    a. The feline leukemia virus subgroup C receptor, FLVCR
       FLVCR1 is the human ortholog of the feline cell surface receptor for Feline leukemia virus subgroup C (FeLV-C).[156] The retrovirus infects all feline hematopoietic cells, impairing feline FLVCR1 function due to binding of the receptor by viral envelope that is continuously synthesized within infected cells. Cats infected with FeLV-C develop a red cell aplasia characterized by a block in erythroid differentiation at the CFU-E/proerythroblast stage. The impairment in differentiation is also observed upon conditional deletion of *flvcr1* in neonatal mice,[157] who develop a severe anemia within 5 weeks of deletion that may be due to erythroid cell apoptosis.[158,159] FLVCR1 functions as a mammalian cell-surface heme exporter that thus appears to protect differentiating early erythroid progenitors from potential heme excesses and subsequent cytotoxicity resulting from any imbalances between heme and globin synthesis.[100,158,159] As noted, erythroid ALAS2 is not subject to transcriptional repression by heme and, importantly, heme oxygenases (HOs) are not normally induced during differentiation of human erythroid progenitors[159,160] or murine erythroid cell lines.[161] It is hypothesized that HO is not induced in order to prevent futile cycles of simultaneous erythroid heme synthesis and catabolism,[158,160] but HO overexpression in FLVCR1-deleted murine erythroid progenitors does not ameliorate the anemia, suggesting either it is not functional in developing erythroblasts or that newly synthesized heme is not accessible by HO.[159] The severity of the anemia in feline and murine FLVCR knockdown models suggests that excess heme synthesis occurs frequently in erythroid cells at the CFU-E/proerythroblast stage (likely prior to initiation of high level globin synthesis). Of interest, knockdown of murine *flvcr1* is embryonic lethal with the embryos displaying a phenotype similar to that of patients with DBA, a congenital red cell aplasia.[162] The most common genetic cause of DBA is haploinsufficiency of large or small ribosomal protein subunits, which results in impairment of erythroid protein (predominantly globin) synthesis, suggesting the anemia is caused by an imbalance of heme and globin synthesis.[163] Recent studies verify the importance of this balance; differentiating erythroid cells from patients with DBA or myelodysplastic syndrome with 5q deletion (del(5q) MDS, where there is haploinsufficiency of another ribosomal protein, RPS14; see Chapter 81) have normal heme synthesis but decreased globin synthesis, resulting in excess heme, oxidative stress, and death of CFU-E/proerythroblasts.[164] Notably, analysis of surviving DBA (or del(5q) MDS) erythroid precursors demonstrates either decreased ALAS2 expression (heme synthesis) and/or increased FLVCR expression (heme export), presumably mitigating the heme:globin imbalance to allow survival. Either inhibition of heme synthesis or facilitating increased heme export during erythroid differentiation ameliorates the anemia in in vitro studies of cells derived from patients with DBA or del(5q) MDS.[164]
    b. GATA1/heme interplay
       As described above, GATA1 is critical for erythroid differentiation; GATA1 initiates heme synthesis by activating two ALAS2 intronic enhancers, with deletion resulting in severe anemia and embryonic lethality in mice.[165] Recent studies indicate heme decreases GATA1 in the later stages of erythropoiesis: in CD71+Ter119lo-hi erythroid cells, heme decreases GATA1, GATA1-target gene, and mitotic spindle gene expression. Thus, as GATA1 initiates heme synthesis, GATA1 and heme together direct globin synthesis and red cell maturation, and heme arrests GATA1 synthesis, there appears to be a GATA1-heme autoregulatory loop. In addition, as excessive heme should prematurely lower GATA1, and impede mitosis, it may explain why these anemias are macrocytic, and why children with GATA1 mutations have DBA-like clinical phenotypes.[166]
    c. The heme-regulated inhibitor of translation, HRI.

As mentioned, HRI, a heme-regulated protein kinase that phosphorylates and inhibits eIF2α, and thus general protein translation, serves as a sensor of intracellular heme and is important for coordinating heme and globin production. Studies of the *Hri* knockout mouse verify the importance of this protective mechanism during high-level hemoglobin synthesis. HRI function appears to be especially important in iron (resulting in heme) deficiency: in these circumstances, the *cessation* of globin production seen in control mice fed an iron-depleted diet does not occur to the same degree in similarly fed *hri*−/− mice, resulting in cytotoxic precipitates of globin protein, ROS production and oxidative stress, and apoptosis of late erythroid precursors.[91] Interestingly, the red cells of iron-deficient *hri*−/− mice are normocytic/hyperchromic (rather than microcytic/hypochromic, as observed in the iron-deficient control mice), and the mice are more anemic. Similarly, mice with combined HRI and severe FECH deficiency (Fech^{m1Pas/m1Pas}, another murine model of heme deficiency) have more severe anemia and globin chain inclusions than control Fech^{m1Pas/m1Pas} mice. Notably, these mice have a 30-fold increase in red cell protoporphyrin IX compared with Fech^{m1Pas/m1Pas} mice, emphasizing that HRI-mediated regulation of erythroid precursor protein synthesis impacts not just globin, but also heme enzyme biosynthesis biosynthesis (presumably through regulation of mTORC1-mediated protein translation[93]), and thus the severity of the porphyria.[136]

HRI-mediated regulation of globin translation also ameliorates the phenotype of β-thalassemia in mice models, minimizing the imbalance in production between α- and β-globins, the accumulation of α-globin aggregates, apoptosis of erythroid precursors, and the resultant ineffective erythropoiesis. This may be related to activation of HRI by the oxidative stress that occurs during erythropoiesis in β-thalassemia or stress erythropoiesis.[92] HRI, by activating the transcription factor ATF4, induces an antioxidant stress response that seems to be important for erythroid differentiation.

Much remains to be discovered regarding the importance of heme in erythropoiesis beyond the paradigm of heme-dependent Bach1 destruction (via proteasome-mediated proteolysis) that derepresses genes containing Bach1 motifs[167] and heme effects on GATA1 levels. A "heme-omics" analysis has been reported recently, demonstrating that a large number of erythroid genes harbor chromosomal heme-sensing hotspots, and describing a DNA motif that demarcates heme regulation independent of Bach1.[168]

(ii) Globin regulation
  a. The alpha-hemoglobin stabilizing protein, AHSP
    The gene encoding this small protein (102 aa) is strongly induced by GATA1 during erythroid differentiation.[169] AHSP primarily binds αHb (i.e., the holoprotein, α-globin-heme), stabilizing it and inhibiting its pro-oxidant properties.[47] It functions as a chaperone, helping newly synthesized apo α-globin chains to fold and promote the refolding of denatured chains, which may be particularly important in heme deficiency.[170] AHSP forms a heterodimer with α globin-heme and when βHb is added to these complexes, AHSP is displaced and tetrameric HbA ($\alpha_2\beta_2$) forms, suggesting that AHSP stabilizes αHb and then passes it to β globin-heme to help form HbA in vivo. Deletion of the gene in mice results in a mild hemolytic anemia with the red cells containing Heinz bodies (eosinophilic inclusions derived from denatured hemoglobin), indicating perhaps that AHSP function is critical only when there is a large imbalance in synthesis between αHb and βHb, such as occurs in β-thalassemia.[171] Interbreeding of AHSP−/− mice with β-thalassemic mice (like the *Hri* knockout above) was indeed shown to worsen the β-thalassemic phenotype.[171]
  b. Proteostasis
    The term "protein quality control mechanisms" has been proposed as a name for a number of cellular posttranslational

mechanisms that serve to stabilize and aid folding of newly forming proteins (e.g., chaperones such as AHSP heat shock protein (Hsp)70, Hsp60, and Hsp90), or recognize misfolded proteins or protein aggregates and either untangle or unfold them or target them for degradation by the ubiquitin proteosome system (UPS) or autophagy.[172] The Hsp70 chaperone system acts early as a sensor of global protein folding status during erythropoiesis, gauging the levels of misfolded or aggregated proteins and determining whether Epo-stimulated erythroid progenitors primed to undergo differentiation should proceed or not.[173] For example, Epo stimulates movement of an Hsp70 family member, HSPA1A, from the cytosol into the nucleus to protect GATA1 from caspase-3–mediated proteolytic cleavage and allow initiation of erythroid differentiation. Insufficient translocation of HSPA1A due to sequestration by cytosolic protein aggregates allows for GATA1 cleavage, preventing differentiation and antiapoptosis signaling by Bcl-X(L), and resulting in cell death.[174] Additionally, during globin synthesis, HRI is regulated by a complex of heme and HSPA8 and, regardless of heme levels, increased protein aggregates sequester HSPA8 allowing activation of HRI and the ISR.[175] Not surprisingly then, given the amount of hemoglobin being produced, these protein quality control mechanisms appear to be particularly important in erythroid precursors during high level hemoglobin synthesis, and when these systems are overwhelmed—for example in severe thalassemias—accumulation of unstable insoluble proteins and cytotoxicity occurs.[176] Notably, drugs targeting UPS or autophagy are being increasingly used in cancer therapies and have the potential to cause anemia.[177]

CONTROL OF ERYTHROPOIESIS

It is evident that a finely regulated mechanism exists that maintains the erythron within "normal" limits and mediates the response to a variety of normal and abnormal situations. In broad outlines, this control system operates in the following manner. Alterations in the concentration of hemoglobin in the blood lead to changes in tissue oxygen tension within the kidney. In response to hypoxia, the kidney secretes the hormone Epo. This hormone induces differentiation of erythroid progenitor cells, expansion of the erythroid marrow, and increased red cell production. This, in turn, leads to an increase in the size of the erythron and an increase in tissue oxygen levels. The major steps in this process are discussed in greater detail in the sections that follow.

Tissue Oxygen

Tissue oxygen tension depends on the relative rates of oxygen supply and demand. Oxygen supply is a complex function of interacting but semiindependent variables, including (a) blood flow to the kidney, (b) blood hemoglobin concentration, (c) hemoglobin oxygen saturation, and (d) hemoglobin oxygen affinity. Each of these functions may be altered to compensate for a deficiency in one of the others. For example, in severe anemia, cardiac output and respiratory rate may increase, and hemoglobin oxygen affinity may be reduced by the red cell allosteric effector, 2,3-biphosphoglycerate (also called 2,3 diphosphoglycerate). Conversely, in hypoxic conditions, secondary polycythemia occurs.

Despite cardiovascular and respiratory adjustments, tissue oxygen tension decreases roughly in proportion to the degree of anemia. Conversely, induced polycythemia of moderate degree leads to normal or increased tissue oxygen tension and an increased tolerance to hypoxia. These changes occur despite the increase in blood viscosity that accompanies polycythemia, suggesting that peripheral vascular resistance decreases to compensate for increased viscosity. However, with advanced degrees of polycythemia, the increase in viscosity may be great enough to negate the advantages of increased oxygen-carrying capacity.

Tissue hypoxia is the fundamental stimulus to erythropoiesis, as first suggested by Miescher in 1893, a concept that has been amply confirmed.[178] However, hypoxia does not exert its effects on erythropoiesis by direct action on the marrow, as Miescher believed, but instead induces Epo. The nature of the tissue oxygen receptors (or oxygen sensor) is still an area for active research. These sensors are located within the kidney and thus Epo production can be induced by renal artery constriction or by hypoxic perfusion of the isolated kidney.

Erythropoietin
Structure of Erythropoietin

Epo is a glycoprotein hormone produced primarily by the kidney, which functions as the major regulator of red cell production. After more than 50 years of effort, the hormone was purified from 2550 L of urine from patients with aplastic anemia, with the *Epo* gene subsequently isolated in 1985. It has a molecular weight (MW) of 34 kD and contains 30% carbohydrate (11% sialic acid, 11% total hexose, and 8% N-acetylglucosamine).[179] The potency of Epo is expressed in units, with one unit defined as the amount present in one tenth of the International Reference Preparation.[180] This unit was originally defined in starved rats as the amount that produced the same erythropoietic response (due to increase in serum Epo level) as treatment with 5 μmol of cobalt.[178] The potency of purified human urinary Epo has been determined to be 70,400 U/mg of protein.[181]

Epo production and regulation by hypoxia inducible factor (HIF) is discussed in detail in Chapter 5.

HIFs are heterodimeric helix-loop-helix transcription factors consisting of two subunits, an oxygen-labile protein, HIF-α and a constitutively expressed, oxygen-insensitive, β subunit, HIF-β.[182] Three genes, HIF1A, HIF2A (or EPAS1), and HIF3A, encoding different isoforms of HIF-α, are present in the human genome—here HIF-α refers to either HIF-1α or HIF-2α. The latter appears to be the primary HIF-α component activating Epo gene expression. The concentration and transcriptional activity of HIF-α geometrically increases upon exposure to hypoxia, provided that cells are iron-replete to prevent IRP1 inhibition of HIF-α translation via binding to a 5' IRE (as for ALAS2 above).[183] Under normoxic conditions, HIF-α mRNA is constitutively expressed, but the protein is then rapidly degraded, via the ubiquitin proteosome complex, following binding by von Hippel-Lindau protein (pVHL). Recognition of HIF-α by pVHL requires prior hydroxylation of specific HIF-α proline residues by prolyl 4-hydroxylase domain (PHD)–containing proteins.[184,185] These PHDs are oxygen- and iron-dependent enzymes. Under hypoxic conditions, little or no proline hydroxylation takes place; thus, pVHL does not bind to HIF-α, which accumulates in the nucleus, heterodimerizes with HIF-β, and recruits the transcriptional coactivators p300/CREB-binding protein, with the whole complex then binding to the *Epo* enhancer to positively influence *Epo* promoter activity and gene transcription. The recruitment of p300/CREB-binding protein to the complex can itself be inhibited by hydroxylation of asparagine-803 in HIF-α, which is catalyzed by asparaginyl hydroxylase (called "factor inhibiting HIF"), another iron and oxygen-sensitive enzyme.[186] It seems that these two amino acid hydroxylases, by virtue of their dependence on normal intracellular oxygen for their function, act as the oxygen sensors in the Epo-producing interstitial cells in the kidney, and, by regulating the function of HIF-α at two distinct points,[187] ultimately control Epo synthesis and production. Not surprisingly, mutations of this pathway may be associated with an increased red cell mass: Chuvash polycythemia is due to a homozygous mutation of *Vhl* that impairs HIF-1α degradation, resulting in a mild increase in Epo levels, while mutations of HIF-2α or PHD2 genes are rarer causes of familial erythrocytosis.[188] Novel PHD inhibitors have recently been developed to enhance Epo and red cell production through stabilization of HIF[189] and are discussed in Chapter 42.

In addition to Epo, a large number of other HIF target genes (e.g., glucose transporters, glycolytic enzymes, iron uptake proteins, vascular endothelial growth factors) are upregulated during hypoxia to aid cells adapt to hypoxic conditions.[190] Apart from the indirect effects of hypoxia on erythropoiesis through HIF-mediated renal Epo production, erythroid progenitor cells in the bone marrow are also subject to the direct cellular effects of hypoxia and HIF production. An analysis of early erythroid progenitor genes upregulated by glucocorticoids (released from the adrenal glands during acute anemia or hypoxic "stress erythropoiesis,"[31,191] as distinct from steady-state red cell production) found that the promoter regions of many of these genes also contain HIF binding sites. Furthermore, in in vitro studies, HIF synergizes with glucocorticoids to dramatically expand erythroid progenitors, perhaps by increasing BFU-E progenitor self-renewal,[31] a HIF effect previously reported during stress erythropoiesis.[192]

Action of Erythropoietin
Epo Receptors

Epo binds to a specific molecule on the cell surface, the EpoR, and expression of both proteins is necessary for adult life. Deletion of either gene in mice results in the identical phenotype of fetal death at embryonic days E11.5 to E13.5 because of a lack of definitive erythropoiesis in the fetal liver and severe anemia.[193] Arguably, the most important control point of erythropoiesis is the interaction of Epo with the receptor for Epo. The activation of EpoR generates an intracellular signal in immature erythroid cells that promotes survival of cells that would otherwise undergo apoptosis. In addition, Epo promotes erythroblast proliferation and differentiation.

EpoR is expressed on hematopoietic cells that respond to Epo, including human and murine erythroid cells, erythroleukemia cell lines, fetal liver tissue rich in erythroid elements, mouse and rat placenta, and on megakaryocytes.[194] EpoR expression on human erythroid cells is relatively low (approximately 1100 molecules per progenitor cell) and correlates with the cell's responsiveness to and dependence on Epo.[194] EpoR are expressed on human BFU-E, increasing in number as BFU-E mature to CFU-E.[19] Erythroid cells at a stage between CFU-E and proerythroblast have the highest expression of EpoR, which decreases as the proerythroblast matures and eventually disappears at the stage of orthochromatic erythroblast.[19,195] The receptor is not expressed on reticulocytes or red cells. The presence of EpoR on megakaryocytes[194,195] explains why Epo at physiological concentrations promotes megakaryocyte differentiation and can thus affect platelet levels. Receptors for Epo are also observed on nonhematopoietic tissues including neurons and cardiac myocytes, endothelial cells, the kidneys, and embryonic muscle. The expression of EpoR in nonerythroid tissues was not believed to be required for normal embryonic development as erythroid tissue–specific EpoR expression (under control of the GATA1 promoter) in EpoR[−/−] embryonic stem cells gives rise to apparently normal mice. However, recent studies indicate that EpoR[−/−] murine embryos develop neural defects, defects in angiogenesis, and cardiac ventricular hypoplasia, which are not a result of generalized hypoxia.[196] In addition, adverse effects observed in patients with certain solid tumors receiving Epo have been ascribed to activation of EpoR expressed on tumor cells.[197]

The human gene is located on chromosome 19p13.2, encodes a protein of 508 aa, and is 68 to 72 kD depending on the degree of glycosylation.[198] Structurally, EpoR is part of a large family of type I cytokine receptors, which includes receptors for IL-2 through -7, and the growth factors G-CSF and Tpo. Type I cytokine receptors share basic structural features and are characterized by four conserved cysteine residues and a tryptophan-serine-x-serine-tryptophan (WSXSW) motif in the extracellular domain, and by conserved box1/box2 regions in the intracytoplasmic domain adjacent to the membrane. While some type I cytokine receptors are heterodimeric and share common subunits, the Epo, Tpo, and G-CSF receptors consist of homodimers.[199] Crystallographic studies confirm that one molecule of Epo simultaneously binds to two EpoR,[200] as is seen with other cytokine-receptor pairs. After binding, both Epo and EpoR are rapidly endocytosed and degraded.[10,194,198,201] Although EpoR activation by Epo can lead to formation of EpoR homodimers,[202] evidence suggests that these dimers exist prior to Epo binding, and that binding shifts and stabilizes an active receptor conformation bringing the two EpoR into closer contact.[203,204]

EpoR signaling pathways are outlined in *Figure 6.6*. Tyrosine phosphorylation of EpoR[10,205] is the first observable event after Epo

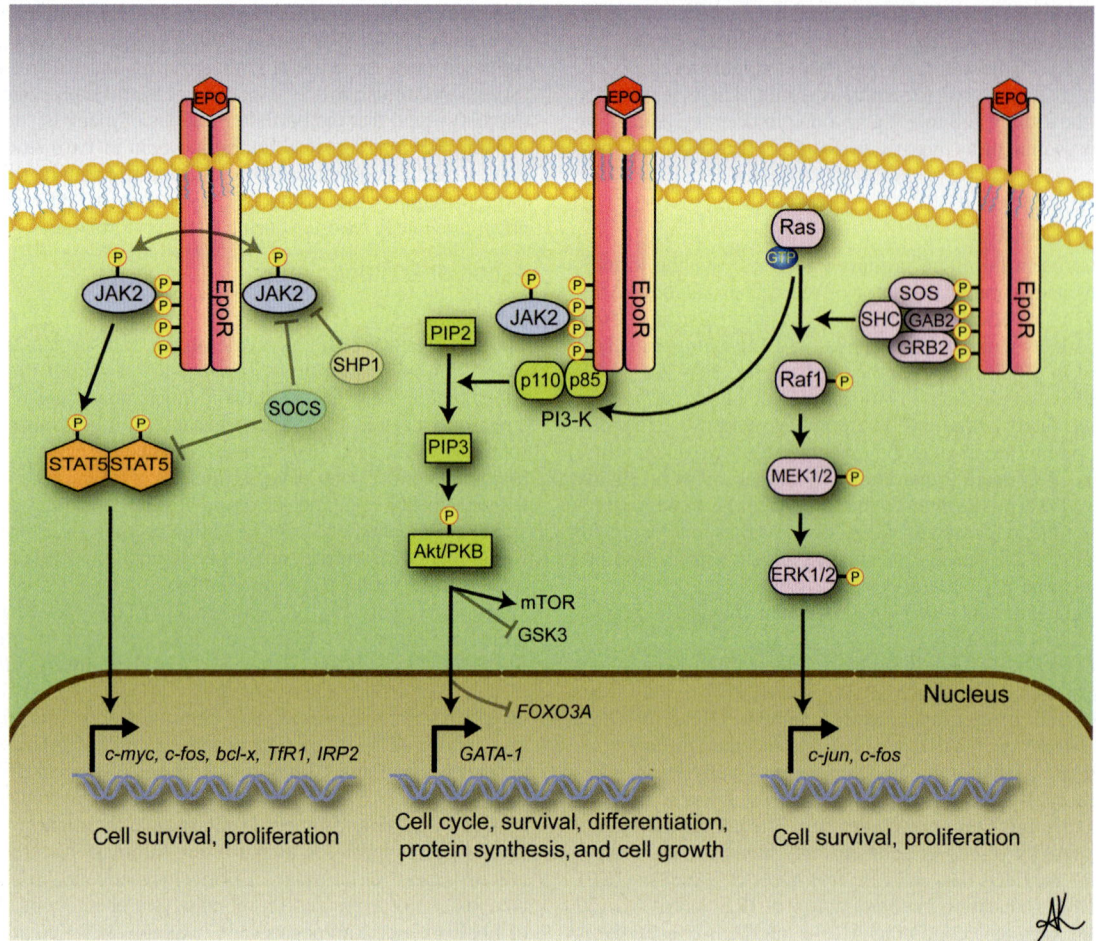

FIGURE 6.6 **Overview of the erythropoietin receptor (EpoR) signaling pathways.** Conformational changes in EpoR dimers induced by Epo binding facilitate the activation of EpoR-associated Jak2 kinases. Jak2 kinase activation results in phosphorylation of several tyrosines in the EpoR cytoplasmic tail that then serve as docking sites for signaling or adaptor proteins containing phosphotyrosine-binding domains. The signaling proteins become phosphorylated and function in numerous downstream signaling cascades. (1) A major target of Jak2 is Stat5, which is phosphorylated, dimerizes, and travels to the nucleus where it activates genes important for cell survival and proliferation. (2) Binding of the regulatory subunit of PI3-kinase, p85, to EpoR phosphotyrosines results in phosphorylation of membrane lipids and the downstream activation of Akt. This kinase regulates cell cycle, cell differentiation, and prosurvival pathways and modulates metabolism and protein translation. (3) The ras/raf/MEK/ERK pathway is activated with binding of the SHC/GRB2/SOS complex to EpoR phosphotyrosines. Activation of the downstream kinase ERK1/2 results in phosphorylation of ELK1, a transcription factor important for cell survival and proliferation (via c-jun and c-fos expression). Negative regulatory proteins are necessary to dampen EpoR signaling. SOCS proteins inhibit Jak2 and Stat5 activation, whereas phosphatases such as SHP1 and SHIP inhibit other phosphorylation-dependent pathways. Note that other EpoR pathways, such as activation of calcium-dependent isoforms of the PKC family of serine/threonine kinases, are not shown (see text for details).

binding. Because EpoR lacks a kinase domain, a tyrosine protein kinase must therefore associate with the receptor. JAK2, a member of the Janus family of cytoplasmic tyrosine kinases, is the primary EpoR-associated kinase and binds to a conserved sequence of amino acids found in a cytoplasmic domain of EpoR (and related receptors). Studies indicate that activation of EpoR through Epo binding initiates a scissor-like rotation of the EpoR dimers, separating the intracellular domains of the two receptor monomers to allow room for the associated Jak2 molecules; in addition, there appears to be a self-rotation of each monomer to allow them to orient properly for transphosphorylation of Jak2.[206] Deletion of the JAK2 gene in mice results in fetal death on E12 to 13, associated with a severe anemia that mirrors the phenotype observed with Epo or EpoR deletion,[207] indicating the importance of Jak2 for Epo signaling. One Epo molecule binds two EpoR molecules, activating JAK2 kinases associated with the juxtamembrane regions (box 1/box 2) of each receptor by physically bringing the inactive (or low-activity) kinases into close proximity during the induced rotational shift in EpoR conformation,[208] such that these kinases cross-phosphorylate each other, gaining full activity.[31,209,210] The activated kinases phosphorylate all eight conserved tyrosine residues of the EpoR cytoplasmic tail. The phosphorylated tyrosine (pY)

residues then serve as docking sites for up to 20 different signaling molecules or adaptor proteins that may be phosphorylated by JAK2 to become active, and leading to various mitogenic, differentiative, and antiapoptotic responses. The signaling molecules and adaptor proteins contain either Src homology 2 (SH2) or other phosphotyrosine-binding domains that mediate recognition of a pY residue in the context of specific adjacent (EpoR) amino acids. The major pathways activated by Epo binding to EpoR include the signal-transducing activator of transcription 5 (STAT5) pathway, and the phosphatidylinositol-3-kinase (PI3-kinase)/Akt and ras/raf/MAPK (mitogen-activated protein kinase) signaling cascades (*Figure 6.6*).

STAT5 Pathway

Upon binding to EpoR, STAT5 is phosphorylated by Jak2,[211] dimerizes, and translocates to the nucleus to mediate gene transcription (e.g., of the mitogenic transcription factor *c-myc*, *Id1*,[212] *TfRC*, *IRP*,[213] and *BCL21.1*). Dissection of the Epo/EpoR/Jak2 signaling axis by targeted deletions of the eight potential pY residues in EpoR has also revealed the importance of pathways downstream of Jak2.[214] Surprisingly, while deletion of all 8 residues results in only mild anemia (hematocrit 75% of that in control mice),[215] restoration solely of Epo/EpoR/Jak2/STAT5 signaling results in near-wild type EpoR activities,[216] and, importantly, STAT5 signaling restores the erythron capacity for proliferative, *stress* erythropoiesis responses. The precise role of STAT5 in EpoR signaling in steady-state erythropoiesis, however, is still unclear. STAT5 is expressed from two very similar genes, STAT5a and STAT5b. In animal studies in which both genes were deleted (STAT5a/b−/− mice), a marked fetal anemia was reported, with lesser but significant anemia in newborn and adult animals.[217] However, Epo weakly activates other STATs in primary erythroid cells, so STAT3[213] and/or STAT1 activation[218] may also partially compensate for STAT5, resulting in a relatively mild inhibition of murine erythropoiesis.[219] Studies suggest Epo acts like a dimmer switch in varying STAT5 activation levels over a wide range as Epo levels increase from the low levels seen with basal state erythropoiesis to the high levels observed during "stress erythropoiesis" that accelerates RBC production.[220]

A potential target of STAT5 is the *BCL2l.1* gene, which encodes an antiapoptotic protein, BCL-X(L), believed to be essential for Epo-dependent survival. Two elegant studies of BCL-X(L)–deficient animals confirmed that expression is required for normal erythropoiesis, but also demonstrate that it promotes the survival of mature erythroid cells that are no longer dependent on Epo for survival.[221,222] Thus, *BCL2l.1* must also be regulated by factors other than Epo-activated STAT5,[218] likely the interplay of GATA1 and Gfi-1B at the *BCL2l.1* promoter.[223] Epo/EpoR signaling may promote survival earlier, at the proerythroblast stage, through upregulation of other antiapoptotic genes such as Pim1, Pim3, Trib3, and the cathepsins inhibitor Serpina3g (Spi2A),[198] as it is cytoprotective for *BCL2l.1*-KO erythroid progenitors.[224]

PI3-kinase Pathway

The distal end of the EpoR cytoplasmic domain and phosphorylation of Y479 are required for activation of the PI3-kinase/Akt and MAP kinase signaling cascades (see *Figure 6.6*). Binding of the p85 regulatory subunit of PI3-kinase to EpoR mediates translocation of the kinase from the cytoplasm to phosphorylate lipids at the cell membrane,[225] resulting in modulation of survival, metabolism, and translation through the subsequent effects of Akt (a kinase directly downstream of PI3-kinase) on mTOR, GSK3, FOXO and GATA1 transcription factors.[226,227] The central role of PI3-kinase in signaling downstream of EpoR is suggested by the ability of a constitutively active Akt to partially rescue erythroid development when expressed in JAK2−/− fetal liver cells.[226] Notably, p85 protein binding also facilitates EpoR endocytosis and degradation to help terminate Epo signaling.

Ras/MAPK Pathway

With regard to the ras/raf/MEK/ERK cascade, Jak2-initiated phosphorylation of tyrosines at the distal end of EpoR allows an *Shc* adaptor protein to associate with the receptor, which then recruits GRB2 and SOS, resulting in activation of erythroid cell membrane–bound K-ras and then Raf activation. This signaling cascade subsequently gives rise (via MEK) to phosphorylation of ERK1/2 which then phosphorylates up to 60 substrates, promoting erythroid cell-cycle progression and proliferation.[228] In contrast to the two pathways described above, however, knockdown (or hyperactivation) of K-ras in erythroid cells, or downstream RAS-modulated targets such as C-Raf, Mek, or Erk have more subtle effects on terminal erythropoiesis.[229] Nonetheless, new drugs targeting the RAS pathway in cancer have the potential to impact erythropoiesis.[230]

Although Epo acts on progenitor cells to promote survival, drive proliferation, and direct erythroid maturation, it is not clear if some downstream intracellular signaling pathways distinctly activate only one of these events. Epo-dependent activation of the PI3-kinase pathway appears important for both cell survival and proliferation, while the MAP kinase pathway appears more important in directing proliferation.[225] It appears more likely, that like for other cytokine receptor signaling, signal pathways are not discrete and there is cross-communication between downstream signaling pathways and perhaps with signaling by other cytokine receptors.[231]

Apart from these three major pathways, there are a number of other well-described mediators of responses downstream of Epo/EpoR that impact erythropoiesis. These include the inositide-specific phospholipase C family (e.g., knockdown of the PLC-γ isoform 1 impedes erythroid development in a STAT5-independent manner[232]) and the protein kinase C pathways (e.g., inhibition of the PKCα isoform impairs Epo-induced differentiation, while PKCε upregulation protects erythroid cells from TRAIL-induced apoptosis[233,234]). In addition, knockdown of the Src family tyrosine kinase Lyn results in attenuated EpoR signaling and decreased erythroblast survival.[214,235,236] The adaptor SH2-containing proteins CrkL (which is phosphorylated by Lyn and indirectly activates Erk1/2), Lnk (which attenuates JAK2 signaling[237]), and Spry1, which appears to downregulate Erk1/2 and Jak2 activation,[238] also appear to be important regulators of EpoR signals. Recent studies have expanded our knowledge of Epo signaling during erythropoiesis, identifying a further 22 novel kinases and phosphatases that are phosphorylated by Epo-EpoR.[239] Surprisingly, a phosphatase, PTPN18, serves to increase EpoR signaling, likely through reversal of phosphorylation of a regulatory molecular adaptor protein, RHEX (regulator of hemoglobinization and erythroid cell expansion) that is found in association with EpoR complexes. Much remains to be learned about this pathway.

Iron availability is intimately involved with the Epo/EpoR signaling pathway at a number of points: for example, regulating HIF and therefore Epo expression through the iron-dependent HIF oxygenases, and HIF translation via the IRE/IRP system; in addition, both TfR1 and TfR2 modulate EpoR signaling. Polymeric IgA (pIgA1-oligomers of IgA joined by their J-chains), secreted in small amounts by bone marrow plasma cells, binds to TfR1 present on the erythroblast cell surface. Binding of pIgA1 or Fe-Tf to TfR1 appears to transmit an intracellular signal that results in activation of erythroblast Akt and ERK1/2, stimulating erythroblast proliferation and differentiation.[240] This pathway may be important to boost erythroid output during stress erythropoiesis, as hypoxia increases pIgA1 levels. TfR2 modulates Epo-dependent erythropoiesis in erythroid precursors, likely by sequestering EpoR, affecting EpoR processing and transport to the cell surface. Bone marrow–specific gene knockout results in increased EpoR expression, Epo sensitivity, and response. These effects are similar to the responses of control marrow erythroid precursors during iron deficiency.[241] In addition, as terminal erythropoiesis is increased, there is heightened release of the TNF cytokine family member, erythroferrone—product of the Epo/EpoR-responsive gene *ERFE*—by these cells. Erythroferrone,[242] the erythroid regulator of systemic iron stores, suppresses liver hepcidin release, thereby decreasing its inhibition of iron efflux from enterocytes, hepatocytes, and macrophages, and allowing for increased erythroid iron availability (Chapter 25).

Finally, as is found with other cell signaling cascades, there is a need for checks and balances in the form of inhibitory or regulatory factors to prevent overstimulation of erythroid cells by Epo/EpoR-mediated growth and survival signals. The distal end of EpoR, for example, acts as a negative regulatory domain to which SH2-containing protein tyrosine phosphatases dock (to pY401, 429, 431) to dephosphorylate substrates such as Jak2 and STAT5 and attenuate Epo signaling. Transgenic animals expressing a truncated human receptor Epo develop severe erythrocytosis, mimicking primary familial and congenital polycythemia (PFCP, see Chapter 45) where patients have elevated red cell mass due to mutations in the EpoR gene.[243] A number of kindreds with PFCP due to mutations in this distal regulatory region of EpoR have since been reported.[244] Identified regulatory phosphatases[245] include the SH2-containing tyrosine phosphatases SHP1, SHP2 (PTPN11[23]), and PTP-1B. Other regulatory factors include the control of EpoR trafficking from the ER by Jak2,[193] EpoR internalization upon interaction with Epo, proteasomal degradation of EpoR (by β-TRCP)[246] and signaling adaptor molecules, and the inducible expression of specific inhibitors such as the suppressor of cytokine signaling (SOCS) protein family members SOCS-1, SOCS-3, and CIS-1 (cytokine inducible SH2-containing protein) by STATs. The SOCS family of proteins downregulate receptor signaling in a negative feedback manner by (1) competing with STAT5 for binding to

EpoR phosphotyrosines and (2) binding and inhibiting the Jak2 kinase activation loop, or (3), ubiquitination and proteosomal targeting of Jak2. Studies indicate VHL directly binds with SOCS1 to ubiquitinate phospho-Jak2, a process impaired in patients with Chuvash polycythemia–associated VHL mutants.[247] The *Epo* gene has been incompletely deleted in 8-week-old mice using a conditional knockout strategy, reducing renal *Epo* gene expression by 95% compared to controls.[248] This animal serves as a model of the Epo/EpoR interactions that likely occur in patients with renal failure, with decreased steady-state erythropoiesis, and a chronic moderate normocytic, normochromic anemia (Hct ~75% of control), related to residual Epo production. Of interest, despite the severe knockdown in Epo expression, the animals appear to have normal stress erythropoiesis responses, as they recover normally from acute hypoxic stress (induced by phenylhydrazine-induced hemolysis), indicating the importance of other mechanisms such as glucocorticoids, hypoxia, BMP4, and SCF in supporting murine stress erythropoiesis.[31,191]

Abnormal Epo/EpoR Signaling

Causes of erythrocytosis include excessive stimulation of Epo production by mutations of HIF-α, or its regulators pVHL, PHD1, or PHD2.[249] (see Chapter 45). In addition, a point mutation of murine EpoR (R129C, a substitution of cysteine for arginine at position 129) that results in constitutive activation of EpoR by homodimerization in the absence of Epo, and erythrocytosis, has been described.[250] Murine EpoR may also be activated by interaction with the Friend spleen focus–forming virus envelope glycoprotein, gp55, promoting EpoR dimerization and polycythemia.[251] Deletions of negative regulatory EpoR domains in humans and mouse models, as noted above, also increase EpoR signaling and result in erythrocytosis, while overexpression of a constitutively active mutant of STAT5A, STAT5A1*6 in human cord blood CD34+ cells favors erythroid over myeloid differentiation in vitro. Building on previous studies,[251] constitutive activation of EpoR in patients with the myeloproliferative disease polycythemia vera was discovered to be due to an activating mutation of Jak2 that encodes a substitution of valine for phenylalanine at position 617 in the protein (discussed in Chapter 84).

Classically it is assumed that cytokines activate downstream signaling through monotonic activation of their cognate receptors. However, a novel homozygous missense variant of the Epo gene was uncovered that results in the substitution R150Q (R = Arginine, Q = glutamine) in the mature protein. Notably, this region of Epo interacts with the high-affinity–binding site (site 1) of EpoR, explaining the mild ~eightfold reduction of EpoR affinity observed with R150Q mutant Epo. Importantly, however, both the measured mutant Epo on-rate ((R150Q) Epo binding to EpoR) and off-rate (dissociation) were significantly higher than with wtEpo-EpoR interactions. Further studies demonstrated the anemia was due to the poor efficacy of (R150Q) Epo signaling in mediating erythroid progenitor proliferation and differentiation. Dissecting the mutant Epo effects, it was shown that while STAT5 stimulation was comparable to that observed with wtEpo, another downstream signaling pathway, the Jak2-mediated phosphorylation of downstream targets, was reduced. Thus, here the biased or partial activation of downstream signaling pathways was due solely to the kinetics of the mutant Epo/EpoR interaction.[252]

Mechanism of Action

Epo is a hormone that promotes erythroid differentiation.[178] Although this has been known for many years, the role of Epo during the very early stages of erythropoiesis is still being defined. Cell lines with features of multipotent hematopoietic progenitor cells[253,254] and purified human blood BFU-E[19] express a small number of EpoR, suggesting a potential role for Epo in mediating their survival and differentiation. Although, in vivo, the BFU-E pool is unaffected by acute changes in serum Epo levels, they can respond to Epo by increasing their cycling, part of the process of erythroid differentiation.[21] Chronic administration of recombinant Epo to humans with end-stage renal disease results in global stimulation of the bone marrow with an increase in the concentration and cycling of all types of hematopoietic progenitors; an

effect that was believed to be indirect. However, more recent studies suggest that Epo can push early hematopoietic progenitors toward an erythroid fate in vivo, altering their transcriptomes to increase erythroid output, at the expense of decreasing myelopoiesis.[255]

The erythroid cell that is the most sensitive to Epo is at a developmental stage between the CFU-E and the proerythroblast, and is the primary target of Epo action. These cells have the highest cell surface expression of EpoR, and are absolutely dependent on Epo for survival.[19,256] Studies on murine splenic erythroid cells infected with the anemia strain of Friend virus[257] have shown that Epo binding is followed by a series of biochemical events, including increased Ca^{2+} uptake, internalization of Epo, a generalized increase in mRNA synthesis, glucose and iron uptake, TfR expression, upregulation of transcription of the heme synthesis enzyme and the α- and β-globin genes, and, eventually, an increase of hemoglobin synthesis as well as synthesis of membrane bands 3 and 4.1.[258] All of these changes result in an increased rate of erythroid differentiation, an increase in reticulocyte production, and an eventual increase in the erythron.

One of the most impressive effects of Epo is the ability of the hormone to maintain the viability of erythroid cells irrespective of any effect on cycling and differentiation.[41,201] Epo retards the DNA cleavage that occurs normally in CFU-E,[19] and, in its absence, DNA cleavage is rapid and proceeds to a cell death characteristic of cells undergoing caspase-mediated apoptosis.[19] In the presence of Epo, cell death is avoided and the erythroid cells differentiate and form mature red cells, suggesting that Epo promotes erythroid differentiation simply by allowing cell survival. This model also suggests that, under normal conditions—due to their variable sensitivities to Epo—a proportion of generated CFU-E undergo apoptosis, and that high Epo levels cause expansion of the erythron simply through allowing survival of more CFU-E, resulting in increased red cell production. Similarly, once the red cell mass is restored to normal, the ensuing decrease of Epo levels leads to a rapid turn-off of erythropoiesis by allowing programmed cell death to occur.[19]

The observation that relatively immature erythroid progenitor cells continue to develop in fetal mice in which either the gene encoding for Epo or EpoR is deleted[259] suggests that Epo acts primarily by promoting survival of more mature erythroid cells and that it has no role, or at least a less significant role, in proliferation of erythroid precursors or in directing the erythroid differentiation of immature hematopoietic cells. The abundant erythroid cells from the spleens of either Epo−/− or EpoR−/− mice (the majority of which are proerythroblasts near the CFU-E stage of erythroid development) undergo apoptosis unless they are either cultured in vitro in Epo (Epo−/− mice) or forced (by transfection with EpoR cDNA) to express EpoR (EpoR−/− mice) and then cultured in the presence of Epo. Thus, neither Epo nor EpoR are necessary for the proliferation and differentiation of stem cells and early progenitor cells into relatively mature erythroid cells (however, as mentioned earlier, Epo at high levels appears to push these stem cells to an erythroid fate[255]). Both Epo and EpoR, however, are absolutely required for erythroid cells to survive the transition from CFU-E/proerythroblasts to mature erythroblasts, suggesting a clear role for Epo in directing the survival of these cells.[220]

Studies of normal murine fetal liver–derived erythroblasts that are transduced with (and thus overexpress) antiapoptotic proteins such as BCL-X(L) or Bcl-2 have emphasized the importance of survival factors at this defined stage of erythropoiesis.[14] These erythroblasts require Epo, SCF, and dexamethasone to allow sustained proliferation; however, with removal of these factors (including Epo), there is initiation of what appears to be normal erythroid differentiation with induction of the erythroid transcription factors (GATA1, KLF1, and NFE2), differentiation divisions, size reduction, hemoglobinization, nuclear condensation, and enucleation. These studies would suggest that Epo-induced survival allows cell-autonomous terminal erythroid differentiation. Interestingly, studies also demonstrate that controlled caspase activation is actually necessary for erythroblast maturation.[260] It is hypothesized that caspase-mediated cleavage of proteins such as lamin B, PARP-1, and acinus is required for terminal maturation, perhaps for initiation of enucleation.[261] In the absence of Epo, there is excessive activation of caspases, resulting in GATA1 cleavage and maturation arrest or apoptosis. However, as described earlier, Epo induces nuclear migration of a molecular chaperone, Hsp70, to protect GATA1 from cleavage during caspase activation.[262] Notably, studies[263] indicate that abrogation of this protective mechanism may be a contributing cause to the ineffective erythropoiesis seen in patients with early myelodysplastic syndrome (see Chapter 80). Newer cancer drugs targeting antiapoptotic proteins such as Bcl-2 or BCL-X(L)[264] have the potential to impact erythropoiesis.

In addition to erythroid cells, Epo has also been shown to affect megakaryocytes and their progenitors CFU-MK. Epo acts as a colony-stimulating factor for murine CFU-MK,[265] whereas in humans, it potentiates the effect of megakaryocyte colony-stimulating factors present in lymphocyte-conditioned medium.[10] It also promotes differentiation of murine megakaryocytes,[266] which express EpoR,[267] and, when injected at high doses into mice, increases platelet production.[268] In patients with renal failure treated with Epo, a minor increase in the platelet count, averaging approximately 30,000/μL, has been noted.[269]

ASSAYS FOR ERYTHROPOIETIN AND ERYTHROPOIETIN LEVELS IN HEALTH AND DISEASE

The presence of Epo in serum, urine, or other body fluids can be detected by bioassays or immunoassays. Bioassays may be in vivo or in vitro and are largely reserved to the research setting. Bioassays typically correlate Epo concentration with some functional measure erythropoiesis such as[59] Fe incorporation into newly produced red cells in mice that have endogenous Epo suppressed by induced polycythemia or[59] Fe or[3] H-thymidine incorporation into erythroid precursors in vitro.[270]

Immunoassays have the advantages of being quick, accurate, relatively inexpensive, and capable of quantifying very low Epo levels ordinarily not detectable by bioassays. Radioimmunoassays have been replaced by enzyme-linked immunosorbent assays. In most cases, immunoassays and bioassays correlate fairly well, although there are exceptions. Immunoassays may detect immunoreactive but not necessarily bioactive hormone. Thus, in renal failure, when serum Epo levels are low or undetectable by bioassays, the immunoassays detect higher levels.[271] Epo concentrations are expressed in international units/L (U/L). Since 1991, the International Reference Standard for Epo to which assays are calibrated has been based on rhEpo. While there is some inter-assay variation, normal immunoassay values typically range from 5 to 25 U/L in healthy nonanemic individuals.[270] The utility of Epo assays in clinical practice is discussed in later chapters in relation to specific clinical syndromes.

THE MATURE RBC

Erythrocytes were first described in detail by Leeuwenhoek in 1674. In 1851, Funke demonstrated that the primary component of the red cell was hemoglobin, and 15 years later Hoppe-Seyler demonstrated that hemoglobin has the property of readily taking up and discharging oxygen, thus defining the major physiologic role of the erythrocytes. More detailed discussion of the evolution of the understanding of erythrocyte structure and function is found in Maxwell Wintrobe's history of hematologic science, *Blood, Pure and Eloquent*.[272] This section provides a description of RBC membrane structure and function, red cell metabolism, and hemoglobin function.

STRUCTURAL FEATURES OF RBCS

Lacking a nucleus, mitochondria, or ribosomes, the red cell is unable to synthesize new protein, carry out the oxidative reactions associated with mitochondria, or undergo mitosis. More than 95% of the cytoplasmic protein is hemoglobin. The remainder includes those enzymes required for energy production and for the maintenance of hemoglobin in a functional, reduced state.

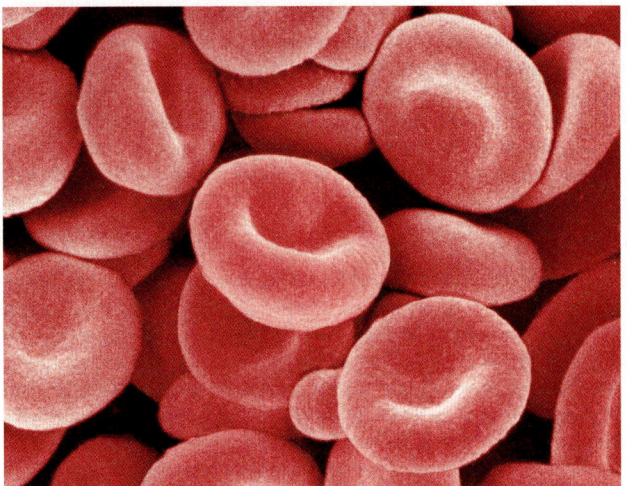

FIGURE 6.7 The normal mature erythrocyte as visualized by the scanning electron microscope. (Susumu Nishinaga/Science Source).

Shape and Dimensions

At rest, the normal human erythrocyte is shaped like a flattened, bilaterally indented sphere, a shape often referred to as a biconcave disc (*Figure 6.7*). In fixed, stained blood smears, only the flattened surfaces are observed; hence, on fixed blood films the erythrocyte appears circular, with a diameter of about 7 to 8 μm and an area of central pallor.

Average values for the mean cellular volume (MCV) in normal subjects range from 80 to 100 fL. The variation in cell size can be documented by means of a frequency distribution curve of red cell volumes generated from the output of a Coulter counter (*Figure 6.8*). The red cell distribution width (RDW) is a measure of the variation in RBC size, and it is a useful measurement when assessing the cause of anemia. In most laboratories, the RDW is defined as the coefficient of variation of the MCV.

It has been proposed that mature red cell size and hemoglobin content are primarily dependent on erythroid precursor cell size at the last cell division during erythropoiesis.[273] Reticulocytes are 24% to 35% larger than mature red cells, although they have similar total hemoglobin content.[274]

The disc shape is well suited to erythrocyte function. The ratio of surface to volume approaches the maximum possible value in such a

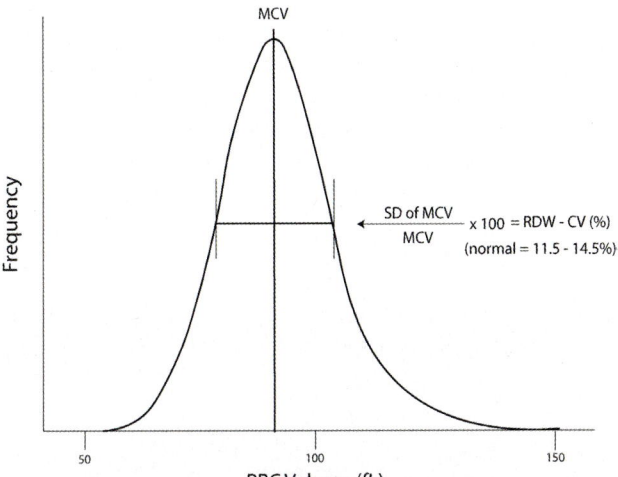

FIGURE 6.8 Frequency distribution curve of erythrocyte volume. Red blood cells (RBCs) are normally distributed about a mean cell volume (MCV) of 90 fL. RBC distribution width (RDW or RDW-CV) is a measure of the range of variation of RBC volume that is reported as part of a standard complete blood count. Normal reference range of RDW-CV in human RBCs is 11.5% to 14.5%. A change in RDW is useful in evaluating the cause of different anemias.

shape,[275] thereby facilitating both gas transfer across the membrane and deformability as the red cell traverses the microcirculation. When red cell movements within small blood vessels are observed by cinemamicrography,[276] the plane of the biconcave disk is oriented in the direction of flow with the leading edge pointed and the trailing edge blunted. When deformed in this way, erythrocytes can pass through vessels of about 4 μm in maximum diameter, significantly smaller than the normal RBC diameter.

Deformability

The erythrocyte is remarkable for its ability to maintain membrane integrity while exhibiting extreme deformability under normal physiologic circumstances.[277] Without undergoing extensive remodeling, the erythrocyte membrane withstands high shear stresses, rapid elongation and folding in the microcirculation, and deformation as the erythrocyte passes through the small fenestrations of the spleen. Cell deformability depends on both the membrane and the cytoplasm; however, it is the elasticity and viscosity of the membrane that are most crucial for deformability.

Among the factors that affect membrane deformability and stability are membrane lipid content, lipid distribution, cytoskeletal proteins, and transmembrane proteins.[278] The cytoskeleton, formed by a lattice-like network of proteins, undoubtedly contributes to the bending energy necessary for assumption of the biconcave shape, as well as to membrane stability.[279] Abnormalities in cytoskeletal proteins cause a variety of pathologically shaped red cells, including spherocytes and elliptocytes (Chapter 29). In addition, proteins adsorbed to the outer surface of the red cell, especially albumin, may also play a role in both maintaining normal cell shape and effecting changes in that shape under some conditions. Red cells suspended in isotonic medium tend toward an echinocytic shape until albumin is added, and increasing amounts of albumin move cells toward the discoid shape.[280]

THE ERYTHROCYTE MEMBRANES AND CYTOSKELETON

The central feature of membrane structure is a matrix formed by a double layer of phospholipids. The lipid bilayer hypothesis was first proposed in 1925[281] and refined by Danielli and Davson a decade later.[282-284] Lipid molecules in the bilayer are oriented with the nonpolar groups directed toward one another, forming hydrophobic interactions. The hydrophilic polar head groups are directed outward, where they interact with the aqueous environment on both the cytoplasmic and plasma surfaces. Within this "sea of lipids" float globular proteins, some that penetrate the membrane completely and others that penetrate the membrane only partially and may be exposed at only one surface. Some proteins appear to have considerable lateral mobility, but in the red cell, many proteins interact with other membrane components, giving them a degree of immobility. Some proteins traverse the lipid bilayer once, whereas others have multiple membrane-spanning domains. On the cytoplasmic side of the membrane is a network of structural proteins that form a cytoskeleton. Certain membrane-spanning proteins interact with various cytoskeletal proteins.[285] Some transmembrane proteins also become covalently linked to lipid,[286] while the glycosylphosphatidylinositol-anchored class of proteins has no membrane-spanning domain but instead has phospholipid "tails" by which they are attached to the membrane.[287]

Much that is known about red cell membranes is derived from studies of the insoluble portion of the cell remaining after hemolysis is induced by osmotic rupture. This material has been called red cell stroma and, if the membrane remains intact after hemolysis, red cell "ghosts." It consists largely of components of the membrane, including the cytoskeleton. Such preparations contain about 52% protein, 40% lipid, and 8% carbohydrate by weight.[288] Most of the carbohydrate is accounted for by the oligosaccharide portion of glycoproteins, with a smaller fraction (about 7%) carried by glycolipids.[288,289]

Lipid Composition

Virtually all of the lipids in the mature erythrocyte are found in the membrane[289-293] (*Table 6.1*). The majority of erythrocyte membrane lipids are phospholipids or unesterified cholesterol, which are present in approximately equimolar quantities. There are four phospholipids: phosphatidylcholine (lecithin), phosphatidylethanolamine, sphingomyelin, and phosphatidylserine. Phospholipids are distributed asymmetrically between the two lipid layers of the membrane.[294,295] Almost all of the aminophosphatides (phosphatidylethanolamine and phosphatidylserine) lie within the inner (cytoplasmic) monolayer, whereas the choline-containing lipids (phosphatidylcholine and sphingomyelin) are the major components of the outer monolayer (*Figure 6.9*). Little or no phosphatidylserine is detectable in the outer lipid layer of normal, nonsenescent red cells. Maintenance of normal asymmetry results in improved mechanical membrane stability under applied shear stress and further appears to supply additional means for cytoskeleton attachment to the lipid bilayer through spectrin-phosphatidylserine interaction.[296] This organization of phospholipids across the bilayer is maintained by transmembrane transporters (flippases).[297]

Table 6.1. *Lipids of the Normal Human Erythrocyte Membrane*

Lipid	Molar Concentration[193]		Weight Concentration[245]	
	μmol/10¹⁰ Cells	Percent of Total	mg/10¹⁰ Cells	Percent of Total
Phospholipids				
Phosphatidylcholine (lecithin)	1.3		1.0	
Phosphatidylethanolamine (cephalin)	1.2		0.9	
Sphingomyelin	1.0		0.8	
Phosphatidylserine	0.6		0.4	
Lysolecithin	0.04			
Others	0.07			
Total phospholipids	4.2	49.5	3.1 (1.7-3.2)ᵃ	69
Cholesterol	4.0	47.1	1.3 (1.1-1.4)ᵃ	29
Glycolipids (globoside)	0.21	3.4	0.1	2
Total lipids	8.41	100	4.5 (3.9-5.2)ᵃ	100

ᵃ*Range in parentheses.*

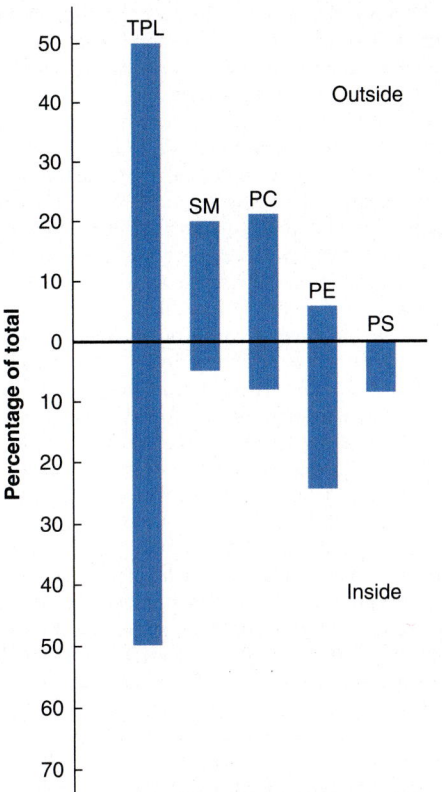

FIGURE 6.9 Distribution of erythrocyte phospholipids between the inner and outer layers of the membrane. PC, phosphatidylcholine; PE, phosphatidylethanolamine; PS, phosphatidylserine; SM, sphingomyelin; TPL, total phospholipids. (From Rothman JE, Lenard J. Membrane asymmetry. *Science.* 1977;195(4280):743-753. Copyright © 1977 by the American Association for the Advancement of Science. Reprinted with permission from AAAS.)

Conditions in which there is loss of asymmetry, in particular the appearance of the anionic phospholipid phosphatidylserine on the external membrane surface, can serve as an early indicator of apoptosis in many cells.[298] In sickle cell anemia, this may be responsible for the shortened RBC survival.[299] The lateral mobility of lipids in the outer membrane layer exceeds that of lipids in the inner layer since lipids in the inner layer may be restricted in their mobility because of interactions of phospholipids with cytoskeletal proteins.[296,300,301]

An additional effect on lipid mobility and membrane deformability may come from the fact that the fatty acids found in erythrocyte phospholipids are also not distributed evenly between the two bilayers.[291,295,302,303] Overall, about one-half of the fatty acids in the membrane are unsaturated. Unsaturated fatty acids, however, and particularly the polyunsaturated acyl chains with four or more double bonds, are a disproportionately large part of the inner leaflet phospholipids, phosphatidylethanolamine and phosphatidylserine. In contrast, phosphatidylcholine, which is predominantly in the outer lipid layer, contains most of the shorter chain saturated fatty acids. Sphingomyelin is especially enriched in fatty acids, with a chain length longer than 20. Membranes rich in sphingomyelin are less "fluid" than those with relatively larger amounts of lecithin.[304] An increased ratio of sphingomyelin to lecithin is found in abetalipoproteinemia and probably accounts for the erythrocyte abnormalities associated with that disorder[302] (see Chapter 29).

The neutral lipid of the erythrocyte consists almost entirely of free, nonesterified cholesterol,[304] and the translocation rate of cholesterol between the two layers is extremely rapid. Cholesterol has a pronounced effect on membrane fluidity.[305,306] It interacts with phospholipids to form what has been called an "intermediate gel state." Thus, compared with pure phospholipid membranes, membranes containing cholesterol are less fluid, that is, more viscous. Relatively modest increases in membrane cholesterol content decrease membrane deformability.[307] Abnormally high levels of cholesterol lead to distortions in red cell

shape; bizarre spicules form ("spur cells"), deformability of the cells is reduced, and they are destroyed in the spleen (Chapter 29).

Lipid Turnover and Acquisition

The mature erythrocyte is unable to synthesize lipids de novo; therefore, any lipid loss must be compensated for by renewal from pathways of interchange with the plasma[303] (*Figure 6.10*). Quantitatively, the most important of these pathways are the transfer of cholesterol and phosphatidylcholine (lecithin) from plasma lipoproteins to red cells (pathways 1 and 3). The rates of transfer are functions of the relative plasma and red cell levels of these lipids and are indirectly affected by the activity of the cholesterol-esterifying enzyme in plasma, lecithin-cholesterol acyltransferase (LCAT).[308] This enzyme catalyzes the reaction in which a fatty acid in the 2 position of lecithin is transferred to free cholesterol, forming cholesterol ester and lysolecithin (*Figure 6.11*, reaction 1A). Neither of the LCAT reaction products can enter the membrane. In patients with congenital LCAT deficiency, membrane cholesterol and lecithin are increased and the red cells are target shaped.[309]

The exchange of cholesterol and lecithin between red cells and plasma is also affected by the plasma bile salt concentration.[310] If erythrocytes are incubated in normal plasma to which bile salts have been added, the cells acquire cholesterol, and this change is accompanied by an increase in surface area and the formation of target cells. Although the mechanism of bile salt action is not fully understood, at least two properties appear to be important: Bile salts inhibit the LCAT reaction and, in addition, they bring about a shift in the distribution of free cholesterol between plasma and cell. Phospholipids also may be added to the membrane.

Membrane Proteins

Early in the history of membrane biochemistry, erythrocytes were used as a model system for the study of plasma membranes because they lacked organelle and nuclear membranes, making the membranes easy to isolate. Solubilization of membrane proteins is accomplished

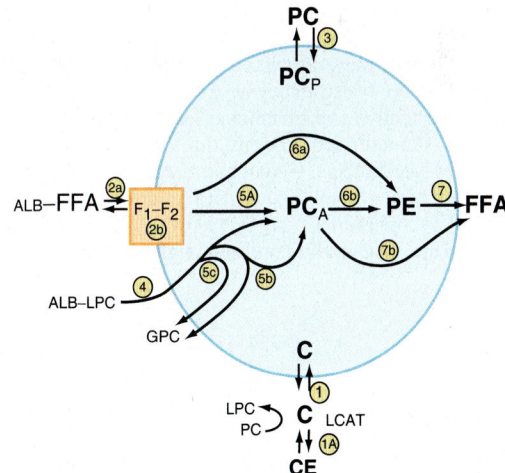

FIGURE 6.10 Pathways of lipid acquisition and turnover in the mature red cell membrane. Reactions and pathways: (1) exchange of cholesterol with plasma lipoprotein; (1A) the LCAT reaction; (2a) transfer of FFA from albumin to membrane; (2b) penetration of FFA to a metabolically active site; (3) exchange of PC with plasma lipoprotein; (4) transfer of LPC from albumin to membrane; (5A) LPC + FFA → PC; (5b) 2LPC → FFA + GPC; (5c) LPC → FFA + GPC; (6a) LPE + FFA → PE; (6b) PC + LPE → LPC + PE; (7) PE → LPE + FFA; (7b) PC → LPC + FFA. Alb, albumin; C, cholesterol; CE, cholesterol ester; FFA, free fatty acid; GPC, glycerylphosphoryl choline; LCAT, lecithin-cholesterol acyltransferase; LPC, lysophosphatidyl choline; LPE, lysophosphatidyl ethanolamine; PC, phosphatidyl choline (lecithin); PE, phosphatidyl ethanolamine. (From Shohet SB. Hemolysis and changes in erythrocyte membrane lipids. *N Engl J Med.* 1972;286(11):577-583. Copyright © 1972 Massachusetts Medical Society. Reprinted with permission from Massachusetts Medical Society.)

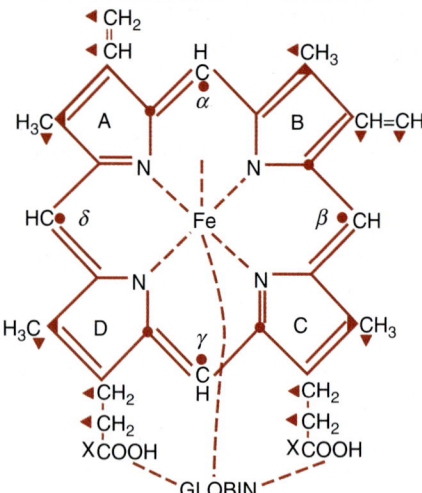

FIGURE 6.11 Chemical structure of heme and its manner of union with globin to form hemoglobin. The carbon atoms derived from the α carbon of glycine are represented by ● ▲, those supplied from the methyl carbon of acetate by ▲, and those derived from the carboxyl group of acetate by ×. The unmarked carbons are those derived either from the methyl carbon atom of acetate or from the carboxyl atom. (Prepared by Dr. G. E. Cartwright.)

by the addition of detergent. Use of an ionic detergent, most commonly sodium dodecyl sulfate (SDS), accomplishes solubilization of essentially all membrane proteins. Proteins extracted from membranes by detergent solubilization can be separated and analyzed with relatively high resolution by means of electrophoresis in polyacrylamide gels.[311,312] Such gels are stained by protein stains, usually Coomassie brilliant blue or by reagents that react with carbohydrate, such as periodic acid-Schiff (PAS).

On Coomassie-stained gels, seven major bands are usually identified, whereas PAS stains four major bands and several minor ones (*Figure 6.12*). Originally, the seven major protein bands were referred to by number. As further refinements in SDS-PAGE produced greater resolution, other bands have been given decimal or alphanumeric designations. Most of these proteins are no longer identified by this numeric nomenclature because they have been given specific names as their chemical structures and membrane function have been defined. The major PAS-stained bands contain three proteins, termed glycophorins or sialoglycoproteins. Glycophorins A and B are proteins that are derived from highly homologous genes and form both homo- and heterodimers. Glycophorins C and D are two proteins produced by a single gene and are structurally unrelated to glycophorins A and B.

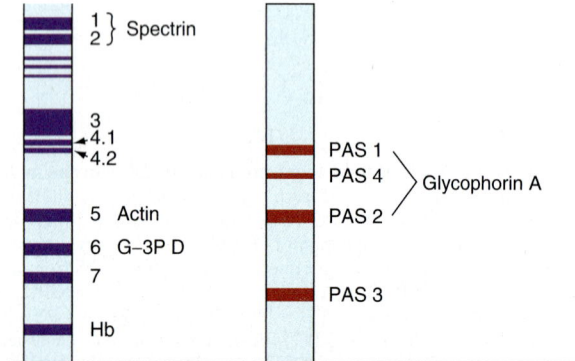

FIGURE 6.12 Schematic of polyacrylamide gel electrophoresis of erythrocyte membrane proteins. In this system, polypeptides migrate according to molecular size, with the smaller molecules moving the farthest. Figure reflects gels stained with Coomassie brilliant blue (left) and periodic acid-Schiff (PAS) reaction (right). (Data from Steck TL. The organization of proteins in the human red blood cell membrane. *J Cell Biol.* 1974;62:1-19.)

With recent advancements in mass spectrometry and the availability of protein databases, the field of proteomics has evolved. The proteome is the entire complement of proteins in a tissue, including all the particular modifications made to a given protein (phosphorylation, glycosylation, acetylation, ubiquitination, etc). The RBC proteome contains hundreds of membrane and soluble proteins. The significance of erythrocyte protein patterns in normal, aging, and RBC disorders is currently an active area of investigation.[313-315]

Historically, as noted above, membrane proteins were first characterized by whether they were stainable by protein-binding or carbohydrate-specific dyes. Now, however, they are classified on the basis of their relationship to the membrane or their functions. One common classification of membrane proteins comprises the categories of integral membrane proteins and peripheral membrane proteins.[316] Integral membrane proteins are most often globular and amphipathic; they have distinct hydrophobic and hydrophilic domains. Of the major Coomassie-stainable proteins, bands 3, 4.5, and 7 are integral membrane proteins. These proteins have one or more membrane-spanning domains. Band 3 has several extracellular domains, of which some are highly glycosylated. Band 4.5 is the glucose transporter. All other Coomassie-stained bands are situated within the cell, either as part of the cytoskeleton or bound in a more or less loose fashion to the inner leaflet of the membrane. All the PAS-stainable proteins are integral membrane proteins. Integral membrane proteins require detergent for removal from the membrane, whereas peripheral membrane proteins can often be extracted from "ghosts" by manipulation of the pH and ion content of buffers and tend to be soluble in neutral aqueous buffers. Proteins attached by phosphatidylinositol anchors to the outer membrane layer also require detergents or other reagents capable of disrupting the lipid bilayer for solubilization.[287]

Transmembrane Proteins

The two predominant erythrocyte transmembrane proteins are GPA and the anion channel (AE1, also known as band 3). AE1 has a number of crucial roles in red cell biology.

Glycophorin A is the principal PAS-stainable glycoprotein of erythrocyte membranes, accounting for approximately 85% of PAS-positive membrane protein. The N terminus of GPA bears the M or N antigen. GPA has also been found to be a binding site for several pathogens, including *Plasmodium falciparum*.[317] Numerous variants of GPA have been described and may cause production of alloantibodies after transfusion. Rarely, some persons lack this protein totally. Although absence of GPA causes no clinically significant hematologic problems, persons with this deficiency may make antibodies that render blood transfusion difficult, given the general unavailability of blood from other GPA-deficient donors.

Glycophorin B, the second most abundant PAS-staining protein, is present on the erythrocyte in one-tenth to one-third the copy number of GPA.[318] Glycophorin B is highly homologous to GPA and the N terminus of glycophorin B carries the "N" amino acid sequence of GPA and always expresses the N antigen.

AE1 is the erythrocyte anion channel or anion-exchange protein. AE1 most likely traverses the membrane 12 times. It has several extracellular domains, but the fourth is the major bearer of carbohydrate. This domain is heavily glycosylated and bears carbohydrate blood group antigens, including I and i and the antigens of the ABO major blood group system. The function of AE1 relates to Cl–HCO$_3$ exchange and it also interacts with the erythroid cytoskeleton by binding ankyrin. Complete absence of erythroid AE1 is rare in humans and has been associated with severe hemolytic anemia and renal tubular acidosis. However, many different mutations of AE1 have been described in association with hereditary spherocytosis and other RBC membrane disorders associated with hemolysis (Chapter 29).

The *Rh proteins* are also important integral membrane proteins. Although they are present in only 100,000 copies per cell,[318] these proteins are clearly important both to erythrocyte biology as well as to transfusion medicine. The RhD protein is the most immunodominant determinant of red cells outside the ABO antigens and is thus the only non-ABO determinant routinely taken into account when blood is selected for nonalloimmunized recipients. Absence of all Rh proteins, as in the Rh$_{null}$ syndrome, is associated with multiple erythrocyte defects and mild hemolytic anemia.[319] The proteins that carry the D, C (or c), and E (or e) Rh antigens are highly homologous to one another and traverse the membrane multiple times.[320] Two Rh genes situated very near each other on chromosome 1 encode the proteins that bear Rh antigens; in the normal situation, one gene encodes the D antigen and the other encodes a protein that bears both the E/e and C/c antigens.[321]

Cytoskeletal Proteins

The most abundant of the peripheral proteins are those that make up the spectrin-actin cytoskeletal complex, accounting for about 35% of the membrane protein. The complex includes large α and β spectrin polypeptide chains (bands 1 and 2 on gel electrophoresis, molecular weight about 240 kD and 225 kD, respectively) and the smaller actin chain corresponding to band 5. The relationship between the integral and peripheral proteins of the membrane is illustrated in *Figure 6.13*.

Spectrin proteins are long, rod-shaped molecules that self-associate into a two-dimensional network with the help of other cytoskeletal proteins.[285] The two forms of spectrin are homologous to each other; however, they are encoded by genes on two different chromosomes, chromosome 1 (α spectrin) and chromosome 14 (β spectrin).[322-324] The α and β spectrin molecules form heterodimers by aligning in antiparallel pairs. These heterodimers then form tetramers by head-to-head association.[285] Incorporation of these tetramers into the latticework of the cytoskeleton occurs with the interaction of other peripheral membrane proteins (*Figure 6.13*).[285]

Erythrocyte actin is an abundant erythrocyte protein of about 45 kD. Actin filaments associate with spectrin tetramers at the ends containing the carboxy terminus of the α-chain and the amino terminus of the β-chain. This association, however, is a low-affinity interaction in the absence of other accessory proteins.

In addition to spectrin and actin, other cytoskeletal proteins are important for membrane stability and maintenance of cell shape. Protein 4.1 contains a spectrin-binding domain and is known to promote spectrin-actin interaction. Ankyrin (Protein 2.1) also serves as a mode of attachment of the cytoskeleton to the membrane.[325] Ankyrin binds to both the anion exchanger band 3 and spectrin. As discussed in

Chapter 29, deficiencies or abnormalities in these cytoskeletal proteins are associated with abnormal erythrocyte shapes, abnormal membrane stability, and hereditary hemolytic anemias.[326]

Membrane Transport Proteins and Membrane Permeability

In general, the membrane acts as a partial barrier to penetration of all solutes. Nonpolar substances diffuse through the membrane at a rate proportional to their solubility in organic solvents. Polar solutes cross the membrane at specialized sites. The erythrocyte membrane has a number of specialized transport proteins, including the anion transporter (AE1, band 3), several cation transporters, a glucose transporter, and a water channel.

The RBC behaves as an osmometer; RBC water always is in osmotic equilibrium. In large part this occurs because erythrocytes have an abundant and highly active water channel protein, aquaporin-1, which contributes as much as 85% of the osmotic water permeability pathway.[327] Aquaporin-1 occurs as a homotetrameric protein that expresses on its extracellular domain both ABH and Colton blood group antigens.[328] Red cells that lack aquaporin-1 have only slightly reduced lifespan in vivo.[327]

There are several pathways that regulate water and solute homeostasis, with one of the major determinants being the monovalent cation content. The erythrocyte membrane is only slightly permeable to the major monovalent cations (Na$^+$ and K$^+$), whereas it is much more permeable to monovalent anions (Cl$^-$ and HCO$_3^-$). Cation concentrations within the erythrocyte are approximately 130 mM K$^+$ and 8 mM Na$^+$, while the plasma contains approximately 140 mM Na$^+$ and 4 mM K$^+$. The steady-state cation concentrations within the erythrocyte are the result of an equilibrium between passive diffusion ("leak") and active transport ("pump"). With respect to sodium, the direction of leak is inward and the direction of pump is outward; in contrast, potassium leaks out and is pumped in. The major cation pump represents a process in which sodium inside the cell is exchanged for potassium on the outside and energy is supplied by ATP. For each molecule of ATP converted to ADP, three sodium ions are pumped out and two potassium ions enter.[329] Active Na$^+$ and K$^+$ transport depends on the activity of the membrane protein Na-K ATPase. Anions cross the membrane by one of two pathways. The first represents an exchange reaction in which an internal anion is exchanged for an external anion. This rapid

The Normal Hematologic System

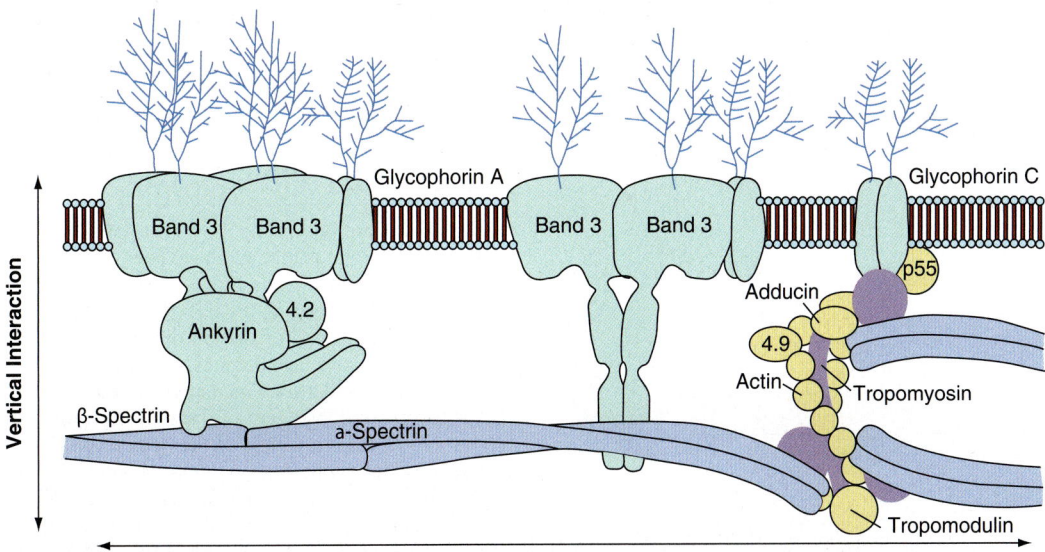

FIGURE 6.13 The erythrocyte membrane. A schematic model of the major proteins of the erythrocyte membrane showing α- and β-spectrin, ankyrin, band 3 (the anion exchanger), 4.1 (protein 4.1) and 4.2 (protein 4.2), actin, and glycophorin. Membrane protein-protein and protein-lipid interactions are often divided into two categories: (1) vertical interactions, which are perpendicular to the plane of the membrane and involve spectrin-ankyrin-band 3-protein 4.2 interactions and weak interactions between spectrin and the negatively charged lipids of the inner half of the membrane lipid bilayer; and (2) horizontal interactions, which are parallel to the plane of the membrane and include interactions between junctional complex proteins and spectrin or other membrane proteins. (From Tse WT, Lux SE. Red blood cell membrane disorders. *Br J Haematol.* 1999;104(1):2-13. Copyright © 1999 Blackwell Science Ltd. Reprinted by permission of John Wiley & Sons, Inc.)

exchange is mediated by the band 3 anion-exchange protein and plays an important role in the chloride-bicarbonate exchanges that occur as the red cell moves between the lungs and tissues (*Figure 6.14*).[330] The second anion pathway represents considerably slower ionic diffusion, accounting for net loss or gain of anions in response to excess K^+ loss or Na^+ entry into the cell, respectively. It should be noted that anions are distributed passively across the cell membrane with steady-state concentrations determined by the Donnan equilibrium. Since the total cation content must equal the total anion charge, the presence of negatively charged impermeant intracellular anions (hemoglobin, 2,3 DPG, adenine nucleotides) influences the RBC monovalent anion content, and thereby explains why concentration of intracellular Cl^- and HCO_3^- is less than the intracellular monovalent cation content. Red cells have two additional monovalent transport processes that specifically result in KCl and water loss with a reduction in cell volume. *KCl cotransport* is stimulated by RBC swelling, leading to K^+ and Cl^- exit from the cell, with an obligatory water loss to maintain isotonicity.[331] This KCl transport pathway is particularly important in regulating cell volume, and is most active in reticulocytes. By decreasing the cell volume of reticulocytes, the hemoglobin concentration is thereby increased to the levels seen in mature red cells. KCl transport is active in sickle and hemoglobin C disorders, and may account for some of the hydration abnormalities seen in these conditions. The *calcium-activated K^+ channel* was first described many years ago by Gardos.[332] Under conditions where Ca^+ accumulates in red cells, there is a rapid loss of K^+ (and Cl^-) without any compensatory Na^+ gain, thus leading to water loss and cellular dehydration. This Gardos effect can be demonstrated in RBC of all ages. The physiologic function of the calcium-activated K^+ channel is not known. It too may be related to some of the RBC hydration changes that are seen in sickle cell anemia.[333] Also, it is now known that the gene encoding this Gardos channel (*KCNN4*) is mutated in some case of hereditary xerocytosis and is responsible for the K loss and cellular dehydration characteristic of this disorder[334] (see Chapter 29). A third regulator of cell volume is the mechanotransduction Piezo1 protein channel. Under the influence of mechanical stresses RBC can become dehydrated. It is now recognized that most cases of hereditary xerocytosis are due to mutations in *FAM38A/PIEZO1*, the gene which encodes PIEZO1.[335]

Glucose enters the erythrocyte by facilitated diffusion, mediated by a transmembrane protein designated the glucose transporter, encoded by the gene *GLUT1*.[336] The transport of glucose into the erythrocyte provides the energy substrate for anaerobic glycolysis; however, the energy requirement of the erythrocyte appears to be relatively low, and the efficiency of glucose transport is relatively high. Therefore, glucose transport is not rate limiting for glycolysis.[337,338] Fructose is not transported under physiologic conditions ($K_m > 200$ mM).

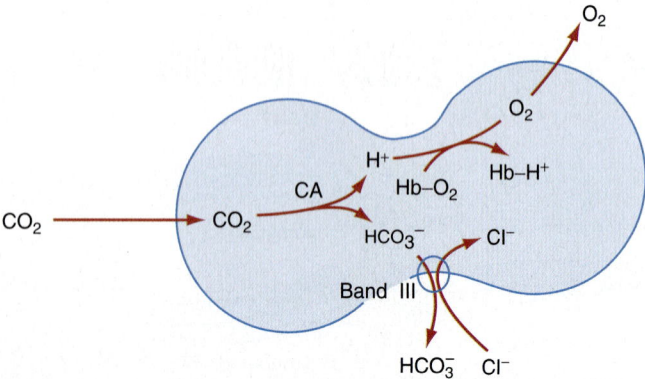

FIGURE 6.14 Role of band 3 in anion and CO_2 transport. The ability of band 3 to accelerate anion transport across the membrane allows rapid equilibration of bicarbonate with the extracellular plasma and concomitant influx of chloride ion. CA, carbonic anhydrase; Hb, hemoglobin. (From Kopito RR, Lodish HF. Structure of the murine anion exchange protein. *J Cell Biochem.* 1985;29(1):1-17. Copyright © 1985 Alan R. Liss, Inc. Reprinted by permission of John Wiley & Sons, Inc.)

Membrane and Membrane-Associated Enzymes

At least 50 enzymes are either membrane proteins or are bound to the erythrocyte membrane in some fashion; certain enzymes are both free in the cytoplasm as well as associated with the membrane. Their functions range from facilitating transport of a variety of molecules necessary to the erythrocyte to playing important roles in producing and using energy from glucose metabolism.

Some erythrocyte enzymes are externally oriented and can therefore react with substrates in the red cell environment. A classic example of an externally oriented enzyme is acetylcholinesterase, first of several membrane proteins discovered to be missing from the affected erythrocytes of patients with paroxysmal nocturnal hemoglobinuria (PNH) (see Chapter 32). It belongs to a class of proteins that are attached to the membrane by a phosphatidylinositol-glycan anchor, so that the entire polypeptide portion of the molecule is extracellular.[287] The role of acetylcholinesterase on the red cell remains obscure[339]; however, some other proteins in this class are complement regulatory proteins; it is the absence of these proteins that causes the characteristic hemolysis of PNH.

Among the enzymes required for the production and use of ATP there are three that form a membrane-bound enzyme complex: aldolase, glyceraldehyde 3-phosphate dehydrogenase (G3PD), and phosphoglycerate kinase. Together, these three enzymes convert fructose diphosphate to 3-phosphoglycerate with the production of ATP. G3PD is the enzyme present in greatest amount in membrane preparations and is seen as band 6 in polyacrylamide gels. G3PD is also found in the erythrocyte cytoplasm and can be demonstrated to bind to a cytoplasmic segment of band 3.

Enzymes that use and degrade ATP are also found in the membrane, although they are not present in large enough quantities to account for bands seen in Coomassie-stained polyacrylamide gels of membrane proteins. Like protein kinases, ATPases phosphorylate membrane proteins, but instead of forming phosphoserine or phosphothreonine bonds, they form acyl bonds as transient intermediates in the catalytic cycle. Important and well-studied ATPases of the erythrocyte membrane include Na^+-K^+ ATPase, Ca^{2+}-Mg^{2+} ATPase, and Mg^{2+} ATPase. The Na^+-K^+ ATPase is also known as the sodium pump or sodium-potassium pump.

Protein kinases are enzymes that phosphorylate other proteins in the presence of ATP by forming phosphoserine or phosphothreonine bonds. Phosphorylation is a major step in the regulation of a variety of target molecules, including structural proteins and enzymes. Both red cell membrane-bound and cytosolic kinases may phosphorylate membrane proteins.[340] In general, phosphorylated structural proteins demonstrate lower-affinity binding to their target proteins than do unphosphorylated proteins. For example, phosphorylation of protein 4.1 leads to a decreased affinity for spectrin and a decreased ability of 4.1 to promote spectrin-actin association.[285]

HEMOGLOBIN AND ERYTHROCYTE FUNCTION

Hemoglobins are one of the most widespread and specialized hemoproteins existing in nature and have been found in prokaryotes, fungi, plants, and animals. These proteins permit the reversible binding of O_2 to heme while keeping the iron in the +2 (ferrous) state. They also facilitate the exchange of carbon dioxide between the lungs and the tissues. Studies have also demonstrated the importance of hemoglobin in control of vascular tone mediated by NO. In vertebrates, hemoglobin is the major constituent of the red cell cytoplasm, accounting for about 90% of the dry weight of the mature cell.

In most invertebrates, oxygen-carrying pigment is transported freely in the plasma rather than within cells. This is an inefficient delivery system. Hemoglobin, as a protein-free in the plasma, would exert an osmotic pressure about five times greater than that produced by the plasma proteins. By the inclusion of hemoglobin in RBCs, the viscosity of the blood can be maintained at a low level, water is not drawn from the tissues by it, and the flow of blood containing such a large amount of protein is made possible. Furthermore, free hemoglobin is not maintained in the circulation and is subject to oxidative denaturation. Attempts to make hemoglobin substitutes have revealed that infusion of free hemoglobin or derivatives causes a significant increase in blood pressure, as a result of the scavenging by free heme of NO produced by vascular endothelium.[341]

In humans at rest, about 250 mL of oxygen are consumed and 200 mL of carbon dioxide are produced per minute. During exercise, these quantities increase 10-fold. If the respiratory gases were carried in physical solution in the plasma, human activity would be restricted to only one-fiftieth of that possible in the presence of hemoglobin-containing red cells. Red cell hemoglobin permits the transportation of 100 times more oxygen than could be carried by the plasma alone.

Evolution and Structure of Hemoglobin

Vertebrate hemoglobin is a conjugated protein with a molecular weight near 64,500 Da. It is a tetramer, consisting of two pairs of similar globin polypeptide chains, covalently attached to a heme complex, ferroprotoporphyrin IX, which is a complex of iron and protoporphyrin[342] (*Figure 6.11*).

Human hemoglobins share a common ancestry with a simpler, single-chain molecule that was similar to myoglobin. The divergence of the invertebrate and vertebrate globin genes occurred more than 670 million years ago, and the divergence of the α and non–α-globin genes probably descended from a common gene more than 450 million years ago.[343] Such an evolution would explain the high degree of homology between the α and non–α-chains, as well as the extraordinary similarities among the non–α-globins. The non-α globin gene family is sometimes designated the β-globin gene family.

Ontogeny of Hemoglobins

Erythroid development is divided into three developmental periods: embryonic, fetal, and adult. In each developmental period, the oxygen delivery requirements are different, and erythroid development has evolved to meet these needs. The genes that encode the α-globin gene family are on chromosome 16 (ζ, α), whereas the genes that encode the members of the non–α-globin gene family (ϵ, γ, β, and δ) are on chromosome 11.[344] These genes are developmentally and coordinately regulated, and through the production of different pairs of globins, different hemoglobins are produced to permit their appropriate expression during different developmental periods. The α-globin gene cluster is capable of producing two types of globins, zeta (ζ) and α. The ζ is an embryonic globin chain produced during the first 8 weeks of fetal development, whereas α is produced during the remainder of the fetal and adult developmental periods. The β-globin gene family members include the embryonic globin ϵ, the fetal globin γ, and two globins expressed primarily during the adult period, β and δ.

The differential pattern of globin gene expression through embryonic and fetal development into adult life leads to the production and assembly of various globins into the specific hemoglobins characteristic of the stage of development (*Figure 6.15*).

Embryonic hemoglobins have oxygen affinity comparable to fetal hemoglobin. The γ chains are encoded by pairs of genes that encode nearly identical proteins: Gγ has a glycine at position 136, whereas Aγ has an alanine.[345] In addition, many Aγ genes also encode a threonine-for-isoleucine substitution at position 75 of the protein.[346] During fetal life, Gγ constitutes about 75% of γ chains, whereas hemoglobin F in adults contains about 60% Aγ chains.[347] This has no known physiologic significance.

Red cells containing hemoglobin F have higher oxygen affinity than adult red cells. This permits the fetus to compete effectively for oxygen in the maternal blood. However, hemoglobin lysates from adult and fetal cells have nearly identical oxygen affinity when they are dialyzed against saline or a neutral buffer.[348] This property of fetal hemoglobin is due to amino acid differences in the amino terminus of the γ chains that impair binding of 2,3-diphosphoglycerate (2,3-DPG, also known as 2,3-bisphosphoglycerate, 2-3-BPG), an allosteric modifier of oxygen binding.[349]

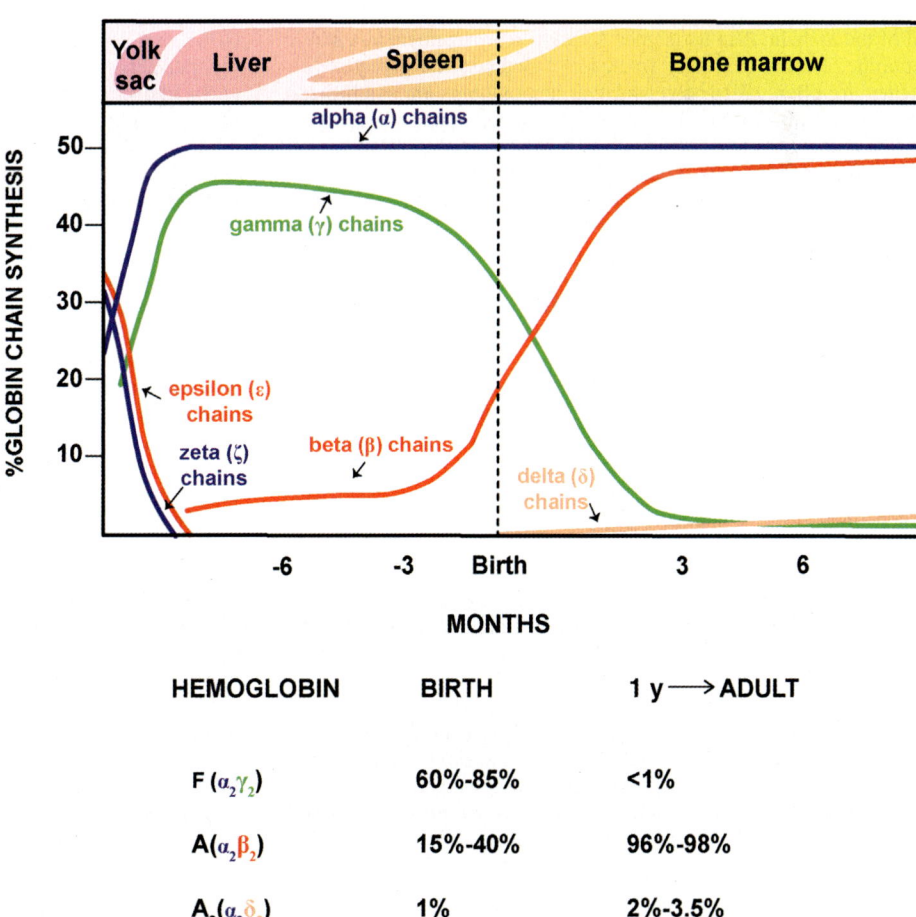

FIGURE 6.15 Fetal, neonatal, and adult erythropoiesis and hemoglobin production. Top: Site of erythropoiesis. Middle: Specific globin chain synthesis. Bottom: Hemoglobin composition at birth and after 1 year of age.

HEMOGLOBIN	BIRTH	1 y ⟶ ADULT
F ($\alpha_2\gamma_2$)	60%-85%	<1%
A ($\alpha_2\beta_2$)	15%-40%	96%-98%
A$_2$ ($\alpha_2\delta_2$)	1%	2%-3.5%

The proportion of the different hemoglobins produced during the different developmental periods is summarized in *Figure 6.15*. At about 20 weeks of fetal development, the site of erythropoiesis begins to switch from the liver and spleen to the bone marrow, where progenitors show increased expression of adult globins, α and β. Beginning at the 30th week and proceeding to the time of birth, a significant switch from fetal to adult erythropoiesis takes place, such that at the time of birth, fetal hemoglobin constitutes approximately 80% of the total hemoglobin. Over the next 25 to 30 weeks following birth, fetal hemoglobin concentration decreases by approximately 10% every 2 weeks until it reaches its normal adult level of <2% by 30 weeks of age.[350] Neonates with hemoglobinopathies or erythropoietic stress can have a greatly prolonged production of hemoglobin F, sometimes extending into adulthood.[351]

Hemoglobin A, $\alpha_2\beta_2$, is the predominant adult hemoglobin and normally constitutes approximately 96% of the total adult hemoglobin. Hemoglobin, A_2, is a minor hemoglobin produced beginning at 35 weeks of gestation but has little physiologic relevance. It normally constitutes <3.5% of hemoglobin; however, it is typically increased in β-thalassemias. Clinically, its major importance is its value in diagnosing β-thalassemias (see Chapter 35).

Modifications of Normal Hemoglobin

Analysis of human red cell hemolysates by cation-exchange chromatography reveals several negatively charged minor hemoglobins that are designated A_{Ia}, A_{Ib}, and A_{Ic}, corresponding to their order of elution. These hemoglobins are formed by the nonenzymatic interaction of glucose with the α-amino groups of valine residues at the N terminus of the β-chains of hemoglobin.[352]

The best characterized of the acquired variants is hemoglobin A_{Ic}, which constitutes about 3.5% of the hemoglobin in normal subjects and may be increased two- to threefold in individuals with diabetes mellitus. Its level is directly proportional to the time-integrated mean blood glucose concentration over the life of the red cell, typically the preceding 2 to 3 months.[353] In the nonenzymatic glycation of hemoglobin A, a molecule of glucose forms a Schiff base with the N terminal of the β-chain, then undergoes Amadori rearrangement to a stable ketamine, 1-amino,1-deoxy fructose.[354] Because the glycated (or, as they are often called, glycosylated) hemoglobins are synthesized throughout the lifespan of the red cell, older cells contain a higher proportion of these modified hemoglobins than younger ones. Preferential destruction of older cells explains the observation that the proportion of this hemoglobin A_{Ic} is reduced in hemolytic anemia.[355] Clinical laboratories currently use a variety of assays to detect and quantify glycated hemoglobins, most commonly, high-pressure liquid chromatography.[356] Hemoglobin F and commonly encountered hemoglobin variants, such as Hb S, Hb C, Hb E, and Hb F, can interfere with these assays, and may help explain discordant assay results.

Laboratory Analysis of Hemoglobins

Normal and variant hemoglobins can be detected and quantified by standard clinical laboratory techniques. Traditionally, cellulose acetate electrophoresis performed at alkaline pH (hemoglobin electrophoresis), which can detect most of the common variants, was the standard laboratory modality.[357] Findings could be confirmed or supplemented by citrate agar electrophoresis or isoelectric focusing. High-performance liquid chromatography (HPLC) and capillary zone electrophoresis (CZE) have largely replaced electrophoresis in large laboratories. Both HPLC and CZE provide a clear separation of hemoglobins A, F, and A_2.

The analysis of hemoglobin A_2 and fetal hemoglobin levels deserves special attention because the levels of these components are indicative of common conditions affecting hemoglobin synthesis. In cases of β-thalassemia trait, hemoglobin A_2 levels are increased from the usual values of less than 3.5%. The subtle increases in hemoglobin A_2 that are characteristic of β-thalassemia trait cannot be quantified accurately by alkaline electrophoretic methods and most laboratories utilize HPLC or CZE[358] (*Figure 6.16*). It is an error to use hemoglobin electrophoresis as the sole method to rule out β-thalassemia.

Hereditary persistence of fetal hemoglobin (HPFH) and $\delta\beta$–thalassemia are types of β-thalassemia caused by deletion of δ- and β-globin

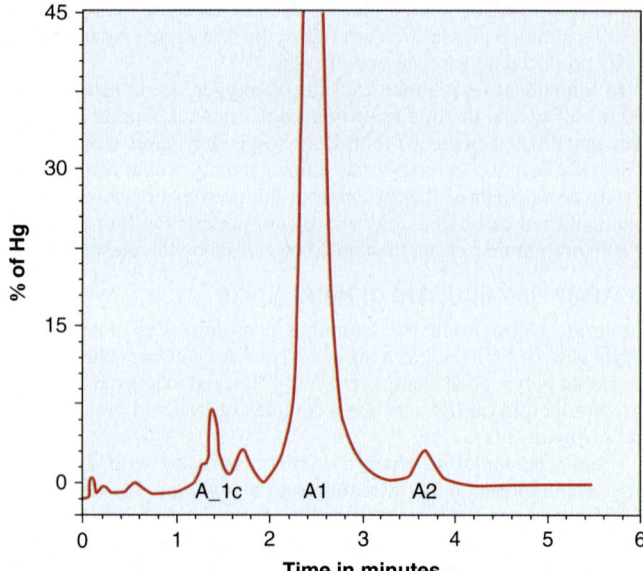

FIGURE 6.16 HPLC showing modified Hb A variants. Hb, hemoglobin; HPLC, high-performance liquid chromatography. (Image provided through the courtesy of the copyright holder, Dr. Edward C. Klatt.)

genes, but distinguished from typical β-thalassemia by more balanced α- and non–α-globin chain synthesis resulting from an increase in γ-globin production resulting in increased hemoglobin F. In both of these thalassemias, Hb A_2 levels are reduced as a result of deletion of δ-globin genes.

Elevated levels of hemoglobin F can be seen in thalassemias, disorders of hematopoiesis, or hereditary disorders of globin synthesis such as HPFH and δ-β–thalassemia.[359] Diagnosis requires the precise measurement of hemoglobin F levels, which can be achieved by either HPLC or CZE. Routine electrophoretic procedures do not completely separate hemoglobin F from A.

In adults, fetal hemoglobin is unevenly distributed in erythrocytes, being restricted to between 0.1% and 7% of total cells.[360] Cells containing fetal hemoglobin are designated F or A/F cells, wherein the hemoglobin F concentration is normally between 14% and 25% of the total hemoglobin.[361] In certain thalassemias and HPFH, the number of F cells is increased. This can be detected by acid treatment of erythrocytes on a glass slide followed by elution of the acid-sensitive hemoglobins (the Kleihauer-Betke technique). Counterstaining can identify hemoglobin F-containing cells among a sea of ghosts.[362]

In normal adult blood, this method demonstrates both colorless cells and light pink cells that vary in intensity containing fetal hemoglobin. By comparison, analysis of cord blood mixed with adult blood demonstrates that true fetal cells in cord blood stain intensely, reflecting the high level of fetal hemoglobin in fetal cells. This assay can be performed on maternal blood to detect feto-maternal hemorrhage or other contamination of the maternal circulation with fetal blood. This can also be tested using flow cytometry with a phycoerythrin-conjugated antiglycophorin antibody to detect feto-maternal hemorrhage.[363]

Structure of Globin

Proteins have at least four levels of structural organization: (1) primary structure, or the linear sequence of amino acids; (2) secondary structure, which describes how the amino acids within segments of the protein are spatially organized, for example, by folding into an α helix or β-pleated sheet; (3) tertiary structure, which refers to the steric relationships of sequence domains separate from each other when analyzed as part of the linear sequence of the protein; and (4) quaternary structure, or the way in which several polypeptide chains join to form a single molecule.

The exact primary structure of all normal globin chains has been determined based on the DNA sequence of the individual globin genes,[364] and the polypeptide chains in hemoglobin differ from one another in amino acid sequence. The α-chain contains 141 amino acids and the non–α-chains, 146. The members of the non–α-chain family are more similar to each other than any member of the non––α-chain family is to any member of the α-chain family. The δ-chain differs from the β-chain in only 10 of the 146 amino acid residues, whereas the γ and β-chains differ by 39 amino acids.

In spite of the differences in the primary structure of α and non–α-globin chains, their secondary structures are remarkably similar. Each has eight helical segments designated by the letters A through H.[365] The helixes of all the non–α-chain members are of identical length; however, a significant difference exists between the α- and non–α-globin chains in the region of the D helix, which contains seven amino acids in the ε, γ, δ, and β-chains, but only two amino acids in the α-chain. Because of the size of the D helix in the α-globin chains, many do not assign it a helix designation. The helixes make up about 75% of the molecule. Interspersed between them are seven nonhelical segments: NA, AB, CD, EF, FG, GH, and HC. This arrangement is important structurally, because the helixes are relatively rigid and linear, whereas the nonhelical segments allow bending.

A given amino acid in a polypeptide chain may be denoted either by its sequential number or by a helical number. In the sequential system, amino acids are numbered from 1 at the N terminus to 141 at the C terminus in the α-chain and from 1 to 146 in the β, γ, and δ-chains. In the helical system, each amino acid is designated by a letter and a number that indicate the helix and the position in the helix, respectively. The helical system is gradually gaining favor, because it illustrates the homology between chains and has more structural significance. For example, the histidine to which heme attaches is amino acid #87 in the α-chain and #92 in the β, γ, and δ-chains; the helical designation for this histidine is the same in all the normal chains, F8.

The tertiary and quaternary structures of hemoglobin have been studied by X-ray diffraction techniques, especially by Perutz and coworkers.[366] In aqueous solutions and in crystals, the polypeptide chains assume a structure in which the polar amino acids face the molecular surface, where they interact with water, rendering the molecule soluble. The groups directed toward the inner core of the molecule are all nonpolar, and the hydrophobic (van der Waals) bonding that occurs between them makes the structure stable. The resulting, roughly spherical, tertiary structure is similar for all the normal hemoglobin polypeptides (*Figure 6.17*) as well as for certain other heme proteins, such as myoglobin.

The heme pocket is the site of many dynamic interactions involving oxygen binding to hemoglobin. Heme is suspended in a nonpolar crevice between the E and F helixes (*Figure 6.17*), and helixes B, G, and H constitute the floor of the pocket. Heme iron forms a covalent bond with the imidazole nitrogen of the "proximal" histidine at F8. In addition, heme forms van der Waals bonds with many other parts of the molecule and in this way makes an important contribution to tertiary structure. If heme is extracted, the central helical regions, C, D, E, and F, unfold with a consequent decrease in solubility.[367] Not surprisingly, some unstable hemoglobins (see Chapter 36) result from amino acid substitutions in the residues that line the heme pocket.[368]

The binding of oxygen to the iron molecule causes the hemoglobin molecule to undergo conformational changes that affect the binding of oxygen to other heme sites.[369] In deoxyhemoglobin, the bond between the imidazole nitrogen of the proximal histidine and iron undergoes considerable strain, displacing iron from the plane of the ring. This strain is conveyed to other parts of the molecule and is in part responsible for the T or tense state of deoxyhemoglobin.[370] The addition of two molecules of oxygen, which is bound to the iron atom in the heme ring by end-on geometry, results in the formation of a hydrogen bond between the oxygen atom that is not bound directly to the iron and the imidazole nitrogen of the histidine at E7 (the "distal" histidine).[370] The binding of oxygen to iron changes the electron spin state of iron and relaxes the covalent bond with the proximal histidine, permitting the iron to move into the plane of the ring and relaxing the molecule, contributing to the R or relaxed state.[371] The overall conformational changes to hemoglobin appear to be the greatest after three molecules of O_2 have been added. In general, proteins that undergo an allosteric change from the tense (T) to a relaxed (R) state are better able to interact with substrate in the relaxed state. As a result, there are two quaternary structures for hemoglobin: one for the oxygenated form and one for the deoxygenated form.

Assembly of Hemoglobin

In general, there is little posttranscriptional regulation of the synthesis of globins, although factors such as the availability of heme can affect translation of globin mRNA.[372] Aside from several variants, such as hemoglobin Lepore, which are synthesized at a slower rate, the synthesis rate of most normal or mutant globins is the same.[373] Nevertheless, individuals with β-chain variants often express less of the variant hemoglobin than hemoglobin A. This observation has been attributed to an increased rate of catabolism of newly synthesized globin chains resulting from decreased solubility, defective heme binding, or abnormal subunit assembly. The best data indicate that the variations seen in most stable hemoglobin variants result from differences in subunit assembly.[374,375]

Following translation of globin mRNA and globin-chain synthesis, heme associates with globins and α-globin chains pair with members of the β-globin family. In large part this binding is a consequence of the different charges on α-globins, which are positively charged (pI = 8.1), and β-globins, which are negatively charged (pI = 6.6).[376] The greater the charge difference, the greater is the electrostatic attraction. Positively charged variants, such as $β_C$ and the uncharged $β_S$, bind to α-globin and assemble into α-β dimers at approximately half the rate of $β_A$ during in vitro mixing experiments.[375] Conversely, more negatively charged variants such as $β_{N-Baltimore}$ bind with a greater association rate. This phenomenon has been suggested as an explanation for the ratio of 60:40 seen for hemoglobin A and hemoglobin S in heterozygotes for $β_S$. Likewise, the percentage of N-Baltimore is increased over that of hemoglobin A.

In conditions of α-globin deficiency, this competition is more pronounced and the percentage of the more positively charged variant is further reduced. Patients who are heterozygous for $β_S$ and α-thalassemia carry percentages of hemoglobin S of approximately 35%, 30%, and 25%, corresponding to one-, two-, or three-gene α-thalassemia.[377]

Hemoglobin A_2 is decreased in certain α-thalassemias and sometimes in iron deficiency, which causes an acquired reduction in α-globin synthesis as a result of decreased heme synthesis. Under these

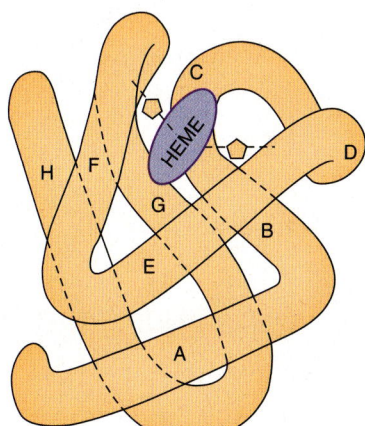

FIGURE 6.17 The tertiary structure of a single globin polypeptide chain. The helical segments, labeled A to H, are relatively linear; bending of the chains occurs between helices. Heme is suspended in a crevice between the E and F helices. (Courtesy of C. A. Finch.)

conditions, the more positively charged δ globin would be expected to compete less well with the normal β-globin. On the contrary, during β-globin deficiency associated with β-thalassemia, δ-globin would be expected to compete more effectively for α-globin chains, and the predicted increase in hemoglobin A_2 is observed.[378]

Oxygen Transport

In order to function as the primary medium of exchange of oxygen and carbon dioxide, hemoglobin must fulfill the four requirements first delineated by Barcroft in the 1920s[379]: It must be capable of transporting a large quantity of oxygen, it must be highly soluble, it must take up and release oxygen at "appropriate pressures," and it must also be a good buffer. Normal hemoglobin fulfills these requirements well, although many abnormal variants fail to meet one or more of these conditions.

Each gram of hemoglobin, when fully saturated, binds 1.39 mL of oxygen. The degree of saturation is related to the oxygen tension (Po_2), which normally ranges from 100 mm Hg in arterial blood to about 35 mm Hg in veins. The relation between oxygen tension and hemoglobin oxygen saturation is described by the oxygen dissociation curve of hemoglobin (*Figure 6.18*). The characteristics of this curve are related in part to properties of hemoglobin itself and in part to the environment within the erythrocyte, with pH, temperature, and concentration of 2,3-DPG being the most important factors affecting oxygen affinity.

Oxygen affinity of a particular hemoglobin is generally expressed in terms of the oxygen tension at which 50% saturation occurs, referred to as the P_{50}. When measured in whole erythrocytes, P_{50} of hemoglobin averages about 26 mm Hg in normal nonsmoking males.[380] When oxygen affinity increases, the dissociation curve shifts leftward, and the value for P_{50} is reduced. Conversely, with decreased oxygen affinity, the curve shifts to the right and P_{50} is increased.

Regulation of Oxygen Affinity

The oxygen dissociation curve of single-subunit heme polypeptides (e.g., myoglobin) is hyperbolic, and oxygen affinity is considerably greater than that of hemoglobin (*Figure 6.18*). In contrast, the oxygen dissociation curve of hemoglobin is sigmoidal; the steepest part of its slope occurs at levels of oxygen tension corresponding to those found in tissues. This difference between the hemoglobin and myoglobin curves is the result of interaction between the four heme-polypeptide units of hemoglobin. Although it was called heme-heme interaction in the past, *subunit cooperativity* better describes the process whereby the binding of oxygen by one subunit increases the oxygen affinity of other subunits; no direct interaction among heme moieties is involved. This allosteric property of hemoglobin permits rapid changes in oxygen affinity during the time the RBC passes through the capillary bed.

The change in oxygen affinity with pH is known as the Bohr effect.[381] Hemoglobin oxygen affinity is reduced as the acidity increases (*Figure 6.18*). Because the tissues are relatively rich in carbon dioxide, and because red cell carbonic anhydrase readily converts carbon dioxide to carbonic acid, the pH is lower there than in arterial blood; therefore, the Bohr effect facilitates transfer of oxygen to tissues. In the lungs, as oxygen is taken up and carbon dioxide is released, the pH rises and the oxygen-affinity curve shifts to the left. This event, termed the alkaline Bohr effect, increases the oxygen affinity of hemoglobin, helping to maximize oxygen uptake. Thus, the Bohr effect links and enhances the transport of both oxygen and carbon dioxide. Hemoglobin F has an enhanced alkaline Bohr effect, increasing oxygen affinity while passing through the fetal pulmonary vasculature.

Another important factor affecting the oxygen affinity of hemoglobin is the concentration of 2,3-DPG,[382-385] which can insert into the pocket between β-globin subunits in tetrameric hemoglobin and thereby reduce oxygen affinity. 2,3-DPG is synthesized from glycolytic intermediates by means of a pathway known as the Rapoport-Luebering shunt (*Figure 6.19*). In the erythrocyte, 2,3-DPG is the predominant phosphorylated compound, accounting for about two thirds of the red cell phosphorus; in contrast, it is present in only trace amounts in other tissues.

The most important function of 2,3-DPG is its effect on the oxygen affinity of hemoglobin. In the deoxygenated state, hemoglobin A can bind 2,3-DPG in a molar ratio of 1:1, a reaction that leads to reduced oxygen affinity and improved oxygen delivery to tissues. The increased oxygen affinity of fetal hemoglobin appears to be related to its lessened ability to bind 2,3-DPG. The increased oxygen affinity of stored blood is accounted for by reduced levels of 2,3-DPG.[386] Transfusion of such blood results in a transient in vivo increase in oxygen affinity that returns toward normal in 7 to 12 hours as the function of the glycolytic pathway is restored.

Changes in 2,3-DPG levels play a significant role in adaptation to hypoxia. In some situations associated with hypoxemia, 2,3-DPG

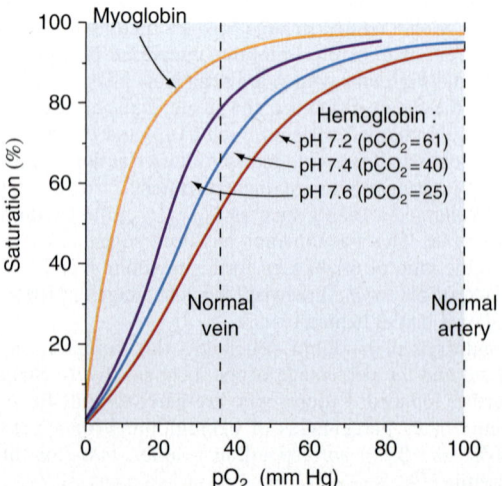

FIGURE 6.18 **Oxygen dissociation curve of hemoglobin, at three values for pH, compared with that of myoglobin.** pCO_2, partial pressure of carbon dioxide; pO_2, partial pressure of oxygen.

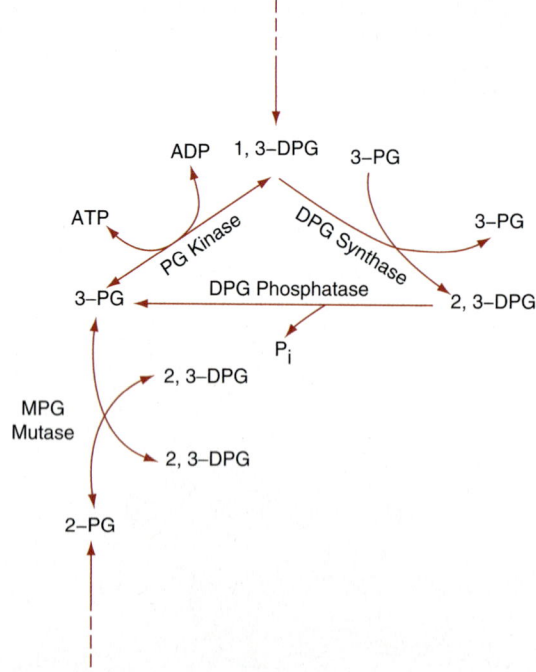

FIGURE 6.19 **Synthesis of 2,3-diphosphoglycerate or 3-phosphoglycerate and ATP from 1,3-diphosphoglycerate by the Rapoport-Luebering shunt.** BPG, bisphosphoglycerate; DPG, diphosphoglycerate; MPG, monophosphoglycerate; PG, phosphoglycerate. (Modified with permission from Cho J, King JS, Qian X, et al. Dephosphorylation of 2,3-bisphosphoglycerate by MIPP expands the regulatory capacity of the Rapoport-Luebering glycolytic shunt. *Proc Natl Acad Sci U S A*. 2008;105(16):5998-6003. Copyright © 2008 National Academy of Sciences, U.S.A.)

levels in red cells increase, oxygen affinity is reduced, and delivery of oxygen to tissues is facilitated. Such situations include abrupt exposure to high altitude, anoxia resulting from pulmonary or cardiac disease, blood loss, and anemia.[387] Increased 2,3-DPG levels also play a role in adaptation to exercise.[388] The compound is not essential to life; however, an individual who lacked the enzymes necessary for 2,3-DPG synthesis was perfectly well except for mild polycythemia (due to increased oxygen affinity). In the completely deoxygenated state, hemoglobin assumes a quaternary structure termed T ("taut" or "tense"). This structure is stabilized by salt bridges involving the carboxy terminals of the peptide chains. The deoxy form is also stabilized by the presence of 2,3-DPG, which joins the β-chains.

Fully oxygenated hemoglobin assumes the R or "relaxed" structure (*Figure 6.20*). Achievement of the R conformation occurs when at least one oxygen molecule is bound on each side of the $\alpha_1\beta_2$ interaction; however, significant subunit cooperativity also exists within each $\alpha_1\beta_1$ dimer of the T-state tetramer. Conversion to the R form is also accompanied by expulsion of the 2,3-DPG and disruption of the salt bridges and hydrophobic interactions at the $\alpha_1\beta_2$ contact point (*Figure 6.20*). Oxygen affinity then becomes much increased, and oxygen is added to the remaining β-chain or chains.

Carbon Dioxide Transport

Transport of carbon dioxide by red cells, unlike that of oxygen, does not occur by direct binding to heme.[389,390] In aqueous solutions, carbon dioxide undergoes a pair of reactions:

$$CO_2 + H_2O \rightarrow H_2CO_3 \rightarrow H^+ + HCO_3^-$$

Carbon dioxide diffuses freely and rapidly into the red cell, where the presence of the enzyme carbonic anhydrase facilitates H_2CO_3 formation. The H^+ liberated is accepted by deoxygenated hemoglobin, a process facilitated by the Bohr effect. The bicarbonate formed in this sequence of reactions diffuses freely across the red cell membrane and a portion is exchanged with plasma Cl^-, a phenomenon called the *chloride* shift (*Figure 6.21*). The bicarbonate is carried in plasma to the lungs, where ventilation keeps the pCO_2 low, resulting in reversal of these reactions and excretion of CO_2 in the expired air. About 85% of tissue carbon dioxide is processed in this way, and 5% is carried in simple solution.

The remainder of the CO_2 is bound to the N-terminal amino group of each polypeptide chain by a carbamino complex, the result of an attack by the electron-poor carbon atom of CO_2 on the electron-rich

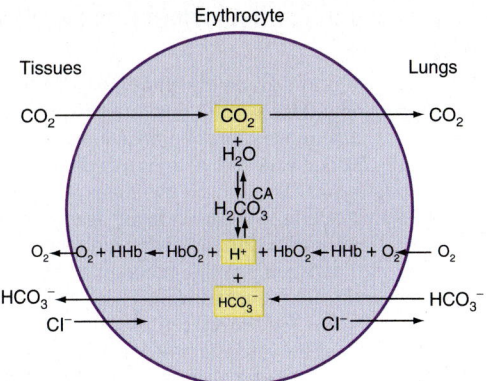

FIGURE 6.21 **Interrelations of oxygen and carbon dioxide transport in the erythrocyte.** Arrows to the left indicate direction of reactions taking place in the tissues; those to the right, in the lungs. In the tissue, CO_2 diffuses into the red cell, and its hydration is catalyzed by carbonic anhydrase (CA). Dissociation of the resulting carbonic acid produces bicarbonate and a proton (H^+). The bicarbonate is exchanged for chloride in the plasma. The proton is accepted by oxyhemoglobin (HbO_2), a reaction that, by means of the Bohr effect, facilitates the dissociation of oxygen. These reactions are reversed in the lungs because of the low pCO_2 and high pO_2. pCO_2, partial pressure of carbon dioxide; pO_2, partial pressure of oxygen.

terminal amino acids. This nonenzymatic process varies directly with pH. Approximately 10% of CO_2 is bound to deoxygenated hemoglobin, forming carbaminohemoglobin (Hb–NH–COO$^-$).

Earlier, the effect of CO_2 on oxygen affinity was noted and attributed to the Bohr effect. An additional, more direct effect results from CO_2 binding to hemoglobin. At a given pH, carbaminohemoglobin has a lower affinity for oxygen than has hemoglobin in the absence of CO_2. This is felt to be a result of the stabilization of the T state through additional bonds, especially involving arginine 141.[391]

The carbon dioxide dissociation curve is analogous to the oxygen dissociation curve, in that it depicts the relationship between CO_2 tension (pCO_2) and CO_2 content. It is somewhat more nearly linear than the oxygen curve, especially in the physiologic range (pCO_2 of 40-60 mm Hg). Because of the Bohr effect, blood containing deoxyhemoglobin has greater affinity for CO_2 than does oxygenated blood. The shift in the CO_2 dissociation curve related to this phenomenon, known as the Haldane effect, facilitates CO_2 binding in the tissues and release in the lungs.

Nitric Oxide: Another Allosteric Effector of Hemoglobin

The recognition of nitric oxide (NO) as an important regulator of vascular and smooth muscle tone has provided many insights into our understanding of vascular physiology. NO is produced by the vascular endothelium and relaxes muscles surrounding vessels, thereby controlling blood pressure. Subsequently, it was determined that free hemoglobin could act as a scavenger of NO and inactivate it, explaining the observation that the infusion of free hemoglobin results in significant elevations of blood pressure.[392] This reaction occurs because the iron in oxygenated heme scavenges NO in a reaction that yields methemoglobin. When free hemoglobin is incubated with NO or S-nitrosothiols, S-nitrosothiols (SNOs) rapidly form on the two 93β cysteines of hemoglobin rather than reacting with the oxygenated heme groups as might be expected. Infusion of the S-nitrosohemoglobin results in no increase in blood pressure.[393]

In the pulmonary circulation, coincident with oxygenation of hemoglobin, NO is added to hemoglobin, and rather than oxidizing the heme iron, it binds to the iron or forms SNO-Hb through the reactive sulfhydryl groups of cysteine 93β of hemoglobin.[394] This role of cysteine 93β may explain why this amino acid is invariant in mammals and birds. Reactivity of NO with the SH groups of cysteine 93β is controlled by the allosteric transition of hemoglobin and the spin state of heme iron. Thus, oxygen binding and conversion to the R state increase reactivity.[395]

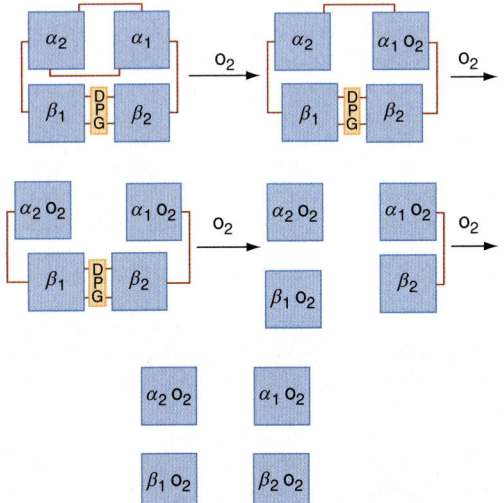

FIGURE 6.20 **Diagrammatic representation of the subunit interaction in hemoglobin as oxygen is added.** Deoxyhemoglobin (upper left), with low oxygen affinity, is in the T (taut) conformation, constrained by salt bridges (interconnecting lines) and the 2,3-DPG molecule. As O_2 is added, salt bridges are broken, and eventually the BPG molecule is expelled, resulting in the R (relaxed) configuration with higher oxygen affinity.

The Normal Hematologic System

Oxidative Denaturation of Hemoglobin: Its Reversibility and Prevention

Oxyhemoglobin in solution gradually undergoes auto-oxidation, becoming methemoglobin ($HbFe^{3+}$). To bind oxygen reversibly, however, the iron in the heme moiety must be maintained in the reduced (ferrous, Fe^{2+}) state, despite exposure to a variety of endogenous and exogenous oxidizing agents. The red cell maintains several metabolic pathways to prevent the action of these oxidizing agents and to reduce hemoglobin iron if it becomes oxidized. Under certain circumstances, these mechanisms fail and hemoglobin becomes nonfunctional. At times, hemolytic anemia supervenes as well. These abnormalities are particularly likely to occur (1) if the red cell is exposed to certain oxidant drugs or toxins, (2) if the intrinsic protective mechanisms of the cell are defective, or (3) if genetic abnormalities of the hemoglobin molecule affect globin stability or the heme crevice (see Chapter 36).

The oxidation of hemoglobin occurs in a stepwise fashion from fully reduced hemoglobin to fully oxidized hemoglobin. In deoxyhemoglobin, the heme iron is in the "high-spin" ferrous state, in which six electrons are in the outer shell, four of which are unpaired. When oxygen is added, one of these electrons is partially transferred to the bound oxygen. Usually, when oxygen is given up, oxyhemoglobin dissociates into partially deoxygenated hemoglobin and molecular oxygen:

$$Hb(O_2)_4 \rightarrow Hb(O_2)_3 + O_2$$

A superoxide anion rather than molecular oxygen may dissociate, however, thus oxidizing the Fe to the ferric state, producing methemoglobin ($HbFe^{3+}$):

$$HbFe^{2+} + O_2 \rightarrow HbFe^{3+}O_2^- \rightarrow HbFe^{3+} + O_2^-$$

This type of dissociation is particularly likely if water gains access to the heme crevice. Methemoglobin formation may also occur in vivo as the result of exposure to superoxide anions:

$$2HbFe^{2+} + O_2 + 2O_2^- + 4H^+ \rightarrow 2HbFe^{3+} + 3O_2 + 2H_2O$$

The formation of methemoglobin may also result from a direct reaction of reduced hemoglobin with the reduction product of the superoxide ion, peroxide:

$$2HbFe^{2+} + 2H_2O_2 \rightarrow 2HbFe^{3+} \cdot H_2O + O_2$$

As a result of these processes, methemoglobin is formed in normal cells at the rate of about 0.5% to 3% per day.[396,397]

Methemoglobin is unable to bind oxygen. It has a distinctive, pH-dependent spectrum (*Figure 6.22*) and, in concentrations >10% of the total hemoglobin, imparts to blood a distinctive brownish hue that does not disappear on vigorous shaking in air. When methemoglobin is present in vivo in concentrations >1.5 to 2.0 g/dL, patients appear visibly cyanotic.[398] Methemoglobin combines readily with cyanide to form cyanomethemoglobin, a pigment so stable that it is used in laboratory procedures for quantifying hemoglobin.

As oxidative denaturation continues, methemoglobin is converted to derivatives known as hemichromes.[399] Hemichromes also may form directly from hemoglobin without methemoglobin as an intermediate. The hemichromes are low-spin, ferric compounds with a greenish hue and a characteristic spectrum (*Figure 6.22*). They are formed when the sixth coordination position of iron becomes covalently attached to a ligand within the globin molecule, a change that requires alteration of tertiary protein structure. Probably, the most common internal ligand is the "distal" histidine at E7. The compound so formed has been called a "reversible" hemichrome, because relatively mild treatment with reducing agents and dialysis under anaerobic conditions converts it to deoxyhemoglobin. It may not be reversible in vivo, however, because it cannot be reduced by methemoglobin reductase.

In contrast, the "irreversible" hemichromes cannot be converted back to normal hemoglobin again in vivo or in vitro, implying that more severe distortions of tertiary protein structure have occurred. In one of

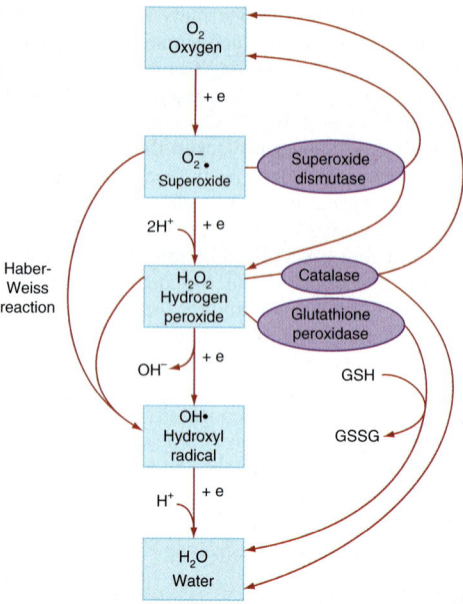

FIGURE 6.22 Steps in the univalent reduction of oxygen and enzymatic pathways affecting the intermediates. The enzymatic pathways, shown on the right, provide the means for processing these intermediates without formation of the highly reactive hydroxyl radical. This potent oxidant can be formed by the reaction shown on the left if superoxide and peroxide concentrations are sufficient and if catalytic quantities of transition metals are present. GSH, glutathione; GSSG, oxidized GSH.

the irreversible hemichromes, the histidine imidazole groups are protonated, that is, they participate in hydrogen bonding. The other irreversible hemichrome is characterized by a mercaptide and nitrogenous linkage at the fifth and sixth positions. Presumably, the mercaptide link is provided by a cysteine residue in the globin chain, perhaps at $\beta93$.

As these changes occur in the vicinity of the heme group, oxidative changes also occur in other parts of the hemoglobin molecule. Once the cell's supply of glutathione (GSH) is exhausted, the titrateable sulfhydryl groups at $\beta93(F9)Cys$ are oxidized, often forming a mixed disulfide with GSH.[400] This change is reversible; however, as further alterations in globin conformation occur, normally protected or "buried" sulfhydryl groups at $\beta112(G14)Cys$ and $\alpha104(G11)Cys$ become exposed and are oxidized, changes that disrupt the $\alpha_1\beta_2$ contacts. These changes facilitate dissociation of polypeptide chains, first into $\alpha\beta$ dimers and finally into monomers.[401] In some instances, heme may dissociate from globin, particularly in the case of certain unstable hemoglobins.

The end products of these changes are precipitated hemichromes and precipitated heme-free globin. In intact erythrocytes, these precipitates take the form of globular inclusions known as Heinz bodies, which are not visible with ordinary Wright stain but can be seen easily after supravital staining with crystal violet or brilliant cresyl blue. Heinz bodies may become attached to the cell membrane and shorten red cell survival.

Another nonfunctional hemoglobin derivative that is occasionally formed during the oxidative denaturation of hemoglobin is sulfhemoglobin. This is a relatively stable pigment and, once formed, cannot be reconverted to hemoglobin in vivo. Instead, it tends to remain within the cell throughout the cell's life. Sulfhemoglobin is bright green and has a distinctive spectrum characterized by an absorption band at about 618 nm. It is a ferrous compound with one sulfur atom attached to each heme group. The sulfur is probably attached to a β carbon in the porphyrin ring, forming a thiochlorin.[400]

Although the exact mode of synthesis of sulfhemoglobin remains to be established, proposed models suggest that methemoglobin is first converted to ferrylhemoglobin in the presence of hydrogen peroxide[402,403]:

$$HbFe^{3+} + H_2O_2 \rightarrow HbFe^{4+}O + H_2O + e^-$$

With the addition of a sulfur-containing compound, such as hydrogen sulfide, the iron in ferrylhemoglobin is reduced and sulfur is incorporated into the porphyrin ring:

$$HbFe^{4+}O + HS^- + 2e^- \rightarrow HbSFe^{2+} + OH^-$$

Although the iron in sulfhemoglobin is reduced, it binds oxygen with an affinity one hundredth that of unmodified hemoglobin.

Known mechanisms for preventing or reversing oxidative denaturation of hemoglobin in the erythrocyte include (1) the methemoglobin reductases, (2) superoxide dismutase, (3) glutathione peroxidase (GPx), and (4) catalase.

Methemoglobin Reduction

Most methemoglobin in erythrocytes is reduced through the action of an enzyme, cytochrome b_5 methemoglobin reductase, which acts in the presence of two electron carriers, cytochrome b_5 and NADH. Only a small amount of methemoglobin is reduced by all other pathways of methemoglobin reduction together. These other pathways involve compounds that cause the reduction of methemoglobin nonenzymatically, ascorbic acid and GSH, as well as a second enzyme, NADPH-flavin reductase. Deficiency of cytochrome b_5 reductase, but not of NADPH-flavin reductase, is associated with methemoglobinemia, confirming that cytochrome b_5 reductase is the most important physiologic means of reducing methemoglobin.[404]

Cytochrome b_5 reductase has been referred to by several other names, including diaphorase I, DPNH dehydrogenase I, NADH dehydrogenase, NADH methemoglobin reductase, and NADH methemoglobin-ferrocyanide reductase. Work in the 1940s established a relationship between the reduction of methemoglobin and the metabolism of lactate to pyruvate, thus implying an important role for NADH.[405] Eventually, two methemoglobin-reducing enzymes were isolated. The NADH-dependent enzyme, which was absent from several patients with methemoglobinemia, has been shown to be a flavoprotein, with one mole of flavin-adenine dinucleotide per mole of apo-enzyme. The reduction of methemoglobin by highly purified cytochrome b_5 reductase in the presence of NADH is extremely slow, implying that another factor is most likely required as an electron carrier. In vitro, this role can be filled by dyes or by ferrocyanide which aid in the laboratory diagnosis. In vivo, cytochrome b_5 acts as the intermediate electron carrier.[406] Erythrocyte cytochrome b_5 greatly accelerates reduction of methemoglobin by cytochrome b_5 reductase. Congenital methemoglobinemia resulting from a deficiency in cytochrome b_5 has been described (see Chapter 36).

A second enzyme system of lesser physiologic importance depends on NADPH for its activity. It probably accounts for only about 5% of the methemoglobin-reducing activity of normal red cells (Table 7.9), and its hereditary deficiency does not lead to methemoglobinemia.[398] The lack of physiologic activity may result from the absence of an intermediate electron carrier analogous to cytochrome b_5. If methylene blue is supplied as the carrier, however, the NADPH-dependent enzyme becomes highly effective in methemoglobin reduction. This property is used in the therapy of methemoglobinemia from various causes.

Enzymes That React With Products of Oxygen Reduction

As molecular oxygen undergoes successive univalent reductions, a variety of reactive species are generated. These species constitute the oxidizing agents most likely to be responsible for the oxidative denaturation of hemoglobin, and they may damage other cellular components as well, especially lipid-containing elements such as the cell membrane.[407] A variety of mechanisms has evolved in respiring organisms to deal with these potential toxins, and some are found within the erythrocyte.

Superoxide anions are produced in biologic tissues from several sources, including oxyhemoglobin itself, as well as oxidative reactions catalyzed by flavin enzymes, such as xanthine oxidase.[408] In addition, many drugs and toxins have oxidant activity and appear to generate superoxide.[409] Once superoxide has been generated in aqueous solution, additional toxic products of oxygen may form spontaneously

(*Figure 6.23*). Thus, superoxide can undergo spontaneous dismutation, yielding peroxide and oxygen:

$$O_2 + O_2 + 2H^+ \rightarrow H_2O_2 + O_2$$

In addition, in the presence of catalytic quantities of transition metals, superoxide and peroxide may react to form the highly reactive hydroxyl radical ($OH\cdot$):

$$O_2 + H_2O_2 \rightarrow OH\cdot + OH^- + O_2$$

Any of these oxygen derivatives may exert toxic effects on cellular components. As previously noted, superoxide induces methemoglobin formation. Hydrogen peroxide is the most stable intermediate in the reduction of oxygen. Although hydrogen peroxide has often been shown to induce the oxidative denaturation of hemoglobin in vitro, whether it does so directly or by giving rise to other products, such as the hydroxyl radical, is not clear.

The hydroxyl radical, one of the most potent redox agents known, may be generated from superoxide and peroxide, as described previously, and from peroxide in the presence of certain metals:

$$Fe^{2+} + H_2O_2 \rightarrow Fe^{3+} + OH^- + OH$$

Thus, enzymes that scavenge superoxide and peroxide may be viewed as mechanisms for preventing the accumulation of these intermediates in sufficient quantities to allow the hydroxyl radical to form.[410]

The superoxide dismutases are enzymes that catalyze the dismutation of superoxide to oxygen and peroxide. Although this reaction occurs spontaneously, the presence of the enzyme speeds the reaction to a rate as much as 109 times faster than the spontaneous rate. In the erythrocyte, superoxide dismutase is a soluble, copper/zinc enzyme with a molecular weight of about 32,000 Da. This enzyme, formerly known as erythrocuprein or hemocuprein, accounts for most of the copper content of the red cell.[411] Once hydrogen peroxide is formed, two enzymes catalyze the decomposition of hydrogen peroxide in erythrocytes. These are GPx and catalase. GPx is a component of the following reaction[412]:

$$H_2O_2 + 2GSH \xrightarrow{GPx} 2HO_2 + GSSG$$

GPx is the major human selenoprotein, which may account for the antioxidant properties of selenium as a micronutrient.[413] Human cells grown in the absence of selenium express significantly reduced GPx activity, despite normal GPx mRNA and transcription levels. It had been proposed that a genetic defect in GPx may lead to a drug-sensitive hemolytic anemia.[414] However, there is doubt that acquired or genetic defects in this enzyme are associated with hemolysis (see Chapter 30).

Catalase, a heme enzyme, decomposes hydrogen peroxide to water and molecular oxygen.[415] It appears to be less important to the red cell than peroxidase, presumably because it is effective only when the peroxide concentration is relatively high. Individuals with hereditary acatalasemia do not develop methemoglobinemia or hemolytic disease.[416]

Glutathione Metabolism

Reduced GSH is a tripeptide (γ-glutamyl-cysteinyl-glycine). Two ATP-dependent enzymatic reactions are required for the de novo synthesis of GSH:

$$\text{glutamic acid} + \text{cysteine} \xrightarrow{\text{glutamyl-cysteine synthetase}} \gamma-\text{glutamyl} - \text{cysteine}$$

$$\gamma-\text{glutamyl} - \text{cysteine} + \text{glycine} \xrightarrow{\text{glutathione synthetase}} \text{GSH}$$

The capacity of normal red cells to synthesize GSH exceeds the rate of turnover by 150-fold. Deficiencies of both of these GSH synthetic enzymes have been associated with hemolytic anemia (see Chapter 30).

In the course of reactions that protect hemoglobin from oxidation, GSH is oxidized, forming oxidized GSH (GSSG), which consists of two GSH molecules joined by a disulfide linkage, and mixed disulfides with hemoglobin. GSSG rapidly leaves the erythrocyte.[417] Thus, maintaining a continuous supply of GSH requires a system to reduce the oxidized forms of GSH. Such a system is provided by glutathione reductase (GR), which catalyzes the reduction of GSSG by NADPH, a product of the pentose phosphate pathway (*Figure 6.23*). GR also catalyzes the reduction of hemoglobin-glutathione disulfides, yielding GSH and hemoglobin.[418]

The gene for GR maps to chromosome 8. This enzyme is a flavoprotein and the activity of GR depends on the dietary intake of riboflavin. Erythrocyte GR activity may be increased by administration of riboflavin, even in apparently normal subjects.[419]

Energy Metabolism

Lacking a storage compound, the normal erythrocyte must have constant access to glucose if its energy metabolism is to be sustained. As previously discussed, glucose enters the cell by means of a facilitated, carrier-mediated transport mechanism. Insulin or other hormones are not required, and transport is not ordinarily the rate-limiting factor in glucose utilization. Without mitochondria, erythrocytes must depend on two less efficient pathways for production of high-energy compounds, the anaerobic glycolytic (Embden-Meyerhof) pathway and

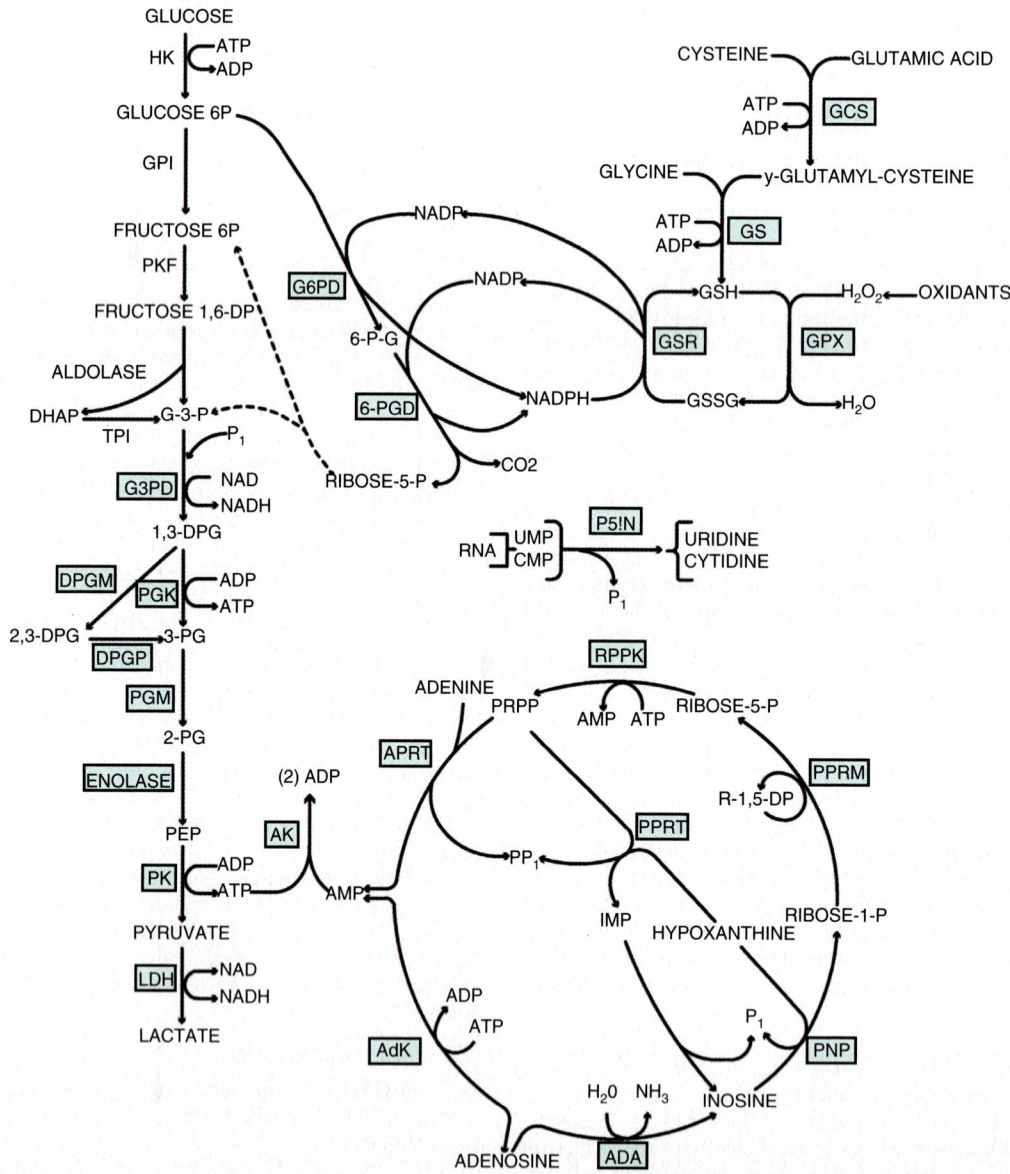

FIGURE 6.23 Metabolic pathways in the erythrocyte. Glycolysis. Enzyme abbreviations: DPGM, 2,3-diphosphoglycerate mutase; DPGP, 2,3-diphosphoglycerate phosphatase; G3PD, glyceraldehyde-3-phosphate dehydrogenase; GPI, glucose phosphate isomerase; HK, hexokinase; LDH, lactate dehydrogenase; PFK, phosphofructokinase; PGK, phosphoglycerate kinase; PGM, phosphoglycerate mutase; PK, pyruvate kinase; TPI, triosephosphate isomerase. Substrate abbreviations: 1,3-DPG, 1,3-diphosphoglycerate; G-3-P, glyceraldehyde-3-phosphate; DHAP, dihydroxyacetone phosphate; (PEP) phosphoenolpyruvate; 2 PG, 2-phosphoglycerate; 3-PG, 3-phosphoglycerate. **HMP shunt and glutathione metabolism.** Enzyme abbreviations: G-6-PD, glucose-6-P dehydrogenase; GCS, gamma glutamyl-cysteine-synthetase; GS, glutathione synthetase; GPx, glutathione peroxidase; GSR, glutathione reductase; 6-PGD, 6-phosphogluconate dehydrogenase. Substrate abbreviations: DHAP, dihydroxyacetone phosphate; G-3-P, glyceraldehyde-3-phosphate; GSH, reduced glutathione; GSSG, oxidized glutathione; 6-PG, 6-phosphogluconate; R-5-P, ribose-5-phosphate. **Purine and pyrimidine metabolism.** Enzyme abbreviations: ADA, adenosine deaminase; AdK, adenosine kinase; AK, adenylate kinase; APRT, adenine phosphoribosyltransferase; PPRM, pyrophosphoribosyl mutase; PPRT, pyrophosphoribosyl transferase; PNP, purine nucleoside phosphorylase; P5!N, pyrimidine 5! Nucleotidase; RPPK, ribopyrophosphoryl kinase. Substrate abbreviations: AMP, adenosine monophosphate; IMP, inosine monophosphate.

the aerobic pentose phosphate pathway, also known as the hexose monophosphate shunt (*Figure 6.23*). Under normal circumstances, about 90% of glucose entering the red cell is metabolized by the anaerobic pathway and 10% by the aerobic pathway.[420] Under conditions of oxidative stress, however, the pentose oxidative pathway may account for up to 90% of glucose consumption.[421]

Three important products are formed by the anaerobic glycolytic pathway: NADH, a cofactor in the methemoglobin reductase reaction; ATP, the major high-energy phosphate nucleotide that powers the cation pump; and 2,3-DPG, a regulator of hemoglobin function (*Figure 6.23*). For each molecule of glucose that enters the pathway, two molecules of NADH are generated. Two molecules of ATP are used in the early steps of glycolysis (*Figure 6.23*), and a maximum of four molecules is produced late in the pathway. Thus, at maximum efficiency, a net yield of two molecules of ATP may be expected for each molecule of glucose catabolized.

Of the 11 enzymes in the glycolytic pathway, three appear to be particularly important in regulation of glycolytic rate. These are hexokinase, phosphofructokinase, and pyruvate kinase (*Figure 6.23*). Hexokinase is the least active enzyme in the series and is therefore often rate limiting. The importance of glycolysis to the red cell is illustrated by the manifestations of inherited glycolytic enzyme deficiencies where the viability of the red cell is reduced and hemolytic anemia results (Chapter 30).

The most important product of the pentose phosphate pathway in erythrocytes is reduced NADPH. In the red cell, NADPH, is a cofactor in the reduction of GSSG, the major reducing agent in the cell and the ultimate source of protection against oxidative attack. The utilization of NADPH is the main stimulus to the utilization of glucose 6-phosphate by the pathway. Redox agents such as methylene blue, cysteine, ascorbate, and others induce up to 20-fold increase in pentose metabolism, presumably by bringing about oxidation of GSH.[422] This metabolic flexibility allows the red cell to respond to unexpected oxidant challenge. The initial reaction of the pentose phosphate pathway is catalyzed by the enzyme G6PD. Hereditary deficiency of red cell G6PD is one of the most common genetic abnormalities in the world associated with hemolysis (Chapter 30). A second function of the pentose pathway is the conversion of hexoses to pentoses. For the most part, the latter are recycled into the glycolytic pathway; however, d-ribose 5-phosphate may be used for nucleotide synthesis.

Mature RBCs are incapable of de novo purine or pyrimidine synthesis, although many enzymes of nucleotide metabolism are present in erythrocytes (*Figure 6.23*). Initial interest in RBC nucleotide metabolism was stimulated by blood bank concerns related to ATP and 2,3-DPG loss during storage of RBCs. Several studies demonstrated that inosine, adenosine, and adenine each could minimize loss of organic phosphates and thereby improve viability of stored blood (Chapter 23). Red cell purine and pyrimidine enzyme disorders also have been associated with inherited hemolytic syndromes, and these cases have further identified an important role of nucleotide metabolism in mature erythrocytes (Chapter 30).

CELL DESTRUCTION

Mechanisms and Site of RBC Destruction

Each day approximately 1% of the body's red cells (3×10^9 cells/kg) die and are replaced by reticulocytes. Why RBCs die after 100 to 120 days is not known. Posited explanations include changes in red cell enzymes and energy depletion with age; alterations in calcium balance; changes in membrane surface charge; oxidative injury; development of autologous antibodies to membrane antigens; and changes in membrane phospholipid asymmetry. While none of these changes explain RBC senescence, and the underlying mechanism remains elusive, aging and death are assumed to be ultimately caused by oxidative stress,[423] with increased stress shown to correlate with reduced life span.[424] However, as not all aged RBCs show evidence of severe oxidative stress, it is likely that other mechanisms are also important. Recent studies have led to the hypothesis that lifespan is determined

by regulation of the interactions of red cells with erythrophagocytic macrophages.[423] This interaction is primarily mediated by phosphatidylserine exposure on the RBC membrane that is a pro-phagocytic or "eat me" signal. This signal *increases* with aging red cells and oxidative stress. Secondarily, membrane expression or function of an antiphagocytic (or "don't eat me" signal) *decreases* as red cells age.[425] The interaction of RBC CD47 with signal regulatory protein α (SIRPα[426]), present on macrophages, inhibits phagocytosis. It has been hypothesized that Epo regulates CD47 expression,[423] and, as EpoRs are present on macrophages, Epo may also modify the phagocytosis threshold, as has been observed following acute hemorrhage; thus, Epo may regulate both life and death of RBCs.

Under normal conditions, 80% to 90% of this normal erythrocyte destruction occurs without release of hemoglobin into plasma.[427,428] Thus, most of the destructive process is considered to be *extravascular*, within reticulo-endothelial macrophages of the spleen and, to a lesser extent, the liver and bone marrow. Approximately 10% to 20% of normal destruction is estimated to occur *intravascularly*.

Extravascular Hemolysis

A number of observations indicate that erythrophagocytosis is the primary mode of physiological extravascular destruction of senescent red cells.[429,430] The HOs responsible for heme degradation (primarily the inducible enzyme, HO-1) are located in the phagocytic cells of the spleen, liver, and bone marrow (and also in hepatocytes). HO-1 knockdown in mice results in a marked loss of these erythrophagocytes in vivo and in in vitro studies, due to heme toxicity following red cell ingestion (see "Iron reutilization function of Heme Oxygenases" section below). In addition, iron derived from heme degradation is largely stored within the macrophage. Likewise, when red cells are damaged in vitro and then reinfused, they are mostly removed from the circulation by macrophages of the spleen and liver.[431] Thus, the evidence indicates that red cell destruction and hemoglobin degradation normally occur within these phagocytes. Studies, however, also indicate an important role for splenic neutrophils in the pathological destruction of allo- or autoantibody opsonized red cells that is observed in the immune-mediated hemolytic anemias (Chapter 31).[432]

The relative importance of the spleen and liver in erythrocyte destruction is influenced by the degree of cell damage[431] Severe red cell damage leads to their destruction in all macrophage-containing organs, but especially in the liver because of its greater blood flow. The spleen, in contrast, preferentially removes minimally damaged erythrocytes.[433] Most senescent red cells are therefore likely destroyed in the spleen; however, after splenectomy, macrophages found in other organs, especially the liver, assume this function, and there is no increase in the survival of normal red cells.[434] Recent studies have attempted to assess mechanisms of splenic sensing and sequestration of spherocytic red cells, as occurs in a number of hemolytic anemias such as hereditary spherocytosis (Chapter 29).

Intravascular Hemolysis

Analysis of haptoglobin (Hp) kinetics in humans suggests 10% to 20% of erythrocyte destruction occurs intravascularly.[427,428] Although both osmotic lysis and red cell fragmentation can cause intravascular destruction, it is unlikely that osmotic lysis plays a role in normal red cell destruction. *Fragmentation* is the loss of part of the cell membrane, usually accompanied by a loss of cellular contents, including hemoglobin. This is the characteristic mode of destruction in the "microangiopathic" hemolytic anemias (Chapters 33, 34, and 50). The blood smear reveals small, misshapen, often triangular or helmet-shaped cells (schistocytes or schizocytes). Fragmentation of red cells is usually due to interactions with injured endothelium, or results from fibrin deposition or increased shear stresses. In response, the cell membrane is capable of limited self-repair. Fragmentation also occurs when reticulocytes are pitted of inclusions, such as residual organelles and hemosiderin granules during passage through the spleen. The enucleation of erythroblasts that normally occurs in the bone marrow may also contribute to hemoglobin release into the circulation, a process which may be increased with ineffective erythropoiesis.

FATE OF INTRAVASCULAR HEMOGLOBIN

Intravascular hemolysis is increased significantly in certain hemolytic anemias (e.g., sickle cell disease, thalassemias, PNH (Chapters 32, 34, and 35)), during infections (e.g., malaria or sepsis due to *Clostridium perfringens*), or trauma. The hemoglobin released into the plasma is pro-oxidant and thus potentially toxic, promoting, for example, the formation of hydroxyl radicals via the Fenton reaction ($H_2O_2 + Fe^{2+} \rightarrow Fe^{3+} + OH\cdot + OH^-$), and oxidative tissue damage.[435] In addition, plasma hemoglobin is a potent scavenger of NO, mediating its nitrosylation to produce methemoglobin and nitrate. NO serves as an important regulator of smooth muscle tone (of especial relevance in small blood vessels), platelet activation and aggregation, and endothelial integrin expression. Intravascular hemolysis may therefore result in smooth muscle dystonias, endothelial dysfunction, and thromboses, problems commonly encountered in sickle cell disease[436,437] and PNH.[438] Fortunately, there are several physiologic mechanisms to remove free hemoglobin from the circulation (*Figure 6.24*).

Haptoglobin

At low rates of release of hemoglobin into the circulation, it is completely bound by Hp, and, once irreversibly bound to Hp, loses its oxidizing ability.[435,439] Once released from red cells into the plasma, tetrameric hemoglobin rapidly dissociates into $\alpha\beta$ dimers that bind Hp tightly in a noncovalent manner (K_d ~1 pM).[440] Heme-free globin (but not heme) can also be bound by Hp.[441] Binding of hemoglobin by Hp prevents H_2O_2-mediated peroxidative modifications to the hemoglobin molecule,[442] Hb translocation across endothelium, and NO scavenging, while allowing productive interactions of the resulting Hp-Hb complex with its receptor, CD163 (see below). The role of Hp as a hemoglobin-binding protein and as the principal factor affecting the apparent "renal threshold" for hemoglobin was originally described by Laurell and Nyman.[443]

Hps are a family of α_2-glycoproteins that bind hemoglobin.[444] The tetrameric molecule is comprised of two dimers of an α-chain (containing a complement control protein or sushi domain) and β-chain (with a serine protease domain) linked in humans by disulfide bonds to form $(\alpha\beta)_2$.[445,446] The gene, located on chromosome 16q22,[447-449] encodes a single polypeptide chain that is cleaved posttranslationally to generate the α and β subunits.[450,451] Transcriptional activity is promoted by IL-1, IL-6, and glucocorticoids as a part of the acute-phase response to systemic inflammation,[452,453] explaining why Hp levels are increased with inflammation.

Human Hp was first described as polymorphic by Smithies et al, who used electrophoresis to separate the various types. There are two major allelic forms of the *hp* gene (*hp1*, *hp2*) that can therefore give rise to three major phenotypes referred to as Hp1-1, Hp2-1, and Hp2-2. These were distinguished using gel electrophoresis according to their different sizes and band patterns (Hp1-1 = 100 kD; Hp2-1 = 120-220 kD; Hp2-2 = 160-500 kD).[454] The β-chain of Hp contains the binding domain for the $\alpha\beta$ hemoglobin dimer; thus, dimeric Hp1-1 binds two hemoglobin dimers, whereas the multimeric Hp2-1 and Hp2-2 may bind several.[455] Differences in the Hp phenotypes observed in different ethnic groups or in association with various diseases (hemochromatosis, diabetes, malaria) have been investigated extensively.[444]

Clinical laboratories measure Hp directly by radial immunodiffusion or immunonephelometric methods, and phenotyping, if performed, now employs monoclonal antibodies and immunoblotting.[456] Normal Hp concentrations differ substantially with technique; ranges such as 0.5 to 1.6 g/L[457] are representative, but each clinical laboratory normally establishes its own reference values. The concentration is influenced by age, with levels very low in newborns, measurable by 3 months of age, and increasing gradually throughout childhood.[458] Decreased Hp concentrations may be observed with hemolytic anemias, ineffective erythropoiesis, severe liver disease, and pregnancy or estrogen therapy. Increased concentrations are seen in diseases where acute-phase proteins are increased, such as infections and malignancies.

Hp is synthesized in hepatocytes.[454] When not bound to hemoglobin, it leaves the plasma with a half-disappearance time of 3.5 to 5 days.[459] The haptoglobin-hemoglobin (Hp-Hb) complex leaves much more rapidly, with a half-disappearance time of 9 to 30 minutes. In hemolytic anemias characterized by intravascular hemolysis, catabolism of Hp may be so rapid that it essentially disappears from the plasma. As there is no compensatory increase in Hp synthesis it may take 5 to 7 days for levels to recover. Hypohaptoglobinemia also occurs in hemolytic states associated with predominantly extravascular hemolysis,[460,461] suggesting hemoglobin may be regurgitated from macrophages when the rate of erythrophagocytosis reaches a maximum.[427]

The Hp-Hb complex is removed from the circulation after high-affinity binding to a scavenger receptor (CD163) found solely on the cell surface of peripheral blood monocytes (to allow immediate uptake[462] and tissue macrophages[462]) and tissue macrophages.[463,464] Hp-Hb complexes may also be taken up by hepatocytes by an unidentified mechanism.[465,466] CD163 is a 130 kD type I transmembrane protein and a member of the scavenger receptor superfamily that functions in binding polyanionic structures such as modified lipoproteins or (bacterial) lipopolysaccharides.[467] In addition to high-affinity binding of Hp-Hb, CD163 is one of five known macrophage cell surface proteins that bind erythroblasts in erythroblastic islands ("nurse cells"[70,468]). After binding to the receptor, Hb-Hp is endocytosed into the macrophage. Subsequently, CD163 recycles to the cell membrane, while the globin moieties of Hp and Hb are degraded within the lysosome, and the heme is released into the cytoplasm to be catabolized by HO-1. Subsequently, the iron is transported back to the bone marrow via transferrin, for synthesis of new hemoglobin.

CD163 expression may be stimulated by the effects of glucocorticoids, IL-6, and IL-10 on a distinct "anti-inflammatory" macrophage population termed "alternatively activated" (or M2-polarized) macrophages that are important for wound healing and chronic inflammation.[469] Notably, recent studies of chronic leg venous ulcers demonstrate that engulfment of extravasated RBCs by tissue macrophages and the release of hemoglobin iron activates a "pro-inflammatory" M1 macrophage population that has anomalous high expression of CD163. These M1 macrophages demonstrate enhanced ROS production and TNF-α release, which perpetuates pro-inflammatory M1 activation and impairs wound healing.[470]

CD163 was knocked out in mice to examine the effects on hemoglobin clearance. Surprisingly, in control animals, hemoglobin was in

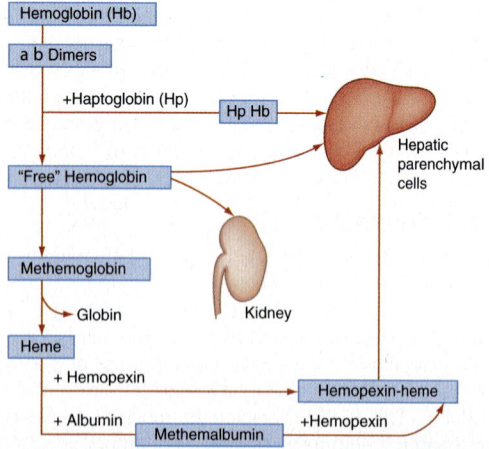

FIGURE 6.24 Pathways for the disposal of hemoglobin in plasma. Hemoglobin freely dissociates into $\alpha\beta$ dimers. These are bound by haptoglobin with subsequent removal of the hemoglobin-haptoglobin complex by hepatic parenchymal cells. Hemoglobin in excess of the haptoglobin-binding capacity circulates as the unbound (free) protein. In this form, it is partially removed by hepatic cells, but it may also follow two other pathways; it may be excreted by the kidney or oxidized to methemoglobin, from which heme is easily dissociated. Heme is initially bound to hemopexin, which transports it to the hepatic parenchymal cell. Heme may also be bound nonspecifically by albumin, forming methemalbumin. This complex probably transfers its heme to hemopexin as the latter becomes available.

fact cleared from the circulation faster than the Hb-Hp complex, while deletion of CD163 had little effect on hepatic Hb-Hp complex uptake, suggesting the presence, at least in mice of another uptake system for Hb-Hp and/or Hb.[471]

Hemoglobin and the Kidney

The Hp-Hb complex is large (~160 kD), and has a negative charge, preventing passage into the glomerular filtrate. Thus, the level of circulating Hp is the most important determinant of the apparent renal threshold.[443] When Hp is saturated, free (unbound) hemoglobin circulates briefly in plasma. As discussed, hepatic parenchymal cells are responsible for removal of some of the free hemoglobin from plasma.[465,466] The dissociation of free hemoglobin into $\alpha\beta$ dimers results in a molecular weight of about 32 kD, which readily pass through the glomerulus.[386] There is a low (<0.6 g/L) renal threshold for free hemoglobin present after Hp saturation related to renal tubular reabsorption through the endocytic receptors megalin and cubilin.[472,473] Once this reabsorption capacity is exceeded, hemoglobin appears in the urine.

Hemoglobinuria, when it is of considerable magnitude, may cause precipitation of heme pigment as casts in the distal tubules, proximal tubule (PT) cell necrosis, and acute renal failure. The mechanism is disputed, but several theories have been proposed: (1) hemoglobin or hemoglobin products are directly toxic to PT cells, (2) precipitation of hemoglobin results in tubular obstruction and renal failure, or (3) direct renal injury by hemoglobin does not occur but instead products of intravascular hemolysis result in systemic or local hypotension (e.g., by scavenging of NO), and these lead to renal failure[474,475] PT dysfunction, including proteinuria, also occurs in the chronic hemolytic diseases such as sickle cell anemia, and leads to chronic kidney disease.[476] Recent studies indicate that hemoglobin can directly compete with filtered albumin for reuptake by PT megalin/cubilin receptors. In sickle cell anemia (HbSS), the resultant albuminuria also contributes to the observed renal disease.[477]

Within the tubular epithelial cell, hemoglobin iron is rapidly extracted by heme-induced HO-1, and stored in the cell as ferritin and hemosiderin.[386] Some tubular epithelial iron may be reused for hemoglobin synthesis, but its mobilization for this purpose occurs at a very slow rate. When iron-laden tubular cells are sloughed into the urine, the urine iron concentration increases and both ferritin and hemosiderin may be detected.[478] Clinically, hemosiderinuria is usually detected by Prussian blue staining of the urinary sediment.[479] Detectable hemosiderin usually does not appear in the urine for 48 hours after a specific episode of hemoglobinuria[479] and may persist for more than a week.[474] In chronic intravascular hemolysis, such as occurs in red cell fragmentation associated with abnormal prosthetic heart valves, or with PNH, hemosiderinuria can result in iron deficiency.[480]

Animal studies of deletion of Hp (or the Hb-Hp receptor, CD163[471]) confirm that the primary function of Hp is not plasma clearance of hemoglobin but rather the diversion of hemoglobin to hepatic and splenic macrophages and the prevention of renal losses of hemoglobin (and thus iron). With time, Hp-deleted animals accumulate hemoglobin-derived iron in the proximal tubular cells of the kidneys.[481] As discussed, Hp is degraded after CD163-mediated endocytosis; thus, Hp is depleted in most patients with chronic hemolytic diseases such as sickle cell disease.

Plasma Heme, Hemopexin, and Methemalbumin
Heme

When the buffering capacity of Hp is exceeded, any free hemoglobin present in plasma is readily oxidized to methemoglobin, which then dissociates nonenzymatically into ferriheme (Fe^{3+}) (also known as hemin) and globin.[482] Apart from intravascular hemolysis, plasma heme may potentially originate from hemoglobin released during normal erythroblast enucleation, or from the breakdown of hemoproteins such as myoglobin, catalases, cytochromes, and neutrophil myeloperoxidase during tissue damage (e.g., rhabdomyolysis). Heme must be chaperoned within the circulation (and likely within cells[483]) as free heme is lipophilic and toxic to cells, promoting lipid peroxidation and

ROS production that can lead to cell membrane injury and apoptosis.[102] In addition, the removal from the circulation and recycling of heme iron both prevents iron loss and, importantly, removes a source of readily available iron for invading micro-organisms.[484] Circulating heme is immediately taken up by the low-density and high-density lipoproteins, LDLs and HDLs, and then rapidly transferred to albumin or the heme-binding glycoprotein, hemopexin, ameliorating the strong oxidative and proinflammatory effects of free heme. Heme is removed from these proteins primarily by hepatocytes.

Hemopexin

Hemopexin, after Hp, forms the second line of defense against hemoglobin-mediated oxidative damage during intravascular hemolysis or internal hemorrhage.[481,485] Hemopexin is a 439 amino acid β_1-glycoprotein, consisting of a single polypeptide chain with a molecular weight of about 70 kD. It binds heme with the highest known affinity of any heme-binding protein (Kd <1 pM) and plays an important role in receptor-mediated hepatocyte heme uptake. Hemopexin is mainly synthesized in the liver,[486] but is also expressed in the kidney, eye, and central nervous system (CNS).[99] The human gene is located at 11p15.4-p15.5, close to the β-globin gene cluster.[487]

The half-life of hemopexin in normal subjects is about 7 days,[488] whereas the heme-hemopexin complex is removed from the circulation with a half-disappearance time of 7 to 8 hours. Hemopexin, like Hp, is an acute-phase reactant and plasma levels rise with an inflammatory stimulus.[489] Hemopexin is also an abundant plasma protein in humans, with levels (0.5-1.5 mg/mL) similar to that of transferrin (2.0-3.6 mg/mL), whereas the heme-hemopexin complex is removed from the circulation with a half-disappearance time of 7 to 8 hours.[480]

Hepatocyte uptake of this complex is by receptor-mediated endocytosis. The receptor, LRP/CD91,[490] is a member of the LDL receptor-related protein superfamily (LRP), also known as CD91. LRP/CD91 is a large protein, 600 kD, with multiple extra-cellular domains, and binds more than 40 different ligands.[491] This receptor is expressed by a variety of cells and heme-hemopexin complexes are taken up by hepatocytes, macrophages, neurons, fibroblasts, and syncytiotrophoblasts. After endocytosis, the receptor recycles to the cell surface, while the heme-hemopexin complex dissociates within the endosome, facilitated by the decrease in pH (and potentially the reduction of ferriheme to ferrous heme), with hemopexin returning to the plasma as an intact protein.[490,492] The heme is discharged into the cytoplasm to undergo catabolism by HO-1. LRP/CD91 is expressed highly by M2-polarized "anti-inflammatory" macrophages that also express CD163 and both receptors are upregulated by glucocorticoids.[493] Similarities between the heme-hemopexin-LRP/CD91 and the Fe-Tf-TfR endocytic transport systems have also been described.[488] Some studies suggest that when large amounts of heme are released into the circulation, recycling of hemopexin becomes saturated and significant amounts are then degraded in the lysosome. Thus, plasma hemopexin levels may decrease following intravascular hemolysis.[489,494] The depletion is less pronounced than that of Hp, and low values imply a relatively severe degree of hemolysis.

Like Hp, hemopexin has been deleted in mice. Interestingly, in animals with deletion of either Hp or hemopexin, the expression of the other protein is upregulated as a compensatory mechanism,[495] perhaps by heme. Animals with deletion of both genes show no obvious alterations in heme catabolism (but see discussion of rodent CD163 gene knockdown in Haptoglobin section above) unless they are subject to acute hemolytic stress when they develop liver inflammation and fibrosis and splenomegaly. Analysis suggests that with acute hemolysis large amounts of hemoglobin and/or heme are deposited in the liver, while the splenomegaly appears to be related to red cell congestion.[495] Of note, in vitro studies indicate a role for hemopexin in the coordinated extracellular uptake of heme exported by the cell surface transporter FLVCR—in the absence of hemopexin there is a marked decrease of FLVCR-mediated export of cytosolic heme.[496] In addition to the importance of FLVCR for proerythroblast survival[157,158] (see above), in vitro studies of FLVCR-deleted bone marrow–derived macrophages suggest FLVCR may also facilitate some recycling of heme from erythrophagocytic macrophages.[100,157]

Methemalbumin

Each mole of human albumin can bind several moles of heme (K_d ~10^{-6}) to form methemalbumin.[497] Heme added to human serum associates primarily with albumin (K_d 5 nM, concentration 35-55 mg/mL) before being transferred to hemopexin (K_d <1 pM, concentration 0.5-1.5 mg/mL), presumably because the molar concentration of albumin is much greater than that of hemopexin.[498] The heme-binding site on albumin can be inhibited in an allosteric or competitive fashion by fatty acids, while increased heme binding to albumin (for example, during an acute hemolytic episode) can decrease the protein binding of medications such as warfarin.[481]

EXTRAVASCULAR HEMOGLOBIN DEGRADATION

The Heme Oxygenase System and the Formation of Bilirubin

The HO system comprises the major physiologically relevant mechanism of heme catabolism.[499] HO is present in humans in two active isoforms, HO-1 and HO-2, encoded by different genes. HO is a mixed function oxidase, that is, it requires molecular oxygen, generating oxidized products and H_2O (*Figure 6.25*). The oxidase catalyzes cleavage of the α-methine bridge of heme—producing iron, CO, and biliverdin IXα—and is the rate-limiting step in the degradation sequence. The concerted activity of NADPH-cytochrome P450 reductase is necessary to

supply electrons and activate oxygen. Biliverdin IXα, a physiological inhibitor of HO function, is rapidly converted to bilirubin IXα by the enzyme BVR. HO and NADPH-cytochrome P450 reductase are present in the endoplasmic reticulum, forming a complex with each other and, at least in vitro, with cytosolic BVR.[500] Bilirubin IXα is in turn conjugated—once it reaches the liver—by uridine diphosphate (UDP)-glucuronyl transferase (UGT) and eventually excreted into the bile. The daily production of bilirubin in man is approximately 400 mg, of which approximately 300 mg is derived from the breakdown of hemoglobin, with the remainder derived from catabolism of other hemoproteins, such as cytochromes and myoglobin.[501]

Studies in mammals initially focused on the role of HO in heme catabolism during breakdown of hemoglobin. However, it has become widely recognized that HO-mediated degradation of heme has various roles in mammals, including antioxidative and iron reutilization functions.[100]

Antioxidative Function of the Heme Oxygenases

Apart from upregulation by heme, the inducible heme oxygenase isoform, HO-1, is activated by more stimuli than perhaps any other gene.[499] Expression is induced by various metals (including sodium arsenite, cobalt, and selenium); hypoxia or hyperoxia; environmental chemicals and UV light; hydrogen peroxide and NO; depletion of intracellular GSH; and heat shock (and thus named HSP32). The enzyme is also induced by hormones, various drugs, fever, starvation,

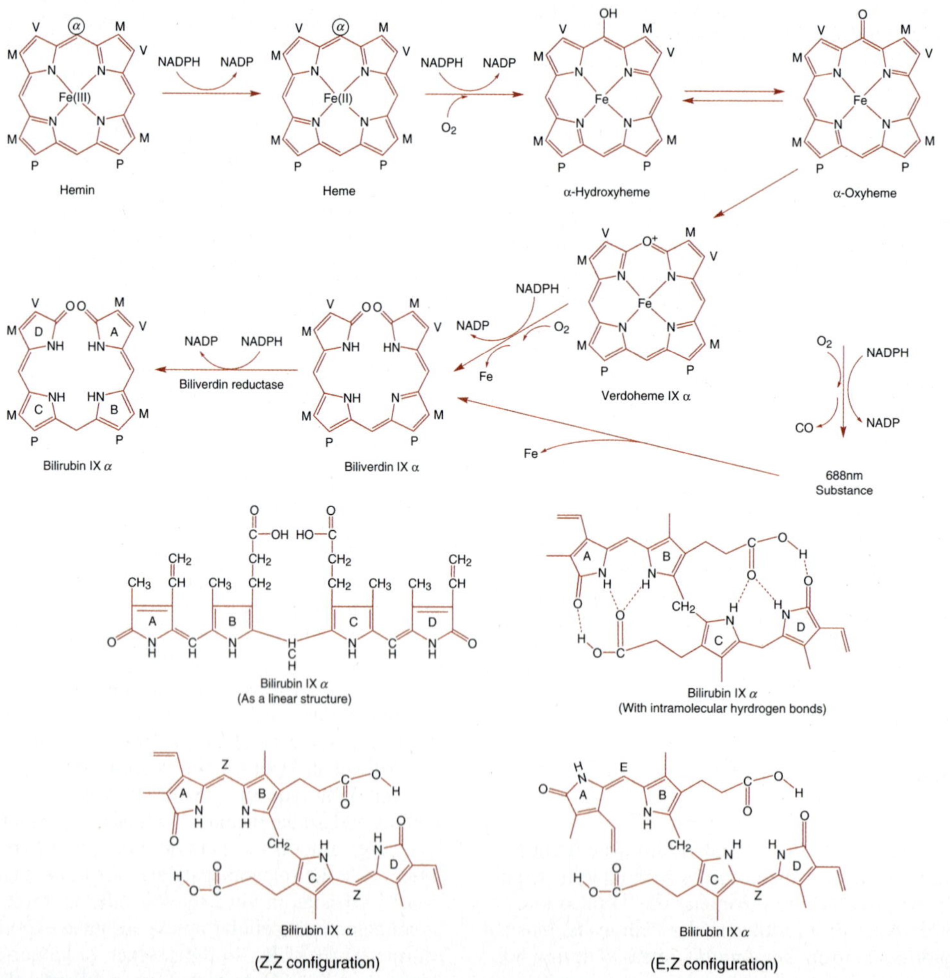

FIGURE 6.25 Formation of bilirubin IXα from heme. The initial reactions are catalyzed by microsomal heme oxygenase and require nicotinamide adenine dinucleotide phosphate (NADPH) as a cofactor. The reaction has a high specificity for the α-methine bridge, and α-oxyheme is a probable intermediate that is oxidized by molecular oxygen to biliverdin. In mammals, biliverdin is converted to bilirubin by biliverdin reductase. At bottom, alternative methods of representing the structure of bilirubin. The intramolecular hydrogen bonding that occurs with the Z,Z configuration is less extensive in the geometric isomers designated E,Z, and E,E (not shown); hence, the latter are more soluble in water.

and stress.[502] Basic leucine zipper "stress-responsive" transcription factors, including members of the ATF family, c-Fos, c-Jun and Nrf2, maf family members, and Bach-1, all regulate HO-1 expression.[94,503] BVR also regulates HO-1. In addition to catalyzing the reduction of biliverdin to bilirubin, BVR has kinase, transcription factor and intracellular heme transport activities. The transport of heme into the nucleus by BVR may increase HO-1 levels as it enables derepression of Bach-1–mediated repression of HO-1 transcription.[94,504,505]

In general, HO-1 expression appears to be rapidly induced in response to cellular oxidative stress and subsequently repressed to low levels once the stimulus is removed. In contrast, HO-2, the predominant HO protein expressed in the brain and testis, is constitutively expressed in all cells, with the promoter responding solely to glucocorticoids.[499] Notably, the N-terminus of HO-2 protein contains HRMs,[506] an ancient motif found in proteins in bacteria, yeast, and mammals that binds heme and serves a regulatory function (e.g., of ALAS-2, Bach-1, and HRI[133,507,508]). In addition, HRMs allow for regulation of HRM-containing proteins by the heme-binding gases. For example, HO-2 binds the vasodilator NO with high affinity and, with less affinity, the potential vasodilator (and neurotransmitter) CO, or O_2.[125] Of interest, a critical HO-2 function is its interaction with the calcium-sensitive potassium (BK) channels that mediate responses of the carotid body (glomus cells) to oxygen levels.[509] In normoxia, HO-2 produces CO from heme to stimulate the channel, while in hypoxic states, CO is not produced from heme, which then binds and inhibits the channel, resulting in cell depolarization and initiation of a cascade of excitatory signals into the CNS to increase ventilation.[510]

The reason for the reduction of biliverdin IXα to bilirubin has been questioned, as the former is water soluble and thus easily excreted, whereas bilirubin is lipid soluble, toxic to the developing brain and requires conjugation to allow efficient excretion in bile.[506] However, being lipophilic, bilirubin also crosses the placenta from fetus to mother and thus the fetus can utilize the mother's hepatobiliary system for excretion. Studies indicate that bilirubin at intracellular nanomolar (i.e., physiological) concentrations functions as a potent antioxidant that protects cells from up to a 10,000-fold excess of H_2O_2; in so doing, it is itself oxidized to biliverdin IXα, which is then recycled back to form bilirubin.[510-512] However, some studies suggest it is less important than, for example, other major intracellular antioxidants such as the GSH system.[513]

Iron Reutilization Function of Heme Oxygenases

Under normal physiological conditions, approximately 25 mg of iron is consumed daily by erythroblasts for heme biosynthesis. With a daily dietary iron intake of only 1 to 2 mg, the recycling of heme-iron from senescent erythrocytes constitutes the main source of iron for erythropoiesis. As mentioned, heme degradation by HO-1 occurs within erythrophagocytic macrophages in the liver, spleen, and bone marrow, releasing iron, which is subsequently exported into the circulation by the sole cell iron exporter ferroportin.[514,515]

A patient with homozygous HO-1 deficiency has been described in detail.[516] The child, who died at age 6 years, had evidence of severe hemolytic anemia with high heme levels, low serum bilirubin, absent hemopexin but *increased* Hp, and hypoferremia. Very high von Willebrand factor and thrombomodulin levels, with evidence of disseminated intravascular coagulation were observed, suggesting widespread endothelial injury. There was iron overload of the liver (involving both Kupffer cells and parenchymal cells) and kidney (PT cells). Asplenia was noted. The child also had hyperlipidemia, and, at autopsy, aortic atheroma was noted. These findings indicate an important role for HO-1–mediated heme breakdown for heme iron reutilization and protection of the vascular endothelium from heme exposure.

Animals with deletion of HO-1 develop hypoferremia, microcytic anemia (hematocrit approximately 30%) and a similar tissue iron overload phenotype.[517,518] More recently, the murine model of HO-1 deficiency has been re-examined from 6 weeks out to 22 months. The animals develop functional hyposplenia.[519] The animals develop asplenia over time, due to splenic fibrosis and loss of the red pulp. Notably, there is a marked loss of the (LRP/CD91- and

CD163-expressing) erythrophagocytes in the liver, spleen, and bone marrow, due to the toxicity of heme released within these macrophages during ingestion of senescent erythrocytes. Thus, the high Hp levels observed in the human subject with HO-1 deficiency are explained by the specific loss of erythrophagocytic macrophages expressing the Hp receptor (whereas hemopexin levels are low as it is also taken up by hepatocytes). With the development of asplenia, senescent red cells undergo intravascular rupture with release of hemoglobin and heme (see above), which is taken up by hepatocytes (via hemopexin) and the proximal renal tubular epithelial cells. These cells thus regulate iron reutilization from erythrocytes in these mice, likely relying on HO-2 function.[519] In sum, these studies in mice and humans demonstrate the importance of erythrophagocytic macrophage and endothelial cell HO-1 function in ameliorating heme toxicity and the need for the HO system for heme iron recycling.

Bilirubin Transport

After release from sites of heme catabolism, bilirubin appears in the plasma. The normal concentration of plasma bilirubin is <1.0 mg/dL. At equilibrium, the concentration is directly related to bilirubin production (mostly from red cell destruction and erythropoiesis (e.g., enucleation)) and inversely related to hepatic clearance[515,516] (*Figure 6.24*).

The structure of the bilirubin IXα molecule is asymmetric and several isomeric forms exist (*Figure 6.25*).[520] In the naturally occurring configuration, all pyrrole rings are similarly rotated, representing the Z,Z or trans configuration. If either outer ring is rotated, then the E,Z or Z,E geometric isomers are formed. Photoisomerization of the Z,Z configuration of bilirubin results in formation of these more soluble photoisomers, which can be excreted without conjugation.[521,522] This is the basis for using phototherapy to prevent neurotoxicity in newborns with hyperbilirubinemia.[523]

Bilirubin is normally present in plasma in several forms.[524,525] Although unconjugated bilirubin is essentially insoluble in water, it combines reversibly with albumin in neutral or alkaline solution. At normal plasma albumin concentrations, the theoretical bilirubin-binding capacity is approximately 70 mg/dL, of which half is tightly bound. These values are reduced by a decrease in plasma albumin concentration or by the presence of organic, anionic substances that compete for albumin-binding sites, such as heme, fatty acids, sulfonamides, and salicylates.[526] When the binding capacity is exceeded, bilirubin readily crosses membranes (for example, the blood-brain barrier, placental and vascular endothelial or hepatocyte membranes) to diffuse into the tissues, and in jaundiced infants the amount of bilirubin outside the vascular circulation exceeds that within it.[523] The tendency of bilirubin to bind to tissues, such as brain, may be due to complex formation with cell membrane polar groups, such as phosphatidylcholine.[526]

In normal adults, <5% of measurable bilirubin is conjugated,[527] but under certain pathologic circumstances, the proportion is greater. This relatively soluble bilirubin derivative may also bind albumin. Most is less tightly bound than the unconjugated form, but a portion is covalently and irreversibly bound.[528] That portion of esterified bilirubin that is reversibly bound to albumin is ultrafilterable. In contrast to the other forms of bilirubin, this complex enters the glomerular filtrate, is not reabsorbed, and excreted in the urine.

Hepatic Bilirubin Metabolism

Processing of bilirubin by the liver is part of a general mechanism whereby plasma protein-bound, organic anions are metabolized and excreted. Hepatic bilirubin metabolism is divided into three distinct phases: Uptake, conjugation, and excretion[496] (*Figure 6.26*). All three phases are necessary for bilirubin to be excreted; however, excretion is normally the slowest, rate-limiting, step.

Within the hepatic sinusoids, the albumin-bilirubin complex dissociates, and bilirubin passes into the hepatocyte where it binds GSH S-transferase and is transferred to the ER. How transport into the hepatocyte occurs remains unclear.[527] It may be a dissociation-limited carrier-independent (diffusion) process,[529] or a bidirectional energy-dependent process.[530] Bidirectional movement of bilirubin appears to

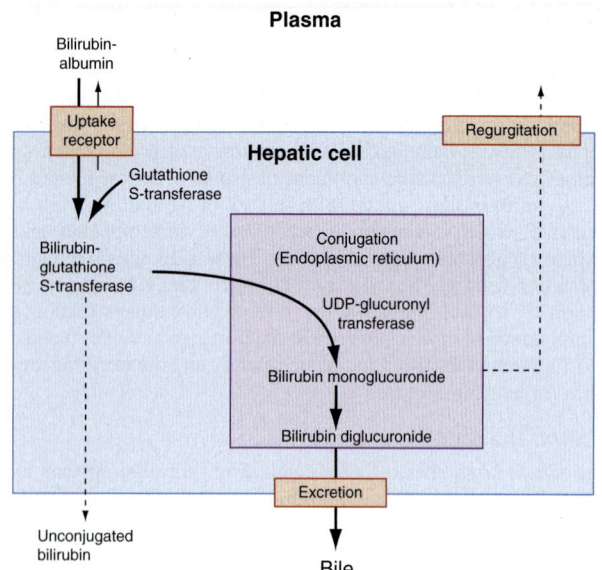

FIGURE 6.26 Normal and abnormal pathways of bilirubin excretion by the hepatic cell. The normal pathways (solid arrows) include uptake and conjugation of bilirubin and excretion of the conjugated derivative. Abnormal pathways (dashed arrows) include regurgitation of bilirubin glucuronide into plasma and excretion of unconjugated bilirubin into bile. UDP, uridine diphosphate.

be extensive.[531] In addition, small amounts formed within the hepatocyte from degradation of hepatic hemoproteins reflux into the plasma in the unconjugated form.[532]

Within the hepatocyte, bilirubin is conjugated with glucuronic acid to form bilirubin diglucuronide, which comprises 80% of the bilirubin present in normal bile; the two monoglucuronide isomers make up most of the remainder.[533] Conjugated bilirubins are more water soluble than unconjugated bilirubin, allowing biliary excretion. Little or no unconjugated bilirubin is found in bile, and if conjugation is impaired, bilirubin content is low. The conjugation reaction is catalyzed by UGT. Hepatocyte UGT exists in several isoforms, catalyzing glucuronidation of various substrates, such as steroid hormones and medications. Bilirubin serves as the substrate for two isoforms (B-UGT 1 and B-UGT 2),[534] but only B-UGT 1 is quantitatively significant in humans.[535] B-UGT activity is also modulated by medications such as phenobarbital, and hormones, such as cortisol and thyroxine.[536]

In hepatocellular disease or biliary obstruction, some conjugated bilirubin may be "regurgitated" into the plasma. Published studies however suggest this may be an exaggeration of a normal physiological transport process.[537] In addition, a small portion of conjugated bilirubin within the hepatocyte is deconjugated and may reflux into the plasma.[532] These pathways explain the increase of both bilirubin fractions in cholestatic liver disease. In other clinical situations, hyperbilirubinemia is mainly due to an increase in unconjugated bilirubin. The most common of these is hemolytic disease, where hemoglobin catabolism and thus bilirubin production are increased. However, inherited disorders may also cause unconjugated hyperbilirubinemia because of an impaired capacity for bilirubin conjugation.

The decreased ability to conjugate bilirubin is the common feature of three inherited disorders: in Crigler-Najjar syndrome type I (CN1; MIM#218800), severe unconjugated hyperbilirubinemia is present from birth and kernicterus is common; in Crigler-Najjar syndrome type II (CN2; MIM#606785), less severe jaundice occurs; and in Gilbert syndrome (GS; MIM#143500), the jaundice is quite mild and often not obvious clinically.[537] These disorders are recessively transmitted, and most patients are therefore homozygous for the mutant gene, *UGT1A1*, although occasionally heterozygotes have minimal jaundice. In CN1 and CN2, the mutation frequently involves exon 1, which confers substrate specificity to the enzyme, resulting in a structurally abnormal protein. In CN1, and in the Gunn rat, an animal

model of this disease, the enzyme is nonfunctional, while in type II, enzyme activity is variably reduced.[530,531,538,539] In GS, the mutation in some patients affects the promoter sequence of exon 1.[535] GS is very common, occurring in up to 10% of the population, but CN1 and CN2 syndromes are rare. In CN1, the HO inhibitor Sn-protoporphyrin may be effective in reducing bilirubin levels. Early orthotopic liver transplantation is curative.[536] No treatment is usually necessary for the other two disorders.

The degree of hyperbilirubinemia seen in children with chronic hemolytic states is influenced by simultaneous inheritance of the gene for GS.[540,541] Infants with hereditary spherocytosis and GS usually require phototherapy for hyperbilirubinemia.[541] The variable hyperbilirubinemia seen in G6PD-deficient neonates may also reflect the presence or absence of GS.[540] In infants known to be G6PD deficient, prevention of severe hyperbilirubinemia by administration of a single intramuscular dose of Sn-mesoporphyrin, another inhibitor of HO, is highly effective and safe.[133,542] Infants with hereditary spherocytosis who also have GS usually require phototherapy for hyperbilirubinemia.[543] The variable hyperbilirubinemia seen in G6PD-deficient neonates may also reflect the presence or absence of the variant form of uridine-diphosphoglucoronylsyl-transferase responsible for GS.[544] In infants known to be G6PD deficient, prevention of severe hyperbilirubinemia by administration of a single intramuscular dose of Sn-mesoporphyrin, another inhibitor of HO, is highly effective and safe.[137,545]

Excretion of conjugated bilirubin from the hepatic cell into the bile canaliculus proceeds against a 40:1 gradient, when concentration in the bile is compared with that in plasma.[546] Animal studies indicated that excretion, normally the rate-limiting step in overall hepatic bilirubin transport, is mediated by an ATP-dependent transport system (ABCC2/MRP2), which is shared by a variety of other organic anions.[534,537] The Dubin-Johnson syndrome (MIM#237500)[542] is an autosomal recessive disorder that is due to homozygous or compound heterozygous mutations in *ABCC2*. It is characterized by mild conjugated hyperbilirubinemia and impaired biliary secretion of non–bile-acid organic anions, but normal bilirubin uptake and conjugation. ABCC2/MRP2 is a member of the multidrug resistance protein subfamily that is localized exclusively to the apical membranes of polarized cells including hepatocytes, renal PTs, and intestinal epithelium.[547,548]

Intestinal Bile Pigment Metabolism

Bilirubin diglucuronide is excreted in bile into the duodenum.[544] There is little intestinal absorption of the conjugated form, although unconjugated bilirubin is readily absorbed. Bilirubin diglucuronide probably remains conjugated during its transit through the small intestine. However, with intestinal stasis, and in newborns, increased deconjugation occurs and intestinal absorption occurs. This enterohepatic circulation of bilirubin may contribute to the severity of jaundice associated with the physiologic hyperbilirubinemia of the newborn.[543] When bilirubin diglucuronide reaches the terminal ileum and colon, it is hydrolyzed by bacterial β-glucuronidases. The methine bridges and usually the vinyl groups are then reduced by bacterial flora forming colorless tetrapyrroles called urobilinogens.[543] Since urobilinogen formation is accomplished by bacteria, it does not occur in newborns, and may be affected by administration of antibiotics. The urobilinogens are easily dehydrogenated to form the orange-yellow pigments, urobilins, which contribute to the color of feces. Up to 20% of the urobilinogen formed in the gut is reabsorbed. The reabsorbed fraction is efficiently excreted by the normal liver without being conjugated.[548] A portion of the reabsorbed pigment may be excreted into the urine. Urobilinogen is filtered by the glomerulus, secreted by the renal tubule, and reabsorbed. If the liver's capacity to excrete urobilinogen is impaired, a disproportionate amount appears in the urine.

Alternate Pathways of Heme and Bilirubin Catabolism

Evidence suggests that some heme may be degraded by pathways other than catabolism by the HOs. On a stoichiometric basis, 35 mg of bilirubin should result from degradation of 1 g of hemoglobin. However, the recovery of fecal urobilinogen is less than expected, suggesting that 20% to 40% of heme may be degraded by some other pathway.[545] Only minimal amounts of unconjugated bilirubin are excreted in the urine; however, excretion of conjugated bilirubin may be substantial when there is complete biliary obstruction. In rats with biliary fistulas, only 60% to 80% of administered radioactive hemoglobin or heme is recovered as bilirubin; a portion of the remainder is found in nonbilirubin fractions of bile.[549] Radioactive bilirubin in patients with prolonged complete biliary obstruction gradually disappears via an unidentified route.[549] Furthermore, in severe inherited defects of bilirubin conjugation, such as those found in infants with CN1 and in the Gunn rat, the alternate pathways appear to be increased.[550] One explanation for these observations is that bilirubin is converted by a series of light-stimulated reactions to a variety of water-soluble derivatives, including hydroxyrubins, bilichrysins, and a dipyrrole.[545] A microsomal P450-dependent mono-oxygenase may contribute to these alternate pathways; in addition, a mitochondrial bilirubin oxygenase has been identified that, in vitro, degrades bilirubin to a variety of products.[551]

Laboratory Evaluation of Hemoglobin Catabolism and Bile Pigments

The serum bilirubin concentration is an important marker of the rate of bilirubin production and of hepatobiliary function. Traditionally, it has been measured by the van den Bergh test in which a mixture of sulfanilic acid, hydrochloric acid, and sodium nitrite (diazo reagent) yields a reddish-violet color with a maximum absorption at 450 nm when added to plasma or other solutions containing bilirubin.[552] A direct reaction, in which the color reaches its maximum intensity at once, indicates conjugated bilirubin, as is seen in plasma or urine from patients with obstructive jaundice. Detection of the unconjugated bilirubin found in plasma of patients with hemolytic disease requires addition of an accelerator, such as alcohol (indirect reaction).

In situations where bilirubin production may be increased and the bilirubin load is likely high, precise measurements of heme catabolism have been determined by measuring endogenous bilirubin production or generation of carbon monoxide (produced in equimolar amounts during heme breakdown). CO production is estimated by measuring blood carboxyhemoglobin levels; end-tidal CO concentration corrected for ambient CO and pulmonary excretion rates of CO are also measured.[553]

References

1. Boycott AE. President's address: the blood as a tissue. Hypertrophy and atrophy of the red corpuscles. *Proc R Soc Med.* 1929;23(1):15-25.
2. Higgins JM. Red blood cell population dynamics. *Clin Lab Med.* 2015;35(1):43-57.
3. Elliott S, Foote MA, Molineux G, eds. *Erythropoietins and Erythropoiesis.* Birkhäuser Verlag; 2006.
4. Thoms JAI, Truong P, Subramanian S, et al. Disruption of a GATA2-TAL1-ERG regulatory circuit promotes erythroid transition in healthy and leukemic stem cells. *Blood.* 2021;138(16):1441-1455.
5. Eaves JC, Eaves AC. Erythropoiesis. In: Golde DW, Takaku F, eds. *Hematopoietic Stem Cells.* Marcel Dekker Inc; 1985.
6. Pellin D, Loperfido M, Baricordi C, et al. A comprehensive single cell transcriptional landscape of human hematopoietic progenitors. *Nat Commun.* 2019;10(1):2395.
7. Gregory CJ, Tepperman AD, McCulloch EA, Till JE. Erythropoietic progenitors capable of colony formation in culture: response of normal and genetically anemic W-W-V mice to manipulations of the erythron. *J Cell Physiol.* 1974;84(1):1-12.
8. Ogawa M, Parmley RT, Bank HL, Spicer SS. Human marrow erythropoiesis in culture. I. Characterization of methylcellulose colony assay. *Blood.* 1976;48(3):407-417.
9. Prchal JF, Adamson JW, Steinmann L, Fialkow PJ. Human erythroid colony formation in vitro: evidence for clonal origin. *J Cell Physiol.* 1976;89(3):489-492.
10. Sawada K, Krantz SB, Kans JS, et al. Purification of human erythroid colony-forming units and demonstration of specific binding of erythropoietin. *J Clin Invest.* 1987;80:357-366.
11. Gregory CJ, Eaves AC. Three stages of erythropoietic progenitor cell differentiation distinguished by a number of physical and biologic properties. *Blood.* 1978;51(3):527-537.
12. Iscove NN. The role of erythropoietin in regulation of population size and cell cycling of early and late erythroid precursors in mouse bone marrow. *Cell Tissue Kinet.* 1977;10(4):323-334.
13. Krantz SB. Erythropoietin. *Blood.* 1991;77(3):419-434.
14. Dolznig H, Habermann B, Stangl K, et al. Apoptosis protection by the Epo target Bcl-X(L) allows factor-independent differentiation of primary erythroblasts. *Curr Biol.* 2002;12(13):1076-1085.
15. Kieran MW, Perkins AC, Orkin SH, Zon LI. Thrombopoietin rescues in vitro erythroid colony formation from mouse embryos lacking the erythropoietin receptor. *Proc Natl Acad Sci U S A.* 1996;93(17):9126-9131.
16. Flygare J, Rayon Estrada V, Shin C, Gupta S, Lodish HF. HIF1alpha synergizes with glucocorticoids to promote BFU-E progenitor self-renewal. *Blood.* 2011;117(12):3435-3444.
17. Clarke BJ, Housman D. Characterization of an erythroid precursor cell of high proliferative capacity in normal human peripheral blood. *Proc Natl Acad Sci U S A.* 1977;74(3):1105-1109.
18. Nathan DG, Chess L, Hillman DG, et al. Human erythroid burst-forming unit: T-cell requirement for proliferation in vitro. *J Exp Med.* 1978;147(2):324-339.
19. Sawada K, Krantz SB, Dai CH, et al. Purification of human blood burst-forming units-erythroid and demonstration of the evolution of erythropoietin receptors. *J Cell Physiol.* 1990;142(2):219-230.
20. Koury ST, Koury MJ, Bondurant MC. Cytoskeletal distribution and function during the maturation and enucleation of mammalian erythroblasts. *J Cell Biol.* 1989;109(6 pt 1):3005-3013.
21. Dessypris EN, Krantz SB. Effect of pure erythropoietin on DNA-synthesis by human marrow day 15 erythroid burst forming units in short-term liquid culture. *Br J Haematol.* 1984;56(2):295-306.
22. Dessypris EN, Graber SE, Krantz SB, Stone WJ. Effects of recombinant erythropoietin on the concentration and cycling status of human marrow hematopoietic progenitors in vivo. *Blood.* 1988;72:2060-2062.
23. Tirelli V, Ghinassi B, Migliaccio AR, et al. Phenotypic definition of the progenitor cells with erythroid differentiation potential present in human adult blood. *Stem Cells Int.* 2011;2011:602483.
24. Yan H, Ali A, Blanc L, et al. Comprehensive phenotyping of erythropoiesis in human bone marrow: evaluation of normal and ineffective erythropoiesis. *Am J Hematol.* 2021;96(9):1064-1076.
25. Mori Y, Chen JY, Pluvinage JV, Seita J, Weissman IL. Prospective isolation of human erythroid lineage-committed progenitors. *Proc Natl Acad Sci U S A.* 2015;112(31):9638-9643.
26. Tanaka Y, Goodman JR. *Electron Microscopy of Human Blood Cells.* Harper & Row; 1972.
27. Killmann SA. On the size of normal human reticulocytes. *Acta Med Scand.* 1964;176:529-533.
28. Socolovsky M, Nam H, Fleming MD, Haase VH, Brugnara C, Lodish HF. Ineffective erythropoiesis in Stat5a(−/−)5b(−/−) mice due to decreased survival of early erythroblasts. *Blood.* 2001;98(12):3261-3273.
29. Zhang J, Socolovsky M, Gross AW, Lodish HF. Role of Ras signaling in erythroid differentiation of mouse fetal liver cells: functional analysis by a flow cytometry-based novel culture system. *Blood.* 2003;102(12):3938-3946.
30. McGrath KE, Catherman SC, Palis J. Delineating stages of erythropoiesis using imaging flow cytometry. *Methods.* 2017;112:68-74.
31. Hattangadi SM, Wong P, Zhang L, Flygare J, Lodish HF. From stem cell to red cell: regulation of erythropoiesis at multiple levels by multiple proteins, RNAs, and chromatin modifications. *Blood.* 2011;118(24):6258-6268.
32. Schumacher HR, Erslev AJ. Bone marrow kinetics. In: Szirmai E, ed. *Nuclear Hematology.* Academic Press; 1956.
33. Simon MC, Pevny L, Wiles MV, Keller G, Costantini F, Orkin SH. Rescue of erythroid development in gene targeted GATA-1-mouse embryonic stem cells. *Nat Genet.* 1992;1(2):92-98.
34. Yu L, Takai J, Otsuki A, et al. Derepression of the DNA methylation machinery of the GATA1 gene triggers the differentiation cue for erythropoiesis. *Mol Cell Biol.* 2017;37(8):e00592-e00616.
35. Hodge D, Coghill E, Keys J, et al. A global role for EKLF in definitive and primitive erythropoiesis. *Blood.* 2006;107(8):3359-3370.
36. Sawado T, Igarashi K, Groudine M. Activation of beta-major globin gene transcription is associated with recruitment of NF-E2 to the beta-globin LCR and gene promoter. *Proc Natl Acad Sci U S A.* 2001;98(18):10226-10231.
37. Kim SI, Bresnick EH. Transcriptional control of erythropoiesis: emerging mechanisms and principles. *Oncogene.* 2007;26(47):6777-6794.
38. Kerenyi MA, Orkin SH. Networking erythropoiesis. *J Exp Med.* 2010;207(12):2537-2541.
39. Anantharaman A, Lin IJ, Barrow J, et al. Role of helix-loop-helix proteins during differentiation of erythroid cells. *Mol Cell Biol.* 2011;31(7):1332-1343.
40. Bondurant MC, Lind RN, Koury MJ, Ferguson ME. Control of globin gene transcription by erythropoietin in erythroblasts from friend virus-infected mice. *Mol Cell Biol.* 1985;5(4):675-683.
41. Koury MJ, Bondurant MC, Atkinson JB. Erythropoietin control of terminal erythroid differentiation: maintenance of cell viability, production of hemoglobin, and development of the erythrocyte membrane. *Blood Cell.* 1987;13(1-2):217-226.
42. Miller BA, Scaduto RC Jr, Tillotson DL, Botti JJ, Cheung JY. Erythropoietin stimulates a rise in intracellular free calcium concentration in single early human erythroid precursors. *J Clin Invest.* 1988;82(1):309-315.
43. Sawyer ST, Krantz SB. Transferrin receptor number, synthesis, and endocytosis during erythropoietin-induced maturation of Friend virus-infected erythroid cells. *J Biol Chem.* 1986;261(20):9187-9195.
44. Gnanapragasam MN, Bieker JJ. Orchestration of late events in erythropoiesis by KLF1/EKLF. *Curr Opin Hematol.* 2017;24(3):183-190.
45. Troadec MB, Warner D, Wallace J, et al. Targeted deletion of the mouse Mitoferrin1 gene: from anemia to protoporphyria. *Blood.* 2011;117(20):5494-5502.
46. Tallack MR, Perkins AC. KLF1 directly coordinates almost all aspects of terminal erythroid differentiation. *IUBMB Life.* 2010;62(12):886-890.
47. Weiss MJ, Zhou S, Feng L, et al. Role of alpha-hemoglobin-stabilizing protein in normal erythropoiesis and beta-thalassemia. *Ann N Y Acad Sci.* 2005;1054:103-117.

48. Saxton RA, Sabatini DM. mTOR signaling in growth, metabolism, and disease. *Cell.* 2017;168(6):960-976.
49. Liu X, Zhang Y, Ni M, et al. Regulation of mitochondrial biogenesis in erythropoiesis by mTORC1-mediated protein translation. *Nat Cell Biol.* 2017;19(6):626-638.
50. Chung J, Bauer DE, Ghamari A, et al. The mTORC1/4E-BP pathway coordinates hemoglobin production with L-leucine availability. *Sci Signal.* 2015;8(372):ra34.
51. Oburoglu L, Tardito S, Fritz V, et al. Glucose and glutamine metabolism regulate human hematopoietic stem cell lineage specification. *Cell Stem Cell.* 2014;15(2):169-184.
52. Burch JS, Marcero JR, Maschek JA, et al. Glutamine via alpha-ketoglutarate dehydrogenase provides succinyl-CoA for heme synthesis during erythropoiesis. *Blood.* 2018;132(10):987-998.
53. Jensen EL, Gonzalez-Ibanez AM, Mendoza P, et al. Copper deficiency-induced anemia is caused by a mitochondrial metabolic reprograming in erythropoietic cells. *Metallomics.* 2019;11(2):282-290.
54. Cui S, Tanabe O, Lim KC, et al. PGC-1 coactivator activity is required for murine erythropoiesis. *Mol Cell Biol.* 2014;34(11):1956-1965.
55. Sen T, Chen J, Singbrant S. Decreased PGC1β expression results in disrupted human erythroid differentiation, impaired hemoglobinization and cell cycle exit. *Sci Rep.* 2021;11(1):17129.
56. Payne EM, Virgilio M, Narla A, et al. L-Leucine improves the anemia and developmental defects associated with Diamond-Blackfan anemia and del(5q) MDS by activating the mTOR pathway. *Blood.* 2012;120(11):2214-2224.
57. Bennani NN, LaPlant BR, Ansell SM, et al. Efficacy of the oral mTORC1 inhibitor everolimus in relapsed or refractory indolent lymphoma. *Am J Hematol.* 2017;92(5):448-453.
58. Stohlman F. Kinetics of erythropoiesis. In: Gordon AS, ed. *Regulation of Hematopoiesis.* Vol 1. Appleton-Century-Crofts; 1970:317.
59. Orlic D. Ultrastructural analysis of erythropoiesis. In: Gordon AS, ed. *Regulation of Hematopoiesis.* Vol 1. Appleton-Century-Crofts; 1970:271.
60. Tooze J, Davies HG. The occurrence and possible significance of haemoglobin in the chromosomal regions of mature erythrocyte nuclei of the newt Triturus cristatus. *J Cell Biol.* 1963;16:501-511.
61. Ji P, Yeh V, Ramirez T, Murata-Hori M, Lodish HF. Histone deacetylase 2 is required for chromatin condensation and subsequent enucleation of cultured mouse fetal erythroblasts. *Haematologica.* 2010;95(12):2013-2021.
62. Ji P, Murata-Hori M, Lodish HF. Formation of mammalian erythrocytes: chromatin condensation and enucleation. *Trends Cell Biol.* 2011;21(7):409-415.
63. Awai M, Okada S, Takebayashi J, Kubo T, Inoue M, Seno S. Studies on the mechanism of denucleation of the erythroblast. *Acta Haematol.* 1968;39(4):193-202.
64. Rind H. Kinetik der erythroblastenentkernung. *Folia Haematol.* 1956;74:262-266.
65. Patel VP, Lodish HF. A fibronectin matrix is required for differentiation of murine erythroleukemia cells into reticulocytes. *J Cell Biol.* 1987;105:3105-3118.
66. Keerthivasan G, Small S, Liu H, Wickrema A, Crispino JD. Vesicle trafficking plays a novel role in erythroblast enucleation. *Blood.* 2010;116(17):3331-3340.
67. Ji P, Jayapal SR, Lodish HF. Enucleation of cultured mouse fetal erythroblasts requires Rac GTPases and mDia2. *Nat Cell Biol.* 2008;10(3):314-321.
68. Chasis JA, Prenant M, Leung A, Mohandas N. Membrane assembly and remodeling during reticulocyte maturation. *Blood.* 1989;74(3):1112-1120.
69. Knutson MD, Oukka M, Koss LM, Aydemir F, Wessling-Resnick M. Iron release from macrophages after erythrophagocytosis is up-regulated by ferroportin 1 overexpression and down-regulated by hepcidin. *Proc Natl Acad Sci U S A.* 2005;102(5):1324-1328.
70. Chasis JA, Mohandas N. Erythroblastic islands: niches for erythropoiesis. *Blood.* 2008;112(3):470-478.
71. Chasis JA. Erythroblastic islands: specialized microenvironmental niches for erythropoiesis. *Curr Opin Hematol.* 2006;13(3):137-141.
72. Zhao G, Yu D, Weiss MJ. MicroRNAs in erythropoiesis. *Curr Opin Hematol.* 2010;17(3):155-162.
73. Zhang L, Flygare J, Wong P, Lim B, Lodish HF. miR-191 regulates mouse erythroblast enucleation by down-regulating Riok3 and Mxi1. *Genes Dev.* 2011;25(2):119-124.
74. Menon V, Ghaffari S. Erythroid enucleation: a gateway into a "bloody" world. *Exp Hematol.* 2021;95:13-22.
75. Tavassoli M, Crosby WH. Fate of the nucleus of the marrow erythroblast. *Science.* 1973;179(4076):912-913.
76. Piva E, Brugnara C, Spolaore F, Plebani M. Clinical utility of reticulocyte parameters. *Clin Lab Med.* 2015;35(1):133-163.
77. Skadberg O, Brun A, Sandberg S. Human reticulocytes isolated from peripheral blood: maturation time and hemoglobin synthesis. *Lab Hematol.* 2003;9(4):198-206.
78. Rees DC, Duley JA, Marinaki AM. Pyrimidine 5' nucleotidase deficiency. *Br J Haematol.* 2003;120(3):375-383.
79. Collins FS, Weissman SM. The molecular genetics of human hemoglobin. *Prog Nucleic Acid Res Mol Biol.* 1984;31:315-462.
80. Schroeder WA, Huisman TH, Shelton JR, et al. Evidence for multiple structural genes for the gamma chain of human fetal hemoglobin. *Proc Natl Acad Sci U S A.* 1968;60(2):537-544.
81. Deisseroth A, Nienhuis A, Turner P, et al. Localization of the human alpha-globin structural gene to chromosome 16 in somatic cell hybrids by molecular hybridization assay. *Cell.* 1977;12(1):205-218.
82. Fritsch EF, Lawn RM, Maniatis T. Molecular cloning and characterization of the human beta-like globin gene cluster. *Cell.* 1980;19(4):959-972.
83. Adamson SD, Herbert E, Godchaux W. Factors affecting the rate of protein synthesis in lysate systems from reticulocytes. *Arch Biochem Biophys.* 1968;125(2):671-683.
84. Bruns GP, London IM. The effect of hemin on the synthesis of globin. *Biochem Biophys Res Commun.* 1965;18:236-242.
85. Lodish HF. Translational control of protein synthesis. *Annu Rev Biochem.* 1976;45:39-72.
86. Balkow K, Mizuno S, Fisher JM, Rabinovitz M. Hemin control of globin synthesis: effect of a translational repressor on Met-tRNAf binding to the small ribosomal subunit and its relation to the activity and alailability of an initiation factor. *Biochim Biophys Acta.* 1973;324(3):397-409.
87. Howard GA, Adamson SD, Herbert E. Studies on cessation of protein synthesis in a reticulocyte lysate cell-free system. *Biochim Biophys Acta.* 1970;213(1):237-240.
88. Kramer G, Cimadevilla JM, Hardesty B. Specificity of the protein kinase activity associated with the hemin-controlled repressor of rabbit reticulocyte. *Proc Natl Acad Sci U S A.* 1976;73(9):3078-3082.
89. Ranu RS, Levin DH, Delaunay J, Ernst V, London IM. Regulation of protein synthesis in rabbit reticulocyte lysates: characteristics of inhibition of protein synthesis by a translational inhibitor from heme-deficient lysates and its relationship to the initiation factor which binds Met-tRNAf. *Proc Natl Acad Sci U S A.* 1976;73(8):2720-2724.
90. Chen JJ. Regulation of protein synthesis by the heme-regulated eIF2alpha kinase: relevance to anemias. *Blood.* 2007;109(7):2693-2699.
91. Han AP, Yu C, Lu L, et al. Heme-regulated eIF2alpha kinase (HRI) is required for translational regulation and survival of erythroid precursors in iron deficiency. *EMBO J.* 2001;20(23):6909-6918.
92. Suragani RN, Zachariah RS, Velazquez JG, et al. Heme-regulated eIF2alpha kinase activated Atf4 signaling pathway in oxidative stress and erythropoiesis. *Blood.* 2012;119(22):5276-5284.
93. Chen JJ, Zhang S. Heme-regulated eIF2α kinase in erythropoiesis and hemoglobinopathies. *Blood.* 2019;134(20):1697-1707.
94. Igarashi K, Sun J. The heme-Bach1 pathway in the regulation of oxidative stress response and erythroid differentiation. *Antioxid Redox Signal.* 2006;8(1-2):107-118.
95. Bottomley SS, Eberhard Muller U. Pathophysiology of heme synthesis. *Semin Hematol.* 1988;25:282-302.
96. Burnham BF. The chemistry of the porphyrins. *Semin Hematol.* 1968;5(4):296-322.
97. Dolphin D. *The Porphyrins.* Vol 1-7. Academic Press; 1978:1979.
98. Lascelles J. *Tetrapyrrole Biosynthesis and its Regulation.* WA Benjamin Inc; 1964.
99. Warren MJ, Smith AG. *Tetrapyrroles: Birth, Life, and Death.* Landes Bioscience, Springer Science & Business Media; 2009.
100. Khan AA, Quigley JG. Control of intracellular heme levels: heme transporters and heme oxygenases. *Biochim Biophys Acta.* 2011;1813(5):668-682.
101. Ponka P. Tissue-specific regulation of iron metabolism and heme synthesis: distinct control mechanisms in erythroid cells. *Blood.* 1997;89(1):1-25.
102. Ryter SW, Tyrrell RM. The heme synthesis and degradation pathways: role in oxidant sensitivity. Heme oxygenase has both pro- and antioxidant properties. *Free Radic Biol Med.* 2000;28(2):289-309.
103. Heinemann IU, Jahn M, Jahn D. The biochemistry of heme biosynthesis. *Arch Biochem Biophys.* 2008;474(2):238-251.
104. Ajioka RS, Phillips JD, Kushner JP. Biosynthesis of heme in mammals. *Biochim Biophys Acta.* 2006;1763(7):723-736.
105. Garcia-Santos D, Schranzhofer M, Bergeron R, Sheftel AD, Ponka P. Extracellular glycine is necessary for optimal hemoglobinization of erythroid cells. *Haematologica.* 2017;102(8):1314-1323.
106. Winter M, Funk J, Körner A, et al. Effects of GlyT1 inhibition on erythropoiesis and iron homeostasis in rats. *Exp Hematol.* 2016;44(10):964-974.e4.
107. Zwifelhofer NM, Cai X, Liao R, et al. GATA factor-regulated solute carrier ensemble reveals a nucleoside transporter-dependent differentiation mechanism. *PLoS Genet.* 2020;16(12):e1009286.
108. Peoc'h K, Nicolas G, Schmitt C, et al. Regulation and tissue-specific expression of δ-aminolevulinic acid synthases in non-syndromic sideroblastic anemias and porphyrias. *Mol Genet Metabol.* 2019;128(3):190-197.
109. Ferreira GC, Dailey HA. Reconstitution of the two terminal enzymes of the heme biosynthetic pathway into phospholipid vesicles. *J Biol Chem.* 1987;262(9):4407-4412.
110. Koch M, Breithaupt C, Kiefersauer R, Freigang J, Huber R, Messerschmidt A. Crystal structure of protoporphyrinogen IX oxidase: a key enzyme in haem and chlorophyll biosynthesis. *EMBO J.* 2004;23(8):1720-1728.
111. Chiabrando D, Marro S, Mercurio S, et al. The mitochondrial heme exporter FLVCR1b mediates erythroid differentiation. *J Clin Invest.* 2012;122(12):4569-4579.
112. Dailey HA, Dailey TA, Wu CK, et al. Ferrochelatase at the millennium: structures, mechanisms and [2Fe-2S] clusters. *Cell Mol Life Sci.* 2000;57(13-14):1909-1926.
113. Jones MS, Jones OT. The structural organization of haem synthesis in rat liver mitochondria. *Biochem J.* 1969;113(3):507-514.
114. Cornah JE, Smith AG. Transformation of uroporphyrinogen III into protohaem. In: Warren MJ, Smith AG, eds. *Tetrapyrroles: Birth, Life and Death.* Landes Bioscience; 2009:74-88.
115. Chen W, Dailey HA, Paw BH. Ferrochelatase forms an oligomeric complex with mitoferrin-1 and Abcb10 for erythroid heme biosynthesis. *Blood.* 2010;116(4):628-630.
116. Shirihai OS, Gregory T, Yu C, Orkin SH, Weiss MJ. ABC-me: a novel mitochondrial transporter induced by GATA-1 during erythroid differentiation. *EMBO J.* 2000;19(11):2492-2502.
117. Chen W, Paradkar PN, Li L, et al. Abcb10 physically interacts with mitoferrin-1 (Slc25a37) to enhance its stability and function in the erythroid mitochondria. *Proc Natl Acad Sci U S A.* 2009;106(38):16263-16268.
118. Yamamoto M, Arimura H, Fukushige T, et al. Abcb10 role in heme biosynthesis in vivo: Abcb10 knockout in mice causes anemia with protoporphyrin IX and iron accumulation. *Mol Cell Biol.* 2014;34(6):1077-1084.
119. Ye H, Rouault TA. Human iron-sulfur cluster assembly, cellular iron homeostasis, and disease. *Biochemistry.* 2010;49(24):4945-4956.

120. Crooks DR, Ghosh MC, Haller RG, Tong WH, Rouault TA. Posttranslational stability of the heme biosynthetic enzyme ferrochelatase is dependent on iron availability and intact iron-sulfur cluster assembly machinery. *Blood*. 2010;115(4):860-869.

121. Piel RB III, Shiferaw MT, Vashisht AA, et al. A novel role for Progesterone receptor membrane component 1 (PGRMC1): a Partner and regulator of ferrochelatase. *Biochemistry*. 2016;55(37):5204-5217.

122. Chung J, Wittig JG, Ghamari A, et al. Erythropoietin signaling regulates heme biosynthesis. *Elife*. 2017;6:e24767.

123. Whitcombe DM, Carter NP, Albertson DG, Smith SJ, Rhodes DA, Cox TM. Assignment of the human ferrochelatase gene (FECH) and a locus for protoporphyria to chromosome 18q22. *Genomics*. 1991;11(4):1152-1154.

124. Magness ST, Tugores A, Brenner DA. Analysis of ferrochelatase expression during hematopoietic development of embryonic stem cells. *Blood*. 2000;95(11):3568-3577.

125. Taketani S, Mohri T, Hioki K, Tokunaga R, Kohno H. Structure and transcriptional regulation of the mouse ferrochelatase gene. *Gene*. 1999;227(2):117-124.

126. Asano H, Li XS, Stamatoyannopoulos G. FKLF-2: a novel Kruppel-like transcriptional factor that activates globin and other erythroid lineage genes. *Blood*. 2000;95(11):3578-3584.

127. Stadtman ER. Allosteric regulation of enzyme activity. *Adv Enzymol Relat Areas Mol Biol*. 1966;28:41-154.

128. Medlock AE, Dailey HA. Regulation of mammalian heme biosynthesis. In: Warren MJ, Smith AG, eds. *Tetrapyrroles: Birth, Life and Death*. Landes Bioscience; 2009:116-127.

129. Gidari AS, Levere RD. Enzymatic formation and cellular regulation of heme synthesis. *Semin Hematol*. 1977;14(2):145-168.

130. Granick S, Urata G. Increase in activity of alpha-aminolevulinic acid synthetase in liver mitochondria induced by feeding of 3,5-dicarbethoxy-1,4-dihydrocollidine. *J Biol Chem*. 1963;238:821-827.

131. Marver HS, Collins A, Tschudy DP, Rechcigl M Jr. Delta-aminolevulinic acid synthetase. II. Induction in rat liver. *J Biol Chem*. 1966;241(19):4323-4329.

132. Sassa S, Granick S. δ-Aminolevulinic acid synthetase and the control of heme and chlorophyll synthesis. In: Vogel JH, ed. *Metabolic Pathways, Vol V, Metabolic Regulation*. Academic Press; 1971.

133. Lathrop JT, Timko MP. Regulation by heme of mitochondrial protein transport through a conserved amino acid motif. *Science*. 1993;259(5094):522-525.

134. De Matteis F. Drug interactions in experimental hepatic porphyria. A model for the exacerbation by drugs of human variegate porphyria. *Enzyme*. 1973;16(1):266-275.

135. De Matteis F, Gibbs AH. Stimulation of the pathway of porphyrin synthesis in the liver of rats and mice by griseofulvin, 3,5-Diethoxycarbonyl-1,4-dihydrocollidine and related drugs: evidence for two basically different mechanisms. *Biochem J*. 1975;146(1):285-287.

136. Handschin C, Lin J, Rhee J, et al. Nutritional regulation of hepatic heme biosynthesis and porphyria through PGC-1alpha. *Cell*. 2005;122(4):505-515.

137. Drummond GS, Kappas A. Chemoprevention of severe neonatal hyperbilirubinemia. *Semin Perinatol*. 2004;28(5):365-368.

138. Vinchi F, Ingoglia G, Chiabrando D, et al. Heme exporter FLVCR1a regulates heme synthesis and degradation and controls activity of cytochromes P450. *Gastroenterology*. 2014;146(5):1325-1338.

139. Fiorito V, Allocco AL, Petrillo S, et al. The heme synthesis-export system regulates the tricarboxylic acid cycle flux and oxidative phosphorylation. *Cell Rep*. 2021;35(11):109252.

140. Fujita H, Yamamoto M, Yamagami T, et al. Sequential activation of genes for heme pathway enzymes during erythroid differentiation of mouse Friend virus-transformed erythroleukemia cells. *Biochim Biophys Acta*. 1991;1090(3):311-316.

141. Taketani S, Inazawa J, Abe T, et al. The human protoporphyrinogen oxidase gene (PPOX): organization and location to chromosome 1. *Genomics*. 1995;29(3):698-703.

142. Houston T, Moore MR, McColl KE, Fitzsimons EJ. Regulation of haem biosynthesis in normoblastic erythropoiesis: role of 5-aminolaevulinic acid synthase and ferrochelatase. *Biochim Biophys Acta*. 1994;1201(1):85-93.

143. Sassa S, Nagai T. The role of heme in gene expression. *Int J Hematol*. 1996;63(3):167-178.

144. Lake-Bullock H, Dailey HA. Biphasic ordered induction of heme synthesis in differentiating murine erythroleukemia cells: role of erythroid 5-aminolevulinate synthase. *Mol Cell Biol*. 1993;13(11):7122-7132.

145. Iacopetta BJ, Morgan EH, Yeoh GC. Transferrin receptors and iron uptake during erythroid cell development. *Biochim Biophys Acta*. 1982;687(2):204-210.

146. Nilsson R, Schultz IJ, Pierce EL, et al. Discovery of genes essential for heme biosynthesis through large-scale gene expression analysis. *Cell Metab*. 2009;10(2):119-130.

147. Sheftel AD, Richardson DR, Prchal J, Ponka P. Mitochondrial iron metabolism and sideroblastic anemia. *Acta Haematol*. 2009;122(2-3):120-133.

148. Hamza I, Dailey HA. One ring to rule them all: trafficking of heme and heme synthesis intermediates in the metazoans. *Biochim Biophys Acta*. 2012;1823(9):1617-1632.

149. Whitman JC, Paw BH, Chung J. The role of ClpX in erythropoietic protoporphyria. *Hematol Transfus Cell Ther*. 2018;40(2):182-188.

150. Kerenyi MA, Grebien F, Gehart H, et al. Stat5 regulates cellular iron uptake of erythroid cells via IRP-2 and TfR-1. *Blood*. 2008;112(9):3878-3888.

151. Schranzhofer M, Schifrer M, Cabrera JA, et al. Remodeling the regulation of iron metabolism during erythroid differentiation to ensure efficient heme biosynthesis. *Blood*. 2006;107(10):4159-4167.

152. Sheftel AD, Zhang AS, Brown C, Shirihai OS, Ponka P. Direct interorganellar transfer of iron from endosome to mitochondrion. *Blood*. 2007;110(1):125-132.

153. Halliwell B, Gutteridge JM. Role of free radicals and catalytic metal ions in human disease: an overview. *Methods Enzymol*. 1990;186:1-85.

154. Balla J, Vercellotti GM, Nath K, et al. Haem, haem oxygenase and ferritin in vascular endothelial cell injury. *Nephrol Dial Transplant*. 2003;18(suppl 5):v8-v12.

155. Rund D, Rachmilewitz E. Pathophysiology of alpha- and beta-thalassemia: therapeutic implications. *Semin Hematol*. 2001;38(4):343-349.

156. Quigley JG, Burns CC, Anderson MM, et al. Cloning of the cellular receptor for feline leukemia virus subgroup C (FeLV-C), a retrovirus that induces red cell aplasia. *Blood*. 2000;95(3):1093-1099.

157. Keel SB, Doty RT, Yang Z, et al. A heme export protein is required for red blood cell differentiation and iron homeostasis. *Science*. 2008;319(5864):825-828.

158. Quigley JG, Yang Z, Worthington MT, et al. Identification of a human heme exporter that is essential for erythropoiesis. *Cell*. 2004;118(6):757-766.

159. Doty RT, Phelps SR, Shadle C, Sanchez-Bonilla M, Keel SB, Abkowitz JL. Coordinate expression of heme and globin is essential for effective erythropoiesis. *J Clin Invest*. 2015;125(12):4681-4691.

160. Alves LR, Costa ES, Sorgine MH, et al. Heme-oxygenases during erythropoiesis in K562 and human bone marrow cells. *PLoS One*. 2011;6(7):e21358.

161. Fujita H, Sassa S. The rapid and decremental change in haem oxygenase mRNA during erythroid differentiation of murine erythroleukaemia cells. *Br J Haematol*. 1989;73(4):557-560.

162. Lipton JM, Ellis SR. Diamond-Blackfan anemia: diagnosis, treatment, and molecular pathogenesis. *Hematol Oncol Clin North Am*. 2009;23(2):261-282.

163. Chiabrando D, Tolosano E. Diamond blackfan anemia at the crossroad between ribosome biogenesis and heme metabolism. *Adv Hematol*. 2010;2010:790632.

164. Yang Z, Keel SB, Shimamura A, et al. Delayed globin synthesis leads to excess heme and the macrocytic anemia of Diamond Blackfan anemia and del(5q) myelodysplastic syndrome. *Sci Transl Med*. 2016;8(338):338ra67.

165. Zhang Y, Zhang J, An W, et al. Intron 1 GATA site enhances ALAS2 expression indispensably during erythroid differentiation. *Nucleic Acids Res*. 2017;45(2):657-671.

166. Doty RT, Yan X, Lausted C, et al. Single-cell analyses demonstrate that a heme–GATA1 feedback loop regulates red cell differentiation. *Blood*. 2019;133(5):457-469.

167. Tanimura N, Miller E, Igarashi K, et al. Mechanism governing heme synthesis reveals a GATA factor/heme circuit that controls differentiation. *EMBO Rep*. 2016;17(2):249-265.

168. Liao R, Zheng Y, Liu X, et al. Discovering how heme controls genome function through heme-omics. *Cell Rep*. 2020;31(13):107832.

169. Gautier EF, Ducamp S, Leduc M, et al. Comprehensive proteomic analysis of human erythropoiesis. *Cell Rep*. 2016;16(5):1470-1484.

170. Weiss MJ, dos Santos CO. Chaperoning erythropoiesis. *Blood*. 2009;113(10):2136-2144.

171. Kong Y, Zhou S, Kihm AJ, et al. Loss of alpha-hemoglobin-stabilizing protein impairs erythropoiesis and exacerbates beta-thalassemia. *J Clin Invest*. 2004;114(10):1457-1466.

172. Khandros E, Weiss MJ. Protein quality control during erythropoiesis and hemoglobin synthesis. *Hematol Oncol Clin North Am*. 2010;24(6):1071-1088.

173. Mathangasinghe Y, Fauvet B, Jane SM, Goloubinoff P, Nillegoda NB. The Hsp70 chaperone system: distinct roles in erythrocyte formation and maintenance. *Haematologica*. 2021;106(6):1519-1534.

174. Gregory T, Yu C, Ma A, Orkin SH, Blobel GA, Weiss MJ. GATA-1 and erythropoietin cooperate to promote erythroid cell survival by regulating bcl-xL expression. *Blood*. 1999;94(1):87-96.

175. Lu L, Han AP, Chen JJ. Translation initiation control by heme-regulated eukaryotic initiation factor 2alpha kinase in erythroid cells under cytoplasmic stresses. *Mol Cell Biol*. 2001;21(23):7971-7980.

176. Khandros E, Thom CS, D'Souza J, Weiss MJ. Integrated protein quality-control pathways regulate free alpha-globin in murine beta-thalassemia. *Blood*. 2012;119(22):5265-5275.

177. Wojcik S. Crosstalk between autophagy and proteasome protein degradation systems: possible implications for cancer therapy. *Folia Histochem Cytobiol*. 2013;51(4):249-264.

178. Krantz SB, Jacobson LO. *Erythropoietin and the Regulation of Erythropoiesis*. University of Chicago; 1970:1-330.

179. Dordal MS, Wang FF, Goldwasser E. The role of carbohydrate in erythropoietin action. *Endocrinology*. 1985;116(6):2293-2299.

180. Cotes PM, Bangham DR. The international reference preparation of erythropoietin. *Bull World Health Organ*. 1966;35(5):751-760.

181. Miyake T, Kung CK, Goldwasser E. Purification of human erythropoietin. *J Biol Chem*. 1977;252(15):5558-5564.

182. Greer SN, Metcalf JL, Wang Y, Ohh M. The updated biology of hypoxia-inducible factor. *EMBO J*. 2012;31(11):2448-2460.

183. Anderson SA, Nizzi CP, Chang YI, et al. The IRP1-HIF-2alpha axis coordinates iron and oxygen sensing with erythropoiesis and iron absorption. *Cell Metab*. 2013;17(2):282-290.

184. Ivan M, Kondo K, Yang H, et al. HIFalpha targeted for VHL-mediated destruction by proline hydroxylation: implications for O_2 sensing. *Science*. 2001;292(5516):464-468.

185. Jaakkola P, Mole DR, Tian YM, et al. Targeting of HIF-alpha to the von Hippel-Lindau ubiquitylation complex by O_2-regulated prolyl hydroxylation. *Science*. 2001;292(5516):468-472.

186. Lando D, Peet DJ, Gorman JJ, Whelan DA, Whitelaw ML, Bruick RK. FIH-1 is an asparaginyl hydroxylase enzyme that regulates the transcriptional activity of hypoxia-inducible factor. *Genes Dev*. 2002;16(12):1466-1471.

187. Bruick RK, McKnight SL. Transcription. Oxygen sensing gets a second wind. *Science*. 2002;295(5556):807-808.

188. Lee FS, Percy MJ. The HIF pathway and erythrocytosis. *Annu Rev Pathol*. 2011;6(1):165-192.

189. Brigandi RA, Johnson B, Oei C, et al. A novel hypoxia-inducible factor-prolyl hydroxylase inhibitor (GSK1278863) for anemia in CKD: a 28-day, phase 2A randomized trial. *Am J Kidney Dis*. 2016;67(6):861-871.

190. Semenza GL. Regulation of mammalian O_2 homeostasis by hypoxia-inducible factor 1. *Annu Rev Cell Dev Biol.* 1999;15:551-578.

191. Paulson RF, Shi L, Wu DC. Stress erythropoiesis: new signals and new stress progenitor cells. *Curr Opin Hematol.* 2011;18(3):139-145.

192. Perry JM, Harandi OF, Paulson RF. BMP4, SCF, and hypoxia cooperatively regulate the expansion of murine stress erythroid progenitors. *Blood.* 2007;109(10):4494-4502.

193. Huang LJ, Constantinescu SN, Lodish HF. The N-terminal domain of Janus kinase 2 is required for Golgi processing and cell surface expression of erythropoietin receptor. *Mol Cell.* 2001;8:1327-1338.

194. Sawyer ST. Receptors for erythropoietin. Distribution, structure, and role in receptor-mediated endocytosis in erythroid cells. In: Harris JR, ed. *Blood Cell Biochemistry.* Vol. I. Plenum Publishing; 1990:365.

195. Berridge MV, Fraser JK, Carter JM, Lin FK. Effects of recombinant human erythropoietin on megakaryocytes and on platelet production in the rat. *Blood.* 1988;72(3):970-977.

196. Pichon A, Jeton F, El Hasnaoui-Saadani R, et al. Erythropoietin and the use of a transgenic model of erythropoietin-deficient mice. *Hypoxia (Auckl).* 2016;4:29-39.

197. Oster HS, Neumann D, Hoffman M, Mittelman M. Erythropoietin: the swinging pendulum. *Leuk Res.* 2012;36(8):939-944.

198. Singh S, Verma R, Pradeep A, et al. Dynamic ligand modulation of EPO receptor pools, and dysregulation by polycythemia-associated EPOR alleles. *PLoS One.* 2012;7(1):e29064.

199. D'Andrea AD, Fasman GD, Lodish HF. A new hematopoietic growth factor receptor superfamily: structural features and implications for signal transduction. *Curr Opin Cell Biol.* 1990;2(4):648-651.

200. Livnah O, Stura EA, Johnson DL, et al. Functional mimicry of a protein hormone by a peptide agonist: the EPO receptor complex at 2.8 A. *Science.* 1996;273(5274):464-471.

201. Koury MJ, Bondurant MC, Graber SE, Sawyer ST. Erythropoietin messenger RNA levels in developing mice and transfer of 125I-erythropoietin by the placenta. *J Clin Invest.* 1988;82(1):154-159.

202. Youssoufian H, Longmore G, Neumann D, Yoshimura A, Lodish HF. Structure, function, and activation of the erythropoietin receptor. *Blood.* 1993;81(9):2223-2236.

203. Livnah O, Stura EA, Middleton SA, Johnson DL, Jolliffe LK, Wilson IA. Crystallographic evidence for preformed dimers of erythropoietin receptor before ligand activation. *Science.* 1999;283(5404):987-990.

204. Kubatzky KF, Ruan W, Gurezka R, et al. Self assembly of the transmembrane domain promotes signal transduction through the erythropoietin receptor. *Curr Biol.* 2001;11(2):110-115.

205. Dusanter-Fourt I, Casadevall N, Lacombe C, et al. Erythropoietin induces the tyrosine phosphorylation of its own receptor in human erythropoietin-responsive cells. *J Biol Chem.* 1992;267(15):10670-10675.

206. Pang X, Zhou HX. A common model for cytokine receptor activation: combined scissor-like rotation and self-rotation of receptor dimer induced by class I cytokine. *PLoS Comput Biol.* 2012;8(3):e1002427.

207. Neubauer H, Cumano A, Muller M, Wu H, Huffstadt U, Pfeffer K. Jak2 deficiency defines an essential developmental checkpoint in definitive hematopoiesis. *Cell.* 1998;93(3):397-409.

208. Remy I, Wilson IA, Michnick SW. Erythropoietin receptor activation by a ligand-induced conformation change. *Science.* 1999;283(5404):990-993.

209. Tsiftsoglou AS, Vizirianakis IS, Strouboulis J. Erythropoiesis: model systems, molecular regulators, and developmental programs. *IUBMB Life.* 2009;61(8):800-830.

210. Ingley E. Integrating novel signaling pathways involved in erythropoiesis. *IUBMB Life.* 2012;64(5):402-410.

211. Damen JE, Wakao H, Miyajima A, et al. Tyrosine 343 in the erythropoietin receptor positively regulates erythropoietin-induced cell proliferation and STAT5 activation. *EMBO J.* 1995;14(22):5557-5568.

212. Wood AD, Chen E, Donaldson IJ, et al. ID1 promotes expansion and survival of primary erythroid cells and is a target of JAK2V617F-STAT5 signaling. *Blood.* 2009;114(9):1820-1830.

213. Zhu BM, McLaughlin SK, Na R, et al. Hematopoietic-specific Stat5-null mice display microcytic hypochromic anemia associated with reduced transferrin receptor gene expression. *Blood.* 2008;112(5):2071-2080.

214. Menon MP, Karur V, Bogacheva O, Bogachev O, Cuetara B, Wojchowski DM. Signals for stress erythropoiesis are integrated via an erythropoietin receptor-phosphotyrosine-343-Stat5 axis. *J Clin Invest.* 2006;116(3):683-694.

215. Zang H, Sato K, Nakajima H, McKay C, Ney PA, Ihle JN. The distal region and receptor tyrosines of the Epo receptor are non-essential for in vivo erythropoiesis. *EMBO J.* 2001;20(12):3156-3166.

216. Sathyanarayana P, Dev A, Fang J, et al. EPO receptor circuits for primary erythroblast survival. *Blood.* 2008;111(11):5390-5399.

217. Socolovsky M, Fallon AE, Wang S, Brugnara C, Lodish HF. Fetal anemia and apoptosis of red cell progenitors in Stat5a−/−5b−/− mice: a direct role for Stat5 in Bcl-X(L) induction. *Cell.* 1999;98(2):181-191.

218. Dolznig H, Grebien F, Deiner EM, et al. Erythroid progenitor renewal versus differentiation: genetic evidence for cell autonomous, essential functions of EpoR, Stat5 and the GR. *Oncogene.* 2006;25(20):2890-2900.

219. Penta K, Sawyer ST. Erythropoietin induces the tyrosine phosphorylation, nuclear translocation, and DNA binding of STAT1 and STAT5 in erythroid cells. *J Biol Chem.* 1995;270(52):31282-31287.

220. Porpiglia E, Hidalgo D, Koulnis M, Tzafriri AR, Socolovsky M. Stat5 signaling specifies basal versus stress erythropoietic responses through distinct binary and graded dynamic modalities. *PLoS Biol.* 2012;10(8):e1001383.

221. Wagner KU, Claudio E, Rucker EB III, et al. Conditional deletion of the Bcl-x gene from erythroid cells results in hemolytic anemia and profound splenomegaly. *Development.* 2000;127(22):4949-4958.

222. Rhodes MM, Kopsombut P, Bondurant MC, Price JO, Koury MJ. Bcl-x(L) prevents apoptosis of late-stage erythroblasts but does not mediate the antiapoptotic effect of erythropoietin. *Blood.* 2005;106(5):1857-1863.

223. Kuo YY, Chang ZF. GATA-1 and Gfi-1B interplay to regulate Bcl-xL transcription. *Mol Cell Biol.* 2007;27(12):4261-4272.

224. Dev A, Byrne SM, Verma R, Ashton-Rickardt PG, Wojchowski DM. Erythropoietin-directed erythropoiesis depends on serpin inhibition of erythroblast lysosomal cathepsins. *J Exp Med.* 2013;210(2):225-232.

225. Sawyer ST, Jacobs-Helber SM. Unraveling distinct intracellular signals that promote survival and proliferation: study of erythropoietin, stem cell factor, and constitutive signaling in leukemic cells. *J Hematother Stem Cell Res.* 2000;9:21-29.

226. Zhao W, Kitidis C, Fleming MD, Lodish HF, Ghaffari S. Erythropoietin stimulates phosphorylation and activation of GATA-1 via the PI3-kinase/AKT signaling pathway. *Blood.* 2006;107(3):907-915.

227. Polak R, Buitenhuis M. The PI3K/PKB signaling module as key regulator of hematopoiesis: implications for therapeutic strategies in leukemia. *Blood.* 2012;119(4):911-923.

228. Steelman LS, Franklin RA, Abrams SL, et al. Roles of the Ras/Raf/MEK/ERK pathway in leukemia therapy. *Leukemia.* 2011;25(7):1080-1094.

229. Zhang J, Lodish HF. Endogenous K-ras signaling in erythroid differentiation. *Cell Cycle.* 2007;6(16):1970-1973.

230. Welsch ME, Kaplan A, Chambers JM, et al. Multivalent small-molecule pan-RAS inhibitors. *Cell.* 2017;168(5):878.e29-889.e29.

231. Bhoopalan SV, Huang LJ, Weiss MJ. Erythropoietin regulation of red blood cell production: from bench to bedside and back. *F1000Res.* 2020;9:F1000.

232. Schnoder TM, Arreba-Tutusaus P, Griehl I, et al. Epo-induced erythroid maturation is dependent on Plcγ1 signaling. *Cell Death Differ.* 2015;22(6):974-985.

233. von Lindern M, Parren-van Amelsvoort M, van Dijk T, et al. Protein kinase C alpha controls erythropoietin receptor signaling. *J Biol Chem.* 2000;275(44):34719-34727.

234. Mirandola P, Gobbi G, Ponti C, Sponzilli I, Cocco L, Vitale M. PKCepsilon controls protection against TRAIL in erythroid progenitors. *Blood.* 2006;107(2):508-513.

235. Ingley E, McCarthy DJ, Pore JR, et al. Lyn deficiency reduces GATA-1, EKLF and STAT5, and induces extramedullary stress erythropoiesis. *Oncogene.* 2005;24(3):336-343.

236. Ingley E. Src family kinases: regulation of their activities, levels and identification of new pathways. *Biochim Biophys Acta.* 2008;1784(1):56-65.

237. Tong W, Zhang J, Lodish HF. Lnk inhibits erythropoiesis and Epo-dependent JAK2 activation and downstream signaling pathways. *Blood.* 2005;105(12):4604-4612.

238. Singh S, Dev A, Verma R, et al. Defining an EPOR- regulated transcriptome for primary progenitors, including Tnfr-sf13c as a novel mediator of EPO- dependent erythroblast formation. *PLoS One.* 2012;7(7):e38530.

239. Held MA, Greenfest-Allen E, Su S, Stoeckert CJ, Stokes MP, Wojchowski DM. Phospho-PTM proteomic discovery of novel EPO- modulated kinases and phosphatases, including PTPN18 as a positive regulator of EPOR/JAK2 Signaling. *Cell Signal.* 2020;69:109554.

240. Coulon S, Dussiot M, Grapton D, et al. Polymeric IgA1 controls erythroblast proliferation and accelerates erythropoiesis recovery in anemia. *Nat Med.* 2011;17(11):1456-1465.

241. Nai A, Lidonnici MR, Rausa M, et al. The second transferrin receptor regulates red blood cell production in mice. *Blood.* 2015;125(7):1170-1179.

242. Kautz L, Jung G, Valore EV, Rivella S, Nemeth E, Ganz T. Identification of erythroferrone as an erythroid regulator of iron metabolism. *Nat Genet.* 2014;46(7):678-684.

243. Divoky V, Liu Z, Ryan TM, Prchal JF, Townes TM, Prchal JT. Mouse model of congenital polycythemia: homologous replacement of murine gene by mutant human erythropoietin receptor gene. *Proc Natl Acad Sci U S A.* 2001;98(3):986-991.

244. Huang LJ, Shen YM, Bulut GB. Advances in understanding the pathogenesis of primary familial and congenital polycythaemia. *Br J Haematol.* 2010;148(6):844-852.

245. Fibach E. Involvement of phosphatases in proliferation, maturation, and hemoglobinization of developing erythroid cells. *J Signal Transduct.* 2011;2011:860985.

246. Meyer L, Deau B, Forejtnikova H, et al. beta-Trcp mediates ubiquitination and degradation of the erythropoietin receptor and controls cell proliferation. *Blood.* 2007;109(12):5215-5222.

247. Russell RC, Sufan RI, Zhou B, et al. Loss of JAK2 regulation via a heterodimeric VHL-SOCS1 E3 ubiquitin ligase underlies Chuvash polycythemia. *Nat Med.* 2011;17(7):845-853.

248. Zeigler BM, Vajdos J, Qin W, Loverro L, Niss K. A mouse model for an erythropoietin-deficiency anemia. *Dis Model Mech.* 2010;3(11-12):763-772.

249. Bento C, Almeida H, Maia TM, et al. Molecular study of congenital erythrocytosis in 70 unrelated patients revealed a potential causal mutation in less than half of the cases (Where is/are the missing gene(s)?). *Eur J Haematol.* 2013;91(4):361-368.

250. Longmore GD, Pharr P, Lodish HF. Mutation in murine erythropoietin receptor induces erythropoietin-independent erythroid proliferation in vitro, polycythemia in vivo. *Leukemia.* 1992;6(suppl 3):130S-134S.

251. Ney PA, D'Andrea AD. Friend erythroleukemia revisited. *Blood.* 2000;96(12):3675-3680.

252. Kim AR, Ulirsch JC, Wilmes S, et al. Functional selectivity in cytokine signaling revealed through a pathogenic EPO mutation. *Cell.* 2017;168(6):1053-1064 e15.

253. Sakaguchi M, Koishihara Y, Tsuda H, et al. The expression of functional erythropoietin receptors on an interleukin-3 dependent cell line. *Biochem Biophys Res Commun.* 1987;146(1):7-12.

254. Tsao CJ, Tojo A, Fukamachi H, et al. Expression of the functional erythropoietin receptors on interleukin 3-dependent murine cell lines. *J Immunol.* 1988;140(1):89-93.

255. Grover A, Mancini E, Moore S, et al. Erythropoietin guides multipotent hematopoietic progenitor cells toward an erythroid fate. *J Exp Med.* 2014;211(2):181-188.

256. Sawada K, Krantz SB, Sawyer ST, Civin CI. Quantitation of specific binding of erythropoietin to human erythroid colony-forming cells. *J Cell Physiol.* 1988;137:337-345.

257. Koury MJ, Sawyer ST, Bondurant MC. Splenic erythroblasts in anemia-inducing Friend disease: a source of cells for studies of erythropoietin-mediated differentiation. *J Cell Physiol.* 1984;121:526-532.

258. Wojchowski DM, He TC. Signal transduction in the erythropoietin receptor system. *Stem Cell.* 1993;11:381-392.

259. Wu H, Liu X, Jaenisch R, Lodish HF. Generation of committed erythroid BFU-E and CFU-E progenitors does not require erythropoietin or the erythropoietin receptor. *Cell.* 1995;83(1):59-67.

260. Carlile GW, Smith DH, Wiedmann M. Caspase-3 has a nonapoptotic function in erythroid maturation. *Blood.* 2004;103(11):4310-4316.

261. Droin N, Cathelin S, Jacquel A, et al. A role for caspases in the differentiation of erythroid cells and macrophages. *Biochimie.* 2008;90(2):416-422.

262. Ribeil JA, Zermati Y, Vandekerckhove J, et al. Hsp70 regulates erythropoiesis by preventing caspase-3-mediated cleavage of GATA-1. *Nature.* 2007;445(7123):102-105.

263. Frisan E, Vandekerckhove J, de Thonel A, et al. Defective nuclear localization of Hsp70 is associated with dyserythropoiesis and GATA-1 cleavage in myelodysplastic syndromes. *Blood.* 2012;119(6):1532-1542.

264. Kodama T, Hikita H, Kawaguchi T, et al. Mcl-1 and Bcl-xL regulate Bak/Bax-dependent apoptosis of the megakaryocytic lineage at multistages. *Cell Death Differ.* 2012;19(11):1856-1869.

265. Clark DA, Dessypris EN. Effects of recombinant erythropoietin on murine megakaryocytic colony formation in vitro. *J Lab Clin Med.* 1986;108(5):423-429.

266. Ishibashi T, Koziol JA, Burstein SA. Human recombinant erythropoietin promotes differentiation of murine megakaryocytes in vitro. *J Clin Invest.* 1987;79(1):286-289.

267. Fraser JK, Tan AS, Lin FK, Berridge MV. Expression of specific high-affinity binding sites for erythropoietin on rat and mouse megakaryocytes. *Exp Hematol.* 1989;17(1):10-16.

268. McDonald TP, Cottrell MB, Clift RE, Cullen WC, Lin FK. High doses of recombinant erythropoietin stimulate platelet production in mice. *Exp Hematol.* 1987;15(6):719-721.

269. Eschbach JW, Abdulhadi MH, Browne JK, et al. Recombinant human erythropoietin in anemic patients with end-stage renal disease. Results of a phase III multicenter clinical trial. *Ann Intern Med.* 1989;111(12):992-1000.

270. Marsden JT. Erythropoietin– measurement and clinical applications. *Ann Clin Biochem.* 2006;43(pt 2):97-104.

271. Sherwood JB, Carmichael LD, Goldwasser E. The heterogeneity of circulating human serum erythropoietin. *Endocrinology.* 1988;122(4):1472-1477.

272. Wintrobe MM, ed. *Blood, Pure and Eloquent.* McGraw Hill; 1980.

273. Lew VL, Raftos JE, Sorette M, Bookchin RM, Mohandas N. Generation of normal human red cell volume, hemoglobin content, and membrane area distributions by "birth" or regulation? *Blood.* 1995;86(1):334-341.

274. D'Onofrio G, Chirillo R, Zini G, Caenaro G, Tommasi M, Micciulli G. Simultaneous measurement of reticulocyte and red blood cell indices in healthy subjects and patients with microcytic and macrocytic anemia. *Blood.* 1995;85(3):818-823.

275. Lenard JG. A note on the shape of the erythrocyte. *Bull Math Biol.* 1974;36(1):55-58.

276. Skalak R, Branemark PI. Deformation of red blood cells in capillaries. *Science.* 1969;164(3880):717-719.

277. Evans EA. Structure and deformation properties of red blood cells: concepts and quantitative methods. *Methods Enzymol.* 1989;173:3-35.

278. Manno S, Takakuwa Y, Mohandas N. Identification of a functional role for lipid asymmetry in biological membranes: phosphatidylserine-skeletal protein interactions modulate membrane stability. *Proc Natl Acad Sci U S A.* 2002;99(4):1943-1948.

279. Chasis JA, Shohet SB. Red cell biochemical anatomy and membrane properties. *Annu Rev Physiol.* 1987;49:237-248.

280. Jay AW. Geometry of the human erythrocyte. I. Effect of albumin on cell geometry. *Biophys J.* 1975;15(3):205-222.

281. Gorter E, Grendel F. On bimolecular layers of lipoids on the chromocytes of the blood. *J Exp Med.* 1925;41(4):439-443.

282. Danielli JF. The thickness of the wall of the red blood corpuscle. *J Gen Physiol.* 1935;19(1):19-22.

283. Adam NK, Askew FA, Danielli JF. Further experiments on surface films of sterols and their derivatives. *Biochem J.* 1935;29(7):1786-1801.

284. Davson H, Danielli JF. Studies on the permeability of erythrocytes: factors in cation permeability. *Biochem J.* 1938;32(6):991-1001.

285. Bennett V. Spectrin: a structural mediator between diverse plasma membrane proteins and the cytoplasm. *Curr Opin Cell Biol.* 1990;2(1):51-56.

286. de Vetten MP, Agre P. The Rh polypeptide is a major fatty acid-acylated erythrocyte membrane protein. *J Biol Chem.* 1988;263(34):18193-18196.

287. Telen MJ. Phosphatidylinositol-linked red blood cell membrane proteins and blood group antigens. *Immunohematol/American Red Cross.* 1991;7(3):65-72.

288. Cooper RA. Lipids of human red cell membrane: normal composition and variability in disease. *Semin Hematol.* 1970;7(3):296-322.

289. Schwartz RS, Chiu DT, Lubin B. Plasma membrane phospholipid organization in human erythrocytes. *Curr Top Hematol.* 1985;5:63-112.

290. Dodge JT, Mitchell C, Hanahan DJ. The preparation and chemical characteristics of hemoglobin-free ghosts of human erythrocytes. *Arch Biochem Biophys.* 1963;100:119-130.

291. Dodge JT, Phillips GB. Composition of phospholipids and of phospholipid fatty acids and aldehydes in human red cells. *J Lipid Res.* 1967;8(6):667-675.

292. Ways P, Hanahan DJ. Characterization and quantification of red cell lipids in normal man. *J Lipid Res.* 1964;5(3):318-328.

293. Lubin BH, Kuypers FA, Chiu DTY, Shohet SB. Analysis of red cell membrane lipids. In: Shohet SB, ed. *Red Cell Membranes.* Churchill Livingstone; 1988:171-202.

294. Rothman JE, Lenard J. Membrane asymmetry. *Science.* 1977;195(4280):743-753.

295. Bretscher MS. Membrane structure: some general principles. *Science.* 1973;181(4100):622-629.

296. Van Dort HM, Knowles DW, Chasis JA, Lee G, Mohandas N, Low PS. Analysis of integral membrane protein contributions to the deformability and stability of the human erythrocyte membrane. *J Biol Chem.* 2001;276(50):46968-46974.

297. Arashiki N, Takakuwa Y. Maintenance and regulation of asymmetric phospholipid distribution in human erythrocyte membranes: implications for erythrocyte functions. *Curr Opin Hematol.* 2017;24(3):167-172.

298. Wang D, Seto E, Shu J, Micieli JA, Fernandes BJ, Denomme GA. Antibody-mediated glycophorin C coligation on K562 cells induces phosphatidylserine exposure and cell death in an atypical apoptotic process. *Transfusion.* 2013;53(10):2134-2140.

299. Kuypers FA, de Jong K. The role of phosphatidylserine in recognition and removal of erythrocytes. *Cell Mol Biol.* 2004;50(2):147-158.

300. Haest CW, Deuticke B. Possible relationship between membrane proteins and phospholipid asymmetry in the human erythrocyte membrane. *Biochim Biophys Acta.* 1976;436(2):353-365.

301. Haest CW, Plasa G, Kamp D, Deuticke B. Spectrin as a stabilizer of the phospholipid asymmetry in the human erythrocyte membrane. *Biochim Biophys Acta.* 1978;509(1):21-32.

302. Cooper RA. Abnormalities of cell-membrane fluidity in the pathogenesis of disease. *N Engl J Med.* 1977;297(7):371-377.

303. Shohet SB. Hemolysis and changes in erythrocyte membrane lipids. I. *N Engl J Med.* 1972;286(11):577-583.

304. Nelson GJ. Composition of neutral lipids from erythrocytes of common mammals. *J Lipid Res.* 1967;8(4):374-379.

305. Bull BS, Brailsford JD. The biconcavity of the red cell: an analysis of several hypotheses. *Blood.* 1973;41(6):833-844.

306. Cooper RA. Influence of increased membrane cholesterol on membrane fluidity and cell function in human red blood cells. *J Supramol Struct.* 1978;8(4):413-430.

307. Tishler RB, Carlson FD. A study of the dynamic properties of the human red blood cell membrane using quasi-elastic light-scattering spectroscopy. *Biophys J.* 1993;65(6):2586-2600.

308. Glomset JA. The plasma lecithins:cholesterol acyltransferase reaction. *J Lipid Res.* 1968;9(2):155-167.

309. Norum KR, Gjone E. Familial serum-cholesterol esterification failure. A new inborn error of metabolism. *Biochim Biophys Acta.* 1967;144(3):698-700.

310. Cooper RA, Jandl JH. Bile salts and cholesterol in the pathogenesis of target cells in obstructive jaundice. *J Clin Invest.* 1968;47(4):809-822.

311. Steck TL. The organization of proteins in the human red blood cell membrane. A review. *J Cell Biol.* 1974;62(1):1-19.

312. Fairbanks G, Steck TL, Wallach DFH. Electrophoretic analysis of the major polypeptides of the human erythrocyte membrane. *Biochemistry.* 1971;10:2606-2617.

313. Goodman SR, Kurdia A, Ammann L, Kakhniashvili D, Daescu O. The human red blood cell proteome and interactome. *Exp Biol Med (Maywood).* 2007;232(11):1391-1408.

314. Pasini EM, Kirkegaard M, Mortensen P, Lutz HU, Thomas AW, Mann M. In-depth analysis of the membrane and cytosolic proteome of red cells. *Blood.* 2006;108(3):791-801.

315. D'Alessandro A, Righetti PG, Zolla L. The red blood cell proteome and interactome: an update. *J Proteome Res.* 2010;9(1):144-163.

316. Singer SJ. A fluid lipid-globular protein mosaic model of membrane structure. *Ann N Y Acad Sci.* 1972;195:16-23.

317. Pasvol G, Wainscoat JS, Weatherall DJ. Erythrocytes deficiency in glycophorin resist invasion by the malarial parasite Plasmodium falciparum. *Nature.* 1982;297(5861):64-66.

318. Anstee DJ. The nature and abundance of human red cell surface glycoproteins. *J Immunogenet.* 1990;17(4-5):219-225.

319. Issitt PD. Null red cell phenotypes: associated biological changes. *Transfus Med Rev.* 1993;7(3):139-155.

320. Cherif-Zahar B, Bloy C, Le Van Kim C, et al. Molecular cloning and protein structure of a human blood group Rh polypeptide. *Proc Natl Acad Sci U S A.* 1990;87(16):6243-6247.

321. Smythe JS, Avent ND, Judson PA, Parsons SF, Martin PG, Anstee DJ. Expression of RHD and RHCE gene products using retroviral transduction of K562 cells establishes the molecular basis of Rh blood group antigens. *Blood.* 1996;87(7):2968-2973.

322. Huebner K, Palumbo AP, Isobe M, et al. The alpha-spectrin gene is on chromosome 1 in mouse and man. *Proc Natl Acad Sci U S A.* 1985;82(11):3790-3793.

323. Prchal JT, Morley BJ, Yoon SH, et al. Isolation and characterization of cDNA clones for human erythrocyte beta-spectrin. *Proc Natl Acad Sci U S A.* 1987;84(21):7468-7472.

324. Winkelmann JC, Leto TL, Watkins PC, et al. Molecular cloning of the cDNA for human erythrocyte beta-spectrin. *Blood.* 1988;72(1):328-334.

325. Lambert S, Bennett V. From anemia to cerebellar dysfunction. A review of the ankyrin gene family. *Eur J Biochem.* 1993;211(1-2):1-6.

326. Delaunay J. The molecular basis of hereditary red cell membrane disorders. *Blood Rev.* 2007;21(1):1-20.

327. Mathai JC, Mori S, Smith BL, et al. Functional analysis of aquaporin-1 deficient red cells. The Colton-null phenotype. *J Biol Chem.* 1996;271(3):1309-1313.

328. Agre P, Preston GM, Smith BL, et al. Aquaporin CHIP: the archetypal molecular water channel. *Am J Physiol.* 1993;265(4 pt 2):F463-F476.

329. Orringer EP, Parker JC. Ion and water movements in red blood cells. *Prog Hematol.* 1973;8:1-23.

330. Tanner MJ. Molecular and cellular biology of the erythrocyte anion exchanger (AE1). *Semin Hematol.* 1993;30(1):34-57.

331. Adragna NC, Di Fulvio M, Lauf PK. Regulation of K-Cl cotransport: from function to genes. *J Membr Biol.* 2004;201(3):109-137.

The Normal Hematologic System

332. Gardos G. The function of calcium in the potassium permeability of human erythrocytes. *Biochim Biophys Acta.* 1958;30(3):653-654.

333. Lew VL, Etzion Z, Bookchin RM. Dehydration response of sickle cells to sickling-induced Ca(++) permeabilization. *Blood.* 2002;99(7):2578-2585.

334. Glogowska E, Lezon-Geyda K, Maksimova Y, Schulz VP, Gallagher PG. Mutations in the Gardos channel (KCNN4) are associated with hereditary xerocytosis. *Blood.* 2015;126(11):1281-1284.

335. Zarychanski R, Schulz VP, Houston BL, et al. Mutations in the mechanotransduction protein PIEZO1 are associated with hereditary xerocytosis. *Blood.* 2012;120(9):1908-1915.

336. Mueckler M, Caruso C, Baldwin SA, et al. Sequence and structure of a human glucose transporter. *Science.* 1985;229(4717):941-945.

337. Baly DL, Horuk R. The biology and biochemistry of the glucose transporter. *Biochim Biophys Acta.* 1988;947(3):571-590.

338. Elbrink J, Bihler I. Membrane transport: its relation to cellular metabolic rates. *Science.* 1975;188(4194):1177-1184.

339. Telen MJ. Erythrocyte blood group antigens: polymorphisms of functionally important molecules. *Semin Hematol.* 1996;33(4):302-314.

340. Plut DA, Hosey MM, Tao M. Evidence for the participation of cytosolic protein kinases in membrane phosphorylation in intact erythrocytes. *Eur J Biochem.* 1978;82(2):333-337.

341. Arnaud F, Scultetus AH, Haque A, et al. Sodium nitroprusside ameliorates systemic but not pulmonary HBOC-201-induced vasoconstriction: an exploratory study in a swine controlled haemorrhage model. *Resuscitation.* 2012;83(8):1038-1045.

342. Hsia CC. Respiratory function of hemoglobin. *N Engl J Med.* 1998;338(4):239-247.

343. Hardison RC. A brief history of hemoglobins: plant, animal, protist, and bacteria. *Proc Natl Acad Sci U S A.* 1996;93(12):5675-5679.

344. Bank A. Understanding globin regulation in beta-thalassemia: it's as simple as alpha, beta, gamma, delta. *J Clin Invest.* 2005;115(6):1470-1473.

345. Bunn HF, Jandl JH. Control of hemoglobin function within the red cell. *N Engl J Med.* 1970;282(25):1414-1421.

346. Schroeder WA, Huisman TH, Efremov GD, et al. Further studies of the frequency and significance of the Tgamma-chain of human fetal hemoglobin. *J Clin Invest.* 1979;63(2):268-275.

347. Jensen M, Attenberger H, Schneider C, Walther JU. The developmental change in the G gamma and A gamma globin. Proportions in hemoglobin F. *Eur J Pediatr.* 1982;138(4):311-314.

348. Allen DW, Wyman J Jr, Smith CA. The oxygen equilibrium of fetal and adult human hemoglobin. *J Biol Chem.* 1953;203(1):81-87.

349. Tyuma I, Shimizu K. Different response to organic phosphates of human fetal and adult hemoglobins. *Arch Biochem Biophys.* 1969;129(1):404-405.

350. Bard H. The postnatal decline of hemoglobin F synthesis in normal full-term infants. *J Clin Invest.* 1975;55(2):395-398.

351. Dover GJ, Boyer SH, Charache S, Heintzelman K. Individual variation in the production and survival of F cells in sickle-cell disease. *N Engl J Med.* 1978;299(26):1428-1435.

352. De Rosa MC, Sanna MT, Messana I, et al. Glycated human hemoglobin (HbA1c): functional characteristics and molecular modeling studies. *Biophys Chem.* 1998;72(3):323-335.

353. Katsiki N, Papanas N, Mikhailidis DP, Fonseca VA. Glycated hemoglobin A(1)c (HbA(1)c) and diabetes: a new era? *Curr Med Res Opin.* 2011;27(suppl 3):7-11.

354. Spicer KM, Allen RC, Hallett D, Buse MG. Synthesis of hemoglobin Aic and related minor hemoglobin by erythrocytes. In vitro study of regulation. *J Clin Invest.* 1979;64(1):40-48.

355. Abraham EC, Cameron BF, Abraham A, Stallings M. Glycosylated hemoglobins in heterozygotes and homozygotes for hemoglobin C with or without diabetes. *J Lab Clin Med.* 1984;104(4):602-609.

356. Bry L, Chen PC, Sacks DB. Effects of hemoglobin variants and chemically modified derivatives on assays for glycohemoglobin. *Clin Chem.* 2001;47(2):153-163.

357. IHIC variants list. International hemoglobin Information center. *Hemoglobin.* 1989;13(3):223-297.

358. Szuberski J, Oliveira JL, Hoyer JD. A comprehensive analysis of hemoglobin variants by high-performance liquid chromatography (HPLC). *Int J Lab Hematol.* 2012;34(6):594-604.

359. Bollekens JA, Forget BG. Delta beta thalassemia and hereditary persistence of fetal hemoglobin. *Hematol Oncol Clin North Am.* 1991;5(3):399-422.

360. Boyer SH, Belding TK, Margolet L, Noyes AN. Fetal hemoglobin restriction to a few erythrocytes (F cells) in normal human adults. *Science.* 1975;188(4186):361-363.

361. Zago MA, Wood WG, Clegg JB, Weatherall DJ, O'Sullivan M, Gunson H. Genetic control of F cells in human adults. *Blood.* 1979;53(5):977-986.

362. Kleihauer E, Braun H, Betke K. Demonstration of fetal hemoglobin in erythrocytes of a blood smear. *Klin Wochenschr.* 1957;35(12):637-638.

363. Farias MG, Dal Bo S, Castro SM, et al. Flow cytometry in detection of fetal red blood cells and maternal F vells to Identify fetomaternal hemorrhage. *Fetal Pediatr Pathol.* 2016;35(6):385-391.

364. Lehmann H, Carrell RW. Variations in the structure of human haemoglobin. With particular reference to the unstable haemoglobins. *Br Med Bull.* 1969;25(1):14-23.

365. Bolton W, Perutz MF. Three dimensional fourier synthesis of horse deoxyhaemoglobin at 2.8 Angstrom units resolution. *Nature.* 1970;228(5271):551-552.

366. Shaanan B. Structure of human oxyhaemoglobin at 2.1 A resolution. *J Mol Biol.* 1983;171(1):31-59.

367. Hrkal Z, Vodrazka Z. A study of the conformation of human globin in solution by optical methods. *Biochim Biophys Acta.* 1967;133(3):527-534.

368. de Castro CM, Devlin B, Fleenor DE, Lee ME, Kaufman RE. A novel beta-globin mutation, beta Durham-NC [beta 114 Leu-->Pro], produces a dominant thalassemia-like phenotype. *Blood.* 1994;83(4):1109-1116.

369. Henry ER, Bettati S, Hofrichter J, Eaton WA. A tertiary two-state allosteric model for hemoglobin. *Biophys Chem.* 2002;98(1-2):149-164.

370. Baldwin J, Chothia C. Haemoglobin: the structural changes related to ligand binding and its allosteric mechanism. *J Mol Biol.* 1979;129(2):175-220.

371. Chance MR, Parkhurst LJ, Powers LS, Chance B. Movement of Fe with respect to the heme plane in the R-T transition of carp hemoglobin. An extended x-ray absorption fine structure study. *J Biol Chem.* 1986;261(13):5689-5692.

372. Kurlekar N, Mehta BC. Haemoglobin A2 levels in iron deficiency anaemia. *Indian J Med Res.* 1981;73:77-81.

373. Forget BG, Cavallesco C, Benz EJ Jr, et al. Studies of globin chain synthesis and globin mRNA content in a patient homozygous for hemoglobin Lepore. *Hemoglobin.* 1978;2(2):117-128.

374. Bunn HF. Subunit assembly of hemoglobin: an important determinant of hematologic phenotype. *Blood.* 1987;69(1):1-6.

375. Shaeffer JR, McDonald MJ, Bunn HF. Assembly of normal and abnormal human hemoglobins. *Trends Biochem Sci.* 1981;6(0):158-161.

376. Bunn HF, McDonald MJ. Electrostatic interactions in the assembly of haemoglobin. *Nature.* 1983;306(5942):498-500.

377. Embury SH, Dozy AM, Miller J, et al. Concurrent sickle-cell anemia and alpha-thalassemia: effect on severity of anemia. *N Engl J Med.* 1982;306(5):270-274.

378. Steinberg MH. Case report: effects of iron deficiency and the -88 C-->T mutation on HbA2 levels in beta-thalassemia. *Am J Med Sci.* 1993;305(5):312-313.

379. Longo LD. Sir Joseph Barcroft: one victorian physiologist's contributions to a half century of discovery. *J Physiol.* 2016;594(5):1113-1125.

380. Humpeler E, Amor H. Sex differences in the oxygen affinity of hemoglobin. *Pflugers Arch.* 1973;343(2):151-156.

381. Jensen FB. Red blood cell pH, the Bohr effect, and other oxygenation-linked phenomena in blood O_2 and CO_2 transport. *Acta Physiol Scand.* 2004;182(3):215-227.

382. Benesch R, Benesch RE. The effect of organic phosphates from the human erythrocyte on the allosteric properties of hemoglobin. *Biochem Biophys Res Commun.* 1967;26(2):162-167.

383. Brewer GJ, Eaton JW. Erythrocyte metabolism: interaction with oxygen transport. *Science.* 1971;171(3977):1205-1211.

384. Marschner JP, Seidlitz T, Rietbrock N. Effect of 2,3-diphosphoglycerate on O_2-dissociation kinetics of hemoglobin and glycosylated hemoglobin using the stopped flow technique and an improved in vitro method for hemoglobin glycosylation. *Int J Clin Pharmacol Ther.* 1994;32(3):116-121.

385. Chanutin A, Curnish RR. Effect of organic and inorganic phosphates on the oxygen equilibrium of human erythrocytes. *Arch Biochem Biophys.* 1967;121(1):96-102.

386. Bunn HF, May MH, Kocholaty WF, Shields CE. Hemoglobin function in stored blood. *J Clin Invest.* 1969;48(2):311-321.

387. Morgan TJ. The oxyhaemoglobin dissociation curve in critical illness. *Crit Care Resusc.* 1999;1(1):93-100.

388. Oski FA, Marshall BE, Cohen PJ, Sugerman HJ, Miller LD. Exercise with anemia. *Ann Intern Med.* 1971;74(1):44-46.

389. Rees SE, Andreassen S. Mathematical models of oxygen and carbon dioxide storage and transport: the acid-base chemistry of blood. *Crit Rev Biomed Eng.* 2005;33(3):209-264.

390. De Rosa MC, Carelli Alinovi C, Galtieri A, Scatena R, Giardina B. The plasma membrane of erythrocytes plays a fundamental role in the transport of oxygen, carbon dioxide and nitric oxide and in the maintenance of the reduced state of the heme iron. *Gene.* 2007;398(1-2):162-171.

391. Arnone A. X-ray studies of the interaction of CO_2 with human deoxyhaemoglobin. *Nature.* 1974;247(437):143-145.

392. Cabrales P, Han G, Nacharaju P, Friedman AJ, Friedman JM. Reversal of hemoglobin-induced vasoconstriction with sustained release of nitric oxide. *Am J Physiol Heart Circ Physiol.* 2011;300(1):H49-H56.

393. Jia L, Bonaventura C, Bonaventura J, Stamler JS. S-nitrosohaemoglobin: a dynamic activity of blood involved in vascular control. *Nature.* 1996;380(6571):221-226.

394. Gow AJ, Luchsinger BP, Pawloski JR, Singel DJ, Stamler JS. The oxyhemoglobin reaction of nitric oxide. *Proc Natl Acad Sci U S A.* 1999;96(16):9027-9032.

395. Lancaster JR Jr. Simulation of the diffusion and reaction of endogenously produced nitric oxide. *Proc Natl Acad Sci U S A.* 1994;91(17):8137-8141.

396. Jaffe ER, Hsieh HS. DPNH-methemoglobin reductase deficiency and hereditary methemoglobinemia. *Semin Hematol.* 1971;8(4):417-437.

397. Mansouri A. Methemoglobin reduction under near physiological conditions. *Biochem Med Metab Biol.* 1989;42(1):43-51.

398. Mansouri A, Lurie AA. Concise review: methemoglobinemia. *Am J Hematol.* 1993;42(1):7-12.

399. Jarolim P, Lahav M, Liu SC, Palek J. Effect of hemoglobin oxidation products on the stability of red cell membrane skeletons and the associations of skeletal proteins: correlation with a release of hemin. *Blood.* 1990;76(10):2125-2131.

400. Berzofsky JA, Peisach J, Blumberg WE. Sulfheme proteins. I. Optical and magnetic properties of sulfmyoglobin and its derivatives. *J Biol Chem.* 1971;246(10):3367-3377.

401. Rachmilewitz EA. Denaturation of the normal and abnormal hemoglobin molecule. *Semin Hematol.* 1974;11(4):441-462.

402. Morell DB, Chang Y. The structure of the chromophore of sulphmyoglobin. *Biochim Biophys Acta.* 1967;136(1):121-130.

403. Berzofsky JA, Peisach J, Horecker BL. Sulfheme proteins. IV. The stoichiometry of sulfur incorporation and the isolation of sulfhemin, the prosthetic group of sulfmyoglobin. *J Biol Chem.* 1972;247(12):3783-3791.

404. Elahian F, Sepehrizadeh Z, Moghimi B, Mirzaei SA. Human cytochrome b5 reductase: structure, function, and potential applications. *Crit Rev Biotechnol.* 2014;34(2):134-143.

405. Gibson QH. The reduction of methaemoglobin in red blood cells and studies on the cause of idiopathic methaemoglobinaemia. *Biochem J.* 1948;42(1):13-23.

406. Hultquist DE, Passon PG. Catalysis of methaemoglobin reduction by erythrocyte cytochrome B5 and cytochrome B5 reductase. *Nature: New biology.* 1971;229(8):252-254.

407. Xiang W, Weisbach V, Sticht H, et al. Oxidative stress-induced posttranslational modifications of human hemoglobin in erythrocytes. *Arch Biochem Biophys.* 2013;529(1):34-44.

408. Clemens MR, Waller HD. Lipid peroxidation in erythrocytes. *Chem Phys Lipids.* 1987;45(2-4):251-268.

409. Winterbourn CC. Free-radical production and oxidative reactions of hemoglobin. *Environ Health Perspect.* 1985;64:321-330.

410. Cimen MY. Free radical metabolism in human erythrocytes. *Clin Chim Acta.* 2008;390(1-2):1-11.

411. Bannister WH. From haemocuprein to copper-zinc superoxide dismutase: a history on the fiftieth anniversary of the discovery of haemocuprein and the twentieth anniversary of the discovery of superoxide dismutase. *Free Radic Res Commun.* 1988;5(1):35-42.

412. Siems WG, Sommerburg O, Grune T. Erythrocyte free radical and energy metabolism. *Clin Nephrol.* 2000;53(1 suppl):S9-S17.

413. Michelson AM. Selenium glutathione peroxidase: some aspects in man. *J Environ Pathol Toxicol Oncol.* 1998;17(3-4):233-239.

414. Necheles TF, Steinberg MH, Cameron D. Erythrocyte glutathione-peroxidase deficiency. *Br J Haematol.* 1970;19(5):605-612.

415. Grune T, Sommerburg O, Siems WG. Oxidative stress in anemia. *Clin Nephrol.* 2000;53(1 suppl):S18-S22.

416. Goth L, Nagy T. Acatalasemia and diabetes mellitus. *Arch Biochem Biophys.* 2012;525(2):195-200.

417. Srivastava SK, Beutler E. The transport of oxidized glutathione from human erythrocytes. *J Biol Chem.* 1969;244(1):9-16.

418. Srivastava SK, Beutler E. Glutathione metabolism of the erythrocyte. The enzymic cleavage of glutathione-haemoglobin preparations by glutathione reductase. *Biochem J.* 1970;119(3):353-357.

419. Hoey L, McNulty H, Strain JJ. Studies of biomarker responses to intervention with riboflavin: a systematic review. *Am J Clin Nutr.* 2009;89(6):1960s-1980s.

420. Murphy JR. Erythrocyte metabolism. I. The equilibration of glucose-C14 between serum and erythrocytes. *J Lab Clin Med.* 1960;55:281-285.

421. Schuster R, Holzhutter HG, Jacobasch G. Interrelations between glycolysis and the hexose monophosphate shunt in erythrocytes as studied on the basis of a mathematical model. *Biosystems.* 1988;22(1):19-36.

422. Gallemann D, Eyer P. Effects of the phenacetin metabolite 4-nitrosophenetol on glycolysis and pentose phosphate pathway in human red cells. *Biol Chem Hoppe Seyler.* 1993;374(1):37-49.

423. Arias CF, Arias CF. How do red blood cells know when to die? *R Soc Open Sci.* 2017;4(4):160850.

424. Marinkovic D, Zhang X, Yalcin S, et al. Foxo3 is required for the regulation of oxidative stress in erythropoiesis. *J Clin Invest.* 2007;117(8):2133-2144.

425. Burger P, Hilarius-Stokman P, de Korte D, van den Berg TK, van Bruggen R. CD47 functions as a molecular switch for erythrocyte phagocytosis. *Blood.* 2012;119(23):5512-5521.

426. Murata Y, Kotani T, Ohnishi H, Matozaki T. The CD47-SIRPα signalling system: its physiological roles and therapeutic application. *J Biochem.* 2014;155(6):335-344.

427. Giblett ER. Recent advances in heptoglobin and transferrin genetics. *Bibl Haematol.* 1968;29:10-20.

428. Noyes WD, Garby L. Rate of haptoglobin in synthesis in normal man. Determinations by the return to normal levels following hemoglobin infusion. *Scand J Clin Lab Invest.* 1967;20(1):33-38.

429. Rifkind RA. Destruction of injured red cells in vivo. *Am J Med.* 1966;41(5):711-723.

430. Bratosin D, Mazurier J, Tissier JP, et al. Cellular and molecular mechanisms of senescent erythrocyte phagocytosis by macrophages. A review. *Biochimie.* 1998;80(2):173-195.

431. Rosse WF, Dourmashkin R, Humphrey JH. Immune lysis of normal human and paroxysmal nocturnal hemoglobinuria (PNH) red blood cells. 3. The membrane defects caused by complement lysis. *J Exp Med.* 1966;123(6):969-984.

432. Meinderts SM, Oldenborg P-A, Beuger BM, et al. Human and murine splenic neutrophils are potent phagocytes of IgG-opsonized red blood cells. *Blood Adv.* 2017;1(14):875.

433. Cooper RA, Shattil SJ. Mechanisms of hemolysis–the minimal red-cell defect. *N Engl J Med.* 1971;285(27):1514-1520.

434. Singer K, Weisz L. The life cycle of the erythrocyte after splenectomy and the problems of splenic hemolysis and target cell formation. *Am J Med Sci.* 1945;210:301-323.

435. Sadrzadeh SM, Graf E, Panter SS, Hallaway PE, Eaton JW. Hemoglobin. A biologic fenton reagent. *J Biol Chem.* 1984;259(23):14354-14356.

436. Wood KC, Hsu LL, Gladwin MT. Sickle cell disease vasculopathy: a state of nitric oxide resistance. *Free Radic Biol Med.* 2008;44(8):1506-1528.

437. Bunn HF, Nathan DG, Dover GJ, et al. Pulmonary hypertension and nitric oxide depletion in sickle cell disease. *Blood.* 2010;116(5):687-692.

438. Pu JJ, Brodsky RA. Paroxysmal nocturnal hemoglobinuria from bench to bedside. *Clin Transl Sci.* 2011;4(3):219-224.

439. Gutteridge JM, Smith A. Antioxidant protection by haemopexin of haem-stimulated lipid peroxidation. *Biochem J.* 1988;256(3):861-865.

440. Okazaki T, Yanagisawa Y, Nagai T. Analysis of the affinity of each haptoglobin polymer for hemoglobin by two-dimensional affinity electrophoresis. *Clin Chim Acta.* 1997;258(2):137-144.

441. McCormick DJ, Atassi MZ. Hemoglobin binding with haptoglobin: delineation of the haptoglobin binding site on the alpha-chain of human hemoglobin. *J Protein Chem.* 1990;9(6):735-742.

442. Buehler PW, Abraham B, Vallelian F, et al. Haptoglobin preserves the CD163 hemoglobin scavenger pathway by shielding hemoglobin from peroxidative modification. *Blood.* 2009;113(11):2578-2586.

443. Laurell CB, Nyman M. Studies on the serum haptoglobin level in hemoglobinemia and its influence on renal excretion of hemoglobin. *Blood.* 1957;12(6):493-506.

444. Carter K, Worwood M. Haptoglobin: a review of the major allele frequencies worldwide and their association with diseases. *Int J Lab Hematol.* 2007;29(2):92-110.

445. Mominoki K, Nakagawa-Tosa N, Morimatsu M, Syuto B, Saito M. Haptoglobin in Carnivora: a unique molecular structure in bear, cat and dog haptoglobins. *Comp Biochem Physiol B Biochem Mol Biol.* 1995;110(4):785-789.

446. Wejman JC, Hovsepian D, Wall JS, Hainfeld JF, Greer J. Structure and assembly of haptoglobin polymers by electron microscopy. *J Mol Biol.* 1984;174(2):343-368.

447. Povey S, Jeremiah SJ, Barker RF, et al. Assignment of the human locus determining phosphoglycolate phosphatase (PGP) to chromosome 16. *Ann Hum Genet.* 1980;43(3):241-248.

448. Robson EB, Polani PE, Dart SJ, Jacobs PA, Renwick JH. Probable assignment of the alpha locus of haptoglobin to chromome 16 in man. *Nature.* 1969;223(5211):1163-1165.

449. Simmers RN, Stupans I, Sutherland GR. Localization of the human haptoglobin genes distal to the fragile site at 16q22 using in situ hybridization. *Cytogenet Cell Genet.* 1986;41(1):38-41.

450. Raugei G, Bensi G, Colantuoni V, et al. Sequence of human haptoglobin cDNA: evidence that the alpha and beta subunits are coded by the same mRNA. *Nucleic Acids Res.* 1983;11(17):5811-5819.

451. Wassler M, Fries E. Proteolytic cleavage of haptoglobin occurs in a subcompartment of the endoplasmic reticulum: evidence from membrane fusion in vitro. *J Cell Biol.* 1993;123(2):285-291.

452. Pajovic S, Jones VE, Prowse KR, Berger FG, Baumann H. Species-specific changes in regulatory elements of mouse haptoglobin genes. *J Biol Chem.* 1994;269(3):2215-2224.

453. Baumann H, Morella KK, Jahreis GP, Marinkovic S. Distinct regulation of the interleukin-1 and interleukin-6 response elements of the rat haptoglobin gene in rat and human hepatoma cells. *Mol Cell Biol.* 1990;10(11):5967-5976.

454. Wassell J. Haptoglobin: function and polymorphism. *Clin Lab.* 2000;46(11-12):547-552.

455. Melamed-Frank M, Lache O, Enav BI, et al. Structure-function analysis of the antioxidant properties of haptoglobin. *Blood.* 2001;98(13):3693-3698.

456. Cox KJ, Thomas AS. The application of immunoblotting to the phenotyping of haptoglobin. *J Forensic Sci.* 1992;37(6):1652-1655.

457. van Rijn HJ, van der Wilt W, Stroes JW, Schrijver J. Is the turbidimetric immunoassay of haptoglobin phenotype-dependent? *Clin Biochem.* 1987;20(4):245-248.

458. Salmi TT. Haptoglobin levels in the plasma of newborn infants with special reference to infections. *Acta Paediatr Scand Suppl.* 1973;241:1-55.

459. Javid J. Human haptoglobins. *Curr Top Hematol.* 1978;1:151-192.

460. Brus I, Lewis SM. The haptoglobin content of serum in haemolytic anaemia. *Br J Haematol.* 1959;5:348-355.

461. Hershko C, Cook JD, Finch CA. Storage iron kinetics. II. The uptake of hemoglobin iron by hepatic parenchymal cells. *J Lab Clin Med.* 1972;80(5):624-634.

462. Schaer CA, Vallelian F, Imhof A, Schoedon G, Schaer DJ. CD163-expressing monocytes constitute an endotoxin-sensitive Hb clearance compartment within the vascular system. *J Leukoc Biol.* 2007;82(1):106-110.

463. Higa Y, Oshiro S, Kino K, Tsunoo H, Nakajima H. Catabolism of globin-haptoglobin in liver cells after intravenous administration of hemoglobin-haptoglobin to rats. *J Biol Chem.* 1981;256(23):12322-12328.

464. Kristiansen M, Graversen JH, Jacobsen C, et al. Identification of the haemoglobin scavenger receptor. *Nature.* 2001;409(6817):198-201.

465. Bissell DM, Hammaker L, Schmid R. Hemoglobin and erythrocyte catabolism in rat liver: the separate roles of parenchymal and sinusoidal cells. *Blood.* 1972;40(6):812-822.

466. Weinstein MB, Segal HL. Uptake of free hemoglobin by rat liver parenchymal cells. *Biochem Biophys Res Commun.* 1984;123(2):489-496.

467. Van Gorp H, Delputte PL, Nauwynck HJ. Scavenger receptor CD163, a Jack-of-all-trades and potential target for cell-directed therapy. *Mol Immunol.* 2010;47(7-8):1650-1660.

468. Rhodes MM, Kopsombut P, Bondurant MC, Price JO, Koury MJ. Adherence to macrophages in erythroblastic islands enhances erythroblast proliferation and increases erythrocyte production by a different mechanism than erythropoietin. *Blood.* 2008;111(3):1700-1708.

469. Biswas SK, Mantovani A. Macrophage plasticity and interaction with lymphocyte subsets: cancer as a paradigm. *Nat Immunol.* 2010;11(10):889-896.

470. Sindrilaru A, Peters T, Wieschalka S, et al. An unrestrained proinflammatory M1 macrophage population induced by iron impairs wound healing in humans and mice. *J Clin Invest.* 2011;121(3):985-997.

471. Etzerodt A, Kjolby M, Nielsen MJ, Maniecki MB, Svendsen P, Moestrup SK. Plasma clearance of hemoglobin and haptoglobin in mice and effect of CD163 gene targeting disruption. *Antioxidants Redox Signal.* 2012;18(17):2254-2263.

472. Lathem W. The renal excretion of hemoglobin: regulatory mechanisms and the differential excretion of free and protein-bound hemoglobin. *J Clin Invest.* 1959;38(4):652-658.

473. Gburek J, Verroust PJ, Willnow TE, et al. Megalin and cubilin are endocytic receptors involved in renal clearance of hemoglobin. *J Am Soc Nephrol.* 2002;13(2):423-430.

474. Zager RA, Gamelin LM. Pathogenetic mechanisms in experimental hemoglobinuric acute renal failure. *Am J Physiol.* 1989;256(3 pt 2):F446-F455.

475. Feola M, Simoni J, Tran R, Canizaro PC. Nephrotoxicity of hemoglobin solutions. *Biomater Artif Cells Artif Organs.* 1990;18(2):233-249.

476. Saraf SL, Zhang X, Kanias T, et al. Haemoglobinuria is associated with chronic kidney disease and its progression in patients with sickle cell anaemia. *Br J Haematol.* 2014;164(5):729-739.

477. Eshbach ML, Kaur A, Rbaibi Y, Tejero J, Weisz OA. Hemoglobin inhibits albumin uptake by proximal tubule cells: implications for sickle cell disease. *Am J Physiol Cell Physiol.* 2017;312(6):C733-c740.

478. Sears DA, Anderson PR, Foy AL, Williams HL, Crosby WH. Urinary iron excretion and renal metabolism of hemoglobin in hemolytic diseases. *Blood.* 1966;28(5):708-725.

479. Marsh GW, Lewis SM. Cardiac haemolytic anaemia. *Semin Hematol.* 1969;6(2):133-149.

480. Muller-Eberhard U. Hemopexin. *N Engl J Med.* 1970;283(20):1090-1094.

481. Ascenzi P, Bocedi A, Visca P, et al. Hemoglobin and heme scavenging. *IUBMB Life.* 2005;57(11):749-759.

482. Altruda F, Poli V, Restagno G, Argos P, Cortese R, Silengo L. The primary structure of human hemopexin deduced from cDNA sequence: evidence for internal, repeating homology. *Nucleic Acids Res.* 1985;13(11):3841-3859.

483. Severance S, Hamza I. Trafficking of heme and porphyrins in metazoa. *Chem Rev.* 2009;109(10):4596-4616.

484. Soares MP, Hamza I. Macrophages and iron metabolism. *Immunity.* 2016;44(3):492-504.

485. Delanghe JR, Langlois MR. Hemopexin: a review of biological aspects and the role in laboratory medicine. *Clin Chim Acta.* 2001;312(1-2):13-23.

486. Morgan WT, Liem HH, Sutor RP, Muller-Ebergard U. Transfer of heme from heme-albumin to hemopexin. *Biochim Biophys Acta.* 1976;444(2):435-445.

487. Naylor SL, Altruda F, Marshall A, Silengo L, Bowman BH. Hemopexin is localized to human chromosome 11. *Somat Cell Mol Genet.* 1987;13(4):355-358.

488. Smith A, Morgan WT. Haem transport to the liver by haemopexin. Receptor-mediated uptake with recycling of the protein. *Biochem J.* 1979;182(1):47-54.

489. Carmel N, Gross J. Hemopexin metabolism in mice with transplantable tumors. *Isr J Med Sci.* 1977;13(12):1182-1190.

490. Hvidberg V, Maniecki MB, Jacobsen C, Hojrup P, Moller HJ, Moestrup SK. Identification of the receptor scavenging hemopexin-heme complexes. *Blood.* 2005;106(7):2572-2579.

491. Lillis AP, Van Duyn LB, Murphy-Ullrich JE, Strickland DK. LDL receptor-related protein 1: unique tissue-specific functions revealed by selective gene knockout studies. *Physiol Rev.* 2008;88(3):887-918.

492. Wu ML, Morgan WT. Conformational analysis of hemopexin by Fourier-transform infrared and circular dichroism spectroscopy. *Proteins.* 1994;20(2):185-190.

493. Wu ML, Morgan WT. Characterization of hemopexin and its interaction with heme by differential scanning calorimetry and circular dichroism. *Biochemistry.* 1993;32(28):7216-7222.

494. Seery VL, Muller-Eberhard U. Binding of porphyrins to rabbit hemopexin and albumin. *J Biol Chem.* 1973;248(11):3796-3800.

495. Potter D, Chroneos ZC, Baynes JW, et al. In vivo fate of hemopexin and heme-hemopexin complexes in the rat. *Arch Biochem Biophys.* 1993;300(1):98-104.

496. Yang Z, Philips JD, Doty RT, et al. Kinetics and specificity of feline leukemia virus subgroup C receptor (FLVCR) export function and its dependence on hemopexin. *J Biol Chem.* 2010;285(37):28874-28882.

497. Mitani K, Fujita H, Sassa S, Kappas A. Heat shock induction of heme oxygenase mRNA in human Hep 3B hepatoma cells. *Biochem Biophys Res Commun.* 1989;165(1):437-441.

498. Thorbecke GJ, Liem HH, Knight S, Cox K, Muller-Eberhard U. Sites of formation of the serum proteins transferrin and hemopexin. *J Clin Invest.* 1973;52(3):725-731.

499. Maines MD, Gibbs PE. 30 some years of heme oxygenase: from a "molecular wrecking ball" to a "mesmerizing" trigger of cellular events. *Biochem Biophys Res Commun.* 2005;338(1):568-577.

500. Yoshinaga T, Sassa S, Kappas A. The occurrence of molecular interactions among NADPH-cytochrome c reductase, heme oxygenase, and biliverdin reductase in heme degradation. *J Biol Chem.* 1982;257(13):7786-7793.

501. Berk PD, Howe RB, Bloomer JR, Berlin NI. Studies of bilirubin kinetics in normal adults. *J Clin Invest.* 1969;48(11):2176-2190.

502. Elbirt KK, Bonkovsky HL. Heme oxygenase: recent advances in understanding its regulation and role. *Proc Assoc Am Physicians.* 1999;111(5):438-447.

503. Kapitulnik J, Maines MD. Pleiotropic functions of biliverdin reductase: cellular signaling and generation of cytoprotective and cytotoxic bilirubin. *Trends Pharmacol Sci.* 2009;30(3):129-137.

504. Kappas A, Drummond GS, Henschke C, Valaes T. Direct comparison of Sn-mesoporphyrin, an inhibitor of bilirubin production, and phototherapy in controlling hyperbilirubinemia in term and near-term newborns. *Pediatrics.* 1995;95(4):468-474.

505. Rizzardini M, Carelli M, Cabello Porras MR, Cantoni L. Mechanisms of endotoxin-induced haem oxygenase mRNA accumulation in mouse liver: synergism by glutathione depletion and protection by N-acetylcysteine. *Biochem J.* 1994;304(pt 2):477-483.

506. Zhang L, Guarente L. Heme binds to a short sequence that serves a regulatory function in diverse proteins. *EMBO J.* 1995;14(2):313-320.

507. Rizzardini M, Terao M, Falciani F, Cantoni L. Cytokine induction of haem oxygenase mRNA in mouse liver. Interleukin 1 transcriptionally activates the haem oxygenase gene. *Biochem J.* 1993;290(pt 2):343-347.

508. Astaldi G, Bagnara GP, Brunelli MA, Topuz UO, Valvassori L, Rizzoli C. Cell separation, cell differential and granulocyte colony frequency in polycythemia vera. *Isr J Med Sci.* 1978;14(11):1157-1161.

509. Zenke-Kawasaki Y, Dohi Y, Katoh Y, et al. Heme induces ubiquitination and degradation of the transcription factor Bach1. *Mol Cell Biol.* 2007;27(19):6962-6971.

510. Williams SE, Wootton P, Mason HS, et al. Hemoxygenase-2 is an oxygen sensor for a calcium-sensitive potassium channel. *Science.* 2004;306(5704):2093-2097.

511. Ogawa K, Sun J, Taketani S, et al. Heme mediates derepression of Maf recognition element through direct binding to transcription repressor Bach1. *EMBO J.* 2001;20(11):2835-2843.

512. de Haro C, Mendez R, Santoyo J. The eIF-2alpha kinases and the control of protein synthesis. *FASEB J.* 1996;10(12):1378-1387.

513. Stocker R, Yamamoto Y, McDonagh AF, Glazer AN, Ames BN. Bilirubin is an antioxidant of possible physiological importance. *Science.* 1987;235(4792):1043-1046.

514. Hentze MW, Muckenthaler MU, Andrews NC. Balancing acts: molecular control of mammalian iron metabolism. *Cell.* 2004;117(3):285-297.

515. Zhang AS, Enns CA. Molecular mechanisms of normal iron homeostasis. *Hematology Am Soc Hematol Educ Program.* 2009:207-214.

516. Yachie A, Niida Y, Wada T, et al. Oxidative stress causes enhanced endothelial cell injury in human heme oxygenase-1 deficiency. *J Clin Invest.* 1999;103:129-135.

517. Brown SB, King RF. The mechanism of haem catabolism. Bilirubin formation in living rats by [18O]oxygen labelling. *Biochem J.* 1978;170(2):297-311.

518. Dore S, Takahashi M, Ferris CD, Hester LD, Guastella D, Snyder SH. Bilirubin, formed by activation of heme oxygenase-2, protects neurons against oxidative stress injury. *Proc Natl Acad Sci U S A.* 1999;96:2445-2450.

519. Kovtunovych G, Eckhaus MA, Ghosh MC, Ollivierre-Wilson H, Rouault TA. Dysfunction of the heme recycling system in heme oxygenase 1 deficient mice: effects on macrophage viability and tissue iron distribution. *Blood.* 2010;116(26):6054-6062.

520. Poss KD, Tonegawa S. Heme oxygenase 1 is required for mammalian iron reutilization. *Proc Natl Acad Sci U S A.* 1997;94(20):10919-10924.

521. Onishi S, Ogino T, Yokoyama T, et al. Biliary and urinary excretion rates and serum concentration changes of four bilirubin photoproducts in Gunn rats during total darkness and low or high illumination. *Biochem J.* 1984;221(3):717-721.

522. Cheng L, Lightner DA. A new photoisomerization of bilirubin. *Photochem Photobiol.* 1999;70(6):941-948.

523. McDonagh AF, Lightner DA. Phototherapy and the photobiology of bilirubin. *Semin Liver Dis.* 1988;8(3):272-283.

524. Itoh S, Onishi S. Kinetic study of the photochemical changes of (ZZ)-bilirubin IX alpha bound to human serum albumin. Demonstration of (EZ)-bilirubin IX alpha as an intermediate in photochemical changes from (ZZ)-bilirubin IX alpha to (EZ)-cyclobilirubin IX alpha. *Biochem J.* 1985;226(1):251-258.

525. Bonnett R, Ioannou S. Phototherapy and the chemistry of bilirubin. *Mol Aspect Med.* 1987;9(5):457-471.

526. Gordon ER, Seligson D, Flye MW. Serum bilirubin pigments covalently linked to albumin. *Arch Pathol Lab Med.* 1996;120(7):648-653.

527. McDonagh AF. Controversies in bilirubin biochemistry and their clinical relevance. *Semin Fetal Neonatal Med.* 2010;15(3):141-147.

528. Reed RG, Davidson LK, Burrington CM, Peters T Jr. Non-resolving jaundice: bilirubin covalently attached to serum albumin circulates with the same metabolic half-life as albumin. *Clin Chem.* 1988;34(10):1992-1994.

529. Zucker SD, Goessling W. Mechanism of hepatocellular uptake of albumin-bound bilirubin. *Biochim Biophys Acta.* 2000;1463(2):197-208.

530. Gollan JL, Schmid R. Bilirubin update: formation, transport, and metabolism. *Prog Liver Dis.* 1982;7:261-283.

531. Zucker SD, Goessling W, Gollan JL. Kinetics of bilirubin transfer between serum albumin and membrane vesicles. Insight into the mechanism of organic anion delivery to the hepatocyte plasma membrane. *J Biol Chem.* 1995;270(3):1074-1081.

532. Kawasaki H, Kuchiba K, Kondo T, Kimura N, Hirayama C. Unconjugated bilirubin kinetics in Dubin-Johnson syndrome. *Clin Chim Acta.* 1979;92(1):87-92.

533. Frydman RB, Tomaro ML, Awruch J, Frydman B. Interconversion of the molecular forms of biliverdin reductase from rat liver. *Biochim Biophys Acta.* 1983;759(3):257-263.

534. Bosma PJ, Seppen J, Goldhoorn B, et al. Bilirubin UDP-glucuronosyltransferase 1 is the only relevant bilirubin glucuronidating isoform in man. *J Biol Chem.* 1994;269(27):17960-17964.

535. Crawford JM, Ransil BJ, Narciso JP, Gollan JL. Hepatic microsomal bilirubin UDP-glucuronosyltransferase. The kinetics of bilirubin mono- and diglucuronide synthesis. *J Biol Chem.* 1992;267(24):16943-16950.

536. Jansen PL, Oude Elferink RP. Hereditary hyperbilirubinemias: a molecular and mechanistic approach. *Semin Liver Dis.* 1988;8(2):168-178.

537. Muraca M, Fevery J, Blanckaert N. Analytic aspects and clinical interpretation of serum bilirubins. *Semin Liver Dis.* 1988;8(2):137-147.

538. Berk PD, Stremmel W. Hepatocellular uptake of organic anions. *Prog Liver Dis.* 1986;8:125-144.

539. Zucker SD, Goessling W, Zeidel ML, Gollan JL. Membrane lipid composition and vesicle size modulate bilirubin intermembrane transfer. Evidence for membrane-directed trafficking of bilirubin in the hepatocyte. *J Biol Chem.* 1994;269(30):19262-19270.

540. Labrune P, Myara A, Hadchouel M, et al. Genetic heterogeneity of Crigler-Najjar syndrome type I: a study of 14 cases. *Hum Genet.* 1994;94(6):693-697.

541. Aono S, Yamada Y, Keino H, et al. Identification of defect in the genes for bilirubin UDP-glucuronosyl-transferase in a patient with Crigler-Najjar syndrome type II. *Biochem Biophys Res Commun.* 1993;197(3):1239-1244.

542. Bosma PJ, Chowdhury JR, Bakker C, et al. The genetic basis of the reduced expression of bilirubin UDP-glucuronosyltransferase 1 in Gilbert's syndrome. *N Engl J Med.* 1995;333(18):1171-1175.

543. Iolascon A, Faienza MF, Moretti A, Perrotta S, Miraglia del Giudice E. UGT1 promoter polymorphism accounts for increased neonatal appearance of hereditary spherocytosis. *Blood.* 1998;91(3):1093.

544. Kaplan M, Algur N, Hammerman C. Onset of jaundice in glucose-6-phosphate dehydrogenase-deficient neonates. *Pediatrics.* 2001;108(4):956-959.

545. Kappas A, Drummond GS, Munson DP, Marshall JR. Sn-Mesoporphyrin interdiction of severe hyperbilirubinemia in Jehovah's Witness newborns as an alternative to exchange transfusion. *Pediatrics.* 2001;108(6):1374-1377.

546. Ritter JK, Yeatman MT, Kaiser C, Gridelli B, Owens IS. A phenylalanine codon deletion at the UGT1 gene complex locus of a Crigler-Najjar type I patient generates a pH-sensitive bilirubin UDP-glucuronosyltransferase. *J Biol Chem*. 1993;268(31):23573-23579.

547. Sampietro M, Iolascon A. Molecular pathology of Crigler-Najjar type I and II and Gilbert's syndromes. *Haematologica*. 1999;84(2):150-157.

548. Jansen PL. Diagnosis and management of Crigler-Najjar syndrome. *Eur J Pediatr*. 1999;158(suppl 2):S89-S94.

549. Nishida T, Gatmaitan Z, Roy-Chowdhry J, Arias IM. Two distinct mechanisms for bilirubin glucuronide transport by rat bile canalicular membrane vesicles. Demonstration of defective ATP-dependent transport in rats (TR-) with inherited conjugated hyperbilirubinemia. *J Clin Invest*. 1992;90(5):2130-2135.

550. Wolkoff AW, Cohen LE, Arias IM. Inheritance of the Dubin-Johnson syndrome. *N Engl J Med*. 1973;288(3):113-117.

551. Toh S, Wada M, Uchiumi T, et al. Genomic structure of the canalicular multi-specific organic anion-transporter gene (MRP2/cMOAT) and mutations in the ATP-binding-cassette region in Dubin-Johnson syndrome. *Am J Hum Genet*. 1999;64(3):739-746.

552. Nies AT, Keppler D. The apical conjugate efflux pump ABCC2 (MRP2). *Pflugers Archiv*. 2007;453(5):643-659.

553. Elder G, Gray CH, Nicholson DC. Bile pigment fate in gastrointestinal tract. *Semin Hematol*. 1972;9(1):71-89.

The Normal Hematologic System

Chapter 7 ■ Neutrophilic Leukocytes

LAURA G. SCHUETTPELZ • DANIEL C. LINK

INTRODUCTION

Neutrophils, also known as polymorphonuclear leukocytes, are central players in the innate immune response. Neutrophils are the most abundant circulating leukocyte in humans and play a critical role in host defense by phagocytizing invading pathogens. Under basal conditions, the production of neutrophils is enormous, with estimates of 800,000 neutrophils produced each second in humans. In the resting uninfected host, the production and elimination of neutrophils are balanced, resulting in a fairly constant concentration of neutrophils in the peripheral blood. When an infection occurs, neutrophil production in the bone marrow and release into the circulation increases, and chemotactic agents are generated that result in migration of neutrophils to the site of the infection and activation of neutrophil defensive functions. Neutrophil number in the blood is tightly regulated. A condition of too few neutrophils (i.e., neutropenia) is associated with profound susceptibility to bacterial infection. On the other hand, too many neutrophils or inappropriate neutrophils activation may result in damage to normal host tissues. This chapter reviews the morphology, production, distribution, and functions of neutrophils.

HISTORY

An important role of pus in infections has been long recognized.[1-3] The antibacterial properties of blood were described by the British surgeon John Hunter around 1761 during the Seven Years' War. He observed that the cellular (buffy coat) component of blood could slow the "spoilage" of blood.[4] In his classic studies, Hunter observed that when blood was allowed to stand, a "buff-colored" layer was visible on top of the red cells. He noted that blood from patients with infected wounds had a thicker "buff-colored inflammatory crust" than that observed in blood from healthy subjects, which we now understand reflects the neutrophilia associated with infection. With time, he noted that blood would "spoil," as determined by the development of an odor typical of spoiled food. Hunter found that the addition of the "buff-colored inflammatory crust" to a blood sample would delay the time to "spoilage," now understood to reflect the antibacterial abilities of neutrophils.

Further insight regarding the cellular components of the inflammatory response and the nature of neutrophils was gained during the 19th and 20th centuries.[1] At one time, the inflammatory cells at sites of infection were thought to be caused by proliferation of connective tissue cells. However, in 1862, Friedrich von Recklinghausen[5] described that many of these cells were capable of locomotion (and called them "amoeboid cells from their resemblance to the amoeba"). In 1841, William Addison suggested that leukocytes in blood could extravasate to tissues,[6] and in 1873, Julius Cohnheim further described the margination and adherence of leukocytes to the vessel followed by the transendothelial migration of the cells to the extravascular tissue.[7] The response to infection by neutrophils in the microvasculature was elegantly described in *An American Text-Book of Surgery* in 1892,[8] where the authors noted the increased blood flow associated with inflammation and the accumulation of white corpuscles on the interior walls of the veins and (to a lesser extent) capillaries. They described that slowing of blood flow was then followed by emigration of these leukocytes from the interior of the veins to the extravascular tissue

via the formation of protuberances from the cell surface that enlarge and guide the leukocyte through the vessel wall. In 1880, the German physician Paul Ehrlich developed staining techniques to facilitate the identification of different leukocyte cell populations in the blood, bone marrow, and tissues.[9] Later, in 1884, the ability of neutrophils to consume foreign substances and attack and destroy bacteria was recognized by the Russian zoologist Élie Metchnikoff, who coined the term "phagocyte" (from Greek, meaning "to eat" and "cell").[10] Together, these early pivotal studies set the stage for advances toward our current understanding of neutrophil activity and function.

NEUTROPHIL DEVELOPMENT

Neutrophils derive from progenitor cells known as the granulocyte-monocyte progenitors (GMPs), which in turn derive from more primitive common myeloid progenitors arising from self-renewing hematopoietic stem cells in the bone marrow. The developmental stages in the granulocyte series and some of their morphologic variations are shown in *Figure 7.1*. Developing neutrophils follow a pattern of proliferation, differentiation, maturation, and storage in the bone marrow and delivery to the blood. In the first three morphologic stages, the myeloblast, promyelocyte, and myelocyte cells are capable of replication, as shown by their uptake of tritiated thymidine (^{3}H-TdR) and the presence of mitoses; in later stages, cells cannot divide but continue to differentiate. The morphologic boundaries of each cell compartment were defined many years ago and were based on criteria such as cell size, ratio of size of nucleus to cytoplasm, fineness of nuclear chromatin, nuclear shape, the presence or absence of nucleoli, the presence and type of cytoplasmic granules, and the cytoplasmic color of stained cells (*Table 7.1*). In this chapter, we will focus on the morphology-based classification of neutrophil development, since it is the standard in the field and widely used in the clinic. However, a recent study used mass cytometry and transcriptome profiling to develop an alternative classification of neutrophil development.[11] Three neutrophil subsets in the bone marrow were identified: (1) pre-neutrophils, a proliferative lineage-committed precursor: (2) immature neutrophils, nonproliferating neutrophils that are normally confined to the bone marrow; and (3) mature neutrophils, which are similar to circulating mature neutrophils (*Figure 7.2*). Of note, flow cytometry panels have been developed to prospectively identify each of these populations in both mice and humans. Although primarily a research tool at this time, this promising approach may yield new insights into the functional heterogeneity of neutrophils.

Transcriptional Regulation of Neutrophil Development

Granulopoiesis is directed by the activity of specific transcription factors, most notably PU.1 and CCAAT-enhancer binding protein α (C/EBPα).[12-14] Other major players include C/EBPß, C/EBPδ, C/EBPζ, C/EBPε,[15] c-Myc,[16] lymphoid enhancer binding factor 1 (Lef-1),[17] and growth factor independent-1 (Gfi-1),[18] among others, and the coordinated expression of these factors is essential for proper granulocytic lineage commitment, differentiation, and maturation (*Figure 7.1*).[19,20]

The transcription factors C/EBPα, PU.1, and c-Myc drive the development of GMP cells from common myeloid progenitors. Thereafter, the relative expression of the transcription factors C/EBPα and PU.1

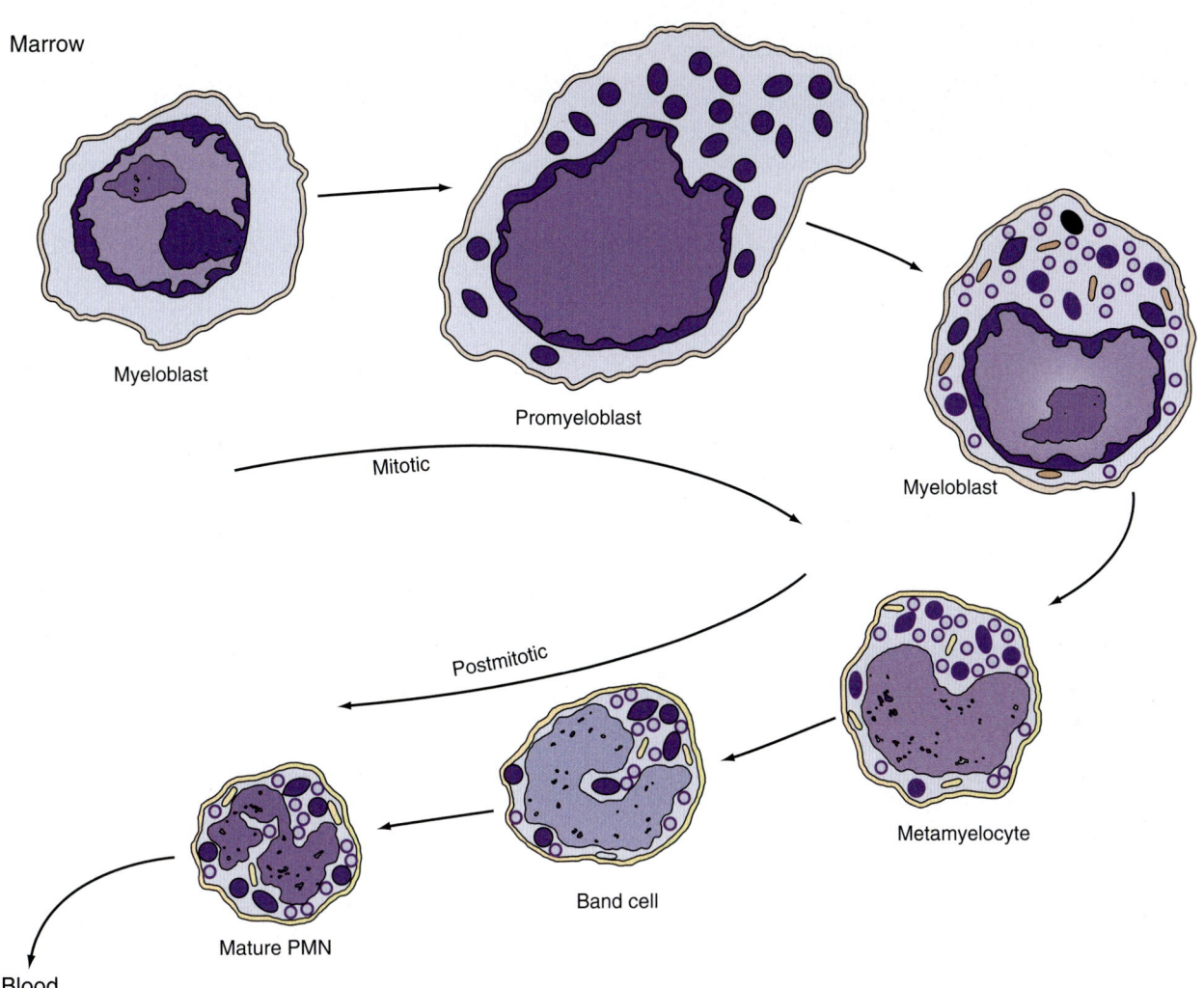

Marrow

Myeloblast

Promyeloblast

Mitotic

Myeloblast

Postmitotic

Metamyelocyte

Band cell

Mature PMN

Blood

FIGURE 7.1 **Neutrophil maturation.** Myeloblasts are undifferentiated cells with a large oval nucleus, large nucleoli, and cytoplasm lacking granules. They originate from a precursor pool of stem cells. Subsequently, there are two stages—the promyelocyte and the myelocyte—each of which produces a distinct type of secretory granule: Azurophils (dark granules) are produced only during the promyelocyte stage, and specific granules (light granules) are produced during the myelocyte stage. The metamyelocyte and band forms are nonproliferating stages that develop into the mature polymorphonuclear neutrophil characterized by a multilobulated nucleus and cytoplasm containing primarily glycogen and granules. Both nonspecific azurophilic granules and specific granules persist throughout these later stages. Also noted are the major transcription factors driving neutrophil lineage commitment and maturation. PMN, polymorphonuclear neutrophil. (Modified from Bainton DF, Ullyot JL, Farquhar MG. The development of neutrophilic PMN leukocytes in human bone marrow: origin and content of azurophilic and specific granules. *J Exp Med.* 1971;134:907.)

The Normal Hematologic System

regulate the commitment of GMPs to the granulocytic lineage.[21,22] While high levels of PU.1, along with that of C/EBPα and interferon regulatory factor 8 (Irf8), promote monocyte development of GMPs,[23] lower levels of PU.1 (along with the activities of the transcription factors C/EBPα, Lef-1, Runx1, and KLF5) favor neutrophil development.[24,25] The transcription factor Gfi-1 also participates in early neutrophil development, repressing PU.1 and Irf8.[26] The expression of C/EBPα and Gfi-1 decreases after the myeloblast stage of development.

Neutrophil terminal differentiation depends on C/EBPε, whose expression is upregulated during granulocytic, but not monocytic, differentiation.[27,28] C/EBPε peaks at the myelocyte stage of development, driving the transition from promyelocytes to myelocytes and promoting the formation of granular and secretory proteins. Furthermore, C/EBPε directly interacts with Rb and E2f1 to repress neutrophil proliferation and promote terminal differentiation. Accordingly, loss of C/EBPε leads to abnormal granulopoiesis with hyposegmented and functionally defective neutrophils.[27,29] Finally, the C/EBP transcription factors E/EBPε, C/EBPß, C/EBPδ, and C/EBPζ, along with Gfi-1, Lef-1, and PU.1, promote further neutrophil maturation.

Stages of Neutrophil Differentiation
Myeloblasts

Myeloblasts are immature cells, derived from more primitive myeloid progenitors, that are typically found in the bone marrow and not in the blood. These cells can divide and give rise to promyelocytes, which in turn give rise to myelocytes. The myeloblast (*Figures 7.1* and *7.3*) has a large nucleus, is round or slightly oval, and has a small amount of cytoplasm. In Wright stain preparations (*Table 7.1*), the nuclear membrane is smooth and even, and is exceedingly thin, with no condensation of chromatin near its inner surface, as noted in lymphoblasts. The chromatin shows an even, diffuse distribution with no aggregation into larger masses, although some condensation may be noted about the nucleoli. The chromatin may appear in the form of fine strands, thus giving the nucleus a sievelike appearance; alternatively, it may have the form of fine dustlike granules, producing a uniform stippled effect. Generally, the myeloblast contains two to five pale, sky blue nucleoli. The cytoplasm is basophilic (blue), and usually, although not invariably, no clear zone is evident about the nucleus. Sometimes, the

Table 7.1. Morphologic Characteristics of Leukocytes (Wright Stain)

| Type of Cell | Nucleus | | | | | | | Cytoplasm | | | |
	Size (μm)	Position	Shape	Color	Chromatin	Nuclear Membrane	Nucleoli	Relative Amount	Color	Perinuclear Clear Zone	Granules
Myeloblast	10-18	Eccentric or central	Round or oval	Light reddish purple	Very fine meshwork	Very fine	2-5	Scanty	Blue	None	None
Promyelocyte	12-20	Eccentric or central	Round or oval	Light reddish purple	Very fine meshwork	Fine	2-5	Moderate	Blue	None	Primary (azurophilic, eosinophilic, or basophilic)
Myelocyte	12-18	Eccentric	Oval or slightly indented	Reddish purple	Fine but becomes gradually coarser	Indistinct	Rare	Moderate	Bluish pink	None	Primary plus, in neutrophils, secondary or specific
Metamyelocyte	10-18	Central or eccentric	Thick horse-shoe or indented	Light purplish blue	Basichromatin and oxychromatin clearly distinguished	Present	None	Plentiful	Pink	None	Neutrophilic, eosinophilic, or basophilic
Juvenile or band form	10-16	Central or eccentric	Band shape of uniform thickness	Light purplish blue	Basichromatin and oxychromatin clearly distinguished	Present	None	Plentiful	Pink	None	Neutrophilic, eosinophilic, or basophilic
Polymorphonuclear neutrophil	10-15	Central or eccentric	2-5 or more distinct lobes	Deep purplish blue	Rather coarse	Present	None	Plentiful	Faint pink	None	Fine, pink, or violet pink

cytoplasm is reticular, spongy, or foamy. By definition, no granules are present in the cytoplasm. Leukemic myeloblasts that contain no perceptible granules often are identified by special stains that demonstrate the presence of myeloperoxidase (MPO) or esterase, thus providing early evidence of differentiation.

Electron microscopy reveals similar findings. The nuclear membrane is thin and indistinct, with minimal or no chromatin condensation. The numerous particles of ribonucleoprotein in the cytoplasm produce deep blue basophilia in stained preparations. Mitochondria

are abundant but small, and the endoplasmic reticulum is flat and appears infrequently. The Golgi apparatus is indistinct, and no cytoplasmic granules are present. EM studies of myeloblasts show peroxidase activity in the rough endoplasmic reticulum and Golgi.[30]

In wet films, myeloblasts appear immobile. In hanging drop preparations, myeloblasts manifest a characteristic snail-like movement.[31,32] Because they are in the process of growth and division, myeloblasts vary in diameter from 10 to 20 μm. In patients with acute leukemia, there may be asynchronous development of the nucleus and

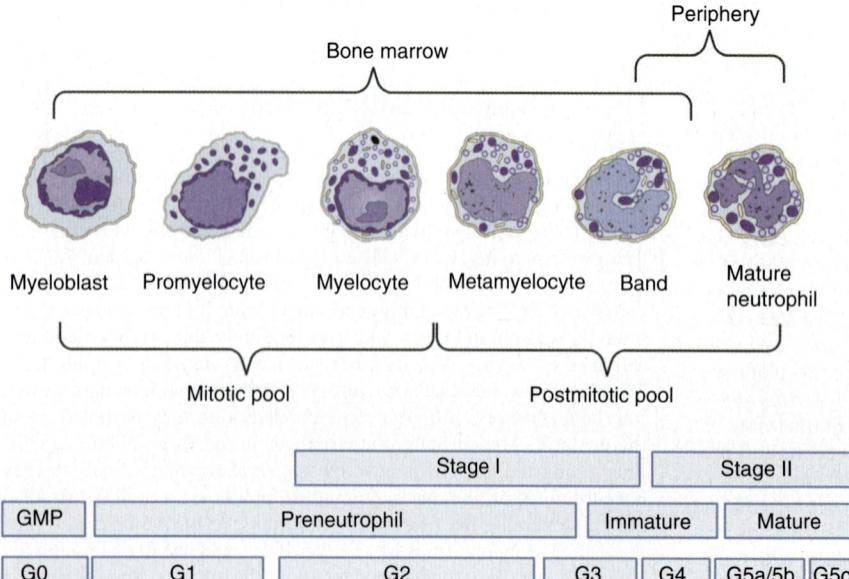

FIGURE 7.2 Neutrophil subsets and nomenclature. Neutrophil lineage cells may be classified morphologically as myeloblasts, promyelocytes, myelocytes, metamyelocytes, band cells, and mature polymorphonuclear neutrophils (see *Figure 7.1*). Earlier forms comprise the mitotic, or dividing, pool, while later forms comprise the nonproliferating postmitotic pool. More recent studies based on single-cell analyses suggest new nomenclatures as indicated.[11,149,378] (Created with BioRender.com.)

cytoplasm; such myeloblasts (sometimes called Rieder cells) suggest more rapid maturation on the part of the nucleus than that of the cytoplasm. Auer bodies, a marker of acute leukemia, are evident in the cytoplasm of cells that otherwise look like myeloblasts.

Neutrophil Promyelocytes

The neutrophil promyelocyte is somewhat larger on average than the myeloblast. It has a round or oval nucleus in which the nuclear chromatin is diffusely distributed, as in the myeloblast; in later stages, slight chromatin condensation is discerned around the nuclear membrane. Nucleoli are present, but as the cell develops, they become less prominent. Compared with the myeloblast, the endoplasmic reticulum in electron microscopic (EM) preparations is more prominent and takes on a dilated, vesicular appearance. EM histochemical and biochemical findings demonstrated that the azurophilic or primary granules first appear and accumulate at the promyelocyte stage and can be identified on fine structural study as characteristic of the neutrophil, eosinophil, or basophil series (*Figure 7.4*).[30] Azurophilic granules contain MPO, an enzyme whose activity is a classic marker of myeloid differentiation. These granules are readily demonstrated by peroxidase staining with light microscopy. Azurophilic granule production ceases at the end of the promyelocyte stage, coincident with the loss of peroxidase activity from the rough endoplasmic reticulum. In early promyelocytes, the few granules present may be difficult to see by using light microscopy; they often lie over the nucleus and are evident only on examination at several focal planes. The primary granules do not transform into specific granules but persist throughout the remainder of the maturation sequence and are seen in all subsequent stages, including the polymorphonuclear forms (*Figure 7.1*).[30,33]

Neutrophil Myelocytes

The neutrophilic myelocyte (*Figure 7.1*) may be defined as the stage in which specific (secondary) granules appear in the cytoplasm and the cell consequently can be identified as belonging to the neutrophilic series when stained and observed to have a pinkish ground-glass background color with the light microscope. The peroxidase-negative specific granules are smaller (approximately 200-nm diameter) than the azurophilic granules (approximately 500-nm diameter) and are near the limit of resolution by light microscopy. These granules are formed in increasing numbers on the convex surface and lateral borders of the somewhat less prominent Golgi apparatus.[30,33] Primary granules persist in myelocytes, but formation of new primary granules is limited

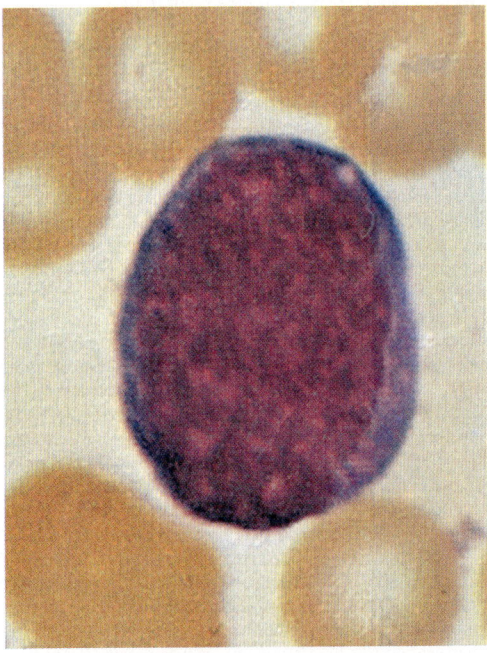

FIGURE 7.3 Myeloblast (×1000, Wright stain).

to the promyelocyte, and each succeeding cell division leads to a decrease in their number in the daughter population.[30,33] The amount of granular endoplasmic reticulum is lower in the myelocyte than in earlier forms, so the cytoplasmic basophilia decreases and disappears. The nucleus of the neutrophilic myelocyte usually is eccentric and round or oval; one side may appear flattened. The nuclear chromatin is somewhat coarse, and nucleoli are small and often not visible, although they are seen clearly with the electron microscope. The mitochondria remain small and are few.

Neutrophil Metamyelocytes

The metamyelocyte is characterized by a clearly indented or horseshoe-shaped nucleus without nucleoli, and the nuclear chromatin is moderately dense, with considerable clumping evident along the nuclear membrane. The cytoplasm is filled with primary, secondary, and tertiary granules, but the secondary granules predominate. The endoplasmic reticulum is sparse, as are polysomes, thus signifying the virtual completion of protein synthesis.

The boundary between the myelocyte and metamyelocyte compartments is best defined physiologically by the fact that myelocytes synthesize DNA, take up ^{3}H-TdR into their nuclear chromatin, divide, and are actively involved in protein synthesis, as evidenced by the presence of nucleoli, abundant endoplasmic reticulum, and polysomes. In classifying cells at this stage, the observer should pay attention to evidence in the nucleus and cytoplasm that protein synthesis has decreased or stopped. This determination is made on the basis of the fact that the nuclear chromatin is coarse and clumped, and that the cytoplasm is faint pink and is essentially the color of the mature cell in stained preparations. These features are also helpful in differentiating metamyelocytes (*Figure 7.5A and B*) from monocytes (*Figure 7.5C*) because in monocytes, nuclear chromatin remains fine, and evidence of protein synthesis persists.

Band Neutrophils

The band stage is characterized by further condensation of nuclear chromatin and transformation of nuclear shapes into sausage or band configurations that have approximately uniform diameters throughout their length (*Figure 7.1*). Subsequently, one or more constrictions begin to develop and progress until the nucleus is divided into two or more lobes connected by filamentous strands of heterochromatin, the polymorphonuclear stage. Some investigators require a clearly visible filamentous strand between lobes (*Figure 7.6A and B*) before classifying a cell as a polymorphonuclear form; anything less clear-cut, whether due to overlapping of nuclear lobes or incomplete constriction, is classified as a band form.[34] Other investigators have regarded a constriction greater than one-half or two-thirds of the nuclear breadth as adequate evidence of lobulation and classify such cells as polymorphonuclear, or use slightly different criteria. Because no clear difference has been shown between band and segmented stages other than nuclear shape and a slightly earlier appearance of ^{3}H-TdR in the band forms, the distinction becomes arbitrary. However, a clear and easily recognizable separation is needed if one wishes to count nuclear lobes for diagnostic purposes, as in the early detection of folic acid deficiency or in assessing marrow release of young forms into the blood.[35] For such purposes, we have chosen the clear separation of nuclear lobes as the criterion for inclusion in the polymorphonuclear category.[34] Cells without this complete formation of distinct lobes (usually connected by a filamentous strand) are classified as band forms.

Polymorphonuclear Neutrophils

In the polymorphonuclear stage, the nucleus in Wright-stained preparations is a deep purplish color and contains coarse, condensed chromatin. The lobes are joined by thin filaments of chromatin, although the filaments may not be easily visible if the lobes are partially superimposed. The cytoplasm is faint pink and contains fine, specific granules that sometimes give only a ground-glass appearance. Because azurophilic granule formation ceases in the promyelocyte stage, and the subsequent myelocyte form is still capable of cell division, the

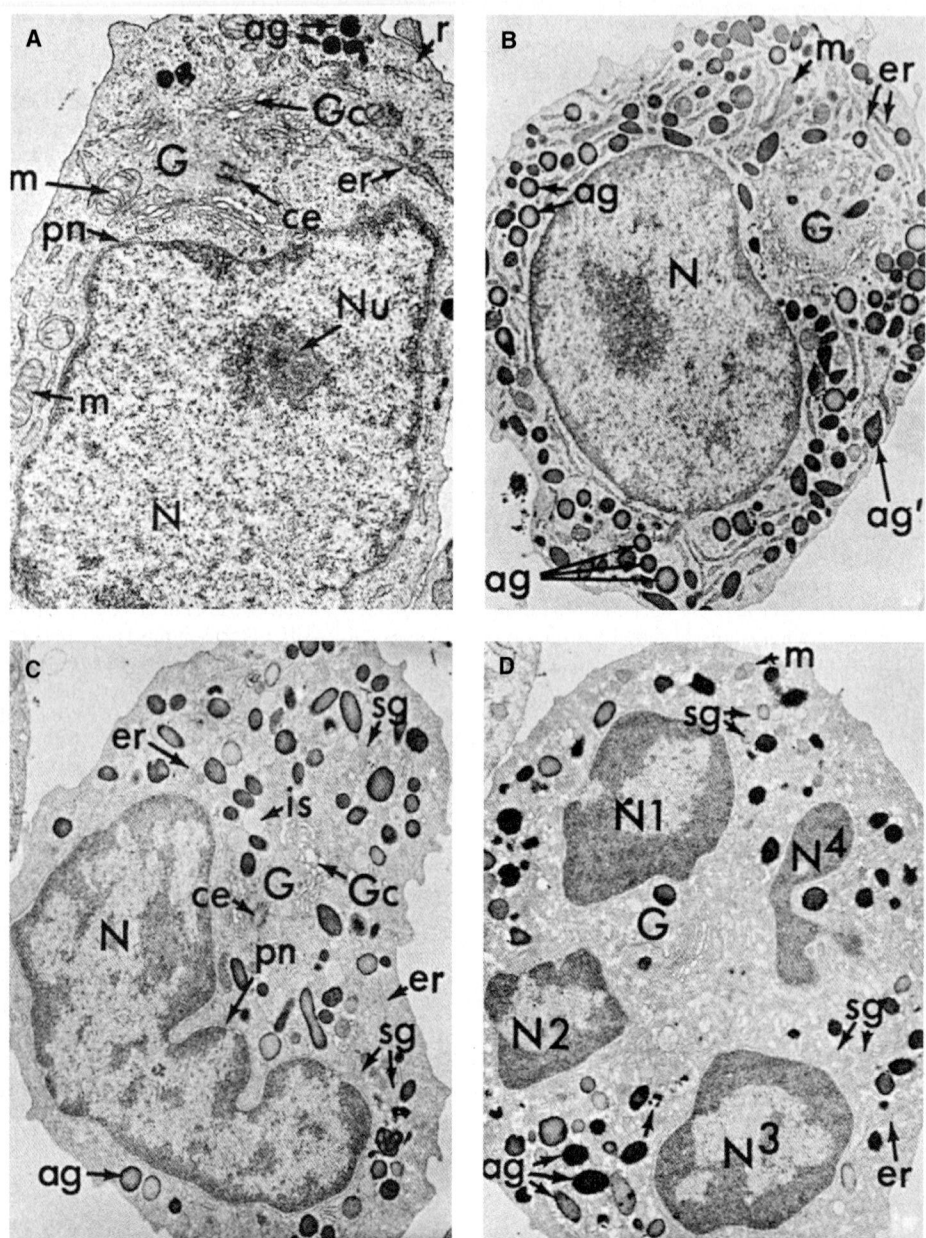

FIGURE 7.4 Early and late promyelocytes, a myelocyte, and a polymorphonuclear neutrophil (PMN) viewed by electron microscopy. A, Early neutrophilic promyelocyte (reacted for peroxidase, 10,500). The nucleus (N) with its prominent nucleolus (Nu) occupies the bulk of this immature cell. The surrounding cytoplasm contains a few azurophilic granules (ag), a large Golgi complex (G), Golgi cisternae (Gc), several mitochondria (m), scanty rough endoplasmic reticulum (er), and many free polysomes (r). A centriole (ce) is present in the Golgi region. All of the azurophilic granules (ag) appear dense because they are strongly reactive for peroxidase. The secretory apparatus, comprising the perinuclear cisterna (pn), rough endoplasmic reticulum (er), and Golgi cisternae (Gc), is also reactive, although less so than the granules. Specimen was fixed in glutaraldehyde for 16 hours at 4 °C, incubated in the peroxidase medium of Graham and Karnovsky for 1 hour at 22 °C, postfixed in osmium tetroxide, treated in block with uranyl acetate, dehydrated in ethanol, infiltrated with propylene oxide, and embedded in Araldite. Section was stained for 1 minute with lead citrate. B, Late neutrophilic promyelocyte (reacted for peroxidase, 7000). This cell is the largest (15 µm) of the neutrophilic series. It has a sizable, slightly indented nucleus (N), a prominent Golgi region (G), and cytoplasm packed with peroxidase-positive azurophilic granules (ag). Note the two general shapes of the azurophilic granules: spherical (ag) and ellipsoid (ag'). Most are spherical, with a homogeneous matrix, but a few ellipsoid forms containing crystalloids also are present. Many of the spherical forms (ag) have a dense periphery and a lighter core, presumably because of incomplete penetration of substrate into the compact centers of mature granules. Peroxidase reaction product is visible (under higher magnification) in less concentrated form within all compartments of the secretory apparatus (endoplasmic reticulum, perinuclear cisterna, and Golgi cisternae). No reaction product is seen in the cytoplasmic matrix, mitochondria, or nucleus. Specimen was fixed in glutaraldehyde for 10 minutes at 4 °C and subsequently processed exactly as was the specimen in (A). C, Neutrophilic myelocyte (reacted for peroxidase, 9000). At this stage, the cell is smaller (10 µm) than the promyelocyte, the nucleus is more indented, and the cytoplasm contains two different types of granules: large, peroxidase-positive azurophils (ag) and the generally smaller specific granules (sg), which do not stain for peroxidase. A number of immature specific granules (is), which are larger, less compact, and more irregular in contour than mature granules, are seen in the Golgi region (G). Note that peroxidase reaction product is present only in azurophilic granules and is not seen in the rough endoplasmic reticulum (er), perinuclear cisterna (pn), and Golgi cisternae (Gc), in keeping with the fact that azurophil production has ceased, and only peroxidase-negative specific granules are produced during the myelocyte stage. D, Mature PMN (reacted for peroxidase, 10 500). The cytoplasm is filled with granules; the smaller peroxidase-negative specific granules (sg) are more numerous, the azurophils (ag) have been reduced in number by cell divisions after the promyelocyte stage. Some small, irregularly shaped azurophilic granule variants are also present (unlabeled arrow). The nucleus is condensed and lobulated (N1-N4), the Golgi region (G) is small and lacks forming granules, the endoplasmic reticulum (er) is scanty, and mitochondria (m) are few. Note that the cytoplasm of this cell has a rather ragged, moth-eaten appearance because the glycogen, which is normally present, has been extracted in this preparation by staining in block with uranyl acetate. (Courtesy of Bainton D, University of California, San Francisco.)

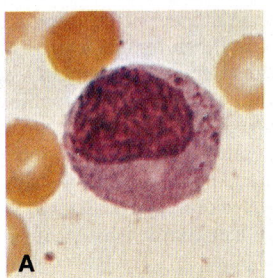 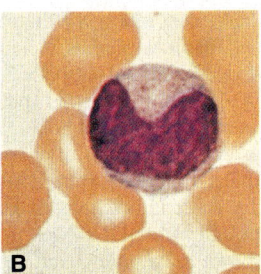

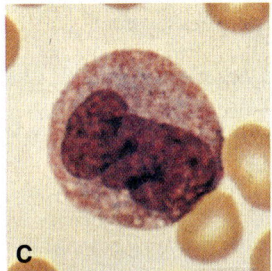

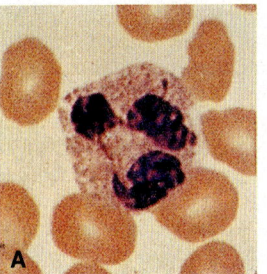 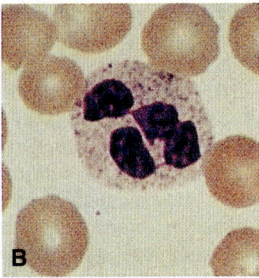

FIGURE 7.6 A and B, Polymorphonuclear neutrophils.

FIGURE 7.5 A, Late myelocyte or early metamyelocyte. B, Metamyelocyte. C, Monocyte (×1000, Wright stain).

density of azurophilic granules is lower in differentiation stages past the promyelocyte. The result is that mature neutrophils contain approximately two specific granules for every azurophilic granule. With maturation, the azurophilic granules, which generate reddish-purple staining in the promyelocytes, lose this metachromasia as they leave the myelocyte stage. This alteration in staining properties is thought to be caused by an increase in acid mucosubstances that complex with basic proteins already present in the azurophilic granules. Thus, in the mature neutrophil, the azurophilic granules appear as light blue-violet granules on Wright-stained smears. Large masses of glycogen become evident for the first time in mature neutrophils; this finding may contribute to their capacity for anaerobic metabolism.

In wet films, marked amoeboid activity of polymorphonuclear neutrophils at physiologic temperatures is characteristic.[36] "Senile" polymorphonuclear leukocytes that are no longer motile and fail to take up neutral red stain have been identified in in vitro preparations.[37] They are seen in small numbers in the blood, where their survival time is short.[38] As discussed much later, significant functional neutrophil development occurs after release from the marrow.

Differential Cell Counting and Normal Values for Leukocytes

Differential cell counting is the enumeration and classification of the leukocytes seen on the blood smear. The usual procedure is to count at least 100 consecutive leukocytes in an area of good cell distribution. A uniformly thin smear of blood on a cover glass is the best preparation for such examination. From the total leukocyte count and the differential count, the absolute concentration of each leukocyte type can be calculated.

Various systems for differential counting have been used. Arneth, for example, painstakingly recorded and tabulated from left to right the number of neutrophilic leukocytes with 1, 2, 3, and so on lobes and made other subdivisions, listing the results in 5 columns, and suggested that cell maturity was directly related to the number of nuclear lobes.[39] Cooke and Ponder modified the Arneth count by classifying neutrophils in five groups based solely on the number of nuclear lobes: Class I, unilobed or lobes joined by a definite band of chromatin, but not a thin filament; Class II, 2 complete lobes with 1 joining filament; Class III, 3 lobes; Class IV, 4 lobes; and Class V, ≥5 lobes.[40] The defining feature of this system was whether the interlobular material was a filament or "band" of nuclear material, thus generating the term "band" for an immature neutrophil. The term *shift to the left* is derived

from this practice and indicates an increase in the proportion of cells with only one or few lobes, whereas *shift to the right* represents an increase in the proportion of multisegmented forms.

From a clinical viewpoint, it is useful to determine whether young forms of neutrophils (band forms and younger) are increased and whether the proportion of multinucleated forms is increased. An increase of younger forms (band cells, metamyelocytes, and myelocytes; shift to the left) suggests increased release of young neutrophils from the bone marrow, which is seen in association with acute infections[35] and inflammation. If a shift to the right is suspected, a neutrophil lobe count may be useful. The chief difficulty associated with this count is clear definition of what constitutes a separate lobe (see "Band Neutrophils" earlier in this chapter). If complete separation of nuclear lobes with or without a connecting filament is the definition used, the normal mean neutrophil lobe count is 2.04, with 95% of normal values falling between 1.66 and 2.42. An increase in mean neutrophil lobe count suggests vitamin B_{12} or folic acid deficiency, congenital hypersegmentation of neutrophils, or a myelodysplastic syndrome.

Alterations in the total number of leukocytes and in their relative proportions are significant as measures of the reactions of the body to noxious agents. The reactions of leukocytes in association with certain diseases are discussed later in this book, as is the presence of abnormal inclusions, such as toxic granulation, Döhle bodies, and various inherited abnormalities in leukocyte morphology.

Physiologic Variation in Neutrophil Values

By the age of 4 to 8 years, the blood differential cell count approaches that seen in the adult. Normal values are presented in *Table 7.2*. Metamyelocytes or myelocytes are not often seen on routine examination of the blood smear, but a few such cells can be found in normal blood after a careful search (3.6/3000 granulocytes)[41]; atypical mononuclear forms and megakaryocyte fragments containing nuclei are also seen in such smears. Although leukocyte concentration is maintained within definite limits in normal humans, fluctuations occur during a single day and from day to day. Light influences the diurnal variation of neutrophils.[42,43] Under conditions of complete physical and mental relaxation, a basal level of 5.0 to 7.0×10^9 cells/L is usual.[44] Ordinary activity may be associated with a moderate increase, and a somewhat higher level is common in the afternoon. Under all these conditions, however, the leukocyte count tends to remain within the normal range.

Climate and altitude have been shown to influence neutrophils. Heat and intense solar radiation are said to cause leukocytosis,[45] while prolonged residence in Antarctica has been reported to cause leukopenia.[46] Acute anoxia, both anoxic and anemic, causes neutrophilic leukocytosis,[47] which does not develop in rats lacking an adrenal gland. In the first few days after a subject has arrived at a high altitude, some leukocytosis, accompanied by lymphopenia and eosinopenia, has been observed, followed quickly by slight lymphocytosis and eosinophilia.[48]

Marked leukocytosis occurs regularly with strenuous exercise. Counts as high as 22.0×10^9/L have been recorded for a runner after an 11-second 100-yard dash, and 35.0×10^9/L has been recorded after completing a quarter-mile run in less than 1 minute.[44] The increment of cells usually consists of segmented neutrophils, but lymphocytosis may be prominent as well. Such leukocytosis recedes to normal in less than 1 hour and, in the neutrophil series, is related to a shift of cells from marginal sites to the circulation.[49] This leukocytosis occurs in the absence of the spleen, suggesting that the spleen is not a major site of cell margination. Leukocyte counts >20.0 × 10⁹/L, mainly neutrophils, are regularly recorded for runners who complete a 26-mile marathon in 2.5 to 3.0 hours; whether a shift to the left, suggesting mobilization of marrow neutrophils, occurs in this circumstance is debatable.[44] Postmarathon leukocytosis subsides slowly over a number of hours and probably reflects a redistribution of granulocytes in the blood, combined with mobilization of cells from the marrow with an increase in total granulocyte pool size. The magnitude of the leukocytosis associated with exercise appears to depend primarily on the intensity of the activity rather than on its duration.[50] Just as exercise can raise the circulating neutrophil count, intense exercise has also been reported to induce neutrophil activation as determined by studies of cell-surface antigen expression.[51]

Convulsive seizures, from whatever cause, are associated with an increase in leukocyte count similar to that noted after violent exercise. Electrically induced convulsions are followed by a reduction in eosinophil and lymphocyte number and an increase in neutrophil number, findings consistent with the effects of adrenal hormone secretion.[52] Epinephrine injection produces leukocytosis, the nature and duration of which appear to vary with the mode of administration. Intramuscular injection causes leukocytosis in two phases.[53] In the first phase, maximal at 17 minutes, the number of neutrophils, lymphocytes, and eosinophils increases and then returns toward normal over several hours. This pattern almost certainly represents a shift leukocytosis. In the second phase, the number of neutrophils rises again at approximately 4 hours, although the number of lymphocytes and eosinophils remains at or below preinjection levels[53]; this phase may reflect an adrenal steroid effect and consists of an absolute neutrophilia. After intravenous injection, leukocytosis peaking at 5 to 10 minutes and of total duration of less than 20 minutes occurs and has been shown to be purely shift neutrophilia.[49,54] The leukocytosis that follows subcutaneous injection is more variable.

Pain, nausea and vomiting, and anxiety may cause leukocytosis in the absence of infection.[55] The paucity of band forms and metamyelocytes indicates that the neutrophilia results from the redistribution of the cells between the marginal and circulating pools.

Slight leukocytosis occurs during pregnancy, and neutrophilia increases as term approaches. The onset of labor is accompanied by neutrophilic leukocytosis, which sometimes is pronounced (34.0 × 10⁹/L). This state continues for 1 day after delivery, receding to normal only after 4 or 5 days. These changes are accompanied by a reduction in the number of circulating eosinophils.[56]

Many of the physiologic variations in leukocytes that have been described can be explained as manifestations of stimulation of the adrenal cortex. The administration of cortisone or hydrocortisone

Table 7.2. Normal Blood Leukocyte Concentrations (95% Confidence Limits)

Subjects (Age)	Sex	No.	Time of Day (h)	WBC	Neutro-phils	Lympho-cytes	Monocytes	Eosinophils	Basophils
Neonates (day 4)		53	Variable, 96 h of life		1981-7553	2200-7100	421-2022	200-1900	
Infants (9-12 mo)									
White		50		5400-24,200	1062-10,890	2178-11,718			
Black		50		4100-14,300	121-6732	900-11,400			
European adults	M	72	0930-1130	3487-9206	1539-5641				
(median age, 25 y)		26	1430-1630	3722-9828	1775-6508				
	F	70	0930-1130	3839-10,135	1861-6821	1158-3460	221-843	25-590	0-140
		29	1430-1630	4450-11,750	2137-7836				
European adults	M	85	0900-1530	3956-9592	2075-6557	962-3784	59-658		
(age, 54-65 y)	F	76	0900-1530	3423-8258	1833-5476	776-3455	59-732		
Pregnant Europeans (third trimester)	F	50	0930-1630	5915-13,962	3656-10,769	1023-3128	349-1140	22-330	0-90
American White adults		226	AM or early PM	4550-10,100	2050-6800	1500-4000	220-950	30-860	0-160
(age, 16-44 y)									
Black American adults	M	65	AM or early PM	3600-10,200	1300-7400	1450-3750	210-1050	30-720	0-100
(age, 16-49 y)									
Black African adults	M	250	0900-1200	2587-9075	775-4131	1012-3876	62-688	47-3371	
(age, 20-45 y)	Mostly M	109		3363-8977					

Values obtained by using a Coulter counter and differential counts of at least 200 cells (except in one African study). Values are expressed in cells 10⁹/L.
Abbreviation: WBC, white blood cell.
Adapted from Bithell TC, Foerster J, Athens JW, Foerster J, Lukens JN, Richard Lee, Kushner J, eds. *Wintrobe's Clinical Hematology.* 9th ed. Lea & Febiger; 1993.

results in increased blood levels of 17-hydroxycorticosteroids that peak at 1 hour and are associated with neutrophilia.[57,58] Eosinopenia and lymphopenia follow, become maximal at 4 to 8 hours, and are proportional to the quantity of hormone administered. Neutrophilia was less constant than the depression in eosinophil and lymphocyte numbers but is probably caused by a steroid hormone–mediated decreased efflux of neutrophils from the blood and increased cell release from the bone marrow.[54,59]

Benign Ethnic Neutropenia

In a study of over 25,000 participants in the 1999 to 2004 National Health and Nutrition Examination Study who were 1 year of age or older, mean leukocyte counts were lower in African Americans compared to Americans of European or Mexican descent.[60] Moreover, the prevalence of neutropenia, defined by a neutrophil count <1500/μL, was 4.5% in Black Americans compared with 0.74% and 0.48% in European Americans and Mexican Americans, respectively. Persistent neutropenia, often moderate (1000-1500/μL), in the absence of other causes, is termed benign ethnic neutropenia. The prevalence of benign ethnic neutropenia in other populations is not well defined, with a reported prevalence of 7% in Black South Africans[61] and 10.7% in Arabs.[62] Genetic studies show benign ethnic neutropenia is strongly associated with a single-nucleotide polymorphism in *ARKR1*, encoding the Duffy antigen.[63,64] A recent longitudinal study of 46 persons with benign ethnic neutropenia confirmed the benign nature of this condition, with stable neutrophil counts and low rates of infections.[65]

NEUTROPHIL STRUCTURE

Neutrophil Granules and Secretory Vesicles

Neutrophil granule production commences between the myeloblast and promyelocyte stages of neutrophil development and continues throughout maturation with a stepwise appearance of granules and secretory vesicles at progressive stages of development (*Figure 7.7*). Neutrophil granules contain proteases and other enzymes that contribute to microbial killing either via fusion with intracellular phagosomes or via extracellular secretion. Although the granules of neutrophils may be viewed as a continuous spectrum, largely resulting from differential production of different granule contents during neutrophil development, studies of neutrophils have operationally defined several types of granules.[66] The four well-defined types of granules in neutrophils are primary granules, secondary granules, tertiary granules, and ficolin-rich granules. Secretory vesicles are distinct organelles that provide a reservoir of membrane proteins required for the earliest stages of neutrophil-mediated responses. Some of the known constituents of these granules and secretory vesicles are listed in *Table 7.3* and described here.

Azurophilic (Primary) Granules

The azurophilic, or primary, granules are formed during the promyelocytic stage of neutrophil development and contain many antimicrobial compounds. These granules fuse with phagocytic vesicles, resulting in the delivery of their contents to the ingested organism. Azurophilic granules are heterogeneous in size and shape. Among the azurophilic granule contents is MPO, a protein that catalyzes the production of hypochlorite (OCl^-) from chloride and hydrogen peroxide produced by the oxidative burst. MPO constitutes approximately 5% of the dry weight of the neutrophil[67] and imparts the greenish coloration to pus. The human neutrophil defensins (HNP-1 to HNP-3), a group of cationic proteins that kill a variety of bacteria, fungi, and viruses,[68] also constitute approximately 5% of total neutrophil protein.[69,70] Other components of azurophilic granules include lysozyme, which degrades bacterial peptidoglycans; bactericidal permeability-increasing protein (BPI), which has antibacterial activity against certain gram-negative bacteria; azurocidin, which has antibacterial as well as antifungal activity against *Candida albicans*; and the serine proteinases—elastase, cathepsin G, proteinase 3, esterase N, and others.[3,66,67,69-74] The granule membrane itself expresses CD63, CD66c, and CD68.[75]

Specific (Secondary) Granules

Specific, or secondary, granules form after primary granules, and are first identified in the myelocytic stage of neutrophil differentiation. Although some specific granules, like azurophilic granules, may fuse with phagosomes, these granules are largely destined for release into the extracellular space. Some of the known contents of specific granules are indicated in *Table 7.3*, and include apolactoferrin, vitamin B_{12}-binding protein, plasminogen activator, collagenase, lysozyme, and others. Release of specific granule contents can modify the inflammatory process. For example, collagenase degrades collagen, thus augmenting movement through collagen and participating in tissue remodeling. Apolactoferrin, by binding iron, may have an antibacterial effect by preventing bacteria from obtaining necessary iron for growth.[76] Iron binding by apolactoferrin may also modify hydroxyl radical formation and cell adhesion.[77] Although the antimicrobial and proinflammatory defensins are stored in azurophilic granules, proHNPs produced at more mature stages of differentiation are not cleaved to the antimicrobial form and are stored in specific granules. ProHNPs are constitutively exocytosed, though their function is unclear.[78] Haptoglobin released from specific granules could also inhibit bacterial growth and inflammation.[79] Specific granules also contain a number of membrane-bound molecules that are expressed on the cell surface, including CD11, CD18, CD66a, CD66b, NB-1 (CD177), f-met-leu-phe (fMLP) receptors, C5a receptors, and cytochrome b_{558}. When cells are stimulated, the surface expression of many of these membrane proteins is increased, and some of the upregulated molecules may be derived from specific granules. The importance of the specific granules in neutrophil function is shown in patients who lack specific granules; these patients are susceptible to repeated skin and respiratory infections and have defective neutrophil chemotaxis and adhesion.[80]

Gelatinase (Tertiary) Granules

Gelatinase, or tertiary, granules, cosediment with specific granules in some subcellular fractionation techniques, and were initially identified as gelatinase-containing granules.[81] They are formed after secondary granules during the metamyelocyte and later stages of neutrophil differentiation. These granules contain gelatinase and other matrix-degrading enzymes. In addition, they express membrane proteins including CDllb/CD18, CD67, CD177, fMLF-R, SCAMP, and VAMP2, which are upregulated to the cell surface with stimulation.

Ficolin-1–Rich Granules

Ficolin-1–rich granules are produced during the terminal stages of neutrophil maturation. They are similar in protein content and function to secretory vesicles, containing primarily albumin, complement receptor (CR) 1, vanin-2 (VNN2), LFA-1, actin, and several cytoskeleton-binding proteins.[82,83] These contents of ficolin-rich granules promote neutrophil adhesion and transendothelial migration.

Secretory Vesicles

Secretory vesicles are distinct from neutrophil granules and are formed during the later stages of neutrophil maturation by a process of endocytosis. Secretory vesicles are located throughout the neutrophil cytoplasm and are significantly smaller than granules. By electron microscopy, they appear as smooth-surfaced vesicles. These vesicles contain membrane-associated receptors such as CR1, CR3, CD10, CD16, and others, as well as alkaline phosphatase, cytochrome b_{558}, and fMLP receptors. Secretory vesicles provide an intracellular reservoir from which membrane proteins can be recruited to the cell surface, and a defining feature of these vesicles is their rapid and complete translocation to the surface membrane with weak stimulation. For example, the secretory vesicle component CR1 can be readily upregulated to the neutrophil surface with minimal stimulation.[84] CR3 (Mac-1), recognized by CD11b antibodies and present in both secretory vesicles and specific granules, is also upregulated to the cell surface with weak stimulation. In contrast to CR1, a more marked upregulation of CR3 is observed with more potent stimulation, demonstrating

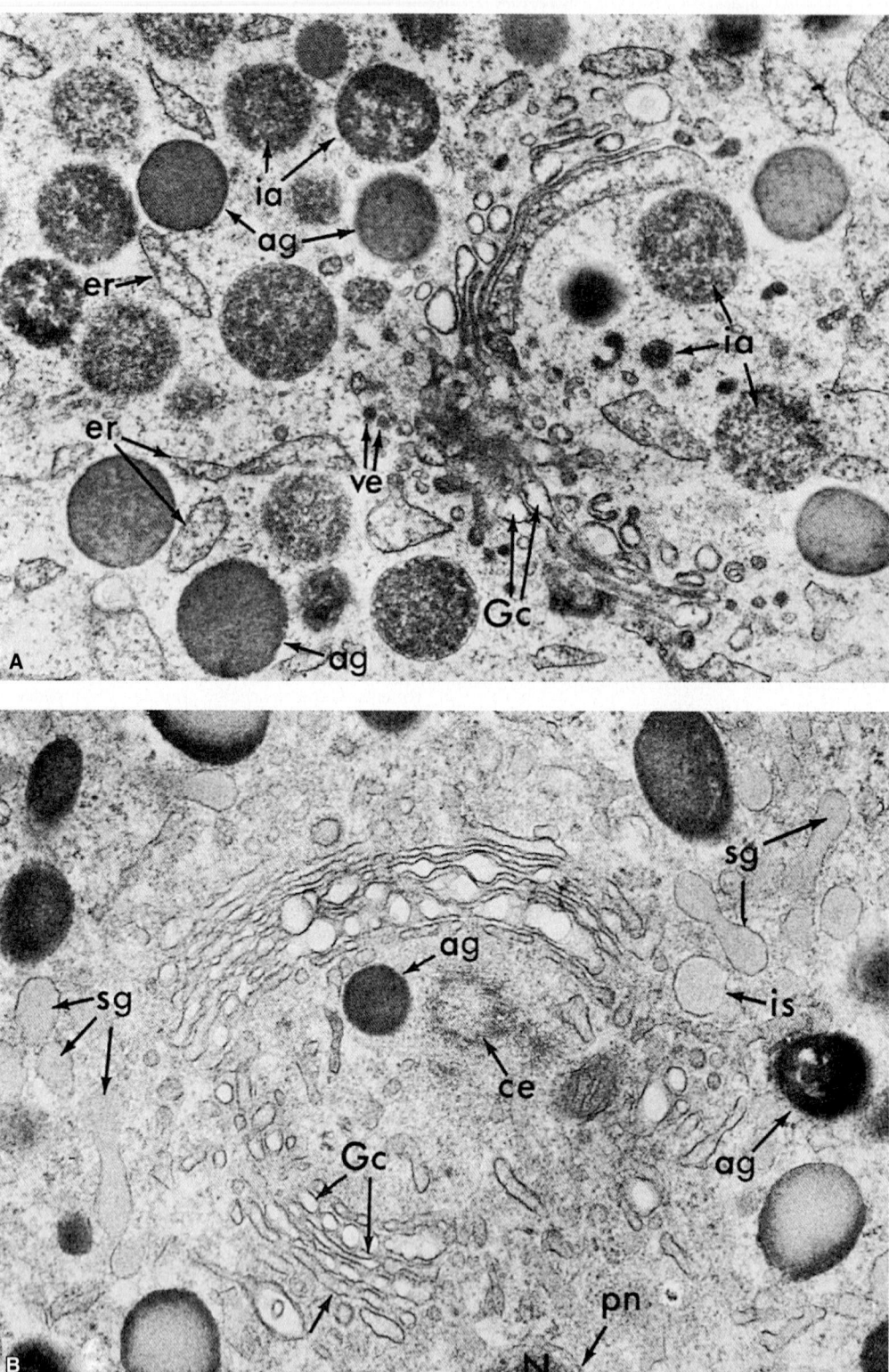

FIGURE 7.7 Granule formation in neutrophil precursors viewed by electron microscopy. A, Golgi region of a neutrophilic promyelocyte reacted for peroxidase (×40,000). At this stage, the peroxidase reaction product is present within the rough endoplasmic reticulum (er), the clusters of smooth vesicles (ve) at the periphery of the Golgi cisternae (Gc), in the Golgi cisternae, and in the immature (ia) and mature (ag) azurophilic granules. The immature granules are larger and less compact than the uniformly dense mature granules. B, Golgi region of a neutrophilic myelocyte reacted for peroxidase (×40,000). Peroxidase-reactive material is seen in the primary or azurophilic granules (ag) but not in the specific (secondary) granules (sg). At this stage (myelocyte), no peroxidase reaction product is seen in the endoplasmic reticulum, Golgi cisternae (Gc), or newly formed, immature specific granules (is). The stacked Golgi cisternae are oriented around the centriole (ce), and the outer cisternae (unlabeled arrow) contain material of intermediate density that is similar to the content of the specific granules, suggesting that the specific granules arise from the convex face of the Golgi complex as in the rabbit. pn, perinuclear cisternae. Courtesy of Bainton D, University of California, San Francisco.

Table 7.3. Contents of Human Neutrophil Granules

Azurophilic (Primary) Granules	Specific (Secondary) Granules	Gelatinase (Tertiary) Granules[a]	Ficolin-1 Rich Granules	Secretory Vesicles
Membrane	**Membrane**	**Membrane**	**Membrane**	**Membrane**
CD63	CD15 antigens	CD11b	CR1	Alkaline phosphatase
CD66c	CD66a	fMLP receptor	Vanin-2	Cytochrome b_{558}[b]
CD68	CD66b	Diacylglycerol deacylating enzyme	LFA-1	CD11b
Matrix	Cytochrome b_{558}[b]	Cytochrome b_{558}[b]		u-PA receptor
Lysozyme	fMLP receptor	Lamin receptor		fMLP receptor
Defensins	Fibronectin receptor	**Matrix**	**Matrix**	CD10, CD13, CD45
Elastase	G-protein α-subunit	Gelatinase[a]	Ficolin-1	CD16
Cathepsin G	Lamin receptor	Acetyltransferase	Albumin	DAF
Proteinase 3	CD11b	Lysozyme		CR1 (CD35)
Esterase N	NB 1 antigen	NRAMP1		**Matrix**
α₁-antitrypsin α-mannosidase Azurocidin Bactericidal permeability-increasing protein	Rap 1, Rap 2 Thrombospondin receptor Tumor necrosis factor receptor Vitronectin receptor u-PA receptor	Ficolin-1		Plasma proteins (including tetranectin and albumin) pro-u-PA/u-PA
β-glycerophosphatase	**Matrix**			
β-glucuronidase	Apolactoferrin			
β-galactosidase	Lysozyme			
β-glucosaminidase	β₂-microglobulin			
α-fucosidase	Collagenase			
Cathepsin B	Gelatinase[a]			
Cathepsin D	Histaminase			
Acid mucopolysaccharide	Heparinase			
Heparin-binding protein	Pro-u-PA			
N-acetyl-β-glucosaminidase	Vitamin B₁₂-binding protein			
Sialidase	Sialidase			
Ubiquitin protein	Protein kinase C inhibitor			
Myeloperoxidase	hCAP-18			
	SGP28			
	PTX3			
	Haptoglobin			
	Prodefensins (proHNPs)			

[a]Gelatinase is present in only a subset of specific granules; most is present in gelatinase granules.
[b]Cytochrome b_{558} is also called b_{245}.
Abbreviations: DAF, decay-accelerating factor; fMLP, f-met-leu-phe; u-PA, urokinase-type plasminogen activator.
Adapted from references Borregaard N, Cowland JB. Granules of the human neutrophilic polymorphonuclear leukocyte. *Blood.* 1997;89:3503-3521; Faurschou M, Kamp S, Cowland JB, et al. Prodefensins are matrix proteins of specific granules in human neutrophils. *J Leukoc Biol.* 2005;78(3):785-793; Theilgaard-Monch K, Jacobsen LC, Neilsen MJ, et al. Haptoglobin is synthesized during granulocyte differentiation, stored in specific granules, and released by neutrophils in response to activation. *Blood.* 2006;108(1):353-361; Rorvig S, Honore C, Larsson LI, et al. Ficolin-1 is present in a highly mobilizable subset of human neutrophil granules and associates with the cell surface after stimulation with fMLP. *J Leukoc Biol.* 2009;86:1439; Borregaard N, Sorensen OE, Theilgaard-Monch K. Neutrophil granules: a library of innate immunity proteins. *Trends Immunol.* 2007;28:340; Borregaard N. Neutrophils, from marrow to microbes. *Immunity.* 2010;33:657; Amulic B, Cazalet C, Hayes G, et al. Neutrophil function: from mechanisms to disease. *Annu Rev Immunol.* 2012;30:459-489; Kolaczkowska E, Kubes P. Neutrophil recruitment and function in health and inflammation. *Nat Rev Immunol.* 2013;13:59-75; Nauseef WM, Borregaard N. Neutrophils at work. *Nat Immunol.* 2014;15:602-611.

that specific granules can also serve as an intracellular reservoir from which membrane proteins can be upregulated to the cell surface.[84] Of note, secretory vesicles can be upregulated to the cell surface in the absence of extracellular calcium, in contrast to specific and gelatinase granules, which require extracellular calcium for release.[84]

Nucleus

Mature neutrophils have a distinct, multilobed nucleus.[85] In addition, they have a unique nuclear envelope composition. Compared to other cells, the nuclear envelope of mature human neutrophils has low levels of lamin A/C and LINC (linker of nucleoskeleton and cytoskeleton), high levels of lamin B receptor and peripheral heterochromatin, and high levels of lamin B2.[86] Together, these features of the neutrophil nucleus may facilitate neutrophil flexibility and deformability for transmigration.[85]

The mechanism and purpose of nuclear lobulation are the subject of speculation. It has been suggested that lobulation facilitates cell deformability and movement through vessel walls and into sites of inflammation; however, experimental evidence supporting this notion is lacking.

The Normal Hematologic System

It was suggested that granulocytes with three or four lobes are more mature than those with only two.[39] However, the number of lobes a neutrophil develops appears to be determined in the band stage (or earlier), and the time of appearance of neutrophils in the blood after pulse labeling with ^{3}H-TdR is unrelated to the number of nuclear lobes.[87] In the past, it was felt that neutrophils, as end-stage cells, undergo little RNA or protein synthesis. Subsequently, it was shown that mature neutrophils can synthesize both RNA and protein. This is likely particularly important when neutrophils migrate into sites of inflammation and begin to synthesize proteins and chemokines that contribute to the activation and resolution of the innate immune response.[3,71-73,88]

Pelger-Huët Anomaly

Pelger-Huët anomaly is a rare, benign anomaly of leukocytes. It is inherited as a non–sex-linked, dominant trait, and involves mutations in the lamin B receptor (*LBR*) gene.[89] It is characterized by distinctive shapes of the nuclei of leukocytes, a reduced number of nuclear segments (best seen in the neutrophils), and coarseness of the chromatin of the nuclei of neutrophils, lymphocytes, and monocytes. The nuclei appear rodlike, dumbbell-shaped, peanut-shaped, and spectacle-like ("pince-nez") with smooth, round, or oval individual lobes (*Figure 7.8*), contrasted with the irregular lobes seen in normal neutrophils. Pelger-Huët cells appear to be normal functionally. Pseudo or acquired Pelger-Huët anomaly may also be seen, in which cells with morphologic changes, such as described previously, have been observed occasionally in association with myxedema, acute enteritis, agranulocytosis, multiple myeloma, malaria, leukemoid reactions secondary to metastases to the bone marrow, drug sensitivity, or chronic lymphocytic leukemia. More commonly, pseudo Pelger-Huët cells are seen in patients with myeloid leukemia or myeloid metaplasia. Pelger-Huët anomaly is discussed further in Chapter 59.

Membrane Receptors and Neutrophil Antigens

Many constituents of the neutrophil plasma membrane have been defined. These include membrane channels, adhesive proteins, receptors for a variety of ligands, ion pumps, and ectoenzymes. Some of the various clusters of differentiation (CD) surface proteins expressed on neutrophils are presented in *Table 7.4*. For example, CD11/CD18 and

CD62L (L-selectin) are involved in neutrophil adhesion. The fMLP- and C5a-receptors sense stimuli and activate neutrophils, whereas aminopeptidase N (CD13) can inactivate interleukin (IL)-8, eliminating its chemotactic activity,[90] and neutrophil endopeptidase (CD10) can inactivate the chemotactic peptide fMLP.[91] CD66a, CD66b, and CD66c can activate neutrophils,[92] and some CD45 antibodies, which recognize a transmembrane protein with tyrosine phosphatase activity in its cytoplasmic domain, inhibit neutrophil chemotaxis.[93] Notably, the components of the membrane are not uniformly distributed. Studies have indicated the presence of differentiated domains in the membrane called *rafts*, which are described in the section "Lipid Rafts."

Table 7.4. Some CD Antigens Expressed on Neutrophils

CD	CD Antigen
CD10	Common acute lymphoid leukemia antigen, neutral endopeptidase
CD11a	Leukocyte factor antigen-1, $\alpha_L\beta_2$
CD11b	Mac-1, $\alpha_M\beta_2$
CD11c	p150, 95, $\alpha_X\beta_2$
CD13	Aminopeptidase N
CD15	Le^x (Ga1β1 → 4G1cNAc(Fucα1 → 3) β1 → 3Ga1β1 → 4G1cNAc → R)
CD15s	sLe^x
CD16	FcRIII
CDw17	LacCer
CD18	β_2-Integrin
CD24	Glycosyl phosphatidylinositol-linked protein
CD31	Platelet endothelial cell adhesion molecule-1
CD32	FcRII
CD43	Leukosialin, sialophorin
CD44	Pgp-1
CD45	Leukocyte common antigen (a protein tyrosine phosphatase)
CD50	Intercellular adhesion molecule-3
CD53	Tetraspanin molecule
CD55	Decay-accelerating factor
CD62 L	L-selectin
CD63	Tetraspan family member
CD64	FcRI
CD65	Ga1β1 → 4G1cNAcβ1 → 3Ga1β1 → G1cNAc(Fucα1 → 3) → R
CD65s	Sialylated CD65
CD66a	CEACAM1 (biliary glycoprotein)
CD66b	CEACAM8 (CGM6)
CD66c	CEACAM6 (NCA)
CD66d	CEACAM3 (CGM1)
CD82	Tetraspan family member
CD88	C5a receptor
CD95	Fas, APO-1
CD114	Granulocyte colony-stimulating factor receptor
CD156	ADAM-8 (a disintegrin and metalloprotease domain)
CD157	Bifunctional ectoenzyme (adenosine diphosphate ribosylase)
CD177	NB1, HNA-2a

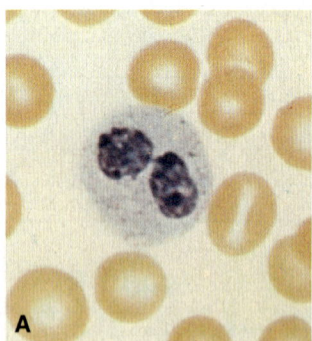

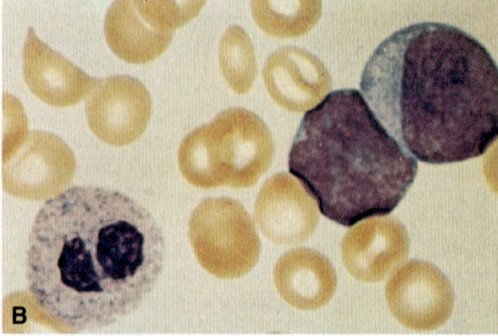

FIGURE 7.8 A and B, Pseudo Pelger-Huët cells, the latter from the blood of a patient with acute myeloblastic leukemia (×1000, Wright stain).

Table 7.5. Neutrophil Antigens

Antigen System	Antigen Name	Old Name	Molecule
HNA-1	HNA-1a	NA1	FCRγIIIb
	HNA-1b	NA2	FCRγIIIb
	HNA-1c	SH	FCRγIIIb
	HNA-1d		FCRγIIIb
HNA-2	HNA-2a	NB1	CD177
HNA-3	HNA-3a	5b	SLC44A2
HNA-4	HNA-4a	Mart	CD11b
HNA-5	HNA-5a	Ond	CD11a

Abbreviation: HNA, human neutrophil antigen.

Antibodies to certain antigens associated with proteins in the plasma membrane have been implicated in transfusion-related acute lung injury (TRALI) and alloimmune and autoimmune neutropenias.[94] These so-called human neutrophil antigens (HNAs) result from polymorphisms in surface glycoproteins. The first clinically relevant neutrophil antigens were described by Lalezari et al[95] and were originally termed NA1 and its allele NA2, and a second antigen was termed NB1. The NA1 and NA2 alleles were found to be present on the glycosyl phosphatidylinositol-linked receptor FcγRIIIB.[95,96] The NB1 antigen[97] is present on a glycosyl phosphatidylinositol-linked protein that is present in secondary granules as well as on the cell surface.[98-100]

Since their original discovery, a new nomenclature for these antigens has been established.[101] In this system, the antigens are termed HNA, for human neutrophil antigen, with the protein/antigen denoted by an integer, and the epitope by a letter. In this system, NA1 became HNA-1a, NA2 became HNA-1b, and NB1 became HNA-2a (Table 7.5). Most clinically relevant alloantibodies and autoantibodies appear to react with the HNA-1 and HNA-2 systems. TRALI is a major cause of transfusion-related mortality and is often due to antibodies against HNA-3a. The HNA-3a antigen results from a nucleotide polymorphism in the choline transporter-like protein-2 gene (SLC44A2).[102,103]

Some differences in neutrophil function have been reported based on HNA phenotype. For example, neutrophils that are homozygous for HNA-1b have a lower affinity for IgG3 and phagocytose targets opsonized with IgG1 and IgG3 at a lower rate than neutrophils homozygous for HNA-1a.[104-106] HNA-1a is typically expressed on about 45% to 65% of circulatory neutrophils[101,107] but on about 90% of circulating neutrophils in healthy people receiving G-CSF for several days.[108] HNA-2a (also known as CD177) is upregulated on the cell surface with stimulation, and also functions as a binding partner for PECAM-1 (CD31) on endothelial cells. Interestingly, the ability of HNA-2a–positive neutrophils to migrate through endothelial cell monolayers correlates with a specific endothelial cell PECAM-1 polymorphism in a region that is the putative binding site of CD177.[109] Thus, CD177/PECAM-1 binding appears to affect neutrophil transmigration across the endothelial lining.

Currently, there are fourteen HNA alleles assigned to five HNA antigen systems.[110] The antigens relevant to blood banking and immune neutropenia are discussed more fully in Chapter 22.

Lipid Rafts

Studies have demonstrated the existence of large noncovalent detergent-resistant complexes in cell extracts that contain important signaling molecules, including protein kinases and many glycosyl phosphatidylinositol-linked membrane proteins capable of transmitting signals.[111,112] These complexes have been termed *lipid rafts*. It is postulated that these complexes or rafts reflect the existence of specific membrane microdomains that have a particular lipid composition and that these clusters of molecules may be important in transmembrane signaling by proteins in the complex. There is evidence that in neutrophils, proteins may enter these rafts when they are translocated to the cell surface. For example, it appears that CD63 and CD11b/CD18 are not present in detergent-resistant complexes when they are intracellular, but they enter such complexes after translocation to the cell surface.[75] These rafts likely play important roles in signaling.

Cytosolic Contents

Although neutrophil cytoplasm contains many components common to all cells, the S100 family members S100A8 (also known as MRP-8) and S100A9 (MRP-14) are particularly abundant in the neutrophil cytoplasm.[113] These are calcium-binding proteins that form both heterodimers and homodimers. They have multiple functions, including regulation of cytoskeletal rearrangement, arachidonic acid metabolism,[114] and modulation of the inflammatory response via stimulation of leukocyte recruitment and cytokine secretion.[115] Notably, the quantity of S100A8 and S100A9 associated with neutrophil plasma membranes increases after stimulation.[113,115] These proteins are also present in secondary and/or tertiary granules, and are released when neutrophils are stimulated.[116] Annexin I or lipocortin I is another abundant neutrophil cytoplasmic protein that comprises approximately 3% of cytosolic protein.[117] Annexin I is partially regulated by glucocorticoids and appears to be a mediator of the anti-inflammatory effects of glucocorticoids.[117] One other notable cytoplasmic constituent is glycogen. Because neutrophils are sometimes required to function in hypoxic conditions, as in an abscess, they are very capable of obtaining energy by glycolysis. The presence of large intracellular glycogen stores gives them the additional ability to function in areas of low extracellular glucose.[118]

Macropolycytes

Macropolycyte is the name applied to giant polymorphonuclear neutrophils with a diameter greater than 16 μm and with 6 to 14 nuclear lobes.[119,120] Such cells are seen only occasionally in healthy subjects (1.3%), but they are found in approximately 5% of people with infections of various types or with intoxications, usually in association with a neutrophilic leukocytosis and myelocytes in the blood.[120] Macropolycytes are commonly seen in association with folic acid or vitamin B$_{12}$ deficiency, as well as in patients recovering from pancytopenia treated with cytotoxic agents, especially hydroxyurea.

Some authors describe cells with hypersegmented nuclei but of a normal size and call them *polycytes* or polylobocytes; similar cells with complex nuclei but without hypersegmentation are called *propolycytes*. The latter forms are seen in approximately 10% of patients recovering from leukocytosis with a marked shift to the left and appear in increasing numbers when anticoagulated blood is allowed to stand in vitro. The mechanism of macropolycyte formation is unknown, but one suggestion is that the skipping of one of the usual cell divisions that occur during maturation results in a hypersegmented cell.

Genetic Sex as Indicated by Leukocytes

Only one X chromosome is essential to the normal activity of a cell; the other in the normal XX female remains condensed and thus is visible as a chromatin body. Sex chromatin (Barr) bodies are present in 80% to 90% of the somatic cells of the normal female subject. The sex chromatin body of the neutrophil of females is a small mass, usually adjacent to the nuclear membrane, that stains deeply with hematoxylin and is approximately 0.7 to 1.2 μm in diameter. It takes the form of a drumstick projecting from one of the nuclear lobes of approximately 2% to 3% (extreme range, 1%-17%) of the segmented neutrophils in the blood.[121] They are well-defined, solid, round projections of chromatin connected to a lobe by a single, fine chromatin strand (*Figure 7.9*). They must be distinguished from small, clubbed or racket-structured nonspecific nodules that may be smaller or larger, as well as irregular in shape or lacking in chromatin, as well as from small (minor) lobes attached to the rest of the nucleus by two strands. Confirmation of the X chromosome in the drumstick has been provided by in situ *hybridization*.[122] Drumsticks are not found in normal male subjects.

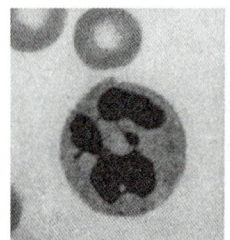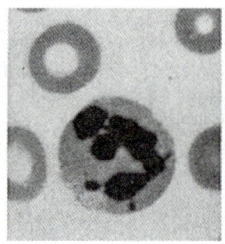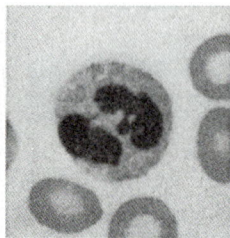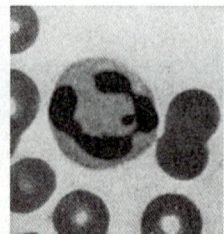

FIGURE 7.9 Granulocytes and sex chromatin patterns. Two cells on the left show the characteristic drumsticks found in the female subjects. The thin strand of chromatin joining the head to a nuclear lobe can be seen clearly. In the two cells on the right, small clubs, such as may be seen in male subjects, should not be confused with drumsticks (Wright stain, ×1300).

The number of chromatin bodies seen in a cell is one less than the number of X chromosomes present. With the increased numbers of X chromosomes found in certain disorders of human development, the number of Barr bodies and drumsticks increases, and isochromosomes formed by duplication of the long arms of the X chromosome give rise to larger drumsticks than are found in the normal female subject. Drumsticks or sessile nodules are seen in chromatin-positive male patients with Klinefelter syndrome and are absent in chromatin-negative female patients with Turner syndrome. Eosinophils and probably basophils also have drumsticks. Drumsticks may be difficult to find in the presence of a marked shift to the left. Double drumsticks or a sessile nodule plus a drumstick in the same neutrophil are rare.

Neutrophil Heterogeneity

Polymorphonuclear neutrophils were first thought to be a homogeneous population of end-stage cells incapable of protein synthesis and of essentially uniform size, granule content, and functional capability. However, recent evidence shows that neutrophils display phenotypic and functional heterogeneity related to factors such as neutrophil age, exposure to microbial products, and microenvironment.

The American anatomist Florence Sabin first suggested potential heterogeneity among neutrophils when she reported in 1923 that myelocytes were less motile than more mature neutrophils.[37] Additionally, a range of rates of motility among neutrophils from a single individual has been observed,[123,124] and Harvath and Leonard suggested the existence of two neutrophil populations based on chemotaxis.[125] Subsequently, several monoclonal antibodies were described that recognize subpopulations of neutrophils, including one that appears to recognize the classic NB1 (HNA-2a) neutrophil antigen, and one that recognizes an activation epitope on CD11/CD18.[126-128] One antibody appears to recognize a neutrophil subset that is more responsive to fMLP as determined by chemotaxis and respiratory burst activity.[126] Neonates have a larger percentage of neutrophils that express low levels of 31D8 antigen.[129] It has been reported that CR2 (CD21), the receptor for C3d, is present on immature neutrophils but not on mature blood neutrophils.[130] One report found that neutrophils from patients with localized juvenile periodontitis express CD21 (CR2) on their surface, whereas normal neutrophils do not.[131] Neutrophil heterogeneity has also been demonstrated in the case of olfactomedin 4 expression, which is highly induced in myeloid progenitors by G-CSF. Although olfactomedin 4 mRNA is expressed in all myelocytes and metamyelocytes, only about 25% of neutrophils in peripheral blood contain olfactomedin 4, which is localized to the specific granules.[132] Subpopulations have also been described based on density, with a population of "low-density granulocytes" that appear to have functional and transcriptional differences from other neutrophils.[133]

Major sources of neutrophil heterogeneity include different stages of development and "activation/priming." Some studies of different populations of polymorphonuclear neutrophils have been interpreted as reflecting maturation or environmental influences,[134] in certain cases possibly reflecting intravascular exposure to stimuli.[135] Earlier studies have shown that neutrophils are more reactive at sites of inflammation; for example, galectin-3 activates the NADPH oxidase of exudated but not peripheral blood neutrophils.[136] Exposure to *Staphylococcus aureus* leads to the development of distinct subsets of neutrophils that differ in cytokine production, macrophage activation potential, and surface antigen expression.[137] In another example, a unique subset of neutrophils with T-cell suppressive activity is found in acute systemic inflammation induced by endotoxin challenge.[138]

Recent work has provided convincing evidence that "aged" neutrophils are antigenically and functionally different from neutrophils recently released from the marrow.[139-141] For example, aged neutrophils display altered expression of multiple surface markers compared to fresh neutrophils. CXCR4 expression increases,[142] along with other surface proteins such as CD11b and CD49, while other proteins such as L-selectin decrease.[143] These alterations likely facilitate clearance of aged neutrophils. In steady-state conditions, aged neutrophils are removed in the bone marrow, liver, and spleen, and their removal by macrophages in the bone marrow exerts a feedback mechanism that has regulatory effects on granulopoiesis.[139,144] In the setting of inflammation, aged neutrophils rapidly home to sites of inflammation where they exhibit a higher phagocytic activity than younger neutrophils that arrive at the site later.[139] Transcriptomic analyses of aged neutrophils reveal alterations in signaling pathways related to cell activation, microbial detection, adhesion, migration, and cell death compared with fresh neutrophils.[140] Experimental data using germ-free mice or mice with genetic defects in microbial detection or antibiotic treatment suggest that neutrophil aging phenotypes are driven, at least in part, by the microbiota.[140] Finally, a recent multiomics study incorporating transcriptomic, metabolomic, lipidomic, and epigenomic datasets of mouse bone marrow neutrophils from both young and old, as well as male and female, animals showed that both sex and age contribute to neutrophil diversity. Notably, males had over 10-fold more significantly differentially expressed genes in their neutrophils with age than females, suggesting that the molecular rate of aging differs between the sexes.[145] Together, these data demonstrate that significant neutrophil development continues to occur after release from the bone marrow, with aging, microbial exposure, and other factors contributing to heterogeneity in their phenotype and function.

There is evidence that circadian oscillations in neutrophil migration and function exist in both mice and humans. Aged neutrophils show diurnal oscillations in the blood, with peak levels of aged neutrophils present in the blood in the daytime.[146] This correlates with diurnal variations in neutrophils reactive oxygen species and phagocytosis, and migration.[147,148] Thus, circadian diversification may contribute to neutrophil heterogeneity.

Neutrophil heterogeneity has been interrogated at the single-cell level using single-cell sequencing. Eight granulocytic populations were identified in mice, including 5 populations that primarily reside in the bone marrow and represent different stages of granulocytic differentiation (*Figure 7.2*).[149] Three major neutrophil subpopulations were identified in the blood and spleen, including a population of CXCR4-high aged neutrophils. Interestingly, the two other mature neutrophil populations in the blood may derive from different granulocytic precursors. Whether these neutrophil populations have distinct functional properties is currently not known. Similar neutrophil populations are present in human blood.

NEUTROPHIL KINETICS

The importance of leukocytes in the defense of the organism is well known. Basic to their roles are cell multiplication, maturation, storage, and delivery to the tissues and sites of infection or cell damage. These processes are called *leukocyte kinetics* and are different for each leukocyte type. To simplify the discussion, each type of leukocyte is considered as a separate system, but these systems constantly interact and complement one another in the defense of the body.

The production, kinetics, and life span of the neutrophil have long been of interest.[144,150-155] A model of these processes in adult humans is shown in *Figure 7.10*. The life cycle of the neutrophil can be divided conveniently into bone marrow, blood, and tissue phases. The assumption is that cells move through the system in an orderly manner as if in a pipeline; this view is supported by the progressive movement of isotopic tracers[156-158] and azurophilic granules[30,33] through the system.

The basal rate of production in the bone marrow is 5 to 10×10^{10} neutrophils/day, with an estimated 62 to 400×10^7 cells/kg passing through the blood each day. Further, the marrow reserve of neutrophils has been estimated to be about 6×10^{11} cells, which suggests a daily turnover rate of approximately 1.7×10^9 cells/kg.[54,151,159] Neutrophil homeostasis is maintained through a balance of granulopoiesis and storage in the bone marrow, release to the intravascular circulation, margination, migration into tissues, clearance, and destruction.[160] Further discussions of these processes related to neutrophil kinetics are provided in the following sections. Notably, the neutrophil system appears to be incompletely developed in premature babies and in early neonatal life; this topic is discussed in the section "Neutrophil Kinetics in the Fetus and Newborn" later in the chapter.

Neutrophil Mitotic and Maturation Compartments

Neutrophil production in normal adult humans takes place only in the bone marrow, and bone marrow neutrophils can be subdivided into the stem cell pool, the mitotic pool, and the postmitotic pool. The myeloblast, promyelocyte, and myelocyte are capable of cell division. These forms, therefore, constitute the mitotic pool (*Figure 7.10*). Simultaneously, they undergo differentiation, as evidenced by the appearance of azurophilic and specific granules in their cytoplasm. The more mature forms of the neutrophil series (metamyelocyte, band, and polymorphonuclear neutrophil) are usually considered incapable of cell division (except perhaps in unusual circumstances),[161] but they do exhibit continuing maturational changes and thus constitute the maturation or postmitotic pool.

Neutrophil production can be estimated either by assessing the production rate in the mitotic compartment or by measuring cell flow through subsequent stages, such as the blood. Labeling studies have estimated the transit time for human neutrophils in the postmitotic pool to be 4 to 6 days. This interval represents the minimum time from DNA synthesis in the previous myelocyte generative cycle until the cell has matured into a segmented neutrophil (or band form) and is released into the blood. Of note, in patients with infection, the transit time is reduced to as little as 48 hours.[162]

Neutrophil Release From the Bone Marrow Into Blood

The bone marrow is the primary site of neutrophil production under basal conditions. The pool of mature postmitotic neutrophils in the bone marrow is estimated at 560×10^7/kg (*Table 7.6*). In contrast, the total blood granulocyte pool (TBGP) in humans under basal conditions is estimated at 61×10^7/kg. Thus, only about 10% of total body neutrophils (ignoring neutrophils in the spleen or other tissues) are present in the blood. This large reservoir of mature neutrophils in the bone marrow is available for release into the circulation in response to stress, providing a rapid means to increase circulating neutrophils.

The mechanisms controlling the release of marrow cells into the blood are only partially understood and discussed in more detail in Chapter 5. Findings of in vitro studies of factors influencing marrow granulocyte migration through membranes demonstrated that pore diameter, morphologic age of cells, and the presence of a chemical attractant are important in marrow cell release.[163] Thus, immature granulocytes (myeloblasts and promyelocytes) could not penetrate membranes with pores smaller than 8 μm and were not responsive to chemoattractants. Mature granulocytes (band and segmented) could penetrate membranes with pores as small as 1 μm, and egress was accelerated by increasing pore size and by use of a chemoattractant.

The Normal Hematologic System

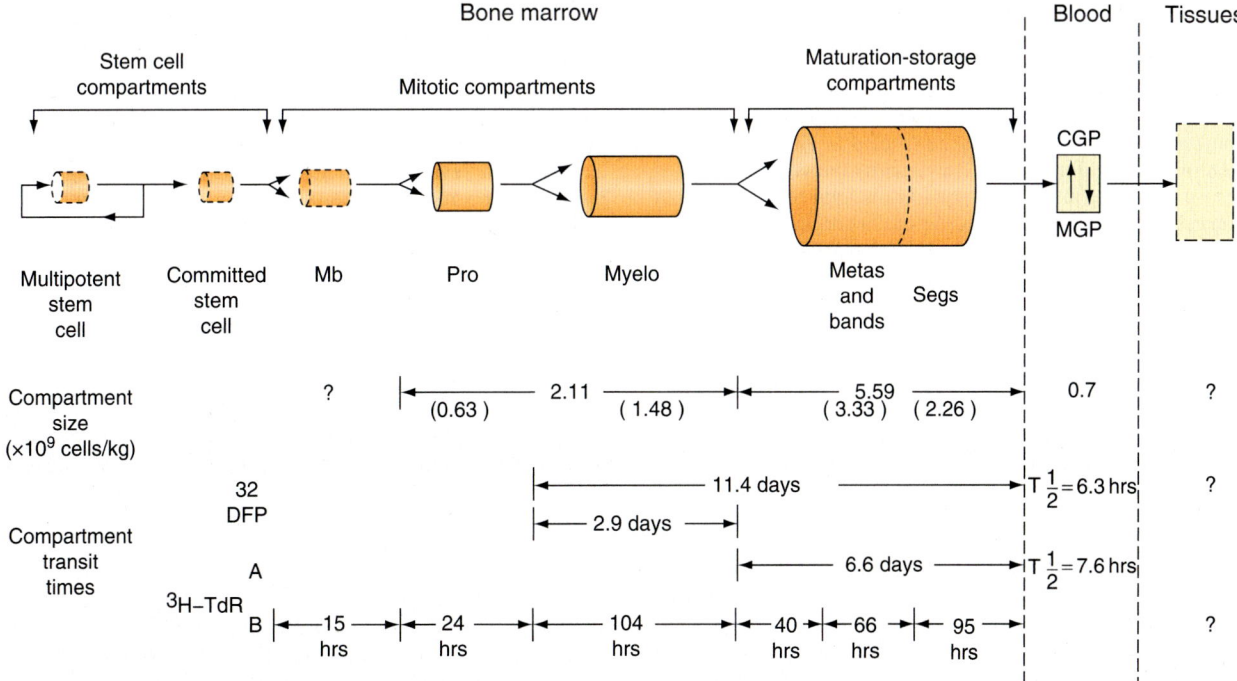

FIGURE 7.10 Model of the production and kinetics of neutrophils in humans. The marrow and blood compartments are drawn to show their relative sizes. In the lower one-third of the figure, the compartment transit times as derived from di-isopropyl fluorophosphate (DF^{32}P) studies[37,379] and from tritiated thymidine (^{3}H-TdR) studies[142,184] are compared. CGP, circulating granulocyte pool; MB, myeloblast; MGP, marginal granulocyte pool; myelo, myelocyte; pro, promyelocyte.

Table 7.6. Blood Neutrophil Parameters in Normal Humans

Parameter	Mean	95% Limits
Total blood granulocyte pool (cells × 10^7/kg)	61	27-128
Circulating blood granulocyte pool (cells × 10^7/kg)	31	13-49
Marginated granulocyte pool (cells × 10^7/kg)	29	8-115
Half-life (hours)	19	13-25
BM cellularity (×10^7/kg)	1300	
BM postmitotic neutrophils (×10^7/kg)	559	
Transit time (days) (27136946)	5.72	
Ratio of blood to BM neutrophils	0.11	

Abbreviation: BM, bone marrow.

Myelocytes and metamyelocytes exhibited intermediate activity. A number of mediators of neutrophil release from the bone marrow have been identified, including tumor necrosis factor (TNF)-α, TNF-β, granulocyte colony-stimulating factor (G-CSF), granulocyte-macrophage colony-stimulating factor (GM-CSF), IL-8, CXCR2, CXCR4, and C5a.[144,164,165] The CXCR4-CXCL12 axis, for example, is a major determinant of neutrophil marrow retention, as demonstrated by patients with WHIM (warts, hypogammaglobulinemia, infection, and myelokathexis) syndrome, in which heterozygous gain-of-function mutations in *CXCR4* lead to enhanced interaction with the ligand CXCL12 and retention of mature neutrophils in the bone marrow.[166,167]

Kinetics in the Blood

Early experiments using cell transfer models and radiotracers suggested a neutrophil half-life of 4.3 to 17.5 hours. However, the radiotracers used in these studies are toxic and any neutrophil manipulation may activate neutrophils, thereby shortening their clearance. A recent study using stable nontoxic labeling methods (using either heavy water or isotope-labeled glucose) has, at least to a degree, overcome these limitations. The study showed that neutrophil half-life in the circulation is 19 hours (*Table 7.6*).[151,168]

Neutrophils in the blood are distributed into two sites: the circulating blood granulocyte pool (CGP) and the marginal granulocyte pool (MGP). These pools were determined using the $DF(^{32})P$ labeling technique, in which neutrophils are labeled in vitro with $DF(^{32})P$ and returned to the donor.[49,54,153] In healthy humans, neutrophils in these two pools are in constant equilibrium, and the pools are of approximately equal size (*Table 7.6*). Various factors can influence the distribution of neutrophils between the CGP and MGP. Brief exercise or epinephrine injection results in demargination of cells, increasing circulating neutrophil numbers by approximately 50%.[49] The distribution of cells in the CGP and MGP can be altered by other means. For example, endotoxin injection induces a transient neutropenia due to a shift from the CGP to MGP.[54] A rapid transient increase in the MGP also has been observed during hemodialysis when Cuprophane membranes are used.[169] This is thought to be mediated by complement activation, resulting in an increase in both neutrophils rolling along small blood vessels and homotypic aggregates of neutrophils.[170-173] This neutrophil margination was transient, being maximal by approximately 15 minutes and resolving by 1 hour of dialysis. Administration of steroids results in an increase of circulating neutrophils, due to both an increase in neutrophil release from the bone marrow and reduced outflow into tissues.[59]

The exact nature of the MGP is not clear. In the past, it was felt to represent transient adhesion to, and rolling along the surface of, endothelial cells, primarily in postcapillary venules. However, a study of the MGP in a patient with leukocyte adhesion deficiency-2 (LAD-2) challenges this model.[174] Patients with LAD-2 lack the ligands for P- and E-selectins, and have a marked decrease in neutrophil rolling in postcapillary venules. Studies of a LAD-2 patient suggested that approximately 20% of neutrophils are in a selectin-independent MGP and approximately 30% are in a selectin-dependent MGP.[174] Surprisingly, this patient's neutrophils had a shorter-than-normal half-life in the circulation, with an increased turnover rate. The inability of CD18 or L-selectin antibodies to shift neutrophils from the MGP to the CGP also suggests that the transient adhesion to endothelial cells manifest as rolling does not fully account for the MGP.[175,176]

Migration Into Tissues and Sites of Destruction

At a local site of tissue damage or infection, adherence of neutrophils to the endothelial cells of the vessel wall and their subsequent migration into the tissues can be seen within minutes. After initial adherence, neutrophils project microscopically visible pseudopods between or through the endothelial cells and force a passage across the endothelial layer.[177] This directed movement, chemotaxis, is induced by the binding of a variety of chemoattractant molecules, such as N-formyl peptides (e.g., fMLP), a cleavage product of the fifth component of complement (C5a), leukotriene B$_4$, and platelet-activating factor (PAF), to specific membrane receptors. Further migration is then delayed by the basement membrane and perivascular cells, and the neutrophils may move parallel to, but beneath, the endothelium until a passage into the surrounding connective tissue is found. Once neutrophils leave the blood, they do not return in significant numbers.[178] The sites into which neutrophils normally disappear are poorly understood. Many neutrophils are removed in the bone marrow by macrophages via CXCR4, where the process produces a feedback inhibition of neutrophil production.[142,144,179,180] Some are also removed in the liver and spleen. Labeled blood neutrophils are found in saliva,[87] but loss into saliva may reflect subclinical infections because few, if any, cells are found in the salivary ducts[181]; the rate at which granulocytes enter the oral cavity has been correlated with the degree of gingivitis.[182] Some cells do penetrate the oral mucosa in healthy subjects, presumably as a result of diapedesis.[181] Loss of leukocytes in the urine also has been demonstrated in normal subjects.[183] In addition, arteriovenous catheterization studies in dogs[184] and in humans[185] provide evidence that suggests leukocytes also are removed in the lungs, liver, and spleen.

Neutrophil Death

After responding to infections or damage signals and performing their effector function, neutrophils initiate mechanisms of cell death. The regulation of neutrophil death is important both to maintain homeostasis under physiological conditions and to optimize the inflammatory response to infection or tissue damage. Neutrophils can undergo several mechanisms of death, including apoptosis, pyroptosis, necroptosis, simple necrosis, and NETosis. Pyroptosis and necroptosis result from activation of pore-induced cell death pathways and are inflammatory processes. In contrast, apoptosis is noninflammatory. NETosis is a form of cell death that involves the release of neutrophil extracellular traps (NETs).[186,187] The type of cell death initiated in neutrophils depends upon the nature and intensity of the stimulus received.[186]

Apoptosis is manifest by characteristic morphologic changes with nuclear condensation and the formation of pyknotic nuclei. Importantly, the cell remains intact and does not release its potentially toxic contents before it is phagocytosed by macrophages and removed. Neutrophils undergo apoptosis in tissue culture (approximately 50% of cells in 24 hours); this process is accompanied by a fall in intracellular pH.[188] The addition of G-CSF, GM-CSF, or IL-1 delays but does not prevent this process.[188] Macrophages phagocytose senescent (apoptotic) neutrophils (as observed more than a century ago), and this is probably one fate of the short-lived blood neutrophil.[8,189] Interestingly, glucocorticoids inhibit neutrophil apoptosis,[190] but they induce it in susceptible lymphocytes. Fas (CD95) is expressed on neutrophils and is capable of inducing apoptosis as it does in other susceptible cells.[190] Neutrophil life span is increased at sites of infection, likely by locally produced cytokines. Neutrophil apoptosis is reversibly inhibited by hypoxia, possibly playing a role in neutrophil survival at sites of inflammation.[191] Neutrophil apoptosis is also delayed in pregnancy, and both estradiol and progesterone can delay neutrophil apoptosis in men and women.[192] As discussed later, in general, diapedesis seems to induce an antiapoptotic state, whereas phagocytosis seems to promote apoptosis, at least partly by upregulating death receptors, thus providing the conditions for resolution of inflammation and avoidance of tissue damage.

NETosis is a more recently described form of cell death that is unique to granulocytes.[187,193] In so-called suicidal NETosis, the nuclear and cellular membranes disintegrate, releasing decondensed chromatin along with granule contents. The loss of intracellular membrane integrity before that of the cell membrane is a characteristic of NETosis. NETs contain DNA strands along with histones and contents of primary, secondary, and tertiary granules and have been suggested to have functions in infection, autoimmune disease, and atherosclerosis.[194] The extracellular chromatin in NETs binds pathogens and forms an antimicrobial matrix along with granule proteins that aid in pathogen killing. NET formation is triggered by pattern recognition and other innate immune receptors, which stimulate the production of reactive oxygen species (ROS) and the activation of MPO, neutrophil elastase, and protein-arginine deiminase type 4 (PAD4) to promote chromatin decondensation.[195]

In many cases, NET formation is followed by cell death (suicidal NETosis); however, neutrophils can also release NETs via vesicular transport without cell death in a process called "vital NETosis." In contrast to suicidal NETosis, vital NETosis, which is stimulated by microorganisms, activated platelets, or complement proteins, is a rapid process that is largely independent of NOX activity and ROS production.[196] This nonlytic type of NET formation involves vesicle-mediated NET formation and the secreted expulsion of DNA, granule proteins, and histones, leaving behind active, anuclear cytoplasts that can crawl and continue to phagocytose microorganisms.[195,197]

Neutrophil Kinetics in the Fetus and Newborn

The fetus exists in a sterile environment and, unlike the adult, does not require antibacterial defenses. However, if the systems ensuring adequate neutrophil production, storage, delivery to tissues, phagocytosis, and bacterial killing are not intact at birth, extrauterine existence is seriously compromised. Maturation of the neutrophil system is not complete in the midgestation fetus, and even the neonate delivered at term has a neutrophil system that in several respects is quantitatively and qualitatively immature. Therefore, newborns, particularly those delivered prematurely, are at risk for serious bacterial infection, with multiple studies showing a strong correlation between prematurity and serious bacterial infection.[198,199] Even babies delivered at term experience a higher incidence of bacterial infection than do older children or adults[200] and, when infected, often display poor resolution of infection despite antibiotic therapy.

Newborn infants, particularly if premature, display many other deficiencies in antibacterial defense, such as low levels of IgG antibody, complement components, fibronectin, and lymphokine production, but only maturational differences in neutrophil kinetics are discussed here. Realizing that the neutrophil system of a fetus is underdeveloped and in a state of maturation, a difference in neutrophil pool sizes and kinetics in this group from those in adults can be expected. In addition, rapid somatic growth in the fetus and newborn places added demands, unique to the neonate, on neutrophil production; cells are needed not only for ongoing antibacterial defense but also for a rapidly increasing body mass.

The investigation of neutrophil kinetics during fetal and neonatal life in humans has been hampered by lack of applicability of the techniques used for such studies in adults. For instance, DF^{32}P and ^{3}H-TdR blood kinetic measurements have not been used in babies because of the radiation exposure and the large volumes of blood required. Nevertheless, the results of clinical studies, coupled with extensive investigation in developing animals, illustrate several developmental differences.

Neutrophil Production and Storage in the Fetus and Newborn

Granulocyte-macrophage progenitor cells (CFU-GM, or granulocyte-macrophage colony-forming unit) have been detected in the human fetal liver as early as 5 to 6 weeks of gestation.[201] Although these early fetal cells produced colonies of mature neutrophils in vitro, mature neutrophils are not detected in the fetus itself until 10 to 11 weeks of gestation when they first appear in the fetal bone marrow.[202] At 14 to 16 weeks of gestation, mature neutrophils are detectable in the fetal peripheral blood.[203,204]

Neutrophil progenitors display robust proliferation in the developing fetus. The proliferative rate of CFU-GM during human gestation, assessed by thymidine suicide, is rapid in the second trimester.[205] Whereas CFU-GM in venous blood of adults displays a thymidine suicide rate ranging from 0% to 7%,[205-207] rates of 45% have been observed in term neonates, and rates of 75% were noted in prematurely born neonates.[205] Similarly, in fetal and neonatal rats, the CFU-GM proliferative rate is high and appears to be near maximal at birth, even in the noninfected state.[208] Unlike in adult animals, no further increase in CFU-GM number or CFU-GM proliferative rate[208] has been detected during either sublethal or lethal bacterial infection, suggesting that the system operates at capacity. The concentration of CFU-GM in blood is higher in the fetus and newborn than that in adults: 20 to 300 CFU-GM/mL of venous blood in adults and approximately 2000 CFU-GM/mL in term neonates.[205,209,210] Even higher venous blood concentrations are found in prematurely delivered infants,[205,210] with the highest values noted in the most premature subjects.[205] The total body pool of CFU-GM has not been measured in human neonates; in rats, the number of CFU-GM/g body weight is small in the fetus ($0.5 \pm 0.1 \times 10^3$ CFU-GM/g) and increases to adult levels ($10.5 \pm 0.2 \times 10^3$/g) at 4 weeks of age.[211]

In the fetus, as in the adult, not only are mature neutrophils stored within the skeletal marrow, but they are also found in the liver and spleen. Techniques that measure the size of the neutrophil storage pool, such as radioisotopic iron labeling, with subsequent liver, spleen, and bone marrow biopsy, have not been applied to normal human neonates. In fetal and neonatal animals, however, the liver and spleen, as well as the long bones, can be removed, and the neutrophils within them can be quantified. Such studies in rats show that the neutrophil storage pool is considerably smaller in prematurely delivered animals (1.0-1.3×10^6 cells/g body weight) than in term (1.3-2.5×10^6 cells/g) and adult animals (4.5-7.5×10^6/g).[212]

During experimental bacterial sepsis in neonatal dogs and rats, the size of the neutrophil storage pool has been serially quantified. Experiments performed with a variety of organisms[208,213] demonstrate depletion of the storage pool and neutropenia before death. Similarly, in human neonates with lethal bacterial sepsis, neutropenia and depletion of the neutrophil storage pool, as assessed by bone marrow aspiration, are nearly universal findings.[204,214,215] Thus, limited storage pools and an inability to accelerate neutrophil production beyond their already high baseline levels predispose neonates (particularly premature newborns) to neutrophil depletion and sepsis with bacterial infection.

Neutrophil Circulating and Marginating Pools in the Newborn

Large fluctuations in the circulating pool of neutrophils are seen shortly after birth, with a marked rise in blood neutrophils occurring in the first 6 to 24 hours of life. Peak levels of circulating neutrophils are observed at 6 to 12 hours of life in term neonates (to an average of 16×10^3 cells/μL) which are followed by a decline to adult levels over the next 72 hours.[216] The neutrophil composition of the peripheral blood of the neonate also differs from adults, with high concentrations of immature neutrophils (metamyelocytes and bands) found immediately following delivery and then falling over the next 3 days.[216]

The Normal Hematologic System

Neutrophil Migration in the Newborn

Many investigators have demonstrated defective neutrophil chemotaxis in neonates. Early investigations using the Rebuck skin window technique in human neonates demonstrated that a preponderance of eosinophils, not neutrophils, was attracted to the abraded dermis. Using the same technique, studies demonstrated that neutrophils in neonates remained at the site of abrasion longer than they did in adults.[217] Using the Boyden chamber method, neutrophils from newborns were found to be less responsive than adult neutrophils in chemotaxis.[218] In addition, factors generated from neonatal serum attracted neutrophils less well than did factors from adult serum. Diminished chemotaxis of cord blood neutrophils was also demonstrated, with reduction to approximately 80% of levels observed with adult neutrophils.[219] In prematurely delivered neonates, neutrophil chemotaxis was even more defective,[220] and the defect persists for a considerable time after birth. A further reduction in chemotaxis of neutrophils from ill neonates compared with healthy neonates and decreased chemotaxis in preterm neonates with bacterial sepsis followed by a return to normal neonatal values (approximately 20% of adult values) with resolution of the infection have been reported.[221] Similar defects have been observed in animal studies, with reduced neonatal neutrophil migration in response to both sterile and infectious stimuli.[222,223] Finally, neutrophils from human neonates irreversibly aggregated after stimulation with either C5a or fMLP, whereas after exposure to the same stimulus, adult neutrophils aggregated and then deaggregated.[224,225]

Multiple differences between neonatal and adult neutrophils contribute to the reduced chemotaxis of the former.[226] For example, impairments in rolling and adhesion of neonatal neutrophils are due in part to reduced expression and shedding of L-selectin, which improves with fetal maturation.[227-229] In addition, neonatal neutrophils have diminished upregulation of CR3 in response to chemotactic stimulation, with adult levels not achieved until 11 months of age.[227] The neonatal vascular endothelium also has reduced ability to upregulate the expression of adhesion molecules following exposure to bacterial lipopolysaccharide (LPS),[228,230] and thus neonatal neutrophils have impaired transmigration through the vascular endothelium due to decreased CR3 as well as reduced chemokine and cytokine release from tissue neutrophils and macrophages.[231,232] Reduced mobilization of intracellular calcium in response to chemoattractants[233] and anomalies in cytoskeletal organization from delayed F-actin induction[234] also contribute to impaired neonatal neutrophil chemotaxis.

Of note, neonatal neutrophils display various functional variations compared to adult neutrophils in addition to reduced chemotaxis. For example, certain granule protein levels are reduced in neonates, including that of BPI, elastase, and lactoferrin.[235,236] In addition, neonatal neutrophils have reduced NET production capabilities compared with adult neutrophils, and they do so via a ROS-independent mechanism.[237,238]

CONTROL MECHANISMS REGULATING NEUTROPHIL PRODUCTION

It is evident that a true steady state of neutrophil kinetics exists only for brief periods. Shifts of cells between marginal and circulating sites may occur without changes in blood neutrophil turnover,[54] but any change in the TBGP size must result from changes in cell inflow or egress. Studies involving leukapheresis have shown that a normal animal replenishes a depleted TBGP by mobilizing cells from the marrow granulocyte reserves.[239] This increase in neutrophil concentration and TBGP size, like that seen with most bacterial infections or after endotoxin or steroid administration, must be triggered by some signal, and some means of stimulating cell production must be available to replenish depleted marrow reserves, whatever the etiology. The nature of these control mechanisms is complex, but several control points exist: recruitment of pluripotent stem cells and their induction into committed myeloid progenitors, stimulation (and perhaps inhibition) of stem cell and myeloid proliferative cell growth, and selective release of cells from the marrow.

Blood cell development is discussed in Chapter 5 and is only briefly discussed here. Pluripotent stem cells are mostly in the G_0 state and must be induced into actively proliferating committed stem cells. Hematopoietic cell growth and development are usually restricted to certain tissues (e.g., bone marrow in adult humans and bone marrow and spleen in mice), and cell differentiation is influenced by organ microenvironment (e.g., erythropoiesis is favored in mouse spleen, but granulocytopoiesis is favored in the bone marrow).

Growth Factors

A large number of growth factors or colony-stimulating factors have been identified that regulate neutrophil production in the bone marrow, as described in Chapter 5. Two of these, G-CSF and GM-CSF, are in clinical use. Exogenous administration of G-CSF expands the granulocyte mitotic pool and decreases the bone marrow transit time of the postmitotic cells without changing the blood neutrophil half-life.[240] G-CSF also markedly increases the release of neutrophils from the bone marrow by decreased bone marrow stromal production of CXCL12.[241] G-CSF not only accelerates the recovery of neutrophil counts after chemotherapy and may decrease associated infectious complications[242,243] but also has effects on mature neutrophils. For example, G-CSF transiently increases CD11b expression,[244] and decreases the surface expression of L-selectin.[245] G-CSF also primes neutrophils for subsequent superoxide production in response to fMLP.[246] Intravenous administration of G-CSF can result in an immediate transient neutropenia,[247,248] similar to the transient increase in the MGP. Evidence of neutrophil degranulation in vivo after administration of G-CSF has also been observed.[249] A number of other cytokines among this class can also activate or prime neutrophils, including TNF-α, IL-6, IL-1, and IL-8.[249-251] The rapid increase in neutrophil production associated with systemic bacterial infection largely reflects a marked increase in G-CSF production. Studies suggest that endothelial cells are the source of the majority of G-CSF production in this setting.[252]

In addition to locally produced stimulators of colony-forming unit stem cell proliferation, inhibitors of proliferation have also been described. Lactoferrin (present in the secondary or specific neutrophil granule) binds to specific receptors on some monocyte macrophages and suppresses release of GM-CSF (and other cytokines), thus inhibiting colony formation. Transferrin also exhibits colony-suppression activity, possibly through inhibition of GM-CSF production by T lymphocytes.[253] Soluble forms of receptors for cytokines may also regulate the response of bone marrow progenitors to growth factors.[254] Neural mechanisms controlling hematopoietic cell proliferation and release have also been demonstrated.[255] As described earlier, many neutrophils are removed in the bone marrow by macrophages via CXCR4, where the process produces a feedback inhibition of neutrophil production.[142,144,179,180]

NEUTROPHIL FUNCTION

The major role of neutrophils is to protect the host against infectious agents. To accomplish this task, the neutrophil must first sense infection, migrate to the site of the infecting organism, and then destroy the infectious agents. Although neutrophils can sense a stimulus in suspension, they can migrate only when in contact with a surface. Thus, although in some cases neutrophils in blood may respond to a stimulus by adhering to other blood cells or foreign bodies, such as bacteria or biomaterials, the usual first step of the neutrophil after sensing an inflammatory stimulus is to adhere more strongly to the blood vessel wall. Usually, this occurs in a postcapillary venule. After adhesion to the endothelial surface, the neutrophil follows a gradient of chemotactic factors to the site of infection and interacts with the organisms. Finally, when the neutrophil reaches the infecting organism, it must destroy it. This destruction is generally accomplished by phagocytosis of the agent followed by release of granules into the phagocytic vesicle, followed by killing of the organism. The mechanisms by which these phenomena occur are very complex and not completely understood.

Neutrophil Chemoattractants

The initial step of the neutrophil response to infection is the detection of an appropriate signal. The interaction of bacteria with blood components, especially antibodies and the complement system, results in the formation of various chemotactic factors. In some instances, the bacteria directly release factors that are chemotactic for neutrophils. The interaction of bacteria or their products with other host cells may also result in the formation of chemotactic factors. The chemotactic factors, or "chemoattractants," provide molecular guidance cues and signal via receptors on the neutrophil to regulate neutrophil trafficking.

Neutrophil chemoattractants belong to four biochemically distinct groups, including chemokines (e.g., CXCL1-CXCL3, CXCL5-CXCL8, CXCL12), chemotactic lipids (e.g., leukotriene B4 or LTB$_4$), formyl peptides (e.g., fMLP), and complement anaphylatoxins (C3a and C5a).[256,257] As described much later, these chemoattractants act through interaction with specific heptathelical G-protein–coupled receptor (GPCRs) on the neutrophil surface. Of note, the different types of chemoattractants, which display temporally and spatially distinct production patterns, appear to play complementary roles during neutrophil trafficking. Neutrophils respond to chemoattractants in a hierarchical manner. These guidance signals can thus be subdivided into "intermediary" and "endtarget" groups, with end target signals being dominant over intermediary chemoattractants.[257] The signaling pathways differ in some ways between these two groups of signals, with intermediary chemoattractants (which include chemokines and chemotactic lipids) signaling through PI3K and PTEN pathways and end target chemoattractants (including formyl peptides and complement anaphylatoxins) generally inducing p38 MAPK phosphorylation.[258]

Chemokines are a large family of chemotactic cytokines.[259] These proteins have four conserved cysteines that form two disulfide bonds. The chemokine family is composed of CXC and CC chemokines. The CXC chemokines have their first two cysteines separated by a single amino acid and stimulate neutrophils, whereas the CC chemokines do not. Among the chemokines, CXCL1 to CXCL3 and CXCL5 to CXCL8 are known intermediary signals for neutrophil chemotaxis, with CXCL8 being the most potent.[260] These chemoattractants are sensed by neutrophils through their receptors CXCR1 and CXCR2. Neutrophils can also be recruited by other chemokines such as CCL3 (also known as macrophage inflammatory protein-a, or MIP-1α) or CCL4 (MIP-ß) via interaction with the CCR1 receptor. In addition, CXCL12 is an important chemokine for the regulation of neutrophil bone marrow storage and release via its receptor CXCR4.[144]

Like the chemokines, lipid chemoattractants are among the intermediary signals for neutrophil chemotaxis. They are derived from arachidonic acid, and the most relevant chemoattractants of this class for neutrophils include leukotriene B4 (LTB4)[261] and PAF. LTB$_4$ is produced by myeloid cells in response to bacterial products (e.g., LPS), cytokines, or other chemoattractants. It interacts with two GPCRs known as BLT1 and BLT2,[262,263] and promotes neutrophil recruitment. PAF is produced by platelets and various immune cells in response to cytokines (e.g., IL-1, IL-6, IL-12, and TNF-a), as well as the hormones angiotensin II and endothelin. It interacts with its receptor PAFR to activate and polarize neutrophils.[264]

Formyl peptides (e.g., fMLP) are among the so-called pathogen-associated and damage-associated molecular patterns (PAMP and DAMPs), produced upon degradation of bacterial components or mitochondria. These chemoattractants were initially identified by studies of the observation that supernatants of bacterial cultures were chemotactic for neutrophils.[265] Subsequent studies identified a number of N-formyl peptides with chemotactic activity,[266] and it was hypothesized that the presence of such a receptor would provide a preimmune receptor for the neutrophil to sense bacterial infections, because bacterial protein synthesis begins with N-formyl methionine, whereas mammalian protein synthesis does not. Interestingly, mammalian mitochondria do synthesize N-formyl methionyl peptides, and these may in some cases also result in neutrophil activation. fMLP

signals through the formyl peptide receptors FPR1 and FPR2 on neutrophils, and is an "end target" chemoattractant promoting neutrophil migration via p38 MAPK activation.[267]

Complement anaphylatoxins are generated through splicing of complement precursors via either the classical, alternative, or lectin-mediated complement activation pathways. C5a is the most potent chemotactic anaphylatoxin,[268] and it signals through the C5aR1 receptor on neutrophils. Like fMLP, C5a is an end target chemoattractant, activating p38 MAPK and providing a strong neutrophil migratory stimulus.

As noted earlier, most chemoattractant receptors are GPCRs that transduce signals via guanine nucleotide–binding heterotrimeric G-proteins.[269] Activation of these GPCRs leads to the exchange of guanosine diphosphate (GDP) for guanosine triphosphate, which in turn leads to the dissociation of the heterotrimeric G-protein into a $G\alpha_i$ subunit and a $G_{\beta\gamma}$ dimer. The $G\alpha_i$ subunit then inhibits adenyl cyclase, reducing intracellular cyclic adenosine monophosphate concentrations. The $G_{\beta\gamma}$ dimer activates both PLCß and PI3Kγ. Activated PLCß then hydrolyzes phosphatidylinositol bisphosphate (PIP$_2$), resulting in the generation of two second messengers, IP$_3$ and 1,2-diacylglycerol, which promote the activation of protein kinase C (PKC). Activated PI3Kγ aids in the conversion of PIP$_2$ to phosphatidylinositol trisphosphate, which leads to the downstream activation of extracellular signal–regulated kinases and phosphokinase B (Akt).

Notably, chemoattractant signaling–induced generation of IP$_3$ promotes an increase in intracellular Ca2+. Experiments suggest that IP$_3$ binds to specific receptors on intracellular membranes, resulting in the release of calcium from intracellular stores, which is rapidly augmented by an influx of extracellular calcium. Thus, shortly after receptor-ligand binding, the intracellular calcium rapidly rises from a resting level of approximately 0.1 to 1 μmol/L.[270] This rise in free intracellular calcium is transient and returns to baseline in approximately 1 to 3 minutes. It appears that the initial rise in intracellular calcium caused by the release of intracellular calcium stores plays a critical part in the alteration of membrane permeability to allow the influx of extracellular calcium. To some extent, variations in intracellular calcium transients may direct specific cellular functions, in that specific granule release occurs at very low (submicromolar) free calcium concentrations, whereas in studies using permeabilized cells, higher (micromolar) levels of free calcium result in release of both specific and azurophilic granules.[271] Although the extracellular calcium influx is critical for many neutrophil responses, it is not critical for all, as degranulation is not blocked by ethylene glycol-bis(2-aminoethyl) tetraacetic acid.[272] Similarly, phagocytosis of particles opsonized with C3bi can occur without apparent intracellular calcium transients.[273]

Although this model of chemotactic signaling via GPCRs explains many observations, it has become clear that signal transduction in neutrophils is far more complex, with both Ca^{2+} and PKC-independent pathways. Tyrosine phosphorylation has been found to play a critical role in signal transduction from various chemotactic factor receptors. Multiple neutrophil proteins are rapidly phosphorylated after activation, including Src family kinases; the Lyn kinase is activated by chemotaxins, increasing its ability to phosphorylate substrates.[269,274] Serine and threonine kinases also appear to be involved in signaling, and some are activated by fMLP. Protein tyrosine phosphatases probably also play a role, as the transmembrane protein phosphatase CD45 has been implicated as a regulator of neutrophil function.[93,275] Chemotactic factors have also been found to activate phospholipase A$_2$ and phospholipase D. Finally, the importance of low-molecular weight guanosine triphosphatases is also being recognized.[276] Knowledge of neutrophil signal transduction is rapidly advancing, and the reader is referred to the current literature.

Finally, physiologic soluble inhibitors of neutrophil function have also been identified. For example, adenosine inhibits neutrophil aggregation, adhesion, chemotaxis, and superoxide production. These inhibitory effects appear to act via A$_2$ receptors without preventing the transient rise in intracellular Ca^{2+}.[277,278]

Neutrophil Priming

"Priming" is an important concept in neutrophil signaling. Signaling in neutrophils is complex and can be initiated by many different stimuli that may share downstream signaling pathways. When neutrophils are exposed to an appropriate low level of a stimulus, they can be primed to a condition such that they display a much more prominent response to a second stimulus than they would if they had not been primed.[3,71-73,279-282] Neutrophils can be primed by one stimulus for a response to a different agonist. Priming occurs at doses that do not result in a rise in cytoplasmic free calcium, but still cause protein tyrosine phosphorylation of signaling molecules. After priming, neutrophils exhibit a more prominent respiratory burst or secretory response to a given stimulus than that would occur if priming had not occurred. This phenomenon may be involved in many physiologic neutrophil responses in vivo. Neutrophil priming can be reversible, with the cells still capable of being reprimed.[282,283]

The mechanism of priming is gradually becoming better understood. In resting neutrophils, the various components of the nicotinamide adenine dinucleotide phosphate (NADPH) oxidase are sequestered within the cell. Following neutrophil stimulation, cytoplasmic components of the NADPH oxidase translocate to the phagosome membrane and assemble to form the active oxidase. This activation process is not "all-or-none." Some stimuli can prime neutrophils, resulting in a state in which agents that normally do not activate neutrophils can stimulate oxidase activity and in which the oxidase response to suboptimal concentrations of agents that do stimulate the oxidase results in a greater-than-expected oxidase response. For example, TNF-α does not stimulate neutrophil NADPH oxidase activity, but fMLP does. However, when neutrophils are pretreated with TNF-α, these primed neutrophils respond to suboptimal concentrations of fMLP with increased oxidase activity. The mechanism of neutrophil priming appears to be the result of a conformational change in p47phox.[282,284] TNF-α priming results in phosphorylation of ser354 in p47phox, which then binds the peptidyl prolyl *cis-trans* isomerase Pin1, resulting in conformational changes in p47phox that result in phosphorylation of other serine residues. This leads to other conformational changes exposing cryptic SH3 sites that can then bind p22phox, resulting in oxidase assembly, making the oxidase more responsive to stimuli.[282,284]

Desensitization

After previous exposure to a stimulus, neutrophils may react less to subsequent stimulation by the same stimulus.[285,286] This phenomenon has been termed *desensitization*. In some cases, the desensitization appears to be specific to the original stimulus, but in other cases, desensitization to different stimuli is also observed (cross-desensitization).[131,285,286]

Desensitization has been observed in patients undergoing hemodialysis, in which exposure of blood to a Cuprophane dialyzer membrane results in the generation of C5a and possibly other factors, which causes a transient neutropenia due to pulmonary leukostasis, as described in Chapter 60.[170,171] Although C5a generation persists throughout dialysis, the neutropenia is transient. In contrast to neutrophils obtained at the start of dialysis, neutrophils obtained after 2 hours of dialysis (after the leukostasis has resolved) do not aggregate in response to plasma leaving the dialyzer membrane, demonstrating desensitization in vivo.[173] A patient with cytomegalovirus infection, whose serum induced granulocyte aggregation (presumably due to C5a), did not experience neutropenia during dialysis, and his neutrophils did not aggregate in response to serum leaving the dialyzer, in contrast to control cells, also demonstrating in vivo desensitization.[173] A similar desensitization was demonstrated in rabbits using the chemotactic peptide fMLP, wherein continuous intravenous infusion of fMLP reproduced a transient neutropenia due to pulmonary sequestration.[287] Neutrophil desensitization may also occur in other pathologic states, including infection, trauma, and multiorgan failure syndrome, and may contribute to neutrophil dysfunction, although the clinical significance of this phenomenon is unclear.

The phenomenon of desensitization has been implicated as the mechanism by which glucocorticoids inhibit neutrophil function. The glucocorticoid-regulated protein annexin 1 (lipocortin 1) can bind a formyl-peptide receptor, induce calcium transients, and desensitize neutrophils to subsequent stimulation by other agents.[288,289] Two formyl-peptide receptors are expressed in neutrophils, the classical FPR1 and the related receptor FPR2. Annexin 1 can bind to FPR2, whereas some peptides derived from annexin 1 may bind both receptors.[288,289] Opiates have been reported to alter many immune functions, including neutrophil functions such as the respiratory burst, in many species,[290] and S00A9 (MRP-14), a prominent component of neutrophils, can inhibit the function of activated macrophages and, possibly by this mechanism, can decrease inflammatory pain.[291]

Neutrophil-Endothelial Cell Adhesion

Both neutrophils and endothelial cells express a variety of adhesive molecules on their cell surface, and the expression and activity of these molecules in many cases can be regulated by stimuli. Some of the known adhesion molecules of neutrophils and endothelial cells are indicated in *Table 7.7*. Approximately one-half of the circulating neutrophils exist in the so-called marginating pool, some of which can be seen microscopically to be rolling along the endothelial surface, maintaining a loose intermittent contact with endothelial cells. The importance of hemodynamic forces, especially of red cells, in directing leukocytes outward from the flowing blood toward the endothelium was described many years ago and subsequently confirmed.[8,292-294] An attractive model of neutrophil-endothelial cell adhesion has been proposed by Springer.[71,295] In this model, selectin molecules on the cell surface are responsible for neutrophil rolling along the vessel wall. This loose adhesion brings the neutrophil in close proximity to the endothelial cell, where chemoattractants can be released or displayed on the cell surface. The interaction of these chemoattractants with neutrophil receptors results in signal transmission and the activation of integrin molecules. These integrins can then bind their ligands on the endothelial cell surface, resulting in a marked increase in adhesion to the endothelial cell and cessation of rolling. After this, the cells sense further chemoattractant gradients and migrate into the tissue where the neutrophils produce compounds that attract other inflammatory cells such as monocytes, lymphocytes, and other neutrophils, as well as promote wound healing. Subsequently, they undergo changes promoting resolution of inflammation.[3,71-73]

Selectins

Three selectins have been identified, and each has an N-terminal domain that is homologous to $Ca^{(2)+}$-dependent lectins (*Figure 7.11*). L-selectin (CD62L) is expressed on the neutrophil surface. The main ligand for L-selectin is the glycoprotein known as *Gly-CAM-1* (glycosylation-dependent cell adhesion molecule-1). Endothelial cells express both E-selectin (CD62E, endothelial-leukocyte adhesion molecule-1) and P-selectin (CD62P, granule membrane protein-140). E-selectin and P-selectin both recognize Lewis^x-related sialylated carbohydrates, mostly on PSGL-1 (P-selectin ligand 1), and also L-selectin. Both PSGL-1 and L-selectin are localized on the tips of neutrophil microvilli, organized by the ERM proteins ezrin, radixin, and moesin, which connect to the actin cytoskeleton.[3,71-73] Expression of E-selectin on the endothelial cell surface can be induced with stimuli such as IL-1 and TNF but requires protein synthesis. In contrast, P-selectin (CD62P) is found in both the Weibel-Palade granules of endothelial cells and the platelet α-granule. Thus, stimulation of endothelial cells with the appropriate stimulus, such as thrombin or histamine, can result in a rapid mobilization of CD62P (P-selectin) to the endothelial cell surface.

Table 7.7. Neutrophil-Endothelial Cell Adhesion Proteins

Neutrophil Integrin		Ligand
$\alpha_L\beta_2$	Leukocyte function antigen-1, CD11a/CD18	ICAM-1 (CD54), CAM-2 (CD102) ICAM-3 (CD50)
$\alpha_M\beta_2$	HMac-1, CD11b/CD18	ICAM-1, iC3b, fibrinogen, factor X
$\alpha_X\beta_2$	p150,95, CD11c/CD18	? iC3b, fibrinogen?
Neutrophil Selectins		**Ligand**
L-selectin	CD62L, leukocyte adhesion molecule-1, Mel-14	Sialylated carbohydrates related to sLe^x (CD15s) and sLe^a on Gly-CAM-1
Endothelial Selectins		**Ligand**
E-selectin	CD62E, ELAM-1	Sialylated carbohydrates
P-selectin	CD62P, granule membrane protein-140, platelet activation–dependent granule-external membrane protein	Sialylated carbohydrates including PSGL-1 on neutrophils
Endothelial Ig Family		**Ligand**
CD54	ICAM-1	CD11a/CD18, CD11b/CD18
CD102	ICAM-2	CD11a/CD18
CD31	PECAM-1	NB1/CD177, CD31
Neutrophil Ig Family		**Ligand**
CD31	PECAM-1	CD31
CD50	ICAM-3	CD11a/CD18
CD66a	CEACAM1 (biliary glycoprotein)	CD66a, CD66c, CD66e
CD66b	CEACAM8 (CGM6)	CD66c
CD66c	CEACAM6 (NCA-50/90)	CD66a, CD66b, CD66c, CD66e
Neutrophil Leukocyte		**Ligand**
Antigen-6 superfamily		
CD177	NB1	CD31 (PECAM-1)

Abbreviations: ELAM, endothelial-leukocyte adhesion molecule; ICAM, intercellular adhesion molecule; Ig, immunoglobulin; PECAM, platelet endothelial cell adhesion molecule; PSGL, P-selectin glycoprotein ligand; ?, not reported.

Integrins

Integrins are noncovalently associated heterodimers of α- and β-subunits, each of which has characteristic structural motifs (*Figures 7.12* and *7.13*). The major integrins of neutrophils are the β_2-integrins made up of $\alpha_L\beta_2$ (leukocyte function antigen-1, CD11a/CD18), $\alpha_M\beta_2$ (HMac-1, CD11b/CD18), and $\alpha_X\beta_2$ (p150,95, CD11c/CD18).[296] Intercellular adhesion molecule (ICAM)-1 (CD54) expressed on the endothelial cell surface is a ligand for both CD11a/CD18 and CD11b/CD18. Other Ig superfamily members are probably also involved in neutrophil-endothelial cell adhesion, including platelet endothelial cell adhesion molecule-1 (CD31), ICAM-3 (CD50; expressed on the neutrophil but not on the endothelial cell), and the CD66 family of neutrophil activation antigens.

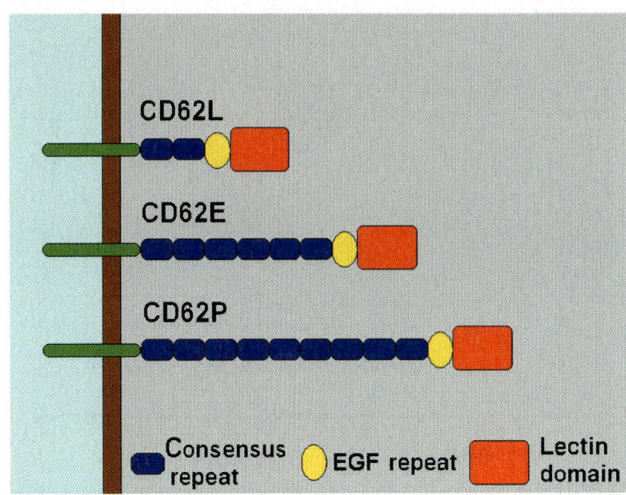

FIGURE 7.11 Schematic of selectin structure. The selectins are attached to the cell via a transmembrane domain with an extracellular domain consisting of a series of short consensus repeats (blue) that form a stalk-like structure linked by an EGF-like domain (yellow) to a carbohydrate-binding C-type lectin domain (red). CD62L contains a membrane-proximal site that is cleaved by a protease after neutrophil activation, resulting in shedding of the extracellular domain. EGF, epidermal growth factor. (From Skubitz A, with permission.)

Sequence of Neutrophil-Endothelial Cell Adhesion

In the Springer model, selectins are responsible for the initial rolling of the neutrophil along the endothelial cell. The association and disassociation constants of selectins for their ligands are very high, and stimulation of neutrophils can result in a rapid increase in L-selectin affinity for its ligand, resulting in tethering of a flowing cell and rolling within a millisecond.[295,297] This increase in affinity is transient, and by 5 minutes after stimulation, much of the L-selectin is shed from the neutrophil surface. The close interaction of the neutrophil with the endothelial cell surface, mediated by the selectins, allows the neutrophils to sense chemoattractants released from or displayed on the endothelial surface. As discussed earlier, these chemoattractants bind to specific receptors on the neutrophil surface, many of which span the membrane seven times, are coupled with G-proteins, and result in transduction of signals that activate integrin-adhesive activity (*Figure 7.13*).

Integrins form a family of adhesive molecules whose affinity for ligand can be rapidly regulated. Stimulation of neutrophils with *N*-formyl peptides or C5a results in rapid upregulation of CD11b/CD18 expression on the neutrophil surface. This increase in expression is

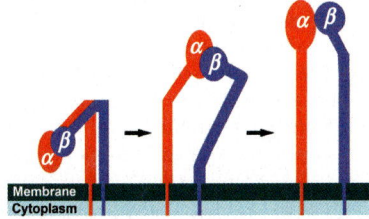

FIGURE 7.12 Schematic of an α,β2-integrin dimer, showing the inactive, low-affinity state (left) and the active, high-affinity state (right). Integrins are heterodimers of α- and β-subunits with a globular "head" region and two "legs." The head of the α-subunit contains EF hand repeats that are divalent metal-binding sites, and a "β propeller" domain with an I domain that contains a binding site for $Mg^{(2)+}$ and $Mn^{(2)+}$. The β-subunit contains an I-like domain. In the low-affinity, inactive state with no ligand bound, the integrin is either bent toward the membrane with a closed headpiece facing toward the membrane or extended with a closed headpiece. With activation, the integrin straightens and rotates the head region outward and the headpiece opens, with an associated change to higher ligand affinity. This change in structure is associated with a separation of the α- and β-subunits. (From Skubitz A, with permission.)

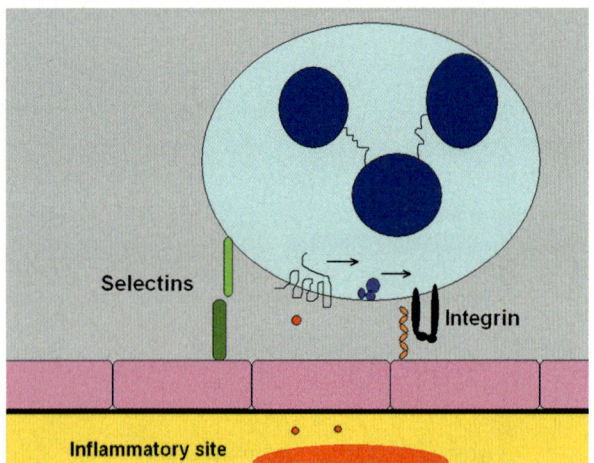

FIGURE 7.13 Neutrophil adhesion to inflamed endothelium follows three sequential steps. First, selectin molecules (green) that recognize carbohydrate ligands bind their ligand and result in tethering and rolling along the vascular wall, bringing the neutrophil in close proximity to the endothelial cell surface. Neutrophils express both CD62L and PSGL-1, and endothelial cells express CD62P and CD62E (P-and E-selectin). Chemotactic agents (red balls) released from the site of inflammation (red) and bound to or released from the endothelial cell surface interact with specific receptors that span the neutrophil membrane seven times and transduce activation signals via G-proteins (purple) that activate integrins (black). These integrins then bind their ligands (immunoglobulin superfamily members, orange) on the endothelial cell surface, resulting in arrest of the neutrophil and subsequent transmigration across the endothelial surface and subsequent chemotaxis to the site of chemoattractant production. (From Skubitz L, with permission.)

caused by fusion of secretory vesicles with the cell membrane. With strong stimulation, it is possible that secondary/tertiary granule fusion contributes as well. However, mere translocation to the cell surface with an increase in cell-surface expression of CD11/CD18 is not sufficient for an increase in adhesiveness. Similarly, studies of cytoplasts have demonstrated that alterations in β_2-integrin–mediated cell adhesion can be manifest without a change in surface expression of CD11b/CD18. Data suggest that alterations in CD11b/CD18-mediated cell adhesiveness are the result of a conformational change of the integrin, causing an alteration in ligand binding.[129,298] Studies have shown that, after activation of neutrophils by chemoattractants, approximately 10% of the surface CD11b/CD18 molecules express an activation epitope recognized by a monoclonal antibody.[129] Cell-surface integrins are in equilibrium between three conformational states. The bent conformation has a closed headpiece, and the two extended conformations have either a closed or open headpiece. The extended open conformation has a much higher affinity for ligand and mediates integrin adhesion.[299,300] During the activation process, following the rise in intracellular calcium concentration, G-protein signaling recruits talins to bind an NPxY domain in the β-integrin chain, resulting in breaking a salt bridge and separation of the α- and β-chains, which results in the extension of the extracellular domain, opening the binding site and generating an intermediate affinity state. Subsequent binding of kindlin-3 to NxxY sites in the β-chain induces the high-affinity conformation.[300] Recent studies suggest that some neutrophil β_2-integrins may acquire an unextended yet high-affinity conformation that inhibits leukocyte adhesion.[301]

As presented in *Table 7.7*, several Ig superfamily members are expressed on endothelial cells and are ligands for leukocyte integrins. CD11b/CD18 binds to a specific site in the third Ig domain of ICAM-1. Leukocyte function antigen-1 (CD11a/CD18) binds to the N-terminal domains of both ICAM-1 and ICAM-2. Thus, the model for neutrophil adhesion and transmigration through vessel walls can be depicted as in *Figures 7.13* and *7.14*. The initial rolling of neutrophils along the vessel wall is mediated by selectins (L-selectin, E-selectin, and P-selectin), and their expression and affinity for ligand can be regulated by inflammatory stimuli. At sites of inflammation,

leukocyte rolling along the vessel wall is increased, and cells may become more closely apposed to the vessel wall, allowing better interaction with chemoattractants released from or presented on the surface of the endothelial cells. Interactions of these chemoattractants with the neutrophil then result in activation of integrin affinity for its ligand, with a resultant firm adhesion of the neutrophil to the endothelial cell surface. Subsequent migration of the neutrophil through the endothelial cell proceeds along the gradient of the chemotactic agent. Extravasation via a transcellular route (through the endothelial cells) has been demonstrated, and the endothelial cell may play a role in this process.[298,300,302] The relative contribution of transcellular and intercellular extravasation is unclear and may depend on the particular tissue and stimuli involved. The presence of multiple adhesion molecules and ligands on both the neutrophil and the endothelial cell, which may vary among endothelial cells in different environments, coupled with the array of chemoattractant agents that may be released locally, provides potentially high specificity for localizing the interaction of a particular type of cell within a particular endothelial environment, based on the large number of combinatorial adhesive molecule-ligand pair combinations available.[295]

This model is supported by elegant studies demonstrating that at physiologic shear stress, neutrophils form rolling adhesions on phospholipid bilayers containing P-selectin but not on those containing ICAM-1. Chemoattractants result in integrin-mediated adhesion to bilayers containing ICAM-1 under static conditions but not under shear conditions. In contrast, neutrophils rolling on bilayers containing both P-selectin and ICAM-1 respond to chemoattractants by spreading and becoming firmly adherent via an integrin-ICAM-1 interaction. Chemoattractants do not increase adhesion or rolling on bilayers containing P-selectin alone.[295] The process of migration through the vascular wall is more complex and not fully understood but involves active interaction by both neutrophil and endothelial cell and utilizes an array of additional adhesion molecules, including junctional adhesion molecules and CD99.[302-304]

The importance of these neutrophil-endothelial interactions to neutrophil recruitment to sites of injury or infection is underscored by the fact that loss of normal production or function of adhesion factors is associated with a group of rare autosomal immunodeficiency disorders known as leukocyte adhesion defects (LADs).[305] These disorders are characterized by blood leukocytosis, nonhealing ulcers, and an absence of pus formation at sites of infection. Loss-of-function mutations in the *ITGB2* gene, encoding CD18, lead to LAD-1.[306] LAD-II results from loss of function mutations in the *SLC35C1* gene, which encodes for a Golgi-localized GDP-fucose transporter. In this disorder, defective fucosylation of selectin ligands leads to defective leukocyte rolling.[307] LAD-III results from mutations in *FERMT3*, which encodes KINDLIN3, an adaptor protein important for integrin activation.[308]

Feedback systems also exist that can inhibit neutrophil rolling and adhesion to endothelial cells (*Figure 7.15*). The pentraxin PTX3 is stored in specific granules. PTX3 can not only bind pathogens and activate complement but can also inhibit neutrophil recruitment to inflammatory sites. Neutrophils can release PTX3 from specific granules, and PTX3 can then bind P-selectin on endothelial cells. The binding of PTX3 to P-selectin inhibits P-selectin binding to PSGL-1 on neutrophils, thus inhibiting rolling.[309] Endothelial cells can release the glycoprotein Del-1, which can bind CD11a/CD18 on neutrophils. Del-1 binding to CD11a/CD18 inhibits CD11a/CD18 binding to ICAM-1, inhibiting neutrophil adhesion.[310,311] CD11/CD18 complexes can also be shed by neutrophils and may further regulate neutrophil function in inflammation.[312]

Neutrophil Aggregation

The increase in polymorphonuclear neutrophil adhesion after stimulation is manifest not only by increased adhesion to endothelial cells but also by neutrophil-neutrophil and neutrophil-platelet adhesion. Although the in vivo formation of neutrophil aggregates was clearly visualized in a rabbit ear model of inflammation in the 1950s,[313] the possibility of neutrophil homotypic aggregation was

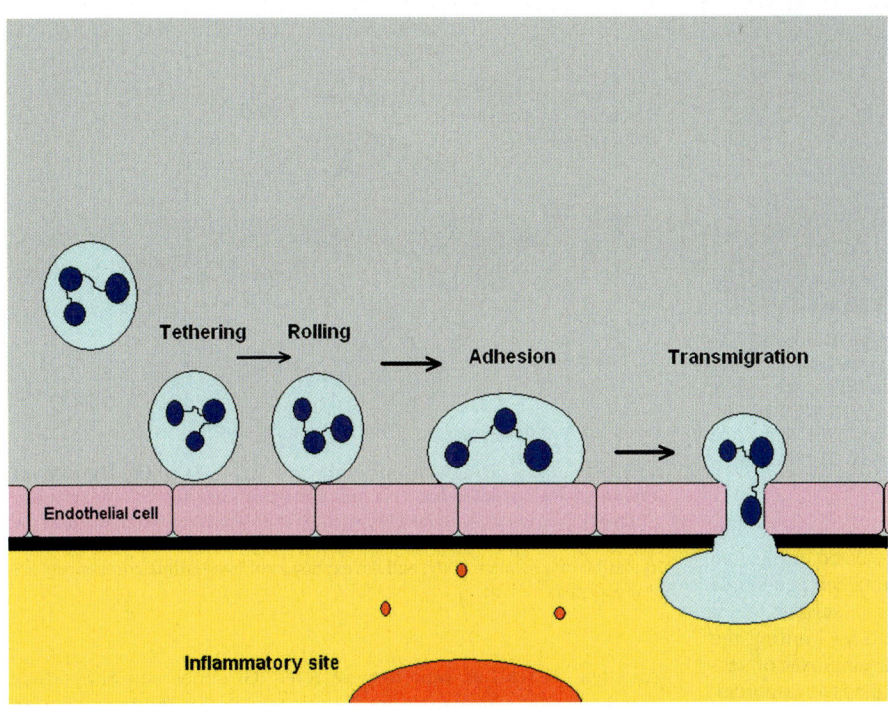

FIGURE 7.14 **Neutrophil adhesion to the vascular wall at a site of inflammation.** Sequential interactions of neutrophils with selectins result in rolling along the vascular wall, followed by sensing chemoattractants (red balls), which activate integrins to cause increased adhesion to the endothelial cells, followed by transmigration through the endothelial cells and basement membrane, followed by chemotaxis to the site of inflammation. (From Skubitz L, with permission.)

considered novel when it was formally demonstrated by Craddock et al.[170,171] Craddock's observations stemmed from earlier descriptions of the phenomenon of hemodialysis neutropenia.[169] The initiation of hemodialysis, using Cuprophane membranes, is followed by a rapid fall in the circulating neutrophil count caused by a transient sequestration of neutrophils in the lung, with a return to the circulation by 1 hour.[169] Craddock demonstrated that neutrophils undergo homotypic aggregation in response to plasma that had been exposed to Cuprophane, largely because of generation of C5a by complement activation.[170-172] Aggregation was also induced by other neutrophil stimuli. Further studies demonstrated that the transient nature of hemodialysis neutropenia was caused by desensitization of neutrophils to the continued infusion of stimulus from the hemodialysis machine, thus demonstrating in vivo the phenomenon of desensitization.[173] This phenomenon, in some clinical situations (e.g., viral infections), may result in neutrophil dysfunction as described later in this book.

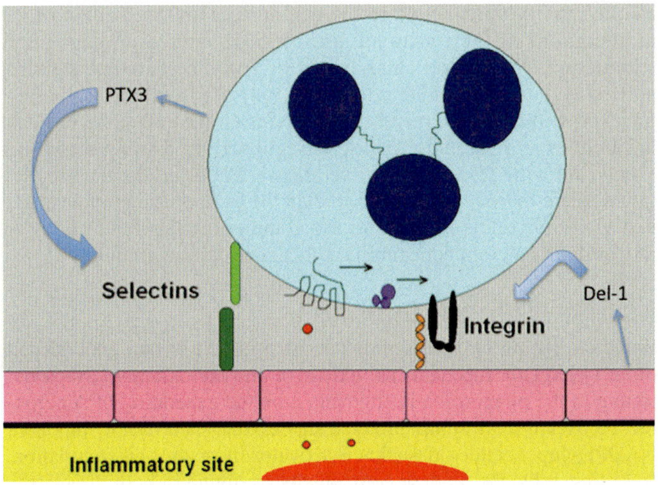

Chemotaxis

The work of von Recklinghausen and Cohnheim described amoeba-like movement of leukocytes more than a century ago.[8] Although the mobility of neutrophils and their concentration in inflammatory lesions were appreciated in early experiments, the development of a two-compartment chamber separated by a leukocyte-permeable membrane permitted quantitation of chemotaxis in vitro and facilitated the investigation of chemotactic factors.[314] Such studies revealed that neutrophils show directional migration under the influence of chemotactic agents, but a concentration gradient is needed for migration to occur. Even in the absence of a gradient, however, in the presence of a chemotactic factor, random migration is enhanced, and localization, or trapping, of the phagocytes occurs.

The neutrophil moves on a surface through a gradient of chemotactic agent by advancing a projection called a *lamellipodium* or *pseudopodium* at the front of the cell. This occurs where the submembranous actin filament network (the cortex) becomes less filamentous. As the cell moves, the pseudopodium ruffles rapidly. Part of the pseudopodium adheres to the underlying surface, and the contents of the cell move forward into the pseudopodium, making it less prominent. This cycle is then repeated with the protrusion of another pseudopodium. Chemotaxis occurs by repetitions of this process, although often the process is so well coordinated as to appear as a continuous gliding motion. The mechanism of these cell movements involves alterations in the polymerization state of actin, regulated by several proteins including the actin-binding protein, gelsolin, and others, as well as adenosine triphosphate–dependent contraction of the actin network mediated by myosin.[315,316] Local contraction of the cytoskeleton moves intracellular components forward into an area where the cortical gel has weakened because of shortening of actin filaments beneath the surface of the advancing pseudopodium. Characteristic contraction waves have been observed in human leukocytes and likened to those seen in amoebae and earthworms (*Figure 7.16*).[32] In leukocytes, the contraction wave appears to originate in the superficial layer of the submembranous organelle-excluding region called the *cortex*, producing a concave area, and the anterior part of the cell stretches or

FIGURE 7.15 **Feedback mechanisms inhibit neutrophil recruitment to inflammatory sites.** Neutrophils can release PTX3 from specific granules, and the PTX3 can then bind P-selectin (CD62P) on endothelial cells. The binding of PTX3 to CD62P inhibits CD62P binding to PSGL-1 on neutrophils, thus inhibiting rolling. Endothelial cells can release the glycoprotein Del-1, which can bind CD11a/CD18 on neutrophils. Del-1 binding to CD11a/CD18 inhibits its CD11a/CD18 binding to ICAM-1, inhibiting neutrophil adhesion. (From Skubitz L, with permission.)

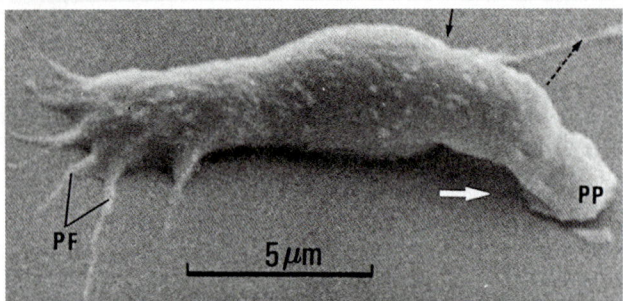

FIGURE 7.16 Scanning electron micrograph of a moving neutrophil. The contraction wave is observed as a concave (black solid arrow) and a convex (black dashed arrow) area. The advancing pseudopodium (PP) is seen being pushed out in the direction of movement (white arrow). Pseudoflagellae (PF) are seen in the rear of the cell. (Reprinted from Senda N, Tamura H, Shibata N, et al. The mechanism of the movement of leucocytes. *Exp Cell Res.* 1975;91(2):393-407. Copyright © 1975 Elsevier. With permission.)

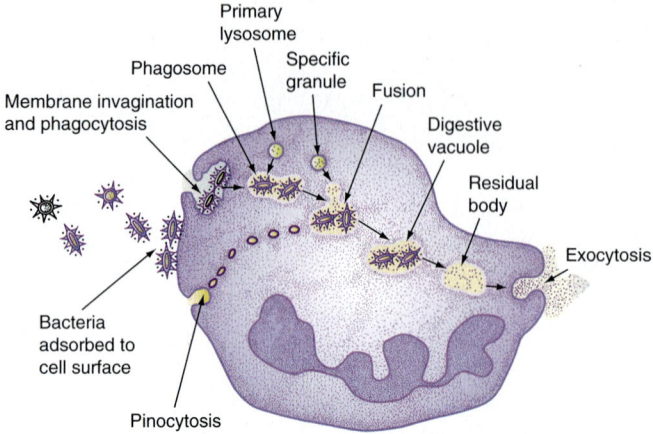

FIGURE 7.17 Diagram of endocytosis; both phagocytosis of immunoglobulin-coated bacteria and pinocytosis are shown. The fusion of a primary lysosome and a specific granule with the phagosome to form the digestive vacuole, the subsequent degradation of the bacteria leading to the formation of a residual body, and the expulsion of indigestible components are also depicted.

is propelled forward as a pseudopodium.[32] How localized changes in the state of actin assembly are established and maintained at a single site in neutrophils during chemotaxis is unclear. Data suggest that a change in plasma membrane tension is the main factor limiting the spread of the leading front and suppressing the development of secondary fronts.[317] While integrin-mediated adhesion plays an important role in migration on a two-dimensional surface, and in crossing tissue barriers such as the endothelium, integrins may be less important in interstitial migration. In studies of migration in three-dimensional environments, elimination of all integrin heterodimers in mouse leukocytes did not affect migration. Thus, the migration in this system was shown to be due solely to the force of changes in the actin network.[315]

Interestingly, mice that express no gelsolin can breed in captivity and have a prolonged bleeding time and abnormal neutrophil chemotaxis.[316] Thus, gelsolin is important in neutrophil chemotaxis, but other proteins can compensate to some extent in its absence. The increase in free calcium that alters the cytoskeleton by activating gelsolin, and thereby decreasing filamentous actin with a resultant decrease in viscosity, may play a role in locomotion; in addition, the transient dissolution of the submembranous cytoskeletal network may allow closer contact of intracellular granules with the plasma membrane, facilitating granule fusion and release.

Phagocytosis

Following their chemotaxis to sites of inflammation, neutrophils come in contact with the foreign material, engulf it, and subject it to the microbicidal and digestive enzymes they contain. This sequence, known as phagocytosis (*Figure 7.17*), was appreciated by Metchnikoff in the 1880s,[10] when he observed the migration of phagocytes into areas of tissue damage in sponges and lower animals. How phagocytes distinguish foreign particles and damaged autologous cells from normal self-components is complex, but this capacity is critical to effective phagocytic function.

Upon encountering a foreign particle or cellular debris, the neutrophil envelops it with pseudopodia, which fuse around it, forming a phagosome that rapidly fuses with azurophilic and specific granules. *Endocytosis* is the process by which material is taken into a cell enclosed within pieces of plasma membrane and therefore never occurs free within the cytoplasm of the cell.[318] Endocytosis is further divided into pinocytosis (drinking by cells) and phagocytosis (eating by cells). Phagocytosis is usually visible by light microscopy, whereas pinocytosis is not, involving ingestion of small particles, such as macromolecules. Both processes proceed through invagination of the cell membrane and the formation of vesicles or vacuoles (phagosomes).

Granule Release

Neutrophils contain four well-defined types of intracellular granules, including azurophilic, specific, gelatinase, and ficolin-1–rich

granules, as well as secretory vesicles. Granules can either fuse with a nascent phagosome to destroy ingested pathogens, or with the plasma membrane, resulting in the release of their contents extracellularly.[66] The azurophilic granules contain many antibacterial compounds, and the fusion of these granules with phagocytic vesicles is important in bacterial killing. Azurophilic granules also contain compounds, such as elastase, that may alter locomotion by hydrolyzing certain extracellular matrix components.[66] The specific granules are more readily released from the cell, suggesting an important function in the extracellular milieu. For example, specific granules contain products that activate the complement cascade.[319] Collagenase may be important in hydrolyzing extracellular matrix proteins and facilitating locomotion. Apolactoferrin, which binds iron, may exert an antibacterial effect by depriving bacteria of iron, altering hydroxyl radical formation, and altering cell adhesion.[76] The gelatinase granules contain gelatinase in addition to other components, and, like collagenase, this enzyme may play a role in extracellular matrix remodeling during locomotion.[81] Finally, both gelatinase granules and the secretory vesicles contain membrane proteins that can be rapidly upregulated to the cell surface and may play a role in alterations of the functional use of these surface proteins after stimulation. Membrane components of specific granules are also upregulated during granule release and may play a role in regulating the expression of these membrane proteins on the cell surface. Each different type of granule release is regulated by distinct signaling events, allowing for their selective release. For example, the specific granules are more readily released than the azurophilic granules, and exocytosis of gelatinase and specific granules is triggered by a lower intracellular calcium concentration than azurophilic granules.[271]

Bacterial Killing and Digestion

Bacterial killing by neutrophils can be ascribed to two general and often synergistic mechanisms: oxidative and nonoxidative. Bacterial killing in the phagosome is augmented by the generation of superoxide. Activated neutrophils produce superoxide via a multicomponent NADPH-dependent oxidase that is activated by neutrophil stimulation. In resting cells, the oxidase components are found in both the plasma membrane and intracellular stores. After stimulation, intracellular components are translocated to the plasma membrane and activated, producing superoxide. Subsequent reactions result in the formation of H_2O_2 and hypochlorous acid (HOCl), which increase bacterial killing. Small amounts of other species (such as singlet oxygen and hydroxyl radical) may also form but are probably of little importance in bacterial killing.

Table 7.8. *Antimicrobial Systems of the Neutrophil*

Oxygen-Dependent
Myeloperoxidase-mediated
Myeloperoxidase-independent
H_2O_2
Superoxide
Oxygen-Independent
Acid
Lysozyme
Lactoferrin
Defensins
Bactericidal permeability-increasing protein

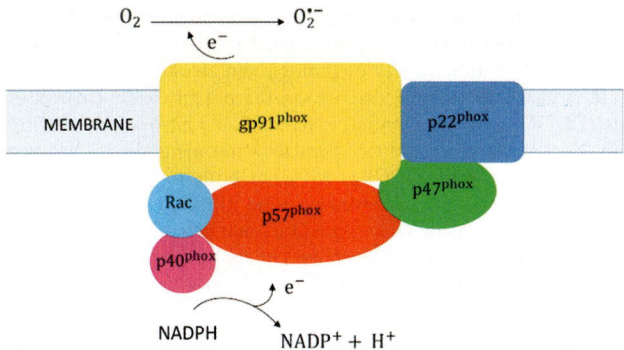

FIGURE 7.18 Model of assembled NADPH oxidase. In the activated phagocyte, the cytosolic components associate at the phagosomal or plasma membrane. With stimulation of the cell, RacGDP dissociates from RhoGDI and undergoes guanine nucleotide exchange, and the RacGTP associates with the membrane and gp91^{phox} (also termed NOX2). p47^{phox}, released from its autoinhibited conformation by multiple phosphorylations in the polybasic region, associates with p22^{phox} and the target membrane, and p67^{phox} associates with RacGTP. The active complex transfers electrons from the cytoplasm to the membrane surface where superoxide is generated. To compensate for the resulting change in membrane potential, protons cross the membrane via specific proton channels. NADPH, nicotinamide adenine dinucleotide phosphate. (Adapted by permission from Springer: Nauseef WM. Assembly of the phagocyte NADPH oxidase. *Histochem Cell Biol.* 2004;122(4):277–291. Copyright © 2004 Springer-Verlag.)

Bacterial killing decreases under anaerobic conditions, whereas phagocytosis does not, so the respiratory burst is important to bactericidal activity. Furthermore, because chronic granulomatous disease is one of the most severe clinical disorders characterized by a defect in bacterial killing, and the defect in this disorder is an inability to develop all of the reactions associated with the respiratory burst, the oxygen-dependent mechanisms appear to be of major importance in bacterial killing.[320-324] However, other bactericidal mechanisms that do not require oxygen also operate within phagocytes (*Table 7.8*).

Oxygen-Dependent Antimicrobial Systems

Neutrophil activation is accompanied by a prominent increase in O_2 use called the *oxidative burst* or *respiratory burst*, described by Baldridge and Gerard in 1932.[321] In 1964, Rossi and Zatti suggested that the respiratory burst is due to an NADPH oxidase,[322] and in 1973, Babior et al reported the production of superoxide by the NADPH oxidase.[323] The oxidative burst is a series of metabolic events that take place when phagocytes are appropriately stimulated, resulting in an increase in oxygen consumption, the production of superoxide (O_2^-), the production of H_2O_2, and an increase in glucose oxidation via the hexose monophosphate shunt.[323,324] Most of the oxidative burst is caused by activation of an NADPH oxidase that catalyzes the one-electron reduction of oxygen to superoxide, using the electron donor NADPH.[323,324]

The NADPH oxidase exists in a latent state consisting of both membrane and cytosolic components in distinct subcellular compartments. Activation involves multiple steps, including assembly at the membrane of two membrane-bound components (gp91^{phox} [NOX2] and p22^{phox}), three cytosolic components (p40^{phox}, p47^{phox}, and p67^{phox}; the term *phox* indicates that the protein is a component of the phagocyte oxidase), and a low-molecular weight G-protein (rac) to form the membrane-bound oxidase complex[323,324] (*Figure 7.18*). The active complex transfers electrons from the cytoplasm to the membrane surface where superoxide is generated. To compensate for the resulting change in membrane potential, protons cross the membrane via specific proton channels. The activated oxidase is readily detected by nitroblue tetrazolium or cytochrome reduction or the production of chemiluminescence. Several mechanisms by which this series of oxygen-dependent reactions may kill bacteria have been postulated (*Table 7.8*). When stimulated by phagocytosis, reactive oxygen metabolites are found localized at the phagosome, and not on parts of the plasma membrane that are not involved in phagocytosis.[324] Although O_2^- has some antibacterial activity, most O_2^- is rapidly converted to H_2O_2 by dismutation, either spontaneously or catalytically by superoxide dismutase.

Of the microbicidal oxidants generated by the respiratory burst, O_2^- and H_2O_2 are not potent microbicides; rather, they function as starting materials to generate more potent oxidizing radicals, such as oxidized halogens and oxidizing radicals.[324]

MPO is present in high concentration in the azurophilic or primary granules of neutrophils and is released into the phagosome during granule-phagosome fusion. MPO, together with H_2O_2 generated during phagocytosis[325,326] and an oxidizable cofactor such as halide (e.g., Cl^- or Br^-), forms oxidized halogens that are potent antimicrobials effective against bacteria, fungi, viruses, mycoplasma, and tumor cells.[325] Several mechanisms that have been proposed to explain bacterial killing by this system include halogenation of the bacterial cell wall, oxidation of various bacterial components, the decarboxylation of bacterial wall amino acids,[320,323-325] and the generation of long-lived chloramines that have antimicrobial activity.[323-326] There is some evidence that reactive nitrogen intermediates may also be produced.[327] Regardless of the mechanisms of killing, the fact that azide inhibition of MPO greatly decreases the microbicidal activity of normal leukocytes provides strong evidence for the importance of this system.[323,324] In patients with MPO deficiency (which is often quantitative rather than qualitative), the activity of other antimicrobial systems is increased, thus partially compensating for the MPO deficiency.[325] This finding may explain the increased susceptibility to infection in only approximately 20% of MPO-deficient patients.[328]

The combination of MPO, halide, and H_2O_2 is efficient in killing bacteria at H_2O_2 concentrations as low as 10 μm, whereas H_2O_2 in the absence of MPO requires 0.5 mmol/L or greater levels to produce similar killing.[323,324] Thus, H_2O_2 alone is a weak antimicrobial. H_2O_2 at high concentrations (>0.5 mmol/L) has antimicrobial activity in the absence of MPO.[320,325] Some organisms are more sensitive than others to H_2O_2, and this sensitivity may depend in part on their ability to degrade it (i.e., catalase or peroxidase content). Certain substances such as iodide or ascorbic acid may enhance the bactericidal action of H_2O_2 or render organisms more sensitive to still other killing mechanisms, such as lysozyme.[320,325]

After the discovery that O_2^- was generated in phagocytes, some authors postulated that O_2^- itself might be microbicidal. The microbicidal activity of O_2^- appears to be weak, however, when compared to that of the H_2O_2 formed from it, especially if MPO is present. Superoxide by itself has minimal bactericidal activity.[320,323-325]

Nitric oxide synthase has been found in primary granules of resting neutrophils, and nitric oxide can be synthesized from arginine by the inducible NO synthase.[329-332] Nitric oxide may interact with neutrophil-derived oxidants to yield other relevant oxidant species, though its role in neutrophil function is unclear.[325] Nitric oxide can react with superoxide to produce reactive nitrogen intermediates that can react with a variety of biologic targets. For example, nitric oxide reacts with superoxide to form the potent oxidant peroxynitrate ($ONOO^-$). MPO potentiates NO-mediated nitrosation.[333] Nitrite (NO_2^-), a major end product of nitric oxide metabolism, has been found to interact with HOCl or MPO, or both, to form nitryl chloride (NO_2Cl) and thus promotes tyrosine nitration.[327,329] Activated neutrophils can convert NO_2^- to NO_2Cl and NO_2 through an MPO-dependent pathway and inactivate endothelial angiotensin-converting enzyme.[327] Thus, neutrophil generation of nitrating and chlorinating species may play important physiologic roles.

Oxygen-Independent Antimicrobial Systems

Because an anaerobic environment does not abolish antimicrobial activity, other mechanisms must be operative, and several have been identified, including the effects of acid, lysozyme, lactoferrin, defensins, cationic proteins, and neutral proteases. The delivery of the wide array of antibacterial compounds to the phagosome by fusion with azurophilic and specific granules generally results in bacterial killing caused by the direct actions of the granule contents. In addition, these effects are potentiated by the acidification of the phagosome, caused partly by the granule contents themselves, as well as by active translocation of H^+ ions into the phagosome by ion pumps. The effectiveness of these mechanisms in the absence of superoxide production is demonstrated by both bacterial killing in anaerobic environments and killing by cells from patients with chronic granulomatous disease, in which catalase-positive organisms have an advantage over catalase-negative species. Nonoxidative killing is of obvious importance in hypoxic environments such as an abscess.

After particle ingestion, the intraphagosomal pH has been reported to decrease to between 3.0 and 6.5.[334,335] Some organisms, such as pneumococci, are sensitive to an acidic pH, whereas others tolerate acid environments without damage. In addition, the acidic environment may enhance the effect of lysosomal hydrolytic enzymes, most of which have optimal activity at acidic pH.

Prominent among the cationic neutrophil granule proteins are the defensins. These small microbicidal peptides kill a variety of bacteria, fungi, and viruses.[68] Defensins exert their effects by forming voltage-dependent ion channels. They are present in very high concentration compared to other stored antibacterial peptides (about 5% of total neutrophil weight).

Lysozyme, a low-molecular weight (14,500 Da) basic protein, is present in both primary and secondary neutrophil granules and is capable of hydrolyzing the cell wall of certain bacteria. Most organisms are resistant to the direct action of lysozyme,[320] although they may become sensitive to its action after exposure to antibody and complement or to H_2O_2 and ascorbic acid.[320] Usually, bacterial death appears to precede the action of lysozyme, so its action may be mostly digestive. The leukocytes of Guernsey and Hereford cattle contain no lysozyme but kill organisms normally.[336]

Lactoferrin is a microbiostatic protein (molecular weight 77,000 Da) that is found in the specific granules of neutrophils as well as in many secretions (e.g., milk and mucus) and exudates. It inhibits bacterial growth by binding the essential nutrient iron (two atoms per molecule), and, in contrast to transferrin, this property is maintained at the low pH values encountered in exudates. A synergistic relationship between lactoferrin and other antimicrobial systems may exist, and lactoferrin may be bactericidal for some organisms.[337]

BPI has antibacterial activity against certain gram-negative bacteria.[74] It also has the property of neutralizing the toxic effects of endotoxin.

Ficolins are soluble molecules that form part of the innate immune system. They can act as pattern recognition molecules and recognize carbohydrates on microorganisms and damaged cells. As part of the innate immune system, ficolins can bind a serine protease and activate the complement system via the lectin pathway. Ficolin-1 has been shown to be present in both gelatinase granules and a readily exocytosable gelatinase-poor granule (the ficolin-1–rich granule).[338] Ficolin-1 becomes associated with the surface membrane following stimulated release.

Other antibacterial granule components include azurocidin[70] and the serine proteinases elastase, cathepsin G, and proteinase 3.[339]

Digestion

Digestion of bacteria is demonstrated both by changes in the morphologic appearance of organisms after phagocytosis and by the release of labeled fragments of bacteria into the surrounding medium.[339] Digestion is thought to result from the action of the acid hydrolytic enzymes released into the phagosome from the primary lysosome. Metabolic blocking agents, such as iodoacetate, cyanide, and arsenite, which inhibit glycolysis and respiration, have no effect on digestion once the bacteria are within the cell.[340] Some bacteria ingested by neutrophils (e.g., certain pneumococci) may be killed and digested slowly, with the undigested material remaining as myelin or residual bodies.

Unsuccessful Ingestion, Killing, or Digestion

Phagocytosis and bacterial killing are not always completed successfully. Some organisms (e.g., certain virulent staphylococci) may survive and multiply within neutrophils and appear to kill them, thus overcoming the defense mechanism.[341] Still other materials ingested by neutrophils, such as the uric acid crystals of gout or the hydroxyapatite crystals of pseudogout, may cause a breakdown of the phagosome wall and release the hydrolytic enzymes into the cytosol. This action may be fatal to the cell, which then lyses and releases its enzymes into the surrounding tissues, where they cause tissue damage and secondary inflammation. In certain streptococcal and other infections, bacterial exotoxins (e.g., streptolysin) are released and damage the phagosomal membrane, thus killing the cell in a similar manner[342]; the infecting organism is freed in the process. Also, certain vitamins (vitamin A) and drugs, when incorporated into phagosomal membranes, render the membranes fragile and readily susceptible to rupture, thereby leading to inflammation.[342]

Secretory Functions of the Neutrophil

Two modes of neutrophil enzyme release or exocytosis are (1) release into phagocytic vacuoles (including release outside the cell during phagocytosis but before the phagosome is sealed off from the exterior of the cell, or release during attempted phagocytosis that cannot be completed because of particle size) and (2) granule content release that is not associated with phagocytosis, that is, true secretion. Whereas the contents of the neutrophil can be released passively as a result of cell lysis, a variety of substances probably are actively secreted by leukocytes in vitro.[3,71-73,88] Most of these substances have been shown to originate from the granule (including secretory vesicle) fraction. Specific granule contents (lactoferrin, B_{12}-binding protein, or both) are released before primary granule contents, and tertiary granules and secretory vesicles are secreted even more rapidly and completely, providing evidence for a differential secretion of granule contents. Because some of these substances are present in plasma normally and the concentration increases in patients with diseases involving the neutrophil system, some authors suggested that neutrophils may serve a secretory function as well as a phagocytic role in vivo.[343-345]

Among the well-studied released granule proteins are the B_{12}-binding proteins or transcobalamins. Granulocytes contain and actively release B_{12}-binding protein.[343] It appears that transcobalamin III is derived from granulocytes; it is unsaturated with B_{12}.[346] Markedly elevated transcobalamin I levels are seen in cases of chronic myelocytic leukemia and myeloid metaplasia; low values occur in patients with chronic leukopenia and aplastic anemia,[343] and good correlation with blood granulocyte pool size has been reported.[344]

Lysozyme is present in primary, secondary, and tertiary granules and is also present in monocytes, serum, and tears, and other secretions.[345,347] Increased concentrations in serum and urine are found in association with monocytic and myeloblastic leukemias. Although it was proposed that serum lysozyme may provide a measure of granulocyte turnover rate (GTR)[347]—lysozyme is present in several cell types, and the GTR does not correlate with serum lysozyme levels in neutropenic patients. In addition, the plasma kinetics of lysozyme do not mirror the kinetics of other neutrophil granule proteins or short-term alterations in the number of circulating neutrophils (in contrast to the kinetics of lactoferrin and gelatinase).[345]

Stimulated neutrophils also synthesize and release a variety of cytokines that may regulate the inflammatory response. For example, neutrophils stimulated with LPSs synthesize IL-1, TNF-α, and IL-1 receptor antagonist, whereas GM-CSF induces synthesis of TNF-α and IL-6. Neutrophil gene expression has two major peaks, one during marrow development when much of the granule content is synthesized and the other when the neutrophil leaves the circulation and enters tissues. On entering the tissue, neutrophils begin to synthesize cytokines and other proteins, including ones that might attract monocytes, lymphocytes, and other neutrophils, and assist in wound healing.[88] In general, diapedesis seems to induce an antiapoptotic state, whereas phagocytosis seems to promote apoptosis, at least partly by upregulating death receptors, thus providing the conditions for resolution of inflammation and avoidance of tissue damage.[88]

Some granule proteins originally viewed as primarily antimicrobial agents may have other effects as well. For example, neutrophil serine proteases may also play a regulatory role in granulopoiesis by antagonizing growth factor effects.[348-350] Mutations in neutrophil elastase result in many cases of cyclic and severe congenital neutropenia.[350] The defensins (HNP-1 to HNP-3) also can regulate lipoprotein metabolism by stimulating the binding of lipoprotein (a) and low-density lipoprotein to vascular cells and can regulate smooth muscle cell contraction.[351]

Immune Cross Talk of Neutrophils

Although historically viewed as cells with limited interaction with the rest of the immune system, recent studies have demonstrated a complex relationship between neutrophils and the adaptive immune system. Such a relationship was implied by the long-recognized fact that neutrophils are among the first to arrive at sites of infection or tissue injury, followed later by monocytes, macrophages, and lymphocytes. The current understanding is limited, but neutrophils can recruit mononuclear leukocytes, regulate macrophage activity, act as an antigen-presenting cell (APC), regulate T-cell differentiation and function, and may transport pathogens/antigens to draining lymph nodes.[3,71-73,88]

Upon reaching a site of inflammation, neutrophils release cytokines such as IL-1ß, signaling to macrophages and other resident cells to produce cytokines that then recruit more neutrophils.[3] Furthermore, leukotriene B4 (LTB4) production by neutrophils and tissue-resident cells promotes the recruitment of additional neutrophils into clusters or "swarms."[352] Within these swarms, neutrophils cluster around pathogens and necrotic tissue, forming a seal with late-recruited monocytes and macrophages to isolate the site of wounding or infection from surrounding viable tissue. Following the killing of invading pathogens and clearance of cellular debris, neutrophil-macrophage interactions promote tissue repair.[353] Macrophages engulf dying neutrophils in a process called efferocytosis, which is stimulated by the expression of "eat me" signals, such as phosphatidylserine and annexin-1, that enhance macrophage phagocytic activity.[354] This process, along with the neutrophil secretion of factors such as macrophage colony-stimulating factor-1 and IL-13, suppress macrophage production of pro-inflammatory cytokines to support the resolution of the inflammatory process.

In addition to migration directly to sites of infection or injury, neutrophils also travel to the spleen and draining lymph nodes where they help to orchestrate the adaptive immune response via interactions with B-lymphocyte and T-lymphocyte subsets. Populations of neutrophils colonize the perimarginal zone (MZ) of the spleen that displays B-cell-helper properties (so-called B-cell-helper neutrophils, N_{BH}).[355] These cells secrete B-cell regulatory factors such as BAFF, APRIL, and IL-21, and in doing so, they promote immunoglobulin class switching, somatic hypermutation, and T-cell–independent antibody production by MZ B cells.[355] Consistent with this role, patients with severe congenital neutropenias were found to have reduced titers of serum immunoglobulins to T-cell independent antigens.[355] Neutrophils also influence B cells in draining lymph nodes in the context of emergency granulopoiesis, where recruited neutrophils secrete BAFF and thus accelerate plasma cell generation and antibody production.[356]

Neutrophils and T cells reciprocally influence one another via contact-dependent and contact-independent mechanisms, and neutrophils can both activate and inhibit the functions of T cells.[357] Activating effects of neutrophils on T cells include both indirect and direct presentation of antigens, as well as activation via direct release of pathogen products. Dendritic cells take up antigens from dying neutrophils, and can then present these as APCs to T cells.[358] Neutrophils may also serve as direct APCs in some circumstances; for example, influenza-infected neutrophils cross-prime CD8+ T cells in an MHC-I–dependent manner.[359] Resting neutrophils do not activate naïve CD4+ T cells in mixed lymphocyte reaction; however, various inflammatory triggers can induce the acquisition of APC characteristics by neutrophils, stimulating the expression of MHC-II and costimulatory molecules.[360-362] Finally, the release of microbial metabolites (e.g., HMB-PP) following their ingestion by neutrophils can activate γδT cells.[363] On the other hand, proteases released during neutrophil degranulation (cathepsin G, elastase) inactivate the T cell-stimulating cytokines IL-2 and IL-6, and catalyze the shedding of their receptors on T cells, thereby inhibiting T-cell activation.[364,365] Similarly, ROS production and arginase release by neutrophils can downregulate TCRg on T cells and inhibit their proliferation.[138,366] Finally, IFNγ-stimulated PD-L1 expression on neutrophils promotes T-cell apoptosis.[367,368]

Neutrophils may also affect tumor growth via immune effects and effects on angiogenesis and may contribute to autoimmune diseases as well, including mediating insulin resistance in mice fed a high-fat diet,[369] though these topics are beyond the scope of this chapter.

Inflammasomes

Innate immunity is typically initiated by recognition of PAMPs, released by invading pathogens, and DAMPs, derived from damaged or dead cells, or in response to cellular stress.[304] IL-1β, a member of the IL-1β family of cytokines, is involved in many inflammatory responses. Toll-like binding to PAMPs results in transcription of the IL-1β precursor pro-IL-1β. Pro-IL-1β is processed by a multimolecular complex termed the *inflammasome*, which converts pro-caspase-1 to its active form, which then cleaves pro-IL-1β to IL-1β.[72] In neutrophils, LPS activates the caspase-1 inflammasome, resulting in IL-1β production.[370] Studies also suggest that other neutrophil proteases, including elastase, proteinase 3, and cathepsin G, can also process pro-IL-1β to its active form.[371] The inflammasome may be an important component of the regulation of gene expression in neutrophils when they extravasate into the tissue at sites of inflammation.

Tissue Damage by Neutrophils

Although neutrophils have multiple mechanisms to kill infectious agents, in some cases, normal host cells may be damaged by the same mechanisms.[372] For example, the tissue damage of acute respiratory distress syndrome, initiated by sepsis, TRALI, or similar events, appears to be largely neutrophil mediated. Neutrophils also appear to have an important role in rheumatoid arthritis, systemic lupus erythematosus, and other autoimmune diseases, as well as inflammation-associated thrombosis.[194,373,374]

Infections That Exhibit Tropism for Neutrophils

Human granulocytic anaplasmosis (previously known as human granulocytic ehrlichiosis) is a tick-borne zoonosis caused by *Anaplasma phagocytophilum*.[375,376] *A. phagocytophilum* is an obligate gram-negative intracellular bacterium that targets and replicates in neutrophils and their progenitors and is related to rickettsia. *A. phagocytophilum* may target neutrophils via α-(1,3) fucosylated PSGL-1, although it may also use other targets, and replicates in vacuoles that do not fuse with lysosomes, forming microcolonies that appear as morulae.[377] Human granulocytic anaplasmosis is an acute febrile illness accompanied by severe myalgias and headaches, usually occurring within 2 weeks of contact with ixodid ticks.[375] Common laboratory findings include leukopenia, thrombocytopenia, and increased transaminases. Although most patients respond promptly to doxycycline, death has been reported to occur in approximately 5% of reported cases, and complications such as pneumonia, renal failure, and central nervous system damage have been reported. Characteristic intracytoplasmic inclusions in neutrophils (morulae) are not always seen or recognized. Human granulocytic anaplasmosis is closely related to the veterinary pathogen *A. phagocytophilum* that infects granulocytes in cattle.

Francisella tularensis, a gram-negative bacterium that causes tularemia, can evade intracellular killing when ingested by neutrophils, in part by disrupting the respiratory burst.[377] In neutrophils infected with live *F. tularensis*, the NADPH oxidase assembly is disrupted and the cells do not generate reactive oxygen species. At the same time, *F. tularensis* also impairs neutrophil activation by heterologous stimuli. Later in infection, the bacteria can escape the phagosome, and persist in the neutrophil cytosol for at least 12 hours.[377]

References

1. Dale DC, Boxer L, Liles WC. The phagocytes: neutrophils and monocytes. *Blood*. 2008;112(4):935-945.
2. Majno G. *The Healing Hand: Man and Wound in the Ancient World*. Harvard University Press; 1975.
3. Kolaczkowska E, Kubes P. Neutrophil recruitment and function in health and inflammation. *Nat Rev Immunol*. 2013;13(3):159-175.
4. Hunter J. *A Treatise on the Blood, Inflammation and Gun-Shot Wounds*. Nicol; 1794.
5. Von Recklinghausen FD. *Die lymphgelfasse und ihre beziehung zum bindegewebe*. A. Hirschwald; 1862.
6. Rather LJ. *Addison and the White Corpuscles: An Aspect of Nineteenth-century Biology*. Cambridge University Press; 1972.
7. Cohnheim JF. Über entzuendung und Eiterung. *Arch für Pathol Anat Physiol für Klin Med*. 1873;40:179-264.
8. Burnett C, Conner PS, Dennis F, et al. *An American Text-Book of Surgery*. Saunders; 1892.
9. Ehrlich P. Methodologische beitrage zur physiologie und pathologie der verschisdenen formen der leukocyten. *Z Klin Med*. 1880;I:553-558.
10. Kaufmann SH. Immunology's foundation: the 100-year anniversary of the Nobel Prize to Paul Ehrlich and Elie Metchnikoff. *Nat Immunol*. 2008;9(7):705-712.
11. Evrard M, Kwok IWH, Chong SZ, et al. Developmental analysis of bone marrow neutrophils reveals populations specialized in expansion, trafficking, and effector functions. *Immunity*. 2018;48(2):364-379 e368.
12. Scott EW, Simon MC, Anastasi J, Singh H. Requirement of transcription factor PU.1 in the development of multiple hematopoietic lineages. *Science*. 1994;265(5178):1573-1577.
13. Heath V, Suh HC, Holman M, et al. C/EBPalpha deficiency results in hyperproliferation of hematopoietic progenitor cells and disrupts macrophage development in vitro and in vivo. *Blood*. 2004;104(6):1639-1647.
14. Hohaus S, Petrovick MS, Voso MT, Sun Z, Zhang DE, Tenen DG. PU.1 (Spi-1) and C/EBP alpha regulate expression of the granulocyte-macrophage colony-stimulating factor receptor alpha gene. *Mol Cell Biol*. 1995;15(10):5830-5845.
15. Wang QF, Friedman AD. CCAAT/enhancer-binding proteins are required for granulopoiesis independent of their induction of the granulocyte colony-stimulating factor receptor. *Blood*. 2002;99(8):2776-2785.
16. Johansen LM, Iwama A, Lodie TA, et al. c-Myc is a critical target for c/EBPalpha in granulopoiesis. *Mol Cell Biol*. 2001;21(11):3789-3806.
17. Skokowa J, Cario G, Uenalan M, et al. LEF-1 is crucial for neutrophil granulocytopoiesis and its expression is severely reduced in congenital neutropenia. *Nat Med*. 2006;12(10):1191-1197.
18. Liu Q, Dong F. Gfi-1 inhibits the expression of eosinophil major basic protein (MBP) during G-CSF-induced neutrophilic differentiation. *Int J Hematol*. 2012;95(6):640-647.
19. Ai Z, Udalova IA. Transcriptional regulation of neutrophil differentiation and function during inflammation. *J Leukoc Biol*. 2020;107(3):419-430.
20. Malengier-Devlies B, Metzemaekers M, Wouters C, Proost P, Matthys P. Neutrophil homeostasis and emergency granulopoiesis: the example of systemic juvenile idiopathic arthritis. *Front Immunol*. 2021;12:766620.
21. Friedman AD. Transcriptional regulation of myelopoiesis. *Int J Hematol*. 2002;75(5):466-472.
22. Dahl R, Walsh JC, Lancki D, et al. Regulation of macrophage and neutrophil cell fates by the PU.1:C/EBPalpha ratio and granulocyte colony-stimulating factor. *Nat Immunol*. 2003;4(10):1029-1036.
23. Kurotaki D, Yamamoto M, Nishiyama A, et al. IRF8 inhibits C/EBPalpha activity to restrain mononuclear phagocyte progenitors from differentiating into neutrophils. *Nat Commun*. 2014;5:4978.
24. Guo H, Ma O, Speck NA, Friedman AD. Runx1 deletion or dominant inhibition reduces Cebpa transcription via conserved promoter and distal enhancer sites to favor monopoiesis over granulopoiesis. *Blood*. 2012;119(19):4408-4418.
25. Shahrin NH, Diakiw S, Dent LA, Brown AL, D'Andrea RJ. Conditional knockout mice demonstrate function of Klf5 as a myeloid transcription factor. *Blood*. 2016;128(1):55-59.
26. Dahl R, Iyer SR, Owens KS, Cuylear DD, Simon MC. The transcriptional repressor GFI-1 antagonizes PU.1 activity through protein-protein interaction. *J Biol Chem*. 2007;282(9):6473-6483.
27. Yamanaka R, Barlow C, Lekstrom-Himes J, et al. Impaired granulopoiesis, myelodysplasia, and early lethality in CCAAT/enhancer binding protein epsilon-deficient mice. *Proc Natl Acad Sci USA*. 1997;94(24):13187-13192.
28. Morosetti R, Park DJ, Chumakov AM, et al. A novel, myeloid transcription factor, C/EBP epsilon, is upregulated during granulocytic, but not monocytic, differentiation. *Blood*. 1997;90(7):2591-2600.
29. Lekstrom-Himes J, Xanthopoulos KG. CCAAT/enhancer binding protein epsilon is critical for effective neutrophil-mediated response to inflammatory challenge. *Blood*. 1999;93(9):3096-3105.
30. Bainton DF, Ullyot JL, Farquhar MG. The development of neutrophilic polymorphonuclear leukocytes in human bone marrow. *J Exp Med*. 1971;134(4):907-934.
31. Rich AR, Wintrobe MM, Lewis MR. The differentiation of myeloblasts from lymphoblasts by their manner of locomotion - a motion picture study of the cells of normal bone marrow and lymph nodes, and of leukemic blood. *Bull Johns Hopkins Hosp*. 1939;65:291-309.
32. Senda N, Tamura H, Shibata N, Yoshitake J, Konko K, Tanaka K. The mechanism of the movement of leucocytes. *Exp Cell Res*. 1975;91(2):393-407.
33. Bainton DF, Farquhar MG. Origin of granules in polymorphonuclear leukocytes. Two types derived from opposite faces of the Golgi complex in developing granulocytes. *J Cell Biol*. 1966;28(2):277-301.
34. Orfanakis NG, Ostlund RE, Bishop CR, Athens JW. Normal blood leukocyte concentration values. *Am J Clin Pathol*. 1970;53(5):647-651.
35. Marsh JC, Boggs DR, Cartwright GE, Wintrobe MM. Neutrophil kinetics in acute infection. *J Clin Invest*. 1967;46(12):1943-1953.
36. Lewis WH. On the locomotion of the polymorphonuclear neutrophiles of the rat in autoplasma cultures. *Bull Johns Hopkins Hosp*. 1934;55:273-279.
37. Sabin FR. Studies of living human blood-cells. *Bull Johns Hopkins Hosp*. 1923;34:277-U241.
38. Fliedner TM, Cronkite EP, Robertson JS. Granulocytopoiesis. I. Senescence and random loss of neutrophilic granulocytes in human beings. *Blood*. 1964;24:402-414.
39. Arneth J. The neutrophile leucocytes during infectious illness. *Deut Med Wochenschr*. 1904;30:54-56.
40. Young CJ. Clinical interpretation of the Arneth count. *Br Med J*. 1935;2(3889):109-111.
41. Efrati P, Rozenszajn L. The morphology of buffy coat in normal human adults. *Blood*. 1960;16:1012-1019.
42. Haus E, Gy N, Lakatua D, Sackett-Lundeen L. Reference values for chronopharmacology. *Annu Rev Chronopharmacol*. 1988;4:333-351.
43. Haus E, Smolensky MH. Biologic rhythms in the immune system. *Chronobiol Int*. 1999;16(5):581-622.
44. Garrey WE, Bryan WR. Variations in the white blood cell counts. *Physiol Rev*. 1935;15:597-638.
45. Kennedy WP, Mackay I. The normal leucocyte picture in a hot climate. *J Physiol*. 1936;87(4):336-344.
46. Muchmore HG, Blackburn AB, Shurley JT, Pierce CM, McKown BA. Neutropenia in healthy men at the South Polar Plateau. *Arch Intern Med*. 1970;125(4):646-648.
47. Cress CH, Clare FB, Gellhorn E. The effect of anoxic and anemic anoxia on the leukocyte count. *Am J Physiol*. 1943;140:299.
48. Verzar F. Lymphocyte and eosinophil count in 1800 and 3450 m altitude. *Schweiz Med Wochenschr*. 1952;82(13):324-327.
49. Athens JW, Raab SO, Haab OP, et al. Leukokinetic studies. III. The distribution of granulocytes in the blood of normal subjects. *J Clin Invest*. 1961;40:159-164.
50. Farris EJ. The blood picture of athletes as affected by intercollegiate sports. *Am J of Anat*. 1943;72:223.
51. Gray AB, Telford RD, Collins M, Baker MS, Weidemann MJ. Granulocyte activation induced by intense interval running. *J Leukoc Biol*. 1993;53(5):591-597.
52. Altschule MD, Altschule LH, Tillotson KJ. Changes in leukocytes of the blood in man after electrically induced convulsions. *Arch Neurol Psychiatr*. 1949;62(5):624-629.
53. Samuels AJ. Primary and secondary leucocyte changes following the intramuscular injection of epinephrine hydrochloride. *J Clin Invest*. 1951;30(9):941-947.
54. Athens JW, Haab OP, Raab SO, et al. Leukokinetic studies. IV. The total blood, circulating and marginal granulocyte pools and the granulocyte turnover rate in normal subjects. *J Clin Invest*. 1961;40:989-995.
55. Milhorat AT, Small SM, Diethelm O. Leukocytosis during various emotional states. *Arch Neurol Psychiatr*. 1942;47:779.
56. Davis ME, Hulit BE. Changes in circulating eosinophils in women during the menstrual cycle and reproduction. *J Clin Endocrinol Metab*. 1949;9(8):714-724.
57. Nelson DH, Sandberg AA, Palmer JG, Tyler FH. Blood levels of 17-hydroxycorticosteroids following the administration of adrenal steroids and their relation to levels of circulating leukocytes. *J Clin Invest*. 1952;31(9):843-849.
58. John TJ. Leukocytosis during steroid therapy. *Am J Dis Child*. 1966;111(1):68-70.
59. Bishop CR, Athens JW, Boggs DR, Warner HR, Cartwright GE, Wintrobe MM. Leukokinetic studies. 13. A non-steady-state kinetic evaluation of the mechanism of cortisone-induced granulocytosis. *J Clin Invest*. 1968;47(2):249-260.

60. Hsieh MM, Everhart JE, Byrd-Holt DD, Tisdale JF, Rodgers GP. Prevalence of neutropenia in the U.S. population: age, sex, smoking status, and ethnic differences. *Ann Intern Med.* 2007;146(7):486-492.
61. Mpofu R, Otwombe K, Mlisana K, et al. Benign ethnic neutropenia in a South African population, and its association with HIV acquisition and adverse event reporting in an HIV vaccine clinical trial. *PLoS One.* 2021;16(1):e0241708.
62. Denic S, Showqi S, Klein C, Takala M, Nagelkerke N, Agarwal MM. Prevalence, phenotype and inheritance of benign neutropenia in Arabs. *BMC Blood Disord.* 2009;9:3.
63. Reiner AP, Lettre G, Nalls MA, et al. Genome-wide association study of white blood cell count in 16,388 African Americans: the continental origins and genetic epidemiology network (COGENT). *PLoS Genet.* 2011;7(6):e1002108.
64. Li J, Glessner JT, Zhang H, et al. GWAS of blood cell traits identifies novel associated loci and epistatic interactions in Caucasian and African-American children. *Hum Mol Genet.* 2013;22(7):1457-1464.
65. Lakhotia R, Aggarwal A, Link ME, Rodgers GP, Hsieh MM. Natural history of benign ethnic neutropenia in individuals of African ancestry. *Blood Cells Mol Dis.* 2019;77:12-16.
66. Borregaard N, Cowland JB. Granules of the human neutrophilic polymorphonuclear leukocyte. *Blood.* 1997;89(10):3503-3521.
67. Schultz J, Kaminker K. Myeloperoxidase of the leucocyte of normal human blood. I. Content and localization. *Arch Biochem Biophys.* 1962;96:465-467.
68. Martin E, Ganz T, Lehrer RI. Defensins and other endogenous peptide antibiotics of vertebrates. *J Leukoc Biol.* 1995;58(2):128-136.
69. Lehrer RI, Ganz T, Selsted ME. Oxygen-independent bactericidal systems. Mechanisms and disorders. *Hematol Oncol Clin North Am.* 1988;2(1):159-169.
70. Gabay JE, Scott RW, Campanelli D, et al. Antibiotic proteins of human polymorphonuclear leukocytes. *Proc Natl Acad Sci USA.* 1989;86(14):5610-5614.
71. Borregaard N. Neutrophils, from marrow to microbes. *Immunity.* 2010;33(5):657-670.
72. Amulic B, Cazalet C, Hayes GL, Metzler KD, Zychlinsky A. Neutrophil function: from mechanisms to disease. *Annu Rev Immunol.* 2012;30:459-489.
73. Nauseef WM, Borregaard N. Neutrophils at work. *Nat Immunol.* 2014;15(7):602-611.
74. Spitznagel JK. Antibiotic proteins of human neutrophils. *J Clin Invest.* 1990;86(5):1381-1386.
75. Skubitz KM, Campbell KD, Iida J, Skubitz AP. CD63 associates with tyrosine kinase activity and CD11/CD18, and transmits an activation signal in neutrophils. *J Immunol.* 1996;157(8):3617-3626.
76. Oram JD, Reiter B. Inhibition of bacteria by lactoferrin and other iron-chelating agents. *Biochim Biophys Acta.* 1968;170(2):351-365.
77. Aruoma OI, Halliwell B. Superoxide-dependent and ascorbate-dependent formation of hydroxyl radicals from hydrogen peroxide in the presence of iron. Are lactoferrin and transferrin promoters of hydroxyl-radical generation? *Biochem J.* 1987;241(1):273-278.
78. Faurschou M, Kamp S, Cowland JB, et al. Prodefensins are matrix proteins of specific granules in human neutrophils. *J Leukoc Biol.* 2005;78(3):785-793.
79. Theilgaard-Monch K, Jacobsen LC, Nielsen MJ, et al. Haptoglobin is synthesized during granulocyte differentiation, stored in specific granules, and released by neutrophils in response to activation. *Blood.* 2006;108(1):353-361.
80. Lekstrom-Himes JA, Dorman SE, Kopar P, Holland SM, Gallin JI. Neutrophil-specific granule deficiency results from a novel mutation with loss of function of the transcription factor CCAAT/enhancer binding protein epsilon. *J Exp Med.* 1999;189(11):1847-1852.
81. Dewald B, Bretz U, Baggiolini M. Release of gelatinase from a novel secretory compartment of human neutrophils. *J Clin Invest.* 1982;70(3):518-525.
82. Rorvig S, Ostergaard O, Heegaard NH, Borregaard N. Proteome profiling of human neutrophil granule subsets, secretory vesicles, and cell membrane: correlation with transcriptome profiling of neutrophil precursors. *J Leukoc Biol.* 2013;94(4):711-721.
83. Lawrence SM, Corriden R, Nizet V. The ontogeny of a neutrophil: mechanisms of granulopoiesis and homeostasis. *Microbiol Mol Biol Rev.* 2018;82(1):e00057-17.
84. Sengelov H, Kjeldsen L, Kroeze W, Berger M, Borregaard N. Secretory vesicles are the intracellular reservoir of complement receptor 1 in human neutrophils. *J Immunol.* 1994;153(2):804-810.
85. Manley HR, Keightley MC, Lieschke GJ. The neutrophil nucleus: an important influence on neutrophil migration and function. *Front Immunol.* 2018;9:2867.
86. Olins AL, Zwerger M, Herrmann H, et al. The human granulocyte nucleus: unusual nuclear envelope and heterochromatin composition. *Eur J Cell Biol.* 2008;87(5):279-290.
87. Fliedner TM, Cronkite EP, Bond VP. A study of the dynamics of proliferation of myelopoiesis with the use of single cell autoradiography. *Folia Haematol.* 1961;6:210-228.
88. Borregaard N, Sorensen OE, Theilgaard-Monch K. Neutrophil granules: a library of innate immunity proteins. *Trends Immunol.* 2007;28(8):340-345.
89. Hoffmann K, Dreger CK, Olins AL, et al. Mutations in the gene encoding the lamin B receptor produce an altered nuclear morphology in granulocytes (Pelger-Huet anomaly). *Nat Genet.* 2002;31(4):410-414.
90. Kanayama N, Kajiwara Y, Goto J, et al. Inactivation of interleukin-8 by aminopeptidase N (CD13). *J Leukoc Biol.* 1995;57(1):129-134.
91. Painter RG, Dukes R, Sullivan J, Carter R, Erdos EG, Johnson AR. Function of neutral endopeptidase on the cell membrane of human neutrophils. *J Biol Chem.* 1988;263(19):9456-9461.
92. Skubitz KM, Campbell KD, Skubitz AP. CD66a, CD66b, CD66c, and CD66d each independently stimulate neutrophils. *J Leukoc Biol.* 1996;60(1):106-117.
93. Harvath L, Balke JA, Christiansen NP, Russell AA, Skubitz KM. Selected antibodies to leukocyte common antigen (CD45) inhibit human neutrophil chemotaxis. *J Immunol.* 1991;146(3):949-957.
94. Flesch BK, Reil A. Molecular genetics of the human neutrophil antigens. *Transfus Med Hemother.* 2018;45(5):300-309.
95. Lalezari P, Nussbaum M, Gelman S, Spaet TH. Neonatal neutropenia due to maternal isoimmunization. *Blood.* 1960;15:236-243.
96. Huizinga TW, Kleijer M, Tetteroo PA, Roos D, von dem Borne AE. Biallelic neutrophil Na-antigen system is associated with a polymorphism on the phospho-inositol-linked Fc gamma receptor III (CD16). *Blood.* 1990;75(1):213-217.
97. Lalezari P, Murphy GB, Allen FH, Jr. NB1, a new neutrophil-specific antigen involved in the pathogenesis of neonatal neutropenia. *J Clin Invest.* 1971;50(5):1108-1115.
98. Stroncek DF, Skubitz KM, McCullough JJ. Biochemical characterization of the neutrophil-specific antigen NB1. *Blood.* 1990;75(3):744-755.
99. Skubitz KM, Stroncek DF, Sun B. Neutrophil-specific antigen NB1 is anchored via a glycosyl-phosphatidylinositol linkage. *J Leukoc Biol.* 1991;49(2):163-171.
100. Goldschmeding R, van Dalen CM, Faber N, et al. Further characterization of the NB 1 antigen as a variably expressed 56-62 kD GPI-linked glycoprotein of plasma membranes and specific granules of neutrophils. *Br J Haematol.* 1992;81(3):336-345.
101. Bux J. Molecular nature of granulocyte antigens. *Transfus Clin Biol.* 2001;8(3):242-247.
102. Greinacher A, Wesche J, Hammer E, et al. Characterization of the human neutrophil alloantigen-3a. *Nat Med.* 2010;16(1):45-48.
103. Curtis BR, Cox NJ, Sullivan MJ, et al. The neutrophil alloantigen HNA-3a (5b) is located on choline transporter-like protein 2 and appears to be encoded by an R>Q154 amino acid substitution. *Blood.* 2010;115(10):2073-2076.
104. Salmon JE, Edberg JC, Kimberly RP. Fc gamma receptor III on human neutrophils. Allelic variants have functionally distinct capacities. *J Clin Invest.* 1990;85(4):1287-1295.
105. Bredius RG, Fijen CA, De Haas M, et al. Role of neutrophil Fc gamma RIIa (CD32) and Fc gamma RIIIb (CD16) polymorphic forms in phagocytosis of human IgG1- and IgG3-opsonized bacteria and erythrocytes. *Immunology.* 1994;83(4):624-630.
106. Nagarajan S, Chesla S, Cobern L, Anderson P, Zhu C, Selvaraj P. Ligand binding and phagocytosis by CD16 (Fc gamma receptor III) isoforms. Phagocytic signaling by associated zeta and gamma subunits in Chinese hamster ovary cells. *J Biol Chem.* 1995;270(43):25762-25770.
107. Matsuo K, Lin A, Procter JL, Clement L, Stroncek D. Variations in the expression of granulocyte antigen NB1. *Transfusion.* 2000;40(6):654-662.
108. Stroncek DF, Jaszcz W, Herr GP, Clay ME, McCullough J. Expression of neutrophil antigens after 10 days of granulocyte-colony-stimulating factor. *Transfusion.* 1998;38(7):663-668.
109. Bayat B, Werth S, Sachs UJ, Newman DK, Newman PJ, Santoso S. Neutrophil transmigration mediated by the neutrophil-specific antigen CD177 is influenced by the endothelial S536N dimorphism of platelet endothelial cell adhesion molecule-1. *J Immunol.* 2010;184(7):3889-3896.
110. Flesch BK, Curtis BR, de Haas M, Lucas G, Sachs UJ. Update on the nomenclature of human neutrophil antigens and alleles. *Transfusion.* 2016;56(6):1477-1479.
111. Stefanova I, Horejsi V, Ansotegui IJ, Knapp W, Stockinger H. GPI-anchored cell-surface molecules complexed to protein tyrosine kinases. *Science.* 1991;254(5034):1016-1019.
112. Cinek T, Horejsi V. The nature of large noncovalent complexes containing glycosyl-phosphatidylinositol-anchored membrane glycoproteins and protein tyrosine kinases. *J Immunol.* 1992;149(7):2262-2270.
113. Odink K, Cerletti N, Bruggen J, et al. Two calcium-binding proteins in infiltrate macrophages of rheumatoid arthritis. *Nature.* 1987;330(6143):80-82.
114. Kerkhoff C, Klempt M, Kaever V, Sorg C. The two calcium-binding proteins, S100A8 and S100A9, are involved in the metabolism of arachidonic acid in human neutrophils. *J Biol Chem.* 1999;274(46):32672-32679.
115. Wang S, Song R, Wang Z, Jing Z, Wang S, Ma J. S100A8/A9 in inflammation. *Front Immunol.* 2018;9:1298.
116. Stroncek DF, Shankar RA, Skubitz KM. The subcellular distribution of myeloid-related protein 8 (MRP8) and MRP14 in human neutrophils. *J Transl Med.* 2005;3:36.
117. Perretti M, Wheller SK, Flower RJ, Wahid S, Pitzalis C. Modulation of cellular annexin I in human leukocytes infiltrating DTH skin reactions. *J Leukoc Biol.* 1999;65(5):583-589.
118. Kumar S, Dikshit M. Metabolic insight of neutrophils in health and disease. *Front Immunol.* 2019;10:2099.
119. Cooke WE. The macropolycyte. *Br Med J.* 1927;1(3443):8.2-13.
120. Kennedy WP, MacKay I. The macropolycyte in health and disease in Iraq. *J Pathol Bacteriol.* 1937;44(3):701-704.
121. Davidson WM, Smith DR. A morphological sex difference in the polymorphonuclear neutrophil leucocytes. *Br Med J.* 1954;2(4878):6-7.
122. Hochstenbach PF, Scheres JM, Hustinx TW, Wieringa B. Demonstration of X chromatin in drumstick-like nuclear appendages of leukocytes by in situ hybridization on blood smears. *Histochemistry.* 1986;84(4-6):383-386.
123. McCutcheon M. Studies on the locomotion of leucocytes I. The normal rate of locomotion of human neutrophilic leucocytes in vitro. *Am J Physiol.* 1923;66:180-195.
124. Howard TH. Quantification of the locomotive behavior of polymorphonuclear leukocytes in clot preparations. *Blood.* 1982;59(5):946-951.
125. Harvath L, Leonard EJ. Two neutrophil populations in human blood with different chemotactic activities: separation and chemoattractant binding. *Infect Immun.* 1982;36(2):443-449.
126. Seligmann B, Malech HL, Melnick DA, Gallin JI. An antibody binding to human neutrophils demonstrates antigenic heterogeneity detected early in myeloid maturation which correlates with functional heterogeneity of mature neutrophils. *J Immunol.* 1985;135(4):2647-2653.
127. Clement LT, Lehmeyer JE, Gartland GL. Identification of neutrophil subpopulations with monoclonal antibodies. *Blood.* 1983;61(2):326-332.

128. Diamond MS, Springer TA. A subpopulation of Mac-1 (CD11b/CD18) molecules mediates neutrophil adhesion to ICAM-1 and fibrinogen. *J Cell Biol.* 1993;120(2):545-556.

129. Krause PJ, Malech HL, Kristie J, et al. Polymorphonuclear leukocyte heterogeneity in neonates and adults. *Blood.* 1986;68(1):200-204.

130. Ross GD. Structure and function of membrane complement receptors. Summary. *Fed Proc.* 1982;41(14):3089-3093.

131. Genco RJ, Van Dyke TE, Levine MJ, Nelson RD, Wilson ME. 1985 Kreshover lecture. Molecular factors influencing neutrophil defects in periodontal disease. *J Dent Res.* 1986;65(12):1379-1391.

132. Clemmensen SN, Bohr CT, Rorvig S, et al. Olfactomedin 4 defines a subset of human neutrophils. *J Leukoc Biol.* 2012;91(3):495-500.

133. Wright HL, Makki FA, Moots RJ, Edwards SW. Low-density granulocytes: functionally distinct, immature neutrophils in rheumatoid arthritis with altered properties and defective TNF signalling. *J Leukoc Biol.* 2017;101(2):599-611.

134. Berkow RL, Baehner RL. Volume-dependent human blood polymorphonuclear leukocyte heterogeneity demonstrated with counterflow centrifugal elutriation. *Blood.* 1985;65(1):71-78.

135. Scott CS, Bynoe AG, Hough D, Roberts BE. C3b receptor-negative peripheral blood neutrophils. A study of normal and haematologically abnormal disorders. *Scand J Haematol.* 1984;32(2):183-189.

136. Karlsson A, Follin P, Leffler H, Dahlgren C. Galectin-3 activates the NADPH-oxidase in exudated but not peripheral blood neutrophils. *Blood.* 1998;91(9):3430-3438.

137. Tsuda Y, Takahashi H, Kobayashi M, Hanafusa T, Herndon DN, Suzuki F. Three different neutrophil subsets exhibited in mice with different susceptibilities to infection by methicillin-resistant *Staphylococcus aureus. Immunity.* 2004;21(2):215-226.

138. Pillay J, Kamp VM, van Hoffen E, et al. A subset of neutrophils in human systemic inflammation inhibits T cell responses through Mac-1. *J Clin Invest.* 2012;122(1):327-336.

139. Uhl B, Vadlau Y, Zuchtriegel G, et al. Aged neutrophils contribute to the first line of defense in the acute inflammatory response. *Blood.* 2016;128(19):2327-2337.

140. Zhang D, Chen G, Manwani D, et al. Neutrophil ageing is regulated by the microbiome. *Nature.* 2015;525(7570):528-532.

141. Rosales C. Neutrophil: a cell with many roles in inflammation or several cell types? *Front Physiol.* 2018;9:113.

142. Casanova-Acebes M, Pitaval C, Weiss LA, et al. Rhythmic modulation of the hematopoietic niche through neutrophil clearance. *Cell.* 2013;153(5):1025-1035.

143. Van Eeden SF, Bicknell S, Walker BA, Hogg JC. Polymorphonuclear leukocytes L-selectin expression decreases as they age in circulation. *Am J Physiol.* 1997;272(1 pt 2):H401-H408.

144. Martin C, Burdon PC, Bridger G, Gutierrez-Ramos JC, Williams TJ, Rankin SM. Chemokines acting via CXCR2 and CXCR4 control the release of neutrophils from the bone marrow and their return following senescence. *Immunity.* 2003;19(4):583-593.

145. Lu RJ, Taylor S, Contrepois K, et al. Multi-omic profiling of primary mouse neutrophils predicts a pattern of sex- and age-related functional regulation. *Nat Aging.* 2021;1:715-733.

146. Adrover JM, Nicolas-Avila JA, Hidalgo A. Aging: a temporal dimension for neutrophils. *Trends Immunol.* 2016;37(5):334-345.

147. Scheiermann C, Kunisaki Y, Lucas D, et al. Adrenergic nerves govern circadian leukocyte recruitment to tissues. *Immunity.* 2012;37(2):290-301.

148. Ella K, Csepanyi-Komi R, Kaldi K. Circadian regulation of human peripheral neutrophils. *Brain Behav Immun.* 2016;57:209-221.

149. Xie X, Shi Q, Wu P, et al. Single-cell transcriptome profiling reveals neutrophil heterogeneity in homeostasis and infection. *Nat Immunol.* 2020;21(9):1119-1133.

150. Boggs DR. The kinetics of neutrophilic leukocytes in health and in disease. *Semin Hematol.* 1967;4(4):359-386.

151. Cartwright GE, Athens JW, Wintrobe MM. The kinetics of granulopoiesis in normal man. *Blood.* 1964;24:780-803.

152. Cronkite EP. Kinetics of granulocytopoiesis. *Clin Haematol.* 1979;8(2):351-370.

153. Mauer AM, Athens JW, Ashenbrucker H, Cartwright GE, Wintrobe MM. Leukokinetic studies. Ii. A method for labeling granulocytes in vitro with radioactive diisopropylfluorophosphate (Dfp). *J Clin Invest.* 1960;39(9):1481-1486.

154. Patt HM. A consideration of myeloid-erythroid balance in man. *Blood.* 1957;12(9):777-787.

155. Warner HR, Athens JW. An analysis of granulocyte kinetics in blood and bone marrow. *Ann N Y Acad Sci.* 1964;113:523-536.

156. Vodopick HA, Athens JW, Warner HR, Boggs DR, Cartwright GE, Wintrobe MM. An evaluation of radiosulfate as a granulocyte label in the dog. *J Lab Clin Med.* 1966;68(1):47-56.

157. Maloney MA, Patt HM. Neutrophil life cycle with tritiated thymidine. *Proc Soc Exp Biol Med.* 1958;98(4):801-803.

158. Bond VP, Fliedner TM, Cronkite EP, Rubini JR, Brecher G, Schork PK. Proliferative potentials of bone marrow and blood cells studied by in vitro uptake of H3-thymidine. *Acta Haematol.* 1959;21(1):1-15.

159. Donohue DM, Reiff RH, Hanson ML, Betson Y, Finch CA. Quantitative measurement of the erythrocytic and granulocytic cells of the marrow and blood. *J Clin Invest.* 1958;37(11):1571-1576.

160. Summers C, Rankin SM, Condliffe AM, Singh N, Peters AM, Chilvers ER. Neutrophil kinetics in health and disease. *Trends Immunol.* 2010;31(8):318-324.

161. Lord BI. Cellular proliferation in normal and continuously irradiated rat bone marrow studied by repeated labelling with tritiated thymidine. *Br J Haematol.* 1965;11:130-143.

162. Fliedner TM, Cronkite EP, Killmann SA, Bond VP. Granulocytopoiesis. Ii. Emergence and pattern of labeling of neutrophilic granulocytes in humans. *Blood.* 1964;24:683-700.

163. Giordano GF, Lichtman MA. Marrow cell egress. The central interaction of barrier pore size and cell maturation. *J Clin Invest.* 1973;52(5):1154-1164.

164. Rother K. Leucocyte mobilizing factor: a new biological activity derived from the third component of complement. *Eur J Immunol.* 1972;2(6):550-558.

165. Terashima T, English D, Hogg JC, van Eeden SF. Release of polymorphonuclear leukocytes from the bone marrow by interleukin-8. *Blood.* 1998;92(3):1062-1069.

166. Zuelzer WW. "Myelokathexis"--a new form of chronic granulocytopenia. Report of a case. *N Engl J Med.* 1964;270:699-704.

167. Hernandez PA, Gorlin RJ, Lukens JN, et al. Mutations in the chemokine receptor gene CXCR4 are associated with WHIM syndrome, a combined immunodeficiency disease. *Nat Genet.* 2003;34(1):70-74.

168. Lahoz-Beneytez J, Elemans M, Zhang Y, et al. Human neutrophil kinetics: modeling of stable isotope labeling data supports short blood neutrophil half-lives. *Blood.* 2016;127(26):3431-3438.

169. Toren M, Goffinet JA, Kaplow LS. Pulmonary bed sequestration of neutrophils during hemodialysis. *Blood.* 1970;36(3):337-340.

170. Craddock PR, Fehr J, Dalmasso AP, Brighan KL, Jacob HS. Hemodialysis leukopenia. Pulmonary vascular leukostasis resulting from complement activation by dialyzer cellophane membranes. *J Clin Invest.* 1977;59(5):879-888.

171. Craddock PR, Hammerschmidt D, White JG, Dalmosso AP, Jacob HS. Complement (C5-a)-induced granulocyte aggregation in vitro. A possible mechanism of complement-mediated leukostasis and leukopenia. *J Clin Invest.* 1977;60(1):260-264.

172. Hammerschmidt DE, Weaver LJ, Hudson LD, Craddock PR, Jacob HS. Association of complement activation and elevated plasma-C5a with adult respiratory distress syndrome. Pathophysiological relevance and possible prognostic value. *Lancet.* 1980;1(8175):947-949.

173. Skubitz KM, Craddock PR. Reversal of hemodialysis granulocytopenia and pulmonary leukostasis: a clinical manifestation of selective down-regulation of granulocyte responses to C5adesarg. *J Clin Invest.* 1981;67(5):1383-1391.

174. Price TH, Ochs HD, Gershoni-Baruch R, Harlan JM, Etzioni A. In vivo neutrophil and lymphocyte function studies in a patient with leukocyte adhesion deficiency type II. *Blood.* 1994;84(5):1635-1639.

175. Jagels MA, Chambers JD, Arfors KE, Hugli TE. C5a- and tumor necrosis factor-alpha-induced leukocytosis occurs independently of beta 2 integrins and L-selectin: differential effects on neutrophil adhesion molecule expression in vivo. *Blood.* 1995;85(10):2900-2909.

176. Jagels MA, Hugli TE. Neutrophil chemotactic factors promote leukocytosis. A common mechanism for cellular recruitment from bone marrow. *J Immunol.* 1992;148(4):1119-1128.

177. Florey HW, Grant LH. Leucocyte migration from small blood vessels stimulated with ultraviolet light: an electron-microscope study. *J Pathol Bacteriol.* 1961;82:13-17.

178. Mauer AM, Athens JW, Warner HR, et al. An analysis of leukocyte radioactivity curves obtained with radioactivce diisopropylfluorophosphate (DFP32). In: Stohlman FJ, ed. *The Kinetics of Cellular Proliferation.* Grune and Stratton; 1959:231-239.

179. Stark MA, Huo Y, Burcin TL, Morris MA, Olson TS, Ley K. Phagocytosis of apoptotic neutrophils regulates granulopoiesis via IL-23 and IL-17. *Immunity.* 2005;22(3):285-294.

180. Rankin SM. The bone marrow: a site of neutrophil clearance. *J Leukoc Biol.* 2010;88(2):241-251.

181. Isaacs RaD AC. A study of the white blood corpuscles appearing in the saliva and their relation to those in the blood. *Am J Med Sci.* 1927;174:70-86.

182. Klinkhamer JM. Quantitative evaluation of gingivitis and periodontal disease. I. The orogranulocytic migratory rate. *Periodontics.* 1968;6(5):207-211.

183. Addis T. The number of formed elements in the urinary sediment of normal individuals. *J Clin Invest.* 1926;2(5):409-415.

184. Ambrus CM, Ambrus JL. Regulation of the leukocyte level. *Ann N Y Acad Sci.* 1959;77:445-486.

185. Bierman HR, Kelly KH, King FW, Petrakis NL. The pulmonary circulation as a source of leucocytes and platelets in man. *Science.* 1951;114(2959):276-277.

186. Perez-Figueroa E, Alvarez-Carrasco P, Ortega E, Maldonado-Bernal C. Neutrophils: many ways to Die. *Front Immunol.* 2021;12:631821.

187. Fuchs TA, Abed U, Goosmann C, et al. Novel cell death program leads to neutrophil extracellular traps. *J Cell Biol.* 2007;176(2):231-241.

188. Gottlieb RA, Giesing HA, Zhu JY, Engler RL, Babior BM. Cell acidification in apoptosis: granulocyte colony-stimulating factor delays programmed cell death in neutrophils by up-regulating the vacuolar H(+)-ATPase. *Proc Natl Acad Sci USA.* 1995;92(13):5965-5968.

189. Savill J, Dransfield I, Hogg N, Haslett C. Vitronectin receptor-mediated phagocytosis of cells undergoing apoptosis. *Nature.* 1990;343(6254):170-173.

190. Liles WC, Dale DC, Klebanoff SJ. Glucocorticoids inhibit apoptosis of human neutrophils. *Blood.* 1995;86(8):3181-3188.

191. Mecklenburgh KI, Walmsley SR, Cowburn AS, et al. Involvement of a ferroprotein sensor in hypoxia-mediated inhibition of neutrophil apoptosis. *Blood.* 2002;100(8):3008-3016.

192. Molloy EJ, O'Neill AJ, Grantham JJ, et al. Sex-specific alterations in neutrophil apoptosis: the role of estradiol and progesterone. *Blood.* 2003;102(7):2653-2659.

193. Brinkmann V, Reichard U, Goosmann C, et al. Neutrophil extracellular traps kill bacteria. *Science.* 2004;303(5663):1532-1535.

194. Grayson PC, Kaplan MJ. At the Bench: neutrophil extracellular traps (NETs) highlight novel aspects of innate immune system involvement in autoimmune diseases. *J Leukoc Biol.* 2016;99(2):253-264.

195. Papayannopoulos V. Neutrophil extracellular traps in immunity and disease. *Nat Rev Immunol.* 2018;18(2):134-147.

196. Pilsczek FH, Salina D, Poon KK, et al. A novel mechanism of rapid nuclear neutrophil extracellular trap formation in response to *Staphylococcus aureus*. *J Immunol*. 2010;185(12):7413-7425.
197. Yipp BG, Petri B, Salina D, et al. Infection-induced NETosis is a dynamic process involving neutrophil multitasking in vivo. *Nat Med*. 2012;18(9):1386-1393.
198. Crosson FJ, Jr, Feder HM, Jr, Bocchini JA, Jr, Hackell JM, Hackell JG. Neonatal sepsis at the Johns Hopkins Hospital, 1969-1975: bacterial isolates and clinical correlates. *Johns Hopkins Med J*. 1977;140(2):37-46.
199. Freedman RM, Ingram DL, Gross I, Ehrenkranz RA, Warshaw JB, Baltimore RS. A half century of neonatal sepsis at Yale: 1928 to 1978. *Am J Dis Child*. 1981;135(2):140-144.
200. Klein JOaM SM. Bacterial sepsis and meningitis. In: Remington JSaK JO, ed. *Infectious Diseases of the Fetus and Newborn Infant*. 1983.
201. Barak Y, Karov Y, Levin S, et al. Granulocyte-macrophage colonies in cultures of human fetal liver cells: morphologic and ultrastructural analysis of proliferation and differentiation. *Exp Hematol*. 1980;8(7):837-844.
202. Slayton WB, Li Y, Calhoun DA, et al. The first-appearance of neutrophils in the human fetal bone marrow cavity. *Early Hum Dev*. 1998;53(2):129-144.
203. Thomas DB, Yoffey JM. Human foetal haemopoiesis. I. The cellular composition of foetal blood. *Br J Haematol*. 1962;8:290-295.
204. Wheeler JG, Chauvenet AR, Johnson CA, et al. Neutrophil storage pool depletion in septic, neutropenic neonates. *Pediatr Infect Dis*. 1984;3(5):407-409.
205. Christensen RD, Harper TE, Rothstein G. Granulocyte-macrophage progenitor cells in term and preterm neonates. *J Pediatr*. 1986;109(6):1047-1051.
206. Rickard KA, Brown RD, Kronenberg H. Studies on the proliferative capacity of the in vitro colony forming cell in normal human bone marrow. *Aust N Z J Med*. 1973;3(4):361-370.
207. Tebbi K, Rubin S, Cowan DH, McCulloch EA. A comparison of granulopoiesis in culture from blood and marrow cells of nonleukemic individuals and patients with acute leukemia. *Blood*. 1976;48(2):235-243.
208. Christensen RD, Hill HR, Rothstein G. Granulocytic stem cell (CFUc) proliferation in experimental group B streptococcal sepsis. *Pediatr Res*. 1983;17(4):278-280.
209. Chervenick PA, Boggs DR. In vitro growth of granulocytic and mononuclear cell colonies from blood of normal individuals. *Blood*. 1971;37(2):131-135.
210. Prindull G, Gabriel M, Prindull B. Circulating myelopoietic stem cells (CFUc): high levels in healthy pre-term infants and reduced levels in sick pre-term infants. *Blut*. 1981;43(2):109-111.
211. Christensen RD, Rothstein G. Pre- and postnatal development of granulocytic stem cells in the rat. *Pediatr Res*. 1984;18(7):599-602.
212. Erdman SH, Christensen RD, Bradley PP, Rothstein G. Supply and release of storage neutrophils. A developmental study. *Biol Neonate*. 1982;41(3-4):132-137.
213. Christensen RD, Rothstein G, Hill HR, Pincus SH. Treatment of experimental group B streptococcal infection with hybridoma antibody. *Pediatr Res*. 1984;18(11):1093-1096.
214. Christensen RD, Rothstein G, Hill HR, Hall RT. Fatal early onset group B streptococcal sepsis with normal leukocyte counts. *Pediatr Infect Dis*. 1985;4(3):242-245.
215. Zeligs BJ, Armstrong CD, Walser JB, Bellanti JA. Age-dependent susceptibility of neonatal rats to group B streptococcal type III infection: correlation of severity of infection and response of myeloid pools. *Infect Immun*. 1982;37(1):255-263.
216. Schmutz N, Henry E, Jopling J, Christensen RD. Expected ranges for blood neutrophil concentrations of neonates: the Manroe and Mouzinho charts revisited. *J Perinatol*. 2008;28(4):275-281.
217. Bullock JD, Robertson AF, Bodenbender JG, Kontras SB, Miller CE. Inflammatory response in the neonate re-examined. *Pediatrics*. 1969;44(1):58-61.
218. Miller ME. Chemotactic function in the human neonate: humoral and cellular aspects. *Pediatr Res*. 1971;5:487-492.
219. Boner A, Zeligs BJ, Bellanti JA. Chemotactic responses of various differentiational stages of neutrophils from human cord and adult blood. *Infect Immun*. 1982;35(3):921-928.
220. Sacchi F, Rondini G, Mingrat G, et al. Different maturation of neutrophil chemotaxis in term and preterm newborn infants. *J Pediatr*. 1982;101(2):273-274.
221. Krause PJ, Herson VC, Boutin-Lebowitz J, et al. Polymorphonuclear leukocyte adherence and chemotaxis in stressed and healthy neonates. *Pediatr Res*. 1986;20(4):296-300.
222. Christensen RD, Rothstein G. Efficiency of neutrophil migration in the neonate. *Pediatr Res*. 1980;14(10):1147-1149.
223. Schuit KE, Homisch L. Inefficient in vivo neutrophil migration in neonatal rats. *J Leukoc Biol*. 1984;35(6):583-586.
224. Mease AD, Burgess DP, Thomas PJ. Irreversible neutrophil aggregation. A mechanism of decreased newborn neutrophil chemotactic response. *Am J Pathol*. 1981;104(1):98-102.
225. Olson TA, Ruymann FB, Cook BA, Burgess DP, Henson SA, Thomas PJ. Newborn polymorphonuclear leukocyte aggregation: a study of physical properties and ultrastructure using chemotactic peptides. *Pediatr Res*. 1983;17(12):993-997.
226. Lawrence SM, Corriden R, Nizet V. Age-appropriate functions and dysfunctions of the neonatal neutrophil. *Front Pediatr*. 2017;5:23.
227. Carr R. Neutrophil production and function in newborn infants. *Br J Haematol*. 2000;110(1):18-28.
228. Nussbaum C, Gloning A, Pruenster M, et al. Neutrophil and endothelial adhesive function during human fetal ontogeny. *J Leukoc Biol*. 2013;93(2):175-184.
229. Anderson DC, Abbassi O, Kishimoto TK, Koenig JM, McIntire LV, Smith CW. Diminished lectin-, epidermal growth factor-, complement binding domain-cell adhesion molecule-1 on neonatal neutrophils underlies their impaired CD18-independent adhesion to endothelial cells in vitro. *J Immunol*. 1991;146(10):3372-3379.
230. Lorant DE, Li W, Tabatabaei N, Garver MK, Albertine KH. P-selectin expression by endothelial cells is decreased in neonatal rats and human premature infants. *Blood*. 1999;94(2):600-609.
231. Carr R, Brocklehurst P, Dore CJ, Modi N. Granulocyte-macrophage colony stimulating factor administered as prophylaxis for reduction of sepsis in extremely preterm, small for gestational age neonates (the PROGRAMS trial): a single-blind, multicentre, randomised controlled trial. *Lancet*. 2009;373(9659):226-233.
232. Anderson DC, Rothlein R, Marlin SD, Krater SS, Smith CW. Impaired transendothelial migration by neonatal neutrophils: abnormalities of Mac-1 (CD11b/CD18)-dependent adherence reactions. *Blood*. 1990;76(12):2613-2621.
233. Weinberger B, Laskin DL, Mariano TM, et al. Mechanisms underlying reduced responsiveness of neonatal neutrophils to distinct chemoattractants. *J Leukoc Biol*. 2001;70(6):969-976.
234. Hilmo A, Howard TH. F-actin content of neonate and adult neutrophils. *Blood*. 1987;69(3):945-949.
235. Levy O, Martin S, Eichenwald E, et al. Impaired innate immunity in the newborn: newborn neutrophils are deficient in bactericidal/permeability-increasing protein. *Pediatrics*. 1999;104(6):1327-1333.
236. Bektas S, Goetze B, Speer CP. Decreased adherence, chemotaxis and phagocytic activities of neutrophils from preterm neonates. *Acta Paediatr Scand*. 1990;79(11):1031-1038.
237. Yost CC, Cody MJ, Harris ES, et al. Impaired neutrophil extracellular trap (NET) formation: a novel innate immune deficiency of human neonates. *Blood*. 2009;113(25):6419-6427.
238. Byrd AS, O'Brien XM, Laforce-Nesbitt SS, et al. NETosis in neonates: evidence of a reactive oxygen species-independent pathway in response to fungal challenge. *J Infect Dis*. 2016;213(4):634-639.
239. Patt HM, Maloney MA, Jackson EM. Recovery of blood neutrophils after acute peripheral depletion. *Am J Physiol*. 1957;188(3):585-592.
240. Price TH, Chatta GS, Dale DC. Effect of recombinant granulocyte colony-stimulating factor on neutrophil kinetics in normal young and elderly humans. *Blood*. 1996;88(1):335-340.
241. Eash KJ, Greenbaum AM, Gopalan PK, Link DC. CXCR2 and CXCR4 antagonistically regulate neutrophil trafficking from murine bone marrow. *J Clin Invest*. 2010;120(7):2423-2431.
242. Rowe JM, Andersen JW, Mazza JJ, et al. A randomized placebo-controlled phase III study of granulocyte-macrophage colony-stimulating factor in adult patients (> 55 to 70 years of age) with acute myelogenous leukemia: a study of the Eastern Cooperative Oncology Group (E1490). *Blood*. 1995;86(2):457-462.
243. Bunn PA, Jr, Crowley J, Kelly K, et al. Chemoradiotherapy with or without granulocyte-macrophage colony-stimulating factor in the treatment of limited-stage small-cell lung cancer: a prospective phase III randomized study of the Southwest Oncology Group. *J Clin Oncol*. 1995;13(7):1632-1641.
244. Yong KL, Linch DC. Differential effects of granulocyte- and granulocyte-macrophage colony-stimulating factors (G- and GM-CSF) on neutrophil adhesion in vitro and in vivo. *Eur J Haematol*. 1992;49(5):251-259.
245. Ohsaka A, Saionji K, Sato N, Mori T, Ishimoto K, Inamatsu T. Granulocyte colony-stimulating factor down-regulates the surface expression of the human leucocyte adhesion molecule-1 on human neutrophils in vitro and in vivo. *Br J Haematol*. 1993;84(4):574-580.
246. Balazovich KJ, Almeida HI, Boxer LA. Recombinant human G-CSF and GM-CSF prime human neutrophils for superoxide production through different signal transduction mechanisms. *J Lab Clin Med*. 1991;118(6):576-584.
247. Morstyn G, Campbell L, Souza LM, et al. Effect of granulocyte colony stimulating factor on neutropenia induced by cytotoxic chemotherapy. *Lancet*. 1988;1(8587):667-672.
248. Lindemann A, Herrmann F, Oster W, et al. Hematologic effects of recombinant human granulocyte colony-stimulating factor in patients with malignancy. *Blood*. 1989;74(8):2644-2651.
249. de Haas M, Kerst JM, van der Schoot CE, et al. Granulocyte colony-stimulating factor administration to healthy volunteers: analysis of the immediate activating effects on circulating neutrophils. *Blood*. 1994;84(11):3885-3894.
250. Borish L, Rosenbaum R, Albury L, Clark S. Activation of neutrophils by recombinant interleukin 6. *Cell Immunol*. 1989;121(2):280-289.
251. Yuo A, Kitagawa S, Kasahara T, Matsushima K, Saito M, Takaku F. Stimulation and priming of human neutrophils by interleukin-8: cooperation with tumor necrosis factor and colony-stimulating factors. *Blood*. 1991;78(10):2708-2714.
252. Boettcher S, Gerosa RC, Radpour R, et al. Endothelial cells translate pathogen signals into G-CSF-driven emergency granulopoiesis. *Blood*. 2014;124(9):1393-1403.
253. Broxmeyer HE, Lu L. Control of myelopoietic growth factor production. *Prog Clin Biol Res*. 1985;184:145-155.
254. Heaney ML, Golde DW. Soluble cytokine receptors. *Blood*. 1996;87(3):847-857.
255. Broome CS, Whetton AD, Miyan JA. Neuropeptide control of bone marrow neutrophil production is mediated by both direct and indirect effects on CFU-GM. *Br J Haematol*. 2000;108(1):140-150.
256. Metzemaekers M, Gouwy M, Proost P. Neutrophil chemoattractant receptors in health and disease: double-edged swords. *Cell Mol Immunol*. 2020;17(5):433-450.
257. Petri B, Sanz MJ. Neutrophil chemotaxis. *Cell Tissue Res*. 2018;371(3):425-436.
258. Heit B, Tavener S, Raharjo E, Kubes P. An intracellular signaling hierarchy determines direction of migration in opposing chemotactic gradients. *J Cell Biol*. 2002;159(1):91-102.
259. Hughes CE, Nibbs RJB. A guide to chemokines and their receptors. *FEBS J*. 2018;285(16):2944-2971.

260. Russo RC, Garcia CC, Teixeira MM, Amaral FA. The CXCL8/IL-8 chemokine family and its receptors in inflammatory diseases. *Expet Rev Clin Immunol.* 2014;10(5):593-619.

261. Subramanian BC, Majumdar R, Parent CA. The role of the LTB4-BLT1 axis in chemotactic gradient sensing and directed leukocyte migration. *Semin Immunol.* 2017;33:16-29.

262. Yokomizo T, Izumi T, Chang K, Takuwa Y, Shimizu T. A G-protein-coupled receptor for leukotriene B4 that mediates chemotaxis. *Nature.* 1997;387(6633):620-624.

263. Yokomizo T, Kato K, Terawaki K, Izumi T, Shimizu T. A second leukotriene B(4) receptor, BLT2. A new therapeutic target in inflammation and immunological disorders. *J Exp Med.* 2000;192(3):421-432.

264. Edwards LJ, Constantinescu CS. Platelet activating factor/platelet activating factor receptor pathway as a potential therapeutic target in autoimmune diseases. *Inflamm Allergy - Drug Targets.* 2009;8(3):182-190.

265. Ward PA, Lepow IH, Newman LJ. Bacterial factors chemotactic for polymorphonuclear leukocytes. *Am J Pathol.* 1968;52(4):725-736.

266. Schiffmann E, Corcoran BA, Wahl SM. N-formylmethionyl peptides as chemoattractants for leucocytes. *Proc Natl Acad Sci USA.* 1975;72(3):1059-1062.

267. Dahlgren C, Gabl M, Holdfeldt A, Winther M, Forsman H. Basic characteristics of the neutrophil receptors that recognize formylated peptides, a danger-associated molecular pattern generated by bacteria and mitochondria. *Biochem Pharmacol.* 2016;114:22-39.

268. Ehrengruber MU, Geiser T, Deranleau DA. Activation of human neutrophils by C3a and C5A. Comparison of the effects on shape changes, chemotaxis, secretion, and respiratory burst. *FEBS Lett.* 1994;346(2-3):181-184.

269. Futosi K, Fodor S, Mocsai A. Neutrophil cell surface receptors and their intracellular signal transduction pathways. *Int Immunopharm.* 2013;17(3):638-650.

270. Theler JM, Lew DP, Jaconi ME, Krause KH, Wollheim CB, Schlegel W. Intracellular pattern of cytosolic Ca2+ changes during adhesion and multiple phagocytosis in human neutrophils. Dynamics of intracellular Ca2+ stores. *Blood.* 1995;85(8):2194-2201.

271. Barrowman MM, Cockcroft S, Gomperts BD. Differential control of azurophilic and specific granule exocytosis in Sendai-virus-permeabilized rabbit neutrophils. *J Physiol.* 1987;383:115-124.

272. Smolen JE, Korchak HM, Weissmann G. The roles of extracellular and intracellular calcium in lysosomal enzyme release and superoxide anion generation by human neutrophils. *Biochim Biophys Acta.* 1981;677(3-4):512-520.

273. Lew DP, Andersson T, Hed J, Di Virgilio F, Pozzan T, Stendahl O. Ca2+-dependent and Ca2+-independent phagocytosis in human neutrophils. *Nature.* 1985;315(6019):509-511.

274. Mocsai A, Jakus Z, Vantus T, Berton G, Lowell CA, Ligeti E. Kinase pathways in chemoattractant-induced degranulation of neutrophils: the role of p38 mitogen-activated protein kinase activated by Src family kinases. *J Immunol.* 2000;164(8):4321-4331.

275. Cui Y, Harvey K, Akard L, et al. Regulation of neutrophil responses by phosphotyrosine phosphatase. *J Immunol.* 1994;152(11):5420-5428.

276. Quinn MT. Low-molecular-weight GTP-binding proteins and leukocyte signal transduction. *J Leukoc Biol.* 1995;58(3):263-276.

277. Cronstein BN, Levin RI, Philips M, Hirschhorn R, Abramson SB, Weissmann G. Neutrophil adherence to endothelium is enhanced via adenosine A1 receptors and inhibited via adenosine A2 receptors. *J Immunol.* 1992;148(7):2201-2206.

278. Skubitz KM, Wickham NW, Hammerschmidt DE. Endogenous and exogenous adenosine inhibit granulocyte aggregation without altering the associated rise in intracellular calcium concentration. *Blood.* 1988;72(1):29-33.

279. Condliffe AM, Chilvers ER, Haslett C, Dransfield I. Priming differentially regulates neutrophil adhesion molecule expression/function. *Immunology.* 1996;89(1):105-111.

280. Brandolini L, Bertini R, Bizzarri C, et al. IL-1 beta primes IL-8-activated human neutrophils for elastase release, phospholipase D activity, and calcium flux. *J Leukoc Biol.* 1996;59(3):427-434.

281. El-Benna J, Dang PM, Gougerot-Pocidalo MA. Priming of the neutrophil NADPH oxidase activation: role of p47phox phosphorylation and NOX2 mobilization to the plasma membrane. *Semin Immunopathol.* 2008;30(3):279-289.

282. Nauseef WM. Pin-ing down PMN priming. *Blood.* 2010;116(26):5788-5789.

283. Brown GE, Reiff J, Allen RC, Silver GM, Fink MP. Maintenance and down-regulation of primed neutrophil chemiluminescence activity in human whole blood. *J Leukoc Biol.* 1997;62(6):837-844.

284. Boussetta T, Gougerot-Pocidalo MA, Hayem G, et al. The prolyl isomerase Pin1 acts as a novel molecular switch for TNF-alpha-induced priming of the NADPH oxidase in human neutrophils. *Blood.* 2010;116(26):5795-5802.

285. O'Flaherty JT, Kreutzer DL, Showell HJ, Vitkauskas G, Becker EL, Ward PA. Selective neutrophil desensitization to chemotactic factors. *J Cell Biol.* 1979;80(3):564-572.

286. Ward PA, Becker EL. The deactivation of rabbit neutrophils by chemotactic factor and the nature of the activatable esterase. *J Exp Med.* 1968;127(4):693-709.

287. Skubitz KM, Craddock PR, Hammerschmidt DE, August JT. Corticosteroids block binding of chemotactic peptide to its receptor on granulocytes and cause disaggregation of granulocyte aggregates in vitro. *J Clin Invest.* 1981;68(1):13-20.

288. Walther A, Riehemann K, Gerke V. A novel ligand of the formyl peptide receptor: annexin I regulates neutrophil extravasation by interacting with the FPR. *Mol Cell.* 2000;5(5):831-840.

289. Hayhoe RP, Kamal AM, Solito E, Flower RJ, Cooper D, Perretti M. Annexin 1 and its bioactive peptide inhibit neutrophil-endothelium interactions under flow: indication of distinct receptor involvement. *Blood.* 2006;107(5):2123-2130.

290. Chadzinska M, Kolaczkowska E, Seljelid R, Plytycz B. Morphine modulation of peritoneal inflammation in Atlantic salmon and CB6 mice. *J Leukoc Biol.* 1999;65(5):590-596.

291. Giorgi R, Pagano RL, Dias MA, Aguiar-Passeti T, Sorg C, Mariano M. Antinociceptive effect of the calcium-binding protein MRP-14 and the role played by neutrophils on the control of inflammatory pain. *J Leukoc Biol.* 1998;64(2):214-220.

292. Blixt A, Jonsson P, Braide M, Bagge U. Microscopic studies on the influence of erythrocyte concentration on the post-junctional radial distribution of leukocytes at small venular junctions. *Int J Microcirc Clin Exp.* 1985;4(2):141-156.

293. Schmid-Schonbein GW, Usami S, Skalak R, Chien S. The interaction of leukocytes and erythrocytes in capillary and postcapillary vessels. *Microvasc Res.* 1980;19(1):45-70.

294. Metchnikoff E. *Lectures on the Comparative Pathology of Inflammation.* Dover; 1968.

295. Springer TA. Traffic signals for lymphocyte recirculation and leukocyte emigration: the multistep paradigm. *Cell.* 1994;76(2):301-314.

296. Langereis JD. Neutrophil integrin affinity regulation in adhesion, migration, and bacterial clearance. *Cell Adhes Migrat.* 2013;7(6):476-481.

297. Alon R, Hammer DA, Springer TA. Lifetime of the P-selectin-carbohydrate bond and its response to tensile force in hydrodynamic flow. *Nature.* 1995;374(6522):539-542.

298. Carman CV, Springer TA. A transmigratory cup in leukocyte diapedesis both through individual vascular endothelial cells and between them. *J Cell Biol.* 2004;167(2):377-388.

299. Springer TA, Dustin ML. Integrin inside-out signaling and the immunological synapse. *Curr Opin Cell Biol.* 2012;24(1):107-115.

300. Zhu J, Zhu J, Springer TA. Complete integrin headpiece opening in eight steps. *J Cell Biol.* 2013;201(7):1053-1068.

301. Fan Z, McArdle S, Marki A, et al. Neutrophil recruitment limited by high-affinity bent beta2 integrin binding ligand in cis. *Nat Commun.* 2016;7:12658.

302. Vestweber D. How leukocytes cross the vascular endothelium. *Nat Rev Immunol.* 2015;15(11):692-704.

303. Ley K, Laudanna C, Cybulsky MI, Nourshargh S. Getting to the site of inflammation: the leukocyte adhesion cascade updated. *Nat Rev Immunol.* 2007;7(9):678-689.

304. Nourshargh S, Alon R. Leukocyte migration into inflamed tissues. *Immunity.* 2014;41(5):694-707.

305. Das J, Sharma A, Jindal A, Aggarwal V, Rawat A. Leukocyte adhesion defect: where do we stand circa 2019? *Genes Dis.* 2020;7(1):107-114.

306. Fischer A, Lisowska-Grospierre B, Anderson DC, Springer TA. Leukocyte adhesion deficiency: molecular basis and functional consequences. *Immunodeficiency Rev.* 1988;1(1):39-54.

307. Frydman M, Etzioni A, Eidlitz-Markus T, et al. Rambam-Hasharon syndrome of psychomotor retardation, short stature, defective neutrophil motility, and Bombay phenotype. *Am J Med Genet.* 1992;44(3):297-302.

308. Mory A, Feigelson SW, Yarali N, et al. Kindlin-3: a new gene involved in the pathogenesis of LAD-III. *Blood.* 2008;112(6):2591.

309. Deban L, Russo RC, Sironi M, et al. Regulation of leukocyte recruitment by the long pentraxin PTX3. *Nat Immunol.* 2010;11(4):328-334.

310. Choi EY, Chavakis E, Czabanka MA, et al. Del-1, an endogenous leukocyte-endothelial adhesion inhibitor, limits inflammatory cell recruitment. *Science.* 2008;322(5904):1101-1104.

311. Eskan MA, Jotwani R, Abe T, et al. The leukocyte integrin antagonist Del-1 inhibits IL-17-mediated inflammatory bone loss. *Nat Immunol.* 2012;13(5):465-473.

312. Gjelstrup LC, Boesen T, Kragstrup TW, et al. Shedding of large functionally active CD11/CD18 Integrin complexes from leukocyte membranes during synovial inflammation distinguishes three types of arthritis through differential epitope exposure. *J Immunol.* 2010;185(7):4154-4168.

313. Allison F, Jr, Smith MR, Wood WB, Jr. Studies on the pathogenesis of acute inflammation. I. The inflammatory reaction as observed in the rabbit ear chamber. *J Exp Med.* 1955;102(6):655-668.

314. Boyden S. The chemotactic effect of mixtures of antibody and antigen on polymorphonuclear leucocytes. *J Exp Med.* 1962;115:453-466.

315. Lammermann T, Bader BL, Monkley SJ, et al. Rapid leukocyte migration by integrin-independent flowing and squeezing. *Nature.* 2008;453(7191):51-55.

316. Stossel TP. The E. Donnall Thomas Lecture, 1993. The machinery of blood cell movements. *Blood.* 1994;84(2):367-379.

317. Houk AR, Jilkine A, Mejean CO, et al. Membrane tension maintains cell polarity by confining signals to the leading edge during neutrophil migration. *Cell.* 2012;148(1-2):175-188.

318. De Duve C, Wattiaux R. Functions of lysosomes. *Annu Rev Physiol.* 1966;28:435-492.

319. Wright DG, Gallin JI. A functional differentiation of human neutrophil granules: generation of C5a by a specific (secondary) granule product and inactivation of C5a by azurophilic (primary) granule products. *J Immunol.* 1977;119(3):1068-1076.

320. Klebanoff SJ. Antimicrobial mechanisms in neutrophilic polymorphonuclear leukocytes. *Semin Hematol.* 1975;12(2):117-142.

321. Baldridge CW, Gerard RW. The extra respiration of phagocytosis. *Am J Physiol.* 1932;103(1):235-236.

322. Rossi F, Zatti M. Biochemical aspects of phagocytosis in polymorphonuclear leucocytes. NADH and NADPH oxidation by the granules of resting and phagocytizing cells. *Experientia.* 1964;20(1):21-23.

323. Babior BM. NADPH oxidase. *Curr Opin Immunol.* 2004;16(1):42-47.

324. Nauseef WM. Assembly of the phagocyte NADPH oxidase. *Histochem Cell Biol.* 2004;122(4):277-291.

325. Klebanoff SJ. Myeloperoxidase: friend and foe. *J Leukoc Biol.* 2005;77(5):598-625.

326. Klebanoff SJ, White LR. Iodination defect in the leukocytes of a patient with chronic granulomatous disease of childhood. *N Engl J Med.* 1969;280(9):460-466.

327. Eiserich JP, Hristova M, Cross CE, et al. Formation of nitric oxide-derived inflammatory oxidants by myeloperoxidase in neutrophils. *Nature.* 1998;391(6665):393-397.

328. Lehrer RI, Cline MJ. Leukocyte myeloperoxidase deficiency and disseminated candidiasis: the role of myeloperoxidase in resistance to Candida infection. *J Clin Invest.* 1969;48(8):1478-1488.

329. Nath J, Powledge A. Modulation of human neutrophil inflammatory responses by nitric oxide: studies in unprimed and LPS-primed cells. *J Leukoc Biol.* 1997;62(6):805-816.

330. Evans TJ, Buttery LD, Carpenter A, Springall DR, Polak JM, Cohen J. Cytokine-treated human neutrophils contain inducible nitric oxide synthase that produces nitration of ingested bacteria. *Proc Natl Acad Sci USA.* 1996;93(18):9553-9558.

331. Wheeler MA, Smith SD, Garcia-Cardena G, Nathan CF, Weiss RM, Sessa WC. Bacterial infection induces nitric oxide synthase in human neutrophils. *J Clin Invest.* 1997;99(1):110-116.

332. Mosser DM, Edwards JP. Exploring the full spectrum of macrophage activation. *Nat Rev Immunol.* 2008;8(12):958-969.

333. Lakshmi VM, Nauseef WM, Zenser TV. Myeloperoxidase potentiates nitric oxide-mediated nitrosation. *J Biol Chem.* 2005;280(3):1746-1753.

334. Jensen MS, Bainton DF. Temporal changes in pH within the phagocytic vacuole of the polymorphonuclear neutrophilic leukocyte. *J Cell Biol.* 1973;56(2):379-388.

335. Mandell GL. Intraphagosomal pH of human polymorphonuclear neutrophils. *Proc Soc Exp Biol Med.* 1970;134(2):447-449.

336. Padgett GA, Hirsch JG. Lysozyme: its absence in tears and leukocytes of cattle. *Aust J Exp Biol Med Sci.* 1967;45(5):569-570.

337. Arnold RR, Cole MF, McGhee JR. A bactericidal effect for human lactoferrin. *Science.* 1977;197(4300):263-265.

338. Rorvig S, Honore C, Larsson LI, et al. Ficolin-1 is present in a highly mobilizable subset of human neutrophil granules and associates with the cell surface after stimulation with fMLP. *J Leukoc Biol.* 2009;86(6):1439-1449.

339. Owen CA, Campbell EJ. The cell biology of leukocyte-mediated proteolysis. *J Leukoc Biol.* 1999;65(2):137-150.

340. Cohn ZA. The fate of bacteria within phagocytic cells. I. The degradation of isotopically labeled bacteria by polymorphonuclear leucocytes and macrophages. *J Exp Med.* 1963;117:27-42.

341. Rogers DE, Tompsett R. The survival of staphylococci within human leukocytes. *J Exp Med.* 1952;95(2):209-230.

342. Zucker-Franklin D. Electron microscope study of the degranulation of polymorphonuclear leukocytes following treatment with streptolysin. *Am J Pathol.* 1965;47:419-433.

343. Corcino J, Krauss S, Waxman S, Herbert V. Release of vitamin B12--binding protein by human leukocytes in vitro. *J Clin Invest.* 1970;49(12):2250-2255.

344. Chikkappa G, Corcino J, Greenerg ML, Herert V. Correlation between varios blood white cell pools and the serum B12-binding capacities. *Blood.* 1971;37(2):142-151.

345. Lollike K, Kjeldsen L, Sengelov H, Borregaard N. Lysozyme in human neutrophils and plasma. A parameter of myelopoietic activity. *Leukemia.* 1995;9(1):159-164.

346. Allen RH. Human vitamin B12 transport proteins. *Prog Hematol.* 1975;9:57-84.

347. Fink ME, Finch SC. Serum neuramidase and granulocyte turnover. *Proc Soc Exp Biol Med.* 1968;127(2):365-367.

348. El Ouriaghli F, Fujiwara H, Melenhorst JJ, Sconocchia G, Hensel N, Barrett AJ. Neutrophil elastase enzymatically antagonizes the in vitro action of G-CSF: implications for the regulation of granulopoiesis. *Blood.* 2003;101(5):1752-1758.

349. Horwitz M, Benson KF, Person RE, Aprikyan AG, Dale DC. Mutations in ELA2, encoding neutrophil elastase, define a 21-day biological clock in cyclic haematopoiesis. *Nat Genet.* 1999;23(4):433-436.

350. Dale DC, Person RE, Bolyard AA, et al. Mutations in the gene encoding neutrophil elastase in congenital and cyclic neutropenia. *Blood.* 2000;96(7):2317-2322.

351. Nassar T, Akkawi S, Bar-Shavit R, et al. Human alpha-defensin regulates smooth muscle cell contraction: a role for low-density lipoprotein receptor-related protein/alpha 2-macroglobulin receptor. *Blood.* 2002;100(12):4026-4032.

352. Lammermann T, Afonso PV, Angermann BR, et al. Neutrophil swarms require LTB4 and integrins at sites of cell death in vivo. *Nature.* 2013;498(7454):371-375.

353. Bouchery T, Harris N. Neutrophil-macrophage cooperation and its impact on tissue repair. *Immunol Cell Biol.* 2019;97(3):289-298.

354. Bosurgi L, Cao YG, Cabeza-Cabrerizo M, et al. Macrophage function in tissue repair and remodeling requires IL-4 or IL-13 with apoptotic cells. *Science.* 2017;356(6342):1072-1076.

355. Puga I, Cols M, Barra CM, et al. B cell-helper neutrophils stimulate the diversification and production of immunoglobulin in the marginal zone of the spleen. *Nat Immunol.* 2011;13(2):170-180.

356. Parsa R, Lund H, Georgoudaki AM, et al. BAFF-secreting neutrophils drive plasma cell responses during emergency granulopoiesis. *J Exp Med.* 2016;213(8):1537-1553.

357. Leliefeld PH, Koenderman L, Pillay J. How neutrophils shape adaptive immune responses. *Front Immunol.* 2015;6:471.

358. Schuster S, Hurrell B, Tacchini-Cottier F. Crosstalk between neutrophils and dendritic cells: a context-dependent process. *J Leukoc Biol.* 2013;94(4):671-675.

359. Hufford MM, Richardson G, Zhou H, et al. Influenza-infected neutrophils within the infected lungs act as antigen presenting cells for anti-viral CD8(+) T cells. *PLoS One.* 2012;7(10):e46581.

360. Wagner C, Iking-Konert C, Hug F, et al. Cellular inflammatory response to persistent localized *Staphylococcus aureus* infection: phenotypical and functional characterization of polymorphonuclear neutrophils (PMN). *Clin Exp Immunol.* 2006;143(1):70-77.

361. Gosselin EJ, Wardwell K, Rigby WF, Guyre PM. Induction of MHC class II on human polymorphonuclear neutrophils by granulocyte/macrophage colony-stimulating factor, IFN-gamma, and IL-3. *J Immunol.* 1993;151(3):1482-1490.

362. Radsak M, Iking-Konert C, Stegmaier S, Andrassy K, Hansch GM. Polymorphonuclear neutrophils as accessory cells for T-cell activation: major histocompatibility complex class II restricted antigen-dependent induction of T-cell proliferation. *Immunology.* 2000;101(4):521-530.

363. Davey MS, Lin CY, Roberts GW, et al. Human neutrophil clearance of bacterial pathogens triggers anti-microbial gammadelta T cell responses in early infection. *PLoS Pathog.* 2011;7(5):e1002040.

364. Bank U, Reinhold D, Schneemilch C, Kunz D, Synowitz HJ, Ansorge S. Selective proteolytic cleavage of IL-2 receptor and IL-6 receptor ligand binding chains by neutrophil-derived serine proteases at foci of inflammation. *J Interferon Cytokine Res.* 1999;19(11):1277-1287.

365. Bank U, Ansorge S. More than destructive: neutrophil-derived serine proteases in cytokine bioactivity control. *J Leukoc Biol.* 2001;69(2):197-206.

366. Rodriguez PC, Quiceno DG, Ochoa AC. L-arginine availability regulates T-lymphocyte cell-cycle progression. *Blood.* 2007;109(4):1568-1573.

367. Chtanova T, Schaeffer M, Han SJ, et al. Dynamics of neutrophil migration in lymph nodes during infection. *Immunity.* 2008;29(3):487-496.

368. de Kleijn S, Langereis JD, Leentjens J, et al. IFN-gamma-stimulated neutrophils suppress lymphocyte proliferation through expression of PD-L1. *PLoS One.* 2013;8(8):e72249.

369. Talukdar S, Oh DY, Bandyopadhyay G, et al. Neutrophils mediate insulin resistance in mice fed a high-fat diet through secreted elastase. *Nat Med.* 2012;18(9):1407-1412.

370. Lu R, Pan H, Shively JE. CEACAM1 negatively regulates IL-1beta production in LPS activated neutrophils by recruiting SHP-1 to a SYK-TLR4-CEACAM1 complex. *PLoS Pathog.* 2012;8(4):e1002597.

371. Netea MG, Simon A, van de Veerdonk F, Kullberg BJ, Van der Meer JW, Joosten LA. IL-1beta processing in host defense: beyond the inflammasomes. *PLoS Pathog.* 2010;6(2):e1000661.

372. Weiss SJ. Tissue destruction by neutrophils. *N Engl J Med.* 1989;320(6):365-376.

373. Sorensen OE, Borregaard N. Neutrophil extracellular traps - the dark side of neutrophils. *J Clin Invest.* 2016;126(5):1612-1620.

374. Nauseef WM, Kubes P. Pondering neutrophil extracellular traps with healthy skepticism. *Cell Microbiol.* 2016;18(10):1349-1357.

375. Bakken JS, Krueth J, Wilson-Nordskog C, Tilden RL, Asanovich K, Dumler JS. Clinical and laboratory characteristics of human granulocytic ehrlichiosis. *JAMA.* 1996;275(3):199-205.

376. Lee HC, Kioi M, Han J, Puri RK, Goodman JL. Anaplasma phagocytophilum-induced gene expression in both human neutrophils and HL-60 cells. *Genomics.* 2008;92(3):144-151.

377. McCaffrey RL, Allen LA. Francisella tularensis LVS evades killing by human neutrophils via inhibition of the respiratory burst and phagosome escape. *J Leukoc Biol.* 2006;80(6):1224-1230.

378. Giladi A, Paul F, Herzog Y, et al. Single-cell characterization of haematopoietic progenitors and their trajectories in homeostasis and perturbed haematopoiesis. *Nat Cell Biol.* 2018;20(7):836-846.

379. Athens J. Neutrophilic granulocyte kinetics and granulocytopoiesis. In: Gordon A, ed. *Regulation of Hematopoiesis.* Appleton-Centruny-Crofts; 1970.

The Normal Hematologic System

Chapter 8 ■ The Human Eosinophil

MANALI MUKHERJEE • PARAMESWARAN NAIR • PAIGE LACY

INTRODUCTION

The eosinophil was first described in 1879 by Paul Ehrlich for its characteristic intracytoplasmic granules exhibiting a high affinity for the negatively charged dye, eosin.[1,2] Although rare in the circulation of healthy individuals, the eosinophil is prominent in peripheral blood and tissue in association with various disease conditions including allergy, inflammatory responses against metazoan helminthic parasites, and certain skin and malignant conditions.[3-8] The eosinophil has received special attention for its potential pathophysiological role in the manifestation of allergic diseases such as asthma, rhinitis, eczema, eosinophilic esophagitis (EE), and Crohn disease. Disorders of the respiratory tract, particularly allergic asthma and rhinitis, exhibit a strong correlation with the number as well as activation status of infiltrating tissue eosinophils. Similarly, many disorders of the gastrointestinal system exhibit prominent eosinophilic inflammation in the mucosa. The presence of eosinophils in the airway and gut mucosa has been associated with both allergic (IgE-dependent) and nonallergic (IgE-independent) manifestations of disease. Although clinically these conditions have been characterized as either allergic or nonallergic, it appears that the mechanisms underlying recruitment and activation of eosinophils in both types of disease are similar. Despite some difficulties in defining the exact immunological role of the eosinophil in disease, there is evidence that the eosinophil remains a major effector cell in many types of allergic and nonallergic inflammation.

Eosinophils are mobile, terminally differentiated granulocytes that arise principally from the bone marrow.[5,9] They are 8 to 10 μm in diameter, and their nuclei are usually bilobed, although three or more lobes are often observed. The eosinophil is characterized by large crystalloid granules, also known as secondary or specific granules, as shown in light microscopy by their bright red staining properties with acidic dyes such as eosin (*Figure 8.1*). As apparent in electron micrographs, the crystalloid granules contain electron-dense crystalline cores surrounded by an electron-lucent granule matrix (*Figure 8.2*). Eosinophils contain up to four other "granule" types: primary granules, small granules, lipid bodies, and small secretory vesicles. Crystalloid granules are membrane bound and contain a number of highly cationic basic proteins. The latter have been implicated in the tissue damage observed in asthma and other similar allergic conditions. Allergen and parasite-induced eosinophilia have been shown to be T cell dependent and are mediated by soluble factors (cytokines) released from sensitized lymphocytes.[10] Recent advances in human eosinophil research have also indicated that eosinophil infiltration into the tissue in allergic-type responses and asthma is regulated by a series of biological events that includes a complex interplay between immunological and inflammatory mechanisms.[3,5]

EOSINOPHIL DIFFERENTIATION

Peripheral blood and tissue eosinophils are derived by hemopoiesis from CD34+ myelocytic progenitors found in the bone marrow and in inflamed tissues. Eosinophils make up approximately 3% of the bone marrow from healthy individuals, of which 37% are fully differentiated and the remainder are promyelocytes/myelocytes and metamyelocytes.[9,11] The appearance of newly matured cells in the blood occurs approximately 2.5 days from the time of the last mitotic division.[9] The turnover of eosinophils is approximately 2.2×10^8 cells/kg/d, and the bone marrow possesses the largest end-differentiated eosinophil reservoir in the healthy body ($9\text{-}14 \times 10^8$ cells/kg).[12] Progenitors differentiate upon exposure to a network of cytokines and chemokines to become committed to the eosinophil/basophil (Eo/B) lineage.[13]

Transcription factors regulate the production of eosinophils in the bone marrow, involving at least three classes: GATA-1 (a zinc finger family member), PU.1, and C/EBP members (CCAAT/enhancer-binding protein family).[14] The fate of distinct lineages is regulated by PU.1, in which low levels induce lymphocytic cells and high levels promote myeloid differentiation.[15] Eosinophil lineage differentiation is synergistically induced by GATA-1 and PU.1.[16] However, GATA-1 is likely the most important transcription factor for eosinophil differentiation, as mice lacking GATA-1 have a specific deficiency in eosinophils.[17]

Eosinophils are more closely related to basophils than neutrophils and monocytes due to lineage differentiation at this stage.[18] In addition, eosinophils retain elements of expression of basophil/mast cell–specific high-affinity Fcε receptor (α subunit),[19] while basophils continue expression of low concentrations of eosinophil major basic protein (MBP).[20] Cytokines and chemokines are soluble factors generated under appropriate stimulation from T cells in the bone marrow. The three key cytokines that are critical for stimulation of bone marrow production of eosinophils are interleukin-3 (IL-3), IL-5, and granulocyte/macrophage colony-stimulating factor (GM-CSF).[21] These three cytokines are also produced by CD4+ and CD8+ T lymphocytes from peripheral blood as well as inflamed tissues.[22] In bone marrow samples, committed eosinophil precursors can be recognized by their expression of the IL-5 receptor (IL-5R) and the C-C chemokine receptor, CCR3, in addition to CD34.[23] It is now well recognized that IL-5 is a key cytokine in terminal differentiation of eosinophils,[24] and expression of the IL-5R on the progenitor cell is one of the first signs of commitment to the eosinophil lineage. The expression of IL-5R is almost exclusively limited to eosinophil progenitors and mature peripheral blood eosinophils, with some expression on basophils but not neutrophils or monocytes. This selectivity in receptor distribution indicates that IL-5 acts primarily as an eosinophilopoietic cytokine. This has resulted in the concept that inhibition of IL-5 with anti-IL-5 antibody therapy will result in the complete loss of eosinophils from the body, thus preventing the manifestation of allergic symptoms (see *Antieosinophil strategies* below). The obligatory role of IL-5 in the differentiation of the eosinophil has been confirmed by numerous studies on transgenic mice in which overexpression of the gene for IL-5 caused marked eosinophilia and increased numbers of eosinophil precursors in their bone marrow.[25,26] Interestingly, eosinophil

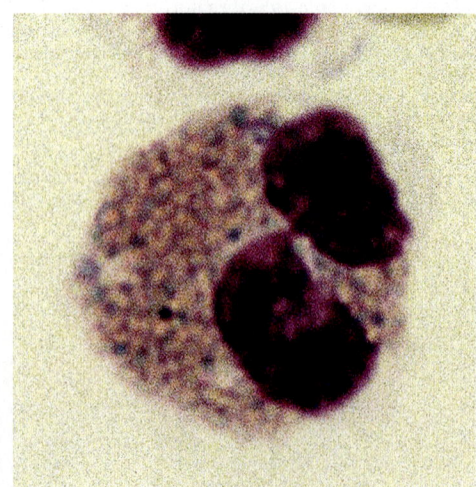

FIGURE 8.1 Photomicrograph of a peripheral blood eosinophil stained with May-Grünwald-Giemsa.

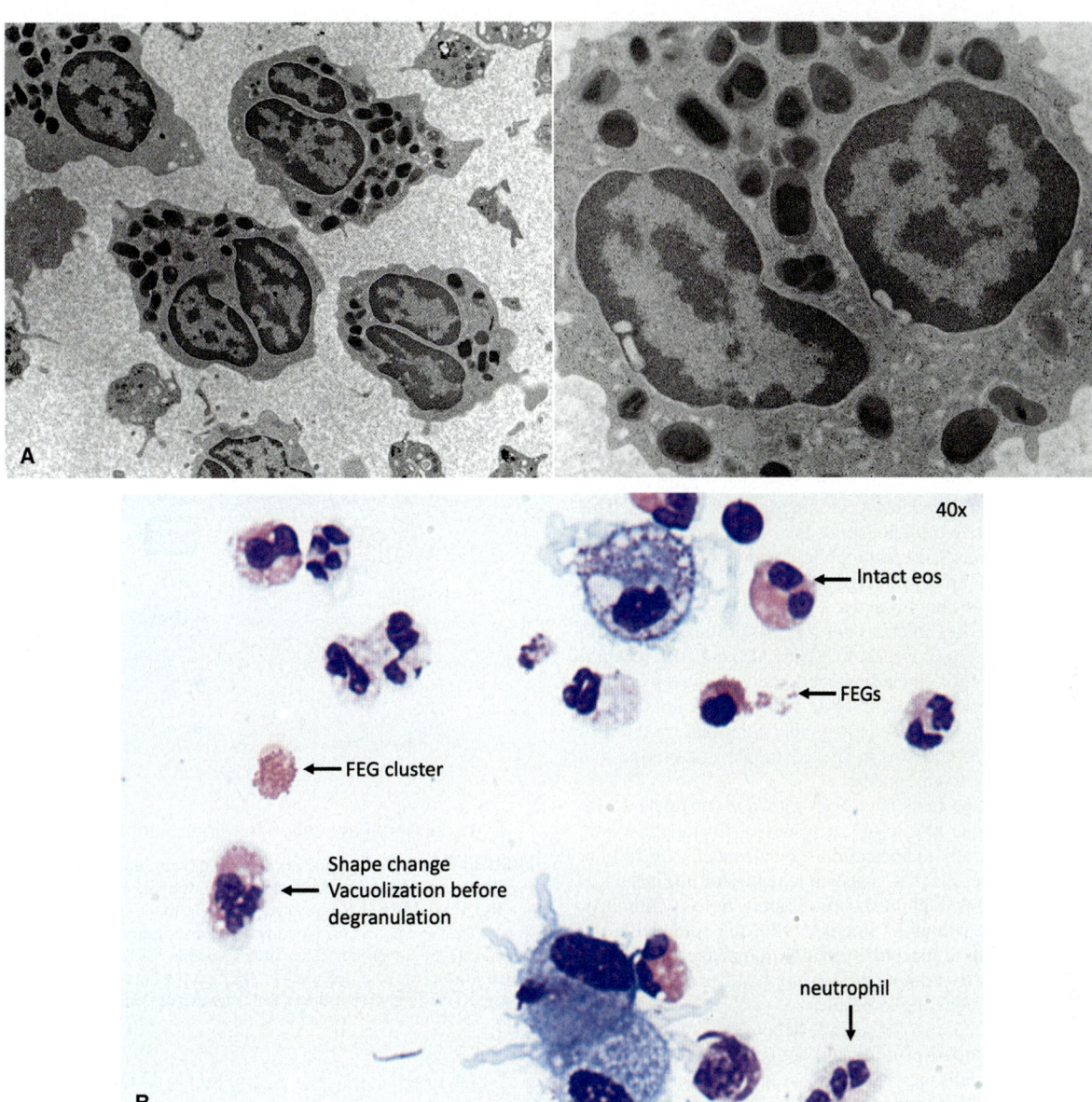

FIGURE 8.2 A, Electron photomicrographs of peripheral blood eosinophils from buffy coat. Original magnification 7655× and 22000×. B, Representative Wright-Giemsa–stained cytospin slide from processed sputum showing eosinophil at different states of degranulation including free eosinophil granules (FEGs), released during cytolysis (40× magnification). (A, Courtesy of Dr. G.E. Quinonez, Department of Pathology, University of Manitoba. B, Hargreave sputum laboratory, Hamilton, ON, Canada.)

differentiation in this transgenic model appeared to be completely independent of IL-3 and GM-CSF, suggesting that IL-5 alone may be sufficient to generate an eosinophilia from stem cell precursors. Gene deletion of IL-5 results in depletion of eosinophils from the circulation, as IL-5 gene-deficient mice exhibit a complete ablation of peripheral blood eosinophils.[27,28] However, although IL-5 gene-deficient mice exhibit almost no eosinophils in their blood, a small pool of apparently IL-5-independent eosinophils persist in the mucosal tissues of these animals.[29]

Additional eosinophilopoietic factors may assist in inducing the differentiation of Eo/B progenitors in the bone marrow, including IL-4, IL-6, IL-11, IL-12, and SCF.[30] C-C chemokines, named for their adjacent cysteine residues in the C-terminal amino acid sequence as distinct from the CXC chemokines, include CCL11/eotaxin and CCL5/RANTES, which have also been shown to be important in the development of eosinophils.[31] CCL11/eotaxin facilitates the efflux of fully mature eosinophils into the peripheral circulation and promotes the recruitment of eosinophils to target tissues. Overall, at the level of

the bone marrow, the early development of Eo/B progenitors is driven by IL-3 and GM-CSF, among other factors, while at later stages, IL-5 regulates the terminal differentiation of eosinophils.

The half-life of eosinophils in the circulation is approximately 18 h with a mean blood transit time of 26 h,[32] although this is extended in eosinophilic conditions, possibly due to the elevation of systemic eosinophil-activating cytokines that promote eosinophil survival. Based on a study of 740 medical students, the normal range of blood eosinophils was shown to be between 0 and 0.5×10^9/L, with counts ranging from 0.015 to 0.65×10^9/L.[33] Circulating eosinophil counts exhibit diurnal variation in humans, in which the lowest and highest levels are seen in the morning and evening, respectively, often exhibiting more than 40% variation within a day.[34] Mild eosinophilia is generally considered to be 0.5 to 1.5×10^9/L, moderate eosinophilia as 1.5 to 5.0×10^9/L, and marked eosinophilia greater than 5.0×10^9/L. Allergy is commonly associated with eosinophilia in the mild range, whereas parasitic infestation is often characterized by a marked eosinophilia.

Eosinophils are predominantly tissue cells, and their major target organs for homing in the healthy individual is the gastrointestinal tract (outside of the esophagus), mammary gland, uterus, thymus, and bone marrow. The gastrointestinal tract is the predominant site of homing for tissue eosinophils in healthy humans.[3,4] In states of disease, eosinophils appear in the lungs, esophagus, skin, and brain (e.g., during strokes). Once they enter target tissues, eosinophils do not return to the blood circulation. Eosinophil numbers can remain high in tissues even when peripheral numbers are low, suggesting that their survival is enhanced upon extravasation. Curiously, pathogen-free laboratory animals have no eosinophils in their blood, while tissue eosinophils are scarce, suggesting that the appearance of eosinophils may be environment or disease related.[11]

Eosinophil Production and Survival in Peripheral Tissue

Eosinophil development and maturation may also occur in situ in peripheral (extramedullary) sites outside of the bone marrow. In this case, Eo/B precursors are released into the bloodstream directly from the bone marrow to circulate to sites where they specifically transmigrate in response to locally produced cytokines and chemokines. This may provide an alternative mechanism for the persistence or accumulation of tissue eosinophils. Like neutrophils, eosinophils are end-stage cells, which, in culture, rapidly undergo cell death by either apoptosis or necrosis. However, eosinophil-active cytokines, such as IL-3, IL-5, and GM-CSF, as well as interferon-γ (IFNγ), prolong eosinophil survival in culture for up to 2 weeks.[35,36] They also enhance receptor expression and cell function, including cytotoxicity against metazoan targets, and mediator release. Local tissue types such as endothelial cells, fibroblasts, and epithelial cells may also contribute to the production of IL-5 and GM-CSF for in situ eosinophil maturation and differentiation in airway or gut mucosa.

Extracellular matrix proteins have been shown to modulate eosinophil responses to soluble physiological stimuli.[37] Eosinophils were shown to adhere specifically to fibronectin,[38] an abundant extracellular matrix protein. Moreover, VLA-4, a known receptor for fibronectin, is involved in mediating eosinophil/fibronectin interactions.[38] Similarly, VLA-6 expressed on eosinophils interacts with the connective tissue protein laminin. These receptors function to enhance eosinophil responses and are likely to promote the activation of tissue eosinophils by cytokines and other signaling molecules.

The eosinophil-specific cytokine, IL-5, delays eosinophil apoptosis and promotes eosinophil priming and activation.[39] IL-5 production by airway CD4+ T cells may be directly stimulated by eosinophils in a paracrine manner to enhance survival of tissue eosinophils.[40] Eosinophil progenitors in nasal explants from atopic patients have been shown to survive and develop into fully mature eosinophils ex vivo using similar mechanisms.[41] Allergen challenge of these explants, as well as lung explants of Brown-Norway rats, was shown to evoke a rapid (6 h) accumulation of MBP-positive cells after allergen challenge.[42] This was shown to be dependent on IL-5 production within the explant, a key cytokine in eosinophil survival.

The IL-5R consists of two subunits, an α subunit of 60 to 80 kDa and a common β_c subunit of between 120 to 140 kDa, which is shared with IL-3R and GM-CSFR. IL-5 interacts with its α subunit specifically but at a lower affinity than the β_c subunit.[43] IL-5 stimulation through the β_c subunit leads to phosphorylation of the tyrosine kinases, Jak2, Lyn, and Syk. While Jak2 signals through the nuclear translocation factor STAT1, Lyn and Syk signal through the mitogenic Ras-Raf1-MEK-ERK pathway (*Figure 8.3*). Tyrosine phosphorylation enhances the expression of the antiapoptotic protein Bcl-x$_L$ in eosinophils and decreases translocation of the proapoptotic signaling molecule Bax, resulting in decreased activation of apoptotic signaling through the caspase family.[44] GM-CSF prolongs the survival of eosinophils bound to tissue sites via α_4 integrin for up to 2 weeks[38] and has also been shown to inhibit eosinophil apoptosis similarly to IL-5. Thus, the growth, maturation, and prolongation of survival of eosinophils in extramedullary tissues may occur in sites other than the bone marrow.

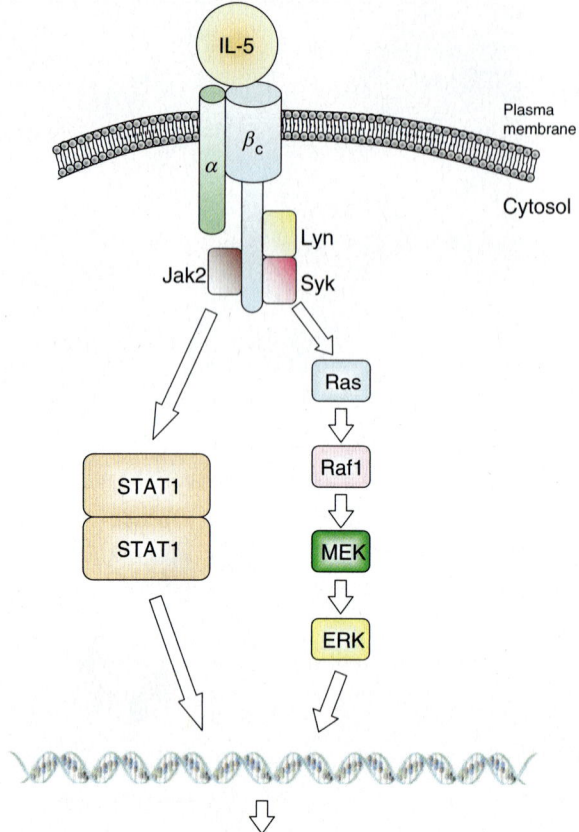

Transcriptional activation leading to antiapoptotic effects

FIGURE 8.3 **Signaling pathway leading from binding of IL-5 to its receptor in the membrane to transcriptional activation in the cell nucleus via the Ras-Raf1-MEK-ERK pathway.** The β subunit of the receptor is also able to activate the Jak2-STAT1 pathway. Transcriptional activation is proposed to generate antiapoptotic effects in eosinophils. ERK, extracellular signal regulated kinase; IL-5, interleukin-5; Jak2, Janus kinase 2; MEK, MAPK/ERK kinase; STAT, signal transducer and activator of transcription protein.

EOSINOPHIL TISSUE ACCUMULATION

Eosinophils migrate predominantly to the gastrointestinal tract during their normal development in healthy subjects,[4] and possibly in response to environmental factors as part of a role in innate defense against parasites. The mechanisms involved in the selective tissue recruitment of eosinophils across the vascular endothelium and into tissues in allergic reactions occur sequentially in four well-defined steps. These include (1) the *tethering* of the eosinophil to the lumenal surface of the vascular endothelium during normal transport through the blood vessel, (2) *rolling* of the eosinophil along the lumenal surface of the activated endothelium in a reversible manner, (3) firm *adhesion* of the eosinophil to endothelial cells, and (4) *transmigration* of the eosinophil through the endothelium into target tissues (*Figure 8.4*). A further, less understood, step-in eosinophil trafficking in the tissues is the in situ differentiation of circulating committed Eo/B precursors. Most migration through endothelium occurs at postcapillary venules.

Each of these steps is controlled by a complex network of chemotactic factors and adhesion molecules, which collectively direct the movement of the eosinophil into the tissues. For eosinophils, L-selectin and $\alpha4$ integrin are thought to be important in tethering and rolling, while $\alpha4$ and $\beta2$ (CD18) integrins mediate firm adhesion. The transmigration step is primarily regulated by $\beta2$ integrins as well as C-C chemokines such as CCL11/eotaxin. Cytokines and chemokines are elaborated by surrounding tissues to modulate the transmigration of eosinophils into tissues. Many of these mechanisms appear to be

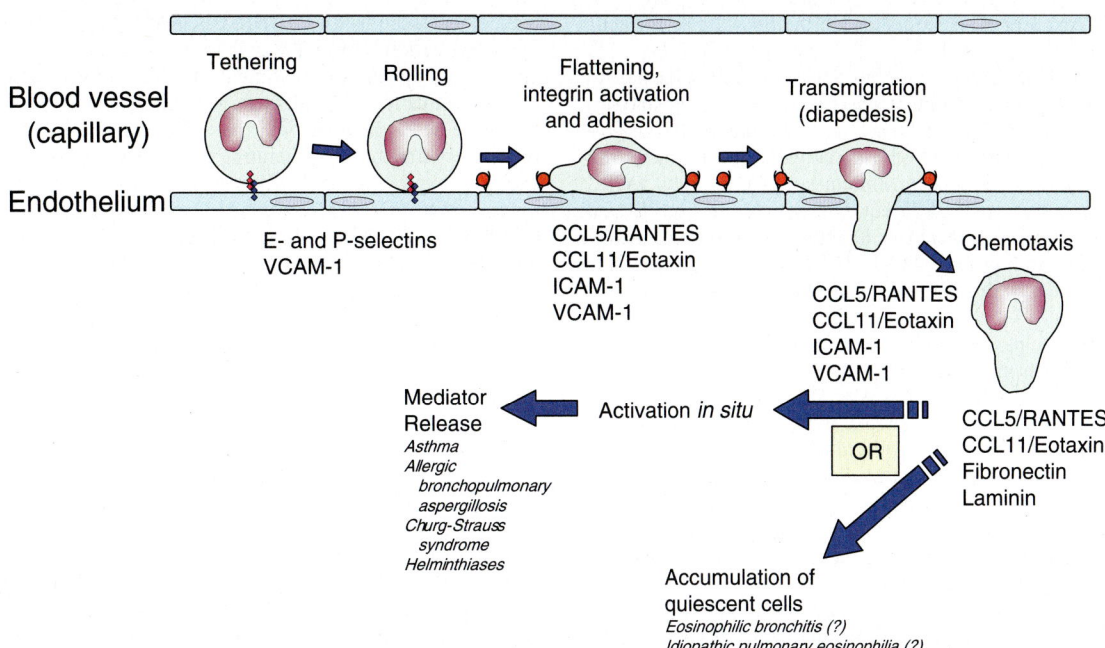

FIGURE 8.4 **Eosinophil tethering, rolling, adhesion, transmigration, and chemotaxis in response to inflammatory signals in tissues.** During chemotaxis, eosinophils may either become activated in response to local inflammation and release mediators, as in asthma and other related conditions, or accumulate in tissues in the apparent absence of mediator release. ICAM-1, intercellular adhesion molecule 1; RANTES, regulated upon activation, normal T-cell expressed and secreted; VCAM-1, vascular cell adhesion molecule 1. ? indicates that it is uncertain whether eosinophilic bronchitis or idiopathic pulmonary eosinophilia show quiescent cells, although when these illnesses resolve, there is very little damage to lung tissues, suggesting that eosinophils are not robustly activated.

controlled at the level of the T-cell response to antigen (allergen)-presenting cells and the subsequent release of cytokines and chemokines, which in turn regulate the activity of eosinophils.

Tethering and Rolling

Our knowledge of the mechanisms involved in eosinophil interactions with the endothelium extends primarily from in vitro assays of leukocyte adhesion to cultured human umbilical vein endothelial cells (HUVECs) both under stable and flow conditions. Antibodies specific for adhesion molecules have been applied in this system and have identified critical regulatory molecules required for adhesion and transmigration of eosinophils. Tethering and rolling of eosinophils on HUVEC cells under flow conditions is regulated by L-selectin (CD62L) expressed on the eosinophil surface interacting with E- and P-selectins (CD62E and CD62P) on endothelial cells.[45] Selectins are characterized by a lectin-binding domain, which is involved in the initial anchoring of inflammatory cells to the venular endothelium. This interaction is enhanced after the release of inflammatory mediators from these cells as well as neighboring tissues. Once tethered, eosinophils roll until they become stimulated by a chemoattractant stimulus (indicating local inflammation), which induces activation of α4 integrin receptors on the leukocyte. In addition, rolling appears to facilitate the subsequent adherence and transmigration of eosinophils into tissues. Eosinophils also express PSGL-1 and the integrins $\alpha4\beta1$ (VLA-4) and $\alpha4\beta7$, which are involved in cell rolling.[45] Eosinophil integrins bind to target sites in the endothelium, primarily ICAM-1 (CD54) and VCAM-1 (CD106), through their Mac-1 (a $\beta2$ integrin, also known as CR3 or CD11b/CD18) and VLA-4 ($\alpha4\beta1$ integrin) receptors, respectively. The constitutive expression of VLA-4 ($\alpha4\beta1$ integrin) is limited to a small number of leukocytes, including eosinophils, monocytes, basophils, and T cells, suggesting that regulated expression of its ligand, VCAM-1, on endothelial cells may be important in selective recruitment of these cells.[46]

Adhesion

The firm adhesion of eosinophils involves the interaction of α4 and β2 integrins with the endothelial layer. Specifically, eosinophils adhere to

TNFα-, IL-1β-, and LPS-activated HUVECs through CR3/ICAM-1 and VLA-4/VCAM-1 interactions.[46-49] Other adhesion molecules that may contribute to this process are LFA-1, VLA-6 ($\alpha4\beta1$), $\alpha4\beta7$ integrin, p150,95, and CD11d. Eosinophils exhibit differential binding properties through VCAM-1 and ICAM-1, which are dependent on their activation status. Freshly prepared unstimulated eosinophils preferentially bind to endothelial VCAM-1 via VLA-4 ($\alpha_4\beta_1$) rather than β_2 to ICAM-1.[31,50] Once activated, eosinophil preference for VCAM-1 shifts to that of endothelial ICAM-1 via β2 integrins.[31,51-53] During extravasation (diapedesis) into tissues, the eosinophil becomes progressively more activated upon contact with extracellular matrix proteins and other stimulated cells. Tissue eosinophils from an antigen challenge model express increased CD11, CD69, and ICAM-1.[54] Eosinophil binding in tissues switches to ICAM-1 and the CS-1 region of tissue fibronectin.[45,51,55] The change in the activation status is also confirmed by the changes in the expression of cell surface molecules seen as the eosinophil goes through tissue. Eosinophils recovered from bronchoalveolar lavage (BAL) express increased ICAM-1, Mac-1, CD69, and decreased L-selectin, suggesting an activated state.[56]

Cytokines such as IL-4 and IL-13 have been shown to upregulate eosinophil adhesion, primarily through upregulation of VCAM-1 on endothelial cells.[57,58] The effects of IL-4 and IL-13 are mediated through Jak3 and the nuclear transcription factor STAT-6.[59,60] Interestingly, a decrease in tissue eosinophilia has been observed in allergen-challenged STAT-6$^{-/-}$ mice, in spite of high levels of VCAM-1 expression.[60] This difference was thought to be due to decreased expression of CCR3 in eosinophils, which is directly controlled by STAT-6.[61] Results from STAT-6$^{-/-}$ mice would suggest that IL-4 and IL-13 also have a role in the induction of CCR3 on eosinophils and T cells. These findings underline the importance of cytokine and chemokine cross talk in the generation of blood eosinophilia and tissue diapedesis.

The switch to ICAM-1-mediated adhesion and transmigration may be associated with facilitation of eosinophil entrance into the tissue. Increased β_1 expression (VCAM-associated) has been shown to slow eosinophil migration compared with ICAM-1/β2.[62] It is important to note that anti-VLA-4 antibodies may not prevent eosinophil migration into tissue if ICAM-1 or P-selectin sites are the first targets for activated eosinophils.[45]

IL-5 also upregulates eosinophil, but not neutrophil, adhesion to unstimulated endothelium, offering a selective pathway of eosinophil adhesion.[63] IL-5 has been shown to activate transendothelial migration of eosinophils through ICAM-1 via decreased β_1 and increased β_2 integrin expression.[63] Similarly, stimulation of eosinophil CCR3 with a chemokine such as CCL11/eotaxin, which can be released from endothelial cells, also increases β_2 integrin expression, resulting in preferential binding to ICAM-1.[64] Thus, numerous cytokines and chemokines have been shown to enhance eosinophil adhesion to endothelium.

Complement proteins are also important in eosinophilic trafficking in tissues. Complement-mediated inflammation, as seen with parasite infection, is associated with the release of C3a and C5a. While C3a increases binding of eosinophil to endothelium but does not increase migration, C5a increases both adhesion and migration.[65] VCAM-1 and ICAM-1 are involved in complement-mediated binding and migration of eosinophils, as this process is blocked by the application of anti-α_4 and β_2 antibodies. These findings illustrate the importance of adhesion molecules VCAM-1 and ICAM-1 in the complement-mediated pathway of anaphylaxis and host defense.

Other more general inflammatory cytokines, such as IL-1 and TNFα, are also released by inflamed tissues and have significant effects on eosinophil migration.[45] Message encoding both IL-1 and TNFα is increased in the airways of symptomatic as opposed to nonsymptomatic asthmatics,[66] and IL-1 is increased in tissues from sites of cutaneous allergy.[67] Antibodies to IL-1 have been shown to decrease the expression of VCAM-1 and ICAM-1 in endothelial cells.[68] Mice deficient in IL-1 expression (IL-1$^{-/-}$) have decreased eosinophil rolling, adhesion, and transmigration.[69] TNFα has also been shown to increase expression of endothelial ICAM-1, VCAM-1, P-selectin, and E-selectin, causing increased eosinophil rolling and adhesion.[70] In addition, TNF$^{-/-}$ mice show decreased eosinophil adhesion and migration into tissue, similar to IL-1$^{-/-}$ mice.[71] These factors may have important roles in allergic asthma where preferential accumulation of eosinophils is a feature of atopic (IgE-dependent) inflammatory conditions.

Transmigration and Chemotaxis

Once eosinophils adhere to vascular endothelium, they commence diapedesis whereby they emerge out of the capillaries and traverse the adjacent connective tissue *en route* to the focus of the inflammatory response. Eosinophils move through the endothelium by extending lamellipodia in the form of a uropod, thus leading to lamellar motion.[45] For cells to move, there must be increased binding forward via the uropod and release of binding to the rear. Changes in the binding affinity for adhesion molecules and extracellular matrix proteins are thought to contribute to cell movement on a substratum. A gradient in binding affinity of eosinophil VLA-4 to fibronectin has been demonstrated,[72] where increased adherence at the leading edge of the cell is followed by deadherence at the rear of the cell, allowing the cell to move on. Cytokines and chemokines also influence the binding of eosinophils to tissue surfaces, such as GM-CSF, which increases the binding affinity of VLA-4 to VCAM-1 or CS-1,[73] and CCL11/eotaxin, which stimulates the reverse reaction.[64] CCL11/eotaxin induces cytoskeletal changes via mitogen-activated protein kinases (MAPKs),[45] Rho guanosine triphosphatases (GTPases), and Rho kinase.[74,75] Eosinophil chemotaxis may be inhibited by CXCL9 (monokine induced by interferon-γ, Mig), a factor that inhibits eotaxin-induced chemotaxis.[76,77] Other chemokines or chemotactic factors, such as CCL5/RANTES, CCL7/monocyte chemoattractant protein-3 (MCP-3), and C5a, may also alter β_1 integrin affinity in eosinophils.[51,78] The balance of these factors determines the rate of eosinophil migration.

Although cytokines (e.g., IL-3, IL-5, and GM-CSF) are essential for the development and proliferation of eosinophils, they are likely to play an immunomodulatory role in priming eosinophils for better chemotactic responses to target tissue sites. The most potent eosinophil chemoattractants include PAF, LTD$_4$, C5a, IL-2, and C-C

chemokines such as CCL11/eotaxin and CCL5/RANTES (Regulated upon Activation, Normal T cell Expressed and Secreted).[79,80] C-C chemokines appear to be essential for inducing the specific migration of eosinophils to inflamed sites. Several distinct families of chemokines have been identified, and the CCR3-binding family in particular plays a crucial role in generating tissue eosinophilia due the nearly exclusive expression of CCR3 in eosinophils.[31] This family of chemokines consists of CCL11/eotaxin (1, 2, and 3), CCL5/RANTES, CCL7, CCL8, CCL12 (MCP-2, 3, and 5), and CCL3/macrophage inhibitory protein (MIP)-1α. Chemokines binding CCR3 may be selective for granulocytes such as eosinophils and basophils, as neutrophils do not express this receptor. CCL11/eotaxin is the only chemokine with potent chemoattractant effects on eosinophils, making it a key ligand for the CCR3 family.[81] CCR3 chemokines are produced by endothelial cells, epithelial cells, parasympathetic nerves, T cells, macrophages, fibroblasts, and eosinophils, among other tissue sources.[82,83]

Basal expression of CCL11/eotaxin in the gut is elevated compared with other tissues in the normal animal.[84] During allergen-induced eosinophilia, CCL11/eotaxin expression is further increased within tissues.[85] Some synergism exists between IL-5 and CCL11/eotaxin, as IL-5 stimulation enhances the eosinophil response to CCL11/eotaxin both in vitro and in vivo.[86,87] In order to define the specific role of CCL11/eotaxin in inflammation, CCL11/eotaxin gene knockout mice have been deployed.[88] These mice produce IL-5 normally and thus continue to develop blood eosinophilia similar to their wild-type heterozygotes. However, CCL11/eotaxin$^{-/-}$ mice do not develop tissue eosinophilia. Thus, the primary role of CCR3 appears to be involved in the homing of circulating eosinophils to target tissues expressing CCL11/eotaxin.

Additional chemokines of the CCR3 family have been shown to exert important effects in situations where CCL11/eotaxin may not be necessarily essential to the response.[45,89] Each chemokine appears to have a unique role in the timing and location of tissue eosinophilia. Peripheral blood levels and cultured mononuclear cells from patients with allergic dermatitis produce increased levels of CCL5/RANTES, CCL2/MCP-1, and CCL3/MIP-1α compared with nonallergic controls.[90] Similarly to CCL11/eotaxin, IL-5-stimulated eosinophils have an increased affinity for CCL5/RANTES. However, unlike CCL11/eotaxin, CCL5/RANTES was specifically associated with exacerbations of eosinophilic bronchitis, thought to be provoked by viral infection. Infections with respiratory syncytial virus leading to eosinophilia have been correlated with increased CCL5/RANTES, CCL2/MCP-1, and CCL3/MIP-1α expression.[91] Children with asthma have large increases in eosinophil-associated MBP, CCL5/RANTES, and CCL3/MIP-1α in their nasal secretions during naturally acquired viral infections.[92] Therefore, the apparently broader range of effects of CCL5/RANTES, CCL3/MIP-1α, and CCL/2MCP-1 may also increase the range of eosinophil activity in disease, even though all of these bind specifically to CCR3 on eosinophils.

Other factors are also produced in mucosal tissues, which are moderately or strongly chemotactic for eosinophils. These include bacterial products (e.g., endotoxin and the tripeptide f-Met-Leu-Phe [fMLF]), the anaphylatoxin complement factor, C5a, opsonized particles (which exert their effect via complement [CR1, CR3] and FcγRII receptors), and other cytokines (IL-4, CXCL8/IL-8, and possibly IL-13). In addition, the lipid-derived mediators, leukotriene B$_4$ (LTB$_4$) and PAF, which are elevated in allergic responses and induce eosinophil respiratory burst and degranulation at higher doses,[30,37,93,94] are also eosinophilotactic. Eosinophil cytokines IL-3, IL-5, and GM-CSF are able to enhance the chemotactic ability of each of these factors. However, PAF antagonists are not sufficient at preventing eosinophilic inflammation in allergy.

EOSINOPHIL MEDIATORS

The eosinophil is considered to be both a factory and a store for a large array of mediators that are released upon activation and are thought to be important in various inflammatory reactions associated with this cell (*Figure 8.5*).

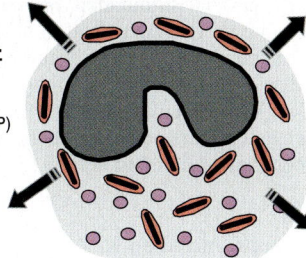

De novo-synthesized lipid mediators
LTC_4, PGE_1, PGE_2, TXB_2, 15-HETE, PAF

Oxidative metabolites
O_2^-, H_2O_2, OH^-, $ONOO^-$

Preformed granule-derived cationic proteins
Major basic protein (MBP)
Eosinophil
    peroxidase (EPX)
Eosinophil cationic
    protein (ECP)
Eosinophil-derived
    neurotoxin (EDN)
Charcot-Leyden
    crystal protein (CLC)

Cytokines, chemokines, and growth factors

IL-1α, IL-2, IL-3, IL-4,
IL-5, IL-6, IL-8, IL-9,
IL-10, IL-12, IL-16,
TGF-α, TGF-β, SCF,
PDGF-B, NGF,
IFN-γ, TNF, GM-CSF,
CCL5/RANTES,
CCL11/eotaxin, MIP-1α

FIGURE 8.5 Mediators released by activated eosinophils. *De novo* synthesized lipid mediators and oxidative metabolites are elaborated directly from the cell membrane or lipid bodies following enzyme activation, while granule-derived cationic proteins and cytokines, chemokines, and growth factors are released following granule-plasma membrane fusion during degranulation. 15-HETE, 15-hydroxyeicosatetraenoic acid; GM-CSF, granulocyte macrophage colony-stimulating factor; IFN, interferon; IL, interleukin; LTC, leukotrienes; MIP, macrophage inhibitory protein; NGF, nerve growth factor; PAF, platelet-activating factor; PDGF, platelet-derived growth factor; $PGE_{1/2}$, prostaglandin $E_{1/2}$; RANTES, regulated upon activation, normal T-cell expressed and secreted; SCF, stem cell factor; TGF, transforming growth factor; TXB_2, thromboxane B_2.

Eosinophil Granule Proteins

The eosinophil contains at least five different populations of phospholipid bilayer membrane-bound granules that appear during various stages of its development from progenitor cells to maturity.

a. Crystalloid granules: these specialized and unique granules measure 0.5 to 0.8 µm in diameter, contain crystalline electron-dense cores (internum) surrounded by an electron-lucent matrix, and can take up acidic dyes avidly due to their cationic nature.[4] They are mainly present in circulating end-differentiated, mature eosinophils, although coreless granules have been observed in immature eosinophils. These granules contain the bulk of highly charged cationic proteins present in eosinophils, including MBP, eosinophil peroxidase (EPX), eosinophil cationic protein (ECP), and eosinophil-derived neurotoxin (EDN). There are approximately 200 crystalloid granules in each cell. The core predominantly comprises crystallized MBP (*Figure 8.6*).

b. Primary granules: these are coreless granules that are enriched with the Charcot-Leyden crystal (CLC) protein, a lysophospholipase, and are present mainly in immature eosinophils, although mature eosinophils have been found to contain primary granules as well. Some authors refer to immature crystalloid granules as primary granules in eosinophil promyelocytes. These measure between 0.1 and 0.5 µm in diameter and are less abundant than crystalloid granules.

c. Small granules: these granules are free of cores, are less than 0.1 µm in diameter, and contain acid phosphatase, arylsulfatase B, catalase, and cytochrome b_{558}.

d. Lipid bodies: there are around five lipid bodies per mature eosinophil, the number of which increases in certain eosinophilic disorders, especially in idiopathic hypereosinophilia. Lipid bodies are enriched in arachidonic acid esterified into glycerophospholipids.

e. Secretory vesicles: eosinophils are densely packed with small secretory vesicles in their cytoplasm. These vesicles appear as dumbbell-shaped structures in cross sections and contain albumin, suggesting an endocytotic origin. These structures are also known as microgranules or tubulovesicular structures.

In these granule subpopulations, eosinophil-derived granule proteins are found in large concentrations. The following sections describe some of the most abundant granule proteins described in eosinophils.

Major Basic Protein

Eosinophil MBP (13.8 kDa) is an arginine-rich 117-amino-acid protein that constitutes a significant proportion of total cell protein in human eosinophils (5-10 pg/cell). MBP was originally named for its abundance in guinea pig eosinophils, which contain as much as 250 pg/cell, making up 50% of the total cellular protein.[95] The high calculated pI point of MBP (11.4) cannot be measured accurately due to the extremely basic nature of the protein.[96] MBP is initially translated as pro-MBP (23-25 kDa) with a calculated pI of 6 to 6.2 in maturing eosinophils.[97,98] The synthesis of MBP is initiated during

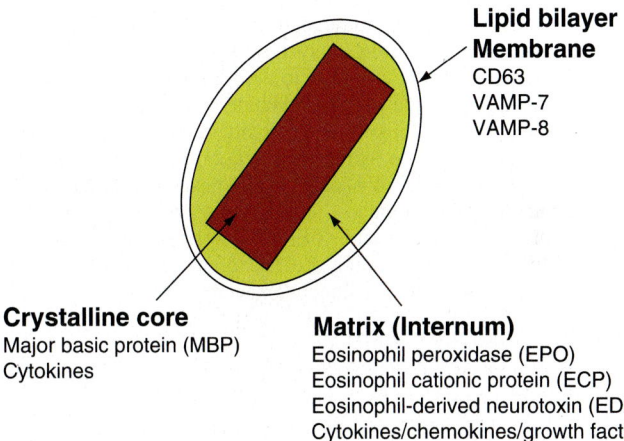

Lipid bilayer Membrane
CD63
VAMP-7
VAMP-8

Crystalline core
Major basic protein (MBP)
Cytokines

Matrix (Internum)
Eosinophil peroxidase (EPO)
Eosinophil cationic protein (ECP)
Eosinophil-derived neurotoxin (EDN)
Cytokines/chemokines/growth factors

FIGURE 8.6 Structure of the eosinophil crystalloid granule. This membrane-bound organelle is a major site of storage of eosinophil cationic granule proteins as well as a number of cytokines, chemokines, and growth factors.

the promyelocytic stage of eosinophil development, characterized by the presence of message encoding this protein, in a neutral pre-pro form that is later processed to form pro-MBP that is subsequently transported to the immature crystalloid granule and cleaved to form MBP.[97,98] The pro- segment of pro-MBP is postulated to protect the cell from cytotoxic effects of MBP during trafficking of pro-MBP from the Golgi apparatus to the crystalloid granule. Mature MBP undergoes condensation from the periphery of immature crystalloid granules to the internum, where it develops a crystalline core as its concentration is increased.[98,99] Once eosinophils have reached full maturity, MBP is no longer transcribed or translated, and detectable messenger RNA encoding MBP disappears from the cell.[98,100]

MBP has been shown to exert cytotoxic effects on helminthic parasites and certain bacteria.[4] It is also cytotoxic to human cells and especially airway tissues, including bronchial epithelial cells and pneumocytes, by disruption of cell membrane lipid bilayers.[101] Such disruption leads to cell permeabilization and lysis and leakage of cell contents to the extracellular milieu. Thus, MBP may be at least partly responsible for tissue damage and neural dysfunction associated with eosinophil infiltration into the bronchial mucosa in asthma.[102] Indeed, airway sections from patients with status asthmaticus exhibit intense MBP-specific immunofluorescence, suggesting that infiltrated eosinophils were fully activated, undergoing extracellular secretion of their contents of MBP.[103] MBP acts on other inflammatory cells, including neutrophils and eosinophils, to induce degranulation and lipid mediator release.[104,105] Parasympathetic ganglia in the airways of patients dying of asthma exhibit eosinophil infiltration, and MBP is an allosteric antagonist for the M2 muscarinic receptor. Loss of M2 receptor function results in airway hyperreactivity.[102] Two homologs of MBP have been described, MBP1 and MBP2, the latter with a calculated pI of 8.7, that possesses similar activities to MBP in cell killing as well as neutrophil and basophil stimulation, but with reduced potency.[106] The nonselective toxicity of MBP within eosinophils is kept at a minimum by its intragranular storage in crystalline cores that lock the protein into a nontoxic conformation.[107] Eosinophil activation induces granule acidification, which then triggers MBP toxicity followed by extracellular aggregation. This process is thought to induce significant damage to pathogens as well as host cells.

Eosinophil Peroxidase

Other eosinophil basic proteins, including EPX, ECP, and EDN, reside in the matrix compartment of the crystalloid granule. EPX is a highly basic (pI of 10.9) heme-containing protein composed of two subunits, a heavy chain of 50 to 57 kDa and a light chain of 11 to 15 kDa. A haloperoxidase enzyme, EPX has 68% sequence identity to neutrophil and monocyte-expressed myeloperoxidase, suggesting that a peroxidase multigene family may have developed through gene duplication.[96,108] Eosinophils store approximately 15 pg/cell of EPX, and this enzyme is important in catalyzing the peroxidative oxidation of halides and pseudohalides, leading to the formation of bactericidal hypohalous acids in reaction with hydrogen peroxide generated during respiratory burst.[109-111] Unlike myeloperoxidase, EPX preferentially uses bromide over chloride, generating hypobromous acid (HOBr) when H_2O_2 is present as its substrate.[112] EPX-generated HOBr kills a variety of microorganisms and also inflicts collateral damage on host tissues such as epithelial cells and other tissue-resident cells, and possesses antitumor activity. Binding of EPX to bacterial and parasitic pathogens also enhances their killing by phagocytic cells.

Eosinophil Cationic Protein

The molecular mass of ECP is 15 kDa, with around 15 pg/cell expressed in human eosinophils. The pI of ECP (10.8) is similar to that of MBP due to a similar arginine-rich sequence. ECP, also known as RNase-3, possesses intrinsic ribonuclease (Rnase) activity and is a member of a subfamily of Rnase A multigenes, with homology to pancreatic Rnase. It is also antiviral and bactericidal, promotes degranulation of mast cells, and is toxic to helminthic parasites.[113,114] The mechanism of action of ECP is thought to involve the formation of pores or channels in the target membrane, which is apparently not dependent on its reversible Rnase activity.[115] ECP is also neurotoxic as derived from its ability to elicit the Gordon phenomenon, involving the destruction of nerve cells.[116]

Eosinophil-Derived Neurotoxin

EDN, another member of the Rnase A multigene family of 18.5 kDa with approximately 100-fold higher Rnase activity than ECP, is less basic than MBP or ECP with a pI of 8.9 due to a relatively smaller number of arginine residues in its sequence. ECP and EDN share a remarkable sequence homology of 67% at the amino acid level for the pre- form of both proteins, suggesting that, evolutionarily, these proteins are derived from the same gene.[117,118] However, EDN has about 100 times more Rnase activity than ECP. Eosinophils express approximately 10 pg/cell of EDN, but there is marked variation between individuals. EDN also induces the Gordon phenomenon.[116] Similar to ECP, EDN also has significant toxicity against viruses, bacteria, and helminths.[119] Messenger RNA encoding EPX, ECP, and EDN has been detected in mature eosinophils, suggesting that these end-differentiated cells have the capacity to continually synthesize these proteins.[100]

The rates of mutation in the gene family expressing ECP and EDN are among the highest in the primate genome, ranking with those of immunoglobulins, T-cell receptors, and major histocompatibility complex (MHC) classes.[118] These genes effectively comprise a superfamily of Rnases expressed in the mammalian genome. Such a high rate of mutation suggests that evolutionary constraints acting on the ECP/EDN superfamily have promoted the acquisition of a specialized antiviral activity that may be important in controlling respiratory virus infections.[120]

Charcot-Leyden Crystal Protein

The CLC protein (17.4 kDa) is produced in eosinophils at very high levels (accounting for 10% of the total cellular protein), although its functional role is still obscure. The CLC protein is a hydrophobic protein with lysophospholipase activity and bears a strong sequence homology to the carbohydrate-binding galectin family of proteins. For this reason, the CLC protein has been designated galectin-10.[121] Electron microscopy has confirmed peripheral periplasmic subcellular localization of galectin-10 within resting eosinophils[122] as opposed to the initial conflicting reports of it being inside the primary granules and nuclear euchromatin.[123,124] Galectin-10 is released in large quantities in the tissues in eosinophilic disorders, which spontaneously autocrystallizes resulting in the formation of distinct, needle-shaped structures. These crystals are colorless and measure 20 to 40 µm in length and 2 to 4 µm across. CLC proteins are abundant in the sputa and feces of patients with severe respiratory and gastrointestinal eosinophilia, which were first observed by Charcot and Robin in 1853.

A list of these and other granule proteins synthesized and stored in eosinophils is presented in *Table 8.1* and published elsewhere.[3,4,30,125,126]

Eosinophil Degranulation

Degranulation is defined as the exocytotic fusion of granules with the plasma membrane during receptor-mediated secretion. During exocytosis, the outer leaflet of the lipid bilayer membrane surrounding the granule encounters the inner leaflet of the plasma membrane, a process known as "docking." The docking step is hypothesized to be regulated by intracellular membrane-associated proteins that act as receptors directing the specificity of granule targeting. After docking, the granule and plasma membrane fuse together and form a reversible structure called the fusion pore, which is also thought to be regulated by similar, or the same, membrane-associated proteins regulating granule docking. Depending on the intensity of the stimulus, the fusion pore may either retreat, leading to reseparation of the granule from the plasma membrane, or expand and allow complete integration of the granule membrane into the plasma membrane as a continuous sheet. The inner leaflet of the granule membrane becomes outwardly exposed, and the granule contents are subsequently expelled to the exterior of the cell.[127,128]

There are four main forms of eosinophil granule release, which have been observed in vitro and in vivo (*Figure 8.7*). The first is the classical sequential release of single crystalloid granules, which was the original hypothesis suggested for a predominant route of degranulation in eosinophils. This type of release is typically seen in vitro and can be elegantly demonstrated electrophysiologically using patch-clamp procedures that measure changes in membrane capacitance, which are directly proportional to increases in the surface area of the cell membrane. During the sequential release of individual crystalloid granules, a step-wise increment in capacitance may be observed as their membranes fuse with that of the cell membrane.[129-132] The second mode of granule release is compound exocytosis, also demonstrated by patch-clamp analysis in which sudden, very large increments in whole cell capacitance occur resulting from individual granules fusing with the cell membrane.[132] Ultrastructural studies of guinea pig eosinophils have also demonstrated evidence for compound exocytosis[133] similar to that observed in rat eosinophils adhering to the outer surface of opsonized parasitic larvae.[134]

The third manner in which eosinophils degranulate is by piecemeal degranulation (PMD). PMD was first characterized by Dvorak and colleagues for the appearance of numerous small vesicles in the cytoplasm coupled with the apparent loss of crystalloid granule core and matrix components, creating a "mottled" appearance in the crystalloid granules by electron microscopy analysis.[135] This was thought to be due to small vesicles budding off from the larger secondary granules and moving to the plasma membrane for fusion, thereby causing gradual emptying of the crystalloid granules to the outside of the cell. PMD was the most commonly observed pattern of degranulation seen in situ in biopsy samples from the upper airways of allergic

Table 8.1. Content of Human Eosinophil Granules and Secretory Vesicles

Crystalloid Granules	Primary Granules	Small Granules	Lipid Bodies	Secretory Vesicles
Core				
Catalase				
Cathepsin D				
Enoyl-CoA-hydrolase				
β-Glucuronidase				
Major basic protein				
Matrix				
Acid phosphatase	Charcot-Leyden crystal protein (galectin-10)	Acid phosphatase	Arachidonic acid	Plasma proteins (Albumin)
Acyl-CoA oxidase		Arylsulfatase B (active)	Cyclooxygenase	
Arylsulfatase B (inactive)		Catalase	Eosinophil peroxidase	
Acid β-glycerophosphatase		Elastase	Esterase	
Bactericidal/permeability-increasing protein		Eosinophil cationic protein	5-Lipoxygenase	
Catalase			15-Lipoxygenase	
Cathepsin D			LTC$_4$ synthase	
Collagenase				
Elastase				
Enoyl-CoA-hydrolase (also in core)				
Eosinophil cationic protein				
Eosinophil-derived neurotoxin				
Eosinophil peroxidase				
Flavin adenine dinucleotide (FAD)				
β-Glucuronidase				
β-Hexosaminidase				
3-Ketoacyl-CoA thiolase				
Lysozyme				
Major basic protein				
Phospholipase A$_2$ (Type II)				
Nonspecific esterases				
Membrane				
CD63		VAMP-7		Cytochrome b$_{558}$ [p22*phox*]
V-type H$^+$-ATPase		VAMP-8		VAMP-2
VAMP-7				VAMP-7
VAMP-8				VAMP-8

Abbreviation: VAMP, vesicle-associated membrane protein.

individuals[136] and is likely to be physiologically the most important mechanism for eosinophil mediator release in allergic disease. An in vitro model for PMD has been established using IFNγ-stimulated eosinophils, in which a piecemeal manner of CCL5/RANTES release was observed.[137] More recent studies have demonstrated that PMD occurs through the formation of tubular structures budding off from crystalloid granules.[138,139] Vesicles associated with PMD are also necessary for the transportation of MBP[140] and eosinophil-derived IL-4.[138,141]

Airway tissue eosinophils in allergic subjects also appear necrotic, which is a fourth pattern of granule release, also termed "cytolysis."[142] This type of release has been previously observed to occur following in vitro stimulation of human eosinophils with the calcium ionophore A23187[143] and appears to be a physiologically relevant event in granule release.

Eosinophil degranulation may be induced by immobilized or soluble stimuli. Degranulation responses to immobilized stimuli have been extensively characterized in eosinophils in view of their role in helminth infections. When incubated with opsonized helminths, eosinophils degranulate onto the surface of the parasite.[134,144] A similar phenomenon occurs when eosinophils are incubated with Sepharose beads coated with antibodies, specifically IgG, IgA, and secretory IgA (sIgA), with sIgA being the most potent inducer of degranulation.[145] Cross-linking of immunoglobulin receptors on eosinophils has been shown to be highly effective at inducing respiratory burst and EDN degranulation in eosinophils, with a hierarchy of effectiveness in degranulation demonstrated to be in the order of secretory IgA (sIgA) = IgA > IgG >> IgE.[145] Eosinophil cytokines such as IL-3, IL-5, and GM-CSF were demonstrated to enhance this process.[146] Allergen-specific IgG$_1$ and IgG$_3$ induce eosinophil degranulation via Fcγ receptor II (CD32).[147]

The Normal Hematologic System

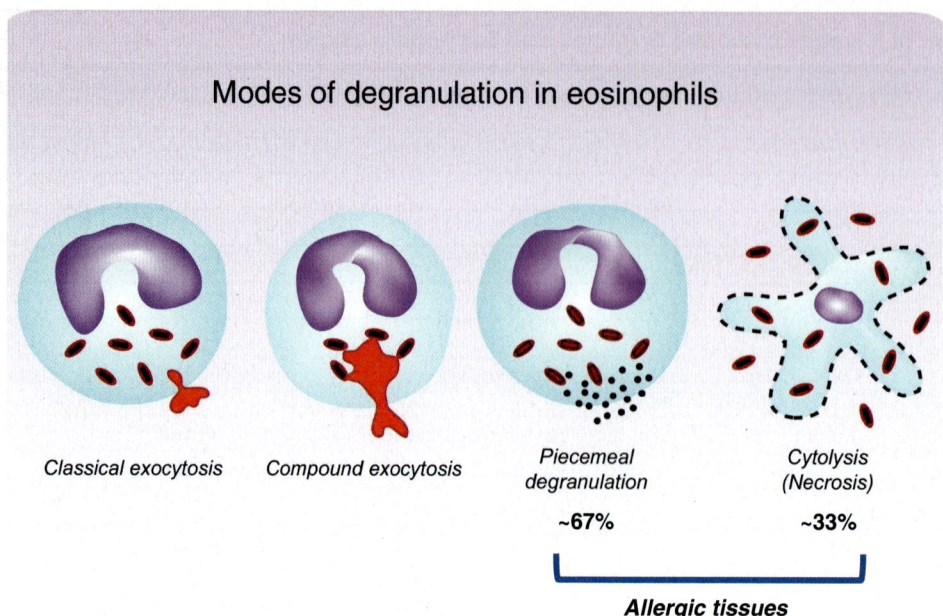

FIGURE 8.7 Four putative physiological modes of eosinophil degranulation. The most commonly observed forms of degranulation in allergic disease are piecemeal degranulation and necrosis (cytolysis). Parasitic and fungal diseases typically exhibit eosinophils undergoing compound exocytosis.

Receptors Expressed by Eosinophils

Eosinophils express a range of receptors for immunoglobulins that may contribute to chemotactic and activation responses in tissues. These include receptors for IgA, IgD, IgE, IgG, and IgM, which may possess up to three chains (α, β, and γ). Human eosinophils express FcαR, which is enhanced in allergic individuals,[148] as well as FcγRII (CD32), but not FcγRI (CD64) or FcγRIII (CD16). Mucosal tissues are enriched in sIgA, potentially as a mechanism against invasive pathogens. IgA, particularly the secretory isoform, is an important mucosal antibody involved in supporting the body's first line of defense. Thus, the sensitivity of the eosinophil to IgA is in agreement with its proposed role in protection against invasive organisms in mucosal tissues. Taken together, these findings along with eosinophil localization in mucosal tissues suggest an important role for sIgA and IgG in mediating the effector functions of eosinophils in vivo.

Some controversy has surrounded the existence of the high-affinity receptor for IgE (FcεRI) on eosinophils. Studies have shown that the α subunit of FcεRI in eosinophils is expressed intracellularly rather than on the cell surface in resting cells, which may be mobilized to the surface and released during activation.[149] Interestingly, although mouse FcεRI contains α, β, and γ subunits, the human homolog lacks the β subunit, suggesting that this subunit is redundant in signaling in cells expressing FcεRI. Eosinophils express an IgE-binding protein, galectin-3 (Mac-2/ε binding protein), as well as the low-affinity FcεRII (CD23), which may have contributed to apparent high-affinity binding for IgE in earlier studies.

Triggers of Degranulation

Degranulation from eosinophils may be induced by a range of stimuli, some that are soluble mediators and others that must be attached or immobilized to an appropriate surface for their effects. The following sections describe the categories of soluble and immobilized stimuli that trigger degranulation in eosinophils.

Soluble Stimuli

Cytokines and chemokines induce eosinophil degranulation, with IL-5 and GM-CSF having a more potent effect than CCL3/MIP-1α or CCL5/RANTES.[80,150,151] Eosinophil granule proteins (MBP and EPX) themselves can cause degranulation, suggesting that eosinophil granule proteins may promote degranulation in an autocrine and paracrine manner.[105]

Many other soluble stimuli can also induce degranulation, including complement fragments C3a and C5a, f-Met-Leu-Phe, PAF, and naturally occurring peptides such as substance P and melittin.[152,153] In particular, PAF is a potent secretagogue for eosinophils, inducing the release of granule proteins, reactive oxygen species, and lipid mediators.[153,154] Furthermore, PAF activates at least two distinct effector pathways in eosinophils, one of which is independent of known PAF receptors.[154,155] In addition, artificial stimuli potently evoke degranulation such as calcium ionophore (A23187) and phorbol myristate acetate (PMA).[143,156] Eosinophils also respond by degranulation to endogenous molecules released by stressed or damaged tissues, including a range of damage-associated molecular patterns (DAMPs). These include uric acid, ATP, high mobility group box (HMGB)-1 protein, and the S100 family of calcium-binding proteins.[157-159] Eosinophils express receptor for advanced glycosylation end products and therefore respond to DAMPs, such as high-mobility group box 1 protein (HMGB1).[160] Eosinophils have also been shown to express a newly discovered seven-transmembrane receptor, the chemoattractant receptor-homologous molecule expressed on Th2 cells (CRTh2),[161] which responds to prostaglandin D_2, a major prostanoid released by mast cells. PGD_2 induces morphological changes, chemokinesis, and degranulation in eosinophils through CRTh2.

A role for eosinophils and their degranulation in the maintenance of innate immunity in response to pathogen-associated membrane patterns has been shown by their expression of Toll-like receptors (TLRs), which serve a role in recognition of conserved motifs in pathogens. Eosinophils express the lipopolysaccharide (LPS)-binding receptor, TLR4, together with CD14,[162] and respond to LPS stimulation. Furthermore, eosinophils constitutively express TLR1, TLR7, TLR9, and TLR10 mRNAs and are activated by the TLR7 ligand.[163] This may represent an important mechanism for eosinophil-mediated host defense against viral and bacterial infections.

Proteolytic enzymes also have the capacity to induce eosinophil degranulation. These are produced by microbes and are also present in various allergens, including house dust mites, fungi, and cockroaches. These enzymes interact with a family of G protein–coupled protease-activated receptors (PARs), and eosinophils constitutively transcribe mRNA for PAR2 and PAR3 but not PAR1 or PAR4.[164] Exposure of eosinophils to trypsin or tryptase, potent serine proteases that serve as agonists for PAR2, induces respiratory burst and degranulation in eosinophils.[165] Eosinophils also degranulate in response to cysteine proteases such as those from cockroaches and *Der f 1* from mite allergens.[166,167] Finally, eosinophils can degranulate in response to aspartate proteases produced by the fungus *Alternaria alternata*.[168] These findings suggest that eosinophils are able to recognize and respond to proteases in the environment and that this results in the release of proinflammatory mediators.

Immobilized Stimuli

Eosinophils also undergo degranulation upon stimulation of Mac-1 β_2 integrin (CD11b/CD18, $\alpha_M\beta_2$) that also serves as a complement receptor (CR3). This molecule has multiple roles in eosinophils; it is important not only in eosinophil adhesion and recruitment but also for activation of eosinophil effector functions. Integrins, and especially Mac-1, play a crucial role in eosinophil activation by immobilized stimuli such as IgG.[169] Degranulation responses induced by soluble stimuli are potently enhanced by adhesion of eosinophils through integrins. Moreover, Mac-1 can directly recognize fungal molecules such as β-glucan, and eosinophils react by degranulation to fungi through this mechanism.[170] Thus, integrins play a major role in recognition of external pathogens and in eosinophil effector functions.

Mechanisms of Degranulation (Exocytosis)

The mechanisms associated with classical exocytosis, compound exocytosis, and PMD, but not cytolysis, are thought to require specific intracellular membrane-associated proteins acting as receptors for granule docking and fusion. These proteins include a family of molecules known as SNAREs (an acronym for *SNAP re*ceptors). The paradigm associated with SNARE molecule function predicts that these proteins are essential for exocytosis. SNAREs were originally described in neuronal tissues and were found to group themselves into two distinct locations, the granule-associated SNAREs (vesicular or v-SNAREs, many of which are known as R-SNAREs for an arginine residue [R] in their associated SNARE motif) and the plasma membrane-associated SNAREs (target or t-SNAREs, many known as Q-SNAREs for the corresponding glutamine [Q] residue).[171] In order for a functional SNARE complex to form during exocytosis, allowing the granule to dock with the plasma membrane, one v-SNARE binds to two t-SNARE molecules. In neuronal cells, a commonly observed v-SNARE is vesicle-associated membrane protein (VAMP)-1 or its isoform VAMP-2. In these cells, the originally described t-SNAREs associating with VAMP-2 were synaptosome-associated protein of 25 kDa (SNAP-25) and syntaxin-1A. These three molecules form a stable detergent-resistant four-helix coiled-coil bundle, which may be regulated by protein phosphorylation.

Nonneuronal cells also express SNAREs, although some isoforms have been identified with high sequence homology to the neuronal SNAREs. At least three SNAP-25 and 16 syntaxin isoforms have been characterized based on detection of homologous SNARE motif messenger RNA sequences. Interestingly, most nonneuronal secretory cells appear to require SNAP-23 and syntaxin-3, syntaxin-4, or syntaxin-6[172,173] for control of exocytosis. Eosinophils have been shown to express the v-SNARE, VAMP-2, in their small secretory vesicles containing CCL5/RANTES, but not their crystalloid granules.[174] Crystalloid granules express mainly VAMP-7 and VAMP-8, the former being important in regulation of crystalloid granule secretion during degranulation responses from permeabilized eosinophils.[175] The t-SNARE isoforms syntaxin-4 and SNAP-23 are expressed in the cell membrane of eosinophils, and these have the potential to act as cognate membrane binding partners for VAMP-2 and VAMP-7 degranulation.[176] The SNARE molecules VAMP-2, SNAP-23, and syntaxin-4 identified in eosinophils are proposed to regulate docking and fusion of CCL5/RANTES-containing small secretory vesicles to elicit exocytosis and mediator secretion (*Figure 8.8*).

SNARE-dependent eosinophil degranulation responses is proposed to be regulated by Rab27a, a vesicle-bound *ras*-related guanosine triphosphatase that is associated with regulation of exocytotic responses in immune cells.[177] Rab27a was shown to be essential for the release of EPX in response to PAF and/or ionomycin.[177] In addition, regulation of SNARE-mediated release of EPX may be controlled by another regulatory protein belonging to the Sec/Munc family, Cdk5 (cyclin-dependent kinase 5), in response to secretory IgA stimulation.[178] These pathways may function in parallel, or in response to specific receptor-mediated signaling mechanisms, to evoke the regulated release of eosinophil granule proteins.

In summary, eosinophil degranulation occurs through finely tuned, highly regulated mechanisms associated with classical and compound exocytosis, as well as piecemeal degranulation involving the transport of small secretory vesicles associated with a tubulovesicular network in activated cells.

Eosinophil Cytolysis (Necrosis)

Several studies have identified a functional capacity for eosinophils to release extracellular membrane-bound intact granules by cytolysis, a major type of degranulation that has been characterized in tissue biopsy eosinophils from patients with eosinophilia.[179,180] Eosinophil cytolysis has also been shown to occur in vitro in response to cytokine withdrawal, leading to the release of intact, membrane-bound EPX$^+$CD63$^+$ granules. Tissues from patients with allergic rhinitis and

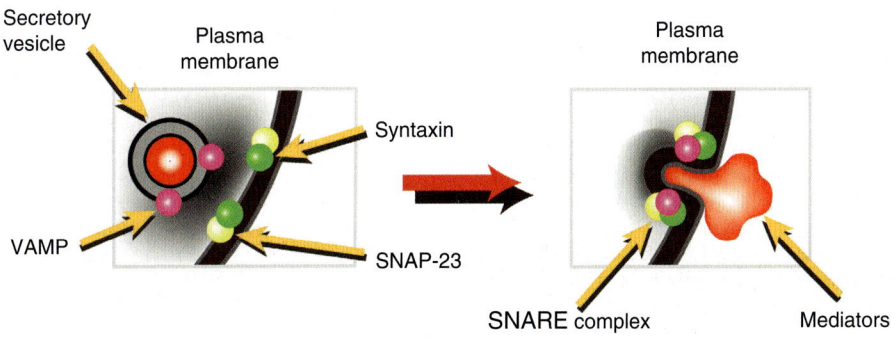

Exocytosis

FIGURE 8.8 Schematic model for molecular regulation of secretory vesicle-plasma membrane fusion proposed to occur in exocytosis in eosinophils. Exocytosis involves membrane fusion between the vesicle and plasma membrane and is a fundamental process associated with classical and compound exocytosis, as well as piecemeal degranulation. In this model, the v-SNARE VAMP is expressed on secretory vesicles, which store mediators, while t-SNAREs, SNAP-23, and syntaxin-4 reside on the inside of the plasma membrane. Following cell activation, v- and t-SNAREs bind together to form a SNARE complex, resulting in fusion and release of inflammatory mediators including CCL5/RANTES. SNAP, synaptosome-associated protein; SNARE, SNAP receptors; VAMP, vesicle-associated membrane protein. (From Lacy P, Logan MR, Bablitz B, Moqbel R. Fusion protein vesicle-associated membrane protein 2 is implicated in IFN-g-induced piecemeal degranulation in human eosinophils from atopic individuals. *J Allergy Clin Immunol.* 2001;107(4):671-678; Logan MR, Lacy P, Bablitz B, Moqbel R. Expression of eosinophil target SNAREs as potential cognate receptors for vesicle-associated membrane protein-2 in exocytosis. *J Allergy Clin Immunol.* 2002;109(2):299-306.)

EE exhibit substantial cytolytic degranulation, with large numbers of free eosinophilic granules evident by transmission electron microscopy analysis of biopsy sections.[180,181] The mechanisms associated with adhesion-induced eosinophil cytolysis takes place via RIPK (receptor-interacting serine/threonine-protein kinase) signaling leading to reactive oxygen species (ROS) production, cytoplasmic vacuolization, and necroptosis.[182] Triggers for eosinophil cytolysis range from complement proteins and IgG[146,169,181,183,184] to the recently demonstrated fibrinogen.[185]

Eosinophil Cytolysis (Extracellular Trap, EETosis)

Several studies using electron and confocal (immunofluorescence) microscopy have identified a unique form of eosinophil cytolysis where histone-coated extracellular DNA traps are released by lytic eosinophils, a phenomenon termed as EETosis.[186,187] Eosinophil extracellular DNA traps (EETs) are formed upon diverse triggers ranging from immobilized immunoglobulins (IgA, IgG), calcium ionophores, platelet activating factor, and complement proteins[186] to fungal antigens.[188] Eosinophils may have evolved this method to trap large multicellular creatures (parasites), similar to how neutrophils trap bacteria. EETs have been shown to reduce the spread of *Haemonchus contortus*, a common livestock parasite, by immobilizing the larvae and preventing them from entering the lungs.[189] EETs with subsequent detection of eosinophilic cationic (cytotoxic) proteins have also been reported in goats with nodular worm (Nematode) infections.[190] Extracellular trap formation from eosinophils appears to fulfill an important immune response against extracellular pathogens, although overproduction of traps is evident in pathologies such as asthma and eosinophilic granulomatosis with polyangiitis (eGPA).[187] Furthermore, EETs are often found in close proximity to eosinophil free granules[191] and CLC proteins,[192] which are classical features of eosinophil activity associated with disease severity and tissue damage.

In summary, mechanisms associated with granule release in eosinophils are critical for effector function of eosinophils. In the absence of degranulation and mediator secretion, the eosinophil is a relatively inert cell and does not affect surrounding tissues, as seen in cases of idiopathic pulmonary eosinophilia and eosinophilic pneumonia. In these conditions, eosinophil numbers are increased in the capillaries and tissues of the lung, but no cellular or structural damage is evident, likely because of the lack of eosinophil degranulation. In contrast, asthmatic patients show profound eosinophil activation in the airways combined with significant tissue destruction, suggesting that, in addition to eosinophilic infiltration, their undergoing degranulation may contribute to mucosal damage in the airways and related symptoms of asthma. Thus, degranulation is a key event in eosinophil-mediated tissue damage.

Membrane-Derived Mediators

Eosinophils produce a wide variety of lipid-derived mediators, which have profound biological activity. The more important products are eicosanoids, which include leukotrienes (especially LTC_4), prostaglandins (particularly PGE_2), thromboxane, and lipoxins (especially LXA_4) as well as PAF. The main substrate for these mediators is arachidonic acid (AA), which is specifically liberated from membrane phospholipids possessing this fatty acid at the *sn*-2 position by phospholipase A_2 (PLA_2) during receptor stimulation. Of the nine known families of PLA_2, two families are expressed in eosinophils, the type IIA and type IV enzymes, which are commonly known as secretory and cytosolic PLA_2, respectively.[193] These enzymes are distinguished by their distribution, size, and sensitivity to Ca^{2+}, where granule-stored $sPLA_2$ (13-15 kDa) requires millimolar amounts of Ca^{2+} for activity while cytosolically localized $cPLA_2$ (85 kDa) is catalytically active in the presence of micromolar amounts of Ca^{2+}. Interestingly, eosinophils express 20- to 100-fold higher levels of secretory PLA_2 in their granules than other circulating leukocytes, suggesting a functional role in inflammatory processes involving eosinophil degranulation.

Eosinophils are a rich source of LTC_4 (5S-hydroxy-6R,S-glutathionyl-7,9,-*trans*-11,14-*cis*-eicosatetraenoic acid).[194,195] Stimulation with the calcium ionophore A23187 generates up to

40 ng/10^6 cells of LTC_4 from normal-density eosinophils, while light-density eosinophils elaborate 70 ng/10^6 cells. Eosinophils produce negligible amounts (6 ng/10^6 cells) of LTB_4 (5S-12R-dihydroxy-6,14-*cis*-8,10-*trans*-eicosatetraenoic acid) compared with up to 200 ng/10^6 cells from neutrophils. LTC_4 generation by human eosinophils was also observed after stimulation with both opsonized zymosan and via an FcγRII-dependent mechanism using Sepharose beads coated with IgG.[196] The production of LTC_4 is dependent upon activation of 5-lipoxygenase, an enzyme that resides in the euchromatin region of the nucleus and translocates to the nuclear membrane upon cell activation, where it activates an 18-kDa protein called FLAP.[197] The substrate for 5-lipoxygenase is AA, which may be released from membrane phospholipids by PLA_2. The first product of this enzyme is an intermediary compound, 5-HPETE, which is transformed into the unstable epoxide LTA_4. At this point, human eosinophils predominantly generate LTC_4 through the action of LTC_4 synthetase.[194,195] Eosinophils are particularly rich in LTC_4 synthetase and account for 70% of all LTC_4 synthetase-positive cells in the airway mucosa of normal and asthmatic individuals.[198] LTC_4 is generated intracellularly in human eosinophils stimulated with the calcium ionophore A23187. LTC_4 is later exported from the cell in a regulated manner.[199]

The production of 15-HETE, a lipid mediator generated via the 15-lipoxygenase pathway, occurs in activated eosinophils. The product 15-HETE has proinflammatory actions and can modulate the chemotactic effects of LTB_4 on neutrophils.[200] The enzyme 15-lipoxygenase may be distinguished from 5-lipoxygenase in that it can modify a larger pool of fatty acid substrates than the latter enzyme and will oxygenate fatty acids that are esterified in phospholipids. Substrates include arachidonic acid, linoleic acid, polyenoic acids, and more complex lipids, such as lipoproteins. Eosinophils are the major cellular source of elevated 15-HETE in asthmatic airways and are capable of generating 100 to 300 times more 15-HETE than neutrophils, endothelial cells, and fibroblasts.[201] Eosinophils also account for 85% of cells positive for 15-lipoxygenase in the airway submucosa of normal and asthmatic subjects.[202,203]

Eosinophils generate large amounts of PAF after stimulation with calcium ionophore, opsonized zymosan or IgG-coated Sepharose beads.[204-207] PAF (1-*O*-alkyl-2-acetyl-*sn*-glycerol-3-phosphocholine) is a potent phospholipid mediator, which causes leukocyte activation. For instance, eosinophils elaborated 25 ng/10^6 cells of PAF after stimulation with calcium ionophore and up to 2 ng/10^6 cells after IgG stimulation. Much of the PAF remained cell associated, possibly acting as an intracellular messenger, or alternatively binding to PAF receptors on eosinophils thus acting as an autocrine agent. As with leukotriene synthesis, eosinophil-derived release of PAF was maximal at 45 minutes. Regulated PAF production is controlled by the release of biologically inactive lyso-PAF from membrane phospholipids by PLA_2, which is later acetylated to form PAF by an acetyltransferase.[205]

The cyclooxygenase pathway is prominent in eosinophils as well, and eosinophils are capable of producing PGE_1 and PGE_2, and thromboxane B_2 from cyclooxygenase acting on free AA. In studies with guinea pig eosinophils, thromboxane B_2 and PGE_2 were shown to be generated following PAF or A23187 stimulation.[208,209]

Many of the enzymes associated with membrane-derived mediator release from eosinophils, including cyclooxygenase and 5-lipoxygenase, are found stored in association with lipid bodies (see *Table 8.1*).[210,211]

Respiratory Burst

Eosinophils undergo respiratory burst concurrently with the release of other mediators during cell activation. The immune function of respiratory burst is to mediate killing of invasive, pathogenic microorganisms; it also has the undesired effect of collateral tissue damage when dysregulated. Respiratory burst is defined as the increase in cell metabolism (measured by the elevated activity of the hexose monophosphate shunt) and oxygen consumption, coupled with the inducible release of ROS in response to specific stimuli. Many stimuli are capable of inducing respiratory burst in eosinophils, including LTB_4, PAF, fMLF, C5a, opsonized particles, and CCL5/RANTES.[30] The principal product of respiratory burst is superoxide ($O_2^{-\bullet}$), a potent oxidant with a highly reactive electron in its outer valence, possessing relatively weak intrinsic microbicidal activity and a very brief half-life. The function of $O_2^{-\bullet}$ is thought to reside in its ability to dismutate rapidly into more reactive ROS, including hydrogen peroxide (H_2O_2) and the hydroxyl radical ($OH^{-\bullet}$), and formation of hypohalous acids (HOBr) upon reaction with EPX produced following eosinophil degranulation. The formation of ROS subsequent to $O_2^{-\bullet}$ generation is dependent upon the presence of a number of catalysts, such as superoxide dismutase, which accelerates the formation of H_2O_2, and the ferrous ion, which induces $OH^{-\bullet}$ production from H_2O_2. $O_2^{-\bullet}$ is also able to react with nitric oxide (NO) produced from nitric oxide synthase enzymes (e.g., iNOS, eNOS) to form the highly reactive peroxynitrite ($ONOO^-$), which alters cell functions and is cytotoxic.

The regulated burst of $O_2^{-\bullet}$ production is mediated through the activation of a membrane-associated enzyme complex, the NADPH oxidase. This enzyme complex is crucial for maintenance of host defense as it is a key mechanism in the destruction of ROS-sensitive organisms. In addition, overactivation of the NADPH oxidase is likely to be cytotoxic to tissues and has been implicated in the pathogenesis of many eosinophil-related disorders including allergic asthma.[4] Interestingly, eosinophils possess the ability to generate up to 10-fold more superoxide than other phagocytes, including neutrophils, in which the mechanisms associated with NADPH oxidase activation have been studied in greater detail.[212] The ability of eosinophils to release more $O_2^{-\bullet}$ is thought to be the result of higher levels of expression of the protein components that make up the NADPH oxidase complex.[213-215] In addition, preferential assembly of NADPH oxidase occurs at the cell membrane in eosinophils, eliciting a predominantly extracellular form of $O_2^{-\bullet}$ release.[216] This is in contrast to neutrophils, which show predominantly intracellular NADPH oxidase assembly during respiratory burst stimulation and bacterial infection.[216,217]

NADPH oxidase is a complex of at least six proteins consisting of phagocytic oxidase (*phox*) subunits, of which two (p22*phox* and gp91*phox*) reside in the membrane as part of the cytochrome b_{558} protein and the remaining proteins (p40*phox*, p47*phox*, p67*phox*, and Rac1 or Rac2) are cytosolic in resting cells.[212] The minimal components of the NADPH oxidase complex were determined using cell-free assays,[218] although several other proteins, such as p40*phox* and Rap1a, also translocate to the membrane-associated oxidase complex during activation and may be involved in "fine-tuning" the activity of the oxidase.[219] Under normal, nonstimulated conditions, the phagocytic oxidases p40*phox*, p47*phox*, and p67*phox* are complexed in the cytosol, while Rac1 or Rac2 are bound to the cytosolic guanine dissociation inhibitor RhoGDI (*Figure 8.9*). Binding between p47*phox* and p67*phox* occurs through the C-terminal SH3 domain of p67*phox* and a proline-rich region (PRR) in p47*phox*. The p67*phox* protein also contains a C-terminal Bem1p (PB1) motif that allows a high-affinity interaction with a C-terminal *phox* and Cdc motif in p40*phox*.[219,220] An SH3 domain also exists in p40*phox* that is capable of interacting with the PRR domain in p47*phox*, although in

vitro binding studies indicate that the affinity of this interaction is lower than that of p40*phox* for p67*phox*.[221,222]

During activation by cell surface receptors engaged by opsonized microbes or inflammatory mediators, p47*phox* is phosphorylated by cellular kinases on multiple serine residues, unmasking tandem SH3 domains to allow binding to p22*phox* in the membrane. Concurrently, p67*phox* and p40*phox*, which are still complexed to p47*phox*, translocate to the cell membrane, and the "activation domain" in p67*phox* promotes electron transfer between NADPH and flavin adenine dinucleotide.[223] Superoxide generation from NADPH oxidase also requires concurrent activation and membrane translocation of Rac1 or Rac2, which binds to tetratricopeptide repeat motifs in the N terminus of p67*phox* and cytochrome b_{558} to induce additional conformational changes necessary for efficient electron transport to O_2.[224] The function of p40*phox* is still uncertain, although it may have a role in activating superoxide production during IgG-mediated phagocytosis.[220]

Rac1 and Rac2 are monomeric guanine triphosphatases (GTPases), which exhibit 92% homology in their amino acid sequence, and are functionally interchangeable in their ability to activate NADPH oxidase, although they differ in their tissue distribution. Rac1 is ubiquitously expressed throughout the body, while neutrophils, eosinophils, and other blood cells predominantly express Rac2, which is mainly expressed in hemopoietic tissues.[216,225,226] These patterns of NADPH oxidase complex formation align with the concept that eosinophils undergo "frustrated phagocytosis" upon encountering large extracellular organisms such as helminthic parasites, while neutrophils preferentially phagocytose smaller microbes for intracellular killing. Eosinophils are partially dependent on Rac2 for the activation of respiratory burst responses, based on findings with Rac2$^{-/-}$ mouse eosinophils, inferring that Rac1 may also be required for NADPH oxidase activation in these cells.[227]

The pathway leading from receptor stimulation to activation of the oxidase is still poorly understood. Many studies on NADPH oxidase activation use phorbol esters, such as PMA, as highly potent artificial stimuli to activate respiratory burst in eosinophils. Phorbol esters are classically known for their ability to directly activate protein kinase C (PKC).[228] The use of pharmacological inhibitors of PKC in respiratory burst has generated paradoxical results, in that PKC inhibitors only partially inhibit agonist-induced H_2O_2 release in guinea pig eosinophils.[229] However, there is a species difference in sensitivity to PMA, as in human eosinophils, where PKC inhibitors actually augment the rate of oxygen consumption in response to opsonized particles.[230] These findings suggest that PKC is not critical for agonist-induced respiratory burst in eosinophils, although stimulation of PKC appears to be able to induce superoxide release on its own.

Taken together, eosinophils generate substantial amounts of $O_2^{-\bullet}$ as part of their role in host defense, and the mechanisms associated with the release of this toxic mediator are under investigation. The release of $O_2^{-\bullet}$ from eosinophils is likely to be a crucial component of the pathophysiological processes underlying eosinophilic inflammation in mucosal tissues.

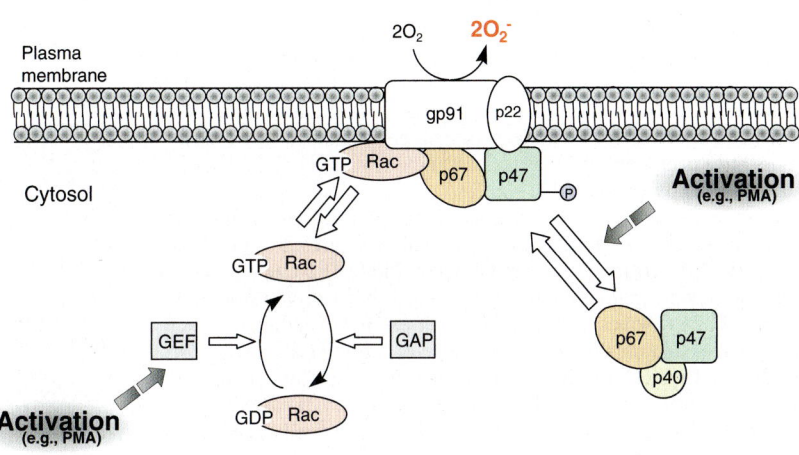

FIGURE 8.9 **Assembly and activation of the NADPH oxidase complex during respiratory burst.** This complex is essential for the inducible release of superoxide for microbicidal reactions and is also present in neutrophils. During cell activation, the GTPase Rac, normally bound to GDP in the resting cell, is activated by a guanine exchange factor (GEF) to bind to GTP. This results in translocation of Rac-GTP to the cell membrane, where other cytosolic proteins p67*phox* and p47*phox* have also translocated, to bind to the two subunits of cytochrome b_{558} (gp91*phox* and p22*phox*). Following the assembly of the oxidase, electrons are transferred from NADPH in the cytosol via flavin adenine dinucleotide (a cofactor) to oxygen molecules to form the highly reactive oxygen intermediate, superoxide. Assembly of this complex is reversed by GTPase-activating protein (GAP), which hydrolyzes GTP on Rac to GDP, and by the dissociation of the *phox* subunits. GTP, guanosine triphosphate; PMA, phorbol myristate acetate.

Eosinophils as Immunoregulatory Cells

The consistent association of eosinophils with a specific pattern of immune response common to helminth infection and atopy suggests that eosinophils may be either a bystander cell or an active component of a complex immune disease. To determine the involvement of eosinophil-derived factors in modulating the immune response, the expression and bioactivity of cytokines released from eosinophils has been explored for their potential physiological effects in immune regulation. Studies have shown that a striking diversity of cytokines and chemokines, including IL-2, IL-4, IL-12, IL-16, GM-CSF, CCL5/RANTES, and TGFβ, are derived from eosinophils and are capable of exerting bioactive effects.[83] For example, IL-2 and IFNγ from CD28-stimulated eosinophils were shown to stimulate proliferation in an IL-2-dependent cell line and MHC class II expression on Colo 205 cells, respectively.[231] The release of IL-4 from eosinophils is important in driving the initiation of a Th2-type response in *Schistosoma mansoni* infection in mice.[232] Eosinophil-derived IL-4 also plays an immunoregulatory role in pulmonary cryptococcosis, as determined in 4get mice (IL-4-IRES-eGFP mice, with eGFP+ IL-4 expressing cells) treated with *Cryptococcus neoformans*, contributing to a susceptibility to Th2-dependent allergic responses during bronchopulmonary mycosis.[233] Secretion of the cytokines APRIL and IL-6 from eosinophils has been shown to be critical for the maintenance of plasma cells in the bone marrow.[234] These studies have demonstrated that eosinophil-derived cytokines and chemokines have the ability to regulate a range of immune and inflammatory responses.

Generally speaking, eosinophils produce significantly smaller amounts of cytokines than T cells, B cells, and other cells. However, in eosinophilic inflammation, eosinophils outnumber T cells in the tissues by as much as a 100-fold. As such, the magnitude of the presence of eosinophils may be a determining factor in regulating immune responses at a local level. The release of eosinophil cytokines often takes place within a much shorter period than the release of cytokines of T cells (which may be several hours), as eosinophil-derived cytokines are stored as preformed mediators in crystalloid granules and may be secreted in response to stimuli in a matter of minutes. The production of cytokines by eosinophils is postulated to contribute to an immunoregulatory role by these cells and may promote an allergic phenotype by influencing the production of Th2 cytokines by T cells.

Allergy is often characterized by a significant polarization of the immune response toward enhanced production of Th2 cytokines and a dramatic increase in allergen-specific and total immunoglobulin E (IgE) levels. Allergic disease is initiated by the generation of allergen-specific CD4+ cells that produce the Th2 cytokines IL-4, IL-5, IL-9, and IL-13. These cytokines are crucial for the maturation, proliferation, survival, and activation of mast cells, basophils, and eosinophils, important effector cells. Th2 cytokines also regulate IgE synthesis by B cells and mucus production by epithelial cells. In contrast, Th1 cells are characterized by the production of the Th1 cytokines IL-2 and IFN-γ. The immunological responses of eosinophils are dependent on an array of cytokines and chemokines that may traditionally be associated with Th1 or Th2 responses. Eosinophils synthesize many of these cytokines and chemokines to which they can also respond. Based on their ability to synthesize, store, and release both Th1 and Th2 cytokines and chemokines, and significant evidence indicating the bioactivity of their released cytokines, eosinophils have been implicated as active components of allergic disease, rather than as bystander cells.

Classically, the Th1 response has been modeled as an immune response that exerts inhibitory effects on Th2 responses. It is therefore paradoxical that eosinophils, as a cell type marking Th2-type responses to allergic diseases or helminthic infections, synthesize and store both Th1 and Th2 cytokines (see *Table 8.2*). For example, binding of CD28 on human eosinophils induced the release of bioactive IL-2 and IFN-γ,[231] both of which are Th1 cytokines, and IL-13, a Th2 cytokine.[235] Since Th1 and Th2 responses are mutually inhibitory, it has been very difficult to dissect the specific roles of eosinophil-derived cytokines in the initiation and effector phases of the allergic immune response. The role of eosinophil-derived Th1 or Th2 cytokines may therefore depend on the timing of eosinophil infiltration into sites of allergic inflammation. Indeed, recent studies using a mouse model of *Nippostrongylus brasiliensis* infection have shown that, while eosinophils may be crucial for secondary Th2 polarized immune response against this parasite, the primary response does not require eosinophil-derived IL-4 or IL-13.[236] However, in the context of viral infections, IFNγ-mediated stimulation of eosinophils leads to the production of CCL5/RANTES that may serve to recruit further immune cells and limit the spread of viruses.[237]

Experimental models that induced eosinophilia in the absence of tissue infiltration of eosinophils have exquisitely demonstrated the importance of the timing and location of chemokine release in recruitment of eosinophils. For example, CCL11/eotaxin gene-knockout (Eo−/−) mice showed decreased tissue eosinophils during the early (but not late) phase of allergic inflammation.[55] Moreover, CCL11/eotaxin-/- mice also showed a significant defect in clearing the larvae of *Trichinella spiralis* from skeletal muscles compared with wild-type animals in spite of similar levels of blood eosinophilia.[238] In terms of eosinophils derived from healthy or diseased humans, migratory response to the three eotaxins (CCL11, CCL24, CCL26) seems to vary. While eosinophils from healthy individuals show comparable migration for all three eotaxins, CCL26 or eotaxin-3 exhibits comparatively higher chemoattractant properties when isolated from asthmatics.[239] Thus, the presence of eosinophils in allergic disease results from a carefully orchestrated process that involves cytokines and chemokines controlling the maturation and recruitment of eosinophils to the site of allergen exposure.

The implications of eosinophil cytokine production are extensive, such as in the case of IL-4, where this cytokine may be released from eosinophils to direct Th2 cell differentiation in local lymph nodes. In support of this possibility, eosinophils have been shown to traffic to paratracheal draining lymph nodes (in a mouse model of asthma), where they were demonstrated to function as antigen-presenting cells expressing MHC class II and costimulatory CD80 and CD86 to stimulate CD4+ T cells.[240] In humans, eosinophils can be induced to express MHC class II and costimulatory molecules following cytokine stimulation and transmigration through endothelial monolayers.[241,242] Moreover, human eosinophils constitutively express a Notch ligand, Jagged1, suggesting that they have the capacity to polarize naïve CD4+ T cells.[243]

During intimate cell-cell contact, the production of IL-4 and IL-13 is not required in abundance to effect important immunoregulatory events, such as enhanced switching of T cells to Th2 phenotype and increased IgE synthesis, both of which are hallmarks of allergic disorders.[244] Mouse eosinophils can process and present antigens to T cells.[245] Under such conditions, antigen-loaded eosinophils, acting as antigen-presenting cells, were found to preferentially initiate the generation of a Th2 response to ovalbumin in an experimental mouse model.[246,247] Furthermore, antigen-pulsed eosinophils were sufficient for expansion of Th2 cells in draining lymph nodes.[247]

Earlier studies suggested that eosinophil recruitment into sites of inflammation was the result of IL-5 and CCL11/eotaxin-1 generation from the adaptive immune response.[3] However, numerous studies in mouse models have shown that the influx of eosinophils into sites of inflammation precedes that of lymphocytes and that it can occur in mice with a deficient adaptive immune system.[232,236,248-250] These studies suggest that eosinophils may be upstream of the adaptive Th2 response and further regulate it in allergic inflammation. A major role for eosinophils in the localized recruitment of effector T cells into the lungs of allergen sensitized and challenged mice has been demonstrated, whereby lung eosinophils elicit the expression of CCL17/thymus- and activation-regulated chemokine and CCL22/macrophage-derived chemokine.[251] Another potential immunomodulatory molecule generated by the eosinophil is the granule protein EDN. In addition to its RNase activity and antiviral properties, EDN is a chemoattractant for dendritic cells[252] and can induce maturation and activation of dendritic cells.[253] In addition, EDN has the capacity to act as an alarmin by enhancing Th2 responses through a TLR2-dependent mechanism.[254] These studies have supported the notion that eosinophils can participate in the generation of allergic immune response through the secretion of a wide diversity of immunomodulatory cytokines, either directly or indirectly through other tissues.

Eosinophils also engage in the maintenance of immune homeostasis by being involved in MHC class I–restricted thymocyte deletion in the thymus.[255] In the thymus, eosinophils express MHC class I and costimulatory molecules CD86 and CD30L and are also positive for CD11b/CD11c, CD25, and CD69, with decreased expression of CD62L, suggestive of an activated phenotype. These eosinophils are anatomically localized within specific compartments of the thymus coinciding with negative selection of double-positive thymocytes. Thus, eosinophils may be associated with MHC class I–restricted thymocyte deletion as part of the maintenance of immune function in early life.

Indeed, abundant numbers of eosinophils were detected in human thymus tissue in infants undergoing open-heart surgery for congenital cardiac disease ranging between the ages of 2 weeks and 12 years. Eosinophils constituted 2% of the total thymic cell count postnatally; the counts were shown to be highest during the early stages of life and declined with age.[256] A fascinating observation was the detection of numerous eosinophils within unique thymic Hassall corpuscles. The latter were suggested to play a major role in regulatory T-cells (Treg) differentiation via the epithelial lining of these corpuscles.[256,257] The lining of Hassall corpuscles synthesizes and releases thymic stromal lymphopoietin (TSLP) that instructs resident thymic dendritic cells to effect the conversion of self-reactive T cells into CD4+CD25+Foxp3+ cells.[258] Indeed, in the mouse, inflammatory Th2-type responses to TSLP were shown to be eosinophil dependent.[259]

Eosinophils are also likely to play a role in long-term maintenance of bone marrow plasma cells, since plasma cell numbers were decreased in the bone marrow of eosinophil-deficient mice, a defect that was reversed by eosinophil reconstitution. Eosinophils supported the survival of plasma cells by secretion of APRIL and IL-6. Subsequent studies revealed that eosinophils play a critical role in maintaining gut homeostasis by promoting T cell–independent IgA class switching and maintaining IgA+ plasma cells in the Peyer patch.[260]

In recent times, single-cell RNA sequencing (scRNA-seq) methods have revealed unique subsets of eosinophils with phenotypic heterogeneity based on the tissue microenvironment and disease/inflammatory states.[261] In addition to heterogeneity, scRNA-seq methods have also revealed myeloid plasticity that is associated with the postinflammatory "resolution" state.[262] Indeed, eosinophils with homeostatic proresolving regulatory function have been described in the lung tissue of healthy individuals[263] as well as in the synovial joints of patients with rheumatoid arthritis in remission.[264] In mice, eosinophils resident in the lung parenchyma have been identified to have IL-5-independent regulatory homeostatic functions compared with those recruited from the periphery (termed as inflammatory). This further translates to human data given, eosinophils isolated from the sputa of healthy individuals have a distinct phenotype (Siglec-8+CD62L+IL-3R^lo) compared with those isolated from asthmatic sputa (Siglec-8+CD62L^lo IL-3R^hi).[263] Eosinophils that suppress T-cell effector functions and modulate Th2 responses to allergens are also described. This CD16+ eosinophil subset encompasses 1% to 5% of total eosinophils in a healthy population and is a stronger suppressor of T-cell proliferation than conventional CD16^neg eosinophils.[265] Furthermore, galectin-10, expressed highly in these CD16+ regulatory eosinophils, was demonstrated to function as the T-cell suppressive molecule.[265,266]

Increased eosinophil infiltrates in solid tumors coupled with an improved prognosis, documented particularly in gastric and colorectal cancers, indicate a plausible homeostatic role of eosinophils in the tumor microenvironment.[8,267] Eosinophils restrict tumor growth by polarizing macrophages into proinflammatory type and inciting infiltration of cytotoxic CD8 T cells[268] and NK cells.[269] Furthermore, GM-CSF directly drives the antitumor activities of eosinophil by activating the IRF5 transcription factor and allowing a robust CD8 T-cell

infiltration.[270] In addition, eosinophil-derived granular proteins may also have direct tumoricidal properties.[158]

In summary, the recognition of the capacity of the eosinophil to synthesize and release a range of immunomodulatory molecules introduced a paradigm shift in understanding the potential of the eosinophil as an effector cell in immune homeostatic mechanisms as well as allergic inflammation and other eosinophil-associated conditions. However, the full capacity of the eosinophil to elaborate mediators including cytokines, the precise microenvironment requirements for such synthesis, the intracellular pattern of production and storage, and the timing of its immunomodulatory function during immune responses remain the subject of intensive investigation.

Eosinophil-Derived Cytokines, Chemokines, and Growth Factors

Human eosinophils have been shown to produce at least 40 different cytokines, chemokines, and growth factors (*Table 8.2*) with the potential to regulate various immune responses.[83] These cytokines have been identified in eosinophils by detecting mRNA and/or protein using reverse transcription–polymerase chain reaction, in situ hybridization, and immunocytochemical staining.[83,137,271-273] In addition, picogram amounts of cytokines, chemokines, and growth factors were measured in supernatants of stimulated eosinophils.[83] These cytokines are likely to act in an autocrine, paracrine, or juxtacrine manner thereby regulating local inflammatory events. Studies have demonstrated that the production of eosinophil-activating cytokines (e.g., IL-3 and GM-CSF) by eosinophils may be important in prolonging the survival of these cells by a putative autocrine loop.[38,272] For instance, adherence of highly purified eosinophils to the extracellular matrix protein, fibronectin, resulted in prolongation of survival of these cells in the absence of exogenous cytokines.[38] Fibronectin-induced eosinophil survival was inhibitable by antibodies against fibronectin and VLA-4 and upregulated by picogram amounts of IL-3 and GM-CSF derived from eosinophils.[38] Observations on eosinophil cytokine release have been mainly studied in vitro, but a few have been confirmed in vivo.[274-277]

A major distinction in cytokine production between eosinophils and T cells is that the former store their cytokines intracellularly as preformed mediators, while the latter produce and release cytokines only following activation. Although many eosinophil-derived cytokines are elaborated at lower concentrations than other leukocytes, eosinophils possess the ability to release these cytokines immediately (within minutes) following stimulation. Stored cytokines include IL-2, IL-4, IL-5, IL-6, IL-10, IL-13, IL-16, GM-CSF, TNFα, CC chemokine ligand 11 (CCL11)/eotaxin, IL-8, CCL5/RANTES, NGF, and TGFα.[83,273] Studies using immunogold electron microscopic analysis or confocal laser scanning microscopy coupled with double immunofluorescence labeling have indicated that several of these cytokines are found in close association with either the crystalline core or matrix of the crystalloid-specific granules of the cell (*Table 8.2*).[137,278-283] For example, CCL5/RANTES was found to be associated predominantly with the matrix compartment of the crystalloid granule in eosinophils (*Figure 8.10*).

Developing eosinophils possess the ability to express cytokine message and protein at early stages of maturation. Eosinophils generated from semisolid culture of cord blood–derived CD34+ cells in the presence of IL-3 and IL-5 were shown to express IL-5 and GM-CSF mRNA after 10 days of culture.[284] Freshly purified CD34+ cells expressed IL-4 and CCL5/RANTES mRNA but not IL-4 and CCL5/RANTES protein. On day 23 of culture, IL-4 and CCL5/RANTES localized to the matrix of MBP+ crystalloid granules as determined by immunofluorescence.[285] In addition, IL-6 protein expression was found in cells after day 16 of culture.[99]

Another site of storage of cytokines and chemokines is within the small secretory vesicle. At least three such proteins were shown to be associated with these vesicles, namely, CCL5/RANTES, IL-4, and TGFα.[137,138,286] These organelles belong to the same group of secretory vesicles identified by electron microscopy analysis as tubulovesicular structures. For example, CCL5/RANTES-positive vesicles are highly sensitive to stimulation by IFNγ and are rapidly mobilized

Table 8.2. Cytokines, Chemokines, and Growth Factors Produced by Human Eosinophils

Cytokine	Products	Stored Protein in Resting Cells (per 10^6 Cells)	Intracellular Site of Storage
Interleukins			
Interleukin-1α	mRNA protein	—	—
Interleukin-1β	mRNA protein	—	—
Interleukin-2	mRNA protein	6 ± 2 pg	Crystalloid granules (core)
Interleukin-3	mRNA protein	—	—
Interleukin-4	mRNA protein	~75 ± 20 pg	Crystalloid granules (core)
Interleukin-5	mRNA protein	—	Crystalloid granules (core/matrix?)
Interleukin-6	mRNA protein	25 ± 6 pg	Crystalloid granules (matrix)
Interleukin-9	mRNA protein	—	—
Interleukin-10	mRNA protein	~25 pg	—
Interleukin-11	mRNA	—	—
Interleukin-12	mRNA protein		
Interleukin-13	mRNA protein	—	—
Interleukin-16	mRNA protein	1.6 ± 0.8 ng	—
Interleukin-17	protein	—	—
Interleukin-25	mRNA protein	—	—
Interferons and Others			
Interferon-γ (IFNγ)	mRNA protein	—	—
APRIL (a proliferation-inducing ligand)	protein	—	—
Granulocyte/macrophage colony-stimulating factor (GM-CSF)	mRNA protein	15.1 ± 0.3 pg	Crystalloid granules (core)
Leukemia inhibitory factor (LIF)	mRNA Protein	—	—
Tumor necrosis factor (TNF)	mRNA protein	—	Crystalloid granules (matrix)
Chemokines			
CCL2/monocyte chemoattractant protein-1 (MCP-1)	Protein	—	—
CCL3/macrophage inflammatory protein-1α (MIP-1α)	mRNA protein	—	—
CCL5/RANTES	mRNA protein	72 ± 15 pg	Crystalloid granules (matrix) and small secretory vesicles
CCL7/MCP-3	mRNA	—	—
CCL11/eotaxin	mRNA protein	19 ± 4 pg	Crystalloid granules
CCL13/MCP-4	mRNA	—	—
CCL17/thymus activation regulated chemokine (TARC)	mRNA protein		
CCL22/macrophage-derived chemokine (MDC)	mRNA protein	—	—

(Continued)

Table 8.2. Cytokines, Chemokines, and Growth Factors Produced by Human Eosinophils (Continued)

Cytokine	Products	Stored Protein in Resting Cells (per 10⁶ Cells)	Intracellular Site of Storage
CCL23/myeloid progenitor inhibitory factor 1 (MPIF-1)	mRNA protein	—	—
CXCL5/epithelial-derived neutrophil-activating peptide 78 (ENA-78)	mRNA protein	1500 pg	—
CXCL8/interleukin-8	mRNA protein	140 pg	Cytoplasmic
CXCL9/monokine induced by gamma interferon (MIG)	mRNA protein	—	—
CXCL10/interferon γ induced protein 10 (IP-10)	mRNA protein	—	—
CXCL11/interferon-inducible T-cell alpha chemoattractant (I-TAC)	mRNA protein	—	—
Growth Factors			
Heparin-binding epidermal growth factor-like binding protein (HB-EGF-LBP)	mRNA	—	—
Nerve growth factor (NGF)	mRNA protein	4 ± 2 pg	—
Platelet-derived growth factor, B chain (PDGF-B)	mRNA	—	—
Stem cell factor (SCF)	mRNA protein	—	Crystalloid granules
Transforming growth factor-α (TGFα)	mRNA protein	22 ± 6 pg	Crystalloid granules (matrix) and small secretory vesicles
Transforming growth factor-β1 (TGFβ1)	mRNA protein	—	—
Vascular endothelial growth factor (VEGF)	mRNA protein	—	Crystalloid granules

The Normal Hematologic System

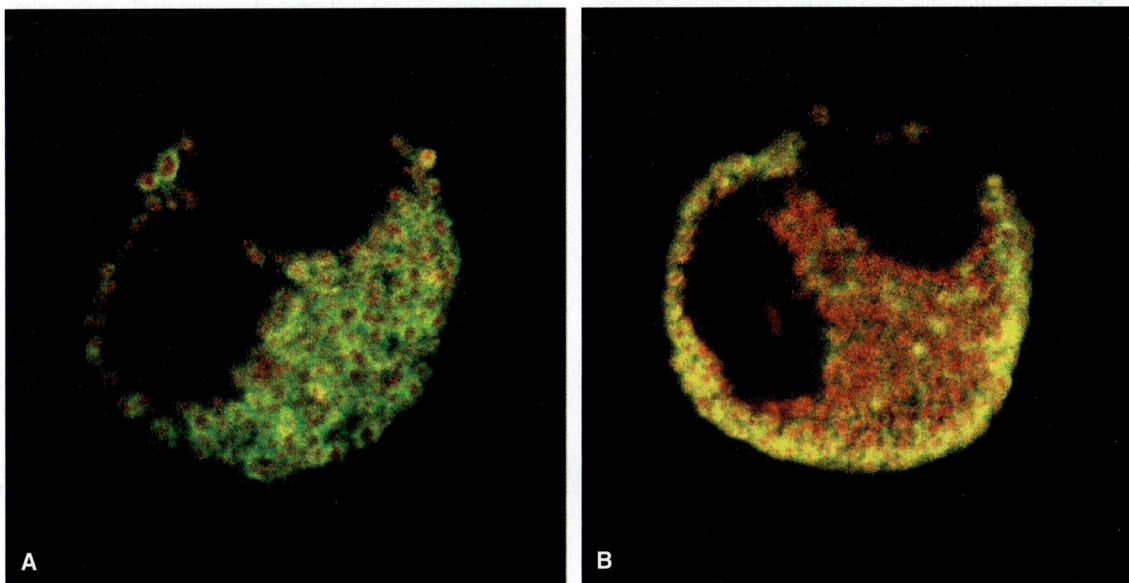

FIGURE 8.10 Translocation of the chemokine CCL5/RANTES in human eosinophils activated by interferon-γ in vitro. Immunoreactivities for CCL5/RANTES (green fluorescence) and eosinophil major basic protein (red fluorescence) are shown in control (A) and IFN-γ-stimulated (10 min, 500 U/mL) (B) cells. The yellow color in (B) resulted from colocalization of green and red immunofluorescence stains. Note that immunoreactivity for MBP remained associated with the cores of the crystalloid granules in both cells, while the green label for CCL5/RANTES translocated toward the cell membrane. CCL5/RANTES was proposed to be released from eosinophils by piecemeal degranulation. (Experimental conditions described in Lacy P, Mahmudi-Azer S, Bablitz B, Hagen SC, Velazquez JR, Man SFP, et al. Rapid mobilization of intracellularly stored RANTES in response to interferon-g in human eosinophils. *Blood*. 1999;94:23-32.)

(within 10 minutes of stimulation) to secrete CCL5/RANTES extracellularly.[137,287] Crystalloid granules, which also contain CCL5/RANTES within their matrix compartment, were found to release this chemokine more slowly in response to IFNγ (1 h), while the majority of MBP remained associated with the core of these granules. These observations suggest that eosinophils have the ability to "shuttle" CCL5/RANTES from the crystalloid granules to the cell exterior and may provide an important in vitro model for eosinophil piecemeal degranulation.

These observations show that eosinophils not only have the ability to synthesize, store, and secrete a diverse array of cytokines, chemokines, and growth factors but are also able to control the release of these important immunomodulatory factors using highly regulated intracellular signaling mechanisms. Indeed, recent studies have highlighted an important contribution by eosinophil-derived cytokines toward the immune development and homeostatic mechanisms.

IMMUNOLOGICAL AND PHYSIOLOGICAL ROLES OF EOSINOPHILS

Perhaps surprisingly, the immunological role of eosinophils has remained elusive since their discovery in the latter half of the 19th century. Eosinophils, or eosinophil-like cells known as heterophils, are widely found throughout the animal kingdom and have been detected in both invertebrates and vertebrates.[160] Their widespread distribution suggests that they evolved through natural selection processes. While they are strongly associated with helminthic parasite infections, evidence for eosinophils having a protective role in parasitic infections is far from certain, at least in mouse models.[6] More recent findings suggest that eosinophils may protect against respiratory virus infections that are prevalent in neonates.[120]

In the healthy organism, eosinophils and their cytokines may be important in establishing homeostatic mechanisms through the production and maintenance of plasma cells in the bone marrow by the production of APRIL cytokine.[234] Moreover, eosinophils may have a central role in the establishment of the metabolic phenotype by promoting insulin responsiveness and decreasing obesity. An intriguing discovery was made that eosinophils respond strongly to the satiety hormone leptin by releasing a range of cytokines,[288] suggesting that eosinophils are involved in metabolic processes associated with fat deposition in a way that extends beyond their perceived role in immunity. Specifically, eosinophil-derived IL-4 has been shown to be essential for the biogenesis of beige fat in the young animal, a type of brown adipose tissue that is present in neonates,[289] by switching monocytes to the alternatively activated macrophage phenotype.[290] The liver is also a site that may depend on eosinophils for normal function. Eosinophil-derived IL-4 was shown to be essential for liver regeneration by promoting hepatocyte proliferation,[291] suggesting an additional function for eosinophils that was not previously recognized. These studies were carried out using transgenic mouse models and have revealed novel roles for eosinophils that were not appreciated until very recently. Future studies will be focused on determining whether these findings from mouse models are translatable to human disease. It is clear from these few studies that there remains to be exciting new developments in the study of the immunological and physiological roles of eosinophils for many years to come.

EOSINOPHILS AND ALLERGIC DISEASE

The association between eosinophils and allergic disease has been known for many years. Eosinophils are a feature of allergic and nonallergic asthma,[292] and large numbers of eosinophils and eosinophil granule products are found in and around the bronchi in patients with asthma.[103,293,294] The gastrointestinal tract is a natural homing site for eosinophils; however, excessive eosinophilia and active secretion in various compartments of the gut result in disease states such as EE,

gastroesophageal reflux disease (GERD), or inflammatory bowel disease.[295] Patients with atopic dermatitis also show strong evidence of eosinophil presence and mediator release.[296,297]

Eosinophils and Asthma

There is a strong correlation between the presence of bronchial hyperresponsiveness (a cardinal clinical feature of asthma) and eosinophilia, particularly activated eosinophils.[293,298] Challenge of the airways with inhaled allergen induces local airway inflammation characterized by influx of both eosinophils and neutrophils. In the late phase of the response, eosinophils are a predominant feature.[299,300] A transient peripheral blood eosinophilia may also occur following these challenges.[299] Challenges with low-molecular-weight occupational compounds such as toluene diisocyanate have also been associated with eosinophilia.[301] Even nonatopic asthma, which appears to lack an IgE-mediated immune response, shows similar increases in airway eosinophils.[301,302]

Eosinophils in the airways may be assessed using bronchial biopsy, BAL, or induced sputum (*Figure 8.2B*). The use of fiberoptic bronchoscopy with biopsy is considered the gold standard for acquiring the best appreciation of eosinophil involvement in asthma.[303,304] A consistent finding in asthmatic airways is the presence of increased numbers of activated eosinophils or their release products, which correlate broadly with the severity of disease as reflected in symptoms, bronchial hyperreactivity, and lung function.[305] Segmental allergen challenge of human subjects' bronchi induces increased eosinophils in the airways[299,300] that were positive for the early activation marker CD69[306] and show upregulation of integrins.[307] Even in mild disease, there may be a significant increase in numbers of eosinophils in the airways of patients, and these are CD69 positive.[302,308]

Eosinophil granule proteins are significantly associated with the incidence of allergy and allergic asthma. As mentioned previously, MBP is found in large amounts in the lung tissues of patients with status asthmaticus, suggesting widespread eosinophil recruitment and degranulation.[103] The analysis of BAL samples from patients with asthma demonstrated that high concentrations of MBP correlate with the severity of bronchial hyperreactivity.[4,103] Intratracheal instillation of MBP and EPX in a primate model provoked bronchoconstriction, and MBP enhanced airway responsiveness to inhaled methacholine. These physiological effects of MBP are likely mediated by its cationic properties, since treatment with polyanionic peptides such as polyglutamic acid reverses the effects of MBP.[309] These studies suggest that eosinophil degranulation is a major feature of allergic asthma.

Sputum analysis offers a noninvasive technique showing correlation of eosinophil numbers with clinical outcomes.[310,311] Increases in sputum eosinophils correlate with the degree of airway responsiveness, asthma symptom scores, and asthma exacerbations.[302,312,313] Monitoring eosinophilic inflammation using induced sputum samples has been suggested as an important adjunct to the clinical management of asthma beyond relying on lung function and symptoms alone.[314] Conversely, a lack of eosinophils in sputum analysis appears to correlate with a lack of response to ICS.[315,316]

One major clinical manifestation of severe/fatal asthma is mucous plugging.[317] Eosinophilia-associated IL-4/IL-13 inflammation contributes to mucous hypersecretion and goblet cell hyperplasia by dysregulating expression of the polymeric mucins MUC5AC and MUC5B.[318] Indeed, mucous plugging (via high-resolution chest tomography) is documented in asthmatics with evidence of sputum eosinophils.[319,320] Moreover, degranulating/lytic eosinophils that release extracellular traps, free granules, and CLC proteins add to the viscosity and tenacity of the luminal mucus.[187] Galectin-10 crystal aggregates can lead to asthma-type pathology in murine models with increased goblet-cell hyperplasia. Antibodies targeted against the galectin-10 conformational epitopes (forming the stacked crystals) ameliorated eosinophilic inflammation and mucus production. In addition, the same antibodies were capable of dissolving CLC proteins present in patient-derived mucus.[321]

The Eosinophil Controversy

Early studies on eosinophil function in the immune response suggested that eosinophils played an immunoprotective role in allergy. For example, eosinophils produce histaminase, which was thought to act by downregulating mast cell–mediated early-phase responses to allergen.[322] However, reports emerging in the latter part of the 20th century suggested that eosinophils had a destructive role in allergic and asthmatic airways, based on the discovery of intensely stained deposits of eosinophil MBP in the airways of individuals who died from fatal asthma.[103] More recent studies then cast this concept back into doubt, including animal models of asthma (IL-5 gene knockouts and anti-IL-5-treated mice) and clinical trials using anti-IL-5, IL-12, and IFNγ.

Mouse Models of Airway Hyperresponsiveness

The roles of IL-5 and eosinophilia have been intensively investigated in numerous mouse models. Depending on the protocol used for sensitization and challenge, it appeared that airway hyperresponsiveness could persist in mice in spite of treatment with an antibody to IL-5 and depletion of blood eosinophils. Animal models of asthma have utilized IL-5$^{-/-}$ mice to determine the contribution of eosinophils to the pathogenesis of airway inflammation induced by allergens. Increased blood and tissue IL-5 levels are typically evident in wild-type mice following allergen challenge.[323] However, several reports showed that airway hyperresponsiveness was not affected in allergen-sensitized and challenged IL-5$^{-/-}$ mice, although blood eosinophil numbers were significantly diminished.[324] Similarly, IL-5$^{-/-}$ mice did not mount a blood or tissue eosinophil response after allergen challenge, nor did they develop airway hyperresponsiveness.[323] Studies using anti-IL-5 injections in mice generated similar observations.[28,325] Restoring IL-5 expression in these animals via vaccinia virus encoding IL-5 reconstituted blood and tissue eosinophilia with an associated development of airway hyperresponsiveness.

In these studies, it appeared that airway hyperresponsiveness could develop during allergen challenge, even though blood eosinophilia was lost. The answer to this dilemma may be in the persistence of tissue eosinophils even during IL-5 depletion. Although IL-5 is important in the differentiation and proliferation of eosinophils in the bone marrow, once they arrive in peripheral mucosal tissues, they may switch to an IL-5-independent mechanism of activation, and possibly recruitment, due to the strongly downregulatory effects of IL-5 on eosinophil IL-5 receptor expression.

The possibility of persistence of IL-5-independent tissue eosinophils has been implicated in results from CCL11/eotaxin$^{-/-}$ mice. Despite developing blood eosinophilia, CCL11/eotaxin$^{-/-}$ mice show reduced but not abolished tissue eosinophilia[40] with associated eosinophil-mediated tissue damage following allergen challenge.[326] However, in IL-5 transgenic mice treated with recombinant CCL11/eotaxin-2, both IL-5 and CCL/eotaxin-2 cooperatively promote eosinophil accumulation in the blood and tissues, leading to increased IL-13 production and enhanced airway hyperresponsiveness during allergen challenge.[29] Neither IL-5 nor CCL11/eotaxin on its own was able to induce these events. These studies indicate that there are distinct roles for eotaxin and IL-5 in eosinophil maturation, proliferation, and homing to target tissues. Thus, while IL-5 is critical for the maturation and proliferation of eosinophils in the bone marrow, eotaxin may be equally essential in a cooperative manner for movement and maintenance of eosinophilia in the tissues. Therefore, a key event in eosinophil-mediated inflammation leading to airway hyperresponsiveness may lie in the persistence of activated eosinophils in the tissue.

Moreover, transgenic mouse models of T cell or lung epithelium-specific expression of IL-5 spontaneously produce severe skin lesions, gastrointestinal dysfunction, splenic enlargement, and airway hyperresponsiveness similar to symptoms associated with human eosinophilic disorders,[327,328] supporting a crucial role for the eosinophil in tissue damage associated with allergy.

Studies in an eosinophil-knockout mouse, generated by linking the diphtheria toxin promoter to the gene expressing EPX (the so-called PHIL mouse), indicate a key role for eosinophils in establishing airway hyperresponsiveness in an acute model of allergic inflammation.[329] In the PHIL mice, eosinophils were depleted in both blood and tissue compartments, and Th2-type airway inflammation and an asthma-like pathology was attenuated upon sensitization and challenge with ovalbumin. These responses were restored by reconstitution of eosinophils[330] or a combination of eosinophils and antigen-specific T cells.[251] Another study showed that GATA-1 promoter disruption in mice (generating the Δdbl-GATA lineage), which also leads to the ablation of eosinophils, had no effect on airway hyperresponsiveness to methacholine challenge in either acute or chronic models of allergic inflammation but showed reduced mucus production and airway remodeling.[17,331] In general, these studies show supportive data for a role for eosinophils in mediating Th2-type inflammatory responses, at least in the mouse model, but with some conflicting details. For example, the Δdbl-GATA mice did not show any significant differences in airway hyperresponsiveness following allergen sensitization and challenge, while PHIL mice exhibited a profound reduction in airway resistance upon challenge with methacholine. Thus, differences are apparent in these eosinophil-lacking mouse models, which prevents a clear interpretation of the role of eosinophils in airway hyperresponsiveness in allergic inflammation.

Indeed, the appropriateness of the mouse as an animal model for investigating airway hyperresponsiveness has been brought into question on numerous occasions. A major limitation of mouse models is that mouse eosinophils seem to be markedly deficient in their ability to undergo respiratory burst[227,332] and degranulate in vivo or in vitro in response to any known eosinophil-specific agonists. As mentioned earlier, eosinophil degranulation appears to be a vital component of the symptoms associated with allergic airway disease, and the use of mouse models to determine the immunological function of eosinophils should be approached with caution.

In conclusion, these findings have important implications for the treatment of asthmatic patients with antieosinophil therapies, such that more specific and targeted treatments may be needed to block either the recruitment or activation of eosinophils at sites of inflammation.

Antieosinophil Strategies in Human Asthma

The role of the eosinophils as a key player in the pathophysiology of asthma has been debated despite evidence that the cells are present and activated in the airway lumen and tissue of patients with current asthma,[333] are increased in number when asthma is uncontrolled[334] or severe,[335] and are decreased when asthma is controlled.[336] Treatment strategies that aim to control airway eosinophilia are significantly more effective and less expensive in improving asthma control[312,313] and decreasing asthma exacerbations compared with guideline-based clinical strategies involving inhaled long-acting β agonists and oral or inhaled glucocorticosteroid treatment.

As mentioned above, cynicism was fueled by observations that, in mouse models of allergic sensitization, airway hyperresponsiveness could be induced without eosinophils.[337] Skepticism grew stronger when therapy using monoclonal antibodies against IL-5, which has no known clinically relevant biologic activity other than on eosinophils, failed to demonstrate improvement in asthma outcomes despite decreasing airway and blood eosinophil numbers.[338] The molecule did not reduce allergen-induced airway constriction or hyperresponsiveness, symptoms, airflow limitation, or exacerbations. The likely explanations for this apparent paradox are either individually, or a combination of, inappropriate methodology, inadequate sample size,[339,340] or an inadequate reduction in bronchial mucosal eosinophil numbers.[341]

This section will describe clinical studies that demonstrated an improvement in asthma control using treatment strategies that aimed to normalize sputum eosinophil count using corticosteroids, critically evaluate clinical trials that failed to demonstrate an improvement in asthma using monoclonal antibodies directed against IL-5. As well, evidence will be presented from a prospective audit of clinical outcomes of patients managed by normalizing sputum cell counts.

Eosinophil-Based Treatment Strategies Using Corticosteroids

Airway eosinophilia can be reliably and relatively noninvasively assessed in sputum.[342] In clinical practice, approximately 30% of patients with asthma attending a tertiary clinic have eosinophilic bronchitis.[343] More severe asthma and more severe airflow limitation correlate with more intense sputum eosinophilia.[344] Two studies in adults and one study in children have evaluated the outcomes of titrating anti-inflammatory treatments with the intention of normalizing eosinophils in sputum. The first single-center, 1-year trial that examined the effect of treating asthma to reduce sputum eosinophils to 2% resulted in a significant reduction of severe exacerbations compared with a control group treated without sputum eosinophil counts.[312] The large number of exacerbations and their severity in the control group was probably a result of the policy at the time to further reduce corticosteroid use if control was maintained for 2 months. The second trial was a multicenter trial conducted over 2 years, and it differed in that the minimum dose of corticosteroid to maintain sputum eosinophils at 3% was determined first and then maintained for the duration of the study.[313] Exacerbations were few and mild compared with the first study and were reduced by about 50% compared with the group treated with the same best-guideline approach to treatment without sputum cell counts. The active treatment reduced eosinophilic exacerbations but had no effect on neutrophilic exacerbations, which were regarded as probably of viral cause. The benefits in both studies were achieved without any increase in corticosteroid dose over that required by the control group. In contrast, a similar study in children showed a nonstatistically significant effect on reducing exacerbations using a sputum strategy that aimed to keep eosinophil levels to below 2.5%.[345] The modest benefit is most likely due to an inadequate control of eosinophils in the treatment arm that was probably related to the inadequate dose of inhaled corticosteroids (ICS) allowed in the study. In addition, the pediatric study was likely underpowered for demonstrating a treatment effect. Most importantly, unlike in adults, majority of exacerbations in children tend to be noneosinophilic, and therefore, an eosinophil-targeted therapy is likely to have only limited clinical benefits. The utility of using sputum eosinophils to decrease exacerbations in adults and children with moderate to severe asthma was recently confirmed in a systematic review and meta-analysis.[314] These findings indicate that, in addition to a significant reduction of exacerbations at a reduced cost,[346] the adverse consequences of new therapies and suboptimal treatment are also possibly avoided.

Anti-IL-5 Clinical Trials

The beneficial effects of corticosteroids are not limited to decreasing eosinophils in the airways.[347] They also reduce the number and activity of other cells such as lymphocytes and mast cells and diminish several markers of remodeling. Thus, it is not possible to definitely conclude the pathobiological role of eosinophils in asthma from those studies using only corticosteroids. The definitive proof would be to reduce eosinophil numbers in the airways using treatments that directly target tissue eosinophils. Recently, the availability of monoclonal antibodies directed against IL-5 has provided us with the opportunity to examine this. In two phase 2 randomized controlled trials on the effect of a humanized monoclonal anti-human IL-5 antibody, mepolizumab,[348,349] and a clinical trial on the effect of another anti-IL-5, reslizumab,[350] both drugs reduced sputum eosinophils to close to zero. This was associated with a reduction of exacerbations compared with the placebo group in the first mepolizumab study[348] and a prednisone-sparing effect and improvement in clinical outcomes in a small sample size in the second.[349] Both studies evaluated a similar intravenous dose of mepolizumab (750 mg). In the larger reslizumab clinical trial,[350] the reduction in sputum eosinophils was associated with improvements in FEV_1 and asthma control over a 5-month period in patients with moderate to severe asthma. Reslizumab was administered as a weight-adjusted dose of 3 mg/kg intravenously. The efficacy of reslizumab has since been confirmed in two replicate phase 3 clinical trials.[351] A total of 953 patients with elevated blood eosinophil counts were randomly assigned to receive either reslizumab (n = 477 [245 in study 1 and 232 in study 2]) or placebo (n = 476 [244 and 232]). In both studies, patients receiving reslizumab had a significant reduction in the frequency of asthma exacerbations (study 1: rate ratio 0.50 [95% confidence interval (CI) 0.37-0.67]; study 2: 0.41 [0.28-0.59]; both P < .0001) compared with those receiving placebo. The results of these studies were in contrast to the negative results of five previous trials, where the effect of the antieosinophil drug was not examined in patients with asthma and current sputum eosinophilia.[316]

The efficacy of mepolizumab has subsequently been confirmed in phase 3 clinical trials. Three doses of mepolizumab (75, 250, and 750 mg) administered intravenously were all effective in reducing exacerbations compared with placebo in a clinical trial of 621 patients with moderate to severe asthma and who had some evidence of "eosinophilic asthma" (DREAM study).[352] This was followed by a second clinical trial of 576 patients aged 12 to 82 years with recurrent asthma exacerbations (at least two in the past year) and evidence of eosinophilic inflammation (at least 150 cells/µL in peripheral blood) despite high doses of ICSs.[353] They were treated every 4 weeks with either one of two doses of mepolizumab (75 mg intravenously [IV] or 100 mg subcutaneously [SC]) or with placebo for 32 weeks. The exacerbation rate was reduced by 47% in the 75 mg IV group and 53% in the 100 mg SC group compared with the placebo group (P < .001 for both comparisons). This suggested that low-dose mepolizumab administered subcutaneously would be effective in patients selected to be eosinophilic asthma based on a single blood eosinophil count.

A post hoc analysis of the DREAM trial showed that there was seasonal variation in the exacerbation rates regardless of whether patients had atopic or nonatopic asthma, and mepolizumab was shown to reduce eosinophils and exacerbation rates in both atopic and nonatopic patients.[354] That is, the benefits of mepolizumab appear to be independent of baseline atopy and seasonality. Another post hoc analysis of the DREAM study suggested that blood eosinophil levels, but not sputum eosinophil levels, were predictors of response to mepolizumab.[355] This inference was drawn from a flawed and underpowered subgroup analysis of 14% of patients in the DREAM study who had both sputum and blood eosinophils enumerated at baseline. The appropriate method to examine whether a sputum eosinophil cutoff of 3% or a blood eosinophil cutoff of 150 cells/µL is a better predictor of response would be to compare the treatment effects (mean difference in number of exacerbations between treatment and placebo on log scale) in both subgroups via an interaction between this subgroup variable and the treatment group variable, which would thus test the significance between the means and not whether one of them is significant while the other is not, based on the confidence intervals being on the same side of unity or not.

Studies also demonstrated that mepolizumab had oral corticosteroid-sparing effects in patients with high sputum or blood eosinophil levels. In a proof-of-concept study of 20 individuals with sputum eosinophilia and airway symptoms despite continued treatment with prednisone, treatment with 5 monthly injections of mepolizumab resulted in a mean reduction in prednisone dose of 83.8% of maximum dose compared with a mean reduction in prednisone dose of 47.7% of maximum dose for the placebo group (P = .04).[349] In a later study, 135 patients with severe eosinophilic asthma,[356] defined by oral corticosteroids (OCS) use in the previous 6 months and a blood eosinophil level of at least 300 cells/µL in the previous 12 months, were treated with six monthly injections of mepolizumab or placebo. Patients receiving mepolizumab were 2.39× more likely to have a reduction in OCS dose than patients receiving placebo (95% CI, 1.25-4.56; P = .008), and patients in the mepolizumab group were also less likely to experience an exacerbation in spite of reductions in OCS dose. However, low doses of mepolizumab (100 mg s/c) do not suppress sputum eosinophilia in approximately 50% of patients and they have more modest exacerbation reduction and prednisone sparing, compared with patients whose sputum eosinophilia is suppressed.[356] This may be due to the inability to suppress in situ eosinophilopoiesis that is likely to be promoted by locally derived IL-5 and IL-13 from ILC2 cells.[357] Eosinophilia that is not suppressed with low-dose mepolizumab can be controlled with higher dose of an anti-IL5 neutralizing antibody, for example, reslizumab administered intravenously.[358]

Inadequate neutralization of airway IL-5 by an anti-IL5 monoclonal antibody can result in a worsening of eosinophilia. The recently demonstrated endogenous autoantibodies in the airway[359] contribute to this phenomenon. Heterocomplexes form between IL-5, the anti-IL5 antibody, and the endogenous IgG antibodies. This may also result in complement activation.[360] These immune complexes could stimulate monocytes and macrophages to secrete danger signals such as TL-1, which could further stimulate ILC2 cells (through receptors such as Death Receptor 3) to secrete more IL-5. Alarmins such as TSLP and IL-33 could upregulate DR3 on the ILC2 cells.[361] Another strategy to reduce eosinophil numbers is to block the IL-5 receptor. Benralizumab is an afucosylated molecule directed against the IL-5R.[362] It reduces exacerbations[363,364] and is effective to reduce the need for prednisone.[365] Benralizumab, by its additional effect of NK cell–mediated antibody-dependent cytotoxicity,[366] causes depletion of eosinophils in tissue and in the airway lumen in both mild[367] and severe asthma.[368] The eosinophil depletion by benralizumab is faster and more profound than with the currently approved doses of mepolizumab.[369]

Other Antieosinophil Treatment Strategies

Corticosteroids are very effective in reducing eosinophil numbers and their activation in the airways of most patients with asthma. Therefore novel treatment strategies such as anti-IL5 should probably be reserved to help taper doses for patients who require high doses of inhaled or regular OCS to control their airway eosinophilia and asthma.[370] Although a larger number of small molecules and monoclonal antibodies and antisense molecules are currently being evaluated to target a number of relevant cytokines or chemoattractants involved in eosinophil recruitment into the airway such as IL-4, IL-13, and eotaxin,[371] none of them have yet been demonstrated to be effective in suppressing an airway eosinophilia that persists despite being treated with prednisone. These are currently being investigated. Dexpramipexole, through mechanisms that are currently not known, have been demonstrated to reduce circulating eosinophil numbers[372] and in nasal polyp tissue.[373] Its effect in asthma is being investigated. While baseline peripheral blood eosinophil numbers seem to be a predictor of response to treatment with anti-IL-13[374] and anti-IL4R monoclonal antibodies such as dupilumab,[375] these treatments are not demonstrated to reduce airway eosinophil numbers (https://clinicaltrials.gov/ct2/show/NCT02573233). Tezepelumab, by blocking the alarmin TSLP, has been demonstrated to reduce blood and airway eosinophil numbers.[376,377] The relative risk reductions of some of these interventions are summarized in *Table 8.3*.

Taken together, these clinical studies confirm that eosinophils are important in the pathophysiology of asthma. Although blood and airway eosinophil numbers are modestly correlated in patients with mild asthma and may predict response to anticosinophil therapies,[378] they are poorly correlated to each other in more severe asthmatic patients who are on high doses of corticosteroids.[379] Moreover, while there is evidence to suggest that airway luminal eosinophil numbers correlate more to clinical indices of asthma control than tissue and blood eosinophils,[336] the role of adjusting antieosinophil therapies guided by measurement of luminal eosinophil activity remains to be proven. Furthermore, with increasing recognition that airway mucus is an important contributor to airflow obstruction, and the role of the eosinophils and EPX in contributing to mucous accumulation,[319] studies are underway to tease apart the interdependence and relative contribution of eosinophil and mucus to asthma severity.

Eosinophilic Esophagitis

Eosinophils are associated with the pathogenesis of gastrointestinal disorders such as EE. Often patients undergoing biopsy for diagnosis of GERD have increased numbers of intraepithelial eosinophils,[380] which appear to clear with effective antireflux therapy.[381] The condition of EE is described as a distinct clinical entity, although the feature of esophageal dysfunction is shared with GERD. The pathogenesis of EE has an allergic basis, and EE has been called asthma of the esophagus. Patients with EE present with increased gastroesophageal reflux and also exhibit choking or food impaction. The clinical symptoms of EE respond well to antiasthma therapy such as systemic corticosteroids,[382] topical corticosteroids,[383,384] and montelukast.[385] Despite therapy, EE appears to be a chronic illness with the potential for relapses.[386] Similar to asthma, a key stimulus for developing exacerbations of EE symptoms is not always food allergen, but inhaled aeroallergen.[387] The mechanism of this surprising observation is not known but may relate back to the shared embryonic origin of the gastrointestinal and respiratory tracts. Recently, lirentelimab, an anti-Siglec-8 antibody that depletes eosinophils and inhibits mast cells has been demonstrated to reduce eosinophilic infiltration in symptomatic patients with eosinophilic gastritis and duodenitis.[388]

EOSINOPHILS IN AUTOIMMUNE DISEASES

Eosinophils have rarely been assigned a causative role in autoimmune diseases. Emerging data show they promote autoimmune responses in the cardiac tissue, lung, and intestines, given their potential to cause tissue damage and perpetuate inflammation.[389,390] Increased peripheral count, infiltration into afflicted tissue, or the presence of eosinophil degranulation products and T2 cytokines are all associatory factors in several systemic and organ-specific autoimmune diseases. For example, blood eosinophilia is characteristic for known autoimmune diseases such as eGPA[391] and bullous pemphigoid.[392] The possible role of eosinophils in bullous pemphigoid is attributed to the recent evidence of EETs confirmed by confocal laser microscopy

Table 8.3. Relative Risk Reduction of Asthma Exacerbations With Monoclonal Antibodies

• Omalizumab (anti-IgE)	25%
• Blood eos >200-400	52%-72%
• Mepolizumab (100 mg SC Q4W) (anti-IL5)	53%
• Blood eos (>150, 300, 400, 500)	52% (59%, 66%, 70%)
• Reslizumab (3 mg/kg IV monthly) (anti-IL5)	
• BREATHE 1	50%
• BREATHE 2	59%
• Benralizumab (30 mg SC Q8W) (anti-IL5R)	
• CALIMA (eos <300, >300)	40%, 28%
• SIROCCO (eos <300, >300)	17%, 51%
• Dupilumab (200/300 mg SC Q2W) (anti-IL4R)	47% (46%)
• Blood eos >300	66%
• Tezepelumab (210 mg SC Q4W) (anti-TSLP)	56%
• Blood eos <300	41%
• Blood eos >450	77%

The Normal Hematologic System

on skin biopsies of patients.[393] For eGPA, despite being a diagnostic criterion, the pathologic role of eosinophils has remained elusive. Recent evidence shows antineutrophil cytoplasmic antibodies characteristic of eGPA causes extensive eosinophil degranulation and EET formation[394] as well as release of galactin-10.[395] As in Crohn disease and ulcerative colitis, increased potential of EPX production ex vivo by eosinophils isolated from patients during active phases of disease compared with stable/controlled state provides evidence of the pathogenic role of eosinophils.[396] Finally, autoantibodies are a hallmark of autoimmune diseases and causality is primarily linked to the source of the self-antigen. That said, the only eosinophil-specific autoantibody that has been described in literature is anti-EPX, reported in the sera of primary biliary cirrhosis[397] and airway secretions from severe eosinophilic asthmatics.[359]

THE EFFECTOR ROLE OF THE EOSINOPHIL IN WORM INFECTIONS

There is a strong relationship between parasitic infection and eosinophilia. Infection with helminths is the most common cause of moderate to marked eosinophilia. Studies in the latter part of the 20th century demonstrated that eosinophils had the capacity to kill parasitic targets and led to the concept that eosinophils were immunoprotective.[398]

As in allergic inflammation, the precise role of eosinophils in the immunopathological changes associated with helminth infections remains ill-understood and rather controversial. Increases in the number of tissue and peripheral blood eosinophils, together with elevations in the levels of total and parasitic-specific IgE and mastocytosis, have been considered for a long time to be hallmarks of infection with parasitic worms,[399] especially during their tissue migratory phases. Much has been published about the inimical role this cell may play in protection against helminths, but there is equally important evidence to suggest that their presence may be a reflection of their participation in the pathology of the disease rather than immunity to the parasitic metazoa. The original observation of Basten and Beeson[10] that helminth-associated eosinophilia is T cell dependent was an important turning point in our current understanding of eosinophil-mediated inflammation in worm infections. The identification and subsequent cloning of GM-CSF, IL-3, and particularly IL-5 helped to explain the T-cell control of eosinophilic response both in terms of eosinophilopoiesis and differentiation as well as priming and activation of the mature cell. The question, however, remains as to why there is a selective increase of eosinophils and what their function is, both locally and systematically, in infected subjects.

In vitro and Mouse Parasitic Helminth Studies

Much has been published on the helminthicidal effects of human, primate, and rodent eosinophils against metazoan targets coated with IgG, IgA, IgE, and/or complement components. In this context, a number of parasitic targets have been studied, including schistosomula of *Schistosoma mansoni*, new-born larvae of *Trichinella spiralis*, and larvae of *Nippostrongylus brasiliensis, Fasciola hepatica,* and others.[400]

Eosinophils adhere readily to appropriately coated larvae and undergo regulated exocytosis, which results in the deposition of the basic and cytotoxic granule-associated proteins. On their own, these preformed products of eosinophils (including MBP, ECP, and EPX) have potent helminthicidal properties at low molar concentrations. The exogenous addition of a number of chemotactic agents, such as LTB_4, PAF, fMLF,[401,402] and cytokines such as GM-CSF, IL-3, TNF-α, and IL-5,[403] to eosinophil preparations enhances their cytotoxic capacity against parasitic larvae. In addition to killing worm larvae, eosinophils that adhere to schistosomula via IgG, IgE, or complement generate substantial amounts of membrane phospholipid-derived mediators. More recent studies have shown that, in IL-5$^{-/-}$ mice, skin implants containing parasites failed to eliminate larval forms of the organisms.[404] The mechanism underlying larval expulsion was shown to be dependent on eosinophils as well as IgM, and the results suggested that the function of eosinophil granule proteins might be

associated with disrupting parasitic larvae to allow processing by antigen-presenting cells, including the eosinophil itself. A recent study using the eosinophil-less PHIL mice demonstrated that infection of these mice with *Schistosoma mansoni* had no effect on traditional measures of disease in this model.[405] However, these findings should be taken with caution as there are many differences in eosinophil functions between mice and humans, and specifically, mouse eosinophils are not as readily activated as their human counterparts.[332]

Helminthiases in Humans and Nonhuman Primates

The precise regulatory and functional roles of eosinophils in human helminthiases during the well-documented inflammatory reaction require urgent and extensive attention. In general, no clear evidence exists of direct contract between eosinophils and adult worms, although accumulation of eosinophils around helminthic parasites has been described. Eosinophils were also found in close contact with the surface tegument of schistosomula of *Schistosoma haematobium* in the cutaneous tissue of immune monkeys, associated with the presence of large number of dead larvae in eosinophil-rich sites.[401] Similar observations were made in other host-parasite systems. Using appropriate antibodies, eosinophil-derived toxic proteins such as MBP have been identified on filarial worm targets in vivo[402] and levels of blood ECP are elevated in patients with filariasis, which may suggest the activation and degranulation of eosinophils.[403]

Thus, the specific role of eosinophils in helminthic parasitic infections is still undetermined, and this remains an area of intense investigation.

CONCLUSIONS

The eosinophil is an enigmatic and fascinating cell that has intrigued biomedical scientists for more than a century. The precise function of this cell in immunology as well as allergic inflammation and asthma remains a matter of debate and requires further study in appropriately designed research projects (see 406 for a more comprehensive assessment of eosinophils and their role in health and disease). However, it is important to recognize that no single cell type, whether the eosinophil, T cell, mast cell, neutrophil, or other lung cell, is on its own responsible for all aspects of the immunopathology and clinical sequelae of airway inflammation in asthma and related diseases. In recognition of this fact, the attention currently focused on the eosinophil is warranted and timely. This relates partially to the overwhelming evidence in favor of a potential effector role of the eosinophil in parasitic helminthic and allergic diseases, including asthma. While the mechanisms of eosinophilia in association with allergic disease are not yet fully understood, they seem likely to be controlled at the level of tissue responses to allergens and the subsequent elaboration of cytokines, which exert both direct and indirect effect on these inflammatory cells. The profile of cytokines generated in allergic reactions, such as allergen-induced late-phase responses in the skin, nose, and lung, appears to conform to a Th2 profile, because mRNA of IL-4 and IL-5, but not IFNγ or IL-2, is expressed or upregulated during these reactions. The release of IL-5 by various cells following stimulation with allergen may, therefore, be responsible for eosinophilia in allergic disease. Thus, a complex network of innate and adaptive immune cells, as well as their cytokine products, may participate in a cascade of events that leads to specific accumulation of eosinophils in sites of allergic inflammation and asthma. Whether tissue damage, a feature of these disease conditions, is the consequence of the activation and exocytosis of these infiltrating cytotoxic cells and the release of their highly basic protein products is yet to be demonstrated unequivocally.

WEBSITES

http://www.annualreviews.org/doi/pdf/10.1146/annurev.immunol.24.
    021605.090720
https://en.wikipedia.org/wiki/Eosinophil
http://en.wikipedia.org/wiki/Eosinophilia
https://apfed.org/

References

1. Kay AB. The early history of the eosinophil. *Clin Exp Allergy.* 2015;45(3):575-582.
2. Gleich GJ. Historical overview and perspective on the role of the eosinophil in health and disease. In: Lee JJ, Rosenberg HF, eds. *Eosinophils in Health and Disease.* Elsevier; 2013:1-11.
3. Rothenberg ME, Hogan SP. The eosinophil. *Annu Rev Immunol.* 2006;24:147-174.
4. Hogan SP, Rosenberg HF, Moqbel R, et al. Eosinophils: biological properties and role in health and disease. *Clin Exp Allergy.* 2008;38(5):709-750.
5. Blanchard C, Rothenberg ME. Biology of the eosinophil. *Adv Immunol.* 2009;101:81-121.
6. Rosenberg HF, Dyer KD, Foster PS. Eosinophils: changing perspectives in health and disease. *Nat Rev Immunol.* 2013;13(1):9-22.
7. Simon D, Simon HU. Eosinophils and skin diseases. In: Lee JJ, Rosenberg HF, eds. *Eosinophils in Health and Disease.* Elsevier, 2013:442-448.
8. Lotfi R, Spada N, Lotze MT. Eosinophils and cancer. In: Lee JJ, Rosenberg HF, eds. *Eosinophils in Health and Disease.* Elsevier; 2013:503-508.
9. Spry CJF. *Eosinophils. A Comprehensive Review and Guide to the Scientific and Medical Literature.* Oxford University Press; 1988.
10. Basten A, Beeson PB. Mechanism of eosinophilia. II. Role of the lymphocyte. *J Exp Med.* 1970;131(6):1288-1305.
11. Spry CJ. The natural history of eosinophils. In: Smith H, Cook RM, eds. *Immunopharmacology of Eosinophils.* Academic Press; 1993:241-243.
12. Walle AJ, Parwaresch MR. Estimation of effective eosinopoiesis and bone marrow eosinophil reserve capacity in normal man. *Cell Tissue Kinet.* 1979;12(3):249-255.
13. Denburg JA, Sehmi R, Saito H, Pil-Seob J, Inman MD, O'Byrne PM. Systemic aspects of allergic disease: bone marrow responses. *J Allergy Clin Immunol.* 2000;106(5 suppl):S242-S6.
14. McNagny K, Graf T. Making eosinophils through subtle shifts in transcription factor expression. *J Exp Med.* 2002;195(11):F43-F7.
15. Walsh JC, DeKoter RP, Lee HJ, et al. Cooperative and antagonistic interplay between PU.1 and GATA-2 in the specification of myeloid cell fates. *Immunity.* 2002;17(5):665-676.
16. Du J, Stankiewicz MJ, Liu Y, et al. Novel combinatorial interactions of GATA-1, PU.1, and C/EBPepsilon isoforms regulate transcription of the gene encoding eosinophil granule major basic protein. *J Biol Chem.* 2002;277(45):43481-43494.
17. Yu C, Cantor AB, Yang H, et al. Targeted deletion of a high-affinity GATA-binding site in the GATA-1 promoter leads to selective loss of the eosinophil lineage in vivo. *J Exp Med.* 2002;195(11):1387-1395.
18. Inman MD, Sehmi R, O'Byrne P, Denburg JA. The role of the bone marrow in allergic disease. In: Denburg JA, ed. *Allergy and Allergic Diseases: The New Mechanisms and Therapeutics.* Humana Press; 1998:85-102.
19. Dombrowicz D, Woerly G, Capron M. IgE receptors on human eosinophils. *Chem Immunol.* 2000;76:63-76.
20. Ackerman SJ, Kephart GM, Habermann TM, Greipp PR, Gleich GJ. Localization of eosinophil granule major basic protein in human basophils. *J Exp Med.* 1983;158(3):946-961.
21. Foster PS. Allergic networks regulating eosinophilia. *Am J Respir Cell Mol Biol.* 1999;21(4):451-454.
22. Hamelmann E, Gelfand EW. IL-5-induced airway eosinophilia--the key to asthma? *Immunol Rev.* 2001;179:182-191.
23. Sutherland DR, Stewart AK, Keating A. CD34 antigen: molecular features and potential clinical applications. *Stem Cell.* 1993;11:50-57.
24. Clutterbuck EJ, Hirst EM, Sanderson CJ. Human interleukin-5 (IL-5) regulates the production of eosinophils in human bone marrow cultures: comparison and interaction with IL-1, IL-3, IL-6, and GMCSF. *Blood.* 1989;73(6):1504-1512.
25. Dent LA, Strath M, Mellor AL, Sanderson CJ. Eosinophilia in transgenic mice expressing interleukin 5. *J Exp Med.* 1990;172(5):1425-1431.
26. Tominaga A, Takaki S, Koyama N, et al. Transgenic mice expressing a B cell growth and differentiation factor gene (interleukin 5) develop eosinophilia and autoantibody production. *J Exp Med.* 1991;173(2):429-437.
27. Foster PS, Hogan SP, Ramsay AJ, Matthaei KI, Young IG. Interleukin 5 deficiency abolishes eosinophilia, airways hyperreactivity, and lung damage in a mouse asthma model. *J Exp Med.* 1996;183(1):195-201.
28. Corry DB, Folkesson HG, Warnock ML, et al. Interleukin 4, but not interleukin 5 or eosinophils, is required in a murine model of acute airway hyperreactivity. *J Exp Med.* 1996;183(1):109-117.
29. Yang M, Hogan SP, Mahalingam S, et al. Eotaxin-2 and IL-5 cooperate in the lung to regulate IL-13 production and airway eosinophilia and hyperreactivity. *J Allergy Clin Immunol.* 2003;112(5):935-943.
30. Giembycz MA, Lindsay MA. Pharmacology of the eosinophil. *Pharmacol Rev.* 1999;51(2):213-339.
31. Bochner BS, Schleimer RP. Mast cells, basophils, and eosinophils: distinct but overlapping pathways for recruitment. *Immunol Rev.* 2001;179:5-15.
32. Steinbach KH, Schick P, Trepel F, et al. Estimation of kinetic parameters of neutrophilic, eosinophilic, and basophilic granulocytes in human blood. *Blut.* 1979;39(1):27-38.
33. Krause JR, Boggs DR. Search for eosinopenia in hospitalized patients with normal blood leukocyte concentration. *Am J Hematol.* 1987;24(1):55-63.
34. Winkel P, Statland BE, Saunders AM, Osborn H, Kupperman H. Within-day physiologic variation of leukocyte types in healthy subjects as assayed by two automated leukocyte differential analyzers. *Am J Clin Pathol.* 1981;75(5):693-700.
35. Rothenberg ME, Owen WF, Jr, Silberstein DS, Soberman RJ, Austen KF, Stevens RL. Eosinophils cocultured with endothelial cells have increased survival and functional properties. *Science.* 1987;237(4815):645-647.
36. Silberstein DS, Austen KF, Owen WF, Jr. Hemopoietins for eosinophils. Glycoprotein hormones that regulate the development of inflammation in eosinophilia-associated disease. *Hematol Oncol Clin North Am.* 1989;3(3):511-533.
37. Dri P, Cramer R, Spessotto P, Romano M, Patriarca P. Eosinophil activation on biologic surfaces. Production of O_2 in response to physiologic soluble stimuli is differentially modulated by extracellular matrix components and endothelial cells. *J Immunol.* 1991;147(2):613-620.
38. Anwar AR, Moqbel R, Walsh GM, Kay AB, Wardlaw AJ. Adhesion to fibronectin prolongs eosinophil survival. *J Exp Med.* 1993;177(3):839-843.
39. Simon HU, Yousefi S, Schranz C, Schapowal A, Bachert C, Blaser K. Direct demonstration of delayed eosinophil apoptosis as a mechanism causing tissue eosinophilia. *J Immunol.* 1997;158(8):3902-3908.
40. Foster PS, Mould AW, Yang M, et al. Elemental signals regulating eosinophil accumulation in the lung. *Immunol Rev.* 2001;179:173-181.
41. Cameron L, Christodoulopoulos P, Lavigne F, et al. Evidence for local eosinophil differentiation within allergic nasal mucosa: inhibition with soluble IL-5 receptor. *J Immunol.* 2000;164(3):1538-1545.
42. Eidelman DH, Minshall E, Dandurand RJ, et al. Evidence for major basic protein immunoreactivity and interleukin 5 gene activation during the late phase response in explanted airways. *Am J Respir Cell Mol Biol.* 1996;15(5):582-589.
43. Miyajima A, Kitamura T, Harada N, Yokota T, Arai K. Cytokine receptors and signal transduction. *Annu Rev Immunol.* 1992;10:295-331.
44. Pazdrak K, Olszewska-Pazdrak B, Stafford S, Garofalo RP, Alam R. Lyn, Jak2, and Raf-1 kinases are critical for the antiapoptotic effect of interleukin 5, whereas only Raf-1 kinase is essential for eosinophil activation and degranulation. *J Exp Med.* 1998;188(3):421-429.
45. Broide D, Sriramarao P. Eosinophil trafficking to sites of allergic inflammation. *Immunol Rev.* 2001;179:163-172.
46. Bochner BS, Luscinskas FW, Gimbrone MA, Jr, et al. Adhesion of human basophils, eosinophils, and neutrophils to interleukin 1-activated human vascular endothelial cells: contributions of endothelial cell adhesion molecules. *J Exp Med.* 1991;173(6):1553-1557.
47. Walsh GM, Hartnell A, Moqbel R, et al. Receptor expression and functional status of cultured human eosinophils derived from umbilical cord blood mononuclear cells. *Blood.* 1990;76(1):105-111.
48. Dobrina A, Menegazzi R, Carlos TM, et al. Mechanisms of eosinophil adherence to cultured vascular endothelial cells. Eosinophils bind to the cytokine-induced ligand vascular cell adhesion molecule-1 via the very late activation antigen-4 integrin receptor. *J Clin Invest.* 1991;88(1):20-26.
49. Weller PF, Rand TH, Goelz SE, Chi-Rosso G, Lobb RR. Human eosinophil adherence to vascular endothelium mediated by binding to vascular cell adhesion molecule 1 and endothelial leukocyte adhesion molecule 1. *Proc Natl Acad Sci U S A.* 1991;88(16):7430-7433.
50. Matsumoto K, Sterbinsky SA, Bickel CA, Zhou DF, Kovach NL, Bochner BS. Regulation of a4 integrin-mediated adhesion of human eosinophils to fibronectin and vascular cell adhesion molecule-1. *J Allergy Clin Immunol.* 1997;99(5):648-656.
51. Weber C, Katayama J, Springer TA. Differential regulation of b1 and b2 integrin avidity by chemoattractants in eosinophils. *Proc Natl Acad Sci U S A.* 1996;93(20):10939-10944.
52. Ebisawa M, Bochner BS, Georas SN, Schleimer RP. Eosinophil transendothelial migration induced by cytokines. I. Role of endothelial and eosinophil adhesion molecules in IL-1b-induced transendothelial migration. *J Immunol.* 1992;149(12):4021-4028.
53. Shahabuddin S, Ponath P, Schleimer RP. Migration of eosinophils across endothelial cell monolayers: interactions among IL-5, endothelial-activating cytokines, and C-C chemokines. *J Immunol.* 2000;164(7):3847-3854.
54. Georas SN, Liu MC, Newman W, Beall LD, Stealey BA, Bochner BS. Altered adhesion molecule expression and endothelial cell activation accompany the recruitment of human granulocytes to the lung after segmental antigen challenge. *Am J Respir Cell Mol Biol.* 1992;7(3):261-269.
55. Rothenberg ME, MacLean JA, Pearlman E, Luster AD, Leder P. Targeted disruption of the chemokine eotaxin partially reduces antigen-induced tissue eosinophilia. *J Exp Med.* 1997;185(4):785-790.
56. Wardlaw AJ, Brightling C, Green R, Woltmann G, Pavord I. Eosinophils in asthma and other allergic diseases. *Br Med Bull.* 2000;56(4):985-1003.
57. Schleimer RP, Sterbinsky SA, Kaiser J, et al. IL-4 induces adherence of human eosinophils and basophils but not neutrophils to endothelium. Association with expression of VCAM-1. *J Immunol.* 1992;148(4):1086-1092.
58. Bochner BS, Klunk DA, Sterbinsky SA, Coffman RL, Schleimer RP. IL-13 selectively induces vascular cell adhesion molecule-1 expression in human endothelial cells. *J Immunol.* 1995;154(2):799-803.
59. Kuperman D, Schofield B, Wills-Karp M, Grusby MJ. Signal transducer and activator of transcription factor 6 (STAT6)-deficient mice are protected from antigen-induced airway hyperresponsiveness and mucus production. *J Exp Med.* 1998;187(6):939-948.
60. Akimoto T, Numata F, Tamura M, et al. Abrogation of bronchial eosinophilic inflammation and airway hyperreactivity in signal transducers and activators of transcription (STAT)6-deficient mice. *J Exp Med.* 1998;187(9):1537-1542.
61. Matsukura S, Stellato C, Georas SN, et al. Interleukin-13 upregulates eotaxin expression in airway epithelial cells by a STAT6-dependent mechanism. *Am J Respir Cell Mol Biol.* 2001;24(6):755-761.
62. Kuijpers TW, Mul EP, Blom M, et al. Freezing adhesion molecules in a state of high-avidity binding blocks eosinophil migration. *J Exp Med.* 1993;178(1):279-284.
63. Werfel SJ, Yednock TA, Matsumoto K, Sterbinsky SA, Schleimer RP, Bochner BS. Functional regulation of b1 integrins on human eosinophils by divalent cations and cytokines. *Am J Respir Cell Mol Biol.* 1996;14(1):44-52.

64. Tachimoto H, Burdick MM, Hudson SA, Kikuchi M, Konstantopoulos K, Bochner BS. CCR3-active chemokines promote rapid detachment of eosinophils from VCAM-1 in vitro. *J Immunol.* 2000;165(5):2748-2754.
65. DiScipio RG, Daffern PJ, Jagels MA, Broide DH, Sriramarao P. A comparison of C3a and C5a-mediated stable adhesion of rolling eosinophils in postcapillary venules and transendothelial migration in vitro and in vivo. *J Immunol.* 1999;162(2):1127-1136.
66. Broide DH, Lotz M, Cuomo AJ, Coburn DA, Federman EC, Wasserman SI. Cytokines in symptomatic asthma airways. *J Allergy Clin Immunol.* 1992;89(5):958-967.
67. Bochner BS, Charlesworth EN, Lichtenstein LM, et al. Interleukin-1 is released at sites of human cutaneous allergic reactions. *J Allergy Clin Immunol.* 1990;86(6 pt 1):830-839.
68. Hirata N, Kohrogi H, Iwagoe H, et al. Allergen exposure induces the expression of endothelial adhesion molecules in passively sensitized human bronchus: time course and the role of cytokines. *Am J Respir Cell Mol Biol.* 1998;18(1):12-20.
69. Broide DH, Campbell K, Gifford T, Sriramarao P. Inhibition of eosinophilic inflammation in allergen-challenged, IL-1 receptor type 1-deficient mice is associated with reduced eosinophil rolling and adhesion on vascular endothelium. *Blood.* 2000;95(1):263-269.
70. Neumann B, Machleidt T, Lifka A, et al. Crucial role of 55-kilodalton TNF receptor in TNF-induced adhesion molecule expression and leukocyte organ infiltration. *J Immunol.* 1996;156(4):1587-1593.
71. Broide DH, Stachnick G, Castaneda D, Nayar J, Sriramarao P. Inhibition of eosinophilic inflammation in allergen-challenged TNF receptor p55/p75- and TNF receptor p55-deficient mice. *Am J Respir Cell Mol Biol.* 2001;24(3):304-311.
72. Masumoto A, Hemler ME. Multiple activation states of VLA-4. Mechanistic differences between adhesion to CS1/fibronectin and to vascular cell adhesion molecule-1. *J Biol Chem.* 1993;268(1):228-234.
73. Sung KL, Li Y, Elices M, Gang J, Sriramarao P, Broide DH. Granulocyte-macrophage colony-stimulating factor regulates the functional adhesive state of very late antigen-4 expressed by eosinophils. *J Immunol.* 1997;158(2):919-927.
74. Adachi T, Vita R, Sannohe S, et al. The functional role of rho and rho-associated coiled-coil forming protein kinase in eotaxin signaling of eosinophils. *J Immunol.* 2001;167(8):4609-4615.
75. Muessel MJ, Scott KS, Friedl P, Bradding P, Wardlaw AJ. CCL11 and GM-CSF differentially use the Rho GTPase pathway to regulate motility of human eosinophils in a three-dimensional microenvironment. *J Immunol.* 2008;180(12):8354-8360.
76. Fulkerson PC, Zimmermann N, Brandt EB, et al. Negative regulation of eosinophil recruitment to the lung by the chemokine monokine induced by IFNg (Mig, CXCL9). *Proc Natl Acad Sci U S A.* 2004;101(7):1987-1992.
77. Fulkerson PC, Zhu H, Williams DA, Zimmermann N, Rothenberg ME. CXCL9 inhibits eosinophil responses by a CCR3- and Rac2-dependent mechanism. *Blood.* 2005;106(2):436-443.
78. Kitayama J, Mackay CR, Ponath PD, Springer TA. The C-C chemokine receptor CCR3 participates in stimulation of eosinophil arrest on inflammatory endothelium in shear flow. *J Clin Invest.* 1998;101(9):2017-2024.
79. Jose PJ, Griffiths-Johnson DA, Collins PD, et al. Eotaxin: a potent eosinophil chemoattractant cytokine detected in a Guinea pig model of allergic airways inflammation. *J Exp Med.* 1994;179(3):881-887.
80. Alam R, Stafford S, Forsythe P, et al. RANTES is a chemotactic and activating factor for human eosinophils. *J Immunol.* 1993;150(8 pt 1):3442-3448.
81. Rothenberg ME. Eotaxin. An essential mediator of eosinophil trafficking into mucosal tissues. *Am J Respir Cell Mol Biol.* 1999;21(3):291-295.
82. Fryer AD, Stein LH, Nie Z, et al. Neuronal eotaxin and the effects of CCR3 antagonist on airway hyperreactivity and M2 receptor dysfunction. *J Clin Invest.* 2006;116(1):228-236.
83. Davoine F, Lacy P. Eosinophil cytokines, chemokines, and growth factors: emerging roles in immunity. *Front Immunol.* 2014;5:570.
84. Zimmermann N, Hogan SP, Mishra A, et al. Murine eotaxin-2: a constitutive eosinophil chemokine induced by allergen challenge and IL-4 overexpression. *J Immunol.* 2000;165(10):5839-5846.
85. Rothenberg ME, Luster AD, Lilly CM, Drazen JM, Leder P. Constitutive and allergen-induced expression of eotaxin mRNA in the Guinea pig lung. *J Exp Med.* 1995;181(3):1211-1216.
86. Collins PD, Marleau S, Griffiths-Johnson DA, Jose PJ, Williams TJ. Cooperation between interleukin-5 and the chemokine eotaxin to induce eosinophil accumulation *in vivo*. *J Exp Med.* 1995;182(4):1169-1174.
87. Mould AW, Ramsay AJ, Matthaei KI, Young IG, Rothenberg ME, Foster PS. The effect of IL-5 and eotaxin expression in the lung on eosinophil trafficking and degranulation and the induction of bronchial hyperreactivity. *J Immunol.* 2000;164(4):2142-2150.
88. Matthews AN, Friend DS, Zimmermann N, et al. Eotaxin is required for the baseline level of tissue eosinophils. *Proc Natl Acad Sci U S A.* 1998;95(11):6273-6278.
89. Gonzalo JA, Lloyd CM, Wen D, et al. The coordinated action of CC chemokines in the lung orchestrates allergic inflammation and airway hyperresponsiveness. *J Exp Med.* 1998;188(1):157-167.
90. Kaburagi Y, Shimada Y, Nagaoka T, Hasegawa M, Takehara K, Sato S. Enhanced production of CC-chemokines (RANTES, MCP-1, MIP-1a, MIP-1b, and eotaxin) in patients with atopic dermatitis. *Arch Dermatol Res.* 2001;293(7):350-355.
91. Harrison AM, Bonville CA, Rosenberg HF, Domachowske JB. Respiratory syncytical virus-induced chemokine expression in the lower airways: eosinophil recruitment and degranulation. *Am J Respir Crit Care Med.* 1999;159(6):1918-1924.
92. Teran LM, Seminario MC, Shute JK, et al. RANTES, macrophage-inhibitory protein 1a, and the eosinophil product major basic protein are released into upper respiratory secretions during virus-induced asthma exacerbations in children. *J Infect Dis.* 1999;179(3):677-681.
93. Palmblad J, Gyllenhammar H, Lindgren JA, Malmsten CL. Effects of leukotrienes and f-Met-Leu-Phe on oxidative metabolism of neutrophils and eosinophils. *J Immunol.* 1984;132(6):3041-3045.
94. Kroegel C, Yukawa T, Dent G, Venge P, Chung KF, Barnes PJ. Stimulation of degranulation from human eosinophils by platelet-activating factor. *J Immunol.* 1989;142(10):3518-3526.
95. Gleich GJ, Loegering DA, Maldonado JE. Identification of a major basic protein in Guinea pig eosinophil granules. *J Exp Med.* 1973;137(6):1459-1471.
96. Hamann KJ, Barker RL, Ten RM, Gleich GJ. The molecular biology of eosinophil granule proteins. *Int Arch Allergy Appl Immunol.* 1991;94(1-4):202-209.
97. Popken-Harris P, McGrogan M, Loegering DA, et al. Expression, purification, and characterization of the recombinant proform of eosinophil granule major basic protein. *J Immunol.* 1995;155(3):1472-1480.
98. Popken-Harris P, Checkel J, Loegering D, et al. Regulation and processing of a precursor form of eosinophil granule major basic protein (ProMBP) in differentiating eosinophils. *Blood.* 1998;92(2):623-631.
99. Mahmudi-Azer S, Velazquez JR, Lacy P, Denburg JA, Moqbel R. Immunofluorescence analysis of cytokine and granule protein expression during eosinophil maturation from cord blood-derived CD34 progenitors. *J Allergy Clin Immunol.* 2000;105(6 Pt 1):1178-1184.
100. Shalit M, Sekhsaria S, Mauhorter S, Mahanti S, Malech HL. Early commitment to the eosinophil lineage by cultured human peripheral blood $CD34^+$ cells: messenger RNA analysis. *J Allergy Clin Immunol.* 1996;98(2):344-354.
101. Abu-Ghazaleh RI, Gleich GJ, Prendergast FG. Interaction of eosinophil granule major basic protein with synthetic lipid bilayers: a mechanism for toxicity. *J Membr Biol.* 1992;128(2):153-164.
102. Adamko DJ, Yost BL, Gleich GJ, Fryer AD, Jacoby DB. Ovalbumin sensitization changes the inflammatory response to subsequent parainfluenza infection. Eosinophils mediate airway hyperresponsiveness, M_2 muscarinic receptor dysfunction, and antiviral effects. *J Exp Med.* 1999;190(10):1465-1478.
103. Filley WV, Holley KE, Kephart GM, Gleich GJ. Identification by immunofluorescence of eosinophil granule major basic protein in lung tissues of patients with bronchial asthma. *Lancet.* 1982;2(8288):11-16.
104. Moy JN, Gleich GJ, Thomas LL. Noncytotoxic activation of neutrophils by eosinophil granule major basic protein. Effect on superoxide anion generation and lysosomal enzyme release. *J Immunol.* 1990;145(8):2626-2632.
105. Kita H, Abu-Ghazaleh RI, Sur S, Gleich GJ. Eosinophil major basic protein induces degranulation and IL-8 production by human eosinophils. *J Immunol.* 1995;154(9):4749-4758.
106. Plager DA, Loegering DA, Checkel JL, et al. Major basic protein homolog (MBP2): a specific human eosinophil marker. *J Immunol.* 2006;177(10):7340-7345.
107. Soragni A, Yousefi S, Stoeckle C, et al. Toxicity of eosinophil MBP is repressed by intracellular crystallization and promoted by extracellular aggregation. *Mol Cell.* 2015;57(6):1011-1021.
108. Ten RM, Pease LR, McKean DJ, Bell MP, Gleich GJ. Molecular cloning of the human eosinophil peroxidase. Evidence for the existence of a peroxidase multigene family. *J Exp Med.* 1989;169(5):1757-1769.
109. Weiss SJ, Test ST, Eckmann CM, Roos D, Regiani S. Brominating oxidants generated by human eosinophils. *Science.* 1986;234(4773):200-203.
110. Mayeno AN, Curran AJ, Roberts RL, Foote CS. Eosinophils preferentially use bromide to generate halogenating agents. *J Biol Chem.* 1989;264(10):5660-5668.
111. Thomas EL, Bozeman PM, Jefferson MM, King CC. Oxidation of bromide by the human leukocyte enzymes myeloperoxidase and eosinophil peroxidase. Formation of bromamines. *J Biol Chem.* 1995;270(7):2906-2913.
112. van Dalen CJ, Kettle AJ. Substrates and products of eosinophil peroxidase. *Biochem J.* 2001;358(pt 1):233-239.
113. Gleich GJ, Loegering DA, Bell MP, Checkel JL, Ackerman SJ, McKean DJ. Biochemical and functional similarities between human eosinophil-derived neurotoxin and eosinophil cationic protein: homology with ribonuclease. *Proc Natl Acad Sci U S A.* 1986;83(10):3146-3150.
114. Lehrer RI, Szklarek D, Barton A, Ganz T, Hamann KJ, Gleich GJ. Antibacterial properties of eosinophil major basic protein and eosinophil cationic protein. *J Immunol.* 1989;142(12):4428-4434.
115. Young JD, Peterson CG, Venge P, Cohn ZA. Mechanism of membrane damage mediated by human eosinophil cationic protein. *Nature.* 1986;321(6070):613-616.
116. Fredens K, Dahl R, Venge P. The Gordon phenomenon induced by the eosinophil cationic protein and eosinophil protein X. *J Allergy Clin Immunol.* 1982;70(5):361-366.
117. Hamann KJ, Ten RM, Loegering DA, et al. Structure and chromosome localization of the human eosinophil-derived neurotoxin and eosinophil cationic protein genes: evidence for intronless coding sequences in the ribonuclease gene superfamily. *Genomics.* 1990;7(4):535-546.
118. Rosenberg HF, Dyer KD, Tiffany HL, Gonzalez M. Rapid evolution of a unique family of primate ribonuclease genes. *Nat Genet.* 1995;10(2):219-223.
119. Domachowske JB, Dyer KD, Bonville CA, Rosenberg HF. Recombinant human eosinophil-derived neurotoxin/RNase 2 functions as an effective antiviral agent against respiratory syncytial virus. *J Infect Dis.* 1998;177(6):1458-1464.
120. Percopo CM, Dyer KD, Ochkur SI, et al. Activated mouse eosinophils protect against lethal respiratory virus infection. *Blood.* 2014;123(5):743-752.
121. Ackerman SJ, Liu L, Kwatia MA, et al. Charcot-Leyden crystal protein (galectin-10) is not a dual function galectin with lysophospholipase activity but binds a lysophospholipase inhibitor in a novel structural fashion. *J Biol Chem.* 2002;277(17):14859-14868.
122. Melo RCN, Wang H, Silva TP, et al. Galectin-10, the protein that forms Charcot-Leyden crystals, is not stored in granules but resides in the peripheral cytoplasm of human eosinophils. *J Leukoc Biol.* 2020;108(1):139-149.

123. Calafat J, Janssen H, Knol EF, Weller PF, Egesten A. Ultrastructural localization of Charcot-Leyden crystal protein in human eosinophils and basophils. *Eur J Haematol*. 1997;58(1):56-66.

124. Dvorak AM, Letourneau L, Login GR, Weller PF, Ackerman SJ. Ultrastructural localization of the Charcot-Leyden crystal protein (lysophospholipase) to a distinct crystalloid-free granule population in mature human eosinophils. *Blood*. 1988;72(1):150-158.

125. Hamann KJ, Douglas I, Moqbel R. Eosinophil mediators. In: Busse WW, Holgate ST, eds. *Asthma and Rhinitis*. 2nd ed. Blackwell Scientific Publications; 2000:394-428.

126. Lacy P, Moqbel R. Immune effector functions of eosinophils in allergic airway inflammation. *Curr Opin Allergy Clin Immunol*. 2001;1(1):79-84.

127. Moqbel R, Lacy P. Exocytotic events in eosinophils and mast cells. *Clin Exp Allergy*. 1999;29(8):1017-1022.

128. Lacy P, Moqbel R. Signaling and degranulation. In: Lee JJ, Rosenberg HF, eds. *Eosinophils in Health and Disease*. Elsevier; 2013:206-219.

129. Nüsse O, Lindau M, Cromwell O, Kay AB, Gomperts BD. Intracellular application of guanosine-5'-O-(3-thiotriphosphate) induces exocytotic granule fusion in Guinea pig eosinophils. *J Exp Med*. 1990;171(3):775-786.

130. Lindau M, Nusse O, Bennett J, Cromwell O. The membrane fusion events in degranulating Guinea pig eosinophils. *J Cell Sci*. 1993;104(pt 1):203-210.

131. Hartmann J, Scepek S, Lindau M. Regulation of granule size in human and horse eosinophils by number of fusion events among unit granules. *J Physiol (Lond)*. 1995;483(pt 1):201-209.

132. Scepek S, Lindau M. Exocytotic competence and intergranular fusion in cord blood-derived eosinophils during differentiation. *Blood*. 1997;89(2):510-517.

133. Newman TM, Tian M, Gomperts BD. Ultrastructural characterization of tannic acid-arrested degranulation of permeabilized Guinea pig eosinophils stimulated with GTP-g-S. *Eur J Cell Biol*. 1996;70(3):209-220.

134. McLaren DJ, Mackenzie CD, Ramalho-Pinto FJ. Ultrastructural observations on the in vitro interaction between rat eosinophils and some parasitic helminths (Schistosoma mansoni, *Trichinella spiralis* and Nippostrongylus brasiliensis). *Clin Exp Immunol*. 1977;30(1):105-118.

135. Dvorak AM, Furitsu T, Letourneau L, Ishizaka T, Ackerman SJ. Mature eosinophils stimulated to develop in human cord blood mononuclear cell cultures supplemented with recombinant human interleukin-5. Part I. Piecemeal degranulation of specific granules and distribution of Charcot-Leyden crystal protein. *Am J Pathol*. 1991;138(1):69-82.

136. Erjefält JS, Andersson M, Greiff L, et al. Cytolysis and piecemeal degranulation as distinct modes of activation of airway mucosal eosinophils. *J Allergy Clin Immunol*. 1998;102(2):286-294.

137. Lacy P, Mahmudi-Azer S, Bablitz B, et al. Rapid mobilization of intracellularly stored RANTES in response to interferon-g in human eosinophils. *Blood*. 1999;94:23-32.

138. Melo RC, Spencer LA, Perez SA, Ghiran I, Dvorak AM, Weller PF. Human eosinophils secrete preformed, granule-stored interleukin-4 through distinct vesicular compartments. *Traffic*. 2005;6(11):1047-1057.

139. Lacy P, Stow JL. Cytokine release from innate immune cells: association with diverse membrane trafficking pathways. *Blood*. 2011;118(1):9-18.

140. Melo RC, Spencer LA, Perez SA, et al. Vesicle-mediated secretion of human eosinophil granule-derived major basic protein. *Lab Invest*. 2009;89(7):769-781.

141. Spencer LA, Melo RC, Perez SA, Bafford SP, Dvorak AM, Weller PF. Cytokine receptor-mediated trafficking of preformed IL-4 in eosinophils identifies an innate immune mechanism of cytokine secretion. *Proc Natl Acad Sci U S A*. 2006;103(9):3333-3338.

142. Persson CG, Erjefalt JS. Eosinophil lysis and free granules: an in vivo paradigm for cell activation and drug development. *Trends Pharmacol Sci*. 1997;18(4):117-123.

143. Fukuda T, Ackerman SJ, Reed CE, Peters MS, Dunnette SL, Gleich GJ. Calcium ionophore A23187 calcium-dependent cytolytic degranulation in human eosinophils. *J Immunol*. 1985;135(2):1349-1356.

144. McLaren DJ, Ramalho-Pinto FJ, Smithers SR. Ultrastructural evidence for complement and antibody-dependent damage to schistosomula of *Schistosoma mansoni* by rat eosinophils in vitro. *Parasitology*. 1978;77(3):313-324.

145. Abu-Ghazaleh RI, Fujisawa T, Mestecky J, Kyle RA, Gleich GJ. IgA-induced eosinophil degranulation. *J Immunol*. 1989;142(7):2393-2400.

146. Kita H, Abu-Ghazaleh RI, Gleich GJ, Abraham RT. Regulation of Ig-induced eosinophil degranulation by adenosine 3',5'- cyclic monophosphate. *J Immunol*. 1991;146(8):2712-2718.

147. Kaneko M, Swanson MC, Gleich GJ, Kita H. Allergen-specific IgG1 and IgG3 through Fc gamma RII induce eosinophil degranulation. *J Clin Investig*. 1995;95(6):2813-2821.

148. Monteiro RC, Hostoffer RW, Cooper MD, Bonner JR, Gartland GL, Kubagawa H. Definition of immunoglobulin A receptors on eosinophils and their enhanced expression in allergic individuals. *J Clin Invest*. 1993;92(4):1681-1685.

149. Seminario MC, Saini SS, MacGlashan DW, Jr, Bochner BS. Intracellular expression and release of FceRIa alpha by human eosinophils. *J Immunol*. 1999;162(11):6893-6900.

150. Rot A, Krieger M, Brunner T, Bischoff SC, Schall TJ, Dahinden CA. RANTES and macrophage inflammatory protein 1 a induce the migration and activation of normal human eosinophil granulocytes. *J Exp Med*. 1992;176(6):1489-1495.

151. Kita H, Weiler DA, Abu-Ghazaleh R, Sanderson CJ, Gleich GJ. Release of granule proteins from eosinophils cultured with IL-5. *J Immunol*. 1992;149(2):629-635.

152. Daffern PJ, Pfeifer PH, Ember JA, Hugli TE. C3a is a chemotaxin for human eosinophils but not for neutrophils. I. C3a stimulation of neutrophils is secondary to eosinophil activation. *J Exp Med*. 1995;181(6):2119-2127.

153. Kernen P, Wymann MP, von T V, et al. Shape changes, exocytosis, and cytosolic free calcium changes in stimulated human eosinophils. *J Clin Invest*. 1991;87(6):2012-2017.

154. Dyer KD, Percopo CM, Xie Z, et al. Mouse and human eosinophils degranulate in response to platelet-activating factor (PAF) and lysoPAF via a PAF-receptor-independent mechanism: evidence for a novel receptor. *J Immunol*. 2010;184(11):6327-6334.

155. Kato M, Kimura H, Motegi Y, et al. Platelet-activating factor activates two distinct effector pathways in human eosinophils. *J Immunol*. 2002;169(9):5252-5259.

156. Egesten A, Gullberg U, Olsson I, Richter J. Phorbol ester-induced degranulation in adherent human eosinophil granulocytes is dependent on CD11/CD18 leukocyte integrins. *J Leukoc Biol*. 1993;53(3):287-293.

157. Rock KL, Kono H. The inflammatory response to cell death. *Annu Rev Pathol*. 2008;3:99-126.

158. Lotfi R, Herzog GI, DeMarco RA, et al. Eosinophils oxidize damage-associated molecular pattern molecules derived from stressed cells. *J Immunol*. 2009;183(8):5023-5031.

159. Kobayashi T, Kouzaki H, Kita H. Human eosinophils recognize endogenous danger signal crystalline uric acid and produce proinflammatory cytokines mediated by autocrine ATP. *J Immunol*. 2010;184(11):6350-6358.

160. Lee JJ, Jacobsen EA, McGarry MP, Schleimer RP, Lee NA. Eosinophils in health and disease: the LIAR hypothesis. *Clin Exp Allergy*. 2010;40(4):563-575.

161. Hirai H, Tanaka K, Yoshie O, et al. Prostaglandin D2 selectively induces chemotaxis in T helper type 2 cells, eosinophils, and basophils via seven-transmembrane receptor CRTH2. *J Exp Med*. 2001;193(2):255-261.

162. Sabroe I, Jones EC, Usher LR, Whyte MK, Dower SK. Toll-like receptor (TLR)2 and TLR4 in human peripheral blood granulocytes: a critical role for monocytes in leukocyte lipopolysaccharide responses. *J Immunol*. 2002;168(9):4701-4710.

163. Nagase H, Okugawa S, Ota Y, et al. Expression and function of Toll-like receptors in eosinophils: activation by Toll-like receptor 7 ligand. *J Immunol*. 2003;171(8):3977-3982.

164. Miike S, McWilliam AS, Kita H. Trypsin induces activation and inflammatory mediator release from human eosinophils through protease-activated receptor-2. *J Immunol*. 2001;167(11):6615-6622.

165. Vliagoftis H, Lacy P, Luy B, et al. Mast cell tryptase activates peripheral blood eosinophils to release granule-associated enzymes. *Int Arch Allergy Immunol*. 2004;135(3):196-204.

166. Miike S, Kita H. Human eosinophils are activated by cysteine proteases and release inflammatory mediators. *J Allergy Clin Immunol*. 2003;111(4):704-713.

167. Wada K, Matsuwaki Y, Yoon J, et al. Inflammatory responses of human eosinophils to cockroach are mediated through protease-dependent pathways. *J Allergy Clin Immunol*. 2010;126(1):169-172.

168. Matsuwaki Y, Wada K, White TA, et al. Recognition of fungal protease activities induces cellular activation and eosinophil-derived neurotoxin release in human eosinophils. *J Immunol*. 2009;183(10):6708-6716.

169. Kaneko M, Horie S, Kato M, Gleich GJ, Kita H. A crucial role for b2 integrin in the activation of eosinophils stimulated by IgG. *J Immunol*. 1995;155(5):2631-2641.

170. Yoon J, Ponikau JU, Lawrence CB, Kita H. Innate antifungal immunity of human eosinophils mediated by a b2 integrin, CD11b. *J Immunol*. 2008;181(4):2907-2915.

171. Söllner T, Whiteheart SW, Brunner M, et al. SNAP receptors implicated in vesicle targeting and fusion. *Nature*. 1993;362(6418):318-324.

172. Brumell JH, Volchuk A, Sengelov H, et al. Subcellular distribution of docking/fusion proteins in neutrophils, secretory cells with multiple exocytic compartments. *J Immunol*. 1995;155(12):5750-5759.

173. Ravichandran V, Chawla A, Roche PA. Identification of a novel syntaxin- and synaptobrevin/VAMP- binding protein, SNAP-23, expressed in non-neuronal tissues. *J Biol Chem*. 1996;271(23):13300-13303.

174. Lacy P, Logan MR, Bablitz B, Moqbel R. Fusion protein vesicle-associated membrane protein 2 is implicated in IFN-g-induced piecemeal degranulation in human eosinophils from atopic individuals. *J Allergy Clin Immunol*. 2001;107(4):671-678.

175. Logan MR, Lacy P, Odemuyiwa SO, et al. A critical role for vesicle-associated membrane protein-7 in exocytosis from human eosinophils and neutrophils. *Allergy*. 2006;61(6):777-784.

176. Logan MR, Lacy P, Bablitz B, Moqbel R. Expression of eosinophil target SNAREs as potential cognate receptors for vesicle-associated membrane protein-2 in exocytosis. *J Allergy Clin Immunol*. 2002;109(2):299-306.

177. Kim JD, Willetts L, Ochkur SI, et al. An essential role for Rab27a GTPase in eosinophil exocytosis. *J Leukoc Biol*. 2013;94(6):1265-1274.

178. Odemuyiwa SO, Ilarraza R, Davoine F, et al. Cyclin-dependent kinase 5 regulates degranulation in human eosinophils. *Immunology*. 2015;144(4):641-648.

179. Erjefalt JS, Persson CG. New aspects of degranulation and fates of airway mucosal eosinophils. *Am J Respir Crit Care Med*. 2000;161(6):2074-2085.

180. Saffari H, Hoffman LH, Peterson KA, et al. Electron microscopy elucidates eosinophil degranulation patterns in patients with eosinophilic esophagitis. *J Allergy Clin Immunol*. 2014;133(6):1728-1734 e1.

181. Erjefalt JS, Greiff L, Andersson M, et al. Allergen-induced eosinophil cytolysis is a primary mechanism for granule protein release in human upper airways. *Am J Respir Crit Care Med*. 1999;160(1):304-312.

182. Radonjic-Hoesli S, Wang X, de Graauw E, et al. Adhesion-induced eosinophil cytolysis requires the receptor-interacting protein kinase 3 (RIPK3)-mixed lineage kinase-like (MLKL) signaling pathway, which is counterregulated by autophagy. *J Allergy Clin Immunol*. 2017;140(6):1632-1642.

183. Kita H, Abu-Ghazaleh R, Sanderson CJ, Gleich GJ. Effect of steroids on immunoglobulin-induced eosinophil degranulation. *J Allergy Clin Immunol*. 1991;87(1 pt 1):70-77.

184. Weiler CR, Kita H, Hukee M, Gleich GJ. Eosinophil viability during immunoglobulin-induced degranulation. *J Leukoc Biol.* 1996;60(4):493-501.

185. Coden ME, Loffredo LF, Walker MT, et al. Fibrinogen is a specific trigger for cytolytic eosinophil degranulation. *J Immunol.* 2020;204(2):438-448.

186. Ueki S, Melo RC, Ghiran I, Spencer LA, Dvorak AM, Weller PF. Eosinophil extracellular DNA trap cell death mediates lytic release of free secretion-competent eosinophil granules in humans. *Blood.* 2013;121(11):2074-2083.

187. Mukherjee M, Lacy P, Ueki S. Eosinophil extracellular traps and inflammatory pathologies-untangling the web!. *Front Immunol.* 2018;9(2763):2763.

188. Muniz VS, Silva JC, Braga YAV, et al. Eosinophils release extracellular DNA traps in response to Aspergillus fumigatus. *J Allergy Clin Immunol.* 2018;141(2):571-585. e7.

189. Muñoz-Caro T, Rubio RMC, Silva LMR, et al. Leucocyte-derived extracellular trap formation significantly contributes to *Haemonchus contortus* larval entrapment. *Parasites Vectors.* 2015;8:607.

190. Anisuzzaman, Anas A, Yasin MG, et al. Natural nodular worm infection in goats induces eosinophil extracellular DNA trap (EET) formation. *Parasitol Int.* 2020;79:102178.

191. Persson C, Ueki S. Lytic eosinophils produce extracellular DNA traps as well as free eosinophil granules. *J Allergy Clin Immunol.* 2018;141(3):1164.

192. Ueki S, Tokunaga T, Melo RCN, et al. Charcot-Leyden crystal formation is closely associated with eosinophil extracellular trap cell death. *Blood.* 2018;132(20):2183-2187.

193. Blom M, Tool AT, Wever PC, et al. Human eosinophils express, relative to other circulating leukocytes, large amounts of secretory 14-kD phospholipase A2. *Blood.* 1998;91(8):3037-3043.

194. Weller PF, Lee CW, Foster DW, Corey EJ, Austen KF, Lewis RA. Generation and metabolism of 5-lipoxygenase pathway leukotrienes by human eosinophils: predominant production of leukotriene C4. *Proc Natl Acad Sci U S A.* 1983;80(24):7626-7630.

195. Shaw RJ, Cromwell O, Kay AB. Preferential generation of leukotriene C4 by human eosinophils. *Clin Exp Immunol.* 1984;56(3):716-722.

196. Shaw RJ, Walsh GM, Cromwell O, Moqbel R, Spry CJ, Kay AB. Activated human eosinophils generate SRS-A leukotrienes following IgG- dependent stimulation. *Nature.* 1985;316(6024):150-152.

197. Cowburn AS, Holgate ST, Sampson AP. IL-5 increases expression of 5-lipoxygenase-activating protein and translocates 5-lipoxygenase to the nucleus in human blood eosinophils. *J Immunol.* 1999;163(1):456-465.

198. Cowburn AS, Sladek K, Soja J, et al. Overexpression of leukotriene C4 synthase in bronchial biopsies from patients with aspirin-intolerant asthma. *J Clin Invest.* 1998;101(4):834-846.

199. Lam BK, Owen WF, Jr, Austen KF, Soberman RJ. The identification of a distinct export step following the biosynthesis of leukotriene C4 by human eosinophils. *J Biol Chem.* 1989;264(22):12885-12889.

200. Nasser SM, Lee TH. Products of 15-lipoxygenase: are they important in asthma? *Clin Exp Allergy.* 2002;32(11):1540-1542.

201. Holtzman MJ, Pentland A, Baenziger NL, Hansbrough JR. Heterogeneity of cellular expression of arachidonate 15-lipoxygenase: implications for biological activity. *Biochim Biophys Acta.* 1989;1003(2):204-208.

202. Bradding P, Redington AE, Djukanovic R, Conrad DJ, Holgate ST. 15-lipoxygenase immunoreactivity in normal and in asthmatic airways. *Am J Respir Crit Care Med.* 1995;151(4):1201-1204.

203. Chu HW, Balzar S, Westcott JY, et al. Expression and activation of 15-lipoxygenase pathway in severe asthma: relationship to eosinophilic phenotype and collagen deposition. *Clin Exp Allergy.* 2002;32(11):1558-1565.

204. Henderson WR, Harley JB, Fauci AS. Arachidonic acid metabolism in normal and hypereosinophilic syndrome human eosinophils: generation of leukotrienes B$_4$, C$_4$, D$_4$ and 15-lipoxygenase products. *Immunology.* 1984;51(4):679-686.

205. Lee T, Lenihan DJ, Malone B, Roddy LL, Wasserman SI. Increased biosynthesis of platelet-activating factor in activated human eosinophils. *J Biol Chem.* 1984;259(9):5526-5530.

206. Cromwell O, Wardlaw AJ, Champion A, Moqbel R, Osei D, Kay AB. IgG-dependent generation of platelet-activating factor by normal and low density human eosinophils. *J Immunol.* 1990;145(11):3862-3868.

207. Burke LA, Crea AE, Wilkinson JR, Arm JP, Spur BW, Lee TH. Comparison of the generation of platelet-activating factor and leukotriene C4 in human eosinophils stimulated by unopsonized zymosan and the calcium ionophore A23187: the effects of nedocromil sodium. *J Allergy Clin Immunol.* 1990;85(1 pt 1):26-35.

208. Sun FF, Czuk CI, Taylor BM. Arachidonic acid metabolism in Guinea pig eosinophils: synthesis of thromboxane B2 and leukotriene B4 in response to soluble or particulate activators. *J Leukoc Biol.* 1989;46(2):152-160.

209. Giembycz MA, Kroegel C, Barnes PJ. Platelet activating factor stimulates cyclo-oxygenase activity in Guinea pig eosinophils. Concerted biosynthesis of thromboxane A2 and E- series prostaglandins. *J Immunol.* 1990;144(9):3489-3497.

210. Dvorak AM, Morgan E, Schleimer RP, Ryeom SW, Lichtenstein LM, Weller PF. Ultrastructural immunogold localization of prostaglandin endoperoxide synthase (cyclooxygenase) to non-membrane-bound cytoplasmic lipid bodies in human lung mast cells, alveolar macrophages, type II pneumocytes, and neutrophils. *J Histochem Cytochem.* 1992;40(6):759-769.

211. Bozza PT, Yu W, Cassara J, Weller PF. Pathways for eosinophil lipid body induction: differing signal transduction in cells from normal and hypereosinophilic subjects. *J Leukoc Biol.* 1998;64(4):563-569.

212. DeLeo FR, Quinn MT. Assembly of the phagocyte NADPH oxidase: molecular interaction of oxidase proteins. *J Leukoc Biol.* 1996;60(6):677-691.

213. Bolscher BG, Koenderman L, Tool AT, Stokman PM, Roos D. NADPH:O$_2$ oxidoreductase of human eosinophils in the cell-free system. *FEBS Lett.* 1990;268(1):269-273.

214. Someya A, Nagaoka I, Iwabuchi K, Yamashita T. Comparison of O$_2^-$-producing activity of Guinea-pig eosinophils and neutrophils in a cell-free system. *Comp Biochem Physiol B.* 1991;100(1):25-30.

215. Yagisawa M, Yuo A, Yonemaru M, et al. Superoxide release and NADPH oxidase components in mature human phagocytes: correlation between functional capacity and amount of functional proteins. *Biochem Biophys Res Commun.* 1996;228(2):510-516.

216. Lacy P, Abdel Latif D, Steward M, Musat-Marcu S, Man SF, Moqbel R. Divergence of mechanisms regulating respiratory burst in blood and sputum eosinophils and neutrophils from atopic subjects. *J Immunol.* 2003;170(5):2670-2679.

217. Carlyon JA, Abdel-Latif D, Pypaert M, Lacy P, Fikrig E. Anaplasma phagocytophilum utilizes multiple host evasion mechanisms to thwart NADPH oxidase-mediated killing during neutrophil infection. *Infect Immun.* 2004;72(8):4772-4783.

218. Abo A, Boyhan A, West I, Thrasher AJ, Segal AW. Reconstitution of neutrophil NADPH oxidase activity in the cell- free system by four components: p67-*phox*, p47-*phox*, p21^{rac1}, and cytochrome *b*-245. *J Biol Chem.* 1992;267(24):16767-16770.

219. Groemping Y, Rittinger K. Activation and assembly of the NADPH oxidase: a structural perspective. *Biochem J.* 2005;386(pt 3):401-416.

220. Suh CI, Stull ND, Li XJ, et al. The phosphoinositide-binding protein p40*phox* activates the NADPH oxidase during FcgIIA receptor-induced phagocytosis. *J Exp Med.* 2006;203(8):1915-1925.

221. Lapouge K, Smith SJ, Groemping Y, Rittinger K. Architecture of the p40-p47-p67*phox* complex in the resting state of the NADPH oxidase. A central role for p67*phox*. *J Biol Chem.* 2002;277(12):10121-10128.

222. Massenet C, Chenavas S, Cohen-Addad C, et al. Effects of p47*phox* C terminus phosphorylations on binding interactions with p40*phox* and p67*phox*. Structural and functional comparison of p40*phox* and p67*phox* SH3 domains. *J Biol Chem.* 2005;280(14):13752-13761.

223. Nisimoto Y, Motalebi S, Han CH, Lambeth JD. The p67*phox* activation domain regulates electron flow from NADPH to flavin in flavocytochrome b$_{558}$. *J Biol Chem.* 1999;274(33):22999-23005.

224. Koga H, Terasawa H, Nunoi H, Takeshige K, Inagaki F, Sumimoto H. Tetratricopeptide repeat (TPR) motifs of p67*phox* participate in interaction with the small GTPase Rac and activation of the phagocyte NADPH oxidase. *J Biol Chem.* 1999;274(35):25051-25060.

225. Didsbury J, Weber RF, Bokoch GM, Evans T, Snyderman R. rac, a novel ras-related family of proteins that are botulinum toxin substrates. *J Biol Chem.* 1989;264(28):16378-16382.

226. Lacy P, Mahmudi-Azer S, Bablitz B, et al. Expression and translocation of Rac2 in eosinophils during superoxide generation. *Immunology.* 1999;98(2):244-252.

227. Lacy P, Willetts L, Kim JD, et al. Agonist activation of F-actin-mediated eosinophil shape change and mediator release is dependent on Rac2. *Int Arch Allergy Immunol.* 2011;156(2):137-147.

228. Petreccia DC, Nauseef WM, Clark RA. Respiratory burst of normal human eosinophils. *J Leukoc Biol.* 1987;41(4):283-288.

229. Rabe KF, Giembycz MA, Dent G, Barnes PJ. Activation of Guinea pig eosinophil respiratory burst by leukotriene B$_4$: role of protein kinase C. *Fundam Clin Pharmacol.* 1992;6(8-9):353-358.

230. van der Bruggen T, Kok PT, Blom M, et al. Transient exposure of human eosinophils to the protein kinase C inhibitors CGP39-360, CGP41-251, and CGP44-800 leads to priming of the respiratory burst induced by opsonized particles. *J Leukoc Biol.* 1993;54(6):552-557.

231. Woerly G, Roger N, Loiseau S, Dombrowicz D, Capron A, Capron M. Expression of CD28 and CD86 by human eosinophils and role in the secretion of type 1 cytokines (interleukin 2 and interferon g): inhibition by immunoglobulin A complexes. *J Exp Med.* 1999;190(4):487-495.

232. Sabin EA, Kopf MA, Pearce EJ. *Schistosoma mansoni* egg-induced early IL-4 production is dependent upon IL-5 and eosinophils. *J Exp Med.* 1996;184(5):1871-1878.

233. Piehler D, Stenzel W, Grahnert A, et al. Eosinophils contribute to IL-4 production and shape the T-helper cytokine profile and inflammatory response in pulmonary cryptococcosis. *Am J Pathol.* 2011;179(2):733-744.

234. Chu VT, Frohlich A, Steinhauser G, et al. Eosinophils are required for the maintenance of plasma cells in the bone marrow. *Nat Immunol.* 2011;12(2):151-159.

235. Woerly G, Lacy P, Younes AB, et al. Human eosinophils express and release IL-13 following CD28-dependent activation. *J Leukoc Biol.* 2002;72(4):769-779.

236. Voehringer D, Reese TA, Huang X, Shinkai K, Locksley RM. Type 2 immunity is controlled by IL-4/IL-13 expression in hematopoietic non-eosinophil cells of the innate immune system. *J Exp Med.* 2006;203(6):1435-1446.

237. Herz U, Lacy P, Renz H, Erb K. The influence of infections on the development and severity of allergic disorders. *Curr Opin Immunol.* 2000;12(6):632-640.

238. Dixon H, Blanchard C, Deschoolmeester ML, et al. The role of Th2 cytokines, chemokines and parasite products in eosinophil recruitment to the gastrointestinal mucosa during helminth infection. *Eur J Immunol.* 2006;36(7):1753-1763.

239. Provost V, Larose M-C, Langlois A, Rola-Pleszczynski M, Flamand N, Laviolette M. CCL26/eotaxin-3 is more effective to induce the migration of eosinophils of asthmatics than CCL11/eotaxin-1 and CCL24/eotaxin-2. *J Leukoc Biol.* 2013;94(2):213-222.

240. Spencer LA, Weller PF. Eosinophils and Th2 immunity: contemporary insights. *Immunol Cell Biol.* 2010;88(3):250-256.

241. Lucey DR, Nicholson-Weller A, Weller PF. Mature human eosinophils have the capacity to express HLA-DR. *Proc Natl Acad Sci U S A.* 1989;86(4):1348-1351.

242. Yamamoto H, Sedgwick JB, Vrtis RF, Busse WW. The effect of transendothelial migration on eosinophil function. *Am J Respir Cell Mol Biol.* 2000;23(3):379-388.

243. Radke AL, Reynolds LE, Melo RC, Dvorak AM, Weller PF, Spencer LA. Mature human eosinophils express functional Notch ligands mediating eosinophil autocrine regulation. *Blood.* 2009;113(13):3092-3101.

244. Wills-Karp M, Luyimbazi J, Xu X, et al. Interleukin-13: central mediator of allergic asthma. *Science.* 1998;282(5397):2258-2261.

245. Padigel UM, Lee JJ, Nolan TJ, Schad GA, Abraham D. Eosinophils can function as antigen-presenting cells to induce primary and secondary immune responses to *Strongyloides stercoralis. Infect Immun.* 2006;74(6):3232-3238.

246. MacKenzie JR, Mattes J, Dent LA, Foster PS. Eosinophils promote allergic disease of the lung by regulating CD4+ Th2 lymphocyte function. *J Immunol.* 2001;167(6):3146-3155.

247. Shi HZ, Xiao CQ, Li CQ, et al. Endobronchial eosinophils preferentially stimulate T helper cell type 2 responses. *Allergy.* 2004;59(4):428-435.

248. Sabin EA, Pearce EJ. Early IL-4 production by non-CD4+ cells at the site of antigen deposition predicts the development of a T helper 2 cell response to *Schistosoma mansoni* eggs. *J Immunol.* 1995;155(10):4844-4853.

249. Shinkai K, Mohrs M, Locksley RM. Helper T cells regulate type-2 innate immunity *in vivo. Nature.* 2002;420(6917):825-829.

250. Voehringer D, Shinkai K, Locksley RM. Type 2 immunity reflects orchestrated recruitment of cells committed to IL-4 production. *Immunity.* 2004;20(3):267-277.

251. Jacobsen EA, Ochkur SI, Pero RS, et al. Allergic pulmonary inflammation in mice is dependent on eosinophil-induced recruitment of effector T cells. *J Exp Med.* 2008;205(3):699-710.

252. Yang D, Rosenberg HF, Chen Q, Dyer KD, Kurosaka K, Oppenheim JJ. Eosinophil-derived neurotoxin (EDN), an antimicrobial protein with chemotactic activities for dendritic cells. *Blood.* 2003;102(9):3396-3403.

253. Yang D, Chen Q, Rosenberg HF, et al. Human ribonuclease A superfamily members, eosinophil-derived neurotoxin and pancreatic ribonuclease, induce dendritic cell maturation and activation. *J Immunol.* 2004;173(10):6134-6142.

254. Yang D, Chen Q, Su SB, et al. Eosinophil-derived neurotoxin acts as an alarmin to activate the TLR2-MyD88 signal pathway in dendritic cells and enhances Th2 immune responses. *J Exp Med.* 2008;205(1):79-90.

255. Throsby M, Herbelin A, Pleau JM, Dardenne M. CD11c+ eosinophils in the murine thymus: developmental regulation and recruitment upon MHC class I-restricted thymocyte deletion. *J Immunol.* 2000;165(4):1965-1975.

256. Tulic MK, Sly PD, Andrews D, et al. Thymic indoleamine 2,3-dioxygenase-positive eosinophils in young children: potential role in maturation of the naive immune system. *Am J Pathol.* 2009;175(5):2043-2052.

257. Tulic MK, Andrews D, Crook ML, et al. Changes in thymic regulatory T-cell maturation from birth to puberty: differences in atopic children. *J Allergy Clin Immunol.* 2012;129(1):199-206.

258. Watanabe N, Wang YH, Lee HK, et al. Hassall's corpuscles instruct dendritic cells to induce CD4+CD25+ regulatory T cells in human thymus. *Nature.* 2005;436(7054):1181-1185.

259. Jessup HK, Brewer AW, Omori M, et al. Intradermal administration of thymic stromal lymphopoietin induces a T cell- and eosinophil-dependent systemic Th2 inflammatory response. *J Immunol.* 2008;181(6):4311-4319.

260. Chu Van T, Beller A, Rausch S, et al. Eosinophils promote generation and maintenance of immunoglobulin-A-expressing plasma cells and contribute to gut immune homeostasis. *Immunity.* 2014;40(4):582-593.

261. Abdala-Valencia H, Coden ME, Chiarella SE, et al. Shaping eosinophil identity in the tissue contexts of development, homeostasis, and disease. *J Leukoc Biol.* 2018;104(1):95-108.

262. Berdnikovs S. The twilight zone: plasticity and mixed ontogeny of neutrophil and eosinophil granulocyte subsets. *Semin Immunopathol.* 2021;43(3):337-346.

263. Mesnil C, Raulier S, Paulissen G, et al. Lung-resident eosinophils represent a distinct regulatory eosinophil subset. *J Clin Invest.* 2016;126(9):3279-3295.

264. Andreev D, Liu M, Kachler K, et al. Regulatory eosinophils induce the resolution of experimental arthritis and appear in remission state of human rheumatoid arthritis. *Ann Rheum Dis.* 2021;80(4):451-468.

265. Lingblom C, Andersson J, Andersson K, Wennerås C. Regulatory eosinophils suppress T cells partly through galectin-10. *J Immunol.* 2017;198(12):4672-4681.

266. Lingblom C, Andersson K, Wennerås C. Kinetic studies of galectin-10 release from eosinophils exposed to proliferating T cells. *Clin Exp Immunol.* 2021;203(2):230-243.

267. Lotfi R, Lee JJ, Lotze MT. Eosinophilic granulocytes and damage-associated molecular pattern molecules (DAMPs): role in the inflammatory response within tumors. *J Immunother.* 2007;30(1):16-28.

268. Carretero R, Sektioglu IM, Garbi N, Salgado OC, Beckhove P, Hämmerling GJ. Eosinophils orchestrate cancer rejection by normalizing tumor vessels and enhancing infiltration of CD8+ T cells. *Nat Immunol.* 2015;16(6):609-617.

269. Lucarini V, Ziccheddu G, Macchia I, et al. IL-33 restricts tumor growth and inhibits pulmonary metastasis in melanoma-bearing mice through eosinophils. *OncoImmunology.* 2017;6(6):e1317420.

270. Arnold IC, Artola-Boran M, Gurtner A, et al. The GM-CSF-IRF5 signaling axis in eosinophils promotes antitumor immunity through activation of type 1 T cell responses. *J Exp Med.* 2020;217(12):e20190706.

271. Moqbel R, Hamid Q, Ying S, et al. Expression of mRNA and immunoreactivity for the granulocyte/macrophage colony-stimulating factor in activated human eosinophils. *J Exp Med.* 1991;174(3):749-752.

272. Kita H, Ohnishi T, Okubo Y, Weiler D, Abrams JS, Gleich GJ. Granulocyte/macrophage colony-stimulating factor and interleukin 3 release from human peripheral blood eosinophils and neutrophils. *J Exp Med.* 1991;174(3):745-748.

273. Lacy P, Moqbel R. Eosinophil cytokines. *Chem Immunol.* 2000;76:134-155.

274. Wong DT, Weller PF, Galli SJ, et al. Human eosinophils express transforming growth factor a. *J Exp Med.* 1990;172(3):673-681.

275. Wong DT, Elovic A, Matossian K, et al. Eosinophils from patients with blood eosinophilia express transforming growth factor b1. *Blood.* 1991;78(10):2702-2707.

276. Desreumaux P, Janin A, Colombel JF, et al. Interleukin 5 messenger RNA expression by eosinophils in the intestinal mucosa of patients with coeliac disease. *J Exp Med.* 1992;175(1):293-296.

277. Broide DH, Paine MM, Firestein GS. Eosinophils express interleukin 5 and granulocyte macrophage-colony- stimulating factor mRNA at sites of allergic inflammation in asthmatics. *J Clin Invest.* 1992;90(4):1414-1424.

278. Beil WJ, Weller PF, Tzizik DM, Galli SJ, Dvorak AM. Ultrastructural immunogold localization of tumor necrosis factor- a to the matrix compartment of eosinophil secondary granules in patients with idiopathic hypereosinophilic syndrome. *J Histochem Cytochem.* 1993;41(11):1611-1615.

279. Dubucquoi S, Desreumaux P, Janin A, et al. Interleukin 5 synthesis by eosinophils: association with granules and immunoglobulin-dependent secretion. *J Exp Med.* 1994;179(2):703-708.

280. Levi-Schaffer F, Lacy P, Severs NJ, et al. Association of granulocyte-macrophage colony-stimulating factor with the crystalloid granules of human eosinophils. *Blood.* 1995;85(9):2579-2586.

281. Moqbel R, Ying S, Barkans J, et al. Identification of messenger RNA for IL-4 in human eosinophils with granule localization and release of the translated product. *J Immunol.* 1995;155(10):4939-4947.

282. Levi-Schaffer F, Barkans J, Newman TM, et al. Identification of interleukin-2 in human peripheral blood eosinophils. *Immunology.* 1996;87(1):155-161.

283. Lacy P, Levi-Schaffer F, Mahmudi-Azer S, et al. Intracellular localization of interleukin-6 in eosinophils from atopic asthmatics and effects of interferon g. *Blood.* 1998;91(7):2508-2516.

284. Gauvreau GM, O'Byrne PM, Moqbel R, et al. Enhanced expression of GM-CSF in differentiating eosinophils of atopic and atopic asthmatic subjects. *Am J Respir Cell Mol Biol.* 1998;19(1):55-62.

285. Velazquez JR, Lacy P, Mahmudi-Azer S, et al. Interleukin-4 and RANTES expression in maturing eosinophils derived from human cord blood CD34+ progenitors. *Immunology.* 2000;101(3):419-425.

286. Egesten A, Calafat J, Knol EF, Janssen H, Walz TM. Subcellular localization of transforming growth factor-a in human eosinophil granulocytes. *Blood.* 1996;87(9):3910-3918.

287. Bandeira-Melo C, Gillard G, Ghiran I, Weller PF. EliCell: a gel-phase dual antibody capture and detection assay to measure cytokine release from eosinophils. *J Immunol Methods.* 2000;244(1-2):105-115.

288. Wong CK, Cheung PF, Lam CW. Leptin-mediated cytokine release and migration of eosinophils: implications for immunopathophysiology of allergic inflammation. *Eur J Immunol.* 2007;37(8):2337-2348.

289. Qiu Y, Nguyen KD, Odegaard JI, et al. Eosinophils and type 2 cytokine signaling in macrophages orchestrate development of functional beige fat. *Cell.* 2014;157(6):1292-1308.

290. Wu D, Molofsky AB, Liang HE, et al. Eosinophils sustain adipose alternatively activated macrophages associated with glucose homeostasis. *Science.* 2011;332(6026):243-247.

291. Goh YP, Henderson NC, Heredia JE, et al. Eosinophils secrete IL-4 to facilitate liver regeneration. *Proc Natl Acad Sci U S A.* 2013;110(24):9914-9919.

292. DeBrosse CW, Rothenberg ME. Allergy and eosinophil-associated gastrointestinal disorders (EGID). *Curr Opin Immunol.* 2008;20(6):703-708.

293. Kim CK, Callaway Z, Kim DW, Kita H. Eosinophil degranulation is more important than eosinophilia in identifying asthma in chronic cough. *J Asthma.* 2011;48(10):994-1000.

294. Grainge CL, Lau LC, Ward JA, et al. Effect of bronchoconstriction on airway remodeling in asthma. *N Engl J Med.* 2011;364(21):2006-2015.

295. Rothenberg ME, Mishra A, Brandt EB, Hogan SP. Gastrointestinal eosinophils. *Immunol Rev.* 2001;179:139-155.

296. Cheng JF, Ott NL, Peterson EA, et al. Dermal eosinophils in atopic dermatitis undergo cytolytic degeneration. *J Allergy Clin Immunol.* 1997;99(5):683-692.

297. Simon D, Braathen LR, Simon HU. Eosinophils and atopic dermatitis. *Allergy.* 2004;59(6):561-570.

298. Horn BR, Robin ED, Theodore J, Van Kessel A. Total eosinophil counts in the management of bronchial asthma. *N Engl J Med.* 1975;292(22):1152-1155.

299. Montefort S, Gratziou C, Goulding D, et al. Bronchial biopsy evidence for leukocyte infiltration and upregulation of leukocyte-endothelial cell adhesion molecules 6 hours after local allergen challenge of sensitized asthmatic airways. *J Clin Invest.* 1994;93(4):1411-1421.

300. Lommatzsch M, Julius P, Kuepper M, et al. The course of allergen-induced leukocyte infiltration in human and experimental asthma. *J Allergy Clin Immunol.* 2006;118(1):91-97.

301. Fabbri LM, Boschetto P, Zocca E, et al. Bronchoalveolar neutrophilia during late asthmatic reactions induced by toluene diisocyanate. *Am Rev Respir Dis.* 1987;136(1):36-42.

302. Bentley AM, Menz G, Storz C, et al. Identification of T lymphocytes, macrophages, and activated eosinophils in the bronchial mucosa in intrinsic asthma. Relationship to symptoms and bronchial responsiveness. *Am Rev Respir Dis.* 1992;146(2):500-506.

303. Wardlaw AJ. Eosinophils in the 1990s: new perspectives on their role in health and disease. *Postgrad Med J.* 1994;70(826):536-552.

304. de BJ, Tillie-Leblond I, Tonnel AB, Jaubert F, Scheinmann P, Gosset P. Difficult asthma in children: an analysis of airway inflammation. *J Allergy Clin Immunol.* 2004;113(1):94-100.

305. Kim CK, Kim SW, Kim YK, et al. Bronchoalveolar lavage eosinophil cationic protein and interleukin-8 levels in acute asthma and acute bronchiolitis. *Clin Exp Allergy.* 2005;35(5):591-597.

306. Julius P, Luttmann W, Knoechel B, Kroegel C, Matthys H, Virchow JC, Jr. CD69 surface expression on human lung eosinophils after segmental allergen provocation. *Eur Respir J.* 1999;13(6):1253-1259.

307. Johansson MW, Kelly EA, Busse WW, Jarjour NN, Mosher DF. Up-regulation and activation of eosinophil integrins in blood and airway after segmental lung antigen challenge. *J Immunol.* 2008;180(11):7622-7635.

308. Hartnell A, Robinson DS, Kay AB, Wardlaw AJ. CD69 is expressed by human eosinophils activated *in vivo* in asthma and *in vitro* by cytokines. *Immunology.* 1993;80(2):281-286.

309. Gundel RH, Letts LG, Gleich GJ. Human eosinophil major basic protein induces airway constriction and airway hyperresponsiveness in primates. *J Clin Invest.* 1991;87(4):1470-1473.

310. Pizzichini E, Pizzichini MM, Efthimiadis A, et al. Indices of airway inflammation in induced sputum: reproducibility and validity of cell and fluid-phase measurements. *Am J Respir Crit Care Med.* 1996;154(2 pt 1):308-317.

311. Lex C, Ferreira F, Zacharasiewicz A, et al. Airway eosinophilia in children with severe asthma: predictive values of noninvasive tests. *Am J Respir Crit Care Med.* 2006;174(12):1286-1291.

312. Green RH, Brightling CE, McKenna S, et al. Asthma exacerbations and sputum eosinophil counts: a randomised controlled trial. *Lancet.* 2002;360(9347):1715-1721.

313. Jayaram L, Pizzichini MM, Cook RJ, et al. Determining asthma treatment by monitoring sputum cell counts: effect on exacerbations. *Eur Respir J.* 2006;27(3):483-494.

314. Petsky HL, Cates CJ, Lasserson TJ, et al. A systematic review and meta-analysis: tailoring asthma treatment on eosinophilic markers (exhaled nitric oxide or sputum eosinophils). *Thorax.* 2012;67(3):199-208.

315. Bacci E, Cianchetti S, Bartoli M, et al. Low sputum eosinophils predict the lack of response to beclomethasone in symptomatic asthmatic patients. *Chest.* 2006;129(3):565-572.

316. Hargreave FE, Nair P. Point: is measuring sputum eosinophils useful in the management of severe asthma? Yes *Chest.* 2011;139(6):1270-1273.

317. Dunican EM, Watchorn DC, Fahy JV. Autopsy and imaging studies of mucus in asthma. Lessons learned about disease mechanisms and the role of mucus in airflow obstruction. *Ann Am Thorac Soc.* 2018;15(suppl 3):S184-S191.

318. Bonser LR, Erle DJ. Airway mucus and asthma: the role of MUC5AC and MUC5B. *J Clin Med.* 2017;6(12):112.

319. Dunican EM, Elicker BM, Gierada DS, et al. Mucus plugs in patients with asthma linked to eosinophilia and airflow obstruction. *J Clin Investig.* 2018;128(3):997-1009.

320. Svenningsen S, Haider E, Boylan C, et al. CT and functional MRI to evaluate airway mucus in severe asthma. *Chest.* 2019;155(6):1178-1189.

321. Persson EK, Verstraete K, Heyndrickx I, et al. Protein crystallization promotes type 2 immunity and is reversible by antibody treatment. *Science.* 2019;364(6442):eaaw4295.

322. Zeiger RS, Colten HR. Histaminase release from human eosinophils. *J Immunol.* 1977;118(2):540-543.

323. Hogan SP, Koskinen A, Matthaei KI, Young IG, Foster PS. Interleukin-5-producing CD4⁺ T cells play a pivotal role in aeroallergen-induced eosinophilia, bronchial hyperreactivity, and lung damage in mice. *Am J Respir Crit Care Med.* 1998;157(1):210-218.

324. Hogan SP, Matthaei KI, Young JM, Koskinen A, Young IG, Foster PS. A novel T cell-regulated mechanism modulating allergen-induced airways hyperreactivity in BALB/c mice independently of IL-4 and IL-5. *J Immunol.* 1998;161(3):1501-1509.

325. Nagai H, Yamaguchi S, Inagaki N, Tsuruoka N, Hitoshi Y, Takatsu K. Effect of anti-IL-5 monoclonal antibody on allergic bronchial eosinophilia and airway hyperresponsiveness in mice. *Life Sci.* 1993;53(15):L243-L7.

326. Hogan SP, Mishra A, Brandt EB, et al. A pathological function for eotaxin and eosinophils in eosinophilic gastrointestinal inflammation. *Nat Immunol.* 2001;2(4):353-360.

327. Lee NA, McGarry MP, Larson KA, Horton MA, Kristensen AB, Lee JJ. Expression of IL-5 in thymocytes/T cells leads to the development of a massive eosinophilia, extramedullary eosinophilopoiesis, and unique histopathologies. *J Immunol.* 1997;158(3):1332-1344.

328. Lee JJ, McGarry MP, Farmer SC, et al. Interleukin-5 expression in the lung epithelium of transgenic mice leads to pulmonary changes pathognomonic of asthma. *J Exp Med.* 1997;185(12):2143-2156.

329. Lee JJ, Dimina D, Macias MP, et al. Defining a link with asthma in mice congenitally deficient in eosinophils. *Science.* 2004;305(5691):1773-1776.

330. Walsh ER, Sahu N, Kearley J, et al. Strain-specific requirement for eosinophils in the recruitment of T cells to the lung during the development of allergic asthma. *J Exp Med.* 2008;205(6):1285-1292.

331. Humbles AA, Lloyd CM, McMillan SJ, et al. A critical role for eosinophils in allergic airways remodeling. *Science.* 2004;305(5691):1776-1779.

332. Kita H. Eosinophils: multifaceted biological properties and roles in health and disease. *Immunol Rev.* 2011;242(1):161-177.

333. Bousquet J, Chanez P, Lacoste JY, et al. Eosinophilic inflammation in asthma. *N Engl J Med.* 1990;323(15):1033-1039.

334. Leuppi JD, Salome CM, Jenkins CR, et al. Predictive markers of asthma exacerbation during stepwise dose reduction of inhaled corticosteroids. *Am J Respir Crit Care Med.* 2001;163(2):406-412.

335. van Veen IH, Ten Brinke A, Gauw SA, Sterk PJ, Rabe KF, Bel EH. Consistency of sputum eosinophilia in difficult-to-treat asthma: a 5-year follow-up study. *J Allergy Clin Immunol.* 2009;124(3):615-617. 7 e1-2.

336. Lemiere C, Ernst P, Olivenstein R, et al. Airway inflammation assessed by invasive and noninvasive means in severe asthma: eosinophilic and noneosinophilic phenotypes. *J Allergy Clin Immunol.* 2006;118(5):1033-1039.

337. Wills-Karp M, Karp CL. Biomedicine. Eosinophils in asthma: remodeling a tangled tale. *Science.* 2004;305(5691):1726-1729.

338. Leckie MJ, ten Brinke A, Khan J, et al. Effects of an interleukin-5 blocking monoclonal antibody on eosinophils, airway hyper-responsiveness, and the late asthmatic response. *Lancet.* 2000;356(9248):2144-2148.

339. O'Byrne PM, Inman MD, Parameswaran K. The trials of interleukin-5, eosinophils and allergic asthma. *J Allergy Clin Immunol.* 2001;108(4):503-508.

340. Lacy P, Weller PF, Moqbel R. A report from the International Eosinophil Society: eosinophils in a tug of war. *J Allergy Clin Immunol.* 2001;108(6):895-900.

341. Flood-Page PT, Menzies-Gow AN, Kay AB, Robinson DS. Eosinophil's role remains uncertain as anti-interleukin-5 only partially depletes numbers in asthmatic airway. *Am J Respir Crit Care Med.* 2003;167(2):199-204.

342. Nair P, Hargreave FE. Measuring bronchitis in airway diseases: clinical implementation and application – airway hyperresponsiveness in asthma – its measurement and clinical significance. *Chest.* 2010;138(2 suppl):38S-43S.

343. D'Silva L, Hassan N, Wang HY, et al. Heterogeneity of bronchitis in airway diseases in tertiary care clinical practice. *Can Respir J J Can Thorac Soc.* 2011;18(3):144-148.

344. ten Brinke A, Zwinderman AH, Sterk PJ, Rabe KF, Bel EH. Factors associated with persistent airflow limitation in severe asthma. *Am J Respir Crit Care Med.* 2001;164(5):744-748.

345. Fleming L, Wilson N, Regamey N, Bush A. Use of sputum eosinophil counts to guide management in children with severe asthma. *Thorax.* 2012;67(3):193-198.

346. D'Silva L, Gafni A, Thabane L, et al. Cost analysis of monitoring asthma treatment using sputum cell counts. *Can Respir J J Can Thorac Soc.* 2008;15(7):370-374.

347. Chakir J, Loubaki L, Laviolette M, et al. Monitoring sputum eosinophils in mucosal inflammation and remodelling: a pilot study. *Eur Respir J.* 2010;35(1):48-53.

348. Haldar P, Brightling CE, Hargadon B, et al. Mepolizumab and exacerbations of refractory eosinophilic asthma. *N Engl J Med.* 2009;360(10):973-984.

349. Nair P, Pizzichini MM, Kjarsgaard M, et al. Mepolizumab for prednisone-dependent asthma with sputum eosinophilia. *N Engl J Med.* 2009;360(10):985-993.

350. Castro M, Mathur S, Hargreave F, et al. Reslizumab for poorly controlled, eosinophilic asthma: a randomized, placebo-controlled study. *Am J Respir Crit Care Med.* 2011;184(10):1125-1132.

351. Castro M, Zangrilli J, Wechsler ME, et al. Reslizumab for inadequately controlled asthma with elevated blood eosinophil counts: results from two multicentre, parallel, double-blind, randomised, placebo-controlled, phase 3 trials. *Lancet Respir Med.* 2015;3(5):355-366.

352. Pavord ID, Korn S, Howarth P, et al. Mepolizumab for severe eosinophilic asthma (DREAM): a multicentre, double-blind, placebo-controlled trial. *Lancet.* 2012;380(9842):651-659.

353. Ortega HG, Liu MC, Pavord ID, et al. Mepolizumab treatment in patients with severe eosinophilic asthma. *N Engl J Med.* 2014;371(13):1198-1207.

354. Ortega H, Chupp G, Bardin P, et al. The role of mepolizumab in atopic and nonatopic severe asthma with persistent eosinophilia. *Eur Respir J.* 2014;44(1):239-241.

355. Katz LE, Gleich GJ, Hartley BF, Yancey SW, Ortega HG. Blood eosinophil count is a useful biomarker to identify patients with severe eosinophilic asthma. *Ann Am Thorac Soc.* 2014;11(4):531-536.

356. Bel EH, Wenzel SE, Thompson PJ, et al. Oral glucocorticoid-sparing effect of mepolizumab in eosinophilic asthma. *N Engl J Med.* 2014;371(13):1189-1197.

357. Sehmi R, Smith SG, Kjarsgaard M, et al. Role of local eosinophilopoietic processes in the development of airway eosinophilia in prednisone-dependent severe asthma. *Clin Exp Allergy.* 2016;46(6):793-802.

358. Mukherjee M, Aleman Paramo F, Kjarsgaard M, et al. Weight-adjusted intravenous reslizumab in severe asthma with inadequate response to fixed-dose subcutaneous mepolizumab. *Am J Respir Crit Care Med.* 2018;197(1):38-46.

359. Mukherjee M, Bulir DC, Radford K, et al. Sputum autoantibodies in patients with severe eosinophilic asthma. *J Allergy Clin Immunol.* 2018;141(4):1269-1279.

360. Mukherjee M, Forero DF, Tran S, et al. Suboptimal treatment response to anti-IL-5 monoclonal antibodies in severe eosinophilic asthmatics with airway autoimmune phenomena. *Eur Respir J.* 2020;56(4):2000117. doi:10.1183/13993003.00117-2020

361. Machida K, Aw M, Salter BMA, et al. The role of the TL1A/DR3 Axis in the activation of group 2 innate lymphoid cells in subjects with eosinophilic asthma. *Am J Respir Crit Care Med.* 2020;202(8):1105-1114.

362. Kolbeck R, Kozhich A, Koike M, et al. MEDI-563, a humanized anti-IL-5 receptor alpha mAb with enhanced antibody-dependent cell-mediated cytotoxicity function. *J Allergy Clin Immunol.* 2010;125(6):1344-1353.e2.

363. Busse WW, Bleecker ER, FitzGerald JM, et al. Long-term safety and efficacy of benralizumab in patients with severe, uncontrolled asthma: 1-year results from the BORA phase 3 extension trial. *Lancet Respir Med.* 2019;7(1):46-59.

364. FitzGerald JM, Bleecker ER, Nair P, et al. Benralizumab, an anti-interleukin-5 receptor α monoclonal antibody, as add-on treatment for patients with severe, uncontrolled, eosinophilic asthma (CALIMA): a randomised, double-blind, placebo-controlled phase 3 trial. *Lancet.* 2016;388(10056):2128-2141.

365. Nair P, Wenzel S, Rabe KF, et al. Oral glucocorticoid-sparing effect of benralizumab in severe asthma. *N Engl J Med.* 2017;376(25):2448-2458.

366. Dagher R, Kumar V, Copenhaver AM, et al. Novel mechanisms of action contributing to Benralizumab's potent anti-eosinophilic activity. *Eur Respir J.* 2022;59(3):2004306.

367. Laviolette M, Gossage DL, Gauvreau G, et al. Effects of benralizumab on airway eosinophils in asthmatic patients with sputum eosinophilia. *J Allergy Clin Immunol.* 2013;132(5):1086-1096.e5.

368. Sehmi R, Lim HF, Mukherjee M, et al. Benralizumab attenuates airway eosinophilia in prednisone-dependent asthma. *J Allergy Clin Immunol.* 2018;141(4):1529-1532 e8.

369. Moran AM, Ramakrishnan S, Borg CA, et al. Blood eosinophil depletion with mepolizumab, benralizumab, and prednisolone in eosinophilic asthma. *Am J Respir Crit Care Med.* 2020;202(9):1314-1316.

370. Smith SG, Chen R, Kjarsgaard M, et al. Increased numbers of activated group 2 innate lymphoid cells in the airways of patients with severe asthma and persistent airway eosinophilia. *J Allergy Clin Immunol.* 2016;137(1):75-86 e8.

371. Nair P. Anti-interleukin-5 monoclonal antibody to treat severe eosinophilic asthma. *N Engl J Med.* 2014;371(13):1249-1251.

372. Panch SR, Bozik ME, Brown T, et al. Dexpramipexole as an oral steroid-sparing agent in hypereosinophilic syndromes. *Blood.* 2018;132(5):501-509.

373. Laidlaw TM, Prussin C, Panettieri RA, et al. Dexpramipexole depletes blood and tissue eosinophils in nasal polyps with no change in polyp size. *Laryngoscope.* 2019;129(2):E61-E66.

374. Hanania NA, Korenblat P, Chapman KR, et al. Efficacy and safety of lebrikizumab in patients with uncontrolled asthma (LAVOLTA I and LAVOLTA II): replicate, phase 3, randomised, double-blind, placebo-controlled trials. *Lancet Respir Med.* 2016;4(10):781-796.

375. Rabe KF, Nair P, Brusselle G, et al. Efficacy and safety of dupilumab in glucocorticoid-dependent severe asthma. *N Engl J Med.* 2018;378(26):2475-2485.

376. Diver S, Khalfaoui L, Emson C, et al. Effect of tezepelumab on airway inflammatory cells, remodelling, and hyperresponsiveness in patients with moderate-to-severe uncontrolled asthma (CASCADE): a double-blind, randomised, placebo-controlled, phase 2 trial. *Lancet Respir Med.* 2021;9(11):1299-1312.

377. Sverrild A, Hansen S, Hvidtfeldt M, et al. The effect of tezepelumab on airway hyperresponsiveness to mannitol in asthma (UPSTREAM). *Eur Respir J.* 2022;59(1):2101296.

378. Bochner BS, Gleich GJ. What targeting eosinophils has taught us about their role in diseases. *J Allergy Clin Immunol.* 2010;126(1):16-25. quiz 6-7.

379. Nair P, O'Byrne PM. Measuring eosinophils to make treatment decisions in asthma. *Chest.* 2016;150(3):485-487.

380. Ruchelli E, Wenner W, Voytek T, Brown K, Liacouras C. Severity of esophageal eosinophilia predicts response to conventional gastroesophageal reflux therapy. *Pediatr Dev Pathol.* 1999;2(1):15-18.

381. Riddell RH. The biopsy diagnosis of gastroesophageal reflux disease, "carditis," and Barrett's esophagus, and sequelae of therapy. *Am J Surg Pathol.* 1996;20(suppl 1):S31-S50.

382. Khan S, Orenstein SR, Di LC, et al. Eosinophilic esophagitis: strictures, impactions, dysphagia. *Dig Dis Sci.* 2003;48(1):22-29.

383. Schroeder S, Fleischer DM, Masterson JC, Gelfand E, Furuta GT, Atkins D. Successful treatment of eosinophilic esophagitis with ciclesonide. *J Allergy Clin Immunol.* 2012;129(5):1419-1421.

384. Lu TX, Sherrill JD, Wen T, et al. MicroRNA signature in patients with eosinophilic esophagitis, reversibility with glucocorticoids, and assessment as disease biomarkers. *J Allergy Clin Immunol.* 2012;129(4):1064-1075.

385. Stumphy J, Al-Zubeidi D, Guerin L, Mitros F, Rahhal R. Observations on use of montelukast in pediatric eosinophilic esophagitis: insights for the future. *Dis Esophagus.* 2011;24(4):229-234.

386. Helou EF, Simonson J, Arora AS. 3-yr-follow-up of topical corticosteroid treatment for eosinophilic esophagitis in adults. *Am J Gastroenterol.* 2008;103(9):2194-2199.

387. Mishra A, Hogan SP, Brandt EB, Rothenberg ME. An etiological role for aeroallergens and eosinophils in experimental esophagitis. *J Clin Invest.* 2001;107(1):83-90.

388. Dellon ES, Peterson KA, Murray JA, et al. Anti-Siglec-8 antibody for eosinophilic gastritis and duodenitis. *N Engl J Med.* 2020;383(17):1624-1634.

389. Diny NL, Rose NR, Čiháková D. Eosinophils in autoimmune diseases. *Front Immunol.* 2017;8:484.

390. Mukherjee M, Nair P. Eosinophils as potential mediators of autoimmunity. In: Jackson D, Wechsler M, eds. *Eosinophilic Lung Diseases.* European Respiratory Society; 2021.

391. Vaglio A, Buzio C, Zwerina J. Eosinophilic granulomatosis with polyangiitis (Churg–Strauss): state of the art. *Allergy.* 2013;68(3):261-273.

392. Hammers CM, Stanley JR. Mechanisms of disease: pemphigus and bullous pemphigoid. *Annu Rev Pathol.* 2016;11:175-197.

393. Simon D, Hoesli S, Roth N, Staedler S, Yousefi S, Simon H-U. Eosinophil extracellular DNA traps in skin diseases. *J Allergy Clin Immunol.* 2011;127(1):194-199.

394. Mukherjee M, Thomas SR, Radford K, et al. Sputum antineutrophil cytoplasmic antibodies in serum antineutrophil cytoplasmic antibody-negative eosinophilic granulomatosis with polyangiitis. *Am J Respir Crit Care Med.* 2019;199(2):158-170.

395. Fukuchi M, Kamide Y, Ueki S, et al. Eosinophil ETosis-mediated release of galectin-10 in eosinophilic granulomatosis with polyangiitis. *Arthritis Rheumatol.* 2021;73(9):1683-1693.

396. Luck W, Becker M, Niggemann B, Wahn U. In vitro release of eosinophil cationic protein from peripheral eosinophils reflects disease activity in childhood Crohn disease and ulcerative colitis. *Eur J Pediatr.* 1997;156(12):921-924.

397. Takiguchi J, Ohira H, Rai T, Abe K, Takahashi A, Sato Y. Anti-eosinophil peroxidase antibodies detected in patients with primary biliary cirrhosis. *Hepatol Res.* 2005;32(1):33-37.

398. Wardlaw AJ, Moqbel R. The eosinophil in allergic and helminth-related inflammatory responses. In: Moqbel R, ed. *Allergy and Immunity to Helminths Common Mechanisms or Divergent Pathways?* Taylor & Francis; 1992:154-186.

399. Kay AB, Moqbel R, Durham SR, et al. Leucocyte activation initiated by IgE-dependent mechanisms in relation to helminthic parasitic disease and clinical models of asthma. *Int Arch Allergy Appl Immunol.* 1985;77(1-2):69-72.

400. Butterworth AE. Cell-mediated damage to helminths. *Adv Parasitol.* 1984;23:143-235.

401. Hsu SY, Hsu HF, Penick GD, Hanson HO, Schiller HJ, Cheng HF. Immunoglobulin E, mast cells, and eosinophils in the skin of rhesus monkeys immunized with x-irradiated cercariae of *Schistosoma japonicum.* *Int Arch Allergy Appl Immunol.* 1979;59(4):383-393.

402. Kephart GM, Gleich GJ, Connor DH, Gibson DW, Ackerman SJ. Deposition of eosinophil granule major basic protein onto microfilariae of Onchocerca volvulus in the skin of patients treated with diethylcarbamazine. *Lab Invest.* 1984;50(1):51-61.

403. Spry CJ. Alterations in blood eosinophil morphology, binding capacity for complexed IgG and kinetics in patients with tropical (filarial) eosinophilia. *Parasite Immunol.* 1981;3(1):1-11.

404. Herbert DR, Lee JJ, Lee NA, Nolan TJ, Schad GA, Abraham D. Role of IL-5 in innate and adaptive immunity to larval *Strongyloides stercoralis* in mice. *J Immunol.* 2000;165(8):4544-4551.

405. Swartz JM, Dyer KD, Cheever AW, et al. *Schistosoma mansoni* infection in eosinophil lineage-ablated mice. *Blood.* 2006;108(7):2420-2427.

406. *Eosinophils in Health and Disease.* Elsevier; 2013. 654.

Chapter 9 ■ Mast Cells and Basophils: Ontogeny, Characteristics, and Functional Diversity

A. DEAN BEFUS • MARIANNA KULKA • KELLY M. MCNAGNY • JUDAH A. DENBURG

INTRODUCTION

In 1965, Selye[1] reviewed the literature on two populations of granulated leukocytes, mast cells and basophils, that contain electron-dense cytoplasmic granules and stain metachromatically with selected basic dyes. These cells have many similarities, but also exhibit intriguing differences. Recent advances in our understanding of their development, contents, biosynthetic activities, and functions are elucidating their relationships and roles in immunity and many inflammatory disorders, including allergy. They produce numerous inflammatory mediators—such as histamine—that are common to both cells, and others that are cell-specific. Both cells express a tetrameric isoform of the high-affinity receptor for immunoglobulin E (IgE). When this receptor is cross-linked by sensitizing allergen or by anti-IgE antibodies, mast cells and basophils can be activated, mediator synthesis and secretion induced, and gene expression is altered, with consequences in many immune and inflammatory events.[2-12]

Classical light microscopic and ultrastructural characteristics of mast cells and basophils are shown in *Figure 9.1A* and *B*. New information and emerging "omic" technologies including immunophenotyping with single-cell mass cytometry (e.g., single-cell RNA-sequencing[12]/transcriptomics and single-cell assay for transposase-accessible chromatin sequencing[13]) and the power of computational biology have transformed our understanding of mast cell and basophil development and hematopoietic relationships, phenotypic heterogeneity, and plasticity (see below). In many ways, the statement by Ehrlich in 1879[1] that basophils are "blood mast cells," and the corollary that mast cells are "tissue basophils," although incorrect, is of some value in thinking about these two cell types. As will be discussed, recent evidence suggests that mast cells, as opposed to basophils, represent a distinct offshoot from other hematopoietic lineages and likely carry out unique roles in tissue homeostasis and disease.

This chapter provides an overview of the developmental biology of these two cell types, comparing and contrasting their physiology, phenotype, activation, and function; lineage commitment and differentiation; and roles in innate and acquired immunity, health, and disease. Continued advances in understanding basophil and mast cell function will lead to new diagnostic and therapeutic strategies for those suffering from allergic and other inflammatory diseases, as well as bone marrow disorders primarily involving these cell types.

GENERAL MORPHOLOGY, MEDIATOR SECRETION, AND RECOVERY

Morphology

Blood smears or preparations of enriched basophils or mast cells from tissues, stained with Wright or May-Grunwald-Giemsa, show similarities in these cell types (*Figure 9.2A* and *B*). The cytoplasm of the cells generally stains pink, the nucleus is purplish or blue, and the cytoplasmic granules are dark blue to purple or even blackish. Basophils in peripheral blood or tissues range in size from 10 to 15 μm, whereas mast cells in tissue sites may appear irregular in shape and up to 20 μm in a long dimension. Ultrastructural analyses not only demonstrate similarities between mast cells and basophils, but also identify distinct differences (*Figure 9.1A* and *B*).[14] In blood, basophils are round, whereas in tissues they can have various shapes. Mast cells can appear round, oval, or elongated in tissues. The most prominent cytoplasmic elements in both cell types are the membrane-bound, electron-dense granules.

Basophils generally possess fewer granules than mast cells and the granules exhibit a more homogeneous ultrastructure than that of mast cells. Basophil granules are often homogeneously electron dense, although dense particles may be interspersed with membrane aggregates and whorls. Charcot-Leyden crystals can be formed in basophils. Mast cell granules may be homogeneously electron dense, or exhibit electron-dense particles, membrane or complex scroll-like patterns, highly organized crystalline structures, or combinations of these. The relationship of these different granule patterns to the tissue site, phase in development, or mediator content is not clear, although Hafez[15] raised the possibility that age may be a component of this heterogeneity. Chen et al[16] conducted a detailed analysis of granule dynamics using soft X-ray tomography and fluorescent microscopy following activation of rat basophilic leukemia cells (a model mast cell) via the IgE receptor. Granule fission and fusion, mitochondrial activation, and giant vesicles containing mitochondria, granules, and lipid bodies indicated multiple morphological alterations following cell activation.

Mast cells produce 30 to 100 nm extracellular membrane vesicles of endocytic origin, called exosomes, that contain mRNA, microRNAs, proteins, and lipids and can transfer these components to other cells and influence their functions.[17] Mast cell production of exosomes has been an exciting topic of investigation (e.g.,[18,19]), and although the mechanisms that control exosome contents and direct them to their target cells are unknown, the composition and cell-to-cell communication functions of exosomes are influenced by activation of mast cells. Basophils likely also produce exosomes, although this has not been well characterized. Basophils contain numerous electron-lucent vesicles of 50 to 70 nm with contents similar to granules that may be associated with a form of mediator exocytosis (see later). Mast cell exosomes contain microRNA that can regulate the function of other cells including microglia,[20] osteoblasts,[21] and stellate cells. Mast cells and basophils also both contain rounded, non–membrane-bound, electron-dense structures called lipid bodies, a rich store of arachidonic acid. Lipid bodies increase in number during cell activation and are thought to be derived from membrane catabolism and the rapid synthesis of lipid mediators such as the cyclo-oxygenase and lipoxygenase derivatives of arachidonic acid.[16] Mast cells also produce larger endosome or plasma membrane–derived structures called extracellular vesicles (~200 nm), which also harbor microRNA and can modify the function of target cells such as group 2 innate lymphoid cells (ILC2).[22]

Mediator Secretion

Mast cells and basophils undergo distinct patterns of granule mediator secretion or synthesis, depending on the stimuli involved in their activation.[5,14,23] *Degranulation or regulated exocytosis,* whereby granules or their contents are released, occurs following stimulation through the IgE receptor or numerous other receptors, such as those for fragments of the complement cascade (see below). Degranulation can be extensive, involving the majority of granules, or it can be more limited. Detailed visualization of mast cell degranulation using different stimuli, IgE-anti-IgE and substance P (cationic ligand of the Mas-related G-protein–coupled receptor [MRGPR]), demonstrated that with stimulation via FcεRI there was membrane fusion of adjacent granules prior to fusion of aggregated granules with the plasma membrane and extracellular release detectable within 10 minutes. By contrast, substance P induces a more rapid release (detectable by 3 minutes) through fusion of individual granules directly with the plasma membrane.[23] Moreover, there were differences in the profiles of mediators secreted following stimulation via each of these pathways; *in vivo* studies in mice showed that anti-IgE stimulation resulted in less plasma exudation compared to substance P at 30 minutes, and greater neutrophil

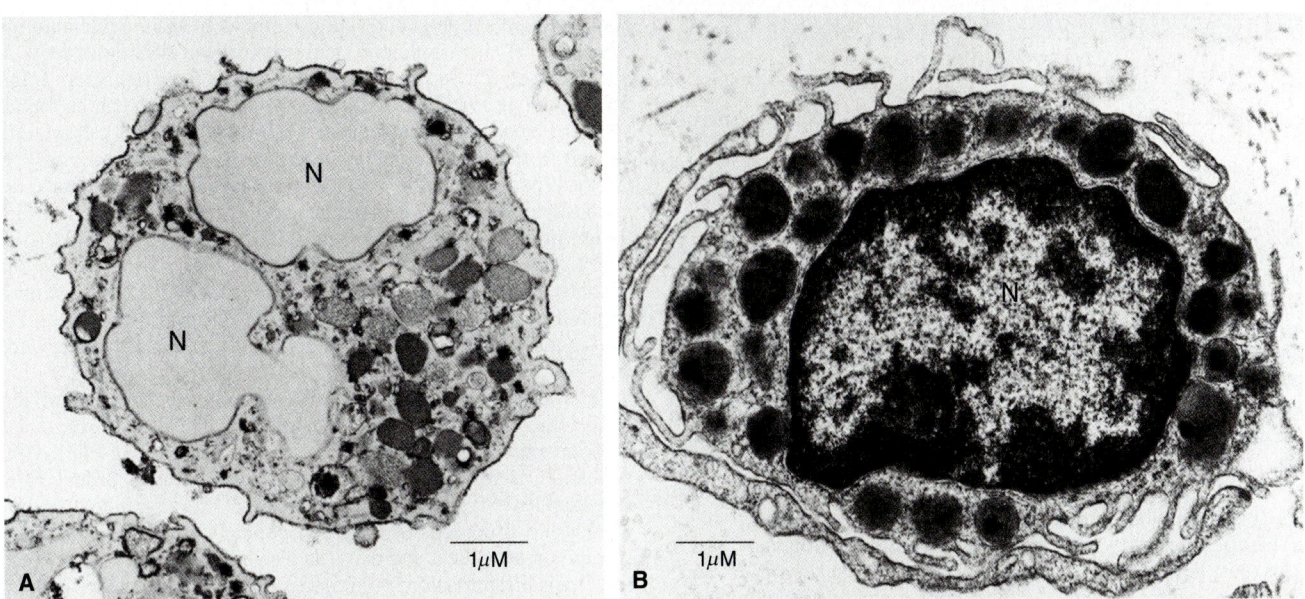

FIGURE 9.1 **A, Basophils are "granulocytes that mature in bone marrow, circulate in the blood, and that can migrate into tissues during inflammatory or immunologic processes.** Mature basophils are round and have electron-dense cytoplasmic granules, prominent aggregates of cytoplasmic glycogen, and short, blunt, irregularly distributed plasma membrane processes." N, nucleus; bar, 1 μm. B, Mast cells normally mature outside of bone marrow or circulation, in many tissues. Immature and mature granules of mast cells and basophils differ distinctively in ultrastructure. Unlike basophils, mast cells generally lack electron-dense aggregates of cytoplasmic glycogen, and have a plasma membrane with uniformly distributed, thin, elongate folds and processes. Mast cell nuclei may appear bilobed, but they generally lack the pattern of peripherally condensed nuclear chromatin characteristic of basophils and other granulocytes. A human skin mast cell is shown with monolobed nucleus with partially condensed chromatin, numerous cytoplasmic granules containing crystalline structures, and thin surface projections. Bar, 1 μm. (A, From Dvorak AM, Warner JA, Fox P, et al. Recovery of human basophils after FMLP-stimulated secretion. *Clin Exp Allergy* 1996;26(3):281-294. Copyright © 1996 Blackwell Science Ltd. Reprinted by permission of John Wiley & Sons, Inc; B, Reprinted by permission from Springer: Dvorak AM. Human mast cells. In: Beck F, Hild W, Kriz W, et al., eds. *Advances in Anatomy, Embryology and Cell Biology*. Springer-Verlag; 1989:114:3-12. Copyright © 1989 Springer-Verlag Berlin Heidelberg.)

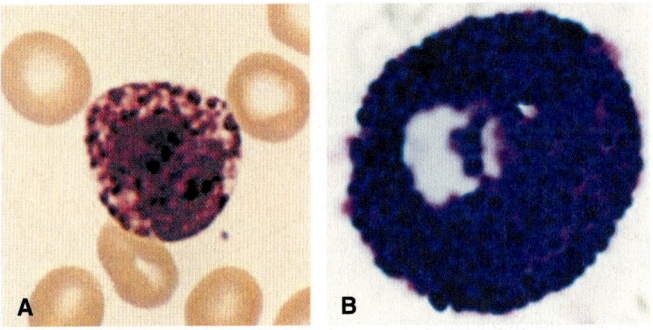

FIGURE 9.2 A, Human peripheral blood basophil stained with Wright stain. B, Rat peritoneal mast cell stained with May-Grunwald-Giemsa stain. (From Lee, Bithell, Foerster, et al., eds. *Wintrobe's Clinical Hematology*, 9th ed. Lea & Febiger; 1993.)

and monocyte infiltration by 6 hours.[23] Interestingly, Gaudenzio et al confirmed earlier work by Kunder et al[24] (2009) that larger, extruded granules released upon anti-IgE activation could traffic to local lymph nodes, perhaps to participate in acquired immune responses. However, smaller granules derived from MRGPR-mediated activation did not show such trafficking. The process is generally similar for basophils via anti-IgE stimulation but, as described below, basophils do not respond to MRGPR-mediated stimuli. In mast cells at least, this degranulation does not lead to extensive cell death, and many cells can recover and degranulate again.[14]

Another form of secretion of stored mediators by mast cells and basophils, as well as by eosinophils, is *piecemeal degranulation*, involving small vesicles arising from granules that shuttle selected granule components to the extracellular milieu.[14] Piecemeal degranulation is the most prevalent form of mast cell and basophil secretion

found in human biopsy material in nonallergic inflammatory conditions; it is associated with secretion of selected mediators, rather than entire contents of the granules. It is postulated that intragranular vesiculotubular networks fuse with the plasma membrane, and discharge their granule contents to the extracellular space in communications between mast cells and neurons in the brain,[25] in psychosocial stress,[26] in acute gastritis,[27] and following Toll-like receptor (TLR) activation.[28] As with anaphylactic degranulation, piecemeal secretion is associated with the ability of mast cells to recharge their granules and respond to stimuli again.

Cytokines and chemokines are also secreted by mast cells through mechanisms independent of degranulation,[5,29] as are arachidonic acid metabolites, prostaglandins, and leukotrienes. Newly synthesized cytokines and chemokines can be secreted by a process called *constitutive exocytosis*. The pathways of secretion of arachidonic acid metabolites as well as that for exosome release are poorly known.[17]

Recovery After Activation

Dvorak[14] summarized the evidence for the ability of mast cells and basophils to recover and regranulate following activation. During this process, mast cells and basophils appear to conserve membrane components and to resynthesize granule and other components, such as rough endoplasmic reticulum, Golgi, and microtubules; this "recovery" generally occurs within 1 to 2 days. In addition to synthesizing these new mediators through transcription/translation, mast cells can also internalize some mediators such as serotonin from the extracellular space via unknown endocytic pathways.[30] Yamada et al[31] identified that several autophagy-associated genes were increased following anti-IgE-mediated mast cell activation, and that RNA-mediated inhibition of some of these genes impaired degranulation and regranulation. Whether death by necrosis or apoptosis is a critical feature of mast cell or basophil activation *in vivo* needs to be more carefully evaluated.

ONTOGENY AND DEVELOPMENTAL BIOLOGY OF MAST CELLS AND BASOPHILS

Clearly defining the progenitors and origins of mast cells and basophils has been a contentious and controversial issue, likely reflecting the fact that this process changes during embryonic and adult development and is susceptible to alterations in environmental and inflammatory cues. An important and emerging concept to consider is that of "layered hematopoiesis" during ontogeny.[32] It is now known that during embryonic and fetal development, a number of hematopoietic lineages colonize developing organs and tissues and thereafter become long-lived, self-renewing tissue-resident cells: macrophages (microglia, Kupffer cells, alveolar and muscle macrophages), mast cells, innate lymphoid cells, and innate and invariant T cells, to name but a few noteworthy examples. These, then, acquire tissue-specific phenotypes, and autonomously carry out specialized immune and homeostatic functions within these tissues, and are rarely replaced by adult bone marrow progenitors unless they are ablated in an inflammatory crisis. It is known that subsets of yolk sac–derived mast cells colonize peripheral tissues very early during embryonic development[33] and appear to be derived from a common erythroid, megakaryocytic, and mast cell progenitor.[34] Thus, it is likely that much of the controversy surrounding the origins and branch points of mast cells and basophils from undifferentiated hematopoietic progenitors has arisen due to a failure to distinguish those tissue-resident precursors that colonized target organs during fetal development from those that are derived from recent adult bone marrow emigrants under steady-state or inflammatory conditions.

With that caveat in mind, studies in adults showed that tissue mast cells and blood basophils are not normally derived *directly* from a common bipotent progenitor but do ultimately share common origins from a CD34+ hematopoietic stem cells, whose differentiation is regulated closely by various marrow and tissue stromal factors (*Figure 9.3*). A unique role is played by CD34 itself—which can be found in some mast cell subpopulations and is involved in mast cell migration as well as tissue inflammatory responses—in these processes.[35] For the most part, basophils and mast cells have distinct ontogenic derivations and markers.[36] In humans and in rodents, mast cell differentiation proceeds from an immature CD34+, CD38+, CD13+, c-kit+, FcεRI-, or FcγRII/III+ cell, or, as recently shown, from a previously uncharacterized immature cell in mouse marrow.[37] More specifically, an adult multipotent, hematopoietic progenitor of both mucosal and serosal mast cell phenotypes can be identified and is characterized as Lin-c-kit+Sca-1-Ly6c-FcεRI-CD27-β7+T1/ST2+ (*Figure 9.3*).[38]

Transcriptionally, mast cell differentiation, heterogeneity, abundance, and functional responses are regulated through the combinatorial activity of several master regulators including PU.1, GATA factors, FOG-1, C/EBP factors, and MITF, as well as through M-Ras and RabGEF1-type signaling molecules.[39,40] As alluded to above, phenotypic alterations of mast cell populations can be governed by specific tissue milieu, and they can also exhibit phenotypic switching and "transdifferentiation,"[1,41] reflecting stochastic processes in peripheral progenitor differentiation.

Identification of the mast cell hematopoietin, stem cell factor (SCF), and its receptor, *c-kit* (CD117), has provided a wealth of insight into the functional role of mast cells in a variety of processes. Mutations in either the ligand ("Steel" locus) or its receptor ("W" locus) render mice largely mast cell deficient, facilitating evaluation of the role of mast cells in a variety of disease models.[4] Mast cells have thus been revealed to be key players not only in allergic inflammation but also in angiogenesis and tumor growth,

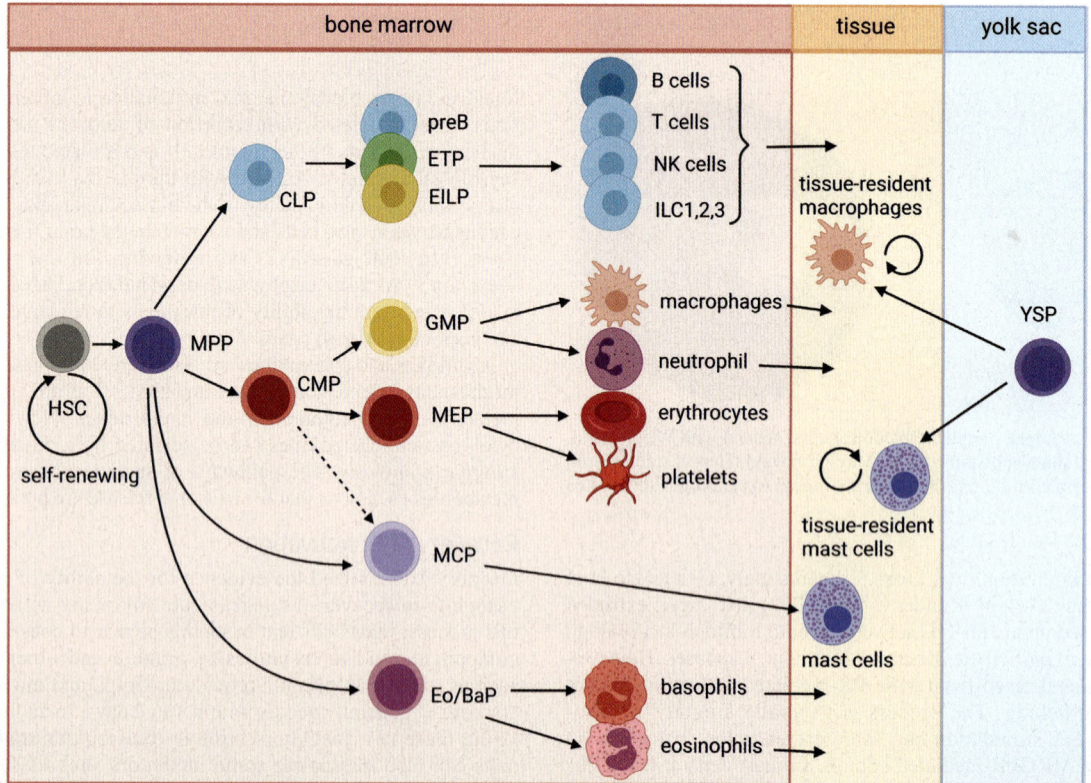

FIGURE 9.3 **Schematic depicting the development of mast cells, basophils, and various lineages from adult HSC and committed progenitors.** CLP, common lymphoid progenitor; CMP, common myeloid progenitor; EILP, early innate lymphoid progenitor; Eo/BaP, eosinophil /basophil precursor; ETP, early thymic progenitor; GMP, granulocyte/macrophage progenitor; HSC, hematopoietic stem cell; ILC, innate lymphoid cell; MCP, mast cell precursor; MEP, megarkaryocyte/erythroid progenitor; MPP, multipotent progenitor; PreB, Pre B cell; YSP, yolk sac progenitor. Dashed arrow indicates residual ambiguity/likely alternate origins of mast cell progenitors. It is noteworthy that recent single-cell sequencing and ontological studies suggest mast cells are most closely related to megakaryocytic and erythroid lineages. (Popescu DM, Botting RA, Stephenson E, et al. Decoding human fetal liver haematopoiesis. *Nature.* 2019;574:365-371). Created with BioRender.com. (Adapted from Chen, et al. *Proc Natl Acad Sci U S A* 2005;102:11129-11130; Wang J, et al. *Curr Drug Targets Inflamm Allergy.* 2003;2:293-302.)

tissue remodeling, metabolic syndrome, graft tolerance, and some autoimmune diseases.[3,4,7,9] However, inasmuch as mutations of the SCF/c-kit gene and many linked loci also affect other hematopoietic lineages and gut function, these studies must be interpreted with some caution. More recent advances in the analysis of mast cell and basophil populations[42] have provided novel insights into their functions and transcriptional regulation of their hematopoietic development.

Mast Cell Growth and Differentiation

Rodent and human mast cells can be grown in vitro from lineage-committed, unipotent or multipotent progenitors. Although interleukin (IL)-3 is known to contribute to murine mast cell and to both human and rodent basophil development,[43] it is SCF/c-kit ligand that uniquely drives human mast cell differentiation. SCF is produced by murine and human fibroblasts, epithelial cells, endothelial cells, and tumor cell lines, and must bind to c-kit to effect differentiation. Mutations in c-kit can result in mast cell deficiency in vivo and in vitro ("loss of function") or, alternately, in autonomous mast cell growth ("gain of function"), generally leading to autophosphorylation.[44] The latter mutations, especially the D-816-V-associated mastocytosis (which can be transferred with similar consequences to the mouse[45]), have formed the basis of newly designed tyrosine kinase inhibitors in some proliferative mast cell and hypereosinophilic disorders.

Recently, it has also been shown that, in response to tissue damage, epithelial and mesenchymal "alarmins" including thymic stromal lymphopoietin (TSLP) and IL-25 or IL-33 can either directly or indirectly influence the activation of tissue-resident mast cells and their progenitors. Mast cells are known to express TSLP and IL-33 receptors permitting direct activation.[2,46] Perhaps more significantly, a newly discovered subset of tissue-resident ILC2s produce enormous amounts of IL-5, IL-9, IL-13 in response to these same alarmins, each of which has the ability to modulate eosinophil, mast cell, and basophil numbers and functions in these tissues.[47-49] *Table 9.1* lists cytokines, growth factors, transcription factors, and signaling molecules that regulate primate/human and rodent mast cell differentiation.

Environmental Activation of Mast Cell and Basophil Progenitors

Mast cell and basophil progenitor pools can expand and contract in blood, bone marrow, and various other tissues in relation to a variety of environmental stimuli, including viruses or nematodes[38], neonatal gut microbiota, or allergens. For example, it has been shown that the gut microbiota regulates a TSLP-induced, IgE-dependent T_H2 response, involving basophil progenitors in rodents and in humans with hyper-IgE syndrome.[50] Similarly, profound decreases in gut flora lead to a B cell–driven overproduction of IgE that binds to its high-affinity receptor on bone marrow progenitors increasing basophilopoiesis, with T_H2 skewed inflammatory responses.[43] More strikingly, it was recently shown that fetal and neonatal mast cell–dependent allergic responses can be induced through the regulated transfer of maternal IgE across the placenta, highlighting a novel mechanism for maternal influences on neonatal hematopoiesis.[51] Previous work on normal, atopic or leukemic/mastocytotic human blood or marrow had identified pure or mixed basophil colonies in semisolid cultures,[52] thus defining a basophil progenitor (termed "CFU-baso" or "CFU-baso/eo").[52] The phenotype and lineage commitment of the basophil progenitor are depicted in *Figure 9.3*.

Basophil Differentiation-Inducing Cytokines

IL-3 is the main cytokine involved in human basophil growth and differentiation,[43] with some evidence for TSLP serving as a cofactor.[43] Granulocyte-macrophage colony-stimulating factor (GM-CSF),[52] IL-4,[53] IL-5,[53] and SCF may also play roles. Cytokines and other factors that modulate basophil or mast cell differentiation are listed in *Table 9.1*.

Table 9.1. Cytokines and Other Factors Involved in Basophil and Mast Cell Growth and Differentiation

Cytokine	Effect
GM-CSF	Basophil growth and differentiation; promotes in vivo basophilia and increases in circulating CFU-baso/eo (primates); basophil activation/survival; downregulates human mast cell differentiation
IL-3	Human basophil growth and differentiation; basophil activation/survival; promotes in vivo basophilia (in primates); mast cell differentiating activity in rodents
IL-5	Primarily eosinophil, but also basophil growth and differentiation; basophil and eosinophil activation/survival
TSLP/IL-33/IL-25	Cofactors in rodent nuocyte (multipotent mucosal progenitor) differentiation and tissue basophilic responses
IL-4/IL-13	Produced by basophils with minimal activity on differentiation
IL-9/IL-10/THPO	Cofactors in rodent mast cell phenotype switching
TGF-β/IFN-α	Negative regulators of basophil differentiation
SCF	Primary mast cell growth factors in mouse and rat; little known effect on basophil differentiation
NGF	Induces mast cell hyperplasia (rodents), human mast cell line (HMC-1), and basophil-eosinophil differentiation in vitro
RA	A mutation in the RA receptor allows for expression of basophil differentiation; may concurrently downregulate human mast cell differentiation
v-erb	Associated with the development of lethal mastocytosis in the rodent
FcγRIIB	Downregulates mast cell growth
Stat5	An essential regulator in vivo of mast cell development
IL-6/TNF/IFN-γ	May play a role in regulating phenotypic direction and lineage commitment of human basophils and mast cell subtypes
IL-18	May play a role in expansion of bone marrow–derived basophils and mast cells

Abbreviations: baso, basophil; CFU, colony forming unit; eo, eosinophil; GM-CSF, granulocyte-macrophage colony-stimulating factor; IFN, interferon; IL, interleukin; NGF, nerve growth factor; RA, retinoic acid; SCF, stem cell factor; TGF, transforming growth factor; THPO, thrombopoietin; TNF, tumor necrosis factor; TSLP, thymic stromal lymphopoietin.

Clinical Relevance of Basophil and Mast Cell Differentiation

Allergic Diseases

The relationship to disease activity, severity, and response to therapy of fluctuations in numbers of human basophil-eosinophil, basophil-mast cell, or mast cell progenitors—including CD34[+] cell subpopulations—in the blood and bone marrow of patients with a variety of allergic disorders, including allergic rhinitis, nasal polyposis, asthma, atopic dermatitis, and drug allergies, has been extensively documented.[54] Mast cell activation syndrome is complex set of diseases and some, based upon presence of kit mutations, share clinical features with mastocytosis syndromes (below). Targeting basophil-eosinophil progenitors with anti-IL-5 or anti-IL-5R monoclonal antibodies leads to maturation arrest or antibody-dependent cellular cytotoxicity, and is accompanied by clinical benefit in patients with eosinophilic bronchitis and asthma.[55] Finally, because IgE binding to FcεRI may lead to basophilopoiesis and increased susceptibility to allergic disease,[50] blocking antibodies directed to IgE, IgE-producing B cells, or the

IgE receptor on basophils have also proven helpful therapeutically in atopic dermatitis, nasal polyposis, and asthma. Given that deletion of genes encoding these receptors (IL-3R, CD34, and FcεRI) in mice has no apparent deleterious effects on development, predictably, therapies targeting these molecules have been well-tolerated. Because recent evidence points to the critical roles of alarmins—IL-25, IL-33, and TSLP—and their receptors in the differentiation and migration of basophils in allergic diseases, targeting this early, innate immune cell–driven axis also offers a number of opportunities for intervention.[43,56,57] A rare population of Lin-CD34+FcεRI+ mast cell progenitors has been identified in poorly controlled human asthmatic subjects that could benefit from such an approach.[58]

Malignancies

In transient leukemias occurring in Down syndrome (trisomy 21), in various hematologic malignancies, as well as in megakaryoblastic leukemia, there is basophilic differentiation (which may also include mast cell proliferation) from leukemic cell progenitors. This could involve aberrant stimulation of basophil or mast cell progenitors by certain transcription factors that also regulate erythroid and megakaryocytic lineages, including GATA factors,[13,59] and likely reflecting a common origin for these cell lineages.[13] Embryonic stem cells or CD34+ progenitors transfected with GATA genes express varying degrees of erythroid/megakaryocytic and basophil/mast cell commitment,[59] whereas mice with mutations in the eosinophil-specific promoter of the GATA-1 gene completely lack eosinophils. Factors such as Gab-2, certain adaptor proteins, signaling molecules, c-kit Lyn and SHP-1, or the flt3 ligand for this tyrosine kinase receptor also can play important roles in basophil and mast cell differentiation. Mutations in bone marrow mesenchymal stem cells have recently been shown to be associated with mastocytosis disease progression.[60]

In addition to mast cell proliferative diseases (mastocytosis of various subtypes, urticaria pigmentosa, and mast cell leukemia),[61] several hematopoietic malignancies exhibit dysregulation of basophil and mast cell lineages, including chronic myeloid leukemia prior to blast crisis, in which the fusion protein bcr-abl may be involved. The biological significance of increased numbers of mast cells in various hematopoietic and lymphatic malignancies, as well as in refractory anemias, may be related to acquisition in the leukemic clone of concomitant *c-kit* mutations. In addition, specific chromosomal abnormalities are found in leukemias associated with basophilia or eosinophilia. Recently and importantly, increases in blood basophils, presumably on the basis of increased basophilopoiesis, have been described in human hyper-IgE syndrome, associated with a DOCK8- polymorphism, paralleling the rodent model.[50] Apart from *c-kit*/SCF, whether other cytokines are involved in malignant basophil or mast cell proliferation in vivo is not known; for example, dysregulated cytokine genes such as those encoding IL-3, IL-4, IL-5, and GM-CSF in 5q-leukemias may play a role in phenotypic expression of leukemic cells.

CHARACTERISTICS OF MAST CELLS AND BASOPHILS

Surface Phenotype and Activation

Much information is available on the surface phenotype of human mast cells and basophils (*Table 9.2*), including identification of receptors for immunoglobulins, complement components, cytokines and chemokines, arachidonic acid metabolites, CD294 (CRTH2, chemoattractant receptor-homologous molecule expressed on T-helper class 2 cells, also known as D prostanoid receptor 2), CD200, vitamin D, and ligands for TLR; as well as integrins and other molecules with or without CD nomenclature.[2,6,62] However, one must be cautious not to generalize about surface marker expression given the heterogeneity and plasticity of mast cells from various tissues and species and the in vivo relevance of various mast cell and basophil-like cell lines.

Table 9.2. Expression of Selected Surface Markers on Human Mast Cells and Basophils

Marker	Mast Cells	Basophils
Fc receptors	FcεRI ($\alpha\beta\gamma2$) FcγRI, IIA, IIB, III (CD64, 32, 16) IgD binding protein complex	FcεRI ($\alpha\beta\gamma2$) FcγRIIA, IIB, IIIB (CD32, 16) IgD binding protein complex (galectin-9 and CD44)
Integrins B_2 family B_1 family	CD11c/18 ($\alpha_D\beta_2$) CD49c/CD29 (α_3B_1) CD49d/CD29 (α_4B_1) CD49e/CD29 (α_5B_1)	CD11a/18 ($\alpha_L\beta_2$) CD11b/18 ($\alpha_M\beta_2$) CD11c/18 ($\alpha_D\beta_2$) CD49d/CD29 ($\alpha_4\beta_1$) CD49e/CD29 ($\alpha_5\beta_1$)
Selectins	N/A	L, P, and E (CD62L, CD162, CD15s)
Chemokine receptors	CCR1,3,4,5,7 CXCR1,2,3,4,6	CCR1,2,3,5,7 CXCR1,2,4,8
Cytokine receptors	c-kit (CD117) IL-3R (CD123) IFNγR IL-1R, IL-10R IL-33R (ST2) TSLPR	IL-2R (CD25) IL-3R (CD123) IL-3/5/GMRβ IL-17RB IL-18R IL-33R (ST2) TSLPR
Cysteinyl leukotriene receptors	cysLT1,2	cysLT1,2
Prostaglandin receptors	CRTH$_2$ (CD294) EP1-3	CRTH$_2$ (CD294)
Toll-like receptors	TLR2,3,4,6,9	TLR1,2,4,5,6,9,10
Complement receptors	C3aR, C5aR	C3aR, C5aR
Other	CD200R3, CD203c, CD300a Vitamin D receptor, Siglec-7 and 8, CD48, MRGPRs, histamine H1 and H4 receptors, cannabinoid receptor (CB1)	CD200R3, CD203c, CD300a, 2D7 antigen, Siglec-7 and 8 Histamine H2 receptor

For a more complete summary of surface markers see: Steiner M, Huber S, Harrer A, Himly M. The evolution of human basophil biology from neglect towards understanding of their immune functions. *Biomed Res Int.* 2016;2016:8232830; Harvima IT, Levi-Schaffer F, Draber P, et al. Molecular targets on mast cells and basophils for novel therapies. *J Allergy Clin Immunol.* 2014;134:530-544; Varricchi G, Raap U, Rivellese F, Marone G, Gibbs BF. Human mast cells and basophils-how are they similar how are they different. *Immunol Rev.* 2018;282:8-34.

One prominent difference is that mature mast cells express CD117 or c-kit (*Table 9.2*), whereas basophils do not. Another important difference lies in expression of Fc receptors that provide key pathways for activation and modulation of function (*Tables 9.2* and *9.3*). Although both mast cells and basophils express high-affinity receptors for IgE, mast cells can express the FcγIR (CD64), II (CD32), and III (CD16),[63] but to date FcγRI (CD64) has not been found on human basophils. Mice deficient in FcγRIIB are highly sensitive to IgG-triggered mast cell degranulation through FcγRIII, and exhibit enhanced passive cutaneous anaphylaxis and elevated immunoglobulin levels in response to antigen stimulation. In addition to inhibition of FcγRIII-mediated activation, FcγRIIB also downregulates FcεRI signaling and is important in the regulation of mast cell and basophil activities.[64] Interestingly, recent studies have shown that basophils and mast cells express a protease-sensitive, IL-3- or IL-4-inducible receptor for IgD that is distinct from receptors for IgG, IgE, and IgA[65-67]

Table 9.3. Selected Mediators of Human Mast Cells and Basophils[a]

Marker	Cell Type	
	Mast Cells	Basophils
Histamine	+	+
Platelet-activating factor (PAF)	+	+
Nitric oxide	+	not known
Proteoglycans	Heparin, chondroitin sulfates	Chondroitin sulfates
Arachidonic acid metabolites	LTB_4, LTC_4, PGD_2, PGF_2, thromboxane A_2	LTB_4, LTC_4
Proteinases	Tryptase, chymase, carboxypeptidase A, cathepsin G-like	
Cytokines/chemokines/growth factors	IL-1,2,3,4,5,6,8 (CXCL8),10,11,13,16, 33 TNF, LT, NGF, TGF-β, GM-CSF, RANTES (CCL5), MCP1 (CCL2), I-309 (CCL1), MIP1α (CCL3), 1β (CCL4), lymphotactin (XCL1), FGF, PDGFAB, VEGF, BDNF	IL-3,4, 6,13,25 MIP-1α (CCL3), RANTES (CCL5), TNF

[a]Mediators selected from more comprehensive lists published by others and recent updates. Abbreviations: BDNF, brain-derived neurotrophic factor; GM-CSF, granulocyte-macrophage colony-stimulating factor; IL, interleukin; LTB_4, leukotriene B_4; LTC_4, leukotriene C_4; NGF, nerve growth factor; PGD_2, prostaglandin D_2; PGF_2, prostaglandin F_2; TGF, transforming growth factor; TNF, tumor necrosis factor; VEGF, vascular endothelial growth factor.
Steiner M, Huber S, Harrer A, Himly M. The evolution of human basophil biology from neglect towards understanding of their immune functions. *Biomed Res Int.* 2016;2016:8232830; Dwyer DF, Barrett NA, Austen KF, Immunological Genome Project Consortium. Expression profiling of constitutive mast cells reveals a unique identity within the immune system. *Nat Immunol.* 2016;17:878-887.

Table 9.4. Factors That Activate Mediator Secretion From Human Basophils and Mast Cells

Stimulation	Mast Cells	Basophils
FcεR and FcγR cross-linkage	+	+
Compound 48/80 and basic polypeptides[a] (includes several neuropeptides and anti-microbial peptides) via MRGPR	SMC only	−
Anaphylatoxins (C3a, C5a)	+	+
fMLP	−	+
Interleukins/chemokines (CC)/histamine-releasing factors (HRF)	MIP-1α (CCL3) IL-1 SCF Ig light chain TSLP	IL-3,5,25,33, MCP1 (CCL-2), MCP2 (CCL-8), MCP3 (CCL-7) MIP-1α (CCL3), RANTES (CCL5) IL-8 (CXCL8), HrHRF CTAPIII/NAP-2 TSLP
TLR ligands	TLR2,3,4	TLR2

[a]Includes adrenocorticotropic hormone, mellitin, substance P, vasoactive intestinal polypeptide, neurotensin, bradykinin, etc.
"+" means that the factor(s) can activate mast cell and/or basophil secretion, whereas "−" means that the factor(s) does not activate secretion.
Abbreviations: fMLP, formyl methionyl leucyl phenylalanine; MRGPR, Mas-related G-protein–coupled receptor; SMC, human skin mast cells; TLR, Toll-like receptor; TSLP, thymic stromal lymphopoietin.
For more details, see Steiner M, Huber S, Harrer A, Himly M. The evolution of human basophil biology from neglect towards understanding of their immune functions. *Biomed Res Int.* 2016;2016:8232830; McNeil BD, Pundir P, Meeker S, et al. Identification of a mast-cell-specific receptor crucial for pseudo-allergic drug reactions. *Nature.* 2015;519:237-241.

and involves interaction of IgD with surface galectin-9 and CD44. Activation of basophils via this IgD induces release of antimicrobial peptides, IL-4 and B cell–activating factor,[63,65,66] but inhibits IgE-mediated degranulation. Indeed, oral immunotherapy in children with milk and egg allergies and natural tolerance in bee keepers were associated with elevated IgD to specific allergens and hyporesponsiveness to allergen challenge.

A number of other stimuli, including anaphylatoxins C3a and C5a, certain lectins, and the bacterial product formyl methionyl leucyl phenylalanine, activate basophils and/or mast cells. It is well known that polycationic substances such as compound 48/80, several drugs associated with pseudoallergic reactions, and numerous basic polypeptides including a spectrum of neuropeptides activate human skin mast cells, but not human mast cells from some other sites, or human basophils. After several decades of not understanding the basis of these reactions, McNeil et al[68] made a major advance when they showed that this human mast cell activation involved a Mas-related G-protein–coupled receptor, MRGPRX2. Recently, Dwyer et al[69] found that mouse mast cells expressed several *Mrgpr* genes, whereas mouse basophils uniquely expressed only one *Mrgpr*. Elucidation of the roles of members of this family of receptors in mast cell and basophil biology is likely to identify other pathways of innate pattern recognition and cell activation important in health and disease.

It is well known that mast cells and nerves have close anatomical relationships.[11,12] Neurogenic vasodilation produced by an axonal reflex in human skin can involve mast cell activation by neuropeptides released from primary afferent nerves. Mast cell–dependent neurogenic inflammation has been described in the respiratory and gastrointestinal tracts and appears to be important in at least some inflammatory and infectious diseases. More recently, the relationship

between mast cells and nerves has been emphasized in the intestine as a component of the gut-brain axis as well as in pain hypersensitivity and hypoxia-ischemia injury and in many other conditions.[11] Recently, neuronal interactions mediated by basophil-derived leukotriene C4 (LTC_4) have been attributed to IgE, in acute flares of itch, highlighting the bidirectional interactions of mast cells and basophils with the nervous system.[70]

In the past, there had been great interest in activation of basophils and mast cells by several ILs, chemokines, and other factors (*Table 9.4*). The significance of these pathways of basophil and mast cell activation in vivo has become increasingly clear, particularly in chronic allergic and parasitic diseases and in bacterial, viral, and fungal infection.[3,4,9,10,28,69,71-74] The CC chemokines appear to be important in basophil activation; however, there is less information for mast cells. SCF appears to be a specific stimulus for mast cells, acting through the CD117 receptor.[75] Redegeld et al[6] made the intriguing observation that highly purified immunoglobulin light chains can sensitize mast cells for antigen-specific activation, providing a molecular mechanism for earlier observations of antigen-specific, but non-antibody-mediated mast cell activation. Additional research on the role of such stimuli for mast cells and/or basophils will shed light on the pathogenesis of inflammatory disorders such as inflammatory bowel disease, rheumatoid arthritis, and allergic airways diseases.[6,76]

Another intriguing difference between mast cells and basophils lies in their expression of selected integrin molecules (*Table 9.2*). Human basophils, but not mast cells, express CD11a/18, CD11b/18, and CD11c/18, which have as their complementary ligands, intercellular adhesion molecule 1/2, C3bi, and fibrinogen, respectively. The latter are expressed on endothelial cells and appear to be involved in the migration of basophils into the tissues during inflammation.

By contrast, mature mast cells and basophils express a repertoire of adhesion molecules designed to interact with the extracellular matrix components, which play significant roles in cell recruitment and activation. In particular, rodent basophils are readily distinguished from mast cells based on their selective expression of the collagen receptor, CD49b/29.[77]

Recent advances in understanding the roles of mast cells in innate immunity, including their expression of TLR and other pattern recognition receptors,[6,9,10] are noteworthy. Basophils express a partially overlapping, but separate repertoire of these types of receptors,[2,62] supporting their distinct role from mast cells in innate immunity. Similarly, although some exciting clues have been uncovered (e.g., ultraviolet B irradiation- and vitamin D receptor-dependent production of IL-*10* by cutaneous mast cells[78]), much is unknown about many other surface molecules on mast cells and basophils, including the vitamin D receptor, CD200R[79] and receptors for IL-33[80] and TSLP[81] (*Table 9.2*).

Mediators

Mast cells and basophils are storehouses of inflammatory mediators that can be released by IgE receptor activation and many other stimuli, and synthesize several other mediators upon activation (*Tables 9.3 and 9.4*). Mediators such as histamine, platelet-activating factor (PAF), arachidonic acid metabolites, and several proteinases have been extensively studied and are important in the inhibition of animal venoms and toxins, in host defenses, pathogenesis of inflammatory diseases, and in tissue injury and repair.[3,4,7,9,11,28,50,62,63,71-74,82] A major distinction between the mast cells and basophils is in several, often abundant serine proteinases in mast cells[28,63,69,72,74,83] which are not major markers of basophils. These proteinases include tryptases, chymases, carboxypeptidase A3, and cathepsin C and G.[69,83] Indeed, proteinases are markers of human mast cell heterogeneity, with two major populations separated by their serine proteinase content, namely, those with tryptase only (MC_T) and those with both tryptase and chymase (MC_{TC}). A limited number of MC_C are also found. Recent work on proteinase-based mast cell heterogeneity in mice has established that even for one previously recognized phenotype, either mucosal mast cells[84] or connective tissue mast cells,[69] there can be tissue-specific differences in proteinase expression. Human basophils can express low levels of tryptases, but little or no chymase.[83] In the mouse, mast cell proteinase 8 (MCP8) and MCP11 are more abundant in basophils than mast cells; indeed, MCP8 has been targeted in two strains of engineered mice to constitutively or conditionally (e.g., diphtheria toxin-mediated) deplete basophils.[74]

Since initial observations in the 1980s, there has been extensive research on cytokine and chemokine production by mast cells and basophils (*Table 9.3*),[2,4,5,7,62,72] though much of this is based only on in vitro cell lines. While cytokine and chemokine mRNA may be detected, actual quantities of the encoded proteins may vary widely. For example, since basophils produce relatively large quantities of IL-4 and IL-13 (hundreds of picograms per 10^6 cells), they are considered important in vivo sources of these cytokines. Interestingly, mast cell granules are a source of both preformed and stored tumor necrosis factor (TNF).[85]

Mast cell–derived chemotactic factors can be important components of host defenses induced by viruses as well as by cancer.[86,87] Many cytokines produced by mast cells can act in an autocrine manner. For example, proinflammatory IL-33 is produced by mast cells[88] and activates mast cell functions,[89] and this pathway has been exploited for novel therapeutics.[90] IL-33 can also facilitate communication between basophils and mast cells,[91] further emphasizing that although basophils and mast cells are etiologically distinct, they may serve cooperative functions during allergic inflammation. Furthermore, the cytokine repertoire of mast cells is broad, representing those associated with both T_H1 and T_H2 phenotypes. It is likely, that in a given population of mast cells, cytokines are differentially expressed in individual cells or at different

times, or that individual mast cells express several functionally distinct cytokines. The control mechanisms that regulate production, secretion, and functions of individual cytokines in mast cells and basophils are not well understood, but can involve epigenetic modifications in the DNA.[92]

Inhibition of Basophil and Mast Cell Activation

Several anti-allergic and anti-inflammatory drugs inhibit the release of histamine and other mediators, including cytokines and chemokines and arachidonic acid metabolites from human basophils and/or mast cells (*Table 9.5*).[93-97] Although many of these drugs are valuable in the treatment of allergies and other inflammatory diseases, their mechanisms of action are diverse; none of the currently used drugs is mast cell–specific or basophil-specific, and the precise targets in vivo can be difficult to define. Furthermore, given the heterogeneity of mast cells at different tissue sites,[69] and perhaps even at different times during the evolution of an inflammatory insult, (e.g., initial injury, repair, chronic, or remodeling phases), agents may vary in the nature or extent of their modulatory effects on basophils and mast cells during the course of an inflammatory response or disease.

There are several promising advances in drug development targeting mast cells and basophils and their roles in allergic and other inflammatory processes. One major advance has been the development of humanized monoclonal antibodies to specific molecular targets such as IgE. Humanized monoclonal antibodies to IgE markedly reduce IgE levels and decrease the density of high-affinity IgE receptors on mast cells and basophils, thus limiting sensitivity to allergens. Because a prominent role has been demonstrated for skin mast cell hyperplasia, and consequent mast cell (and basophil) activation in the pathogenesis, diagnosis, and treatment of chronic spontaneous and induced urticaria, newer generation (nonsedating) antihistaminics and anti-IgE biologics are of proven benefit in these disorders.[94,96] Anti-IgE has also been reported to be effective and safe in the treatment of moderate to severe allergic asthma, some cases of atopic dermatitis, and persistent allergic rhinitis and is a promising new adjunctive treatment for food allergy.[94-97] Moreover, from this pioneering approach numerous other humanized monoclonal

Table 9.5. Inhibition of Mediator Secretion from Mast Cells and Basophils

Existing Drugs
β_2 Adrenergic agonists
Methylxanthines (nonselective phosphodiesterase inhibitors)
Antihistamines (H1–H4)
Sulfasalazine (or metabolites)
Corticosteroids
Cyclosporine A/Fk506
Ketotifen
Monoclonal antibodies (e.g., anti-IgE, anti-IL-5)
Sodium cromoglycate/nedocromil sodium (inhibit mast cells but not basophils)
Drugs in Development
Flavonoids (e.g., Quercetin)
Inhibitors of Syk, Bruton, and other kinases
Monoclonal antibodies to several biologic targets Chimeric or fusion proteins
Agonism of inhibitory receptors (eg, FcγRIIB, Siglec-8, CD300a, MRGPRs, LILRB$_4$; see text)

Abbreviations: IgE, immunoglobulin E; IL, interleukin.
For further details see, Harvima IT, Levi-Schaffer F, Draber P, et al. Molecular targets on mast cells and basophils for novel therapies. *J Allergy Clin Immunol.* 2014;134:530-544

antibody targets are being used in the clinic, including monoclonal antibodies to IL-4, IL-5, and/or their receptors, and others are in various phases of clinical testing, e.g., antibodies to IL-13 and TSLP.[95-98] The mechanisms of action of these antibodies are complex and in part likely involve direct or indirect effects on mast cells and basophils.

Other promising targets for drugs that would inhibit mast cell and basophil function include Bruton tyrosine kinase, Syk, and other kinases; the prostaglandin D_2 receptor CRTH2; c-kit, antiproteinases, and several inhibitory molecules expressed by mast cells and basophils that have immunoreceptor tyrosine-based inhibitory motifs, such as FcγRIIB, leukocyte Ig-like receptor B4, sialic acid–binding immunoglobulin-like lectin 8 (Siglec-8), CD200R; and CD300.[83,93,99-101] Interestingly, several mediators including IL-10, interferons, transforming growth factor (TGF)-ß, histamine, CD203c, and arachidonic acid metabolites produced by mast cells and basophils appear to have autocrine regulatory roles that could also be targeted to modulate the functions of these cells.[102]

Other approaches include the design of chimeric proteins for targeted elimination of FcεRI-expressing cells, selective initiation of inhibitory signaling pathways, and targeted ligation of surface inhibitor receptors such as FcγRIIb.[103] Although these strategies have proven effective at inhibiting mast cell activation in vitro, it is unclear whether they would be effective in a clinical setting. Small molecule inhibitors of mast cells and basophils have been extensively studied and many of these compounds are phytochemicals such as quercetin, resveratrol, and various phenolics and terpenes. Recently, inhibitors of non-IgE activation of mast cells through the MrgprX2 receptor have gained significant interest.[104]

BASOPHIL AND MAST CELL FUNCTIONS

Inflammatory Injury and Host Defenses

Basophils and mast cells are central players in allergic inflammation as they express high-affinity receptors for IgE and produce several mediators in common, each with potential to initiate inflammatory cascades and complex cellular and molecular networks involved in injury and repair (*Figure 9.4*). In early phases of allergic responses, the pool of circulating mature basophils and the large tissue repository of mast cells are important. However, basophils and mast cells are not restricted to these sites, because under certain circumstances a large influx of basophils can occur into local tissues (e.g., cutaneous basophilic hypersensitivity,[28] asthma[62]), and the numbers of mast cell progenitors in the circulation and in selected tissues can be increased

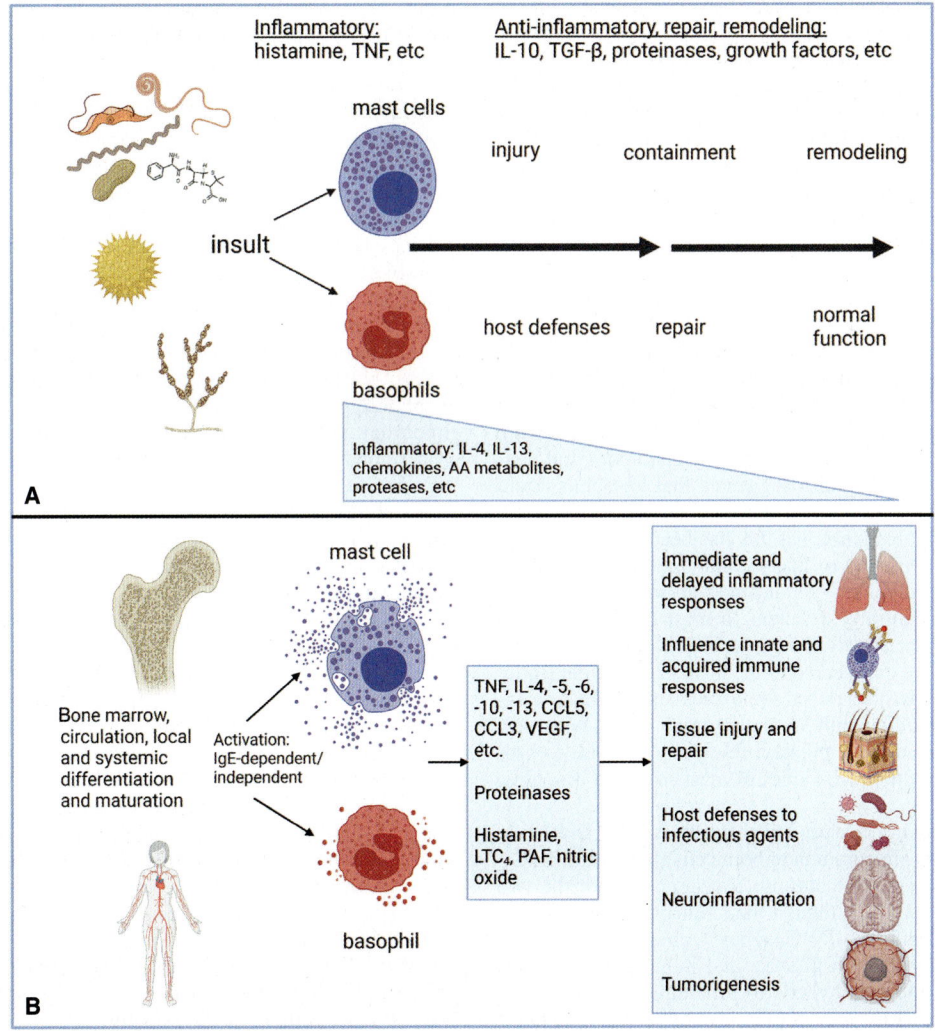

FIGURE 9.4 A, Model of activities of mast cells and basophils in the sequential responses of tissue injury, containment, repair, and remodeling. B, Summary of the activation of mast cells (MC) and basophils (Ba), the mediators they produce, and the spectrum of their actions in host defenses and tissue injury. AA, arachidonic acid; IL, interleukin; LTC_4, leukotriene C_4; PAF, platelet-activating factor; TGF, transforming growth factor; TNF, tumor necrosis factor; VEGF, vascular endothelial growth factor. Created with BioRender.com.

and differentiate.[7] Mast cells and basophils are important in allergic reactions such as food allergy, but it must also be noted that other cell types such as classical phagocytes also play roles.[105,106]

The roles of basophils and mast cells in inflammation differ with regard to some of the stimuli that are important for cell activation. Some mast cell populations respond to a number of basic secretagogues, including several neuropeptides, through newly recognized family of G-protein–coupled receptors MRGPR[68]; and given the close anatomical association between mast cells and nerves[11,107] and abundant evidence for their functional interdependence, it is likely that mast cell–dependent neurogenic pathways are important.[11] There is much less evidence for nerve-basophil interactions, although a recent study demonstrated the role of basophil-nerve communication in mast cell–independent acute itch.[70] It is intriguing that IgE receptors exist on neurons,[108] and although the clinical significance of this observation is unknown, the implications are considerable. For example, depending upon the distribution of IgE receptors on neurons in the central nervous system as well as peripherally, allergens could communicate directly with the nervous system and impact sensory pathways, central processing, or efferent responses, as well[2] as cognition and behavior. Such pathways might help explain associations between stress, depression and allergy.[109,110]

Since early the earliest reports of the role of mast cells in innate antimicrobial immunity, there has been great interest in expression and function of TLRs on mast cells and basophils.[2,9,71,72] There is increasing evidence that the profiles of mediators produced by these pathways differ from those following IgE-mediated activation; knowledge of such differences will help elucidate the distinct roles of these two cell types in host defenses and inflammatory diseases.[72,111] For example, recent evidence that mast cells produce extracellular DNA traps as part of their antimicrobial repertoire raises critical questions about the activation and signaling pathways involved and the potential therapeutic opportunities that such knowledge might uncover.[112] Similarly, the pathways involved in antiviral activities by mast cells and potentially by basophils are beginning to be unraveled.[9,10] Interestingly, there is a growing literature about the use of mast cell activators as adjuvants for vaccination, enhancing primary antimicrobial responses.[113]

The role of mast cells and basophils in the development and expression of adaptive immunity has also been an exciting area of new knowledge, albeit with some controversy.[72,111] Both mast cells and basophils can enter draining lymph nodes[111] and mast cells are well known to induce dendritic cell traffic to lymph nodes and dendritic cell priming.[111] Initial studies suggested that basophils could act as dendritic cells, especially in responses to protease-containing allergens eliciting a T_H2 response, but this has been challenged and the published effects attributed to likely contamination of enriched basophils with dendritic cells.[72] As outlined above, the use of W mutant mice that are naturally deficient in mast cells has been a powerful tool to study mast cell functions, but recent work in two additional strains of mice engineered to be mast cell deficient (independent of mutations in *kit*) has raised some questions about the conclusions from earlier studies with W mutant mice.[114,115] With new and powerful tools and models, the next few years promise to provide more clarity about the precise roles of mast cells and basophils in immunity.[74,116]

A spectrum of mediators is produced by mast cells and basophils. Several mediators are common to both cells (histamine, LTC_4, PAF, etc), whereas the cytokine and proteinase profiles of the two cells types are distinct (above), though their functional significance remains to be fully clarified.[83,115] Caughey[83] nicely reviewed the association of MCPs with both allergic and nonallergic diseases ranging from asthma and anaphylaxis to inflammatory bowel disease, autoimmune arthritis, atherosclerosis, hypertension, heart failure, and fibrotic conditions of the lungs and other organs.[117] Knockout of MCPs in mouse models has rapidly expanded our knowledge of some of the functions of these abundant and diverse enzymes. For example, mouse MCP4 has an anti-inflammatory effect in allergic asthma but is proinflammatory in models of bullous pemphigoid.[83,118] Mouse MCP4 and mast cell carboxypeptidase A3 are important in degradation of several animal toxins, for example, snake, Gila monster, and scorpion venom.[115] Basophil-derived MCP11 induces microvascular leakage in mice, independent of mast cells.[119] Since mast cells release all of their granule contents, it has been suggested that even lysosomal enzymes serve an important function in bacterial infection.[120]

Containment of Injury, Initiation of Repair, Remodeling, and Normal Function

Following initial insult and injury, the inflammatory response elaborates mediators and pathways that minimize the extent of the tissue damage and begin repair processes. In addition to early activation, mast cell and basophil mediators are involved in these phases of the response. Histamine, arachidonic acid metabolites, and several cytokines, particularly, IL-1, IL-6, IL-10, TNF, and TGF-β, have several effects on endothelial, epithelial, mesenchymal, and inflammatory cells. Such effects include influences on epithelial and endothelial integrity and function, regulation of blood flow and vascular permeability, tissue edema, fibroblast proliferation and biochemical phenotype, and others. The involvement of mast cells in tissue injury, repair, and remodeling has been studied in several conditions,[121-125] and it is obvious that the pathways involved are multifactorial. As murine knockout models are more widely employed to address these questions, we will begin to better understand the role of mast cells and basophils in this "containment and repair phase" of inflammatory injury.

Once the site of injury is contained and repair processes have begun, mast cells and perhaps basophils are likely to be involved in the remodeling of the tissues and the return to normal function. The numerous proteinases of mast cells have distinct substrate specificities, and restructuring of the extracellular matrix in the local environment is very likely to be among their functions. Cytokines such as TGF-β, IL-1, IL-6, and IL-13 that influence the activities of fibroblasts are likely to be important candidates for this remodeling phase in the responses to injury. Given the life span and normal distribution of mast cells and basophils, an attractive hypothesis is that basophils play a particularly important role in the injury phase, but their importance in the latter phases (containment and remodeling) is minimal. By contrast, mast cells are undoubtedly important not only in the injury phase but also in the containment and remodeling phases. Given the multiplicity of mast cell phenotypes, it may be that there is a general pattern of expression of functionally linked clusters of mast cell genes[69] that, in a carefully orchestrated manner, facilitates the evolving roles of local mast cell populations in the three phases of injury, containment, and repair/remodeling.[126]

Dynamic Equilibrium and Homeostasis

In addition to the evolving mast cell phenotype outlined above, some subsets of mast cells are involved in normal tissue homeostasis, such as neurogenic and endocrine responses.[127-129] Although these aspects of mast cell function are not well understood, there is a diverse, largely correlative, literature on mast cell involvement in such processes as sexual behavior, implantation, parturition, neuroendocrine signaling, the hypothalamic-pituitary-adrenal axis, gastric acid secretion, bone metabolism, and myelopoiesis. Furthermore, given the prominent anatomical association between mast cells and the vasculature, and the effects of mast cell products on blood flow, permeability, and leukocyte adhesion and diapedesis in inflammation,[130] it is widely held that one normal physiologic role of mast cells is in the dynamic regulation of tissue perfusion and the chemical and cellular composition of extravascular spaces. To date, little direct evidence exists that basophils exhibit similar functions within tissues; rather, the basophil appears to be mostly involved in a rapid, circulating response with potential for recruitment to sites of injury and involvement in host defenses and their regulation. The application of selected, conditional knockout models to these processes will help clarify the roles of mast cells and basophils. In addition, exciting advances in cell and molecular biology, such as the role of exosomes and microRNAs in cell communication and regulation,[17-21] will likely take our knowledge and its potential application into novel directions.

References

1. Selye H. *The Mast Cells.* Butterworths; 1965.
2. Varricchi G, Raap U, Rivellese F, Marone G, Gibbs BF. Human mast cells and basophils—How are they similar how are they different? *Immunol Rev.* 2018;282:8-34.
3. Olivera A, Rivera J. Paradigm shifts in mast cell and basophil biology and function: an emerging view of immune regulation in health and disease. In: Gibbs B, Falcone F, eds. *Basophils and Mast Cells. Methods in Molecular Biology.* Vol 2163. Humana; 2020:3-31.
4. Galli SJ, Gaudenzio N, Tsai M. Mast cells in inflammation and disease: recent progress and ongoing concerns. *Annu Rev Immunol.* 2020;38:49-77.
5. Moon TC, Befus AD, Kulka M. Mast cell mediators: their differential release and the secretory pathways involved. *Front Immunol.* 2014;5:569.
6. Redegeld FA, Yu Y, Kumari S, Charles N, Blank U. Non-IgE mediated mast cell activation. *Immunol Rev.* 2018;282:87-113.
7. Dahlin JS, Maurer M, Metcalfe DD, Pejler G, Sagi-Eisenberg R, Nilsson G. The ingenious mast cell: contemporary insights into mast cell behavior and function. *Allergy.* 2022;77(1):83-99. doi:10.1111/all.14881.
8. Valent P, Akin C, Hartmann K, et al. Mast cells as a unique hematopoietic lineage and cell system: from Paul Ehrlich's visions to precision medicine concepts. *Theranostics.* 2020;10:10743-10768.
9. Marshall JS, Portales-Cervantes L, Leong E. Mast cell responses to viruses and pathogen products. *Int J Mol Sci.* 2019;20(17):4241.
10. Jimenez M, Cervantes-Garcia D, Cordova-Davalos LE, Perez-Rodriguez MJ, Gonzalez-Espinosa C, Salinas E. Responses of mast cells to pathogens: beneficial and detrimental roles. *Front Immunol.* 2021;12:685865.
11. Forsythe P. Mast cells in neuroimmune interactions. *Trends Neurosci.* 2019; 42:43-55.
12. Plum T, Wang X, Rettel M, Krijgsveld J, Feyerabend TB, Rodewald HR. Human mast cell proteome reveals unique lineage, putative functions, and structural basis for cell ablation. *Immunity.* 2020;52:404-416 e405.
13. Ranzoni AM, Tangherloni A, Berest I, et al. Integrative single-cell RNA-seq and ATAC-seq analysis of human developmental hematopoiesis. *Cell Stem Cell.* 2021;28:472-487 e477.
14. Dvorak AM. Ultrastructural studies of human basophils and mast cells. *J Histochem Cytochem.* 2005;53:1043-1070.
15. Abdel Hafez SMN. Age related changes in the dermal mast cells and the associated changes in the dermal collagen and cells: A histological and electron microscopy study. *Acta Histochem.* 2019;121:619-627.
16. Chen HY, Chiang DM, Lin ZJ, et al. Nanoimaging granule dynamics and subcellular structures in activated mast cells using soft X-ray tomography. *Sci Rep.* 2016;6:34879.
17. Valadi H, Ekstrom K, Bossios A, Sjostrand M, Lee JJ, Lotvall JO. Exosome-mediated transfer of mRNAs and microRNAs is a novel mechanism of genetic exchange between cells. *Nat Cell Biol.* 2007;9:654-659.
18. Veerappan A, Thompson M, Savage AR, et al. Mast cells and exosomes in hyperoxia-induced neonatal lung disease. *Am J Physiol Lung Cell Mol Physiol.* 2016;310:L1218-1232.
19. Canas JA, Rodrigo-Munoz JM, Gil-Martinez M, Sastre B, del Pozo V. Exosomes: a key piece in asthmatic inflammation. *Int J Mol Sci.* 2021;22:963.
20. Hu L, Si L, Dai X, et al. Exosomal miR-409-3p secreted from activated mast cells promotes microglial migration, activation and neuroinflammation by targeting Nr4a2 to activate the NF-kappaB pathway. *J Neuroinflammation.* 2021;18:68.
21. Kim DK, Bandara G, Cho YE, et al. Mastocytosis-derived extracellular vesicles deliver miR-23a and miR-30a into pre-osteoblasts and prevent osteoblastogenesis and bone formation. *Nat Commun.* 2021;12:2527.
22. Toyoshima S, Sakamoto-Sasaki T, Kurosawa Y, et al. miR103a-3p in extracellular vesicles from FcepsilonRI-aggregated human mast cells enhances IL-5 production by group 2 innate lymphoid cells. *J Allergy Clin Immunol.* 2021;147:1878-1891.
23. Gaudenzio N, Sibilano R, Marichal T, et al. Different activation signals induce distinct mast cell degranulation strategies. *J Clin Invest.* 2016;126:3981-3998.
24. Kunder CA, St John AL, Li G, et al. Mast cell-derived particles deliver peripheral signals to remote lymph nodes. *J Exp Med.* 2009;206:2455-2467.
25. Sandhu JK, Kulka M. Decoding mast cell-microglia communication in neurodegenerative diseases. *Int J Mol Sci.* 2021;22(2):1093.
26. Vicario M, Guilarte M, Alonso C, et al. Chronological assessment of mast cell-mediated gut dysfunction and mucosal inflammation in a rat model of chronic psychosocial stress. *Brain Behav Immun.* 2010;24:1166-1175.
27. Caruso RA, Parisi A, Crisafulli C, et al. Intraepithelial infiltration by mast cells in human Helicobacter pylori active gastritis. *Ultrastruct Pathol.* 2011;35:251-255.
28. Schwartz C, Eberle JU, Voehringer D. Basophils in inflammation. *Eur J Pharmacol.* 2016;778:90-95.
29. Blank U, Madera-Salcedo IK, Danelli L, et al. Vesicular trafficking and signaling for cytokine and chemokine secretion in mast cells. *Front Immunol.* 2014;5:453.
30. Ferjan I, Lipnik-Stangelj M. Chronic pain treatment: the influence of tricyclic antidepressants on serotonin release and uptake in mast cells. *Mediators Inflamm.* 2013;2013:340473.
31. Yamada T, Ushio H, Niyonsaba F, Okumura K, Ikeda S, Ogawa H. Roles of autophagy in degranulation and regranulation of mast cells. *J Derm Sci.* 2016;84:e75.
32. Elsaid R, Soares-da-Silva F, Peixoto M, et al. Hematopoiesis: a layered organization across chordate species. *Front Cell Dev Biol.* 2020;8:606642.
33. Gentek R, Ghigo C, Hoeffel G, et al. Hemogenic endothelial fate mapping reveals dual developmental origin of mast cells. *Immunity.* 2018;48:1160-1171 e1165.
34. Popescu DM, Botting RA, Stephenson E, et al. Decoding human fetal liver haematopoiesis. *Nature.* 2019;574:365-371.
35. Drew E, Huettner CS, Tenen DG, McNagny KM. CD34 expression by mast cells: of mice and men. *Blood.* 2005;106:1885-1887.
36. Arinobu Y, Iwasaki H, Gurish MF, et al. Developmental checkpoints of the basophil/mast cell lineages in adult murine hematopoiesis. *Proc Natl Acad Sci U S A.* 2005;102:18105-18110.
37. Franco CB, Chen CC, Drukker M, Weissman IL, Galli SJ. Distinguishing mast cell and granulocyte differentiation at the single-cell level. *Cell Stem Cell.* 2010;6:361-368.
38. Rodewald HR, Dessing M, Dvorak AM, Galli SJ. Identification of a committed precursor for the mast cell lineage. *Science.* 1996;271:818-822.
39. Cantor AB, Iwasaki H, Arinobu Y, et al. Antagonism of FOG-1 and GATA factors in fate choice for the mast cell lineage. *J Exp Med.* 2008;205:611-624.
40. Walsh JC, DeKoter RP, Lee HJ, et al. Cooperative and antagonistic interplay between PU.1 and GATA-2 in the specification of myeloid cell fates. *Immunity.* 2002;17:665-676.
41. Nakano T, Sonoda T, Hayashi C, et al. Fate of bone marrow-derived cultured mast cells after intracutaneous intraperitoneal and intravenous transfer into genetically mast cell-deficient W/Wv mice. Evidence that cultured mast cells can give rise to both connective tissue type and mucosal mast cells. *J Exp Med.* 1985;162:1025-1043.
42. Leslie M. Immunology. Mouse studies challenge rare immune cell's powers. *Science.* 2010;329:1595.
43. Hui CC, McNagny KM, Denburg JA, Siracusa MC. In situ hematopoiesis: a regulator of TH2 cytokine-mediated immunity and inflammation at mucosal surfaces. *Mucosal Immunol.* 2015;8:701-711.
44. Grootens J, Ungerstedt JS, Ekoff M, et al. Single-cell analysis reveals the KIT D816V mutation in haematopoietic stem and progenitor cells in systemic mastocytosis. *EBioMedicine.* 2019;43:150-158.
45. Zappulla JP, Dubreuil P, Desbois S, et al. Mastocytosis in mice expressing human Kit receptor with the activating Asp816Val mutation. *J Exp Med.* 2005;202:1635-1641.
46. Babina M, Wang Z, Franke K, Zuberbier T. Thymic stromal lymphopoietin promotes MRGPRX2-triggered degranulation of skin mast cells in a STAT5-dependent manner with further support from JNK. *Cells.* 2021;10(1):102.
47. Siracusa MC, Saenz SA, Hill DA, et al. TSLP promotes interleukin-3-independent basophil haematopoiesis and type 2 inflammation. *Nature.* 2011;477:229-233.
48. Ziegler SF, Artis D. Sensing the outside world: TSLP regulates barrier immunity. *Nat Immunol.* 2010;11:289-293.
49. Roediger B, Weninger W. Group 2 innate lymphoid cells in the regulation of immune responses. *Adv Immunol.* 2015;125:111-154.
50. Hill DA, Siracusa MC, Abt MC, et al. Commensal bacteria-derived signals regulate basophil hematopoiesis and allergic inflammation. *Nat Med.* 2012;18:538-546.
51. Msallam R, Balla J, Rathore APS, et al. Fetal mast cells mediate postnatal allergic responses dependent on maternal IgE. *Science.* 2020;370:941-950.
52. Denburg JA, Telizyn S, Messner H, et al. Heterogeneity of human peripheral blood eosinophil-type colonies: Evidence for a common basophil-eosinophil progenitor. *Blood.* 1985;66:312-318.
53. Denburg JA. Basophil and mast cell lineages in vitro and in vivo. *Blood.* 1992;79:846-860.
54. Denburg JA, Telizyn S, Belda A, Dolovich J, Bienenstock J. Increased numbers of circulating basophil progenitors in atopic patients. *J Allergy Clin Immunol.* 1985;76:466-472.
55. Menzies-Gow A, Flood-Page P, Sehmi R, et al. Anti-IL-5 (mepolizumab) therapy induces bone marrow eosinophil maturational arrest and decreases eosinophil progenitors in the bronchial mucosa of atopic asthmatics. *J Allergy Clin Immunol.* 2003;111:714-719.
56. Salter BM, Oliveria JP, Nusca G, et al. IL-25 and IL-33 induce Type 2 inflammation in basophils from subjects with allergic asthma. *Respir Res.* 2016;17:5.
57. Tsuzuki H, Arinobu Y, Miyawaki K, et al. Functional interleukin-33 receptors are expressed in early progenitor stages of allergy-related granulocytes. *Immunology.* 2017;150:64-73.
58. Dahlin JS, Malinovschi A, Ohrvik H, et al. Lin- CD34hi CD117int/hi FcepsilonRI+ cells in human blood constitute a rare population of mast cell progenitors. *Blood.* 2016;127:383-391.
59. Martin DIK, Zon LI, Mutter G, Orkin SH. Expression of an erythroid transcription factor in megakaryocytic and mast cell lineages. *Nature.* 1990;344:444-447.
60. Garcia-Montero AC, Jara-Acevedo M, Alvarez-Twose I, et al. KIT D816V-mutated bone marrow mesenchymal stem cells in indolent systemic mastocytosis are associated with disease progression. *Blood.* 2016;127:761-768.

The Normal Hematologic System

61. Theoharides TC, Valent P, Akin C. Mast cells, mastocytosis, and related disorders. *N Engl J Med.* 2015;373:163-172.

62. Schroeder JT. Basophils beyond effector cells of allergic inflammation. *Adv Immunol.* 2009;101:123-161.

63. Daeron M. Innate myeloid cells under the control of adaptive immunity: the example of mast cells and basophils. *Curr Opin Immunol.* 2016;38:101-108.

64. Kanagaratham C, El Ansari YS, Lewis OL, Oettgen HC. IgE and IgG antibodies as regulators of mast cell and basophil functions in food allergy. *Front Immunol.* 2020;11:603050.

65. Chen K, Xu W, Wilson M, et al. Immunoglobulin D enhances immune surveillance by activating antimicrobial, proinflammatory and B cell-stimulating programs in basophils. *Nat Immunol.* 2009;10:889-898.

66. Shan M, Carrillo J, Yeste A, et al. Secreted IgD amplifies humoral T Helper 2 cell responses by binding basophils via galectin-9 and CD44. *Immunity.* 2018;49:709-724 e708.

67. Zhai GT, Wang H, Li JX, et al. IgD-activated mast cells induce IgE synthesis in B cells in nasal polyps. *J Allergy Clin Immunol.* 2018;142:1489-1499 e1423.

68. McNeil BD, Pundir P, Meeker S, et al. Identification of a mast-cell-specific receptor crucial for pseudo-allergic drug reactions. *Nature.* 2015;519:237-241.

69. Dwyer DF, Barrett NA, Austen KF; Immunological Genome Project Consortium. Expression profiling of constitutive mast cells reveals a unique identity within the immune system. *Nat Immunol.* 2016;17:878-887.

70. Wang F, Trier AM, Li F, et al. A basophil-neuronal axis promotes itch. *Cell.* 2021;184:422-440 e417.

71. Reber LL, Sibilano R, Mukai K, Galli SJ. Potential effector and immunoregulatory functions of mast cells in mucosal immunity. *Mucosal Immunol.* 2015;8:444-463.

72. Steiner M, Huber S, Harrer A, Himly M. The evolution of human basophil biology from neglect towards understanding of their immune functions. *BioMed Res Int.* 2016;2016:8232830.

73. Ohnmacht C, Schwartz C, Panzer M, Schiedewitz I, Naumann R, Voehringer D. Basophils orchestrate chronic allergic dermatitis and protective immunity against helminths. *Immunity.* 2010;33:364-374.

74. Karasuyama H, Mukai K, Obata K, Tsujimura Y, Wada T. Nonredundant roles of basophils in immunity. *Annu Rev Immunol.* 2011;29:45-69.

75. Saito H, Hatake K, Dvorak AM, et al. Selective differentiation and proliferation of hematopoietic cells induced by recombinant human interleukins. *Proc Natl Acad Sci U S A.* 1988;85:2288-2292.

76. Groot Kormelink T, Askenase PW, Redegeld FA. Immunobiology of antigen-specific immunoglobulin free light chains in chronic inflammatory diseases. *Curr Pharm Des.* 2012;18:2278-2289.

77. Bochner BS, Schleimer RP. Mast cells, basophils, and eosinophils: distinct but overlapping pathways for recruitment. *Immunol Rev.* 2001;179:5-15.

78. Biggs L, Yu C, Fedoric B, Lopez AF, Galli SJ, Grimbaldeston MA. Evidence that vitamin D(3) promotes mast cell-dependent reduction of chronic UVB-induced skin pathology in mice. *J Exp Med.* 2010;207:455-463.

79. Gorczynski RM, Chen Z, Khatri I, Yu K. Graft-infiltrating cells expressing a CD200 transgene prolong allogeneic skin graft survival in association with local increases in Foxp3(+)Treg and mast cells. *Transpl Immunol.* 2011;25:187-193.

80. Cho KA, Suh JW, Sohn JH, et al. IL-33 induces Th17-mediated airway inflammation via mast cells in ovalbumin-challenged mice. *Am J Physiol: Lung Cell Mol Physiol.* 2012;302:L429-L440.

81. Roan F, Bell BD, Stoklasek TA, Kitajima M, Han H, Ziegler SF. The multiple facets of thymic stromal lymphopoietin (TSLP) during allergic inflammation and beyond. *J Leukoc Biol.* 2012;91:877-886. doi:10.1189/jlb.1211622.

82. Virk H, Arthur G, Bradding P. Mast cells and their activation in lung disease. *Transl Res.* 2016;174:60-76.

83. Caughey GH. Mast cell proteases as pharmacological targets. *Eur J Pharmacol.* 2016;778:44-55.

84. Xing W, Austen KF, Gurish MF, Jones TG. Protease phenotype of constitutive connective tissue and of induced mucosal mast cells in mice is regulated by the tissue. *Proc Natl Acad Sci U S A.* 2011;108:14210-14215.

85. Gordon JR, Galli SJ. Mast cells as a source of both preformed and immunologically inducible TNF-alpha/cachectin. *Nature.* 1990;346:274-276.

86. Oldford SA, Haidl ID, Howatt MA, Leiva CA, Johnston B, Marshall JS. A critical role for mast cells and mast cell-derived IL-6 in TLR2-mediated inhibition of tumor growth. *J Immunol.* 2010;185:7067-7076.

87. McAlpine SM, Issekutz TB, Marshall JS. Virus stimulation of human mast cells results in the recruitment of CD56 T cells by a mechanism dependent on CCR5 ligands. *FASEB J.* 2012;26:1280-1289.

88. Hsu CL, Neilsen CV, Bryce PJ. IL-33 is produced by mast cells and regulates IgE-dependent inflammation. *PLoS One.* 2010;5:e11944.

89. Kato Y, Morikawa T, Kato E, et al. Involvement of activation of mast cells via IgE signaling and epithelial cell-derived cytokines in the pathogenesis of pollen food allergy syndrome in a murine model. *J Immunol.* 2021;206(12):2791-2802.

90. Okragly AJ, Corwin KB, Elia M, et al. Generation and characterization of torudokimab (LY3375880): a monoclonal antibody that neutralizes Interleukin-33. *J Inflamm Res.* 2021;14:3823-3835.

91. Hsu CL, Chhiba KD, Krier-Burris R, et al. Allergic inflammation is initiated by IL-33-dependent crosstalk between mast cells and basophils. *PLoS One.* 2020;15:e0226701.

92. Monticelli S, Lee DU, Nardone J, Bolton DL, Rao A. Chromatin-based regulation of cytokine transcription in Th2 cells and mast cells. *Int Immunol.* 2005;17:1513-1524.

93. Harvima IT, Levi-Schaffer F, Draber P, et al. Molecular targets on mast cells and basophils for novel therapies. *J Allergy Clin Immunol.* 2014;134:530-544.

94. Zhao ZT, Ji CM, Yu WJ, et al. Omalizumab for the treatment of chronic spontaneous urticaria: A meta-analysis of randomized clinical trials. *J Allergy Clin Immunol.* 2016;137:1742-1750 e1744.

95. Pelaia C, Crimi C, Vatrella A, Tinello C, Terracciano R, Pelaia G. Molecular targets for biological therapies of severe asthma. *Front Immunol.* 2020;11:603312.

96. Kolkhir P, Altrichter S, Munoz M, Hawro T, Maurer M. New treatments for chronic urticaria. *Ann Allergy Asthma Immunol.* 2020;124:2-12.

97. Paranjape A, Tsai M, Mukai K, et al. Oral immunotherapy and basophil and mast cell reactivity in food allergy. *Front Immunol.* 2020;11:602660.

98. Canonica GW, Senna G, Mitchell PD, O'Byrne PM, Passalacqua G, Varricchi G. Therapeutic interventions in severe asthma. *World Allergy Organ J.* 2016;9:40.

99. Dispenza MC, Krier-Burris RA, Chhiba KD, Undem BJ, Robida PA, Bochner BS. Bruton's tyrosine kinase inhibition effectively protects against human IgE-mediated anaphylaxis. *J Clin Invest.* 2020;130:4759-4770.

100. Kupczyk M, Kuna P. Targeting the PGD2/CRTH2/DP1 signaling pathway in asthma and allergic disease: current status and future perspectives. *Drugs.* 2017;77:1281-1294.

101. Gebremeskel S, Schanin J, Coyle KM, et al. Mast cell and eosinophil activation are associated with COVID-19 and TLR-mediated viral inflammation: implications for an anti-Siglec-8 antibody. *Front Immunol.* 2021;12:650331.

102. Tsai SH, Kinoshita M, Kusu T, et al. The ectoenzyme E-NPP3 negatively regulates ATP-dependent chronic allergic responses by basophils and mast cells. *Immunity.* 2015;42:279-293.

103. Zhang K, Zhu D, Kepley C, Terada T, Saxon A. Chimeric human fcgamma-allergen fusion proteins in the prevention of allergy. *Immunol Allergy Clin North Am.* 2007;27:93-103.

104. Roy S, Chompunud Na Ayudhya C, Thapaliya M, Deepak V, Ali H. Multifaceted MRGPRX2: new insight into the role of mast cells in health and disease. *J Allergy Clin Immunol.* 2021;148:293-308.

105. Arias K, Chu DK, Flader K, et al. Distinct immune effector pathways contribute to the full expression of peanut-induced anaphylactic reactions in mice. *J Allergy Clin Immunol.* 2011;127:1552-1561 e1551.

106. Reber LL, Marichal T, Mukai K, et al. Selective ablation of mast cells or basophils reduces peanut-induced anaphylaxis in mice. *J Allergy Clin Immunol.* 2013;132:881-888 e881-811.

107. Dong H, Wang Y, Zhang X, et al. Stabilization of brain mast cells alleviates LPS-induced neuroinflammation by inhibiting microglia activation. *Front Cell Neurosci.* 2019;13:191.

108. van der Kleij H, Charles N, Karimi K, et al. Evidence for neuronal expression of functional Fc (epsilon and gamma) receptors. *J Allergy Clin Immunol.* 2010;125:757-760.

109. Van Lieshout RJ, Bienenstock J, MacQueen GM. A review of candidate pathways underlying the association between asthma and major depressive disorder. *Psychosom Med.* 2009;71:187-195.

110. Tao R, Fu Z, Xiao L. Chronic food antigen-specific IgG-mediated hypersensitivity reaction as a risk factor for adolescent depressive disorder. *Genomics Proteomics Bioinformatics.* 2019;17:183-189.

111. Abraham SN, St John AL. Mast cell-orchestrated immunity to pathogens. *Nat Rev Immunol.* 2010;10:440-452.

112. Elieh Ali Komi D, Kuebler WM. Significance of mast cell formed extracellular traps in microbial defense. *Clin Rev Allergy Immunol.* 2022;62(1):160-179. doi:10.1007/s12016-021-08861-6.

113. Johnson-Weaver BT, Choi HW, Yang H, et al. Nasal immunization with small molecule mast cell activators enhance immunity to co-administered subunit immunogens. *Front Immunol.* 2021;12:730346.

114. Katz HR, Austen KF. Mast cell deficiency, a game of kit and mouse. *Immunity.* 2011;35:668-670.

115. Galli SJ, Tsai M, Marichal T, Tchougounova E, Reber LL, Pejler G. Approaches for analyzing the roles of mast cells and their proteases in vivo. *Adv Immunol.* 2015;126:45-127.

116. Feyerabend TB, Gutierrez DA, Rodewald HR. Of mouse models of mast cell deficiency and metabolic syndrome. *Cell Metab.* 2016;24:1-2.

117. Krystel-Whittemore M, Dileepan KN, Wood JG. Mast cell: a multi-functional master cell. *Front Immunol.* 2015;6:620.

118. Lin L, Bankaitis E, Heimbach L, et al. Dual targets for mouse mast cell protease-4 in mediating tissue damage in experimental bullous pemphigoid. *J Biol Chem.* 2011;286:37358-37367.

119. Yamagishi H, Mochizuki Y, Hamakubo T, et al. Basophil-derived mouse mast cell protease 11 induces microvascular leakage and tissue edema in a mast cell-independent manner. *Biochem Biophys Res Commun.* 2011;415:709-713.

120. Fukuishi N, Murakami S, Ohno A, et al. Does beta-hexosaminidase function only as a degranulation indicator in mast cells? The primary role of beta-hexosaminidase in mast cell granules. *J Immunol.* 2014;193:1886-1894.

121. Garbuzenko E, Nagler A, Pickholtz D, et al. Human mast cells stimulate fibroblast proliferation, collagen synthesis and lattice contraction: a direct role for mast cells in skin fibrosis. *Clin Exp Allergy.* 2002;32:237-246.

122. Margulis A, Nocka KH, Brennan AM, et al. Mast cell-dependent contraction of human airway smooth muscle cell-containing collagen gels: influence of cytokines, matrix metalloproteases, and serine proteases. *J Immunol.* 2009;183:1739-1750.

123. Monument MJ, Hart DA, Salo PT, Befus AD, Hildebrand KA. Neuroinflammatory mechanisms of connective tissue fibrosis: targeting neurogenic and mast cell contributions. *Adv Wound Care (New Rochelle)*. 2015;4:137-151.

124. Tellechea A, Leal EC, Kafanas A, et al. Mast cells regulate wound healing in diabetes. *Diabetes*. 2016;65:2006-2019.

125. Arbi S, Eksteen EC, Oberholzer HM, Taute H, Bester MJ. Premature collagen fibril formation, fibroblast-mast cell interactions and mast cell-mediated phagocytosis of collagen in keloids. *Ultrastruct Pathol*. 2015;39:95-103.

126. Ud-Din S, Wilgus TA, Bayat A. Mast cells in skin scarring: a review of animal and human research. *Front Immunol*. 2020;11:552205.

127. Befus D. Reciprocal interactions between mast cells and the endocrine system. In: Freier S, ed. *The Neuroendocrine-immune Network*. CRC Press; 1990: 39-52.

128. Maurer M, Theoharides T, Granstein RD, et al. What is the physiological function of mast cells? *Exp Dermatol*. 2003;12:886-910.

129. Loewendorf AI, Matynia A, Saribekyan H, Gross N, Csete M, Harrington M. Roads less traveled: sexual dimorphism and mast cell contributions to migraine pathology. *Front Immunol*. 2016;7:140.

130. Gaboury JP, Niu XF, Kubes P. Nitric oxide inhibits numerous features of mast cell-induced inflammation. *Circulation*. 1996;93:318-326.

The Normal Hematologic System

Chapter 10 ■ Monocytes, Macrophages, and Dendritic Cells

MATTHEW COLLIN • VENETIA BIGLEY • FLORENT GINHOUX

ABBREVIATIONS (IN ORDER OF APPEARANCE)

DC	dendritic cell(s)
RES	reticuloendothelial system
MPS	mononuclear phagocyte system
LC	Langerhans cell
GMP	granulocyte-macrophage progenitors
SLAN	sulfo LacNAc
LPS	lipopolysaccharide
CNS	central nervous system
IFN	interferon
EMP	erythromyeloid progenitors
HSC	hematopoietic stem cell
LMPP	lymphoid-primed multipotent progenitors
CLR	C-type lectin
PRR	Pattern recognition receptor
TLR	Toll-like receptor
NLR	NOD-like receptor
RLR	RIG-I-like receptor
LCH	Langerhans cell histiocytosis
ECD	Erdheim-Chester disease
RDD	Rosai Dorfman disease
HLH	hemophagocytic lymphohistiocytosis
GVHD	graft-vs-host disease

Gene symbols have been adopted with commonly used alternative names in parentheses, with the exception of the following where the more common name is used:

CD11b	ITGAM
CD11c	ITGAX
CD16	FCGR3A
CD13	ANPEP
CD123	IL3RA
CD169	SIGLEC1
CD141	THBD
M-CSF	CSF1
GM-CSF	CSF2
IL-12	IL12A/B heterodimer
RANK ligand	TNFSF11

INTRODUCTION

Monocytes, macrophages, and dendritic cells are myeloid cells that play fundamental roles in host defense, immune regulation, development, and tissue homeostasis. The earliest macrophages appear in the yolk sac of the embryo and colonize tissues widely including the hematopoietic and lymphoid organs, developing brain, and epidermis. Some of these populations remain stable, slowly self-renewing for the life of an organism. Monocytes are produced by fetal liver and bone marrow hematopoiesis and circulate in the peripheral blood. They have a prominent ability to respond rapidly to inflammatory insults, amplifying the recruitment of neutrophils and lymphoid cells in acute and chronic inflammation. They also migrate into tissues where they replenish some populations of tissue macrophages in the steady state. During inflammation, monocytes and their derivatives play a prominent role in phagocytosis, antigen presentation, and, ultimately, resolution and healing. Dendritic cells (DC) formed by definitive hematopoiesis are found in the blood, epithelial tissues, and lymphoid organs. They form a bridge between innate and adaptive immune systems by capturing antigen and presenting epitopes to

T cells governing tolerance, immunity, and the polarity of responses. Owing to the prominence of infection, inflammation, and immunity in pathology, monocytes, macrophages, and DC are involved in a wide range of clinical disorders (*Figure 10.1*).

Historical Perspective

The Reticuloendothelial System

The ability of macrophages to phagocytose foreign bodies was observed in the late nineteenth century and correctly surmised, by Metchnikoff, to be a form of host defense. Phagocytosis was an early hallmark of "cellular" immunity and was initially pitted against "humoral" immunity as the dominant form of resistance to infectious organisms. Early in the twentieth century, two discoveries reconciled these positions: the ability of antibody or complement to opsonize a particle and to accelerate phagocytosis and the dependency of antibody formation upon the uptake and presentation of antigens by phagocytes.[1] Macrophages of mammals are components of the reticuloendothelial system (RES), defined, by Aschoff in 1922, as the network of cells able to take up vital dyes injected intravenously or into tissues. The wider RES encompassed endothelium and fibroblasts; however, the most marked uptake of dye was observed in phagocytes. These techniques identified prominent populations of macrophages in the red pulp and sinuses of the spleen, bone marrow, lymph nodes, liver, adrenals, hypophysis, and connective tissues. Independent studies subsequently added the microglia of the brain and alveolar macrophages. This work defined many of the macrophage populations that are relevant today and was important in forming the basis of the mononuclear phagocyte system (MPS).

The Mononuclear Phagocyte System

The MPS was proposed by van Furth and Cohn in the 1960s to clarify the distinction between the leukocyte and endothelial or fibroblast components of the RES. It was postulated that the key phagocytic capacity of the RES was due to tissue macrophages that were derived from monocytes, together comprising a unified system.[2] Proponents of the MPS were careful to maintain a distinction between monocyte-derived "free" macrophages and other populations of "fixed" macrophages that were proliferative in situ and had a less certain origin. However, promoted by the observation that monocytes readily differentiate into macrophages in vitro, the MPS concept soon broadened to encompass all macrophage populations. It is only in recent years, using lineage-tracing techniques, that long-lived macrophages have been rediscovered and their origins mapped to prenatal hematopoiesis.[3-5] Many tissues thus contain fixed self-renewing macrophage populations that are only replaced by bone marrow–derived cells after significant perturbation. Notably, microglia, Langerhans cells (LC) of the epidermis, alveolar macrophages, and Kupffer cells of the liver show almost complete bone marrow independence in the steady state, but interstitial dermis, gut, and serosal surfaces replenish their macrophages through continual monocyte recruitment. Thus, the MPS is now considered to have multiple origins and variable dependence upon the bone marrow during adult life (*Figure 10.2*).

The Discovery of Dendritic Cells

The discovery of DC, a myeloid cell with some of the properties traditionally associated with macrophages, required a further modification of the MPS as originally conceived.[6] Sceptics initially argued that DC were just another phenotype of macrophage and that the antigen presenting function of DC was already intrinsic to the role of the MPS. However, parallel lineage tracing techniques and conditional ablation models revealed that DC arise from a specific branch of hematopoiesis

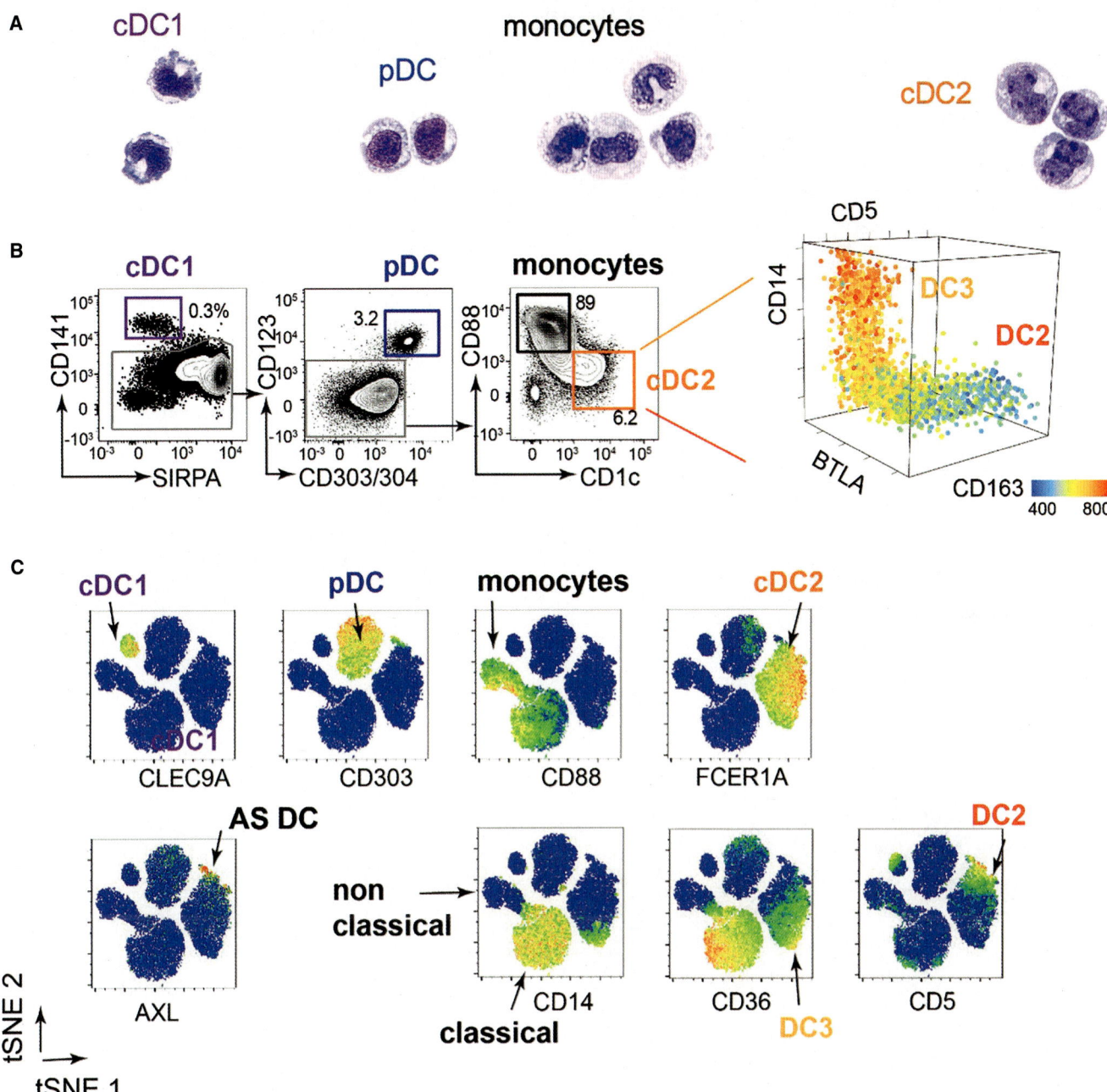

FIGURE 10.1 Monocytes and DC. A, Giemsa-stained cytopsins of purified human blood DC and classical monocytes. B, Fluorescence cytometry of human blood mononuclear cells showing gating for DC1, pDC, monocytes (using CD88), and cDC2, which are now further split into DC2 and DC3 by BTLA and CD5 (DC2), and CD14 and CD164 (DC3). Note AXL[+] SIGLECT[+] DC have been pregated and do not contaminate pDC in this example. C, Mass cytometry of human blood mononuclear cells depicted with tSNE showing clear separation of monocyte and DC populations, with the exception of the graded boundaries of classical and nonclassical monocytes and subsets of cDC2, DC2, and DC3. Note the small AXL[+] SIGLEC[+] population annexed to DC2 for which it is a potential precursor population.

that is traceable from lymphomyeloid progenitors through specific compartments of granulocyte-macrophage progenitors (GMPs) that is completely distinct from the developmental trajectories of monocytes and macrophages.[7,8]

DIVERSITY AND CLASSIFICATION

Like nearly all immune cells that have been described, monocytes, macrophages, and DC achieve a high level of functional specialization through diversification of gene expression and surface phenotype under the control of a network of transcription factors. Aided by cross-species comparisons and more recently by single cell transcriptomics,

the functional boundaries of discrete populations are now relatively well defined in the steady state and increasingly so in perturbed states and inflammation (*Table 10.1*; *Figure 10.1*).

Monocytes

Monocytes are blood-borne myeloid mononuclear cells. They are rounded cells, 10 to 15 μm in size, with oval, kidney-shaped, or indented nuclei, a rim of heterochromatin, and mostly euchromatic nucleoplasm. Their cytoplasm is relatively abundant, compared with nonactivated lymphocytes, containing granules with myeloperoxidase, lysozyme, nonspecific esterases, and lysosomes. They migrate from the circulation and enter tissues in the steady state and are rapidly

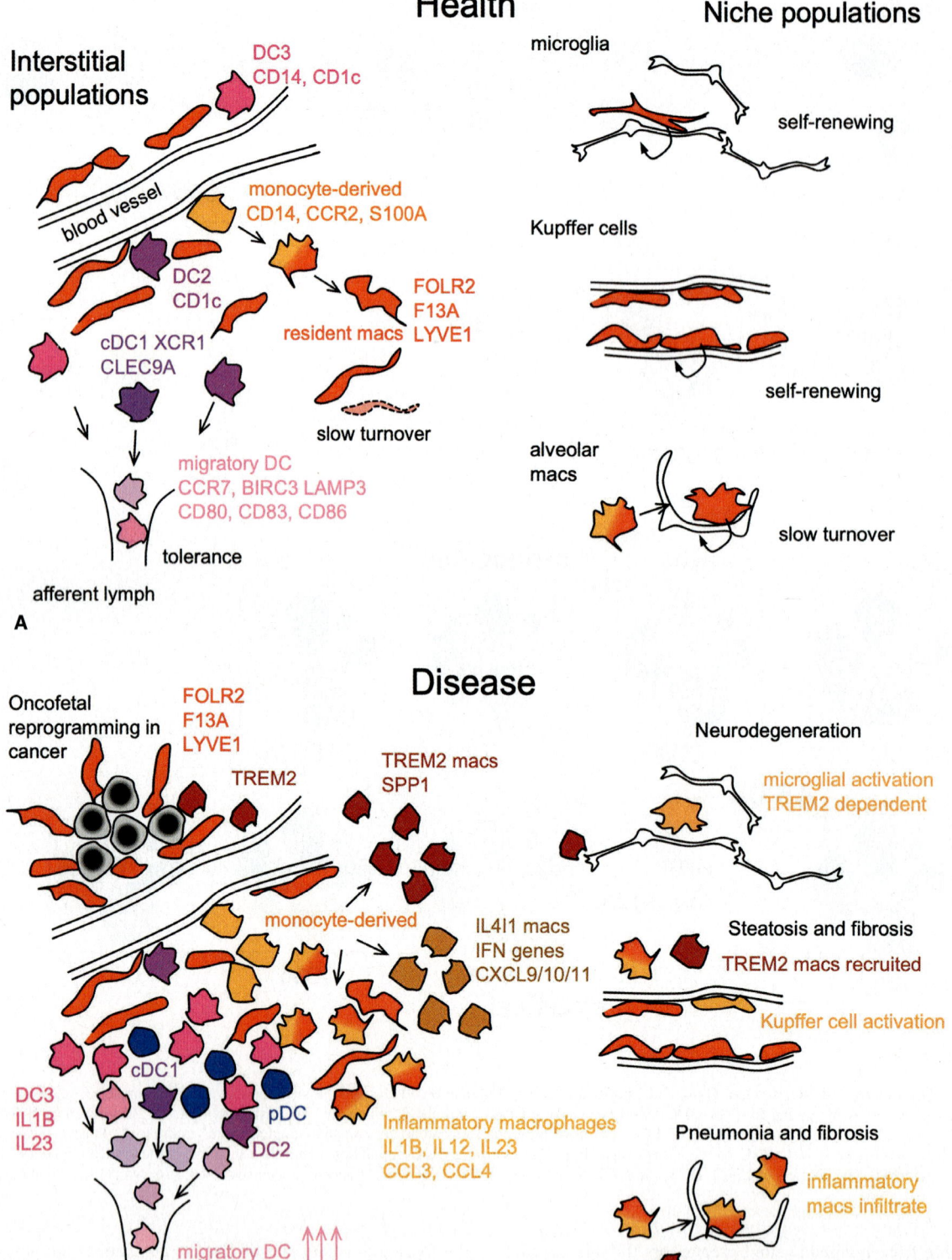

FIGURE 10.2 Tissue populations in health and disease. A, A highly generalized overview of steady-state populations comprising monocyte-derived cells that contribute to resident macrophages in many interstitial tissues, and myeloid DC. Resident macrophages have a conserved signature in most tissues. A small population of migratory DC showing evidence of maturation is usually detectable. Niche macrophages are present in special anatomic sites. B, In disease states such as infection, autoimmunity, or cancer witness a significant expansion of cells including many monocyte-derived populations that diversify into multiple functional subsets, some of which are shown. There is often recruitment of DC, including pDC, which are not usually found in healthy tissues, and expansion of migratory DC populations. In cancer, tumor-associate macrophages comprise populations with a resident signature associated with oncofetal reprogramming and TREM2+ cells. In other niche sites, specialized macrophages may become activated and become supplemented or replaced by incoming monocyte-derived cells, which serve a range of tissue-specific pathological functions.

Table 10.1. Overview of Classification

Subset	Markers	Distribution	Function
Classical monocyte	HLA-DR, CD11c CD88 CD14 (CD16 negative)	Blood Recruited to inflamed tissues	Precursor of inflammatory macs, DC, and some resident macs
Nonclassical monocyte	HLA-DR, CD11c CD88 CD16, SLAN (CD14 low)	Blood Patrolling vessels Prominent related population in lung	Endothelial homeostasis?
Monocyte-derived macrophage	HLA-DR, CD11c CD14 CCR2 S100A8/9 SIRPA CD209	Steady-state interstitial tissues Recruited and diversified in inflammation into multiple functional subsets	Immune phagocytosis Bacterial killing Secretion of IL1B, cytokines, and chemokines Antigen processing
Resident tissue macrophage	FOLR2 FXIIIA LYVE-1 CD163 MRC1 HES1	Interstitial tissues Localized to perivascular and perineural locations Induced by oncofetal reprogramming	Maintenance of epithelial, vascular, and neuronal health
pDC	CD123 (CD11c negative) CD45RA BTLA CLEC4C NRP1	Blood Lymphoid organs Recruited in inflammation	Production of type I infection
DC1	HLA-DR, CD11c low (CD88 negative) BTLA CLEC9A XCR1	Blood Most tissues, lymphoid organs	Uptake of dying cells Cross-presentation of intracellular antigen Production of type III interferon
DC2	HLA-DR, CD11c (CD88 negative) CD1c FCER1A CD2 CLEC10A	Blood Most tissues, lymphoid organs	Indirect antigen presentation Production of IL-12
DC3	HLA-DR, CD11c, CD11b (CD88 negative) CD14 CD163 CD36	Blood Most tissues, lymphoid organs Promoted by GM-CSF in inflammation	Indirect antigen presentation Production of IL-23 Stimulation of resident memory T cells
AXL⁺SIGLEC6⁺ DC	HLA-DR, CD123 (CD11c negative) AXL SIGLEC2 SIGLEC6	Blood Inflamed tissues Contaminate pDC preparations gated on CD123	Pre-DC2? Transitional function between pDC and DC2?
Migratory DC	CCR7 CD83 LAMP3 IDO BIRC3	Inflamed tissues Tumors	Migration to the lymph node to induce immune activation or tolerance
Langerhans cells	Langerin CD1a EpCAM E-Cadherin	Epidermis	Migration to the lymph node to induce immune activation or tolerance Regulation of commensals?

The Normal Hematologic System

recruited in inflammation. *In vitro*, they adhere strongly to native and artificial substrates by a range of adhesion receptors. Mammalian monocytes are heterogeneous.[9,10] The majority, bearing CD14 in humans and Ly6C in mice, behave as classical inflammatory mononuclear cells that extravasate during inflammation and display a wide range of differentiation potentials. Minor populations of nonclassical monocytes include cells expressing the Fc receptor FCGR3A (CD16) and the glycosyl residue 6-sulfo LacNAc (SLAN) that show less phenotypic plasticity and are generally lower in inflammatory potential.

Classical Monocytes

Classical monocytes express CD14, which allows them to sense lipopolysaccharide (LPS) and CCR2, a receptor that is required for them

to exit the bone marrow and enter tissue in response to inflammatory chemokines. They also express CCR1 and CCR5, and recruitment via these receptors is implicated in chronic inflammatory conditions including atherosclerosis, rheumatoid arthritis, and multiple sclerosis. Classical monocytes may adopt a great many phenotypic states depending upon stimulus[11,12] and are likely to act as steady-state precursors of tissue macrophage populations that show BM dependence, such as the dermis and intestine.[8,13]

Nonclassical Monocytes

Nonclassical monocytes express CD16 and a low level of CD14. They may arise from classical monocytes by peripheral conversion, although not all evidence agrees with this.[14] They express higher

CX3CR1 and lower CCR2 than classical monocytes. The majority express SLAN[15,16] and have been described by some authors as a type of DC. Although their gene expression is slightly shifted toward DC, they cluster with monocytes and there is no evidence to suggest that they are developmentally related to DC.[17] In mice, a population of nonclassical monocytes exhibit the ability to patrol vascular endothelium[18,19] but a discrete function in human immunity remains elusive.

Intermediate Monocytes

The bivariate plot of CD14 versus CD16 has a "knee" containing double-positive cells, which have been classified as "intermediate" monocytes. Certain properties such as expression of MHC class II, costimulatory molecules CD80 and CD86, and cytokine secretion are highest in this region, but almost all other phenotypic markers are distributed continuously between classical and nonclassical monocytes, and the literature is fraught with inconsistencies of gating.[20] Classical monocytes express CD16 when stimulated, so many inflammatory states witness an apparent increase in monocytes occupying the intermediate region. Single cell RNA sequencing suggests that intermediate monocytes are activated classical monocytes.[21]

Monocyte-Derived Cells in Steady-State Tissues

Nonlymphoid tissues, including the skin, lung, and intestine, contain steady-state populations of smaller CD14+ cells that appear to form a continuum with classical monocytes.[13,22-28] In some tissues, notably the lung, CD16+ cells are also evident. These cells are mobile and migrate from explanted organs, but their physiological role is unclear. Although they lack CCR7, the chemokine receptor for lymph node homing, they may drain to the lymph node and contribute to subcapsular macrophage populations or return to the bloodstream. A proportion may eventually become fixed macrophages, contributing to those interstitial populations that are known to be bone marrow derived.

Monocyte-Derived Macrophages

The recruitment of classical monocytes to inflamed tissues and their differentiation into activated inflammatory macrophages is a paradigm of cellular immunology.[29-33] Inflammatory macrophages have characteristic ruffled borders with extensive, dynamic plasma membrane processes and lamellipodia. The cytoplasm is rich in synthetic organelles and endocytic vesicles, often containing debris and residues of phagocytosis in abundant lysosomes. The process of monocyte differentiation in vitro has also been intensively studied. Monocytes respond to a huge array of stimuli to generate macrophages with a wide range of phenotypes. "Classical" macrophage activation was first demonstrated through the ability of IFNγ and LPS to enhance antimicrobial resistance to bacille Calmette-Guerin and *Listeria monocytogenes* in animal models. The critical role of IFNγ, IL-12 (IL12A/B), and associated intracellular signaling pathways in mediating resistance to intracellular infection has also been elegantly demonstrated in humans by studies of genetic susceptibility to mycobacteria.[34]

The M1/M2 Paradigm

In addition to classical immune activation (M1 phenotype), monocytes can adopt a state of "alternative" activation, induced by exposure to IL4 or IL13 (M2). For several decades, this bipolar model of monocyte differentiation dominated the landscape of macrophage biology.[35] With the advent of high-resolution single cell analysis, the M1/M2 paradigm is rapidly becoming obsolete.[11,36-38] The concept that M2 macrophages have a "resident" gene expression signature is being replaced by more sophisticated analysis of tissue populations in which it is now possible to separate macrophages with different origins and kinetics of renewal.[8] Although the signature genes of M1 and M2 show some correlation with recruited and resident populations, this is only an approximation.[28]

Macrophages

Macrophages are tissue cells. They are larger than monocytes and can be stellate, with two or more processes, or fibroblastoid in vivo. They are found in almost all organs in the interstitial spaces where their

microscopic appearance matches the classical description of "histiocytes." They are typically found adjacent to lamina propria, and in perivascular and perineural locations.[39-41] They also occupy multiple highly specialized niches in different organs including the brain, lung, liver, and spleen where they are specifically identified as microglia, alveolar macrophages, Kupffer cells, among others. The specification of different macrophage populations is strongly anatomical and occurs early in development.[42,43]

Profiling active chromatin in macrophages isolated from different organs reveals a common macrophage enhancer landscape shaped by lineage determining transcription factors such as SPI1 (PU.1). This creates many poised enhancer sites that are differentially occupied by signal-dependent transcription factors according to anatomical location.[44,45] A range of secondary tissue-specific transcription factors have emerged such as RARA/B for peritoneal macrophages, RUNX3 for intestinal macrophages, LXRA for Kupffer cells and kidney macrophages, and MEF2C and SALL1 for microglia.[5,46,47] These regulators determine the unique properties and functions of specific populations.

Differentiation of Resident Macrophages From Monocytes and DC

Single cell transcriptomics have provided new insights into the identification of resident tissue macrophages within complex populations of myeloid cells that include monocyte-derived cells and DC[28,38](*Figure 10.2*). By overlaying expression profiles from human fetal macrophages, and long-term resident murine macrophages, it is possible to identify adult human macrophage clusters that have a strong "resident" signature and are potentially derived during fetal life (see section III). This signature includes the well-known macrophage marker F13A (Factor XIIIA), the hyaluronin receptor LYVE1, folate receptor FOLR2, and basic hemophagocytic lymphohistiocytosis (HLH) protein HES1, involved in notch signaling.[28,38] Resident macrophages also elaborate CCL18, complement C1Q components, and lipid metabolism pathways, although these are shared with other populations.[28] In contrast, recruited monocyte-derived cells retain expression of monocyte signature genes including CD14, SIRPA (CD172a) S100A8/9, and CCR2.[29,32] In addition, they activate a range of immune-related transcripts including CD40, CD38, LAMP3, SPP1 (osteopontin) CCL8, CXCL8,9,10, tetraspanins, CD9, and CD63, in addition to regulatory molecules TREM2, IL-4 induced IL4I1, CD274 (PDL1), and IDO (indoleamine 2,3-dioxygenase).[28] Within this group of cells, it is possible to identify more DC-like populations marked by CD1 antigens, the Fc Epsilon receptor FCER1A (FCER1A), CLEC10A, and higher expression of MHC class II and costimulatory antigens CD80 and CD86.

Microglia

Microglia are a unique population of brain resident macrophages that appear early in embryogenesis from yolk sac progenitors and remain self-renewing and independent from the bone marrow for the life on an organism.[3] During development and under physiological conditions, microglia are specifically adapted to requirements of the central nervous system (CNS) and play key roles in programmed cell death, removal of newborn neurons, and modification of synapses by pruning, elimination, and maturation.[48-50] In response to CNS insults they become morphologically activated, increase in number, and upregulate new transcriptomic programs.[51,52] There is much interest in the role of microglia in aging and neurodegenerative disease. TREM2 and APOE appear to play a major role in their activation in Alzheimer disease.[52,53] Genome-wide association with neurodegeneration identifies many transcripts upregulated in activated microglia.[54] Although it is difficult to establish causation in humans, germline mutations in key microglial genes cause neurodegenerative disease. Nasu-Hakola disease is associated with mutation of *TREM2* or *DAP12*.[55] Pigmented orthochromatic leukodystrophy and hereditary diffuse leukoencephalopathy with spheroids are both associated with *CSF1R* mutation.[56] Finally, mice with microglia carrying MAP kinase pathway mutation (*BRAF*V600E) cause a neurodegenerative disease that has similarity with the late effects of neurodegenerative histiocytosis.[57] This raises the interesting possibility that somatic mutation in early embryonic precursors could contribute to cognitive dysfunction.

Kupffer Cells

Kupffer cells were described in 1876 by Karl Wilhelm von Kupffer. They line the luminal surface of the hepatic sinusoidal endothelium and comprise the largest population of resident macrophages in the body. Kupffer cells are exposed to the portal blood, clearing pathogens and responding to metabolites from the gut. They express multiple receptors for bacterial ligands, complement components including C3a and C5a receptors, CD11b (ITGAM) and CD11c (ITGAX) and Fc receptors. Production of IL6 in response to inflammatory challenge is critical in the induction of acute phase proteins, such as C-reactive protein, serum amyloid protein, complement, and fibrinogen. They play a key role in hepatic steatosis through CD36, a receptor for oxidized LDL.[58] A high-fat diet induces Kupffer cell turnover and replacement with monocyte-derived cells that diversify from the resting Kupffer cell transcriptional program and promote inflammation.[59,60]

Alveolar Macrophages

Alveolar macrophages are a unique population occupying a niche of the respiratory epithelium exposed to the external environment. They are found in bronchoalveolar lavage and are therefore relatively easy to study in humans where they are characterized as large cells with high phagocytic activity and low immunostimulatory capacity. Alveolar macrophages play an essential role in the metabolism of surfactant proteins, and failure of their homeostasis results in pulmonary alveolar proteinosis.[61] In humans, this may occur in association with antibodies to GM-CSF, which is required for the terminal development of macrophages or with *GATA2* mutation, which causes an absolute monocytopenia.[62] In lung transplant recipients, donor alveolar macrophages persist for at least 2 years implying local self-renewal or a long lifespan.[63] In some mouse models alveolar macrophages are completely independent of the bone marrow in the steady state[64]; in others, there is a slow turnover from monocyte precursors.[8] Macrophages can even be engrafted into the lung by direct inoculation into the airways.[65] It is possible to dissect a number of interstitial macrophage and monocyte-derived populations from lung tissue, some of which may serve as precursors to the alveolar resident macrophage.[66-68] In mouse models, migration of prealveolar macrophages into the alveolar space requires the cytoskeletal protein L-plastin and induction of the transcription factor PPARG.[69]

Intestinal Macrophages

The gut contains an abundant population of lamina propria macrophages and DC.[27,70-72] The macrophage population is closely associated with the epithelium and is uniquely anergic to stimulation by bacterial Toll-like receptor (TLR) ligands while maintaining high phagocytic and bactericidal capacity.[71] Other macrophages are found deeper in the submucosa associated with vessels, nerves, and the serosal surface, where they play critical roles in maintaining epithelial, vascular, and neuroenteric health.[73-76] In the mouse, about 80% of intestinal macrophages are continually derived from monocytes, while the remainder associated with nerves, blood vessels, Peyer patches, and Paneth cells are long-lived and self-renewing.[8,70,73] Studies in human transplantation indicate that intestinal macrophages are renewed with kinetics that appear to define a series of differentiation steps from monocytes.[13]

Osteoclasts

Osteoclasts are multinucleated giant cells found at the margins of bone matrix where they secrete proteolytic enzymes to resorb bone, forming small excavations known as Howship lacunae. They share expression of myeloid and macrophage antigens such as CD13 and CD68 and were included in the original definition of the mononuclear phagocyte system.[2] It has been shown by parabiosis and lineage tracing that osteoclasts are initially formed by embryonic macrophages and continually expanded by fusion of bone marrow–derived monocytes.[77] Multinucleated giant cells with bone-resorbing capacity can be made

from classical monocytes cultured with RANK ligand (TNFSF11) and M-CSF (CSF1) or IL4/IL13. Both express tartrate-resistant acid phosphatase, DC-STAMP, and can digest mineral hydroxyapatite. *Bona fide* osteoclasts are said to be induced by RANK ligand rather than IL4/IL13 and have fewer nuclei and greater capacity to digest the matrix components of bone through expression of cathepsin K.[78] When osteoclast development from CD34+ progenitor fractions is studied in vitro, a common monocyte, DC, osteoclast precursor has been proposed.[79]

Faulty osteoclast metabolism is one of the causes of osteopetrosis, a failure of bone resorption leading to excessive bone formation and secondary bone marrow failure. Genetic ablation of osteoclasts leads to an osteopetrotic phenotype in mice.[77] In humans, many different genes are associated with loss of function or absence of osteoclasts. Mutations in *TCIRG1*, *CLCN7*, *OSTM1*, and *PLEKHM1* cause osteopetrosis by disrupting the trafficking of acidic vesicles. Osteoclast-poor osteopetrosis is associated with mutations in the osteoclast growth factors M-CSF and RANK ligand or their receptors.[80]

Vascular Macrophages

Atherosclerosis is now well recognized as a modified form of inflammation in which monocytes and macrophages are major drivers of plaque formation and thrombosis. Macrophage accumulation involves an initial step of monocyte recruitment followed by local proliferation in situ, at least partially dependent upon the macrophage scavenger receptor MSR1.[81] Many risk factors for atherogenesis appear to act by modifying monocyte homeostasis or function.[82] Long-lived macrophages associated with vessels and nerves appear to play critical roles in the maintenance of vascular integrity.[39,40]

Genitourinary Tract

Interstitial populations of macrophage in the kidney are closely apposed to the peritubular capillaries and receive trans-cytosed particles with high efficiency, approaching that of the Kupffer cell and splenic red pulp macrophage.[83] It has been proposed that this population of macrophages is intimately associated with immune activation leading to nephritis in immune complex disease.[84] Macrophages also play important roles in the testis and ovary where they participate in the removal of apoptotic sperm and in follicular atresia.[85]

Bone Marrow

Macrophages are important components of the hematopoietic stem cell niche and interact with both osteoblasts and mesenchymal stem cells to retain hematopoietic stem cells within the bone marrow.[86] Developing erythroblasts are also in contact with a central macrophage that handles iron stores and efferocytosis of erythroblast nuclei (pyrenocytes). Adhesion between erythroblasts and macrophages is initially mediated by VACM1 and alpha4beta1 integrin. This is superseded by MERTK-Protein S-dependent uptake following enucleation.[87] Depletion of CD169+ (SIGLEC1) bone marrow macrophages does not result in overt anemia but reduces the capacity of erythropoiesis to respond to stress.[88]

Lymph Nodes

Macrophages play carefully choreographed roles in the induction of immune responses. In the subcapsular spaces of lymph nodes, CD169+ macrophages are positioned to capture antigen from afferent lymph and transport it to B cells in the follicles.[89,90] This function is one of many examples of monocyte and macrophages providing direct help to B cells through presentation of intact antigen and elaboration of maturation and class-switching factors including BAFF and APRIL. Surrounding the follicles, a capsule of marginal zone macrophages is specialized to engulf apoptotic B cells that fail to receive survival stimuli and achieve maturation in the germinal centers.[91]

Spleen

The spleen is rich in diverse populations of macrophages.[92] The red pulp contains a major population bearing CD36, CD163, and SIRPA, involved in the uptake of senescent red cells and iron recycling. The marginal zone contains two more populations: outer marginal zone macrophages involved in uptake of blood-borne pathogens and inner marginal zone metallophilic macrophages that efferocytose lymphocyte nuclei from the white pulp. The outer zone macrophages express the scavenger receptor MARCO and the C-type lectin CD209, while the inner zone metallophilic cells are rich in CD169 and are homologous to subcapsular macrophages of the lymph node. Mouse knockouts suggest that marginal zone macrophages contribute to resistance to infection by communicating with B cells[90] and may also play a role in tolerance.

Thymus

Several populations of macrophages are distributed throughout the thymus.[93] One of their best described roles is the efferocytosis or apoptotic thymocytes. The population responsible for this activity is controlled by the transcription factor NR4A1.[94] Thymic DC play an integral role in central T cell tolerance by positive selection of T cells in the cortex.

Dendritic Cells

The classification of mammalian DC is now well established.[95-97] Two major classes exist, myeloid DC, bearing CD33, CD13 (ANPEP), CD11b, and CD11c (in common with monocytes), and plasmacytoid DC (pDC), which lack these antigens but express the naïve T-cell marker CD45RA and high levels of CD123 (IL3RA). In mice, myeloid DC are also commonly known as conventional or classical DC (DC). Myeloid DC comprise three subsets DC1 (previously cDC1), DC2, and DC3. Myeloid (or conventional classical) DC1 express the lectin CLEC9A for apoptotic cell uptake and the unique chemokine receptor XCR1. They are characterized as cross-presenting DC critical for responses to virus-infected cells, intracellular pathogens, and tumors. DC2 and DC3 are closely related and were previously known collectively as cDC2.[97] These DC correspond to the "indeterminate cell" that inhabits interstitial tissues, expressing lower CD1a than Langerhans cells and almost no Langerin. Both DC2 and DC3 express CD1c, CD2, FCER1A, and CLEC10A and are more abundant than DC1 in blood and tissues. DC2 express some antigens found on DC1, such as BTLA, while DC3 share monocyte antigens including CD14 and CD163.[21,98,99] DC3 have greater expression of inflammatory gene modules and are selectively expanded in inflammatory and autoimmune disease.[100-102] In some publications they are referred to as inflammatory cDC2[98,100,101] or "monocyte-derived DC."[103] The latter simply reflects the expression of monocyte-like traits by DC3 and is not based on evidence of a monocyte origin. In the resting state, all DC populations are distinguishable from monocytes by their lack of expression of CD88, among other antigens.[98-100] During inflammation, it becomes more difficult to assign a precise origin as maturation leads to convergent expression of activation and migration transcriptional modules.[101]

Morphology and Distribution

Blood DC are smaller than monocytes and may be found in the lymphoid gates of flow cytometry analyses. In the tissues, they are smaller than macrophages and less extensively arborized with multiple short processes. During migration through the afferent lymph they mature into "veiled cells" with extensive macropinocytic processes. In lymph nodes they form a population of highly motile "interdigitating cells" that transit rapidly between lymphocytes until a cognate antigen is detected by T cells. In vitro they are lightly or nonadherent compared with monocytes or macrophages, a property that was exploited in their original isolation from mouse spleen.[6] The process of DC maturation is intimately linked to their function in promoting both tolerance and immunity.[104] More recently, attention has been drawn to the potential for tumors to subvert this process and evade immune responses by stimulating the development of mature DC with regulatory function ("mregDC").[105]

Plasmacytoid Dendritic Cells

Plasmacytoid dendritic cells were first identified in human blood and tonsil as interferon-producing cells with eccentric nuclei and prominent endoplasmic reticulum (resembling a plasma cell). They do not express the myeloid antigens CD11c, CD33, CD11b, or CD13[106-108] but retain expression of the GMP markers CD123 and CD45RA. Like all human DC they express CD4, but at a higher level than myeloid DC.[109] In addition, pDC have an array of surface receptors that regulate the production of type I interferon. These include CLEC4C (CD303, BDCA-2), NRP1 (neuropilin, CD304, BDCA-4), the inhibitory receptors LILRA4 (CD85g; ILT7) and LILRB4 (CD85k, ILT3), and more recently characterized antigens FCER1A, BTLA, TNFRSF21 (DR6, CD358), and CD300A.[110,111] Transcriptional profiling has also added FAM129C, CUX2, and GZMB.[112] Several recent papers have described a small subset of CD123+ pDC that express CD2 or CD5.[99,113]

Plasmacytoid DC are specialized to sense and respond to viral infection by the rapid secretion of interferons and cytokines.[111,114] TLR7 and TLR9 are the key endosomal pattern recognition receptors that sense single-stranded RNA and double-stranded DNA, respectively.[111] STING1 has also been reported as playing a role in DNA sensing.[115] Depending upon the nature of the nucleic acid cargo and mode of delivery, interferon and cytokine production may be differentially regulated.[116] IRF7 is the major transducer of type I interferon production in pDC,[117] while production of TNF and IL-6 is dependent upon the NF-κB pathway. Many signaling molecules participate in and regulate this process including MYD88 and DOCK2 (reviewed in 111,114). Ligation of surface receptors modulates activation or tolerance through the regulation of the IRF7 and NF-κ pathways. CD300A transmits enhancing signals through an ITIM domain[110] while ligation of FCER1A, I LILRA4 (ILT7), and CLEC4C (BDCA2) inhibits IFNα production via ITAM signaling (reviewed in 111). TNFRSF21 (DR6, CD358) is a specific marker of human pDC, and knockdown in pDC cell lines impairs IRF7 translocation to the nucleus.[118] Sphingosine-1-phosphate signaling interacts with LILRA4 to limit TLR-induced interferon production[119] and with IFNAR to terminate the IFNα response.[120] The importance of IRF7 in regulating IFNα production in humans was underscored by the severe susceptibility to influenza and demonstrable lack of IFNα production by pDC in a patient with compound heterozygous *IRF7* mutation.[121] Deficiency of MYD88 and IRAK4 are predicted to affect pDC while DOCK8 deficiency is known to be associated with decreased pDC number and function.[122] In addition to being studied in acute viral infection, pDC have been studied in chronic infections. Early production of IFNα by gut pDC appears to be beneficial in HIV elite controllers,[123] but in chronic hepatitis, persistence may be promoted by attenuated pDC responses and pDC-mediated induction of T cell tolerance.[124,125] The prominent role of type I interferon production and signaling and potential of pDC to sensing self-nucleic acids[126] have implicated pDC in the pathogenesis of psoriasis,[127] lupus,[128] and other autoimmune diseases. Many potential therapeutic targets are presented by the factors that modulate IFNα release by pDC. Conflicting roles for pDC have been reported in allergy.[129,130] Tolerogenic pDC under the influence of GM-CSF have also been proposed to contribute to tumor progression.[131]

DC1

Human DC1 were originally described as a subset of myeloid blood DC with high expression of CD141 (THBD, thrombomodulin, BDCA-3) and are found at approximately one-tenth the frequency of DC2 and DC3 in steady-state blood and tissues.[95,106,108,112,132-134] In common with myeloid DC2/3, they express CD13 and CD33 but differ by low CD11c and little CD11b or SIRPA (CD172a). CLEC9A, the C-type lectin receptor for exposed actin[135,136]; the cell adhesion molecule CADM1; and the chemokine receptor XCR1 are highly specific across all mammalian species.[95] IDO and the antigen BTLA are also highly expressed.[112] Human DC1 are found in blood and among resident DC of lymph node (LN), tonsil, spleen, and BM[112,134,137-140] and nonlymphoid tissues, skin, lung, intestine, and liver.[24-27,95,112,133,134,141,142]

DC1 have a high intrinsic capacity to cross-present antigens via MHC class I to activate CD8+ T cells and to promote Th1 and NK response through IL-12.[133,137,138,143] Although they are perhaps less polarized toward this role in humans than in mice, conserved mechanisms are evident that mediate efficient recognition of viral and intracellular antigens, transport of antigen to the appropriate endosomal compartments, and production of type III interferon (IFNl).[144] They are also intrinsically resistant to productive viral infection.[104,145] CLEC9A is a highly functional marker because it directs cell-associated antigens into the cross-presentation pathway.[146,147] DC1 express higher TLR3, 9, and 10 than other DC.[21,148,149] TLR3 plays an important role in the recognition of dsRNA and production of type I interferons via IRF3.[150] Defects in the TLR3/IRF3 axis in humans are associated with specific susceptibility to HSV1 encephalitis.[151] TLR9 is potentially also important in interferon responses to DNA, as in pDC. DC1 accumulation in hepatitis C infection has been linked to the beneficial role of type III interferon in viral clearance.[141] The XCR1 chemokine receptor enables close interaction with XCL-producing activated T cells and NK cells and may assist their positioning in peripheral tissues. Several recent studies indicate the importance of this axis in coordinating peripheral Th1 and cytotoxic responses[152,153] in reciprocity with the action of DC-derived CXCL9/10 upon activated T cells.[154]

DC2

The major population of myeloid DC in human blood, tissues, and lymphoid organs expresses CD1c, CD2, FCER1A, CLEC10A, and the myeloid antigens CD11b, CD11c, CD13, and CD33.[112] This population was treated as a homogenous entity (cDC2) until recent evidence clearly defined two phenotypic and functional subpopulations, DC2 and DC3. DC2 are more "DC-like" with higher expression of CD5, BTLA, CD1c, HLA-DQ, and IRF4.[21,98,155] Their origin is more closely linked with DC1 precursors through lineage trajectories marked by high IRF8 and CD123 expression.[99,100]

Single cell transcriptomics are now being used to dissect the relative contribution of DC2 and DC3 to CD1c[+] DC in the dermis,[156] lung,[24-26] intestine,[27] and liver of humans.[95,134,142] Interdigitating cells of the T-cell areas in lymph node, tonsil, and spleen may also be mapped to DC2 or DC3.[112,134,138,139,157] CD5[+] DC2 are more active than CD5[−] DC3 in CCR7-dependent migration, naïve T cell proliferation, and priming of Th2, Th17, Th22, and Tregs.[21,155]

DC3

DC3 express myeloid DC antigens CD1c, CD2, FCER1A, and CLEC10A in common with DC2 but are distinguished by higher expression of CD14, CD32, CD36, CD163, CD206, SIRPA, and MAFB compared with DC2.[21,155] As an approximation, the expression of CD14 on a cell with otherwise bona fide DC antigen expression suggests the existence of DC3 and likely accounts for significant populations of myeloid DC in inflamed tissues.[102] The origin of DC3 is distinct from monocytes but does not pass through a high IRF8 pathway like pDC, DC1, and DC2.[99] Their production is stimulated by GM-CSF independently of other DC and monocytes.[100]

In vivo models suggest that DC3 play a particular role in stimulating and positioning resident memory T cells in the tissues.[100] When stimulated, there is convergence of the activated phenotypes of DC2 and DC3, and the relative contributions of these subsets to activities previously ascribed to cDC2 (both subsets combined) have not been unraveled. Both subsets may use CD1 antigens to present the glycolipid antigens of mycobacteria.[158] Among the lectins, CLEC4A, CLEC10A, CLEC12A, and the asialoglycoprotein receptor ASGR1/2 are highly expressed. In common with monocytes, TLR2, 4, 5, 6, and 8 are present with notable expression of NOD2, NLRP1, NLRP3, and NAIP. DC3 with lower CD5 are less active in proliferation assays and produce mainly Th1[21,155] and differ in their production of TNFα, IL-6, IL-10, and IL-23 in response to TLR ligation.[155,159] Under inflammatory conditions it is likely that DC3 are the highest producers of IL-12 and can become excellent cross-presenting cells.[101,144,157,160]

AXL[+] SIGLEC6[+] DC

Single cell transcriptomic analysis of human blood has identified a small fraction of immature DC, marked by the expression of AXL and SIGLEC6 and a transitional phenotype between pDC and DC2.[21,99,113,161] These "AS" or "transitional" DC readily differentiate into DC2 in vitro and account for many historical reports of myeloid DC developing from pDC; essentially pDC preparations also contained myeloid DC precursors.[162] The function of these cells remains unclear. Their development into DC2 suggests that they are simply "pre-DC2."[99,113] According to this view, their proximity to the pDC trajectory may reflect suppression of the DC1 program that results in transient activation of pDC gene expression modules. Alternatively, they have been characterized as a unique subset of DC that may play a subtle role in tuning immune responses.[21,161] DC3 are uniquely susceptible to infection by HIV-1 in a SIGLEC1-dependent manner, a unique functional feature that might indicate a relationship with immunity to viruses.[163]

Migratory DC

A long-cherished view is that tissue DC mature and migrate to lymph nodes where they contribute to lymphoid DC populations and exercise tolerogenic functions in the steady state or immunogenic activation during antigen challenges.[104] Through single cell transcriptomics it has been possible to identify these itinerant populations of DC that have matured and are expressing lymph node homing functions including CD83, LAMP3, IDO, BIRC3, and CCR7. These migratory DC or mature regulatory "mReg" DC offer fascinating insights into immunoregulation in the steady state, inflammation, and tumor microenvironments.[102,105,164-166]

Langerhans Cells

LC inhabit the basal epidermis and other stratified squamous epithelia. They express the C-type lectin Langerin (CD207) and the invariant MHC class I molecule CD1a. Originally described as nerve cells by Paul Langerhans in 1868, a series of studies in the 1970s confirmed their leukocyte origin and expression of MHC class II molecules. Close integration of LC within the epithelial layer is mediated by E-Cadherin (CDH1), EPCAM (TROP1), TACSTD2 (TROP2), AXL, and tight junction proteins claudin, occludin, and TJP1 (ZO-1).[167,168] Multiple lines of evidence show that human LC proliferate at about 2% to 3%, consistent with a self-renewing, BM-independent compartment that persists in conditions of absolute monocytopenia[169,170] and limb transplantation.[171] Although they are distinct from all other DC by their origin from prenatal monocyte precursors and self-renewing capacity, in common with myeloid cDC2, LC express high levels of FCER1A and CD39 (ATPase). They also share some attributes with DC1 including high MHC class I–related gene expression and functional cross-presentation capacity.[172-175] LC migrate to skin-draining LN where they appear in the T-cell areas as DC2-like populations expressing langerin, CD1a, and CD1c. EpCAM and other epithelial markers are downregulated. Differences between inflamed and noninflamed skin-draining nodes[176] and between skin-draining nodes and tonsil[177] have been used to highlight the contribution of migratory LC to nodal DC populations.

When the skin becomes inflamed, local production of TNFα and IL1β stimulates LC to lose their connections with the surrounding epithelium and migrate across the basement membrane into the afferent lymphatics. Although LC were the primary model of migratory myeloid DC, their nonredundant function in immunity has been surprisingly difficult to pin down. In humans, LC-like cells can be differentiated in vitro into potent cross-presenting DC with high IL-15 production and the ability to present mycobacterial glycolipid antigens and stimulate CD8 T cells.[172,173] Transgenic expression of human CD1a on murine LC licensed them for presentation of lipid antigens to Th17 and Th22 cells resulting in skin inflammation.[178] However, it has also been reported that LC lack critical TLRs[179] and can induce Tregs and IL-22 production through CD1a-restricted antigens to autologous T cells.[180] Overall, the role of LCs is related to maintaining epidermal health and tolerance to commensals, with the ability to respond to selected intracellular pathogens and viruses under inflammatory conditions.[181]

The Normal Hematologic System

ORIGIN

Prenatal Macrophage Populations

Erythromyeloid Progenitors From the Yolk Sac

Mammalian hematopoiesis develops through successive waves beginning extraembryonically in the yolk sac blood islands where primitive erythromyeloid progenitors (EMPs) generate erythroblasts, megakaryocytes, and macrophages. EMPs are dependent upon RUNX1, SPI1 (PU.1), IRF8, and CSF1R but are independent of MYB and FLT3. A second wave of transient definitive hematopoiesis also originates in the yolk sac but has greater differentiation potential and requires MYB.[182-184] The differential transcription factor requirements of primitive and definitive hematopoiesis together with judiciously timed activation of lineage tracing markers have been used to dissect the relative contributions of different waves of hematopoiesis to macrophage populations[3-5,185] (*Figure 10.3*). The earliest yolk sac macrophages migrate through the embryo prior to vascularization and begin the process of populating the tissues.[3,42,186] Yolk sac–derived macrophages give rise to long-lived populations of microglia, LC, and initiate formation of Kupffer cells and other macrophages that can persist into adult life.[42,185,186] *MYB* and *FTL3* knockout mice, which lack definitive hematopoiesis, are able to sustain tissue macrophages from this primitive wave; however, when definitive hematopoiesis is allowed to proceed, fetal liver monocytes make a substantial contribution to many tissue macrophage populations as outlined below. Macrophages differentiated from induced pluripotential stem cells retain the features of yolk sac macrophages and are able to colonize the brain and lung to form microglia and alveolar macrophages, respectively.[187] In humans, this source of cells is a valuable experimental tool for examining primitive macrophage biology.[188,189]

Fetal Liver Hematopoiesis

Following the initial colonization of tissue by yolk sac macrophages, a wave of fetal liver monocytes enters nearly all organs and differentiates into resident macrophages. As a result of closure of the blood-brain barrier soon after, the brain becomes isolated and microglia remain exclusively yolk sac derived for life.[3] LC retain some yolk sac origin but are mainly derived from fetal liver monocytes.[190] Fetal liver monocytes are initially derived from transient definitive hematopoiesis arising from late yolk sac EMP[191] but are MYB-dependent, like true definitive hematopoiesis.[4,182] This wave is soon replaced by monocytes arising from definitive hematopoiesis, which expand into tissue macrophage populations during rapid growth of the fetal organs. Although the yolk sac is sufficient to provide tissue macrophages when it is the sole source of hematopoietic potential, the majority of tissue macrophages are derived via fetal liver monocytes.[4] In the mouse, the alveolar macrophage niche has been used to test the ability of successive waves of precursors to give rise to tissue macrophages. While all sources can replace alveolar macrophages, fetal liver monocytes are the most prolific on a per-cell basis.[64]

Definitive Hematopoiesis

Definitive hematopoietic stem cells (HSCs) arise in the aorta-gonad-mesonephros region at day 32 in humans (day 9 in the mouse) and migrate first to the fetal liver and then to the bone marrow. Ultimately, these HSC provide monocytes and DC for the remainder of the life of an organism through developmental pathways that are dependent upon RUNX1, GATA2, SPI1, IRF8, CSF1R, MYB, and FLT3. At birth, a small fraction of LC and variable percentages of all tissue macrophages can be traced to definitive HSC. The tissues that depend upon continual renewal from monocytes during adult life (gut, skin, and interstitial tissues) show a higher proportion of HSC-derived macrophages at birth.[8,70,192,193] In general, most interstitial macrophages are renewed by monocytes.[194] At the other end of the spectrum, populations with specialized tissue niches (microglia, LC, alveolar macrophages, and Kupffer cells) are usually self-renewing and do not require BM-derived precursors, unless disrupted.[195] If this occurs, then BM-derived cells are recruited to fill the empty niches in the epidermis, hepatic parenchyma, and alveolar spaces.[64,196,197] The ability of HSC-derived cells to replace LC, alveolar macrophages, and Kupffer cells has been formally demonstrated in human BM transplant recipients.[198-201]

Fetal Macrophages and Dendritic Cells

Fetal macrophages and DC have been isolated from brain, skin, lung, gut, spleen, LN, and thymus.[186,202-205] Conventional DC1 and DC2 can be identified in tissues and migratory fractions of LN DC. Although they can respond to TLR ligation, fetal DC1 strongly promote regulatory T-cell induction and inhibit the production of TNF by T cells through the expression of arginase-2 activity. It has been suggested that these unique properties play an important role in homeostatic immune-suppressive responses during gestation.[204] Early tissue macrophages retain gene expression signatures of EMP but already show evidence of tissue specification especially in the brain and liver, compared with the lung and skin.[186]

Differences Between Primitive and Definitive Origin Macrophages

The fact that most tissue macrophage populations present at birth have a dual contribution from primitive yolk sac hematopoiesis (pre-HSC) or definitive waves of hematopoiesis (HSC derived) has led many investigators to postulate that these are programs significant functional differences.[206] However, LC, Kupffer cells, and alveolar macrophage populations can be ablated and replaced by definitive origin cells without any perceptible changes to gene expression or function, once homeostasis is restored.[64,197,207,208] In the heart and serosal cavity, it is possible to distinguish between resident and more recently recruited macrophages,[193,209] possibly because of time-dependent variables or because these sites have weaker niche signals than the epidermis, liver, and lung. Under conditions of chronic perturbation, it is possible that resident and recruited cells maintain strong functional differences.[210,211]

Monocyte, Macrophage, and DC Development in the Adult

Lineage Priming in Hematopoiesis

Monocytes and DC have finite life spans of days to weeks after entering the periphery and are replenished by independent lineages of lymphomyeloid hematopoiesis.[14] It is now thought that progenitors are primed at an early stage of development and follow predestined pathways to give rise to mature cells.[212] This model has largely replaced the classical hierarchical descriptions of hematopoiesis in which there are sequential bifurcations of cell potential. It is now thought that previously defined progenitor fractions such as granulocyte-macrophage progenitors (GMPs) do not contain homogeneous multipotent cells, but a cross-section of distinct developmental pathways that share a common, transient phenotype.[213,214] Similarly, the entities macrophage-dendritic cell progenitor (MDP) and common dendritic cell progenitor (CDP) are phenotypic annotations that contain a higher density of related cell fates; they do not signify a discrete developmental stage where fate suddenly bifurcates. Although bipotential and tripotential cells exist, profiling of more than 2000 clonal outputs from the entire range of human progenitors does not reveal any significant populations corresponding to human MDP or CDP.[215,216]

Lymphomyeloid Progenitors

In addition to lineage priming, it now appears that the classical dichotomy between lymphoid and myeloid potential is not the initial restriction of cell fate. The most significant early partitioning occurs when megakaryocyte and erythroid potentials separate from lymphomyeloid potential.[213,214,216] Granulocytes, monocytes, DC, and lymphoid lineages all descend through lineage-primed pathways from lymphoid-primed multipotent progenitors (LMPPs). Regions previously defined as common myeloid progenitors have been resolved into mixtures of megaerythroid and myeloid precursors that are parallel rather than

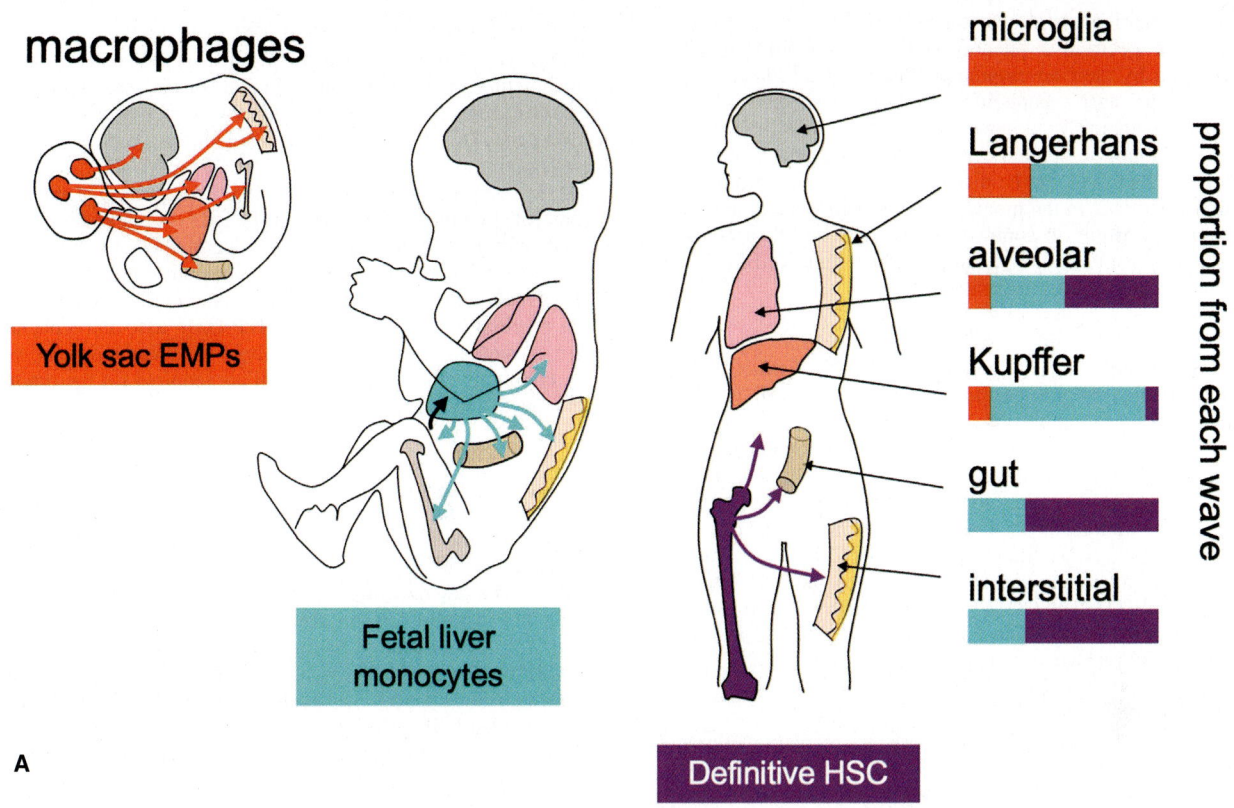

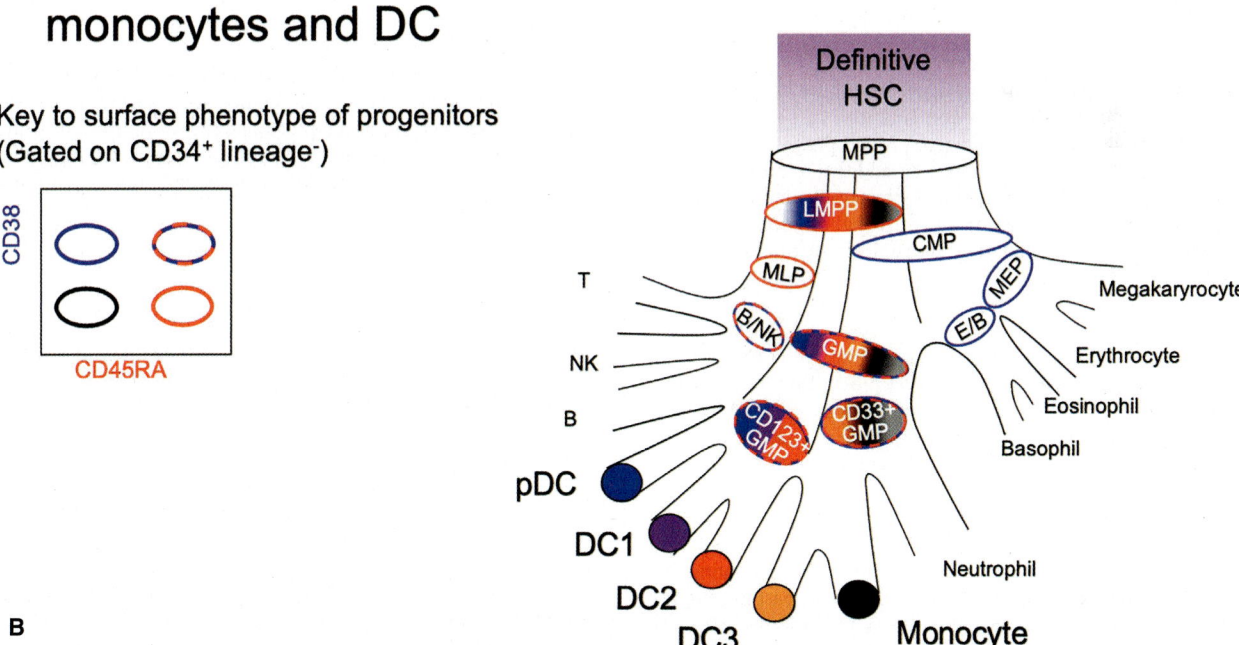

FIGURE 10.3 **Origins.** A, Macrophages. Schematic depicting three waves of macrophage development described in the mouse from yolk sac early myeloid progenitors (EMP; red), fetal liver monocytes (blue), and definitive hematopoietic stem cells (HSC; purple). Bars on the right-hand side show the estimated contribution of each wave based on mouse data. B, Monocytes and DC. Schematic showing the development of human DC from lymphoid-primed multipotent progenitors (LMPP), via granulocyte-macrophage progenitors (GMP) according to contemporary lineage-primed models of hematopoiesis. B/NK, progenitors of B and NK cells; CMP, common myeloid progenitors; E/B, eosinophil and basophil progenitors; MEP, megakaryocyte erythroid progenitors; MLP, multilymphoid progenitors. The inset is a key to the surface phenotype of each progenitor compartment depicted by the color of its border in the main figure (blue for CD38+ and red for CD45RA+).

The Normal Hematologic System

antecedent to other regions of hematopoiesis. DC and monocytes can be ordered as a spectrum of phenotypes from lymphoid to myeloid that is mirrored by their developmental pathways.[215] Plasmacytoid DC (pDC) are the most "lymphoid" with RAG, rearranged IgH loci, and CD45RA. Myeloid DC express myeloid antigens; DC1 are easy to separate from monocyte-derived cells but DC2 and DC3 share many antigens in common and can be difficult to dissociate entirely from monocyte-derived DC. In the mouse, it is commonly stated that pDC have a lymphoid origin, in contrast to other DC.[217,218] In humans, markers have not yet been discovered to resolve primitive LMPP into components that mirror this observation.[99]

Granulocyte Macrophage Progenitor Fractions

In the GMP compartment it is possible to identify distinct regions enriched for monocyte and DC lineages. High M-CSFR (CD115) expression marks a region enriched for monocyte and myeloid DC potential (MDP-like), which may be further fractionated by high expression of CLEC12A and CD64 into common monocyte progenitors.[219] High CD123 expression defines another region of GMP containing mainly unipotent progenitors for the classical DC lineages pDC, DC1, and DC2 (CDP-like).[99,113,215] In the CD123-low fraction of GMP, DC and monocyte potential may be separated by differential expression of CD33 and CD117.[99] At the single cell level, another study reports that the CD123 high fraction of KIT+ FLT3+ cells identifies monocyte, DC, and osteoclast potential.[79]

The Role of Growth Factors

In common with all lineages of hematopoiesis, the regulation of monocyte, macrophage, and DC development depends upon the coordinated regulation of gene expression orchestrated by networks of transcription factors (TFs) and extrinsic growth factor signals acting through growth factor receptors (*Figure 10.4*). There is considerable interest in the use of growth factors to augment production or activity of monocytes and DC, particularly in the field of vaccination and cancer therapy where FLT3 ligand and GM-CSF have been given as a means of expanding DC populations. Conversely, growth factors such as G-CSF that enhance production of immature myeloid cells may lead to immunosuppressive effects. Many different approaches have also been taken to producing tolerogenic DC with combinations of growth factors, cytokines, and immunosuppressive agents. Macrophage production is primarily controlled by the M-CSF axis. In addition to administration of M-CSF to expand monocyte and macrophage populations, specific drugs have also been developed to target signaling via the M-CSF receptor with the aim of attenuating macrophage recruitment during inflammation.

Stem Cell Factor

Stem cell factor (SCF) is an early hematopoietic growth factor that binds to KIT (CD117), which is highly expressed by early LMPP and monocytic and granulocytic precursor regions of the GMP. SCF is widely added to in vitro hematopoietic culture systems to promote overall cell production and is usually retained for the production of DC and monocytes.[220]

Thrombopoietin

Thrombopoietin (TPO) is also an early growth factor promoting the formation of megakaryocytes that has been used in the past to generate myeloid cells in vitro. It does not specifically promote monocyte or DC generation, and more recent studies have dispensed with it.[113,215]

Interleukin-3

High expression of the IL3 receptor CD123 characterizes regions of GMP with DC-restricted potential.[99,113,215] However, the function of IL3 is less clear during the development of DC as it is not essential for hematopoiesis in mice or the production of DC by in vitro cultures. High levels of IL3 are associated with sepsis and the inflammatory response.[221]

Fms-Like Tyrosine Kinase-3 Ligand

Fms-like tyrosine kinase-3 ligand (FLT3LG) is frequently described as a DC-poietin from the observation in mice that knockout leads to failure of DC production. In keeping with this, injection in human volunteers expands DC production and FLT3LG increases production of DC from progenitors cultured in vitro.[215,220] However, the receptor FLT3 (CD135) is highly expressed on all LMPP suggesting a more fundamental role in human hematopoiesis. FLT3LG is markedly elevated in patients with low progenitor cell mass due to *GATA2* mutation, aplastic anemia, or following recovery from chemotherapy.[222] Activation of FLT3 signaling by internal tandem duplication is a common feature of acute myeloid leukemia with an LMPP-GMP associated phenotype. These considerations highlight the role of FLT3 in the development of early lymphomyeloid progenitors that are required for the production of monocyte and DC lineages.

GM-CSF (CSF2)

GM-CSF is secreted by T cells and epithelial cells and came to prominence as a key factor in promoting the differentiation of monocytes into DC in vitro.[223] Recent observations suggest that GM-CSF is required for the differentiation of DC3 in xenografts in in vitro culture and that it is a key mediator of interactions between resident memory T cells and myeloid cells in graft-versus-host disease (GVHD) and cancer.[100,224] The absolute requirement of alveolar macrophages for GM-CSF is also shown by patients who develop pulmonary alveolar proteinosis because of antibodies to GM-CSF. Therapeutic antibodies to GM-CSF have shown promising results in early-phase clinical trials in the treatment of inflammatory responses including COVID infection, possibly through the attenuation of inflammatory macrophages.[225,226]

M-CSF (CSF1)

M-CSF is widely produced by endothelial cells, stromal cells, and smooth muscle and is detectable in plasma and serum. It is a critical factor in promoting the differentiation of monocytes, macrophages, and inflammatory DC. The M-CSF receptor, CD115, is widely used to define monocytes and their derivatives in mice.[7] Knockout mice lacking either the receptor or growth factor have a severe defect of macrophage production and develop osteopetrosis as a result of osteoclast deficiency. Owing to the role of macrophages in promoting inflammatory disease and neoplasia, there is considerable interest in inhibition of the M-CSF axis for therapeutic gain.[225,227]

Interleukin 34

IL-34 is an alternative ligand for M-CSFR[228] accounting for the ability of LCs and microglia to persist in M-CSF knockout mice.[229,230] New roles for IL-34 are emerging in the differential regulation of LC and macrophages in the steady state and inflammation[231-233] and in the regulation of tolerance through its production by Tregs.[234]

Interleukin 4

IL-4 is well known for two key aspects in monocyte, macrophage, and DC biology: the specification of "alternatively activated" (M2) macrophages[235] and the induction of monocyte-derived DC.[37,223] IL-4 induced transcripts also include DC-STAMP, a critical regulator of cell fusion, linking responses to IL-4 with giant cell formation.[78] IL-4 is also linked to macrophage proliferation induced under conditions of Th2 immunity.[236]

RANK Ligand (TNFSF11)

RANK ligand is a critical inducer of osteoclast formation. A distinction is usually drawn between osteoclasts generated with IL-4 and MGCs formed in the presence of IL-4 and IL-13, although they share a great many properties in common.[78] RANK ligand is highly expressed in the bone marrow and is found in soluble and a membrane-bound form expressed on stromal cells.

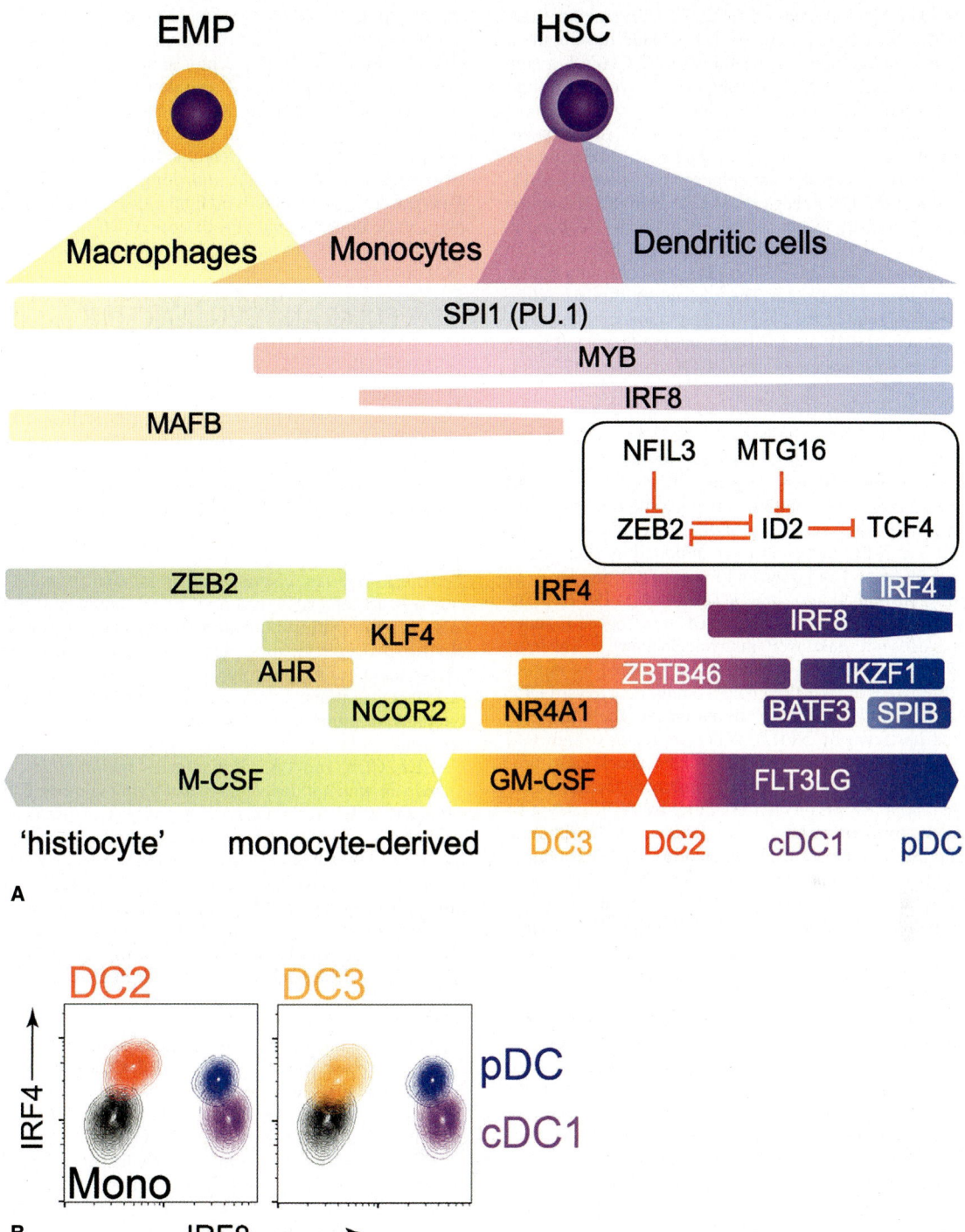

FIGURE 10.4 Regulation of development. A, Macrophages and monocyte-derived cells differentiate under the influence of transcription factors that include SPI1 (PU.1), MAFB, zinc finger E-box-binding homeobox 2 (ZEB2), and Kruppel-like factor 4 (KLF-4). Aryl hydrocarbon receptor (AHR), NCOR2, and NR4A1 also play a role in monocyte differentiation. Critical negative feedback loops that mutually exclude alternate DC fates between DC2, cDC1/DC1, and pDC are shown in the box. ZBTB46, Basic leucine zipper transcriptional factor ATF-like 3 (BATF3), and Ikaros family zinc finger 1 (IKZF1) also play key roles. B, Early lineage priming and late differentiation between pDC, cDC1/DC1, DC2, and alternate fates also critically depends upon the balance of interferon response factors IRF4 and IRF8, as illustrated in the 2D plot showing their expression in blood classical monocytes and DC by intracellular fluorescence cytometry.

Regulation of Development by Transcription Factors

Monocyte, macrophage, and DC development in mammals is guided by many transcription factors (TFs) that facilitate lymphomyeloid differentiation and ultimately lead to the specification of an array of distinct phenotypes.[237,238] Several factors are known to act at multiple stages in development first as pioneer factors making chromatin accessible, then as lineage-determining factors specifying a gene expression program, and finally as response elements in mature cells. Cooperation

and mutual antagonism both exist and may mirror regulatory networks observed in other cell types such as lymphocytes.

Pioneer Factors in the Early Stem Cell Compartment

SPI1 (PU.1) is an ets-related factor operating in early progenitors to antagonize GATA1 and direct development away from megakaryocyte-erythroid differentiation. It is required for the development of LMPP and subsequently of all monocytes and DC. Downstream targets of

SPI1 include the key myeloid genes *CSF1R* (M-CSF receptor) and *ITGAM* (CD11b), and it is required for macrophage development from both primitive and definitive hematopoiesis.[185] GATA2, a zinc finger protein, is also essential for the development of lymphomyeloid progenitors, and haploinsufficiency in humans compromises almost all mononuclear cells.[62,169,222,239] A specific role in DC development has been documented in mice.[240] IRF8 also appears to govern lineage priming at an early stage and acts as a pioneer factor within SPI1-primed cells to direct the DC lineage.[215] MAFB is highly expressed in myelomonocytic progenitors and monocytes. It assists PU.1 in the repression of erythroid differentiation and remains at high levels in monocytes, macrophages, and LC.[241] It is also detectable at a higher level in DC3 compared with DC2.[21] The zinc finger E-box binding protein ZEB2 is also required for the priming of monocyte development and expression of CSF1R at early stages in development. It plays a key role in the later specification of myeloid DC.

The ID2-ZEB2-TCF4 Axis

Inhibitor of DNA binding (ID) proteins are key regulators of stem cell potential, controlling myeloid bias during early lineage commitment by blocking binding of basic HLH proteins including TCF3 (E2A) and TCF4 (E2-2). ZEB2 is also differentially active in primitive and definitive hematopoiesis.[242] The specification of pDC is completely dependent upon TCF4 and ZEB2 and is strongly inhibited by ID2, which directs development away from pDC and toward DC1 and DC2. In humans, heterozygous mutation or loss of TCF4 causes Pitt-Hopkins syndrome in which mature IFNα-secreting pDC are reduced in number, although this does not cause overt immunodeficiency.[113] The level of ID2 activity in classical DC progenitors is regulated by mutual antagonism with ZEB2.[243,244] ID2 promotes commitment toward DC1 while high ZEB2 indirectly favors pDC development. The ID2-ZEB2 axis is regulated upstream by NFIL3, which promotes a high ID2 state[245] and MTG16, which enhances ZEB2.[246] Feedback loops promote stability and eventually permit full commitment to either DC1 or pDC lineages. Suppression of DC1 potential by ZEB2 may also be required for the formation of DC2, at a later point.[244] Although mature DC1 and DC2 are more closely related to each other than to pDC, the common antagonism of DC1 fate brings the DC2 and pDC developmental trajectories very close and probably explains the pDC-like qualities of pre-DC2 (also known as AXL$^+$ SIGLEC6$^+$ or "transitional" DC).

IRF4, IRF8, and BATF3

The interferon regulatory factors IRF4 and IRF8 play important roles in monocyte, macrophage, and DC development. High IRF8 expression defines the classical DC pathway through which pDC, DC1, and DC2 develop. Activation of specific enhancer elements of IRF8 by the ID2-ZEB2-TCF4 axis recruits BATF3 and IRF8 to an autoregulatory loop that maintains high IRF8 and defines the DC1 fate.[247] At alternative IRF8 enhancers, transcription factor activation permits the formation of pDC and DC2. Mature pDC express both IRF8 and IRF4, whereas DC2 pass through a transient high IRF8 state and express more IRF4 as mature cells. Expression of both is lower in DC3 and not present in monocytes.

IRF8 mutation impairs monocyte and DC development in humans.[170,248] Gene dosage is a critical determinant in understanding the effect of IRF8 variants upon hematopoiesis. Biallelic mutation ablates all monocyte and DC production, diverting hematopoietic output toward neutrophils.[170] The importance of IRF8 in DC1 development is underscored by the ability to generate DC1-like cells from human fibroblasts using only expression of SPI1, IRF8, and BATF3.[249]

Some populations of murine DC2 require IRF4 for their development and expression of Th2 and Th17 functions, depending on the model.[250,251] In humans, monocytes require IRF4 to differentiate toward a DC phenotype.[36]

Terminal Differentiation Factors

Commitment to a particular lineage activates additional factors that stabilize the transcriptome. In pDC, SPIB, BCL11A, and RUNX1 enter a feed-forward loop with TCF4 to maintain the pDC transcriptome. ZBTB46 is expressed in both DC1 and DC2 during terminal differentiation, and populations of DC2 in the mouse require either KLF4 or NOTCH receptor signals.[252] KLF4 is also required for monocyte development[253] and downregulation of KLF4 by notch signaling allows monocytes to differentiate into LC, a property inherent in DC2.[254,255] Subsets of DC2 have been described in mice and human spleen that have differential expression of TBX21 (T-BET)/RUNX3, and RORC/CEBPA, mirroring the terminal differentiation of T-helper cells and innate lymphoid cells.[256] IKZF1 (IKAROS) also plays a role in determining the balance of DC maturation, and humans with IKZF1 mutation have selective pDC deficiency with increased DC1 production.[257]

MOLECULAR AND CELLULAR FUNCTIONS

Chemotaxis

Chemotaxis, the movement of cells in response to chemical gradients, plays a major part in the steady-state positioning and inflammatory recruitment of leukocytes within tissues. Matrix-bound gradients may also mediate "haptotaxis." Chemotactic receptors are commonly seven spanning G protein–coupled receptors related to the environment-sensing retinal rhodopsins and olfactory receptors.

Chemotactins

The most important chemotactins in inflammation are N-formylated peptides, a chemical signature of the N terminus of prokaryotic proteins, together with complement components C3a and C5a (the "anaphylatoxins"), chemokines, and leukotrienes. Chemokines consist of a large family of related polypeptides that also mediate the movement of leukocytes in the steady state and are frequently also involved in lymphocyte migration. Chemokines are divided into subclasses on the basis of the spacing of the N-terminal cysteine residues. CCL#, CXCL#, CL#, and CX3CL# refer to four families of chemokine ligands, in which # denotes the identifying number, C denotes a cysteine, and X denotes a noncysteine amino acid. Many are angiogenic, marked by an additional ELR (Glu-Leu-Arg) sequence prior to the CC motif.[258] Ligand binding leads to integrin activation and polarization of the actin cytoskeleton. Together these processes facilitate adhesion, directional sensing, and migration through the classical mechanisms of actin polymerization and F-actin formation at the leading edge, driven by accumulation of small GTPases, RAC, CDC42, and PI3K while RHO GTPase and its effectors accumulate at the trailing edge.

Chemokines

Broadly speaking, chemokine receptors may be divided into inflammatory receptors, such as CCR1, CCR2, CCR3, and CCR5, that have multiple ligands, and receptors that control the positioning of lymphocytes and monocytes in tissues. These include CCR7 (CCL19,20), XCR1 (XCL1,2), CCR6 (CCL20), CCR9 (CCL25), and several CXCR receptors that have 1 to 2 specific ligand pairings (*Figure 10.5*). Negative regulation is achieved through nonsignaling decoy receptors. Viruses may also express both ligands and receptors to manipulate the immune response. Under conditions of inflammation, monocytes are recruited to tissues by CCL2 (MCP-1), CCL3 (MIP1a), and CCL5 (RANTES) acting through CCR1, CCR2, and CCR5. Attempts to inhibit inflammatory cell recruitment have been challenging, owing to the abundance of potential ligands for a particular receptor.[259] Experts in the field have noted that functional specificity is much greater when spatiotemporal factors are considered and that the system should be regarded as exquisitely balanced, rather than just simply redundant.[258]

Differential Chemokine Usage by Monocytes and DC

Migration dependent upon CCR2 is a hallmark of classical monocyte recruitment and contributes to steady-state populations of macrophages in the dermis, gut, and serosal surfaces.[70,192,193] It is not clear which ligands are responsible for homeostatic recruitment among the candidates CCL2, 7, 8,12, and 13. Classical monocytes have higher expression of CCR2, while CX3CR1 is a marker of the nonclassical subset, conserved between species. The latter is more selective, binding only CX3CL1 (fractalkine). CCR7 is an important receptor in positioning

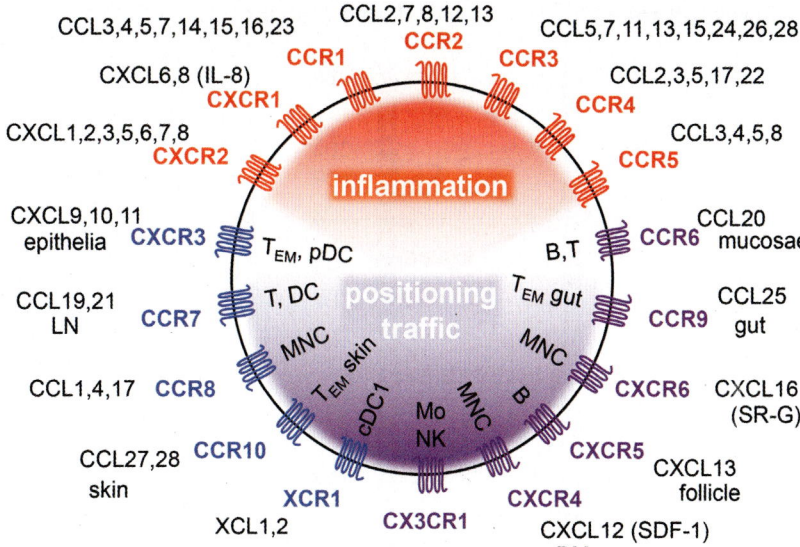

FIGURE 10.5 Chemokines and their receptors. Chemokines and their receptors, depicted as seven spanning membrane proteins, involved in inflammatory recruitment and in the positioning and trafficking of mononuclear cells. Receptors in red have many ligands and are mainly implicated in inflammation. Blue receptors are selective for 2 to 3 ligands and have more specialized roles such as the recruitment of cells to lymph nodes or imprinting of memory T cells to skin. Purple receptors are the most selective with specific ligands. CXCL8 is IL-8, CXCL16 is macrophages scavenger receptor G (SR-G) when surface bound, and CXCL12 is stromal cell–derived factor (SDF-1).

migratory DC and lymphocytes in the lymph node, under the influence of gradients in CCL19 and CCL21.[260] The two chemokines have complementary functions in guiding cells to the correct location. CCL21 may be immobilized and directs migratory cells to the surface of the afferent lymphatics and HEV. CCL19 is expressed in soluble form in the lymph node and downregulates CCR7 expression thus helping to terminate the chemotactic signal. Monocytes and macrophages do not express CCR7, but it may be upregulated on monocyte-derived DC. Expression of CCR7 is often used as a surrogate marker of the ability of a cell to traffic to lymph nodes. XCR1 highly restricted to the DC1 subset of DC as discussed below.

Surface Receptors

Monocytes, macrophages, and dendritic cells are able to interact with a staggering array of extracellular signals through the expression of many different classes of receptors. Among the key processes mediated by surface receptors are pathogen sensing, phagocytosis, adhesion, and transendothelial migration, antigen presentation, and regulation of metabolism. Many plasma membrane glycoproteins are shed into the circulation by alternative splicing or proteolytic cleavage. These may act as decoy receptors or inhibitors, and many provide biomarkers for macrophage activation in pathology.

Integrins

Integrins are large heterodimeric glycoproteins that connect the extracellular matrix to the cytoskeleton and mediate bidirectional signaling to control cell-cell and cell-matrix interactions.[261] Integrin specificity and function is determined by an assortment of 24 different α and β subunit pairs that are divided into four families: fibronectin/vitronectin-binding, collagen receptors, laminin receptors, and receptors restricted to leukocytes (*Figure 10.6*). The group of leukocyte receptors formed by the β2 (CD18) subunit comprises the family of CD11 proteins among which CD11a (LFA-1) and the complement receptors CD11b (complement receptor 3; CR3) and CD11c (complement receptor 4; CR4) play critical roles in monocyte and DC biology. CD11 integrins recognize Ig-like intercellular adhesion molecules ICAM-1 and ICAM-2 and CD49d/VLA4 binds to vascular cell adhesion molecule (VCAM), α4β7 to MAdCAM, and αEβ7 to E-cadherin. Integrins are critically required for transendothelial migration, following activation of selectins and endothelial rolling. Firm adhesion is mediated by interactions between β1 and β2 integrins expressed on leukocytes with VCAM-1 and ICAM-1 on the endothelium. There is considerable interest in targeting these proteins with monoclonal antibodies to attenuate leukocyte recruitment in inflammation.[262]

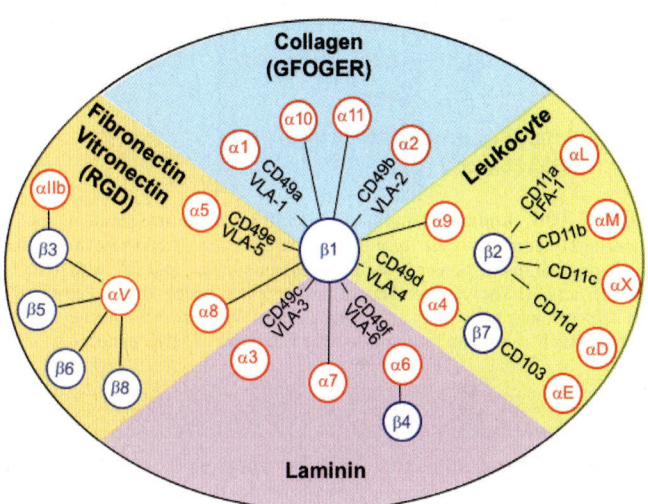

FIGURE 10.6 Integrins. Integrins consist of two chains (alpha and beta) that may be expressed in combinatorial fashion to give receptor complexes with different ligand specificities. Beta 1 is widely distributed on mammalian cells and is the partner for very late antigens (VLA 1-6; CD49a-f) so named for their delayed induction after T-cell activation. Beta 2 (CD18) is restricted to leukocytes and is the partner for all of the CD11 alpha chains L, M, X, and D that form LFA-1 (CD11a) and the complement receptors C3 (CD11b) and C4 (CD11c). The collagen receptors recognize a sequence GFOGER. The fibronectin and vitronectin receptors bind to RGD.

Immunoglobulin Superfamily Molecules

Proteins with immunoglobulin domains are extremely abundant forming the basis of multiple key recognition systems in immunity. The immunoglobulin fold is a modular building block that may be assembled into many different array configurations and is involved in several distinct types of homotypic and heterotypic interactions (*Figure 10.7*). MHC molecules; coreceptors (CD3, CD4, CD8, CD19, CD79); costimulatory antigens (CD28, CD80, CD86); inhibitory receptors (CD200, SIRPA); cell adhesion molecules, including the CD2 and SLAM family of homotypic receptors (CD2, CD48, CD54/ICAM-1, CD58/LFA-3, CD150, CD229, CD244); and growth factor and cytokine receptors (CD117, PDGFR, MSCFR, IL-1R) all contain Ig superfamily domains. The Ig superfamily adhesion molecules VCAM-1 and ICAM-1 expressed on endothelium interact with leukocyte integrins, to mediate firm adhesion, a key step in transendothelial migration.

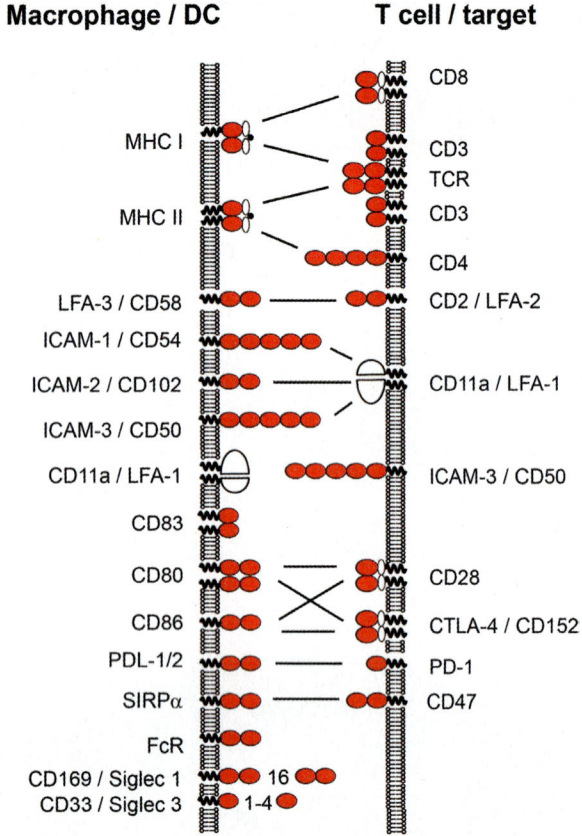

FIGURE 10.7   Immunoglobulin superfamily interactions. Immunoglobulin superfamily domains (red) form the structure of many important molecules mediating the interactions of macrophages, monocytes, and DC with T cells or other targets. The key members of this large and widely distributed family are depicted, together with their binding partners. White ovoids indicate non-Ig domains such as integrin receptors and the N termini of MHC molecules.

Fc and Complement Receptors

The expression of immunoglobulin Fc receptors is a cardinal property of mononuclear phagocytes allowing them to take up particles opsonized by antibody and to receive signals from the humoral immune milieu.[263] Fc receptors are members of the Ig superfamily and may be activatory or inhibitory. They are abundant on monocytes, macrophages, and DC with a greater enrichment for inhibitory receptor expression on DC. Recent evidence suggests that the therapeutic benefit of monoclonal antibody therapy is dependent upon macrophage-mediated cytotoxicity to opsonized cells.[264] Myeloid cells express multiple receptors for complement, including the anaphylatoxin C3a and C5a receptors, complement receptors 1 (CD35) and 2 (CD21), and the integrin complement receptors CD11b (CR3) and CD11c (CR4).

Scavenger Receptors

Macrophages express a wide range of scavenger receptors that include well-known macrophage antigens, macrophage scavenger receptor 1 (MSR1), macrophage receptor with collagenous structure (MARCO), CD36, CD68, and CD163. Although these are structurally diverse, consensus has assembled scavenger receptors into a supergroup of classes A to J (*Figure 10.8*), which overlaps with some other biochemical classifications by including, for example, a number of C-type lectins in group E (LOX1 and DECTIN 1).[265,266] Scavenger receptors are united by their ability to recognize common polyionic ligands including lipoproteins, apoptotic cells, cholesterol ester, phospholipids, proteoglycans, ferritin, and carbohydrates. The most well-known scavenger receptors recognize oxidized LDL: the B class proteins SR-B1 and SR-B2 (CD36) and E class C-type lectin, SR-E1 (LOX1). SR-I1 (CD163) is the main receptor for haptoglobin and hemoglobin

complexes. Scavenger receptors are highly expressed by splenic macrophages and Kupffer cells.

C-Type Lectins

C-type lectins receptors (CLRs) are a heterogeneous superfamily of soluble and transmembrane proteins so named because they require calcium ions for ligand binding. They are important as scavenger receptors, pattern recognition receptors, and adhesion molecules.[267] Recognition of fungal pathogens involves CLRs belonging to the Dectin-1 (CLEC7A) and Dectin-2 (CLEC4N) clusters of receptors. Recent screening of fungal antigen libraries with chimeric Fc proteins has identified that the melanin-binding lectin CLEC1A (MelLec) mediates protection against *Aspergillus fumigatus*.[268] Other well-known CLRs include DEC-205 (CD205), macrophage mannose receptor (CD206), Langerin (CD207), DC-LAMP (CD208), and DC-SIGN (CD209). Most of these function as pattern recognition receptors for viruses and fungi.

The selectins P-selectin, E-selectin, and L-selectin are CLRs that predominantly recognize the sialyl Lewis x (sLex) tetrasaccharide modification present on mucin-like glycoproteins. P-selectin is stored in the Weibel-Palade bodies of endothelial cells and in platelet α-granules, and its main ligand, P-selectin glycoprotein ligand-1 (PSGL-1), is expressed by all circulating leukocytes. Upregulation of P-selectin is a major mechanism initiating the rolling of leukocytes in inflammation. E-selectin is found on skin endothelial cells in the steady state but can be induced on most endothelial cells by inflammatory stimuli. Ligands for E-selectin include the leukocyte surface markers CD34 and CD44. L-selectin is constitutively expressed by leukocytes and controls the homing of monocytes and DC to lymphoid organs via peripheral node addressin (PNAd) and to mucosal tissue via the mucosal addressin, cell adhesion molecule-1 (MAdCAM-1). Activation of selectin binding mediates tethering and rolling on the surface of activated endothelial cells, the first step in transendothelial migration.

Siglecs

Siglecs are sialic acid–binding immunoglobulin-type lectins involved in a range of recognition and regulation processes. Siglec 1 (CD169; Sialoadhesin), siglec 2 (CD22), siglec 4 (MAG), and siglec 15 are structurally related and conserved between species. Siglec 3 (CD33) is part of a large family of related molecules that are more diverse between species.[267,269] Siglecs frequently contain intracellular ITIM domains and may transmit regulatory signals in cis by binding sialic acid on neighboring surface proteins.

TAM Receptors

The three TAM receptors, TYRO3, AXL, and MER, are members of a distinct protein tyrosine kinase group involved in recognition of apoptotic cells and downregulation of cytokine production by myeloid cells engaged in efferocytosis. Their ligands Gas6 and protein S are optimally bound in the presence of exposed phosphatidyl serine and calcium. Deletion of the TAM receptors results in autoimmunity, blindness, and sterility as a direct result of the failure of phagocytes to remove apoptotic cells causing overproduction of inflammatory cytokines.[270]

Regulatory Receptors: TREM, CD200R, and SIRPA

The receptors TREM1-4 (triggering receptor expressed on myeloid cells) are members of the Ig superfamily that signal via DAP12 to activate a variety of processes including antigen presenting cell function.[271]

The CD200R receptor is an inhibitory receptor restricted to myeloid cells that binds CD200 on a range of cellular targets. Ligation of the receptor inhibits the production of TNF, interferon, and NO and is implicated in scenarios of immune evasion by pathogens and malignant cells.[272]

SIRPA (signal regulatory protein alpha) is highly expressed on monocytes and macrophages and interacts with CD47 on target cells to transmit a phagocytosis checkpoint signal. This system plays a major role in maintenance of the HSC niche and in protecting red cells

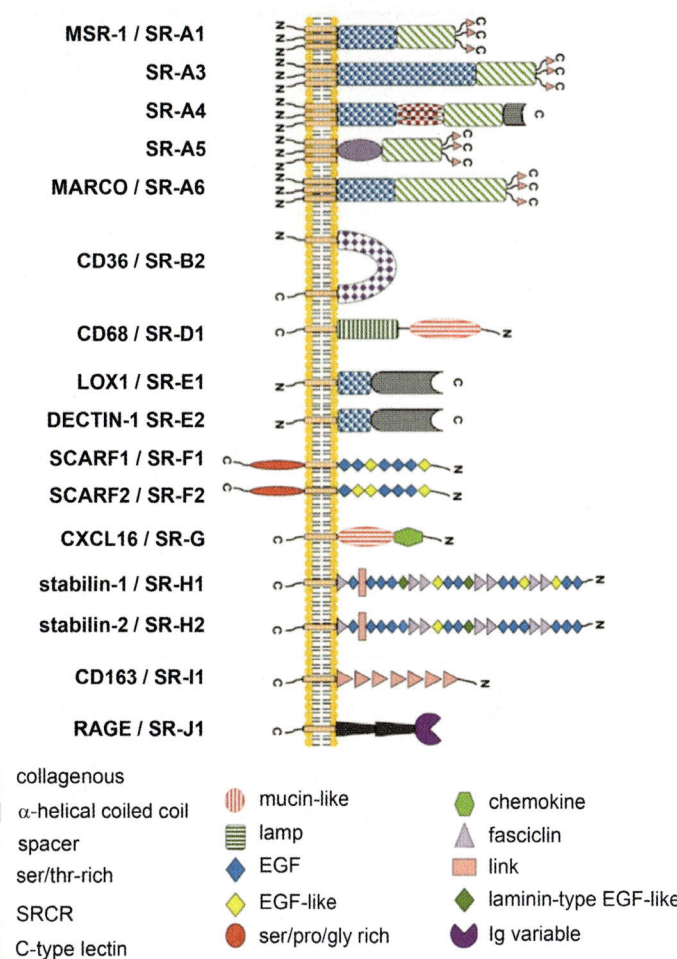

FIGURE 10.8 Scavenger receptors. Scavenger receptors are widely expressed by phylogenetically distant organisms and have been assembled into a structurally diverse super-group of molecules consisting of classes A to J. Class C is not expressed in mammals and therefore not shown. Abbreviations: MSR, macrophage scavenger receptor; MARCO, macrophage receptor with collagenous structure; LOX, oxidized low-density lipoprotein; SCARF, scavenger receptor class F; RAGE, receptor for advanced glycation end products; SRCR, scavenger receptor cysteine-rich domain. (Adapted from Zani IA, Stephen SL, Mughal NA, et al. Scavenger receptor structure and function in health and disease. *Cells.* 2015;4(2):178-201. http://creativecommons.org/licenses/by/4.0/)

from phagocytosis by splenic macrophages.[273,274] Owing to the role of macrophages in therapeutic antibody-mediated uptake of target cells, there is considerable interest in blocking SIRPA interactions to enhance efficacy.[275]

Pattern Recognition Receptors

Pattern recognition receptors (PRRs) bind to microbial and host-derived molecules present during infection or inflammation to activate innate immunity.[276] The main classes include CLRs (see above), toll-like receptors (TLRs), NOD-like receptors (NLRs), and RIG-I-like receptors (RLRs). Some PRRs are present on epithelial and stromal cells, but the most diverse arrays are found in macrophages and DC and are linked directly to signal transduction mechanisms that elicit rapid focused responses.

Toll-Like Receptors

Humans have 10 TLRs consisting of an ectodomain with leucine-rich repeats, a transmembrane domain, and a cytoplasmic Toll/IL-1 receptor (TIR) domain that initiates intracellular signaling.[277,278] TLRs 1, 2, 4, 5, and 6 are located on the plasma membrane while the intracellular TLRs 3, 7, 8, and 9 are found in endosomes. Cell surface TLRs recognize microbial membrane lipids, lipoproteins, and proteins. TLR4 recognizes LPS; TLR1/2/6 bind to lipoproteins, peptidoglycans, lipotechoic acids, zymosan, mannan, and tGPI-mucin. TLR5 is specific for bacterial flagellin and TLR10, and TLR2 recognizes ligands from *Listeria*. Intracellular TLRs bind to nucleic acids derived from bacteria and viruses: TLR3: double-stranded RNA; TLR7: single-stranded RNA; TLR9: unmethylated CpG and hemozoin, a crystalline by-product of the malarial parasite *Plasmodium falciparum*; TLR8: viral and bacterial RNA. It has recently been demonstrated that antimicrobial

peptides act to focus and amplify pathogen binding to PRRs.[279] TLR signaling involves TIR domain–containing adaptor proteins such as MyD88 and TRIF that initiate signal transduction culminating in the activation of NF-κB, IRFs, and MAP kinases. Combinatorial stimuli that activate both TLR signaling and parallel recognition systems, such as Fc receptor binding, are strongly synergistic through the coordinated recruitment of signal transduction pathways.[280]

NOD-Like Receptors, RIG-I-Like Receptors, and Intracellular DNA Sensors

Phylogenetically ancient systems mediate cytosolic recognition of pathogenic nucleic acids through a range of nucleotide-binding domains and helicase structures. There are 22 human NLRs, 3 RLRs, and a range of other oligonucleotide-binding proteins such as AIM2 and GAS.[150,281,282] Binding of these sensor molecules is involved in a multitude of innate immune signaling pathways, including the upregulation of NF-κB and MAP kinase signaling, induction of MHC expression, interferon production, and assembly of the inflammasome, a protein complex that activates caspases, necessary for the production of IL-1β and IL-18.[283] Dysregulation of inflammasome function is the underlying cause of many autoinflammatory disorders.[284]

Phagocytosis

Monocytes, macrophages, and DC are able to internalize and ingest small particles or microbes by phagocytosis[285] (*Figure 10.9*). Actin rearrangement to engulf a particle relies on the signaling of RHO family GTPases, specifically RHOA. A phagocytic synapse has been described in which antigen-binding receptors such as DECTIN-1 achieve a critical density to trigger signaling by clustering together and excluding the inhibitory phosphatases CD45 and CD148.[286]

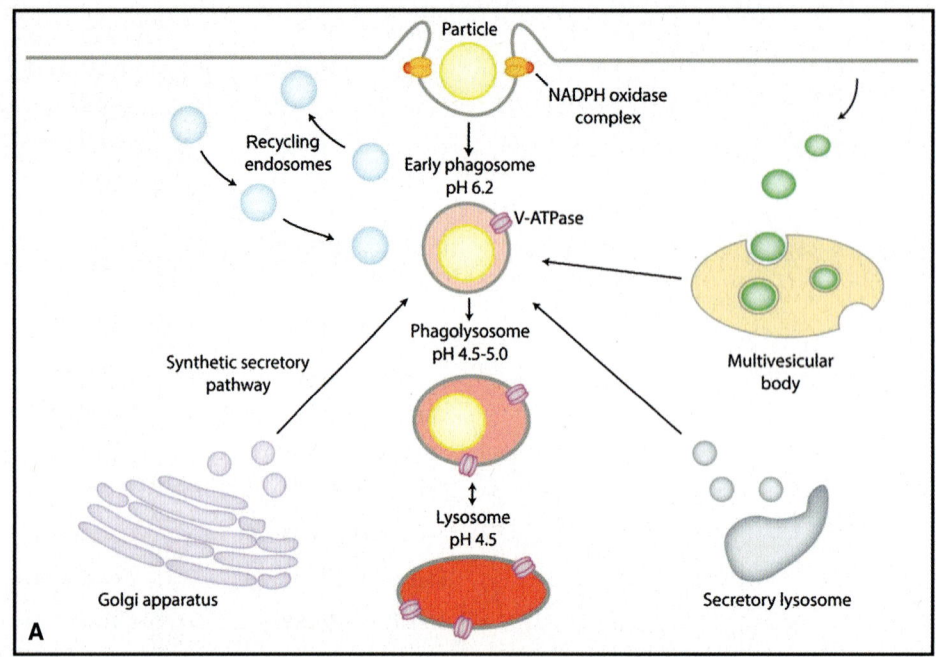

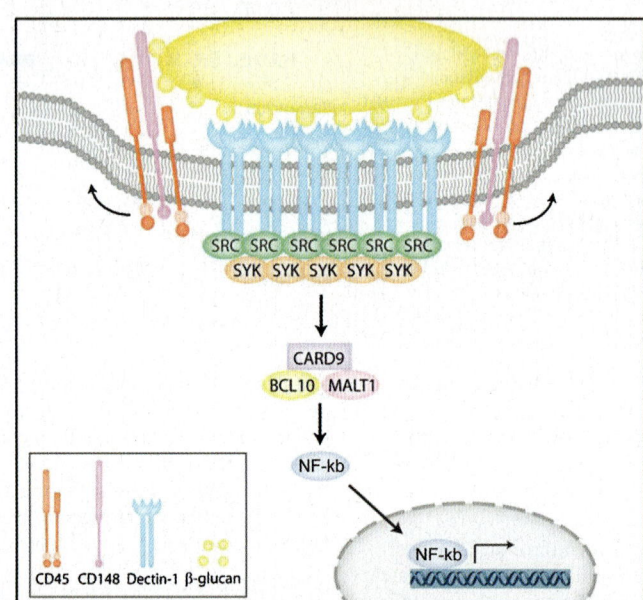

FIGURE 10.9 Phagocytosis. A, The uptake of exogenous particles results in a dynamic, integrated sequence of plasma membrane fusion and fission with intracellular vesicular membranes. The progressive acidification and maturation of phagosomes intersecting with vesicles from the biosynthetic and secretory pathway culminates in phagolysosomal fusion and digestion. B, The phagocytic synapse illustrated by dectin binding to β-glucan. The regulatory phosphatases CD45 and CD148 are excluded by a zone of integrins resulting in recruitment of SRC and SYK family kinases that activate cytoskeletal reorganization, actin polymerization, and membrane recycling, leading to the engulfment of the particle. NADPH, nicotinamide adenine dinucleotide phosphate. (Reproduced with permission from Gordon S. Phagocytosis: an immunobiologic process. *Immunity.* 2016;44:463-475.)

The resulting intracellular vesicle is termed a phagosome, which subsequently matures through step-wise fusion of endosomes and lysosomes, driven by RAB GTPase, to become a phagolysosome. Acidification continues to a pH of nearly 4, which, combined with hydrolytic and catabolic enzymes, leads to the destruction of microbes.

Phagocytic Receptors

Opsonic receptors including Fc receptors and complement receptors mediate phagocytosis of microbial particles bound by immunoglobulin and complement, respectively. Other molecules may function as opsonins, including fibronectin, mannose-binding lectin, and milk fat globulin (lactadherin). Platelets too may opsonize larger particles and direct them to phagocytic and antigen presenting pathways. Opsonic

phagocytosis is not always proinflammatory, however, as illustrated by the role of complement in synaptic pruning by microglia during development. This process may become subverted and proinflammatory in neurodegenerative disease.[287] Nonopsonic receptors engage in direct recognition and include many classes already discussed such as scavenger receptors, CLRs, and siglecs.

Macropinocytosis by Dendritic Cells

Macropinocytosis is a major mechanism of antigen uptake by DC.[288] The large lamellipodia that led to the description of afferent lymphatic DC as "veiled cells" allow the cell to internalize macropinosomes equivalent to its own volume within an hour. This activity depends upon actin ruffling, CDC42, and RAC. Most of the fluid taken up by macropinocytosis in DC is rapidly exocytosed. When pathogens are sensed, lysosomal signaling downregulates macropinocytosis and triggers cytoskeleton reorganization in preparation for migration and antigen presentation. The release of lysosomal calcium via the ion channel TRPML1 (transient receptor potential cation channel, mucolipin subfamily, member 1) plays a direct role in the activation of myosin II.[289]

Autophagy

Autophagy allows lysosomes containing MHC class II to access antigens derived from the cytosolic compartment. Approximately 20% to 30% of MHC class II ligands originate from intracellular cytosolic and nuclear proteins. Deliberately targeting phagophores (the precursors of autophagosomes) by fusing antigens to the N terminus of LC3B enhances MHC class II presentation up to 20-fold. Autophagy is thought to be critical in defense against viruses and intracellular infection such as *Listeria*.[290]

Efferocytosis

The engulfment of apoptotic cells is known as efferocytosis.[291] The receptors that recognize an apoptotic cell and mediate efferocytosis are distinct from those that mediate phagocytosis, and the process is closer mechanistically to macropinocytosis. During efferocytosis, RHOA activity is suppressed and RAC1 coordinates the engulfment of the apoptotic body and formation of an "efferosome." Although progressive vesicle fusion leads to the formation of a low-pH compartment similar to a phagolysosome, the activation of different signaling pathways ensures that the event is nonimmunogenic under physiological conditions. Macrophages play a prominent role in efferocytosis in the bone marrow and spleen where they, respectively, coordinate the removal of erythrocyte nuclei and effete red cells.

Antigen Processing and Presentation

The capacity of macrophages and DC to present antigens to T cells was first recognized in classical experiments describing the requirement for "accessory" cells in order to generate lymphocyte proliferation and antibody production in vitro. Accessory cell function is now known to encompass antigen uptake, processing, and presentation as an MHC-bound peptide complex. Both macrophages and DC are able to perform this function, but DC are naturally equipped to stimulate the proliferation of naive T cells with approximately 100-fold greater potency than macrophages.[292]

Activation of Antigen Presentation Pathways

Specific pathways of antigen processing and presentation are activated, depending on the receptor mediating endocytosis and the combinatorial binding of TLRs and other pathogen receptors. Myeloid DC and monocyte-derived DC are competent to present externally acquired antigen to maturing MHC class II dimers in the late endosomes. A complex pathway involving invariant chain and HLA-DM maintains MHC class II in an open configuration for peptide binding. Conventional DC1 express high levels of the lectin CLEC9A that recognizes exposed actin filaments and directs antigen into the cross-presentation pathway.[135,136,293] Cross-presentation can be achieved by DC2/3 and monocyte-derived DC in the context of additional TLR ligation.[160] In this manner, macrophages and DC integrate molecular information derived from pathogens during the initial contact, to determine the route of antigen handling and subsequent polarity of downstream immune responses.[294] In vivo depletion models have confirmed that efficient T-cell priming is dependent upon DC but not macrophages.[295] The superior ability of DC in T-cell priming is linked to higher expression of MHC and costimulatory molecules and lack of inhibitory receptor ligand pairing. Although proficient monocyte-derived antigen-presenting cells are rapidly formed at sites of inflammation, DC presumably improve the fitness of the immune system to generate rapid anamnestic responses and may have evolved under the selective pressure of a relatively small number of highly virulent pathogens.

Adaptive Immunity and T-Cell Polarization
Immune Regulatory Molecules

Macrophages are highly active secretory cells, producing an enormous variety of molecules when stimulated. These include a wide array of chemokines (CCL1, 11, 22, 24, CXCL9-11), cytokines (IL-1β, TNF-α, IL-6, IL10, IL-1, IL-23), type 1 interferons, transforming growth factor-β, angiogenic factors (PDGF, VEGF), and growth factors (CSF-1 and GM-CSF). Activation induces macrophages to synthesize large quantities of leukotrienes from lipo-oxygenase-mediated metabolism of arachidonic acid.

T-Cell Polarizing Signals

Secretion is important for the polarization and imprinting of T cells. Following TCR ligation (signal 1) and costimulation (signal 2), polarizing signals (signal 3) include IL-12 for the initiation of TH1 responses, IL-4 for generation of TH2 cells, and IL-23 for TH-17 cells.[296] Mature DC also provide homing instructions to activated T cells in order to navigate the T cells to the tissue from which the DC originated. The exact mechanism of this "signal 4" is not clear, but upregulation of skin-targeting receptors CLA and CCR10 or gut targeting receptors α4β7 and CCR9 endows T cells with specific tissue homing properties. It has been shown that DC possess the enzymes to metabolize sunlight-induced vitamin D3 into the active form 1,25-dihydroxyvitamin D3, which induces CCR10 on T cells and concomitantly suppresses gut-homing receptors α4β7 and CCR9. Vitamin A metabolites may exert a reciprocal effect on gut resident T cells.

Immune Effector Functions
Reactive Oxygen and Nitrogen Species

The ability to kill phagocytosed bacteria is a major defense function of macrophages.[297] Maturation of phagolysosomes is associated with recruitment of antimicrobial effectors, including reactive oxygen and nitrogen, proteases, antimicrobial peptides, and lysozyme. NADPH phagocyte oxidase (also known as phox) and inducible nitric oxide synthase (iNOS/NOS2) generate superoxide (O2-•) and nitric oxide (NO•) radicals, respectively. Both require NADPH and oxygen and may function together, although they are separate enzyme complexes with independent regulation. The respiratory burst of human neutrophils and activated monocytes/macrophages is defective in many inborn errors that give rise to chronic granulomatous disease.[298] Questions still remain about exactly how bacteria are killed or resist killing in phagolysosomes. The ability of classically activated macrophages to generate NO from arginine contrasts with the alternative catabolism of this amino acid to L-ornithine, via arginase, in alternatively activated macrophages.

Extracellular Vesicles and Exosomes

The production of extracellular vesicles from the plasma membrane and exosomes from the endosomal compartment facilitates a wide variety of communication between cells including the transfer of membrane proteins and mRNA.[299] Macrophages and dendritic cells produce exosomes bearing MHC molecules that are able to transfer antigen-presentation capacity to bystander cells.[300] After radiation injury, macrophages can also enhance healing and repair by the transfer of WNT ligands to stem cells.[301]

Tissue Homeostasis, Repair, and Fibrosis

In recent years, it has been appreciated that the resolution of inflammation is an active process stimulated by specific mediators, rather than a simple waning or dilution of proinflammatory factors. Following an inflammatory event, monocytes and macrophages undergo phenotypic and functional changes that orchestrate this process. Many proinflammatory signals generate feedback inhibition to promote resolution, including Fc receptors, TLRs, purine nucleosides, and metabolites of the respiratory burst. Regulatory circuits involving Tregs, B cells, and stromal cells are activated, and specialized pro-resolving mediators are secreted by macrophages.

Specialized Pro-resolving Mediators

Resolvins are lipid metabolites of omega-3 fatty acids block neutrophil influx and stimulate clearance of debris by efferocytosis. Several families are synthesized by macrophages: E-series resolvins are derived from the omega-3 fatty acid EPA and D-series resolvins, protectins, and maresins are synthesized from DHA.[302] Their action is mediated by G protein–coupled receptors and has been shown to be beneficial in a wide range of animal models of inflammation, wound healing, and organ protection.

Repair

Macrophages entering the tissues during the resolution of inflammation display a wound healing phenotype characterized by the production of growth factors such as PDGF, TGF-β1, IGF-1, and VEGF-α and extracellular matrix components. These promote the differentiation of recruited and local tissue fibroblasts into myofibroblasts to stimulate angiogenesis and achieve wound closure.[303] A severe injury may also result in the recruitment and activation of additional stem cell and local progenitor cell populations by macrophages. During the repair phase macrophages secrete inhibitory mediators IL-10 and TGF-β1 and express cell surface receptors PD-L1 and PD-L2 to suppress adaptive immune responses. There is much interest in the subversion of these healing mechanisms by malignant cells to promote angiogenesis and attenuate immunosurveillance.[304]

Fibrosis

Failure to terminate the inflammatory response leads to chronic inflammation and fibrosis, largely stimulated by a feedback loop between macrophages and fibroblasts.[305] Macrophages produce IL-13, PDGF, and TGF-β, stimulating fibroblasts, which in turn provide reciprocal M-CSF. Both cells continue to elaborate extracellular matrix ultimately resulting in dense collagen deposition punctuated by entrapped fixed macrophages and fibroblasts.

Regulation of Metabolism

The activity of macrophages is intimately connected with many metabolic processes. Bone marrow macrophages, Kupffer cells, and splenic red pulp macrophages are responsible for iron recycling and contain the largest store of iron outside the red cell mass. Iron is acquired by uptake of transferrin through receptor-mediated endocytosis of the transferrin receptor (CD71), and iron-laden macrophages can be easily observed in conditions of iron overload such as genetic hemochromatosis and multiple transfusions. In more recent studies, a prominent role for macrophages in promoting obesity and insulin resistance has also been described, through their recruitment to adipose tissue and production of TNF, IL-6, and interferon.[306] A genetic screen in *Drosophila* identified CCR2-dependent monocyte-derived macrophages acting via PDGFC as the key regulators of adipocyte hypertrophy.[307] Adipose tissue–associated macrophages expressing TREM2 also have profound effects on adipocyte homeostasis.[308] In the liver, a subpopulation of stable resident Kupffer cells is poised to deliver steatotic signals dependent on the lipid receptor CD36 and growth factor–binding protein IGFBP7, when challenged with a high-fat diet.

Cell Fusion and Giant Cell Formation

The acquisition of a fusion-competent phenotype by macrophages is necessary to form osteoclasts and multinucleated giant cells. Cytokines M-CSF, RANKL, and IL-4 and surface receptors TREM/DAP12 activate NF-κB, NFATc1, STAT6, and SYK, which in turn induce DC-STAMP and OC-STAMP, E-Cadherin, and matrix metalloproteinase MMP9.[309,310] CCL2 is also involved in coalescence. Membrane apposition is facilitated by CD44, CD36, SIRPA, and CD200 while RAC1 and DOCK180 are required for cytoskeletal reorganization. The tetraspanins CD9 and CD81 appear to exert a regulatory role. The release of ATP via P2X7 and recognition of adenosine by its receptor (ADORA1) is also required. The role of TLR ligation in giant cell formation has recently been highlighted by genetic studies implicating TLR4 polymorphism in idiopathic granulomatous disorders.[311] An alternative mechanism of giant cell formation involving atypical mitosis, rather than cell fusion, has been proposed in the context of chronic TLR2 stimulation.[312]

ROLE IN DISEASE

Monocyte and Dendritic Cell Deficiency

In common with specific defects of lymphocyte and granulocyte development and function, a number of inborn errors of immunity (IEIs) have now been described in monocytes and dendritic cells.[313] *GATA-2* mutation causes a failure of LMPP and mononuclear cell development resulting in absolute DC and monocyte deficiency with loss of B cells and NK cells (DCML deficiency or monoMAC syndrome).[222] Biallelic *IRF8* mutation also causes complete loss of monocytes and DC.[170] Heterozygous dominant negative or recessive *IRF8* mutation is associated with stage-specific interruption of DC development that reveals the different trajectories of DC2, DC3, and monocyte hematopoiesis.[99] *IKZF1* mutation, known for causing failure of B-cell development, also skews the development of DC toward DC1 at the expense of pDC.[257] Severe functional impairment of DC2 and pDC was also revealed in patients with SPPL2A and IRF7 deficiency, respectively.[121,314] Patients with DC and monocyte loss or dysfunction typically have impaired immunity to mycobacteria, viruses, and intracellular pathogens. There is often autoimmunity implying dysregulation of tolerance failure and an increased risk of malignancy presumably through failure of immunosurveillance.

Histiocytic Neoplasms

Histiocytic disorders are caused by activating mutations of the MAP kinase pathway.[315,316] The most common mutation, *BRAF^V600E*, accounts for just over half of all cases of Langerhans cell histiocytosis (LCH), Erdheim-Chester disease (ECD), juvenile xanthogranuloma (JXG), and Rosai Dorfman disease (RDD). Each type of histiocytosis is characterized by accumulation of a distinct phenotype of abnormal myeloid cells with a specific pattern of tissue tropism. LCH cells express langerin and CD1a and have Birbeck granules, similar to Langerhans cells, and typically cause lytic bone lesions, skin rash and affect hematopoietic organs in high-risk cases.[315,317] In contrast, ECD and JXG are characterized by foamy macrophages, with no clear neoplastic phenotype, promoting bone sclerosis, perinephric fibrosis, vasculitis, and serositis.[318] RDD is linked to sinus macrophages and has nodal and extranodal forms.[319] Histiocytic neoplasms can destroy the posterior pituitary leading to diabetes insipidus and promote neurodegeneration with devastating consequences.

Hemophagocytic Lymphohistiocytosis

Hyperinflammation mediated by cytokines, notably IFNγ, can induce extreme activation of macrophages resulting in profound cytopenia, hepatosplenomegaly, hyperferritinemia, hypertriglyceridemia, and hypofibrinogenemia. This condition is known as macrophage activation syndrome or HLH and is rapidly fatal owing to profound cytopenia and metabolic disturbances.[320,321] Congenital deficiency of perforin, munc, or syntaxin proteins, resulting in uncontrolled viral infection and expansion of frustrated effector T cells, is a recognized cause of HLH presenting in infancy. Older children and adults may have compound heterozygosity or hypomorphic mutations of related genes combined with other risks and triggers including herpesvirus infection, mycobacterial infection, and malignancy, notably lymphoma. Recognition of "hyperinflammation" as a process associated with chimeric antigen receptor T-cell therapy and SARS-CoV2 infection has led to an increasing awareness of HLH. Improvements in diagnosis and management have followed, notably the use of the HScore for clinical assessment and biologics to break the feed-forward cycle of inflammation.[322,323]

Lysosomal Storage Diseases

Lysosomal storage disorders are a heterogeneous group of diseases arising from genetic deficiency of a catabolic lysosomal enzyme.[324,325] Gaucher disease, caused by β-glucocerebrosidase deficiency, is the most common and results in sphingolipid accumulation and the formation of foamy Gaucher macrophages. These accumulate in sheets causing end organ damage and failure in the bone marrow, spleen, liver, lung, kidneys, and brain. Other lysosomal storage disorders exhibiting foamy macrophages are Fabry disease, GM1 gangliosidosis, and Wolman/cholesterol ester storage disorder. In Niemann-Pick A and B the macrophages have a distinctly blue appearance and are described as "sea blue histiocytes."

Infection

Myeloid cells are critical in host defense to pathogens as outlined in the preceding paragraphs, describing their anatomical positioning, mechanisms of antigen sensing and update, ability to prime adaptive immunity, and role as effector cells. Granuloma formation is one of the cardinal roles of macrophages. Recent high-resolution analysis has highlighted the surprising regulatory role of granuloma macrophages, which express high levels of CD274 (PD-L1), IDO, and TGFB. The COVID pandemic has triggered a series of detailed investigations into the blood myeloid cell compartment describing left-shifted myelopoiesis, loss of DC, and skewing of monocyte populations, typically found in many viral infections.[326-328] Alveolar cells have also come under scrutiny revealing abundant proinflammatory macrophages in severe disease.[329]

Cancer

The concept of tumor-associated macrophages (TAMs) promoting tumor progression and metastasis has been widely studied for several decades.[330] Single-cell approaches are now providing an unprecedented level of detail in terms of population architecture, new surface markers, and specific functional attributes in many different tumors.[165,331-334] Common features emerge including the identification of significant populations of resident-type macrophages expressing F13A and FOLR2, together with proinflammatory monocyte-derived cells. The de novo appearance of macrophages with resident markers coincident with more primitive endothelial cells has been described as oncofetal reprogramming.[331] FOLR2$^+$ macrophages have a perivascular location and are associated anatomically and numerically with lymphocyte infiltration. In contrast to the conventional story of TAMs promoting tumor progression, a greater density of FOLR2$^+$ macrophages is associated with improved survival in breast cancer.[335]

Atherosclerosis

Atherosclerosis is a lipid-driven inflammatory disease characterized by intravascular plaques containing lipid-laden macrophages or "foam cells." These arise from monocytes recruited in response to endothelial damage and participate in the complex milieu of immune cells, tissue damage, and plaque progression that characterize advanced disease. Recent advances through single cell analysis have revealed multiple populations of resident and recruited macrophages, dendritic cells, and other myeloid cells in addition to classical foam cells.[336] Murine atherosclerosis models show an influx of recruited monocyte-derived cells that supplement resident macrophages as disease progresses. These include inflammatory clusters expressing IL1B and chemokines and alternately activated cells enriched in TREM2 expression, lipid metabolism genes, and signatures that overlap with osteoclasts, hinting at a role in calcification.[337] Similar studies in human atheroma reveal LYVE1$^+$ F13A$^+$ FOLR2$^+$ resident macrophages, inflammatory cells elaborating IL1B and TNFA, interferon activated cells, and TREM2$^+$ foamy macrophages.[338,339] Many complex cell-cell interactions are traceable and highlight cooperativity between myeloid cells and T cells (which are prominent). Risk loci identified by genome-wide association also feature among the genes expressed by disease-specific populations.

Autoimmunity

Myeloid cells play a major role in immune-mediated inflammatory disease by promoting local immune cell recruitment, antigen presentation, T-cell activation, tissue damage, and fibrosis. Macrophages are a major component of the inflammatory "pannus" in rheumatoid arthritis. Animal models suggest that resident macrophages play a regulatory role and restrict immune activation[340] while recruited monocyte-derived cells are the source of IL1B, cytokines, and growth factors that promote lymphocyte activation, fibroblast proliferation, and joint destruction.[341,342] The immune architecture of inflammatory bowel disease has also received close attention. Here, inflammatory monocytes and DC2 were found to produce oncostatin M, a proinflammatory mediator that is not suppressed by TNF-directed therapy, which potentially explains treatment failure in some patients.[342] In psoriasis, a DC3 population and some inflammatory macrophages coproduce IL1B and IL23A.[102] Many other inflammatory diseases are under investigation with similar techniques.

Transplantation

Allograft rejection and GVHD have long been known to involve cell-mediated immunity promoted by myeloid cells.[344] There is renewed interest in donor myeloid cells in GVHD, particularly with the demonstration that they potentially stimulate host resident T cells.[345,346] Single cell approaches are providing many new insights into allograft rejection including the recognition that donor-derived resident macrophages dominate in nonrejecting kidneys but are become massively outnumbered by recipient inflammatory macrophages during rejection, leading to activation of cytotoxic and fibrosis pathways.[344] In the mouse it has also been elegantly demonstrated that monocytes are capable of recognizing MHC mismatches directly through paired immunoglobulin-like receptors.[347]

CONCLUSION

Monocytes, macrophages, and DC, cells of the mononuclear phagocytes system are among the phylogenetically most ancient defensive components of multicellular organisms. Their ability to sense a huge array of stimuli and to respond in many different ways is critical to the maintenance of immunocompetence, tissue homeostasis, and metabolic integrity. Almost every pathological process of medical significance involves mononuclear phagocytes, presenting a rich vein of opportunity for therapeutic exploitation accelerated by the advent of single cell technologies.

References

1. Cavaillon JM. The historical milestones in the understanding of leukocyte biology initiated by Elie Metchnikoff. *J Leukoc Biol.* 2011;90:413-424.
2. van Furth R, Cohn ZA, Hirsch JG, Humphrey JH, Spector WG, Langevoort HL. The mononuclear phagocyte system: a new classification of macrophages, monocytes, and their precursor cells. *Bull World Health Organ.* 1972;46:845-852.
3. Ginhoux F, Greter M, Leboeuf M, et al. Fate mapping analysis reveals that adult microglia derive from primitive macrophages. *Science.* 2010;330:841-845.
4. Ginhoux F, Guilliams M. Tissue-resident macrophage ontogeny and homeostasis. *Immunity.* 2016;44:439-449.
5. Perdiguero EG, Geissmann F. The development and maintenance of resident macrophages. *Nat Immunol.* 2016;17:2-8.
6. Steinman RM, Cohn ZA. Identification of a novel cell type in peripheral lymphoid organs of mice. I. Morphology, quantitation, tissue distribution. *J Exp Med.* 1973;137:1142-1162.
7. Guilliams M, Ginhoux F, Jakubzick C, et al. Dendritic cells, monocytes and macrophages: a unified nomenclature based on ontogeny. *Nat Rev Immunol.* 2014;14:571-578.
8. Liu Z, Gu Y, Chakarov S, et al. Fate mapping via Ms4a3-expression history traces monocyte-derived cells. *Cell.* 2019;178:1509-1525.e19.
9. Guilliams M, Mildner A, Yona S. Developmental and functional heterogeneity of monocytes. *Immunity.* 2018;49:595-613.
10. Kapellos TS, Bonaguro L, Gemünd I, et al. Human monocyte subsets and phenotypes in major chronic inflammatory diseases. *Front Immunol.* 2019;10:2035.
11. Xue J, Schmidt SV, Sander J, et al. Transcriptome-based network analysis reveals a spectrum model of human macrophage activation. *Immunity.* 2014;40:274-288.
12. Ginhoux F, Schultze JL, Murray PJ, Ochando J, Biswas SK. New insights into the multidimensional concept of macrophage ontogeny, activation and function. *Nat Immunol.* 2016;17:34-40.

The Normal Hematologic System

13. Bujko A, Atlasy N, Landsverk OJB, et al. Transcriptional and functional profiling defines human small intestinal macrophage subsets. *J Exp Med.* 2018;215:441-458.

14. Patel AA, Zhang Y, Fullerton JN, et al. The fate and lifespan of human monocyte subsets in steady state and systemic inflammation. *J Exp Med.* 2017;214:1913-1923.

15. Schakel K, von Kietzell M, Hansel A, et al. Human 6-sulfo LacNAc-expressing dendritic cells are principal producers of early interleukin-12 and are controlled by erythrocytes. *Immunity.* 2006;24:767-777.

16. Hofer TP, Zawada AM, Frankenberger M, et al. slan-defined subsets of CD16-positive monocytes: impact of granulomatous inflammation and M-CSF receptor mutation. *Blood.* 2015;126:2601-2610.

17. Calzetti F, Tamassia N, Micheletti A, Finotti G, Bianchetto-Aguilera F, Cassatella MA. Human dendritic cell subset 4 (DC4) correlate to a subset of CD14dim/-CD16++ monocytes. *J Allergy Clin Immunol.* 2018;141(6):2276-2279.e3.

18. Auffray C, Fogg D, Garfa M, et al. Monitoring of blood vessels and tissues by a population of monocytes with patrolling behavior. *Science.* 2007;317:666-670.

19. Cros J, Cagnard N, Woollard K, et al. Human CD14dim monocytes patrol and sense nucleic acids and viruses via TLR7 and TLR8 receptors. *Immunity.* 2010;33:375-386.

20. Thomas GD, Hamers AAJ, Nakao C, et al. Human blood monocyte subsets: a new gating strategy defined using cell surface markers identified by mass cytometry. *Arterioscler Thromb Vasc Biol.* 2017;37:1548-1558.

21. Villani AC, Satija R, Reynolds G, et al. Single-cell RNA-seq reveals new types of human blood dendritic cells, monocytes, and progenitors. *Science.* 2017;356:eaah4573.

22. Haniffa M, Ginhoux F, Wang XN, et al. Differential rates of replacement of human dermal dendritic cells and macrophages during hematopoietic stem cell transplantation. *J Exp Med.* 2009;206:371-385.

23. McGovern N, Schlitzer A, Gunawan M, et al. Human dermal CD14+ cells are a transient population of monocyte-derived macrophages. *Immunity.* 2014;41:465-477.

24. Desch AN, Gibbings SL, Goyal R, et al. Flow cytometric analysis of mononuclear phagocytes in nondiseased human lung and lung-draining lymph nodes. *Am J Respir Crit Care Med.* 2016;193:614-626.

25. Baharom F, Thomas S, Rankin G, et al. Dendritic cells and monocytes with distinct inflammatory responses reside in lung mucosa of healthy humans. *J Immunol.* 2016;196:4498-4509.

26. Patel VI, Booth JL, Duggan ES, et al. Transcriptional classification and functional characterization of human airway macrophage and dendritic cell subsets. *J Immunol.* 2017;198:1183-1201.

27. Watchmaker PB, Lahl K, Lee M, et al. Comparative transcriptional and functional profiling defines conserved programs of intestinal DC differentiation in humans and mice. *Nat Immunol.* 2014;15:98-108.

28. Mulder K, Patel AA, Kong WT, et al. Cross-tissue single-cell landscape of human monocytes and macrophages in health and disease. *Immunity.* 2021;54:1883-1900.e5.

29. Eguíluz-Gracia I, Bosco A, Dollner R, et al. Rapid recruitment of CD14(+) monocytes in experimentally induced allergic rhinitis in human subjects. *J Allergy Clin Immunol.* 2016;137:1872-1881.e12.

30. Beitnes AC, Raki M, Brottveit M, Lundin KE, Jahnsen FL, Sollid LM. Rapid accumulation of CD14+CD11c+ dendritic cells in gut mucosa of celiac disease after in vivo gluten challenge. *PLoS One.* 2012;7:e33556.

31. Bain CC, Scott CL, Uronen-Hansson H, et al. Resident and pro-inflammatory macrophages in the colon represent alternative context-dependent fates of the same Ly6Chi monocyte precursors. *Mucosal Immunol.* 2013;6:498-510.

32. Liao CT, Andrews R, Wallace LE, et al. Peritoneal macrophage heterogeneity is associated with different peritoneal dialysis outcomes. *Kidney Int.* 2017;91:1088-1103.

33. Amorim A, De Feo D, Friebel E, et al. IFNγ and GM-CSF control complementary differentiation programs in the monocyte-to-phagocyte transition during neuroinflammation. *Nat Immunol.* 2022;23:217-228.

34. Casanova JL, Abel L. Genetic dissection of immunity to mycobacteria: the human model. *Annu Rev Immunol.* 2002;20:581-620.

35. Mantovani A, Sica A, Locati M. Macrophage polarization comes of age. *Immunity.* 2005;23:344-346.

36. Goudot C, Coillard A, Villani AC, et al. Aryl hydrocarbon receptor controls monocyte differentiation into dendritic cells versus macrophages. *Immunity.* 2017;47:582-596.e6.

37. Sander J, Schmidt SV, Cirovic B, et al. Cellular differentiation of human monocytes is regulated by time-dependent interleukin-4 signaling and the transcriptional regulator NCOR2. *Immunity.* 2017;47:1051-1066.e12.

38. Dick SA, Wong A, Hamidzada H, et al. Three tissue resident macrophage subsets coexist across organs with conserved origins and life cycles. *Sci Immunol.* 2022;7:eabf7777.

39. Lim HY, Lim SY, Tan CK, et al. Hyaluronan receptor LYVE-1-expressing macrophages maintain arterial tone through hyaluronan-mediated regulation of smooth muscle cell collagen. *Immunity.* 2018;49:326-341.e7.

40. Chakarov S, Lim HY, Tan L, et al. Two distinct interstitial macrophage populations coexist across tissues in specific subtissular niches. *Science.* 2019;363:eaau0964.

41. Ydens E, Amann L, Asselbergh B, et al. Profiling peripheral nerve macrophages reveals two macrophage subsets with distinct localization, transcriptome and response to injury. *Nat Neurosci.* 2020;23(5):676-689.

42. Mass E, Ballesteros I, Farlik M, et al. Specification of tissue-resident macrophages during organogenesis. *Science.* 2016;353:aaf4238.

43. Guilliams M, Thierry GR, Bonnardel J, Bajenoff M. Establishment and maintenance of the macrophage niche. *Immunity.* 2020;52:434-451.

44. Lavin Y, Winter D, Blecher-Gonen R, et al. Tissue-resident macrophage enhancer landscapes are shaped by the local microenvironment. *Cell.* 2014;159:1312-1326.

45. Gosselin D, Link VM, Romanoski CE, et al. Environment drives selection and function of enhancers controlling tissue-specific macrophage identities. *Cell.* 2014;159:1327-1340.

46. Blériot C, Chakarov S, Ginhoux F. Determinants of resident tissue macrophage identity and function. *Immunity.* 2020;52:957-970.

47. Utz SG, See P, Mildenberger W, et al. Early fate defines microglia and non-parenchymal brain macrophage development. *Cell.* 2020;181(3):557-573.e18.

48. Crotti A, Ransohoff RM. Microglial physiology and pathophysiology: insights from genome-wide transcriptional profiling. *Immunity.* 2016;44:505-515.

49. Masuda T, Sankowski R, Staszewski O, et al. Spatial and temporal heterogeneity of mouse and human microglia at single-cell resolution. *Nature.* 2019;566:388-392.

50. Thion MS, Ginhoux F, Garel S. Microglia and early brain development: an intimate journey. *Science.* 2018;362:185-189.

51. Keren-Shaul H, Spinrad A, Weiner A, et al. A unique microglia type associated with restricting development of Alzheimer's disease. *Cell.* 2017;169:1276-1290.e17.

52. Krasemann S, Madore C, Cialic R, et al. The TREM2-APOE pathway drives the transcriptional phenotype of dysfunctional microglia in neurodegenerative diseases. *Immunity.* 2017;47:566-581.e9.

53. Zhou Y, Song WM, Andhey PS, et al. Human and mouse single-nucleus transcriptomics reveal TREM2-dependent and TREM2-independent cellular responses in Alzheimer's disease. *Nat Med.* 2020;26:131-142.

54. Gosselin D, Skola D, Coufal NG, et al. An environment-dependent transcriptional network specifies human microglia identity. *Science.* 2017;356:eaal3222.

55. Paloneva J, Manninen T, Christman G, et al. Mutations in two genes encoding different subunits of a receptor signaling complex result in an identical disease phenotype. *Am J Hum Genet.* 2002;71:656-662.

56. Nicholson AM, Baker MC, Finch NA, et al. CSF1R mutations link POLD and HDLS as a single disease entity. *Neurology.* 2013;80:1033-1040.

57. Mass E, Jacome-Galarza CE, Blank T, et al. A somatic mutation in erythro-myeloid progenitors causes neurodegenerative disease. *Nature.* 2017;549(7672):389-393.

58. Blériot C, Barreby E, Dunsmore G, et al. A subset of Kupffer cells regulates metabolism through the expression of CD36. *Immunity.* 2021;54:2101-2116.e6.

59. Ramachandran P, Dobie R, Wilson-Kanamori JR, et al. Resolving the fibrotic niche of human liver cirrhosis at single-cell level. *Nature.* 2019;575:512-518.

60. Seidman JS, Troutman TD, Sakai M, et al. Niche-specific reprogramming of epigenetic landscapes drives myeloid cell diversity in nonalcoholic steatohepatitis. *Immunity.* 2020;52:1057-1074.e7.

61. Suzuki T, Trapnell BC. Pulmonary alveolar proteinosis syndrome. *Clin Chest Med.* 2016;37:431-440.

62. Collin M, Dickinson R, Bigley V. Haematopoietic and immune defects associated with GATA2 mutation. *Br J Haematol.* 2015;169:173-187.

63. Eguíluz-Gracia I, Schultz HH, Sikkeland LI, et al. Long-term persistence of human donor alveolar macrophages in lung transplant recipients. *Thorax.* 2016;71:1006-1011.

64. van de Laar L, Saelens W, De Prijck S, et al. Yolk sac macrophages, fetal liver, and adult monocytes can colonize an empty niche and develop into functional tissue-resident macrophages. *Immunity.* 2016;44:755-768.

65. Suzuki T, Arumugam P, Sakagami T, et al. Pulmonary macrophage transplantation therapy. *Nature.* 2014;514:450-454.

66. Vieira Braga FA, Kar G, Berg M, et al. A cellular census of human lungs identifies novel cell states in health and in asthma. *Nat Med.* 2019;25:1153-1163.

67. Reyfman PA, Walter JM, Joshi N, et al. Single-cell transcriptomic analysis of human lung provides insights into the pathobiology of pulmonary fibrosis. *Am J Respir Crit Care Med.* 2019;199:1517-1536.

68. Peters JM, Blainey PC, Bryson BD. *Consensus Transcriptional States Describe Human Mononuclear Phagocyte Diversity in the Lung across Health and Disease.* Cold Spring Harbor Laboratory Press; 2020.

69. Todd EM, Zhou JY, Szasz TP, et al. Alveolar macrophage development in mice requires L-plastin for cellular localization in alveoli. *Blood.* 2016;128:2785-2796.

70. Bain CC, Bravo-Blas A, Scott CL, et al. Constant replenishment from circulating monocytes maintains the macrophage pool in the intestine of adult mice. *Nat Immunol.* 2014;15:929-937.

71. Bain CC, Mowat AM. Macrophages in intestinal homeostasis and inflammation. *Immunol Rev.* 2014;260:102-117.

72. James KR, Gomes T, Elmentaite R, et al. Distinct microbial and immune niches of the human colon. *Nat Immunol.* 2020;21:343-353.

73. De Schepper S, Verheijden S, Aguilera-Lizarraga J, et al. Self-maintaining gut macrophages are essential for intestinal homeostasis. *Cell.* 2018;175:400-415.e13.

74. Shaw TN, Houston SA, Wemyss K, et al. Tissue-resident macrophages in the intestine are long lived and defined by Tim-4 and CD4 expression. *J Exp Med.* 2018;215:1507-1518.

75. Matheis F, Muller PA, Graves CL, et al. Adrenergic signaling in muscularis macrophages limits infection-induced neuronal loss. *Cell.* 2020;180:64-78.e16.

76. Chikina AS, Nadalin F, Maurin M, et al. Macrophages maintain epithelium integrity by limiting fungal product absorption. *Cell.* 2020;183:411-428.e16.

77. Jacome-Galarza CE, Percin GI, Muller JT, et al. Developmental origin, functional maintenance and genetic rescue of osteoclasts. *Nature.* 2019;568:541-545.

78. ten Harkel B, Schoenmaker T, Picavet DI, Davison NL, de Vries TJ, Everts V. The foreign body giant cell cannot resorb bone, but dissolves hydroxyapatite like osteoclasts. *PLoS One.* 2015;10:e0139564.

79. Xiao Y, Palomero J, Grabowska J, et al. Macrophages and osteoclasts stem from a bipotent progenitor downstream of a macrophage/osteoclast/dendritic cell progenitor. *Blood Adv.* 2017;1:1993-2006.

80. Penna S, Capo V, Palagano E, Sobacchi C, Villa A. One disease, many genes: implications for the treatment of osteopetroses. *Front Endocrinol.* 2019;10:85.

81. Robbins CS, Hilgendorf I, Weber GF, et al. Local proliferation dominates lesional macrophage accumulation in atherosclerosis. *Nat Med.* 2013;19:1166-1172.
82. Tabas I, Lichtman AH. Monocyte-macrophages and T cells in atherosclerosis. *Immunity.* 2017;47:621-634.
83. Stamatiades EG, Tremblay ME, Bohm M, et al. Immune monitoring of trans-endothelial transport by kidney-resident macrophages. *Cell.* 2016;166:991-1003.
84. Viehmann SF, Böhner AMC, Kurts C, Brähler S. The multifaceted role of the renal mononuclear phagocyte system. *Cell Immunol.* 2018;330:97-104.
85. Mossadegh-Keller N, Sieweke MH. Testicular macrophages: guardians of fertility. *Cell Immunol.* 2018;330:120-125.
86. Chow A, Lucas D, Hidalgo A, et al. Bone marrow CD169+ macrophages promote the retention of hematopoietic stem and progenitor cells in the mesenchymal stem cell niche. *J Exp Med.* 2011;208:261-271.
87. Toda S, Segawa K, Nagata S. MerTK-mediated engulfment of pyrenocytes by central macrophages in erythroblastic islands. *Blood.* 2014;123(25):3963-3971.
88. Chow A, Huggins M, Ahmed J, et al. CD169(+) macrophages provide a niche promoting erythropoiesis under homeostasis and stress. *Nat Med.* 2013;19:429-436.
89. Junt T, Moseman EA, Iannacone M, et al. Subcapsular sinus macrophages in lymph nodes clear lymph-borne viruses and present them to antiviral B cells. *Nature.* 2007;450:110-114.
90. Saunderson SC, Dunn AC, Crocker PR, McLellan AD. CD169 mediates the capture of exosomes in spleen and lymph node. *Blood.* 2014;123:208-216.
91. Bellomo A, Gentek R, Bajénoff M, Baratin M. Lymph node macrophages: scavengers, immune sentinels and trophic effectors. *Cell Immunol.* 2018;330:168-174.
92. A-Gonzalez N, Castrillo A. Origin and specialization of splenic macrophages. *Cell Immunol.* 2018;330:151-158.
93. Liu LT, Lang ZF, Li Y, et al. Composition and characteristics of distinct macrophage subpopulations in the mouse thymus. *Mol Med Rep.* 2013;7:1850-1854.
94. Tacke R, Hilgendorf I, Garner H, et al. The transcription factor NR4A1 is essential for the development of a novel macrophage subset in the thymus. *Sci Rep.* 2015;5:10055.
95. Guilliams M, Dutertre CA, Scott CL, et al. Unsupervised high-dimensional analysis aligns dendritic cells across tissues and species. *Immunity.* 2016;45:669-684.
96. Collin M, Bigley V. Human dendritic cell subsets: an update. *Immunology.* 2018;154:3-20.
97. Ginhoux F, Guilliams M, Merad M. Expanding dendritic cell nomenclature in the single-cell era. *Nat Rev Immunol.* 2022;22(2):67-68.
98. Dutertre CA, Becht E, Irac SE, et al. Single-cell analysis of human mononuclear phagocytes reveals subset-defining markers and identifies circulating inflammatory dendritic cells. *Immunity.* 2019;51:573-589.e8.
99. Cytlak U, Resteu A, Pagan S, et al. Differential IRF8 transcription factor requirement defines two pathways of dendritic cell development in humans. *Immunity.* 2020;53:353-370.e8.
100. Bourdely P, Anselmi G, Vaivode K, et al. Transcriptional and functional analysis of CD1c⁺ human dendritic cells identifies a CD163⁺ subset priming CD8⁺CD103⁺ T cells. *Immunity.* 2020;53:335-352.e8.
101. Bosteels C, Neyt K, Vanheerswynghels M, et al. Inflammatory type 2 cDCs acquire features of cDC1s and macrophages to orchestrate immunity to respiratory virus infection. *Immunity.* 2020;52:1039-1056.e9.
102. Nakamizo S, Dutertre CA, Khalilnezhad A, et al. Single-cell analysis of human skin identifies CD14+ type 3 dendritic cells co-producing IL1B and IL23A in psoriasis. *J Exp Med.* 2021;218:e20202345.
103. Reynolds G, Vegh P, Fletcher J, et al. Developmental cell programs are co-opted in inflammatory skin disease. *Science.* 2021;371(6527):eaba6500.
104. Ardouin L, Luche H, Chelbi R, et al. Broad and largely concordant molecular changes characterize tolerogenic and immunogenic dendritic cell maturation in thymus and periphery. *Immunity.* 2016;45:305-318.
105. Maier B, Leader AM, Chen ST, et al. A conserved dendritic-cell regulatory program limits antitumour immunity. *Nature.* 2020;580:257-262.
106. Dzionek A, Fuchs A, Schmidt P, et al. BDCA-2, BDCA-3, and BDCA-4: three markers for distinct subsets of dendritic cells in human peripheral blood. *J Immunol.* 2000;165:6037-6046.
107. Dzionek A, Sohma Y, Nagafune J, et al. BDCA-2, a novel plasmacytoid dendritic cell-specific type II C-type lectin, mediates antigen capture and is a potent inhibitor of interferon alpha/beta induction. *J Exp Med.* 2001;194:1823-1834.
108. MacDonald KP, Munster DJ, Clark GJ, Dzionek A, Schmitz J, Hart DN. Characterization of human blood dendritic cell subsets. *Blood.* 2002;100:4512-4520.
109. Jardine L, Barge D, Ames-Draycott A, et al. Rapid detection of dendritic cell and monocyte disorders using CD4 as a lineage marker of the human peripheral blood antigen-presenting cell compartment. *Front Immunol.* 2013;4:495.
110. Ju X, Zenke M, Hart DN, Clark GJ. CD300a/c regulate type I interferon and TNF-alpha secretion by human plasmacytoid dendritic cells stimulated with TLR7 and TLR9 ligands. *Blood.* 2008;112:1184-1194.
111. Bao M, Liu YJ. Regulation of TLR7/9 signaling in plasmacytoid dendritic cells. *Protein Cell.* 2013;4:40-52.
112. Heidkamp GF, Sander J, Lehmann CHK, et al. Human lymphoid organ dendritic cell identity is predominantly dictated by ontogeny, not tissue microenvironment. *Sci Immunol.* 2016;1(6):eaai7677.
113. See P, Dutertre CA, Chen J, et al. Mapping the human DC lineage through the integration of high-dimensional techniques. *Science.* 2017;356(6342):eaag3009.
114. Swiecki M, Colonna M. The multifaceted biology of plasmacytoid dendritic cells. *Nat Rev Immunol.* 2015;15:471-485.
115. Bode C, Fox M, Tewary P, et al. Human plasmacytoid dendritic cells elicit a Type I Interferon response by sensing DNA via the cGAS-STING signaling pathway. *Eur J Immunol.* 2016;46:1615-1621.
116. Bruni D, Chazal M, Sinigaglia L, et al. Viral entry route determines how human plasmacytoid dendritic cells produce type I interferons. *Sci Signal.* 2015;8:ra25.
117. Honda K, Yanai H, Negishi H, et al. IRF-7 is the master regulator of type-I interferon-dependent immune responses. *Nature.* 2005;434:772-777.
118. Li J, Du Q, Hu R, et al. Death receptor 6 is a novel plasmacytoid dendritic cell-specific receptor and modulates type I interferon production. [letter]. *Protein Cell.* 2016;7(4):291-294.
119. Dillmann C, Ringel C, Ringleb J, et al. S1PR4 signaling attenuates ILT 7 internalization to limit IFN-α production by human plasmacytoid dendritic cells. *J Immunol.* 2016;196:1579-1590.
120. Teijaro JR, Studer S, Leaf N, et al. S1PR1-mediated IFNAR1 degradation modulates plasmacytoid dendritic cell interferon-α autoamplification. *Proc Natl Acad Sci U S A.* 2016;113:1351-1356.
121. Ciancanelli MJ, Huang SX, Luthra P, et al. Infectious disease. Life-threatening influenza and impaired interferon amplification in human IRF7 deficiency. *Science.* 2015;348:448-453.
122. Keles S, Jabara HH, Reisli I, et al. Plasmacytoid dendritic cell depletion in DOCK8 deficiency: rescue of severe herpetic infections with IFN-α 2b therapy. *J Allergy Clin Immunol.* 2014;133:1753-1755.e3.
123. Li H, Goepfert P, Reeves RK. Short communication: plasmacytoid dendritic cells from HIV-1 Elite Controllers maintain a gut-homing phenotype associated with immune activation. *AIDS Res Hum Retroviruses.* 2014;30:1213-1215.
124. Yonkers NL, Rodriguez B, Milkovich KA, et al. TLR ligand-dependent activation of naive CD4 T cells by plasmacytoid dendritic cells is impaired in hepatitis C virus infection. *J Immunol.* 2007;178:4436-4444.
125. Woltman AM, Op den Brouw ML, Biesta PJ, Shi CC, Janssen HL. Hepatitis B virus lacks immune activating capacity, but actively inhibits plasmacytoid dendritic cell function. *PLoS One.* 2011;6:e15324.
126. Lande R, Ganguly D, Facchinetti V, et al. Neutrophils activate plasmacytoid dendritic cells by releasing self-DNA-peptide complexes in systemic lupus erythematosus. *Sci Transl Med.* 2011;3:73ra19.
127. Ganguly D, Chamilos G, Lande R, et al. Self-RNA-antimicrobial peptide complexes activate human dendritic cells through TLR7 and TLR8. *J Exp Med.* 2009;206:1983-1994.
128. Berggren O, Alexsson A, Morris DL, et al. IFN-alpha production by plasmacytoid dendritic cell associations with polymorphisms in gene loci related to autoimmune and inflammatory diseases. *Hum Mol Genet.* 2015;24:3571-3581.
129. Froidure A, Vandenplas O, D'Alpaos V, Evrard G, Pilette C. Defects in plasmacytoid dendritic cell expression of inducible costimulator ligand and IFN-α are associated in asthma with disease persistence. [letter]. *Am J Respir Crit Care Med.* 2015;192(3):392-395.
130. Pritchard AL, Carroll ML, Burel JG, White OJ, Phipps S, Upham JW. Innate IFNs and plasmacytoid dendritic cells constrain Th2 cytokine responses to rhinovirus: a regulatory mechanism with relevance to asthma. *J Immunol.* 2012;188:5898-5905.
131. Ghirelli C, Reyal F, Jeanmougin M, et al. Breast cancer cell-derived GM-CSF licenses regulatory Th2 induction by plasmacytoid predendritic cells in aggressive disease subtypes. *Cancer Res.* 2015;75:2775-2787.
132. Ziegler-Heitbrock L, Ancuta P, Crowe S, et al. Nomenclature of monocytes and dendritic cells in blood. *Blood.* 2010;116:e74-80.
133. Haniffa M, Shin A, Bigley V, et al. Human tissues contain CD141hi cross-presenting dendritic cells with functional homology to mouse CD103+ nonlymphoid dendritic cells. *Immunity.* 2012;37:60-73.
134. Granot T, Senda T, Carpenter DJ, et al. Dendritic cells display subset and tissue-specific maturation dynamics over human life. *Immunity.* 2017;46:504-515.
135. Ahrens S, Zelenay S, Sancho D, et al. F-actin is an evolutionarily conserved damage-associated molecular pattern recognized by DNGR-1, a receptor for dead cells. *Immunity.* 2012;36:635-645.
136. Zhang JG, Czabotar PE, Policheni AN, et al. The dendritic cell receptor Clec9A binds damaged cells via exposed actin filaments. *Immunity.* 2012;36:646-657.
137. Jongbloed SL, Kassianos AJ, McDonald KJ, et al. Human CD141+ (BDCA-3)+ dendritic cells (DCs) represent a unique myeloid DC subset that cross-presents necrotic cell antigens. *J Exp Med.* 2010;207:1247-1260.
138. Poulin LF, Salio M, Griessinger E, et al. Characterization of human DNGR-1+ BDCA3+ leukocytes as putative equivalents of mouse CD8alpha+ dendritic cells. *J Exp Med.* 2010;207:1261-1271.
139. Mittag D, Proietto AI, Loudovaris T, et al. Human dendritic cell subsets from spleen and blood are similar in phenotype and function but modified by donor health status. *J Immunol.* 2011;186:6207-6217.
140. Segura E, Valladeau-Guilemond J, Donnadieu MH, Sastre-Garau X, Soumelis V, Amigorena S. Characterization of resident and migratory dendritic cells in human lymph nodes. *J Exp Med.* 2012;209:653-660.
141. Yoshio S, Kanto T, Kuroda S, et al. Human blood dendritic cell antigen 3 (BDCA3) (+) dendritic cells are a potent producer of interferon-λ in response to hepatitis C virus. *Hepatology.* 2013;57:1705-1715.
142. Kelly A, Fahey R, Fletcher JM, et al. CD141⁺ myeloid dendritic cells are enriched in healthy human liver. *J Hepatol.* 2014;60:135-142.
143. Bachem A, Guttler S, Hartung E, et al. Superior antigen cross-presentation and XCR1 expression define human CD11c+CD141+ cells as homologues of mouse CD8+ dendritic cells. *J Exp Med.* 2010;207:1273-1281.
144. Cohn L, Chatterjee B, Esselborn F, et al. Antigen delivery to early endosomes eliminates the superiority of human blood BDCA3+ dendritic cells at cross presentation. *J Exp Med.* 2013;210:1049-1063.
145. Silvin A, Yu CI, Lahaye X, et al. Constitutive resistance to viral infection in human CD141(+) dendritic cells. *Sci Immunol.* 2017;2(13):eaai8071.

146. Schreibelt G, Klinkenberg LJ, Cruz LJ, et al. The C-type lectin receptor CLEC9A mediates antigen uptake and (cross-)presentation by human blood BDCA3+ myeloid dendritic cells. *Blood*. 2012;119:2284-2292.

147. Li J, Ahmet F, Sullivan LC, et al. Antibodies targeting Clec9A promote strong humoral immunity without adjuvant in mice and non-human primates. *Eur J Immunol*. 2015;45:854-864.

148. Hemont C, Neel A, Heslan M, Braudeau C, Josien R. Human blood mDC subsets exhibit distinct TLR repertoire and responsiveness. *J Leukoc Biol*. 2013;93:599-609.

149. Colletti NJ, Liu H, Gower AC, Alekseyev YO, Arendt CW, Shaw MH. TLR3 signaling promotes the induction of unique human BDCA-3 dendritic cell populations. *Front Immunol*. 2016;7:88.

150. Liu S, Cai X, Wu J, et al. Phosphorylation of innate immune adaptor proteins MAVS, STING, and TRIF induces IRF3 activation. *Science*. 2015;347:aaa2630.

151. Lafaille FG, Pessach IM, Zhang SY, et al. Impaired intrinsic immunity to HSV-1 in human iPSC-derived TLR3-deficient CNS cells. *Nature*. 2012;491:769-773.

152. Brewitz A, Eickhoff S, Dähling S, et al. CD8(+) T cells orchestrate pDC-XCR1(+) dendritic cell spatial and functional cooperativity to optimize priming. *Immunity*. 2017;46:205-219.

153. Ohta T, Sugiyama M, Hemmi H, et al. Crucial roles of XCR1-expressing dendritic cells and the XCR1-XCL1 chemokine axis in intestinal immune homeostasis. *Sci Rep*. 2016;6:23505.

154. Alexandre YO, Ghilas S, Sanchez C, Le Bon A, Crozat K, Dalod M. XCR1+ dendritic cells promote memory CD8+ T cell recall upon secondary infections with Listeria monocytogenes or certain viruses. *J Exp Med*. 2016;213:75-92.

155. Yin X, Yu H, Jin X, et al. Human blood CD1c+ dendritic cells encompass CD5high and CD5low subsets that differ significantly in phenotype, gene expression, and functions. *J Immunol*. 2017;198:1553-1564.

156. Alcántara-Hernández M, Leylek R, Wagar LE, et al. High-Dimensional phenotypic mapping of human dendritic cells reveals interindividual variation and tissue specialization. *Immunity*. 2017;47:1037-1050.e6.

157. Segura E, Durand M, Amigorena S. Similar antigen cross-presentation capacity and phagocytic functions in all freshly isolated human lymphoid organ-resident dendritic cells. *J Exp Med*. 2013;210:1035-1047.

158. Van Rhijn I, Ly D, Moody DB. CD1a, CD1b, and CD1c in immunity against mycobacteria. *Adv Exp Med Biol*. 2013;783:181-197.

159. Bakdash G, Buschow SI, Gorris MA, et al. Expansion of a BDCA1+CD14+ myeloid cell population in melanoma patients may attenuate the efficacy of dendritic cell vaccines. *Cancer Res*. 2016;76:4332-4346.

160. Nizzoli G, Krietsch J, Weick A, et al. Human CD1c+ dendritic cells secrete high levels of IL-12 and potently prime cytotoxic T-cell responses. *Blood*. 2013;122:932-942.

161. Leylek R, Alcántara-Hernández M, Lanzar Z, et al. Integrated cross-species analysis identifies a conserved transitional dendritic cell population. *Cell Rep*. 2019;29:3736-3750.e8.

162. Zhang H, Gregorio JD, Iwahori T, et al. A distinct subset of plasmacytoid dendritic cells induces activation and differentiation of B and T lymphocytes. *Proc Natl Acad Sci U S A*. 2017;114:1988-1993.

163. Ruffin N, Gea-Mallorquí E, Brouiller F, et al. Constitutive Siglec-1 expression confers susceptibility to HIV-1 infection of human dendritic cell precursors. *Proc Natl Acad Sci U S A*. 2019;116:21685-21693.

164. Zhang Q, He Y, Luo N, et al. Landscape and dynamics of single immune cells in hepatocellular carcinoma. *Cell*. 2019;179:829-845.e20.

165. Zilionis R, Engblom C, Pfirschke C, et al. Single-cell transcriptomics of human and mouse lung cancers reveals conserved myeloid populations across individuals and species. *Immunity*. 2019;50:1317-1334.e10.

166. Chen YL, Gomes T, Hardman CS, et al. Re-evaluation of human BDCA-2+ DC during acute sterile skin inflammation. *J Exp Med*. 2020;217(3):jem.20190811.

167. Bauer T, Zagorska A, Jurkin J, et al. Identification of Axl as a downstream effector of TGF-beta1 during Langerhans cell differentiation and epidermal homeostasis. *J Exp Med*. 2012;209:2033-2047.

168. Hieronymus T, Zenke M, Baek JH, Sere K. The clash of Langerhans cell homeostasis in skin: should I stay or should I go? *Semin Cell Dev Biol*. 2015;41:30-38.

169. Bigley V, Haniffa M, Doulatov S, et al. The human syndrome of dendritic cell, monocyte, B and NK lymphoid deficiency. *J Exp Med*. 2011;208:227-234.

170. Bigley V, Maisuria S, Cytlak U, et al. Biallelic interferon regulatory factor 8 mutation: a complex immunodeficiency syndrome with dendritic cell deficiency, monocytopenia, and immune dysregulation. *J Allergy Clin Immunol*. 2018;141:2234-2248.

171. Kanitakis J, Morelon E, Petruzzo P, Badet L, Dubernard JM. Self-renewal capacity of human epidermal Langerhans cells: observations made on a composite tissue allograft. *Exp Dermatol*. 2011;20:145-146.

172. Romano E, Cotari JW, Barreira da Silva R, et al. Human Langerhans cells use an IL-15R-α/IL-15/pSTAT5-dependent mechanism to break T-cell tolerance against the self-differentiation tumor antigen WT1. *Blood*. 2012;119:5182-5190.

173. Banchereau J, Thompson-Snipes L, Zurawski S, et al. The differential production of cytokines by human Langerhans cells and dermal CD14(+) DCs controls CTL priming. *Blood*. 2012;119:5742-5749.

174. Artyomov MN, Munk A, Gorvel L, et al. Modular expression analysis reveals functional conservation between human Langerhans cells and mouse cross-priming dendritic cells. *J Exp Med*. 2015;212:743-757.

175. Carpentier S, Vu Manh TP, Chelbi R, et al. Comparative genomics analysis of mononuclear phagocyte subsets confirms homology between lymphoid tissue-resident and dermal XCR1(+) DCs in mouse and human and distinguishes them from Langerhans cells. *J Immunol Methods*. 2016;432:35-49.

176. Geissmann F, Dieu-Nosjean MC, Dezutter C, et al. Accumulation of immature Langerhans cells in human lymph nodes draining chronically inflamed skin. *J Exp Med*. 2002;196:417-430.

177. De Monte A, Olivieri CV, Vitale S, et al. CD1c-Related DCs that express CD207/langerin, but are distinguishable from langerhans cells, are consistently present in human tonsils. *Front Immunol*. 2016;7:197.

178. Kim JH, Hu Y, Yongqing T, et al. CD1a on Langerhans cells controls inflammatory skin disease. *Nat Immunol*. 2016;17:1159-1166.

179. van der Aar AM, Sylva-Steenland RM, Bos JD, Kapsenberg ML, de Jong EC, Teunissen MB. Loss of TLR2, TLR4, and TLR5 on Langerhans cells abolishes bacterial recognition. *J Immunol*. 2007;178:1986-1990.

180. Seneschal J, Clark RA, Gehad A, Baecher-Allan CM, Kupper TS. Human epidermal Langerhans cells maintain immune homeostasis in skin by activating skin resident regulatory T cells. *Immunity*. 2012;36:873-884.

181. Kashem SW, Igyarto BZ, Gerami-Nejad M, et al. Candida albicans morphology and dendritic cell subsets determine T helper cell differentiation. *Immunity*. 2015;42:356-366.

182. Hoeffel G, Chen J, Lavin Y, et al. C-myb(+) erythro-myeloid progenitor-derived fetal monocytes give rise to adult tissue-resident macrophages. *Immunity*. 2015;42:665-678.

183. McGrath KE, Frame JM, Fegan KH, et al. Distinct sources of hematopoietic progenitors emerge before HSCs and provide functional blood cells in the mammalian embryo. *Cell Rep*. 2015;11:1892-1904.

184. Ivanovs A, Rybtsov S, Ng ES, Stanley EG, Elefanty AG, Medvinsky A. Human haematopoietic stem cell development: from the embryo to the dish. *Development*. 2017;144:2323-2337.

185. Schulz C, Gomez Perdiguero E, Chorro L, et al. A lineage of myeloid cells independent of Myb and hematopoietic stem cells. *Science*. 2012;336:86-90.

186. Bian Z, Gong Y, Huang T, et al. Deciphering human macrophage development at single-cell resolution. *Nature*. 2020;582:571-576.

187. Takata K, Kozaki T, Lee CZW, et al. Induced-pluripotent-stem-cell-derived primitive macrophages provide a platform for modeling tissue-resident macrophage differentiation and function. *Immunity*. 2017;47:183-198.e6.

188. Buchrieser J, James W, Moore MD. Human induced pluripotent stem cell-derived macrophages share ontogeny with MYB-independent tissue-resident macrophages. *Stem Cell Rep*. 2017;8:334-345.

189. Lee CZW, Kozaki T, Ginhoux F. Studying tissue macrophages in vitro: are iPSC-derived cells the answer? *Nat Rev Immunol*. 2018;18:716-725.

190. Hoeffel G, Wang Y, Greter M, et al. Adult Langerhans cells derive predominantly from embryonic fetal liver monocytes with a minor contribution of yolk sac-derived macrophages. *J Exp Med*. 2012;209:1167-1181.

191. Gomez Perdiguero E, Klapproth K, Schulz C, et al. Tissue-resident macrophages originate from yolk-sac-derived erythro-myeloid progenitors. *Nature*. 2015;518:547-551.

192. Tamoutounour S, Guilliams M, Montanana Sanchis F, et al. Origins and functional specialization of macrophages and of conventional and monocyte-derived dendritic cells in mouse skin. *Immunity*. 2013;39:925-938.

193. Bain CC, Hawley CA, Garner H, et al. Long-lived self-renewing bone marrow-derived macrophages displace embryo-derived cells to inhabit adult serous cavities. *Nat Commun*. 2016;7:ncomms11852.

194. Yona S, Kim KW, Wolf Y, et al. Fate mapping reveals origins and dynamics of monocytes and tissue macrophages under homeostasis. *Immunity*. 2013;38:79-91.

195. Hashimoto D, Chow A, Noizat C, et al. Tissue-resident macrophages self-maintain locally throughout adult life with minimal contribution from circulating monocytes. *Immunity*. 2013;38:792-804.

196. Ginhoux F, Tacke F, Angeli V, et al. Langerhans cells arise from monocytes in vivo. *Nat Immunol*. 2006;7:265-273.

197. Scott CL, Zheng F, De Baetselier P, et al. Bone marrow-derived monocytes give rise to self-renewing and fully differentiated Kupffer cells. *Nat Commun*. 2016;7:10321.

198. Collin MP, Hart DN, Jackson GH, et al. The fate of human Langerhans cells in hematopoietic stem cell transplantation. *J Exp Med*. 2006;203:27-33.

199. Mielcarek M, Kirkorian AY, Hackman RC, et al. Langerhans cell homeostasis and turnover after nonmyeloablative and myeloablative allogeneic hematopoietic cell transplantation. *Transplantation*. 2014;98:563-568.

200. Thomas ED, Ramberg RE, Sale GE, Sparkes RS, Golde DW. Direct evidence for a bone marrow origin of the alveolar macrophage in man. *Science*. 1976;192:1016-1018.

201. Gale RP, Sparkes RS, Golde DW. Bone marrow origin of hepatic macrophages (Kupffer cells) in humans. *Science*. 1978;201:937-938.

202. Schuster C, Vaculik C, Fiala C, et al. HLA-DR+ leukocytes acquire CD1 antigens in embryonic and fetal human skin and contain functional antigen-presenting cells. *J Exp Med*. 2009;206:169-181.

203. Schuster C, Mildner M, Mairhofer M, et al. Human embryonic epidermis contains a diverse Langerhans cell precursor pool. *Development*. 2014;141:807-815.

204. McGovern N, Shin A, Low G, et al. Human fetal dendritic cells promote prenatal T-cell immune suppression through arginase-2. *Nature*. 2017;546:662-666.

205. Park JE, Jardine L, Gottgens B, Teichmann SA, Haniffa M. Prenatal development of human immunity. *Science*. 2020;368:600-603.

206. Gomez Perdiguero E, Geissmann F. Myb-independent macrophages: a family of cells that develops with their tissue of residence and is involved in its homeostasis. *Cold Spring Harb Symp Quant Biol*. 2013;78:91-100.

207. Sere K, Baek JH, Ober-Blobaum J, et al. Two distinct types of Langerhans cells populate the skin during steady state and inflammation. *Immunity*. 2012;37:905-916.

208. Nagao K, Kobayashi T, Moro K, et al. Stress-induced production of chemokines by hair follicles regulates the trafficking of dendritic cells in skin. *Nat Immunol*. 2012;13:744-752.

209. Dick SA, Macklin JA, Nejat S, et al. Self-renewing resident cardiac macrophages limit adverse remodeling following myocardial infarction. *Nat Immunol*. 2019;20:29-39.

210. Vannella KM, Barron L, Borthwick LA, et al. Incomplete deletion of IL-4Ralpha by LysM(Cre) reveals distinct subsets of M2 macrophages controlling inflammation and fibrosis in chronic schistosomiasis. *PLoS Pathog.* 2014;10:e1004372.

211. Zhu Y, Herndon JM, Sojka DK, et al. Tissue-resident macrophages in pancreatic ductal adenocarcinoma originate from embryonic hematopoiesis and promote tumor progression. *Immunity.* 2017;47:323-338.e6.

212. Lin DS, Kan A, Gao J, Crampin EJ, Hodgkin PD, Naik SH. DiSNE Movie visualization and assessment of clonal kinetics reveal multiple trajectories of dendritic cell development. *Cell Rep.* 2018;22:2557-2566.

213. Velten L, Haas SF, Raffel S, et al. Human haematopoietic stem cell lineage commitment is a continuous process. *Nat Cell Biol.* 2017;19:271-281.

214. Karamitros D, Stoilova B, Aboukhalil Z, et al. Single-cell analysis reveals the continuum of human lympho-myeloid progenitor cells. *Nat Immunol.* 2018;19(1):85-97.

215. Lee J, Zhou YJ, Ma W, et al. Lineage specification of human dendritic cells is marked by IRF8 expression in hematopoietic stem cells and multipotent progenitors. *Nat Immunol.* 2017;18:877-888.

216. Lai S, Xu Y, Huang W, et al. *Mapping Human Hematopoietic Hierarchy at Single Cell Resolution by Microwell-Seq.* Biorxiv; 2018.

217. Dress RJ, Dutertre CA, Giladi A, et al. Plasmacytoid dendritic cells develop from Ly6D$^+$ lymphoid progenitors distinct from the myeloid lineage. *Nat Immunol.* 2019;20:852-864.

218. Rodrigues PF, Alberti-Servera L, Eremin A, Grajales-Reyes GE, Ivanek R, Tussiwand R. Distinct progenitor lineages contribute to the heterogeneity of plasmacytoid dendritic cells. *Nat Immunol.* 2018;19:711-722.

219. Kawamura S, Onai N, Miya F, et al. Identification of a human clonogenic progenitor with strict monocyte differentiation potential: a counterpart of mouse cMoPs. *Immunity.* 2017;46:835-848.e4.

220. Fadilah SA, Vuckovic S, Khalil D, Hart DN. Cord blood CD34+ cells cultured with FLT3L, stem cell factor, interleukin-6, and IL-3 produce CD11c+CD1a-/c- myeloid dendritic cells. *Stem Cells Dev.* 2007;16:849-855.

221. Weber GF, Chousterman BG, He S, et al. Interleukin-3 amplifies acute inflammation and is a potential therapeutic target in sepsis. *Science.* 2015;347:1260-1265.

222. Dickinson RE, Milne P, Jardine L, et al. The evolution of cellular deficiency in GATA2 mutation. *Blood.* 2014;123:863-874.

223. Sallusto F, Lanzavecchia A. Efficient presentation of soluble antigen by cultured human dendritic cells is maintained by granulocyte/macrophage colony-stimulating factor plus interleukin 4 and downregulated by tumor necrosis factor alpha. *J Exp Med.* 1994;179:1109-1118.

224. Komuczki J, Tuzlak S, Friebel E, et al. Fate-mapping of GM-CSF expression identifies a discrete subset of inflammation-driving T helper cells regulated by cytokines IL-23 and IL-1β. *Immunity.* 2019;50(5):1289-1304.e6.

225. Ushach I, Zlotnik A. Biological role of granulocyte macrophage colony-stimulating factor (GM-CSF) and macrophage colony-stimulating factor (M-CSF) on cells of the myeloid lineage. *J Leukoc Biol.* 2016;100:481-489.

226. Mariano VJ, Mylonakis E. In inpatients with COVID-19 who need supplemental oxygen, lenzilumab increased ventilation-free survival. *Ann Intern Med.* 2022;175(4):JC39.

227. Mun SH, Park PSU, Park-Min KH. The M-CSF receptor in osteoclasts and beyond. *Exp Mol Med.* 2020;52:1239-1254.

228. Felix J, Elegheert J, Gutsche I, et al. Human IL-34 and CSF-1 establish structurally similar extracellular assemblies with their common hematopoietic receptor. *Structure.* 2013;21(4):528-539.

229. Wang Y, Szretter KJ, Vermi W, et al. IL-34 is a tissue-restricted ligand of CSF1R required for the development of Langerhans cells and microglia. *Nat Immunol.* 2012;13:753-760.

230. Greter M, Lelios I, Pelczar P, et al. Stroma-derived interleukin-34 controls the development and maintenance of langerhans cells and the maintenance of microglia. *Immunity.* 2012;37:1050-1060.

231. Wang Y, Bugatti M, Ulland TK, Vermi W, Gilfillan S, Colonna M. Nonredundant roles of keratinocyte-derived IL-34 and neutrophil-derived CSF1 in Langerhans cell renewal in the steady state and during inflammation. *Eur J Immunol.* 2016;46:552-559.

232. Baek JH, Zeng R, Weinmann-Menke J, et al. IL-34 mediates acute kidney injury and worsens subsequent chronic kidney disease. *J Clin Invest.* 2015;125:3198-3214.

233. Yamane F, Nishikawa Y, Matsui K, et al. CSF-1 receptor-mediated differentiation of a new type of monocytic cell with B cell-stimulating activity: its selective dependence on IL-34. *J Leukoc Biol.* 2014;95:19-31.

234. Bézie S, Picarda E, Ossart J, et al. IL-34 is a Treg-specific cytokine and mediates transplant tolerance. *J Clin Invest.* 2015;125:3952-3964.

235. Martinez FO, Helming L, Milde R, et al. Genetic programs expressed in resting and IL-4 alternatively activated mouse and human macrophages: similarities and differences. *Blood.* 2013;121:e57-69.

236. Jenkins SJ, Ruckerl D, Thomas GD, et al. IL-4 directly signals tissue-resident macrophages to proliferate beyond homeostatic levels controlled by CSF-1. *J Exp Med.* 2013;210:2477-2491.

237. Nutt SL, Chopin M. Transcriptional networks driving dendritic cell differentiation and function. *Immunity.* 2020;52:942-956.

238. Anderson DA, Dutertre CA, Ginhoux F, Murphy KM. Genetic models of human and mouse dendritic cell development and function. *Nat Rev Immunol.* 2021;21:101-115.

239. Dickinson RE, Griffin H, Bigley V, et al. Exome sequencing identifies GATA-2 mutation as the cause of dendritic cell, monocyte, B and NK lymphoid deficiency. *Blood.* 2011;118:2656-2658.

240. Onodera K, Fujiwara T, Onishi Y, et al. GATA2 regulates dendritic cell differentiation. *Blood.* 2016;128:508-518.

241. Wu X, Briseño CG, Durai V, et al. Mafb lineage tracing to distinguish macrophages from other immune lineages reveals dual identity of Langerhans cells. *J Exp Med.* 2016;213:2553-2565.

242. Huang X, Ferris ST, Kim S, et al. Differential usage of transcriptional repressor Zeb2 enhancers distinguishes adult and embryonic hematopoiesis. *Immunity.* 2021;54:1417-1432.e7.

243. Wu X, Briseño CG, Grajales-Reyes GE, et al. Transcription factor Zeb2 regulates commitment to plasmacytoid dendritic cell and monocyte fate. *Proc Natl Acad Sci U S A.* 2016;113:14775-14780.

244. Scott CL, Soen B, Martens L, et al. The transcription factor Zeb2 regulates development of conventional and plasmacytoid DCs by repressing Id2. *J Exp Med.* 2016;213:897-911.

245. Bagadia P, Huang X, Liu TT, et al. An Nfil3-Zeb2-Id2 pathway imposes Irf8 enhancer switching during cDC1 development. *Nat Immunol.* 2019;20:1174-1185.

246. Ghosh HS, Ceribelli M, Matos I, et al. ETO family protein Mtg16 regulates the balance of dendritic cell subsets by repressing Id2. *J Exp Med.* 2014;211:1623-1635.

247. Durai V, Bagadia P, Granja JM, et al. Cryptic activation of an Irf8 enhancer governs cDC1 fate specification. *Nat Immunol.* 2019;20:1161-1173.

248. Hambleton S, Salem S, Bustamante J, et al. IRF8 mutations and human dendritic-cell immunodeficiency. *N Engl J Med.* 2011;365:127-138.

249. Rosa FF, Pires CF, Kurochkin I, et al. Direct reprogramming of fibroblasts into antigen-presenting dendritic cells. *Sci Immunol.* 2018;3:eaau4292.

250. Persson EK, Uronen-Hansson H, Semmrich M, et al. IRF4 transcription-factor-dependent CD103(+)CD11b(+) dendritic cells drive mucosal T helper 17 cell differentiation. *Immunity.* 2013;38:958-969.

251. Schlitzer A, McGovern N, Teo P, et al. IRF4 transcription factor-dependent CD11b+ dendritic cells in human and mouse control mucosal IL-17 cytokine responses. *Immunity.* 2013;38:970-983.

252. Tussiwand R, Everts B, Grajales-Reyes GE, et al. Klf4 expression in conventional dendritic cells is required for T helper 2 cell responses. *Immunity.* 2015;42:916-928.

253. Feinberg MW, Wara AK, Cao Z, et al. The Kruppel-like factor KLF4 is a critical regulator of monocyte differentiation. *EMBO J.* 2007;26:4138-4148.

254. Milne P, Bigley V, Gunawan M, Haniffa M, Collin M. CD1c+ blood dendritic cells have Langerhans cell potential. *Blood.* 2015;125:470-473.

255. Jurkin J, Krump C, Köffel R, et al. Human skin dendritic cell fate is differentially regulated by the monocyte identity factor KLF4 during steady state and inflammation. *J Allergy Clin Immunol.* 2017;139(6):1873-1884.e10.

256. Brown CC, Gudjonson H, Pritykin Y, et al. Transcriptional basis of mouse and human dendritic cell heterogeneity. *Cell.* 2019;179:846-863.e24.

257. Cytlak U, Resteu A, Bogaert D, et al. Ikaros family zinc finger 1 regulates dendritic cell development and function in humans. *Nat Commun.* 2018;9:1239.

258. Zlotnik A, Yoshie O. The chemokine superfamily revisited. *Immunity.* 2012;36:705-716.

259. Schall TJ, Proudfoot AE. Overcoming hurdles in developing successful drugs targeting chemokine receptors. *Nat Rev Immunol.* 2011;11:355-363.

260. Schumann K, Lammermann T, Bruckner M, et al. Immobilized chemokine fields and soluble chemokine gradients cooperatively shape migration patterns of dendritic cells. *Immunity.* 2010;32:703-713.

261. Barczyk M, Carracedo S, Gullberg D. Integrins. *Cell Tissue Res.* 2010;339:269-280.

262. Ley K, Rivera-Nieves J, Sandborn WJ, Shattil S. Integrin-based therapeutics: biological basis, clinical use and new drugs. *Nat Rev Drug Discov.* 2016;15:173-183.

263. Guilliams M, Bruhns P, Saeys Y, Hammad H, Lambrecht BN. The function of Fcγ receptors in dendritic cells and macrophages. *Nat Rev Immunol.* 2014;14:94-108.

264. Weiskopf K, Weissman IL. Macrophages are critical effectors of antibody therapies for cancer. *mAbs.* 2015;7:303-310.

265. Prabhudas M, Bowdish D, Drickamer K, et al. Standardizing scavenger receptor nomenclature. *J Immunol.* 2014;192:1997-2006.

266. Zani IA, Stephen SL, Mughal NA, et al. Scavenger receptor structure and function in health and disease. *Cells.* 2015;4:178-201.

267. Macauley MS, Crocker PR, Paulson JC. Siglec-mediated regulation of immune cell function in disease. *Nat Rev Immunol.* 2014;14:653-666.

268. Stappers MHT, Clark AE, Aimanianda V, et al. Recognition of DHN-melanin by a C-type lectin receptor is required for immunity to Aspergillus. *Nature.* 2018;555:382-386.

269. Pillai S, Netravali IA, Cariappa A, Mattoo H. Siglecs and immune regulation. *Annu Rev Immunol.* 2012;30:357-392.

270. Lemke G, Rothlin CV. Immunobiology of the TAM receptors. *Nat Rev Immunol.* 2008;8:327-336.

271. Ford JW, McVicar DW. TREM and TREM-like receptors in inflammation and disease. *Curr Opin Immunol.* 2009;21:38-46.

272. Vaine CA, Soberman RJ. The CD200-CD200R1 inhibitory signaling pathway: immune regulation and host-pathogen interactions. *Adv Immunol.* 2014;121:191-211.

273. Oldenborg PA, Zhelznyak A, Fang YF, Lagenaur CF, Gresham HD, Lindberg FP. Role of CD47 as a marker of self on red blood cells. *Science.* 2000;288:2051-2054.

274. Burger P, Hilarius-Stokman P, de Korte D, van den Berg TK, van Bruggen R. CD47 functions as a molecular switch for erythrocyte phagocytosis. *Blood.* 2012;119:5512-5521.

275. Veillette A, Chen J. SIRPα-CD47 immune checkpoint blockade in anticancer therapy. *Trends Immunol.* 2018;39:173-184.

276. Iwasaki A, Medzhitov R. Regulation of adaptive immunity by the innate immune system. *Science.* 2010;327:291-295.

277. Kang JY, Lee JO. Structural biology of the toll-like receptor family. *Annu Rev Biochem.* 2011;80:917-941.

278. Kawasaki T, Kawai T. Toll-like receptor signaling pathways. *Front Immunol.* 2014;5:461.

279. Lee EY, Lee MW, Wong GCL. Modulation of toll-like receptor signaling by antimicrobial peptides. *Semin Cell Dev Biol.* 2018;88:173-184.
280. Lennartz M, Drake J. Molecular mechanisms of macrophage Toll-like receptor-Fc receptor synergy. *F1000Res.* 2018;7:21.
281. Kanneganti TD, Lamkanfi M, Nunez G. Intracellular NOD-like receptors in host defense and disease. *Immunity.* 2007;27:549-559.
282. Goubau D, Deddouche S, Reis e Sousa C. Cytosolic sensing of viruses. *Immunity.* 2013;38:855-869.
283. Lamkanfi M, Dixit VM. Inflammasomes and their roles in health and disease. *Annu Rev Cell Dev Biol.* 2012;28:137-161.
284. de Jesus AA, Canna SW, Liu Y, Goldbach-Mansky R. Molecular mechanisms in genetically defined autoinflammatory diseases: disorders of amplified danger signaling. *Annu Rev Immunol.* 2015;33:823-874.
285. Gordon S. Phagocytosis: an immunobiologic process. *Immunity.* 2016;44:463-475.
286. Goodridge HS, Reyes CN, Becker CA, et al. Activation of the innate immune receptor Dectin-1 upon formation of a "phagocytic synapse." *Nature.* 2011;472:471-475.
287. Lui H, Zhang J, Makinson SR, et al. Progranulin deficiency promotes circuit-specific synaptic pruning by microglia via complement activation. *Cell.* 2016;165:921-935.
288. Bretou M, Kumari A, Malbec O, et al. Dynamics of the membrane-cytoskeleton interface in MHC class II-restricted antigen presentation. *Immunol Rev.* 2016;272:39-51.
289. Bretou M, Sáez PJ, Sanséau D, et al. Lysosome signaling controls the migration of dendritic cells. *Sci Immunol.* 2017;2(16):eaak9573.
290. Mintern JD, Macri C, Chin WJ, et al. Differential use of autophagy by primary dendritic cells specialized in cross-presentation. *Autophagy.* 2015;11:906-917.
291. Macrophages M. Clean up: efferocytosis and microbial control. *Curr Opin Microbiol.* 2014;17:17-23.
292. Steinman RM, Lustig DS, Cohn ZA. Identification of a novel cell type in peripheral lymphoid organs of mice. 3. Functional properties in vivo. *J Exp Med.* 1974;139:1431-1445.
293. Segura E, Amigorena S. Cross-presentation in mouse and human dendritic cells. *Adv Immunol.* 2015;127:1-31.
294. Underhill DM, Goodridge HS. Information processing during phagocytosis. *Nat Rev Immunol.* 2012;12:492-502.
295. Bedoui S, Whitney PG, Waithman J, et al. Cross-presentation of viral and self antigens by skin-derived CD103+ dendritic cells. *Nat Immunol.* 2009;10:488-495.
296. Kapsenberg ML. Dendritic-cell control of pathogen-driven T-cell polarization. *Nat Rev Immunol.* 2003;3:984-993.
297. Fang FC. Antimicrobial reactive oxygen and nitrogen species: concepts and controversies. *Nat Rev Microbiol.* 2004;2:820-832.
298. de Oliveira-Junior EB, Bustamante J, Newburger PE, Condino-Neto A. The human NADPH oxidase: primary and secondary defects impairing the respiratory burst function and the microbicidal ability of phagocytes. *Scand J Immunol.* 2011;73:420-427.
299. Raposo G, Stoorvogel W. Extracellular vesicles: exosomes, microvesicles, and friends. *J Cell Biol.* 2013;200:373-383.
300. Wakim LM, Bevan MJ. Cross-dressed dendritic cells drive memory CD8+ T-cell activation after viral infection. *Nature.* 2011;471:629-632.
301. Saha S, Aranda E, Hayakawa Y, et al. Macrophage-derived extracellular vesicle-packaged WNTs rescue intestinal stem cells and enhance survival after radiation injury. *Nat Commun.* 2016;7:13096.
302. Serhan CN. Pro-resolving lipid mediators are leads for resolution physiology. *Nature.* 2014;510:92-101.
303. Wynn TA, Vannella KM. Macrophages in tissue repair, regeneration, and fibrosis. *Immunity.* 2016;44:450-462.
304. Noy R, Pollard JW. Tumor-associated macrophages: from mechanisms to therapy. *Immunity.* 2014;41:49-61.
305. Zhou X, Franklin RA, Adler M, et al. Circuit design features of a stable two-cell system. *Cell.* 2018;172:744-757.e17.
306. Thomas D, Apovian C. Macrophage functions in lean and obese adipose tissue. *Metabolism.* 2017;72:120-143.
307. Cox N, Crozet L, Holtman IR, et al. Diet-regulated production of PDGFcc by macrophages controls energy storage. *Science.* 2021;373:eabe9383.
308. Jaitin DA, Adlung L, Thaiss CA, et al. Lipid-associated macrophages control metabolic homeostasis in a trem2-dependent manner. *Cell.* 2019;178:686-698.e14.
309. Aguilar PS, Baylies MK, Fleissner A, et al. Genetic basis of cell-cell fusion mechanisms. *Trends Genet.* 2013;29:427-437.
310. Helming L, Gordon S. Molecular mediators of macrophage fusion. *Trends Cell Biol.* 2009;19:514-522.
311. O'Neill L, Molloy ES. The role of toll like receptors in giant cell arteritis. *Rheumatology.* 2016;55:1921-1931.
312. Herrtwich L, Nanda I, Evangelou K, et al. DNA damage signaling instructs polyploid macrophage fate in granulomas. *Cell.* 2016;167:1264-1280.e18.
313. Bigley V, Collin M. Insights from patients with dendritic cell immunodeficiency. *Mol Immunol.* 2020;122:116-123.
314. Kong XF, Martinez-Barricarte R, Kennedy J, et al. Disruption of an antimycobacterial circuit between dendritic and helper T cells in human SPPL2a deficiency. *Nat Immunol.* 2018;19(9):973-985.
315. Allen CE, Beverley PCL, Collin M, et al. The coming of age of Langerhans cell histiocytosis. *Nat Immunol.* 2020;21:1-7.
316. McClain KL, Bigenwald C, Collin M, et al. Histiocytic disorders. *Nat Rev Dis Prim.* 2021;7:73.
317. Goyal G, Tazi A, Go RS, et al. Expert consensus recommendations for the diagnosis and treatment of Langerhans cell histiocytosis in adults. *Blood.* 2022;139(17):2601-2621. doi:10.1182blood.2021014343
318. Goyal G, Heaney ML, Collin M, et al. Erdheim-Chester disease: consensus recommendations for evaluation, diagnosis, and treatment in the molecular era. *Blood.* 2020;135:1929-1945.
319. Abla O, Jacobsen E, Picarsic J, et al. Consensus recommendations for the diagnosis and clinical management of Rosai-Dorfman-Destombes disease. *Blood.* 2018;131:2877-2890.
320. Jordan MB, Allen CE, Greenberg J, et al. Challenges in the diagnosis of hemophagocytic lymphohistiocytosis: recommendations from the north American consortium for histiocytosis (NACHO). *Pediatr Blood Cancer.* 2019;66(11):e27929.
321. Knaak C, Nyvlt P, Schuster FS, et al. Hemophagocytic lymphohistiocytosis in critically ill patients: diagnostic reliability of HLH-2004 criteria and HScore. *Crit Care.* 2020;24:244.
322. Fardet L, Galicier L, Lambotte O, et al. Development and validation of the HScore, a score for the diagnosis of reactive hemophagocytic syndrome. *Arthritis Rheumatol.* 2014;66:2613-2620.
323. Locatelli F, Jordan MB, Allen C, et al. Emapalumab in children with primary hemophagocytic lymphohistiocytosis. *N Engl J Med.* 2020;382:1811-1822.
324. Platt FM, d'Azzo A, Davidson BL, Neufeld EF, Tifft CJ. Lysosomal storage diseases. *Nat Rev Dis Prim.* 2018;4:27.
325. Sun A. Lysosomal storage disease overview. *Ann Transl Med.* 2018;6:476.
326. Silvin A, Chapuis N, Dunsmore G, et al. Elevated calprotectin and abnormal myeloid cell subsets discriminate severe from Mild COVID-19. *Cell.* 2020;182:1401-1418.e18.
327. Kvedaraite E, Hertwig L, Sinha I, et al. Major alterations in the mononuclear phagocyte landscape associated with COVID-19 severity. *Proc Natl Acad Sci U S A.* 2021;118:e2018587118.
328. Yoshida M, Worlock KB, Huang N, et al. Local and systemic responses to SARS-CoV-2 infection in children and adults. *Nature.* 2022;602:321-327.
329. Liao M, Liu Y, Yuan J, et al. Single-cell landscape of bronchoalveolar immune cells in patients with COVID-19. *Nat Med.* 2020;26:842-844.
330. Wynn TA, Chawla A, Pollard JW. Macrophage biology in development, homeostasis and disease. *Nature.* 2013;496:445-455.
331. Sharma A, Seow JJW, Dutertre CA, et al. Onco-fetal reprogramming of endothelial cells drives immunosuppressive macrophages in hepatocellular carcinoma. *Cell.* 2020;183:377-394.e21.
332. Lee HO, Hong Y, Etlioglu HE, et al. Lineage-dependent gene expression programs influence the immune landscape of colorectal cancer. *Nat Genet.* 2020;52:594-603.
333. Molgora M, Esaulova E, Vermi W, et al. TREM2 modulation remodels the tumor myeloid landscape enhancing anti-PD-1 immunotherapy. *Cell.* 2020;182:886-900.e17.
334. Katzenelenbogen Y, Sheban F, Yalin A, et al. Coupled scRNA-seq and intracellular protein activity reveal an immunosuppressive role of TREM2 in cancer. *Cell.* 2020;182:872-885.e19.
335. Nalio Ramos R, Missolo-Koussou Y, Gerber-Ferder Y, et al. Tissue-resident FOLR2+ macrophages associate with CD8+ T cell infiltration in human breast cancer. *Cell.* 2022;185:1189-1207.e25.
336. Willemsen L, de Winther MP. Macrophage subsets in atherosclerosis as defined by single-cell technologies. *J Pathol.* 2020;250:705-714.
337. Cochain C, Vafadarnejad E, Arampatzi P, et al. Single-cell RNA-seq reveals the transcriptional landscape and heterogeneity of aortic macrophages in murine atherosclerosis. *Circ Res.* 2018;122:1661-1674.
338. Fernandez DM, Rahman AH, Fernandez NF, et al. Single-cell immune landscape of human atherosclerotic plaques. *Nat Med.* 2019;25:1576-1588.
339. Vallejo J, Cochain C, Zernecke A, Ley K. Heterogeneity of immune cells in human atherosclerosis revealed by scRNA-Seq. *Cardiovasc Res.* 2021;117:2537-2543.
340. Culemann S, Grüneboom A, Nicolás-Ávila JÁ, et al. Locally renewing resident synovial macrophages provide a protective barrier for the joint. *Nature.* 2019;572:670-675.
341. Zhang F, Wei K, Slowikowski K, et al. Defining inflammatory cell states in rheumatoid arthritis joint synovial tissues by integrating single-cell transcriptomics and mass cytometry. *Nat Immunol.* 2019;20:928-942.
342. Kuo D, Ding J, Cohn IS, et al. HBEGF+ macrophages in rheumatoid arthritis induce fibroblast invasiveness. *Sci Transl Med.* 2019;11(491):eaau8587.
343. Smillie CS, Biton M, Ordovas-Montanes J, et al. Intra- and inter-cellular rewiring of the human colon during ulcerative colitis. *Cell.* 2019;178:714-730.e22.
344. Malone AF. Monocytes and macrophages in kidney transplantation and insights from single cell RNA-seq studies. *Kidney360.* 2021;2:1654-1659.
345. Divito SJ, Aasebø AT, Matos TR, et al. Peripheral host T cells survive hematopoietic stem cell transplantation and promote graft-versus-host disease. *J Clin Invest.* 2020;130:4624-4636.
346. Jardine L, Cytlak U, Gunawan M, et al. Donor monocyte-derived macrophages promote human acute graft-versus-host disease. *J Clin Invest.* 2020;130:4574-4586.
347. Dai H, Lan P, Zhao D, et al. PIRs mediate innate myeloid cell memory to nonself MHC molecules. *Science.* 2020;368:1122-1127.

Chapter 11 ■ Lymphocytes and Lymphatic Organs

CHRISTOPHER Y. PARK • MATTHEW M. KLAIRMONT

LYMPH NODES AND LYMPHOID TISSUE

Lymphoid cells represent one of the two major branches of hematopoiesis originating from hematopoietic stem cells (HSCs) and arise from a common lymphoid committed precursor that is present in the bone marrow (BM) in postnatal life. Central or primary lymphoid organs, including the BM and thymus, develop first during ontogeny and represent anatomic sites of antigen-independent lymphoid development. Eventually, developing lymphocytes leave these sites to populate peripheral or secondary lymphoid tissues such as the spleen, lymph nodes (LNs), and mucosa-associated lymphoid tissues (e.g., the Waldeyer ring [tonsils and adenoids] or Peyer patches [PPs]), where they undergo antigen-dependent differentiation in specialized environments in order to undergo terminal differentiation and become specialized immune effector cells. B cells arise from common lymphoid progenitors (CLPs) in the BM that give rise to committed B-cell progenitors that differentiate into naïve B cells initially, but then undergo affinity maturation in secondary tissues upon exposure to specific antigens, where they can give rise to plasma cells or memory B cells (see Chapter 12). Following seeding of the thymus by T-cell precursors, T cells develop into CD4$^+$ or CD8$^+$ T cells following negative and positive selection based on the strength of their interactions with self-antigens (see Chapter 13). In contrast to B cells, T cells do not need to undergo affinity maturation but are activated in secondary lymphoid tissues and proliferate upon exposure to antigenic stimulation. Natural killer (NK) cells, one type of innate lymphoid cell (ILC), also develop from precursors in the BM and complete maturation in peripheral lymphoid tissues (see Chapter 14). Both primary and secondary lymphoid tissues represent highly organized microenvironments composed of heterogeneous cellular and stromal components that help orchestrate normal lymphocyte development and activation, both during the antigen-independent and antigen-dependent stages of maturation. The microenvironment in the secondary lymphoid tissues promotes the selective interactions between lymphocytes and antigens that allow for the initiation and expansion of functional immune responses. Through this choreographed process of lymphocyte development, the cellular immune system has evolved to generate sufficient numbers of lymphocytes to recognize the large diversity of foreign antigens that might be encountered while maintaining immune tolerance to self.

PRIMARY (CENTRAL) LYMPHOID TISSUES

Bone Marrow

BM is distributed inside the different long, short, and flat bones and constitutes one of the largest organs in humans, accounting for 4% to 5% of total body weight[1,2] exceeding other organs such as the brain (2%), liver (2.6%), heart (0.5%), or the entire network of secondary lymphoid organs (SLOs) (1%-1.5%).[3] In a "standard" 70-kg adult human, BM tissues weigh approximately 3 kg and occupy a volume of 1.5 to 3 L. The BM is the most prominent source of de novo cellular generation, reaching rates of 4×10^{11} to 5×10^{11} cells/day in adult humans (0.5-1.5×10^9 in mice),[4-7] which outnumber those of other tissues of high turnover such as intestinal epithelium (10^{11} cells/d)[8] or testis (100-300×10^6 spermatozoids/d). To achieve this, it is estimated that the BM delivers approximately half of its total cellular content to the systemic circulation daily, although only approximately one-fourth of produced cells are nucleated.[9]

The BM is the source of self-renewing HSCs as well as early common lymphoid precursors that give rise to T cells, B cells, and NK cells. Although hematopoiesis initially arises in the yolk sac and then moves to the fetal liver, following birth, the BM is the major site of hematopoiesis throughout adulthood.[10] The two major branches of the hematopoietic system—the lymphoid and myeloid branches—are initiated when multipotent progenitors give rise to the common lymphoid and myeloid progenitors. While the common myeloid progenitors give rise to committed progenitor cells that give rise to all the myeloid lineages including granulocytes, monocytes, erythroid cells, megakaryocytes, as well as a subset of dendritic cells (DCs), the CLP gives rise to committed B-cell progenitors that mature into B cells in the BM as well as a precursor cell that egresses from the BM to seed the thymus to give rise to T-cell progenitors that complete their differentiation program in the thymus. The BM also is an important site for cellular immunity because long-lived plasma cells migrate back to the BM to set up long-term residence after being generated in peripheral lymphoid organs and tissues.

In addition to the hematopoietic cells in the BM, nonhematopoietic cells including endothelial, mesenchymal, and neural cells are important cellular constituents in the BM, providing important growth and survival signals, in some cases providing unique microenvironments, or niches, that allow orderly maturation of hematopoietic cell types.[11-13] The number of these cells has been difficult to estimate because they are difficult to dissociate viably, but studies using fluorescent reporters or immunophenotypic signatures have shown that mesenchymal and vascular cells account for less than 1% of the total mononuclear cellular pool in the mouse BM.[14-18] Direct imaging studies have shown that even these quantifications underestimate the frequency of these cell types,[18,19] a limitation worth taking into account when drawing conclusions regarding the physiologic relevance of stromal subsets.[3] Hematopoiesis can occur in both trabecular bone (mostly present in flat and irregular bones, as well as the epiphysis and metaphysis of long bones)[20] and cortical bone (found in the diaphysis, or shafts, of long bones). Although trabecular bone exhibits a greater degree of bone remodeling, shows an increased endosteal/BM volume ratio, and is more densely vascularized than cortical bone, only minor variations in hematopoietic content and physiology have been described.[19,21,22]

Cellular "niches" in BM have been reported for hematopoietic stem and progenitor cells (HSPCs), CLPs, B-cell progenitors, erythrocytes, regulatory T cells (Tregs), CD4$^+$/CD8$^+$ memory T cells, and plasma cells, among others.[12,23] Many of the niches are located around diverse microvessel types that distinctly regulate access to nutrients, oxygen, and metabolites derived from circulating blood.[23,24] Previously, HSCs were thought to reside in paratrabecular areas in specialized niches with B-cell precursors located more centrally, but this view has been challenged by numerous studies in model organisms such as the mouse, where specific HSC niches have been identified.[12,25] It is now thought that osteoblasts provide a paratrabecular HSC niche upon marrow ablation, but that under steady-state conditions, they provide a niche not for HSCs but early lymphoid progenitors, since ablation of osteoblasts led to acute depletion of lymphoid progenitors but not HSCs.[26,27] While these data suggest that hematopoietic development is characterized by a centripetal movement away from bone surfaces toward deeper regions of the BM, this conceptually attractive hypothesis is challenged by studies directly visualizing progenitors.

First, a spatial analysis of the tissue distribution adopted by CLPs suggested these progenitors localize in bone-distal regions in close interaction with interleukin (IL)-7-expressing CXCL12-abundant reticular cells.[28] Second, global mapping of thousands of genetically labeled HSPCs within intact three-dimensional marrow plugs revealed their significant accumulation in central BM zones.[19] Thus, it is not clear whether hierarchical organization of the hematopoietic compartment is reflected in the microanatomical organization of the BM. One important caveat to these studies, however, is that these findings regarding HSPC niches/localization are almost entirely based on evaluation of the mouse BM, and therefore, the relevance of these findings to humans remains to be confirmed.

In humans, the earliest B-cell precursors can be recognized by their expression of the B-cell surface antigen CD19, as well as CD34, a marker of immaturity, and these cells later acquire CD10. These cells express terminal deoxynucleotidyl transferase (TdT), RAG1, and RAG2, which are involved in immunoglobulin gene rearrangements. CD19 is expressed throughout the entire B-cell differentiation program, whereas CD34 and CD10 are eventually lost at the same time the B-cell marker CD20 is expressed, the immunoglobulin gene is rearranged, and both are expressed on the surface of the cell. The earliest T cell–committed progenitor is not well defined in humans, but these precursors are thought to exit the BM to seed the thymus to complete their developmental program in the specialized environment of the thymus. Precursor lymphocytes or lymphoblasts are not easily identified in BM biopsies but can be more readily identified in Wright-Giemsa–stained aspirate smears, where they exhibit round nuclei with dispersed chromatin, small nucleoli, and scant cytoplasm. These B-cell precursors, or hematogones, are commonly increased in regenerating BM, especially in children, and can be misidentified as neoplastic lymphoid cells in samples drawn from patients with acute lymphoblastic leukemia.[29,30]

Cytokines and chemokines influence B-cell differentiation and trafficking in the BM. One of the major players is CXC-chemokine ligand 12 (CXCL12), also known as stromal cell–derived factor-1 (SDF1), and its receptor CXCR4. Immediately after commitment to the B lineage, precursors become dependent on CXCL12 and its receptor CXCR4, demonstrated by severe disruption of normal B-cell precursor development in CXCL12 (SDF1) knockout, but not IL-7 knockout embryos.[31] CXCL12 is expressed by osteoblasts, BM stromal cells, and endothelial cells (ECs). CXCR4 is present in HSCs and in early stages of B-cell differentiation, whereas it is downregulated in pre–B cells and mature B cells in peripheral lymphoid organs. It is upregulated again after antigen stimulation and plasma cell differentiation, which may explain the homing of these cells back to the BM. Other important molecules for early B-cell development include early B-cell factors and the FLT3 ligand, essential at the pre–pro-B and pro-B stages.[32] B cells complete their maturation in the BM to give rise to naïve B cells. For a more complete description of B-cell development, please see Chapter 12.

Thymus

The thymus is located in the anterior superior mediastinum and is the site where immature precursors that migrate from the BM undergo maturation and selection to become mature, naïve T cells capable of responding to antigen (*Figure 11.1*). The thymus is critical to the development of a normal T-cell repertoire in early life, and there is evidence that it continues to function in T-cell development throughout life.[33,34] The embryonic origins of the thymus are controversial,[35] with one view holding that the thymic primordium arises from the third pharyngeal pouch (endoderm) as well as the pharyngeal crest (ectoderm)[36] and the other supporting an exclusively endodermal origin.[37] It is also clear that the neural crest also contributes to the mature thymus, including the perivascular mesenchyme of the thymus.[38] Early during development, neural crest cells migrate into the thymus, surround the epithelial rudiments, and give rise to the connective tissue capsule and trabecular septa that give rise to the lobules.

The thymus consists of two lobes connected by an isthmus that are covered by a fibrous capsule and is divided into lobules that are separated by trabeculae that extend from the capsule to penetrate the parenchyma. The thymus has a central lymphoid compartment—the thymic epithelial space—and a peripheral compartment—the perivascular space.[34] The thymic epithelial space is divided into a cortex, which includes the peripheral cortex containing an outer or subcapsular cortex, the inner or deep cortex, and the central medulla. The anatomic differences correspond to distinct microenvironments supporting distinct phases of thymocyte development, with the superficial cortex containing large, proliferating precursors, whereas the deep cortex is composed predominantly of nondividing, small thymocytes. The cortex and medulla are each characterized by specialized epithelium and accessory cells that provide specialized microenvironments for T-cell maturation (see "Thymic Epithelium").

In hematoxylin-eosin–stained sections, the cortex appears dark because it is mostly composed of lymphocytes, whereas the medulla appears eosinophilic and paler because of predominance of epithelial cells that include keratinized Hassall corpuscles, which are clusters of concentrically arranged epithelial cells characterized by a well-developed framework of tonofilaments that form an uninterrupted epithelial structure together with other epithelial components of the inner parts of the thymic parenchyma.[39] Hassall corpuscles are solid or cystic and of unclear origin, but monoclonal antibodies for high-molecular-weight keratins that react with skin epithelial cells also bind to Hassall corpuscles.[40,41]

The cortex is the site in which positive and negative selection occurs. Cortical thymocytes include medium-sized cells with dispersed chromatin and nucleoli in the outer cortex and smaller, more mature-appearing round lymphocytes in the inner cortex. Phagocytic histiocytes are also present in the cortex, where they both present antigen and phagocytize apoptotic thymocytes. Most cortical thymocytes represent precursor T cells that are "double positive" (DP) for both CD4 and CD8 (TdT$^+$, CD1a$^+$, CD4$^+$, and CD8$^+$). The cortex also contains cortical epithelial cells, which are large cells with vesicular chromatin, prominent nucleoli, and pale cytoplasm that form a reticular supporting meshwork.

Medullary thymocytes are small, mature lymphocytes with round to slightly irregular nuclei and inconspicuous nucleoli. Medullary thymocytes represent later stages in T-cell development and exhibit the immunophenotype of mature, "single-positive (SP)" T cells expressing CD4 or CD8 (TdT$^-$, CD1a$^-$, CD3$^+$, CD4$^+$, or CD8$^+$). The thymic medulla also contains a unique population of mature B cells with dendritic morphology that expresses B-cell markers CD23, CD37, CD72, CD76, immunoglobulin (Ig) M, and IgD. These cells form rosettes with non-B cells and have been called asteroid cells. The close relationship of these cells with T cells and epithelial thymic cells suggests that they may play a functional role in T-cell differentiation.[42-44] It also has been suggested that they may be the cell of origin for primary mediastinal large B-cell lymphoma. Medullary epithelial cells are smaller and spindle shaped and include Hassall corpuscles. The medulla contains DCs that are similar to cutaneous Langerhans cells and LN interdigitating DCs.

Epithelial cells interact with migrating T-cell precursors from the BM to organize the thymus, with prothymocytes regulating induction of the cortical microenvironment[45] and mature thymocytes (TCR$^+$) organizing medullary thymic epithelial cells (mTECs).[46] In the outer cortex, thymocytes and epithelial cells interact to form lymphoepithelial complexes known as nurse cells that are composed of large clusters of lymphocytes surrounded by a cell membrane and appear to reside within the cell body of the epithelial cell. These complexes are located within the corticomedullary junction, where they are thought to be involved in thymocyte selection.[47]

Overview of Thymic T-Cell Development

T-cell commitment occurs in a spatially organized manner in the thymus with early T-cell progenitors (ETPs) derived from HSCs in the fetal liver or adult BM first arriving at the corticomedullary junction.[48] Developing double negative-2 (DN2) and DN3 thymocytes migrate through the cortex toward the subcapsular region, and DP thymocytes are generated in the outer cortex.[49] ETPs are CD4/CD8 DN and transit through DN1 (CD44$^+$CD25$^-$), DN2 (CD44$^+$CD25$^+$), DN3 (CD44$^-$CD25$^+$), and DN4 (CD44$^-$CD25$^-$) stages. During the

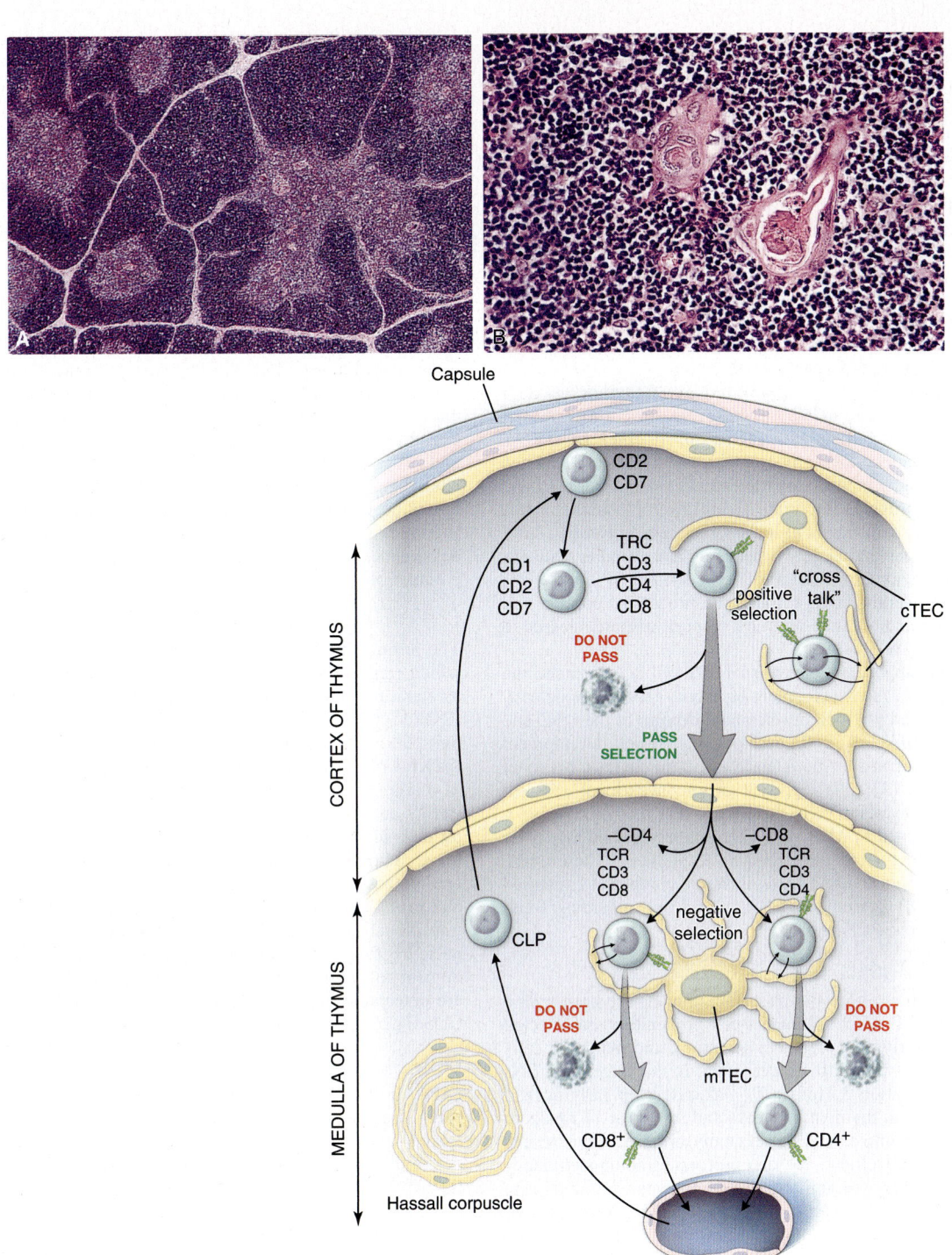

FIGURE 11.1 A, Normal infant human thymus. The thymus is surrounded by dense connective tissue capsule (not pictured) and is organized into adjacent lobules separated by connective tissue extending from the capsule to form trabeculae. At low-power magnification, one can appreciate the lobular architecture with clear separation between the dark-stained cortex and the lighter medulla, which contains keratinized Hassall corpuscles. The medulla is a continuous tissue that extends throughout the thymus and is surrounded by the cortex, and thus it cannot be appreciated in a single section. B, Medulla. Higher magnification. Normal Hassall (thymic) corpuscles show characteristic concentric arrangement of keratinizing epithelial cells. They are composed of tightly packed, concentrically arranged, type IV endothelioreticular cells with flattened nuclei. The central mass is composed of keratinized cells. C, T-cell development in the thymus. Schematic drawing of the major steps in thymic education. The process of T-cell differentiation likely originates with seeding of thymus by common lymphoid progenitors (CLP) and is accomplished by the expression and deletion of specific surface CD antigens. CLPs enter the medulla of the thymus via a postcapillary venule and then migrate to the periphery of the thymic lobule. The presence of CD2 and CD7 on the cell surface indicates an early stage of differentiation. This is followed by expression of the CD1 molecule. As maturation progresses, the cells express TCRs, CD3, CD4, and CD8. These cells are then presented with self and foreign antigens by cortical thymic epithelial cells (cTECs). If the lymphocyte recognizes self MHC and self- or foreign antigen, then it will survive the selection (positive selection); if not, death of the cell will occur. Cells that pass the positive selection test leave the cortex and enter the medulla. Here they undergo another selection process in which cells directed to self-antigen displayed by self-MHC by medullary thymic epithelial cells (mTECs) are eliminated (negative selection). Cells that survive that selection then become either cytotoxic CD8+ T lymphocytes or helper CD4+ T lymphocytes. These cells are now ready for the immune response; they leave the thymus from the medulla and enter the blood circulation. Hormonal substances secreted by epithelioreticular cells within the thymic (Hassall) corpuscle promote the process of thymic cell education. (Parts A and B reprinted with permission from Mills SE. *Histology for Pathologists*. 4th ed. Wolters Kluwer Health/Lippincott Williams & Wilkins; 2013. Part C adapted with permission from Pawlina W. *Histology: A Text and Atlas*. Wolters Kluwer; 2016.)

DN2 and DN3 stages, V(D)J rearrangements at the TCRγ, δ, and β loci occur. Production of a successfully rearranged T-cell receptor (TCR) β-chain leads to further differentiation into the DN4 stage. This process, called "β selection," ensures commitment to the αβT-cell lineage, and DN4 thymocytes proliferate and express CD4 and CD8 coreceptors, giving rise to CD4/CD8 DP thymocytes.

In the cortex, DP thymocytes undergo TCRα-VJ rearrangement and express αβTCR on the cell surface. Interaction of αβTCR with peptide major histocompatibility complex (pMHC) presented in the cortical microenvironment regulates the fate of DP thymocytes. While DP thymocytes that receive low avidity TCR interactions with self-pMHC survive and differentiate into CD4SP or CD8SP thymocytes, thereby undergoing positive selection, DP thymocytes expressing TCR strongly reactive to self-pMHC (self-reactive cells) die by apoptosis in a process referred to as negative selection.

Following positive selection, CD4SP or CD8SP thymocytes relocate to the medulla, where mTECs express and present a variety of peripheral tissue-restricted antigens (TRAs) or in which DCs do so indirectly. In the medulla, SP thymocytes reactive to TRAs are deleted by negative selection or induced to differentiate into Foxp3$^+$ T$_{regs}$, and thus, the medulla provides important T-cell developmental controls that are crucial for establishment of self-tolerance and preventing autoimmunity in a process that largely depends on autoimmune regulator (Aire), a nuclear factor expressed in mTECs. Mature SP thymocytes that express self-tolerant TCRs through the process of cortical and medullary positive and negative selection, respectively, are released to the circulation as naïve T cells.

In addition to supporting conventional αβT-cell development, the thymus also supports the development of unconventional (nonclassical) T cells. αβT- and γδT-cell development diverge at the DN2 and DN3 stages, and unlike αβT-cell development, γδT-cell development does not require antigen-specific interactions in the thymus. Invariant natural killer T (iNKT) cells represent an unconventional αβT-cell subset expressing invariant Vα14-Jα18 TCR that recognizes glycolipid antigens presented by MHC-like CD1d molecules and play roles in controlling innate and adaptive immune responses.[50] These iNKT cells are positively selected by CD1d/glycolipid complexes expressed on the surface of DP thymocytes.[51] For more details regarding T-cell development, please see Chapter 13.

Ontogeny of the Thymus

Unlike mice, which are born lymphopenic, humans are born with a full complement of T cells.[52] Human T-cell progenitors are detected in fetal thymi as early as 9 weeks of gestation, and mature T cells appear in the thymus by 12 to 13 weeks and in the spleen and LNs by 24 weeks of gestation.[53] Human T$_{regs}$ also develop early in fetal life and are detected in thymi at 12 weeks and in LNs at 14 weeks of gestation.[54,55] Unlike in neonatal thymectomy in mice, which results in defects in T-cell development[56] and profound immunodeficiency and multiorgan lymphocytic infiltration,[57,58] patients who underwent neonatal thymectomy, often performed during surgery to repair congenital cardiac abnormalities, remain healthy into adulthood and do not exhibit increased incidence of infections,[59,60] autoimmunity, or allergy.[61] This is likely because they maintain normal blood T$_{reg}$ frequencies and numbers,[62] even though they do exhibit more extensive declines in naïve T-cell frequencies with age than nonthymectomized individuals.[63,64]

Thymic Epithelium

The thymus provides a specialized microenvironment that allows for proper spatiotemporal regulation of T-cell development to establish the T-cell repertoire and ensure proper formation of the adaptive immune system. This process requires the interplay between developing T cells with a variety of nonhematopoietic stromal cells including TECs, ECs, and fibroblasts, as well as hematopoietic stromal cells such as DCs. TECs play a major role in thymocyte development and can be divided into two functionally distinct groups: cortical TECs (cTECs) and mTECs. These TECs provide multiple signals to guide the differentiation, migration, proliferation, survival, and death of developing

thymocytes.[65,66] Both cTECs and mTECs are derived from endodermal epithelium, yet they serve distinct roles in T-cell development. cTECs induce positive selection of diverse and functionally distinct T cells by virtue of unique antigen-processing systems, whereas mTECs help establish T-cell tolerance via ectopic expression of peripheral TRAs and cooperation with DCs. Finally, the roles of cTECs and mTECs are expanding because it is now known that they are important for the development not only of conventional T cells but also of unconventional T cells that bridge innate and adaptive immunity.

Generation of Thymic Epithelium

TECs are derived from endodermal epithelium from the third pharyngeal pouch.[67] Early TEC development is controlled by transcription factors including FoxN1 (Whn), Tbx1, and Pax1.[68,69] FoxN1 is a major mediator of TEC development and function because FoxN1 deficiency completely disrupts thymic T-cell development in animals and human as a result of its transcriptional regulation of various genes essential for T-cell development, including cytokines, chemokines, and Notch ligands.[70-73] While FoxN1 is required for TECs during embryogenesis, it likely is not required for the maintenance and function of postnatal TECs.[74,75] Other factors that are required for the proliferation and maintenance of both cTECs and mTECs during TEC development include the transcription factor p63 and its interacting partner Polycomb protein Cbx4.[76-78]

Cortical Thymic Epithelium Development

The stroma in the thymic cortex is mainly composed of cTECs, which can be identified based on their expression of proteins such as Keratin-8, Keratin-18, cerebellar degeneration-related antigen 1 (CDR1), CD205, CD249 (Ly51), IL-7, the thymoproteasome subunit β5t, and the atypical nonsignaling chemokine receptor CCRL1/ACKR4 (CCX-CKR1). In contrast, mTECs express a different set of markers including Keratin-5, Keratin-14, CD80, and Aire. Both cTECs and mTECs are derived from common endodermal progenitor cells identified in the third pharyngeal pouch[79,80] that require the transcription factor FoxN1 for proper TEC development[81,82] and generation of a transitional progenitor stage that gives rise to both cTECs and mTECs, including the Aire$^+$ subset.[81,83,84] While generation of transitional TEC progenitors does not require lymphocyte-derived signals,[85,86] functional maturation of cTECs requires thymocyte development beyond the DN1 stage because mature MHC class II^{hi} cTECs are detectable in Rag1-deficient mice (arrested at DN3) but not in CD3eTg26 mice (arrested at DN1).[82]

Early T-Cell Development and Migration in the Cortex

cTECs are the predominant source for multiple factors required for early T-cell development. Expression of the delta-like canonical Notch ligand 4 (Dll4) by cTECs is essential and sufficient for T-lineage determination of early lymphoid progenitors.[87-89] cTECs also produce IL-7,[90] which promotes survival, proliferation, and differentiation of thymocytes.[91-93] Migration of DN thymocytes from the corticomedullary junction to the subcapsular region is mediated by multiple signals. For example, chemokines produced by cTECs, including CCL25 and CXCL12, interact with their receptors CCR9 and CXCR4, respectively, on DN thymocytes.[94-97] CXCL12-CXCR4 signaling also promotes β selection.[98] Outward migration of DN thymocytes is regulated by CCRL1/ACKR4,[99,100] an atypical nonsignaling chemokine receptor highly expressed in cTECs,[101] as well as vascular cell adhesion molecule 1 (VCAM-1) expressed by cTECs that interacts with its receptor integrins α4β1 and α4β7 on DN thymocytes.[102] DN thymocytes turn back inward and differentiate into DP thymocytes at the subcapsular region, where transforming growth factor (TGF)-β is expressed and exerts negative feedback on the DN to DP transition.[103]

Positive Selection in the Cortex

The major function of cTECs is the induction of T-cell–positive selection. As described earlier, low-affinity TCR engagement by pMHC complexes induces positive selection of functional T cells, whereas high-affinity TCR-pMHC interactions lead to negative selection of self-reactive T cells. Recent studies support the idea that cTECs can specifically induce positive selection because of their unique proteolytic and antigen-processing capabilities that allow them to produce MHC-associating peptides that are essential for positive selection. For the MHC class I system, cTECs are equipped with a specialized type of proteasome called a "thymoproteasome" that contains the β5t subunit,[104,105] unlike most somatic cells that express "standard proteasomes" containing β5 subunits.[106,107] In mice deficient for β5t, cTECs express β5- and β5i-containing proteasomes and display a spectrum of MHC class I–associating peptides that are different from those in β5t-sufficient cTECs.[108,109] In these mice, positive selection of MHC class I–restricted thymocytes is substantially reduced, leading to a marked reduction (20% of wild type) and altered repertoire of CD8+ T cells, indicating that optimal positive selection of CD8+ T cells requires the β5t-dependent peptide repertoire in cTECs. A recent study identified unique cleavage motifs in β5t-dependent MHC class I–associating peptides that confer low-affinity TCR interaction and capabilities to efficiently induce positive selection,[110] suggesting that β5t exhibits unique peptide cleavage preferences from subunits β5 and β5i.[104,110] Thus, these studies suggest that cTECs regulate positive selection of CD8+ T cells by producing a unique set of MHC class I–associating peptides that exhibit low affinity for TCR.[111]

It is likely that cTECs have unique protein degradation and antigen-processing machineries that allow presentation of unique MHC class II–associating peptides to induce positive selection of CD4+ T cells as well. Multiple lines of evidence support this model. First, cTECs highly express lysosomal proteases cathepsin L and thymus-specific serine protease (TSSP).[112-114] Second, mice deficient for cathepsin L show a reduced positive selection of polyclonal CD4+ T cells.[115,116] Third, TSSP-deficient mice show a defective positive selection of CD4+ T cells with certain TCR specificities,[117,118] including diabetogenic self-reactive CD4+ T cells.[119] Finally, mice with defective macroautophagy, a cellular process that facilitates loading of endogenously generated peptides onto MHC class II molecules, specifically in TECs, showed altered repertoire selection of certain CD4+ T cells.[120] Despite these data supporting the presence of unique machineries on cTECs for inducing positive selection of CD4+ T cells, the nature of MHC class II–associating peptides produced by cTECs is unknown.

Negative Selection in the Cortex

The thymic cortex also is the site where self-reactive thymocytes are deleted by negative selection. However, unlike for their roles in positive selection, cTEC-specific peptides are not required for cortical negative selection because negative selection was observed to be normal in β5t-deficient[108] and TSSP-deficient mice.[117] Instead, resident DCs appear to be responsible for negative selection in the cortex.[121]

Thymic Nurse Cells

Thymic nurse cells (TNCs) were first recognized when large TECs that had engulfed multiple (up to 50) living lymphocytes within their intracellular vesicles were identified in enzymatically dissociated thymus tissue.[122,123] This study and others led many to hypothesize that TNCs provide a unique microenvironment for T-cell selection, although the precise cell lineage and function of TNC-forming thymic epithelium remained elusive.[124] Supporting this model, recent reports have shown that formation of TNCs requires normal development of cTECs[125,126] and that approximately 10% to 15% of β5t-expressing cTECs, but not mTECs, form thymocyte-wrapping complexes in the thymus of adult mice that are identical to the previously described TNCs.[127] Most TNC-enveloped lymphocytes are long-lived, unselected DP thymocytes undergoing secondary TCRα-VJ rearrangements. Thus, TNCs appear to be formed upon persistent interactions between cTEC and DP thymocytes and serve to facilitate secondary TCRα rearrangements. Given that the efficiency of secondary TCRα rearrangements is controlled by DP thymocyte survival,[128] the microenvironments within intra-TNC vesicles may ensure survival of enclosed DP thymocytes, thereby increasing the opportunities for positive selection and maximizing the developmental efficiency of functional T cells.[129] However, numerous important unanswered questions remain, including the

mechanisms by which unselected thymocytes are enclosed in TNCs, how intra-TNC microenvironments promote survival and/or continued TCR rearrangement in DP thymocytes, and how positively selected thymocytes are released from the TNC complexes.

More recent data suggest that cTECs also regulate unconventional T-cell development. A spontaneous mutant mouse line, called TN, exhibits an almost complete loss of mature cTECs, yet only a modest effect on mTECs[125] because of a missense mutation in the gene encoding β5t, resulting in substantial loss of β5t[high] mature cTECs and accumulation of β5t[low] transitional TEC progenitors. In TN mutant mice, the frequency of total thymic γδT cells was unaltered, whereas the proportion of γδT17 cells was greatly increased, the TCR repertoire of γδT17 cells was markedly skewed from Vγ 4 to Vγ6, and γδT17-dependent inflammatory responses in peripheral tissues were markedly perturbed.[125] Thus, normal cTEC development contributes to optimal repertoire formation of conventional αβT cells as well as unconventional "innate type" γδT cells.

mTEC Development

mTECs emerge from TEC progenitors expressing cTEC-associated genes, including Keratin-5, Keratin-14, CD80, Aire, Claudin-3, and Claudin-4, and react with the fucose-binding lectin *Ulex europaeus* agglutinin 1.[130,131] mTECs are further classified into two subsets on the basis of their expression of MHC class II and CD80—mTEChi (MHC class IIhi CD80hi) and mTEClo (MHC class IIlo CD80lo), with the mTEChi cells representing functionally mature mTECs expressing Aire.[130]

Numerous studies have demonstrated that mTEC cells and thymocytes depend on one another for their induction and survival, sometimes referred to as "thymic cross talk." Early studies indicated that thymic medulla formation is defective in mice with T-cell development arrested at early stages.[119] Mice deficient for positive selection showed a marked reduction of thymic medullary regions and mTEC cellularity without affecting overall thymus size or cortical architecture, indicating that the positively selected SP thymocytes induce the development of mTECs, which, in turn, provide a microenvironment for selection and maturation of SP thymocytes.[130,132-134]

It is now clear that the signaling pathways for the activation of nuclear factor-κB (NF-κB) are required for mTEC development because mice deficient in multiple components of this pathway, including tumor necrosis factor (TNF) receptor-associated factor 6, NF-κB–inducing kinase, IκB-kinase α, Bcl-3, NF-κB2 (p52), or RelB, exhibit defective development of Aire+ mTECs and thymic medulla formation in an mTEC-autonomous manner.[135-143] These NF-κB pathways are activated by TNF superfamily (TNFSF) receptors, receptor for activating NF-κB (RANK), CD40, and lymphotoxin β receptor (LTβR), expressed on mTECs that interact with their respective TNFSF ligands RANKL, CD40L, and lymphotoxins (LTs), which are expressed mostly by SP thymocytes.[144-147] These interactions thus represent another example of thymic cross talk between mTECs and developing thymocytes via receptor-ligand interactions. In addition, TNFSF ligand-mediated mTEC development is ensured by TCR-ligand interactions between self-reactive SP thymocytes and mTECs.[148-152]

RANKL is a critical mediator of mTEC development produced by lymphoid tissue inducer (LTi) cells and γδT cells in the embryonic thymus and by SP thymocytes and iNKT cells in the postnatal thymus.[146,147,153,154] The TNFSF ligands CD40L and LTs are expressed predominantly by SP thymocytes[144,147,154] and have cooperative as well as distinct functions in mTEC development. While RANKL and CD40L synergistically promote development and proliferation of Aire+ mTECs,[144,146] LTs regulate the development of CCL21-expressing mTECs.[155-157] LT signals also regulate the expression of RANK in mTECs[158] to influence mTEC terminal differentiation.[159] RANKL signaling in mTECs leads to increased expression of some TRAs, costimulatory molecules, and osteoprotegerin (OPG).[160] OPG serves as an inhibitory decoy receptor for RANKL and represses RANKL-mediated mTEC development and expansion.[146,160,161] The presence of a RANKL-OPG negative feedback system that requires mTEC interactions with SP thymocytes indicates that mTEC numbers and function must be properly adjusted in order to ensure that self-reactive SP thymocytes can be moderately, but not excessively, deleted in the thymic medulla. mTEC development has also been shown to be promoted by coordination between RANKL and type I interferon (IFN) signals[162] and negatively regulated by TGF-β signaling.[163] microRNA miR-29a has also been reported to be essential for postnatal maintenance of mTECs.[164,165]

Medulla Migration and Emigration of Thymocytes

DP thymocytes that received positive selection signals differentiate into CD4SP or CD8SP thymocytes and express the chemokine receptor CCR7 on the cell surface.[166] CCR7-expressing SP thymocytes are attracted from the cortex to the medulla[166-168] by the CCR7 ligand chemokines, CCL19 and CCL21, which are produced by mTECs[166] and medullary fibroblasts.[169] During their time in the medulla, which is estimated to be 4 to 5 days,[170] SP thymocytes are exposed to antigens presented by mTECs and DCs. CCR7-mediated medullary migration is required to ensure negative selection of self-reactive SP thymocytes,[157,171] and the importance of this interaction was demonstrated in mice deficient for CCR7 or CCR7 ligand chemokines, which exhibit organ-specific autoimmunity.[167,172,173] CCR7 signals also direct the migration of γδT cells to the medulla.[174] mTECs produce another chemokine XCL1 that mediates medullary accumulation of thymus-resident DCs.[175]

SP thymocytes that have successfully completed developmental programs and repertoire selection are exported from the thymus into the circulation by chemotactic signaling mediated by sphingosine-1 phosphate (S1P) and its receptor S1PR1. Mature SP thymocytes express high levels of S1PR1 and then migrate toward a gradient of S1P,[167,176,177] which is provided by neural crest-derived perivascular cells (pericytes) in the corticomedullary junction[178] as well as the circulating blood.[179] Although it is not entirely clear what mechanism ensures the timing of SP thymocyte emigration such that only mature yet self-tolerant SP thymocytes exit the thymus, one potential explanation is that the increased levels of S1PR1 needed for thymocyte egress may only be induced upon cessation of TCR signaling after completion of self-reactivity screening and downregulation of CD69, which serves as an inhibitor of S1PR1 surface expression. This would render SP thymocytes responsive to S1P and primed for thymic exit.[180]

TRA Expression by mTECs

In a phenomenon referred to as "promiscuous gene expression," a diverse array of TRAs, defined as antigens whose expression is primarily restricted to peripheral tissues, are also transcribed in mTECs, particularly in mTEC^hi cells.[181-184] This allows SP thymocytes reactive to these TRAs to be deleted from the conventional T-cell pool by negative selection or differentiation into Foxp3+ Tregs (see mTEC-DC Interactions for Central Tolerance). The importance of mTECs in establishing central tolerance is supported by many studies that show that T cells produced in mice lacking normal mTEC development caused autoimmune disorders.[135,137,138,140-145,147,181,185] In order to ensure maximal number and sufficient epitope density of TRAs to SP thymocytes, each TRA protein is expressed in only 1% to 3% of mTECs,[66] and a single mTEC expresses a set of *TRA* genes, which are clustered in chromosomes and colocalized to nuclear subdomains.[186] A substantial fraction of TRAs is controlled by the nuclear protein Aire,[187] which is predominantly expressed in mTECs.[188-190] The critical role of Aire-driven TRA expression in the establishment of self-tolerance through negative selection of TRA-reactive SP thymocytes[191-193] and generation of Foxp3+ Tregs[194-196] has been established by studies in humans with genetic deficiency of Aire, resulting in autoimmune polyendocrinopathy syndrome type 1 or autoimmune polyendocrinopathy-candidiasis-ectodermal dystrophy,[197] as well as in mice with similar organ-specific autoimmune disorders,[187,198,199] indicating that Aire is essential for establishment of self-tolerance. Aire does not appear to bind DNA directly[200,201] but instead appears to epigenetically regulate transcriptional elongation and pre-mRNA processing of target *TRA* genes. Given that Aire deficiency causes abnormal medulla organization and mTEC development in mice[202-207] as

well as defective T-cell tolerance against transcriptionally unrepressed TRAs,[191,198] some have posited that Aire controls TRA expression in mTEC but that deficiencies in the establishment of tolerance are caused by alterations in mTEC differentiation. This may be because Aire also regulates expression of a large number of non-TRA proteins, such as cytokines, chemokines, MHC class II peptide-loading factors, posttranslational modifiers, and proteases.[175,191,208-210] Regardless, it should be noted that additional transcriptional or epigenetic mechanisms are responsible for the induction of TRAs because more than half of total TRAs[210,211] expressed in mTECs are Aire independent.[181,187] Some of these Aire-independent TRAs are regulated by LTβR signaling.[156,212]

Although mTEC-dependent tolerance induction protects against autoimmunity through education of SP thymocytes on TRA-expressing cells, this system likely has unintended consequences on antitumor immunity because self-antigens expressed in mTECs also include tumor-associated antigens, resulting in the deletion of tumor-specific T cells.[195,213-215] Thus, manipulations that reduce deletion of tumor-specific T cells may be expected to confer a benefit against tumors. Indeed, it has been shown that suppression of RANKL-mediated mTEC development and maintenance can rescue tumor-specific T cells from medullary deletion and attenuate tumor progression in mice.[160,161] These studies suggest that new therapies that modulate T-cell tolerance centrally may be used to increase antitumor immunity.

mTEC-DC Interactions for Central Tolerance

While mTECs play a major role in inducing T-cell tolerance, thymic DCs also play a significant role in inducing T-cell tolerance through their ability to directly present endogenously expressed antigens or by indirectly presenting antigens expressed by other cells. Thymic DCs are predominantly localized in the medulla[168,174]; therefore, they contribute to T-cell tolerance by inducing negative selection of self-antigen. For example, thymic DCs can present Mtv-encoded superantigens, TRAs expressed by mTECs, and blood-borne antigens to developing thymocytes to induce negative selection.[216-219] In addition, peripheral DCs presenting peripheral antigens can be recruited to the thymic medulla to induce negative selection.[220-222]

mTECs and thymic DCs are also important for protection from autoimmunity because of their ability to induce development of T_regs through their antigen presentation function.[223,224] Several lines of evidence establish the importance of mTEC TRA expression and Foxp3+ T_reg generation. First, mice deficient for mTEC development or expression of MHC class II on mTECs exhibit impaired thymic development of Foxp3+ T_regs.[135,137,142,225] Second, studies evaluating T_reg generation in neo–self-antigen transgenic mice or in response to endogenous self-antigens showed that Foxp3+ T_regs specific for these antigens were generated because of their interactions with Aire+ mTECs.[194-196,226] Indirect presentation of TRAs by thymic DCs has been estimated to account for approximately half of Aire-dependent negative selection and T_reg development.[227] Thymic DCs can also induce development of Foxp3+ T_regs reactive to blood-borne antigens.[216,220] It is thought that Hassall corpuscles, which are composed of terminally differentiated mTECs, may provide the microenvironment for the generation of T_regs through their production of thymic stromal lymphopoietin,[228] which has been shown to activate immature thymic DCs to express costimulatory molecules[229,230] and induce differentiation of CD4SP thymocytes into Foxp3+ T_regs.[228]

Unconventional T-Cell Development in the Medulla

Recent studies indicate that the thymic medulla is an important site that supports the development of several types of unconventional T cells. mTECs play a distinct role from cTECs in the development of γδT cells. This is thought to be because of mTECs expression of Skint1, a B7-family protein expressed in the fetal thymus that promotes intrathymic maturation of Vγ5Vδ1+ epidermal γδT cells.[231-233] Skint1 is thought to induce strong, agonist-like signals to Vγ5Vδ1 TCR and induce a differentiation program toward an IFNγ-producing lineage.[234] Given differences in mechanisms of antigen presentation in cTECs and mTECs, it is possible that cTECs and mTECs provide a distinct set of ligands or selecting molecules that regulate the development of distinct subpopulations of γδT cells. Supporting this model, in fetal mouse thymus it has been shown that Vγ5Vδ1+ γδT cells closely associate with mTECs and promote Aire+ mTEC development,[233,234] supporting a model in which there is bidirectional cross talk between RANKL-expressing γδT cells and Skint1-expressing mTECs.

Similar cross talk interactions may occur between iNKT cells and mTECs because it was also shown that mTECs were required for optimal maturation of iNKT cells and that developing iNKT cells express RANKL and CD40L to promote development of Aire+ mTECs.[153] Mature iNKT cells express the chemokine receptor CXCR3, which is required for thymic retention in response to its ligand CXCL10 produced in the medulla.[235]

The thymic medulla also supports the development of natural IL-17-producing T-helper (nT_H17) cells, a recently described unconventional CD4+ αβT-cell subset.[236] RelB-dependent Aire+ mTECs appear to be required for nT_H17 cell development.[237] Given the likely role of these cells in protective and pathologic inflammatory responses, these data identify a novel mechanism by which mTECs regulate inflammatory and autoimmune responses.

Thymic Involution

The thymus is largest at birth, but with age begins to atrophy. The thymic epithelial space begins to atrophy as early as age 1 year, although it was previously thought to begin starting at puberty. This space shrinks by about 3% per year through middle age and then 1% per year thereafter,[34] and with the loss of cortical lymphocytes and atrophy of epithelial cells and replacement by fat, more than 50% of the thymus is replaced by adipose tissue by the age of 40 to 45 years. The "fatty infiltration" noted in the adult thymus occurs in the perivascular (extraparenchymal) space, separated from the remaining lymphoepithelial complex by the epithelial basement membrane and the sheet of epithelial cells.[238-243] Because the fat merely takes the place of the normal thymus parenchyma, the organ's shape and volume remain unchanged.[39] The mechanisms regulating age-related involution are not entirely clear, but involution is associated with decreased potential of intrathymic progenitors to maintain the level of mature thymocytes,[244] and this results in a smaller number of naïve T cells.[245] There are well-documented decreases in new thymic emigrants in peripheral blood T cells as individuals age.[246-248] The persistent decrease in the number of epithelial cells and thymocytes is likely not the only event

responsible for age-related thymic involution because there is an even more pronounced decrease in medullary interdigitating DCs.[249] It is also clear that the thymus may undergo acute involution as a result of stress, which is mediated by adrenal corticosteroids, and which can be mimicked by injections of glucocorticoids, which can eliminate as many as 75% of the thymocytes within 2 to 3 days, preferentially affecting the cortex owing to the sensitivity of cortical thymocytes to cortisone.

Despite the continuous reduction in thymic epithelial space, more recent studies suggest that the greatest decline in the generation of new T cells occurs later in life. In human thymic tissue obtained from organ donors aged several months to greater than 70 years, DP thymocytes (indicating ongoing selection) were detected at the expected frequency (60%-80%) in thymus tissue from donors aged less than 40 years, whereas few DP thymocytes were detected in adults aged greater than 40 years.[250] Similarly, new T-cell emigrants in the human blood, spleen, and LNs were markedly reduced in individuals over 40 years.[246,250] Despite this significant decline in T-cell production in middle age, residual thymic activity can persist beyond the fifth decade of life, as shown by the observation that recent thymic emigrants can be detected in the peripheral blood in this age group[247] as well as in renal transplant recipients after T-cell depletion therapy.[251] Together, these findings indicate that, although thymic function ceases after the fourth decade of life for the most part, residual thymus tissue may be present in some individuals and, therefore, provide a substrate for potential therapies to rejuvenate the human immune system.

LYMPH NODES

LNs are bean-shaped encapsulated lymphoid organs measuring from only a few millimeters in the longest dimension up to 1 cm (*Figure 11.2*). LNs are present throughout the body but are most frequent in the axillary, cervical, and inguinal regions as well as the mediastinum and retroperitoneum. They arise from the budding of groups of cells from large vessels of the lymphatic system that are subsequently infiltrated by connective tissue and lymphatic vessels. Given their origins as outgrowths of lymphatic vessels, LNs are located at branches of the lymphatic system and therefore are optimally positioned to capture antigens and encounter chemokines present in lymph drained from most organs via the afferent lymphatics (*Figures 11.2-11.6*).

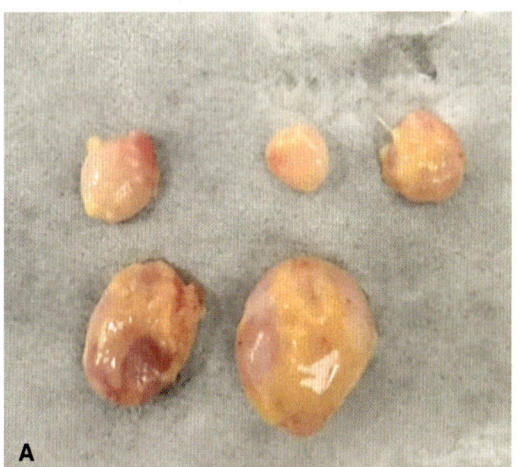 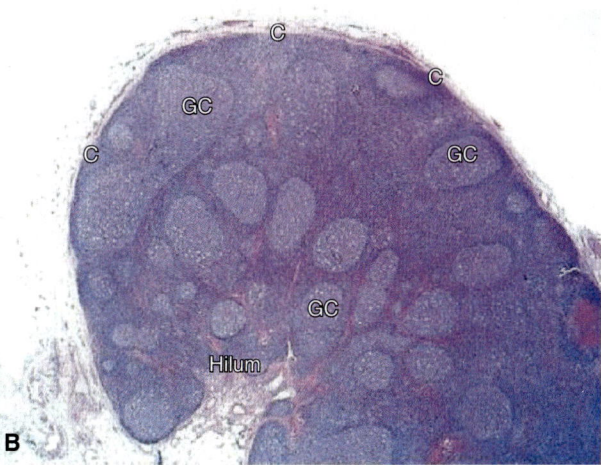

FIGURE 11.2 A, Freshly excised resting LNs (top) and reactive LNs (bottom). In the resting state, LNs typically measure only a few millimeters in the longest dimension; however, upon antigenic stimulation, reactive changes can cause the LN to expand to approximately 1 cm. B, Low-magnification hematoxylin and eosin section of reactive LN. Lymph nodes have a capsule (C), a cortex, a medulla, and sinuses (subcapsular, cortical, and medullary). The capsule is a thin connective tissue covering. Lymphatics penetrate the capsule and enter the subcapsular sinus. The sinuses contain histiocytes (macrophages), which take up and process antigen, which is then presented to lymphocytes. The cortex is composed of adjacent lymphoid nodules, usually with fine connective tissue trabecula extending from the capsule separating the nodules. Each nodule contains a germinal center (GC) that stains lighter than the outer mantle zone because of the proliferating medium-sized and large lymphocytes with less dense staining properties. The medulla is composed of interconnecting medullary cords composed of lymphocytes and interspersed light staining channels, the medullary sinuses. This section is almost entirely composed of cortex. (Reprinted with permission from Ioachim HL, Medeiros LJ. *Ioachim's Lymph Node Pathology*. 4th ed. Wolters Kluwer Health/Lippincott Williams & Wilkins; 2009.)

FIGURE 11.3 **Schematic drawing of normal lymph node.** Lymphatics vessels (LVs) penetrate the capsule and enter the subcapsular sinus. The cortex is composed of adjacent lymphatic nodules, usually with fine connective tissue trabecula extending from the capsule separating the nodules. The cortex contains lymphoid follicles (tan ovals) composed of small lymphocytes (centrocytes) or germinal centers. Follicles are organized by underlying follicular dendritic cells (FDCs) that reorganize in the context of the germinal center reaction. The medulla is composed of interconnecting medullary cords composed of lymphocytes and interspersed medullary sinuses. Lymph flows from the afferent lymphatic ducts into the subcapsular sinus down the trabecular sinuses through the conduit system, which is created by extracellular matrix proteins produced by fibroblastic reticular cells that allow antigen to be samples at the T/B-cell boundary zone. Lymph then flows into the medullary sinuses and exits the node via efferent lymphatics at the hilum. Migration of lymphocytes is regulated by chemokines such as CCL19, CCL21, and CXCL13. Please see section entitled Lymphocyte Migration into Lymphoid Tissues for a discussion of HEV—high endothelial venule, DC—dendritic cell. (Adapted with permission of American Society for Clinical Investigation from Ruddle NH. Lymphatic vessels and tertiary lymphoid organs. *J Clin Invest.* 2014;124(3):953-959; permission conveyed through Copyright Clearance Center, Inc.)

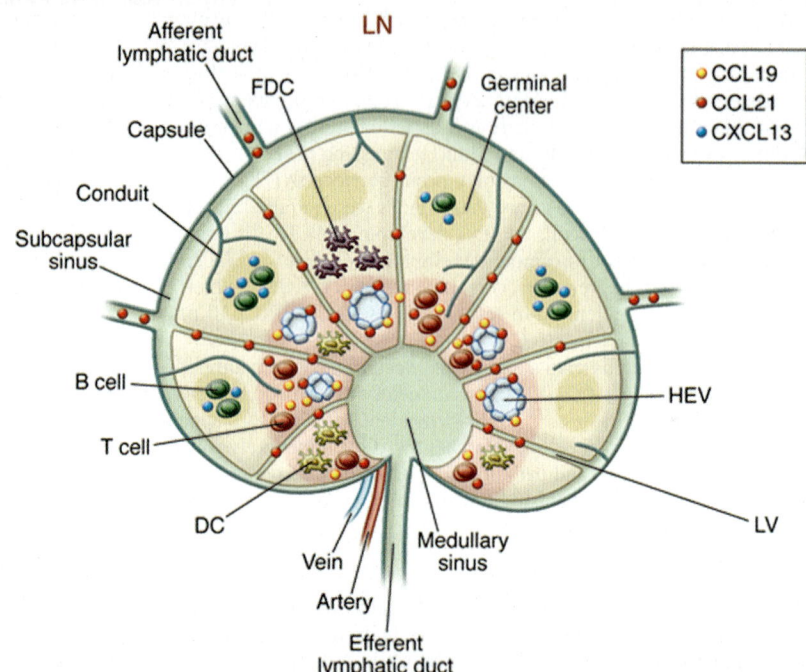

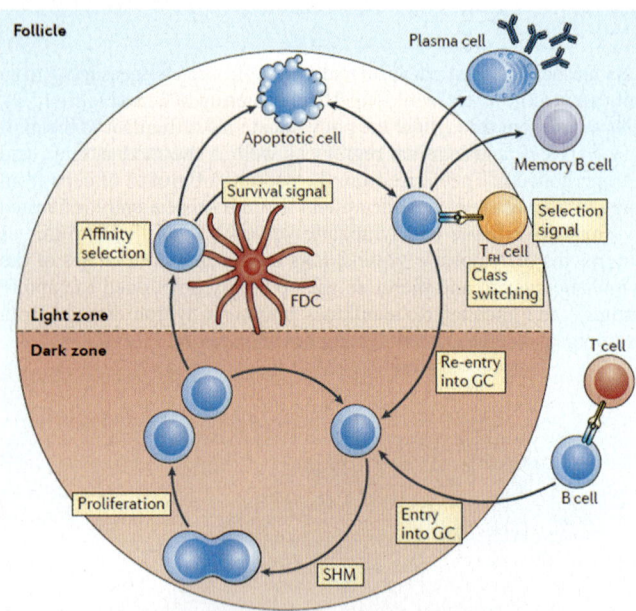

FIGURE 11.4 **The germinal center reaction.** Simplified schematic of affinity maturation in the germinal center (GC). At the T cell–B cell border of the lymph node, B cells present antigen to T-helper cells and receive costimulatory signals. The selected cells enter the dark zone of the GC and undergo somatic hypermutation (SHM) by upregulating components of the SHM machinery, including activation-induced deaminase (AID). After one cycle (or possibly more) or proliferation and SHM, the B cells migrate to the light zone, In the light zone, the mutated BCRs that are the product of SHM are now exposed to antigens that are incorporated into immune complexes on the follicular dendritic cells (FDCs). If the affinity of the BCR is very low, the B cell will not receive survival signals and will undergo apoptosis. The remaining B cells need to compete for limited T cell help, which favors the higher-affinity B cells and forces the others to undergo apoptosis. Surviving B cells can then undergo one of three fates: they can reenter the dark zone and undergo further proliferation and SHM, they can exit the GC as plasma cells, or they can exit as memory B cells. Reentry will allow for further affinity maturation. It is thought that FDCs might influence affinity maturation by regulating the amount of antigen on their surface. (Reprinted by permission from Nature: Heesters BA, Myers RC, Carroll MC. Follicular dendritic cells: dynamic antigen libraries. *Nat Rev Immunol.* 2014;14:495-504. Copyright © 2014 Springer Nature.)

Histologically, the LN is composed of three discrete, but not separated, regions—the cortex, paracortex, and medulla. The superficial cortex is located immediately underneath the fibrous capsule and contains most of the B cells in the LN organized in nodules, or follicles, the formation of which relies on the presence of underlying follicular dendritic cells (FDCs). When B cells in follicles are stimulated to proliferate by antigen, they form germinal centers (GCs), which are composed predominantly of B cells and also contain CD3[+] T cells, which serve to promote B-cell differentiation and immunoglobulin production as well as play a role in preventing autoimmunity by limiting T cell–dependent B-cell stimulation. The paracortex, or deep cortex, is located toward the center of the node and contains predominantly T cells and T-cell antigen-presenting cells (APCs) such as macrophages and DCs. The medulla represents the innermost area of the LN and contains B cells, T cells, plasma cells, macrophages, and DCs.

LNs are surrounded by a thin external fibrotic capsule from which internal prolongations penetrate the parenchyma to form septae that provide a basic supportive framework for the organization of the LN. Nodal arteries enter and leave the LN through the hilum. Nodal arteries branch into arterioles in the medulla and capillaries in the paracortex before giving rise to highly specialized postcapillary venules in the T-cell zone known as high endothelial venules (HEVs), which are composed of characteristic plump, cuboidal-to-cylindrical ECs with a single large, round nucleus and abundant cytoplasm. These vessels follow the fibrous septae and form capillary networks that connect to postcapillary venules. These specialized postcapillary vessels play an important role in the recruitment of circulating lymphocytes into the LN parenchyma with important roles for nepmucin and autotoxin, which are expressed by HEVs, as well as chemokines and chemoattractants including CCR7.

T cells enter the paracortex after passing through the HEV to encounter antigen-presenting interdigitating cells or can enter from the lymph into the marginal sinus after activation in tissues. Chemokines such as CCL19 and CCL21 that can bind to CCR7 and LFA1 on activated T cells are critical for T-cell transport through the HEV. S1P receptor signaling also promotes this process.[252] Expression of CCR5 and LFA1 on B cells and follicular T-helper (T$_{FH}$) cells are critical for their recruitment by FDCs by CXCL13, intracellular adhesion molecule 1 (ICAM-1), and VCAM-1.[253] Interactions are different in the spleen, which lacks HEV, but red pulp cord sinuses express similar molecules.[254] This process is described in greater detail below.

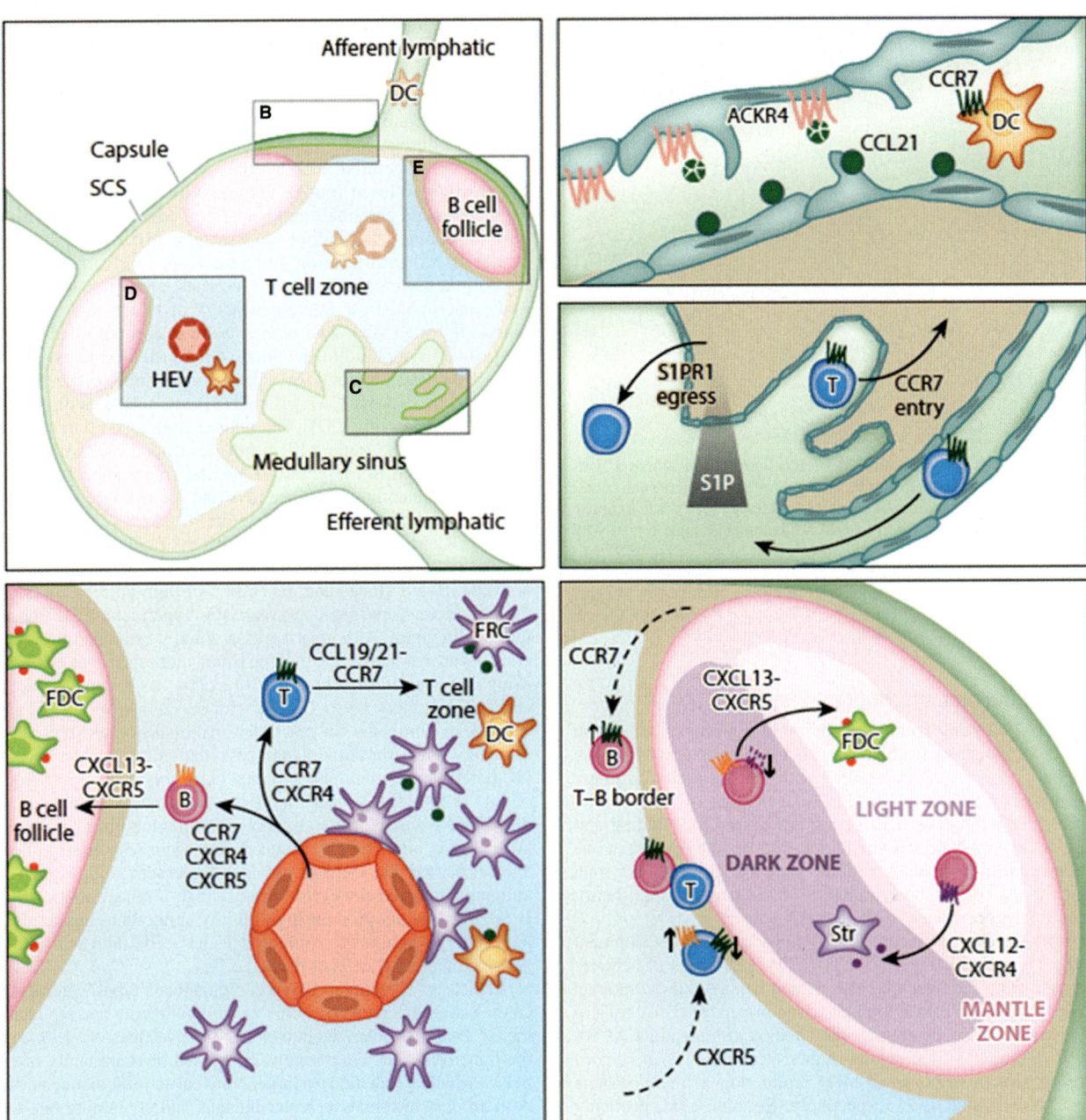

FIGURE 11.5 A-E, Chemokine-guided migration and positioning in the lymph node. B, Lymphatic endothelial cells in the SCS floor produce CCR7 ligands. DCs derived via afferent lymph express CCR7. Lymphatic endothelial cells in the SCS ceiling express the atypical chemokine receptor CCRL1/ACKR4, which can sequester the CCR7 ligand CCL21 and generate functional gradients. C, Medullary sinuses are sites of lymphocyte egress. Egress is guided by S1P and its receptor, S1PR1. T cells entering the medullary sinuses from afferent lymph can enter the LN in a CCR7-dependent manner. D, Lymphocytes enter the LN via HEVs in a manner dependent on CCR7, CXCR4, and CXCR5 (for B cells). CXCL13-CXCR5 interactions guide incoming B cells into their compartments and CCL19/CCL21-CCR7 interactions do the same for T cells. Stromal cells in the respective regions are important producers of positioning chemokines. E, Activated B cells upregulate CCR7 and relocate to the T cell–B cell border. A subset of activated CD4+ T cells acquire CXCR5 and migrate toward the B-cell follicle. B-cell positioning within the emerging germinal center is guided by CXCR4, which mediates localization to the dark zone, and CXCR5, which mediates localization to the light zone. CXCR4 downregulation is another mechanism that contributes to B-cell migration into the light zone. For more detailed descriptions, please see text. DC, dendritic cell; FDC, follicular dendritic cell; FRC, fibroblastic reticular cell; HEV, high endothelial venule; LN, lymph node; S1P, sphingosine-1-phosphate; SCS, subcapsular sinus; Str, stromal cell. (Used with permission of Annual Reviews, Inc. from Schulz O, Hammerschmidt SI, Moschovakis GL, et al. Chemokines and chemokine receptors in lymphoid tissue dynamics. *Annu Rev Immunol.* 2016;34:203-242; permission conveyed through Copyright Clearance Center, Inc.)

Afferent lymphatics reach the LN at its convex margin and empty into the subcapsular sinus. Lymph then moves through the cortical sinuses into the medullary sinuses, which eventually converge to give rise to one efferent lymphatic vessel in the hilar region. Thus, the sinus network constitutes an irrigation system, relating each afferent lymphatic to a well-defined functional compartment. The sinuses are bordered by a discontinuous monolayer of sinus lining cells that stretch into the lumen to prevent the sinus walls from collapsing, and intercellular gaps in the sinus lining allow unimpeded contact between the luminal contents and surrounding tissue. Sinus lining cells possess long dendrites and are connected to neighbors through well-developed desmosomes, and they are also intimately associated with reticulin fibers from the sinus cavity. These components of the fibrous network supporting the sinuses, typically composed of type IV collagen, are engulfed by slender protrusions extending from the cell's body.[255,256]

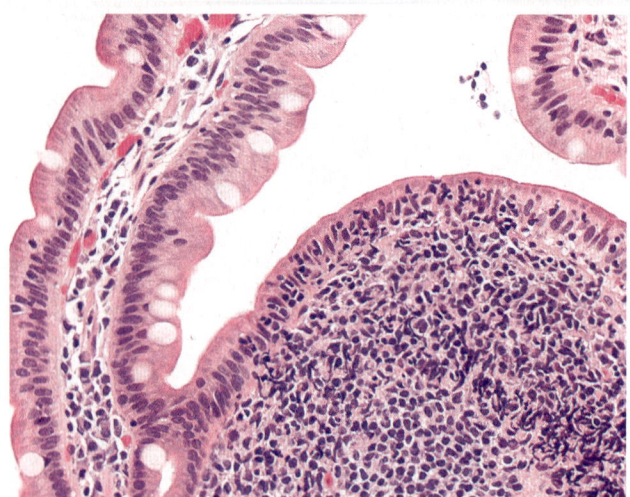

FIGURE 11.6 High magnification of surface epithelium above a lymphoid nodule within a Peyer patch. The polymorphous germinal center (below) is surrounded by monotonous, small round lymphocytes that comprise the nodule's mantle zone. Above this lies the subepithelial dome region with lymphocytes, plasma cells, and macrophages. The follicle-associated epithelium characteristically has few, if any, goblet cells; ultrastructurally and phenotypically, most of these epithelial cells would be identified as M cells. (Reprinted with permission from Mills SE. *Histology for Pathologists.* 4th ed. Wolters Kluwer Health/Lippincott Williams & Wilkins; 2013.)

Ontogeny of Secondary Lymphoid Tissue

The LN and PP develop from the budding of a group of cells from large vessels of lymph sacs, which are penetrated by connective tissue and lymphatic vessels interconnecting with other vessels forming a network. This is regulated by the *PROX1* gene that is expressed on lymphatic endothelial cells (LECs) and is required for budding and sprouting of the lymphatic endothelium.[257] The budding occurs in one spot in the anterior cardinal veins of the neck and generates a lymph sac, which gives rise to the lymphatics of the neck, thorax, heart, lungs, and forelegs regulated by the *PROX1* gene.[258]

Following the establishment of the lymphatics, SLO development is initiated when circulating CD3⁻CD4⁺CD45⁺ LTi cells of hematopoietic origin from the liver (the site of fetal hematopoiesis) interact with mesenchymal-derived lymphoid tissue organizer (LTo) cells at the LN anlagen. LTi cells express the chemokine receptor CXCR5 and IL-7R (CD127), which results in their accumulation at sites of LN development in response to local production of their cognate ligands, CXCL13 and IL-7, respectively. Retinoic acid, probably derived from nerve fibers, induces the expression of CXCL13 in stromal cells. Recruited LTi cells accumulate in response to local expression of CXCL13 to form the first cell clusters. In response to IL-7 and TNFSF11 (also known as RANKL or TRANCE), LTi cells are induced to secrete LTα1β2, which stimulates stromal LTo cells expressing the LTβ receptor (LTβR) to produce the chemokines CXCL13, CCL19, and CCL21 and to initiate the recruitment of hematopoietic cells. Chemokines CCL19 and CCL21 interact with their receptor CCR7 to recruit T cells and DCs, and chemokine CXCL13 interacts with the chemokine receptor CXCR5 to recruit B cells to the follicles.

LTo cells also express adhesion molecules including ICAM-1, VCAM-1, and mucosal vascular addressin cell adhesion molecule 1 (MAdCAM-1) to aid in the retention of lymphocytes,[259] as well as growth factors such as vascular endothelial growth factor C (VEGF-C), fibroblast growth factor-2, and hepatocyte growth factor to promote development of the lymphatic vasculature and HEVs.[260,261] Finally, LTo cells differentiate into multiple stromal cell types including FDCs as well as fibroblastic reticular cells (FRCs) and marginal reticular cells (MRCs), which form scaffolding networks supporting cellular migration.[262-264] Once initiated, the expression of chemokines (CXCL13, CCL19, CCL21, and CXCL12) by LTo cells continues to recruit more LTi cells and lymphocytes to establish a positive feedback loop, thereby

ensuring maintenance of lymphoid organ development by providing a sustained source of LTo cell stimulation through the LTβR.

Cortex

Primary lymphoid follicles are present in the cortex and composed of aggregates of naïve B cells expressing IgM, IgD, CD21, and CD23 associated with a small network of FDCs, which are not easily visible on routine hematoxylin and eosin sections. The lymphoid cells are small and round and contain nuclei with dense chromatin and scant cytoplasm. Antigen stimulation induces follicular B-cell proliferation and expansion to give rise to secondary follicles, which include mantle zones, a GC containing tingible body macrophages, a dense meshwork of FDCs, and sometimes a marginal zone (MZ). The mantle zone is composed of B cells of the primary lymphoid follicle that were pushed aside during expansion of the GC, and therefore, like primary follicle B cells, mantle zone B cells express IgM, IgD, CD21, and CD23, with occasional B cells coexpressing CD5. The mantle zone also contains memory B cells when the outer MZ is not developed. MZs are typically more prominent in mesenteric LNs, the spleen, and PPs and typically less demarcated in other LNs and intermingle with the small lymphocytes of the outer mantle zone.[265]

The GC is the compartment in which the T cell–dependent immune response occurs by sustaining the proliferative expansion of antigen-activated B-cell clones and generation of high-affinity antibodies by the induction of antigen-driven somatic hypermutation of the immunoglobulin genes. Although it was originally estimated that each GC contains an average of one to three B-cell clones per mature GC,[266-269] using more sensitive techniques, it recently has become apparent that each GC contains 10 to 100s of clones.[270] In response to primary immune response, the GC reaction is maximally reached by days 10 to 12, and without further antigenic stimulation, GCs wane by 21 days. GC B cells undergo immunoglobulin class or isotype switch from IgM or IgD to IgG, IgA, or IgE; however, this process is not exclusive to the GCs because B cells undergo immunoglobulin class or isotype switching in other sites in T cell–independent responses, although to a lesser degree. The GC also provides a microenvironment that selects antigen-stimulated clones that produce high-affinity antibody, whereas B cells that do not produce high-affinity antibody to the inciting antigen undergo apoptosis. Antigen-selected cells then exit the GC to become memory B cells or plasma cells.

The early GC contains two predominant cell types: centrocytes and centroblasts. After several hours or days following antigen challenge, the GC becomes polarized into two distinctive areas: the dark zone and the light zone. The dark zone is composed predominantly of centroblasts, which are medium to large, noncleaved follicular center B cells with an oval to round vesicular nucleus and containing one to three small nucleoli and a narrow rim of basophilic cytoplasm. Centrocytes, which are cleaved follicular center cells with dense chromatin, inconspicuous nucleoli, and scant cytoplasm, are also present in the dark zone. The dark appearance is caused by the close packing of cells with limited cytoplasm in a small area; mitotic figures are common in this area. The light zone contains predominantly quiescent centrocytes with more cytoplasm that results in the paler staining seen in the light zone. GC cells lack expression of the antiapoptotic protein BCL-2 and express the transcription factor BCL-6, which is required for controlling the proliferation and differentiation of B cells in the GC[271-273]; BCL-6 expression is confined to B cells in follicles in nonneoplastic lymphoid tissues, and therefore, its presence outside the follicles is abnormal. The lack of BCL-2 expression favors B-cell death following activation unless rescued by high-affinity interactions between their antigen receptor and a given antigen. After undergoing apoptosis, cell remnants and nuclear debris are phagocytosed by tingible body macrophages, which can be recognized by light microscopy.[256,274]

The light zone also contains a high concentration of FDCs, which are difficult to appreciate in unstimulated follicles but can be recognized in GCs based on their vesicular and often double nuclei with small nucleoli. Contrary to other DCs, FDCs are derived from mesenchymal cells and are important organizers of the GCs and the T cell–dependent immune response. These cells express a profile of molecules that attract B and T cells and facilitate the antigen-presenting process. Most important among these is CXCL13, a chemokine that recruits B and T cells expressing CXCR5. FDCs also express CD23, the adhesion molecules ICAM-1 and VCAM-1, and complement receptors (CD21 and CD35) that stably present antigens in the form of immunocomplexes.

Both centroblasts and centrocytes express mature B-cell antigens (CD19, CD20, CD22, and CD79) as well as the GC markers BCL-6 and CD10. Centroblasts lack surface immunoglobulin or express it at low levels because the immunoglobulin gene undergoes somatic hypermutation and class switch in these cells under the selective pressure of antigen affinity, and therefore when surface immunoglobulin is reexpressed, the centrocytes have a higher affinity for the driving antigen.[238-243] BCL-6 is an essential nuclear zinc-finger transcription factor required for GC formation and the T cell–dependent immune response. It is expressed in GC B cells but not in naïve B cells, mantle zone B cells, memory B cells, or plasma cells.[225-230] CD10 is a membrane-associated molecule (common acute lymphoblastic leukemia antigen) that is also expressed in early pro–B cells in the BM, lost in naïve cells, and then reexpressed in GC cells. Its function is not well known, but it seems to be indispensable for GC formation. CD10+ mature lymphoid cells are restricted to GCs, and their identification outside this compartment suggests the presence of a follicular lymphoid neoplasm. An important functional phenotypic change in GC cells is the downregulation of the antiapoptotic molecule BCL-2, constitutively expressed in naïve and memory lymphoid cells.[238-243] Thus, these cells are susceptible to death through apoptosis, and only the clones encountering the specific antigens will be rescued and survive in this microenvironment. GC B cells also express surface molecules involved in cell interactions with FDCs and T cells. In particular, CD40, CD86, and CD71 facilitate the association with T cells,[238-243] whereas CD11a/CD18 and CD29/CD49d recognize the FDC ligands CD44, ICAM-1, and VCAM-1. Similarly, GC lymphoid cells express receptors for the FDC molecules CD86D and IL-15, providing proliferative signals and B cell–activating factor (BAFF), which triggers survival signals that facilitate the rescue of BCL-2− cells from apoptosis.[275-279]

GCs also contain significant numbers of specialized subpopulations of T cells that play important roles in the regulation of the B-cell differentiation process and T cell–mediated immune response. T_{FH} cells are mainly localized to the light zone and the mantle zone.[280] T_{FH} cells express CD4, CD57, ICOS, PD-1 (programmed death-1, or CD279), and CXCR5, the receptor for the FDC secreted chemokine CXCL13. T_{FH} cells promote B-cell differentiation, including activation-induced cytidine deaminase, immunoglobulin class switch, and immunoglobulin production. GCs also contain CD4+, CD25+, and Foxp3+ T_{regs} that play a role in preventing autoimmunity and limiting T cell–dependent B-cell stimulation. They also appear to directly suppress B-cell immunoglobulin production and class switch.[281] T_{regs} are also found in interfollicular areas.

MZs are sometimes seen around follicles in LNs, particularly in mesenteric LNs, but are prominent in the spleen. MZ B cells resemble centrocytes but contain more abundant pale cytoplasm. These cells represent a mixture of naïve and memory B cells and are associated with a unique phenotype, expressing pan–B-cell markers and surface IgM, but lacking CD5, CD10, or CD23, and express little or no IgD. They also express CD21, CD25, and alkaline phosphatase. In some reactive conditions, clusters of slightly larger B cells with even more abundant pale to eosinophilic cytoplasm, so-called monocytoid B cells, appear between the mantle zone and cortical sinuses. Similar to MZ B cells, they represent a mixture of naïve and memory B cells.

Paracortex

While much is known about the specialized microenvironments in which B cells reside and undergo activation and selection as well as class switching and somatic hypermutation, much less is known about the T-cell area, which predominantly resides in the paracortex, also sometimes referred to as the interfollicular T-cell zone. Given that T cells cannot be activated by soluble antigen and require contact of their TCR with antigen peptides presented in the context of autologous MHC molecules on APCs—MHC class I for CD8+ T cells and MHC class II for CD4+ T cells—T cells are intimately associated with APCs in the paracortex. These APCs are derived from BM monocytes and express markers such as CD80 and CD97 and are sometimes referred to as interdigitating DCs because their cytoplasmic processes establish a three-dimensional network that envelopes T cells and create a unique microenvironment for T-cell activation and proliferation.[282] Interdigitating DCs are unique from FDCs, which contain desmosomes on their dendritic processes at points of contact between FDCs, because they form interdigitations with their cellular extensions. These cells contain abundant, pale-staining cytoplasm and a large, elongated, bizarre characteristic nucleus. Cell outlines show several deep clefts and folds, and the nuclei show delicate chromatin and inconspicuous nucleoli.[283] DCs also express CD11c, the DEC-205 multilectin receptor for antigen expression, high levels of MHC classes I and II, and accessory molecules such as CD40, CD54, and CD86.[284] Thus, DCs are able to support the expansion and survival of CD8+ cytotoxic T cell and CD4+ T_H cells.

Although much attention is paid to the GC with respect to the generation of antigen-dependent responses, it is important to note that initial contact with antigen occurs mostly outside the follicle. HEVs, which are specially differentiated vessels and postcapillary venules, present in SLOs allow extravasation and egress of naïve and central memory lymphocytes or other immune cells, including DCs, from the circulation into the LN.[285-288] HEVs can be recognized by their plump ECs whose nuclei often appear to virtually occlude the lumen. In order to allow recruitment of immune cells into the LN, HEVs specifically express and produce addressins, which serve as tissue-specific recognition molecules, including sulfated carbohydrate ligands, L-selectin ligands, and some adhesion molecules such as ICAM-1, VCAM-1, or MAdCAM-1.[285-287,289-294] These addressins bind to L-selectin and α4β7 integrins on lymphocytes. In contrast, postcapillary venules in other tissues do not express lymphocyte adhesion molecules unless stimulated by inflammatory mediators.[295] In addition, it should be noted that HEV cells do not express lymphoid chemokines (CCL19, CCL21, and CXCL13) but present them at luminal surfaces through binding to scaffold molecules. Chemokines CCL19 and CCL21 are necessary for the recruitment and disposition of T cells and DCs within lymphoid tissue, and chemokine CXCL13 functions in the recruitment and disposition of B cells. These chemokines are also involved in lymphoid neogenesis.[260,296-300] Thus, HEVs are necessary for active and functional lymphoid organs. For a more detailed description of the mechanisms that regulate lymphocyte ingress and egress from LNs, please see the Lymph Node Vasculature and Conduit System section.

Several studies have revealed that continuous engagement of LTβR on HEVs by LTα1β2+ cells is critical for the induction and maintenance of HEV gene expression and HEV cell morphology.[301,302] In mice, the major sources of LTα1β2 for HEV regulation in lymphoid tissues are CD11c+ DCs and B cells.[303-305] CD11c+ cells and activated B cells contribute to an increase in VEGF production, resulting in proliferation of ECs in LNs.

Lymph Node Vasculature and Conduit System

The interaction among the lymph, blood, and the different cellular components of the LN is facilitated by a highly organized vascular system. Arteries arrive at the hilus and branch to reach the subcapsular area and paracortex, where the capillaries form loops and specialize into postcapillary HEVs. Lymph arrives through the afferent lymphatic vessels at the opposite pole of the node, which opens to the subcapsular sinus and flows through the trabecular and medullary sinuses toward the efferent lymph vessels at the hilus. Macrophages in the subcapsular sinuses capture large antigens, immune complexes, and viruses and may present them to nearby B cells in the cortical areas. Small soluble antigens may diffuse through the sinus wall and reach the cortical areas.[306]

While uptake and transport via migratory DCs is the major avenue of antigen delivery from nonlymphoid tissues into LNs, soluble antigen can also freely drain via the afferent lymph. Upon arriving at the LN, smaller antigens with a hydrodynamic radius of less than ~4 nm (or molecular weight <70 kDa) rapidly permeate the LN cortex through the nodal conduit system, which is a specialized structure that connects the lymphatic sinuses with the walls of the blood vessels, particularly the HEVs in the paracortex, allowing rapid movement of small antigenic particles and cytokines from the afferent lymph deep into the portal of entry of lymphocytes to the nodal parenchyma.[307] This structure consists of small conduits composed of a core of types I and III collagen fibers associated with cross-linked microfibrils of fibromodulin and decorin, all of them surrounded by a basal membrane of laminin and type IV collagen. The conduit system is completely wrapped by the cytoplasm of FRCs. At certain places not totally covered by FRCs, DCs contact the basal membrane and reach inside the conduit to capture antigens. The FRC-formed conduits make these antigens readily accessible to resident DCs, cognate B cells, and FDCs that are in close contact to the FRC network.[307-309] In contrast, larger particles such as viruses are physically excluded from the conduit network and are instead captured by medullary and subcapsular sinus macrophages[310] that transfer them to B cells in the

LN cortex.[311-313] Recent evidence suggests that LECs residing along the subcapsular sinus may also capture and store free antigen under inflammatory conditions.[314]

Lymph Node Stroma

The LN structure is supported by numerous nonhematopoietic stromal cell types that are critical for LN organization and providing important signals to promote proper immune responses to antigenic challenge (*Figure 11.7*). These stromal cells represent multiple cell types with differing function and are characterized by heterogeneous expression of a number of antigens, including CD31 (PECAM) and podoplanin (GP38 in mice, GP36 in humans).[315] These stromal cell types include LECs and blood ECs, but we will focus our discussion on FDCs, FRCs, and MRCs, which have been distinguished on the basis of their morphology, immunophenotypic features, and function.

Follicular Dendritic Cells

FDCs are nonhematopoietic stromal cells that originate from perivascular precursors and are critical for efficient GC formation and

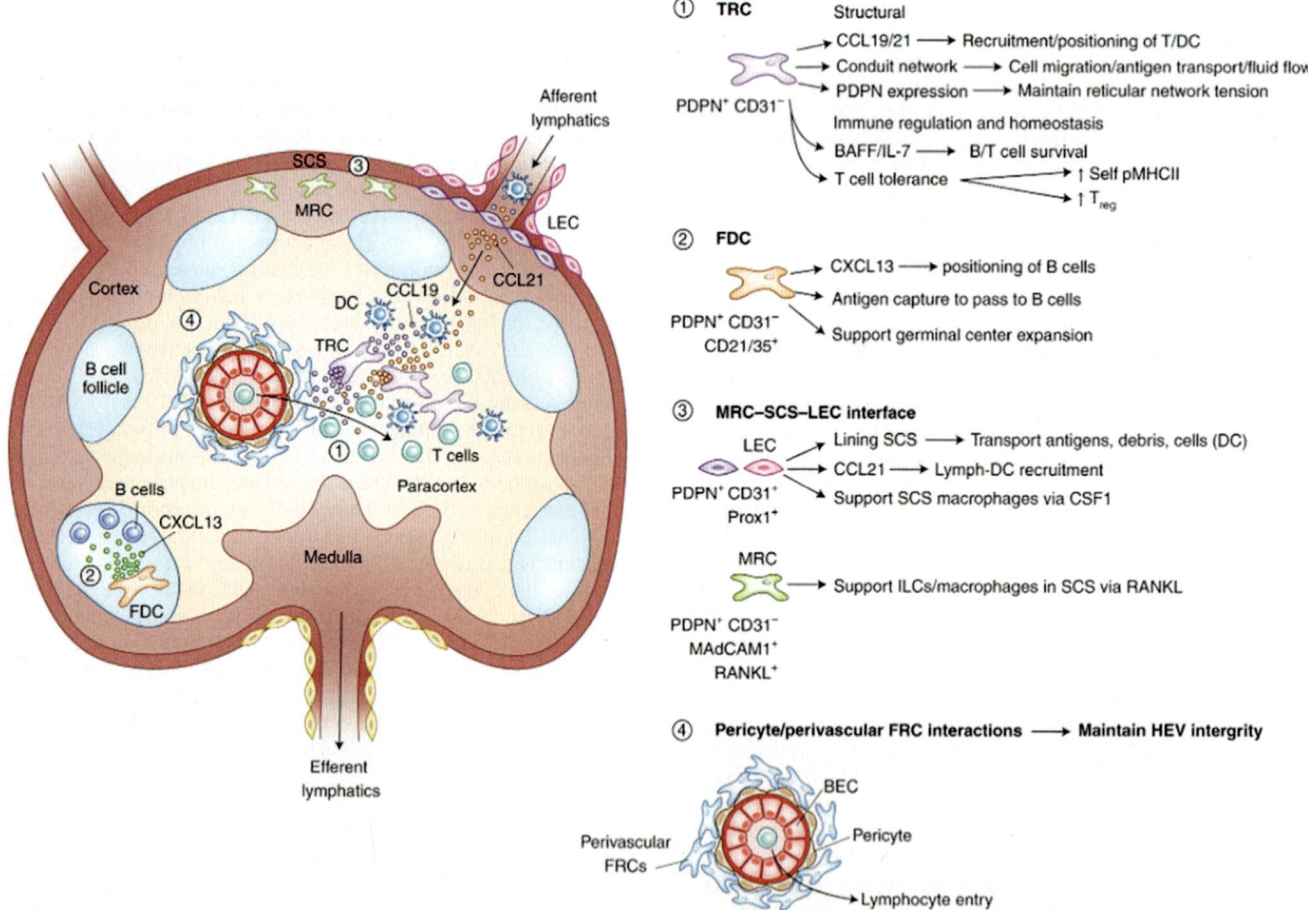

FIGURE 11.7 Lymph node stromal cell subtypes. The lymph node stromal compartment is composed of multiple nonhematopoietic (CD45⁻) cell populations that maintain LN homeostasis. Fibroblastic reticular cells (FRCs) express podoplanin and encompass multiple subtypes including T zone reticular cells (TRCs), marginal reticular cells, and medullary reticular cells. TRCs (PDPN⁺, CD31⁻) are situated in the paracortical and interfollicular regions of the LN where they form a conduit network with structural and immunoregulatory functions. 1. TRCs facilitate cell motility, transportation of antigens, maintenance of reticular networks, and localization of T cells and dendritic cells through the formation of CCL19/21 gradients. 2. Follicular dendritic cells (FDCs) (PDPN⁺, CD31⁻, CD21⁺, CD35⁺) are key antigen-presenting cells that recruit naïve B cells through the expression of CXCL13 and facilitate reactive germinal center formation. 3. Marginal reticular cells (PDPN⁺, CD31⁻, MAdCAM1⁺, RANKL⁺) are found at the periphery of cortical B-cell follicles and promote macrophage and innate lymphoid cell (ILC) homeostasis through expression of RANKL. Lymphatic endothelial cells (LECs) (PDPN⁺, CD31⁺) line the subcapsular sinuses (SCS) where they secrete chemokines that facilitate LN leukocyte trafficking and promote macrophage and ILC homeostasis through the expression of CSF1. 4. Blood endothelial cells (BECs) (PDPN⁻, CD31⁺) form high endothelial venules (HEVs), which express adhesion molecules that facilitate lymphocyte recruitment. Pericytes and perivascular FRCs line HEVs where they form tight junctions that support the integrity of the vascular barrier and secrete lymphocyte chemotactic factors. BAFF, B-cell activating factor; ILC, innate lymphoid cell; PDPN, podoplanin; SCS, subcapsular sinus. (Reprinted by permission from Nature: Krishnamurty AT, Turley SJ. Lymph node stromal cells: cartographers of the immune system. *Nat Immunol.* 2020;21(4):369-380. Copyright © 2020 Springer Nature America, Inc.)

the production of high-affinity antibodies[316-320] (*Figures 11.7 and 11.8*). FDCs are difficult to identify by routine light microscopy but can be identified based on their immunophenotypic features. FDCs express the monocytic marker CD14, three types of complement receptors, CD35 (CR1), the long isoform of CD21 (CR2), and CD11b (CR3); VCAM1, which facilitates leukocyte adhesion; immunoglobulin Fc receptor CD32; surface PD-L1; and multiple TLRs including TLR4, which respond to pathogen-associated molecular patterns and upon activation increase FDC antigen presentation.[316,318,319,321] A subset of FDCs in the light zone additionally express CD23, the low-affinity receptor for IgE, and one of the ligands for CD21, allowing binding of complexes containing CD21 with higher affinity and to interact with IgE. In the absence of complement component C3 or following the deletion of the Cr2 locus (which encodes CR1 and CR2 in mice), FDCs are unable to retain antigen and GCs are reduced.[322] Although affinity maturation can occur outside of GCs, the depletion of FDCs, the disruption of antigen binding, or the ablation of CD35 or CD21 on FDCs results in the loss of GC maintenance and severely impairs somatic hypermutation responses.[322-324]

Electron microscopy has revealed that FDCs contain one or more large, irregularly shaped nuclei with vesicular chromatin and long cytoplasmic dendrites connected by desmosomes, which together form an intricate network of processes seeded with lymphocytes. Along the slender protrusions, small globular structures, or iccosomes, representing immune complex-coated bodies, are observed. FDCs function by trapping immune complexes in recycling endosomal compartments, thereby protecting the antigen from degradation.[325] This allows them to present intact antigens integrated in large immune complexes to activated GC B cells for long periods of time, allowing these B cells to receive survival signals and undergo affinity maturation, leading to the formation of the memory B-cell pool.[310,326-329]

FDCs maintain normal follicular structures by producing the B-cell chemotactic cue CXC-chemokine ligand 13 (CXCL13), which signals via CXC-chemokine receptor 5 (CXCR5) to attract B cells and specific subsets of T cells to the follicles.[330] While FDCs are dispensable for resting B-cell homeostasis,[324] they play important roles in the GC reaction. Primary B-cell follicles contain light zone (LZ) and dark zone (DZ) FDC subtypes. Both arise from a common CXCL13+ precursor and differentiate into distinct subtypes that polarize during the germinal center reaction to orchestrate formation of the GC light and dark zones[318,319,331] (*Figure 11.8*). Activated B cells migrate to the T cell–B cell border of the follicle where they present antigen to T helper cells and receive costimulation. Selected B cells then migrate to the center of the follicle, where they start a cycle of proliferation and hypermutation in the dark zone before undergoing antigen-driven selection by LZ FDCs. LZ and DZ FDCs coordinate these events by producing CXCL12, CXCL13, as well as BAFF, APRIL, and other survival factors.[318,319,324,332] Following selection by FDCs, B cells can either undergo cycles of affinity maturation or exit the GC as memory B cells or plasma cells.[333] These cell fate decisions are influenced in part by the availability of IL-4 and are modulated by FDCs through the expression of IL4Ra, upregulation of which limits B-cell IL-4 exposure and enhances memory cell differentiation. By contrast, IL4Ra deficiency results in increased B-cell IL4 availability and, consequently, reduction of the memory B-cell compartment.[331]

FDC maturation requires LT and TNF signaling for maturation, and disruption of these pathways results in the loss of FDCs.[334-336] Mice lacking FDCs fail to maintain proper segregation of B- and T-cell zones and were unable to support germinal center formation upon immune activation. Interestingly, loss of FDCs was found to result in encroachment of CCL21-expressing FRCs into the B cell–rich areas, which might suggest that FDCs may additionally contribute

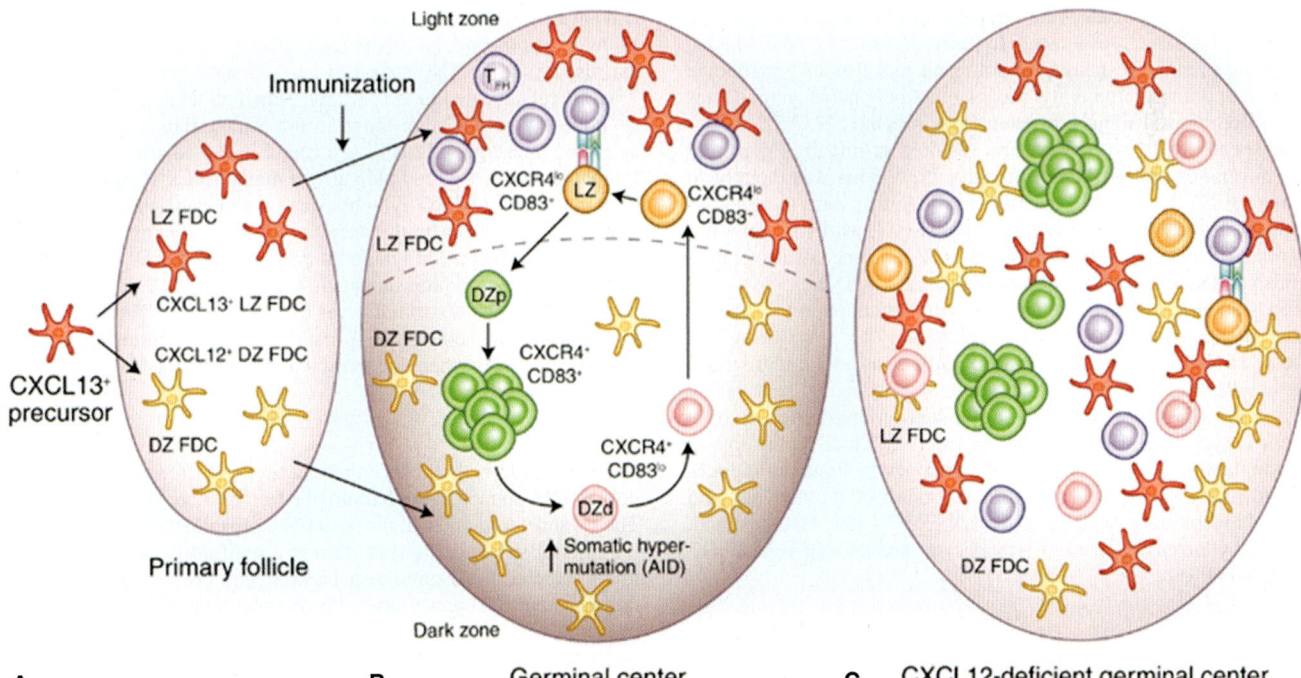

FIGURE 11.8 Distinct light zone and dark zone follicular dendritic cell subtypes facilitate germinal center B-cell differentiation. A, Follicular dendritic cells (FDCs) arise from a common CXCL13+ precursor and differentiate into CXCL13+ light zone (LZ) and CXCL12+ dark zone (DZ) FDCs, both of which are present in steady state primary B-cell follicles. **B,** Upon immunization, LZ and DZ FDCs polarize to orchestrate the formation of germinal center light and dark zones. During affinity maturation, follicular helper T-cell (T_FH) signaling recruits LZ B cells into the DZ where they differentiate into proliferating DZ B cells (DZp). DZp B cells undergo somatic hypermutation mediated by activation-induced deaminase (AID) to become differentiating DZ B cells (DZb) which reenter the LZ and differentiate into LZ B cells. **C,** Genetic ablation of FDC CXCL12 prevents the polarization of LZ and DZ FDCs and the formation of discrete GC light and dark zones, resulting in impaired T cell–dependent humoral immunity. (Reprinted by permission from Nature: Muppidi J.R., Klein U. Directing traffic in the germinal center roundabout. *Nat Immunol.* 2020;21(6):599-601. Copyright © 2020 Springer Nature America, Inc.)

to maintenance of strict follicle borders through repression of T-cell chemotactic cues or by repelling FRCs that are typically outside of follicles in the T cell–rich paracortical areas.[324]

Lineage tracing experiments have shown that splenic FDCs, FRCs, and MRCs originate from a common precursor that expresses homeobox protein NKX2-5 and insulin gene enhancer protein ISL1; the origins of other stromal cell types have not been resolved.[337] Unlike FDCs from the spleen, only cultured FDCs from the lymph node are able to form B-cell clusters, suggesting developmental and functional differences. Recent reports indicate that the additional FDCs generated during GC formation can originate from both perivascular mesenchymal cells and the local differentiation of MRCs.[263,317]

Fibroblastic Reticular Cells

FRCs are PDPN+ contractile myofibroblasts that are essential for the regulation of LN structure, physiology, and immune cell homeostasis and responses.[338-340] FRCs encompass multiple subtypes including T-zone reticular cells (TRCs), which comprise the major mesenchymal stromal cell network in the T cell zone, and MRCs, which are found at the periphery of cortical B-cell follicles and promote macrophage and ILC homeostasis (*Figure 11.7*).

TRCs delineate the T-cell zone boundaries by secreting chemokines such as CCL19 and CCL21, which facilitate T-cell and dendritic-cell recruitment and migration.[262,341,342] At steady state, TRCs secrete interleukin (IL)-7 and BAFF, the main survival factors for T and B cells, respectively.[343,344] T-zone FRCs produce extracellular matrix and sheath the conduit system, a network that transports the lymph throughout the T-cell zone.[309,345,346] FRCs are also able to induce peripheral tolerance by facilitating presentation of peripheral tissue-restricted antigens.[347] (*Figure 11.7*).

The importance of FRCs in both organizing lymphocyte position and maintaining cell homeostasis and viability in LNs has been demonstrated by studies in which specific ablation of FRCs in vivo via administration of diphtheria toxin was performed. FRC-depleted LNs lost segregation of B- and T-cell compartments, failed to maintain normal T-cell numbers, and were incapable of mounting virus-specific CD4+ and CD8+ T-cell responses. However, depletion of FRCs during an ongoing immune response did not result in a loss of lymphocyte activation or antiviral immunity, showing that only naïve lymphocytes require FRC-derived signals for retention within the LN.[343,348]

Unexpectedly, loss of FRCs also resulted in impaired germinal center formation and humoral immunity.[343,349] This was thought to be due to FRCs localized to the B-cell follicle that were to be major producers of the B-cell survival factor BAFF. Thus, FRCs may not only organize and maintain the paracortical T-cell zone but also help to establish and maintain B-cell homeostasis in the follicle.

FRCs undergo significant changes during inflammation to accommodate the massive influx of naïve leukocytes.[346,350-352] During this process, Th17-mediated IL-17 signaling drives metabolic reprogramming of FRCs to support their activation, expansion, and survival.[349] The initial FRC swelling phase is dependent on migrating DCs that express C-type lectin-like receptor (CLEC)-2, which is the ligand for podoplanin expressed on FRCs.[353] Podoplanin signaling induces FRCs to relax, thereby decreasing the tension of the network and allowing concomitant swelling of the LN.[353,354] Later, FRCs expand, regulated by the engagement of lymphocyte- and DC-derived LIGHT and LTaß on FRCs.[355-357]

Marginal Reticular Cells

MRCs are the second major mesenchymal cell population present in primary B-cell follicles (*Figure 11.7*). While FDCs occupy the center of the follicles,[262,324,332,333] MRCs are located in the outer follicle, just below the subcapsular sinus, and have been shown to produce BAFF and CXCL13[264,358]; however, failure to maintain B-cell homeostasis in the absence of FRCs suggests that MRC-derived BAFF and CXCL13 alone are not sufficient for maintaining B-cell follicles. While little is known about the functional contributions of MRCs to LN biology, fate-mapping studies have suggested that this population gives rise to FDCs and thus may serve as an important stromal cell progenitor.[263]

Other studies have suggested that MRCs represent adult counterparts of the lymphoid tissue organizer (LTo) cells, but their exact functions in quiescent LNs remain elusive.[264]

SPLEEN

The spleen is an SLO that is responsible for generating blood-borne immune responses, and it also serves as a blood filter for damaged or senescent formed elements of the blood. The spleen is covered by a connective tissue capsule, which is several millimeters thick, and in humans, it contains only a few muscle cells and is not capable of marked contractions. The internal surface of the capsule is the point of origin of an extensive network of trabeculae that divides the organ into communicating compartments, with a sponge-like appearance and spaces containing the parenchyma, or pulp tissue. The capsule is indented on the medial surface where the blood vessels, lymphatics, and nerves enter and leave. The orphan homeobox gene-11 *HOX11*, or *TLX1*, regulates splenic development[359] as shown in Tlx1-deficient mice, which lack spleens but in which other SLOs develop normally. The deficient spleen has two major compartments that can be distinguished histologically and morphologically—red pulp and white pulp. These differences are caused by the distinct cellular components that make up each section. The white pulp is composed of aggregates of lymphocytes, and its organization is similar to that of the lymphoid tissue of LNs, although B-cell follicles are associated with prominent MZs (*Figure 11.9*). The white pulp stains dark blue to purple because of the predominance of small lymphocytes on histologic sections. The red pulp appears red grossly and histologically because of the predominance of blood-filled sinuses (*Figure 11.9*). The spleen is an SLO, but it serves several other functions unrelated to the immune system and affects all blood cells throughout their life span by providing the microenvironment for the final differentiation of reticulocytes, platelets, and monocytes. It is also a reservoir for erythrocytes and granulocytes and removes aged or deformed red blood cells.[360] Because the spleen filters blood, this means that pathogens or antigens enter the MZ and are screened, allowing immediate innate or longer-lasting adaptive immune responses, and this is facilitated by numerous cell types that can also be seen in LNs, including macrophages, monocytes, DCs, and T and B cells located in the MZ, red pulp, and white pulp.

Follicles and GCs are found in the Malpighian corpuscles, and T cells and interdigitating cells are found in the adjacent periarteriolar lymphoid sheath. The red pulp also contains APCs, lymphocytes (particularly a subset of γδT lymphocytes), and plasma cells. A distinctive feature of the spleen is the presence of a prominent MZ encircling white pulp composed of lymphoid cells with abundant pale cytoplasm and macrophages, which surrounds both the B- and T-cell zones[361,362] and also contains a stromal layer of MRCs.[358,363] These MRCs are most prominent adjacent to B-cell follicles but interrupted at MZ bridging channels where the marginal sinus connects directly to T-cell areas.[364]

White Pulp

The white pulp is the main lymphoid tissue of the spleen and is composed of the supporting reticulum, the free cells, and the blood vessels. The B- and T-cell areas in the spleen are organized around the branching arterial vessels. The reticulum is a scaffolding made of reticular fibers secreted from spindle-shaped reticular cells, runs circumferentially around the central artery to provide support for free cells and blood vessels, and is pronounced at the periphery of the white pulp, where the reticular cells extend concentric sheets of membranes.[265,266] The central artery gives off secondary branches that radiate through the white pulp with different destinations, some terminating before they reach the edges of the white pulp, whereas others terminate in the MZ or extend even further into the red pulp. In the human spleen, some branches curve back from the red pulp to form a delicate network around lymphatic follicles located at the periphery of the white pulp, where T lymphocytes are usually found in intimate contact with the interdigitating cells.[367] The central artery is surrounded by tightly packed lymphocytes, which follow the artery, becoming eventually a

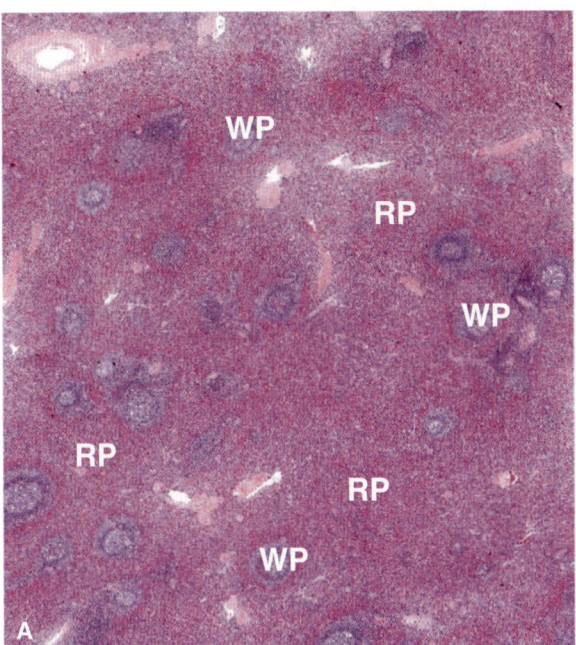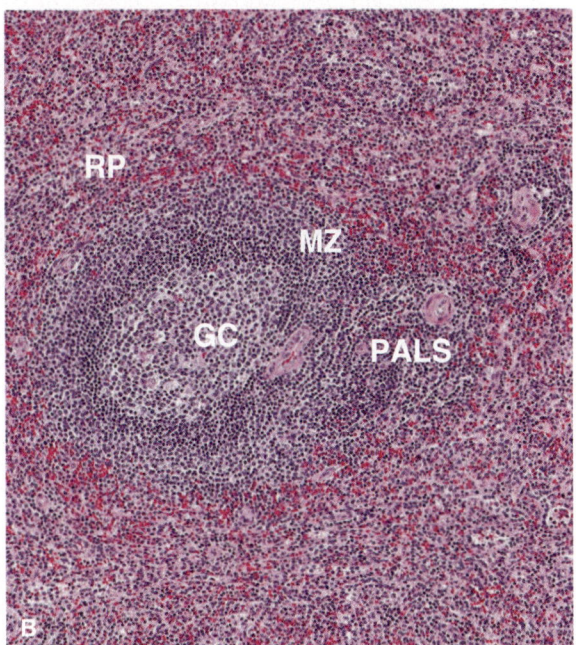

FIGURE 11.9 Normal human spleen. A, The splenic tissue is composed of red and white pulp. The red pulp (RP) contains venous sinuses separated by cords of red cells (cords of Billroth), which are not visible in this low-power micrograph. The white pulp (WP) contains reactive follicles with germinal centers and a T-cell zone; both are surrounded by a pale-staining marginal zone composed of medium-sized cells with abundant pale cytoplasm that separates white pulp from red pulp. The T-cell zone has an appearance similar to that of the nodal paracortex with interdigitating dendritic cells present in a background of small lymphocytes. B, Higher magnification of white pulp. The white pulp is composed of lymphoid aggregates with germinal centers (GC) that are encircled by an inner darker staining mantle zone (MC) and a prominent outer marginal zone (MZ) that separates the white pulp from red pulp (RP). The lymphatic nodules largely consist of B lymphocytes. Thick-walled central arteries are usually evident penetrating the white pulp. The T cell–rich periarteriolar lymphoid sheath (PALS) surrounds the central artery. (Modified with permission from Orazi A, Weiss LM, Foucar K, et al. *Knowles' Neoplastic Hematopathology.* 3rd ed. Wolters Kluwer Health/Lippincott Williams & Wilkins; 2014.)

diffuse thin sheath as the artery divides into small arterioles known as the periarteriolar lymphatic sheath (PALS). The PALS is divided into the central and peripheral areas, the former consisting of tightly packed T lymphocytes and interdigitating cells, seen in the T cell–dependent area, or paracortex of the LN. The periphery of the PALS lacks the interdigitating cells and contains B and T lymphocyte collections known as follicles and blast-like cells in the GC of the secondary follicle. No FDCs are located in the central section of PALS, and their presence in the mantle of the nodules, facing the MZ, places them in a strategic location to capture foreign substances entering the spleen. Foreign antigens are localized first in the MZ and then cross the marginal sinus to lodge in the mantle of the nodules, forming a crescentic cap. The nodules of the peripheral section of PALS constitute the B cell–dependent regions of the spleen (*Figure 11.9*).

Similar to LNs, the T- and B-cell compartments are recruited and maintained by specific chemokines. CCL19 and CCL21 are produced mainly by stromal cells in the T-cell areas, and the FDCs secrete CXCL13; these chemokines recruit cells expressing the receptors CCR7 and CXCR5, respectively. T cells surround the arterioles in a discontinuous manner, whereas B-cell follicles may be found adjacent to the T-cell sheaths or directly attached to the arteriole without a T-cell layer.[367]

A distinctive area of the splenic white pulp is the MZ, which is more evident in follicles with an expanded GC. This area comes into contact with large quantities of circulating blood because many arterial vessels terminate in this region and some of them, with funnel-shaped orifices, empty their contents into the interstices of the MZ, which, unlike the red pulp, has no sinuses. Although a marginal sinus separates the MZ from the white pulp in rodents, human spleen lacks a marginal sinus. The marginal sinus does not have the tall ECs that direct traffic in the LNs (HEVs), and some authors speculate that this function is performed by splenic macrophages located in the marginal sinus. These cells have distinct phagocytic and morphologic properties, which distinguish them from macrophages in other locations of the spleen, including the ability to bind lymphocytes.[368] This anatomic

relationship between an open blood area and the MZ seems to facilitate direct contact between blood-borne antigens and B cells.[361,362] B cells in the MZ have slightly irregular nuclei, resembling those of centrocytes but with more abundant pale cytoplasm. These cells express CD21 and IgM, but contrary to mantle cells, IgD expression is negative or weak. These cells predominantly surround the follicles but are almost absent from the T-cell regions. Some studies in human spleen distinguish between an inner and outer MZ separated by a shell-like accumulation of CD4+ T cells and a layer of peculiar fibroblasts that extend to the T-cell areas as a meshwork. These cells express smooth muscle a-actin and myosin, MAdCAM-1, VCAM-1, and VAP-1.[367]

Red Pulp

The red pulp is composed of sinuses and cords, which are composed of a meshwork of reticular fibers and cells.[369,370] The red pulp sinuses are tortuous vascular channels 35 to 40 μm in diameter, lined with elongated ECs arranged with their long axes parallel to that of the vessels. The sinuses form an interconnected meshwork and are surrounded by annular fibers of extracellular matrix that can be appreciated on periodic acid–Schiff staining. Through the fenestrations of this network, blood cells pass from the cords to the sinuses. The ECs have three distinctive morphologic features: (a) micropinocytotic vesicles, (b) loosely organized cytoplasmic filaments, and (c) tightly organized filaments along the basal side, which provide the cell with rigidity and contractility. Slitlike gaps between the ECs allow passage of blood cells from the cordal spaces into the lumen, but the slits never exceed 0.2 to 0.5 μm in width because the intraendothelial filaments run parallel to the slits and restrict their opening.[371] Adventitial cells cover the sinus wall from the cordal side and contribute to blood flow regulation by covering or exposing the interendothelial slits. Although normal red blood cells are flexible and capable of passing through the slits, the presence of rigid inclusions, such as Heinz bodies, interferes with their passage.

The reticular cells extend membranous processes into the interstices and contact those of adjacent cells, forming cavernous spaces.

The large reticular cells have microfilaments that endow them with the capacity to retract and extend and thus determine the available space thereby regulating blood flow and the passage of blood cells. These cordal spaces receive blood directly from the arterial vessels because the central artery gives off many branches, which terminate in slender, straight, nonanastomosing arterioles that enter the cords of the red pulp but not the sinuses. Some of the arterioles divide into arterial capillaries, which are enveloped by a sheath of phagocytic cells. These sheaths were called ellipsoids, but now they are called periarterial macrophage sheaths, which, in the human spleen, are not well developed. The periarterial macrophage sheath functions as a major source of phagocytic cells and may also regulate blood flow. The cords represent a unique vascular space, with regulation by the cordal reticular cells of its flow, which removes old or damaged red cells. Sinusoidal blood flows into the venous system. The sinusoidal cells express endothelial markers such as factor VIII, but they are also positive for CD8. The red pulp cords also contain plasmablasts and plasma cells. Upregulation of CXCR4 in these cells may play a role in this movement because it binds to the CXCL12 expressed in the red pulp; in contrast, CXCR5 and CCR7, which bind to the white pulp chemokines CXCL13, CCL19, and CCL21, are downregulated in these cells.[361]

Ontogeny of the Spleen

Spleen development can be viewed as occurring in two distinct stages. In the initial phase, primitive red pulp formation occurs during embryonic spleen development independently of LT signaling and instead relies on the expression of homeobox transcription factors including *TLX1* and *PBX1*.[372] White pulp and MZ formation occur in the postnatal setting and, similar to LN organogenesis, in an LT-dependent manner.[373]

Unlike the formation of LNs and PPs, which depend on stromal LTo cells (VCAM-1+ICAM-1+MAdCAM-1+), hematopoietic CD3−CD4+IL-7Ra+ LTi cells,[374,375] and LTα1ß2,[376-378] embryonic spleen development occurs in the absence of LT signaling. LTi cells are also dispensable because the absence of LTi cells as a result of *RORg* gene knockout leads to the lack of embryonic LNs but not spleen organogenesis.[379] Dependencies on LT signaling appear to be developmentally regulated because embryonic LTa-/- spleen grafts retain their ability to regenerate spleen,[380] whereas neonatal spleen stromal grafts do not.[381]

Although specialized subsets of LTo cells guide LN and PP development,[374,375,382] it appears that the spleen requires a unique group of spleen organizer (SPo) cells for neonatal spleen regeneration,[363] which may not be surprising because the spleen is unique from LNs both structurally and functionally and embryonic spleen development can occur in the absence of LT signaling.[376-379] The role of stromal cell types during development can similarly be seen to occur in embryonic and early postnatal phases. In the embryonic stage, spleen mesenchymal cells and formation of the splenic anlage commences (E10.5 in mice).[372,376] Nkx2-5+Islet1+ mesenchymal progenitors give rise to the majority of mesenchymal stromal lineages in the spleen, including GP38+ FRCs, CD35+ FDCs, and NG2+ pericytes.[383] LTo cells can also arise from this pool of multipotent stromal cells[367] and are likely PDGFRß+ cells.[374,384] LTi of their precursors emerge by E12 to E13 in the fetal spleen,[369] and at E16.5, these cells are present surrounding CD31+ or VE-cadherin (CD144+) central arterioles in close proximity to MAdCAM-1+VE-cadherin+ ECs,[384-386] thus localizing in all areas where white pulp will develop,[358,387] and this localization is independent of LT up to at least E15.[379,380] Eventually, LT becomes essential for organization of white pulp compartments, and NF-κB signaling is critical for LTo cell maturation and function,[388] beginning at E17.5 in mouse.[388,389] The importance of LT signaling increases from this point onward, and increased numbers of LTi begin to express LTα1β2 after birth,[386] and these signals are likely enhanced by the combination of LTi and mature B cells, which colocalize around central arterioles and functionally express LT.[386,390,391]

Following establishment of white pulp formation, formation of the MZ occurs and is critical for establishment of immune competence, but the events underlying this transition are not entirely clear. The origins

of the MZ are thought to depend on MRCs, which may represent adult SPo cells.[358] Upregulation of VCAM-1 and ICAM-1 on stromal cells surrounding the central arteriole in spleen occurs post birth[385,386] when mature B cells begin to enter nascent white pulp,[363,386] and these events do not occur in LTα−/− mice,[392,393] and thus, these events are similar to LNs, in which the positive feedback loop initiated by LTi engagements leads to the maturation of stromal organizer cells and upregulation of CXCL13 as well as the adhesion molecules VCAM-1, ICAM-1, and MAdCAM-1.[363,386,394,395]

MUCOSA-ASSOCIATED LYMPHOID TISSUE

Specialized, nonencapsulated lymphoid tissue is found in association with certain epithelium embedded directly in the submucosa of the organs in which they are found, in particular, the gastrointestinal tract (gut-associated lymphoid tissue—PPs of the distal ileum and mucosal lymphoid aggregates in the colon and rectum), the nasopharynx and oropharynx (Waldeyer ring—adenoids and tonsils), and, in some species, the lung (bronchus-associated lymphoid tissue; BALT). Collectively, these are known as mucosa-associated lymphoid tissue (MALT). MALT comprises four lymphoid compartments: organized mucosal lymphoid tissue, lamina propria, intraepithelial lymphocytes, and regional (mesenteric) LNs.

Organized lymphoid tissue is structurally and immunophenotypically similar to the follicles found in LNs, although the MZ is expanded and may reach the superficial epithelium, exemplified by the PPs of the terminal ileum and in Waldeyer ring, and MZ T cells are morphologically similar to those found in the spleen. The interfollicular areas are occupied by T cells and interdigitating DCs. The mucosal lamina propria contains mature plasma cells, macrophages, and occasional B and T lymphocytes. These plasma cells secrete mainly dimeric IgA, but small populations producing IgM, IgG, and IgE are also present. The dimeric IgA and pentameric IgM are secreted into the intestinal lumen bound to the secretory component, a glycoprotein produced by the enterocytes. The T lymphocytes in the lamina propria are composed of a mixed population of CD4+ and CD8+ T cells and present in similar ratios to the peripheral blood, with a slight predominance (2:1-3:1) of CD4+ T cells. Intraepithelial lymphocytes are composed of a heterogeneous population of T cells. CD3+, CD5+, and CD8+ cells predominate, whereas 10% to 15% are CD3+ and DN for CD4 and CD8. CD3+ and CD4+ cells are a minority, and only rare cells are CD56+.[358,396] Most of the T cells express the αβ form of the TCR, and around 10% of the cells are TCRγδ+.

The epithelium above the PPs contains clusters of B cells and specialized epithelial cells called membranous or microfold cells (M cells), which originate from a common precursor present on the follicle-associated epithelium side of the crypt that also differentiates into the absorptive enterocytes.[392] These cells are also found in other parts of the gastrointestinal tract and other mucosal sites, particularly in the epithelium overlying lymphoid follicles.[393] M cells serve as immunologic sentinels by capturing luminal antigens and delivering them to the underlying immune cells.[397-400] A distinct layer of DCs is found immediately below the dome epithelium,[401] and many of these cells are enfolded within the basolateral pocket of M cells, where they receive antigens transported from the mucosal surface by the M cells. B-cell follicles fill the dome region of mucosal lymphoid organs, and the T-cell zone is typically found to the sides of the B-cell follicles or between follicles (*Figure 11.1*). Like encapsulated LNs, the HEVs of mucosal lymphoid organs surround the B-cell follicles and are in the T-cell zone. Also, like LNs, mucosal lymphoid organs such as PPs and colonic patches have efferent lymphatics, which are used as a point of egress for activated or recirculating cells. The basic structure of mesenteric LNs is similar to that of other LNs, but the MZ surrounding the follicles is usually expanded and visible.

The organization of the immune system in mucosal sites is orchestrated by the coordinated action of several adhesion molecules, chemokines, and their respective receptors. Lymphoid cells that respond to antigen in the MALT acquire homing properties that enable them to return to these tissues.[402,403] This homing is mediated, in part, by expression of high levels of α4β7 integrin, which binds to MAdCAM-1 on HEVs in gut-associated lymphoid tissue.[295] In addition, the MALT immune cells express αEβ7 integrin (CD103), whose ligand E-cadherin is expressed on the basolateral surface of the epithelial cells. Epithelial cells also secrete CCL25, which recruits immune cells expressing its receptor CCR9.[404]

Although individual mucosal lymphoid tissues develop following the same general program, each has unique characteristics. For example, the development of SLOs is temporally regulated—mesenteric LNs in mice begin to develop on embryonic day E9 to E10, brachial LNs on E13, axillary LNs on E15, inguinal LNs on E16, and popliteal LNs on E17. In contrast, PPs are still developing up until birth,[405] and the tear duct-associated lymphoid tissue (TALT) and nasal-associated lymphoid tissue (NALT) develop after birth.[406,407] In addition to the developmentally programmed lymphoid organs, ectopic lymphoid tissues like BALT only develop following infection or inflammation.[408-410]

As described earlier, the LT-driven expression of homeostatic chemokines like CXCL13 is important for the development of essentially all lymphoid tissues.[330] However, submucosal lymphoid tissues like PPs, isolated lymphoid follicles (ILFs), and NALT express additional homeostatic chemokines such as CCL20 and CCL9[411] that attract populations of DCs and B cells to the subepithelial dome region. Like other homeostatic chemokines, CCL20 expression in the dome epithelium requires LT signaling.[412] In addition, mice lacking CCR6, the receptor for CCL20, is required on B cells for the proper maturation of ILFs from cryptopatches in the small intestine.[413,414] While CCR6 is also expressed on putative LTi cells in cryptopatches,[415] CCR6 expression on LTi cells is not critical for cryptopatch formation.[415-417] Interestingly, the requirement for the various chemokines in ILF formation is distinct between the small intestine and the colon; ILFs do not form in the absence of CCL20 or CXCL13 in the small intestine, but they are present in the colon of mice in which CCL20 or CXCL13 signaling is disrupted.[416,417]

Most lymphoid organs develop during embryogenesis in a sterile environment. However, some mucosal lymphoid organs complete or even initiate their development after birth and are markedly influenced by exposure to commensal microbiota.[418] For example, PPs, NALT, TALT, and cryptopatches all develop in germ-free mice.[374,407,416] However, the cryptopatches mature in response to microbial colonization of the gut and accumulate B cells and ultimately transform into ILFs.[417,419] The requirements for the transition from cryptopatches to ILFs are different between the small and the large intestine: counterintuitively, the maturation of ILFs in the small intestine depends on the microbiota, whereas the maturation of ILFs in the colon, where the microbial density should be the highest, occurs in a microbiota-independent, yet MyD88-dependent manner.[416,417] Similarly, environmental exposure helps the maturation of NALT.[420] In part, exposure to antigen causes some level of inflammation that leads to immune reactivity and expands GCs, just as it would in conventional lymphoid organs. However, microbial triggers also promote M-cell differentiation and maturation in both the gut[421,422] and the airways.[423,424] Given the interactions between M and B cells, it is not surprising that microbial exposure leads to the accumulation of B cells, the differentiation of a dome epithelium, and, ultimately, to the maturation of mucosal lymphoid tissues.

TERTIARY LYMPHOID ORGANS

Although SLOs such as the spleen, LNs, and MALTs develop in predetermined locations throughout the body to monitor self- and non–self-antigens as they drain from peripheral tissues, it is becoming increasingly clear that antigen-specific responses may also be generated at other sites. Tertiary lymphoid tissue refers to highly ordered structures that exhibit a cellular composition similar to that of lymphoid follicles observed in the LNs and spleen (*Figures 11.10* and *11.11*). Tertiary lymphoid organs (TLOs) are most commonly observed in tissues affected by nonresolving inflammation

due to infection, autoimmunity, cancer, chronic allograft rejection, or environmental irritants.[425,426] These follicles show variable degrees of organization, ranging from simple T- and B-cell aggregates to highly organized structures with distinct B- and T-cell zones, FDCs associated with GCs, and HEVs, although they are not encapsulated or supplied by afferent lymphatics. Recent studies have shown that the development and function of these structures are regulated by novel immune cell subsets and that these structures may be associated with beneficial or deleterious outcomes depending on the clinical context.

TLOs have a structure similar to that of LNs or PPs. In addition to the histology, the constituent cells of TLOs and the molecules they express are quite similar to those in SLOs, as would be expected.[427-429] T-cell zones are CD62L+ and mainly central memory CD4+ T cells or naïve T cells that accumulate via HEVs from the bloodstream. The T-cell area also contains immature and CD208+ mature DCs. The density of HEVs is strongly correlated with the density of CD3+ T cells, CD8+ T cells, CD20+ B cells, and CD208+ mature DCs.[430] The B-cell follicle is composed of a mantle of naïve B cells surrounding a GC that is composed of highly proliferating B cells and a network of CD21+ FDCs.

Like SLOs, TLOs also rely on homeostatic chemokines (e.g., CXCL13, CCL19, CCL21, CXCL12) and lymphoneogenic cytokines (e.g., LTαβ) for their development.[412] However, unlike SLOs, they do not require LTi cells. For example, mice deficient in the nuclear hormone receptor retinoic acid–related orphan receptor-(RORγ t) and the transcriptional repressor Id2 still retain the capacity to develop TLOs at inflammatory sites, despite lacking LTi cells.[410,431-433] Thus, while the initiation of TLO development relies on an inducible inflammatory trigger, SLOs are developmentally preprogrammed. In fact, immune cells may substitute for LTi cells in the formation of TLO. The critical importance of T_H cells, particularly IL-17-secreting CD4+ (T_H17) T cells have recently been described because blocking antibodies to IL-17 inhibited the formation of inducible BALT (iBALT) tissue, although IL-17 was dispensable for the maintenance of established lymphoid clusters,[416] and adoptive transfer of in vitro–generated T_H17 cells into an experimental mouse model of multiple sclerosis was sufficient to induce TLOs; T_H1, T_H2, and T_H9 cells failed to induce this phenotype.[434-437] Data supporting a role for podoplanin have also been described, with increased numbers of podoplanin-positive T cells in TLOs in experimental inflammatory arthritis models[438] as well as in patients with rheumatoid arthritis, multiple sclerosis, renal allograft rejection, and giant-cell arteritis.[438-442] Thus, it has been speculated that similar to the role of podoplanin and its ligand CLEC-2 in LN development,[259,435,443] podoplanin expression on T cells may support the recruitment and retention of leukocytes within TLOs. In separate studies, roles for IL-21 and IL-22 produced by T cells have also been described in the formation of TLOs.[438,439,442,444-446] Roles for other immune cells in TLO regulation have also been described, including innate immune cells such as neutrophils[447] as well as ILCs including innate lymphoid cell-3 (ILC3) and γδT cells,[448-450] which share characteristics with activated T_H17 cells and LTi cells.

T_H17, γδT cells expressing IL-17A, or ILC3 may substitute for LTi cells for development of TLOs[448,451] by virtue of their common features with LTi cells, especially the production of common cytokines such as IL-17A, IL-22, LTβ, TNF, and granulocyte-macrophage colony-stimulating factor (GM-CSF).

T_{FH} cells expressing CXCL13 are also implicated in the regulation of TLOs, representing a key initiator of lymphoid organogenesis that functions upstream of LTβR signaling, promoting B-cell activities, and supporting the generation of high-affinity antibodies in GCs.[448,451] Instead of STo cells, stromal tissue cells such as synovial fibroblasts (e.g., in rheumatoid arthritis) contribute to TLO formation. CXCL13 can be produced by MRCs, T_{FH}, and FDCs, as well as some monocytes/macrophages, a subset of memory T cells, activated B cells, some ECs, stromal cells, or epithelial cells in inflammatory foci. Chemokines, CXCL13, CCL19, CCL21, and CXCL12, are involved in not only the initiation of TLO development but also maintenance

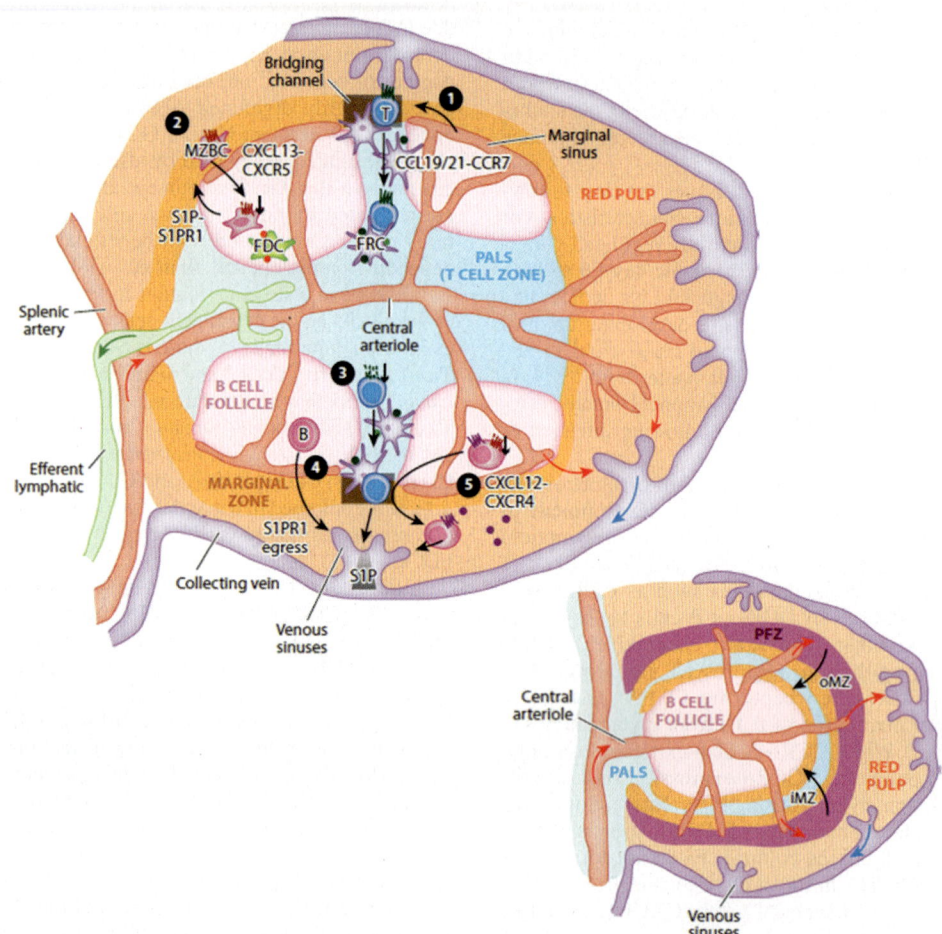

FIGURE 11.10 **Chemokine-guided migration and positioning in the spleen.** A, In mice and rats, lymphocytes and DCs leave the bloodstream from the marginal sinus, which is located between the white pulp and the marginal zone. Marginal zone bridging channels promote further transit to the white pulp by FRCs producing CCL21. Marginal zone B cells shuttle between the marginal zone and B-cell follicles. This shuttling behavior is controlled by reciprocal regulation of CXCR5 and S1PR1 expression. Newly generated CD8[+] effector T cells migrate from the T-cell zone (also known as the periarteriolar lymphoid sheath, or PALS) to the red pulp via bridging channels. Downregulation of CCR7 is required to release effector cells from the spleen. Follicular B cells leave the follicle via the marginal zone. Lymphocyte egress from the spleen depends on S1PR1. Efferent lymphatics closely associated with large arteries are also observed in the spleen, but it is not clear to what extent they participate in lymphocyte egress. Plasma blasts translocate from the follicles to the red pulp via the bridging channels. They downregulate CXCR5 and CCR7, concomitantly upregulate CXCR4, and are then attracted toward CXCL12, which is expressed in the red pulp. Further egress from the red pulp to venous sinuses is S1P driven. Red and blue arrows indicate the direction of blood flow. B, In contrast to rodents, humans lack marginal sinuses. Instead, an additional compartment, the perifollicular zone, is present between the marginal zone and the red pulp. Like the red pulp, this zone contains blood-filled spaces without an endothelial lining. Thus, it is assumed that, in humans, lymphocytes enter the marginal zone from the open circulation of the perifollicular zone and then transmigrate to the white pulp.[246] B, B cell; DC, dendritic cell; FRC, fibroblastic reticular cell; iMZ, inner marginal zone; MZBC, marginal zone B cell; oMZ, outer marginal zone; PFZ, perifollicular zone; S1PR1, sphingosine-1-phosphate receptor 1; T, T cell. (Used with permission of Annual Reviews, Inc. from Schulz O, Hammerschmidt SI, Moschovakis GL, et al. Chemokines and chemokine receptors in lymphoid tissue dynamics. *Annu Rev Immunol*. 2016;34:203-242; permission conveyed through Copyright Clearance Center, Inc.)

of the highly organized cellular architecture of established SLOs and TLOs.

ILCs have been shown to be present in TLOs, but their role in tertiary lymphoneogenesis has not been resolved. For example, while ILCs and NK cells produce IL-22 that supports TLO development in salivary glands,[444] the predominant sources of IL-22 in this model are αβ and γδT cells. Similarly, while LTi cells have been found in inflamed lungs that develop iBALT, the development of lymphoid aggregates in these sites did not depend on LTi cell activity,[410] and intestinal TLOs can develop in response to microbiota in RORγt-deficient mice that lack LTi cells.[432] Similar to ILC3s, γδT cells can also share effector characteristics with activated T_H17 cells, including the secretion of IL-17A, IL-17F, IL-22, IL-21, and GM-CSF.[451] In mice displaying iBALT in response to *Pseudomonas aeruginosa* infection, γδT cells were the main source of IL-17 that triggered stromal cell differentiation into podoplanin[+] follicular cells expressing CXCL12, supporting a role for γδT cells in TLO development.[446] While γδT cells facilitated the development of iBALT, αβT cells formed larger areas of lymphoid aggregates. Thus, it has been proposed that an early innate γδT-cell

response initiates the development of iBALT but that this process is later maintained by infiltrating αβT cells.[410,452] A similar role for γδT cells may occur in TLOs in salivary glands, where an early prominent IL-22-producing γδT-cell response is later replaced by αβT cells.[444]

While there is still much to understand about the mechanisms driving the formation of TLOs, accumulating evidence suggests that they can influence disease outcomes because TLOs can promote antigen-specific responses to promote antitumor and antipathogen immunity,[453] can play a protective role in atherosclerosis,[454] and can promote disease by supporting local autoantibody responses in autoimmune diseases, such as rheumatoid arthritis. Thus, it is likely that future studies will further clarify the roles of TLOs in chronic inflammatory disease states.

TLOs have been described in melanoma, MALT lymphoma, non–small cell lung carcinoma, as well as breast, colorectal, rectal, ovarian, and germ cell cancers, where they can be located peritumorally or intratumorally.[455] Intratumoral TLOs are much rarer than peritumoral TLOs in common types of cancer, but the frequency of intratumoral TLOs varies depending on the tissue of cancer origin and the tumor

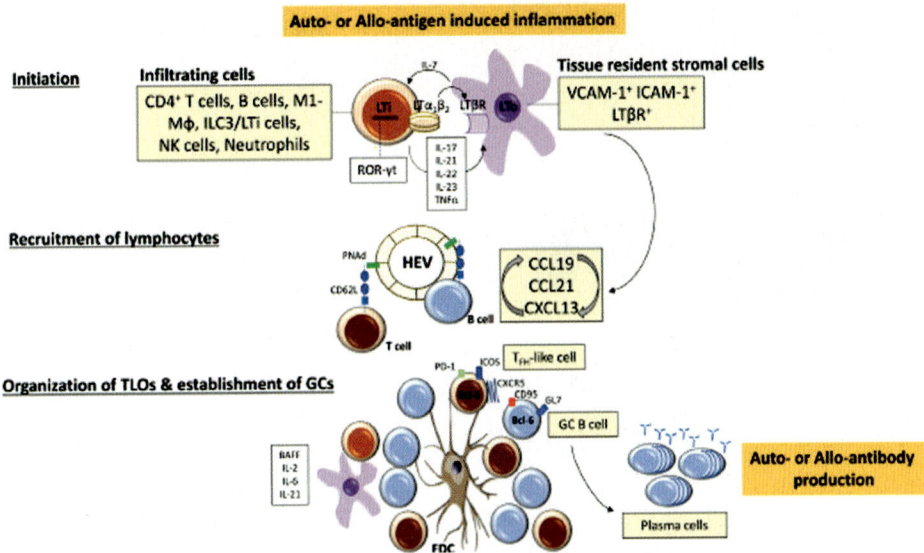

FIGURE 11.11 Tertiary lymphoid organ (TLO) initiation and formation. A, TLO-initiating immune cells (among which are lymphoid tissue inducer [LTi]-like cells) accumulate at sites of inflammation and interact with stromal mesenchymal lymphoid tissue organizing (LTo) cells. The binding of $LT\alpha1\beta2$ on LTi cells with $LT\beta R$ on LTo cells leads to the release of chemokines CCL19, CCL21, and CXC-chemokine ligand 13 (CXCL13) that mediate further immune cell recruitment and spatial organization within the forming TLO. B, Similarly, local release of homeostatic chemokines drives the formation of high endothelial venules (HEVs) and lymphangiogenesis, leading to homing of (auto- or alloreactive) naïve and memory B and T cells. A well-organized TLO is composed of compartmentalized T- and B-cell areas, follicular dendritic cells (FDCs), dendritic cells, HEVs, and lymphatic vessels. C, Under the influence of $LT\alpha1\beta2$, stromal cells acquire the phenotypic and functional properties of FDCs, which facilitate persistent antigen presentation within TLOs, and CD4+ T cells acquire follicular helper (TFH)-like effector characteristics (CXCR5hiPD-1hiICOShi) to drive activation of B cells. Cytokines, such as B-cell activating factor (BAFF), IL-21, and IL-6, contribute to the survival and maintenance of TFH cells and germinal center (GC) B cells, which subsequently differentiate into antibody-secreting plasma cells. (From Alsughayyir J, Pettigrew GJ, Motallebzadeh R. Spoiling for a fight: B lymphocytes as initiator and effector populations within tertiary lymphoid organs in autoimmunity and transplantation. *Front Immunol.* 2017;8:1639. http://creativecommons.org/licenses/by/4.0/)

type. The presence of TLOs in cancer tissues has been reported to be a favorable prognostic indicator,[429,455-474] although some studies have concluded that this is not always the case,[458,463] or may only apply to exceptional cancers such as renal cell carcinoma.[465] The majority of cancer-associated TLOs develop in peritumoral areas at the invasive front (or invasive margin) and form a wall around the cancer tissue. Peritumoral TLOs are positioned just outside the cancer tissue or in the periphery of the cancer (within the cancer-invasive area). Evidence from both experimental mouse models and human cancers show that TLOs are functional. For example, in a mouse model of melanoma, tumor-infiltrating lymphocytes developed TLOs and displayed clonal expansion of T cells reactive to melanoma tumor antigens and showed antitumor effects through the release of IFNγ.[475,476] Similar activities were also observed in LTα-deficient mice lacking peripheral LNs, suggesting that T-cell responses are primed locally within the tissue.[475] In human non–small cell lung carcinoma, TLOs are associated with improved patient survival, with enhanced antitumor immunity associated with increased frequencies of follicular B cells and plasma cells that display antibody specificity to tumor-associated antigens.[477-479] Therefore, TLO development in tumors may promote GC reactions and antitumor immunity. This is supported by the finding that the density of GCs in lung and breast cancers significantly correlates with patient outcome.[429,464,467] In addition to lymphoid chemokines (CCL19, CCL21, and CXCL13) and adhesion molecules (ICAM-2, ICAM-3, VCAM-1, and MAdCAM-1), CCL17, CCL22, and IL16 are found in TLOs.[429,464,470] One interesting feature in lung cancer is that, unlike in LNs where NK cells and DCs colocalized, no NKp46+ NK cells are detected in TLOs, which would abrogate NK-cell proliferation, IFNγ secretion, and cytotoxic function, as well as DC maturation.[428]

Lymphocyte Migration Into Lymphoid Tissues

Migration of leukocytes across the vascular endothelium is a complex multistep process, which involves different types of endothelia for different leukocytes, as well as a variety of adhesion molecules (*Figures 11.12* and *11.13*). When B and T lymphocytes complete their maturation in the BM and thymus, respectively (primary

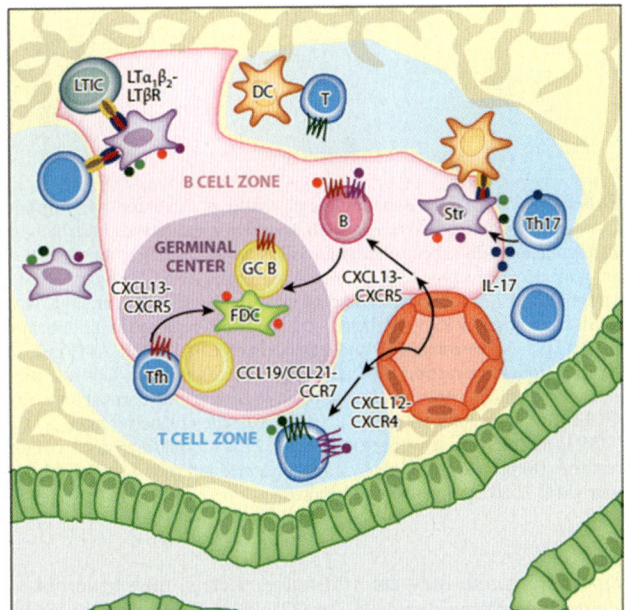

FIGURE 11.12 Chemokines in TLO dynamics. Lymphocytes are recruited into emerging TLOs through extravasation from HEVs. CCL21, CCL19, CXCL12, and CXCL13 produced by stromal cells promote TLO organization and the segregation of distinct B- and T-cell zones. DCs, T cells, and classical LTi cells (LTICs) probably induce chemokine secretion in stromal cells by LTβR signaling and IL-17 secretion in the case of TH17 cells. FDCs enable the formation of GCs in TLOs through CXCL13 secretion and the attraction of CXCR5-expressing B cells and TFH cells. DC, dendritic cell; FDC, follicular dendritic cell; GC B, germinal center B cell; HEV, high endothelial venule; LTIC, lymphoid tissue inducer cell; Str, stromal cell; TFH cell, T follicular helper cell; TH17, T helper 17 cell; TLO, tertiary lymphoid organ. (Used with permission of Annual Reviews, Inc. from Schulz O, Hammerschmidt SI, Moschovakis GL, et al. Chemokines and chemokine receptors in lymphoid tissue dynamics. *Annu Rev Immunol.* 2016;34:203-242; permission conveyed through Copyright Clearance Center, Inc.)

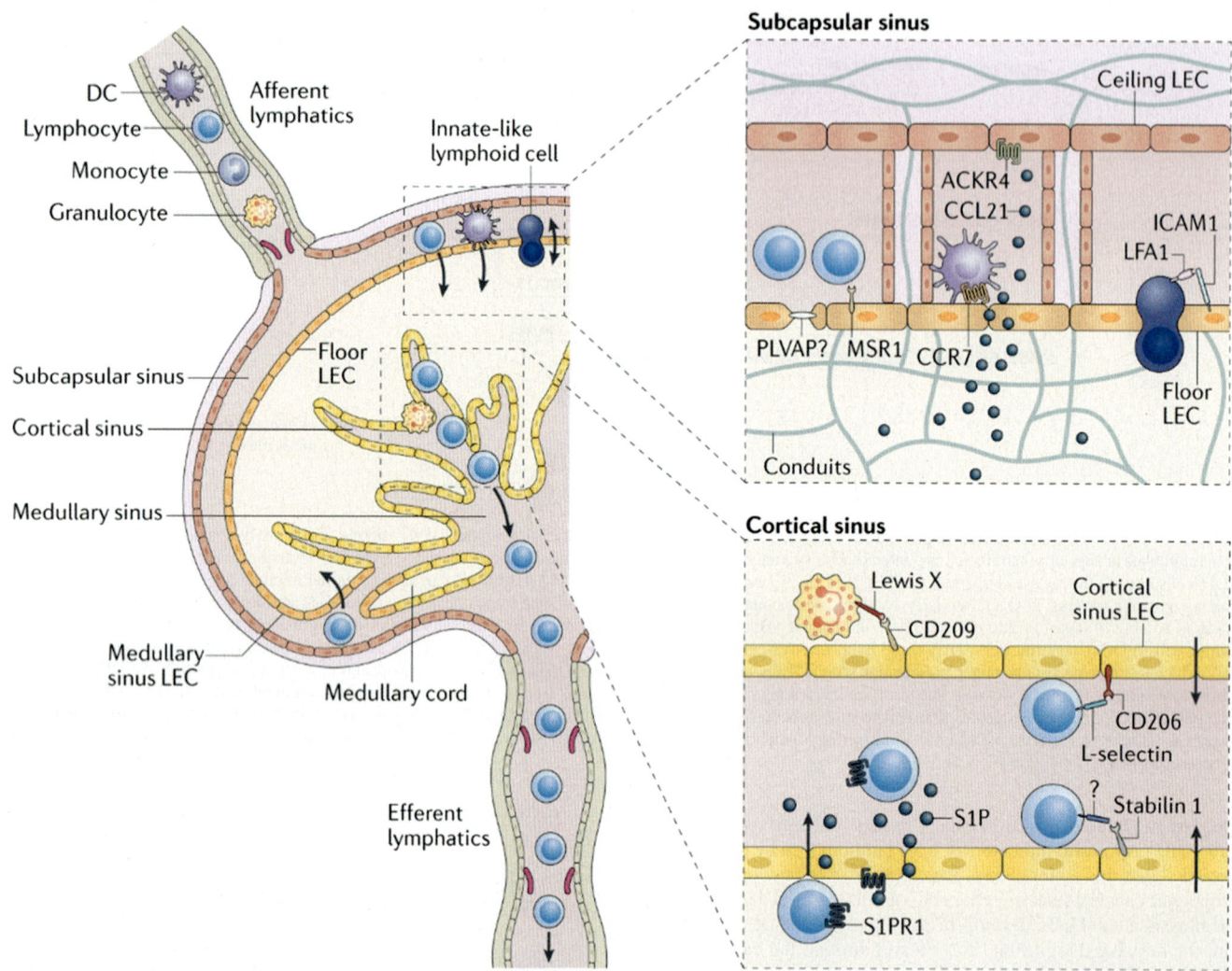

FIGURE 11.13 Lymph node leukocyte traffic is mediated by lymphatic endothelial cells. Chemokine gradients established by lymphatic endothelial cells (LECs) guide incoming leukocytes from the afferent lymphatics into the lymph node parenchyma. Dendritic cells (DCs) and T cells (when in the presence of DCs) transmigrate through subcapsular sinus LECs while T cells in the absence of DCs migrate through medullary sinus LECs. Subcapsular sinus LECs express the chemokine decoy receptor ACKR4, which scavenges the CCR7 ligands CCL19 and CCL21 from the subcapsular sinus and creates a chemokine gradient that guides the migration of incoming dendritic cells and T cells. Subcapsular sinus lymphocyte transmigration into the LN parenchyma is also facilitated by LEC expression of MSR1 and possibly PLVAP. Innate-like lymphoid cells patrol the subcapsular sinus lumen and the parenchyma beneath floor LECs; their transmigration is facilitated by LEC expression of S1P and dependent on LFA1 and ICAM1 interaction. Neutrophils localize to medullary sinus LECs, which express CD209, facilitating adhesion through interaction with neutrophil Lewis X (CD15). Cortical sinus LECs express S1P, which guides lymphocyte exit from the lymph node via efferent lymphatics. Lymphocytes exit the lymph node through the cortical sinuses, which is mediated by LEC expression of S1P. ACKR4, atypical chemokine receptor 4; CCL21, CC-chemokine ligand 21; CCR7, CC-chemokine receptor 7; ICAM1, intercellular adhesion molecule 1; LFA1, leukocyte function-associated antigen 1; MSR1, macrophage scavenger receptor 1; PLVAP, plasmalemma vesicle-associated protein; S1P, sphingosine-1-phosphate; S1PR1, sphingosine-1-phosphate receptor 1. (Reprinted by permission from Nature: Jalkanen S, Salmi M. Lymphatic endothelial cells of the lymph node. *Nat Rev Immunol.* 2020;20(9):566-578. Copyright © 2020 Springer Nature Limited.)

lymphoid organs), they are still naïve, that is, they have not yet encountered antigenic stimulation. The migration patterns of naïve lymphocytes differ from those of activated (or memory) lymphocytes. Naïve lymphocytes enter the SLOs (homing) and settle in specific (T-dependent or T-independent) compartments. Antigen-activated or memory lymphocytes migrate specifically to sites where they have encountered antigen. Thus, memory T lymphocytes tend to accumulate in extranodal tissues where they have previously been antigenically stimulated. These lymphoid accumulations represent TLOs and are associated with epithelial surfaces, such as the gut, respiratory tree, and sites of inflammation in the skin and synovium. In some of these accumulations, however, there are also small numbers of naïve lymphocytes.

Naïve (i.e., mature, nonactivated) lymphocytes migrate from the peripheral blood into SLOs such as LNs and PPs by interacting with

the specialized endothelium of HEVs. These postcapillary venules consist of characteristic tall and cuboidal ECs surrounded by a thick basal lamina and a prominent perivascular sheath and are abundant in the T cell–dependent areas of the LN and are used as entry sites for both T and B lymphocytes.[253,480-482] The ECs of HEVs interact with lymphocytes and selectively allow lymphocyte adherence and migration between HEV EC junctions.[262] HEVs are found in LNs and other extranodal locations, such as PPs, tonsils, adenoids of the pharynx, appendix, and lymphocyte aggregates of the stomach and small intestine.

In contrast, flat-walled venules support leukocyte extravasation in nonlymphoid tissues including the skin, but unlike HEVs, the extent of extravasation is much smaller, and they mainly allow memory-type lymphocytes and DCs to extravasate.[286,288] Relatively, little is known about the molecular mechanisms underlying leukocyte extravasation through these flat-walled venules, although both adhesion molecules and chemokines appear to play important roles.

Molecules Regulating Lymphocyte Migration Across Blood Vessels

a. HEVs in peripheral LNs. Circulating lymphocytes are able to selectively recognize and adhere to the lumen of HEVs. At steady state, approximately 40% of the lymphocytes interacting with the HEV ECs are in the process of transmigrating, but this number goes up to about 90% in mice in which circulating lymphocytes were depleted by thoracic duct cannulation.[483] Intravenously injected lymphocytes in lymphocyte-depleted mice rapidly adhere to and penetrate the HEV wall faster than in normal mice.[483] Together, these data show that trafficking across HEVs is homeostatically regulated by the number of lymphocytes in the blood.[483] Lymphocyte interactions with HEV ECs are directed by a site-specific adhesion cascade involving several specific molecules and chemokines that act in sequence.[286,288,484] This adhesion cascade is initiated by leukocyte tethering/rolling, followed by the firm arrest of rolling lymphocytes and finally by transvenular migration (extravasation) of lymphocytes.[286,485,486] This entire process is very similar to that observed in the lumen of inflamed blood vessels,[487] although some distinct and specific molecules are used in HEVs, as detailed below.

i. Tethering/rolling. As naïve lymphocytes flow into HEVs, they rapidly decelerate and interact weakly and transiently via adhesive interactions (tethering) with the HEV ECs, resulting in their rolling along the inner surface of the HEV wall. This process is mediated by CD62L (L-selectin) expressed on lymphocytes and by sialomucins on HEV ECs. L-selectin is a lectin-type cell adhesion molecule expressed on all leukocytes that recognizes sugars. It binds to specific O-glycans expressed on HEV sialomucins, a group of heavily glycosylated proteins (mucins) whose carbohydrate moieties contain sialic acid. The critical recognition determinant on the O-glycans is 6-sulfo sialyl Lewis X (sLex), which serves as a capping structure on core-2 and extended core-1 branches, and is specifically recognized by the MECA-79 monoclonal antibody. HEVs in the peripheral LNs express at least five different sialomucins, including GlyCAM-1,[488] CD34,[489] podocalyxin,[490] endomucin,[491] and nepmucin/CD300g.[492] To synthesize the L-selectin–binding MEC-79–reactive sLex structures, HEV ECs express a set of glycosyltransferases, including 1,3-fucosyltransferases IV and VII, Core1-O3GlcNAcT (also known as O3GlcNAcT-3 or Core1-GlcNAcT), Core2-O1,6-GlcNAcT (Core2-GlcNAcT), GlcNAc6ST-1, and GlcNAc6ST-2.[493]

In order for L-selectin to mediate primary adhesion (i.e., rolling), it must be located on the tips of HEV microvilli in peripheral LNs.[494,495] Homing of naïve lymphocytes to SLOs or the PPs of the gut requires L-selectin interaction with integrin, but it is not required for activated T lymphocytes, which lack expression of L-selectin.[496] The critical importance of L-selectin in mediating lymphocyte adhesion to HEV has been shown in gene knockout mice as well as by the observation that L-selectin antibodies block 99% of lymphocyte migration to the LN.[497] Rolling by L-selectin requires its linkage to cytoskeletal proteins such as actinin, vinculin, and talin through its carboxy terminal 11 amino acids.[498] This enables leukocytes to reduce their speed and sense chemoattractants, which activate firm adhesion. The HEV sialomucins are also called peripheral node addressins (PNAds) because they function as an "address code." These sialomucins share a common sugar epitope, that is, the 6-sulfo sLex structure mentioned previously. Binding of the MECA-79 antibody to this epitope abrogates L-selectin–PNAd interactions. In mesenteric LN HEVs, MAdCAM-1, a sialomucin bearing two immunoglobulin-like domains[499] serves as a vascular addressin, and α4β7 integrin serves as the cognate lymphocyte receptor that mediates rolling and adhesion.[494] Within

the HEV lumen, all L-selectin–expressing leukocytes undergo rolling/tethering, but only lymphocytes firmly adhere to HEV ECs.[286]

ii. Firm arrest/adhesion. After tethering/rolling, lymphocytes further decelerate and undergo a shear-resistant firm arrest/adhesion to the HEV wall in preparation for transendothelial migration. Arrest is primarily mediated by interactions between β2 integrin LFA-1 (CD11a/CD18) on lymphocytes and ICAM-1/ICAM-2 on HEV ECs. While L-selectin is constitutively active, integrins generally need to be activated to mediate adhesion. Integrin activation is induced by G protein–coupled receptor (GPCR) signaling in the lymphocytes at HEVs, which is initiated by lymphocyte interaction with chemokines displayed on ECs via specific receptors. Chemokines are generally positively charged and, therefore, bind to negatively charged molecules such as certain glycosaminoglycan chains that are abundantly expressed on HEV ECs, thereby preventing the chemokines from being washed away by the blood flow.[286,500] In the peripheral LNs, LFA-1 on T cells becomes activated when HEV-associated chemokines including CCL21/CCL19 and CXCL12 interact with their specific receptors on T cells, CCR7, and CXCR4, respectively, whereas LFA-1 on B cells is activated by interactions with CXCL13 via CXCR5. CCL21 (secondary lymphoid tissue chemokine) induces arrest of naïve T cells to ICAM-1[501] with 6-fold higher efficiency for naïve than for memory T cells.[502] Because these chemokine receptors are expressed preferentially on lymphocytes, only lymphocytes exhibit firm adhesion via activated LFA-1, which then binds to the immunoglobulin-like domain containing adhesion molecules, ICAM-1 and ICAM-2, on the surface of HEV ECs.

iii. Intraluminal crawling and transmigration. Upon undergoing firm adhesion, naïve lymphocytes crawl along the luminal HEV surface (intraluminal crawling), migrate to distant emigration sites, and then transmigrate between adjacent ECs at certain hot spots along the HEV wall where the HEV basal lamina has numerous pores to reach the abluminal side of HEVs.[262] The basal lamina consists of type IV collagen, fibronectin, and laminin, which allow chemokine immobilization mainly via electrostatic interactions. The HEV basal lamina binds locally produced lymphoid chemokines, including CCL21, CCL19, CXCL12, and CXCL13, creating a chemokine-rich environment. The HEV basal lamina also facilitates directional trafficking of lymphocytes from HEVs into the lymphoid tissue parenchyma by serving as a guidance structure.[286] Other adhesion molecules expressed on HEV ECs such as CD31, VCAM-1, JAM-A, JAM-B, JAM-C, ESAM, VE-cadherin, and nepmucin (CD300g) are thought to contribute to lymphocyte transmigration, but their specific roles and their modes of action have not been defined.[503]

Lysophosphatidic acid (LPA) plays a critical role in regulating lymphocyte transmigration across HEVs. LPA is a lysophospholipid that is mainly generated by the enzymatic action of lysophospholipase D, autotaxin (ATX), expressed in HEV ECs, which converts plasma lysophosphatidylcholine into LPA.[504,505] Local inhibition of the ATX/LPA axis substantially blocks the lymphocyte transmigration across HEVs, whereas a local administration of LPA abrogates this effect, likely because of its ability to promote lymphocyte deadhesion (or release) from ECs.[506] At the HEV lumen, LPA acts directly on HEV ECs via its receptors LPA4 and LPA6, which are both GPCRs, but each of these receptors mediate different effects because LPA4 deficiency comprises lymphocyte transmigration across the HEV wall to a greater extent than LPA6 deficiency.[507]

iv. Migration of nonlymphoid cells across HEVs. Under physiologic conditions, not only naïve lymphocytes but also DC precursors, plasmacytoid DCs (pDCs), and central memory T cells enter LNs by extravasating across HEVs. Although DC precursor cells rely on similar mechanisms as naïve lymphocytes to

The Normal Hematologic System

migrate into LNs,[508] this process has not been fully elucidated. However, it has been shown that pDCs robustly transmigrate underneath HEV ECs but not non-HEV ECs.[509] Like memory T cells, pDCs require CCR7 to enter the LNs via HEVs,[510,511] and similar to naïve T cells, pDCs cells express high levels of L-selectin and CCR7, which they use to interact with HEV ECs. However, it is not clear whether HEV-associated lysophospholipid LPA is required for their transmigration.

Neutrophils are prevented from entering LNs via HEVs normally, but they can rapidly migrate into draining LNs when sterile inflammation occurs locally. Neutrophil migration across HEVs occurs only after IL-17-producing lymphocytes initially migrate into the draining LNs, resulting in production of CXCL2, a chemokine ligand for CXCR2, by HEVs, which, in turn, induces migration of CXCR2-expressing neutrophils from the blood into the draining LNs. The effect of IL-17 on CXCL2 depends on IL-1b, which is also enhanced by IL-17.[512]

b. HEVs in intestinal lymphoid tissues. Lymphocyte trafficking to the small intestine is mediated by adhesion pathways that depend on whether or not the lymphocyte has encountered antigen. Naïve lymphocyte interactions mainly depend on lymphocyte L-selectin and HEV-expressed sialomucins/PNAds, whereas lymphocytes that have been exposed to antigen-experienced DCs in the small intestine depend on interactions between lymphocyte integrin $\alpha4\beta7$ and the vascular cell adhesion molecule MAdCAM-1. Naïve lymphocytes upregulate expression of integrin $\alpha4\beta7$ and the chemokine receptor CCR9 after migrating into the small intestine and being exposed to high concentrations of DC-derived retinoic acid.[513] The $\alpha4\beta7$ specifically binds MAdCAM-1, and CCR9 is the receptor for the chemokine CCL25 secreted by small intestinal venules. Thus, these lymphocytes are recruited because of small intestinal EC expression of MAdCAM-1 and CCL25. In contrast, the orphan chemokine receptor GPR15 has been shown to control the localization of T effector cells in the colon.[514]

c. Flat ECs in peripheral tissues. Flat ECs found in nonspecialized postcapillary venules in the skin can also mediate immune cell trafficking under steady-state conditions, but they are much less efficient at doing so than HEV ECs. Flat ECs support leukocyte rolling under noninflamed conditions,[515] which is largely determined by P-selectin with E-selectin playing a smaller role, but L-selectin is not involved.[494] Most skin T cells express the P-selectin–binding molecule cutaneous lymphocyte antigen (CLA), which is derived from the glycosylation of a lymphocyte sialomucin PSGL-1, as well as chemokine receptor CCR8, whose expression is induced by keratinocyte-derived factors.[516] Upon binding to EC-displayed selectins, CLA-expressing T cells extravasate from dermal venules. The engagement of lymphocyte CCR8 with constitutively expressed CCL1 in the dermal venules is thought to promote extravasation by activating lymphocyte integrins. Skin T cells also express the chemokine receptor CCR4, whose engagement with dermal venule–expressed CCL17 promotes T-cell migration into the skin. In inflamed skin, activated T cells express high levels of CCR10, which engages CCL27, which is produced by keratinocytes and is highly displayed on inflamed venules.[517] One mechanism for CCR10 induction in skin T cells is via skin DC production of the active vitamin D3 metabolite 1,25(OH)2D3 from sunlight-induced vitamin D3, which upregulates CCR10 expression in T cells.[518] Supporting the importance of CCR10 in T-cell recruitment into inflamed but not normal skin, CCR10 is largely absent from T cells in uninflamed skin.[516,519]

Recent studies indicate that T cells are abundant in the skin and exhibit unique immunologic properties.[520] It has been approximated that 2×10^{10} T cells exist in the skin, which is almost twice the number of T cells in the entire circulation.[521] Most skin T cells exhibit the phenotype of effector memory T cells, and some are central memory T cells. The prevailing hypothesis is that effector memory T cells that arise upon the antigenic stimulation of naïve as well as central memory T cells in LNs migrate into peripheral tissues via venules bearing

flat ECs and return to the LNs via lymphatics, whereas the central memory T cells that also arise in LNs recirculate between the blood vascular and lymphatic vascular systems using HEVs, just like naïve T cells.[522,523] However, the presence of CLA-expressing central memory (L-selectin$^+$CCR7$^+$) T cells in the skin (~20% of normal skin T cells) in humans[524] indicates that not all central memory T cells recirculate via the conventional route; some of them migrate into the periphery and then move to the LNs via lymphatics. On the other hand, a substantial proportion of memory T cells in the skin does not appear to leave the tissue and, therefore, are called tissue-resident memory T cells (TRMs) because of their inability to respond to the exit cue provided by S1P and because they express low levels of the transcription factor KLF2 and of S1PR1 as well as high expression of the C-type lectin CD69.[525] TRMs can thus provide effective protection against local antigen rechallenge.

T_{reg} cells are also found in the skin, where they comprise 10% to 20% of skin T cells.[521,526] They constitutively migrate to the draining LNs via lymphatics[527] but show increased migration during cutaneous immune responses and eventually return to the skin upon reexposure to antigen. Migrating T_{regs} have a stronger immunosuppressive effect than LN-residing T_{regs} and appear to help downregulate cutaneous immune responses,[527] but the molecular mechanism underlying their migration from the skin to LNs remains unclear.

Recent studies have shown that DCs also continuously migrate from the skin to draining LNs at steady state.[527] DCs do not require $\beta2$ integrins for their migration because DC migration in CD18$^{-/-}$ mice deficient in the $\beta2$ integrin subunit does not show defects in migration from the blood to normal or inflamed skin, or from the skin to draining LNs.[528] They are guided into lymphatics by a tissue-immobilized gradient of CCL21 in an integrin-independent, but CCR7-dependent, manner.[529]

ILCs are non–T, non–B lymphocytes that are important in innate immune responses and in the regulation of inflammation.[530] Group 2 ILCs are relatively abundant in the skin, but it is unknown whether these cells are recruited to the skin or whether they migrate from the skin into the draining LNs.[531]

Molecules Regulating DC Migration Into Lymphatics

a. Chemokines and their receptors. The trafficking of lymphocytes and DCs into the lymphatic vessels is an active process that requires chemokines presented on lymphatic ECs to attract and guide cells into lymphatics. For example, the CCR7 ligand chemokine, CCL21, is abundantly expressed on lymphatic capillaries and induces the migration and entry of CCR7-expressing DCs to the lymphatics. CCL21 expressed on the lymphatic basal lamina, binds the lymphatic EC marker podoplanin with high affinity, and can be shed into the perivascular stroma,[532] which may lead to the generation of a perilymphatic CCL21 concentration gradient. In addition, a chemokine-scavenging molecule, CCRL1/ACKR4, is expressed by lymphatic ECs that line the ceiling but not the floor of the subcapsular sinus.[533] CCRL1/ACKR4 sequesters and induces CCL21 degradation, which is thought to contribute to the formation of a CCL21 concentration gradient from the sinus toward the LN parenchyma, which helps direct DCs to migrate toward the inner areas of LNs. Indeed, DCs have been shown to require the lymphatic EC-displayed CCL21 to enter the lumen of lymphatics in a CCR7-dependent manner.[534,535]

In addition, CCR7 can be upregulated by molecules released from damaged or inflamed cells, including prostaglandin E2[536,537] and extracellular NAD$^+$.[536] Notably, however, while DC migration across the subcapsular sinus lymphatic EC layer is CCR7 dependent, T-cell migration across the sinus lymphatic ECs is completely independent of CCR7 signaling.[538] Thus, the CCL21-CCR7 axis does not appear to be the only regulator of immune cell trafficking across the LN subcapsular sinus.

Under inflammatory conditions, the chemokine CX3CL1 (fractalkine) appears on lymphatic ECs and is actively secreted, and soluble rather than membrane-anchored chemokine promotes

DC migration toward lymphatics and transmigration across lymphatic ECs.[539] Inflammation also induces CXCL12 on the surface of lymphatic ECs, allowing DCs to migrate across these cells in a CXCL12/CXCR4-dependent manner.[540] In lymphocytes, CXCL12 acts in synergy with CCR7 ligands to promote cell migration by sensitizing the cells through CXCR4, thus enabling them to respond to lower concentrations of CCR7 ligands.[541] Given that mature DCs also express both CCR7 and CXCR4 at levels comparable with those on lymphocytes, chemokine-induced synergy may also enhance DC recruitment into lymphatics under certain conditions. CCL1 expressed by the subcapsular sinus lymphatic ECs of skin-draining LNs promotes DC migration into the LN parenchyma, but not by capillary lymphatic vessels in the skin, and inhibition of the CCL1/CCR8 interaction leads to impaired DC migration into the LN parenchyma.[542]

b. Adhesion molecules and their receptors. As previously mentioned, integrins are not required for DC migration into afferent lymphatics at steady state.[543] Podoplanin expressed on lymphatic ECs can capture CCL21 and also binds the lectin-type molecule CLEC-2. Podoplanin binding to CLEC-2 promotes the formation of actin-rich protrusions on DCs, which allow them to spread along stromal scaffolds and support DC motility.[544] Although ICAM-1 and VCAM-1 are expressed at low levels in lymphatic ECs, they are strongly upregulated during inflammation and, therefore, can interact with β2 integrins (LFA-1 and Mac-1)[545] and β1 integrin VLA-4, respectively, to contribute to DC migration.[546] Lymphatic ECs promote DC transmigration by producing the immunomodulatory molecule semaphorin 3A, which binds plexin A1 on DCs to promote actomyosin contraction as well as, possibly, to induce the disassembly of adhesive components at the trailing edge of DCs.[547]

Lymphocyte Migration Across the Lymphoid Tissue Parenchyma

Once lymphocytes have entered the LNs, they search for antigen by moving in the cell-dense, highly constrained parenchyma. Integrin-independent, Rho-dependent interstitial T-cell motility has been shown to be regulated by ATX produced by LN stromal cells.[548] ATX on the cell surface of FRCs generates LPA through its enzymatic activity, and LPA enhances lymphocyte motility through the densely packed reticular network with high levels of biologically relevant LPA species expressed in the LN paracortex at sites that are either close to or distant from HEVs.[549] Intravital two-photon microscopic analysis showed that T-cell migration in the parenchyma is significantly attenuated in the conditional ATX-deficient mice compared with control mice and that T-cell motility and Rho-ROCK-myosin II pathway activation in response to LPA depends on LPA receptor LPA2 expression on the T-cell surface.[549] Together, these results suggest that the LPA generated by FRCs acts locally on T cells via LPA2, thereby regulating T-cell contractility and motility in the LN reticular network.

In addition, chemokines direct naïve lymphocytes to their compartmental homing, that is, T cells to the paracortex and B cells to the follicles once they have crossed the HEV. CCL21 is expressed not only on HEVs but also by stromal cells within the T-cell areas of LNs, spleen, and PPs. A second ligand for CCR7 is CCL19 (ELC, Epstein-Barr virus–induced molecule-1 ligand chemokine), which is also expressed in T-cell areas and is made by macrophages and the DCs of the paracortex. In vitro, the CCL21 and CCL19 attract T cells effectively and B cells weakly. This process is described in more detail in Chapter 13. In summary, CCL21 and CCL19 chemokines bind to their receptor CCR7 and stimulate T-cell crossing of the HEV, whereas B cells cross the HEV using more than one chemokine/receptor system.

Lymphocyte Egress From Lymphoid Tissues

Egress of lymphocytes from lymphoid tissues is currently thought to be regulated primarily by S1P, which is structurally similar to LPA. S1P acts on a family of five GPCRs (S1P1-S1P5) and is rapidly degraded into a biologically inactive form by S1P phosphatases and S1P lyase in vivo.[550]

S1P regulates lymphocyte migration through its differential expression in tissues, resulting in a chemotactic gradient. The concentration of S1P is high in the peripheral blood owing to its release from erythrocytes and vascular ECs. In contrast, S1P levels are low in lymphoid tissues because of an abundance of S1P lyase. Thus, the differential concentration of S1P between the blood and lymphoid tissue is thought to drive lymphocyte emigration from lymphoid tissues. Lymphocytes within the lymphoid tissues express high levels of the S1P receptor, S1P1, and thus migrate in response to the S1P gradient. In contrast, peripheral blood lymphocytes express low levels of S1P1, as a result of downregulation by internalization in response to the high S1P concentration in the blood. When blood-borne lymphocytes enter lymphoid tissues, S1P1 is upregulated because of the lack of S1P in the tissue. Within the LNs, the lymphocytes are then transported to the cortical sinuses, the medullary sinus, and finally to the efferent lymphatics, by sensing the S1P concentration gradient in an S1P1-dependent manner. This cyclical change in lymphocyte S1P1 expression, which has been proposed to direct lymphocyte egress from the LNs, has been proposed to similarly regulate lymphocyte egress from the thymus.[551] Although this model of lymphocyte egress is currently favored, a number of findings do not entirely support this model. First, S1P1 transcripts are also abundant in the ECs and vascular smooth muscle cells surrounding blood vessels, and strong S1P1 activation is detected in both the lymphatic and vascular ECs in lymphoid tissues, where most lymphocytes show no evidence of S1P1 activation under homeostatic conditions.[552] Second, despite S1P1 also being expressed at high levels on other cell types such as macrophages, DCs, and NK cells, only lymphocytes exit the LNs in response to physiologic concentrations of S1P. This could be because of cell type–specific effects, but these findings also indicate that S1P's role in regulating lymphocyte egress likely is more complex than currently conceived.

S1P also appears to regulate the barrier function of HEVs in antigen-stimulated LNs. Studies in mesenteric LNs have shown that platelets migrate across HEVs together with lymphocytes in mesenteric LNs and are activated by specific interactions between the platelet cell surface lectin CLEC-2 and podoplanin, expressed on the surrounding FRCs,[553] resulting in secretion of S1P, which stimulates the HEVs to maintain their vascular integrity. Because the effect of the podoplanin-CLEC-2 interaction on HEV integrity has only been detected in mesenteric LNs where exogenous antigens are abundant and in peripheral LNs only in the context of immunization, these findings suggest that this mechanism is important under inflammatory conditions.

LYMPH NODE ALTERATIONS IN LYMPHOMA

Lymphomas involving LNs and other sites show characteristic histologic changes that inform their classification. Frequently, lymphoma cells are accompanied by distinct inflammatory infiltrates with characteristic cellular compositions, particularly in tumors such as Hodgkin lymphoma, certain peripheral T-cell lymphomas such as angioimmunoblastic T-cell lymphoma (AITL), and polymorphic posttransplant lymphoproliferative disorders. Other lymphomas, such as marginal zone lymphoma, mantle cell lymphoma, and follicular lymphoma (FL), can show features that retain or recapitulate normal LN architecture. In others such as Burkitt lymphoma, diffuse large B-cell lymphoma, and anaplastic large cell lymphoma, the normal tissue architecture is characteristically effaced by sheets of lymphoma cells and the accompanying microenvironment populations are relatively less abundant (*Figure 11.14*). Regardless of the specific cellular or architectural alteration in lymphomas, similar to many nonhematopoietic malignancies, growing evidence supports a model in which lymphoma cells engage in novel interactions, associations, and interdependencies with the immune and stromal cells of the tumor microenvironment that supply essential prolymphoma survival and proliferation signals and modulate host antitumor immunity.[320,554-571]

B-cell lymphomas provoke a host of changes to the composition, distribution, and transcriptional activity of the normal lymph node cellularity (*Figure 11.14*). In the Hodgkin lymphomas, infrequent large

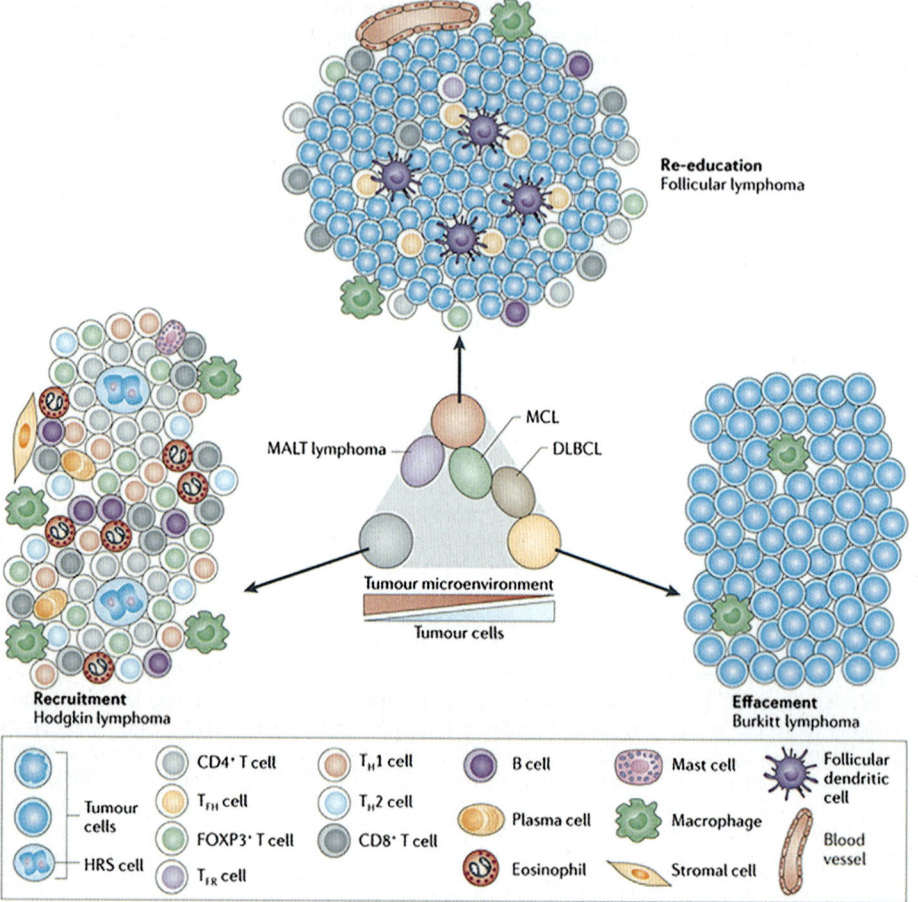

FIGURE 11.14 Spectrum of lymph node alterations in B-cell lymphomas. B-cell lymphomas induce a broad spectrum of changes to the composition and distribution of the normal lymph node cellularity. In classic Hodgkin lymphoma, infrequent tumor cells (e.g., Hodgkin cells) recruit a polymorphous inflammatory infiltrate that comprises the vast majority of the tumor cellularity. In follicular lymphoma, neoplastic B cells reprogram the transcriptional activity of normal lymph node leukocyte and stromal cell populations (e.g., FDCs) in order to support lymphomagenesis and FL cell survival. In Burkitt lymphoma, the normal nodal architecture and cellularity is effaced by sheets of high-grade neoplastic B cells. FOXP3, forkhead box protein P3; MALT, mucosa-associated lymphoid tissue; MCL, mantle cell lymphoma; TFH, follicular T helper; TFR, follicular regulatory T. (Reprinted by permission from Nature: Scott DW, Gascoyne RD. The tumour microenvironment in B cell lymphomas. *Nat Rev Cancer.* 2014;14(8):517-534. Copyright © 2014 Springer Nature.)

neoplastic lymphoid cells can recruit a dense infiltrate of reactive immune and stromal cells that can comprise over 95% of the tumor cellularity. In nodular lymphocyte predominant Hodgkin lymphoma, scattered large lymphoma cells are admixed with large nodules of small reactive B cells (*Figure 11.15B*). By contrast, most classic Hodgkin lymphoma (cHL) histologic subtypes recruit a more polymorphous inflammatory infiltrate consisting of T cells, neutrophils, eosinophils, plasma cells, histiocytes, fibroblasts, and other cell types.[572] The orchestration of these distinctive tumor microenvironments is facilitated by the secretion of numerous chemokines and cytokines directly by the transformed lymphoid cells and by the microenvironment populations with which they interact. In cHL, for example, Hodgkin/Reed-Sternberg (HRS) cells secrete colony-stimulating factor 1 (CSF1) and CX3CL1, which likely help to recruit macrophages. Because the CSF1 receptor-enriched microenvironment is associated with worse survival, this signaling axis provides a potential therapeutic target.[572] Macrophages, in turn, produce IL-8, which recruits neutrophils into the tumor tissue, whereas IL-5 production by HRS cells attracts eosinophils.[556] HRS cells also express CD30, allowing them to interact with CD30 ligand expressed on eosinophils and mast cells.[573,574] HRS cells produce TGF-ß, IL-10, galectin-1, and prostaglandin E2 and express PD-L1, which collectively can promote T-cell anergy.[575] In EBV+ cases of cHL, the latency type II pattern includes the expression of Latent Membrane Protein 1 (LMP1), LMP2, and Epstein-Barr nuclear antigen-1. Oncogene LMP1 mimics CD40 activation, whereas LMP2 mimics BCR signaling.[576,577] CD40, in turn, interacts with surrounding T cells expressing CD40 ligand, leading to prosurvival signaling.[578-582]

In some lymphomas, nonhematopoietic stromal cell populations are essential for lymphomagenesis. Follicular lymphoma, which primarily occurs in lymph nodes and manifests as B-cell aggregates

associated with FDCs, is a paradigmatic example of the critical bidirectional cross talk between lymphoma cells and certain LN stromal cell subtypes, namely, FDCs and FRCs, whose transcriptional activity is reprogrammed to promote the competitive fitness of the neoplastic clone. In a murine model of early *EZH2*[Y641]-driven follicular lymphomagenesis, FL-associated FDCs were found to support the survival and expansion of neoplastic centrocytes in a T_{FH} cell–independent fashion, which, in contrast to wild-type centrocytes, was diminished in the presence of FDC blockade with recombinant lymphotoxin-β receptor.[320] In addition to FDCs, FL-associated FRCs are also important, if not essential, for FL pathogenesis as suggested by in vitro studies in which FRCs were able to sustain the survival and proliferation of FL centrocytes but not normal germinal center centrocytes.[558] These interactions are mediated at least in part through bidirectional TNF and TGFβ cross talk between FL cells and FDCs or FRCs, leading to transcriptional alterations that support FL survival and expansion, including expression of *CXCL12, CCL19*, and *CCL21* (*Figure 11.15*). Other changes observed in FL include increased numbers of T_{regs} and decreased effector T cells compared with normal LNs, with lesions showing a follicular pattern of Foxp3+ T cells showing increased risk of transformation and shorter survival than those who had a diffuse pattern.[583] The presence of PD-1+ T cells in follicles also is associated with longer time to transformation.[584]

FL cells not only benefit from tumor-promoting properties of recruited and reeducated nonmalignant cellular elements but also manage to escape immune surveillance. When FL cells are incubated with autologous T cells, defects of T-cell synapse formation are observed.[585] Furthermore, CREBBP mutations have been associated with reduced expression of MHC class II,[586] whereas B2M mutations, resulting in loss of MHC class I, are more typical of transformed FL.[587,588] Overall, these findings suggest that FL is not just a passive colonizer of existing

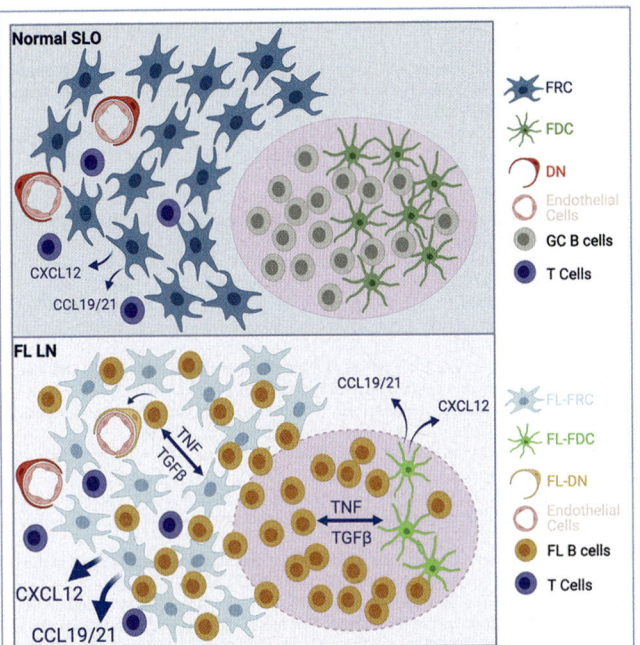

FIGURE 11.15 Transcriptional remodeling of FL-associated lymph node stromal cells (LNSCs). FL B cells and LNSCs engage in TNF and TGF-B-mediated bidirectional cross talk. These interactions prompt alterations in FRC and FDC transcriptional activity, which support FL pathogenesis such as increased expression of CCL19, CCL21, and CXCL12. FL-FRC, follicular lymphoma-associated fibroblastic reticular cell; FDC, follicular lymphoma-associated follicular dendritic cell; FL-DN, follicular lymphoma-associated double-negative (PDPN-/CD31-) lymph node stromal cell. (Reprinted from Mourcin F, Verdière L, Roulois D, et al. Follicular lymphoma triggers phenotypic and functional remodeling of the human lymphoid stromal cell landscape. *Immunity.* 2021;54(8):1788-1806.e7. Copyright © 2021 Elsevier. With permission.)

secondary lymphoid structure, but instead "reeducates" or "reprograms" the tumor microenvironment to promote its own growth and survival while simultaneously escaping immune surveillance.[586] The observation that the vast majority of FLs express surface immunoglobulin (sIg) despite ongoing somatic hypermutation implies positive selection for sIg expression.[589-592] Unlike other B-cell malignancies, the usage of IGHV genes is not stereotyped, suggesting that antigen selection may not play a major role in the expansion of FL cells. While self-antigen recognition was documented to occur in FL,[590,591] a more common explanation underlying continuing sIg expression may reside in frequent N-glycosylation motifs that are introduced during somatic hypermutation and are characteristic of FL, being present in 80% of cases, while these motifs are uncommon in other B-cell malignancies and in normal B cells.[592] Such motifs are relevant because they allow for the addition of unusual, high-mannose terminated glycans in V regions, whereas constant regions are fully glycosylated.[593] Mannosylated sIg binds C-type lectins such as DC-SIGN or the mannose receptor,[594] resulting in activation of intracellular signaling pathways.[595] Lectins are expressed, for example, by tumor-associated macrophages that can be found in the TME to varying extents.[596] In summary, high mannose in sIg represents an additional mechanism by which FL cells thrive in a tumor-supportive milieu.

In the case of T-cell lymphomas, the role of the microenvironment is perhaps best illustrated by AITL, which is characterized by arborizing HEVs, irregular perivascular proliferation of FDCs in close contact with neoplastic cells and vessels, and a polymorphic cellular infiltrate. The lymphoproliferation itself usually shows a characteristic diffuse morphologic pattern (pattern III), with a smaller number of lesions showing pattern I (hyperplastic follicles) or pattern II (depleted follicles).[597,598] These changes can be understood given the presumptive derivation of AITL from T_{FH} cells, which normally reside in GCs where they interact with GC B cells to promote

B-cell survival, Ig class-switch recombination, and somatic hypermutation.[599] Consistent with their T_{FH} derivation, AITL cells show high expression of CXCL13 and IL-21,[600-603] which are critical for B-cell recruitment into GCs and subsequent activation. AITL cells also express T_{FH}-associated antigens, including costimulatory models such as PD-1, CD200, ICOS, and CD40L, which favor strong interactions with B cells and consequently B-cell responses. AITL cells also express SAP, c-MAF,[604,605] and CXCR5 (the CXCL13 receptor), which promote T_{FH} localization to GCs, as well as LTβ,[606,607] which, based on its role in normal LNs, likely induces the FDC proliferation that characterizes these lesions. AITL cells also promote the formation of the prominent vascularization that gives this disease its name through their production of VEGF and angiopoietin 1.[608,609] Interestingly, when increased numbers of AITL cells accumulate, parallel decreases in the accompanying inflammatory infiltrate and/or FDC cells are frequently observed, giving rise to a morphologic picture that can mimic peripheral T-cell lymphoma.[610] Thus, while AITL initially appears to depend on supportive signals from FDCs like other GC-derived lymphomas, AITL cell growth may become independent of interactions with the microenvironment with disease progression.

References

1. Ellis RE. The distribution of active bone marrow in the adult. *Phys Med Biol.* 1961;5:255-258.
2. Woodard HQ, Holodny E. A summary of the data of mechanik on the distribution of human bone marrow. *Phys Med Biol.* 1960;5:57-59.
3. Nombela-Arrieta C, Manz MG. Quantification and three-dimensional microanatomical organization of the bone marrow. *Blood Adv.* 2017;1(6):407-416.
4. Dancey JT, Deubelbeiss KA, Harker LA, Finch CA. Neutrophil kinetics in man. *J Clin Invest.* 1976;58(3):705-715.
5. Harker LA, Finch CA. Thrombokinetics in man. *J Clin Invest.* 1969;48(6):963-974.
6. Kaushansky K. Lineage-specific hematopoietic growth factors. *N Engl J Med.* 2006;354(19):2034-2045.
7. Palis J. Primitive and definitive erythropoiesis in mammals. *Front Physiol.* 2014;5:3.
8. Potten CS, Loeffler M. Stem cells: attributes, cycles, spirals, pitfalls and uncertainties. Lessons for and from the crypt. *Development.* 1990;110(4):1001-1020.
9. Sender R, Fuchs S, Milo R. Revised estimates for the number of human and bacteria cells in the body. *PLoS Biol.* 2016;14(8):e1002533.
10. Lichtman MA. The ultrastructure of the hemopoietic environment of the marrow: a review. *Exp Hematol.* 1981;9(4):391-410.
11. Mercier FE, Ragu C, Scadden DT. The bone marrow at the crossroads of blood and immunity. *Nat Rev Immunol.* 2011;12(1):49-60.
12. Crane GM, Jeffery E, Morrison SJ. Adult haematopoietic stem cell niches. *Nat Rev Immunol.* 2017;17(9):573-590.
13. Itkin T, Gur-Cohen S, Spencer JA, et al. Distinct bone marrow blood vessels differentially regulate haematopoiesis. *Nature.* 2016;532(7599):323-328.
14. Casanova-Acebes M, Pitaval C, Weiss LA, et al. Rhythmic modulation of the hematopoietic niche through neutrophil clearance. *Cell.* 2013;153(5):1025-1035.
15. Kunisaki Y, Bruns I, Scheiermann C, et al. Arteriolar niches maintain haematopoietic stem cell quiescence. *Nature.* 2013;502(7473):637-643.
16. Kusumbe AP, Ramasamy SK, Itkin T, et al. Age-dependent modulation of vascular niches for haematopoietic stem cells. *Nature.* 2016;532(7599):380-384.
17. Smith-Berdan S, Schepers K, Ly A, Passegue E, Forsberg EC. Dynamic expression of the robo ligand Slit2 in bone marrow cell populations. *Cell Cycle.* 2012;11(4):675-682.
18. Zhou BO, Yue R, Murphy MM, Peyer JG, Morrison SJ. Leptin-receptor-expressing mesenchymal stromal cells represent the main source of bone formed by adult bone marrow. *Cell Stem Cell.* 2014;15(2):154-168.
19. Acar M, Kocherlakota KS, Murphy MM, et al. Deep imaging of bone marrow shows non-dividing stem cells are mainly perisinusoidal. *Nature.* 2015;526(7571):126-130.
20. Clarke B. Normal bone anatomy and physiology. *Clin J Am Soc Nephrol.* 2008;3(suppl 3):S131-S139.
21. Kiel MJ, Iwashita T, Yilmaz OH, Morrison SJ. Spatial differences in hematopoiesis but not in stem cells indicate a lack of regional patterning in definitive hematopoietic stem cells. *Dev Biol.* 2005;283(1):29-39.
22. Lassailly F, Foster K, Lopez-Onieva L, Currie E, Bonnet D. Multimodal imaging reveals structural and functional heterogeneity in different bone marrow compartments: functional implications on hematopoietic stem cells. *Blood.* 2013;122(10):1730-1740.
23. Spencer JA, Ferraro F, Roussakis E, et al. Direct measurement of local oxygen concentration in the bone marrow of live animals. *Nature.* 2014;508(7495):269-273.
24. Nombela-Arrieta C, Silberstein LE. The science behind the hypoxic niche of hematopoietic stem and progenitors. *Hematology Am Soc Hematol Educ Program.* 2014;2014(1):542-547.
25. Morrison SJ, Scadden DT. The bone marrow niche for haematopoietic stem cells. *Nature.* 2014;505(7483):327-334.
26. Visnjic D, Kalajzic Z, Rowe DW, Katavic V, Lorenzo J, Aguila HL. Hematopoiesis is severely altered in mice with an induced osteoblast deficiency. *Blood.* 2004;103(9):3258-3264.
27. Zhu J, Garrett R, Jung Y, et al. Osteoblasts support B-lymphocyte commitment and differentiation from hematopoietic stem cells. *Blood.* 2007;109(9):3706-3712.

The Normal Hematologic System

28. Cordeiro Gomes A, Hara T, Lim V Y, et al. Hematopoietic stem cell niches produce lineage-instructive signals to control multipotent progenitor differentiation. *Immunity.* 2016;45(6):1219-1231.

29. Loken MR, Shah VO, Dattilio KL, Civin CI. Flow cytometric analysis of human bone marrow. II. Normal B lymphocyte development. *Blood.* 1987;70(5):1316-1324.

30. Longacre TA, Foucar K, Crago S, et al. Hematogones: a multiparameter analysis of bone marrow precursor cells. *Blood.* 1989;73(2):543-552.

31. Egawa T, Kawabata K, Kawamoto H, et al. The earliest stages of B cell development require a chemokine stromal cell-derived factor/pre-B cell growth-stimulating factor. *Immunity.* 2001;15(2):323-334.

32. Sitnicka E, Brakebusch C, Martensson IL, et al. Complementary signaling through flt3 and interleukin-7 receptor alpha is indispensable for fetal and adult B cell genesis. *J Exp Med.* 2003;198(10):1495-1506.

33. Delves PJ, Roitt IM. The immune system. Second of two parts. *N Engl J Med.* 2000;343(2):108-117.

34. Haynes BF, Markert ML, Sempowski GD, Patel DD, Hale LP. The role of the thymus in immune reconstitution in aging, bone marrow transplantation, and HIV-1 infection. *Annu Rev Immunol.* 2000;18:529-560.

35. Hollander G, Gill J, Zuklys S, Iwanami N, Liu C, Takahama Y. Cellular and molecular events during early thymus development. *Immunol Rev.* 2006;209:28-46.

36. Varga I, Pospisilova V, Jablonska-Mestanova V, Galfiova P, Polak S. The thymus: picture review of human thymus prenatal development. *Bratisl Lek Listy.* 2011;112(7):368-376.

37. Le Douarin NM, Jotereau FV. Tracing of cells of the avian thymus through embryonic life in interspecific chimeras. *J Exp Med.* 1975;142(1):17-40.

38. Dupin E, Creuzet S, Le Douarin NM. The contribution of the neural crest to the vertebrate body. *Adv Exp Med Biol.* 2006;589:96-119.

39. Kendall MD, Johnson HR, Singh J. The weight of the human thymus gland at necropsy. *J Anat.* 1980;131(pt 3):483-497.

40. Haynes BF. The human thymic microenvironment. *Adv Immunol.* 1984;36:87-142.

41. Lobach DF, Scearce RM, Haynes BF. The human thymic microenvironment. Phenotypic characterization of Hassall's bodies with the use of monoclonal antibodies. *J Immunol.* 1985;134(1):250-257.

42. Fend F, Nachbaur D, Oberwasserlechner F, Kreczy A, Huber H, Muller-Hermelink HK. Phenotype and topography of human thymic B cells. An immunohistologic study. *Virchows Arch B Cell Pathol Incl Mol Pathol.* 1991;60(6):381-388.

43. Hofmann WJ, Momburg F, Moller P, Otto HF. Intra- and extrathymic B cells in physiologic and pathologic conditions. Immunohistochemical study on normal thymus and lymphofollicular hyperplasia of the thymus. *Virchows Arch A Pathol Anat Histopathol.* 1988;412(5):431-442.

44. Isaacson PG, Norton AJ, Addis BJ. The human thymus contains a novel population of B lymphocytes. *Lancet.* 1987;2(8574):1488-1491.

45. Hollander GA, Wang B, Nichogiannopoulou A, et al. Developmental control point in induction of thymic cortex regulated by a subpopulation of prothymocytes. *Nature.* 1995;373(6512):350-353.

46. Ritter MA, Boyd RL. Development in the thymus: it takes two to tango. *Immunol Today.* 1993;14(9):462-469.

47. Hendrix TM, Chilukuri RV, Martinez M, et al. Thymic nurse cells exhibit epithelial progenitor phenotype and create unique extra-cytoplasmic membrane space for thymocyte selection. *Cell Immunol.* 2010;261(2):81-92.

48. Bhandoola A, Sambandam A, Allman D, Meraz A, Schwarz B. Early T lineage progenitors: new insights, but old questions remain. *J Immunol.* 2003;171(11):5653-5658.

49. Takahama Y. Journey through the thymus: stromal guides for T-cell development and selection. *Nat Rev Immunol.* 2006;6(2):127-135.

50. Kronenberg M, Engel I. On the road: progress in finding the unique pathway of invariant NKT cell differentiation. *Curr Opin Immunol.* 2007;19(2):186-193.

51. Gapin L, Matsuda JL, Surh CD, Kronenberg M. NKT cells derive from double-positive thymocytes that are positively selected by CD1d. *Nat Immunol.* 2001;2(10):971-978.

52. Burt TD. Fetal regulatory T cells and peripheral immune tolerance in utero: implications for development and disease. *Am J Reprod Immunol.* 2013;69(4):346-358.

53. Haynes BF, Martin ME, Kay HH, Kurtzberg J. Early events in human T cell ontogeny. Phenotypic characterization and immunohistologic localization of T cell precursors in early human fetal tissues. *J Exp Med.* 1988;168(3):1061-1080.

54. Cupedo T, Nagasawa M, Weijer K, Blom B, Spits H. Development and activation of regulatory T cells in the human fetus. *Eur J Immunol.* 2005;35(2):383-390.

55. Michaelsson J, Mold JE, McCune JM, Nixon DF. Regulation of T cell responses in the developing human fetus. *J Immunol.* 2006;176(10):5741-5748.

56. Sakaguchi S, Sakaguchi N, Asano M, Itoh M, Toda M. Immunologic self-tolerance maintained by activated T cells expressing IL-2 receptor alpha-chains (CD25). Breakdown of a single mechanism of self-tolerance causes various autoimmune diseases. *J Immunol.* 1995;155(3):1151-1164.

57. Dalmasso AP, Martinez C, Sjodin K, Good RA. Studies on the role of the thymus in immunobiology; reconstitution of immunologic capacity in mice thymectomized at birth. *J Exp Med.* 1963;118:1089-1109.

58. Sakaguchi S, Takahashi T, Nishizuka Y. Study on cellular events in postthymectomy autoimmune oophoritis in mice. I. Requirement of Lyt-1 effector cells for oocytes damage after adoptive transfer. *J Exp Med.* 1982;156(6):1565-1576.

59. Mancebo E, Clemente J, Sanchez J, et al. Longitudinal analysis of immune function in the first 3 years of life in thymectomized neonates during cardiac surgery. *Clin Exp Immunol.* 2008;154(3):375-383.

60. Wells WJ, Parkman R, Smogorzewska E, Barr M. Neonatal thymectomy: does it affect immune function? *J Thorac Cardiovasc Surg.* 1998;115(5):1041-1046.

61. Silva SL, Albuquerque A, Amaral AJ, et al. Autoimmunity and allergy control in adults submitted to complete thymectomy early in infancy. *PLoS One.* 2017;12(7):e0180385.

62. Silva SL, Albuquerque AS, Serra-Caetano A, et al. Human naive regulatory T-cells feature high steady-state turnover and are maintained by IL-7. *Oncotarget.* 2016;7(11):12163-12175.

63. Prelog M, Keller M, Geiger R, et al. Thymectomy in early childhood: significant alterations of the CD4(+)CD45RA(+)CD62L(+) T cell compartment in later life. *Clin Immunol.* 2009;130(2):123-132.

64. van den Broek T, Delemarre EM, Janssen WJ, et al. Neonatal thymectomy reveals differentiation and plasticity within human naive T cells. *J Clin Invest.* 2016;126(3):1126-1136.

65. Anderson G, Takahama Y. Thymic epithelial cells: working class heroes for T cell development and repertoire selection. *Trends Immunol.* 2012;33(6):256-263.

66. Klein L, Kyewski B, Allen PM, Hogquist KA. Positive and negative selection of the T cell repertoire: what thymocytes see (and don't see). *Nat Rev Immunol.* 2014;14(6):377-391.

67. Gordon J, Wilson VA, Blair NF, et al. Functional evidence for a single endodermal origin for the thymic epithelium. *Nat Immunol.* 2004;5(5):546-553.

68. Anderson G, Lane PJ, Jenkinson EJ. Generating intrathymic microenvironments to establish T-cell tolerance. *Nat Rev Immunol.* 2007;7(12):954-963.

69. Boehm T. Thymus development and function. *Curr Opin Immunol.* 2008;20(2):178-184.

70. Blackburn CC, Augustine CL, Li R, et al. The nu gene acts cell-autonomously and is required for differentiation of thymic epithelial progenitors. *Proc Natl Acad Sci U S A.* 1996;93(12):5742-5746.

71. Nehls M, Kyewski B, Messerle M, et al. Two genetically separable steps in the differentiation of thymic epithelium. *Science.* 1996;272(5263):886-889.

72. Nehls M, Pfeifer D, Schorpp M, Hedrich H, Boehm T. New member of the winged-helix protein family disrupted in mouse and rat nude mutations. *Nature.* 1994;372(6501):103-107.

73. Vigliano I, Gorrese M, Fusco A, et al. FOXN1 mutation abrogates prenatal T-cell development in humans. *J Med Genet.* 2011;48(6):413-416.

74. Itoi M, Tsukamoto N, Amagai T. Expression of Dll4 and CCL25 in Foxn1-negative epithelial cells in the post-natal thymus. *Int Immunol.* 2007;19(2):127-132.

75. Zuklys S, Gill J, Keller MP, et al. Stabilized beta-catenin in thymic epithelial cells blocks thymus development and function. *J Immunol.* 2009;182(5):2997-3007.

76. Candi E, Rufini A, Terrinoni A, et al. DeltaNp63 regulates thymic development through enhanced expression of FgfR2 and Jag2. *Proc Natl Acad Sci U S A.* 2007;104(29):11999-12004.

77. Liu B, Liu YF, Du YR, et al. Cbx4 regulates the proliferation of thymic epithelial cells and thymus function. *Development.* 2013;140(4):780-788.

78. Senoo M, Pinto F, Crum CP, McKeon F. p63 Is essential for the proliferative potential of stem cells in stratified epithelia. *Cell.* 2007;129(3):523-536.

79. Bleul CC, Corbeaux T, Reuter A, Fisch P, Monting JS, Boehm T. Formation of a functional thymus initiated by a postnatal epithelial progenitor cell. *Nature.* 2006;441(7096):992-996.

80. Rossi SW, Jenkinson WE, Anderson G, Jenkinson EJ. Clonal analysis reveals a common progenitor for thymic cortical and medullary epithelium. *Nature.* 2006;441(7096):988-991.

81. Baik S, Jenkinson EJ, Lane PJ, Anderson G, Jenkinson WE. Generation of both cortical and Aire(+) medullary thymic epithelial compartments from CD205(+) progenitors. *Eur J Immunol.* 2013;43(3):589-594.

82. Shakib S, Desanti GE, Jenkinson WE, Parnell SM, Jenkinson EJ, Anderson G. Checkpoints in the development of thymic cortical epithelial cells. *J Immunol.* 2009;182(1):130-137.

83. Ohigashi I, Zuklys S, Sakata M, et al. Aire-expressing thymic medullary epithelial cells originate from beta5t-expressing progenitor cells. *Proc Natl Acad Sci U S A.* 2013;110(24):9885-9890.

84. Ribeiro AR, Rodrigues PM, Meireles C, Di Santo JP, Alves NL. Thymocyte selection regulates the homeostasis of IL-7-expressing thymic cortical epithelial cells in vivo. *J Immunol.* 2013;191(3):1200-1209.

85. Klug DB, Carter C, Conti GC, Richie ER. Cutting edge: thymocyte-independent and thymocyte-dependent phases of epithelial patterning in the fetal thymus. *J Immunol.* 2002;169(6):2842-2845.

86. Ripen AM, Nitta T, Murata S, Tanaka K, Takahama Y. Ontogeny of thymic cortical epithelial cells expressing the thymoproteasome subunit beta5t. *Eur J Immunol.* 2011;41(5):1278-1287.

87. Calderon L, Boehm T. Synergistic, context-dependent, and hierarchical functions of epithelial components in thymic microenvironments. *Cell.* 2012;149(1):159-172.

88. Hozumi K, Mailhos C, Negishi N, et al. Delta-like 4 is indispensable in thymic environment specific for T cell development. *J Exp Med.* 2008;205(11):2507-2513.

89. Koch U, Fiorini E, Benedito R, et al. Delta-like 4 is the essential, nonredundant ligand for Notch1 during thymic T cell lineage commitment. *J Exp Med.* 2008;205(11):2515-2523.

90. Hara T, Shitara S, Imai K, et al. Identification of IL-7-producing cells in primary and secondary lymphoid organs using IL-7-GFP knock-in mice. *J Immunol.* 2012;189(4):1577-1584.

91. Boudil A, Matei IR, Shih HY, et al. IL-7 coordinates proliferation, differentiation and Tcra recombination during thymocyte beta-selection. *Nat Immunol.* 2015;16(4):397-405.

92. Moore TA, von, Freeden-Jeffry U, Murray R, Zlotnik A. Inhibition of gamma delta T cell development and early thymocyte maturation in IL-7 -/- mice. *J Immunol.* 1996;157(6):2366-2373.

93. Shitara S, Hara T, Liang B, et al. IL-7 produced by thymic epithelial cells plays a major role in the development of thymocytes and TCRgammadelta+ intraepithelial lymphocytes. *J Immunol.* 2013;190(12):6173-6179.

94. Ara T, Itoi M, Kawabata K, et al. A role of CXC chemokine ligand 12/stromal cell-derived factor-1/pre-B cell growth stimulating factor and its receptor CXCR4 in fetal and adult T cell development in vivo. *J Immunol.* 2003;170(9):4649-4655.

95. Benz C, Heinzel K, Bleul CC. Homing of immature thymocytes to the subcapsular microenvironment within the thymus is not an absolute requirement for T cell development. *Eur J Immunol.* 2004;34(12):3652-3663.

96. Misslitz A, Pabst O, Hintzen G, et al. Thymic T cell development and progenitor localization depend on CCR7. *J Exp Med.* 2004;200(4):481-491.

97. Plotkin J, Prockop SE, Lepique A, Petrie HT. Critical role for CXCR4 signaling in progenitor localization and T cell differentiation in the postnatal thymus. *J Immunol.* 2003;171(9):4521-4527.

98. Trampont PC, Tosello-Trampont T., Shen Y, et al. CXCR4 acts as a costimulator during thymic beta-selection. *Nat Immunol.* 2010;11(2):162-170.

99. Bunting MD, Comerford I, Seach N, et al. CCX-CKR deficiency alters thymic stroma impairing thymocyte development and promoting autoimmunity. *Blood.* 2013;121(1):118-128.

100. Lucas B, White AJ, Ulvmar MH, et al. CCRL1/ACKR4 is expressed in key thymic microenvironments but is dispensable for T lymphopoiesis at steady state in adult mice. *Eur J Immunol.* 2015;45(2):574-583.

101. Rode I, Boehm T. Regenerative capacity of adult cortical thymic epithelial cells. *Proc Natl Acad Sci U S A.* 2012;109(9):3463-3468.

102. Prockop SE, Palencia S, Ryan CM, Gordon K, Gray D, Petrie HT. Stromal cells provide the matrix for migration of early lymphoid progenitors through the thymic cortex. *J Immunol.* 2002;169(8):4354-4361.

103. Takahama Y, Letterio JJ, Suzuki H, Farr AG, Singer A. Early progression of thymocytes along the CD4/CD8 developmental pathway is regulated by a subset of thymic epithelial cells expressing transforming growth factor beta. *J Exp Med.* 1994;179(5):1495-1506.

104. Murata S, Sasaki K, Kishimoto T, et al. Regulation of CD8+ T cell development by thymus-specific proteasomes. *Science.* 2007;316(5829):1349-1353.

105. Tomaru U, Ishizu A, Murata S, et al. Exclusive expression of proteasome subunit {beta}5t in the human thymic cortex. *Blood.* 2009;113(21):5186-5191.

106. Kloetzel PM. Antigen processing by the proteasome. *Nat Rev Mol Cell Biol.* 2001;2(3):179-187.

107. Tanaka K, Kasahara M. The MHC class I ligand-generating system: roles of immunoproteasomes and the interferon-gamma-inducible proteasome activator PA28. *Immunol Rev.* 1998;163:161-176.

108. Nitta T, Murata S, Sasaki K, et al. Thymoproteasome shapes immunocompetent repertoire of CD8+ T cells. *Immunity.* 2010;32(1):29-40.

109. Xing Y, Jameson SC, Hogquist KA. Thymoproteasome subunit-beta5T generates peptide-MHC complexes specialized for positive selection. *Proc Natl Acad Sci U S A.* 2013;110(17):6979-6984.

110. Sasaki K, Takada K, Ohte Y, et al. Thymoproteasomes produce unique peptide motifs for positive selection of CD8(+) T cells. *Nat Commun.* 2015;6:7484.

111. Takahama Y, Nitta T, Mat Ripen A, Nitta S, Murata S, Tanaka K. Role of thymic cortex-specific self-peptides in positive selection of T cells. *Semin Immunol.* 2010;22(5):287-293.

112. Bowlus CL, Ahn J, Chu T, Gruen JR. Cloning of a novel MHC-encoded serine peptidase highly expressed by cortical epithelial cells of the thymus. *Cell Immunol.* 1999;196(2):80-86.

113. Honey K, Rudensky AY. Lysosomal cysteine proteases regulate antigen presentation. *Nat Rev Immunol.* 2003;3(6):472-482.

114. Viret C, Leung-Theung-Long S, Serre L, et al. Thymus-specific serine protease controls autoreactive CD4 T cell development and autoimmune diabetes in mice. *J Clin Invest.* 2011;121(5):1810-1821.

115. Honey K, Nakagawa T, Peters C, Rudensky A. Cathepsin L regulates CD4+ T cell selection independently of its effect on invariant chain: a role in the generation of positively selecting peptide ligands. *J Exp Med.* 2002;195(10):1349-1358.

116. Nakagawa T, Roth W, Wong P, et al. Cathepsin L: critical role in Ii degradation and CD4 T cell selection in the thymus. *Science.* 1998;280(5362):450-453.

117. Gommeaux J, Gregoire C, Nguessan P, et al. Thymus-specific serine protease regulates positive selection of a subset of CD4+ thymocytes. *Eur J Immunol.* 2009;39(4):956-964.

118. Viret C, Lamare C, Guiraud M, et al. Thymus-specific serine protease contributes to the diversification of the functional endogenous CD4 T cell receptor repertoire. *J Exp Med.* 2011;208(1):3-11.

119. Shores EW, Van Ewijk W, Singer A. Disorganization and restoration of thymic medullary epithelial cells in T cell receptor-negative scid mice: evidence that receptor-bearing lymphocytes influence maturation of the thymic microenvironment. *Eur J Immunol.* 1991;21(7):1657-1661.

120. Stritesky GL, Xing Y, Erickson JR, et al. Murine thymic selection quantified using a unique method to capture deleted T cells. *Proc Natl Acad Sci U S A.* 2013;110(12):4679-4684.

121. McCaughtry TM, Baldwin TA, Wilken MS, Hogquist KA. Clonal deletion of thymocytes can occur in the cortex with no involvement of the medulla. *J Exp Med.* 2008;205(11):2575-2584.

122. Wekerle H, Ketelsen UP, Ernst M. Thymic nurse cells. Lymphoepithelial cell complexes in murine thymuses: morphological and serological characterization. *J Exp Med.* 1980;151(4):925-944.

123. Wekerle H, Ketelsen UP. Thymic nurse cells--Ia-bearing epithelium involved in T-lymphocyte differentiation? *Nature.* 1980;283(5745):402-404.

124. Pezzano M, Samms M, Martinez M, Guyden J. Questionable thymic nurse cell. *Microbiol Mol Biol Rev.* 2001;65(3):390-403.

125. Nitta T, Muro R, Shimizu Y, et al. The thymic cortical epithelium determines the TCR repertoire of IL-17-producing gammadeltaT cells. *EMBO Rep.* 2015;16(5):638-653.

126. Nitta T, Suzuki H. Thymic stromal cell subsets for T cell development. *Cell Mol Life Sci.* 2016;73(5):1021-1037.

127. Nakagawa Y, Ohigashi I, Nitta T, et al. Thymic nurse cells provide microenvironment for secondary T cell receptor alpha rearrangement in cortical thymocytes. *Proc Natl Acad Sci U S A.* 2012;109(50):20572-20577.

128. Guo J, Hawwari A, Li H, et al. Regulation of the TCRalpha repertoire by the survival window of CD4(+)CD8(+) thymocytes. *Nat Immunol.* 2002;3(5):469-476.

129. Ni PP, Solomon B, Hsieh CS, Allen PM, Morris GP. The ability to rearrange dual TCRs enhances positive selection, leading to increased Allo- and Autoreactive T cell repertoires. *J Immunol.* 2014;193(4):1778-1786.

130. Gray DH, Seach N, Ueno T, et al. Developmental kinetics, turnover, and stimulatory capacity of thymic epithelial cells. *Blood.* 2006;108(12):3777-3785.

131. Hamazaki Y, Fujita H, Kobayashi T, et al. Medullary thymic epithelial cells expressing Aire represent a unique lineage derived from cells expressing claudin. *Nat Immunol.* 2007;8(3):304-311.

132. Negishi I, Motoyama N, Nakayama K, et al. Essential role for ZAP-70 in both positive and negative selection of thymocytes. *Nature.* 1995;376(6539):435-438.

133. Philpott KL, Viney JL, Kay G, et al. Lymphoid development in mice congenitally lacking T cell receptor alpha beta-expressing cells. *Science.* 1992;256(5062):1448-1452.

134. Surh CD, Ernst B, Sprent J. Growth of epithelial cells in the thymic medulla is under the control of mature T cells. *J Exp Med.* 1992;176(2):611-616.

135. Akiyama T, Maeda S, Yamane S, et al. Dependence of self-tolerance on TRAF6-directed development of thymic stroma. *Science.* 2005;308(5719):248-251.

136. Burkly L, Hession C, Ogata L, et al. Expression of relB is required for the development of thymic medulla and dendritic cells. *Nature.* 1995;373(6514):531-536.

137. Kajiura F, Sun S, Nomura T, et al. NF-kappa B-inducing kinase establishes self-tolerance in a thymic stroma-dependent manner. *J Immunol.* 2004;172(4):2067-2075.

138. Kinoshita D, Hirota F, Kaisho T, et al. Essential role of IkappaB kinase alpha in thymic organogenesis required for the establishment of self-tolerance. *J Immunol.* 2006;176(7):3995-4002.

139. Naspetti M, Aurrand-Lions M, DeKoning J, et al. Thymocytes and RelB-dependent medullary epithelial cells provide growth-promoting and organization signals, respectively, to thymic medullary stromal cells. *Eur J Immunol.* 1997;27(6):1392-1397.

140. Weih F, Carrasco D, Durham SK, et al. Multiorgan inflammation and hematopoietic abnormalities in mice with a targeted disruption of RelB, a member of the NF-kappa B/Rel family. *Cell.* 1995;80(2):331-340.

141. Zhang B, Wang Z, Ding J, Peterson P, Gunning WT, Ding HF. NF-kappaB2 is required for the control of autoimmunity by regulating the development of medullary thymic epithelial cells. *J Biol Chem.* 2006;281(50):38617-38624.

142. Zhang X, Wang H, Claudio E, Brown K, Siebenlist U. A role for the IkappaB family member Bcl-3 in the control of central immunologic tolerance. *Immunity.* 2007;27(3):438-452.

143. Zhu M, Chin RK, Christiansen PA, et al. NF-kappaB2 is required for the establishment of central tolerance through an Aire-dependent pathway. *J Clin Invest.* 2006;116(11):2964-2971.

144. Akiyama T, Shimo Y, Yanai H, et al. The tumor necrosis factor family receptors RANK and CD40 cooperatively establish the thymic medullary microenvironment and self-tolerance. *Immunity.* 2008;29(3):423-437.

145. Boehm T, Scheu S, Pfeffer K, Bleul CC. Thymic medullary epithelial cell differentiation, thymocyte emigration, and the control of autoimmunity require lympho-epithelial cross talk via LTbetaR. *J Exp Med.* 2003;198(5):757-769.

146. Hikosaka Y, Nitta T, Ohigashi I, et al. The cytokine RANKL produced by positively selected thymocytes fosters medullary thymic epithelial cells that express autoimmune regulator. *Immunity.* 2008;29(3):438-450.

147. Rossi SW, Kim MY, Leibbrandt A, et al. RANK signals from CD4(+)3(-) inducer cells regulate development of Aire-expressing epithelial cells in the thymic medulla. *J Exp Med.* 2007;204(6):1267-1272.

148. Irla M, Guenot J, Sealy G, Reith W, Imhof BA, Serge A. Three-dimensional visualization of the mouse thymus organization in health and immunodeficiency. *J Immunol.* 2013;190(2):586-596.

149. Irla M, Guerri L, Guenot J, et al. Antigen recognition by autoreactive CD4(+) thymocytes drives homeostasis of the thymic medulla. *PLoS One.* 2012;7(12):e52591.

150. Irla M, Hugues S, Gill J, et al. Autoantigen-specific interactions with CD4+ thymocytes control mature medullary thymic epithelial cell cellularity. *Immunity.* 2008;29(3):451-463.

151. Jenkinson SR, Williams JA, Jeon H, et al. TRAF3 enforces the requirement for T cell cross-talk in thymic medullary epithelial development. *Proc Natl Acad Sci U S A.* 2013;110(52):21107-21112.

152. Williams JA, Zhang J, Jeon H, et al. Thymic medullary epithelium and thymocyte self-tolerance require cooperation between CD28-CD80/86 and CD40-CD40L costimulatory pathways. *J Immunol.* 2014;192(2):630-640.

153. White AJ, Jenkinson WE, Cowan JE, et al. An essential role for medullary thymic epithelial cells during the intrathymic development of invariant NKT cells. *J Immunol.* 2014;192(6):2659-2666.

154. White AJ, Withers DR, Parnell SM, et al. Sequential phases in the development of Aire-expressing medullary thymic epithelial cells involve distinct cellular input. *Eur J Immunol.* 2008;38(4):942-947.

155. Lkhagvasuren E, Sakata M, Ohigashi I, Takahama Y. Lymphotoxin beta receptor regulates the development of CCL21-expressing subset of postnatal medullary thymic epithelial cells. *J Immunol.* 2013;190(10):5110-5117.

The Normal Hematologic System

156. Seach N, Ueno T, Fletcher AL, et al. The lymphotoxin pathway regulates Aire-independent expression of ectopic genes and chemokines in thymic stromal cells. *J Immunol.* 2008;180(8):5384-5392.

157. Zhu M, Chin RK, Tumanov AV, Liu X, Fu YX. Lymphotoxin beta receptor is required for the migration and selection of autoreactive T cells in thymic medulla. *J Immunol.* 2007;179(12):8069-8075.

158. Mouri Y, Yano M, Shinzawa M, et al. Lymphotoxin signal promotes thymic organogenesis by eliciting RANK expression in the embryonic thymic stroma. *J Immunol.* 2011;186(9):5047-5057.

159. White AJ, Nakamura K, Jenkinson WE, et al. Lymphotoxin signals from positively selected thymocytes regulate the terminal differentiation of medullary thymic epithelial cells. *J Immunol.* 2010;185(8):4769-4776.

160. Akiyama N, Shinzawa M, Miyauchi M, et al. Limitation of immune tolerance-inducing thymic epithelial cell development by Spi-B-mediated negative feedback regulation. *J Exp Med.* 2014;211(12):2425-2438.

161. Khan IS, Mouchess ML, Zhu ML, et al. Enhancement of an anti-tumor immune response by transient blockade of central T cell tolerance. *J Exp Med.* 2014;211(5):761-768.

162. Otero DC, Baker DP, David M. IRF7-dependent IFN-beta production in response to RANKL promotes medullary thymic epithelial cell development. *J Immunol.* 2013;190(7):3289-3298.

163. Hauri-Hohl M, Zuklys S, Hollander GA, Ziegler SF. A regulatory role for TGF-beta signaling in the establishment and function of the thymic medulla. *Nat Immunol.* 2014;15(6):554-561.

164. Papadopoulou AS, Dooley J, Linterman MA, et al. The thymic epithelial microRNA network elevates the threshold for infection-associated thymic involution via miR-29a mediated suppression of the IFN-alpha receptor. *Nat Immunol.* 2011;13(2):181-187.

165. Zuklys S, Mayer CE, Zhanybekova S, et al. MicroRNAs control the maintenance of thymic epithelia and their competence for T lineage commitment and thymocyte selection. *J Immunol.* 2012;189(8):3894-3904.

166. Ueno T, Saito F, Gray DH, et al. CCR7 signals are essential for cortex-medulla migration of developing thymocytes. *J Exp Med.* 2004;200(4):493-505.

167. Kurobe H, Liu C, Ueno T, et al. CCR7-dependent cortex-to-medulla migration of positively selected thymocytes is essential for establishing central tolerance. *Immunity.* 2006;24(2):165-177.

168. Kwan J, Killeen N. CCR7 directs the migration of thymocytes into the thymic medulla. *J Immunol.* 2004;172(7):3999-4007.

169. Gray DH, Tull D, Ueno T, et al. A unique thymic fibroblast population revealed by the monoclonal antibody MTS-15. *J Immunol.* 2007;178(8):4956-4965.

170. McCaughtry TM, Wilken MS, Hogquist KA. Thymic emigration revisited. *J Exp Med.* 2007;204(11):2513-2520.

171. Nitta T, Nitta S, Lei Y, Lipp M, Takahama Y. CCR7-mediated migration of developing thymocytes to the medulla is essential for negative selection to tissue-restricted antigens. *Proc Natl Acad Sci U S A.* 2009;106(40):17129-17133.

172. Davalos-Misslitz AC, Rieckenberg J, Willenzon S, et al. Generalized multi-organ autoimmunity in CCR7-deficient mice. *Eur J Immunol.* 2007;37(3):613-622.

173. Hopken UE, Wengner AM, Loddenkemper C, et al. CCR7 deficiency causes ectopic lymphoid neogenesis and disturbed mucosal tissue integrity. *Blood.* 2007;109(3):886-895.

174. Reinhardt A, Ravens S, Fleige H, et al. CCR7-mediated migration in the thymus controls gammadelta T-cell development. *Eur J Immunol.* 2014;44(5):1320-1329.

175. Lei Y, Ripen AM, Ishimaru N, et al. Aire-dependent production of XCL1 mediates medullary accumulation of thymic dendritic cells and contributes to regulatory T cell development. *J Exp Med.* 2011;208(2):383-394.

176. Allende ML, Dreier JL, Mandala S, Proia RL. Expression of the sphingosine 1-phosphate receptor, S1P1, on T-cells controls thymic emigration. *J Biol Chem.* 2004;279(15):15396-15401.

177. Matloubian M, Lo CG, Cinamon G, et al. Lymphocyte egress from thymus and peripheral lymphoid organs is dependent on S1P receptor 1. *Nature.* 2004;427(6972):355-360.

178. Zachariah MA, Cyster JG. Neural crest-derived pericytes promote egress of mature thymocytes at the corticomedullary junction. *Science.* 2010;328(5982):1129-1135.

179. Pappu R, Schwab SR, Cornelissen I, et al. Promotion of lymphocyte egress into blood and lymph by distinct sources of sphingosine-1-phosphate. *Science.* 2007;316(5822):295-298.

180. Love PE, Bhandoola A. Signal integration and crosstalk during thymocyte migration and emigration. *Nat Rev Immunol.* 2011;11(7):469-477.

181. Derbinski J, Gabler J, Brors B, et al. Promiscuous gene expression in thymic epithelial cells is regulated at multiple levels. *J Exp Med.* 2005;202(1):33-45.

182. Derbinski J, Schulte A, Kyewski B, Klein L. Promiscuous gene expression in medullary thymic epithelial cells mirrors the peripheral self. *Nat Immunol.* 2001;2(11):1032-1039.

183. Klein L, Klugmann M, Nave KA, Tuohy VK, Kyewski B. Shaping of the autoreactive T-cell repertoire by a splice variant of self protein expressed in thymic epithelial cells. *Nat Med.* 2000;6(1):56-61.

184. Klein L, Kyewski B. "Promiscuous" expression of tissue antigens in the thymus: a key to T-cell tolerance and autoimmunity? *J Mol Med (Berl).* 2000;78(9):483-494.

185. Metzger TC, Khan IS, Gardner JM, et al. Lineage tracing and cell ablation identify a post-Aire-expressing thymic epithelial cell population. *Cell Rep.* 2013;5(1):166-179.

186. Pinto S, Michel C, Schmidt-Glenewinkel H, et al. Overlapping gene coexpression patterns in human medullary thymic epithelial cells generate self-antigen diversity. *Proc Natl Acad Sci U S A.* 2013;110(37):E3497-E3505.

187. Anderson MS, Venanzi ES, Klein L, et al. Projection of an immunological self shadow within the thymus by the aire protein. *Science.* 2002;298(5597):1395-1401.

188. Heino M, Peterson P, Kudoh J, et al. Autoimmune regulator is expressed in the cells regulating immune tolerance in thymus medulla. *Biochem Biophys Res Commun.* 1999;257(3):821-825.

189. Heino M, Peterson P, Sillanpaa N, et al. RNA and protein expression of the murine autoimmune regulator gene (Aire) in normal, RelB-deficient and in NOD mouse. *Eur J Immunol.* 2000;30(7):1884-1893.

190. Zuklys S, Balciunaite G, Agarwal A, Fasler-Kan E, Palmer E, Hollander GA. Normal thymic architecture and negative selection are associated with Aire expression, the gene defective in the autoimmune-polyendocrinopathy-candidiasis-ectodermal dystrophy (APECED). *J Immunol.* 2000;165(4):1976-1983.

191. Anderson MS, Venanzi ES, Chen Z, Berzins SP, Benoist C, Mathis D. The cellular mechanism of Aire control of T cell tolerance. *Immunity.* 2005;23(2):227-239.

192. Liston A, Gray DH, Lesage S, et al. Gene dosage—limiting role of Aire in thymic expression, clonal deletion, and organ-specific autoimmunity. *J Exp Med.* 2004;200(8):1015-1026.

193. Liston A, Lesage S, Wilson J, Peltonen L, Goodnow CC. Aire regulates negative selection of organ-specific T cells. *Nat Immunol.* 2003;4(4):350-354.

194. Aschenbrenner K, D'Cruz LM, Vollmann EH, et al. Selection of Foxp3+ regulatory T cells specific for self antigen expressed and presented by Aire+ medullary thymic epithelial cells. *Nat Immunol.* 2007;8(4):351-358.

195. Malchow S, Leventhal DS, Nishi S, et al. Aire-dependent thymic development of tumor-associated regulatory T cells. *Science.* 2013;339(6124):1219-1224.

196. Yang S, Fujikado N, Kolodin D, Benoist C, Mathis D. Immune tolerance regulatory T cells generated early in life play a distinct role in maintaining self-tolerance. *Science.* 2015;348(6234):589-594.

197. Nagamine K, Peterson P, Scott HS, et al. Positional cloning of the APECED gene. *Nat Genet.* 1997;17(4):393-398.

198. Kuroda N, Mitani T, Takeda N, et al. Development of autoimmunity against transcriptionally unrepressed target antigen in the thymus of Aire-deficient mice. *J Immunol.* 2005;174(4):1862-1870.

199. Ramsey C, Winqvist O, Puhakka L, et al. Aire deficient mice develop multiple features of APECED phenotype and show altered immune response. *Hum Mol Genet.* 2002;11(4):397-409.

200. Giraud M, Jmari N, Du L, et al. An RNAi screen for Aire cofactors reveals a role for Hnrnpl in polymerase release and Aire-activated ectopic transcription. *Proc Natl Acad Sci U S A.* 2014;111(4):1491-1496.

201. Waterfield M, Khan IS, Cortez JT, et al. The transcriptional regulator Aire coopts the repressive ATF7ip-MBD1 complex for the induction of immunotolerance. *Nat Immunol.* 2014;15(3):258-265.

202. Dooley J, Erickson M, Farr AG. Alterations of the medullary epithelial compartment in the Aire-deficient thymus: implications for programs of thymic epithelial differentiation. *J Immunol.* 2008;181(8):5225-5232.

203. Gillard GO, Dooley J, Erickson M, Peltonen L, Farr AG. Aire-dependent alterations in medullary thymic epithelium indicate a role for Aire in thymic epithelial differentiation. *J Immunol.* 2007;178(5):3007-3015.

204. Gillard GO, Farr AG. Contrasting models of promiscuous gene expression by thymic epithelium. *J Exp Med.* 2005;202(1):15-19.

205. Gray D, Abramson J, Benoist C, Mathis D. Proliferative arrest and rapid turnover of thymic epithelial cells expressing Aire. *J Exp Med.* 2007;204(11):2521-2528.

206. Nishikawa Y, Nishijima H, Matsumoto M, et al. Temporal lineage tracing of Aire-expressing cells reveals a requirement for Aire in their maturation program. *J Immunol.* 2014;192(6):2585-2592.

207. Yano M, Kuroda N, Han H, et al. Aire controls the differentiation program of thymic epithelial cells in the medulla for the establishment of self-tolerance. *J Exp Med.* 2008;205(12):2827-2838.

208. Laan M, Kisand K, Kont V, et al. Autoimmune regulator deficiency results in decreased expression of CCR4 and CCR7 ligands and in delayed migration of CD4+ thymocytes. *J Immunol.* 2009;183(12):7682-7691.

209. Ruan QG, Tung K, Eisenman D, et al. The autoimmune regulator directly controls the expression of genes critical for thymic epithelial function. *J Immunol.* 2007;178(11):7173-7180.

210. St-Pierre C, Trofimov A, Brochu S, Lemieux S, Perreault C. Differential features of AIRE-induced and AIRE-independent promiscuous gene expression in thymic epithelial cells. *J Immunol.* 2015;195(2):498-506.

211. Sansom SN, Shikama-Dorn N, Zhanybekova S, et al. Population and single-cell genomics reveal the Aire dependency, relief from Polycomb silencing, and distribution of self-antigen expression in thymic epithelia. *Genome Res.* 2014;24(12):1918-1931.

212. Chin RK, Zhu M, Christiansen PA, et al. Lymphotoxin pathway-directed, autoimmune regulator-independent central tolerance to arthritogenic collagen. *J Immunol.* 2006;177(1):290-297.

213. Bos R, van Duikeren S, van Hall T, et al. Expression of a natural tumor antigen by thymic epithelial cells impairs the tumor-protective CD4+ T-cell repertoire. *Cancer Res.* 2005;65(14):6443-6449.

214. Cloosen S, Arnold J, Thio M, Bos GM, Kyewski B, Germeraad WT. Expression of tumor-associated differentiation antigens, MUC1 glycoforms and CEA, in human thymic epithelial cells: implications for self-tolerance and tumor therapy. *Cancer Res.* 2007;67(8):3919-3926.

215. Zhu ML, Nagavalli A, Su MA. Aire deficiency promotes TRP-1-specific immune rejection of melanoma. *Cancer Res.* 2013;73(7):2104-2116.

216. Atibalentja DF, Byersdorfer CA, Unanue ER. Thymus-blood protein interactions are highly effective in negative selection and regulatory T cell induction. *J Immunol.* 2009;183(12):7909-7918.

217. Ferrero I, Anjuere F, MacDonald HR, Ardavin C. In vitro negative selection of viral superantigen-reactive thymocytes by thymic dendritic cells. *Blood.* 1997;90(5):1943-1951.

218. Gallegos AM, Bevan MJ. Central tolerance to tissue-specific antigens mediated by direct and indirect antigen presentation. *J Exp Med.* 2004;200(8):1039-1049.

219. Moore NC, Anderson G, McLoughlin DE, Owen JJ, Jenkinson EJ. Differential expression of Mtv loci in MHC class II-positive thymic stromal cells. *J Immunol.* 1994;152(10):4826-4831.

220. Baba T, Badr Mel S, Tomaru U, Ishizu A, Mukaida N. Novel process of intrathymic tumor-immune tolerance through CCR2-mediated recruitment of Sirpalpha+ dendritic cells: a murine model. *PLoS One.* 2012;7(7):e41154.

221. Bonasio R, Scimone ML, Schaerli P, Grabie N, Lichtman AH, von Andrian UH. Clonal deletion of thymocytes by circulating dendritic cells homing to the thymus. *Nat Immunol.* 2006;7(10):1092-1100.

222. Hadeiba H, Lahl K, Edalati A, et al. Plasmacytoid dendritic cells transport peripheral antigens to the thymus to promote central tolerance. *Immunity.* 2012;36(3):438-450.

223. Josefowicz SZ, Lu LF, Rudensky AY. Regulatory T cells: mechanisms of differentiation and function. *Annu Rev Immunol.* 2012;30:531-564.

224. Sakaguchi S, Miyara M, Costantino CM, Hafler DA. Foxp3+ regulatory T cells in the human immune system. *Nat Rev Immunol.* 2010;10(7):490-500.

225. Cowan JE, Parnell SM, Nakamura K, et al. The thymic medulla is required for Foxp3+ regulatory but not conventional CD4+ thymocyte development. *J Exp Med.* 2013;210(4):675-681.

226. Hinterberger M, Aichinger M, Prazeres da Costa O, Voehringer D, Hoffmann R, Klein L. Autonomous role of medullary thymic epithelial cells in central CD4(+) T cell tolerance. *Nat Immunol.* 2010;11(6):512-519.

227. Perry JSA, Lio CJ, Kau AL, et al. Distinct contributions of Aire and antigen-presenting-cell subsets to the generation of self-tolerance in the thymus. *Immunity.* 2014;41(3):414-426.

228. Watanabe N, Wang YH, Lee HK, et al. Hassall's corpuscles instruct dendritic cells to induce CD4+CD25+ regulatory T cells in human thymus. *Nature.* 2005;436(7054):1181-1185.

229. Hanabuchi S, Ito T, Park WR, et al. Thymic stromal lymphopoietin-activated plasmacytoid dendritic cells induce the generation of Foxp3+ regulatory T cells in human thymus. *J Immunol.* 2010;184(6):2999-3007.

230. Watanabe N, Hanabuchi S, Soumelis V, et al. Human thymic stromal lymphopoietin promotes dendritic cell-mediated CD4+ T cell homeostatic expansion. *Nat Immunol.* 2004;5(4):426-434.

231. Barbee SD, Woodward MJ, Turchinovich G, et al. Skint-1 is a highly specific, unique selecting component for epidermal T cells. *Proc Natl Acad Sci U S A.* 2011;108(8):3330-3335.

232. Boyden LM, Lewis JM, Barbee SD, et al. Skint1, the prototype of a newly identified immunoglobulin superfamily gene cluster, positively selects epidermal gammadelta T cells. *Nat Genet.* 2008;40(5):656-662.

233. Roberts NA, White AJ, Jenkinson WE, et al. Rank signaling links the development of invariant gammadelta T cell progenitors and Aire(+) medullary epithelium. *Immunity.* 2012;36(3):427-437.

234. Turchinovich G, Hayday AC. Skint-1 identifies a common molecular mechanism for the development of interferon-gamma-secreting versus interleukin-17-secreting gammadelta T cells. *Immunity.* 2011;35(1):59-68.

235. Drennan MB, Franki AS, Dewint P, et al. Cutting edge: the chemokine receptor CXCR3 retains invariant NK T cells in the thymus. *J Immunol.* 2009;183(4):2213-2216.

236. Kim JS, Garvin SG., Koretzky GA, Jordan MS. The requirements for natural Th17 cell development are distinct from those of conventional Th17 cells. *J Exp Med.* 2011;208(11):2201-2207.

237. McCarthy NI, Cowan JE, Nakamura K, et al. Osteoprotegerin-mediated homeostasis of Rank+ thymic epithelial cells does not limit Foxp3+ regulatory T cell development. *J Immunol.* 2015;195(6):2675-2682.

238. Durie FH, Foy TM, Masters SR, Laman JD, Noelle RJ. The role of CD40 in the regulation of humoral and cell-mediated immunity. *Immunol Today.* 1994;15(9):406-411.

239. Engel P, Gribben JG, Freeman GJ, et al. The B7-2 (B70) costimulatory molecule expressed by monocytes and activated B lymphocytes is the CD86 differentiation antigen. *Blood.* 1994;84(5):1402-1407.

240. Freeman GJ, Freedman AS, Segil JM, Lee G, Whitman JF, Nadler LM. B7, a new member of the Ig superfamily with unique expression on activated and neoplastic B cells. *J Immunol.* 1989;143(8):2714-2722.

241. Freeman GJ, Gribben JG, Boussiotis VA, et al. Cloning of B7-2: a CTLA-4 counter-receptor that costimulates human T cell proliferation. *Science.* 1993;262(5135):909-911.

242. Munro JM, Freedman AS, Aster JC, et al. In vivo expression of the B7 costimulatory molecule by subsets of antigen-presenting cells and the malignant cells of Hodgkin's disease. *Blood.* 1994;83(3):793-798.

243. Splawski JB, Fu SM, Lipsky PE. Immunoregulatory role of CD40 in human B cell differentiation. *J Immunol.* 1993;150(4):1276-1285.

244. Min H, Montecino-Rodriguez E, Dorshkind K. Reduction in the developmental potential of intrathymic T cell progenitors with age. *J Immunol.* 2004;173(1):245-250.

245. Calder AE, Hince MN, Dudakov JA, Chidgey AP, Boyd RL. Thymic involution: where endocrinology meets immunology. *Neuroimmunomodulation.* 2011;18(5):281-289.

246. Douek DC, McFarland RD, Keiser PH, et al. Changes in thymic function with age and during the treatment of HIV infection. *Nature.* 1998;396(6712):690-695.

247. Jamieson BD, Douek DC, Killian S, et al. Generation of functional thymocytes in the human adult. *Immunity.* 1999;10(5):569-575.

248. Junge S, Kloeckener-Gruissem B, Zufferey R, et al. Correlation between recent thymic emigrants and CD31+ (PECAM-1) CD4+ T cells in normal individuals during aging and in lymphopenic children. *Eur J Immunol.* 2007;37(11):3270-3280.

249. Nakahama M, Mohri N, Mori S, Shindo G, Yokoi Y, Machinami R. Immunohistochemical and histometrical studies of the human thymus with special emphasis on age-related changes in medullary epithelial and dendritic cells. *Virchows Arch B Cell Pathol Incl Mol Pathol.* 1990;58(3):245-251.

250. Thome JJ, Grinshpun B, Kumar BV, et al. Longterm maintenance of human naive T cells through in situ homeostasis in lymphoid tissue sites. *Sci Immunol.* 2016;1(6):eaah6506.

251. Gurkan S, Luan Y, Dhillon N, et al. Immune reconstitution following rabbit antithymocyte globulin. *Am J Transplant.* 2010;10(9):2132-2141.

252. Davis MD, Kehrl JH. The influence of sphingosine-1-phosphate receptor signaling on lymphocyte trafficking: how a bioactive lipid mediator grew up from an "immature" vascular maturation factor to a "mature" mediator of lymphocyte behavior and function. *Immunol Res.* 2009;43(1-3):187-197.

253. Mora JR, von Andrian UH. T-cell homing specificity and plasticity: new concepts and future challenges. *Trends Immunol.* 2006;27(5):235-243.

254. van Krieken JH, Te Velde J, Kleiverda K, Leenheers-Binnendijk L, van de Velde CJ. The human spleen; a histological study in splenectomy specimens embedded in methylmethacrylate. *Histopathology.* 1985;9(6):571-585.

255. Castenholz A. Architecture of the lymph node with regard to its function. *Curr Top Pathol.* 1990;84(pt 1):1-32.

256. Wacker HH, Frahm SO, Heidebrecht HJ, Parwaresch R. Sinus-lining cells of the lymph nodes recognized as a dendritic cell type by the new monoclonal antibody Ki-M9. *Am J Pathol.* 1997;151(2):423-434.

257. Kiefer F, Adams RH. Lymphatic endothelial differentiation: start out with Sox--carry on with Prox. *Genome Biol.* 2008;9(12):243.

258. Wigle JT, Harvey N, Detmar M, et al. An essential role for Prox1 in the induction of the lymphatic endothelial cell phenotype. *EMBO J.* 2002;21(7):1505-1513.

259. Peduto L, Dulauroy S, Lochner M, et al. Inflammation recapitulates the ontogeny of lymphoid stromal cells. *J Immunol.* 2009;182(9):5789-5799.

260. van de Pavert SA, Mebius RE. New insights into the development of lymphoid tissues. *Nat Rev Immunol.* 2010;10(9):664-674.

261. Vondenhoff MF, Greuter M, Goverse G, et al. LTbetaR signaling induces cytokine expression and up-regulates lymphangiogenic factors in lymph node anlagen. *J Immunol.* 2009;182(9):5439-5445.

262. Bajenoff M, Egen JG, Koo LY, et al. Stromal cell networks regulate lymphocyte entry, migration, and territoriality in lymph nodes. *Immunity.* 2006;25(6):989-1001.

263. Jarjour M, Jorquera A, Mondor I, et al. Fate mapping reveals origin and dynamics of lymph node follicular dendritic cells. *J Exp Med.* 2014;211(6):1109-1122.

264. Katakai T. Marginal reticular cells: a stromal subset directly descended from the lymphoid tissue organizer. *Front Immunol.* 2012;3:200.

265. van Krieken JH, von Schilling C, Kluin PM, Lennert K. Splenic marginal zone lymphocytes and related cells in the lymph node: a morphologic and immunohistochemical study. *Hum Pathol.* 1989;20(4):320-325.

266. Jacob J, Kassir R, Kelsoe G. In situ studies of the primary immune response to (4-hydroxy-3-nitrophenyl)acetyl. I. The architecture and dynamics of responding cell populations. *J Exp Med.* 1991;173(5):1165-1175.

267. Jacob J, Kelsoe G. In situ studies of the primary immune response to (4-hydroxy-3-nitrophenyl)acetyl. II. A common clonal origin for periarteriolar lymphoid sheath-associated foci and germinal centers. *J Exp Med.* 1992;176(3):679-687.

268. Jacob J, Miller C, Kelsoe G. In situ studies of the antigen-driven somatic hypermutation of immunoglobulin genes. *Immunol Cell Biol.* 1992;70(pt 2):145-152.

269. Liu YJ, Johnson GD, Gordon J, MacLennan IC. Germinal centres in T-cell-dependent antibody responses. *Immunol Today.* 1992;13(1):17-21.

270. Tas JM, Mesin L, Pasqual G, et al. Visualizing antibody affinity maturation in germinal centers. *Science.* 2016;351(6277):1048-1054.

271. Dent AL, Shaffer AL, Yu X, Allman D, Staudt LM. Control of inflammation, cytokine expression, and germinal center formation by BCL-6. *Science.* 1997;276(5312):589-592.

272. Pittaluga S, Ayoubi TA, Wlodarska I, et al. BCL-6 expression in reactive lymphoid tissue and in B-cell non-Hodgkin's lymphomas. *J Pathol.* 1996;179(2):145-150.

273. Ye BH, Cattoretti G, Shen Q, et al. The BCL-6 proto-oncogene controls germinal-centre formation and Th2-type inflammation. *Nat Genet.* 1997;16(2):161-170.

274. Kroese FG, Timens W, Nieuwenhuis P. Germinal center reaction and B lymphocytes: morphology and function. *Curr Top Pathol.* 1990;84(pt 1):103-148.

275. Freedman AS. Expression and function of adhesion receptors on normal B cells and B cell non-Hodgkin's lymphomas. *Semin Hematol.* 1993;30(4):318-328.

276. Freedman AS, Munro JM, Rice GE, et al. Adhesion of human B cells to germinal centers in vitro involves VLA-4 and INCAM-110. *Science.* 1990;249(4972):1030-1033.

277. Hase H, Kanno Y, Kojima M, et al. BAFF/BLyS can potentiate B-cell selection with the B-cell coreceptor complex. *Blood.* 2004;103(6):2257-2265.

278. Li L, Zhang X, Kovacic S, et al. Identification of a human follicular dendritic cell molecule that stimulates germinal center B cell growth. *J Exp Med.* 2000;191(6):1077-1084.

279. Park CS, Yoon SO, Armitage RJ, Choi YS. Follicular dendritic cells produce IL-15 that enhances germinal center B cell proliferation in membrane-bound form. *J Immunol.* 2004;173(11):6676-6683.

280. Vinuesa CG, Tangye SG, Moser B, Mackay CR. Follicular B helper T cells in antibody responses and autoimmunity. *Nat Rev Immunol.* 2005;5(11):853-865.

281. Lim HW, Hillsamer P, Banham AH, Kim CH. Cutting edge: direct suppression of B cells by CD4+ CD25+ regulatory T cells. *J Immunol.* 2005;175(7):4180-4183.

282. Crivellato E, Baldini G, Basa M, Fusaroli P. The three-dimensional structure of interdigitating cells. *Ital J Anat Embryol.* 1993;98(4):243-258.

283. van der Valk P, Meijer CJ. The histology of reactive lymph nodes. *Am J Surg Pathol.* 1987;11(11):866-882.

284. Inaba K, Pack M, Inaba M, Sakuta H, Isdell F, Steinman RM. High levels of a major histocompatibility complex II-self peptide complex on dendritic cells from the T cell areas of lymph nodes. *J Exp Med.* 1997;186(5):665-672.

285. Girard JP, Moussion C, Forster R. HEVs, lymphatics and homeostatic immune cell trafficking in lymph nodes. *Nat Rev Immunol.* 2012;12(11):762-773.

286. Miyasaka M, Tanaka T. Lymphocyte trafficking across high endothelial venules: dogmas and enigmas. *Nat Rev Immunol.* 2004;4(5):360-370.

287. Rosen SD. Ligands for L-selectin: homing, inflammation, and beyond. *Annu Rev Immunol.* 2004;22:129-156.

288. von Andrian UH, Mempel TR. Homing and cellular traffic in lymph nodes. *Nat Rev Immunol.* 2003;3(11):867-878.

289. Hiraoka N, Kawashima H, Petryniak B, et al. Core 2 branching beta1,6-N-acetylglucosaminyltransferase and high endothelial venule-restricted sulfotransferase collaboratively control lymphocyte homing. *J Biol Chem.* 2004;279(4):3058-3067.

290. Hiraoka N, Petryniak B, Nakayama J, et al. A novel, high endothelial venule-specific sulfotransferase expresses 6-sulfo sialyl Lewis(x), an L-selectin ligand displayed by CD34. *Immunity.* 1999;11(1):79-89.

291. Kawashima H, Petryniak B, Hiraoka N, et al. N-acetylglucosamine-6-O-sulfotransferases 1 and 2 cooperatively control lymphocyte homing through L-selectin ligand biosynthesis in high endothelial venules. *Nat Immunol.* 2005;6(11):1096-1104.

292. Mitoma J, Bao X, Petryanik B, et al. Critical functions of N-glycans in L-selectin-mediated lymphocyte homing and recruitment. *Nat Immunol.* 2007;8(4):409-418.

293. Uchimura K, Gauguet JM, Singer MS, et al. A major class of L-selectin ligands is eliminated in mice deficient in two sulfotransferases expressed in high endothelial venules. *Nat Immunol.* 2005;6(11):1105-1113.

294. Yeh JC, Hiraoka N, Petryniak B, et al. Novel sulfated lymphocyte homing receptors and their control by a Core1 extension beta 1,3-N-acetylglucosaminyltransferase. *Cell.* 2001;105(7):957-969.

295. von Andrian UH, Mackay CR. T-cell function and migration. Two sides of the same coin. *N Engl J Med.* 2000;343(14):1020-1034.

296. Aloisi F, Pujol-Borrell R. Lymphoid neogenesis in chronic inflammatory diseases. *Nat Rev Immunol.* 2006;6(3):205-217.

297. Carragher DM, Rangel-Moreno J, Randall TD. Ectopic lymphoid tissues and local immunity. *Semin Immunol.* 2008;20(1):26-42.

298. Drayton DL, Liao S, Mounzer RH, Ruddle NH. Lymphoid organ development: from ontogeny to neogenesis. *Nat Immunol.* 2006;7(4):344-353.

299. Hayasaka H, Taniguchi K, Fukai S, Miyasaka M. Neogenesis and development of the high endothelial venules that mediate lymphocyte trafficking. *Cancer Sci.* 2010;101(11):2302-2308.

300. Huang HY, Luther SA. Expression and function of interleukin-7 in secondary and tertiary lymphoid organs. *Semin Immunol.* 2012;24(3):175-189.

301. Browning JL, Allaire N, Ngam-Ek A, et al. Lymphotoxin-beta receptor signaling is required for the homeostatic control of HEV differentiation and function. *Immunity.* 2005;23(5):539-550.

302. Drayton DL, Ying X, Lee J, Lesslauer W, Ruddle NH. Ectopic LT alpha beta directs lymphoid organ neogenesis with concomitant expression of peripheral node addressin and a HEV-restricted sulfotransferase. *J Exp Med.* 2003;197(9):1153-1163.

303. Kumar V, Scandella E, Danuser R, et al. Global lymphoid tissue remodeling during a viral infection is orchestrated by a B cell-lymphotoxin-dependent pathway. *Blood.* 2010;115(23):4725-4733.

304. Liao S, Ruddle NH. Synchrony of high endothelial venules and lymphatic vessels revealed by immunization. *J Immunol.* 2006;177(5):3369-3379.

305. Moussion C, Girard JP. Dendritic cells control lymphocyte entry to lymph nodes through high endothelial venules. *Nature.* 2011;479(7374):542-546.

306. Batista FD, Harwood NE. The who, how and where of antigen presentation to B cells. *Nat Rev Immunol.* 2009;9(1):15-27.

307. Roozendaal R, Mebius RE, Kraal G. The conduit system of the lymph node. *Int Immunol.* 2008;20(12):1483-1487.

308. Roozendaal R, Mempel TR, Pitcher LA, et al. Conduits mediate transport of low-molecular-weight antigen to lymph node follicles. *Immunity.* 2009;30(2):264-276.

309. Sixt M, Kanazawa N, Selg M, et al. The conduit system transports soluble antigens from the afferent lymph to resident dendritic cells in the T cell area of the lymph node. *Immunity.* 2005;22(1):19-29.

310. Nossal GJ, Abbot A, Mitchell J, Lummus Z. Antigens in immunity. XV. Ultrastructural features of antigen capture in primary and secondary lymphoid follicles. *J Exp Med.* 1968;127(2):277-290.

311. Carrasco YR, Batista FD. B cells acquire particulate antigen in a macrophage-rich area at the boundary between the follicle and the subcapsular sinus of the lymph node. *Immunity.* 2007;27(1):160-171.

312. Junt T, Moseman EA, Iannacone M, et al. Subcapsular sinus macrophages in lymph nodes clear lymph-borne viruses and present them to antiviral B cells. *Nature.* 2007;450(7166):110-114.

313. Phan TG, Grigorova I, Okada T, Cyster JG. Subcapsular encounter and complement-dependent transport of immune complexes by lymph node B cells. *Nat Immunol.* 2007;8(9):992-1000.

314. Tamburini BA, Burchill MA, Kedl RM. Antigen capture and archiving by lymphatic endothelial cells following vaccination or viral infection. *Nat Commun.* 2014;5:3989.

315. Malhotra D, Fletcher AL, Turley SJ. Stromal and hematopoietic cells in secondary lymphoid organs: partners in immunity. *Immunol Rev.* 2013;251(1):160-176.

316. Tew JG, Kosco MH, Burton GF, Szakal AK. Follicular dendritic cells as accessory cells. *Immunol Rev.* 1990;117:185-211.

317. Krautler NJ, , Kana V, Kranich J, et al. Follicular dendritic cells emerge from ubiquitous perivascular precursors. *Cell.* 2012;150(1):194-206.

318. Heesters BA, van Megesen K, Tomris I, et al. Characterization of human FDCs reveals regulation of T cells and antigen presentation to B cells. *J Exp Med.* 2021;218(10):e20210790.

319. Pikor NB, Mörbe U, Lütge M, et al. Remodeling of light and dark zone follicular dendritic cells governs germinal center responses. *Nat Immunol.* 2020;21(6):649-659.

320. Béguelin W, Teater M, Meydan C, et al. Mutant EZH2 induces a pre-malignant lymphoma niche by reprogramming the immune response. *Cancer Cell.* 2020;37(5):655-673.e11.

321. Dijkstra CD, Van den Berg TK. The follicular dendritic cell: possible regulatory roles of associated molecules. *Res Immunol.* 1991;142(3):227-231.

322. Fischer MB, Goerg S, Shen L, et al. Dependence of germinal center B cells on expression of CD21/CD35 for survival. *Science.* 1998;280(5363):582-585.

323. Matsumoto M, Fu YX, Molina H, et al. Distinct roles of lymphotoxin alpha and the type I tumor necrosis factor (TNF) receptor in the establishment of follicular dendritic cells from non-bone marrow-derived cells. *J Exp Med.* 1997;186(12):1997-2004.

324. Wang X, Cho B, Suzuki K, et al. Follicular dendritic cells help establish follicle identity and promote B cell retention in germinal centers. *J Exp Med.* 2011;208(12):2497-2510.

325. Heesters BA, Chatterjee P, Kim YA, et al. Endocytosis and recycling of immune complexes by follicular dendritic cells enhances B cell antigen binding and activation. *Immunity.* 2013;38(6):1164-1175.

326. Kaplan ME, Coons AH, Deane HW. Localization of antigen in tissue cells; cellular distribution of pneumococcal polysaccharides types II and III in the mouse. *J Exp Med.* 1950;91(1):15-30. 4 pl.

327. Kelsoe G. Life and death in germinal centers (redux). *Immunity.* 1996;4(2):107-111.

328. MacLennan IC. Germinal centers. *Annu Rev Immunol.* 1994;12:117-139.

329. Szakal AK, Gieringer RL, Kosco MH, Tew JG. Isolated follicular dendritic cells: cytochemical antigen localization, Nomarski, SEM, and TEM morphology. *J Immunol.* 1985;134(3):1349-1359.

330. Ansel KM, Ngo VN, Hyman PL, et al. A chemokine-driven positive feedback loop organizes lymphoid follicles. *Nature.* 2000;406(6793):309-314.

331. Duan L, Liu D, Chen H, et al. Follicular dendritic cells restrict interleukin-4 availability in germinal centers and foster memory B cell generation. *Immunity.* 2021;54(10):2256-2272.e6.

332. Cyster JG, Ansel KM, Reif K, et al. Follicular stromal cells and lymphocyte homing to follicles. *Immunol Rev.* 2000;176:181-193.

333. Allen CD, Cyster JG. Follicular dendritic cell networks of primary follicles and germinal centers: phenotype and function. *Semin Immunol.* 2008;20(1):14-25.

334. Alimzhanov MB, Kuprash DV, Kosco-Vilbois MH, et al. Abnormal development of secondary lymphoid tissues in lymphotoxin beta-deficient mice. *Proc Natl Acad Sci U S A.* 1997;94(17):9302-9307.

335. Endres R, Alimzhanov MB, Plitz T, et al. Mature follicular dendritic cell networks depend on expression of lymphotoxin beta receptor by radioresistant stromal cells and of lymphotoxin beta and tumor necrosis factor by B cells. *J Exp Med.* 1999;189(1):159-168.

336. Pasparakis M, Alexopoulou L, Douni E, Kollias G. Tumour necrosis factors in immune regulation: everything that's interesting is..new!. *Cytokine Growth Factor Rev.* 1996;7(3):223-229.

337. Castagnaro L, Lenti E, Maruzzelli S, et al. Nkx2-5(+)islet1(+) mesenchymal precursors generate distinct spleen stromal cell subsets and participate in restoring stromal network integrity. *Immunity.* 2013;38(4):782-791.

338. Choi SY, Bae H, Jeong SH, et al. YAP/TAZ direct commitment and maturation of lymph node fibroblastic reticular cells. *Nat Commun.* 2020;11(1):519.

339. Lütge M, Pikor NB, Ludewig B. Differentiation and activation of fibroblastic reticular cells. *Immunol Rev.* 2021;302(1):32-46.

340. Perez-Shibayama C, Islander U, Lütge M, et al. Type I interferon signaling in fibroblastic reticular cells prevents exhaustive activation of antiviral CD8(+) T cells. *Sci Immunol.* 2020;5(51):eabb7066.

341. Katakai T, Hara T, Sugai M, Gonda H, Shimizu A, et al. Lymph node fibroblastic reticular cells construct the stromal reticulum via contact with lymphocytes. *J Exp Med.* 2004;200(6):783-795.

342. Krishnamurty AT, Turley SJ. Lymph node stromal cells: cartographers of the immune system. *Nat Immunol.* 2020;21(4):369-380.

343. Cremasco V, Woodruff MC, Onder L, et al. B cell homeostasis and follicle confines are governed by fibroblastic reticular cells. *Nat Immunol.* 2014;15(10):973-981.

344. Link A, Vogt TK, Favre S, et al. Fibroblastic reticular cells in lymph nodes regulate the homeostasis of naive T cells. *Nat Immunol.* 2007;8(11):1255-1265.

345. Gretz JE, Anderson AO, Shaw S. Cords, channels, corridors and conduits: critical architectural elements facilitating cell interactions in the lymph node cortex. *Immunol Rev.* 1997;156:11-24.

346. Martinez VG, Pankova V, Krasny L, et al. Fibroblastic reticular cells control conduit matrix deposition during lymph node expansion. *Cell Rep.* 2019;29(9):2810-2822.e5.

347. Fletcher AL, Lukacs-Kornek V, Reynoso ED, et al. Lymph node fibroblastic reticular cells directly present peripheral tissue antigen under steady-state and inflammatory conditions. *J Exp Med.* 2010;207(4):689-697.

348. Denton AE, , Roberts EW, Linterman MA, Fearon DT. Fibroblastic reticular cells of the lymph node are required for retention of resting but not activated CD8+ T cells. *Proc Natl Acad Sci U S A.* 2014;111(33):12139-12144.

349. Majumder S, Amatya N, Revu S, et al. IL-17 metabolically reprograms activated fibroblastic reticular cells for proliferation and survival. *Nat Immunol.* 2019;20(5):534-545.

350. Gregory JL, Walter A, Alexandre YO, et al. Infection programs sustained lymphoid stromal cell responses and shapes lymph node remodeling upon secondary challenge. *Cell Rep.* 2017;18(2):406-418.

351. Li L, Wu J, Abdi R, Jewell CM, Bromberg JS. Lymph node fibroblastic reticular cells steer immune responses. *Trends Immunol.* 2021;42(8):723-734.

352. Severino P, Palomino DT, Alvarenga H, et al. Human lymph node-derived fibroblastic and double-negative reticular cells alter their chemokines and cytokines expression profile following inflammatory stimuli. *Front Immunol.* 2017;8:141.

353. Astarita JL, Cremasco V, Fu J, et al. The CLEC-2-podoplanin axis controls the contractility of fibroblastic reticular cells and lymph node microarchitecture. *Nat Immunol.* 2015;16(1):75-84.

354. Acton SE, Farrugia AJ, Astarita JL, et al. Dendritic cells control fibroblastic reticular network tension and lymph node expansion. *Nature.* 2014;514(7523):498-502.

355. Benahmed F, Chyou S, Dasoveanu D, et al. Multiple CD11c+ cells collaboratively express IL-1beta to modulate stromal vascular endothelial growth factor and lymph node vascular-stromal growth. *J Immunol.* 2014;192(9):4153-4163.

356. Chyou S, Ekland EH, Carpenter AC, et al. Fibroblast-type reticular stromal cells regulate the lymph node vasculature. *J Immunol.* 2008;181(6):3887-3896.

357. Kumar V, Dasoveanu DC, Chyou S, et al. A dendritic-cell-stromal axis maintains immune responses in lymph nodes. *Immunity.* 2015;42(4):719-730.

358. Katakai T, Suto H, Sugai M, et al. Organizer-like reticular stromal cell layer common to adult secondary lymphoid organs. *J Immunol.* 2008;181(9):6189-6200.

359. Roberts CW, Shutter JR, Korsmeyer SJ. Hox11 controls the genesis of the spleen. *Nature.* 1994;368(6473):747-749.

360. Lewis SM. The spleen—mysteries solved and unresolved. *Clin Haematol.* 1983;12(2):363-373.

361. Mebius RE, Kraal G. Structure and function of the spleen. *Nat Rev Immunol.* 2005;5(8):606-616.

362. van Krieken JH, te Velde J. Normal histology of the human spleen. *Am J Surg Pathol.* 1988;12(10):777-785.

363. Tan JK, Watanabe T. Stromal cell subsets directing neonatal spleen regeneration. *Sci Rep.* 2017;7:40401.

364. Bajenoff M, Glaichenhaus N, Germain RN. Fibroblastic reticular cells guide T lymphocyte entry into and migration within the splenic T cell zone. *J Immunol.* 2008;181(6):3947-3954.

365. Weiss L. The structure of the normal spleen. *Semin Hematol.* 1965;2:205-228.

366. Weiss L. A scanning electron microscopic study of the spleen. *Blood.* 1974;43(5):665-691.

367. Steiniger B, Ruttinger L, Barth PJ. The three-dimensional structure of human splenic white pulp compartments. *J Histochem Cytochem.* 2003;51(5):655-664.

368. Lyons AB, Parish CR. Are murine marginal-zone macrophages the splenic white pulp endothelial analog of high endothelial venules? *Eur J Immunol.* 1995;25(11):3165-3172.

369. Chen LT, Weiss L. Electron microscopy of the red pulp of human spleen. *Am J Anat.* 1972;134(4):425-457.

370. Weiss L. The red pulp of the spleen: structural basis of blood flow. *Clin Haematol.* 1983;12(2):375-393.

371. Chen LT, Weiss L. The role of the sinus wall in the passage of erythrocytes through the spleen. *Blood.* 1973;41(4):529-537.

372. Brendolan A, Rosado MM, Carsetti R, Selleri L, Dear TN. Development and function of the mammalian spleen. *Bioessays.* 2007;29(2):166-177.

373. Pabst R, Westermann J, Rothkotter HJ. Immunoarchitecture of regenerated splenic and lymph node transplants. *Int Rev Cytol.* 1991;128:215-260.

374. Honda K, Nakano H, Yoshida H, et al. Molecular basis for hematopoietic/mesenchymal interaction during initiation of Peyer's patch organogenesis. *J Exp Med.* 2001;193(5):621-630.

375. Cupedo T, Vondenhoff MFR, Heeregrave EJ, et al. Presumptive lymph node organizers are differentially represented in developing mesenteric and peripheral nodes. *J Immunol.* 2004;173(5):2968-2975.

376. Banks TA, Rouse BT, Kerley MK, et al. Lymphotoxin-alpha-deficient mice. Effects on secondary lymphoid organ development and humoral immune responsiveness. *J Immunol.* 1995;155(4):1685-1693.

377. De Togni P, Goellner J, Ruddle NH, et al. Abnormal development of peripheral lymphoid organs in mice deficient in lymphotoxin. *Science.* 1994;264(5159):703-707.

378. Futterer A, Mink K, Luz A, Kosco-Vilbois MH, Pfeffer K. The lymphotoxin beta receptor controls organogenesis and affinity maturation in peripheral lymphoid tissues. *Immunity.* 1998;9(1):59-70.

379. Sun Z, Unutmaz D, Zou YR, et al. Requirement for RORgamma in thymocyte survival and lymphoid organ development. *Science.* 2000;288(5475):2369-2373.

380. Glanville SH, Bekiaris V, Jenkinson EJ, et al. Transplantation of embryonic spleen tissue reveals a role for adult non-lymphoid cells in initiating lymphoid tissue organization. *Eur J Immunol.* 2009;39(1):280-289.

381. Tan JK, Watanabe T. Murine spleen tissue regeneration from neonatal spleen capsule requires lymphotoxin priming of stromal cells. *J Immunol.* 2014;193(3):1194-1203.

382. Onder L, Danuser R, Scandella E, et al. Endothelial cell-specific lymphotoxin-beta receptor signaling is critical for lymph node and high endothelial venule formation. *J Exp Med.* 2013;210(3):465-473.

383. Fremont RD, Rice TW. Splenosis: a review. *South Med J.* 2007;100(6):589-593.

384. Brendolan A, Caamano JH. Mesenchymal cell differentiation during lymph node organogenesis. *Front Immunol.* 2012;3:381.

385. Withers DR, Kim M-Y, Bekiaris V, et al. The role of lymphoid tissue inducer cells in splenic white pulp development. *Eur J Immunol.* 2007;37(11):3240-3245.

386. Vondenhoff MF, Desanti GE, Cupedo T, et al. Separation of splenic red and white pulp occurs before birth in a LTalphabeta-independent manner. *J Leukoc Biol.* 2008;84(1):152-161.

387. Kim MY, McConnell FM, Gaspal FMC, et al. Function of CD4+CD3- cells in relation to B- and T-zone stroma in spleen. *Blood.* 2007;109(4):1602-1610.

388. Dejardin E, Droin NM, Delhase M, et al. The lymphotoxin-beta receptor induces different patterns of gene expression via two NF-kappaB pathways. *Immunity.* 2002;17(4):525-535.

389. Weih F, Caamano J. Regulation of secondary lymphoid organ development by the nuclear factor-kappaB signal transduction pathway. *Immunol Rev.* 2003;195:91-105.

390. Ngo VN, Cornall RJ, Cyster JG. Splenic T zone development is B cell dependent. *J Exp Med.* 2001;194(11):1649-1660.

391. Tumanov A, Kuprash DV, Lagarkova MA, et al. Distinct role of surface lymphotoxin expressed by B cells in the organization of secondary lymphoid tissues. *Immunity.* 2002;17(3):239-250.

392. Sierro F, Pringault E, Assman PS, Kraehenbuhl JP, Debard N. Transient expression of M-cell phenotype by enterocyte-like cells of the follicle-associated epithelium of mouse Peyer's patches. *Gastroenterology.* 2000;119(3):734-743.

393. Miller H, Zhang J, Kuolee R, Patel GB, Chen W. Intestinal M cells: the fallible sentinels? *World J Gastroenterol.* 2007;13(10):1477-1486.

394. Cupedo T, Mebius RE. Cellular interactions in lymph node development. *J Immunol.* 2005;174(1):21-25.

395. Mebius RE. Organogenesis of lymphoid tissues. *Nat Rev Immunol.* 2003;3(4):292-303.

396. Bagdi E, Diss TC, Munson P, Isaacson PG. Mucosal intra-epithelial lymphocytes in enteropathy-associated T-cell lymphoma, ulcerative jejunitis, and refractory celiac disease constitute a neoplastic population. *Blood.* 1999;94(1):260-264.

397. Corr SC, Gahan CC, Hill C. M-cells: origin, morphology and role in mucosal immunity and microbial pathogenesis. *FEMS Immunol Med Microbiol.* 2008;52(1):2-12.

398. Kraehenbuhl JP, Neutra MR. Molecular and cellular basis of immune protection of mucosal surfaces. *Physiol Rev.* 1992;72(4):853-879.

399. Neutra MR, Frey A, Kraehenbuhl JP. Epithelial M cells: gateways for mucosal infection and immunization. *Cell.* 1996;86(3):345-348.

400. Neutra MR, Pringault E, Kraehenbuhl JP. Antigen sampling across epithelial barriers and induction of mucosal immune responses. *Annu Rev Immunol.* 1996;14:275-300.

401. Iwasaki A, Kelsall BL. Localization of distinct Peyer's patch dendritic cell subsets and their recruitment by chemokines macrophage inflammatory protein (MIP)-3alpha, MIP-3beta, and secondary lymphoid organ chemokine. *J Exp Med.* 2000;191(8):1381-1394.

402. Butcher EC. Warner-Lambert/Parke-Davis Award lecture. Cellular and molecular mechanisms that direct leukocyte traffic. *Am J Pathol.* 1990;136(1):3-11.

403. Gowans JL, Knight EJ. The route of Re-circulation of lymphocytes in the rat. *Proc R Soc Lond B Biol Sci.* 1964;159:257-282.

404. Agace WW. T-cell recruitment to the intestinal mucosa. *Trends Immunol.* 2008;29(11):514-522.

405. Rennert PD, Browning JL, Mebius R, Mackay F, Hochman PS. Surface lymphotoxin alpha/beta complex is required for the development of peripheral lymphoid organs. *J Exp Med.* 1996;184(5):1999-2006.

406. Fukuyama S, Hiroi T, Yokota Y, et al. Initiation of NALT organogenesis is independent of the IL-7R, LTbetaR, and NIK signaling pathways but requires the Id2 gene and CD3(-)CD4(+)CD45(+) cells. *Immunity.* 2002;17(1):31-40.

407. Nagatake T, Fukuyama S, Kim DY, et al. Id2-, RORgammat-, and LTbetaR-independent initiation of lymphoid organogenesis in ocular immunity. *J Exp Med.* 2009;206(11):2351-2364.

408. GeurtsvanKessel CH, Willart MAM, Bergen IM, et al. Dendritic cells are crucial for maintenance of tertiary lymphoid structures in the lung of influenza virus-infected mice. *J Exp Med.* 2009;206(11):2339-2349.

409. Halle S, Dujardin HC, Bakocevic N, et al. Induced bronchus-associated lymphoid tissue serves as a general priming site for T cells and is maintained by dendritic cells. *J Exp Med.* 2009;206(12):2593-2601.

410. Rangel-Moreno J, Carragher DM, de la Luz Garcia-Hernandez M, et al. The development of inducible bronchus-associated lymphoid tissue depends on IL-17. *Nat Immunol.* 2011;12(7):639-646.

411. Zhao X, Sato A, Dela Cruz CS, et al. CCL9 is secreted by the follicle-associated epithelium and recruits dome region Peyer's patch CD11b+ dendritic cells. *J Immunol.* 2003;171(6):2797-2803.

412. Rangel-Moreno J, Moyron-Quiroz J, Kusser K, Hartson L, Nakano H, Randall TD. Role of CXC chemokine ligand 13, CC chemokine ligand (CCL) 19, and CCL21 in the organization and function of nasal-associated lymphoid tissue. *J Immunol.* 2005;175(8):4904-4913.

413. Ebisawa M, Hase K, Takahashi D, et al. CCR6hiCD11c(int) B cells promote M-cell differentiation in Peyer's patch. *Int Immunol.* 2011;23(4):261-269.

414. McDonald KG, McDonough JS, Wang C, Kucharzik T, Williams IR, Newberry RD. CC chemokine receptor 6 expression by B lymphocytes is essential for the development of isolated lymphoid follicles. *Am J Pathol.* 2007;170(4):1229-1240.

415. Lugering A, Ross M, Sieker M, et al. CCR6 identifies lymphoid tissue inducer cells within cryptopatches. *Clin Exp Immunol.* 2010;160(3):440-449.

416. Baptista AP, Olivier BJ, Goverse G, et al. Colonic patch and colonic SILT development are independent and differentially regulated events. *Mucosal Immunol.* 2013;6(3):511-521.

417. Bouskra D, Brézillon C, Bérard M, et al. Lymphoid tissue genesis induced by commensals through NOD1 regulates intestinal homeostasis. *Nature.* 2008;456(7221):507-510.

418. Round JL, Mazmanian SK. The gut microbiota shapes intestinal immune responses during health and disease. *Nat Rev Immunol.* 2009;9(5):313-323.

419. Pabst O, Herbrand H, Worbs T, et al. Cryptopatches and isolated lymphoid follicles: dynamic lymphoid tissues dispensable for the generation of intraepithelial lymphocytes. *Eur J Immunol.* 2005;35(1):98-107.

420. Krege J, Seth S, Hardtke S, Davalos-Misslitz ACM, Förster R. Antigen-dependent rescue of nose-associated lymphoid tissue (NALT) development independent of LTbetaR and CXCR5 signaling. *J Immunol.* 2009;39(10):2765-2778.

421. Jeong KI, Suzuki H, Nakayama H, Doi K. Ultrastructural study on the follicle-associated epithelium of nasal-associated lymphoid tissue in specific pathogen-free (SPF) and conventional environment-adapted (SPF-CV) rats. *J Anat.* 2000;196(pt 3):443-451.

422. Terahara K, Yoshida M, Igarashi O, et al. Comprehensive gene expression profiling of Peyer's patch M cells, villous M-like cells, and intestinal epithelial cells. *J Immunol.* 2008;180(12):7840-7846.

423. Teitelbaum R, Schubert W, Gunther L, et al. The M cell as a portal of entry to the lung for the bacterial pathogen *Mycobacterium tuberculosis. Immunity.* 1999;10(6):641-650.

424. Wang J, Gusti V, Saraswati A, Lo DD. Convergent and divergent development among M cell lineages in mouse mucosal epithelium. *J Immunol.* 2011;187(10):5277-5285.

The Normal Hematologic System

425. Pitzalis C, Jones GW, Bombardieri M, Jones SA. Ectopic lymphoid-like structures in infection, cancer and autoimmunity. *Nat Rev Immunol.* 2014;14(7):447-462.

426. Jones GW, Hill DG, Jones SA. Understanding immune cells in tertiary lymphoid organ development: it is all starting to come together. *Front Immunol.* 2016;7:401.

427. de Chaisemartin L, Goc J, Damotte D, et al. Characterization of chemokines and adhesion molecules associated with T cell presence in tertiary lymphoid structures in human lung cancer. *Cancer Res.* 2011;71(20):6391-6399.

428. Germain C, Gnjatic S, Dieu-Nosjean MC. Tertiary lymphoid structure-associated B cells are key players in anti-tumor immunity. *Front Immunol.* 2015;6:67.

429. Martinet L, Filleron T, Le Guellec S, Rochaix P, Garrido I, Girard JP. High endothelial venule blood vessels for tumor-infiltrating lymphocytes are associated with lymphotoxin beta-producing dendritic cells in human breast cancer. *J Immunol.* 2013;191(4):2001-2008.

430. Martinet L, Le Guellec S, Filleron T, et al. High endothelial venules (HEVs) in human melanoma lesions: major gateways for tumor-infiltrating lymphocytes. *OncoImmunology.* 2012;1(6):829-839.

431. Cherrier M, Sawa S, Eberl G. Notch, Id2, and RORgammat sequentially orchestrate the fetal development of lymphoid tissue inducer cells. *J Exp Med.* 2012;209(4):729-740.

432. Lochner M, Ohnmacht C, Presley L, et al. Microbiota-induced tertiary lymphoid tissues aggravate inflammatory disease in the absence of RORgamma t and LTi cells. *J Exp Med.* 2011;208(1):125-134.

433. Sawa S, Cherrier M, Lochner M, et al. Lineage relationship analysis of RORgammat+ innate lymphoid cells. *Science.* 2010;330(6004):665-669.

434. McGeachy MJ, Chen Y, Tato CM, et al. The interleukin 23 receptor is essential for the terminal differentiation of interleukin 17-producing effector T helper cells in vivo. *Nat Immunol.* 2009;10(3):314-324.

435. Peters A, Pitcher LA, Sullivan JM, et al. Th17 cells induce ectopic lymphoid follicles in central nervous system tissue inflammation. *Immunity.* 2011;35(6):986-996.

436. Stritesky GL, Yeh N, Kaplan MH. IL-23 promotes maintenance but not commitment to the Th17 lineage. *J Immunol.* 2008;181(9):5948-5955.

437. Grogan JL, Ouyang W. A role for Th17 cells in the regulation of tertiary lymphoid follicles. *Eur J Immunol.* 2012;42(9):2255-2262.

438. Jones GW, Bombardieri M, Greenhill CJ, et al. Interleukin-27 inhibits ectopic lymphoid-like structure development in early inflammatory arthritis. *J Exp Med.* 2015;212(11):1793-1802.

439. Canete JD, Celis R, Yeremenko N, et al. Ectopic lymphoid neogenesis is strongly associated with activation of the IL-23 pathway in rheumatoid synovitis. *Arthritis Res Ther.* 2015;17:173.

440. Chaitanya GV, Omura S, Sato F, et al. Inflammation induces neuro-lymphatic protein expression in multiple sclerosis brain neurovasculature. *J Neuroinflammation.* 2013;10:125.

441. Ciccia F, Rizzo A, Maugeri R, et al. Ectopic expression of CXCL13, BAFF, APRIL and LT-beta is associated with artery tertiary lymphoid organs in giant cell arteritis. *Ann Rheum Dis.* 2017;76(1):235-243.

442. Deteix C, Attuil-Audenis V, Duthey A, et al. Intragraft Th17 infiltrate promotes lymphoid neogenesis and hastens clinical chronic rejection. *J Immunol.* 2010;184(9):5344-5351.

443. Benezech C, Nayar S, Finney BA, et al. CLEC-2 is required for development and maintenance of lymph nodes. *Blood.* 2014;123(20):3200-3207.

444. Barone F, Nayar S, Campos J, et al. IL-22 regulates lymphoid chemokine production and assembly of tertiary lymphoid organs. *Proc Natl Acad Sci U S A.* 2015;112(35):11024-11029.

445. Bombardieri M, Barone F, Lucchesi D, et al. Inducible tertiary lymphoid structures, autoimmunity, and exocrine dysfunction in a novel model of salivary gland inflammation in C57BL/6 mice. *J Immunol.* 2012;189(7):3767-3776.

446. Fleige H, Ravens S, Moschovakis GL, et al. IL-17-induced CXCL12 recruits B cells and induces follicle formation in BALT in the absence of differentiated FDCs. *J Exp Med.* 2014;211(4):643-651.

447. Foo SY, Zhang V, Lalwani A, et al. Regulatory T cells prevent inducible BALT formation by dampening neutrophilic inflammation. *J Immunol.* 2015;194(9):4567-4576.

448. Carrega P, Loiacono F, Di Carlo E, et al. NCR(+)ILC3 concentrate in human lung cancer and associate with intratumoral lymphoid structures. *Nat Commun.* 2015;6:8280.

449. Meier D, Bornmann C, Chappaz S, et al. Ectopic lymphoid-organ development occurs through interleukin 7-mediated enhanced survival of lymphoid-tissue-inducer cells. *Immunity.* 2007;26(5):643-654.

450. Schmutz S, Bosco N, Chappaz S, et al. Cutting edge: IL-7 regulates the peripheral pool of adult ROR gamma+ lymphoid tissue inducer cells. *J Immunol.* 2009;183(4):2217-2221.

451. Jones GW, Jones SA. Ectopic lymphoid follicles: inducible centres for generating antigen-specific immune responses within tissues. *Immunology.* 2016;147(2):141-151.

452. Zhu M, Fu Y. Proinflammatory IL-17 induces iBALT development. *Cell Mol Immunol.* 2012;9(2):101-102.

453. Dieu-Nosjean MC, Goc J, Giraldo NA, Sautès-Fridman C, Fridman WH. Tertiary lymphoid structures in cancer and beyond. *Trends Immunol.* 2014;35(11):571-580.

454. Hu D, Mohanta SK, Yin C, et al. Artery tertiary lymphoid organs control aorta immunity and protect against atherosclerosis via vascular smooth muscle cell lymphotoxin beta receptors. *Immunity.* 2015;42(6):1100-1115.

455. Hiraoka N, Ino Y, Yamazaki-Itoh R, Kanai Y, Kosuge T, Shimada K. Intratumoral tertiary lymphoid organ is a favourable prognosticator in patients with pancreatic cancer. *Br J Cancer.* 2015;112(11):1782-1790.

456. Barone F, Bombardieri M, Rosado MM, et al. CXCL13, CCL21, and CXCL12 expression in salivary glands of patients with Sjogren's syndrome and MALT lymphoma: association with reactive and malignant areas of lymphoid organization. *J Immunol.* 2008;180(7):5130-5140.

457. Behr DS, Peitsch WK, Hametner C, et al. Prognostic value of immune cell infiltration, tertiary lymphoid structures and PD-L1 expression in Merkel cell carcinomas. *Int J Clin Exp Pathol.* 2014;7(11):7610-7621.

458. Bento DC, Jones E, Junaid S, et al. High endothelial venules are rare in colorectal cancers but accumulate in extra-tumoral areas with disease progression. *OncoImmunology.* 2015;4(3):e974374.

459. Cipponi A, Mercier M, Seremet T, et al. Neogenesis of lymphoid structures and antibody responses occur in human melanoma metastases. *Cancer Res.* 2012;72(16):3997-4007.

460. Coppola D, Nebozhyn M, Khalil F, et al. Unique ectopic lymph node-like structures present in human primary colorectal carcinoma are identified by immune gene array profiling. *Am J Pathol.* 2011;179(1):37-45.

461. Di Caro G, Bergomas F, Grizzi F, et al. Occurrence of tertiary lymphoid tissue is associated with T-cell infiltration and predicts better prognosis in early-stage colorectal cancers. *Clin Cancer Res.* 2014;20(8):2147-2158.

462. Dieu-Nosjean MC, Antoine M, Danel C, et al. Long-term survival for patients with non-small-cell lung cancer with intratumoral lymphoid structures. *J Clin Oncol.* 2008;26(27):4410-4417.

463. Figenschau SL, Fismen S, Fenton KA, et al. Tertiary lymphoid structures are associated with higher tumor grade in primary operable breast cancer patients. *BMC Cancer.* 2015;15:101.

464. Germain C, Gnjatic S, Tamzalit F, et al. Presence of B cells in tertiary lymphoid structures is associated with a protective immunity in patients with lung cancer. *Am J Respir Crit Care Med.* 2014;189(7):832-844.

465. Giraldo NA, Becht E, Pagès F, et al. Orchestration and prognostic significance of immune checkpoints in the microenvironment of primary and metastatic renal cell cancer. *Clin Cancer Res.* 2015;21(13):3031-3040.

466. Goc J, Germain C, Vo-Bourgais TKD, et al. Dendritic cells in tumor-associated tertiary lymphoid structures signal a Th1 cytotoxic immune contexture and license the positive prognostic value of infiltrating CD8+ T cells. *Cancer Res.* 2014;74(3):705-715.

467. Gu-Trantien C, Loi S, Garaud S, et al. CD4(+) follicular helper T cell infiltration predicts breast cancer survival. *J Clin Invest.* 2013;123(7):2873-2892.

468. Lee HJ, Kim JY, Park IA, et al. Prognostic significance of tumor-infiltrating lymphocytes and the tertiary lymphoid structures in HER2-positive breast cancer treated with adjuvant trastuzumab. *Am J Clin Pathol.* 2015;144(2):278-288.

469. Lee HJ, Park IA, Song IH, et al. Tertiary lymphoid structures: prognostic significance and relationship with tumour-infiltrating lymphocytes in triple-negative breast cancer. *J Clin Pathol.* 2016;69(5):422-430.

470. Martinet L, Garrido I, Filleron T, et al. Human solid tumors contain high endothelial venules: association with T- and B-lymphocyte infiltration and favorable prognosis in breast cancer. *Cancer Res.* 2011;71(17):5678-5687.

471. Vayrynen JP, Sajanti SA, Klintrup K, et al. Characteristics and significance of colorectal cancer associated lymphoid reaction. *Int J Cancer.* 2014;134(9):2126-2135.

472. Willis SN, Mallozzi SS, Rodig SJ, et al. The microenvironment of germ cell tumors harbors a prominent antigen-driven humoral response. *J Immunol.* 2009;182(5):3310-3317.

473. Wirsing AM, Rikardsen OG, Steigen SE, Uhlin-Hansen L, Hadler-Olsen E. Characterisation and prognostic value of tertiary lymphoid structures in oral squamous cell carcinoma. *BMC Clin Pathol.* 2014;14:38.

474. Zhu W, Germain C, Liu Z, et al. A high density of tertiary lymphoid structure B cells in lung tumors is associated with increased CD4(+) T cell receptor repertoire clonality. *OncoImmunology.* 2015;4(12):e1051922.

475. Kirk CJ, Hartigan-O'Connor D, Mule JJ. The dynamics of the T-cell antitumor response: chemokine-secreting dendritic cells can prime tumor-reactive T cells extranodally. *Cancer Res.* 2001;61(24):8794-8802.

476. Schrama D, thor Straten P, Fischer WH, et al. Targeting of lymphotoxin-alpha to the tumor elicits an efficient immune response associated with induction of peripheral lymphoid-like tissue. *Immunity.* 2001;14(2):111-121.

477. Ladanyi A, Kiss J, Somlai B, et al. Density of DC-LAMP(+) mature dendritic cells in combination with activated T lymphocytes infiltrating primary cutaneous melanoma is a strong independent prognostic factor. *Cancer Immunol Immunother.* 2007;56(9):1459-1469.

478. Breitfeld D, Ohl L, Kremmer E, et al. Follicular B helper T cells express CXC chemokine receptor 5, localize to B cell follicles, and support immunoglobulin production. *J Exp Med.* 2000;192(11):1545-1552.

479. Schaerli P, Willimann K, Lang AB, Lipp M, Loetscher P, Moser B. CXC chemokine receptor 5 expression defines follicular homing T cells with B cell helper function. *J Exp Med.* 2000;192(11):1553-1562.

480. Ebert LM, Schaerli P, Moser B. Chemokine-mediated control of T cell traffic in lymphoid and peripheral tissues. *Mol Immunol.* 2005;42(7):799-809.

481. Kim CH. The greater chemotactic network for lymphocyte trafficking: chemokines and beyond. *Curr Opin Hematol.* 2005;12(4):298-304.

482. Sackstein R. The lymphocyte homing receptors: gatekeepers of the multistep paradigm. *Curr Opin Hematol.* 2005;12(6):444-450.

483. Yamaguchi K, Schoefl GI. Blood vessels of the Peyer's patch in the mouse: III. High-endothelium venules. *Anat Rec.* 1983;206(4):419-438.

484. Butcher EC, Picker LJ. Lymphocyte homing and homeostasis. *Science.* 1996;272(5258):60-66.

485. von Andrian UH. Intravital microscopy of the peripheral lymph node microcirculation in mice. *Microcirculation.* 1996;3(3):287-300.

486. Janssen GH, Tangelder GJ, Oude Egbrink MG, Reneman RS. Spontaneous leukocyte rolling in venules in untraumatized skin of conscious and anesthetized animals. *Am J Physiol.* 1994;267(3 pt 2):H1199-H1204.

487. Springer TA. Traffic signals on endothelium for lymphocyte recirculation and leukocyte emigration. *Annu Rev Physiol.* 1995;57:827-872.

488. Lasky LA, Singer MS, Dowbenko D, et al. An endothelial ligand for L-selectin is a novel mucin-like molecule. *Cell.* 1992;69(6):927-938.

489. Baumheter S, Singer MS, Henzel W, et al. Binding of L-selectin to the vascular sialomucin CD34. *Science.* 1993;262(5132):436-438.

490. Sassetti C, Tangemann K, Singer MS, Kershaw DB, Rosen SD. Identification of podocalyxin-like protein as a high endothelial venule ligand for L-selectin: parallels to CD34. *J Exp Med.* 1998;187(12):1965-1975.

491. Kanda H, Tanaka T, Matsumoto M, et al. Endomucin, a sialomucin expressed in high endothelial venules, supports L-selectin-mediated rolling. *Int Immunol.* 2004;16(9):1265-1274.

492. Umemoto E, Tanaka T, Kanda H, et al. Nepmucin, a novel HEV sialomucin, mediates L-selectin-dependent lymphocyte rolling and promotes lymphocyte adhesion under flow. *J Exp Med.* 2006;203(6):1603-1614.

493. Uchimura K, Rosen SD. Sulfated L-selectin ligands as a therapeutic target in chronic inflammation. *Trends Immunol.* 2006;27(12):559-565.

494. Berlin C, Bargatze RF, Campbell JJ, et al. Alpha 4 integrins mediate lymphocyte attachment and rolling under physiologic flow. *Cell.* 1995;80(3):413-422.

495. von Andrian UH, Hasslen SR, Nelson RD, Erlandsen SL, Butcher EC. A central role for microvillous receptor presentation in leukocyte adhesion under flow. *Cell.* 1995;82(6):989-999.

496. Bargatze RF, Jutila MA, Butcher EC. Distinct roles of L-selectin and integrins alpha 4 beta 7 and LFA-1 in lymphocyte homing to Peyer's patch-HEV in situ: the multistep model confirmed and refined. *Immunity.* 1995;3(1):99-108.

497. Arbones ML, Ord DC, Ley K, et al. Lymphocyte homing and leukocyte rolling and migration are impaired in L-selectin-deficient mice. *Immunity.* 1994;1(4):247-260.

498. Pavalko FM, Walker DM, Graham L, Goheen M, Doerschuk CM, Kansas GS. The cytoplasmic domain of L-selectin interacts with cytoskeletal proteins via alpha-actinin: receptor positioning in microvilli does not require interaction with alpha-actinin. *J Cell Biol.* 1995;129(4):1155-1164.

499. Briskin MJ, McEvoy LM, Butcher EC. MAdCAM-1 has homology to immunoglobulin and mucin-like adhesion receptors and to IgA1. *Nature.* 1993;363(6428):461-464.

500. Shulman Z, Shinder V, Klein E, et al. Lymphocyte crawling and transendothelial migration require chemokine triggering of high-affinity LFA-1 integrin. *Immunity.* 2009;30(3):384-396.

501. Campbell JJ, Hedrick J, Zlotnik A, Siani MA, Thompson DA, Butcher EC. Chemokines and the arrest of lymphocytes rolling under flow conditions. *Science.* 1998;279(5349):381-384.

502. Tangemann K, Gunn MD, Giblin P, Rosen SD. A high endothelial cell-derived chemokine induces rapid, efficient, and subset-selective arrest of rolling T lymphocytes on a reconstituted endothelial substrate. *J Immunol.* 1998;161(11):6330-6337.

503. Umemoto E, Hayasaka H, Bai Z, et al. Novel regulators of lymphocyte trafficking across high endothelial venules. *Crit Rev Immunol.* 2011;31(2):147-169.

504. Kanda H, Newton R, Klein R, Morita Y, Gunn MD, Rosen SD. Autotaxin, an ectoenzyme that produces lysophosphatidic acid, promotes the entry of lymphocytes into secondary lymphoid organs. *Nat Immunol.* 2008;9(4):415-423.

505. Nakasaki T, Tanaka T, Okudaira S, et al. Involvement of the lysophosphatidic acid-generating enzyme autotaxin in lymphocyte-endothelial cell interactions. *Am J Pathol.* 2008;173(5):1566-1576.

506. Bai Z, Cai L, Umemoto E, et al. Constitutive lymphocyte transmigration across the basal lamina of high endothelial venules is regulated by the autotaxin/lysophosphatidic acid axis. *J Immunol.* 2013;190(5):2036-2048.

507. Hata E, Sasaki N, Takeda A, et al. Lysophosphatidic acid receptors LPA4 and LPA6 differentially promote lymphocyte transmigration across high endothelial venules in lymph nodes. *Int Immunol.* 2016;28(6):283-292.

508. Liu K, Victora GD, Schwickert TA, et al. In vivo analysis of dendritic cell development and homeostasis. *Science.* 2009;324(5925):392-397.

509. Matsutani T, Tanaka T, Tohya K, et al. Plasmacytoid dendritic cells employ multiple cell adhesion molecules sequentially to interact with high endothelial venule cells--molecular basis of their trafficking to lymph nodes. *Int Immunol.* 2007;19(9):1031-1037.

510. Seth S, Oberdörfer L, Hyde R, et al. CCR7 essentially contributes to the homing of plasmacytoid dendritic cells to lymph nodes under steady-state as well as inflammatory conditions. *J Immunol.* 2011;186(6):3364-3372.

511. Umemoto E, Otani K, Ikeno T, et al. Constitutive plasmacytoid dendritic cell migration to the splenic white pulp is cooperatively regulated by CCR7- and CXCR4-mediated signaling. *J Immunol.* 2012;189(1):191-199.

512. Brackett CM, Muhitch JB, Evans SS, Gollnick SO. IL-17 promotes neutrophil entry into tumor-draining lymph nodes following induction of sterile inflammation. *J Immunol.* 2013;191(8):4348-4357.

513. Iwata M, Hirakiyama A, Eshima Y, Kagechika H, Kato C, Song SY. Retinoic acid imprints gut-homing specificity on T cells. *Immunity.* 2004;21(4):527-538.

514. Nguyen LP, Pan J, Dinh TT, et al. Role and species-specific expression of colon T cell homing receptor GPR15 in colitis. *Nat Immunol.* 2015;16(2):207-213.

515. Weninger W, Ulfman LH, Cheng G, et al. Specialized contributions by alpha(1,3)-fucosyltransferase-IV and FucT-VII during leukocyte rolling in dermal microvessels. *Immunity.* 2000;12(6):665-676.

516. McCully ML, Ladell K, Hakobyan S, Mansel RE, Price DA, Moser B. Epidermis instructs skin homing receptor expression in human T cells. *Blood.* 2012;120(23):4591-4598.

517. Reiss Y, Proudfoot AE, Power CA, Campbell JJ, Butcher EC. CC chemokine receptor (CCR)4 and the CCR10 ligand cutaneous T cell-attracting chemokine (CTACK) in lymphocyte trafficking to inflamed skin. *J Exp Med.* 2001;194(10):1541-1547.

518. Sigmundsdottir H, Pan J, Debes GF, et al. DCs metabolize sunlight-induced vitamin D3 to "program" T cell attraction to the epidermal chemokine CCL27. *Nat Immunol.* 2007;8(3):285-293.

519. Homey B, Alenius H, Müller A, et al. CCL27-CCR10 interactions regulate T cell-mediated skin inflammation. *Nat Med.* 2002;8(2):157-165.

520. Clark RA. Resident memory T cells in human health and disease. *Sci Transl Med.* 2015;7(269):269rv1.

521. Clark RA, Chong B, Mirchandani N, et al. The vast majority of CLA+ T cells are resident in normal skin. *J Immunol.* 2006;176(7):4431-4439.

522. Mackay CR, Marston WL, Dudler L. Naive and memory T cells show distinct pathways of lymphocyte recirculation. *J Exp Med.* 1990;171(3):801-817.

523. Sallusto F, Geginat J, Lanzavecchia A. Central memory and effector memory T cell subsets: function, generation, and maintenance. *Annu Rev Immunol.* 2004;22:745-763.

524. Clark RA, Watanabe R, Teague JE, et al. Skin effector memory T cells do not recirculate and provide immune protection in alemtuzumab-treated CTCL patients. *Sci Transl Med.* 2012;4(117):117ra7.

525. Schenkel JM, Masopust D. Tissue-resident memory T cells. *Immunity.* 2014;41(6):886-897.

526. Sather BD, Treuting P, Perdue N, et al. Altering the distribution of Foxp3(+) regulatory T cells results in tissue-specific inflammatory disease. *J Exp Med.* 2007;204(6):1335-1347.

527. Tomura M, Honda T, Tanizaki H, et al. Activated regulatory T cells are the major T cell type emigrating from the skin during a cutaneous immune response in mice. *J Clin Invest.* 2010;120(3):883-893.

528. Grabbe S, Varga G, Beissert S, et al. Beta2 integrins are required for skin homing of primed T cells but not for priming naive T cells. *J Clin Invest.* 2002;109(2):183-192.

529. Weber M, Hauschild R, Schwarz J, et al. Interstitial dendritic cell guidance by haptotactic chemokine gradients. *Science.* 2013;339(6117):328-332.

530. Artis D, Spits H. The biology of innate lymphoid cells. *Nature.* 2015;517(7534):293-301.

531. Roediger B, Kyle R, Yip KH, et al. Cutaneous immunosurveillance and regulation of inflammation by group 2 innate lymphoid cells. *Nat Immunol.* 2013;14(6):564-573.

532. Kerjaschki D, Regele HM, Moosberger I, et al. Lymphatic neoangiogenesis in human kidney transplants is associated with immunologically active lymphocytic infiltrates. *J Am Soc Nephrol.* 2004;15(3):603-612.

533. Ulvmar MH, Werth K, Braun A, et al. The atypical chemokine receptor CCRL1 shapes functional CCL21 gradients in lymph nodes. *Nat Immunol.* 2014;15(7):623-630.

534. Forster R, Schubel A, Breitfeld D, et al. CCR7 coordinates the primary immune response by establishing functional microenvironments in secondary lymphoid organs. *Cell.* 1999;99(1):23-33.

535. Ohl L, Mohaupt M, Czeloth N, et al. CCR7 governs skin dendritic cell migration under inflammatory and steady-state conditions. *Immunity.* 2004;21(2):279-288.

536. Partida-Sanchez S, Goodrich S, Kusser K, et al. Regulation of dendritic cell trafficking by the ADP-ribosyl cyclase CD38: impact on the development of humoral immunity. *Immunity.* 2004;20(3):279-291.

537. Scandella E, Men Y, Gillessen S, Förster R, Groettrup M. Prostaglandin E2 is a key factor for CCR7 surface expression and migration of monocyte-derived dendritic cells. *Blood.* 2002;100(4):1354-1361.

538. Braun A, Worbs T, Moschovakis GL, et al. Afferent lymph-derived T cells and DCs use different chemokine receptor CCR7-dependent routes for entry into the lymph node and intranodal migration. *Nat Immunol.* 2011;12(9):879-887.

539. Johnson LA, Jackson DG. The chemokine CX3CL1 promotes trafficking of dendritic cells through inflamed lymphatics. *J Cell Sci.* 2013;126(pt 22):5259-5270.

540. Kabashima K, Shiraishi N, Sugita K, et al. CXCL12-CXCR4 engagement is required for migration of cutaneous dendritic cells. *Am J Pathol.* 2007;171(4):1249-1257.

541. Bai Z, Hayasaka H, Kobayashi M, et al. CXC chemokine ligand 12 promotes CCR7-dependent naive T cell trafficking to lymph nodes and Peyer's patches. *J Immunol.* 2009;182(3):1287-1295.

542. Qu C, Edwards EW, Tacke F, et al. Role of CCR8 and other chemokine pathways in the migration of monocyte-derived dendritic cells to lymph nodes. *J Exp Med.* 2004;200(10):1231-1241.

543. Lammermann T, Bader BL, Monkley SJ, et al. Rapid leukocyte migration by integrin-independent flowing and squeezing. *Nature.* 2008;453(7191):51-55.

544. Acton SE, Astarita JL, Malhotra D, et al. Podoplanin-rich stromal networks induce dendritic cell motility via activation of the C-type lectin receptor CLEC-2. *Immunity.* 2012;37(2):276-289.

545. Johnson LA, Clasper S, Holt AP, Lalor PF, Baban D, Jackson DG. An inflammation-induced mechanism for leukocyte transmigration across lymphatic vessel endothelium. *J Exp Med.* 2006;203(12):2763-2777.

546. Teijeira A, Rouzaut A, Melero I. Initial afferent lymphatic vessels controlling outbound leukocyte traffic from skin to lymph nodes. *Front Immunol.* 2013;4:433.

547. Takamatsu H, Takegahara N, Nakagawa Y, et al. Semaphorins guide the entry of dendritic cells into the lymphatics by activating myosin II. *Nat Immunol.* 2010;11(7):594-600.

548. Katakai T, Kondo N, Ueda Y, Kinashi T. Autotaxin produced by stromal cells promotes LFA-1-independent and Rho-dependent interstitial T cell motility in the lymph node paracortex. *J Immunol.* 2014;193(2):617-626.

549. Takeda A, Kobayashi D, Aoi K, et al. Fibroblastic reticular cell-derived lysophosphatidic acid regulates confined intranodal T-cell motility. *Elife.* 2016;5:e10561.

550. Takeda A, Sasaki N, Miyasaka M. The molecular cues regulating immune cell trafficking. *Proc Jpn Acad Ser B Phys Biol Sci.* 2017;93(4):183-195.

551. Cyster JG, Schwab SR. Sphingosine-1-phosphate and lymphocyte egress from lymphoid organs. *Annu Rev Immunol.* 2012;30:69-94.

552. Kono M, Tucker AE, Tran J, Bergner JB, Turner EM, Proia RL. Sphingosine-1-phosphate receptor 1 reporter mice reveal receptor activation sites in vivo. *J Clin Invest.* 2014;124(5):2076-2086.

The Normal Hematologic System

553. Herzog BH, Fu J, Wilson SJ, et al. Podoplanin maintains high endothelial venule integrity by interacting with platelet CLEC-2. *Nature*. 2013;502(7469):105-109.

554. Nicholas NS, Apollonio B, Ramsay AG. Tumor microenvironment (TME)-driven immune suppression in B cell malignancy. *Biochim Biophys Acta*. 2016;1863(3):471-482.

555. Xu ML, Fedoriw Y. Lymphoma microenvironment and immunotherapy. *Surg Pathol Clin*. 2016;9(1):93-100.

556. Lackraj T, Goswami R, Kridel R. Pathogenesis of follicular lymphoma. *Best Pract Res Clin Haematol*. 2018;31(1):2-14.

557. Gaulard P, de Leval L. The microenvironment in T-cell lymphomas: emerging themes. *Semin Cancer Biol*. 2014;24:49-60.

558. Mourcin F, VerdièreL, Roulois D, et al. Follicular lymphoma triggers phenotypic and functional remodeling of the human lymphoid stromal cell landscape. *Immunity*. 2021;54(8):1901.

559. Burger JA, Gribben JG. The microenvironment in chronic lymphocytic leukemia (CLL) and other B cell malignancies: insight into disease biology and new targeted therapies. *Semin Cancer Biol*. 2014;24:71-81.

560. Aoki T, Chong LC, Takata K, et al. Single-cell transcriptome analysis reveals disease-defining T-cell subsets in the tumor microenvironment of classic Hodgkin lymphoma. *Cancer Discov*. 2020;10(3):406-421.

561. Bagaev A, Kotlov N, Nomie K, et al. Conserved pan-cancer microenvironment subtypes predict response to immunotherapy. *Cancer Cell*. 2021;39(6):845-865.e7.

562. Cader FZ, Hu X, Goh WL, et al. A peripheral immune signature of responsiveness to PD-1 blockade in patients with classical Hodgkin lymphoma. *Nat Med*. 2020;26(9):1468-1479.

563. Dheilly E, Battistello E, Katanayeva N, et al. Cathepsin S regulates antigen processing and T cell activity in non-Hodgkin lymphoma. *Cancer Cell*. 2020;37(5):674-689.e12.

564. Fiore D, Cappelli LV, Broccoli A, Zinzani PL, Chan WC, Inghirami G. Peripheral T cell lymphomas: from the bench to the clinic. *Nat Rev Cancer*. 2020;20(6):323-342.

565. Kotlov N, Bagaev A, Revuelta MV, et al. Clinical and biological subtypes of B-cell lymphoma revealed by microenvironmental signatures. *Cancer Discov*. 2021;11(6):1468-1489.

566. Mourcin F, Verdière L, Roulois D, et al. Follicular lymphoma triggers phenotypic and functional remodeling of the human lymphoid stromal cell landscape. *Immunity*. 2021;54(8):1788-1806.e7.

567. Roider T, Seufert J, Uvarovskii A, et al. Dissecting intratumour heterogeneity of nodal B-cell lymphomas at the transcriptional, genetic and drug-response levels. *Nat Cell Biol*. 2020;22(7):896-906.

568. Ruella M, Klichinsky M, Kenderian SS, et al. Overcoming the immunosuppressive tumor microenvironment of Hodgkin lymphoma using chimeric antigen receptor T cells. *Cancer Discov*. 2017;7(10):1154-1167.

569. Steen CB, Luca BA, Esfahani MS, et al. The landscape of tumor cell states and ecosystems in diffuse large B cell lymphoma. *Cancer Cell*. 2021;39(10):1422-1437.e10.

570. Scott DW, Steidl C. The classical Hodgkin lymphoma tumor microenvironment: macrophages and gene expression-based modeling. *Hematology Am Soc Hematol Educ Program*. 2014;2014(1):144-150.

571. Scott DW, Gascoyne RD. The tumour microenvironment in B cell lymphomas. *Nat Rev Cancer*. 2014;14(8):517-534.

572. Kuppers R. The biology of Hodgkin's lymphoma. *Nat Rev Cancer*. 2009;9(1):15-27.

573. Steidl C, Lee T, Shah SP, et al. Tumor-associated macrophages and survival in classic Hodgkin's lymphoma. *N Engl J Med*. 2010;362(10):875-885.

574. Steidl C, Connors JM, Gascoyne RD. Molecular pathogenesis of Hodgkin's lymphoma: increasing evidence of the importance of the microenvironment. *J Clin Oncol*. 2011;29(14):1812-1826.

575. Fhu CW, Graham AM, Yap CT, et al. Reed-Sternberg cell-derived lymphotoxin-a activates endothelial cells to enhance T-cell recruitment in classical Hodgkin lymphoma. *Blood*. 2014;124(19):2973-2982.

576. Martin-Moreno AM, Roncador G, Maestre L, et al. CSF1R protein expression in reactive lymphoid tissues and lymphoma: its relevance in classical Hodgkin lymphoma. *PLoS One*. 2015;10(6):e0125203.

577. Locatelli SL, Careddu G, Serio S, et al. Targeting cancer cells and tumor microenvironment in preclinical and clinical models of Hodgkin lymphoma using the dual PI3Kd/? Inhibitor RP6530. *Clin Cancer Res*. 2019;25(3):1098-1112.

578. Aoki T, Chong LC, Takata K, et al. Single-cell profiling reveals the importance of CXCL13/CXCR5 axis biology in lymphocyte-rich classic Hodgkin lymphoma. *Proc Natl Acad Sci U S A*. 2021;118(41):e2105822118.

579. Pinto A, Aldinucci D, Gloghini A, et al. Human eosinophils express functional CD30 ligand and stimulate proliferation of a Hodgkin's disease cell line. *Blood*. 1996;88(9):3299-3305.

580. Chemnitz JM, Eggle D, Driesen J, et al. RNA fingerprints provide direct evidence for the inhibitory role of TGFbeta and PD-1 on CD4+ T cells in Hodgkin lymphoma. *Blood*. 2007;110(9):3226-3233.

581. Kilger E, Kieser A, Baumann M, Hammerschmidt W. Epstein-Barr virus-mediated B-cell proliferation is dependent upon latent membrane protein 1, which simulates an activated CD40 receptor. *EMBO J*. 1998;17(6):1700-1709.

582. Mancao C, Hammerschmidt W. Epstein-Barr virus latent membrane protein 2A is a B-cell receptor mimic and essential for B-cell survival. *Blood*. 2007;110(10):3715-3721.

583. Tzankov A, Meier C, Hirschmann P, Went P, Pileri SA, Dirnhofer S. Correlation of high numbers of intratumoral FOXP3+ regulatory T cells with improved survival in germinal center-like diffuse large B-cell lymphoma, follicular lymphoma and classical Hodgkin's lymphoma. *Haematologica*. 2008;93(2):193-200.

584. Smeltzer JP, Jones JM, Ziesmer SC, et al. Pattern of CD14+ follicular dendritic cells and PD1+ T cells independently predicts time to transformation in follicular lymphoma. *Clin Cancer Res*. 2014;20(11):2862-2872.

585. Ramsay AG, Clear AJ, Kelly G, et al. Follicular lymphoma cells induce T-cell immunologic synapse dysfunction that can be repaired with lenalidomide: implications for the tumor microenvironment and immunotherapy. *Blood*. 2009;114(21):4713-4720.

586. Green MR, Kihira S, Liu CL, et al. Mutations in early follicular lymphoma progenitors are associated with suppressed antigen presentation. *Proc Natl Acad Sci U S A*. 2015;112(10):E1116-E1125.

587. Kridel R, Chan FC, Mottok A, et al. Histological transformation and progression in follicular lymphoma: a clonal evolution study. *PLoS Med*. 2016;13(12):e1002197.

588. Pasqualucci L, Khiabanian H, Fangazio M, et al. Genetics of follicular lymphoma transformation. *Cell Rep*. 2014;6(1):130-140.

589. Bahler DW, Levy R. Clonal evolution of a follicular lymphoma: evidence for antigen selection. *Proc Natl Acad Sci U S A*. 1992;89(15):6770-6774.

590. Cha SC, Qin H, Kannan S, et al. Nonstereotyped lymphoma B cell receptors recognize vimentin as a shared autoantigen. *J Immunol*. 2013;190(9):4887-4898.

591. Sachen KL, Strohman MJ, Singletary J, et al. Self-antigen recognition by follicular lymphoma B-cell receptors. *Blood*. 2012;120(20):4182-4190.

592. Zhu D, McCarthy H, Ottensmeier CH, Johnson P, Hamblin TJ, Stevenson FK. Acquisition of potential N-glycosylation sites in the immunoglobulin variable region by somatic mutation is a distinctive feature of follicular lymphoma. *Blood*. 2002;99(7):2562-2568.

593. Radcliffe CM, Arnold JN, Suter DM, et al. Human follicular lymphoma cells contain oligomannose glycans in the antigen-binding site of the B-cell receptor. *J Biol Chem*. 2007;282(10):7405-7415.

594. Coelho V, Krysov S, Ghaemmaghami AM, et al. Glycosylation of surface Ig creates a functional bridge between human follicular lymphoma and microenvironmental lectins. *Proc Natl Acad Sci U S A*. 2010;107(43):18587-18592.

595. Linley A, Krysov S, Ponzoni M, Johnson PW, Packham G, Stevenson FK. Lectin binding to surface Ig variable regions provides a universal persistent activating signal for follicular lymphoma cells. *Blood*. 2015;126(16):1902-1910.

596. Kridel R, Xerri L, Gelas-Dore B, et al. The prognostic impact of CD163-positive macrophages in follicular lymphoma: a study from the BC cancer agency and the lymphoma study association. *Clin Cancer Res*. 2015;21(15):3428-3435.

597. Attygalle A, Al-Jehani R, Diss TC, et al. Neoplastic T cells in angioimmunoblastic T-cell lymphoma express CD10. *Blood*. 2002;99(2):627-633.

598. Ree HJ, Kadin ME., Kikuchi M, et al. Angioimmunoblastic lymphoma (AILD-type T-cell lymphoma) with hyperplastic germinal centers. *Am J Surg Pathol*. 1998;22(6):643-655.

599. McHeyzer-Williams LJ, Pelletier N, Mark L, Fazilleau N, McHeyzer-Williams MG. Follicular helper T cells as cognate regulators of B cell immunity. *Curr Opin Immunol*. 2009;21(3):266-273.

600. Dupuis J, Boye K, Martin N, et al. Expression of CXCL13 by neoplastic cells in angioimmunoblastic T-cell lymphoma (AITL): a new diagnostic marker providing evidence that AITL derives from follicular helper T cells. *Am J Surg Pathol*. 2006;30(4):490-494.

601. Grogg KL, Attygalle AD, Macon WR, Remstein ED, Kurtin PJ, Dogan A. Angioimmunoblastic T-cell lymphoma: a neoplasm of germinal-center T-helper cells? *Blood*. 2005;106(4):1501-1502.

602. Grogg KL, Attygale AD, Macon WR, Remstein ED, Kurtin PJ, Dogan A. Expression of CXCL13, a chemokine highly upregulated in germinal center T-helper cells, distinguishes angioimmunoblastic T-cell lymphoma from peripheral T-cell lymphoma, unspecified. *Mod Pathol*. 2006;19(8):1101-1107.

603. Ortonne N, Dupuis J, Plonquet A, et al. Characterization of CXCL13+ neoplastic t cells in cutaneous lesions of angioimmunoblastic T-cell lymphoma (AITL). *Am J Surg Pathol*. 2007;31(7):1068-1076.

604. Bisig B, Thielen C, Herens C, et al. c-Maf expression in angioimmunoblastic T-cell lymphoma reflects follicular helper T-cell derivation rather than oncogenesis. *Histopathology*. 2012;60(2):371-376.

605. Gaulard P, de Leval L. Follicular helper T cells: implications in neoplastic hematopathology. *Semin Diagn Pathol*. 2011;28(3):202-213.

606. Foss HD, Anagnostopoulos I, Herbst H, et al. Patterns of cytokine gene expression in peripheral T-cell lymphoma of angioimmunoblastic lymphadenopathy type. *Blood*. 1995;85(10):2862-2869.

607. de Leval L, Rickman DS, Thielen C, et al. The gene expression profile of nodal peripheral T-cell lymphoma demonstrates a molecular link between angioimmunoblastic T-cell lymphoma (AITL) and follicular helper T (TFH) cells. *Blood*. 2007;109(11):4952-4963.

608. Konstantinou K, Yamamoto K, Ishibashi F, et al. Angiogenic mediators of the angiopoietin system are highly expressed by CD10-positive lymphoma cells in angioimmunoblastic T-cell lymphoma. *Br J Haematol*. 2009;144(5):696-704.

609. Piccaluga PP, Agostinelli C, Califano A, et al. Gene expression analysis of angioimmunoblastic lymphoma indicates derivation from T follicular helper cells and vascular endothelial growth factor deregulation. *Cancer Res*. 2007;67(22):10703-10710.

610. Attygalle AD, Cabeçadas J, Gaulard P, et al. Peripheral T-cell and NK-cell lymphomas and their mimics; taking a step forward—report on the lymphoma workshop of the XVIth meeting of the European Association for Haematopathology and the Society for Hematopathology. *Histopathology*. 2014;64(2):171-199.

Chapter 12 ■ B Lymphocytes

JEFFREY J. BEDNARSKI II

ONTOGENY

Pluripotent stem cells give rise to all hematopoietic lineages through asymmetric division in which one daughter cell undergoes differentiation and the other remains as a self-renewing stem cell. Interaction with stromal cells, as well as growth and differentiation factors, directs stem cell differentiation into various lineages including B and T lymphocytes. For example, exposure to the thymic microenvironment stimulates T-cell differentiation, whereas contact with bone marrow stromal cells supports differentiation into B lymphocytes or myeloid cells. Multiple checkpoints ensure proper development of B lymphocytes, and several of these have been found disrupted in patients with primary immunodeficiency. The differentiation of the B cell involves critical processes divided into two periods (*Figure 12.1*). Early differentiation from stem cell to immature B cell is antigen independent and occurs in the bone marrow. The first period can be subdivided into two stages: from stem cell to progenitor B (pro-B) cell and from pro-B cell to immature B cell. Later stages of differentiation from immature B cell to plasma cell is antigen dependent and occurs primarily in peripheral lymphoid organs.

GENERATION OF A DIVERSE LYMPHOCYTE REPERTOIRE

Lymphocytes traverse functionally distinct stages as they develop into mature B and T lymphocytes. To complete development, all lymphocytes must express a functional, nonautoreactive antigen receptor. In B cells, two copies of the immunoglobulin heavy chain (IgH) combine with two copies of the immunoglobulin light chain (IgL) to generate a mature antigen receptor, known as the B-cell receptor (BCR). Each B cell expresses a unique BCR that recognizes a distinct epitope on a foreign antigen. Expression of a BCR is tightly regulated during B lymphocyte maturation by unique transcription factors and signals from various surface receptors.

IMMUNOGLOBULIN GENE ASSEMBLY

Among the seminal discoveries in immunology was the characterization of the structure and mechanism of assembly of the immunoglobulin genes.[1] In humans, the IgH chain gene is located on chromosome 14.[2] There are two distinct *IgL* genes: *IgLκ* is located on chromosome 2 and *IgLλ* is on chromosome 22.[3-5] The first two exons of all the Ig genes encode the variable region (V), which recognizes antigen. The second exon is assembled in developing lymphocytes from component variable (V), joining (J), and, in some cases, diversity (D) gene segments through the process of V(D)J recombination, which requires the generation and repair of DNA double-stranded breaks (DSBs).[6,7] The assembly of different V, D, and J gene segments (combinatorial diversity) and the imprecision of the assembly process (junctional diversity) together provide the basis for the adaptive immune system to recognize a vast diversity of foreign antigens. Downstream of the V, D, and J segments lie constant region (C) gene segments (*Figure 12.2*). The IgL chain loci have a single C region, whereas the IgH chain locus has a series of nine C regions, each corresponding to a different immunoglobulin isotype. Each C gene segment in the IgH locus is bordered by switch regions that function as breakpoints during class switching in mature B cells. Successful assembly of the genes encoding the appropriate antigen receptor heterodimer is essential for normal B- and T-cell development.

Immunoglobulin Gene Structure

The heavy chain gene is encoded by variable (V_H), diversity (D), joining (J_H), and constant (C) region gene segments. The IgH locus contains 100 to 200 V_H gene segments in the 5′ region of the locus followed by approximately 30 D_H and 6 J_H gene segments.[8,9] Of the available V_H genes only a portion are functional, and an even smaller portion is available for rearrangement.[10,11] The V_H segment encodes two of the three complementarity-determining regions (CDRs), which together determine the antigen-binding site. The third CDR is encoded by the 3′ end of the V_H segment, the D gene segment, and the DJ_H junctional area. The joining of the V_H, D, and J_H segments proceeds in two steps (*Figure 12.2*). First, a D segment joins a J_H segment to form a DJ_H complex. A V_H segment then joins to the DJ_H to make a complete exon.

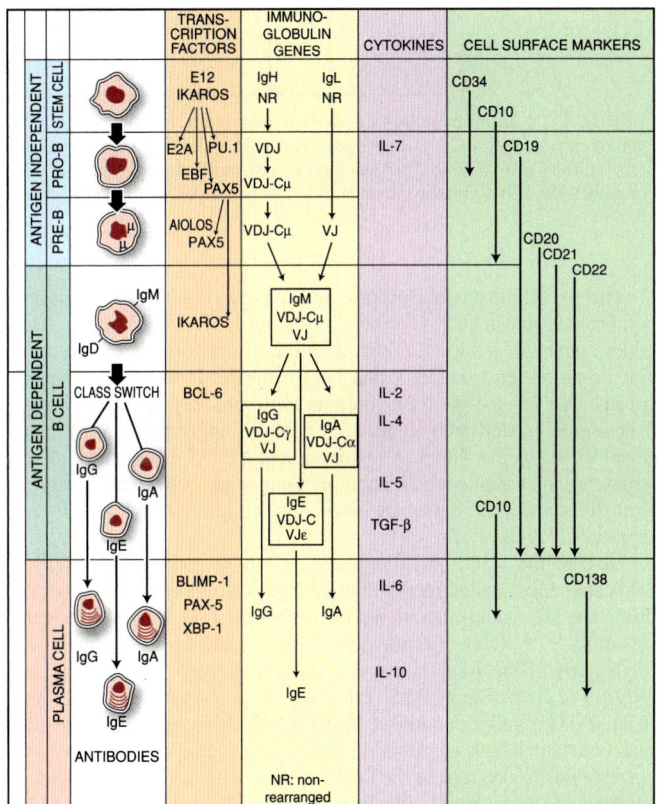

FIGURE 12.1 B-cell differentiation. The first stage (blue) of B-cell development is antigen independent and takes place in the bone marrow. Normal development of lymphopoiesis depends on the IKAROS family of transcription factors, which form multimeric complexes with other members, that is, AIOLOS and HELIOS. These complexes induce a second wave of transcription factors, that is, PU.1, E2A, EBF, and PAX5, which in turn induce expression of B-cell lineage-specific genetic program. During this early stage of development the IgH and IgL genes are assembled resulting in expression of surface IgM. The B cell subsequently egresses from the bone marrow to peripheral lymphoid organs where antigen-dependent development continues (green). This stage includes class switch recombination and affinity maturation of the assembled immunoglobulin receptors (Ig). Interaction of sIg with antigen and helper T cells triggers antibody secretion and terminal B-cell differentiation to plasma cells (red). V, variable; D, diversity; J, joining.

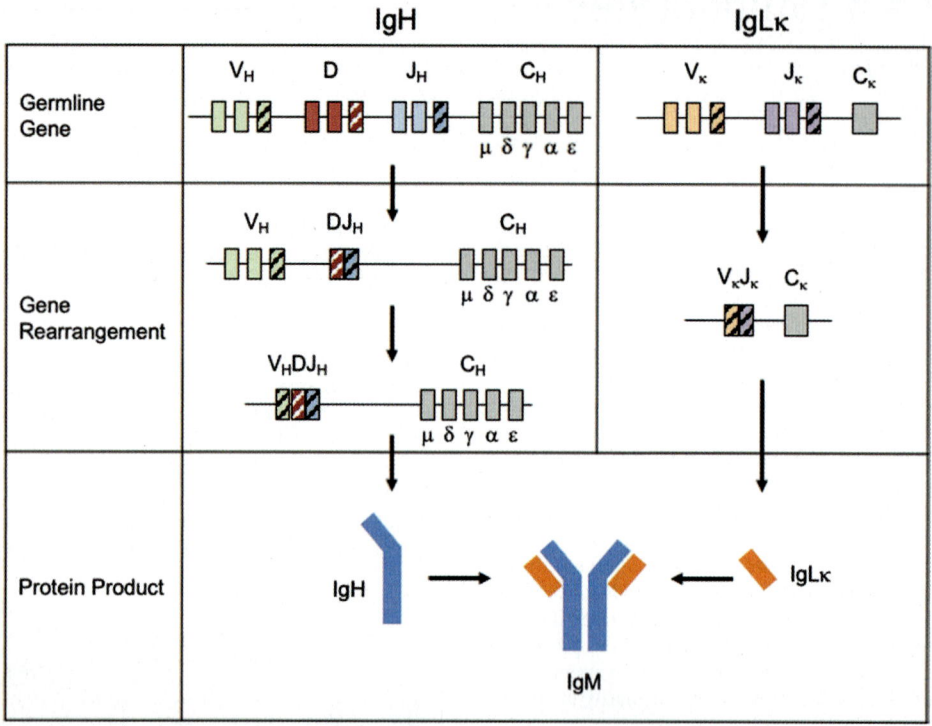

FIGURE 12.2 Immunoglobulin gene rearrangement. IgH and IgL immunoglobulin genes are rearranged through VDJ recombination to assemble the second exon of each gene from V, D, and J gene segments. Following completion of V(D)J recombination of the IgH chain, the IgLκ chain rearranges, and, if successful, pairs with the IgH chain to form a complete IgM molecule. If both IgLκ alleles rearrange unsuccessfully, the IgLλ gene rearranges and pairs with IgH to form a complete IgM. If both IgLλ genes cannot rearrange successfully, the cell dies by apoptosis.

The two light chain isotypes, IgLκ (kappa) and IgLλ (lambda), comprise approximately 60% and 40% of all BCRs, respectively. Both genes consist of a variable domain and a constant domain. The variable domain is encoded by V and J segments (no D segments are present in either *IgL* locus). *IgL*κ contains approximately 76 Vκ segments, 5 Jκ segments, and a Cκ gene. *IgL*κ contains approximately 30 functional Vκ segments, 4 to 5 Jλ segments, and 4 to 5 Cλ genes, which are structured such that each Jλ gene segment is adjacent to a Cλ region. Both *IgL*κ and *IgL*λ genes are assembled by joining of V and J gene segments (*Figure 12.2*).

Next to the V, D, and J segments of all Ig genes are conserved DNA sequences called recombination signal sequences (RSSs), which guide the DNA rearrangements necessary for immunoglobulin gene assembly.[12-14] RSSs are attached to the 3′ side of the V segments, the 5′ side of the J segments, and on both sides of the D segments (*Figure 12.3*). Each RSS consists of a conserved heptamer (CACAGTG) and a nonamer (ACAAAAACC) separated by a spacer of a constant length of either 12 or 23 base pairs. The 12-bp spacer corresponds to one turn of the DNA α-helix, whereas the 23-bp spacer corresponds to two turns. This way, the recombining segments are juxtaposed on the same side of the DNA helix, so that they can be recognized by the enzymes of the recombination machinery.[14,15] Joining of the various segments is limited between an RSS with a 12-bp spacer and one with 23 bp (the 12/23 rule).[16,17] The pattern of the RSS at each locus is uniform. For example, in the IgH locus, all V_H and J_H segments have a 23-bp spacer, whereas all J_H segments have a 12-bp spacer (*Figure 12.3*). Recombination strictly follows the 12/23 rule of spacers, which prevents inappropriate recombination of a V_H segment joining directly to a J_H segment.[16,17] The RSS sequences are the only ones that are required for recombination, whereas the coding sequences (V, D, or J) can be replaced by other DNA, but the joining still occurs only if the 12/23 rule is satisfied. The multiple copies of each gene segment (V, D, and J) and the different combinations used in recombination reactions (combinatorial diversity) account for a substantial part of the diversity of Ig receptors.

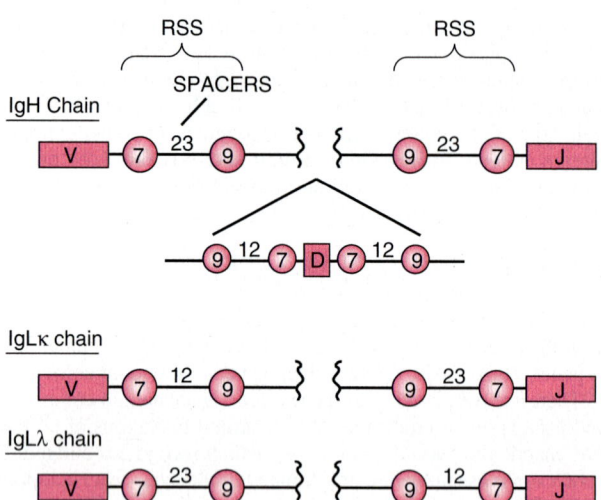

FIGURE 12.3 Structure of recombination signal sequences (RSS). The coding sequences of the immunoglobulin genes are flanked by a 7-nucleotide sequence (heptamer) followed by either 12- or 23-nucleotide spacer and then by a 9-nucleotide sequence (nonamer). This order allows rearrangements only between a segment in which the heptamer/nonamer sequences are separated by a 12-mer spacer and another segment in which they are separated by a 23-mer spacer. This is known as the 12/23 rule. D, diversity; J, joining; V, variable.

RAG1 and RAG2 Proteins

Immunoglobulin gene assembly requires the generation of DNA DSBs at the border of the V, D, and J segments, excision of the intervening DNA segment and subsequent joining of the broken DNA ends.[7,18] The generation of DNA breaks (*Figure 12.4*) is mediated by two enzymes known as recombinase activating genes 1 and 2 (RAG1 and RAG2).[13] The expression of RAG1 and RAG2 is limited to developing lymphocytes that are actively engaged in assembling immunoglobulin

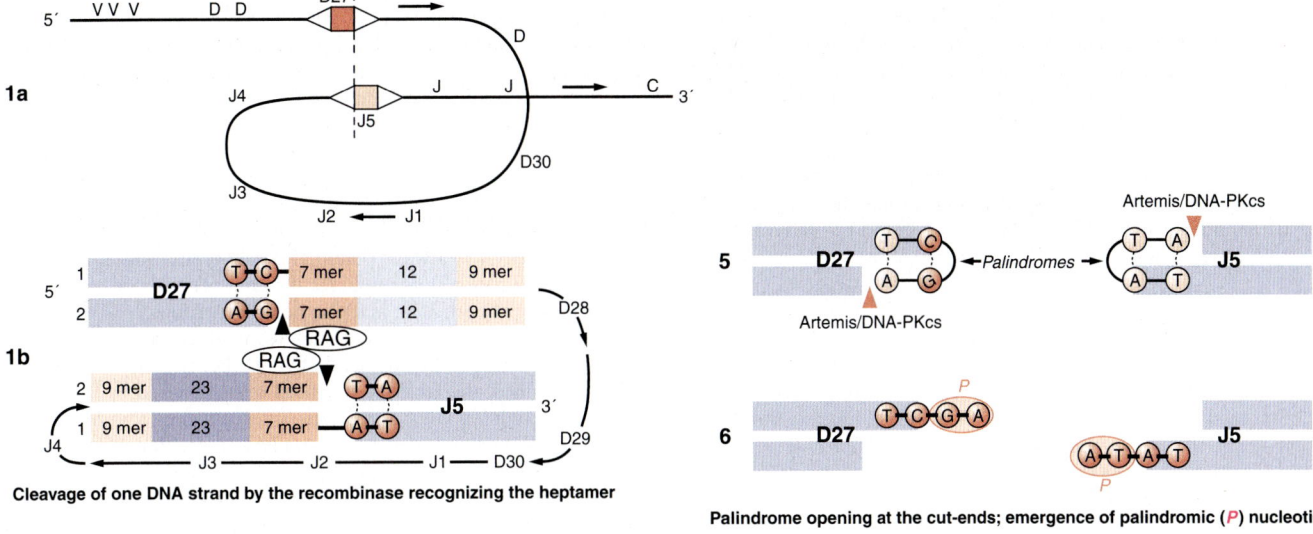

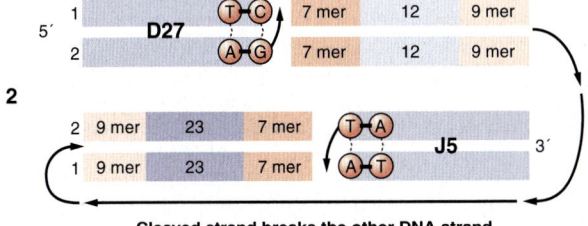

Cleavage of one DNA strand by the recombinase recognizing the heptamer

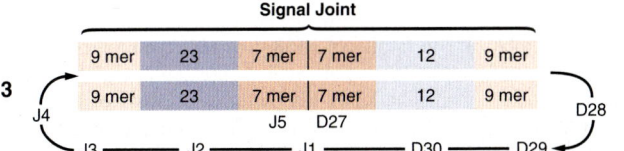

Cleaved strand breaks the other DNA strand

Signal Joint

Signal joint and intervening sequences form a circular structure to be discarded

Palindrome (hairpin) formation at the cut-ends

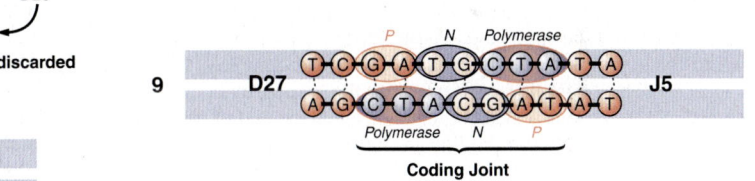

Palindrome opening at the cut-ends; emergence of palindromic (*P*) nucleotides

TdT adds non-templated (no-existent in the genome) nucleotides (*N*)

DNA repair: Exonuclease removes improperly paired nucleotides

Coding Joint

DNA repair: 1) Polymerase adds complementary nucleotides
2) Ligase completes the coding joint

FIGURE 12.4 V(D)J recombination. Shown is the recombination of two hypothetical segments, D27 and J5. Recombination begins with the RAG endonuclease (comprising RAG1 and RAG2 proteins) recognizing the heptamers and nonamers (Panel 1). RAG cuts one strand at the junction between the heptamer and the coding sequence. The other strand is cut by a nucleophile attack from the cut end resulting in a hairpin sealed coding end (Panel 2). The two blunt ends of the heptamers join to form a signal joint (Panel 3), while a hairpin seals the cut coding ends (Panel 4). The hairpin is nicked open by the Artemis/DNA-PKcs complex (Panels 5 and 6). The opening is usually asymmetric and creates overhangs, with the nucleotides at the end of the overhang being derived from the complementary opposite strand. These are known as palindromic (*P*) nucleotides (Panels 5 and 6). The DNA double-stranded breaks of the coding ends can have nucleotides added to their ends by TdT (known as *N-nucleotides*; Panel 7). Improperly paired nucleotides are removed (Panel 8), and the coding joint is completed with the addition of missing nucleotides (Panel 9). The P- and N-nucleotides added to the coding joint constitute the junctional diversity. The joining of different D and J gene segments constitutes combinatorial diversity. D, diversity; DNA-PKcs, DNA-dependent protein kinase catalytic subunit; J, joining; TdT, terminal deoxynucleotidyl transferase; V, variable.

receptor genes. The RAG1 and RAG2 proteins are believed to have evolved from DNA transposons, which are mobile DNA elements that encode their own transposase, enzymes that excise DNA from one location and re-insert it elsewhere in the genome.

Both RAG proteins are required for V(D)J recombination and, thus, for development of B and T lymphocytes. Deficiency of either RAG1 or RAG2 in mice[19,20] or humans[21] results in severe combined immune deficiency (SCID), which is characterized by absent lymphocytes and increased risk of lethal infections. Both RAG1 and RAG2 contain core domains that retain the recombinase activity that is necessary and sufficient for carrying out V(D)J recombination. For RAG1, the core is located in the sequence 384 to 1008 from a total of 1040 amino acids, and for RAG2 in amino acids 1 to 383 of a total of 527. The core of RAG1 contains a nonamer-binding domain, a dimerization and DNA-binding domain, and the endonuclease domain, which depends on zinc binding for catalytic activity. The non-core N-terminal region of RAG1 contains a RING finger domain that has ubiquitin ligase activity and domains that determine subnuclear localization. The RAG2 core domain contains six repeats, each consisting of an antiparallel β-sheet, formed by four β-strands. The repeats are arranged in a circular formation like blades of a propeller, a structure that is known to mediate protein–protein interactions.[22] The C-terminus of RAG2 contains a Plant Homeodomain (PHD) finger motif, usually present in chromatin-associated proteins. The PHD of RAG2 binds to tri-methylated lysine-4 on histone H3 and regulates differential access to sites of recombination.[23] The PHD finger of *RAG2* modulates V(D)J recombination, and mutations of this region result in immune deficiencies.[24,25] Two RAG1 and two RAG2 proteins combine to form an active heterotetramer complex.[26] Each RAG1 binds a separate RAG2. The crystal structure of the RAG complex shows a Y-shaped structure with the nonamer binding domains of RAG1 forming the stem and the catalytic amino acids of RAG1 in the crevice of the Y.[27] RAG2 stabilizes the binding of RAG1 to the heptamer elements.

V(D)J Recombination Reaction: Formation of the Coding and Signal Joints

V(D)J recombination and assembly of immunoglobulin receptor genes proceeds in three steps.[26,28-30] In the first step, the RAG1 and RAG2 proteins together with HMGB1 or HMGB2 bind to and align the two RSSs that will undergo rearrangement (*Figure 12.4*, Panel 1).[31-33] RAG1 binds to both the nonamer, which acts as an anchoring platform, and the heptamer, which stabilizes the complex in the presence of RAG2. HMGB1 and HMGB2 are sequence-nonspecific DNA-binding proteins that support binding of the RAG complex to the RSSs and enhance DNA cleavage.[32] The RAG2 C-terminus interacts directly with histones to stabilize the RAG1/RAG2 complex and direct binding to specific signal sequences.[23]

In the second step the recombinase makes a single strand DNA break (also known as a nick) just 5′ of the heptamer of the RSS, that is between the last nucleotide of the coding sequence and the first nucleotide of the RSS (*Figure 12.4*, Panel 1). The free 3′-OH group of the nicked DNA strand invades the phosphodiester bond of the opposite DNA strand resulting in a double-stranded DNA break. The cleavage leaves a blunt phosphorylated signal end and a hairpin-sealed coding end (*Figure 12.4*, Panels 2 and 3). Formation of the hairpin requires significant bending of one or both DNA strands (*Figure 12.4*, Panel 4). This process occurs at each gene segment being joined and, thus, generates four DNA ends: two hairpin-sealed ends (termed coding ends) and two blunt ends (termed signal ends).

In the third step, the broken DNA ends must be reannealed to form an intact gene and chromosome. The RAG proteins continue to be bound to the signal and coding ends in a four-end complex, known as a cleaved signal complex, at least while the coding ends are still processed.[34] The hairpin-sealed coding ends are at the end of the gene segments that will be joined (coding joint) to form in the final gene product and remain in the chromosome. If the signal ends are in the same orientation, they are joined (signal joint) to form a circular, extrachromosomal DNA (deletional recombination). Alternatively, if the segments are in inverse orientation, the signal joint along with the coding joint is retained in the chromosome (inversional recombination). For coding joint formation, the hairpins must be opened, which is accomplished by the DNA-PK/Artemis complex.[35,36] Because the nicking may not be exactly in the center of the hairpin, the opening creates an overhang in one strand formed by the nucleotides from the other strand (*Figure 12.4*, Panels 5 and 6). These are known as P-nucleotides, which come from the opposite or complementary end of the hairpin or palindrome. Most of the coding ends detected in normal lymphoid precursors have 3′ overhangs.[37] TdT adds nucleotides known as N-nucleotides (nongermline) to the strand with the missing nucleotides (*Figure 12.4*, Panels 7 and 8). Disruption of TdT drastically lowers junctional insertions. The alterations in the coding joint as a result of P- and N-nucleotides are the basis for junctional diversity (*Figure 12.4*, Panel 9). RSSs in coding joints are assumed to be lost in coding joints as a consequence of the end processing. In contrast, signal joints are precisely joined without any sequence modifications and in inversional recombination are retained in the chromosome.

The imprecision in the joints between variable gene segments by the above processes increases Ig diversity by at least 100-fold. However, one of the consequences of the imprecision of V(D)J recombination is a change in the reading frame at the junction between the two gene segments, causing the segments to join out of phase, so that the triplet reading frame for translation is not preserved. In this case the rearrangement results in nonproductive V(D)J combinations with introduction of stop codons that interrupt translation. Productive rearrangements occur when the junction lies within a codon and the resulting amino acid is encoded by nucleotides from both gene segments involved. One in three recombination attempts are productive. Difference in mRNA stability allows pro-B and pre-B cells to distinguish between productive and nonproductive Ig gene rearrangements.

DNA Repair Mechanisms

Cleavage of DNA is always potentially dangerous, and although the recombinase function is essential for the integrity and normal function of the immune system, it is, at the same time, perilous.[6,7,38] The V(D)J recombination, as well as class switch recombination (CSR), are necessary processes, but they demand DNA DSBs. If genetic integrity is to be maintained, the DNA breaks need to be repaired.[6,7,39] A highly conserved, complex DNA repair machinery ensures rejoining of the broken DNA ends and continued lymphocyte development. Double-stranded DNA breaks activate a signaling cascade in which sensors of the broken DNA trigger transducers, which in turn initiate effector proteins to manage diverse cellular programs, including DSB repair, cell cycle arrest, and cell death.[40] The coding and signal joints generated by RAG cleavage are repaired by nonhomologous end joining (NHEJ) proteins.[6,7,35,41] An important sensor is the MRN complex, consisting of a nuclease (MRE11), the chromosome protein (RAD50), and the protein NBS1 (NBN).[41-43] The MRN complex is rapidly assembled at DSBs and recruits the kinase ATM (ataxia telangiectasia mutated), which is the primary signal transducer in NHEJ.[6,7,44-46] ATM is a member of the phosphoinositol 3-kinase (PI3K)-like family of serine-threonine protein kinases and phosphorylates numerous substrates needed in the DNA repair pathway and cell cycle checkpoint.[47-50] ATM also initiates a diverse genetic program involved in B-cell differentiation, including activation of nuclear factor-κB (NF-κB) and associated survival programs.[51,52] DNA-PK (DNA-dependent protein kinase), another member of the family of PI3K-like serine-threonine kinases, is also recruited in the DSBs generated during immunoglobulin gene recombination.[6,7,35,36] The DNA-PK complex consists of a catalytic subunit (DNA-PKcs) together with two DNA-binding proteins, KU70 and KU80. KU70 and KU80 form a stable heterodimer, which binds altered DNA ends regardless of sequence composition, such as DSBs, nicks, or hairpin loops.[7,53] The heterodimer forms a complex with DNA-PKcs, which phosphorylates many DNA-binding proteins near the DSB, including the KU components, to regulate NHEJ. ATM and DNA-PK phosphorylate hundreds of proteins, including p53, to coordinate a diverse cellular response to DSBs.[50] The DNA-PK complex recruits ARTEMIS (DCLRE1C) to the broken DNA ends generated during V(D)J recombination.[54] ARTEMIS is a metallo-β-lactamase enzyme that hydrolyzes covalent bonds and is required for efficient opening of hairpin-sealed coding ends generated by the RAG recombinase.[36,55-57] Mutation or loss of ARTEMIS results in block in B- and T-cell development and severe immunodeficiency.[41,57,58]

Allelic Exclusion

Ig gene rearrangements follow a defined sequence for the various loci and only rearrange one gene/allele at any given time.[59] This hierarchical ordering of rearrangement is termed allelic exclusion. *IgH* is rearranged in pro-B cells followed by rearrangements of *IgL* genes in pre-B cells.[60] The *IgLκ* gene is rearranged first, and if both alleles fail to rearrange productively, the *IgLλ* gene is rearranged. The process of allelic exclusion ensures that each cell produces only a single productive *IgH* and *IgL* chain gene and, thus, is only reactive to a single antigen. In addition, allelic exclusion permits only one allele of each gene (i.e., *IgH*, *IgLκ*, *IgLλ*) to be rearranged at a given time, thereby limiting DNA breaks to a single chromosome and promoting genomic stability. Recent work has demonstrated that ATM-dependent DNA damage responses initiate feedback mechanisms that modulate allele accessibility and control allelic exclusion.[61,62] In early B cells, RAG DSBs on one allele cause nuclear repositioning and inhibition of DNA break generation on the other allele.[61,62] At the end of its early developmental stage, the B cell emerges with the expression on its surface of a unique antigen receptor (*Figure 12.2*).[63]

Regulation of V(D)J Recombination

Initiation of rearrangements by the recombinase requires that the gene must be accessible, that is, the locus must be able to act as a template for the recombinase. In cells competent for rearrangement it was found that *IgH* or *IgL* genes are transcribed prior to V(D)J recombination. These germline mRNA transcripts are incapable of encoding the protein. Transcription likely alters the chromatin structure of the locus permitting the recombinase to recognize the RSS or, alternatively, enhancers may establish altered chromatin regions where both the recombinase and the transcription machinery have access.[15,64] Enhancers and promoters function as accessibility control elements, which regulate V(D)J recombination. The enhancer of the IgM heavy chain (Eμ) is located within the intron between the J$_H$ segments and the Cμ gene and is associated with matrix attachment regions, which improve gene recombination.[65] There are three additional enhancers within the *IgH* locus. One of them (DQ52) competes more efficiently in conferring accessibility to the J$_H$ region. Interaction between DQ52 and Eμ is likely responsible for ordered rearrangement, that is, D to J$_H$ followed by V$_H$-to-DJ$_H$ complex.[66] The *IgLκ* chain intronic enhancer is active only in mature B cells and plasmacytomas, and its stage restriction is dictated by a single motif that binds the transcription of NF-κB. The enhancer between the Jκ and Cκ genes becomes transcriptionally active in the transition from the pre-B to B cell stage.[67] Despite the promiscuity and redundancy of regulatory sequences, transcription is specific for tissue lineage and even stage of development. Several transcription factors and other signals lead to changes in expression levels.

BCR V Gene Repertoire

The total number of *IgH* and *IgL* V gene segments defines the available repertoire. However, not all genes are equally functional, and as a result, the expressed repertoire is biased. Some of the V segments are utilized with a significantly higher frequency than would be expected if all had an equal chance for rearrangement. The bias of the expressed repertoire shows striking association with certain diseases. For example, the V$_H$4-21, a member of the V$_H$4 family, is found in cold agglutinins.[68] This unbalanced expression affects all V, D, and J gene segments. For example, the J$_H$4 segment (one of the existing six), on the basis of equal opportunity among all five segments, should be detected in 17% of B cells but is found in 32% of B clones from fetal liver and in 42% of pre-B cell leukemia.[69] Also, the frequency of N-nucleotide additions in leukemic blasts differs in children less than 3 years of age (12.5%) compared with children greater than 3 years old (89%).[69] Interestingly, fetal B lymphocytes have a lower frequency of N-nucleotide additions, which suggests that the transforming event causing leukemia in the younger age group may occur in fetal life. In chronic lymphocytic leukemia (CLL) and non-Hodgkin lymphoma, the use of V segments is also restricted.[70,71]

GENETIC DEFECTS IN V(D)J RECOMBINATION

V(D)J recombination is necessary for immune diversity and survival, but this objective can be achieved only through DNA DSBs, which threaten genomic stability. Two fundamental processes operate in V(D)J recombination: the generation of DNA DSBs and the subsequent repair of the broken DNA ends. Errors in either of these processes result in failure to generate functional Ig receptors and a severe combined immune deficiency (SCID) with loss of both B and T lymphocytes.[72-74] All patients with SCID have increased susceptibility to severe infections, which are invariably fatal unless treated with hematopoietic stem cell transplant to reconstitute the immune system. Genetic mutations that affect DNA break generation during V(D)J recombination have isolated defects in lymphocytes as this recombinase machinery is specific to developing immune cells. In contrast, DNA repair disorders have manifestations in both lymphoid and nonlymphoid cells.[75] Impaired repair pathways lead to errant

resolution of DNA breaks as translocations, which trigger malignant transformation. Consequently, patients with DNA repair disorders have hypersensitivity to DNA-damaging agents, termed radiosensitive SCID, and an increased incidence of leukemia and other malignancies.[75]

RAG1 and RAG2 Mutations

Disruption of either the *RAG1* or *RAG2* gene prevents V(D)J recombination resulting in a block of lymphocyte development and a lack of mature B and T lymphocytes.[19,20,76] *RAG* mutations in humans are a prominent cause of SCID associated with absence of circulating B and T cells but normal NK cell population (termed T$^-$B$^-$NK$^+$ SCID).[76] Moreover, hypomorphic mutations (i.e., mutations that reduce but do not abolish recombinase activity) in *RAG1* and *RAG2* cause Omenn syndrome, a disease characterized by immune dysregulation and oligoclonal T-cell expansion (see below). Mutations have been identified throughout the entire *RAG1* and *RAG2* genes.[76] In both *RAG1* and *RAG2*, most mutations are clustered in the core domains, resulting in decreased nuclease activity. In *RAG1*, mutations are frequently found in the nonamer-binding domain, the catalytic domain, and the zinc-binding domain. Mutations have also been identified in the noncore regions of both genes. Most of these are nonsense or frameshift mutations that result in a truncated, inactive protein. However, conservative, missense mutations in noncore regions have been identified in patients with Omenn syndrome. These mutations result in attenuated function of the RAG complex.[76] Interesting, some of these mutations in RAG1 and RAG2 do not affect the initiation of V(D)J recombination but severely impair the coding and signal joint formation (DNA repair).[77,78]

Omenn Syndrome

Omenn syndrome is an inherited disorder characterized by generalized erythroderma, lymphadenopathy, hepatosplenomegaly, diarrhea, eosinophilia, and hypogammaglobulinemia with increased serum IgE.[79] Overall, the clinical condition of Omenn syndrome resembles graft-versus-host disease. The immunologic hallmark of Omenn syndrome is the expansion and activation of an oligoclonal population of autoreactive T cells, which infiltrate tissues. These T cells are typically skewed to a T helper 2 (T$_H$2) phenotype and secrete cytokines that stimulate eosinophilia and increased IgE levels.[80] The expanded population of T cells expresses a limited and distinct repertoire of T-cell receptor specificities suggesting self-antigen (autoimmune)-driven proliferation and a critical defect in T-cell development.[81] Omenn syndrome describes a constellation of clinical symptoms and signs that define an inflammatory condition that can be associated with various genetic defects.[82] V(D)J recombination is impaired but not abolished, which leads to the generation of a few T cells that expand in the periphery and infiltrate target organs.[83] The most common cause of Omenn syndrome is hypomorphic mutations in *RAG1* and *RAG2*.[84-86] Mutations have also been described in other genes involved in V(D)J recombination (that is, *DCLRE1C* (*ARTEMIS*), DNA ligase 4) and lymphocyte development (i.e., IL2RA, IL7R, and adenosine deaminase).[82,87,88] Not all patients with these mutations develop Omenn syndrome, which suggests that additional factors, such as an autoantigen or an external antigen possibly from a recent infection, may be necessary to incite the inflammatory state.

DNA-PKcs Mutations

The original *scid* mutation was discovered in mice before the characterization of the recombinase complex and was subsequently identified as a mutation in DNA-PKcs.[89,90] Mutations in KU70 and KU80, the other components of the DNA-PK complex, have also been identified in immune deficiencies.[91,92] Mice and humans with deficiency of DNA-PK lack mature lymphocytes and have agammaglobulinemia.[93,94] The few lymphocytes that do accumulate have long P-nucleotides. In addition to the lack of rearrangements, there is an inability to repair damage from irradiation due to the role of DNA-PK in the repair of DNA breaks outside of the immune system.

Ataxia Telangiectasia

Ataxia telangiectasia (AT) is an autosomal recessive disorder caused by mutations in the ATM protein kinase, which mediates repair to DSBs generated during V(D)J recombination or from DNA-damaging agents.[6,7,40,95] AT is characterized by immunodeficiency, progressive cerebellar ataxia, oculocutaneous telangiectasias, radiosensitivity, chromosomal instability, and elevated risk for development of lymphoid malignancies. AT cells have a DNA repair defect and cannot efficiently rejoin broken DNA.[96,97] Indeed, one of the hallmarks of AT is the generation of aberrant rearrangements during V(D)J recombination, such as translocations, large chromosomal deletions, and inversions. Immunodeficiency in AT affects both T and B cells. Patients with AT display irradiation sensitivity and defects in cell-cycle checkpoint control (i.e., inability to arrest at the G_1-S and S-phase checkpoints), which underscores the diverse cellular processes controlled by ATM in response to DNA breaks.

Nijmegen Breakage Syndrome and Ataxia Telangiectasia–Like Disorder

Nijmegen breakage syndrome is a rare autosomal disorder due to hypomorphic mutations in NBS1 (*NBN*) with clinical features overlapping with those of AT.[98] Mutations in NBS1 result in defective humoral and cellular immunity, radiosensitivity, chromosomal instability, and predisposition to cancer. Patients have recurrent bacterial sinopulmonary infections, hypogammaglobulinemia, and impaired antibody responses to antigens. Mutations in *MRE11* also result in a similar clinical disorder termed ataxia telangiectasia–like disorder.[99] NBS1 and MRE11 recruit ATM to sites of DNA damage and, thus, deficiencies of these proteins result in similar abnormalities as mutations in ATM.[98,99]

Defects of Ligases

Joining of processed DNA ends to form appropriate coding and signal joints requires DNA ligases. Ligase IV (*LIG4*) is the primary ligase involved in NHEJ during V(D)J recombination.[6,7] Mutations in *LIG4* result in a rare disorder characterized by pancytopenia, immune deficiency, microcephaly, developmental delay, growth delay, and radiation sensitivity.[100] Furthermore, mutations in XLF/Cerrunos (*NHEJ1*), which cooperates with Ligase IV to ensure proper DNA break repair, also results in radiation-sensitive immune deficiency and microcephaly.[101] Owing to the general defect in DNA repair mechanisms, both of these syndromes have an increased risk of malignant transformation and development of lymphoid malignancies.

EARLY STAGES OF B-CELL DEVELOPMENT

The study of early B-cell development in normal human bone marrow is hampered by the relative paucity of these cells. Therefore, the majority of information on these early stages has come from mouse models, patients with immune deficiency, and study of leukemias. Because aberrant phenotypes in acute leukemias have been identified the applicability of the results from these studies should be interpreted with caution.[102,103] Investigations have used normal adult bone marrow[104] or fetal bone marrow and fetal liver[105,106] as a source of B-cell precursors in cultures or after injection into mice.[107,108]

The development of B cells can be separated into three stages according to phenotype: (a) precursor B cells (which includes pro-B cells and pre-B cells), (b) immature B cells, and (c) mature B cells (*Figure 12.1*). Markers defining the precursor B cell stage are CD19, the surrogate light chain (SLC, see below), and occasionally some other promiscuous markers, such as CD2 or CD7. The expression of CD2 has been detected on biphenotypic acute lymphoblastic leukemia (ALL) cells and also on their normal counterparts in human fetal hematopoietic tissues.[109,110] Another useful phenotypic marker for precursors of B cells is the nuclear enzyme TdT,[111,112] the DNA polymerase that adds *N*-nucleotides at the DNA ends generated during V(D)J recombination. CD24 is also expressed at a very early stage and at a higher density compared with mature surface IgM+ B cells.[113]

Entrance into the immature B cell stage is defined by expression of surface IgM (representing a mature BCR), which includes both IgH and IgL (κ or λ) chains. Thus, Ig gene rearrangements are complete at this stage. The immature B cell stage is characterized by expression of only IgM without IgD. CD10 is expressed at high density on immature B cells.[104]

The hallmark of mature B cells is expression of a mature BCR or surface immunoglobulin. Early mature B cells are mostly IgM+IgD+ and later undergo class switching to express IgG or IgA. Maturation of B lymphocytes is associated with a change in the density of the two isotypes from IgM^high^IgD^low^ eventually to IgM^low^IgD^high^. New markers appear on B lymphocytes with the expression of IgM (*Figure 12.1*), such as CD21, which is present in more than 90% of the cells.[104,114] During the transition to mature B cells, expression of CD34 and TdT disappears, CD10 is downregulated, and cells express first CD22 and later CD20.[104] Activation triggers loss of CD21 and CD22, while CD23 is expressed and is upregulated by interleukin (IL) 4.[115] Expression of CD24 decreases with B-cell maturation and, in combination with expression of CD45, it can be used to identify the mature stage of B cells, which is useful in B-cell neoplasms.[116] CD45 expression varies with B-cell maturation and is low in the most immature precursors in the bone marrow. It is upregulated as normal B-cell differentiation progresses and then declines at the terminal stages of differentiation as plasma cells become negative for CD45.[117]

Probably the most important application of the B-cell surface marker phenotype is in classification of B-cell malignancies. Incorporation of immunophenotype into traditional morphologic features resulted in the revised classification of well-defined disease entities by the World Health Organization.[118,119]

STEM CELL TO PROGENITOR B CELL

Transcriptional Regulation

Hematopoiesis is coordinated by several genes that orchestrate cell interactions as well as release of growth and differentiation factors. Specific cell lineages have been identified that differentiate from pluripotent stem cells guided through a well-defined hierarchical sequence to mature functional cells.[120] During fetal life, lymphopoiesis takes place in the yolk sac and liver and after birth in the bone marrow. "Master" transcription factors regulate differentiation of lineages through activation of target genes to progressively narrow cellular differentiation potential to specific lineages.[120-125] A common progenitor gives rise to separate myeloid and lymphoid progenitors and then latter to lymphocytic lineages: B, T, natural killer, and dendritic cells.

IKAROS

Normal development of lymphopoiesis depends on the IKAROS family of transcription factors, which selectively regulate lymphocytic development. IKAROS (*IKZF1*) is a zinc finger protein, which functions as transcription factor during different stages of B- and T-cell differentiation.[126] The *Ikaros*^−/−^ mice have a complete block of B-cell differentiation, including an absence of pro-B and precursor B (pre-B) cells in fetal liver and bone marrow.[127,128] *Ikaros* is highly conserved in humans and mice and has significant functions in hematopoiesis, including lymphocyte development. *Ikaros* is expressed in hematopoietic stem cell subsets, particularly at two stages: (a) long-term self-renewing stem cells and (b) multipotent progenitors, which are not self-renewing but able to differentiate into lymphoid-committed progenitors.[129] The *Ikaros* gene can generate eight different protein isoforms by alternative splicing.[129] The isoforms detected in hematopoietic stem cells differ from those detected in lymphoid progenitors. Other members of the IKAROS family include AIOLOS and HELIOS, which encode transcription factors that have important functions in B-cell differentiation and function.[130-132] All family members can form multimeric complexes with each other. *Ikaros* is required not only for the early stages of lymphocytic differentiation but also for late stages, especially in T-cell maturation. It exerts multiple regulatory functions by recruiting repressor complexes, also known as chromatin remodeling machines. *IKAROS* is also needed for the maintenance of B cells by regulating BCR signaling and functions as a tumor suppressor in ALL, especially forms of the disease associated with poor prognosis.[133]

PU.1

The transcription factor PU.1 also acts at the pluripotent level of myeloid-lymphoid progenitors, and its expression maintains the hematopoietic progenitor pool by supporting the generation of the earliest lymphoid and myeloid progenitors.[134] PU.1 is essential for early B-cell development and regulates expression of the *IL7Rα* gene, rendering B-cell progenitors responsive to appropriate differentiation signals, and thus promoting differentiation to the pro-B cell stage.[135-137] Among the three main B-cell populations, B-1, B-2 (follicular), and marginal zone B cells, PU.1 directs differentiation toward the B-2 subpopulation and enhances the activity of other transcription factors, including the interferon (IFN)-regulatory factor.[138-140]

TCF3

TCF3 (previously E2A) is important for lymphocytic differentiation and encodes two proteins, E12 and E47, of the basic helix-loop-helix (HLH) family by differential splicing. These proteins bind as homodimers and are essential for the coordination of *Ig* gene rearrangements.[141-143] In the absence of *TCF3* B-cell differentiation is blocked prior to the pro-B cell stage.[143] The basic region of TCF3 mediates DNA binding, whereas the HLH domain is required for protein dimerization.[143] E12 directs differentiation along B lineage while blocking myeloid differentiation by regulating expression of other transcription factors, including early B-cell factor (*EBF*) and *Pax5*.[144,145] TCF3 proteins are also required for the IL-7-dependent expansion of pro-B cells, progression to the pre-B cell stage, and regulation of *IgLκ* gene rearrangements.[146-148] In mature B cells, *TCF3* promotes IgH isotype switching and somatic hypermutation (SHM) by recruiting AID to the Ig loci.[148]

PAX5

Pax5 encodes a paired domain DNA-binding protein and is expressed in early, but not late, stages of B-cell development.[145] PAX5 directs differentiation of a common myeloid/lymphoid progenitor to lymphocytic programs by suppressing response to myeloid growth factors and repressing genes inappropriately expressed at the pro-B cell stage.[149,150] In early B cells, PAX5 binds to the 3′-*IgH* enhancer and regulates IgH gene rearrangements, which are necessary for generation of the pre-B cell receptor (pre-BCR) and transition to the pre-B cell developmental stage.[151] PAX5 also controls transcription of several other genes in B cells, including *CD19*, *VPREB1*, *IGLL1* (lambda-5), and several intronic sites of the C_H gene segment.[152] In the absence of PAX5, pro-B cells develop normally but further maturation is blocked.[153,154] Another gene target for PAX5 is the adaptor protein B-cell linker protein (BLNK), which acts as a scaffold linking the tyrosine kinase SYK with downstream signaling proteins (i.e., BTK, PLCγ2) to transduce signals from the pre-BCR. Therefore, PAX5 regulation of *BLNK* gene expression controls the pro-B to pre-B transition and mediates constitutive signaling of the pre-BCR in cell proliferation, growth factor responsiveness, and V(D)J recombination.

EBF

Early B-cell factor (*EBF*) is also essential for early B-lymphocyte development. EBF regulates expression of the CD79A and CD79B coreceptors, which are necessary for pre-BCR signaling.[155,156] EBF also activates transcription of other B cell–specific genes, including other transcriptional regulators (such as *Pax5*) that direct the early stages of B-cell lymphopoiesis.[157,158] Consequently, loss of *EBF* arrests B-cell development at a stage earlier than that of *PAX5* deficiency.[157]

In summary, the targets of IKZF1 are the genes of the transcription factors TCF3 (E2A), PU.1, EBF, and PAX5, all of which regulate B-cell differentiation before the expression of Ig genes. The three transcription factors PAX5, TCF3 (E2A), and EBF form a cross-regulatory network, with TCF3 being the most potent B-cell regulator, essential for expression of PAX5 and EBF.

CELL INTERACTIONS IN EARLY B-CELL DEVELOPMENT

Study of B-cell differentiation has become feasible with the development of long-term bone marrow culture techniques. This approach has helped to define the cells that are essential for B-cell development and the factors that support B-cell growth and differentiation. The bone marrow stroma, which consists of adventitial reticular cells, adipocytes, fibroblasts, and sinus endothelial cells, makes critical contributions to hematopoietic differentiation.[159,160] Stromal cells express several adhesion molecules and cytokines to support differentiation of hematopoietic stem cells toward the B-cell lineage.

Several adhesion molecules have critical functions in mediating the interactions between B-cell progenitors and stromal cells. Common lymphoid progenitors express very late antigen-4 (VLA-4), which adheres to vascular cell adhesion molecule-1 (VCAM1) on stromal cells.[161,162] This interaction promotes binding of the receptor tyrosine kinase KIT (CD117) on the surface of early B cells to stem-cell factor (SCF) on marrow stromal cells, which stimulates KIT and induces proliferation of B-cell progenitors. B cells remain in contact with stromal cells throughout the early stages of differentiation. As they mature B cells migrate to the central sinuses, and following expression of a mature surface IgM receptor (immature B cell stage), they exit the bone marrow and complete maturation in the peripheral lymphoid organs.[163]

Bone marrow stromal cells also secrete cytokines and chemokines that promote early B-cell development. Among cytokines with a wide range of functions is IL-7, which acts on common lymphoid progenitors to mediate growth and differentiation of lymphocytes in the bone marrow.[164] IL-7 is essential for the growth and survival of B cells in mice but may be dispensable for human B-cell development.[165] IL-7 secreted by stromal cells binds to the IL-7 receptor (IL-7R) on B cells, which is composed of the IL-7Rα chain in combination with the common cytokine receptor γ chain (*IL2RG*).[166] Mice lacking IL-7, IL-7Rα, or IL2RG have a severe block in B-cell development.[164,167-170] IL-7 exerts changes in gene expression, which effect differentiation of pro-B cells to pre-B cells, especially in concert with other growth factors.[167,171] It synergizes with FMS-like tyrosine kinase 3 ligand (*FLT3LG*) and induces expansion of fetal B cells.[172] IL-7R has been detected on human B-cell progenitors, with a pro-B cell phenotype, which lack expression of CD19 and clonogenic capacity; are CD34+; have messenger RNAs (mRNAs) for CD79B, *RAG1*, *PAX5*; and are TdT+.[173] IL7Rα-deficient stem cells do not differentiate in short-term cultures into pro-B cells; therefore, its expression defines an entry into a stage characterized by upregulation of multiple B lymphoid–associated markers.

IL-7 modulates EBF expression, which activates target genes that are specific for B-cell differentiation programs.[158] In addition, IL-7 stimulates association of the V_H segments to the recombinase complex.[174] Even though the block from IL-7 deficiency is after the pro-B cell stage, these cells have certain abnormalities, such as failure to upregulate terminal deoxynucleotidyl transferase (TdT) and the high-affinity IL-7R chain.[167] The net result of IL-7 deficiency is lack of expression of the IgH chain and the pre-BCR, events that are critical for advancement from the pro-B cell to pre-B cell stage.

Thymic stroma-derived lymphopoietin (TSLP) resembles IL-7 and can assume a host of functions in the absence of IL-7, including regulation of the development of IgM+ B cells from IgM− precursors.[175,176] TSLP binds to a receptor that includes IL-7Rα but not IL2RG. TSLP may promote B-cell development in the fetal liver and in the bone marrow of newborn mice.

Another essential signaling molecule produced by bone marrow stromal cells is the chemokine CXCL12. CXCL12 is constitutively produced by stromal cells and binds to its cognate receptor, CXCR4, on early B cells. CXCR4 is only on hematopoietic progenitors once they are committed to B-cell development.[177,178] CXCR4 expression is induced after rearrangement of the IgH chain and by signals from the pre-BCR.[139] CXCL12 induces intracellular actin polymerization in lymphocytes, a process that is a prerequisite for cell motility.[179] Indeed, CXCR4-expressing B-cell precursors migrate to different regions of the bone marrow, specifically away from IL-7-producing stromal cells.[139,163,180]

PRO-B CELL TO IMMATURE B CELL

Early B-cell differentiation is divided into two stages: the pro-B and the pre-B cells. Molecular definition of the stages of early B-cell development identified cells with IgH chains in the cytoplasm without IgL chains and no mature IgM molecules on the cell surface (*Figure 12.1*).[181,182] In pro-B cells the IgH chain gene is assembled and pairs with surrogate light chains (SLCs) to generate a pre-BCR (*Figure 12.5*). Expression of the pre-BCR signals transition to the pre-B cell stage, where *IgL* chain genes are assembled. Pairing of IgL with the IgH results in expression of surface IgM (i.e., mature BCR) and transition to the immature B lymphocyte stage. This developmental hierarchy of IgH and IgL gene rearrangement segregates *IgH* and *IgL* gene rearrangement and ensures that each immature B cell expresses only one unique antigen receptor (i.e., one copy each of IgH and IgL).

The IgH chain gene is rearranged first at the pro-B cell stage. D to J_H segments of IgH are rearranged followed by V_H to DJ_H rearrangement (*Figure 12.2*). If productive, an IgH chain is expressed on the cell surface in complex with SLC to form the pre-BCR (*Figure 12.5*).[183-185] The SLC consists of two noncovalently associated proteins, VPREB1 and λ5 (*Figure 12.5*).[186,187] The λ5 chain resembles the constant domain of the conventional light chain, and VPREB1 is the equivalent of the variable region.[188] The SLC is linked by a disulfide bond between the IgH chain and the constant domain of λ5 protein.[189] Importantly, not all IgH chains can pair with the SLC, since some V_H segments have structural features that prevent their association.[190]

Once expressed, the paired IgH and SLC assemble with CD79A and CD79B to form the complete pre-BCR.[191] Oligomerization of the pre-BCR through ligand-dependent (i.e., heparan sulfate[192] or

galectin-1[193]) or -independent mechanisms[194] activates the SYK tyrosine kinase leading to phosphorylation of the adaptor protein BLNK, which then activates additional downstream effector proteins, including BTK (Bruton tyrosine kinase).[191,195-197] Immediately after its expression, the pre-BCR synergizes with signals from the IL-7R to drive proliferation, suppress IgH rearrangement and inhibit RAG1/RAG2 expression (pre-BI stage).[191,196-199] At this point, the *RAG1, RAG2,* and *DNTT* (encodes TdT) genes are turned off, thus preventing further IgH rearrangements and securing allelic exclusion. Ultimately, pre-BCR signaling transitions and initiates cell-cycle arrest. Pre-BCR signaling suppresses IL-7R signals through inhibition of AKT, a key kinase downstream of the IL-7R.[191,200] In addition, pre-BCR signals induce CXCR4, which triggers migration of pre-B cells away from IL-7-producing stromal cells.[139] Finally, activation of RAS by the pre-BCR promotes cell cycle exit.[201]

Arrest of cell cycle triggers transition to small pre-B cells (pre-BII stage) and results in reexpression of RAG1/RAG2 and initiation of *IgL* chain gene rearrangement.[196] Loss of IL-7R signaling leads to increased SYK and BLNK expression, which reenforces pre-BCR signaling.[200] Pre-BCR signals through BLNK and BTK to induce expression of IRF4, which together with PU.1, promotes *IgLκ* germline transcription and rearrangement.[139,140,196] Pre-B cells can undergo multiple, sequential *IgL* rearrangements as they attempt to generate a functional IgL chain gene.[202] Several cellular mechanisms ensure that only one *IgL* chain allele is rearranged at a given time (allelic exclusion) in order to maintain monoallelic expression of IgH and IgL chains in a single B cell.[59,196,203] Expression of a functional IgL chain leads to expression of surface IgM and formation of a complete mature BCR, which signals transition to immature B cell and migration out of the bone marrow.

In conclusion, the pre-BCR plays a major role in the expansion of pre-B cells, allelic exclusion, repertoire selection, activation of V(D)J recombination, and developmental progression to IgM+ B cells. The importance of pre-BCR signaling for progression from pro-B cell to pre-B cell stages and beyond is emphasized by the fact that deficiencies of any component of the pre-BCR or downstream signaling molecules blocks developmental progression of B cells at the pro-B or pre-B stage.[204-207]

GENETIC DEFECTS OF EARLY B-CELL DEVELOPMENT

Failure of B-cell development may result from defects in signaling through the pre-BCR.[191,204] Immune deficiencies resulting from arrest of B-cell development are usually associated clinically with recurrent bacterial infections, laboratory findings of markedly reduced numbers of B cells, and hypogammaglobulinemia.

Mutations of *CD79A* and *CD79B*

CD79A and CD79B contain immunoreceptor tyrosine-based activation motifs (ITAMs) on their cytoplasmic domains, which are critical for transduction of pre-BCR signals.[208] These ITAMs act as docking sites for SYK kinase and trigger its activation.[209] Deficiency of the CD79B chain abolishes formation of the CD79A-CD79B dimer and blocks assembly of the SLC, resulting in arrest of differentiation at the pro-B cell stage.[210] A patient with mutation in CD79A had failure to thrive with chronic diarrhea in the first month of life and bronchitis and neutropenia later in life.[211] She had severe hypogammaglobulinemia and absent B cells with a block of B-cell development at the pro-B cell stage.

Mutations of λ5

The SLC is formed from two components: VPREB1 and λ5. A boy with mutations in both alleles of the λ5 genes presented with recurrent infections, hypogammaglobulinemia, and lack of B cells at an early age.[212] In contrast to this patient, mice that are deficient in λ5 have a leaky block at the pro-B cell stage and still maintain 10% to 20% of the B cells.[206]

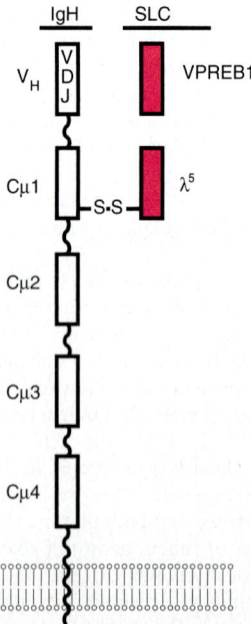

FIGURE 12.5 Structure of the pre-B cell receptor. The pre-B cell receptor (pre-BCR) is composed of an IgH chain and a surrogate light chain that consists of two components, λ5 and VPREB1. The IgH chain is linked by a disulfide bond to the λ5 component, whereas the VPREB is noncovalently attached. IgH, immunoglobulin heavy chain.

Mutations of the *IgH*

Defects in IgH have been associated with agammaglobulinemia.[213,214] The defects consist of a large deletion of a 75- to 100-kb segment (including D, J_H, and μ constant region), a base-pair substitution in the alternative splice site (with inhibition of the synthesis of the membrane form of Ig), or insertional mutation at the beginning of the μ constant region, which resulted in premature codon and absence of the IgH chain. Mutations of the IgH chain are inherited in an autosomal recessive fashion.

Mutations of *BLNK*

BLNK acts as a scaffold and recruits BTK (and other signaling molecules) to the pre-BCR.[215] In response to pre-BCR activation, BLNK is phosphorylated by SYK and, in turn, activates several downstream cellular programs.[215] A 20-year-old man with absent B cells and hypogammaglobulinemia was found to have a mutation in *BLNK* that altered the position of the splice-donor site for intron-1 and resulted in a marked decrease of *BLNK* transcripts and BLNK protein.[216] The patient had recurrent infections, undetectable serum Ig, and less than 0.01% of CD19+ cells in the blood. In contrast to this profound block in B-cell differentiation, mice with loss of *Blnk* have a leaky block of B-cell differentiation.[215]

Mutations of BTK: Bruton Agammaglobulinemia

BTK has critical functions in B-cell development due to its essential role in pre-BCR and BCR signaling.[217] BTK is recruited to the pre-BCR and BCR through BLNK and is subsequently phosphorylated by SYK.[195,218,219] BTK regulates numerous downstream signaling molecules, such as PLCG2, a linkage essential for Ca^{2+} signals.[220] In 1952, Bruton described the first patient with mutations in BTK and association immune deficiency.[221] This severe immune deficiency was found to be inherited in an X-linked pattern and became known as X-linked agammaglobulinemia (XLA, also known as Bruton agammaglobulinemia).[222] Patients have very low serum Ig levels, no response to immunization, markedly decreased B cells (0.3% of normal levels), and no germinal centers (GCs).[223-227] More than 400 mutations in *BTK* have been characterized to date.[228] The BTK protein has a catalytic kinase domain, protein interaction domains, a pleckstrin homology domain that binds phosphatidylinositol-3,4,5-triphosphate (PIP_3), and a Tec homology domain that contains the zinc-binding BTK motif. Mutations in all of these regions of the *BTK* gene have been identified and produce variable degrees of immunodeficiency, depending on which domain is affected.[229] Evidence from the bone marrow of patients with XLA shows expansion of pro-B cells and negligible numbers of mature B cells consistent with a block in the transition to pre-B cells.[230]

MATURE B LYMPHOCYTES AND SURFACE IMMUNOGLOBULIN

The expression of surface immunoglobulin (sIg), or a mature BCR, is the hallmark of mature B lymphocytes, which settle in the primary lymphoid follicles. sIg on B lymphocytes serves as the receptor for antigen. The first Ig to appear on B lymphocytes is IgM. In subsequent developmental processes, the constant region of IgH can be changed from IgM to other Ig classes. Each B lymphocyte contains on an average 50,000 to 100,000 molecules of Ig, although the density of surface Ig varies among individual B cells.[231] Ig is distributed on the surface in small clusters.[232,233] In human B lymphocytes the clusters are separated from each other by a few thousand angstroms of bare membrane, indicating restriction in the free distribution of sIg (*Figure 12.6*).

BCR Complex: Structure and Signaling

The surface Ig (sIg) of the B lymphocyte, or BCR, forms a complex with several components assembled into two structurally and functionally distinct modules: an antigen-recognition module (sIg) and a signal-transducer module, which is the heterodimer of the CD79A/CD79B polypeptide chains (*Figure 12.7*).[234-236] sIg provides the specificity for antigen recognition through its antigen-binding sites. However, the cytoplasmic tails of the heavy chains of surface IgM consist of only three amino acids and, therefore, are not suitable for signal transduction. Consequently, IgM associates with two other proteins that carry out this function: CD79A and the CD79B. The transmembrane region of $C\mu$ is required for binding to the CD79A/CD79B heterodimer. Upon antigen binding to sIg and receptor clustering, the CD79A/CD79B heterodimer initiates and controls BCR intracellular signaling, ultimately triggering an effector response. The signaling capacity of CD79A is contained within its ITAM motif.[237] Following the binding of the ligand by the BCR, the ITAMs are phosphorylated by specific protein tyrosine kinases (PTKs), which provides binding sites for recruitment of other proteins and initiation of signal transduction to coordinate cellular responses, such as proliferation and differentiation of the B cell. The *CD79A* and *CD79B* genes are active only in the B lineage. The expression of sIg requires association with the CD79A/CD79B heterodimer.

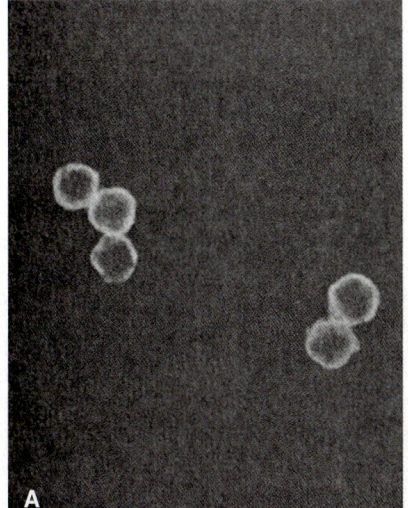
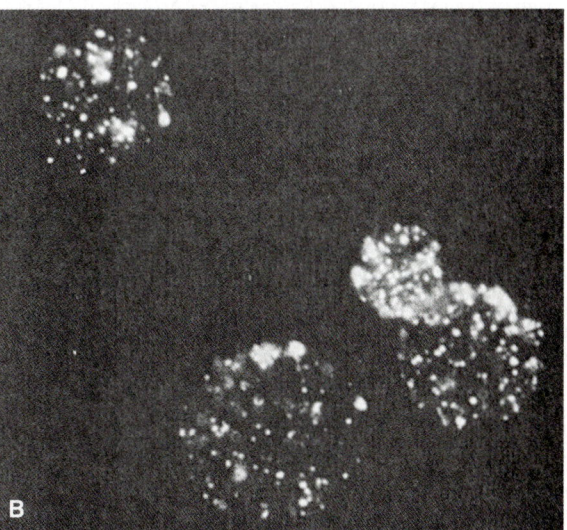

FIGURE 12.6 Distribution of surface immunoglobulin (Ig) on B cells. Immunofluorescence of sIgM on normal B cells. (A) In resting B cells (at 4 °C) sIgM is distributed in a uniform ring around the periphery of the cell. (B) Upon activation (at 37 °C), sIgM forms discrete patches uniformly dispersed over the cell surface. (Reprinted with permission from Zucker-Franklin D, Greaves MF, Grossi CE, Marmont AM. *Atlas of Blood Cells: Function and Pathology.* 2nd ed. Lea & Febiger; 1988.)

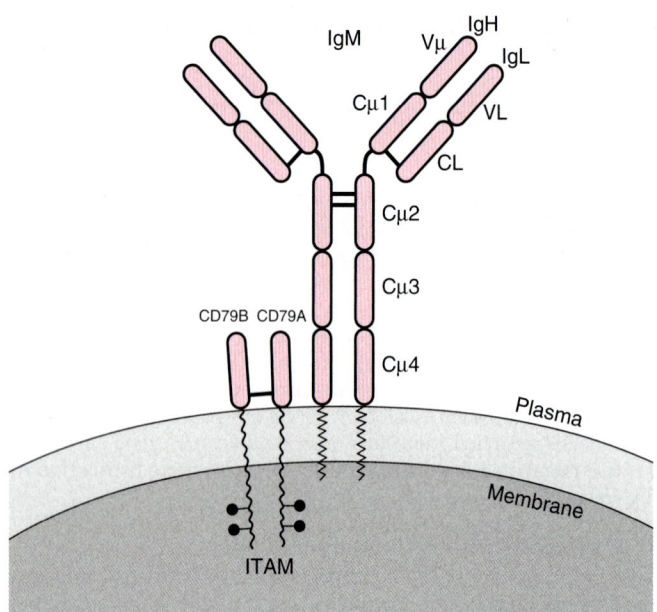

FIGURE 12.7 Structure of the B-cell receptor (BCR). Surface immunoglobulin Ig (IgM is shown) constitutes the antigen-specific component of BCR. It is composed of two IgH and two IgL chains, which are noncovalently associated with a heterodimer consisting of CD79A and CD79B. The CD79A/CD79B heterodimer constitutes the signal transduction component. ITAM, immunoreceptor tyrosine-based activation motif.

B-Cell Receptor and Lipid Rafts

Ligand binding changes the orientation of the BCR molecules so that the ITAMs become accessible to phosphorylation, which causes signal spreading.[238] Signal spreading results in assembly of arrays of BCRs in close proximity. These early events of BCR reorganization provide a mechanism for detecting low concentrations of antigens. Cross-linking of BCR by antigen leads to a series of morphologic and molecular events that are interrelated, that is, BCR aggregation and its loading to lipid rafts, signaling, and finally internalization and antigen presentation.

In the resting state the BCR floats on the cell membrane as monomer, but at the time of signal spreading they form oligomers and gather in specialized membrane microdomains referred to as lipid rafts.[239] Lipid rafts are dynamic assemblies of proteins and lipids that float freely within the liquid-disordered bilayer of cellular membranes, and they can also cluster to form larger, ordered platforms that regulate membrane function in eukaryotic cells.[240] Lipid rafts are estimated to represent 30% to 40% of the cell surface in lymphocytes and have a role in B-cell activation as platforms for BCR signaling and antigen trafficking.[239] Cross-linking of the BCR with antigen enhances its transfer to lipid rafts, while the pre-BCR is constitutively located on lipid rafts.[239-243] Lipid rafts regulate BCR signaling by facilitating its association with coreceptors and with cosignaling molecules, that is, SYK, LYN, BTK, and BLNK.[239] They can also exclude molecules that inhibit BCR signaling such as CD22. Furthermore, in anergic or tolerized B cells, the BCR is unable to enter lipid rafts, indicating that inclusion of BCR within these microdomains is an absolute requirement for initiation of signaling.[244] Similarly, localization of BCR within the rafts occurs only in mature, but not immature, B cells.[245] The CD21/CD19 complex coreceptor, which markedly enhances BCR activation, stabilizes the residence of BCR within the rafts and thus prolongs B-cell activation.[246] In contrast, the FcγRII, which inhibits B-cell activation, destabilizes BCR-raft association.[247] On lipid rafts, B cells divert captured antigen to the endocytic pathway for further processing and presentation to T cells.[242]

After translocation of BCR (or other immune receptors) onto lipid rafts, the rafts form clusters, which leads to the formation of the immunological synapse, a highly ordered membrane structure in which immune receptors, signaling molecules, and cell adhesion molecules are locally associated.[248] Within the synapse, immune receptors are ringed by adhesion molecules as well as several signaling molecules and cytoskeletal components on the cytoplasmic side. Synapse formation occurs in both T cells and B cells suggesting that this is a unique mechanism associated with foreign antigen capturing for processing and handling by the immune system to secure a cellular response.[249] Presentation of antigen by antigen-presenting cells (such as dendritic cells) triggers formation of the synapse on B cells. During the close encounter between the B cell and antigen-presenting cell, the B cell samples and gathers antigen for internalization and processing.

B-CELL RECEPTOR SIGNALING

BCR signaling is initiated by the ITAM motifs of the CD79A/CD79B heterodimer and the PTKs and subsequently can be divided into three major pathways: (a) initial interactions, (b) phosphoinositide (PI3-K) pathways, and (c) the RAS pathway (*Figure 12.8*).[250,251]

Initiation Pathway

BCR uses several distinct families of cytoplasmic PTKs. Three distinct types of PTKs are activated on BCR engagement: (a) the SRC-PTKs (LYN, BLK, and FYN), (b) SYK, and (c) BTK.[250,251] Activation of LYN is one of the earliest events in BCR-induced signaling. LYN localizes in the cell membrane and is responsible for the initial phosphorylation of the ITAMs on CD79A and CD79B. The SYK kinase is recruited to the phosphorylated ITAMs and is subsequently phosphorylated by LYN or by an autophosphorylation mechanism.[252] This phosphorylation step activates SYK, which can then recruit BLNK.[253] BLNK is a linker protein that functions as a scaffold to assemble macromolecular complexes that include PLCG2, VAV, and BTK.[254,255] BTK is then phosphorylated by LYN or SYK and coordinates several cellular programs critical for B-cell function.[218]

Phosphoinositide Pathways

The lipid-metabolizing enzymes PLCG2 and PIK3CA hydrolyze membrane-bound inositol-containing phospholipids to generate signaling intermediates, including inositol triphosphate (IP3), PIP3, and diacylglycerol (DAG). PLCG2 is activated through several pathways in B cells.[256] Association with BLNK results in PLCG2 activation by SYK kinase. BTK also contributes to PLCG2 activation.[257] PIP_3, the product of PIK3CA activation, binds to PLCG2, thus providing another pathway for PLCG2 activation. PLCG2 activation leads to generation of IP_3 and DAG. IP_3 binds to receptors on the endoplasmic reticulum, leading to release of calcium (Ca^{2+}) into the cytosol. Cytoplasmic calcium stimulates calmodulin and calcineurin resulting in activation of the NFAT transcription factor.[258,259] DAG activates RAS and protein kinase C, which in turn regulate several other transcription factors, including NF-κB and AP-1.

PIK3CA is activated by at least two pathways downstream of the BCR. BCR engagement phosphorylates both c-CBL and the CD19/CD21 coreceptor complex, both of which can then bind to PIK3CA.[260-262] PIK3CA can also bind to LYN and FYN, further enhancing its activation. PIK3CA activation results in generation of PIP3, which recruits proteins to the plasma membrane where they can be activated by the BCR signaling complex. For example, the phosphoinositides generated by PIK3CA bind to the AKT1 kinase.[263] AKT1 activation is mediated by the serine/threonine kinase PDK1, which is stimulated by PIP_3 and phosphorylates AKT1. Activation of AKT1 controls a variety of cellular programs, including survival, proliferation, migration, and metabolism.

The RAS Pathway

BCR cross-linking leads to activation of RAS. RAS is a guanine nucleotide–binding protein, which cycles between a guanosine diphosphate (GDP)-bound (inactive) and a GTP-bound (active) state. RAS activity is controlled by the balance between GDP- and GTP-bound states through (1) guanine nucleotide exchange factors (GEFs) that

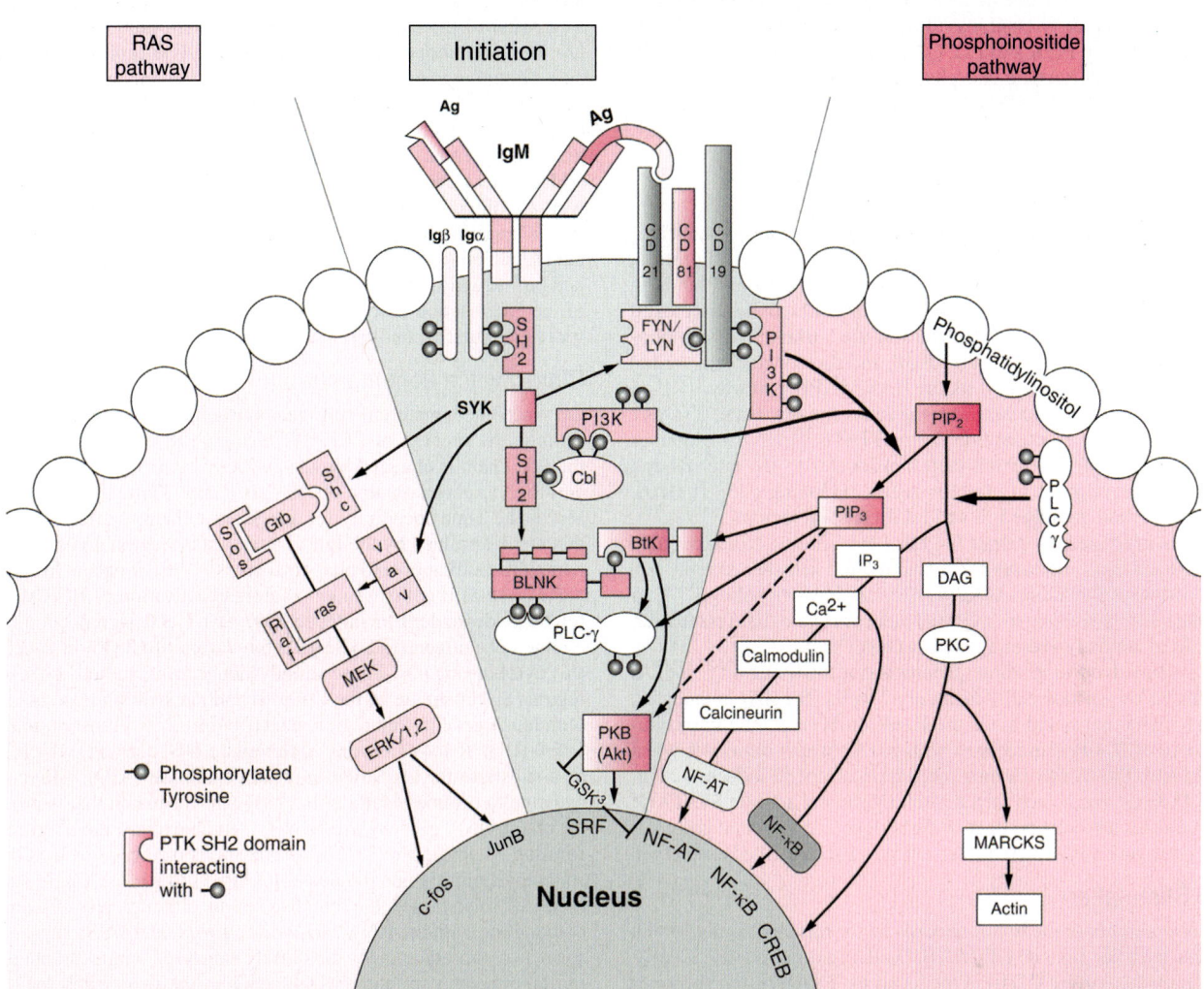

FIGURE 12.8 B-cell receptor signaling. Engagement of the B-cell receptor (BCR) initiates a highly complex signal transduction program. The three main signaling pathways are displayed. *Initiation* (gray shaded area): Antigen (Ag) binding to the BCR activates protein tyrosine kinases (PTK) such as LYN, FYN, and SYK, which then triggers assembly of adapter proteins such as BLNK and CBL to initiate downstream kinases, including BTK and AKT. *Phosphoinositide signaling* (dark pink shaded area): Activation of PI3K and PLCγ results in generation of inositol phosphatides, which activate calcium signaling and PKC. *RAS pathway* (light pink shaded area). The MAPK pathway is activated through adapter proteins GRB, SHC, and SOS. Cumulatively, these three pathways trigger downstream signaling molecules, including AKT, calcineurin, and ERK1/2, to activate transcription factors (NFAT, NF-κB, CREB, C-FOS, and others). BLNK, B-cell linker; BTK, Bruton tyrosine kinase; CBL, casitas B-lineage lymphoma; DAG, diacylglycerol; ERK, extracellular signal–regulated kinase; MAPK, mitogen-activated protein kinase; NFAT, nuclear factor-AT; NF-κB, nuclear factor-κB; PIP3, phosphatidylinositol-3,4,5 triphosphate; PKC, protein kinase C; PLC, phospholipase C.

The Normal Hematologic System

promote the transition from a GDP- to a GTP-bound state and (2) guanosine triphosphatase (GTPase)-activating proteins, which stimulate the hydrolysis of GTP to GDP.[264] One pathway of RAS activation is through the adapter protein SHC1, which is phosphorylated after BCR engagement. SHC1 binds to a second adapter protein GRB2, which in turn binds to SOS, one of the GEFs for RAS.[265,266] Another GEF protein, VAV, is also recruited to phosphorylated SYK.[267] A negative regulator of the RAS pathway is CBL (casitas B-lineage lymphoma), which competes for binding to SOS. Binding of SOS and CBL to GRB2 is mutually exclusive.[268] Activated RAS triggers a three-kinase signaling cascade that ends in activation of the mitogen-activated protein kinase (MAPK). RAS-GTP phosphorylates a MAPK kinase kinase (MAP3K) called RAF1, which is the first kinase of the cascade. RAF1 phosphorylates and activates the MAPK kinases (MAP2K) MEK1 and MEK2, which in turn phosphorylates the MAPK proteins ERK1 and ERK2. Phosphorylated ERKs form dimers and are translocated to the nucleus, where they phosphorylate transcription factors c-FOS and JUN members of the ETS family.

Adapter Molecules: Plasticity and Diversity of Signaling

Adapter proteins possess domains that mediate protein-protein or protein-lipid interactions, but they have no intrinsic enzymatic activity. Adapter proteins assemble multimolecular signaling complexes and direct their formation to specific cellular locations.[269-271] The cytosolic adapter protein BLNK connects BTK to SYK and brings PLCG2 on the lipid rafts. BLNK is required for the translocation of PLCG2 from the cytosol to the plasma membrane and its subsequent activation. BLNK is essential in pre-B cell development and, with BTK, induces cell proliferation.

Coreceptor Complexes

The coreceptor complex CD19/CD21 activates associated protein kinases, which induce phosphorylation of tyrosine residues on CD19.[114] These phosphorylated tyrosines then recruit additional PI3Ks to augment BCR signaling. BCR activation of BTK is dependent on CD19, whereas activation of LYN and SYK is independent of CD19.[272]

CD22 is also associated with BCR. CD22 contains ITAMs and four immunoreceptor tyrosine-based inhibition motifs (ITIMs) in the cytoplasmic region. PI3K and PLCG1 associate with the ITAM motif, whereas the protein tyrosine phosphatase SHP-1 binds to its ITIMs.[273] As a result of multiple ITIMs, CD22 likely functions as a negative regulator of B-cell activation.

CYTOKINE STIMULATION OF B CELLS

Several cytokines act on B cells to stimulate diverse functions, including antibody production, class-switch recombination, proliferation, and differentiation. IL-4 is produced by helper T cells and binds to its transmembrane receptor (IL-4 receptor), which is complexed with common gamma chain (IL2RG) on the surface of B lymphocytes.[274-276] IL-4 binding activates PI3K and the downstream serine/threonine kinase AKT as well as the RAS/MAPK pathway.[277] IL-4 stimulation of B cells also activates the Janus kinases 1 and 3 (JAK1 and JAK3) and the transcription factor STAT6.[278,279] IL-4 induces dimerization of STAT6, which then translocates to the nucleus and stimulates transcription of effector genes, including class II HLA, *CD23*, *IL-4R*, and germline IgE and IgG1 constant regions.[280]

IL-5 is produced by helper T cells, and binding to its cognate receptor on B cells increases BTK activity and activates several signaling pathways, including JAK2/STAT5 and RAS signaling.[281] IL-5 stimulates class switching to IgG1 and induces terminal differentiation of B cells to antibody-secreting plasma cells.[281]

IL-6 is involved in terminal differentiation of B cells.[282,283] IL-6 is produced by various cells, including T cells, B cells, monocytes, and endothelial cells, and binds the IL-6R on B cells. The intracellular domain of IL-6R is associated with gp130, which dimerizes when IL-6 binds to the IL-6R. Homodimerization of gp130 induces activation of JAK kinases, which then phosphorylate and activate STAT3.[284] IL-6 stimulates antibody production (IgM, IgA, and IgG) and promotes helper T-cell function, which further activates B-cell antibody secretion.

CD40 Stimulation

CD40 is a member of the tumor necrosis factor receptor family, which interacts with its ligand, CD154 (CD40L), expressed on T cells. Signal transduction by CD40 is mediated by TRAF (tumor necrosis factor receptor activation factor) proteins that bind to its cytoplasmic region.[285,286] Five different TRAFs (TRAF1, TRAF2, TRAF3, TRAF5, and TRAF6) associate with CD40 and initiate signaling cascades. Engagement of CD40 by its ligand also activates the SRC kinases LYN and FYN and BTK. Signaling follows the RAS pathway via the nucleotide exchanging factor SOS, leading to JNK and ERK activation. The functional outcome of CD40 depends on the state of activation of B cells and the intensity of stimulation. On naive B cells CD40 stimulation induces proliferation and Ig production, but on memory B cells it induces apoptosis. These different cellular programs are coordinated by the type of TRAF associated with CD40. For example, trimers of TRAF2 mediate apoptosis, whereas trimers of TRAF6 or TRAF5 mediate proliferation.[285] TRAF6 plays a role in class switch. GC formation and Ig class switch are hallmarks of CD40-mediated (namely, T cell–dependent) B-cell responses.

Polyclonal Activation

B lymphocytes can be activated in an antigen-independent manner by polyclonal B-cell activators. These substances stimulate all B cells regardless of their antigen specificity and are primarily microbial cell constituents, such as lipopolysaccharide (LPS), staphylococcal protein A, streptolysin O, and pneumococcal polysaccharide III. A prototypical is LPS, which binds to CD14 and stimulates B-cell proliferation and Ig class switching.[287]

ANTIBODY EFFECTOR FUNCTIONS

Germinal Center Reaction

Following assembly of the BCR in the bone marrow, immature B cells exit the bone marrow and migrate to secondary lymphoid organs (spleen and lymph nodes). Upon antigen encounter, B cells proliferate and form GCs. GCs are composed of proliferating B cells, antigen-specific T cells, and follicular dendritic cells. GCs are formed as a result of the expansion of one or a small number of B cells and are therefore monoclonal or oligoclonal. The rapidly expanding B cells (dividing ~ every 6 hours) have low sIg and are termed centroblasts.[288,289] They expand in the dark zone of the GC, termed based on the high density of cells in this region.[289] The dividing centroblasts give rise to centrocytes that reexpress sIg and migrate to the light zone, which is less densely packed.[289] Centrocytes reencounter antigen as well as follicular helper T cells and follicular dendritic cells. During the GC reaction, B cells undergo modification of the immunoglobulin genes, including SHM to improve antigen affinity and CSR to link antigen recognition to different antibody functions. The consequence of the GC reaction is selective expansion of B cells with high affinity for the stimulating antigen.

Class Switch Recombination

Once activated, mature B cells generate antibodies of different isotypes through the process of CSR.[290] During CSR, the constant region of the IgH chain is changed but the antibody retains the entire IgL chain and the variable domains of the IgH chain. Thus, the antibody preserves the same specificity for antigen but changes effector functions that are determined by the IgH chain constant region domains, such as complement fixation and phagocytosis.[291,292] CSR occurs in the GC in naïve, mature B cells through (i) antigen activation of BCR signaling (either T dependent or independent), (ii) T cell signals alone in the absence of antigen (i.e., CD40L stimulation of CD40 on B cells), or (iii) cytokine signals. These stimuli induce transcription of the switch region (Sμ) upstream of the Cμ exon and the switch region associated with the target constant region gene (*Figure 12.9*). Transcription forms DNA-RNA R-loops on the nontemplate DNA strand, which serves as a substrate for activation-induced deaminase (AID). AID converts cytosine to uridine resulting in a base pair mismatch that is processed by uracil-DNA glycosylase (UNG), which excises the aberrant base forming an abasic site.[290] The abasic site is further processed by apurinic/apyrimidinic endonuclease 1 (APE1) to form a single-stranded nick. AID also targets the template strand, although less efficiently, in conjunction with the RNA exosome complex, and DSBs subsequently form as a consequence of the closely staggered single-stranded nicks on the opposing strands.[293] DNA ends in the two switch regions are then joined by NHEJ placing the new C region exon downstream of the IgH variable region exons (*Figure 12.9*).[290,294,295]

Antibody Functions

There are five main classes of Ig: IgM, IgD, IgG, IgE, and IgA, which have distinct functions (*Table 12.1*).

IgM can form pentamers in its secreted form, which results in 10 antigen recognition sites per macromolecule. IgM primarily functions in complement activation. IgM antibodies are the first to be produced in a primary immune response and are subsequently replaced by IgG antibodies.

IgD primarily functions as a surface receptor on B cells and plays a role in antigen recognition and B-cell activation. It is expressed during certain periods of B-cell differentiation.

IgG is the major Ig in humans and is present at the highest concentration in serum. IgG molecules have a long half-life of 21 days. There are four isotypic subclasses of IgG (IgG1, IgG2, IgG3, and IgG4) that differ by variations in amino acid sequences of the carboxy-terminal parts of the constant regions. IgG primarily functions in opsonization whereby the constant region of the antibody binds to receptors on macrophages and granulocytes resulting in internalization of antigen and/or activation of cell-mediated killing of bacteria or viral-infected cells. IgG also functions in complement activation. Notably, IgG is the only subclass that transfers across the placenta, thereby giving a measure of protection to the newborn.[296]

IgE has a high affinity for receptors on mast cells and basophils. When antigen binds IgE, the mast cell is triggered to degranulate, thereby releasing vasoactive substances, including histamine, which are responsible for such clinical manifestations of allergies and anaphylactic reactions. IgE also has functions in immunologic responses to parasitic infections.

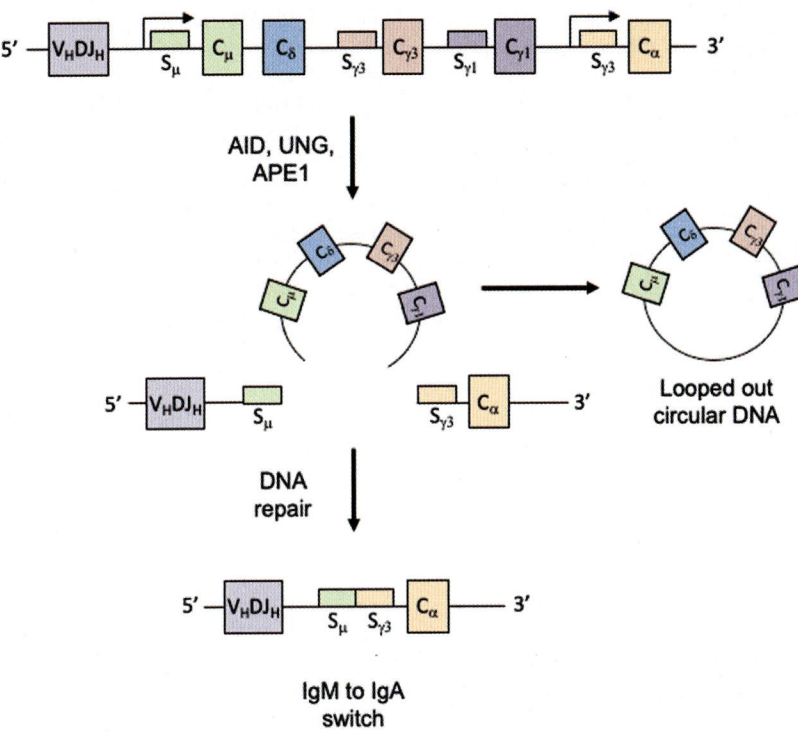

FIGURE 12.9 Class switch recombination. In class switch recombination, the IgH variable region is linked to a different constant region, which results in a change in effector function with preservation of antigen recognition. All IgH chains are initially generated using the Cμ constant region to generate IgM. In the germinal-center reaction, different stimuli (BCR, cytokines, CD40, T-cell help) activate transcription of distinct switch regions (S) location just upstream of constant region (C) exons. Activation-induced deaminase (AID), uracil-DNA glycosylase (UNG), and apurinic/apyrimidinic endonuclease 1 (APE1) generate DNA double-stranded breaks in the transcribed S regions. Subsequently, the broken DNA ends in the switch region join, placing the new C exon downstream of the variable region.

Table 12.1. Antibody Effector Functions

Properties	Properties of Immunoglobulins				
	IgM	**IgG**	**IgA**	**IgD**	**IgE**
Subclasses	2	4	2	–	–
Molecular weight (kDa)	950	150	150-300	185	190
Heavy chain	μ	γ	α	δ	ε
Light chain	κ, λ	κ, λ	κ, λ	κ, λ	κ, λ
Percent carbohydrates	10-12	4	10	12	12
Survival ($t_{1/2}$ days)	5	21	6	3	2
Complement fixation					
Classical	+++	+	–	–	–
Alternative	–	–	+	+	+
Cross placenta	–	+	–	+	+
External secretions	+	+	+++	–	+
Cytophilic for:					
Macrophages	±	+++	–	–	–
Mast cells	–	±	–	–	+++
Serum concentration (g/L)	1.5	11.0	2.4	0.03	<0.005
Percent of total Ig	5	80	15	–	–

Abbreviations: –, negative; +, weak; +++, strong; ±, borderline; Ig, immunoglobulin.

IgA exists as monomers in serum, but it can also form dimers. IgA dimers function principally in mucosal immunity. IgA is generated by B cells near mucosal barriers, and the dimeric form is transcytosed by epithelial cells to luminal surfaces where it binds bacteria and prevents adherence to mucosal surfaces, thereby blocking colonization.

Somatic Hypermutation

The variable region of the IgH and IgL chains undergo further diversification during the GC reaction. This process is known as somatic hypermutation (SHM) and proceeds through introduction of new point mutations in the variable regions of the IgH and IgL chains.[291] The antigen specificity of the BCR is not changed but the sequence variance alters antigen affinity, thus contributing to affinity maturation of the antigen-reactive B cells. SHM only occurs in antigen-stimulated B cells in the context of T-cell help. AID, which functions in CSR, also introduces DNA nicks in the variable region that are essential for SHM.[291] The mutations generated during SHM occur principally in the CDRs, which contact antigen directly. Mutations are introduced at a rate of ~10^{-3} mutations per base pair per division. SHM occurs during the period in which B cells undergo a high rate of divisions in the dark zone of GCs.[297] B cells can undergo several rounds of SHM during the GC reaction as cells with higher affinity for target antigen are iteratively selected for continued expansion and maturation.

Secreted Antibodies

Each of the immunoglobulins can be expressed as membrane-bound receptor or secreted antibodies. The ratio of secreted Ig to membrane-bound Ig increases with maturation from resting B cells to plasma cells. The transmembrane and secreted forms are encoded by the same gene. Utilization of different polyadenylation sites at the end of each constant region gene determines which form is generated (*Figure 12.10*). Termination at the first polyadenylation site generates a carboxy terminus with hydrophobic transmembrane domain. In contrast, the second polyadenylation site produces a carboxy terminus with a hydrophilic secretory tail.

TERMINAL STAGES OF B-CELL DIFFERENTIATION

Memory B Cell

Following the GC reaction, affinity selected B cells can differentiate to memory B cells or plasma cells. Memory B cells are long lived and divide very slowly. They express sIg but do not secrete antibody. However, upon rechallenge with antigen, memory B cells expand clonally and produce 7 to 10 times more antibody than the antigen-inexperienced B cells as part of the secondary antibody response.[298] Since memory B cells are derived from a GC reaction, their Ig genes have the somatic mutations and class switch properties established during the selective process in the GC. The mechanism that maintains the memory B-cell pool is unknown.

Plasma Cell Differentiation

GC B cells can also differentiate into plasma cells. Plasma cells have very long life spans and migrate to the bone marrow, which is essential for their continued survival. Plasma cells do not express surface Ig but continue to secrete antibody and, thus, are a source of long-lasting high-affinity, antigen-specific antibody production. Compared with other B cells, plasma cells have a very distinct cellular morphology with round or oval shape and an eccentrically located nucleus with chromatin arranged in pyramidal blocks against the nuclear membrane, giving the characteristic "cartwheel" appearance (*Figure 12.11*).[299,300] Plasma cells also have an expansive endoplasmic reticulum that fills the entire cytoplasm and sustains production of antibody (*Figure 12.12*).[301-306]

Plasma cell differentiation requires the transcriptional repressor PRDM1 (BLMP1).[307,308] PRDM1 suppresses *MYC* transcription, resulting in cessation of the cell cycle, and also represses *PAX5*, which is required for lineage commitment of B-cell development

and for isotype switching in GCs.[309] PRDM1 promotes plasmacytic differentiation by extinguishing expression of genes that are important for BCR signaling, GC function, and proliferation, but allowing the expression of XBP1 (X-box binding protein). XBP1 is required for terminal differentiation of B lymphocytes to plasma cells.[310] A small subpopulation of GC cells in the light zone express PRDM1, suggesting that these cells have survived the selection process and are probably destined to become plasma cells. A negative feedback loop operates in the GCs between PRDM1 and BCL6, which blocks PRDM1 expression and plasma cell differentiation irreversibly.[311,312] Maturation into a plasma cell results in downregulation of the BCR, the major histocompatibility complex class II, CD19, and CD20 along with increased surface expression of syndecan-1 (CD138) and CD38.

B-1 B Cells

A subset of B cells called B-1 B cells, are part of the innate immune system. This subpopulation of B cells expresses the CD5 antigen, which is ordinarily present on T cells.[313] B-1 B cells possess unique properties, that is, they are phenotypically identical to conventional B cells, but they are larger and in mice they have 10 times more surface IgM with λ chains.[314] These B cells are predominately located in peritoneal and pleural cavities and are only found in small numbers in secondary lymphoid organs. B-1 B cells produce antibodies that recognize capsular polysaccharide antigens and are important in early immune responses to infection. The majority of the circulating antibodies present prior to any infection are produced by B-1 B cells. B-1 cells may have different antibody repertoires (e.g., have few N-region insertions in their rearranged V genes), and the V_H repertoire is biased toward V gene families proximal to J_H, whereas in conventional B cells it is more randomized. B-1 B cells specificities are directed against several pathogens and are important in mucosal immunity.[315] The B-1 B cell subpopulation may therefore play an important role in the development of B-cell repertoire related to natural immunity, which develops in the absence of an encounter with exogenous antigens. However, the precise function of these cells is still uncertain.

B-1 B cells originate from a lineage distinct from that of conventional B lymphocytes.[316-318] They develop early in ontogeny from progenitor cells found in fetal liver but not in adult bone marrow. In contrast, conventional B-cell progenitors are found in both fetal liver

FIGURE 12.10 Alternative mRNA processing determines expression of membrane versus secreted immunoglobulin. There are two polyadenylation (polyA) sites in each IgH chain, one for secreted and one for membrane-bound forms. Cμ1–Cμ4 are the exons of IgM. mRNA, messenger RNA; TM, transmembrane region.

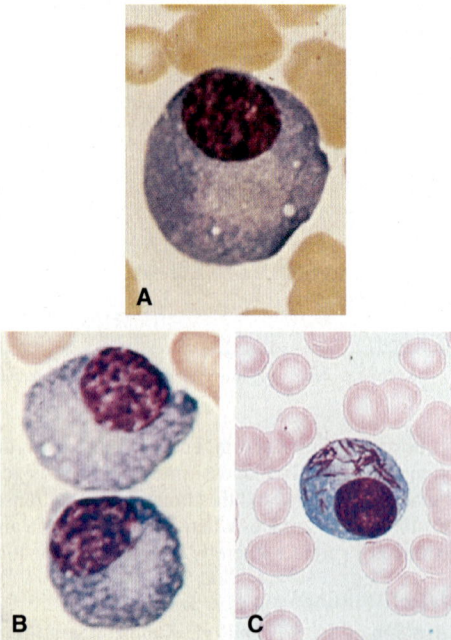

FIGURE 12.11 Histology of plasma cells. A, Normal plasma cell. B and C, Plasmablasts with vacuoles from the bone marrow of a patient with infection and arthritis.

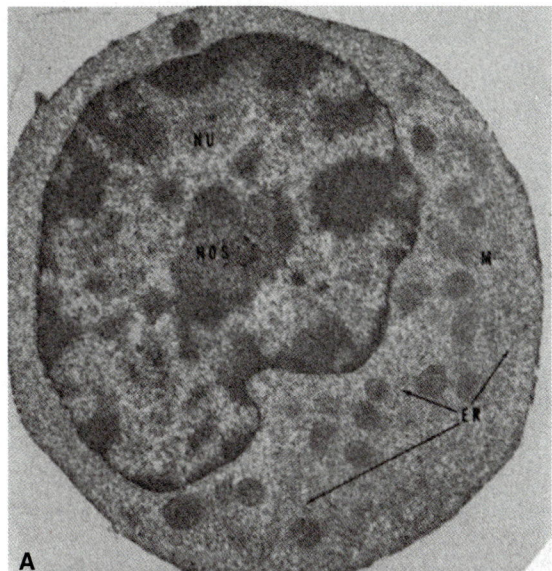

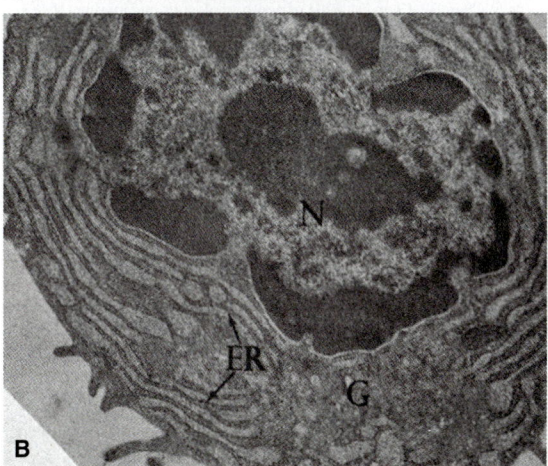

FIGURE 12.12 Morphology of endoplasmic reticulum in plasma cell.
Terminal B-cell differentiation into plasma cells is characterized morphologically by an extensive expansion of the endoplasmic reticulum. A, An antibody-producing B cell with sparse endoplasmic reticulum (ER). B, Mature plasma cell displaying well-organized ER and distinct Golgi apparatus (G). (A, Reprinted with permission from Harris TN, Hummeler K, Harris S. Electron microscopic observations on antibody-producing lymph node cells. *J Exp Med.* 1966;123(1):161-172. Originally published in *Journal of Experimental Medicine.* https://doi.org/10.1084/jem.123.1.161. Copyright © 1966 by The Rockefeller University Press. B, Reprinted with permission from Gudat FG, Harris TN, Harris S, et al. Studies on antibody-producing cells. I. Ultrastructure of 19S and 7S antibody-producing cells. *J Exp Med.* 1970;132(3):448-474. Originally published in *Journal of Experimental Medicine.* https://doi.org/10.1084/jem.132.3.448. Copyright © 1970 by The Rockefeller University Press.)

and adult bone marrow. B-1 B cells are present in high numbers in fetal and neonatal life (50% of all IgM⁺ B cells) but progressively diminish in number after birth and are present in small numbers (less than 10%-30% of B cells) in adult spleen, lymph nodes, and peripheral blood.[319-322] Their proliferative capacity is high, and as a result, they give rise spontaneously to cell lines that demonstrate *MYC* amplification.[323] In adults, B-1 B cells are self-renewing and, thus, they do not arise from undifferentiated progenitors.

Increased numbers of B-1 B cells are found in patients with rheumatoid arthritis, Sjögren syndrome, and progressive systemic sclerosis but not in patients with systemic lupus erythematosus.[324-327] Numbers of B-1 B cells are also increased after bone marrow transplantation.[328] In 95% of patients with B-cell CLL (B-CLL), the leukemic cells express the CD5 antigen.[329] CD5 is also detected on cells from other B-cell lymphomas.

GENETIC PROFILES OF B-CELL ACTIVATION AND DIFFERENTIATION

Every B cell is characterized by its own unique Ig receptor that is maintained through its life and is transferred to all members of its progeny throughout differentiation. While the Ig gene is conserved throughout maturation, B cells have genetic profiles that are unique to each developmental stage or functional state. The full transcriptome of cell populations can be characterized by gene expression microarrays and RNA sequencing techniques. Using this approach, groups of genes that are characteristic of a lineage or a specific stage of differentiation can be identified. Each group of genes, then, defines a signature of a cell type or a particular function. The Immunological Genome Project (www.immgen.org), a consortium of immunology and computational biology laboratories, has compiled gene expression and regulatory network data for all immune cells.[330] Comparison of the transcriptional profiles has identified gene signatures unique to each stage of B-cell development.[331]

Comparison of naive B cells, B cells activated by a foreign antigen, and B cells tolerant against "self" showed that the naive or resting state is maintained by several inhibitory genes.[332,333] B-cell activation is associated with loss of expression of some of the inhibitory genes rather than the induction of genes that regulate entry into the cell cycle. Self-tolerant B cells have increased expression of more inhibitory genes at the same time that they maintain the expression of the basal inhibitory gene profile. In addition, the gene profile of activated B cells differs from that of GC B cells, which are activated by T cells.[334] GC B cells differ from naive B cells in the expression of hundreds of genes.[335] Plasma cells, which represent the end stage of B-cell differentiation, have a cohort of genes that are differently expressed compared with other B cells.[336]

B-Cell Malignancies

Malignancies arise from a single cell at a specific state of differentiation. Therefore, B-cell malignancies inherit a unique Ig rearrangement (in other words, they are a monoclonal population) and also have a gene expression signature that resembles the cell line from which they originated. Gene expression profiling on B-cell leukemias and lymphomas has provided extensive insight into the similarities and differences between malignant cells and their related normal B-cell equivalents.[337]

Diffuse large B-cell lymphomas (DLBCLs) have been shown to have two different gene profiles.[337,338] One subtype has a gene expression profile that resembles GC B cells (GCB DLBCL), whereas the second subtype more closely resembles activated B cells (ABC DLBCL). These two subtypes have distinct genetic signatures. For example, GCB DLBCL has retained the hypermutation machinery, but ABC DLBCL does not express the genes necessary for SHM.[339] The GCB DLBCL closely resembles follicular lymphoma.[338] Based on shared gene expression profiles it has been suggested that ABC DLBCL may arise from a cell in its transition to becoming a plasma cell. These two different types of DLBCL, which are distinguishable by gene expression profiling, have very disparate overall survival rates in response to standard treatment regimens.[338] Therefore, gene expression profiles are molecular predictors of survival after chemotherapy for DLBCL.[338,340]

B-CLL can be phenotypically separated into two groups depending on whether they have germline or somatically mutated Ig genes, with the former having distinctly worse prognosis.[341] Gene expression profiling, though, demonstrates that these two subgroups share a common gene expression signature suggesting that they both arise from a common cell of origin, likely a memory B cell.[341,342] This is consistent with the active SHM machinery in CLL blasts, which could play a role in intraclonal diversification development.[343] Gene expression arrays also identified altered apoptotic signaling in B-CLL cases resistant to DNA damaging agents (i.e., chemotherapy).[344]

In Hodgkin lymphoma, the Hodgkin and Reed-Sternberg (HRS) cells are primarily derived from B cells based on recombination of IgH and IgL genes.[345] However, HRS cells have a distinct gene expression profile that is similar to that of Epstein-Barr virus–transformed B cells.[346] HRS cells have a complex network of deregulated transcription factors (i.e., *GATA3, MSC/ABF-1, NR2F1/EAR-3,* and *NFE2L3/NRF3*), which alter cell differentiation and support proliferation. Several of the genes normally active in B cells are downregulated in HRS cells.[347]

These studies in gene expression signatures have been instrumental in advancing the understanding of oncogenesis and in delineating the molecular basis underlying divergent treatment responses for phenotypically similar malignancies. These findings provide a platform for designing more targeted and personalized treatment strategies.

References

1. Hozumi N, Tonegawa S. Evidence for somatic rearrangement of immunoglobulin genes coding for variable and constant regions. *Proc Natl Acad Sci U S A.* 1976;73(10):3628-3632.
2. Watson CT, Breden F. The immunoglobulin heavy chain locus: genetic variation, missing data, and implications for human disease. *Gene Immun.* 2012;13(5):363-373.
3. Lefranc MP. Nomenclature of the human immunoglobulin genes. *Curr Protoc Immunol.* 2001. Appendix 1:Appendix 1P. doi:10.1002/0471142735.ima01ps40.
4. Erikson J, Martinis J, Croce CM. Assignment of the genes for human lambda immunoglobulin chains to chromosome 22. *Nature.* 1981;294(5837):173-175.
5. McBride OW, Hieter PA, Hollis GF, Swan D, Otey MC, Leder P. Chromosomal location of human kappa and lambda immunoglobulin light chain constant region genes. *J Exp Med.* 1982;155(5):1480-1490.
6. Alt FW, Zhang Y, Meng FL, Guo C, Schwer B. Mechanisms of programmed DNA lesions and genomic instability in the immune system. *Cell.* 2013;152(3):417-429.
7. Helmink BA, Sleckman BP. The response to and repair of RAG-mediated DNA double-strand breaks. *Annu Rev Immunol.* 2012;30:175-202.
8. Pascual V, Capra JD. Human immunoglobulin heavy-chain variable region genes: organization, polymorphism, and expression. *Adv Immunol.* 1991;49:1-74.
9. Matsuda F, Honjo T. Organization of the human immunoglobulin heavy-chain locus. *Adv Immunol.* 1996;62:1-29.
10. Matsuda F, Shin EK, Nagaoka H, et al. Structure and physical map of 64 variable segments in the 3'0.8-megabase region of the human immunoglobulin heavy-chain locus. *Nat Genet.* 1993;3(1):88-94.
11. Tomlinson IM, Walter G, Marks JD, Llewelyn MB, Winter G. The repertoire of human germline VH sequences reveals about fifty groups of VH segments with different hypervariable loops. *J Mol Biol.* 1992;227(3):776-798.
12. Sakano H, Huppi K, Heinrich G, Tonegawa S. Sequences at the somatic recombination sites of immunoglobulin light-chain genes. *Nature.* 1979;280(5720):288-294.
13. Fugmann SD, Lee AI, Shockett PE, Villey IJ, Schatz DG. The RAG proteins and V(D)J recombination: complexes, ends, and transposition. *Annu Rev Immunol.* 2000;18:495-527.
14. Gellert M. Recent advances in understanding V(D)J recombination. *Adv Immunol.* 1997;64:39-64.
15. Sleckman BP, Gorman JR, Alt FW. Accessibility control of antigen-receptor variable-region gene assembly: role of cis-acting elements. *Annu Rev Immunol.* 1996;14:459-481.
16. Tonegawa S. Somatic generation of antibody diversity. *Nature.* 1983;302(5909):575-581.
17. Bassing CH, Alt FW, Hughes MM, et al. Recombination signal sequences restrict chromosomal V(D)J recombination beyond the 12/23 rule. *Nature.* 2000;405(6786):583-586.
18. Gellert M. V(D)J recombination: RAG proteins, repair factors, and regulation. *Annu Rev Biochem.* 2002;71:101-132.
19. Mombaerts P, Iacomini J, Johnson RS, Herrup K, Tonegawa S, Papaioannou VE. RAG-1-deficient mice have no mature B and T lymphocytes. *Cell.* 1992;68(5):869-877.
20. Shinkai Y, Rathbun G, Lam KP, et al. RAG-2-deficient mice lack mature lymphocytes owing to inability to initiate V(D)J rearrangement. *Cell.* 1992;68(5):855-867.
21. Schwarz K, Gauss GH, Ludwig L, et al. RAG mutations in human B cell-negative SCID. *Science.* 1996;274(5284):97-99.
22. Callebaut I, Mornon JP. The V(D)J recombination activating protein RAG2 consists of a six-bladed propeller and a PHD fingerlike domain, as revealed by sequence analysis. *Cell Mol Life Sci.* 1998;54(8):880-891.
23. West KL, Singha NC, De Ioannes P, et al. A direct interaction between the RAG2 C terminus and the core histones is required for efficient V(D)J recombination. *Immunity.* 2005;23(2):203-212.
24. Elkin SK, Ivanov D, Ewalt M, et al. A PHD finger motif in the C terminus of RAG2 modulates recombination activity. *J Biol Chem.* 2005;280(31):28701-28710.
25. Akamatsu Y, Monroe R, Dudley DD, et al. Deletion of the RAG2 C terminus leads to impaired lymphoid development in mice. *Proc Natl Acad Sci U S A.* 2003;100(3):1209-1214.
26. Bailin T, Mo X, Sadofsky MJ. A RAG1 and RAG2 tetramer complex is active in cleavage in V(D)J recombination. *Mol Cell Biol.* 1999;19(7):4664-4671.
27. Kim MS, Lapkouski M, Yang W, Gellert M. Crystal structure of the V(D)J recombinase RAG1-RAG2. *Nature.* 2015;518(7540):507-511.
28. Eastman QM, Leu TM, Schatz DG. Initiation of V(D)J recombination in vitro obeying the 12/23 rule. *Nature.* 1996;380(6569):85-88.
29. Hiom K, Gellert M. A stable RAG1-RAG2-DNA complex that is active in V(D)J cleavage. *Cell.* 1997;88(1):65-72.
30. Hiom K, Gellert M. Assembly of a 12/23 paired signal complex: a critical control point in V(D)J recombination. *Mol Cell.* 1998;1(7):1011-1019.
31. Bergeron S, Madathiparambil T, Swanson PC. Both high mobility group (HMG)-boxes and the acidic tail of HMGB1 regulate recombination-activating gene (RAG)-mediated recombination signal synapsis and cleavage in vitro. *J Biol Chem.* 2005;280(35):31314-31324.
32. Dai Y, Wong B, Yen YM, Oettinger MA, Kwon J, Johnson RC. Determinants of HMGB proteins required to promote RAG1/2-recombination signal sequence complex assembly and catalysis during V(D)J recombination. *Mol Cell Biol.* 2005;25(11):4413-4425.
33. Mundy CL, Patenge N, Matthews AG, Oettinger MA. Assembly of the RAG1/RAG2 synaptic complex. *Mol Cell Biol.* 2002;22(1):69-77.
34. Besmer E, Mansilla-Soto J, Cassard S, et al. Hairpin coding end opening is mediated by RAG1 and RAG2 proteins. *Mol Cell.* 1998;2(6):817-828.
35. Lieber MR. The mechanism of double-strand DNA break repair by the nonhomologous DNA end-joining pathway. *Annu Rev Biochem.* 2010;79:181-211.
36. Ma Y, Pannicke U, Schwarz K, Lieber MR. Hairpin opening and overhang processing by an Artemis/DNA-dependent protein kinase complex in nonhomologous end joining and V(D)J recombination. *Cell.* 2002;108(6):781-794.
37. Schatz DG, Swanson PC. V(D)J recombination: mechanisms of initiation. *Annu Rev Genet.* 2011;45:167-202.
38. Jeggo PA, Concannon P. Immune diversity and genomic stability: opposite goals but similar paths. *J Photochem Photobiol B.* 2001;65(2-3):88-96.
39. Casali P, Pal Z, Xu Z, Zan H. DNA repair in antibody somatic hypermutation. *Trends Immunol.* 2006;27(7):313-321.
40. Shiloh Y. The ATM-mediated DNA-damage response: taking shape. *Trends Biochem Sci.* 2006;31(7):402-410.
41. Burma S, Chen BP, Chen DJ. Role of non-homologous end joining (NHEJ) in maintaining genomic integrity. *DNA Repair.* 2006;5(9-10):1042-1048.
42. Wen J, Cerosaletti K, Schultz KJ, Wright JA, Concannon P. NBN phosphorylation regulates the accumulation of MRN and ATM at sites of DNA double-strand breaks. *Oncogene.* 2013;32(37):4448-4456.
43. Xu Y. DNA damage: a trigger of innate immunity but a requirement for adaptive immune homeostasis. *Nat Rev Immunol.* 2006;6(4):261-270.
44. Chen HT, Bhandoola A, Difilippantonio MJ, et al. Response to RAG-mediated VDJ cleavage by NBS1 and gamma-H2AX. *Science.* 2000;290(5498):1962-1965.
45. D'Amours D, Jackson SP. The Mre11 complex: at the crossroads of dna repair and checkpoint signalling. *Nat Rev Mol Cell Biol.* 2002;3(5):317-327.
46. Deriano L, Stracker TH, Baker A, Petrini JH, Roth DB. Roles for NBS1 in alternative nonhomologous end-joining of V(D)J recombination intermediates. *Mol Cell.* 2009;34(1):13-25.
47. Khanna KK, Keating KE, Kozlov S, et al. ATM associates with and phosphorylates p53: mapping the region of interaction. *Nat Genet.* 1998;20(4):398-400.
48. Matsuoka S, Huang M, Elledge SJ. Linkage of ATM to cell cycle regulation by the Chk2 protein kinase. *Science.* 1998;282(5395):1893-1897.
49. Savitsky K, Bar-Shira A, Gilad S, et al. A single ataxia telangiectasia gene with a product similar to PI-3 kinase. *Science.* 1995;268(5218):1749-1753.
50. Matsuoka S, Ballif BA, Smogorzewska A, et al. ATM and ATR substrate analysis reveals extensive protein networks responsive to DNA damage. *Science.* 2007;316(5828):1160-1166.
51. Bredemeyer AL, Helmink BA, Innes CL, et al. DNA double-strand breaks activate a multi-functional genetic program in developing lymphocytes. *Nature.* 2008;456(7223):819-823.
52. Bednarski JJ, Sleckman BP. At the intersection of DNA damage and immune responses. *Nat Rev Immunol.* 2019;19(4):231-242.
53. Jeggo PA. Identification of genes involved in repair of DNA double-strand breaks in mammalian cells. *Radiat Res.* 1998;150(5 suppl):S80-S91.
54. Brandt VL, Roth DB. Artemis: guarding small children and, now, the genome. *J Clin Invest.* 2003;111(3):315-316.
55. Chu G. Double strand break repair. *J Biol Chem.* 1997;272(39):24097-24100.
56. Lieber MR. The biochemistry and biological significance of nonhomologous DNA end joining: an essential repair process in multicellular eukaryotes. *Gene Cell.* 1999;4(2):77-85.
57. Moshous D, Callebaut I, de Chasseval R, et al. Artemis, a novel DNA double-strand break repair/V(D)J recombination protein, is mutated in human severe combined immune deficiency. *Cell.* 2001;105(2):177-186.
58. Moshous D, Pannetier C, Chasseval RR, et al. Partial T and B lymphocyte immunodeficiency and predisposition to lymphoma in patients with hypomorphic mutations in artemis. *J Clin Invest.* 2003;111(3):381-387.
59. Brady BL, Steinel NC, Bassing CH. Antigen receptor allelic exclusion: an update and reappraisal. *J Immunol.* 2010;185(7):3801-3808.
60. Ehlich A, Schaal S, Gu H, Kitamura D, Muller W, Rajewsky K. Immunoglobulin heavy and light chain genes rearrange independently at early stages of B cell development. *Cell.* 1993;72(5):695-704.
61. Hewitt SL, Yin B, Ji Y, et al. RAG-1 and ATM coordinate monoallelic recombination and nuclear positioning of immunoglobulin loci. *Nat Immunol.* 2009;10(6):655-664.
62. Skok JA, Brown KE, Azuara V, et al. Nonequivalent nuclear location of immunoglobulin alleles in B lymphocytes. *Nat Immunol.* 2001;2(9):848-854.
63. Reth M, Hombach J, Wienands J, et al. The B-cell antigen receptor complex. *Immunol Today.* 1991;12(6):196-201.
64. Sen R, Oltz E. Genetic and epigenetic regulation of IgH gene assembly. *Curr Opin Immunol.* 2006;18(3):237-242.
65. Harraghy N, Buceta M, Regamey A, Girod PA, Mermod N. Using matrix attachment regions to improve recombinant protein production. *Methods Mol Biol.* 2012;801:93-110.

66. Kottmann AH, Zevnik B, Welte M, Nielsen PJ, Kohler G. A second promoter and enhancer element within the immunoglobulin heavy chain locus. *Eur J Immunol.* 1994;24(4):817-821.

67. Atchison ML, Perry RP. The role of the kappa enhancer and its binding factor NF-kappa B in the developmental regulation of kappa gene transcription. *Cell.* 1987;48(1):121-128.

68. Pascual V, Victor K, Spellerberg M, Hamblin TJ, Stevenson FK, Capra JD. VH restriction among human cold agglutinins. The VH4-21 gene segment is required to encode anti-I and anti-i specificities. *J Immunol.* 1992;149(7):2337-2344.

69. Wasserman R, Galili N, Ito Y, Reichard BA, Shane S, Rovera G. Predominance of fetal type DJH joining in young children with B precursor lymphoblastic leukemia as evidence for an in utero transforming event. *J Exp Med.* 1992;176(6):1577-1581.

70. Friedman DF, Cho EA, Goldman J, et al. The role of clonal selection in the pathogenesis of an autoreactive human B cell lymphoma. *J Exp Med.* 1991;174(3):525-537.

71. Zelenetz AD, Chen TT, Levy R. Clonal expansion in follicular lymphoma occurs subsequent to antigenic selection. *J Exp Med.* 1992;176(4):1137-1148.

72. O'Driscoll M, Jeggo P. Immunological disorders and DNA repair. *Mutat Res.* 2002;509(1-2):109-126.

73. Schwarz K, Bartram CR. V(D)J recombination pathology. *Adv Immunol.* 1996;61:285-326.

74. Fischer A, Cavazzana-Calvo M, De Saint Basile G, et al. Naturally occurring primary deficiencies of the immune system. *Annu Rev Immunol.* 1997;15:93-124.

75. Gennery AR, Cant AJ, Jeggo PA. Immunodeficiency associated with DNA repair defects. *Clin Exp Immunol.* 2000;121(1):1-7.

76. Notarangelo LD, Kim MS, Walter JE, Lee YN. Human RAG mutations: biochemistry and clinical implications. *Nat Rev Immunol.* 2016;16(4):234-246.

77. Qiu JX, Kale SB, Yarnell Schultz H, Roth DB. Separation-of-function mutants reveal critical roles for RAG2 in both the cleavage and joining steps of V(D)J recombination. *Mol Cell.* 2001;7(1):77-87.

78. Yarnell Schultz H, Landree MA, Qiu JX, Kale SB, Roth DB. Joining-deficient RAG1 mutants block V(D)J recombination in vivo and hairpin opening in vitro. *Mol Cell.* 2001;7(1):65-75.

79. Omenn GS. Familial reticuloendotheliosis with eosinophilia. *N Engl J Med.* 1965;273:427-432.

80. Lev A, Simon AJ, Amariglio N, Rechavi G, Somech R. Selective clinical and immune response of the oligoclonal autoreactive T cells in Omenn patients after cyclosporin A treatment. *Clin Exp Immunol.* 2012;167(2):338-345.

81. Rieux-Laucat F, Bahadoran P, Brousse N, et al. Highly restricted human T cell repertoire in peripheral blood and tissue-infiltrating lymphocytes in Omenn's syndrome. *J Clin Invest.* 1998;102(2):312-321.

82. Marrella V, Maina V, Villa A. Omenn syndrome does not live by V(D)J recombination alone. *Curr Opin Allergy Clin Immunol.* 2011;11(6):525-531.

83. Villa A, Santagata S, Bozzi F, et al. Partial V(D)J recombination activity leads to Omenn syndrome. *Cell.* 1998;93(5):885-896.

84. Corneo B, Moshous D, Gungor T, et al. Identical mutations in RAG1 or RAG2 genes leading to defective V(D)J recombinase activity can cause either T-B-severe combined immune deficiency or Omenn syndrome. *Blood.* 2001;97(9):2772-2776.

85. Noordzij JG, Verkaik NS, Hartwig NG, de Groot R, van Gent DC, van Dongen JJ. N-terminal truncated human RAG1 proteins can direct T-cell receptor but not immunoglobulin gene rearrangements. *Blood.* 2000;96(1):203-209.

86. Wada T, Takei K, Kudo M, et al. Characterization of immune function and analysis of RAG gene mutations in Omenn syndrome and related disorders. *Clin Exp Immunol.* 2000;119(1):148-155.

87. Ege M, Ma Y, Manfras B, et al. Omenn syndrome due to ARTEMIS mutations. *Blood.* 2005;105(11):4179-4186.

88. Gennery AR, Hodges E, Williams AP, et al. Omenn's syndrome occurring in patients without mutations in recombination activating genes. *Clin Immunol.* 2005;116(3):246-256.

89. Bosma GC, Custer RP, Bosma MJ. A severe combined immunodeficiency mutation in the mouse. *Nature.* 1983;301(5900):527-530.

90. Blunt T, Finnie NJ, Taccioli GE, et al. Defective DNA-dependent protein kinase activity is linked to V(D)J recombination and DNA repair defects associated with the murine scid mutation. *Cell.* 1995;80(5):813-823.

91. Nussenzweig A, Chen C, da Costa Soares V, et al. Requirement for Ku80 in growth and immunoglobulin V(D)J recombination. *Nature.* 1996;382(6591):551-555.

92. Gu Y, Seidl KJ, Rathbun GA, et al. Growth retardation and leaky SCID phenotype of Ku70-deficient mice. *Immunity.* 1997;7(5):653-665.

93. Taccioli GE, Amatucci AG, Beamish HJ, et al. Targeted disruption of the catalytic subunit of the DNA-PK gene in mice confers severe combined immunodeficiency and radiosensitivity. *Immunity.* 1998;9(3):355-366.

94. van der Burg M, Ijspeert H, Verkaik NS, et al. A DNA-PKcs mutation in a radiosensitive T-B- SCID patient inhibits Artemis activation and nonhomologous end-joining. *J Clin Invest.* 2009;119(1):91-98.

95. Lavin MF, Shiloh Y. The genetic defect in ataxia-telangiectasia. *Annu Rev Immunol.* 1997;15:177-202.

96. Jeggo PA, Carr AM, Lehmann AR. Splitting the ATM: distinct repair and checkpoint defects in ataxia-telangiectasia. *Trends Genet.* 1998;14(8):312-316.

97. Bredemeyer AL, Sharma GG, Huang CY, et al. ATM stabilizes DNA double-strand-break complexes during V(D)J recombination. *Nature.* 2006;442(7101):466-470.

98. van der Burgt I, Chrzanowska KH, Smeets D, Weemaes C. Nijmegen breakage syndrome. *J Med Genet.* 1996;33(2):153-156.

99. Taylor AM, Groom A, Byrd PJ. Ataxia-telangiectasia-like disorder (ATLD)-its clinical presentation and molecular basis. *DNA Repair.* 2004;3(8-9):1219-1225.

100. Enders A, Fisch P, Schwarz K, et al. A severe form of human combined immunodeficiency due to mutations in DNA ligase IV. *J Immunol.* 2006;176(8): 5060-5068.

101. Buck D, Malivert L, de Chasseval R, et al. Cernunnos, a novel nonhomologous end-joining factor, is mutated in human immunodeficiency with microcephaly. *Cell.* 2006;124(2):287-299.

102. Hurwitz CA, Loken MR, Graham ML, et al. Asynchronous antigen expression in B lineage acute lymphoblastic leukemia. *Blood.* 1988;72(1):299-307.

103. Ross CW, Stoolman LM, Schnitzer B, Schlegelmilch JA, Hanson CA. Immunophenotypic aberrancy in adult acute lymphoblastic leukemia. *Am J Clin Pathol.* 1990;94(5):590-599.

104. Loken MR, Shah VO, Dattilio KL, Civin CI. Flow cytometric analysis of human bone marrow. II. Normal B lymphocyte development. *Blood.* 1987;70(5):1316-1324.

105. Ryan D, Kossover S, Mitchell S, Frantz C, Hennessy L, Cohen H. Subpopulations of common acute lymphoblastic leukemia antigen-positive lymphoid cells in normal bone marrow identified by hematopoietic differentiation antigens. *Blood.* 1986;68(2):417-425.

106. Uckun FM, Ledbetter JA. Immunobiologic differences between normal and leukemic human B-cell precursors. *Proc Natl Acad Sci U S A.* 1988;85(22):8603-8607.

107. DiGiusto D, Chen S, Combs J, et al. Human fetal bone marrow early progenitors for T, B, and myeloid cells are found exclusively in the population expressing high levels of CD34. *Blood.* 1994;84(2):421-432.

108. Pontvert-Delucq S, Breton-Gorius J, Schmitt C, et al.. Characterization and functional analysis of adult human bone marrow cell subsets in relation to B-lymphoid development. *Blood.* 1993;82(2):417-429.

109. Uckun FM. Regulation of human B-cell ontogeny. *Blood.* 1990;76(10):1908-1923.

110. Uckun FM, Muraguchi A, Ledbetter JA, et al. Biphenotypic leukemic lymphocyte precursors in CD2+CD19+ acute lymphoblastic leukemia and their putative normal counterparts in human fetal hematopoietic tissues. *Blood.* 1989;73(4):1000-1015.

111. Bollum FJ. Terminal deoxynucleotidyl transferase as a hematopoietic cell marker. *Blood.* 1979;54(6):1203-1215.

112. Janossy G, Bollum FJ, Bradstock KF, McMichael A, Rapson N, Greaves MF. Terminal transferase-positive human bone marrow cells exhibit the antigenic phenotype of common acute lymphoblastic leukemia. *J Immunol.* 1979;123(4):1525-1529.

113. Duperray C, Boiron JM, Boucheix C, et al. The CD24 antigen discriminates between pre-B and B cells in human bone marrow. *J Immunol.* 1990;145(11):3678-3683.

114. Tedder TF, Zhou LJ, Engel P. The CD19/CD21 signal transduction complex of B lymphocytes. *Immunol Today.* 1994;15(9):437-442.

115. Defrance T, Aubry JP, Rousset F, et al. Human recombinant interleukin 4 induces Fc epsilon receptors (CD23) on normal human B lymphocytes. *J Exp Med.* 1987;165(6):1459-1467.

116. Lavabre-Bertrand T, Duperray C, Brunet C, et al. Quantification of CD24 and CD45 antigens in parallel allows a precise determination of B-cell maturation stages: relevance for the study of B-cell neoplasias. *Leukemia.* 1994;8(3):402-408.

117. Caldwell CW, Patterson WP. Relationship between CD45 antigen expression and putative stages of differentiation in B-cell malignancies. *Am J Hematol.* 1991;36(2):111-115.

118. Harris NL, Jaffe ES, Stein H, et al. A revised European-American classification of lymphoid neoplasms: a proposal from the International Lymphoma Study Group. *Blood.* 1994;84(5):1361-1392.

119. Swerdlow SH, Campo E, harris NL, et al. *WHO Classification of Tumours of Haematopoietic and Lymphoid Tissues.* 4th ed. International Agency for Research on Cancer; 2008.

120. Orkin SH. Diversification of haematopoietic stem cells to specific lineages. *Nat Rev Genet.* 2000;1(1):57-64.

121. Busslinger M. Transcriptional control of early B cell development. *Annu Rev Immunol.* 2004;22:55-79.

122. Hagman J, Lukin K. Transcription factors drive B cell development. *Curr Opin Immunol.* 2006;18(2):127-134.

123. Medina KL, Singh H. Genetic networks that regulate B lymphopoiesis. *Curr Opin Hematol.* 2005;12(3):203-209.

124. Rothenberg EV, Pant R. Origins of lymphocyte developmental programs: transcription factor evidence. *Semin Immunol.* 2004;16(4):227-238.

125. Shivdasani RA, Orkin SH. The transcriptional control of hematopoiesis. *Blood.* 1996;87(10):4025-4039.

126. Sellars M, Kastner P, Chan S. Ikaros in B cell development and function. *World J Biol Chem.* 2011;2(6):132-139.

127. Georgopoulos K, Bigby M, Wang JH, et al. The Ikaros gene is required for the development of all lymphoid lineages. *Cell.* 1994;79(1):143-156.

128. Wang JH, Nichogiannopoulou A, Wu L, et al. Selective defects in the development of the fetal and adult lymphoid system in mice with an Ikaros null mutation. *Immunity.* 1996;5(6):537-549.

129. Klug CA, Morrison SJ, Masek M, Hahm K, Smale ST, Weissman IL. Hematopoietic stem cells and lymphoid progenitors express different Ikaros isoforms, and Ikaros is localized to heterochromatin in immature lymphocytes. *Proc Natl Acad Sci U S A.* 1998;95(2):657-662.

130. Kelley CM, Ikeda T, Koipally J, et al. Helios, a novel dimerization partner of Ikaros expressed in the earliest hematopoietic progenitors. *Curr Biol.* 1998;8(9):508-515.

131. Ma S, Pathak S, Mandal M, Trinh L, Clark MR, Lu R. Ikaros and Aiolos inhibit pre-B-cell proliferation by directly suppressing c-Myc expression. *Mol Cell Biol.* 2010;30(17):4149-4158.

132. Thompson EC, Cobb BS, Sabbattini P, et al. Ikaros DNA-binding proteins as integral components of B cell developmental-stage-specific regulatory circuits. *Immunity.* 2007;26(3):335-344.

133. Payne KJ, Dovat S. Ikaros and tumor suppression in acute lymphoblastic leukemia. *Crit Rev Oncog.* 2011;16(1-2):3-12.

134. Iwasaki H, Somoza C, Shigematsu H, et al. Distinctive and indispensable roles of PU.1 in maintenance of hematopoietic stem cells and their differentiation. *Blood.* 2005;106(5):1590-1600.

The Normal Hematologic System

135. DeKoter RP, Schweitzer BL, Kamath MB, et al. Regulation of the interleukin-7 receptor alpha promoter by the Ets transcription factors PU.1 and GA-binding protein in developing B cells. *J Biol Chem.* 2007;282(19):14194-14204.

136. McKercher SR, Torbett BE, Anderson KL, et al. Targeted disruption of the PU.1 gene results in multiple hematopoietic abnormalities. *EMBO J.* 1996;15(20):5647-5658.

137. Scott EW, Simon MC, Anastasi J, Singh H. Requirement of transcription factor PU.1 in the development of multiple hematopoietic lineages. *Science.* 1994;265(5178):1573-1577.

138. Ye M, Ermakova O, Graf T. PU.1 is not strictly required for B cell development and its absence induces a B-2 to B-1 cell switch. *J Exp Med.* 2005;202(10):1411-1422.

139. Johnson K, Hashimshony T, Sawai CM, et al. Regulation of immunoglobulin light-chain recombination by the transcription factor IRF-4 and the attenuation of interleukin-7 signaling. *Immunity.* 2008;28(3):335-345.

140. Pongubala JM, Nagulapalli S, Klemsz MJ, McKercher SR, Maki RA, Atchison ML. PU.1 recruits a second nuclear factor to a site important for immunoglobulin kappa 3' enhancer activity. *Mol Cell Biol.* 1992;12(1):368-378.

141. Markus M, Benezra R. Two isoforms of protein disulfide isomerase alter the dimerization status of E2A proteins by a redox mechanism. *J Biol Chem.* 1999;274(2):1040-1049.

142. Riley RL, Blomberg BB, Frasca D. B cells, E2A, and aging. *Immunol Rev.* 2005;205:30-47.

143. Kee BL, Quong MW, Murre C. E2A proteins: essential regulators at multiple stages of B-cell development. *Immunol Rev.* 2000;175:138-149.

144. Kee BL, Murre C. Induction of early B cell factor (EBF) and multiple B lineage genes by the basic helix-loop-helix transcription factor E12. *J Exp Med.* 1998;188(4):699-713.

145. Nera KP, Kohonen P, Narvi E, et al. Loss of Pax5 promotes plasma cell differentiation. *Immunity.* 2006;24(3):283-293.

146. Lazorchak A, Jones ME, Zhuang Y. New insights into E-protein function in lymphocyte development. *Trends Immunol.* 2005;26(6):334-338.

147. Lazorchak AS, Wojciechowski J, Dai M, Zhuang Y. E2A promotes the survival of precursor and mature B lymphocytes. *J Immunol.* 2006;177(4):2495-2504.

148. Schoetz U, Cervelli M, Wang YD, Fiedler P, Buerstedde JM. E2A expression stimulates Ig hypermutation. *J Immunol.* 2006;177(1):395-400.

149. Chiang MY, Monroe JG. BSAP/Pax5A expression blocks survival and expansion of early myeloid cells implicating its involvement in maintaining commitment to the B-lymphocyte lineage. *Blood.* 1999;94(11):3621-3632.

150. Delogu A, Schebesta A, Sun Q, Aschenbrenner K, Perlot T, Busslinger M. Gene repression by Pax5 in B cells is essential for blood cell homeostasis and is reversed in plasma cells. *Immunity.* 2006;24(3):269-281.

151. Zhang Z, Espinoza CR, Yu Z, et al. Transcription factor Pax5 (BSAP) transactivates the RAG-mediated V(H)-to-DJ(H) rearrangement of immunoglobulin genes. *Nat Immunol.* 2006;7(6):616-624.

152. O'Brien P, Morin P, Jr, Ouellette RJ, Robichaud GA. The Pax-5 gene: a pluripotent regulator of B-cell differentiation and cancer disease. *Cancer Res.* 2011;71(24):7345-7350.

153. Schaniel C, Gottar M, Roosnek E, Melchers F, Rolink AG. Extensive in vivo self-renewal, long-term reconstitution capacity, and hematopoietic multipotency of Pax5-deficient precursor B-cell clones. *Blood.* 2002;99(8):2760-2766.

154. Thevenin C, Nutt SL, Busslinger M. Early function of Pax5 (BSAP) before the pre-B cell receptor stage of B lymphopoiesis. *J Exp Med.* 1998;188(4):735-744.

155. Akerblad P, Rosberg M, Leanderson T, Sigvardsson M. The B29 (immunoglobulin beta-chain) gene is a genetic target for early B-cell factor. *Mol Cell Biol.* 1999;19(1):392-401.

156. Gisler R, Jacobsen SE, Sigvardsson M. Cloning of human early B-cell factor and identification of target genes suggest a conserved role in B-cell development in man and mouse. *Blood.* 2000;96(4):1457-1464.

157. Hagman J, Lukin K. Early B-cell factor 'pioneers' the way for B-cell development. *Trends Immunol.* 2005;26(9):455-461.

158. Treiber T, Mandel EM, Pott S, et al. Early B cell factor 1 regulates B cell gene networks by activation, repression, and transcription- independent poising of chromatin. *Immunity.* 2010;32(5):714-725.

159. Anthony BA, Link DC. Regulation of hematopoietic stem cells by bone marrow stromal cells. *Trends Immunol.* 2014;35(1):32-37.

160. Dorshkind K. Regulation of hemopoiesis by bone marrow stromal cells and their products. *Annu Rev Immunol.* 1990;8:111-137.

161. Moreau I, Duvert V, Caux C, et al. Myofibroblastic stromal cells isolated from human bone marrow induce the proliferation of both early myeloid and B-lymphoid cells. *Blood.* 1993;82(8):2396-2405.

162. Ryan DH, Nuccie BL, Abboud CN, Winslow JM. Vascular cell adhesion molecule-1 and the integrin VLA-4 mediate adhesion of human B cell precursors to cultured bone marrow adherent cells. *J Clin Invest.* 1991;88(3):995-1004.

163. Beck TC, Gomes AC, Cyster JG, Pereira JP. CXCR4 and a cell-extrinsic mechanism control immature B lymphocyte egress from bone marrow. *J Exp Med.* 2014;211(13):2567-2581.

164. von Freeden-Jeffry U, Vieira P, Lucian LA, McNeil T, Burdach SE, Murray R. Lymphopenia in interleukin (IL)-7 gene-deleted mice identifies IL-7 as a nonredundant cytokine. *J Exp Med.* 1995;181(4):1519-1526.

165. Puel A, Ziegler SF, Buckley RH, Leonard WJ. Defective IL7R expression in T(-)B(+)NK(+) severe combined immunodeficiency. *Nat Genet.* 1998;20(4):394-397.

166. Corcoran AE, Smart FM, Cowling RJ, Crompton T, Owen MJ, Venkitaraman AR. The interleukin-7 receptor alpha chain transmits distinct signals for proliferation and differentiation during B lymphopoiesis. *EMBO J.* 1996;15(8):1924-1932.

167. Wei C, Zeff R, Goldschneider I. Murine pro-B cells require IL-7 and its receptor complex to up-regulate IL7R alpha, terminal deoxynucleotidyltransferase, and c mu expression. *J Immunol.* 2000;164(4):1961-1970.

168. Corcoran AE, Riddell A, Krooshoop D, Venkitaraman AR. Impaired immunoglobulin gene rearrangement in mice lacking the IL-7 receptor. *Nature.* 1998;391(6670):904-907.

169. Cao X, Shores EW, Hu-Li J, et al. Defective lymphoid development in mice lacking expression of the common cytokine receptor gamma chain. *Immunity.* 1995;2(3):223-238.

170. DiSanto JP, Muller W, Guy-Grand D, Fischer A, Rajewsky K. Lymphoid development in mice with a targeted deletion of the interleukin 2 receptor gamma chain. *Proc Natl Acad Sci U S A.* 1995;92(2):377-381.

171. Dittel BN, LeBien TW. The growth response to IL-7 during normal human B cell ontogeny is restricted to B-lineage cells expressing CD34. *J Immunol.* 1995;154(1):58-67.

172. Namikawa R, Muench MO, de Vries JE, Roncarolo MG. The FLK2/FLT3 ligand synergizes with interleukin-7 in promoting stromal-cell-independent expansion and differentiation of human fetal pro-B cells in vitro. *Blood.* 1996;87(5):1881-1890.

173. Ryan DH, Nuccie BL, Ritterman I, Liesveld JL, Abboud CN, Insel RA. Expression of interleukin-7 receptor by lineage-negative human bone marrow progenitors with enhanced lymphoid proliferative potential and B-lineage differentiation capacity. *Blood.* 1997;89(3):929-940.

174. Chowdhury D, Sen R. Regulation of immunoglobulin heavy-chain gene rearrangements. *Immunol Rev.* 2004;200:182-196.

175. Levin SD, Koelling RM, Friend SL, et al. Thymic stromal lymphopoietin: a cytokine that promotes the development of IgM+ B cells in vitro and signals via a novel mechanism. *J Immunol.* 1999;162(2):677-683.

176. Zhang Y, Zhou B. Functions of thymic stromal lymphopoietin in immunity and disease. *Immunol Res.* 2012;52(3):211-223.

177. Deichmann M, Kronenwett R, Haas R. Expression of the human immunodeficiency virus type-1 coreceptors CXCR-4 (fusin, LESTR) and CKR-5 in CD34+ hematopoietic progenitor cells. *Blood.* 1997;89(10):3522-3528.

178. Ishii T, Nishihara M, Ma F, et al. Expression of stromal cell-derived factor-1/pre-B cell growth-stimulating factor receptor, CXC chemokine receptor 4, on CD34+ human bone marrow cells is a phenotypic alteration for committed lymphoid progenitors. *J Immunol.* 1999;163(7):3612-3620.

179. Vicente-Manzanares M, Cabrero JR, Rey M, et al. A role for the Rho-p160 Rho coiled-coil kinase axis in the chemokine stromal cell-derived factor-1alpha-induced lymphocyte actomyosin and microtubular organization and chemotaxis. *J Immunol.* 2002;168(1):400-410.

180. Fistonich C, Zehentmeier S, Bednarski JJ, et al. Cell circuits between B cell progenitors and IL-7(+) mesenchymal progenitor cells control B cell development. *J Exp Med.* 2018;215(10):2586-2599.

181. Raff MC, Megson M, Owen JJ, Cooper MD. Early production of intracellular IgM by B-lymphocyte precursors in mouse. *Nature.* 1976;259(5540):224-226.

182. Osmond DG, Rolink A, Melchers F. Murine B lymphopoiesis: towards a unified model. *Immunol Today.* 1998;19(2):65-68.

183. Lemmers B, Gauthier L, Guelpa-Fonlupt V, Fougereau M, Schiff C. The human (PsiL+mu-) proB complex: cell surface expression and biochemical structure of a putative transducing receptor. *Blood.* 1999;93(12):4336-4346.

184. Meffre E, Fougereau M, Argenson JN, Aubaniac JM, Schiff C. Cell surface expression of surrogate light chain (psi L) in the absence of mu on human pro-B cell lines and normal pro-B cells. *Eur J Immunol.* 1996;26(9):2172-2180.

185. Sanz E, de la Hera A. A novel anti-Vpre-B antibody identifies immunoglobulin-surrogate receptors on the surface of human pro-B cells. *J Exp Med.* 1996;183(6):2693-2698.

186. Karasuyama H, Rolink A, Melchers F. Surrogate light chain in B cell development. *Adv Immunol.* 1996;63:1-41.

187. Mattei MG, Fumoux F, Roeckel N, Fougereau M, Schiff C. The human pre-B-specific lambda-like cluster is located in the 22q11.2-22q12.3 region, distal to the IgC lambda locus. *Genomics.* 1991;9(3):544-546.

188. Burrows PD, Stephan RP, Wang YH, Lassoued K, Zhang Z, Cooper MD. The transient expression of pre-B cell receptors governs B cell development. *Semin Immunol.* 2002;14(5):343-349.

189. Gauthier L, Lemmers B, Guelpa-Fonlupt V, Fougereau M, Schiff C. Mu-surrogate light chain physicochemical interactions of the human preB cell receptor: implications for VH repertoire selection and cell signaling at the preB cell stage. *J Immunol.* 1999;162(1):41-50.

190. Melchers F. Fit for life in the immune system? Surrogate L chain tests H chains that test L chains. *Proc Natl Acad Sci U S A.* 1999;96(6):2571-2573.

191. Herzog S, Reth M, Jumaa H. Regulation of B-cell proliferation and differentiation by pre-B-cell receptor signalling. *Nat Rev Immunol.* 2009;9(3):195-205.

192. Bradl H, Wittmann J, Milius D, Vettermann C, Jack HM. Interaction of murine precursor B cell receptor with stroma cells is controlled by the unique tail of lambda 5 and stroma cell-associated heparan sulfate. *J Immunol.* 2003;171(5):2338-2348.

193. Gauthier L, Rossi B, Roux F, Termine E, Schiff C. Galectin-1 is a stromal cell ligand of the pre-B cell receptor (BCR) implicated in synapse formation between pre-B and stromal cells and in pre-BCR triggering. *Proc Natl Acad Sci U S A.* 2002;99(20):13014-13019.

194. Bannish G, Fuentes-Panana EM, Cambier JC, Pear WS, Monroe JG. Ligand-independent signaling functions for the B lymphocyte antigen receptor and their role in positive selection during B lymphopoiesis. *J Exp Med.* 2001;194(11):1583-1596.

195. Tsukada S, Baba Y, Watanabe D. Btk and BLNK in B cell development. *Adv Immunol.* 2001;77:123-162.

196. Clark MR, Mandal M, Ochiai K, Singh H. Orchestrating B cell lymphopoiesis through interplay of IL-7 receptor and pre-B cell receptor signalling. *Nat Rev Immunol.* 2014;14(2):69-80.

197. Rickert RC. New insights into pre-BCR and BCR signalling with relevance to B cell malignancies. *Nat Rev Immunol.* 2013;13(8):578-591.

198. Melchers F, ten Boekel E, Yamagami T, Andersson J, Rolink A. The roles of preB and B cell receptors in the stepwise allelic exclusion of mouse IgH and L chain gene loci. *Semin Immunol.* 1999;11(5):307-317.

199. Grawunder U, Leu TM, Schatz DG, et al. Down-regulation of RAG1 and RAG2 gene expression in preB cells after functional immunoglobulin heavy chain rearrangement. *Immunity.* 1995;3(5):601-608.

200. Ochiai K, Maienschein-Cline M, Mandal M, et al. A self-reinforcing regulatory network triggered by limiting IL-7 activates pre-BCR signaling and differentiation. *Nat Immunol.* 2012;13(3):300-307.

201. Mandal M, Powers SE, Ochiai K, et al. Ras orchestrates exit from the cell cycle and light-chain recombination during early B cell development. *Nat Immunol.* 2009;10(10):1110-1117.

202. Casellas R, Shih TA, Kleinewietfeld M, et al. Contribution of receptor editing to the antibody repertoire. *Science.* 2001;291(5508):1541-1544.

203. Geier JK, Schlissel MS. Pre-BCR signals and the control of Ig gene rearrangements. *Semin Immunol.* 2006;18(1):31-39.

204. Conley ME, Rohrer J, Rapalus L, Boylin EC, Minegishi Y. Defects in early B-cell development: comparing the consequences of abnormalities in pre-BCR signaling in the human and the mouse. *Immunol Rev.* 2000;178:75-90.

205. Mundt C, Licence S, Shimizu T, Melchers F, Martensson IL. Loss of precursor B cell expansion but not allelic exclusion in VpreB1/VpreB2 double-deficient mice. *J Exp Med.* 2001;193(4):435-445.

206. Kitamura D, Kudo A, Schaal S, Muller W, Melchers F, Rajewsky K. A critical role of lambda 5 protein in B cell development. *Cell.* 1992;69(5):823-831.

207. Kitamura D, Roes J, Kuhn R, Rajewsky K. A B cell-deficient mouse by targeted disruption of the membrane exon of the immunoglobulin mu chain gene. *Nature.* 1991;350(6317):423-426.

208. Papavasiliou F, Jankovic M, Suh H, Nussenzweig MC. The cytoplasmic domains of immunoglobulin (Ig) alpha and Ig beta can independently induce the precursor B cell transition and allelic exclusion. *J Exp Med.* 1995;182(5):1389-1394.

209. Kurosaki T. Genetic analysis of B cell antigen receptor signaling. *Annu Rev Immunol.* 1999;17:555-592.

210. Kurosaki T. Functional dissection of BCR signaling pathways. *Curr Opin Immunol.* 2000;12(3):276-281.

211. Minegishi Y, Coustan-Smith E, Rapalus L, Ersoy F, Campana D, Conley ME. Mutations in Igalpha (CD79a) result in a complete block in B-cell development. *J Clin Invest.* 1999;104(8):1115-1121.

212. Minegishi Y, Coustan-Smith E, Wang YH, Cooper MD, Campana D, Conley ME. Mutations in the human lambda5/14.1 gene result in B cell deficiency and agammaglobulinemia. *J Exp Med.* 1998;187(1):71-77.

213. Yel L, Minegishi Y, Coustan-Smith E, et al. Mutations in the mu heavy-chain gene in patients with agammaglobulinemia. *N Engl J Med.* 1996;335(20):1486-1493.

214. Schiff C, Lemmers B, Deville A, Fougereau M, Meffre E. Autosomal primary immunodeficiencies affecting human bone marrow B-cell differentiation. *Immunol Rev.* 2000;178:91-98.

215. Pappu R, Cheng AM, Li B, et al. Requirement for B cell linker protein (BLNK) in B cell development. *Science.* 1999;286(5446):1949-1954.

216. Minegishi Y, Rohrer J, Coustan-Smith E, et al. An essential role for BLNK in human B cell development. *Science.* 1999;286(5446):1954-1957.

217. Desiderio S. Role of Btk in B cell development and signaling. *Curr Opin Immunol.* 1997;9(4):534-540.

218. Kurosaki T, Kurosaki M. Transphosphorylation of Bruton's tyrosine kinase on tyrosine 551 is critical for B cell antigen receptor function. *J Biol Chem.* 1997;272(25):15595-15598.

219. Satterthwaite AB, Li Z, Witte ON. Btk function in B cell development and response. *Semin Immunol.* 1998;10(4):309-316.

220. Kurosaki T, Tsukada S. BLNK: connecting Syk and Btk to calcium signals. *Immunity.* 2000;12(1):1-5.

221. Bruton OC. Agammaglobulinemia. *Pediatrics.* 1952;9(6):722-728.

222. Janeway CA, Apt L, Gitlin D. Agammaglobulinemia. *Trans Assoc Am Phys.* 1953;66:200-202.

223. Siegal FP, Pernis B, Kunkel HG. Lymphocytes in human immunodeficiency states: a study of membrane-associated immunoglobulins. *Eur J Immunol.* 1971;1(6):482-486.

224. Conley ME, Parolini O, Rohrer J, Campana D. X-linked agammaglobulinemia: new approaches to old questions based on the identification of the defective gene. *Immunol Rev.* 1994;138:5-21.

225. Parolini O, Hejtmancik JF, Allen RC, et al. Linkage analysis and physical mapping near the gene for X-linked agammaglobulinemia at Xq22. *Genomics.* 1993;15(2):342-349.

226. Tsukada S, Saffran DC, Rawlings DJ, et al. Deficient expression of a B cell cytoplasmic tyrosine kinase in human X-linked agammaglobulinemia. *Cell.* 1993;72(2):279-290.

227. Vetrie D, Vorechovsky I, Sideras P, et al. The gene involved in X-linked agammaglobulinaemia is a member of the src family of protein-tyrosine kinases. *Nature.* 1993;361(6409):226-233.

228. Conley ME, Mathias D, Treadaway J, Minegishi Y, Rohrer J. Mutations in btk in patients with presumed X-linked agammaglobulinemia. *Am J Hum Genet.* 1998;62(5):1034-1043.

229. Vihinen M, Brandau O, Branden LJ, et al. BTKbase, mutation database for X-linked agammaglobulinemia (XLA). *Nucleic Acids Res.* 1998;26(1):242-247.

230. Nomura K, Kanegane H, Karasuyama H, et al. Genetic defect in human X-linked agammaglobulinemia impedes a maturational evolution of pro-B cells into a later stage of pre-B cells in the B-cell differentiation pathway. *Blood.* 2000;96(2):610-617.

231. Scher I, Sharrow SO, Wistar R, Jr, Asofsky R, Paul WE. B-lymphocyte heterogeneity: ontogenetic development and organ distribution of B-lymphocyte populations defined by their density of surface immunoglobulin. *J Exp Med.* 1976;144(2):494-506.

232. de Petris S, Raff MC. Distribution of immunoglobulin on the surface of mouse lymphoid cells as determined by immunoferritin electron microscopy. Antibody-induced, temperature-dependent redistribution and its implications for membrane structure. *Eur J Immunol.* 1972;2(6):523-535.

233. Lejonc RJ, Gourdin MF, Mannoni P, Dreyfus B, Reyes F. The surface morphology of human B lymphocytes as revealed by immunoelectron microscopy. *J Exp Med.* 1975;141(2):392-410.

234. Cambier JC, Bedzyk W, Campbell K, et al. The B-cell antigen receptor: structure and function of primary, secondary, tertiary and quaternary components. *Immunol Rev.* 1993;132:85-106.

235. Pleiman CM, D'Ambrosio D, Cambier JC. The B-cell antigen receptor complex: structure and signal transduction. *Immunol Today.* 1994;15(9):393-399.

236. van Noesel CJ, van Lier RA. Architecture of the human B-cell antigen receptors. *Blood.* 1993;82(2):363-373.

237. Cambier JC. Antigen and Fc receptor signaling. The awesome power of the immunoreceptor tyrosine-based activation motif (ITAM). *J Immunol.* 1995;155(7):3281-3285.

238. Treanor B. B-cell receptor: from resting state to activate. *Immunology.* 2012;136(1):21-27.

239. Pierce SK. Lipid rafts and B-cell activation. *Nat Rev Immunol.* 2002;2(2):96-105.

240. Simons K, Ehehalt R. Cholesterol, lipid rafts, and disease. *J Clin Invest.* 2002;110(5):597-603.

241. Aman MJ, Ravichandran KS. A requirement for lipid rafts in B cell receptor induced Ca(2+) flux. *Curr Biol.* 2000;10(7):393-396.

242. Cheng PC, Dykstra ML, Mitchell RN, Pierce SK. A role for lipid rafts in B cell antigen receptor signaling and antigen targeting. *J Exp Med.* 1999;190(11):1549-1560.

243. Guo B, Kato RM, Garcia-Lloret M, Wahl MI, Rawlings DJ. Engagement of the human pre-B cell receptor generates a lipid raft-dependent calcium signaling complex. *Immunity.* 2000;13(2):243-253.

244. Weintraub BC, Jun JE, Bishop AC, Shokat KM, Thomas ML, Goodnow CC. Entry of B cell receptor into signaling domains is inhibited in tolerant B cells. *J Exp Med.* 2000;191(8):1443-1448.

245. Chung JB, Baumeister MA, Monroe JG. Cutting edge: differential sequestration of plasma membrane-associated B cell antigen receptor in mature and immature B cells into signaling-competent and -incompetent glycosphingolipid-enriched domains. *J Immunol.* 2001;166(2):736-740.

246. Cherukuri A, Cheng PC, Sohn HW, Pierce SK. The CD19/CD21 complex functions to prolong B cell antigen receptor signaling from lipid rafts. *Immunity.* 2001;14(2):169-179.

247. Dykstra M, Cherukuri A, Pierce SK. Rafts and synapses in the spatial organization of immune cell signaling receptors. *J Leukoc Biol.* 2001;70(5):699-707.

248. Bromley SK, Burack WR, Johnson KG, et al. The immunological synapse. *Annu Rev Immunol.* 2001;19:375-396.

249. Batista FD, Iber D, Neuberger MS. B cells acquire antigen from target cells after synapse formation. *Nature.* 2001;411(6836):489-494.

250. DeFranco AL. The complexity of signaling pathways activated by the BCR. *Curr Opin Immunol.* 1997;9(3):296-308.

251. Reth M, Wienands J. Initiation and processing of signals from the B cell antigen receptor. *Annu Rev Immunol.* 1997;15:453-479.

252. Kurosaki T, Takata M, Yamanashi Y, et al. Syk activation by the Src-family tyrosine kinase in the B cell receptor signaling. *J Exp Med.* 1994;179(5):1725-1729.

253. Chiu CW, Dalton M, Ishiai M, Kurosaki T, Chan AC. BLNK: molecular scaffolding through 'cis'-mediated organization of signaling proteins. *EMBO J.* 2002;21(23):6461-6472.

254. Fu C, Turck CW, Kurosaki T, Chan AC. BLNK: a central linker protein in B cell activation. *Immunity.* 1998;9(1):93-103.

255. Yablonski D, Weiss A. Mechanisms of signaling by the hematopoietic-specific adaptor proteins, SLP-76 and LAT and their B cell counterpart, BLNK/SLP-65. *Adv Immunol.* 2001;79:93-128.

256. Falasca M, Logan SK, Lehto VP, Baccante G, Lemmon MA, Schlessinger J. Activation of phospholipase C gamma by PI 3-kinase-induced PH domain-mediated membrane targeting. *EMBO J.* 1998;17(2):414-422.

257. Fluckiger AC, Li Z, Kato RM, et al. Btk/Tec kinases regulate sustained increases in intracellular Ca2+ following B-cell receptor activation. *EMBO J.* 1998;17(7):1973-1985.

258. Dolmetsch RE, Lewis RS, Goodnow CC, Healy JI. Differential activation of transcription factors induced by Ca2+ response amplitude and duration. *Nature.* 1997;386(6627):855-858.

259. Rao A, Luo C, Hogan PG. Transcription factors of the NFAT family: regulation and function. *Annu Rev Immunol.* 1997;15:707-747.

260. Kim TJ, Kim YT, Pillai S. Association of activated phosphatidylinositol 3-kinase with p120cbl in antigen receptor-ligated B cells. *J Biol Chem.* 1995;270(46):27504-27509.

261. Marshall AJ, Niiro H, Yun TJ, Clark EA. Regulation of B-cell activation and differentiation by the phosphatidylinositol 3-kinase and phospholipase Cgamma pathway. *Immunol Rev.* 2000;176:30-46.

262. Tuveson DA, Carter RH, Soltoff SP, Fearon DT. CD19 of B cells as a surrogate kinase insert region to bind phosphatidylinositol 3-kinase. *Science.* 1993;260(5110):986-989.

263. Chan TO, Rittenhouse SE, Tsichlis PN. AKT/PKB and other D3 phosphoinositide-regulated kinases: kinase activation by phosphoinositide-dependent phosphorylation. *Annu Rev Biochem.* 1999;68:965-1014.

264. Genot E, Cantrell DA. Ras regulation and function in lymphocytes. *Curr Opin Immunol.* 2000;12(3):289-294.

The Normal Hematologic System

265. Harmer SL, DeFranco AL. Shc contains two Grb2 binding sites needed for efficient formation of complexes with SOS in B lymphocytes. *Mol Cell Biol.* 1997;17(7):4087-4095.

266. Lankester AC, van Schijndel GM, Rood PM, Verhoeven AJ, van Lier RA. B cell antigen receptor cross-linking induces tyrosine phosphorylation and membrane translocation of a multimeric Shc complex that is augmented by CD19 co-ligation. *Eur J Immunol.* 1994;24(11):2818-2825.

267. Deckert M, Tartare-Deckert S, Couture C, Mustelin T, Altman A. Functional and physical interactions of Syk family kinases with the Vav proto-oncogene product. *Immunity.* 1996;5(6):591-604.

268. Deckert M, Elly C, Altman A, Liu YC. Coordinated regulation of the tyrosine phosphorylation of Cbl by Fyn and Syk tyrosine kinases. *J Biol Chem.* 1998;273(15):8867-8874.

269. Kelly ME, Chan AC. Regulation of B cell function by linker proteins. *Curr Opin Immunol.* 2000;12(3):267-275.

270. Kurosaki T. Regulation of B-cell signal transduction by adaptor proteins. *Nat Rev Immunol.* 2002;2(5):354-363.

271. Leo A, Schraven B. Adapters in lymphocyte signalling. *Curr Opin Immunol.* 2001;13(3):307-316.

272. Buhl AM, Cambier JC. Phosphorylation of CD19 Y484 and Y515, and linked activation of phosphatidylinositol 3-kinase, are required for B cell antigen receptor-mediated activation of Bruton's tyrosine kinase. *J Immunol.* 1999;162(8):4438-4446.

273. Tedder TF, Tuscano J, Sato S, Kehrl JH. CD22, a B lymphocyte-specific adhesion molecule that regulates antigen receptor signaling. *Annu Rev Immunol.* 1997;15:481-504.

274. Keegan AD, Nelms K, Wang LM, Pierce JH, Paul WE. Interleukin 4 receptor: signaling mechanisms. *Immunol Today.* 1994;15(9):423-432.

275. Nelms K, Keegan AD, Zamorano J, Ryan JJ, Paul WE. The IL-4 receptor: signaling mechanisms and biologic functions. *Annu Rev Immunol.* 1999;17:701-738.

276. Russell SM, Keegan AD, Harada N, et al. Interleukin-2 receptor gamma chain: a functional component of the interleukin-4 receptor. *Science.* 1993;262(5141):1880-1883.

277. Wills-Karp M, Finkelman FD. Untangling the complex web of IL-4- and IL-13-mediated signaling pathways. *Sci Signal.* 2008;1(51):pe55.

278. Ihle JN, Witthuhn BA, Quelle FW, Yamamoto K, Silvennoinen O. Signaling through the hematopoietic cytokine receptors. *Annu Rev Immunol.* 1995;13:369-398.

279. Schindler C, Darnell JE, Jr. Transcriptional responses to polypeptide ligands: the JAK-STAT pathway. *Annu Rev Biochem.* 1995;64:621-651.

280. Takeda K, Tanaka T, Shi W, et al. Essential role of Stat6 in IL-4 signalling. *Nature.* 1996;380(6575):627-630.

281. Takatsu K, Kouro T, Nagai Y. Interleukin 5 in the link between the innate and acquired immune response. *Adv Immunol.* 2009;101:191-236.

282. Akira S, Yoshida K, Tanaka T, Taga T, Kishimoto T. Targeted disruption of the IL-6 related genes: gp130 and NF-IL-6. *Immunol Rev.* 1995;148:221-253.

283. Kishimoto T, Akira S, Narazaki M, Taga T. Interleukin-6 family of cytokines and gp130. *Blood.* 1995;86(4):1243-1254.

284. Mihara M, Hashizume M, Yoshida H, Suzuki M, Shiina M. IL-6/IL-6 receptor system and its role in physiological and pathological conditions. *Clin Sci (Lond).* 2012;122(4):143-159.

285. Grammer AC, Lipsky PE. CD40-mediated regulation of immune responses by TRAF-dependent and TRAF-independent signaling mechanisms. *Adv Immunol.* 2000;76:61-178.

286. Bishop GA, Moore CR, Xie P, Stunz LL, Kraus ZJ. TRAF proteins in CD40 signaling. *Adv Exp Med Biol.* 2007;597:131-151.

287. Wright SD, Ramos RA, Tobias PS, Ulevitch RJ, Mathison JC. CD14, a receptor for complexes of lipopolysaccharide (LPS) and LPS binding protein. *Science.* 1990;249(4975):1431-1433.

288. Camacho SA, Kosco-Vilbois MH, Berek C. The dynamic structure of the germinal center. *Immunol Today.* 1998;19(11):511-514.

289. Mesin L, Ersching J, Victora GD. Germinal center B cell dynamics. *Immunity.* 2016;45(3):471-482.

290. Chaudhuri J, Alt FW. Class-switch recombination: interplay of transcription, DNA deamination and DNA repair. *Nat Rev Immunol.* 2004;4(7):541-552.

291. Honjo T, Kinoshita K, Muramatsu M. Molecular mechanism of class switch recombination: linkage with somatic hypermutation. *Annu Rev Immunol.* 2002;20:165-196.

292. Stavnezer J. Antibody class switching. *Adv Immunol.* 1996;61:79-146.

293. Basu U, Meng FL, Keim C, et al. The RNA exosome targets the AID cytidine deaminase to both strands of transcribed duplex DNA substrates. *Cell.* 2011;144(3):353-363.

294. Chang HHY, Pannunzio NR, Adachi N, Lieber MR. Non-homologous DNA end joining and alternative pathways to double-strand break repair. *Nat Rev Mol Cell Biol.* 2017;18(8):495-506.

295. Boboila C, Alt FW, Schwer B. Classical and alternative end-joining pathways for repair of lymphocyte-specific and general DNA double-strand breaks. *Adv Immunol.* 2012;116:1-49.

296. Morell A, Skvaril F, van Loghem E, Kleemola M. Human IgG subclasses in maternal and fetal serum. *Vox Sang.* 1971;21(6):481-492.

297. Bachl J, Carlson C, Gray-Schopfer V, Dessing M, Olsson C. Increased transcription levels induce higher mutation rates in a hypermutating cell line. *J Immunol.* 2001;166(8):5051-5057.

298. McHeyzer-Williams MG, Ahmed R. B cell memory and the long-lived plasma cell. *Curr Opin Immunol.* 1999;11(2):172-179.

299. Bessis M. *Living Blood Cells and Their Ultrastructure.* Springer-Verlag; 1973.

300. Murphy MJ, Hay JB, Morris B, Bessis MC. Ultrastructural analysis of antibody synthesis in cells from lymph and lymph nodes. *Am J Pathol.* 1972;66(1):25-42.

301. Gudat FG, Harris TN, Harris S, Hummeler K. Studies on antibody-producing cells. 3. Identification of young plaque-forming cells by thymidine- 3 H labeling. *J Exp Med.* 1971;134(5):1155-1169.

302. Bosman C, Feldman JD, Pick E. Heterogeneity of antibody-forming cells. An electron microscopic analysis. *J Exp Med.* 1969;129(5):1029-1044.

303. Gudat FG, Harris TN, Harris S, Hummeler K. Studies on antibody-producing cells. I. Ultrastructure of 19S and 7S antibody-producing cells. *J Exp Med.* 1970;132(3):448-474.

304. Gudat FG, Harris TN, Harris S, Hummeler K. Studies on antibody-producing cells. II. Appearance of 3 H-thymidine-labeled rosette-forming cells. *J Exp Med.* 1971;133(2):305-320.

305. Harris TN, Hummeler K, Harris S. Electron microscopic observations on antibody-producing lymph node cells. *J Exp Med.* 1966;123(1):161-172.

306. Hummeler K, Harris TN, Tomassini N, Hechtel M, Farber MB. Electron microscopic observations on antibody-producing cells in lymph and blood. *J Exp Med.* 1966;124(2):255-262.

307. Shaffer AL, Lin KI, Kuo TC, et al. Blimp-1 orchestrates plasma cell differentiation by extinguishing the mature B cell gene expression program. *Immunity.* 2002;17(1):51-62.

308. Angelin-Duclos C, Cattoretti G, Lin KI, Calame K. Commitment of B lymphocytes to a plasma cell fate is associated with Blimp-1 expression in vivo. *J Immunol.* 2000;165(10):5462-5471.

309. Lin KI, Angelin-Duclos C, Kuo TC, Calame K. Blimp-1-dependent repression of Pax-5 is required for differentiation of B cells to immunoglobulin M-secreting plasma cells. *Mol Cell Biol.* 2002;22(13):4771-4780.

310. Reimold AM, Iwakoshi NN, Manis J, et al. Plasma cell differentiation requires the transcription factor XBP-1. *Nature.* 2001;412(6844):300-307.

311. Shaffer AL YX, He Y, Boldrick J, Chan EP, Staudt LM. BCL-6 represses genes that function in lymphocyte differentiation, inflammation, and cell cycle control. *Immunity.* 2000;13(2):199-212.

312. Tunyaplin C, Shaffer AL, Angelin-Duclos CD, Yu X, Staudt LM, Calame KL. Direct repression of prdm1 by Bcl-6 inhibits plasmacytic differentiation. *J Immunol.* 2004;173(2):1158-1165.

313. Caligaris-Cappio F, Gobbi M, Bofill M, Janossy G. Infrequent normal B lymphocytes express features of B-chronic lymphocytic leukemia. *J Exp Med.* 1982;155(2):623-628.

314. Gadol N, Ault KA. Phenotypic and functional characterization of human Leu1 (CD5) B cells. *Immunol Rev.* 1986;93:23-34.

315. Berland R, Wortis HH. Origins and functions of B-1 cells with notes on the role of CD5. *Annu Rev Immunol.* 2002;20:253-300.

316. Braun J, Citri Y, Baltimore D, et al. B-Ly1 cells: immortal Ly-1+ B lymphocyte cell lines spontaneously arising in murine splenic cultures. *Immunol Rev.* 1986;93:5-21.

317. Herzenberg LA, Kantor AB. B-cell lineages exist in the mouse. *Immunol Today.* 1993;14(2):79-83. discussion 88-90.

318. Kantor AB, Herzenberg LA. Origin of murine B cell lineages. *Annu Rev Immunol.* 1993;11:501-538.

319. Antin JH, Emerson SG, Martin P, Gadol N, Ault KA. Leu-1+ (CD5+) B cells. A major lymphoid subpopulation in human fetal spleen: phenotypic and functional studies. *J Immunol.* 1986;136(2):505-510.

320. Hardy RR, Hayakawa K. Development and physiology of Ly-1 B and its human homolog, Leu-1 B. *Immunol Rev.* 1986;93:53-79.

321. Hayakawa K, Hardy RR. Development and function of B-1 cells. *Curr Opin Immunol.* 2000;12(3):346-353.

322. Montecino-Rodriguez E, Dorshkind K. B-1 B cell development in the fetus and adult. *Immunity.* 2012;36(1):13-21.

323. Herzenberg LA, Stall AM, Lalor PA, et al. The Ly-1 B cell lineage. *Immunol Rev.* 1986;93:81-102.

324. Hayakawa K, Hardy RR, Honda M, Herzenberg LA, Steinberg AD, Herzenberg LA. Ly-1 B cells: functionally distinct lymphocytes that secrete IgM autoantibodies. *Proc Natl Acad Sci U S A.* 1984;81(8):2494-2498.

325. Plater-Zyberk C, Maini RN, Lam K, Kennedy TD, Janossy G. A rheumatoid arthritis B cell subset expresses a phenotype similar to that in chronic lymphocytic leukemia. *Arthritis Rheum.* 1985;28(9):971-976.

326. Dauphinee M, Tovar Z, Talal N. B cells expressing CD5 are increased in Sjogren's syndrome. *Arthritis Rheum.* 1988;31(5):642-647.

327. Hardy RR, Hayakawa K, Shimizu M, Yamasaki K, Kishimoto T. Rheumatoid factor secretion from human Leu-1+ B cells. *Science.* 1987;236(4797):81-83.

328. Ault KA, Antin JH, Ginsburg D, et al. Phenotype of recovering lymphoid cell populations after marrow transplantation. *J Exp Med.* 1985;161(6):1483-1502.

329. Boumsell L, Coppin H, Pham D, et al. An antigen shared by a human T cell subset and B cell chronic lymphocytic leukemic cells. Distribution on normal and malignant lymphoid cells. *J Exp Med.* 1980;152(1):229-234.

330. Heng TS, Painter MW, Immunological Genome Project C. The Immunological Genome Project: networks of gene expression in immune cells. *Nat Immunol.* 2008;9(10):1091-1094.

331. Painter MW, Davis S, Hardy RR, Mathis D, Benoist C, Immunological Genome Project C. Transcriptomes of the B and T lineages compared by multiplatform microarray profiling. *J Immunol.* 2011;186(5):3047-3057.

332. Glynne R, Ghandour G, Rayner J, Mack DH, Goodnow CC. B-lymphocyte quiescence, tolerance and activation as viewed by global gene expression profiling on microarrays. *Immunol Rev.* 2000;176:216-246.

333. Glynne RJ, Watson SR. The immune system and gene expression microarrays--new answers to old questions. *J Pathol.* 2001;195(1):20-30.

334. Staudt LM, Brown PO. Genomic views of the immune system*. *Annu Rev Immunol.* 2000;18:829-859.

335. Ma C, Staudt LM. Molecular definition of the germinal centre stage of B-cell differentiation. *Philos Trans R Soc Lond B Biol Sci.* 2001;356(1405):83-89.

336. Underhill GH, George D, Bremer EG, Kansas GS. Gene expression profiling reveals a highly specialized genetic program of plasma cells. *Blood.* 2003;101(10):4013-4021.

337. Staudt LM. Gene expression profiling of lymphoid malignancies. *Annu Rev Med.* 2002;53:303-318.

338. Alizadeh AA, Eisen MB, Davis RE, et al. Distinct types of diffuse large B-cell lymphoma identified by gene expression profiling. *Nature.* 2000;403(6769):503-511.

339. Lossos IS, Alizadeh AA, Eisen MB, et al. Ongoing immunoglobulin somatic mutation in germinal center B cell-like but not in activated B cell-like diffuse large cell lymphomas. *Proc Natl Acad Sci U S A.* 2000;97(18):10209-10213.

340. Rosenwald A, Wright G, Chan WC, et al. The use of molecular profiling to predict survival after chemotherapy for diffuse large-B-cell lymphoma. *N Engl J Med.* 2002;346(25):1937-1947.

341. Rosenwald A, Alizadeh AA, Widhopf G, et al. Relation of gene expression phenotype to immunoglobulin mutation genotype in B cell chronic lymphocytic leukemia. *J Exp Med.* 2001;194(11):1639-1647.

342. Klein U, Tu Y, Stolovitzky GA, et al. Gene expression profiling of B cell chronic lymphocytic leukemia reveals a homogeneous phenotype related to memory B cells. *J Exp Med.* 2001;194(11):1625-1638.

343. Gurrieri C, McGuire P, Zan H, et al. Chronic lymphocytic leukemia B cells can undergo somatic hypermutation and intraclonal immunoglobulin V(H)DJ(H) gene diversification. *J Exp Med.* 2002;196(5):629-639.

344. Vallat L, Magdelenat H, Merle-Beral H, et al. The resistance of B-CLL cells to DNA damage-induced apoptosis defined by DNA microarrays. *Blood.* 2003;101(11):4598-4606.

345. Kuppers R, Rajewsky K. The origin of Hodgkin and Reed/Sternberg cells in Hodgkin's disease. *Annu Rev Immunol.* 1998;16:471-493.

346. Kuppers R, Klein U, Schwering I, et al. Identification of Hodgkin and Reed-Sternberg cell-specific genes by gene expression profiling. *J Clin Invest.* 2003;111(4):529-537.

347. Schwering I, Brauninger A, Klein U, et al. Loss of the B-lineage-specific gene expression program in Hodgkin and Reed-Sternberg cells of Hodgkin lymphoma. *Blood.* 2003;101(4):1505-1512.

The Normal Hematologic System

Chapter 13 ■ T Lymphocytes

JUSTIN C. BOUCHER • RAWAN G. FARAMAND • MARCO L. DAVILA

T-LYMPHOCYTE MORPHOLOGY

The T lymphocyte is 5 to 8 μm in diameter, with a high nucleocy-toplasmic ratio. Aided by routine staining and visualized with light microscopy, the nucleus is purple with densely packed chromatin, and the cytoplasm forms a narrow light-blue rim. By transmission electron microscopy, the nucleus has shallow indentations with dense heterochromatin along the nuclear membrane and euchromatin occupying most of the remaining nuclear surface. One or two nucleoli are visible. The cytoplasm shows a few organelles, such as mitochondria and a small Golgi apparatus. By scanning electron microscopy, the surface of the T lymphocytes is either smooth or shows short microvilli, depending on the method of preparation and the state of activation.[1]

T-LYMPHOCYTE DEVELOPMENT

Thymic Microenvironment

The thymus gland is a multilobed organ located behind the sternum. Each lobe of the thymus can be divided into a central medulla and a peripheral cortex, surrounded by an outer capsule. The cortex is heavily infiltrated with developing T lymphocytes and a few epithelial and mesenchymal cells, whereas the medulla is composed of more epithelial cells but fewer lymphocytes. Epithelial cells, also called "nurse cells," constitute the framework of the thymus and are functionally essential for the maturation of T lymphocytes. The critical role of the epithelial component of the thymic stroma for intrathymic T-cell development is most dramatically illustrated by the phenotype of nude mice. In nude mice, disruption of the forkhead transcription factor Foxn1 blocks epithelial differentiation and leads to loss of intrathymic T-cell development and severe immunodeficiency.[2]

The human thymus becomes fully differentiated by approximately the 15th week of gestation and early migrants contribute to the development of the thymic microenvironment. T-cell maturation is directed in different microenvironments within the thymus, and their differentiation is coupled with highly coordinated T-cell migration between distinct regions of the thymus. T-cell precursors enter the subcapsular cortical areas, where they encounter networks of cortical epithelial stroma. In the cortical area, cortical thymus epithelial cells (TECs) support early T-cell-progenitor commitment and differentiation. They also play a central role in T-cell receptor (TCR) rearrangement, positive selection (PS), and negative selection (Figure 13.1). As they differentiate, they move from the cortex toward the medulla of the thymus.[3] Medullary TECs, in conjunction with dendritic cells (DCs), support negative selection of T-cell precursors.[4]

T-Cell Progenitors

T-cell progenitors derive from the liver during fetal development, whereas in adults, they derive from the bone marrow. The thymus is populated by hematopoietic multipotent progenitors from the bone marrow.[5] Recruitment of T-cell progenitors involves the chemokines CCL21 (or SLC, secondary lymphoid tissue chemokine) and CCL25 produced by the fetal thymus, which attract CD4⁻/CD8⁻/CD25⁻/CD44⁺ thymocytes.[6]

Notch, Cytokines, and T-Cell Commitment

Signaling through the Notch receptor is a crucial factor for T-cell commitment.[7-10] Notch plays a pivotal role in determining T-/B--lineage choice, and signaling through Notch drives the commitment of lymphoid precursors to the T lineage.[11-13] Notch belongs to a family of conserved proteins that function as cell-surface receptors

and direct regulators of gene transcription.[14] It was first isolated as a gene involved in chromosomal translocations in a subset of human T-cell acute lymphoblastic leukemia cases. Ligands for Notch include Delta, Serrate, and several other molecules corresponding to these two classes.[15]

In cells of the immune system, there are two Notch receptors, NOTCH1 and NOTCH2.[16] The pleiotropic signaling by Notch regulates differentiation, proliferation, and cell death, but it is not clear which function most precisely determines cell fate and ultimately directs T-cell commitment.[17] With Notch inactivation, double-negative T cells diminish in the thymus, whereas B-cell precursors increase, probably from a more efficient production of B cells within the thymus.[18] On the other hand, transgenic expression of Notch in the bone marrow permits the accumulation of CD4⁺ T cells or CD8⁺ T cells (CTLs). Notch is also needed in later stages for TCR gene rearrangements, PS, and CD4/CD8 lineage choice.[19]

Of the cytokines implicated in T-cell differentiation interleukin (IL)-7 is essential.[20] Mice genetically deficient in the IL7 receptor have a profound reduction of T and B lymphocytes, and thymocyte development is blocked at a very early stage before the induction of CD25 and Tcrb gene rearrangements.[21] IL7 is produced constitutively by epithelial cells, and it induces proliferation of DN thymocytes[22] and/or maintains their viability.[23] CD34⁺ thymocytes cultured with IL7 start to express CD8 and CD4 but remain CD3 and TCR negative, indicating that other stimuli are essential for generating CD3⁺/CD4⁺/CD8⁺ cells. IL7 also induces Tcrβ gene rearrangements.[24] IL7 regulation is tightly coordinated during T-cell maturation for thymocyte survival, as IL7 is essential for the postselection expansion of positively selected thymocytes.[25]

Other cytokines, such as IL1, IL2, and IL4, have also been shown to play a role in thymocyte differentiation.[20] In the thymus, IL1 enhances thymocyte proliferation and is necessary for maturation and CD4⁺CD8⁺ differentiation. IL2 plays an important role in developing regulatory T cells (Tregs) in the thymus. It is produced by mature self-reactive CD4 T cells residing in the thymus[26] and prevents deletion of thymocytes poised to develop into Tregs. IL4 drives CD8⁺ single-positive (SP) thymocytes into a memory-like state called innate CTLs and can also promote the development of Tregs.

T-Cell-αβ vs T-Cell-γδ Selection

Distinguished by their surface TCR expression, T cells can be subdivided into two major populations, αβ and γδ T cells. Both αβ and γδ T cells differentiate from multipotent CD4⁻CD8⁻ double-negative (DN) precursors in the thymus. T-precursor cells undergo extensive DNA rearrangements at the β, γ, and δ TCR loci, thus generating two distinct characteristics and functions of T-cell subsets.[27] αβ T cells generally express CD4 or CD8 lineage markers and primarily develop into helper or cytotoxic subsets, respectively. However, most γδ T cells lack CD4 and CD8 and share several markers associated with natural killer (NK) cells or antigen-presenting cells (APCs).[27,28]

αβ and γδ T cell populations show distinct anatomical localization, antigen specificity, and function. After egress from the thymus, naïve αβ T cells home to the lymph nodes and to the T-cell zones of the spleen where they encounter vast numbers of DCs presenting nonself and pathogen-encoded antigens. MHC molecules restrict the recognition of peptide fragments by αβ T cells. Thus, αβ T cells contribute primarily to the antigen-specific killing and memory phases of immune protection from pathogens.[27,28] γδ T cells do not require antigen processing and major histocompatibility complex (MHC) presentation of peptides. These cells are believed to have a prominent role in the recognition of lipid antigens. γδ T cells combine conventional adaptive features (inherent in their TCRs and pleiotropic effector functions) with rapid, innate-like responses (expression of toll-like receptors (TLRs) and share NK cell markers). Thus, γδ T cells play an important role in the initiation of immune reactions.[28]

CD4/CD8 Lineage Commitment

Double-positive (DP) thymocytes differentiate into phenotypically and functionally distinct lineages of αβ T cells, CD4+ and CD8+ SP T cells. Typically, thymocyte development proceeds through a well-understood series of steps (CD4−CD8− DN T cell → CD4+CD8+ DP T cell → CD4+ or CD8+ SP T cell), which are broadly characterized by coreceptor expression of CD4 and CD8, as well as TCR gene rearrangement and expression (*Figure 13.1*). When progenitor cells begin to express CD2 but have not yet rearranged their TCR genes, they are DN for CD4 and CD8 (CD4−CD8−). After TCR gene rearrangement, thymocytes upregulate both CD4 and CD8, which serve as coreceptor to bind MHC II and MHC I, and are involved in the positive selection of CD4+CD8+ thymocyte cells. Further, CD4+CD8+ thymocytes undergo lineage commitment, maturing into a CD8+ or a CD4+ T cell. Lineage commitment occurs at the late stage of positive selection and works by downregulation of CD4 and CD8 (reducing the signal from the TCR) and then upregulation of CD4 only.

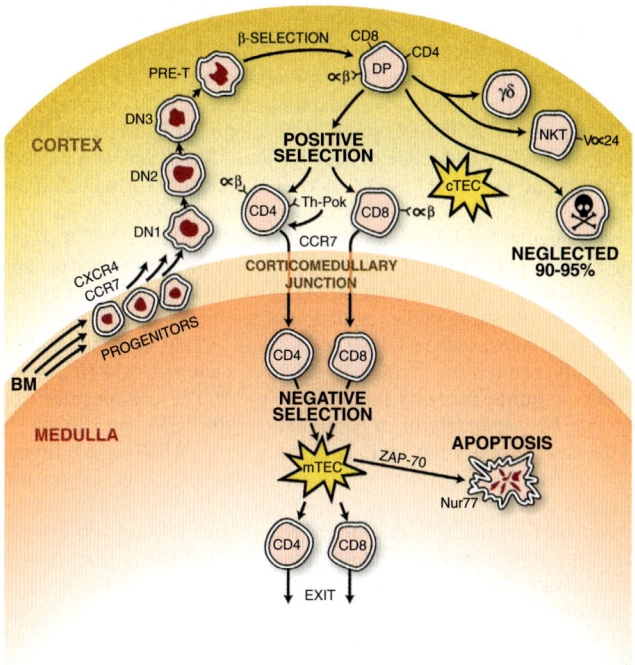

FIGURE 13.1 The first migrants from the bone marrow arrive and settle in the corticomedullary junction. They lack expression of CD4 and CD8, and are known as double negatives (DN). These new immigrants begin to move to the outer cortex and, depending on certain markers, are distinguished in three stages: DN1, DN2, and DN3. The migration is supported through interactions between P-selectin (thymic epithelium) and its ligand (progenitor cells). In the outer cortex, they become double positive (DP; i.e., CD4+/CD8+), and at the DN3 stage, they undergo gene rearrangements with expression of the T-cell receptor (TCR)-β gene (β selection). Signals provided by the CCR-7 chemokine receptor guide the positively selected thymocytes that have already separated into the CD4 or CD8 lineages back to the medulla. A final screening for the "affinity" of their TCR binding to autoantigens takes place in the medulla (NS). It is triggered by contacts of their TCR with tissue-restricted self-antigens (TRAs) on medullary thymic endothelial cells (mTECs). Promiscuous gene expression (pGE), for autoantigens, regulated by the AIRE gene (see chapter text for details), controls central tolerance. The thymic medullary epithelium ultimately allows survival of the "useful," and it ignores the "useless" and "destroys" the harmful.[128] Exit of mature T cells from the thymus is regulated by the G-protein-coupled receptor, sphingosine-1-phosphate receptor 1 (S1P-1), as well as the very late antigen (VLA-) and lymphotoxin-β receptor.

The TCRs of CD4+ cells interact with peptides bound to class II MHC molecules, whereas the TCRs of CD8+ cells recognize peptide-class I MHC complexes. The mechanism by which the lineages diverge from DP thymocytes into SP thymocytes is unknown.[29,30] The *instructive* model proposes that thymocytes carrying an MHC class I restricted TCR differentiate to CD8+ cells, whereas engagement of TCR with class II MHC induces commitment to CD4. An alternative model, known as stochastic (or selective), proposes that DP thymocytes are already committed randomly to a lineage regardless of MHC specificity of their TCR.

The cytoplasmic region of CD4 may direct CD4 lineage commitment. A chimeric construct, for example, made of the cytoplasmic region of CD4 and the extracellular and transmembrane region of CD8a supports the development of cells with the CD4+/CD8a− phenotype, but with a class I restricted TCR.[31] The cytoplasmic tail of CD4 is preferentially associated with tyrosine kinase LCK. Therefore, CD4 is likely to deliver stronger signals than the coengagement of TCR and CD8.[32,33] Therefore, the strength of signal model suggests that strong signals dictated by the frequency of the available ligand induce CD4 differentiation, whereas weak signals induce CD8. Another aspect of signaling evaluated was the duration of signals. When the interaction is limited to a few hours, the cells become CD8+, but exposure for longer periods of time result in CD4+ lineage commitment.[34] Accordingly, TCR of a DP thymocyte initiates downregulation of CD8 and produces a CD4+/CD8− intermediate cell. At this stage, the duration of signaling determines the final outcome. That is, short signaling produces CTLs, whereas persistent signaling in the CD4+/CD8− intermediate cell causes CD4+ differentiation.[35]

Variation of LCK function seems to be the single most important parameter in CD4/CD8 lineage decision. Constitutively active LCK promotes CD4 differentiation, even in the presence of class I MHC–restricted TCR. On the other hand, when LCK is catalytically inactivated, all thymocytes, including those with class II MHC–restricted TCR, become CD8+.[36,37] Also, in the absence of LCK, cross-linking of CD3 induces CD8 differentiation.[38] The LCK-dependent regulation of lineage commitment is not only phenotypic but also functional because the class II MHC–restricted CD8+ cells behave as killer cells, whereas class I restricted CD4+ cells upregulate CD40 ligand, which is characteristic of helper T cells.[36] These experimental results suggest that CD4 differentiation is a default pathway.[39] The multiplicity of the models entertained and the ambiguity of some of the results are evidence that the precise mechanism of T-cell lineage commitment remains elusive.[30,40]

More recently, a transcription factor Th-POK (T-helper-inducing POK factor) was found to be necessary and sufficient for CD4 lineage commitment and the absence of Th-POK results in the development of CTLs.[41] The existence of this factor was suspected as a result of studies of the spontaneous recessive mutant mouse with helper deficient cells (i.e., CD4+ T cells).[42] Th-POK belongs to the POK family of transcription factors characterized by two motifs, a regulatory POZ/BTB domain (for interaction with other transcription factors) and a Zn-finger DNA-binding domain.

Positive and Negative Selection

The random nature of TCR gene rearrangements determines the specificities directed not only against foreign antigens but also against self-antigens. Self-reactive T cells are harmful if they exit the thymus. Therefore, mechanisms have been developed to allow the thymus to select only those deemed useful, neglect useless TCRs, and delete potentially dangerous TCRs.[43] Selection begins at the DP stage when the TCR is expressed at low levels.[44-47] If a TCR recognizes a self-peptide presented by MHC molecules, the ensuing options for each DP thymocyte are determined by the TCR and MHC-peptide (pMHC) ligand interaction. If the affinity of interaction is weak, the cell is positively selected, whereas a T cell having a high-affinity TCR is negatively selected.[48] Cells with TCRs that do not bind with sufficient avidity are neglected and die by apoptosis, whereas in the positively selected cell the expression of *RAG*, which encodes the proteins regulating V(D)J recombination, and *PTCRA* (pre-TCR) genes is turned off and the expression of CD4 and CD8 is partially downregulated. The cell then moves from the cortex to the medulla, where one of the coreceptors is re-expressed and cell lineage is defined.[49,50] Signaling by LCK regulates positive and negative selection, and in its absence, the selection mechanisms are compromised.[51] LCK interacts with the coreceptors CD4 and CD8 through two cysteines in the cytoplasmic region of each coreceptor and two cysteines in LCK.[52]

Hematopoietic components of the thymic stroma are radiosensitive, whereas the epithelial components are radioresistant. These differences allowed the construction of chimeric thymuses composed of epithelial and hematopoietic elements with different MHC backgrounds. These studies indicated that the thymic cortical epithelium is responsible for PS and hematopoietic stromal cells are inducers of NS.[53] Cortical epithelial cells have weak MHC expression and developing DP thymocytes have low TCR expression, so their interactions are of the low avidity required by PS. Similarly, hematopoietic cells in the corticomedullary junction express MHC molecules at a higher density and the T cells have upregulated their TCRs. As a result, the interactions in this anatomic location are appropriate for NS. PS is driven by peptides with varying affinities; however, by increasing the peptide concentration, even low-affinity ligands can positively select.[54] Other parameters of a pMHC complex, such as the conformation[55] and the concentration[56] of the peptide, contribute to repertoire selection. Despite the evidence that each pMHC complex selects more than one TCR, the immense diversity of the fully developed T-cell repertoire depends on a large number of pMHCs[57] as well as on the quantity and quality of the stromal cells.[58] Peptide diversity during selection seems to have a greater effect on NS than on PS. In thymus organ cultures, testing with a diverse array of peptides, the addition of 1% of DCs reduced the number of CD4+ T cells selected by 80% compared to that of the controls in the absence of DCs. Thus, the quantity and quality of the selecting stromal cells have a significant impact on the selected repertoire by multiple peptides.[58]

An important selection force in these cellular interactions is the strength of the interaction, which determines the outcome. Strong interactions lead to deletion, whereas intermediate strength induces PS. This may explain the increase of PS following the blocking of CD28/B7 interactions.[59] Removal of strong self-reactive cells is the sole purpose of NS. Such clones may initiate autoimmunity if they exit to the periphery. An estimated 2000 to 3000 tissue-specific antigens are expressed in human or murine medullary thymic endothelial cells (mTECs)[60,61]; about 500 of these genes may be AIRE (autoimmune regulator) dependent. Using hen egg lysozyme as a reporter for the insulin promoter, it was shown that expression of antigen in the thymic stroma is necessary and sufficient for deletion.[62]

Expression of tissue-restricted self-antigens by mTECs results from promiscuous gene expression (pGE) by the mTECs.[60] Some of the genes are expressed by both mTECs and cortical thymic endothelial cells (cTECs; pool 1), whereas others are expressed only by mTECs (pool 2), and finally, others are expressed only in the more mature mTECs (i.e., strongly positive for MHC class II; pool 3). Depending on the stage of differentiation of mTECs, two models have been proposed for pGE: (1) in the developmental, or progressive restriction model, pGE is detected in immature and perhaps pluripotent progenitor cells, and (2) in the terminal differentiation model, pGE is mutated in mTECs of a mature phenotype.[63] The pGE is regulated by AIRE, the gene mutated in the rare autoimmune disorder known as autoimmune polyglandular syndrome type 1 (APS-1).[64] AIRE has a nuclear localization signal and several potential DNA-binding and protein interaction domains. In cooperation with transcription factor CREB-binding protein, it transactivates the transcription of other genes, although it is still a mystery how a single molecule controls the transcription of such an array of genes.

The pGE is conserved across species barriers, as a study with thymic cTECs and mTECs has recently shown the AIRE gene has the highest enrichment in mTECs and the promiscuously overexpressed genes are remarkably well conserved among species.[65] In humans, a set of 443 genes have been detected overexpressed in mTECs (comparable to 555 in mice). This is an underestimate, as most were detected

by polymerase chain reaction. These genes show no preference for any chromosome. Another interesting finding is the clustering of non-homologous genes. This clustering has been suggested to result from the juxtaposition of genes involved in the formation of a particular tissue. Because the promiscuously expressed genes do not all share such a function, the clustering results from epigenetic mechanisms of regulation. They become accessible to mTECs as a result of belonging to the same "gene neighborhood." pGE is not only sufficient for self-tolerance but also likely essential for genetic propagation, since infertility as a result of gonad-specific autoimmunity is highly prevalent in APS-1[66] and Aire−/− mice.[67] In addition to genetic control, self-tolerance may be regulated by epigenetic mechanisms.

Self-tolerance is mediated by NS or clonal deletion,[68] but some self-reactive T-cells are also submitted to nondeletional central tolerance and give rise to immunosuppressive CD4+ T cells, also known as natural Tregs.[69] Tregs are T cells with medium to high affinity for self-antigens. However, they escape NS and are positively selected by a subset of DCs that have been educated by a thymic stromal lymphopoietin (TSLP) produced by Hassall corpuscles.[70] Other evidence suggests that CD4+ Tregs are positively selected by thymic epithelial cells expressing self-antigens but not by bone-marrow-derived DCs.[71]

The binding of TCR to its ligand induces phosphorylation of the three immunoreceptor tyrosine-based activation motifs (ITAMs) of the ζ chain and the single ITAM in each of the CD3 ε, δ, and γ chains. The ζ chain is constitutively associated in thymocytes with the ZAP70 kinase, suggesting that a low level of activation, or tonic signaling, takes place continuously.[72] ZAP70 is indispensable for PS and NS because both processes are abrogated in ZAP70-deficient mice.[73] However, the SRC-like adaptor protein (SLAP) downregulates TCR expression at the DP stage of development and rescues T-cell development in the absence of ZAP70. Thus, SLAP acts as a negative regulator and probably "marks" activated receptors for retention and degradation.[74] The main downstream signaling pathway for PS is the Ras/mitogen-activated protein kinase (MAPK) cascade.[75] TCR signaling alone is not sufficient to induce selection for survival or death.[76] The costimulatory interaction of CD40/CD40L is a master regulator of NS, usually acting in the regulation of the ligands of other costimulatory molecules, such as CD80 and CD86.[77] CD40 may induce other costimuli required for thymocyte deletion, such as CD54 (ICAM-1), FASL, or tumor necrosis factor (TNF).[78-80] These molecules may regulate NS separately or in combination with CD5 and CD28. The CD28 costimulatory molecule engaged with the TCR signals thymocytes to undergo apoptosis or maturation, depending on the intensity of costimulation.[81]

Stimulation of maturation of DP thymocytes follows activation of the extracellular signal–regulated kinase ERK/MAPK pathway and upregulation of the anti-apoptotic protein BCL2. Apoptosis is triggered by the expression of the Nur77 family of transcription factors and occurs only if TCR engagement is accompanied by costimulation. Ca2+ fluxes in mature T lymphocytes regulate proliferation, differentiation, and survival. Some of the functions of Ca2+ are mediated by the Ca2+-dependent phosphatase calcineurin, which is disrupted by cyclosporin A and FK506 and block the initial steps of PS.[82,83] However, intracellular chelators reduce deletion,[84] which suggests that interference of Ca2+ fluxes and function exerts several effects on thymocyte selection.

All signaling pathways end up targeting regulation of transcription factors, and various studies have examined the roles of nuclear factor of activated T cells (NFAT) and nuclear factor-κB (NF-κB), but only members of the Nur77 family have been clearly shown to be involved in selection, with a major role in apoptosis of thymocytes.[85] It has been estimated that 90% to 95% of thymocytes die in the thymus and the appearance of vast numbers of dead cells on histologic sections is why histopathologists call the thymus the "graveyard" of T cells. The timing of PS versus NS has been challenging to define, but it is believed that NS occurs relatively late because TCR affinity increases with time and it is the high affinity of the TCR that triggers NS. At the end of selection, mature T lymphocytes exit the thymus and traffic to secondary lymphoid organs.

THE T-CELL RECEPTOR

The α/β T-Cell-Receptor Complex

The αβ TCR is formed by two chains, α and β (*Figure 13.2*), each consisting of a constant domain, Cα and Cβ, and a variable domain, Vα and Vβ. The Vα domain is encoded by two gene segments, Vα and Jα, and is homologous to the V domain of the Ig light chain. The Vβ domain is formed by three polypeptides, Vβ, Dβ, and Jβ. The constant domains correspond to the Ig C domains, but the Cα-Cβ interface is highly polar, and the CL-CH1 interface is hydrophobic. Cβ has a large loop, which extends out to the side of the domain, and it may interact with the coreceptors. The Cα domain has several structural deviations from the C-type Ig domain. The V domains are very similar to the V domains of an antibody. They contribute to forming the TCR-combining site, which comprises hypervariable loops or complementarity-determining regions (CDR) 1, 2, and 3 from the α and β chains and another loop termed HV-4, which exhibits some hypervariability. The CDR1 and CDR2 are formed by the V segments, which are less polymorphic in the TCR than in *IGH* because fewer V segments are available for TCR, whereas the CDR3 is polymorphic as a result of the larger number of J segments available for the β chain contributing to CDR3.

The loops of Vβ that contribute to the antigen-binding site of the TCR are similarly placed as in the *IGH* V region. A disulfide bond links the chains, and the heterodimer is anchored to the cell membrane by the transmembrane region, ending in the cytoplasm by a short (three- to five-amino acid) cytoplasmic tail. Crystallization of the TCR shows that it resembles the Fab fragment of Ig.[86] However, TCR-αβ is extensively glycosylated with up to seven N-linked sites distributed between the α and β chains. The combining site is usually flat, similar to anti-protein antibodies, and consistent with the TCR's function of binding to the surface of the pMHC.[87] The diversity of CDR3 is much higher, implying that the function of CDR3 is in peptide discrimination, whereas CDR1 and 2 interact with more conserved structural elements of the MHC. The TCR contains many more J segments and thus can increase V-Jα and V-D-Jβ junctional diversity in the CDR3.[88] The

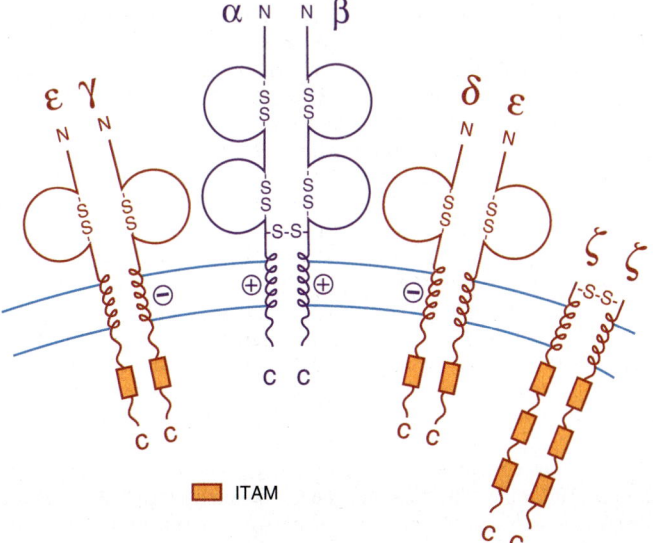

FIGURE 13.2 T-cell-receptor complex. The T-cell receptor complex consists of two components: ligand binding (antigen recognition) and signal transduction. The antigen recognition component consists of two polypeptide chains, α and β. Because of their short intracytoplasmic tails, they cannot link themselves to the signal transduction cascade. The signal transduction component consists of the CD3 proteins γ, δ, and ε, members of the immunoglobulin superfamily, and two other proteins forming either a homodimer (two ζ proteins) or a heterodimer (ζ-η). The γ, δ, and ε chains have one immunoreceptor tyrosine-based activation motif each, and the ζ chain has three. See chapter text for details. ITAM, immunoreceptor tyrosine-based activation motif.

TCR residues that contact the pMHC are always in the apices of the CDR (i.e., for CDR1α, residues 27-30; for CDR2α, residues 50-52; for CDR1β, residues 27-30; and for CDR2β, residues 52 and 53).

TCRs interact with peptides bound to MHC molecules. The amino-terminal domains, α₁ and α₂ of the MHC class I heavy chain, form the binding site for the peptide. The site consists of a floor of eight strands of antiparallel β-pleated sheets, which support two α helices, one contributed by the α₁ domain and the other by the α₂ domain aligned in an antiparallel orientation. This arrangement forms a groove, on the floor of which lies the peptide from an antigen to be presented to the TCR. The floor of the groove is supported by two Ig domains from below; one is the α₃ domain of the heavy chain and the other the β₂-microglobulin. Some of the peptide residues are exposed above the groove and interact directly with the TCR, whereas others point to the groove floor. Depressions in the floor of the groove, known as pockets A through F, interact with some side chains of the bound peptide.[89]

Several TCR-pMHCs have been analyzed to clarify the contributions of Vα for the buried surface area (i.e., the interface between the TCR and the pMHC). The contribution of Vα is on average 57% and that of Vβ 43%.[90] The orientation of the TCR over the pMHC is diagonal rather than orthogonal.[91] It is more likely that the TCR turns around the MHC molecule by approximately 35° and also varies in its roll in a range of 19° (range 30°).[92] X-ray crystallography reveals that the initiation of T-cell signaling is favored by a diagonal binding position of the TCR with the supramolecular assembly. This form of interaction of the TCR with its target contrasts with antibodies, which use different binding positions even with the same antigen. The diagonal approach of the TCR to the MHC-peptide complex evolved to facilitate the initiation of T-cell signaling, since different TCRs can recognize the same MHC-bound antigen. The diagonal binding geometry has implications for the mechanism of initiation of T-cell signaling because it places the TCR in an orientation that facilitates the positioning of the CDR1 and CDR2 loops over the α₁/α₂ helices of MHC class I and the α₁/β₁ helices for class II molecules.

The Vα domain is critical in setting up these orientations, facilitating the readout of the peptide sequence. Thus, the CDR1 and CDR2 interactions of Vα are conserved[93] and provide the basic affinity of the TCR. The CDR3 loop is positioned to contact the peptide in the peptide-binding groove, while the Vβ interaction is more variable in the C-terminal half of the peptide. The contribution of the individual CDR loops to the interaction varies. CDR1β and CDR2β contribute little or nothing to the interaction, whereas the CDR3β loops are centrally located and usually dominate the interactions.[90] The contribution of the peptide to the interactions with the TCR varies, but usually two to five side chains of the peptide make direct contact with the TCR. These contact points, known as hot spots, are peptide residues that bulge out of the groove, which is more prominent and sometimes profound as in MHC class I.[94] In MHC class II interactions with the TCR, the peptide side chains are more uniformly dispersed and slightly deeper in the MHC binding groove.[94] In delineating the roles of V-region loops of the TCR, the CDR1 and CDR2 loops provide the basic affinity in the interaction, while CDR3 provides the specificity.[90] The residues of the peptide that protrude highest from the groove provide the basis for discrimination of peptide and for altering affinity or half-life of the TCR-pMHC interaction. An important insight from crystallographic studies is the role of water that fills the TCR-pMHC interface. Water molecules provide additional complementarity by filling the interface's cavities and mediate contact between TCR and pMHC.[95]

Overall, the consistent feature of the TCR-pMHC interaction is that the peptide contributes a smaller portion of the binding interface (21%-34%) and a smaller proportion of contacts (26%-47%) than MHC. The central positions of the peptide play a critical role and define the peptides as agonists, partial agonists, and antagonists.[96] The binding of TCR to the pMHC results in T-cell activation and usually there is a correlation among affinity, half-life, and function.[97] Mutational analysis of the role of the centrally located residues indicates that in some systems, biologic activity increases.[98] Yet, in others, the peptide is converted from an agonist to an antagonist[99]; nevertheless, the affinities of the pMHC for TCR change only marginally. Contacts on certain hot spots are very sensitive in changing the functional read-out but are not based on changes in the affinity of binding or half-life differences in TCR-pMHC complexes. It has been argued that affinities are measured in isolated TCR-pMHC complexes and true affinity measurement may require the presence of coreceptors and signaling components and need to be measured by cellular assays.[99]

The TCR is not alone in its interaction with the pMHC but is also associated with coreceptors such as CD4, CD8, and CD3 chains. The monomorphic CD3 γ, δ, ε, and ζ chains, together with the $\alpha\beta$ heterodimer, form the TCR complex. CD4 or CD8 act as assistants to the TCRs in helper and cytotoxic function, respectively. Therefore, they have been known as coreceptors.[100] Current evidence suggests that CD4 binds to the same MHC II as the TCR of the CD4+ T cell and similarly the CD8 binds to the same MHC I as the TCR of the CTL. The binding of the coreceptors occurs with another site of the MHC molecule than that involved in TCR binding. The TCR binds to the pMHC surface at an angle of 45° to 80° relative to the axis of the two α helices of MHC,[101] which excludes the possibility for direct association of the coreceptors with a TCR that binds the same pMHC. One possibility is that coreceptors could be linked with TCR in the cytoplasm through signaling molecules (i.e., ZAP70 and LCK).[102] Another is that the coreceptor associated with a TCR binds to a different pMHC to which a second TCR binds, forming a pseudodimer.[103]

CD8 is a dimer that includes either two α chains or one α chain and one β chain, whereas CD4 is a monomer with four Ig-like domains. Both CD8 chains consist of an Ig-like V domain and a long mucin-like stalk. The Ig-like domain binds to the $\alpha 3$ domain of MHC,[104] forming some hydrogen bonds with the α_2 domain and the $\beta_2 M$ chain away from the peptide interface. In CD4, only the fourth Ig-like domain binds to the pMHC. The ternary complex (TCR-pMHC-CD4/CD8) within the T-cell-APC interface of the immune synapse[105] has a V shape[106] (*Figure 13.3*). Although the CD8α stalk is longer than CD8β, it reaches only 50 to 60 Å, which is not long enough to traverse the distance of approximately 100 Å to the TCR-pMHC complex. As a result, the TCR-pMHC has to tilt for CD8 to reach the MHC. The stalk of CD8 is heavily glycosylated, and changes in glycosylation (which occur after T-cell activation) result in a decrease of binding to MHC.[107] The coreceptors enhance TCR signaling by strengthening the stability of the TCR-pMHC complex.[108] The V-shaped ternary complex accepts the coreceptors that bind to the same pMHC as the TCR,[106] while the CD3 proteins probably lie inside the V-shaped structure. Such an arrangement makes possible the association of signaling molecules such as ZAP-70, LCK, and SRC kinases with CD4 and CD8.

CD2 binds to CD58 (LFA-3) in humans based on electrostatic complementarity with the CD2 surface heavily populated by basic residues, whereas CD58 is acidic. The interactions span approximately 134 Å, very similar to that of the TCR-pMHC. Therefore, the CD2/CD58 interaction in the contact zone between T cell and the APC would facilitate the scanning of the pMHC by the TCR and lower the threshold for TCR triggering in vitro and T-cell activation in vivo.[109] CD28 and CTLA4 (CD152) are type I membrane proteins consisting of one moderately to heavily glycosylated V Ig-like domain and are expressed as disulfide-linked homodimers. Their counterreceptors B7-1 (CD80) and B7-2 (CD86) consist of two Ig-like domains, a membrane-proximal C-2 type and a membrane-distal V type. B7-2 binds CD28 more effectively than CTLA4 and enhances costimulatory effects when CD28 and CTLA4 are coexpressed. In contrast, B7-1 binds preferentially CTLA4, and its inhibitory effect would not be affected in the presence of CD28. Delayed expression of B7-1 on APCs appears to be timed to enhance the inhibitory function of CTLA4. During an immune response the CD28/B7-2-activating complexes are 10,000-fold less stable than the inhibitory complexes formed later by CTLA4/B7-1.[110]

The Signal Transduction Component of the TCR

TCR-$\alpha\beta$ is accompanied by five other polypeptide chains, collectively known as the CD3 accessory proteins: γ, δ, ε, ζ, and η. They form

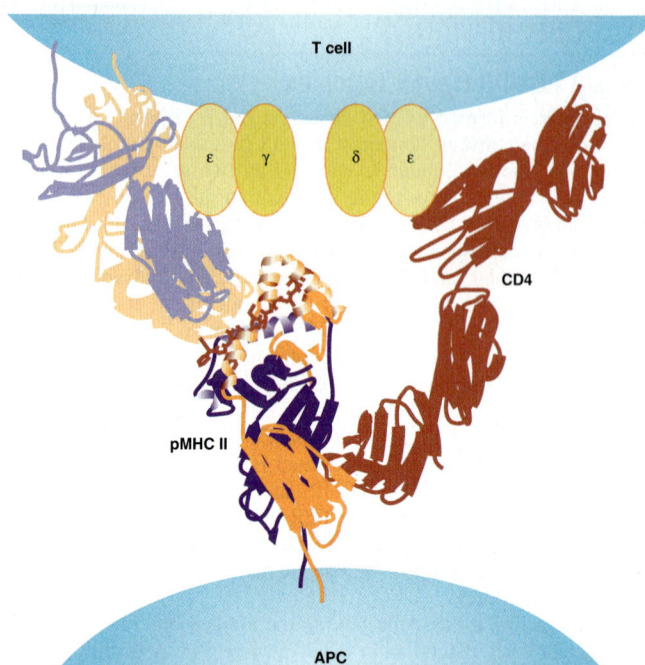

FIGURE 13.3 T-cell receptor (TCR)-major histocompatibility complex (MHC) coreceptor interaction. The CD4 and CD8 are coreceptors of the TCR (i.e., "assistants" in the interaction of the TCR with the peptide-MHC complex [pMHC]). In this function, the N-terminal domain of CD4 (D1) makes contact with the α_2 and β_2 domains of MHC II. In the CD8, the CD8α subunit of the CD8$\alpha\beta$ heterodimer contributes the binding energy, interacting with both the α_2 and α_3 domains of pMHC I, and CD8β binds only to α_3. Therefore, both coreceptors recognize different sites of MHC from the TCR. The length of each receptor is not long enough to reach the MHC-binding site, traversing alongside the TCR-MHC complex. It is proposed that TCR-MHC complex has to tilt for the coreceptor to reach the MHC, forming a V-shaped ternary complex. The CD3 components of the TCR (γ, δ, ε) probably are located inside the V-shaped structure. APC, T-cell antigen-presenting cell. (Courtesy of Dr. G. F. Gao.)

disulfide-linked heterodimers, such as $\delta\varepsilon$ and $\gamma\varepsilon$ or $\zeta\zeta$[111] (*Figure 13.2*). The γ, δ, and ε proteins show a significant degree of similarity to one another and include an Ig-like domain similar to a C domain, with an intrachain disulfide bond. The extracellular region of ζ is composed of only nine amino acids and contains the only cysteine of the molecule, which forms the disulfide bond with another ζ or with an η chain. In the transmembrane region, the γ, δ, and ε proteins have negatively charged amino acids complementary to the positively charged amino acids of the transmembrane region of the TCR-$\alpha\beta$. The cytoplasmic regions of γ, δ, and ε chains are long, ranging from 40 to 80 amino acids, whereas ζ is longer with 113 amino acids. The η chain is a splice variant of the ζ chain and like a heterodimer with the ζ chain exists only in a small number of T-cells. CD3 proteins have a dual mission in the TCR: escorting the receptor to the cell membrane and mediating signals generated by the TCR-pMHC complex. The complex is assembled in the endoplasmic reticulum, transported to the Golgi apparatus, and transferred to the plasma membrane. The numbers of ζ chain are the rate-limiting step of synthesis of the TCR because it is synthesized at only 10% of the level of the other TCR complex and regulates the degradation of the vast majority of newly synthesized α, β, or CD3 components within 4 hours of their synthesis. The remaining nondegraded chains are long-lived and form complete TCR-CD3 complexes with a limiting role by ζ. The TCR-CD3 complex lacking ζ migrates through the endoplasmic reticulum and Golgi apparatus intact and is transported to the lysosomes where it is degraded. A lysosome-targeting motif has been identified in the δ and γ chains and consists of a dileucine-based motif (DKQTLL) and tyrosine-based motif in the carboxy-terminal region.[112]

In the completed complex, the TCR α chain pairs with CD3 δ and ε, and TCR β pairs with CD3 γ and ε. The ζ chain joins the TCR and the CD3 chains in the last stage of the assembly. Two TCR αβ heterodimers are associated with one each of γε and δε heterodimers and one ζζ homodimer. Signal transduction by the CD3 accessory proteins is based on ITAM domains located in the γ, δ, and ε proteins (one ITAM domain in each) or the ζ chain (three ITAM domains). An ITAM consists of two YXXY/L sequences separated by six to eight amino acids (Y = tyrosine, X = any amino acid, and L = leucine).[113] Phosphorylation of tyrosine allows the ITAM motifs to serve as binding sites for protein tyrosine kinases via their SH2 domain. An important protein tyrosine kinase in T-cell activation is ZAP70, which is recruited to the ITAM motifs of ζ. The multiplicity of ITAM motifs in the cytoplasmic tails of the CD3 proteins results in signal amplification and increases the sensitivity of the TCR to ligand stimulation. Triplication of a single ITAM motif significantly enhances Ca^{2+} mobilization, association with ZAP70, and transcriptional activity in the NFAT complex involved in *IL2* gene regulation.[114] Cross-linking of a single isolated ITAM results in approximately threefold induction in NFAT-regulated activity, and cross-linking of a triplicated motif results in an approximately eightfold increase in NFAT-regulated activity.

T-CELL ACTIVATION

Topology of Immune Recognition

The αβ-TCR recognizes short peptides (i.e., eight to ten amino acids) for class I-restricted TCRs or 13 to 25 amino acids for class II-restricted TCRs. However, approximately only nine amino acids contact the TCR. The peptide is embedded in a groove formed by the α_1-α_2 domains of MHC I or the α_1-β_1 domains of MHC II (*Figure 13.4*). Interaction of TCRs initiates signal transduction, leading to transcription of genes encoding cytokines in CD4+ T cells or assembling and mobilizing the machinery of CTLs needed to kill cells recognized as infected, malignant, or foreign. The crystal structure of the αβ-TCR has been solved including several of them in complex with their cognate pMHC.[91,92,95,115-117] Data support the docking model of the TCR-ligand interaction, in which the TCR approaches the peptide held by an MHC. In this model, the Vα domain of the TCR is closest to the N-terminal residues of the peptide, whereas the Vβ domain of the TCR is closest to the C-terminal end of the peptide. In this orientation, the TCR Vβ domain contacts the MHC I α_1 domain, while the TCR Vα domain interacts with the α_2 of MHC I. The TCR orientation relative to the long axis of the MHC platform varies between 45° and 80° (i.e., the angle formed between a line passing through the centers of the Vα and Vβ domains of the TCR and a second line defined by the peptide on the MHC platform).[118]

The peptides in all MHC I structures have their N- and C-termini anchored into two fixed pockets approximately 20 Å apart in the MHC I platform. Longer peptides usually bulge in the center. In MHC II, the peptides assume an extended conformation, and the middle portion is smooth and concaves away from the TCR. Residues 1 and 5 of the peptide (p-1, p-5) in MHC II point toward the TCR and are critical in TCR recognition. The coreceptors bind to the same pMHC ligand as the TCR, but coreceptor binding is independent of TCR binding and is severalfold weaker.[119,120] The TCR, pMHC, and coreceptor form a ternary complex that assumes a V shape, with the pMHC II at the apex and the TCR and CD4 as the two arms. Overall, crystallography of TCR with pMHC suggests that MHC docking involves residues that are conserved within CDR1 and CDR2 of the TCR and provide a basal level of stabilizing energy in the formation of the complex.[121]

The Immune Synapse

TCR interactions with the pMHC take place in an intercellular junction between the T-cell and the APC. In this junction, signal 1 (TCR) and signal 2 (costimulation) are processed. This interface reveals a dramatic reorganization of signaling components, forming the immune synapse,[105] a term borrowed from Sherrington's turn-of-the-century definition of the interconnections of neurons as synapses.[122] In the absence of antigen, the T cell maintains its motility and continues to crawl around the APC and may even leave for another partner. Some receptors on the APC may convey a "danger signal" for the T cell to pay particular attention and explore the APC in search of antigen.[123]

The immune synapse (IS) relays information across the cell junction in both directions[124] and is organized into two major compartments. The central supramolecular activation cluster (cSMAC), enriched in TCRs and CD28, and the peripheral supramolecular activation cluster (pSMAC), which contains the LFA1 molecule and talin[125] (*Figure 13.5*). On the APC, the cSMAC contains the pMHC and CD80 (ligand for CD28), and the pSMAC contains ICAM-1 (counterreceptor for LFA1) and CD58, which is the ligand for CD2. The IS develops over a period of minutes after interactions of the T cell and the APC. The central area of the T cell closest to the APC includes the bulk of the TCRs, which are surrounded by integrins farther away.[125,126] The final arrangement defines the mature IS or the bull's-eye[125] (i.e., the cSMAC, a central area 1 to 3 μm in diameter that contains TCR, CD28, and C-2), surrounded by pSMAC, an adhesion ring that contains the LFA1 and talin. The formation of a mature IS with APCs (instead of artificial lipid bilayers) shows that TCR signaling precedes the completion of the mature IS.[127] Bull's-eye IS also has been observed with CTLs during recognition and killing of target cells.[128] Granule secretion occurs after microtubule-organizing center polarization in cSMAC where membrane fusion occurs followed by disruption and blebbing of the target cell membrane.[129]

The kinetics of the IS from its early beginnings are coordinated and organized by the cytoskeleton.[125] T-cell activation is accompanied by a dynamic reorganization of cortical actin with an increase of filamentous actin. These cytoskeletal changes are accompanied by progressive morphologic changes of the T cells, which become round and spread.[130] The TCR-pMHC can only interact at a distance of 15 nm, significantly below the thick glycocalyces of the 2 cells that separate their membranes by a 50- to 100-nm distance. Adhesion molecules, such as L-selectin, located on the tip of microvilli, may initiate the

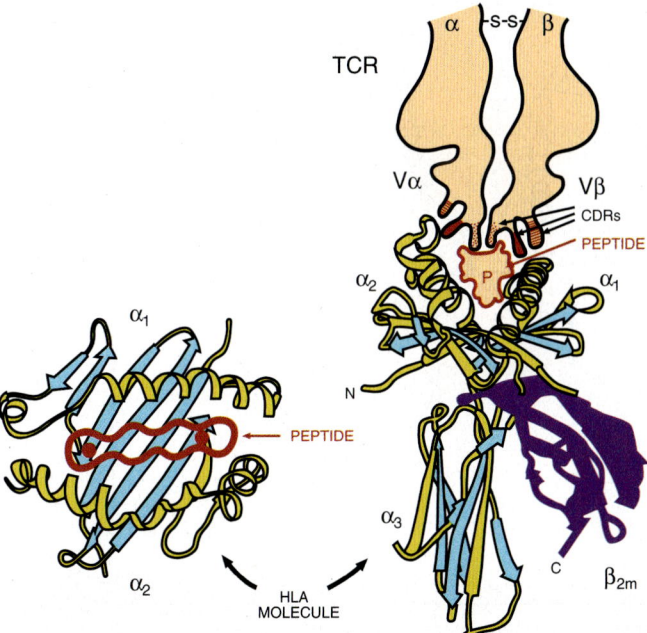

FIGURE 13.4 T-cell receptor (TCR) interaction with HLA-peptide complex. Crystallographic studies of the HLA class I molecule have shown that the two variable domains (α_1 and α_2) form a groove that binds the peptide that is released as a result of antigen processing. The peptide groove is formed by the helices of the α_1 and α_2 domains (A). Binding of the peptide is mediated through anchor amino acids near both ends of the peptide (in A). The TCR binds to both the major histocompatibility complex molecule and the peptide. The complementarity-determining region (CDR) 3 of both the α and β chains interacts with amino acids of the peptide, whereas the CDR1 and CDR2 interact with the major histocompatibility complex molecule (B). HLA, human leukocyte antigen.

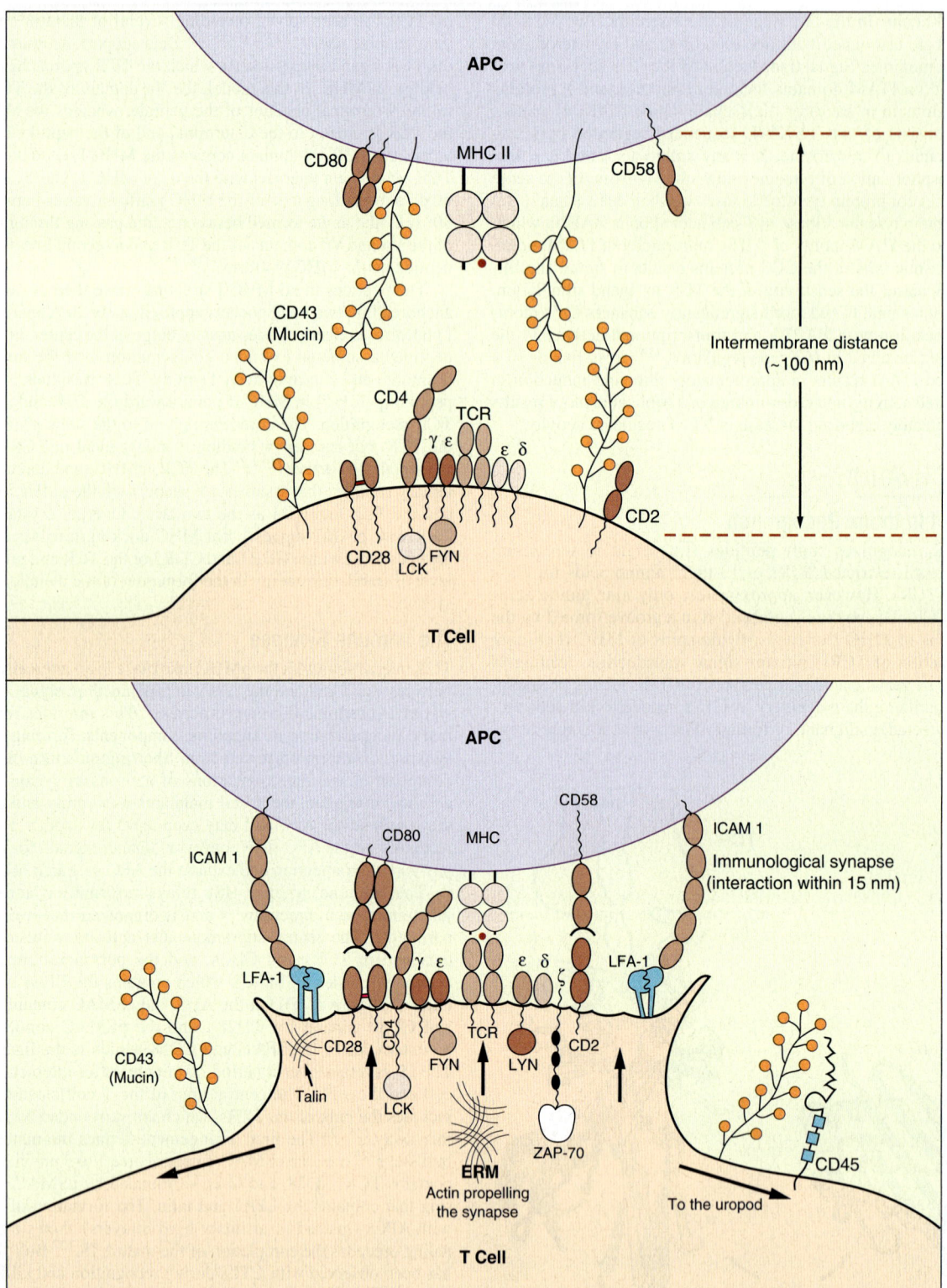

FIGURE 13.5 The structure of the immunologic synapse. The immunologic synapse is formed between T cell and an antigen-presenting cell (APC; in the case of the CD4+ T cell) or with a target cell (in the case of the CD81 T cell). Immunologic synapse formation is a multistep process. A thick glycocalyx on both cells, made predominantly from the mucin molecule CD43, comes in conflict with the approaching T cell and APC. This distance (50-100 nm) is too long for the T-cell receptor (TCR) peptide to interact with major histocompatibility complex (MHC), as the interaction occurs at 15 nm. The integrin lymphocyte function molecule (LFA)-1 and its counterreceptor, intercellular adhesion molecule (ICAM), which interact at 40 nm, may bring the cells for an initial contact. More importantly, chemokine signaling that activates heterotrimeric G proteins activates myosin II, and the cortical cytoskeleton collapses, disanchoring CD43 by the ERM (ezrin/radixin/moesin) adaptor proteins. With loss of the cell rigidity, a new F-actin network creates a pseudopod that propels the leading edge of the T cell toward the APC. This approach at an intercellular distance of 15 nm prevents CD43 reentry in the central area of T-cell-APC contact. Concomitantly, talin (a large cytoskeletal protein with attachment to integrins) maintains LFA-1 immobilized in a ring around the central part of the synapse. Although LFA-1/ICAM-1 interacts initially at a distance of 40 nm (extended LFA-1 form), after activation it assumes a bent form (high affinity) that brings the cell membranes closer ("ratchet"-like effect). Multiple other adhesion molecules of low affinity, such as between seen CD2 and CD58, contribute to the alignment of the 2 cell surfaces at a 15-nm distance, allowing the TCR to sample the small numbers of the peptide-MHC complex ("proofreading"). The final mature immunologic synapse ("bull's-eye") consists of a central supramolecular activation cluster and a peripheral integrin-rich zone. (From Dustin ML, Cooper JA. The immunological synapse and the actin cytoskeleton: molecular hardware for T-cell signaling. *Nat Immunol*. 2000;1:23-29; Delon J, Stelon S, Germain RN, et al. Imaging of T-cell interactions with antigen-presenting cells in culture and in intact lymphoid tissue. *Immunol Rev*. 2002;189:51–63.)

T-cell-APC interaction, until LFA1, lying on flat surfaces of the membrane, is released from its inhibitory state by activating signals delivered by chemokines. These signals also result in forming myosin II thick filaments, disrupting and pulling the thick network of polymerized actin away. In this clearing, new actin polymerization pushes forward new filopodia and lamellipodia (i.e., the cell becomes motile). Once the T cell is polarized, long interfering molecules of glycocalyx, such as CD43 and CD45, are pulled to the rear end, or uropod, of the cell. In the meantime, activated high-affinity LFA1 released from inhibition stabilizes the contact area between the cells, moving laterally and forming strong bonds with ICAM-1 across the cell junction.[131] In the membrane clearing created and stabilized by LFA1 adhesion, the TCRs sample the MHC on the APC surface for complementary peptides. Paradoxically, a large cluster of TCRs is pulled to the rear of the cell, but through the mediation of myosin II is brought to the front, reinforcing the frontal cluster.[132] TCR links with the cytoskeleton further stabilize the nascent IS. These links are mediated by some of the components of CD3 (i.e., ζ chain), which, through its phosphorylated ITAMs, induces actin polymerization.

The first stage of IS formation contact is antigen independent and mediated by CD28 on the T cell and CD80/CD-86 on the APC, which are more abundant (>10)[133] than the pMHC (approximately 100-200). The CD28 affinity for CD80 is at least two orders of magnitude above that determined for the TCR-pMHC. These interactions of CD28 preceding TCR are contrary to the original definition of the costimulatory function of CD28 believed to parallel or follow TCR signaling. The second stage of IS formation is antigen dependent, and the T cell extends large cytoplasmic, pulsatile protrusions toward the APC.[134,135] Tyrosine-phosphorylated Vav-1 and tyrosine-phosphorylated LCP2 (SLP76) assemble with the p21-activated kinase (PAK1) via the adaptor protein NCK1.[136-138] The T-cell-APC complex is stabilized in the third stage, which is regulated by increases of intracellular Ca^{2+}. By the end of the third phase, the supramolecular activation cluster is in place with all the receptors and signaling molecules held together with clusters of glycolipid-enriched membranes (ie, lipid rafts) on the surface and an elaborate cytoskeleton scaffolding underneath.

T-Cell Receptor Signaling

We organize TCR signaling into three phases: (1) initiation, (2) generation of phosphoinositides, and (3) the Ras pathway (*Figure 13.6*). Signaling is initiated by activation of LCK, which is regulated by two tyrosines: Tyr 394 in the activation loop and Tyr 505 in the C-terminus. LCK is kept inactive or "closed" by two intramolecular bonds. One is between Tyr 505, which is phosphorylated by the C-terminal SRC kinase, and the SH2 domain of LCK. The other bond is formed between the SH3 domain of LCK and a sequence connecting the SH2 and kinase domains. For activation of LCK, Tyr 505 needs to be dephosphorylated by CD45, a protein tyrosine phosphatase,[139] whereas Tyr 394 is autophosphorylated and activates the kinase domain. The large-sized CD45 isoforms are excluded from the IS,[140,141] but some move back to cSMAC adjacent to the TCRs.[142] LCK, recruited by CD4, is maintained in the activated state by CD28[143] and phosphorylates the ITAMs of the ζ chain of the TCR in a sequential and ordered manner, establishing thresholds of T-cell activation.[144] This mechanism determines whether a sufficient number of tyrosines are phosphorylated for full activation and supports the kinetic proofreading model of T-cell activation, which examines the relationship between kinetics of TCR-ligand interaction and intensities of T-cell activation.[145-148] ZAP70 is recruited to the phosphorylated ITAMs of the ζ chain and, in turn, activates the adaptor protein LAT. LAT has a short extracellular and long intracellular region and possesses a central position in T-cell activation because it assembles other adaptor molecules and signaling proteins.

There are two groups of adaptor proteins: transmembrane adaptor proteins and cytosolic adaptor proteins.[149] LAT (a transmembrane adaptor protein) is located in lipid rafts and is phosphorylated by ZAP70. As a result, it recruits PLCG1, phosphoinositide 3-kinase (PI3-K), IL-2-inducible T-cell kinase (ITK),

adaptor proteins GRB2 and GADS (GRAP2), and, indirectly, Vav and LCP2 (SLP76).[150-152] LCP2 is a cytosolic adaptor protein with three protein-binding motifs and plays an essential role in signaling pathways required for IL2 secretion.[153] It is expressed on thymocytes, T cells, mast cells, NK cells, and platelets. Through Gads, it binds indirectly to LAT after TCR ligation. Also, LAT and LCP2 function as mutually dependent intermolecular scaffolds that recruit crucial signaling regulators to sites of raft aggregation. In mice deficient in LCP2 (or LAT), thymocyte development is arrested at the stage where the TCR β chain is coupled to the pre-Tα chain. Also, LCP2 recruits ITK to lipid rafts and allows for optimal phosphorylation of PLCG1, which also associates with ZAP70.

Regulation of T-Cell Activation: Costimulation and Inhibition

T-cell activation depends on signals delivered by the TCR engaged with the pMHC. However, additional signaling is needed, and this function is known as costimulation. Costimulatory signals are delivered to the T cell through CD28, CTLA4, ICOS, 4-1BB, and/or OX40 proteins reacting with ligands (counterreceptors) on APCs. These receptors do not act independently but modify the responses mediated by TCRs.

The CD28 consists of one Ig-like domain of V-type, whereas the two ligands contain two Ig domains, one V type and the other C type. It has a short 41aa cytoplasmic tail that contains several signaling motifs, including YMNM and proline-rich PRRP and PYAP motifs. These signaling motifs provide docking sites for PI3K, GRB2, ITK, and LCK, which transduce signals downstream, resulting in activation and costimulatory functions. CD28 is constitutively expressed on T cells (all CD4+ and approximately 50% of CD8+). The TCR and CD28 have been found to be in close proximity within the cSMAC, and the YMNM and PYAP motifs are essential for IS formation. The central role of CD28 function is to stimulate cell cycle progression and prevent apoptosis. It also enhances the production of various cytokines, such as IL1, IL2, IL4, IL5, and interferon (IFN)-γ, and plays a fundamental role in Th1-Th2 differentiation. CD28/B7 interactions also play a critical role in B-cell stimulation. Another receptor, CTLA4 (CD152), shares approximately 30% identity with CD28; it is not detected in naïve T cells but is induced after T-cell activation. Both CD28 and CTLA4 share the same ligands. The importance of the CD28/B7 costimulation pathway was established with a mouse transplantation study in which blockade of the pathway by CTLA4-Ig prolonged cardiac graft survival and prevented the development of vascular lesions associated with chronic rejection.[154]

ICOS (inducible costimulator) is another costimulatory receptor homologous to CD28 and CTLA4. It is a disulfide-linked homodimer that lacks the extracellular motif present in CD28, which is implicated in binding with the B7 molecules. The ligand for ICOS (ICOS-L or B7h) is a B7-like molecule expressed constitutively on B cells and macrophages, and inducibly expressed on activated but not resting T cells. ICOS augments T-cell proliferative responses and cytokine secretion, particularly IL10.[155] Costimulation by ICOS promotes germinal center reaction and isotype switching. ICOS and CD28 regulate Th2 responses; whereas CD28 is critical in the priming stage to induce Th-2 differentiation, ICOS plays a role in regulating Th2 effector functions.[156] Furthermore, activation of the ICOS pathway of costimulation initiates acute and chronic graft rejection, which indicates that the ICOS costimulatory pathway also regulates Th1 responses.[157]

4-1BB is a tumor necrosis factor receptor (TNFR) superfamily member and is an important mediator of T-cell survival signaling, especially in CD8 T cells. The protein is transiently expressed early after antigen-induced activation. When costimulatory signals are abundant, 4-1BB is primarily involved in T cells survival by recruitment of TRAFs that result in NFκB and MAP kinase activation.[158] However, when other costimulatory signals are limited, 4-1BB can drive T-cell proliferation and effector function.

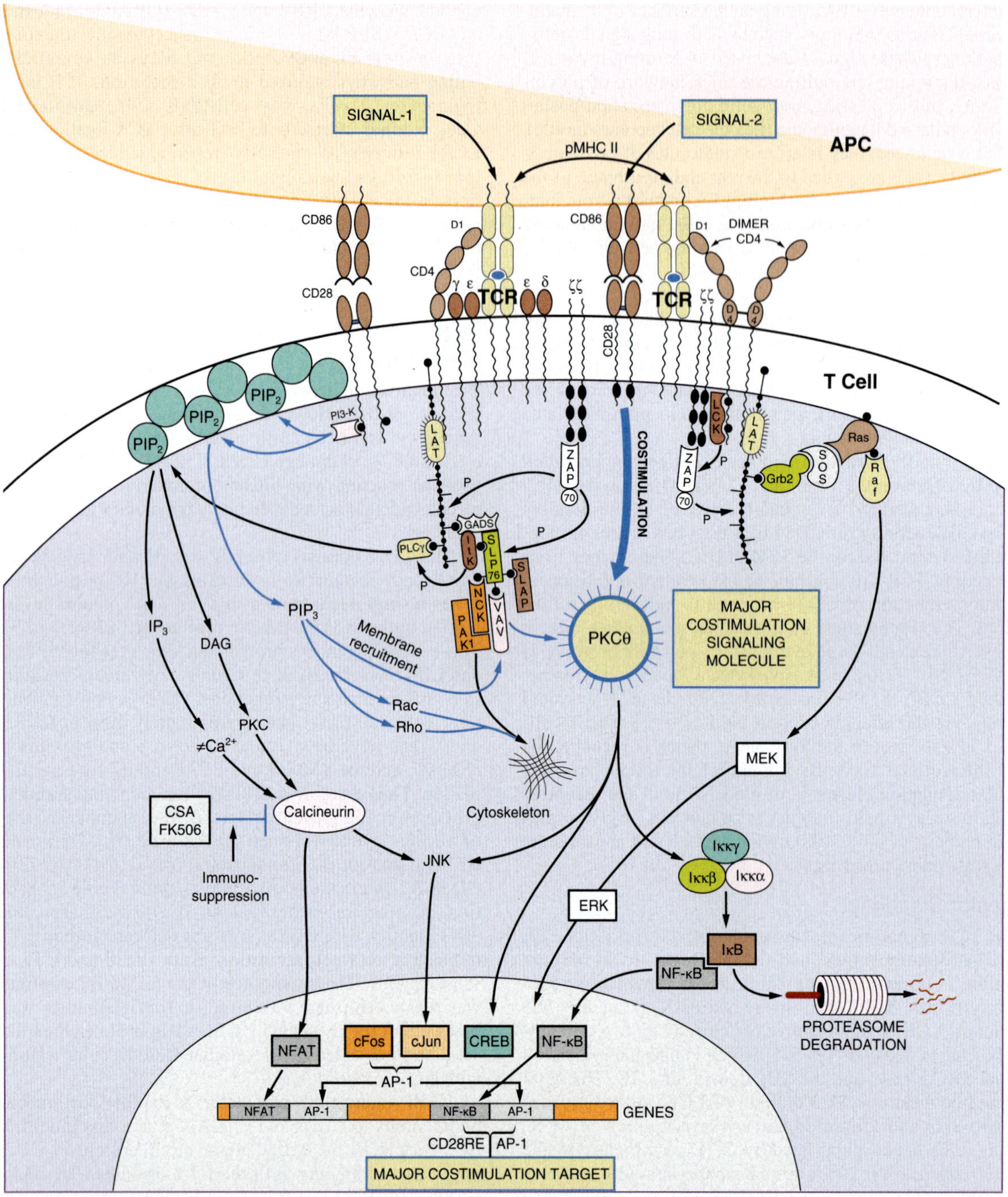

FIGURE 13.6 T-cell activation. T cells are activated by two signals: Signal 1 is delivered by the T-cell receptor (TCR) interacting with the peptide-major histocompatibility complex (pMHC), and signal 2, or costimulatory signal, by CD28 interacting with CD80/CD86. A number of adaptor proteins (i.e., proteins acting as scaffolding) assemble a supramolecular signaling complex. Foremost among them are LAT (linker for activated T cells) and SLP-76 (SH2 domain–containing leukocyte-specific phosphoprotein of 76 kDa). LAT expression is limited to T cells, natural killer (NK) cells, platelets, and mast cells and is not expressed on B cells or monocytes. LAT is a membrane adaptor protein as compared to SLP-76, which is cytoplasmic. Engagement of TCR activates Lck, which is associated with the coreceptor (CD4 or CD8). Lck phosphorylates ZAP-70 (ζ-chain-associated protein). ZAP-70 in turn phosphorylates LAT, which at this point makes the transition between proximal and downstream signaling events initiated by TCR. LAT is also associated with the coreceptor, competing in the binding with Lck. LAT and Lck are linked to individual coreceptors, rather than both of them being linked to the same molecule. LAT as an adaptor protein is a scaffolding that is associated with several downstream molecules: phospholipase (PLC)-γ generates phosphoinositides and increases Ca2+, which activates protein kinase C (PKC) and calcineurin, respectively. Another cluster is formed with Gads (Grb-related protein), SLP-76, Vav, and so forth that regulates the cytoskeleton together with the PIP3 product of phosphoinositide-3-kinase (PI3-K). The other signaling pathway linked to LAT is through the Ras activation, linking to the activation of MAPK/ERK kinase (MEK) and extracellular signal-regulated kinase (ERK). A central position in T-cell signaling is occupied by the novel PKC isoform, PKCθ, which is selectively expressed in T lymphocytes and is recruited to the immunologic synapse. It induces essential activation signals for interleukin-2 synthesis in cooperation with calcineurin. It is a master inducer of NF-κB activation and its translocation to the nucleus. PI3-K associated with CD28 generates PIP3 that recruits Vav and PKCθ to the membrane. APC, antigen-presenting cell; CREB, cyclic adenosine monophosphate response element–binding protein; DAG, diacylglycerol; NF-κB, nuclear factor-κB; NFAT, nuclear factor of activated T cells; PIP3, phosphatidylinositol (3, 4, 5)-triphosphate; SLAP, SRC-like adaptor protein. (Important information from Bosselut R, Zhang W, Ashe JM, et al. Association of the adaptor molecule LAT with CD4 and CD8 co-receptors identifies a new co-receptor function in T cell receptor signal transduction. *J Exp Med.* 1999;190:1517–1525; Myung PS, Boerthe NJ, Koretzky GA. Adapter proteins in lymphocyte antigen-receptor signaling. *Curr Opin Immunol.* 2000;12:256–266; Koretzky GA, Myzeng PS. Positive and negative regulation of T cell activation by adaptor proteins. *Nat Rev Immunol.* 2001;1:95–107; Cantrell DA. T-cell antigen receptor signal transduction. *Immunology.* 2002;105:369–374.)

CD4 T LYMPHOCYTES

Naïve CD4+ T cells can be further differentiated into different subsets upon activation (e.g., Th1, Th2, Th17, Th9, Th22, and Tregs), which are characterized by distinct cytokine profiles[159-164] (*Figure 13.7*). The generation of these effector T-cell subsets is driven primarily by the stimulatory cytokines present in the microenvironment during activation; these cytokines induce transcription factors that prime naïve precursor cells for differentiation.[165] In the classical Th1/Th2 balance disease induction model, the equilibrium between the T-helper subsets was considered the critical component for the pathogenesis of immune-mediated inflammatory conditions such as allergic diseases and autoimmune diseases.[166] More recently, the pathogenic T-helper population disease induction model proposes that it is a pathogenic subpopulation of T-helper cells that are the key component in immune-mediated inflammatory diseases.[167]

Th1 CD4+ T Cells

The most prominent factor for Th1 differentiation is IL-12. If an APC secretes IL-12, naïve CD4+ T cells differentiate into Th1 effectors. The major effector of IL-12 receptor signaling is the transcription factor STAT4, which promotes the expression of multiple Th1-cell genes, including the IFNγ gene.[168] IL-12 is an important Th1 driving cytokine, but not all Th1 responses require IL-12. For example, Th1 responses to certain viruses are not dependent on IL-12.[169,170] During the early Th1 polarizing signaling, the critical transcription factor for

Th1 development is T-bet.[168,171] The importance of T-bet in Th1 differentiation is underscored by the spontaneous development of asthma in T-bet-targeted deletion mice.[172] Th1 cells are crucial for host defense against intracellular pathogens including *Leishmania major*, *Mycobacterium tuberculosis*, and viruses.[169,170,173] IFN-γ-producing Th1 cells also are known to contribute to the pathogenicity of organ-specific autoimmune diseases including autoimmune type 1 diabetes and multiple sclerosis.[174,175] For instance, the pathogenic roles of Th1 cells have been well described in several mouse disease models, including experimental autoimmune encephalomyelitis (EAE), which is a mouse model of multiple sclerosis.[175] The adoptive transfer of Th1 cells was found to exacerbate EAE.[176] Moreover, the genetic abrogation of T-bet, which is a key transcription factor for Th1 cell differentiation, resulted in resistance to EAE.[177]

Th2 CD4+ T Cells

Innate cytokines IL-25, IL-33, and TSLP are critical for developing Th2 immune responses.[178] Th2 cells are characterized by the secretion of IL-4, IL-5, and IL-13, as well as IL-9 and IL-10.[179] The addition of exogenous IL-4 to in vitro cultures promotes Th2 differentiation. The key transcription factor for Th2 differentiation is GATA3, which is induced in the early stages of Th2 signaling.[180] In vitro Th2 differentiation depends on activation of the transcription factor STAT6, which sequentially enhances GATA3 expression.[181] GATA3 translocates to the nucleus, reorganizing the chromatin structure of the Th2-locus encompassing the IL-4, IL-5, and IL-13 genes.[181] In addition, GATA3

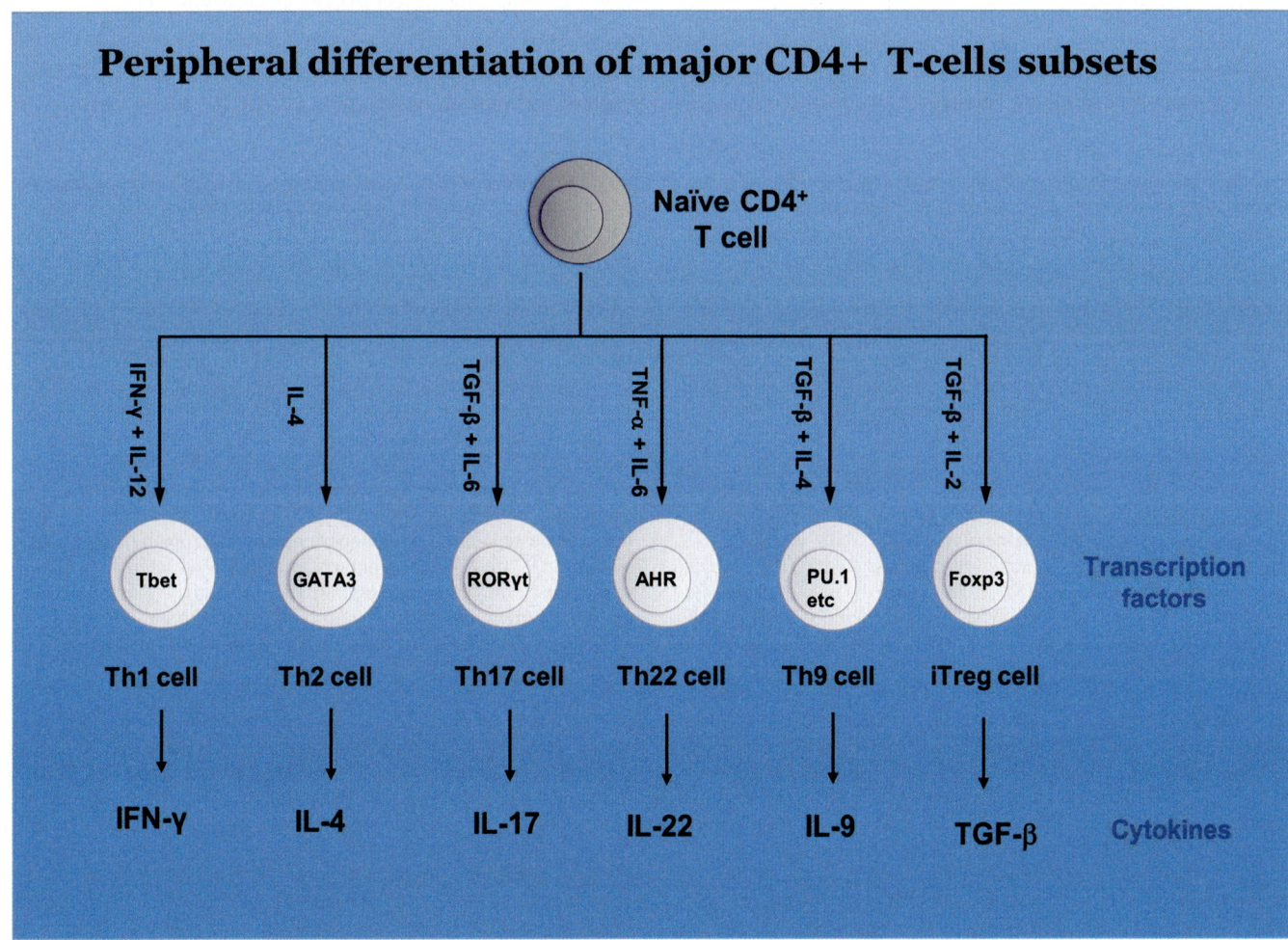

Peripheral differentiation of major CD4+ T-cells subsets

FIGURE 13.7 Differentiation of CD4+ T cells. Upon T-cell receptor (TCR) stimulation, naïve CD4+ T cells can differentiate into functionally distinct effector cell subsets depending on the specific inflammatory conditions present. This differentiation is driven by key transcriptional regulators, including Tbet for T_H1, GATA-binding protein 3 (GATA3) for T_H2 differentiation and RAR-related orphan receptor γ (RORγt) for T_H17 differentiation, aryl hydrocarbon receptor (AHR) for T_H22 cells, transcription factor PU.1 for T_H9, and forkhead box P3 (FoxP3) for iT_{reg} differentiation. IFN, interferon; TGF-β, transforming growth factor-β; TNF-α, tumor necrosis factor alpha; IL, interleukin.

opposes Th1 differentiation by inhibiting the expression of the IL-12 receptor β chain and STAT4.[181]

Th2 cells play an important role in host defense against multicellular parasites, allergies, and atopic diseases.[182-184] Th2 cells direct the killing of parasites in the tissues and expulse them from the intestine. Th2 cells stimulate the development of M2 macrophages and protect the host against damage mediated by these large extracellular parasites, which contribute to the rapid resolution of tissue damage in parasite infection.[183] Th2 cells involved in the allergy response contribute to a complex inflammatory response to stimulate and recruit specialized subsets of immune cells, such as eosinophils and basophils, to the site of infection or in response to allergens or toxins, leading to tissue eosinophilia and mast cell hyperplasia.[184] It results in mucus production, goblet cell metaplasia, and airway hyperresponsiveness. Th2 cells also regulate B cell class switching to IgE. Because they influence the production of antibodies and allergic responses, overactivation of Th2 plays a critical role in the pathogenesis of allergic response.[184] Th2 cells function in epithelial tissues, mainly in the intestinal tract and lungs, and are intimately regulated by innate and epithelial cell types that inhabit these tissues.[182] Th2 cells are also associated with the pathology of several different autoimmune diseases including systemic lupus erythematosus, experimental autoimmune myocarditis, and so on,[185] particularly those associated with humoral immune responses. Indeed, studies have demonstrated that aberrant and continued IL-4 expression in vivo can rescue autoreactive B cells from apoptosis, enhance their survival, and induce activation of autoreactive B cells and thereby promote autoimmune disease.[186]

Th17 CD4+ T Cells

IL-17-producing T cells were classified as a new distinct CD4 T-cell subset.[161,187] Th17 CD4+ T cells are a critical regulator of immunity and are commonly found in the intestine. In the periphery, particularly in the gut, where the production of IL-17 is important for the recruitment of other immune cells and the production of other factors to promote pathogen clearance.[188] Th17 cells are linked with the proinflammatory cytokine IL-23 because IL-23-deficient (p19⁻/⁻) mice contain very few Th17 cells.[189] A further study proved that IL-23 is involved in Th17-mediated immune pathology but is not required to differentiate Th17 from naïve CD4 T cells. Also, transforming growth factor β (TGF-β) and IL-6 have been identified as factors responsible for differentiation of Th17 from naïve T cells.[190] The development of autoimmune diseases such as multiple sclerosis, psoriasis, type I diabetes, primary Sjögren syndrome, asthma, and rheumatoid arthritis underscores the role of Th17-driven inflammation.[191-193]

Th22 CD4+ T Cells

Th22 cells are characterized by the CCR10+CCR6+CCR4+ immune phenotype and aryl hydrocarbon receptor as its key transcription factor. Th22 subsets can produce cytokines such as IL-22, IL-26, and IL-13, of which IL-22 is the most important functional cytokine.[194,195] Recent studies indicate that IL-6 and TNF-α, along with the help of plasmacytoid DCs, promote the Th22 phenotype.[195] IL-22 secretion by Th22 cells primarily affects epithelial and stromal cells rather than other hematopoietic cells, which lack a functional IL-22 receptor. Expression of the skin-homing receptors CCR4 and CCR10 on Th22 cells suggests that these cells can migrate to the skin, where they have a role in host defense against microbial pathogens and tissue repair or remodeling. Multiple studies indicate that Th22 cells may also be involved in the pathogenesis of inflammatory skin disorders such as psoriasis, atopic eczema, and allergic contact dermatitis.[196] IL-22 has a protective and regenerative effect on epithelial cells by multiple mechanisms.[197] In addition to the induction of antimicrobial peptides, IL-22 inhibits terminal differentiation of keratinocytes, induces the production of matrix metalloproteinases 1 and 3 linked to tissue degradation, and recruits neutrophils through the induction of chemokine production.[198]

Moreover, many studies found that Th22 cells are a critical component of protecting the mucosal barrier in human disease as well as in mouse models of colitis.[199-201] Basu et al. showed that the adoptive transfer of Th22 cells plays a protective role during adaptive phases of

a response in the intestinal mucosa.[199] Likewise, the adoptive transfer of IL-22-producing CD4+ T cell protects mice from inflammatory bowel disease (IBD).

Th9 CD4+ T Cells

The initial description of polarized IL-9-secreting Th cells was made from experiments with T cells cultured in the presence of IL-2, IL-4, and TGF-β.[202] Fully differentiated IL-4-producing Th2 cells cultured in the presence of TGF-β subsequently produce IL-9.[203] Th9 cell development requires integrating multiple signals, which are also involved in other Th subset development. The balance of cytokine signals is therefore critical for optimal IL-9 production and Th9 cell development. Several transcription factors, including PU.1, STAT, IRF1, IRF4, NF-κB, Bcl6, and the Smad/Notch complex, have been reported to be involved in Th9 differentiation. They directly interact with the Il9 gene promoter to increase IL-9 production.[204]

Th9 cells have protective or pathological functions in immune-mediated diseases, such as allergic diseases, autoimmune diseases, infection, and antitumor immunity.[204] Th9 cell-derived IL-9 exacerbates immune responses by enhancing antibody production and increasing immune cell infiltration and activity within the respiratory tract. Th9 cells can impair the tissue repair processes, increase intestinal permeability, and enhance pro-inflammatory Th-cell responses. Underlying mechanisms show Th9 cells can increase lymphocyte infiltration into the tumor and enhance the antitumor activity of mast cells. Furthermore, Th9 cell-derived IL-21 can limit tumor growth by stimulating antitumor activity of lymphocytes, and Th9 cell-derived IL-3 promotes DC survival, potentially enhancing the antitumor adaptive immune responses.[203,204]

Regulatory T Cells

Tregs constitute about 5% to 10% of peripheral CD4+ T cells and express the immune phenotype CD4+/CD25+ (the α chain of the IL2 receptor). They are CTLA4+ (costimulatory molecule cytotoxic T-lymphocyte antigen-4) and GITR+ (glucocorticoid-induced TNFR family–related protein).[69] Differentiation of CD4+ Tregs is mediated by interactions of CD4+ thymocytes with stromal cells. Tregs are enriched in autoreactive cells[205] but are resistant to deletion by NS, as compared to conventional CD4+ thymocytes.[206] The TCR of Tregs is of relatively high affinity for autoantigens, which facilitates their reactivation in the periphery by self-antigens. However, their affinity is still below the level required to trigger NS. These fundamental differences between the TCRs of Tregs and other thymocytes, in terms of specificity (MHC II vs. peripheral tissue antigens), affinity, and the nature of the selecting cell, provide an additional protection mechanism against autoimmunity and are a form of peripheral tolerance. The selection of Tregs is mediated by bone-marrow-derived APCs,[207] and their development and function depend on the transcription factor FOXP3.[208] Mutations of the human gene *FOXP3* lead to immune dysregulation polyendocrinopathy enteropathy and X-linked syndrome,[209] an X-linked immunodeficiency associated with autoimmunity involving endocrine organs; IBD; and atopic dermatitis. Once exiting the thymus, Tregs depend on DCs, which present them with autoantigens for their survival, preservation, and function.[210] In the periphery, CD4+/CD25+ Tregs may also arise from CD4+/CD25⁻ T cells upon stimulation of TCR and costimulation with TGF-β.[211]

Tregs play an essential role in maintaining host immune homeostasis. Treg-mediated suppression serves as a vital mechanism of negative regulation of immune-mediated inflammation and features prominently in autoimmune and autoinflammatory disorders, allergy, acute and chronic infections, cancer, and metabolic inflammation.[212,213] So far, at least four basic mechanisms have been described for Tregs to suppress immune responses: modulation of the maturation and function of APCs, the killing of target cells, disruption of metabolic pathways, and the production of anti-inflammatory cytokines.[214] Also, maintaining lineage stability is critical for Tregs to ensure tolerance and tissue homeostasis.[215] However, in some settings such as inflammation, Tregs display lineage plasticity and switch their cell fate to various effector T-cell types. Some Tregs can downregulate Foxp3 expression and/or acquire effector T-helper-cell–like phenotypes.[216]

Plasticity of CD4 T-Cell Subsets

The identification and naming of these CD4 T-cell subsets disguise that these populations are not all terminally differentiated cells and that the majority are plastic. The tissue microenvironment and immune responses can affect the differentiation and stability of CD4 T-cell subsets, but the exact mechanisms are unclear. Antigen-experienced T cells tend to be less flexible, and some are fully differentiated, but others can remain plastic and gain new cytokine-producing capabilities after antigen restimulation.[217] This is demonstrated by the fact that Th1 cell clones could be induced to secrete IL10, a hallmark cytokine of Th2 cells, after stimulation with IL12.[218] Central memory T cells, in particular, are able to acquire properties and functional abilities during the immune response. Th1 memory cells respond to IL4 by gaining IL4-producing capacities after TCR stimulation while maintaining their ability to produce IFNγ.[219] Th17 cells are also heterogeneous and secrete many effector cytokines in addition to IL17. These include IL4, IL9, and IL22, which are also produced by Th2, Th9, and Th22 cells, respectively. In chronic immune responses, Th17 cells can completely switch to IFNγ-producing Th1 cells.

CD8⁺ T LYMPHOCYTES

CTLs produce primarily type 1 cytokines because CTLs have no requirement for STAT4 signaling via IL12 to develop into Tc1 effectors. The Tc1/Tc2 regulation is mediated by TGF-β with IL4 promoting Tc1 development and cytotoxicity in the presence of TGF-β.[220] There is some cross-regulation between CD4⁺ T cells and CTLs. CTLs produce relatively high levels of IFN-γ and, as a result, enhance Th1 immunity. On the other hand, Th2-cell-derived IL4 stimulates the development of Tc2 cells in allergic states.

For the CTL to become an active effector, the precursor cell must be stimulated by the antigen to undergo proliferation and differentiation.[221] Activation results from the interaction of the naïve CTL with professional APCs. Granules are not always visible before activation, but the killing machinery (i.e., perforin, granzymes, and FasL) is delivered immediately upon priming.[222,223] The granule is 0.5 to 1.0 μm in diameter and is heterogeneous in structure.[224] The core is homogeneous, and sometimes it is surrounded by double membranes containing the perforin enclosed by a thin membrane.[225] Multiple small vesicles surround the core toward the periphery of the granule. Depending on the preponderance of these two components, granules have been distinguished as type I (dominated by the cores) or type II (with dominant multivesicular component but no cores), and other granules in terms of content are intermediate between types I and II. The granules are similar to late endosomes and have the properties of two usually separate organelles: those of the secretory type and those of lysosomes.[226] Similarities with lysosomes include the acidic pH, the mannose-6-phosphate receptor (MPR), and the lysosomal marker, lysosome-associated membrane protein. Endocytic components carrying CD3/TCR, CD8, and MHC molecules reach the perforin-containing granule and are displayed in the outer leaflet of the membrane.

The Role of Perforin

Perforin was the name given to a protein within the granules that perforate the cell membrane and opens pores, which were believed to be the cause of lysis and cell death. The C-terminal domain of perforin is the Ca^{2+}-binding site that initiates the insertion of the molecule into the cell membrane.[227] The insertion is mediated by exposure of several aspartate residues after cleavage of the C-terminus to yield a 60-kD active form. These residues are presumed to become approximated in three dimensions and bind Ca^{2+}, and the molecule becomes highly reactive for lipids from exposure to amphipathic domains. At 37 °C, perforin inserts into the membrane and approximately 20 perforin monomers form a tubular structure (16 nm wide) with a torus in the upper ring,[228] similar to that formed by the C9 component of complement. Purified perforin causes cell lysis but not the DNA fragmentation and condensation associated with apoptosis, a hallmark of target cell lysis by CTLs.[229] Target cell death requires the combined action of perforin and granule-associated granzymes. However, mice deficient in perforin suffer more serious consequences of lack of or diminished cytolytic functions[230] than mice deficient in granzymes A and B.[231] It has been assumed that granzymes enter passively through perforin pores (*Figure 13.8*). Large pores that allow passive diffusion of granzymes are formed only with large concentrations of perforin.

The Normal Hematologic System

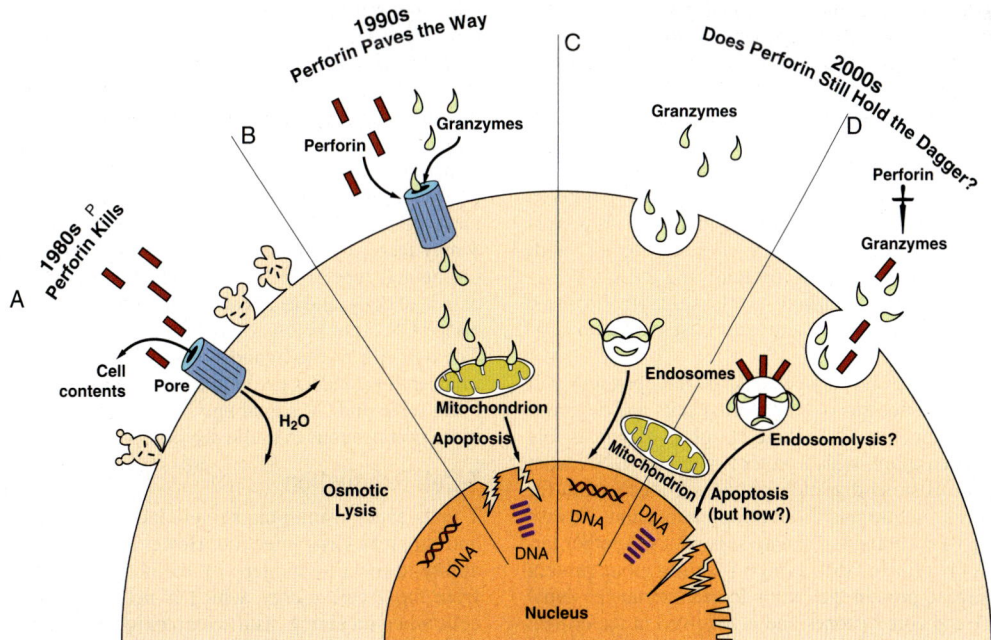

FIGURE 13.8 What is the role of perforin in cell lysis? The perforin lesion used to be considered the cause of cell death by osmotic lysis (as with complement) (A). When the granzymes were implicated in the cause of cell death by the apoptotic pathway, it was believed that the pores of perforin allow the entrance of the granzymes into the cell (B). Granzymes, however, can still enter the cell without perforin; however, by themselves, they cannot cause cell death (C). Because granzymes enter the cell by endocytosis and are within endocytic vesicles, it is argued that perforin is needed to release them in the cytosol by punching holes in the vesicles (endosomolytic mechanism; D). At this point, it is known that cytotoxic T lymphocytes kill their targets, and for this function, they need at least two of the contents of the granules: the granzymes and the perforin. The exact mechanism, however, is still strongly debated.

The pore size formed by small concentrations of perforin does not permit the diffusion of proteins larger than 8 kD. However, even under these conditions, granzymes (32-65 kD) have access to the cytosol, although not by direct diffusion through perforin pores.

The entrance of granzyme B into the cell at low perforin concentrations is suggested to occur probably due to endocytosis ("facilitated access" hypothesis). Perforin endocytosed together with granzyme disrupts the endocytic pathway and releases granzyme for delivery to the nucleus. Support for this interpretation comes from the observation that brefeldin, which interferes with the redistribution of proteins out of the endosomal system, inhibited the perforin-induced release of granzyme B, blocked its translocation to the nucleus, and inhibited cell death.[232] Granzyme B is therefore able to enter the interior of the cell autonomously in the absence of perforin. However, apoptotic death does not occur, unless perforin is present.[233] Endocytosis follows the binding to the receptor, and granzyme B is detected first within Rab5-positive endocytic vesicles and subsequently in Rab5-negative endocytic compartments.[234] Granzyme B is released to the cytoplasm by a second signal provided by perforin. From the cytoplasm, granzyme B reaches the nucleus, initiating the apoptotic pathway. The localization in the nucleus occurs before the nuclear events of apoptosis, suggesting that nuclear translocation of granzyme B transmits an apoptotic signal.[235]

The Role of Granzymes

At least four granzymes are present ubiquitously in human cytotoxic cells (i.e., A, G, H, and K). After synthesis, the granzymes undergo posttranslational modifications and, as a result, assume an active conformation. First, the signal peptide is removed, and subsequently, they are glycosylated and then sorted by MPR in the Golgi apparatus on the way to the granules.[236] Granzyme B is a serine protease and is the only granzyme with the preference for proteolytic cleavage of aspartate residues. In this respect, it has a specificity similar to caspases and has an extended substrate specificity with nine amino acids contacting the substrate.[237] Cleavage of target cell caspases results in the activation of the cellular apoptotic cascade. Granzyme B activates apoptosis by two distinct pathways: that is, by directly cleaving its substrates, caspase 3 or caspase 8,[238] or by a caspase-independent pathway through mitochondria. Mitochondrial factors enhance extramitochondrial caspase activation and play a central role in the execution of apoptosis, involving disruption of electron transport, energy metabolism, production of reactive oxygen radicals, and the release of apoptotic proteins, such as cytochrome-c.[239,240]

BCL2 can rescue cells from granzyme-B-mediated cell death, specifically blocking mitochondrial membrane depolarization and inhibiting the release of cytochrome c and apoptosis-inducing factors into the cytosol.[241] The mitochondrial apoptotic pathway is triggered by direct cleavage of BID (BH-3 interacting domain)[242]; it results in the translocation of BID to mitochondria where it interacts with its receptors, BAX (BCL2-associated X protein) and BAK (BCL2-antagonist killer), triggering cytochrome-c release. Cytochrome c then activates the apoptosome, which activates caspase 9 and ultimately caspase 3.[243]

Granzyme A is a tryptase and induces caspase-independent cell death. It concentrates in the nucleus of the targeted cells and degrades histone H1 into small fragments.[244] Histone H1 plays a critical role in chromatin hypercondensation, which protects genomic DNA from endonuclease digestion. Histone digestion provides a mechanism for unfolding compacted chromatin and facilitating endogenous DNase access to DNA during T-cell-granule–mediated apoptosis. Another target for granzyme A is the protein HMG2 (high-mobility group protein 2). HMG2 is a nonhistone protein that binds to the internucleosomal linker region of DNA and core histones and is involved in the critical steps of DNA replication and transcription. It binds preferentially to distorted DNA and unwinds damaged DNA for its repair. It facilitates the assembly of higher-order nucleoprotein structures by bending and looping DNA or by stabilizing underwound DNA. However, HMG2 is cleaved by granzyme A and thus opens up chromatin and blocks the de novo transcription required for cellular repair responses. Opening

up chromatin probably contributes to the observed synergy of granzyme A with granzyme B in the induction of oligonucleosomal DNA fragmentation during CTL lysis.[245] Both granzyme A and B directly cleave lamin B,[246] a member of the lamin family of proteins that maintain the integrity of the nuclear envelope. The entry of granzyme A into the nucleus requires the signal from perforin, and once inside the nucleus, it binds to insoluble factors because it does not leak out even after the nuclear membrane is permeabilized.[247]

Despite the wealth of information on the mechanism of this critical pathway, several areas are not well understood. Perforin has an indispensable role in the delivery of granzyme B, but certainly not simply as a pore-forming molecule. On the other hand, granzymes induce the nuclear changes affecting DNA (i.e., by apoptosis), but even if they enter the cell in the absence of perforin, they cannot be translocated to the nucleus without perforin.[248] The mechanism of granzyme delivery by perforin is not clear. It has been postulated that the intracellular delivery of granzymes is through an endosomolytic mechanism.[249] Translocation of a fluorescent probe from the target cell membrane to interior membranes, including the nuclear envelope and mitochondria, is supportive of this prediction.[250]

Homozygous loss-of-function defect in the human perforin gene is associated with several clinical manifestations, mainly due to uncontrolled T-cell and macrophage activation with overproduction of inflammatory cytokines. The syndrome is known as familial hemophagocytic lymphohistiocytosis (FHL).[251] The disease is mapped in chromosome 10q21-22 (i.e., the location of the perforin gene). Overall, the incidence of the mutation is approximately 20% in all FHL patients. For the development of FHL syndrome, a viral infection or a defect of an additional pathway that controls lymphocyte homeostasis is required. Mice deficient in granzyme B lose the ability to induce DNA fragmentation, even though perforin causes membrane damage. Deficiency of both granzymes A and B causes susceptibility to ectromelia infection,[252] although cytotoxic lymphocytes with the same deficiency and inability to cause DNA fragmentation can exert a potent antitumor effect.[253]

Death Receptor Pathway

Cytotoxic lymphocytes use two pathways for killing their targets: the exocytosis pathway (perforin-granzyme) and a death receptor pathway. Although multiple receptors on the cell surface can initiate an apoptotic cascade, they converge at one point downstream to a common final pathway. The point of confluence is the adaptor molecule FADD (fas-associated death domain). These alternate apoptotic pathways may be considered as the FADD pathway.[254] The pathways that converge to FADD are initiated by FAS (CD95), physiologically the most important receptor in the family of TNFRs. FADD binds and recruits caspase 8, which stands at the apex of the cascade of all caspases[255] and forms the DISC (death-inducing signaling complex).[256] Caspase 8 may target the mitochondria through BID or caspase 3, depending on the cell type.[257,258] In the FADD pathway, FASL is not stored in activated cells, and as a result, it requires the induction of a new ligand after TCR stimulation, which requires 1 to 2 hours after stimulation. The half-life of the ligand is long (2-3 hours), and the CTL can kill innocent bystanders (as long as they express the appropriate receptor, FAS) without TCR signaling.[259] In this respect, the FADD pathway is more promiscuous than the perforin pathway.

T-Cell Exhaustion

T cells execute immune surveillance to eliminate transformed cells and suppress virus infection. However, cognate T cells may lose their ability to react to antigens by the mechanism of exhaustion. Distinct from the T-cell anergy, which is defined as a tolerance status of T cells when receiving insufficient antigen activation and costimulation, T-cell exhaustion is a state of T-cell dysfunction that arises during repeated antigen stimulation. T-cell exhaustion was initially observed in mice chronically infected with the lymphocytic choriomeningitis virus (LCMV)[260] and subsequently reported in human chronic viral infections and cancer.[261] In the setting of T-cell exhaustion, decreased IL-2 production as well as high proliferative capacity happened in the

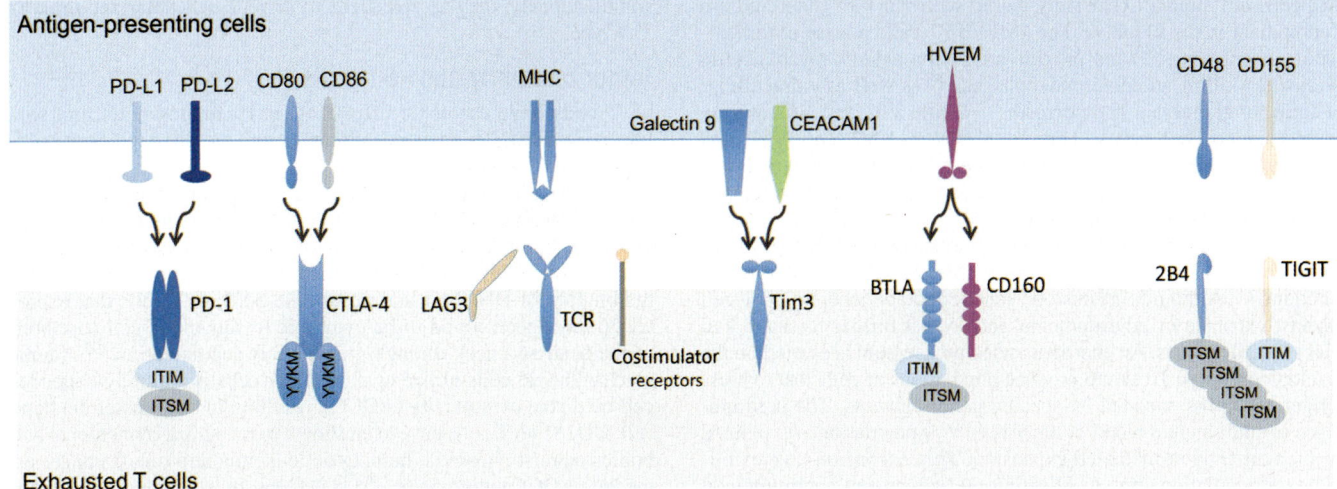

FIGURE 13.9 **Inhibitory receptors and their corresponding ligands.** Schematic overview of inhibitory and costimulatory receptors expressed by T cells interacting with their counterpart on antigen-presenting cells (APCs). Many inhibitory receptors have immunoreceptor tyrosine-based inhibitory motifs (ITIMs) and/or immunoreceptor tyrosine-based switch motifs (ITSMs) in their intracellular domains; however, some receptors have specific motifs, such as YVKM for cytotoxic T lymphocyte antigen 4 (CTLA4). BTLA, B and T lymphocyte attenuator; CEACAM1, carcinoembryonic antigen-related cell adhesion molecule 1; HVEM, herpes virus entry mediator; MHC, major histocompatibility complex; PD1, programmed cell death protein 1; PDL1, PD1 ligand 1; TCR, T-cell receptor; TIGIT, T-cell immunoreceptor with immunoglobulin and ITIM domains; Tim3, T-cell immunoglobulin and mucin domain–containing protein 3.

early stage, which is followed by defects in the production of IFNγ, TNF, and chemokines, as well as in degranulation. Characteristically, T-cell exhaustion is also accompanied by a progressive increase in the amount and diversity of inhibitory receptors that are expressed, including PD1 (programmed cell death protein 1), LAG3 (lymphocyte activation gene 3 protein), 2B4, BTLA (B and T lymphocyte associated), CD160, Tim3, and TIGIT (T cell immunoreceptor with immunoglobulin and ITIM domains) (*Figure 13.9*). Ultimately, if the severity or duration of the infection is high or prolonged, exhausted T cells can be programmed to death.[262]

The underlying mechanism contributing to T-cell exhaustion can be classified into three general categories[262]: (1) cell-to-cell signals including prolonged TCR engagement (signal 1) and costimulatory and/or coinhibitory signals (signal 2); (2) soluble factors such as excessive levels of inflammatory cytokines including type I interferons and suppressive cytokines IL-10 and TGF-β; (3) tissue and microenvironmental influences such as oxygen tension, pH, nutrient levels, and surrounding immune cells and stromal cells.

Higher and sustained expression of inhibitory receptors is a hallmark of exhausted T cells. Typically, the higher the number of inhibitory receptors coexpressed by exhausted T cells, the more severe the exhaustion. Indeed, coexpression of multiple inhibitory receptors is a cardinal feature. These coexpression patterns are mechanistically relevant, as simultaneous blockade of multiple inhibitory receptors results in synergistic reversal of T-cell exhaustion. This concept was demonstrated for PD1 and LAG3 in chronic LCMV infection[263] and for PD1 and CTLA4 in HIV infection[264] and cancer.[265] Several mechanisms by which inhibitory receptors might regulate T-cell function[262] are as follows: (1) by ectodomain competition: Inhibitory receptors sequester target receptors or ligands and/or prevent the optimal formation of microclusters and lipid rafts (e.g., CTLA4); (2) through modulation of intracellular mediators: It causes local and transient intracellular attenuation of positive signals from activating receptors such as the TCR and costimulatory receptors; and (3) through the induction of inhibitory genes: It has been known the intracellular domain of PD1 contains an immunoreceptor tyrosine-based inhibitory motif (ITIM) and an immunoreceptor tyrosine-based switch motif (ITSM). ITSM can transmit inhibitory signaling by recruiting the tyrosine-protein phosphatase SHP1 (also known as PTPN6) and/or SHP2 (also known as PTPN11). CTLA4 contains cytoplasmic YVKM motif, which, through binding to phosphatidylinositol 3-kinase, SHP-2, and the AP-1/AP-2 clathrin adaptor complexes, optimizes CTLA4 function (*Figure 13.9*).

Furthermore, some evidence also implicates PD1 signaling can modulate the expression of effector genes, such as *BATF*, which encodes the activator protein 1 (AP-1) family member basic leucine zipper transcription factor, ATF-like.

In addition to inhibitory receptors, it has become clear that costimulatory receptors are also involved in T-cell exhaustion.[266] The signaling adaptor TNFR-associated factor 1 (TRAF1) is downregulated in exhausted T cells in HIV progressors and chronic LCMV infection. Adoptive transfer of CTLs expressing TRAF1 effectively controls chronic LCMV infection compared with transfer of TRAF1-deficient CTLs. It indicates a crucial role for TRAF1-dependent costimulatory pathways in this setting.[267] It has also been possible to exploit the potential beneficial role of costimulation to reverse exhaustion by combining agonistic antibodies to positive costimulatory pathways with blockade of inhibitory pathways. 4-1BB is a TNFR family member and positive costimulatory molecule, which is expressed on activated T cells. Combining PD1 blockade and treatment with an agonistic antibody to 4-1BB dramatically improved exhausted T-cell function and viral control.[268]

γδ T CELLS

γδ T cells are innate-like T lymphocytes that have a TCR from rearranged γ and δ genes and account for between 1% and 20% of all circulating T cells.[269] These cells can quickly identify pathogens in an MHC-independent manner and act as a first line of defense for the immune system.[270] Initially, the γδ TCR repertoire is small, since it involves rearrangements of a small number of V segments so that the junctional diversity is limited. In human embryos between 8.5 and 15.0 weeks of gestation, the most common V fragments are Vδ2 joined to Dδ3 and Vγ1-8 or Vγ9 with Jγ1. These cells are referred to as the Vδ2 cells. Rearrangements after birth at approximately 4 to 6 months of age involve the joining of other γδ segments such as Vδ1 to Dδ1 and Dδ2, and the Vγ1 family with the Jγ2 cluster. Postnatally in the thymus, the Vδ2 subset represents 15% and the Vδ1 85% of the γδ cells, and these proportions remain relatively constant throughout adult life.

Vδ1 and Vδ2 cells are believed to represent separate lineages with different developmental pathways and tissue distribution.[271] Most of the γδ T cells with intraepithelial localization are Vδ1, whereas Vδ2 are detected in peripheral blood. Vδ1 T cells make up less than 30% of circulating γδ T cells and have a diversity of paired Vγ chains, while

Vδ2 cells are almost exclusively paired with the Vγ9 chain and are predominant in the blood.[272] The Vγ9/Vδ2 T cells release proinflammatory chemokines[273] and provide protection against mycobacteria by directly killing infected macrophages,[274] as well as extracellular bacteria by granulysin and perforin.[275] While Vδ1 and Vδ2 are the predominant γδ cell types, there are also Vδ3, Vδ4, Vδ6, Vδ7, and Vδ8 T cells that have been found in the peripheral blood of lymphoma patients; however, further study is required to determine their γ chain pairings and how they are activated.[276]

It has, however, been questioned whether two distinct γδ T-cell subsets exist or one V9V2 T-cell population exerts multiple effector functions.[277] Although intrinsic or genetic factors generate γδ T-cell subsets, extrinsic or environmental factors act further to shape and select specific clones. An enormous selective pressure is exerted on the development of γδ T cells to produce populations of cells that express antigen receptors encoded by specific gene segments. The predominance in adult human blood of the Vδ2 to Vγ9 population is explained by such an antigen-mediated expansion. This expansion creates oligoclonal populations due to selection pressures from environmental microbes and certain edible plants. In contrast to the Vγ2/Vδ2 (Vγ2 is the same as Vγ9) T cells, which are a major circulating population, the Vδ1 cells account for the vast majority of the γδ T cells in tissues such as intestine and spleen.[278]

γδ T-Cell Receptor: Structure and Antigen Recognition

Antigen recognition by the γδ TCR resembles recognition by antibodies.[279] The V and C domains are organized into "Ig folds" (approximately seven β strands packed face to face in two antiparallel β sheets, constrained by intradomain disulfide bonding). The V regions are subdivided into framework and hypervariable regions, which have three CDRs. The orientations of Vγ and Vδ are similar to the relative orientations between the V domains in the Fab Ig fragment or the αβ TCR. However, the CDR3 of Vδ is diverse in length and composition (8-21 amino acids), a range similar only to IGH (3-25). Furthermore, the CDR3 loops of the γδ TCR protrude above the rest of the molecule, creating clefts. These distinguish them from the equivalent loops of the αβ TCR, which are flat and bind to the pMHC, and from the antibodies that bind large proteins.[280]

The γδ TCR exists as a complex with CD3 polypeptides and recognizes antigens with a wide distribution, by a mechanism fundamentally different from that of αβ TCRs, since antigens are not processed and not MHC restricted.[279-282] Costimulation of Vγ9Vδ2 cells has been shown to occur through TLRs and NK receptors in combination with TCR stimulation.[283] Vγ9+ T cells respond to superantigens, such as staphylococcal enterotoxin A.[284] Some mucosal γδ T cells interact with MHC-encoded proteins, MICA and MICB,[285] through the NKG2D C-type lectin receptor.[286] MICA and MICB class I molecules identify stressed cells and have a very restricted pattern of expression primarily limited to the intestine. MICA and MICB do not present peptides because the peptide-binding groove is of limited size.[287] These molecules may function in innate immunity as important targets for Vδ1+ cells to eliminate stressed cells.[278] Unique to Vδ1 T cells is the ability to recognize the tumor-associated antigen B7-H6, allowing these cells to have antitumor effects.[288] Some Vδ1+ cells recognize the nonpolymorphic CD1c member of the CD1 family of molecules, expressed on APCs presenting lipid and glycolipid foreign antigens to T cells.[289] These γδ cells activated in response to CD1c produce IFN-γ and direct αβ T cells to Th1 differentiation. Furthermore, they are cytotoxic, express granulysin, and can lyse infected DCs via the perforin pathway and kill released bacteria by granulysin. Therefore, their role is significant in host defense before antigen-specific T cells have differentiated.[290]

Direct recognition of CD1c may represent a bridge between innate and adaptive immunity in a fashion similar to the recognition of CD1d by murine and human NK+ αβ T cells,[291] which polarize T cells to a Th2 phenotype. The CD1C-restricted γδ T cells promote the maturation of myeloid-derived DCs, which can present antigens to CD4+ T cells. This function of γδ T cells is important because they stimulate the rapid accumulation of mature DCs during microbial invasion[292];

simultaneously, they secrete IL12 to drive T-cell polarization to the Th1 type.

Tumor Immunity and γδ T Cells

γδ T cells have cytotoxic effects against hematopoietic and solid tumors in an MHC-independent manner and are not dependent on the expression of a particular antigen. One mechanism through which γδ T cells provide their antitumor effects is receptor-ligand interactions. NKG2D on Vγ9Vδ2 cells can bind to MICA/B on hematopoietic and epithelial tumor cells to induce cytotoxicity.[293] Vγ9Vδ2 T cells can also secrete IFNγ and kill hepatocellular carcinoma cells through the binding of DNAM-1 and nectin-like-5.[294] γδ T cells that express CD56 have been found to be cytotoxic to squamous cell carcinoma of the head and neck through granzyme B degranulation.[295] Another mechanism γδ cells utilize against tumor cells is antibody-dependent cell-mediated cytotoxicity (ADCC), resulting in the lysis of the tumor cell. CD16+ γδ T cells have been shown to recognize monoclonal antibodies against chronic lymphocytic leukemia and breast cancer and mediate ADCC cytotoxicity.[296] One recent study has suggested that γδ and αβ T cells could be activated together to fight tumor cells cooperatively. This was done using an antibody directed against butyrophilin family member BTN3A1 to redirect γδ T cells to attack tumor cells while also increasing the activity of tumor-specific αβ T cells.[297]

T-CELL ADOPTIVE TRANSFER FOR CANCER IMMUNOTHERAPY

T lymphocytes play an important role in tumor immunity as evidenced by a more favorable prognosis for patients with tumor-infiltrating T cells. These accomplishments reflect decades of work that translated findings of T-cell biology to patients. The earliest application of adoptive T-cell therapies for patients occurred in the laboratory of Dr. Steven Rosenberg at the National Cancer Institute.[298] They developed laboratory procedures to isolate and expand tumor-infiltrating lymphocytes (TILs) from patient's metastases with the rationale that they would be enriched for tumor-reactive T cells and could mediate antitumor responses.[299] Indeed, after a few months of expansion, they infused the TILs back into patients and reported complete responses in approximately 20% of patients with stage IV metastatic melanoma, an incurable solid tumor malignancy. However, the labor-intensive and lengthy TIL production limited the effort of Rosenberg and colleagues to adapt this technology to a broader number of patients. TILs also allowed the Rosenberg group to identify tumor-reactive TCRs that they used to create TCRαβ genetic constructs.[300] These TCR genetic constructs were used to genetically modify autologous T cells with a monoclonal antitumor TCR and infuse them back into patients. They again observed a complete remission (CR) rate of approximately 20% for patients with metastatic melanoma.

An important demonstration from these TCR gene therapy trials was that they could produce a bulk collection of tumor-reactive T cells within a few weeks vs. the few months required for TIL isolation and expansion. However, several disadvantages remained by using the TCR for tumor targeting. Two major disadvantages include MHC restriction, which precludes the use of a TCR in the majority of patients, and MHC class I downregulation, which is a mechanism of immune escape. A major advance in antitumor T-cell therapy was the development of the chimeric antigen receptor,[301] which is a hybrid protein that includes the intracellular signaling elements of the TCR, such as CD3ζ, paired to the antigen-binding domains of an antibody.[302,303] Since antigen recognition is MHC independent, it can be applied to all patients regardless of MHC haplotype. Transduction of T cells with chimeric antigen receptors (CARs) allows genetic retargeting of a bulk, polyclonal population of T cells to a monoclonal antitumor specificity in as short a time as 1 week.[304]

CARs are a type of adoptive cell therapy that has revolutionized the treatment paradigm of relapsed/refractory (R/R) hematologic malignancies. Based on the results of the pivotal ELIANA study, CD19-targeted CAR T cells for the treatment of R/R B acute lymphoblastic leukemia (B-ALL) were the first cell-based therapeutic approach approved by the US Food and Drug Administration (FDA) in 2017. In this study of pediatric and young adults with R/R B-ALL, 82% achieved CR.[305] Since then, there have been four more FDA approvals of CAR T products to treat hematologic malignancies. Axicabtagene ciloleucel, tisagenlecleucel, brexucabtagene autoleucel, and lisocabtagene maraleucel are approved for the treatment of R/R aggressive non-Hodgkin Lymphoma with CR rates of 58%, 40%, 53%, and 67%, respectively.[306-309] For patients with follicular lymphoma, axicabtagene ciloleucel was FDA approved based on the results of the Zuma 2 trial with a CR rate of 80% and an overall survival of 93% at 12 months.[310] The most recent approval that targets the B-cell maturation antigen has led to objective responses of 73% in patients with relapsed and/or refractory multiple myeloma, leading to the FDA approval of idecabtagene vicleucel (Ide-cel).[311]

While this unique immunotherapy has generated exciting responses, it has also generated a constellation of immune-related and novel toxicities. These include cytokine release syndrome (CRS) and neurologic toxicity. CRS is a widespread inflammatory disorder causing high-grade fevers, cardiovascular toxicities, and respiratory insufficiency, which is initiated by the en masse activation of CAR T cells, leading to a large release of cytokines.[312,313] Risk factors for CRS development include disease burden, underlying disease, pro-inflammatory tumor microenvironment, costimulatory domain, and lymphodepleting chemotherapy.[314] Treatment of mild CRS includes supportive care and management of constitutional symptoms. However, some patients develop severe CRS requiring escalation of care to include tocilizumab and steroids in addition to intensive care unit supportive measures.[315] Patients can also develop neurologic toxicities including seizures, aphasia, amnesia, and, in severe cases, cerebral edema. It is believed that these neurologic toxicities are related in part to the CAR T cells, since they have been identified in the cerebrospinal fluid of treated patients.[312,316] Similar to CRS, patients with mild neurotoxicity are managed with supportive care with corticosteroids reserved for patients with severe toxicity.[315]

In addition to CRS and neurotoxicity, patients can develop on-target off-tumor toxicity including B-cell aplasia and prolonged cytopenias which can lead to infectious complications. B-cell aplasia is related to the tissue distribution of CD19 expression.[317] CAR T cells kill all CD19+ cells, malignant and normal, so B-cell aplasia results in many patients, which is managed with antibiotics and/or gamma globulin.[315] Another challenge for CAR T-cell therapy is relapse due to antigen escape. In global CD19 CAR trial against B-ALL, 94% of relapses were from CD19− disease.[305] Despite the success of autologous CAR T cells, this approach has several disadvantages. Autologous CAR T cells require leukapheresis of every patient, which can delay treatment due to the manufacturing process as well as manufacturing failure in some patients. One way to address these issues is by using allogeneic "off-the-shelf" T cells manufactured from healthy donors. Disadvantages of allogeneic CAR T cells include the potential of developing graft-vs.-host disease and rapid elimination of the CAR T cells by the host immune system. Novel approaches to enhance allogeneic CAR T cells are currently being studied in ongoing clinical trials and include gene editing, γδ T cells, and NK cells.[318]

The clinical success of CAR T cells has served as the culmination of decades of work of optimizing and refining adoptive T-cell therapies. It has also stimulated significant commercial interest in other T-cell therapies with TILs and TCR gene therapies undergoing extensive clinical evaluation for many solid tumor malignancies. Considering the clinical efficacy of using checkpoint inhibitors to reverse T-cell exhaustion and induce antitumor responses has resulted in numerous approvals for solid tumor malignancies as well, the pantheon of modern oncology treatment that includes surgery, radiation, and chemotherapy now also includes T-cell therapies. As further insights into T-cell biology are developed, they will hopefully be applied again to adoptive T-cell therapies and to enhance antitumor efficacy and allow adaption to even more cancers.

References

1. Polliack A, Lampen N, Clarkson BD, et al. Identification of human B and T lymphocytes by scanning electron microscopy. *J Exp Med.* 1973;138(3):607-624.
2. Boehm T, Bleul CC, Schorpp M. Genetic dissection of thymus development in mouse and zebrafish. *Immunol Rev.* 2003;195:15-27.
3. Lind EF, Prockop SE, Porritt HE, Petrie HT. Mapping precursor movement through the postnatal thymus reveals specific microenvironments supporting defined stages of early lymphoid development. *J Exp Med.* 2001;194(2):127-134.
4. Derbinski J, Schulte A, Kyewski B, Klein L. Promiscuous gene expression in medullary thymic epithelial cells mirrors the peripheral self. *Nat Immunol.* 2001;2(11):1032-1039.
5. Ikuta K, Uchida N, Friedman J, Weissman IL. Lymphocyte development from stem cells. *Annu Rev Immunol.* 1992;10:759-783.
6. Liu C, Ueno T, Kuse S. The role of CCL21 in recruitment of T-precursor cells to fetal thymi. *Blood.* 2005;105(1):31-39.
7. Harman BC, Jenkinson EJ, Anderson G. Entry into the thymic microenvironment triggers Notch activation in the earliest migrant T cell progenitors. *J Immunol.* 2003;170(3):1299-1303.
8. Anderson G, Pongracz J, Parnell S, Jenkinson EJ. Notch ligand-bearing thymic epithelial cells initiate and sustain Notch signaling in thymocytes independently of T cell receptor signaling. *Eur J Immunol.* 2001;31(11):3349-3354.
9. Deftos ML, Bevan MJ. Notch signaling in T cell development. *Curr Opin Immunol.* 2000;12(2):166-172.
10. Allman D, Aster JC, Pear WS. Notch signaling in hematopoiesis and early lymphocyte development. *Immunol Rev.* 2002;187:75-86.
11. Allman D, Punt JA, Izon DJ, Aster JC, Pear WS. An invitation to T and more: notch signaling in lymphopoiesis. *Cell.* 2002;109(suppl):S1-S11.
12. Mumm JS, Kopan R. Notch signaling: from the outside in. *Dev Biol.* 2000;228(2):151-165.
13. Koch U, Lacombe TA, Holland D, et al. Subversion of the T/B lineage decision in the thymus by lunatic fringe-mediated inhibition of Notch-1. *Immunity.* 2001;15(2):225-236.
14. Milner LA, Bigas A. Notch as a mediator of cell fate determination in hematopoiesis: evidence and speculation. *Blood.* 1999;93(8):2431-2448.
15. Rebay I, Fleming RJ, Fehon RG, Cherbas L, Cherbas P, Artavanis-Tsakonas S. Specific EGF repeats of Notch mediate interactions with Delta and Serrate: implications for Notch as a multifunctional receptor. *Cell.* 1991;67(4):687-699.
16. Artavanis-Tsakonas S, Rand MD, Lake RJ. Notch signaling: cell fate control and signal integration in development. *Science.* 1999;284(5415):770-776.
17. Robey E, Regulation of T cell fate by Notch. *Annu Rev Immunol.* 1999;17:283-295.
18. Wilson A, MacDonald HR, Radtk F. Notch 1-deficient common lymphoid precursors adopt a B cell fate in the thymus. *J Exp Med.* 2001;194(7):1003-1012.
19. Rothenberg EV, Taghon T. Molecular genetics of T cell development. *Annu Rev Immunol.* 2005;23:601-649.
20. Carding SR, Hayday AC, Bottomly K. Cytokines in T-cell development. *Immunol Today.* 1991;12(7):239-245.
21. Peschon JJ, Morrissey PJ, Grabstein KH, et al. Early lymphocyte expansion is severely impaired in interleukin 7 receptor-deficient mice. *J Exp Med.* 1994;180(5):1955-1960.
22. Groh V, Fabbi M, Strominger JL. Maturation or differentiation of human thymocyte precursors in vitro? *Proc Natl Acad Sci U S A.* 1990;87(15):5973-5977.
23. Suda T, Zlotnik A. IL-7 maintains the T cell precursor potential of CD3-CD4-CD8- thymocytes. *J Immunol.* 1991;146(9):3068-3073.
24. Muegge K, Vila MP, Durum SK. Interleukin-7: a cofactor for V(D)J rearrangement of the T cell receptor beta gene. *Science.* 1993;261(5117):93-95.
25. Munitic I, Williams JA, Yang Y, et al. Dynamic regulation of IL-7 receptor expression is required for normal thymopoiesis. *Blood.* 2004;104(13):4165-4172.
26. Hemmers S, Schizas M, Azizi E, et al. IL-2 production by self-reactive CD4 thymocytes scales regulatory T cell generation in the thymus. *J Exp Med.* 2019;216(11):2466-2478.
27. Taghon T, Yui MA, Pant R, Diamond RA, Rothenberg EV. Developmental and molecular characterization of emerging beta- and gammadelta-selected pre-T cells in the adult mouse thymus. *Immunity.* 2006;24(1):53-64.
28. Vantourout P, Hayday A. Six-of-the-best: unique contributions of gammadelta T cells to immunology. *Nat Rev Immunol.* 2013;13(2):88-100.
29. Singer A, Bosselut R, Bhandoola A. Signals involved in CD4/CD8 lineage commitment: current concepts and potential mechanisms. *Semin Immunol.* 1999;11(4):273-281.
30. Germain RN. T-cell development and the CD4-CD8 lineage decision. *Nat Rev Immunol.* 2002;2(5):309-322.
31. Itano A, Salmon P, Kioussis D, Tolaini M, Corbella P, Robey E. The cytoplasmic domain of CD4 promotes the development of CD4 lineage T cells. *J Exp Med.* 1996;183(3):731-741.
32. Veillette A, Bookman MA, Horak EM, Bolen JB. The CD4 and CD8 T cell surface antigens are associated with the internal membrane tyrosine-protein kinase p56lck. *Cell.* 1988;55(2):301-308.
33. Wiest DL, Yuan L, Jefferson J, et al. Regulation of T cell receptor expression in immature CD4+CD8+ thymocytes by p56lck tyrosine kinase: basis for differential signaling by CD4 and CD8 in immature thymocytes expressing both coreceptor molecules. *J Exp Med.* 1993;178(5):1701-1712.
34. Yasutomo K, Doyle C, Miele L, Germain RN. The duration of antigen receptor signalling determines CD4+ versus CD8+ T-cell lineage fate. *Nature.* 2000;404(6777):506-510.

The Normal Hematologic System

35. Bosselut R, Feigenbaum L, Sharrow SO, Singer A. Strength of signaling by CD4 and CD8 coreceptor tails determines the number but not the lineage direction of positively selected thymocytes. *Immunity*. 2001;14(4):483-494.

36. Hernandez-Hoyos G, Sohn SJ, Rothenberg EV, Alberola-Ila J. Lck activity controls CD4/CD8 T cell lineage commitment. *Immunity*. 2000;12(3):313-322.

37. Sohn SJ, Forbush KA, Pan XC, Perlmutter RM. Activated p56lck directs maturation of both CD4 and CD8 single-positive thymocytes. *J Immunol*. 2001;166(4):2209-2217.

38. Basson MA, Bommhardt U, Mee PJ, Tybulewicz VLJ, Zamoyska R. Molecular requirements for lineage commitment in the thymus—antibody-mediated receptor engagements reveal a central role for lck in lineage decisions. *Immunol Rev*. 1998;165:181-194.

39. Cibotti R, Punt JA, Dash KS, Sharrow SO, Singer A. Surface molecules that drive T cell development in vitro in the absence of thymic epithelium and in the absence of lineage-specific signals. *Immunity*. 1997;6(3):245-255.

40. Chan S, Correia-Neves M, Benoist C, Mathis D. CD4/CD8 lineage commitment: matching fate with competence. *Immunol Rev*. 1998;165:195-207.

41. He X, Kappes DJ. CD4/CD8 lineage commitment: light at the end of the tunnel? *Curr Opin Immunol*. 2006;18(2):135-142.

42. He X, He X, Dave VP, et al. The zinc finger transcription factor Th-POK regulates CD4 versus CD8 T-cell lineage commitment. *Nature*. 2005;433(7028):826-833.

43. von Boehmer H, Teh HS, Kisielow P. The thymus selects the useful, neglects the useless and destroys the harmful. *Immunol Today*. 1989;10(2):57-61.

44. Bevan MJ. In thymic selection, peptide diversity gives and takes away. *Immunity*. 1997;7(2):175-178.

45. Amsen D, Kruisbeek AM. Thymocyte selection: not by TCR alone. *Immunol Rev*. 1998;165:209-229.

46. Anderson G, Hare KJ, Jenkinson EJ. Positive selection of thymocytes: the long and winding road. *Immunol Today*. 1999;20(10):463-468.

47. Jameson SC, Hogquist KA, Bevan MJ. Positive selection of thymocytes. *Annu Rev Immunol*. 1995;13:93-126.

48. Sprent J, Webb SR. Function and specificity of T cell subsets in the mouse. *Adv Immunol*. 1987;41:39-133.

49. Bommhardt U, Basson MA, Krummrei U, Zamoyska R. Activation of the extracellular signal-related kinase/mitogen-activated protein kinase pathway discriminates CD4 versus CD8 lineage commitment in the thymus. *J Immunol*. 1999;163(2):715-722.

50. Jameson SC, Bevan MJ. T-cell selection. *Curr Opin Immunol*. 1998;10(2):214-219.

51. Trobridge PA, Forbush KA, Levin SD. Positive and negative selection of thymocytes depends on Lck interaction with the CD4 and CD8 coreceptors. *J Immunol*. 2001;166(2):809-818.

52. Turner JM, Brodsky MH, Irving BA, Levin SD, Perlmutter RM, Littman DR. Interaction of the unique N-terminal region of tyrosine kinase p56lck with cytoplasmic domains of CD4 and CD8 is mediated by cysteine motifs. *Cell*. 1990;60(5):755-765.

53. Benoist C, Mathis D. Positive selection of the T cell repertoire: where and when does it occur? *Cell*. 1989;58(6):1027-1033.

54. Liu CP, Crawford F, Marrack P, Kappler J. T cell positive selection by a high density, low affinity ligand. *Proc Natl Acad Sci U S A*. 1998;95(8):4522-4526.

55. Barton GM, Beers C, deRoos P, et al. Positive selection of self-MHC-reactive T cells by individual peptide-MHC class II complexes. *Proc Natl Acad Sci U S A*. 2002;99(10):6937-6942.

56. Lee DS, Ahn C, Ernst B, Sprent J, Surh CD. Thymic selection by a single MHC/peptide ligand: autoreactive T cells are low-affinity cells. *Immunity*. 1999l;10(1):83-92.

57. Surh CD, Lee DS, Fung-Leung WP, Karlsson L, Sprent J. Thymic selection by a single MHC/peptide ligand produces a semidiverse repertoire of CD4+ T cells. *Immunity*. 1997;7(2):209-219.

58. Anderson G, Partington KM, Jenkinson EJ. Differential effects of peptide diversity and stromal cell type in positive and negative selection in the thymus. *J Immunol*. 1998;161(12):6599-6603.

59. Vacchio MS, Williams JA, Hodes RJ. A novel role for CD28 in thymic selection: elimination of CD28/B7 interactions increases positive selection. *Eur J Immunol*. 2005;35(2):418-427.

60. Derbinski J, Gäbler J, Brors B, et al. Promiscuous gene expression in thymic epithelial cells is regulated at multiple levels. *J Exp Med*. 2005;202(1):33-45.

61. Siggs OM, Makaroff LE, Liston A. The why and how of thymocyte negative selection. *Curr Opin Immunol*. 2006l;18(2):175-183.

62. Liston A, Lesage S, Gray DHD, Boyd RL, Goodnow CC. Genetic lesions in T-cell tolerance and thresholds for autoimmunity. *Immunol Rev*. 2005;204:87-101.

63. Kyewski B, Klein L. A central role for central tolerance. *Annu Rev Immunol*. 2006;24:571-606.

64. Pitkanen J, Peterson P. Autoimmune regulator: from loss of function to autoimmunity. *Genes Immun*. 2003;4(1):12-21.

65. Gotter J, Brors B, Hergenhahn M, Kyewski B. Medullary epithelial cells of the human thymus express a highly diverse selection of tissue-specific genes colocalized in chromosomal clusters. *J Exp Med*. 2004;199(2):155-166.

66. Vogel A, Strassburg CP, Obermayer-Straub P, Brabant G, Manns MP. The genetic background of autoimmune polyendocrinopathy-candidiasis-ectodermal dystrophy and its autoimmune disease components. *J Mol Med (Berl)*, 2002. 80(4):201-211.

67. von Boehmer H, Aifantis I, Gounari F, et al. Thymic selection revisited: how essential is it? *Immunol Rev*. 2003;191:62-78.

68. Starr TK, Jameson SC, Hogquist KA. Positive and negative selection of T cells. *Annu Rev Immunol*. 2003;21:139-176.

69. Sakaguchi S. Naturally arising CD4+ regulatory t cells for immunologic self-tolerance and negative control of immune responses. *Annu Rev Immunol*. 2004;22:531-562.

70. Liu YJ. A unified theory of central tolerance in the thymus. *Trends Immunol*. 2006;27(5):215-221.

71. Ribot J, Romagnoli P, van Meerwijk JP. Agonist ligands expressed by thymic epithelium enhance positive selection of regulatory T lymphocytes from precursors with a normally diverse TCR repertoire. *J Immunol* 2006;177(2):1101-1107.

72. van Oers NS, Killeen N, Weiss A. ZAP-70 is constitutively associated with tyrosine-phosphorylated TCR zeta in murine thymocytes and lymph node T cells. *Immunity*. 1994;1(8):675-685.

73. Negishi I, Motoyama N, Nakayama K, et al. Essential role for ZAP-70 in both positive and negative selection of thymocytes. *Nature*. 1995;376(6539):435-438.

74. Sosinowski T, Killeen N, Weiss A. The Src-like adaptor protein downregulates the T cell receptor on CD4+CD8+ thymocytes and regulates positive selection. *Immunity*. 2001;15(3):457-466.

75. Alberola-Ila J, Hernandez-Hoyos G. The Ras/MAPK cascade and the control of positive selection. *Immunol Rev*. 2003;191:79-96.

76. Page DM, Kane LP, Allison JP, Hedrick SM. Two signals are required for negative selection of CD4+CD8+ thymocytes. *J Immunol*. 1993;151(4):1868-1880.

77. Li R, Page DM. Requirement for a complex array of costimulators in the negative selection of autoreactive thymocytes in vivo. *J Immunol*. 2001;166(10): 6050-6056.

78. Dautigny N, Le Campion A, Lucas B. Timing and casting for actors of thymic negative selection. *J Immunol*. 1999;162(3):1294-1302.

79. Page DM. Cutting edge: thymic selection and autoreactivity are regulated by multiple coreceptors involved in T cell activation. *J Immunol*. 1999;163(7):3577-3581.

80. Kishimoto H, Sprent J. Several different cell surface molecules control negative selection of medullary thymocytes. *J Exp Med*. 1999;190(1):65-73.

81. McKean DJ, Huntoon CJ, Bell MP, et al., Maturation versus death of developing double-positive thymocytes reflects competing effects on Bcl-2 expression and can be regulated by the intensity of CD28 costimulation. *J Immunol*. 2001;166(5):3468-3475.

82. Wang CR, Hashimoto K, Kubo S, et al. T cell receptor-mediated signaling events in CD4+CD8+ thymocytes undergoing thymic selection: requirement of calcineurin activation for thymic positive selection but not negative selection. *J Exp Med*. 1995;181(3):927-941.

83. Urdahl KB, Pardoll DM, Jenkins MK. Cyclosporin A inhibits positive selection and delays negative selection in alpha beta TCR transgenic mice. *J Immunol*. 1994;152(6):2853-2859.

84. Kane LP, Hedrick SM. A role for calcium influx in setting the threshold for CD4+CD8+ thymocyte negative selection. *J Immunol*. 1996;156(12):4594-4601.

85. Zhou T, Cheng J, Yang P, et al. Inhibition of Nur77/Nurr1 leads to inefficient clonal deletion of self-reactive T cells. *J Exp Med*. 1996;183(4):1879-1892.

86. Fields BA, Mariuzza RA. Structure and function of the T-cell receptor: insights from X-ray crystallography. *Immunol Today*. 1996;17(7):330-336.

87. Madden DR. The three-dimensional structure of peptide-MHC complexes. *Annu Rev Immunol*. 1995;13:587-622.

88. Davis MM, Bjorkman PJ. T-cell antigen receptor genes and T-cell recognition. *Nature*. 1988;334(6181):395-402.

89. Bjorkman PJ, Saper MA, Samraoui B, Bennett WS, Strominger JL, Wiley DC. Structure of the human class I histocompatibility antigen, HLA-A2. *Nature*. 1987;329(6139):506-512.

90. Rudolph MG, Wilson IA. The specificity of TCR/pMHC interaction. *Curr Opin Immunol*. 2002;14(1):52-65.

91. Garboczi DN, Ghosh P, Utz U, Fan QR, Biddison WE, Wiley DC. Structure of the complex between human T-cell receptor, viral peptide and HLA-A2. *Nature*. 1996;384(6605):134-141.

92. Reinherz EL, Tan K, Tang L, et al. The crystal structure of a T cell receptor in complex with peptide and MHC class II. *Science*. 1999;286(5446):1913-1921.

93. Garcia KC, Teyton L, Wilson IA, Structural basis of T cell recognition. *Annu Rev Immunol*. 1999;17:369-397.

94. Speir JA, Stevens J, Joly E, Butcher GW, Wilson IA. Two different, highly exposed, bulged structures for an unusually long peptide bound to rat MHC class I RT1-Aa. *Immunity*. 2001;14(1):81-92.

95. Hennecke J, Carfi A, Wiley DC. Structure of a covalently stabilized complex of a human alphabeta T-cell receptor, influenza HA peptide and MHC class II molecule, HLA-DR1. *EMBO J*. 2000;19(21):5611-5624.

96. Sloan-Lancaster J, Allen PM. Altered peptide ligand-induced partial T cell activation: molecular mechanisms and role in T cell biology. *Annu Rev Immunol*. 1996;14:1-27.

97. Davis MM, Boniface JJ, Reich Z. Ligand recognition by alpha beta T cell receptors. *Annu Rev Immunol*. 1998;16:523-544.

98. Udaka K, Wiesmüller KH, Kienle S, Jung G, Walden P. Self-MHC-restricted peptides recognized by an alloreactive T lymphocyte clone. *J Immunol*. 1996;157(2):670-678.

99. Sykulev Y, Vugmeyster Y, Brunmark A, Ploegh HL, Eisen HN. Peptide antagonism and T cell receptor interactions with peptide-MHC complexes. *Immunity*. 1998;9(4):475-483.

100. Janeway CA Jr. The T cell receptor as a multicomponent signalling machine: CD4/CD8 coreceptors and CD45 in T cell activation. *Annu Rev Immunol*. 1992;10:645-674.

101. Hennecke J, Wiley DC. T cell receptor-MHC interactions up close. *Cell*. 2001;104(1):1-4.

102. Thome M, Germain V, Disanto JP, Acuto O. The p56lck SH2 domain mediates recruitment of CD8/p56lck to the activated T cell receptor/CD3/zeta complex. *Eur J Immunol*. 1996;26(9):2093-2100.

103. Irvine DJ, Purbhoo MA, Krogsgaard M, Davis MM. Direct observation of ligand recognition by T cells. *Nature*. 2002;419(6909):845-849.

104. Gao GF, Jakobsen BK. Molecular interactions of coreceptor CD8 and MHC class I: the molecular basis for functional coordination with the T-cell receptor. *Immunol Today*. 2000;21(12):630-636.

105. Maltais S, Côté S, Drolet G, Falardeau P. Cellular colocalization of dopamine D1 mRNA and D2 receptor in rat brain using a D2 dopamine receptor specific polyclonal antibody. *Prog Neuro-Psychopharmacol Biol Psychiatry*. 2000;24(7):1127-1149.

106. Gao GF, Rao Z, Bell JI. Molecular coordination of alphabeta T-cell receptors and coreceptors CD8 and CD4 in their recognition of peptide-MHC ligands. *Trends Immunol*. 2002;23(8):408-413.

107. Moody AM, Chui D, Reche PA, Priatel JJ, Marth JD, Reinherz EL. Developmentally regulated glycosylation of the CD8alphabeta coreceptor stalk modulates ligand binding. *Cell*. 2001;107(4):501-512.

108. van der Merwe PA, Davis SJ. Molecular interactions mediating T cell antigen recognition. *Annu Rev Immunol*. 2003;21:659-684.

109. Bachmann MF, Barner M, Kopf M. CD2 sets quantitative thresholds in T cell activation. *J Exp Med*. 1999;190(10):1383-1392.

110. Collins AV, Brodie DW, Gilbert RJC, et al. The interaction properties of costimulatory molecules revisited. *Immunity*. 2002;17(2):201-210.

111. Clevers H, Alarcon B, Wileman T, Terhorst C. The T cell receptor/CD3 complex: a dynamic protein ensemble. *Annu Rev Immunol*. 1988;6:629-662.

112. Letourneur F, Klausner RD. A novel di-leucine motif and a tyrosine-based motif independently mediate lysosomal targeting and endocytosis of CD3 chains. *Cell*. 1992;69(7):1143-1157.

113. Cambier JC. Antigen and Fc receptor signaling. The awesome power of the immunoreceptor tyrosine-based activation motif (ITAM). *J Immunol*. 1995;155(7):3281-3285.

114. Irving BA, Chan AC, Weiss A. Functional characterization of a signal transducing motif present in the T cell antigen receptor zeta chain. *J Exp Med*. 1993;177(4):1093-1103.

115. Garcia KC, Degano M, Stanfield RL. An alphabeta T cell receptor structure at 2.5 A and its orientation in the TCR-MHC complex. *Science*. 1996;274(5285):209-219.

116. Ding YH, Smith KJ, Garboczi DN, Utz U, Biddison WE, Wiley DC. Two human T cell receptors bind in a similar diagonal mode to the HLA-A2/Tax peptide complex using different TCR amino acids. *Immunity*. 1998;8(4):403-411.

117. Teng MK, Smolyar A, Tse AGD, et al. Identification of a common docking topology with substantial variation among different TCR-peptide-MHC complexes. *Curr Biol*. 1998;8(7):409-412.

118. Wang JH, Reinherz EL. Structural basis of T cell recognition of peptides bound to MHC molecules. *Mol Immunol*. 2002;38(14):1039-1049.

119. Xiong Y, Kern P, Chang HC, Reinherz EL. T cell receptor binding to a pMH-CII ligand is kinetically distinct from and independent of CD4. *J Biol Chem*. 2001;276(8):5659-5667.

120. Wyer JR, Willcox BE, Gao GF, et al. T cell receptor and coreceptor CD8 alphaalpha bind peptide-MHC independently and with distinct kinetics. *Immunity*. 1999;10(2):219-225.

121. Mazza G, Housset D, Piras C, et al. Glimpses at the recognition of peptide/MHC complexes by T-cell antigen receptors. *Immunol Rev*. 1998;163:187-196.

122. Sherrington CS. *The Integrative Action of the Nervous System*. 1906; Yale University Press.

123. Matzinger P. An innate sense of danger. *Semin Immunol*. 1998;10(5):399-415.

124. Bromley SK, Burack WR, Johnson KG, et al. The immunological synapse. *Annu Rev Immunol*. 2001;19:375-396.

125. Monks CR, Freiberg BA, Kupfer H, Sciaky N, Kupfer A. Three-dimensional segregation of supramolecular activation clusters in T cells. *Nature*. 1998;395(6697):82-86.

126. Grakoui A, Bromley SK, Sumen C, et al. The immunological synapse: a molecular machine controlling T cell activation. *Science*. 1999;285(5425):221-227.

127. Lee KH, Holdorf AD, Dustin ML, Chan AC, Allen PM, Shaw AS. T cell receptor signaling precedes immunological synapse formation. *Science*. 2002;295(5559):1539-1542.

128. Stinchcombe JC, Bossi G, Booth S, Griffiths GM. The immunological synapse of CTL contains a secretory domain and membrane bridges. *Immunity*. 2001;15(5):751-761.

129. Liepins A, Faanes RB, Lifter J, Choi YS, de Harven E. Ultrastructural changes during T-lymphocyte-mediated cytolysis. *Cell Immunol*. 1977;28(1):109-124.

130. Acuto O, Cantrell D. T cell activation and the cytoskeleton. *Annu Rev Immunol*. 2000;18:165-184.

131. Sedwick CE, Morgan MM, Jusino L, Cannon JL, Miller J, Burkhardt JK. TCR, LFA-1, and CD28 play unique and complementary roles in signaling T cell cytoskeletal reorganization. *J Immunol*. 1999;162(3):1367-1375.

132. Wulfing C, Davis MM. A receptor/cytoskeletal movement triggered by costimulation during T cell activation. *Science*. 1998;282(5397):2266-2269.

133. Meijer CJ, van der Loo EM, van Vloten WA, van der Velde EA, Scheffer E, Cornelisse CJ. Early diagnosis of mycosis fungoides and Sezary's syndrome by morphometric analysis of lymphoid cells in the skin. *Cancer*. 1980;45(11):2864-2871.

134. Donnadieu E, Bismuth G, Trautmann A. Antigen recognition by helper T cells elicits a sequence of distinct changes of their shape and intracellular calcium. *Curr Biol*. 1994;4(7):584-595.

135. Negulescu PA, Krasieva TB, Khan A, Kerschbaum HH, Cahalan MD. Polarity of T cell shape, motility, and sensitivity to antigen. *Immunity*. 1996;4(5):421-430.

136. Tuosto L, Michel F, Acuto O. p95vav associates with tyrosine-phosphorylated SLP-76 in antigen-stimulated T cells. *J Exp Med*. 1996;184(3):1161-1166.

137. Wu J, Motto DG, Koretzky GA, Weiss A. Vav and SLP-76 interact and functionally cooperate in IL-2 gene activation. *Immunity*. 1996;4(6):593-602.

138. Bubeck Wardenburg J, Pappu R, Bu JY, et al. Regulation of PAK activation and the T cell cytoskeleton by the linker protein SLP-76. *Immunity*. 1998;9(5):607-616.

139. Mustelin T, Coggeshall KM, Altman A. Rapid activation of the T-cell tyrosine protein kinase pp56lck by the CD45 phosphotyrosine phosphatase. *Proc Natl Acad Sci U S A*. 1989;86(16):6302-6306.

140. Anton van der Merwe P, Davis SJ, Shaw AS, Dustin ML. Cytoskeletal polarization and redistribution of cell-surface molecules during T cell antigen recognition. *Semin Immunol*. 2000;12(1):5-21.

141. Leupin O, Zaru R, Laroche T, Müller S, Valitutti S. Exclusion of CD45 from the T-cell receptor signaling area in antigen-stimulated T lymphocytes. *Curr Biol*. 2000;10(5):277-280.

142. Johnson KG, Bromley SK, Dustin ML, Thomas ML. A supramolecular basis for CD45 tyrosine phosphatase regulation in sustained T cell activation. *Proc Natl Acad Sci U S A*. 2000;97(18):10138-10143.

143. Holdorf AD, Lee KH, Burack WR, Allen PM, Shaw AS. Regulation of Lck activity by CD4 and CD28 in the immunological synapse. *Nat Immunol*. 2002;3(3):259-264.

144. Kersh EN, Shaw AS, Allen PM. Fidelity of T cell activation through multistep T cell receptor zeta phosphorylation. *Science*. 1998. 281(5376):572-575.

145. Kersh GJ, Allen PM. Essential flexibility in the T-cell recognition of antigen. *Nature*. 1996;380(6574):495-498.

146. McKeithan TW. Kinetic proofreading in T-cell receptor signal transduction. *Proc Natl Acad Sci U S A*. 1995;92(11):5042-5046.

147. Rabinowitz JD, Beeson C, Lyons DS, Davis MM, McConnell HM. Kinetic discrimination in T-cell activation. *Proc Natl Acad Sci U S A*. 1996;93(4):1401-1405.

148. Lanzavecchia A, Iezzi G, Viola A. From TCR engagement to T cell activation: a kinetic view of T cell behavior. *Cell*. 1999;96(1):1-4.

149. Leo O, Wienands J, Baier G, Horejsi V, Schraven B. Adapters in lymphocyte signaling. *J Clin Invest*. 2002;109(3):301-309.

150. Zhang W, Sloan-Lancaster J, Kitchen J, Trible RP, Samelson LE. LAT: the ZAP-70 tyrosine kinase substrate that links T cell receptor to cellular activation. *Cell*. 1998;92(1):83-92.

151. Samelson LE. Signal transduction mediated by the T cell antigen receptor: the role of adapter proteins. *Annu Rev Immunol*. 2002;20:371-394.

152. Sims TN, Dustin ML. The immunological synapse: integrins take the stage. *Immunol Rev*. 2002;186:100-117.

153. Koretzky GA, Myung PS. Positive and negative regulation of T-cell activation by adaptor proteins. *Nat Rev Immunol*. 2001;1(2):95-107.

154. Larsen CP, Elwood ET, Alexander DZ, et al., Long-term acceptance of skin and cardiac allografts after blocking CD40 and CD28 pathways. *Nature*. 1996;381(6581):434-438.

155. Carreno BM, Collins M. The B7 family of ligands and its receptors: new pathways for costimulation and inhibition of immune responses. *Annu Rev Immunol*. 2002;20:29-53.

156. Gonzalo JA, Tian J, Delaney T, et al. ICOS is critical for T helper cell-mediated lung mucosal inflammatory responses. *Nat Immunol*. 2001;2(7):597-604.

157. Ozkaynak E, Gao W, Shemmeri N, et al. Importance of ICOS-B7RP-1 costimulation in acute and chronic allograft rejection. *Nat Immunol*. 2001;2(7):591-596.

158. Jang IK, Lee ZH, Kim YJ, Kim SH, Kwon BS. Human 4-1BB (CD137) signals are mediated by TRAF2 and activate nuclear factor-kappa B. *Biochem Biophys Res Commun*. 1998;242(3):613-620.

159. Murphy KM, Reiner SL. The lineage decisions of helper T cells. *Nat Rev Immunol*. 2002;2(12):933-944.

160. Hori S, Nomura T, Sakaguchi S. Control of regulatory T cell development by the transcription factor Foxp3. *Science*. 2003;299(5609):1057-1061.

161. Harrington LE, Hatton RD, Mangan PR, et al. Interleukin 17-producing CD4+ effector T cells develop via a lineage distinct from the T helper type 1 and 2 lineages. *Nat Immunol*. 2005;6(11):1123-1132.

162. Kaplan MH. Th9 cells: differentiation and disease. *Immunol Rev*. 2013;252(1):104-115.

163. Soroosh P, Doherty TA. Th9 and allergic disease. *Immunology*. 2009;127(4):450-458.

164. Wolk K, Witte E, Witte K, Warszawska K, Sabat R. Biology of interleukin-22. *Semin Immunopathol*. 2010;32(1):17-31.

165. O'Shea JJ, Paul WE. Mechanisms underlying lineage commitment and plasticity of helper CD4+ T cells. *Science*. 2010;327(5969):1098-1102.

166. Mosmann TR, Coffman RL. TH1 and TH2 cells: different patterns of lymphokine secretion lead to different functional properties. *Annu Rev Immunol*. 1989;7:145-173.

167. Endo Y, Hirahara K, Yagi R, Tumes DJ, Nakayama T. Pathogenic memory type Th2 cells in allergic inflammation. *Trends Immunol*. 2014;35(2):69-78.

168. Mullen AC, High FA, Hutchins AS, et al. Role of T-bet in commitment of TH1 cells before IL-12-dependent selection. *Science*. 2001;292(5523):1907-1910.

169. Schijns VE, Haagmans BL, Wierda CM, et al. Mice lacking IL-12 develop polarized Th1 cells during viral infection. *J Immunol*. 1998;160(8):3958-3964.

170. Oxenius A, Karrer U, Zinkernagel RM, Hengartner H. IL-12 is not required for induction of type 1 cytokine responses in viral infections. *J Immunol*. 1999;162(2):965-973.

171. Afkarian M, Sedy JR, Yang J, et al. T-bet is a STAT1-induced regulator of IL-12R expression in naive CD4+ T cells. *Nat Immunol*. 2002;3(6):549-557.

172. Finotto S, Neurath MF, Glickman JN, et al. Development of spontaneous airway changes consistent with human asthma in mice lacking T-bet. *Science*. 2002;295(5553):336-338.

173. Reiner SL, Locksley RM. The regulation of immunity to Leishmania major. *Annu Rev Immunol*. 1995;13:151-177.

174. Christen U, von Herrath MG. Manipulating the type 1 vs type 2 balance in type 1 diabetes. *Immunol Res*. 2004;30(3):309-325.

175. Sospedra M, Martin R. Immunology of multiple sclerosis. *Annu Rev Immunol*. 2005;23:683-747.

The Normal Hematologic System

176. Ito A, Matejuk A, Hopke C, et al. Transfer of severe experimental autoimmune encephalomyelitis by IL-12- and IL-18-potentiated T cells is estrogen sensitive. *J Immunol*. 2003;170(9):4802-4809.

177. Bettelli E, Sullivan B, Szabo SJ, Sobel RA, Glimcher LH, Kuchroo VK. Loss of T-bet, but not STAT1, prevents the development of experimental autoimmune encephalomyelitis. *J Exp Med*. 2004;200(1):79-87.

178. Saenz SA, Taylor BC, Artis D. Welcome to the neighborhood: epithelial cell-derived cytokines license innate and adaptive immune responses at mucosal sites. *Immunol Rev*. 2008;226:172-190.

179. Vahedi G, CPoholek A, Hand TW, et al: Helper T-cell identity and evolution of differential transcriptomes and epigenomes. *Immunol Rev*. 2013;252(1):24-40.

180. Zheng W, Flavell RA. The transcription factor GATA-3 is necessary and sufficient for Th2 cytokine gene expression in CD4 T cells. *Cell*. 1997;89(4):587-596.

181. Ansel KM, Djuretic I, Tanasa B, Rao A. Regulation of Th2 differentiation and Il4 locus accessibility. *Annu Rev Immunol*. 2006;24:607-656.

182. Licona-Limon P, Kim LK, Palm NW, Flavell RA. TH2, allergy and group 2 innate lymphoid cells. *Nat Immunol*. 2013;14(6):536-542.

183. Allen JE, Sutherland TE. Host protective roles of type 2 immunity: parasite killing and tissue repair, flip sides of the same coin. *Semin Immunol*, 2014;26(4):329-340.

184. Wynn TA. Type 2 cytokines: mechanisms and therapeutic strategies. *Nat Rev Immunol*. 2015;15(5):271-282.

185. Raphael I, Nalawade S, Eagar TN, Forsthuber TG. T cell subsets and their signature cytokines in autoimmune and inflammatory diseases. *Cytokine*. 2015;74(1):5-17.

186. Illera VA, Perandones CE, Stunz LL, Mower DA, Ashman RF. Apoptosis in splenic B lymphocytes. Regulation by protein kinase C and IL-4. *J Immunol*. 1993;151(6):2965-2973.

187. Park H, Li Z, Yang XO, et al. A distinct lineage of CD4 T cells regulates tissue inflammation by producing interleukin 17. *Nat Immunol*. 2005;6(11):1133-1141.

188. Korn T, Bettelli E, Oukka M, Kuchroo VK. IL-17 and Th17 cells. *Annu Rev Immunol*. 2009;27:485-517.

189. Langrish CL, Chen Y, Blumenschein WM, et al. IL-23 drives a pathogenic T cell population that induces autoimmune inflammation. *J Exp Med*. 2005;201(2):233-240.

190. Veldhoen M, Hocking RJ, Atkins CJ, Locksley RM, Stockinger B. TGFbeta in the context of an inflammatory cytokine milieu supports de novo differentiation of IL-17-producing T cells. *Immunity*. 2006;24(2):179-189.

191. Alunno A, Carubbi F, Bartoloni E, et al. Unmasking the pathogenic role of IL-17 axis in primary Sjogren's syndrome: a new era for therapeutic targeting? *Autoimmun Rev*. 2014;13(12):1167-1173.

192. Luchtman DW, Ellwardt E, Larochelle C, Zipp F. IL-17 and related cytokines involved in the pathology and immunotherapy of multiple sclerosis: current and future developments. *Cytokine Growth Factor Rev*. 2014;25(4):403-413.

193. Singh RP, Hasan S, Sharma S, et al. Th17 cells in inflammation and autoimmunity. *Autoimmun Rev*. 2014;13(12):1174-1181.

194. Trifari S, Kaplan CD, Tran EH, Crellin NK, Spits H. Identification of a human helper T cell population that has abundant production of interleukin 22 and is distinct from T(H)-17, T(H)1 and T(H)2 cells. *Nat Immunol*. 2009;10(8):864-871.

195. Duhen T, Geiger R, Jarrossay D, Lanzavecchia A, Sallusto F. Production of interleukin 22 but not interleukin 17 by a subset of human skin-homing memory T cells. *Nat Immunol*. 2009;10(8):857-863.

196. Mirshafiey A, Simhag A, El Rouby NMM, Azizi G. T-helper 22 cells as a new player in chronic inflammatory skin disorders. *Int J Dermatol*. 2015;54(8):880-888.

197. Eyerich S, Eyerich K, Cavani A, Schmidt-Weber C. IL-17 and IL-22: siblings, not twins. *Trends Immunol*. 2010;31(9):354-361.

198. Wolk K, Witte E, Wallace E, et al. IL-22 regulates the expression of genes responsible for antimicrobial defense, cellular differentiation, and mobility in keratinocytes: a potential role in psoriasis. *Eur J Immunol*. 2006;36(5):1309-1323.

199. Basu R, O'Quinn DB, Silberger DJ, et al. Th22 cells are an important source of IL-22 for host protection against enteropathogenic bacteria. *Immunity*. 2012;37(6):1061-1075.

200. Leung JM, Davenport M, Wolff MJ, et al. IL-22-producing CD4+ cells are depleted in actively inflamed colitis tissue. *Mucosal Immunol*. 2014;7(1):124-133.

201. Broadhurst MJ, Leung JM, Kashyap V, et al. IL-22+ CD4+ T cells are associated with therapeutic trichuris trichiura infection in an ulcerative colitis patient. *Sci Transl Med*. 2010;2(60):60ra88.

202. Schmitt E, Germann T, Goedert S, et al. IL-9 production of naive CD4+ T cells depends on IL-2, is synergistically enhanced by a combination of TGF-beta and IL-4, and is inhibited by IFN-gamma. *J Immunol*.1994;153(9):3989-3996.

203. Kaplan MH, Hufford MM, Olson MR. The development and in vivo function of T helper 9 cells. *Nat Rev Immunol*. 2015;15(5):295-307.

204. Li Y, Yu Q, Zhang Z, et al. TH9 cell differentiation, transcriptional control and function in inflammation, autoimmune diseases and cancer. *Oncotarget*. 2016;7(43):71001-71012.

205. Romagnoli P, Hudrisier D, van Meerwijk JP. Preferential recognition of self antigens despite normal thymic deletion of CD4(+)CD25(+) regulatory T cells. *J Immunol*. 2002;168(4):1644-1648.

206. van Santen HM, Benoist C, Mathis D. Number of T reg cells that differentiate does not increase upon encounter of agonist ligand on thymic epithelial cells. *J Exp Med*. 2004;200(10):1221-1230.

207. Romagnoli P, Hudrisier D, van Meerwijk JP. Molecular signature of recent thymic selection events on effector and regulatory CD4+ T lymphocytes. *J Immunol*. 2005;175(9):5751-5758.

208. Brunkow ME, Jeffery EW, Hjerrild KA, et al. Disruption of a new forkhead/winged-helix protein, scurfin, results in the fatal lymphoproliferative disorder of the scurfy mouse. *Nat Genet*. 2001;27(1):68-73.

209. Chatila TA, Blaeser F, Ho N, et al. JM2, encoding a fork head-related protein, is mutated in X-linked autoimmunity-allergic disregulation syndrome. *J Clin Invest*. 2000;106(12):R75-R81.

210. Yamazaki S, Iyoda T, Tarbell K, et al. Direct expansion of functional CD25+ CD4+ regulatory T cells by antigen-processing dendritic cells. *J Exp Med*. 2003;198(2):235-247.

211. Zheng SG, Wang JH, Gray JD, Soucier H, Horwitz DA. Natural and induced CD4+CD25+ cells educate CD4+CD25– cells to develop suppressive activity: the role of IL-2, TGF-beta, and IL-10. *J Immunol*. 2004;172(9):5213-5221.

212. Sakaguchi S. Regulatory T cells: history and perspective. *Methods Mol Biol*. 2011;707:3-17.

213. Josefowicz SZ, Lu LF, Rudensky AY. Regulatory T cells: mechanisms of differentiation and function. *Annu Rev Immunol*. 2012;30:531-564.

214. Vignali DA, Collison LW, Workman CJ. How regulatory T cells work. *Nat Rev Immunol*. 2008;8(7):523-532.

215. Hori S. Lineage stability and phenotypic plasticity of Foxp3(+) regulatory T cells. *Immunol Rev*. 2014;259(1):159-172.

216. Zhou X, Bailey-Bucktrout S, Jeker LT, Bluestone JA. Plasticity of CD4(+) FoxP3(+) T cells. *Curr Opin Immunol*. 2009;21(3):281-285.

217. Sallusto F, Geginat J, Lanzavecchia A. Central memory and effector memory T cell subsets: function, generation, and maintenance. *Annu Rev Immunol*. 2004;22:745-763.

218. Gerosa F, Paganin C, Peritt D, et al. Interleukin-12 primes human CD4 and CD8 T cell clones for high production of both interferon-gamma and interleukin-10. *J Exp Med*. 1996;183(6):2559-2569.

219. Messi M, Giacchetto I, Nagata K, Lanzavecchia A, Natoli G, Sallusto F. Memory and flexibility of cytokine gene expression as separable properties of human T(H)1 and T(H)2 lymphocytes. *Nat Immunol*. 2003;4(1):78-86.

220. Erard F, Garcia-Sanz JA, Moriggl R, Wild MT. Presence or absence of TGF-beta determines IL-4-induced generation of type 1 or type 2 CD8 T cell subsets. *J Immunol*. 1999;162(1):209-214.

221. Mescher MF. Molecular interactions in the activation of effector and precursor cytotoxic T lymphocytes. *Immunol Rev*. 1995;146:177-210.

222. Bossi G, Griffiths GM. Degranulation plays an essential part in regulating cell surface expression of Fas ligand in T cells and natural killer cells. *Nat Med*. 1999;5(1):90-96.

223. Blott EJ, Bossi G, Clark R, Zvelebil M, Griffiths GM. Fas ligand is targeted to secretory lysosomes via a proline-rich domain in its cytoplasmic tail. *J Cell Sci*. 2001;114(pt 13):2405-2416.

224. Peters PJ, Borst J, Oorschot V, et al. Cytotoxic T lymphocyte granules are secretory lysosomes, containing both perforin and granzymes. *J Exp Med*. 1991;173(5):1099-1109.

225. Tschopp J, Nabholz M. Perforin-mediated target cell lysis by cytolytic T lymphocytes. *Annu Rev Immunol*. 1990;8:279-302.

226. Peters PJ, Geuze HJ, van der Donk HA, Borst J. A new model for lethal hit delivery by cytotoxic T lymphocytes. *Immunol Today*. 1990;11(1):28-32.

227. Uellner R, Zvelebil MJ, Hopkins J, et al. Perforin is activated by a proteolytic cleavage during biosynthesis which reveals a phospholipid-binding C2 domain. *EMBO J*. 1997;16(24):7287-7296.

228. Dourmashkin RR, Deteix P, Simone CB, Henkart P. Electron microscopic demonstration of lesions in target cell membranes associated with antibody-dependent cellular cytotoxicity. *Clin Exp Immunol*. 1980;42(3):554-560.

229. Duke RC, Persechini PM, Chang S, Liu CC, Cohen JJ, Young JD. Purified perforin induces target cell lysis but not DNA fragmentation. *J Exp Med*. 1989. 170(4):1451-1456.

230. Bhakdi S, Tranum-Jensen J. Alpha-toxin of *Staphylococcus aureus*. *Microbiol Rev*. 1991;55(4):733-751.

231. Ebnet K, Hausmann M, Lehmann-Grube F, et al. Granzyme A-deficient mice retain potent cell-mediated cytotoxicity. *EMBO J*. 1995;14(17):4230-4239.

232. Browne KA, Blink E, Sutton VR, Froelich CJ, Jans DA, Trapani JA. Cytosolic delivery of granzyme B by bacterial toxins: evidence that endosomal disruption, in addition to transmembrane pore formation, is an important function of perforin. *Mol Cell Biol*. 1999;19(12):8604-8615.

233. Shi L, Mai S, Israels S, Browne K, Trapani JA, Greenberg AH. Granzyme B (GraB) autonomously crosses the cell membrane and perforin initiates apoptosis and GraB nuclear localization. *J Exp Med*. 1997;185(5):855-866.

234. Pinkoski MJ, Hobman M, Heibein JA, et al. Entry and trafficking of granzyme B in target cells during granzyme B-perforin-mediated apoptosis. *Blood*. 1998;92(3):1044-1054.

235. Trapani JA, Jans P, Smyth MJ, et al. Perforin-dependent nuclear entry of granzyme B precedes apoptosis, and is not a consequence of nuclear membrane dysfunction. *Cell Death Differ*. 1998;5(6):488-496.

236. Griffiths GM. Protein sorting and secretion during CTL killing. *Semin Immunol*. 1997;9(2):109-115.

237. Darmon AJ, Nicholson DW, Bleackley RC. Activation of the apoptotic protease CPP32 by cytotoxic T-cell-derived granzyme B. *Nature*. 1995;377(6548):446-448.

238. Barry M, Bleackley RC. Cytotoxic T lymphocytes: all roads lead to death. *Nat Rev Immunol*. 2002;2(6):401-409.

239. Heibein JA, Barry M, Motyka B, Bleackley RC. Granzyme B-induced loss of mitochondrial inner membrane potential (Delta Psi m) and cytochrome c release are caspase independent. *J Immunol*. 1999;163(9):4683-4693.

240. MacDonald G, Shi L, Velde CV, Lieberman J, Greenberg AH. Mitochondria-dependent and -independent regulation of Granzyme B-induced apoptosis. *J Exp Med*. 1999;189(1):131-144.

241. Susin SA, Zamzami N, Castedo M, et al. Bcl-2 inhibits the mitochondrial release of an apoptogenic protease. *J Exp Med*. 1996;184(4):1331-1341.

242. Sutton VR, Davis JE, Cancilla M, et al. Initiation of apoptosis by granzyme B requires direct cleavage of bid, but not direct granzyme B-mediated caspase activation. *J Exp Med*. 2000;192(10):1403-1414.

243. Alimonti JB, Shi L, Baijal PK, Greenberg AH. Granzyme B induces BID-mediated cytochrome c release and mitochondrial permeability transition. *J Biol Chem.* 2001;276(10):6974-6982.

244. Zhang D, Pasternack MS, Beresford PJ, Wagner L, Greenberg AH, Lieberman J. Induction of rapid histone degradation by the cytotoxic T lymphocyte protease Granzyme A. *J Biol Chem.* 2001;276(5):3683-3690.

245. Fan Z, Beresford PJ, Zhang D, Lieberman J. HMG2 interacts with the nucleosome assembly protein SET and is a target of the cytotoxic T-lymphocyte protease granzyme A. *Mol Cell Biol.* 2002;22(8):2810-2820.

246. Zhang D, Beresford PJ, Greenberg AH, Lieberman J. Granzymes A and B directly cleave lamins and disrupt the nuclear lamina during granule-mediated cytolysis. *Proc Natl Acad Sci U S A.* 2001;98(10):5746-5751.

247. Jans DA, Briggs LJ, Jans P, et al. Nuclear targeting of the serine protease granzyme A (fragmentin-1). *J Cell Sci.* 1998;111 (pt 17):2645-2654.

248. Trapani JA, Smyth MJ. Functional significance of the perforin/granzyme cell death pathway. *Nat Rev Immunol.* 2002;2(10):735-747.

249. Froelich CJ, Dixit VM, Yang X. Lymphocyte granule-mediated apoptosis: matters of viral mimicry and deadly proteases. *Immunol Today.* 1998;19(1):30-36.

250. Kawasaki Y, Saito T, Shirota-Someya Y, et al. Cell death-associated translocation of plasma membrane components induced by CTL. *J Immunol.* 2000;164(9):4641-4648.

251. Stepp SE, Dufourcq-Lagelouse R, Deist FL, et al. Perforin gene defects in familial hemophagocytic lymphohistiocytosis. *Science.* 1999;286(5446):1957-1959.

252. Mullbacher A, Waring P, Tha Hla R, et al. Granzymes are the essential downstream effector molecules for the control of primary virus infections by cytolytic leukocytes. *Proc Natl Acad Sci U S A.* 1999;96(24):13950-13955.

253. Davis JE, Smyth MJ, Trapani JA. Granzyme A and B-deficient killer lymphocytes are defective in eliciting DNA fragmentation but retain potent in vivo anti-tumor capacity. *Eur J Immunol.* 2001;31(1):39-47.

254. Russell JH, Ley TJ. Lymphocyte-mediated cytotoxicity. *Annu Rev Immunol.* 2002;20:323-370.

255. Juo P, Kuo CJ, Yuan J, Blenis J. Essential requirement for caspase-8/FLICE in the initiation of the Fas-induced apoptotic cascade. *Curr Biol.* 1998;8(18):1001-1008.

256. Kischkel FC, Hellbardt S, Behrmann I, et al. Cytotoxicity-dependent APO-1 (Fas/CD95)-associated proteins form a death-inducing signaling complex (DISC) with the receptor. *EMBO J.* 1995;14(22):5579-5588.

257. Waterhouse NJ, Trapani JA. CTL: caspases Terminate Life, but that's not the whole story. *Tissue Antigens.* 2002;59(3):175-183.

258. Fesik SW. Insights into programmed cell death through structural biology. *Cell.* 2000;103(2):273-282.

259. Wang R, Rogers AM, Ratliff TL, Russell JH. CD95-dependent bystander lysis caused by CD4+ T helper 1 effectors. *J Immunol.* 1996;157(7):2961-2968.

260. Moskophidis D, Lechner F, Pircher H, Zinkernagel RM. Virus persistence in acutely infected immunocompetent mice by exhaustion of antiviral cytotoxic effector T cells. *Nature.* 1993;362(6422):758-761.

261. Zarour HM. Reversing T-cell dysfunction and exhaustion in cancer. *Clin Cancer Res.* 2016;22(8):1856-1864.

262. Wherry EJ, Kurachi M. Molecular and cellular insights into T cell exhaustion. *Nat Rev Immunol.* 2015;15(8):486-499.

263. Blackburn SD, Shin H, Haining WN, et al. Coregulation of CD8+ T cell exhaustion by multiple inhibitory receptors during chronic viral infection. *Nat Immunol.* 2009;10(1):29-37.

264. Kaufmann DE, Kavanagh DG, Pereyra F, et al. Upregulation of CTLA-4 by HIV-specific CD4+ T cells correlates with disease progression and defines a reversible immune dysfunction. *Nat Immunol.* 2007;8(11):1246-1254.

265. Wolchok JD, Kluger H, Callahan MK, et al. Nivolumab plus ipilimumab in advanced melanoma. *N Engl J Med.* 2013;369(2):122-133.

266. Odorizzi PM, Wherry EJ. Inhibitory receptors on lymphocytes: insights from infections. *J Immunol.* 2012;188(7):2957-2965.

267. Wang C, McPherson AJ, Jones RB, et al. Loss of the signaling adaptor TRAF1 causes CD8+ T cell dysregulation during human and murine chronic infection. *J Exp Med.* 2012;209(1):77-91.

268. Vezys V, Penaloza-MacMaster P, Barber DL, et al. 4-1BB signaling synergizes with programmed death ligand 1 blockade to augment CD8 T cell responses during chronic viral infection. *J Immunol.* 2011;187(4):1634-1642.

269. Ravens S, Schultze-Florey C, Raha S, et al. Human gammadelta T cells are quickly reconstituted after stem-cell transplantation and show adaptive clonal expansion in response to viral infection. *Nat Immunol.* 2017;18(4):393-401.

270. Chien YH, Meyer C, Bonneville M. Gammadelta T cells: first line of defense and beyond. *Annu Rev Immunol.* 2014;32:121-155.

271. De Rosa SC, Mitra DK, Watanabe N, Herzenberg LA, Herzenberg LA, Roederer M. Vdelta1 and Vdelta2 gammadelta T cells express distinct surface markers and might be developmentally distinct lineages. *J Leukoc Biol.* 2001;70(4):518-526.

272. Wesch D, Hinz T, Kabelitz D. Analysis of the TCR Vgamma repertoire in healthy donors and HIV-1-infected individuals. *Int Immunol.* 1998;10(8):1067-1075.

273. Cipriani B, Borsellino G, Poccia F, et al. Activation of C-C beta-chemokines in human peripheral blood gammadelta T cells by isopentenyl pyrophosphate and regulation by cytokines. *Blood.* 2000;95(1):39-47.

274. Dieli F, Troye-Blomberg M, Ivanyi J, et al. Vgamma9/Vdelta2 T lymphocytes reduce the viability of intracellular *Mycobacterium tuberculosis. Eur J Immunol.* 2000;30(5):1512-1519.

275. Dieli F, Troye-Blomberg M, Ivanyi J, et al. Granulysin-dependent killing of intracellular and extracellular *Mycobacterium tuberculosis* by Vgamma9/Vdelta2 T lymphocytes. *J Infect Dis.* 2001;184(8):1082-1085.

276. Wang L, Xu M, Wang C, et al. The feature of distribution and clonality of TCR gamma/delta subfamilies T cells in patients with B-cell non-Hodgkin lymphoma. *J Immunol Res.* 2014;2014:241246.

277. Bottino C, Tambussi G, Ferrini S, et al. Two subsets of human T lymphocytes expressing gamma/delta antigen receptor are identifiable by monoclonal antibodies directed to two distinct molecular forms of the receptor. *J Exp Med.* 1988;168(2):491-505.

278. Falini B, Flenghi L, Pileri S, et al. Distribution of T cells bearing different forms of the T cell receptor gamma/delta in normal and pathological human tissues. *J Immunol.* 1989;143(8):2480-2488.

279. Hayday AC. [gamma][delta] cells: a right time and a right place for a conserved third way of protection. *Annu Rev Immunol.* 2000;18:975-1026.

280. Allison TJ, Garboczi DN. Structure of gammadelta T cell receptors and their recognition of non-peptide antigens. *Mol Immunol.* 2002;38(14):1051-1061.

281. Carding SR, Egan PJ. Gammadelta T cells: functional plasticity and heterogeneity. *Nat Rev Immunol.* 2002;2(5):336-345.

282. Born W, Cady C, Jones-Carson J, Mukasa A, Lahn M, O'Brien R. Immunoregulatory functions of gamma delta T cells. *Adv Immunol.* 1999;71:77-144.

283. Rincon-Orozco B, Kunzmann V, Wrobel P, Kabelitz D, Steinle A, Herrmann T. Activation of V gamma 9V delta 2 T cells by NKG2D. *J Immunol.* 2005;175(4):2144-2151.

284. Morita CT, Li H, Lamphear JG, et al. Superantigen recognition by gammadelta T cells: SEA recognition site for human Vgamma2 T cell receptors. *Immunity.* 2001;14(3):331-344.

285. Groh V, Steinle A, Bauer S, Spies T. Recognition of stress-induced MHC molecules by intestinal epithelial gammadelta T cells. *Science.* 1998;279(5357):1737-1740.

286. Bauer S, Groh V, Wu J, et al. Activation of NK cells and T cells by NKG2D, a receptor for stress-inducible MICA. *Science.* 1999;285(5428):727-729.

287. Li P, Willie ST, Bauer S, Morris DL, Spies T, Strong RK. Crystal structure of the MHC class I homolog MIC-A, a gammadelta T cell ligand. *Immunity.* 1999;10(5):577-584.

288. Li Y, Wang Q, Mariuzza RA. Structure of the human activating natural cytotoxicity receptor NKp30 bound to its tumor cell ligand B7-H6. *J Exp Med.* 2011;208(4):703-714.

289. Beckman EM, Melián A, Behar SM, et al. CD1c restricts responses of mycobacteria-specific T cells. Evidence for antigen presentation by a second member of the human CD1 family. *J Immunol.* 1996;157(7):2795-2803.

290. Spada FM, Grant EP, Peters PJ, et al. Self-recognition of CD1 by gamma/delta T cells: implications for innate immunity. *J Exp Med.* 2000;191(6):937-948.

291. Exley M, Garcia J, Balk SP, Porcelli S. Requirements for CD1d recognition by human invariant Valpha24+ CD4-CD8- T cells. *J Exp Med.* 1997;186(1):109-120.

292. Leslie DS, Vincent MS, Spada FM, et al. CD1-mediated gamma/delta T cell maturation of dendritic cells. *J Exp Med.* 2002;196(12):1575-1584.

293. Kong Y, Cao W, Xi X, Ma C, Cui L, He W. The NKG2D ligand ULBP4 binds to TCRgamma9/delta2 and induces cytotoxicity to tumor cells through both TCRgammadelta and NKG2D. *Blood.* 2009;114(2):310-317.

294. Toutirais O, Cabillic F, Le Friec G, et al. DNAX accessory molecule-1 (CD226) promotes human hepatocellular carcinoma cell lysis by Vgamma9Vdelta2 T cells. *Eur J Immunol.* 2009;39(5):1361-1368.

295. Alexander AA, Maniar A, Cummings JS, et al. Isopentenyl pyrophosphate-activated CD56+ {gamma}{delta} T lymphocytes display potent antitumor activity toward human squamous cell carcinoma. *Clin Cancer Res.* 2008;14(13):4232-4240.

296. Seidel UJ, Vogt F, Grosse-Hovest L, Jung G, Handgretinger R, Lang P. Gammadelta T cell-mediated antibody-dependent cellular cytotoxicity with CD19 antibodies assessed by an impedance-based label-free real-time cytotoxicity assay. *Front Immunol.* 2014;5:618.

297. Payne KK, Mine JA, Biswas S, et al. BTN3A1 governs antitumor responses by coordinating alphabeta and gammadelta T cells. *Science.* 2020;369(6506):942-949.

298. Rosenberg SA, Packard BS, Aebersold PM, et al. Use of tumor-infiltrating lymphocytes and interleukin-2 in the immunotherapy of patients with metastatic melanoma. A preliminary report. *N Engl J Med.* 1988;319(25):1676-1680.

299. Dudley ME, Wunderlich JR, Shelton TE, Even J, Rosenberg SA. Generation of tumor-infiltrating lymphocyte cultures for use in adoptive transfer therapy for melanoma patients. *J Immunother.* 2003;26(4):332-342.

300. Morgan RA, Dudley ME, Wunderlich JR, et al. Cancer regression in patients after transfer of genetically engineered lymphocytes. *Science.* 2006;314(5796):126-129.

301. Kloss CC, Condomines M, Cartellieri M, Bachmann M, Sadelain M. Combinatorial antigen recognition with balanced signaling promotes selective tumor eradication by engineered T cells. *Nat Biotechnol.* 2013;31(1):71-75.

302. Gross G, Waks T, Eshhar Z. Expression of immunoglobulin-T-cell receptor chimeric molecules as functional receptors with antibody-type specificity. *Proc Natl Acad Sci U S A.* 1989;86(24):10024-10028.

303. Eshhar Z, Waks T, Gross G, Schindler DG. Specific activation and targeting of cytotoxic lymphocytes through chimeric single chains consisting of antibody-binding domains and the gamma or zeta subunits of the immunoglobulin and T-cell receptors. *Proc Natl Acad Sci U S A.* 1993;90(2):720-724.

304. Lee DW, Kochenderfer JN, Stetler-Stevenson M, et al. T cells expressing CD19 chimeric antigen receptors for acute lymphoblastic leukaemia in children and young adults: a phase 1 dose-escalation trial. *Lancet.* 2015;385(9967):517-528.

305. Maude SL, Laetsch TW, Buechner J, et al. Tisagenlecleucel in children and young adults with B-cell lymphoblastic leukemia. *N Engl J Med.* 2018;378(5):439-448.

306. Neelapu SS, Locke FL, Bartlett NL, et al. Axicabtagene ciloleucel CAR T-cell therapy in refractory large B-cell lymphoma. *N Engl J Med.* 2017;377(26):2531-2544.

307. Schuster SJ, Bishop MR, Tam CS, et al. Tisagenlecleucel in adult relapsed or refractory diffuse large B-cell lymphoma. *N Engl J Med.* 2018;380(1):45-56.

The Normal Hematologic System

308. Wang M, Munoz J, Goy A, et al. KTE-X19 CAR T-cell therapy in relapsed or refractory mantle-cell lymphoma. *N Engl J Med.* 2020;382(14):1331-1342.

309. Abramson JS, Palomba ML, Gordon LI, et al. Lisocabtagene maraleucel for patients with relapsed or refractory large B-cell lymphomas (TRANSCEND NHL 001): a multicentre seamless design study. *Lancet.* 2020;396(10254):839-852.

310. Jacobson CJ, Segal A, William B, et al. Primary analysis of zuma-5: a phase 2 study of axicabtagene ciloleucel (Axi-Cel) in patients with relapsed/refractory (R/R) indolent non-Hodgkin lymphoma (iNHL). *Blood.* 2020;136:40-41.

311. Munshi NC, Anderson LD, Shah N, et al. Idecabtagene vicleucel in relapsed and refractory multiple myeloma. *N Engl J Med.* 2021;384(8):705-716.

312. Davila ML, Riviere I, Wang X, et al. Efficacy and toxicity management of 19-28z CAR T cell therapy in B cell acute lymphoblastic leukemia. *Sci Transl Med.* 2014;6(224):224ra25.

313. Lee DW, Santomasso BD, Locke FL, et al. ASBMT consensus grading for cytokine release syndrome and neurologic toxicity associated with immune effector cells. *Biol Blood Marrow Transplant.* 2019;25(4):625-638.

314. Faramand RG, Jain M, Staedtke V, et al. Tumor microenvironment composition and severe Cytokine Release Syndrome (CRS) influence toxicity in patients with large b cell lymphoma treated with axicabtagene ciloleucel. *Clin Cancer Res.* 2020;26(18):4823-4831.

315. Neelapu SS, Tummala S, Kebriaei P, et al. Chimeric antigen receptor T-cell therapy—assessment and management of toxicities. *Nat Rev Clin Oncol.* 2018;15(1):47-62.

316. Santomasso BD, Park JH, Salloum D, et al. Clinical and biologic correlates of neurotoxicity associated with CAR T cell therapy in patients with B-Cell Acute Lymphoblastic Leukemia (B-ALL). *Cancer Discov.* 2018;8(8):958-971.

317. Maude SL, Frey N, Shaw PA, et al. Chimeric antigen receptor T cells for sustained remissions in leukemia. *N Engl J Med.* 2014;371(16):1507-1517.

318. Depil S, Duchateau P, Grupp SA, Mufti G, Poirot L. 'Off-the-shelf' allogeneic CAR T cells: development and challenges. *Nat Rev Drug Discov.* 2020;19(3):185-199.

Chapter 14 ■ Natural Killer and Innate Lymphoid Cells

MATTHEW R. LORDO • TODD A. FEHNIGER • BETHANY L. MUNDY-BOSSE • AHARON G. FREUD

The Normal Hematologic System

OVERVIEW

Natural killer (NK) cells are cytotoxic lymphocytes of the innate immune system that play a critical role in the control of viral infection and malignancy, and represent the founding member of an expanding family of innate lymphoid cells (ILCs). Human NK cells are identified via non–NK-restricted surface antigens: CD56 (neural cell adhesion molecule) or NKp46 (activating receptor) expression and a lack of CD3 (a marker of T cells). NK cells are readily identifiable in the peripheral blood, where they comprise approximately 10% of circulating lymphocytes. In addition, NK cells are found in secondary lymphoid tissues (e.g., lymph nodes, spleen), bone marrow, liver, uterus, and skin, among other tissues. NK cells are heterogeneous and exist within a range of maturation and functional states, delineated by the expression of distinct surface markers. In addition, the precise complement of activating and inhibitory receptors expressed on NK cells, which permits the discrimination of target cells from normal tissue, varies from NK cell to NK cell. Thus, NK cells constitute a diverse population of effector cells, even in the absence of germ line DNA-rearranged antigen-specific receptors.

NK cells were originally described based on their function: they are large granular lymphocytes that kill target cells "naturally," that is, without prior exposure and in a non–major histocompatibility complex (MHC)-dependent fashion. As knowledge about NK cells has expanded, however, it has become clear that NK cells function in far more than spontaneous cytotoxicity. NK cells are robust cytokine and chemokine producers and are thus capable of modulating the function of other immune cells. In addition, despite being originally classified as members of the innate immune system, recent work has shown that NK cells can display "adaptive" or memory-like properties in response to numerous stimuli, including specific haptens, viruses, or combined cytokine activation. Thus, NK cells are unique cytotoxic and immunomodulatory "first responder" cells that can both form a bridge to the adaptive immune response and participate in it directly. Here, we provide an overview of NK cell development, function, and highlight their role in the treatment of hematologic diseases.

Additional non–NK innate cells known collectively as ILCs were discovered recently, and a formal classification system that summarized these findings was proposed in 2013. At that time, ILCs were organized into three groups: Group 1—consisting of cytotoxic NK cells and the helper ILC1 subset, Group 2—ILC2s, and Group 3—consisting of ILC3s and lymphoid tissue inducer (LTi) cells.[1] Each group is distinct with respect to its functional and immunophenotypic repertoire, mirroring the diversity and organization of T-cell subsets such as the adaptive CD8+ cytotoxic T cells and the CD4+ T helper type 1 (T_H1), T_H2, and T_H17 counterparts, respectively. Developmentally, however, ILCs lack specific attributes that define adaptive cells such as receptor gene rearrangement and thus represent a distinct developmental lineage.

Since ILCs were discovered, our ability to track and understand how they develop and influence the balance of health and disease has continued to expand. The vast majority of initial studies defining the roles and development of ILCs were performed in mice; however, more recent work includes additional characterizations of human ILC subsets. Although most ILC attributes are complementary between the two systems, some important differences have been appreciated and are discussed and highlighted throughout the chapter.

NATURAL KILLER CELL AND INNATE LYMPHOID CELL DEVELOPMENT AND TISSUE LOCALIZATION

ILCs are descendants of the common lymphoid progenitor (CLP),[2] a relationship first suggested by studies with Ikaros and common γ-chain knockout mice, which were deficient in B, T, and NK cells.[3,4] It was proven thereafter with the discovery of a CLP capable of producing B, T, and NK cells.[5,6] Differentiation of ILCs from the CLP has been the focus of many research efforts and has resulted in a model of distinct developmental intermediates with progressive commitment toward individual ILC subsets, similar to adaptive immune cell development (*Figure 14.1*).

Murine Innate Lymphoid Cell Development

In mice, the early innate lymphoid progenitor (EILP) is the first ILC lineage–specified progenitor downstream of the CLP. The EILP is capable of producing both cytotoxic and helper ILC lineages,

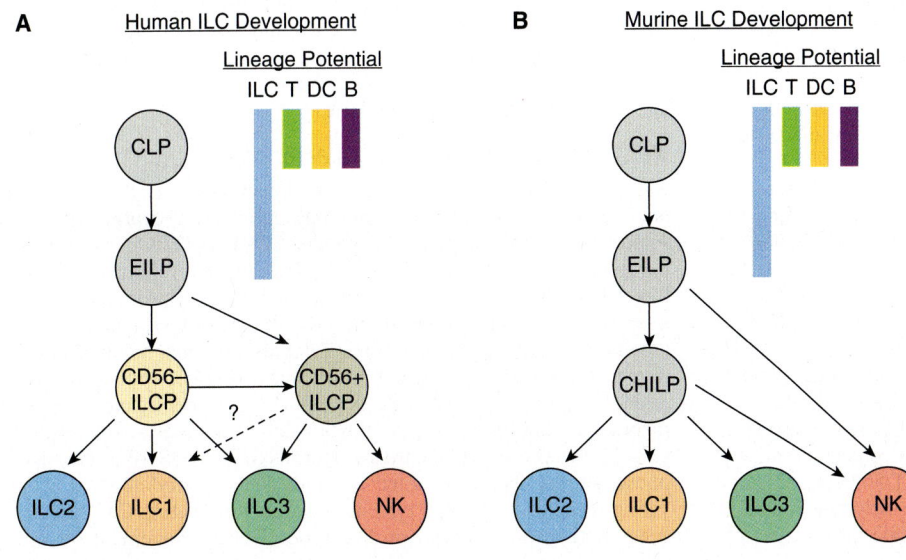

A Human ILC Development
B Murine ILC Development

FIGURE 14.1 Models of innate lymphoid cells (ILC) development. A, Human ILC development derives through the multipotent common lymphoid progenitor (CLP) which also has T, B, and DC potential. The CLP matures into an early innate lymphoid progenitor (EILP), at which point it is restricted to the ILC lineage. The EILP further matures into an ILC precursor (ILCP), which gives rise to all NK and helper ILC subsets. Note the divergent developmental pathway of ILC2s from NK cells. B, Murine ILC development similarly proceeds through the CLP. The EILP and common helper ILP (CHILP) are downstream progenitors that are ILC restricted. The question mark (?) indicates the current uncertainty of ILC1 development from the CD56+ ILCP in humans.

309

including LTi cells, but no other innate or adaptive lineages.[7] The EILP was originally identified immunophenotypically as a lineage antigen (Lin)⁻Thy1.2⁻IL-7Rα⁻α₄β₇⁺ derivative of the CLP that expresses high levels of the intracellular T-cell factor 1 (Tcf-1, encoded by the *Tcf7* gene), an HMG (high mobility group) box-containing transcription factor essential for T-cell development.[7] Furthermore, mice deficient in Tcf-1 lack all ILC populations, including NK cells and helper ILCs, as well as T cells, but they have normal amounts of B cells.

A more restricted ILC progenitor that is capable of helper ILC and LTi cell differentiation but lacks NK cell potential was initially identified and termed the common helper innate lymphoid progenitor (CHILP). It was identified as Lin⁻Id2⁺IL-7Rα⁺CD25⁻α₄β₇⁺ and was discovered with the assistance of an Id-2 GFP reporter.[8] Additional studies have shown that the transcription factor PLZF is heterogeneously expressed by CHILPs and that PLZF⁻ cells are capable of all helper ILC differentiation including LTi cells, whereas the PLZF⁺ subset is restricted to non–LTi helper ILCs.[9] PLZF expression at this stage of development is associated with surface PD-1 expression allowing for surface identification in mice.[10] Identification of the CHILP combined with reports of a Lin⁻flk2⁻CD27⁺CD244⁺IL-7Rα⁺CD122⁻ committed NK cell progenitor (NKP) in mice initially supported a model wherein the NK cell lineage diverges from helper ILCs early in development.[11] However, the discovery of the NKP preceded our knowledge of ILCs, and more recent studies utilizing high-sensitivity reporter mice challenge this model by demonstrating NK cell development from the CHILP.[12,13] Altogether, these more recent findings suggest that previous notions of a divergence between NK cell and helper ILC development in mice may not occur as early as previously thought.

Once committed to the NK lineage, NK cells in mice can be divided into four major developmental stages based on the expression of CD27 and CD11b following the acquisition of NK1.1. The least mature NK cells lack both CD27 and CD11b. Acquisition of CD27 occurs first and is associated with the ability to secrete interferon (IFN)-γ, followed by acquisition of CD11b, the expression of which correlates with cytotoxic potential. Following the formation of CD27⁺CD11b⁺ NK cells, CD27 is downregulated on the cell surface, producing terminally mature cytotoxic CD27⁻CD11b⁺ NK cells.[14]

Human Innate Lymphoid Cell Development

The murine-based model of NK cells originating from a CLP was supported in humans when a CD34⁺CD45RA⁺CD10⁺ CLP was identified and demonstrated the ability to generate B, T, NK cells, and dendritic cells (DCs) in vitro.[5] Other non–NK ILC lineages have also been confirmed to originate through this common pathway.[1] Emerging data continue to reveal similarities between developmental pathways in mice and humans, although slight differences have been reported in the human setting and are described here.

Much of what we know about human ILC development originates from work that defined stepwise NK cell developmental intermediates (NKDI) prior to the identification and characterization of human ILCs.[15] These NKDIs range from multipotent stage 1 progenitors (downstream of the CLP) to stage 6 mature cytotoxic NK cells and are distinguished based on the differential expression of the surface markers CD34, CD117, CD94, NKp80, CD16, and CD57.[16] Although development begins in the bone marrow, terminal NK cell development in humans largely occurs in peripheral tissues, including the tonsil, spleen, and lymph nodes.[17] Stage 1 cells in these tissues are multipotent progenitors with the potential to give rise to NK, T, and DCs but not B cells. Stage 2 cells are developmentally distinct based on their ability to proliferate and differentiate into mature NK cells in vitro with IL-15 alone, and more recently, it was shown that the stage 2 NKDI population contains a common ILC progenitor (similar to the EILP in mice) capable of generating all ILCs and NK cells, but not other white blood cell types.[17] Stage 3 NKDIs are also ILC/NK cell restricted, and recently, two distinct ILC precursor subsets were described within the stage 3 population: CD56⁻ stage 3 cells, which are capable of differentiating into all ILCs including NK cells, and CD56⁺ stage 3 cells, which cannot differentiate into ILC2s.[18,19]

Stage 4 cells are further committed to the NK cell lineage. These cells express high levels of CD56 and CD94, and are potent producers of IFN-γ, particularly the stage 4B (NKp80⁺) subset, with minimal cytotoxicity (hereafter referred to as CD56^bright NK cells). Lastly, stage 5 and 6 cells, which predominate in the blood, are notable for dim CD56 and high CD16 expression as well as potent cytotoxic abilities (hereafter referred to as CD56^dim NK cells).[20]

Not only has research delineated the pathways associated with human NK cell development, but current research efforts are also uncovering the importance of local tissue microenvironments in influencing NK cell subset distribution, maturation, and function. Mature and terminally differentiated NK cells largely reside in the blood, bone marrow, spleen, and lungs, and share transcriptional programs across sites. In contrast, immature NK cells and precursor populations with reduced effector capacity populate lymph nodes and intestine, and exhibit tissue-resident signatures and site-specific adaptations.[21] Recent research has also identified surface markers that can be used to distinguish tissue-resident NK cells from circulating NK cells, including expression of chemokine receptors such as CXCR6 or integrins like CD103 and CD49a. Studying tissue-resident NK cell phenotypes in the context of other ILCs (discussed in more detail later in the chapter) is an active area of research. Furthermore, the influence of local tissue microenvironments on NK cell plasticity is a burgeoning area in the field. Inflammatory states seen in the context of autoimmune disease or infection in addition to microenvironments created by cancer cells have been found to mold NK cell and ILC phenotypes.[22] Thus, understanding how these cells develop in healthy and diseased states is important to ultimately understanding how their functions may be manipulated therapeutically.

RECEPTORS ON NATURAL KILLER CELLS: TARGET-CELL RECOGNITION AND CYTOKINE SIGNALING

NK cell target recognition is a tightly regulated process that integrates activating and inhibitory receptor signals with the activation state of the NK cell to determine the functional response (*Figure 14.2*). Unlike adaptive T and B lymphocytes, the diversity and specificity of NK cell responses do not arise from the rearrangement of DNA sequences that encode a predominant, antigen-specific receptor. Instead, NK cells express a variety of germ line DNA-encoded, invariant activating and inhibitory receptors whose signals integrate to govern NK cell functional responses.[23] As a general rule, NK cell inhibitory receptors recognize MHC class I molecules, immunologic markers of "self." Reduced or absent MHC class I expression, which may be seen on an infected or malignant transformed cell, does not on its own result in NK cell activation. NK cell triggering does not classically occur without signals from activating receptors, which typically recognize cell stress–induced ligands or antibody constant regions that may be found on an opsonized target. In addition, through the constitutive expression of cytokine receptors, the surrounding milieu can further tune the signals arising from activating and inhibitory receptor engagement by altering the NK cell's activation state.

Natural Killer Cell Inhibitory Receptors

The predominant NK cell inhibitory receptors are CD94/NKG2A and a family of killer cell immunoglobulin-like receptors (KIRs; *Figure 14.3*).[23] The evolutionarily older CD94/NKG2A is the principal inhibitory receptor of CD56^bright NK cells and relatively immature CD56^dim cells, whereas KIR acquisition is a property of the more mature CD56^dim population. NK cell inhibitory receptors share a common signaling motif in their cytoplasmic domains, the immunoreceptor tyrosine-based inhibitory motif (ITIM), defined by the amino acid sequence (I/L/V/S) XYXX (L/V). Upon ligand engagement by an inhibitory receptor, the tyrosine in this motif is phosphorylated by an Src family kinase and recruits SHP-1 or SHP-2 (tyrosine phosphatases). These recruited enzymes dephosphorylate local activating receptor-associated tyrosine kinases, terminating Ca^{2+} influx, functional responses, and proliferation. Thus, engagement of any

	Receptor Name	Ligand
Inhibitory	KIRs	HLA class I
	CD94/NKG2A	HLA-E
	LIR-1	HLA class I & nonclassical HLA class I
Activating	FcγRIIIa (CD16)	IgG Fc region
	NKp46	Viral hemagglutinins, unknown
	NKp30	Viral hemagglutinins, B7-H6, BAG6, unknown
	NKp44*	Viral hemagglutinins, unknown
	NKp80	Activation-induced C-type lectin (AICL)
	CD94/NKG2C	HLA-E
	KIRs	HLA class I
	NKG2D	*MICA/B, ULBP1-6*
	DNAM-1	*CD155 (Necl5), CD112 (Nectin-2)*
	SFR	*2B4, Ly9, CRACC, CD48, SLAM, CD84, NTB-A*
Cytokine	IL-2R	IL-2
	IL-12R	IL-12
	IL-15R	IL-15
	IL-18R	IL-18
	IL-21R	IL-21
	IFNAR	IFN-α
	TGFβRI/II	TGF-β
	IL-10R	IL-10

FIGURE 14.2 Selected natural killer (NK) cell activating, inhibitory, and cytokine receptors and their ligands. Italic denotes activating receptor that does not signal via ITAMs. Asterisk denotes induced expression. HLA, human leukocyte antigen; IFN, interferon; Ig, immunoglobulin; ITAMs, immunoreceptor tyrosine-based activation motifs; TGF, transforming growth factor.

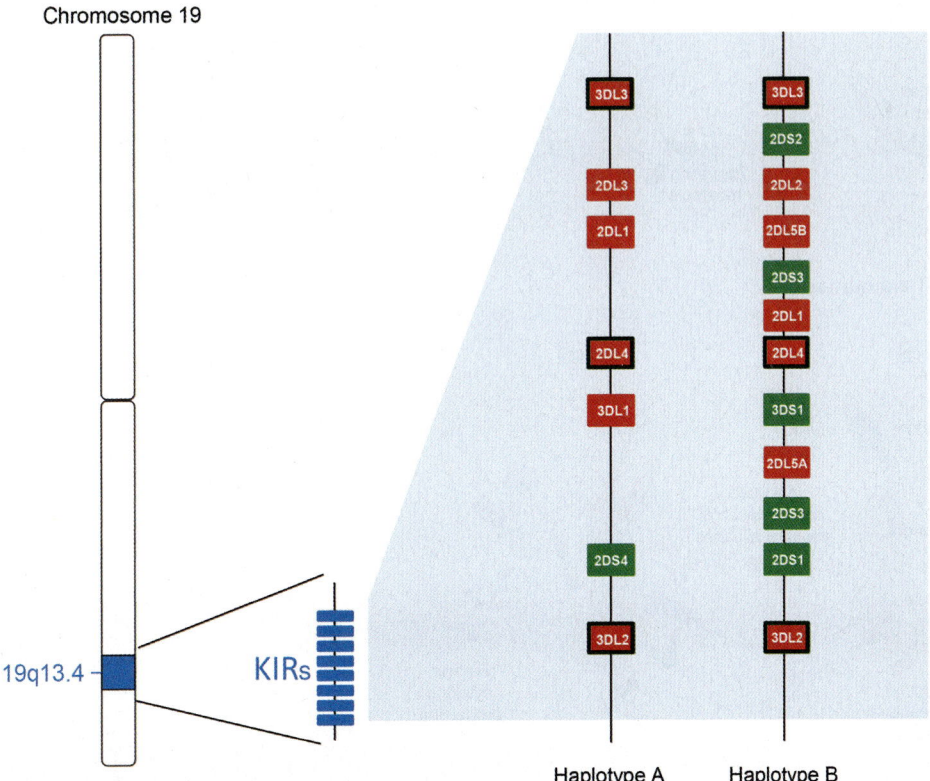

FIGURE 14.3 The killer cell immunoglobulin-like receptor (KIR) gene locus and major haplotypes. Their human KIR locus is located on chromosome 19 and consists of 13 highly polymorphic genes and 2 pseudogenes. KIRs are activating (shown in green) or inhibitory (red) in nature, though some, such as 2DL4, can function as both. Two broad KIR haplotypes have been defined that differ in their gene content, with haplotype A consisting almost exclusively of inhibitory KIRs and haplotype B consisting of both inhibitory and activating KIRs. Haplotypes are further subtyped based on the exact KIR genes present, with representative A and B haplotypes shown. Both haplotypes contain three conserved framework genes (outlined in black) that define the centromeric and telomeric regions of the KIR locus. KIR pseudogenes not shown.

inhibitory receptor reduces the potential of most activating receptors to stimulate a response.

CD94/NKG2A is a heterodimeric, type II transmembrane C-type lectin receptor expressed on both human and murine NK cells. CD94 also associates with other NKG2 receptors, including the activating NKG2C, and itself has no cytoplasmic domain. Instead, inhibitory signals are transmitted by the two ITIMs contained within the cytoplasmic tail of NKG2A. CD94/NKG2A recognizes the nonclassical MHC class I molecule HLA-E, which is widely expressed on normal tissue and presents the leader sequences of other class I molecules (HLA-A, HLA-B, HLA-C). In contrast, KIRs are a family of monomeric type I transmembrane proteins encoded by 14 different genes (KIR 2DL1-5, 3DL1-3, 2DS1-5, 3DS1) that are only expressed on human NK cells.[24] The first number in KIR nomenclature represents the number of extracellular immunoglobulin-like domains (2 or 3), and L or S represent the length of the cytoplasmic tail (L for long, S for short). KIRs can be either activating or inhibitory, and all inhibitory receptors have long (L), ITIM-containing cytoplasmic tails. KIRs recognize MHC class I molecules, and different KIRs recognize distinct MHC subsets. KIR2DL1 recognizes HLA-C2 molecules, KIR2DL2/3 recognizes HLA-C1, and KIR3DL1 recognizes HLA-Bw4. KIR sequences and expression patterns generate a pool of NK cells with unique inhibitory properties. This is achieved in several different ways. First, a given NK cell expresses only a subset of available KIR genes. In addition, KIRs are inherited as haplotypes that vary in their proportion of activating and inhibitory KIRs (Haplotype A = more inhibitory, B = more activating). Finally, several alleles exist for each KIR which modulate surface expression density and MHC affinity. Specific KIR alleles have been linked to susceptibility to certain autoimmune disease, viruses, and cancer, as well as to allogeneic hematopoietic cell transfer outcomes, highlighting the biological importance of KIR-KIR ligand interactions and NK cell functional modulation. Finally, NK cells also express the inhibitory leukocyte immunoglobulin-like receptor 1, which recognizes both classical and nonclassical MHC class I molecules.

In addition to constitutively expressed inhibitory receptors, NK cells, like other immune cells, upregulate inhibitory receptors upon activation as a means of controlling the magnitude and duration of an immune response and limiting activation-induced cell death. These induced inhibitory checkpoint molecules, which include T-cell Ig and ITIM domain, PD-1, and LAG-3, typically bind ligands expressed on target cells such as tumors.[25] Thus, one strategy for improving NK cell immunotherapy outcomes involves blockade of these induced checkpoint receptors, tipping the balance of NK cell signaling toward activation.

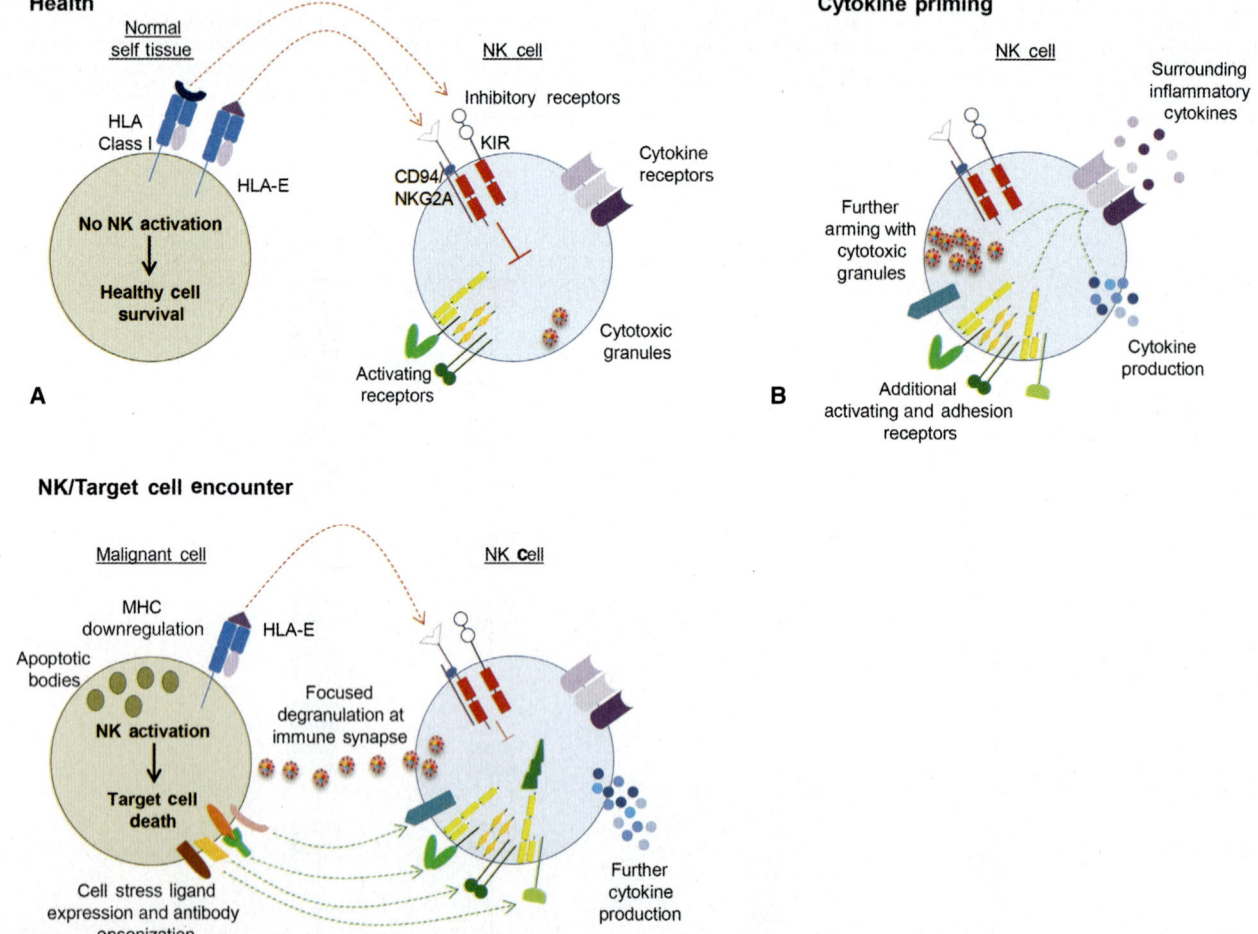

FIGURE 14.4 Natural killer (NK) cell activation—the response to target cells depends on an integration of signals. A, In the healthy state, non–cytokine-primed NK cells encounter self tissue expressing major histocompatibility complex (MHC) class I, which delivers inhibitory signals to NK cells via killer cell immunoglobulin-like receptors (KIRs) and CD94/NKG2A, preventing NK cell activation. B, Under inflammatory conditions, pro-inflammatory cytokines bind NK cells via constitutively expressed receptors. In NK cells, these cytokine signals promote cytokine production and upregulation of activating and adhesion receptors, further arming them with cytotoxic granules and effector molecules that prime the NK cell for an encounter with a target cell. C, Virally infected or malignantly transformed cells downregulate MHC class I and upregulate cell stress ligands. Thus, when an NK cell encounters such a target, activating receptor signals outweigh inhibitory ones, tipping the balance in favor of NK cell activation and promoting enhanced cytokine production and focused degranulation toward the target cell.

Natural Killer Cell Activating Receptors

The pool of NK cell activating receptors is more diverse than that of the inhibitory ones (*Figure 14.4*). Most NK cell activating receptors are associated with immunoreceptor tyrosine-based activation motif (ITAM)-bearing signaling adapters. Different signaling adapters possess different numbers of ITAMs (3 in CD3ξ, 2 in DAP12, and 1 in FcεRI), and ITAMs are defined by YXXL/I motifs separated by six to eight amino acids. The binding of an activating receptor to its ligand results in the phosphorylation of ITAM tyrosine residues by Src family kinases. These phosphorylated tyrosines recruit additional tyrosine kinases and scaffolding proteins that activate a variety of different signaling pathways.[23] Some of the most notable NK cell activating receptors that associate with ITAM-bearing signaling adapters are FcRγIIIa (CD16), the natural cytotoxicity (NCR) receptors, CD94/NKG2C, and activating KIR. CD94/NKG2C and activating KIR recognize the same ligands as their inhibitory counterparts. Although CD94/NKG2C is usually expressed on only a minor subset of NK cells, this subset has been shown to expand preferentially in the setting of human CMV infection, generating adaptive NK cells.[26]

FcγRIIIa is one of several Fc receptors that bind antibody constant domains. Fc receptors are subclassified based on the type of antibody that they recognize.[27] FcγRIIIa is one of several IgG-recognizing Fcγ receptors. Fcγ receptors are expressed on monocytes, macrophages, and DCs, among others, where they are important mediators of phagocytosis. FcγRIIIa is a low-affinity receptor, primarily expressed on NK cells, that signals via CD3ξ or FcRγ. Although signals from several activating receptors are usually required to activate an NK cell, signals from FcγRIIIa alone are potent enough to result in antibody-dependent cytokine release and cytotoxicity. FcγRIIIa, then, allows for specific NK cell targeting to cells expressing an antigen of interest.[28] This is relevant not only physiologically in the context of a mixed immune response but also therapeutically. Indeed, combination therapy involving NK cells and monoclonal antibodies directed against tumor antigens is under active investigation.

NK cell NCRs include NKp30, NKp44, NKp46, and NKp80.[23] With the exception of NKp80, a C-type lectin, NCRs are type I transmembrane proteins with extracellular immunoglobulin domains responsible for ligand binding, and a transmembrane portion bearing a positively charged amino acid that mediates association with signaling adaptors. NKp30, NKp46, and NKp80 show constitutive NK cell expression, whereas NKp44 is induced upon NK activation. NKp30 and NKp46 associate with CD3ξ and FcRγ, and NKp44 with DAP12. NKp80 signals through a hemi-ITAM sequence that is part of its cytoplasmic domain. The identities of all NCR ligands have not been elucidated. NKp30, 44, and 46 have been shown to bind viral hemagglutinins. With regard to tumor ligands, NKp30 binds B7-H6 and BAG6, present on multiple different tumor cell lines, but specific tumor ligands for the other NCRs remain unknown. NKp80 is genetically linked to its ligand, activation-induced C-type lectin, expressed on a variety of malignant cells as well as activated, nonmalignant tissues.

Two important NK cell activating receptors that do not signal via ITAMs are NKG2D and DNAX accessory molecule (DNAM-1).[23] Unlike other NKG2 family receptors, NKG2D exists as a homodimer and signals via the adaptor DAP10. DAP10 does not have ITAMs and, instead, has a YXXM motif in its cytoplasmic tail that recruits PI3K. NKG2D binds a variety of different ligands that, for the most part, are induced by cellular stress and resemble MHC class I, such as MIC-A/B, and ULBP1-6. DNAM-1 is an Ig-like adhesion molecule whose cytoplasmic domain has three sites that can be phosphorylated upon binding to its ligands, the nectin proteins Necl5 and Nectin-2. These ligands are expressed on a wide variety of tumor cells, and DNAM-1 plays an important role in tumor immunosurveillance. Indeed, activating signals from DNAM-1 synergize with those from other NK cell receptors to promote IFN-γ production.[29]

An additional family of receptors important in activating NK cells is the signaling lymphocyte activating molecule (SLAM) family receptors (SFRs), which are solely detected on hematopoietic cells. This family of receptors consists of 7 members, including 2B4, Ly9, CRACC, CD48, SLAM, CD84, and NTB-A. All of the SFRs are expressed on mature NK cells, except SLAM. The members of this family are able to recognize each other and thus mediate homotypic interactions between cells of the hematopoietic lineage. These interactions have been found to be important in NK cell education (discussed later in the chapter). They signal through cytoplasmic immunoreceptor tyrosine switch motifs, which then recruit a family of SH2-domain-only–containing adapters, including SLAM-associated protein (SAP).[30] Studies in SLAM-deficient mice have demonstrated severe NK cell functional defects and suggest this family of receptors can be activating or inhibitory depending on the presence or absence of SAP family adapters.[31] Furthermore, loss-of-function mutations in SAP have been described in patients with X-linked lymphoproliferative disease.

Natural Killer Cell Cytokine Receptors

NK cell cytotoxicity and cytokine production in response to a target cell is modulated by cytokines present in the local environment as a result of constitutive NK cell expression of cytokine receptors. Cytokines such as IFN-α and interleukin (IL)-2, IL-12, IL-15, IL-18, and IL-21, produced by early innate immune responders like DCs and macrophages, are potent inducers of NK cell activation and cytotoxicity.[32] For instance, IL-15, the central cytokine in NK cell development and homeostasis, enhances NK cell cytotoxicity along with promoting survival and proliferation. Part of the IL-15 receptor (β/γ subunit) is also utilized by IL-2, and, as a result, IL-2 exerts similar biologic effects. IL-12 stimulates both NK cell cytokine production and cytotoxicity, and IL-18 synergizes with IL-12 and IL-15 to promote IFN-γ production. The effects of IL-21 on NK cells are not fully understood and may depend on synergistic signals from other cytokines like IL-15, in the presence of which IL-21 appears to promote NK cell cytotoxicity and maturation. NK cell functional responses and cytotoxicity can also be diminished by immunosuppressive cytokines like IL-10 and transforming growth factor (TGF) β.

Human CD56^{dim} NK cells are cytotoxic at rest, but the CD56^{bright} population is not and, as such, typically thought to function almost exclusively in cytokine production. In addition to physiologic levels of cytokines that can enhance NK cell cytotoxicity, high doses of IL-2 promote NK cell proliferation and lymphokine-activated killer (LAK) cell generation. LAK cells, used in early NK cell immunotherapy, are robustly cytotoxic and lyse a broader array of targets than do conventional NK cells, yet the high systemic doses of IL-2 required for their generation can result in significant toxicity. CD56^{bright} NK cells can be rendered cytotoxic through LAK cell generation. However, this NK cell subset appears to be more plastic than previously thought, since recent reports have demonstrated marked enhancement of CD56^{bright} NK cell cytotoxicity and antitumor function after brief culture in low-dose IL-15. Such IL-15-based enhancement of CD56^{bright} NK cell antitumor responses was also observed to occur in vivo in cancer patients treated with an IL-15/IL-15Rα superagonist complex or repeated IL-15 dosing.[33,34]

NATURAL KILLER CELL SELF TOLERANCE VIA EDUCATION

In light of their potent cytotoxicity, a critical feature of NK cells is self tolerance. A major mechanism for T- and B-cell tolerance is the deletion, during development, of cells with receptors specific for self antigens. Given that NK cells lack a predominant antigen-specific receptor, they must distinguish healthy self cells from target cells via alternative mechanisms. KIRs and MHC class I allele inheritance are not linked, and a given NK cell expresses only a fraction of the KIR alleles it possesses. As a result, a small proportion of human NK cells exist that lack CD94/NKG2A and express only KIRs without cognate ligands present in that individual, yet autoimmunity does not occur. This is the result of NK cell "licensing" or education, whereby NK cells that fail to signal through an inhibitory receptor during development are functionally anergic.[35] Thus, inhibitory receptors have a paradoxical role in that they also enable NK cell functional responses.

Furthermore, it is becoming clear that licensing is not purely a developmental process. In transplant scenarios, populations of previously licensed NK cells without a cognate ligand in the recipient lose their capacity for functional responses, whereas previously unlicensed NK cells can acquire functional competence.[36] Licensing, then, appears to be a dynamic process, with inhibitory receptor signals continually tuning the ability of an NK cell to respond to a target. Although both KIRs and CD94/NKG2A can license NK cells, licensing through KIRs has been demonstrated to confer enhanced function compared to licensing through CD94/NKG2A.[37] The mechanism for NK cell licensing has not been fully elucidated. It is not clear whether licensing is the result of NK cell "arming" or "disarming." In the arming hypothesis, inhibitory receptor signals themselves confer the ability to respond to activating receptors. However, the disarming model posits that unlicensed NK cells are hyporesponsive as a result of continuous signaling through a self-specific activating receptor. Here, inhibitory signals provide a counterbalance to this activation-induced anergy. The molecular mechanisms that underlie the licensing process are not well described but may involve increasing basal mTOR/Akt pathway activation.[38] In support of this, NK cell education and licensing have been linked to changes in metabolic activity. It has been shown that resting NK cells have low levels of oxidative phosphorylation and glycolysis, which are upregulated upon NK activation, suggesting a role for these pathways in NK cell function. Increased metabolism has been associated with increased granzyme B production, suggesting NK cell effector functions and metabolic activity are closely linked.[39] Furthermore, initial studies have demonstrated increased glucose metabolism in educated NK cells compared to uneducated NK cells. Among educated NK cells, those educated through NKG2A have superior metabolic function and higher metabolic resilience compared to NK cells educated via KIRs.[40]

NATURAL KILLER CELL FUNCTIONS

NK cells are critical for host defense against viral infection, malignant transformation, and certain intracellular bacteria and fungi. Specifically, NK cells play a central role in immunity against herpes viruses, and impaired NK cell function has been associated with an increased likelihood of cancer development.[41] As members of the innate immune system, NK cells are involved in the first wave of defense against pathogens and tumor initiation and can recruit additional innate and adaptive immune cells as required. NK cells mediate these important functions through two primary effector mechanisms: cytotoxicity and cytokine production.

Natural Killer Cell Cytotoxicity

As implied by their name, NK cells kill targets "naturally" or without prior sensitization (*Figure 14.5*). NK cells kill via the release of cytotoxic granules or by expressing ligands for death receptors, though the granule exocytosis pathway predominates. NK cell degranulation is a multistep, highly regulated process that results in directed granule release toward the target.[42] Completion of the first stage, initiation, depends on the balance of activating and inhibitory receptor signals transmitted to the NK cell upon "sampling" a target within the tissue or tumor environment. A small percentage of NK cells express open (activated) conformation of lymphocyte function–associated antigen-1 (LFA-1) at rest, an integrin that likely enables short-term engagement with target cells during this sampling phase before additional activating receptor signals are delivered. Secondary signals from activating receptors like NKG2D, DNAM-1, or the costimulatory CD2 likely further activate LFA-1, promoting tight adhesion with the target cell and immune synapse formation. Upon ligand binding, LFA-1 delivers signals that activate protein kinases, promote F-actin polymerization and reorganization, and arrest migration. These signals, in addition to those from activating receptors, promote lytic granule convergence upon the microtubule organizing center (MTOC) and granule

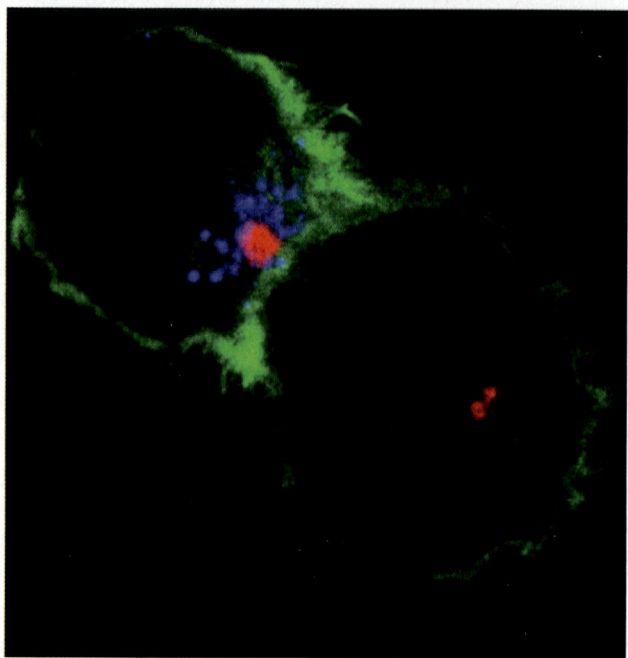

MTOC
Perforin
F-actin

FIGURE 14.5 **Natural killer (NK) cell and tumor target cell cytotoxic synapse.** Immunofluorescence photomicrograph of a primary human NK cell (top) conjugated to a tumor target (K562 leukemia, bottom cell), creating a cytotoxic synapse. After recognition of the target and triggering of the NK cell, granules with perforin (blue) and granzymes mobilize to the cytotoxic synapse at the microtubule-organizing center (MTOC, red), prior to their release at the target cell. This is followed by induction of an apoptotic-like cell death of the target by granzymes. F-actin: green. (Used with permission of Emily M. Mace, PhD.)

polarization to the immune synapse. More importantly, the initiation phase of lytic granule release can be reversed by signals from inhibitory receptors.

During the next effector stage, the NK cell is committed to degranulation. Here, the de novo F-actin polymerization that began in the initiation stage brings about significant cytoskeletal rearrangements as well as firm adhesion to the target cell. NK cells at the effector stage take on a characteristic, flattened shape that extends the diameter of the immune synapse, where a lytic cleft forms. Lytic granules are then delivered to the synapse, and a subset is released across the cleft toward the target. The final stage, termination, involves detachment from the target cell and either the return to a resting state or engagement with a new target cell. Interestingly, NK cell cytotoxic kinetics are such that when an NK cell chooses to engage with additional targets rather than retuning to rest, subsequent kills occur more rapidly.

NK cell degranulation onto a target results in death by apoptosis. NK cell granules contain cytotoxic proteins such as perforin and granzyme B that act in concert to kill target cells. Perforin forms holes in target cell membranes that permit entry of granzyme proteins, serine proteases that cleave caspase proteins to trigger apoptosis. Expression of death receptor ligands such as tumor necrosis factor (TNF)-related apoptosis-inducing ligand (TRAIL) and Fas ligand also results in caspase-dependent apoptosis of cells that express the cognate receptors.

Natural Killer Cell Cytokine Production

In addition to degranulation, NK cells also produce cytokines that modulate other members of the immune system. Although robust NK cell degranulation typically occurs in the setting of activating receptor ligation (either by antibody binding or by target cell engagement), cytokine production occurs in response to both cytokines and activating receptor stimulation. NK cells constitutively express receptors for cytokines such as IFN-α, IL-2, IL-12, IL-15, IL-18, and IL-21. In response to these cytokines, NK cells produce cytokines such as IFN-γ, TNF, and granulocyte macrophage colony–stimulating factor, and chemokines such as macrophage inflammatory protein (MIP)-1α, MIP-1β, XCL1, and CCL5 (RANTES, ie, regulated upon activation, normal T cell expressed and secreted) which have been shown to be important in the recruitment of anticancer DCs to tumor sites.[43] Stimulation with individual cytokines typically does not suffice to induce robust cytokine production by NK cells. However, stimulation with combinations of cytokines (e.g., IL-12 and IL-18 or IL-12 and IL-15) does, especially by the CD56[bright] subset, which is particularly cytokine-responsive. Like other immune cell types, overstimulation of NK cells leads to activation-induced cell death, which may also prevent unchecked persistent NK activation in the setting of inflammation. Tumor cell engagement or activating receptor ligation induces cytokine and chemokine production by both CD56[bright] and CD56[dim] NK cells. Release of chemokines (MIP-1α/β, RANTES) in response to activating receptor engagement typically occurs more rapidly than IFN-γ or TNF production. In addition, engagement of individual receptors can suffice for chemokine release, whereas the engagement of multiple receptors is generally required for IFN-γ and TNF production.[44]

Functional Immune Cross Talk: Natural Killer Cells Interact With a Broad Array of Immune Partners

NK cells interact with other members of the immune system either indirectly, via the release of cytokines and chemokines, or directly, via cell-cell interactions.[45] NK cells interact directly with DCs, macrophages, and T cells. NK cells are activated by mature DC–derived cytokines and cellular contact in the paracortical areas of lymphoid tissue. In addition, NK cells appear to have a role in DC editing and can selectively kill immature DCs, likely as a result of their lower MHC class I expression. Similarly, macrophages secrete pro-inflammatory cytokines that stimulate NK cells, and activated NK cells can edit the macrophage pool, selectively killing M0 and M2 macrophages but sparing M1. In addition to interacting with other innate immune cells, there is also cross talk between NK and T cells. NK cells contribute to the resolution of adaptive immune responses by killing activated T cells that upregulate NKG2D ligands. In addition, NK cells are principal producers of IFN-γ, which promotes T$_H$1 polarization, along with other important immune functions like MHC class II upregulation and macrophage activation. Other NK cell-derived cytokines and chemokines that modulate the immune system are MIP-1α and β, which activate and recruit granulocytes along with promoting the synthesis of pro-inflammatory cytokines, RANTES, which is chemotactic for T cells, basophils, and eosinophils, and TNF, which participates in multiple antitumor and antiviral functions along with mediating systemic inflammatory responses.

Natural Killer Cell Memory

Immunologic memory, or the ability to respond more quickly and robustly upon re-exposure to a target, is typically not a property attributed to innate immune cells (*Figure 14.6*). However, recently, paradigm-shifting evidence has emerged demonstrating that NK cells can indeed display memory-like properties in response to certain stimuli. The first such evidence came from mouse models, where murine NK cells were shown to display antigen-specific memory-like responses following stimulation with specific haptens or viruses, and

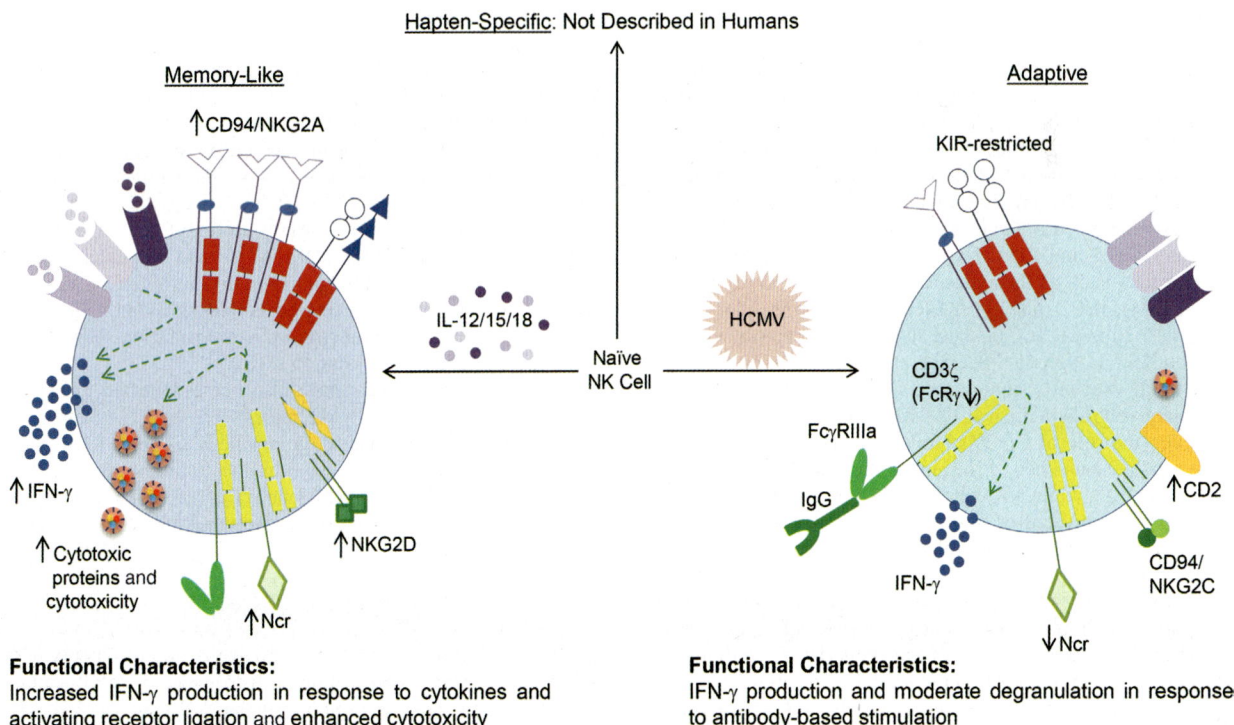

Functional Characteristics:
Increased IFN-γ production in response to cytokines and activating receptor ligation and enhanced cytotoxicity

Functional Characteristics:
IFN-γ production and moderate degranulation in response to antibody-based stimulation

FIGURE 14.6 **Types of human natural killer (NK) cell memory.** Human NK cells have been shown to display memory-type responses following infection with human cytomegalovirus (HCMV) or combined cytokine preactivation. HCMV infection expands mature, NKG2C+ NK cells with a restricted killer cell immunoglobulin-like receptor (KIR) repertoire. These cells show increased expression of CD2 but decreased expression of natural cytotoxicity receptors (NKp30, NKp46) and downregulate the intracellular adaptor FcRγ. Functionally, HCMV-adaptive NK cells appear specialized toward interferon (IFN)-γ production in response to antibody-dependent stimulation. In contrast, IL-12/15/18 preactivation results in the differentiation of cytokine-induced memory-like NK cells, which show increased CD94/NKG2A expression, along with increased levels of numerous different activating receptors. Memory-like NK cells produce enhanced IFN-γ in response to cytokine or activating receptor stimulation than naïve NK cells and are more robustly cytotoxic. Promising results have been identified in early-phase clinical trials.[46] IL, interleukin.

non–antigen-specific responses following combined cytokine preactivation.[47] Similar properties have more recently been described for human NK cells and are described in more detail here.

Human cytokine-induced memory-like NK cells differentiate following short-term stimulation with the cytokines IL-12, 15, and 18. These memory-like cells are long-lived and display enhanced cytokine production as well as cytotoxicity upon restimulation with tumor targets in vitro and in vivo.[46,48] Furthermore, the enhanced responsiveness of these memory-like cells is preserved with cell division. Cytokine-induced memory-like NK cells appear to be less sensitive to KIR-based inhibitory signaling but show increased levels of the inhibitory receptor NKG2A. Memory-like NK cells also upregulate certain activating receptors, including NKG2D, NKp46, and NKp30.

A different type of NK cell memory has been described in response to human cytomegalovirus (HCMV) infection.[26] These HCMV-adaptive NK cells are phenotypically mature, KIR-restricted, and usually express the activating receptor NKG2C. Adaptive NK cells also express higher levels of the costimulatory molecule CD2 but lower levels of activating receptors like NKp46 and NKp30. In addition, adaptive NK cells express altered levels of intracellular signaling adapters, which appears to bias them toward FcγRIIIa responsiveness and toward IFN-γ production over cytotoxicity. A similar population has also been described in mice in response to murine cytomegalovirus (MCMV) infection, whereby the Ly49H receptor on a subset of murine NK cells (analogous to KIRs on human NK cells) binds to the m157 viral protein encoded by MCMV, leading to NK cell activation and a memory-like response upon re-exposure to MCMV infection.[49] The physiological roles, developmental biology, and molecular regulation of both types of memory-like NK cells are subjects of ongoing investigation, and their therapeutic potential is being actively explored.

TYPE 1 INNATE LYMPHOID CELLS

Group 1 ILCs are defined by their ability to produce IFN-γ and shared dependence on Tbx21 (TBET, i.e., T-box expressed in T cells) for appropriate maturation and function.[1] Unlike NK cells, however, ILC1s, in general, do not depend on EOMES or express perforin and granzymes—and are largely noncytotoxic helper ILCs.[50] Among all of the ILCs, human ILC1s are perhaps the most challenging to identify due to the lack of at least one specific marker that can consistently positively distinguish them from NK cells or other helper ILC subsets. In lieu of a positive identifier, ILC1s in humans are generally recognized as Lin− cells expressing the common ILC surface proteins CD161 and CD127 but lacking all other ILC subset-specific identifiers such as those used for NK cells (CD16, NKp80, KIRs, and CD94), ILC2 (CD294, KLRG1), and ILC3 (CD117, IL-1R1, NKp44).[51] In mice, ILC1s share many cell receptors with NK cells, such as NK1.1, NKp46, NKG2D, and Ly49, making their distinction difficult. Recently, the surface marker CD200r1 has been shown to selectively distinguish ILC1s from NK cells in the murine liver; however, the role of CD200r1 in the identification of human ILC1s is yet to be established.[52] In some instances, ILC1s have been described as CD49a+, while NK cells are CD49b+; but, as CD49a can be upregulated on activated or tissue-resident NK cells, this is not entirely specific and is likely not a reliable marker for distinguishing between NK cells and ILC1s in many disease settings.[16,50] Within the murine liver, a CD49a+CD49b−Eomes− population identified as ILC1s was also shown to not be able to give rise to Eomes+ tissue-resident NK cells.[53] Interestingly, these cells did have cytotoxic potential largely through TRAIL-mediated killing, but these cells also expressed granzymes and perforin. Similar subsets of ILC1s were also discovered in salivary glands and could be identified by CD103 expression.[54]

Clinically, ILC1s have been shown to be expanded and activated in chronic obstructive pulmonary disease (COPD), inflammatory bowel diseases such as Crohn, and acute myeloid leukemia (AML).[55,56] Two distinct locations and types of human ILC1s have been described in the gut, including a CD161+CD127+NKp44− subset

that exists in the lamina propria and a separate intraepithelial NKp44+CD103+CD127− subset.[57] Tissue obtained from Crohn patients has shown expansion of ILC1s within the lamina propria which correlated with disease severity.[58] Patients with COPD similarly showed elevated numbers of ILC1s.[59] In both COPD and Crohn, the expansion of ILC1s seemed to correlate with simultaneous decreases of ILC2s in COPD and NCR+ ILC3s in the setting of Crohn disease.[60] These observations led to the discovery that ILC2s and ILC3s are plastic and can differentiate into ILC1s with the assistance of IL-12, IL-15, or IL-18 stimulation.[34] In patients with AML, ILC1s (Lin−CD56+CD94+CD16−TBET+EOMES^Lo/−) were found to be enriched and hypofunctional in the leukemic bone marrow, which was recapitulated using AML mouse models.[56] Similarly, synergism between IL-15 and TGFβ signaling has been shown to promote an ILC1 phenotype in part through intratumoral conversion of mature NK cells into ILC1-like cells, which promotes tumor immune evasion in solid tumor models.[61-63] Thus, ILC1s may possess some pro-tumorigenic functions, although separating direct pro-tumorigenic functions of ILC1s from the effects of reduced immunosurveillance through NK cell inhibition requires further investigation. Promotion of NK cell conversion into an ILC1-like phenotype has also been observed in nonalcoholic fatty liver disease (NAFLD). Patients with NAFLD demonstrated reduced degranulation of the CD3−CD56+TBET^HiEOMES^Lo population upon exposure to tumor targets. The degree of hypofunctionality correlated with the level of inflammation and steatosis present. The TGFβ pathway was also implicated in promoting conversion in this disease setting.[64]

Aside from their potential roles in pathological states, the physiological importance of ILC1s has been well established in mice, with liver-resident ILC1s having been shown to be critical for the clearance of MCMV infection.[52] Mice deficient in Zfp683 (encoding the transcription factor Hobit, leading to loss of liver ILC1s) had significantly higher viral titers of MCMV and worse overall survival compared to WT mice or mice who lacked NK cells but retained ILC1s.

ILC1s also play an important role in providing host protection against multiple intestinal organisms. TBET-deficient mice that lack ILC1s and have normal NK cell numbers were shown to be susceptible to *Toxoplasma gondii* infection.[8] These results suggest a critical role in ILC1s in defending against Toxoplasma, although due to impairment of NK cell migration, the phenotype cannot be exclusively attributed to ILC1s. Acute responses against *Clostridium difficile* were shown to be ILC dependent as Rag1−/−IL-2Rγ−/− mice were much more susceptible to *C. difficile* than Rag1−/− alone mice.[60] In addition, both Rag1−/−TBET−/− and Rag1−/−IFN-γ−/− mice had much more severe disease and higher mortality compared to controls. ILC1-derived IFN-γ also serves to protect murine hosts against Salmonella infections, likely by stimulating protective mucus formation. However, these mice also had enterocolitis due to IFN-γ.[65]

CD103+CD49a+ ILC1s have also been identified to expand and regulate tumor growth in PyMT mice.[66] These ILC1s expressed cytolytic granules such as perforin, granzyme B, C, and TRAIL, and were able to mediate tumor cell lysis. Similar to the hepatic ILC1s, these developed independent of Nfil-3 but required IL-15. Overexpression of IL-15 was able to slow tumor growth, whereas IL-15 depletion accelerated it.

TYPE 2 INNATE LYMPHOID CELLS

ILC2s are identified by their specific expression of CD294 (CRTH2) and KLRG1 in addition to common ILC markers CD161 (in humans) and CD127 (in both mice and humans).[1] ILC2s are dependent on the transcription factors GATA-3 and RAR-related orphan receptor (ROR)α for proper development and functional maturation. ILC2s are classically stimulated by IL-25 and IL-33 to produce primarily IL-5, TSLP, and IL-13. Consistent with their original discovery in murine gut, ILC2s were initially proven to be an important immune mediator in generating an appropriate anti-helminth response as was demonstrated against *Nippostrongylus brasiliensis*.[67]

Subsequent to their identification in gut, ILC2s have now been described in skin, liver, adipose tissue, and lung with unique functions.[68] In the lungs and airway-associated soft tissues, ILC2s contribute to the pathology underlying asthma, COPD, sinusitis, fibrosis, and even epithelial repair following viral infections such as with respiratory syncytial virus. Elevated IL-33 and IL-25 in addition to increased numbers of ILC2s, both in humans and mice, have been shown to be an important component of inflammation in asthma.[69] Rag2$^{-/-}$IL-2R$\gamma^{-/-}$ mice had less inflammation compared to Rag2$^{-/-}$ mice alone. Furthermore, the inflammatory response was rescued in the Rag2$^{-/-}$IL-2R$\gamma^{-/-}$ mice when ILC2s were reconstituted.[55]

Allergen-provoked reactions are also ILC2 mediated, as mice deficient in ILC2s were unable to mount a response to the allergen papain.[70] Part of these responses are thought to be due to ILC2-mediated recruitment of activated DCs that drive T$_H$2 cell differentiation and recruitment through CC-chemokine ligand 17 (CCL17) release.[70] Patients with chronic sinusitis showed higher levels of ILC2s compared to nonallergic donors, further suggesting their involvement in reactive airway diseases.[71] Activated ILC2s and elevated IL-13 levels within the lung tissue have been linked to lung inflammation and fibrosis. Indeed, bronchial alveolar lavage fluid from patients with idiopathic pulmonary fibrosis was shown to have more ILC2s than that from healthy controls.[72] Similarly, patients with systemic sclerosis with pulmonary involvement had higher numbers of peripheral blood ILC2s.[73]

In the skin, ILC2s have been implicated in atopic dermatitis and wound healing. The number of circulating and blister-resident ILC2s in patients with atopic dermatitis was increased in addition to the ILC2-activating cytokines TSLP, IL-33, and IL-25.[74] In Rag1$^{-/-}$ mice, treatment with MC903, an agent capable of mimicking atopic dermatitis reactions, induced elevated levels of activated intradermal ILC2s. ILC2s were proven to be an important component of this inflammatory response, as mice treated with ILC2-depleting antibodies had a significantly impaired skin thickening and ILC2 cytokine response.[75] ILC2-derived IL-33 is an important factor in cutaneous wound healing, as IL-33-deficient mice were shown to have impaired wound closure.[76] Addition of exogenous IL-33 was able to restore proper wound healing through ILC2 activation in the skin.

In the liver, ILC2s have also been shown to be a component of hepatitis in both chemical and infectious models. In particular, hepatic inflammation induced by concanavalin A caused increased IL-33 and ILC2 expansion.[77] Depletion of ILC2s attenuated hepatic injury, whereas adoptive transfer of ILC2s strengthened the inflammatory response in the liver. Chronic hepatitis causes fibrosis, and recent studies have suggested that ILC2-propagated IL-13 may be a critical catalyst to this reaction by causing transdifferentiation of stellate cells needed for pathologic remodeling and fibrosis.[78]

ILC2s, particularly those that produce IL-5, are also an important regulator of metabolism in adipose tissue. These ILCs have the capacity to recruit macrophages and eosinophils that help to promote conversion of white adipose tissue to beige adipose tissue, resulting in the thermogenic release of energy as opposed to storage.[79] Collectively, the coordinated efforts of ILC2s appear to be protective against obesity and obesity-related morbidities such as insulin resistance and type 2 diabetes. Indeed, mice lacking ILC2s and fed a high-fat diet were much more susceptible to insulin resistance and increased white adipose tissue.[80]

TYPE 3 INNATE LYMPHOID CELLS

ILC3s are defined in humans by their surface expression of CD117 (c-kit), IL-1R1, CD161, CD127, NKp44, and the absence of CD94.[1] It was previously believed that both NKp44$^+$ and NKp44$^-$ ILC3s existed in humans; however, emerging data now suggest that NKp44$^+$ ILC3s represent a bona fide ILC3 population whereas "NKp44$^-$ ILC3s" in humans contain a mix of cell populations including precursors and NK cell subsets.[22,81,82] Heterogeneous populations of ILC3s have been identified by their expression of NKp46 in mice (NCR+ ILC3s), the expression of which correlates with TBET and

IFN-γ expression in addition to signature ILC3 transcription factors and cytokines.[57] ILC3s have been defined as expressing high levels of the transcription factors RORγt and the aryl hydrocarbon receptor (AHR). In response to IL-1β and IL-23, ILC3s produce IL-17A and IL-22. They exist most extensively in secondary lymphoid tissues such as Peyer's patches and intestinal lymphoid follicles, and functionally ILC3s help to maintain healthy gut flora in addition to having roles in the airway and skin.[68]

Within the intestines, ILC3s act through IL-22 to stimulate intestinal stem cells to regenerate epithelial cells.[83] This relationship has proven to be essential in patients with damaged epithelium secondary to chemotherapy or methotrexate. In addition, IL-22 promotes tolerance of commensal flora in humans and mice. Indeed, mice deficient in IL-22 producing ILC3s resulted in compromised epithelial protection and dissemination of *Alcaligenes xylosoxidans* that was reversed with exogenous IL-22 administration.[84] Murine ILC3s have also been shown to be protective against *Citrobacter rodentium*, although this role is not unique and has been shown to be similar to responses by T cells.[85] Human ILC3s can also help to protect against Helicobacter sp., *C. difficile*, and even *Candida albicans*.[55]

ILC3s have an important and nonredundant role in noninfectious inflammatory bowel diseases. IL-17A-producing NCR-ILC3s have been shown to be more abundant in patients with Crohn disease.[58] Contrary to expectations, IL-17A has actually been shown to have a protective role in the gut. Indeed, clinical studies in patients with Crohn disease of an IL-17A-neutralizing antibody, secukinumab, showed that those who received the drug were susceptible to inflammatory and infectious adverse events compared to those receiving placebo.[86] Thus, it is possible that ILC3s actually are increased to promote intestinal health in the face of the pathologic and inflammatory processes in Crohn, although this has yet to be tested. Recently, ILC3s have been shown to promote gut tolerance via secretion of IL-2, leading to stimulation of regulatory T cell (Treg) populations that are important in limiting autoimmune T-cell responses. ILC3-derived IL-2 was found to be decreased in the gut of Crohn disease patients, which correlated with lower Treg frequency and increased auto-inflammation.[87]

Intradermal ILC3s are also an important component of psoriasis, with plaques and lesions enriched with inflammatory infiltrates. Peripheral blood of patients with psoriasis has been notable for elevated numbers of ILC3s that correspondingly decrease following anti-inflammatory treatments such as with TNF neutralizing agents.[88,89] ILC3s are certainly not alone in this disease process, as $\gamma\delta$ T cells have also been demonstrated to release IL-17A, IL-17F, and IL-22 that are crucial to the disease progression.[28] Mechanistically, these cytokines are thought to recruit neutrophils that are a primary component of the inflammatory process. Psoriatic disease can also include an arthritic component, and synovial fluid from joints of affected patients showed increased numbers of ILC3s, further suggesting their role in the disease process.[90]

CLINICAL RELEVANCE AND APPLICATIONS OF NATURAL KILLER CELLS AND INNATE LYMPHOID CELLS IN HEMATOLOGY

The clinical importance of NK cells in hematologic malignancies has been well established. A subset of patients with AML have been found to possess developmentally inhibited and hypofunctional peripheral NK cells, marked by low levels of KIR and CD57 expression, which correlate with faster disease progression and lower overall survival compared with patients with intact NK development.[91] This developmental blockade has been found to be the result, at least in part, of aberrant activation of the AHR pathway in NK cell precursors by AML-derived AHR agonists, leading to induction of microRNAs that negatively regulate many of the genes and transcription factors required for normal NK cell development.[92] Furthermore, the NK cells of AML patients often have increased expression of the inhibitory receptor NKG2A, leading to functional suppression, which correlates with worse prognosis.[93] The finding of dysfunctional or dysregulated NK cells is not unique to patients with AML; it has also been described in other hematologic malignancies including CLL and multiple myeloma.[94,95] Thus, studying the pathways utilized by cancer cells to evade NK cell killing in order to design targeted therapies to restore the functional NK cell pool is an active area of research.

The inherent antitumor function of NK cells has been actively utilized clinically, first in the setting of allogeneic hematopoietic cell transplantation (HCT), and more recently in the form of adoptive cellular therapy. Although T cells are also critical mediators of graft-vs-leukemia responses, they can also cause graft-vs-host disease (GVHD), wherein allogeneic T cells attack normal host tissues. More importantly, NK cells do not directly cause GVHD and may even protect against this immune reaction.[96] Initial evidence for NK cell graft-vs-leukemia responses in vivo arose from MHC-haploidentical, T-cell-depleted HCT for AML therapy. Here, NK cell alloreactivity against AML blasts was associated with improved long-term disease-free survival.[97,98] Since then, several studies have conclusively demonstrated that donor KIR haplotype influences long-term HCT outcomes in AML patients.[99-101] Specifically, the KIR B haplotype, which contains a predominance of activating KIR, contributes to relapse protection and improved survival compared to the largely inhibitory A haplotype.[100] Subsequent studies identified specific activating KIRs (KIR2DS1) that are protective against AML relapse.[101]

In addition to administering NK cells in the form of HCT, several groups are investigating the clinical potential of adoptive NK cell therapy. Early studies in patients with relapsed/refractory AML consisted of enriched related-donor allogeneic (MHC-haploidentical) NK cell infusions supported by exogenous IL-2 administration. These studies demonstrated the safety, feasibility, and preliminary ability of such NK cell products to induce complete remissions.[102,103] These studies stimulated interest in NK cell therapy, and several groups are actively investigating strategies to enhance the in vivo antitumor functionality of adoptively transferred NK cells. One approach involves combined cytokine preactivation of NK cells prior to infusion, leading to the generation of memory-like NK cells with enhanced antitumor responses in vivo.[46] Alternately, other groups are seeking to expand adaptive NK cells, akin to those that expand in response to CMV, for infusion into patients. Activating and expanding NK cells by incubating them with K562 feeder cells expressing membrane-bound IL-21 before adoptive transfer has also been explored for NK cell therapy in phase 1 clinical trials with low incidences of infusion related reactions observed.[104] The promising results from this trial has led to a phase 2 clinical trial with CSTD002, a product derived from haploidentical donor NK cells and expanded ex vivo using plasma membrane (PM21) nanoparticles bearing membrane-bound IL-21 and 4-1BBL.[105] Clinical outcomes from these and other studies will be of substantial interest to the field. Moreover, a number of immunostimulatory cytokine strategies have been promising in preclinical studies (IL-12, IL-15, IL-18, IL-21), and safe in early-phase clinical trials (IL-15), and can expand, once activated, and restore function to endogenous NK cells.[32,106]

Besides modifying an adoptively transferred NK cell's inherent threshold for antitumor activity, antitumor responses can also be enhanced by modulating activating and inhibitory receptor signals received in vivo. Ongoing clinical trials are investigating the use of antibodies against NK cell inhibitory receptors (KIR and NKG2A). With reduced inhibitory signals, NK cells would be biased toward activation upon encountering a target cell expressing activating receptor ligands. With regards to activating receptors, FcγRIIIa is highly useful clinically since its ligation alone can activate NK cell effector functions, and it can also be used to target NK cells toward antibody-opsonized targets. The combination of NK cells and tumor antigen-targeting antibodies is also being actively investigated in the clinical setting. Next-generation protein-engineering strategies are

also being tested, including bispecific killer cell engagers, which, similar to bispecific T-cell engagers, link NK cell activation via activating receptors (e.g., CD16) to a tumor-restricted marker (e.g., CD19). Finally, NK cells can be engineered to express chimeric antigen receptors (CARs), another way to specifically target them to a cell of interest. CARs consist of an extracellular region recognizing a specific antigen (single-chain functional variable fragment, or scFv; Chapter 13), a transmembrane domain, and an intracellular portion with NK-cell-activating signaling domains such as CD3ζ (with newer-generation CARs also containing additional costimulatory signaling domains such as CD28, 4-1BB, or OX40). CD33-CAR NK-92 cells have been engineered and tested in phase 1 clinical trials for patients with relapsed/refractory AML, with no dose-limiting toxicities observed at up to 5 billion cells per patient.[107] Additionally, CD19-CAR NK cells derived from cord blood have shown promising results in patients with CD19-expressing B-cell malignancies, such as CLL or DLBCL, and also did not demonstrate dose-limiting toxicities.[108,109] Although the clinical effectiveness of CAR NK cells requires additional investigation in phase 2 and 3 trials, NK cells thus far have shown less toxicity compared with counterpart T-cell therapies and theoretically should have reduced CAR escape secondary to activating NK cell receptor expression. Thus, NK cell-based cancer immunotherapy is a rapidly expanding and highly promising field, fueled by the intricate and flexible nature of the NK cell anticancer program. Strategies to enhance NK cell anticancer responses are shown in *Figure 14.7*, and several concurrent NK cell immunotherapy strategies will likely be needed to optimize NK cells as anticancer effectors.

Although rare, hematologic malignancies with an NK cell origin have been described. According to the classification of NK cell disorders from the World Health Organization, there are five main NK-cell malignancies: NK-lymphoblastic leukemia/lymphoma, chronic lymphoproliferative disorder of NK cells, aggressive NK cell leukemia, Epstein-Barr virus (EBV)-positive NK cell lymphoproliferative disease of childhood, and extranodal NK/T cell lymphoma nasal type. Many of these NK cell malignancies are driven by prior infection of the EBV and are most prevalently found in Asia and South America for currently unknown reasons. The prognosis for patients with EBV-associated NK malignancies is poor, and the paucity of cases has resulted in poorly defined standards of care, although chemotherapy and frontline radiotherapy have shown some degree of efficacy in early-stage disease.[122] Thus, much more research must be done to understand the biology of these diseases to design and test targeted therapies.

The clinical importance of non-NK cell ILCs in hematology is a burgeoning topic in the field that has garnered great interest among researchers.[82] TGFβ has been found to functionally impair ILC1-like cells in patients with AML that is restored upon disease remission.[123] Furthermore, another study found enrichment of ILC1s, which also exhibited hypofunctional activity, in the bone marrow of AML patients and mouse models.[56] Studies have demonstrated that ILC2s can promote progression of AML or APL via secretion of IL-5 or IL-13, which stimulate activity of Tregs and myeloid-derived suppressor cells (MDSCs), respectively.[124,125] Cancer or mesenchymal-derived prostaglandin D2 was found to be responsible for activation of ILC2s in this context via binding to the CRTH2 receptor on ILC2s. Other examples implicate ILCs in protection from GVHD that develops after allogeneic HCT.[126] Studies have identified that ILC3 production of IL-22 protects intestinal stem cells from immune-mediated tissue damage, thereby regulating the sensitivity to GVHD.[127] It has also been demonstrated that ILC2s are protective from acute GVHD by suppressing T_H1 and T_H17 responses via MDSC and Treg activation.[128] Additional studies show a role for ILCs in preserving T-cell development during experimental GVHD, and a correlation between activated ILCs and attenuated susceptibility to GVHD.[126,129] Ongoing studies will continue to unravel the role of ILCs in hematologic and immune diseases, and potential for ILC-based therapeutics.

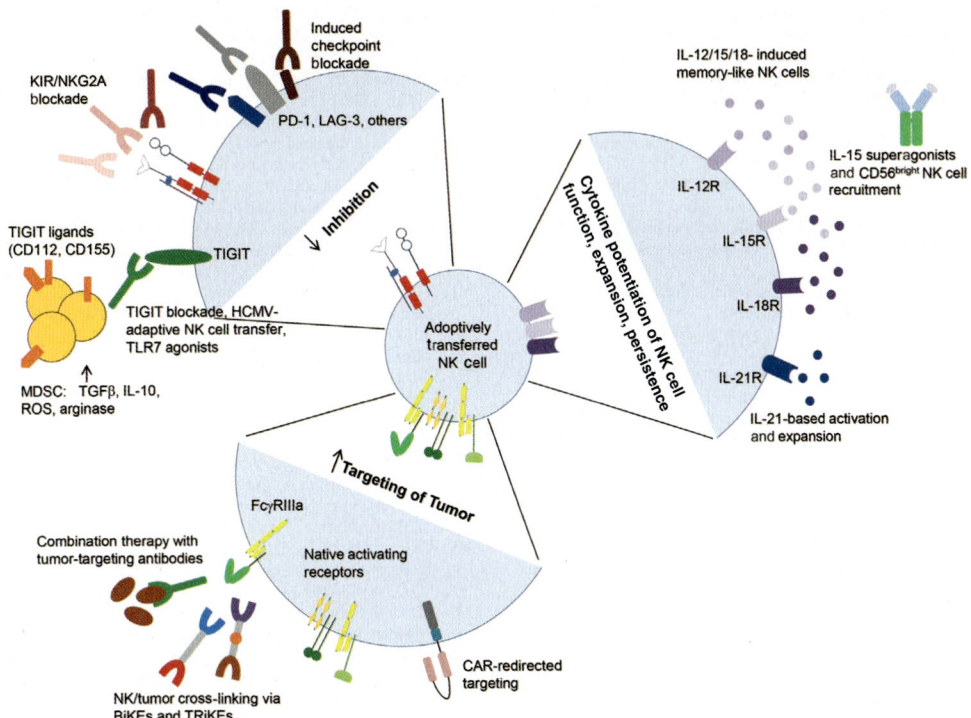

FIGURE 14.7 Strategies to enhance natural killer (NK) cell therapy for hematologic malignancies. Several strategies have been studied to enhance NK cell antitumor function in the clinical setting, including enhancing functional status (via cytokines and coactivating receptors), augmenting target cell recognition (targeting), and blockade of inhibition. One such strategy involves using cytokines to activate, expand, and promote the survival of adoptively transferred NK cells. This can be accomplished by IL-12/15/18 preactivation, leading to the generation of memory-like NK cells, currently under investigation in clinical trials (NCT01898793, NCT02782546).[46] In addition, cytokines like IL-15 can be used to enhance the cytotoxicity of typically noncytotoxic NK cell populations, such as CD56[bright] NK cells.[33,34] Since IL-15 is the key cytokine for NK cell homeostasis and function, efforts have also been made to design enhanced IL-15 drugs with improved in vivo potency and persistence. Additional cytokines such as IL-21 are also being explored for their potential to expand NK cells with preserved, enhanced antitumor function.[110] A second strategy involves limiting NK cell inhibitory signals. This can be accomplished via blockade of endogenously expressed inhibitory receptors like KIRs and NKG2A via antibodies such as monalizumab (anti-NKG2A) and lirilumab (anti-KIR2DL), whose promising preclinical studies have prompted several clinical trials (NCT02643550, NCT02557516, NCT02671435, NCT01714739).[111] In addition to endogenously expressed inhibitory receptors, NK cells upregulate inhibitory receptors such as PD-1, LAG-3, and TIM-3 upon activation to prevent uncontrolled immune responses. Blockade of induced checkpoint molecules is another approach to enhance NK responses, akin to recent successes with T-cell checkpoint blockade.[112-115] Finally, myeloid-derived suppressor cells and regulatory T cells within the tumor environment can suppress innate and adaptive immune cells via several mechanisms.[116-118] A third strategy centers on enhancing the ability of NK cells to effectively recognize and become activated by tumor targets. One approach is to guide NK cell antibody–dependent cellular cytotoxicity by administering therapeutic antibodies recognizing tumor-expressed ligands.[119] In addition, using bispecific and trispecific killer engagers (BiKEs, TRiKEs) that recognize FcγRIIIa as well as tumor antigens, NK cells can be specifically redirected toward tumor targets.[120] Finally, NK cells can be engineered to target an antigen of interest using chimeric antigen receptors, which consist of an extracellular antibody single-chain variable fragment fused to multiple intracellular signaling domains.[121] These trigger-enhancing strategies, whether alone or in combination, promise to enhance NK cell immunotherapeutic outcomes. CAR, chimeric antigen receptor; HCMV, human cytomegalovirus; KIRs, killer cell immunoglobulin-like receptors; MDSC, myeloid derived suppressor cells; ROS, reactive oxygen species; TGF, transforming growth factor; TIGIT, T-cell Ig and immunoreceptor tyrosine-based inhibitory motif domain.

ACKNOWLEDGMENTS

We acknowledge and thank the coauthors of the prior edition, Julia A. Wagner and Steven D. Scoville.

References

1. Spits H, Artis D, Colonna M, et al. Innate lymphoid cells–a proposal for uniform nomenclature. *Nat Rev Immunol.* 2013;13(2):145-149.
2. Diefenbach A, Colonna M, Koyasu S. Development, differentiation, and diversity of innate lymphoid cells. *Immunity.* 2014;41(3):354-365.
3. Georgopoulos K, Bigby M, Wang JH, et al. The Ikaros gene is required for the development of all lymphoid lineages. *Cell.* 1994;79(1):143-156.
4. Cao X, Shores EW, Hu-Li J, et al. Defective lymphoid development in mice lacking expression of the common cytokine receptor gamma chain. *Immunity.* 1995;2(3):223-238.
5. Galy A, Travis M, Cen D, et al. Human T, B, natural killer, and dendritic cells arise from a common bone marrow progenitor cell subset. *Immunity.* 1995;3(4):459-473.
6. Kondo M, Weissman IL, Akashi K. Identification of clonogenic common lymphoid progenitors in mouse bone marrow. *Cell.* 1997;91(5):661-672.
7. Yang Q, Li F, Harly C, et al. TCF-1 upregulation identifies early innate lymphoid progenitors in the bone marrow. *Nat Immunol.* 2015;16(10):1044-1050.
8. Klose CSN, Flach M, Möhle L, et al. Differentiation of type 1 ILCs from a common progenitor to all helper-like innate lymphoid cell lineages. *Cell.* 2014;157(2):340-356.
9. Constantinides MG, McDonald BD, Verhoef PA, et al. A committed precursor to innate lymphoid cells. *Nature.* 2014;508(7496):397-401.
10. Seillet C, Mielke LA, Amann-Zalcenstein DB, et al. Deciphering the innate lymphoid cell transcriptional program. *Cell Rep.* 2016;17(2):436-447.
11. Renoux VM, Zriwil A, Peitzsch C, et al. Identification of a human natural killer cell lineage-restricted progenitor in fetal and adult tissues. *Immunity.* 2015;43(2):394-407.
12. Xu W, Cherrier DE, Chea S, et al. An Id2(RFP)-Reporter mouse redefines innate lymphoid cell precursor potentials. *Immunity.* 2019;50(4):1054-1068.e1053.
13. Walker JA, Clark PA, Crisp A, et al. Polychromic reporter mice reveal unappreciated innate lymphoid cell progenitor heterogeneity and elusive ILC3 progenitors in bone marrow. *Immunity.* 2019;51(1):104-118.e107.
14. Mundy-Bosse BL, Scoville SD, Chen L, et al. MicroRNA-29b mediates altered innate immune development in acute leukemia. *J Clin Invest.* 2016;126(12):4404-4416.
15. Freud AG, Caligiuri MA. Human natural killer cell development. *Immunol Rev.* 2006;214:56-72.
16. Freud AG, Mundy-Bosse BL, Yu J, et al. The broad spectrum of human natural killer cell diversity. *Immunity.* 2017;47(5):820-833.
17. Freud AG, Becknell B, Roychowdhury S, et al. A human CD34(+) subset resides in lymph nodes and differentiates into CD56bright natural killer cells. *Immunity.* 2005;22(3):295-304.
18. Chen L, Youssef Y, Robinson C, et al. CD56 expression marks human group 2 innate lymphoid cell divergence from a shared NK cell and group 3 innate lymphoid cell developmental pathway. *Immunity.* 2018;49(3):464-476.e464.
19. Lim AI, Li Y, Lopez-Lastra S, et al. Systemic human ILC precursors provide a substrate for tissue ILC differentiation. *Cell.* 2017;168(6):1086-1100.e1010.

20. Cooper MA, Fehniger TA, Caligiuri MA. The biology of human natural killer-cell subsets. *Trends Immunol.* 2001;22(11):633-640.

21. Dogra P, Rancan C, Ma W, et al. Tissue determinants of human NK cell development, function, and residence. *Cell.* 2020;180(4):749-763.e713.

22. Bal SM, Golebski K, Spits H. Plasticity of innate lymphoid cell subsets. *Nat Rev Immunol.* 2020;20(9):552-565.

23. Long EO, Kim HS, Liu D, et al. Controlling natural killer cell responses: integration of signals for activation and inhibition. *Annu Rev Immunol.* 2013;31:227-258.

24. Manser AR, Weinhold S, Uhrberg M. Human KIR repertoires: shaped by genetic diversity and evolution. *Immunol Rev.* 2015;267(1):178-196.

25. Davis ZB, Vallera DA, Miller JS, et al. Natural killer cells unleashed: checkpoint receptor blockade and BiKE/TriKE utilization in NK-mediated anti-tumor immunotherapy. *Semin Immunol.* 2017;31:64-75.

26. Rölle A, Brodin P. Immune adaptation to environmental influence: the case of NK cells and HCMV. *Trends Immunol.* 2016;37(3):233-243.

27. Nimmerjahn F, Ravetch JV. Fcgamma receptors as regulators of immune responses. *Nat Rev Immunol.* 2008;8(1):34-47.

28. Seidel UJ, Schlegel P, Lang P. Natural killer cell mediated antibody-dependent cellular cytotoxicity in tumor immunotherapy with therapeutic antibodies. *Front Immunol.* 2013;4:76.

29. de Andrade LF, Smyth MJ, Martinet L. DNAM-1 control of natural killer cells functions through nectin and nectin-like proteins. *Immunol Cell Biol.* 2014;92(3):237-244.

30. Chen S, Yang M, Du J, et al. The self-specific activation receptor SLAM family is critical for NK cell education. *Immunity.* 2016;45(2):292-304.

31. Dong Z, Davidson D, Pérez-Quintero LA, et al. The adaptor SAP controls NK cell activation by regulating the enzymes Vav-1 and SHIP-1 and by enhancing conjugates with target cells. *Immunity.* 2012;36(6):974-985.

32. Romee R, Leong JW, Fehniger TA. Utilizing cytokines to function-enable human NK cells for the immunotherapy of cancer. *Scientifica (Cairo).* 2014;2014:205796.

33. Wagner JA, Rosario M, Romee R, et al. CD56bright NK cells exhibit potent antitumor responses following IL-15 priming. *J Clin Invest.* 2017;127(11):4042-4058.

34. Dubois S, Conlon KC, Müller JR, et al. IL15 infusion of cancer patients expands the subpopulation of cytotoxic CD56(bright) NK cells and increases NK-cell cytokine release capabilities. *Cancer Immunol Res.* 2017;5(10):929-938.

35. Jonsson AH, Yokoyama WM. Natural killer cell tolerance licensing and other mechanisms. *Adv Immunol.* 2009;101:27-79.

36. Foley B, Felices M, Cichocki F, et al. The biology of NK cells and their receptors affects clinical outcomes after hematopoietic cell transplantation (HCT). *Immunol Rev.* 2014;258(1):45-63.

37. Yu J, Heller G, Chewning J, et al. Hierarchy of the human natural killer cell response is determined by class and quantity of inhibitory receptors for self-HLA-B and HLA-C ligands. *J Immunol.* 2007;179(9):5977-5989.

38. Marçais A, Marotel M, Degouve S, et al. High mTOR activity is a hallmark of reactive natural killer cells and amplifies early signaling through activating receptors. *Elife.* 2017;6:e26423.

39. Wang Z, Guan D, Wang S, et al. Glycolysis and oxidative phosphorylation play critical roles in natural killer cell receptor-mediated natural killer cell functions. *Front Immunol.* 2020;11:202.

40. Highton AJ, Diercks BP, Möckl F, et al. High metabolic function and resilience of NKG2A-educated NK cells. *Front Immunol.* 2020;11:559576.

41. Imai K, Matsuyama S, Miyake S, et al. Natural cytotoxic activity of peripheral-blood lymphocytes and cancer incidence: an 11-year follow-up study of a general population. *Lancet.* 2000;356(9244):1795-1799.

42. Mace EM, Dongre P, Hsu HT, et al. Cell biological steps and checkpoints in accessing NK cell cytotoxicity. *Immunol Cell Biol.* 2014;92(3):245-255.

43. Böttcher JP, Bonavita E, Chakravarty P, et al. NK cells stimulate recruitment of cDC1 into the tumor microenvironment promoting cancer immune control. *Cell.* 2018;172(5):1022-1037.e1014.

44. Fauriat C, Long EO, Ljunggren HG, et al. Regulation of human NK-cell cytokine and chemokine production by target cell recognition. *Blood.* 2010;115(11):2167-2176.

45. Malhotra A, Shanker A. NK cells: immune cross-talk and therapeutic implications. *Immunotherapy.* 2011;3(10):1143-1166.

46. Romee R, Rosario M, Berrien-Elliott MM, et al. Cytokine-induced memory-like natural killer cells exhibit enhanced responses against myeloid leukemia. *Sci Transl Med.* 2016;8(357):357ra123.

47. Min-Oo G, Kamimura Y, Hendricks DW, et al. Natural killer cells: walking three paths down memory lane. *Trends Immunol.* 2013;34(6):251-258.

48. Romee R, Schneider SE, Leong JW, et al. Cytokine activation induces human memory-like NK cells. *Blood.* 2012;120(24):4751-4760.

49. Min-Oo G, Lanier LL. Cytomegalovirus generates long-lived antigen-specific NK cells with diminished bystander activation to heterologous infection. *J Exp Med.* 2014;211(13):2669-2680.

50. Spits H, Bernink JH, Lanier L. NK cells and type 1 innate lymphoid cells: partners in host defense. *Nat Immunol.* 2016;17(7):758-764.

51. Scoville SD, Freud AG, Caligiuri MA. Modeling human natural killer cell development in the era of innate lymphoid cells. *Front Immunol.* 2017;8:360.

52. Weizman OE, Adams NM, Schuster IS, et al. ILC1 confer early host protection at initial sites of viral infection. *Cell.* 2017;171(4):795-808.e712.

53. Cortez VS, Colonna M. Diversity and function of group 1 innate lymphoid cells. *Immunol Lett.* 2016;179:19-24.

54. Fuchs A, Vermi W, Lee JS, et al. Intraepithelial type 1 innate lymphoid cells are a unique subset of IL-12- and IL-15-responsive IFN-γ-producing cells. *Immunity.* 2013;38(4):769-781.

55. Ebbo M, Crinier A, Vély F, et al. Innate lymphoid cells: major players in inflammatory diseases. *Nat Rev Immunol.* 2017;17(11):665-678.

56. Lordo MR, Wu KC, Altynova E, et al. Acute myeloid leukemia alters group 1 innate lymphoid cell differentiation from a common precursor. *J Immunol.* 2021;207(6):1672-1682.

57. Mjösberg J, Spits H. Human innate lymphoid cells. *J Allergy Clin Immunol.* 2016;138(5):1265-1276.

58. Bernink JH, Peters CP, Munneke M, et al. Human type 1 innate lymphoid cells accumulate in inflamed mucosal tissues. *Nat Immunol.* 2013;14(3):221-229.

59. Silver JS, Kearley J, Copenhaver AM, et al. Inflammatory triggers associated with exacerbations of COPD orchestrate plasticity of group 2 innate lymphoid cells in the lungs. *Nat Immunol.* 2016;17(6):626-635.

60. Abt MC, Lewis BB, Caballero S, et al. Innate immune defenses mediated by two ILC subsets are critical for protection against acute *Clostridium difficile* infection. *Cell Host Microbe.* 2015;18(1):27-37.

61. Gao Y, Souza-Fonseca-Guimaraes F, Bald T, et al. Tumor immunoevasion by the conversion of effector NK cells into type 1 innate lymphoid cells. *Nat Immunol.* 2017;18(9):1004-1015.

62. Cortez VS, Ulland TK, Cervantes-Barragan L, et al. SMAD4 impedes the conversion of NK cells into ILC1-like cells by curtailing non-canonical TGF-beta signaling. *Nat Immunol.* 2017;18(9):995-1003.

63. Hawke LG, Mitchell BZ, Ormiston ML. TGF-Beta and IL-15 synergize through MAPK pathways to drive the conversion of human NK cells to an innate lymphoid cell 1-like phenotype. *J Immunol.* 2020;204(12):3171-3181.

64. Cuff AO, Sillito F, Dertschnig S, et al. The obese liver environment mediates conversion of NK cells to a less cytotoxic ILC1-like phenotype. *Front Immunol.* 2019;10:2180.

65. Klose CS, Kiss EA, Schwierzeck V, et al. A T-bet gradient controls the fate and function of CCR6-RORgammat+ innate lymphoid cells. *Nature.* 2013;494(7436):261-265.

66. Dadi S, Chhangawala S, Whitlock BM, et al. Cancer immunosurveillance by tissue-resident innate lymphoid cells and innate-like T cells. *Cell.* 2016;164(3):365-377.

67. Moro K, Yamada T, Tanabe M, et al. Innate production of T(H)2 cytokines by adipose tissue-associated c-Kit(+)Sca-1(+) lymphoid cells. *Nature.* 2010;463(7280):540-544.

68. Ignacio A, Breda CNS, Camara NOS. Innate lymphoid cells in tissue homeostasis and diseases. *World J Hepatol.* 2017;9(23):979-989.

69. Kim HY, Umetsu DT, Dekruyff RH. Innate lymphoid cells in asthma: will they take your breath away? *Eur J Immunol.* 2016;46(4):795-806.

70. Halim TY, Krauss RH, Sun AC, et al. Lung natural helper cells are a critical source of Th2 cell-type cytokines in protease allergen-induced airway inflammation. *Immunity.* 2012;36(3):451-463.

71. Mjösberg JM, Trifari S, Crellin NK, et al. Human IL-25- and IL-33-responsive type 2 innate lymphoid cells are defined by expression of CRTH2 and CD161. *Nat Immunol.* 2011;12(11):1055-1062.

72. Hams E, Armstrong ME, Barlow JL, et al. IL-25 and type 2 innate lymphoid cells induce pulmonary fibrosis. *Proc Natl Acad Sci U S A.* 2014;111(1):367-372.

73. Wohlfahrt T, Usherenko S, Englbrecht M, et al. Type 2 innate lymphoid cell counts are increased in patients with systemic sclerosis and correlate with the extent of fibrosis. *Ann Rheum Dis.* 2016;75(3):623-626.

74. Salimi M, Barlow JL, Saunders SP, et al. A role for IL-25 and IL-33-driven type-2 innate lymphoid cells in atopic dermatitis. *J Exp Med.* 2013;210(13):2939-2950.

75. Kim BS, Siracusa MC, Saenz SA, et al. TSLP elicits IL-33-independent innate lymphoid cell responses to promote skin inflammation. *Sci Transl Med.* 2013;5(170):170ra116.

76. Rak GD, Osborne LC, Siracusa MC, et al. IL-33-Dependent group 2 innate lymphoid cells promote cutaneous wound healing. *J Invest Dermatol.* 2016;136(2):487-496.

77. Neumann K, Karimi K, Meiners J, et al. A proinflammatory role of type 2 innate lymphoid cells in murine immune-mediated hepatitis. *J Immunol.* 2017;198(1):128-137.

78. McHedlidze T, Waldner M, Zopf S, et al. Interleukin-33-dependent innate lymphoid cells mediate hepatic fibrosis. *Immunity.* 2013;39(2):357-371.

79. Flach M, Diefenbach A. Adipose tissue: ILC2 crank up the heat. *Cell Metabol.* 2015;21(2):152-153.

80. Brestoff JR, Kim BS, Saenz SA, et al. Group 2 innate lymphoid cells promote beiging of white adipose tissue and limit obesity. *Nature.* 2015;519(7542):242-246.

81. Vivier E, Artis D, Colonna M, et al. Innate lymphoid cells: 10 years on. *Cell.* 2018;174(5):1054-1066.

82. Lordo MR, Scoville SD, Goel A, et al. Unraveling the role of innate lymphoid cells in acute myeloid leukemia. *Cancers (Basel).* 2021;13(2):320.

83. Aparicio-Domingo P, Romera-Hernandez M, Karrich JJ, et al. Type 3 innate lymphoid cells maintain intestinal epithelial stem cells after tissue damage. *J Exp Med.* 2015;212(11):1783-1791.

84. Sonnenberg GF, Monticelli LA, Alenghat T, et al. Innate lymphoid cells promote anatomical containment of lymphoid-resident commensal bacteria. *Science.* 2012;336(6086):1321-1325.

85. Rankin LC, Girard-Madoux MJ, Seillet C, et al. Complementarity and redundancy of IL-22-producing innate lymphoid cells. *Nat Immunol.* 2016;17(2):179-186.

86. Hueber W, Sands BE, Lewitzky S, et al. Secukinumab, a human anti-IL-17A monoclonal antibody, for moderate to severe Crohn's disease: unexpected results of a randomised, double-blind placebo-controlled trial. *Gut.* 2012;61(12):1693-1700.

87. Zhou L, Chu C, Teng F, et al. Innate lymphoid cells support regulatory T cells in the intestine through interleukin-2. *Nature.* 2019;568(7752):405-409.

88. Villanova F, Flutter B, Tosi I, et al. Characterization of innate lymphoid cells in human skin and blood demonstrates increase of NKp44+ ILC3 in psoriasis. *J Invest Dermatol.* 2014;134(4):984-991.

89. Teunissen MBM, Munneke JM, Bernink JH, et al. Composition of innate lymphoid cell subsets in the human skin: enrichment of NCR(+) ILC3 in lesional skin and blood of psoriasis patients. *J Invest Dermatol.* 2014;134(9):2351-2360.

90. Leijten EF, van Kempen TS, Boes M, et al. Brief report: enrichment of activated group 3 innate lymphoid cells in psoriatic arthritis synovial fluid. *Arthritis Rheumatol.* 2015;67(10):2673-2678.

91. Chretien AS, Fauriat C, Orlanducci F, et al. Natural killer defective maturation is associated with adverse clinical outcome in patients with acute myeloid leukemia. *Front Immunol.* 2017;8:573.

92. Scoville SD, Nalin AP, Chen L, et al. Human AML activates the aryl hydrocarbon receptor pathway to impair NK cell development and function. *Blood.* 2018;132(17):1792-1804.

93. Stringaris K, Sekine T, Khoder A, et al. Leukemia-induced phenotypic and functional defects in natural killer cells predict failure to achieve remission in acute myeloid leukemia. *Haematologica.* 2014;99(5):836-847.

94. MacFarlane AW, Jillab M, Smith MR, et al. NK cell dysfunction in chronic lymphocytic leukemia is associated with loss of the mature cells expressing inhibitory killer cell Ig-like receptors. *OncoImmunology.* 2017;6(7):e1330235.

95. Pittari G, Vago L, Festuccia M, et al. Restoring natural killer cell immunity against multiple myeloma in the era of new drugs. *Front Immunol.* 2017;8:1444.

96. Olson JA, Leveson-Gower DB, Gill S, et al. NK cells mediate reduction of GVHD by inhibiting activated, alloreactive T cells while retaining GVT effects. *Blood.* 2010;115(21):4293-4301.

97. Ruggeri L, Capanni M, Urbani E, et al. Effectiveness of donor natural killer cell alloreactivity in mismatched hematopoietic transplants. *Science.* 2002;295(5562):2097-2100.

98. Velardi A, Ruggeri L, Mancusi A, et al. Natural killer cell allorecognition of missing self in allogeneic hematopoietic transplantation: a tool for immunotherapy of leukemia. *Curr Opin Immunol.* 2009;21(5):525-530.

99. Cooley S, Trachtenberg E, Bergemann TL, et al. Donors with group B KIR haplotypes improve relapse-free survival after unrelated hematopoietic cell transplantation for acute myelogenous leukemia. *Blood.* 2009;113(3):726-732.

100. Cooley S, Weisdorf DJ, Guethlein LA, et al. Donor selection for natural killer cell receptor genes leads to superior survival after unrelated transplantation for acute myelogenous leukemia. *Blood.* 2010;116(14):2411-2419.

101. Venstrom JM, Pittari G, Gooley TA, et al. HLA-C-dependent prevention of leukemia relapse by donor activating KIR2DS1. *N Engl J Med.* 2012;367(9):805-816.

102. Rubnitz JE, Inaba H, Ribeiro RC, et al. NKAML: a pilot study to determine the safety and feasibility of haploidentical natural killer cell transplantation in childhood acute myeloid leukemia. *J Clin Oncol.* 2010;28(6):955-959.

103. Miller JS, Soignier Y, Panoskaltsis-Mortari A, et al. Successful adoptive transfer and in vivo expansion of human haploidentical NK cells in patients with cancer. *Blood.* 2005;105(8):3051-3057.

104. Ciurea SO, Schafer JR, Bassett R, et al. Phase 1 clinical trial using mbIL21 ex vivo-expanded donor-derived NK cells after haploidentical transplantation. *Blood.* 2017;130(16):1857-1868.

105. Vasu S, Bejanyan N, Devine S, et al. BMT CTN 1803: haploidentical natural killer cells (CSTD002) to prevent post-transplant relapse in AML and MDS (NK-REALM). *Blood.* 2019;134(suppl 1):1955.

106. Romee R, Cooley S, Berrien-Elliott MM, et al. First-in-human phase 1 clinical study of the IL-15 superagonist complex ALT-803 to treat relapse after transplantation. *Blood.* 2018;131(23):2515-2527.

107. Tang X, Yang L, Li Z, et al. First-in-man clinical trial of CAR NK-92 cells: safety test of CD33-CAR NK-92 cells in patients with relapsed and refractory acute myeloid leukemia. *Am J Cancer Res.* 2018;8(6):1083-1089.

108. Liu E, Marin D, Banerjee P, et al. Use of CAR-transduced natural killer cells in CD19-positive lymphoid tumors. *N Engl J Med.* 2020;382(6):545-553.

109. Liu E, Tong Y, Dotti G, et al. Cord blood NK cells engineered to express IL-15 and a CD19-targeted CAR show long-term persistence and potent antitumor activity. *Leukemia.* 2018;32(2):520-531.

110. Granzin M, Stojanovic A, Miller M, et al. Highly efficient IL-21 and feeder cell-driven ex vivo expansion of human NK cells with therapeutic activity in a xenograft mouse model of melanoma. *OncoImmunology.* 2016;5(9):e1219007.

111. McWilliams EM, Mele JM, Cheney C, et al. Therapeutic CD94/NKG2A blockade improves natural killer cell dysfunction in chronic lymphocytic leukemia. *OncoImmunology.* 2016;5(10):e1226720.

112. Stojanovic A, Fiegler N, Brunner-Weinzierl M, et al. CTLA-4 is expressed by activated mouse NK cells and inhibits NK Cell IFN-γ production in response to mature dendritic cells. *J Immunol.* 2014;192(9):4184-4191.

113. Callahan MK, Postow MA, Wolchok JD. Targeting T cell Co-receptors for cancer therapy. *Immunity.* 2016;44(5):1069-1078.

114. Huang BY, Zhan YP, Zong WJ, et al. The PD-1/B7-H1 pathway modulates the natural killer cells versus mouse glioma stem cells. *PLoS One.* 2015;10(8):e0134715.

115. Benson DM, Jr, Bakan CE, Mishra A, et al. The PD-1/PD-L1 axis modulates the natural killer cell versus multiple myeloma effect: a therapeutic target for CT-011, a novel monoclonal anti-PD-1 antibody. *Blood.* 2010;116(13):2286-2294.

116. Sarhan D, Cichocki F, Zhang B, et al. Adaptive NK cells with low TIGIT expression are inherently resistant to myeloid-derived suppressor cells. *Cancer Res.* 2016;76(19):5696-5706.

117. Liu LL, Pfefferle A, Yi Sheng VO, et al. Harnessing adaptive natural killer cells in cancer immunotherapy. *Mol Oncol.* 2015;9(10):1904-1917.

118. Spinetti T, Spagnuolo L, Mottas I, et al. TLR7-based cancer immunotherapy decreases intratumoral myeloid-derived suppressor cells and blocks their immunosuppressive function. *OncoImmunology.* 2016;5(11):e1230578.

119. Wang W, Erbe AK, Hank JA, et al. NK cell-mediated antibody-dependent cellular cytotoxicity in cancer immunotherapy. *Front Immunol.* 2015;6:368.

120. Felices M, Lenvik TR, Davis ZB, et al. Generation of BiKEs and TriKEs to improve NK cell-mediated targeting of tumor cells. *Methods Mol Biol.* 2016;1441:333-346.

121. Bollino D, Webb TJ. Chimeric antigen receptor-engineered natural killer and natural killer T cells for cancer immunotherapy. *Transl Res.* 2017;187:32-43.

122. Kwong YL. Natural killer-cell malignancies: diagnosis and treatment. *Leukemia.* 2005;19(12):2186-2194.

123. Salome B, Gomez-Cadena A, Loyon R, et al. CD56 as a marker of an ILC1-like population with NK cell properties that is functionally impaired in AML. *Blood Adv.* 2019;3(22):3674-3687.

124. Trabanelli S, Chevalier MF, Martinez-Usatorre A, et al. Tumour-derived PGD2 and NKp30-B7H6 engagement drives an immunosuppressive ILC2-MDSC axis. *Nat Commun.* 2017;8(1):593.

125. Wu L, Lin Q, Ma Z, et al. Mesenchymal PGD(2) activates an ILC2-Treg axis to promote proliferation of normal and malignant HSPCs. *Leukemia.* 2020;34(11):3028-3041.

126. Munneke JM, Björklund AT, Mjösberg JM, et al. Activated innate lymphoid cells are associated with a reduced susceptibility to graft-versus-host disease. *Blood.* 2014;124(5):812-821.

127. Hanash AM, Dudakov JA, Hua G, et al. Interleukin-22 protects intestinal stem cells from immune-mediated tissue damage and regulates sensitivity to graft versus host disease. *Immunity.* 2012;37(2):339-350.

128. Bruce DW, Stefanski HE, Vincent BG, et al. Type 2 innate lymphoid cells treat and prevent acute gastrointestinal graft-versus-host disease. *J Clin Invest.* 2017;127(5):1813-1825.

129. Dudakov JA, Mertelsmann AM, O'Connor MH, et al. Loss of thymic innate lymphoid cells leads to impaired thymopoiesis in experimental graft-versus-host disease. *Blood.* 2017;130(7):933-942.

The Normal Hematologic System

Chapter 15 ■ Major Histocompatibility Complex

QIUHENG JENNIFER ZHANG • MICHELLE HICKEY • MAXIM ROSARIO • NWE NWE SOE • CARRIE L. BUTLER • REBECCA A. SOSA • J. MICHAEL CECKA • ELAINE F. REED

INTRODUCTION

The major histocompatibility complex (MHC) is a tightly linked cluster of genes that appear to have evolved to maintain the individuality of members of vertebrate species. The genes and their products are key to the development of an adaptive immune response. The preservation of the gene complex through evolution suggests that there is a survival advantage to having these genes in close proximity to one another. Although the gene complex may serve functions that have yet to be described, its discovery through studies of tumor transplantation between inbred mouse strains initially focused investigators on its role in compatibility between cells (histocompatibility). The importance of the MHC in the field of human organ and tissue transplantation provided much of the early impetus for study, but new dimensions of infection, autoimmune disease, cancer, vaccine development, and more have propelled broader interests.

The human MHC encompasses approximately 3.6 Mb on chromosome 6p21.3 and contains about 253 functional genes and pseudogenes.[1,2] Nearly 40% of the genes and encoded molecules are involved in aspects of the immune response. MHC genes play an important role in regulating inflammation, the complement cascade, and the adaptive immune response. MHC alleles have been associated with more than 100 autoimmune diseases, including multiple sclerosis, type 1 diabetes, systemic lupus erythematosus, ulcerative colitis, celiac disease, Crohn disease, and rheumatoid arthritis. Many MHC genes are highly polymorphic, and differences in MHC molecules between a transplant or transfusion recipient and donor often provoke T-cell, B-cell, and NK-cell responses. Thus, MHC molecules are key targets of immune responses in transplantation and transfusion medicine. Matching human leukocyte antigens (HLAs) of the donor and recipient prolongs graft survival in most solid organ and all stem cell transplants. Patients exposed to allogeneic HLA antigens expressed on transfused blood cells, transplanted tissues, or through pregnancy may produce antibodies to HLAs, which are a major obstacle to transplantation of stem cells and solid organs. In this chapter, we review MHC genetics, polymorphism, structure, and function, with special focus on some of the lesser known, nonclassical MHC genes and antigens; the roles they may play; and their interactions with other genes and molecules of the human MHC.

GENETICS OF THE MAJOR HISTOCOMPATIBILITY COMPLEX

The mammalian MHC can be physically divided into three regions: MHC class I (telomeric) genes, MHC class II (centromeric) genes, and MHC class III genes.[3,4] In humans, the classical MHC antigens are called HLAs. The HLA class I region spans 1.6 Mb of DNA and is composed of highly polymorphic classical class I genes (*HLA-A, -B,* and *-C*), nonclassical class I genes (*HLA-E, -F,* and *-G*), class I–like genes (*MICA, MICB*), and other genes apparently not related to the immune system (*Figure 15.1*).

The HLA class II region spans 0.7 Mb DNA and contains genes that encode antigen-presenting molecules (*HLA-DR, -DQ,* and *-DP*), antigen-processing molecules (*HLA-DM* and *-DO*), immune proteasome genes (*LMP*), and TAP transporters associated with classical class I antigen loading. HLA-DR, DQ, and DP molecules present antigens to CD4 T lymphocytes. The *DM* and *DO* genes are not expressed on the cell surface but form heterotetrameric complexes involved in peptide exchange and loading onto DR, DQ, and DP molecules. The HLA-DR region contains one functional gene for the α chain (*DRA*) but has one or two functional genes for the β chain (*DRB1, DRB3, DRB4, DRB5*), depending on the *HLA-DRB1* allele type (*Figure 15.2*). The highly polymorphic *DRB1* alleles are present in all haplotypes. Based on the *DRB1* allele type and the *DRB3/4/5* gene content, human MHC haplotypes are grouped into four types. Individuals expressing *DRB1*15* or *DRB1*16* coexpress a *DRB5* gene encoding DR51. Individuals expressing *DRB1*11, DRB1*12, DRB1*13, DRB1*14,* or *DRB1*03* express a *DRB3* gene encoding DR52. Individuals expressing *DRB1*04, DRB1*07,* or *DRB1*09* express a *DRB4* gene encoding DR53. *DRB1*01, DRB1*08,* and *DRB1*10* are not usually associated with a second expressed DRB gene (*Figure 15.2*).

The HLA class III region located between the class I and class II regions is the most "gene-dense" region of the human genome and contains 75 loci with 0.9 Mb of DNA with many immune- and nonimmune-related genes that are highly conserved. The HLA class III region encodes proteins (C4, C2, CFB) that are essential for the complement activation pathways of the humoral immune responses. The tumor necrosis factor family (TNF, lymphotoxin α-LTα, lymphotoxin β-LTβ), which plays an important role in inflammation and infection, is also encoded in the class II region. Heat-shock proteins, a family of molecular chaperones induced by environmental stresses that provide a protective role for ischemia injury, oxidation stress, and inflammation are also encoded here.

Human Leukocyte Antigen Gene Polymorphism and Nomenclature

The human MHC is the most polymorphic region known to date in humans. MHC polymorphism results in a diverse array of antigen-presenting molecules within individuals and within the population and confers the ability to mount appropriate immune responses to pathogens. Early population studies using serologic typing methods identified an unprecedented number of HLAs at each locus. However, DNA sequencing has revealed an even more extensive polymorphism as the serologically defined antigens include multiple allelic variants that differ at one or more nucleotide residues. To date, 22,436 distinct HLA class I alleles and 8462 class II alleles have been recognized (IMGT/HLA database, version 3.45, July 2021).

The differences between HLA proteins are localized primarily to the extracellular region of these molecules, which bind peptides and interact with T-cell receptors. The high degree of HLA polymorphism is likely the result of positive selection for human survival by enhancing the diversity in the repertoire of HLA-bound peptides. HLA class I polymorphisms are predominantly found in the first 180 amino acids of the heavy chain, and the HLA class II polymorphisms are found in the first 90 to 95 amino acids of the α and/or β chains. The extensive allelic diversity at these loci is generated by point mutation, recombination, and gene conversion. Many substitutions are shared by more than one HLA allele and thus demonstrate a patchwork pattern of sequence polymorphisms, suggesting segmental exchanges may also play a role in generating diversity.

The HLA nomenclature can be daunting as the change from serological typing (which defines antigens) to DNA typing (which defines alleles) has resulted in some conflicts. The standard DNA nomenclature is illustrated in *Figure 15.3* and includes four fields (separated by a colon): the antigen (first field), allele group (second field), designation for silent substitutions (those that do not result in a change in the protein third field), and differences in noncoding regions (fourth field). In addition to the unique allele number, there are additional optional suffixes that may be added to an allele to indicate its expression status.

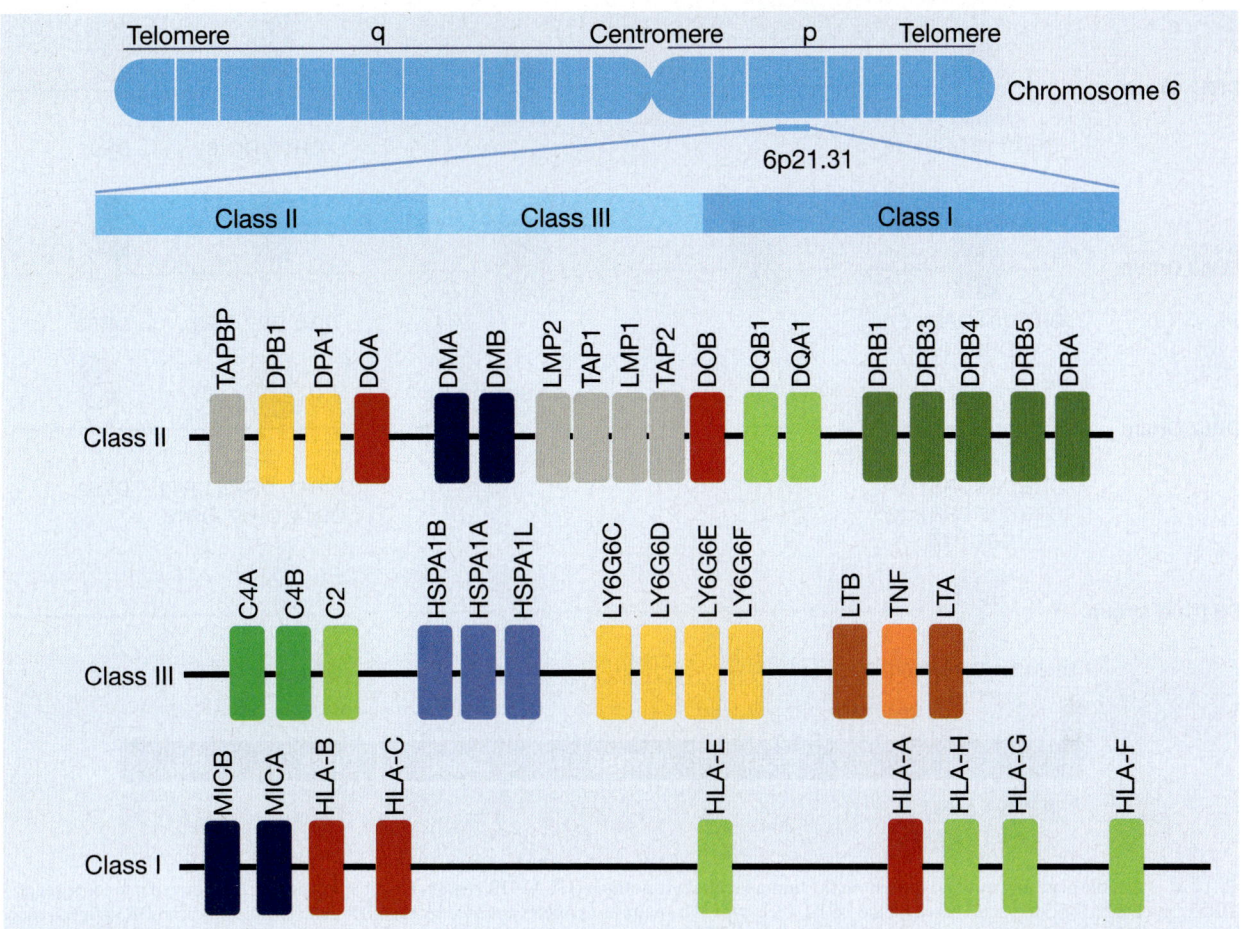

FIGURE 15.1 Genetic map of the human MHC (HLA) region. The human MHC is located on chromosome 6p21.3 and includes MHC class I genes (telomeric) and class II genes (centromeric) separated by MHC class III genes. HLA, human leukocyte antigen; LTA, lymphotoxin α; LTB, lymphotoxin β; MHC, major histocompatibility complex.

Alleles that are not expressed—"Null" alleles—have been given the suffix "**N**." Alleles that are alternatively expressed may have the suffix L (**L**ow), S (**S**ecreted), C (**C**ytoplasm), A (**A**berrant expression), or Q (**Q**uestionable). In the clinical setting, HLA typing for hematopoietic stem cell transplants requires high-resolution typing, minimally to the allele level (e.g., *A*24:02*), whereas for solid organ transplants HLA types have been reported at the antigen level (A24). This usually is the first two digits after the asterisk, but because the DNA nomenclature uses allele groups that are related by nucleotide sequence similarities, there are a few exceptions (*Table 15.1*).

HLAs were initially defined using serologic microcytotoxicity techniques that relied on the availability of viable lymphocyte preparations and a battery of carefully selected antisera that recognized distinct HLAs. During the past 20 years, DNA-based typing techniques have replaced serologic methods in clinical applications. DNA typing methods provide a more precise definition of the HLA system and improve the reliability of the typing. The three methods most widely used for HLA typing and histocompatibility testing are sequence-specific priming (SSP), sequence-specific oligonucleotide probes (SSO), and Sanger sequence–based typing.[5] However, these assays are primarily limited to sequence analysis of the HLA antigen recognition site due to relatively low throughput and high cost. Recently, long-range polymerase chain reaction–based massive parallel sequencing, or next-generation sequencing (NGS) typing, has emerged as a useful tool to amplify the entire length of HLA genes followed by shotgun fragmentation and sequencing. Using this strategy, final assembly of randomly sequenced fragments permits in-phase linkage of reads across the entire gene region. More important, full-length sequence

data are now being used to interrogate the biologic and clinical relevance of introns, additional exons, promoters, and regulatory regions of HLA genes.[6]

Human Leukocyte Antigen Haplotypes and Inheritance

The MHC alleles present on each parental chromosome are called an HLA haplotype, and these are codominantly expressed and inherited in a Mendelian fashion (*Figure 15.4*). Each parental chromosome 6 provides a haplotype or linked set of MHC genes to the offspring. The child carries one representative HLA antigen from each of the class I and class II loci of each parent. A child is, by definition, a one-haplotype match to each parent unless recombination has occurred. Statistically, there is a 25% chance that siblings will share the same parental haplotypes (two-haplotype match or HLA-identical), a 50% chance that they will share one haplotype (one-haplotype match), and a 25% chance that neither haplotype will be the same (zero-haplotype match). Haplotypes are usually inherited intact from each parent, although crossover between the A and B loci occurs in about 2% of offspring, resulting in a recombination. The HLA region demonstrates strong linkage disequilibrium across *HLA-A*, *B*, *C*, *DR*, *DQ*, and *DP* alleles. Linkage disequilibrium is a phenomenon where alleles at adjacent HLA loci are inherited together more often than would be expected by chance. For example, if *HLA-A1* and *HLA-B8* occur at gene frequencies of 16% and 10%, respectively, in a population, the probability of finding them together should be 1.6%. However, the observed occurrence of the *HLA-A1-B8* combination is significantly higher than the predicted incidence (about 8%). Existing data suggest that positive selection is operating on the haplotype and that the linked loci confer a particular selective advantage for the host.

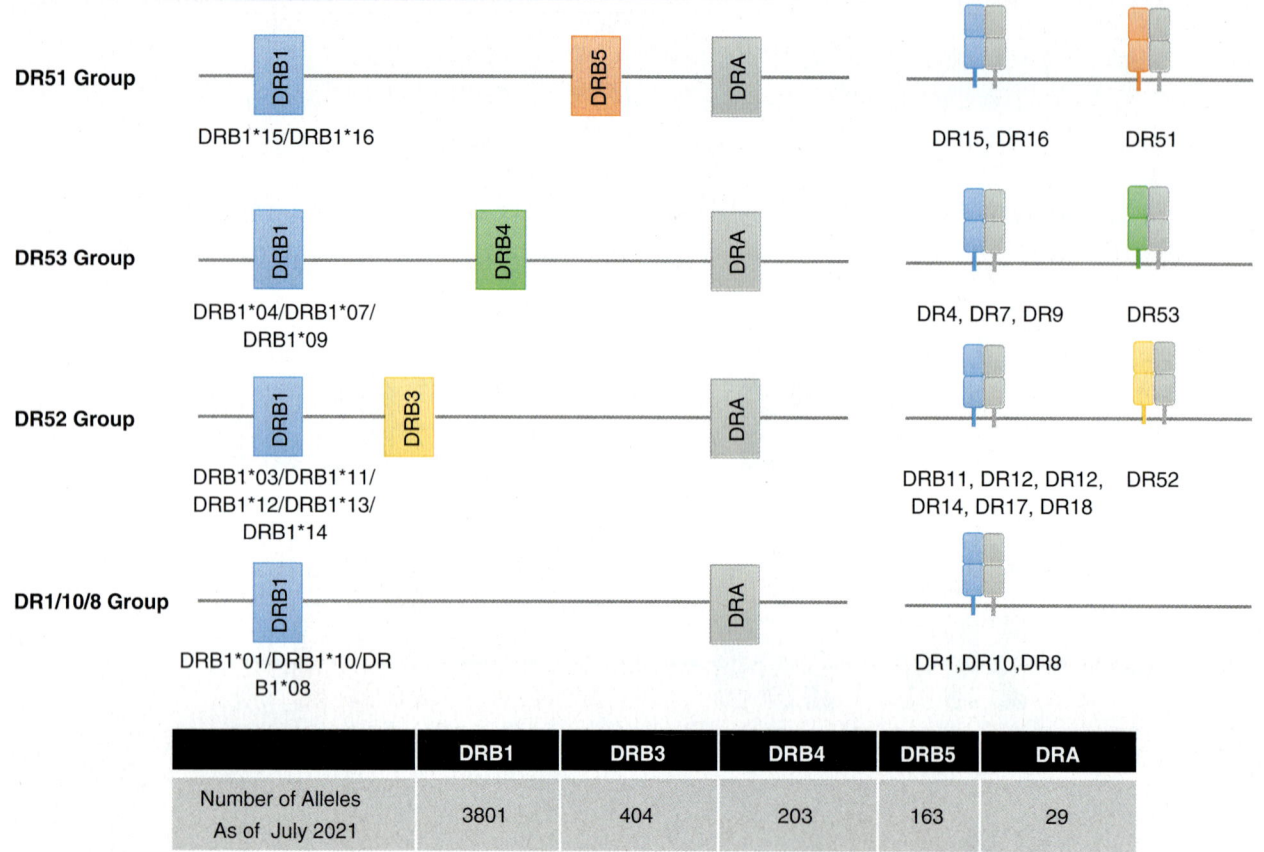

FIGURE 15.2 **Variable gene and antigen content in the human leukocyte antigen (HLA)-DR region.** HLA haplotypes are categorized into four groups: DR51, DR52, DR53, and DR1/10/8 (left panel) based on the DRB1 allele type. The number of alleles encoded by each DR gene is indicated. The DR antigens encoded by the different haplotypes are shown to the right. (From EMBL-EBI. IMGT/HLA database. http://www.ebi.ac.uk/imgt/hla/stats.html. Accessed July 2021.)

STRUCTURE AND FUNCTION OF HUMAN LEUKOCYTE ANTIGEN MOLECULES

HLA class I and class II molecules are expressed on distinct cell populations. The HLA class I molecules are expressed by all nucleated cells in the body. They present endogenous peptides (such as viral peptides) to CD8+ cytotoxic T cells that in turn respond to the infected cells. However, the level of HLA class I expression varies by locus, as well as among alleles at a locus. Furthermore, expression of class I molecules can be downregulated by pathologic events such as malignant transformation, viral infections, and stress conditions and upregulated by proinflammatory cytokines. HLA class II molecules, on the other hand, present exogenous peptides (such as bacterial peptides) to CD4+ helper T cells, which regulate the effector function of other immune cells. Thus, HLA class II molecules are expressed on selected cell types, especially on antigen-presenting cells (APCs), such as B lymphocytes, dendritic cells, and macrophages. Class II molecules can also be constitutively expressed in some parenchymal cells such as peritubular capillaries in human kidney. The expression levels of both class I and class II HLA molecules and expression of HLA class II molecules on other cell types can be induced in response to cytokines including TNF-α and INF-γ.

*The basic structure of HLAs appears to have evolved to perform antigen presentation functions. The HLA class I molecule is a heterodimer of a membrane-spanning 44-kDa heavy α chain (encoded by an *HLA-A*, *-B*, or *-C* gene) that is bound noncovalently to a 12-kDa β_2-microglobulin (β_2m) light chain, a non-MHC gene located in chromosome 15 (*Figure 15.5*).[7] The β_2m is not a transmembrane protein. The α chain folds into three domains: α_1, α_2, and α_3. The α_3 domain and β_2m show similarities in amino acid sequence to immunoglobulin C domains and have similar folded structures, whereas the α_1 and α_2 domains fold together into a single structure consisting of two segmented α_1 helices lying on a sheet of eight antiparallel β strands. The folding of the α_1 and α_2 domains creates a long cleft or groove, which is the site into which endogenous or exogenous peptides are loaded. Usually, HLA-A and HLA-B exhibit higher expression levels than HLA-C. HLA-C is poorly expressed and has been reported to have transcriptional and/or posttranscriptional control by microRNAs[8] and a more restricted peptide repertoire that limits assembly.[9]

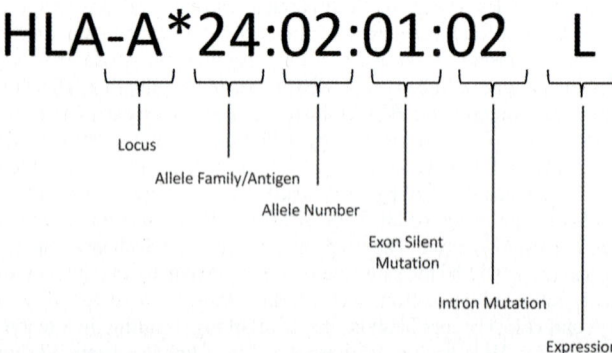

FIGURE 15.3 **Human leukocyte antigen (HLA) nomenclature.** Each HLA allele is named with a unique number separated by colons (:) into four fields. The first field specifies a group of alleles and is equivalent to the serologically defined antigen. The number used in the first field directly corresponds to the antigen name with some exceptions because the DNA nomenclature uses allele groups that are related by nucleotide sequence similarities. The second field specifies a group of alleles that encode a distinct HLA protein. The third field denotes synonymous mutations within the coding region of the gene. The fourth field represents genetic variations in noncoding regions. A modifier can be added to designate an expression variant.

Table 15.1. Summary of Common HLA Alleles With Different Antigen Names

HLA Class I		HLA Class II	
Allele	Antigen	Allele	Antigen
B*14:01	B64	DRB1*03:01	DR17
B*14:02	B65	DRB1*03:02	DR18
B*15/01/04/05/06/07/15	B62	DQB1*03:01	DQ7
B*15:02/08/11	B75	DQB1*03:02	DQ8
B*15:03	B72	DQB1*03:03	DQ9
B*15:09	B70		
B*15:10	B71		
B*15:12/14	B76		
B*40:01	B60		
B*40:02	B61		
C*03:02	Cw10		
C*03:03	Cw9		

Abbreviation: HLA, human leukocyte antigen.

The HLA class II molecule is composed of two transmembrane glycoprotein chains, α (33-35 kDa encoded by *DRA*, *DQA1*, or *DPA1*) and β (26-28 kDa encoded by *DRB*, *DQB1*, or *DPB1*). Each chain has two domains, and the two chains together form a compact four-domain structure grossly similar to that of HLA class I molecule. The α_2 and β_2 domains, like the α_3 and β_2m domains of the HLA class I molecule, have amino acid sequence and structural similarities to immunoglobulin C domains. The α_1 and β_1 domains of class II molecules form the peptide-binding cleft.

A major difference between HLA class I and class II is that the ends of the peptide-binding grove are more open in HLA class II molecules than in HLA class I molecules. As a result, the HLA class I can accommodate short peptides (~9 amino acids long) and the ends of the peptide are substantially buried within the class I molecule. In contrast, the class II groove has open ends and can accommodate much longer peptides (12-20 amino acids long). The fine structure within the groove includes pockets that accommodate peptides with certain characteristics (*Figure 15.5*). Accommodation of different amino acid side chains serves to anchor residues with specific characteristics, which confers a rudimentary specificity to the HLA allele. Not all HLAs can bind the same peptides. The T-cell receptor recognizes this compound ligand, making contacts with both the HLA molecule and with peptide antigen fragment. Geographically diverse pathogens

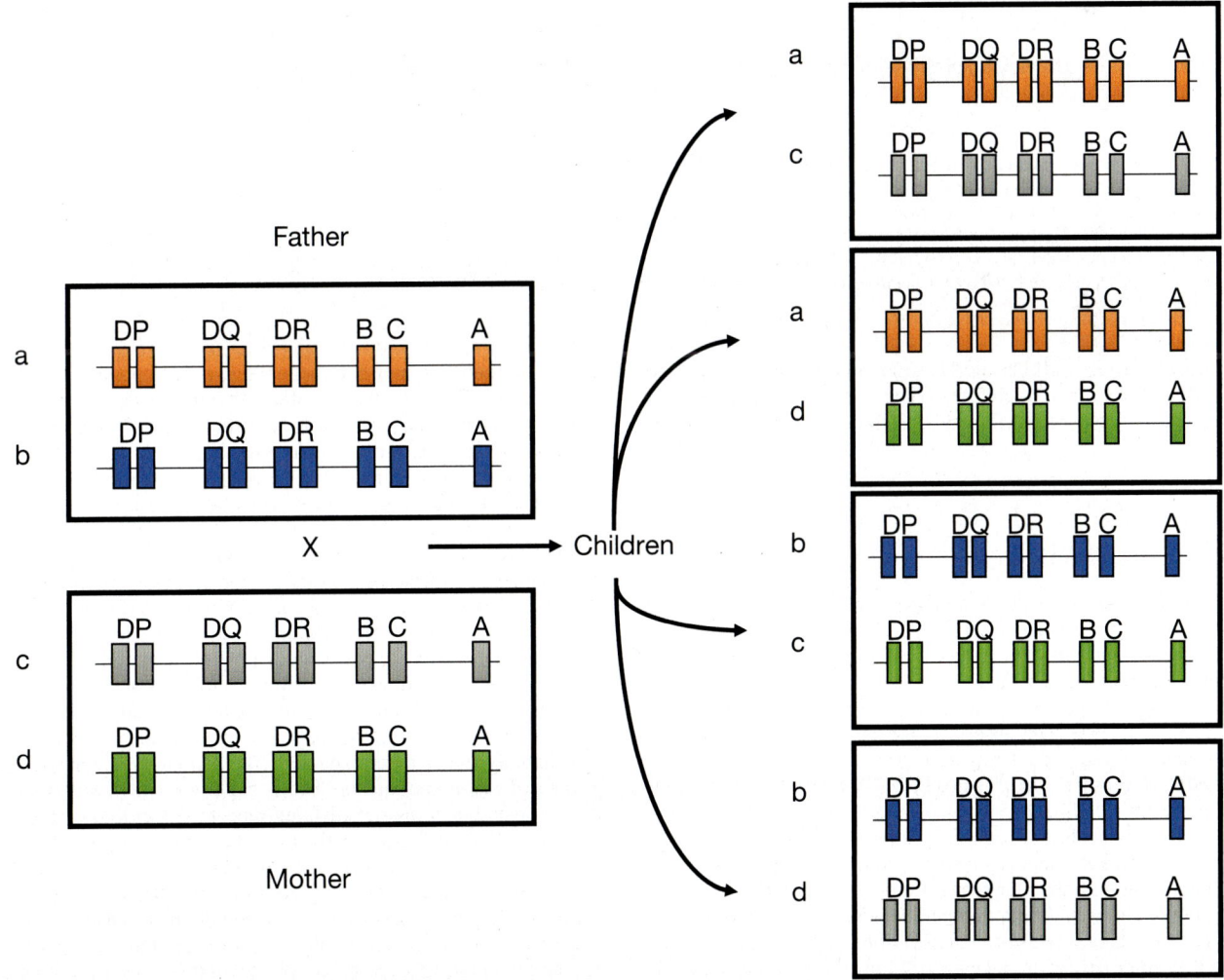

FIGURE 15.4 **Human leukocyte antigen (HLA) haplotype segregation in a family.** Each child inherits one HLA haplotype from each parent. Because each parent has two different haplotypes (paternal = ab and maternal = cd), four different haplotypic combinations are possible in the offspring (ac, ad, bc, and bd). Therefore, a child has 25% chance of having HLA-identical or two haplotype-matched sibling donors and a 50% chance of having a one-haplotype-matched sibling donor. All children have one haplotype matched to each parent unless recombination has occurred.

The Normal Hematologic System

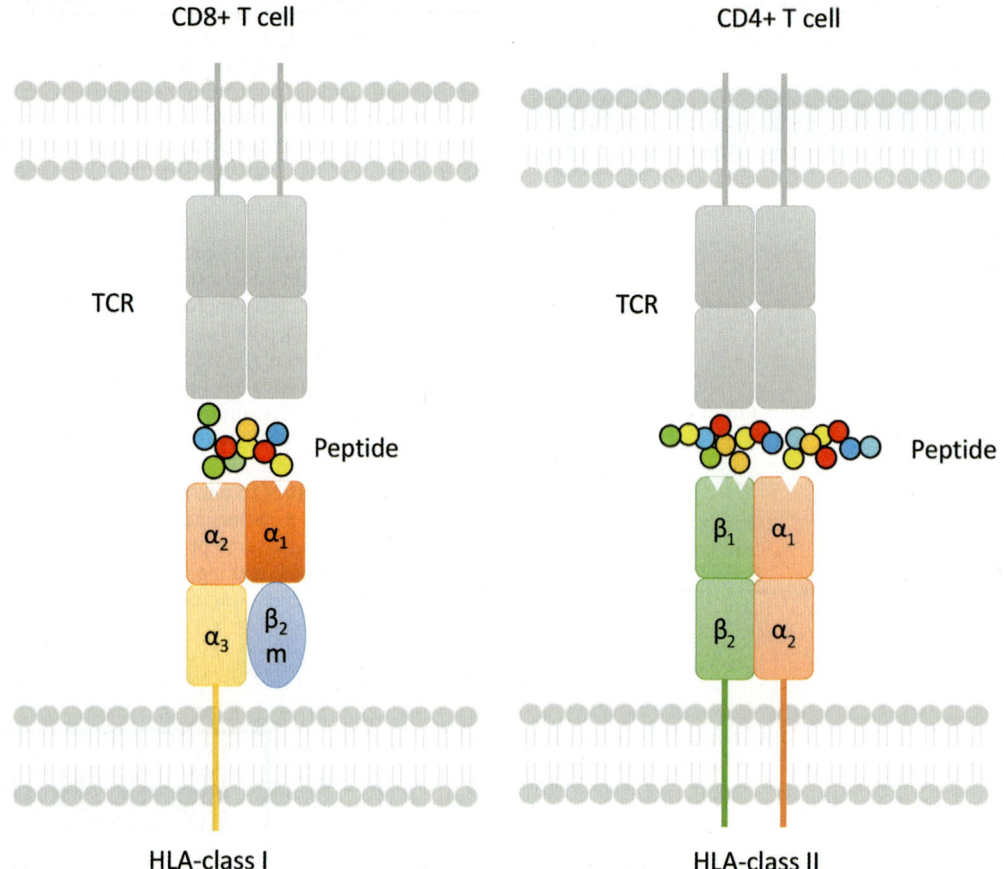

FIGURE 15.5 Schematic structure of human leukocyte antigen (HLA) molecules, bound peptides, and T cell–antigen receptor interactions. HLA class I and class II molecules present peptide antigens to CD8+ and CD4+ T cells, respectively. The α1 and α2 domains of HLA class I molecule form a peptide-binding cleft and display the complex at the cell surface. Similarly, the α1 and β1 domains of HLA class II molecules form the peptide-binding cleft. The major difference between class I and class II is that the ends of the peptide-binding grove are more open in HLA class II molecules than in HLA class I molecules. As a result, the HLA class I can accommodate only short peptides (~9 amino acids long) and the ends of the peptide are substantially buried within the class I molecule. In contrast, the class II groove has open ends and can accommodate longer peptides (12-20 amino acids long). The T-cell receptor (TCR) recognizes the complex of HLA and its bound peptide.

have probably driven and selected HLA polymorphisms that provide a survival advantage, and, therefore, ethnic populations from distinct geographical regions show different constellations of common HLA allotypes.

CELLULAR RESPONSES TO HUMAN LEUKOCYTE ANTIGEN ALLOANTIGENS

Allogeneic HLAs provoke strong immune responses. It has been estimated that the engagement of T cells by allogeneic HLAs may be hundreds of times greater than engagement of nominal pathogen-derived antigens. These strong responses make HLAs the major barrier to transplantation of tissues and organs between individuals. Two basic types of response have been observed, one involving "direct" presentation of donor HLAs to the recipient's T cells by donor cells and the other "indirect" presentation of donor HLAs that have been processed by the recipient's cells and presented to the recipient's T cells via recipient HLA molecules (*Figure 15.5*). Direct presentation is possible because of the marked similarity between different HLAs that permits direct interaction with the recipient's T-cell receptors. "Alloreactive" T cells are not removed during thymic selection. Indirect presentation proceeds in the same way as presentation of exogenous nominal antigens in that donor HLAs are taken up by host dendritic cells, monocytes, or B cells and broken down and antigenic peptides are loaded into the recipient's HLA class II molecules for presentation to CD4+ T cells. Antigen processing and presentation are described in greater detail under "HLA Antigen Presentation."

In addition to T and B lymphocytes, a third population of lymphocytes, NK cells, have been recently implicated in alloimmune responses. Historically, NK cells were thought of as components of innate immunity based on their intrinsic ability to spontaneously kill target cells independent of HLA antigen restriction. However, it is now clear that NK cells are quite sophisticated and use a highly specific target cell recognition receptor system consisting of a multitude of inhibitory and activating receptors. NK cell function is regulated by a number of surface receptors during development, priming, and cell-to-cell interactions. Killer cell immunoglobulin-like receptors (KIRs) derive diversity from the presence or absence of KIR genes, copy number, and allelic polymorphism. To date, 16 distinct *KIR* have been identified, including eight inhibitory *KIR*, six activating *KIR*, and two pseudogenes. The number and type of *KIR* genes present varies substantially between individuals. Based on KIR gene content, two KIR haplotypes have been defined. The A haplotype contains seven genes and two pseudo genes. The B haplotypes vary widely in gene contest and contain more activating receptors than the A haplotypes. Inhibitory KIR recognize distinct motifs of polymorphic HLA class I (HLA-A, -B, or -C) molecules. Upon engagement of their specific HLA class I ligands, inhibitory KIR dampen NK-cell reactivity. In contrast, activating KIR are believed to stimulate NK-cell reactivity when they sense their cognate ligands. Although most of the receptors for the activating KIR are unknown, the best characterized KIR2DS1 is known to bind HLA-C C2 allotypes albeit with lower affinity than its inhibitory counterpart KIR2DL1.[10] KIR and HLA gene families map to different human chromosomes (19 and 6, respectively), and their independent segregation produces a wide diversity in the number and type of inherited KIR-HLA combinations, likely contributing to overall immune competency. Since NK cells circulate in a state that can spontaneously deliver lethal effector function, it is critical that they do not attack healthy cells. Under normal homeostatic conditions, individual NK cells express at least one inhibitory receptor to a self-HLA class I molecule to prevent detrimental autoimmune responses to self.

In allogeneic transplantation, recipient NK cells expressing an inhibitory receptor can be activated to mediate target cell killing when the allograft lacks the relevant HLA class I ligand for that inhibitory receptor—a phenomenon of the "missing-self" hypothesis. Furthermore, the allograft may express stress-induced proteins that could serve as ligands for other activating receptors and enhance NK response—"induced-self" killing. The expression of CD16 (Fc-γ R III), an Fc receptor for IgG, allows NK cells to trigger antibody-dependent cell-mediated cytotoxicity ADCC against specific targets. Note that polymorphisms in this receptor have been described[11] and that they can have clinical consequences.[12] If the recipient produces donor-specific HLA antibodies, the recipient NK cells can elicit specific cytolysis against the allograft through the antibody-mediated NK-cell recognition. Because NK can exhibit graft-versus-leukemia effect in HSCT, KIR genotyping becomes an important component for donor selection. KIR typing can be determined using SSP, SSO, or NGS methods. The KIR-HLA mismatch and NK-cell alloreactivity can be predicted from the recipient's KIR types, recipient's HLA class I types, and donor's HLA class I types. In HLA-matched kidney transplant patients, NK alloreactivity is associated with poor graft outcomes.

ANTI–HUMAN LEUKOCYTE ANTIGEN ANTIBODIES

Sensitization to allogeneic HLAs occurs through pregnancies, prior transplantation, or blood transfusions and other exposures. Sensitization to HLA limits access to organ and platelet donors and to successful organ transplantation.[13] HLA antibodies are produced against epitopes, also known as antigenic determinates. Although HLA antibody can be produced against epitopes that are unique to a particular HLA antigen, antibodies may also be directed against epitopes that are shared by several HLAs. Groups of HLAs that are frequently reactive with an alloantiserum are called cross-reacting groups (CREGs). Amino acid sequence data fitted with three-dimensional structural information on HLAs suggests that many of these CREGs share structural features that might explain their cross-reactivity. Recently, epitope matching that predicts similarities of HLA antigenic determinants between donors and recipients has been adapted in kidney transplantations to reduce humoral immune responses.[14]

Two types of assays are commonly used to detect HLA antibodies: crossmatch and solid phase immunoassays. In the early 1960s, several groups recognized that patients with circulating antibodies against donor HLAs experienced irreversible hyperacute rejection of their transplanted kidney.[15] The "CDC" crossmatch test mixed patient serum with donor lymphocytes and complement to detect the presence or absence of antibody-mediated complement-dependent donor cell death. The crossmatch test nearly eliminated hyperacute rejection of transplanted organs by 1972. In the 1980s, the indirect flow cytometric crossmatch was introduced to detect donor HLA antibodies, increasing the sensitivity of the crossmatch test. The development of microparticles that incorporate fluorescent dyes into different beads that can be distinguished in a flow cytometer or Luminex platform permits very precise identification of HLA antibodies, even in broadly reactive sera. Luminex single antigen (SAB) test is considered as a semi-qualitative assay that provides the measurement of fluorescent intensities of the beads that correlate with the concentration of HLA antibodies and can be reported as median fluoresce intensity. The Luminex SAB assay is highly sensitive and specific and made "virtual" prediction of physical crossmatches possible for most patients. The virtual crossmatch compares the antibody specificities present in the patient's serum with the donor's HLA type to assess crossmatch compatibility. The Organ Procurement and Transplantation Network has established a mechanism to enter "unacceptable" HLAs for transplant candidates based on

antibody identification using solid-phase tests, which are used to virtually crossmatch donors for organ allocation in the United States.[16] The virtual crossmatch prevents allocation of incompatible deceased donor kidneys to sensitized patients with known donor-specific antibodies. By comparing the constellation of HLA-reactive antibodies in the sensitized patient with the HLA types of historical kidney donors, we can estimate the percentage of organ donors who would be incompatible with a transplant candidate, and the difficulty in finding a compatible donor in the United States.

High-dose posttransplantation cyclophosphamide (PTCy) treatment opens up a number of patients for stem cell transplant who would otherwise be ineligible for transplant.[17,18] As the number of HLA mismatches increase between the donor and recipient, the risk of graft-versus-host disease (GVHD) and graft rejection increases. Given that most patients without HLA matching donors will have a haploidentical donor available, PTCy prophylaxis is a novel treatment that allows for haploidentical and even HLA-mismatched unrelated T-cell replete donors.[19] HLA-mismatched donation raises the problem of sensitization in the recipient. Approximately 20% to 25% of patients who have undergone hematopoietic stem cell transplantation are sensitized to HLA.[20-22] Donor-specific HLA antibodies (DSAs) also pose a risk in hematopoietic stem cell transplantation (HSCT) as the number of HLA-mismatched donors (cord blood transplants and haploidentical HSCT) is increasing. Preformed HLA DSA is associated with a two- to 10-fold increase of engraftment failure of mismatched HSCT.[23] HLA DSA–mediated engraftment failure after HSCT can occur either by antibody-dependent cell-mediated cytotoxicity or by complement-mediated cytotoxicity.[24] Limited donor options and an urgent need to proceed to allogeneic transplant have led transplant centers to develop desensitization protocols to permit successful donor stem cell engraftment. Commonly used desensitization protocols include intravenous immune globulin, plasma exchange, bortezomib, and rituximab and have demonstrated successful DSA reduction.[25]

NONCLASSICAL HUMAN LEUKOCYTE ANTIGEN CLASS I GENES AND MOLECULES

The nonclassical MHC I genes include *HLA-E, -F, -G,* and *-H.* They are expressed at the cell surface in a limited distribution of cells as heterodimers with β_2m (*Figure 15.6*). Compared with *A, -B,* and *-C* they are less polymorphic and have shorter intracellular tails.

HLA-E, -F, -G, -H

To date *HLA-E* is the most studied of the nonclassical MHC class I genes.[26] The gene is located on chromosome 6 downstream from *HLA-C.* It encodes eight exons. The first is a leader sequence followed by three exons that encode α_1, α_2, and α_3 extracellular domains. Exon 5 encodes a transmembrane domain, and exons 6 and 7 encode the intracellular tail (https://www.ncbi.nlm.nih.gov/gene). HLA-E is expressed on lymphocytes and endothelial cells from most tissues in the human body. It is also upregulated by proinflammatory cytokines.[27] Although there are eight known protein-coding alleles (HLA Nomenculature@ hla.alleles.org), two alleles—*HLA-E*01:01* and *-E*01:03*—dominate in human populations.[28] They differ by an arginine-to-glycine mutation at codon 107, which lies outside the peptide-binding region. The known ligands for HLA-E peptide complexes are the heterodimer-inhibitory and -activating CD94-NKG2 receptors found on NK cells.[29] These receptors have different affinities for HLA-E depending on the presented peptide.[30]

HLA-E binds a restricted set of peptides derived from the signal peptides of HLA-A, -B, -C, and -G antigens. NK cells utilize the CD94/NKG2A receptor to bind HLA-E molecules to generate inhibitory signals that prevent NK cells from eliciting killing activities. HLA-E provides a means by which NK cells can survey for proper MHC class I expression and TAP functioning. Like the HLA-A, -B, and -C molecules, HLA-E presents peptide at the surface of the cell. Unlike the classical class I molecules, the peptide-binding groove of HLA-E contains five conserved hydrophobic pockets, which impose

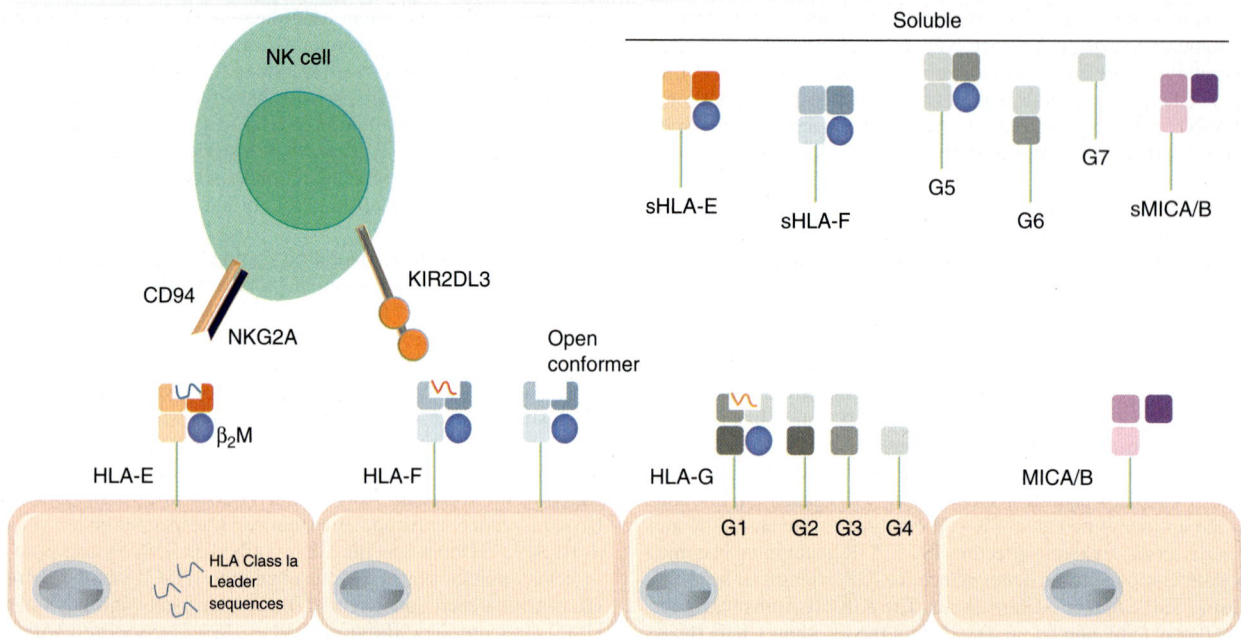

FIGURE 15.6 **Nonclassical human leukocyte antigen (HLA)-E, -F, -G, and MHC class I chain–related protein A/B (MICA/MICB).** HLA-E, F, G, and MICA/B can be presented on a varied distribution of cells and are not exclusive. HLA-E can present leader peptide sequences from major histocompatibility complex (MHC) class I processing and interact with CD94-NKG2A. HLA-F can present peptide and interact with the KIR2DL3 receptor or be expressed at the cell surface as a peptide-independent open conformer. MICA surface expression is not associated with β2-microglobulin or peptide presentation. Functional roles for membrane-bound and soluble forms of HLA-G, as well as sHLA-E, sHLA-F, and sMICA/B, are still being discovered.

strict sequence restriction on the peptides that it presents.[31] Certain leader sequences of classical class I molecules can be presented at the cell surface in context with HLA-E.[32] Therefore, depending on the peptide bound to HLA-E, and its presence at the cell surface, the interaction between HLA-E and its cognate NK-cell receptor will trigger inhibitory or activating signals.[33,34]

HLA-E is a conduit between the innate and adaptive immune system. In addition to binding NK-cell receptors, HLA-E can present a variety of peptides to CD8 T cells. These include virally derived HIV, EBV, and CMV protein sequences along with autoimmune peptides derived from gliadin and human heat-shock proteins.[35] Because of the relative monomorphic nature of HLA-E, it could be a pivotal molecule in the design of treatments for some diseases.[36,37] Proinflammatory cytokines can upregulate HLA-E in ECs and induce its secretion providing protection from NK-cell lysis.[27] When sHLA-E is decreased in patients after HSCT it is associated with severe acute and long-term chronic GVHD and lower overall rates of survival.[38] How important these interactions are to the outcomes of other pathogenic process is still under study. HLA-F, first described by Lee et al in 1990, is the least studied of the MHC Ib genes. To date, its expression has predominantly been found on B cells, activated lymphocytes,[39] and extravillous trophoblasts at the maternal-fetal interface.[40] HLA-F is differentiated from the other MHC class I genes in that it may be expressed at the cell surface independent of bound peptide.[41] These stable molecules lacking bound peptide have been referred to as "open conformers." HLA-F displays very low-level polymorphism coding for six distinct proteins (http://www.ebi.ac.uk/ipd/imgt/hla/) and is predicted to present a very restricted peptide repertoire.[42] HLA-F binds heavy chains of HLA-I and facilitates their migration to the cell surface.[41] HLA-G molecules are expressed on the trophoblast and can inhibit NK cell–mediated cell lysis, through interaction with the receptors leukocyte immunoglobulin-like receptor 2 (LIR1/ILT2) and 4 (LIR2/ILT4). For example, *KIR2DL3* is a highly polymorphic inhibitory framework gene expressed by NK cells, hinting at an important role in immune surveillance. HLA-F is known to interact with KIR2DL3.[43] Also, it has recently been discovered that open conformers of HLA-F interact with KIR3DS1,[44] a relatively monomorphic-activating receptor that is found in all modern humans and may have originated more than 3

million years ago.[45] KIR3DS1 elicits an antiviral response to inhibit HIV replication. Recently it was shown that HLA-F can also associate with beta-2 microglobulin (β₂m) and bind a diverse (>2000) set of peptides between 7 and 30 residues long and be recognized by LIR1/ILT2.[46]

HLA-G is another member of the nonclassical HLA family.[47] In humans, the gene maps to the short arm of chromosome 6. It consists of eight exons. Exon 1 encodes a signal peptide; exons 2, 3, and 4 encode the extracellular domains α₁, α₂, and α₃, respectively; exons 5 and 6 encode the transmembrane and cytoplasmic domains, whereas exon 7 is not transcribed due to a stop codon in exon 6. This premature termination alters the exposure of amino acid sequence signals for recycling protein motifs resulting in the expression of mostly high-affinity peptides with longer surface half-lives.[48] HLA-G is the most polymorphic of the nonclassical HLA I genes. Unlike the classical MHC I genes, the 61 known allelic polymorphisms (http://www.ebi.ac.uk/ipd/imgt/hla/) recorded to date are distributed among the α₁, α₂, and α₃ domains rather than the peptide groove and is not constitutively expressed. Alternative spicing of the gene's mRNA encodes four membrane-bound and three soluble protein isoforms.[49] In addition, several other structures of HLA-G associated as multimers and linked by disulfide bridges with and without β₂m have been described.[50-52] HLA-G exerts an inhibitory immunomodulatory effect by binding to CD160, CD8, KIR2DL4, LIR1/ILT2, and LIR2/ILT4. These receptors are found on B cells, monocytes, dendritic cells, and subsets of NK, CD4⁺, and CD8⁺ T cells. The mechanism of action of HLA-G on these lymphocytes is under investigation and is believed to be diverse ranging from downregulation of chemokine receptors to affecting maturation and proliferation in both the innate and adaptive immune settings.[53] HLA-G is known to play an important role in parasitic infections.[54]

The pathophysiologic effect of HLA-G has been most intensively studied during pregnancy where dividing extravillous trophoblast cells express and secrete different isoforms of HLA-G at the maternal-fetal interface initiating a complex cross talk necessary for a successful pregnancy.[55] When the leader sequence of HLA-G is expressed bound to HLA-E, the complex preferentially interacts with CD94/NKG2C, thus activating NK-cell lysis.[33] Because HLA-G is highly expressed on invading trophoblastic cells at the maternal-fetal interface, it is believed that this is one mechanism by which the immune system can fine-tune the connection between the fetus and the mother during pregnancy.

HLA-G and HLA-E are coexpressed on many cell types during physiologic conditions and both may act to induce anergy in activated immune effector cells.[56] However, during pathologic conditions such as cancer this cooperation may break down.[56] An intriguing finding is that HLA-G can modulate HLA-E expression. Cells transfected with isoforms HLA-G1 and HLA-G3 differentially increase the expression of HLA-E on their surface.[57] The outcome of how tumor cells subvert HLA-G and HLA-E expression is complex and differs between tumor types.[56]

The expression of HLA-G may also occur on other tissues, including cornea, thymus, inflamed bowel, and various tumor types. Expression of HLA-G on these tissues is controversial and must be interpreted with caution because lymphocytes can bind the Fc receptor of HLA-G-labeling antibodies and HLA-G antibodies may themselves cross-react with other MHC class I heavy chains.[58]

HLA-H was originally predicted to lack function due to its deletion from chromosomes carrying specific alleles of HLA-A but is now known to represent a transcribed pseudogene with mRNA expression levels similar to HLA-G.[59] Recently an unexpectedly high worldwide genetic diversity of HLA-H alleles was described,[60] suggesting its functional importance. To date, there is no validated antibody to detect HLA-H, significantly hindering studies to explore potential physiological and/or pathological roles. HLA-H has been proposed to be responsible for genetic hemochromatosis, with >80% of tested patients with the disease having a mutation.[61-63]

MICA and MICB

MHC class I chain–related (MIC) genes were first described in the mid-1990s.[64,65] Seven *MIC* genes have been identified, *MICA-MICG*. Only *MICA* and *MICB* encode expressed transcripts, and the rest are pseudogenes. The MICA gene is located at a close proximity centromeric to the HLA-B locus resulting in a very strong linkage disequilibrium effect between the two.[66] Similar to classical MHC I genes, *MICA* and *MICB* express a leader sequence, three extracellular domains, a transmembrane segment, and a cytoplasmic tail. MIC genes are polymorphic with 119 known *MICA* alleles and 43 *MICB* alleles (http://www.ebi.ac.uk/ipd/imgt/hla/). They carry a conserved recognition site, and similar MIC genes are observed in numerous animal species.[64] *MICA* and *MICB* are associated with autoimmune disease, transplantation pathology, cancer, and infectious complications.[67] Expression of MIC protein has been demonstrated on many human tissues, including lung, liver, colon, thymus, and kidney but not lymphocytes or central nervous system tissues.[68,69]

The extracellular domains of MICA and MICB share up to 30% homology with classical MHC class I genes.[64] MICA and MICB are highly glycosylated proteins that do not associate with β_2m[70] or CD8.[64] They do not present bound peptides and are independent of classical MHC I processing.[70] Also, unlike classical MHC class I proteins, the putative peptide-binding cleft of MICA bends over such that the molecule's underside is exposed to the extracellular space.[71]

MICA and MICB expression are notably upregulated on epithelial cells and are an indicator of cellular stress.[70] Stress-induced MICA and MICB bind the activating NKG2D receptors expressed on NK and T cells, which respond against stressed or damaged cells. In the intestinal epithelium, stress-induced expression of MICA serves as a ligand for γδ T-cell recognition and killing.[72] This interaction elicits a cytolytic response and therefore provides a first line of defense against intracellular pathogens and tumor-stressed cells. The importance of the MIC-NKG2D interaction is exemplified by the fact that viruses target MICA and MICB through ubiquitination and micro-RNA,[73,74] and tumors can shed MICA to hinder recognition via NKG2D.[75] Soluble forms of MICA or MICB (sMICA/sMICB) released from cancer cells may constitute an immune escape mechanism that systemically impairs antitumor immunity,[76,77] which may be useful for staging of cancer disease.

NONCLASSICAL MAJOR HISTOCOMPATIBILITY COMPLEX CLASS II MOLECULES

Nonclassical HLA-DM and HLA-DO molecules are produced by genes in the MHC class II region. Nonclassical MHC class II molecules mainly reside in endosomal/lysosomal compartments where they regulate peptide editing for MHC II molecules.

HLA-DM

The human HLA-DM is a heterodimeric protein that consists of α and β chains. It has one α-chain gene (*DMA*) and one β-chain gene (*DMB*; *Figure 15.1*). Both *DM* genes have limited polymorphism.[78] There are 7 *DMA* alleles resulting in 4 proteins and 13 *DMB* alleles resulting in 7 different proteins (HLA Nomenculature@hla.alleles.org). Allele frequency studies show that more than 95% have *DMA*01:01* and *DMB*01:01* alleles, 28% to 29% have *DMA*01:02* and *DMB*01:02* alleles, and 1% to 10% have other allelic variants (http://www.allele-frequencies.net). Haplotype analysis suggests a strong positive linkage disequilibrium between *DMA* and *DMB* alleles.[79] The amino acid sequences of DM molecules are about 30% similar to those of other human MHC II molecules, whereas the DR, DQ, DP, and DO molecules are about 63% to 69% homologous.[78,80-82] The majority of amino acid differences are located in β chain. DM is expressed in all class II–expressing APCs. The DM molecule is found primarily in late endosomal/lysosomal compartments of APCs. However, DM can be detected at low levels on the surface of B cells and dendritic cells, as well.[83,84] The transcription and expression levels of DM are generally lower than that of other class II molecules. The Class II MHC Transactivator (CIITA) and Regulatory Factor X (RFX-5), which control the transcription of classical MHC II molecules, are required for DM gene transcription. Interferon-γ, a known activator of the transcription of classical MHC-II genes, upregulates the transcription and expression of *DM* genes.[83,85]. Upon synthesis, DM exits from the endoplasmic reticulum (ER) to the endosomal MHC II peptide-loading compartment (MIIC) that is mediated by a tyrosine-based localization motif (YTPL) on the cytoplasmic tail of the DM β chain.[86-89]

DM does not bind peptides because its peptide-binding groove is closed.[90] Despite its lack of peptide-loading ability, it has a major role in MHC II antigen presentation machinery (*Figure 15.7*) by serving as a chaperone and a peptide editor.[91,92] MHC class II molecules are unstable in the absence of peptide and have a strong tendency to aggregate.[93,94] Following transcription and translation, MHC II molecules assemble in the ER and make a complex with the invariant chain (Ii). The flexible region of Ii can bind the peptide-binding groove and stabilize the complex as it translocates into MIIC, which is rich in antigenic peptides. Once the MHC II-Ii complex reaches MIIC, lysosomal enzyme proteases degrade Ii into class II invariant chain peptides (CLIP). The MHC-CLIP complex has a larger hydrophobic surface that attracts DM to bind to the complex. DM binding to the complex induces MHC II conformational change and dissociates CLIP from the peptide-binding groove.[95,96] Following dissociation of CLIP, DM still associates with MHC II molecule functioning as a chaperone to stabilize the empty MHC II molecule in a peptide-perceptive conformation.[97] DM also assists DO, another nonclassical MHC II molecule, to stabilize and accumulate in the endosomal compartment. The DO molecule is unstable and is rapidly degraded if it is not transported out of the ER.[98] In fact, DO forms a complex with DM in the ER that stabilizes the DO heterodimer and enables DO to exit the ER.[88]

In addition, DM plays an important peptide-editing function in antigen presentation. Peptides bind to the MHC II molecule by forming hydrogen bonds between the α and β chains and the carboxyl group of the peptide backbone, and the other side is formed by the interaction between the binding-groove pocket and peptide side chain.[99] The DM binding near the N terminus of the MHC II peptide-binding grove alters the conformation of the MHC II molecule and disrupts hydrogen bond interaction.[100,101] The **conformational** alteration prevents the binding of weakly bound low-affinity peptide and favors strongly bound high-affinity peptide binding.[102] The strongly bound peptide–MHC II complexes are more stable and resistant to DM editing (DM resistance) compared with weakly bound peptide (DM sensitive). Several studies have shown that the DM-mediated peptide-editing function is pH dependent and its maximum action is at acidic pH of 4.5 to 5.5 in late endosomal/lysosomal compartment.[103,104]

DM polymorphism has a profound impact on peptide loading to MHC II molecules.[105] The *DMA*01:03* allele has lower catalytic efficiency and peptide release velocity than that of the *DMA*01:01* allele. As a consequence, *DMA*01:03* increases the half-life of autoimmune-related peptide and MHC II binding. This study gives a clue that DM polymorphism might contribute to autoimmune diseases. Certain DMA or DMB alleles and classical MHC II combination is correlated with autoimmune disease such as rheumatoid arthritis (RA) and type 1 diabetes (T1D).[106] Of interest, some studies have shown that single-nucleotide polymorphism (SNP) on DM gene is correlated with disease association. SNP *rs151719-G* located on the intron region of *DMB* gene is protective to RA and T1D, whereas it increases the risk of multiple sclerosis and autoimmune thyroid disease.[107] A recently published paper shows that SNP *rs1063478-T* on DMA gene has a strong protective effect on hepatitis C virus (HCV) infection and clearance and response to interferon/Ribavirin in patients with chronic HCV type 1 infection.[108,109] In addition, an intronic SNP *rs6902982* on *DMB* gene is linked with HIV-mediated Kaposi sarcoma formation.[110] However, the mechanistic role of DM SNP in the pathogenesis of immune disease is still unclear and has yet to be investigated.

It is well documented that MHC molecules modulate tumor immunity. A recent study shows that high DMB mRNA and protein expression in the tumor cells of advanced-stage serous ovarian cancer are directly related to increased numbers of the infiltrating and activating CD8 T lymphocytes into tumor epithelium. High DMB expression was associated with improved patient survival.[111] Another study by Jastaniah et al[91] observed higher expression of DM and DR and low expression of CLIP molecules in ETV6-AML1–positive precursor-B acute lymphoblastic leukemia (ALL) compared with ETV6-AML1–negative ALL. In fact, ETV6-AML1–positive ALL was associated with long-term remission and survival and a low relapse rate.[91] These antitumor effects of DM molecules indicate that the higher DM expression favors better immune response and patient outcome. In addition, one study addresses the low level of DM expression detected in patients with RA.[112] Taken together, these findings suggest that the DM expression level makes a substantial contribution to the immune response in disease. In hematopoietic cell transplantation, HLA-DPB1 immunogenicity is based on T-cell epitope alloreactivity between the donor and recipient. Peptide antigens presented on the cell surface called immunopeptidome of DPB1 allotypes determines T-cell alloreactivity. HLA-DM plays a peptide editing role in immunopeptidome diversity and guides T-cell alloreactivity in DPB1 permissive and nonpermissive alloresponse. Therefore, DM is a potential target to modulate immunopeptidome diversity and immunotherapy in HSCT.[113]

HLA-DO

Human HLA-DO is a heterodimer molecule with α and β chains. It is encoded by one α-chain gene (*DOA*) and one β-chain gene (*DOB*) that are separated from each other unlike other class II α- and β-chain genes that are positioned as pairs (*Figure 15.1*). Twelve *DOA* allelic variants produce three proteins. There is one null allele. *DOB* has 13 allelic variants that produce 5 different proteins (HLA Nomenclature@hla.alleles.org). There is no linkage disequilibrium between the *DOA* and *DOB* genes. However, strong linkage disequilibrium was seen between *DOB*01:02* and *DRB1*15:02*.[114] DO is expressed mainly in B lymphocytes, mature dendritic cell, and thymus medullary epithelial cell raising the possibility that DO expression is controlled by specific factors in those cells.[115,116] Transcription of the *DOA* gene is regulated by transcription coactivator CIITA, whereas the *DOB* gene transcription is regulated by CIITA-dependent and -independent mechanisms.[116,117] Interferon-γ induces transcription of the *DOA* gene but not of the *DOB* gene.[85,118]

Despite the structural similarity between DO and classical MHC II molecules, DO does not bind peptides. Amino acid changes in the DO α chain preclude hydrogen bond formation between the peptide

and the peptide-binding groove. DO is a known modulator of DM function by engaging as a cochaperone of DM molecule (*Figure 15.7*). DO physically associates with DM (to form a complex that inhibits DM-mediated peptide repertoire selection of immunodominant epitopes).[100,119,120] DO also affects DM-mediated stability of the empty MHC II molecules.[121] Some studies show that DO-DM association is maximum at near-neural pH in the early endosomes.[98,121,122] The DO/DM ratio also affects DM peptide selection activity.[101] Overexpression of DO leads to an increased DR-CLIP accumulation and a decreased peptide–MHC II presentation at the cell surface. A low DO/DM ratio favors the peptide-editing action of DM molecules and induces CLIP dissociation from MHC II.[123] Overall, the expression level of DM is higher than that of DO, so free DM (active) is more abundant than the DO-DM complex (inactive) in cells. Approximately 50% of DM is associated with DO in peripheral B cells, which favors functionally active DM regulation of peptide loading and antigen presentation function.[124,125]

Several studies demonstrate that DO polymorphisms are correlated with immune system dysregulation. The allele G at the SNP *rs9296068* locus located on the 5′UTR region of *DOA* gene is correlated with higher intragraft B lymphocytes in pediatric liver grafts that contribute to acute liver rejection.[126] The SNP *rs929068G* represses *DOA* exon and decreases DOA gene expression. The dysfunctional DOA is one cause of the enhanced response of intragraft B cells. *DOA rs2284191G* had a protective effect on HCV infection and clearance, and *DOB rs7383287G* was associated with a decreased risk of HCV chronicity.[108] In addition, the expression level of DO molecules and disease association was observed in several studies. One study finds that B-cell chronic lymphocytic leukemia (CLL) has higher DOB expression that is correlated with the expression of DM-sensitive antigens in malignant cells. As a result, antitumor CD4 T cells strongly recognize DM-sensitive antigens presented on malignant cells.[127] This finding suggests that overexpression of DO in certain diseases might be used as a therapeutic target. Another study by Souwer et al shows that the DOA mRNA level was significantly upregulated in malignant cells of patients with CLL. This upregulated DOA mRNA is correlated with poor prognosis and unfavorable clinical outcome.[128] Collectively, DO has been proven as a critical modulator of DM function to tune antigen presentation and immune response.

HUMAN LEUKOCYTE ANTIGEN PRESENTATION

In the most classical sense, antigen presentation is the process by which foreign proteins are processed and presented by APCs to cells of the adaptive immune system to control pathogens. The well-studied endogenous and exogenous pathways of antigen processing and presentation at the surface of the cell in the context of HLA class I and II molecules are summarized follows. In addition, we discuss various alternative mechanisms of antigen presentation, cross-presentation, and cross-dressing.

Endogenous Pathway

Protein antigens from pathogens that gain access to the intracellular space are processed and presented in the context of HLA class I via the endogenous pathway (*Figure 15.8A*). Once inside the cell, pathogen proteins are degraded in the proteasome[129] and then trimmed by the amino-terminal peptidase known as ER-associated aminopeptidase 1 (ERAP1).[130] Peptides then enter the ER via the transporter associated with antigen-processing (TAP) 1 or 2 transporters[131] and come into the vicinity of the MHC class I loading complex that includes Calnexin, Calreticulin, and Tapasin.[132] These chaperone proteins support the HLA class I molecule until it assembles with a high-affinity binding peptide also known as "best-fit" peptide and β_2m in a process known as peptide editing.[133] Peptides that bind to HLA class I molecules are generally about 8 to 10 amino acids long.[134] The MHC:Peptide:β_2m is then exported to the cell membrane via the secretory pathway and functions to present foreign peptide to CD8$^+$ T cells. MHC class I molecules are expressed on all nucleated cells.

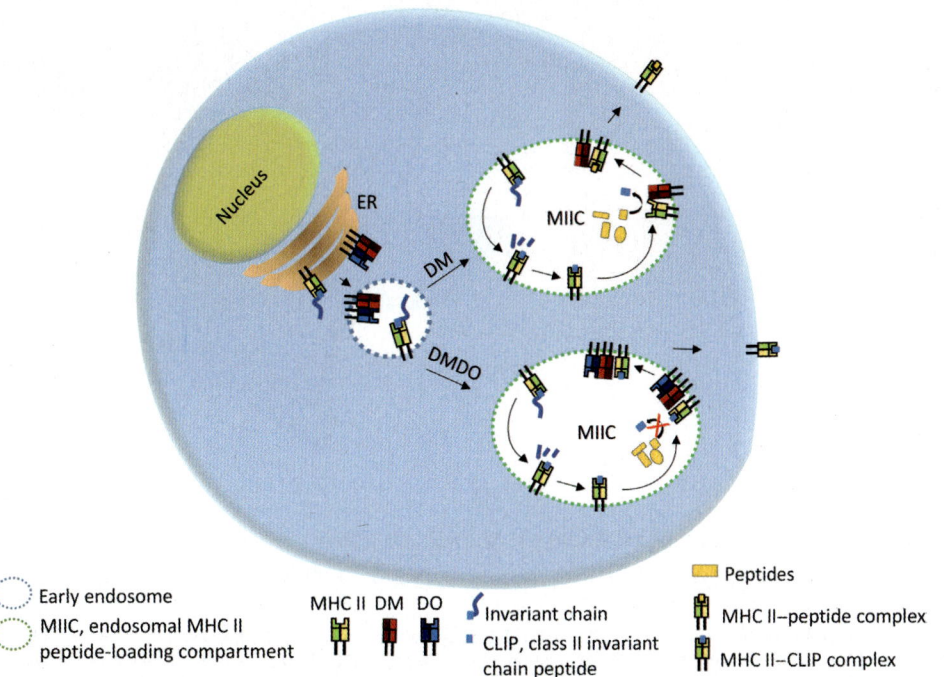

FIGURE 15.7 **The role of HLA-DM and DO in peptide editing.** HLA-DM molecules complex with HLA-DO molecules (DMDO). DMDO and uncomplexed DM exit the endoplasmic reticulum (ER) and move to early endosomes where they interact with HLA class II molecule-invariant chain complexes (MIIC). Ii is degraded into class II variant chain peptide (CLIP) forming an MHC II–CLIP complex. In the absence of DO, DM binding to MHC II changes its conformation to release CLIP. DM stabilizes MHC II in a peptide-receptive conformation (chaperone function). DM-MHC II favors high-affinity peptide binding (peptide-editing function). In the presence of DO, the DMDO complex inhibits the chaperone and peptide-editing function of DM, resulting in MHC II-CLIP being presented at the cell surface.

The efficiency of HLA-A, -B, and -C molecules binding to the MHC class I loading complex as well as the pace of peptide loading and translocation to the cell surface differ between molecules of the different loci. HLA-A and -C molecules bind to the complex more efficiently than HLA-B molecules, whereas peptide loading and translocation of HLA-B molecules to the cell surface occur more rapidly than for HLA-A and -C molecules.[135,136] Furthermore, HLA-B molecules at the cell surface are more likely to be ubiquitously loaded with peptides, whereas a portion of HLA-A and -C molecules lack peptides.[135]

Exogenous Pathway

Antigen presentation of pathogens that do not directly invade the cell requires endocytosis (*Figure 15.8B*). APCs engulf the extracellular space in endosomes that fuse with lysosomes forming phagolysosomes. These compartments are known for their relatively acidic pH and protease activity that allows for protein degradation.

In the ER, HLA class II molecules are present and bound to a protein called the invariant chain (Ii, CD74) that prevents antigenic peptides formed through the endogenous pathway from binding. The HLA class II:Ii complex is transported to a late endosomal compartment that contains the proteases cathepsin S and L and the nonclassical HLA-DM molecule. The compartment is known as the MHC class II compartment (MIIC).[137] The invariant chain is digested by the proteases into the class II–associated Ii peptide (CLIP).[138] HLA-DM then facilitates the exchange of the CLIP protein for a "best-fit" peptide and the HLA class II:peptide translocates to the cell surface and functions to present antigen to CD4+ T cells.[96] Peptides presented by HLA class II molecules are generally 12 to 20 amino acids long as the peptide-binding groove on class II molecules is open at either end, accommodating longer peptides than class I molecules.[139,140]

The nonclassical HLA-DO molecule is a cochaperone that strongly pairs with HLA-DM[88] in DC, B cells, and medullary thymic epithelial cells. HLA-DO functions to inhibit DM-mediated peptide loading in B cells resulting in the presentation of an altered repertoire of peptides internalized by the B-cell receptor.[141]

Cross-Presentation

Cross-presentation describes the ability of APC, primarily DC, to present peptides from exogenously acquired antigens in the context of HLA class I without being directly infected with the pathogen.[142] APCs that cross-present antigens are then able to cross-prime CD8+ T cells. The process is also relevant for the cross-presentation of tumor antigens and cross-priming of antitumor CD8+ T cells.[143] There are two pathways by which cross-presentation of exogenous antigen occurs—the cytosolic and vacuolar pathways (*Figure 15.9*).

The Cytosolic Pathway

In the cytosolic pathway, considered the principal pathway for cross-presentation of exogenous antigens,[144] peptide processing is thought to be dependent on the proteasome as it is abolished with the addition of proteasome inhibitors.[145] Phagocytosed extracellular proteins are translocated from the phagosome to the cytosol (P2C), processed through the proteasome where they are hydrolyzed into oligopeptides, and then transported by TAP to MHC I molecules through the ER. Challenging this dogma is recent evidence that peptides may import back into the phagosomes and there bind MHC I in a "phagosome to cytosol to phagosome" P2C2P mechanism.[146-149]

The processes by which extracellular proteins are translocated from the phagosome to the cytosol and then, after proteolytic digestion, back into the phagosome are areas of intense study. In support of the P2C2P model is convincing evidence for the recruitment of ER components Sec61, Sec22a, TAP, and MHC I from the ER to the phagosome membrane by a small GTPase Rab39a that serves to alter the molecular composition and function of phagosomes into peptide-loading compartments.[146,147,150-153] Interestingly, MHC I molecules found in proteasomes are in a peptide-empty conformation and are capable of binding peptides and transmigrating to the cell surface through incompletely understood mechanisms.

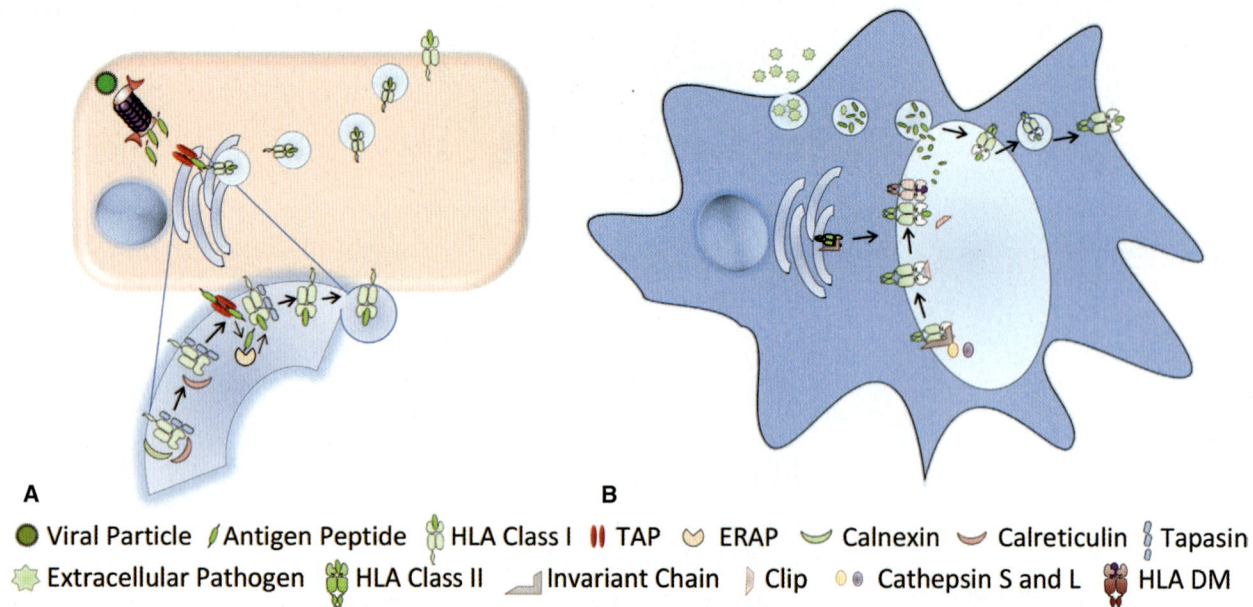

● Viral Particle ∕ Antigen Peptide ⊞ HLA Class I ▌▌ TAP ◡ ERAP ◡ Calnexin ◡ Calreticulin ⦚ Tapasin
⬡ Extracellular Pathogen ⊛ HLA Class II ◢ Invariant Chain ◗ Clip ◦◦ Cathepsin S and L ⬤ HLA DM

FIGURE 15.8 The endogenous and exogenous pathways of peptide loading and presentation. Pathogens that enter the cell are processed into peptides through the proteasome in the endogenous pathway of antigen presentation (A). Peptides then enter the ER through the TAP transporter and are trimmed by the aminopeptidase ERAP1. The MHC class I loading complex, including the human leukocyte antigen (HLA) class I molecule, Calnexin, Calreticulin, and Tapasin, is present in the ER. HLA class I molecules are loaded with the "best-fit" peptide and exported to the cell membrane via the secretory pathway. In the exogenous pathway of antigen presentation (B), extracellular pathogens are engulfed by the cell and degraded into peptides in the high-pH environment of the phagolysosome. HLA class II molecules associated with the invariant chain (Ii) are transported from the ER to a late endosomal compartment that contains the proteolytic enzymes cathepsin S and L and the nonclassical HLA-DM molecule. Ii is cleaved leaving behind the CLIP fragment of the protein. HLA-DM then facilitates the exchange of the CLIP protein for the best-fit peptide. The HLA class II molecule then translocates to the cell membrane.

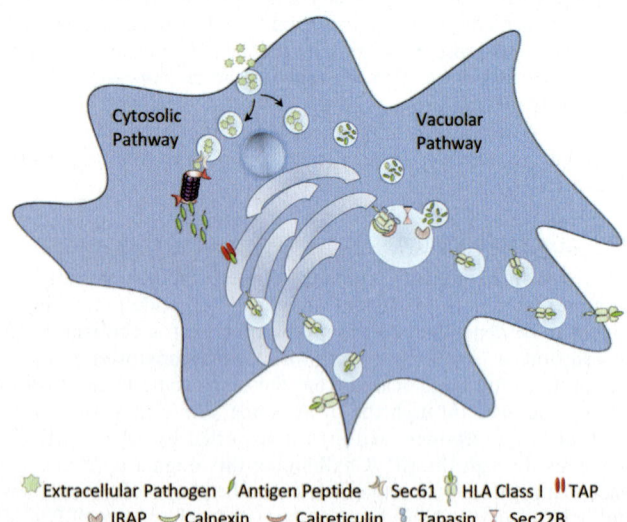

⬡ Extracellular Pathogen ∕ Antigen Peptide ◀ Sec61 ⊞ HLA Class I ▌▌ TAP
◡ IRAP ◡ Calnexin ◡ Calreticulin ⦚ Tapasin ⟏ Sec22B

FIGURE 15.9 Cross-presentation of antigens. Cross-presentation of antigens derived from extracellular pathogens in the context of human leukocyte antigen (HLA) class I can occur via the cytosolic or vacuolar pathways. In the cytosolic pathway, extracellular pathogens are engulfed by the cell and transported into the cytosol through the Sec61 translocon where they are then processed through the proteasome. Processed antigens then gain access to the ER through TAP, and antigen presentation proceeds similarly to the endogenous pathway. In the vacuolar pathway, engulfed extracellular pathogens are degraded in the high-pH environment of the endosome. Peptide loading of HLA class I is thought to occur in endocytic vesicles that are targeted to phagosomes via SEC22B. Class I molecules are loaded with peptides after they are trimmed by the aminopeptidase IRAP and are then transported to the cell membrane.

The Vacuolar Pathway

In the vacuolar pathway, cross-presentation is generally independent of TAP and resistant to proteasome inhibition and sensitive to lysosomal proteolysis with cathepsin S inhibitors,[154,155] suggesting that both antigen processing and loading onto HLA class I molecules occur in endocytic compartments. The presence of endosomes that also contain ER resident proteins such as calnexin and calreticulin[156] and that the ER membrane is in close contact with forming phagosomes[157] indicate that the ER contributes MHC class I loading machinery to the forming phagosome at the plasma membrane in support of cross-presentation.[148,150,157-159] Furthermore, the recruitment of ER proteins to the phagosomes is dependent on SEC22B, as knockdown of this molecule significantly impeded cross-presentation but not presentation of endogenous or class II–restricted antigen presentation.[29]

The peptide repertoire generated through TAP-independent proteolysis in the endocytic compartment differs from that generated through proteosomal hydrolysis in the cytosol. The two mechanisms, thus, require an element of chance that class I molecules will ultimately be loaded with immune-dominate peptide products able to prime T cells. Recently, this was elegantly addressed by Sengupta et al,[160] who provide evidence for the presence of active proteasomes in the endosomal compartment capable of proteolytic antigen hydrolysis followed by peptide loading of MHC I- an intraphagosome, TAP-independent mechanism of cross-presentation.

Class II Molecule Origin and Peptide Loading in Cross-Presentation

The source of class I molecules for cross-presentation and the cellular compartment where peptide loading occurs is currently under study. Class I molecules have been shown to be recycled from the membrane to endosomes per the function of a conserved tyrosine residue in the cytoplasmic tail essential for cross-presentation (*Figure 15.9*).[161,162] Other evidence shows that they can also originate from the ER and be targeted to endosomes via a signal in the Ii protein, thereby linking the cross/endogenous and exogenous pathways of antigen presentation as CD74 is classically considered essential in the process for loading of peptides onto HLA class II molecules.[163,164]

Peptide loading of the class I molecule during cross-presentation is thought to occur in the late secretory pathway, where class I molecules come into close contact with peptide antigens and the peptide-trimming insulin-responsive aminopeptidase (IRAP)[150,159,165,166] in TAP-containing vesicles beyond the ER. In support of this hypothesis are data showing that IRAP is found in close association and in fact can be coprecipitated with HLA class I molecules from intracellular vesicles.[165] There is also evidence for this process to occur in a TAP-independent manner via another, as yet, undescribed transporter.[167] In the proteasome and TAP-independent vacuolar pathway, peptide loading has been shown also to occur using newly synthesized and suboptimally loaded class I molecules exported through a novel secretory pathway that is independent of SEC22B and Ii.[164]

Cross-Dressing

Cross-dressing involves the transfer of intact, functional, antigen-presenting HLA molecules from one cell to another without antigen processing (*Figure 15.10*).[168,169] Generally, this process is described in the context of allogeneic organ transplant where recipient and donor tissues are found in close proximity. After transplantation, the recipient cells acquire intact donor HLA class I:peptide complexes through three distinct cell-cell mechanisms: trogocytosis (or membrane exchange), uptake of exosomes,[170-172] and tunneling nanotubes (TNTs) (*Figure 15.10*). Given that it is impossible to selectively block the three processes, it is difficult to determine the contribution of each to the transfer of specific membrane components.

Trogocytosis

Trogocytosis, also known as membrane exchange, is described as being a fast exchange of membrane sections from one cell to another.[139] Occurring within minutes, the process does not allow for antigen processing and is distinct from exosomal uptake (described in the following). Transferred membrane proteins retain their structure and function, and organized clusters of proteins such as those found at the immune synapse or lipid rafts have been observed and are dependent on HLA:TCR interactions.[173,174] Trogocytosis is often described between immune cells,[175] but the transfer of membrane proteins from recipient hematopoietic cells to donor APCs after bone marrow transplant has also been shown to lead to immune synapse formation in mice.[176]

Functional immunomodulation through cross-dressing by trogocytosis has been demonstrated. Hematologic tumor cells were found to be able to capture the inhibitory molecule HLA G from allogeneic or autologous cells allowing for immune escape mechanisms.[177] HLA G binds receptors LILRB1/ILT2 and LILRB2/ILT4 expressed on NK, T, and B cells, and myeloid APC resulting in the inhibition of effector immune cell functions and the induction of immune inhibitory or regulatory functionality.[174,178] Paradoxically, the innate immune cell component is also involved in immune activation in the context of hematopoietic tumors as activated NK cells that are recently degranulated in patients with hematologic cancer have been shown to display non–NK tumor cell antigens on their surface that are hypothesized to be the result of trogocytosis between the tumor and NK cell.[179]

Exosome Uptake

Extracellular vesicles, such as exosomes, are secreted from cells as a form of intercellular communication.[172] Preformed, functional HLA loaded with peptide antigens can be found in exosomes.[161-164] Secretion of exosomes has been reported in numerous cell types.[170,180]

Secreted exosomes were found to be captured and presented preferentially by mouse CD8+ DC without internalization and reprocessing.[181] Uptake of exosomes by this subset of immune cells was dependent on LFA-1 receptor expression on the CD8+ DC and ICAM-1 expression by the exosomes[181]; however, the authors of this study do not show that presented HLA:peptide complexes were functionally capable of stimulating T cells. In another study, exosomal transfer between mouse DCs was dependent on cell-cell interactions, and the exosomes served to transfer peptide but not intact HLA:peptide complexes. Peptides transferred to the recipient DC via the exosome were loaded onto the recipient cells' endogenously generated HLA class I molecules and elicited an antigen-specific T-cell response.[182] Concurrently, transfer of peptide-bound HLA molecules to recipient DC was accomplished via trogocytosis. In contrast to the described study, CD8a− DCs were more efficient at antigen presentation via cross-dressing than CD8a+ DCs. The differing protocols for DC maturation used in these two studies could potentially contribute

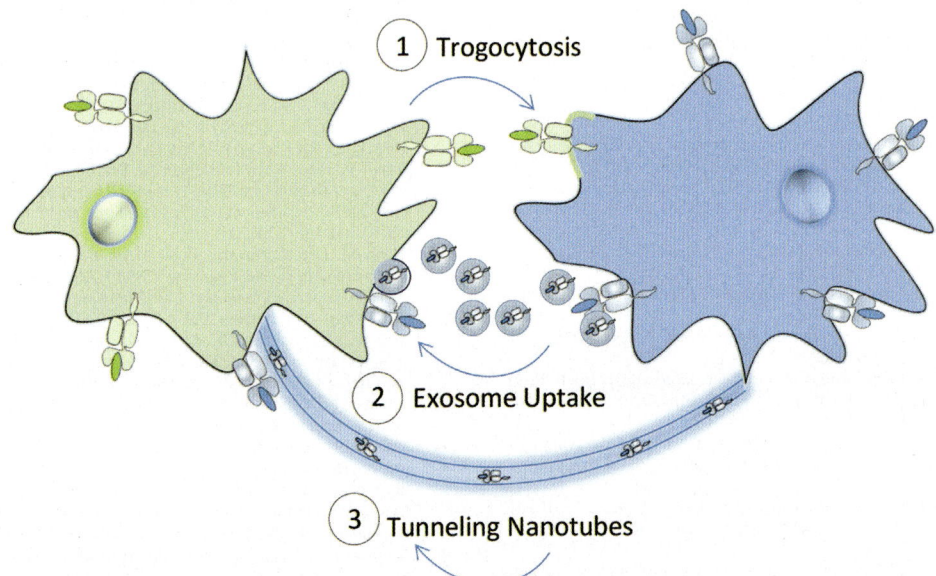

FIGURE 15.10 Cross-dressing of antigens. Cross-dressing has been shown to occur by three different mechanisms. (1) Trogocytosis, also called membrane exchange, is the fast exchange of a section of membrane from one cell to another. (2) The intercellular transfer of proteins can also occur by exosome secretion and uptake or through (3) membranous channels called tunneling nanotubes that form between cells. The direction of the arrows indicates the direction of intracellular protein transfer.

(1) Trogocytosis
(2) Exosome Uptake
(3) Tunneling Nanotubes

The Normal Hematologic System

to the differences in DC types that are preferentially cross-dressed to present antigen.[183]

Recipient APCs displaying donor allogeneic HLA originating from endosomes are capable of initiating a direct alloimmune response resulting in transplant rejection in animal models of skin and heart transplantation.[184] A study by Liu et al employed an allogeneic heterotopic mouse heart transplant model to study the mechanism by which presentation of donor antigen initiates an alloreactive T-cell response resulting in acute rejection in the recipient.[185] The authors showed that a small number of donor DCs transplanted with the donor heart migrate to the recipient's lymphoid tissue and transfer donor HLA and APC activating signals to the recipient's conventional DC (cDC) via clusters of CD9+CD63+ extracellular vesicles. In this form of cross-dressing, the vesicles were internalized or remained attached, but did not fuse, to the recipient's cDC, resulting in activation of the cDC and downstream activation of T cells.[185] Recipient DC presentation of donor MHC antigens via exosome uptake is persistent and may be a primary driver of CD8 T cell–mediated alloimmune response even late after transplantation.[186]

Tunneling Nanotubes

TNTs are long, thin, F-actin-based membranous channels connecting cells.[187] TNTs allow for the intercellular signaling or the transfer of vesicles, organelles, and molecules between cells and are described to connect various types of immune and nonimmune cells.[188] Transfer of HLA class I molecules via TNTs is described between HeLa cells[189] and B cells.[190] Transfer of HLA class II molecules was shown between endothelial cells in vitro, and the cross-dressed endothelial cells were capable of presenting antigen and eliciting the production of IL-2 from T cells.[191] However, in this paper, the intercellular transfer of class II molecules was not definitively shown to be via TNTs, as first, TNTs were not identified by classical F-actin staining, and second, the class II transfer and T-cell activation experiments were done independently.[191]

SUMMARY

This chapter covers the basic background and current clinically relevant knowledge on the genetics, structure, and function of the human MHC (HLA) molecules and their role in antigen presentation. HLA plays an important role in both solid organ and HSCT transplantation; however, the mechanisms of allograft rejection and GVHD are not fully understood. With studies at the genome, proteome, and transcriptome levels of the MHC region, our knowledge of MHC in autoimmune diseases, inflammation, and transplantation immunology will be further elucidated.

References

1. Complete sequence and gene map of a human major histocompatibility complex. The MHC sequencing consortium. *Nature.* 1999;401:921-923. doi:10.1038/44853
2. Shiina T, Hosomichi K, Inoko H, Kulski JK. The HLA genomic loci map: expression, interaction, diversity and disease. *J Hum Genet.* 2009;54:15-39. doi:10.1038/jhg.2008.5
3. Klein J, Sato A. The HLA system. First of two parts. *N Engl J Med.* 2000;343:702-709. doi:10.1056/NEJM200009073431006
4. Klein J, Sato A. The HLA system. Second of two parts. *N Engl J Med.* 2000;343:782-786. doi:10.1056/NEJM200009143431106
5. Erlich H. HLA DNA typing: past, present, and future. *Tissue Antigens.* 2012;80:1-11. doi:10.1111/j.1399-0039.2012.01881.x
6. Lan JH, Zhang Q. Clinical applications of next-generation sequencing in histocompatibility and transplantation. *Curr Opin Organ Transplant.* 2015;20:461-467. doi:10.1097/MOT.0000000000000217
7. Bjorkman PJ, Saper MA, Samraoui B, Bennett WS, Strominger JL, Wiley DC. Structure of the human class I histocompatibility antigen, HLA-A2. *Nature.* 1987;329:506-512. doi:10.1038/329506a0
8. Kulkarni S, Savan R, Qi Y, et al. Differential microRNA regulation of HLA-C expression and its association with HIV control. *Nature.* 2011;472:495-498. doi:10.1038/nature09914
9. Neijssen J, Herberts C, Drijfhout JW, et al. Cross-presentation by intercellular peptide transfer through gap junctions. *Nature.* 2005;434:83-88. doi:10.1038/nature03290
10. Pende D, Falco M, Vitale M, et al. Killer Ig-like Receptors (KIRs): their role in NK cell modulation and developments leading to their clinical exploitation. *Front Immunol.* 2019;10:1179.
11. Carton G, Dacheux L, Salles G, et al. Therapeutic activity of humanized anti-CD20 monoclonal antibody and polymorphism in IgG Fc receptor FcgammaRIIIa gene. *Blood.* 2002;99(3):754-758.
12. Treon SP, Hansen M, Branagan AR, et al. Polymorphisms in FcgammaRIIIA (CD16) receptor expression are associated with clinical response to rituximab in Waldenström's macroglobulinemia. *J Clin Oncol.* 2005;23(3):474-481.
13. Terasaki PI, Cai J. Humoral theory of transplantation: further evidence. *Curr Opin Immunol.* 2005;17:541-545. doi:10.1016/j.coi.2005.07.018
14. Tambur AR. HLA-epitope matching or eplet risk stratification: the devil is in the details. *Front Immunol.* 2018;9:2010. doi:10.3389/fimmu.2018.02010
15. Terasaki PI, McClelland JD. Microdroplet assay of human serum cytotoxins. *Nature.* 1964;204:998-1000. doi:10.1038/204998b0
16. Cecka JM, Kucheryavaya AY, Reinsmoen NL, Leffell MS. Calculated PRA: initial results show benefits for sensitized patients and a reduction in positive crossmatches. *Am J Transplant.* 2011;11:719-724. doi:10.1111/j.1600-6143.2010.03340.x
17. Luznik L, O'Donnell PV, Symons HJ, et al. HLA-haploidentical bone marrow transplantation for hematologic malignancies using nonmyeloablative conditioning and high-dose, posttransplantation cyclophosphamide. *Biol Blood Marrow Transplant.* 2008;14:641-650. doi:10.1016/j.bbmt.2008.03.005
18. Jones RJ. Is post-transplant cyclophosphamide a true game-changer in allogeneic transplantation: the struggle to unlearn. *Best Pract Res Clin Haematol.* 2019;32:101112. doi:10.1016/j.beha.2019.101112
19. Rappazzo KC, Zahurak M, Bettinotti M, et al. Nonmyeloablative, HLA-mismatched unrelated peripheral blood transplantation with high-dose post-transplantation cyclophosphamide. *Transplant Cell Ther.* 2021;27(11):909.e1-909.e6.
20. Ciurea SO, Thall PF, Wang X, et al. Donor-specific anti-HLA Abs and graft failure in matched unrelated donor hematopoietic stem cell transplantation. *Blood.* 2011;118:5957-5964. doi:10.1182/blood-2011-06-362111
21. Yoshihara S, Maruya E, Taniguchi K, et al. Risk and prevention of graft failure in patients with preexisting donor-specific HLA antibodies undergoing unmanipulated haploidentical SCT. *Bone Marrow Transplant.* 2012;47:508-515. doi:10.1038/bmt.2011.131
22. Huo MR, Xu YJ, Zhai SZ, et al. Prevalence and risk factors of antibodies to human leukocyte antigens in haploidentical stem cell transplantation candidates: a multi-center study. *Hum Immunol.* 2018;79:672-677. doi:10.1016/j.humimm.2018.06.003
23. Brand A, Doxiadis IN, Roelen DL. On the role of HLA antibodies in hematopoietic stem cell transplantation. *Tissue Antigens.* 2013;81:1-11. doi:10.1111/tan.12040
24. Kongtim P, Cao K, Ciurea SO. Donor specific anti-HLA antibody and risk of graft failure in haploidentical stem cell transplantation. *Adv Hematol.* 2016;2016:4025073. doi:10.1155/2016/4025073
25. Gladstone DE, Bettinotti MP. HLA donor-specific antibodies in allogeneic hematopoietic stem cell transplantation: challenges and opportunities. *Hematology Am Soc Hematol Educ Program.* 2017;2017:645-650. doi:10.1182/asheducation-2017.1.645
26. Fauchet R, Boscher M, Bouhallier O, et al. New class I in man: serological and molecular characterization. *Hum Immunol.* 1986;17:3-20. doi:10.1016/0198-8859(86)90069-8
27. Coupel S, Moreau A, Hamidou M, Horejsi V, Soulillou JP, Charreau B. Expression and release of soluble HLA-E is an immunoregulatory feature of endothelial cell activation. *Blood.* 2007;109:2806-2814. doi:10.1182/blood-2006-06-030213
28. Grimsley C, Ober C. Population genetic studies of HLA-E: evidence for selection. *Hum Immunol.* 1997;52:33-40. doi:10.1016/S0198-8859(96)00241-8
29. Braud VM, Allan DSJ, O'Callaghan CA, et al. HLA-E binds to natural killer cell receptors CD94/NKG2A, B and C. *Nature.* 1998;391:795-799. doi:10.1038/35869
30. Petrie EJ, Clements CS, Lin J, et al. CD94-NKG2A recognition of human leukocyte antigen (HLA)-E bound to an HLA class I leader sequence. *J Exp Med.* 2008;205:725-735. doi:10.1084/jem.20072525
31. O'Callaghan CA, Tormo J, Willcox BE, et al. Structural features impose tight peptide binding specificity in the nonclassical MHC molecule HLA-E. *Mol Cell.* 1998;1:531-541. doi:10.1016/s1097-2765(00)80053-2
32. Braud V, Jones EY, McMichael A. The human major histocompatibility complex class Ib molecule HLA-E binds signal sequence-derived peptides with primary anchor residues at positions 2 and 9. *Eur J Immunol.* 1997;27:1164-1169. doi:10.1002/eji.1830270517
33. Llano M, Lee N, Navarro F, et al. HLA-E-bound peptides influence recognition by inhibitory and triggering CD94/NKG2 receptors: preferential response to an HLA-G-derived nonamer. *Eur J Immunol.* 1998;28:2854-2863. doi:10.1002/(SICI)1521-4141(199809)28:09<2854::AID-IMMU2854>3.0.CO;2-W
34. Sullivan LC, Clements CS, Rossjohn J, Brooks AG. The major histocompatibility complex class Ib molecule HLA-E at the interface between innate and adaptive immunity. *Tissue Antigens.* 2008;72:415-424. doi:10.1111/j.1399-0039.2008.01138.x
35. Kraemer T, Blaszczyk R, Bade-Doeding C. HLA-E: a novel player for histocompatibility. *J Immunol Res.* 2014;2014:352160. doi:10.1155/2014/352160
36. Walters LC, Harlos K, Brackenridge S, et al. Pathogen-derived HLA-E bound epitopes reveal broad primary anchor pocket tolerability and conformationally malleable peptide binding. *Nat Commun.* 2018;9(1):3137.
37. Bansal A, Gehre MN, Qin K, et al. HLA-E-restricted HIV-1-specific CD8+ T cell responses in natural infection. *J Clin Invest.* 2021;131(16):e148979.
38. Kordelas L, Schwich E, Lindemann M, et al. Decreased soluble human leukocyte antigen E levels in patients after allogeneic hematopoietic stem cell transplantation are associated with severe acute and extended chronic graft-versus-host disease and inferior overall survival. *Front Immunol.* 2019;10:3027. doi:10.3389/fimmu.2019.03027
39. Lee N, Ishitani A, Geraghty DE. HLA-F is a surface marker on activated lymphocytes. *Eur J Immunol.* 2010;40:2308-2318. doi:10.1002/eji.201040348

40. Ishitani A, Sageshima N., Lee N., et al. Protein expression and peptide binding suggest unique and interacting functional roles for HLA-E, F, and G in maternal-placental immune recognition. *J Immunol.* 2003;171:1376-1384. doi:10.4049/jimmunol.171.3.1376

41. Goodridge JP, Burian A, Lee N, Geraghty DE. HLA-F complex without peptide binds to MHC class I protein in the open conformer form. *J Immunol.* 2010;184:6199-6208. doi:10.4049/jimmunol.1000078

42. Wainwright SD, Biro PA, Holmes CH. HLA-F is a predominantly empty, intracellular, TAP-associated MHC class Ib protein with a restricted expression pattern. *J Immunol.* 2000;164:319-328. doi:10.4049/jimmunol.164.1.319

43. Kollnberger S. The role of HLA-class I heavy-chain interactions with killer-cell immunoglobulin-like receptors in immune regulation. *Crit Rev Immunol.* 2016;36:269-282. doi:10.1615/CritRevImmunol.2016017965

44. Garcia-Beltran WF, Hölzemer A, Martrus G, et al. Open conformers of HLA-F are high-affinity ligands of the activating NK-cell receptor KIR3DS1. *Nat Immunol.* 2016;17:1067-1074. doi:10.1038/ni.3513

45. Parham P, Norman PJ, Abi-Rached L, Guethlein LA. Variable NK cell receptors exemplified by human KIR3DL1/S1. *J Immunol.* 2011;187:11-19. doi:10.4049/jimmunol.0902332

46. Dulberger CL, McMurtrey CP, Hölzemer A, et al. Human leukocyte antigen F presents peptides and regulates immunity through interactions with NK cell receptors. *Immunity.* 2017;46:1018-1029 e1017. doi:10.1016/j.immuni.2017.06.002

47. Geraghty DE, Koller BH, Orr HT. A human major histocompatibility complex class I gene that encodes a protein with a shortened cytoplasmic segment. *Proc Natl Acad Sci U S A.* 1987;84:9145-9149. doi:10.1073/pnas.84.24.9145

48. Park B, , Lee S, Kim E, Chang S, Jin M, Ahn K. The truncated cytoplasmic tail of HLA-G serves a quality-control function in post-ER compartments. *Immunity.* 2001;15:213-224. doi:10.1016/s1074-7613(01)00179-0

49. Paul P, Adrian Cabestre F, Ibrahim EC, et al. Identification of HLA-G7 as a new splice variant of the HLA-G mRNA and expression of soluble HLA-G5, -G6, and -G7 transcripts in human transfected cells. *Hum Immunol.* 2000;61:1138-1149. doi:10.1016/s0198-8859(00)00197-x

50. Carosella ED, Favier B, Rouas-Freiss N, Moreau P, Lemaoult J. Beyond the increasing complexity of the immunomodulatory HLA-G molecule. *Blood.* 2008;111:4862-4870. doi:10.1182/blood-2007-12-127662

51. Boyson JE, Erskine R, Whitman MC, et al. Disulfide bond-mediated dimerization of HLA-G on the cell surface. *Proc Natl Acad Sci U S A.* 2002;99:16180-16185. doi:10.1073/pnas.212643199

52. Morales PJ, Pace JL, Platt JS, Langat DK, Hunt JS. Synthesis of beta(2)-microglobulin-free, disulphide-linked HLA-G5 homodimers in human placental villous cytotrophoblast cells. *Immunology.* 2007;122:179-188. doi:10.1111/j.1365-2567.2007.02623.x

53. Menier C, Rouas-Freiss N, Favier B, et al. Recent advances on the non-classical major histocompatibility complex class I HLA-G molecule. *Tissue Antigens.* 2010;75:201-206. doi:10.1111/j.1399-0039.2009.01438.x

54. Sabbagh A, Sonon P, Sadissou I, et al. The role of HLA-G in parasitic diseases. *HLA.* 2018;91:255-270. doi:10.1111/tan.13196

55. Gregori S, Amodio G, Quattrone F, Panina-Bordignon P. HLA-G Orchestrates the early interaction of human trophoblasts with the maternal Niche. *Front Immunol.* 2015;6:128. doi:10.3389/fimmu.2015.00128

56. Morandi F, Pistoia V. Interactions between HLA-G and HLA-E in physiological and pathological conditions. *Front Immunol.* 2014;5:394. doi:10.3389/fimmu.2014.00394

57. Teklemariam T, Zhao L, Hantash BM. Full-length HLA-G1 and truncated HLA-G3 differentially increase HLA-E surface localization. *Hum Immunol.* 2012;73:898-905. doi:10.1016/j.humimm.2012.06.007

58. Apps R, Gardner L, Moffett A. A critical look at HLA-G. *Trends Immunol.* 2008;29:313-321. doi:10.1016/j.it.2008.02.012

59. Jordier F, Gras D, De Grandis M, et al. HLA-H: transcriptional activity and HLA-E Mobilization. *Front Immunol.* 2019;10:2986. doi:10.3389/fimmu.2019.02986

60. Paganini J, Abi-Rached L, Gouret P, Pontarotti P, Chiaroni J, Di Cristofaro J. HLAIb worldwide genetic diversity: new HLA-H alleles and haplotype structure description. *Mol Immunol.* 2019;112:40-50. doi:10.1016/j.molimm.2019.04.017

61. Feder JN, Gnirke A, Thomas W, et al. A novel MHC class I-like gene is mutated in patients with hereditary haemochromatosis. *Nat Genet.* 1996;13:399-408. doi:10.1038/ng0896-399

62. Jouanolle AM, Gandon G, Jézéquel P, et al. Haemochromatosis and HLA-H. *Nat Genet.* 1996;14:251-252. doi:10.1038/ng1196-251

63. Jazwinska EC, Cullen LM, Busfield F, et al. Haemochromatosis and HLA-H. *Nat Genet.* 1996;14:249-251. doi:10.1038/ng1196-249

64. Bahram S, Bresnahan M, Geraghty DE, Spies T. A second lineage of mammalian major histocompatibility complex class I genes. *Proc Natl Acad Sci U S A.* 1994;91:6259-6263. doi:10.1073/pnas.91.14.6259

65. Leelayuwat C, Townend DC, Degli-Esposti MA, Abraham LJ, Dawkins RL. A new polymorphic and multicopy MHC gene family related to nonmammalian class I. *Immunogenetics.* 1994;40:339-351. doi:10.1007/BF01246675

66. Baranwal AK, Mehra NK. Major histocompatibility complex class I chain-related A (MICA) molecules: relevance in solid organ transplantation. *Front Immunol.* 2017;8:182. doi:10.3389/fimmu.2017.00182

67. Choy MK, Phipps ME. MICA polymorphism: biology and importance in immunity and disease. *Trends Mol Med.* 2010;16:97-106. doi:10.1016/j.molmed.2010.01.002

68. Stephens HA. MICA and MICB genes: can the enigma of their polymorphism be resolved?. *Trends Immunol.* 2001;22:378-385. doi:10.1016/s1471-4906(01)01960-3

69. Schrambach S, Ardizzone M, Leymarie V, Sibilia J, Bahram S. In vivo expression pattern of MICA and MICB and its relevance to auto-immunity and cancer. *PLoS One.* 2007;2:e518. doi:10.1371/journal.pone.0000518

70. Groh V, Bahram S, Bauer S, Herman A, Beauchamp M, Spies T. Cell stress-regulated human major histocompatibility complex class I gene expressed in gastro-intestinal epithelium. *Proc Natl Acad Sci U S A.* 1996;93:12445-12450. doi:10.1073/pnas.93.22.12445

71. Strong RK. Class (I) will come to order—not. *Nat Struct Biol.* 2000;7:173-176. doi:10.1038/73254

72. Groh V, Steinle A, Bauer S, Spies T. Recognition of stress-induced MHC molecules by intestinal epithelial gammadelta T cells. *Science (New York, N.Y.).* 1998;279:1737-1740. doi:10.1126/science.279.5357.1737

73. Thomas M, Wills M, Lehner PJ. Natural killer cell evasion by an E3 ubiquitin ligase from Kaposi's sarcoma-associated herpesvirus. *Biochem Soc Trans.* 2008;36:459-463. doi:10.1042/BST0360459

74. Stern-Ginossar N, Elefant N, Zimmermann A, et al. Host immune system gene targeting by a viral miRNA. *Science (New York, N.Y.).* 2007;317:376-381. doi:10.1126/science.1140956

75. Groh V, Wu J, Yee C, Spies T. Tumour-derived soluble MIC ligands impair expression of NKG2D and T-cell activation. *Nature.* 2002;419:734-738. doi:10.1038/nature01112

76. Holdenrieder S, Stieber P, Peterfi A, Nagel D, Steinle A, Salih HR. Soluble MICA in malignant diseases. *International journal of cancer. Journal international du cancer.* 2006;118:684-687. doi:10.1002/ijc.21382

77. Holdenrieder S, Stieber P, Peterfi A, Nagel D, Steinle A, Salih HR. Soluble MICB in malignant diseases: analysis of diagnostic significance and correlation with soluble MICA. *Cancer Immunol Immunother.* 2006;55:1584-1589. doi:10.1007/s00262-006-0167-1

78. Alfonso C, Karlsson L. Nonclassical MHC class II molecules. *Annu Rev Immunol.* 2000;18:113-142. doi:10.1146/annurev.immunol.18.1.113

79. Feng ML, Liu RZ, Shen T, Zhao YL, Zhu ZY, Liu DZ. Analysis of HLA-DM polymorphisms in the Chinese Han population. *Tissue Antigens.* 2012;79:157-164. doi:10.1111/j.1399-0039.2012.01838.x

80. Kelly AP, Monaco JJ, Cho SG, Trowsdale J. A new human HLA class II-related locus, DM. *Nature.* 1991;353:571-573. doi:10.1038/353571a0

81. Cho SG, Attaya M, Monaco JJ. New class II-like genes in the murine MHC. *Nature.* 1991;353:573-576. doi:10.1038/353573a0

82. Servenius B, Rask L, Peterson PA. Class II genes of the human major histocompatibility complex. The DO beta gene is a divergent member of the class II beta gene family. *J Biol Chem.* 1987;262:8759-8766.

83. Andersson T, Patwardhan A, Emilson A, Carlsson K, Scheynius A. HLA-DM is expressed on the cell surface and colocalizes with HLA-DR and invariant chain in human Langerhans cells. *Arch Dermatol Res.* 1998;290:674-680. doi:10.1007/s004030050372

84. Arndt SO, Vogt AB, Markovic-Plese S, et al. Functional HLA-DM on the surface of B cells and immature dendritic cells. *EMBO J.* 2000;19:1241-1251. doi:10.1093/emboj/19.6.1241

85. Ting JP, Trowsdale J. Genetic control of MHC class II expression. *Cell.* 2002;109(suppl):S21-S33. doi:10.1016/s0092-8674(02)00696-7

86. Lindstedt R, Liljedahl M, Peleraux A, Peterson PA, Karlsson L. The MHC class II molecule H2-M is targeted to an endosomal compartment by a tyrosine-based targeting motif. *Immunity.* 1995;3:561-572. doi:10.1016/1074-7613(95)90127-2

87. Marks MS, Roche PA, van Donselaar E, Woodruff L, Peters PJ, Bonifacino JS. A lysosomal targeting signal in the cytoplasmic tail of the beta chain directs HLA-DM to MHC class II compartments. *J Cell Biol.* 1995;131:351-369. doi:10.1083/jcb.131.2.351

88. Liljedahl M, Kuwana T, Fung-Leung WP, Jackson MR, Peterson PA, Karlsson L. HLA-DO is a lysosomal resident which requires association with HLA-DM for efficient intracellular transport. *EMBO J.* 1996;15:4817-4824.

89. Potter PK, Copier J, Sacks SH, et al. Accurate intracellular localization of HLA-DM requires correct spacing of a cytoplasmic YTPL targeting motif relative to the transmembrane domain. *Eur J Immunol.* 1999;29:3936-3944. doi:10.1002/(SICI)1521-4141(199912)29:12<3936::AID-IMMU3936>3.0.CO;2-K

90. Mosyak L, Zaller DM, Wiley DC. The structure of HLA-DM, the peptide exchange catalyst that loads antigen onto class II MHC molecules during antigen presentation. *Immunity.* 1998;9:377-383. doi:10.1016/s1074-7613(00)80620-2

91. Jastaniah WA, Alessandri AJ, Reid GS, Schultz KR. HLA-DM expression is elevated in ETV6-AML1 translocation-positive pediatric acute lymphoblastic leukemia. *Leuk Res.* 2006;30:487-489. doi:10.1016/j.leukres.2005.08.013

92. Pos W, Sethi DK, Wucherpfennig KW. Mechanisms of peptide repertoire selection by HLA-DM. *Trends Immunol.* 2013;34:495-501. doi:10.1016/j.it.2013.06.002

93. Germain RN, Hendrix LR. MHC class II structure, occupancy and surface expression determined by post-endoplasmic reticulum antigen binding. *Nature.* 1991;353:134-139. doi:10.1038/353134a0

94. Stern LJ, Wiley DC. The human class II MHC protein HLA-DR1 assembles as empty alpha beta heterodimers in the absence of antigenic peptide. *Cell.* 1992;68:465-477. doi:10.1016/0092-8674(92)90184-e

95. Blum JS, Wearsch PA, Cresswell P. Pathways of antigen processing. *Annu Rev Immunol.* 2013;31:443-473. doi:10.1146/annurev-immunol-032712-095910

96. Denzin LK, Cresswell P. HLA-DM induces CLIP dissociation from MHC class II alpha beta dimers and facilitates peptide loading. *Cell.* 1995;82:155-165. doi:10.1016/0092-8674(95)90061-6

97. Kropshofer H, Arndt SO, Moldenhauer G, Hammerling GJ, Vogt AB. HLA-DM acts as a molecular chaperone and rescues empty HLA-DR molecules at lysosomal pH. *Immunity.* 1997;6:293-302. doi:10.1016/s1074-7613(00)80332-5

98. Liljedahl M, Winqvist O, Surh CD, et al. Altered antigen presentation in mice lacking H2-O. *Immunity.* 1998;8:233-243. doi:10.1016/s1074-7613(00)80475-6

99. Jensen PE, Weber DA, Thayer WP, Westerman LE, Dao CT. Peptide exchange in MHC molecules. *Immunol Rev.* 1999;172:229-238. doi:10.1111/j.1600-065x.1999.tb01368.x

100. van Ham SM, Tjin EPM, Lillemeier BF, et al. HLA-DO is a negative modulator of HLA-DM-mediated MHC class II peptide loading. *Curr Biol.* 1997;7:950-957. doi:10.1016/s0960-9822(06)00414-3

101. Pathak SS, Lich JD, Blum JS. Cutting edge: editing of recycling class II:peptide complexes by HLA-DM. *J Immunol.* 2001;167:632-635. doi:10.4049/jimmunol.167.2.632

102. Painter CA, Stern LJ. Structural Insights into HLA-DM mediated MHC II peptide exchange. *Curr Top Biochem Res.* 2011;13:39-55.

103. Sloan VS, Cameron P, Porter G, et al. Mediation by HLA-DM of dissociation of peptides from HLA-DR. *Nature.* 1995;375:802-806. doi:10.1038/375802a0

104. Nicholson MJ, Moradi B, Seth NP, et al. Small molecules that enhance the catalytic efficiency of HLA-DM. *J Immunol.* 2006;176:4208-4220. doi:10.4049/jimmunol.176.7.4208

105. Alvaro-Benito M, Wieczorek M, Sticht J, Kipar C, Freund C. HLA-DMA polymorphisms differentially affect MHC class II peptide loading. *J Immunol.* 2015;194:803-816. doi:10.4049/jimmunol.1401389

106. Alvaro-Benito M, Morrison E, Wieczorek M, Sticht J, Freund C. Human leukocyte Antigen-DM polymorphisms in autoimmune diseases. *Open Biol.* 2016;6(8):160165. doi:10.1098/rsob.160165

107. Sirota M, Schaub MA, Batzoglou S, Robinson WH, Butte AJ. Autoimmune disease classification by inverse association with SNP alleles. *PLoS Genet.* 2009;5:e1000792, doi:10.1371/journal.pgen.1000792

108. Huang P, Dong L, Lu X, et al. Genetic variants in antigen presentation-related genes influence susceptibility to hepatitis C virus and viral clearance: a case control study. *BMC Infect Dis.* 2014;14:716. doi:10.1186/s12879-014-0716-8

109. Chen H, Yao Y, Wang Y, et al. Polymorphisms of HLA-DM on treatment response to interferon/Ribavirin in patients with chronic hepatitis C virus type 1 infection. *Int J Environ Res Public Health.* 2016;13. doi:10.3390/ijerph13101030

110. Aissani B, Boehme AK, Wiener HW, Shrestha S, Jacobson LP, Kaslow RA. SNP screening of central MHC-identified HLA-DMB as a candidate susceptibility gene for HIV-related Kaposi's sarcoma. *Genes Immun.* 2014;15:424-429. doi:10.1038/gene.2014.42

111. Callahan MJ, Nagymanyoki Z, Bonome T, et al. Increased HLA-DMB expression in the tumor epithelium is associated with increased CTL infiltration and improved prognosis in advanced-stage serous ovarian cancer. *Clin Cancer Res.* 2008;14:7667-7673. doi:10.1158/1078-0432.CCR-08-0479

112. Louis-Plence P, Kerlan-Candon S, Morel J, et al. The down-regulation of HLA-DM gene expression in rheumatoid arthritis is not related to their promoter polymorphism. *J Immunol.* 2000;165:4861-4869. doi:10.4049/jimmunol.165.9.4861

113. Meurer T, Crivello P, Metzing M, et al. Permissive HLA-DPB1 mismatches in HCT depend on immunopeptidome divergence and editing by HLA-DM. *Blood.* 2021;137:923-928. doi:10.1182/blood.2020008464

114. Naruse TK, Kawata H, Inoko H, et al. The HLA-DOB gene displays limited polymorphism with only one amino acid substitution. *Tissue Antigens.* 2002;59:512-519. doi:10.1034/j.1399-0039.2002.590608.x

115. Karlsson L, Surh CD, Sprent J, Peterson PA. A novel class II MHC molecule with unusual tissue distribution. *Nature.* 1991;351:485-488. doi:10.1038/351485a0

116. Chen X, Jensen PE. The expression of HLA-DO (H2-O) in B lymphocytes. *Immunol Res.* 2004;29:19-28. doi:10.1385/IR:29:1-3:019

117. Nagarajan UM, Lochamy J, Chen X, et al. Class II transactivator is required for maximal expression of HLA-DOB in B cells. *J Immunol.* 2002;168:1780-1786. doi:10.4049/jimmunol.168.4.1780

118. Walter W, Scheuer C, Lingnau K, et al. H2-M, a facilitator of MHC class II peptide loading, and its negative modulator H2-O are differentially expressed in response to proinflammatory cytokines. *Immunogenetics.* 2000;51:794-804 doi:10.1007/s002510000210

119. Poluektov YO, Kim A, Sadegh-Nasseri S. HLA-DO and its role in MHC class II antigen presentation. *Front Immunol.* 2013;4:260. doi:10.3389/fimmu.2013.00260

120. Denzin LK, Sant'Angelo DB, Hammond C, Surman MJ, Cresswell P. Negative regulation by HLA-DO of MHC class II-restricted antigen processing. *Science (New York, N.Y.).* 1997;278:106-109. doi:10.1126/science.278.5335.106

121. Kropshofer H, Vogt AB, Thery C, et al. A role for HLA-DO as a co-chaperone of HLA-DM in peptide loading of MHC class II molecules. *EMBO J.* 1998;17:2971-2981. doi:10.1093/emboj/17.11.2971

122. Jiang W, Strohman MJ, Somasundaram S, et al. pH-susceptibility of HLA-DO tunes DO/DM ratios to regulate HLA-DM catalytic activity. *Sci Rep.* 2015;5:17333. doi:10.1038/srep17333

123. Glazier KS, Hake SB, Tobin HM, Chadburn A, Schattner EJ, Denzin LK et al. Germinal center B cells regulate their capability to present antigen by modulation of HLA-DO. *J Exp Med.* 2002;195:1063-1069. doi:10.1084/jem.20012059

124. Kropshofer H, Hammerling GJ, Vogt AB. The impact of the non-classical MHC proteins HLA-DM and HLA-DO on loading of MHC class II molecules. *Immunol Rev.* 1999;172:267-278. doi:10.1111/j.1600-065x.1999.tb01371.x

125. Chen X, Laur O, Kambayashi T, et al. Regulated expression of human histocompatibility leukocyte antigen (HLA)-DO during antigen-dependent and antigen-independent phases of B cell development. *J Exp Med.* 2002;195:1053-1062. doi:10.1084/jem.20012066

126. Sindhi R, Higgs BW, Weeks DE, et al. Genetic variants in major histocompatibility complex-linked genes associate with pediatric liver transplant rejection. *Gastroenterology.* 2008;135:830-839. 839 e831-810. doi:10.1053/j.gastro.2008.05.080

127. Kremer AN, van der Meijden ED, Honders MW, et al. Human leukocyte antigen-DO regulates surface presentation of human leukocyte antigen class II-restricted antigens on B cell malignancies. *Biol Blood Marrow Transplant.* 2014;20:742-747. doi:10.1016/j.bbmt.2014.02.005

128. Souwer Y, Chamuleau MED, van de Loosdrecht AA, et al. Detection of aberrant transcription of major histocompatibility complex class II antigen presentation genes in chronic lymphocytic leukaemia identifies HLA-DOA mRNA as a prognostic factor for survival. *Br J Haematol.* 2009;145:334-343. doi:10.1111/j.1365-2141.2009.07625.x

129. Cascio P, Hilton C, Kisselev AF, Rock KL, Goldberg AL. 26S proteasomes and immunoproteasomes produce mainly N-extended versions of an antigenic peptide. *EMBO J.* 2001;20:2357-2366. doi:10.1093/emboj/20.10.2357

130. Saveanu L, Carroll O, Lindo V, et al. Concerted peptide trimming by human ERAP1 and ERAP2 aminopeptidase complexes in the endoplasmic reticulum. *Nat Immunol.* 2005;6:689-697. doi:10.1038/ni1208

131. Reits E, Griekspoor A, Neijssen J, et al. Peptide diffusion, protection, and degradation in nuclear and cytoplasmic compartments before antigen presentation by MHC class I. *Immunity.* 2003;18:97-108. doi:10.1016/s1074-7613(02)00511-3

132. Wearsch PA, Cresswell P. The quality control of MHC class I peptide loading. *Curr Opin Cell Biol.* 2008;20:624-631. doi:10.1016/j.ceb.2008.09.005

133. Elliott T, Williams A. The optimization of peptide cargo bound to MHC class I molecules by the peptide-loading complex. *Immunol Rev.* 2005;207:89-99. doi:10.1111/j.0105-2896.2005.00311.x

134. Rock KL, Goldberg AL. Degradation of cell proteins and the generation of MHC class I-presented peptides. *Annu Rev Immunol.* 1999;17:739-779. doi:10.1146/annurev.immunol.17.1.739

135. Neefjes JJ, Ploegh HL. Allele and locus-specific differences in cell surface expression and the association of HLA class I heavy chain with beta 2-microglobulin: differential effects of inhibition of glycosylation on class I subunit association. *Eur J Immunol.* 1988;18:801-810. doi:10.1002/eji.1830180522

136. Neisig A, Wubbolts R, Zang X, Melief C, Neefjes J. Allele-specific differences in the interaction of MHC class I molecules with transporters associated with antigen processing. *J Immunol.* 1996;156:3196-3206.

137. Hartman IZ, Kim A, Cotter RJ, et al. A reductionist cell-free major histocompatibility complex class II antigen processing system identifies immunodominant epitopes. *Nat Med.* 2010;16:1333-1340. doi:10.1038/nm.2248

138. Unanue ER, Turk V, Neefjes J. Variations in MHC class II antigen processing and presentation in Health and disease. *Annu Rev Immunol.* 2016;34:265-297. doi:10.1146/annurev-immunol-041015-055420

139. Joly E, Hudrisier D. What is trogocytosis and what is its purpose? *Nat Immunol.* 2003;4:815. doi:10.1038/ni0903-815

140. Stern LJ, Brown JH, Jardetzky TS, et al. Crystal structure of the human class II MHC protein HLA-DR1 complexed with an influenza virus peptide. *Nature.* 1994;368:215-221. doi:10.1038/368215a0

141. Denzin LK, Fallas JL, Prendes M, Yi W. Right place, right time, right peptide: DO keeps DM focused. *Immunol Rev.* 2005;207:279-292. doi:10.1111/j.0105-2896.2005.00302.x

142. Jung S, Unutmaz D, Wong P, et al. In vivo depletion of CD11c+ dendritic cells abrogates priming of CD8+ T cells by exogenous cell-associated antigens. *Immunity.* 2002;17:211-220.

143. Joffre OP, Segura E, Savina A, Amigorena S. Cross-presentation by dendritic cells. *Nat Rev Immunol.* 2012;12:557-569. doi:10.1038/nri3254

144. Sigal LJ, Rock KL. Bone marrow-derived antigen-presenting cells are required for the generation of cytotoxic T lymphocyte responses to viruses and use transporter associated with antigen presentation (TAP)-dependent and -independent pathways of antigen presentation. *J Exp Med.* 2000;192:1143-1150.

145. Kovacsovics-Bankowski M, Rock KL. A phagosome-to-cytosol pathway for exogenous antigens presented on MHC class I molecules. *Science (New York, N.Y.).* 1995;267:243-246.

146. Ackerman AL, Kyritsis C, Tampe R, Cresswell P. Early phagosomes in dendritic cells form a cellular compartment sufficient for cross presentation of exogenous antigens. *Proc Natl Acad Sci U S A.* 2003;100:12889-12894. doi:10.1073/pnas.1735556100

147. Zehner M, Marschall AL, Bos E, et al. The translocon protein Sec61 mediates antigen transport from endosomes in the cytosol for cross-presentation to CD8(+) T cells. *Immunity.* 2015;42:850-863. doi:10.1016/j.immuni.2015.04.008

148. Ackerman AL, Giodini A, Cresswell P. A role for the endoplasmic reticulum protein retrotranslocation machinery during crosspresentation by dendritic cells. *Immunity.* 2006;25:607-617. doi:10.1016/j.immuni.2006.08.017

149. Lawand M, Abramova A, Manceau V, Springer S, van Endert P. TAP-dependent and -independent peptide import into dendritic cell phagosomes. *J Immunol.* 2016;197:3454-3463. doi:10.4049/jimmunol.1501925

150. Houde M, Bertholet S, Gagnon E, et al. Phagosomes are competent organelles for antigen cross-presentation. *Nature.* 2003;425:402-406. doi:10.1038/nature01912

151. Cruz FM, Colbert JD, Rock KL. The GTPase Rab39a promotes phagosome maturation into MHC-I antigen-presenting compartments. *EMBO J.* 2020;39:e102020. doi:10.15252/embj.2019102020

152. Cebrian I, Visentin G, Blanchard N, et al. Sec22b regulates phagosomal maturation and antigen crosspresentation by dendritic cells. *Cell.* 2011;147:1355-1368. doi:10.1016/j.cell.2011.11.021

153. Friedman JR, Dibenedetto JR, West M, Rowland AA, Voeltz GK. Endoplasmic reticulum-endosome contact increases as endosomes traffic and mature. *Mol Biol Cell.* 2013;24:1030-1040. doi:10.1091/mbc.E12-10-0733

154. Bertholet S, Goldszmid R, Morrot A, et al. Leishmania antigens are presented to CD8+ T cells by a transporter associated with antigen processing-independent pathway in vitro and in vivo. *J Immunol.* 2006;177:3525-3533.

155. Shen L, Sigal LJ, Boes M, Rock KL. Important role of cathepsin S in generating peptides for TAP-independent MHC class I crosspresentation in vivo. *Immunity.* 2004;21:155-165. doi:10.1016/j.immuni.2004.07.004

156. Muller-Taubenberger A, Lupas AN, Li H, Ecke M, Simmeth E, Gerisch G. Calreticulin and calnexin in the endoplasmic reticulum are important for phagocytosis. *EMBO J.* 2001;20:6772-6782. doi:10.1093/emboj/20.23.6772

157. Gagnon E, Duclos S, Rondeau C, et al. Endoplasmic reticulum-mediated phagocytosis is a mechanism of entry into macrophages. *Cell.* 2002;110:119-131.

158. Burgdorf S, Scholz C, Kautz A, Tampe R, Kurts C. Spatial and mechanistic separation of cross-presentation and endogenous antigen presentation. *Nat Immunol.* 2008;9:558-566. doi:10.1038/ni.1601

159. Guermonprez P, Saveanu L, Kleijmeer M, Davoust J, van Endert P, Amigorena S. ER-phagosome fusion defines an MHC class I cross-presentation compartment in dendritic cells. *Nature.* 2003;425:397-402. doi:10.1038/nature01911

160. Sengupta D, Graham M, Liu X, Cresswell P. Proteasomal degradation within endocytic organelles mediates antigen cross-presentation. *EMBO J.* 2019;38:e99266. doi:10.15252/embj.201899266

161. Lizee G, Basha G, Tiong J, et al. Control of dendritic cell cross-presentation by the major histocompatibility complex class I cytoplasmic domain. *Nat Immunol.* 2003;4:1065-1073. doi:10.1038/ni989

162. Basha G, Lizée G, Reinicke AT, Seipp RP, Omilusik KD, Jefferies WA. MHC class I endosomal and lysosomal trafficking coincides with exogenous antigen loading in dendritic cells. *PLoS One.* 2008;3:e3247 doi:10.1371/journal.pone.0003247

163. Basha G, Omilusik K, Chavez-Steenbock A, et al. A CD74-dependent MHC class I endolysosomal cross-presentation pathway. *Nat Immunol.* 2012;13:237-245. doi:10.1038/ni.2225

164. Ma W, Zhang Y, Vigneron N, et al. Long-peptide cross-presentation by human dendritic cells occurs in Vacuoles by peptide exchange on Nascent MHC class I molecules. *J Immunol.* 2016;196:1711-1720. doi:10.4049/jimmunol.1501574

165. Saveanu L, Carroll O, Weimershaus M, et al. IRAP identifies an endosomal compartment required for MHC class I cross-presentation. *Science (New York, N.Y.).* 2009;325:213-217. doi:10.1126/science.1172845

166. Firat E, Saveanu L, Aichele P, et al. The role of endoplasmic reticulum-associated aminopeptidase 1 in immunity to infection and in cross-presentation. *J Immunol.* 2007;178:2241-2248.

167. Merzougui N, Kratzer R, Saveanu L, van Endert P. A proteasome-dependent, TAP-independent pathway for cross-presentation of phagocytosed antigen. *EMBO Rep.* 2011;12:1257-1264. doi:10.1038/embor.2011.203

168. Campana S, De Pasquale C, Carrega P, Ferlazzo G, Bonaccorsi I. Cross-dressing: an alternative mechanism for antigen presentation. *Immunol Lett.* 2015;168:349-354. doi:10.1016/j.imlet.2015.11.002

169. Smyth LA, Afzali B, Tsang J, Lombardi G, Lechler RI. Intercellular transfer of MHC and immunological molecules: molecular mechanisms and biological significance. *Am J Transplant.* 2007;7:1442-1449. doi:10.1111/j.1600-6143.2007.01816.x

170. Herrera OB, Golshayan D, Tibbott R, et al. A novel pathway of alloantigen presentation by dendritic cells. *J Immunol.* 2004;173:4828-4837. doi:10.4049/jimmunol.173.8.4828

171. Smyth LA, Herrera OB, Golshayan D, Lombardi G, Lechler RI. A novel pathway of antigen presentation by dendritic and endothelial cells: implications for allorecognition and infectious diseases. *Transplantation.* 2006;82:S15-S18. doi:10.1097/01.tp.0000231347.06149.ca

172. Benichou G, Wang M, Ahrens K, Madsen JC. Extracellular vesicles in allograft rejection and tolerance. *Cell Immunol.* 2020;349:104063. doi:10.1016/j.cellimm.2020.104063

173. He T, Zong S, Wu X, Wei Y, Xiang J. CD4+ T cell acquisition of the bystander pMHC I colocalizing in the same immunological synapse comprising pMHC II and costimulatory CD40, CD54, CD80, OX40L, and 41BBL. *Biochem Biophys Res Commun.* 2007;362:822-828. doi:10.1016/j.bbrc.2007.08.072

174. LeMaoult J, Caumartin J, Daouya M, et al. Immune regulation by pretenders: cell-to-cell transfers of HLA-G make effector T cells act as regulatory cells. *Blood.* 2007;109:2040-2048. doi:10.1182/blood-2006-05-024547

175. Ahmed KA, Munegowda MA, Xie Y, Xiang J. Intercellular trogocytosis plays an important role in modulation of immune responses. *Cell Mol Immunol.* 2008;5:261-269. doi:10.1038/cmi.2008.32

176. Markey KA, Koyama M, Gartlan KH, et al. Cross-dressing by donor dendritic cells after allogeneic bone marrow transplantation contributes to formation of the immunological synapse and maximizes responses to indirectly presented antigen. *J Immunol.* 2014;192:5426-5433. doi:10.4049/jimmunol.1302490

177. LeMaoult J, Caumartin J, Daouya M, et al. Trogocytic intercellular membrane exchanges among hematological tumors. *J Hematol Oncol.* 2015;8:24. doi:10.1186/s13045-015-0114-8

178. Caumartin J, Favier B, Daouya M, et al. Trogocytosis-based generation of suppressive NK cells. *EMBO J.* 2007;26:1423-1433. doi:10.1038/sj.emboj.7601570

179. Krzywinska E, Allende-Vega N, Cornillon A, et al. Identification of anti-tumor cells carrying natural killer (NK) cell antigens in patients with hematological cancers. *EBioMedicine.* 2015;2:1364-1376. doi:10.1016/j.ebiom.2015.08.021

180. Fevrier B, Raposo G. Exosomes: endosomal-derived vesicles shipping extracellular messages. *Curr Opin Cell Biol.* 2004;16:415-421. doi:10.1016/j.ceb.2004.06.003

181. Segura E, Guerin C, Hogg N, Amigorena S, Thery C. CD8+ dendritic cells use LFA-1 to capture MHC-peptide complexes from exosomes in vivo. *J Immunol.* 2007;179:1489-1496.

182. Wakim LM, Bevan MJ. Cross-dressed dendritic cells drive memory CD8+ T-cell activation after viral infection. *Nature.* 2011;471:629-632. doi:10.1038/nature09863

183. Smyth LA, Harker N, Turnbull W, et al. The relative efficiency of acquisition of MHC:peptide complexes and cross-presentation depends on dendritic cell type. *J Immunol.* 2008;181:3212-3220.

184. Marino J, Babiker-Mohamed MH, Crosby-Bertorini P, et al. Donor exosomes rather than passenger leukocytes initiate alloreactive T cell responses after transplantation. *Sci Immunol.* 2016;1(1):aaf8759. doi:10.1126/sciimmunol.aaf8759

185. Liu Q, Rojas-Canales DM, Divito SJ, et al. Donor dendritic cell-derived exosomes promote allograft-targeting immune response. *J Clin Invest.* 2016;126:2805-2820. doi:10.1172/JCI84577

186. Smyth LA, Lechler RI, Lombardi G. Continuous acquisition of MHC:peptide complexes by recipient cells contributes to the generation of anti-graft CD8(+) T cell immunity. *Am J Transplant.* 2017;17:60-68. doi:10.1111/ajt.13996

187. Rustom A, Saffrich R, Markovic I, Walther P, Gerdes HH. Nanotubular highways for intercellular organelle transport. *Science (New York, N.Y.).* 2004;303:1007-1010. doi:10.1126/science.1093133

188. Abounit S, Zurzolo C. Wiring through tunneling nanotubes—from electrical signals to organelle transfer. *J Cell Sci.* 2012;125:1089-1098. doi:10.1242/jcs.083279

189. Schiller C, Huber JE, Diakopoulos KN, Weiss EH. Tunneling nanotubes enable intercellular transfer of MHC class I molecules. *Hum Immunol.* 2013;74:412-416. doi:10.1016/j.humimm.2012.11.026

190. Osteikoetxea-Molnar A, Szabó-Meleg E, Tóth EA, et al. The growth determinants and transport properties of tunneling nanotube networks between B lymphocytes. *Cell Mol Life Sci.* 2016;73:4531-4545. doi:10.1007/s00018-016-2233-y

191. Millet V, Naquet P, Guinamard RR. Intercellular MHC transfer between thymic epithelial and dendritic cells. *Eur J Immunol.* 2008;38:1257-1263. doi:10.1002/eji.200737982

The Normal Hematologic System

Chapter 16 ■ Complement System

ROBERT A. BRODSKY • EVAN M. BRAUNSTEIN

INTRODUCTION

The name complement was introduced by Paul Ehrlich and J. Morgenroth, because it was thought to complete the activity of the antibodies from which it could be distinguished by its particular properties. Complement is an evolutionary ancient immune defense system that is present in vertebrates and invertebrates. It serves as a guardian of the intravascular space and tissues, enabling the host to recognize and clear invading pathogens (eg, bacteria, viruses) and altered host cells while at the same time protecting healthy host cells and tissues. It is now recognized that complement represents a multimolecular system and is activated by three different pathways—the classical, the alternative, and the lectin—with the final lytic or effector function being carried out by a common pathway. This final common pathway leads to the formation of the membrane attack complex (MAC). In humans, this system is formed through the interaction of more than 30 plasma proteins and cell surface receptors.

CLASSICAL PATHWAY

The classical pathway is initiated by two functional units: the recognition unit, which consists of three proteins, C1q, C1r, and C1s, and the activation unit, which consists of C2, C3, and C4[1] (Figure 16.1). The MAC is activated by the classical pathway by the generation of three complex enzymes with proteolytic activity, the formation of which requires the association of two or more proteins.[2] Not all Ig classes are capable of binding to C1q; IgG1 and IgG3 bind readily, whereas IgG4 does not bind at all. Complement binding to the IgG subclasses is determined by the flexibility of the hinge that prevents steric interference between Fab and C1q binding. IgG3, with the longest hinge region, is the most efficient of all IgG subclasses. Exposure of the C1q-binding site of IgM molecules is optimal when the molecule assumes the staple configuration as it binds to the antigen (Figure 16.2). This site is hidden in the native form of IgM by the closeness of the subunits. IgM has the strongest binding ability because one C1q molecule that is bound to one IgM antibody is capable of lysing an erythrocyte. IgG normally exists in a monomeric state in which C1q-binding sites are exposed but affinity is too low to allow adequate C1 binding. Sequential antigen and Fc-Fc binding by IgG leads to formation of hexamers that bind C1q with high avidity and activate complement.[3] Ig antibodies that are bound to independent epitopes can activate the complement cascade in this way. Depending on the epitope density, activation occurs when at least 800 IgG molecules bind to the cell. For this reason, IgM antibodies are considerably more efficient lysins.

C1 Esterase (C1)

C1 esterase is a complex that is assembled from three proteins: C1q (recognition subunit), C1r, and C1s (catalytic complex).[4] Although most complement factors are synthesized in the liver, C1 components are synthesized in the local environment by monocytes, macrophages, epithelial cells, and fibroblasts.[5]

C1q: Recognition Unit of C1s

All activators of the complement cascade recognize C1q, which consists of a total of 18 polypeptide chains, 6 of each of the 3 different types, A, B, and C.[6-8] All polypeptide chains are equal in length, and each comprises a short N-terminal region that is involved in the formation of A-B and C-C interchain disulfide bonds. It is followed by collagen-like sequences, which consist of repeating triplets X-Y-Gly, a collagen-like motif (X is often a proline; Y is usually hydroxyproline or hydroxylysine). These sequences are not found in human serum

proteins but are present in collagen fibrils. At the beginning, three heterotrimers (each consisting of A, B, and C polypeptide chains) associate, forming a stalk. Because of the interruption of the collagen sequence, the triplets dissociate into six radiating arms (Figure 16.3A). At the C-terminal end, each arm ends in a globular head, which consists of heterotrimers of protein domains known as C1q modules. When viewed by electron microscopy, the C1q resembles a bouquet of flowers (Figure 16.3B).

Modules of the C1

gC1q Module

Most of the C1 activators, such as immune complexes, β-amyloid fibrils, and HIV, are recognized by the globular heads of C1q.[9] The C1q globular heads are also integral for recognition of apoptotic cells via phosphatidylserine binding.[10,11] Each head is composed of trimers of the gC1q domain, which is detected not only in C1q but also in type VIII and type X collagens and several other proteins.[6] The gC1q modules bear structural features that are seen in members of the TNF family.[12]

CUB Module: C1r-C1s Uegf Bone Morphogenic Protein 1 Module

The acronym CUB (for complement C1r/Cr1s, Uegf, and the human bone morphogenetic protein 1) is a structural motif found almost exclusively in extracellular and plasma membrane–associated proteins. The CUB modules of C1r and C1s surround the single epidermal growth factor (EGF) module and a pair of complement control protein (CCP) modules. CUB modules are detected in proteins that are involved in developmental processes. They contain four cysteine residues, forming two disulfide bonds, except the N-terminal CUB module of C1r and C1s, which has only two cysteines.

Epidermal Growth Factor Module: Epidermal Growth Factor-Like Modules

EGF-like modules are detected in diverse proteins that are involved in processes such as blood coagulation and cell adhesion. They have six cysteines that form three disulfide bonds. In C1r and C1s, the EGF module has characteristic consensus sequences with residues Asp and Asn that are hydroxylated and are involved in Ca^{2+} binding.

Complement Control Protein Module

The CCP module is detected in complement receptors and other CCPs. Their consensus sequence consists of aromatic and hydrophobic residues and four cysteines. The crystal structure has been solved and shows six β strands around a hydrophobic core.[13] The modules are ellipsoidal with the β strands aligned along their long axis, with N and C termini at opposite ends.

Serum Protease Domain

The target bonds in the substrates for cleavage by the C1 esterase have one Arg residue. Indicative of its trypsin-like enzymatic specificity is the Asp residue that is found close to the substrate-binding site. Arginyl bonds, such as Arg-isoleucine (Ile), are the targets in the autoactivation of C1r and in the activation of C1s by C1r. Arg-containing bonds are also cleaved in C4 and C2 by the active C1s. C1s' esterase activity is expressed only by the multimolecular complex, which is a tetramer that is formed by two C1r and two C1s. Therefore, the enzymatic activity depends on protein-protein interactions among the four components of the esterase, which are facilitated by Ca^{2+}.[14] Ca^{2+} brings together one CUB and one EGF module to form a compact structure.[15] During the formation of the tetramer, interactions are flexible to allow a single C1r to cleave the neighboring and the distant C1s.[16]

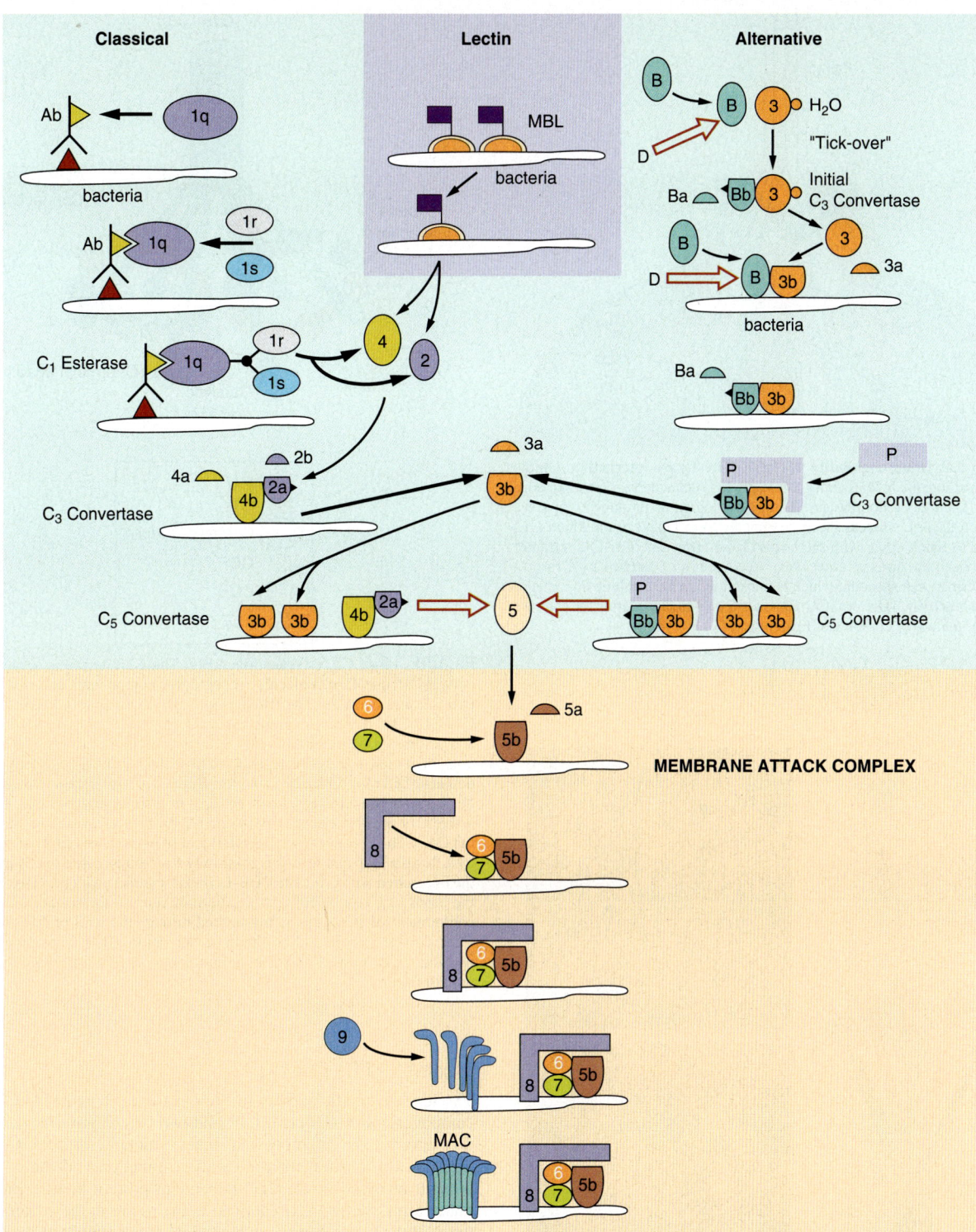

FIGURE 16.1 The complement © pathways. The hemolytic function of C is activated by three pathways, which converge to the same final common pathway (see the text for details). The classical pathway uses C1q as the recognition molecule, which generates sequentially three enzymatic functions: C1 esterase, C3 convertase, and C5 convertase. The alternative pathway initiates activation by a "tick-over" mechanism in the absence of antibody and again generates similar enzymatic functions as the classical pathway. The lectin pathway is triggered by a receptor, mannose-binding lectin (MBL), which, through carbohydrate binding, activates the MBL-associated serine protease (MASP) esterases. An MASP cleaves C4 and C2, generating the same C3 convertase as the classical pathway, which it joins at this point. All pathways converge to the same membrane attack complex (MAC) pathway, which they initiate by cleaving C5.

The Normal Hematologic System

C1r and C1s

The C1r and C1s are single polypeptide chains of approximately 85 kDa, with serine protease activity. In the proenzyme form, they are single glycoproteins, which are activated by cleavage of a single Arg-Ile bond, forming a two-chain active enzyme. They are composed of two CUB modules,[17] an EGF-like module, two CCP modules, and a C-terminal chymotrypsin-like serine protease domain (*Figure 16.4*).

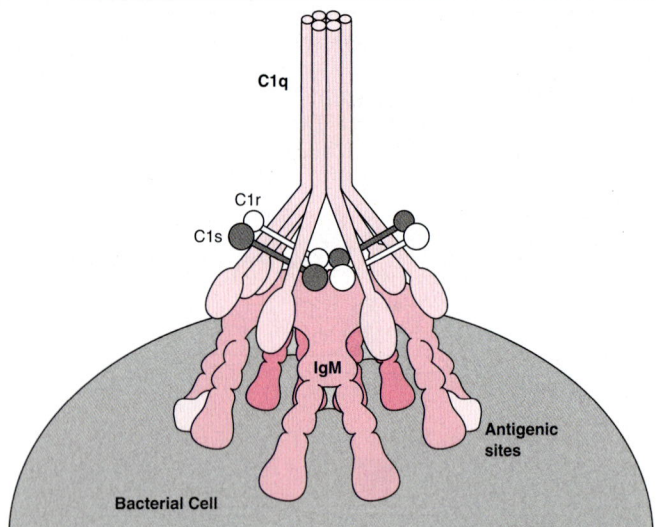

FIGURE 16.2 **Immunoglobulin M (IgM)-C1 esterase interaction.** On the surface of pathogens, IgM assumes the staple (as seen sideways) or crab conformation. The Fabs touch the surface of a pathogen, or immune complexes deposited on tissues, whereas the Fc fragments form a plateau on which C1q finds space to touch down with the heads of the arms. The C1r-C1s tetramer weaves between the arms as a necklace. Recognition of patterns by C1q creates a conformational shakeup, which is transmitted to the catalytic domains of C1r, which is activated. In turn, C1r activates C1s, which performs the esterase functions of the whole complex, C1 esterase.

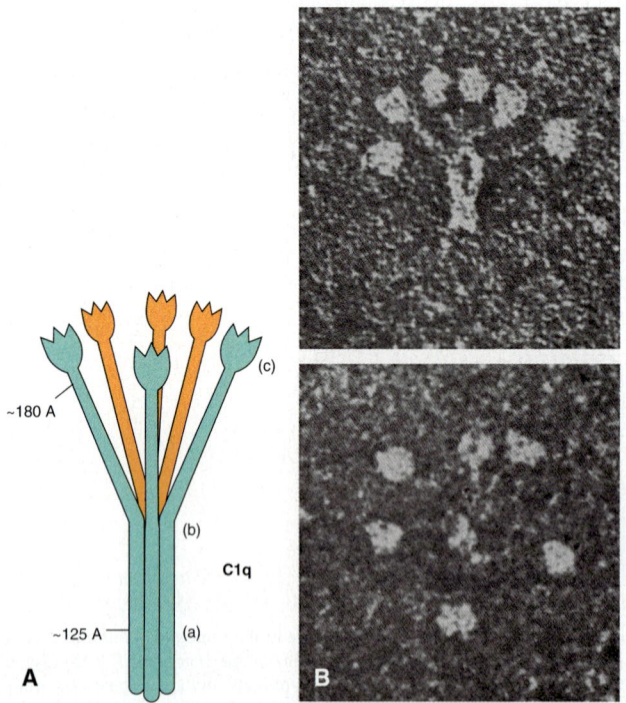

FIGURE 16.3 A, C1q molecule. Each of the six subunits is made of three polypeptide chains that form a triple helical strand. The N-terminal ends have a collagen-like structure and are packed together, forming a central stalk *(a)*; halfway, they bend and separate from each other *(b)* to end at the C-terminal end in a globular domain *(c)* that binds to the immunoglobulin. B, Electron micrographs of the C1q molecule (upper) and bird's eye view (lower). (B, From Knobel HR, Villiger W, Isliker H. Chemical analysis and electron microscopy studies of human C1q prepared by different methods. *Eur J Immunol.* 1975;5(1):78-82. Copyright © 1975 WILEY-VCH Verlag GmbH & Co. KGaA, Weinheim. Reprinted by permission of John Wiley & Sons, Inc.)

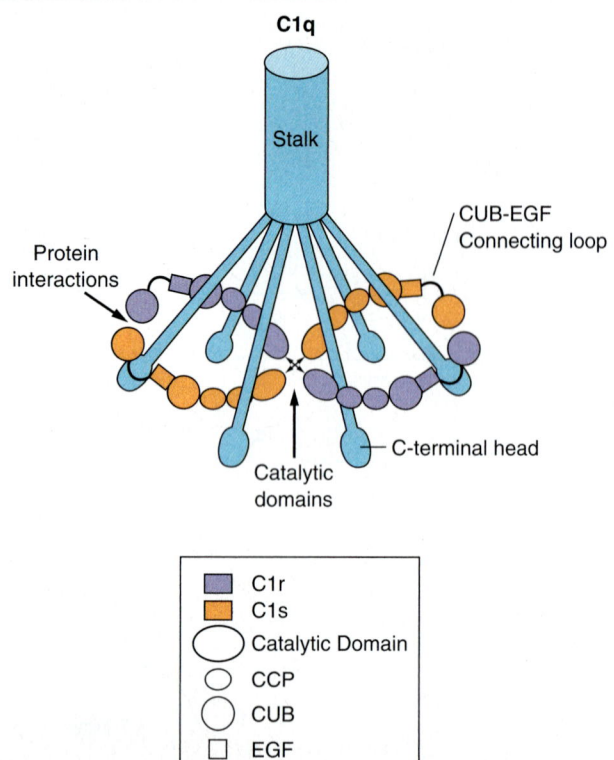

FIGURE 16.4 **C1, esterase assembly.** The C1 esterase is a complex that consists of one C1q molecule (recognition component) and a tetramer of two C1r and two C1s. The tetramer in isolation assumes a linear form: C1s-C1r-C1r-C1s. It weaves among the arms of the C1q in a necklace-like way and assumes a figure of "8." This arrangement allows access of the catalytic domain of the C1 in the zymogen form to be in contact with the active catalytic domain of C1r for C1s to be activated. Both C1rs have access to both C1s. The flexibility of the tetramer allows changes in their relative position, so that the active C1s sites have access to C4 and C2 for their cleavage and formation of the C4a-C2b C3 convertase. The CUB and EGF modules of C1r are connected by a flexible loop and form a high-affinity Ca^{2+}-binding site that is involved in the interaction with C1s. The CUB-EGF pair interacts with the C1q arm. When the heads of C1q interact with a pattern of sites on the surface of a target, a conformational stress that is transmitted through the arms of C1q triggers the C1r catalytic domain and results in its activation. CCP, complement control protein; CUB, C1r-C1s Uegf bone morphogenic protein 1; EGF, epidermal growth factor.

Assembly of C1 Esterase

The first enzymatic activity of the C cascade is assembled from five components, one C1q, two C1r, and two C1s (*Figure 16.4*). The C1r-C1s tetramer, in isolation, is a linear structure, with the C-terminal domains responsible for the catalytic function and the N-terminal domain involved in the Ca^{2+}-dependent protein interactions. In the linear form, the two C1r catalytic domains are in the center, whereas those of the C1s are at the two ends. In the assembly of the C1 esterase, which is the first enzymatic activity of the classical complement cascade, the linear tetramer assumes a compact figure-eight conformation. In this configuration, all four catalytic domains of C1r and C1s are brought into juxtaposition under the cone that is formed by the arms of the C1q. The protein interaction domains are located outside the arms of C1q.[7,8]

Activation of C1 esterase occurs upon recognition by the globular heads of C1q of pattern target sites (eg, antibody bound to pathogen surfaces, immune complexes). This binding generates transient conformational changes, which activate C1r by disrupting the C1r homodimer. Activated C1r in turn breaks an Arg-Ile bond, activating C1s.[14] These transient "earthquakes" do not bring about the collapse of the elaborate C1 esterase edifice, because C1r and C1s are associated tightly with the C1q collagen arms by the CUB-EGF modules that were discussed previously.

C1s is a highly specific enzyme, but, within the mechanical constraints that are imposed by the superstructure of the whole assembly, it requires some degree of freedom of mobility for its interaction with the substrate. These requirements are provided by the CCP modules, especially CCP-2, which is linked by a flexible hinge to the CCP-1 module. This allows CCP-2 to act as a handle and a spacer, to amplify the shift that is required for the serine protease domain.[7,13]

C1q-Binding Proteins

In addition to its function in C activation, C1q binds to other proteins that are sometimes called receptors, mediating other C1q functions.[18,19] There are two types of surface proteins that bind to C1q. One binds to the collagenous portion of C1q (cC1q receptor), and the other binds to the globular heads (gC1q receptor). Some of these proteins are transmembrane, whereas others are intracellular, such as calreticulin (CALR) and the gC1q-binding protein (gC1qR, now known as C1QBP). The C1q structure bears similarity to the proteins of the collectin family, which includes the mannose-binding lectin (MBL), the pulmonary surfactant protein A, and conglutinin. However, the collectins are C-type lectins and bind carbohydrates, whereas the heads of C1q recognize protein patterns on immune complexes.

The term C1qR has been used loosely, sometimes without hard evidence that the receptor triggers cell signaling that leads to some cellular functions.[19] The gC1qR is expressed on myeloid cells[20] and microglial cells,[21] in which it mediates chemotaxis and phagocytosis, and in platelets,[22] modulating their function in injured vascular sites. Calreticulin is a Ca^{2+}-binding protein that is located primarily in the ER of most nucleated cells. It has been found that calreticulin binds C1q and therefore qualifies as cC1qR, but the significance of this interaction remains elusive. Interestingly, *Trypanosoma cruzi* calreticulin also inhibits the lectin pathway of complement.[23]

C4 and C2 Complex: C3 Convertase

C3 convertase is formed by the interaction of two fragments from the C4 and C2 components of complement. Complement component 4 circulates in the blood as a disulfide-linked heterotrimer that consists of α (93 kDa), β (75 kDa), and γ (33 kDa) chains. C3 and C5 components share a similar structure that is considered to be evolutionarily derived from one ancestral gene. The C3 and C4 components share an internal thioester bond, which is formed between a cysteine and a glutamine, which are two residues apart.[24]

C4 is synthesized as a single polypeptide chain but is later hydrolyzed, giving rise to the three constituent chains. C1s activates C4 by splitting the α chain, releasing the C4a fragment from the N-terminal end of the chain. The thioester bond, which is normally hidden in the C4b fragment, is exposed, reacts with an NH_2 or OH group of the surrounding molecules, and deposits C4b on the surface of potential targets for C attack.

C2 is a single-chain protein of approximately 100 to 110 kDa, with a distinct structure that consists of three globular regions: three N-terminal CCP domains, a single von Willebrand factor (vWF) domain in the center, and a serine protease domain in the C terminus.[25] CCP modules are highly compact structures, folding independently into a β barrel (eg, two interacting antiparallel β sheets), that form an ellipsoid structure. Loops that connect the β strands protrude from the module and may function as the ligand-binding sites. The vWF type A module consists of five parallel β strands and a short antiparallel strand that form a central twisted core, which is surrounded by seven amphipathic α helices.[26] Cleavage of C2 by C1s occurs in the N-terminal region of the vWF domain, which results in the generation of two fragments, a larger (70 kDa) C2a, consisting of most of vWF and SP domains, and a smaller (30 kDa) C2b fragment (CCP-1, CCP-2, and CCP-3). Fragmentation of C2 exposes a C4b-binding site that is located on the C2a fragment, which interacts with C4b. C4b-C2a complex formation depends on Mg^{2+} ions, which are coordinated by residues in the metal ion–binding MIDAS (metal ion–dependent

adhesion site) motif of the vWF modules, which is also present in several integrins (see Appendix A, CD61). By electron microscopy, the C2a fragment appears as a two-lobed structure that links the C4b and C3b fragments in the final C5 convertase (see the following discussion). The C4b-C2a complex is a serine esterase with an esterolytic activity and with the C3 as the natural substrate.[27]

C3b-C4b-C2a Complex: C5 Convertase
C3 Component

The C3 component of the complement is the most abundant in the serum (1.2 mg/mL) and occupies the most critical position in all three C cascades. The prevailing hypothesis is that a gene that was common for all three components, C3, C4, and C5, originated from an ancestral $α_2$-macroglobulin gene. Subsequent duplication formed the *C4* and *C3–C5* genes, and a second duplication formed separate *C3* and *C5* genes.

C3 comprises an α chain (110 kDa) and a β chain (75 kDa), which are connected covalently by a single disulfide bond. It is synthesized as a single protein and is modified posttranslationally by a furin-like enzyme, which removes a sequence of four arginines.[28]

Another disulfide bond within the α chain connects the N and C termini (*Figure 16.5*). C3 convertase cleaves the α chain at a site that is close to the N terminus, generating two fragments: a small C3a (9 kDa) and a large C3b (176 kDa). The C3b consists of the remaining α chain, which is linked by the disulfide bond to the intact β chain. Cleavage of the α chain of C3 by the C3 convertase exposes the thioester bond, which, in the intact molecule, is well protected within a pocket in the α chain, with a half-life of 231 hours. In the metastable C3b fragment, the bond is exposed, with a half-life of 60 μs. These differences strikingly express the extraordinary reactivity of the thioester bond for certain groups on the cell surfaces. The thioester bond participates in a chemical transacylation reaction that results in the attachment of C3b on OH or NH_2 groups on cell surfaces, complex carbohydrates, or immune complexes that are within a radius of 600 Å from the point at which it was generated. Attachment of C3b is not discriminatory between self- and non-self surfaces but is regulated by CCPs (see the following discussion). The selection, however, of the OH groups on the sites of binding is quite restricted.[29] C3b expresses multiple sites for binding to other complement proteins that determine its fate. C3b is deposited on and around the C4b-C2a complex, binding through the thioester bond. The deposition produces an enzyme with a change in the specificity from C3 to C5, generating the C5 convertase.[30] C3b is also deposited on other previously deposited C3b molecules, forming C3b-C3b dimers. The C3b-C4b and C3b-C3b dimers form high-affinity binding sites for C5, and probably the role of these dimers is to hold the substrate in a rigid position for efficient cleavage of C5. It also appears that the C3b-C3b-IgG complexes function as better precursors of convertases than monomeric C3b.

There is also evidence for C5 activation in the absence of the C5 convertase. Surfaces densely populated with C3b or C4b are able to prime C5 for activation by the C3 convertase, in effect bypassing the C5 convertase and leading to formation of the MAC.[31]

C3 Fragmentation

C3 is fragmented by several enzymes that generate a variety of functionally active fragments (*Figure 16.5*). The activation of C3 by the C3 convertase cleaves the peptide bond between residues 726 and 727 (Arg-Ser) and generates a small C3a (9 kDa) and a large C3b (176 kDa) fragment. C3a is the N terminus of the α chain that functions as anaphylatoxin. C3b consists of the remaining α chain (α′) and the entire β chain, which are linked by the disulfide bond. C3b is inactivated by further proteolysis by factor I and one of the cofactors. The first cleavage occurs between residues 1281 and 1282 of the α′ chain and generates the inactivated C3b or $iC3b_2$, which is the ligand for CD11b-CD18 integrin (see Appendix A). A second cleavage by factor I separates a small fragment C3f (2 kDa) from the α′ chain and yields another inactivated C3b or $iC3b_2$. Factor I, with CR1 or factor H as cofactor, cleaves the α chain once more, at residues 932 and 933, to

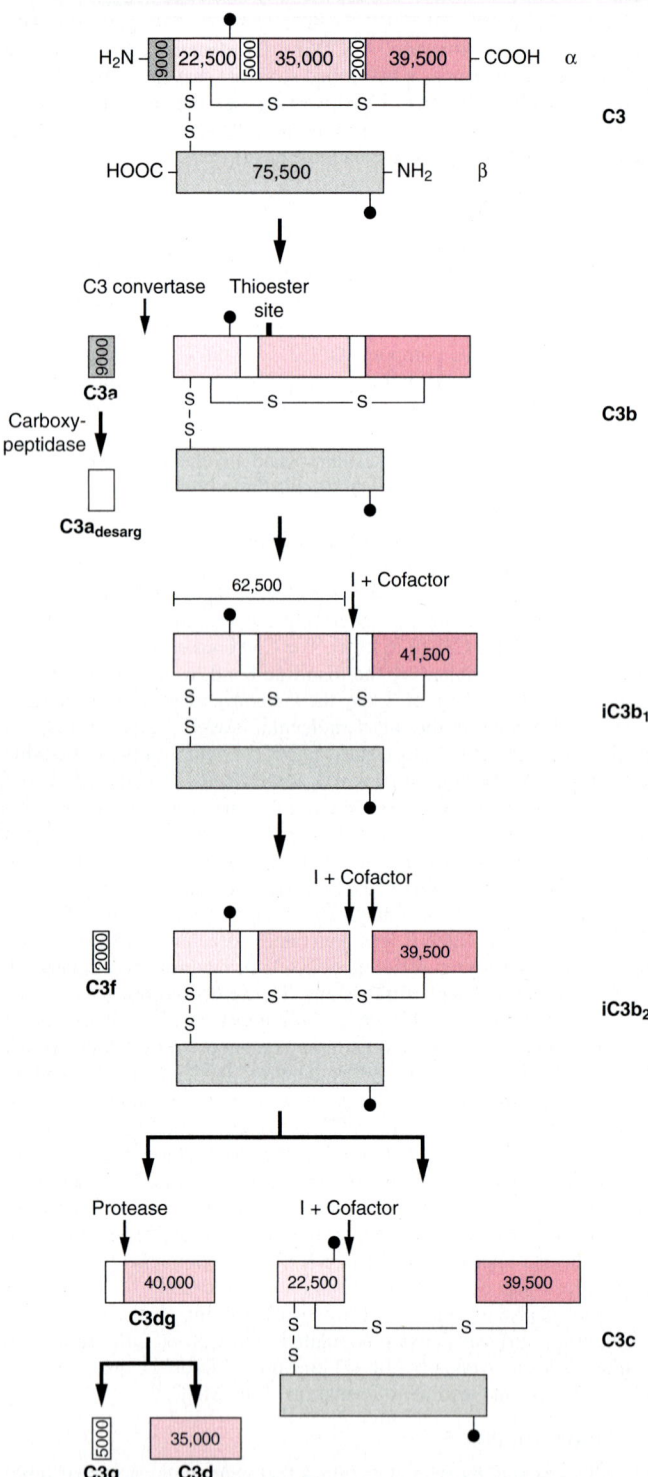

FIGURE 16.5 C3 degradation. The C3 component not only contributes to the classical pathway in the formation of the C5 convertase but also, as a result of fragmentation, provides parts of its molecule for other important functions. For example, C3a serves as an anaphylatoxin, C3b serves as a ligand for the CR1 receptor (CD35), C3d serves as a ligand for CR2 receptor (CD21), and iC3b serves as a ligand for CR3 receptor (lymphocyte function–associated antigen-1 integrin, CD11b/CD18) and for CD11c/CD18 integrin. (From Sahu A, Lambris JD. Structure and biology of complement protein C3, a connecting link between innate and acquired immunity. *Immunol Rev.* 2001;180(1):35-48. Copyright © 2001 Munksgaard. Reprinted by permission of John Wiley & Sons, Inc.)

yield C3dg and C3c. The C3dg fragment is a ligand for CD21 (CR2), a component of the coreceptor CD19-CD21-CD81 complex on B cells (see Chapter 12). C3dg is cleaved by a protease into C3g and C3d fragments.

ALTERNATIVE PATHWAY

The alternative complement pathway represents an important natural defense mechanism that is independent of the immune response (*Figure 16.1*). Activation of the alternative pathway involves three components: C3, B factor, and D factor. Polysaccharides (zymosan), bacterial products, aggregated human IgA, cobra venom factor, and many other substances are activators of the alternative C cascade. The mechanisms that initiate this pathway have been the subject of much debate. The enzyme that cleaves C3 contains C3b as one of its components, which is the product of a previous C3 cleavage. The origin of the first C3b becomes a puzzling problem. Normally, C3 continuously generates a low level of a functionally C3b-like form by a "tick-over" mechanism. The mechanism for the tick-over is not a proteolytic process but involves the spontaneous hydrolysis of the thioester bond by H_2O and the formation of a metastable C3 (H_2O). The hydrolysis occurs in vitro at 37 °C at a rate of 0.005% per minute.[32] The C3 (H_2O) is an uncleaved C3 molecule and yet has the conformation and function of a C3b in the presence of Mg^{2+}, which provides a site for binding of the B factor.

Factor B

Factor B (90 kDa) has a structure that is similar to C2: It consists of three CCP modules, a vWF type A module, and a serine protease domain that are all connected by short amino acid sequences. By electron microscopy, it appears as a three-lobed structure, presumably with each module corresponding to one of the lobes.

Factor D

Factor D is a serine protease with only one known substrate, factor B. The single Arg^{233}-Lys^{234} bond of factor B becomes susceptible to the enzymatic activity of factor D only when it forms an Mg^{2+}-dependent complex with C3b. It is the only enzyme in blood that is able to catalyze this reaction and is therefore absolutely required for alternative-pathway activation.

The concentration of factor D in the blood is 1.8 ± 0.4 μg/mL, the lowest of any complement protein, which makes factor D the limiting factor in the activation of the alternative pathway. It is a single-chain protein (24 kDa) and is structurally similar to pancreatic serine proteases. It circulates in blood in a zymogen or profactor form[33] converted to the mature enzyme as a result of conformational changes. However, this first step generates a "resting" enzyme because of an inhibitory sequence loop, which prevents its activation. The active enzyme conformation is induced after binding to the substrate in a second step.

Factor D has a structure that is similar to other members of the serine proteases: The polypeptide chain is folded into two antiparallel β barrels. Each barrel consists of six β strands with the same topology in all members.[33] Efficient catalysis requires three amino acids, Asp^{103}, His^{58}, and Ser^{195}, forming the "catalytic triad," and the positioning of the three residues is crucial for the synergistic action that is required for hydrolysis of the target bond. In the bottom of the substrate specificity pocket is an Asp residue, which places factor D in the category of the trypsin subfamily of serine proteases and cleaves an Arg-Lys bond of its single natural substrate, factor B.

Properdin

Properdin is one of six plasma glycoproteins that collectively comprise the alternative pathway of complement (APC). It was first described by Pillemer et al.[34] as a novel plasma protein that activated complement in the absence of immune complexes. Properdin consists of a single chain (53 kDa), which by electron microscopy appears as a rodlike structure that forms cyclic dimers, trimers, and tetramers.[35] The monomer consists of an N-terminal region of no known homology, followed by six thrombospondin type 1 repeats (TSRs) of approximately 60 amino acids.[36] Repeats of this type have been identified in the cell adhesion molecule thrombospondin and in a variety of other proteins, including thrombospondin types 1 and 2 (TSP-1 and TSP-2), C6 to C9, and the circumsporozoite protein of malaria parasites.[37]

Removal of TSR5 prevents binding to C3b and sulfatide, whereas, with the removal of TSR4, properdin is unable to stabilize the C3b-Bb complex but is still able to bind C3b and sulfatide,[38,39] while it exists only as a monomer or a dimer. Absence of TSR3 does not affect any of the functions of properdin, including the formation of the polymers. TSR5 is important for polymer formation, because, in its absence, no cyclic polymers are detected. Properdin, as does thrombospondin, binds sulfated glycoconjugates and sulfatide with especially high affinity when it is activated. Properdin significantly contributes to linking innate and adaptive immunity. It is synthesized by endothelial cells, especially under turbulent blood flow conditions,[40] and mRNA has been detected in neutrophils, monocytes, and T cells. In response to chemoattractants C5a or IL8, neutrophils discharge their properdin content promptly, as well as C3 and factor B, which they store within their granules. Factor D is supplied locally by blood, which completes the list of the components that are essential for activation of the alternative pathway. T cells and monocytes participate in the process because they also secrete properdin, factor B, and C3. Activation-produced fragments C3d and iC3b are essential B-cell activation factors,[41] thus linking with the adaptive immune system.

Activation of the Alternative Pathway of Complement

In the presence of Mg^{2+}, C3 (H_2O; also referred to as iC3) binds factor B, which is cleaved by factor D into a large Bb and a small Ba fragment (*Figure 16.1*). The Bb forms a complex with the iC3, which is termed the initial C3 convertase. Although the iC3-Bb complex is destroyed on host surfaces by factor H and factor I (see the following discussion), C3b fragments that are deposited on foreign surfaces associate with factor B in the presence of Mg^{2+}. The C3b-B complex activates factor D, which cleaves factor B into Bb and Ba fragments. The distinction between activator and nonactivator surfaces is not clear. An activator surface is one that allows binding of factor B to C3b in preference of factor H (see the following discussion), thus activating the alternative pathway, and the opposite is true for nonactivators. Nonactivators can be converted to activators by removing sialic acid. A widely used activator is cobra venom factor, which binds to factor B and forms a stable C3 convertase. The factor is functionally analogous to C3b but is related structurally to C3c. It is used to deplete serum of C3 in a variety of experimental situations and is resistant to inactivation by factors H and I.

The C3b-Bb complex is stabilized by the serum protein properdin, which amplifies the cleavage and deposition of more C3b molecules[42,43] to form the C5 convertase. The serine protease activity of the C3b-Bb complex, which is located in the Bb component, accelerates deposition of C3b fragments (C3b amplification), a unique feature of the alternative pathway, on and around the C3b-Bb complex. Some will form C3b-C3b dimers, which have a high affinity for C5 self-amplified C5 convertase,[43] and switch cleavage from C3 to C5, thus initiating the formation of the cytolytic C5b-9 complex. As the activation continues, at the outer ring of this circle, monomeric C3bs form more C3 convertases with factor B, which in turn deposits a new crop of C3bs, forming a new generation of C3b-C3b dimers, that is, C5 convertases. These cycles of successive outward deposition of C3 and C5 convertase activities continue until all surfaces are covered or the supply of individual components is exhausted.

LECTIN COMPLEMENT PATHWAY

The lectin pathway is an important humoral mechanism of innate immunity. It is activated by pattern recognition receptors, such as MBL, which interacts with carbohydrates[44] (*Figure 16.1*).

MBL is a member of the collectin family, which includes the lung surfactant proteins, SP-A and SP-D, and a protein that is localized in the hepatic cell cytosol, CL-L1. Collectins are composed of a C-terminal lectin domain (carbohydrate recognition domain) and a neck region that connects to the collagen-like region, followed by a short cross-linking region that contains two to three cysteines. The neck region forms an α-helical coiled-coil structure, which initiates the formation of a trimer. In blood, MBL is found as multimers (ie, dimers to hexamers). MBL is a C-type lectin, as it requires Ca^{2+} for binding to a carbohydrate ligand.

Associated with MBL are four serine proteases that are known as MBL-associated serine proteases (MASPs): MASP1, MASP2, MASP3,[45] and sMAP or MAp-19, a truncated form of MASP2. MASP2 and sMAP are encoded by a single gene, but two different mRNAs are generated by alternative splicing.[46] All MASP proteases have a modular structure that is identical to C1r-C1s: a CUB domain, an EGF-like domain, a second CUB domain, two CCP domains, and a serine protease domain. The serine protease domain is homologous to the chymotrypsinogen family. An Asp residue in the substrate specificity pocket indicates trypsin-like substrate specificity. MASP's association with MBL is mediated by the CUB-EGF domain and is Ca^{2+} dependent.[46] The MASP proteases are activated when MBL binds to conserved pathogen-associated sugar arrays that form molecular patterns, which are shared by broad classes of pathogens.[47]

When MASP is activated, it cleaves C4 and C2, and the C4b fragment binds covalently to the microbial surface or the lectin itself and becomes the focus for C2 binding and activation. The remaining cascade is identical to that of the classical pathway (*Figure 16.1*).

MBL binds mannose-acetyl glucosamine and GlcNAc, which are also ligands for other types of GlcNAc-binding lectins, which are termed ficolins and are present in the serum. Ficolins contain collagen-like and fibrinogen-like domains. They bind to GlcNAc through the fibrinogen-like domain. They are associated with MASPs and sMAP and have the capacity to activate the lectin pathway.[48] In the serum, there are two types of ficolins, which are named L-ficolin and H-ficolin (Hakata antigen).[49,50]

The recognition that is mediated by MBL and ficolins in complement activation is detected as far back in evolution as the ascidians, our closest invertebrate relatives. It indicates that the lectin pathway has been important in innate immunity since before the evolution of adaptive immune systems in jawed vertebrates.

MEMBRANE ATTACK COMPLEX

C5

C5 (191 kDa) consists of two polypeptide chains, α (115 kDa) and β (75 kDa). C5 convertase selectively cleaves an Arg74-Leu75 bond of the α chain, generating C5a, a potent leukocyte chemotactic peptide that consists of 74 amino acids and has considerable structural homology with C3a and C4a, the other two anaphylatoxins. The remaining larger fragment, C5b, in its nascent state constitutes the nucleus for the MAC. It possesses a metastable binding site with specificity for C6. By electron microscopy, C5 has the shape of a heart or of an ellipse, but the heart-shaped form is related to the elliptical type by rotation.[51] The binding sites for C6 and C7 are located in the α chain of C5b. Interaction with C5b involves the C terminus of C6, specifically the C6c fragment that consists of two factor I modules (FIMs).

C6

C6 is a single polypeptide chain (104 kDa), which, by trypsin digestion, can be separated into an N-terminal region (C6a) with some homology to C8 and C9 and a C-terminal region (C6b) with homology to factor H and factor I. Several disulfide bonds separate discrete segments of C6, which is structurally homologous to a variety of other proteins. Overall, the primary sequence is a patchwork, with several modules that are involved in protein-protein interactions (*Figure 16.6*). Starting from the N terminus, there are several domains: two tandem TSP-1s, a class A low-density lipoprotein receptor (LDLR), an extended central segment that is referred to as the membrane attack complex perforin (MACPF) domain with homology to perforin, an EGF, a third TSP-1, two CCPs, and two FIMs, which are related to those in the H

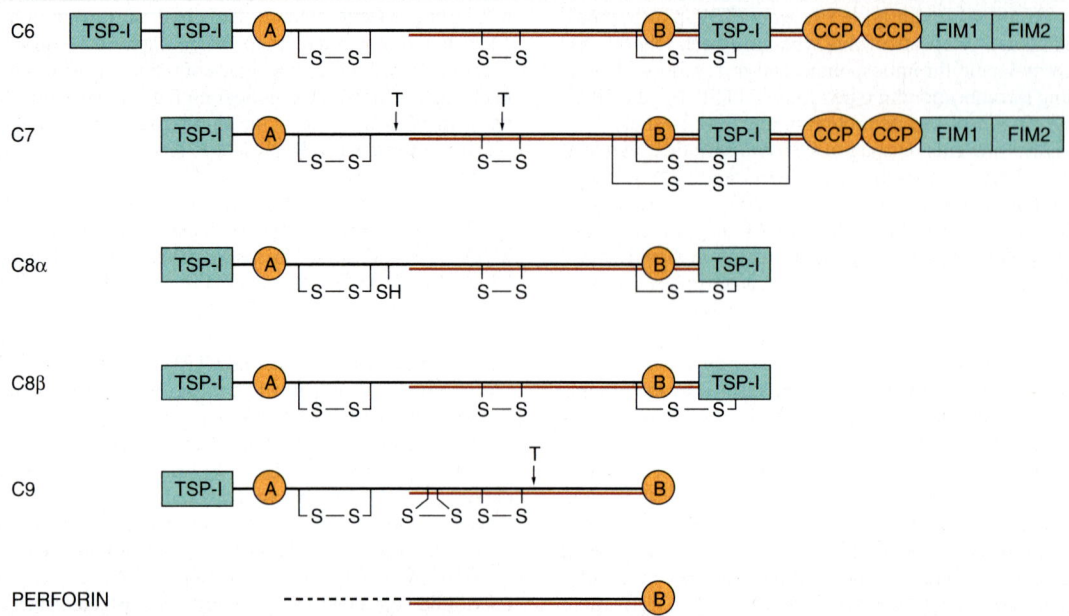

FIGURE 16.6 **Structural organization of the complement components C6 to C9.** The last five complement components (C6-C9) are structurally and genetically related proteins and form the membrane attack complex (MAC) family. They all have a similar modular structure. In the middle of each molecule is a sequence-designated MAC perforin (MACPF) to emphasize its similarity with perforin. MACPF is the portion of the molecule that is inserted in the membrane to form the pore. C8g is the sixth component, which is not modular and differs structurally from the others. It is considered that the perforin gene gave rise first to the C9 gene, which evolved in retrograde, followed by the appearance of the genes for the other proteins. The modules in C6 and C7, which are not shared by C8 and C9 (ie, complement control protein [CCP] and factor I module [FIM]), are used to interact with C5. A, low-density lipoprotein receptor class A; B, low-density lipoprotein receptor class B (or epidermal growth factor precursor module); TSP-1, thrombospondin 1.

chain of the complement control factor I.[52] The FIMs are specific C5-binding modules, and yet they are not absolutely necessary, probably because other hydrophobic interactions also contribute to the C5-C6 interactions. As devices that facilitate C5-C6 interactions, FIMs make a greater contribution to the classical pathway in which C5b density is not as high as it is in the alternative pathway, because fewer C5bs are formed in the classical pathway and C5b half-life is shorter.[53]

The secondary structure of C6 is a mixture of α helices and β sheets. The α helices reside in MACPF, which is free of disulfide bonds. By transmission electron microscopy, C6 appears as a sickle.

C7

C7 is a single polypeptide (97 kDa), which, like C6, is a mosaic of several modules that are found in other proteins. Starting from the N terminus, C7 has one TSP1, one LDLR type A (LDLRA), a second TSP1, two CCPs, and two FIMs. Its secondary structure is high in β sheets (38%), and, by electron microscopy, it appears as a flexible elongated molecule (151-59-43 Å).[54] The three components C5-C6-C7 in a fluid phase form rosettes as a consequence of radial aggregation. However, the complexes on a phospholipid area insert themselves, anchoring by the stalk, whereas the Cys-rich segments fasten the complex for the assembly of the MAC. The C5b-7 complex does not traverse the phospholipid membrane and does not cause lysis. The long flexible stalk of C7 provides greater surface area for interaction within the membrane.

C8

The C8 component consists of three chains: α (64 kDa), β (64 kDa), and γ (22 kDa), all being encoded by separate genes. The C8α and C8γ are linked by a single disulfide bond, and the C8α-C8$\beta\gamma$ heterodimer is associated noncovalently with C8β through a binding site on the C8α chain.[55] The α chain interacts with C9, directs the insertion into the membrane of the first C9 in the formation of MAC, and interacts with lipids, thus becoming accessible to MAC formation. Note that, together with the membrane protein CD59, they inhibit MAC formation in homologous cells and protect them from lysis.

The C8β chain has three binding sites for C8α, the C5b-7 complex, and membrane lipids. For binding of C8β to the C8α-γ complex, the

N-terminal TSP1, LDLRA, and the MACPF segment are most important, and, furthermore, they mediate the incorporation of C8 into the MAC.[56]

The C8 α and β chains are structurally related and are members of the MAC family, whereas the C8γ chain is a member of the lipocalin family, which is unrelated to the MAC family.[57] The lipocalins are widely distributed proteins that are involved in the transport of small lipophilic substances, such as retinol and pheromones, but C8 does not bind retinol. They all share the same folding pattern, which is known as the lipocalin fold. Strikingly, C8γ is the only protein from a different family among the 35 proteins of the complement system. Furthermore, C8γ is not absolutely required for the expression of C8 activity by the α and β chains, but it enhances their function.[58] The crystal structure of C8γ has been solved and confirms its lipocalin fold and, furthermore, identifies its structural relationship to the neutrophil gelatinase, a protein that is released from the granules of activated neutrophils.[59] Overall, it forms a calyx with a distinct large hydrophobic cavity at the base of the calyx for ligand binding.

C9

Complement component C9 is a single polypeptide chain (71 kDa) that has a modular structure that is similar to that of the other members of the MAC family: an N-terminal TSP1; an LDLRA; the extended central sequence MACPF, which is homologous to perforin[60]; and an EGF module in the C-terminal end. C9 is endowed with the capacity to polymerize spontaneously in a circular fashion and to create tubules.

MEMBRANE ATTACK COMPLEX FORMATION

The C5b-7 complex binds to the cell membrane, and, although it inflicts no harm on the cell, it marks it for subsequent assault by C8 (*Figure 16.1*). The C5b-8 complex appears foliaceous by electron microscopy, with branched structures radiating from the central pedicle, but, on smaller phospholipid vesicles, C5b-8 monomers appear as long, rod-like structures that are 250 Å wide.[61] The C8α chain mediates binding and self-polymerization of C9 to form MAC.[62] The N-terminal TSP1 and LDLRA modules are the principal binding sites for C9 with the cooperative function of the MACPF domain. MACs are heterogeneous in size, probably as a result of their composition, and the number of the C9 subunits may vary from 1 to 18, whereas all other components contribute only one molecule.[63]

The final molecular weight of the MAC therefore varies between 66 and 1850 kDa. The average C9 binding capacity per C8 molecule is 15.4 molecules. C9 polymerizes spontaneously, but the C5b-8-induced rate of C9 polymerization is 10,000-fold greater. Self-associating C9 complexes develop new antigenic determinants that are not present in the monomer. C9 is inserted into the membrane through its C-terminal region, and disulfide bonds stabilize the complex. Electron microscopically, the polymerized C9 appears as a cylinder that extends 120 Å above the cell surface. The extracellular hydrophilic end terminates in an annulus that is 30 Å thick, with an inner diameter of approximately 100 Å[61] (*Figure 16.7*). The C5b-8 complex is attached firmly to the C9 cylinder and actually extends 160 to 180 Å above the annulus. The annulus, which is seen with computer-assisted programs, appears to be made of whorls[64] (*Figure 16.7*).

Because the height of the monomeric C9 is only 80 Å, and the poly C9 cylinder is 160 Å, the C9 must be unfolding and must transform into a rod-like structure. Thus, the formation of the cylinder by polymerization of C9 molecules involves the transformation of a hydrophilic C9 monomer into an amphiphilic C9 polymer.

The N-terminal part of C9 does not participate directly in polymerization and is located in the upper rim of the cylinder.[64] The MACPF domain traverses across the thickness of the cell membrane, forming the wall of the cylinder. The C-terminal part of C9 returns back up near the rim, indicating that polymerization transforms a straight ellipsoid C9 into a U shape.[65]

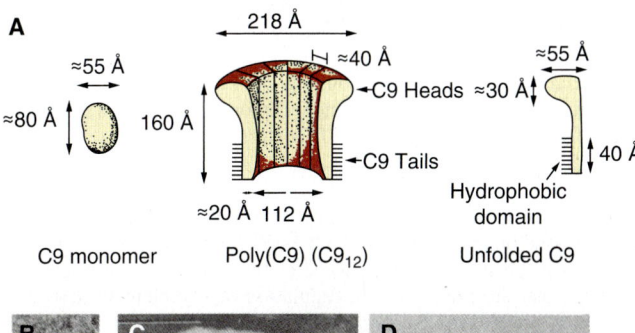

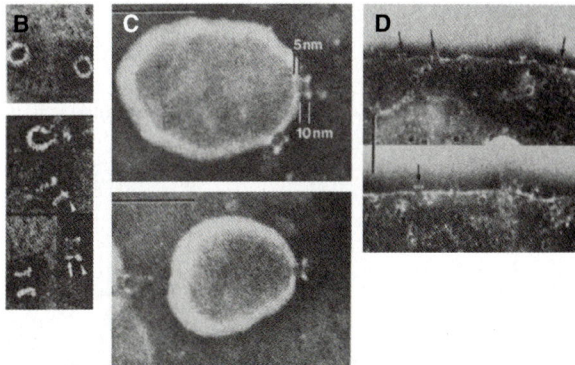

FIGURE 16.7 A, C9 molecule in its monomeric form, folded (left) or unfolded (right) and in its polymerized form (center) as a tubular structure that is seen on cell membranes. B, Poly C9 as ring structures (top view) or tubules (side view). C, Lipid vesicle with a typical cylinder that is formed from polymerization of C9 (side view). The cylinder penetrates the wall and protrudes to the outside, above the surface of the vesicle. D, Lesions that are induced by complement on sheep red blood cell membranes clearly show cylindric structures of the membrane attack complex and its penetration into the membrane (arrows). (A and B, Courtesy of Dr. E. R. Podack. From Podack ER, Tschopp J. Polymerization of the ninth component of complement (C9): formation of poly(C9) with a tubular ultrastructure resembling the membrane attack complex of complement. *Proc Natl Acad Sci U S A*. 1982;79:574-578; C and D, Courtesy of Dr. S. Bhakdi. From Bhakdi S, Tranum-Jensen J. Molecular nature of the complement lesion. *Proc Natl Acad Sci U S A*. 1978;75:5655-5659.)

C9 aligns with other molecules side by side, like staves of a barrel forming a volute-like structure (ie, a capital of an Ionian-style Greek column). Not all agree with the cylinder model of MAC. Others suggest that MAC proteins cause a distortion of the phospholipid bilayer, thus creating "leaky patches."[66]

REGULATION OF COMPLEMENT ACTIVATION

A large number of proteins, known as CCPs, are involved in the regulation of complement activation (*Table 16.1*). This complex regulatory system is best understood if we consider the stages of complement activation that are regulated or whether CCPs exist in fluids versus cellular surfaces. CCPs exert regulation mainly by accelerating dissociation of the convertases, a function that is known as decay-accelerating activity (DAA), or by acting as cofactors to the serine protease factor I, a function that is known as cofactor activity (CA). Some regulators are able to serve as both decay accelerators and cofactors, such as factor H, C4-binding protein (C4bp), and complement receptor 1 (CD35).

Control of the Initiation Step
C1 Inhibitor

C1 inhibitor (C1 INH) is a heavily glycosylated α-globulin with a molecular weight of 105 kDa. It is synthesized in the liver and by blood monocytes. Its gene is located on chromosome 11. C1 INH belongs to the superfamily of serpin proteins (serine protease inhibitors).[67] The inhibitor possesses a site that is structurally similar to the substrate, and, when a protease binds to this site and cleaves a peptide bond, it forms a covalent bond that results in a stable complex between the inhibitor and the enzyme. C1 INH inhibits activation of the classical and alternative pathways. It binds to C1r and C1s, forming stable complexes that prevent them from acting as an esterase. It also binds to the

Table 16.1. Regulatory Proteins of Complement

Factor	Location	Function
Initiation Step		
C1 inhibitor	Serum	Inactivates C1r and C1s
Amplification Step		
Factor I	Serum	Fragmentation of C3b and C4b
Membrane cofactor protein	Membrane	Cofactor for factor I in degradation of C3b
		Prevents C3 convertase formation
Decay-accelerating factor	Membrane	Dissociates preformed C3 and C5 convertases
C4-binding protein	Serum	Accelerates decay of C4b as cofactor for factor I
		Impairs uptake of factor B by C3
Factor H	Serum	Cofactor for factor I in C3b cleavage
		Promotes cleavage of C3b
		Impairs uptake of factor B by C3b
Complement receptor 1	Membrane	Displaces Bb from C3b
Properdin	Serum	Stabilizes C3 convertases
Membrane Attack		
S protein	Serum	Blocks fluid-phase membrane attack complex
CD59	Membrane	Blocks membrane attack complex on cells

Adapted from Uszewski MK, Farries TC, Lublin DM, et al. Control of the complement system. *Adv Immunol*. 1996;61:201-283. Copyright © 1996 Academic Press, Inc. With permission.

C1r-C1s complex and causes rapid dissociation of the C1 esterase. In the alternative pathway, it prevents factor B from binding to immobilized C3b. Cleavage of factor B by factor D is markedly inhibited when C3b is incubated with C1 INH.[68,69] A genetically inherited deficiency of C1 INH is manifested by recurrent acute attacks of circumscribed edema. Hereditary angioneurotic edema (HAE) may cause death from laryngeal edema. The mortality rate that is associated with this condition has been reduced with androgen therapy. This disease assumes two forms. In most (85%) cases (type 1 HAE), the inhibitor is present in reduced concentrations, whereas in the second form (type 2 HAE), it is present in normal concentrations but is biologically inactive.

Control of C3 and C5 Convertases

The C3 convertase cleaves C3 to C3b and C3a, whereas the C5 convertase cleaves C5 and initiates the final stage that ends with the formation of MAC. These amplification steps are regulated by seven proteins: three of them are present in the serum (C4BP, factor H, and factor I), and four are cell membrane proteins (MCP, decay-accelerating factor [DAF or CD55], CR1, and CR2). The overall function of these proteins is to prevent formation of the two convertases on self-cells. Except for factor I, all other proteins belong to a structurally related family of proteins that is known as the CCPs. The genes are clustered on the long arm of chromosome 1q32.

A striking structural feature that is common to these proteins is the multiple homologous cysteine-rich domains, a 60-amino-acid sequence referred to as CCP repeats.[70] The CCP module or repeat has four invariant cysteines, an invariant tryptophan, and highly conserved prolines, glycines, and hydrophobic residues.[71] The number of CCP domains is 30 in CR1, 20 in factor H, and 4 in CD55. The 60-amino-acid unit represents an ancestral domain that gave rise to the complement genes through duplication and splicing. The CCP domains are found in other complement proteins, such as C1r, C1s, C2, and factor B, as well as in noncomplement proteins, such as IL-2 receptor, haptoglobin, and coagulation factor XIII. Each CCP domain has a hydrophobic core that is interlaced with β strands connected by protruding loops, possessing a privileged position for interactions with other proteins. The control of the convertases is achieved by two mechanisms: (a) by dissociating the convertase to its individual components (DAA) and (b) by proteolytic degradation of C4b or C3b components as a result of the CA of the RCA proteins that act as cofactors for the serine protease, factor I. Some proteins have DAA and CA activity in the serum (C4BP, factor H) or cell surface (CR1), whereas others possess only one activity for the C4b and C3b components.

Regulators on Cell Surfaces
Membrane Cofactor Protein (CD46)

The extracellular region of membrane cofactor protein (MCP) consists of four CCP domains that contain the binding site for C3b and C4b and a region that is rich in serines, threonines, and prolines. The serine, threonine, and proline region is *O*-glycosylated and provides protection from proteolysis. A portion of this region may be removed by alternative splicing, which generates two of the four MCP isoforms. Two alternate forms of cytoplasmic regions contribute to the formation of another two MCP isoforms. MCP is present in almost all cells examined, except for red blood cells. Sites for C3b binding are in CCP2, CCP3, and CCP4 domains. The C3b and C4b binding sites have residues that bind to both complement components and others that are specific for each component.[72] MCP acts as cofactor for the serine protease factor I for inactivation of C4b that is deposited on self-tissues.[73] MCP in the maternal-fetal interface protects the fetal tissue from attack by the maternal complement. It is found on the inner membrane of the spermatozoa and may play a role in protecting the sperm against C3b deposition. MCP is a receptor for several pathogens. The measles virus binds to an extended surface of MCP that encompasses the area from the top of CCP1 to the bottom of CCP2.[74] The measles virus binding to CD46 is more like that of polio virus to its receptor: a wider open area that is flexibly hinged between CCP1 and CCP2 domains.[75] This leaves the virus still exposed to immune attack. It contrasts with the narrow, recessed binding site or canyon in the case of HIV and rhinoviruses.[76] The M-protein of *Streptococcus pyogenes*,[77] which causes serious suppurative skin infections (eg, cellulitis, necrotizing fasciitis), binds directly to CCP3 and CCP4 domains at a site that is distinct from the C3b-binding site. MCP mediates adherence of group A streptococci to keratinocytes.[78] HHV-6 also uses CD46 as a receptor and binds to CCP2 and CCP3.[79]

Decay-Accelerating Factor (CD55)

DAF contains four CCP domains and is attached to the membrane by a GPI anchor. Its molecular weight is between 70 and 80 kDa, depending on its glycosylation. Soluble forms exist in body fluids that may arise from the action of a phospholipase on the membrane form. It is expressed on all hematopoietic cells, endothelial and epithelial cells, and cells of the gastrointestinal, genitourinary, and central nervous systems. Erythrocytes possess approximately 3000 DAF molecules, and, among the lymphoid cells, the natural killer (NK) cells appear to be deficient in DAF. Neutrophil activation results in enhanced expression of DAF (from 10,000-20,000 molecules per cell). It is present in a soluble form in many body fluids, including plasma, tears, saliva, urine, synovial fluid, and cerebrospinal fluid.

DAF accelerates the decay of C3 convertase for the classical and alternative pathways and prevents its formation (*Figure 16.8*). Regulation by DAF involves separate sites for the two convertases as well as common sites for both.[80] For the alternative C3 convertase, DAF acts on the type A domain (vWF type A domain) of the Bb component.[81] Classical C3 convertase is regulated by a site that is located in the CCP2-CCP3 domain junction, which consists of three consecutive lysines and a hydrophobic patch.[82,83] DAF is used as receptor by many pathogens, such as several types of echoviruses, enteroviruses, and *Escherichia coli*. It constitutes a functional component of the LPS receptor complex.[84] CD55 is the ligand of CD97, the prototype of a large seven-span transmembrane family (as many as 2000 members) with variable numbers of EGF domains and sequence homology to the G protein–coupled peptide hormone receptors.[85,86] CD97 is associated with inflammation and is detected in malignancies.

Complement Receptor 1

Receptors for complement components or their breakdown products are expressed on many cells and tissues. They mediate various effector functions listed in *Table 16.2*. Some of the functions of complement receptors that are related to the regulation of complement activation are briefly reviewed. The complement receptor type 1 (CR1, C3b/

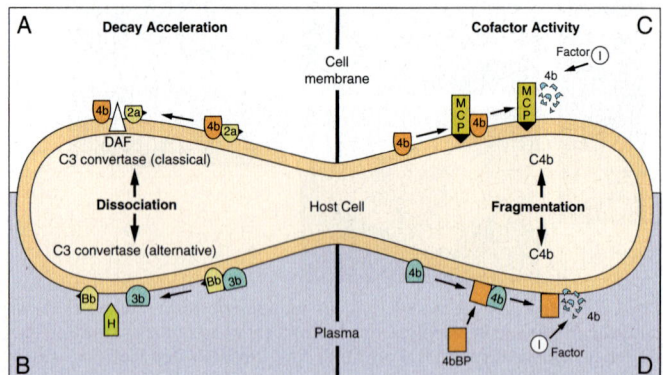

FIGURE 16.8 A and B, Decay activity on cell surfaces. A, Decay accelerating factor (DAF, CD55) is a GPI-anchored protein, which dissociates formed C3 convertase complex as well as prevents its formation. B, Factor H is a serum protein that expresses DA activity by attacking C3 convertases on self-surfaces. It binds to the C3b-Bb complex and displaces factor B irreversibly. C and D, Cofactor activity. C, Membrane cofactor protein (MCP, CD46) is a cell membrane protein that contains binding sites for C3b and C4b. It acts as cofactor for factor I to cleave both proteins. It is also the measles virus receptor. D, C4b-binding protein (C4BP) is a serum protein that acts as a cofactor for factor I for cleaving C4b.

Table 16.2. Cellular Distribution and Function of Receptors for Complement Components

Receptor	Cell type	Functions
C1q	Neutrophils	Respiratory burst
	Monocytes	—
	B cells	—
	NK cells	Enhanced antibody-dependent cell-mediated cytotoxicity
CR1	Macrophages	Enhanced phagocytosis
	Neutrophils	Same as macrophages
	B cells	—
	T cells	—
	Red blood cells	—
	Eosinophils	—
	Epithelial cells: kidney	—
CR2	B cells	Activation
CR3	Similar to CR1	Similar to CR1
Factor H	B cells	Secretion of factor I
	Monocytes	Respiratory burst
	Neutrophils	—
C5a	Mast cells	Histamine release
	Neutrophils	Chemotaxis, increased adhesiveness
		Enhancement of CR1 expression
	Macrophages	—
C3a/C4a	Mast cells	Histamine release

Used with permission of Annual Reviews, Inc. From Fearon DT, Wong WW. Complement ligand-receptor interactions that mediate biological responses. *Annu Rev Immunol.* 1983;1:243-271; permission conveyed through Copyright Clearance Center, Inc.

C4b receptor, CD35) was the first to be discovered as the receptor for immune adherence, a fundamental event in the initiation of the immune response. It is a polymorphic membrane protein of 190 to 280 kDa composed of 2039 residues and present on all peripheral blood cells except platelets, NK cells, and most T cells.[87] CR1 is expressed on kidney podocytes and FDCs. Cell membrane expression of CR1 is upregulated by chemotactic peptides, such as C5a, endotoxin, and cytokines. Blood cells at resting state express only 5% to 10% of the total cellular CR1 at the plasma membrane, whereas the remaining CR1 is found intracellularly. The red blood cells express 100 to 400 receptors per cell, and the leukocytes have 10,000 to 50,000 receptors per cell. However, because the number of red cells is approximately 1000 times more than white cells, they possess more than 85% of the total CR1 that is available in the blood.

CR1 contains 30 CCP domains with three sites for C4b binding and two sites for C3b binding. The CCP15 domain is critical for C4b binding and, together with the CCP16 domain, is required for C3b binding. The CCP domains are arranged in larger domains that are known as long homologous repeats, with each one containing seven CCPs. It is likely that this arrangement facilitates the binding of CR1 with clusters of its ligands. There are four allotypes of CR1 (A-D). CR1, one of the most versatile RCAs, possesses DAA and CA, which are restricted to reducing the complement activity on cells that have absorbed immune complexes. The DAA of CD35 is mediated by CCP1 to CCP3 domains for the classical and alternative pathways.[88] In the classical pathway, CR1 inhibits the uptake of C2 by C4b as well as displaces C2a from C4b2a C3 convertase and from C4b2a3b C5 convertase. It also promotes the cleavage of C4b to C4c and C4d by factor I and the cleavage

of C3b to iC3b (ligand of CR3) and C3dg (ligand of CR2) by factor I. In the alternative pathway, the CR1 impairs uptake of factor B by C3b and displaces Bb from C3bBb C3 convertase. Complexes that are bound to erythrocytes are eliminated in the spleen. Conversion of C3b to fragments leads to binding of the complexes to macrophages and monocytes that possess CR3 or to lymphoid follicular areas in which all three CRs are expressed.

CR1 has the capacity to inhibit complement activation on cells and tissues other than those in which it is expressed (extrinsic protection), whereas DAF and MCP protect only the cells on which they are expressed (intrinsic protection). CR1 facilitates phagocytosis, which in the absence of other ligands does not occur with resting neutrophils or monocytes. However, activation of these cells upregulates CR1 expression and alters its function, so that phagocytosis of C3b-coated particles may occur. Soluble human CR1 inhibits complement-dependent tissue damage and reduces inflammatory responses.

Regulators in Body Fluids
Factor H

Factor H is a soluble glycoprotein that is present in blood at concentrations of 0.3 to 0.5 mg/L. It is a single polypeptide chain of 150 kDa with a highly elongated shape. It is composed of 1213 amino acids that are assembled in 20 CCP domains. Factor H synthesis in the liver and in other extrahepatic sites (myeloblasts) is regulated by IL6.[89]

The main functions of factor H are (a) binding to the α chain of C3b, blocking the amplification cycle in the alternative pathway (tick-over), and preventing the generation of C3 convertase, C3bBb; (b) binding to the C3bBb enzyme and irreversibly displacing the Bb component (DA activity); and (c) acting as cofactor for factor I and enhancing its affinity for C3b. By these three activities, factor H prevents the formation of the C5 convertase and, thus, generation of MACs by the alternative pathway. Factor H possesses an impressive number of discriminatory functional sites. Its 20 CCP domains and long and flexible structure allow factor H to scan a large surface area. The affinity of factor H for C3b is affected by the properties of the cell or tissue surface. Carbohydrate-rich polymers that are found on yeast and bacterial cells prevent binding of factor H to C3b, thus enabling the complement activation to react against these pathogens. Removal of sialic acid from sheep erythrocytes prevents binding of factor H to C3b and allows activation of complement. Sialic acids are also critical for factor H–mediated complement regulation on endothelial cells, erythrocytes, and platelets.[90]

Factor H binds to polyanions, and blocking of this site enhances its affinity for C3b.[91] The propensity of factor H to bind on polyanions, such as heparin on host tissues, may function as a protective mechanism against the alternative CP.[92] The discriminatory ability of factor H depends on its differential binding to various types of surfaces to which C3b has been initially deposited. The nonactivating surfaces have sialic acid and other negatively charged glycosaminoglycans to which factor H binds through domain CCP20. The same domain is important for binding within approximately 30 Å from the C3d attachment site, indicating that the binding sites of factor H for polyanion and C3d overlap.[93] It is possible that discrimination by factor H occurs by a joint recognition of C3 and polyanions. The CCP11 to CCP20 domains are important for binding to activator surfaces,[94] but the DAA or CA varies among these CCPs, depending on the nature of the surface on which C3b has been deposited. It appears that factor H uses different CCP domains, individually or in combinations, for recognition of C3, host, or foreign tissues. The CCP1 to CCP4 domains are used to bind intact C3b, the CCP6 to CCP8 domains bind to the cell surface via heparin sulfate, and the CCP19 and CCP20 domains bind to C3b and to polyanions (mostly sialic acid) on the cell surface that forms a ternary complex that facilitates factor I–mediated inactivation of C3b to iC3b and accelerated decay of C3bBb (*Figure 16.9*).[95]

Factor H germline variants are the most common predisposing lesion underlying sporadic and familial cases of complement-mediated hemolytic uremic syndrome (cmHUS).[96,97] HUS is characterized by microangiopathic hemolytic anemia, thrombocytopenia, and acute

The Normal Hematologic System

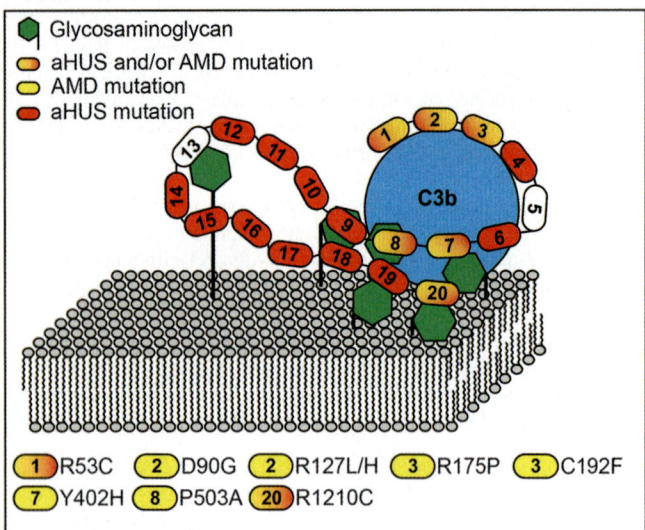

FIGURE 16.9 Factor H is composed of 20 CCP domains. CCP domains 1 to 4 and 19 to 20 mediate interactions with C3b, with an additional minor site between CCP6, 7, and 8 or CCP12, 13, and 14. Several FH regions mediate interactions with glycosaminoglycans (green hexagons), and binding is additive with adjacent CCP domains: CCP16 to 20 bind heparin, dextran sulfate, hyaluronic acid, and chondroitin sulfate A, B, & C; CCP8 to 14 bind heparin, dextran sulfate, hyaluronic acid, and chondroitin sulfate C; CCP1 to 7 bind heparin, dextran sulfate, and hyaluronic acid. While the individual CCP domains responsible for glycosaminoglycan binding have been mapped to CCP7 to 9, 13, and CCP19 to 20, CCP domains 19-20 are the principal domains responsible for FH localization to cell membranes and glycosaminoglycan binding. Missense mutations observed in aHUS are primarily located in CCP domains 19-20, but have been found in other domains (red). Some aHUS mutations occur in domains reported to contain AMD associated variants (orange). Of the 8 reported FH variants in AMD, only R53C and R1210C also occur in aHUS (orange), while the remaining 6 are only reported in AMD (yellow). The FH variant with the highest AMD-associated risk (R1210C) occurs in CCP20, while the most common AMD risk allele (Y402H) is located in CCP7 and displays diminished binding to glycosaminoglycan within Bruch's membrane. Note: because of the large number of aHUS associated mutations they are not listed in this figure.

renal failure in affected individuals, but other organs (brain, heart, gut, etc.) may also be affected. cmHUS may be sporadic or familial. The majority of cases are driven by overactivation of the alternative pathway.[98,99] Factor H germline variants are also found in a significant portion of patients with macular degeneration.[100]

A set of 12 missense variants in the CCP domains between CCP16 and CCP20 are associated with cmHUS. Nine of them are in CCP20 and are inferred to lead to a functional defect.[101] The positions of these variants correspond to basic residues that are involved in binding to heparin. It is suggested that these variants result in impairment of the normal function of factor H to prevent the activation of the alternative CP due to reduced binding to sulfated glycosaminoglycans. These experiments of nature strongly imply that the host-versus-foreign discrimination property of factor H resides in CCP20 and is lost as a consequence of these variants.[102] Lack of host recognition results in uncontrolled complement activation and, eventually, renal failure.

Mice that are deficient in factor H develop membranoproliferative glomerulonephritis as a result of uncontrolled activation of the alternative CP.[103] Factor H belongs to a protein family of several members; factor H–like protein 1 (FHL-1) or reconectin shares the complement regulatory functions with factor H and interacts with heparin. It contains the first 7 of 20 CCP domains of factor H and has 4 unique residues that are attached to the terminal end.[104] Both factor H and FHL-1 are synthesized by the same gene, but their transcripts are differentially regulated. They are produced by the liver, monocytes, and neuronal cells. Other members of the family are factor H–related (FHR) proteins 1 to 5,[105]

which bind to C3b and particularly to the C3d fragment.[106] These proteins normally do not increase complement activation because they lack the ability to bind sialic acid on the cell surface. However, germline variants in FHR-1 have been shown to gain this function, leading to pathologic complement activation due to attraction of C3 to the cell surface and competitive blocking of factor H.[107]

C4B-Binding Protein

The C4b-binding protein (C4BP) is a regulator of the classical CP C3 convertase. C4BP possesses CA and DAA. It consists of eight subunits that radiate from a central core in a spider-like formation (*Figure 16.10*). The peripheral end of each subunit is capable of binding one C4 molecule. Each of the seven subunits known as α chains has a molecular weight of 75 kDa, and the eighth subunit, known as a β chain, is 45 kDa. They are flexible, 33 nm in length, and linked together by disulfide bonds near the carboxy termini. In addition to the most common form of C4BP, $\alpha_7:\beta_1$, there are two other minor forms, $\alpha_7:\beta_0$ and $\alpha_6:\beta_1$. The α chains are composed of 549 amino acids divided into 8 CCP domains, with 58 residues left in the C terminus to form the disulfide bond with the other α chains in the core region. The β chains have three CCP domains and are attached by a disulfide bond in a similar way to the α chains. The genes for C4BP are within the gene cluster of the other RCA proteins. The C4b-binding site is localized in the CCP1 and CCP2 domains of the α chain, in a cluster of positively charged amino acids.[108] The same region is also important for binding to heparin, *Bordetella pertussis*, and the M-protein of *S. pyogenes*, *Neisseria gonorrhoeae*, and *E. coli*.

C4BP is synthesized in the liver under stimulation of IL6 and TNF-α and is present in the blood at a concentration of 0.2 mg/L. The mechanism of control of the classical pathway by C4BP depends on the binding to C4b and the displacement of C2a from the C4b2a convertase (DAA), as well as its function as a cofactor for cleavage of C4b by factor I. Dissociation of C2a from the classical pathway C3 convertase destroys its activity and prevents rebinding of the C2a to C4b. C4BP acts also as cofactor for cleavage of C3b by factor I.[109]

Protein S binds with high affinity to the β chain of C4BP.[110] Protein S of the coagulation pathway is a vitamin K–dependent anticoagulant protein. It acts as the cofactor for activated protein C that inactivates factor Va and is also the direct inhibitor of factor Xa. The concentration of free protein S is determined by the concentration of C4BP, as 50% or more of protein S is bound to C4BP. Protein S that is bound to C4BP is unable to participate in the anticoagulant protein C system. It is critical that the balance between free and C4BP-bound protein S is maintained stable, because lack of free protein S leads to thrombosis. Protein S–bound C4BP is probably localized on negatively charged surfaces that are found in platelets and apoptotic cells. Conditions with elevated C4BP (autoimmune diseases) may be associated with increased clotting tendency as a result of increased binding of protein S to C4BP.

Factor I

Factor I is a serine protease that mediates proteolytic degradation of C3b, iC3b, and C4b only if a cofactor binds to the substrate to promote the binding of the enzyme. These cofactors for C3 and C4 degradation on host cells are MCP (*Figure 16.8*), and, to a lesser extent, CR1, whereas in plasma the cofactors are C4BP and factor H (*Figures 16.8 and 16.9*). Factor I is constitutively active and essential for control of the fluid and cellular complement reactions. Genetic deficiency of factor I leaves the generation of C3 convertases uncontrolled, leading to incapacitation of the complement system as a result of the continuous low-level conversion of C3. Fragmentation by factor I of C3 and C4 determines the specificity of their derivatives for CR1, CR2, and CR3. Factor I is a two-chain disulfide-linked protein that is synthesized from a single-chain precursor. The H chain is 50 kDa, and the L chain is 38 kDa in molecular mass and has the serine esterase domain. The H chain is composed of three different types of modules that are derived from different gene superfamilies. One module, which is also found in C6 and C7, is from members of the follistatin family of the

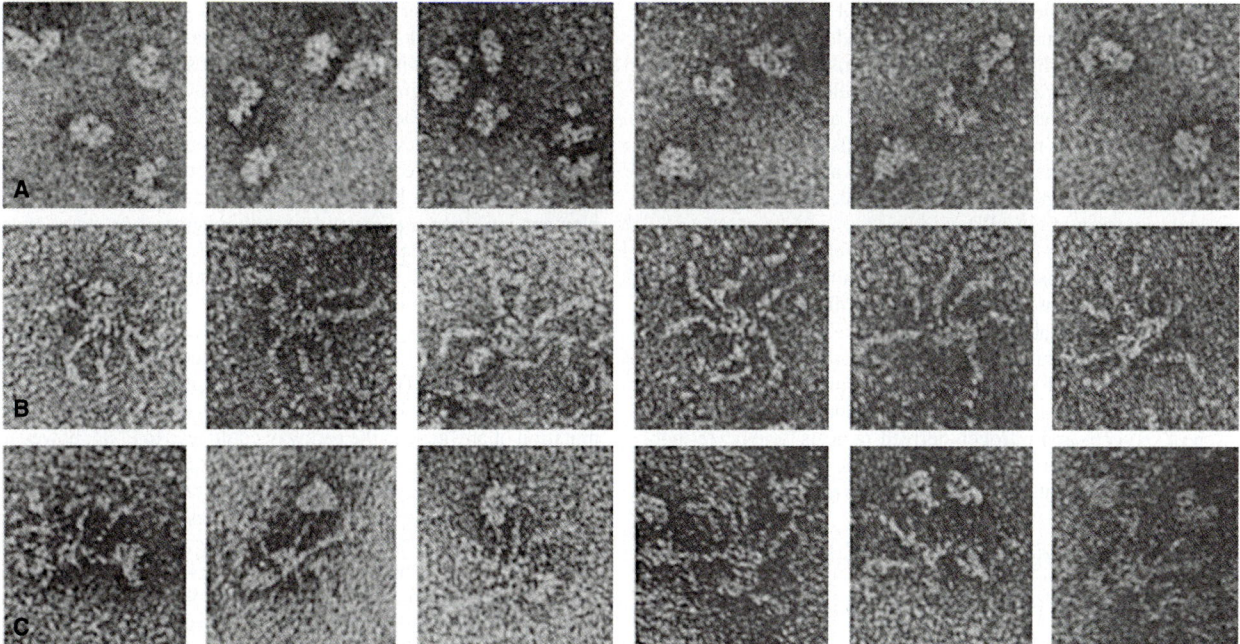

FIGURE 16.10 Electron micrographs of the C4b (A) and the C4b-binding protein (B) that form complexes with C4b (C). (Courtesy of Dr. Björn Dahlbäck. From Dahlback B, Smith CA, Muller-Eberhard HJ. Visualization of human C4b-binding protein and its complexes with vitamin K-dependent protein S and complement protein C4b. *Proc Natl Acad Sci U S A*. 1983;80:3461-3465.)

extracellular matrix; a second type is a scavenger-receptor cysteine-rich module; and the third type constitutes two LDLR-A modules.

The only known substrates for factor I are C3b and C4b. C3b is cleaved at Arg^{1303}-Ser^{1304} and Arg^{1320}-Ser^{1321}. For this cleavage, the cofactors are factor H, MCP, and CR1. C4BP acts as a cofactor for cleavage of C4b and C3b. C4b is cleaved at Arg^{1336}-Asn^{1337}. In general, for C3b and C4b and all subsequent fragments, factor I acts on the C-terminal side of an Arg.

Control of the Membrane Attack Complex Assembly

Protein S

Protein S is identical to vitronectin (serum-spreading factor). It is a 75- to 80-kDa protein that is synthesized from a single polypeptide chain that is subsequently cleaved to give the mature polypeptide as a single- or double-chain protein. At the NH_2 terminus, there is a somatomedin B domain (containing eight cysteines) followed by a linear sequence, which contains the RGD sequence that is responsible for the binding of integrins. Two domains of the S protein have homology to hemopexin. The C terminus is rich in basic residues that mediate the binding of S protein with sulfated polysaccharides.

Protein S binds to the metastable C5b-7 complex and prevents the formation of MAC. Because MAC in the process of its formation can be inserted on any cell membrane, the most important function of S protein is the protection of the cells of the body that may be attacked by MAC as innocent bystanders. Protein S acts through its heparin-binding site, which prevents the polymerization of C9. Protein S is important in cell-matrix interactions, and, through its multiple binding sites, it participates in several functions of adherence, phagocytosis, and the coagulation cascade in which it interacts with thrombin.

Clusterin (Cytolysis Inhibitor)

Clusterin is an 80-kDa protein composed of two chains (α and β). The gene is located on chromosome 8p21-p12. It is present in a variety of tissues and in the serum at concentrations of 35 to 105 μg/L. It forms complexes with lipoproteins and binds to C7, C8b, and C9, to inhibit MAC formation.[111]

Clusterin is involved in several other poorly understood functions. It has been found to be upregulated in injured tissues and in Alzheimer disease, as well as in tissues undergoing apoptosis.

Control of Deposited MAC: CD59

CD59 is an 18- to 20-kDa protein that inhibits MAC formation.[112] It has been known by a variety of other names, such as homologous restriction factor 20, membrane inhibitor of reactive lysis, and protectin. It is a GPI-anchored protein and is widely distributed in human tissues and most body fluids (see the following discussion). Somatic mutations that result in the loss of GPI-anchored proteins, including CD59, are characteristically found in blood cells of patients with paroxysmal nocturnal hemoglobinuria (PNH).[99,113]

Conclusion

The RCA proteins exert several important functions in the regulation of complement activity: (a) they prevent complement activation in the blood (factor H and C4BP); (b) they interfere with the assembly and function of convertase activity on cell membranes (DAF and MCP), protecting the cells of the body from complement attack; (c) they transport and clear immune complexes (CR1); and (d) they mediate transmembrane and intracellular trafficking (CR1) and transmembrane signaling (CR2).

The CCP units that are characteristic of the members of the proteins of the RCA gene cluster are present also in C1r, C6, C7, factor B, properdin, and noncomplement proteins, such as coagulation factor XIII and IL2 receptor. The 60-amino-acid unit represents an ancestral domain that gave rise to the complement genes through duplication and splicing with domains from the serine protease gene family.

ANAPHYLATOXINS

Activation of the complement cascade leads to the release of important inflammatory factors that are known as anaphylatoxins: the C3a, C4a, and C5a molecules. Their amino acid sequence varies from 74 to 78 residues. The cysteines are conserved in all anaphylatoxins and form three disulfide bonds that stabilize the conformation and form the core of the molecule. The C terminus forms the active site, with the C-terminal Arg being essential for function. Under physiologic conditions, the molecule is folded or compact.

The C-terminal end protrudes from the core and is considered to be the active site of the molecule that mediates biologic activities. Removal of the last Arg (C5a desArg) results in a loss of spasmogenic activity, but the chemotactic and other neutrophil activation functions are retained. The N-terminal region of C5a binds to its high-affinity receptor on neutrophils, which spans the membrane seven times with the N terminus on the extracellular side.[114] It belongs to the rhodopsin family of receptors, the members of which are linked to G proteins. Binding of C5a to its receptor on neutrophils induces a variety of responses, depending on its concentration, such as chemotaxis, granule secretion, upregulation of adhesion molecules, changes of cytoskeleton, and activation of NADPH oxidase.

All anaphylatoxins are cleaved rapidly in the serum by carboxypeptidase-N, an enzyme that removes the C-terminal Arg that is found on all three anaphylatoxins. The main biologic function of anaphylatoxins is related to their ability to increase vascular permeability as a result of mast cell degranulation. Anaphylatoxins also cause serious lung injury because of their capacity to recruit and sequester leukocytes in the pulmonary circulation. Anaphylatoxins also mediate production of oxygen- and nitrogen-derived radicals, leukocyte margination, release of granule-associated proteolytic enzymes, and capillary leakage, all components of an inflammatory response.

COMPLEMENT COMPONENT DEFICIENCIES

C1 Esterase Inhibitor: Hereditary Angioedema

HAE is an autosomal dominant disease with an estimated prevalence of 1 in 50,000; it afflicts persons of all races with no sex predominance.[115] It manifests as recurrent attacks of intense, massive localized edema without pruritus and in the absence of any identifiable initiating event. Gastrointestinal and respiratory systems are most commonly involved with upper airways symptoms, including risk of asphyxiation. There are two types of HAE: type 1 (80%-85% of cases) caused by decreased production of C1 INH and type 2 (15%-20%) caused by a functionally impaired C1 INH (C1 esterase inhibitor).

C1 INH belongs to the same family as α_1-antitrypsin; antithrombin, IFN-γ, and IL6 stimulate its synthesis and release from the liver and monocytes. The main function of C1 INH is prevention of autoactivation of the complement cascade. It also inactivates coagulation factors XIIa, XIIf, and XId and activated kallikrein. The mechanism of action involves formation of irreversible covalent bonds with the substrates.

Under physiologic conditions, small quantities of factor XII are autoactivated to factor XIIa and trigger the contact system, which cleaves pre-kallikrein to kallikrein; this cleaves kininogen, generating excessive release of kinins, especially bradykinin. This pathway normally is blocked by C1 INH, which inhibits factor XIIa. In the absence of the normal control function of C1 INH, not only is factor XIIa not inhibited but kallikrein also generates plasmin from plasminogen, activating factor XIIa for more kallikrein as well as activation of the C1 esterase. Symptomatic attacks of hereditary angioedema can be mitigated by intravenous administration of recombinant human C1-esterase (rhC1INH). A phase 3, randomized, placebo-controlled trial showed that intravenous administration of rhC1INH is safe and effective in providing rapid and sustained symptom improvement compared with placebo.[116]

Deficiency of Other Early Complement Components

Homozygous deficiencies of the early components of the classical pathway are associated with SLE, and the severity of the associated disease is greatest with C1q deficiency. This is caused by failure of C1q synthesis or synthesis of a dysfunctional molecule. C4 deficiency is associated with early onset of severe SLE. C2 deficiency is the most common homozygous complement deficiency in whites; C3 deficiency is associated with recurrent pyogenic infections, and deficiency of factor H has been associated with membranoproliferative glomerulonephritis.

Paroxysmal Nocturnal Hemoglobinuria

PNH is an acquired hemolytic anemia that results from the expansion of hematopoietic stem cells with a severe deficiency or absence of GPI, a glycolipid moiety that anchors more than a dozen different proteins to the cell surface of blood cells.[113] In most cases, GPI anchor deficiency in PNH results from a somatic mutation in *PIGA*, an X-linked gene whose product is required for the first step in GPI anchor biosynthesis. This results in the absence of complement regulatory proteins CD55 and CD59, leading to chronic complement-mediated hemolysis of the PNH erythrocytes. Hemolysis in PNH is chronic because of a continuous state of complement activation through tick-over, but paroxysms resulting in brisk hemolysis coincide with increases in complement activation that may occur with inflammatory states or surgery. The most common clinical manifestations include fatigue, dyspnea, hemoglobinuria, and abdominal pain,[117] but thrombosis is the leading cause of death in PNH.[118]

GPI biosynthesis is a posttranslational event that occurs in the endoplasmic reticulum.[119] There are over 10 steps and more than 20 gene products required. The PIGA gene product is one of seven proteins involved in the first step of GPI anchor biosynthesis. Theoretically, a mutation of any gene in the pathway could lead to PNH; however, most cases are caused by *PIGA* mutations. This is because *PIGA* is on the X chromosome; therefore, a single mutation in a hematopoietic stem cell will result in GPI anchor protein deficiency (males have a single X chromosome and females have only one active X chromosome due to lyonization). The remaining known genes in the GPI anchor biosynthetic pathway are on autosomes; thus, two "hits" disrupting function on both alleles would be necessary to interrupt GPI anchor synthesis.

The absence of CD59 is most responsible for the clinical manifestations in PNH. Accordingly, rare cases of inherited mutations in CD59 leading to loss of CD59 on the cell surface have been well documented.[120,121] The phenotype of these patients mimics PNH in that they manifest chronic intravascular hemolysis with paroxysmal flares of hemolysis and a propensity for thrombosis. Unlike PNH, pedigrees with inherited CD59 deficiency also present with relapsing immune-mediated peripheral neuropathy. In classical PNH, the CD59 deficiency is only found on the blood cells; in patients with germline CD59 mutations, CD59 is deficient in all cells in the body. Thus, germline CD59 deficiency may be associated with demyelination via activation of terminal complement.

There are three drugs (eculizumab, ravulizumab, and pegcetacoplan) approved by the US Food and Drug Administration (FDA) to treat PNH. Eculizumab and ravulizumab are humanized monoclonal antibodies that block terminal complement by binding to C5.[122-125] Both eculizumab and ravulizumab (C5 inhibitors) require intravenous administration, but the half-life of ravulizumab is four times longer allowing for every 8-week maintenance infusion.[126] Eculizumab and ravulizumab block formation of the MAC and in doing so compensate for the CD59 deficiency of patients with PNH. These drugs are highly effective in reducing thrombosis risk in PNH to baseline, highlighting the interplay between complement activation and thrombosis.[127,128] They do not compensate for the CD55 deficiency; thus, eculizumab and ravulizumab abrogate the intravascular hemolysis in PNH, but most patients with PNH on C5 inhibitors will continue to experience mild to moderate extravascular hemolysis due to C3 fragment deposition on the PNH red cells.[129] This explains why more than 50% of patients with PNH treated with C5 inhibitors develop a positive direct antiglobulin test (C3 positive but IgG negative) in conjunction with a mild to moderate anemia and elevated reticulocyte count.[130] The most serious risk of terminal complement blockade is life-threatening *Neisseria* infections (roughly 0.5% per year). Thus, all patients treated with complement inhibitors should be vaccinated against *Neisseria*.

The majority of patients with classical PNH respond well to C5 inhibitors; however, the hemoglobin response is highly variable and may depend on underlying bone marrow failure, concurrent inflammatory conditions, genetic factors, and the size of the PNH red cell clone following therapy.[131] In fact, up to 20% of patients continue to require red cell transfusions despite treatment with eculizumab. The most common reason for continued transfusions is extravascular hemolysis. An increase in the percentage of PNH red cells after eculizumab therapy correlates not only with response but also with extravascular hemolysis. The PNH red cells that are protected by eculizumab are CD55 deficient and thus are susceptible to opsonization by C3 fragments and premature removal in the spleen and liver.[129] Pharmacogenetics has also been shown to influence response to therapy. Polymorphisms in the complement receptor 1 (CR1) gene are associated with response to eculizumab. CR1, through binding C3b and C4b, enhances the decay of the C3 and C5 convertases.[132] The density of CR1 on the surface of red cells modulates binding of C3 fragments to the GPI-negative red cells when C5 is inhibited. Patients with PNH with polymorphisms in CR1 that lead to low CR1 levels (L/L genotype) are more likely to be suboptimal responders to eculizumab than patients with intermediate (H/L genotype) or high (H/H genotype) levels of CR1. More recently, it has been discovered that a single missense C5 heterozygous mutation, c.2654G → A, prevents binding and blockade by eculizumab while retaining the functional capacity to cause hemolysis.[133] The c.2654G → A polymorphism is present in 3.5% of the Japanese population and accounts for the poor response to eculizumab in patients who carry the mutation.

Pegcetacoplan is a pegylated peptide that targets C3. Drug administration is every 3 days by subcutaneous infusion over 15 minutes. Pegcetacoplan was FDA approved to treat PNH in 2021 based on a phase 3 open-label, controlled trial showing pegcetacoplan was superior to eculizumab in improving hemoglobin and other hematologic outcomes by preventing intravascular and extravascular hemolysis.[134] There were 41 patients in the pegcetacoplan arm compared with 39 in the eculizumab arm and follow-up was reported at 16 weeks; thus, more experience will be needed to determine long-term safety and efficacy of this promising agent. Many other complement inhibitors that block at C5 (crovalimab) or upstream of C5 (iptacopan and danicopan) are in last-stage clinical trials but not yet approved by the FDA.

Atypical Hemolytic Uremic Syndrome (aka Complement-Mediated Hemolytic Uremic Syndrome)

The atypical hemolytic uremic syndrome (aHUS) is a life-threatening disease characterized by thrombocytopenia, microangiopathic hemolytic anemia, and acute renal failure.[135,136,] Other manifestations include seizures, stroke, mental status changes, hypertension, and diarrhea. End-organ damage is due to microvascular thrombosis in the arterioles and capillaries, termed thrombotic microangiopathy (TMA). The majority of cases are caused by inherited variants that dysregulate the APC.[137,138] These variants involve gene products that cause downregulation of alternative pathway inhibitors (eg, factor H, factor I) or increase the half-life of alternative pathway activators (eg, C3, factor B). Environmental factors (eg, infections, pregnancy, surgery) are also required to trigger the disease by increasing complement activation. Thus, "two hits" (a genetic variant that leads to APC dysregulation and environmental stressor that increases complement activity) are necessary to cause the disease. A minority of cases are also caused by autoantibodies to factor H. Complications of aHUS are primarily due to complement-mediated damage to the microvascular endothelium, especially in the kidney, or other organ systems. Eculizumab and ravulizumab are FDA approved to treat aHUS and are highly effective.[139] Differentiating aHUS from other TMAs and especially thrombotic thrombocytopenic purpura (TTP) is difficult due to overlapping clinical manifestations. In patients presenting with TMAs it is important to obtain ADAMTS13 levels and screen for Shiga toxin before instituting definitive therapy. Plasma exchange is often initiated before the results of these assays return, due to the aggressiveness of TMAs. If ADAMTS13 activity is less than 10%, a diagnosis of TTP is established and daily plasma exchange is continued. If ADAMTS13 activity is greater than 10% and Shiga toxin assay is negative, a diagnosis of aHUS and treatment with a C5 inhibitor must be considered.[140] Genetic testing for variants that lead to increased activation of the alternative CP should be pursued but is informative in approximately 50% of cases.[141,142,] Even when variants in the alternative CP are uncovered, their pathologic significance is often uncertain.[143] Serum-based assays to test for complement activation are in development but are not yet available for clinical decision making.[98] Many patients with aHUS are able to discontinue treatment with C5 inhibitors after achieving a complete remission; however, those with germline variants in complement regulatory genes are more likely to relapse.[144,145]

Shiga Toxin–Associated Hemolytic Uremic Syndrome–Hemolytic Uremic Syndrome

The clinical manifestations of Shiga toxin–associated (STEC) HUS span a wide spectrum, with some patients mildly affected with minimal symptoms to others having a severe clinical course resulting in renal failure, substantial neurologic consequences, and even death. The care of patients with STEC-HUS remains supportive, with no therapies available to directly treat the underlying pathophysiology. Evidence from human[146,147] and animal[148,149] models have suggested that complement activation may play a role in the course of STEC HUS, although this has not been fully characterized. Eculizumab has been used in STEC-HUS with reports suggesting some benefit[150,151] and others stating no benefit.[152,153]

HELLP Syndrome

A severe form of preeclampsia characterized by Hemolysis, Elevated Liver enzymes, and Low Platelets (HELLP) poses risk of serious morbidity and mortality to both the mother and fetus during pregnancy.[154] Patients with HELLP syndrome have clinical manifestations similar to aHUS, including thrombotic microangiopathy, renal dysfunction, hypertension, seizures, and altered mental states. Complement has been implicated in its pathogenesis.[155,156] An increased frequency of genetic variants in complement regulatory genes similar to those found in patients with aHUS, including *CFH*, *CFI*, and *CD46*, has been reported in women with preeclampsia,[157] HELLP,[158,159] and pregnancy-associated HUS.[160] In addition, a study evaluating a cohort of women with HELLP syndrome found that nearly 80% of the patients had detectable systemic complement activation; addition of eculizumab to serum of patients with HELLP blocked complement-mediated killing in vitro.[156]

Age-Related Macular Degeneration

Age-related macular degeneration (AMD), the most frequent etiology of blindness in the Western world, is characterized by drusen accumulation between the retinal pigment epithelium and Brusch membrane. The resultant inflammation and complement deposition lead to loss of photoreceptors (macular atrophy) and/or abnormal blood vessel growth (choroidal neovascularization) causing blindness. Heritable factors represent approximately half of AMD risk, with major contributions from complement loci (CFH, C2-CFB, C3).[161] The data for CFH are particularly noteworthy. The CFH Y402H variant is found in 30% of Caucasians, presumably due to evolutionary infectious selection, and is associated with AMD odds ratio of 2.3 per allele.[162] The uncommon CFH R1210C variant found in 1.4% of AMD cases has an associated AMD odds ratio of 23 and has also been observed in patients with aHUS.[163-165] CFH R1210C occurs in CCP domain 20, which mediates CFH interactions with glycosaminoglycans, C3b, and cell membranes.[90] Other rare CFH variants associated with AMD include R53C, D90G, R127L, R127H, R175P, C192F, and P503A.[166]

Cold-Agglutinin Disease

Cold-agglutinin disease (CAD) is an antibody- and complement-mediated hemolytic anemia that leads to extravascular and intravascular hemolysis with a propensity for thrombosis. CAD is classified as primary or secondary. Primary CAD is a clonal B-cell lymphoproliferative disorder that is now referred to as "primary cold agglutinin-associated lymphoproliferative disease"; it is distinct from lymphoplasmacytic lymphoma (MYD88 L265P negative), marginal-zone lymphoma, and other low-grade lymphoproliferative diseases.[167] Secondary CAD is a syndrome associated with a variety of infectious (*Mycoplasma pneumoniae*) and neoplastic disorders (eg, aggressive lymphomas, Hodgkin lymphoma, carcinomas). Cold agglutinins are autoantibodies (typically IgM) that agglutinate RBCs at 4 °C, but they may also act at warmer temperatures. Most pathogenic cold agglutinins are of the IgM class, have a thermal amplitude that exceeds 28 °C to 30 °C, and are present at a titer of 1:256 or greater.

Cold agglutinins with a thermal amplitude of greater than room temperature bind to red cells in acral parts of the circulation (fingers, toes, ears, etc.) and are commonly directed against the I antigen. Binding of IgM activates the classical CP. C1 esterase activates C4 and C2, ultimately generating the C3 convertase that cleaves C3 to C3a and C3b. Upon return to central portions of the circulation (approximately 37 °C) the IgM-CA dissociates from the cell surface but C3b remains bound to the cell. The C3b-coated red cells bind to complement receptors on macrophages of the reticuloendothelial system, predominantly in the liver (extravascular hemolysis). C3b of the surviving red cells is eventually cleaved, leaving a high number of circulating red cells with C3d on the surface. Thus, patients with CAD have a direct antiglobulin test that is strongly positive for C3d but negative for IgG and IgM. The CP activity does not proceed to activate the terminal pathway in most cases, due to the expression of CD55 and CD59 on the red cell membrane; however, in more severe cases, usually in association with an inflammatory state (infection, surgery, etc.), intravascular hemolysis resulting from terminal activation may occur.

Rituximab is the most common first-line therapy.[168] It leads to remission (median duration of 1 year) in roughly 50% of patients. Relapsed patients may respond to subsequent rituximab therapy. Fludarabine plus rituximab has a 75% response rate (median duration over 5 years) but significantly more toxicity.[169] Rituximab plus bendamustine is better tolerated and also very effective.[170] There are case reports of eculizumab therapy in the occasional patient with CAD with intravascular hemolysis, and there is evidence that a monoclonal antibody that targets C1s can help to control extravascular hemolysis.[171] However, complement inhibitors are not yet approved by FDA for use in CAD. In patients with secondary CAD, treatment should target the underlying cause.

COVID-19

COVID-19, the disease caused by severe acute respiratory syndrome coronavirus-2 (SARS-CoV-2) caused a severe pandemic starting in late 2019 resulting in millions of deaths. Severe disease and end-organ damage in COVID-19 is the result of a dysregulated host immune response, and significant evidence suggests that complement is a major contributor.[172,173] Deposition of terminal complement and thrombotic microangiopathy has been observed in lung, kidney, and heart tissue of patients with severe COVID-19 disease,[174] and numerous studies have demonstrated high rates of both arterial and venous thrombosis ranging from 10% to 30%.[175] The SARS-CoV-2 spike protein leads to dysregulation of the APC by binding to heparan sulfate and competing with factor H for binding to the cell.[176] Whether pharmacologic inhibition can effectively treat COVID-19 is under investigation.

Pharmacologic Complement Inhibitors

Eculizumab, ravulizumab, and recombinant human C1INH (rhC1INH) are currently the only FDA-approved complement inhibitors. The number of approved complement inhibitors will grow in the coming years and the indications for complement inhibitors will likely expand. There are more than a dozen novel complement inhibitors in preclinical/clinical development.[177] Many of these compounds target C5 since terminal complement blockade is proven to be safe and effective in humans but upstream complement inhibitors are increasingly being studied in clinical trials.

Deficiencies of Terminal Complement Components

Deficiencies of the terminal complement components, such as C7, have been detected in several countries, whereas C6 has been detected primarily in blacks in the United States and in South Africa, and the majority of C9 deficiencies have been found in Japan.[178–180] C6 deficiency has been defined as quantitatively zero C6 (C6Q0) or subtotal C6 (C6SD), when C6 is structurally abnormal but hemolytically active.[181]

Deficiencies are due to single-base deletions or mutations that lead to premature stop codons. In C6 deficiency there is a tendency for mutations in exon 6[180] with defects in an area that is adjacent to a sequence that contains seven Gs and a string of six Ts.[182] Carboxy-terminally truncated C6, which results in a shorter dysmorphic but

functionally active, molecule, has been detected in South African families.[183] Complement component C6 deficiency is associated with *Neisseria* infections often being recurrent.[184]

Infections with serogroup B are a major problem in these patients; these infections limit the usefulness of the available vaccine, which is not directed against this group. Other infections have also been detected in homozygous C6 deficiency, such as SLE, Still disease, and glomerulosclerosis.[185]

ACKNOWLEDGMENTS

We would like to acknowledge the contribution of Frixos Paraskevas, who wrote a previous version of this chapter, as many parts of this previous version remain in the current version.

References

1. Muller-Eberhard HJ. Molecular organization and function of the complement system. *Annu Rev Biochem.* 1988;57:321-347.
2. Reid KB, Porter RR. The proteolytic activation systems of complement. *Annu Rev Biochem.* 1981;50:433-464.
3. Diebolder CA, Beurskens FJ, de Jong RN, et al. Complement is activated by IgG hexamers assembled at the cell surface. *Science.* 2014;343(6176):1260-1263.
4. Reid KB, Day AJ. Structure-function relationships of the complement components. *Immunol Today.* 1989;10(6):177-180.
5. Ghebrehiwet B, Hosszu KH, Peerschke EI. C1q as an autocrine and paracrine regulator of cellular functions. *Mol Immunol.* 2017;84:26-33.
6. Kishore U, Reid KB. C1q: structure, function, and receptors. *Immunopharmacology.* 2000;49(1-2):159-170.
7. Arlaud GJ, Gaboriaud C, Thielens NM, et al. Structural biology of C1: dissection of a complex molecular machinery. *Immunol Rev.* 2001;180:136-145.
8. Arlaud GJ, Gaboriaud C, Thielens NM, Budayova-Spano M, Rossi V, Fontecilla-Camps JC. Structural biology of the C1 complex of complement unveils the mechanisms of its activation and proteolytic activity. *Mol Immunol.* 2002;39(7-8):383-394.
9. Tacnet-Delorme P, Chevallier S, Arlaud GJ. Beta-amyloid fibrils activate the C1 complex of complement under physiological conditions: evidence for a binding site for A beta on the C1q globular regions. *J Immunol.* 2001;167(11):6374-6381.
10. Ramirez-Ortiz ZG, Pendergraft WFIII, Prasad A, et al. The scavenger receptor SCARF1 mediates the clearance of apoptotic cells and prevents autoimmunity. *Nat Immunol.* 2013;14(9):917-926.
11. Paidassi H, Tacnet-Delorme P, Garlatti V, et al. C1q binds phosphatidylserine and likely acts as a multiligand-bridging molecule in apoptotic cell recognition. *J Immunol.* 2008;180(4):2329-2338.
12. Shapiro L, Scherer PE. The crystal structure of a complement-1q family protein suggests an evolutionary link to tumor necrosis factor. *Curr Biol.* 1998;8(6):335-338.
13. Gaboriaud C, Rossi V, Bally I, Arlaud GJ, Fontecilla-Camps JC. Crystal structure of the catalytic domain of human complement c1s: a serine protease with a handle. *EMBO J.* 2000;19(8):1755-1765.
14. Budayova-Spano M, Lacroix M, Thielens NM, Arlaud GJ, Fontecilla-Camps C., Gaboriaud C. The crystal structure of the zymogen catalytic domain of complement protease C1r reveals that a disruptive mechanical stress is required to trigger activation of the C1 complex. *EMBO J.* 2002;21(3):231-239.
15. Thielens NM, Enrie K, Lacroix M, et al. The N-terminal CUB-epidermal growth factor module pair of human complement protease C1r binds Ca2+ with high affinity and mediates Ca2+-dependent interaction with C1s. *J Biol Chem.* 1999;274(14):9149-9159.
16. Lorincz Z, Gal P, Dobo J, et al. The cleavage of two C1s subunits by a single active C1r reveals substantial flexibility of the C1s-C1r-C1r-C1s tetramer in the C1 complex. *J Immunol.* 2000;165(4):2048-2051.
17. Bork P, Beckmann G. The CUB domain. A widespread module in developmentally regulated proteins. *J Mol Biol.* 1993;231(2):539-545.
18. Eggleton P, Reid KB, Tenner AJ. C1q—how many functions? How many receptors?. *Trends Cell Biol.* 1998;8(11):428-431.
19. Eggleton P, Tenner AJ, Reid KB. C1q receptors. *Clin Exp Immunol.* 2000;120(3):406-412.
20. Leigh LE, Ghebrehiwet B, Perera TP, et al. C1q-mediated chemotaxis by human neutrophils: involvement of gClqR and G-protein signalling mechanisms. *Biochem J.* 1998;330(pt 1):247-254.
21. Webster SD, Park M, Fonseca MI, Tenner AJ. Structural and functional evidence for microglial expression of C1qR(P), the C1q receptor that enhances phagocytosis. *J Leukoc Biol.* 2000;67(1):109-116.
22. Peerschke EI, Ghebrehiwet B. Human blood platelet gC1qR/p33. *Immunol Rev.* 2001;180:56-64.
23. Sosoniuk E, Vallejos G, Kenawy H, et al. Trypanosoma cruzi calreticulin inhibits the complement lectin pathway activation by direct interaction with L-Ficolin. *Mol Immunol.* 2014;60(1):80-85.
24. Tack BF. The beta-Cys-gamma-Glu thiolester bond in human C3, C4, and alpha 2-macroglobulin. *Springer Semin Immunopathol.* 1983;6(4):259-282.
25. Jenkins PV, Pasi KJ, Perkins SJ. Molecular modeling of ligand and mutation sites of the type A domains of human von Willebrand factor and their relevance to von Willebrand's disease. *Blood.* 1998;91(6):2032-2044.
26. Hinshelwood J, Perkins SJ. Metal-dependent conformational changes in a recombinant vWF-A domain from human factor B: a solution study by circular

dichroism, Fourier transform infrared and (1)H NMR spectroscopy. *J Mol Biol.* 2000;298(1):135-147.

27. Arlaud GJ, Volanakis JE, Thielens NM, Narayana SV, Rossi V, Xu Y. The atypical serine proteases of the complement system. *Adv Immunol.* 1998;69:249-307.

28. Sahu A, Lambris JD. Structure and biology of complement protein C3, a connecting link between innate and acquired immunity. *Immunol Rev.* 2001;180:35-48.

29. Sahu A, Kozel TR, Pangburn MK. Specificity of the thioester-containing reactive site of human C3 and its significance to complement activation. *Biochem J.* 1994;302(pt 2):429-436.

30. Pangburn MK, Rawal N. Structure and function of complement C5 convertase enzymes. *Biochem Soc Trans.* 2002;30(pt 6):1006-1010.

31. Mannes M, Dopler A, Zolk O, et al. Complement inhibition at the level of C3 or C5: mechanistic reasons for ongoing terminal pathway activity. *Blood.* 2021;137(4):443-455.

32. Pangburn MK, Schreiber RD, Muller-Eberhard HJ. Formation of the initial C3 convertase of the alternative complement pathway. Acquisition of C3b-like activities by spontaneous hydrolysis of the putative thioester in native C3. *J Exp Med.* 1981;154(3):856-867.

33. Volanakis JE, Narayana SV. Complement factor D, a novel serine protease. *Protein Sci.* 1996;5(4):553-564.

34. Pillemer L, Blum L, Lepow I, Ross O, Todd E, Wardlaw A. The properdin system and immunity: demonstration and isolation of a new serum protein, properdin, and its role in immune phenomena. *Science.* 1954;120:279-285.

35. Pangburn MK. Analysis of the natural polymeric forms of human properdin and their functions in complement activation. *J Immunol.* 1989;142(1):202-207.

36. Smith CA, Pangburn MK, Vogel CW, Muller-Eberhard HJ. Molecular architecture of human properdin, a positive regulator of the alternative pathway of complement. *J Biol Chem.* 1984;259(7):4582-4588.

37. Goundis D, Reid KB. Properdin, the terminal complement components, thrombospondin and the circumsporozoite protein of malaria parasites contain similar sequence motifs. *Nature.* 1988;335(6185):82-85.

38. Higgins JM, Wiedemann H, Timpl R, Reid KB. Characterization of mutant forms of recombinant human properdin lacking single thrombospondin type I repeats. Identification of modules important for function. *J Immunol.* 1995;155(12):5777-5785.

39. Perdikoulis MV, Kishore U, Reid KB. Expression and haracterization of the thrombospondin type I repeats of human properdin. *Biochim Biophys Acta.* 2001;1548(2):265-277.

40. Bongrazio M, Pries AR, Zakrzewicz A. The endothelium as physiological source of properdin: role of wall shear stress. *Mol Immunol.* 2003;39(11):669-675.

41. Schwaeble WJ, Reid KB. Does properdin crosslink the cellular and the humoral immune response? *Immunol Today.* 1999;20(1):17-21.

42. Xu Y, Narayana SV, Volanakis JE. Structural biology of the alternative pathway convertase. *Immunol Rev.* 2001;180:123-135.

43. Rawal N, Pangburn MK. Structure/function of C5 convertases of complement. *Int Immunopharm.* 2001;1(3):415-422.

44. Petersen SV, Thiel S, Jensenius JC. The mannan-binding lectin pathway of complement activation: biology and disease association. *Mol Immunol.* 2001;38(2-3):133-149.

45. Thielens NM, Cseh S, Thiel S, et al. Interaction properties of human mannan-binding lectin (MBL)-associated serine proteases-1 and-2, MBL-associated protein 19, and MBL. *J Immunol.* 2001;166(8):5068-5077.

46. Stover CM, Thiel S, Thelen M, et al. Two constituents of the initiation complex of the mannan binding lectin activation pathway of complement are encoded by a single structural gene. *J Immunol.* 1999;162(6):3481-3490.

47. Jack DL, Klein NJ, Turner MW. Mannose-binding lectin: targeting the microbial world for complement attack and opsonophagocytosis. *Immunol Rev.* 2001;180:86-99.

48. Matsushita M, Fujita T. Ficolins and the lectin complement pathway. *Immunol Rev.* 2001;180:78-85.

49. Matsushita M, Kuraya M, Hamasaki N, Tsujimura M, Shiraki H, Fujita T. Activation of the lectin complement pathway by H-ficolin (Hakata antigen). *J Immunol.* 2002;168(7):3502-3506.

50. Fujita T. Evolution of the lectin-complement pathway and its role in innate immunity. *Nat Rev Immunol.* 2002;2(5):346-353.

51. DiScipio RG. Formation and structure of the C5b-7 complex of the lytic pathway of complement. *J Biol Chem.* 1992;267(24):17087-17094.

52. Haefliger JA, Tschopp J, Vial N, Jenne DE. Complete primary structure and functional characterization of the sixth component of the human complement system. Identification of the C5b-binding domain in complement C6. *J Biol Chem.* 1989;264(30):18041-18051.

53. DiScipio RG, Linton SM, Rushmere NK. Function of the factor I modules (FIMS) of human complement component C6. *J Biol Chem.* 1999;274(45):31811-31818.

54. DiScipio RG, Chakravarti DN, Muller-Eberhard HJ, Fey GH. The structure of human complement component C7 and the C5b-7 complex. *J Biol Chem.* 1988;263(1):549-560.

55. Sodetz JM. Structure and function of C8 in the membrane attack sequence of complement. *Curr Top Microbiol Immunol.* 1989;140:19-31.

56. Musingarimi P, Plumb ME, Sodetz JM. Interaction between the C8 alpha-gamma and C8 beta subunits of human complement C8: role of the C8 beta N-terminal thrombospondin type 1 module and membrane attack complex/perforin domain. *Biochemistry.* 2002;41(37):11255-11260.

57. Schreck SF, Parker C, Plumb ME, Sodetz JM. Human complement protein C8 gamma. *Biochim Biophys Acta.* 2000;1482(1-2):199-208.

58. Parker CL, Sodetz JM. Role of the human C8 subunits in complement-mediated bacterial killing: evidence that C8 gamma is not essential. *Mol Immunol.* 2002;39(7-8):453-458.

59. Ortlund E, Parker CL, Schreck SF, et al. Crystal structure of human complement protein C8gamma at 1.2 A resolution reveals a lipocalin fold and a distinct ligand binding site. *Biochemistry.* 2002;41(22):7030-7037.

60. Shinkai Y, Takio K, Okumura K. Homology of perforin to the ninth component of complement (C9). *Nature.* 1988;334(6182):525-527.

61. Tschopp J, Podack ER, Muller-Eberhard HJ. Ultrastructure of the membrane attack complex of complement: detection of the tetramolecular C9-polymerizing complex C5b-8. *Proc Natl Acad Sci U S A.* 1982;79(23):7474-7478.

62. Scibek JJ, Plumb ME, Sodetz JM. Binding of human complement C8 to C9: role of the N-terminal modules in the C8 alpha subunit. *Biochemistry.* 2002;41(49):14546-14551.

63. Muller-Eberhard HJ. The membrane attack complex of complement. *Annu Rev Immunol.* 1986;4:503-528.

64. DiScipio RG, Berlin C. The architectural transition of human complement component C9 to poly(C9). *Mol Immunol.* 1999;36(9):575-585.

65. DiScipio RG. The size, shape and stability of complement component C9. *Mol Immunol.* 1993;30(12):1097-1106.

66. Esser AF. Big MAC attack: complement proteins cause leaky patches. *Immunol Today.* 1991;12(9):316-318, discussion 321.

67. Davis AE3rd. C1 inhibitor and hereditary angioneurotic edema. *Annu Rev Immunol.* 1988;6:595-628.

68. Jiang H, Wagner E, Zhang H, Frank MM. Complement 1 inhibitor is a regulator of the alternative complement pathway. *J Exp Med.* 2001;194(11):1609-1616.

69. DeZern AE, Uknis M, Yuan X, et al. Complement blockade with a C1 esterase inhibitor in paroxysmal nocturnal hemoglobinuria. *Exp Hematol.* 2014;42(10):857-861.e1.

70. Liszewski MK, Farries TC, Lublin DM, Rooney IA, Atkinson JP. Control of the complement system. *Adv Immunol.* 1996;61:201-283.

71. Kirkitadze MD, Barlow PN. Structure and flexibility of the multiple domain proteins that regulate complement activation. *Immunol Rev.* 2001;180:146-161.

72. Liszewski MK, Leung M, Cui W, et al. Dissecting sites important for complement regulatory activity in membrane cofactor protein (MCP; CD46). *J Biol Chem.* 2000;275(48):37692-37701.

73. Barilla-LaBarca ML, Liszewski MK, Lambris JD, Hourcade D, Atkinson JP. Role of membrane cofactor protein (CD46) in regulation of C4b and C3b deposited on cells. *J Immunol.* 2002;168(12):6298-6304.

74. Casasnovas JM, Larvie M, Stehle T. Crystal structure of two CD46 domains reveals an extended measles virus-binding surface. *EMBO J.* 1999;18(11):2911-2922.

75. Manchester M, Naniche D, Stehle T. CD46 as a measles receptor: form follows function. *Virology.* 2000;274(1):5-10.

76. Manchester M, Liszewski MK, Atkinson JP, Oldstone MB. Multiple isoforms of CD46 (membrane cofactor protein) serve as receptors for measles virus. *Proc Natl Acad Sci U S A.* 1994;91(6):2161-2165.

77. Okada N, Liszewski MK, Atkinson JP, Caparon M. Membrane cofactor protein (CD46) is a keratinocyte receptor for the M protein of the group A streptococcus. *Proc Natl Acad Sci U S A.* 1995;92(7):2489-2493.

78. Giannakis E, Jokiranta TS, Ormsby RJ, et al. Identification of the streptococcal M protein binding site on membrane cofactor protein (CD46). *J Immunol.* 2002;168(9):4585-4592.

79. Greenstone HL, Santoro F, Lusso P, Berger EA. Human Herpesvirus 6 and Measles Virus employ distinct CD46 domains for receptor function. *J Biol Chem.* 2002;277(42):39112-39118.

80. Brodbeck WG, Kuttner-Kondo L, Mold C, Medof ME. Structure/function studies of human decay-accelerating factor. *Immunology.* 2000;101(1):104-111.

81. Hourcade DE, Mitchell L, Kuttner-Kondo LA, Atkinson JP, Medof ME. Decay-accelerating factor (DAF), complement receptor 1 (CR1), and factor H dissociate the complement AP C3 convertase (C3bBb) via sites on the type A domain of Bb. *J Biol Chem.* 2002;277(2):1107-1112.

82. Williams P, Chaudhry Y, Goodfellow IG, et al. Mapping CD55 function. The structure of two pathogen-binding domains at 1.7 A. *J Biol Chem.* 2003;278(12):10691-10696.

83. Uhrinova S, Lin F, Ball G, et al. Solution structure of a functionally active fragment of decay-accelerating factor. *Proc Natl Acad Sci U S A.* 2003;100(8):4718-4723.

84. Heine H, Ulmer AJ, El-Samalouti VT, Lentschat A, Hamann L. Decay-accelerating factor (DAF/CD55) is a functional active element of the LPS receptor complex. *J Endotoxin Res.* 2001;7(3):227-231.

85. McKnight AJ, Gordon S. The EGF-TM7 family: unusual structures at the leukocyte surface. *J Leukoc Biol.* 1998;63(3):271-280.

86. Lea S. Interactions of CD55 with non-complement ligands. *Biochem Soc Trans.* 2002;30(pt 6):1014-1019.

87. Krych-Goldberg M, Atkinson JP. Structure-function relationships of complement receptor type 1. *Immunol Rev.* 2001;180:112-122.

88. Krych-Goldberg M, Hauhart RE, Subramanian VB, et al. Decay accelerating activity of complement receptor type 1 (CD35). Two active sites are required for dissociating C5 convertases. *J Biol Chem.* 1999;274(44):31160-31168.

89. Schlaf G, Demberg T, Beisel N, Schieferdecker HL, Gotze O. Expression and regulation of complement factors H and I in rat and human cells: some critical notes. *Mol Immunol.* 2001;38(2-3):231-239.

90. Hyvarinen S, Meri S, Jokiranta TS. Disturbed sialic acid recognition on endothelial cells and platelets in complement attack causes atypical hemolytic uremic syndrome. *Blood.* 2016;127(22):2701-2710.

91. Meri S, Pangburn MK. Discrimination between activators and nonactivators of the alternative pathway of complement: regulation via a sialic acid/polyanion binding site on factor H. *Proc Natl Acad Sci U S A.* 1990;87(11):3982-3986.

92. Meri S, Pangburn MK. Regulation of alternative pathway complement activation by glycosaminoglycans: specificity of the polyanion binding site on factor H. *Biochem Biophys Res Commun.* 1994;198(1):52-59.

The Normal Hematologic System

93. Hellwage J, Jokiranta TS, Friese MA, et al. Complement C3b/C3d and cell surface polyanions are recognized by overlapping binding sites on the most carboxyl-terminal domain of complement factor H. *J Immunol.* 2002;169(12):6935-6944.

94. Pangburn MK, Pangburn KL, Koistinen V, Meri S, Sharma AK. Molecular mechanisms of target recognition in an innate immune system: interactions among factor H, C3b, and target in the alternative pathway of human complement. *J Immunol.* 2000;164(9):4742-4751.

95. Conway EM. Sweeteners for factor H. *Blood.* 2016;127(22):2656-2658.

96. Fremeaux-Bacchi V, Fakhouri F, Garnier A, et al. Genetics and outcome of atypical hemolytic uremic syndrome: a nationwide French series comparing children and adults. *Clin J Am Soc Nephrol.* 2013;8(4):554-562.

97. Nester CM, Barbour T, de Cordoba SR, et al. Atypical aHUS: state of the art. *Mol Immunol.* 2015;67(1):31-42.

98. Gavriilaki E, Yuan X, Ye Z, et al. Modified Ham test for atypical hemolytic uremic syndrome. *Blood.* 2015;125(23):3637-3646.

99. Brodsky RA. Complement in hemolytic anemia. *Blood.* 2015;126(22):2459-2465.

100. Fritsche LG, Fariss RN, Stambolian D, Abecasis GR, Curcio CA, Swaroop A. Age-related macular degeneration: genetics and biology coming together. *Annu Rev Genom Hum Genet.* 2014;15:151-171.

101. Perkins SJ, Goodship TH. Molecular modelling of the C-terminal domains of factor H of human complement: a correlation between haemolytic uraemic syndrome and a predicted heparin binding site. *J Mol Biol.* 2002;316(2):217-224.

102. Pangburn MK. Cutting edge: localization of the host recognition functions of complement factor H at the carboxyl-terminal—implications for hemolytic uremic syndrome. *J Immunol.* 2002;169(9):4702-4706.

103. Pickering MC, Cook HT, Warren J, et al. Uncontrolled C3 activation causes membranoproliferative glomerulonephritis in mice deficient in complement factor H. *Nat Genet.* 2002;31(4):424-428.

104. Zipfel PF, Jokiranta TS, Hellwage J, Koistinen V, Meri S. The factor H protein family. *Immunopharmacology.* 1999;42(1-3):53-60.

105. Friese MA, Hellwage J, Jokiranta TS, et al. FHL-1/reconectin and factor H: two human complement regulators which are encoded by the same gene are differently expressed and regulated. *Mol Immunol.* 1999;36(13-14):809-818.

106. Hellwage J, Jokiranta TS, Koistinen V, Vaarala O, Meri S, Zipfel PF. Functional properties of complement factor H-related proteins FHR-3 and FHR-4: binding to the C3d region of C3b and differential regulation by heparin. *FEBS Lett.* 1999;462(3):345-352.

107. Merinero HM, Subias M, Pereda A, Gomez-Rubio E, et al. Molecular bases for the association of FHR-1 with atypical hemolytic uremic syndrome and other diseases. *Blood.* 2021;137(25):3484-3494.

108. Blom AM, Kask L, Dahlback B. Structural requirements for the complement regulatory activities of C4BP. *J Biol Chem.* 2001;276(29):27136-27144.

109. Blom AM, Kask L, Dahlback B. CCP1-4 of the C4b-binding protein alpha-chain are required for factor I mediated cleavage of complement factor C3b. *Mol Immunol.* 2003;39(10):547-556.

110. Nelson RM, Long GL. Solution-phase equilibrium binding interaction of human protein S with C4b-binding protein. *Biochemistry.* 1991;30(9):2384-2390.

111. Tschopp J, Chonn A, Hertig S, French LE. Clusterin, the human apolipoprotein and complement inhibitor, binds to complement C7, C8 beta, and the b domain of C9. *J Immunol.* 1993;151(2):2159-2165.

112. Farkas I, Baranyi L, Ishikawa Y, et al. CD59 blocks not only the insertion of C9 into MAC but inhibits ion channel formation by homologous C5b-8 as well as C5b-9. *J Physiol.* 2002;539(pt 2):537-545.

113. Brodsky RA. Paroxysmal nocturnal hemoglobinuria. *Blood.* 2014;124(18):2804-2811.

114. Gerard C, Gerard NP. C5A anaphylatoxin and its seven transmembrane-segment receptor. *Annu Rev Immunol.* 1994;12:775-808.

115. Zuraw BL. Clinical practice. Hereditary angioedema. *N Engl J Med.* 2008;359(10):1027-1036.

116. Riedl MA, Bernstein JA, Li H, et al. Recombinant human C1-esterase inhibitor relieves symptoms of hereditary angioedema attacks: phase 3, randomized, placebo-controlled trial. *Ann Allergy Asthma Immunol.* 2014;112(2):163-169.e1.

117. Schrezenmeier H, Muus P, Socie G, et al. Baseline characteristics and disease burden in patients in the International Paroxysmal Nocturnal Hemoglobinuria Registry. *Haematologica.* 2014;99(5):922-929.

118. Hill A, Kelly RJ, Hillmen P. Thrombosis in paroxysmal nocturnal hemoglobinuria. *Blood.* 2013;121(25):4985-4996. quiz 5105.

119. Fujita M, Kinoshita T. GPI-anchor remodeling: potential functions of GPI-anchors in intracellular trafficking and membrane dynamics. *Biochim Biophys Acta.* 2012;1821(8):1050-1058.

120. Yamashina M, Ueda E, Kinoshita T, et al. Inherited complete deficiency of 20-kilodalton homologous restriction factor (CD59) as a cause of paroxysmal nocturnal hemoglobinuria. *N Engl J Med.* 1990;323(17):1184-1189.

121. Nevo Y, Ben-Zeev B, Tabib A, et al. CD59 deficiency is associated with chronic hemolysis and childhood relapsing immune-mediated polyneuropathy. *Blood.* 2013;121(1):129-135.

122. Hill A, Hillmen P, Richards SJ, et al. Sustained response and long-term safety of eculizumab in paroxysmal nocturnal hemoglobinuria. *Blood.* 2005;106(7):2559-2565.

123. Rother RP, Rollins SA, Mojcik CF, Brodsky RA, Bell L. Discovery and development of the complement inhibitor eculizumab for the treatment of paroxysmal nocturnal hemoglobinuria. *Nat Biotechnol.* 2007;25(11):1256-1264.

124. Hillmen P, Young NS, Schubert J, et al. The complement inhibitor eculizumab in paroxysmal nocturnal hemoglobinuria. *N Engl J Med.* 2006;355(12):1233-1243.

125. Brodsky RA, Young NS, Antonioli E, et al. Multicenter phase 3 study of the complement inhibitor eculizumab for the treatment of patients with paroxysmal nocturnal hemoglobinuria. *Blood.* 2008;111(4):1840-1847.

126. Brodsky RA. How I treat paroxysmal hemoglobinuria. *Blood.* 2021;137(10):1304-1309.

127. Hillmen P, Muus P, Duhrsen U, et al. Effect of the complement inhibitor eculizumab on thromboembolism in patients with paroxysmal nocturnal hemoglobinuria. *Blood.* 2007;110(12):4123-4128.

128. Emadi A, Brodsky RA. Successful discontinuation of anticoagulation following eculizumab administration in paroxysmal nocturnal hemoglobinuria. *Am J Hematol.* 2009;84(10):699-701.

129. Risitano AM, Notaro R, Marando L, et al. Complement fraction 3 binding on erythrocytes as additional mechanism of disease in paroxysmal nocturnal hemoglobinuria patients treated by eculizumab. *Blood.* 2009;113(17):4094-4100.

130. Hill A, Rother RP, Arnold L, et al. Eculizumab prevents intravascular hemolysis in patients with paroxysmal nocturnal hemoglobinuria and unmasks low-level extravascular hemolysis occurring through C3 opsonization. *Haematologica.* 2010;95(4):567-573.

131. Kulasekararaj AG, Brodsky RA, Hill A. Monitoring of patients with paroxysmal nocturnal hemoglobinuria on a complement inhibitor. *Am J Hematol.* 2021;96(7):E232-E235.

132. Rondelli T, Risitano AM, Peffault de Latour R, et al. Polymorphism of the complement receptor 1 gene correlates with hematological response to eculizumab in patients with paroxysmal nocturnal hemoglobinuria. *Haematologica.* 2014;99(2):262-266.

133. Nishimura J, Yamamoto M, Hayashi S, et al. Genetic variants in C5 and poor response to eculizumab. *N Engl J Med.* 2014;370(7):632-639.

134. Hillmen P, Szer J, Weitz I, et al. Pegcetacoplan versus eculizumab in paroxysmal nocturnal hemoglobinuria. *N Engl J Med.* 2021;384(11):1028-1037.

135. Wada H, Matsumoto T, Yamashita Y. Natural history of thrombotic thrombocytopenic purpura and hemolytic uremic syndrome. *Semin Thromb Hemost.* 2014;40(8):866-873.

136. Sperati CJ, Moliterno AR. Thrombotic microangiopathy: focus on atypical hemolytic uremic syndrome. *Hematol Oncol Clin N Am.* 2015;29(3):541-559.

137. Rodriguez de Cordoba S, Hidalgo MS, Pinto S, Tortajada A. Genetics of atypical hemolytic uremic syndrome (aHUS). *Semin Thromb Hemost.* 2014;40(4):422-430.

138. Legendre CM, Licht C, Muus P, et al. Terminal complement inhibitor eculizumab in atypical hemolytic-uremic syndrome. *N Engl J Med.* 2013;368(23):2169-2181.

139. Barbour T, Scully M, Ariceta G, et al. Long-term efficacy and safety of the long-acting complement C5 inhibitor ravulizumab for the treatment of atypical hemolytic uremic syndrome in adults. *Kidney Int Rep.* 2021;6(6):1603-1613.

140. Cataland SR, Holers VM, Geyer S, Yang S, Wu HM. Biomarkers of terminal complement activation confirm the diagnosis of aHUS and differentiate aHUS from TTP. *Blood.* 2014;123(24):3733-3738.

141. Maga TK, Nishimura CJ, Weaver AE, Frees KL, Smith RJ. Mutations in alternative pathway complement proteins in American patients with atypical hemolytic uremic syndrome. *Hum Mutat.* 2010;31(6):E1445-E1460.

142. Noris M, Remuzzi G. Genetics and genetic testing in hemolytic uremic syndrome/thrombotic thrombocytopenic purpura. *Semin Nephrol.* 2010;30(4):395-408.

143. Bu F, Borsa NG, Jones MB, et al. High-throughput genetic testing for thrombotic microangiopathies and C3 glomerulopathies. *J Am Soc Nephrol.* 2016;27(4):1245-1253.

144. Chaturvedi S, Dhaliwal N, Hussain S, Dane K, et al. Outcomes of a clinician-directed protocol for discontinuation of complement inhibition therapy in atypical hemolytic uremic syndrome. *Blood Adv.* 2021;5(5):1504-1512.

145. Fakhouri F, Fila M, Hummel A, Ribes D, et al. Eculizumab discontinuation in children and adults with atypical hemolytic-uremic syndrome: a prospective multicenter study. *Blood.* 2021;137(18):2438-2449.

146. Thurman JM, Marians R, Emlen W, et al. Alternative pathway of complement in children with diarrhea-associated hemolytic uremic syndrome. *Clin J Am Soc Nephrol.* 2009;4(12):1920-1924.

147. Orth D, Khan AB, Naim A, et al. Shiga toxin activates complement and binds factor H: evidence for an active role of complement in hemolytic uremic syndrome. *J Immunol.* 2009;182(10):6394-6400.

148. Keepers TR, Psotka MA, Gross LK, Obrig TG. A murine model of HUS: Shiga toxin with lipopolysaccharide mimics the renal damage and physiologic response of human disease. *J Am Soc Nephrol.* 2006;17(12):3404-3414.

149. Zoja C, Locatelli M, Pagani C, et al. Lack of the lectin-like domain of thrombomodulin worsens Shiga toxin-associated hemolytic uremic syndrome in mice. *J Immunol.* 2012;189(7):3661-3668.

150. Dinh A, Anathasayanan A, Rubin LM. Safe and effective use of eculizumab in the treatment of severe Shiga toxin Escherichia coli-associated hemolytic uremic syndrome. *Am J Health Syst Pharm.* 2015;72(2):117-120.

151. Lapeyraque AL, Malina M, Fremeaux-Bacchi V, et al. Eculizumab in severe shiga-toxin-associated HUS. *N Engl J Med.* 2011;364(26):2561-2563.

152. Menne J, Nitschke M, Stingele R, et al. Validation of treatment strategies for enterohaemorrhagic Escherichia coli O104:H4 induced haemolytic uraemic syndrome: case-control study. *BMJ.* 2012;345:e4565.

153. Travert B, Dossier A, Jamme M, et al. ShigaToxin-associated hemolytic uremic syndrome in adults, France, 2009-2017. *Emerg Infect Dis.* 2021;27(7):1876-1885.

154. Weinstein L. Syndrome of hemolysis, elevated liver enzymes, and low platelet count: a severe consequence of hypertension in pregnancy. *Am J Obstet Gynecol.* 1982;142(2):159-167.

155. Fang CJ, Richards A, Liszewski MK, Kavanagh D, Atkinson JP. Advances in understanding of pathogenesis of aHUS and HELLP. *Br J Haematol.* 2008;143(3):336-348.

156. Vaught AJ, Gavriilaki E, Hueppchen N, et al. Direct evidence of complement activation in HELLP syndrome: a link to atypical hemolytic uremic syndrome. *Exp Hematol.* 2016;44(5):390-398.

157. Salmon JE, Heuser C, Triebwasser M, et al. Mutations in complement regulatory proteins predispose to preeclampsia: a genetic analysis of the PROMISSE cohort. *PLoS Med*. 2011;8(3):e1001013.

158. Vaught AJ, Braunstein EM, Jasem J, et al. Germline mutations in the alternative pathway of complement predispose to HELLP syndrome. *JCI Insight*. 2018;3(6):e99128.

159. Fakhouri F, Jablonski M, Lepercq J, et al. Factor H, membrane cofactor protein, and factor I mutations in patients with hemolysis, elevated liver enzymes, and low platelet count syndrome. *Blood*. 2008;112(12):4542-4545.

160. Fakhouri F, Roumenina L, Provot F, et al. Pregnancy-associated hemolytic uremic syndrome revisited in the era of complement gene mutations. *J Am Soc Nephrol*. 2010;21(5):859-867.

161. Fritsche LG, Igl W, Bailey JN, et al. A large genome-wide association study of age-related macular degeneration highlights contributions of rare and common variants. *Nat Genet*. 2016;48(2):134-143.

162. Sofat R, Casas JP, Webster AR, et al. Complement factor H genetic variant and age-related macular degeneration: effect size, modifiers and relationship to disease subtype. *Int J Epidemiol*. 2012;41(1):250-262.

163. Zhan X, Larson DE, Wang C, et al. Identification of a rare coding variant in complement 3 associated with age-related macular degeneration. *Nat Genet*. 2013;45(11):1375-1379.

164. Raychaudhuri S, Iartchouk O, Chin K, et al. A rare penetrant mutation in CFH confers high risk of age-related macular degeneration. *Nat Genet*. 2011;43(12):1232-1236.

165. Caprioli J, Castelletti F, Bucchioni S, et al. Complement factor H mutations and gene polymorphisms in haemolytic uraemic syndrome: the C-257T, the A2089G and the G2881T polymorphisms are strongly associated with the disease. *Hum Mol Genet*. 2003;12(24):3385-3395.

166. Wagner EK, Raychaudhuri S, Villalonga MB, et al. Mapping rare, deleterious mutations in factor H: association with early onset, drusen burden, and lower antigenic levels in familial AMD. *Sci Rep*. 2016;6:31531.

167. Randen U, Troen G, Tierens A, et al. Primary cold agglutinin-associated lymphoproliferative disease: a B-cell lymphoma of the bone marrow distinct from lymphoplasmacytic lymphoma. *Haematologica*. 2014;99(3):497-504.

168. Berentsen S, Ulvestad E, Gjertsen BT, et al. Rituximab for primary chronic cold agglutinin disease: a prospective study of 37 courses of therapy in 27 patients. *Blood*. 2004;103(8):2925-2928.

169. Berentsen S, Randen U, Vagan AM, et al. High response rate and durable remissions following fludarabine and rituximab combination therapy for chronic cold agglutinin disease. *Blood*. 2010;116(17):3180-3184.

170. Berentsen S. How I treat cold agglutinin disease. *Blood*, 2021;137(10):1295-1303.

171. Röth A, Barcellini W, D'Sa S, et al. Sutimlimab in cold agglutinin disease. *N Engl J Med*. 2021;384(14):1323-1334.

172. Gavriilaki E, Brodsky RA. Severe COVID-19 infection and thrombotic microangiopathy: success does not come easily. *Br J Haemotol*. 2020;189(6):e227-e230.

173. Risitano AM, Mastellos DC, Huber-Lang M, et al. Complement as a target in COVID-19? *Nat Rev Immunol*. 2020;20(6):343-344.

174. Ackermann M, Verleden SE, Kuehnel M, et al. Pulmonary vascular endothelialitis, thrombosis, and angiogenesis in Covid-19. *N Engl J Med*. 2020;383(2):120-128.

175. Bilaloglu S, Aphinyanaphongs, Jones S, et al. Thrombosis in hospitalized patients with COVID-19 in a New York city health system. *JAMA*. 2020;324(8):799-801.

176. Yu J, Yuan X, Chen H, Chaturvedi S, et al. Direct activation of the alternative complement pathway by SARS-CoV-2 spike proteins is blocked by factor D inhibition. *Blood*. 2020;136(18):2080-2089.

177. Risitano AM, Marotta S. Therapeutic complement inhibition in complement-mediated hemolytic anemias: past, present and future. *Semin Immunol*. 2016;28(3):223-240.

178. Morgan BP, Walport MJ. Complement deficiency and disease. *Immunol Today*. 1991;12(9):301-306.

179. Orren A. Molecular mechanisms of complement component C6 deficiency; a hypervariable exon 6 region responsible for three of six reported defects. *Clin Exp Immunol*. 2000;119(2):255-258.

180. Orren A, O'Hara AM, Morgan BP, Moran AP, Wurzner R. An abnormal but functionally active complement component C9 protein found in an Irish family with subtotal C9 deficiency. *Immunology*. 2003;108(3):384-390.

181. Hobart MJ, Fernie BA, Fijen KA, Orren A. The molecular basis of C6 deficiency in the Western Cape, South Africa. *Hum Genet*. 1998;103(4):506-512.

182. Zhu Z, Atkinson TP, Hovanky KT, et al. High prevalence of complement component C6 deficiency among African-Americans in the south-eastern USA. *Clin Exp Immunol*. 2000;119(2):305-310.

183. Wurzner R, Hobart MJ, Fernie BA, et al. Molecular basis of subtotal complement C6 deficiency. A carboxy-terminally truncated but functionally active C6. *J Clin Invest*. 1995;95(4):1877-1883.

184. Orren A, Potter PC, Cooper RC, du Toit E. Deficiency of the sixth component of complement and susceptibility to Neisseria meningitidis infections: studies in 10 families and five isolated cases. *Immunology*. 1987;62(2):249-253.

185. Dragon-Durey MA, Fremeaux-Bacchi V, Blouin J, Barraud D, Fridman WH, Kazatchkine MD. Restricted genetic defects underlie human complement C6 deficiency. *Clin Exp Immunol*. 2003;132(1):87-91.

The Normal Hematologic System

Chapter 17 ■ Megakaryocytes

WILLIAM VAINCHENKER • NAJET DEBILI • HANA RASLOVA

INTRODUCTION

Platelets are the smallest anucleated blood cells in mammals. They were first described in 1865 by a German pathologist, Max Shultze, as little spherules, but he did not further investigate their origins and functions.[1] However, it was believed that these spherules were erythrocyte precursors or particles derived from leukocytes or even more artifacts. Their real description was attributed to Giulio Bizzozero, who called them piastrine in Italian, plaquettes in French, and Bluplättchen in German.[1] They were further called platelets in English. In fact, the complete description was made by James Homer Wright, who established that platelets are anucleated cell fragments, which derive from bone marrow giant cells called megakaryocytes (MKs), thus discovering the MK/platelet axis.[2] This discovery led to the paradox that the smallest blood cells originate from the biggest bone marrow cells.

Platelets play a central role in hemostasis and have several recently discovered other functions such as wound healing and the regulation of inflammation, angiogenesis, and immune response. In pathology, they are not only involved in hemostasis and thrombosis, but also in atherosclerosis, metastasis and viral infection.[3-5] In human, their level is relatively constant in normal individuals, and is not as tightly regulated as for erythrocytes, with a large interindividual heterogeneity. The number of platelets ranges from 1.5 to $4.5 \times 10^5/\mu L$ in humans, the mean platelet volume being more strictly regulated. This interindividual variability may be dependent of single nucleotide polymorphisms (SNPs) in genes involved in platelet production.[6] Platelets have a short life between 7 and 10 days and must be constantly renewed by a very dynamic process called megakaryopoiesis, which produces 10^{11} platelets per day in man.[7-9]

As all the other hematopoietic lineages, the MKs and platelets are derived from the hematopoietic stem cells (HSCs). Until the discovery of its major extracellular cue, thrombopoietin (TPO) and the development of in vitro cultures, megakaryopoiesis has been quite ignored due to the rarity of MKs in the bone marrow.

Megakaryopoiesis is one of the most original cellular processes in the organism. It includes several steps, the two first ones concern the early steps of differentiation: the commitment of HSC toward the MK lineage and the proliferation of committed progenitors, two processes which are not basically different from those of other hematopoietic lineages although there are some similarities between the HSC and MK programs with the description of a MK/platelet-biased HSC.[10] The two other subsequent steps are very specific to the MK differentiation. The first consists in a mechanism of polyploidization, which is called endomitosis and leads to a giant cell, the MK. It is this cell that will further mature by increasing synthesis of platelet proteins before giving rise to platelets. The second and last step consists of a dynamic cytoplasmic fragmentation. In human of adult age, the entire process takes place in the marrow, except for platelet release, which occurs in the blood flow.

Regulation of the megakaryopoiesis is operated both by cell autonomous processes such as transcriptional regulation and by extracellular cues dominated by TPO that binds to its receptor MPL (myeloproliferative leukemia)/TPOR and activates a downstream cascade entirely dependent on janus kinase 2 (JAK2). The formation of platelets by itself is controlled by profound dynamic changes in the cytoskeleton regulated by the MK interaction with the bone marrow environment in closeness, proximity to vessels. Recent reports suggest that the MK population in the bone marrow is heterogeneous and that all MKs may not be involved in platelet production. Some of them may be essentially involved in bone marrow remodeling and in the regulation of HSC quiescence.[11-14] Others in the bone marrow but predominantly in the lung are antigen-presenting cells (APCs) and thus close to dendritic cells or monocytes.[12-16]

Acquired or hereditary diseases of the MK/platelet lineages involve mainly deregulations of the transcriptional regulation and of the TPO/MPL signaling as well as defects in cytoskeleton organization (Tables 17.1 and 17.2).

In this chapter, we will describe the different steps of differentiation, the transcriptional regulation, the cytokine regulation, and the changes in cytoskeleton, which lead to generation of platelets through proplatelet formation, as well as the different pathologies associated with alterations in these processes.

THE DIFFERENT STEPS OF MEGAKARYOPOIESIS

The different steps of hematopoiesis can be studied by different approaches. At the beginning stages of differentiation are HSC/progenitors (HSCPs). These immature cells cannot be identified by cytology and were initially characterized by biological assays only: HSCs on their capacity to reconstitute hematopoiesis in irradiated recipients and HSCPs on their capacity to give rise to colonies composed of mature cells in clonal assays. These clonal assays are performed essentially in vitro for hematopoietic progenitors, but the colony-forming unit (CFU) assay in the spleen was the first to allow in vivo identification and quantification of a subpopulation of HSCs called CFU-S.[102] Later, the different steps of hematopoiesis were characterized using a panel of differentiation markers (CD) defined by monoclonal antibodies.[103] Finally, new techniques based on single cell gene profiling or tracking are presently used to better identify the heterogeneity of the HSCP compartment.[104,105]

Hematopoietic Stem Cell and Megakaryocyte Commitment

The MK/platelet lineage is derived from the multipotent HSC, which gives rise to all hematopoietic lineages including the lymphoid and myeloid lineages. HSCs are comprised in a heterogeneous compartment of quiescent cells with different reconstitution activities after irradiation. They have been classified in two main subpopulations, that is, the long-term reconstitution HSC (LT-HSC) and the short-term reconstitution HSC (ST-HSC), according to their self-renewal capacities.[103,106] Till recently, it was assumed that the homeostatic hematopoiesis was sustained mainly by LT-HSCs; however, there is increasing evidence using new techniques of cell tracking that ST-HSCs and hematopoietic progenitors mainly contribute to the hematopoietic production in mice during several months.[104]

Using differentiation markers coupled with biological assays, a quite strict hematopoietic hierarchy has been defined in mouse (see Figure 17.1).[103] At the top of this hierarchy are the LT-HSCs. A population that is enriched with more than 50% of LT-HSC has been defined by a combination of differentiation markers. These LT-HSCs give rise to ST-HSCs, which then will produce multipotent progenitors (MPPs) capable to differentiate toward all the lymphoid and myeloid lineages including MKs. Although multipotent, the MPP has restricted self-renewal capacities in comparison to HSC. In this classical model of

Table 17.1. Primary Thrombocytosis

Disorder	Gene Mutations	Type of Mutations	Reference	Mechanism	Clinical Characteristics
Acquired *BCR-ABL* MPN					
CML	BCR-ABL1	Translocation t(9;22) (q34;q11) Gene fusion	17 18 19	Signaling activation (STAT5/PI3K)	Associated with hyperleukocytosis Spontaneous constant progression to acute leukemia
***BCR-ABL* negative MPN**					
ET	JAK2 (60%) CALR (25%) MPL (3%) No driver (12%)	V617F Frameshift exon 9 W515L/K/R S505N S204P/S Y591N/F	20 21 22 23 24 25 26 27	MPL/JAK2/STAT	Risk of thrombosis and bleeding Possibility to progress to myelofibrosis and acute myelogenous leukemia (AML)
PMF	Similar mutations as in ET	Mutations as in ET usually associated with other mutations (epigenetics, splicing, transcription factor)	28	MPL/JAK2/STAT	Progression to cytopenia and thrombocytopenia Frequent progression to AML
MPN/MDS					
RARS-T	Similar mutations as in ET but rare mutation in CALR	Association with SF3B1 mutations and eventually TET2 and ASXL1 mutations	29 30 31 32 33 34	MPL/JAK2/STAT	Risk of thrombosis Better prognosis than RARS
MDS					
5q- syndrome	Haploinsufficiency for miR-145 and miR-146a	Haploinsufficiency for *RPS14, CSNK1A1, DIAPH1*	35 36 37 38	*FLI1* overexpression? *DIAPH1* haploinsufficiency	Progression to AML
Familial thrombocytosis					
	THPO	Exon 3: splice donor intron 2 T > C	39 40 41	TPO/MPL/JAK2/STAT	Autosomal dominant
	JAK2: Gain of function	V617I R564Q H608N R867Q S735R/R938Q	42 43 44 45 45	MPL/JAK2/STAT	Autosomal dominant
	MPL: Gain of function	MPLS505N	46	MPL/JAK2/STAT	Autosomal dominant
		MPLW515R	Vilaine and Hermouet unpublished		
	MPL: Trafficking defect	MPLK53N MPLP106L	47 48 49 50	TPO/MPL/JAK2/STAT	Autosomal dominant with incomplete penetrance Autosomal recessive - ? Autosomal dominant with incomplete penetrance?

Table 17.2. Inherited Thrombocytopenia

platelet's Size	Disease	Abbreviation, OMIM,[(ref)]	Affected Gene, Cellular Function	Type of Defect
small	Wiskott-Aldrich syndrome	WAS, 301000,[51]	*WAS*, cytoskeleton reorganization	defect in MK migration and in platelet formation
	X-linked thrombocytopenia	XLT, 313900,[52]	*WAS*, cytoskeleton reorganization	defect in MK migration and in platelet formation
	FYB-related thrombocytopenia	FYB-RT, na,[53]	*FYB*, signaling, cytoskeleton reorganization	defect in MK maturation, in platelet formation and increased platelet clearance
normal	*ANKRD26*-related thrombocytopenia	THC2, 313900,[54]	*ANKRD26*, signaling	defect in platelet formation

(continued)

The Normal Hematologic System

Table 17.2. Inherited Thrombocytopenia (Continued)

platelet's Size	Disease	Abbreviation, OMIM,[ref]	Affected Gene, Cellular Function	Type of Defect
	Familial platelet disorder with predisposition to acute myeloid leukemia	FPD/AML, 601399,[55]	RUNX1, transcription factor	dysmegakaryopoiesis and defect in platelet formation
	ETV6-related thrombocytopenia	THC5, 616216,[56-59]	*ETV6*, transcription factor	dysmegakaryopoiesis and defect in platelet formation
	Congenital amegakaryocytic thrombocytopenia	CAMT, 604498,[60,61,541]	*MPL*, signaling	dysmegakaryopoiesis
	Radioulnar synostosis with amegakaryocytic thrombocytopenia	RUSAT, 605432,[62]	*HOXA11*, transcription factor	dysmegakaryopoiesis
			MECOM, transcription factor	dysmegakaryopoiesis
	Thrombocytopenia with absent radii	TAR, 274000,[63]	*RBM8A*, translation factor	dysmegakaryopoiesis
	CYCS-related thrombocytopenia	THC4, 612004,[64]	*CYCS*, electron transport, apoptosis	defect in platelet formation
	THPO-related disease	THPO-RD, na,[65]	*THPO*, signaling	dysmegakaryopoiesis
large	Paris-Trousseau thrombocytopenia	TCPT, 188025,[66]	11q23 deletion including FLI1, transcription factor	dysmegakaryopoiesis and defect in platelet formation
	Jacobsen syndrome	JBS, 147791,[67]	11q23 deletion including *FLI1*, transcription factor	dysmegakaryopoiesis and defect in platelet formation
	FLI1-related thrombocytopenia	FLI1-RT, na,[68]	*FLI1*, transcription factor	dysmegakaryopoiesis and defect in platelet formation
	X-linked thrombocytopenia with thalassemia	XLTT, 314050,[69]	*GATA1*, transcription factor	dysmegakaryopoiesis and defect in platelet formation
	X-linked thrombocytopenia with dyserythropoietic anemia	XLTDA, 300367[70-75]	*GATA1*, transcription factor	dysmegakaryopoiesis and defect in platelet formation
	Gray platelet syndrome	GPS, 139090,[76,77-79]	*GATA1*, transcription factor	dysmegakaryopoiesis and defect in platelet formation
			NBEAL2, granule biogenesis	defect in the biogenesis of alpha granules
	GFI1b-related thrombocytopenia (GPS)	GFI1b-RT, 187900,[80,81]	*GFI1b*, transcription factor	dysmegakaryopoiesis
	Bi- and mono-allelic Bernard-Soulier	BSS, 231200,[82]	*GPIBA, GPIBB, GP9*, signaling	defect in platelet formation
	Di George or velocardiofacial syndromes	Di George syndrome, 188400; VCF, 192430,[83]	22q11.2 deletion including *GPIBB*, signaling	defect in platelet formation
	MYH9-related disease	MYH9-RD, na,[84]	*MYH9*, cytoskeleton reorganization	defect in platelet formation
	Sitosterolaemia	STSL, 210250,[85]	*ABCG5, ABCG8*, molecule transporters	microenvironment abnormality
	Platelet-type von Willebrand disease	PT-VWD, 177820,[86]	*GPIBA*, signaling	shortened platelet survival
	ITGA2/ITGB3-related thrombocytopenia	*ITGA2/ITGB3*-RT, 187800,[87]	*ITGA2, ITGB3*, signaling	defect in platelet formation
	TUBB1-related thrombocytopenia	*TUBB1*-RT, 613112,[88,89]	*TUBB1*, cytoskeleton reorganization	defect in platelet formation
	FLNA-related thrombocytopenia	FLNA-RT, na,[90]	*FLNA*, cytoskeleton reorganization	defect in platelet formation
	SRC-related thrombocytopenia	THC6, 616937,[91]	*SRC*, signaling	dysmegakaryopoiesis and defect in platelet formation
	PRKACG-related thrombocytopenia	PRKACG-RT, 616176,[92]	*PRKACG*, signaling	defect in platelet formation
	GNE-related thrombocytopenia	GNE-RT, na,[93]	*GNE*, enzyme in the sialic acid biosynthetic pathway	likely increased platelet destruction
	ACTN1-related thrombocytopenia	ACTN1-RT, 615193,[94]	*ACTN1*, cytoskeleton reorganization	defect in platelet formation
	SLFN14-related thrombocytopenia	SLFN14-RT, na,[95]	*SLFN14*, nk	unknown mechanism
	TPM4-related thrombocytopenia	TPM4-RT, na,[96]	*TPM4*, cytoskeleton reorganization	defect in platelet formation
	G6B-related thrombocytopenia	G6B-RT, na,[97]	*C6orf25*, signaling	likely defect in MK differentiation and platelet formation
	DIAPH1-related disease	DIAPH1-RT, na,[98]	*DIAPH1*, cytoskeleton reorganization	defect in platelet formation
	TRPM7-related disease	TRPM7-RT, na,[99]	*TRPM7*, cytoskeleton reorganization	defect in platelet formation
nonspecified	Stormorken syndrome	STRMK, 185070,[100]	*STIM1*, Ca(2+) sensor	unknown mechanism
heterogenous	York platelet syndrome	YPS, na,[101]	*STIM1*, Ca(2+) sensor	unknown mechanism

na, not available; nk, not known.

hematopoiesis, the MPP is the point of segregation between the lymphoid and myeloid lineages and will commit by giving two types of oligopotent progenitors, one called CLP (common lymphoid progenitor) and the other CMP (common myeloid progenitor). Concerning the myeloid series, the CMP will give birth to two more restricted progenitors, the GMP (granulocyte-macrophage progenitor) and the MEP (megakaryocyte-erythroid progenitor) underscoring the proximity between the MK and erythroid lineages. Finally, the MEP will differentiate to produce an erythroid progenitor and a MK progenitor (MK-P), the first cell committed to the MK lineage. In humans a similar hierarchy has also been defined using other cell markers.

However, in these last years, this model of hematopoiesis has been challenged and recent results suggest that it is an oversimplistic model of hematopoiesis:

- Combining biological assays with surface markers, Adolfsson et al have identified a lymphoid-primed multipotent progenitor, which has lost the MK/erythroid potential and kept the lymphoid and GM potentials (*Figure 17.1*). This suggests that the MK and erythroid lineages could emerge directly from an HSC.[107] Although this result remains controversial, it was shown that the MPP population was itself heterogeneous with three types of MPP (MPP2, MPP3, and MPP4), the MPP2 being biased to the erythroid/MK differentiation, the MPP1 belonging to the HSC compartment.[108]
- Using a barcoding technique, it was shown that the CMP is not really an oligopotent progenitor with several myeloid potentials, but rather its immune phenotype corresponds to different committed progenitors directly emerging from a MPP.[109]
- RNA-seq experiments performed on single cells also demonstrate that the MEP defined by surface markers was essentially an erythroid progenitor nearly completely devoid of MK potential.[110,111] This result does not exclude the presence of a bipotent MK/erythroid progenitor, but probably not at the stage corresponding to the previously defined MEP. In humans, it was demonstrated that in the fetus and cord blood, the MEP emerges mostly directly from the HSC and MPP compartments. In the adult bone marrow, in contrary to the fetus, a majority of progenitors are unipotent and MK-P

may emerge directly from the HSC compartment.[112] In addition, using biological assays, this study has confirmed that what was defined as a MEP in humans was essentially a unipotent erythroid progenitor[112] (*Figure 17.1*). This is in agreement with the original description of a MEP that was enriched in the CD34+CD38[low] cell population.[113] It has been more recently shown that the Lin−CD34+CD38[mid]CD45RA−FLT3−MPL+CD36−CD41− cell population has both an erythroid and MK phenotype.[114] This cell type may be close to the PreMegE in the mouse.[115]

- Finally, these last years saw the emergence of the concept of a MK/platelet-biased mouse HSC. It has been shown that HSC expressing von Willebrand Factor (vWF) (identified with green fluorescent protein expressed under the control of the vWF promoter) was at the top of the HSC hierarchy and was able to give rise to an accelerated platelet reconstitution in transplantation assays.[10] Similarly, it was shown that HSCs expressing high level of Kit also led to a rapid platelet reconstitution. Further experiments have shown that Lin−Sca+Kit+ CD41+cells are multipotent but myeloid-biased HSCs[116,117] and are capable to efficiently give rise to monopotent MK-P that can also express the CD42+ antigen in stress conditions (CD42 being considered as a later marker of MK differentiation than the CD41 antigen, see below).[118] A MK-biased HSC has also been detected in human using single RNA-seq (scRNAseq).[119,120]

Thus, it remains unclear how MK commitment occurs in the hematopoietic hierarchy.[121] Current results can be biased by the fact the MK and HSC have many common transcription regulators and are also regulated by the TPO/MPL axis. Thus, many markers used to define HSC may be also expressed during MK differentiation. Inversely, MK/platelet-restricted proteins such as the CD41 and the vWF are also expressed by HSC, as underscored by the fact that during ontogeny, CD41 is one of the first markers to define the birth of HSC and the hematopoietic differentiation derived from embryonic stem/induced pluripotent stem (ES/iPS) cells (see below).[122] Presently, it is considered that MK-P may emerge by two different pathways: one directly from HSC, this pathway being privileged in stress or inflammatory conditions because it may not require a mitosis for MK commitment,

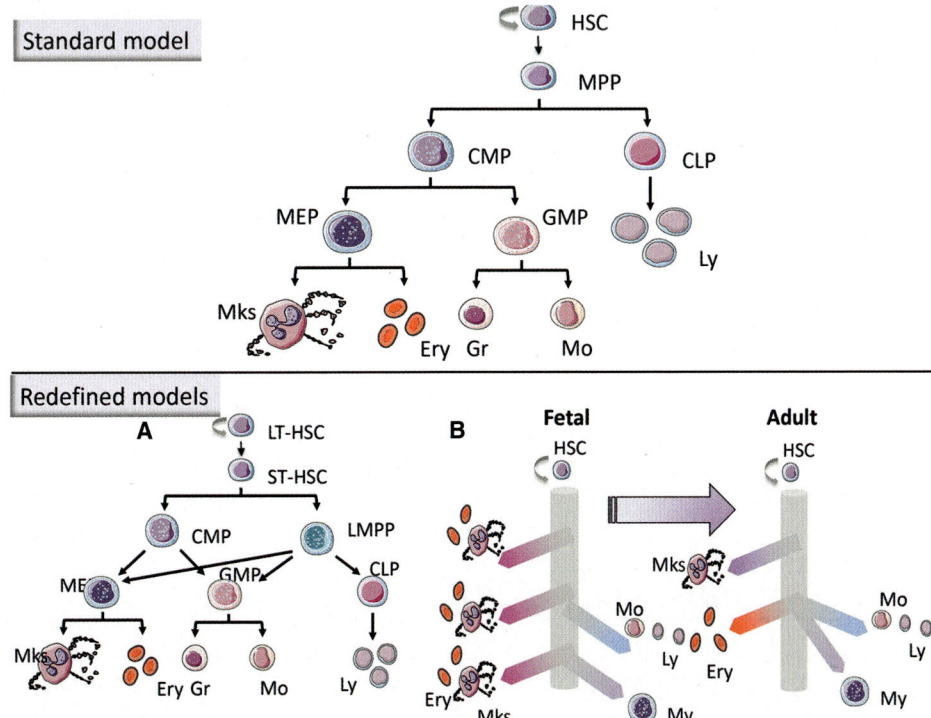

FIGURE 17.1 **Different models of hematopoietic hierarchy and megakaryocyte commitment.** The Standard model is derived from the work of the team of I Weissman,[12] model that is the most usual. 'Two alternative models: one described by Adolfsson et al[16] in mice (A) and the other by the team of J Dick[106] in humans (B).

The Normal Hematologic System

and thus it is a rapid pathway to produce platelets in emergency,[118] the other through the classical hierarchical pathway of hematopoiesis. It is considered that around 30% of the platelet production arises from the first pathway and 70% by the second pathway. Whether this direct commitment of MK-P from an HSC requires a mitosis step remains to be determined.

Megakaryocyte Progenitors

MK-Ps have been identified by their capacity to give rise to MK colonies in semi solid medium. Technically, the certain identification of MKs in culture requires the use of markers: the revelation of acetylcholinesterase by an enzymatic reaction in the mouse and the expression of certain platelet proteins such as CD41 or vWF revealed by specific antibodies in the human setting. For these reasons, cultures are usually performed in collagen or in fibrin clot, allowing these labeling steps. Two main types of progenitors have been initially identified: high proliferative progenitors called Burst Forming Unit-MKs and more mature progenitors called CFU-MKs. Presently, all the MK-Ps defined by biological assays are called CFU-MKs that are eventually subclassified based on the size of the colonies they give rise to. It remains controversial if colonies composed of two cell clusters or eventually individual MKs can be considered as defining as arising from an MK-P. However, the cells defined as MK-Ps by their phenotype can give rise to individual MKs in single cell experiments. Indeed, a polyploid MK can be considered as the equivalent of a CFU-E if the number of DNA replication is taken into consideration.

MK-Ps have been enriched in the Lin⁻Kit⁺IL3-Rα⁻FcγRII/III^{lo}Sca1⁻of the CD150⁺CD9^{hi}endoglin^{lo} cell fraction.[123,124] These

MK-Ps also express CD41 at high level.[115] In contrast, a low level of CD41 is expressed on some HSCs and other progenitors.

In humans, the equivalent of the mouse MK-P corresponds to CD34⁺CD38⁺CD41⁺MPL⁺⁺⁺ or of a CMP expressing CD41 (CD34⁺CD38⁺CD41⁺IL3Rα⁺CD45RA⁻).[114,125] However, a fraction of human MK-Ps do not express CD41 at high level and can be also detected in the CD34⁺CD38$^{low/medium}$ cell fraction (*Figure 17.2*).

Later Steps of Megakaryocyte Differentiation and Differentiation Markers

The later stages of differentiation are characterized by cytological approaches including ultrastructure and confocal microscopy and by differentiation markers.

The MK-Ps are 2N cells without specific cytological features that proliferate by mitosis. They undergo further differentiation to give rise to MKs that will polyploidize and acquire important cytoplasmic changes.

Historically, a transitional cell between the MK-P and the MK/megakaryoblast has been defined as a promegakaryoblast. This cell is still a 2N cell that is essentially capable to polyploidize and has been characterized in the mouse setting by the acetylcholinesterase staining[126] and in the human setting by ultrastructural studies coupled to the revelation of the platelet peroxidase.[127] This small cell (same size as a lymphocyte) may already contain some immature α−granules and exhibit the first membrane invagination, the precursor of the demarcation membrane system (DMS) also called invaginated membrane system (IMS).[128] This stage of differentiation is particularly important because it corresponds to the stage where the MK differentiation is

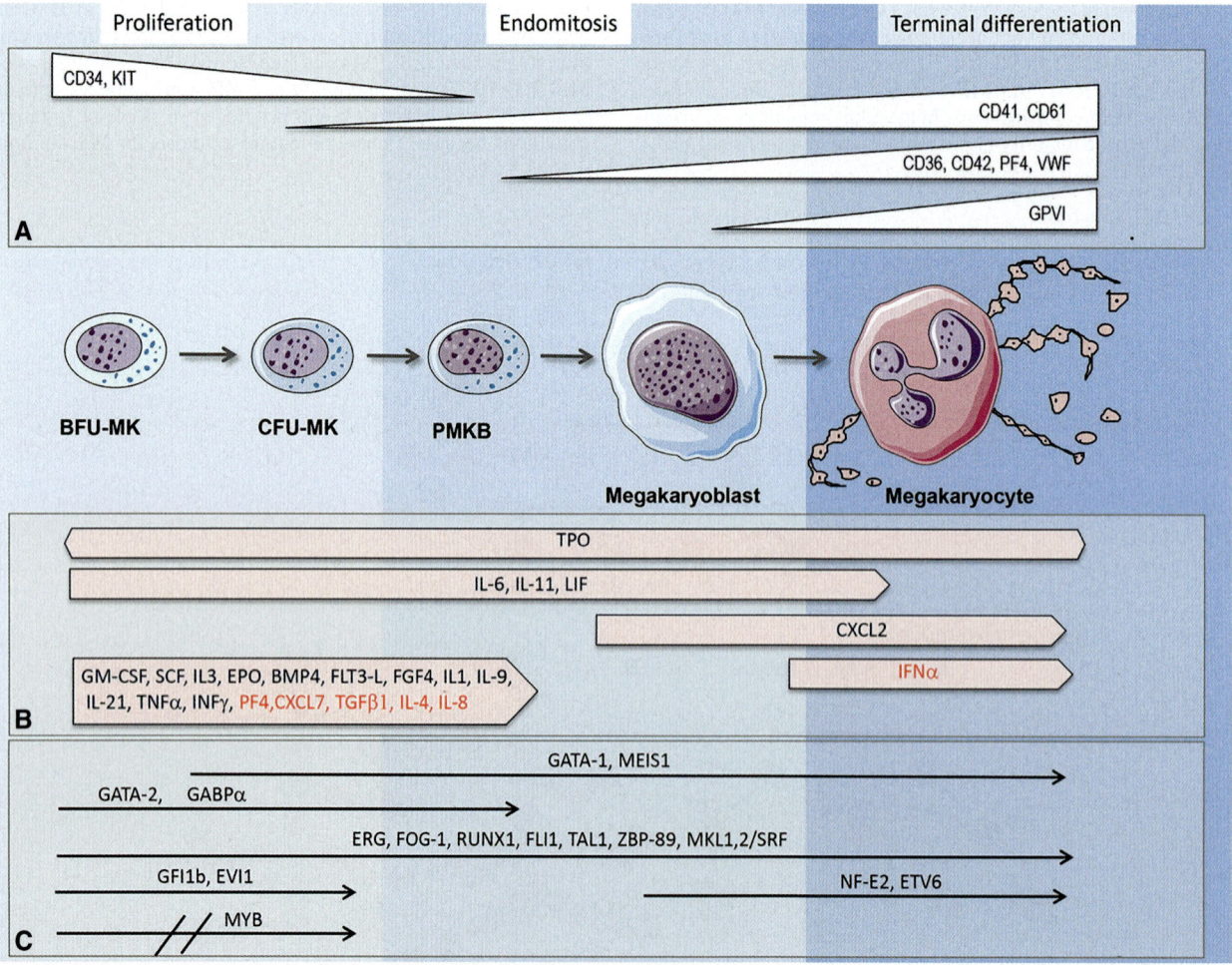

FIGURE 17.2 Schematic illustration of megakaryocyte differentiation. Differentiation antigens, growth factors, and transcription factors. A, Kinetics of different markers through MK differentiation. B, Extrinsic regulation of MK differentiation. C, Intrinsic regulation of MK differentiation.

blocked in acute megakaryoblastic leukemia (AMKL).[127] Later stages of differentiation have been classified in megakaryoblast, proMK, and MK. This classification, which is less frequently used, is based on the size of the cell, the aspect of the nucleus, and the cytoplasm development. At the end of maturation, mature MKs are usually large cells (40-120 μm in diameter) with an abundant cytoplasm and a single polylobulated nucleus.

MK differentiation is characterized by differentiation markers[7,8] (*Figure 17.2A*). In human, the three main differentiation markers that are used are the CD34, CD41, and CD42. CD34 is an adhesion protein that is used as a marker for HSC and hematopoietic progenitors. CD41 overall indicates the integrin α2b/β3, also called GPIIb/IIIa, and is subclassified into the CD41a (GPIIb/IIIa complex) and the CD41b (GPIIb), whose expression is restricted to the MK/platelet lineage, the CD61 being the GPIIIa/β3 integrin, which is more widely expressed. The CD41 is the receptor for many proteins of the extracellular matrix (ECM), but more particularly for fibrinogen. Its deficiency is associated with a platelet disorder, the Glanzmann thrombasthenia. Some rare activating mutations in β3 integrin can also lead to a macrothrombocytopenia through a defect in proplatelet formation.[129] The CD42 is a complex of four proteins: GPIbα, GPIbβ, GPIX, and GPV, the complex of the three first proteins being necessary for membrane localization. GPIbα is a heavily O-glycosylated protein, which can be cleaved by protease to give the glycocalicin. The CD42 is the platelet receptor for the vWF and its deficiency leads to the Bernard-Soulier syndrome.

In the adult, the CD41 expression permits to define the different stages of MK maturation from MK-P to platelets. The CD42 is expressed slightly later, from the onset of polyploidization to platelets. Schematically, the CD34+CD41+CD42- phenotype permits to define a fraction of MK-Ps, while CD34+CD41+CD42+ corresponds to the transitional cell (promegakaryoblast). Further maturation is characterized by a CD34-CD41+CD42+ phenotype with the expression of CD41 and CD42 increasing with MK maturation, the more mature MKs being CD34-CD41+++CD42+++.[7] It has been suggested that PTPRJ (CD148) was only expressed during late stages of megakaryopoiesis.[14]

Other markers are also used such as the KIT receptor (receptor for the stem cell factor [SCF]) and the KIT+CD41+ phenotype defines cells close to the CD34+CD41+ cells. Markers such as the CD36 or GPVI are expressed simultaneously with the CD42.

Proteins contained in the α-granules, more particularly the vWF, also permitted to study the MK maturation. vWF is expressed at low level on some promegakaryoblasts and its expression increased during MK maturation with a granular pattern of staining.[130,131] Antibodies against vWF are frequently used to identify and quantify MKs on histological sections.

We will focus on the two most important features of MK maturation: polyploidization and changes in MK maturation, which will lead to MK fragmentation through proplatelet formation.

Megakaryocyte and Polyploidization

MKs are one of the rare mammalian cells to be polyploid in the absence of any stress. MK polyploidization is an intrinsic step of the differentiation process.[132] It begins simultaneously with the synthesis of platelet-specific proteins just after the promegakaryoblast stage (*Figure 17.2*). This polyploidization leads to cells with a 2^XN ploidy ranging from 2N to 128N, with a modal ploidy at of 16N both in human and mouse.[133] At the end of polyploidization, MKs increase their cytoplasmic maturation with a possible coupling of the DMS development with polyploidization.[134] However, polyploidization is not indispensable for terminal MK maturation and some 2N and 4N MKs, called micro-MKs, can be fully mature and give rise to platelets. They are rare in the normal BM, but are more frequent in the fetal liver and in culture, more particularly in cord blood cells as well as in the fetal liver.[135-137] The main role of polyploidization is to increase cell size. As platelets arise from MK cytoplasmic fragmentation, polyploidization increases the number of platelets produced per MK. This process may be more efficient for platelet production than proliferation by classical mitosis. Indeed, it is expected that the number of platelets will increase by the power of 2 during each division (cell number) and by the power of 3 at each cycle of endomitosis (cell size

is dependent of the volume).[138] For example, micro-MKs may produce one or two platelets, whereas a 16N MK will produce a mean of 2500 platelets (1000-5000). Therefore, platelet production is dependent on two parameters: the size of the MKs correlated to the ploidy level and the number of MKs. Polyploidization rapidly increases under the control of TPO, permitting to quickly respond to the platelet demand. Then, the number of MKs in the marrow increases as a secondary response. However, polyploidization may induce other advantageous characteristics: (1) all the alleles of the polylobulated nucleus remain functional[139]; thus, polyploidization is a manner to increase mRNA synthesis and to increase the metabolic activity; (2) cells are more resistant to a genotoxic stress due to multiple functional alleles and are also less sensitive than 2N cells to a haploinsufficiency due to germline or acquired mutations.[132]

The mechanism of MK polyploidization has been called endomitosis because it was initially thought that it was a mitosis, but without nuclear membrane rupture.[133] The process of endomitosis has been now well described due to the possibility to study in vitro the endomitotic cultured MKs in real time. Endomitosis is a normal mitosis with a defect in late cytokinesis.[140,141] In the transition from 2N to 4N, the two daughter cells are nearly separated, but with persistence of nucleoplasmic bridges. Thereafter, due to the absence of cytokinesis, the two incompletely separated daughter cells, as well as the two nuclei, fuse together to give a polyploid cell with a single bilobulated nucleus.[142-144] A similar phenomenon occurs in the transition from 4N to 8N and to higher ploidy, but with less pronounced separation of the daughter cells. However, it has been described that certain 4N cells may divide again with a true cytokinesis.[145]

Endomitosis represents a succession of G1-S-G2-M cycles with defect of cytokinesis explaining the 2^XN ploidy level.[133,146] Polyploid MKs enter mitosis with a multipolar spindle and a segregation of chromosomes to the different poles, but in contrast to mitosis, the segregation can be asymmetrical.[147] The cell cycle is similarly regulated as in mitosis, but with some differences. The endomitotic cell cycle requires high level of cyclin D, more particularly cyclin D3, while cyclin E is indispensable.[146,148] In contrast to a normal mitosis, Aurora A and Aurora B are dispensable.[149,150] Importantly, Polo-kinase1 that regulates the centrosome, like Aurora A, is indispensable.[151] Interestingly, Aurora A inhibition increases differentiation and polyploization and could be a manner to restore a normal MK differentiation in AMKL (M7) and in myelofibrosis.[142,152,153] Clinical trials with Aurora A kinase inhibitors are presently ongoing.[154] In the endomitotic cell cycle, cyclin B1 whose precise level has been a subject of debate[133,140] must be degraded by CDC20. The absence of CDC20 leads to an endomitotic arrest and eventually apoptosis.[155] Interestingly, the MK cell cycle could be reprogrammed from endomitosis to endocycle (succession of G1/S/G2 cell cycles without mitosis entry) by rescuing the absence of CDC20 by cyclin-dependent kinase (CDK)1 and CDK2 depletion leading to high ploidy in MKs producing normal platelet levels through proplatelet formation.[155]

In the endomitotic process, the failure of cytokinesis is related to a "physiologic" defect in the cleavage furrow with either a normal formation with its subsequent regression at the 2N/4N stage or its ingression at higher ploidy level.[144,156,157] This appears to be the result of a defect in myosin II accumulation, which powers the forces of the cleavage furrow in mitotic cells and allows cytokinesis. In immature MKs, two types of myosin II are present: myosin IIA (MYH9) and myosin IIB (MYH10). This myosin II accumulation defect is related to two mechanisms: first a silencing of the *MYH10* gene by RUNX1 and friend leukemia virus–induced erythroleukemia-1 (FLI1) during differentiation[158] and the absence of MYH9 accumulation due to a defect in RhoA activity at the cleavage furrow.[158,159] This decrease in RhoA activity is related to the downregulation of two Rho-GEF, GEF-H1 at the 2N/4N transition, and ECT2 at higher ploidy levels.[157]

Finally, MKs are capable to escape the tetraploid checkpoint, which is normally regulated by the Rho/Hippo/p53 pathway, by impeding tetraploid cells to enter a new cycle of replication.[160-162] The basis of this escape has not been elucidated, but the same tetraploid MKs can respond to a genotoxic stress by inducing p53, which arrests the endomitotic cell cycle.[162-164]

The Normal Hematologic System

Gene expression and DNA methylation have been studied during polyploidization and both approaches have shown that the processes of polyploidization and maturation were intertwined.[165,166] However, using scRNAseq, it has been shown that high ploidy MKs have a transcriptional profile redirected toward translation and posttranslational modifications of proteins.[167]

Megakaryocyte Cytoplasmic Maturation

Three types of cytoplasmic modifications are responsible of the MK maturation associated with the increased synthesis of platelet proteins: the DMS (also called IMS), the development of granules, more particularly α-granules, dense granules and lysosomes, and the reorganization of the cytoskeleton leading to a marginal zone responsible for the spheroid shape of mature MKs before proplatelet formation (*Figure 17.3*).

Demarcation Membranes or Invaginated Membrane System

The demarcation membranes correspond to an extensive membrane system (DMS) inside the MK cytoplasm, which develops during MK maturation (*Figure 17.3*). It progressively extends to completely dissect the cytoplasm of the more mature MKs. At the ultrastructural level, DMS delineate platelet territories. It is why it was initially suggested that platelets were already preformed in the cytoplasm and the rupture of the DMS led to the formation of the blood platelets. Later, it was demonstrated that platelets usually arise from proplatelet formation and that in this model, DMS only functions as a membrane reservoir. For this reason, some authors have renamed the DMS and called it the IMS.[168] Indeed it was shown that the DMS originates from the invagination of the cell membrane.[169,170] Then, the system extends in the cytoplasm leading to a complex folded structure dissecting the MK cytoplasm organized in an intertwined tubular system.[171] This system is in continuity with the extracellular space explaining the emperipolesis, where cells, usually granulocyte precursors but also lymphocytes, are trapped and migrate inside the DMS with a possible exchange of membrane,[172] but not really inside the MK cytoplasm.[128] The DMS contains the same proteins as the plasma membrane and will form the future platelet plasma membrane. Recently, the existence of a pre-DMS has been shown due to the invagination of the plasma membrane during endomitosis, at the site of furrow formation. Thus, the pre-DMS accumulates between the different lobes of the multilobulated nucleus.[134,171] The development of the DMS is not only due to the continuous invagination of the plasma membrane, but also to the direct incorporation of glycoproteins through the Golgi and lipids from the smooth endoplasmic reticulum (ER), but without continuity between the different membrane systems.[134] Therefore, the DMS appears as a complex convoluted membrane system with multiple connections with the cell surface and is not totally derived from an invagination of the plasma membrane.

Granules and Mitochondria

There are three types of granules, the most abundant being α-granules.

α-Granules

α-granules are secretory granules that arise from both the secretory and the endocytic pathways.[173] They have a very typical ultrastructural morphology evoking a bull's eye due to the presence of a dense

nucleoid[128] (*Figure 17.3*). During MK maturation, the number of α-granules largely increases. They are localized in the indentation of the nucleus close to the Golgi apparatus in immature MKs, and later in the cytoplasm at the exception of the marginal zone.[171] Many different proteins contained in α-granules are synthesized in the ER and migrate to the Golgi and the trans-Golgi network before being sorted in the α-granules. They include membrane proteins such as P-selectin or soluble proteins. The proteoglycan serglycin permits to store basic soluble proteins such as PF4 or platelet-derived growth factor (PDGF).[174,175] Other proteins such as vWF may aggregate in the α-granules. Many proteins arrive and are packaged in α-granules by a clathrin-dependent endocytosis, through their interaction with a surface receptor.[176] The best example is the fibrinogen, which is incorporated in α-granules after binding to the GPIIb/IIIa, meaning that a fraction of this integrin is active in MKs.[177,178] The GPIIb/IIIa and the fibrinogen are subsequently incorporated in the α-granules. Other proteins such as albumin can be also incorporated by pinocytosis. The α-granules contain hundreds of proteins involved in numerous functions: mainly in hemostasis, such as vWF and fibrinogen that form a hemostatic plug. α-Granules proteins are also implicated in angiogenesis; inflammation; and bone marrow remodeling mediated by growth factors (PDGF, basic fibroblast growth factor [bFGF], transforming growth factor [TGF]-β1), chemokines (PF4, CCL5/Rantes) and ECM. The α-granules proteins are either secreted after platelet activation or, for the glycoproteins, incorporated into the cell membrane. The existence of a system of packaging of proteins in different types of α-granules has been suggested, with in particular some granules that would contain angiogenic factors (vascular endothelial growth factor) and others that would gather antiangiogenic factors (thrombospondin, endostatin).[179] In addition, the different proteins are differentially distributed inside the α-granules.[180]

As stated above, the α-granules are formed by two pathways: one is the direct emergence from the trans-Golgi network and the main pathway concerns the multivesicular bodies (MVBs), an endosomal structure that serves as an intermediate structure to sort the different granules in MKs.[181]

Defects in the formation or the release of α-granules leads to the gray platelet syndrome (GPS), a disorder characterized by a macrothrombocytopenia, which may progress to myelofibrosis and an increased emperipolesis.[182-184] It is a heterogeneous disorder related in most cases to germline mutations in the *NBEAL2* (neurobeachin-like 2) gene,[77-79] but mutations in *GFI1b* and *GATA-1* have also been associated with this syndrome.[80,81] The absence of α-granules has been described in the arthrogryposis, renal dysfunction and cholestasis syndrome, which is associated with bleeding.[185] This syndrome is caused by mutations in trafficking proteins VPS33b or VIPAR forming the same functional complex that may sort some cargos from the trans-Golgi to MVB.[186,187] The absence of the complex leads to a quasi absence of α-granule formation and a defect in MVB maturation.[188]

Platelet Dense Granules (δ-Granules)

Platelet dense granules are mainly involved in hemostasis and contain high concentrations of small molecules, such as serotonin, adenosine triphosphate, adenosine diphosphate, and Ca^{2+}.[189] They are revealed by mepacrine staining and by specific ultrastructural studies. Dense

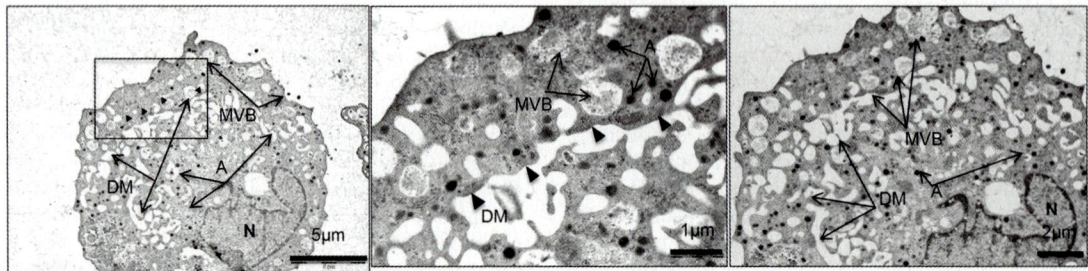

FIGURE 17.3 Ultrastructural illustration of a mature megakaryocyte. A, α-granules; DM, Demarcation membranes; MVB, Multivesicular body.

bodies only originate from the endosomal compartment, mainly from MVB.[190-192] Some extracellular molecules are concentrated by specific transporters using the endocytic pathway. For serotonin, the serotonin transporter and the vesicular monoamine transporter (VMAT2) are used for endocytosis and concentration in platelet dense granules. Others are synthesized by MKs, and using the secretory pathway, they traffic to early endosomes and to MVB and dense granules or directly to dense granules through the AP3/Rab32/38b pathway.[189,191] Therefore, the dense granules belong to the lysosome-related organelles such as melanosomes, which can be also affected in storage pool disease, such as the Hermansky-Pudlak syndrome. There are several different storage pool disorders that are associated with a deficiency in dense bodies and all lead to a bleeding disorder underscoring the role of dense granules in platelet aggregation. The Chediak-Higashi syndrome, one of the storage pool diseases, is related to a mutation in *CHS1/LYST*, a gene belonging to the BEACH domain–containing proteins as *NBEAL2* in GPS.[193]

Lysosomes

Lysosomes are prominent structures in the cytoplasm of MKs. Their synthesis begins very early during differentiation.[192] They are more heterogeneous than the other platelet/MK granules. They contain the same proteins as lysosomes of other cell types such as LAMP1-3, acid hydrolases, and cathepsin D and E.[192] Interestingly, they might arise via a common path as the α-granules and dense granules from MVB, but the precise mechanisms are not known.

In addition, *mitochondria* are present in MKs. The mitochondria mass increases with ploidy probably by fission, but with smaller mitochondria.[162] In immature MKs, they are localized in the perinuclear region.[162] There is indirect evidence that by regulating the energy, mitochondria play an important role in MK maturation and proplatelet formation. This could be related to the formation of mitochondrial reactive oxygen species (ROS), which are indispensable for late stages of megakaryopoiesis.[194] The mitochondria mass is regulated by both the Wnt and Hippo pathways.[162,195]

Cytoskeleton

During maturation, MKs develop an important cytoskeleton, which plays an essential role in maintaining the cellular organization. This cytoskeleton is the principal determinant at the end of maturation and the formation of proplatelets (see next chapter).[196]

During maturation, one major characteristic of the MK cytoplasm is to be organized in three zones[171]: the first zone is the perinuclear region with the Golgi complex, the second one comprises a central region where DMS and granules are localized, and the third one is a marginal zone devoid of organelles. This latest region corresponds to a microtubule network and actomyosin filaments, which provide the cortical force and permits to keep the DMS tightly folded in the central zone. This marginal zone nearly disappears at the end of maturation, when proplatelets are formed.

The cytoskeleton is also involved in the organization of the central zone. The distribution of organelles is regulated by myosin IIA, and in its absence, the organelles are clustered in the cytoplasm due to the role of the actomyosin cytoskeleton in the mobility of organelles.[197] The spectrin-actin cytoskeleton is indispensable for the development of the DMS, including the invagination of the plasma membrane.[198] The DMS is associated to the F-actin cytoskeleton, probably through spectrin, in a complex tubular network. In addition, PI(4.5)P2 accumulation in DMS is responsible for F-actin polymerization through the Wasp/Wave/Arp2/3 pathway that is necessary for proper DMS development.[199]

Megakaryocyte and Platelet Formation
Proplatelet Formation and MK Rupture

The first evidence that MKs give platelets through long cytoplasmic extensions comes from the pioneering work of Thiery et al showing that mature MKs take an octopus shape during cultures.[200] It was Radley who provided the seminal hypothesis that the long extensions called "proplatelets" were responsible for platelet production.[201] It

was further demonstrated that proplatelet extension was dependent upon microtubules and DMS.[202] The complete description of this process was performed using in vitro cultures, by demonstrating that the microtubule forces power the elongation of proplatelets by unwinding the DMS.[203,204] Along these extensions, there are several swelling regions, which could delineate future platelets. It was subsequently suggested that platelets arise only from the tip of the proplatelets as the microtubules bundles loop back in the proplatelet shaft.[204] *In vivo*, the mechanisms of proplatelet formation may be slightly different with a less important role of microtubules in the elongation process.[205] Proplatelets extend though the vessel wall and platelets are formed in the sinusoid vessel.[201,206] Imaging has demonstrated that proplatelets, or a fragment of proplatelets, are detached from MKs by the blood shear in vivo and that in vitro this rupture is facilitated by shear forces.[207,208] In the circulation, these detached proplatelets will give rise to an intermediate structure called preplatelets (discoid structure with a 2 to 10 μm diameter) that will convert into barbell proplatelets to donate two individual platelets.[209,210] This transition from preplatelets to platelets is also powered by microtubule forces.[209] The platelet formation occurs in the circulation, but preplatelets or proplatelets can be trapped in the microcirculation, more particularly in the lung where they can fragment into platelets.

Alternatively it has also been shown that an entire MK can migrate in the circulation and form platelets, more particularly in the pulmonary circulation.[206,211,212] Using two-photon intravital microscopy it has been demonstrated the presence of MK originating from the bone marrow and the spleen in the lung circulation of mice. These MKs were forming proplatelets and preplatelets. Moreover, the authors demonstrate that HSC, MPPs, MK-Ps, and immature MKs are present in the parenchyma of the lung and that were capable of repopulating the bone marrow space and of completely correcting a thrombocytopenia. This suggests that the lung is an important organ in platelet biogenesis as well as a hematopoietic organ specialized in platelet production.[213] However, a recent study has shown that MKs in the lung parenchyma are a specialized population of immune cells. They are 2N cells that express platelet proteins such as CD41 and CD42, but also CD11c, major histocompatibility complex (MHC) class II or CD11b.[15] A close population of immune MKs has been identified in the bone marrow.[12] It remains unclear whether this specific population is capable of producing platelets.

The microtubules play a central role in the elongation of proplatelets and β-1 tubulin (*TUBB1*) and α-4 tubulin are the major components of the MK tubulin,[214,215] explaining that some variants in the *TUBB1* gene are responsible of macrothrombocytopenia or worsened the phenotype of other thrombocytopenias[88,89] (*Figure 17.4*).

Microtubule elongation at their + ends occurs not by polymerization, but by a sliding process that involves the microtubule motor protein dynein.[216] In addition, organelles such as granules and mitochondria are redistributed from the cell body along the proplatelet.[217] These movements are facilitated by the bipolar arrangement of the microtubules and are powered by the microtubule motor kinesin. The number of centrosomes increases with the level of ploidy, which regulates both the pre-DMS and the number of microtubule extensions to control the number of proplatelets formed by individual MKs. The microtubule stability and dynamic are important determinants for their motor function. They are mainly controlled by posttranslational modifications of the different tubulin isoforms such as tyrosination, glutamylation, and acetylation that are implicated in proplatelet formation.[218,219]

However, at least in vitro, proplatelets are a complex structure with numerous branching. It has been shown that these branching are regulated by the F-actin cytoskeleton,[204] but it is not yet clear if these branched structures exist in vivo. However, the F-actin cytoskeleton plays a central role upstream the proplatelet formation by being implicated together with GPIb in the development of the DMS.[199]

Recently, it has been suggested that an alternative mechanism of platelet production may occur. In stress conditions, platelets may be formed by MK rupture, a very efficient and rapid cytoplasmic fragmentation occurring in blood vessels.[220] This new form of platelet release

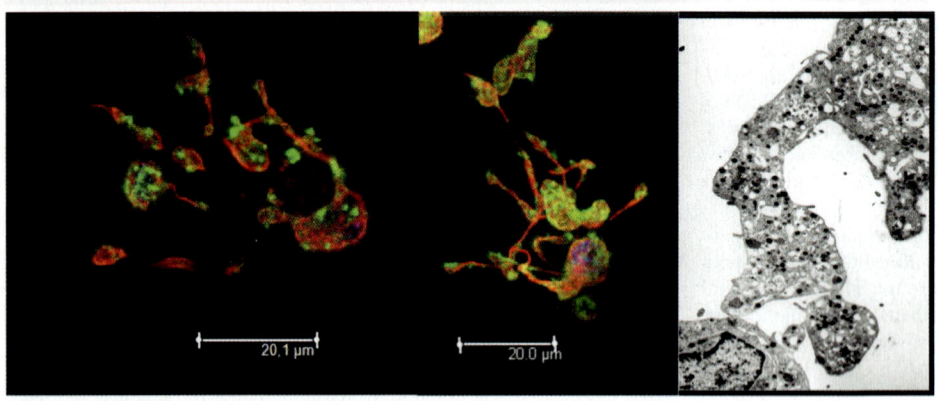

FIGURE 17.4 Proplatelet formation studied by confocal microscopy and transmission electron microscopy. Blue: nuclear labeling by DAPI, Green: F-vWF, Red: tubulin.

is only observed in acute platelet need. It is induced by inflammatory cytokines, more particularly through interleukin (IL)-1α-IL-1R1 signaling.[220] In addition, it has been suggested that the majority of platelet production in basal conditions occurs by budding and not by proplatelet formation.[221] However, whether these MK buds are really platelets is controversial. Recent evidence suggests that they are more MK microvesicles devoid of organelles than true platelets.[222]

Role of the Marrow Environment in Platelet Production

There is increasing evidence that proplatelet formation is a cell autonomous process as it occurs in culture, even in the absence of TPO or other cytokines. However, this process must be tightly regulated because platelets cannot be produced in the marrow environment, as they do not have the properties to transmigrate. Thus, platelets must be produced in the blood flow. Immature MKs are localized near the cortical bone close to osteoblasts (forming the endosteal niche), and at the end of maturation, they migrate toward the vessels (vascular niche). Mature MKs are located in the subendothelium region of the marrow sinusoids.[206,223,224] There is some recent evidence that the entire megakaryopoiesis takes place in the perisinusoidal region where HSCs are also localized.[225] Thus, there could only be limited migration to bring MKs in direct contact with endothelial cells. This migration is mediated by a gradient of CXCL12/SDF1 leading to a signaling through its receptor CXCR4.[223] When MKs are relocalized in contact to the endothelial cells, they begin to form proplatelets extending through the sinusoid vessel. It has been suggested that CXCL12 by itself could regulate late stages of MK differentiation including the formation of proplatelets[226,227] although there is some evidence that CXCR4 signaling is abrogated by RGS16 in the more mature MKs.[228] MK proplatelet formation may be also regulated by an autocrine stimulation by insulin-like growth factor binding protein-2, migration inhibitory factor, and nardilysin induced by turbulence in the blood flow.[229] It was also evidenced that proplatelet formation is regulated by inhibition. Indeed, in the cavity of the bone marrow, the collagen type I is predominant in the environment and inhibits proplatelet formation.[230,231] When MKs migrate to the vessels, the high local concentration of collagen IV relieves the inhibitory effects of collagen type I.[231] This effect is mediated through signaling by GPVI and α2β1,[230,231] but the role of GPVI may be predominant. It has been also suggested that other ECMs, such as vWF, laminin, and fibrinogen through GPIIb/IIIa favor proplatelet formation.[232] A recent study has underscored the role of the β1 integrin in the process of MK adhesion to the osteoblastic niche. It has been shown that *βGalt1*[-/-] mice have a severe thrombocytopenia in part related to a defective megakaryopoiesis. Indeed, MKs are dysplastic with an absence of DMS development and are located in the endosteal niche.[233] The βGalt1 deficiency leads to an activation of the β1 integrin increasing the adhesive properties of MKs. The β1 integrin knockout rescues this defect in thrombopoiesis.[233]

MKs are capable to form podosomes, a complex structure composed of F-actin and vinculin as well as metalloproteases, cortactin, and myosin IIA.[234] These structures are regulated by the WASP family and the Arp2/3 complex and play an important role in MK migration

as well as in ECM degradation, allowing the formation of transendothelial pores and then permitting the transendothelial passage of the proplatelets.[234-236] Myosin IIA is dispensable for the development of this process, but plays a role in their distribution and their size.[236]

CDC42 and RHOA together with GPIB play an important role in MK polarization and transendothelial passage of MKs and proplatelets in the marrow sinusoids.[237]

Role of Cytoskeleton in the Regulation of Platelet Production

The elongation of proplatelets as well as the reversible transition of preplatelets to barbell proplatelets is regulated by microtubule forces. However, except for β1 tubulin variants or mutations,[238,239] most human hereditary thrombocytopenia affect genes of the spectrin/actin/myosin cytoskeleton such as α-actinin 1 or *MYH9* or their regulators *DIAPH1*, *SRC*, and *WAS*. In addition, mutations in genes encoding GPIb (*GP1BB, GP1BA, GP9*) and filamin A (*FLNA*), linking the actin cytoskeleton to the membrane, also lead to macrothrombocytopenia.[240,241]

The spectrin/actin/myosin cytoskeleton plays a central role in the early proplatelet formation by regulating the DMS development and its proper organization, as well as by regulating the cortical forces. For example, *Myh9* knockout leads to a premature proplatelet formation, probably related to a decrease in adhesion and cortical forces due to the quasi disappearance of the marginal zone.[242] Similarly pharmacologic inhibition of myosin II activity increases by more than two fold the formation of proplatelets.[243,244] Furthermore, the forces necessary for abscission of proplatelets into platelets are not only mediated by microtubules, but also by actomyosin. It has been shown that the shear activates myosin IIA activity inducing cytofission, a mechanism close to cytokinesis.[245] Thus, the activity of myosin IIA must be timely regulated to ensure an adequate proplatelet formation and platelet release. This explains why most mutations in genes of the actomyosin pathway induce a macrothrombocytopenia. In addition, the actin cytoskeleton plays an important role in the migration of MKs and in the protrusion of proplatelets in the basement membrane.[234] Such a defect may partially explain the thrombocytopenia of the WAS (Wiskott-Aldrich syndrome).[235]

The actin cytoskeleton is regulated by the Rho family of GTPases, namely RhoA, Rac1, and Cdc42. In the human system, the in vitro activation of RhoA decreases polyploidy and proplatelet formation and inhibition of RhoA acts inversely.[244] Furthermore, in mice, protein kinase C-ε (PKCε) regulates proplatelet formation by modulating RhoA activity. However, *RhoA* knockout induces a macrothrombocytopenia.[246] The macrothrombocytopenia was related to changes in the stiffness of the cell membrane, in platelet defects with their rapid clearance from the circulation, and to an increased MK migration with abnormal proplatelet formation in the sinusoids.[237,247] RhoA has several effectors that regulate MK differentiation. The inhibition of Rock reproduces in vitro the same effects on ploidy and proplatelet formation than RhoA inhibition, meaning that Rock is the main effector.[248] This effect of Rock on proplatelet formation is mediated through the phosphorylation of the myosin light chain and activation of myosin IIA.[244,248]

Interestingly, pharmacological or genetic inhibition of the proteasome leads to a thrombocytopenia both in human and mouse related to an activation of the RhoA/Rock pathway.[249] More recently, it has been shown in human setting, but not in mouse, that DIAPH1 (mDia1) is also an effector of RhoA on proplatelet formation.[250] Indeed, DIAPH1 inhibits human proplatelet formation by inducing F-actin polymerization and altering microtubule stability showing that the RhoGTPase may control both the actin and the microtubule cytoskeletons.[250] These in vitro studies were further confirmed by the discovery of gain-of-function mutations in *DIAPH1* in two families with a macrothrombocytopenia.[98] A last effector could be the LIM kinase/cofilin pathway that may also be activated by RhoA as well as by Cdc42 and Rac1 and that leads to a defect in proplatelet formation.[251]

In many cell systems, Cdc42 and Rac1 play an opposite role than RhoA. For instance, in vitro inhibition of Cdc42 and to a lesser extent of Rac1 inhibits proplatelet formation by disrupting the DMS, whereas activation of Cdc42 increases proplatelet formation.[252,253] Strikingly, this effect is mainly mediated by Pak1/2 in mice,[253] whereas it is mediated by N-WASP, but neither by WASP or PAKs in humans.[252] In mice, the individual knockout of *Cdc42* and *Rac1* has a low or no effect on the platelet level.[254] However, the double knockout induces a macrothrombocytopenia associated with very abnormal MKs characterized by the absence of a marginal zone and their fragmentation in the bone marrow. In culture, there is an absence of proplatelet formation. This MK defect is associated with an impaired tubulin organization and a resulting loss of interaction with actin. It was suggested that this defect is mediated by the LIMK/cofilin pathway.[254] Double *Cdc42* and *RhoA* knockout mice have also been generated and exhibited a profound macrothrombocytopenia related to the absence of proplatelet formation due a major defect in MK maturation and a defect in transmigration.[255] Apart of this both being related to a defect in serum response factor (Srf)/Mkl1 activation.[255]

All these results suggest that there is an important interplay between the actin and microtubule cytoskeletons regulated by the Rho GTPase. However, it appears that there are also some differences between human and mouse. One of these differences concerns the role of WASP with the *Wasp* knockout mice presenting a moderate thrombocytopenia with a normal platelet size, whereas patients lacking WASP have a profound microthrombocytopenia.[235] Interestingly, a knockout of profilin 1 (PFN1), a protein that promotes actin filament elongation, gives rise to a very similar phenotype than WAS patients. It was shown to be due to a premature release of platelets in the bone marrow, as previously shown for *Wasp* knockout mice. *Pfn1* knockout also induces a disorganization of microtubules in platelets with the presence of stable hyperacetylated microtubules.[256] Microtubules are also disorganized in platelets of WAS patients, and as PFN1 may interact with WASP, it was suggested that a defect in PFN1 localization was responsible of the thrombocytopenia of WAS patients.[256]

Pan-histone deacetylase (HDAC) inhibitors induce a thrombocytopenia by several mechanisms including the induction of hematopoietic progenitor apoptosis. *In vitro* proplatelet formation is inhibited with some disorganization in the cytoskeleton.[257-259] It has been suggested that this may be due to HDAC6 inhibition because HDAC6 regulates the acetylation of microtubules.[257,260] However, there is also evidence that cortactin, an actin nucleation–promoting factor whose activity is regulated by acetylation, plays a major role in the defect of proplatelet formation induced by HDAC6 inhibition only in human setting.[261]

Role of Apoptosis in the Regulation of Platelet Production

At the end of maturation, after the release of proplatelets, the MK body dies by apoptosis and is engulfed by macrophage.[262] It was assumed that in some ways MK fragmentation may mimic an apoptotic death. However, when forming proplatelets, MKs need to inhibit apoptosis.[263] In MKs, there is an equilibrium between different members of the BCL-2 family: MCL-1 and BCL-X$_L$ (antiapoptotic) restrain the activity of BAK and BAX (proapoptotic).[263,264] Furthermore, platelet survival depends on the equilibrium between BCL-X$_L$ and BAK1/BAX. The platelet lifespan is limited by the decrease in the level of BCL-X$_L$ after few days (5 days in the mouse) leading to an excess

of BAK1 and BAX and apoptosis although platelets are anucleated cells.[264] BAK1 plays a more important role than BAX in the platelet senescence. Deletion of BCL-X$_L$ and MCL-1 totally inhibits MK development, whereas the single deletion of BCL-X$_L$ permits a normal MK differentiation, but with a nearly complete defect in proplatelet formation in mice. This result clearly establishes that the intrinsic pathway of apoptosis must be inhibited to produce platelets. It also shows that the thrombocytopenia induced by BH3 mimetics may be related to BCL-X$_L$ inhibition.[265] Furthermore, it was shown that activation of the extrinsic pathway of apoptosis by Fas-L also decreases platelet production and that caspase-8 deletion has no impact on baseline platelet production extending the concept that classical apoptosis is not involved in platelet production.[266]

However, it was shown before these genetic experiments that in vivo overexpression of BCL-2 or a BIM deficiency leads to a thrombocytopenia and overexpression of BCL-X$_L$ in a defect of proplatelet formation.[267-269] In culture systems, the pan-caspase inhibitor zVAD-FMK:carbobenzoxy-valyl-alanyl-aspartyl-[O-methyl]-fluoromethylketone inhibits proplatelet formation.[270,271] The presence of active caspase-3 was identified in discrete parts of maturing MK cytoplasm, suggesting a compartmentalized activation of caspase contrasting with the diffuse staining observed in apoptotic MKs although cytochrome c was released, without detectable DNA fragmentation.[271]

Accordingly, an autosomal dominant form of thrombocytopenia was detected in members of a family with a constitutive variant form of cytochrome *c* (G41S) with enhanced ability to activate caspases through an enhanced affinity for apoptotic protease activating factor-1. It was suggested that this thrombocytopenia was related to an accelerated platelet formation leading to the release of platelets in the bone marrow rather than in the blood stream.[64] However, the disorder was recently shown to be associated with two types of platelets: platelets in the circulation with a normal microtubule coil and platelets in the marrow looking more like MK cytoplasmic fragments. This suggests that the thrombocytopenia may rather be related to a MK rupture in the marrow.[272]

Taken together, there is no strong argument to sustain the initial hypothesis that mature MKs may undergo classical apoptosis in order to promote platelet shedding through proplatelet formation. This conclusion does not rule out the possibility that caspases could be activated in mature MKs to induce platelet release through so far unidentified molecular and cellular mechanisms, independently of any cell death program. Recently, an alternative pathway of platelet release was identified, which is defined by a rapid cytoplasmic fragmentation in blood vessels by MK rupture. This new form of platelet release is only observed under stress and is not dependent on TPO, but on the IL-1α-IL-1R1 signaling and caspase-3 activation leading to deregulated tubulin expression and decreased membrane stability.[220] This new mechanism seems to be different from apoptosis. Thus, it will be important to determine what the precise caspase-3 target proteins in MKs are and where caspase-3 may be activated in the cytoplasm.

MEGAKARYOCYTE AND BONE MARROW MICROENVIRONMENT

Surprisingly, it has been shown these last years that MKs play an important role in the regulation of HSC, both after irradiation and in steady state conditions. After irradiation, MKs migrate close to the endosteum due to a TPO signaling through MPL and to adhesion by CD41. By secreting PDGF-β they induce the proliferation of the osteoblast niche and facilitate HSC engraftment.[273] In steady state conditions and after an injury, MKs can also directly regulate HSC quiescence through the secretion of TGF-β1 and PF4.[274,275] More recently, it was shown that this effect could be also mediated by the synthesis of TPO by MKs. Indeed, MKs and osteoblasts interact through Clec2 (MK) and podoplanin (osteoblast). This interaction induces Clec2 signaling and the synthesis of important HSC regulators by MKs such as TPO, PF4, CXCL12, and angiopoietin 1.[276] However, future studies have shown that the synthesis of TPO protein by MKs could not be detected whereas TPO transcripts were present.[277] Thus,

MKs may have two different functions: in transplantation they favor the homing and proliferation of HSC, and in the absence of stress they are an important regulator of HSC quiescence.

In addition, MKs are able to remodel the bone marrow environment by secreting TGF-β1, different ECMs such as collagen and fibronectin and metalloproteases, as well as the bone itself through the synthesis of PGDF-β, lysyl oxidase, and TGF-β1 that stimulate osteoblast differentiation and proliferation and also by inhibiting osteoclasts.[278,279] In addition, adhesion of JAK2V617F MKs to fibronectin may induce their proliferation in myeloproliferative neoplasms.[280]

A subset of MKs could be specialized in bone marrow remodeling and regulation of HSC as recently shown by scRNAseq.[12,14]

This important role of MKs in bone marrow and bone remodeling explains that several hereditary or malignant disorders involving the MK lineage are associated with a myelofibrosis and/or an osteosclerosis.

MEGAKARYOCYTES AS IMMUNE CELLS

Platelets have an important immune function not only by secreting several cytokines or chemokines (IL-1, TGF-β1, CXCL1), but by also expressing CD62P and CD40L.[281] In addition, platelets express nearly all Toll like receptors (TLRs) and are capable to cross-present exogenous proteins via MHC class I to CD8 T cells.[282] In addition, platelets may be the targets of numerous viruses such as the HIV, dengue virus, and SARS-CoV-2.[283] It has been shown that mature MKs have the same properties that are transmitted to platelets and can also be infected by several viruses.[284,285]

However, recent studies have shown that a subset of MKs could have an important immune function and may be an immune cell:

First, it has been shown that murine bone marrow MKs can be reprogrammed in the lung by IL-33 to APC expressing both class I and class II MHC capable to activate both CD8+ and CD4+ lymphocytes.[15] This study underscores the MK plasticity and explains the platelet heterogeneity.

Second, it has been shown that a population of immune cells close to dendritic cells or monocytes is considered as MKs due to the expression of several genes associated with the MK lineage as those encoding the GPIb complex, PF4, and the CD41.[12,13] However, these cells are hypoploid (essentially 2N). Although they are regulated by TPO/MPL, their transcriptional program is not regulated by GATA1, but by PU.1 and IRF8.[12] Furthermore, it is unclear whether these immune MKs can produce platelets and, even if they could, their low ploidy mitigates their contribution to platelet production. It will be important in the future to determine the phylogeny of these immune MKs.

MEGAKARYOCYTE ONTOGENY

The development of the hematopoietic system emerges mostly by two waves: one in the yolk sac, which is mainly HSC independent and called primitive hematopoiesis, and another that is HSC dependent. It is called definitive hematopoiesis and is first localized in the fetal liver and then in the bone marrow in neonate and adult.[286,287]

The development of megakaryopoiesis has been essentially studied in mice. Early stages corresponding to the yolk sac hematopoiesis have been investigated in the human system, mostly through ES and iPS cell differentiation.

The first platelets are detected as early as E9.5 in mouse peripheral blood of the mouse and their number increases rapidly after E10.5. In human setting, platelets are also detected early in the blood. In mice, the first platelets originate from a first wave of MKs, which derives from a monopotent precursor detected at E8.5 in the yolk sac. This precursor gives rise to only diploid MKs (diploid platelet precursor cell), whose differentiation is independent on TPO.[288,289] These diploid MKs were capable to form proplatelets and thus to produce platelets within less than 3 days of differentiation.[289] Almost simultaneously, true hematopoietic progenitors are detected including CFU-MKs that give rise to polyploid MKs, but with a lower ploidy than in the adult. In the yolk sac, all the progenitors (MK or non-MK) express CD41 with MK precursors expressing higher levels of CD41.[289]

Definitive hematopoiesis is HSC dependent. HSCs emerge in the AGM (aorta-gonad-mesonephros) and express also the CD41.[286] Subsequently, they migrate into the fetal liver, which becomes the site of hematopoiesis with an MK differentiation leading to polyploid MKs.

In humans, it is much more difficult to study this process, but the differentiation of ES and iPS cells mimics the yolk sac hematopoiesis. There is a first wave, with the presence of bipotent (MEP) or tripotent (E/MK/monocyte) progenitors with low proliferative capacities and a CD45−CD41+GPA+ phenotype.[290,291] The MKs deriving from this wave exhibit a low ploidy (2N and 4N). A second wave can be observed without true HSCs, but with CD45low hematopoietic progenitors with higher proliferative capacities. However, MKs remain mainly of low ploidy with a minority of 8N MKs. In the fetal liver, MKs are cytologically close to marrow MKs, but there are MKs with a low ploidy (2N and 4N) with frequently two nuclei. Cord blood megakaryopoiesis shares many similarities with the fetal one.

Gene profiling has identified major changes in gene expression between the ES-derived and adult MKs and in fetal liver and neonate MKs.[292] For example, *MYCN* and *LIN28b* are downregulated during MK development, whereas CXCR4 is only expressed at high level in adult MKs.[292,293] This could be related to the differential expression of the micro RNA miR9.[294] It has been suggested that the human fetal to adult transition is mediated by IGF2BP3, which regulates positive transcription elongation factor b activation.[295]

These studies have shown that although different from adult, the platelets produced from the induced pluripotent stem cell (iPSC) and embryonic stem cell (ESC) differentiation are functional meaning that in the future ESC and iPSC can be used to produce platelets in large quantities.[296-298] It has been shown that neonate platelets have a longer lifespan than adult platelets, probably due to an increased level of BCL-2, but not of BCL-X$_L$, the main antiapoptotic member of the BCL-2 family in adult platelets.[299]

TRANSCRIPTIONAL REGULATION OF MEGAKARYOPOIESIS

Hematopoietic differentiation into all blood cell types is dependent on stage-specific regulators, including noncoding RNAs, epigenetic regulators, morphogenic signals, and transcription factors (TFs).[300] Megakaryopoiesis is tightly regulated by a cooperation of different TFs, some of them being involved in other transcriptional complexes regulating other hematopoietic lineages (*Figure 17.2C*). As an example, MKs derive from a MEP and their development is regulated by several TFs common to both MK and erythroid cells, such as GATA-binding protein 1 (GATA-1), T-cell acute lymphoblastic leukemia 1 (TAL1 or stem cell leukemia [SCL]), friend of GATA-1 (FOG) family member 1 (FOG-1), GFI1b, and nuclear factor erythroid 2 (NF-E2). In contrast, FLI1, RUNX1, and GABPα on one side and Krüppel-like factor 1 (KLF1) on the other side drive mono-lineage production of MKs and erythroid cells, respectively.[301,302]

These TFs regulate gene expression by binding to specific cis element motifs in promoters and enhancers. Most of them globally activate or repress gene transcription to promote terminal maturation and suppress alternate lineages. RUNX1 promotes MK and lymphoblastic differentiation at the expense of myelopoiesis. Similarly, GATA-1 favors MK/E differentiation by activating its own promoter, but simultaneously inhibits PU.1 gene regulation thus leading to the repression of myelopoiesis.

During the last decade, efforts were made to decipher gene transcription networks regulating the early stages of hematopoietic differentiation. In MKs, the first cooperations described were between GATA-1 and RUNX1[303] and between GATA-1 and FLI1.[304] Later, in 2011, genome wide analysis revealed combinatorial interactions between GATA-1, GATA-2, RUNX1, FLI1, and TAL1.[302] More recently, the cooperation between RUNX1, FLI1, and NF-E2 in later stages of megakaryopoiesis was reported.[305]

GATA-1 and GATA-2 are zinc finger (ZF) DNA–binding proteins belonging to the GATA family. They recognize the WGATAR motif through two ZFs.[306] The C-terminal ZF binds to the GATA consensus sites, whereas the N-terminal ZF promotes the interaction between GATA and specific DNA sequences through stabilizing the association with ZF protein cofactors.[306,307] GATA-1 is required for the erythroid and MK commitment during hematopoiesis, while GATA-2 is crucial for the proliferation and survival of early hematopoietic cells. However, GATA-2 is also involved in lineage-specific transcriptional regulation as a dynamic partner of GATA-1: in the absence of GATA-1, GATA-2 contributes to cell cycle progression and the maintenance of MK identity of GATA-1–deficient cells, including GATA-1short (GATA-1s) (see below), expressing fetal MK-Ps.[308]

GATA-1 and FOG-1

GATA-1 is an X-linked TF containing N-terminal activation domain (NAD) and the above-mentioned N- and C-terminal ZFs that bind to WGATAR motif in the regulatory region of several genes encoding for MK-specific proteins such as GPIIb, PF4, GPIbα, GPIbβ, β-thromboglobulin, GPIX, or GPV and MPL. MK-specific gene promoters also possess, in tandem with the GATA motifs, DNA consensus sequence for the Ets family (GGA/T) that is absent from erythroid genes.

In mouse model, *GATA-1* deletion in ESCs leads to the arrest of erythroid maturation at the proerythroblast stage inducing lethal anemia at embryonic day 10.5 and 11.5 of gestation.[309] The selective loss of GATA-1 expression in MKs leads to hyperproliferation of small hypoploid MKs, impaired cytoplasmic maturation, and marked decrease in platelet count. These defects are accompanied by a decrease in the expression of MK-specific genes such as GPIbα, GPIbβ, PF4, and MPL, as well as p45[NF-E2,310,311] and underline the multiple functions of GATA-1 in MK development. In human, different mutations in N- and C-terminal ZFs induce distinct and overlapping phenotypes. The germline N-terminal ZF mutation V205M causes severe anemia and macrothrombocytopenia.[70] Valine at position 205 is crucial for the interaction between GATA-1 and its cofactor FOG-1 required for terminal maturation of both MK and erythroid cells.[71] Other germline GATA-1 mutations affecting interaction with FOG-1 were reported to lead to anemia and macrothrombocytopenia, G208S,[72] D218G, D218Y,[73,74] G208R,[75] or to GPS, R216Q.[76] The C-terminal GATA-1 X414R mutation was reported in a family with the rare X-linked blood group (Lu(a-b-) phenotype) and mild macrothrombocytopenia.[312] Acquired mutations leading to the loss of NAD contribute to the Down syndrome (DS)–associated transient myeloproliferative disorder (TMD) or AMKL. These mutations result in the expression of only a shortened isoform of GATA-1, GATA-1s, lacking exon 2, and amino acids 1 to 83.[301] Interestingly, patients with germline GATAs-type mutations, usually by modifying the splicing of the exon 2, present no signs of TMD or AMKL, but develop hypoplastic anemia close to Diamond-Blackfan anemia.[301]

GATA-1 activates or represses target genes depending upon chromosomal context and this activation or repression occurs via FOG-1–dependent and -independent mechanisms.

The absence of FOG-1 leads to a phenotype similar to that of GATA-1 in the erythroid lineage, but with profound additional abnormalities in the MK lineage (i.e., absence of MK-P). This phenotype is due to the loss in the interaction between FOG-1 and GATA-2 in the early stages of the MK lineage. The interaction between FOG-1 and GATA-1 is specifically required for late stages of MK maturation, but not early MK development suggesting that GATA-1 and -2 are functionally interchangeable only at early stages in MK development.[313] FOG-1 interacts also with subunits of the nucleosome and the histone deacetylase (NuRD) complex through a specific motif located at its N-terminus. Disruption of FOG-1/NuRD interaction leads to splenomegaly, extramedullary erythropoiesis, granulocytosis, and thrombocytopenia secondary to a block in MK maturation.[314] The preservation of GATA-1/FOG-1/NuRD complex is necessary for maintaining lineage fidelity by constraining lineage-inappropriate gene expression throughout erythroid/MK development.[315] Krüppel-type ZF TF ZBP-89 was also identified as being a component of multiprotein complexes involving GATA-1 and FOG-1. As for FOG-1 and GATA-1, functional

ZBP-89 is required for normal megakaryopoiesis and definitive erythropoiesis but not for primitive erythropoiesis.[316]

GATA-2

GATA-2 plays an essential role in proliferation and survival of HSCP compartments[317] and is required for mast cell formation but not for erythroid and myeloid terminal differentiation.[318] Genetic complementation studies in *GATA-1*-null cells showed that GATA-1 rapidly displaces GATA-2, which is coupled to transcriptional repression. In erythroid lineage, GATA-1 disrupts the positive autoregulation of GATA-2 expression[319] and it cannot be excluded that this kind of regulation also exists in MKs. GATA-2 promotes megakaryopoiesis by driving progenitor cell proliferation and MK lineage gene expression while suppressing myeloid gene expression. In late megakaryopoiesis, GATA-2 plays an extensive role as a transcriptional repressor at loci defined by a specific DNA signature.[320] Furthermore, by using a mouse model of human GATA-1 DS-AMKL, it was shown that GATA-2 overexpression contributes to dysregulated MK proliferation in the absence of full-length GATA-1. GATA-2 is a critical TF that coordinates cellular proliferation and maintains MK identity in GATA-1-deficient or mutant cells.[308]

T-Cell Acute Lymphocytic Leukemia 1

TAL1, also called SCL, is a basic helix-loop-helix TF that acts as an activator or as a repressor. It is expressed at both early and late stages of hematopoietic development and is essential for normal HSC generation. In addition, it is indispensable, like GATA-1, for the development of the erythroid, MK, and mast cells.[321-323] TAL1 is critical for MK proliferation, ploidization, cytoplasmic maturation, and platelet release by direct regulation of *NF-E2*,[324] *MEF2C*,[325] and *p21* (*CDKN1A*) genes.[326] It was previously demonstrated that TAL1 and its heterodimeric partner, E2A, recognize the E-box (CANNTG) located near the WGATAR motif. However, in vivo studies showed that TAL1 does not require its DNA-binding region for its developmental functions.[327] More recently, it was shown, that TAL1 is not primarily guided by binding an E-box, but rather by its interaction with a GATA factor that is strongly bound to its DNA-binding site motif. In the presence of a GATA factor, a structure with TAL1-E2A bound upstream from GATA may serve as a platform for the recruitment of activators and coactivators. Once the GATA factor is no longer present, the remaining TAL1 may assume a different position or conformation that interferes with the recruitment of positive regulators, leading to a loss of induction.[328] TAL1 core complex (TAL1, LMO2, LDB1, E2A) interacts with GATA-1 when activating E-genes.[329,330] In absence of GATA-1, TAL1 cooperates with ETO2 in a repressor complex. The repressor TAL1/ETO2 complex interacts with GFI1b in erythroid cells but not in MKs.[331] In primary MKs, TAL1 is present in a multiprotein complex with RUNX1, FLI1, GATA-1, and GATA-2[302] and its redundancy with Lyl-1 was shown in murine megakaryopoiesis.[332]

RUNX1 (Also Called AML1, CBFA2, PEBP2αB)

RUNX1 is the core-binding factor (CBF)α subunit of the CBF complex and a master regulator of hematopoiesis. It is essential for induction of definitive hematopoiesis during embryogenesis. In adult mouse hematopoiesis, RUNX1 negatively regulates the in vivo long-term HSC activity, the number of different lineage immature progenitors, and myeloid progenitors and positively regulates megakaryopoiesis and B and T lymphopoiesis.[333] RUNX1 contains a conserved Runt domain responsible for DNA binding and CBFβ and a transactivation domain. CBFβ enhances the DNA-binding ability and protects RUNX1 from proteasomal degradation. RUNX1 has also CBFβ-independent functions and interacts with many others cofactors and chromatin modifiers to both activate and repress a broad range of hematopoietic genes according to the cellular context. It binds to the DNA consensus sequence TG(T/C)GGT that is found in proximity of ETS, and WGATAR sites in MK genes. RUNX1 regulates different steps of megakaryopoiesis, such as, the MK generation from HSC by direct negative regulation of NOTCH4,[334] the endomitosis entry by direct negative regulation of MYH10,[158,335] the arrest of polyploidization by direct positive regulation of p19INK4D[336] and the proplatelet formation via positive regulation of myosin chains MYL9[337,338] and MYH9,[338] and the negative regulation of ANKRD26.[339] It also regulates platelet functions via positive regulation of ALOX12,[340] PKCθ,[341] PF4,[342] and NF-E2 involved in terminal MK differentiation.[343] RUNX1 can also act as a transactivator or a repressor of the same genes depending on the cell context; for example, MPL is repressed by RUNX1 in hematopoietic progenitors, but is activated in MKs.[344]

Germline *RUNX1* mutations are found in familial platelet disorders with predisposition to acute myelogenous leukemia (FPD/AML). This very rare condition is characterized by thrombocytopenia, platelet dysfunction, and a 35% lifetime risk of developing myelodysplasia and/or AML.[345] The mutations are located either in the Runt domain or in the transactivation C-ter domain. Heterozygous deletions and frameshifts mimicking haploinsufficiency often lead to isolated thrombocytopenia, while missense and nonsense mutations may also inhibit wild-type RUNX1 (so-called dominant negative mutants), creating a higher propensity to develop leukemia.[346] Inhibition of JNK and TGF-β1 pathways was shown to correct the in vitro MK defect linked to the RUNX1 haploinsufficiency.[347]

ETS Family

ETS family of TFs includes more than 13 different proteins. The members of the ETS family share an evolutionarily conserved DNA-binding domain of 85 amino acids with a winged-helix-turn-helix configuration that allows binding to GGAA/T core sequences. Three members of ETS family, ETS1, GAPBα (GA-binding protein α), and FLI1, have been shown to transactivate MK-specific genes, the most important being, however, FLI1. Indeed, *ETS1* knockout mice have a marked defect in lymphoid lineages, but normal megakaryopoiesis. However, its expression increases during MK maturation and its overexpression promotes MK differentiation and enhances the upregulation of GATA-2 and MK-specific genes.[348] GABPα expression level is more important during early stages of megakaryopoiesis. Accordingly, GABPα preferentially occupies ETS elements of early MK-specific genes such as *ITGA2B* (GPIIB) and *MPL*, whereas FLI1 binds both early and late MK-specific genes (*GPIBA, GPIX,* and *PF4*).[349] Interestingly, some ETS sites in promoters of MK-specific genes could be occupied by both GABPα and FLI1, but at different stages of megakaryopoiesis, as this was shown for *PF4*.[350] The mice with conditional deletion of *GABPα* in hematopoietic cells display reduced number of myeloid progenitor cells as a result of reduced expression of the transcriptional repressor GFI-1, without affecting erythroid lineage.[351] However, no data on MK lineage were reported; thus, the precise role of GABPα in megakaryopoiesis has to be clarified.

FLI1 directs the commitment toward MK lineage at the stage of MEP, while EKLF (FLI1 antagonist) to the erythroid lineage.[352] Moreover, it was recently shown, that the interaction between FLI1 and GATA-1 selectively regulates a distinct MK-specific set of genes that are expressed at a low level in HSC/progenitor and further induced during MK differentiation, but silenced in the erythroid lineage.[320] The *Fli1*[-/-] mice died at embryonic stage due to a defect in vascular development and in megakaryopoiesis. They display an increase in small, immature MKs and abnormal α granule biosynthesis. Disorganization of platelet DMS is also detected. The defects on megakaryopoiesis lead to a marked thrombocytopenia, with an excess of small immature MKs undergoing apoptosis.[353] These abnormalities are related to those observed in the Jacobsen syndrome or Paris-Trousseau thrombocytopenia characterized by a deletion in 11q23.3 to 24 region involving both *ETS1* and *FLI1*. Overexpression of FLI1 in patient hematopoietic progenitors partially restores the dysmegakaryopoiesis linked to this syndrome.[354] More recently, point mutations in *FLI1* were reported in inherited thrombocytopenia. The loss of the C-terminal regulatory domain of FLI1 leads to a reduced platelet count and impaired platelet aggregation and activation.[355] As already mentioned, FLI1 cooperates with other MK-specific TFs such as GATA-1/2, FOG-1, RUNX1, and TAL1 to transcriptionally activate (*GPIX, GPIBA, PF4*) or repress (*MYH10, ANKRD26*) genes at a precise stage of MK maturation and promotes chromatin looping between enhancers and promoters

through LDB1 complex.[356] It should be noted here that the presence/absence of MK-specific TFs in multiprotein complex depends on the differentiation stage and on target gene.

The role of ETS family transcriptional repressor ETS variant 6, ETV6 (also called *TEL*), in megakaryopoiesis was previously underlined in mice with the erythroid/MK conditional *ETV6* knockout. These mice are thrombocytopenic, and homozygous knockout leads to the absence of MK colony formation.[357] Only recently, germline mutations in *ETV6* gene, encoding a transcription repressor, were described to induce thrombocytopenia predisposing to hematopoietic malignancies in human. All described germline mutations result in impairment of ETV6 function and induce a defect in proplatelet formation.[56-59] This defect was linked to impaired cytoskeleton organization caused by a decreased expression of CDC42 and RHOA.[59] Interestingly, ETV6 absence also leads to an upregulation of proinflammatory transcripts suggesting that ETV6 negatively regulates the generation of MK with an "immune-like" phenotype.[358]

Finally, *ETS*-related gene (*ERG*, chr21) that plays a crucial role in establishing definitive hematopoiesis is also required for normal megakaryopoiesis. Its endogenous repression is required for the proliferation and maintenance of AMKL cell lines and it strongly cooperates with GATA-1s in DS AMKL to immortalize MK-Ps.[359] This overexpression of ERG blocks AKT-induced death of megakaryoblasts.[360] Simultaneous heterozygous alterations in *FLI1* and *ERG* lead to the more pronounced phenotype than simple mutations including a loss of HSCs with a reduction in the number of committed hematopoietic progenitors, a decrease in MK number, and severe thrombocytopenia. These results suggest that these TFs may coregulate common target genes.[361]

GFI1B

As previously mentioned, FLI1 and EKLF play important roles in the bifurcation of MEP toward erythroid or MK lineage. Two other TFs, GFI1b and MYB, also act in the MEP. GFI1b is a transcriptional repressor required for the development of both erythroid and MK lineages. GFI1b binds to DNA-specific sites and is associated with LSD1 (KDM1A), a histone demethylase to induce gene repression. It can also activate some genes through PRMT1. *Gfi1b* knockout is lethal in the embryo, where major abnormalities in the erythroid and MK differentiation lead to fatal anemia and thrombocytopenia. Fetal liver progenitors from *Gfi1b* knockout mice give rise to small MK colonies with a decreased level of GPIIb, MPL, and NF-E2 compared to wild-type cells.[362] This phenotype could be a consequence of an increased expression of type III TGF-β receptor in MEP. Indeed, in human MEP, GFI1b binds to the proximal TGFBR3 promoter leading to the repression of TGFBR3. After GFI1B inhibition, deregulated TGF-β signaling deeply alters proliferation and differentiation of MEP.[363] Moreover, in complex with β-catenin and LSD1, GFI1b regulates Wnt/β-catenin signaling pathway involved in spreading of MKs on integrin substrates.[364]

MYB

The basic helix-turn-helix TF MYB negatively regulates megakaryopoiesis at the stage of definitive MEP, while primitive erythropoiesis and megakaryopoiesis are MYB independent. Suboptimal levels of MYB favor the differentiation of MKs and macrophages, while high levels are important for erythropoiesis and lymphopoiesis.[365] In MEP, TPO downmodulates MYB expression through induction of miR-150.[366] Mice bearing loss-of-function mutations of *MYB* exhibit excessive megakaryopoiesis and thrombocytosis by a TPO-independent mechanism[367] and point mutations in *MYB* are found in human myelofibrosis or AMKL. Furthermore, depletion in *MYB* corrects the thrombocytopenia of *Mpl*[-/-] mice.

NF-E2

NF-E2 TF is a heterodimer composed of the large p45[NF-E2] and the small MAF (MAFF, MAFG, and MAFK) subunits. The basic leucine zipper bZIP domains of NF-E2 and of the small MAFs mediate their DNA binding and dimerization. The sequence recognized by the NF-E2/small MAF heterodimer is an extended AP-1 motif (T/C)GCTGA(C/G)TCA(T/C).[368] In MKs, p45[NF-E2] is regulated by GATA-1, TAL1, and RUNX1 TFs.[324,343,369] p45[NF-E2] knockout mice die at birth from severe thrombocytopenia resulting from an increased MK number with marked maturation defects, especially in the development of the DMS and in the distribution of α-granules.[370] A deep defect in the proplatelet formation was also observed in vitro.[371] The decreased number of CFU-MKs in p45[NF-E2] knockout mice, and, when NF-E2 is overexpressed in murine bone marrow cells, the inverse increased number of CFU-MKs, enhanced MK maturation and higher release of platelets suggest that NF-E2 is crucial not only in terminal MK development, but also plays an important role in its early steps.[372,373] The critical partner of p45[NF-E2] in MKs is MAFG, which not only mediates DNA binding through its bZIP domain, but also targets the NF-E2/MAFG heterodimer to a specific subnuclear localization, since deletion of the C-terminal domain of the small MAF factor does recapitulate the platelet phenotype observed in p45[NF-E2] knockout mice.[374] NF-E2 is a key TF in MK regulating genes involved in MK maturation and in the biogenesis and functions of platelets. The first direct target of p45[NF-E2] in MKs to be identified was the gene coding for thromboxane synthase,[375] which is important for platelet function, but not for proplatelet formation. Several other target genes of p45[NF-E2] such as *TUBB1* are involved in the process of proplatelet formation.[371] TUBB1 is restricted to the MK lineage and is expressed at late stages of differentiation. *Tubb1* knockout mice display a thrombocytopenia with abnormal-shaped platelets (i.e., absence of a discoid shape).[376] Other p45[NF-E2] targets were identified such as caspase-12[377]; Rab27b, a small G protein involved in vesicle/granule trafficking[378]; 3beta-hydroxysteroid dehydrogenase, a key enzyme for the synthesis of estrogen[379]; and the adaptor protein LIM and senescent cell antigen–like domains 1 implicated in cell migration and spreading.[380] The combination of NF-E2, GATA-1, and ETS1 proteins plays a critical role in regulating expression of the α isoform of the human thromboxane A_2 receptor (TPα) during different stages of MK differentiation and in platelets. The prostanoid thromboxane A_2 acts as a potent mediator of platelet aggregation and vasoconstriction.[381] MK maturation is closely related to the cellular response to oxidative stress in bone marrow and it was demonstrated that NF-E2 regulates cytoprotective genes that are common targets of p45 and Nrf2, in contrary to platelet genes that are regulated only by p45. The functional domination of p45 over Nrf2 favors ROS accumulation by limiting the expression level of cytoprotective genes. This ROS accumulation promotes the full activation of platelet genes such as *Txas, Gp6, Selp,* and *Slamf1*.[382] Combined analysis of ChIP-seq and microarrays performed in p45[NF-E2] null MKs identified 49 and 10 genes that were p45[NF-E2] activated and p45[NF-E2] repressed, respectively. Among the 49 genes, 15 are known for a role in platelet formation and function (for example, *Selp, Myl9*).[383] Recent work emphasizes the importance of RUNX1, FLI1, and NF-E2 cooperation at late stage of MK differentiation. Indeed, these 3 TFs co-occupy late-acting cis-elements and show evidence for additive activity at genes responsible for platelet assembly and release.[305]

Serum Response Factor and Its Coactivator MKL1

The importance of **SRF** and its co-activator **MKL1** (also called **MAL or MRTFA**) in megakaryopoiesis was highlighted after the identification of t(1;22) translocation leading to the fusion protein between two TFs OTT (RBM15) and MAL (MKL1) in neonate AMKL.[384] MKL1 is associated with G-actin in the cytoplasm of nonactivated cell. After activation of Rho pathway, G-actin is sequestered and MKL1 is translocated to the nucleus. In combination with SRF, it activates components of the cytoskeleton dynamics (*Tpm1, Actb, Flna*) and cellular motility (*Mmp9* and *Myl9*) required for MK migration and platelet biogenesis.[385,386] MKL2, a homologue of MKL1, is also critical for MK maturation and platelet formation. The double *Mkl1/Mkl2* knockout mice have a more extreme thrombocytopenia than mice lacking SRF suggesting that MKL1 and MKL2 have both SRF-dependent and SRF-independent activity in megakaryopoiesis.[63]

Other Transcription Factors

The role of some other TFs in megakaryopoiesis was suggested after identification of their mutations in thrombocytopenia. Radio-ulnar synostosis associated with amegakaryocytic thrombocytopenia (RUSAT) is a rare autosomal dominant inherited thrombocytopenia characterized by severe thrombocytopenia due to an absence or a significant reduction in MKs. It might evolve into aplastic anemia, necessitating bone marrow or umbilical cord stem cell transplantation. Till recently, only the mutation in TF *HOXA11* has been known in RUSAT. Recently, mutations in *MECOM* encoding for the transcriptional regulator protein EVI1 were also identified in the eighth ZF motif in the C-terminal domain.[387] This oligomerization domain is involved in interactions with EVI1 itself and RUNX1.[388] Thus, these mutations might alter not only protein-DNA binding but also protein-protein interactions in transcriptional regulation. In normal human cells, MECOM is expressed in HSCs and plays an important function in hematopoiesis and stem cell self-renewal. High MECOM expression is observed in 3q21q26 syndrome leukemias representing 5%-10% of all cases of AML and characterized by dysmorphic MKs and increased platelet counts. In HEL cells induced to MK differentiation, the enforced EVI1 expression inhibits MK differentiation by blocking endomitosis through downregulation of CDK2. These results suggested that ectopic EVI1 expression contributes to a defective MK differentiation and thus contributes to the phenotype observed in 3q21q26 syndrome leukemia.[389] The potential role of EVI1 in megakaryopoisis was also supported by its recent implication in mechanism leading to thrombocytopenia with absent radii syndrome (TAR). Indeed, in individuals with TAR, EVI1 represses RBM8A gene expression by binding with increased affinity to a site created by a pathogenic variant in the 5′ untranslated region of RBM8A.[63] The TAR patients display low number of MKs in bone marrow with a defect in their maturation.

The role of HOXA11 in megakaryopoiesis is not well understood; however, the HOX protein activity requires interaction with MEIS and PBX homeodomain subfamilies. MEIS1 was shown to be essential for MK development. Inactivation of *Meis1* in mice leads to the lack of MKs and platelets and to the localized defects in vascular patterning that may cause hemorrhages.[390] The complex MEIS1/PBXs (PBX1B and PBX2) was shown to bind to regulatory element TME (tandem repeat of MEIS1 binding element) and interact with GATA-1 and ETS1 in the regulation of megakaryocytic gene expression.[391] Its main target was shown to be FLI1.[392]

More recently, the role IKAROS family in megakaryopoiesis was underlined. Indeed, Helios (IKZF3) was shown to regulate the HSCP multipotency and to repress the MK priming.[393] Germline mutations in *IKZF5* (Pegasus) were reported to cause inherited thrombocytopenia.[394] Ikaros (IKZF1) negatively regulates MK specification, but its concomitant loss with GATA1 inhibits MK maturation.[395,396]

Finally, ZF protein ZNF648 was recently identified to be required for both erythroid and megakaryocytic differentiation.[397]

EPIGENETIC REGULATION OF MEGAKARYOPOIESIS

The promoter activity regulation in the mechanisms leading to cell type–specific gene expression is closely associated with epigenetic modifications leading to the reorganization of the chromatin. Different genes exhibit alternative promoters and a switch in their usage needs to take place during development. As an example, RUNX1 is expressed under two functionally distinct promoters, P1 and P2 resulting in different protein isoforms with different functions. Some P2-derived splice variants lack the transcriptional activation domain and can act in a dominant negative manner that would affect the regulation of RUNX1 target genes.[398] More recently, it was shown that both *Itga2b* and *Mpl* genes encoding, respectively, for CD41 and MPL exhibit also alternative promoters in HSCs and MKs. Itga2b expression is controlled by lineage-specific networks associated with H4K8ac in MKs or H3K27me3 in the multipotential hematopoietic cell line HPC7. The changing patterns of histone modifications are dependent on enzymes including histone acetyl transferases (HAT), HDACs, methylase transferases, and demethylases. During the commitment to MK differentiation, the decrease in H3K27me3 at the *Itga2b* locus is related to the upregulation of H3K27 demethylase Jmjd3. In a similar manner, the *Mpl* expression is also dependent on Jmjd3 expression level. Overall these results clearly demonstrate that the upregulation of the H3K27 demethylase Jmjd3 during megakaryopoiesis participates in the transition in expression of Itga2b and *Mpl* from HSC/HPC to MK.[399]

The CBP/p300 family of HAT interacts with different hematopoietic TFs including PU.1, GATA-1, and GATA-2. The binding of GATA-2 and PU.1 to the *Itga2b* promoter was shown to be limited to the uncommitted cells, while GATA-1, which is specifically upregulated during megakaryopoiesis, can induce cell type–specific histone acetylation including its own acetylation. Therefore, during megakaryopoiesis, changes in the transcriptional network would facilitate histone acetylation and the implementation of the H4K8ac lineage-specific pattern on the *Itga2b* promoter.[399]

We already mentioned that at the bipotent MK/E stage, the KLF1 induces the erythroid lineage commitment, while FLI1 and RUNX1 induce the MK commitment. In a recent work, it was nicely demonstrated that RUNX1 binds to the *KLF1* promoter. This binding increases during MK differentiation and results in the recruitment of co-repressors and in an increase of repressive histone marks. By this mechanism, RUNX1 epigenetically represses KLF1 and increases the proportion of FLI1 thus balancing the switch toward MK lineage.[400]

Whether a TF will act as an activator or repressor depends on the promoter context, its expression level, its posttranslational modifications, and protein-protein interactions. RUNX1 can be modified by several posttranslational modifications such as phosphorylation, acetylation, and methylation. The tyrosine phosphorylation of RUNX1 by Src family kinases negatively regulates activity of RUNX1 in MKs and T lymphocytes.[401] Moreover, the methylation of RUNX1 by the arginine methyltransferase PRMT1 abrogates its association with SIN3A corepressor complex and promotes the transcription of CD41.[402] The SIN3A complex functions as a corepressor by recruiting HDACs. HAT- and HDAC-mediated acetylation/deacetylation modulates the function of histone and nonhistone proteins including TFs (GATA-1, RUNX1),[403] but also act on nonhistone proteins such as the chaperone HSP90, tubulin, and p53. **The HDAC inhibitors** are frequently used in clinics in cancer treatment but with thrombocytopenia as a constant side effect. In the mouse, simultaneous inactivation of *Hdac1* and *Hdac2* induces MK apoptosis and thrombocytopenia.[404] In human setting, the in vitro use of pan-histone deacetylase inhibitor (HDACi) abexinostat inhibits human MK differentiation by inducing progenitor and precursor apoptosis through silencing of some DNA repair genes such as RAD51. This leads, similar to *HDAC1/2* knockout mouse, to the accumulation of DNA double strand breaks and the induction of p53. A p53-independent defect in proplatelet formation was also found.[258] This last effect could be due to the changes in the cytoskeleton mediated by HDAC6 inhibition (see above).

Polycomb repressive complexes 1 and 2 (PRCs 1 and 2) are also involved in the epigenetic regulation of megakaryopoiesis. PRC1 represses the transcription of genes through monoubiquitination at H2AK119 (H2AK119ub1) and PRC2 through trimethylation at H3K27 (H3K27me3). In the canonical pathway, PRC2 initiates gene silencing by catalyzing H3K27me3 modification. PRC1 is then recruited to the target regions by binding to H3K27me3 through the CBX component of PRC1 and catalyzes the monoubiquitination of H2AK119 to maintain gene silencing. However, PRC1 can be recruited independently of H3K27me3. Indeed, Bmi1, a core component of PRC1, binds directly to the Runx1/CBFβ TF complex and a significant chromatin occupancy overlap between the PRC1 core component Ring1b and Runx1/CBFβ, as well as functional regulation of a fraction of commonly bound genes, was demonstrated in MK cells. These findings indicate that Runx1 and CBFβ contribute to direct PRC1 recruitment at some sites in MKs, independently of PRC2.[405] *Bmi1* knockout in mice induces abnormal megakaryopoiesis accompanied by marked extramedullary hematopoiesis resulting in lethal myelofibrosis. This phenotype was linked to the derepression of some genes including the oncogene Hmga2 that is overexpressed in primary myelofibrosis (PMF).[406]

PRC2 complex contains the core components EZH2, SUZ12, JARID2, and EED and is implicated in stem cell maintenance and lymphocyte homeostasis. It catalyzes the methylation of histone 3 at lysine 27 (H3K27me). Inactivating mutations in *EZH2* and other PRC2 members are found in up to 10% of MPNs and more particularly in PMF. The PRC2-related gene ASXL1 is also frequently mutated in patients with PMF suggesting that EZH2 and ASXL1 could be involved in the regulation of megakaryopoiesis. Interestingly, *Ezh2* knockout leads to thrombocytosis in adult mice, and to a deep defect in erythropoiesis in fetal liver, suggesting differential roles of PRC2 during ontogenesis.[407] EZH2 regulates the MK polyploidization by directly inhibiting p21^{cip1} expression and indirectly the expression of p19^{INK4D}. In addition, it regulates the actin cytoskeleton and proplatelet formation.[408] ASXL1 plays an important role in the recruitment (via its interaction with EZH2) and/or the stability of PRC2 and is also associated with BAP1 protein to form a polycomb deubiquitinase complex that removes monoubiquitin from histone H2A lysine 119 (H2AK119Ub). Hematopoietic-specific *Asxl1* knockout in mice leads to progressive, multilineage cytopenias and dysplasia with increased numbers of HSC/progenitors.[409] ASXL1 loss/decrease also hampers erythroid development, while its role in megakaryopoiesis remains to be defined.[410] *Asxl2* knockout induces a thrombocytopenia in mouse with a defect in MK lineage. A possible mechanism is the coregulation of a set of genes with RUNX1.[411] Interestingly, thrombocytopenia with giant platelets and myeloid transformation are detected in *Bap1* knockout mice.[412]

Mutations have been identified in genes of epigenetic regulators such as DNA methylation regulators (*TET2, DNMT3A*) and splicing factors (*SF3B1, SRSF2, U2AF1*) in MPNs including PMF, suggesting their role in the control of MK differentiation. TET2 is the enzyme catalyzing active demethylation through oxidation of 5mC into 5hmC and loss-of-function mutations are found in MPNs. The *Tet2* knockout in mice leads to a phenotypic and functional amplification and a competitive advantage of HSC/progenitors and to the alteration of several mature hematopoietic lineages including the MK lineage as attested by a decreased platelet count.[413] Mild thrombocytopenia is also observed in some mice transplanted with *Dnmt3a*-knockout HSCs predisposing to malignant transformation.[414]

The hematopoietic-specific depletion of *Srsf2* has shown that immature hematopoietic cells are more susceptible to the loss of SRSF2 than the differentiated cell populations. However, a significant decrease in platelet count suggests that SRSF2 could be involved in the regulation of MK differentiation.[415]

As we previously mentioned, RBM15 (OTT) is translocated to MKL1 in AMKL. RBM15 is an RNA-binding protein that binds to pre–messenger RNA intronic regions of MK genes such as *GATA-1, RUNX1, TAL1,* and *MPL*. The binding of RBM15 to specific intronic regions allows the recruitment of SF3B1 to the same sites for alternative splicing. RBM15 expression is regulated by PRMT1 that methylates RBM15 at a residue R578 causing RBM15 degradation via ubiquitylation. Interestingly, overexpression of PRMT1 in AMKL cell lines blocks MK terminal differentiation by downregulation of RBM15 protein level. Thus, PRMT1 may represent a drugable target for the treatment of AMKL. Once RBM15 level is reduced, the alternative spliced isoforms RUNX1a, GATA-1s, and MPL-exon9 will be produced, contributing to the blockage of MK differentiation.[56]

Different stages of megakaryopoiesis are also regulated by different *small noncoding RNAs (microRNAs or miRNAs or miR)* binding to the 3′UTR region of target mRNAs. They modulate protein expression by degrading mRNA or repressing translation.

During MK differentiation, numerous miRNAs are downregulated with a simultaneous upregulation of their target genes necessary for MK differentiation, while other miRNAs are upregulated to silence non-MK genes. They are involved in lineage commitment, in proliferation or in maturation and we focus only on some of them. miR-130A regulates MAFB, a TF that is upregulated during MK differentiation and that synergizes with GATA and ETS to activate transcription from GPIIb promoter upon ERK activation. Downregulation of miR-155 leads to upregulation of ETS1 and MEIS1 and to enhanced MK differentiation[416] and miR-22 promotes MK differentiation through GFI1 repression.[417] Other downregulated miRNAs such as miR-101, miR-20, let-7D, miR-181C, and B miR-17 are putative regulators of RUNX1[418] and a regulatory loop between miR-27A and RUNX1 was shown in the erythroid/megakaryocytic lineage determination.[419] The commitment of MEP toward MK lineage is also enhanced by the reduction of MYB expression that is controlled by three different miRs, miR-150,[366] miR34A,[420] and miR-105.[421]

TPO/MPL signaling is also regulated by different miRNAs. Both MPL and MAPK1 (MEK/ERK pathway) are regulated by miR28A and aberrant miR28A overexpression may contribute to MPL downregulation in some PV and PMF patients.[422] In PMF, the overexpression of miR-155-5p and the resulting downregulation of JARID2 were also shown to potentially contribute to MK hyperplasia.[423]

miRs are also involved in MK ploidization. MCM7 is a member of Minichromosome maintenance protein complex required for initiation of DNA replication. During MK endomitosis, the expression of MCM7 and its intronic miR-106b-25 cluster was found to be uncoupled; downregulation of MCM7 simultaneously with increased expression of miR-106b-25 cluster was detected in polyploid MK.[424] A cell cycle negative regulator p19^{INK4D} that is responsible for the arrest of endomitosis was shown to be directly regulated by miR-125B[425] and more recently, a repression of the TF ARID3A by the same miR was shown be to a crucial event in megakaryoblastic leukemia (AMKL) pathogenesis.[426]

Other miRNAs are involved in MK maturation: overexpression of miR-25 promotes megakaryopoiesis by inhibiting PTEN[424]; genetic ablation of miR-142 causes impaired MK maturation, inhibition of polyploidization, abnormal proplatelet formation, and thrombocytopenia due to disorganized actin filament homeostasis[427]; and inhibition of miR-146A transcription by PLZF results in an increased CXCR4 level.[428] Recently, let-7B was shown to regulate mitochondrial biogenesis during MK ontogenesis through Wnt.[429]

Finally, drastic decrease in the miR-10A and -10B levels in the late stage of megakaryopoiesis is required to allow the expression of human GPIα and the formation of the GPIb-IX-V complex.[430]

In contrast, very few are known on the role of the **long noncoding RNAs (lncRNAs)** expressed during megakaryopoiesis, but most of them are transcribed from conventional gene promoters by GATA-1, GATA-2, FLI1, and TAL.[431] The antisense RBM15 lncRNA increases the translation of RBM15, a protein that plays an important role in normal and leukemic megakaryopoiesis (see above).[432]

CYTOKINE REGULATION OF MEGAKARYOPOIESIS AND SIGNALING

The regulation of megakaryopoiesis is dominated by TPO and the cascade of signaling is induced by its receptor MPL and initiated by JAK2. TPO can be considered as important for the MK lineage as erythropoietin (EPO) is for the erythroid lineage. However, a significant production of platelets is TPO independent in the mouse. In contrast, platelet production is completely dependent of the TPO/MPL/JAK2 in the human setting explaining that defects in this axis are implicated in both inherited and acquired disorders of platelet production (thrombocytopenia or thrombocytosis). Many other cytokines can act on the MK lineage, but mainly synergize with TPO (*Figure 17.2B*).

The Thrombopoietin/Myeloproliferative Leukemia Axis
Thrombopoietin and Its Identification

Since 1958, the existence of a hormonal factor regulating the platelet production has been postulated to be present in the serum in cases of thrombocytopenia, following the model of regulation of erythropoiesis by EPO.[433] All the attempts to purify this factor from the sera of thrombocytopenic animals failed. In addition, studies of the formation of MK colonies in vitro suggested the existence of two types of factors: the first was called MK-CSF and the second synergistic or potentiator factor. It was believed that MK-CSF was not a unique cytokine, but several cytokines such as IL-3 and the synergistic factor

were thought to correspond to TPO as it was defined in vivo.[434,435] As cytokines of the IL-6 family (IL-6, IL-11, LIF) also behave as synergistic factors, it was uncertain whether TPO really exists.[436,437] A major advance on the road to TPO was the discovery of *v-mpl*. F. Wendling et al isolated a new replication defective retrovirus, which induces a lethal myeloproliferative disease in the mouse.[438] The genome of this virus contains an oncogenic sequence *v–mpl* in phase (same open reading frame) with the virus envelope sequence. This fusion protein harbors the sequence of *v-mpl* sharing a homology with an hematopoietic cytokine receptor truncated in its extracellular domain.[439] The proto-oncogene (*c-mpl*) was cloned and its sequence confirmed that it belongs to the hematopoietic cytokine family with a duplication of the cytokine receptor module. Therefore, the *c-mpl* product called Mpl was an orphan hematopoietic cytokine receptor. Further studies demonstrate that *MPL* was mainly expressed in human MKs and platelets. By using an antisense strategy, it was demonstrated that *MPL* knockdown induces an inhibition of MK colony formation by aplastic sera (a presumed source of TPO).[440] Thus, it was hypothesized that the ligand of MPL was the putative TPO. Two teams using MPL as a bait purified its ligand from sera of irradiated animals.[441,442] Another team used a more complex strategy by expressing MPL in a factor–dependent cell line, treating these cells by a mutagenic agent, and factor-independent clones through an autocrine loop were isolated and the *TPO* cDNA was cloned by a functional strategy.[443] The MPL ligand was subsequently called TPO by most teams when it was established that it regulates MK differentiation in *vitro* and platelet production in vivo and MPL was renamed TPO-R by some authors for simplification.

The gene encoding for TPO, now called *THPO*, was mapped to human chromosome 3q2. It contains 6 exons and encodes for a peptide of 332 amino acids excluding a 21 amino acid peptide signal with a 36-kD molecular weight.[444] The recombinant and natural TPO is a 60 to 70 kD protein due to several sites of N- and O-glycosylations.[445]

The protein contains two domains: the N-terminal domain also called the cytokine domain (153 amino acids) binds to MPL and exhibits homology with EPO (20% of identical amino acids and 25% conservative substitution), both having four α helices (A-D) organized in two antiparallel helical pairs and four conserved cysteines in the N-terminal domains, which are important for TPO bioactivity.[446,447] A similar organization is found for EPO. However, there is no cross-binding of EPO to MPL or TPO to EPO-R. The C-terminal domain (179 amino acids) is very specific to TPO. It is heavily N- and O-glycosylated permitting to increase the half-life of the molecule in circulation and also to facilitate secretion.[448] The function analysis of TPO structure has shown that interaction of TPO with MPL is dependent on helix A and helix D.[449] Interestingly, certain residues such as R10 may be involved not in receptor binding, but in receptor activation.

TPO is mainly synthesized by the liver. Its transcript is detected in many other organs and cells such as the kidney, smooth muscle, stromal cells, and also MKs,[450] but the protein is nearly exclusively present in the liver.[277] Thus, overall as EPO, TPO behaves essentially as an hormone.

Thrombopoietin and Its Biological Effects

Before its cloning, it was suggested that TPO was a growth factor only regulating late stages of megakaryopoiesis including polyploidization, cell size, and platelet formation.[433,445] The great surprise was that the recombinant TPO acts on all stages of megakaryopoiesis, except proplatelet formation, but including progenitors[445] (*Figure 17.2B*). Furthermore TPO is also a main regulator of HSC, more particularly of LT-HSC by inducing their quiescence and stimulating DNA repair.[445]

In vitro the recombinant TPO induces the formation of MK colonies from MK-Ps, even from purified progenitors.[451-453] However this response does not reach a maximal efficiency and an optimal growth requires addition of other cytokines such as the SCF.[454] TPO increases MK polyploidization and improves their differentiation with a more developed DMS and a well distribution of the α-granules in the cytoplasm.[203,453,455] This leads to a marked improvement in the number of MKs forming proplatelets.[452,456] However, this late stage is TPO independent because TPO-starved mature MKs are capable to form proplatelets.[452,457] In human, TPO is not indispensable for in vitro MK differentiation because cocktails of cytokines such as SCF, IL-3, and IL-6 give a very similar growth and differentiation of purified CD41+ progenitors, but are less effective for proplatelet formation.[452] This implies that TPO is the only cytokine, which allows a complete MK maturation.[455] *Thpo* as well as *Mpl* knockout results in thrombocytopenia without altering other blood cells; nevertheless, this thrombocytopenia is not extremely profound (15% of the normal platelet count) and is not lethal.[458-460] This TPO-independent platelet production has been the subject of numerous investigations.[461,462] There is some evidence that in *Thpo*[-/-] mice the platelet level is corrected by the combination of SDF1/CXCL12 and bFGF and this is related to the relocalization of MKs to the vascular bone marrow niche allowing an efficient thrombopoiesis.[224] This raises the possibility that the bone marrow environment through cell-cell and cell-ECM interaction was responsible of the TPO-independent platelet production.

The most surprising result was that *Thpo*[-/-] and *Mpl*[-/-] mice have a 10-fold decrease in HSC and in immature progenitors (see in more detailed the paragraph on MPL).[463-466] When transplantation of normal bone marrow cells was performed into *Thpo*[-/-] recipient mice, 10- to 20-fold decrease in the expansion of HSC was observed.[460,463] In addition, TPO acts directly in vitro on HSC and immature progenitors.[467] This means that TPO is one of the major regulators of HSC in the mouse.[468] This was confirmed in humans when it was demonstrated that congenital amegakaryocytic thrombocytopenia (CAMT), an inherited disease characterized by profound thrombocytopenia and progressing to aplastic anemia, was due to loss-of-function mutations of both *MPL* alleles[469,470] and more recently with the discovery in patients with aplastic anemia of a germline *THPO* mutation that generates a new cysteine, which is predicted to inhibit TPO binding to MPL.[65] Patients with such a heterozygous mutation had a mild thrombocytopenia, whereas patients with a homozygous mutation display an aplastic anemia.[65]

The role of TPO on the functions of platelets that naturally express MPL is not well determined. TPO does not significantly modify platelet lifespan.[471] *In vivo*, the effects on platelet function are moderate and it has been suggested that TPO primes platelets and favors platelet adhesion to vWF.[472,473] The *BCR-ABL1*-negative MPNs are associated with a marked increased risk in thrombosis. All *BCR-ABL1*-negative MPNs lead to a slight constitutive activation of the MPL signaling and a TPO hypersensitivity.[474] However, presently there is no evidence that platelets play an important role in the increased thrombosis risk.[475,476]

MPL: Structure/Function

MPL, the TPO receptor, is a homodimeric type I cytokine receptor with homology with EPO-R and G-CSF-R[477,478] (*Figure 17.5*). In humans, the gene is located on 1p34 and contains 12 exons.[479] There are four different transcripts (*MPL-P, MPL-K, MPL-Tr,* and *MPL-Del*). The predominant form is *MPL-P*. The role of the other different forms is controversial although *MPL-K* and *MPL-Tr* behave as dominant-negative forms and *MPL-Del* is implicated in a different signaling.[480-482] *OTT* (*RBM15*), a gene present in the OTT-MAL fusion responsible of some pediatric AMKL, regulates *MPL* splicing.[384,483] The protein resulting from *MPL-P*, subsequently called MPL, is an N-glycosylated protein with four sites of glycosylation. It has an 85 to 92 kD molecular weight with an extracellular domain of 490 amino acids, a transmembrane domain of 22 amino acids with a single membrane spanning helix, and an intracytoplasmic domain of 122 amino acids that is noncovalently associated with one of two members of the JAK family, JAK2 or TYK2.[484] A MPL homodimer binds one TPO molecule. Introduction of a cystein residue in a conserved extracellular dimer interface domain leads to the formation of a constitutively active covalent disulfide bonded dimer,[485] similar to the R129C activating mutation of EPO-R.[486] The precise structure of MPL is currently unknown, due to the absence of X-ray structure of the TPO/MPL complex. For other cytokine receptors, it has been possible to determine the amino acids implicated in ligand binding by mutagenesis. Such an approach has been performed for MPL and has shown that the amino acids implicated in TPO binding include F104, found mutated in rare cases of CAMT,[487] and other residues located in proximity to F104 such as F45, L103, and L257.[60]

As in other type I cytokine receptors, the minimum functional region in the intracellular domain contains three regions: a switch region with an hydrophobic motif necessary for signaling, a Box 1 characterized by a proline-rich motif (PXXPXP) that is the site for JAK2 (or TYK2) binding, and a Box 2 required for maximum growth and also involved in JAK2 binding.[488-491]

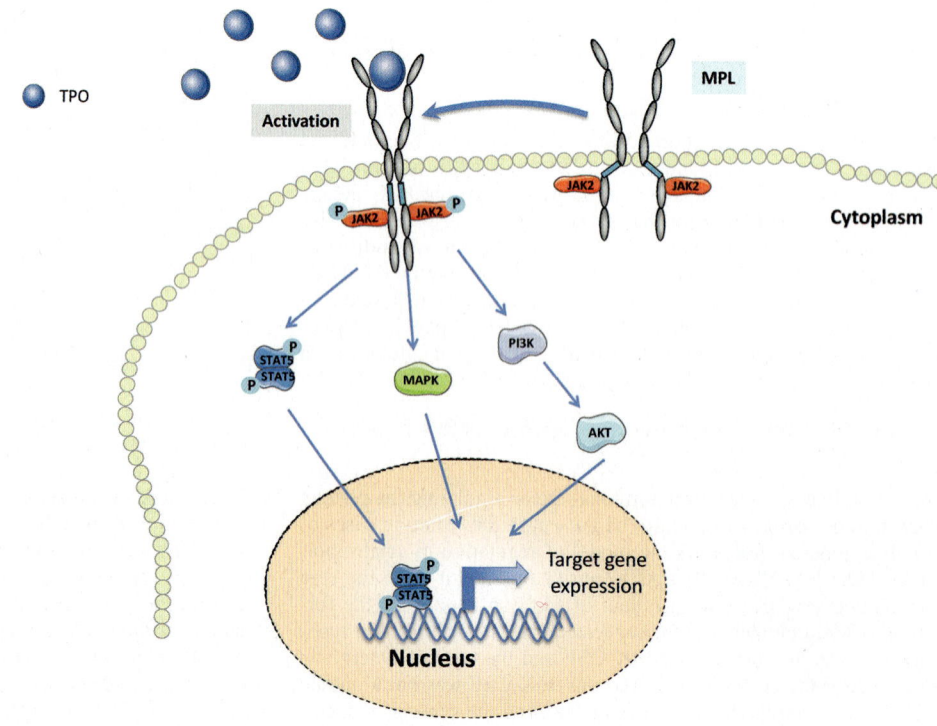

FIGURE 17.5 Schematic illustration of MPL activation by TPO and the downstream signaling.

On the other hand, MPL has two unique properties in comparison to other cytokine receptors:

- The extracellular domain is duplicated, with two cytokine receptor homology module (CRMs) with a D1-D2, D3-D4 structure, and the distal CRM binds TPO.[492] Furthermore, deletion of the membrane-distal domain causes constitutive activation.[493]
- Following the transmembrane domain, there is an amphipathic domain of 5 amino acids (RWQFP) that prevents dimerization of the receptor in the absence of ligand.[494] All substitutions of W515, except W515C and W515P, lead to the activation of MPL in the absence of TPO and activate JAK2.[495,496] In MPNs, a somatic mutation on W515, usually W515L or W515K, is found in 3% to 5% of ET or PMF.[23,474,497]

It has been shown that EPO-R is a preformed homodimeric receptor that contacts JAK2 intracellularly and is exposed at the cell surface as an inactive homodimer to be activated by EPO through conformation changes[486,498,499] although a recent study suggests that it dimerization is induced by EPO.[500] MPL is mainly present on the cell surface as a monomer, probably in a monomer-dimer equilibrium.[495,501] TPO binding leads to the formation of dimers and activates MPL by triggering conformational changes in the extracellular domain.[502,503] This allows modifications of the transmembrane helix favoring active dimerization and conformational changes in the intracellular domain of MPL, which leads to JAK2 activation. In contrast to EPO-R,[504] MPL can be activated under several conformation interfaces.[502,503] Human and mouse MPL differ by several amino acids. Among them, histidine H499 located in the transmembrane region is involved in binding of the small molecule eltrombopag and prevents an active dimerization of the receptor that may be induced by mutations to asparagine (N).[505] However, the S505N mutation found in both inherited thrombocytosis (germline) and in ET (somatic mutation)[24,25,506] induces an active dimerization of the human receptor, even in presence of H499.[46]

MPL: Expression and Function

MPL is expressed by all MK cells from progenitors to platelets.[507] The presence of MPL on the platelet membrane plays a central role in TPO clearance.[508-511] However, MPL is expressed on other hematopoietic cells such as HSCs and immature progenitors of all myeloid lineages.[512] It has to be underscored that the precise study of MPL expression on human cells has been hampered until recently due to the absence of specific antibodies.[513] MPL has also been identified on endothelial cells, hepatocytes, and colon cancer–initiating cells.[514-516]

The phenotype of the constitutive *Mpl* knockout mice phenocopies that of *Thpo* knockout, the only differences being that *Mpl*$^{+/-}$ mice have a slight increase in platelets.[458,459,517] As with *Tpo*$^{-/-}$ mice, a marked decrease in the HSC and immature progenitors (around 5-10-fold decrease) is present in *Mpl*$^{-/-}$ mice with a marked loss of reconstitution capacity.[463] There is evidence that TPO is synthesized in the bone marrow niche by osteoblasts, but also by MKs themselves.[276] It is strongly suggested that, in this environment, TPO induces HSC quiescence. Indeed, *Mpl* knockout HSCs are cycling due to the downregulation of the two CDKi p57^{KIP2} and p19^{INK4D}.[465,466] This effect of TPO may be direct, but also indirect by increasing the interaction of the HSC with the niche through the β1-integrin.[465] However, in transplantation assays, TPO induces a proliferation of LT-HSCs and not their quiescence.[518,519] Thus, TPO exerts two opposite effects on HSCs. It has been suggested that the effect on quiescence is restricted to the most primitive HSCs and the proliferative effects to the other HSCs and immature progenitors.[464] Such regulation would prevent HSC exhaustion in case of high TPO level due to a thrombocytopenia.[464] An alternative hypothesis is that at low dose, TPO will induce a quiescence and at a high dose a proliferative effect through self-renewal mitosis in the HSC compartment.[520] An opposite dose effect of TPO has been observed in cells (cell lines or MKs) expressing high level of JAK2 and MPL, with a proliferative effect at low dose and antiproliferative effect leading to cell cycle arrest and senescence at high dose.[521-523] In addition, TPO is able to induce a rapid commitment of HSC toward the MK lineage by a metabolic reprogramming with highly active mitochondria.[524]

There is evidence that the effects of TPO/MPL on HSC are partially mediated by the HOX genes. In cell lines, TPO induces *HOXB4*, a gene involved in the self-renewal of HSCs as well as an increase in the *MEIS 1* transcript (see above).[525] TPO signaling also induces the nuclear localization of HOXA9.[526] The TPO/MPL axis is involved in the survival of HSCs by regulating Bcl-X$_L$ and MCL-1.[527] Furthermore, TPO/MPL regulates DNA repair of HSC through the DNA-PK–dependent non–homologous end-joining (NHEJ) pathway.[528]

Overall, the defect in HSCs in *Thpo*$^{-/-}$ and *Mpl*$^{-/-}$ mice is quite similar to that of JAK2- or STAT5-deficient mice, suggesting that most effects are mediated through JAK2/STAT5 signaling[529,530] although the effects of TPO on NHEJ DNA repair are mediated by the MAPK/ERK and NFκB pathways.[531]

TPO/MPL axis is a regulator of adult HSCs. However, there is evidence that this axis does not play a major role in the emergence of HSC in the embryo.[532] The TPO/MPL axis amplifies LT-HSCs in the fetal liver, but is dispensable for the hematopoiesis of the fetus.[463]

Intracellular Trafficking of MPL

MPL is synthesized in the ER and associates with JAK2 and TYK2 that behave as chaperones by preventing the mature protein from being degraded by the proteasome (*Figure 17.6*). This chaperone function is independent of the kinase activity as it is mediated by the N-terminal FERM domains of JAK2 or TYK2 in a similar manner as for EPO-R.[491,533] The form present in the ER is N-glycosylated on the four extracellular asparagines and can be detected as high mannose N-glycosylation that is sensitive to endoglycosidase H.[534] The complex oligosaccharide glycosylation takes place in the Golgi apparatus. In the ER, calreticulin is a chaperone of MPL, controlling its proper folding and allowing its trafficking to the Golgi. Calreticulin and calnexin are likely binding to the 4 N-glycosylation residues located in the extracellular domain.[535] Then, MPL follows the canonical secretory pathway to traffic to the cell membrane (*Figure 17.6*). Recently, an alternative pathway has been described by which the immature form of MPL traffics to the cell surface from the ER by the autophagosome pathway, thus avoiding the Golgi processing enzymes.

After binding to TPO, MPL is internalized via a clathrin-dependent endocytosis pathway. MPL can be recycled back to the cell surface[523,536] and a fraction is degraded via the proteasome and lysosome pathways[536] (*Figure 17.6*). A knockout of *Dnm2* (dynamin 2 encoding gene), a GTPase related to the clathrin pathway, in the MK/platelet lineage leads to a profound macrothrombocytopenia and a myelofibrosis. This arises from defects in MK differentiation, more particularly of DMS development, but also in MPL endocytosis leading to high TPO plasma level and a constitutive JAK2 activation.[537] Casitas B-lineage lymphoma (CBL) proto oncogene through binding to SHP2 can ubiquitinate MPL on the lysines (K) 553 and 573 and induce the degradation of MPL by the proteasome.[538] In addition, the motif Y$_8$RRL in the intracellular domain allows a lysosome-mediated degradation. Thus, Y521 (Y8) can promote MPL degradation through the lysosomal pathway.[539] Y591 (Y78) is a negative regulator of MPL by promoting the endocytosis of the receptor via the AP2 complex and decreasing signaling via the MAPK/ERK pathway.[540]

The MPL recycling does not seem to occur in platelets or, if it does, it must occur at low level.

The MPL intracellular trafficking plays a central role in the regulation of the platelet production, as we will see further, by regulating the level of plasma TPO, but also of signaling. A defect of MPL trafficking has been observed in numerous inherited or acquired disorders:

- In CAMT, most missense mutations lead to a defect in MPL trafficking to the cell membrane with a complete blockage in the ER for the most frequent mutation R102P.[60,61,541] Interestingly, a partial blockage of MPL P106L or MPL K39N in the ER leads to a paradoxical thrombocytosis.[47,48,61,541] This is due to the dual function of MPL in signaling and in TPO clearance (see next chapter), two functions that do not require the same amounts of membrane MPL; much less MPL is required for signaling, especially in early progenitors.[541]

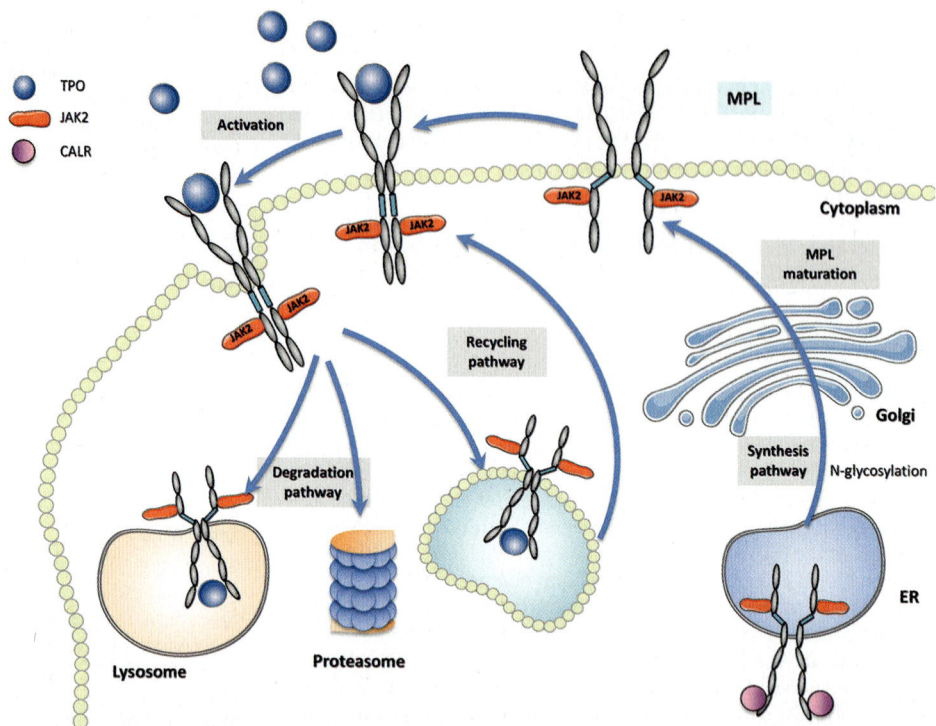

FIGURE 17.6 Schematic illustration of MPL trafficking.

- In MPNs, JAK2V617F induces a downregulation of MPL plasma membrane localization by several mechanisms including decreased chaperone activity and recycling together with increased proteasome activation.[523] In platelets and cell lines, an excess of the immature form is detected.[49,50] Initially, it was suggested that the increased immature form was due to a blockage in the ER, but it could also be due to trafficking through the autophagosome pathway.[542] In around 30% of ET and PMF, acquired mutations of *CALR* are present and all of them are located in the exon 9 leading to a +1 frameshift and the synthesis of a new C-terminal peptide positively charged and devoid of the ER retention signal KDEL.[21,22] This mutated calreticulin binds to MPL, specifically to the extracellular MPL region around N117 and behaves as an abnormal chaperone inducing the migration of the immature form of MPL from the ER to the plasma membrane where it activates MPL by dimerization.[535,543-545]
- In addition, in triple-negative ET, rare mutations at cytosolic Y591 can be found leading to an increased level of MPL on the membrane.[26,27] Finally, loss-of-function mutations of *CBL* that may induce a decrease in the degradation of MPL and other cytokine receptors have been found in several types of myeloid malignancies.[28,546]

Regulation of Thrombopoietin Plasma Level

The normal TPO levels in the plasma are below 30 pg/mL and 1000 pg/mL in human and mouse, respectively. The plasma level of TPO is inversely correlated with the number of platelets, with some exceptions in pathology.[547,548] This increased level of TPO in thrombocytopenia is essentially observed when the defect is due to a decrease of MKs in the bone marrow, like it is the case in aplastic anemia or CAMT, reaching levels above 2 ng/mL. The TPO level is extremely high in *Mpl*$^{-/-}$ mice as in CAMT in human.[458,549,550]

It was initially thought that TPO synthesis in the liver was regulated by the platelet mass through a sensor (*Figure 17.7*). This was based on the model of erythropoiesis where the synthesis of EPO is regulated by kidney hypoxia. However, no increase in the *THPO* transcripts both in the liver or kidney was observed in animals rendered thrombocytopenic either by irradiation, chemotherapy, or antiplatelet antibodies.[510,551] An increase in *THPO* transcripts has been detected in the stroma in case of thrombocytopenia in mouse and in human, with a correlation between the level of transcripts and the TPO plasma level.[552,553] The TPO of liver origin may represent more than 60% of the synthesized TPO,[450] and in steady state regulates the platelet level as well as the HSC quiescence.[277] However, the precise contribution of the stroma-derived TPO in stress conditions remains unknown.

Therefore, it was hypothesized by Kuter and Rosenberg and Fielder et al that the TPO level was mainly regulated by its clearance.[508,509,547,553] Platelets and MKs are the two main cell types to express MPL on the cell surface and to bind TPO. It was shown after TPO binding that platelets and MKs internalize the TPO/MPL complex and degrade TPO.[509] Therefore, the TPO plasma level is regulated in normal and pathologic conditions by the platelet/MK mass, but more specifically by the level of MPL expressed on platelet and MK cell surface (*Figure 17.7*). The MPL level present on endothelial cells does not participate in the TPO clearance.[554]

In favor of the clearance hypothesis, it was further shown that a partial retroviral rescue of Mpl level in *Mpl*$^{-/-}$ mice induces a thrombocytosis due to high TPO levels.[555] A similar rescue of *Mpl*$^{-/-}$ mice by an Mpl transgene expressed at low level in mature MKs and platelets leads to thrombocytosis, but with normal TPO plasma level probably due to the increased number of MK precursors in the marrow.[556] Furthermore, it was shown that the specific knockout of *Mpl* or *JAK2* during MK differentiation leads to an important thrombocytosis associated with an increased number of MK precursors and MKs, but normal TPO plasma level.[557,558] This normal level of TPO was explained by the increased number of MK precursors expressing MPL and the thrombocytosis by the fact that late stages of MK differentiation could be TPO independent. An alternative hypothesis is that the TPO/MPL/JAK2 induces an arrest of proliferation during MK differentiation and its relieve leads to thrombocytosis.[521-523]

These mouse models have been important to understand human pathology. For instance, the two inherited MPL mutations, MPLP106L and MPLK39N, induce a thrombocytosis with high TPO level associated with a low expression of MPL on MKs and platelets.[47,61,541]

Until recently, it was considered that the liver and the kidney were producing constitutive levels of TPO, and the high TPO transcript level associated with a low protein level was thought to be due to an inefficient translation. Indeed, the *THPO* gene has an unusual 5'untranslated structure, which contains several AUG initiation codons. They inhibit the initiation of translation at the eighth AUG sequence located in the third exon.[39] Some splicing mutations release this inhibition and can cause hereditary thrombocytosis resulting from an excess of TPO synthesis[39-41] (*Table 17.1*).

However, there is evidence that in a context of inflammation, IL-6 induces an increase in TPO synthesis in the liver that is in great part responsible for the thrombocytosis of inflammatory diseases.[559,560] More recently Grozovsky et al have demonstrated that the Ashwell-Morell receptor that binds desialylated platelets and remove them from the circulation increases TPO synthesis.[561] Thus, there is a link between the platelet destruction and TPO synthesis because aged platelets are desialylated and their rate of removal increases TPO synthesis by a JAK2/STAT3-dependent mechanism. This molecular mechanism is closely related to the induction of TPO synthesis by IL-6/IL-6 receptor activation of the JAK1/STAT3 pathway[561] (*Figure 17.7*). The mechanism of regulation of TPO synthesis by desialylated platelets must be important to increase platelet production during sepsis or to control the TPO synthesis in homeostasis.[562] Furthermore it has been shown that platelets from MPN have an abnormal expression of the glycan structure β4-N-acetyllactosamine (Galβ1,4GlcNAc) that leads to an increased TPO synthesis contributing to the thrombocytosis.[563]

TPO/MPL and the Signaling Cascade in Megakaryocytes

MPL belongs to the hematopoietic cytokine family and lacks a catalytic domain. The JAK family of kinases plays this role. They are constitutively bound to the cytoplasmic domain of the receptor and become activated through conformational changes of the receptor to induce the signaling cascade.

TYK2 and JAK2 bind to MPL, but only JAK2 is indispensable because TPO does not induce a signaling in *Jak2* knockout cells.[564] However, it is not known whether TYK2 could contribute to the signaling through TYK2/JAK2 heterodimer.

When TPO binds to MPL, it induces the dimerization of the receptor and conformation changes of the dimer by modifying the rotation of the transmembrane helix leading to an activation of JAK2 probably by transphosphorylation.[494,503]

Janus Kinase 2

JAK2 is associated with three "myeloid" homodimeric type I receptors (EPO-R, G-CSF-R, and MPL) and as all the other members of the JAK family contains two kinase domains, one catalytically active at the C-terminus, and one catalytically inactive or very weakly active that precedes the kinase domain called the pseudokinase domain.[565,566] The pseudokinase domain has important structural roles in regulating cytokine-dependent activation and in preventing self-activation of the kinase domain. At the N-terminus, JAKs possess a FERM-like domain (homologous to protein four point one, ezrin, radixin, moesin) that binds to Box 1 and a Src Homology 2 (SH2)-like domain, which may bind to Box 2 of MPL.[445,567]

*JAK2*V617F is the predominant mutation in *BCR-ABL1*-negative MPNs and is associated with three diseases: polycythemia vera (>92% of cases), essential thrombocythemia (60% of the cases), and PMF (60% of the cases). PV is essentially a disease of the erythroid lineage, and ET and PMF of the MK lineages.[28,568] This single mutation gives rise to several phenotypes because it abnormally activates more or less the three myeloid receptors; among them, MPL plays a central role in the pathogenesis.[569] *JAK2*V617F is a mutation in the pseudokinase domain, which on one hand relieves the pseudokinase inhibitory function on the kinase domain and on the other hand changes the conformation of the pseudokinase domain and induces activation of the kinase domain via a specific circuit involving conserved phenylalanines, the SH2-JH2 linker, and the kinase domain.[570] Thus, JAK2V617F behaves as a preactivated JAK2.[571]

Other mutations affecting the platelet production are found in inherited thrombocytosis. These mutations are usually located in the pseudokinase domain, but can also affect the kinase domain.[42-45]

When activated, JAK2 phosphorylates the five tyrosines (Y) in the intracellular domain of MPL (Y521, Y542, Y591, Y626, and Y631).[540,572] Y521 (Y8) and Y591 (Y78) are negative regulators as previously seen.[539,540] In contrast, Y626 (Y112) and Y631 (Y117) are positive regulator sites. Y626 is the most important tyrosine for signaling including for oncogenic mutant MPL[573] and is essential for the recruitment of the SHC adaptor to activate the RAS/MAPK pathway, STAT5, STAT3, and probably STAT1, but also SHIP, GRB2, SOS, VAV, and CBL.[572]

STATS

After binding to MPL, the different STATs are phosphorylated by JAK2.[574] Tyrosine phosphorylation of STATs is essential for their parallel dimerization, which is based on the affinity that the SH2 domain of one STAT exerts for the phosphorylated tyrosine residue in the C-terminal transactivation domain of another STAT.[575] These dimers bind to sites on both strands of DNA. Importantly, after being regulated by phosphorylated STATs, some promoters require binding of unphosphorylated STATs (U-STATs) for maintaining high levels of transcription for longer time.[576] STAT5 and STAT1 appear to be the

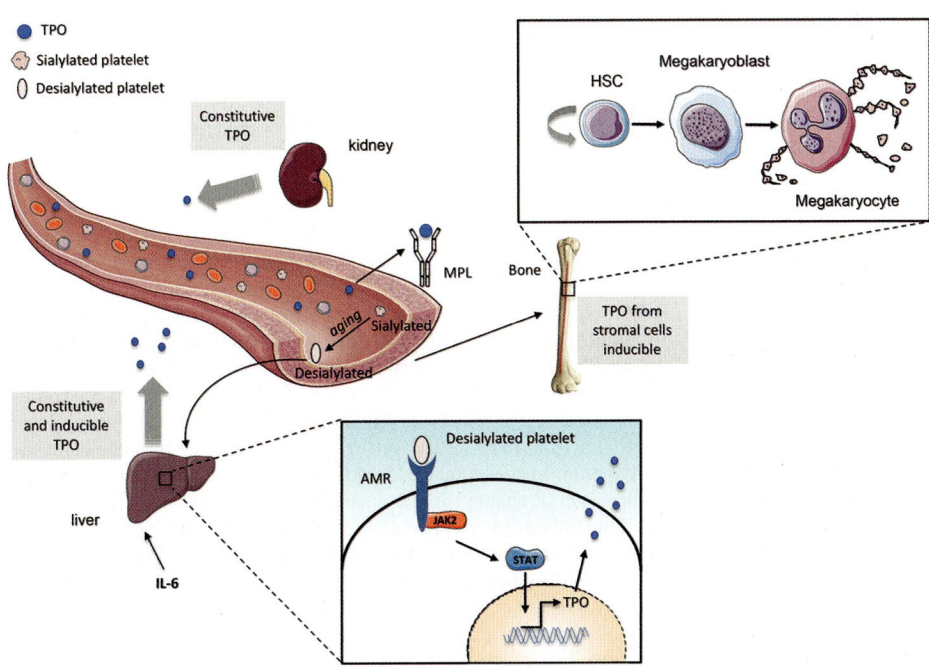

FIGURE 17.7 Regulation of plasma TPO level by synthesis and clearance.

The Normal Hematologic System

most important STATs for MK differentiation.[577] Phospho-STAT5A/B regulates numerous genes involved in survival, proliferation, or signaling, such as *BCL-X$_L$, cyclins D, PIM1,* and *SOCS*, but not genes involved in differentiation.[577] This model has been recently challenged by showing that U-STAT5 colocalizes with major MK TFs and acts as a repressor of the MK differentiation program suggesting that U-STAT5 is actively regulating cell fate and is not only acting after specific STAT5 activation. In this model, TPO induces the phosphorylation and the activation of STAT5 delocalizes the binding of U-STAT5 from MK promoters to release their inhibition allowing the induction of a MK differentiation program.[578]

The important role of STAT5 on megakaryopoiesis has been demonstrated by genetic studies. Mice deficient in Stat5A and B are thrombocytopenic[577] and a STAT5 deficiency inhibits the development of thrombocytosis by JAK2V617F or CALR mutant in mice.[579,580] STAT1 seems also to favor the MK differentiation[581] and has been described to act downstream of GATA-1 favoring polyploidization.[582] The role of STAT3 is more controversial[583] and recent studies suggest that it operates more as a brake in the MK differentiation.[584] Its deficiency in the *JAK2*V617F mouse model increases thrombocytosis.[584]

The PI3K Pathway

The PI3K pathway is the second pathway induced by TPO and by many other cytokines that play an important role in megakaryopoiesis. PI3K is a heterodimeric lipid kinase composed of a 110-kD kinase subunit (p110) and an 85-kD (p85) regulatory subunit. P85 does not interact directly with MPL.[585] Therefore, MPL activates the PI3K through a complex that includes the SHP2 phosphatase, the scaffold protein GAB/IRS, and p85 leading to tyrosine phosphorylation of p85.[585,586] An alternative pathway involves the binding of tensin 2 on Y631 of MPL, its phosphorylation by JAK2 to recruit the p85 subunit.[587]

When activated, the p110 subunit of PI3K catalyzes the formation of the membrane phospholipid PIP3 that recruits proteins with a pleckstrin homology (PH) domain such as PDK-1 or AKT. PDK-1 phosphorylates and partially activates important substrates, including AKT, ribosomal protein p70S6 kinase, and PKC. Phospho-AKT plays a central role by inducing cell survival, and the entry in cell cycle, by inhibiting the TF FOXO3a through its sequestration in the cytoplasm, and by inducing degradation of BAD and inhibition of GSK-3β.[588] More particularly, TPO promotes downregulation of p27 in MKs through a PI3K/AKT/FOXO3a pathway.[589]

Downstream of AKT, the serine-threonine kinase mTOR (mTORC1) plays an important role in regulating proliferation, cell size, ploidy, and late differentiation including proplatelet formation by activating p70S6K and eukaryotic translation initiation factor 4E-binding protein.[590-592] mTOR signaling is more activated in MKs derived from cord blood cells than from adult CD34$^+$ cells.[135] In addition, the mTOR pathway plays an important role in aging and autophagy. The increased ROS production during aging in mice induces the mTOR pathway leading to an increase in the size of MKs and in the mean platelet volume, as well as in platelet activation favoring venous thromboembolism.[593] Initially, it was shown that blocking autophagy by a *Let7* knockout in the hematopoietic system impedes MK differentiation.[594] However, when the *Let7* knockout was restricted to the MK lineage, there was no defect in MK differentiation but in platelet activation.[595]

The RAS-RAF-MEK-ERK Pathway

The RAS-RAF-MEK-ERK pathway is also involved in megakaryopoiesis, but its effects are more controversial and/or dependent on the cell models. The adapter molecule SHC is recruited to the P-Y626 of MPL and becomes phosphorylated by JAK2. P-SHC recruits GRB2 that activates RAS *via* the guanine exchange factor SOS. Activated guanosine triphosphate (GTP)-bound RAS activates RAF1 that in turn phosphorylates MEK1/2 that activates the MAPK, ERK1/2.[574,596] However, one characteristic of TPO signaling, compared to all the other cytokines, is the prolonged MAPK activation. In the UT-7 cell line, this sustained activation is dependent on RAP1 and B-RAF.[597] The activated ERK1/2 is translocated to the nucleus

where they phosphorylate several TFs on serine and threonine such as ELK-1, STAT3, and RUNX1.

In cell lines like UT-7 with two (erythroid and MK) lineage potentials, activation of the MAPK pathway induces MK differentiation at the expense of the erythroid differentiation.[598] In mouse primary cells, inhibition of the MAPK pathway with chemical inhibitors leads to an inhibition of MK differentiation, polyploidization, and proplatelet formation, as well as MK migration in a CXCL12/SDF1 gradient.[293,599] However *Raf-1* deficient mice have no defect in megakaryopoiesis.[600] *B-Raf* knockout leads to an embryonic lethality. Thus, its role on MK differentiation was studied using *B-Raf* knockout ES cells presenting a decreased cell proliferation, without significant effect on differentiation.[601] In human, results may depend on the stage of ontogenesis. In the neonate, low doses of inhibitors increase proliferation and inhibit differentiation.[602] In adult, several reports show that inhibition of MAPK favors MK differentiation markedly increasing polyploidization and proplatelet formation.[339,590] Inversely, the use of an active MEK inhibits proplatelet formation.[339] Thus, these results contrast to what has been observed in cell lines and mouse MKs, possibly because these cells express high levels of MPL that might not be relevant in vivo. Furthermore, CXCL12-dependent migration of human MKs relies more on the PI3K pathway than on the MAPK pathway. Unexpectedly, activation of ERK also appears to induce senescence of MK, a phenomenon that might be coupled with differentiation.[521] Indeed, there is evidence that activation of MAPK must be switched off at the end of differentiation to obtain an efficient proplatelet formation in vitro.[339] It was recently shown that the thrombocytopenia associated with *ANKRD26* mutations is the consequence of a sustained MAPK activation during late differentiation.[339]

TPO also activates JNK and p38 in primary MKs. It has been suggested that JNK is involved in the response of MKs to shear force and induces their differentiation.[603] p38 plays an important role by negatively regulating the late stages of megakaryopoiesis. It is inactivated by the dual phosphatase DUSP4. DUSP4 is methylated by PRMT1, a methylation that leads to its ubiquitinylation and its subsequent degradation.[604] An increase in PRMT1 may be responsible of the thrombocytopenia in myelodysplastic syndromes.[604]

Other signaling pathways that are activated by TPO/MPL play important roles in the regulation of megakaryopoiesis, but are regulated at a higher level by other cues such as cell interaction and ECM though integrins.

The SRC Family Kinases and SYK Kinase

Members of Src kinase (SFK) family are usually considered as negative regulators of megakaryopoiesis. MKs and platelets express several SFKs, more particularly FYN, LYN, and SRC, as well as the SYK kinase.[605] FYN and LYN are activated by TPO and FYN expression increases during MK differentiation. LYN binds to Y626 (Y112) of MPL upon activation by TPO and is considered as the most important member of the SFK family implicated in MK differentiation.[606,607] In mouse, pharmacological and genetic inhibition of *Lyn* leads to MKs with an increased ploidy, suggesting a negative regulation of MAPK and AKT pathways by LYN.[606] In addition, there is a link between the activation of LYN by TPO and the focal adhesion kinase (FAK).[608] There is no TPO induction of Lyn phosphorylation in Fak-deficient MKs, confirming that FAK is a regulator of TPO/MPL signaling.[608] Sphingosine 1-phosphate (S1P) plays an important role in the release of proplatelets in the blood stream by guiding MK elongations through the bone marrow sinusoid.[609] In MKs S1P is synthesized by sphingosin kinase 2 (Sphk2) and MKs deficient in *Sphk2* exhibit a loss of SFK function and a defect in the fragmentation of proplatelet in the circulation. In consequence, *Sphk2$^{-/-}$* mice exhibit a mild thrombocytopenia without changes in the other blood cell level.[610]

The induction of proplatelet formation by the αIIbβ3 integrin involved the signaling through SFK and Syk to PLCγ2.[611] Deleting SHP2 in MKs induces a moderate macrothrombocytopenia due to a decrease in the activation of both the RAS-ERK and the SFK/SYK/PLCγ2 signaling pathways. The double knockout of *Shp1* and *Shp2* leads to a more severe macrothrombocytopenia with major defect in

MK maturation and ploidization associated with a poor response to TPO. A similar defect in MK differentiation is observed in the *G6b-B* knockout, suggesting that this immunoreceptor tyrosine-based inhibitory motif (ITIM)-containing receptor, known to interact with Shp1/2, acts upstream to regulate thrombopoiesis.[612,613] In human germline biallelic mutations of *G6b-B* lead to a macrothrombocytopenia with a focal myelofibrosis.[614]

In human, chemical inhibition of SFK leads to an increased cell proliferation associated with a defect in proplatelet formation.[615] It was recently shown that SFK may regulate proplatelet formation by activating N-WASP by phosphorylation.[252] Furthermore, inhibition of SFK induces a defect in MK migration in SDF1/CXCL12 gradient that may be related to an inhibition of podosome formation. It has also been shown that SFK can negatively regulate the transcriptional activity of RUNX1 in MKs through tyrosine phosphorylation.[401] SHP2 dephosphorylates RUNX1 and restores a RUNX1 activity. Additionally, MAPK activates RUNX1 by serine phosphorylation.[401] Thus, SFK may have a double role on megakaryopoiesis: inhibiting early stages through RUNX1 inactivation and favoring the late stages of differentiation by phosphorylating the WASP family. This complex effect may depend on the specific SFK members that are activated in MKs.

A dominant gain-of-function mutation in SRC has been described in a pedigree with an inherited thrombocytopenia and a myelofibrosis. Major defects in MK maturation with a reduction of proplatelet formation and increased podosome formation were observed in these patients. These defects were corrected in vitro by a SRC inhibitor.[91]

Protein Kinase C

The PKC family of serine/threonine kinases can be activated by TPO in a PI3K pathway–dependent manner. The classical PKC, PKCα, inhibits proplatelet formation and polyploidy.[616] An increased ploidy and proplatelet formation was detected in *Prkca-/-* mice. Two new members of this family, PKCε and PKCδ, also regulate megakaryopoiesis.[616] PKCε is downregulated during normal MK differentiation. Overexpression of this kinase isoform inhibits terminal differentiation, more particularly proplatelet formation.[617] In contrast, PKCδ is expressed at a constant level during MK differentiation and PKCδ downregulation inhibits MK differentiation including proplatelet formation.[618] These effects are mediated by changes in the equilibrium between BAD and Bcl-XL or possibly by the phosphorylation of MARCKS.[619]

Negative Regulation of TPO/MPL/JAK2 Signaling

After binding to MPL, the signaling cascade induced by TPO is transient, due to a negative regulation. One major pathway downregulating MPL signaling is the endocytosis of the receptor, as we saw above.

Other mechanisms exist, involving the binding of negative regulators to the phosphorylated MPL or JAK2. As mentioned above, LYN and SYK bind to MPL and behave as negative regulators. However, the main molecules that are directly involved in the downregulation of active MPL are the SOCS proteins, the JAK2 inhibitor LNK, phosphatases that eliminate the p-Y on MPL and JAK2, and other inhibitors of the downstream signal, such as PIAS for the activated STATs and different phosphatases for the MAPK or PI3K pathways. We will focus on the SH2 domain–containing SOCS and LNK proteins that target JAK2 P-Y, more particularly the dityrosine motif found in its activation loop.

SOCS Family

The SOCS family members inhibit JAKs, cytokine receptors, or JAK/cytokine receptor complexes.[620-622] They are involved in a feedback inhibition of cytokine receptor signaling because they are induced by STATs. Three of them, CIS, SOCS1 and SOCS3, are involved in the negative regulation of MPL/JAK2.[620] The inhibition of signaling is complex, but the main mechanism is related to a degradation of the phosphorylated protein (JAK2 or the complex) by the proteasome following ubiquitination. The SOCSs, through their SOCS box, behave as E3 ubiquitin ligases after binding to phosphorylated targets via their SH2 domain. In addition, SOCS3 may directly inhibit JAK2 kinase activity through its kinase inhibitory region. One important characteristic is that the SOCS proteins are involved in a cross-talk between different receptors. For example, interferon (IFN) α induces SOCS1, which can subsequently inhibit the MPL/JAK2 signaling.[623]

In MPNs, the promoters of *SOCS1, 2,* and *3* can be methylated, resulting in an increase in the signaling induced by JAK2, CALR, or MPL mutants.[624,625] However, it has been described that SOCS3 cannot negatively regulate but may eventually increase the JAK2V617F signaling.[626]

LNK

LNK (SH2B3) belongs to a family of three proteins with SH2-B (SH2B1) and APS (SH2B2) that contain three domains including a SH2 domain and a PH domain. In contrast to the other members of this family, LNK specifically inhibits JAK2 and more particularly EPO-R and MPL signaling.[627,628] It binds on p-Y813 of JAK2 located between the pseudokinase and kinase domains. *Lnk-/-* mice develop a myeloproliferative disorder with a thrombocytosis, splenomegaly, and myelofibrosis, but also an excess of B cells.[629] The *Lnk-/-* mice present a MK hyperplasia and an excess of HSCs with increased properties of self-renewal and quiescence,[630] resulting from an increased signaling by TPO/MPL.[627] Inversely, overexpression of LNK inhibits megakaryopoiesis and the activation of STAT3 and MAPK.

Mutations of *LNK* have been initially identified in *JAK2*V617F-negative ET and PMF.[631] These mutations are loss-of-functions mutations on one allele and are often localized in the PH domain. It was suggested that *LNK* mutations were the drivers of MPNs. However, in most cases, somatic *LNK* mutations occur as secondary events in *BCR-ABL*-negative MPNs.[28,632] In addition, some mutations are germline variants that predispose to MPNs[633] or induce erythrocytosis.[634] *JAK2*V617F MPNs are often associated with a downregulation of LNK.[635]

Phosphatases

The main phosphatases that may target JAK2 include SHP1 and SHP2 (PTPN6 and PTPN11, respectively), PTP1B (also known as PTPN1), TCPTP (T-cell protein tyrosine phosphatase, PTPN2), CD45, and indirectly SHIP1. SHP2 plays an important role in TPO signaling not as phosphatase but as a positive regulator of the ERK/MAPK activation by a mechanism, which remains to be determined (see SFK and signaling).[636] A *Ship1* knockout leads to an increase in MK-Ps, but with normal number of MKs that are relocalized in the spleen and a slight decrease in platelet number. Although STAT3, ERK1/2 and AKT phosphorylation were increased, most abnormalities may be related to a defect in CXCR4 signaling.[637]

The TPO/MPL Axis and Therapy

When TPO was cloned, it was immediately assumed that it would have a major clinical interest for increasing platelet production, as EPO for red blood cells, and also for increasing the number of HSCs. The full length TPO was difficult to produce due to its glycan terminal domain although recombinant human TPO produced in CHO cells and the pegylated cytokine domain called *PEG-rHuMGDF* (Amgen) were used in clinical trials. The results were relatively moderate; only a slight shortening of the thrombocytopenic period was observed after chemotherapy. The best and unexpected indication was immune thrombocytopenic purpura (ITP). PEG-MGDF was subsequently used in platelet apheresis donors to increase the platelet yield. Some of them developed neutralizing antibodies cross-reacting with the natural TPO leading to a profound thrombocytopenia and very severe bleeding. All trials with either recombinant TPO or PEG-MGDF were stopped in 2002 before the development of a second generation of less immunogene TPO mimetics.[638]

Two molecules with no homology with TPO and behaving as TPO agonists are now used in clinics.[548,638] *Romiplostim* (Amgen) is composed of 14 amino acids attached to 2 disulfide-bonded human immunoglobulin G1 kappa heavy chain constant regions by glycine bridges.

The romiplostim contains two TPO mimetic peptides that bind to MPL with high affinity on the same site as TPO and activate the receptor. *Eltrombopag* (GlaxoSmithKline and now developed by Novartis) is a member of the biarylhydrazone class, which is rapidly absorbed following oral administration. It binds to MPL at its extracellular juxtamembrane end at residue H499, activating the conformation of the dimer.[505]

Romiplostim and eltrombopag are essentially used in ITP where they increase platelet production stimulating megakaryopoiesis and inhibiting the apoptosis of MKs mediated by antiplatelet antibodies.[639] They are also used in thrombocytopenia and severe liver diseases that are in great part due to a defect in TPO synthesis.[548,638,640] Recently, it has been shown that some aplastic anemia responds to both molecules.[641-643] It is unknown if the aplastic anemia is due to mutations in the *THPO* gene. Clinical trials are being developed in thrombocytopenia of myelodysplastic syndrome (MDS) or chronic myelo-monocytic leukemia (CMML).[644] However, Romiplostim and eltrombopag are not exactly redundant molecules. In ITP, there is no clear cross-resistance between romiplostim and eltrombopag.[645] This may be the consequence of two different mechanisms—the binding of romiplostim to MPL is in competition with endogenous TPO, while it is not the case for eltrombopag. Thus, romiplostim may be less effective if the level of plasma TPO is normal or already high—these two MPL agonists do not induce exactly the same signaling pathways and in vitro eltrombopag promotes proplatelet formation at a higher level than romiplostim.[646]

More recently, *MPL antagonists* have been developed to decrease the signaling in MPNs, more particularly to target HSCs in MPNs. LCP4 is a 20-amino acid cyclic peptide, which was capable to inhibit the effects of TPO on hematopoietic progenitors from PMF.[647] This effect is more pronounced that on progenitors from healthy controls suggesting that such an approach might be efficient in targeting the mutated cells.

Other Cytokines Involved in the Positive or Negative Regulation of Platelet Production

Many other cytokines play a role in vitro, but their precise role in the homeostatic regulation of platelet production is not demonstrated except for the SCF/KIT ligand and SDF1/CXCL12. Inflammatory cytokines may play an important role on platelet production in stress conditions and pathology (*Figure 17.2*). In addition, several negative regulators of MK differentiation are present in α-granules of MKs and platelets.

Positive Regulators

Stem Cell Factor/KIT Ligand

SCF is one of the most important cytokines that regulate hematopoiesis, more particularly for the erythroid and mast cell lineages, but also for HSCs and all immature progenitors. It binds to the tyrosine kinase receptor KIT and activates the PI3K at high level. *In vitro,* SCF is synergistic with numerous cytokines including TPO, to induce MK colony formation and differentiation.[452,454,648,649] KIT is expressed at high level on MK/platelet-biased HSCs and is downregulated during MK differentiation.[650] SCF mainly increases the proliferative effect of TPO and may also enhance the quality of MK maturation induced by TPO. Kit deficiency leads to a decrease in MK production in vivo and in the rebound thrombocytosis after 5-FU treatment in mouse.[651] Mice deficient in SCF also present a thrombocytopenia.[652] However, the thrombocytopenia could be the consequence of a deficiency in immature progenitors and not the result of a direct effect on MK differentiation.

Cytokines of the IL-6 Family

IL-6 was the first cytokine family member with a function in both inflammation and development that was shown to play a role in megakaryopoiesis. This cytokine family binds to heterodimer receptors that use GP130 as signaling chain. GP130 is associated with JAK1 and eventually JAK2 and principally activates STAT3.

The effects of IL-6, LIF, and IL-11 have been studied in details because it was initially suggested that they were important regulators of the homeostatic production of platelets.[653-657] *In vitro*, none of the

cytokines are individually able to induce MK colony formation[658] but they have some synergistic activity with the GM-CSF, IL-3, and SCF. A combination of SCF, IL-3, and IL-6 is as efficient as TPO in inducing the formation of MK colonies.[659] IL-6, LIF, and IL-11 mainly improved MK terminal differentiation in cultures stimulated by GM-CSF or IL-3.[656] For this reason, before identification of TPO, IL-6 and TPO were believed to be the same molecule.[436,437]

IL-11 exerts a more pronounced effect than the other members of the family. IL-11 was tested in clinical trials to correct thrombocytopenia, but had minor effects.[660-662] Furthermore, knockout of the different genes of the IL-6 family and of their cognate receptors did not modify the platelet level in normal or in *Mpl⁻/⁻* mice.[461] Thus, their role to regulate platelet level in vivo is minor. However, they may be responsible of the thrombocytosis observed during inflammation because IL-6 upregulates TPO synthesis in the liver (see above).

Other inflammatory cytokines also play a role in megakaryopoiesis, more particularly IL-1α that increases the number of cytokine receptors on hematopoietic progenitors and acts directly on MKs to induce platelet production by MK rupture (see above). IL-1β may have the same function. TNF alpha also induces MK differentiation. CCL5 (RANTES) directly induces MK polyploidization and proplatelet formation.[663] It may be implicated in the thrombocytosis associated with colitis in mice.[663] In addition, activation of TLRs during infection may increase platelet production.

GM-CSF and IL-3

Before the identification of SCF and TPO, IL-3 and at a lower extent GM-CSF were the main colony-stimulating factors for the MK lineage.[657,664] Their effects are synergistic with SCF. However, their relevance in vivo is uncertain because their knockout had no effects on megakaryopoiesis and platelet production in normal and *Mpl⁻/⁻* mice.[665] Their in vivo administration had only minor effects on platelet production.

Erythropoietin

The erythroid and MK lineages are close at both the cellular and the molecular levels. EPO-R was detected on the MK lineage,[666] and initially EPO was used to induce MK colony formation.[667-669] Some synergy between TPO and EPO has been described.[670] However, administration of EPO has a minor effect on platelet level except when the TPO/MPL axis is abrogated.[671] EPO appears to be the growth factor responsible of the TPO-independent platelet production in mice.[671]

SDF1/CXCL12

CXCL12 is not a cytokine, but a chemokine that acts through the 7 transmembrane G protein–coupled receptor CXCR4. CXCL12 plays an important role in megakaryopoiesis, but most of its effects are indirect (migration, cell, or ECM interaction) although some direct effects on proplatelet formation and ploidization have been described. Surprisingly, the use of a CXCR4 antagonist stimulates megakaryopoiesis and platelet formation.[672]

Other Cytokines and Pathways

Other cytokines exert an effect in stimulating megakaryopoiesis in vitro, among them IL-9, IL-21, FLT3-L, and FGF4. Their physiological role seems minor but may be involved in the thrombocytosis of inflammation. However, they are presently used in cocktail of cytokines to produce high number of polyploid MKs from CD34⁺ cells in vitro and functional platelets in large quantities, with the ultimate goal to use them for transfusion.[673] IL33 regulates in part the differentiation of immune MKs in the lung.[15]

Two signaling pathways not induced by cytokines play a role in MK differentiation, more particularly in pathology.

Notch and its signaling are implicated in the biology of numerous cell types, more particularly for cell specification. In hematopoiesis, Notch is important in T-cell development and HSC biology. The effect of the Notch pathway on megakaryopoiesis has been studied in details because OTT, a compound of the fusion protein OTT-MAL responsible for some AMKL, may interfere with the Notch pathway.[674] It was initially shown that Notch favors murine MK differentiation by increasing the specification of HSCs toward the MK lineage.[675] However, the effects of Notch signaling can be more complex since it may increase erythroid differentiation at the level of MEPs. In contrast, it increases the proliferation of MK-Ps in the presence of SCF.[676] In human progenitors, Notch signaling inhibits MK terminal differentiation.[677] Thus, Notch signaling increases the proliferation of MK-Ps, but delays or inhibits MK terminal differentiation.

The Wnt pathway also regulates the differentiation and proliferation of numerous cell types, more particularly stem cells including HSCs. There was some evidence that the Wnt pathway is a negative regulator of early and late stages of megakaryopoiesis because inhibition of GSK-3β increases megakaryopoiesis in vitro.[678] In contrast to these results, it was shown that the canonical Wnt pathway favors MK terminal differentiation, including proplatelet formation[679] and this effect may be related to an increase in mitochondrial mass.

Negative Regulators

Some emphasis has been made on the negative regulators of MK differentiation because in vitro MK colony formation was inhibited by increasing the concentration of serum, but not by platelet-poor plasma.[680,681] This indicated that some platelet substances could inhibit the growth of MK-Ps, suggesting a feedback regulation by platelets. Several growth factors/chemokines stored in platelets have been shown to negatively regulate megakaryopoiesis.

Transforming Growth Factor-β

TGF-β is a family of five proteins TGF-β1-5. Platelets are the most important sources of TGF-β1 in the organism that is synthesized by MKs and stored in α-granules.[682] TGF-β1 plays a central role in cell biology by regulating the proliferation and differentiation of many cell types. It is usually an inhibitor of cell proliferation, but in some conditions it can be a growth factor. It is implicated in numerous pathologies including malignancies and fibrosis. In the hematopoiesis, TGF-β1 acts on all cell types and more particularly on HSCs by inducing their quiescence and on the immune system by inhibiting autoreactive cells. MKs are particularly sensitive to the inhibitory effects of TGF-β1 both on the proliferation of progenitors and on ploidization.[681,683-686] In contrast, TGF-β1 can accelerate cell differentiation for instance in erythropoiesis.[687] TGF-β1 secreted by MKs plays a pivotal role in the pathogenesis of myelofibrosis.[688,689] Surprisingly, it was suggested that a member of the TGF-β family, BMP4, is induced by TPO and stimulates megakaryopoiesis making an autocrine loop.[690]

PF4 Also Called CXCL4

PF4 also called CXCL4 is a 7.8-kDa chemokine[691] essentially synthesized by MKs and stored in the α-granules. PF4 also acts on many cell types, more particularly on endothelial cells. It inhibits MK-P proliferation and differentiation through the low-density lipoprotein-related protein 1.[691-693] There is some evidence that PF4 acts as an autocrine regulator of megakaryopoiesis in vivo.[694]

CXCL7

The CXCL7 chemokine, close to PF4, is also synthesized and stored in MKs. CXCL7 is translated into a propeptide that is subsequently cleaved in several molecules. It has been shown that two cleaved forms, β-thromboglobulin and NAP2, can inhibit megakaryopoiesis.[695,696]

Other Regulators

Other cytokines such as IL-4 and IL-8 can also inhibit megakaryopoiesis.[697,698] Before the cloning of the different IFNs, it was believed that purified IFNs inhibit megakaryopoiesis.[699,700] Later experiments showed that IFN-γ may increase megakaryopoiesis by acting on hematopoietic progenitors in synergy with SCF and may induce MK differentiation.[701] This may be related to the activation of STAT1. In contrast, IFN-α inhibits platelet production, but on late stages of megakaryopoiesis, more particularly at the stage of proplatelet formation.[702,703] However, it may also inhibit megakaryopoiesis through induction of SOCS.[623] IFN-α is presently one of the treatments of ETs and of other *BCR-ABL*-negative MPNs.[704]

Iron deficiency is associated with an increased platelet production and a thrombocytosis. Recent evidence suggests that iron deficiency induces a MK bias of MEP as a consequence of an attenuated ERK signaling.[705]

PRINCIPAL PATHOLOGIES ASSOCIATED WITH A PRIMARY DEFECT IN MEGAKARYOPOIESIS

All along this chapter we have discussed the pathogenesis of the main pathologies associated with a platelet defect. The main pathologies are summarized in *Table 17.1* (thrombocytosis) and 2 (inherited thrombocytopenia).

Briefly, acquired disorders of the megakaryopoiesis are essentially malignant diseases. Pediatric AMKL are diseases associated with alterations in TFs, resulting in fusion proteins such as OTT-MAL and ETO2-GLIS2. They can also result from *GATA-1* mutation associated with mutations affecting other pathways (epigenetic, signaling) in trisomy 21.[384,706-709] *BCR-ABL1*-negative MPNs are signaling disorders related to a constitutive JAK2 activation as a consequence of acquired somatic mutations (*JAK2*V617F, *MPL*, and *CALR* mutations) and lead to a MK hyperplasia and a thrombocytosis.[28] Thrombocytosis can also be observed in CML (*BCR-ABL1*-positive MPNs).[19] MDS are associated with a dysmegakaryopoiesis and usually a thrombocytopenia. Thrombocytopenia can result from mutations in genes involved in epigenetic regulators and/or in splicing more particularly *SRSF2*, *U2AF1*, and *ZRSR2*. In rare MPN/MDS (RARS-T) or MDS (5q-syndrome), a thrombocytosis can be observed.[710] In the former as in MPNs, the thrombocytosis is due to *JAK2*V617F mutation in the majority of cases, but associated with a *SF3B1* mutation (gene of the spliceosome) responsible of the sideroblastic anemia.[29-32] In the latter, the mechanism of the thrombocytosis is not completely understood, but could be due to an haploinsufficiency in miR-145 and miR-146A that leads to an FLI1 overexpression.[37] However, it cannot be excluded that haploinsufficiency in other sequences such as the *DIAPH1* gene could be involved in the pathogenesis of the thrombocytosis.

Inherited thrombocytosis is related to an activation of the TPO/MPL/JAK2 axis with mutations in *THPO*, *MPL*, or *JAK2*[39,48,711] (see *Table 17.1*). Inherited thrombocytopenia represents a more heterogeneous group of diseases. Thrombocytopenia with an absence or a marked decrease in MKs is either loss-of-function mutations in the TPO/MPL/JAK2 axis such as CAMT (mutations in MPL) or related disorders leading to aplastic anemia with mutations in *THPO* or *MPL* or in genes involved in transcription such as *RBM8A* (TAR syndrome), and *MECOM* and *HOXA11* (RUSAT).[712] Close to these two last syndromes, some inherited disorders leading to aplastic anemia can be revealed by a thrombocytopenia such as Fanconi anemia (disease of DNA replication and DNA repair/chromosome fragility) and Shwachman-Diamond syndrome (ribosomopathy).

Inherited macrothrombocytopenia are very heterogeneous diseases.[241,387,712,713] (see *Table 17.2*). They are mainly related to mutations in genes of the actin-myosin cytoskeleton such as *MYH9*, of the GPIb complex (Bernard-Soulier), *ACTIN*, and *FLNA* (X-linked transmission) or regulators of actomyosin such as *SRC* and *DIAPH1*, but more rarely in TFs such as *GATA-1* (X-linked transmission). Inherited thrombocytopenia with normal platelet size can be the consequences of mutations in TFs such as mutations in *RUNX1* (FPD/AML, thrombocytopenia with a predisposition to leukemia), in *ETV6* (THC5), and of mutations or deletion in *FLI1* (Jacobsen syndrome or Paris-Trousseau thrombocytopenia). Mutations in the 5′ UTR of *ANKRD26* (THC2) lead to changes in expression of the protein and also to thrombocytopenia. Inherited microthrombocytopenia are found in WAS (X-linked transmission) and in autosomal recessive thrombocytopenia with mutation in *FYB* gene.

ACKNOWLEDGMENTS

We thank Stefan Constantinescu, Isabelle Plo, and Caroline Marty for their help improving the manuscript and Laure Gilles for editing the figures.

References

1. Brewer DB. Max Schultze (1865), G. Bizzozero (1882) and the discovery of the platelet. *Br J Haematol.* 2006;133(3):251-258.
2. Wright JH, Minot GR. The VISCOUS metamorphosis of the blood platelets. *J Exp Med.* 1917;26(3):395-409.
3. Ozaki Y, Tamura S, Suzuki-Inoue K. New horizon in platelet function: with special reference to a recently-found molecule, CLEC-2. *Thromb J.* 2016;14(suppl 1):27.
4. Thomas MR, Storey RF. The role of platelets in inflammation. *Thromb Haemostasis.* 2015;114(3):449-458.
5. Deppermann C, Kubes P. Platelets and infection. *Semin Immunol.* 2016;28:536-545.
6. Gieger C, Radhakrishnan A, Cvejic A, et al. New gene functions in megakaryopoiesis and platelet formation. *Nature.* 2011;480(7376):201-208.
7. Bluteau D, Lordier L, Di Stefano A, et al. Regulation of megakaryocyte maturation and platelet formation. *J Thromb Haemost.* 2009;7(suppl 1):227-234.
8. Deutsch VR, Tomer A. Advances in megakaryocytopoiesis and thrombopoiesis: from bench to bedside. *Br J Haematol.* 2013;161(6):778-793.
9. Guo T, Wang X, Qu Y, Yin Y, Jing T, Zhang Q. Megakaryopoiesis and platelet production: insight into hematopoietic stem cell proliferation and differentiation. *Stem Cell Invest.* 2015;2:3.
10. Sanjuan-Pla A, Macaulay IC, Jensen CT, et al. Platelet-biased stem cells reside at the apex of the haematopoietic stem-cell hierarchy. *Nature.* 2013;502(7470):232-236.
11. Norozi F, Shahrabi S, Hajizamani S, Saki N. Regulatory role of megakaryocytes on hematopoietic stem cells quiescence by CXCL4/PF4 in bone marrow niche. *Leuk Res.* 2016;48:107-112.
12. Sun S, Jin C, Si J, et al. Single-cell analysis of ploidy and transcriptome reveals functional and spatial divergency in murine megakaryopoiesis. *Blood.* 2021;138(14):1211-1224.
13. Wang H, He J, Xu C, et al. Decoding human megakaryocyte development. *Cell Stem Cell.* 2021;28(3):535-549.e8.
14. Liu C, Wu D, Xia M, et al. Characterization of cellular heterogeneity and an immune subpopulation of human megakaryocytes. *Adv Sci.* 2021;8(15):e2100921.
15. Pariser DN, Hilt ZT, Ture SK, et al. Lung megakaryocytes are immune modulatory cells. *J Clin Invest.* 2021;131(1):e137377.
16. Yeung AK, Villacorta-Martin C, Hon S, Rock JR, Murphy GJ. Lung megakaryocytes display distinct transcriptional and phenotypic properties. *Blood Adv.* 2020;4(24):6204-6217.
17. Rowley JD. Letter: a new consistent chromosomal abnormality in chronic myelogenous leukaemia identified by quinacrine fluorescence and Giemsa staining. *Nature.* 1973;243(5405):290-293.
18. Rowley JD. Human oncogene locations and chromosome aberrations. *Nature.* 1983;301(5898):290-291.
19. Deininger MW, Goldman JM, Melo JV. The molecular biology of chronic myeloid leukemia. *Blood.* 2000;96(10):3343-3356.
20. James C, Ugo V, Le Couedic JP, et al. A unique clonal JAK2 mutation leading to constitutive signalling causes polycythaemia vera. *Nature.* 2005;434(7037):1144-1148.
21. Klampfl T, Gisslinger H, Harutyunyan AS, et al. Somatic mutations of calreticulin in myeloproliferative neoplasms. *N Engl J Med.* 2013;369(25):2379-2390.
22. Nangalia J, Massie CE, Baxter EJ, et al. Somatic CALR mutations in myeloproliferative neoplasms with nonmutated JAK2. *N Engl J Med.* 2013;369(25):2391-2405.
23. Pikman Y, Lee BH, Mercher T, et al. MPLW515L is a novel somatic activating mutation in myelofibrosis with myeloid metaplasia. *PLoS Med.* 2006;3(7):e270.
24. Ding J, Komatsu H, Wakita A, et al. Familial essential thrombocythemia associated with a dominant-positive activating mutation of the c-MPL gene, which encodes for the receptor for thrombopoietin. *Blood.* 2004;103(11):4198-4200.
25. Beer PA, Campbell PJ, Scott LM, et al. MPL mutations in myeloproliferative disorders: analysis of the PT-1 cohort. *Blood.* 2008;112(1):141-149.
26. Milosevic Feenstra JD, Nivarthi H, Gisslinger H, et al. Whole-exome sequencing identifies novel MPL and JAK2 mutations in triple-negative myeloproliferative neoplasms. *Blood.* 2016;127(3):325-332.
27. Cabagnols X, Favale F, Pasquier F, et al. Presence of atypical thrombopoietin receptor (MPL) mutations in triple-negative essential thrombocythemia patients. *Blood.* 2016;127(3):333-342.
28. Vainchenker W, Kralovics R. Genetic basis and molecular pathophysiology of classical myeloproliferative neoplasms. *Blood.* 2016;129(6):667-679.
29. Broseus J, Alpermann T, Wulfert M, et al. Age, JAK2(V617F) and SF3B1 mutations are the main predicting factors for survival in refractory anaemia with ring sideroblasts and marked thrombocytosis. *Leukemia.* 2013;27(9):1826-1831.
30. Malcovati L, Cazzola M. Refractory anemia with ring sideroblasts. *Best Pract Res Clin Haematol.* 2013;26(4):377-385.
31. Patnaik MM, Tefferi A. Refractory anemia with ring sideroblasts and RARS with thrombocytosis. *Am J Hematol.* 2015;90(6):549-559.
32. Visconte V, Rogers HJ, Singh J, et al. SF3B1 haploinsufficiency leads to formation of ring sideroblasts in myelodysplastic syndromes. *Blood.* 2012;120(16):3173-3186.
33. Szpurka H, Jankowska AM, Makishima H, et al. Spectrum of mutations in RARS-T patients includes TET2 and ASXL1 mutations. *Leuk Res.* 2010;34(8):969-973.
34. Schmitt-Graeff AH, Teo SS, Olschewski M, et al. JAK2V617F mutation status identifies subtypes of refractory anemia with ringed sideroblasts associated with marked thrombocytosis. *Haematologica.* 2008;93(1):34-40.
35. Van den Berghe H. The 5q- syndrome. *Scand J Haematol Suppl.* 1986;45:78-81.
36. Ebert BL, Pretz J, Bosco J, et al. Identification of RPS14 as a 5q- syndrome gene by RNA interference screen. *Nature.* 2008;451(7176):335-339.
37. Starczynowski DT, Kuchenbauer F, Argiropoulos B, et al. Identification of miR-145 and miR-146a as mediators of the 5q- syndrome phenotype. *Nat Med.* 2010;16(1):49-58.
38. Schneider RK, Adema V, Heckl D, et al. Role of casein kinase 1A1 in the biology and targeted therapy of del(5q) MDS. *Cancer Cell.* 2014;26(4):509-520.
39. Wiestner A, Schlemper RJ, van der Maas AP, Skoda RC. An activating splice donor mutation in the thrombopoietin gene causes hereditary thrombocythaemia. *Nat Genet.* 1998;18(1):49-52.
40. Liu K, Kralovics R, Rudzki Z, et al. A de novo splice donor mutation in the thrombopoietin gene causes hereditary thrombocythemia in a Polish family. *Haematologica.* 2008;93(5):706-714.
41. Zhang B, Ng D, Jones C, et al. A novel splice donor mutation in the thrombopoietin gene leads to exon 2 skipping in a Filipino family with hereditary thrombocythemia. *Blood.* 2011;118(26):6988-6990.
42. Mead AJ, Chowdhury O, Pecquet C, et al. Impact of isolated germline JAK2V617I mutation on human hematopoiesis. *Blood.* 2013;121(20):4156-4165.
43. Etheridge SL, Cosgrove ME, Sangkhae V, et al. A novel activating, germline JAK2 mutation, JAK2R564Q, causes familial essential thrombocytosis. *Blood.* 2014;123(7):1059-1068.
44. Rumi E, Harutyunyan AS, Casetti I, et al. A novel germline JAK2 mutation in familial myeloproliferative neoplasms. *Am J Hematol.* 2014;89(1):117-118.
45. Marty C, Saint-Martin C, Pecquet C, et al. Germ-line JAK2 mutations in the kinase domain are responsible for hereditary thrombocytosis and are resistant to JAK2 and HSP90 inhibitors. *Blood.* 2014;123(9):1372-1383.
46. Ding J, Komatsu H, Iida S, et al. The Asn505 mutation of the c-MPL gene, which causes familial essential thrombocythemia, induces autonomous homodimerization of the c-Mpl protein due to strong amino acid polarity. *Blood.* 2009;114(15):3325-3328.
47. Moliterno AR, Williams DM, Gutierrez-Alamillo LI, Salvatori R, Ingersoll RG, Spivak JL. Mpl Baltimore: a thrombopoietin receptor polymorphism associated with thrombocytosis. *Proc Natl Acad Sci U S A.* 2004;101(31):11444-11447.
48. El-Harith el HA, Roesl C, Ballmaier M, et al. Familial thrombocytosis caused by the novel germ-line mutation p.Pro106Leu in the MPL gene. *Br J Haematol.* 2009;144(2):185-194.
49. Moliterno AR, Hankins WD, Spivak JL. Impaired expression of the thrombopoietin receptor by platelets from patients with polycythemia vera. *N Engl J Med.* 1998;338(9):572-580.
50. Moliterno AR, Spivak JL. Posttranslational processing of the thrombopoietin receptor is impaired in polycythemia vera. *Blood.* 1999;94(8):2555-2561.
51. Massaad MJ, Ramesh N, Geha RS. Wiskott-Aldrich syndrome: a comprehensive review. *Ann N Y Acad Sci.* 2013;1285:26-43.
52. Albert MH, Bittner TC, Nonoyama S, et al. X-linked thrombocytopenia (XLT) due to WAS mutations: clinical characteristics, long-term outcome, and treatment options. *Blood.* 2010;115(16):3231-3238.
53. Levin C, Koren A, Pretorius E, et al. Deleterious mutation in the FYB gene is associated with congenital autosomal recessive small-platelet thrombocytopenia. *J Thromb Haemost.* 2015;13(7):1285-1292.
54. Noris P, Perrotta S, Seri M, et al. Mutations in ANKRD26 are responsible for a frequent form of inherited thrombocytopenia: analysis of 78 patients from 21 families. *Blood.* 2011;117(24):6673-6680.
55. Song WJ, Sullivan MG, Legare RD, et al. Haploinsufficiency of CBFA2 causes familial thrombocytopenia with propensity to develop acute myelogenous leukaemia. *Nat Genet.* 1999;23(2):166-175.
56. Zhang MY, Churpek JE, Keel SB, et al. Germline ETV6 mutations in familial thrombocytopenia and hematologic malignancy. *Nat Genet.* 2015;47(2):180-185.
57. Topka S, Vijai J, Walsh MF, et al. Germline ETV6 mutations confer susceptibility to acute lymphoblastic leukemia and thrombocytopenia. *PLoS Genet.* 2015;11(6):e1005262.
58. Noetzli L, Lo RW, Lee-Sherick AB, et al. Germline mutations in ETV6 are associated with thrombocytopenia, red cell macrocytosis and predisposition to lymphoblastic leukemia. *Nat Genet.* 2015;47(5):535-538.
59. Poggi M, Canault M, Favier M, et al. Germline variants in ETV6 underlie reduced platelet formation, platelet dysfunction and increased levels of circulating CD34+ progenitors. *Haematologica.* 2017;102(2):282-294.
60. Varghese LN, Zhang JG, Young SN, et al. Functional characterization of c-Mpl ectodomain mutations that underlie congenital amegakaryocytic thrombocytopenia. *Growth Factors.* 2014;32(1):18-26.
61. Stockklausner C, Klotter AC, Dickemann N, et al. The thrombopoietin receptor P106L mutation functionally separates receptor signaling activity from thrombopoietin homeostasis. *Blood.* 2015;125(7):1159-1169.
62. Niihori T, Ouchi-Uchiyama M, Sasahara Y, et al. Mutations in MECOM, encoding oncoprotein EVI1, cause radioulnar synostosis with amegakaryocytic thrombocytopenia. *Am J Hum Genet.* 2015;97(6):848-854.
63. Albers CA, Paul DS, Schulze H, et al. Compound inheritance of a low-frequency regulatory SNP and a rare null mutation in exon-junction complex subunit RBM8A causes TAR syndrome. *Nat Genet.* 2012;44(4):435-439. S1-2.
64. Morison IM, Cramer Borde EM, Cheesman EJ, et al. A mutation of human cytochrome c enhances the intrinsic apoptotic pathway but causes only thrombocytopenia. *Nat Genet.* 2008;40(4):387-389.
65. Dasouki MJ, Rafi SK, Olm-Shipman AJ, et al. Exome sequencing reveals a thrombopoietin ligand mutation in a Micronesian family with autosomal recessive aplastic anemia. *Blood.* 2013;122(20):3440-3449.
66. Favier R, Douay L, Esteva B, et al. A novel genetic thrombocytopenia (Paris-Trousseau) associated with platelet inclusions, dysmegakaryopoiesis and chromosome deletion At 11q23. *Comptes rendus de l'Academie des sciences Serie III, Sciences de la vie.* 1993;316(7):698-701.
67. Jacobsen P, Hauge M, Henningsen K, Hobolth N, Mikkelsen M, Philip J. An (11;21) translocation in four generations with chromosome 11 abnormalities in the offspring. A clinical, cytogenetical, and gene marker study. *Hum Hered.* 1973;23(6):568-585.
68. Stevenson WS, Rabbolini DJ, Beutler L, et al. Paris-Trousseau thrombocytopenia is phenocopied by the autosomal recessive inheritance of a DNA-binding domain mutation in FLI1. *Blood.* 2015;126(17):2027-2030.

69. Yu C, Niakan KK, Matsushita M, Stamatoyannopoulos G, Orkin SH, Raskind WH. X-linked thrombocytopenia with thalassemia from a mutation in the amino finger of GATA-1 affecting DNA binding rather than FOG-1 interaction. *Blood.* 2002;100(6):2040-2045.

70. Nichols KE, Crispino JD, Poncz M, et al. Familial dyserythropoietic anaemia and thrombocytopenia due to an inherited mutation in GATA1. *Nat Genet.* 2000;24(3):266-270.

71. Crispino JD, Lodish MB, MacKay JP, Orkin SH. Use of altered specificity mutants to probe a specific protein-protein interaction in differentiation: the GATA-1:FOG complex. *Mol Cell.* 1999;3(2):219-228.

72. Mehaffey MG, Newton AL, Gandhi MJ, Crossley M, Drachman JG. X-linked thrombocytopenia caused by a novel mutation of GATA-1. *Blood.* 2001;98(9):2681-2688.

73. Freson K, Devriendt K, Matthijs G, et al. Platelet characteristics in patients with X-linked macrothrombocytopenia because of a novel GATA1 mutation. *Blood.* 2001;98(1):85-92.

74. Freson K, Matthijs G, Thys C, et al. Different substitutions at residue D218 of the X-linked transcription factor GATA1 lead to altered clinical severity of macrothrombocytopenia and anemia and are associated with variable skewed X inactivation. *Hum Mol Genet.* 2002;11(2):147-152.

75. Del Vecchio GC, Giordani L, De Santis A, De Mattia D. Dyserythropoietic anemia and thrombocytopenia due to a novel mutation in GATA-1. *Acta Haematol.* 2005;114(2):113-116.

76. Tubman VN, Levine JE, Campagna DR, et al. X-linked gray platelet syndrome due to a GATA1 Arg216Gln mutation. *Blood.* 2007;109(8):3297-3299.

77. Albers CA, Cvejic A, Favier R, et al. Exome sequencing identifies NBEAL2 as the causative gene for gray platelet syndrome. *Nat Genet.* 2011;43(8):735-737.

78. Gunay-Aygun M, Falik-Zaccai TC, Vilboux T, et al. NBEAL2 is mutated in gray platelet syndrome and is required for biogenesis of platelet alpha-granules. *Nat Genet.* 2011;43(8):732-734.

79. Kahr WH, Hinckley J, Li L, et al. Mutations in NBEAL2, encoding a BEACH protein, cause gray platelet syndrome. *Nat Genet.* 2011;43(8):738-740.

80. Aminkeng F. GFI1B mutation causes autosomal dominant gray platelet syndrome. *Clin Genet.* 2014;85(6):534-535.

81. Monteferrario D, Bolar NA, Marneth AE, et al. A dominant-negative GFI1B mutation in the gray platelet syndrome. *N Engl J Med.* 2014;370(3):245-253.

82. Savoia A, Kunishima S, De Rocco D, et al. Spectrum of the mutations in Bernard-Soulier syndrome. *Hum Mutat.* 2014;35(9):1033-1045.

83. Rosa RF, Rosa RC, Dos Santos PP, Zen PR, Paskulin GA. Hematological abnormalities and 22q11.2 deletion syndrome. *Rev Bras Hematol Hemoter.* 2011;33(2):151-154.

84. Balduini CL, Pecci A, Savoia A. Recent advances in the understanding and management of MYH9-related inherited thrombocytopenias. *Br J Haematol.* 2011;154(2):161-174.

85. Lu K, Lee MH, Carpten JD, Sekhon M, Patel SB. High-resolution physical and transcript map of human chromosome 2p21 containing the sitosterolaemia locus. *Eur J Hum Genet.* 2001;9(5):364-374.

86. Miller JL, Cunningham D, Lyle VA, Finch CN. Mutation in the gene encoding the alpha chain of platelet glycoprotein Ib in platelet-type von Willebrand disease. *Proc Natl Acad Sci U S A.* 1991;88(11):4761-4765.

87. Nurden AT, Pillois X, Fiore M, Heilig R, Nurden P. Glanzmann thrombasthenia-like syndromes associated with Macrothrombocytopenias and mutations in the genes encoding the alphaIIbbeta3 integrin. *Semin Thromb Hemost.* 2011;37(6):698-706.

88. Basciano PA, Bussel J, Hafeez Z, Christos PJ, Giannakakou P. The beta 1 tubulin R307H single nucleotide polymorphism is associated with treatment failures in immune thrombocytopenia (ITP). *Br J Haematol.* 2013;160(2):237-243.

89. Bodie K, Gagne GD, Sramek MK, Desmond DJ, Abel SJ, Fagerland JA. Asymptomatic macrothrombocytopenia in a young pure-bred beagle dog: a case report. *Toxicol Pathol.* 2011;39(6):980-987.

90. Nurden P, Debili N, Coupry I, et al. Thrombocytopenia resulting from mutations in filamin A can be expressed as an isolated syndrome. *Blood.* 2011;118(22):5928-5937.

91. Turro E, Greene D, Wijgaerts A, et al. A dominant gain-of-function mutation in universal tyrosine kinase SRC causes thrombocytopenia, myelofibrosis, bleeding, and bone pathologies. *Sci Transl Med.* 2016;8(328):328ra30.

92. Manchev VT, Hilpert M, Berrou E, et al. A new form of macrothrombocytopenia induced by a germ-line mutation in the PRKACG gene. *Blood.* 2014;124(16):2554-2563.

93. Zhen C, Guo F, Fang X, Liu Y, Wang X. A family with distal myopathy with rimmed vacuoles associated with thrombocytopenia. *Neurol Sci.* 2014;35(9):1479-1481.

94. Kunishima S, Okuno Y, Yoshida K, et al. ACTN1 mutations cause congenital macrothrombocytopenia. *Am J Hum Genet.* 2013;92(3):431-438.

95. Fletcher SJ, Johnson B, Lowe GC, et al. SLFN14 mutations underlie thrombocytopenia with excessive bleeding and platelet secretion defects. *J Clin Invest.* 2015;125(9):3600-3605.

96. Pleines I, Woods J, Chappaz S, et al. Mutations in tropomyosin 4 underlie a rare form of human macrothrombocytopenia. *J Clin Invest.* 2017;127(3):814-829.

97. Melhem M, Abu-Farha M, Antony D, et al. Novel G6B gene variant cause familial autosomal recessive thrombocytopenia and anemia. *Eur J Haematol.* 2017;98(3):218-227.

98. Stritt S, Nurden P, Turro E, et al. A gain-of-function variant in DIAPH1 causes dominant macrothrombocytopenia and hearing loss. *Blood.* 2016;127(23):2903-2914.

99. Stritt S, Nurden P, Favier R, et al. Defects in TRPM7 channel function deregulate thrombopoiesis through altered cellular Mg(2+) homeostasis and cytoskeletal architecture. *Nat Commun.* 2016;7:11097.

100. Nesin V, Wiley G, Kousi M, et al. Activating mutations in STIM1 and ORAI1 cause overlapping syndromes of tubular myopathy and congenital miosis. *Proc Natl Acad Sci U S A.* 2014;111(11):4197-4202.

101. Markello T, Chen D, Kwan JY, et al. York platelet syndrome is a CRAC channelopathy due to gain-of-function mutations in STIM1. *Mol Genet Metabol.* 2015;114(3):474-482.

102. Becker AJ, Mc CE, Till JE. Cytological demonstration of the clonal nature of spleen colonies derived from transplanted mouse marrow cells. *Nature.* 1963;197:452-454.

103. Kondo M, Wagers AJ, Manz MG, et al. Biology of hematopoietic stem cells and progenitors: implications for clinical application. *Annu Rev Immunol.* 2003;21:759-806.

104. Hofer T, Rodewald HR. Output without input: the lifelong productivity of hematopoietic stem cells. *Curr Opin Cell Biol.* 2016;43:69-77.

105. Perie L, Duffy KR. Retracing the in vivo haematopoietic tree using single-cell methods. *FEBS Lett.* 2016;590(22):4068-4083.

106. Morrison SJ, Uchida N, Weissman IL. The biology of hematopoietic stem cells. *Annu Rev Cell Dev Biol.* 1995;11:35-71.

107. Adolfsson J, Mansson R, Buza-Vidas N, et al. Identification of Flt3+ lympho-myeloid stem cells lacking erythro-megakaryocytic potential a revised road map for adult blood lineage commitment. *Cell.* 2005;121(2):295-306.

108. Pietras EM, Reynaud D, Kang YA, et al. Functionally distinct subsets of lineage-biased multipotent progenitors control blood production in normal and regenerative conditions. *Cell Stem Cell.* 2015;17(1):35-46.

109. Kokkaliaris KD, Lucas D, Beerman I, Kent DG, Perie L. Understanding hematopoiesis from a single-cell standpoint. *Exp Hematol.* 2016;44(6):447-450.

110. Paul F, Arkin Y, Giladi A, et al. Transcriptional heterogeneity and lineage commitment in myeloid progenitors. *Cell.* 2015;163(7):1663-1677.

111. Psaila B, Barkas N, Iskander D, et al. Single-cell profiling of human megakaryocyte-erythroid progenitors identifies distinct megakaryocyte and erythroid differentiation pathways. *Genome Biol.* 2016;17:83.

112. Notta F, Zandi S, Takayama N, et al. Distinct routes of lineage development reshape the human blood hierarchy across ontogeny. *Science.* 2016;351(6269):aab2116.

113. Debili N, Coulombel L, Croisille L, et al. Characterization of a bipotent erythro-megakaryocytic progenitor in human bone marrow. *Blood.* 1996;88(4):1284-1296.

114. Sanada C, Xavier-Ferrucio J, Lu YC, et al. Adult human megakaryocyte-erythroid progenitors are in the CD34+CD38mid fraction. *Blood.* 2016;128(7):923-933.

115. Pronk CJ, Rossi DJ, Månsson R, et al. Elucidation of the phenotypic, functional, and molecular topography of a myeloerythroid progenitor cell hierarchy. *Cell Stem Cell.* 2007;1(4):428-442.

116. Gekas C, Graf T. CD41 expression marks myeloid-biased adult hematopoietic stem cells and increases with age. *Blood.* 2013;121(22):4463-4472.

117. Miyawaki K, Arinobu Y, Iwasaki H, et al. CD41 marks the initial myelo-erythroid lineage specification in adult mouse hematopoiesis: redefinition of murine common myeloid progenitor. *Stem Cells.* 2015;33(3):976-987.

118. Haas S, Hansson J, Klimmeck D, et al. Inflammation-induced emergency megakaryopoiesis driven by hematopoietic stem cell-like megakaryocyte progenitors. *Cell Stem Cell.* 2015;17(4):422-434.

119. Psaila B, Mead AJ. Single-cell approaches reveal novel cellular pathways for megakaryocyte and erythroid differentiation. *Blood.* 2019;133(13):1427-1435.

120. Psaila B, Wang G, Rodriguez-Meira A, et al. Single-cell analyses reveal megakaryocyte-biased hematopoiesis in myelofibrosis and identify mutant clone-specific targets. *Mol Cell.* 2020;78(3):477-492.e8.

121. Woolthuis CM, Park CY. Hematopoietic stem/progenitor cell commitment to the megakaryocyte lineage. *Blood.* 2016;127(10):1242-1248.

122. Mitjavila-Garcia MT, Cailleret M, Godin I, et al. Expression of CD41 on hematopoietic progenitors derived from embryonic hematopoietic cells. *Development.* 2002;129(8):2003-2013.

123. Nakorn TN, Miyamoto T, Weissman IL. Characterization of mouse clonogenic megakaryocyte progenitors. *Proc Natl Acad Sci U S A.* 2003;100(1):205-210.

124. Ng AP, Kauppi M, Metcalf D, Di Rago L, Hyland CD, Alexander WS. Characterization of thrombopoietin (TPO)-responsive progenitor cells in adult mouse bone marrow with in vivo megakaryocyte and erythroid potential. *Proc Natl Acad Sci U S A.* 2012;109(7):2364-2369.

125. Nishikii H, Kanazawa Y, Umemoto T, et al. Unipotent megakaryopoietic pathway bridging hematopoietic stem cells and mature megakaryocytes. *Stem Cells.* 2015;33(7):2196-2207.

126. Long MW, Williams N, McDonald TP. Immature megakaryocytes in the mouse: in vitro relationship to megakaryocyte progenitor cells and mature megakaryocytes. *J Cell Physiol.* 1982;112(3):339-344.

127. Breton-Gorius J, Reyes F, Duhamel G, Najman A, Gorin NC. Megakaryoblastic acute leukemia: identification by the ultrastructural demonstration of platelet peroxidase. *Blood.* 1978;51(1):45-60.

128. Breton-Gorius J, Reyes F. Ultrastructure of human bone marrow cell maturation. *Int Rev Cytol.* 1976;46:251-321.

129. Ghevaert C, Salsmann A, Watkins NA, et al. A nonsynonymous SNP in the ITGB3 gene disrupts the conserved membrane-proximal cytoplasmic salt bridge in the alphaIIbbeta3 integrin and cosegregates dominantly with abnormal proplatelet formation and macrothrombocytopenia. *Blood.* 2008;111(7):3407-3414.

130. Rabellino EM, Levene RB, Leung LL, Nachman RL. Human megakaryocytes. II. Expression of platelet proteins in early marrow megakaryocytes. *J Exp Med.* 1981;154(1):88-100.

131. Vinci G, Tabilio A, Deschamps JF, et al. Immunological study of in vitro maturation of human megakaryocytes. *Br J Haematol.* 1984;56(4):589-605.

132. Pandit SK, Westendorp B, de Bruin A. Physiological significance of polyploidization in mammalian cells. *Trends Cell Biol.* 2013;23(11):556-566.

133. Ravid K, Lu J, Zimmet JM, Jones MR. Roads to polyploidy: the megakaryocyte example. *J Cell Physiol.* 2002;190(1):7-20.

134. Eckly A, Heijnen H, Pertuy F, et al. Biogenesis of the demarcation membrane system (DMS) in megakaryocytes. *Blood.* 2014;123(6):921-930.

The Normal Hematologic System

135. Liu ZJ, Italiano J, Jr, Ferrer-Marin F, et al. Developmental differences in megakaryo-cytopoiesis are associated with up-regulated TPO signaling through mTOR and elevated GATA-1 levels in neonatal megakaryocytes. *Blood.* 2011;117(15):4106-4117.

136. Hegyi E, Navarro S, Debili N, et al. Regulation of human megakaryocytopoiesis: analysis of proliferation, ploidy and maturation in liquid cultures. *Int J Cell Clon.* 1990;8(4):236-244.

137. Vainchenker W, Guichard J, Breton-Gorius J. Differentiation of human megakaryocytes in culture starting from the primordial circulating cells in the newborn. *C R Hebd Seances Acad Sci Ser D Sci Nat.* 1978;287(3):177-179.

138. Winkelmann M, Pfitzer P, Schneider W. Significance of polyploidy in megakaryocytes and other cells in health and tumor disease. *Klin Wochenschr.* 1987;65(23):1115-1131.

139. Raslova H, Roy L, Vourc'h C, et al. Megakaryocyte polyploidization is associated with a functional gene amplification. *Blood.* 2003;101(2):541-544.

140. Vitrat N, Cohen-Solal K, Pique C, et al. Endomitosis of human megakaryocytes are due to abortive mitosis. *Blood.* 1998;91(10):3711-3723.

141. Nagata Y, Muro Y, Todokoro K. Thrombopoietin-induced polyploidization of bone marrow megakaryocytes is due to a unique regulatory mechanism in late mitosis. *J Cell Biol.* 1997;139(2):449-457.

142. Lordier L, Jalil A, Aurade F, et al. Megakaryocyte endomitosis is a failure of late cytokinesis related to defects in the contractile ring and Rho/Rock signaling. *Blood.* 2008;112(8):3164-3174.

143. Lordier L, Pan J, Naim V, et al. Presence of a defect in karyokinesis during megakaryocyte endomitosis. *Cell Cycle.* 2012;11(23):4385-4389.

144. Geddis AE, Fox NE, Tkachenko E, Kaushansky K. Endomitotic megakaryocytes that form a bipolar spindle exhibit cleavage furrow ingression followed by furrow regression. *Cell Cycle.* 2007;6(4):455-460.

145. Leysi-Derilou Y, Robert A, Duchesne C, Garnier A, Boyer L, Pineault N. Polyploid megakaryocytes can complete cytokinesis. *Cell Cycle.* 2010;9(13):2589-2599.

146. Wang Z, Zhang Y, Kamen D, Lees E, Ravid K. Cyclin D3 is essential for megakaryocytopoiesis. *Blood.* 1995;86(10):3783-3788.

147. Roy L, Coullin P, Vitrat N, et al. Asymmetrical segregation of chromosomes with a normal metaphase/anaphase checkpoint in polyploid megakaryocytes. *Blood.* 2001;97(8):2238-2247.

148. Eliades A, Papadantonakis N, Ravid K. New roles for cyclin E in megakaryocytic polyploidization. *J Biol Chem.* 2010;285(24):18909-18917.

149. Lordier L, Chang Y, Jalil A, et al. Aurora B is dispensable for megakaryocyte polyploidization, but contributes to the endomitotic process. *Blood.* 2010;116(13):2345-2355.

150. Goldenson B, Kirsammer G, Stankiewicz MJ, Wen QJ, Crispino JD. Aurora kinase A is required for hematopoiesis but is dispensable for murine megakaryocyte endomitosis and differentiation. *Blood.* 2015;125(13):2141-2150.

151. Trakala M, Partida D, Salazar-Roa M, et al. Activation of the endomitotic spindle assembly checkpoint and thrombocytopenia in Plk1-deficient mice. *Blood.* 2015;126(14):1707-1714.

152. Wen Q, Goldenson B, Silver SJ, et al. Identification of regulators of polyploidization presents therapeutic targets for treatment of AMKL. *Cell.* 2012;150(3):575-589.

153. Wen QJ, Yang Q, Goldenson B, et al. Targeting megakaryocytic-induced fibrosis in myeloproliferative neoplasms by AURKA inhibition. *Nat Med.* 2015;21(12):1473-1480.

154. Payton M, Cheung HK, Ninniri MSS, et al. Dual targeting of Aurora kinases with AMG 900 exhibits potent preclinical activity against acute myeloid leukemia with distinct post-mitotic outcomes. *Mol Cancer Therapeut.* 2018;17(12):2575-2585.

155. Trakala M, Rodriguez-Acebes S, Maroto M, et al. Functional reprogramming of polyploidization in megakaryocytes. *Dev Cell.* 2015;32(2):155-167.

156. Geddis AE, Kaushansky K. Endomitotic megakaryocytes form a midzone in anaphase but have a deficiency in cleavage furrow formation. *Cell Cycle.* 2006;5(5):538-545.

157. Gao Y, Smith E, Ker E, et al. Role of RhoA-specific guanine exchange factors in regulation of endomitosis in megakaryocytes. *Dev Cell.* 2012;22(3):573-584.

158. Lordier L, Bluteau D, Jalil A, et al. RUNX1-induced silencing of non-muscle myosin heavy chain IIB contributes to megakaryocyte polyploidization. *Nat Commun.* 2012;3:717.

159. Roy A, Lordier L, Mazzi S, et al. Differential activity of nonmuscle myosin II isoforms determines their localization at the cleavage furrow of megakaryocytes. *Blood.* 2016;128(26):3137-3145.

160. Zhao B, Guan KL. Hippo pathway key to ploidy checkpoint. *Cell.* 2014;158(4):695-696.

161. Ganem NJ, Cornils H, Chiu SY, et al. Cytokinesis failure triggers hippo tumor suppressor pathway activation. *Cell.* 2014;158(4):833-848.

162. Roy A, Lordier L, Pioche-Durieu C, et al. Uncoupling of the Hippo and Rho pathways allows megakaryocytes to escape the tetraploid checkpoint. *Haematologica.* 2016;101(12):1469-1478.

163. Iancu-Rubin C, Mosoyan G, Glenn K, Gordon RE, Nichols GL, Hoffman R. Activation of p53 by the MDM2 inhibitor RG7112 impairs thrombopoiesis. *Exp Hematol.* 2014;42(2):137-145 e5.

164. Fuhrken PG, Apostolidis PA, Lindsey S, Miller WM, Papoutsakis ET. Tumor suppressor protein p53 regulates megakaryocytic polyploidization and apoptosis. *J Biol Chem.* 2008;283(23):15589-15600.

165. Raslova H, Kauffmann A, Sekkai D, et al. Interrelation between polyploidization and megakaryocyte differentiation: a gene profiling approach. *Blood.* 2007;109(8):3225-3234.

166. Farlik M, Halbritter F, Muller F, et al. DNA methylation dynamics of human hematopoietic stem cell differentiation. *Cell Stem Cell.* 2016;19(6):808-822.

167. Choudry FA, Bagger FO, Macaulay IC, et al. Transcriptional characterization of human megakaryocyte polyploidization and lineage commitment. *J Thromb Haemost.* 2021;19(5):1236-1249.

168. Radley JM, Haller CJ. The demarcation membrane system of the megakaryocyte: a misnomer? *Blood.* 1982;60(1):213-219.

169. Behnke O. An electron microscope study of the megacaryocyte of the rat bone marrow. I. The development of the demarcation membrane system and the platelet surface coat. *J Ultra Res.* 1968;24(5):412-433.

170. Nakao K, Angrist AA. Membrane surface specialization of blood platelet and megakaryocyte. *Nature.* 1968;217(5132):960-961.

171. Ru YX, Zhao SX, Dong SX, Yang YQ, Eyden B. On the maturation of megakaryocytes: a review with original observations on human in vivo cells emphasizing morphology and ultrastructure. *Ultrastruct Pathol.* 2015;39(2):79-87.

172. Cunin P, Bouslama R, Machlus KR, et al. Megakaryocyte emperipolesis mediates membrane transfer from intracytoplasmic neutrophils to platelets. *Elife.* 2019;8:e44031.

173. Blair P, Flaumenhaft R. Platelet alpha-granules: basic biology and clinical correlates. *Blood Rev.* 2009;23(4):177-189.

174. Schick BP, Pestina TI, San Antonio JD, Stenberg PE, Jackson CW. Decreased serglycin proteoglycan size is associated with the platelet alpha granule storage defect in Wistar Furth hereditary macrothrombocytopenic rats. Serglycin binding affinity to type I collagen is unaltered. *J Cell Physiol.* 1997;172(1):87-93.

175. Woulfe DS, Lilliendahl JK, August S, et al. Serglycin proteoglycan deletion induces defects in platelet aggregation and thrombus formation in mice. *Blood.* 2008;111(7):3458-3467.

176. Handagama P, Rappolee DA, Werb Z, Levin J, Bainton DF. Platelet alpha-granule fibrinogen, albumin, and immunoglobulin G are not synthesized by rat and mouse megakaryocytes. *J Clin Invest.* 1990;86(4):1364-1368.

177. Handagama P, Scarborough RM, Shuman MA, Bainton DF. Endocytosis of fibrinogen into megakaryocyte and platelet alpha-granules is mediated by alpha IIb beta 3 (glycoprotein IIb-IIIa). *Blood.* 1993;82(1):135-138.

178. Harrison P, Wilbourn B, Debili N, et al. Uptake of plasma fibrinogen into the alpha granules of human megakaryocytes and platelets. *J Clin Invest.* 1989;84(4):1320-1324.

179. Italiano JE, Jr, Battinelli EM. Selective sorting of alpha-granule proteins. *J Thromb Haemost.* 2009;7(suppl 1):173-176.

180. Cramer EM, Meyer D, le Menn R, Breton-Gorius J. Eccentric localization of von Willebrand factor in an internal structure of platelet alpha-granule resembling that of Weibel-Palade bodies. *Blood.* 1985;66(3):710-713.

181. Heijnen HF, Debili N, Vainchencker W, Breton-Gorius J, Geuze HJ, Sixma JJ. Multivesicular bodies are an intermediate stage in the formation of platelet alpha-granules. *Blood.* 1998;91(7):2313-2325.

182. Nurden AT, Nurden P. Should any genetic defect affecting alpha-granules in platelets be classified as gray platelet syndrome? *Am J Hematol.* 2016;91(7):714-718.

183. Raccuglia G. Gray platelet syndrome. A variety of qualitative platelet disorder. *Am J Med.* 1971;51(6):818-828.

184. Breton-Gorius J, Vainchenker W, Nurden A, Levy-Toledano S, Caen J. Defective alpha-granule production in megakaryocytes from gray platelet syndrome: ultrastructural studies of bone marrow cells and megakaryocytes growing in culture from blood precursors. *Am J Pathol.* 1981;102(1):10-19.

185. Gissen P, Tee L, Johnson CA, et al. Clinical and molecular genetic features of ARC syndrome. *Hum Genet.* 2006;120(3):396-409.

186. Gissen P, Johnson CA, Morgan NV, et al. Mutations in VPS33B, encoding a regulator of SNARE-dependent membrane fusion, cause arthrogryposis-renal dysfunction-cholestasis (ARC) syndrome. *Nat Genet.* 2004;36(4):400-404.

187. Cullinane AR, Straatman-Iwanowska A, Zaucker A, et al. Mutations in VIPAR cause an arthrogryposis, renal dysfunction and cholestasis syndrome phenotype with defects in epithelial polarization. *Nat Genet.* 2010;42(4):303-312.

188. Bem D, Smith H, Banushi B, et al. VPS33B regulates protein sorting into and maturation of alpha-granule progenitor organelles in mouse megakaryocytes. *Blood.* 2015;126(2):133-143.

189. Ambrosio AL, Di Pietro SM. Storage pool diseases illuminate platelet dense granule biogenesis. *Platelets.* 2016;28(2):1-9.

190. Youssefian T, Cramer EM. Megakaryocyte dense granule components are sorted in multivesicular bodies. *Blood.* 2000;95(12):4004-4007.

191. Ambrosio AL, Boyle JA, Di Pietro SM. Mechanism of platelet dense granule biogenesis: study of cargo transport and function of Rab32 and Rab38 in a model system. *Blood.* 2012;120(19):4072-4081.

192. King SM, Reed GL. Development of platelet secretory granules. *Semin Cell Dev Biol.* 2002;13(4):293-302.

193. Whiteheart SW. alpha-Granules at the BEACH. *Blood.* 2013;122(19):3247-3248.

194. Poirault-Chassac S, Nivet-Antoine V, Houvert A, et al. Mitochondrial dynamics and reactive oxygen species initiate thrombopoiesis from mature megakaryocytes. *Blood Adv.* 2021;5(6):1706-1718.

195. Undi RB, Gutti U, Gutti RK. LiCl regulates mitochondrial biogenesis during megakaryocyte development. *J Trace Elem Med Biol.* 2017;39:193-201.

196. Machlus KR, Italiano JE, Jr. The incredible journey: from megakaryocyte development to platelet formation. *J Cell Biol.* 2013;201(6):785-796.

197. Pertuy F, Eckly A, Weber J, et al. Myosin IIA is critical for organelle distribution and F-actin organization in megakaryocytes and platelets. *Blood.* 2014;123(8):1261-1269.

198. Patel-Hett S, Wang H, Begonja AJ, et al. The spectrin-based membrane skeleton stabilizes mouse megakaryocyte membrane systems and is essential for proplatelet and platelet formation. *Blood.* 2011;118(6):1641-1652.

199. Schulze H, Korpal M, Hurov J, et al. Characterization of the megakaryocyte demarcation membrane system and its role in thrombopoiesis. *Blood.* 2006;107(10):3868-3875.

200. Thiery JP, Bessis M. Genesis of blood platelets from the megakaryocytes in living cells. *Comptes rendus hebdomadaires des seances de l'Academie des sciences.* 1956;242(2):290-292.

201. Radley JM, Scurfield G. The mechanism of platelet release. *Blood.* 1980;56(6):996-999.

202. Leven RM, Tablin F. Extracellular matrix stimulation of Guinea pig megakaryocyte proplatelet formation in vitro is mediated through the vitronectin receptor. *Exp Hematol.* 1992;20(11):1316-1322.

203. Cramer EM, Norol F, Guichard J, et al. Ultrastructure of platelet formation by human megakaryocytes cultured with the Mpl ligand. *Blood.* 1997;89(7):2336-2346.

204. Italiano JE, Jr, Lecine P, Shivdasani RA, Hartwig JH. Blood platelets are assembled principally at the ends of proplatelet processes produced by differentiated megakaryocytes. *J Cell Biol.* 1999;147(6):1299-1312.

205. Bornert A, Boscher J, Pertuy F, et al. Cytoskeletal-based mechanisms differently regulate in vivo and in vitro proplatelet formation. *Haematologica.* 2021;106(5):1368-1380.

206. Tavassoli M. Megakaryocyte--platelet axis and the process of platelet formation and release. *Blood.* 1980;55(4):537-545.

207. Junt T, Schulze H, Chen Z, et al. Dynamic visualization of thrombopoiesis within bone marrow. *Science.* 2007;317(5845):1767-1770.

208. Dunois-Larde C, Capron C, Fichelson S, Bauer T, Cramer-Borde E, Baruch D. Exposure of human megakaryocytes to high shear rates accelerates platelet production. *Blood.* 2009;114(9):1875-1883.

209. Thon JN, Macleod H, Begonja AJ, et al. Microtubule and cortical forces determine platelet size during vascular platelet production. *Nat Commun.* 2012;3:852.

210. Thon JN, Montalvo A, Patel-Hett S, et al. Cytoskeletal mechanics of proplatelet maturation and platelet release. *J Cell Biol.* 2010;191(4):861-874.

211. Martin JF, Slater DN, Trowbridge EA. Abnormal intrapulmonary platelet production: a possible cause of vascular and lung disease. *Lancet.* 1983;1(8328):793-796.

212. Zucker-Franklin D, Philipp CS. Platelet production in the pulmonary capillary bed: new ultrastructural evidence for an old concept. *Am J Pathol.* 2000;157(1):69-74.

213. Lefrancais E, Ortiz-Munoz G, Caudrillier A, et al. The lung is a site of platelet biogenesis and a reservoir for haematopoietic progenitors. *Nature.* 2017;544(7648):105-109.

214. Lecine P, Italiano JE, Jr, Kim SW, Villeval JL, Shivdasani RA. Hematopoietic-specific beta 1 tubulin participates in a pathway of platelet biogenesis dependent on the transcription factor NF-E2. *Blood.* 2000;96(4):1366-1373.

215. Strassel C, Magiera MM, Dupuis A, et al. An essential role for α4A-tubulin in platelet biogenesis. *Life Sci Alliance.* 2019;2(1):e201900309.

216. Bender M, Thon JN, Ehrlicher AJ, et al. Microtubule sliding drives proplatelet elongation and is dependent on cytoplasmic dynein. *Blood.* 2015;125(5):860-868.

217. Richardson JL, Shivdasani RA, Boers C, Hartwig JH, Italiano JE, Jr. Mechanisms of organelle transport and capture along proplatelets during platelet production. *Blood.* 2005;106(13):4066-4075.

218. Khan AO, Slater A, Maclachlan A, et al. Post-translational polymodification of β1-tubulin regulates motor protein localisation in platelet production and function. *Haematologica.* Published online 2020.

219. van Dijk J, Bompard G, Cau J, et al. Microtubule polyglutamylation and acetylation drive microtubule dynamics critical for platelet formation. *BMC Biol.* 2018;16(1):116.

220. Nishimura S, Nagasaki M, Kunishima S, et al. IL-1alpha induces thrombopoiesis through megakaryocyte rupture in response to acute platelet needs. *J Cell Biol.* 2015;209(3):453-466.

221. Potts KS, Farley A, Dawson CA, et al. Membrane budding is a major mechanism of in vivo platelet biogenesis. *J Exp Med.* 2020;217(9):e20191206.

222. Italiano JE, Bender M, Merrill-Skoloff G, Ghevaert C, Nieswandt B, Flaumenhaft R. Microvesicles, but not platelets, bud off from mouse bone marrow megakaryocytes. *Blood.* 2021;138(20):1998-2001.

223. Niswander LM, Fegan KH, Kingsley PD, McGrath KE, Palis J. SDF-1 dynamically mediates megakaryocyte niche occupancy and thrombopoiesis at steady state and following radiation injury. *Blood.* 2014;124(2):277-286.

224. Avecilla ST, Hattori K, Heissig B, et al. Chemokine-mediated interaction of hematopoietic progenitors with the bone marrow vascular niche is required for thrombopoiesis. *Nat Med.* 2004;10(1):64-71.

225. Stegner D, vanEeuwijk JMM, Angay O, et al. Thrombopoiesis is spatially regulated by the bone marrow vasculature. *Nat Commun.* 2017;8(1):127.

226. Lane WJ, Dias S, Hattori K, et al. Stromal-derived factor 1-induced megakaryocyte migration and platelet production is dependent on matrix metalloproteinases. *Blood.* 2000;96(13):4152-4159.

227. Hamada T, Mohle R, Hesselgesser J, et al. Transendothelial migration of megakaryocytes in response to stromal cell-derived factor 1 (SDF-1) enhances platelet formation. *J Exp Med.* 1998;188(3):539-548.

228. Berthebaud M, Riviere C, Jarrier P, et al. RGS16 is a negative regulator of SDF-1-CXCR4 signaling in megakaryocytes. *Blood.* 2005;106(9):2962-2968.

229. Ito Y, Nakamura S, Sugimoto N, et al. Turbulence activates platelet biogenesis to enable clinical scale ex vivo production. *Cell.* 2018;174(3):636-648.e18.

230. Sabri S, Jandrot-Perrus M, Bertoglio J, et al. Differential regulation of actin stress fiber assembly and proplatelet formation by alpha2beta1 integrin and GPVI in human megakaryocytes. *Blood.* 2004;104(10):3117-3125.

231. Semeniak D, Kulawig R, Stegner D, et al. Proplatelet formation is selectively inhibited by collagen type I through Syk-independent GPVI signaling. *J Cell Sci.* 2016;129(18):3473-3484.

232. Larson MK, Watson SP. Regulation of proplatelet formation and platelet release by integrin alpha IIb beta3. *Blood.* 2006;108(5):1509-1514.

233. Giannini S, Lee-Sundlov MM, Rivadeneyra L, et al. β4GALT1 controls β1 integrin function to govern thrombopoiesis and hematopoietic stem cell homeostasis. *Nat Commun.* 2020;11(1):356.

234. Schachtner H, Calaminus SD, Sinclair A, et al. Megakaryocytes assemble podosomes that degrade matrix and protrude through basement membrane. *Blood.* 2013;121(13):2542-2552.

235. Sabri S, Foudi A, Boukour S, et al. Deficiency in the Wiskott-Aldrich protein induces premature proplatelet formation and platelet production in the bone marrow compartment. *Blood.* 2006;108(1):134-140.

236. Eckly A, Scandola C, Oprescu A, et al. Megakaryocytes use in vivo podosome-like structures working collectively to penetrate the endothelial barrier of bone marrow sinusoids. *J Thromb Haemost.* 2020;18(11):2987-3001.

237. Dütting S, Gaits-Iacovoni F, Stegner D, et al. A Cdc42/RhoA regulatory circuit downstream of glycoprotein Ib guides transendothelial platelet biogenesis. *Nat Commun.* 2017;8:15838.

238. Freson K, De Vos R, Wittevrongel C, et al. The TUBB1 Q43P functional polymorphism reduces the risk of cardiovascular disease in men by modulating platelet function and structure. *Blood.* 2005;106(7):2356-2362.

239. Kunishima S, Kobayashi R, Itoh TJ, Hamaguchi M, Saito H. Mutation of the beta1-tubulin gene associated with congenital macrothrombocytopenia affecting microtubule assembly. *Blood.* 2009;113(2):458-461.

240. Balduini CL, Savoia A. Genetics of familial forms of thrombocytopenia. *Hum Genet.* 2012;131(12):1821-1832.

241. Favier R, Raslova H. Progress in understanding the diagnosis and molecular genetics of macrothrombocytopenias. *Br J Haematol.* 2015;170(5):626-639.

242. Eckly A, Strassel C, Freund M, et al. Abnormal megakaryocyte morphology and proplatelet formation in mice with megakaryocyte-restricted MYH9 inactivation. *Blood.* 2009;113(14):3182-3189.

243. Shin JW, Swift J, Spinler KR, Discher DE. Myosin-II inhibition and soft 2D matrix maximize multinucleation and cellular projections typical of platelet-producing megakaryocytes. *Proc Natl Acad Sci U S A.* 2011;108(28):11458-11463.

244. Chang Y, Aurade F, Larbret F, et al. Proplatelet formation is regulated by the Rho/ROCK pathway. *Blood.* 2007;109(10):4229-4236.

245. Spinler KR, Shin JW, Lambert MP, Discher DE. Myosin-II repression favors pre/proplatelets but shear activation generates platelets and fails in macrothrombocytopenia. *Blood.* 2015;125(3):525-533.

246. Pleines I, Hagedorn I, Gupta S, et al. Megakaryocyte-specific RhoA deficiency causes macrothrombocytopenia and defective platelet activation in hemostasis and thrombosis. *Blood.* 2012;119(4):1054-1063.

247. Suzuki A, Shin JW, Wang Y, et al. RhoA is essential for maintaining normal megakaryocyte ploidy and platelet generation. *PLoS One.* 2013;8(7):e69315.

248. Avanzi MP, Goldberg F, Davila J, Langhi D, Chiattone C, Mitchell WB. Rho kinase inhibition drives megakaryocyte polyploidization and proplatelet formation through MYC and NFE2 downregulation. *Br J Haematol.* 2014;164(6):867-876.

249. Shi DS, Smith MC, Campbell RA, et al. Proteasome function is required for platelet production. *J Clin Invest.* 2014;124(9):3757-3766.

250. Pan J, Lordier L, Meyran D, et al. The formin DIAPH1 (mDia1) regulates megakaryocyte proplatelet formation by remodeling the actin and microtubule cytoskeletons. *Blood.* 2014;124(26):3967-3977.

251. Kauskot A, Poirault-Chassac S, Adam F, et al. LIM kinase/cofilin dysregulation promotes macrothrombocytopenia in severe von Willebrand disease-type 2B. *JCI Insight.* 2016;1(16):e88643.

252. Palazzo A, Bluteau O, Messaoudi K, et al. The cell division control protein 42-Src family kinase-neural Wiskott-Aldrich syndrome protein pathway regulates human proplatelet formation. *J Thromb Haemostasis.* 2016;14(12):2524-2535.

253. Antkowiak A, Viaud J, Severin S, et al. Cdc42-dependent F-actin dynamics drive structuration of the demarcation membrane system in megakaryocytes. *J Thromb Haemost.* 2016;14(6):1268-1284.

254. Pleines I, Dutting S, Cherpokova D, et al. Defective tubulin organization and proplatelet formation in murine megakaryocytes lacking Rac1 and Cdc42. *Blood.* 2013;122(18):3178-3187.

255. Heib T, Hermanns HM, Manukjan G, et al. RhoA/Cdc42 signaling drives cytoplasmic maturation but not endomitosis in megakaryocytes. *Cell Rep.* 2021;35(6):109102.

256. Bender M, Stritt S, Nurden P, et al. Megakaryocyte-specific Profilin1-deficiency alters microtubule stability and causes a Wiskott-Aldrich syndrome-like platelet defect. *Nat Commun.* 2014;5:4746.

257. Iancu-Rubin C, Gajzer D, Mosoyan G, Feller F, Mascarenhas J, Hoffman R. Panobinostat (LBH589)-induced acetylation of tubulin impairs megakaryocyte maturation and platelet formation. *Exp Hematol.* 2012;40(7):564-574.

258. Ali A, Bluteau O, Messaoudi K, et al. Thrombocytopenia induced by the histone deacetylase inhibitor abexinostat involves p53-dependent and -independent mechanisms. *Cell Death Dis.* 2013;4:e738.

259. Bishton MJ, Harrison SJ, Martin BP, et al. Deciphering the molecular and biologic processes that mediate histone deacetylase inhibitor-induced thrombocytopenia. *Blood.* 2011;117(13):3658-3668.

260. Li L, Yang XJ. Tubulin acetylation: responsible enzymes, biological functions and human diseases. *Cell Mol Life Sci.* 2015;72(22):4237-4255.

261. Messaoudi K, Ali A, Ishaq R, et al. Critical role of the HDAC6-cortactin axis in human megakaryocyte maturation leading to a proplatelet-formation defect. *Nat Commun.* 2017;8(1):1786.

262. Radley JM, Haller CJ. Fate of senescent megakaryocytes in the bone marrow. *Br J Haematol.* 1983;53(2):277-287.

263. Josefsson EC, James C, Henley KJ, et al. Megakaryocytes possess a functional intrinsic apoptosis pathway that must be restrained to survive and produce platelets. *J Exp Med.* 2011;208(10):2017-2031.

264. White MJ, Kile BT. Apoptotic processes in megakaryocytes and platelets. *Semin Hematol.* 2010;47(3):227-234.

265. Kile BT. The role of apoptosis in megakaryocytes and platelets. *Br J Haematol.* 2014;165(2):217-226.

266. Josefsson EC, Burnett DL, Lebois M, et al. Platelet production proceeds independently of the intrinsic and extrinsic apoptosis pathways. *Nat Commun.* 2014;5:3455.

267. Bouillet P, Metcalf D, Huang DC, et al. Proapoptotic Bcl-2 relative Bim required for certain apoptotic responses, leukocyte homeostasis, and to preclude autoimmunity. *Science*. 1999;286(5445):1735-1738.
268. Kaluzhny Y, Yu G, Sun S, et al. BclxL overexpression in megakaryocytes leads to impaired platelet fragmentation. *Blood*. 2002;100(5):1670-1678.
269. Ogilvy S, Metcalf D, Print CG, Bath ML, Harris AW, Adams JM. Constitutive Bcl-2 expression throughout the hematopoietic compartment affects multiple lineages and enhances progenitor cell survival. *Proc Natl Acad Sci U S A*. 1999;96(26):14943-14948.
270. Clarke MC, Savill J, Jones DB, Noble BS, Brown SB. Compartmentalized megakaryocyte death generates functional platelets committed to caspase-independent death. *J Cell Biol*. 2003;160(4):577-587.
271. De Botton S, Sabri S, Daugas E, et al. Platelet formation is the consequence of caspase activation within megakaryocytes. *Blood*. 2002;100(4):1310-1317.
272. Ong L, Morison IM, Ledgerwood EC. Megakaryocytes from CYCS mutation-associated thrombocytopenia release platelets by both proplatelet-dependent and -independent processes. *Br J Haematol*. 2016;176(2):268-279.
273. Olson TS, Caselli A, Otsuru S, et al. Megakaryocytes promote murine osteoblastic HSC niche expansion and stem cell engraftment after radioablative conditioning. *Blood*. 2013;121(26):5238-5249.
274. Nakamura-Ishizu A, Takubo K, Fujioka M, Suda T. Megakaryocytes are essential for HSC quiescence through the production of thrombopoietin. *Biochem Biophys Res Commun*. 2014;454(2):353-357.
275. Bruns I, Lucas D, Pinho S, et al. Megakaryocytes regulate hematopoietic stem cell quiescence through CXCL4 secretion. *Nat Med*. 2014;20(11):1315-1320.
276. Nakamura-Ishizu A, Takubo K, Kobayashi H, Suzuki-Inoue K, Suda T. CLEC-2 in megakaryocytes is critical for maintenance of hematopoietic stem cells in the bone marrow. *J Exp Med*. 2015;212(12):2133-2146.
277. Decker M, Leslie J, Liu Q, Ding L. Hepatic thrombopoietin is required for bone marrow hematopoietic stem cell maintenance. *Science*. 2018;360(6384):106-110.
278. Malara A, Currao M, Gruppi C, et al. Megakaryocytes contribute to the bone marrow-matrix environment by expressing fibronectin, type IV collagen, and laminin. *Stem Cells*. 2014;32(4):926-937.
279. Ravid K, Karagianni A. Myeloproliferative disorders and its effect on bone homeostasis: the role of megakaryocytes. *Blood*. 2022;139(21):3127-3137.
280. Matsuura S, Thompson CR, Ng SK, et al. Adhesion to fibronectin via α5β1 integrin supports expansion of the megakaryocyte lineage in primary myelofibrosis. *Blood*. 2020;135(25):2286-2291.
281. Semple JW, Italiano JE, Jr, Freedman J. Platelets and the immune continuum. *Nat Rev Immunol*. 2011;11(4):264-274.
282. Shiraki R, Inoue N, Kawasaki S, et al. Expression of Toll-like receptors on human platelets. *Thromb Res*. 2004;113(6):379-385.
283. Flaujac C, Boukour S, Cramer-Bordé E. Platelets and viruses: an ambivalent relationship. *Cell Mol Life Sci*. 2010;67(4):545-556.
284. Zufferey A, Speck ER, Machlus KR, et al. Mature murine megakaryocytes present antigen-MHC class I molecules to T cells and transfer them to platelets. *Blood Adv*. 2017;1(20):1773-1785.
285. Quirino-Teixeira AC, Andrade FB, Pinheiro MBM, Rozini SV, Hottz ED. Platelets in dengue infection: more than a numbers game. *Platelets*. 2021;33(2):1-8.
286. Cumano A, Godin I. Ontogeny of the hematopoietic system. *Annu Rev Immunol*. 2007;25:745-785.
287. Palis J. Hematopoietic stem cell-independent hematopoiesis: emergence of erythroid, megakaryocyte, and myeloid potential in the mammalian embryo. *FEBS Lett*. 2016;590(22):3965-3974.
288. Potts KS, Sargeant TJ, Dawson CA, et al. Mouse prenatal platelet-forming lineages share a core transcriptional program but divergent dependence on MPL. *Blood*. 2015;126(6):807-816.
289. Potts KS, Sargeant TJ, Markham JF, et al. A lineage of diploid platelet-forming cells precedes polyploid megakaryocyte formation in the mouse embryo. *Blood*. 2014;124(17):2725-2729.
290. Chou ST, Byrska-Bishop M, Tober JM, et al. Trisomy 21-associated defects in human primitive hematopoiesis revealed through induced pluripotent stem cells. *Proc Natl Acad Sci U S A*. 2012;109(43):17573-17578.
291. Klimchenko O, Mori M, Distefano A, et al. A common bipotent progenitor generates the erythroid and megakaryocyte lineages in embryonic stem cell-derived primitive hematopoiesis. *Blood*. 2009;114(8):1506-1517.
292. Bluteau O, Langlois T, Rivera-Munoz P, et al. Developmental changes in human megakaryopoiesis. *J Thromb Haemost*. 2013;11(9):1730-1741.
293. Mazharian A, Watson SP, Severin S. Critical role for ERK1/2 in bone marrow and fetal liver-derived primary megakaryocyte differentiation, motility, and proplatelet formation. *Exp Hematol*. 2009;37(10):1238-1249.e5.
294. Ferrer-Marin F, Gutti R, Liu ZJ, Sola-Visner M. MiR-9 contributes to the developmental differences in CXCR-4 expression in human megakaryocytes. *J Thromb Haemostasis*. 2014;12(2):282-285.
295. Elagib KE, Lu CH, Mosoyan G, et al. Neonatal expression of RNA-binding protein IGF2BP3 regulates the human fetal-adult megakaryocyte transition. *J Clin Invest*. 2017;127(6):2365-2377.
296. Nakamura S, Takayama N, Hirata S, et al. Expandable megakaryocyte cell lines enable clinically applicable generation of platelets from human induced pluripotent stem cells. *Cell Stem Cell*. 2014;14(4):535-548.
297. Liu Y, Wang Y, Gao Y, et al. Efficient generation of megakaryocytes from human induced pluripotent stem cells using food and drug administration-approved pharmacological reagents. *Stem Cells Transl Med*. 2015;4(4):309-319.
298. Lu SJ, Li F, Yin H, et al. Platelets generated from human embryonic stem cells are functional in vitro and in the microcirculation of living mice. *Cell Res*. 2011;21(3):530-545.
299. Liu ZJ, Hoffmeister KM, Hu Z, et al. Expansion of the neonatal platelet mass is achieved via an extension of platelet lifespan. *Blood*. 2014;123(22):3381-3389.
300. Rowe RG, Mandelbaum J, Zon LI, Daley GQ. Engineering hematopoietic stem cells: lessons from development. *Cell Stem Cell*. 2016;18(6):707-720.
301. Crispino JD, Weiss MJ. Erythro-megakaryocytic transcription factors associated with hereditary anemia. *Blood*. 2014;123(20):3080-3088.
302. Tijssen MR, Cvejic A, Joshi A, et al. Genome-wide analysis of simultaneous GATA1/2, RUNX1, FLI1, and SCL binding in megakaryocytes identifies hematopoietic regulators. *Dev Cell*. 2011;20(5):597-609.
303. Elagib KE, Racke FK, Mogass M, Khetawat R, Delehanty LL, Goldfarb AN. RUNX1 and GATA-1 coexpression and cooperation in megakaryocytic differentiation. *Blood*. 2003;101(11):4333-4341.
304. Eisbacher M, Holmes ML, Newton A, et al. Protein-protein interaction between Fli-1 and GATA-1 mediates synergistic expression of megakaryocyte-specific genes through cooperative DNA binding. *Mol Cell Biol*. 2003;23(10):3427-3441.
305. Zang C, Luyten A, Chen J, Liu XS, Shivdasani RA. NF-E2, FLI1 and RUNX1 collaborate at areas of dynamic chromatin to activate transcription in mature mouse megakaryocytes. *Sci Rep*. 2016;6:30255.
306. Trainor CD, Omichinski JG, Vandergon TL, Gronenborn AM, Clore GM, Felsenfeld G. A palindromic regulatory site within vertebrate GATA-1 promoters requires both zinc fingers of the GATA-1 DNA-binding domain for high-affinity interaction. *Mol Cell Biol*. 1996;16(5):2238-2247.
307. Martin DI, Orkin SH. Transcriptional activation and DNA binding by the erythroid factor GF-1/NF-E1/Eryf 1. *Genes Dev*. 1990;4(11):1886-1898.
308. Huang Z, Dore LC, Li Z, et al. GATA-2 reinforces megakaryocyte development in the absence of GATA-1. *Mol Cell Biol*. 2009;29(18):5168-5180.
309. Fujiwara Y, Browne CP, Cunniff K, Goff SC, Orkin SH. Arrested development of embryonic red cell precursors in mouse embryos lacking transcription factor GATA-1. *Proc Natl Acad Sci U S A*. 1996;93(22):12355-12358.
310. Shivdasani RA, Fujiwara Y, McDevitt MA, Orkin SH. A lineage-selective knockout establishes the critical role of transcription factor GATA-1 in megakaryocyte growth and platelet development. *EMBO J*. 1997;16(13):3965-3973.
311. Vyas P, Ault K, Jackson CW, Orkin SH, Shivdasani RA. Consequences of GATA-1 deficiency in megakaryocytes and platelets. *Blood*. 1999;93(9):2867-2875.
312. Singleton BK, Roxby DJ, Stirling JW, et al. A novel GATA1 mutation (Stop414Arg) in a family with the rare X-linked blood group Lu(a-b-) phenotype and mild macrothrombocytic thrombocytopenia. *Br J Haematol*. 2013;161(1):139-142.
313. Chang AN, Cantor AB, Fujiwara Y, et al. GATA-factor dependence of the multitype zinc-finger protein FOG-1 for its essential role in megakaryopoiesis. *Proc Natl Acad Sci U S A*. 2002;99(14):9237-9242.
314. Gao Z, Huang Z, Olivey HE, Gurbuxani S, Crispino JD, Svensson EC. FOG-1-mediated recruitment of NuRD is required for cell lineage re-enforcement during haematopoiesis. *EMBO J*. 2010;29(2):457-468.
315. Gregory GD, Miccio A, Bersenev A, et al. FOG1 requires NuRD to promote hematopoiesis and maintain lineage fidelity within the megakaryocytic-erythroid compartment. *Blood*. 2010;115(11):2156-2166.
316. Woo AJ, Moran TB, Schindler YL, et al. Identification of ZBP-89 as a novel GATA-1-associated transcription factor involved in megakaryocytic and erythroid development. *Mol Cell Biol*. 2008;28(8):2675-2689.
317. Tsai FY, Keller G, Kuo FC, et al. An early haematopoietic defect in mice lacking the transcription factor GATA-2. *Nature*. 1994;371(6494):221-226.
318. Tsai FY, Orkin SH. Transcription factor GATA-2 is required for proliferation/survival of early hematopoietic cells and mast cell formation, but not for erythroid and myeloid terminal differentiation. *Blood*. 1997;89(10):3636-3643.
319. Grass JA, Boyer ME, Pal S, Wu J, Weiss MJ, Bresnick EH. GATA-1-dependent transcriptional repression of GATA-2 via disruption of positive autoregulation and domain-wide chromatin remodeling. *Proc Natl Acad Sci U S A*. 2003;100(15):8811-8816.
320. Pimkin M, Kossenkov AV, Mishra T, et al. Divergent functions of hematopoietic transcription factors in lineage priming and differentiation during erythro-megakaryopoiesis. *Genome Res*. 2014;24(12):1932-1944.
321. Hall MA, Curtis DJ, Metcalf D, et al. The critical regulator of embryonic hematopoiesis, SCL, is vital in the adult for megakaryopoiesis, erythropoiesis, and lineage choice in CFU-S12. *Proc Natl Acad Sci U S A*. 2003;100(3):992-997.
322. Mikkola HK, Klintman J, Yang H, et al. Haematopoietic stem cells retain long-term repopulating activity and multipotency in the absence of stem-cell leukaemia SCL/tal-1 gene. *Nature*. 2003;421(6922):547-551.
323. Salmon JM, Slater NJ, Hall MA, et al. Aberrant mast-cell differentiation in mice lacking the stem-cell leukemia gene. *Blood*. 2007;110(10):3573-3581.
324. McCormack MP, Hall MA, Schoenwaelder SM, et al. A critical role for the transcription factor Scl in platelet production during stress thrombopoiesis. *Blood*. 2006;108(7):2248-2256.
325. Gekas C, Rhodes KE, Gereige LM, et al. Mef2C is a lineage-restricted target of Scl/Tal1 and regulates megakaryopoiesis and B-cell homeostasis. *Blood*. 2009;113(15):3461-3471.
326. Chagraoui H, Kassouf M, Banerjee S, et al. SCL-mediated regulation of the cell-cycle regulator p21 is critical for murine megakaryopoiesis. *Blood*. 2011;118(3):723-735.
327. Porcher C, Liao EC, Fujiwara Y, Zon LI, Orkin SH. Specification of hematopoietic and vascular development by the bHLH transcription factor SCL without direct DNA binding. *Development*. 1999;126(20):4603-4615.
328. Han GC, Vinayachandran V, Bataille AR, et al. Genome-wide organization of GATA1 and TAL1 determined at high resolution. *Mol Cell Biol*. 2016;36(1):157-172.
329. Kerenyi MA, Orkin SH. Networking erythropoiesis. *J Exp Med*. 2010;207(12):2537-2541.
330. Tripic T, Deng W, Cheng Y, et al. SCL and associated proteins distinguish active from repressive GATA transcription factor complexes. *Blood*. 2009;113(10):2191-2201.

331. Schuh AH, Tipping AJ, Clark AJ, et al. ETO-2 associates with SCL in erythroid cells and megakaryocytes and provides repressor functions in erythropoiesis. *Mol Cell Biol.* 2005;25(23):10235-10250.

332. Chiu SK, Orive SL, Moon MJ, et al. Shared roles for Scl and Lyl1 in murine platelet production and function. *Blood.* 2019;134(10):826-835.

333. Ichikawa M, Yoshimi A, Nakagawa M, Nishimoto N, Watanabe-Okochi N, Kurokawa M. A role for RUNX1 in hematopoiesis and myeloid leukemia. *Int J Hematol.* 2013;97(6):726-734.

334. Li Y, Jin C, Bai H, et al. Human NOTCH4 is a key target of RUNX1 in megakaryocytic differentiation. *Blood.* 2018;131(2):191-201.

335. Antony-Debre I, Bluteau D, Itzykson R, et al. MYH10 protein expression in platelets as a biomarker of RUNX1 and FLI1 alterations. *Blood.* 2012;120(13):2719-2722.

336. Gilles L, Guieze R, Bluteau D, et al. P19INK4D links endomitotic arrest and megakaryocyte maturation and is regulated by AML-1. *Blood.* 2008;111(8):4081-4091.

337. Jalagadugula G, Mao G, Kaur G, Goldfinger LE, Dhanasekaran DN, Rao AK. Regulation of platelet myosin light chain (MYL9) by RUNX1: implications for thrombocytopenia and platelet dysfunction in RUNX1 haplodeficiency. *Blood.* 2010;116(26):6037-6045.

338. Bluteau D, Glembotsky AC, Raimbault A, et al. Dysmegakaryopoiesis of FPD/AML pedigrees with constitutional RUNX1 mutations is linked to myosin II deregulated expression. *Blood.* 2012;120(13):2708-2718.

339. Bluteau D, Balduini A, Balayn N, et al. Thrombocytopenia-associated mutations in the ANKRD26 regulatory region induce MAPK hyperactivation. *J Clin Invest.* 2014;124(2):580-591.

340. Kaur G, Jalagadugula G, Mao G, Rao AK. RUNX1/core binding factor A2 regulates platelet 12-lipoxygenase gene (ALOX12): studies in human RUNX1 haplodeficiency. *Blood.* 2010;115(15):3128-3135.

341. Jalagadugula G, Mao G, Kaur G, Dhanasekaran DN, Rao AK. Platelet protein kinase C-theta deficiency with human RUNX1 mutation: PRKCQ is a transcriptional target of RUNX1. *Arterioscler Thromb Vasc Biol.* 2011;31(4):921-927.

342. Aneja K, Jalagadugula G, Mao G, Singh A, Rao AK. Mechanism of platelet factor 4 (PF4) deficiency with RUNX1 haplodeficiency: RUNX1 is a transcriptional regulator of PF4. *J Thromb Haemost.* 2011;9(2):383-391.

343. Glembotsky AC, Bluteau D, Espasandin YR, et al. Mechanisms underlying platelet function defect in a pedigree with familial platelet disorder with a predisposition to acute myelogenous leukemia: potential role for candidate RUNX1 targets. *J Thromb Haemost.* 2014;12(5):761-772.

344. Satoh Y, Matsumura I, Tanaka H, et al. AML1/RUNX1 works as a negative regulator of c-Mpl in hematopoietic stem cells. *J Biol Chem.* 2008;283(44):30045-30056.

345. Owen CJ, Toze CL, Koochin A, et al. Five new pedigrees with inherited RUNX1 mutations causing familial platelet disorder with propensity to myeloid malignancy. *Blood.* 2008;112(12):4639-4645.

346. Michaud J, Wu F, Osato M, et al. In vitro analyses of known and novel RUNX1/AML1 mutations in dominant familial platelet disorder with predisposition to acute myelogenous leukemia: implications for mechanisms of pathogenesis. *Blood.* 2002;99(4):1364-1372.

347. Estevez B, Borst S, Jarocha D, et al. RUNX-1 haploinsufficiency causes a marked deficiency of megakaryocyte-biased hematopoietic progenitor cells. *Blood.* 2021;137(19):2662-2675.

348. Lulli V, Romania P, Morsilli O, et al. Overexpression of Ets-1 in human hematopoietic progenitor cells blocks erythroid and promotes megakaryocytic differentiation. *Cell Death Differ.* 2006;13(7):1064-1074.

349. Pang L, Xue HH, Szalai G, et al. Maturation stage-specific regulation of megakaryopoiesis by pointed-domain Ets proteins. *Blood.* 2006;108(7):2198-2206.

350. Okada Y, Nobori H, Shimizu M, et al. Multiple ETS family proteins regulate PF4 gene expression by binding to the same ETS binding site. *PLoS One.* 2011;6(9):e24837.

351. Yang ZF, Drumea K, Cormier J, Wang J, Zhu X, Rosmarin AG. GABP transcription factor is required for myeloid differentiation, in part, through its control of Gfi-1 expression. *Blood.* 2011;118(8):2243-2253.

352. Bouilloux F, Juban G, Cohet N, et al. EKLF restricts megakaryocytic differentiation at the benefit of erythrocytic differentiation. *Blood.* 2008;112(3):576-584.

353. Hart A, Melet F, Grossfeld P, et al. Fli-1 is required for murine vascular and megakaryocyte development and is hemizygously deleted in patients with thrombocytopenia. *Immunity.* 2000;13(2):167-177.

354. Raslova H, Komura E, Le Couedic JP, et al. FLI1 monoallelic expression combined with its hemizygous loss underlies Paris-Trousseau/Jacobsen thrombopenia. *J Clin Invest.* 2004;114(1):77-84.

355. Moussa O, LaRue AC, Abangan RS, Jr, et al. Thrombocytopenia in mice lacking the carboxy-terminal regulatory domain of the Ets transcription factor Fli1. *Mol Cell Biol.* 2010;30(21):5194-5206.

356. Giraud G, Kolovos P, Boltsis I, et al. Interplay between FLI-1 and the LDB1 complex in murine erythroleukemia cells and during megakaryopoiesis. *iScience.* 2021;24(3):102210.

357. Hock H, Meade E, Medeiros S, et al. Tel/Etv6 is an essential and selective regulator of adult hematopoietic stem cell survival. *Genes Dev.* 2004;18(19):2336-2341.

358. Fisher MH, Kirkpatrick GD, Stevens B, et al. ETV6 germline mutations cause HDAC3/NCOR2 mislocalization and upregulation of interferon response genes. *JCI Insight.* 2020;5(18):e140332.

359. Salek-Ardakani S, Smooha G, de Boer J, et al. ERG is a megakaryocytic oncogene. *Cancer Res.* 2009;69(11):4665-4673.

360. Stankiewicz MJ, Crispino JD. AKT collaborates with ERG and Gata1s to dysregulate megakaryopoiesis and promote AMKL. *Leukemia.* 2013;27(6):1339-1347.

361. Kruse EA, Loughran SJ, Baldwin TM, et al. Dual requirement for the ETS transcription factors Fli-1 and Erg in hematopoietic stem cells and the megakaryocyte lineage. *Proc Natl Acad Sci U S A.* 2009;106(33):13814-13819.

362. Saleque S, Cameron S, Orkin SH. The zinc-finger proto-oncogene Gfi-1b is essential for development of the erythroid and megakaryocytic lineages. *Genes Dev.* 2002;16(3):301-306.

363. Randrianarison-Huetz V, Laurent B, Bardet V, Blobe GC, Huetz F, Dumenil D. Gfi-1B controls human erythroid and megakaryocytic differentiation by regulating TGF-beta signaling at the bipotent erythro-megakaryocytic progenitor stage. *Blood.* 2010;115(14):2784-2795.

364. Shooshtarizadeh P, Helness A, Vadnais C, et al. Gfi1b regulates the level of Wnt/β-catenin signaling in hematopoietic stem cells and megakaryocytes. *Nat Commun.* 2019;10(1):1270.

365. Tober J, McGrath KE, Palis J. Primitive erythropoiesis and megakaryopoiesis in the yolk sac are independent of c-myb. *Blood.* 2008;111(5):2636-2639.

366. Barroga CF, Pham H, Kaushansky K. Thrombopoietin regulates c-Myb expression by modulating micro RNA 150 expression. *Exp Hematol.* 2008;36(12):1585-1592.

367. Metcalf D, Carpinelli MR, Hyland C, et al. Anomalous megakaryocytopoiesis in mice with mutations in the c-Myb gene. *Blood.* 2005;105(9):3480-3487.

368. Andrews NC, Kotkow KJ, Ney PA, Erdjument-Bromage H, Tempst P, Orkin SH. The ubiquitous subunit of erythroid transcription factor NF-E2 is a small basic-leucine zipper protein related to the v-maf oncogene. *Proc Natl Acad Sci U S A.* 1993;90(24):11488-11492.

369. Takayama M, Fujita R, Suzuki M, et al. Genetic analysis of hierarchical regulation for Gata1 and NF-E2 p45 gene expression in megakaryopoiesis. *Mol Cell Biol.* 2010;30(11):2668-2680.

370. Shivdasani RA, Rosenblatt MF, Zucker-Franklin D, et al. Transcription factor NF-E2 is required for platelet formation independent of the actions of thrombopoietin/MGDF in megakaryocyte development. *Cell.* 1995;81(5):695-704.

371. Lecine P, Villeval JL, Vyas P, Swencki B, Xu Y, Shivdasani RA. Mice lacking transcription factor NF-E2 provide in vivo validation of the proplatelet model of thrombocytopoiesis and show a platelet production defect that is intrinsic to megakaryocytes. *Blood.* 1998;92(5):1608-1616.

372. Levin J, Peng JP, Baker GR, et al. Pathophysiology of thrombocytopenia and anemia in mice lacking transcription factor NF-E2. *Blood.* 1999;94(9):3037-3047.

373. Fock EL, Yan F, Pan S, Chong BH. NF-E2-mediated enhancement of megakaryocytic differentiation and platelet production in vitro and in vivo. *Exp Hematol.* 2008;36(1):78-92.

374. Motohashi H, Fujita R, Takayama M, et al. Molecular determinants for small Maf protein control of platelet production. *Mol Cell Biol.* 2011;31(1):151-162.

375. Deveaux S, Cohen-Kaminsky S, Shivdasani RA, et al. p45 NF-E2 regulates expression of thromboxane synthase in megakaryocytes. *EMBO J.* 1997;16(18):5654-5661.

376. Schwer HD, Lecine P, Tiwari S, Italiano JE, Jr, Hartwig JH, Shivdasani RA. A lineage-restricted and divergent beta-tubulin isoform is essential for the biogenesis, structure and function of blood platelets. *Curr Biol.* 2001;11(8):579-586.

377. Kerrigan SW, Gaur M, Murphy RP, Shattil SJ, Leavitt AD. Caspase-12: a developmental link between G-protein-coupled receptors and integrin alphaIIbbeta3 activation. *Blood.* 2004;104(5):1327-1334.

378. Tiwari S, Italiano JE, Jr, Barral DC, et al. A role for Rab27b in NF-E2-dependent pathways of platelet formation. *Blood.* 2003;102(12):3970-3979.

379. Nagata Y, Yoshikawa J, Hashimoto A, Yamamoto M, Payne AH, Todokoro K. Proplatelet formation of megakaryocytes is triggered by autocrine-synthesized estradiol. *Genes Dev.* 2003;17(23):2864-2869.

380. Chen Z, Hu M, Shivdasani RA. Expression analysis of primary mouse megakaryocyte differentiation and its application in identifying stage-specific molecular markers and a novel transcriptional target of NF-E2. *Blood.* 2007;109(4):1451-1459.

381. Narumiya S, Sugimoto Y, Ushikubi F. Prostanoid receptors: structures, properties, and functions. *Physiol Rev.* 1999;79(4):1193-1226.

382. Motohashi H, Kimura M, Fujita R, et al. NF-E2 domination over Nrf2 promotes ROS accumulation and megakaryocytic maturation. *Blood.* 2010;115(3):677-686.

383. Fujita R, Takayama-Tsujimoto M, Satoh H, et al. NF-E2 p45 is important for establishing normal function of platelets. *Mol Cell Biol.* 2013;33(14):2659-2670.

384. Mercher T, Coniat MB, Monni R, et al. Involvement of a human gene related to the Drosophila spen gene in the recurrent t(1;22) translocation of acute megakaryocytic leukemia. *Proc Natl Acad Sci U S A.* 2001;98(10):5776-5779.

385. Gilles L, Bluteau D, Boukour S, et al. MAL/SRF complex is involved in platelet formation and megakaryocyte migration by regulating MYL9 (MLC2) and MMP9. *Blood.* 2009;114(19):4221-4232.

386. Ragu C, Boukour S, Elain G, et al. The serum response factor (SRF)/megakaryocytic acute leukemia (MAL) network participates in megakaryocyte development. *Leukemia.* 2010;24(6):1227-1230.

387. Savoia A. Molecular basis of inherited thrombocytopenias: an update. *Curr Opin Hematol.* 2016;23(5):486-492.

388. Senyuk V, Sinha KK, Li D, Rinaldi CR, Yanamandra S, Nucifora G. Repression of RUNX1 activity by EVI1: a new role of EVI1 in leukemogenesis. *Cancer Res.* 2007;67(12):5658-5666.

389. Kilbey A, Alzuherri H, McColl J, Cales C, Frampton J, Bartholomew C. The Evi1 proto-oncoprotein blocks endomitosis in megakaryocytes by inhibiting sustained cyclin-dependent kinase 2 catalytic activity. *Br J Haematol.* 2005;130(6):902-911.

390. Azcoitia V, Aracil M, Martinez AC, Torres M. The homeodomain protein Meis1 is essential for definitive hematopoiesis and vascular patterning in the mouse embryo. *Dev Biol.* 2005;280(2):307-320.

391. Okada Y, Nagai R, Sato T, et al. Homeodomain proteins MEIS1 and PBXs regulate the lineage-specific transcription of the platelet factor 4 gene. *Blood.* 2003;101(12):4748-4756.

392. Wang H, Liu C, Liu X, et al. MEIS1 regulates hemogenic endothelial generation, megakaryopoiesis, and thrombopoiesis in human pluripotent stem cells by targeting TAL1 and FLI1. *Stem Cell Rep.* 2018;10(2):447-460.

393. Cova G, Taroni C, Deau MC, et al. Helios represses megakaryocyte priming in hematopoietic stem and progenitor cells. *J Exp Med*. 2021;218(10):e20202317.

394. Lentaigne C, Greene D, Sivapalaratnam S, et al. Germline mutations in the transcription factor IKZF5 cause thrombocytopenia. *Blood*. 2019;134(23):2070-2081.

395. Malinge S, Thiollier C, Chlon TM, et al. Ikaros inhibits megakaryopoiesis through functional interaction with GATA-1 and NOTCH signaling. *Blood*. 2013;121(13):2440-2451.

396. Liu A, Li S, Donnenberg V, et al. Immunomodulatory drugs downregulate IKZF1 leading to expansion of hematopoietic progenitors with concomitant block of megakaryocytic maturation. *Haematologica*. 2018;103(10):1688-1697.

397. Ferguson DCJ, Mokim JH, Meinders M, et al. Characterization and evolutionary origin of novel C$_2$H$_2$ zinc finger protein (ZNF648) required for both erythroid and megakaryocyte differentiation in humans. *Haematologica*. Published online 2020.

398. Pozner A, Lotem J, Xiao C, et al. Developmentally regulated promoter-switch transcriptionally controls Runx1 function during embryonic hematopoiesis. *BMC Dev Biol*. 2007;7:84.

399. Dumon S, Walton DS, Volpe G, et al. Itga2b regulation at the onset of definitive hematopoiesis and commitment to differentiation. *PLoS One*. 2012;7(8):e43300.

400. Kuvardina ON, Herglotz J, Kolodziej S, et al. RUNX1 represses the erythroid gene expression program during megakaryocytic differentiation. *Blood*. 2015;125(23):3570-3579.

401. Huang H, Woo AJ, Waldon Z, et al. A Src family kinase-Shp2 axis controls RUNX1 activity in megakaryocyte and T-lymphocyte differentiation. *Genes Dev*. 2012;26(14):1587-1601.

402. Zhao X, Jankovic V, Gural A, et al. Methylation of RUNX1 by PRMT1 abrogates SIN3A binding and potentiates its transcriptional activity. *Genes Dev*. 2008;22(5):640-653.

403. Yan B, Yang J, Kim MY, et al. HDAC1 is required for GATA-1 transcription activity, global chromatin occupancy and hematopoiesis. *Nucl Acids Res*. 2021;49(17):9783-9798.

404. Wilting RH, Yanover E, Heideman MR, et al. Overlapping functions of Hdac1 and Hdac2 in cell cycle regulation and haematopoiesis. *EMBO J*. 2010;29(15):2586-2597.

405. Yu M, Mazor T, Huang H, et al. Direct recruitment of polycomb repressive complex 1 to chromatin by core binding transcription factors. *Mol Cell*. 2012;45(3):330-343.

406. Oguro H, Yuan J, Tanaka S, et al. Lethal myelofibrosis induced by Bmi1-deficient hematopoietic cells unveils a tumor suppressor function of the polycomb group genes. *J Exp Med*. 2012;209(3):445-454.

407. Mochizuki-Kashio M, Mishima Y, Miyagi S, et al. Dependency on the polycomb gene Ezh2 distinguishes fetal from adult hematopoietic stem cells. *Blood*. 2011;118(25):6553-6561.

408. Mazzi S, Dessen P, Vieira M, et al. Dual role of EZH2 on megakaryocyte differentiation. *Blood*. 2021;138(17):1603-1614.

409. Abdel-Wahab O, Gao J, Adli M, et al. Deletion of Asxl1 results in myelodysplasia and severe developmental defects in vivo. *J Exp Med*. 2013;210(12):2641-2659.

410. Shi H, Yamamoto S, Sheng M, et al. ASXL1 plays an important role in erythropoiesis. *Sci Rep*. 2016;6:28789.

411. Micol JB, Pastore A, Inoue D, et al. ASXL2 is essential for haematopoiesis and acts as a haploinsufficient tumour suppressor in leukemia. *Nat Commun*. 2017;8:15429.

412. Dey A, Seshasayee D, Noubade R, et al. Loss of the tumor suppressor BAP1 causes myeloid transformation. *Science*. 2012;337(6101):1541-1546.

413. Quivoron C, Couronne L, Della Valle V, et al. TET2 inactivation results in pleiotropic hematopoietic abnormalities in mouse and is a recurrent event during human lymphomagenesis. *Cancer Cell*. 2011;20(1):25-38.

414. Mayle A, Yang L, Rodriguez B, et al. Dnmt3a loss predisposes murine hematopoietic stem cells to malignant transformation. *Blood*. 2015;125(4):629-638.

415. Komeno Y, Huang YJ, Qiu J, et al. SRSF2 is essential for hematopoiesis, and its myelodysplastic syndrome-related mutations dysregulate alternative pre-mRNA splicing. *Mol Cell Biol*. 2015;35(17):3071-3082.

416. Romania P, Lulli V, Pelosi E, Biffoni M, Peschle C, Marziali G. MicroRNA 155 modulates megakaryopoiesis at progenitor and precursor level by targeting Ets-1 and Meis1 transcription factors. *Br J Haematol*. 2008;143(4):570-580.

417. Weiss CN, Ito K. microRNA-22 promotes megakaryocyte differentiation through repression of its target, GFI1. *Blood Adv*. 2019;3(1):33-46.

418. Garzon R, Pichiorri F, Palumbo T, et al. MicroRNA fingerprints during human megakaryocytopoiesis. *Proc Natl Acad Sci U S A*. 2006;103(13):5078-5083.

419. Ben-Ami O, Pencovich N, Lotem J, Levanon D, Groner Y. A regulatory interplay between miR-27a and Runx1 during megakaryopoiesis. *Proc Natl Acad Sci U S A*. 2009;106(1):238-243.

420. Navarro F, Gutman D, Meire E, et al. miR-34a contributes to megakaryocytic differentiation of K562 cells independently of p53. *Blood*. 2009;114(10):2181-2192.

421. Kamat V, Paluru P, Myint M, French DL, Gadue P, Diamond SL. MicroRNA screen of human embryonic stem cell differentiation reveals miR-105 as an enhancer of megakaryopoiesis from adult CD34+ cells. *Stem Cells*. 2014;32(5):1337-1346.

422. Girardot M, Pecquet C, Boukour S, et al. miR-28 is a thrombopoietin receptor targeting microRNA detected in a fraction of myeloproliferative neoplasm patient platelets. *Blood*. 2010;116(3):437-445.

423. Norfo R, Zini R, Pennucci V, et al. miRNA-mRNA integrative analysis in primary myelofibrosis CD34+ cells: role of miR-155/JARID2 axis in abnormal megakaryopoiesis. *Blood*. 2014;124(13):e21-e32.

424. Haldar S, Roy A, Banerjee S. Differential regulation of MCM7 and its intronic miRNA cluster miR-106b-25 during megakaryopoiesis induced polyploidy. *RNA Biol*. 2014;11(9):1137-1147.

425. Qu M, Fang F, Zou X, et al. miR-125b modulates megakaryocyte maturation by targeting the cell-cycle inhibitor p19INK4D. *Cell Death Dis*. 2016;7(10):e2430.

426. Alejo-Valle O, Weigert K, Bhayadia R, et al. The megakaryocytic transcription factor ARID3A suppresses leukemia pathogenesis. *Blood*. 2022;139(5):651-665.

427. Chapnik E, Rivkin N, Mildner A, et al. miR-142 orchestrates a network of actin cytoskeleton regulators during megakaryopoiesis. *Elife*. 2014;3:e01964.

428. Labbaye C, Spinello I, Quaranta MT, et al. A three-step pathway comprising PLZF/miR-146a/CXCR4 controls megakaryopoiesis. *Nat Cell Biol*. 2008;10(7):788-801.

429. Undi RB, Gutti U, Gutti RK. Role of let-7b/Fzd4 axis in mitochondrial biogenesis through wnt signaling: in neonatal and adult megakaryocytes. *Int J Biochem Cell Biol*. 2016;79:61-68.

430. Zhang Z, Ran Y, Shaw TS, Peng Y. MicroRNAs 10a and 10b regulate the expression of human platelet glycoprotein Ibalpha for normal megakaryopoiesis. *Int J Mol Sci*. 2016;17(11):1873.

431. Paralkar VR, Mishra T, Luan J, et al. Lineage and species-specific long noncoding RNAs during erythro-megakaryocytic development. *Blood*. 2014;123(12):1927-1937.

432. Tran NT, Su H, Khodadadi-Jamayran A, et al. The AS-RBM15 lncRNA enhances RBM15 protein translation during megakaryocyte differentiation. *EMBO Rep*. 2016;17(6):887-900.

433. Cserhati I, Kelemen E. Acute prolonged thrombocytosis in mice induced by thrombocythaemic sera; a possible human thrombopoietin; a preliminary communication. *Acta Med Acad Sci Hungar*. 1958;11(4):473-475.

434. Sparrow RL, Williams N. Megakaryocyte colony stimulating factor: its identity to interleukin-3. *Prog Clin Biol Res*. 1986;215:123-128.

435. Williams N, Eger RR, Jackson HM, Nelson DJ. Two-factor requirement for murine megakaryocyte colony formation. *J Cell Physiol*. 1982;110(1):101-104.

436. Williams N. Is thrombopoietin interleukin 6? *Exp Hematol*. 1991;19(7):714-718.

437. Straneva JE, van Besien KW, Derigs G, Hoffman R. Is interleukin 6 the physiological regulator of thrombopoiesis? *Exp Hematol*. 1992;20(1):47-50.

438. Wendling F, Vigon I, Souyri M, Tambourin P. Myeloid progenitor cells transformed by the myeloproliferative leukemia virus proliferate and differentiate in vitro without the addition of growth factors. *Leukemia*. 1989;3(7):475-480.

439. Souyri M, Vigon I, Penciolelli JF, Heard JM, Tambourin P, Wendling F. A putative truncated cytokine receptor gene transduced by the myeloproliferative leukemia virus immortalizes hematopoietic progenitors. *Cell*. 1990;63(6):1137-1147.

440. Methia N, Louache F, Vainchenker W, Wendling F. Oligodeoxynucleotides antisense to the proto-oncogene c-mpl specifically inhibit in vitro megakaryocytopoiesis. *Blood*. 1993;82(5):1395-1401.

441. de Sauvage FJ, Hass PE, Spencer SD, et al. Stimulation of megakaryocytopoiesis and thrombopoiesis by the c-Mpl ligand. *Nature*. 1994;369(6481):533-538.

442. Bartley TD, Bogenberger J, Hunt P, et al. Identification and cloning of a megakaryocyte growth and development factor that is a ligand for the cytokine receptor Mpl. *Cell*. 1994;77(7):1117-1124.

443. Lok S, Kaushansky K, Holly RD, et al. Cloning and expression of murine thrombopoietin cDNA and stimulation of platelet production in vivo. *Nature*. 1994;369(6481):565-568.

444. Gurney AL, Kuang WJ, Xie MH, Malloy BE, Eaton DL, de Sauvage FJ. Genomic structure, chromosomal localization, and conserved alternative splice forms of thrombopoietin. *Blood*. 1995;85(4):981-988.

445. Kaushansky K. Thrombopoietin and its receptor in normal and neoplastic hematopoiesis. *Thromb J*. 2016;14(suppl 1):40.

446. Park H, Park SS, Jin EH, et al. Identification of functionally important residues of human thrombopoietin. *J Biol Chem*. 1998;273(1):256-261.

447. Hou J, Zhan H. Expression of active thrombopoietin and identification of its key residues responsible for receptor binding. *Cytokine*. 1998;10(5):319-330.

448. Linden HM, Kaushansky K. The glycan domain of thrombopoietin enhances its secretion. *Biochemistry*. 2000;39(11):3044-3051.

449. Song JS, Park H, Hong HJ, Yu MH, Ryu SE. Homology modeling of the receptor binding domain of human thrombopoietin. *J Comput Aided Mol Des*. 1998;12(5):419-424.

450. Qian S, Fu F, Li W, Chen Q, de Sauvage FJ. Primary role of the liver in thrombopoietin production shown by tissue-specific knockout. *Blood*. 1998;92(6):2189-2191.

451. Kaushansky K, Lok S, Holly RD, et al. Promotion of megakaryocyte progenitor expansion and differentiation by the c-Mpl ligand thrombopoietin. *Nature*. 1994;369(6481):568-571.

452. Norol F, Vitrat N, Cramer E, et al. Effects of cytokines on platelet production from blood and marrow CD34+ cells. *Blood*. 1998;91(3):830-843.

453. Debili N, Wendling F, Katz A, et al. The Mpl-ligand or thrombopoietin or megakaryocyte growth and differentiative factor has both direct proliferative and differentiative activities on human megakaryocyte progenitors. *Blood*. 1995;86(7):2516-2525.

454. Rasko JE, O'Flaherty E, Begley CG. Mpl ligand (MGDF) alone and in combination with stem cell factor (SCF) promotes proliferation and survival of human megakaryocyte, erythroid and granulocyte/macrophage progenitors. *Stem Cells*. 1997;15(1):33-42.

455. Kaushansky K, Broudy VC, Lin N, et al. Thrombopoietin, the Mpl ligand, is essential for full megakaryocyte development. *Proc Natl Acad Sci U S A*. 1995;92(8):3234-3238.

456. Choi ES, Nichol JL, Hokom MM, Hornkohl AC, Hunt P. Platelets generated in vitro from proplatelet-displaying human megakaryocytes are functional. *Blood*. 1995;85(2):402-413.

457. Choi ES, Hokom MM, Chen JL, et al. The role of megakaryocyte growth and development factor in terminal stages of thrombopoiesis. *Br J Haematol*. 1996;95(2):227-233.

458. Gurney AL, Carver-Moore K, de Sauvage FJ, Moore MW. Thrombocytopenia in c-mpl-deficient mice. *Science*. 1994;265(5177):1445-1447.

459. de Sauvage FJ, Carver-Moore K, Luoh SM, et al. Physiological regulation of early and late stages of megakaryocytopoiesis by thrombopoietin. *J Exp Med*. 1996;183(2):651-656.

460. Kimura S, Roberts AW, Metcalf D, Alexander WS. Hematopoietic stem cell deficiencies in mice lacking c-Mpl, the receptor for thrombopoietin. *Proc Natl Acad Sci U S A*. 1998;95(3):1195-1200.
461. Gainsford T, Nandurkar H, Metcalf D, Robb L, Begley CG, Alexander WS. The residual megakaryocyte and platelet production in c-mpl-deficient mice is not dependent on the actions of interleukin-6, interleukin-11, or leukemia inhibitory factor. *Blood*. 2000;95(2):528-534.
462. Gainsford T, Roberts AW, Kimura S, et al. Cytokine production and function in c-mpl-deficient mice: no physiologic role for interleukin-3 in residual megakaryocyte and platelet production. *Blood*. 1998;91(8):2745-2752.
463. Alexander WS, Roberts AW, Nicola NA, Li R, Metcalf D. Deficiencies in progenitor cells of multiple hematopoietic lineages and defective megakaryocytopoiesis in mice lacking the thrombopoietic receptor c-Mpl. *Blood*. 1996;87(6):2162-2170.
464. de Graaf CA, Metcalf D. Thrombopoietin and hematopoietic stem cells. *Cell Cycle*. 2011;10(10):1582-1589.
465. Yoshihara H, Arai F, Hosokawa K, et al. Thrombopoietin/MPL signaling regulates hematopoietic stem cell quiescence and interaction with the osteoblastic niche. *Cell Stem Cell*. 2007;1(6):685-697.
466. Qian H, Buza-Vidas N, Hyland CD, et al. Critical role of thrombopoietin in maintaining adult quiescent hematopoietic stem cells. *Cell Stem Cell*. 2007;1(6):671-684.
467. Zeigler FC, de Sauvage F, Widmer HR, et al. In vitro megakaryocytopoietic and thrombopoietic activity of c-mpl ligand (TPO) on purified murine hematopoietic stem cells. *Blood*. 1994;84(12):4045-4052.
468. Solar GP, Kerr WG, Zeigler FC, et al. Role of c-mpl in early hematopoiesis. *Blood*. 1998;92(1):4-10.
469. Ihara K, Ishii E, Eguchi M, et al. Identification of mutations in the c-mpl gene in congenital amegakaryocytic thrombocytopenia. *Proc Natl Acad Sci U S A*. 1999;96(6):3132-3136.
470. Ballmaier M, Germeshausen M, Schulze H, et al. c-mpl mutations are the cause of congenital amegakaryocytic thrombocytopenia. *Blood*. 2001;97(1):139-146.
471. Lebois M, Dowling MR, Gangatirkar P, et al. Regulation of platelet lifespan in the presence and absence of thrombopoietin signaling. *J Thromb Haemost*. 2016;14(9):1882-1887.
472. Harker LA, Roskos LK, Marzec UM, et al. Effects of megakaryocyte growth and development factor on platelet production, platelet life span, and platelet function in healthy human volunteers. *Blood*. 2000;95(8):2514-2522.
473. Chen J, Herceg-Harjacek L, Groopman JE, Grabarek J. Regulation of platelet activation in vitro by the c-Mpl ligand, thrombopoietin. *Blood*. 1995;86(11):4054-4062.
474. Vainchenker W, Constantinescu SN, Plo I. Recent advances in understanding myelofibrosis and essential thrombocythemia. *F1000Res*. 2016;5:F1000.
475. Vannucchi AM. Insights into the pathogenesis and management of thrombosis in polycythemia vera and essential thrombocythemia. *Intern Emerg Med*. 2010;5(3):177-184.
476. Falanga A, Marchetti M. Thrombosis in myeloproliferative neoplasms. *Semin Thromb Hemost*. 2014;40(3):348-358.
477. Vigon I, Mornon JP, Cocault L, et al. Molecular cloning and characterization of MPL, the human homolog of the v-mpl oncogene: identification of a member of the hematopoietic growth factor receptor superfamily. *Proc Natl Acad Sci U S A*. 1992;89(12):5640-5644.
478. Skoda RC, Seldin DC, Chiang MK, Peichel CL, Vogt TF, Leder P. Murine c-mpl: a member of the hematopoietic growth factor receptor superfamily that transduces a proliferative signal. *EMBO J*. 1993;12(7):2645-2653.
479. Mignotte V, Vigon I, Boucher de Crevecoeur E, Romeo PH, Lemarchandel V, Chretien S. Structure and transcription of the human c-mpl gene (MPL). *Genomics*. 1994;20(1):5-12.
480. Millot GA, Feger F, Garcon L, Vainchenker W, Dumenil D, Svinarchuk F. MplK, a natural variant of the thrombopoietin receptor with a truncated cytoplasmic domain, binds thrombopoietin but does not interfere with thrombopoietin-mediated cell growth. *Exp Hematol*. 2002;30(2):166-175.
481. Coers J, Ranft C, Skoda RC. A truncated isoform of c-Mpl with an essential C-terminal peptide targets the full-length receptor for degradation. *J Biol Chem*. 2004;279(35):36397-36404.
482. Li J, Sabath DF, Kuter DJ. Cloning and functional characterization of a novel c-mpl variant expressed in human CD34 cells and platelets. *Cytokine*. 2000;12(7):835-844.
483. Xiao N, Laha S, Das SP, Morlock K, Jesneck JL, Raffel GD. Ott1 (Rbm15) regulates thrombopoietin response in hematopoietic stem cells through alternative splicing of c-Mpl. *Blood*. 2015;125(6):941-948.
484. Sattler M, Durstin MA, Frank DA, et al. The thrombopoietin receptor c-MPL activates JAK2 and TYK2 tyrosine kinases. *Exp Hematol*. 1995;23(9):1040-1048.
485. Alexander WS, Metcalf D, Dunn AR. Point mutations within a dimer interface homology domain of c-Mpl induce constitutive receptor activity and tumorigenicity. *EMBO J*. 1995;14(22):5569-5578.
486. Watowich SS, Yoshimura A, Longmore GD, Hilton DJ, Yoshimura Y, Lodish HF. Homodimerization and constitutive activation of the erythropoietin receptor. *Proc Natl Acad Sci U S A*. 1992;89(6):2140-2144.
487. Fox NE, Lim J, Chen R, Geddis AE. F104S c-Mpl responds to a transmembrane domain-binding thrombopoietin receptor agonist: proof of concept that selected receptor mutations in congenital amegakaryocytic thrombocytopenia can be stimulated with alternative thrombopoietic agents. *Exp Hematol*. 2010;38(5):384-391.
488. Tanner JW, Chen W, Young RL, Longmore GD, Shaw AS. The conserved box 1 motif of cytokine receptors is required for association with JAK kinases. *J Biol Chem*. 1995;270(12):6523-6530.
489. Tong W, Sulahian R, Gross AW, Hendon N, Lodish HF, Huang LJ. The membrane-proximal region of the thrombopoietin receptor confers its high surface expression by JAK2-dependent and -independent mechanisms. *J Biol Chem*. 2006;281(50):38930-38940.
490. Constantinescu SN, Huang LJ, Nam H, Lodish HF. The erythropoietin receptor cytosolic juxtamembrane domain contains an essential, precisely oriented, hydrophobic motif. *Mol Cell*. 2001;7(2):377-385.
491. Royer Y, Staerk J, Costuleanu M, Courtoy PJ, Constantinescu SN. Janus kinases affect thrombopoietin receptor cell surface localization and stability. *J Biol Chem*. 2005;280(29):27251-27261.
492. Deane CM, Kroemer RT, Richards WG. A structural model of the human thrombopoietin receptor complex. *J Mol Graph Model*. 1997;15(3):170-178. 85-88.
493. Sabath DF, Kaushansky K, Broudy VC. Deletion of the extracellular membrane-distal cytokine receptor homology module of Mpl results in constitutive cell growth and loss of thrombopoietin binding. *Blood*. 1999;94(1):365-367.
494. Staerk J, Lacout C, Sato T, Smith SO, Vainchenker W, Constantinescu SN. An amphipathic motif at the transmembrane-cytoplasmic junction prevents autonomous activation of the thrombopoietin receptor. *Blood*. 2006;107(5):1864-1871.
495. Defour JP, Itaya M, Gryshkova V, et al. Tryptophan at the transmembrane-cytosolic junction modulates thrombopoietin receptor dimerization and activation. *Proc Natl Acad Sci U S A*. 2013;110(7):2540-2545.
496. Defour JP, Chachoua I, Pecquet C, Constantinescu SN. Oncogenic activation of MPL/thrombopoietin receptor by 17 mutations at W515: implications for myeloproliferative neoplasms. *Leukemia*. 2016;30(5):1214-1216.
497. Pardanani AD, Levine RL, Lasho T, et al. MPL515 mutations in myeloproliferative and other myeloid disorders: a study of 1182 patients. *Blood*. 2006;108(10):3472-3476.
498. Livnah O, Stura EA, Middleton SA, Johnson DL, Jolliffe LK, Wilson IA. Crystallographic evidence for preformed dimers of erythropoietin receptor before ligand activation. *Science*. 1999;283(5404):987-990.
499. Constantinescu SN, Keren T, Socolovsky M, Nam H, Henis YI, Lodish HF. Ligand-independent oligomerization of cell-surface erythropoietin receptor is mediated by the transmembrane domain. *Proc Natl Acad Sci U S A*. 2001;98(8):4379-4384.
500. Mohan K, Ueda G, Kim AR, et al. Topological control of cytokine receptor signaling induces differential effects in hematopoiesis. *Science*. 2019;364(6442):eaav7532.
501. Cui L, Moraga I, Lerbs T, et al. Tuning MPL signaling to influence hematopoietic stem cell differentiation and inhibit essential thrombocythemia progenitors. *Proc Natl Acad Sci U S A*. 2021;118(2):e2017849118.
502. Matthews EE, Thevenin D, Rogers JM, et al. Thrombopoietin receptor activation: transmembrane helix dimerization, rotation, and allosteric modulation. *Faseb J*. 2011;25(7):2234-2244.
503. Staerk J, Defour JP, Pecquet C, et al. Orientation-specific signalling by thrombopoietin receptor dimers. *EMBO J*. 2011;30(21):4398-4413.
504. Seubert N, Royer Y, Staerk J, et al. Active and inactive orientations of the transmembrane and cytosolic domains of the erythropoietin receptor dimer. *Mol Cell*. 2003;12(5):1239-1250.
505. Leroy E, Defour JP, Sato T, et al. His499 regulates dimerization and prevents oncogenic activation by asparagine mutations of the human thrombopoietin receptor. *J Biol Chem*. 2016;291(6):2974-2987.
506. Chaligne R, Tonetti C, Besancenot R, et al. New mutations of MPL in primitive myelofibrosis: only the MPL W515 mutations promote a G1/S-phase transition. *Leukemia*. 2008;22(8):1557-1566.
507. Debili N, Wendling F, Cosman D, et al. The Mpl receptor is expressed in the megakaryocytic lineage from late progenitors to platelets. *Blood*. 1995;85(2):391-401.
508. Fielder PJ, Gurney AL, Stefanich E, et al. Regulation of thrombopoietin levels by c-mpl-mediated binding to platelets. *Blood*. 1996;87(6):2154-2161.
509. Fielder PJ, Hass P, Nagel M, et al. Human platelets as a model for the binding and degradation of thrombopoietin. *Blood*. 1997;89(8):2782-2788.
510. Cohen-Solal K, Villeval JL, Titeux M, Lok S, Vainchenker W, Wendling F. Constitutive expression of Mpl ligand transcripts during thrombocytopenia or thrombocytosis. *Blood*. 1996;88(7):2578-2584.
511. Cohen-Solal K, Vitrat N, Titeux M, Vainchenker W, Wendling F. High-level expression of Mpl in platelets and megakaryocytes is independent of thrombopoietin. *Blood*. 1999;93(9):2859-2866.
512. Petit Cocault L, Fleury M, Clay D, Larghero J, Vanneaux V, Souyri M. Monoclonal antibody 1.6.1 against human MPL receptor allows HSC enrichment of CB and BM CD34(+)CD38(-) populations. *Exp Hematol*. 2016;44(4):297-302.e1.
513. Abbott C, Huang G, Ellison AR, et al. Mouse monoclonal antibodies against human c-Mpl and characterization for flow cytometry applications. *Hybridoma*. 2010;29(2):103-113.
514. Cardier JE, Dempsey J. Thrombopoietin and its receptor, c-mpl, are constitutively expressed by mouse liver endothelial cells: evidence of thrombopoietin as a growth factor for liver endothelial cells. *Blood*. 1998;91(3):923-929.
515. Hino M, Nishizawa Y, Tagawa S, Yamane T, Morii H, Tatsumi N. Constitutive expression of the thrombopoietin gene in a human hepatoma cell line. *Biochem Biophys Res Commun*. 1995;217(2):475-481.
516. Wu Z, Wei D, Gao W, et al. TPO-induced metabolic reprogramming drives liver metastasis of colorectal cancer CD110+ tumor-initiating cells. *Cell Stem Cell*. 2015;17(1):47-59.
517. Alexander WS, Roberts AW, Maurer AB, Nicola NA, Dunn AR, Metcalf D. Studies of the c-Mpl thrombopoietin receptor through gene disruption and activation. *Stem Cells*. 1996;14(suppl 1):124-132.
518. Abkowitz JL, Chen J. Studies of c-Mpl function distinguish the replication of hematopoietic stem cells from the expansion of differentiating clones. *Blood*. 2007;109(12):5186-5190.
519. Fox N, Priestley G, Papayannopoulou T, Kaushansky K. Thrombopoietin expands hematopoietic stem cells after transplantation. *J Clin Invest*. 2002;110(3):389-394.
520. Hirao A. TPO signal for stem cell genomic integrity. *Blood*. 2014;123(4):459-460.
521. Besancenot R, Chaligne R, Tonetti C, et al. A senescence-like cell-cycle arrest occurs during megakaryocytic maturation: implications for physiological and pathological megakaryocytic proliferation. *PLoS Biol*. 2010;8(9).

522. Besancenot R, Roos-Weil D, Tonetti C, et al. JAK2 and MPL protein levels determine TPO-induced megakaryocyte proliferation vs differentiation. *Blood.* 2014;124(13):2104-2115.

523. Pecquet C, Diaconu CC, Staerk J, et al. Thrombopoietin receptor down-modulation by JAK2 V617F: restoration of receptor levels by inhibitors of pathologic JAK2 signaling and of proteasomes. *Blood.* 2012;119(20):4625-4635.

524. Nakamura-Ishizu A, Matsumura T, Stumpf PS, et al. Thrombopoietin metabolically primes hematopoietic stem cells to megakaryocyte-lineage differentiation. *Cell Rep.* 2018;25(7):1772-1785.e6.

525. Kirito K, Fox N, Kaushansky K. Thrombopoietin stimulates Hoxb4 expression: an explanation for the favorable effects of TPO on hematopoietic stem cells. *Blood.* 2003;102(9):3172-3178.

526. Kirito K, Fox N, Kaushansky K. Thrombopoietin induces HOXA9 nuclear transport in immature hematopoietic cells: potential mechanism by which the hormone favorably affects hematopoietic stem cells. *Mol Cell Biol.* 2004;24(15):6751-6762.

527. Chou FS, Griesinger A, Wunderlich M, et al. The thrombopoietin/MPL/Bcl-xL pathway is essential for survival and self-renewal in human preleukemia induced by AML1-ETO. *Blood.* 2012;120(4):709-719.

528. de Laval B, Pawlikowska P, Petit-Cocault L, et al. Thrombopoietin-increased DNA-PK-dependent DNA repair limits hematopoietic stem and progenitor cell mutagenesis in response to DNA damage. *Cell Stem Cell.* 2013;12(1):37-48.

529. Akada H, Akada S, Hutchison RE, Sakamoto K, Wagner KU, Mohi G. Critical role of Jak2 in the maintenance and function of adult hematopoietic stem cells. *Stem Cells.* 2014;32(7):1878-1889.

530. Bradley HL, Hawley TS, Bunting KD. Cell intrinsic defects in cytokine responsiveness of STAT5-deficient hematopoietic stem cells. *Blood.* 2002;100(12):3983-3989.

531. de Laval B, Pawlikowska P, Barbieri D, et al. Thrombopoietin promotes NHEJ DNA repair in hematopoietic stem cells through specific activation of Erk and NF-kappaB pathways and their target, IEX-1. *Blood.* 2014;123(4):509-519.

532. Petit-Cocault L, Volle-Challier C, Fleury M, Peault B, Souyri M. Dual role of Mpl receptor during the establishment of definitive hematopoiesis. *Development.* 2007;134(16):3031-3040.

533. Huang LJ, Constantinescu SN, Lodish HF. The N-terminal domain of Janus kinase 2 is required for Golgi processing and cell surface expression of erythropoietin receptor. *Mol Cell.* 2001;8(6):1327-1338.

534. Albu RI, Constantinescu SN. Extracellular domain N-glycosylation controls human thrombopoietin receptor cell surface levels. *Front Endocrinol.* 2011;2:71.

535. Chachoua I, Pecquet C, El-Khoury M, et al. Thrombopoietin receptor activation by myeloproliferative neoplasm associated calreticulin mutants. *Blood.* 2016;127(10):1325-1335.

536. Dahlen DD, Broudy VC, Drachman JG. Internalization of the thrombopoietin receptor is regulated by 2 cytoplasmic motifs. *Blood.* 2003;102(1):102-108.

537. Bender M, Giannini S, Grozovsky R, et al. Dynamin 2-dependent endocytosis is required for normal megakaryocyte development in mice. *Blood.* 2015;125(6):1014-1024.

538. Saur SJ, Sangkhae V, Geddis AE, Kaushansky K, Hitchcock IS. Ubiquitination and degradation of the thrombopoietin receptor c-Mpl. *Blood.* 2010;115(6):1254-1263.

539. Hitchcock IS, Chen MM, King JR, Kaushansky K. YRRL motifs in the cytoplasmic domain of the thrombopoietin receptor regulate receptor internalization and degradation. *Blood.* 2008;112(6):2222-2231.

540. Sangkhae V, Saur SJ, Kaushansky A, Kaushansky K, Hitchcock IS. Phosphorylated c-Mpl tyrosine 591 regulates thrombopoietin-induced signaling. *Exp Hematol.* 2014;42(6):477-486.e4.

541. Favale F, Messaoudi K, Varghese LN, et al. An incomplete trafficking defect to the cell-surface leads to paradoxical thrombocytosis for human and murine MPL P106L. *Blood.* 2016;128(26):3146-3158.

542. Cleyrat C, Darehshouri A, Steinkamp MP, et al. Mpl traffics to the cell surface through conventional and unconventional routes. *Traffic.* 2014;15(9):961-982.

543. Pecquet C, Chachoua I, Roy A, et al. Calreticulin mutants as oncogenic rogue chaperones for TpoR and traffic-defective pathogenic TpoR mutants. *Blood.* 2019;133(25):2669-2681.

544. Elf S, Abdelfattah NS, Baral AJ, et al. Defining the requirements for the pathogenic interaction between mutant calreticulin and MPL in MPN. *Blood.* 2018;131(7):782-786.

545. Masubuchi N, Araki M, Yang Y, et al. Mutant calreticulin interacts with MPL in the secretion pathway for activation on the cell surface. *Leukemia.* 2020;34(2):499-509.

546. Grand FH, Hidalgo-Curtis CE, Ernst T, et al. Frequent CBL mutations associated with 11q acquired uniparental disomy in myeloproliferative neoplasms. *Blood.* 2009;113(26):6182-6192.

547. Kuter DJ, Rosenberg RD. The reciprocal relationship of thrombopoietin (c-Mpl ligand) to changes in the platelet mass during busulfan-induced thrombocytopenia in the rabbit. *Blood.* 1995;85(10):2720-2730.

548. Kuter DJ. The biology of thrombopoietin and thrombopoietin receptor agonists. *Int J Hematol.* 2013;98(1):10-23.

549. King S, Germeshausen M, Strauss G, Welte K, Ballmaier M. Congenital amegakaryocytic thrombocytopenia: a retrospective clinical analysis of 20 patients. *Br J Haematol.* 2005;131(5):636-644.

550. Ballmaier M, Germeshausen M. Congenital amegakaryocytic thrombocytopenia: clinical presentation, diagnosis, and treatment. *Semin Thromb Hemost.* 2011;37(6):673-681.

551. Stoffel R, Wiestner A, Skoda RC. Thrombopoietin in thrombocytopenic mice: evidence against regulation at the mRNA level and for a direct regulatory role of platelets. *Blood.* 1996;87(2):567-573.

552. McCarty JM, Sprugel KH, Fox NE, Sabath DE, Kaushansky K. Murine thrombopoietin mRNA levels are modulated by platelet count. *Blood.* 1995;86(10):3668-3675.

553. Li J, Xia Y, Kuter DJ. Interaction of thrombopoietin with the platelet c-mpl receptor in plasma: binding, internalization, stability and pharmacokinetics. *Br J Haematol.* 1999;106(2):345-356.

554. Geddis AE, Fox NE, Kaushansky K. The Mpl receptor expressed on endothelial cells does not contribute significantly to the regulation of circulating thrombopoietin levels. *Exp Hematol.* 2006;34(1):82-86.

555. Lannutti BJ, Epp A, Roy J, Chen J, Josephson NC. Incomplete restoration of Mpl expression in the mpl-/- mouse produces partial correction of the stem cell-repopulating defect and paradoxical thrombocytosis. *Blood.* 2009;113(8):1778-1785.

556. Tiedt R, Coers J, Ziegler S, et al. Pronounced thrombocytosis in transgenic mice expressing reduced levels of Mpl in platelets and terminally differentiated megakaryocytes. *Blood.* 2009;113(8):1768-1777.

557. Meyer SC, Keller MD, Woods BA, et al. Genetic studies reveal an unexpected negative regulatory role for Jak2 in thrombopoiesis. *Blood.* 2014;124(14):2280-2284.

558. Ng AP, Kauppi M, Metcalf D, et al. Mpl expression on megakaryocytes and platelets is dispensable for thrombopoiesis but essential to prevent myeloproliferation. *Proc Natl Acad Sci U S A.* 2014;111(16):5884-5889.

559. Kaser A, Brandacher G, Steurer W, et al. Interleukin-6 stimulates thrombopoiesis through thrombopoietin: role in inflammatory thrombocytosis. *Blood.* 2001;98(9):2720-2725.

560. Wolber EM, Jelkmann W. Interleukin-6 increases thrombopoietin production in human hepatoma cells HepG2 and Hep3B. *J Interferon Cytokine Res.* 2000;20(5):499-506.

561. Grozovsky R, Begonja AJ, Liu K, et al. The Ashwell-Morell receptor regulates hepatic thrombopoietin production via JAK2-STAT3 signaling. *Nat Med.* 2015;21(1):47-54.

562. Grozovsky R, Giannini S, Falet H, Hoffmeister KM. Regulating billions of blood platelets: glycans and beyond. *Blood.* 2015;126(16):1877-1884.

563. Di Buduo CA, Giannini S, Abbonante V, Rosti V, Hoffmeister KM, Balduini A. Increased B4GALT1 expression is associated with platelet surface galactosylation and thrombopoietin plasma levels in MPNs. *Blood.* 2021;137(15):2085-2089.

564. Drachman JG, Millett KM, Kaushansky K. Thrombopoietin signal transduction requires functional JAK2, not TYK2. *J Biol Chem.* 1999;274(19):13480-13484.

565. Bandaranayake RM, Ungureanu D, Shan Y, Shaw DE, Silvennoinen O, Hubbard SR. Crystal structures of the JAK2 pseudokinase domain and the pathogenic mutant V617F. *Nat Struct Mol Biol.* 2012;19(8):754-759.

566. Ungureanu D, Wu J, Pekkala T, et al. The pseudokinase domain of JAK2 is a dual-specificity protein kinase that negatively regulates cytokine signaling. *Nat Struct Mol Biol.* 2011;18(9):971-976.

567. Vainchenker W, Constantinescu SN. JAK/STAT signaling in hematological malignancies. *Oncogene.* 2013;32(21):2601-2613.

568. Grinfeld J, Nangalia J, Green AR. Molecular determinants of pathogenesis and clinical phenotype in myeloproliferative neoplasms. *Haematologica.* 2016;102(1):7-17.

569. Sangkhae V, Etheridge SL, Kaushansky K, Hitchcock IS. The thrombopoietin receptor, MPL, is critical for development of a JAK2V617F-induced myeloproliferative neoplasm. *Blood.* 2014;124(26):3956-3963.

570. Leroy E, Dusa A, Colau D, et al. Uncoupling JAK2 V617F activation from cytokine-induced signalling by modulation of JH2 alphaC helix. *Biochem J.* 2016;473(11):1579-1591.

571. Silvennoinen O, Hubbard SR. Molecular insights into regulation of JAK2 in myeloproliferative neoplasms. *Blood.* 2015;125(22):3388-3392.

572. Drachman JG, Kaushansky K. Dissecting the thrombopoietin receptor: functional elements of the Mpl cytoplasmic domain. *Proc Natl Acad Sci U S A.* 1997;94(6):2350-2355.

573. Pecquet C, Staerk J, Chaligne R, et al. Induction of myeloproliferative disorder and myelofibrosis by thrombopoietin receptor W515 mutants is mediated by cytosolic tyrosine 112 of the receptor. *Blood.* 2010;115(5):1037-1048.

574. Drachman JG, Rojnuckarin P, Kaushansky K. Thrombopoietin signal transduction: studies from cell lines and primary cells. *Methods.* 1999;17(3):238-249.

575. Reich NC. STATs get their move on. *JAK-STAT.* 2013;2(4):e27080.

576. Cheon H, Stark GR. Unphosphorylated STAT1 prolongs the expression of interferon-induced immune regulatory genes. *Proc Natl Acad Sci U S A.* 2009;106(23):9373-9378.

577. Kirito K, Kaushansky K. Transcriptional regulation of megakaryopoiesis: thrombopoietin signaling and nuclear factors. *Curr Opin Hematol.* 2006;13(3):151-156.

578. Park HJ, Li J, Hannah R, et al. Cytokine-induced megakaryocytic differentiation is regulated by genome-wide loss of a uSTAT transcriptional program. *EMBO J.* 2016;35(6):580-594.

579. Walz C, Ahmed W, Lazarides K, et al. Essential role for Stat5a/b in myeloproliferative neoplasms induced by BCR-ABL1 and JAK2(V617F) in mice. *Blood.* 2012;119(15):3550-3560.

580. Yan D, Hutchison RE, Mohi G. Critical requirement for Stat5 in a mouse model of polycythemia vera. *Blood.* 2012;119(15):3539-3549.

581. Duek A, Lundberg P, Shimizu T, et al. Loss of Stat1 decreases megakaryopoiesis and favors erythropoiesis in a JAK2-V617F-driven mouse model of MPNs. *Blood.* 2014;123(25):3943-3950.

582. Huang Z, Richmond TD, Muntean AG, Barber DL, Weiss MJ, Crispino JD. STAT1 promotes megakaryopoiesis downstream of GATA-1 in mice. *J Clin Invest.* 2007;117(12):3890-3899.

583. Kirito K, Osawa M, Morita H, et al. A functional role of Stat3 in in vivo megakaryopoiesis. *Blood.* 2002;99(9):3220-3227.

584. Grisouard J, Shimizu T, Duek A, et al. Deletion of Stat3 in hematopoietic cells enhances thrombocytosis and shortens survival in a JAK2-V617F mouse model of MPN. *Blood.* 2015;125(13):2131-2140.

585. Miyakawa Y, Rojnuckarin P, Habib T, Kaushansky K. Thrombopoietin induces phosphoinositol 3-kinase activation through SHP2, Gab, and insulin receptor substrate proteins in BAF3 cells and primary murine megakaryocytes. *J Biol Chem.* 2001;276(4):2494-2502.

586. Bouscary D, Lecoq-Lafon C, Chretien S, et al. Role of Gab proteins in phosphatidylinositol 3-kinase activation by thrombopoietin (Tpo). *Oncogene.* 2001;20(18):2197-2204.

587. Jung AS, Kaushansky A, Macbeath G, Kaushansky K. Tensin2 is a novel mediator in thrombopoietin (TPO)-induced cellular proliferation by promoting Akt signaling. *Cell Cycle.* 2011;10(11):1838-1844.

588. Geddis AE, Fox NE, Kaushansky K. Phosphatidylinositol 3-kinase is necessary but not sufficient for thrombopoietin-induced proliferation in engineered Mpl-bearing cell lines as well as in primary megakaryocytic progenitors. *J Biol Chem.* 2001;276(37):34473-34479.

589. Nakao T, Geddis AE, Fox NE, Kaushansky K. PI3K/Akt/FOXO3a pathway contributes to thrombopoietin-induced proliferation of primary megakaryocytes in vitro and in vivo via modulation of p27(Kip1). *Cell Cycle.* 2008;7(2):257-266.

590. Guerriero R, Parolini I, Testa U, et al. Inhibition of TPO-induced MEK or mTOR activity induces opposite effects on the ploidy of human differentiating megakaryocytes. *J Cell Sci.* 2006;119(pt 4):744-752.

591. Raslova H, Baccini V, Loussaief L, et al. Mammalian target of rapamycin (mTOR) regulates both proliferation of megakaryocyte progenitors and late stages of megakaryocyte differentiation. *Blood.* 2006;107(6):2303-2310.

592. Drayer AL, Olthof SG, Vellenga E. Mammalian target of rapamycin is required for thrombopoietin-induced proliferation of megakaryocyte progenitors. *Stem Cells.* 2006;24(1):105-114.

593. Yang J, Zhou X, Fan X, et al. mTORC1 promotes aging-related venous thrombosis in mice via elevation of platelet volume and activation. *Blood.* 2016;128(5):615-624.

594. Cao Y, Cai J, Zhang S, et al. Loss of autophagy leads to failure in megakaryopoiesis, megakaryocyte differentiation, and thrombopoiesis in mice. *Exp Hematol.* 2015;43(6):488-494.

595. Ouseph MM, Huang Y, Banerjee M, et al. Autophagy is induced upon platelet activation and is essential for hemostasis and thrombosis. *Blood.* 2015;126(10):1224-1233.

596. Rojnuckarin P, Drachman JG, Kaushansky K. Thrombopoietin-induced activation of the mitogen-activated protein kinase (MAPK) pathway in normal megakaryocytes: role in endomitosis. *Blood.* 1999;94(4):1273-1282.

597. Garcia J, de Gunzburg J, Eychene A, Gisselbrecht S, Porteu F. Thrombopoietin-mediated sustained activation of extracellular signal-regulated kinase in UT7-Mpl cells requires both Ras-Raf-1- and Rap1-B-Raf-dependent pathways. *Mol Cell Biol.* 2001;21(8):2659-2670.

598. Rouyez MC, Boucheron C, Gisselbrecht S, Dusanter-Fourt I, Porteu F. Control of thrombopoietin-induced megakaryocytic differentiation by the mitogen-activated protein kinase pathway. *Mol Cell Biol.* 1997;17(9):4991-5000.

599. Severin S, Ghevaert C, Mazharian A. The mitogen-activated protein kinase signaling pathways: role in megakaryocyte differentiation. *J Thromb Haemost.* 2010;8(1):17-26.

600. Kamata T, Pritchard CA, Leavitt AD. Raf-1 is not required for megakaryocytopoiesis or TPO-induced ERK phosphorylation. *Blood.* 2004;103(7):2568-2570.

601. Kamata T, Kang J, Lee TH, Wojnowski L, Pritchard CA, Leavitt AD. A critical function for B-Raf at multiple stages of myelopoiesis. *Blood.* 2005;106(3):833-840.

602. Fichelson S, Freyssinier JM, Picard F, et al. Megakaryocyte growth and development factor-induced proliferation and differentiation are regulated by the mitogen-activated protein kinase pathway in primitive cord blood hematopoietic progenitors. *Blood.* 1999;94(5):1601-1613.

603. Luff SA, Papoutsakis ET. Megakaryocytic maturation in response to shear flow is mediated by the activator protein 1 (AP-1) transcription factor via mitogen-activated protein kinase (MAPK) mechanotransduction. *J Biol Chem.* 2016;291(15):7831-7843.

604. Su H, Jiang M, Senevirathne C, et al. Methylation of dual-specificity phosphatase 4 controls cell differentiation. *Cell Rep.* 2021;36(4):109421.

605. Lannutti BJ, Shim MH, Blake N, Reems JA, Drachman JG. Identification and activation of Src family kinases in primary megakaryocytes. *Exp Hematol.* 2003;31(12):1268-1274.

606. Lannutti BJ, Drachman JG. Lyn tyrosine kinase regulates thrombopoietin-induced proliferation of hematopoietic cell lines and primary megakaryocytic progenitors. *Blood.* 2004;103(10):3736-3743.

607. Lannutti BJ, Minear J, Blake N, Drachman JG. Increased megakaryocytopoiesis in Lyn-deficient mice. *Oncogene.* 2006;25(23):3316-3324.

608. Hitchcock IS, Fox NE, Prevost N, Sear K, Shattil SJ, Kaushansky K. Roles of focal adhesion kinase (FAK) in megakaryopoiesis and platelet function: studies using a megakaryocyte lineage specific FAK knockout. *Blood.* 2008;111(2):596-604.

609. Zhang L, Orban M, Lorenz M, et al. A novel role of sphingosine 1-phosphate receptor S1pr1 in mouse thrombopoiesis. *J Exp Med.* 2012;209(12):2165-2181.

610. Zhang L, Urtz N, Gaertner F, et al. Sphingosine kinase 2 (Sphk2) regulates platelet biogenesis by providing intracellular sphingosine 1-phosphate (S1P). *Blood.* 2013;122(5):791-802.

611. Mazharian A, Thomas SG, Dhanjal TS, Buckley CD, Watson SP. Critical role of Src-Syk-PLC{gamma}2 signaling in megakaryocyte migration and thrombopoiesis. *Blood.* 2010;116(5):793-800.

612. Mazharian A, Wang YJ, Mori J, et al. Mice lacking the ITIM-containing receptor G6b-B exhibit macrothrombocytopenia and aberrant platelet function. *Sci Signal.* 2012;5(248):ra78.

613. Geer MJ, van Geffen JP, Gopalasingam P, et al. Uncoupling ITIM receptor G6b-B from tyrosine phosphatases Shp1 and Shp2 disrupts murine platelet homeostasis. *Blood.* 2018;132(13):1413-1425.

614. Hofmann I, Geer MJ, Vögtle T, et al. Congenital macrothrombocytopenia with focal myelofibrosis due to mutations in human G6b-B is rescued in humanized mice. *Blood.* 2018;132(13):1399-1412.

615. Mazharian A, Ghevaert C, Zhang L, Massberg S, Watson SP. Dasatinib enhances megakaryocyte differentiation but inhibits platelet formation. *Blood.* 2011;117(19):5198-5206.

616. Williams CM, Harper MT, Poole AW. PKCalpha negatively regulates in vitro proplatelet formation and in vivo platelet production in mice. *Platelets.* 2014;25(1):62-68.

617. Gobbi G, Mirandola P, Sponzilli I, et al. Timing and expression level of protein kinase C epsilon regulate the megakaryocytic differentiation of human CD34 cells. *Stem Cells.* 2007;25(9):2322-2329.

618. Carubbi C, Masselli E, Martini S, et al. Human thrombopoiesis depends on Protein kinase Cdelta/protein kinase Cepsilon functional couple. *Haematologica.* 2016;101(7):812-820.

619. Machlus KR, Wu SK, Stumpo DJ, et al. Synthesis and dephosphorylation of MARCKS in the late stages of megakaryocyte maturation drive proplatelet formation. *Blood.* 2016;127(11):1468-1480.

620. Babon JJ, Lucet IS, Murphy JM, Nicola NA, Varghese LN. The molecular regulation of Janus kinase (JAK) activation. *Biochem J.* 2014;462(1):1-13.

621. Linossi EM, Nicholson SE. Kinase inhibition, competitive binding and proteasomal degradation: resolving the molecular function of the suppressor of cytokine signaling (SOCS) proteins. *Immunol Rev.* 2015;266(1):123-133.

622. Starr R, Willson TA, Viney EM, et al. A family of cytokine-inducible inhibitors of signalling. *Nature.* 1997;387(6636):917-921.

623. Wang Q, Miyakawa Y, Fox N, Kaushansky K. Interferon-alpha directly represses megakaryopoiesis by inhibiting thrombopoietin-induced signaling through induction of SOCS-1. *Blood.* 2000;96(6):2093-2099.

624. Teofili L, Martini M, Cenci T, et al. Epigenetic alteration of SOCS family members is a possible pathogenetic mechanism in JAK2 wild type myeloproliferative diseases. *Int J Cancer.* 2008;123(7):1586-1592.

625. Oh ST, Gotlib J. JAK2 V617F and beyond: role of genetics and aberrant signaling in the pathogenesis of myeloproliferative neoplasms. *Expet Rev Hematol.* 2010;3(3):323-337.

626. Hookham MB, Elliott J, Suessmuth Y, et al. The myeloproliferative disorder-associated JAK2 V617F mutant escapes negative regulation by suppressor of cytokine signaling 3. *Blood.* 2007;109(11):4924-4929.

627. Tong W, Lodish HF. Lnk inhibits Tpo-mpl signaling and Tpo-mediated megakaryocytopoiesis. *J Exp Med.* 2004;200(5):569-580.

628. Tong W, Zhang J, Lodish HF. Lnk inhibits erythropoiesis and Epo-dependent JAK2 activation and downstream signaling pathways. *Blood.* 2005;105(12):4604-4612.

629. Velazquez L, Cheng AM, Fleming HE, et al. Cytokine signaling and hematopoietic homeostasis are disrupted in Lnk-deficient mice. *J Exp Med.* 2002;195(12):1599-1611.

630. Bersenev A, Wu C, Balcerek J, Tong W. Lnk controls mouse hematopoietic stem cell self-renewal and quiescence through direct interactions with JAK2. *J Clin Invest.* 2008;118(8):2832-2844.

631. Oh ST, Simonds EF, Jones C, et al. Novel mutations in the inhibitory adaptor protein LNK drive JAK-STAT signaling in patients with myeloproliferative neoplasms. *Blood.* 2010;116(6):988-992.

632. McMullin MF, Cario H. LNK mutations and myeloproliferative disorders. *Am J Hematol.* 2016;91(2):248-251.

633. Rumi E, Harutyunyan AS, Pietra D, et al. LNK mutations in familial myeloproliferative neoplasms. *Blood.* 2016;128(1):144-145.

634. Lasho TL, Pardanani A, Tefferi A. LNK mutations in JAK2 mutation-negative erythrocytosis. *N Engl J Med.* 2010;363(12):1189-1190.

635. Bersenev A, Wu C, Balcerek J, et al. Lnk constrains myeloproliferative diseases in mice. *J Clin Invest.* 2010;120(6):2058-2069.

636. Mazharian A, Mori J, Wang YJ, et al. Megakaryocyte-specific deletion of the protein-tyrosine phosphatases Shp1 and Shp2 causes abnormal megakaryocyte development, platelet production, and function. *Blood.* 2013;121(20):4205-4220.

637. Perez LE, Desponts C, Parquet N, Kerr WG. SH2-inositol phosphatase 1 negatively influences early megakaryocyte progenitors. *PLoS One.* 2008;3(10):e3565.

638. Kuter DJ, Gernsheimer TB. Thrombopoietin and platelet production in chronic immune thrombocytopenia. *Hematol Oncol Clin N Am.* 2009;23(6):1193-1211.

639. Molineux G, Newland A. Development of romiplostim for the treatment of patients with chronic immune thrombocytopenia: from bench to bedside. *Br J Haematol.* 2010;150(1):9-20.

640. Dusheiko G. Thrombopoietin agonists for the treatment of thrombocytopenia in liver disease and hepatitis C. *Clin Liver Dis.* 2009;13(3):487-501.

641. Olnes MJ, Scheinberg P, Calvo KR, et al. Eltrombopag and improved hematopoiesis in refractory aplastic anemia. *N Engl J Med.* 2012;367(1):11-19.

642. Gill H, Leung GM, Lopes D, Kwong YL. The thrombopoietin mimetics eltrombopag and romiplostim in the treatment of refractory aplastic anaemia. *Br J Haematol.* 2016;176(6):991-994.

643. Desmond R, Townsley DM, Dumitriu B, et al. Eltrombopag restores trilineage hematopoiesis in refractory severe aplastic anemia that can be sustained on discontinuation of drug. *Blood.* 2014;123(12):1818-1825.

644. Bussel JB. The new thrombopoietic agenda: impact on leukemias and MDS. *Best Pract Res Clin Haematol.* 2014;27(3-4):288-292.

645. D'Arena G, Guariglia R, Mansueto G, et al. No cross-resistance after sequential use of romiplostim and eltrombopag in chronic immune thrombocytopenic purpura. *Blood.* 2013;121(7):1240-1242.

646. Di Buduo CA, Currao M, Pecci A, Kaplan DL, Balduini CL, Balduini A. Revealing eltrombopag's promotion of human megakaryopoiesis through AKT/ERK-dependent pathway activation. *Haematologica.* 2016;101(12):1479-1488.

647. Wang X, Haylock D, Hu CS, et al. A thrombopoietin receptor antagonist is capable of depleting myelofibrosis hematopoietic stem and progenitor cells. *Blood.* 2016;127(26):3398-3409.

648. Debili N, Masse JM, Katz A, Guichard J, Breton-Gorius J, Vainchenker W. Effects of the recombinant hematopoietic growth factors interleukin-3, interleukin-6, stem cell factor, and leukemia inhibitory factor on the megakaryocytic differentiation of CD34+ cells. *Blood.* 1993;82(1):84-95.

649. Avraham H, Vannier E, Cowley S, et al. Effects of the stem cell factor, c-kit ligand, on human megakaryocytic cells. *Blood.* 1992;79(2):365-371.

650. Shin JY, Hu W, Naramura M, Park CY. High c-Kit expression identifies hematopoietic stem cells with impaired self-renewal and megakaryocytic bias. *J Exp Med.* 2014;211(2):217-231.

651. Hunt P, Zsebo KM, Hokom MM, et al. Evidence that stem cell factor is involved in the rebound thrombocytosis that follows 5-fluorouracil treatment. *Blood.* 1992;80(4):904-911.

652. Arnold J, Ellis S, Radley JM, Williams N. Compensatory mechanisms in platelet production: the response of Sl/Sld mice to 5-fluorouracil. *Exp Hematol.* 1991;19(1):24-28.

653. Burstein SA, Mei RL, Henthorn J, Friese P, Turner K. Leukemia inhibitory factor and interleukin-11 promote maturation of murine and human megakaryocytes in vitro. *J Cell Physiol.* 1992;153(2):305-312.

654. Metcalf D, Hilton D, Nicola NA. Leukemia inhibitory factor can potentiate murine megakaryocyte production in vitro. *Blood.* 1991;77(10):2150-2153.

655. Bruno E, Briddell RA, Cooper RJ, Hoffman R. Effects of recombinant interleukin 11 on human megakaryocyte progenitor cells. *Exp Hematol.* 1991;19(5):378-381.

656. Kimura H, Ishibashi T, Uchida T, Maruyama Y, Friese P, Burstein SA. Interleukin 6 is a differentiation factor for human megakaryocytes in vitro. *Eur J Immunol.* 1990;20(9):1927-1931.

657. Bruno E, Hoffman R. Effect of interleukin 6 on in vitro human megakaryocytopoiesis: its interaction with other cytokines. *Exp Hematol.* 1989;17(10):1038-1043.

658. Taguchi K, Saitoh M, Arai Y, et al. Disparate effects of interleukin 11 and thrombopoietin on megakaryocytopoiesis in vitro. *Cytokine.* 2001;15(5):241-249.

659. Debili N, Breton-Gorius J, Vainchenker W. Hematopoietic growth factors and human megakaryocyte differentiation. *Bone Marrow Transplant.* 1992;9(suppl 1):11-15.

660. Kurzrock R. rhIL-11 for the prevention of dose-limiting chemotherapy-induced thrombocytopenia. *Oncology.* 2000;14(9 suppl 8):9-11.

661. Kaye JA. Clinical development of recombinant human interleukin-11 to treat chemotherapy-induced thrombocytopenia. *Curr Opin Hematol.* 1996;3(3):209-215.

662. Hao J, Sun L, Huang H, et al. Effects of recombinant human interleukin 11 on thrombocytopenia and neutropenia in irradiated rhesus monkeys. *Radiat Res.* 2004;162(2):157-163.

663. Machlus KR, Johnson KE, Kulenthirarajan R, et al. CCL5 derived from platelets increases megakaryocyte proplatelet formation. *Blood.* 2016;127(7):921-926.

664. Kavnoudias H, Jackson H, Ettlinger K, Bertoncello I, McNiece I, Williams N. Interleukin 3 directly stimulates both megakaryocyte progenitor cells and immature megakaryocytes. *Exp Hematol.* 1992;20(1):43-46.

665. Scott CL, Robb L, Mansfield R, Alexander WS, Begley CG. Granulocyte-macrophage colony-stimulating factor is not responsible for residual thrombopoiesis in mpl null mice. *Exp Hematol.* 2000;28(9):1001-1007.

666. Zhang H, Wang S, Liu D, et al. EpoR-tdTomato-Cre mice enable identification of EpoR expression in subsets of tissue macrophages and hematopoietic cells. *Blood.* 2021;138(20):1986-1997.

667. Vainchenker W, Bouguet J, Guichard J, Breton-Gorius J. Megakaryocyte colony formation from human bone marrow precursors. *Blood.* 1979;54(4):940-945.

668. Vainchenker W, Guichard J, Breton-Gorius J. Growth of human megakaryocyte colonies in culture from fetal, neonatal, and adult peripheral blood cells: ultrastructural analysis. *Blood Cells.* 1979;5(1):25-42.

669. McLeod DL, Shreve MM, Axelrad AA. Induction of megakaryocyte colonies with platelet formation in vitro. *Nature.* 1976;261(5560):492-494.

670. Papayannopoulou T, Brice M, Farrer D, Kaushansky K. Insights into the cellular mechanisms of erythropoietin-thrombopoietin synergy. *Exp Hematol.* 1996;24(5):660-669.

671. Hacein-Bey-Abina S, Estienne M, Bessoles S, et al. Erythropoietin is a major regulator of thrombopoiesis in thrombopoietin-dependent and -independent contexts. *Exp Hematol.* 2020;88:15-27.

672. Abraham M, Weiss ID, Wald H, et al. Sequential administration of the high affinity CXCR4 antagonist BKT140 promotes megakaryopoiesis and platelet production. *Br J Haematol.* 2013;163(2):248-259.

673. Pineault N, Cortin V, Boyer L, et al. Individual and synergistic cytokine effects controlling the expansion of cord blood CD34(+) cells and megakaryocyte progenitors in culture. *Cytotherapy.* 2011;13(4):467-480.

674. Mercher T, Raffel GD, Moore SA, et al. The OTT-MAL fusion oncogene activates RBPJ-mediated transcription and induces acute megakaryoblastic leukemia in a knockin mouse model. *J Clin Invest.* 2009;119(4):852-864.

675. Mercher T, Cornejo MG, Sears C, et al. Notch signaling specifies megakaryocyte development from hematopoietic stem cells. *Cell Stem Cell.* 2008;3(3):314-326.

676. Weiss-Gayet M, Starck J, Chaabouni A, Chazaud B, Morle F. Notch stimulates both self-renewal and lineage plasticity in a subset of murine CD9High committed megakaryocytic progenitors. *PLoS One.* 2016;11(4):e0153860.

677. Poirault-Chassac S, Six E, Catelain C, et al. Notch/Delta4 signaling inhibits human megakaryocytic terminal differentiation. *Blood.* 2010;116(25):5670-5678.

678. Ono M, Matsubara Y, Shibano T, Ikeda Y, Murata M. GSK-3beta negatively regulates megakaryocyte differentiation and platelet production from primary human bone marrow cells in vitro. *Platelets.* 2011;22(3):196-203.

679. Macaulay IC, Thon JN, Tijssen MR, et al. Canonical Wnt signaling in megakaryocytes regulates proplatelet formation. *Blood.* 2013;121(1):188-196.

680. Vainchenker W, Chapman J, Deschamps JF, et al. Normal human serum contains a factor(s) capable of inhibiting megakaryocyte colony formation. *Exp Hematol.* 1982;10(8):650-660.

681. Mitjavila MT, Vinci G, Villeval JL, et al. Human platelet alpha granules contain a nonspecific inhibitor of megakaryocyte colony formation: its relationship to type beta transforming growth factor (TGF-beta). *J Cell Physiol.* 1988;134(1):93-100.

682. Fava RA, Casey TT, Wilcox J, Pelton RW, Moses HL, Nanney LB. Synthesis of transforming growth factor-beta 1 by megakaryocytes and its localization to megakaryocyte and platelet alpha-granules. *Blood.* 1990;76(10):1946-1955.

683. Ishibashi T, Miller SL, Burstein SA. Type beta transforming growth factor is a potent inhibitor of murine megakaryocytopoiesis in vitro. *Blood.* 1987;69(6):1737-1741.

684. Kuter DJ, Gminski D, Rosenberg RD. Platelets contain several inhibitors of megakaryocyte growth and ploidization. *Prog Clin Biol Res.* 1990;356:245-257.

685. Bruno E, Miller ME, Hoffman R. Interacting cytokines regulate in vitro human megakaryocytopoiesis. *Blood.* 1989;73(3):671-677.

686. Greenberg SM, Chandrasekhar C, Golan DE, Handin RI. Transforming growth factor beta inhibits endomitosis in the Dami human megakaryocytic cell line. *Blood.* 1990;76(3):533-537.

687. Zermati Y, Fichelson S, Valensi F, et al. Transforming growth factor inhibits erythropoiesis by blocking proliferation and accelerating differentiation of erythroid progenitors. *Exp Hematol.* 2000;28(8):885-894.

688. Chagraoui H, Komura E, Tulliez M, Giraudier S, Vainchenker W, Wendling F. Prominent role of TGF-beta 1 in thrombopoietin-induced myelofibrosis in mice. *Blood.* 2002;100(10):3495-3503.

689. Le Bousse-Kerdiles MC, Martyre MC. Involvement of the fibrogenic cytokines, TGF-beta and bFGF, in the pathogenesis of idiopathic myelofibrosis. *Pathol Biol.* 2001;49(2):153-157.

690. Jeanpierre S, Nicolini FE, Kaniewski B, et al. BMP4 regulation of human megakaryocytic differentiation is involved in thrombopoietin signaling. *Blood.* 2008;112(8):3154-3163.

691. Gewirtz AM, Zhang J, Ratajczak J, et al. Chemokine regulation of human megakaryocytopoiesis. *Blood.* 1995;86(7):2559-2567.

692. Han ZC, Sensebe L, Abgrall JF, Briere J. Platelet factor 4 inhibits human megakaryocytopoiesis in vitro. *Blood.* 1990;75(6):1234-1239.

693. Lambert MP, Wang Y, Bdeir KH, Nguyen Y, Kowalska MA, Poncz M. Platelet factor 4 regulates megakaryopoiesis through low-density lipoprotein receptor-related protein 1 (LRP1) on megakaryocytes. *Blood.* 2009;114(11):2290-2298.

694. Lambert MP, Rauova L, Bailey M, Sola-Visner MC, Kowalska MA, Poncz M. Platelet factor 4 is a negative autocrine in vivo regulator of megakaryopoiesis: clinical and therapeutic implications. *Blood.* 2007;110(4):1153-1160.

695. Oda M, Kurasawa Y, Todokoro K, Nagata Y. Thrombopoietin-induced CXC chemokines, NAP-2 and PF4, suppress polyploidization and proplatelet formation during megakaryocyte maturation. *Gene Cell.* 2003;8(1):9-15.

696. Han ZC, Bellucci S, Walz A, Baggiolini M, Caen JP. Negative regulation of human megakaryocytopoiesis by human platelet factor 4 (PF4) and connective tissue-activating peptide (CTAP-III). *Int J Cell Clon.* 1990;8(4):253-259.

697. Sonoda Y, Kuzuyama Y, Tanaka S, et al. Human interleukin-4 inhibits proliferation of megakaryocyte progenitor cells in culture. *Blood.* 1993;81(3):624-630.

698. Emadi S, Clay D, Desterke C, et al. IL-8 and its CXCR1 and CXCR2 receptors participate in the control of megakaryocytic proliferation, differentiation, and ploidy in myeloid metaplasia with myelofibrosis. *Blood.* 2005;105(2):464-473.

699. Dukes PP, Izadi P, Ortega JA, Shore NA, Gomperts E. Inhibitory effects of interferon on mouse megakaryocytic progenitor cells in culture. *Exp Hematol.* 1980;8(8):1048-1056.

700. Ganser A, Carlo-Stella C, Greher J, Volkers B, Hoelzer D. Effect of recombinant interferons alpha and gamma on human bone marrow-derived megakaryocytic progenitor cells. *Blood.* 1987;70(4):1173-1179.

701. Tsuji K, Muraoka K, Nakahata T. Interferon-gamma and human megakaryopoiesis. *Leuk Lymphoma.* 1998;31(1-2):107-113.

702. Pozner RG, Ure AE, Jaquenod de Giusti C, et al. Junin virus infection of human hematopoietic progenitors impairs in vitro proplatelet formation and platelet release via a bystander effect involving type I IFN signaling. *PLoS Pathog.* 2010;6(4):e1000847.

703. Yamane A, Nakamura T, Suzuki H, et al. Interferon-alpha 2b-induced thrombocytopenia is caused by inhibition of platelet production but not proliferation and endomitosis in human megakaryocytes. *Blood.* 2008;112(3):542-550.

704. Vannucchi AM, Harrison C. Emerging treatments for classical myeloproliferative neoplasms. *Blood.* 2016;129(6):693-703.

705. Xavier-Ferrucio J, Scanlon V, Li X, et al. Low iron promotes megakaryocytic commitment of megakaryocytic-erythroid progenitors in humans and mice. *Blood.* 2019;134(18):1547-1557.

706. Gruber TA, Downing JR. The biology of pediatric acute megakaryoblastic leukemia. *Blood.* 2015;126(8):943-949.

707. Thiollier C, Lopez CK, Gerby B, et al. Characterization of novel genomic alterations and therapeutic approaches using acute megakaryoblastic leukemia xenograft models. *J Exp Med.* 2012;209(11):2017-2031.

708. Wechsler J, Greene M, McDevitt MA, et al. Acquired mutations in GATA1 in the megakaryoblastic leukemia of Down syndrome. *Nat Genet.* 2002;32(1):148-152.

709. Yoshida K, Toki T, Okuno Y, et al. The landscape of somatic mutations in down syndrome-related myeloid disorders. *Nat Genet.* 2013;45(11):1293-1299.

710. Sperling AS, Gibson CJ, Ebert BL. The genetics of myelodysplastic syndrome: from clonal haematopoiesis to secondary leukaemia. *Nat Rev Cancer.* 2017;17(1):5-19.

711. Hong WJ, Gotlib J. Hereditary erythrocytosis, thrombocytosis and neutrophilia. *Best Pract Res Clin Haematol.* 2014;27(2):95-106.

712. Johnson B, Fletcher SJ, Morgan NV. Inherited thrombocytopenia: novel insights into megakaryocyte maturation, proplatelet formation and platelet lifespan. *Platelets.* 2016;27(6):519-525.

713. Nurden AT, Freson K, Seligsohn U. Inherited platelet disorders. *Haemophilia.* 2012;18(suppl 4):154-160.

Chapter 18 ■ Platelet Structure

ELISABETH M. BATTINELLI • KATIE MAURER

STRUCTURAL AND FUNCTIONAL ANATOMY

The pool of healthy platelets serves critical functions in maintaining endothelial homeostasis, sealing leaky capillary beds, and coordinating and propagating coagulation. Platelets also contribute to wound healing by delivering and concentrating phospholipids and coagulation factors, as well as growth factors and cytokines. Platelets adapt their responses through residual RNA to react to various systemic states, including acute or chronic inflammation. The structure and function of platelets are tightly interrelated and efficient. Despite their small size, platelets are densely packed and serve an integral role in circulatory maintenance and systems of defense in the human body.

Light Microscopy

Platelets are seen on Wright-stained smears by light microscopy as small fragments lacking a nucleus (i.e., anucleate) with occasional granules (*Figure 18.1*). Although there is considerable variation in the size and shape of platelets, they typically measure 2 μm in diameter with a volume of 8 fL.[1] Young platelets (i.e., recently released from the marrow) are referred to as *reticulated*, given their RNA content and as an analogy to reticulocytes (young red cells).[2] About 30% of platelets may have a procoagulant phenotype after being stimulated with collagen and thrombin, leading to high expression levels of α-granule proteins and phosphatidylserine (PS) on their surface.[3] These "procoagulant platelets" have been associated with inflammatory states, such as thrombotic events.

Electron Microscopy and Subcellular Features

Resting and activated platelets differ morphologically and biochemically. The resting state is marked by baseline homeostatic metabolic activity, while the activated state results from stimulation of the platelet by an agonist (e.g., thrombin). Circulating platelets in the resting state appear as flat discs with smooth contours by scanning electron microscopy (*Figure 18.2*). They exhibit rare spiny filopodia and invaginations throughout the surface, indicative of a channel system known as the surface-connected canalicular system (SCCS). The SCCS is the conduit through which granule contents exocytose after simulation.[4] Transmission electron microscopy demonstrates a complex platelet surface as well as cytoplasm packed with numerous substructures and organelles, although platelets lack a nucleus. These elements—platelet membrane, canalicular system, and contractile apparatus—are essential to achieving hemostasis (*Figure 18.2*). Platelet structure can be classified into surface, membrane structures, cytoskeleton, and granules, with each component playing a critical role in platelet structure and function.

Platelet Surface

Plasma Membrane

The platelet plasma membrane is a 20-nm-thick trilaminar structure[5] and is similar in appearance to that of other blood cells.[6] The membrane incorporates glycoproteins (GPs) and lipids into its phospholipid bilayer and has a complex composition, distribution, and function. Most platelet functions are carried out by the membrane, which integrates both intra- and extraplatelet events including permeability, adhesion, response to stimulation, activation/secretion, and aggregation. The membrane surface serves as the site of blood coagulation,

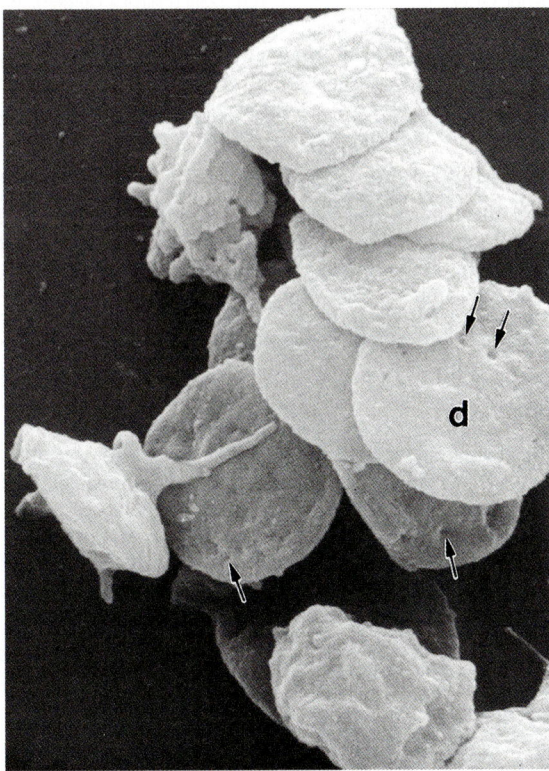

FIGURE 18.2 Unstimulated human platelet visualized by electron microscopy. The majority are discoid (d) in shape with surface indentations (arrows) corresponding to openings of the surface-connected canalicular system to the external milieu. Magnification × 15,000. (Reprinted by permission from Springer: Stenberg PE, Shuman MA, Levine SP, et al. Optimal techniques for the immunocytochemical demonstration of β-thromboglobulin, platelet factor 4, and fibrinogen in the alpha granules of unstimulated platelets. *Histochem J.* 1984;16(9):983-1001. Copyright © 1984 Springer Nature.)

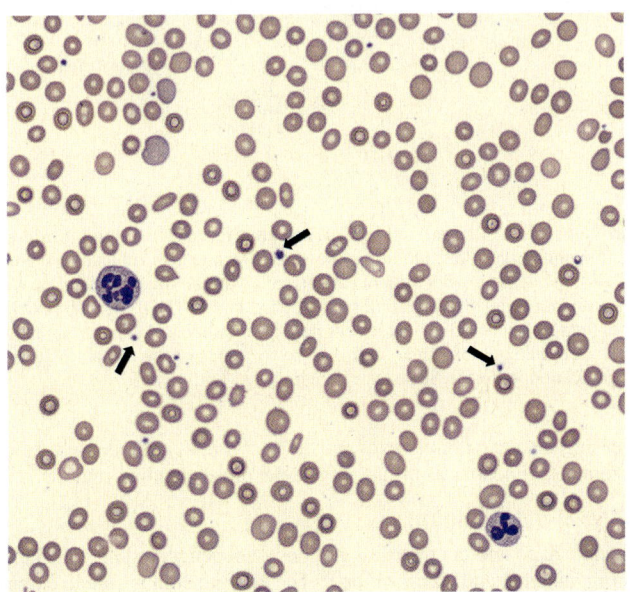

FIGURE 18.1 A human peripheral blood smear stained with Wright-Giemsa. Small round platelets (arrows) are scattered between erythrocytes and leukocytes. The bluish cytoplasm contains purple-red granules. (Original magnification of a 35-mm slide ×100.)

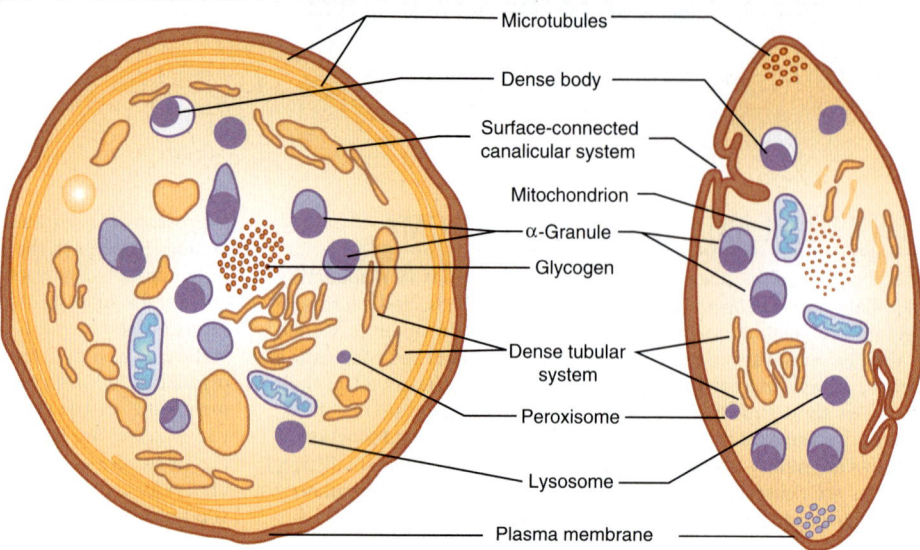

FIGURE 18.3 Schematic of a human platelet with major components seen by electron microscopy and cytochemistry. Membrane components include the plasma membrane, surface-connected canalicular system, and dense tubular system. In addition, platelets contain mitochondria, microtubules, glycogen, and four types of storage organelles (α-granules, dense bodies, microperoxisomes, and lysosomes). Microperoxisomes and lysosomes are only visible by cytochemical stains, whereas α-granules and dense bodies can be seen morphologically. (From Bentfeld-Barker ME, Bainton DF. Identification of primary lysosomes in human megakaryocytes and platelets. *Blood.* 1982;59:472-481, with permission.)

acting as a surface upon which soluble proteins are attracted and assembled in complexes for generation of thrombin and fibrin.

In unstimulated resting platelets, membrane lipids are distributed asymmetrically, with the outer layer composed primarily of neutral species and the inner layer concentrated with anionic forms such as PS.[7] Resting platelets are essentially nonreactive (i.e., in terms of thrombin generation), a feature that may be attributable to this sequestration of PS on the inner membrane.[8] PS is a critical component and accelerator of plasma coagulation. PS contributes to assembly of membrane-dependent enzyme cofactor functions of coagulation factors VIII and V, and as such, it is a critical component and accelerator of plasma coagulation.[9] When stimulated, activated platelets play a key role in thrombin formation (i.e., the "thrombin burst") by concentrating PS and coagulation factors in "cap" structures.[8,10,11] The platelet plasma membrane also maintains ionic homeostasis through distribution of sodium and calcium adenosine triphosphatase (ATPase) pumps.[12]

Platelet Membranous Systems

High actin content in platelets underlie key contractile responses during activation, a feature reminiscent of muscle-related cells. Similarly, the two membranous systems of platelets, the SCCS and the dense tubular system, resemble muscle-like transverse tubules and sarcotubules.[13]

Surface-Connected Canalicular System

The SCCS, also known as the *open canalicular system*, is a fenestrated and contiguous network throughout the surface plasma membrane[3,14,15] (*Figure 18.3*). The SCCS functions as an internal reservoir of surplus membrane that facilitates platelet expansion and filopodia formation for adhesion.[16] It also serves as a storage reservoir for membrane GPs, including $\alpha_{IIb}\beta_3$ (GPIIb-IIIa), which increase upon the surface following activation.[16] The SCCS also serves as a conduit for granule release in the secretory phase of activated platelets[4] as well as an avenue of entry and exit for translocation of molecules between platelet and plasma. The SCCS may have a role in host defense against bacteria by "covering" organisms or debris at wound sites and promoting the local immune response.[17,18]

Dense Tubules

In contrast to the SCCS, the *dense tubular system* is a closed-channel network composed of membrane-limited narrow tubules measuring 40 to 60 nm in diameter[19] (*Figures 18.3* and *18.4*). The dense tubular system contains residual smooth endoplasmic reticulum retained from the megakaryocyte,[20,21] peroxidase,[22-24] glucose 6-phosphatase,[25] adenylate cyclase, and Ca^{2+}- and Mg^{2+}-activated ATPases.[26] In some animals (e.g., cat, rat, mouse) but not humans, this system also contains acetylcholinesterase.[27] The dense tubular system functions to regulate intracellular calcium transport by selectively binding, sequestering, and

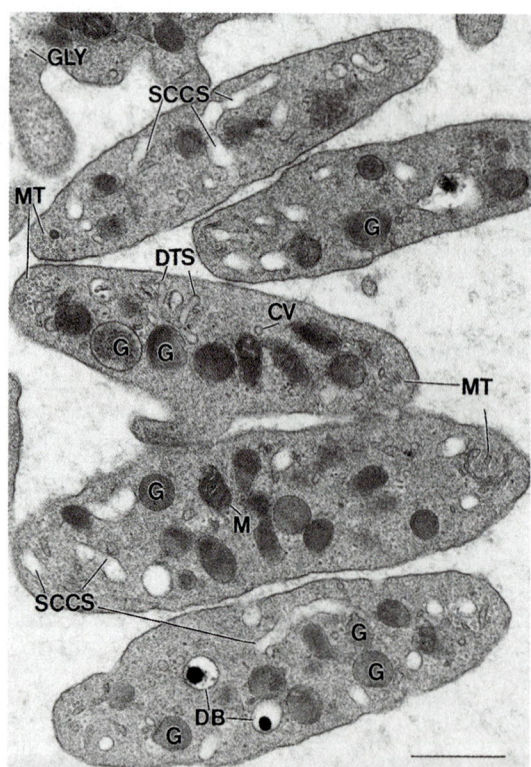

FIGURE 18.4 Ultrastructure of an unstimulated human platelet. Membranous organelles, including the surface-connected canalicular system (SCCS) and dense tubular system (DTS), and cytoplasmic organelles, including mitochondria (M), α-granules (G), dense bodies (DB), coated vesicles (CV), and glycogen (GLY), are identified. Microtubules (MT) are present as cross-sectional and longitudinal profiles at the poles of the discoid platelets. Magnification × 46,000. Scale bar = 0.5 μm.

releasing divalent cations after activation.[26] Finally, the dense tubular system also functions as the site of platelet prostaglandin synthesis.[28,29]

Platelet Cytoskeleton

Platelet shape and contractile function are dependent upon cytoskeletal organization and composition.[30] The cytoskeleton is able to extend extracellular protrusions, collect and extrude secretory granules, and impact surface reactivity, all of which can directly change platelet shape (*Figure 18.5*). Three distinct structures are responsible for execution of these functions: the membrane skeleton, which supports the inner plasma membrane leaflet; the mass of actin and intermediate filaments filling the cytoplasm; and finally the microtubule band, which encircles the platelet producing the classical disc-like form at rest.[30,31] The overall network is composed of three filaments/tubules, including the 5- to 6-nm-diameter actin microfilaments,[32,33] the 10- to 12-nm desmin and vimentin intermediate filaments,[34,35] and the 25-nm microtubules primarily composed of tubulin.[36-38] The combination of these three filaments comprises approximately 30% to 50% of total platelet protein, depending on the activation state.

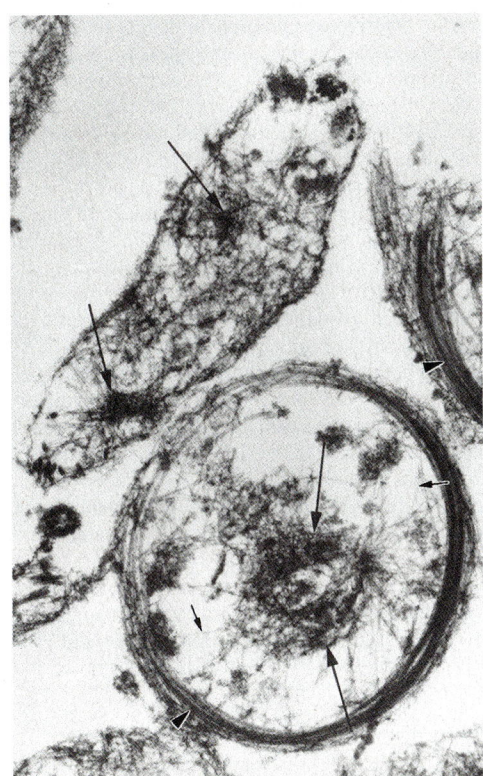

FIGURE 18.5 Human platelet cytoskeletons (prepared with fixation and lysis in Triton X-100 detergent). Single actin filaments (short arrows) are seen throughout the cytoplasm. Clusters of filaments (long arrows) are seen as well. Microtubule coils are present at the peripheries (arrowheads). Magnification × 30,000. (Reprinted with permission from Boyles J, Fox JE, Phillips DR, Stenberg PE. Organization of the cytoskeleton in resting, discoid platelets: preservation of actin filaments by a modified fixation that prevents osmium damage. *J Cell Biol.* 1985;101:1463-1472. Originally published in *Journal of Cell Biology.* https://doi.org/10.1083/jcb.101.4.1463. Copyright © 1985 by The Rockefeller University Press.)

Membrane Skeleton

The platelet membrane skeleton was first characterized in 1969 using electron microscopy[39,40] and later underwent biochemical analysis by detergent lysis with Triton X-100.[30,41] The membrane skeleton comprises short actin filaments connecting surface receptors with cytoplasmic actin filaments.[32] One component, Filamin-A, links the cytoplasmic domain of GPIbα to actin filaments and binds integrins. Other membrane skeleton components are involved in structural integrity and signaling, including spectrin, talin, migfilin, Src, and other small GTPase family members (*Table 18.1*).[30,31] These membrane skeleton components function together to facilitate platelet sensing and response to environmental cues.

Cytoplasmic Actin and Intermediate Filaments

The majority of the platelet cytoskeleton is composed of actin (M_r = 42,000), which makes up approximately 25% of the total platelet protein.[42] Other cytoskeletal proteins tropomyosin and α-actinin account for about 2% to 5% of total platelet protein.[43-46] Actin is present in soluble, monomeric (G-actin), and filamentous (F-actin) forms and functions to connect both to membrane skeleton and microtubules.[31] In the resting state, 40% of actin is in microfilaments dispersed throughout the cytoplasm.[47] Intermediate actin filaments are more stable structures due to high vimentin content and bear tension in the cytoplasm.[35]

Stimulation of platelets induces significant changes in the organization of the cytoskeleton. The discoid resting shape transforms into a more rounded shape with extension of filopodia.[48,49] Upon activation, intracellular calcium concentration rises, as does the proportion of F-actin (up to 60% to 70%).[49] Monomers of actin polymerize into filaments at the periphery,[48,50] and filaments bundle together to constitute the burgeoning filopodia.[51-53] Myosin light chain phosphorylation leads to binding to actin,[54-56] which creates the necessary tension for granule centralization and filopodia retraction.[57] The structure is further remodeled by accumulation of talin and surface $\alpha_{IIb}\beta_3$ proteins that associate with the actin filaments, along with a calcium-dependent protease, calpain.[58] The formation of these protein complexes plays a key role in platelet secretion, clot retraction, and spreading (filopodia and lamellipodia extension) associated with platelet activation.

Microtubules

The discoid form of the platelet is maintained by a circumferential microtubule band.[36,37] Composed of two nonidentical subunits of α- and β-tubulin, this 25-nm-diameter microtubule coil is situated adjacent to but not in contact with the plasma membrane.[59] In unstimulated platelets, 13 protofilaments of αβ tubulin dimers are polymerized; upon activation, microtubules disassemble and later reassemble, resulting in changes to platelet shape.[59] Evidence suggests that microtubules play a key role in determining platelet size, and their disorganization may account for giant platelet disorders.[60-62] For example, the

Table 18.1. Major Platelet Cytoskeletal Proteins

Protein	Molecular Weight (kDa)	Main Known Function
Actin	42	~30% of platelet protein; primary component of microfilaments; F-actin binds myosin
Myosin II	500	4% of platelet protein; light chain phosphorylation contracts microfilaments; binds actin
Talin	235	2% of platelet protein; interacts with α-actinin and vinculin
Actin-binding protein (filamin 1)	260	Cross-links actin filaments; links glycoprotein Ib-IX complex with membrane skeleton
Vinculin	130	Links actin; interacts with talin
α-Actinin	102	Promotes actin polymerization; dimers cross-link F-actin
Thymosin β_4	5	Binds to G-actin monomers to inhibit polymerization
Profilin	15.2	Binds to G-action to inhibit polymerization; adds adenosine triphosphate (ATP)
Myosin light-chain kinase	105	Phosphorylates myosin to activate its ATPase leading to contraction
Tropomyosin	28	Binds specific F-actins
Calmodulin	17	Binds Ca^{2+}; activates myosin light-chain kinase

May-Hegglin anomaly is an autosomal dominant disorder in which the MYH9 gene encoding nonmuscle myosin heavy chain II (NMMHCII) is mutated leading to increased numbers of single tubules and coils of tubules in a disorganized fashion, resulting in large platelets.[61]

Platelet Granules and Organelles

In order to appropriately respond to stimuli and environmental cues, platelets contain secretory granules and mechanisms for release of cargo. A variety of granules are found in platelets, including α- and dense granules, lysosomes, and peroxisomes. Cargo release (e.g., fibrinogen and adenosine diphosphate [ADP]) upon stimulation is primarily mediated by α-granules and dense bodies.

Platelet granule secretion is triggered by an increase in metabolic activity initiated by a surge of calcium release and increased adenosine triphosphate (ATP) production.[63] Upon platelet stimulation, a "contractile ring" appears around centralized granules, which then fuse with surface membranes and extrude their contents.[5,6,64] The mechanisms for granule docking, fusion, and extrusion are shared between platelets and other similar cellular systems.[65,66] Platelets can adapt the strength of granule secretion to the nature of the original stimulus. For example, strong signals of activation including thrombin and collagen result in more granule secretion compared with weak signals such as ADP and epinephrine.[66]

α-Granules

α-Granules, spherical in shape and approximately 300 nm in diameter, are the predominant platelet granules at approximately 50 granules per platelet.[67] An outer membrane encloses two distinct intragranular zones that are variable in electron density. The larger, denser region is typically eccentrically placed and contains a nucleoid material rich in platelet-specific proteins (e.g., β-thromboglobulin).[68] The second zone with a lower electron density is situated peripherally adjacent to the granule membrane. This zone contains tubular structures with adhesive GPs (e.g., von Willebrand factor [vWF] and multimerin) as well as factor V.[69-71] α-Granules also store plasma proteins taken up by platelets[72-74] (*Table 18.2*).

α-Granules acquire protein contents in three distinct ways: from megakaryocytes, through endocytosis during platelet circulation in the peripheral blood, and through translation of residual mRNA that is retained or endocytosed by the platelet itself. Some of the proteins synthesized in megakaryocytes include β-thromboglobulin, PF4, and thrombospondin. β-Thromboglobulin and PF4, both in the CXC family of chemokines, share amino acid sequence homology and heparin-binding properties, and both localize in the dense nucleoid of α-granules.[15,75-79] Representing about 5% of total platelet proteins, these proteins are also frequently used as serum or plasma markers of platelet activation.[80,81] Thrombospondin is released in response to thrombin and is thought to contribute to multiple biologic processes.[82,83]

vWF, also synthesized in megakaryocytes, is contained in tubular structures of the peripheral zone α-granules (reminiscent of its localization to Weibel-Palade bodies in vascular endothelial cells).[70,84] Factor V and multimerin (a factor V/Va-binding protein) are found with vWF in platelets.[71,85] Fibrinogen is actively incorporated in α-granules from plasma rather than synthesized de novo from megakaryocytes.[73] Other plasma proteins may also be taken up into α-granules, including immunoglobulin G (IgG), albumin, β-amyloid protein precursor, and fibronectin.[84,86-88] α-Granules also contain signaling molecules that may drive mitogenic activity, including growth factors (e.g., platelet-derived growth factor, transforming growth factor-β₁ [TGF-β1], and vascular endothelial growth factor [VEGF]).[89,90] α-Granules contain both pro- and anti-angiogenesis proteins (e.g., VEGF and endostatin, respectively, but how angiogenesis regulatory proteins are selectively stored and released is incompletely characterized).[91-96] A role for platelet-derived TGF-β1 in fibrotic conditions, including cardiac fibrosis, has been described.[97,98]

The protein $α_{IIb}β_3$ is contained in platelet α-granules and contributes to fibrinogen receptors on the surface of activated platelets.[99-101] P-selectin (granule membrane protein-140), an α-granule membrane protein, translocates to the plasma membrane upon platelet activation.[102,103] Finally, other surface proteins on α-granules include CD9, Rap1b, platelet endothelial cell adhesion molecular-1 (PECAM-1), GPIb-IX-V, and osteonectin.[104-106] In a disorder termed gray platelet

Table 18.2. Platelet Granule Components Secreted Upon Activation

Granule Protein	Amount per 10⁹ Platelets	Functions/Comments
Platelet-Specific Proteins		
Platelet factor 4	12 μg	Marker of platelet activation
β-Thromboglobulin	10–20 μg	Marker of platelet activation
Coagulant Proteins		
Fibrinogen	140 μg	Platelet aggregation
Factor V	4 μg	Critical cofactor for coagulation
Mitogenic and Angiogenic Factors		
Platelet-derived growth factor	30–100 ng	Smooth muscle mitogen
Vascular endothelial growth factor		High concentrations in platelets
Transforming growth factor-β		Binds thrombospondin; complex activation pathway
α-Granule Membrane-Specific Proteins and Adhesive Glycoproteins		
Thrombospondin	40 μg	Multiple complexes
von Willebrand factor	0.3 μg	Critical role in adhesion
P-selectin	20,000 copies on activated platelets	Mediates platelet-leukocyte binding
Multimerin		Binds factor V
Dense Granule Components		
Adenosine triphosphate	440 nmol/mg	40% released with activation
Adenosine diphosphate	630 nmol/mg	Mediator of aggregation; 95% secreted with activation
Serotonin	100 nmol/mg	95% released with activation
Calcium	2630 nmol/mg	70% secreted with activation

syndrome, platelets have reduced numbers of α-granules and some proteins, perhaps due to incorrect targeting of α-granule proteins in the megakaryocyte.[107,108]

Dense Bodies

There are approximately five dense bodies per platelet, so named due to a distinctive electron-dense "bull's eye" appearance by electron microscopy, which are 250-nm-diameter granules containing a reservoir of ADP, a key agonist for platelet activation that acts by amplifying effects of other stimuli.[109-111] Dense bodies also contain ATP, calcium, pyrophosphate, and serotonin (5-hydroxytryptamine), along with smaller amounts of guanosine triphosphate (GTP), guanosine diphosphate (GDP), and magnesium.[78] Serotonin is taken up from plasma by circulating platelets and packaged in dense granules, while adenine nucleotides are synthesized by megakaryocytes.[112-114] P-selectin and granulophysin are also contained in the dense granule membrane.[115]

Lysosomes

Lysosomes, with a diameter of 200 nm and pH of 3.5 to 5.5, are small vesicles containing acid hydrolases including cathepsins, β-glucuronidase, β-hexosaminidase, β-galactosidase, aryl sulfatase, β-glycerophosphatase, and heparitinase.[116] Other lysosomal proteins expressed on the plasma membrane after activation include cathepsin D and the lysosome-associated membrane proteins (LAMP-1/LAMP-2).[117,118] Release of lysosomal contents requires stronger agonists (e.g., thrombin or collagen) compared with α-granules or dense-body contents, and they are released more slowly and incompletely (at most 60% of the granules).

Organelles: Microperoxisomes, Coated Vesicles, Mitochondria, and Glycogen

Peroxisomes are 90-nm-diameter relatively rare granules with catalase activity that may contribute to platelet-activating factor synthesis.[119,120] Alkaline diaminobenzidine can be used to identify these structures.

A platelet may contain approximately seven mitochondria, which are smaller than those found in other cell types. As in other cells, the mitochondria facilitate the citric acid cycle and respiratory chain activities.[121] Glycogen, essential for platelet metabolism, is found in small particles or in masses of closely associated particles in platelets.[122]

BIOCHEMISTRY AND METABOLISM

Composition

By dry weight, the platelet consists of approximately 60% protein, 15% lipid, and 8% carbohydrates. Platelets contain several vitamins and minerals including vitamin B_{12}, folic acid, ascorbic acid, calcium, magnesium, potassium, and zinc.[123] The intraplatelet sodium concentration is 39 mEq, and the potassium concentration is 138 mEq.[124] This gradient is maintained by an active ion pump deriving energy from membrane ATPase (ouabain-sensitive Na^+/K^+-dependent type and appears to be contained in two separate metabolic compartments).[125]

Resting/unstimulated platelets limit Ca^{2+} transport from plasma and promote active Ca^{2+} efflux in order to maintain low cytoplasmic concentration of 100 to 500 nmol/L.[126] Platelets contain two distinct calcium pools: a cytosolic pool with rapid turnover regulated by a plasma membrane sodium-calcium antiporter and a slower exchanging pool sequestered in the dense tubular system regulated by Ca^{2+}/Mg^+-ATPase.[127] Platelets transport calcium either against a gradient into the extracellular space or by sequestering it in the dense tubular system.

Energy Metabolism and Generation of Adenosine Triphosphate

Platelets are similar to skeletal muscle in usage of active glycolysis and glycogen synthesis for energy metabolism, as well as use of actomyosin-like ATPase for intracellular energy.[128] The platelet is adapted metabolically to expend energy rapidly during aggregation, release, and clot retraction.

Glucose taken up from plasma serves as the main energy source for platelets. In the resting state, half of absorbed glucose provides energy for synthetic function or is converted to glycogen. The citric acid cycle, NAD-NADH (nicotinamide adenine dinucleotide–nicotinamide adenine dinucleotide) system, and glycolytic pathway (including its regulatory enzymes phosphorylase, pyruvate kinase, hexokinase, phosphofructokinase, and glyceraldehyde 3-phosphate dehydrogenase) are all active in platelets.[128] Up to 98% of pyruvate contained in platelets is converted to lactate, which then exits the platelet.[129-131] Platelets also contain enzymes for carrying out fatty acid oxidation and oxidative phosphorylation (*Figure 18.3*).[132,133]

In unstimulated platelets, most ATP is produced by oxidative phosphorylation through fatty acid β-oxidation.[122] Other mechanisms of ATP production, including hexose monophosphate shunt, glycogen turnover, and the citric acid cycle are quiescent in the resting platelet.[131] Glycolysis can compensate for reduced ATP production if oxidative phosphorylation is inhibited. In unstimulated platelets, ATP energy maintains homeostatic levels of ions including H^+, K^+, Na^{2+}, and Ca^{2+}.[12,134] Upon platelet stimulation, there is a major increase in metabolic activity including glycogenolysis, glycolysis, and oxidation.[128,135,136] These pathways synthesize ATP to an approximately equal amount, although oxidation provides greater ATP yield per mole of glucose.[129,133]

Nucleotide Metabolism and the Nonmetabolic Role for Adenosine Diphosphate

Adenine nucleotides are separated into at least two distinct pools and make up 90% of free platelet nucleotides.[103] About 40% of total adenine nucleotides contribute to the metabolic (cytoplasmic) pool used for maintenance and homeostasis of energy-consuming platelet functions. This metabolic pool undergoes constant turnover, demonstrated by rapid incorporation of (^{14}C)-adenine and (^{32}P)-phosphate into ATP. In resting platelets, the enzyme adenylate kinase maintains relative concentrations of AMP, ADP, and ATP.[137]

Dense bodies contain another storage pool of adenine nucleotides (mainly ATP and ADP), constituting about two-thirds of total platelet nucleotides. This pool is not metabolically active, does not rapidly take up exogenous phosphate or adenine, and undergoes slow equilibration with the metabolic pool.[138] The storage pool extrudes nucleotides from the platelet during the release reaction but is not replenished after release. Conversion of G-actin to F-actin requires ATP hydrolysis, and the resulting ADP associates with F-actin. This actin-bound ADP makes up one-third of platelet nucleotides.[139] Up to 40% of ATP produced by platelets is used during actin treadmilling[111] and up to 7% is consumed by phosphoinositides (PIP and PIP_2) turnover.[112]

When ATP is broken down for energy generation for the release reaction, it is irreversibly degraded to hypoxanthine and diffuses out of the platelet rather than being rephosphorylated.[140] In normal stored platelets this reaction proceeds slowly. Hypoxanthine can then be reincorporated from the plasma by the salvage pathway into metabolic AMP (*Figure 18.6*).[113,141] Upon stimulation, various ATP-producing pathways are activated, resulting in a decrease in steady-state levels of ATP and accumulation of hypoxanthine. Activated platelets also transiently increase their phosphate uptake.[115] While platelet stimulation is known to activate ATP-requiring pathways, the mechanisms by which these pathways are linked to platelet signaling processing is unknown.

Lipid Composition and Metabolism and the Generation of Arachidonic Acid

Approximately 80% of total platelets comprise phospholipids, while the remaining 20% are neutral lipids and glycolipids.[142] Human platelets contain five major subtypes of phospholipids: phosphatidylcholine (38% of total), phosphatidylethanolamine (PE, 27%), sphingomyelin (17%), PS (10%), and phosphatidylinositol (PI, 5%).[8] Platelet fractionation demonstrates that 57% of platelet phospholipid is contained

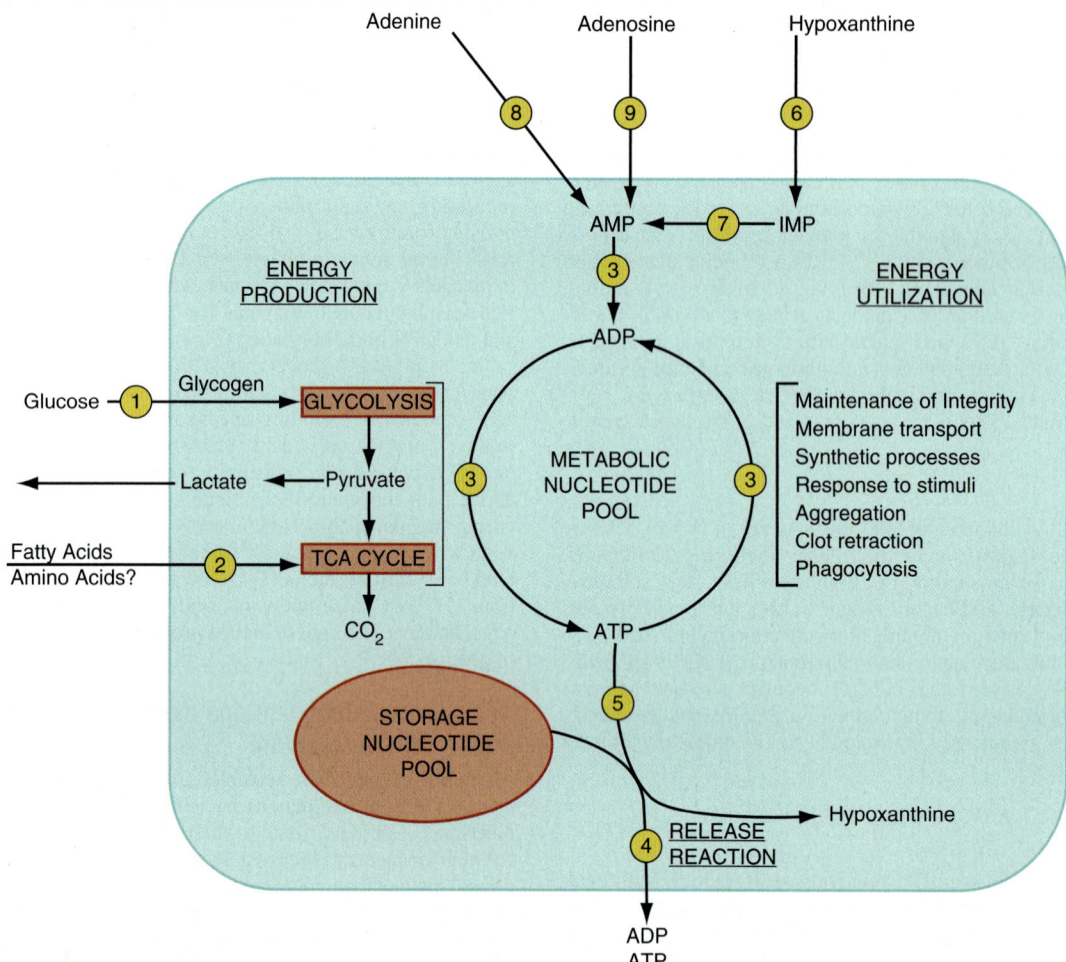

FIGURE 18.6 Schematic of platelet metabolism. Most of the platelet energy is derived from glucose metabolism, with a smaller proportion derived from fatty acid metabolism. Glycolysis and the citric acid cycle contribute approximately equally to energy production. Platelet energy reserve is provided by the metabolic pool of platelet nucleotides. This energy is used for maintenance of platelet structural integrity and in reactions of platelet response to stimuli. The granule-bound storage (nonmetabolic) nucleotide pool is discharged during the release reaction. ADP, adenosine diphosphate; AMP, adenosine monophosphate; ATP, adenosine triphosphate; IMP, inosine monophosphate; TCA, tricarboxylic acid. (Adapted from Hirsh J, Doery JCG. Platelet function in health and disease. *Prog Hematol.* 1972;7:185-234. Copyright © 1972 Elsevier. With permission.)

in the plasma membrane.[143] The inner leaflet contains mostly negatively charged phospholipids (PE, PI, PS), which prevents inappropriate coagulation by clustering phospholipids that accelerate coagulation (e.g., PS) away from the surface of the platelet.[144,145] Platelet activation results in reversal of this asymmetric arrangement, when the phospholipids that interact with coagulation proteins (PS and PE) redistribute and are exposed on the platelet surface to promote clot formation.[11,146,147] Membrane scramblase enzymes appear to maintain this asymmetric distribution of surface phospholipids, while a flippase reverses the asymmetry upon platelet activation.[148]

The majority of platelet fatty acids are esterified as phospholipids, with very few in the free form. Platelet phospholipids are enriched in the precursor of prostaglandins, arachidonate, at the "sn-2" position.[149] Upon activation, phospholipase A_2 activity increases, resulting in release of arachidonic acid from membrane phospholipids.[150-152] Once released, arachidonic acid is oxygenated and forms PGH_2, the cyclic endoperoxide intermediate, by cyclo-oxygenase-1, leading to TXA_2 formation.[149] A small proportion of arachidonate metabolism is accounted for by the lipoxygenase pathway, which produces 12-hydroxyeicosatetraenoic acid (12-HETE). Genetic alterations in TXA_2 generation have been associated with clinical bleeding syndromes.[153]

About 28% of total platelet lipids comprise neutral lipids, mostly cholesterol, which is a major component of the platelet membrane as

well as being present in the cytoskeleton.[154] Cholesterol is not synthesized by platelets but rather is made by megakaryocytes. Other neutral lipids such as ceramides, glycolipids, and gangliosides have been found in platelets.[155]

MICROPARTICLES AND KINETICS

Microparticles

Platelet microparticles, generated during platelet activation, are small structures rich in PS that contribute to acceleration of plasma coagulation by enhancing factor Xa and thrombin generation.[156] Microparticle composition is variable depending on stimulus (thrombin, tissue factor, shear, C5b-9, ionophor A23187).[157,158] They have been shown to bind to different factors including Xa, VIII, Va, and protein S.[159,160] Microparticles have been suggested to have a key procoagulant role, as patients deficient in these structures have associated clinical bleeding disorders.[161,162]

Platelet Heterogeneity

The normal human platelet count is approximately 150,000 to 400,000/μL, with a typical mean platelet volume between 7.5 and 10.5 fL. Long proplatelet extensions from megakaryocytes release young platelets into blood, which tend to be larger and more dense, undergoing remodeling in circulation by shedding some surface components.[163]

Disruptions in the steps of platelet production may give rise to macrothrombocytopenias,[164] and characteristics of large platelets may reflect unique properties of recently released platelets from the marrow or production of proplatelets under acerated or abnormal conditions.

Platelet Distribution and Survival Kinetics

Lifespan

Platelet lifespan in humans is estimated at approximately 8 to 12 days, which has been ascertained by time required to clear platelets labeled with (^{51})Cr (chromate) and widely validated with other labeling assays including (^{111})In (indium), 8-hydroxyquinoline chelation, and (^{68})Ga (gallium).[165-167]

Platelet turnover is estimated to be 1.2 to 1.5×10^{11} per day at steady state (i.e., when production is equal to destruction/consumption).[168,169] The Panel on Diagnostic Application of Radioisotopes in Hematology and International Committee for Standardization in Hematology have published recommendations for platelet lifespan estimation, and multiple models have been proposed.[169,170]

Platelet survival and programmed death are regulated by Bcl02 proteins.[171,172] Bcl-x(L) in platelets maintains a survival signal by suppression of Bak. Bak activation leads to classical apoptosis resulting in mitochondrial damage, caspase activation, and PS exposure.[173] Animals deficient in Bak have longer-lived platelets compared with normal, demonstrating a predetermined platelet death program.[173]

Distribution

Approximately two-thirds of the total platelet pool is present in circulating blood, with one-third pooling in the spleen, although the two pools appear to exchange freely.[168,174] In splenectomized patients, 100% of the platelet pool exists in circulation. Administration of epinephrine results in platelet evacuation out of the spleen and an increase in the circulating platelet count but 30% to 50%,[175] whereas platelet counts in asplenic patients are unsurprisingly unaffected by epinephrine. There is some evidence to suggest that the splenic platelet pool contains the largest, youngest platelets. Longer transit time through splenic cords is thought to underlie splenic platelet sequestration, versus binding to splenic reticular and endothelial cells by platelets.[176] Various pathophysiologic states can increase platelet sequestration in the spleen to 80% to 90% of total platelet mass, leading to peripheral thrombocytopenia. Intracardiac epinephrine administration has also been reported to result in platelet release from the lungs.[177] Vigorous exercise also leads to rise in platelet count, and this observation is not affected by prior splenectomy.[177]

INTERACTIONS BEYOND PLATELETS: THE COAGULATION SYSTEM

Platelet Interactions With the Plasma Coagulation System

Thrombin generation is accelerated by platelet activation, wherein production of factor Xa and thrombin results in activation of the coagulation "cascade" during which a series of calcium-dependent complexes are generated by both the extrinsic and intrinsic pathways.[140] Phospholipid surfaces serve as the primary sites for this complex development.[178,179] On the surface of activated platelets, soluble factor Xa binds to Va, which suggests that activated platelet surfaces are a major site for coagulation reactions; however, the precise elements involved are incompletely described.[180] Factor VIIIa bound to platelets may bind to IXa, and the effector cell protease receptor-1 (EPR-1) has been described as a binding site for factors Va and Xa. It remains unclear whether there are specific receptors for VIIIa and Va. Also yet to be established is whether factor VIII is contained within platelets in the resting state. While platelets actively take up fibrinogen from plasma, they do not appear to take up much plasma vWF with bound factor VIII.[74]

Factor XI can be activated by thrombin, especially on the surface of platelets or when proteoglycans are present.[181,182] In this setting,

thrombin is generated through tissue factor produced due to cellular injury, which then activates factor XI. Factor XI is bound to platelets when prothrombin is present, and this in turn activates factor IX and leads to downstream increased thrombin production.[183,184] This process may conserve a small portion of the initial thrombin by linking it to protein substrates immobilized on platelet surface away from plasma inhibitors.[11,185] Clinically, the amount of platelet-associated factor XI, but not plasma factor XI, is the main determinant of bleeding severity in factor-deficient patients.[186,187]

Platelets have multiple functions in coagulation and are capable of regulating their resting and activated states.[187] These processes are facilitated by both platelet microparticles as well as whole platelets themselves. Coagulation factor binding to high-affinity receptors located on platelet membranes concentrates those factors and facilitates ongoing coagulation. Surface binding of coagulation factors also serves to protect them from plasma inhibitors[187] and also facilitates rapid delivery of coagulant and agonist to sites of vessel injury to achieve hemostasis.

Platelet Forms of Plasma Proteins

Fibrinogen, vWF, and factor V are three factors found in platelet α-granules that have a major contribution to coagulation. Platelets have large amounts of fibrinogen and less vWF (which they synthesize). Factor V is both incorporated from plasma and synthesized de novo in megakaryocytes. About 20% of total factor V in blood is located within α-granules. Factor Va (the thrombin-activated form) is the main secreted platelet phosphoprotein.[11,188] That factor V plays a key role in hemostasis is emphasized by the observation that in two families of factor V Quebec and α-granule factor V defects (but not plasma factor V) the condition leads to severe clinical bleeding diathesis. This is thought to be due to excessive proteolysis in the granules.[189,190] Platelet fibrinogen composes nearly 10% of total protein in the platelet.[191,192] vWF is present in large amounts in α-granules and is thought to play a role in subendothelial platelet adherence.[193]

Other Platelet-Associated Coagulation Factors

Numerous platelet proteins contribute to coagulation, as noted in *Table 18.3*, in addition to several other plasma coagulation factors (and inhibitors) associated with platelets. FXIII, an active subunit A of plasma factor XIII, is found in the cytosol rather than in association with an organelle. FXIII comprises half of total blood factor XIII activity.[194,195] α-Granules contain high-molecular-weight kininogen, which is secreted and expressed on the plasma membrane after activation by thrombin.[196,197] About 2.5% of all protein S in blood is contained in platelets. Protein S is synthesized by megakaryocytes, stored in α-granules, and released upon thrombin stimulation.[196] Dense granules contain polyphosphate (concentration ~130 mM), an anionic polymer that is released after platelet activation. Polyphosphate has a key role in activating the contact pathway, enhancing Va activation and accelerating thrombin generation.[198,199] Polyphosphates may also alter clot structure by incorporation into fibrin clots.[199]

Protease Inhibitors

Platelet α-granules also contain all known plasma protease inhibitors,[200] including α$_1$-protease inhibitor, C1 inhibitor, α$_2$-macroglobulin, plasminogen activator inhibitor-1, lipoprotein-associated coagulation inhibitor, α$_2$-antiplasmin, protease nexin I (thrombin inhibitor), and protease nexin II (factors IXa and XIa inhibitors).

Clot Retraction

Blood placed in a glass tube at ambient temperature for several hours to clot will express clear serum from the fibrin-red cell mass as platelets exert their contractile potential.[57] In vitro clot retraction requires surface integrin α$_{IIb}$β$_3$ (or GPIIb-IIIa) and contractile proteins (actin, myosin, nonmuscle myosin heavy chain IIA).[201,202] Talin activates integrin, which is required for clot retraction.[203,204] Although this phenomenon is well described in the laboratory, how this process proceeds in vivo remains a largely open question.

Table 18.3. Platelet-Associated Coagulation Factors

Protein	Subcellular Localization	Mechanism of Release	Proposed Function
Fibrinogen			
Total			
Surface	Membrane	Not released	Platelet aggregation by adenosine diphosphate
Intracellular	α-Granules	Secreted	Platelet aggregation by thrombin
Factor V	α-Granules	Secreted	Factor Xa receptor
von Willebrand factor	α-Granules	Secreted	Platelet adhesion
Factor XI	Membrane	Unknown	Intrinsic coagulation initiation
Factor XIII	Cytosol	Not released	Cross-links fibrin upon activation
High-molecular-weight kininogen	α-Granules	Secreted	Contact activation of coagulation

Clinical Impacts

Normal platelet physiology is a highly regulated, interconnected series of processes and pathways that requires efficient and effective communication and response to carry out platelet functions. In some inherited or acquired defects, these mechanisms can go awry with a range of clinical consequences. For example, Glanzmann thrombasthenia is an autosomal recessive disorder characterized by defective platelet glycoprotein (GP)IIb/IIIa, which as noted above is the primary platelet receptor for fibrinogen.[62] The result of this defect is absence of fibrinogen bridging of platelets leading to prolonged bleeding time. In many cases, the clinical phenotype may be mild bleeding, but significant bleeds, including intracranial bleeds, can occur.[205] Scott syndrome is a rare inherited bleeding disorder in which there is a defect in translocation of PS to the outer platelet membrane upon platelet activation, leading to impairment in thrombin formation.[206] The exact mechanism underlying this defect remains unclear.

References

1. Frojmovic MM, Panjwani R. Geometry of normal mammalian platelets by quantitative microscopic studies. *Biophys J.* 1976;16:1071-1089.
2. Tong M, Seth P, Penington DG. Proplatelets and stress platelets. *Blood.* 1987;69(2):522-528.
3. Handtke S, Steil L, Greinacher A, Thiele T. Toward the relevance of platelet subpopulations for transfusion medicine. *Front Med (Lausanne).* 2018;5:17.
4. White JG. Electron microscopic studies of platelet secretion. *Prog Hemost Thromb.* 1974;2:49-98.
5. White JG, Clawson GC. Overview article: biostructure of blood platelets. *Ultrastruct Pathol.* 1980;1:533-558.
6. White JG. Anatomy and structural organization of the platelet. In: Colman RW, Hirsh J, Marder VJ, Salzman EW, eds. *Hemostasis and Thrombosis. Basic Principles and Clinical Practice.* 2nd ed. JB Lippincott; 1987:537-554.
7. Bevers EM, Comfurius JP, van Rijn JL, Hemker HC, Zwaal RF. Generation of prothrombin-converting activity and the exposure of phosphatidylserine at the outer surface of platelets. *Eur J Biochem.* 1982;122:429-437.
8. Miletich JP, Jackson CM, Majerus PW. Properties of the factor Xa binding site on human platelets. *J Biol Chem.* 1978;253:6908-6916.
9. Schick PK. The organization of aminophospholipids in human platelet membranes: selective changes induced by thrombin. *J Lab Clin Med.* 1978;91:802-811.
10. Scandura JM, Ahmad S, Walsh PN. A binding site expressed on the surface of activated human platelets is shared by factor X and prothrombin. *Biochemistry.* 1996;35:8890-8902.
11. Podoplelova N, Sveshnikova A, Kotova Y, et al. Coagulation factors bound to procoagulant platelets concentrate in cap structures to promote clotting. *Blood.* 2016;128(13):1745-1755.
12. Simons ER, Greenberg-Sperssky SM. Transmembrane non-covalent cation gradients. In: Holmsen H, ed. *Platelet Responses and Metabolism.* 3rd ed. CRC Press; 1987:31-49.
13. White JG. Is the canalicular system the equivalent of the muscle sarcoplasmic reticulum?. *Hemostasis.* 1975;4:185-191.
14. White JG, Clawson CC. The surface-connected canalicular system of blood platelets—a fenestrated membrane system. *Am J Pathol.* 1980;101:353-364.
15. Stenberg PE, Shuman MA, Levine SP, Bainton DF. Redistribution of alpha granules and their contents in thrombin-stimulated platelets. *J Cell Biol.* 1984;98:748-760.
16. Kieffer N, Guichard J, Breton-Gorius J. Dynamic redistribution of major surface receptors after contact-induced platelet activation and spreading: an immunoelectron microscopic study. *Am J Pathol.* 1992;40:57-73.
17. Middleton E, Rondina M. Platelets in infectious disease. *Hematol Am Soc Hematol Educ Program.* 2016;2016(1):256-261.
18. White J. Platelets are covercytes, no phagocytes: uptake of bacteria involves channels of the open canalicular sytem. *Platelets.* 2005;16(2):121-131.
19. Behnke O. The morphology of blood platelet systems. *Ser Haematol.* 1970;3:3-16.
20. Behnke O. An electron microscope study of the rat megakaryocyte. II. Some aspects of platelet release and microtubules. *J Ultrastruct Res.* 1969;26:111-129.
21. Daimon T, Gotoh Y. Cytochemical evidence of the origin of the dense tubular system in the mouse platelet. *Histochemistry.* 1982;76:189-196.
22. Breton-Gorius J, Guichard J. Ultrastructural localization of peroxidase activity in human platelets and megakaryocytes. *Am J Pathol.* 1972;66:277-286.
23. Breton-Gorius J. The value of cytochemical peroxidase reactions at the ultrastructural level in hematology. *Histochem J.* 1980;12:127-137.
24. White JG. Interaction of membrane systems in blood platelets. *Am J Pathol.* 1972;66:295-312.
25. Nichols BA, Setzer PY, Bainton DF. Glucose-6-phosphatase as a cytochemical marker of endoplasmic reticulum in human leukocytes and platelets. *J Histochem Cytochem.* 1984;32:165-171.
26. Cutler L, Rodan G, Feinstein MB. Cytochemical localization of adenylate cyclase and of calcium ion, magnesium ion–activated ATPases in the dense tubular system of human blood platelets. *Biochim Biophys Acta.* 1978;542:357-371.
27. Tranum-Jensen J, Behnke O. Acetylcholinesterase in the platelet–megakaryocyte system. II. Structural localization in megakaryocytes of the rat, mouse, and cat. *Eur J Cell Biol.* 1981;24:281-286.
28. Gerrard JM, White JG, Rao GHR, Townsend E. Localization of platelet prostaglandin production in the platelet dense tubular system. *Am J Pathol.* 1976;83:283-298.
29. Gerrard JM, White JG, Peterson DA. The platelet dense tubular system: its relationship to prostaglandin synthesis and calcium flux. *Thromb Haemost.* 1978;40:224-231.
30. Fox JEB. Platelet cytoskeleton. In: Colman RW, Hirsh J, Marder VJ, Clowes AW, George JN, eds. *Thrombosis and Hemostasis. Basic Principles and Clinical Practice.* 4th ed. Lippincott Williams & Wilkins; 2001:429-446.
31. Cramer EM. Platelets and megakaryocytes: anatomy and structural organization. In: Colman RW, Hirsh J, Marder VJ, Clowes AW, George JN, eds. *Thrombosis and Hemostasis. Basic Principles and Clinical Practice.* 4th ed. Lippincott Williams & Wilkins; 2001:411-428.
32. Fox JEB, Boyles JK, Reynolds CC, Phillips DR. Actin filament content and organization in unstimulated platelets. *J Cell Biol.* 1984;98:1985-1991.
33. White JG. Arrangements of actin filaments in the cytoskeleton of human platelets. *Am J Pathol.* 1984;117:207-217.
34. Tablin F, Taube D. Platelet intermediate filaments: detection of a vimentin like protein in human and bovine platelets. *Cell Motil Cytoskeleton.* 1987;8:61-67.
35. Muzbek L, Adany R, Glukhova MA, Frid MG, Kabakov AE, Koteliansky VE. The identification of vimentin in human blood platelets. *Eur J Cell Biol.* 1987;43:501-504.
36. Sixma JJ, Molenaar I. Microtubules and microfibrils in human platelets. *Thromb Diath Haemorrh.* 1966;16:153-162.
37. Behnke O. Further studies on microtubules. A marginal bundle in human and rat thrombocytes. *J Ultrastruct Res.* 1965;13:469-477.
38. Castle AG, Crawford N. Platelet microtubule subunit proteins. *Thromb Haemost.* 1979;42:1630-1633.
39. White JG. The submembrane filaments of blood platelets. *Am J Pathol.* 1969;56:267-277.
40. Hartwig JH, DeSisto M. The cytoskeleton of the resting human blood platelet: structure of the membrane skeleton and its attachment to actin filaments. *J Cell Biol.* 1991;112:407-425.
41. Fox JEB, Boyles JK, Berndt MC, Steffen PK, Anderson LK. Identification of a membrane skeleton in platelets. *J Cell Biol.* 1988;106:1525-1538.
42. Fox JEB, Reynolds CC, Morrow JS, Phillips DR. Spectrin is associated with membranebound actin filaments in platelets and is hydrolyzed by the Ca²⁺-dependent protease during platelet activation. *Blood.* 1987;69:537-545.

43. Niederman R, Pollard T. Human platelet myosin. II. In vitro assembly and structure of myosin filaments. *J Cell Biol*. 1975;67:72-92.
44. O'Halloran T, Beckerle MC, Burridge K. Identification of talin as a major cytoplasmic protein implicated in platelet activation. *Nature*. 1985;317:449-451.
45. Koteliansky VE, Gneushev GN, Glukhova MA, Venyaminov SY, Muszbek L. Identification and isolation of vinculin from platelets. *FEBS Lett*. 1984;165:26-30.
46. Schollmeyer JV, Rao GHR, White JG. An actin-binding protein in human platelets. Interactions with alpha-actinin on gelation of actin and the influence of cytochalasin B. *Am J Pathol*. 1978;93:433-446.
47. Nachmias VT. Cytoskeleton of human platelets at rest and after spreading. *J Cell Biol*. 1980;86:795-802.
48. Jennings LK, Fox JEB, Edwards HH, Phillips DR. Changes in the cytoskeletal structure of human platelets following thrombin activation. *J Biol Chem*. 1981;256:6927-6932.
49. Carlsson L, Markey F, Blikstad I, Persson T, Lindberg U. Reorganization of actin in platelets stimulated by thrombin as measured by the DNase I inhibition assay. *Proc Natl Acad Sci U S A*. 1979;76:6376-6380.
50. Dingus J, Hwo S, Bryan J. Identification by monoclonal antibodies and characterization of human platelet caldesmon. *J Cell Biol*. 1986;102:1748-1757.
51. Casella JF, Flanagan MD, Lin S. Cytochalasin D inhibits actin polymerization of actin filaments formed during platelet shape change. *Nature*. 1981;293:302-305.
52. Hartwig JH. Mechanism of actin rearrangements mediating platelet activation. *J Cell Biol*. 1992;118:1421-1442.
53. Karlsson R, Lassing I, Hoglund AS, Lindberg U. The organization of microfilaments in spreading platelets: a comparison with fibroblasts and glial cells. *J Cell Physiol*. 1984;121:96-113.
54. Fox JEB, Phillips DR. Role of phosphorylation in mediating the association of myosin with the cytoskeletal structures of human platelets. *J Biol Chem*. 1982;257:4120-4126.
55. Nachmias VT, Kavaler J, Jacubowitz S. Reversible association of myosin with the platelet cytoskeleton. *Nature*. 1985;313:70-72.
56. Hathaway DR, Adelstein RS. Human platelet myosin light chain kinase requires the calcium-binding protein calmodulin for activity. *Proc Natl Acad Sci U S A*. 1979;76:1653-1657.
57. Pollard TD, Fujiwara K, Handin R, Weiss G. Contractile proteins in platelet activation and contraction. *Ann N Y Acad Sci*. 1977;283:218-236.
58. Fox JEB, Reynolds CC, Phillips DR. Calcium-dependent proteolysis occurs during platelet activation. *J Biol Chem*. 1983;258:9973-9979.
59. Behnke O, Zelander T. Substructure in negatively stained microtubules of mammalian blood platelets. *Exp Cell Res*. 1967;43:236-243.
60. Thon JN, Macleod H, Begonja AJ. Microtubule and cortical forces determine platelet size during vascular platelet production. *Nat Commun*. 2012;3:852.
61. White JG, Sauk JJ. The organization of microtubules and microtubule coils in giant platelet disorders. *Am J Pathol*. 1984;116:514-522.
62. Bury L, Falcinelli E, Chiasserini D, et al. Cytoskeletal perturbation leads to platelet dysfunction and thrombocytopenia in variant forms of Glanzmann thrombasthenia. *Haematologica*. 2016;101(1):46-56.
63. Verhoeven AJ, Mommersteeg ME, Akkerman JW. Quantification of energy consumption in platelets during thrombin-induced aggregation and secretion: tight coupling between platelet responses and the increment in energy consumption. *Biochem J*. 1984;221:777-786.
64. White JG. Exocytosis of secretory organelles from blood platelets incubated with cationic polypeptides. *Am J Pathol*. 1972;69:41-53.
65. Lemons PP, Chen D, Bernstein AM, Bennett MK, Whiteheart SW. Regulated secretion in platelets: identification of elements of the platelet exocytosis machinery. *Blood*. 1997;90:1490-1500.
66. Blair P, Flaumenhaft R. Platelet alpha-granules: basic biology and clinical correlates. *Blood Rev*. 2009;23:177-189.
67. Harrison P, Cramer EM. Platelet alpha granules. *Blood Rev*. 1993;7:52-65.
68. Holt JC, Niewiarowski S. Biochemistry of alpha granule proteins. *Semin Hematol*. 1985;22:151-168.
69. White JG. Tubular elements in platelet granules. *Blood*. 1968;32:148-156.
70. Cramer EM, Meyer D, Menn RL, Breton-Gorius J. Eccentric localization of von Willebrand factor in an internal structure of platelet alpha-granule resembling that of Weibel-Palade bodies. *Blood*. 1985;66:710-713.
71. Hayward CP, Furmaniak-Kazmierczak E, Cieutat AM, et al. Factor V is complexed with multimerin in resting platelet lysates and colocalizes with multimerin in platelet alpha-granules. *J Biol Chem*. 1995;270:19217-19226.
72. Zucker-Franklin D.. Endocytosis by human platelets: metabolic and freeze-fracture studies. *J Cell Biol*. 1981;91:706-715.
73. Harrison P, Wilbourn B, Debili N, et al. Uptake of plasma fibrinogen into the alpha granules of human megakaryocytes and platelets. *J Clin Invest*. 1989;84(4):1320-1324.
74. Handagama PJ, George JN, Shuman MA, McEver RP, Bainton DF. Incorporation of a circulating protein into megakaryocyte and platelet granules. *Proc Natl Acad Sci U S A*. 1987;84(3):861-865.
75. Sander HJ, Slot JW, Bouma BN, Bolhuis PA, Pepper DS, Sixma JJ. Immunocytochemical localization of fibrinogen, platelet factor 4, and beta thromboglobulin in thin frozen sections of human blood platelets. *J Clin Invest*. 1983;72(4):1277-1287.
76. Hegyi E, Nakeff A. Ultrastructural localization of platelet factor 4 in rat megakaryocytes and platelets by gold-labeled antibody detection. *Exp Hematol*. 1989;17(3):223-228.
77. Walz A, Dewald B, von Tscharner V, Baggiolini M. Effects of the neutrophil-activating peptide NAP-2, platelet basic protein, connective tissue-activating peptide III and platelet factor 4 on human neutrophils. *J Exp Med*. 1989;70:1745-1758.
78. Rollins BJ. Chemokines. *Blood*. 1997;90:909-922.

79. Etulain J, Mena H, Negrotto S, Schattner M. Stimulation of PAR-1 or PAR-4 promotes similar pattern of VEGF and endostatin release and pro-angiogenic responses mediated by human platelets. *Platelets*. 2015;26(8):799-804.
80. Rucinski B, Niewiarowski S, James P, Walz DA, Budzynski AZ. Antiheparin proteins secreted by human platelets: purification and characterization and radioimmunoassay. *Blood*. 1979;53:47-58.
81. Kaplan KL, Nossel HL, Drillings M, Lesznik G. Radioimmunoassay of platelet factor 4 and b-thromboglobulin: development and application to studies of platelet release in relation to human platelet factor 4. *Thromb Res*. 1977;11:673-681.
82. Baenziger NL, Brodie GN, Majerus PW. A thrombin-sensitive protein of human platelet membranes. *Proc Natl Acad Sci U S A*. 1971;68:240-243.
83. Bornstein P. The thrombospondins: structure and regulation of expression. *FASEB J*. 1992;6:3290-3300.
84. Wencel-Drake JD, Painter RG, Zimmerman TS, Ginsberg MH. Ultrastructural localization of human platelet thrombospondin, fibrinogen, fibronectin, and von Willebrand factor in frozen thin section. *Blood*. 1985;74:929-938.
85. Chiu HC, Schick P, Colman RW. Biosynthesis of factor V in isolated guinea pig megakaryocytes. *J Clin Invest*. 1985;75:339-346.
86. George JN. Platelet immunoglobulin G: its significance for the evaluation of thrombocytopenia and for understanding the origin of alpha-granule proteins. *Blood*. 1990;76:859-870.
87. Li QX, Berndt MC, Bush AI, et al. Membrane-associated forms of the betaA4 amyloid protein precursor of Alzheimer's disease in human platelet and brain: surface expression on the activated human platelet. *Blood*. 1994;84:133-142.
88. Schmaier AH, Dahl LD, Hasan AA, Cines DB, Bauer KA, Van Nostrand WE. Factor IXa inhibition by protease nexin-2/amyloid beta-protein precursor on phospholipid vesicles and cell membranes. *Biochemistry*. 1995;34:1171-1179.
89. Assoian RK, Komoriya AK, Meyers CA, Miller DM, Sporn MB. Transforming growth factor-b in human platelets: identification of a major storage site, purification, and characterization. *J Biol Chem*. 1983;258:7155-7163.
90. Mohle R, Green D, Moore MA, Nachman RL, Rafii S. Constitutive production and thrombin-induced release of vascular endothelial growth factor by human megakaryocytes and platelets. *Proc Natl Acad Sci U S A*. 1997;94:663-667.
91. Italiano J, Richardson JL, Patel-Hett S, et al. Angiogenesis is regulated by a novel mechanism: pro- and antiangiogenic proteins are organized into separate platelet alpha granules and differentially released. *Blood*. 2008;111:1227-1233.
92. Battinelli EM, Markens BA, Italian JE, Jr. Release of angiogenesis regulatory proteins from platelet alpha granules: modulation of physiologic and pathologic angiogenesis. *Blood*. 2011;118:1359-1369.
93. Klement GL, Yip TT, Cassiola F. Platelets actively sequester angiogenesis regulators. *Blood*. 2009;113:2835-2842.
94. Chatterjee M, Huang Z, Zhang W. Distinct platelet packaging, release, and surface expression of proangiogenic and antiangiogenic factors on different platelet stimuli. *Blood*. 2011;117:3907-3911.
95. Ma L, Perini R, McKnight. Proteinase-activated receptors 1 and 4 counter-regulate endostatin and VEGF release from human platelets. *Proc Natl Acad Sci U S A*. 2005;102:216-220.
96. Lambert M, Meng R, Xiao L, et al. Intramedullary megakaryocytes internalize released platelet factor 4 and store it in alpha granules. *J Thromb Haemost*. 2015;13(10):1888-1899.
97. Meyer A, Wang W, Qu J. Platelet TGF-β1 contributions to plasma TGF-β1, cardiac fibrosis, and systolic dysfunction in a mouse model of pressure overload. *Blood*. 2012;119:1064-1074.
98. Ahamed J, Burg N, Yoshinaga K, Janczak CA, Rifkin DB, Coller BS. In vitro and in vivo evidence for shear-induced activation of latent transforming growth factor-betal. *Blood*. 2008;112:3650-3660.
99. Suzuki H, Nakamura S, Itoh Y, Tanaka T, Yamazaki H, Tanoue K. Immunocytochemical evidence for the translocation of a-granule membrane glycoprotein IIb/IIIa (integrin aIIbb3) of human platelets to the surface membrane during the release reaction. *Histochemistry*. 1992;97:381-388.
100. Cramer EM, Savidge GF, Vainchenker W, et al. Alpha-granule pool of glycoprotein IIb-IIIa in normal and pathologic platelets and megakaryocytes. *Blood*. 1990;75:1220-1227.
101. Wencel-Drake JD, Plow EF, Kunicki TJ, Woods VL, Keller DM, Ginsberg MH. Localization of internal pools of membrane glycoproteins involved in platelet adhesive responses. *Am J Pathol*. 1986;124:324-334.
102. Stenberg PE, McEver RP, Shuman MA, Jacques YV, Bainton DF. A platelet alpha-granule membrane protein (GMP-140) is expressed on the plasma membrane after activation. *J Cell Biol*. 1985;101:880-886.
103. Metzelaar MJ, Heijnen HFG, Sixma JJ, Nieuwenhuis HK. Identification of a 33-Kd protein associated with the a-granule membrane (GMP33) that is expressed on the surface of activated platelets. *Blood*. 1992;79:372-379.
104. Cramer EM, Berger G, Berndt MC. Platelet a-granule and plasma membrane share two new components: CD9 and PECAM-1. *Blood*. 1994;84:1722-1730.
105. Berger G, Masse JM, Cramer EM. Alpha-granule membrane mirrors the platelet plasma membrane and contains the glycoproteins Ib, IX, and V. *Blood*. 1996;87:1385-1395.
106. Breton-Gorius J, Clezardin P, Guichard J, et al. Localization of platelet osteonectin at the internal face of the alphagranule membranes in platelets and megakaryocytes. *Blood*. 1992;79:936-941.
107. Rosa JP, George JN, Bainton DF, et al. Gray platelet syndrome. Demonstration of alpha granule membranes that can fuse with the cell surface. *J Clin Invest*. 1987;80:1138-1146.
108. Cramer EM, Vainchenker W, Vinci G, Guichard J, Breton-Gorius J. Gray platelet syndrome: immunoelectron microscopic localization of fibrinogen and von Willebrand factor in platelets and megakaryocytes. *Blood*. 1985;66:1309-1316.

109. Fukami MH, Salganicoff L. Human platelet storage granules—a review. *Thromb Haemost.* 1977;38:963-974.

110. McNicol A, Israels SJ. Platelet dense granules: structure, function and implications for hemostasis. *Thromb Res.* 1999;95:1-13.

111. Daniel JL, Molish IR, Robkin L, Holmsen H. Nucleotide exchange between cytosolic ATP and F-actin-bound ADP may be a major ATP-utilizing process in unstimulated platelets. *Eur J Biochem.* 1986;156:677-684.

112. Verhoeven AJM, Tysnes OB, Aarbakke GM, Cook CA, Holmsen H. Turnover of the phospho-monoester groups of polyphosphoinositol lipids in unstimulated platelets. *Eur J Biochem.* 1987;166:3-9.

113. Rivard GE, McLaren JD, Brunst RF. Incorporation of hypoxanthine into adenine and guanine nucleotides by human platelets. *Biochim Biophys Acta.* 1975;381:144-156.

114. Akkerman JWN, Verhoeven AJM. Energy metabolism and function. In: Holmsen H, ed. *Platelet Responses and Metabolism. Vol 3: Response-Metabolism Relationships.* CRC Press; 1987:69-99.

115. Verhoeven AJM, Tysnes OB, Horvli O, Cook CA, Holmsen H. Stimulation of phosphate uptake in human platelets by thrombin and collagen. Changes in specific ^{32}P-labeling of metabolic ATP and polyphosphoinositides. *J Biol Chem.* 1987;262:7047-7052.

116. White JG. Platelet secretory granules and associated proteins. *Lab Invest.* 1993;68:497-498.

117. Febbraio M, Silverstein RL. Identification and characterization of LAMP-1 as an activation-dependent platelet surface glycoprotein. *J Biol Chem.* 1990;265:18531-18537.

118. Silverstein RL, Febbraio M. Identification of lysosome-associated membrane protein-2 as an activation-dependent platelet surface glycoprotein. *Blood.* 1992;80:1470-1478.

119. de Duve C. Biochemical studies on the occurrence, biogenesis, and life history of mammalian peroxisomes. *J Histochem Cytochem.* 1973;21:941-948.

120. Van den BH, de Vet EC, Zomer AS. The role of peroxisomes in ether lipid synthesis. Back to the roots of PAF. *Adv Exp Med Biol.* 1996;416:33-41.

121. Akkerman JWN, Gorter G, Soons H, Holmsen H. Close correlation between platelet responses and adenylate energy charge during transient substrate depletion. *Biochim Biophys Acta.* 1983;760:34-42.

122. Holmsen H, Farstad M. *Platelet Responses and Metabolism*, Vol. 2. CRC Press; 1987:245-282. *Energy metabolism.*

123. Weiss HJ, Kelly A, Herbert V. Vitamin B$_2$12 and folate activity in normal human platelets. *Blood.* 1968;31:258-262.

124. Cooley MH, Cohen P. Potassium transport in human blood platelets. *J Lab Clin Med.* 1967;70:69-79.

125. Brass LF. The effect of Na$^+$ on Ca^{2+} homeostasis in unstimulated platelets. *J Biol Chem.* 1984;259:12571-12575.

126. Enouf J, Bredoux R, Bourdeau N, Levy-Toledano S. Two different Ca^{2+} transport systems are associated with plasma and intracellular human platelet membranes. *J Biol Chem.* 1987;262:9293-9297.

127. Karpatkin S, Charmatz A, Langer RM. Glycogenesis and glyconeogenesis in human platelets. Incorporation of glucose, pyruvate, and citrate into platelet glycogen, glycogen synthetase and fructose1,6 diphosphatase activity. *J Clin Invest.* 1970;49:140-149.

128. Akkerman JWN. Regulation of glycolytic flux in human platelets: relationship between energy produced by glyco(geno)lysis and energy consumption. *Biochim Biophys Acta.* 1978;541:241-250.

129. Karpatkin S. Studies on human platelet glycolysis. Effect of glucose, cyanide, insulin, citrate, and agglutination and contraction on platelet glycolysis. *J Clin Invest.* 1967;46:409-417.

130. Karpatkin S, Charmatz A. Heterogeneity of human platelets. III. Glycogen metabolism in platelets of different sizes. *Br J Haematol.* 1970;19:135-143.

131. Akkerman JWN. Regulation of carbohydrate metabolism in platelets. A review. *Thromb Haemost.* 1978;39:712-724.

132. Cohen P, Derksen A, Van den Bosch H. Pathways of fatty acid metabolism in human platelets. *J Clin Invest.* 1970;49:128-139.

133. Doery JC, Hirsh J, Cooper I. Energy metabolism in human platelets: interrelationship between glycolysis and oxidative metabolism. *Blood.* 1970;36:159-168.

134. Dean WL. Structure, function, and subcellular localization of a human platelet Ca^{2+}-ATPase. *Cell Calcium.* 1989;10:289-297.

135. Marcus AJ. Pathways of oxygen utilization by stimulated platelets and leukocytes. *Semin Hematol.* 1979;16:188-195.

136. Gear ARL, Schneider W. Control of platelet glycogenolysis; activation of phosphorylase kinase by calcium. *Biochim Biophys Acta.* 1975;392:111-120.

137. Holmsen H, Day HJ, Storm E. Adenine nucleotide metabolism of blood platelets. VI. Subcellular localization of nucleotide pools with different functions in the platelet release reaction. *Biochim Biophys Acta.* 1969;186:254-266.

138. Reimers HJ, Packham MA, Mustard JF. Labeling of the releasable adenine nucleotides of washed human platelets. *Blood.* 1977;49:89-99.

139. Holmsen H. Energy metabolism and platelet responses. *Vox Sang.* 1981;40:1-7.

140. Davie EW, Ratnoff OD. Waterfall sequence for intrinsic blood clotting. *Science.* 1964;145:1310-1312.

141. Holmsen H, Salganicoff L, Fukami MH. Platelet behaviour and biochemistry. In: Ogston D, Bennett P, eds. *Haemostasis: Biochemistry, Physiology, and Pathology.* Wiley-Liss; 1977:239-319.

142. Schick PK. Platelet and megakaryocyte lipids. In: Colman RW, Hirsh J, Marder VJ, et al. eds. 4th ed. *Hemostasis and Thrombosis: Basic Principles and Clinical Practice.* Lippincott Williams & Wilkins; 2001:521-534.

143. Perret B, Chap HJ, Douste-Blazy L. Asymmetric distribution of arachidonic acid in the plasma membrane of human platelets: a determination using purified phospholipases and a rapid method for membrane isolation. *Biochim Biophys Acta.* 1979;556:434-446.

144. Schick PK, Kurica KB, Chacko GK. Location of phosphatidylethanolamine and phosphatidylserine in the human platelet plasma membrane. *J Clin Invest.* 1976;57:1221-1226.

145. Bevers EM, Comfurius P, Zwaal RF. Changes in membrane phospholipid distribution during platelet activation. *Biochim Biophys Acta.* 1983;736:57-66.

146. Sims PJ, Wiedmer T. Unraveling the mysteries of phospholipid scrambling. *Thromb Haemost.* 2001;86:266-275.

147. Comfurius P, Williamson P, Smeets EF, Schlegel RA, Bevers EM, Zwaal RF. Reconstitution of phospholipid scramblase activity from human blood platelets. *Biochemistry.* 1996;35:7631-7634.

148. Nagata S, Sakuragi T, Segawa K. Flippase and scramblase for phosphatidylserine exposure. *Curr Opin Immunol.* 2020 Feb;62:31-38. Epub 2019 Dec 11. PMID: 31837595. doi: 10.1016/j.coi.2019.11.009.

149. Marcus AJ. The role of lipids in platelet function: with particular reference to the arachidonic acid pathway. *J Lipid Res.* 1976;9:793-826.

150. Clark JD, Schievella AR, Nalefski EA, Lin LL. Cytosolic phospholipase A2. *J Lipid Mediat Cell Signal.* 1995;12:83-117.

151. Riendeau D, Gray J, Weech PK, et al. Arachidonyl trifluoromethyl ketone, a potent inhibitor of 85-kDa phospholipase A2, blocks production of arachidonate and 12-hydroxyeicosatetraenoic acid by calcium ionophore-challenged platelets. *J Biol Chem.* 1994;269:15619-15624.

152. Dennis EA. The growing phospholipase A2 superfamily of signal transduction enzymes. *Trends Biochem Sci.* 1997;22:1-2.

153. Nance D, Campbell R, Rowley J, et al. Combined variants in factor VIII and prostaglandin synthetase-1 amplify hemorrhage severity across three generations of descendents. *J Thromb Haemostasis.* 2016;14(11):2230-2240.

154. Schick PK, Tuszynski GP, Woort PWV. Human platelet cytoskeletons: specific content of glycolipids and phospholipids. *Blood.* 1983;61:163-166.

155. Rapaport SI, Proctor RR, Patch MJ, Yettra M. The mode of inheritance of PTA deficiency: evidence for the existence of a major PTA deficiency and a minor PTA deficiency. *Blood.* 1961;18:149-155.

156. Barry OP, FitzGerald GA. Mechanisms of cellular activation by platelet microparticles. *Thromb Haemost.* 1999;82:794-808.

157. Sims PJ, Faioni EM, Wiedmer T, Shattil SJ. Complement proteins C5b-9 cause release of membrane vesicles from the platelet surface that are enriched in the membrane receptor for coagulation factor Va and express prothrombinase activity. *J Biol Chem.* 1988;263:18205-18212.

158. Thiagarajan P, Tait JF. Collagen-induced exposure of anionic phospholipid in platelets and platelet-derived microparticles. *J Biol Chem.* 1991;266:24302-24307.

159. Dahlback B, Wiedmer T, Sims PJ. Binding of anticoagulant vitamin K dependent protein S to platelet-derived microparticles. *Biochemistry.* 1992;31:12769-12777.

160. Gilbert GE, Sims PJ, Wiedmer T, Furie B, Furie BC, Shattil SJ. Platelet-derived microparticles express high affinity receptors for factor VIII. *J Biol Chem.* 1991;266:17261-17268.

161. Sims PJ, Wiedmer T, Esmon CT, Weiss HJ, Shattil SJ. Assembly of the platelet prothrombinase complex is linked to vesiculation of the platelet plasma membrane. Studies in Scott syndrome: an isolated defect in platelet procoagulant activity. *J Biol Chem.* 1989;264:17049-17057.

162. Weiss HJ. Scott syndrome: a disorder of platelet coagulant activity. *Semin Hematol.* 1994;31:312-319.

163. Thon JN, Italiano JE. Platelets: production, morphology and ultrastructure. *Handb Exp Pharmacol.* 2012;210:3-22.

164. Thon JN, Italiano JE, Jr. Does size matter in platelet production?. *Blood.* 2012;120:1552-1561.

165. Kummer H, Von Muhlenen A, Laissue J. Survival of labeled and non-labeled platelets in the lethally irradiated dog: an evaluation of the ^{51}Cr-chromium method. *Helv Med Acta.* 1969;35:226-235.

166. Welch MJ, Thakur ML, Coleman RE, Patel M, Siegel BA, Ter-Pogossian M. Gallium-68 labeled red cells and platelets: new agents for positron tomography. *J Nuclear Med.* 1977;18:558-562.

167. Aster RH. The study of platelet kinetics with ^{51}Cr-labeled platelets. In: Paulus JM, ed. *Platelet Kinetics.* North-Holland; 1971:317-323.

168. Harker LA, Finch CA. Thrombokinetics in man. *J Clin Invest.* 1969;48:963-974.

169. Lewis SM, Recommended methods for radioisotope platelet survival studies: by the Panel on Diagnostic Application of Radioisotopes in Hematology, International Committee for Standardization in Hematology. *Blood.* 1977;50:1137-1144.

170. Lotter MG, Heyns AD, Badenhorst PN, et al. Evaluation of mathematic models to assess platelet kinetics. *J Nuclear Med.* 1986;27:1192-1201.

171. Josefsson EC, White MJ, Dowling MR. Platelet life span and apoptosis. *Methods Mol Biol.* 2012;788:59-71.

172. Mason KD, Carpinelli MR, Flethcer JI. Programmed anuclear cell death delimits platelet life span. *Cell.* 2007;128:1173-1186.

173. Freedman M, Altszuler N, Karpatkin S. Presence of a nonsplenic platelet pool. *Blood.* 1977;50:419-425.

174. Aster RH. Pooling of platelets in the spleen: role in the pathogenesis of "hypersplenic" thrombocytopenia. *J Clin Invest.* 1966;45:645-657.

175. Shulman NR, Watkins SP, Jr, Itscoitz SB, Students AB. Evidence that the spleen retains the youngest and hemostatically most effective platelets. *Trans Assoc Am Physicians.* 1968;81:302-313.

176. Weiss L. A scanning electron microscopic study of the spleen. *Blood.* 1974;43:665-691.

177. Bierman HR, Kelly KH, Cordes FL, Byron RL, Jr, Polhemus JA, Rappoport S. The release of leukocytes and platelets from the pulmonary circulation by epinephrine. *Blood.* 1952;7:683-692.

178. Mann KG, Bopvill EG, Srishnaswamy S. Surface-dependent reactions of the vitamin K-dependent enzyme complexes. *Blood.* 1991;76:1-16.

179. Walsh PN. Platelet coagulant activities and hemostasis: a hypothesis. *Blood.* 1974;43:597-605.

180. Miletich JP, Jackson CM, Majerus PW. Interaction of coagulation factor Xa with human platelets. *Proc Natl Acad Sci U S A.* 1977;74:4033-4036.

181. Gailani D, Broze GJ, Jr. Factor XI activation in a revised model of blood coagulation. *Science.* 1991;253:909-912.

182. Naito K, Fujikawa K. Activation of human blood coagulation factor XI independent of factor XII. Factor XI is activated by thrombin and factor XIa in the presence of negatively charged surfaces. *J Biol Chem.* 1991;266:7353-7358.

183. Walsh PN, Griffin JH. Contributions of human platelets to the proteolytic activation of blood coagulation factors XII and XI. *Blood.* 1981;57:106-118.

184. Sinha D, Seaman FS, Walsh PN. Role of calcium ions and the heavy chain of factor XIa in the activation of human coagulation factor IX. *Biochemistry.* 1987;26:3768-3775.

185. Baglia FA, Badellino KO, Ho DH, Dasari VR, Walsh PN. A binding site for the kringle II domain of prothrombin in the apple I domain of factor XI. *J Biol Chem.* 2000;275:31954-31962.

186. Shirk RA, Konkle BA, Walsh PN. Nonsense mutation in exon V of the factor XI gene does not abolish platelet factor XI expression. *Br J Haematol.* 2000;111:91-95.

187. Walsh PN, Sinha D, Kueppers F, Seaman FS, Blankstein KB. Regulation of factor XIa activity by platelets and alpha I-protease inhibitor. *J Clin Invest.* 1987;80:1578-1586.

188. Chesney CM, Pifer D, Colman RW. Subcellular localization and secretion of factor V from human platelets. *Proc Natl Acad Sci U S A.* 1981;78:5180-5184.

189. Rand MD, Kalafatis M, Mann KG. Platelet coagulation factor Va: the major secretory phosphoprotein. *Blood.* 1994;83:2180-2190.

190. Tracy PB, Giles AR, Mann KG, Eide LL, Hoogendoorn H, Rivard GE. Factor V (Quebec): a bleeding diathesis associated with a qualitative platelet factor V deficiency. *J Clin Invest.* 1984;74:1221-1228.

191. Hayward CP, Cramer EM, Kane WH, et al. Studies of a second family with the Quebec platelet disorder: evidence that the degradation of the α-granule membrane and its soluble contents are not secondary to a defect in targeting proteins to α-granules. *Blood.* 1997;89:1243-1253.

192. Louache F, Debili N, Cramer E, Breton-Gorius J, Vainchenker W. Fibrinogen is not synthesized by human megakaryocytes. *Blood.* 1991;77:311-316.

193. Nachman RL, Marcus AJ, Zucker-Franklin D. Immunological studies of proteins associated with subcellular fractions of normal human platelets. *J Lab Clin Med.* 1967;69:651-668.

194. Jenkins CS, Phillips DR, Clemetson KJ, Meyer D, Larrieu MJ, Lüscher EF. Platelet membrane glycoproteins implicated in ristocetin-induced aggregation. Studies of the proteins on platelets from patients with Bernard-Soulier syndrome and von Willebrand's disease. *J Clin Invest.* 1976;57:112-124.

195. Kappelmayer J, Bacsko B, Birinyi L, Zákány R, Kelemen E, Adány R. Consecutive appearance of coagulation factor XIII subunit A in macrophages, megakaryocytes, and liver cells during early human development. *Blood.* 1995;86:2191-2197.

196. Schmaier AH, Smith RM, Purdon AD, White JG, Colman RW. High molecular weight kininogen: localization in unstimulated and activated platelets; and activation by platelet calpain(s). *Blood.* 1986;67:119-130.

197. Schwarz HP, Heeb MJ, Wencel-Drake D, Griffin JH. Identification and quantitation of protein S in human platelets. *Blood.* 1985;66:1452-1455.

198. Smith SA, Mutch NJ, Baskar D, Rohloff P, Docampo R, Morrissey JH. Polyphosphate modulates blood coagulation and fibrinolysis. *Proc Natl Acad Sci U S A.* 2006;103:903-908.

199. Müller F, Mutch NJ, Schenk WA. Platelet polyphosphates are proinflammatory and procoagulant mediators in vivo. *Cell.* 2009;139:1143-1156.

200. Morrissey JH, Choi SH, Smith SA. Polyphosphate: an ancient molecule that links platelets, coagulation, and inflammation. *Blood.* 2012;119:5972-5979.

201. Schmaier AH, Dahl LD, Rozemuller AJM, et al. Protease nexin-2/amyloid β protein precursor. A tight-binding inhibitor of coagulation factor IXa. *J Clin Invest.* 1993;92:2540-2545.

202. Rooney MM, Farrell DH, van Hemel BM, de Groot PG, Lord ST. The contribution of the three hypothesized integrin-binding sites in fibrinogen to platelet-mediated clot retraction. *Blood.* 1998;92:2374-2381.

203. Léon C, Eckly A, Hechler B, et al. Megakaryocyte-restricted MYH9 inactivation dramatically affects hemostasis while preserving platelet aggregation and secretion. *Blood.* 2007;110:3183-3191.

204. Haling JR, Monkley SJ, Critchley DR, Petrich BG. Talin-independent integrin activation is required for fibrin clot retraction by platelets. *Blood.* 2011;117:1719-1722.

205. Botero JP, Lee K, Branchford BR, et al. ClinGen platelet disorder variant curation expert panel. Glanzmann thrombasthenia: genetic basis and clinical correlates. *Haematologica.* 2020;105(4):888-894.

206. Toti F, Satta N, Fressinaud E, Meyer D, Freyssinet JM. Scott syndrome, characterized by impaired transmembrane migration of procoagulant phosphatidylserine and hemorrhagic complications, is an inherited disorder. *Blood.* 1996 Feb 15;87(4):1409-1415.

Chapter 19 ■ Platelet Function in Hemostasis and Thrombosis

DAVID C. CALVERLEY

PLATELET ADHESION AND ACTIVATION

Primary hemostasis and arterial thrombosis are the results of a complex series of cell-cell, cell-protein, and protein-protein reactions that involve platelets, leukocytes, endothelium, subendothelial matrix, and plasma proteins, such as fibrinogen and von Willebrand factor (vWF). The consequences of arterial thrombosis include events such as myocardial infarction (MI), unstable angina, and stroke. These clinicopathologic entities and their associated cellular physiologic mechanisms that are outlined in this chapter collectively account for the largest cause of morbidity and mortality in the Western world.

Platelet adhesion to exposed subendothelium is a complex, multistep process that involves a diverse array of adhesive ligands (vWF, collagen, fibrinogen/fibrin, fibronectin, thrombospondin, laminin, and vitronectin) and surface receptors (GPIb/V/IX, GPVI, integrins $\alpha_{IIb}\beta_3$, $\alpha_2\beta_1$, $\alpha_5\beta_1$, and $\alpha_6\beta_1$)[1–13] (Figure 19.1). The specific ligand/receptor players in primary platelet adhesion are largely dependent on the arterial flow conditions present.[5,14] As such, in larger arteries and veins, platelet adhesion to the vessel wall is thought to involve fibrillar collagen, fibronectin, and laminin. There are at least 25 forms of collagen, and several of these are present in the blood vessel wall, whereas one (type IV) is present in the subendothelial basement membrane.[15] In the high-shear conditions present in smaller arteries, platelet tethering is dependent on the unique shear-dependent interaction between GPIb/V/IX and subendothelial vWF. The subsequent rapid platelet deceleration allows for other ligand-receptor interactions such as collagen and $\alpha_2\beta_1$ that have slower binding kinetics and take on the role of mediating firm platelet adhesion. A metalloprotease, ADAMTS13, cleaves vWF; this cleavage prevents the accumulation of ultrahigh-molecular-weight multimers that would otherwise cause spontaneous platelet clumping and arterial thrombosis.

Following initial platelet adhesion, subsequent platelet-platelet interaction (aggregation) is mediated by two receptors, GPIb/V/IX and $\alpha_{IIb}\beta_3$, and their respective contributions are dependent on the flow conditions present. In high-shear stress conditions, GPIb/V/IX receptor and vWF ligand action are predominant, with fibrinogen playing a stabilizing role. At low-shear conditions, fibrinogen is thought to be the primary ligand supporting platelet plug formation through its interaction with $\alpha_{IIb}\beta_3$. It has been shown that thrombus formation can take place in the absence of vWF and fibrinogen, and this supports the idea that a third ligand directed to the $\alpha_{IIb}\beta_3$ receptor may also exist in vivo.[16]

Platelet Glycoprotein Ib Complex-von Willebrand Factor Interaction and Signaling

It has long been recognized that the interaction of the platelet glycoprotein (GP) Ib "complex" (including the single-chain polypeptides GPIbα, GPIbβ, GPIX, and GPV) with its primary ligand, vWF, is the receptor-ligand pairing that initiates platelet adhesion followed by a cascade of events leading to pathologic thrombosis or physiologic hemostasis. A unique aspect of this receptor-ligand interaction is that it requires the presence of high arterial shear rates to take place, thus explaining the predisposition of platelet-rich "white clots" in the arterial circulation over clots found in the venous circulation, with its relatively lower shear forces, in which clot formation takes place independent of the GPIb complex.

Using a parallel-plate flow cytometer, platelet interaction with subendothelial vWF has been characterized as occurring in a biphasic fashion.[4] In this respect, the rate of translocation of platelets from blood to the endothelial cell surface increased linearly up to wall shear rates of 1500/s, whereas the translocation rate remained relatively constant with the wall shear rate between 1500 and 6000/s. This ability to

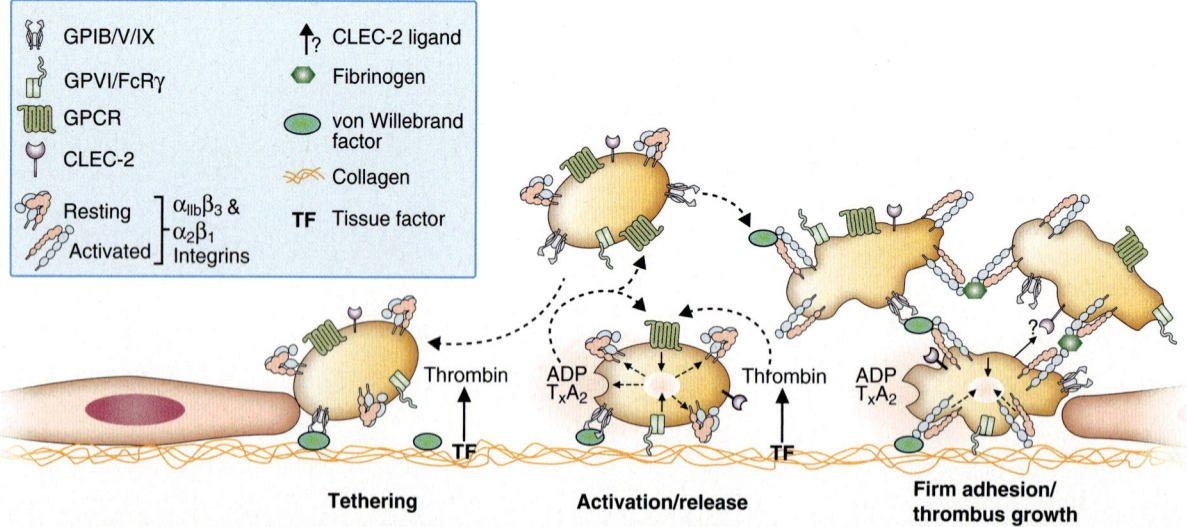

FIGURE 19.1 **Model for platelet adhesion to the subendothelial matrix at sites of vascular injury and subsequent thrombus formation.** The initial contact (tethering) to the ECM is mediated predominantly by GPIb-vWF interactions. In the second step, GPVI-collagen interactions initiate cellular activation followed by the shift of integrins to a high-affinity state and the release of second-wave agonists, most importantly ADP, ATP, and TXA$_2$. In parallel, exposed tissue factor locally triggers the formation of thrombin, which, in addition to GPVI, mediates cellular activation. Finally, firm adhesion of platelets to collagen through activated $\alpha_2\beta_1$ (directly) and $\alpha_{IIb}\beta_3$ (indirectly via vWF or other ligands) results in sustained GPVI signaling, enhanced release of soluble agonists, and procoagulant activity. Released ADP, ATP, and TXA$_2$ amplify integrin activation on adherent platelets and mediate thrombus growth by activating additional platelets. The forming thrombus is stabilized by signaling through CLEC-2, whose ligands are podoplanin and possibly CLEC-2 itself, and other receptors. CLEC-2, C-type lectin receptor 2; GP, glycoprotein; GPCR, G protein–coupled receptors; TXA$_2$, thromboxane A$_2$. (Reprinted by permission from Springer: Stegner D, Nieswandt B. Platelet receptor signaling in thrombus formation. *J Mol Med.* 2011;89(2):109-121. Copyright © 2010 Springer-Verlag.)

mediate translocation or rolling of the platelet on vWF is contingent on the GPIb complex, and mammalian cells expressing either the full complex or a complex lacking the GPV subunit were able to roll onto vWF in a GPIbα chain–dependent manner.[17,18]

It is clear that arterial thrombus formation is contingent on both the presence of high wall shear rates and interaction between the GPIb complex and vWF. Studies involving the endpoint of real-time thrombus formation that involved comparison of blood from both patients with Bernard-Soulier syndrome (which lacks the platelet-GPIb complex) and severe (type 3) von Willebrand disease versus normal blood led to the conclusion that GPIb-vWF interaction was required for platelet-surface interaction at high shear rates (>1210/s), whereas normal thrombus formation at lower shear rates (<340/s) was possible with blood deficient in either GPIb or vWF.[19] In normal blood, thrombus formation was accelerated as shear rate increased, and this served to verify the unique shear-flow dependence of this receptor-ligand interaction.

The GPIb complex consists of four transmembrane subunits, each of which is a member of the leucine-rich repeat protein superfamily that participates in cell-matrix interactions throughout nature. Each of the four subunits contains one or more tandem, 24-amino-acid leucine-rich repeats flanked by conserved disulfide loop structures at both the N and C termini of the repeats.[20] GPIbα is covalently associated with the GPIbβ chain through disulfide linkage of cysteine residues, and both of these chains are noncovalently associated with GPIX in a 1:1 ratio and with GPV in a 2:1 ratio[21–23] (*Figure 19.2*).

vWF is a large multimeric glycoprotein that circulates in plasma and is also found in platelets and the Weibel-Palade bodies of endothelial cells. Mature vWF is a 2050-amino-acid subunit that is disulfide linked into large multimers. It contains three adjacent A domains

in the N-proximal half of the peptide that collectively regulate the adhesion of platelets to subendothelial matrix. In this respect, the A_1 and A_3 domains bind to different matrix collagens, whereas the A_1 domain contains the binding site for the GPIb complex.[24] The A_1 domain is the primary role player in platelet adhesion because this part of the molecule is believed to change its conformation in response to immobilization and high shear forces, thus making it a high-affinity ligand for the GPIb complex receptor.[25,26] It has also been suggested that shear stresses may induce conformational changes in the GPIb complex that may be important in increasing its affinity for vWF.[27] Through the simultaneous binding of collagen and platelets, vWF can serve as a molecular bridge between platelets and the subendothelial matrix mediating platelet adhesion to the vessel wall. Thus, by associating with matrix proteins, vWF mediates rapid and reversible platelet adhesion that promotes the rolling of these cells along the surface of vascular injury.

The binding interaction between vWF and GPIb appears to involve at least three distinct regions within the N-terminal 282 residues of GPIb. Each of these regions appears to be responsible for either direct binding to vWF or modulating its affinity for the ligand.[28] In this respect, one region (His 1 to Glu 282), which includes a cluster between residues Asp 252 and Arg 293 containing sulfated tyrosine residues and important anionic residues, appears to be predominantly responsible for vWF-GPIb complex interaction in the presence of botrocetin over ristocetin.[29–31]

The second region contains the disulfide loop between Cys 209 and Cys 248 along with two naturally occurring mutations (Gly 233 to Val and Met 239 to Val) and two additional mutation sites identified in the laboratory (Asp 235 to Val and Lys 237 to Val) that can individually lead to expression of the pseudo- or platelet-type von Willebrand disease phenotype.[29] This disorder is associated with a gain-of-function GPIbα on platelets that adheres to vWF in the presence of lower concentrations of ristocetin (0.3-0.5 mg/mL) than are required for the wild-type phenotype (1.5 g/mL). It is analogous to type 2B von Willebrand disease, in which high-molecular-weight vWF multimers are absent from the plasma, and similar gain-of-function mutations have been localized to the Cys 509 to Cys 695 disulfide loop of vWF exon 28.

The third region includes the N-terminal flanking sequence of the leucine-rich repeat (LRG) motifs and the LRGs themselves. Mutations involving single amino acid residues within these LRGs account for some cases of the congenital bleeding disorder, Bernard-Soulier syndrome, in which the GPIb complex binds poorly or not at all to vWF. Evidence using mammalian Chinese hamster ovary cells expressing loss-of-function proteins and anti-GPIbα monoclonal antibodies has suggested that N-terminal LRGs may play a more direct role in the interaction with vWF.[32]

Glycoprotein Ib Complex Interaction With Thrombin

Recent studies have examined the potential role of the GPIb complex in thrombin-mediated platelet activation. The physiologic significance of the interaction of thrombin with the GPIb complex has remained relatively controversial. GPIbα contains a well-characterized high-affinity binding site for thrombin, and thrombin is also capable of cleaving GPV near the surface to release a soluble fragment.[33]

Recent studies have suggested that a relationship exists between thrombin binding to the GPIb complex and cleavage of the seven-transmembrane G protein–coupled protease-activated thrombin receptor—protease-activated receptor (PAR)-1 (see section "Platelet Thrombin [Protease-Activated] Receptors and Signaling") and that accelerated coagulation on the surface of a developing thrombus is a downstream consequence of thrombin-GPIb interaction that takes place due to enhanced phospholipid exposure.[34,35] These studies support a procoagulant role of this thrombin-GPIb pairing, and this activity also plays an important role in the generation of platelet microparticles.[36,37] In contrast, studies using GPV-null mice have suggested that the GPV subunit may act as a negative regulator of thrombin-mediated platelet activation, whereas data from another study suggest that thrombin-GPIb interaction leads to conformational changes in thrombin that reduce its cleavage of fibrinogen.[38,39]

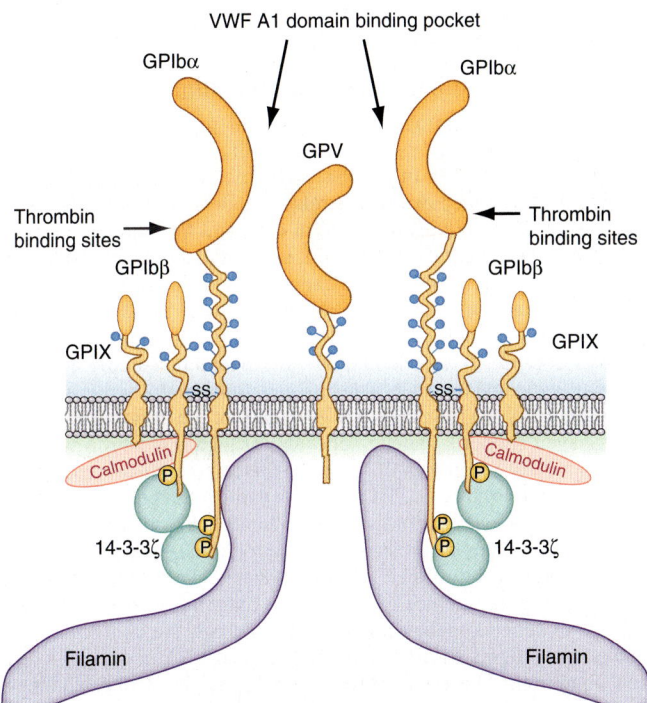

FIGURE 19.2 Schematic illustration of the glycoprotein (GP) Ib/V/IX complex and associated proteins. The N-terminal domain of GPIbα contains binding sites for von Willebrand factor (vWF) and thrombin. The cytoplasmic domain of GPIbα contains the phosphorylation-dependent 14-3-3 binding sites and also the binding site for filamin that links GPIb-IX to the actin cytoskeleton underlining the membrane. The cytoplasmic domain of GPIbβ is phosphorylated by protein kinase A (PKA), and this phosphorylation is required for 14-3-3 binding. The membrane proximal region in the cytoplasmic domain of GPIbβ and GPIX contains calmodulin-binding sites. (Reprinted with permission from Du X. Signaling and regulation of the platelet glycoprotein Ib-IX-V complex. *Curr Opin Hematol.* 2007;14(3):262-269.)

Whether thrombin-mediated platelet activation is upregulated or downregulated (or both) by thrombin-GPIb interaction, one relatively recent study suggests that mutual cooperativity between thrombin-induced GPIb-IX signaling and PAR signaling is required for optimal platelet response.[40] The synergy of both receptors greatly enhances platelet sensitivity to low concentrations of thrombin, and this mutually dependent cooperativity requires a GPIb-IX-specific 14-3-3-Rac1-LIMK1 signaling pathway.[40]

The phenotype of a GPIbα knockout mouse has been reported and was similar in many ways to human Bernard-Soulier syndrome.[41] This mouse was then capable of having the wild-type phenotype restored by a human GPIbα transgene. Future use of this mouse model might be helpful toward further elucidation of the physiologic role of platelet-GPIb complex interaction with thrombin.[42] In the meantime, the current data extend further support for the role of the GPIb complex as a thrombin receptor on platelets, whereas, recent insights notwithstanding, elucidation of the downstream consequences of that interaction with respect to platelet activation and thrombus formation will remain the subject of further investigation.

Studies have focused on the interaction of the GPIb complex with activated intact endothelium through ligands other than vWF adherent to subendothelial matrix. These include a study of a reversible association of GPIb with endothelial cell P-selectin, which is examined in more detail in the section "Platelets and Endothelium." The interaction of platelet-GPIb with the neutrophil adhesion receptor Mac-1 is discussed in the section "Platelets and Immune Cells." These interactions may contribute more to inflammatory responses than platelet thrombus formation.

Glycoprotein Ib Complex Signaling

When the GPIb complex interacts with its vWF ligand under conditions of elevated shear stress, there is abundant evidence that signaling pathways are activated that lead to (a) elevation of intracellular calcium; (b) activation of a tyrosine kinase signaling pathway that incorporates nonreceptor tyrosine kinases such as Src, Fyn, Lyn, and Syk; phospholipase C (PIC)γ2; and adaptor proteins such as SHC, LAT, and SLP-76; (c) GTPase-activating protein; (d) tyrosine phosphatases (PTP-1B and SHPTP10); (e) inside-out signaling through the $\alpha_{IIb}\beta_3$ integrin followed by platelet aggregation[28]; and (f) activation of protein kinase C (PKC), protein kinase G (PKG), and phosphoinositide 3-kinase (PI3K). vWF binding also upregulates integrin $\alpha_{IIb}\beta_3$ affinity indirectly through stimulation of adenosine diphosphate (ADP) secretion.[29] Other downstream players and events that play roles after GPIb receptor occupancy include (a) the homodimeric signaling protein 14-3-3 and calmodulin, (b) receptor cross-linking, and (c) the immunoreceptor tyrosine-based activation motif (ITAM)-containing proteins Fcγ receptor IIA (FcγRIIA) and Fc receptor (FcR) γ chain. In addition to these components, the effect of shear force itself on GPIb signaling, including the affinity and number of bonds between vWF and GPIb, can play a potentially important role.[30,31]

Evidence has also been presented suggesting that indirect mechanisms may also be involved in GPIb signaling, which are linked to ADP release and/or thromboxane A$_2$ (TXA$_2$) generation.[29,30] The increase in intracellular calcium prompted by vWF-GPIb interaction promotes dense granule secretion of ADP, which then activates integrin $\alpha_{IIb}\beta_3$ through the P2Y$_1$ and P2Y$_{12}$ purinergic receptors (see section "Platelet P2Y$_1$ and P2Y$_{12}$ Receptor Roles in Adenosine Diphosphate–Mediated Activation").

14-3-3ζ is among the 10 isoforms of the 14-3-3 family of proteins that is named according to its electrophoretic gel migration position. Functionally, this family has a wide range of activities, including participating as a DNA damage, cell-cycle checkpoint protein; regulation of PKC activity; and formation of heterotrimers with the signaling kinase Raf and the guanosine triphosphate exchange factor Ras.[43–45] Binding sites for 14-3-3 have been identified in the cytoplasmic domains of GPIbα, GPIbβ, GPIX, and GPV. In this respect, peptide fragments corresponding to overlapping cytoplasmic sequences of the four subunits demonstrated binding in vitro, whereas yeast two-hybrid studies documented in vivo interaction between 14-3-3ζ and both

GPIbα and GPIbβ.[46,47] Site-directed mutagenesis and protein-binding experiments confirmed the need for phosphorylation of Ser 166 of the 14-3-3 consensus sequence in the GPIbβ cytoplasmic domain to permit high-affinity 14-3-3 binding.[47,48] Findings that have evolved in lieu of the preceding observations include the binding of fibrinogen to mammalian cell–transfected $\alpha_{IIb}\beta_3$ in response to vWF binding to cotransfected GPIb-IX that was inhibited when the 14-3-3–binding domain was deleted from the GPIb-IX transfectant.[49] Also, the lipid kinase PI3K has been found to play a role in this GPIb-IX dependence of $\alpha_{IIb}\beta_3$ activation through its participation in complex formation with the GPIb complex and 14-3-3.[50] The reason for these associations would be to regulate, in short order, the formation of inositols phosphorylated in the 3-position within the reorganizing cytoskeleton in response to platelet activation (see section "Role of Cytoskeletal Rearrangement in Platelet Activation").[28]

Many adhesion receptors initiate signaling through cross-linking, and there is evidence to suggest that the GPIb complex may also use this mechanism. The GPV subunit surface expression on platelets is roughly half that of the other three subunits (12,000 vs. 25,000 copies per cell). It has also been suggested that two or more GPIbα subunits cluster into a complex with the other glycoprotein subunits.[51] The fact that there is one GPV subunit available in this complex for every two of the other subunits and that both actin-binding protein (ABP or filamin; a membrane skeleton protein that associates with GPIbα; see later in the chapter) and 14-3-3 exist as dimers lends support to the concept of a complex consisting of a pair of GPIbα-GPIbβ-GPIX trimers joined noncovalently by a single GPV monomer (*Figure 19.2*).

Once vWF binds to GPIb/V/IX, signaling complexes form in the vicinity of the GPIbα cytoplasmic tail consisting of cytoskeletal proteins such as 14-3-3ζ as well as signaling proteins such as Src and PI 3-kinase. This process leads to Syk activation, protein tyrosine phosphorylation, and recruitment of other cytoplasmic proteins with pleckstrin homology (PH) domains that can support interactions with 3-phosphorylated phosphoinositides.[30,52–55]

Platelet-Collagen Interaction and Signaling

Collagens are very important activators of platelets in the vascular subendothelium and vessel wall and, thus, are prime targets for therapeutic intervention in patients experiencing a pathologic arterial thrombotic event such as MI or stroke. Platelets have two major surface receptors for collagen—integrin $\alpha_2\beta_1$ and the immunoglobulin superfamily member GPVI. In addition to binding collagen with high affinity, $\alpha_2\beta_1$ binds laminins, E-cadherins, matrix metalloproteins, C1q, echovirus, and rotavirus. In addition to these two surface receptors, the GPIb complex can also be considered an indirect collagen receptor because its subendothelial vWF ligand essentially acts as a bridging molecule between platelets and collagen by fixing itself to the latter, which, in turn, acts as scaffolding for the multimers.

Collagen supports platelet adhesion through interaction with the integrin surface receptor $\alpha_2\beta_1$, although this interaction alone does not support platelet activation.[56] Laboratory evidence suggests that GPVI and the 14-kDa FcRγ-chain signaling subunit (FcRγ chain) with which GPVI forms a complex are both required for collagen-mediated platelet adhesion and activation.[55–67] Thus, platelet adhesion to collagen is a multistep process. Once exposed to an injured vascular wall, vWF adheres to subendothelial collagen and undergoes a conformational change allowing its A1 domain to bind to GPIb/V/IX under high-shear flow conditions. This rapidly formed bond is quickly broken and reestablished, and this leads to the platelet rolling along the vascular wall. This in turn slows down the platelet and allows the signaling receptor GPVI to bind collagen, more specifically the repeating sequence Gly-Pro-Hyp (where Hyp is hydroxyproline). Both receptors can signal, but the role of GPVI is considered predominant in this respect.[68]

Notwithstanding the preceding scenarios, of the many receptors studied only $\alpha_2\beta_1$ and GPVI have a defined role in platelet-collagen interactions; however, in spite of extensive studies, their relative importance with respect to both adhesion and activation continues to be debatable. Problems associated with the isolation of collagen from extracellular matrices and possible but poorly understood differences between human ex vivo and mouse in vivo experimental systems explain these ongoing unresolved issues.[68]

In contrast to soluble platelet agonists, collagen is an insoluble component of the vessel wall and extravascular tissue. Its contribution to platelet signaling is therefore limited to platelets in contact with damaged vessel walls and those that seep into the extravascular space. The contribution of respective surface receptors involved with in vitro collagen-activated platelet signaling in experimental models is therefore dependent on the mechanism and extent of injury, and this may explain the debate noted above regarding their respective roles.[69,70] While collagen is seen as a potent activator in vitro, its role in vivo is likely more context dependent than other platelet agonists like thrombin.

$\alpha_2\beta_1$ Receptor

The platelet-collagen receptor to be first identified and characterized was the integrin $\alpha_2\beta_1$ receptor, also known as *GPIa/IIa*, and on lymphocytes as *VLA-2*.[71] Integrins are a family of α-β heterodimers on the surface of cells that carry out diverse interactions between the cell surface and its environment that ultimately lead to changes in cell behavior in response to the ligand-receptor interaction. In all α subunits of integrins, seven tandem repeats are localized to the N-terminal end and folded into a seven-bladed β-propeller structure.[72] The α_2 subunit also contains an I domain between the second and third repeats that includes a metal coordination site for Mg^{2+} that is critical for interaction with collagen.[71] Similar domains are found on the β subunit, although less is known about these, and it appears that the interaction of $\alpha_2\beta_1$ with collagen involves only the I domain of α_2. The β_1 subunit exhibits a cysteine-rich domain containing CGXC sequences that is close to the membrane surface. This region has protein disulfide isomerase activity responsible for regulating conformational changes of the β_1 subunit (which, in turn, alters α_2 conformation, increasing its avidity for collagen) in response to inside-out signaling through the cytoplasmic domain.[73,74]

The role of integrin $\alpha 2\beta 1$ in hemostasis and thrombosis has been controversial for a long time. Early publications suggested the integrin to be the central platelet collagen receptor that is essential for shear-resistant adhesion to the extracellular matrix, although studies on mice lacking either the $\alpha 2$- or the $\beta 1$-subunit failed to show a major hemostatic defect. It is now accepted that $\alpha 2\beta 1$ plays a significant but not essential role for the adhesion process as other receptors, most notably integrin $\alpha IIb\beta 3$, are also able to mediate shear-resistant platelet attachment to the extracellular matrix.[75]

Glycoprotein VI Receptor

Although the GPVI receptor was identified on the surface of platelets in 1982, its role in collagen-mediated platelet activation was not appreciated until much later.[76] The human and murine genes were cloned and characterized, and GPVI was found to be a member of the immunoglobulin superfamily.[67,74,77,78] The expression of GPVI in platelets is very closely associated with that of the 14-kDa FcRγ chain, which also serves as the signaling subunit for GPVI.[79,80] Expression of GPVI on mouse platelets appears to be dependent on FcRγ chain expression, and the latter has also been found to be critical for collagen-mediated platelet activation.[62,80] GPVI has two Ig C2 loops, and the N-terminal loop likely contains the collagen-binding domain.[68] It appears that GPVI has a requirement for the quaternary structure of collagen to be in a triple-helical conformation for the two to associate.[81]

Following the cloning of GPVI, mouse knockout studies have suggested GPVI may be the primary receptor involved in collagen-mediated platelet activation.[82–84] Further studies have enabled the collagen-binding site on GPVI to be characterized.[85]

Studies incorporating collagen-related peptides (arranged in triple-helical structures with sequences similar to collagen) and the snake venom convulxin as agonists have shown them to signal by clustering GPVI molecules on the surface.[59,64,86] However, the idea of GPVI receptor clustering as a platelet activation mechanism applicable to collagen is tempered by consideration of the theoretically much greater distances that would exist between adjacent GPVI-binding

sites along fibrillar collagen compared with the larger, noncovalently linked structures of convulxin, in which GPVI-binding site distribution is much different.[87]

Platelet-Collagen Signaling

Many of the early signaling events that follow GPVI stimulation have been characterized, although synergism between these GPVI mediators and those related to other adhesion receptors such as GPIb/V/IX and soluble agonists released by activated platelets further complicates full elucidation of the players and pathways associated with platelet-collagen signaling.

The GPVI signaling pathway has been found to be essential for collagen-mediated platelet activation, and mouse platelet studies have shown a central role for this receptor in promoting platelet-collagen interaction.[88] Integrin $\alpha_2\beta_1$ also contributes to platelet adhesion through amplification of signals from GPVI.[89,90] As noted in the previous section, exposure of platelets to collagen surfaces is thought to result in GPVI clustering that in turn triggers the tyrosine phosphorylation of the FcRγ chain.[79] GPVI signaling may be influenced by its association with glycolipid-enriched microdomains (membrane rafts) in the plasma membrane, although it is unclear whether GPVI is constitutively associated with the rafts or is recruited.[91,92] The GPVI/FcRγ chain complex leads to platelet activation through a pathway that has many aspects in common with signaling by immune receptors, such as the FcR receptor family (of which FcγRIIA is the lone family member found in platelets) and the B- and T-cell antigen receptors. Much of what we know about GPVI signaling has been based on earlier work related to immunoreceptor signaling.[93,94]

Immunoreceptors such as the FcRs and the FcRγ chain all have the ITAM in common. Tyrosine phosphorylation of the ITAM by Lyn and Fyn of the Src family of tyrosine kinases takes place after activation of GPVI. The phosphorylated Src kinase, in turn, leads to activation of the tyrosine kinase Syk after its autophosphorylation.[95] Syk then initiates a downstream signaling cascade involving the LAT and SLP-76 adapter proteins, which leads to formation of a signaling complex by virtue of its multiple phosphorylation sites that also act as docking sites, leading to recruitment of additional proteins to the plasma membrane.[96] Transport to the signaling complex and activation of the cytosolic second messenger–producing enzymes PI3K and PLCγ2 is also facilitated by tyrosine-phosphorylated LAT.[97] PI3K leads to the generation of PI3,4P3 and PI3,4,5P3 (PIP3), and this, in turn, supports recruitment of proteins to the membrane signalosome complex with specific PH domains including a member of the Tec kinase family, Btk, along with PLCγ2.[98,99] Syk is critical for collagen-mediated platelet activation through the GPVI/FcRγ chain complex, and knockout mouse studies have shown that absence of this enzyme leads to loss of phosphorylation of LAT, the adapter SLP-76, and PLCγ2.[99,100]

Adapters such as LAT are modular proteins without enzyme activity that support protein-protein interaction. Many adapter proteins appear to participate in the regulation of PLCγ2. These proteins appear to come together in T lymphocytes along with PLCγ1 to form a LAT/SLP-76 signalosome that is essential for activation of PLCγ2.[101] SLP-76 is thought to be especially important among adapters in the regulation of PLCγ2, because its loss results in reduced phosphorylation of PLCγ2.[100,102]

Along with the adapter proteins noted earlier, PI3K and its associated second messenger pathway also play a very important role in the regulation of PLCγ2 through activation of other signaling proteins such as protein kinase B (PKB; also known as Akt).[101,103] One of the two PKB isoforms, PKBβ (Akt2), is important for normal platelet function and thrombus formation and leads to impaired α and dense granule secretion along with impaired $\alpha_{IIb}\beta_3$ activation when absent.[101] Integrin-linked kinase (ILK) is another PI3K downstream effector that interacts with β_1 and β_3 integrin subunit cytoplasmic tails and is considered important in the bidirectional signaling of $\alpha_2\beta_1$ and $\alpha_{IIb}\beta_3$.[104,105] It may also be playing a role in regulating PKB.[106] Using PI3K inhibitors such as wortmannin and LY294002, studies have demonstrated significantly reduced PLCγ2 activation through GPVI.[107–109] These inhibitors have also been shown to block platelet activation through the FcγRIIA immunoreceptor, and this demonstrates an additional similarity between signaling pathways of this receptor and the FcRγ chain.[110]

PlCγ2 is known to play a critical role in aggregation and secretion responses to collagen, as demonstrated in PlCγ2 knockout mice and in other studies.[111,112] The major role of PlC isoforms is concerned with the generation of the second messengers inositol 1,4,5-triphosphate and 1,2-diacylglycerol (DAG), which participate in intracellular calcium homeostasis and activation of many isoforms of PKC. The former process culminates in a robust calcium signal that promotes efficient platelet activation. The PKC isoforms make possible the regulatory serine/threonine phosphorylation events needed for activation of $\alpha_2\beta_1$ as well as $\alpha_{IIb}\beta_3$, and interaction of these two integrins with their ligands facilitates a second round of signaling that includes some of the same molecules downstream of GPVI, such as Syk, SLP-76, and PlCγ2.[113]

Research has led to increased knowledge about $\alpha_2\beta_1$ receptor signaling. The use of $\alpha_2\beta_1$-selective ligands has demonstrated calcium-dependent spreading and tyrosine phosphorylation of several proteins when interaction with platelets takes place, including Src, Syk, SLP-76, PLCγ2, p38 MAP kinase, ILK, Rac, and PAK.[108,114,115] It appears likely that only GPVI and GPIb/V/IX are able to bind collagen and vWF, respectively, without prior platelet activation. Once activation starts, $\alpha_2\beta_1$ and $\alpha_{IIb}\beta_3$ are able to bind their respective ligands as well.

The C-type lectin receptor CLEC-2 is highly expressed on platelets and has a hem(ITAM) motif (one YxxL sequence) that signals through Syk. CLEC-2 clustering leads to similar signaling events to GPVI that involve SFK, Syk, and Tec family kinases.[116] Platelet activation through CLEC-2 leads to release of secondary mediators ADP and TXA$_2$. CLEC-2 ligands include the transmembrane protein podoplanin (widely expressed outside the vasculature) and possibly CLEC-2 itself.[117] A mouse model that lacks platelet CLEC-2 has impaired thrombus formation suggesting the ligand is in platelets or plasma.[117]

Other Platelet Adhesion Receptors

Other adhesive proteins present in the extracellular matrix and involved in the interaction between platelets and the subendothelium include fibronectin, thrombospondin, laminin, and vitronectin. Fibronectin is stored in platelet α granules and secreted upon thrombin-mediated platelet activation. Thrombospondin is also stored in platelet α granules. It interacts with fibrinogen, fibrin, fibronectin, and collagen on the platelet membrane, and its release during platelet activation might relate to its capability to overcome the antithrombotic activity of physiologic nitric oxide (NO). Laminin is a large glycoprotein and can amplify platelet activation through GPVI binding. Recent data suggest that laminin may also interact with vWF and the GPIb/V/IX complex thereby supporting platelet adhesion under high-shear flow conditions.[118] The extracellular adhesive protein vitronectin can bind to platelet receptor $\alpha_{IIb}\beta_3$ or the integrin $\alpha_v\beta_3$ and appears to be functionally similar to fibronectin.

Physiologic Inhibition of Platelet Adhesion

Negative regulation of platelets is essential to set the stimulus threshold for thrombus formation, determine final clot size and stability, and prevent uncontrolled thrombosis. The mechanisms behind the negative regulation of platelet activation are described later in the chapter, and in this respect, roles of players such as NO and prostacyclin have been well characterized. Platelet activation and aggregation can also be inhibited by signaling through the platelet–endothelial cell adhesion molecule (PECAM)-1 (CD31), carcinoembryonic antigen cell adhesion molecule (CEACAM)-1, carcinoembryonic antigen cell adhesion molecule (CEACAM)-2, G6b-B, and L1LRB2/paired immunoglobulin-like receptor B (PIRB).[119–121] These molecules are expressed on a number of blood cells and endothelial cells and have a wide array of regulatory functions in processes such as apoptosis and cell activation. PECAM-1 becomes tyrosine phosphorylated following platelet stimulation by a diverse set of agonists, which suggests that it has a negative feedback role in this setting. Its main ligand is itself, so

it has been proposed that interactions between platelet and endothelial PECAM-1 might serve to restrict thrombus growth through the signaling mechanisms described as follows; this is supported by studies involving PECAM-1-knockout mice.[122,123]

Following homophilic interactions and/or clustering, PECAM-1 is tyrosine phosphorylated in its cytoplasmic-tail ITIM domain (immunoreceptor tyrosine-based inhibition motif) by Src family kinases, and this engenders recruitment of tyrosine, serine/threonine, or lipid phosphatases with resultant kinase-dependent signaling inhibition.[120,124] The net result is reduced total platelet tyrosine phosphorylation, calcium mobilization, and signaling through PI3K.[120] ITIM-mediated signaling inhibition through the ITAM domain is not the only mechanism by which PECAM-1 dampens platelet adhesion because low-density lipoprotein and thrombin-dependent signaling pathways also appear to be downregulated by PECAM-1.[120,124] Negative effects have also been documented with GPIb signaling and platelet FcγRIIA-mediated responses.[125,126] In addition, ITIM-containing proteins have been found to have inhibitory regulatory roles following stimulation by G protein–coupled receptor (GPCR) agonists and in the regulation of $\alpha_{IIb}\beta_3$ function suggesting their role is not solely limited to inhibition of ITAM signaling.[121]

vWF multimer size and, thus also vWF activity, is mainly regulated by the metalloprotease ADAMTS13, and recently other factors have been found to cleave vWF, including plasmin and leukocyte proteases.[127,128] ADAMTS13 cleaves released large vWF multimers into smaller fragments. Different circumstances can induce vWF unfolding, thereby exposing the ADAMTS13 cleavage site. These include high-shear flow conditions, denaturing agents such as urea, and mutations seen in von Willebrand disease type 2A. In contrast, reduced ADAMTS13 activity may lead to insufficient vWF processing, causing a prothrombotic state such as thrombotic thrombocytopenic purpura (see Chapter 49).

Platelet Thrombin (Protease-Activated) Receptors and Signaling

PARs are GPCRs that use a unique mechanism to convert an extracellular protein cleavage event into an intracellular activation signal. In this case, the ligand is already part of the receptor per se, by virtue of the fact that it is represented by the amino acid sequence SFLLRN (residues 42-47) and is unmasked as a new amino terminus after thrombin cleaves the peptide bond between Arg 41 and Ser 42. This "tethered ligand" then proceeds to dock irreversibly with the body of its own receptor to effect transmembrane signaling.

Thrombin signaling in platelets is mediated, at least in part, by four members of a family of G protein–coupled PARs (PAR-1, -2, -3, and -4; see previous section for a discussion of the GPIb complex as a thrombin receptor).[129] Human platelets express PAR-1 and PAR-4, and activation of either is sufficient to trigger platelet aggregation.[130,131] Mouse platelets express PAR-3 and PAR-4.[132] PAR-1, -3, and -4 can be activated by thrombin, whereas PAR-2 can be activated by trypsin, tryptase, and coagulation factors VIIa and Xa but not thrombin.[133–135] Presumably, other proteases are capable of recognizing the active sites of these receptors and can thus also trigger PAR signaling.

PAR-1 is the prototype family member and was the first to be cloned and characterized in the human and hamster.[130,136] A synthetic peptide that mimics the PAR-1-tethered ligand (SFLLRN) is capable of functioning as an agonist by activating the receptor independent of cleavage of the 41-residue N-terminal exodomain.

The mechanism by which GPCRs, such as PAR-1, signal through the G proteins is shown in *Figure 19.3*. PAR-1 is capable of coupling to members of the G12/13, Gq, and Gi/z families and, thus, is connected to a significant number of intracellular signaling pathways. The α subunits of G12 and G13 are believed to be involved in mediating rearrangement of the actin cytoskeleton and platelet shape change,[137] and downstream signaling mediators include Rho family members, among others. The α subunit of Gq is needed for platelet secretion and aggregation and participates in the activation of PlCβ that leads to calcium mobilization and PKC activation.[138,139] The α subunit of Gz is a

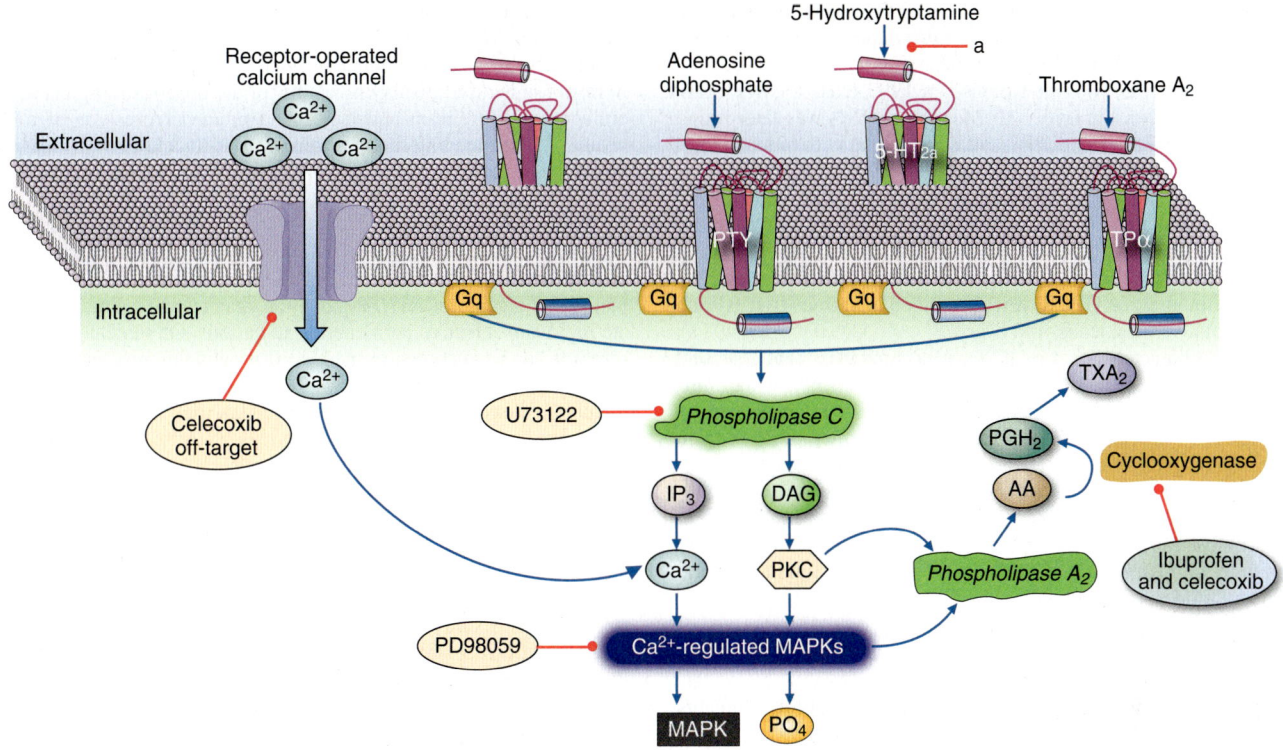

FIGURE 19.3 **GPCRs signaling networks in human platelets.** 5-HT receptor blockers (a): cyproheptadine and ketanserin. 5-HT, 5-hydroxytryptamine; AA, arachidonic acid; DAG, diacylglycerol; IP_3, inositol triphosphate; MAPKs, mitogen-activated protein kinases; PGH_2, prostaglandin H_2; PKC, protein kinase C; TXA_2, thromboxane A_2. (From Khan N, Dar Farroq A, Sadek B. Investigation of cyclooxygenase and signaling pathways involved in human platelet aggregation mediated by synergistic interaction of various agonists. *Drug Des Devel Ther.* 2015;9:3497-3506. Originally published by and used with permission from Dove Medical Press Ltd.)

G_i family member that has been speculated to play an epinephrine-like role in human platelets through inhibition of adenylate cyclase.[30,140]

The β-γ subunit counterparts of G proteins involved in PAR-1 signaling are involved in a plethora of activities, including activation of protein kinases, channels, and lipid-modifying enzymes, such as PI3K, which provides attachment for multiple signaling protein complexes close to the inner leaflet of the cell membrane.[141–143] Thus, this vast network of signaling pathways mediated through several G protein families is in keeping with the pleiotropic roles that thrombin has been shown to exhibit in cellular homeostasis, which extends beyond platelet activation to include endothelial cells, leukocytes, smooth muscle cells, and T lymphocytes, along with physiologic processes such as tissue injury, inflammation, angiogenesis, and embryonic development.[41]

Once activated, PAR-1 is rapidly uncoupled from signaling and internalized into the cell.[144–146] It is then transported to lysosomes and degraded.[145,147–149] Platelets presumably have no need for a thrombin-receptor recycling mechanism, because once activated, they are irreversibly incorporated into blood clots. Conversely, in cell lines with characteristics similar to megakaryocytes (MKs), new protein synthesis is needed for recovery of PAR-1 signaling,[145,147] and, in endothelial cells, sensitivity to thrombin is maintained by delivery of naïve PAR-1 to the cell surface from a preformed intracellular pool.[147]

Physiologic differences exist between PAR-1 and PAR-4 on human platelets. When antibodies to the thrombin interaction site of PAR-1 are used, platelet activation is blocked at low, as opposed to high, thrombin concentrations.[148,149] Antibodies that blocked PAR-4 alone had no effect on thrombin-mediated platelet activation. If both receptors were blocked, platelet activation was blocked at both low and high thrombin concentrations,[132] and so PAR-1 appears to be most efficient at mediating platelet activation at low concentrations of thrombin, whereas PAR-4 functions in the absence of PAR-1 but only at high thrombin concentrations. Because PAR-1 is capable of

mediating platelet activation at low thrombin concentrations, the exact role of PAR-4 in human platelet function remains speculative. It has been shown that the rate of platelet activation through PAR-4 is significantly slower and more sustained than that through PAR-1.[41,150,151] Given the importance of this system with respect to normal hemostasis, PAR-4 may serve as a redundant backup receptor to PAR-1, or it may serve as an important receptor for one or more proteases other than thrombin.

Platelet Adenosine Diphosphate (Purinergic) Receptors and Signaling

Evidence that ADP plays an important role in both formation of the platelet plug and the pathogenesis of arterial thrombosis has been accumulating since its initial characterization in 1960 as a factor derived from red blood cells that influences platelet adhesion.[152] ADP is present in high (molar) concentrations in platelet-dense granules and is released when platelet stimulation takes place with other agonists, such as collagen; thus, ADP serves to amplify further the biochemical and physiologic changes associated with platelet activation and aggregation. Inhibitors of this ADP-associated aggregation include commonly used clinical agents such as clopidogrel that have proven to be very effective antithrombotic drugs.[153,154]

Adenine nucleotides interact with P2 receptors that are ubiquitous among different cell types and have been found to regulate a wide range of physiologic processes. They are divided into two groups, the G protein–coupled or "metabotropic" superfamily named *P2Y* and the ligand-gated ion channel or "ionotropic" superfamily termed *P2X*.[155] Two G protein–coupled (P2Y) receptors contribute to platelet aggregation. The $P2Y_1$ receptor initiates aggregation through mobilization of calcium stores, and the $P2Y_{12}$ receptor is coupled to inhibition of adenylate cyclase and is essential for a full aggregation response to ADP with stabilization of the platelet plug. $P2X_1$ is a third ADP receptor present in platelets and has been shown to contribute to aggregation in response to collagen. Both the $P2Y_{12}$ and $P2X_1$ receptors have been shown to play key roles in platelet activation and aggregation under flow conditions characterized by high shear stress.[156,157]

The $P2Y_1$ receptor was first cloned in 1993 from a chick brain complementary DNA library.[158–160] Messenger RNA was later found in MK-like cell lines, such as HEL and K562, along with human platelets.[161] It was also established that the purported agonist effects of purified triphosphate nucleotides were, in fact, due to their transformation into diphosphate analogs by the ectonucleotidases present at the cell surface of the platelets and brain capillary endothelial cells being studied.[161,162] The $P2Y_1$ receptor has 373 amino acid residues and the prototype structure of a GPCR. It is distributed in various tissues such as heart, blood vessels, testis, and ovary.[159]

After the characterization of $P2Y_1$, it became clear that a second platelet ADP receptor had to exist that was responsible for the inhibition of cAMP production by ADP that, in turn, was unaffected by blocking $P2Y_1$.[163–168] The $P2Y_{12}$ receptor was cloned in 2001 from human and rat platelet complementary DNA libraries using *Xenopus* oocytes.[169] The receptor indeed showed the ability to display ADP-mediated inhibition of platelet cyclic AMP (cAMP) formation that was not blocked by $P2Y_1$ antagonists. The receptor has been localized to certain regions of the brain, such as the substantia nigra and thalamus, in addition to platelets.[169]

Platelet $P2Y_1$ and $P2Y_{12}$ Receptor Roles in Adenosine Diphosphate–Mediated Activation

Even at high concentrations, ADP is a weak activator of PlC. Thus, its role in platelet activation is based more on its ability to activate other pathways. Inhibition of either of the $P2Y_1$ or $P2Y_{12}$ receptors is sufficient to block ADP-mediated platelet aggregation, and coactivation of both receptors is therefore necessary, through the G proteins G_q and G_i, respectively, for ADP to activate and aggregate the platelet.[170] A series of studies involving the use of selective $P2Y_1$ and $P2Y_{12}$ receptor antagonists, a cAMP inhibitor, gene targeting, and G_q and G_i protein agonists that would theoretically activate the two main G protein pathways associated with ADP stimulation (see the following) have led to the conclusion that a signaling event downstream from G_i is required for the conformational change and subsequent aggregation associated with the $\alpha_{IIb}\beta_3$ receptor.[166,168,171–177]

Studies done with platelets from patients who manifest defective $P2Y_{12}$, along with experiments involving the study of $P2Y_1$ receptor function in platelet-rich plasma that has high fibrinogen concentrations, have demonstrated that the $P2Y_1$ receptor has roles in activation and aggregation in addition to shape change and that it is fully capable of mounting an aggregation response that is nonetheless transient in nature.[166,178,179] The $P2Y_1$ receptor is an absolute requirement for ADP-mediated aggregation based on knockout mouse studies, as evidenced by the demonstration that platelets can become refractory to ADP due to desensitization of the $P2Y_1$ receptor and the observation that adrenaline (which activates the G protein G_i that mediates inhibition of adenylate cyclase) does not restore aggregation in the presence of $P2Y_1$ selective antagonists.[174–179] Platelet shape change is dependent on two separate G signaling pathways, a G_q-linked release of calcium from internal stores, and a G_{12}/G_{13} link to activation of Rho kinases and Rho guanine nucleotide exchange factors that activate small G proteins.[137,180,181] The primary role of the $P2Y_{12}$ receptor in platelet activation and aggregation is to amplify and complete the aggregation response to ADP as well as to other agonists.[163–167] In the presence of a high ADP concentration, the receptor is also capable of mediating partial platelet aggregation on its own in $P2Y_1$ and G_q knockout mice, thus proving that $\alpha_{IIb}\beta_3$ conformational change followed by aggregation can actually take place in the absence of calcium mobilization and PKC activation.[175,181] In general terms, it appears that $P2Y_{12}$ is responsible for acting as an ADP costimulus receptor in the presence of low concentrations of other agonists, such as collagen, thrombin, chemokines, or IgG, whereas the $P2Y_1$ receptor has a specific role early in platelet activation.[170,182,183] Another role for the $P2Y_{12}$ receptor is the potentiation of platelet secretion.[182,184] Because of its central role in the formation and stabilization of thrombi, the $P2Y_{12}$ receptor is a well-established target of antithrombotic drugs such as clopidogrel.[182,185]

Platelets from $P2Y_{12}$-deficient mice aggregate poorly or not at all in response to ADP displaying a shift in the dose-response curves for collagen and thrombin and lack ADP-induced repression of cAMP levels.[186] The bleeding time of homozygous knockouts was markedly prolonged compared with near-normal results in heterozygotes.[187]

$P2X_1$ Receptor

$P2X_1$ was first discovered in platelets using polymerase chain reaction of transcripts from platelets and MK-like cell lines.[187–191] This third platelet P2 receptor is an ATP-gated ion channel and is known to mediate rapid and selective permeability to cations. On platelets, the $P2X_1$ receptor has been shown to mediate fast calcium entry stimulated by ADP.[192] $P2X_1$ is a 399-amino-acid protein composed of two transmembrane domains, intracellular N and C termini, and an extracellular loop with 10 conserved cysteine residues.[155] At least three P2X subunits are required to constitute a membrane pore, and these receptors are typically expressed on excitable cells, such as neurons.

Although activation of the $P2X_1$ receptor alone cannot induce platelet aggregation, it contributes to aggregation in response to collagen.[193,194] The role of $P2X_1$ in platelet function seems to be particularly relevant under flow conditions characterized by high shear stress.[194–196] A study of $P2X_1$-deficient ($P2X_1^{/}$) mice has further indicated that this receptor contributes to the thrombosis of small arteries. $P2X_1^{-/-}$ mice display resistance to the localized arterial thrombosis of mesenteric arterioles triggered by laser-induced vessel wall injury and to the acute systemic thromboembolism induced by infusion of a mixture of collagen and adrenaline.[194] Conversely, increased systemic thrombosis has been reported in mice overexpressing the human $P2X_1$ receptor.[197]

Adenosine Diphosphate Receptor Signaling

ADP is considered a weak agonist compared with collagen or thrombin, for example. Aggregation is typically reversible when platelets are stimulated by ADP alone. In addition, low concentrations of ADP serve to amplify the effects of both strong and weaker agonists, the latter including serotonin and adrenaline.[130,131] As noted in the preceding paragraphs, ADP signal transduction downstream from the $P2Y_1$ receptor leads to a transient rise in free cytoplasmic calcium as a result of mobilization from internal stores, and this is followed by secondary store–mediated influx, whereas a concomitant inhibition of adenylate cyclase is initiated by ADP stimulation of the $P2Y_{12}$ receptor. The G protein family member responsible for signaling through $P2Y_1$ to PlCβ is G_q, whereas the member responsible for signaling through $P2Y_{12}$ to inhibit adenylate cyclase is G_i. The G_i family member associated with $P2Y_{12}$ appears to be primarily Gi_2 inasmuch as Gi_2 knockout mice have an impaired response to ADP and those lacking $G_{i3}\alpha$ and $G_z\alpha$ do not.[140,198,199] ADP also induces a rapid influx of calcium from the external media through ligand-gated calcium channels.[200,201] Although partial platelet aggregation without shape change can be seen in $P2Y_1$ and G_q knockout mice in the presence of high ADP concentrations, the fact that aggregation is not seen at lower concentrations suggests that the G_q-dependent PlCβ pathway leading to phosphoinositide hydrolysis and PKC activation is necessary to mobilize calcium after ADP stimulation and is essential for full platelet aggregation to take place in response to ADP.[138,175,202,203]

Although ADP-mediated platelet activation via the $P2Y_1$ receptor incorporates the G_q-dependent PlC-β second messenger pathway, the $P2Y_{12}$ receptor mediates its postoccupancy signaling through G_i-dependent PI3 kinase activation and subsequent repression of cAMP levels. In addition to the PI3K role, several groups have reported a role for Rap1B in $P2Y_{12}$ signal transduction. Rap1B is a small GTPase that is highly expressed in platelets, and its ADP-stimulated increased activation is abolished by $P2Y_{12}$ antagonists and G_i knockout mice.[204–206] Rap1B activation through other receptors such as FcγRIIA and GPVI also appears to have a $P2Y_{12}$ component.[205,206] Evidence suggests that ADP-induced Rap1B activation lies downstream of PI3K, because

PI3K inhibitors have been shown to inhibit Rap1B activation, although evidence differs as to which isoform is involved.[204,206]

The same G_i protein–associated signaling pathway used by platelet ADP receptors has been found to act in a synergistic fashion when it is triggered either through other platelet receptors or through key downstream players triggered by other receptors, such as PlCγ2.[207,208] It has been suggested that concomitant signaling through the G proteins and tyrosine kinases of other receptor pathways may potentially be seen as a general mechanism in which ADP contributes to efficient platelet activation and aggregation.[182,209] For example, ADP in platelets has been proposed to be an important cofactor of PI3 kinase activation that is stimulated through the PAR-1 thrombin receptor.[210] It is interesting that there is a difference in the ability of ADP to potentiate aggregation through the two platelet thrombin receptors (PAR-1 and PAR-4), in that PAR-1 is more dependent on secreted ADP acting through P2Y$_{12}$ than PAR-4.[211,212] Collagen-induced platelet aggregation is similarly facilitated by P2Y$_{12}$.[186,213,214]

ADP has been implicated as an important cofactor of platelet activation seen in the settings of experimental cross-linking of the FcγRIIA immunoreceptor and in patients with heparin-induced thrombocytopenia.[215] The latter is a disorder in which platelet activation and often serious thrombotic sequelae take place as a consequence of administration of the anticoagulant heparin or low-molecular-weight heparin. In susceptible patients, an autoantibody is generated by the immune system that is directed to a complex on the platelet membrane formed by the heparin molecule and platelet factor 4. The Fc portion of the autoantibody is then capable of activating the platelet through its interaction with the FcγRIIA receptor. Activation of PI3K has been shown to be a central player in these two settings.

P2Y$_{12}$ activation has been found to play an important role in the activation of α$_{IIb}$β$_3$. Using P2Y$_{12}$ knockout mice, Andre et al. noted that platelets activated with PAR-4 or ADP were defective in binding soluble fibrinogen relative to wild-type mice.[190] Similarly, in humans it has been observed that P2Y$_{12}$ antagonists such as clopidogrel inhibit P-selectin expression and platelet-leukocyte conjugate formation, whereas aspirin does not.[216]

Platelet Activation by Soluble Agonists

α$_2$-Adrenergic Receptors and Epinephrine

Epinephrine is unique among platelet agonists because it is considered to be capable of stimulating secretion and aggregation but not cytoskeletal reorganization responsible for shape change. Furthermore, generation of the key signaling enzyme PlC through epinephrine stimulation appears to be dependent on TXA$_2$ and can thus be blocked with aspirin.[217] It is interesting, however, that epinephrine stimulation in the presence of aspirin is still capable of leading to the conformational change in the α$_{IIb}$β$_3$ receptor that precedes fibrinogen binding and platelet aggregation.[218,219] Similarly, the thrombin inhibitor hirudin has been found to block epinephrine-associated aggregation of washed platelets in one study, suggesting that an element of thrombin costimulation of platelets may be necessary to enhance the effects of epinephrine.[220] In low doses, epinephrine is thought to prime platelets for activation with other agonists, and the resulting stimulation is stronger than with either agonist alone.

Platelet responses to epinephrine are mediated through α$_2$-adrenergic receptors,[221,222] and these responses have been found to vary among individuals, with some donors with otherwise normal platelets manifesting delayed or absent responses.[223] Potentiation is typically attributed to cAMP formation inhibition.

Arachidonic Acid, Thromboxane A$_2$, and Thromboxane Receptors

After platelet stimulation by a number of agonists, arachidonic acid is generated directly by phospholipase A from its membrane phospholipid precursors (PC, PS, and PI) and indirectly by PlC generation of DAG followed by DAG lipase action (*Figure 19.4*). Most platelet agonists are believed to activate this pathway. Three known eicosanoid subsets of biochemical compounds are known to be derived from

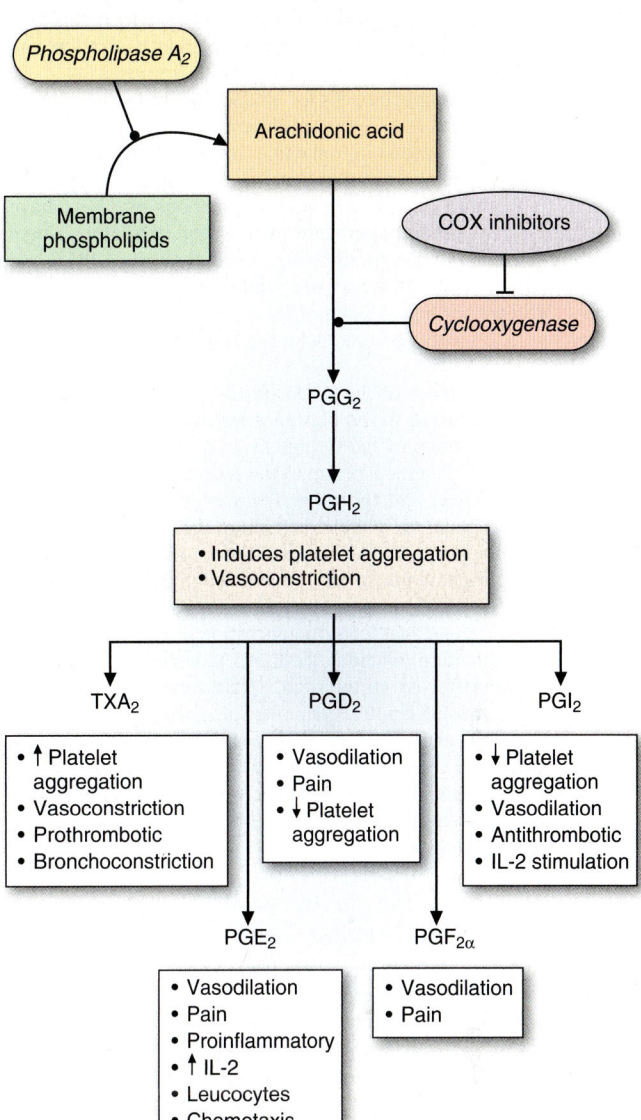

FIGURE 19.4 Cascade of metabolism of arachidonic acid by COX pathways. COX, cyclooxygenase; IL-2, interleukin 2; PGD$_2$, prostaglandin D$_2$; PGE$_2$, prostaglandin E$_2$; PGF$_{2a}$, prostaglandin F$_{2a}$; PGG$_2$, prostaglandin G$_2$; PGH$_2$, prostaglandin H$_2$; PGI$_2$, prostaglandin I$_2$; TXA$_2$, thromboxane A$_2$. (From Khan N, Dar Farroq A, Sadek B. Investigation of cyclooxygenase and signaling pathways involved in human platelet aggregation mediated by synergistic interaction of various agonists. *Drug Des Devel Ther.* 2015;9:3497-3506. Originally published by and used with permission from Dove Medical Press Ltd.)

the formation of arachidonic acid: the prostanoids, leukotrienes, and epoxides. The prostanoids are formed by the cyclooxygenase pathway and include endoperoxides and thromboxanes along with prostaglandins. The leukotrienes are formed by the lipoxygenase pathway and the epoxides by the cytochrome P450 epoxygenase pathway. Although all three of these pathways are present in platelets, most arachidonic acid ends up being metabolized to TXA$_2$.[224]

TXA$_2$ is produced in platelets from arachidonic acid through the generation of PGH$_2$ by the enzyme cyclooxygenase, which is irreversibly inhibited by aspirin through acetylation of a serine residue near its C terminus.[225,226] PGH$_2$ is the parent compound for both biologically active prostaglandins, such as PGE$_2$ and PGI$_2$, and TXA$_2$. The former two compounds act to inhibit platelet activation by generating intracellular cAMP, whereas TXA$_2$ activates platelets. Although prostaglandin and thromboxane pathways can be present in the same cell, platelets primarily synthesize thromboxane, and endothelial cells mainly synthesize prostaglandins such as PGI_2, which acts as a local vasodilator and thus indirectly opposes platelet activation and vasoconstriction.[226]

Like ADP and epinephrine, TXA_2 is also capable of activating nearby platelets after its release into plasma. It has a very short half-life of 30 s before its conversion to the inactive metabolite TXB_2 prevents widespread platelet activation beyond the vicinity of thrombus formation.[227,228] Both arachidonic acid and analogs of TXA_2 have been found to activate and aggregate platelets by mediating shape change and phosphorylation of signaling enzymes, such as PlCβ and PKC.[229,230] Signaling events associated with stimulation of the TXA_2 receptor (TXR) farther downstream of PlCβ and PKC include activation of p38 mitogen-activated protein kinase and the small heat-shock protein hsp27.[231]

The TXR is a member of the seven-transmembrane GPCR family and has been localized to the plasma membrane. The receptor is coupled to the α subunits of the G_q and G_{12}/G_{13} members of the G protein family.[140,232,233] One isoform of the receptor has been cloned from placenta (TXRα) and the other from endothelium (TXRβ). Both are found in platelets; platelet activation through the G_q pathway has been found to activate PlCβ, and the G_{12}/G_{13} pathway regulates myosin light-chain phosphorylation through activation of Rho kinase.[140,232,234] In addition, the α receptor is associated with activation of adenylate cyclase that leads to generation of cAMP, known to inhibit platelet activation, whereas the β receptor inhibits adenylate cyclase activation after its stimulation.[234] Because TXA_2 is a net agonist, the effects of PlCβ activation must somehow outweigh those of adenylate cyclase activation, or MK and platelet TXRβ receptor expression levels may outweigh those of TXRα receptor expression levels.[234] TXR knockout mice have a prolonged bleeding time, do not aggregate in response to TXA_2 agonists, and show delayed aggregation with collagen.[235]

Coordination Between Platelet Adhesion Events and Soluble Agonist Stimulation in Thrombus Growth

The mechanism by which soluble agonists coordinate their actions with platelet adhesion–related processes is an important consideration in the context of the steps required to facilitate thrombus growth.[236] The constraint imposed by blood flow on these prothrombotic processes represents the primary means by which platelet adhesion and activation are negatively regulated. These arterial high-shear forces have complex effects on platelet-vWF matrix interactions that are both pro- and antithrombotic in nature. Rapid blood flow also has complex

and poorly characterized effects on the formation and clearance of soluble agonists such as TXA_2.

One model to explain these relationships incorporates intra- and intercellular calcium signaling phenomena as a central unifying process.[236] In this model, the initial platelet/vessel wall interaction is characterized by contact between platelet-GPIb and matrix vWF with subsequent early platelet $α_{IIb}β_3$ conformational change, all leading to weak platelet activation. Costimulation of platelets by these adhesion events and soluble agonist receptors is then needed to potentiate and sustain activation signals initiated by the early GPIb/vWF/$α_{IIb}β_3$ interactions, and this costimulation leads to deceleration and arrest of platelet movement as the nidus of the thrombus develops. Platelet intracellular calcium is proposed to be the primary second messenger mediating these events, based on evidence suggesting an inverse correlation between calcium flux and platelet translocation behavior under flow conditions.[31] Intercellular calcium-related signaling between platelets is then thought to lead to ADP release at the site of contact between platelets, which in turn sustains these $α_{IIb}β_3$-derived calcium signals by a $P2Y_{12}$-linked signaling mechanism.[237]

REGIONAL ARCHITECTURE OF THE PLATELET PLUG AND REGULATION OF PLATELET ACTIVATION IN VIVO

The above sections describe individual signaling pathway components and the interactions between these components and pathways involved with platelet activation, and this information has been derived from characterization of bleeding disorders resulting from genetic or acquired defects of their molecular components. Recent studies in vivo suggest this model may in fact be a little simplistic. Rather than a nidus of uniformly activated platelets contained in a fibrin meshwork, in vivo platelet plugs develop a regional architecture where not all platelets are activated in the same way, and fibrin is distinctly localized. Based on intravital imaging studies in the microcirculation, plug architecture has been described as consisting of a core of highly activated, densely packed, degranulated platelets that express P-selectin sitting inside a shell of less activated, loosely associated platelets that do not express P-selectin[238,239] (*Figure 19.5*). Fibrin sits at the base of the core in the extravascular space. This heterogeneous platelet activation within a plug is due to interplay between platelet agonists and the plug's physical microenvironment that results in existence of gradients of soluble agonists like thrombin, ADP, and TXA_2. Thus, individual platelets are exposed to differing agonist combinations that

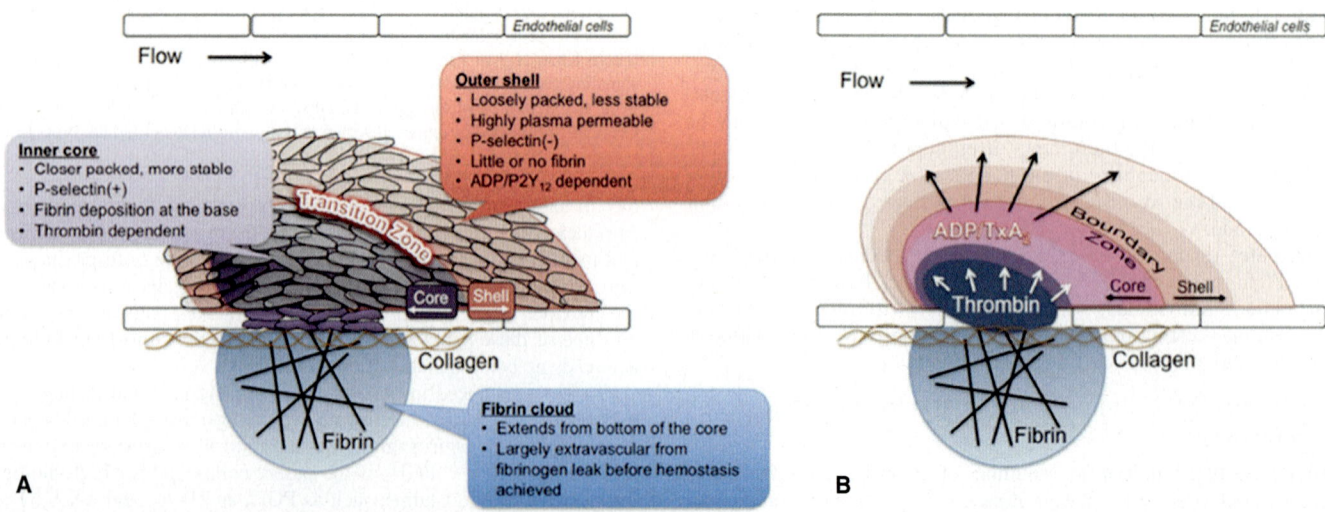

FIGURE 19.5 Regional architecture of a hemostatic plug. A. The properties of the core and shell regions of a hemostatic plug are described. **B.** The core and shell architecture develops as a result of local platelet agonist gradients that are shaped by physical forces within the platelet mass microenvironment. (Reprinted from Tomaiuolo M, Brass LF, Stalker TJ. Regulation of platelet activation and coagulation and its role in vascular injury and arterial thrombosis. *Interv Cardiol Clin.* 2017;6(1):1-12. Copyright © 2016 Elsevier. With permission.)

vary over time and space. A high concentration of thrombin sits inside the core and, as the plug becomes more porous, a gradient of ADP and thromboxane A_2 develops. It can also be concluded based on this that signaling pathway-specific pharmacological inhibitors such as aspirin and clopidogrel would be expected to have distinct effects on platelet plug architecture.

In addition to the molecular mechanisms of platelet-leukocyte interaction described in the section on platelet-cell interactions later in this chapter, with respect to platelet plug regional architecture it can also be said that the relatively more porous outer shell of the platelet plug may also facilitate recruitment of leukocytes needed for injury repair or elimination of pathogens. In low-shear stress venous injury sites, thrombin plays a key role in this respect—activation/cleavage of the platelet thrombin receptor PAR4 promotes leukocyte recruitment and migration while platelet P-selectin also enables leukocyte interaction with the thrombus.[240,241] Inhibition of this movement is afforded by both thrombin-mediated fibrin generation leading to physical barriers to leukocyte recruitment along with GPIb binding of thrombin that in turn lessens its effect on leukocyte trafficking.[240]

Rather than being a series of binary "on/off" processes, platelet activation is a graded sequence of events, some reversible and others irreversible. Reversible steps include shape change from discoid to other shapes, $\alpha_{IIb}\beta_3$ integrin activation leading to platelet aggregation, and TXA_2 formation. Subsequent irreversible steps include dense and alpha granule secretion, phosphatidylserine exposure supporting coagulation factor complex assembly, and membrane blebbing and microparticle formation.

Platelet activation is heterogeneous within a platelet plug, and that leads to a mass with a gradient of platelet activation extending from the injury site.[238] How this gradient develops is presently an unanswered question. Platelets with different degrees of activation may represent subpopulations with distinct characteristics, although a leading theory would suggest agonist distribution is the primary factor involved as depicted in *Figure 19.5*.

KEY REGULATORS OF PLATELET ACTIVATION

Platelet adhesion and activation is ultimately contingent on stimuli that regulate a core set of signaling mediators. Three central mediator families of platelet activation are PLC, PKC, and PI3K, and these mediators underlie two of the critical events in platelet activation, namely, secretion of secondary mediators and activation of $\alpha_{IIb}\beta_3$ (*Figure 19.6*). These are not the only critical regulators of platelet function, but they represent key nodes in the complex network of platelet signaling.[121]

PLC activation is important because it catalyzes the cleavage of phosphatidylinositol 4,5-bisphosphate (PIP2) to generate DAG, which activates PKC, and IP3, which binds to IP3 receptors on the dense tubular system of platelets to activate calcium flux into the cytosol. Studies that have utilized broad-spectrum inhibitors and mice deficient in one of the several individual isoforms of PKC have identified an overall positive role for the PKC family in the regulation of granule secretion, TXA_2 synthesis, integrin activation, aggregation, and thrombus formation.[242] Negative regulatory roles have also been identified, including roles in receptor desensitization and calcium release. All class I PI3K isoforms phosphorylate PIP2 to generate PIP3 that enables signaling to or recruitment of proteins containing PH domains to the plasma membrane. In turn, this is thought to localize signaling kinases to within close proximity of their downstream effectors.

Platelet activation leads to exposure of phosphatidylserine on the outer leaflet of the plasma membrane, which in turn confers procoagulant activity on this platelet subpopulation by increasing assembly of complexes of coagulation cascade proteases and their cofactors (e.g., the prothrombinase complex that leads to thrombin generation). This phosphatidylserine exposure is mediated by intracellular and mitochondrial accumulation of calcium that in turn facilitates cyclophilin D–mediated formation of the mitochondrial transition pore and the disruption of the inner mitochondrial membrane.[243,244] In addition to agonist-mediated stimulation, activation of platelet apoptotic pathways also leads to membrane outer leaflet phosphatidylserine exposure

through inner mitochondrial membrane disruption.[245] Exposure of phosphatidylserine also requires activation of phospholipid scramblases that also transfers it from the inner membrane leaflet to the outer leaflet.

A long-established negative regulator of platelet activation, the nitric oxide (NO)-cyclic guanylyl monophosphate (cGMP) pathway (as described in the next section), has relatively recently been found to in fact play biphasic roles in platelet activation through several receptor signaling pathways including platelet pattern-recognition receptor signaling pathways, which are discussed further in the section on platelets and immune cells. Low concentrations of NO and cGMP synthesized in platelet activation promote platelet activation and significantly increase platelet sensitivity to low concentrations of platelet agonists to receptors like GPIb-IX and GPCR receptors.[246,247] On the other hand, complete deficiency of endothelial and inducible NO synthase along with pharmacological inhibitors of the NO-cGMP pathway have been shown to inhibit platelet activation in response to these low-dose agonists.[246,247] Similarly, high concentrations of NO and cGMP analogs also are inhibitory to platelet activation through cGMP-dependent elevation of cAMP and activation of cAMP-dependent protein kinase.[247] The important stimulatory roles of the NO-cGMP pathway in platelet activation signaling mediated by TLR pattern recognition receptor family members native to platelets such as TLR2, 4, and 9 have been reported by different groups.[248]

Physiologic Inhibition of Platelet Activation

One of the many remarkable features of platelets is their ability to remain in a physiologic resting state and resist becoming activated while navigating the heart, arterial and venous circulations, and splenic microcirculation for an average of 10 days (*Figure 19.7*). Over this time, platelets can be expected to remain in a quiescent state while they encounter high-shear forces, what must be frequent collisions with other circulating cells as well as normal endothelium, and relatively profound turbulence associated with arterial branch points

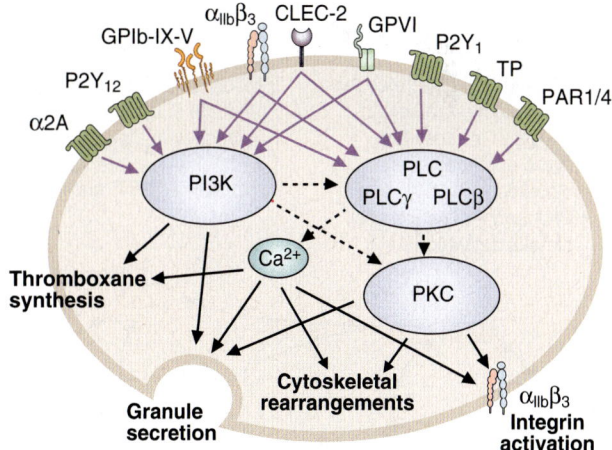

FIGURE 19.6 Phospholipase C (PLC), protein kinase C (PKC), and phosphatidylinositide-3-kinase (PI3K) are key mediators of platelet activation. All main activating platelet agonist receptors identified to date activate at least one of the following key activatory signaling mediators: PLC, PKC, or PI3K. These signaling nodes underlie several key processes required for platelet activation, including secretion of secondary mediators and activation of integrin $\alpha_{IIb}\beta_3$, facilitating fibrinogen binding and platelet aggregation, and also cytoskeletal rearrangements, which enable platelet shape change and spreading. α_2A, adrenergic receptor; $\alpha_{IIb}\beta_3$, receptor for fibrinogen; CLEC-2, C-type lectin receptor 2; GPVI, glycoprotein VI (collagen receptor); GPIb-IX-V, glycoprotein Ib-IX-V (von Willebrand factor receptor); PAR, protease-activated receptor; $P2Y_1/P2Y_{12}$, ADP receptors; TP, thromboxane A_2 receptor. (From Bye AP, Unsworth AJ, Gibbins JM. Platelet signaling: a complex interplay between inhibitory and activatory networks. *J Thromb Haemost.* 2016;14(5):918-930. http://creativecommons.org/licenses/by/4.0/)

and diseased yet physically intact arteries and arterioles. Indeed, the pathologic consequences associated with widespread inappropriate platelet activation are life- and limb-threatening when associated with well-characterized clinical disorders such as thrombotic thrombocytopenic purpura and heparin-induced thrombocytopenia. The mechanisms responsible for maintaining the fine balance of keeping platelets in a resting state until they encounter a genuine need to undergo adhesion, activation, and aggregation at the site of vascular injury are almost as diverse as those responsible for mediating these physiologic phenomena.

The inhibitory signaling pathways are few in number but suppress several key nodes in the platelet signaling network that function in activation.[121] Some general mechanisms involved in physiologic inhibition of platelet activation include phenomena such as (a) generation of negative-regulating molecules by the platelet (e.g., cAMP), endothelium (e.g., PGI_2, NO, heparan sulfate), and at distant sites (e.g., antithrombin); (b) direct contact of circulating platelets with collagen prevented by a barrier of endothelial cells; (c) generation of an ecto-ADPase (CD39) by endothelial cells that will metabolize ADP secreted from activated platelets and, thus, is intended to limit further activation; (d) tendency for blood flow to wash away unbound thrombin from the site of platelet plug formation and, hence, limit the extent of clot formation; (e) brief half-life of certain key platelet activators such as TXA_2; (f) ability to alter the conformation of a receptor such that it is then able to interact with a specific proaggregatory ligand, as happens with $\alpha_{IIb}\beta_3$ and plasma fibrinogen; and (g) the ability to inactivate switched-on receptors associated with activation through biochemical modifications such as phosphorylation or their removal from the platelet surface.

In addition to negative regulators such as ITIM-containing proteins discussed in the section on platelet adhesion inhibition earlier that are thought to reduce activation of key players like PLC and PI3K, other endogenous inhibitory mechanisms include (a) endothelial cell-selective adhesion molecule (ESAM), (b) Wnt-β-catenin and semaphorin 3A (Sema3A) that negatively regulate integrin $\alpha_{IIb}\beta_3$ activity, (c) phosphatases that limit phosphorylation-dependent mechanisms, (d) receptor desensitization that limits the response to secondary mediator signaling, and (e) intracellular nuclear receptors with different mechanisms of action such as peroxisome proliferator-activating receptor (PPAR) α.[249]

Biochemical modification leads to receptor desensitization and occurs with GPCRs present on the surface of platelets, with the notable exception of PAR-1 because thrombin requires an intact N terminus to activate the receptor.[250] Desensitization of GPCRs is normally mediated through phosphorylation of serine and threonine residues associated with the cytoplasmic side of the receptor by GPCR kinases.[251] The role of phosphorylation of these residues is to uncouple them from their G proteins and then lay the groundwork for internalization of the receptor through the binding of arrestin proteins.[252,253] Some of the physiologic and biochemical phenomena related to inhibition of platelet activation are described in the following.

Inhibitory Prostaglandins

PGE_2 and PGI_2, along with PGE_1, are examples of prostaglandins generated through the arachidonic acid pathway that inhibit platelet activation and aggregation, which are processes mediated in part by other prostaglandins and thromboxanes derived from the same pathway. The inhibitors carry this out through GPCRs that regulate adenylate cyclase–mediated generation of cAMP, which in turn activates PKA (or A kinases) and protein kinase G.[254] Many substrates of PKA and PKG are yet to be well characterized, although there is considerable overlap in these established targets such as Rap1b, Gα13, and GPIbβ.[130] Mouse platelets deficient in PKG have a prothrombotic phenotype and increased intravascular adhesion and aggregation after ischemia.[255]

The receptors of prostaglandins believed to increase cAMP levels in platelets such as PGI_2 have been described as being coupled

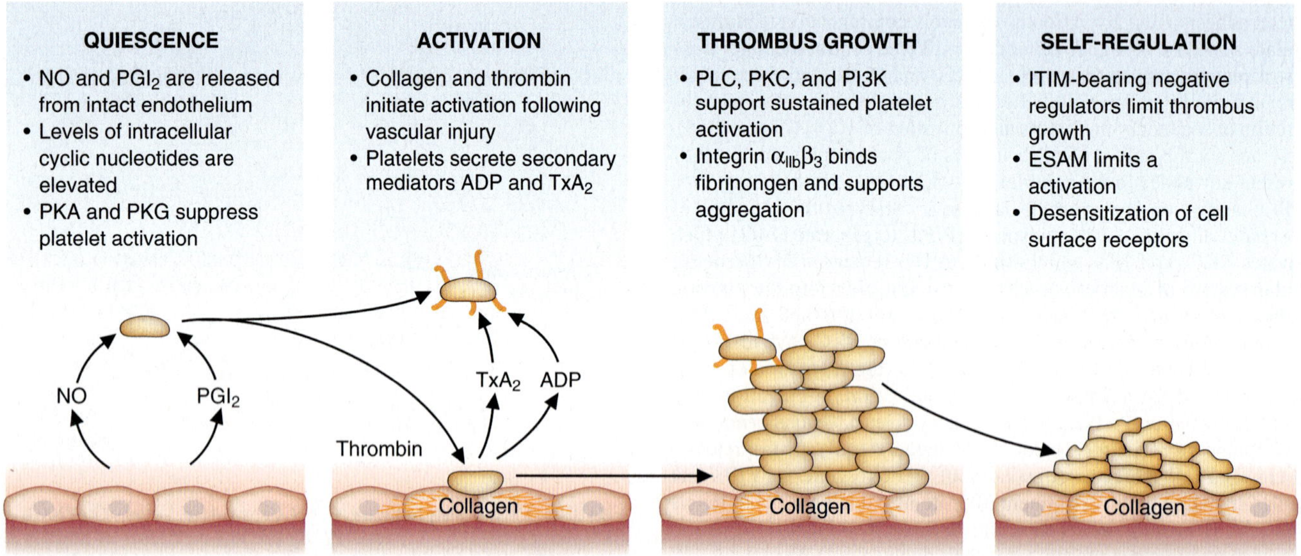

QUIESCENCE	ACTIVATION	THROMBUS GROWTH	SELF-REGULATION
• NO and PGI_2 are released from intact endothelium • Levels of intracellular cyclic nucleotides are elevated • PKA and PKG suppress platelet activation	• Collagen and thrombin initiate activation following vascular injury • Platelets secrete secondary mediators ADP and TxA_2	• PLC, PKC, and PI3K support sustained platelet activation • Integrin $\alpha_{IIb}\beta_3$ binds fibrinongen and supports aggregation	• ITIM-bearing negative regulators limit thrombus growth • ESAM limits a activation • Desensitization of cell surface receptors

FIGURE 19.7 Stages of platelet activation and thrombus formation. Platelets in the circulation are kept in a quiescent state by nitric oxide (NO) and prostacyclin (prostaglandin I_2; PGI_2), which are released by the vascular endothelium. In platelets, NO and PGI_2 increase the levels of cGMP and cAMP and suppress platelet activity by the activation of protein kinase A (PKA) and protein kinase G (PKG). Following vessel injury, components of the subendothelial matrix are exposed, including collagen, which provides an adhesive surface for platelets to attach to and initiate signaling events and platelet activation. Local production of thrombin and secretion of secondary mediators also contribute to the initiation of platelet activation. Key components of platelet signaling pathways are activated, including phospholipase C (PLC), protein kinase C (PKC), and phosphatidylinositide-3-kinase (PI3K), supporting sustained platelet activation and thrombus formation through the initiation of cytoskeletal rearrangements, granule secretion, and activation of integrin $\alpha_{IIb}\beta_3$. So as to limit thrombus growth and prevent the formation of occlusive thrombi, platelets contain self-regulating negative feedback mechanisms that counteract positive signaling. These negative regulators include immunoreceptor tyrosine-based inhibition motif (ITIM)-containing receptors; endothelial cell-selective adhesion molecule (ESAM), which negatively regulates integrin $\alpha_{IIb}\beta_3$ activity; phosphatases that counteract phosphorylation-dependent positive signaling; and receptor desensitization, which reduces the platelets' response to secondary mediator signaling. TXA_2, thromboxane A_2. (From Bye AP, Unsworth AJ, Gibbins JM. Platelet signaling: a complex interplay between inhibitory and activatory networks. *J Thromb Haemost.* 2016;14(5):918-930. http://creativecommons.org/licenses/by/4.0/)

to the α subunits of G$_s$. Conversely, most platelet agonists suppress cAMP formation by inhibiting adenylate cyclase via one or more of the G$_i$ family members that are expressed in platelets.[256] In addition to these considerations, cAMP levels in platelets are also governed by the activity of phosphodiesterase, the enzyme responsible for cAMP metabolism. This enzyme activity is inhibited by drugs such as the weak antiplatelet agent dipyridamole, the bronchodilator theophylline, and sildenafil, used to treat erectile dysfunction in men.

Raising cAMP levels causes a number of specific changes in platelet function. These include limitation of phosphoinositide hydrolysis, which is believed to occur through blockade of the inositol 1,4,5-triphosphate receptor and inhibition of the resynthesis of the phosphatidylinositol 4,5-biphosphate precursor of DAG formation. There is also a smaller increase in the cytosolic free Ca^{2+} concentration in response to agonists and an accelerated uptake of Ca^{2+} into the dense tubular system.[257,260] The targets through which cAMP and PKA reduce platelet reactivity are incompletely understood. They include ABP (filamin), myosin light chain, vasodilator-stimulated phosphoprotein (VASP), and Rap1B. Another PKA substrate is the β subunit of the GPIb complex, and this phosphorylation may in turn reduce platelet activation through its increased interaction with the 14-3-3ζ protein.[47,48] The 14-3-3 family of proteins exist as homodimers and modulate effector pathways in diverse cell types through interaction with key signaling enzymes.[44]

Pleckstrin and Protein Kinase C Inhibition

PKC is an important serine-threonine kinase with protean effector manifestations in platelet signaling. PKC is the receptor for the lipid second messenger DAG and is a key enzyme in the signaling events that follow activation of receptors coupled to PlC. PKC isozymes phosphorylate multiple cellular proteins at serine and threonine residues. PKC is actually a family of structurally related molecules, and platelets contain at least the α, β, δ, ε, η, θ, and perhaps ζ and λ isozymes.[261]

Once activated, PKC appears to mediate individual roles that, in some respects, may be considered contradictory in nature. These include positive effects such as mediating secretion and aggregation as well as negative effects that can be observed when platelets are incubated with phorbol esters before agonist stimulation. Under these circumstances, the agonist effector-mediated responses are reduced or do not occur, particularly if they are mediated by effectors downstream from phosphoinositide hydrolysis, and this phenomenon may represent a form of negative feedback.[262–264] This is speculated as possibly being due to a shorter duration of signaling for calcium release.[265]

Several platelet proteins are known PKC substrates, and these include Pleckstrin (P47), myosin light chain (P20), ABP, and the α subunits of the G proteins G$_z$, G$_{12}$, and G$_{13}$. The precise role of Pleckstrin in platelets is unknown, although its first and last 100 residues are homologous with domains in molecules with roles in signal transduction. These so-called Pleckstrin homology domains are speculated to play roles in protein-protein interactions, and so phosphorylated Pleckstrin may have a role in the negative regulation of PKC. One study suggests that phosphorylated Pleckstrin may be accomplishing negative regulation of PKC through inhibiting phosphoinositide hydrolysis and the activity of the lipid kinase, PI3K.[266] Reduced activity of PI3K leads to reduced phosphorylation of PI-4,5-P2 to PI-3,4,5-P3, a molecule that, in turn, is involved in the activation of the PKC isoforms.[267]

Other Inhibitory Processes of Platelet Activation

The α$_{IIb}$β$_3$ receptor on the surface of activated and resting platelets along with the fibrinogen that binds to stimulated platelets expressing the activated form of α$_{IIb}$β$_3$ has been observed to undergo rapid internalization into MK and platelet α-granules.[268–270] It has been speculated that this may represent a mechanism by which platelets not involved in clot formation may be able to return to a resting state.[271] The in vivo evidence supporting this unique platelet-inhibitory process is included in a paper describing the transfusion of plasma into an afibrinogenemic patient followed by the demonstration that platelet fibrinogen could be restored faster than new platelets could be produced in the bone marrow.[272]

NO is generated by endothelial cells and platelets from L-arginine in response to shear stress forces and other platelet agonists, such as thrombin and ADP. This molecule works to inhibit platelet activation through the cyclic guanosine monophosphate second messenger generated by guanylate cyclase activation. Endothelial NO synthase activity is enhanced during platelet activation, presumably as an additional means for limiting platelet aggregation. As detailed in the above section on regulation of platelet activation, a relatively recent new concept in platelet NO-cGMP pathway signaling concerns its biphasic nature with respect to platelet activation rather than what had previously been considered a strictly inhibitory role for many years.

Platelet junctional adhesion molecule A (JAM-A) is a member of the immunoglobulin superfamily of surface membrane proteins and is thought to prevent platelet aggregation through inactivation of integrin α$_{IIb}$β$_3$.[121] In quiescent platelets, it is phosphorylated and associates with α$_{IIb}$β$_3$ to allow recruitment of C-terminal Src kinase (Csk) that in turn regulates autoinhibition of c-Src, thus preventing c-Src-dependent phosphorylation and activation of α$_{IIb}$β$_3$. Mice deficient in JAM-A have hyperreactive platelets.[273]

Two members of the nuclear receptor subfamily 1 of transcription factors, FXR (farnesoid X receptor) and LXR (liver X receptor), and the associated RXR (retinoid X receptor), are expressed in platelets with the latter forming heterodimers with the other two.[274] These transcription factors have been found to play an interesting role in inhibition of platelet activation in that platelet stimulation with FXR, LXR, or RXR ligands inhibits both platelet aggregation and granule release.[274–276] Aggregation was impaired by inhibition of α$_{IIb}$β$_3$ integrin activation and outside-in signaling.[276] In mice platelet accumulation at vascular injury sites was likewise impaired by FXR and LXR ligand infusions.[274,275]

Platelet Secretion

The extent of secretion of α-, dense-, and lysosomal granule contents is dependent on the strength of the agonist, occurs in association with platelet activation, and is one of the many downstream consequences mediated by the activation of and transport to the internal leaflet of the plasma membrane of PKC. Granule contents that are involved in enhancing activation and aggregation of both their own and other platelets in the vicinity include ADP, vWF, fibrinogen, and calcium ions. Platelets contain three types of granules: dense granules contain agonists that amplify platelet activation, α granules contain proteins that enhance adhesion, and lysosomal granules contain glycosidases and proteases with largely unknown function.

The strongest responses a platelet can mount to agonist stimulation include activation, secretion, and aggregation. The granule secretory (release) phase is most readily documented in vitro by the "secondary wave" that denotes a second surge of aggregation activity of a fixed number of platelets in response to release of proaggregatory granule contents. These platelets are exposed to an agonist under the controlled in vitro conditions associated with platelet aggregation studies in which clinical defects in primary hemostasis due to platelet perturbations are further characterized. The secondary wave is typically seen best when the agonist is a weaker one, such as epinephrine, or is a relatively lower concentration of another relatively weak agonist, ADP. These two agonists require both cyclooxygenase activity and a primary wave of aggregation to induce secretion at low calcium concentrations.[277]

Although platelets are anucleate, they contain mRNA and are capable of synthesizing a restricted group of proteins mainly related to inflammation and apoptosis.[278,279] In addition to this, as described below in the section on platelet RNA transfer, microparticles, and miRNA transfer, vesicles are secreted from the membranes of stimulated platelets referred to as platelet microparticles that are enriched with specific membrane proteins that make them significantly procoagulant in settings such as heparin-induced thrombocytopenia, peripheral artery disease, and MI.[280]

Several studies suggest that the mechanism by which platelet granules (vesicles) fuse with the cell membrane to release their granule contents involves soluble *N*-ethylmaleimide-sensitive factor attachment protein (SNAP) receptor (SNARE) complexes that are formed between vesicle-associated membrane proteins (VAMPs; v-SNAREs) and proteins in the target membranes (different members of the syntaxin, SNAP-25, and VAMP gene families; t-SNAREs) in a lock-and-key form of docking.[281,282] Many lines of evidence show that these SNARE complexes are crucial for membrane trafficking and fusion events such as secretion and exocytosis. There is evidence that suggests the specific isoforms VAMP-3 and VAMP-8 form SNARE complexes with platelet syntaxin 4 and that these specific complexes mediate platelet secretion.[282,283] Simultaneous with the exocytosis of platelet granules, it is apparent that there is also inward (centripetal) movement of other intracellular contents, and this may play a role in transporting proaggregatory proteins away from the membrane surface and thus serve as another counterbalancing mechanism for limiting the extent of thrombus formation. Examples of this phenomenon include the internalization of fibrinogen from the surface of activated platelets, along with GPIIbIIIa receptors from the surface of resting and activated platelets, as noted earlier.[274]

PLATELET AGGREGATION: $\alpha_{IIb}\beta_3$ RECEPTOR AND ITS SIGNALING MECHANISMS

Platelet aggregation is a complex phenomenon that is the end result of a series of adhesion- and activation-related processes. The molecular mechanisms involved in platelet aggregation continue to be an area of very active research that also periodically reminds us that there is still much to be characterized about this important aspect of platelet function. Essential components of this process include an agonist, calcium, and the adhesive proteins, fibrinogen and vWF. Divalent cations, such as calcium and magnesium, are required for platelet aggregation in trace amounts, and these alter the specificity of the integrin $\alpha_{IIb}\beta_3$ for its ligands.[283] Fibrinogen and vWF play dominant roles in platelet aggregation through binding to $\alpha_{IIb}\beta_3$ and also by the ability of the former to generate polymerized fibrin as support for the platelets in a thrombus.[284,285] The multivalent nature of fibrinogen and vWF allows them to cross-link platelets on binding to $\alpha_{IIb}\beta_3$ on stimulated platelets to initiate platelet aggregation.

The molecular basis of integrin signaling that occurs in platelet $\alpha_{IIb}\beta_3$ is an integral part of thrombus formation and is important in understanding this process. GPIIb (α_{IIb}) and GPIIIa (β_3) were identified as the abnormal proteins present in patients with Glanzmann thrombasthenia in the 1970s.[286,287] They represent the most abundant receptor on the platelet surface. Like all integrin receptors, this complex is composed of noncovalently linked subunits. Each subunit is encoded by separate genes on the long arm of chromosome 17. Both subunits consist of a large extracellular domain and very short cytoplasmic domains, and together they form a heterodimer. Within their combined extracellular domains is the ligand-binding pocket, with surrounding subunit domains conferring specificity.[288] Equally important are the short cytoplasmic domains critical for transmembrane signaling. These domains act to anchor the receptor to the cytoskeletal elements.[289–291]

The signaling pathways of GP$\alpha_{IIb}\beta_3$ are complex and have been extensively studied (*Figure 19.8*). Central concepts of the signaling pathway include inside-out signaling, which involves the processes termed *affinity* and *avidity modulation*,[273,292] and outside-in signaling in which messages are transmitted to the inside of the platelet via the events occurring outside the membrane through $\alpha_{IIb}\beta_3$ activation. Knowledge regarding these complex pathways has been reviewed.[288,289,293]

Normally, undisturbed endothelium possesses nonthrombogenic properties that can inactivate activated coagulation factors, increase blood flow, inhibit platelet aggregation, and modulate fibrinolysis. Substances that inhibit platelet activation released by the endothelium

include PGI$_2$, NO, and ADPase. In addition, platelets release PGE$_2$ that acts to prevent its own activation. These molecules act via the Gs protein pathway that stimulates protein kinases to modulate various enzymes involved in platelet receptor $\alpha_{IIb}\beta_3$ activation.[293] They may also act to phosphorylate and inactivate various protein receptor agonists.[294,295]

Primary platelet agonists such as ADP, thrombin, and matrix proteins—collagen and vWF—affect platelet aggregation through a process known as *inside-out signaling*. This term denotes an integrin property that involves the binding action of agonists and extracellular matrix ligands to their receptors, leading to activation of numerous platelet functions, including the conformational change of $\alpha_{IIb}\beta_3$ to a high-affinity state, referred to as *affinity modulation*. The relative contribution of soluble and extracellular matrix stimuli to inside-out signaling likely varies with flow conditions and other factors related to vascular perturbation. For example, GPIb/V/IX function is most relevant under high-shear stress conditions such as those associated with arterioles and capillaries and in stenotic arteries. Ligand binding is initially reversible and later becomes irreversible in nature.[296] Therefore, one of the effects of inside-out signaling on $\alpha_{IIb}\beta_3$ is exposure of the fibrinogen-binding site through signal transduction involving the cytoplasmic domains (*Figure 19.8*).[294,297] Various regulatory intracellular or transmembrane proteins participate in this process. Overall, the data provide strong evidence that association between subunit cytoplasmic tails and possibly also between integrin subunit transmembrane domains works to maintain the $\alpha_{IIb}\beta_3$ complex in a resting nonadhesive conformation, and disruption of this state causes separation of the tails with consequent changes in the extracellular domains to increase $\alpha_{IIb}\beta_3$ affinity.[298,299] Evidence currently suggests that any role for extracellular or transmembrane molecules in affinity modulation is secondary to $\alpha_{IIb}\beta_3$ regulation by intracellular proteins, in particular a 270-kDa dimer named talin that interacts with the integrin cytoplasmic tail and a required integrin coactivator protein kindlin-3.[293,300] The complexity of the mechanisms by which inside-out signaling triggers $\alpha_{IIb}\beta_3$ activation is significant.[301,302]

Talin is a large protein that has been implicated as a trigger of integrin activation and binds to two sites in the β_3 cytoplasmic tail: the NPLY sequence in the midsegment of the cytoplasmic tail and a sequence in the membrane proximal region.[303] Its binding to the latter region may follow the former and may trigger separation of β_3 from the α_{IIb} cytoplasmic tail resulting in activation. Other proteins bind to the NPLY sequence and whether these function as coactivators or suppressors remains to be determined.[304,305] Talin must also be activated to accomplish this, and multiple activation pathways have been described. The small GTPase Rap1 is an important regulator of $\alpha_{IIb}\beta_3$ activation and is the integrating point of many platelet-activating signals.[121]

Avidity modulation, the less dominant action, acts to cluster the $\alpha_{IIb}\beta_3$ heterodimers into oligomers through lateral diffusion.[306,307] These conversions are critical in allowing $\alpha_{IIb}\beta_3$ to engage soluble adhesive ligands. These ligands contain the classical integrin recognition sequence RGD, Arg-Gly-Asp, which acts as a bridge between adjacent platelets allowing aggregation to proceed.[308] In addition, more $\alpha_{IIb}\beta_3$ translocates to the platelet surface membrane from the degranulating α-granule pool, where additional receptor is stored. These changes facilitate irreversible binding to fibrinogen. An important role for tyrosine kinase– and phosphatase-associated phosphorylation-dephosphorylation in integrin activation exists as assessed by the blockade of fibrinogen binding and platelet aggregation by enzyme inhibitors.[309,310]

After ligand binding occurs, a multitude of intracellular signals are generated that are collectively referred to as *outside-in signaling*. This "contact-dependent signaling" determines the extent to which platelets will spread on a vascular matrix and how resistant to detachment they are.[311,312] Outside-in signaling occurs in a discrete pattern in which ligand binding initiates integrin clustering and assembly of a "nascent" signaling complex proximal to the $\alpha_{IIb}\beta_3$ cytoplasmic tails, and this is followed by the growth of a larger "actin-based" signaling complex. It can be envisioned that the nascent complex is characterized

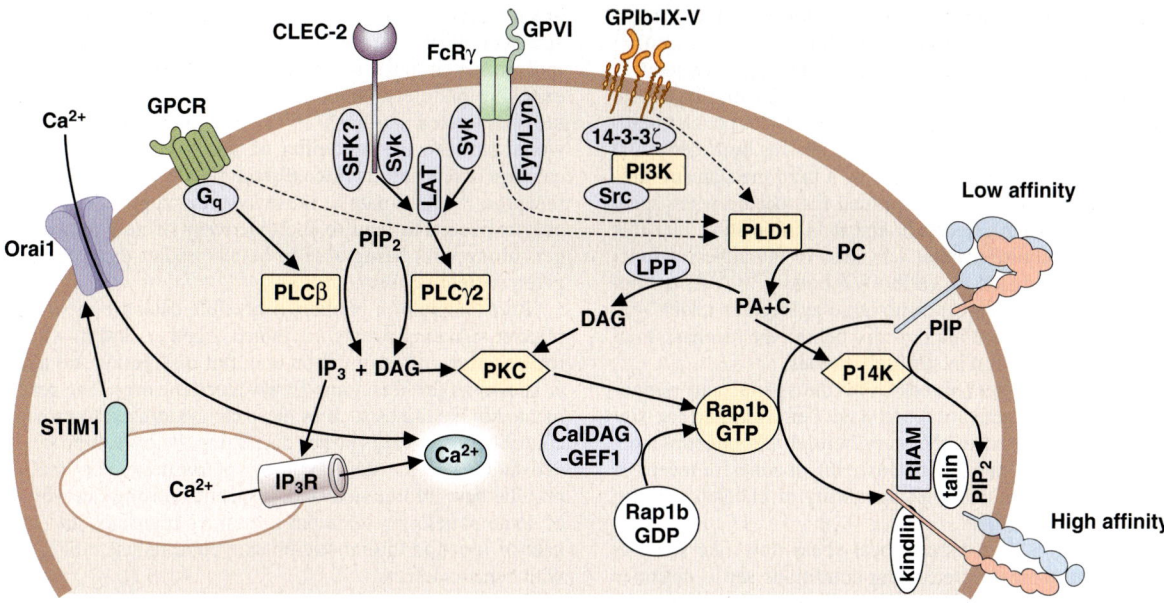

FIGURE 19.8 Common signaling mechanisms linking platelet receptors to integrin activation. The pathway how glycoprotein (GP)-Ib triggers direct integrin activation is poorly understood, but the involvement of phosphoinositol-3-kinase (PI3K) and phospholipase (PL) D1 has been proposed. Cross-linking of GPVI or C-type lectin receptor (CLEC-2) activates the immunoreceptor tyrosine-based activation motif (ITAM) signaling pathway leading to PLCγ2 activation, whereas stimulation of G protein–coupled receptors triggers PLCβ activation via the Gq pathway. Both PLC isoforms hydrolyze phosphatidylinositol-4,5-bisphosphate (PIP$_2$) to inositol-1,4,5-trisphosphate (IP$_3$) and diacylglycerol (DAG). IP$_3$ releases Ca^{2+} from the intracellular stores and in turn STIM1 opens Orai1 channels in the plasma membrane, a process called store-operated calcium entry. DAG activates protein kinase C (PKC), whereas elevated Ca^{2+} activates Ca^{2+} and diacylglycerol-regulated guanine nucleotide exchange factor I (CalDAG-GEF1) and, subsequently, Rap1b. Activation of Rap1b leads to recruitment of its effector, Rap1-GTP-interacting adaptor molecule (RIAM), and its binding partner, talin1, to the plasma membrane. This enables talin1 binding to the β$_3$ integrin tail and talin-induced activation of α$_{IIb}$β$_3$ integrin. Kindlin3 is equally essential for this process and interacts with the cytoplasmic tail of β integrins. The hypothetical involvement of PLD1 during integrin activation is depicted here as well. PLD1 becomes activated downstream of GPCRs, GPIb, and GPVI and hydrolyzes phosphatidylcholine (PC) to phosphatidic acid (PA) and choline (C). PA can be converted into DAG via lipid phosphate phosphatase-1 (LPP) and thereby stimulates PKC. In addition, PA activates phosphoinositol-4-phosphate kinase (PI4K), which converts phosphatidylinositol-4-phosphate (PIP) into PIP$_2$, which itself is required for talin1 recruitment to the plasma membrane. (Reprinted by permission from Springer: Stegner D, Nieswandt B. Platelet receptor signaling in thrombus formation. *J Mol Med.* 2011;89(2):109-121. Copyright © 2010 Springer-Verlag.)

temporally by (a) activation of Src kinases bound to the β$_3$ cytoplasmic tail by fibrinogen engaging and facilitating integrin clustering, then (b) recruitment and activation of Syk by Src, then (c) Src and/or Syk phosphorylation of various substrates, including adaptor proteins SLP-76 and c-Cbl along with the Rac GTPase Vav, and these substrates in turn act by participating in signaling to the actin cytoskeleton.[293] As the nascent complex assembles, many additional proteins are recruited that can influence actin reorganization, including Rac, the adaptor Nck, PAK, PI3-kinase, and VASP, an actin-bundling protein.[294] All these signaling events during platelet aggregation are further supported by release of granules induced by the binding of adhesive proteins to the extracellular domain of β$_3$. This complex series of events serve as a determinant of the final clot size.

Activation of α$_{IIb}$β$_3$ by agonists is very rapid, and the platelet can become fully competent to bind fibrinogen/vWF via the receptor within seconds after its initial encounter with agonist. Once full spreading and aggregation of platelets occurs, usually within several minutes, focal adhesion kinase is phosphorylated.[313–315] The PI3K system is activated once α$_{IIb}$β$_3$ is engaged, leading to generation of D3 phosphoinositides.[316] These proteins act to prevent the depolymerization of the actin cytoskeleton, with the result that the platelet aggregate is stabilized.[317] The end result of this outside-in signaling is a stable platelet clot.

In addition to outside-in signaling, following binding of fibrinogen to α$_{IIb}$β$_3$, one or more of a number of other events can be postulated to occur that facilitate platelet aggregation. These include the formation of a dimeric fibrinogen bridge between α$_{IIb}$β$_3$ receptors on adjacent platelets, conformational changes in bound fibrinogen and/or occupied α$_{IIb}$β$_3$, and additional interactions of bound receptor with cytoskeletal elements.[318–321]

Although fibrinogen is the dominant ligand, other RGD-containing peptides also bind to α$_{IIb}$β$_3$, including vWF, collagen, fibronectin, and vitronectin. Because vWF binds to GPIb/V/IX, it is close to α$_{IIb}$β$_3$ that may facilitate their interaction. Thus, α$_{IIb}$β$_3$ may also play a role in platelet adhesion, particularly in stabilizing cell-matrix interactions.[322] Other platelet membrane proteins have also been shown to associate with α$_{IIb}$β$_3$, including CD9 and Gas6,[323] and these may play a role in modulating α$_{IIb}$β$_3$ function. Not only does the α$_{IIb}$β$_3$ receptor have important roles with respect to platelet function, but it also affects coagulation and the inflammatory process. It acts to promote the formation of the prothrombinase complex[324] and mediates the adhesion of leukocytes to the platelet membrane and endothelium (i.e., vascular inflammation).[325–328] This receptor may also have a role in cell proliferation. In this respect, antagonists to α$_V$β$_3$ or to both α$_{IIb}$β$_3$ and α$_V$β$_3$ significantly inhibited intimal hyperplasia after vascular injury in all but one of at least 12 animal studies.[329]

Platelet Aggregation and Arterial Shear Flow

Platelet aggregation was once considered to be comparatively straightforward involving just α$_{IIb}$β$_3$ interacting with fibrinogen as described in the preceding paragraphs. With the ability to analyze in vivo platelet aggregate formation in real time, though, it has become apparent that this process is much more complex than previously thought. Platelet aggregation now appears to represent a series of adhesion reactions involving multiple receptors and adhesive ligands such as vWF, fibrinogen, and fibronectin with the contribution of individual receptor-ligand interactions dependent on prevailing blood flow conditions. It has been postulated that at least three distinct mechanisms can initiate aggregation with each mechanism working over a specific arterial shear range in vivo.[330] Under low-shear conditions (<1000/second) the predominant mechanism is thought to involve fibrinogen and $\alpha_{IIb}\beta_3$ exclusively, and this occurs independent of GPIb/vWF interaction.[331] Subsequent stimulation by locally generated soluble agonists induces platelet shape change and an increase in $\alpha_{IIb}\beta_3$ affinity for fibrinogen. At shear rates between 1000 and 10,000/second platelet-platelet interactions become more vWF dependent with roles for both GPIb and $\alpha_{IIb}\beta_3$ in promoting platelet aggregates. Now a third mechanism initiating platelet aggregation has been identified that occurs when shear rates are very high (>10,000/second), and it is interesting that this mechanism does not require platelet activation or the adhesive function of $\alpha_{IIb}\beta_3$ and is mediated by GPIb/vWF bonds.[289,332] This finding that nonactivated platelets can form large aggregates under very high shear may have important implications behind the mechanism of pathologic thrombus formation in stenosed arteries.

Advanced microscopy techniques show the spatial and temporal regulation of integrin activation and have demonstrated the signaling cascades are just part of the story behind this phenomenon. Coordination of the cytoskeleton with clustering of adhesive receptors and mediators of activation underlies the ability of platelets to form stable aggregates under shear stress.[121]

Presence of features that disrupt local shear flow like stenosis or aneurysms can exacerbate preexisting conditions set to optimize platelet recruitment and activation. These areas generate zones of fluid acceleration and deceleration.[333,334] Antiplatelet agents that block TXA_2 and ADP signaling pathways prevent shear-dependent aggregation that occurs in deceleration zones, which indicates that platelet activation is a necessary component of the deposition process.[333]

Aneurysms lead to flow disturbances often associated with intramural thrombi, and their presence is associated with distinct mechanisms such as release of degenerative enzymes, flow-induced hypoxia, and changes in wall stress distribution that further deteriorate local conditions.[335–337] These mechanisms lead to vessel wall weakening, which in turn leads to aneurysmal growth, rupture, and mortality.

Thus, collectively these studies suggest that flow disturbances affect platelet deposition and that platelet deposition in turn causes flow disturbances—this explains the existence of thrombus forming on top of atherosclerotic plaques, which in turn leads to events such as MI and strokes. Under conditions of significant nonphysiologic shear flow such as left ventricular assist and other such artificial devices, evidence suggests vWF fibers actually become resistant to tissue plasminogen activator and ADAMTS-13 and are capable of supporting platelet aggregation independent of platelet activation.[332,338]

PLATELET SIGNALING AS A GLOBAL INTERLINKED NETWORK

It is now clear that platelet signaling is best viewed as a heavily interlinked network rather than a series of linear, arrow-based signaling schema of pathways explaining cellular responses (*Figure 19.9*). The fact that platelet surface receptors in an activating environment are the recipients of simultaneous multiple agonists implies that these signaling pathways also act in synergy. This is because the interlinked and simultaneously activated platelet signaling pathways downstream from adhesion receptors and GPCRs are primarily driven by the extent of intracellular calcium rise as one of the main parameters.[339] Significant advances in platelet function screening have meant that the high-throughput technologies of pharmaceutical research have been harnessed to also shed more light on the signaling behind platelet function in the context of diagnosis of platelet disorders.[340] Flow cytometry is one technology that has been particularly useful in this regard.[341]

Systems approaches have also played a major role recently in platelet biology research, and these incorporate two aspects: a top-down approach in which the properties of intact and complex systems are modeled and a reductionist approach that involves modeling relatively few aspects of platelet signaling or function, but in greater detail.[121] As noted in the earlier section on regional platelet architecture, the former approach has recently led to better insight into how platelet thrombi contain a core of phosphatidylserine-exposing platelets surrounded by a more loosely packed and partially activated shell.[238,239,342] An example of the latter approach would involve the modeling of processes that regulate cytosolic calcium levels and its release from the dense tubular system via IP3 receptors.[343] Ultimately, these systems approaches can be reasonably expected to lead to the discovery of new antithrombotic targets along with being able to better predict thrombotic risk within given patient cohorts.

An example of a publicly accessible database in which molecular platelet signaling events are joined together, and in which biochemical reactions of coagulation and clot dissolution are also provided, is known as the Reactome (www.reactome.org). The reactions documented in databases such as these can be utilized to provide weighted contributions toward further discerning the overall process of platelet activation. These systems biology approaches are optimally situated to provide new information with respect to sorting out why dysfunction of some platelet proteins but not others translates into a bleeding or gain-of-function thrombotic phenotype in mouse models and humans with genetic defects.

ROLE OF CYTOSKELETAL REARRANGEMENT IN PLATELET ACTIVATION

Platelet activation is associated with significant changes in the actin cytoskeleton that initially support shape change followed by facilitating platelet spreading once they come into contact with adhesive surfaces like exposed subendothelial collagen or other platelets. The first events in shape change include pseudopodia formation to increase surface area, and this is mediated BY cytosolic calcium increase through Gq or G13 activation that couples to the small GTPase Rho. Rho in turn mediates activation of myosin light-chain kinase in order to facilitate cytoskeletal reorganization. This reorganization leads to relocalization of platelet granules and organelles to the platelet center, short-term filopodia formation, and sustained lamellipodia formation that enables secretion and spreading over the area of blood vessel damage.[344] Spreading is dependent on phospholipase C activation, intracellular calcium mobilization, and integrin $\alpha_{IIb}\beta_3$ activation. Rapid actin cytoskeleton reorganization is characterized by uncapping, severing, and nucleation of the actin filaments along with interaction with activated myosin II. These events are regulated by Rho GTPases, Rac, Cdc42, RhoA, VASP, and PKC.

PLATELET-CELL INTERACTIONS

Platelets and Endothelium

The mechanisms behind platelet interaction with vWF, collagen, and other subendothelial matrix molecules exposed as a result of damaged endothelium have been well studied and described in earlier sections of this chapter. In addition to these platelet–subendothelial interaction paradigms, evidence has emerged that circulating unactivated platelets have the capacity (as do neutrophils) to roll on intact activated endothelium in vivo and then reversibly adhere to it in a process that is dependent on endothelial cell expression of P-selectin.[345–348] This sequence of molecular interactions is a well-controlled multistep process involving platelet tethering and interaction of platelet P-selectin glycoprotein ligand-1 (PSGL-1) or GPIbα with endothelial P-selectin ("rolling"), followed by subsequent "firm adhesion" to the vascular wall mediated through β_3 integrins. GPIbα and PSGL-1 have structural similarities, including similar ligand-binding domains. P-selectin is also expressed on the surface of activated platelets and is an α-granule component in resting platelets. Endothelial P-selectin is rapidly expressed on the surface in response to inflammatory stimuli by translocating from membranes of storage granules (Weibel-Palade bodies) to the plasma membrane within seconds.

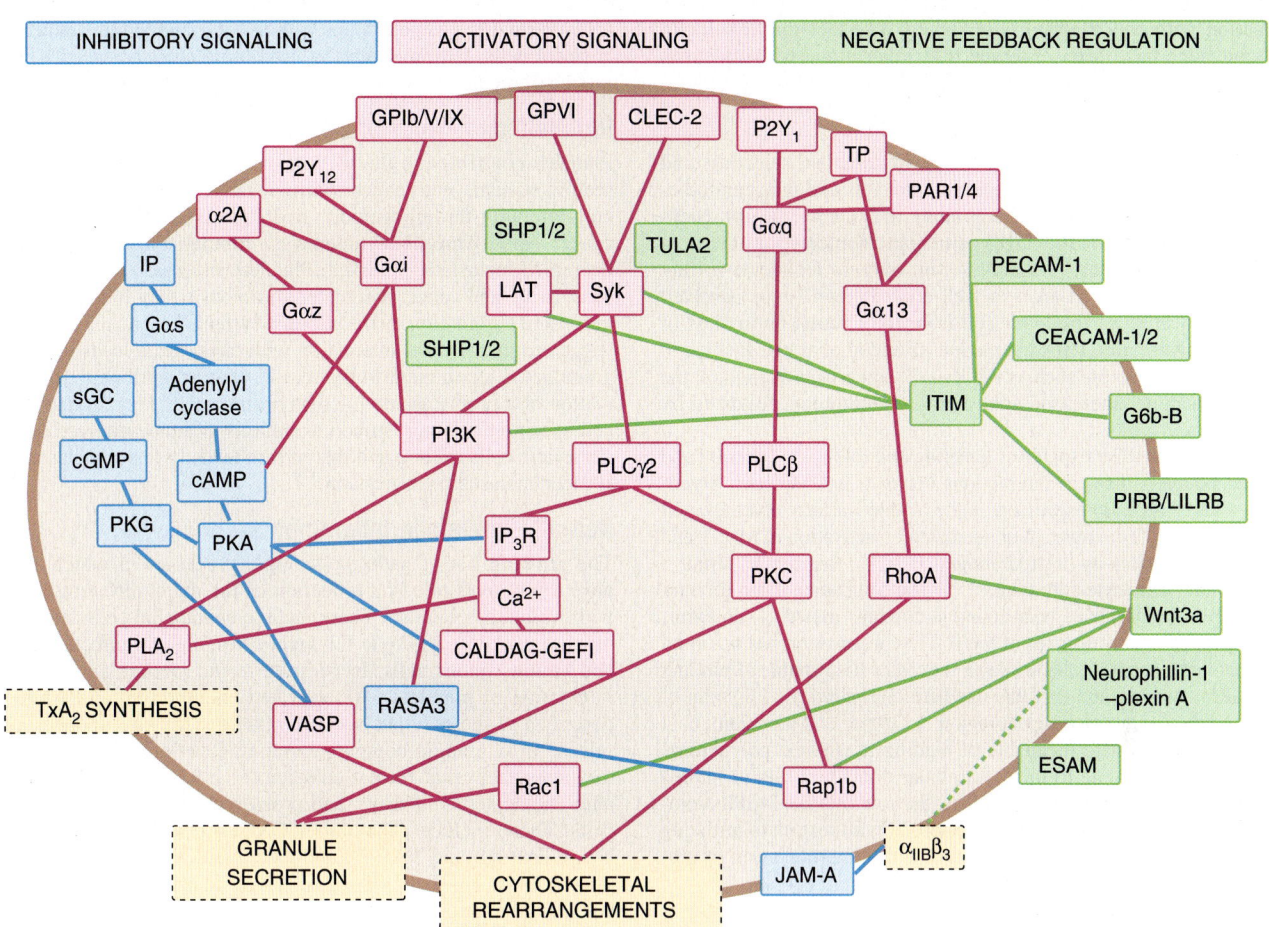

FIGURE 19.9 Complexity of platelet signaling networks. Platelet signaling models frequently describe signaling pathways activated by individual agonists; however, platelet signaling in vivo is highly complex and involves simultaneous activation by multiple agonists and negative regulators, which form a complex signaling network. Several key signaling molecules, that is, phospholipase C (PLC), protein kinase C (PKC), and phosphatidylinositide-3-kinase (PI3K), are common between the different pathways and form key nodes of platelet regulation. Blue boxes and lines represent mediators of inhibitory signaling that act to suppress platelet function in the absence of platelet activators in the healthy endothelium. Red boxes and lines represent mediators of activatory signaling following platelet activation by platelet agonists. Green boxes and lines represent mediators of negative feedback and inhibitory signaling that act to limit platelet activation following stimulation by platelet agonists. α_2A, adrenergic receptor; CALDAG-GEFI, Ca^{2+}-dependent Rap1 guanine nucleotide exchange factor; CEACAM-1/2, carcinoembryonic antigen cell adhesion molecule-1/2; CLEC-2, C-type lectin receptor 2; ESAM, endothelial cell-selective adhesion molecule; GP, glycoprotein; IP, prostaglandin receptor; IP_3R, inositol trisphosphate receptor; ITIM, immunoreceptor tyrosine-based inhibition motif; JAM-A, junctional adhesion molecule A; LAT, linker of activated T cells; PAR, protease-activated receptor; PECAM-1, platelet–endothelial cell adhesion molecule-1; PIRB, paired immunoglobulin-like receptor B; PKA, protein kinase A; PKG, protein kinase G; PLA_2, phospholipase A_2; sGC, soluble guanyl cyclase; TULA2, T-cell ubiquitin ligand-2; TXA_2, thromboxane A_2; VASP, vasodilator-stimulated phosphoprotein. (From Bye AP, Unsworth AJ, Gibbins JM. Platelet signaling: a complex interplay between inhibitory and activatory networks. *J Thromb Haemost.* 2016;14(5):918-930. http://creativecommons.org/licenses/by/4.0/)

As noted in an earlier section, there are multiple general mechanisms at play in inhibition of platelet activation that involve intact endothelium. It is increasingly recognized that inflammatory stimuli facilitate sustained platelet-endothelial interaction by perturbing these antiadhesion and activation mechanisms and increasing the surface expression of endothelial molecules. Adhesion of platelets to inflamed endothelium involves a similar coordinated multistep process as occurs in hemostasis and thrombosis, including platelet tethering, surface translocation, and firm adhesion.[349] In atherosclerosis, accumulation of modified oxidized lipoprotein particles in the setting of hyperlipidemia leads to surface expression of endothelial P- and E-selectin as well as endothelial vWF.[349,350]

Along with endothelial P-selectin, it is not surprising that vWF expressed on activated venous endothelium has also been implicated in platelet adhesion and translocation.[351] The precise nature of the relationships between these two endothelial cell molecules and the platelet-GPIb complex and the role different shear forces may play in determining which ligand GPIb may preferentially associate with remain to be determined. As noted in the section on "Platelet"

Aggregation and Arterial Shear Flow," aggregation is currently considered to consist of a series of adhesion reactions involving multiple receptors and adhesive ligands such as vWF, fibrinogen, and fibronectin with the contribution of individual receptor-ligand interactions dependent on prevailing blood flow conditions. Studies using intravital microscopy have confirmed that platelet-endothelium adhesion takes place even under high shear stress in vivo.[352,353] Platelets rolling on activated endothelium can be inhibited by both anti-P-selectin and anti-GPIbα antibodies, and this suggests that platelet-GPIb/V/IX mediates platelet adhesion to both the subendothelial matrix and the intact endothelium.[354] PSGL-1 on platelets has also been shown to mediate platelet rolling on the endothelial cell monolayer under high shear stress.[355]

Platelet firm adhesion to intact endothelial cells following rolling is a process dependent on $\alpha_{IIb}\beta_3$ bridging to endothelium that involves endothelial receptors such as $\alpha_V\beta_3$ and intercellular adhesion molecule (ICAM)-1 interacting with platelet-bound fibrinogen, fibronectin, and vWF.[326,347,356,357] This firm adhesion induces platelet surface P-selectin expression, and whether this selectin plays any role in their interaction with endothelium is unknown. The fact that P-selectin knockout mice have been observed to display impaired hemostasis suggests a potential role in this respect.[358]

Platelets and Immune Cells

In addition to the participation of the GPIb complex, selectins, and the β_3 integrin in the interaction between platelets and intact endothelium described earlier, these proteins along with the β_2 integrin receptor Mac-1 ($\alpha_M\beta_2$ or CD11b/CD18) participate in interactions between platelets and leukocytes.[359] Platelets contribute to leukocyte rolling and extravasation, which are two well-characterized steps involved in the translocation of the latter cell from the circulation to sites of infection.[360] Normally, after interaction of endothelial cell P-selectin with leukocyte receptors such as PSGL-1, β_2 integrin activation on the leukocyte mediates increased adhesion to endothelium, followed by extravasation.

Neutrophils are also capable of tethering and rolling on adherent and activated platelets through interactions between its P-selectin glycoprotein 1 and P-selectin expressed on the platelet surface, and they will subsequently display extravasation mediated by activation of Mac-1 and lymphocyte function–associated antigen 1 ($\alpha_L\beta_2$) that are required to mediate stable leukocyte adhesion.[361–363] The α subunits of certain integrins, such as Mac-1, have been found to contain "insert" (I) domains, homologous to the A_1 domain of vWF. This observation has taken on added interest since it has been shown that Mac-1 is capable of binding to the GPIb complex and that this interaction required the I domain of Mac-1 and the leucine-rich repeat region of GPIbα.[364] Mac-1 knockout mouse neutrophils were incapable of binding to isolated polypeptide fragments corresponding to the extracellular domain of GPIbα (called *glycocalicin*). For this reason and others, the role of Mac-1-GPIb complex interaction could turn out to be important with respect to initiating and propagating inflammation associated with the progression of atherosclerotic, purely thrombotic, or atherothrombotic processes.

Mac-1 has also been found to associate with other receptors of the platelet membrane, including the junctional adhesion molecule-3, ICAM-2, fibrinogen bound to $\alpha_{IIb}\beta_3$, and high-molecular-weight kininogen bound to GPIbα.[365–369] These associations have been characterized individually; however, their downstream signaling partners along with any coordinated actions that may exist between the ligand-receptor pairs in vivo remain to be determined. During this adhesive process, the association of platelet membrane PSGL-1 and Mac-1 stimulates the release of inflammatory cytokines from platelets, which in turn induces inflammatory cascades in monocytes.[370,371] This integrin, selectin, and cytokine-based set of coordinated reactions linking neutrophils, platelets, and monocytes lead to circulating activated platelets and platelet–white cell aggregates that promote formation of atherosclerotic lesions.[372]

Platelets have been found to contain mRNA transcripts for all TLR1 to TLR10 (Toll-like) receptors.[373,374] TLRs are pathogen-associated molecular pattern recognition receptors that have important roles regulating initiation of the innate immune response to foreign organisms. Platelets express functional TLR4, TLR2, and TLR9 and, in conjunction with their innate immune response and inflammation role, these can all also initiate concordant thrombotic responses of varying intensities.[375] Others mediate or alter interactions with neutrophils and trigger alpha-granule release.

In addition to the above platelet roles in innate immunity, platelets also participate in adaptive immunity through their interactions with and activation of dendritic cells (DCs).[376] Through the CD40-CD154 axis they can induce DCs to present antigens to T cells, and platelet/DC interaction can also be mediated through the P-selectin/PSGL1 axis.[377] This recruitment and activation of DCs is followed by their phagocytosis of the platelets.

Platelet-mediated immune activation described above differs from their hemostatic responses. Scanning electron micrographs of platelets alone versus with leukocytes point toward a distinct morphological shape change dependent on their function.[378] While thrombin-mediated platelet shape change involves conversion of the discoid shape to long, intertwined pseudopodia, TLR7 stimulation leads to smaller platelet groups with fewer pseudopodia connecting to adjacent cells. Different platelet activation levels are needed for formation of the hemostatic plug or recruitment of leukocytes.

Platelets and Metastatic Cells

Platelets contribute to the well-described increased thrombotic risk seen in patients with cancer with elevated platelet counts known to correlate with thrombogenicity and decreased survival in numerous cancer types. Thrombocytopenia by comparison is associated with decreased metastatic potential. Platelet/cancer cell interaction in the vasculature and cancer-associated thrombosis may block their recognition and elimination by the immune system. Recent animal data have suggested that platelet interaction with tumor cells leads to increased granulocyte recruitment to the tumor, which contributes to early formation of a prometastatic microenvironment.[379] Platelet depletion by cell-specific depleting antibodies inhibits granulocytic recruitment to metastatic cells in lung and this in turn leads to fewer metastases and reduced metastatic progression.[379]

Role of Platelets in Inflammation

The growing list of pathophysiologic processes in which platelets have a proposed role is a reflection of the many different cell types with which they interact. These include endothelial cells, neutrophils, monocytes, DCs, cytotoxic T lymphocytes, malaria-infected red cells, and various tumor cells. In addition to the mechanisms behind the interaction of platelets with activated endothelium and white cells described in the previous section, platelet activation induces a local release of α granule contents containing various potent inflammatory substances that further enhance the inflammatory response and alter chemotactic, adhesive, and proteolytic properties of endothelial cells. These include chemokines CXCL4 (PF-4), CXCL7 (PBP, β-TG, CTAP-III, and NAP-2), and CCL5 (RANTES), platelet-derived growth factor, IL-1β, CD40 ligand, TXA$_2$, leukotriene B$_4$, and platelet-activating factor.

The interaction between platelets, leukocytes, and the vascular wall can occur in various sequences.[380] First, platelets can form aggregates with leukocytes that promote leukocyte recruitment either by activating leukocyte adhesion receptors or by directly serving as a bridging molecule between leukocytes and the endothelium. When adhered to the vessel wall, platelets can attract leukocytes by releasing chemoattractants and providing an adhesive surface for leukocyte adhesion. Thus, platelets, leukocytes, and endothelial cells all become activated in a cascade-like fashion.

A key receptor-ligand interaction in these processes includes P-selectin and PSGL-1 (as noted earlier) that was initially found to be important in rolling interactions between leukocytes and the vessel wall and later found to be important in the recruitment of tissue factor bearing microparticles in thrombosis as well.[357,381] Using apolipoprotein E-deficient mice, it has been shown that platelet P-selectin plays a critical role in atherosclerosis by promoting leukocyte recruitment on atherosclerosis-prone endothelium.[382] Disruption of platelet/leukocyte interactions through genetic deficiency of P-selectin or anti-P-selectin antibodies decreases leukocyte recruitment and atherogenesis.[106,383]

A second key interaction involves platelet CD40 ligand, which is related to the tumor necrosis family, and CD40. Once on the activated platelet surface, CD40L increases the release of attractants for neutrophils and monocytes and triggers outside-in signaling by inducing $\alpha_{IIb}\beta_3$ phosphorylation and enhancing thrombus stability.[325,384] High levels of soluble CD40L are released from platelets in response to thrombosis that then functions as a primary platelet agonist in an autocrine loop with $\alpha_{IIb}\beta_3$ as the primary agonist receptor.

Platelet RNA Transfer, Microparticles, and miRNA Transfer

While communication between platelets, immune cells, and endothelial cells through receptor signaling, protein interactions, and released granule content has been long established, more recently other means of communication have been described including bidirectional RNA transcript transfer.[385] These experiments have included demonstration of bidirectional transfer of mRNA between endothelial and monocyte cell lines incubated with platelet-like particles along with in vivo transfer of platelet TLR2 mRNA to mice with TLR2-deficient mononuclear leukocytes.[385,386]

In addition to the resultant hemostatic and immune activation described in the above sections, platelet activation also leads to formation of microparticles that contain all the proteins related to their hemostatic and immune roles.[387] Platelet microparticle roles are protean and include such diverse examples as promotion of monocyte recruitment to atherosclerotic plaques, promotion of atherosclerosis progression in diabetes, and increased release in response to influenza and dengue.[375] In addition to containing proteins, platelet microparticles contain various forms of RNA including microRNA (miRNA), which are small, noncoding RNAs that function in posttranscriptional regulation of gene expression. Platelets are thus capable of affecting neighboring cells by microparticle miRNA transfer. Examples of this include thrombin-stimulated platelets releasing microparticles that in turn transfer miR-320b to endothelial cells with resultant decreased ICAM-1 expression,[388] miR-223 to cancer cells that leads to cancer progression,[389] and miR-24 to solid tumor cells that results in disrupted mitochondrial function, tumor cell death, and decreased proliferation.[390]

ROLE OF PLATELETS IN ATHEROGENESIS AND ATHEROTHROMBOSIS

Atherosclerosis is the major cause of vascular occlusive disorders such as coronary artery disease, stroke, and peripheral arterial disease. The instability associated with atherosclerotic plaque progression enhances vulnerability to disruption or ulceration, and this is associated with secondary deep vessel wall injury and thrombus formation.[391–393] Based on extensive laboratory and clinical experience, it is clear that platelet activation and aggregation play an integral role on two fronts: (a) in the cytokine-driven local inflammatory changes associated with plaque formation and growth, followed by (b) thrombus associated with plaque instability (rupture or ulceration) (*Figure 19.10*).

Platelets in Atherogenesis

The importance of the role of both arterial wall and systemic inflammation in atherogenesis and its later clinical manifestations, along with the molecular interface between inflammation and thrombosis, has been the subject of much attention in the literature.[394–396] An increased number of links between thrombosis and inflammatory mediators have been observed, and new roles for platelets in inflammation are now apparent.[397]

Many of the molecular players mediating leukocyte-endothelium interactions have also been found to play important roles coordinating leukocyte attachment and transmigration across layers of platelets adherent to injured vascular intima.[364,398] In addition, the binding of platelets to leukocytes influences important white cell effector responses, such as cell activation, signaling associated with integrin activation, and chemokine synthesis. Thus, it has become clear that inflammation is capable of leading to local thrombosis, and thrombosis is capable of initiating and propagating inflammation.

As noted in the section "Platelets and Endothelium," platelet adhesion to intact endothelium (as opposed to exposed subendothelium following vascular injury) has been well characterized using intravital microscopy and atherosclerosis animal models, and in some cases, adhesion has been shown to occur even before detectable atherosclerotic lesions are manifested.[116,399] Animal models have provided strong evidence linking platelets to early events of atherogenesis. An atherosclerosis mouse model lacking α_{IIb} exhibited substantial reduction in atherosclerotic lesion formation.[400] The importance of P-selectin in atherosclerosis lesion formation has been well described.[104,105,383] Similarly, platelets play a key role in recruitment of inflammatory effector myeloid and immune cells, including neutrophils, monocytes, and lymphocytes. Activated platelets interact with endothelial cells of inflamed

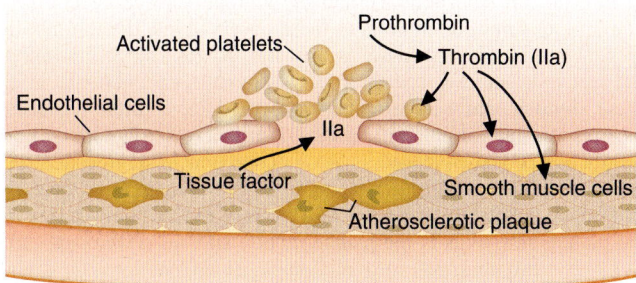

FIGURE 19.10 **Platelet adherence to the endothelium occurs at the site of vascular injury, often in an area of atherosclerosis.** Damage/erosion of the endothelial surface or rupture/ulceration of an underlying atherosclerotic plaque exposes subendothelial matrix to which platelets adhere and are activated. Tissue factor may also be present and result in the generation of thrombin (IIa). In addition, thrombin can be generated along the surface of activated platelets or released microparticle (not depicted). Thrombin, in turn, can elicit effects on platelets and endothelial or smooth muscle cells in the area. (From Wallace EL, Smyth SS. Targeting platelet thrombin receptor signaling to prevent thrombosis. *Pharmaceuticals (Basel)*. 2013;6(8):915-928. http://creativecommons.org/licenses/by/3.0/)

or atherosclerotic arteries and deposit platelet-derived cytokines such as chemokine (C-C motif) ligand 5 (CCL5) or chemokine (C-X-C motif) ligand 4 (CXCL4) onto the surface of endothelial cells that in turn facilitates leukocyte recruitment into the lesions.[401] Platelet-leukocyte aggregates are in fact an independent risk factor for atherothrombotic disease and promote atherogenesis in mouse models.[106] Platelet-leukocyte interactions could potentially impact atherosclerosis and atherothrombosis by modulating NETosis ("neutrophil extracellular traps" that promote venous and arterial thrombosis in animal models) since this appears to require P-selectin/P-selectin glycoprotein ligand 1 interaction.[402,403] Thus, activated platelets could potentially promote atherosclerosis through facilitating NET generation.

Platelet adhesion has been found to activate endothelial cell nuclear factor-κB (NF-κB) and its regulated genes, many of which play key roles in platelet-leukocyte-endothelium-extracellular matrix molecular events that support inflammatory and proatherogenic phenotypes. This includes events that contribute to lesion maturation such as smooth muscle cell and fibroblast proliferation and promotion of collagen synthesis.[404–406] Inhibition of COX-1, an enzyme with expression restricted to platelets, in turn inhibited lesion formation in an atherosclerosis mouse model.[407] Another atherosclerosis mouse model demonstrated that prolonged antibody blockade of GPIbα leads to reduced arterial leukocyte accumulation in carotid arterial intima and subsequent reduced atherosclerosis lesion formation.[106] This suggests that vWF may also have a role in atherogenesis.[408]

In contrast to animal data, conclusions regarding the role of human platelets in atherogenesis are not nearly as extensive. Mouse data cannot be unequivocally applied to humans because mouse platelets differ from human with respect to expression levels of certain surface receptors. Systemic platelet activation in humans has been described in a variety of atherosclerosis disease presentations. However, antiplatelet agents have not been found to influence disease progression when applied in the secondary disease prevention setting in humans in whom atherosclerosis is likely advanced, as opposed to the possibly preventable progression of early lesions that are present before an initial atherosclerosis clinical event.[349] With respect to the role of NF-κB noted in the preceding paragraph, one study of patients revealed a marked elevation of NF-κB in those with unstable as compared with stable angina.[409]

The Normal Hematologic System

Platelets in Atherothrombosis

The interior of intact atherosclerotic plaques is rich in components that are highly thrombogenic (e.g., collagen types I and III, fibrinogen/fibrin, thrombospondin), and the luminal surface is relatively nonthrombogenic. In contrast to these observations, the thrombotic response to plaque disruption is dynamic. In this respect, thrombosis, repeat thrombosis, and thrombolysis along with embolization all occur simultaneously in many patients with ACS, and this is considered responsible for intermittent flow obstructions.[410] The initial flow obstruction is acknowledged as being due to platelet aggregation, but subsequent fibrin stabilization is important to the longevity of the early and fragile platelet thrombus.[411] As a result of reduced flow caused by the platelet thrombus at the plaque-rupture site, an erythrocyte- and fibrin-rich thrombus may form and propagate up and down the artery in both directions.[410]

Normally, blood flow is laminar with adjacent fluid layers traveling parallel to each other but at different velocities due to fluid drag exerted by the vessel wall and this leads to shear forces between adjacent fluid planes. However, at arterial branch points, curvatures, and areas of stenosis, these flow profiles develop alterations leading to shear gradients, turbulence, flow separation, and eddy formation, and these will influence atherogenesis. Progression of the lesion exacerbates these flow disturbances, and so a dangerous cycle of shear-dependent atherosclerosis acceleration can occur.[412] The rate of fluctuation in blood flow has been quoted as the major parameter altering endothelial function, and, as such, cell function responds to flow changes through a variety of mechanotransduction mechanisms.[413] These mechanosensory signaling mechanisms are very sensitive to changes in wall shear stress leading to alterations in cell morphology, gene expression profiles, and increased adhesiveness. Thus, at high shear rates as occurs in stenosed atherosclerotic arteries (>5000/second), shear will directly induce platelet activation and aggregation as noted in the section "Platelet Aggregation and Arterial Shear Flow," and recent evidence suggests this can occur independently of ADP and TXA_2, which implies shear gradients can promote platelet deposition and initial thrombus growth even in the presence of aspirin and a $P2Y_{12}$ inhibitor.[414]

There is evidence that alteration of the endothelium such as may occur with early atherogenesis (particularly when under the influence of atherosclerosis risk factors) or plaque disruption may cause the endothelium to generate more mediators that enhance constriction, such as endothelin-1, and fewer mediators that enhance dilation, such as PGI_2 and NO.[411,415–417] Coronary angioplasty data collected at the time of ACS have shown that transient vasoconstriction often accompanies plaque disruption or fissuring, and thrombosis.[418] This vasoconstriction occurs with significant vessel wall damage and is dependent on both platelets and thrombin, with platelet dependence shown to be mediated by serotonin and TXA_2.[418,419]

References

1. Agbanyo FR, Sixma JJ, de Groot PG, Languino LR, Plow EF. Thrombospondin–platelet interactions. Role of divalent cations, wall shear rate, and platelet membrane glycoproteins. *J Clin Invest.* 1993;92:288-296.
2. Hindriks G, Ijsseldijk MJ, Sonnenberg A, Sixma JJ, de Groot PG. Platelet adhesion to laminin: role of Ca^{2+} and Mg^{2+} ions, shear rate, and platelet membrane glycoproteins. *Blood.* 1992;79:928-935.
3. Nievelstein PF, D'Alessio PA, Sixma JJ. Fibronectin in platelet adhesion to human collagen types I and III. Use of nonfibrillar and fibrillar collagen in flowing blood studies. *Arteriosclerosis.* 1988;8:200-206.
4. Savage B, Saldivar E, Ruggeri ZM. Initiation of platelet adhesion by arrest onto fibrinogen or translocation on von Willebrand factor. *Cell.* 1996;84:289-297.
5. Savage B, Almus-Jacobs F, Ruggeri ZM. Specific synergy of multiple substrate–receptor interactions in platelet thrombus formation under flow. *Cell.* 1998;94:657-666.
6. Bonnefoy A, Harsfalvi J, Pfliegler G, Fauvel-Lafève F, Legrand C. The subendothelium of the HMEC-1 cell line supports thrombus formation in the absence of von Willebrand factor and collagen types I, III and VI. *Thromb Haemost.* 2001;85:552-559.
7. Houdijk WP, Sakariassen KS, Nievelstein PF, Sixma JJ. Role of factor VIII–von Willebrand factor and fibronectin in the interaction of platelets in flowing blood with monomeric and fibrillar human collagen types I and III. *J Clin Invest.* 1985;75:531-540.
8. Moroi M, Jung SM, Shinmyozu K, Tomiyama Y, Ordinas A, Diaz-Ricart M. Analysis of platelet adhesion to a collagen-coated surface under flow conditions: the involvement of glycoprotein VI in the platelet adhesion. *Blood.* 1996;88:2081-2092.
9. Turitto VT, Weiss HJ, Zimmerman TS, Sussman,. Factor VIII/von Willebrand factor in subendothelium mediates platelet adhesion. *Blood.* 1985;65:823-831.
10. Denis C, Methia N, Frenette PS, et al. A mouse model of severe von Willebrand disease: defects in hemostasis and thrombosis. *Proc Natl Acad Sci U S A.* 1998;95:9524-9529.
11. Beumer S, IJsseldijk MJ, de Groot PG, Sixma JJ. Platelet adhesion to fibronectin in flow: dependence on surface concentration and shear rate, role of platelet membrane glycoproteins GP IIb/IIIa and VLA-5, and inhibition by heparin. *Blood.* 1994;84:3724-3733.
12. Kroll MH, Hellums JD, McIntire LV, Schafer AI, Moake JL. Platelets and shear stress. *Blood.* 1996;88:1525-1541.
13. Beumer S, Heijnen HF, IJsseldijk MJ, Orlando E, de Groot PG, Sixma JJ. Platelet adhesion to fibronectin in flow: the importance of von Willebrand factor and glycoprotein Ib. *Blood.* 1995;86:3452-3460.
14. Sakariassen KS, Nievelstein PF, Coller BS, Sixma JJ. The role of platelet membrane glycoproteins Ib and IIb-IIIa in platelet adherence to human artery subendothelium. *Br J Haematol.* 1986;63:681-691.
15. Barnes MJ, Farndale RW. Collagens and atherosclerosis. *Exp Gerontol.* 1999;34:513-525.
16. Ni H, Yuen PS, Papalia JM, et al. Plasma fibronectin promotes thrombus growth and stability in injured arterioles. *Proc Natl Acad Sci U S A.* 2003;100:2415-2419.
17. Fredrickson BJ, Dong JF, McIntire LV, Lopez JA. Shear-dependent rolling on von Willebrand factor of mammalian cells expressing the platelet glycoprotein Ib-IX-V complex. *Blood.* 1998;92:3684-3693.
18. Cranmer SL, Ulsemer P, Cooke BM, et al. Glycoprotein (GP) Ib-IX-transfected cells roll on a von Willebrand factor matrix under flow. Importance of the GPIb/actin-binding protein (ABP-280) interaction in maintaining adhesion under high shear. *J Biol Chem.* 1999;274:6097-6106.
19. Tsuji S, Sugimoto M, Miyata S, Kuwahara M, Kinoshita S, Yoshioka A. Real-time analysis of mural thrombus formation in various platelet aggregation disorders: distinct shear-dependent roles of platelet receptors and adhesive proteins under flow. *Blood.* 1999;94:968-975.
20. Roth GJ. Developing relationships: arterial platelet adhesion, glycoprotein Ib, and leucine-rich glycoproteins. *Blood.* 1991;77:5-19.
21. Berndt MC, Gregory C, Kabral A, Zola H, Fournier D, Castaldi PA. Purification and preliminary characterization of the glycoprotein Ib complex in the human platelet membrane. *Eur J Biochem.* 1985;151:637-649.
22. Du X, Beutler L, Ruan C, Castaldi PA, Berndt MC. Glycoprotein Ib and glycoprotein IX are fully complexed in the intact platelet membrane. *Blood.* 1987;69:1524-1527.
23. Modderman PW, Admiraal LG, Sonnenberg A, von dem Borne AE. Glycoproteins V and Ib-IX form a noncovalent complex in the platelet membrane. *J Biol Chem.* 1992;267:364-369.
24. Ruggeri ZM. Structure and function of von Willebrand factor. *Thromb Haemost.* 1999;82:576-584.
25. Miyata S, Goto S, Federici AB, Ware J, Ruggeri ZM. Conformational changes in the A1 domain of von Willebrand factor modulating the interaction with platelet glycoprotein Ibα. *J Biol Chem.* 1996;271:9046-9053.
26. Siedlecki CA, Lestini BJ, Kottke-Marchant KK, Eppell SJ, Wilson DL, Marchant RE. Shear-dependent changes in the three-dimensional structure of human von Willebrand factor. *Blood.* 1996;88:2939-2950.
27. Peterson DM, Stathopoulos NA, Giorgio TD, Hellums JD, Moake JL. Shear-induced platelet aggregation requires von Willebrand factor and platelet membrane glycoproteins Ib and IIb-IIIa. *Blood.* 1987;69:625-628.
28. Berndt MC, Shen Y, Dopheide SM, Gardiner EE, Andrews RK. The vascular biology of the glycoprotein Ib-IX-V complex. *Thromb Haemost.* 2001;86:178-188.
29. Moake JL, Turner NA, Stathopoulos NA, Nolasco L, Hellums JD. Shear-induced platelet-aggregation can be mediated by vWF released from platelets, as well as by exogenous large or unusually large vWF multimers, requires adenosine-diphosphate, and is resistant to aspirin. *Blood.* 1988;71:1366-1374.
30. Mazzucato M, Pradella P, Cozzi MR, De Marco L, Ruggeri ZM. Sequential cytoplasmic calcium signals in a 2-stage platelet activation process induced by the glycoprotein Ibα mechanoreceptor. *Blood.* 2002;100:2793-2800.
31. Nesbitt WS, Kulkarni S, Giuliano S, et al. Distinct glycoprotein Ib/V/IX and integrin $\alpha_{IIb}\beta_2$-3-dependent calcium signals cooperatively regulate platelet adhesion under flow. *J Biol Chem.* 2002;277:2965-2972.
32. Marchese P, Murata M, Mazzucato M, et al. Identification of three tyrosine residues of glycoprotein Ibα with distinct roles in von Willebrand factor and α-thrombin binding. *J Biol Chem.* 1995;270:9571-9578.
33. Dong JF, Hyun W, Lopez JA. Aggregation of mammalian cells expressing the platelet glycoprotein (GP) Ib-IX complex and the requirement for tyrosine sulfation of GP Ibα. *Blood.* 1995;86:4175-4183.
34. Murata M, Ware J, Ruggeri ZM. Site-directed mutagenesis of a soluble recombinant fragment of platelet glycoprotein Ibα demonstrating negatively charged residues involved in von Willebrand factor binding. *J Biol Chem.* 1991;266:15474-15480.
35. Miller JL, Cunningham D, Lyle VA, Finch CN. Mutation in the gene encoding the α chain of platelet glycoprotein Ib in platelet-type von Willebrand disease. *Proc Natl Acad Sci U S A.* 1991;88:4761-4765.
36. Celikel R, McClintock RA, Roberts JR, et al. Modulation of alpha-thrombin function by distinct interactions with platelet glycoprotein Ibα. *Science.* 2003;301:218.
37. Dumas JJ, Kumar R, Seehra J, Somers WS, Mosyak L. Crystal structure of the GpIbα-thrombin complex essential for platelet aggregation. *Science.* 2003;301:222.

38. Shen Y, Romo GM, Dong JF, et al. Requirement of leucine-rich repeats of glycoprotein (GP) Ibα for shear-dependent and static binding of von Willebrand factor to the platelet membrane GP Ib-IX-V complex. *Blood.* 2000;95:903-910.
39. Berndt MC, Phillips DR. Interaction of thrombin with platelets: purification of the thrombin substrate. *Ann N Y Acad Sci.* 1981;370:87-95.
40. Estevez B, Kim K, Delaney MK, et al. Signaling-mediated cooperativity between glycoprotein Ib-IX and protease-activated receptors in thrombin-induced platelet activation. *Blood.* 2016;127:626-636.
41. Ware J, Russell S, Ruggeri ZM. Generation and rescue of a murine model of platelet dysfunction: the Bernard-Soulier syndrome. *Proc Natl Acad Sci U S A.* 2000;97:2803-2808.
42. Coughlin SR. Protease-activated receptors in vascular biology. *Thromb Haemost.* 2001;86:298-307.
43. Robinson K, Jones D, Patel Y, et al. Mechanism of inhibition of protein kinase C by 14-3-3 isoforms. *Biochem J.* 1994;299:853-861.
44. Muslin AJ, Tanner JW, Allen PM, Shaw AS. Interaction of 14-3-3 with signaling proteins is mediated by the recognition of phosphoserine. *Cell.* 1996;84:889-897.
45. Morrison D. 14-3-3: modulators of signaling proteins? *Science.* 1994;266:56-57.
46. Andrews RK, Harris SJ, McNally T, Berndt MC. Binding of purified 14-3-3ζ signaling protein to discrete amino acid sequences within the cytoplasmic domain of the platelet membrane glycoprotein Ib-IX-V complex. *Biochemistry.* 1998;37:638-647.
47. Calverley DC, Kavanagh TJ, Roth GJ. Human signaling protein 14-3-3ζ interacts with platelet glycoprotein Ib subunits Ibα and Ibβ. *Blood.* 1998;91:1295-1303.
48. Feng S, Christodoulides N, Resendiz JC, Berndt MC, Kroll MH. Cytoplasmic domains of GpIbα and GpIbβ regulate 14-3-3ζ binding to GpIb/IX/V. *Blood.* 2000;95:551-557.
49. Gu M, Xi X, Englund GD, Berndt MC, Du X. Analysis of the roles of 14-3-3 in the platelet glycoprotein Ib-IX-mediated activation of integrin $\alpha_{II}b\beta_{2}3$ using a reconstituted mammalian cell expression model. *J Cell Biol.* 1999;147:1085-1096.
50. Munday AD, Berndt MC, Mitchell CA. Phosphoinositide 3-kinase forms a complex with platelet membrane glycoprotein Ib-IX-V complex and 14-3-3ζ. *Blood.* 2000;96:577-584.
51. Lopez JA. The platelet glycoprotein Ib-IX complex. *Blood Coagul Fibrinolysis.* 1994;5:97-119.
52. Kasirer-Friede A, Ware J, Leng LJ, Marchese P, Ruggeri ZM, Shattil SJ. Lateral clustering of platelet GP Ib-IX complexes leads to up-regulation of the adhesive function of integrin $\alpha_{II}b\beta_{2}3$. *J Biol Chem.* 2002;277:11949-11956.
53. Yap CL, Anderson KE, Hughan SC, Dopheide SM, Salem HH, Jackson SP. Essential role for phosphoinositide 3-kinase in shear-dependent signaling between platelet glycoprotein Ib/V/IX and integrin $\alpha_{II}b\beta_{2}3$. *Blood.* 2002;99:151-158.
54. Feng S, Resendiz JC, Lu X, Kroll MH. Filamin binding to the cytoplasmic tail of glycoprotein Ibα regulates von Willebrand factor-induced platelet activation. *Blood.* 2003;102:2122-2129.
55. Wu Y, Asazuma N, Satoh K, et al. Interaction between von Willebrand factor and glycoprotein Ib activates Src kinases in human platelets: the role of phosphoinositide 3-kinase. *Blood.* 2003;101:3469-3476.
56. Santoro SA, Walsh JJ, Staatz WD, Baranski KJ. Distinct determinants on collagen support $\alpha_{2}2\beta_{2}1$ integrin-mediated platelet adhesion and platelet activation. *Cell Regul.* 1991;2:905-913.
57. Moroi M, Jung SM. Platelet receptors for collagen. *Thromb Haemost.* 1997;78:439-444.
58. Ryo R, Yoshida A, Sugano W, et al. Deficiency of P62, a putative collagen receptor, in platelets from a patient with defective collagen-induced platelet aggregation. *Am J Hematol.* 1992;39:25-31.
59. Morton LF, Hargreaves PG, Farndale RW, Young RD, Barnes MJ. Integrin $\alpha_{2}2\beta_{2}1$-independent activation of platelets by simple collagen-like peptides: collagen tertiary (triple-helical) and quaternary (polymeric) structures are sufficient alone for $\alpha_{2}2\beta_{2}1$-independent platelet reactivity. *Biochem J.* 1995;306:337-344.
60. Gibbins J, Asselin J, Farndale R, Barnes M, Law CL, Watson SP. Tyrosine phosphorylation of the Fc receptor γ-chain in collagen-stimulated platelets. *J Biol Chem.* 1996;271:18095-18099.
61. Asselin J, Gibbins JM, Achison M, et al. A collagen-like peptide stimulates tyrosine phosphorylation of Syk and phospholipase Cγ2 in platelets independent of the integrin $\alpha_{2}2\beta_{2}1$. *Blood.* 1997;89:1235-1242.
62. Gibbins JM, Okuma M, Farndale R, Barnes M, Watson SP. Glycoprotein VI is the collagen receptor in platelets which underlies tyrosine phosphorylation of the Fc receptor γ-chain. *FEBS Lett.* 1997;413:255-259.
63. Ichinohe T, Takayama H, Ezumi Y, Yanagi S, Yamamura H, Okuma M. Cyclic AMP-insensitive activation of c-Src and Syk protein-tyrosine kinases through platelet membrane glycoprotein VI. *J Biol Chem.* 1995;270:28029-28036.
64. Polgar J, Clemetson JM, Kehrel BE, et al. Platelet activation and signal transduction by convulxin, a C-type lectin from *Crotalus durissus terrificus* (tropical rattlesnake) venom via the p62/GPVI collagen receptor. *J Biol Chem.* 1997;272:13576-13583.
65. Arai M, Yamamoto N, Moroi M, Akamatsu N, Fukutake K, Tanoue K. Platelets with 10% of the normal amount of GPVI have an impaired response to collagen that results in a mild bleeding tendency. *Br J Haematol.* 1995;89:124-130.
66. Ichinohe T, Takayama H, Ezumi Y, et al. Collagen-stimulated activation of syk but not c-src is severely compromised in human platelets lacking membrane glycoprotein VI. *J Biol Chem.* 1997;272:63-68.
67. Clemetson JM, Polgar J, Magnenat E, Wells TN, Clemetson KJ. The platelet collagen receptor glycoprotein VI is a member of the immunoglobulin superfamily closely related to FcαR and the natural killer receptors. *J Biol Chem.* 1999;274:29019-29024.
68. Ruggeri ZM, Mendolicchio GL. Adhesion mechanisms in platelet function. *Circ Res.* 2007;100:1673-1685.
69. Mangin P, Yap CL, Nonne C, et al. Thrombin overcomes the thrombosis defect associated with platelet GPVI/FcRgamma deficiency. *Blood.* 2006;107:4346-4353.
70. Dubois C, Panicot-Dubois L, Merrill-Skoloff G, Furie B, Furie BC. Glycoprotein VI-dependent and -independent pathways of thrombus formation in vivo. *Blood.* 2006;107:3902-3906.
71. Staatz WD, Rajpara SM, Wayner EA, Carter WG, Santoro SA. The membrane glycoprotein Ia-IIa (VLA-2) complex mediates the Mg^{++}-dependent adhesion of platelets to collagen. *J Cell Biol.* 1989;108:1917-1924.
72. Springer TA. Folding of the N-terminal, ligand-binding region of integrin α-subunits into a β-propeller domain. *Proc Natl Acad Sci U S A.* 1997;94:65-72.
73. Lahav J, Gofer-Dadosh N, Luboshitz J, Hess O, Shaklai M. Protein disulfide isomerase mediates integrin-dependent adhesion. *FEBS Lett.* 2000;475:89-92.
74. Miura Y, Ohnuma M, Jung SM, Moroi M. Cloning and expression of the platelet-specific collagen receptor glycoprotein VI. *Thromb Res.* 2000;98:301-309.
75. Varga-Szabo D, Pleines I, Nieswandt B. Cell adhesion mechanisms in platelets. *Arterioscler Thromb Vasc Biol.* 2008;28:403-412.
76. Clemetson KJ, McGregor JL, James E, Dechavanne M, Lüscher EF. Characterization of the platelet membrane glycoprotein abnormalities in Bernard-Soulier syndrome and comparison with normal by surface-labeling techniques and high-resolution two-dimensional gel electrophoresis. *J Clin Invest.* 1982;70:304-311.
77. Jandrot-Perrus M, Busfield S, Lagrue AH, et al. Cloning, characterization, and functional studies of human and mouse glycoprotein VI: a platelet-specific collagen receptor from the immunoglobulin superfamily. *Blood.* 2000;96:1798-1807.
78. Ezumi Y, Uchiyama T, Takayama H. Molecular cloning, genomic structure, chromosomal localization, and alternative splice forms of the platelet collagen receptor glycoprotein VI. *Biochem Biophys Res Commun.* 2000;277:27-36.
79. Tsuji M, Ezumi Y, Arai M, Takayama H. A novel association of Fc receptor γ-chain with glycoprotein VI and their co-expression as a collagen receptor in human platelets. *J Biol Chem.* 1997;272:23528-23531.
80. Nieswandt B, Bergmeier W, Schulte V, Rackebrandt K, Gessner JE, Zirngibl H. Expression and function of the mouse collagen receptor glycoprotein VI is strictly dependent on its association with the FcRγ chain. *J Biol Chem.* 2000;275:23998-24002.
81. Kehrel B, Wierwille S, Clemetson KJ, et al. Glycoprotein VI is a major collagen receptor for platelet activation: it recognizes the platelet-activating quaternary structure of collagen, whereas CD36, glycoprotein IIb/IIIa, and von Willebrand factor do not. *Blood.* 1998;91:491-499.
82. Kato K, Kanaji T, Russell S, et al. The contribution of glycoprotein VI to stable platelet adhesion and thrombus formation illustrated by targeted gene deletion. *Blood.* 2003;102:1701-1707.
83. Massberg S, Gawaz M, Gruner S, et al. A crucial role of glycoprotein VI for platelet recruitment to the injured arterial wall in vivo. *J Exp Med.* 2003;197:41-49.
84. Schulte V, Rabie T, Prostredna M, Aktas B, Grüner S, Nieswandt B. Targeting of the collagen-binding site on glycoprotein VI is not essential for in vivo depletion of the receptor. *Blood.* 2003;101:3948-3952.
85. Smethurst PA, Joutsi-Korhonen L, O'Connor MN, et al. Identification of the primary collagen-binding surface on human glycoprotein VI by site-directed mutagenesis and by a blocking phage antibody. *Blood.* 2004;103:903-911.
86. Chen JC, Diacovo TG, Grenache DG, Santoro SA, Zutter MM. The $\alpha_{2}2$ integrin subunit-deficient mouse—a multifaceted phenotype including defects of branching morphogenesis and hemostasis. *Am J Pathol.* 2002;161:337-344.
87. Nieswandt B, Schulte V, Bergmeier W, et al. Long-term antithrombotic protection by in vivo depletion of platelet glycoprotein VI in mice. *J Exp Med.* 2001;193:459-469.
88. Nieswandt B, Brakebusch C, Bergmeier W, et al. Glycoprotein VI but not $\alpha_{2}2\beta_{2}1$ integrin is essential for platelet interaction with collagen. *EMBO J.* 2001;20:2120-2130.
89. Kuijpers MJE, Schulte V, Bergmeier W, et al. Complementary roles of platelet glycoprotein VI and integrin $\alpha_{2}2\beta_{2}1$ in collagen-induced thrombus formation in flowing whole blood ex vivo. *FASEB J.* 2003;17:U372-U394.
90. Kahn ML, Diacovo TG, Bainton DF, Lanza F, Trejo J, Coughlin SR. Glycoprotein V-deficient platelets have undiminished thrombin responsiveness and do not exhibit a Bernard-Soulier phenotype. *Blood.* 1999;94:4112-4121.
91. Ramakrishnan V, Reeves PS, DeGuzman F, et al. Increased thrombin responsiveness in platelets from mice lacking glycoprotein V. *Proc Natl Acad Sci U S A.* 1999;96:13336-13341.
92. Locke D, Chen H, Liu Y, Liu C, Kahn M. Lipid rafts orchestrate signaling by the platelet receptor glycoprotein VI. *J Biol Chem.* 2002;277:18801-18809.
93. Myung PS, Boerthe NJ, Koretzky GA. Adapter proteins in lymphocyte antigen-receptor signaling. *Curr Opin Immunol.* 2000;12:256-266.
94. Tomlinson MG, Lin J, Weiss A. Lymphocytes with a complex: adapter proteins in antigen signaling. *Immunol Today.* 2000;21:584-591.
95. Watson SP, Asazuma N, Atkinson B, et al. The role of ITAM- and ITIM-coupled receptors in platelet activation by collagen. *Thromb Haemost.* 2001;86:276-288.
96. Clements JL, Lee JR, Gross B, et al. Fetal hemorrhage and platelet dysfunction in SLP-76-deficient mice. *J Clin Invest.* 1999;103:19-25.
97. Gross BS, Melford SK, Watson SP. Evidence that phospholipase C-2 interacts with SLP-76, syk, lyn, LAT and the Fc receptor γ-chain after stimulation of the collagen receptor glycoprotein VI in human platelets. *Eur J Biochem.* 1999;263:612-623.
98. Bobe R, Wilde JI, Maschberger P, et al. Phosphatidylinositol 3-kinase-dependent translocation of phospholipase Cγ2 in mouse megakaryocytes is independent of Bruton's tyrosine kinase translocation. *Blood.* 2001;97:678-684.
99. Pasquet JM, Gross B, Quek L, et al. LAT is required for tyrosine phosphorylation of phospholipase Cγ2 and platelet activation by the collagen receptor GPVI. *Mol Cell Biol.* 1999;19:8326-8334.

100. Gross B, Lee JR, Clements JL, et al. Tyrosine phosphorylation of SLP-76 is downstream of Syk following stimulation of the collagen receptor GPVI in platelets. *J Biol Chem.* 1999;274:5963-5971.

101. Woulfe D, Jiang H, Morgans A, Monks R, Birnbaum M, Brass LF. Defects in secretion, aggregation, and thrombus formation in platelets from mice lacking Akt2. *J Clin Invest.* 2004;113:441-450.

102. Leo L, di Paola J, Judd BA, Koretzky GA, Lentz SR. Role of the adapter protein SLP-76 in GPVI-dependent platelet procoagulant responses to collagen. *Blood.* 2002;100:2839-2844.

103. Barry FA, Gibbins JM. Protein kinase B is regulated in platelets by the collagen receptor glycoprotein VI. *J Biol Chem.* 2002;277:12874-12878.

104. Dong ZM, Chapman SM, Brown AA, Frenette PS, Hynes RO, Wagner DD. The combined role of P- and E-selectins in atherosclerosis. *J Clin Invest.* 1998;102:145-152.

105. Dong ZM, Brown AA, Wagner DD. Prominent role of P-selectin in the development of advanced atherosclerosis in ApoE-deficient mice. *Circulation.* 2000;101:2290-2295.

106. Massberg S, Brand K, Gruner S, et al. A critical role of platelet adhesion in the initiation of atherosclerotic lesion formation. *J Exp Med.* 2002;196(7):887-896.

107. Pasquet JM, Noury M, Nurden AT. Evidence that the platelet integrin $\alpha_{IIb}\beta_3$ is regulated by the integrin-linked kinase, ILK, in a PI3-kinase dependent pathway. *Thromb Haemost.* 2002;88:115-122.

108. Stevens JM, Jordan PA, Sage T, Gibbins JM. The regulation of integrin-linked kinase in human platelets: evidence for involvement in the regulation of integrin $\alpha_2\beta_1$. *J Thromb Haemost.* 2004;2:1443-1452.

109. Falet H, Barkalow KL, Pivniouk VI, Barnes MJ, Geha RS, Hartwig JH. Roles of SLP-76, phosphoinositide 3-kinase, and gelsolin in the platelet shape changes initiated by the collagen receptor GPVI/FcRγ-chain complex. *Blood.* 2000;96:3786-3792.

110. Pasquet JM, Bobe R, Gross B, et al. A collagen-related peptide regulates phospholipase Cγ2 via phosphatidylinositol 3-kinase in human platelets. *Biochem J.* 1999;342:171-177.

111. Gratacap MP, Payrastre B, Viala C, Mauco G, Plantavid M, Chap H. Phosphatidylinositol 3,4,5-trisphosphate-dependent stimulation of phospholipase C-γ2 is an early key event in FcγRIIA-mediated activation of human platelets. *J Biol Chem.* 1998;273:24314-24321.

112. Wang D, Feng J, Wen R, et al. Phospholipase Cγ2 is essential in the functions of B cell and several Fc receptors. *Immunity.* 2000;13:25-35.

113. Fujita H, Hashimoto Y, Russell S, Zieger B, Ware J. In vivo expression of murine platelet glycoprotein Ibα. *Blood.* 1998;92:488-495.

114. Inoue O, Suzuki-Inoue K, Dean WL, Frampton J, Watson SP. Integrin $\alpha_2\beta_1$ mediates outside-in regulation of platelet spreading on collagen through activation of Src kinases and PLC-γ2. *J Cell Biol.* 2003;160:769-780.

115. Sundaresan P, Farndale RW. Platelet p38 MAP kinase phosphorylation is required by $\alpha_2\beta_1$ through Src family kinases and protein phosphatases. *Platelets.* 2003;13:361.

116. Watson SP, Herbert JM, Pollitt AY. GPVI and CLEC-2 in hemostasis and vascular integrity. *J Thromb Haemost.* 2010;8:1456-1467.

117. Suzuki-Inoue K, Inoue O, Ozaki Y. Novel platelet activation receptor CLEC-2: from discovery to prospects. *J Thromb Haemost.* 2011;9(suppl 1):44-55.

118. Inoue O, Suzuki-Inoue K, Ozaki Y. Redundant mechanism of platelet adhesion to laminin and collagen under flow: involvement of von Willebrand factor and glycoprotein Ib-IX-V. *J Biol Chem.* 2008;283(24):16279-16282.

119. Patil S, Newman DK, Newman PJ. Platelet endothelial cell adhesion molecule-1 serves as an inhibitory receptor that modulates platelet responses to collagen. *Blood.* 2001;97:1727-1732.

120. Cicmil M, Thomas JM, Leduc M, et al. Platelet endothelial cell adhesion molecule-1 signaling inhibits the activation of human platelets. *Blood.* 2002;99:137-144.

121. Bye AP, Unsworth AJ, Gibbins JM. Platelet signaling: a complex interplay between inhibitory and activatory networks. *J Thromb Haemost.* 2016;14:918-930.

122. Albelda SM, Muller WA, Buck CA, Newman PJ. Molecular and cellular properties of PECAM-1 (endoCAM/CD31): a novel vascular cell–cell adhesion molecule. *J Cell Biol.* 1991;114:1059-1068.

123. Falati S, Patil S, Gibbins J, et al. Opposing effects of P-selectin and PECAM-1 on arterial thrombus growth and stability in vivo. *J Thromb Haemost.* 2003;1(suppl 1):OC054.

124. Relou IAM, Gorter G, Ferreira IA, van Rijn HJ, Akkerman JW. Platelet endothelial cell adhesion molecule-1 (PECAM-1) inhibits low density lipoprotein-induced signaling in platelets. *J Biol Chem.* 2003;278:32638-32644.

125. Rathore V, Stapleton MA, Hillery CA, et al. PECAM-1 negatively regulates GPIb/V/IX signaling in murine platelets. *Blood.* 2003;102:3658-3664.

126. Thai LM, Ashman LK, Harbour SN, Hogarth PM, Jackson DE. Physical proximity and functional interplay of PECAM-1 with the Fc receptor FcγRIIa on the platelet plasma membrane. *Blood.* 2003;102:3637-3645.

127. Bernardo A, Ball C, Nolasco L, Moake JF, Dong JF. Effects of inflammatory cytokines on the release and cleavage of the endothelial cell-derived ultralarge von Willebrand factor multimers under flow. *Blood.* 2004;104:100-106.

128. Raife TJ, Cao W, Atkinson BS, et al. Leukocyte proteases cleave von Willebrand factor at or near the ADAMTS13 cleavage site. *Blood.* 2009;114:1666-1674.

129. Coughlin SR. How the protease thrombin talks to cells. *Proc Natl Acad Sci U S A.* 1999;96:11023-11027.

130. Vu T-KH, Hung DT, Wheaton VI, Coughlin SR. Molecular cloning of a functional thrombin receptor reveals a novel proteolytic mechanism of receptor activation. *Cell.* 1991;64:1057-1068.

131. Xu WF, Andersen H, Whitmore TE, et al. Cloning and characterization of human protease-activated receptor 4. *Proc Natl Acad Sci U S A.* 1998;95:6642-6646.

132. Kahn ML, Nakanishi-Matsui M, Shapiro MJ, Ishihara H, Coughlin SR. Protease-activated receptors 1 and 4 mediate activation of human platelets by thrombin. *J Clin Invest.* 1999;103:879-887.

133. Molino M, Barnathan ES, Numerof R, et al. Interactions of mast cell tryptase with thrombin receptors and PAR-2. *J Biol Chem.* 1997;272:4043-4049.

134. Camerer E, Røttingen JA, Iversen JG, Prydz H. Coagulation factors VII and X induce Ca^{2+} oscillations in Madin-Darby canine kidney cells only when proteolytically active. *J Biol Chem.* 1996;271:29034-29042.

135. Camerer E, Huang W, Coughlin SR. Tissue factor- and factor X-dependent activation of PAR2 by factor VIIa. *Proc Natl Acad Sci U S A.* 2000;97:5255-5260.

136. Rasmussen UB, Vouret-Craviari V, Jallat S, et al. cDNA cloning and expression of a hamster α-thrombin receptor coupled to Ca^{2+} mobilization. *FEBS Lett.* 1991;288:123-128.

137. Klages B, Brandt U, Simon MI, Schultz G, Offermanns S. Activation of G12/G13 results in shape change and rho/rho kinase-mediated myosin light chain phosphorylation in mouse platelets. *J Cell Biol.* 1999;144:745-754.

138. Offermanns S, Toombs CF, Hu YH, Simon MI. Defective platelet activation in G α(q)-deficient mice. *Nature.* 1997;389:183-186.

139. Taylor S, Chae H, Rhee SG, Exton J. Activation of the B1 isozyme of phospholipase C by α subunits of the Gq class of G proteins. *Nature.* 1991;350:516-518.

140. Yang J, Wu J, Kowalska MA, et al. Loss of signaling through the G protein, Gz, results in abnormal platelet activation and altered responses to psychoactive drugs. *Proc Natl Acad Sci U S A.* 2000;97:9984-9989.

141. Stoyanov B, Volinia S, Hanck T, et al. Cloning and characterization of a G protein-activated human phosphoinositide-3 kinase. *Science.* 1995;269:690-693.

142. Clapham DE, Neer EJ. G protein β γ subunits. *Annu Rev Pharmacol Toxicol.* 1997;37:167-203.

143. Leevers SJ, Vanhaesebroeck B, Waterfield MD. Signalling through phosphoinositide 3-kinases: the lipids take centre stage. *Curr Opin Cell Biol.* 1999;11:219-225.

144. Lefkowitz RJ, Pitcher J, Krueger K, Daaka Y. Mechanisms of β-adrenergic receptor desensitization and resensitization. *Adv Pharmacol.* 1998;42:416-420.

145. Hoxie JA, Ahuja M, Belmonte E, Pizarro S, Parton R, Brass LF. Internalization and recycling of activated thrombin receptors. *J Biol Chem.* 1993;268:13756-13763.

146. Ishii K, Chen J, Ishii M, et al. Inhibition of thrombin receptor signaling by a G protein-coupled receptor kinase. Functional specificity among G protein-coupled receptor kinases. *J Biol Chem.* 1994;269:1125-1130.

147. Hein L, Ishii K, Coughlin SR, Kobilka BK. Intracellular targeting and trafficking of thrombin receptors: a novel mechanism for resensitization of a G protein-coupled receptor. *J Biol Chem.* 1994;269:27719-27726.

148. Hung DT, Vu TK, Wheaton VI, Ishii K, Coughlin SR. Cloned platelet thrombin receptor is necessary for thrombin-induced platelet activation. *J Clin Invest.* 1992;89:1350-1353.

149. Brass LF, Vassallo RJ, Belmonte E, Ahuja M, Cichowski K, Hoxie JA. Structure and function of the human platelet thrombin receptor. Studies using monoclonal antibodies directed against a defined domain within the receptor N terminus. *J Biol Chem.* 1992;267:13795-13798.

150. Shapiro MJ, Weiss EJ, Faruqi TR, Coughlin SR. Protease-activated receptors 1 and 4 are shut off with distinct kinetics after activation by thrombin. *J Biol Chem.* 2000;275:25216-25221.

151. Covic L, Gresser AL, Kuliopulos A. Biphasic kinetics of activation and signaling for PAR1 and PAR4 thrombin receptors in platelets. *Biochemistry.* 2000;39:5458-5467.

152. Gaarder A, Jonsen L, Laland S, Hellem A, Owren PA. Adenosine diphosphate in red cells as a factor in the adhesiveness of human blood platelets. *Nature.* 1961;192:531-532.

153. Savi P, Herbert JM. Pharmacology of ticlopidine and clopidogrel. *Haematologica.* 2000;85:73-77.

154. Humphries RG. Pharmacology of AR-C69931MX and related compounds: from pharmacological tools to clinical trials. *Haematologica.* 2000;85:66-72.

155. Ralevic V, Burnstock G. Receptors for purines and pyrimidines. *Pharmacol Rev.* 1998;50:413-492.

156. Turner NA, Moake JL, McIntire LV. Blockade of adenosine diphosphate receptors P2Y$_{12}$ and P2Y$_1$ is required to inhibit platelet aggregation in whole blood under flow. *Blood.* 2001;98:3340-3345.

157. Remijn JA, Wu YP, Jeninga EH, et al. Role of ADP receptor P2Y12 in platelet adhesion and thrombus formation in flowing blood. *Arterioscler Thromb Vasc Biol.* 2002;22:686-691.

158. Webb TE, Simon J, Krishek BJ, et al. Cloning and functional expression of a brain G-protein-coupled ATP receptor. *FEBS Lett.* 1993;324:219-225.

159. Léon C, Vial C, Cazenave JP, Gachet C. Cloning and sequencing of a human cDNA encoding endothelial P2Y$_1$ purinoceptor. *Gene.* 1997;171:295-297.

160. Ayyanathan K, Webb TE, Sandhu AK, et al. Cloning and chromosomal localization of the human P2Y$_1$ purinoceptor. *Biochem Biophys Res Commun.* 1996;218:783-788.

161. Léon C, Hechler B, Vial C, Leray C, Cazenave JP, Gachet C. The P2Y$_1$ receptor is an ADP receptor antagonized by ATP and expressed in platelets and megakaryoblastic cells. *FEBS Lett.* 1997;403:26-30.

162. Hechler B, Vigne P, Léon C, Breittmayer JP, Gachet C, Frelin C. ATP derivatives are antagonists of the P2Y$_1$ receptor: similarities with the platelet ADP receptor. *Mol Pharmacol.* 1998;53:727-733.

163. Daniel JL, Dangelmaier C, Jin J, Ashby B, Smith JB, Kunapuli SP. Molecular basis for ADP-induced platelet activation. I. Evidence for three distinct ADP receptors on human platelets. *J Biol Chem.* 1998;273:2024-2029.

164. Geiger J, Honig-Liedl P, Schanzenbacher P, Walter U. Ligand specificity and ticlopidine effects distinguish three human platelet ADP receptors. *Eur J Pharmacol.* 1998;351:235-246.

165. Fagura MS, Dainty IA, McKay GD, et al. $P2Y_21$-receptors in human platelets which are pharmacologically distinct from $P2Y_{ADP}$-receptors. *Br J Pharmacol.* 1998;124:157-164.
166. Hechler B, Eckly A, Ohlmann P, Cazenave JP, Gachet C. The $P2Y_11$ receptor, necessary but not sufficient to support full ADP-induced platelet aggregation, is not the target of the drug clopidogrel. *Br J Haematol.* 1998;103:858-866.
167. Jantzen HM, Gousset L, Bhaskar V, et al. Evidence for two distinct G-protein-coupled ADP receptors mediating platelet activation. *Thromb Haemost.* 1999;81:111-117.
168. Léon C, Vial C, Gachet C, et al. The $P2Y_21$ receptor is normal in a patient presenting a severe deficiency of ADP-induced platelet aggregation. *Thromb Haemost.* 1999;81:775-781.
169. Hollopeter G, Jantzen HM, Vincent D, et al. Identification of the platelet ADP receptor targeted by antithrombotic drugs. *Nature.* 2001;409:202-207.
170. Jarvis GE, Humphries RG, Roberston MJ, Leff P. ADP can induce aggregation of human platelets via both $P2Y_21$ and P_2T receptors. *Br J Pharmacol.* 2000;129:275-282.
171. Jin J, Kunapuli SP. Coactivation of two different G protein-coupled receptors is essential for ADP-induced platelet aggregation. *Proc Natl Acad Sci U S A.* 1998;95:8070-8074.
172. Jin J, Daniel JL, Kunapuli SP. Molecular basis for ADP-induced platelet activation. II. The $P2Y_21$ receptor mediates ADP-induced intracellular calcium mobilization and shape change in platelets. *J Biol Chem.* 1998;273:2030-2034.
173. Savi P, Beauverger P, Labouret C, et al. Role of $P2Y_21$ purinoceptor in ADP-induced platelet activation. *FEBS Lett.* 1998;422:291-295.
174. Fabre JE, Nguyen M, Latour A, et al. Decreased platelet aggregation, increased bleeding time and resistance to thromboembolism in $P2Y_21$-deficient mice. *Nat Med.* 1999;5:1199-1202.
175. Léon C, Hechler B, Freund M, et al. Defective platelet aggregation and increased resistance to thromboembolism in purinergic $P2Y_21$ receptor null mice. *J Clin Invest.* 1999;104:1731-1737.
176. Savi P, Pflieger M, Herbert JM. cAMP is not an important messenger for ADP-induced platelet aggregation. *Blood Coagul Fibrinolysis.* 1996;7:249-252.
177. Daniel JL, Dangelmaier C, Jin J, Kim YB, Kunapuli SP. Role of intracellular signaling events in ADP-induced platelet aggregation. *Thromb Haemost.* 1999;82:1322-1326.
178. Cattaneo M, Lecchi A, Randi AM, McGregor JL, Mannucci PM. Identification of a new congenital defect of platelet function characterized by severe impairment of platelet responses to adenosine diphosphate. *Blood.* 1992;80:2787-2796.
179. Nurden P, Savi P, Heilmann E, et al. An inherited bleeding disorder linked to a defective interaction between ADP and its receptor on platelets. *J Clin Invest.* 1995;95:1612-1622.
180. Paul BZ, Daniel JL, Kunapuli SP. Platelet shape change is mediated by both calcium-dependent and-independent signalling pathways. *J Biol Chem.* 1999;274:28293-28300.
181. Bauer M, Retzer M, Wilde JI, et al. Dichotomous regulation of myosin phosphorylation and shape change by Rho-kinase and calcium in intact human platelets. *Blood.* 1999;94:1665-1672.
182. Gachet C. ADP receptors of platelets and their inhibition. *Thromb Haemost.* 2001;86:222-232.
183. Storey RF, Sanderson HM, White AE, May JA, Cameron KE, Heptinstall S. The central role of the P22T receptor in amplification of human platelet activation, aggregation, secretion and procoagulant activity. *Br J Haematol.* 2000;110:925-934.
184. Hechler B, Cattaneo M, Gachet C. The P2 receptors in platelet function. *Semin Thromb Haemost.* 2005;31:150-161.
185. Savi P, Labouret C, Delesque N, Guette F, Lupker J, Herbert JM. $P2Y_212$, a new platelet ADP receptor, target of clopidogrel. *Biochem Biophys Res Commun.* 2001;283:379-383.
186. Foster CJ, Prosser DM, Agans JM, et al. Molecular identification and characterization of the platelet ADP receptor targeted by thienopyridine antithrombotic drugs. *J Clin Invest.* 2001;107:1591-1598.
187. Andre P, Delaney SM, LaRocca T, et al. $P2Y_212$ regulates both platelet adhesion/activation, thrombus growth and thrombus stability in injured arteries. *J Clin Invest.* 2003;112:398-406.
188. Vial C, Hechler B, Léon C, Cazenave JP, Gachet C. Presence of $P2X_21$ purinoceptors in human platelets and megakaryoblastic cell lines. *Thromb Haemost.* 1997;78:1500-1504.
189. Sun B, Li J, Okahara K, Kambayashi J. $P2X_21$ purinoceptor in human platelets. Molecular cloning and functional characterization after heterologous expression. *J Biol Chem.* 1998;273:11544-11547.
190. Scase TJ, Heath MF, Allen JM, Sage SO, Evans RJ. Identification of a $P2X_21$ purinoceptor expressed on human platelets. *Biochem Biophys Res Commun.* 1998;242:525-528.
191. Clifford EE, Parker K, Humphreys BD, Kertesy SB, Dubyak GR. The $P2X_21$ receptor, an adenosine triphosphate-gated cation channel, is expressed in human platelets but not in human blood leucocytes. *Blood.* 1998;91:3172-3181.
192. MacKenzie A, Mahaut-Smith Smith, Sage SO. Activation of receptor-operated cation channels via $P2X_21$ not P_2T purinoceptors in human platelets. *J Biol Chem.* 1996;271:2879-2881.
193. Oury C, Toth-Zsamboki E, Thys C, Tytgat J, Vermylen J, Hoylaerts MF. The ATP-gated $P2X_21$ ion channel acts as a positive regulator of platelet responses to collagen. *Thromb Haemost.* 2001;86:1264-1271.
194. Hechler B, Lenain N, Marchese P, et al. A role of the fast ATP-gated $P2X_21$ cation channel in thrombosis of small arteries in vivo. *J Exp Med.* 2003;198:661-667.
195. Cattaneo M, Marchese P, Jacobson KA, Ruggeri ZM. New insights into the role of $P2X_21$ in platelet function. *Haematologica.* 2002;87:13-14.
196. Oury C, Sticker E, Cornelissen H, et al. ATP augments von Willebrand factor-dependent shear-induced platelet aggregation through Ca^{2+}-calmodulin and myosin light chain kinase activation. *J Biol Chem*;279:26266-26273. 2004.
197. Oury C, Kuijpers MJ, Toth-Zsamboki E, De Vos R, Vermylen J, Hoylaerts MF. Overexpression of the platelet $P2X_21$ ion channel in transgenic mice generates a novel prothrombotic phenotype. *Blood.* 2003;101:3969-3976.
198. Murata T, Ushikubi F, Matsuoka T, et al. Altered pain perception and inflammatory response in mice lacking prostacyclin receptor. *Nature.* 1997;388:678.
199. Jantzen H-M, Milstone DS, Gousset L, Conley PB, Mortensen RM. Impaired activation of murine platelets lacking Galphai2. *J Clin Invest.* 2001;108:477.
200. Sage SO, Rink TJ. Kinetic differences between thrombin induced and ADP induced calcium influx and release from internal stores in fura-2 loaded human platelets. *Biochem Biophys Res Commun.* 1986;136:1124-1129.
201. Mahaut-Smith MP, Sage SO, Rink TJ. Rapid ADP evoked currents in human platelets recorded with the nystatin permeabilized patch technique. *J Biol Chem.* 1992;267:3060-3065.
202. Yang X, Sun L, Ghosh S, Rao AK. Human platelet signaling defect characterized by impaired production of inositol-1,4,5-triphosphate and phosphatidic acid and diminished Pleckstrin phosphorylation: evidence for defective phospholipase C activation. *Blood.* 1996;88:1676-1683.
203. Gabbetta J, Yang X, Kowalska MA, Sun L, Dhanasekaran N, Rao AK. Platelet signal transduction defect with Gα subunit dysfunction and diminished Gαq in a patient with abnormal platelet responses. *Proc Natl Acad Sci U S A.* 1997;94:8750-8755.
204. Woulfe D, Jiang H, Mortensen R, Yang J, Brass LF. Activation of Rap1B by G_i family members in platelets. *J Biol Chem.* 2002;277:23382-23390.
205. Lova P, Paganini S, Sinigaglia F, Balduini C, Torti M. A G_i-dependent pathway is required for activation of the small GTPase Rap1B in human platelets. *J Biol Chem.* 2002;277:12009-12015.
206. Larson MK, Chen H, Kahn ML, et al. Identification of $P2Y_212$-dependent and independent mechanisms of glycoprotein VI-mediated Rap1 activation in platelets. *Blood.* 2003;101:1409-1415.
207. Nieswandt B, Bergmeier W, Eckly A, et al. Evidence for cross-talk between GPVI and Gi coupled receptors during collagen-induced platelet aggregation. *Blood.* 2001;97:3829-3835.
208. Gratacap MP, Hérault JP, Viala C, et al. FcγRIIA requires a Gi-dependent pathway for an efficient stimulation of phosphoinositide 3-kinase, calcium mobilization, and platelet aggregation. *Blood.* 2000;96:3439-3446.
209. Payrastre B, Gratacap MP, Trumel C, et al. ADP: an important cofactor of PI 3-kinase activation in human blood platelets. *Haematologica.* 2000;85:32-36.
210. Trumel C, Payrastre B, Plantavid M, et al. A key role of adenosine diphosphate in the irreversible platelet aggregation induced by the PAR1-activating peptide through the late activation of phosphoinositide 3-kinase. *Blood.* 1999;94:4156-4165.
211. Covic L, Singh C, Smith H, Kuliopulos A. Role of PAR4 thrombin receptor in stabilizing platelet-platelet aggregates as revealed by a patient with Hermansky-Pudlak syndrome. *Thromb Haemost.* 2002;87:722-727.
212. Kim S, Foster C, Lecchi A, et al. Protease-activated receptors 1 and 4 do not stimulate G_i signaling pathways in the absence of secreted ADP and cause human platelet aggregation independently of G_i signaling. *Blood.* 2002;99:3629-3636.
213. Quinton TM, Ozdener F, Dangelmaier C, Daniel JL, Kunapuli SP. Glycoprotein VI-mediated platelet fibrinogen receptor activation occurs through calcium-sensitive and PKC-sensitive pathways without a requirement for secreted ADP. *Blood.* 2002;99:3228-3234.
214. Jung SM, Moroi M. Platelet collagen receptor integrin $\alpha_22\beta_21$ activation involves differential participation of ADP-receptor subtypes $P2Y_21$ and $P2Y_212$ but not intracellular calcium. *Eur J Biochem.* 2001;268:3513-3522.
215. Polgar J, Eichler P, Greinacher A, Clemetson KJ. Adenosine diphosphate (ADP) and ADP receptor play a major role in platelet activation/aggregation induced by sera from heparin-induced thrombocytopenia patients. *Blood.* 1998;91:549-554.
216. Storey RF, Judge HM, Wilcox RG, Heptinstall S. Inhibition of ADP-induced P-selectin expression and platelet-leukocyte conjugate formation by clopidogrel and the $P2Y_212$ receptor antagonist AR-C69931MX but not aspirin. *Thromb Haemost.* 2002;88:488-494.
217. Siess W, Weber PC, Lapetina EG. Activation of phospholipase C is dissociated from arachidonate metabolism during platelet shape change induced by thrombin or platelet-activating factor: epinephrine does not induce phospholipase C activation or platelet shape change. *J Biol Chem.* 1984;259:8286-8292.
218. Bennett JS, Vilaire G, Burch JW. A role for prostaglandins and thromboxanes in the exposure of platelet fibrinogen receptors. *J Clin Invest.* 1981;68:981-987.
219. Peerschke EI. Induction of human platelet fibrinogen receptors by epinephrine in the absence of released ADP. *Blood.* 1982;60:71-77.
220. Lanza F, Beretz A, Stierlé A, Hanau D, Kubina M, Cazenave JP. Epinephrine potentiates human platelet activation but is not an aggregating agent. *Am J Physiol.* 1988;255:H1276-H1288.
221. Regan JW, Nakata H, DeMarinis RM, Caron MG, Lefkowitz RJ. Purification and characterization of the human platelet α_22-adrenergic receptor. *J Biol Chem.* 1986;261:3894-3900.
222. Kobilka BK, Matsui H, Kobilka TS, et al. Cloning sequencing and expression of the gene coding for the platelet α_22-adrenergic receptor. *Science.* 1987;238:650-656.
223. Scrutton MC, Clare KC, Hutton RA, Bruckdorfer KR. Depressed responsiveness to adrenaline in platelets from apparently normal human donors: a familial trait. *Br J Haematol.* 1981;49:303-314.
224. Smith WL. The eicosanoids and their biochemical mechanisms of action. *Biochem J.* 1989;259:315-324.
225. Smith JB, Willis AL. Aspirin selectively inhibits prostaglandin production in human platelets. *Nature.* 1971;231:235-237.
226. Roth GJ, Calverley DC. Aspirin, platelets, and thrombosis: theory and practice. *Blood.* 1994;83:885-898.
227. FitzGerald GA. Mechanisms of platelet activation: thromboxane A_22 as an amplifying signal for other agonists. *Am J Cardiol.* 1991;68:11B-15B.

228. Hamberg M, Svensson J, Samuelsson B. Thromboxanes: a new group of biologically active compounds derived from prostaglandin endoperoxides. *Proc Natl Acad Sci U S A*. 1975;72:2994-2998.

229. Gerrard JM, Carroll RC. Stimulation of protein phosphorylation by arachidonic acid and endoperoxide analog. *Prostaglandins*. 1981;22:81-94.

230. Pulcinelli FM, Ashby B, Gazzaniga PP, Daniel JL. Protein kinase C activation is not a key step in ADP-mediated exposure of fibrinogen receptors on human platelets. *FEBS Lett*. 1995;364:87-90.

231. Saklatvala J, Rawlinson L, Waller RJ, et al. Role for p38 mitogen-activated protein kinase in platelet aggregation caused by collagen or a thromboxane analogue. *J Biol Chem*. 1996;271:6586-6589.

232. Offermanns S, Laugwitz KL, Spicher K, Schultz G. G proteins of the G12 family are activated via thromboxane A2 and thrombin receptors in human platelets. *Proc Natl Acad Sci U S A*. 1994;91:504-508.

233. Raychowdhury MK, Yukawa M, Collins LJ, McGrail SH, Kent KC, Ware JA. Alternative splicing produces a divergent cytoplasmic tail in the human endothelial thromboxane A2 receptor. *J Biol Chem*. 1995;270:7011.

234. Hirata T, Ushikubi F, Kakizuka A, Okuma M, Narumiya S. Two thromboxane $A_2$2 receptor isoforms in human platelets. Opposite coupling to adenylyl cyclase with different sensitivity to Arg60 to Leu mutation. *J Clin Invest*. 1996;97:949-956.

235. Thomas DW, Mannon RB, Mannon PJ, et al. Coagulation defects and altered hemodynamic responses in mice lacking receptors for thromboxane A2. *J Clin Invest*. 1998;102:1994.

236. Jackson SP, Nesbitt WS, Kulkarni S. Signaling events underlying thrombus formation. *J Thromb Haemost*. 2003;1:1602-1612.

237. Nesbitt WS, Giuliano S, Kulkarni S, Dopheide SM, Harper IS, Jackson SP. Intercellular calcium communication regulates platelet aggregation and thrombus growth. *J Cell Biol*. 2003;160:1151-1161.

238. Stalker TJ, Traxler EA, Wu J, et al. Hierarchical organization in the hemostatic response and its relationship to the platelet-signaling network. *Blood*. 2013;121:1875-1885.

239. Tomaiuolo M, Brass LF, Stalker TJ. Regulation of platelet activation and coagulation and its role in vascular injury and arterial thrombosis. *Interv Cardiol Clin*. 2017;6:1-12.

240. Kaplan ZS, Zarpellon A, Alwis I, et al. Thrombin-dependent intravascular leukocyte trafficking regulated by fibrin and the platelet receptors GPIb and PAR4. *Nat Commun*. 2015;6:7835.

241. Ghasemzadeh M, Kaplan ZS, Alwis I, et al. The CXCR1/2 ligand NAP-2 promotes directed intravascular leukocyte migration through platelet thrombi. *Blood*. 2013;121:4555-4566.

242. Harper MT, Poole AW. Diverse functions of protein kinase C isoforms in platelet activation and thrombus formation. *J Thromb Haemost*. 2010;8:454-462.

243. Jobe SM, Wilson KM, Leo L, et al. Critical role for the mitochondrial permeability transition pore and cyclophilin D in platelet activation and thrombosis. *Blood*. 2008;111:1257-1265.

244. Choo HJ, Saafir TB, Mkumba L, et al. Mitochondrial calcium and reactive oxygen species regulate agonist-initiated platelet phosphatidylserine exposure. *Arterioscler Thromb Vasc Biol*. 2012;32:2946-2955.

245. Choo HJ, Kholmukhamedov A, Zhou C, et al. Inner mitochondrial membrane disruption links apoptotic and agonist-initiated phosphatidylserine externalization in platelets. *Arterioscler Thromb Vasc Biol*. 2017;37:1503-1512.

246. Yin H, Liu J, Li Z, Berndt MC, et al. Src family tyrosine kinase Lyn mediates VWF/GPIb-IX-induced platelet activation via the cGMP signaling pathway. *Blood*. 2008;112:1139-1146.

247. Zhang G, Xiang B, Dong A, et al. Biphasic roles for soluble guanylyl cyclase (sGC) in platelet activation. *Blood*. 2011;118:3670-3679.

248. Zhang G, Han J, Welch EJ, et al. Lipopolysaccharide stimulates platelet secretion and potentiates platelet aggregation via TLR4/MyD88 and the cGMP-dependent protein kinase pathway. *J Immunol*. 2009;182:7997-8004.

249. Senis YA. Protein-tyrosine phosphatases: a new frontier in platelet signal transduction. *J Thromb Haemost*. 2013;11:1800-1813.

250. Brass LF, Molino M. Protease-activated G protein-coupled receptors on human platelets and endothelial cells. *Thromb Haemost*. 1997;78:234-241.

251. Premont RT, Ingles J, Lefkowitz RJ. Protein kinases that phosphorylate activated G protein-coupled receptors. *FASEB J*. 1995;9:175-182.

252. Ferguson SS, Barak LS, Zhang J, Caron MG. G-protein-coupled receptor regulation: role of G-protein-coupled receptor kinesis and arrestins. *Can J Physiol Pharmacol*. 1996;74:1095-1110.

253. Goodman OB, Krupnick JG, Santini F, et al. β-Arrestin acts as a clathrin adaptor in endocytosis of the β$_2$-adrenergic receptor. *Nature*. 1996;383:447-450.

254. Smolenski A. Novel roles of cAMP/cGMP-protects from thrombosis by suppressing integrin αIIbβ3-dependent outside-in signaling in platelets.dependent signaling in platelets. *J Thromb Haemost*. 2012;10:167-176.

255. Massberg S, Sausbier M, Klatt P, et al. Increased adhesion and aggregation of platelets lacking cyclic guanosine 3′,5′-monophosphate kinase I. *J Exp Med*. 1999;189:1255-1264.

256. Brass LF. Molecular basis of platelet activation. In *Hematology: Basic Principles and Practice*, Hoffman R, Benz EJ, Shattil SJ, et al., 3rd ed. Churchill-Livingstone; 2000:1753-1770.

257. Cavallini L, Coassin M, Borean A, Alexandre A. Prostacyclin and sodium nitroprusside inhibit the activity of the platelet inositol 1,4,5-triphosphate receptor and promote its phosphorylation. *J Biol Chem*. 1996;271:5545-5551.

258. Nishimura T, Yamamoto T, Komuro Y, Hara Y. Antiplatelet functions of a stable prostacyclin analog, SM-10906 are exerted by its inhibitory effect on inositol 1,4,5-triphosphate production and cytosolic Ca^{2+} increase in rat platelets stimulated by thrombin. *Thromb Res*. 1995;79:307-317.

259. Lapetina EG. Incorporation of synthetic 1,2-diacylglycerol into platelet phosphatidylinositol is increased by cyclic AMP. *FEBS Lett*. 1986;195:111-114.

260. de Chaffoy de Courcelles D, Roevens P, van Belle H. Agents that elevate platelet cAMP stimulate the formation of phosphatidylinositol 4-phosphate in intact human platelets. *FEBS Lett*. 1986;195:115-118.

261. Abrams CS, Kazanietz MG. Platelet signalling: protein kinase C. In *Platelets in Thrombotic and Non-Thrombotic Disorders*: Gresele P, Page C, Fuster V, Vermylen J, Cambridge University Press; 2002:272.

262. Watson SP, Lapetina EG. 1,2 Diacylglycerol and phorbol ester inhibit agonist-induced formation of inositol phosphates in human platelets: possible implications for negative feedback regulation of inositol phospholipid hydrolysis. *Proc Natl Acad Sci U S A*. 1985;82:2623-2626.

263. Zavoico GB, Halenda SP, Sha'afi RI, Feinstein MB. Phorbol myristate acetate inhibits thrombin-stimulated Ca^{2+} mobilization and phosphatidylinositol 4,5-bisphosphate hydrolysis in human platelets. *Proc Natl Acad Sci U S A*. 1985;82:3859-3862.

264. MacIntyre DE, McHicol A, Drummond AH. Tumour-promoting phorbol esters inhibit agonist-induced phosphatidate formation and Ca^{2+} flux in human platelets. *FEBS Lett*. 1985;180:160-164.

265. Connolly TM, Lawing WJ, Jr, Majerus PW. Protein kinase C phosphorylates human platelet inositol trisphosphate 5′-phosphomonoesterase, increasing the phosphatase activity. *Cell*. 1986;46:951-958.

266. Abrams CS, Wu H, Zhao W, et al. Pleckstrin inhibits phosphoinositide hydrolysis initiated by G-protein-coupled and growth factor receptors: a role for Pleckstrin's PH domains. *J Biol Chem*. 1995;270:14485-14492.

267. Nakinishi H, Brewer KA, Exton JH. Activation of the ζ isozyme of protein kinase C by phosphatidylinositol 3,4,5-trisphosphate. *J Biol Chem*. 1993;268:13-16.

268. George JN. Platelet immunoglobulin G: its significance for the evaluation of thrombocytopenia and for understanding the origin of α-granule proteins. *Blood*. 1990;76:859-870.

269. Handagama P, Scarborough RM, Shuman MA, Bainton DF. Endocytosis of fibrinogen into megakaryocyte and platelet α-granules is mediated by α$_{II}$bβ$_2$3 (glycoprotein IIb-IIIa). *Blood*. 1993;82:135-138.

270. Wencel-Drake JD. Plasma membrane GPIIb-IIIa: evidence for a cycling receptor pool. *Am J Pathol*. 1990;136:61-70.

271. Wencel-Drake JD, Boudignon-Proudhon C, Dieter MG, Criss AB, Parise LV. Internalization of bound fibrinogen modulates platelet aggregation. *Blood*. 1996;87:602-612.

272. Harrison P, Wilbourn BR, Cramer EM, et al. The influence of therapeutic blocking of Gp IIb/IIIa on platelet α-granular fibrinogen. *Br J Haematol*. 1992;82:721-728.

273. Naik MU, Stalker TJ, Brass LF, Naik UP. JAM-A protects from thrombosis by suppressing integrin αIIbβ3-dependent outside-in signaling in platelets. *Blood*. 2012;119:3352-3360.

274. Spyridon M, Moraes LA, Jones CI, et al. LXR as a novel antithrombotic target. *Blood*. 2011;117:5751-5761.

275. Moraes LA, Unsworth AJ, Vaiyapuri S, et al. Farnesoid X receptor and its ligands inhibit the function of platelets. *Arterioscler Thromb Vasc Biol*. 2016;36:2324-2333.

276. Unsworth AJ, Bye AP, Tannetta DS, et al. Farnesoid X receptor and liver X receptor ligands initiate formation of coated platelets. *Arterioscler Thromb Vasc Biol*. 2017;37:1482-1493.

277. Banga HS, Simons ER, Brass LF, Rittenhouse SE. Activation of phospholipases A and C in human platelets exposed to epinephrine: role of glycoproteins IIb/IIIa and dual role of epinephrine. *Proc Natl Acad Sci U S A*. 1986;83:9197-9201.

278. Denis MM, Tolley ND, Bunting M, et al. Escaping the nuclear confines: signal-dependent pre-mRNA splicing in anucleate platelets. *Cell*. 2005;122:379.

279. Weyrich A, Dixon DA, Pabla R, et al. Signal-dependent translation of a regulatory protein, Bcl-3, in activated human platelets. *Proc Natl Acad Sci U S A*. 1998;95:5556.

280. van der Zee PM, Biro E, Ko Y, et al. P-selectin-and CD63-exposing platelet microparticles reflect platelet activation in peripheral arterial disease and myocardial infarction. *Clin Chem*. 2006;52:657.

281. Lemons PP, Chen D, Bernstein AM, Bennett MK, Whiteheart SW. Regulated secretion in platelets: identification of elements of the platelet exocytosis machinery. *Blood*. 1997;90:1490-1500.

282. Bernstein AM, Whiteheart SW. Identification of a cellubrevin/vesicle associated membrane protein 3 homologue in human platelets. *Blood*. 1999;93:571-579.

283. Polgár J, Chung SH, Reed GL. Vesicle-associated membrane protein 3 (VAMP-3) and VAMP-8 are present in human platelets and are required for granule secretion. *Blood*. 2002;100:1081-1083.

284. Carrell NA, Fitzgerald LA, Steiner B, Erickson HP, Phillips DR. Structure of human platelet membrane glycoproteins IIb and IIIa as determined by electron microscopy. *J Biol Chem*. 1985;260:1743-1749.

285. Weisel JW, Nagaswami C, Vilaire G, Bennett JS. Examination of the platelet membrane glycoprotein IIb-IIIa complex and its interaction with fibrinogen and other ligands by electron microscopy. *J Biol Chem*. 1992;267:16637-16643.

286. Phillips DR, Agin PP. Platelet membrane defects in Glanzmann's thrombasthenia: evidence for decreased amounts of two major glycoproteins. *J Clin Invest*. 1977;60:535-545.

287. Nurden AT, Caen JP. An abnormal platelet glycoprotein pattern of three cases of Glanzmann's thrombasthenia. *Br J Haematol*. 1974;253:253-260.

288. Casserly IP, Topol EJ. Glycoprotein IIb/IIIa antagonists—from bench to practice. *Cell Mol Life Sci*. 2002;59:478-500.

289. Jackson SP. The growing complexity of platelet aggregation. *Blood*. 2007;109:5087-5295.

290. Patil S, Jedsadayanmata A, Wencel-Drake D., Wang W, Knezevic I, Lam SC. Identification of a talin-binding site in the integrin β$_2$3 subunit distinct from the NPLY regulatory motif of post-ligand binding functions: the talin N-terminal head domain interacts with the membrane-proximal region of the β$_2$3 cytoplasmic tail. *J Biol Chem*. 1999;274:28575-28583.

291. Calderwood DA, Shattil SJ, Ginsberg MH. Integrins and actin filaments: reciprocal regulation of cell adhesion and signaling. *J Biol Chem*. 2000;275:22607-22610.

292. Shattil SJ, Kashiwagi H, Pampori N. Integrin signaling: the platelet paradigm. *Blood*. 1998;91:2645-2657.

293. Shattil SJ, Newman PJ. Integrins: dynamic scaffolds for adhesion and signaling in platelets. *Blood*. 2004;104:1606-1615.

294. Manganello JM, Djellas Y, Borg C, Antonakis K, Le Breton GC. Cyclic AMP-dependent phosphorylation of thromboxane A$_2$2 receptor-associated G$\alpha_2$13. *J Biol Chem*. 1999;274:28003-28010.

295. Wang GR, Zhu Y, Halushka PV, Lincoln TM, Mendelsohn ME. Mechanism of platelet inhibition by nitric oxide: in vivo phosphorylation of thromboxane receptor by cyclic GMP-dependent protein kinase. *Proc Natl Acad Sci U S A*. 1998;95:4888-4893.

296. Peerschke EI. Regulation of platelet aggregation by post-fibrinogen binding events. *Thromb Haemost*. 1995;73:862-867.

297. O'Toole TE, Ylanne J, Culley BM. Regulation of integrin affinity states through an NPXY motif in the β subunit cytoplasmic domain. *J Biol Chem*. 1995;270:8553-8558.

298. Vinogradova O, Vaynberg J, Kong X, Haas TA, Plow EF, Qin J. Membrane-mediated structural transitions at the cytoplasmic face during integrin activation. *Proc Natl Acad Sci U S A*. 2004;101:4094-4099.

299. Kim M, Carman CV, Springer TA. Bidirectional transmembrane signaling by cytoplasmic domain separation in integrins. *Science*. 2003;301:1720-1725.

300. Moser M, Nieswandt B, Ussar S, Pozgajova M, Fassler R. Kindlin-3 is essential for integrin activation and platelet aggregation. *Nat Med*. 2008;14:325-330.

301. Calderwood DA, Ginsberg MH. Talin forges the links between integrins and actin. *Nat Cell Biol*. 2003;5:694.

302. Han J, Lim CJ, Watanabe N, et al. Reconstructing and deconstructing agonist-induced activation of integrin alphaIIbbeta3. *Curr Biol*. 2006;16:1796.

303. Wegener KL, Partridge AW, Han J, et al. Structural basis of integrin activation by talin. *Cell*. 2007;128:171.

304. Kiema T, Lad Y, Jiang P, et al. The molecular basis of filamin binding to integrins and competition with talin. *Mol Cell*. 2006;21:337.

305. Ma YQ, Qin J, Plow EF. Platelet integrin alpha(IIb)beta(3): activation mechanisms. *J Thromb Haemost*. 2007;5:1345.

306. Bennett JS, Zigmond S, Vilaire G, Cunningham ME, Bednar B. The platelet cytoskeleton regulates the affinity of the integrin α$_{II}$bβ$_2$3 for fibrinogen. *J Biol Chem*. 1999;274:25301-25307.

307. Kucik DF. Rearrangement of integrins in avidity regulation by leukocytes. *Immunol Res*. 2002;26:199-206.

308. Bennett JS, Vilaire G. Exposure of platelet fibrinogen receptors by ADP and epinephrine. *J Clin Invest*. 1979;64:1393-1401.

309. Jackson SP, Schoenwaelder SM, Yuan YP, Salem HH, Cooray P. Non-receptor protein tyrosine kinases and phosphatases in human platelets. *Thromb Haemost*. 1996;76:640-650.

310. Lerea KM, Tonks NK, Krebs EG, Fischer EH, Glomset JA. Vanadate and molybdate increase tyrosine phosphorylation in a 50-kilodalton protein and stimulate secretion in electropermeabilized platelets. *Biochemistry*. 1989;28:9286-9292.

311. Savage B, Shattil SJ, Ruggeri ZM. Modulation of platelet function through adhesion receptors. A dual role for glycoprotein IIb-IIIa mediated by fibrinogen and glycoprotein Ib-von Willebrand factor. *J Biol Chem*. 1992;267:11300-11306.

312. Prevost N, Woulfe D, Tognolini M, Brass LF. Contact-dependent signaling during the late events of platelet activation. *J Thromb Haemost*. 2003;1:1613-1627.

313. Law DA, Phillips DR. Glycoprotein IIb/IIIa in platelet aggregation and acute arterial thrombosis. In: *Platelet Glycoprotein IIb/IIIa Inhibitors in Cardiovascular Disease*, Lincoff AM, Topol EJ, Humana Press; 1999:35-66.

314. Naik MU, Naik UP. Calcium and integrin-binding protein regulates focal adhesion kinase activity during platelet spreading on immobilized fibrinogen. *Blood*. 2003;102:3629-3636.

315. Parsons JT. Focal adhesion kinase: the first ten years. *J Cell Sci*. 2003;116:1409-1416.

316. Downes CP, Currie RA. Lipid signaling. *Curr Biol*. 1998;8:R865-R867.

317. Kovacsovics TJ, Bachelot C, Toker A, et al. Phosphoinositide 3-kinase inhibitors spares actin assembly in activating platelets but reverses platelet aggregation. *J Biol Chem*. 1995;270:11358-11366.

318. Gawaz MP, Loftus JC, Bajt ML, Frojmovic MM, Plow EF, Ginsberg MH. Ligand bridging mediates integrin alpha IIb beta 3 (platelet GPIIB-IIIA) dependent homotypic and heterotypic cell–cell interactions. *J Clin Invest*. 1991;88:1128.

319. Zamarron C, Ginsberg MH, Plow EF. A receptor-induced binding site in fibrinogen elicited by its interaction with platelet membrane glycoprotein IIb-IIIa. *J Biol Chem*. 1991;266:16193.

320. Frelinger AL,III, Lam SC, Plow EF, Smith MA, Loftus JC, Ginsberg MH. Occupancy of an adhesive glycoprotein receptor modulates expression of an antigenic site involved in cell adhesion. *J Biol Chem*. 1988;263:12397.

321. Tuszynski GP, Kornecki E, Cierniewski C, et al. Association of fibrin with the platelet cytoskeleton. *J Biol Chem*. 1984;259:5247.

322. Phillips DR, Jennings LK, Prasanna HR. Ca^{2+}−mediated association of glycoprotein G (thrombinsensitive protein, thrombospondin) with human platelets. *J Biol Chem*. 1980;255:11629.

323. Brass LF, Jiang H, Wu J, Stalker TJ, Zhu L. Contact-dependent signaling events that promote thrombus formation. *Blood Cells Mol Dis*. 2006;36:157.

324. Swords NA, Tracy PB, Mann KG. Intact platelet membranes, not platelet-released microvesicles, support the procoagulant activity of adherent platelets. *Arterioscler Thromb*. 1993;13:1613-1622.

325. Henn V, Slupsky JR, Grafe M, et al. CD40 ligand on activated platelets triggers an inflammatory reaction of endothelial cells. *Nature*. 1998;391:591-594.

326. Bombeli T, Schwartz BR, Harlan JM. Adhesion of activated platelets to endothelial cells: evidence for a GP-IIb/IIIa-dependent bridging mechanism and novel roles for endothelial intercellular adhesion molecule 1 (ICAM-1), α$_V$β$_2$3 integrin, and GPIbα. *J Exp Med*. 1998;187:329-339.

327. Buttrum SM, Hatton R, Nash GB. Selectin-mediated rolling of neutrophils on immobilized platelets. *Blood*. 1993;82:1165-1174.

328. Weber C, Springer TA. Neutrophil accumulation on activated, surface-adherent platelets in flow is mediated by interaction of Mac-1 with fibrinogen bound to α$_{II}$bβ$_2$3 and stimulated by platelet-activating factor. *J Clin Invest*. 1997;100:2085-2093.

329. Smyth SS, Reis ED, Zhang W, Fallon JT, Gordon RE, Coller BS. β$_2$3-Integrin-deficient mice but not P-selectin-deficient mice develop intimal hyperplasia after vascular injury: correlation with leukocyte recruitment to adherent platelets 1 hour after injury. *Circulation*. 2001;103:2501-2507.

330. Maxwell MJ, Westein E, Nesbitt WS, Giuliano S, Dopheide SM, Jackson SP. Identification of a 2-stage platelet aggregation process mediating shear-dependent thrombus formation. *Blood*. 2007;109:566-567.

331. Chauhan AK, Kisucka J, Lamb CB, Bergmeier W, Wagner DD. von Willebrand factor and factor VIII are independently required to form stable occlusive thrombi in injured veins. *Blood*. 2006;109:2424-2429.

332. Ruggeri ZM, Orje JN, Habermann R, Federici AB, Reininger AJ. Activation-independent platelet adhesion and aggregation under elevated shear stress. *Blood*. 2006;108(6):1903-1910.

333. Jain A, Graveline A, Waterhouse A, et al. A shear gradient-activated microfluidic device for automated monitoring of whole blood haemostasis and platelet function. *Nat Commun*. 2016;7:10176.

334. Westein E, van der Meer AD, Kuijpers MJ, et al. Atherosclerotic geometries exacerbate pathological thrombus formation poststenosis in a von Willebrand factor-dependent manner. *Proc Natl Acad Sci U S A*. 2013;110:1357-1362.

335. Fontaine V, Jacob MP, Houard X, et al. Involvement of the mural thrombus as a site of protease release and activation in human aortic aneurysms. *Am J Pathol*. 2002;161:1701-1710.

336. Vorp DA, Lee PC, Wang DH, et al. Association of intraluminal thrombus in abdominal aortic aneurysm with local hypoxia and wall weakening. *J Vasc Surg*. 2001;34:291-299.

337. Wang DH, Makaroun MS, Webster MW, Vorp DA. Effect of intraluminal thrombus on wall stress in patient-specific models of abdominal aortic aneurysm. *J Vasc Surg*. 2002;36:598-604.

338. Herbig BA, Diamond SL. Pathological von Willebrand factor fibers resist tissue plasminogen activator and ADAMTS13 while promoting the contact pathway and shear-induced platelet activation. *J Thromb Haemost*. 2015;13:1699-1708.

339. Versteeg HH, Heemskerk JW, Levi M, Reitsma PH. New fundamentals in hemostasis. *Physiol Rev*. 2013;93:327-358.

340. Lordkipanidze M, Lowe GC, Kirkby NS, UK Genotyping and Phenotyping of Platelets Study Group, et al. Characterization of multiple platelet activation pathways in patients with bleeding as a high-throughput screening option: use of 96-well Optimul assay. *Blood*. 2014;123:e11-e22.

341. de Witt SM, Swieringa F, Cavill R, et al. Identification of platelet function defects by multi-parameter assessment of thrombus formation. *Nat Commun*. 2014;5:4257.

342. Tomaiuolo M, Stalker TJ, Welsh JD, Diamond SL, Sinno T, Brass LF. A systems approach to hemostasis: 2. Computational analysis of molecular transport in the thrombus microenvironment. *Blood*. 2014;124:1816-1823.

343. Dolan AT, Diamond SL. Systems modeling of Ca(2+) homeostasis and mobilization in platelets mediated by IP3 and store-operated Ca(2+) entry. *Biophys J*. 2014;106:2049-2060.

344. Hartwig JH. The platelet cytoskeleton. In *Platelets*: Michelson A, 3rd ed. Academic Press; 2013:145-168.

345. Kansas GS. Selectins and their ligands: current concepts and controversies. *Blood*. 1996;88:3259-3287.

346. Frenette PS, Johnson RC, Hynes RO, Wagner DD. Platelets roll on stimulated endothelium in vivo: an interaction mediated by endothelial P-selectin. *Proc Natl Acad Sci U S A*. 1995;92:7450-7454.

347. Frenette PS, Moyna C, Hartwell DW, Lowe JB, Hynes RO, Wagner DD. Platelet–endothelial interactions in inflamed mesenteric venules. *Blood*. 1998;91:1318-1324.

348. Katayama T, Ikeda Y, Handa M, et al. Immunoneutralization of glycoprotein Ibα attenuates endotoxin-induced interactions of platelets and leukocytes with rat venular endothelium in vivo. *Circ Res*. 2000;86:1031-1037.

349. Gawaz M, Langer H, May AE. Platelets in inflammation and atherogenesis. *J Clin Invest*. 2005;115:3378-3384.

350. Wagner DD, Frenette PS. The vessel wall and its interactions. *Blood*. 2008;111:5271-5281.

351. Andre P, Denis CV, Ware J, et al. Platelets adhere to and translocate on von Willebrand factor presented by endothelium in stimulated veins. *Blood*. 2000;96:3322-3328.

352. Massberg S, Gruner S, Konrad I, et al. Enhanced in vivo platelet adhesion in vasodilator-stimulated phosphoprotein (VASP)-deficient mice. *Blood*. 2004;103:136-142.

353. Massberg S, Enders G, Matos FC, et al. Fibrinogen deposition at the postischemic vessel wall promotes platelet adhesion during ischemia-reperfusion in vivo. *Blood*. 1999;94:3829-3838.

354. Romo GM, Dong JF, Schader A, et al. The glycoprotein Ib-IX-V complex is a platelet counterreceptor for P-selectin. *J Exp Med*. 1999;190:803-814.

355. Frenette PS, Denis CV, Weiss L, et al. P-Selectin glycoprotein ligand 1 (PSGL-1) is expressed on platelets and can mediate platelet–endothelial interactions in vivo. *J Exp Med*. 2000;191:1413-1422.

356. D'Souza SE, Byers-Ward VJ, Gardiner EE, Wang H, Sung SS. Identification of an active sequence within the first immunoglobulin domain of intercellular cell adhesion molecule-1 (ICAM-1) that interacts with fibrinogen. *J Biol Chem*. 1996;271:24270-24277.

357. Falati S, Liu Q, Gross P, et al. Accumulation of tissue factor into developing thrombi in vivo is dependent upon microparticle P-selectin glycoprotein ligand 1 and platelet P-selectin. *J Exp Med*. 2003;197:1585-1598.

The Normal Hematologic System

358. Subramaniam M, Frenette PS, Saffaripour S, Johnson RC, Hynes RO, Wagner DD. Defects in haemostasis in P-selectin-deficient mice. *Blood*. 1996;87:1238-1242.

359. McEver RP. Adhesive interactions of leukocytes, platelets, and the vessel wall during hemostasis and inflammation. *Thromb Haemost*. 2001;86:746-756.

360. Springer TA. Traffic signals for lymphocyte recirculation and leukocyte emigration: the multistep paradigm. *Cell*. 1994;76:301-314.

361. Diacovo TG, Roth SJ, Buccola JM, Bainton DF, Springer TA. Neutrophil rolling, arrest, and transmigration across activated, surface adherent platelets via sequential action of P-selectin and the β2-integrin CD11b/CD18. *Blood*. 1996;88:146-157.

362. Evangelista V, Manarini S, Sideri R, et al. Platelet/polymorphonuclear leukocyte interaction: P-selectin triggers protein-tyrosine phosphorylation-dependent CD11b/CD18 adhesion—role of PSGL-1 as a signaling molecule. *Blood*. 1999;93:876-885.

363. Yang J, Furie BC, Furie B. The biology of P-selectin glycoprotein ligand-1: its role as a selectin counterreceptor in leukocyte-endothelial and leukocyte-platelet interaction. *Thromb Haemost*. 1999;81:1-7.

364. Simon DI, Chen Z, Xu H, et al. Platelet glycoprotein Ibα is a counterreceptor for the leukocyte integrin Mac-1 (CD11b/CD18). *J Exp Med*. 2000;192:193-204.

365. Santoso S, Sachs UJ, Kroll H, et al. The junctional adhesion molecule 3 (JAM-3) on human platelets is a counterreceptor for the leukocyte integrin Mac-1. *J Exp Med*. 2002;196:679-691.

366. Diacovo TG, deFougerolles AR, Bainton DF, Springer TA. A functional integrin ligand on the surface of platelets: intercellular adhesion molecule-2. *J Clin Invest*. 1994;94:1243-1251.

367. Wright SD, Weitz JI, Huang AJ, Levin SM, Silverstein SC, Loike JD. Complement receptor type three (CD11b/CD18) of human polymorphonuclear leukocytes recognizes fibrinogen. *Proc Natl Acad Sci U S A*. 1988;85:7734-7738.

368. Altieri DC, Bader R, Mannucci PM, Edgington TS. Oligospecificity of the cellular adhesion receptor Mac-1 encompasses an inducible recognition specificity for fibrinogen. *J Cell Biol*. 1988;107:1893-1900.

369. Chavakis T, Santoso S, Clemetson KJ, et al. High molecular weight kininogen regulates platelet–leukocyte interactions by bridging Mac-1 and glycoprotein Ib. *J Biol Chem*. 2003;278:45375-45381.

370. Weyrich AS, Elstad MR, McEver RP, et al. Activated platelets signal chemokine synthesis by human monocytes. *J Clin Invest*. 1996;97:1525-1534.

371. Neumann FJ, Marx N, Gawaz M, et al. Induction of cytokine expression in leukocytes by binding of thrombin-stimulated platelets. *Circulation*. 1997;95:2387-2394.

372. Huo Y, Schober A, Forlow SB, et al. Circulating activated platelets exacerbate atherosclerosis in mice deficient in apolipoprotein E. *Nat Med*. 2003;9:61-67.

373. Koupenova M, Mick E, Mikhalev E, et al. Sex differences in platelet toll-like receptors and their association with cardiovascular risk factors. *Arterioscler Thromb Vasc Biol*. 2015;35:1030-1037.

374. Cognasse F, Nguyen KA, Damien P, et al. The inflammatory role of platelets via their TLRs and siglec receptors. *Front Immunol*. 2015;6:83.

375. Koupenova M, Clancy L, Corkrey HA. Circulating platelets as mediators of immunity, inflammation, and thrombosis. *Circ Res*. 2018;122:337-351.

376. Semple JW, Italiano JE, Jr, Freedman J. Platelets and the immune continuum. *Nat Rev Immunol*. 2011;11:264-274.t.

377. Langer HF, Daub K, Braun G, et al. Platelets recruit human dendritic cells via Mac-1/JAM-C interaction and modulate dendritic cell function in vitro. *Arterioscler Thromb Vasc Biol*. 2007;27:1463-1470.

378. Koupenova M, Vitseva O, MacKay CR, et al. Platelet-TLR7 mediates host survival and platelet count during viral infection in the absence of platelet-dependent thrombosis. *Blood*. 2014;124:791-802.

379. Labelle M, Begum S, Hynes RO. Platelets guide the formation of early metastatic niches. *Proc Natl Acad Sci U S A*. 2014;111:E3053-E3061.

380. Lowenberg EC, Meijers JC, Levi M. Platelet-vessel wall interaction in health and disease. *Neth J Med*. 2010;68:242-251.

381. Falati S, Gross P, Merrill-Skoloff G, Furie BC, Furie B. Real-time in vivo imaging of platelets, tissue factor and fibrin during arterial thrombus formation in the mouse. *Nat Med*. 2002;8:1175-1181.

382. Li G, Sanders JM, Phan ET, Ley K, Sarembock IJ. Arterial macrophages and regenerating endothelial cells express P-selectin in atherosclerosis-prone apolipoprotein E-deficient mice. *Am J Pathol*. 2005;167:1511-1518.

383. Burger PC, Wagner DD. Platelet P-selectin facilitates atherosclerotic lesion development. *Blood*. 2003;101(7):2661-2666.

384. Prasad KS, Andre P, He M, Bao M, Manganello J, Phillips DR. Soluble CD40 ligand induces β3 integrin tyrosine phosphorylation and triggers platelet activation by outside-in signaling. *Proc Natl Acad Sci U S A*. 2003;100:12367-12371.

385. Risitano A, Beaulieu LM, Vitseva O, Freedman JE. Platelets and platelet-like particles mediate intercellular RNA transfer. *Blood*. 2012;119:6288-6295.

386. Clancy L, Beaulieu LM, Tanriverdi K, Freedman JE. The role of RNA uptake in platelet heterogeneity. *Thromb Haemost*. 2017;117:948-961.

387. Morrell CN, Aggrey AA, Chapman LM, et al. Emerging roles for platelets as immune and inflammatory cells. *Blood*. 2014;123:2759-2767.

388. Gidlöf O, van der Brug M, Ohman J, et al. Platelets activated during myocardial infarction release functional miRNA, which can be taken up by endothelial cells and regulate ICAM1 expression. *Blood*. 2013;121:3908-3917, S1-26.

389. Liang H, Yan X, Pan Y, et al. MicroRNA-223 delivered by platelet-derived microvesicles promotes lung cancer cell invasion via targeting tumor suppressor EPB41L3. *Mol Cancer*. 2015;14:58.

390. Michael JV, Wurtzel JGT, Mao GF, et al. Platelet microparticles infiltrating solid tumors transfer miRNAs that suppress tumor growth. *Blood*. 2017;130:567-580.

391. Falk E. Plaque rupture with severe pre-existing stenosis precipitating coronary thrombosis: characteristics of coronary atherosclerotic plaques underlying fatal occlusive thrombi. *Br Heart J*. 1983;50:127-134.

392. Davies MJ, Thomas AC. Plaque fissuring: the cause of acute myocardial infarction, sudden ischaemic death, and crescendo angina. *Br Heart J*. 1985;53:363-373.

393. Burke AP, Farb A, Malcolm GT, Liang Y, Smialek JE, Virmani R. Plaque rupture and sudden death related to exertion in men with coronary artery disease. *JAMA*. 1999;281:921-926.

394. Ross R. Atherosclerosis—an inflammatory disease. *N Engl J Med*. 1999;340:115-126.

395. Libby P, Ridker PM, Maseri A. Inflammation and atherosclerosis. *Circulation*. 2002;105:1135-1143.

396. Borissoff JI, Spronk HM, ten Cate H. The hemostatic system as a modulator of atherosclerosis. *N Engl J Med*. 2011;364:1746-1760.

397. Libby P, Simon DI. Inflammation and thrombosis—the clot thickens. *Circulation*. 2001;103:1718-1720.

398. Ostrovsky L, King AJ, Bond S, et al. A juxtacrine mechanism for neutrophil adhesion on platelets involves platelet-activating factor and a selectin-dependent activation process. *Blood*. 1998;91:3028-3036.

399. Theilmeier G, Michiels C, Spaepen E, et al. Endothelial von Willebrand factor recruits platelets to atherosclerosis-prone sites in response to hypercholesterolemia. *Blood*. 2002;99:4486-4493.

400. Massberg S, Schurzinger K, Lorenz M, et al. Platelet adhesion via glycoprotein IIb integrin is critical for atheroprogression and focal cerebral ischemia: an in vivo study in mice lacking glycoprotein IIb. *Circulation*. 2005;112:1180-1188.

401. Koenen RR, von Hundelshausen P, Nesmelova IV, et al. Disrupting functional interactions between platelet chemokines inhibits atherosclerosis in hyperlipidemic mice. *Nat Med*. 2009;15(1):97-103.

402. Warnatsch A, Ioannou M, Wang Q, Papayannopoulos V. Inflammation. Neutrophil extracellular traps license macrophages for cytokine production in atherosclerosis. *Science*. 2015;349(6245):316-320.

403. Etulain J, Martinod K, Wong SL, Cifuni SM, Schattner M, Wagner DD. P-selectin promotes neutrophil extracellular trap formation in mice. *Blood*. 2015;126(2):242-246.

404. Mach F, Schonbeck U, Sukhova GK, Atkinson E, Libby P. Reduction of atherosclerosis in mice by inhibition of CD40 signalling. *Nature*. 1998;394:200-203.

405. Chi H, Messas E, Levine RA, Graves DT, Amar S. Interleukin-1 receptor signaling mediates atherosclerosis associated with bacterial exposure and/or a high-fat diet in a murine apolipoprotein E heterozygote model: pharmacotherapeutic implications. *Circulation*. 2004;110:1678-1685.

406. Kirii H, Niwa T, Yamada Y, et al. Lack of interleukin-1β decreases the severity of atherosclerosis in ApoE-deficient mice. *Arterioscler Thromb Vasc Biol*. 2003;23:656-660.

407. Belton OA, Duffy A, Toomey S, Fitzgerald DJ. Cyclooxygenase isoforms and platelet vessel wall interactions in the apolipoprotein E knockout mouse model of atherosclerosis. *Circulation*. 2003;108:3017-3023.

408. Methia N, Andre P, Denis CV, Economopoulos M, Wagner DD. Localized reduction of atherosclerosis in von Willebrand factor-deficient mice. *Blood*. 2001;98:1424-1428.

409. Ritchie ME. Nuclear factor-κB is selectively and markedly activated in humans with unstable angina pectoris. *Circulation*. 1998;98:1707-1713.

410. Falk E. Coronary thrombosis: pathogenesis and clinical manifestations. *Am J Cardiol*. 1991;68(suppl B):28B-35B.

411. Falk E. Advanced lesions and acute coronary syndromes: a pathologist's view. In *Syndromes of Atherosclerosis: Correlations of Clinical Imaging and Pathology*: Fuster V, Futura; 1996:81-104.

412. Nesbitt WS, Mangin P, Salem HH, Jackson SP. The impact of blood rheology on the molecular and cellular events underlying arterial thrombosis. *J Mol Med*. 2006;84:989-995.

413. Lehoux S, Tedgui A. Cellular mechanics and gene expression in blood vessels. *J Biomech*. 2003;36:631-643.

414. Nesbitt WS, Westein E, Tovar-Lopez J, et al. A shear gradient-dependent platelet aggregation mechanism drives thrombus formation. *Nat Med*. 2009;15:665-673.

415. Reddy KG, Nair RN, Sheehan HM, Hodgson JM. Evidence that selective endothelial dysfunction may occur in the absence of angiographic or ultrasound atherosclerosis in patients with risk factors for atherosclerosis. *J Am Coll Cardiol*. 1994;23:833-843.

416. Bogaty P, Hackett D, Davies G, Maseri A. Vasoreactivity of the culprit lesion in unstable angina. *Circulation*. 1994;90:5-11.

417. Yanagisawa M, Kurihara H, Kimura S, et al. A novel potent vasoconstrictor peptide produced by vascular endothelial cells. *Nature*. 1988;332:411-415.

418. Fuster V. Mechanisms leading to myocardial infarction: insights from studies of vascular biology. *Circulation*. 1994;90:2126-2146.

419. Willerson JT, Golino P, Eidt J, Campbell WB, Buja LM. Specific platelet mediators and unstable coronary artery lesions: experimental evidence and potential clinical implications. *Circulation*. 1989;80:198-205.

Chapter 20 ■ Blood Coagulation and Fibrinolysis

STEPHEN J. EVERSE • THOMAS ORFEO • KATHLEEN E. BRUMMEL-ZIEDINS • KENNETH G. MANN

INTRODUCTION

The opposing forces of fibrin clot formation and dissolution maintain hemostasis and preserve vascular function and integrity. Procoagulant events (platelet adhesion/activation, α-thrombin generation, and cross-linked fibrin clot formation) protect the vasculature from perforating injury and excessive blood loss in a process tightly regulated by plasma and cellular inhibition systems. Subsequent activation of the fibrinolytic system removes the clot, restores blood flow, and initiates tissue repair and regeneration. Hemostasis thus refers to multiple discrete processes that collectively culminate in preservation of vascular integrity. Circulating and adherent cells collaborate with plasma and cell membrane–associated proteins to carry out key roles in both pathways. Hemostasis is not a passive but a continuously active process in maintaining vascular integrity. With vascular perforation, focal interactions initiate procoagulant and fibrinolytic events and initiate tissue repair. Each process must operate in a cooperative fashion, or the entire system is compromised. Thus, balance between the procoagulant, anticoagulant, fibrinolytic, and antifibrinolytic processes is required to prevent extravascular blood loss, or undesirable intravascular thrombosis.[1]

Much of our knowledge of hemostasis has been gleaned and validated from observations of hemostatic and thrombotic pathology; however, much is still not well understood. Epidemiologic studies have expanded our knowledge about key factors that determine risk for venous and arterial thrombosis; however, vascular thrombosis is still the primary cause of death in the United States and Western Europe.[2] Thus, although the present information base is formidable, investigators continue to examine the processes that contribute to blood coagulation and fibrinolysis. The current concepts governing the roles of protein and cellular components, their structures, functions, and regulations are summarized in the following sections.

ESSENTIAL FEATURES OF COAGULATION

MacFarlane[3] and Davie and Ratnoff[4] provided the first integrated descriptions of the coagulation system. They proposed a "cascade" or "waterfall" sequence of events in which the reactions occur in a defined series leading to prothrombin activation and fibrin clot formation. Each reaction shares a similar mechanism in which an inactive zymogen is converted to an active enzyme. Although some facets of these initial descriptions are still valid, the emerging concept of coagulation and fibrinolysis centers on a complex network of highly interwoven collections of simultaneously occurring processes. Procoagulant, anticoagulant, and fibrinolytic processes occur with many positive and negative feedback loops regulating the processes. These overlapped reactions can be operationally described as five distinct phases: *initiation* of coagulation, *propagation* of α-thrombin formation, *termination* of the procoagulant response, *elimination* of the fibrin clot, and tissue *repair* and regeneration. The reactions involved in these five phases share several key features and the nomenclature used to describe the protein components of the reactions is similar.

The proteolytic enzymes and their zymogen precursors are mostly members of the serine protease family that includes chymotrypsin and trypsin with the zymogen and enzyme forms distinguished by an "α" to signify the active enzyme. For example, *factor Xa* is the active enzyme and *factor X* is the corresponding zymogen. Factor II, most commonly referred to as prothrombin, is the zymogen that upon activation becomes factor αIIa or α-thrombin. The nonzymogen procofactors factors V and VIII also share this nomenclature, in which the proteolytically activated fully functional cofactor forms are designated

factors Va and *VIIIa;* conversely, the inactivated forms are designated with an "i" subscript (factor Va_i). The protein cofactors that are cell associated, tissue factor and thrombomodulin, primarily exist in one form and designation. The mechanisms of the individual procoagulant reactions are likewise similar. In each case, a complex consisting of a serine protease, a cofactor protein and Ca^{2+} is assembled on a membrane surface. Each complex enzyme cleaves a zymogen to an enzyme.[5] The progression from complex to complex results in amplification of product formation.[6] In blood, the membrane surface is provided by platelets and by other circulating cells and microparticles. The vessel wall also contributes cofactors and membrane to support complex formation. The common features of these membrane-cofactor-protease complexes include target recognition, reaction amplification, regulation, and localization. The response to injury is rapid and ordinarily modulated to ensure a sufficient but not excessive response to the injury.

The initiation of the antihemorrhagic response occurs when the vascular wall is perforated and the antithrombotic nature of the vessel wall is overcome to achieve a prothrombotic state. Membrane surface and subcellular elements, including tissue factor, are presented and initiate the subsequent phases of coagulation. The assembly of the multicomponent procoagulant complexes on membrane surfaces triggers propagation of the coagulation response. The net result of the activities of these complexes (the intrinsic and extrinsic tenase and prothrombinase complexes) is an explosive local expression of α-thrombin. The initial burst of α-thrombin sustains the procoagulant response by activating circulating platelets, the procofactors V and VIII, and the zymogen factors VII and XI.[7-16] Thrombin cleaves the fibrinopeptides from fibrinogen and activates factor XIII (to factor XIIIa),[17] a protransglutaminase that, when activated, cross-links (to fXIIIa) and stabilizes the fibrin clot. Tight regulation by antithrombin, tissue factor pathway inhibitor (TFPI), and the dynamic protein C system (thrombin-thrombomodulin) ensures that the response is appropriate to the stimulating injury. The thrombin-activatable fibrinolysis inhibitor (TAFI),[18,19] a procarboxypeptidase zymogen, thrombin-activated as TAFIa, protects the fibrin clot by downregulating the fibrinolytic system. The propagation phase thus stems blood loss by producing a platelet-rich cross-linked fibrin clot.[20] Ultimately, inhibition of the procoagulant enzyme complexes by direct inhibition of the serine proteases and proteolytic inactivation of the cofactor proteins restores homeostasis by limiting coagulation to the site of vascular damage and preventing excessive clot formation.

The plasma proenzyme plasminogen is activated to plasmin by proteases associated with the vascular endothelial cells. Plasmin cleaves the cross-linked fibrin matrix to produce soluble peptides including D-dimer.[21,22] The mechanism by which plasmin is generated is complex and involves several proteins with key roles throughout the hemostatic response. The solubilization and removal of the fibrin scaffolding of the hemostatic plug is coordinated with the processes of tissue repair and regeneration in part triggered by products of the processes. The extracellular matrix is degraded to allow for cell migration into the damaged area. Vascular cells repopulate the site and recreate the elements necessary to restore the vessel to its (relatively) previously unperturbed state.

These steps occur rapidly and in a precise choreographed manner and must be localized to the site of injury. Localization presents challenges because the hemostatic response occurs under conditions of highly variable flow in vascular tubes of various diameters.[23] Localization is controlled on several levels. Endothelial cells actively inhibit coagulation by constitutively synthesizing various anticoagulants and platelet activation inhibitors. Furthermore, the surfaces of inactivated, undamaged blood and vascular cells are not conducive to the assembly and function of the procoagulant protein complexes. Thus, surface availability for procoagulant complex assembly is ordinarily limited by vascular pathology. The activated cell/damaged membrane surfaces may also provide for rapid transfer of intermediate products between complexes; such two-dimensional transfer of intermediates between complexes would increase the rates of complex formation and provide protection from the abundant plasma inhibitors. The essential features of the hemostatic response (recognition, amplification, regulation, and localization) ensure that the response is localized to the injury, amplified appropriately according to the severity of the injury, and attenuated to block a systemic reaction.[24,25]

In contrast to hemostasis, thrombosis is invoked by the presentation of intravascular tissue factor either by damaged endothelium or by an inflammatory cell. The resulting coagulation process is invoked, but in this instance results in the pathology of thrombosis. Vascular thrombotic occlusions composed of platelets and fibrin are significantly influenced by vascular architecture, vascular cell biology, and flow biophysics. In arterial thrombosis, high shear rates make platelet-rich clots (white clots) more apparent, while in the low-shear venous circulation, fibrin-rich clots (red clots) are observed. However, it is likely that, in both vascular environments, events similar to those associated with the hemostatic process occur.

OVERVIEW OF PROCOAGULANT PATHWAYS: PRIMARY (EXTRINSIC) AND ACCESSORY (INTRINSIC) PATHWAYS

Two procoagulant pathways have been identified that converge at the "intrinsic" fXase (fIXa·fVIIIa) complex (*Figure 20.1*). The contact or "intrinsic" pathway is activated by the interaction of blood with a foreign surface. This pathway is activated by the factor XIIa–high-molecular-weight kininogen (HMWK)–prekallikrein complex in association with foreign surfaces including glass, dextran sulfate, or kaolin. The complex catalyst activates factor XI leading to the factor XIa–HMWK complex, which activates fIX to fIXa. The "intrinsic" fXase rapidly cleaves fX to fXa.

Factor Xa is directly but less effectively produced by the "extrinsic" fXase, which is composed of plasma-derived fVIIa and tissue factor and expressed when the latter is exposed to blood. The "extrinsic" fXase also activates fIX to fIXa as the reaction progresses, with suppression of the quaternary complex occurring by TFPI. The "intrinsic" fXase complex is kinetically superior and ultimately produces the majority of fXa.

Since bleeding pathology is not ordinarily associated with defects of the initiation protein complexes of the contact pathway, most investigations conclude that the "extrinsic" pathway is not the primary provider for hemostasis. The "intrinsic" pathway, however, has been implicated in some forms of thrombosis. The primary ("extrinsic") and accessory ("intrinsic") pathways, initiated by independent routes, both lead to the activation of factor IX and converge at the "intrinsic" fXase complex (*Figure 20.1*). Regardless of the path, the outcome is the formation of the prothrombinase complex and thrombin generation. Each reaction of the primary pathway of coagulation involves the vitamin K–dependent zymogens and serine proteases, cofactor proteins, and Ca^{2+} ions assembled on membranes. The complexes display reaction rates 10^5 to 10^9 times greater than the respective serine proteases alone.[5]

Clinical laboratory tests differentiate between the pathways. The activated partial thromboplastin time (aPTT) initiates coagulation through the accessory pathway, whereas the prothrombin time (PT) assay initiates coagulation through the primary pathway.[26-28] The designations of primary and accessory pathways are based on clinical evidence of bleeding diseases. Deficiencies of proteins associated with the "intrinsic" or accessory pathway (factor XII, prekallikrein, and HMWK) exist but are not associated with abnormal bleeding events, even after surgical challenge.[29-31] However, deficiencies of the protein components of the "extrinsic" or primary pathway (prothrombin and factors

V, VII, VIII, IX, and X) can lead to severe bleeding diatheses.[16,32-35] Factor XI deficiency may also result in bleeding episodes subsequent to trauma or surgery.[20,36] The role of the accessory pathway is therefore not clearly understood. Factor XI appears to play a role in coagulation,[21,37] most likely unrelated to its activity in the "intrinsic" pathway, with the contribution of factor XI to hemostasis thought to be due to its activation by α-thrombin. Factor XIa then functions in the propagation phase of α-thrombin generation in association with the primary pathway.[7,22]

Factor XII, prekallikrein, and HMWK are required for activity of the contact or accessory pathway, and deficiencies are reported by the aPTT. Factor XII and prekallikrein are zymogens that are activated to serine proteases, while HMWK is a cofactor. The accessory pathway factors are hypothesized to play a role in disseminated intravascular coagulation (DIC) associated with the systemic inflammatory response syndrome[38,39] and may also be involved in the promotion of thrombus stability.[5,24,40,41] The accessory pathway may also be important in cardiopulmonary bypass because of contact between blood components and synthetic surfaces.[39]

The importance of the membrane component in coagulation was initially identified by kinetic studies of the prothrombinase complex. In the absence of the membrane surface, the cofactor (factor Va)-enzyme (factor Xa) interaction is relatively weak, with a dissociation constant (K_d) of 800 nmol/L.[42-44] The factor Va–lipid interaction (K_d = 3 nmol/L) and factor Xa–lipid interaction (K_d = 110 nmol/L)[45] show higher affinity. However, all of the components must be present to generate the high-affinity factor Va–factor Xa–Ca^{2+} membrane complex, with a K_d of 1 nmol/L.[46] The fully assembled complex is stabilized through factor Va–factor Xa, factor Va–lipid, and factor Xa–lipid interactions.[14,47,48] Similar properties have been observed for the fIXa/fVIIIa, TF/fVIIa, and Tm/fIIa complexes.[42]

The primary pathway of coagulation is initiated or triggered by the interaction of circulating factor VIIa with its cofactor tissue factor.[49-51] In general, the serine proteases associated with hemostasis circulate in their zymogen or inactive forms; however, low levels of circulating factor VIIa are present in blood.[52] This factor VIIa binds to tissue factor expressed by pathology and initiates the procoagulant response. Free factor VIIa is a poor enzyme with virtually no proteolytic activity but as a consequence is protected from interacting with the circulating inhibitors in the absence of tissue factor. Tissue factor, an integral membrane protein not normally expressed on vascular cell surfaces, is constitutively expressed on extravascular cellular surfaces[53-58] and thus becomes exposed upon damage to the endothelial cell layer. Tissue factor is also expressed on peripheral blood cells and endothelial cells stimulated by inflammatory cytokines.[59,60]

Upon interaction of plasma factor VIIa and the injury/pathology presented, tissue factor, the "extrinsic" fXase complex (factor VIIIa–tissue factor) is formed and initiates coagulation by activating factors IX and X. Factor IXa forms a complex with its cofactor, factor VIIIa, to generate the intrinsic "fXase" complex, and factor Xa combines with factor Va to form the prothrombinase complex. The factor VIIIa–factor IXa complex more efficiently activates factor X to factor Xa, providing a robust source of the enzyme component (factor Xa) of the prothrombinase complex.

Deficiencies of the "intrinsic" fXase components factor VIIIa (hemophilia A) and factor IXa (hemophilia B) illustrate the significance of the factor IX activation by the fVIIa/TF complex and the enhanced rate of factor X activation by the intrinsic fXase and the inhibition of the extrinsic fXase by TFPI. Hemophilia A and B are detected using the aPTT. From inspection of *Figure 20.1*, it would appear that activation of factor X by the "extrinsic" fXase should compensate for the lack of factor X activation by the "intrinsic" fXase in hemophilias A and B. However, this compensatory mechanism only occurs during clinical administration of supraphysiologic concentrations of recombinant factor VIIa during replacement therapy for hemophilia with inhibitors. The natural physiologic levels of factor VIIa are not able to provide sufficient levels of factor Xa to support normal coagulation. Factor Xa generation is suppressed to approximately half the level observed when factor X is the only substrate presented.[61,62]

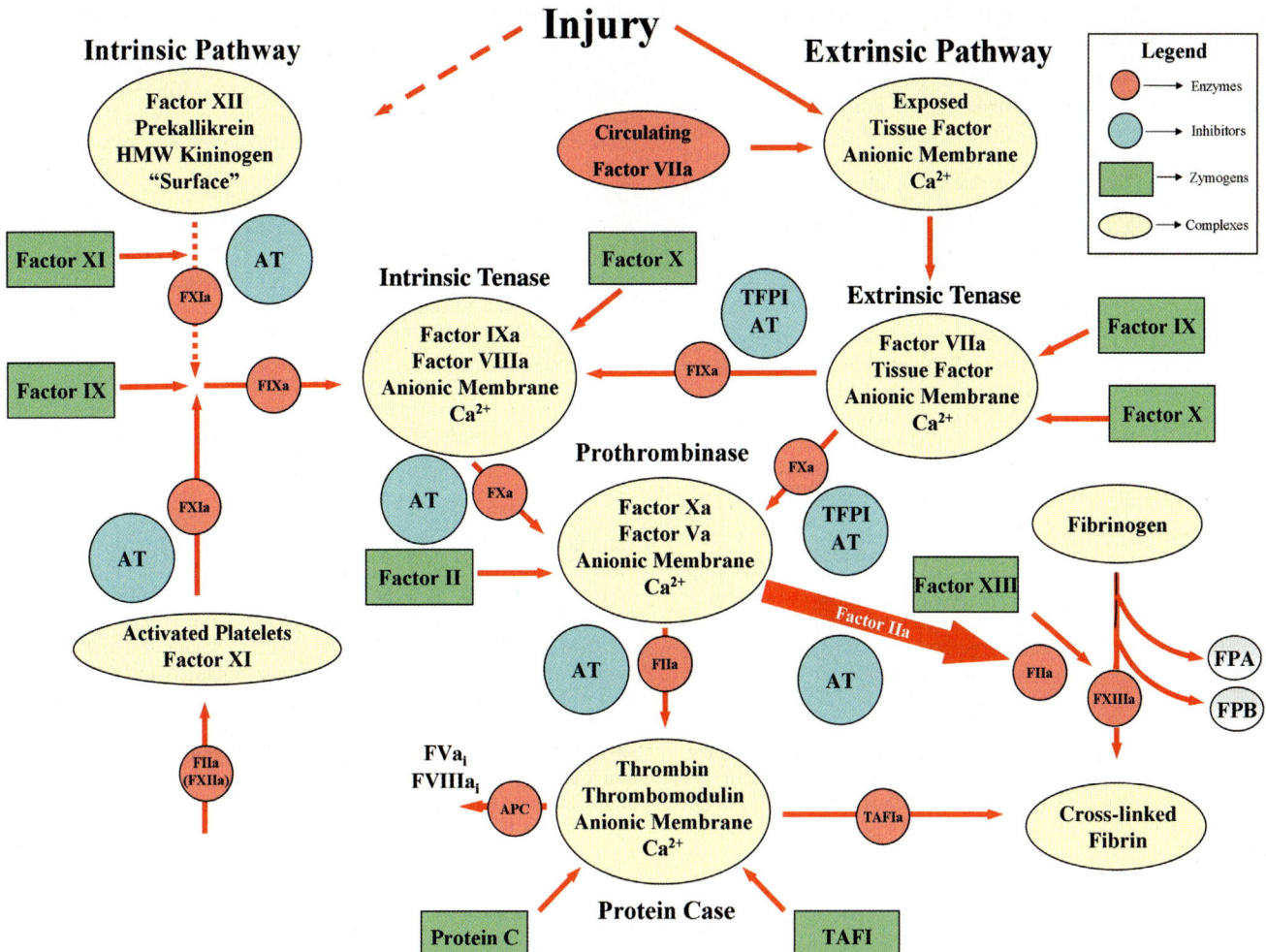

FIGURE 20.1 Overview of hemostasis. There are two pathways to initiate coagulation: the primary extrinsic pathway (shown on right) and the intrinsic (also called the contact pathway) (shown on left). The components of these multistep processes are illustrated as follows: enzymes (*pink circles*), inhibitors (*blue circles*), zymogens (*green boxes*), or complexes (*cream ovals*). The intrinsic pathway has no known bleeding etiology associated with it; thus, this path is considered accessory to hemostasis. On injury to the vessel wall, tissue factor, a membrane-bound cofactor, is exposed to circulating factor VIIa, forming the extrinsic tenase, a vitamin K–dependent complex. Factor IX and factor X are converted to the serine proteases factor IXa (FIXa) and factor Xa (FXa), which are the enzymatic components of the intrinsic tenase and the prothrombinase complexes. The combined actions of the intrinsic and extrinsic tenase and the prothrombinase complexes lead to an explosive burst of the enzyme thrombin (FIIa). In addition to its multiple procoagulant roles, thrombin also acts in an anticoagulant capacity when combined with the cofactor thrombomodulin in the protein Case complex. The product of the protein Case reaction, activated protein C (APC), inactivates the cofactors factors Va and VIIIa. The cleaved species, factors Va_i (FVa_i) and $VIIIa_i$ ($FVIIIa_i$), no longer support the respective procoagulant activities of the prothrombinase and intrinsic tenase complexes. Once thrombin is generated through procoagulant mechanisms, thrombin cleaves fibrinogen (releasing fibrinopeptides A and B [FPA and FPB, respectively]) and activates factor XIII to form a cross-linked fibrin clot. Thrombin-thrombomodulin also activates thrombin-activatable fibrinolysis inhibitor (TAFI) that slows down fibrin degradation by plasmin. The procoagulant response is downregulated by the stoichiometric inhibitors tissue factor pathway inhibitor (TFPI) and antithrombin (AT). TFPI serves to attenuate the activity of the extrinsic tenase, the trigger of coagulation. AT directly inhibits thrombin, FIXa, and FXa. The intrinsic pathway provides an alternate route for the generation of factor IXa. Thrombin has also been shown to activate factor XI. The fibrin clot is eventually degraded by plasmin yielding soluble fibrin peptides (see *Figure 20.23*). HMW, high molecular weight.

Factor IX, not factor X, appears to be the preferred substrate of the extrinsic fXase. In addition, factor IXα, the intermediate species in factor IX activation, is generated more rapidly in the presence of factor X. Factor IXα activation to the final product factor IXa occurs at a higher rate than factor IX activation, thereby providing a burst of factor IXa to form the intrinsic fXase complex. The low level of factor Xa generated by the tissue factor–factor VIIa complex most likely functions in the activation of factor IX. A model of extrinsic fXase behavior suggests that factor IX is converted to factor IXα by the extrinsic fXase or factor Xa–phospholipid complex. Factor IXα is then rapidly converted to factor IXa by the extrinsic fXase.[61,62] The factor VIIIa–factor IXa complex subsequently activates the major fraction of factor X to factor Xa and provides the enzyme component for the prothrombinase complex. Measurements of second-order rate constants for factor Xa generation by the intrinsic and extrinsic fXase complexes

also support this model. The rate of factor Xa generation by the tissue factor–factor VIIa complex is 1/50th the rate of factor Xa generation by the factor VIIIa–factor IXa complex.[61-63] Both complexes thus have distinct roles in the procoagulant response.

In summary, the procoagulant response is triggered upon the interaction of factor VIIa with tissue factor, when the latter is exposed and/or expressed as a result of vascular perturbation. The extrinsic fXase generates low levels of factors IXa and Xa during the initiation phase of coagulation. Factor Xa–phospholipid complexes also assist in the activation of factor IX. Factor IXa combines with factor VIIIa on the membrane surface, and the intrinsic fXase accelerates factor Xa generation 50-fold over the extrinsic fXase. The burst of factor Xa overcomes circulating levels of factor Xa inhibitors and initiates maximal levels of prothrombinase complex activity. Prothrombinase activity subsequently leads to a burst of α-thrombin generation and propagation of the procoagulant response.[61,62]

PROCOAGULANT PROTEINS: ACCESSORY PATHWAY FACTORS AND FACTOR XI

The procoagulant proteins that make up the intrinsic or accessory pathway consist of factor XII, plasma prekallikrein, HMWK, and factor XI. These proteins are responsible for the contact activation of blood coagulation. The physiologic role of the intrinsic pathway is not clearly understood, but it does not appear to be essential for hemostasis because individuals deficient in factor XII, plasma prekallikrein, or HMWK do not manifest abnormal bleeding. However, evidence from animal studies indicate that contact pathway factors contributes to thrombosis. For example, factor XII–deficient mice have shown resistance to atrial and venous thrombosis formation.[40,64-66] Pharmacologic targeting of contact pathway enzymes has been shown to provide protection from thrombosis.[67-70] Factor XI appears to play a more prominent role, unrelated to its activities in the intrinsic pathway, after activation by thrombin.[7,37] Each of these proteins is described in terms of its gene structure and expression, biochemistry, activation, function, and regulation in regard to hemostasis (*Figure 20.2*).

Factor XII (Hageman Factor, Contact Factor)

Factor XII, or *Hageman factor* (HF), is the zymogen precursor of the serine protease factor XIIa. Factor XII is also known as *contact factor* for its role in the initiation of coagulation on contact with substances such as glass or kaolin. The contact pathway is the basis for the activated partial thromboplastin time clotting assay. Factor XII circulates in plasma at an average concentration of 40 μg/mL (500 nmol/L)[76,77] (*Table 20.1*). Increased levels of factor XII are seen in postmenopausal women using estrogen replacement therapy and during pregnancy. Animal studies also demonstrate enhanced expression of factor XII by estrogen and prolactin.[78-80] Since a deficiency of factor XII is not associated with any bleeding abnormality, its precise role in hemostasis is at present unknown. Studies show that mice lacking factor XII are protected against arterial thrombosis and stroke.[40,41,81,82]

This suggests that the intrinsic pathway of coagulation is essential for thrombus stability. The components of the contact pathway are also believed to provide a link between coagulation and inflammation,[83] with the multifunctional cellular protein gC1q-R/p33 postulated to play a central bridging role between these two processes.[84] Misfolded protein aggregates have been implicated in activating factor XII.[85]

Gene Structure and Expression

Human factor XII is produced by a single gene located on chromosome 5q35.3[86,87] (*Table 20.2*). The gene for factor XII spans approximately 12 kilobases (kb) and is composed of 13 introns and 14 exons.[88] The intron/exon gene structure is similar to the gene structures of tissue plasminogen activator (t-PA) and urokinase-type plasminogen activator (u-PA).[88] The promoter does not contain the CAAT or TATA sequences common in other genes, but it does contain two LF-A1 transcription elements characteristic of genes with liver-specific expression. The promoter also contains one estrogen-responsive element.[88,89]

Biochemistry

Human factor XII is synthesized as a precursor protein with a 19-residue signal peptide. The mature factor XII molecule is a 596-amino acid single-chain β-globulin with a molecular weight of approximately 80 kDa.[90-94] It circulates at a concentration of 40 μg/mL (500 nmol/L) with a half-life ($t_{1/2}$) of 2 to 3 days (*Table 20.1*). The factor XII molecule is composed of two domains: an NH_2-terminal heavy chain and a COOH-terminal light chain. The heavy chain contains several domain structures: fibronectin type I and type II domains, two epidermal growth factor (EGF)-like domains, a kringle domain, and a proline-rich region (residues 277-330) (*Figure 20.3*). The light chain contains the serine protease catalytic domain, a region homologous to the B-chain of the enzyme plasmin. The mature factor XII molecule contains approximately 17% carbohydrate. Glycosylation consists of an O-linked fucose at Thr[95] in the first EGF domain[95];

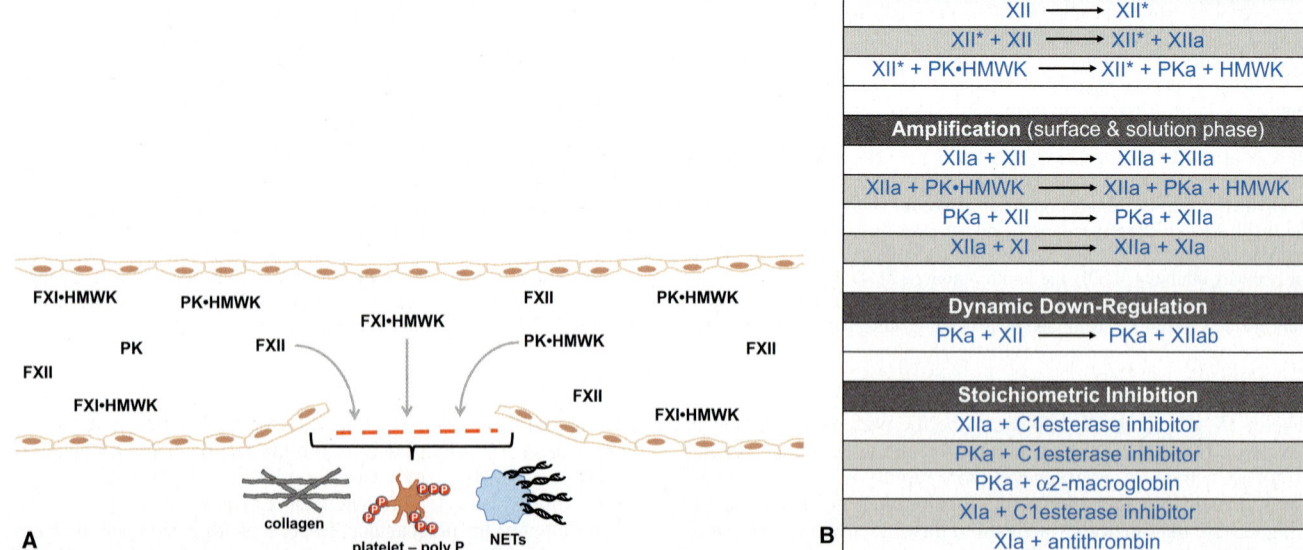

FIGURE 20.2 Ruptured atheromas: an example of physiologically relevant sites of contact pathway activation. A, Physiologic factor XII (FXII)-dependent coagulation has been reported to involve the exposure of blood to negatively charged, insoluble structures displaying phosphate rich polymers as a primary component. Activated platelet–derived/associated aggregates of polyphosphate and divalent metal ions (Ca^{2+}, Mg^{2+}, and Zn^{2+} ions)[71] and neutrophil-extruded strands of DNA/protein complexes (NETs)[72,73] have been shown individually and in concert to support FXII-dependent coagulation.[71] Type 1 collagen has also been reported to support FXII-dependent coagulation.[74] Most of the factor XI (FXI, ≥95% or ~30 nM) and prekallikrein (PK) (~75%, or ~360 nM) in blood is bound to high-molecular-weight kininogen (HMWK), with surface binding of both complexes mediated by a domain on HMWK. B, Initial FXII autoactivation (FXII→FXII*) upon surface binding appears to involve a conformational transition of the single-chain zymogen to a more active conformation rather than autoproteolyis to yield the two-chain FXIIa enzyme.[75] Central reactions defining surface-dependent initiation, amplification, and downregulation of FXII-dependent coagulation are shown. The production of FXIa is the required event for contact pathway–dependent coagulation to occur. FXIa efficiently catalyzes the activation of factor IX (FIX), with a catalytic efficiency comparable with that of the extrinsic tenase for FIX.

Table 20.1. Biochemical Properties of Blood Coagulation Proteins

Protein	Molecular Weight (Da)	Plasma Concentration		Plasma Half-Life (days)	Carbo-Hydrate (%)	Clinical Phenotype[a]		Functional Classification
		(nmol/L)	(μg/mL)			H	T	
Intrinsic Pathway Proteins								
Factor XII	80,000	500	40	2-3	17	–		Protease zymogen
Prekallikrein	85/88,000	486	42		15			Protease zymogen
High-molecular-weight kininogen	120,000	670	80		42	–		Cofactor
Low-molecular-weight kininogen	66,000	1300	90		30			Cofactor
Factor XI	160,000	30	5	2.5-3.3	5	±		Protease zymogen
Extrinsic Pathway Proteins								
Tissue factor	44,000							Cell-associated cofactor
Factor VII	50,000	10	0.5	0.25	13	+	±	VKD protease zymogen
Factor VIIa	50,000			0.1	13			VKD serine protease
Factor X	59,000	170	10	1.5	15	+		VKD protease zymogen
Factor Xa	48,000				3			VKD serine protease
Factor IX	55,000	90	5	1	17	+		VKD protease zymogen
Factor IXa	45,000							VKD serine protease
Factor V	330,000	20	6.6	0.5	13-25	+		Soluble procofactor
Factor Va	180,000				8			Cofactor
Factor VIII	280,000	0.7	0.2	0.3-0.5	4	+		Soluble procofactor
Factor VIIIa	170,000							Cofactor
von Willebrand factor	255,000 (monomer)	Varies	10		10-15	+		Platelet adhesion, carrier for factor VIII
Prothrombin	72,000	1400	100	2.5	8	+		VKD protease zymogen
α-Thrombin	37,000				5			VKD serine protease
Fibrinogen	340,000	7400	2500	3-5	3	+	±	Structural protein, cell adhesion
Aα	66,500							
Bβ	52,000							
γ	46,500							
Factor XIII	320,000	93	30	9-10		+		Transglutaminase zymogen
A-chain	83,200							
B-chain	79,700				5			

+, presence of phenotype; –, absence of phenotype; ±, some individuals present with the phenotype and others do not; H, hemorrhagic disease/hemophilia; T, thrombotic disease/thrombophilia; VKD, vitamin K dependent.
[a]Clinical phenotype: the expression of either H or T phenotype in deficient individuals.

N-linked carbohydrates at Asn^{230} and Asn^{414} in the kringle and catalytic domains, respectively; and six O-linked carbohydrates in the proline-rich region.[96] The factor XII molecule also contains four zinc ion (Zn^{2+})-binding sites.[97] Zn^{2+} binding to factor XII likely induces a conformation change that promotes activation of factor XII associated with negatively charged surfaces.[98-100]

Activation

Factor XII undergoes autoactivation on interaction with negatively charged surfaces such as glass, kaolin, dextran sulfate, ellagic acid, celite, or bismuth subgallate[101-111] and on interaction with hydrophobic surfaces.[112] This is likely only an in vitro event triggered by the artificial surfaces used in studies of the contact pathway, although research is ongoing. Although factor XII associates with many physiologically relevant anionic surfaces, including negatively charged phospholipids,[113-125] the autoactivation of factor XII induced by these surfaces in vitro does not appear to represent the mechanism for factor

XII activation in vivo.[126] Instead, factor XII is most likely activated by a cell membrane–associated proteinase.[127,128] When factor XII, prekallikrein, and HMWK form a complex on anionic phospholipids of the cell membrane, prekallikrein is cleaved, forming the enzyme kallikrein. Kallikrein then activates factor XII (plasmin activates factor XII as well) via a single cleavage at Arg^{353}-Val^{354} to generate an 80-kDa two-chain enzyme, α-factor XIIa (factor XIIa, α-HFa, or HFa), composed of an NH_2-terminal heavy chain (relative molecular weight [M_r] = 52,000) and a COOH-terminal light chain (M_r = 28,000) held together by a disulfide bond (Cys^{340}-Cys^{467}) (*Figure 20.3*). This cleavage is essential for exposure of the active site in factor XIIa.[129] Factor XIIa can then bind negatively charged surfaces and activate factor XI and prekallikrein.[130,131] Two secondary cleavages can also occur on factor XII: one outside the disulfide bond (Arg^{334}-Asn^{335}) and one inside the disulfide loop (Arg^{343}-Leu^{344}), generating β-factor XIIa ($FXII_f$, HF_f).[132-135] β-Factor XIIa has no surface-binding capabilities but is able to activate prekallikrein.[101,136,137]

Table 20.2. Molecular Genetics of Blood Coagulation Proteins

Protein	Molecular Weight (Da)	Gene Location: Chromosome	Gene Size (kb)	Gene Organization: # of Exons	Messenger RNA Size (kb)	UNIPROT Accession Number[a]
Intrinsic pathway proteins						
Factor XII	80,000	5q35.3	12	15	2.0	P00748
Prekallikrein	85/88,000	4q35.2	31	17	2.2	P03952
High-molecular-weight kininogen	120,000	3q27.3	27.1	10	3.5	P01042
Low-molecular-weight kininogen	66,000	3q27.3				P01042
Factor XI	160,000	4q35	23	15	2.1	P03951
Extrinsic pathway proteins						
Tissue factor	44,000	1p21.3	12.6	6	2.1	P13726
Factor VII	50,000	13q34	14.9	10	2.5	P08709
Factor VIIa	50,000					
Factor X	59,000	13q34	26.7	8	1.5	P00742
Factor Xa	48,000					
Factor IX	55,000	Xq27.1	32.7	8	2.8	P00740
Factor IXa	45,000					
Factor V	330,000	1q24.2	74.5	25	6.9	P12259
B region	150,000					
Factor Va	180,000					
Factor VIII	280,000	Xq28	186	27	9.0	P00451
Factor VIIIa	170,000					
von Willebrand factor (monomer)	255,000	12p13.31	175.8	52	8.6	P04275
Prothrombin	72,000	11p11.2	20.3	14	1.9	P00734
α-Thrombin	37,000					
Fibrinogen	340,000					
Aα	66,500	4q31.3	5.4	6	2.2	P02671
Bβ	52,000	4q31.3	9.8	8	1.9	P02675
γ	46,500	4q32.1	8.5	10	1.5	P02679
Factor XIII	320,000					
A-chain	83,200	6p25.1	176.6	15	3.8	P00488
B-chain	79,700	1q31.3	28.5	12	2.2	P05160

[a]https://www.uniprot.org.

Function

Factor XIIa is a serine protease that activates factor XI and prekallikrein by mechanisms dependent on anionic surfaces and the cofactor HMWK.[130,138] Factor XIIa also activates the C1 component of the complement system.[139] In addition, factor XIIa downregulates the Fc receptor on monocytes and macrophages,[140] induces release of interleukin (IL)-1 and IL-6 from monocytes and macrophages,[141] and stimulates neutrophils.[142] Although these roles have no apparent impact on normal coagulation, factor XII/XIIa may be an important link between coagulation and inflammation[143] (for review, see Ref. 136). Factor XIIa also activates plasminogen to plasmin, linking the contact pathway to fibrinolysis.[144]

Regulation

C1 inhibitor is the major inhibitor of both factor XIIa and β-factor XIIa and irreversibly inhibits both enzymes.[145-148] Antithrombin and plasminogen activator inhibitor (PAI)-1 also inhibit factor XIIa.[149-151] Endothelial cells and eosinophils are reported to produce proteins that inhibit factor XII activation but not factor XIIa activity.[152-154] Amyloid

precursor protein likewise is reported to inhibit factor XII activation but not factor XIIa.[155]

Plasma Prekallikrein (Fletcher Factor)

Plasma prekallikrein, or *Fletcher factor,* is the zymogen form of the enzyme kallikrein. Prekallikrein circulates in plasma at an average concentration of 42 μg/mL (486 nmol/L)[156,157] (*Table 20.1*). Approximately 75% circulates in a noncovalent complex with HMWK,[158,159] and the remaining 25% circulates as free prekallikrein. Like factor XII, prekallikrein is a component of the intrinsic or accessory pathway and serves as a link between coagulation and inflammation. Prekallikrein is also linked to fibrinolytic events. Plasma prekallikrein deficiency is rare and is not associated with hemostatic defects except perhaps in deficient individuals with other cardiovascular risk factors.[160,161]

Gene Structure and Expression

The human prekallikrein gene is located on chromosome 4q35.2, close to the factor XI gene[162] (*Table 20.2*). The human plasma prekallikrein gene spans 30 kb and contains 15 exons and 14 introns.[163] A total of

Factor XII: 80 kDa

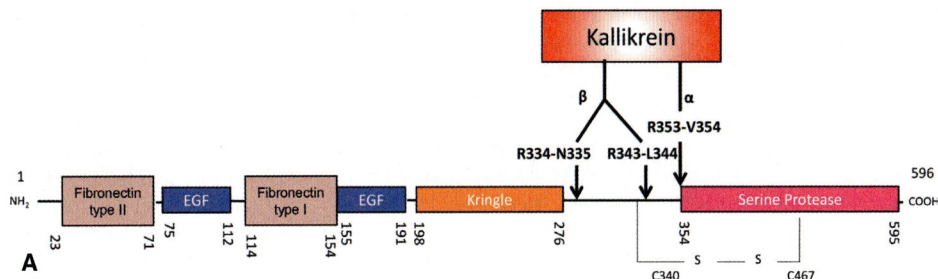

Prekallikrein: 85/88 kDa

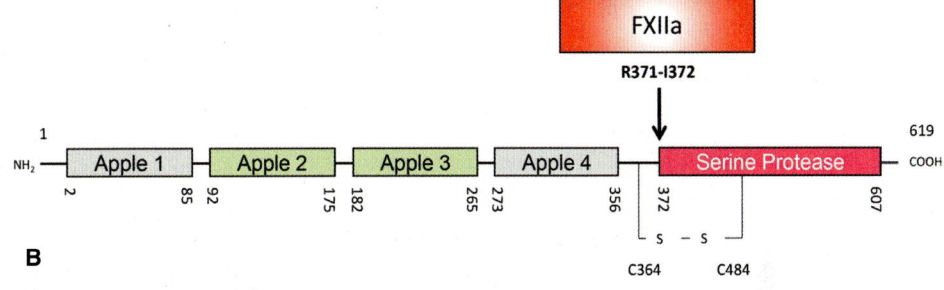

HMW Kininogen: 120 kDa
LMW Kininogen: 66 kDa

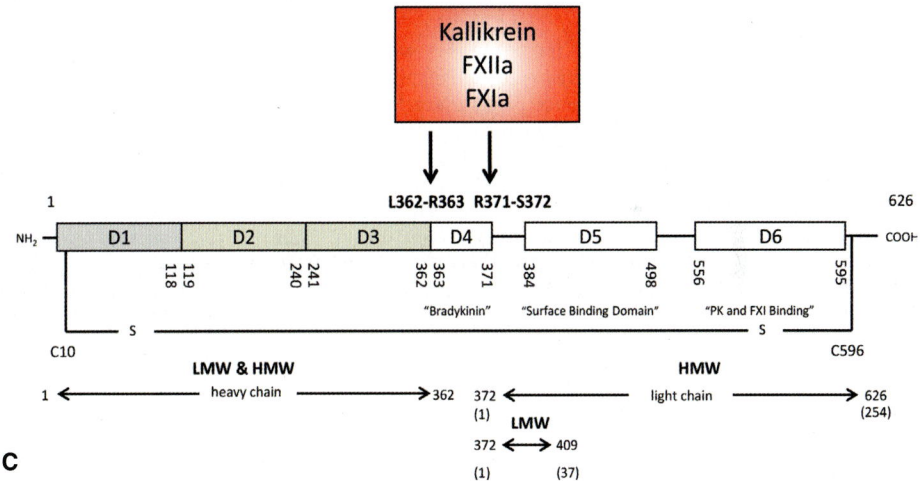

Factor XI: 160 kDa

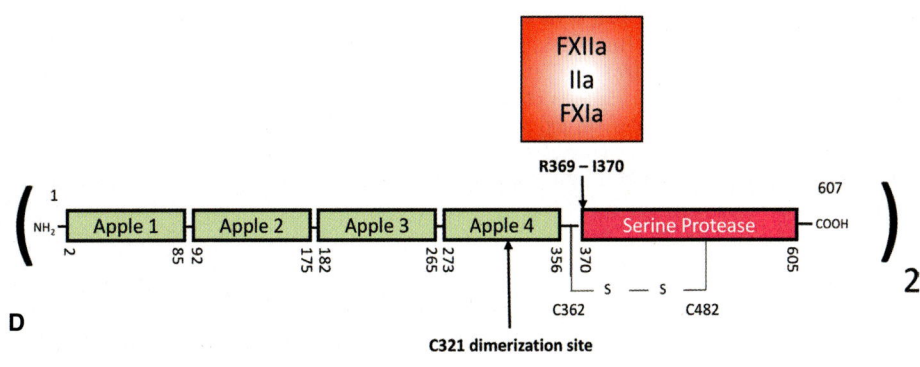

FIGURE 20.3 Schematic representation of the intrinsic pathway (contact) proteins. Factor XII (FXII), prekallikrein (PK), high-molecular-weight (HMW) kininogen, low-molecular-weight (LMW) kininogen, and factor XI (FXI) are shown with their various domains depicted as blocks. Activating proteases are placed in a box above the cleavage sites with the specific amino acid residues of the site shown directly underneath. Key interchain disulfide bonds (S-S) are included. For the kininogens, horizontal arrows indicate the amino acid residues defining heavy and light chain regions of the activated forms of the cofactors. Factor XI is illustrated as a monomer. EGF, epidermal growth factor.

12 allelic variants have been identified in the 5′ proximal promoter and in 7 of the exons. A common polymorphism (30% of the population) leads to an Asn124Ser replacement in the heavy chain of the apple 2 domain of prekallikrein. Two other polymorphisms in the coding region of the protein, His189Pro in the apple 3 domain of the heavy chain and His183Gln, were identified.[163] Prekallikrein and factor XI are highly homologous, and both human and rat factor XI prekallikrein genes are located on chromosome 4, suggesting a gene duplication event from a common ancestor.[164] Prekallikrein mRNA has been detected in human kidney, adrenal gland, placenta, and brain, but the liver is considered to be the major site of synthesis.[165-167]

Biochemistry

Human plasma prekallikrein is synthesized as a precursor with a 19-amino acid signal peptide. The mature form of the protein, appearing as a doublet of 85 and 88 kDa when analyzed by sodium dodecyl sulfate–polyacrylamide gel electrophoresis (SDS-PAGE), is a single-chain fast γ-globulin of 619 amino acids (*Table 20.1*).[144,168,169] Prekallikrein contains 15% carbohydrate with five N-linked sugar moieties.[165] Structurally, prekallikrein contains four tandem repeats, called *apple domains,* in the NH$_2$-terminal portion of the molecule (*Figure 20.3*). Each apple domain consists of 90 to 91 amino acid residues including six to eight cysteines that are disulfide bonded to form the distinct domain structure.[165,170] The apple 1 and apple 4 domains mediate the binding of prekallikrein to HMWK.[171,172] The apple domains of prekallikrein are highly homologous to the apple domains of factor XI. Apple domains have been found only in these two proteins, lending support to a gene duplication event from a common ancestor.[162,170] The COOH-terminal region of prekallikrein contains the catalytic site.

Activation

Prekallikrein is activated by factor XIIa in complex with the cofactor HMWK on an anionic surface (*Figure 20.3*). Prekallikrein is also activated by β-factor XII in the absence of a surface.[173] The factor XIIa–HMWK complex or β-factor XII catalyzes the cleavage of the Arg^{371}-Ile^{372} bond in prekallikrein. This cleavage is also reported to occur in the absence of factor XIIa when prekallikrein is bound to HMWK on the endothelial cell surface.[127,174] The enzyme kallikrein is a two-chain molecule composed of an NH$_2$-terminal heavy chain (M$_r$ = 53,000) containing the four apple domains and a COOH-terminal light chain (M$_r$ = 36,000 or 33,000) containing the active site.[144,165,175,176]

Function

Kallikrein is a member of the trypsin family of serine proteases. In the presence of an appropriate anionic surface and the cofactor HMWK, kallikrein activates factor XII to factor XIIa and proteolyzes factor XIIa to β-factor XIIa. Kallikrein also undergoes autoproteolysis at Lys^{145}-Ala^{146} to yield β-kallikrein.[177,178] Enzyme activity is significantly reduced on conversion of kallikrein to β-kallikrein.[176] Kallikrein cleaves HMWK at two sites to generate the vasoactive nonapeptide bradykinin.[179,180] Bradykinin is a potent vasodilator and stimulates endothelial cell prostacyclin synthesis, resulting in hypotension.[181,182] Kallikrein is also an activator of fibrinolytic zymogens and converts both plasminogen to plasmin and pro–u-PA to u-PA.[144,183,184] In addition, kallikrein has been reported to activate neutrophils and stimulate elastase release as part of the hemostatic and inflammatory responses.[185]

Regulation

C1 inhibitor and α_2-macroglobulin are the major inhibitors of kallikrein.[186,187] C1 inhibitor forms a 1:1 stoichiometric complex with kallikrein and abolishes its proteolytic and amidolytic activities.[187-190] α_2-Macroglobulin inhibits the ability of kallikrein to generate bradykinin and partially inhibits amidolytic activity.[190] C1 inhibitor and α_2-macroglobulin each inhibit equivalent amounts of kallikrein in plasma, but C1 inhibitor acts much more rapidly and plays the major role in reducing kallikrein activity.[191] Antithrombin and antithrombin-heparin are slow inhibitors of kallikrein although the antithrombin-heparin-HMWK complex is an effective inhibitor.[192-194] Protein C inhibitor also inhibits kallikrein.[195-197]

High-Molecular-Weight Kininogen (Fitzgerald Factor, Williams Factor)

HMWK, also known as *Fitzgerald factor* or *Williams factor,* circulates in plasma at an average concentration of 80 μg/mL (670 nmol/L)[198,199] (*Table 20.1*). HMWK acts as a cofactor for the activation of factor XII and prekallikrein and is the precursor of the vasoactive peptide bradykinin. A second form of kininogen, low-molecular-weight kininogen (LMWK), is also found in plasma. LMWK can be cleaved to yield bradykinin but has no procoagulant activity. LMWK circulates at an average concentration of 90 μg/mL (1300 nmol/L).[200] Deficiencies of HMWKs and LMWKs are rare and are not associated with bleeding diatheses.[201] The major established function of the kininogens is to serve as a source of bradykinin and thereby to contribute to a number of vascular events regulated by bradykinin.[202]

Gene Structure and Expression

The two forms of kininogen, HMWK and LMWK, are the products of a single gene[203,204] located on chromosome 3q27.3[205] (*Table 20.2*). The kininogen gene consists of 10 introns and 11 exons and spans 27 kb.[204] The gene produces messenger RNAs (mRNAs) for the two different forms of kininogen by alternative splicing.[204] HMWK and LMWK share the coding region of the first nine exons and the portion of exon 10 containing the bradykinin sequence and the first 12 amino acids following the COOH terminus of bradykinin. Exon 10 also codes for a 56-kDa light chain unique to HMWK, whereas exon 11 codes for a 4-kDa light chain unique to LMWK. Human liver contains mRNAs for both HMWK and LMWK[203,204]; only HMWK is expressed and secreted by human umbilical vein endothelial cells.[206] Estrogen administration[207] and pregnancy[208] increase HMWK levels. Conversely, progesterone treatment reduces kininogen gene expression and plasma kininogen levels.[209]

Biochemistry

Human HMWKs and LMWKs are synthesized as precursor proteins containing 18 amino acid signal peptides. The mature form of HMWK is a 120-kDa single-chain α-globulin of 626 residues, whereas the LMWK form is a 66-kDa single-chain β-globulin composed of 409 residues.[199,200,209] Glycosylation at a number of shared sites (Asn^{151}, Asn^{187}, Asn^{276}, and Asn^{383}) and sites unique to HMWK (Thr^{515}, Thr^{521}, Thr^{528}, Thr^{539}, Thr^{553}, Thr^{559}, Thr^{575}, and Thr^{610}) presumably accounts for the substantial increase over the masses predicted from the amino acid compositions (70,000 for HMWK and 46,000 for LMWK). The NH$_2$-terminal heavy chains (residues 1-362) of the two forms are identical and consist of three consecutive regions designated domains 1, 2, and 3 (D1, D2, and D3) (*Figure 20.3*). Domain 1 has a low-affinity Ca^{2+}-binding site.[210] Domains 2 and 3 share homology with cysteine protease inhibitors.[211] Both HMWK and LMWK are potent inhibitors of cysteine proteases such as calpain.[198,212] Domain 3 also contains a cell-binding region[213-217] and is reported to inhibit α-thrombin activity[214,216,218] and platelet activation.[216,218,219] The central domain of both kininogens, domain 4 (D4), is the bradykinin region. Domain 4 also contains a cell-binding region[220] and a region that inhibits α-thrombin activity.[221] The two forms of kininogen have different COOH-terminal light-chain regions. The light chain of LMWK (residues 372-409) consists of a single domain, domain 5$_L$ (D5$_L$), with no known function. The light chain of HMWK (residues 372-626) is composed of two regions, domain 5$_H$ (D5$_H$) and domain 6$_H$ (D6$_H$). Domain 5$_H$ contains additional cell-binding regions[213,214,217,222,223] and mediates HMWK binding to anionic surfaces, heparin, and Zn^{2+}.[192,193,224,225] Domain 6$_H$ has binding sites for prekallikrein and factor XI.[226-228]

Activation

Kallikrein, factor XIIa, and factor XIa cleave HMWK to release bradykinin (residues 363-371) (*Figure 20.3*). Kallikrein also cleaves LMWK to release bradykinin. Bradykinin release from HMWK yields a two-chain protein composed of the heavy-chain (D1, D2, and D3) disulfide linked (Cys^{10}-Cys^{596}) to the light chain ($D5_H$ and $D6_H$). This molecule retains procoagulant activity, binding to prekallikrein, factor XI, and anionic surfaces via light-chain interactions[226,229,230] and induces apoptosis in endothelial cells.[231]

Function

The major role proposed for the kininogens is as a source of bradykinin. Bradykinin release provides a key vasoactive agent with a variety of roles and directly links the contact pathway to vascular repair processes. HMWK also functions as a nonenzymatic cofactor in the contact pathway of coagulation. HMWK binds anionic surfaces, prekallikrein, and factor XI, thus enhancing their activation by surface-associated factor XIIa. Although most studies of contact activation make use of artificial surfaces, cell membranes may provide appropriate sites for contact activation in vivo. Many cells contain kininogens and express kininogen-binding sites.[199,206,232-237] There is some evidence to support cell membrane–associated contact activation. Prekallikrein bound to HMWK on platelets or endothelial cells can result in the generation of kallikrein by a factor XIIa–dependent[127,184] or –independent mechanism.[127] However, factor XI bound to HMWK on the surface of platelets is not activated to factor Xia.[238] HMWK and its cleaved form exert anticoagulant effects via their inhibitory action on platelet adhesion[239] and aggregation.[240]

Factor XI (Plasma Thromboplastin Antecedent)

Factor XI, also known as *plasma thromboplastin antecedent*, circulates as a homodimer at an average concentration of 5 µg/mL (30 nmol/L)[241] in complex with HMWK[242] (*Table 20.1*). Factor XI is also found in human platelets, and the platelet form accounts for approximately 0.5% of the factor XI antigen in blood.[243-247] Factor XI is the zymogen precursor of the enzyme factor XIa. Unlike the other members of the accessory or contact pathway, factor XIa has an established role in coagulation as part of a positive feedback loop enhancing α-thrombin generation.[7,16] Although rare in the general population (~1 in 100,000 individuals),[248] factor XI deficiency is common in the Ashkenazi (European) Jewish population, with approximately 1 in 200 individuals affected by factor XI deficiency.[249-253] Factor XI deficiency can be associated with severe bleeding tendencies[254] after injury or surgical trauma. Spontaneous hemorrhage is not common. Factor XI deficiency is unusual in that bleeding abnormalities vary considerably and range from a complete absence of symptoms to life-threatening hemorrhage.[255] The severity of the bleeding complications is also not related to the severity of factor XI deficiency. Individuals with mild deficiency may experience severe hemorrhagic events, whereas individuals with severe deficiency may have no abnormal bleeding.[249,251,253,256-260]

Gene Structure and Expression

The gene for human factor XI is located on chromosome 4q35 and spans 23 kb (*Table 20.2*). The gene contains 14 introns and 15 exons.[168,261] Although mRNA for human plasma factor XI has been found in liver, pancreas, and kidney,[262] evidence suggests that the primary site of synthesis is the liver: plasma factor XI levels decrease in liver disease, and a patient with no history of factor XI deficiency developed a deficiency subsequent to a liver transplant from a factor XI-deficient donor.[263] Platelet factor XI is exclusively synthesized in the megakaryocyte.[264] Human platelet factor XI lacks exon 5 and may be an alternative splicing product of the plasma factor XI gene or a product of a gene specific to megakaryocytes.[264]

There are three major types of genetic mutations associated with factor XI deficiency: (a) intronic point mutations that interrupt exon splicing[251,265]; (b) exonic point mutations that lead to mutations in specific amino acids and result in premature polypeptide termination, disruption of dimerization, or reduced protein secretion[251,265-269]; and (c) nucleotide deletions that lead to decreased protein synthesis.[270,271] Two specific exonic point mutations account for the majority of the cases of factor XI deficiency in the Ashkenazi Jewish population. An E117X mutation in exon 5 (type II mutation) introduces a stop codon and results in premature polypeptide termination. The type II mutation

accounts for approximately 52% of the cases of factor XI deficiency in the Ashkenazi Jewish population. An F283L mutation in exon 9 (type III mutation) that accounts for 36% of the cases is believed to prevent intracellular dimer formation and protein secretion. These mutations are less frequent in the general population.[250,251,265,269] Approximately 150 mutations have been identified in the factor XI gene with four exhibiting founder effects in specific populations.[272]

Biochemistry

Human factor XI is found in plasma and in platelets. The two forms of the protein are somewhat different and may have different functions as well. Plasma factor XI accounts for most of the factor XI antigen in the human system and is a disulfide-linked homodimer ($M_r = 160,000$), with approximately 5% of its mass made up by carbohydrate (*Table 20.1*). Each of the two identical polypeptide chains is synthesized with an 18-amino-acid signal peptide. The mature polypeptide chain ($M_r = 80,000$) consists of 607 amino acid residues[243-245] and has five potential glycosylation sites, although only Asn^{72}, Asn^{108}, Asn^{432}, and Asn^{473} are glycosylated.[273] Exons 3 to 10 of the plasma factor XI gene encode four NH_2-terminal tandem sequences termed *apple domains* (apple 1 to apple 4, *Figure 20.3*). The apple domains are homologous to the apple domains in human plasma prekallikrein.[273] Exons 11 to 15 encode the COOH-terminal catalytic domain. Human platelet factor XI lacks exon 5 and amino acids Ala^{91}-Arg^{144} in the NH_2 terminus of the apple 2 domain. The mature platelet polypeptide chain ($M_r = 55,000$) may form a disulfide-linked tetramer of identical subunits ($M_r = 220,000$) or may be disulfide linked to a platelet plasma membrane protein.[244,257,264] Plasma factor XI circulates in complex with HMWK.[242] Formation of this complex, mediated by the apple 1 domain of factor XI, is required for factor XI to associate with anionic surfaces.[274] The apple 1 domain also contains binding sites for α-thrombin[275] and prothrombin.[260] The apple 2, apple 3, or both domains mediate the binding of factor IX, the substrate of factor Xia.[260,276-279] In addition to potentially mediating the factor XIa–factor IX interaction, the apple 3 domain contains binding sites for platelets and heparin.[280-282] The apple 4 domain contains the site (Cys^{321}) involved in the dimerization process. Dimerization is required for efficient intracellular processing and protein secretion.[266] Factor XIIa associates with a region of the apple 4 domain as well.[283] Polyphosphates have also been proposed as a natural cofactor for factor XI activation in plasma.[284,285]

Activation

Plasma factor XI is cleaved at an internal Arg^{369}-Ile^{370} bond to yield a disulfide-linked two-chain activated serine protease (*Figure 20.3*). The factor XI homodimer yields two disulfide-linked heavy chains containing the apple domains and two light chains containing the active sites.[286-288] Activation of factor XI can be accomplished by factor XIIa and α-thrombin and by autoactivation by factor XIa itself. Activation of factor XI by factor XIIa requires HMWK and an anionic surface. However, deficiencies of factor XII and HMWK do not result in bleeding diatheses, whereas factor XI deficiency is associated with hemorrhage. This suggests that factor XIIa–dependent activation of factor XI, a part of the contact pathway, is not likely to be the primary route of factor XIa generation in hemostasis. The physiologically relevant pathway for factor XI activation in coagulation is believed to involve α-thrombin.[7,16,289] Factor XI in complex with HMWK binds to the platelet surface via the apple 3 domain.[280] The rate of α-thrombin activation of factor XI on the platelet surface is greater than the rates of platelet-supported factor XIIa activation and factor XIa autoactivation.[290] Although platelets appear to play a key role in providing the surface for factor XI activation, the precise mechanism of activation of platelet factor XI and its function remain unclear.[291]

Function

Subsequent to activation, factor XIa remains bound to the surface. Factor XIa is a trypsin-like serine protease that cleaves and activates factor IX in a Ca^{2+}-dependent fashion.[292-294] Factor IXa is the enzyme component of the intrinsic tenase complex that provides the burst of factor Xa necessary for normal coagulation. As part of a positive feedback loop, α-thrombin activates factor XI. In turn, factor XIa generates factor IXa, contributing to the high levels of factor Xa that ensure efficient α-thrombin generation.[7] Factor XI as an antithrombotic target is being explored.[295,296]

Regulation

Factor XIa is regulated by four serine protease inhibitors or serpins: antithrombin, α_1-protease inhibitor, C1 inhibitor, and α_2-antiplasmin.[145,287,297-307] Factor XIa is also reported to be inhibited by PAI-1 and protein C inhibitor.[151,308] In addition, platelets secrete several factor XIa inhibitors,[309-313] including protease nexin-2 (PN2). PN2 is a truncated form of the Alzheimer β-amyloid protein precursor and contains a Kunitz-type serine protease inhibitor domain. Platelet-bound factor XIa is protected from inactivation by PN2[292]; however, heparin enhances PN2 inactivation of factor XIa. Factor XIa bound to the surface of endothelial cells that secrete heparan sulfate glycosaminoglycans (GAGs) may be readily inactivated by PN2.[314]

PROCOAGULANT PROTEINS: VITAMIN K–DEPENDENT PROTEIN FAMILY

The first identification/description of vitamin K–dependent proteins was introduced by Henrik Dam et al at the University of Copenhagen in the late 1920s.[315-317] They demonstrated that chickens fed a lipid-free diet exhibited a hemorrhagic condition. The addition of alfalfa meal or a lipid extract of alfalfa prevented this condition. The active compound, 2-methyl-3-phytyl-1,4-naphthoquinone (phylloquinone), was subsequently isolated from green plants. Further work performed by Doisy et al[318] in the 1930s showed that vitamin K activity in bacteria is also present as a series of menaquinones, 2-methyl-1,4-naphthoquinones substituted at the 3 position with an unsaturated polyisoprenoid chain. The Nobel Prize was awarded to Dam and Doisy in 1941 for their discovery of the fat-soluble vitamin K.

Simultaneously with the discovery of the vitamin, a naturally occurring antagonist, bishydroxycoumarin (dicumarol), was described. This naturally occurring vitamin K antagonist was identified as a toxic agent in spoiled sweet clover causing hemorrhage in cattle. The increase in clotting time was later identified as a function of decreased prothrombin time.[319] This led to the synthesis of several oral anticoagulant analogs and coumarin derivatives, including warfarin.

Vitamin K is essential in the biosynthesis of functional clotting factors. It is the required cofactor for the enzyme catalyzing the conversion of 9 to 13 NH_2-terminal glutamic acid residues to γ-carboxy glutamic acid residues (Gla). The enzyme required for this conversion uses a reduced form of vitamin K.

This specific posttranslational modification allows the vitamin K–dependent proteins to interact with Ca^{2+} and a membrane surface to exert their effect. The modification was initially identified and characterized in bovine prothrombin.[320-323] Gla residues were missing or present in decreased amounts in prothrombin isolated from cattle treated with coumarin derivatives. The vitamin K–dependent proteins present in plasma after treatment with anticoagulants lacked biologic activity due to decreased Ca^{2+}-dependent phospholipid binding. Therefore, preventing the formation of Gla residues became a basis for anticoagulant therapy.

Recently, two cDNAs were identified that encode proteins with NH_2-terminal Gla domains.[324] Both appear to be integral membrane proteins but bear no other similarity to the vitamin K–dependent proteins beyond the Gla domain. Mineralized tissues contain two proteins with Gla residues.[325] Matrix Gla protein is produced within vascular smooth muscle cells and inhibits vascular calcification by binding extracellular calcium.[326,327] Gla has also been found as a component of the toxin peptides from the marine snail *Conus*.[328-330] The biologic activity of the toxins has been found to depend on the Gla residue(s). The identification of Gla in invertebrates suggests that vitamin K has a much wider range of biologic functions than previously thought. Gas

6 is a novel member of the vitamin K–dependent family of proteins, and when bound to the receptor tyrosine kinase Axl it has been shown to mediate cell survival. γ-Carboxylation of Gas 6 is necessary for its function.[331]

The vitamin K–dependent proteins can be divided into two classes: procoagulant (factors II, VII, IX, and X; *Figure 20.4A*) and anticoagulant (protein C, protein S, and protein Z; *Figure 20.4B*). The vitamin K–dependent proteins are part of a family of serine proteinases (except for protein S and protein Z) related to the trypsin/chymotrypsin superfamily. Sequence homology exists between the proteins at both the gene and the protein level, possibly due to a common ancestral gene.[332,333] Congenital deficiencies of factors II, VII, IX, and X are associated with bleeding tendencies, whereas protein C and protein S deficiencies are associated with thrombotic tendencies. These proteins are composed of separate domains, each of which is characterized by highly conserved regions that fold, independently from the rest of the molecule, into a characteristic three-dimensional shape. The domains of the vitamin K–dependent proteins are illustrated in *Figure 20.4*. NH_2-terminal Gla domains (containing from 9 to 13 Gla residues) are followed by either a kringle domain in factor II or an EGF-like domain (EGF) in factor VII, factor IX, factor X, protein C, protein S, and protein Z. Protein S contains a thrombin-sensitive region before the EGF domain. The active site is contained within the serine protease domain for factor II, factor VII, factor IX, factor X, and protein C and becomes functional on specific peptide bond cleavages. Protein S is not a serine protease precursor and instead contains a sex hormone–binding globulin-like domain in the COOH terminus. Protein Z contains a "pseudo-catalytic domain" in the COOH terminus and does not function as a serine protease enzyme.

The synthesis of these proteins occurs primarily in the liver followed by secretion into circulation. However, recently, a functional prothrombin gene product has been found to be synthesized by human kidney cells.[334] The concentration of circulating zymogens in plasma varies 200-fold from 100 µg/mL for prothrombin to 0.5 µg/mL for factor VII (*Table 20.1*). Levels present in plasma can be affected by polymorphisms in the promoter or coding region,[335-337] and aberrant levels are considered a risk factor for ischemic heart disease.[338] Cholesterol and triglyceride levels have also been correlated with plasma concentrations of the vitamin K–dependent proteins.[339-341] Liver function in the synthesis of the clotting factors, dietary intake/adsorption of vitamin K, and drug interactions can affect individuals on anticoagulant therapy.[342,343]

Clearance ($t_{1/2}$) of the vitamin K–dependent proteins varies from approximately 6 hours for factor VII to 2.5 days for prothrombin (*Table 20.1*). Once the zymogen is activated to its serine protease form, it is then inactivated by inhibitors and the complex cleared from the blood.

These activated forms of the vitamin K–dependent proteins are key components in the formation of the vitamin K–dependent coagulation complexes: the *extrinsic tenase* (factor VIIa–tissue factor); the *intrinsic tenase* (factor IXa–factor VIIIa); *prothrombinase* (factor Xa–factor Va); and *protein Case* (thrombin-thrombomodulin) (*Figure 20.5*). When all the components for each complex are assembled on the appropriate membrane surfaces (e.g., activated platelets, monocytes, blood cells, or endothelium), the specific reactions occur with rates enhanced by 10^4- to 10^9-fold over enzyme-substrate alone[5] (*Table 20.3*). A simple calculation can illustrate the importance of the rate enhancements achieved through complex assembly (vitamin K–dependent serine protease-cofactor-membrane-Ca^{2+}): if blood takes 4 minutes to clot in a normal person, then in the absence of membrane and cofactor, blood clot formation would take approximately 3.8 years.

Gene Structure and Expression

The family of vitamin K–dependent proteins is mainly synthesized in the liver by hepatocytes. Decreased levels of the vitamin K–dependent proteins are indicators of liver dysfunction.[346,347] Liver transplantation has been shown either to treat vitamin K deficiency[348] or to bring

Factor VII: 50 kDa

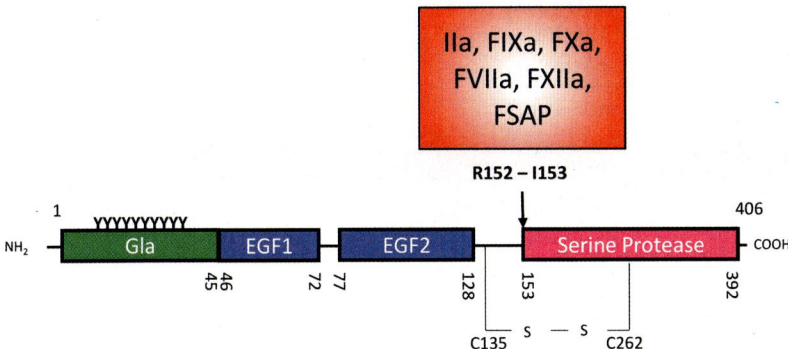

Factor IX: 55 kDa

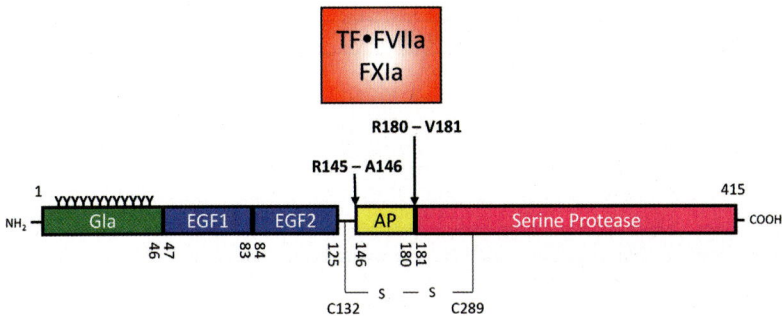

Factor X: 59 kDa

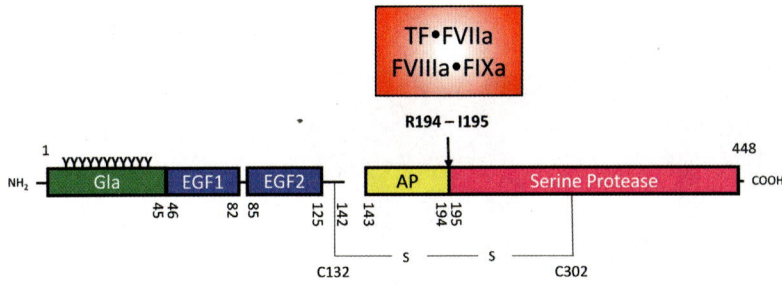

Prothrombin: 72 kDa

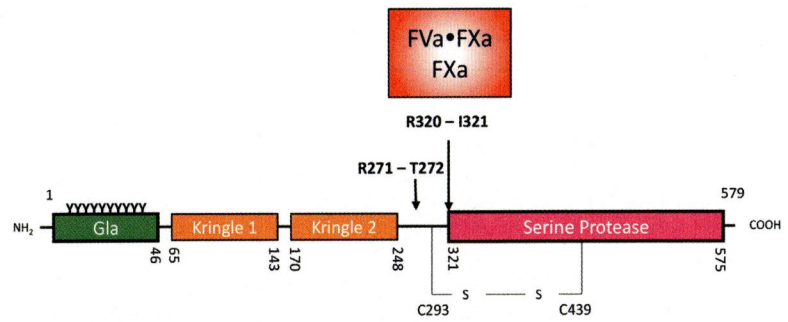

A

FIGURE 20.4 Schematic representation of the vitamin K–dependent proteins. The building blocks for these proteins include an NH$_2$-terminal Gla domain with 9 to 13 Gla residues followed by either an epidermal growth factor (EGF)-like domain in factor VII (FVII), factor IX (FIX), factor X (FX), protein C, protein S, and protein Z or a kringle domain in prothrombin. Protein S contains a thrombin-sensitive region (TSR) before the EGF domain. Active sites are contained within the serine protease domain. Cleavage sites for the conversion of zymogens to their active forms are designated by arrows; activating proteases are placed in boxes above the arrows. Factor IX, factor X, and protein C are activated by proteolytic removal of an activation peptide (AP). Protein S is not a serine protease precursor and instead contains a sex hormone–binding globulin–like domain (SHGB) in the COOH terminus. Protein Z also contains a "pseudo catalytic domain" in the COOH terminus and does not function as a serine protease. For reference, the molecular weight for each zymogen is listed, and disulfide bonds (-S-S-) critical to the integrity of the two-chain zymogens or active forms are presented. A, Panel illustrates the procoagulant vitamin K–dependent proteins factor VII, factor IX, factor X, and prothrombin. B, Panel illustrates the anticoagulant proteins, protein C, protein S, and protein Z. C, Structural ribbon diagram of factor IXa (PDB: 1PFX). FSAP, factor VII–activating protease; mIIa, meizothrombin; TF, tissue factor.

Protein C: 62 kDa

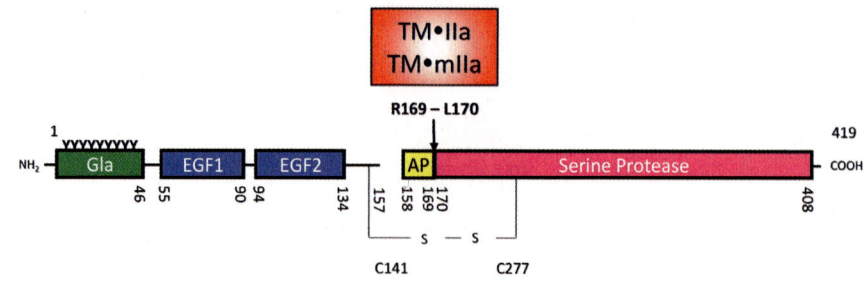

Protein S: 69 kDa

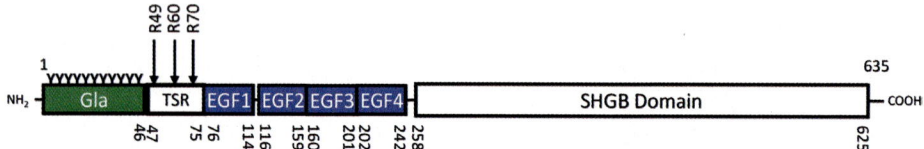

Protein Z: 62 kDa

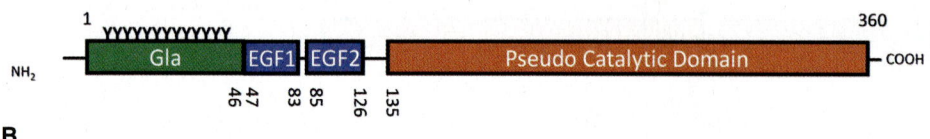

B

Factor IXa

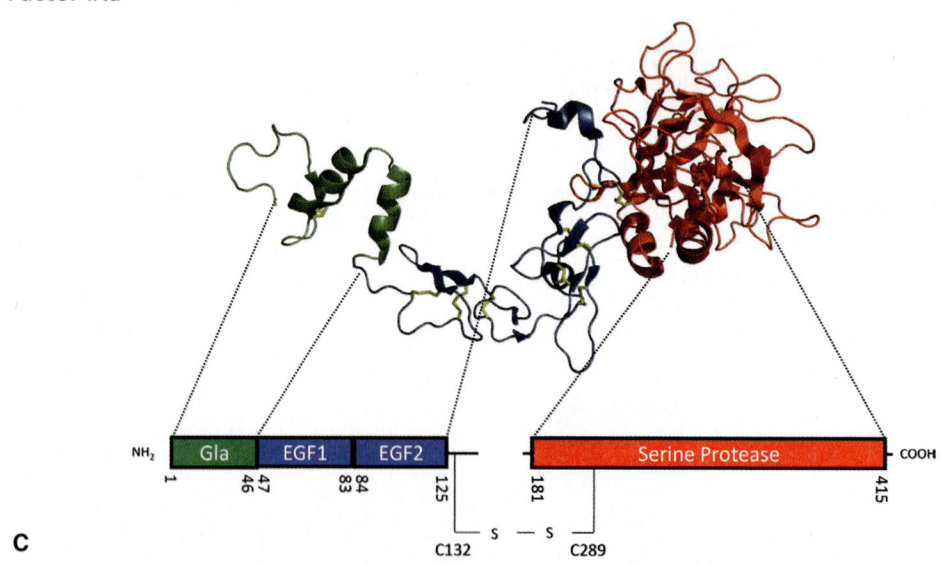

C

FIGURE 20.4 Continued

about vitamin K deficiency.[349] The genes encoding all of the vitamin K–dependent coagulation proteins have been sequenced and are seen in *Table 20.2*. The difference between the vitamin K–dependent protein genes and most other eukaryotic genes is that the 5′-flanking regions lack TATA boxes. Binding sites for liver-enriched or liver-specific (or both) transcription factors, which are important for hepatic expression of these proteins, are contained within the regulatory region of these genes. A common pentanucleotide motif that occurs in a similar location in the regulatory region of the genes encoding factor VII, factor IX, and factor X may be important in their possible coordinate expression.

Posttranslational Processing

The vitamin K–dependent proteins are synthesized in the liver as preprozymogens in a process that requires a dietary intake of vitamin K. They are modified posttranslationally at glutamic acid (γ-carboxylation to form γ-carboxy glutamic acid)[321] and at aspartic acid and asparagine (β-hydroxylation to form erythro-β-hydroxy aspartic acid [Hya] and erythro-β-hydroxy asparagine [Hyn])[91,350,351]; they are also modified by sulfation at tyrosine residues as well as the addition of sugar moieties (glycosylation).[350,351] This high degree of posttranslational processing is necessary for the biologic activity of the mature vitamin K–dependent proteins.

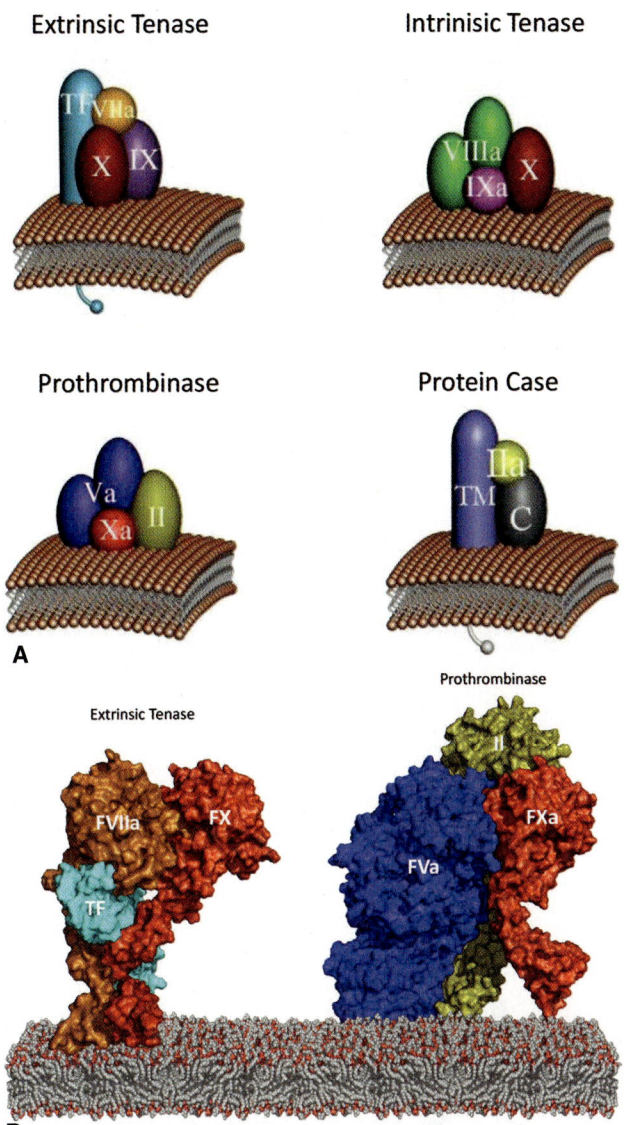

Extrinsic Tenase **Intrinisic Tenase**

Prothrombinase **Protein Case**

A

Extrinsic Tenase

Prothrombinase

B

FIGURE 20.5 Vitamin K–dependent complexes. A, Three procoagulant complexes (extrinsic tenase, intrinsic tenase, and prothrombinase) and one anticoagulant complex (protein Case) are illustrated. Each membrane complex consists of a vitamin K–dependent serine protease (factor VIIa [VIIa], factor IXa [Ixa], factor Xa [Xa], or thrombin [IIa]) and a soluble or cell surface–associated cofactor (factor VIIIa, factor Va, tissue factor [TF], or thrombomodulin [TM]). Each serine protease is shown in association with the appropriate cofactor protein and zymogen substrate(s) on the membrane surface. The membrane serves as a scaffold for the coagulation reactants, enhancing the reaction rates by 10^4- to 10^9-fold. When vascular damage or inflammatory cytokine activation occurs, TF becomes exposed to flowing blood carrying low levels of factor VIIa. The formed extrinsic tenase complex activates the circulating serine protease zymogens factors IX and X. Factor IXa becomes the serine protease for the intrinsic tenase complex, which, with its cofactor factor VIIIa, activates factor X to its active protease form factor Xa. Factor Xa formed primarily from the intrinsic tenase combines with its cofactor factor Va to activate II to IIa on the prothrombinase complex. Cofactor regulation occurs when IIa released from the prothrombinase complex binds to endothelial cell surface protein TM to form the protein Case anticoagulant complex. This complex generates activated protein C, which then proteolytically inactivates factors Va and VIIIa. B, Structural models of extrinsic tenase[344] and prothrombinase.[345] (A, From Mann KG. *Coagulation Explosion.* Vermont Business Graphics; 1997.)

Proteolytic Maturation

The vitamin K–dependent proteins are synthesized in the liver as a single-chain precursor that contains a prepro sequence followed by the polypeptide region. The hydrophobic signal peptide (prepeptide) gets the protein to the endoplasmic reticulum, the first compartment in the

secretory pathway. For the vitamin K–dependent proteins to become mature, the polypeptide is translocated out of the first compartment in the endoplasmic reticulum across the lipid bilayer into the lumen of the endoplasmic reticulum. The signal peptide is then removed by a signal peptidase. The propeptide, which plays a role in docking vitamin K–dependent carboxylase,[352] is removed by an endoproteinase. The release of the propeptide coincides with γ-carboxylation (Gla formation)[353] (*Figure 20.6A*). Removal of an internal di- or tripeptide in single-chain factor X and protein C occurs, which converts them to their mature two-chain zymogen form. Several studies describe the endoproteinase that cleaves the propeptide and the internal bonds as furin/paired basic amino acid cleaving enzyme.[355-357]

Carboxylation and Vitamin K–Dependent Carboxylase

The γ-carboxylation reaction is catalyzed by the enzyme γ-glutamyl carboxylase. This enzyme is located in the rough endoplasmic reticulum and requires the reduced form of vitamin K, oxygen, and carbon dioxide.[322] The carboxylation mechanism involves proton abstraction of the γ-hydrogen of the glutamate residues near the NH_2 terminus of the nascent prepro protein (*Figure 20.6B*). The generated carbanion at each glutamic acid residue then reacts with free CO_2, forming γ-carboxy glutamic acid. It is this Gla region that mediates the Ca^{2+}-dependent binding of the protein to anionic phospholipid surfaces, thereby ensuring close proximity and interaction with other components of the coagulation sequence and with cell receptors for vitamin K–dependent ligands. Without vitamin K, the coagulation protein precursors continue to be synthesized but are not γ-carboxylated. In this form, they are still secreted into plasma but are nonfunctional.

The cDNA for the human γ-carboxylase gene was cloned and sequenced by Wu et al.[358] The open reading frame predicts a molecular weight of approximately 87.5 kDa. Glycosylation of the carboxylase probably accounts for its decreased mobility on SDS-PAGE (94 kDa). Vitamin K–dependent carboxylase has been identified in many cell types.[359] This supports the notion that vitamin K has a wide range of biologic functions.

The presence of vitamin K is essential to maintain the γ-carboxylation reaction. Vitamin K_1 (phylloquinone) is primarily found in leafy green vegetables and vegetable oils. Additional K activity may be provided by vitamin K_2 (menaquinones) synthesized by intestinal Gram-negative bacteria. Synthetic vitamin K_3 (menadione) has no intrinsic activity until it undergoes in vivo transformation to the active menaquinone form. These K vitamins are 2-methyl-1,4-naphthoquinones with repeating five-carbon prenyl units at position 3. In vivo, vitamin K is recycled in a microsomal oxidation-reduction system for continued use in the γ-carboxylation reaction. To perform the γ-carboxylation reaction, vitamin K has to be present in its reduced hydroquinone form. As the precursor proteins are carboxylated, vitamin K is oxidized to the epoxide.[360] The epoxide in the presence of 2,3-epoxide reductase, using thiols as the reducing

Table 20.3. Rate Enhancement by Vitamin K–Dependent Complexes

Complex[a]	Substrates	Fold Enhancement[b]
FVIIa/TF/PCPS/Ca^{2+}	FIX	$>1 \times 10^{9c}$
FVIIa/TF/PCPS/Ca^{2+}	FX	3×10^4
FIXa/FVIIIa/PCPS/Ca^{2+}	FX	1×10^9
FXa/FVa/PCPS/Ca^{2+}	FII	3×10^5
FIIa/TM/PCPS/Ca^{2+}	PC	1×10^5

Abbreviations: F, factor; PC, phosphatidylcholine; PS, phosphatidylserine; TF, tissue factor; TM, thrombomodulin.
[a]Complexes are assembled on membranes composed of PC and PS (3:1 molar ratio PC/PS).
[b]Rate enhancement is derived from the ratio of catalytic efficiency (number of catalytic events per unit time/Michaelis constant [k_{cat}/K_m]) for the complex to the catalytic efficiency of the free serine protease for a given substrate.
[c]No measurable activation of FIXa by FVIIa without TF and the membrane. The catalytic efficiency of the extrinsic tenase toward FIX is reduced relative to FX.

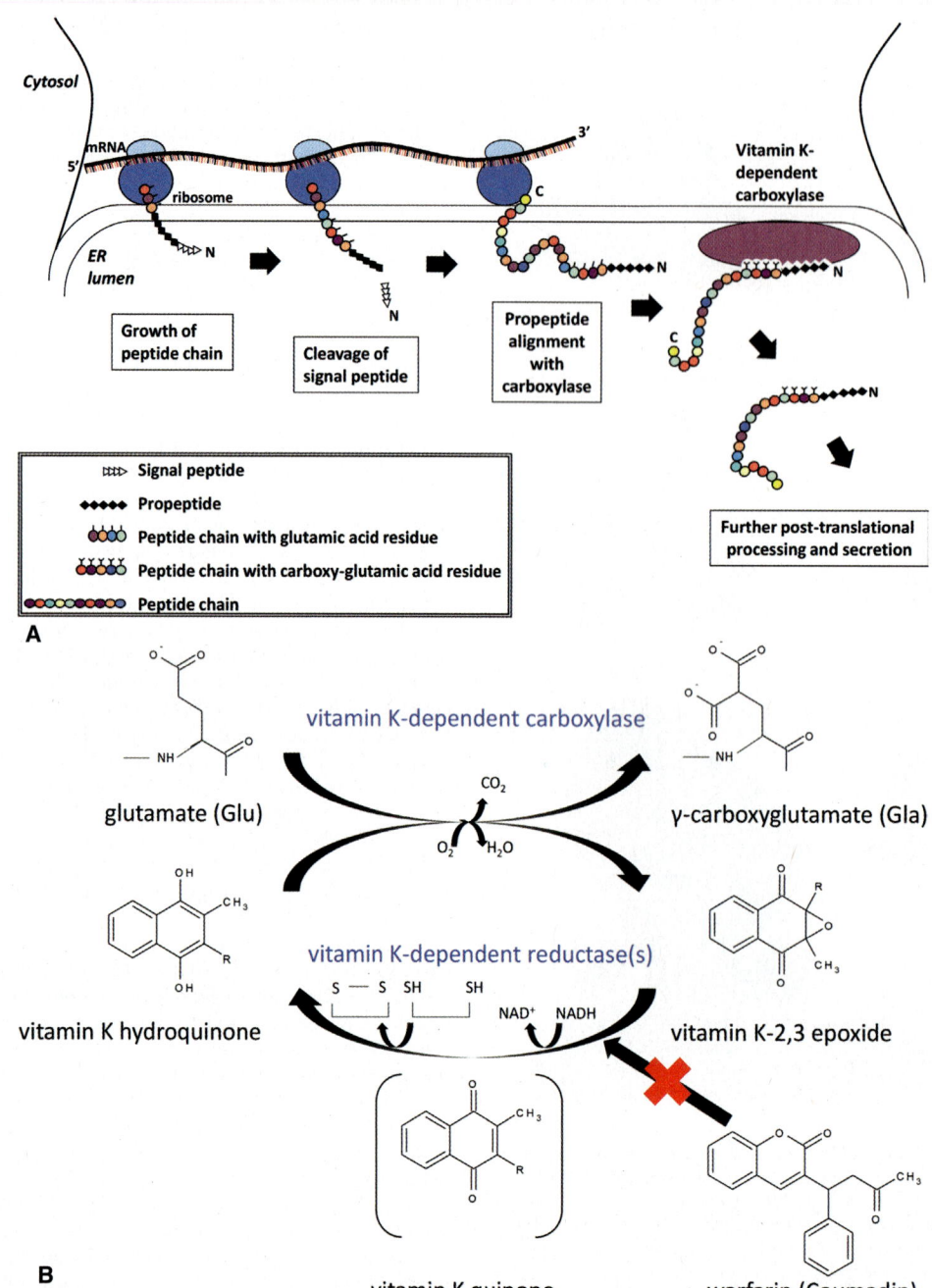

FIGURE 20.6 Vitamin K–dependent processes. A, Schematic representation of the synthesis and posttranslational carboxylation pathway of vitamin K–dependent proteins in the endoplasmic reticulum. B, The mechanism of γ-carboxy glutamate (Gla) generation by a vitamin K–dependent reaction cycle is illustrated. The regeneration of vitamin K hydroquinone by the vitamin K–dependent reductases is inhibited by anticoagulants, as illustrated by Coumadin. (A, Reprinted from Bovill EG, Malhotra OP, Mann KG. Mechanisms of vitamin K antagonism. *Baillieres Clin Haematol.* 1990;3(3):555-581. Copyright © 1990 Elsevier. With permission.)

agent, yields the quinone form of vitamin K.[361] A subsequent nicotinamide adenine dinucleotide phosphate- or nicotinamide adenine dinucleotide-dependent quinone reductase reaction resynthesizes the hydroquinone form. The cycle can thus begin again.

One important target for anticoagulant therapy is the process required for the regeneration of reduced hydroquinone vitamin K. Anticoagulants that effectively block this reaction include warfarin (Coumadin), dicumarol, and phenprocoumon (*Figure 20.6B*). These oral anticoagulants are structurally similar to the quinone form of vitamin K, thereby targeting the reductase enzyme and inhibiting the reduction to the requisite hydroquinone form. The affinity of the anticoagulants for the reductase enzymes determines the efficacy of the drug.[12,362] In the United States, the most widely used oral anticoagulant warfarin (Coumadin) is also used as rat poison. It acts as

a competitive inhibitor of oxidized vitamin K and interferes with its reduction. Without the regeneration of the reduced form of vitamin K, the vitamin K–dependent protein carboxylase is unable to convert glutamate to γ-carboxy glutamate. Thus, these drugs indirectly affect carboxylation and can be overcome with excess vitamin K. The level of competitive inhibition achieved in Coumadin therapy among individuals taking the same dose regimen is variable. Factors affecting the efficacy of treatment include liver function in the synthesis of the clotting factors, enhancement of effect from other medications, and dietary intake/adsorption of vitamin K.[363] Therefore, proper monitoring of oral anticoagulant therapy is essential with frequently measured PT and corrected assay sensitivity using the international normalized ratio.[364,365] Several lines of evidence indicate that vitamin K antagonists inhibit not only posttranslational modification on coagulation factors but also the synthesis of functional extrahepatic vitamin K–dependent proteins potentially resulting in vascular calcification.[366,367]

Hydroxylation

Hydroxylation in the context of vitamin K–dependent proteins refers to the addition of a hydroxyl group (–OH) to aspartic acid and asparagine residues present in the EGF-like domains. The EGF-1 domains of human factors IX and X, protein C, and protein S contain a homologous aspartic acid residue that is hydroxylated to form erythro-β-hydroxy aspartic acid (Hya).[91,368,369] Protein S also contains asparagine residues in EGF-2 and EGF-4 domains that are hydroxylated to form erythro-β-hydroxy asparagine residues (Hyn).[370] This posttranslational modification to Hya and Hyn occurs by a β-hydroxylase enzyme, a 2-oxo-glutarate–dependent dioxygenase.[351,371] The mechanism of action involves the recognition of a consensus sequence Cys-X-Asp/Asn-X-X-X-X-Tyr/Phe-X-Cys-X-Cys.[370] The reason for this modification to Hya and Hyn is unclear. No effect has been found on the overall fold of the EGF-1 domain, its affinity, or specificity for calcium.[372] These modifications also appear to have no relevance to the biologic activity or macromolecular interactions of the vitamin K–dependent proteins.[373,374]

Glycosylation

The addition of a carbohydrate moiety as a posttranslational modification to proteins is referred to as *glycosylation*. The vitamin K–dependent proteins contain significant amounts of carbohydrate (*Tables 20.1* and *20.4*). Carbohydrate adducts on Asn, Ser, and Thr residues are found in key domains of these proteins, including the activation peptide of factor IX and factor X; the EGF domains in factor VII, factor IX, and protein Z; and the kringle domain in prothrombin. In most cases, the purpose of these modifications remains unknown. However,

differences in the properties of the carbohydrate variants of protein C have been noted.[375,376]

General Structure/Function Features

The vitamin K–dependent proteins, both procoagulant and anticoagulant, share a common protein domain structure. Each has a tripartite design: an NH$_2$-terminal γ-carboxy glutamic acid (Gla) domain, a linker region (kringle domains, EGF-like domains [EGF], or a thrombin-sensitive finger region, or all three), and a COOH-terminal domain usually consisting of a serine protease domain (factors II, VII, IX, and X and protein C) (*Figure 20.4*). The Gla domain is involved in the Ca^{2+} ion-dependent binding of vitamin K–dependent proteins to anionic phospholipid membranes. The number of domains in the linker region is variable, and, in general, they are involved in protein-protein interactions. The COOH-terminal catalytic domain seen in factors II, VII, IX, and X and protein C is homologous to the pancreatic serine proteases, trypsin, and chymotrypsin. The nonserine protease domain seen in protein S (a cofactor of activated protein C [APC]) is homologous to sex hormone–binding globulin.[377] Protein Z is an enzymatically inactive homolog of factors VII, IX, and X and protein C.[378] A separate review of the Gla, EGF, and serine protease domains is presented below.

The importance of each of the domains has been uncovered through studies from natural variants that occur in patients with either familial bleeding (i.e., factor IX deficiency/hemophilia B) or thrombotic disease (i.e., protein C deficiency). The situations that can cause a disease state are either deficiency in the level of protein present (cross-reactive material [CRM]–negative) or expressed protein that is present but nonfunctional (CRM$^+$). Defects have diverse causes, including mutations that lead to amino acid substitutions in one or more domains, defects in posttranslational modifications, or mutations that introduce stop codons resulting in either no expression or expression of

Table 20.4. Biochemical Properties of Human Anticoagulant Proteins and Inhibitors

Protein	Molecular Weight (Da)	Plasma Concentration (nmol/L)	Plasma Concentration (µg/mL)	Plasma Half-Life (days)	Carbohydrate (%)	Clinical Phenotype[a] H	Clinical Phenotype[a] T	Protein Family	Functional Classification
Protein C	62,000	65	4	0.33	23		+	VKD	Proteinase zymogen
Protein S	69,000	300	20	1.75	7		+	VKD	Inhibitor/cofactor
Protein Z	62,000	47	2.9	2.5			±	VKD	Cofactor
Thrombomodulin	100,000								Cofactor/modulator
α_2-Macroglobulin	735,000	2700-4000	2000-3000	0.002				Complement	Proteinase inhibitor
Tissue factor pathway inhibitor	40,000	1-4	0.1	6.4×10^{-4} -1.4×10^{-3}				Kunitz	Proteinase inhibitor
Antithrombin	58,000	2400	140	2.5-3.0	15			Serpin	Proteinase inhibitor
Heparin cofactor II	66,000	500-1400	33-90	2.5	10			Serpin	Proteinase inhibitor
α_1-Proteinase inhibitor	53,000	28,000	1500–3500	6	12			Serpin	Proteinase inhibitor
C1 esterase inhibitor	104,000	962	100	0.07	35			Serpin	Proteinase inhibitor
Protein C inhibitor	57,000	90	5	1	23		+	Serpin	Proteinase inhibitor
Protein Z inhibitor	72,000	60	4.3	0.46			+	Serpin	Proteinase inhibitor

Abbreviations: +, presence of phenotype; ±, some individuals present with phenotype and others do not; H, hemorrhagic disease/hemophilia; T, thrombotic disease/thrombophilia; VKD, vitamin K-dependent.
[a]Clinical phenotype: the expression of either H or T phenotype in deficient individuals.

truncated proteins. In the case of combined vitamin K deficiency, a rare hereditary bleeding disorder,[379,380] two studies have identified a missense mutation in the γ-carboxylase gene that results in a defective γ-glutamyl carboxylase and thus incomplete processing of the vitamin K–dependent proteins.[381,382]

When a hemostatic disorder characterized by a dysfunctional protein (CRM$^+$) is identified, it is through the combination of techniques including protein isolation, in vitro studies, and DNA technology that the root of the defect is elucidated. The importance of domains as functional units and of specific amino acid interactions can be uncovered using recombinant DNA technology. Single amino acid substitutions can be introduced into domains or entire domains removed to determine where the intra- and interprotein interactions take place. Structural information through nuclear magnetic resonance spectroscopy and x-ray crystallography provides amino acid assignments and tertiary structure, thus allowing for precise approaches to site-directed mutagenesis studies. The combination of all these techniques results in a map of how the domains are aligned and interact. Furthermore, using computational molecular dynamics, one can predict conformational changes associated with protein-protein, protein-ligand, and protein-surface interactions. Identifying residues directly involved in binding to membranes, metal ions, or small substrates can lead to new drug therapies.

The first x-ray crystal structure of a vitamin K–dependent protein was obtained by Tulinsky's laboratory for prothrombin fragment 1 (factor II, residues 1-155) in the presence[383] and absence of calcium.[384,385] These results provided information regarding the entire Gla domain, the connector peptide, and kringle 1. In the absence of calcium, only the connector peptide and the kringle can be visualized in the resulting x-ray crystal analysis. Prothrombin is the only vitamin K–dependent protein with a kringle domain. It is likely that organization of the polypeptide chains of the Gla domain is similar for all vitamin K–dependent proteins. To date, several other vitamin K–dependent protein structures have been elucidated[386-396] (see *Table 20.5*). Many studies on the individual vitamin K–dependent proteins have been conducted and are detailed under each protein subsection.

All the vitamin K–dependent proteins contain an NH$_2$-terminal Gla domain, and only factors II, VII, IX, and X and protein C contain a serine protease domain. Factors IX, X, and VII; protein C; and protein S contain EGF domains. Several recent reviews have been written on vitamin K–dependent proteins.[397-400]

Gla Domain

The Gla domain constitutes the first approximately 50 residues of the vitamin K–dependent proteins (*Figure 20.4*). The negative charge elicited from the string of Gla residues (9-13) contributes to the binding to Ca^{2+} and the generation of the conformation required for binding to anionic phospholipid membranes. This surface in vivo is supplied by activated platelets or other blood cells in response to vascular damage through exposure of the internal face of their cell membranes where it is phosphatidylserine (PS) rich.[383,401] In vitro systems that attempt to mimic coagulation mainly use natural or synthetic preparations of PS and phosphatidylcholine, often at a 1:3 molar ratio. Studies have shown that PS exposure is crucial for cells to support the membrane-bound

Table 20.5. Highest Resolution Structures of Human Procoagulant, Anticoagulant, Fibrinolytic Proteins, and Their Inhibitors

Protein	Structure	Resolution (Å)	PDB Code
Procoagulant Proteins–			
Intrinsic Pathway			
Factor XII	Catalytic domain	2.1	4XDE
	Fibronectin-EGF2	1.6	4BDX
Prekallikrein	Plasma kallikrein	1.4	6I44
HMW Kininogen	N/A		
LMW Kininogen	N/A		
Factor XI	XI zymogen	2.9	2F83
	XIa + inhibitor	1.2	6TS4
	XI + HMW kininogen peptide	2.9	5I25
Vitamin K Dependent			
Factor VII	VII zymogen (des Gla-EGF1)	2.0	1JBU
	VIIa (des Gla-EGF1) + inhibitor	1.4	5PAG
	VIIa + TF extracellular domain + inhibitor	1.3	6R2W
Factor IX	IXa (des Gla-EGF1) + inhibitor	1.3	5JB9
	Gla domain (bovine)	1.6	1J34
	IXa (porcine)	3.0	1PFX
	IXa (des Gla-EGF1) + AT + pentasaccharide	1.7	3KCG
Factor X	Xa (des Gla-EGF1)	1.3	2JKH
	Xa (des Gla)	1.9	3K9X
	Gla domain + snake factor X binding protein	2.3	1IOD
	Xa (des Gla-EGF1) + AT + pentasaccharide	3.3	2GD4
	Prothrombinase (Xa + Va from snake venom)	3.3	4BXS
Factor II	Prothrombin	4.1	6C2W
	Prethrombin 1	2.2	3NXP
	Prethrombin 2 + fragment 2	1.9	3K65
	Prethrombin 2	1.9	3SQE
	Meizothrombiun (desF1)	2.1	3E6P
	α-IIa	1.6	3U69
	α-IIa + inhibitor (small molecule)	1.1	5AFY
	α-IIa + inhibitor (hirudin fragment)	1.3	2UUF

(Continued)

Table 20.5. Highest Resolution Structures of Human Procoagulant, Anticoagulant, Fibrinolytic Proteins, and Their Inhibitors (Continued)

Protein	Structure	Resolution (Å)	PDB Code
Cofactors			
Tissue factor	Extracellular domain	1.7	2HFT
	TF extracellular domain + VIIa + inhibitor	1.3	6R2W
Factor V	V	3.3	7KVE
	C2 domain	1.9	1CZT
	Va-inactive (bovine)	2.8	1SDD
	Prothrombinase (Va + Xa from snake venom)	3.3	4BXS
Factor VIII	VIIIa	3.6	3MF2
	VIIIa chimera (human + porcine) membrane bound VIIIa	3.2	6MF0
		15	3J2S
vWf	A1 domain mutant	1.6	5BV8
	A1 domain mutant + GP1bα	2.1	4C2A
	A2 domain	1.7	3ZQK
	A3 domain	1.8	1ATZ
	A3 domain + collagen	2.8	4DMU
Anticoagulant Proteins–			
Dynamic Inhibition			
Protein C	APC (des Gla)	2.8	1AUT
	APC (des Gla) + Fab	2.2	6M3B
	Gla Domain of APC + PC receptor	1.6	1LQV
Protein S	EGF3-EGF4		1Z6C
Protein Z	PZ (des Gla-EGF1) + PZI	2.3	3F1S
Thrombomodulin	EGF 4-6 of thrombomodulin + IIa	2.3	1DX5
Proteinase Inhibitors			
α₂-Macroglobin	α₂-M	4.2	6TAV
TFPI	TFPI (1st Kunitz domain)	2.5	4BQD
	TFPI (2nd Kunitz domain) + antibody	1.8	4DTG
	TFPI (3rd Kunitz domain)		1IRH
Antithrombin	AT plasma α-AT	2.8	2B4X
	Plasma ß-AT	2.6	1E05
	ATIII + IIa + heparin	2.6	1E04
	AT + IXa (des Gla-EGF1) + pentasaccharide	2.5	1TB6
	AT + Xa (des Gla-EGF1) + pentasaccharide	1.7	3KCG
		3.3	2GD4
Heparin cofactor II	Heparin cofactor II	2.4	1JMJ
	Heparin cofactor II + IIa	2.2	1JMO
α₁-Antitrypsin	α₁-AT	1.8	3NE4
	α₁-AT + trypsin	2.6	1EZX
C1 esterase inhibitor	C1-inh	2.1	5DU3
Protein C inhibitor	PCI	2.0	2OL2
	PCI + IIa + heparin	1.6	3B9F
Protein Z–dependent inhibitor	PZI	2.1	4AFX
	PZI + PZ (des Gla-EGF1)	2.3	3F1S
Proteins of Clot Formation			
Factor XIII	XIII zymogen	2.0	1EVU
	XIIIa	2.0	4KTY
Fibrinogen	Fibrinogen	2.9	3GHG
	Fibrinogen (chicken)	2.7	1M1J
	Fragment E	1.4	1JY2
	Fragment E + IIa	3.7	2A45
	Alpha domain from fibrinogen-420	2.1	1FZD
Fibrin	D-dimer	2.3	1FZC
Fibrinolytic System–			
Proteins			
Plasminogen	Plasminogen	2.5	4DUR
	Angiostatin (Kringles 1-3)	1.8	1KI0
	Plasmin + streptokinase	2.8	1BML

Table 20.5. Highest Resolution Structures of Human Procoagulant, Anticoagulant, Fibrinolytic Proteins, and Their Inhibitors (Continued)

Protein	Structure	Resolution (Å)	PDB Code
t-PA	Single-chain + inhibitor	3.4	1BDA
	Two-chain + inhibitor	2.3	1RTF
	t-PA + PAI-1	3.2	5BRR
u-PA	Two-chain + inhibitor	1.4	6XVD
	NH$_2$-terminal fragment + receptor + antibody u-PA + PAI-1	1.9	2FD6
		2.3	3PB1
Factor VII Activating Protease	N/A		
Inhibitors			
TAFI	TAFIa	1.6	1KWM
	TAFIa + inhibitor	2.0	4P10
PAI-1	Latent form	1.8	1LJ5
	Active form	2.4	1DVM
	Active form + inhibitor	1.8	7AQF
	PAI-1 + t-PA	3.2	5BRR 3PB1
	PAI-1 + u-PA	2.3	
PAI-2	Stabilized mutant	1.6	2JRR
α$_2$-Antiplasmin	α$_2$-AP (mouse)	2.7	2R9Y

Abbreviations: AT, antithrombin; EGF, epidermal growth factor; HMW, high molecular weight; LMW, low molecular weight; N/A, not currently available; PAI, plasminogen activator inhibitor; t-PA, tissue plasminogen activator; TAFI, thrombin-activatable fibrinolysis inhibitor; TFPI, tissue factor pathway inhibitor; u-PA, urokinase-type plasminogen activator.
Updated: Feb 2022.

enzymatic reactions and that PS is more effective than other equally charged lipids.[5,402,403] The striking degree of homology among the Gla domains of the vitamin K–dependent clotting factors suggests that the affinity of the calcium-Gla complexes for phospholipids would also be very similar. However, this turns out not to be the case. The dissociation constants for binding to phosphatidylcholine and PS-containing vesicles vary, with K$_d$ values in the range of 50 nmol/L for protein Z and protein S,[404] 100 to 300 nmol/L for factor X and prothrombin,[405] 15 nmol/L for protein C,[404] and 17,000 nmol/L for factor VII.[404,406] A systematic analysis of the sequence/structural basis for these divergent membrane-binding properties is available.[394,404]

The mode of interaction between the Gla domain–containing coagulation factors and biologic membranes has been difficult to study and is still a subject for debate. Two models of binding have been presented. One involves the bridging of calcium between specific Gla residues and the negative anionic phospholipid membrane components.[406,407] A second model involves a major hydrophobic contribution to the membrane binding. X-ray crystallographic[384,408-410] and nuclear magnetic resonance studies[411] have been conducted to elucidate the conformational changes, in the absence and presence of calcium, that occur on Gla domain binding to a lipid membrane. In the absence of calcium, the negatively charged Gla residues appear exposed to the solution, and the hydrophobic residues of the Gla domain are buried in its interior.[411] On Ca^{2+} binding to the Gla domain, the conformation is altered to expose the hydrophobic residues, making possible their insertion into the lipid membrane. The hydrophobic patch in prothrombin fragment 1 surrounding the first pair of Gla residues was determined to be Phe^4, Leu^5, and Val^8. Site-directed mutagenesis studies of protein C determined these residues (Phe^4, Leu^5, and Leu^8) to be important in membrane interactions.[412-414] The actual mechanism of membrane binding is still under active investigation.

Epidermal Growth Factor Domain

The Gla domain is followed by two tandem EGF domains (EGF-1 and EGF-2) in factor VII, factor IX, factor X, and protein C and four EGF domains (EGF-1 to EGF-4) in protein S[415] (*Figure 20.4*). The first EGF domain (EGF-1) contains the posttranslationally modified amino acid β-hydroxy aspartic acid in the case of factors IX and X and β-hydroxy asparagine in the case of protein S.[350,368,370,416-418] An EGF-like domain consists of 40 to 50 amino acids, including six cysteine residues involved in disulfide bond formation. The EGF domains have been evaluated by nuclear magnetic resonance spectroscopy.[400,419-423] The EGF-2 domains of factor Xa,[392] factor VIIa,[394] activated protein C,[396] and factor IXa[424] have been evaluated by x-ray crystallography. The EGF-like domains are found widely distributed in extracellular and membrane proteins. Proteins containing these domains are involved in blood coagulation, fibrinolysis, complement activation, and microfibril formation in connective tissue and in signal transduction.[370,425,426] These domains are similar to the archetypal protein, EGF, which contains nine of these domains and is derived from a membrane-bound precursor.

The structure of the EGF-like domains is dominated by β sheets and β turns. Several point mutations in the EGF domain of factor IX have been identified that cause hemophilia B.[427] Calcium-binding sites have been identified in the NH$_2$-terminal EGF-like domains isolated from factors VII, IX, and X and proteins C and Z, with K$_d$ values ranging from 1 to 5 mm. This Ca^{2+}-binding site is functionally important because vitamin K–dependent proteins that have missense mutations in EGF-1 that disrupt the Ca^{2+}-binding site have reduced biologic activity. In these proteins, the second EGF domain does not appear to bind calcium. The NH$_2$-terminal EGF domain of protein S does not appear to bind Ca^{2+}.

The function of the EGF domain is still unclear. One hypothesis is that it serves as a spacer. A consistent elongation of the molecules of factors VII, IX, and X and protein C and protein S has been noted. The distance between the membrane-binding Gla domain and the serine protease domain is crucial to the placement of the active site in an appropriate position relative to the target peptide bond in its substrate.[428] Calcium binding serves a role in the function of these domains. For example, it has been proposed that, for appropriate docking of factor VIIa to tissue factor, Ca^{2+} binding to the EGF domain is required.[429] Calcium binding to the EGF domains in non-vitamin K–dependent proteins has been observed in the Notch protein[430] and fibrillin.[431]

Serine Protease Domain

The serine protease domain accounts for approximately half the mass of each protein. Peptide bond cleavage at specific sites converts the vitamin K–dependent zymogens to their active serine protease forms (*Figure 20.4*). These enzymes are serine proteases in the same family as trypsin and chymotrypsin. The mechanism of proteolysis by chymotrypsin involves a catalytic triad, composed of Asp^{102}, His^{57}, and Ser^{195} (chymotrypsin numbering). The nucleophilic attack is carried out by the hydroxyl group of Ser^{195} with the imidazole ring of His^{57} taking up the liberated proton and the carboxylate ion of Asp^{102} stabilizing the developing charge. More extensive elements of structure (i.e., calcium-, membrane-, and cofactor-binding sites) are required for interactions of enzymes and substrates in the coagulation process.

The serine protease domains of all the Gla-containing factors show a high degree of sequence identity with each other and to trypsin and chymotrypsin, cleaving almost specifically at arginyl residues. However, unlike trypsin, which shows little specificity beyond the requirement for arginyl or lysyl residues at the cleavage site, the activated coagulation factors have extended substrate specificity pockets where only a small number of amino acid sequences are recognized by each activated factor. Despite a high degree of structural similarity between the protease domains of protein C and factors II, VII, IX, and X, each of these factors has a highly specific function in coagulation. Some of this discrimination may be mediated by surface loops and other domains away from the substrate-binding pocket that are not highly homologous.

Factor VII (Proconvertin, Convertin)

The vitamin K–dependent single-chain zymogen factor VII (M_r = 50,000), also known as *proconvertin*, circulates in plasma at a concentration of 0.5 µg/mL, or 10 nmol/L[432,433] (*Table 20.1*). It is synthesized primarily in the liver. The activated two-chain serine protease form, factor VIIa, circulates in plasma at approximately 1% the concentration of its precursor, or 0.1 nmol/L.[52] The mechanism for the initial activation of this zymogen is unclear. One recently identified candidate is the factor VII–activating protease (FSAP; see section on factor VII–activating protease). The function of factor VIIa is to serve as an initiator of the extrinsic pathway of coagulation when bound to its membrane cofactor, tissue factor. Factor VII has the shortest $t_{1/2}$ of all the clotting factor zymogens (~3-6 hours).[434] Its activated form factor VIIa has a $t_{1/2}$ of 2.4 hours.[435,436]

Factor VII deficiency is an autosomal recessive disorder with wide phenotypic and genotypic variability.[437-440] Its incidence in the general population is approximately 1 in 500,000. In a large French-Canadian kindred, the incidence is approximately 1 in 335.[441] Bleeding phenotypes can range from mild to severe and include bruising, epistaxis, postsurgical hemorrhage, and cerebral hemorrhage. Severe bleeding is most commonly associated with plasma factor VII levels that are <1%.[442] Patients have prolonged PTs, and the final diagnosis is established by plasma factor VII coagulant activity (VII:C) using factor VII–deficient plasma and animal thromboplastins, immunologic quantitation of factor VII antigen, or both.[433,443] Treatment of these individuals includes the use of fresh frozen plasma, prothrombin complex concentrates,[444] factor VII concentrates (plasma-derived or recombinant),[445] and liver transplantation.[446] Owing to its short $t_{1/2}$ (~3-6 hours), therapy with factor VII concentrates is difficult. Recently, the use of recombinant factor VII as a safe and effective treatment for factor VII deficiency has been evaluated.[447-449] During the last decade, supraphysiologic concentrations of recombinant factor VIIa have been used clinically for treatment of patients with hemophilia A or B (factor VIII or factor IX deficiency, respectively) and patients undergoing surgical procedures.[450-455] Recombinant factor VIIa has been suggested for treatment of almost all bleeding disorders.[456] The mechanism of hemostasis by recombinant factor VIIa is not fully understood, although several hypotheses have been proposed.[457-460]

Studies on the molecular basis for factor VII deficiency have led to the identification of several mutations in the factor VII gene. These mutations have been identified in the splice site,[461] the promoter region,[462] the EGF domain,[463] and numerous single base pair (bp) mutations.[464,465] For more detail, there is a factor VII mutation database available at europium.csc.mrc.ac.uk.[466] Factor VII deficiency in mice is not lethal at the embryonic stage, but factor VII$^{-/-}$ neonates die from hemorrhage within the first days after birth.[467,468]

Gene Structure and Expression

The factor VII gene is located on chromosome 13q34, consists of nine exons, and spans 12.8 kb[469-471] (*Table 20.2*). It is located approximately 2.8 kb upstream from the factor X gene. The mRNA encodes a 2.5-kb message.[472] Alternative splicing of the factor VII gene yields two gene transcripts. One gene transcript contains eight segments as exons, and the second gene transcript contains nine segments as exons. The additional exon, which is unique among the vitamin K–dependent proteins, is in the prepro leader sequence. Factor VII mRNA expression is localized in the liver,[473] where its expression is 6% of the factor X mRNA level.[474] Extrahepatic synthesis of factor VII has been observed in human atherosclerotic vessels.[475] The 5′-flanking region of the factor VII gene contains binding sites for the liver-enriched transcription factor hepatic nuclear factor (HNF)-4.[476] Three potential activation peptide-1–binding sites are also contained in this region. Both genetic and epigenetic modifications in the promoter region of the factor VII gene have been shown to affect plasma factor VIIa levels.[477]

Biochemistry

Factor VII circulates in plasma as a single-chain zymogen of a molecular weight of 50,000.[432,470,478,479] Its 406-amino-acid structure consists of an NH_2-terminal Gla domain containing 10 γ-carboxy glutamate residues, β-hydroxy aspartic acid at position 63,[369] an aromatic residue–rich α-helical region, two EGF domains, and a serine protease domain (*Figure 20.4*). The NH_2 terminus, along with the serine protease domain, is involved in the metal binding properties of the protein and its interaction with its cofactor tissue factor.[480-482] The COOH terminus of factor VII is important in its interactions with factor X.[483] Structures of factors VII[484] and VIIa[395] and the extrinsic tenase[485] have been determined and have been utilized in a variety of ways to enhance our understanding of this protein.

Activation

The single-chain zymogen factor VII is activated to its two-chain serine protease form, factor VIIa, through a single peptide bond cleavage between Arg^{152}-Ile^{153} (*Figure 20.4*). The resulting protease consists of an NH_2-terminal light chain (M_r = 20,000) containing the membrane-binding Gla domain (10 Gla residues), linked by a single disulfide bond between Cys^{135} and Cys^{262} to a COOH-terminal heavy chain (M_r = 30,000) that contains the catalytic domain. A small amount of activated factor VII (10-100 pmol/L) already circulates in the cleaved active two-chain form.[486] This small portion of plasma factor VIIa has very poor catalytic efficiency in the absence of its cofactor, tissue factor.[487,488] The cleavage of factor VII to factor VIIa is catalyzed by several proteases, including α-thrombin,[8] factor IXa,[489] factor Xa,[8] autoactivation by factor VIIa,[490] factor XIIa,[491] and FSAP.[492] The endothelial cell protein C receptor has been reported to bind factor VII and suppress its activation by factor Xa.[493]

Function

Factor VII is a crucial zymogen in blood coagulation and can bind to tissue factor with a subnanomolar K_d and become activated by a number of proteases. Once converted to its active serine protease form and bound to its cofactor, the integral membrane protein tissue factor, it forms the extrinsic tenase complex[494,495] (*Figure 20.5*). The enzyme complex is so named because it contains a protein, tissue factor, normally extrinsic to the plasma environment. The extrinsic tenase complex (factor VIIa–tissue factor–membrane surface–Ca^{2+}) activates a fraction of the circulating vitamin K–dependent zymogens, factors IX and X, to their serine protease forms.[43,496-498] Thus, it serves to initiate the formation of the intrinsic tenase (factor IXa–factor VIIIa–membrane–Ca^{2+}) and the prothrombinase complexes (factor Xa–factor Va–membrane–Ca^{2+}). In vitro studies have shown that the rate of activation by the extrinsic tenase complex is significantly greater (~100,000-fold) than the rate of substrate (factors IX and X) activation by the enzyme factor VIIa alone.[499,500] Factor Xa bound to a membrane surface can activate additional factor VII in a positive feedback loop.[8,501]

Regulation

Free factor VIIa, unlike other serine proteases of the coagulation cascade,[488] is not readily inhibited by circulating protease inhibitors, including the antithrombin-heparin complex.[502,503] This is most likely because of its poor catalytic efficiency when not bound to its cofactor tissue factor. However, when factor VIIa is bound to tissue factor, antithrombin-heparin exhibits significant inhibition of factor VIIa.[504-506] Thus, regulation of tissue factor expression is the primary means to control factor VIIa activity. Paradoxically, in normal hemostasis, factor VII (10 nmol/L) is an effective competitor of factor VIIa (0.1 nmol/L) for binding to tissue factor. This competition downregulates the level of enzymatically active complex (factor VIIa–tissue factor), thus suppressing initiation of the clotting cascade. Once the extrinsic tenase complex (factor VIIa–tissue factor–Ca^{2+}–membrane) activates factor X to factor Xa, tissue factor pathway inhibitor (TFPI) can form a quaternary complex (factor VIIa–tissue factor–factor Xa–TFPI) with no enzymatic activity[507] (*Figure 20.7*).

Factor IX (Plasma Thromboplastin Component, Christmas Factor, Hemophilia B Factor)

The zymogen factor IX is a single-chain vitamin K–dependent procoagulant glycoprotein synthesized in the liver, which has also been referred to as *plasma thromboplastin component, Christmas factor,* or *hemophilia B factor*. It circulates in plasma ($t_{1/2}$ = 24 hours)[508] at a mean concentration of 5 μg/mL, or 90 nmol/L, with a relative molecular weight of 55,000[509] (*Table 20.1*). In addition, there may be a pool of noncirculating factor IX, which is readily available to the intravascular space, systemically distributed and sequestered either to the endothelial surface[510] or subendothelial components, specifically collagen IV.[511-513] High levels of factor IX have been correlated with an increased risk of venous thrombosis.[514]

Deficiency of this glycoprotein, known as *hemophilia B,* is considered one of the most common inherited coagulation disorders. The factor IX gene, found on the X chromosome, is a sex-linked recessive bleeding disorder that is found in males. The frequency of this disorder in the general population is approximately 1 in 30,000 males.[509,515] It rarely affects females, but several cases have been identified involving a mutation on the factor IX gene.[516,517] Acquired hemophilia can also occur due to the generation of autoantibodies.[518] Many mutations, including large deletions, small deletions, point mutations, and missense mutations, have been identified in factor IX that appear to reduce activity in the presence of normal antigen levels (CRM$^+$) or impair synthesis resulting in reduction of both activity and antigen (CRM$^-$).[519,520] Several specific cases and studies are noted: X translocation,[521] links to factor V^{Leiden},[522] population studies,[523-526] and factor IX Denver.[527] The point mutation called *factor IX Denver* results in a 100-fold decrease in the binding affinity of factor IXa Denver for factor VIIIa (K_d = 9.9 nmol/L) compared with normal factor IXa.[527] Mutations in the EGF-1-like domain of factor IX, specifically at Gly^{48}, have also been identified in CRM$^+$ individuals with hemophilia B.[528] Molecular insights into hemophilia B, as well as hemophilia A, have been formatted in reviews with references to accession numbers and locus identification.[529,530]

Hemophiliacs experience prolonged bleeding episodes that can be life threatening and lead to chronic disabilities. The clinical presentation or phenotype is not homogeneous. Severe disease is associated with <1% functional factor IX, moderate disease with 1% to 5%, and mild disease with 5% to 25%. Female carriers usually have approximately 20% to 50% functional factor IX. Traditionally, treatment for hemophilia B involves plasma-derived or recombinant factor IX.[531,532] One problem with this therapy is the development of inhibitory antibodies. There is a North American Immune Tolerance Registry to study immune tolerance in hemophiliacs.[533] An alternative treatment in the last decade has been the use of recombinant factor VIIa at

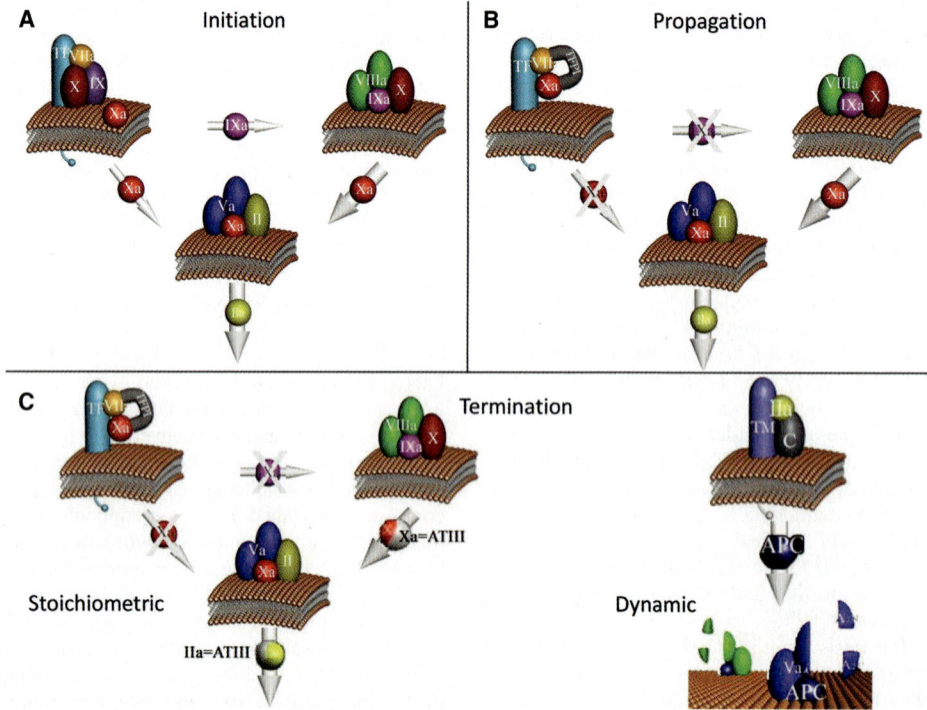

FIGURE 20.7 Regulation of the procoagulant response. Four vitamin K–dependent complexes are illustrated: the extrinsic tenase, the intrinsic tenase, prothrombinase, and protein Case. The procoagulant response is regulated by the stoichiometric inhibitors antithrombin (AT) and tissue factor pathway inhibitor (TFPI). AT inhibits thrombin, factor Xa, and factor IXa that are free in solution. TFPI inhibits both factor Xa and the factor VIIa–tissue factor (TF)–factor Xa complex. Activated protein C (APC) generated from the protein Case complex (thrombomodulin [TM]-thrombin [IIa]) inactivates FVa and FVIIIa by proteolysis of their heavy chains. A, Initiation phase; B, Propagation; C, Termination. (Adapted from Mann KG. *Coagulation Explosion.* Vermont Business Graphics; 1997.)

supraphysiologic concentrations (~90 µg/kg). These therapies eliminate the immediate danger of bleeding but do not constitute a cure for the patients. The potential for gene-based therapy for the treatment of hemophilia has become a new avenue for investigation.[534-537] To date, transgene therapy has proved successful in animal models, and human trials have been initiated as well.[538-546]

Gene Structure and Expression

The gene for factor IX is located on the X chromosome at position q27.1, near the factor VIII gene.[547-549] The gene contains eight exons and seven introns and has an overall size of 33 kb.[550,551] Five *cis*-acting elements have been identified in the promoter region of the factor IX gene.[552,553] These include binding sites for transcription factor C/EBP,[554] an HNF-1-binding site,[555] an HNF-4-binding site,[556] and a site for the D-box binding protein.[557] Two essential age-regulatory elements, AE5′ and AE3′, have been identified in the 5′ upstream region of the gene encoding factor IX in transgenic mice.[558] Together, these elements identify the advancing age-associated increase in factor IX gene expression.

Single point mutations in the factor IX promoter region have been correlated with a rare form of hemophilia B termed *hemophilia B Leyden*.[552,559,560] Hemophilia B Leyden is characterized by an altered developmental expression of blood coagulation factor IX.[552] These individuals have increasing levels of factor IX after puberty, or after administration of testosterone, resulting in decreased bleeding instances.[561,562] Studies in mice support the role of androgen receptor binding to the factor IX promoter in regulating the developmental expression of factor IX.[563]

Biochemistry

The structure of human factor IX consists of 415 amino acids that are separated into a Gla domain (12 Gla residues), two tandem EGF domains (EGF-1 [residues 46-84] and EGF-2 [residues 85-127]), an activation peptide region, and a serine protease domain[294,551,564] (*Figure 20.4*). Glycosylation in the form of O-linked and N-linked oligosaccharides makes up 17% by weight of the factor IX protein—specifically, O-linked oligosaccharides at Ser[53] and Ser[61] in the EGF-1 domain and O-linked and N-linked oligosaccharides at Asn[157], Asn[167], Thr[159], and Thr[169] in the activation peptide region.[565-568] The Gla domains are crucial for binding to anionic lipid membranes through Ca^{2+} interactions. The x-ray crystal structure of human factor IX with Ca^{2+} has shown that EGF-1 binds a single Ca^{2+} with residues Asp[47], Gly[48], Gln[50], Asp[64], and Asp[65] functioning as the ligands.[424,569] Hydrophobic interactions[570] and a salt bridge (Glu[78]-Arg[94])[571] between the carboxy end of EGF-1 and EGF-2 have also been identified.[393] Ca^{2+} binding and hydrophobic interactions lock the domains in a manner that ensures biologic activity. Several point mutations in the EGF domain give rise to hemophilia B.[427]

Activation

Factor IX activation to its serine protease form, factor IXa, is a two-stage process requiring sequential cleavages at Arg[145] and Arg[180], releasing a 35-residue activation peptide with an approximate molecular weight of 11,000[572,573] (*Figure 20.4*). Physiologic activators of factor IX are either tissue factor–factor VIIa (extrinsic tenase complex)[496,574] or factor XIa.[575-577] The first step in activation is the cleavage by its physiologic activators at the Arg[145]-Ala[146] bond, resulting in factor IXα. This cleavage has been shown to be important in its affinity for its cofactor factor VIIIa[578] and has been identified as a molecular defect in factor IX$_{Chapel Hill}$.[579] The second step is cleavage at the Arg[180]-Val[181] bond, resulting in factor IXa b, the active form, also known as *factor IXa*. Both cleavages are required for full biologic activity of factor IXa.[573] In vitro, factor IX has also been shown to be cleaved by factor Xa at Arg[145] on phospholipid membrane surfaces,[61] producing the inactive precursor factor IXα and increasing the overall rate of factor IXa production by tissue factor–factor VIIa. Both cleavage sites, Arg[145] and Arg[180], have been identified as single point mutations in hemophilia B.[580] The x-ray crystal structure of porcine factor IXa has also been solved.[393]

The active serine protease ($M_r = 45,000$) structure is composed of a heavy chain ($M_r = 28,000$) and a light chain ($M_r = 17,000$) covalently associated through a disulfide bond. Factor IXa forms the intrinsic tenase complex with its cofactor factor VIIIa, Ca^{2+}, and a membrane surface primarily supplied by platelets (*Figure 20.5*). On formation of this complex, factor X is activated to its serine protease form, factor Xa. Factor IXa (the enzyme) alone without its cofactor (factor VIIIa) has poor amidolytic and proteolytic activity (10^7-fold less activity).

Function

The main role for factor IXa in blood coagulation is to form the intrinsic tenase complex, which efficiently activates factor X to factor Xa. The complex is so named because the components, including the cofactor, are intrinsic to circulating blood, unlike tissue factor, the cofactor for the extrinsic tenase complex. Both complexes activate factor X to factor Xa. The extrinsic tenase complex (factor VIIa-tissue factor-Ca^{2+}-membrane) catalyzes the initial formation (picomolar amounts) of factor Xa, which ultimately participates in prothrombinase complex assembly and the resulting conversion of prothrombin to thrombin, allowing clot formation to occur. The intrinsic tenase complex (factor IXa-factor VIIIa-Ca^{2+}-membrane) generates the second burst of factor Xa that results in the propagation phase of the activation of prothrombin to thrombin (*Figure 20.8*).[583] The intrinsic tenase complex is kinetically more efficient than the extrinsic tenase complex in generating factor Xa. Factor Xa generation by tissue factor–factor VIIa occurs at only 1/50th the rate of factor X activation by the factor IXa–factor VIIIa complex.[61-63] Without the intrinsic complex being formed, as occurs in situations like hemophilia A or B, factor Xa is not generated in levels sufficient to produce the propagation phase of thrombin generation (*Figure 20.8*).[460,581,582]

When the competitive substrates factors IX and X are simultaneously presented to the extrinsic tenase complex, factor IXa generation is increased, whereas factor Xa generation is suppressed.[61,62] This occurs because the factor Xa initially produced cleaves factor IX at Arg[145], producing factor IXα. Factor IXα is a better substrate for factor VIIa–tissue factor than factor IX; the intermediate is converted to factor IXab (factor IXa) by cleavage at Arg[180] by factor VIIa–tissue factor. This cooperative enzymatic action results in factor IX being an improved substrate for the extrinsic tenase complex, whereas factor X activation is suppressed.

Regulation

Plasma factor IXa is primarily inhibited by antithrombin[584] (*Figure 20.7*). In vitro experiments conducted on phospholipid vesicles and cell membranes showed that PN2/amyloid β-protein precursor (PN-2/APP) can also inhibit factor IXa.[585] Interestingly, an insect salivary protein, Prolixin-S, has been shown to inhibit factor IXa generation and the intrinsic tenase complex formation.[586]

One strategy to improve existing antithrombotic therapies has been to develop factor IXa inhibitors,[587] including the use of monoclonal antibodies that target factor IX/factor IXa[588,589] or aptamers targeting factor IXa.[590,591] Currently, problems exist in using direct thrombin inhibitors to regulate thrombin activity. Targeting the end product of an amplifying cascade results in a narrow window of therapeutic dose, which is difficult to achieve in clinical practice.[592-594] The advantages of regulating events upstream (factor IX/factor IXa; the intrinsic tenase complex) as an approach to antithrombotic therapy would be to potentially produce a partial reduction in the magnitude of thrombin formation.[595,596]

Factor X (Stuart Factor)

The *zymogen factor X*, or *Stuart factor*, is a vitamin K–dependent glycoprotein that is synthesized in the liver.[574,597] It circulates in plasma at a mean concentration of 10 µg/mL or 170 nmol/L and has a $t_{1/2}$ of approximately 1.5 days[508,598,599] (*Table 20.1*). In the Leiden Thrombophilia study, a population-based case control study on venous thrombosis, high levels of factor X alone predicted the risk of thrombosis but were not a risk factor for venous thrombosis when the levels of other vitamin K–dependent proteins were taken into account.[600]

The Normal Hematologic System

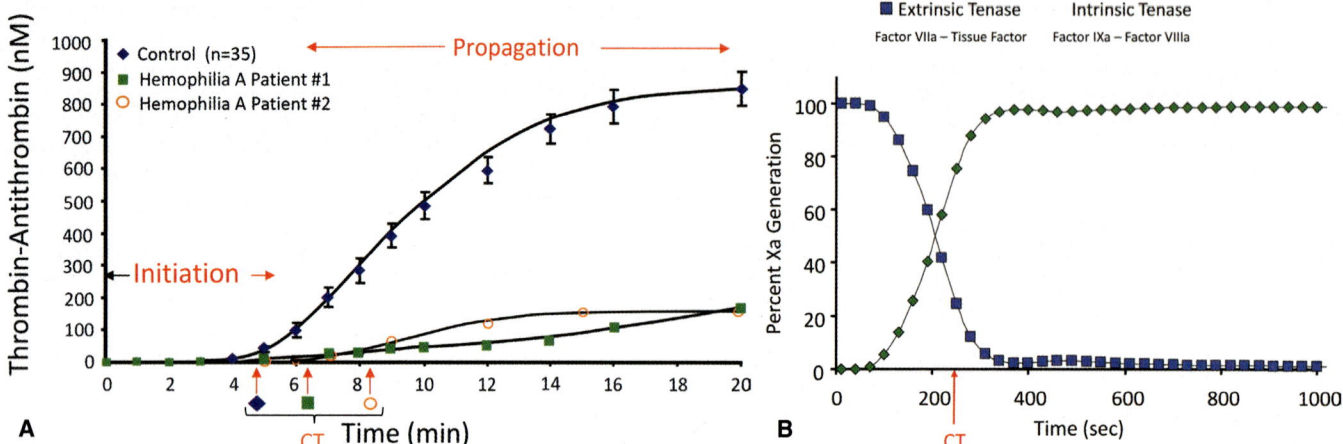

FIGURE 20.8 **Profiles of thrombin and factor Xa generation.** A, Empirical time course (x-axis: 0-20 minutes) of thrombin-antithrombin formation (y-axis: nmol/L thrombin-antithrombin complex) during whole blood coagulation initiated with 5 pmol/L tissue factor.[581] Data represent means plus or minus standard error of the means for 35 individuals; thrombin-antithrombin levels reach maximum levels of 900 nmol/L (blue diamonds) in this group of normal individuals. Clot time (CT) is shown below with the symbols for each curve. Thrombin generation is divided into two phases: an initiation phase and a propagation phase. When two patients with hemophilia A were studied (green squares, red circles), CT was delayed, and the propagation phase of thrombin generation was not present.[460,582] By not having factor VIIIa present, the intrinsic tenase complex is unable to generate the additional factor Xa that is required for the burst or propagation phase of thrombin generation. B, Computer simulation of the time course of factor Xa generation on activation of the factor VIIa–tissue factor pathway.[583] Concentrations are expressed as the relative percentage of factor Xa produced by each catalyst at each time point. The factor Xa that is initially produced is via the extrinsic tenase complex. After CT, the majority of factor Xa generated is via the intrinsic Xase. The clot time represents the time point in the computer simulation at which calculated thrombin levels are comparable with thrombin levels (~10 nmol/L) measured in clotting whole blood (see *Figure 20.13B*).

Factor X deficiency is a rare autosomal recessive disorder with varied phenotype and genotype. Homozygous factor X deficiency has an incidence of 1 in 1 million in the general population.[601,602] Heterozygotes are often clinically asymptomatic, whereas the most severely affected homozygous individuals exhibit extensive bleeding early in life. Multiple factor X deficiency cases have been identified, and the gene defects have been elucidated in individuals with bleeding tendencies[603-609] and in an individual without a bleeding tendency,[610] although mutations within the catalytic domain are not always consistent with the phenotype of the individual.[611] As with most deficiencies, the level of factor X expression is indicative of the bleeding response. When factor X levels are approximately 1%, bleeding can include hemarthrosis, soft tissue hemorrhage, and menorrhagia. With functional levels above 15%, bleeding is infrequent and usually mild. Acquired factor X deficiency is rare and is usually associated with light-chain amyloidosis.[612-614] In amyloidosis, factor X is thought to be adsorbed onto extracellular amyloid fibrils, thereby decreasing the circulating factor X level and increasing bleeding. In these cases, replacement with factor X products is not as effective a therapy for deficiency because it is continuously removed from plasma. Treatment of bleeding from factor X deficiency can involve the administration of fresh frozen plasma or prothrombin complex concentrates. No sure venous or arterial thrombotic event has ever been reported in congenital factor X deficiency.[615]

The importance of factor X generation is illustrated by transgenic mice with a total deficiency of factor X. Homozygous deficiency (−/−) results in partial embryonic lethality with signs of massive bleeding.[467,616] Those mice that survive to term die within 5 to 20 days from fatal neonatal bleeding. The lethality of factor X knockout genotype in mice supports the significance of factor X function in hemostasis.

Gene Structure and Expression

The gene for factor X spans 27 kb, is located on chromosome 13 bands q34, and yields a 1.5-kb mRNA[469,617-619] (*Table 20.2*). The gene for factor X is located near the gene for factor VII. Studies to elucidate the liver-specific expression of factor X have included the characterization of the human[620] and murine factor X promoter.[621] Using a hepatoma cell line that expresses factor X, the first 279 bp of the 5′-flanking sequence upstream of the first AUG proved to be sufficient to confer maximal promoter activity.[620] From mutagenesis studies, two protein-binding sites within the 279-bp fragment were identified that are critical for promoter activity: CCAAT (at −120 to −116) and ACTTTG (at −56 to −51).[620] Factor X also lacks a typical TATA box. In the human factor X promoter, the binding proteins HNF-4 (at −73),[622] nuclear factor-Y (at −128),[622] GATA-4 (GATA element at −96),[623] and the Sp family of transcription factors I footprinted sites (at −165 and −195)[623] have been identified as playing crucial roles in modulating the activity of the proximal promoter of factor X.

Biochemistry

Human factor X is a vitamin K–dependent glycoprotein of molecular weight 59,000 that circulates in plasma (10 μg/mL or 170 nmol/L) as a two-chain molecule composed of a disulfide-linked light chain ($M_r = 16,500$) and heavy chain ($M_r = 42,000$)[624,625] (*Table 20.1*). Its structure contains an NH_2-terminal light chain consisting of a Gla domain (11 Gla residues), with a single β-hydroxy aspartic acid residue and two EGF-like domains (EGF-1 and EGF-2) (*Figure 20.4*). The COOH-terminal heavy chain consists of an activation peptide region and a catalytic (serine protease) domain. Most of the carbohydrate moieties (~15%) are located within the heavy chain[598] in the activation peptide domain.[626] Ca^{2+} binding in the first EGF domain has been proposed to enhance the structural rigidity of the factor X molecule.[422] Numerous structures of factor Xa (des Gla)[392] have been deposited in the Protein Data Bank, the majority of which are bound to inhibitors and have provided insight into specificity and function.[627]

Activation

Factor X is activated to its serine protease form factor Xa through a cleavage of the activation peptide at Arg^{194}-Ile^{195} (Arg^{52}-Ile^{53} of the heavy chain) (*Figure 20.4*). A 52-amino-acid activation peptide is released with a relative molecular mass of 12,000. The resulting catalytic serine protease, factor Xa, has a molecular weight of 48,000 and is composed of a light chain ($M_r = 18,000$) and a disulfide-linked heavy chain ($M_r = 30,000$). The activation of factor X is catalyzed by factor VIIa–tissue factor (the extrinsic tenase complex)[497] and factor IXa–factor VIIIa (the intrinsic tenase complex).[628] In vitro studies have determined that factor X has to be bound to the membrane before activation.[45,629]

Function

The main function of factor Xa is to form the prothrombinase complex (factor Xa–factor Va–membrane–Ca^{2+}) (*Figure 20.5*). Factor Xa is the serine protease enzyme in the prothrombinase complex that catalytically activates prothrombin to thrombin, the key enzyme in blood coagulation. The prothrombinase complex activates prothrombin to thrombin 10^5-fold faster than factor Xa alone.[42] Factor Xa is a unique regulatory enzyme in that it is formed through both the extrinsic tenase and intrinsic tenase complexes (as mentioned in the section on factor IX). During the initial stages of the hemostatic event, low levels of both factor Xa and factor IXa are generated. Once generated, the limited amounts of factor Xa produced by extrinsic tenase bind to available membrane sites and convert picomolar amounts of prothrombin to thrombin[37,630,631] (*Figure 20.8B*). This thrombin then activates factor VIII[632] and factor V,[633] allowing the initial formation of the intrinsic tenase and prothrombinase complexes. Thus, the time period in which factor Xa directly generates picomolar amounts of thrombin is referred to as the *initiation phase of blood coagulation*. The burst or propagation phase of thrombin generation is then obtained from additional factor Xa generated via the intrinsic tenase complex (factor IXa–factor VIIIa–Ca^{2+}–membrane) (*Figure 20.8*). The intrinsic tenase complex activates factor X at a 50- to 100-fold higher rate than the extrinsic tenase complex.[61-63] This burst in factor Xa levels overcomes the levels of factor Xa inhibitors, such as TFPI, and achieves maximal prothrombinase activity and propagation of the procoagulant event.

There is evidence that factor Xa can also trigger intracellular signaling events by increasing endothelial cell cytosolic Ca^{2+} and the release of endothelial cell mitogens.[634] Mitogenic activity toward smooth muscle cells[635] and lymphocytes[636] has also been identified. Both factor X and factor Xa have been shown to provoke PAR-2-dependent protective signaling responses in endothelial cells.[637] An alternative initiation of factor X to factor Xa has been identified on stimulated cells of monocytic and myeloid differentiation involving the specific adhesive receptor Mac-1.[638] A novel factor Xa receptor, effector cell protease receptor-1, has been identified on the surface of a monocytic cell line.[639] A platelet factor Xa receptor has been described as important in mediating prothrombin binding via factor Xa binding to platelet factor Va.[640]

Regulation

Once assembled, the extrinsic tenase (factor VIIa-tissue factor-Ca^{2+}-membrane) is rapidly inactivated along with its product factor Xa through the action of TFPI (*Figure 20.7*). The factor Xa active site associates with the COOH terminus of TFPI[641,642] to localize the TFPI to the membrane. Once localized, the factor Xa–TFPI complex rapidly inactivates tissue factor–factor VIIa, forming a stable quaternary complex, tissue factor–factor VIIa–TFPI–factor Xa. The factor Xa–TFPI complex has been shown to be elevated in patients with cancer.[643]

Factor Xa is also inhibited by antithrombin[644] when not in complex with prothrombinase.[645,646] Its inhibition is enhanced through the use of heparin, which increases the reactivity of antithrombin with its targets (i.e., factor Xa).

Because factor Xa is a major player in the coagulation cascade, it is a target for regulation by synthetic inhibitors in treating ischemic heart disease and cerebrovascular disease. Many studies are currently underway to develop a new class of antithrombotic agents that target factor Xa.[647-653]

Factor II (Prothrombin)

Factor II, or *prothrombin*, is a single-chain vitamin K–dependent zymogen that, when activated, yields factor IIa (thrombin), the key enzyme in blood coagulation. The zymogen prothrombin (M_r = 72,000, 8% carbohydrate) is the most abundant of the vitamin K–dependent proteins and circulates in plasma at a mean concentration of 1.4 μmol/L or 100 μg/mL[654-656] (*Table 20.1*). Prothrombin is primarily synthesized in the liver with a $t_{1/2}$ of approximately 2.5 days. Low levels of prothrombin expression have been identified in other tissues including brain, diaphragm, stomach, kidney, spleen, intestine,

uterine, placental, and adrenal.[657,658] Increased prothrombin levels have been associated with an increased risk of venous thrombosis.

Human prothrombin deficiency, first described by Quick in 1943,[27] is rare because of the autosomal nature of its expression. Prothrombin deficiencies are classified as either hypoprothrombinemia or dysprothrombinemia and occur due to genetic disorders affecting either transcriptional regulation or protein function.[659,660] These disorders are characterized by variable pathologies extending from mild bruising to clinically severe bleeding.[661] Homozygotes are characterized by severe bleeding, and heterozygotes either have mild bleeding or are asymptomatic. Prothrombin complex concentrates have been used for prophylaxis and bleeding episodes in individuals with prothrombin deficiency.[444] The importance of α-thrombin to hemostasis is demonstrated in prothrombin-deficient mice, which experience embryonic and neonatal lethality.[662-664]

Gene Structure and Expression

The 21-kb human prothrombin gene is located on chromosome 11 bands p11.2 and has been extensively studied.[665-668] The prothrombin gene contains 14 exons and 13 introns[666] and is transcribed as a pre-propeptide of 622 amino acids.[667,668] The 43-amino acid propeptide mediates posttranslational processing to generate the mature protein of 579 amino acids. The promoter region of the prothrombin gene lacks a TATA box.

Many studies have been conducted on prothrombin gene polymorphisms to determine their relationships to thrombophilia. One common polymorphism is the G20210A transition in the 3′-untranslated region of the promoter. This mutation has been linked to familial thrombosis. The G20210A polymorphism of the prothrombin gene has been associated with elevated prothrombin levels and an increased risk for venous thrombosis.[669] It is one of the most commonly identified genetic risk factors for thrombosis. An additional polymorphism, A19911G, in the prothrombin gene has been identified that can modulate the risk of the G20210A polymorphism in developing deep vein thrombosis.[670] Several reviews have been written on the influence of genetic polymorphisms (including the prothrombin G20210A) and the laboratory diagnosis of thrombophilia.[671-673]

Biochemistry

Initial observations about the structure/function relationship of the prothrombin molecule came about from the partial primary structures of bovine and human prothrombins. Subsequently, the complete primary structure of human prethrombin 2 (residues 272-579), which is the precursor of thrombin, was determined.[674] Finally, the primary structure for bovine prothrombin[675] and human prothrombin[668] were deduced from isolated cDNAs. The elucidated structure of human prothrombin is characterized by an NH_2-terminal Gla domain (residues 1-40 with 10 Gla residues), followed by two kringle domains (kringle 1, residues 65-143; kringle 2, residues 170-248) and the serine protease precursor domain (residues 272-579). Human prothrombin has three N-linked sugar chains—two in the first kringle domain and one in the catalytic domain.[676,677]

The first x-ray crystal structure of a blood coagulation protein fragment, bovine prothrombin kringle 1, was determined in Tulinsky's laboratory in 1986.[385] Kringles have been identified as common motifs in many plasma proteins, including prothrombin, plasminogen, t-PA, urokinase, factor XII, and apolipoprotein A.[677,678] The kringle 1 domain contains four cysteine residues participating in two disulfide bonds. The role of the kringle 1 domain of prothrombin is still unclear, but it has been suggested that it is involved with the interaction of prothrombin and factor Va in the prothrombinase complex.[679,680] The NH_2-terminal Gla domain and the first kringle domain together are referred to as *prothrombin fragment 1*. The kringle 2 domain of human prothrombin, located in prothrombin fragment 2 (residues 156-271), is similar in sequence and presumably in structure. The kringle 2 domain also binds Ca^{2+} and appears to be the primary region in prothrombin that mediates the interaction of the prothrombin molecule with factor Va in the prothrombinase complex.[681,682] This latter interaction has been suggested to initiate conformational changes that make reaction sites accessible for enzymatic cleavage of prothrombin.[683] The sequence of the enzyme α-thrombin is contained within prethrombin 2 (residues 272-579).

Activation

Prothrombin is activated to the procoagulant α-thrombin by two cleavages: one at Arg[271]-Thr[272] and another at Arg[320]-Ile[321] by the prothrombinase complex (factor Xa–factor Va–phospholipid membrane–Ca[2+]) (*Figure 20.4*). Membrane-bound factor Va serves as the receptor for factor Xa, the catalytic serine protease. The rate of α-thrombin generation by prothrombinase is 3×10^5-fold faster than the rate for factor Xa alone at potential physiologic concentrations of the proteins.[42] Recent studies have indicated that the order of these two cleavages differs depending on the cell surface upon which prothrombinase is assembled.[684,685]

On synthetic phospholipid vesicles, the activation of prothrombin by prothrombinase proceeds through an initial cleavage of prothrombin at Arg([320])-Ile([321]), giving rise to meizothrombin, a two-chain disulfide-linked molecule (*Figure 20.9*; pathway A, cleavage at 1).[686] The probable mechanism involves meizothrombin dissociating from prothrombinase with a subsequent rebinding step and conversion to α-thrombin.[686,687] Meizothrombin expresses some of the activities of α-thrombin. However, meizothrombin has impaired fibrinogen clotting ability compared with α-thrombin.[688] Meizothrombin is subsequently cleaved at Arg([271])-Thr([272]) (*Figure 20.9*; pathway A, cleavage at 2), yielding the NH$_2$-terminal half of the molecule, consisting of the Gla domain and two kringle domains (prothrombin fragment 1.2: residues 1-271) and α-thrombin. α-Thrombin consists of an NH$_2$-terminal 49-residue A-chain (residues 272-320) disulfide-linked to a COOH-terminal 259-residue B-chain (residues 321-579) containing the catalytic triad.

An alternative cleavage pathway occurs when factor Xa alone acts on prothrombin or when prothrombinase is assembled on washed platelets.[684] In the presence of factor Xa, Ca[2+], and an appropriate membrane surface, the initial cleavage occurs at Arg[271]-Thr[272] and gives rise to prothrombin fragment 1.2 and prethrombin 2 (*Figure 20.9*; pathway B, cleavage at 2). Cleavage at Arg[320] in prethrombin 2 (*Figure 20.9*; pathway B, cleavage at 2) yields α-thrombin. In contrast to the meizothrombin pathway, the prethrombin 2 intermediate appears not to dissociate from prothrombinase.[689] Prothrombin fragment 1.2 remains noncovalently associated with α-thrombin. In vitro, α-thrombin is associated ($K_d = 10$ nmol/L) with prothrombin fragment 2,[690] the latter's precursor prothrombin fragment 1.2, or both.[691] In contrast to other vitamin K–dependent proteins, the phospholipid-binding region is no longer covalently attached to the serine protease domain after prothrombin conversion to thrombin.

Thrombin and meizothrombin catalyze cleavage at Arg[155] of prothrombin, yielding a truncated molecule called *prethrombin 1* (residues 156-579) that lacks the Gla domain. Thrombin can also cleave at Arg[284], yielding a truncated α-thrombin species (residues 284-579), which is the form of thrombin found in commercial preparations.

The membrane surface that supports the prothrombinase complex in vivo has traditionally been assumed to be primarily provided by platelets, but it can also be provided by other circulating blood cells, such as monocytes and lymphocytes, and by vascular endothelial cells.[692] Since prothrombin activation on platelets proceeds through the prothrombin 2 pathway and meizothrombin formation has been observed in clotting blood,[685,693] it appears that prothrombin activation in blood involves both pathways. Prothrombin activation through the meizothrombin pathway has been reported to occur on the subpopulation of red blood cells that express phosphatidylserine on their surface.[685]

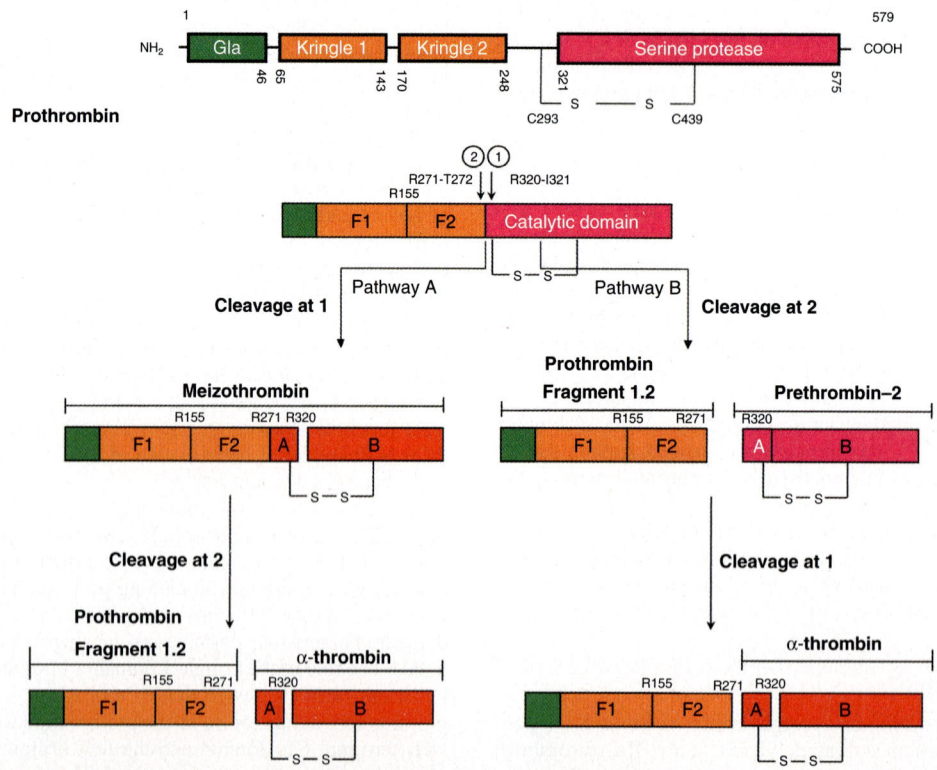

FIGURE 20.9 **Schematic representation of the pathways for prothrombin activation.** The generation of α-thrombin from its zymogen precursor prothrombin, by factor Xa involves the cleavage of two peptide bonds. The reaction begins either via step 1 (cleavage at R320-I321) or step 2 (cleavage at R271-T272). Cleavage at 1 (R320), pathway A, produces meizothrombin. Meizothrombin is composed of a prothrombin fragment consisting of fragment 1 (F1, residues 1-155: Gla domain + kringle 1), fragment 2 (F2, residues 156-271: kringle 2), and residues 272 to 320 (A-chain) linked by a disulfide bond to the catalytic domain (B-chain). Subsequent cleavage at R271 (cleavage at 2, pathway A) generates prothrombin fragment 1.2 (F1 and F2) and the disulfide-linked heterodimer α-thrombin (A- and B-chains). In pathway B cleavage occurs first at 2 (R271), generating prothrombin fragment 1.2 (F1 and F2) and prethrombin-2. Subsequent cleavage at R320 produces the A- and B-chains of α-thrombin.

Function

α-Thrombin can be considered the central enzyme in blood coagulation in that it contributes to reactions at all levels, allowing for the overall maintenance of vascular fidelity. Its main role is in stemming blood loss through fibrin clot formation.[694] The series of events that leads up to and occurs after fibrin formation also involves protein activation by α-thrombin. This includes activation of platelets,[695] factor VII,[8] factor V,[696] factor VIII,[697] factor XI,[7] and factor XIII.[17] α-Thrombin activity also extends from the procoagulant process to anticoagulation and suppression of fibrinolytic reactions. For example, α-thrombin-thrombomodulin activates the anticoagulant protein, protein C,[698] and the antifibrinolytic protein, TAFI.[36]

Relatively minute concentrations of thrombin are generated during the initiation phase of blood coagulation, primarily due to the factor Xa generated from the extrinsic tenase complex (*Figure 20.8*). These levels of thrombin, in the range of 0.5 to 2.0 nmol/L, have been shown to be sufficient for the initiation of rapid activation of platelets, factor XIII and factor V, and fibrin formation in an ex vivo whole blood model.[581] All of these processes occur before the major burst of thrombin generation during the propagation phase of the reaction.

α-Thrombin's role continues into the tissue repair and remodeling phase that is necessary to regenerate damaged vascular tissue. α-Thrombin is a potent mitogen[699,700] and stimulates cell division in macrophages,[701] smooth muscle cells,[702] and endothelial cells.[703] α-Thrombin also appears to be involved in the growth and metastasis of tumors by promoting angiogenesis,[704,705] possibly through vascular endothelial growth factor.[706] The roles that thrombin plays in coagulation and beyond are outlined in a recent review.[707]

Regulation

In vivo, the activity of the prothrombinase complex has to be tightly regulated to ensure that adequate but limited levels of α-thrombin are generated. If too much α-thrombin is continuously generated, localized clot formation can lead to occlusion or systemic thrombosis. Equally, if too little α-thrombin is generated, hemorrhagic conditions result. Two reaction systems, one covalent and one proteolytic, regulate α-thrombin generation. Antithrombin-heparin (or heparan sulfate) is a potent inhibitor of blood coagulation and inhibits both α-thrombin and factor Xa via covalent interactions.[708,709] α-Thrombin also participates in its own downregulation by binding to thrombomodulin on the vascular cell surface and converting protein C to APC. This anticoagulant serine protease then cleaves factors Va and VIIIa. These cofactors for the vitamin K–dependent complexes are no longer available for ongoing reactions, thereby eliminating α-thrombin generation. In ex vivo models of blood coagulation, prothrombin levels and antithrombin appear to have the most significant impact on α-thrombin generation.[710] Increased levels of antithrombin reduce α-thrombin generation by inhibiting α-thrombin activity and preventing positive feedback.[710] Decreased levels of antithrombin allow for higher levels of prothrombin activation and prolongation of α-thrombin generation.[710]

PROCOAGULANT PROTEINS: PROCOAGULANT COFACTOR PROTEINS

There are two categories of cofactor proteins: the plasma-derived soluble procoagulant procofactors factors V and VIII (and their circulating carrier von Willebrand factor [vWF]) and the cell-associated coagulation cofactor, tissue factor. Factors V and VIII are highly homologous (40% identity), sharing many structural and functional similarities. Tissue factor is a single-chain transmembrane protein that is composed of extracellular, transmembrane, and cytoplasmic domains.

Tissue Factor (Tissue Thromboplastin, CD142, Coagulation Factor III)

Tissue factor, also known as *tissue thromboplastin, CD142,* and *coagulation factor III*, is a transmembrane protein that functions as a nonenzymatic cofactor for factor VIIa in the extrinsic tenase complex. In the absence of injury or stimulus, tissue factor is not ordinarily expressed on cellular surfaces in direct contact with circulating blood.

Presentation of tissue factor to the circulation is the event that triggers the procoagulant primary pathway of coagulation (*Figure 20.1*). There are no known mutations or deficiencies of human tissue factor, leading to the speculation that tissue factor is essential for life. In mice, inactivation of the tissue factor gene to create homozygous tissue factor–null mice proves to be lethal during embryonic development.[711-714]

Gene Structure and Expression

The tissue factor gene is located on chromosome 1p21.3[715,716] and spans 12.4 kb (*Table 20.2*). The gene contains five introns and six exons.[717] Tissue factor expression can be induced in a number of cultured cell types. Fibroblasts express tissue factor on exposure to serum or mitogenic cytokines,[718,719] as do vascular smooth muscle cells and keratinocytes.[720,721] Monocytic cells and monocytes isolated from peripheral blood also express tissue factor when stimulated by bacterial endotoxin or other proinflammatory agents.[720,721] The presence of these cells may be associated with DIC.[722] In vitro, certain leukemic cell lines constitutively express low levels of tissue factor.[723-725] Tissue factor expression by circulating, nonvascular cells and microparticles/microvesicles plays key roles in cancer, sepsis, and perhaps atherosclerotic plaque formation.[56,726-733] However, tissue factor in the subendothelial cell layer is proposed to trigger coagulation on exposure to the circulation. Cultured vascular endothelial cells express tissue factor on stimulation by IL-1, tumor necrosis factor (TNF)-α, and bacterial endotoxin.[720,721] In vivo, there is little or no detectable tissue factor expression on unstimulated endothelial cells. Certain conditions such as sepsis, placental villitis, and graft rejection induce tissue factor expression on endothelial cells in vivo.[722,734-736] The mechanism governing tissue factor expression under nonpathologic conditions is presently unknown. Studies of transcriptional control of tissue factor expression in various cell lines have demonstrated that Sp1 sites are important in basal transcription of the tissue factor gene. EGR-1, activation peptide-1, and NF-kb sites mediate tissue factor expression in response to pathologic stimulation.[713,737-741]

Biochemistry

Tissue factor is a single-chain glycoprotein ($M_r = 44,000$)[742] of 261 or 263 amino acids (*Table 20.1*). It is synthesized with a signal peptide of 32 amino acids. The variability in protein size is due to heterogeneity at the NH_2 terminus.[715,743,744] Tissue factor is a member of the class 2 cytokine receptor superfamily[745] and a type I integral membrane protein. The type I designation refers to the location of the NH_2 and COOH termini. The NH_2 terminus of tissue factor (residues 1-219) is extracellular, whereas the COOH terminus of the protein is intracellular (residues 243-263). Tissue factor also contains a hydrophobic membrane-spanning domain (residues 220-242) (*Figure 20.10*). This domain appears to function solely to anchor tissue factor in the membrane.[749] The NH_2-terminal domain of tissue factor is composed of two fibronectin type III domains and is glycosylated at Asn^{11}, Asn^{124}, and Asn^{137}.[750] X-ray crystal structures of tissue factor show that the two fibronectin type III domains are joined at an angle of approximately 120°.[746,751-755] There are two disulfide bonds (Cys^{49}-Cys^{57} and Cys^{186}-Cys^{209}) in the extracellular region of which the second exists in a RHStaple configuration (characteristic of allosteric disulfides).[756,757] This disulfide is responsible for the cryptic (reduced) and procoagulant (oxidized) forms of tissue factor discussed in the literature.[758-761] A role for glycosylation remains controversial[747,750,762,763] while other posttranslational modifications[764,765] play important roles in modulating tissue factor biological activities. The COOH-terminal cytoplasmic domain is quite short and contains a single cysteine residue (Cys^{245}) that is linked to a palmitate or stearate fatty acyl chain via a thioester bond.[756] The COOH terminus also contains a serine that may be phosphorylated.[766] The function of the COOH terminus and the importance of these two modifications are not clear, as deletion of this domain has no significant effect on tissue factor procoagulant activity.[749]

Function

The nonenzymatic cofactor tissue factor can bind either factor VII or factor VIIa in a Ca^{2+}-dependent manner and form a high-affinity

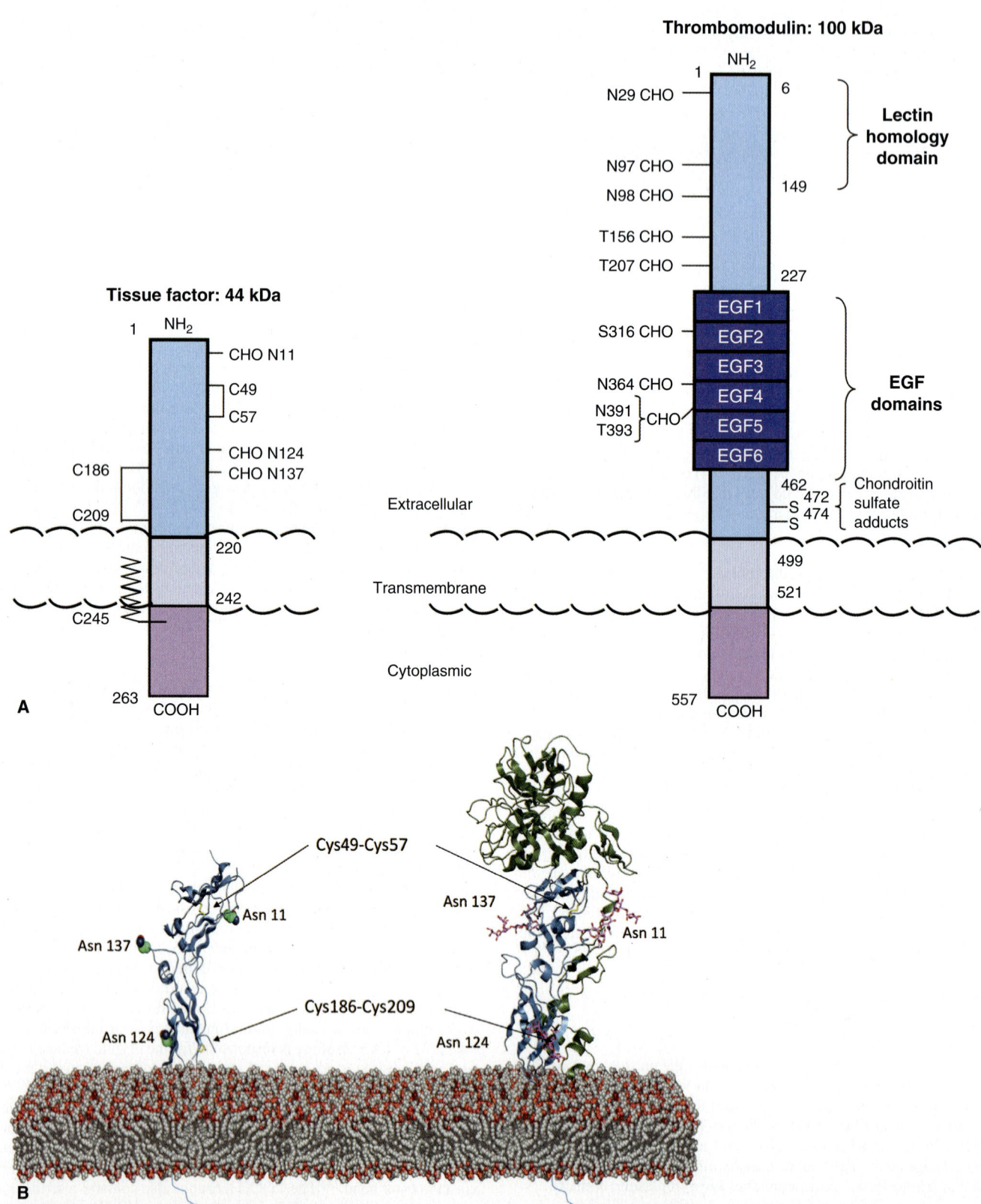

FIGURE 20.10 **Transmembrane cofactors.** A, Schematics of tissue factor and thrombomodulin. Tissue factor is composed of an extracellular domain (residues 1-219), a transmembrane domain (residues 220-242), and a cytoplasmic domain (residues 243-263). Two disulfide bonds (S-S) and the sites of the three carbohydrate moieties (CHO) are identified by amino acid residue. One cysteine (C245) contains a thiol ester linkage to a fatty acid. Tissue factor is the cofactor for factor VIIa in the extrinsic tenase complex and is exposed on the subendothelial surface after injury. Thrombomodulin is an endothelial cell-surface glycoprotein composed of five distinct domains. The domain structures include a lectin-like domain (residues 6-149), a domain containing six epidermal growth factor (EGF)-like regions (residues 227-462), a small extracellular domain rich in threonine and serine residues (two residues, S472 and S474, have been identified as sites of chondroitin sulfate adducts), a membrane-spanning region (residues 499-521), and a cytoplasmic tail (residues 522-557). There are nine known glycosylation sites (CHO) on the thrombomodulin molecule. Thrombomodulin functions as the cofactor in the protein Case complex and assists in the generation of activated protein C. B, Structural ribbon diagram of tissue factor (blue) (PDB: 2HFT)[746] and tissue factor and factor VIIa (green) (PDB: 1DAN).[485] The tissue factor carbohydrate side chains have been added to the structure.[747,748]

1:1 complex. Once bound to tissue factor, the zymogen factor VII is rapidly converted to an active enzyme via limited proteolysis.[767] The tissue factor–factor VIIa, or extrinsic tenase complex, activates factors IX and X. When tissue factor is exposed or expressed, or both, subsequent to vascular perturbation, low levels of circulating factor VIIa bind to tissue factor and the extrinsic tenase triggers the procoagulant cascade. Factor VII bound to tissue factor is converted to factor VIIa, augmenting factors IXa and Xa generation. The primary role of the complex is to provide factor IXa and low levels of factor Xa, which serve to promote factor IXa production[61-63,501] and to directly catalyze the conversion of trace amounts of prothrombin to thrombin.

In the absence of tissue factor, factor VIIa is relatively inert. Once bound to tissue factor, the catalytic activity of factor VIIa is increased 20- to 100-fold with low-molecular-weight substrates[490,768-770] and approximately 10^4-fold with its macromolecular substrates factors X and IX.[768,770,771] Tissue factor alters the active site of factor VIIa, thus functioning as an allosteric activator of the enzyme.

Although the cofactor is necessary for enzymatic activity, complex formation between tissue factor and factor VIIa does not share the same requirements for an anionic phospholipid membrane surface as the other procoagulant complexes. The membrane dependency of the extrinsic tenase complex arises from membrane-mediated substrate delivery. Both factors X and IX bind to anionic membrane surfaces for efficient two-dimensional transfer to the extrinsic tenase.

An additional role for tissue factor–factor VIIa beyond its activation of the coagulation cascade involves triggering signaling through the G protein–coupled, protease-activated receptor 2, which is relevant to inflammation and angiogenesis.[758,772]

Regulation

Tissue factor activity is mainly regulated by controlling its presentation. The commonly accepted source of functional tissue factor is through exposure of the subendothelium on vascular damage, although its presentation on microparticles/microvesicles is strongly linked with pathologies.[773-777] Tissue factor function is under the control of an allosteric disulfide bond.[757-761,778] Once the tissue factor–factor VIIa complex is formed in the vicinity of an injury, the extrinsic tenase activity is then modulated by TFPI and antithrombin reduction of enzymatic activity.

Factor VIII (Antihemophilic Factor, Factor VIII:Antigen, Factor VIII:Coagulant)

Factor VIII, or *antihemophilic factor*, is a nonenzymatic procofactor that circulates in plasma in complex with the large multimeric protein vWF. Initially, factor VIII and vWF were thought to be a single entity, and early reports on factor VIII were actually measuring facets of vWF structure and function. The factor VIII protein is designated as *factor VIII:Ag* (antigen; VIII:Ag is vWF), and its procoagulant function is designated *factor VIII:C* (coagulant).[779] Factor VIII circulates at an average concentration of 0.2 μg/mL (0.7 nmol/L; *Table 20.1*). The ratio of factor VIII to vWF is fairly constant and in the range of 1 molecule of factor VIII to 50 to 100 molecules of vWF monomeric units.[780,781] vWF acts to regulate the plasma concentration of factor VIII. Desmopressin (1-Deamino-8-D-arginine vasopressin) administration elicits an increase in the plasma concentration of vWF and, in turn, increases the plasma level of factor VIII.[782] vWF also stabilizes factor VIII in plasma. Factor VIII in complex with vWF has a plasma $t_{1/2}$ of approximately 12 hours, whereas factor VIII alone undergoes rapid clearance and has a $t_{1/2}$ of approximately 2 hours.[783-786] Deficiency of factor VIII, or hemophilia A, is a well-characterized bleeding disorder linked to the X chromosome. Hemophilia A, therefore, occurs almost exclusively in males and occurs at a frequency of 1:5000 to 1:10,000 males. Females with one abnormal factor VIII gene are unaffected carriers. The severity of bleeding in patients with hemophilia A is correlated with the level of functional factor VIII in plasma.[787,788] Approximately 50% to 60% of hemophilia A cases are severe, with factor VIII coagulant activity <1% of normal. Severe hemophilia A is manifested in frequent episodes of spontaneous bleeding into joints, muscles, and internal organs. Factor VIII coagulant

activity in the range of 1% to 5% of normal (25%-30% of patients) results in moderate hemophilia A. In the moderate form, abnormal bleeding is generally linked to any trauma, including minor injury. The remaining patients have 6% to 30% of normal factor VIII activity and exhibit mild hemophilia A. In the mild form, factor VIII deficiency results in bleeding events only subsequent to significant trauma or surgery.[789]

Gene Structure and Expression

The factor VIII gene has been mapped to the long arm of the X chromosome in band q28.[790-794] The factor VIII gene is 186 kb in length and contains 25 introns and 26 exons.[9,792,795] The liver and spleen are thought to be the primary sites of factor VIII biosynthesis,[796-802] although factor VIII mRNA has been detected in other cell types as well.[802]

Biochemistry

Human factor VIII has a relative molecular weight in the range of 280,000 (*Table 20.1*). The heterogeneity in molecular weight is due to proteolysis of the protein in circulation, processing,[8] or both. It is a glycoprotein of 2351 amino acids that is synthesized as a precursor molecule with a 19-amino-acid signal peptide.[9,803] The sequence of factor VIII is highly homologous to that of factor V.[804] The procofactors factors VIII and V are organized into discrete structural domains. The NH2-terminal heavy chains of both proteins contain the A1 and A2 domains (*Figure 20.11*). The COOH-terminal light chains contain the A3, C1, and C2 domains. The heavy and light chains are separated by the B domain. The three A domains of factor VIII are homologous to each other and to the A domains of factor V and ceruloplasmin.[803,804,806,807] The two C domains of factor VIII are homologous to each other and to the C domains of factor V. The C domains are also homologous to milk fat globule protein and the A-, C-, and D-chains of discoidin 1.[808,809] The B domain of factor VIII is not homologous to the factor V B domain, nor do the B domains of either protein share homology with any known proteins.

The factor VIII molecule is secreted as a two-chain heterodimer as a result of intracellular proteolysis at the B-A3 junction (Arg[1649]). Additional cleavages within the B-chain yield A1-A2-B fragments that are variable in length.[810-813] The B domain (residues 741-1649) contains 19 of the 25 potential N-linked glycosylation sites in factor VIII and is highly glycosylated. The murine factor VIII B-chain is also heavily glycosylated, suggesting that glycosylation of the B-chain may be important for protein expression or function, or both.[813] The B domains of factors VIII and V are excised during activation of the proteins to generate the cofactor molecules factors VIIIa and Va.

Factor VIII shares homology with the copper ion (Cu+)-binding protein ceruloplasmin and contains a Cu+-binding site in the A1 domain.[814,815] This site is important for protein function. A similar Cu+-binding site in the A3 domain does not appear to play a role in protein function.

Factor VIII also contains binding sites for vWF, anionic phospholipids, factor IXa, and, potentially, factor X. Factor VIII interaction with vWF requires the NH2 and COOH termini of the factor VIII light chain (A3, C1, and C2 domains), although a specific vWF-binding site has been identified at residues 1673 to 1684 on the light chain.[780,816-818] The vWF-binding site is removed from the factor VIII protein by α-thrombin cleavage at Arg[1689]. A phospholipid-binding region has been identified on the factor VIII C2 domain between residues 2303 to 2332,[819] although both the C1 and C2 domains are important in binding to a phospholipid surface.[820] High-affinity factor IXa binding is mediated by the light chain of the factor VIII molecule. The A3 domain contains a high-affinity site for factor IXa localized at residues Glu[1811] to Lys[1818].[821,822] Residues 552 to 565 in the A2 domain of the factor VIII heavy chain may also play a role in factor VIII interaction with factor IXa.[823-825] Mutations within this region have been documented in the hemophilia A mutation database.[826] Specifically, Ser558Phe, Val559Ala, Asp560Ala, and Gln565Arg have been described as CRM+ with defective activity resulting in mild hemophilia A. These residues have been shown to be essential for the catalytic efficiency of the factor VIIIa–factor IXa complex while not affecting the binding affinity between the two species.[827] X-ray crystal structures of factor VIII are now available[806,828] as well as cryo-electron microscopy structures of factor VIII interacting with a membrane surface.[829,830] Homology modeling using these and other structures have generated models of the intrinsic tenase complex.[831,832] The factor IXa-binding sites in the A2 and A3 domains are likely located in close proximity on the same side of the factor VIIIa molecule.[833,834] A factor X–binding site may exist on the COOH terminus of the factor VIII A1 domain.[835,836]

Factor VIII also contains several tyrosine residues modified by the addition of sulfate.[837] The tyrosine sulfate residues enhance α-thrombin cleavage of the procofactor.[838] In addition, factor VIII contains biantennary complex-type sugar chains with blood group A or H, or both, determinants.[839]

Function

The procofactor factor VIII is activated by α-thrombin to generate the cofactor factor VIIIa. Activation by α-thrombin involves cleavages at Arg[372] (the A1-A2 junction), Arg[740] (the A2-B junction), and Arg[1689] in the light chain (*Figure 20.11*). The resulting molecule contains three separate polypeptide chains: a light-chain region (A3-C1-C2) bound to the NH_2 region of the heavy chain (A1) in a Ca^{2+}-dependent manner and the noncovalently associated A2 region of the heavy chain. Once formed, the cofactor factor VIIIa binds its serine protease enzyme factor IXa to form the Ca^{2+}- and membrane-dependent complex, the intrinsic tenase (*Figure 20.5*). This complex is homologous to the prothrombinase complex. The intrinsic tenase complex catalyzes factor X conversion to factor Xa at a rate several orders of magnitude greater than the enzyme factor IXa alone.[840,841] Factor Xa generated via the intrinsic tenase complex (factor IXa–factor VIIIa–Ca^{2+}–membrane) yields the propagation phase of α-thrombin generation by raising the factor Xa concentration approximately 100-fold over that achieved by the extrinsic tenase complex (*Figure 20.8B*).[583] Without formation of the intrinsic complex, as occurs in a situation like that of hemophilia A or B, factor Xa is not generated at a level sufficient to produce the propagation phase of α-thrombin generation (*Figure 20.8A*).[460,581,582]

Like the prothrombinase complex, the cofactor (factor VIIIa) interaction with the enzyme (factor IXa) in the presence of divalent cations and an anionic phospholipid surface is a high-affinity interaction with a K_d of 2 nmol/L. The interaction of factor IXa with phospholipid in the absence of its cofactor is of approximately 100-fold lower affinity.[841,842] Binding of factor IXa, factor VIII, or factor X (substrate) to the resting platelet is negligible[843-845]; however, on the activated platelet approximately 600 sites/platelet exist for factor IXa ($K_d \sim$ 2.5 nmol/L alone converting to 0.5 nmol/L in the presence of factor VIIIa and factor X[846]) and 1000 high-affinity sites/platelet appear for factor VIIIa ($K_d \sim$ 0.8 nmol/L) and factor X ($K_d \sim$ 5-10 nmol/L).[847]

Regulation

Factor VIIIa function is primarily regulated by dissociation of a fragment (residues 373-740) containing the A2 subunit from the heterotrimer. Once the A2 subunit is displaced, factor VIIIa loses all cofactor function. Dissociation is spontaneous and occurs rapidly under physiologic conditions. Factor IXa stabilizes factor VIIIa, delaying dissociation of the heterotrimer and prolonging the transient activity of factor VIIIa.[848,849] Factor VIIIa is also regulated by limited proteolysis. Factor IXa cleaves the factor VIIIa A1 subunit at Arg[336] and eliminates factor VIIIa function.[849-851] In addition to factor IXa, the A1 subunit of factor VIIIa is cleaved by factor Xa and α-thrombin.[11,837,849,852] APC is a key anticoagulant enzyme that likewise cleaves the A1 subunit at Arg[336]. APC also cleaves the factor VIIIa A2 subunit at Arg.[11,570,853] The APC cleavages occur sequentially with the A1 cleavage first and the A2 cleavage second.[854] Factor IXa protects factor VIIIa from APC cleavage at Arg[562]; however, protein S blocks the protective effect.[855] Although factor VIIIa is proteolytically inactivated by a number of enzymes, spontaneous dissociation is the key regulator of cofactor function.

Factor V (Labile Factor)

Factor V was first recognized as an unstable plasma component necessary for the generation of α-thrombin.[27] *Factor V* is a large single-chain glycoprotein that circulates in plasma at an average concentration of 6.6 μg/mL (20 nmol/L) (*Table 20.1*). Factor V is also contained in the α-granules of human platelets, with approximately 18% to 25% of the total factor V present in platelets.[856] The identification, role in coagulation, and overall importance of factor V in hemostasis has been discussed in recent reviews.[857-860]

Congenital factor V deficiency, or *parahemophilia*, is an extremely rare disorder inherited in an autosomal recessive manner. Patients can exhibit severe bleeding diatheses. Although complete lack of factor V in humans does not appear to be lethal, factor V–deficient mice experience fatal hemorrhage in utero.[861] Combined deficiencies of factors V and VIII have also been observed. Interestingly, combined cofactor deficiencies occur more commonly than factor V deficiency alone.[862,863] The gene for ERGIC-53, a calcium-dependent lectin that serves as a glycoprotein-sorting receptor between the endoplasmic reticulum and the Golgi complex, has been linked to combined factors V and VIII deficiency.[864,865] Mutations in this gene in patients with combined hemophilia have been described. Factor V deficiency becomes even more complex when platelet factor V is taken into consideration. Patients have been identified with normal functional levels of plasma factor V, but deficiencies of platelet factor V that result in bleeding disorders.[856,866-868] Lack of platelet α-granules and their contents in storage pool disorders leads to deficiency of platelet factor V.[866,867] Factor V^Quebec is an autosomal dominant bleeding disorder characterized by mild thrombocytopenia, normal levels of plasma factor V, and degraded platelet factor V with very low activity.[856,868] The LOVD (Leiden Open Variation Database, https://www.lovd.nl/3.0/home) includes a factor V mutation database as well as information on many other coagulation linked genes.[869]

Gene Structure and Expression

The human factor V gene is located on chromosome 1 bands q24.2[870] (*Table 20.2*). The gene spans approximately 80 kb and consists of 24 introns and 25 exons. Transcription and processing yield an mRNA species of 6.8 kb. The intron-exon structure of the factors V and VIII genes are quite similar, and the genes likely evolved from a common ancestor. The liver appears to be the primary site of factor V biosynthesis.[804,871,872] While human megakaryocytes express factor V,[873-875] platelet factor V is modified after endocytosis from circulating liver-derived plasma factor V.[876-880] Bovine aortic endothelial cells[881] and vascular smooth muscle cells[882] also have been reported to express factor V.

Biochemistry

Human factor V (M_r 330,000)[883-886] is a single-chain glycoprotein of 2196 amino acids derived from a precursor molecule with a signal peptide (*Table 20.1* and *Figure 20.11*). Factor V consists of an NH_2-terminal heavy chain (residues 1-709: A1-A2 domains), a central B domain (residues 710-1545), and a COOH-terminal light chain (residues 1546-2196: A3-C1-C2 domains). The A domains are homologous to those found in factor VIII and plasma ceruloplasmin; the C domains are homologous to the slime mold protein discoidin.[804] Like factor VIII and ceruloplasmin, factor V is also a copper-binding protein.[887]

Factor V undergoes extensive posttranslational modification, including phosphorylation, sulfation, glycosylation, and formation of mixed disulfides between its five free cysteine residues and circulating thiols like cysteine and homocysteine.[888] Phosphorylation occurs at sites in the heavy chain, B region, and light chain. Phosphorylation at Ser[692] affects the rate of inactivation of factor Va by APC.[889] Factor V is sulfated at a number of sites in the heavy chain (Tyr[665], Tyr[696], and Tyr[698]), the B region (Tyr[1494], Tyr[1510], and Tyr[1515]), and the light chain (Tyr[1565]). The sulfation status of factor V has been related to its function.[890,891] Carbohydrate accounts for 13% to 25% of the mass of factor V.[892] The heavy chain has nine potential N-linked glycosylation sites. In the B region, 25 asparagine residues are candidates for

Factor VIII: 280 kDa

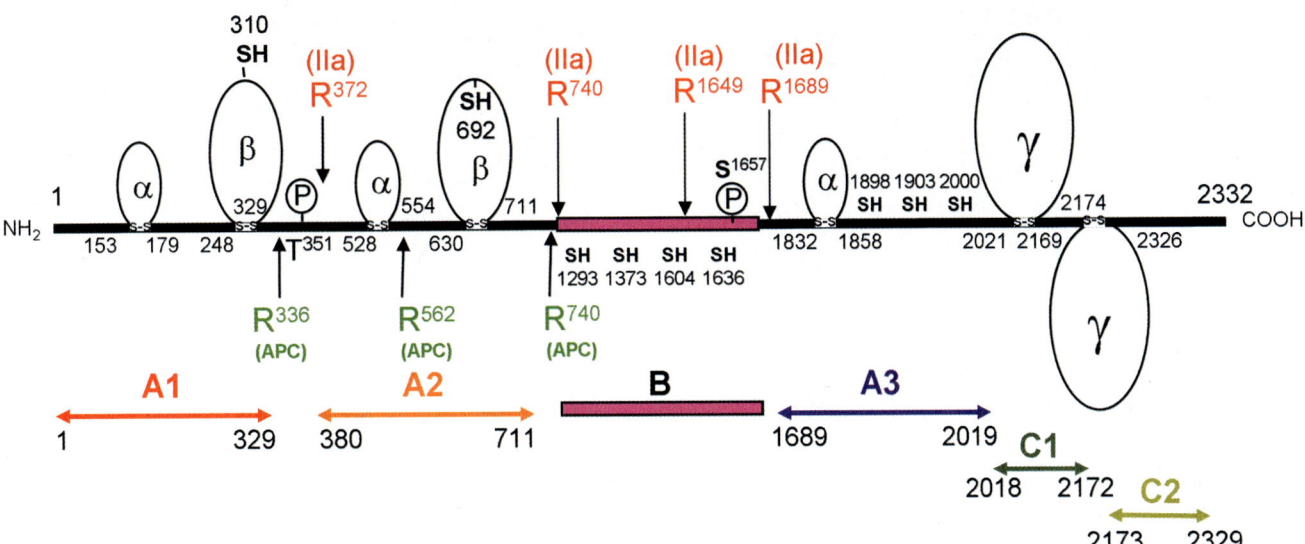

Factor V: 330 kDa

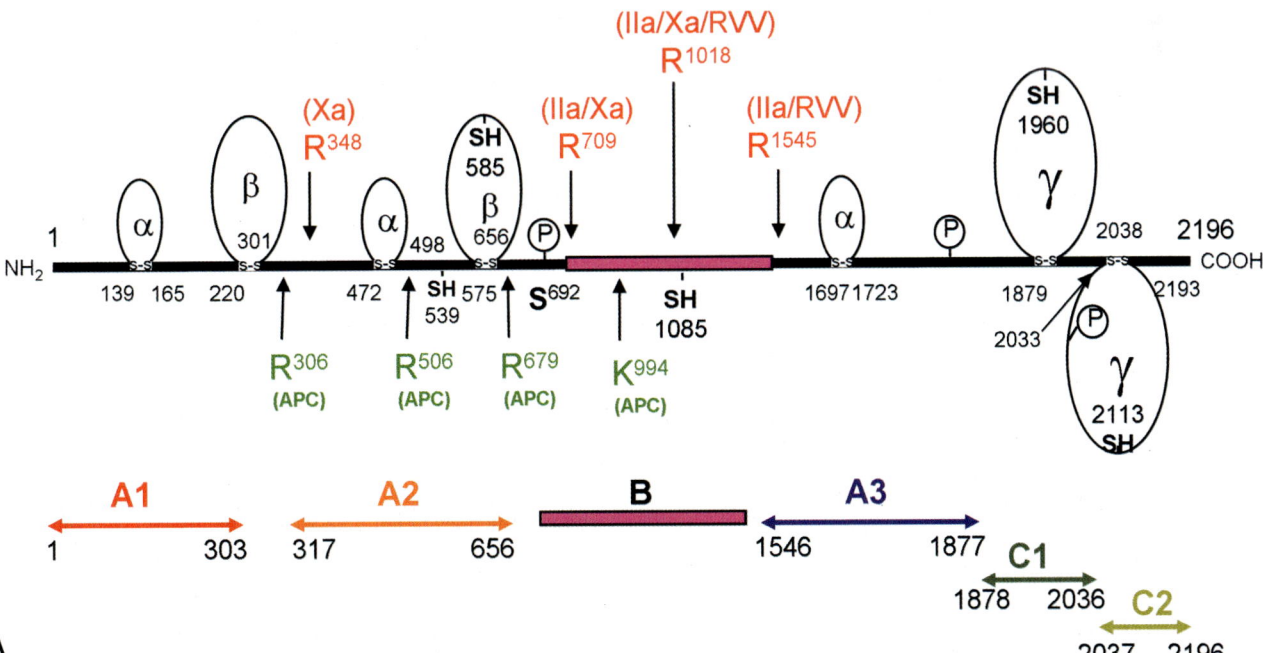

FIGURE 20.11 Soluble procofactors. A, Domain structures of the soluble procofactors factor VIII and factor V. The disulfide loop structures of factor VIII and factor V defining the α, ß, and γ loops are illustrated as bubbles. α-Thrombin (IIa), activated protein C (APC), factor Xa, and Russell viper venom (RVV) cleavage sites are shown with vertical arrows. The linear domain structures (A1-A2-A3-C1-C2) are illustrated with horizontal arrows bracketed by the beginning and ending amino acid number. The B regions (factor V, residues 710-1545; factor VIII, residues 741-1649) are represented by the crosshatched regions. Phosphorylation sites are illustrated by a P inscribed in a circle and the phosphoamino acid, serine (S) or threonine (T), illustrated above or below it. Free cysteine thiols are represented by SH and identified by residue number. B, Crystal structures. Bovine factor Va des-A2 (PDB: 1SDD)[805] and human factor VIIIa (PDB: 2R7E).[806]

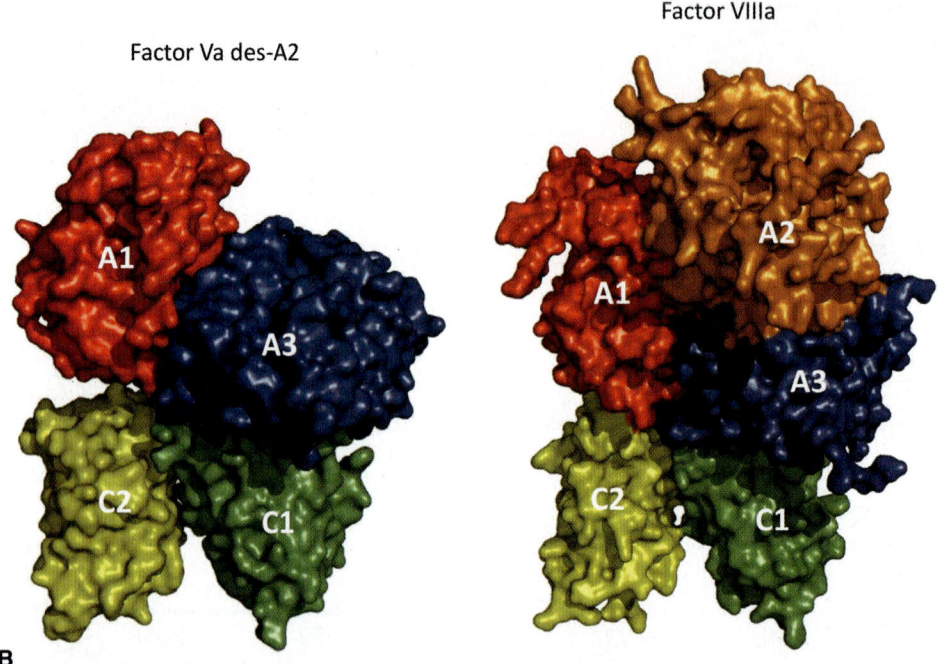

FIGURE 20.11 Continued

modification with carbohydrate; carbohydrate accounts for approximately 50% of the mass of the B region. The light chain of factor V has three N-linked glycosylation sites. Differential glycosylation of Asn[2182] in the C2 domain is reported to be responsible for the factor V1 and factor V2 variants observed in plasma. The two variants have slightly different molecular masses and charges.[893] Factors Va1 and Va2 are distinguished by functional differences as well. Factor Va1 does not appear to bind to anionic phospholipid as efficiently as factor Va2 and is not as competent a cofactor in the prothrombinase complex as factor Va2.[892,894-896] The presence of an oligosaccharide at Asn[2182] apparently reduces the affinity of factor Va1 for the phospholipid surface and interferes with prothrombinase complex assembly and function. The COOH-terminal fragment of the factor Va light chain (residues 1753-2183) that contains the Asn[2182] glycosylation site is one of the two regions that mediate membrane association.[897]

The crystal structure of APC-inactivated bovine factor Va (factor Va$_i$),[805] which includes the A1 domain from the heavy chain and the entire light chain, showed a domain organization quite different from early models of either factor V or factor VIII.[898,899] The recent crystal structure of the prothrombinase complex from the venom of Australian Eastern Brown snake (*Pseudonaja textilis*) supports the domain organization of the bovine factor Va$_i$ structure.[900] Most notably, the structure places the C1 and C2 domains in a "side-by-side" orientation, in which both C domains can interact with the phospholipid surface. This model has been supported by biochemical experiments.[901-903] From these structures, homology models have been generated for the prothrombinase complex[904,905] and the ternary complex (prothrombinase + prothrombin).[906]

Activation

The procofactor factor V does not bind factor Xa and is essentially completely inactive.[42] Limited proteolysis of the factor V molecule yields the active cofactor factor Va. Factor Va functions as both a factor Xa receptor and a positive modulator of factor Xa catalytic potential in the prothrombinase complex. Rate enhancements of 300,000-fold derive from the participation of factor Va in the process of factor Xa activation of prothrombin.[594]

α-Thrombin is the primary catalyst of factor V activation in vivo. α-Thrombin cleaves factor V at Arg[709], Arg[1018], and Arg[1545].[795] (*Figure 20.11*). The α-thrombin-generated form of factor Va is a

heterodimer consisting of an NH$_2$-terminal heavy chain (M_r = 105,000 [A1-A2 domains]) linked noncovalently to a COOH-terminal light chain (M_r = 73,000 [A3-C1-C2 domains]).[885,907-910] The association of the heavy and light chains of factor Va shows a divalent cation dependence. The B domain is excised during proteolysis.[16,907,909]

Factor Xa cleaves factor V at Arg[709], Arg[1018], and Arg[1545], producing a factor Va molecule similar to the factor Va produced by α-thrombin cleavage.[633,911] Factor Xa cleavage of factor V is less efficient than α-thrombin cleavage,[633,911] although factor V released from stimulated platelets is partially activated and is more efficiently cleaved by factor Xa than plasma factor V.[912]

Other enzymes may also activate or partially activate factor V. Platelet calpain,[913] cathepsin G, and human neutrophil elastase[914,915] partially activate factor V. The fibrinolytic enzyme plasmin both activates and inactivates factor V.[916-918] Plasmin cleavage and inactivation of factor V are hypothesized to play a role in hemorrhage subsequent to thrombolytic therapy by decreasing the level of factor Va cofactor activity.[919]

Function

Activation of the procofactor factor V yields the functional form factor Va. Factor Va acts as a cofactor for the serine protease factor Xa in the prothrombinase complex. Factor Va forms at least part of the receptor for factor Xa on platelets and serves to anchor factor Xa to the membrane surface.[857] Factor Va stabilizes the prothrombinase complex and enhances prothrombin activation.[5,696] Anticoagulant roles of factor V have also been reported, including (1) functioning as a cofactor with protein S in the downregulation of factor VIIIa by APC[860,920,921] and (2) functions in multiple ways in the tissue factor inhibitor pathway[922,923] (*Figure 20.12*).

Factor Va Regulation and Factor V[Leiden]

Factor Va is regulated by proteolytic inactivation by APC. An anionic membrane surface is required for complete cleavage and full inactivation of the cofactor; in the absence of phospholipid, factor Va cleavage is not complete, and the cofactor retains some activity. Protein S, a suggested cofactor for APC, only functions in the presence of a phospholipid bilayer as well. In the presence of a membrane surface, APC cleaves factor Va sequentially at three sites: Arg,[514] Arg,[311] and Arg.[687] Factor Va is initially cleaved at Arg.[514] Subsequently, the

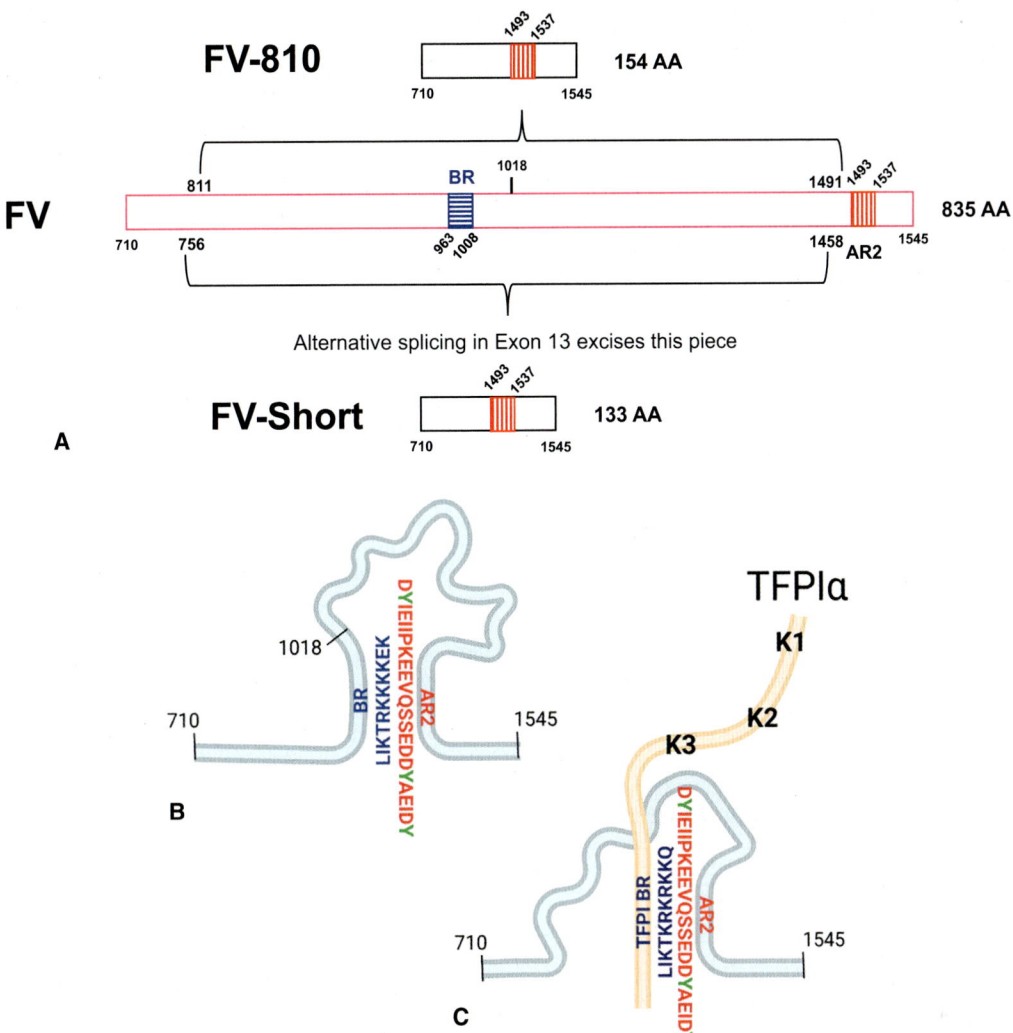

FIGURE 20.12 Structure Function Features of the FV B Domain that regulate its coagulant and anticoagulant mechanisms. FV is synthesized as a single chain molecule, which is converted to an active, noncovalently associated, two-chain cofactor (FVa) by the proteolytic removal of a linker region (B domain: residues 710-1545). Converging lines of research over the last 2 decades have led to insights into the way the B domain structural elements function to regulate coagulation. These studies include (1) FV deletion mutants engineered to lack either a basic region (FV810) located within the N-terminal region of the B domain (BR: residues 963-1008) or an acidic region at the C terminus of the B domain (AR-2: residues 1493-1537) yield derivatives of single chain FV with cofactor activity.[924-926] These data support a structural model in which binding between the BR and AR-2 regions within the B domain is essential to blocking cofactor activity by the full-length single chain molecule; (2) families with a moderately severe bleeding phenotype[927-931] have been shown to share an extensive deletion of the B domain (600-700 residues) that includes the BR region. These deletions are precipitated by mutations in exon 13 that promote alternative splicing. Individuals with this truncated form of FV, termed FV-short, were also observed to have elevated levels of TFPIα[928-931]; (3) the exposed AR-2 domain in FV-short binds TFPIα with high affinity (K_d = ~1 nM)[932]; (4) the FV-short TFPIα complex binds to protein S with high affinity and this ternary complex functions as an effective inhibitor of FXa[933,934]; (5) production of FV-short occurs at low frequency (~1%) in the absence of the potentiating mutations and thus is present in healthy individuals; and (6) TFPIα does not bind to the full-length FV B domain[932] so FV-short is the physiologically relevant FV species in the ternary complex that inhibits FXa. A, Comparison between recombinant (FV810) and naturally occurring (FV-short) B domain variants and the full-length FV B domain; B, schematic depicting high-affinity interaction between BR and AR-2 domains within the normal full-length B domain. Sequence of BR domain is in blue and that of AR-2 domain in red (created with BioRender.com); and C, schematic of FV-short showing sequences involved in the interaction site between AR-2 of FV-short B domain (red) and the basic region (BR, blue) located on the C-terminal tail of TFPIα (created with BioRender.com).

membrane-dependent cleavage at Arg[311] results in complete loss of factor Va cofactor activity. An additional APC-mediated cleavage of factor Va fragments occurs at Arg.[687] Loss of cofactor activity coincides with dissociation of the A2 domain of APC-cleaved factor Va in a process similar to the spontaneous dissociation of factor VIIIa.[935-937]

The importance of this regulatory mechanism is demonstrated by the "APC resistance" syndrome associated with factor V[Leiden].[938] Individuals with factor V[Leiden] have a G to A substitution at nucleotide 1691 in the factor V gene that results in an Arg[506]→Gln mutation at the protein level.[939] Factor Va[Leiden] has normal cofactor activity as part of the prothrombinase complex. However, unlike normal factor Va, factor Va[Leiden] is not readily inactivated by APC. The Arg[506]→Gln mutation hinders the first step in the sequential series of inactivating

cleavages by APC. Factor Va[Leiden] retains cofactor activity and continues to promote α-thrombin generation for an extended period of time. Inactivation of factor Va[Leiden] by cleavage of the Arg[306] bond occurs eventually but is markedly slower than normal factor Va.[940] The prevalence of the factor V[Leiden] mutation is approximately 5% in whites.[941] Individuals heterozygous for factor V[Leiden] have a 7-fold greater risk of thrombosis than normal individuals, whereas individuals homozygous for factor V[Leiden] have an 80-fold greater risk of thrombosis.[942] The risk of thrombosis in individuals with factor V[Leiden] is also exacerbated by other genetic and acquired risk factors such as protein C or protein S deficiency, or both, and use of oral contraceptives.[857,943] The effects of factor V[Leiden] are of considerable interest, as factor V[Leiden] is the most common prothrombotic risk factor yet identified.[944-946]

von Willebrand Factor (von Willebrand Factor: Antigen, Ristocetin Cofactor, von Willebrand Factor Ristocetin: Cofactor)

vWF is a multifunctional protein with several key roles in coagulation. vWF circulates in plasma at an average concentration of 10 μg/mL[947] (*Table 20.1*) and is also contained in the α-granules of human platelets.[948] ABO blood type has a significant influence on vWF levels, with individuals of types A, B, or AB blood having much higher levels of vWF than individuals with type O blood.[949,950] vWF is also known for its role in ristocetin-induced platelet aggregation,[951,952] which is the basis of clinical assays. vWF was first recognized as the missing or defective factor in a severe autosomal dominant bleeding disorder.[953-956] von Willebrand disease is fairly common and is estimated to occur in 1% to 2% of the general population.[957-960] vWF is also an acute-phase reactant; levels are elevated as a result of stress, pregnancy, or surgical trauma,[961-964] and it is a key player in hemostasis.[965]

Gene Structure and Expression

The vWF gene is located on chromosome 12 band p13.31 and is 178 kb long with 51 introns and 52 exons[966-968] (*Table 20.2*). A pseudogene with approximately 98% homology to the vWF gene has been mapped to chromosome 22.[967,968] vWF is expressed only by endothelial cells and megakaryocytes.[969-971] vWF is stored in Weibel-Palade bodies in endothelial cells and in α-granules in platelets.[972-974] There are several regulatory elements that control vWF expression including GATA-binding consensus sequences in the promoter region.[975] Endothelial cell-specific expression appears to be regulated by NF1 and Oct-1-binding sites.[972,975-978] vWF expression is also regulated by complex signaling pathways that are directed by specific cellular environments.[976,979-981] In addition, vWF plasma levels can be regulated through release of vWF from endothelial cell and platelet storage compartments. Platelet activation results in the release of vWF, and endothelial cell vWF release is induced by histamine and 1-deamino-8-d-arginine vasopressin.[982-984]

Biochemistry

vWF is a large adhesive glycoprotein that circulates in plasma as a heterogeneous mixture of disulfide-linked multimers. The biocycle of vWF comprises a series of steps ranging from regulated expression of the vWF gene in endothelial cells and megakaryocytes to its clearance from the blood.[985] vWF is synthesized as a prepro molecule containing a 22-amino-acid signal peptide, a propeptide of 741 amino acids, and the mature vWF protein of 2050 amino acids.[986-991] The prepro vWF molecule comprises internally repeated A, B, C, and D domains arranged in the sequence D1-D2-D′-D3-A1-A2-A3-D4-B-C1-C2. The A repeats share homology with complement factor B, collagen type IV, chicken cartilage matrix protein, and the I domain of the integrin α-subunit.[992,993] Portions of the C domains are homologous to sequences in procollagen and thrombospondin.[994] Prepro vWF undergoes extensive posttranslational modification to yield the mature vWF protein lacking the D1 and D2 domains. The large vWF propolypeptide copurifies with factor VIII and vWF and is designated *vWF antigen-II*. The mature vWF monomer has a molecular weight of approximately 255,000 based on protein sequence and carbohydrate content.[986,987,990,991,995] The disulfide-linked multimers range in size from dimers ($M_r = 600,000$) to extremely large multimers of 20 million D. vWF has binding sites for factor VIII, heparin, collagen, platelet glycoprotein (gp) Ib, and platelet gpIIb-IIIa.[996-1009]

Function

vWF has multiple functions in hemostasis. vWF stabilizes factor VIII and protects it from inactivation by APC,[197,1010] thus significantly prolonging factor VIII half-life in circulation.[783,785,786] vWF is a structural protein and is part of the subendothelial matrix. vWF also acts as a bridge between platelets and promotes platelet aggregation. The primary platelet-binding site for vWF is the gpIb-IX-V receptor complex. gpIb-IX-V is an active receptor on unstimulated platelets and serves to promote platelet aggregation and adhesion to vWF in the absence of platelet activation.[414] This is likely a key element in the procoagulant

response serving to recruit and localize platelets to the site of damage before the events that induce platelet activation.[1011] Subsequent platelet activation also induces expression of another receptor complex, gpIIb-IIIa. The gpIIb-IIIa complex recognizes a number of adhesive proteins including vWF. gpIIb-IIIa receptor binding of these adhesive proteins creates a strong network of platelets, other cells, and matrix components.

Endothelial cells secrete vWF multimers, which are larger than those found circulating in plasma.[1012] The function of these large multimeric forms of vWF is to bind to and agglutinate blood platelets under high shear rates. These large multimers of vWF are degraded by a specific metalloprotease called a disintegrin-like and metalloprotease domain with thrombospondin in type I motifs (ADAMTS)-13.[1013-1015] In familial and acquired thrombotic thrombocytopenic purpura, ultra-large vWF multimers are correlated to defective ADAMTS-13 activity.[1016]

PROCOAGULANT PROTEINS: THROMBIN (FACTOR IIA)

The enzyme α-thrombin, or factor IIa, is the central enzyme in blood coagulation and plays myriad roles in hemostasis[23] as well as roles in tissue repair, development, and pathogenic processes.[663,701,1017-1019] α-Thrombin is the most potent activator of circulating platelets, thus providing the requisite surface for procoagulant activities. α-Thrombin cleaves fibrinogen to generate the fibrin clot,[694,1020-1022] converts factor XIII to factor XIIIa to cross-link and stabilize the clot,[17,1023] and, in association with thrombomodulin, activates TAFI, which delays dissolution of the fibrin clot.[36,1024] α-Thrombin also acts directly and indirectly to amplify its own production. The procofactors V and VIII are activated by α-thrombin[696,697,804,1025] as are factor XI[7] and, potentially, factor VII.[8] In an analysis of a whole blood model of coagulation, a time course of α-thrombin generation and of the protein products of its catalytic activities illustrates that most procoagulant responses to α-thrombin occur during the initiation phase before fibrin formation (*Figure 20.13*).[581] Less than 0.2% of the final α-thrombin produced is required to achieve the activation of its primary substrates in blood. After fibrin clot formation, during the propagation phase, the bulk of α-thrombin is formed (~95%).

In addition, α-thrombin also acts as a mitogen in a variety of cell types[699-703,1026-1030]; induces the release of cytokines,[1031-1035] vasoactive compounds,[1036-1038] and chemoattractants[1039] as part of the response to vascular damage; and stimulates events that initiate tissue repair.[1040-1044]

α-Thrombin acts to indirectly inhibit its own generation through the protein C anticoagulation pathway, a dynamic inhibitory system. α-Thrombin forms the protein Case complex with its cofactor thrombomodulin and activates protein C to APC.[948,1045] APC cleaves factors Va and VIIIa, thus inhibiting prothrombinase and intrinsic tenase function and blocking α-thrombin formation. The binding of α-thrombin to thrombomodulin both produces a potent anticoagulant and alters α-thrombin reactivity. Once bound to thrombomodulin, α-thrombin no longer recognizes fibrinogen as a substrate and no longer acts in a procoagulant capacity.[1046,1047]

α-Thrombin generation must be tightly regulated to ensure that localized, adequate levels of the enzyme are produced. Markedly decreased levels of α-thrombin due to hypoprothrombinemia or reduced α-thrombin activity due to genetic mutation (dysprothrombinemia) are often characterized by bleeding diatheses.[1048,1049] Conversely, elevated levels of α-thrombin promote the risk of thrombosis. A G→A transition at nucleotide position 20,210 (G20210A) in the 3′-untranslated region of the prothrombin gene results in elevated plasma levels of prothrombin[669] and is strongly associated with venous thrombotic events.[1050-1053]

Roles in Coagulation

On phospholipids, membrane activation to α-thrombin proceeds through the obligate intermediate meizothrombin. In contrast, on platelets, the reaction has been reported to proceed through prothrombin 2 (see *Figure 20.9*).[684] Both meizothrombin and α-thrombin possess

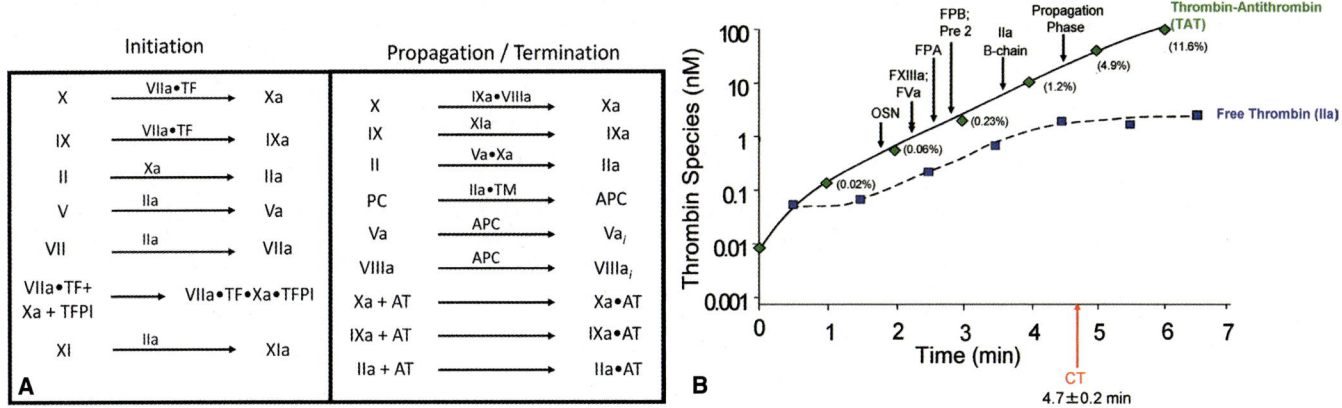

FIGURE 20.13 **Initiation, propagation, and termination of thrombin generation and the procoagulant response.** A, Low levels of thrombin are required to initiate clot formation (initiation phase) and trigger the coagulation cascade response (propagation phase). The enzymes, cofactors, and inhibitors act together to generate a hemostatic response that can be divided into an initiation phase and a propagation/termination phase. During the initiation phase, factors X and IX are converted to their respective serine proteases factor Xa and factor IXa; low levels of thrombin are subsequently generated by factor Xa. This thrombin then can activate platelets and the procofactors factors V and VIII, which stimulate further thrombin generation during the propagation phase. Thrombin generation is attenuated by shutting down the initiation phase by means of the stoichiometric inhibitor of the extrinsic tenase complex, tissue factor pathway inhibitor (TFPI), followed by antithrombin (AT), which directly inhibits thrombin and factors Xa and IXa. B, Time course of early thrombin-antithrombin (TAT) complex formation from whole blood coagulation of 35 individuals is presented: y-axis, TAT (solid line [green diamonds]) and free thrombin (dashed line [blue squares]) concentrations (nmol/L) are shown on a log scale; x-axis, time in minutes. Arrows indicate the time and TAT concentration at which each of the indicated events (osteonectin [OSN] release, a marker of platelet activation, factor XIII activation [fXIIIa], fibrinopeptide A [FPA] release, fibrinopeptide B [FPB] release, and prothrombin activation) has entered a phase of rapid activation. The percentage of total TAT present at the point of activation is shown in parentheses. APC, activated protein C; CT, clot time; PC, protein C; TF, tissue factor. (Reprinted from Brummel KE, Paradis SG, Butenas S, et al. Thrombin functions during tissue factor-induced blood coagulation. *Blood.* 2002;100(1):148-152. Copyright © 2002 American Society of Hematology. With permission.)

catalytic activity and cleave a variety of substrates. Although meizothrombin is a short-lived intermediate in the activation process, it appears to play several important roles in coagulation. Meizothrombin is a potent vasoactive agent and acts on the adrenergic receptor to induce vascular constriction. The vasoactive potency of meizothrombin is five to seven times greater than that of α-thrombin.[1054,1055] However, the ability of meizothrombin to activate platelets and cleave fibrinogen is greatly reduced compared with that of α-thrombin.[687,1056] These are major roles for α-thrombin in promoting an efficient and effective procoagulant response. α-Thrombin has long been recognized as the most potent platelet agonist.[695] α-Thrombin induces release of platelet α-granule contents, including a number of procoagulant and adhesive proteins,[199,948,1057-1065] and of adenosine diphosphate from the platelet-dense granules. α-Thrombin also triggers the translocation of anionic phospholipid to the outer leaflet of the platelet membrane. α-Thrombin thus provides a cross-linked platelet mesh and an anionic surface appropriate for procoagulant complex assembly and function.

In addition, α-thrombin generates and stabilizes the fibrin clot. α-Thrombin cleaves the Arg^{16}-Gly^{17} bond in the Aα-chain and the Arg^{14}-Gly^{15} bond in the Bβ-chain of fibrinogen, releasing fibrinopeptide A (FPA) and fibrinopeptide B (FPB), respectively.[694] FPA and FPB release allows formation of overlapping fibrin strands.[1020-1022] α-Thrombin cleavage of the 37-residue NH$_2$-terminal activation peptide of factor XIII generates the transglutaminase factor XIIIa.[17,1023] Factor XIIIa cross-links and stabilizes the fibrin clot by catalyzing the formation of intermolecular γ-glutamyl α-lysyl isopeptide bonds between fibrin molecules.[17] TAFI, also known as *plasma carboxypeptidase B* or *carboxypeptidase U,* is likewise activated in an α-thrombin-dependent manner to provide activated TAFI (TAFIa).[36,1024] TAFIa has carboxypeptidase B–like activity and is a key link between the coagulation and fibrinolytic cascades. TAFIa prevents premature clot lysis by cleaving COOH-terminal lysine and arginine residues on fibrin, rendering it a less suitable cofactor in t-PA-dependent plasminogen activation.[1066] At elevated concentrations, TAFIa also directly inhibits plasmin and therefore clot lysis.[1066] In addition, TAFI is a substrate for factor XIIIa and is cross-linked to fibrin and incorporated into the fibrin clot.[1067] The α-thrombin-dependent processes involved in clot formation and stabilization likely occur simultaneously to generate a mature clot that effectively reduces blood loss.[1068]

α-Thrombin has other key roles in procoagulant events as well. α-Thrombin activates factor XI[7,631] and the procofactors factor V, factor VIII,[696,697,804,1025] and potentially factor VII.[8] Meizothrombin likewise is an efficient activator of factor XI[1069] and possibly factor V.[1070] Meizothrombin is thought to function to enhance α-thrombin generation by activating factor XI before its final processing to form α-thrombin.

Roles in Anticoagulation

Although α-thrombin is the central enzyme in the procoagulant response, it is also a key mediator of anticoagulant events as well.[1071] When α-thrombin binds to the cell membrane–associated cofactor thrombomodulin, the reactivity of α-thrombin is altered. α-Thrombin bound to thrombomodulin no longer cleaves fibrinogen or acts as a procoagulant enzyme.[1046,1047] Instead, the α-thrombin-thrombomodulin complex, or protein Case, cleaves protein C to generate the enzyme APC. APC is a potent anticoagulant and inactivates the cofactors factor Va and factor VIIIa.[1046,1072] α-Thrombin activation of platelets also induces the release of anticoagulant and inhibitory proteins from the α-granules.[310,1073-1075]

Roles in Tissue Repair and Regeneration

Tissue repair and regeneration is the final phase of the hemostatic response to injury. Subsequent to lysis of the fibrin clot, multiple cell types choreograph the restructuring of the damaged vasculature. Vascular permeability is increased, and inflammatory cells accumulate at the site of injury. Smooth muscle cells, fibroblasts, and endothelial cells migrate to the site and proliferate. Cellular differentiation, as well as production and remodeling of the extracellular matrix, restores the vascular tissue. α-Thrombin contributes to these processes through a variety of interactions with different cell types. α-Thrombin is a potent mitogen[699,700,1026-1029] and stimulates proliferation of smooth muscle cells,[700,702,1030] macrophages,[701] and endothelial cells.[701,703] The mitogenic effects of α-thrombin are due to direct activation of cellular proliferation or α-thrombin-induced secretion of a variety of growth factors, or both. Platelet activation, an early event in the procoagulant response, results in the release of a plethora of α-granule proteins that regulate cell growth, vascular permeability, and chemotaxis.[321,1076-1083] α-Thrombin thus mediates multiple aspects of the hemostatic response to vascular injury from the formation and stabilization of the initial fibrin plug to the final stages of tissue repair and regeneration.

Thrombin Receptors

Many of the effects of α-thrombin on platelets and cells are elicited through α-thrombin interaction with receptor molecules in which α-thrombin binds to a receptor and initiates a signal transduction mechanism. The interaction between α-thrombin and the human platelet thrombin receptor, protease-activated receptor (PAR)-1, however, is characterized by a more unusual mechanism in which the receptor is also a substrate for α-thrombin.[1044,1084,1085] PAR-1 is a 425-amino acid transmembrane protein with a large NH_2-terminal extracellular domain.[1044,1085] α-Thrombin cleaves the extracellular region of the receptor at Arg,[41] producing a "tethered ligand." The new NH_2 terminus binds back to and activates the receptor.[1044,1085] PAR-1 is also found on T lymphocytes, monocytes, and endothelial cells and mediates the α-thrombin-induced responses of these cells as well.

Two additional α-thrombin receptors homologous to PAR-1 have also been identified: PAR-3 and PAR-4. PAR-3 is expressed on human platelets and endothelial cells, although at much lower levels than PAR-1.[1086] PAR-3 is required for normal α-thrombin-dependent platelet activation in mice,[755] but in the human system, the role of PAR-3 appears to be primarily in cellular development. PAR-3 is expressed at high levels on human megakaryocytes, the precursor cells of platelets.[755] PAR-4, however, is believed to act in combination with PAR-1 as a dual mechanism to elicit the multiple effects of α-thrombin on human platelets. A signaling-mediated cooperativity between PARs and GP1b-IX has also been identified to drive platelet activation at low concentrations of thrombin.[1087]

Structure/Function Relationships

In vivo, α-thrombin is derived from proteolytic cleavage of prothrombin by the prothrombinase complex (see *Figures 20.4* and *20.9*). Cleavage of the Arg^{320}-Ile^{321} bond in prothrombin yields meizothrombin. Subsequent cleavage of the Arg^{271}-Thr^{272} bond gives rise to fragment 1.2 and α-thrombin. Human α-thrombin cleaves its own NH_2 terminus at Arg^{284}-Thr^{285} to generate a stable α-thrombin molecule. The initial form of human α-thrombin has an NH_2-terminal A-chain of 49 residues, whereas the autocatalytically generated stable protein has an A-chain of 36 residues. The COOH-terminal B-chain of α-thrombin has 259 amino acid residues including the catalytic triad residues His^{363}, Asp^{419}, and Ser^{525}.

α-Thrombin is subject to further degradation resulting in stable, degraded thrombin molecules with reduced reactivity.[1088-1090] These degraded forms are designated β- and γ-thrombin. The degradation of α-thrombin may be autocatalytic or may be due to proteolysis by enzymes other than α-thrombin. Human β-thrombin is generated by cleavage at Arg^{382} and Arg^{393}, which deletes a segment of the α-thrombin B-chain.[1091,1092] Cleavage of β-thrombin at Arg^{443} and Lys^{474} deletes an additional segment of the B-chain and results in formation of γ-thrombin. β- and γ-thrombin retain some activity toward small peptide substrates,[1055,1093] factor XIII,[1094] antithrombin,[1095] prothrombin,[1096] and factor XI.[1097] However, both β- and γ-thrombin have no significant ability to cleave fibrinogen or protein C.[654,1095,1098] These proteolyzed forms of α-thrombin have been identified as products of the blood clotting reaction in vivo,[693] but their mechanism of production and function is unknown.

The stable form of human α-thrombin possesses at least five distinct binding sites for substrates, inhibitors, cofactors, apolar molecules, and sodium ions (Na^+). The apolar binding site is located near the catalytic center of α-thrombin.[1099] The Na^+ binding site is in the B-chain, in a cavity formed by three antiparallel β sheets, and appears to play a role in determining whether α-thrombin acts as a procoagulant or an anticoagulant. In the presence of Na^+, α-thrombin recognizes fibrinogen as a substrate and acts as a procoagulant. In the absence of Na^+, α-thrombin has increased specificity for protein C and functions in an anticoagulant capacity.[1100,1101] The binding of Na^+ therefore appears to mediate the dual nature of α-thrombin as both a procoagulant and an anticoagulant.

Exosite I, the fibrinogen-binding site, is an anion-binding, electropositive site distinct from, but acting in concert with, the active site of the α-thrombin molecule.[1101] In addition to fibrinogen, exosite I also recognizes the COOH-terminal domain of hirudin, the hirudin-like region of PAR-1, and the fifth and sixth EGF-like domains of thrombomodulin.[1101] Detailed information about exosite I is available from the x-ray crystal structure of the α-thrombin-hirudin complex. In solution, the COOH-terminal domain of hirudin is disordered.[1102,1103] However, in the α-thrombin-hirudin complex, the COOH terminus of hirudin inserts into the large groove in the α-thrombin molecule to interact with exosite I. Hirudin also inserts into the active site of α-thrombin.[1104-1106] The high-affinity interaction ($K_d = 2 \times 10^{-14}$ mol/L) between α-thrombin and the inhibitor hirudin is thus stabilized by electrostatic, polar, and hydrophobic interactions.[1104,1107]

Exosite II is a second electropositive, anion-binding site located on the opposite side of the α-thrombin molecule compared with exosite I. Exosite II recognizes the COOH-terminal region of the B-chain of thrombin and sulfated polysaccharides such as heparin and the chondroitin sulfate moiety of thrombomodulin.[1101]

The active site of α-thrombin is responsible for mediating interactions with substrate molecules including fibrinogen, protein C, and antithrombin.[1101] The active site of α-thrombin is similar to the active sites of trypsin and chymotrypsin. However, unlike the relatively nonspecific pancreatic enzymes, α-thrombin also has secondary binding sites, exosites I and II, that confer specificity to α-thrombin. For substrates such as fibrinogen, there may be multiple secondary binding sites.[1108]

Regulation

α-Thrombin regulates its own production through complex formation with thrombomodulin and activation of protein C (*Figure 20.7*). α-Thrombin enzymatic activity is mediated mainly by antithrombin. The inhibitory activity of antithrombin is potentiated in vivo by cell-expressed heparan sulfate GAGs or by pharmaceutical heparins.[708,709] Antithrombin inhibits α-thrombin through formation of a covalent complex with the active site of α-thrombin.[1109] α-Thrombin-antithrombin (TAT) complexes are rapidly cleared from the circulation by the liver.[1110]

α-Thrombin is also inhibited by α_2-macroglobulin, a broad specificity proteinase inhibitor. α_2-Macroglobulin does not appear to be a primary inhibitor of α-thrombin but rather functions as a secondary inhibitor.[1055] Unlike antithrombin, α_2-macroglobulin does not complex with the active site of its target enzymes. Enzymes in complex with α_2-macroglobulin retain the ability to cleave small peptidyl substrates, although they are unable to cleave large substrates.[1111] α-Thrombin interaction with α_2-macroglobulin involves limited proteolysis of α_2-macroglobulin. Subsequent to cleavage, α_2-macroglobulin undergoes a conformation change that traps the enzyme inside the α_2-macroglobulin molecule.[1112,1113] The α_2-macroglobulin-enzyme complexes are rapidly cleared from circulation.[1114,1115] A recent review discusses the structural features of thrombin and its inhibition.[1116]

ANTICOAGULANT PROTEINS: DYNAMIC INHIBITORY SYSTEM

The protein C pathway provides a dynamic inhibitory system to regulate α-thrombin production.[1117-1119] The activity of this anticoagulant pathway is directly dependent on the level of α-thrombin production. The protein C activating complex, or protein Case, is a membrane-dependent multiprotein complex similar to the membrane-dependent procoagulant complexes (see *Figures 20.5* and *20.7*). The key proteins in the protein C pathway are α-thrombin, thrombomodulin, protein C, and protein S.

Protein C

Protein C, first identified as a thrombin inhibitory activity or autoprothrombin II-A,[1120] is the zymogen form of the enzyme APC. Protein C circulates at a concentration of 4 μg/mL (65 nmol/L) with a $t_{1/2}$ of 8 to

10 hours[1121-1123] (*Table 20.4*). The $t_{1/2}$ of protein C is markedly shorter than most other members of the vitamin K–dependent protein family and is the likely basis of the transient hypercoagulable state subsequent to administration of coumarin-based anticoagulants.[1124-1128] Homozygous protein C deficiency is associated with severe thrombotic tendencies and can result in fatal neonatal thrombotic events.[1129] Heterozygous protein C deficiency is associated with increased risk of thrombosis.[1130-1132] The mutation in factor V[Leiden], which blocks a key APC cleavage site in factor Va[Leiden], is another defect leading to an alteration in the protein C anticoagulant pathway and predisposition to thrombosis.

Gene Structure and Expression

The protein C gene is located on chromosome 2 bands q14.3 and spans 11 kb with eight introns and nine exons[1133,1134] (*Table 20.6*). The promoter region contains HNF-1-, HNF-3-, and Sp1-binding sites that promote gene expression.[1135,1136] HNF-3 is a liver-specific transcription factor.

Biochemistry

Protein C is synthesized in the liver as a single-chain polypeptide with a prepro sequence of 42 amino acids. The prepro protein is subsequently processed to remove the leader sequence and the dipeptide Lys[156]-Arg[157]. Thus, in plasma, most protein C circulates as a heterodimer consisting of a disulfide-linked (Cys[141]-Cys[277]) heavy and light chain.[1137-1142] However, approximately 5% to 10% of circulating protein C is the single-chain form.[375] The two-chain form of human protein C (M_r = 62,000) is a 419-amino acid glycoprotein with approximately 23% carbohydrate (*Table 20.4* and *Figure 20.4B*). The NH$_2$-terminal light chain (residues 1-155; M_r = 21,000) contains the Gla domain (residues 6-29; nine Gla residues) and a hydrophobic region that connects the Gla domain to two EGF domains (residues 55-90 and 94-134). The COOH-terminal heavy chain (residues 158-419; M_r = 41,000) contains the serine protease domain. Residues 158 to 169 constitute the activation peptide domain. A β-hydroxy aspartate residue (Asp[71]) in the first EGF domain is required for Ca^{2+}-dependent alterations in protein C. Ca^{2+} binding is mediated by the first EGF domain as well as the Gla domain and the serine protease domain.[368,412,416,1143-1148] Leu[5] in the NH$_2$ terminus is important in mediating phospholipid binding.[406] There are several glycosylation variants (Asn[97], Asn[248], Asn[313], and Asn[329]) with two to four N-linked carbohydrate chains.[375] The major forms, α-protein C and β-protein C, have four and three carbohydrate moieties, respectively. All the protein C carbohydrate variants can be activated but appear to have different anticoagulant properties and rates of activation.[376] An x-ray crystal structure has been determined for Gla-domainless activated protein C.[396]

Activation

Protein C is the zymogen form of the enzyme APC. Protein C is cleaved at the Arg[169]-Leu[170] bond, releasing its activation peptide from the heavy chain to generate the active enzyme.[1149,1150] The α-thrombin-thrombomodulin complex is likely the major physiologic activator of protein C.[1151] There are other activators as well. Plasmin activates and then inactivates protein C.[1125,1152] Meizothrombin also binds thrombomodulin and can efficiently activate protein C.[688,1153] Factor Xa has likewise been reported to bind to thrombomodulin and activate protein C[1154]; however, this mechanism has not been confirmed in subsequent studies.[1155,1156] Glycosaminoglycans have been shown to potentiate factor Xa–mediated protein C activation.[1157] Copperhead snake venom also contains a protein C activator.[1158] The erythrocyte-derived microparticle surface has been shown to support APC-mediated regulation of blood coagulation.[1159]

Function

APC is a serine protease with key anticoagulant functions. The most important anticoagulant role for the protein C pathway is the proteolytic inactivation of factor Va. APC inactivates factor Va via a series of proteolytic cleavages, thus inhibiting the generation of α-thrombin. APC also cleaves and inactivates factor VIIIa, although the

spontaneous dissociation of the factor VIIIa A2 domain is the probable physiologic regulator of factor Xa generation. Full inactivation of factor Va by APC requires an anionic phospholipid surface, and the rates of APC inactivation of factors Va and VIIIa are enhanced by protein S.[1160]

APC also has a profibrinolytic effect. This effect is due to TAFI. TAFI is activated by the α-thrombin-thrombomodulin complex and acts to prolong clot lysis. APC cleavage of factor Va inhibits α-thrombin generation, thus reducing α-thrombin-thrombomodulin-mediated TAFI activation.[1161] The prolongation of clot lysis by TAFIa likely contributes to the prothrombotic tendencies associated with factor V[Leiden].[1162]

The endothelial cell protein C receptor provides cell-specific binding sites for both protein C and APC.[1163,1164] However, two other coagulation proteases, factors VIIa and Xa, have been shown to bind to this receptor.[1165] Endothelial cell protein C receptor is downregulated by TNF-α.[1164] Monocytes appear to express specific binding sites for APC that are distinct from endothelial cell protein C receptor.[1166,1167] The cell-expressed binding sites may be important in the anti-inflammatory properties of APC.[1168] APC blocks the septic shock response in animal models[1169,1170] and has shown clinical success in patients with severe sepsis.[1171,1172] Recent mouse studies identify APC-induced PAR-1 biased dependent signaling as central to APC's in vivo benefits in sepsis and stroke.[1173] APC reduces the levels of inflammatory cytokines such as TNF-α.[1170,1174] The anti-inflammatory properties of APC are also due to inhibition of α-thrombin generation and, therefore, inhibition of the proinflammatory properties of α-thrombin.

Regulation

Protein C activation and APC activity are controlled on several levels. Inflammatory agents such as endotoxin, IL-1β, transforming growth factor-β (TGF-β), and TNF-α regulate protein C activation on endothelial cells.[1175-1184] TNF-α is responsible for downregulation of thrombomodulin on the endothelial cell surface.[1178,1181-1184] There are multiple other factors that downregulate thrombomodulin as well. APC activity is regulated mainly by the protein C inhibitor or PAI-3.[1185-1187]

Protein S

Protein S is a vitamin K–dependent protein that is not a serine protease precursor. Protein S circulates at a plasma concentration of 20 µg/mL (300 nmol/L)[1188,1189] (*Table 20.4*). Approximately 40% of protein S circulates in the free form, and the remaining 60% circulates as a 1:1 complex with C4b-binding protein (C4bBP), a regulatory protein of the complement system.[1188] Protein S is thought to function as a cofactor for APC in the inactivation of factors Va and VIIIa.[197,1190-1195] Heterozygous deficiency of protein S increases the risk for developing thrombosis; however, the diagnosis is complicated.[1196-1198] The protein S cofactor effect is minimal, however, and does not correlate with the thrombotic pathologies manifested in protein S–deficient patients.[1199-1205] Protein S has also been reported to inhibit prothrombin activation through several mechanisms.[710,1206-1208] Although the precise function of protein S is not clear, protein S is important in anticoagulation.

Gene Structure and Expression

The gene for protein S is located on chromosome 3 at band q11.1 and spans at least 80 kb[1209,1210] (*Table 20.6*). The gene contains 15 exons and 14 introns.[1209,1211,1212] A second copy of the protein S gene has also been identified; however, this second gene is likely a pseudogene.[1213,1214] The pseudogene spans approximately 55 kb and differs from the protein S gene in that it lacks exon 1 and has multiple nucleotide substitutions. Protein S is synthesized in the liver[1215,1216] and by a variety of other cell types including endothelial cells,[1217-1219] osteoclasts,[1220] and lymphoid cells.[1221] Protein S is also found in the α-granules of platelets.[1074]

Biochemistry

Protein S (M_r = 69,000) is a single-chain glycoprotein with approximately 8% carbohydrate and 11 Gla residues[598,1222] (*Table 20.4* and *Figure 20.4B*). Protein S is synthesized with a signal sequence and propeptide

The Normal Hematologic System

region of 41 amino acids.[1211,1212,1216,1223] The mature form of the protein has 635 amino acids and is organized into eight domains: an NH_2-terminal Gla domain (residues 1-45), an aromatic stack, a 29-residue thrombin-sensitive domain (residues 46-75), four EGF domains (residues 76-242), and a COOH-terminal domain homologous to the sex hormone–binding globulin and androgen-binding protein.[1224,1225] The Gla domain and EGF domains mediate Ca^{2+} binding.[1226] The Gla domain is also involved in interactions with phospholipid membranes.[1227] C4bBP binds to the COOH-terminal sex hormone–binding globulin domain.[1228,1229] Protein S reversibly self-associates in the absence of Ca^{2+}.[1230] The protein S enhancement of TPFI is dependent on a direct interaction involving $Glu^{231,1231}$ and $Arg^{204,1232}$ within the TFPI K3 domain and the sex hormone–binding globulin domain of protein S.[1233,1234]

Function

The precise function of protein S in the protein C inhibitory pathway is not clearly defined. Protein S enhances APC inactivation of factors Va and VIIIa in a phospholipid-dependent fashion.[197,1190-1195] The interaction between protein S and APC alters the structure of APC and moves the APC active site closer to the membrane surface.[1235] Protein S may also serve directly in an anticoagulant capacity. Protein S has been reported to bind to factor Xa,[1206] factor VIII,[1236] and factor Va[1206] to compete for prothrombinase-binding sites on the membrane surface,[710,1208] serving as a cofactor to stimulate the inhibition of factor Xa by TFPI[1231,1237,1238] and the inhibition of factor Xa activation by tissue factor-fVIIa.[1239] These interactions serve to inhibit prothrombin activation in vitro.[1240] The C4bBP–protein S complex may inhibit factor X activation as well.[1241]

Protein S also has additional potential roles outside of anticoagulation. Protein S interaction with T cells promotes T-cell aggregation and proliferation and may serve to regulate inflammatory processes.[1242]

Regulation

α-Thrombin cleavage of protein S at Arg^{49}, Arg^{60}, or Arg^{70} in the thrombin-sensitive domain inhibits the ability of protein S to act as a cofactor for APC.[1194,1243-1245] Protein S activity is also regulated by interaction with C4bBP. The 1:1 complex between protein S and C4bBP neutralizes the anticoagulant capacity of protein S. Approximately 60% of plasma protein S circulates bound to C4bBP.

Protein Z

Protein Z, a vitamin K–dependent glycoprotein, is an enzymatically inactive homolog of factors VII, IX, and X, and protein C.[378] Protein Z was first identified in bovine plasma by Prowse and Esnouf in 1977[1246] and later in human plasma by Broze and Miletich in 1984.[1247] The name protein Z came about from its being the last of the vitamin K–dependent proteins to elute during anion exchange chromatography.[1248] Protein Z circulates in plasma in a complex with protein Z–dependent protease inhibitor (ZPI).[1249] This inhibitor, ZPI, has been identified as a 72-kDa member of the serpin superfamily.

Reports suggest that protein Z behaves as a negative acute-phase reactant.[1250,1251] Protein Z levels have been found to be low in newborn infants[1252,1253] and in individuals with DIC,[1254] liver disease,[1255] and amyloidosis.[1256] High plasma levels have been found in individuals on chronic hemodialysis and with idiopathic thrombocytopenic purpura.[1257] Protein Z levels also appear to be more susceptible to warfarin therapy than other vitamin K–dependent proteins.[1258]

Gene Structure and Expression

The gene for protein Z is located on chromosome 13 at band q34 (*Table 20.6*). It spans approximately 14 kb and consists of nine exons, including one alternative exon.[378] The gene organization is similar to that of the other vitamin K–dependent proteins, factors VII, IX, and X, and protein C.

Homozygous and heterozygous protein Z–deficient mice showed no abnormalities in growth and development. Protein Z deficiency has been reported to be prothrombotic in nature in factor V^{Leiden} mice.[1259] In general, evidence supports the anticoagulant role of the complex between protein Z and the serpin ZPI and the thrombotic consequences of its deficiency.[1260-1262] Protein Z–deficient mice crossed with factor V^{Leiden} mice did not have viable progeny. Several clinical studies identified diminished levels of plasma protein Z in patients with unidentified bleeding disorders.[1263,1264] Protein Z has also been identified in liver disease,[1255] atherosclerosis,[1265] and reproductive biology.[1266]

Biochemistry

Protein Z has a molecular weight of 62,000 and circulates in plasma at a mean concentration of 2.9 ± 1.0 μg/mL[1247,1258] (*Table 20.4*). The plasma $t_{1/2}$ of protein Z is 2.5 days.[1258] Structurally, protein Z is similar to factors VII, IX, and X, and protein C, containing a Gla domain (13 residues) and two EGF domains at its NH_2 terminus, consisting of 360 amino acids[378,1267,1268] (*Figure 20.4B*). However, like protein S, protein Z does not function as a protease. The COOH terminus contains a region homologous to the catalytic domains present in the serine protease zymogens. The catalytic triad is not present in protein Z, except for the conserved Asp residue.[1267,1268]

Table 20.6. Molecular Genetics of Human Anticoagulant Proteins and Their Inhibitors

Protein	Molecular Weight (Da)	Gene Location: Chromosome	Gene Size (kb)	Gene Organization: # of Exons	mRNA Size (kb)	UNIPROT Accession Number[a]
Protein C	62,000	2q14.3	11.8	8	1.8	P04070
Protein S	69,000	3q11.1	100.7	16	2.3	P07225
Protein Z	62,000	13q34	13.7	9	1.5	P22891
Thrombomodulin	100,000	20p11.21	4	Intronless	4	P07204
α_2-Macroglobulin	735,000	12p13.31	48.2	36	4.6	P01023
Tissue factor pathway inhibitor	40,000	2q32.1	90.2	8	3.8	P10646
Antithrombin	58,000	1q25.1	13.5	7	1.5	P01008
Heparin cofactor II	66,000	22q11.21	13.6	5	2.2	P05546
α_1-Proteinase inhibitor	53,000	14q32.13	12.2	7	1.4	P01009
C1 esterase inhibitor	104,000	11q12.1	17.2	8	1.8	P05155
Protein C inhibitor	57,000	14q32.1	11.7	6	2.1	P05154
Protein Z inhibitor	72,000	14q32.13	12.8	7	2.5	Q9UK55

[a]https://www.uniprot.org.

Function

Protein Z is a vitamin K–dependent protein that does not function as a serine protease enzyme. Protein Z circulates in plasma in complex with ZPI. The main role of protein Z appears to be an anticoagulant effect through the inactivation of factor Xa by forming a Ca^{2+}-dependent complex with factor Xa bound to phospholipid with the help of ZPI.[1249] Originally, it was reported that ZPI can also inhibit factor IXa, although subsequent studies did not confirm this,[1269] and instead it was shown that there is a 39-loop that restricts the ZPI specificity of factor IXa.[1270] More recent studies of protein Z have focused on a potential mechanism by which protein Z acts as a cofactor in the modulation of the activity of ZPI. This includes direct interaction of protein Z with both factor Xa and ZPI at phospholipid surfaces, forming the complex factor Xa–ZPI–protein Z at the phospholipid surface[1271] and forming a Gla-Gla interaction between protein Z and factor Xa to accelerate the inhibition rate.[1272,1273] Protein Z has also been suggested to induce structural changes in ZPI that aligns the inhibitory site of ZPI with the active site of factor Xa.[1273] These interactions can alter the secretion, localization, and clearance of ZPI.[1200] In vitro, protein Z has also been shown to have a weak interaction ($K_d = 8.9$ μmol/L) with thrombin that facilitates the binding of thrombin to phospholipid surfaces.[1274] It is also consumed, like all other coagulation factors and inhibitors, during the course of DIC.

Thrombomodulin

Thrombomodulin is a type 1 transmembrane protein constitutively expressed on the surface of vascular endothelial cells (*Figure 20.10*). It is an essential that displays a range of anti-inflammatory, anticoagulant, and antifibrinolytic properties.[1275] Thrombomodulin is a high-affinity receptor for α-thrombin and acts as a cofactor for the α-thrombin-dependent activation of protein C and TAFI. Thrombomodulin activity on the surface of endothelial cells is decreased by inflammatory cytokines and may contribute to the hypercoagulation characteristic of inflammatory states. Thrombomodulin is expressed widely during fetal development.[1276] Homozygous thrombomodulin-deficient mice die in utero before the formation of the cardiovascular system, suggesting a potential role for thrombomodulin in mammalian development.[1277]

Gene Structure and Expression

The human thrombomodulin gene is located on chromosome 20 band p11.21 and spans 3.7 kb[1278,1279] (*Table 20.6*). The gene is unusual in that it lacks introns.[1280,1281] Thrombomodulin expression has been reported in a variety of cell types, including vascular endothelial cells,[1282,1283] neutrophils,[1284] monocytes,[1285,1286] platelets,[1263] synovial cells,[1287] and squamous epithelial cells.[1288-1290] Vascular expression is limited to endothelial cells. Thrombomodulin activity on the surface of endothelial cells is decreased by homocysteine, lipopolysaccharide, IL-1β, and TNF-α.[1175,1176,1291-1293] Many of these same inflammatory agents that downregulate thrombomodulin also upregulate tissue factor, contributing to the hypercoagulation associated with inflammation. Hypoxia also downregulates thrombomodulin expression.[1294] Likewise, thrombomodulin expression is decreased by glucose-modified albumin, which may provide a link to diabetic thrombotic complications.[1295] Conversely, dibutyl cyclic adenosine monophosphate, retinoic acid, shear stress, and increased temperature (42 °C) upregulate thrombomodulin activity on endothelial cells.[1296-1300] Upregulation of thrombomodulin expression by TNF-α may involve a consensus sequence of a cyclic adenosine monophosphate response element in the 3'-untranslated region of the thrombomodulin gene.[1301] Increased thrombomodulin gene transcription due to elevated temperature is mediated by consensus sequence recognition sites for a heat shock element in the 5'-promoter region.[1300] Upregulation of thrombomodulin expression in response to elevated temperature may be a protective mechanism to compensate for the procoagulant effects of the inflammatory mechanism.

Biochemistry

Human thrombomodulin is synthesized with an 18-amino acid signal sequence followed by a 557-residue polypeptide chain of the mature protein.[1278,1280,1281,1302] Thrombomodulin has five different domain structures: an NH_2-terminal domain having weak homology to lectins (residues 6-149) such as the asialoglycoprotein receptor,[1303] 6 EGF-like domains (residues 227-462), a 34-residue region rich in serine and threonine corresponding to potential O-linked glycosylation sites (residues 463-497), a 23-residue hydrophobic transmembrane region (residues 499-521), and a COOH-terminal domain (residues 522-557) containing several potential phosphorylation sites and one free cysteine residue (Cys^{536}) (*Figure 20.10*). The fifth and sixth EGF domains support α-thrombin association.[1304] The region required for efficient protein C activation extends from the linker region between EGF domains 3 and 4 through EGF-6.[1305-1308] Ser^{472} and Ser^{474} in the serine- and threonine-rich region are potential sites for chondroitin sulfate addition.[1309] The presence of chondroitin sulfate increases the affinity for α-thrombin more than 10-fold,[1310] thus increasing the ability of thrombomodulin to block fibrinogen cleavage and platelet activation by α-thrombin.[1311,1312] The chondroitin sulfate moiety also enhances inactivation of α-thrombin by antithrombin[1311,1313] and modulates the Ca^{2+} dependence of protein C activation.[1310,1313] The O-linked sugar domain of thrombomodulin is required for APC generation on cellular surfaces. This domain is extended and rigid and rises approximately perpendicular to the membrane surface. The O-linked sugar domain likely functions to elevate α-thrombin from the membrane surface.[1314] The active site of α-thrombin bound to thrombomodulin is located approximately 65 Å from the membrane surface.[1315]

Although no consensus sequence for internalization via coated pit-mediated endocytosis is found in thrombomodulin, coated and non-coated pit-mediated endocytosis has been observed.[1316] Internalization appears to be mediated by the NH_2-terminal lectin-like domain.[1317]

Function

Thrombomodulin functions as a cofactor for α-thrombin in the activation of protein C and TAFI. Production of APC by the α-thrombin-thrombomodulin complex is approximately 1000 times faster than by equivalent concentrations of protein C and thrombin. Once bound to thrombomodulin, α-thrombin's procoagulant activities are neutralized. The high-affinity α-thrombin-thrombomodulin interaction is mediated mainly by exosite I on the α-thrombin molecule. Exosite I also binds fibrinogen, and the interaction of α-thrombin with thrombomodulin therefore blocks fibrinogen binding and cleavage. In addition, thrombomodulin induces conformational changes in α-thrombin.[1318-1323] Overall, the changes that occur on α-thrombin interaction with thrombomodulin reduce the ability of α-thrombin to generate fibrin, and to activate factor V and platelets,[1324,1325] while increasing the rate of inactivation of α-thrombin by antithrombin.[1326-1328] α-Thrombin-thrombomodulin, or protein Case, functions solely in an anticoagulant and antifibrinolytic capacity.

Regulation

There are several potential mechanisms of thrombomodulin regulation on the cell surface. Thrombomodulin expression is downregulated by endotoxin and inflammatory cytokines.[1181] Shear stress, homocysteine, and hypoxia likewise downregulate thrombomodulin expression.[1293,1294,1299,1329] α-Thrombin may also regulate thrombomodulin activity, although evidence is somewhat controversial. Thrombomodulin-dependent α-thrombin internalization has been reported.[1330-1332] However, the α-thrombin-thrombomodulin complex appears to be stable under some conditions.[1072,1333] In addition, thrombomodulin activity can be regulated proteolytically, mainly by neutrophil elastase.[1334,1335] Neutrophils decrease thrombomodulin activity via oxidation as well.[1336]

ANTICOAGULANT PROTEINS: PROTEINASE INHIBITORS

Proteinases, enzymes that hydrolyze peptide bonds, are found in a wide array of biologic systems, including the blood coagulation process (clot formation and fibrinolysis), the digestive system, apoptotic cascades, and the immune system. To keep these systems in balance between

The Normal Hematologic System

activation and inhibition, a complex system of proteinase inhibitors has evolved. In blood, proteinase inhibitors constitute a significant percentage of circulating proteins. In general, proteinases that activate the coagulation and fibrinolytic cascades have highly defined substrate specificities. Coagulation is kept in check through the action of several specific and broad-spectrum proteinase inhibitors. Specific clot formation inhibitors are antithrombin and TFPI. Fibrinolysis-specific inhibitors are PAI-1 and α_2-antiplasmin. Together, specific and broad-spectrum inhibitors function to localize, limit, and control hemostasis.

α_2-Macroglobulin

α_2-Macroglobulin is a nonspecific proteinase inhibitor that targets a broad spectrum of protease substrates.[1337] It is present in human plasma at concentrations ranging from 2 to 4 µmol/L (2-3 mg/mL) (*Table 20.4*). α_2-Macroglobulin can also be found at higher concentrations in extravascular fluids.[1338] This protease inhibitor can be produced in a variety of cells including hepatocytes, fibroblasts, and macrophages.[1114,1339] α_2-Macroglobulin is also found in several species including the horseshoe crab.[1340]

Reduced levels of serum α_2-macroglobulin in humans have been observed in individuals with chronic obstructive lung disease[1341] and cancer metastasis.[1342] In humans, no absolute deficiency has been reported to date, leading to the suggestion that such a congenital deficiency is incompatible with survival. The inactivation of the mouse α_2-macroglobulin gene results in viable mice that produce normal-sized litters but are more resistant to endotoxin challenge.[1343] In a later study, it was suggested that this phenotype in mice functions as a neutralizer of transforming growth factor-β and as an inducer of nitric oxide synthesis.[1344]

Gene Structure and Expression

The gene encoding human α_2-macroglobulin spans approximately 48 kb and consists of 36 exons and 35 introns[1345] (*Table 20.6*). It is located on chromosome 12p13.31.[1346-1348] The α_2-macroglobulin gene is a single-copy gene in the human genome. α_2-Macroglobulin is synthesized in the liver as a pro-α_2-macroglobulin, which contains a 23-residue signal peptide. Three transcription initiation sites, including a TATA box, a TATA-like structure (ATAAA), and a potential HP-1-binding site, have been identified in the liver.[1345]

Biochemistry

Human α_2-macroglobulin circulates in plasma as a tetramer with four identical single-chain subunits with an individual relative molecular weight of 180,000 and a total relative molecular weight of 735,000.[1346,1349,1350] An unusual feature of this protein is that multiple forms may be found in various species and may appear only during acute-phase reactions.[1114,1338,1339] A dimeric form termed *pregnancy zone protein* has been found in human plasma at peak levels during the last trimester. Therefore, this protein may be found in human plasma composed of either two or four identical subunits.[1351,1352]

α_2-Macroglobulin has a unique mechanism by which it achieves broad specificity.[1353] The initial step involves the "bait region" of α_2-macroglobulin.[1113] This region consists of a 25-amino acid sequence that has sequence motifs appropriate for many proteases.[1354] After proteolysis in this bait region, α_2-macroglobulin undergoes conformational changes that trap the proteinase inside the molecule.[1113] The crystal structure of human α_2-macroglobulin displays a large central cavity capable of containing one or two average-sized proteases.[1355] These conformational changes have been referred to as a *slow to fast transition*.[1112,1113] The active site of the substrate proteinase is not found in complex with the inhibitor. Studies have shown that the entrapped proteinase is no longer able to interact with macromolecular substrates, inhibitors, and antibodies but still appears to retain its ability to react with small substrates and inhibitors.[1113] These complexes are rapidly cleared from the circulation by the endocytic α_2-macroglobulin receptor also known as the *low-density lipoprotein receptor-related protein* (LRP). This receptor is found on most mast cells and tissues. The proteinase inhibitor complex has an approximate $t_{1/2}$ of 2 to 5 minutes.[1114]

Another important feature of α_2-macroglobulin is the presence of a β-cysteinyl-γ-glutamyl thiol ester.[1356,1357] Studies have shown that these thiol esters may directly react with small nucleophiles, such as ammonia or methylamine; induce a conformational change; and prevent proteinase binding.[1358] The conformational changes associated with proteolysis of the bait region generate a thiol ester more susceptible to nucleophilic attack, with the result that surface Lys residues of the trapped proteinase can react with it and become covalently linked to α_2-macroglobulin. Binding studies in vitro have identified specific high-affinity receptors for α_2-macroglobulin-proteinase complexes on many cell types, including fibroblasts, macrophages, and hepatocytes.[1115]

Function

One role for α_2-macroglobulin is to inhibit a broad range of proteinases. It is distinctive in its capacity to inhibit members from each of four mechanistic classes of proteinases (serine, cysteine, and aspartic proteinases, and metalloproteinases). α_2-Macroglobulin functions as a secondary inhibitor to serine proteinases in plasma by inhibiting thrombin, kallikrein, and plasmin.[1359,1360] It may also be important in preventing thromboembolic events when there is a congenital deficiency of antithrombin or sepsis.[1361,1362] α_2-Macroglobulin also inhibits various growth factors and cytokines, including TGF-β,[1363] IL-1β,[1364] IL-6,[1365] acidic fibroblast growth factor,[1366] basic fibroblast growth factor,[1366] TNF-α,[1367] and IL-2.[1368] Polymorphisms identified in α_2-macroglobulin have been thought to play a role in Alzheimer disease.[1369-1371] Overall, the biologic role of α_2-macroglobulin in vivo is still being elucidated.

Tissue Factor Pathway Inhibitor

TFPI, formerly called *extrinsic pathway inhibitor* or *lipoprotein-associated coagulation inhibitor*, is a multivalent, Kunitz-type plasma proteinase inhibitor. TFPI modulates tissue factor–dependent coagulation in vivo by rapidly inhibiting the extrinsic tenase complex (factor VIIa–tissue factor) as soon as it is formed[1372-1374] (*Figure 20.7*). It circulates in plasma at approximately 0.1 µg/mL[1375] as a heterogeneous collection of partially proteolyzed forms[328,1376] (*Table 20.4*). Ninety percent of circulating TFPI is found associated with lipoproteins, primarily low-density lipoprotein.[1377-1379] Parenteral TFPI is cleared from the circulation primarily by the liver and has an unusually short $t_{1/2}$ (minutes) compared with other proteinase inhibitors.

Many reviews of TFPI have been published.[1380-1384] The importance of TFPI in blood coagulation has been best illustrated through transgenic mice that have a complete deficiency (–/–) of TFPI. This deficiency is incompatible with birth and survival.[1385] However, this lethality in mice can be rescued by heterozygous or homozygous factor VII deficiency.[1386] This implies that diminishing the level of factor VII lessens the need for TFPI-mediated inhibition of the factor VIIa–tissue factor coagulation pathway during embryogenesis.[1386] When mice are generated that have a combined heterozygous TFPI deficiency and homozygous apolipoprotein E deficiency, they exhibit a greater atherosclerotic burden.[1387] These observations suggest a role for TFPI in protection from atherosclerosis and as a potential regulator of thrombosis.

To date, there are no known human TFPI-deficient individuals described, which suggests that human embryos with the TFPI$^{-/-}$ genotype fail to develop. A role for TFPI in preventing thrombosis and other cardiovascular diseases is currently under intensive clinical and in vitro investigation.[1388] One application for recombinant TFPI is in the area of sepsis in which patients frequently have reduced TFPI levels.[1389,1390]

Gene Structure and Expression

The human TFPI gene has been localized to chromosome 2 band q32.1[1391-1393] (*Table 20.6*). It spans 85 kb, over half of which consists of the 5′ noncoding region. The coding region is distributed over nine exons[1394]; mature TFPI contains three Kunitz domains that are encoded on separate exons. The gene specifies a protein of 304 amino acids; the first 28 residues comprise a signal peptide. Two variants of TFPI (isoforms α and β) arising from alternative splicing have been identified; the variable region involves residues 210 to 251 of the primary gene product, spanning a large portion of the third Kunitz domain. TFPI is expressed constitutively by cultured endothelial cells, and its level of synthesis is hardly affected by endotoxin or inflammatory cytokines.[1395,1396] TFPI is not expressed by hepatocytes. TFPI is found bound to low- and high-density lipoproteins located within platelets or noncovalently associated with endothelial cell heparin sulfate proteoglycans.[1375] TFPI is catabolized in the liver and kidney by uptake/degradation via the low-density LRP or its homologs.[1397]

Biochemistry

TFPI ($M_r = 40,000$) is a single-chain glycoprotein of the Kunitz proteinase inhibitor family.[1398,1399] As isolated, the COOH terminus of TFPI displays some degradation. Structurally, mature full-length TFPI (276 amino acids in the α isoform) consists of an acidic NH_2-terminal region, three tandem Kunitz-like serine protease inhibitor domains (K1 to K3), and a positively charged COOH-terminal region[1397,1398] (*Figure 20.14A*). The tandem Kunitz domains are essential for the function of TFPI.[1400] The Kunitz 1 inhibitor domain (residues 26-76) binds factor VIIa–tissue factor. The second Kunitz domain (residues 97-147) of TFPI binds the factor Xa active site. The Kunitz 3 domain (residues 189-239) of TFPIα binds protein S, and the protein S–mediated potentiation of factor Xa inhibition by TFPIα involves protein S–Kunitz 3 interaction.[1232] Heparin binds at two heparin-binding sites: a high-affinity site in the COOH-terminal basic region and a low-affinity site between Gly^{212} and Phe^{243} in the third Kunitz domain.[641,642,1401]

TFPI contains three potential N-linked glycosylation sites (Asn^{117}, Asn^{167}, and Asn^{228}), with one or more of these oligosaccharides sulfated during expression by cultured endothelial cells.[1402] Two O-linked glycosylation sites have also been identified (Ser^{202} and Thr^{203}). A significant proportion of TFPI molecules in the blood is truncated to variable extents at the COOH-terminal end (some lacking most of the third Kunitz domain) and has compromised inhibitory activity.[1403] In contrast, TFPI released by heparin infusion is full length and more active than the truncated forms.[1399] The inhibitory activity of TFPI is enhanced by heparin.

The normal plasma concentration of TFPI is 0.1 μg/mL. TFPIα is found either associated with lipoproteins, such as low- and high-density lipoproteins or lipoprotein(a), complexed noncovalently to endothelial cell heparan sulfate proteoglycans,[1375] or associated with endothelial cell surfaces via a glycosyl-phosphatidyl-inositol (GPI) anchor.[1381,1382] On heparin administration, TFPI is released from endothelial cells, primarily microvascular, causing a 2- to 10-fold increase in circulating TFPI levels.[1399,1404,1405] TFPI release on heparin therapy is responsible for the observed elevation in PT and

Tissue factor pathway inhibitor (TFPI): 40 kDa

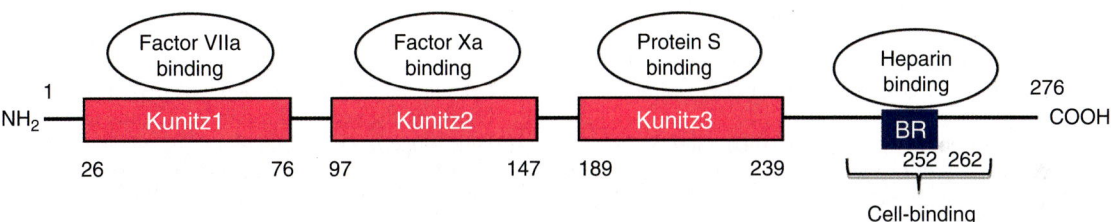

Antithrombin (AT): 58 kDa

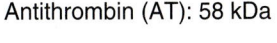

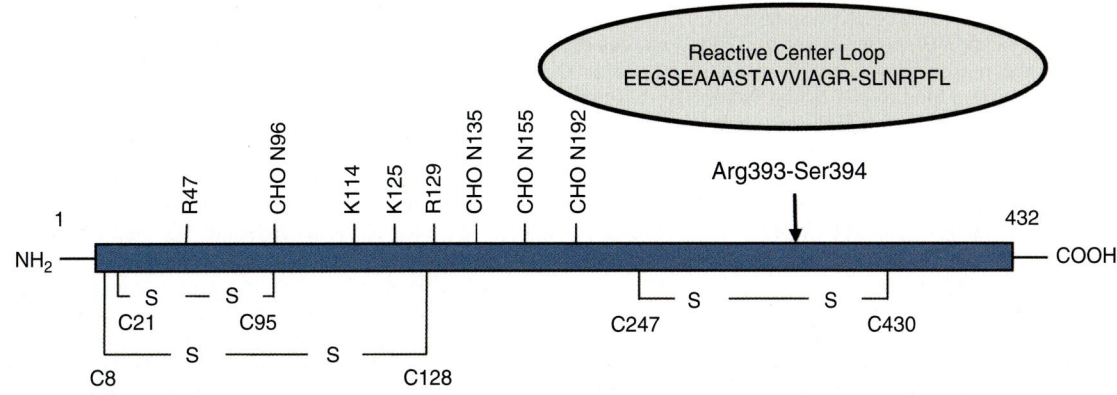

FIGURE 20.14 Soluble stoichiometric inhibitors. Tissue factor pathway inhibitor (TFPI) contains three Kunitz domains. TFPI inhibits the serine protease factor Xa (FXa) directly and tissue factor–factor VIIa complex in a factor Xa–dependent mechanism, shutting down the extrinsic pathway of coagulation. Kunitz 1 domain binds factor VIIa, Kunitz 2 domain binds factor Xa, and Kunitz 3 binds protein S with this interaction reported to enhance the activity of TFPI.[1232] The COOH terminus of TFPI contains a basic region (BR), the cell-binding domain, which binds to heparin, factor V-short, and partially activated factor V species. Antithrombin (AT) contains two intrachain disulfide bonds (-S-S-) in its NH_2 terminus and one in its COOH terminus with a carbohydrate-rich domain (CHO) in between. Asn^{135} is not glycosylated in the b form of AT. The region of interaction between the active sites of target proteases and AT is illustrated as a circle (reactive center loop) above the reactive site bond R^{393}-S^{394}. Heparin binding occurs in the NH_2 terminus involving interactions with residues R^{47}, K^{114}, K^{125}, and R^{129} and enhances the rate of inhibition of certain serine proteases.

raises the possibility that a portion of the antithrombotic effect of the polysaccharide may be mediated by TFPI. GPI-anchored TFPIα is not released by heparin therapy and represents the largest in vivo pool of TFPI. A minor pool of TFPI (~10% of total TFPI in blood) is located within platelets and is released after dual stimulation by collagen and thrombin.[1075] TFPIβ has Kunitz 1 and Kunitz 2 domains and a unique C-terminal region that contains a GPI-anchor sequence.[1382]

The qualitative and quantitative properties of TFPI can be altered both by the genotype of an individual and by environmental factors. This is illustrated by in vitro experiments in which factor V^Leiden is combined with reduced levels of TFPI. Factor V^Leiden, when combined with TFPI levels that are at the low end (50%) of the normal range, can produce an unregulated propagation phase of thrombin generation in a synthetic plasma system.[1406] In a control with normal factor V, the propagation phase of thrombin generation is attenuated substantially at the tissue factor concentrations used in this experiment (i.e., it is near threshold). With factor V^Leiden and low normal TFPI, the propagation phase of thrombin generation is equivalent to a situation in which the protein C regulatory system is totally dysfunctional. This observation suggests the risk of thrombotic pathology. An in vivo parallel to this in vitro experiment has been reported by Eitzman et al,[1407] who showed that factor V^Leiden (+/+) mice with reduced levels of TFPI (+/−) died of thrombosis.

Function

TFPI is the principal stoichiometric inhibitor of the extrinsic pathway (factor VIIa–tissue factor) of coagulation (*Figure 20.7*). The extrinsic pathway generates low levels of the serine proteases, factor IXa (~1 pmol/L), and factor Xa (~10 pmol/L).[583] As soon as the proteases are formed, factor Xa can activate prothrombin to generate thrombin and factor IXa can combine with its cofactor factor VIIIa and form the intrinsic tenase complex to generate more factor Xa. This is followed by the formation of the prothrombinase complex (factor Xa–factor Va), which converts prothrombin to thrombin. The TFPI mechanism allows the factor VIIa–tissue factor complex to initiate factor Xa formation but then suppresses high levels of factor Xa product formation by this complex. TFPI is the principal regulator of the initiation phase of thrombin generation[583] (*Figure 20.13*).

The actual mechanism involves a rapid interaction between the second Kunitz domain of TFPI with the factor Xa active site; localization of the complex to the membrane surface is mediated by the Gla domain of factor Xa.[642,1408,1409] Once surface bound, the factor Xa–TFPI complex rapidly inactivates tissue factor–factor VIIa. This complex formation depends on the binding of the first Kunitz domain of TFPI to the factor VIIa active site. These interactions together form a stable quaternary complex, tissue factor–factor VIIa–TFPI–factor Xa. Ethylenediaminetetraacetic acid can readily dissociate this inhibited quaternary complex. Protein S enhances TFPIα inhibition of factor Xa[1237]; although whether this affects TFPIα suppression of the factor VIIa–tissue factor complex is controversial.[1410]

Inhibition of factor VIIa–tissue factor by TFPI is not completely dependent on the presence of factor Xa because the factor IXa–TFPI complex can also bind to and inhibit factor VIIa–tissue factor. However, the binding affinity of TFPI for factor IXa is significantly less than for factor Xa. The physiologic relevance of this route of inhibition is thus debatable because high plasma concentrations of TFPI are required. At normal plasma concentrations, this multicomponent interaction of TFPI allows basal function of the factor VIIa–tissue factor complex but inhibits it after more extensive activation occurs.

When combined with the stoichiometric inhibitor antithrombin, a synergistic regulatory effect of blood coagulation occurs by inducing kinetic "thresholds" such that the initiating tissue factor stimulus must achieve a significant magnitude to propel thrombin generation.[1411] Tissue factor concentrations below the threshold concentration are ineffective in promoting robust thrombin generation because of the cooperative influence of the inhibitors; concentrations in excess of the threshold yield robust and almost equivalent thrombin generation. In a similar fashion, TFPI and the dynamic protein C–thrombomodulin–thrombin system cooperate to provide a threshold-limited, synergistic inhibition of thrombin production.[1412] In this instance, TFPI slows the

initiation phase, whereas the APC system reduces the availability of the cofactors factors Va and VIIIa, thereby shutting down the propagation phase of thrombin generation (*Figure 20.13*).

Regulation

TFPI administered intravenously to rats and mice is cleared rapidly from the circulation by liver hepatocytes, which recognize its COOH-terminal region (third Kunitz domain and basic COOH terminus).[1413-1415] TFPI is cleared by the promiscuous endocytic receptor, low-density LRP. Several lines of evidence suggest that TFPI binding to heparin-like sites on the cell surface may precede its catabolism by LRP. In addition, TFPI appears to be important for factor Xa catabolism. TFPI-factor Xa complexes are cleared by a liver receptor that is distinct from LRP.

ANTICOAGULANT PROTEINS: SERINE PROTEASE INHIBITOR SUPERFAMILY (SERPIN)

Inhibitory serpins are irreversible covalent suicide protease inhibitors. These inhibitors target serine proteases, a family of proteolytic enzymes sharing common active site architectures and common catalytic mechanisms. Key features of these enzymes include a nucleophilic serine hydroxyl moiety that attacks the carbonyl group of the targeted bond and the formation of a transient acyl-enzyme intermediate between the enzyme and the NH2-terminal part of the substrate polypeptide. In vivo, when a serpin successfully reacts with a protease, catalysis of serpin proteolysis is arrested at the acyl-enzyme stage and the serpin-enzyme complex is cleared from the circulation by specific receptor-mediated processes. Members of this multigene inhibitor family include antithrombin, heparin cofactor II, α1-proteinase inhibitor (also known as α1-*antitrypsin*), C1 esterase inhibitor, protein C inhibitor, PAI-1, α2-antiplasmin, protein Z–dependent protease inhibitor, and protease nexin-1. Plasminogen activator-1 and α2-antiplasmin are discussed in detail in the section Inhibitors of the Fibrinolytic System, and protein Z–dependent protease inhibitor is discussed briefly in the section Protein Z. Serpins function in diverse physiologic processes including blood coagulation, fibrinolysis, complement activation, angiogenesis, apoptosis, inflammation, neoplasia, and viral pathogenesis[1416-1418] (*Table 20.7*). When a member of the serpin family is either deficient or dysfunctional, several biologic disorders are evidenced, including thrombosis,[1419,1420] emphysema,[1421] lupus erythematosus,[1422] liver disease,[1423] and dementia.[1424]

In the past 2 decades, advances have been made to further understand the mechanism of action of serpins.[1109,1425-1436] Serpins in uncleaved states (native or latent) and cleaved states have been crystallized.[1433,1437,1438] Achievement of the first crystal structure for a serpin-protease complex (α1-antitrypsin-trypsin)[1439] has confirmed the physical displacement of the tethered protease: the conformation of α1-antitrypsin in the complex is superimposable with that of the isolated cleaved α1-antitrypsin. The crystal structure also revealed that the translocated, tethered protease has undergone an overall 37% loss of structure with its catalytic site radically disrupted.

Inhibitory serpins share a similar backbone structure but expose a variable reactive site loop. This loop binds to the catalytic groove of the target proteases. Serpin specificity derives in part from the sequence of the reactive site loop and also from secondary binding sites.[1440,1441] Initially, the reaction of a serpin and serine protease involves formation of a noncovalent Michaelis complex between the exposed reactive site loop and the protease active site. Exosite interactions between the two molecules, or in some cases, exosite binding of a cofactor, induce structural changes that increase the availability of the reactive site loop. Reversible complex formation is followed by reaction of the active site serine residue of the protease with the serpin "bait" peptide bond to form an acyl-enzyme intermediate. Trapping of this covalent complex between the reactive site loop and the protease appears to involve a process that both physically translocates the reactive loop-protease complex approximately 71 Å from the initial docking site and induces a general disordering of the protease's

Table 20.7. Inhibitors

Serpin	System(s) Regulated	Target Protease(s)	Deficiency State
Antithrombin	Coagulation	Thrombin, FXa, FIXa, kallikrein,[a] FXIa, and FVIIa[b]	Thrombosis
Heparin cofactor II	Coagulation	Thrombin	Thrombosis in some individuals
Protein C inhibitor	Coagulation	APC, kallikrein	None reported
α_1-Proteinase inhibitor	Inflammation	Elastase	Pulmonary emphysema
	Tissue remodeling	Cathepsin G	—
	Coagulation	APC, FXIa, and FXa	—
Plasminogen activator inhibitor-1	Fibrinolysis	Tissue-type plasminogen activator, urokinase-type plasminogen activator	Bleeding
α_2-Antiplasmin	Fibrinolysis	Plasmin	Bleeding
C1 esterase inhibitor	Complement	C1r, C1s	Angioedema
	Contact factors	FXIIa, kallikrein	—
	Coagulation	FXIa	—
Protease nexin-1	Coagulation	Thrombin	None reported

Abbreviations: APC, activated protein C; F, factor.
[a]Reaction also requires the presence of high-molecular-weight kininogen.
[b]Antithrombin-heparin inhibits factor VIIa only when bound to tissue factor.

conformation with consequent loss of any further catalytic activity.[1439] The energy for translocation and structural alteration of the protease derives from the insertion of the proteolytically released reactive site loop of the serpin into β sheet A of its central core. A kinetic partitioning of serpin-protease reactions between stable inhibited complexes and mixtures of regenerated enzyme and proteolyzed serpin reflects the relative rates of reactive site loop insertion versus deacylation.[1442] A number of recent reviews have been written on the known serpin conformations and their biologic significance.[1416,1443-1450]

Antithrombin

Antithrombin is a member of the serpin proteinase inhibitory family and circulates in blood as a single-chain glycoprotein[307] (*Table 20.4*). Its $t_{1/2}$ is approximately 61 to 72 hours.[1451,1452] Other names for antithrombin include *antithrombin–heparin cofactor* and *heparin cofactor*. Despite its name, antithrombin inhibits not only thrombin but also many of the other enzymes in the coagulation pathway.

Congenital antithrombin deficiency exhibits an autosomal dominant pattern of inheritance, with an incidence of 1:2000 to 1:5000.[1453] The complete absence of antithrombin is lethal. Individuals with this deficiency have partial expression of antithrombin and are prone to thromboembolic disease.[1454] Inherited deficiency is categorized by either quantitative defect with a reduction in antigen and activity (type I) or qualitative with reduced antithrombin functional activity and normal antigen levels (type II).[1455] These defects are caused by a variety of mutations that include insertions, deletions, and missense mutations.[1456-1458] Function can be compromised by mutations in the thrombin-binding domain or the heparin-binding domain. Unstable variants of antithrombin have been identified in families with severe episodic thrombotic disease. Acquired antithrombin deficiency occurs in patients with sepsis or severe traumatic shock.[1459,1460] Therefore, studies are being conducted on the use of antithrombin as an agent for treating coagulation abnormalities associated with sepsis or other inflammation disorders.[1461,1462]

Gene Structure and Expression

The gene encoding antithrombin is located on chromosome 1 at band q25.1[1463] and spans 13.5 kb of genomic DNA[1464] (*Table 20.6*). The gene is composed of seven exons and six introns.[1464] The mechanisms underlying antithrombin gene expression are not well established. It is primarily expressed in the liver with low levels detected in the brain and kidney. *Cis*-acting elements and *trans*-acting factors have been identified that regulate constitutive expression of the human antithrombin gene.[1465]

Biochemistry

Human antithrombin is a single-chain glycoprotein ($M_r = 58,000$) that circulates in blood at a concentration of approximately 140 µg/mL (2.4 µmol/L)[307,1466]. It circulates as two glycoforms, α and β variants, that contain identical polypeptide backbones but differ in carbohydrate content and heparin affinity.[1467] The antithrombin α variant is the predominant form (~90%).[1468] The structure of antithrombin α consists of 432 amino acid residues, with three disulfide bonds and four sialylated oligosaccharides at Asn^{96}, Asn^{135}, Asn^{155}, and Asn^{192} (*Figure 20.14B*). The carbohydrate residues account for 15% of the total mass.[1468-1471] The antithrombin β variant is not glycosylated at Asn^{135}. Antithrombin β binds heparin more tightly than does antithrombin α and is observed to preferentially accumulate on the vessel wall when heparan sulfate proteoglycans are exposed.[1472] The reactive site peptide bond is Arg^{393}-Ser^{394}.

The first x-ray crystal structure of antithrombin that was determined was a cleaved form that diffracted to 3.2 Å resolution.[1473] Significant differences between structures of antithrombin and another serpin, α_1-antitrypsin, were identified in the NH_2-terminal region that defines the heparin-binding site. Since then, several x-ray crystal structures of intact antithrombin have been solved to 2.6 to 3.0 Å.[1474-1476]

Function

Antithrombin has a broad spectrum of inhibitory activity with most of its target proteases participating in the coagulation cascade. It is primarily an inhibitor of the serine protease thrombin as well as factor Xa, factor IXa, factor VIIa–tissue factor, factor XIa, factor XIIa, and plasma kallikrein.[1477-1479] Antithrombin plays a key role in maintaining hemostasis. Antithrombin also displays antiproliferative and anti-inflammatory properties that primarily derive from its ability to inhibit thrombin. In addition, latent or cleaved forms of antithrombin have antiangiogenic activities.[1480] Heparins and heparan sulfates potentiate these reactions and are used in the treatment of thrombosis.[1481] When antithrombin is complexed with heparin, its rate of inhibition of several coagulation proteases is accelerated by up to 10,000-fold.

In general, binding of heparins to antithrombin improves its reactivities with proteases in two ways: (1) by inducing conformational changes in antithrombin, including better presentation both of the reactive center loop and of exosites on antithrombin that interact with target enzymes; and (2) by enabling a template effect, whereby binding of enzyme and antithrombin to the same heparin molecule improves the likelihood of the interaction.

The mechanism of inhibition involves reaction of the active site of the enzyme with a peptide loop structure (reactive center loop, *Figure 20.14B*) of the serpin to form a tight, equimolar (1:1) complex. Inactivation is suspected to proceed through covalent bond formation between antithrombin and the protease, followed by inactivating structural rearrangements of both antithrombin and the protease. However, the exact mechanism of inhibition of serine proteases by antithrombin is uncertain. In the case of factor Xa inhibition, crystallographic data indicate that heparin-induced conformational change in antithrombin permits contacts between antithrombin and the active site and two exosites of factor Xa.[1482]

Heparin Cofactor II (Leuserpin 2)

Heparin cofactor II, also called *leuserpin 2,* is a member of the serpin family.[1483] Like antithrombin, heparin cofactor II inhibits thrombin in a reaction that is accelerated more than 1000-fold by heparin.[1484] However, heparin cofactor II is unique in that it is also stimulated by the proteoglycan dermatan sulfate. The plasma concentration of heparin cofactor II is 0.5 to 1.4 μmol/L[1485,1486] (*Table 20.4*). Its plasma $t_{1/2}$ is approximately 2.5 days. The physiologic role of heparin cofactor II is uncertain at the present time. Low levels of thrombin–heparin cofactor II complexes are detected in normal plasma samples; elevated levels were detected in patients with DIC.[1487] Although inherited deficiency of heparin cofactor II has been associated with thrombosis, this is not always the case.[1488-1490] The incidence of heparin cofactor II deficiency in patients with thromboembolytic disorders appears to be similar to that in the normal population.[1491]

Gene Structure and Expression

The gene encoding human heparin cofactor II, consisting of five exons and four introns, spans approximately 14 kb on chromosome 22 at band q11.21 proximal to the breakpoint cluster region.[1492,1493] The human heparin cofactor II gene is expressed exclusively in the liver and by a hepatoma-derived cell line.[1494,1495]

Biochemistry

Human heparin cofactor II ($M_r = 66,000$) circulates as a single-chain protein of 480 amino acid residues that contains 10% carbohydrate (*Figure 20.15*).[1485,1493,1494] It is glycosylated at Asn^{30}, Asn^{169}, and Asn^{368} and is sulfated at Tyr^{60} and Tyr^{73}. It has three cysteines with no identified disulfide bonds. A cationic region of the molecule encompassing residues 163 to 194 constitutes the GAG-binding site; dermatan sulfate and heparin bind to heparin cofactor II at nonidentical but overlapping sites in this region.[1496,1497] Residues Lys^{173}, Arg^{184}, Lys^{185}, Arg^{189}, Arg^{192}, and Arg^{193} have been specifically implicated in heparin binding.[1498] The NH_2-terminal region of heparin cofactor II contains a cluster of acidic residues that are thought to interact with the positively charged GAG-binding site.[1499,1500] This "acidic" tail of heparin cofactor II contains two so-called hirudin domains—$Glu^{56}AspAspAspTyrLeuAsp^{62}$ and $Glu^{69}AspAspAspTyrIleAsp^{75}$; in each, the Tyr residue is sulfated. It has been proposed that the NH_2-terminal "acidic" tail is constrained in the native structure through association with the highly cationic heparin-binding region. In the presence of GAG, the acidic region is displaced from the heparin-binding site, thus making it available for binding to the anion-binding exosite I of thrombin.[1501] However, crystallographic studies of heparin cofactor II indicate that the acidic tail of heparin cofactor II is flexible in the crystal and not associated with the heparin-binding site.[1433] Other functionally important regions of heparin cofactor II include a chemotactic peptide harbored between residues Asp^{49} and Tyr^{60} that is released by leukocyte proteases.[1502] Residues Phe^{456} to Ile^{460} constitute a pentapeptide recognition motif for the hepatic serpin-enzyme complex receptor that may be involved in clearance of heparin cofactor II–enzyme complexes.[1503]

The domain of heparin cofactor II with homology to other serpins is at the COOH terminus of the protein. It exhibits approximately 30% homology to antithrombin and other serpins. The reactive site peptide bond is Leu^{444}-Ser^{445}.[1504] This reactive center loop sequence is consistent for an inhibitor with specificity for proteases with a preference for nonpolar residues with relatively bulky side chains in the P1 position. Two such proteases, chymotrypsin and cathepsin G, do react with heparin cofactor II. Thrombin reactivity with heparin cofactor II is unusual because thrombin generally prefers substrates with arginine in the P1 position. Exosite binding interactions, such as that between the hirudin-like sequences of heparin cofactor II and exosite I of thrombin, compensate for the less-than-ideal structure of the P1 residue and allow thrombin to form a productive Michaelis complex with heparin cofactor II.[1433,1505]

Function

The only coagulation enzyme inhibited by heparin cofactor II appears to be thrombin.[1506] However, the rate of thrombin inhibition by heparin cofactor II in the absence or presence of GAGs is significantly slower than by antithrombin under similar conditions. Considering that the plasma concentration of heparin cofactor II is 25% to 50% that of antithrombin and that low levels of heparin cofactor II are not strongly associated with thrombosis,[1507] the physiologic role of heparin cofactor II as a systemic thrombin inhibitor has been questioned. In vitro, heparin cofactor II inhibition of thrombin is stimulated by dermatan sulfate proteoglycans synthesized by fibroblasts and vascular smooth muscle cells.[1508] Thus, heparin cofactor II may be uniquely suited to regulate extravascular thrombin in areas of vascular endothelium disruption, in which heparin cofactor II would be exclusively stimulated by dermatan sulfate in the subendothelial

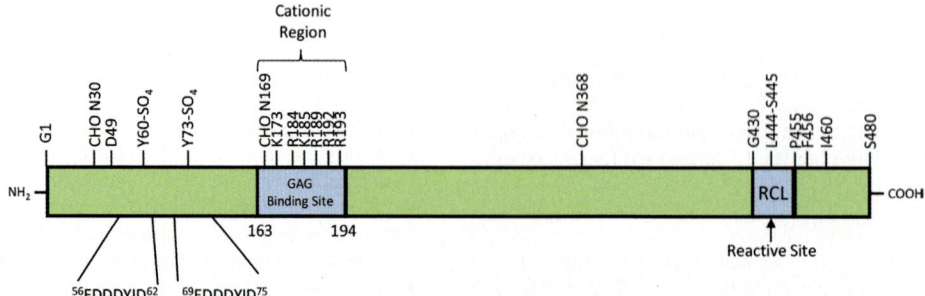

Heparin cofactor II (leuserpin-2): 66 kDa

FIGURE 20.15 Schematic of Heparin cofactor II (leuserpin 2). The protein is a serine protease inhibitor targeting a-thrombin. Both dermatan sulfate and heparin enhance its rate of inhibition of α-thrombin. Key structural features of the NH_2 terminus of the molecule include two "hirudin-like" acidic domains, each containing a sulfated tyrosine residue, which mediate binding interaction with exosite 1 of thrombin, and a highly cationic cluster of amino acids expressing overlapping binding sites for heparin and dermatan sulfate. Key structural features of the COOH terminus of the molecule include a reactive center loop (RCL) containing the reactive site peptide bond (L444-S445) and a recognition motif for hepatic serpin-enzyme complex receptor (P456-I460).

layers.[1509] In addition, heparin cofactor II may participate in regulation of acute inflammation and wound healing by harboring a peptide chemotactic for neutrophils and monocytes that is released by leukocyte proteolysis.[1502]

Heparin cofactor II may also have a role in protection from thrombosis during pregnancy. Increased levels of dermatan sulfate in the maternal and fetal circulation[1510] along with increased levels of heparin cofactor II in pregnant women have been reported.[1511,1512] Heparin cofactor II has also been reported to potentiate the activation of endothelial cells and promote angiogenesis.[1513]

α_1-Proteinase Inhibitor (α_1-Antitrypsin)

α_1-Proteinase inhibitor is the most abundant circulating inhibitor of the serpin family. It is a single-chain glycoprotein that circulates in blood at a concentration of 1.5 to 3.5 mg/mL with a relative molecular weight of 53,000[1339,1514] (*Table 20.4*). It is synthesized predominantly in the liver and has a $t_{1/2}$ of 6 days.[1515] α_1-Proteinase inhibitor is considered an acute-phase reactant.[1516]

Deficiency in α_1-proteinase inhibitor is a common autosomal recessive disorder (1:1600-1:1800) that can potentially be lethal.[1517,1518] It is found associated with emphysema,[1421] liver cirrhosis,[1423] and hepatocellular carcinoma.[1423] Treatment for α_1-proteinase inhibitor deficiency relies on infusions of human plasma-derived α_1-proteinase inhibitor.[1519] Progress is under way to develop a therapy based on gene repair[1520-1522] or strategies to block aberrant conformational transitions.[1518,1519,1523]

Gene Structure and Expression

The gene for α_1-proteinase inhibitor is located on chromosome 14 band q32.13, is approximately 5 kb long,[1524] and contains seven exons and six introns[1524-1527] (*Table 20.6*). Uniquely, α_1-antichymotrypsin, corticosteroid-binding globulin, kallistatin, and protein C inhibitor also map to the same region on chromosome 14.[1526,1528,1529] These genes are actively transcribed in the liver and cultured hepatoma cells. However, a few other cell types (macrophages and intestinal epithelial cells) express some of these serpin genes.[1530] Hepatocyte nuclear factor-1α and hepatocyte nuclear factor-4 play important roles in expression of the α_1-proteinase inhibitor gene in hepatic, intestinal, and pulmonary epithelial cells.[1531]

Biochemistry

α_1-Proteinase inhibitor is the most studied of the serpins, with high-resolution crystal structures achieved for the inhibitor by itself and in complex with a target protease.[1418] The 394-amino-acid sequence for human α_1-proteinase inhibitor shows 1 cysteine and 3 glucosamine-based carbohydrate chains (*Figure 20.16*).[1532,1533] The reactive site bond that is targeted by serine proteinases is between Met(358) and Ser(359).[1534] Studies using (13)C nuclear magnetic resonance spectroscopy of the complex between human 13Cmethionine-labeled α_1-proteinase inhibitor and porcine pancreatic elastase have shown that a tetrahedral intermediate complex is formed during the serpin-proteinase interactions.[1535] The three-dimensional x-ray crystal structure of cleaved α_1-proteinase inhibitor identified that, for activity, α_1-proteinase inhibitor requires the insertion of a single residue, Thr345, into β sheet A.[1536] This was supported by the x-ray crystal structures of α_1-proteinase inhibitor complexed with synthetic peptides that correspond to the unprimed NH2-terminal side of the active site loop.[1537] The five-stranded β sheet A of α_1-proteinase inhibitor undergoes conformational changes that facilitate and stabilize the insertion into sheet A of the reactive center loop after cleavage by its target serine proteases. The solution structure of α_1-proteinase inhibitor has also been characterized by high-flux neutron scattering and by synchrotron x-ray scattering.[1538]

Function

α_1-Proteinase inhibitor can inhibit a wide range of serine proteases. Its primary physiologic target is the inhibition of neutrophil elastase to protect the elastin fibers of the lung. The role of α_1-proteinase inhibitor in blood coagulation is minimal. It has been shown to inhibit factor XIa in vivo[1539,1540] to be an important inhibitor of factor Xa in purified and plasma systems.[644] APC complexes with α_1-proteinase inhibitor have also been detected by enzyme-linked immunosorbent assay in patients with DIC.[1541] Inhibition by α_1-proteinase inhibitor is heparin independent.

C1 Esterase Inhibitor

C1 esterase inhibitor is a member of the serpin proteinase inhibitor family that is present at 170 µg/mL in blood[1542] (*Table 20.4*). It is predominantly synthesized in the liver. When complexed with a protease (e.g., factor XIa), it has a $t_{1/2}$ of 95 to 104 minutes.[1540] Targets for C1 esterase inhibitor are found in the complement cascade and the coagulation cascade.

Deficiency in C1 esterase inhibitor can result in hereditary angioedema[1543] and has been identified in a patient with lupus erythematosus.[1422] Cases of acquired C1 esterase inhibitor deficiency have been reported associated with splenic lymphoma.[1544,1545] C1 esterase inhibitor-deficient mice show no obvious phenotypic abnormality,[1546] although, in conjunction with a bradykinin type 2 receptor knockout, diminished vascular permeability was observed.[1546] The C1 esterase inhibitor is used in the treatment of hereditary angioedema[1547,1548] and sepsis.[1549] Its potential use in reducing ischemia reperfusion injury is being investigated.[1550]

α_1-proteinase inhibitor (α_1-antitrypsin) – 53 kDa

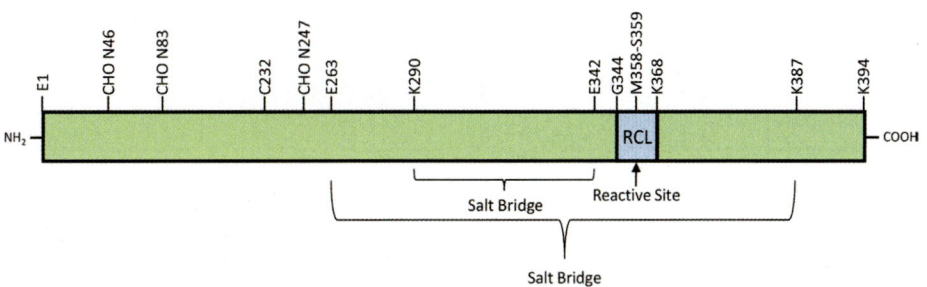

FIGURE 20.16 Schematic of α_1-proteinase inhibitor (α_1-PI): α_1-PI or α_1-antitrypsin is a member of the serine protease inhibitor family A, which also includes protein C inhibitor and protein Z inhibitor. Its primary physiologic target appears to be neutrophil elastase. Mutations in α_1-PI gene resulting in misfolding, accumulation of misfolded protein polymers, or decreases in secreted, functional molecules have been strongly associated with disease pathogenesis.[1532] Key structural features of the protein include three N-linked carbohydrate chains at N46, N83, and N247, as well as two important salt bridges E342-K290 and E263-K387. Mutations that disrupt either salt bridge result in decreased plasma levels with pathologic consequences in homozygous carriers,[1532,1533] no disulfide bonds with single cysteine (C232), and a reactive center loop (RCL) containing the reactive site peptide bond (M358-S359).

Gene Structure and Expression

The primary structure of human C1 esterase inhibitor was initially determined by peptide and DNA sequencing.[1551] The only proteolytic processing that occurs is that a 22-residue signal peptide required for secretion is cleaved. The C1 esterase inhibitor gene is located on chromosome 11 band p12.1[1551] (*Table 20.6*). The C1 esterase inhibitor gene consists of eight exons and seven introns and is approximately 17 kb in length.[1552] In vivo, androgens enhance expression of C1 esterase inhibitor. In vitro studies show that C1 esterase inhibitor mRNA and protein levels increase after stimulation with γ- and α-interferon, TNF-α, IL-6, and monocyte colony-stimulating factor.[1552]

The molecular defects found associated with C1 esterase inhibitor deficiency include *Alu* repeat-mediated deletions, missense mutations, frame shifts, stop codon mutations, promoter variants, splice site mutations, or deletions of a few amino acids.[1553,1554] The clinical manifestation of this deficiency is predominantly angioedema.

Biochemistry

C1 esterase inhibitor is a single-chain glycoprotein containing 478 amino acid residues that circulates with an apparent molecular mass of 104,000 when analyzed by SDS-PAGE (*Figure 20.17*). The amino acids account for only 51% of the apparent molecular mass of the circulating protein, with 35% of the remaining mass accounted for by carbohydrate moieties.[1542] Neutron scattering, x-ray crystal structure determinations, (^{1})H nuclear magnetic resonance spectroscopy, and Fourier transform infrared spectroscopy have been used to study the structure of C1 esterase inhibitor, revealing a two-domain structure.[1559-1561] The NH$_2$ terminus, containing 113 amino acids, is heavily glycosylated with 3 N-linked and 7 O-linked oligosaccharides. The COOH terminus contains 365 amino acids with 3 N-linked oligosaccharides. When C1 esterase reacts with target proteases, the serpin undergoes changes in its whole secondary structure—not only the reactive site loop.

Function

C1 esterase inhibitor is a member of the serpin inhibitor family. It plays an important role in the regulation of the classic complement pathway, specifically as the sole regulator of the activities of C1r and C1s.[1562] C1 esterase inhibitor's role in coagulation is mainly targeted to the contact activation pathway through the regulation of kallikrein,[145,188] factor XII,[146] factor XIIa,[148] and factor XIa.[297,304,1492,1493,1563] Unlike other serpin inhibitors, such as antithrombin, protein C inhibitor, or PAI-1, the activity of C1 esterase inhibitor is not affected by heparin.[1564]

Protein C Inhibitor (Plasminogen Activator Inhibitor-3)

Protein C inhibitor is a member of the serine proteinase inhibitor family. It is also known as *PAI-3*. Protein C inhibitor is considered nonspecific in that its targets range from procoagulant, anticoagulant, and fibrinolytic enzymes to plasma and tissue kallikreins, the sperm protease acrosin, and prostate-specific antigen.[1565,1566] It circulates in blood at a concentration of 5 µg/mL[1567,1568] (*Table 20.4*) and is cleared from the circulation with a $t_{1/2}$ of 1 day. When in complex with a target (e.g., APC), it is cleared from circulation with a $t_{1/2}$ of 20 minutes.[1569] Hereditary or acquired protein C inhibitor deficiency has not been documented to date.[1570] A case control study of thrombophilia showed that high levels of protein C inhibitor might constitute a mild risk factor for venous thrombosis. Protein C inhibitor–deficient mice (–/–) show impaired spermatogenesis and male infertility.[1571]

Gene Structure and Expression

The gene for protein C inhibitor has been mapped to chromosome 14 band q32.1 (*Table 20.6*). It is 11.5 kb in length and consists of five exons separated by four introns.[1572,1573] The organization and location of this gene are similar to those of the genes for α_1-antitrypsin and α_1-antichymotrypsin, suggesting a common ancestor for these genes.[1572,1574,1575] Human protein C inhibitor is mainly synthesized in the liver,[1568] but it has also been identified in platelets and megakaryocytes,[1576,1577] the kidney,[1578] and the testes, seminal vesicle, and prostate.[1578]

Biochemistry

Human protein C inhibitor in blood has a relative molecular weight of 57,000.[1567,1574] The mature protein contains 387 amino acids; a 19-amino-acid signal peptide is present before secretion (*Figure 20.18*). Five potential N-linked glycosylation sites were found in the mature

C1 esterase inhibitor: 104 kDa

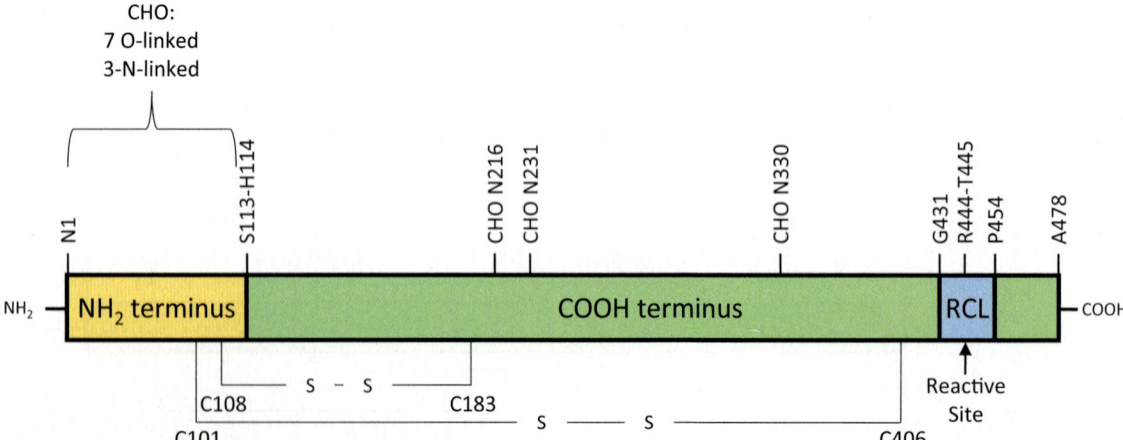

FIGURE 20.17 Schematic of C1 esterase inhibitor. C1 esterase inhibitor is a multifunctional serpin, functioning as the primary plasma inhibitor of complement activation and of contact pathway activation of coagulation.[1555] Two important functional domains are depicted: the reactive center loop and reactive site bond R444-T445 localized at the C terminus of the molecule and the heavily glycosylated N-terminal domain. The two disulfide bridges linking the N-terminal region to the C-terminal region appear to stabilize the RCL in its reactive conformation thereby maintaining its interaction kinetics with target proteases.[1556] The N-terminal domain has no homology with other members of the serpin family; removal of residues 1 to 98 from C1 esterase had no effect on its inhibitory properties.[1556,1557] The N-terminal region appears to mediate the interaction of C1 esterase inhibitor with cells and extracellular matrix; potential roles for C1 esterase inhibitor that are independent of its role in inhibiting complement and coagulation proteases are under investigation.[1558]

Protein C Inhibitor (PCI, PAI-3): 57 kDa

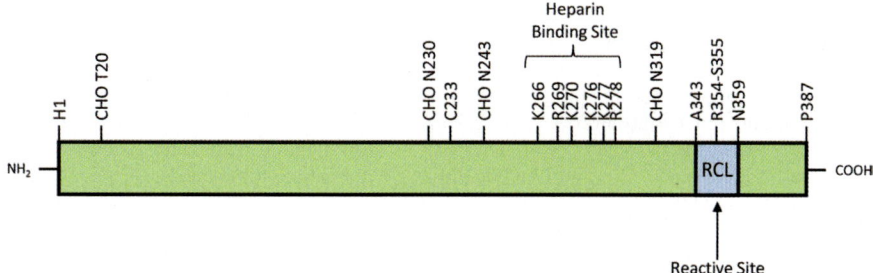

FIGURE 20.18 Schematic of Protein C inhibitor (PCI). The protein is a relatively nonspecific serine protease inhibitor and functions as the primary plasma protein inhibitor of activated protein C (APC) and as an efficient inhibitor of the thrombin-thrombomodulin complex, the catalyst that converts protein C to APC. It is present in platelet alpha granules and when released during platelet activation appears to localize to the platelet surface. PCI isolates appear highly heterogeneous because of differences in N-glycan structures, N-glycosylation occupancy, and N-terminal sequence.[1579] Key structural features include a cluster of cationic residues that mediate PCI binding to heparin, a free thiol (C233), a reactive center loop (RCL) containing the reactive site peptide bond (R354-S355), and three asparagine-linked glycans that appear to modulate PCI reactivity with serine proteases.[1580]

protein,[1574] and their roles in protein C inhibitor activity have been studied by mutational analysis.[1580] The reactive site bond is located at Arg^{354}-Ser^{355}, and a stable 1:1 molar complex is formed between protein C inhibitor and its target proteinases. Protein C inhibitor binds heparin, and its activity is accelerated when in complex with heparin[1581]; unlike other related heparin-binding serpins such as antithrombin, heparin cofactor II, and protease nexin, the primary heparin-binding site of protein C inhibitor is in the H helix, not the D helix.[1582] A recent crystal structure of this inhibitor provides a structural basis for understanding its multiple functions.[1583]

Function

Protein C inhibitor is a nonspecific inhibitor of serine proteinases and inhibits APC, thrombin, thrombin-thrombomodulin, factor Xa, u-PA,[1584-1586] and t-PA.[1587,1588] The major target of protein C inhibitor, as its name suggests, is APC,[1569,1589,1590] although from a kinetic point of view, the reaction with thrombin-thrombomodulin is the most favorable.[1588] This is the physiologically most important inhibitor of APC. Protein C inhibitor has been shown to regulate TAFI activation by inhibiting the thrombin-thrombomodulin complex.[1584] Its importance as a dual regulator of coagulation and fibrinolysis remains unresolved.[1591] The importance of the regulation of APC by protein C inhibitor is evident by the use of this complex as a marker for detection of deep vein thrombosis.[1592] Other targets for protein C inhibitor include human kallikrein,[195] factor Xia,[195] factor Xa, and thrombin. Because there are no documented patients with a deficiency to date, the actual function of protein C inhibitor in vivo is yet to be elucidated.

PROTEINS OF CLOT FORMATION

Early efforts to understand how blood clots form were directed at dissecting the vertebrate coagulation system and determining its components. This work revealed the central event in blood coagulation to be the conversion of soluble fibrinogen (factor I) to insoluble fibrin. Basically, this is accomplished when the coagulation enzyme thrombin (factor IIa) removes small polar peptides (termed *fibrinopeptides*) from each fibrinogen molecule, forming fibrin. These fibrin molecules noncovalently interact with each other, forming a fibrin web. Fibrin stabilization is accomplished by the action of a second coagulation enzyme (factor XIIIa) that introduces numerous covalent cross-links between these fibrin molecules. The resulting fibrin web is able to capture platelets and red blood cells, effectively sealing the wound and stemming plasma loss.

Factor XIII (Fibrin Stabilizing Factor)

The first apparent suggestion of cross-linked fibrin by factor XIII came in 1923 from Barkan and Gaspar, who reported that fibrinogen

preparations, when clotted in the presence of Ca^{2+}, generated clots that were insoluble in weak bases.[1593,1594] Later, in the 1940s, work by Robbins,[1595] Laki and Lorand,[1596] and Lorand[1597] confirmed the presence of a serum factor that caused the transition to an insoluble clot and termed it *fibrin stabilizing factor*. It was not until 1963 that the International Committee on Blood Clotting Factors acknowledged fibrin stabilizing factor as a clotting factor and termed it *factor XIII*.[1598] Recommended terms and abbreviations for factor XIII have been established.[1594]

Factor XIII functions as a transglutaminase that can form cross-linked amide bonds between specific glutamine and lysine residues on polypeptide chains. It plays an important role in hemostasis and thrombosis as well as participates in physiologic processes of cell proliferation and cell migration. Factor XIIIa has multiple substrates including fibrin(ogen), fibronectin, α_2-plasmin inhibitor, collagen, vitronectin, vWF, actin, myosin, factor V, and thrombospondin.[1599-1607] Recent reviews discuss the role of factor XIII in blood clotting,[1608] angiogenesis,[1609] cellular function,[1610] inflammation,[1611] and cardiac and vascular diseases.[1612]

Gene Structure and Expression

Plasma factor XIII circulates as a heterotetramer composed of two A-chains and two B-chains. The genes are located on different chromosomes. The gene for the factor XIII A subunit is located on chromosome 6 band p25.1[1613,1614] and spans approximately 160 kb[1615] (*Table 20.2*). The gene has 15 exons specifying a mature protein of 731 amino acids. The circulating product of the B subunit gene is a protein of 641 amino acids. The gene is located on chromosome 1 band q31.3,[1616] spans approximately 28 kb, and has 12 exons[1617] (*Table 20.2*). Ten short homologous units, termed *sushi* or *glycoprotein-1 domains*, are coded for by exons 2 to 11 in the B subunit gene.[1618,1619] Proteins associated with regulation of the complement system also contain sushi domains.[1620,1621]

Factor XIII deficiency is autosomal recessive and is a rare bleeding disorder. It has a frequency in the general population of 1 in 2 million.[1622,1623] The phenotype displays varying degrees of bleeding and is typically associated with the absence of cross-linking of fibrin monomers and impaired cross-linking of α_2-antiplasmin inhibitor to fibrin.[1624] Mutations have been identified in both the A and B subunits,[1625] with the latter being the least common. Reviews by Loewy et al[1624] and Ariens et al[1626] describe the deficiency mutations and polymorphisms for both gene products that have been identified to date.

Five common polymorphisms in the A subunit have been identified. Three of these (Val34Leu, Pro564Leu, and Glu651Gln) have allele frequencies >0.2. Adverse effects have not been associated with the Glu651Gln variation; however, young women with the Leu564/Leu564 genotype may be at increased risk of hemorrhagic stroke.[1627] The (Val34→Leu) polymorphism in the A subunit is found in approximately 25% of the population.[1628] This Val to Leu replacement takes place three amino acids away from the thrombin cleavage site at Arg[37]-Gly[38].[1628] Owing to its close proximity to the thrombin cleavage site, it has been postulated that this mutation might modulate factor XIII activation. Studies suggest that this polymorphism is a determining factor in arterial and venous thrombosis.[1629-1634] This polymorphism has been suggested to be associated with a protective effect against myocardial infarction.[1629,1635] The Leu encoding allele occurs at a lower frequency in patients exhibiting myocardial infarction, deep vein thrombosis, and cerebral infarction. Studies also showed that the Leu[34] mutation accelerates factor XIII activation by thrombin and affects fibrin cross-linking.[1636-1639] This acceleration has been proposed to account for the wide reference range reported for factor XIII activity. A study by Undas et al[1640] demonstrated in a bleeding time blood model that aspirin has a more pronounced effect on factor XIII activation when individuals are carriers of the Leu[34] allele. The mechanism underlying the lower risk for myocardial infarction observed in the Leu[34] carriers, despite faster factor XIII activation, is still unclear.

Biochemistry

There are two pools of factor XIII—a plasma pool and an intracellular platelet pool. Plasma factor XIII circulates as a 320-kDa A_2B_2 heterotetramer composed of two identical A-chains (M_r = 83.2 kDa) and two B-chains (M_r = 79.7 kDa)[1641] (*Table 20.1*). The A- and B-chains associate noncovalently with an apparent binding constant of 0.4 μmol/L.[1642] Plasma concentration of factor XIII is approximately 30 μg/mL (94 nmol/L),[1643] with a reference interval in the population of 66% to 134%.[1644] The A subunit contains 731 residues, is not glycosylated, and contains three important functional sites: the catalytic site (Cys[314]-His[373]-Asp[396]), a calcium-binding site, and the activation peptide.[1645,1646] The A subunit is arranged into five distinct structural domains: the activation peptide (residues 1-37); the β sandwich (residues 38-184); the catalytic core (residues 185-515); barrel 1 (residues 516-628); and barrel 2 (629-731). The activation peptide of one A subunit limits access to the active site cysteine of the other A subunit of the dimer. The B subunit contains 641 residues, is glycosylated, and contains 10 sushi domain repeats.[1618] Each sushi domain repeat contains approximately 60 amino acids and is stabilized by two disulfide bonds. By electron microscopy, the B domain appears as strands that are thin, flexible, and kinked.[1647] The B-chain has no enzymatic activity and has been thought to function as a carrier of the A subunit.[1022,1648,1649]

Several x-ray crystal structures of the zymogen factor XIII A_2 subunit have been solved up to 2.0 Å.[1023,1650] These studies revealed a catalytic triad of Cys[314]-His[373]-Asp[396] similar in structure to that observed in cysteine proteases. Crystal structures of thrombin-activated factor XIII have been solved with[1651] and without Ca^{2+}.[1652-1654]

The bone marrow is the primary site of synthesis for the plasma factor XIII A-chain.[1655-1657] Intracellular factor XIII is present in platelets, megakaryocytes, and monocytes as the 160-kDa A_2 homodimer.[1658-1661] The intracellular A_2 dimer, located in the cell cytosol, does not contain a leader sequence or carbohydrate, and its amino terminus is acetylated. How the A_2 dimer is transferred out of the cell and which cell type is the primary source of plasma A_2 are not clearly understood.[1662] Secretion may be accomplished by the same pathway used by other nonclassically secreted proteins in blood, including fibroblast growth factor[1663] and the interleukins.[1664] Approximately 50% of the total potential factor XIII A-chain activity in human blood is found in platelets.[1658]

During fibrin formation, platelet A_2 can be expressed on the platelet surface and plays an important role in fibrin cross-linking. Plasma factor XIII A-chains can also bind to thrombin-activated platelets.[1665,1666] This binding is enhanced by thrombin cleavage of the A-chains as well as the thrombin-dependent activation of the platelet. The association of the factor XIIIa molecule with the activated platelet surface allows it to participate at the platelet-fibrin interface, thereby

stabilizing hemostatic plugs. The factor XIIIa binding site on platelets can be degraded by plasmin.[1665] The B subunit is solely synthesized in the hepatocyte[1656,1667] and is secreted as a monomer.[1667] After being secreted, the A and B subunits associate, becoming an A_2B_2 tetrameric molecule in the blood.

Activation

Activation of the zymogen by thrombin occurs in the NH_2 terminus of the A-chains at Arg[37]-Gly[38] and releases a 37-amino-acid activation peptide from each of the A-chains[1668] (*Figure 20.19*). Whether immediate dissociation of the activation peptide from the rest of the molecule is part of the activation process is not clear, because crystals of thrombin-activated FXIII showed no change in the location and conformation of the activation peptides.[1651] This was also seen in the ion-bound structures,[1652-1654] in which the active site residues remained inaccessible to solvent and substrate. These combined results suggest that exposure of the catalytic residues is likely to occur on substrate binding.[1624] Calcium is required for factor XIIIa to expose its active site cysteine.[1673-1675] Catalytic activity is expressed only after the A-chain dimer is dissociated from the B-chain through a Ca^{2+}-dependent process after thrombin proteolysis.[1648,1649] Fibrin and fibrinogen play important roles as cofactors in the dissociation of the B-chains from thrombin-cleaved factor XIII.[1657,1663] The intracellular form of factor XIII only contains the A-chain; therefore, it does not require the dissociation of the B-chain, but it still requires a calcium-dependent thrombin proteolysis.

The process of factor XIII activation in whole blood has been correlated with fibrin formation,[1068] while in hemophilia this coordination is disrupted.[1676] This creates a carefully regulated system that has cross-linked polymers occurring as soon as fibrin is being formed. The rate of thrombin cleavage of plasma factor XIII has been shown to be greatly accelerated by the presence of fibrin polymers.[1677,1678] This positive feedback network between thrombin, fibrin(ogen), and factor XIIIa ensures that a stable clot can form rapidly to maintain hemostasis.

Function

Activated factor XIII is essential for normal hemostasis and performs numerous functions in pathologic processes.[1599,1624] Being a transglutaminase, activated factor XIII forms isopeptide bonds between the γ-carboxylamide and -amino groups of glutamyl and lysyl residues, respectively. Factor XIIIa is the only enzyme in the blood coagulation cascade that uses a cysteine for catalysis. To date, no known endogenous inhibitor has been described to regulate this important enzyme. Substrates for factor XIII include fibrin(ogen), fibronectin, $α_2$-plasmin inhibitor, collagen, vitronectin, vWF, actin, myosin, factor V, and thrombospondin.[1599-1607]

Fibrin is the main physiologic substrate for factor XIIIa. The basic mechanism involves γ-chain dimerization and α-chain polymerization by creating isopeptide cross-links. The structural specificity for this reaction remains poorly defined. It appears to reside within the primary amino acid sequence surrounding the surface-exposed glutamine residues.[1679,1680] How clot stabilization occurs in fibrin formation is covered in the section on Polymerization (Fibrin Formation).

Fibrinogen (Factor I) and Fibrin

This section focuses on the gene structure, structure/function relationships, and regulation of fibrinogen and its insoluble counterpart fibrin. These topics, although extensively discussed within this section, have also been the subject of several comprehensive reviews,[1681-1685] as well as a 2000 New York Academy of Sciences symposium.[1686]

Fibrinogen is composed of six polypeptide chains (two Aα-chains, two Bβ-chains, and two γ-chains); after posttranslational modification, the mature protein circulates in the blood with an average molecular weight of 340,000 Da (*Table 20.1*). The polypeptide chains are distributed into two symmetric half-molecules, each containing one Aα-, one Bβ-, and one γ-chain with the NH_2 and COOH termini oriented in the same direction. The half-molecules are linked by noncovalent and disulfide bonds at their amino termini, yielding a linear arrangement

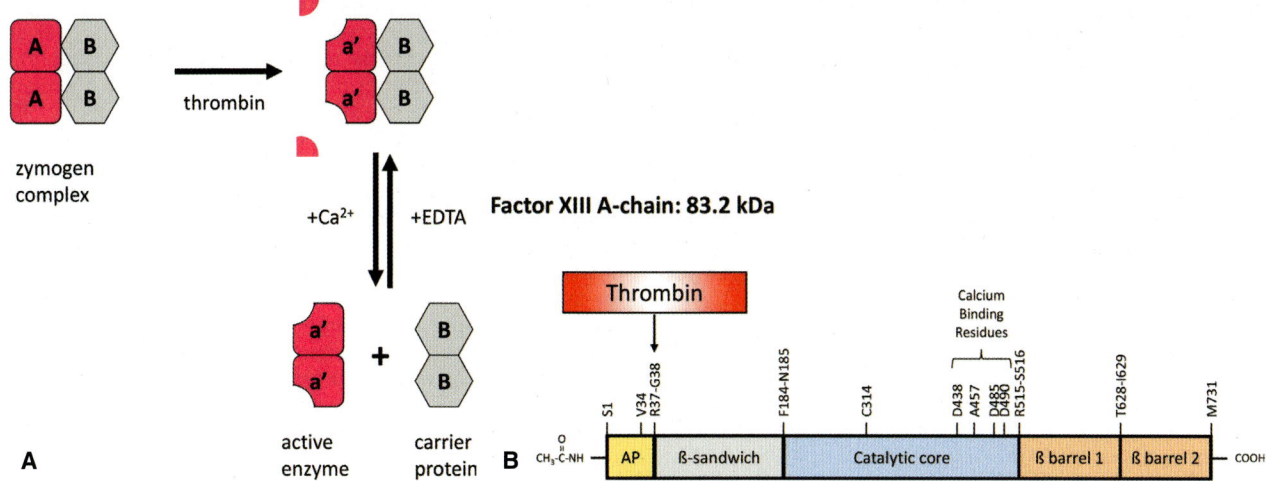

FIGURE 20.19 Plasma factor XIII. A, The thrombin-catalyzed activation of plasma factor XIII (A$_2$B$_2$; 320,000 Da) occurs in two steps. In the first step, thrombin cleaves the (R^{37}–G^{38}) bond. This releases the activation peptides (residues 1-37) from the A-chains, producing the inactive intermediate a'$_2$B$_2$. Fibrinogen interactions promote this event. In the second Ca^{2+}-dependent step, the B-chains dissociate from the a'$_2$B$_2$ intermediate, exposing the active site cysteine, Cys^{314}, of the a' subunits. These chains can reassociate in the presence of divalent cation chelators like ethylenediaminetetraacetic acid (EDTA). The enzyme a'$_2$ is now capable of catalyzing the formation of isopeptide bonds between glutamine residues and lysine residues of adjoining polypeptide chains. In this model, the a'-chains are oriented in such a way as to promote cross-linking of fibrin polymers in an antiparallel configuration. B, Plasma FXIII is a protransglutaminase composed of four noncovalently associated molecules: two identical transglutaminase precursors (A-chains) and two identical molecules (B-chains) that function as carriers. Platelet FXIII unlike plasma FXIII is a dimer of the FXIII-A chain. During plasma FXIII activation, α-thrombin cleaves off the activation peptide (AP) from FXIII-A; dissociation of the dimeric FXIIIa molecule from the B-chains appears required to permit the structural rearrangements required to yield the functional transglutaminase.[1669] Beyond the formation of γ-γ chain α-α chain isopeptide bonds between fibrin monomers, plasma factor FXIIIa has been shown to covalently incorporate at least 48 different proteins into the fibrin clot.[1670] Key structural regions of the A-chain include the N-terminal AP, β sandwich region, catalytic core, β-barrel 1, and β-barrel 2. Each AP in the dimer occupies the opposing A-chain active site, thus functioning both to block transglutaminase activity and contribute to stabilizing the A-chain dimer prior to activation.[1671] The β-barrel domains have been proposed as sites of interaction with the B-chains.[1672] The catalytic core region contains the catalytic triad (C314, H373, D396) and the Ca^{2+}-binding site, occupancy of which is necessary for enzymatic activity. C314 functions as nucleophile, forming a thioester linkage to the carboxamide group of a glutamine residue in one protein substrate, which is then displaced by the epsilon amino group of a lysine residue in the other protein substrate.

of three nodular structures. The outside two domains, formed by the carboxyl-terminal regions of the Bβ- and γ-chains of fibrinogen, are designated D, whereas the central domain that contains the amino termini of all the chains is designated E. Between 1.7 and 5.0 g of fibrinogen is synthesized per day by the liver,[1687,1688] with approximately 75% of this fibrinogen secreted into the plasma and the remainder distributed between the lymph and interstitial fluids.[1688] This translates into a mean plasma level of 2.5 mg/mL with a normal $t_{1/2}$ of 3 to 5 days.[1689,1690] Fibrinogen is considered to be an acute-phase reactant, and as such, it is upregulated 2- to 10-fold in response to a variety of physiologic stresses including trauma, pregnancy, and tissue inflammation.[1691]

Fibrinogen has been found in the blood plasma of all vertebrates, including the most primitive vertebrate, the lamprey. Early phylogenetic work on fibrinogen began with protein sequences obtained for various fibrinopeptides.[1692,1693] It was immediately obvious that, although these peptides were exceptionally variable, certain features were conserved; without exception, they all contained an arginyl-glycine bond required for thrombin cleavage.[1694] Determination of the protein sequences for all three chains revealed that they were homologous and were evolved from a common ancestor.[1695] The β- and γ-chains share the most identity (42%) in their COOH-terminal domains, although they share no homology with the C-terminal α-chain.[1696-1699] In fact, the C-terminal α-chain varies greatly between species (molecular weight ranges from 60 to 120 kDa).

Sequence data, especially the detailed work determining intron/exon junctures, support the hypothesis that all three fibrinogen genes evolved from a common ancestor through a series of duplications that began approximately 1 billion years ago.[1700-1704] At this point, the ancestral gene duplicated to form both the Aα-chain and a β/γ-chain precursor gene. Then, sometime before the last time lampreys and mammals shared a common ancestor (450 million years ago), the β/γ gene duplicated, forming today's β- and γ-chains. There is now

a growing collection of proteins that share more than 30% sequence identity with both the β- and γ-chains, including α$_E$C domains,[1705-1707] chicken cytotactin,[1708] mouse T-cell protein,[1708] sea cucumber,[1709] and scabrous gene product from the fruit fly.[1710]

Gene Structure and Expression

The fibrinogen locus is composed of three closely linked genes (specifying the polypeptides Aα, Bβ, and γ) found as single copies in a region of approximately 50 kb (bands q31.3-32.1) of chromosome 4[1711-1716] (*Table 20.2*). Both the Aα- and γ-chains are transcribed from the same DNA strand, whereas the Bβ-chain is transcribed from the opposing strand.[1700] The Aα gene contains 6 exons, whereas the Bβ has 8 and the γ-chain has 10.[1717-1719] The expression of all three genes appears to share a common regulatory mechanism, potentially via their 5'-flanking regions.[1720,1721] Therefore, expression for the three chains is coordinately controlled and, at least for the hepatocyte, results in almost equal levels of mRNA for each chain in the cell.[1703,1715,1718,1722]

A single transcription initiation event at the promoter of each chain produces multiple mRNAs due to alternative polyadenylation site selection in all three chains, as well as alternative splicing for both Aα- and γ-chains.[1705,1723-1725] In the case of the γ-chain, normal processing results in a polypeptide chain ending at Valγ^{411} (human numbering); however, approximately 10% of the time during splicing, the last intron is retained as an exon, resulting in a new chain, γ', which ends at Leuγ^{427}.[1715,1726] Sometimes the α-chain also fails to remove the last intron, producing a translated protein product that is 27-kDa larger.[1705-1707,1727] The resulting larger form of fibrinogen is called *fibrinogen-420* (1%-2% of circulating human molecules), and the α-chain extension is called α$_E$C.[1728] Interestingly, this new domain shares as much sequence identity (~40%) with the COOH-terminal domain of the β- and γ-chains as the two share with each other.[1727]

Common polymorphisms of the fibrinogen genes are associated with plasma fibrinogen concentrations as well as susceptibility to, or severity of, atherothrombotic disease.[1729] Epidemiologic studies have shown a strong association between two polymorphisms of the fibrinogen β-chain gene and fibrinogen plasma concentration.[1730,1731] However, the majority of the studies did not find any relation with fibrinogen polymorphisms and cardiovascular disease.[1730,1731] The effect of these polymorphisms and vascular disease still remains in question because environmental or intermediate conditions of the phenotype can influence the outcome. This supports the notion of individualized susceptibility to disease, which is determined by the genotype and environmental risk factors.

Afibrinogenemia

Inherited or *congenital afibrinogenemia* is an autosomal recessive disorder characterized by a total lack of fibrinogen in the plasma. This disorder, originally described in 1920, now affects more than 150 families, putting the estimated prevalence in the general population at approximately 1 in 1 million.[1715,1732,1733] It is usually detected at birth with uncontrollable bleeding from the umbilical cord. The phenotype varies from mild to severe with some patients experiencing spontaneous intracranial hemorrhage and splenic rupture throughout life, as well as bleeding after minor trauma.[1734,1735] It has been suggested that the presence of functional vWF, which allows platelet thrombus formation in the absence of fibrin, may be responsible for the phenotypic variation observed.[1736,1737] Most patients respond well to replacement therapy.[1738] To date, 86% of all afibrinogenemia results from a truncation mutation in the fibrinogen Aα gene.[1732]

Investigation of the roles that both fibrinogen and fibrin play in vivo has been greatly enhanced by the creation of transgenic mice either lacking fibrinogen[1739] or expressing a modified form of fibrinogen.[1740] The fibrinogen-deficient mice (Fib Aα$^{-/-}$) were often able to survive to sexual maturity, even though they had no immunologically detectable levels of any chain (Aα, Bβ, γ) in circulation.[1739] As expected, plasma from these deficient mice was unable to clot in vitro even when combined with exogenous thrombin. In addition, the plasma did not support platelet aggregation in vitro. This is consistent with the view that fibrinogen bridges platelets via activated receptors (e.g., $\alpha_{IIb}\beta_3$).[1741] However, in vivo, these mice are able to form platelet thrombi and are often able to withstand spontaneous bleeding episodes.[1737] The resilience of the Fib Aα$^{-/-}$ mice is probably due to the fact that all factors required for thrombin generation and platelet activation are present and that platelets have alternative ligands for their activated receptors that are capable of supporting adhesion and thrombus formation.[1733]

Breeding experiments crossing fibrinogen-deficient mice with other mice deficient in a hemostatic factor are providing insights into the roles fibrinogen and fibrin play in vivo. For example, mice with combined deficiency in both fibrinogen and vWF were found to form stable thrombi, although platelet deposition was found to be delayed and unstable.[1737] However, crossbreeding plasminogen-deficient mice (Plg$^{-/-}$) with Aα$^{-/-}$ mice eliminated many of the spontaneous pathologies[1742,1743] (conjunctivitis, pulmonary lesions, terminal vessel thrombosis, ulceration, or prolapse of the rectum and wasting) normally associated with the Plg$^{-/-}$ genotype, including death at 6 months. In addition, the delayed tissue repair observed in Plg$^{-/-}$ mice after arterial challenge,[1744] corneal damage,[1745,1746] or skin incision were all corrected by the removal of fibrinogen. These data, in combination with other data not discussed here, support the concept that the physiologic role for the plasminogen activation system is fibrin lysis.[1747]

Hereditary Dysfibrinogenemias

Like many of the other coagulation disorders, classic dysfibrinogenemias were frequently recognized by the mother when her child bled abnormally. These disorders are associated with prolonged thrombin times usually caused by a point mutation in one of the chains, but clinically, the patient presents with normal plasma fibrinogen concentrations. Hypofibrinogenemias, on the other hand, are associated with low plasma fibrinogen concentrations (<1.5 mg/mL) due to a mutation(s) that can affect transcription, mRNA processing, translation,

chain processing, and assembly, excretion, or stability of the mature protein.[1748] Hypofibrinogenemias can be classified into four groups according to the effect of the mutation: mutations that affect (a) intracellular processing, (b) retention in the endoplasmic reticulum, (c) intracellular assembly, and (d) Aα-chain truncations.[1734,1735,1748]

Dysfibrinogenemias can be divided into five groups based on their specific action: (a) mutations that impair or impede thrombin, (b) defects in the construction of protofibrils, (c) impaired lateral association of protofibrils, (d) defects in interactions with other substances, and (e) other unknown mechanisms.[1748] Thus, most common mutations are those that impede conversion of fibrinogen to fibrin by thrombin, which catalyzes the hydrolysis of the bonds between Argα^{16}-Glyα^{17} and Argβ^{14}-Glyβ^{15}, releasing FPA and FPB, respectively. The active site of thrombin is highly specific for an Arg in the P1 position as observed by the human variant replacement of Argα^{16} by His, which leads to delayed release of FPA[1749] or Cys, resulting in no release of FPA.[1750,1751] In the case of Argβ^{14}, only a Cys variant (fibrinogen Christchurch[1752]) has been observed.

The identification of these mutations, originally through protein chemistry methods and now using DNA technology, has provided unique insights into the structural/function relationships of fibrinogen and fibrin. These mutants were originally gathered and published in the *Index of Variant Human Fibrinogen*,[1753] but with the advent of the Web, the material has been converted to a dynamic database (http://www.geht.org).[1754] As of January 2012 (Release 37), 617 molecular abnormalities were present in the database, with 356 found in the Aα-chain (99 were Argα(^{16}) mutations), 82 in the Bβ-chain, and 176 in the γ-chain.

Biosynthesis

Pulse chase experiments in a human hepatic carcinoma line have shown that there is a large intercellular pool of both Aα- and γ-chains, but it is the Bβ-chain synthesis that limits assembly in the rough endoplasmic reticulum.[1755,1756] However, in both chicken and rat hepatocytes, it seems to be the Aα-chain that limits fibrinogen assembly.[1756,1757] In addition, several extrahepatic sites of fibrinogen synthesis have been identified, including human cervical epithelial cells[1758] and lung alveolar epithelial cells.[1759] γ-Chain-only synthesis has been observed in vivo in the brain, lung, and bone marrow.[1760,1761] A physiologic role remains to be determined.

A number of posttranslational modifications (*Table 20.8*) must occur after synthesis but before secretion. These include removal of the signal peptides from all three chains during or after passage across the membrane[1762]; a biantennary carbohydrate (M$_r$ ~ 2500 Da) being added to Asnγ^{52} on the γ-chain much earlier than the Asnβ^{364} on the Bβ-chain[1760,1763-1766]; and when synthesized, fibrinogen being fully phosphorylated (Serα^3 and Ser3α^{46})—but in its circulating form, only 20% to 30% of these sites remain phosphorylated.[1767] The first residue on the Bβ-chain is also posttranslationally modified to form pyroglutamic acid, thus removing its free amino terminus.

Biochemistry and Activation

The fibrinogen molecule contains two copies of three separate polypeptide chains designated Aα, Bβ, and γ (*Table 20.8*). These are arranged into two identical half-molecules in an elongated structure composed of three globules. In the central globule all six NH$_2$ termini of the polypeptides reside, and thus it has been referred to as the *N-disulfide knot*.[1692,1768] There are 11 disulfide bonds in this region, three of which link the two half-molecules. Experiments in which one or more of the 29 intra- and interchain disulfides were removed or small deletions made have shown that for dimer formation both disulfide bonds and the noncovalent interactions of the amino termini are important.[1769-1773] The common form of the Aα-chain contains 610 amino acid residues with an M$_r$ of 66,500 Da and two phosphorylation sites (Serα^3 and Serα^{346}), and thrombin cleavage of the Argα^{16}-Glyα^{17} bond releases FPA. The Aα-chain of fibrinogen has sites appropriate for factor XIIIa-catalyzed formation of cross-links,[1774] t-PA enhancement site (residues 148-160) found in fibrin,[1775] as well as consensus integrin recognition sites (residues 95-98 and 572-575). The Bβ-chain

Table 20.8. Key Features of Human Fibrinogen Chains

	Aα	αEC	Bβ	γ	γ′
Total number of residues	610	236	461	411	427
Expression level (%)	98	2	100	90	10
Fibrinopeptide length	16		14		
Thrombin cleavage site	Arg^{16}-Gly^{17}		Arg^{14}-Gly^{15}		
Newly exposed N termini	Gly^{17}-Pro-Arg-Val		Gly^{15}-His-Arg-Pro		
Cross-linking sites					
Acceptor (Gln)	328, 366			398	
Donor (Lys)	508-584			406	
Number of calcium-binding sites	?	1	2	1	1
Carbohydrate linkage site		667	364	52	52
Phosphorylation site	3, 346				

? indicates literature disagreement over the value.

is composed of 461 amino acids, displays an M$_r$ of 52,000 Da and has a single glycosylation site (Asnβ^{364}) and a Ca^{2+}-binding site (residues 381-385). Thrombin cleavage of the Argβ^{14}-Glyβ^{15} bond releases FPB. The γ-chain of fibrinogen is made up of 411 amino acids with an M$_r$ of 46,500 Da, is glycosylated at Asnγ^{52}, and has a Ca^{2+}-binding site (residues 318-324), a t-PA enhancement site (residues 320-324) in fibrin, and both donor (Glnγ^{398}) and acceptor (Lysγ^{406}) sites for cross-link formation.

A comprehensive history of early fibrinogen and fibrin structure/function relationships can be found in an excellent review by Blomback.[1686] In the first recorded structural experiment, Bailey et al[1776] placed both a concentrated solution of fibrinogen (which forms a viscous strand) and a fibrin thread in an x-ray beam. The resulting patterns were indistinguishable not only from each other but also from the patterns of keratin and myosin. They all showed a characteristic 5.1-Å-repeat spacing that was later determined to be due to supercoiled α helices.[1777] Around this same time, a different physiochemical "picture" of fibrinogen was emerging. Techniques including electrophoresis, ultracentrifugation, viscosity measurements, and light scattering were coming into vogue and determined that fibrinogen was a prolate ellipsoid with a length between 500 and 700 Å, an axial ratio between 5 and 20 Å, and a molecular weight near 340 kDa.[421,1778-1780]

Hall and Slayter[1781] produced shadow-cast photographs of fibrinogen and observed three unconnected globules in a line. The center globule was the smallest, with a diameter of approximately 50 Å; the terminal globules were found to be of equivalent size, approximately 60 Å. The total molecular length was estimated to be 475 Å; thus, the connections between the globules were approximated to 150 Å, and Cohen[1782] suggested that these globules could be linked by α helices, which would explain the characteristic α-helix 5.1-Å-repeat spacing observed in the fiber diffraction. This trinodular structure has become known as the *Hall and Slayter model of fibrinogen.*

The reconstruction of fibrinogen from both enzymatic and chemical fragmentation products has allowed an exact picture of the structure and function of fibrinogen to emerge. Many fragments were subjected to protein sequencing and the sequences reassembled until the whole structure was determined. These fragments also gave insights into the polymerization process as well as the shape of fibrinogen. Because plasmin is the natural protease for fibrin removal, it was the obvious choice for initial fragmentation. Nussenzweig et al[1783] characterized such a fibrinogen lysate that was chromatographed using a diethylaminoethyl cellulose column. The resulting peaks were denoted *A* through *E,* and it was determined that the pools D and E contained the bulk of the material, with an approximate mass ratio of 2:1. This coordinated well with the Hall and Slayter model in which pool E would represent the center globule and be called *fragment E,* and the terminal globules

would be found in pool D and called *fragment D.*[1784] Thus, fibrinogen is a symmetric molecule, with a dyad axis drawn through fragment E.

Much effort has been expended in trying to crystallize fibrinogen. The first view was an 18-Å structure of a modified bovine fibrinogen,[1785] later refined to approximately 4 Å.[1786] The modification was a partial proteolysis that predominantly removed the C-terminal α-chains. However, the density for the central domain was "poorly defined." The first look at an unmodified fibrinogen was the 5.5-Å followed by 2.7-Å structures of chicken fibrinogen.[1787,1788] Chicken fibrinogen was chosen as a target because it has the shortest α-chains that lack a series of repeated sequences found in most other species[1707,1789,1790] (*Figure 20.20*). This structure provided the first atomic resolution view of the central domain of fibrinogen, although the α domains were too disordered to allow the chain to be traced. A 35-kDa digestion product of fragment E (FE$_5$) was solved at 1.4 Å,[1792] which correlates well with the observed fragment E region in the 2.7-Å chicken fibrinogen structure.

The first atomic resolution structure in the fibrinogen field was for a human recombinant γ-chain.[1793] As predicted, the fold of the γ-chain was unique and not represented in any of the structural databases.[1699] The next advance came with the 2.9-Å structure of human fragment D,[1794] displaying the two globular β and γ domains forming the furrow. As expected, the β and γ COOH-terminal domains share the same fold[1793,1795] and are oriented approximately 130° apart. These observations have been confirmed in a structure of lamprey fragment D[1796] and a recombinant human fragment D.[1797,1798] To date, a crystal structure of intact human fibrinogen has not been solved.

Polymerization (Fibrin Formation)

The goal of a polymerization is to build a scaffold of sufficient mechanical strength to serve as a hemostatic plug. Interestingly, only 20% of a "clot" is actually protein—the remainder is solvent.[1799] In 1952, Ferry[1800] proposed a half-staggered overlap model to explain the polymerization process. This model can be expressed succinctly in terms of "knobs" and "holes."[1695] When thrombin removes the fibrinopeptides, it creates new amino termini on the α- and β-chains called *knobs.* Because the knobs are located in the central globule (fragment E) of the Hall and Slayter model, the holes for them to fit into must be present on the terminal domains (fragment D). To accommodate the half-staggered overlap model, the knobs on one molecule interact with holes in two different molecules. Reciprocally, a knob from each of these molecules fits into the holes on the first molecule's fragment D. The binding sites of the α and β knobs were localized to the γ- and β-chains, respectively, using fragment D digested to different extents.[1801] To identify the polymerization hole in the γ-chain, recombinant γ-chain crystals were soaked in a solution containing a peptide mimic of the knob.[1795] As was expected, the hole was preformed

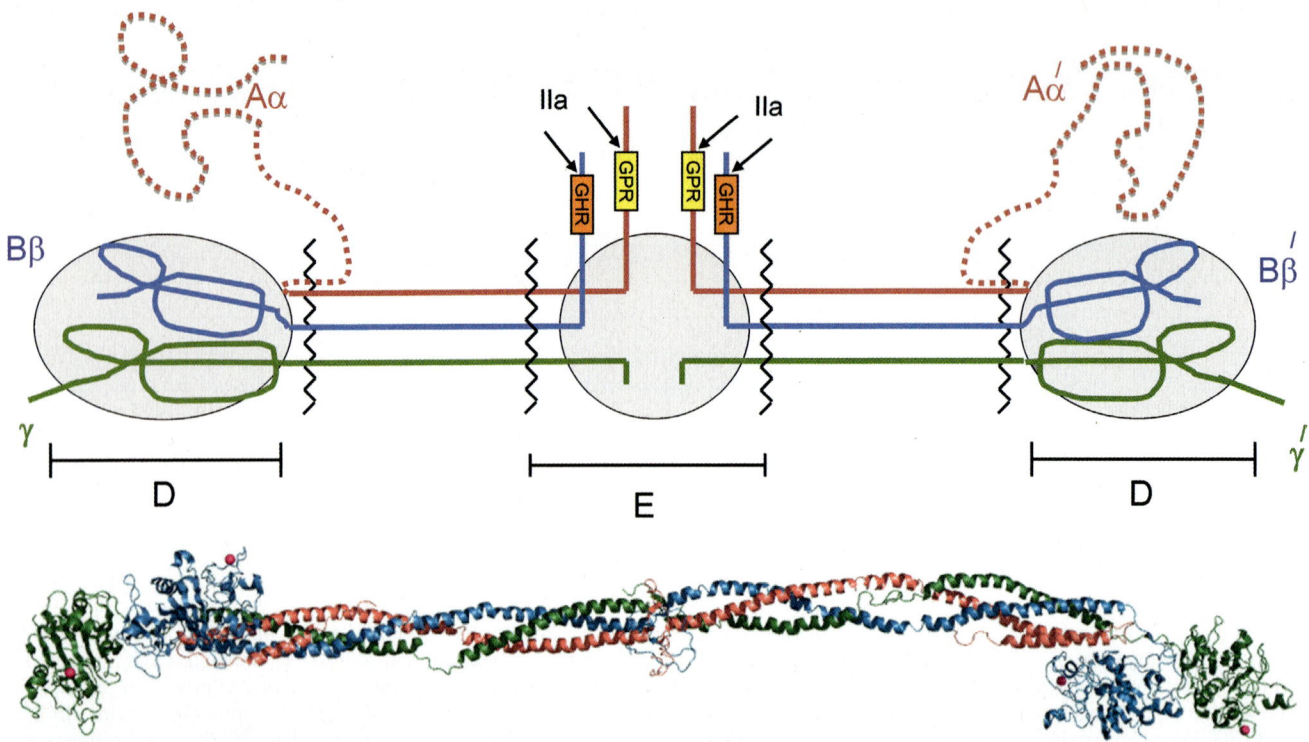

FIGURE 20.20 **A schematic and crystal structure of human fibrinogen (PDB: 3GHG).**[1791] All six NH$_2$ termini are gathered together in the central or E domain. Three chains (α-, β-, and γ-) extend out from this domain through coiled coils in either direction forming the terminal or D domains. α-Thrombin (IIa) cleavage sites at the N termini of the Aα and Bβ are indicated, with the new N termini that associate with "holes" in the D domains to form fibrin depicted in the boxes. Pink spheres indicate the four Ca^{2+} sites. Note: the carboxy termini of the α-chains are not visible in the crystal structure.

and contained a strong electronegative potential that was neutralized on the binding of the doubly positively charged peptide. The binding interaction was noncovalent and composed of only ionic and hydrogen bonds. Using laser tweezers, the strength of this interaction has been measured between 125 and 130 pN, which is the majority of the force holding fibrin polymer together at this early stage.[1802]

The existence of a β-chain hole and that this hole binds the β-chain knob were confirmed with a double-D x-ray crystal structure in which peptide knobs for the α- and β-chains were present.[1803] As would be expected, the β-chain knob also binds with a combination of ionic and hydrogen bonds to the β-chain hole, although it contributes only 15 to 20 pN to the interaction.[1802] In another study using combinations of peptide knobs, it was determined that the β hole is not fully formed until the knob is present[1804] and is much less discriminating in peptide acceptance.[1805] This conformational change may be the basis for the acceleration of fibrin formation observed in the presence of the peptide ligand GHRP.[1685,1801] No evidence has been found for an analogous mechanism with the γ hole; rather, the γ hole seems always ready to accept an α knob, although in the absence of an α knob, the β knob readily binds to both holes.[1804] A single example of an α knob peptide (GPRVVE) has been observed occupying a β hole,[1806] but recent experiments using laser tweezers have demonstrated that this interaction is not physiologically relevant.[1802]

The conversion of fibrinogen to fibrin can be separated into three congruent processes: (a) removal of the fibrinopeptides, (b) assembly, and (c) covalent stabilization. We examine each in depth in the following sections.

Fibrinopeptide Release

Many early investigators tried to determine the differences between fibrinogen and fibrin. Their molecular weights were identical, and fibrinogen was the more electronegative of the two.[1807] In the conversion of fibrinogen to fibrin, thrombin catalyzes the hydrolysis of Arg-Gly bonds, removing small, polar aminoterminal pieces (fibrinopeptides) from the α- and β-chains.[1808,1809] Cleavage of Argα^{16} by

thrombin releases FPA and forms fibrin I. The release of two FPA peptides exposes a site in fragment E that aligns with a complementary site in fragment D to form overlapping fibrils. Subsequent cleavage by thrombin at Argβ^{14} releases FPB and leads to the formation of fibrin II, presumably increasing lateral aggregation of the protofibrils. FPA and FPB vary in length (between 13 and 21 amino acids in various mammals) and constitute <2% of the total mass.[1810]

Early studies in citrated plasmas or purified fibrinogen found that FPA and FPB are released at very different rates, with FPA being released first.[1809,1811-1813] A sequential model for release has been postulated in which thrombin binds equally to both chains, but the presence of FPA hinders the release of FPB because thrombin is unable to undergo a required conformation change.[1814-1817] As the polymerization process proceeds, the FPB release rate continues to increase, suggesting that a polymerization-induced structure change facilitates its release.[1814,1815,1818] When the fibrinogen to fibrin conversion is studied in a nonanticoagulated whole blood system, the pattern of fibrin formation based on fibrinopeptide release is different from that seen in citrated plasma or purified fibrinogen.[1068]

Bettelheim and Bailey[1819] first hypothesized that, on FPA and FPB release, these newly exposed amino termini (knobs) must be the principal contact sites during polymerization. In human fibrinogen, the α-chain knob, after FPA release, begins with the sequence GPRVV, whereas the β-chain, after FPB release, starts with GHRPL. Synthetic peptide GPR derivatives based on the β knob were found to bind to both fibrinogen and fragment D and inhibit fibrin monomer polymerization.[1801] Peptides based on the β knob also bound to both fibrinogen and fragment D but were unable to inhibit fibrin monomer polymerization. In analogous studies, venoms can be used to selectively remove only FPA without activating factor XIII, and fibrin will still form.[1820,1821] Although it appears morphologically the same, this type of fibrin lacks the normal strength of fibrin.[1822-1824] Removal of only FPB (without FPA release) results in fibrin formation in lampreys,[1694] but human fibrinogen clots only if the temperature is maintained below 15 °C.[1824]

Fibrin Assembly

The release of the FPAs from fibrinogen results in the formation of an intermediate termed *fibrin monomer*, which is all but indistinguishable from fibrinogen, and leads to the formation of the fibrin dimer through the noncovalent charge-charge (salt links) and hydrogen bonds between the knobs and the holes.[1825] As fibrin monomers continue to be generated, the dimer elongates from both ends as a two-stranded molecule until it reaches approximately 30 monomers, when it becomes a protofibril.[1811,1826,1827]

The second step in fibrin assembly is the lateral association of protofibrils into thicker fibrin fibers.[1826,1827] These fibers are formed from the association of between 14 and 22 protofibrils.[1828] Because protofibrils, not dimers, are required for this step, it is believed that the forces involved in lateral association are weak and, therefore, only become "strong" in large numbers. Fragment D, specifically the

β-chain, is likely responsible for this aspect of fiber growth.[1021,1829,1830] Clots are known to branch, although how this is accomplished is not clear. For example, perhaps a protofibril can attach and form a link between two growing fibers,[1021,1682,1831] or perhaps this is the role for the C-terminal region of the α-chains.[1832,1833] The presence or absence of carbohydrates also seems to affect branching.[1766]

The description of fibrinogen activation and fibrin assembly has been based on studies using citrated plasmas, purified proteins, or both. To understand the in vivo process of fibrin formation, a system with nonanticoagulated blood has been used; in this experimental model, the pattern of fibrin formation based on fibrinopeptide release is different from systems using citrated plasma or purified fibrinogen[1068] (*Figure 20.21*). In this study, cleavage of FPA and subsequent clot formation occur just before the propagation phase of thrombin

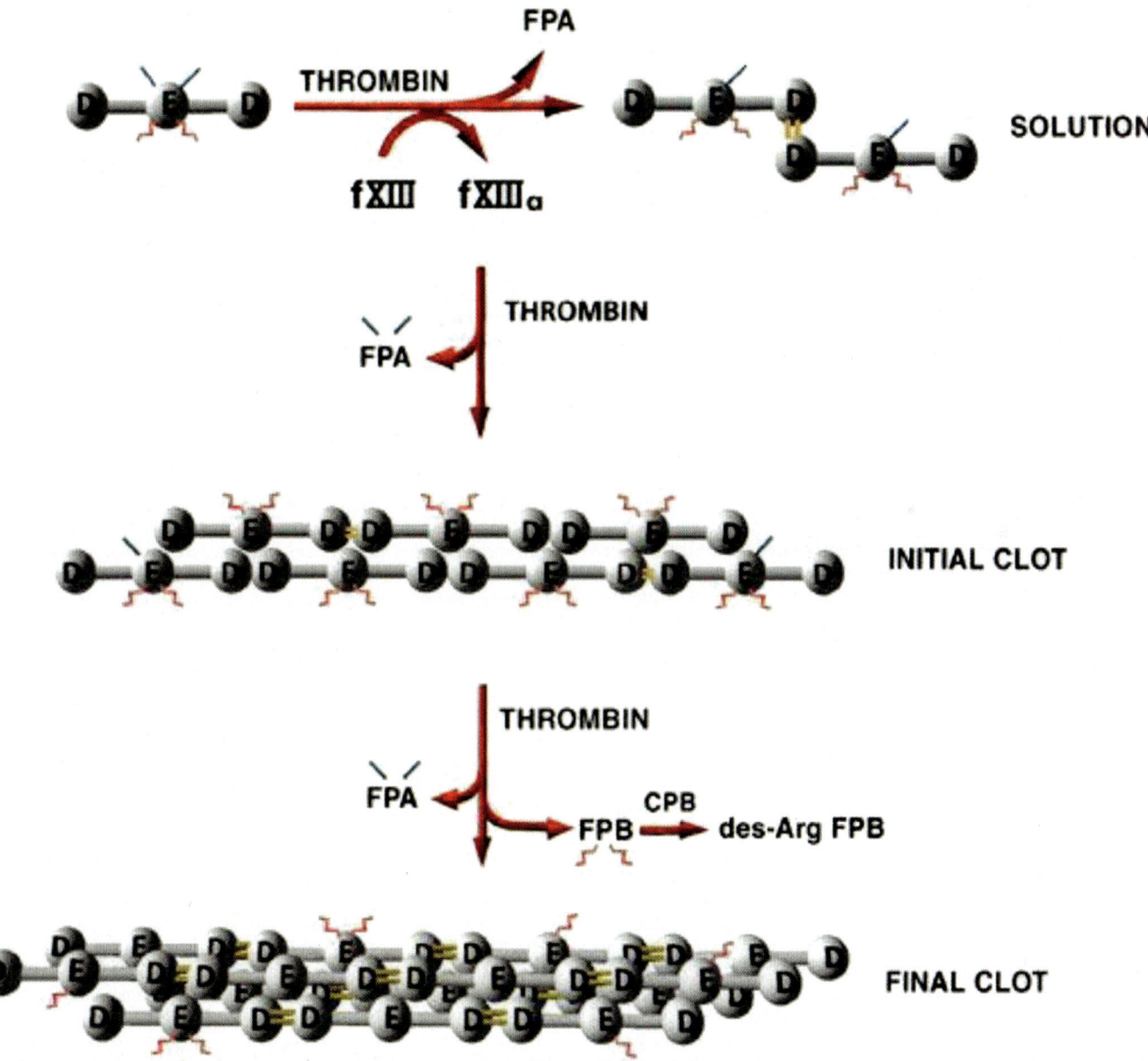

FIGURE 20.21 **Schematic representation of whole blood fibrin formation.** α-Thrombin at the beginning of clot formation simultaneously acts on fibrinogen (D-E-D) and factor XIII (FXIII). A portion (~40%) of fibrinopeptide A (FPA) is released from fibrinogen, and an initial clot is formed from the complementary overlap of the exposed sites between the E and D domains of adjacent molecules. Activated factor XIII (FXIIIa) simultaneously cross-links adjacent D domains (D = D). Thus, the initial soluble fibrin clot is composed of fibrinogen, fibrin, and g-g dimers (double yellow lines) with fibrinopeptide B (FPB) still attached. The initial clot is continuously acted on by thrombin, releasing the remaining FPA and some of the FPB to yield a final clot with the majority of FPB still attached. The released FPB is selectively acted on by a carboxypeptidase B–like enzyme (CPB) cleaving the carboxyl terminal arginine to produce des-Arg FPB. The significance of this cleavage is still unclear. (From Brummel KE, Butenas S, Mann KG. An integrated study of fibrinogen during blood coagulation. *J Biol Chem.* 1999;274(32):22862-22870. http://creativecommons.org/licenses/by/4.0/)

generation. At the point of visual clot formation, virtually all fibrinogen (and some product already cross-linked) disappears from the fluid phase of the reaction. Thus, the "clot" appears to be a mixture composed of fibrin I and fibrinogen. The insoluble material present in the fibrin clot is virtually all cross-linked by factor XIIIa, whose activation is nearly simultaneous with FPA removal. Therefore, the transglutaminase factor XIIIa is available to cross-link the γ-chains of the initial fibrinogen/fibrin I clot. In purified systems, it has been observed that FPB removal precedes the cross-linking reaction. However, in the whole blood clotting model, the FPB antigen epitope is found associated with the β-chain after clot formation has occurred. FPB release proceeds at a slower rate than FPA release, occurs after γ-γ dimer formation, and only reaches approximately 38% of its theoretical maximum value. Doolittle and Pandi[1834] have recently proposed that interaction of the β-knob with the β-hole generates a conformational change and exposes t-PA-binding sites, which ultimately hasten a clot's removal.

Fibrin Cross-Linking

To strengthen the "weak" (noncovalent) interactions holding the dimers and protofibrils together, factor XIII (a transglutaminase found circulating in the plasma) is activated to factor XIIIa by thrombin in the presence of Ca^{2+} to link the side chains of lysyl and glutamyl residues by isopeptide bonds. Thrombin activation of factor XIII has been shown to coincide with FPA release during the initiation phase of thrombin generation.[581,1068] The concentrations of thrombin (based on thrombin-antithrombin complex) needed for factor XIII activation, FPA release, and FPB release have been calculated to be 0.8 ± 0.3 nmol/L, 1.3 ± 0.4 nmol/L, and 1.7 ± 0.5 nmol/L, respectively.[581]

It has been proposed that as many as six cross-links can form between a fibrin monomer and its neighbors[1835,1836] and that the presence of these cross-links increases the strength, chemical resistance to urea, and lysis by plasmin.[1595,1596,1837-1841] Early in fibrin assembly, factor XIIIa has been shown to link $Gln\gamma^{398}$ and $Lys\gamma^{406}$ in reciprocal cross-links between adjacent C-terminal γ-chains.[1602,1842] Once the majority of γ-chain cross-links are inserted, then a much slower process begins to insert multiple cross-links between neighboring α-chains.[1843] Because each α-chain has two glutamyl acceptor sites and five potential lysine donor sites, a complex cross-linked network can result.[1844] The result is cross-linked fibrin, which is more resistant to clot lysis.[1841,1845] Factor XIIIa also covalently attaches α_2-plasmin inhibitor (the principal fibrinolytic inhibitor) to α-chains in the clot, thereby increasing resistance to degradation.[1846,1847]

Function

Fibrinogen functions in hemostasis to stem blood loss. It serves as a molecular bridge to support interplatelet aggregation, and it is the precursor of fibrin, which is the main component of the protein scaffolding of the forming hemostatic plug. Platelet aggregation critically depends on fibrinogen binding to activated platelets via the platelet fibrinogen receptor gpIIb-IIIa as well as fibrin adhesion. Fibrinogen/fibrin also regulates thrombin activity by interactions that include the proteolytic cleavage by thrombin of fibrinopeptides to form a fibrin clot and thrombin exosite binding to fibrin, which potentially limits the diffusion of thrombin and thereby regulates clot propagation. The structure, stability, and duration of the insoluble counterpart fibrin are controlled by an interplay between fibrin formation and fibrinolysis, which includes other molecular and cellular components. An important enzyme for the structure and stability of the fibrin clot is the transglutaminase factor XIIIa. Its function is to cross-link fibrin and other adhesive proteins including integrin receptors, providing a stable network. Once activated, the fibrinolysis inhibitor called *TAFI* functions to attenuate fibrinolysis by removing C-terminal lysines from fibrin. This appears to be critical in the stabilization of the fibrin clot by reducing the number of sites available for plasminogen binding, thus reducing the rate of plasmin generation with consequent prolongation of fibrin dissolution.[1070,1848] TAFI has also been shown to play a role in the premature lysis of clots from hemophilic plasma.[1849]

Fibrinogen is primarily recognized for its role in hemostasis, but it is also required for competent inflammatory reactions. Fibrinogen is an acute-phase reactant, with levels increasing during inflammation. During these situations, fibrinogen functions as a bridging molecule in cell-cell interactions. Fibrin and fibrinogen constitute a matrix that can allow for the modulation of cellular responses through a variety of different cell types, including endothelial cells, epithelial cells, leukocytes, platelets, and fibroblasts. Cellular receptors that can bind fibrinogen and fibrin include the integrins $\alpha_{IIb}\beta_3$, $\alpha_V\beta_3$, and $\alpha_5\beta_1$, and the cellular adhesion molecules intercellular adhesion molecule-1 and vascular endothelial cadherin.

Although the function of fibrinogen and fibrin as a barrier to stemming blood loss through the dense fibrin network appears central to hemostasis, the findings from fibrinogen-deficient mice suggest that compensating mechanisms exist. Homozygous Aα-chain–deficient mice are born with normal appearance and without elevated fetal mortality.[1739] These mice have no detectable levels of the Aα-, Bβ-, and γ-chains in their blood.[1739] Therefore, the maintenance of hemostasis in these animals is most likely derived from normal thrombin generation and the support of platelet aggregation and adhesion by vWF.

Most clinical assays use fibrin formation as a means to assess hemostasis (PT and activated partial thromboplastin time). The formation of a visible fibrin clot occurs during the initiation phase of coagulation at very low levels of thrombin, approximately 3% to 5% of the total amount of thrombin produced.[581,630] The majority of thrombin ($\sim$95%) is generated after clot formation during the propagation phase, which is overlooked when a fibrin endpoint assay is used.[581] In congenital hemophilia A and B, only a slight prolongation of clot time is observed; the major impairment is in thrombin generation during the propagation phase of the reaction (see *Figure 20.8*).[936] Thus, most catalyst and thrombin formation is ignored using the current technology for evaluating clinical hemorrhagic risk or thrombosis. The survivability of the afibrinogenemic genotype in mice and male patients also supports this concept that critically important events are taking place beyond the endpoint of fibrin formation.

Regulation of Fibrin Lysis

The coagulation system prevents blood loss at the site of injury, filling one role in hemostasis. However, there must also exist mechanisms to limit the coagulation system and processes to remove a clot once it is no longer needed. This role is filled by the fibrinolytic system that uses elements from plasma, platelets, tissue, and other blood cells to regulate the degradation of fibrin. The main player is the zymogen plasminogen that on activation becomes plasmin, a serine protease, whose primary physiologic role is the degradation of the fibrin clot and extracellular matrix molecules. Even though the plasmin cleavage sites are similar for both fibrinogen and fibrin, we consider them separately for clarity.

Fibrinogenolysis

Marder[1850,1851] proposed a scheme for fragmentation of fibrinogen based on his own detailed studies and the work of others.[1852,1853] In the first step, fibrinogen is converted to fragment X ($M_r \sim 247,000$) by the removal of the C-terminal α-chain as well as the first 42 amino acids of the β-chain[1854,1855] (*Figure 20.22*). Fragment X remains clottable before it is split asymmetrically, forming fragment Y ($M_r \sim 150,000$), fragment D ($M_r \sim 88,000$), and some small detritus relating to the coiled-coil region. Finally, fragment Y is further split into fragment D and fragment E ($M_r \sim 50,000$), and some more detritus is released.

Fibrinolysis

Differences observed in the degradation products between fibrinogen and fibrin are due to the presence of the cross-links, not a change in the specificity of plasmin, which predominantly attacks the coiled-coil region between fragment E and fragment D. Degradation of cross-linked fibrin is much slower than fibrinogen, in large part because of the inaccessibility of the plasmin cleavage sites.[1854,1856,1857] The first step in degrading cross-linked fibrin is the removal of the α-chains

Fibrinogenolysis

Fibrinolysis

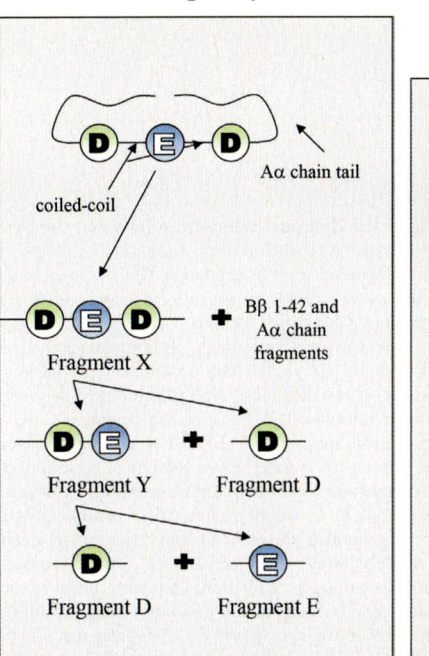

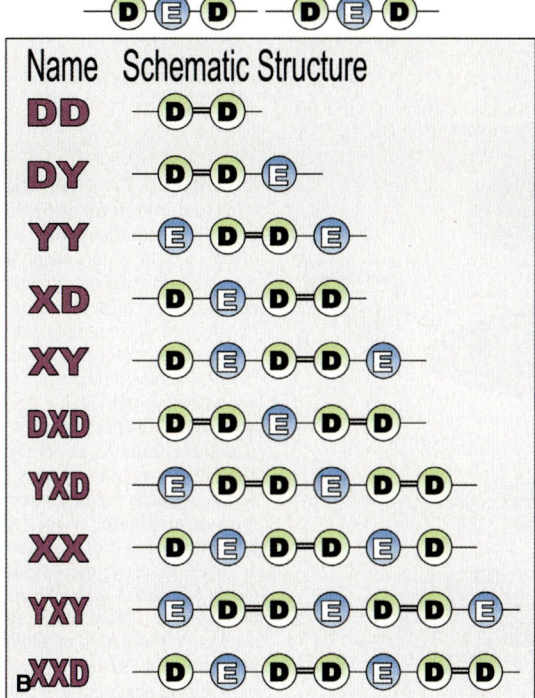

FIGURE 20.22 Fibrinogenolysis and fibrinolysis. A, Fibrinogen is represented as a trinodular structure (D-E-D domains). Each E-domain and D-domain is separated by a coiled-coil domain. The Aα-chain tail is shown as a line. Plasmin digests fibrinogen, yielding various fragments, the largest of which is fragment X. Fragment X contains the two D domains, the E domain, and the α-helical coiled coils but lacks the C termini of the Aα-chains and the peptide Bβ-chains. Fragment Y consists of the central E domain connected by the coiled coil to one of the terminal D domains. Fragment Y can be further degraded by cleavage of the coiled-coil domain to release a second D domain and fragment E. B, The domain composition of the monomer units of degraded fibrin is indicated by the circles containing a D or an E. Intermolecular cross-links between the γ-chains are shown as thicker lines connecting the D regions. The structures of the various-sized fragments of cross-linked fibrin monomers resulting from plasmin proteolysis of fibrin are presented.

so that the coiled-coils are exposed. As the coiled-coils are cleaved, different-sized fragments are released.[1858] The smallest of these degradation products are double-D ($M_r \sim 180,000$), also known as *D-dimer,* a soluble fragment in which the two D fragments are linked by two isopeptide linkages, and a fragment with the stoichiometry D_2E (termed *DY;* $M_r \sim 235,000$), a double-D and a fragment E held in place by strong, noncovalent bonding.[1859,1860] A large number of intermediate-sized fibrin degradation products arising from cleavages between the fragment D and fragment E regions are also generated (*Figure 20.22*). The largest of these fragments is the XXD (two fragment Xs and a fragment D) with a mass in the range of 595 kDa. Some of these complexes (e.g., D-dimer) have been identified in the blood of patients with various thrombotic or thrombolytic disorders.

PROTEINS OF THE FIBRINOLYTIC SYSTEM

Clot formation is integrated with clot dissolution to maintain hemostasis. The biochemical mechanisms of clot dissolution center on fibrin-specific activation of plasminogen to plasmin. The key proteins involved are plasminogen, plasminogen activators (t-PA and u-PA), PAI-1, α_2-antiplasmin, and TAFI (*Figure 20.23*).

Plasminogen

Plasminogen is the inactive precursor of the enzyme plasmin, which is the primary catalyst of fibrin degradation. Hereditary plasminogen deficiency has been described as either a deficiency of plasminogen antigen and activity (type I) or as a normal antigen level but reduced activity (type II, dysplasminogenemia).[1861] Thrombophilia and ligneous conjunctivitis are clinical manifestations associated with homozygous deficiency; the impact of heterozygous deficiency remains in dispute. Homozygous plasminogen-deficient mice are viable but exhibit severe thrombosis with systemic fibrin deposition and die prematurely.[1862,1863]

Gene Structure and Expression

The plasminogen gene is located on the long arm of chromosome 6 at band q26[1864,1865] (*Table 20.9*). It spans 52.5 kb of DNA with 19 exons. It is in close proximity to two genes for apolipoprotein A and for the plasminogen-related genes A and B.[1866-1868] The first exon codes for the signal sequence; each of the five kringle domains is encoded by two exons, as is the activation peptide. Plasminogen expression is normally stable, with the regulation of the activity of the fibrinolytic system occurring mainly via the regulation of the plasminogen activators and their inhibitors. However, plasminogen is an acute-phase reactant protein.[1774,1865] Two sequence elements common to acute-phase reactant genes have been located at positions 76 to 81 and −553 to −558.[1865] Other potential regulatory transcriptional elements have been identified, including HNF-1, AP-1, CREB, and GATA.[1868]

Biochemistry

Plasminogen is synthesized in the liver and is present in a wide variety of tissues and body fluids, including saliva, lacrimal gland secretions, seminal vesicle fluid, and prostate secretions.[1869] Plasminogen circulates in plasma at an approximate concentration of 200 mg/L (2 μmol/L; *Table 20.10*). It has a circulating $t_{1/2}$ of 2.2 days.[1870] The $t_{1/2}$ in disease states, in which the fibrinolytic system is activated, can be shortened dramatically.

Human plasminogen is a single-chain glycoprotein of a relative molecular weight of 88,000 containing 2% carbohydrate (*Table 20.10* and *Figure 20.24*). Two major carbohydrate variants of plasminogen are found in roughly equal amounts in human plasma: plasminogen variant 1 is glycosylated at two sites, Asn^{289} and Thr^{346}, whereas plasminogen variant 2 is glycosylated only at Thr^{346}. Isoelectric focusing of either of these major carbohydrate variants, even when the proteins are isolated from a single plasma donor, reveals additional heterogeneity derived from variable sialic acid content.[1871-1874] Heterogeneity in the primary sequence of plasminogen has also been observed, reflecting the presence of two high-incidence polymorphisms and a number of low-incidence polymorphisms in the human population. Functional differences between the two major carbohydrate forms have been reported.[1875-1879] An additional glycosylation site at Ser^{249} containing a trisaccharide has been identified.[1880]

The primary structure of plasminogen contains 791 amino acids segregated into an NH_2-terminal activation peptide domain (residues Glu^1-Lys^{77}), a region containing five kringles (K1-K5;

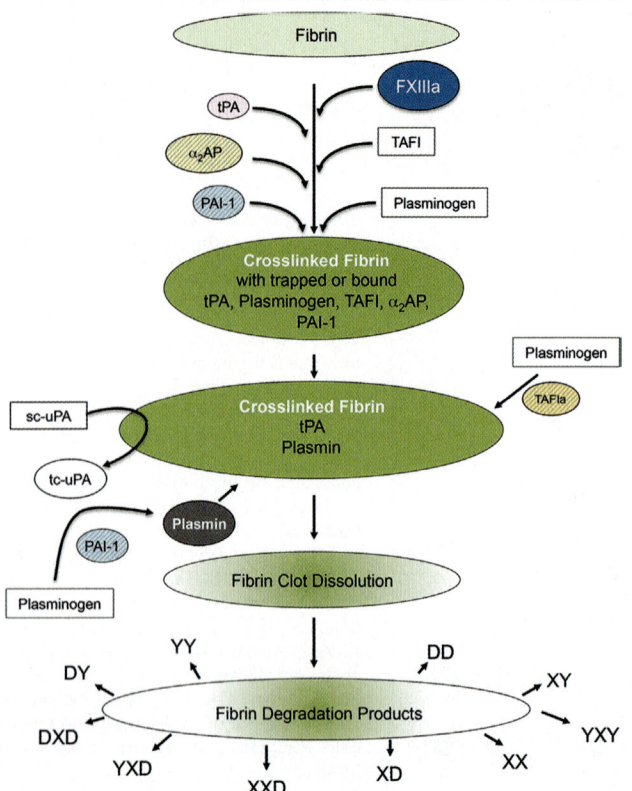

FIGURE 20.23 Schematic of the dynamic interaction between the proteins and inhibitors of fibrinolysis. Cross-linked fibrin formation is integrated with fibrin clot dissolution and degradation of its products. The enzymes (*dark blue ovals*), inhibitors (*light blue ovals*), zymogens (*open boxes*), and complexes (*large green ovals*) are illustrated in a simplified form to show this multicomponent process. The key proteins involved are plasminogen, plasminogen activators (tissue-type plasminogen activator [tPA], single-chain urokinase-type plasminogen activator [scu-PA], and two-chain urokinase-type plasminogen activator [tcu-PA]), plasminogen activator inhibitor-1 (PAI-1), α_2-antiplasmin (α_2-AP), and thrombin-activatable fibrinolysis inhibitor (TAFI). t-PA and plasminogen both bind to the fibrin surface where t-PA is an effective catalyst of plasminogen activation. Initially, plasmin proteolysis of fibrin generates new, higher-affinity binding sites for plasminogen, setting up an amplifying loop of plasminogen activation. Reinforcing this process, generated plasmin can convert the single-chain form of urokinase, an ineffective catalyst, to its active form, thus increasing the concentration of available plasminogen activation. Opposing these events are antifibrinolytic mechanisms. α_2-AP, both soluble and cross-linked to fibrin, forms complexes with plasmin, rendering it inactive. PAI-1 rapidly reacts with both t-PA and two-chain urokinase, reducing the concentration of plasminogen activators. Formation of activated TAFI (TAFIa) results in removal of plasmin-generated COOH-terminal lysine residues, thus suppressing the rate of fibrin lysis. Fibrin degradation occurs by cleavage at the D-E-D domains of fibrin polymers by plasmin to yield a variety of polymers as illustrated (see *Figure 20.22*).

residues Lys^{78}-Arg^{541}), and a catalytic domain (residues Val^{562}-Asn^{791})[1864,1881,1882] (*Figure 20.24*). As secreted into the blood, plasminogen has a glutamic acid at its NH$_2$ terminus, referred to as Glu-plasminogen. Proteolysis by plasmin at one of several potential sites in the NH$_2$-terminal region results in a degraded form of plasminogen; the most common product is Lys^{78}-plasminogen. Removal of the NH$_2$-terminal peptide region results in a major structural change in the plasminogen molecule, yielding a species of plasminogen that has a higher affinity than Glu-plasminogen for fibrin and is a better substrate for plasminogen activators.[1883] The primary site for Lys-plasminogen formation is at the fibrin clot; the $t_{1/2}$ of Lys-plasminogen is shorter than the full-length molecule ($t_{1/2}$ = 0.8 days). Each kringle domain contains 78 to 80 amino acids. The K1 and K4 kringle domains have been identified as containing sites that are responsible for regulating the binding of plasminogen to fibrin,[1884,1885] α_2-antiplasmin,[1886] histidine-rich glycoprotein,[1887] the kininogens,[1888] thrombospondin,[1889] and cell surface receptors. These sites on the plasminogen kringles (called *lysine-binding sites*) bind lysyl residues in the target molecules; COOH-terminal lysyl residues are bound more avidly. Lysine analogs (i.e., â-aminocaproic acid and tranexamic acid) can compete with lysyl residues in proteins for binding to plasminogen and, hence, are useful inhibitors of fibrinolysis.[1890,1891] The conformational change associated with the removal of the NH$_2$-terminal activation peptide also occurs on binding of lysine or its analogs to the appropriate kringles in Glu-plasminogen.[1891-1893] The shape of the Glu-plasminogen molecule changes from a prolate ellipsoid of axial ratio 2.6 to a more random coil-type structure of axial ratio >5, similar in dimension to Lys-plasminogen.[1894,1895] A fragment of plasminogen comprising K1-K4, also known as *angiostatin,* has been shown to inhibit angiogenesis.[1896] The catalytic domain of plasminogen

(Val^{562}-Asn^{791}) shows considerable homology to trypsin and other serine proteases and includes the catalytic triad (His^{603}, Asp^{646}, and Ser^{741}) typical of these proteases.[1897]

Function

Plasminogen is a zymogen devoid of enzymatic activity until converted to the serine protease plasmin by cleavage of the Arg^{561}-Val^{562} peptide bond by plasminogen activators such as u-PA and t-PA (*Figure 20.25*). In plasma or bound to fibrin in a blood clot, cleavage of this peptide bond by either t-PA or u-PA converts Glu-plasminogen into Glu-plasmin, a two-chain enzyme that can degrade fibrin, fibrinogen, and a number of other molecules. Plasmin is composed of a heavy chain (kringle domains) and a light chain (catalytic domain) that are attached by two disulfide bonds. Glu-plasmin can autodigest by cleaving itself, most commonly at Lys^{77} to generate Lys-plasmin.[1898,1899] Inhibition of plasmin by α_2-antiplasmin is the primary route for regulation of plasmin's hemostatic function; suppression of plasmin activity beyond the locale of fibrin deposition is imperative if fibrinogenolysis is to be prevented. Plasmin bound through its lysine-binding sites to fibrin reacts more slowly with α_2-antiplasmin than when free in solution. This differential reactivity effectively localizes plasmin activity to the fibrin surface.

Plasminogen Activators

The process of plasminogen activation can occur through three distinct pathways: (a) the intrinsic activator system (analogous to the contact system of blood coagulation), (b) the extrinsic activators (t-PA and u-PA), and (c) an exogenous activator system involving pharmacologic agents (thrombolytic drugs). The pathway used in vivo appears to be the extrinsic pathway. However, both the intrinsic and exogenous activator systems could play an important role in human disease.

Table 20.9. Proteins and Inhibitors of the Fibrinolytic System: Molecular Genetics

Name	Molecular Weight (Da)	Gene Location: Chromosome	Gene Size (kb)	Gene Organization: # of Exons	mRNA Size (kb)	UNIPROT Accession Number[a]
Plasminogen	88,000	6q26	52.5	19	2.9	P00747
Tissue-type plasminogen activator	70,000	8p11.21	32.7	14	2.7	P00750
Urokinase-type plasminogen activator	54,000	10q22.2	6.4	11	2.4	P00749
Thrombin-activatable fibrinolysis inhibitor	58,000	13q14.13	48	11	1.8	Q96IY4
PAI-1	50,000	7q22.1	12.2	9	3.2	P05121
PAI-2	60,000	18q21.33-q22.1	16.5	8	1.9	P05120
α_2-Antiplasmin	70,000	17p13.3	16	10	2.2	P08697
Factor VII–activating protease	64,000	10q25.3	35	13	3.0	Q14520

Abbreviation: PAI, plasminogen activator inhibitor.
[a]http://www.uniprot.org.

Intrinsic Activators

The body has evolved a mechanism to recognize invasion by foreign substances. Many of these foreign substances contain negatively charged surfaces that allow for the activation of the intrinsic (contact) pathway (factor XII, prekallikrein, HMWK, and factor XI). Plasminogen can interact with this intrinsic pathway of blood coagulation to generate plasmin. There is continued debate as to the extent to which the intrinsic pathway functions in regulating normal fibrinolysis. It has been estimated that this pathway contributes only approximately 15% of the total fibrinolytic activity in human plasma.[1900] Several studies have established that kallikrein and factors IXa and XIIa can directly activate plasminogen to plasmin.[1901-1904] At this time, it is best to conclude that the physiologic significance and relevance of the contact system in fibrinolysis are not entirely clear. It has been suggested that individuals with factor XII deficiency as well as deficiencies in some of the other intrinsic coagulation factors may have a subtle, but potentially significant, defect in fibrinolysis under certain clinical conditions. Additional studies are needed to address this controversial subject.

Extrinsic Activator: Tissue Plasminogen Activator

There are two dominant extrinsic activator systems in the body: t-PA and u-PA. These activators have unique structures and properties that affect the specificity and rate of plasmin generation.

The t-PA molecule is predominantly a product of endothelial cells[1905-1909]; it is also produced by vascular smooth muscle cells,[1910] neuronal cells,[1911] megakaryocytes,[1912,1913] mast cells,[1914,1915] monocytes,[1916] and fibroblasts.[1917] Factors that regulate its secretion and release from the endothelium are important mediators of blood clotting or inflammation. These include thrombin, histamine, acetylcholine, bradykinin, epinephrine, ILs, shear stress, and vaso-occlusion.[1918,1919] t-PA antigen is present in normal plasma at approximately 5 µg/L (70 pmol/L; *Table 20.10*).[1920-1924] Functional concentrations have been reported to be <20 pmol/L with the remainder of the t-PA antigen found in complex with PAI-1.[1921,1925,1926] The $t_{1/2}$ in plasma is quite short, with pharmacokinetic modeling indicating a $t_{1/2}$ of 2.4 minutes for active t-PA and 5 minutes for the t-PA/PAI-1 complex.[1927,1928] The t-PA molecule and the t-PA/PAI-1 complex are cleared from the

Table 20.10. Proteins and Inhibitors of the Fibrinolytic System: Biochemical Properties

Name	Molecular Weight (Da)[a]	Amino Acid Number	Plasma Concentration (nmol/L)	Plasma Concentration (mg/L)	Half-Life	Carbohydrates (%)
Plasminogen	88,000	791	2000	200	2.2 days	2
Tissue-type plasminogen activator	70,000	527	0.07	0.005	2.4 min	7/13
Urokinase-type plasminogen activator	54,000	411	0.04	0.002	5 min	7
Thrombin-activatable fibrinolysis inhibitor	58,000	401	75	4.5	10 min[a]	23[b]
Plasminogen activator inhibitor-1	50,000	379	0.2	0.01	<10 min	13
Plasminogen activator inhibitor-2	60,000	415	<0.07	<0.005	—	22[b]
α_2-Antiplasmin	70,000	464	1000	70	2.6 d	13
Factor VII–activating protease	64,000	537	190	12	—	5

[a]Activated form.
[b]Estimated value calculated from difference of molecular weight determined by sodium dodecyl sulfate–polyacrylamide gel electrophoresis and weight of sum of amino acids derived from complementary DNA.

Plasminogen

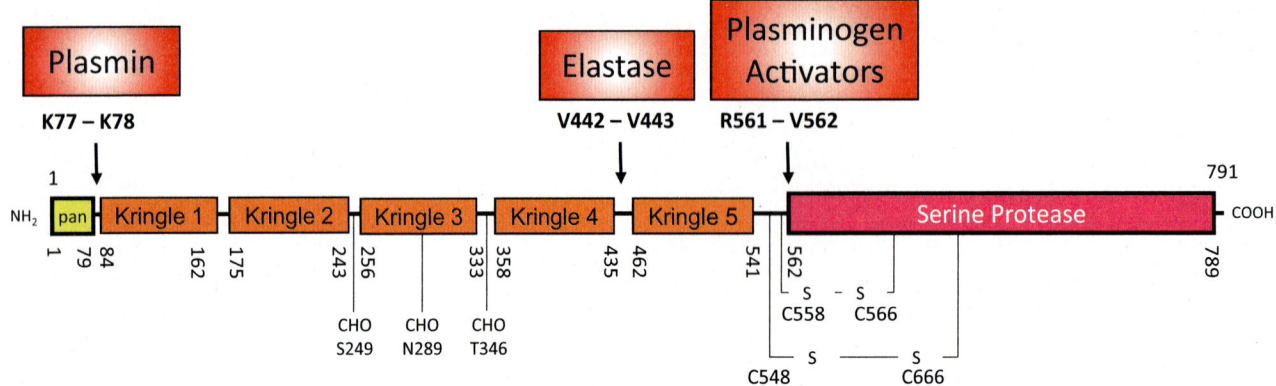

FIGURE 20.24 Schematic of plasminogen. Plasminogen is the inactive precursor of the enzyme plasmin, which is the primary catalyst of fibrin degradation. Human plasminogen is a single-chain glycoprotein containing 2% carbohydrate (CHO). CHO variants are shown for plasminogens 1 and 2. The primary structure of plasminogen contains 791 amino acids segregated into an NH$_2$-terminal activation peptide domain (pan), a region containing five kringles, and a catalytic domain. Proteolysis by plasmin at one of several potential sites in this NH$_2$-terminal region results in a degraded form of plasminogen; the most common product is K78-plasminogen. Cleavage by plasminogen activators at R561-V562 results in plasmin.

plasma by two specific cell receptor systems in the liver as well as receptor-mediated clearance by endothelial cells[1929] (for review see[1851,1930,1931]).

Gene Structure and Expression

The human gene for t-PA is found on chromosome 8 band p11.21 and spans 32.7 kb[1932] (*Table 20.9*). There are 14 exons with distinct structural motifs encoded by individual exons.[1933-1935] The processed transcript codes for a protein product of 562 amino acids: residues 1 to 23 comprise the signal peptide, whereas residues 24 to 32 function as a propeptide region. Further processing removes residues 32 to 35 to yield the circulating protein product. The 5′-flanking region of the t-PA gene extends more than 9500 bp with a functional retinoic acid response element identified at −7300 bp[1936] and a multihormone responsive enhancer localized to the region −7145 to −9758 bp.[1937-1939] A number of *cis*-acting elements have been identified in the proximal promoter region. A transcription initiation site 209 bp upstream of the translation start site was initially identified. A consensus TATA sequence was identified 22 bp upstream of this transcription start site.[1934,1935] Subsequently, a TATA-independent transcript initiation site 99 bp upstream of the translation start site was identified as the primary site of transcription initiation in fibroblasts[1940] and endothelial cells.[1941] The significance of t-PA transcripts with different-length 5′-untranslated regions is not established; deletion of the entire 5′-untranslated region of t-PA was observed to increase the stability of the t-PA transcript.[1942] Translational control of t-PA gene expression has been observed in some cell types, implicating a regulatory role for the 3′-untranslated region of the t-PA transcript.[1943,1944]

A number of polymorphisms of the t-PA gene have been identified. A 311-bp *Alu* insertion/deletion polymorphism within the eighth intron of the t-PA gene has been extensively studied.[1945-1950] A similar polymorphism in the angiotensin-converting enzyme gene has been linked to plasma levels of this enzyme.[1951] In contrast, no correlation of plasma t-PA levels with its *Alu* polymorphism has been observed.[1947-1949] With one exception,[1945] clinical studies have indicated no correlation between this polymorphism and the incidence of

stroke or myocardial infarction.[1947-1949] A single nucleotide polymorphism (−7351 C/T) in an Sp1-binding site in the far upstream enhancer element of the t-PA gene has been linked to the vascular release rate of t-PA in vivo[1952] and to the frequency of occurrence of first myocardial infarction.[1953]

No cases of congenital deficiency of t-PA have been reported. Transgenic mice lacking a functional t-PA gene developed normally and displayed a normal basal hemostatic phenotype.[1954] Mice in which both the t-PA and u-PA genes were disabled had shortened lifespans and experienced severe, spontaneous thrombotic episodes.[1954,1955]

Biochemistry

The t-PA molecule is a serine proteinase with a molecular weight of 70 kDa[1956] (*Table 20.10* and *Figure 20.26*). It was originally isolated as a single polypeptide chain of 527 amino acids[1957] with an NH$_2$-terminal serine residue; full-length t-PA has an NH$_2$-terminal extension of three amino acids (Gly-Ala-Arg).[1958-1960] Numbering in this chapter is based on Ser^1-t-PA, the most extensively studied form because of its availability as a recombinant product.

The single-chain t-PA molecule is an efficient plasminogen activator in the presence of fibrin[1961-1964] and is converted into a somewhat more active two-chain molecule by cleavage of the peptide bond between Arg^{275} and Ile^{276}.[1872,1962-1965] This cleavage is performed primarily by the action of plasmin during fibrinolysis; factor Xa and kallikrein can also catalyze this conversion. The t-PA molecule divides structurally and functionally into two major regions with the Arg^{275}-Ile^{276} bond as the boundary: the 38-kDa NH$_2$-terminal portion (Ser^1-Arg^{275}), called the *heavy* or *A-chain* in the two-chain molecule, contains structures involved in fibrin binding, fibrin-specific plasminogen activation, and plasma clearance mechanisms; and the 28-kDa catalytic region (Ile^{276}-Pro^{527}), called the *light* or *B-chain,* is homologous to the proteolytic domain of other serine proteases. Specifically, the A-chain contains a fibronectin fingerlike domain,[1966] an EGF-like domain,[1967] and two kringle domains.[383,1968] The finger domain extends from residues 4 to 50 and is involved in the binding of t-PA to fibrin.[1969,1970] The binding of the finger region to fibrin is not blocked by â-aminocaproic acid.[1971] The finger domain of

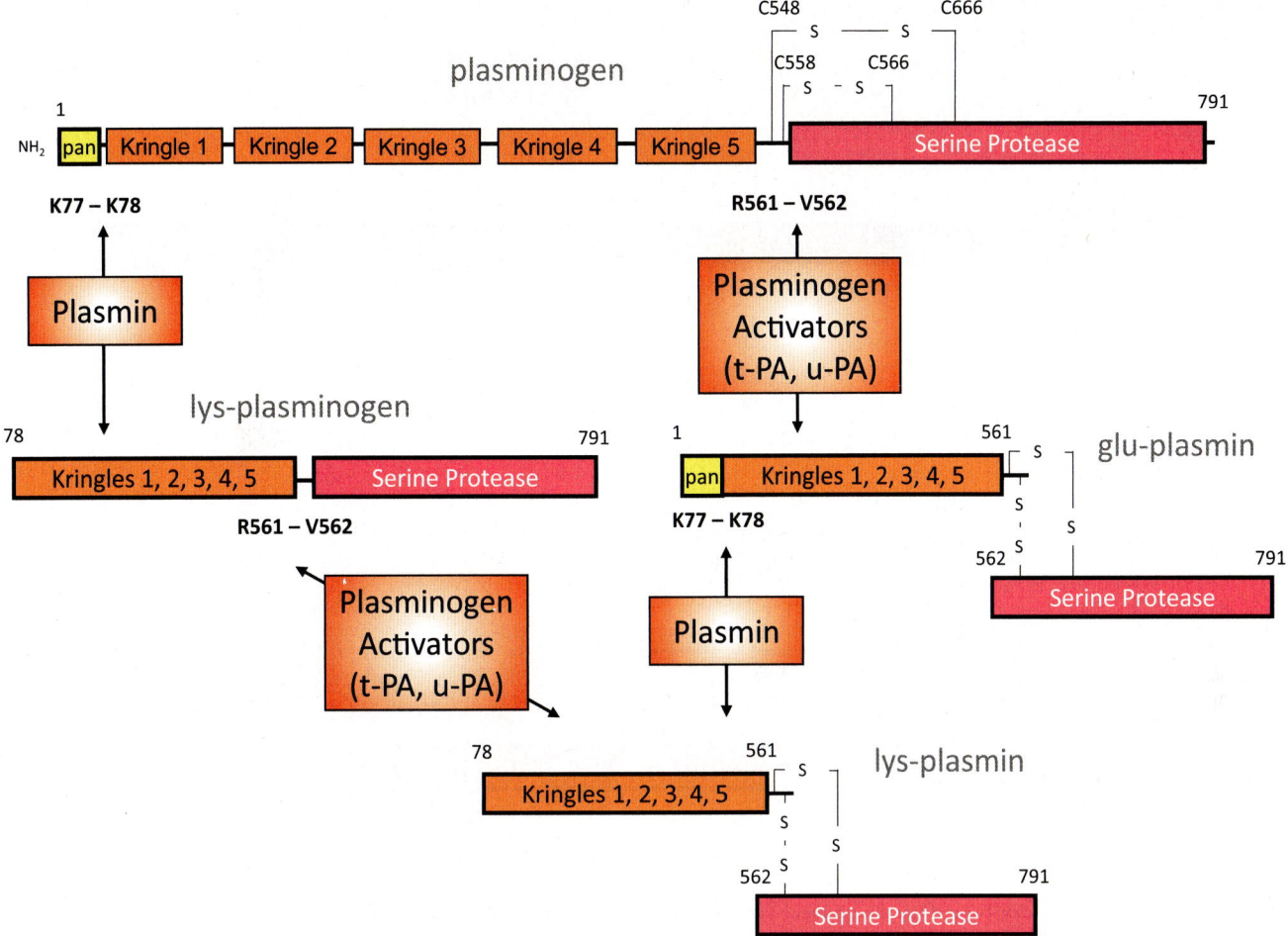

FIGURE 20.25 Molecular forms of plasmin(ogen). Plasminogen in its native form has a glutamic acid at residue 1 and is referred to as glu-plasminogen. Glu-plasminogen has a molecular weight of 88,000 Da and contains 791 amino acids. Cleavage at R561-V562 in glu-plasminogen by plasminogen activators (tissue-type plasminogen activator [t-PA] and urokinase-type plasminogen activator [u-PA]) yields glu-plasmin. Glu-plasmin consists of an NH_2-terminal heavy chain linked by two disulfide bonds to a catalytic domain. At the localized clot level, plasmin that is formed can cleave glu-plasminogen at the NH_2-terminal bond K77-K78 to yield lys-plasminogen. Lys-plasminogen can be activated by plasminogen activators that hydrolyze the R561-V562 bond to yield lys-plasmin.

t-PA has sequence homology and structural homology[1972] to similar structures found in fibronectin. Selected mutations in the finger or the EGF domain have been shown to result in prolonged half-lives in vivo for the modified t-PA molecules, indicating a role for these regions in uptake mechanisms.[1973,1974] The kringle domains of t-PA span residues 87 to 176 (kringle 1) and residues 176 to 262 (kringle 2). The biologic role of kringle 1 remains undiscovered.[1969-1971] The kringle 2 domain is involved in the binding of t-PA to fibrin.[1969,1970] This binding interaction is blocked by lysine and its analogs such as â-aminocaproic acid,[1969] indicating the presence of a plasminogen-like lysine-binding pocket. The overall crystal structure of t-PA kringle 2[1975] resembles that of kringle 4 of plasminogen, although differences are observed in the arrangement of residues forming the lysine-binding sites.[1975-1978] The light or B-chain of t-PA contains the active site catalytic triad of this serine protease (His[322], Asp[371], and Ser[478]).[677,1957,1979] Both the single- and two-chain forms of t-PA cleave plasminogen at Arg[561]-Val[562] to yield the enzyme plasmin. The catalytic efficiency of single-chain t-PA toward plasminogen in solution and toward tripeptide paranitroanilide substrates is lower than the two-chain form.[1962,1964,1980] Both forms have been crystallized[1981,1982] and exhibit enhanced and roughly equivalent rates of proteolysis of plasminogen when fibrin is present.[1962]

The t-PA molecule has three potential N-linked glycosylation sites and one O-linked site. The O-linked site is found at Thr[61] in the EGF domain.[1983] The presence of a fucose at this site appears to facilitate the uptake of t-PA by hepatocytes.[1984] Two major carbohydrate variants of t-PA have been identified. Type I is glycosylated at Asn[117] (kringle 1), Asn[184] (kringle 2), and Asn[448] (catalytic domain), whereas type II is glycosylated only at Asn[117] and Asn[448].[1985,1986] The presence of carbohydrate at Asn[184] appears to downregulate the fibrinolytic activity of type I t-PA by interfering with the association between the lysine-binding site of its kringle 2 domain and fibrin.

Regulation

Regulation of t-PA activity in blood is accomplished by three primary mechanisms: control of its catalytic potential via the fibrin dependence of plasminogen activation; control of systemic levels of functional t-PA by the concerted processes of rapid t-PA removal by hepatic clearance and of inhibition by the circulating serpin PAI-1; and control of t-PA activity levels at the site of injury by the competing processes of increased t-PA secretion by traumatized and recruited cells versus PAI-1 release by activated platelets. T-PA manifests its full fibrinolytic potential only when bound to fibrin.[1987-1989] This binding interaction aligns t-PA and plasminogen on the fibrin surface so that the catalytic efficiency of t-PA is enhanced several hundredfold. This is vital to the localization of plasmin generation at the site of fibrin deposition. Systemic t-PA levels in blood are under highly dynamic control characterized by maintenance of relatively low levels of the protein (70 pmol/L) with a high clearance rate ($t_{1/2}$ = 2.4 minutes) and by maintenance of an extremely effective

t-PA: 70 kDa

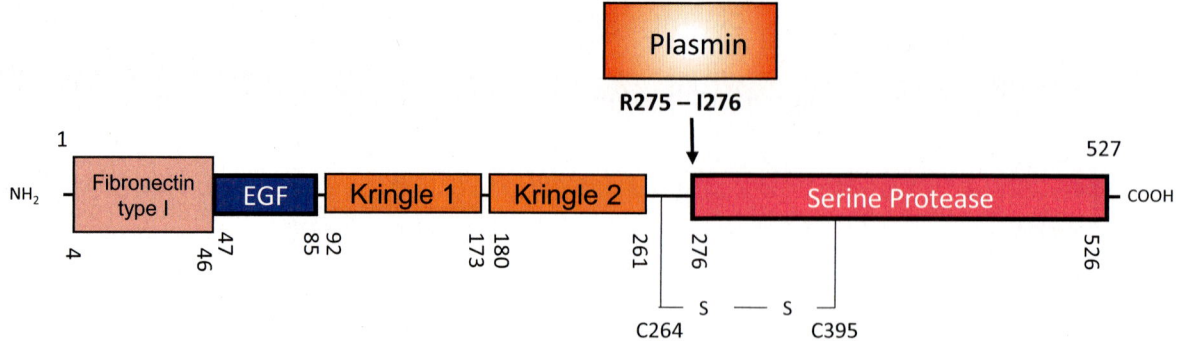

sc-uPA: 54 kDa

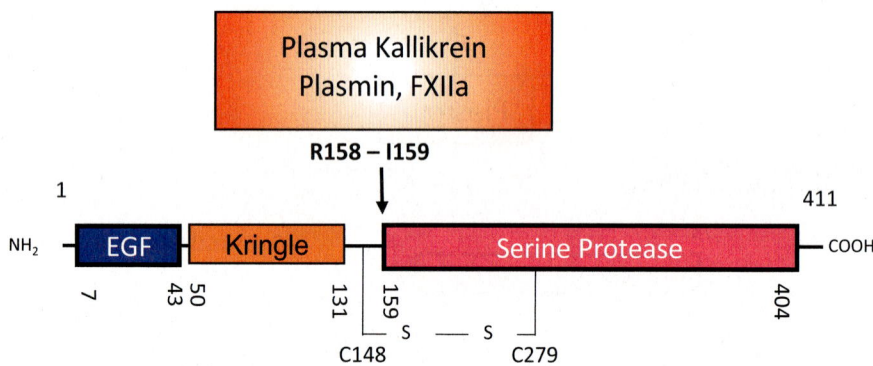

FIGURE 20.26 **Fibrinolytic proteins tissue-type plasminogen activator (t-PA) and single-chain urokinase-type plasminogen activator (sc-uPA).** The single-chain t-PA molecule is an efficient plasminogen activator in the presence of fibrin and is converted into a somewhat more active two-chain molecule by cleavage of the peptide bond between R275 and I276. This cleavage is performed primarily by the action of plasmin during fibrinolysis. Structurally t-PA contains a fibronectin type I domain, an epidermal growth factor (EGF)-like domain, and two kringle domains, and a serine protease-type catalytic domain. The kringle 2 domain and the fibronectin domain of t-PA are involved in the binding of t-PA to fibrin. sc-uPA is an ineffective catalyst. Plasmin or plasma kallikrein can hydrolyze the K158–I159 peptide bond, converting sc-uPA into the fully active two-chain form (two-chain urokinase-type plasminogen activator). u-PA is composed of an EGF domain (EGF), a single kringle domain, and the serine protease-type catalytic domain. One glycosylation site (CHO) is present in the serine protease domain.

inhibitor, PAI-1 (second-order rate constant for complex formation = 10^7 to 10^8 M^{-1} s^{-1}), at a circulating concentration severalfold higher than that of t-PA. The release of t-PA from the vessel wall is another important regulator of fibrinolysis.[1990,1991] The rate at which clots lyse is dependent on how rapidly t-PA is secreted by the relevant cells in the vicinity of an injury.[1992,1993] For example, activated platelets secrete serotonin that can induce endothelial cells to release t-PA; they also release PAI-1 from their α-granules. Although only a fraction of this PAI-1 is in the active form, it functions to downregulate plasminogen activation.[1994-1996]

Extrinsic Activator: Urokinase Plasminogen Activator

The other major extrinsic activator in the blood is u-PA. This activator was first identified in the urine,[1997-1999] where it is present at relatively high concentrations (40-80 μg/L).[1999,2000] It was subsequently detected in the media of cultured human kidney cells, endothelial cells, malignant cell lines, and tumors and in plasma.[2001-2004] u-PA is a serine protease and is synthesized as a single-chain molecule called *prourokinase* or *single-chain u-PA* (scu-PA). The plasma concentration of scu-PA ranges from 2 to 4 ng/mL (37-74 pmol/L; *Table 20.10*)[2005]; the $t_{1/2}$ of scu-PA is quite short, approximately 5 minutes, and metabolism occurs in both the liver and the kidney. scu-PA has a very low level of proteolytic activity.[2006] Plasmin can hydrolyze the Lys[158]-Ile[159] peptide bond, converting scu-PA into the two-chain form (tcu-PA).[1997,2007-2009] The mechanism in blood by which scu-PA is converted into tcu-PA still remains poorly defined. It has been postulated that, within a thrombus, t-PA initially activates plasminogen bound to fibrin to form plasmin, and that it is this fibrin-localized plasmin that then converts scu-PA into tcu-PA.[2010-2012] This process results in an amplification of the rate of plasmin formation. The main site of urokinase-driven plasminogen activation appears to be extravascular, where it has an important role in promoting degradation of extracellular matrix by triggering the activation of plasminogen and, possibly, matrix metalloproteinases.[2013] Regulation of urokinase is important to normal and pathologic processes including embryogenesis, wound healing, tumor cell invasion, and metastasis.[2014-2016] Inhibitors of urokinase have been shown to suppress the growth of primary tumors and to interfere with metastasis of tumor cells.[2017-2023]

Gene Structure and Expression

The human u-PA gene spans 6.4 kb with 11 exons[2024] and is located on chromosome 10, band q22.2[2025] (*Table 20.9*). The overall intron-exon arrangement is similar to that of the t-PA gene. The primary amino acid sequence of the purified, intact two-chain molecule has been determined,[1997,1998,2026] and the cDNA has been isolated and sequenced[2027]: the gene specifies a protein of 431 amino acids, with the first 20 residues constituting a signal peptide.

The Normal Hematologic System

The disruption of the urokinase gene (u-PA$^{-/-}$) in mice is not lethal.[1954] These mice did not display spontaneous thrombi in their vasculature. The phenotype of u-PA$^{-/-}$ mice included occasional minor fibrin deposits in the liver and intestine, excessive fibrin deposits in chronic nonhealing skin lesions, and increased susceptibility to bacterial infections.[1954,2028-2030]

Biochemistry

u-PA is a single-chain glycoprotein containing 411 amino acids (M_r = 54,000; *Table 20.10*; *Figure 20.26*). It has 12 disulfide bonds with one (Cys^{148}-Cys^{279}) serving to link the catalytic domain (B-chain) to the NH$_2$-terminal domain (A-chain). Posttranslational modifications include glycosylation at Asn$^{(302)}$, addition of a single fucose residue at Thr^{18},[2031] and regulatory phosphorylation at Ser^{138}/Ser^{303}.[2032] u-PA is composed of an EGF domain (residues 7-43), a single kringle domain (residues 50-131), a connecting peptide region (residues 132-157), and the serine protease-type catalytic domain (residues 159-411). The EGF domain contains the residues essential for urokinase binding to the urokinase receptor[2033] and appears to be the domain responsible for the ability of urokinase to induce cellular proliferation and differentiation.[2034-2036] The function of the kringle domain of urokinase remains to be established. It displays no binding affinity for fibrin. Recent evidence indicates that the kringle domain may have a role in mediating the process by which urokinase stimulates smooth muscle migration.[2037-2039] Residues His^{204}, Asp^{255}, and Ser^{356} form the catalytic triad of urokinase; unlike the single-chain form of t-PA, they are not properly positioned for efficient catalysis. scu-PA does not form complexes with PAI-1 or react with peptidyl chloromethylketones that inhibit the two-chain form; scu-PA-catalyzed hydrolysis of tripeptide paranitroanilide substrates proceeds with 0.1% to 0.4% the efficiency of tcu-PA,[2040,2041] and plasminogen activation by scu-PA appears to be equally inefficient when compared with tcu-PA.[2012,2042]

The urokinase molecule is asymmetric in shape with the growth factor, kringle, and catalytic domains arranged like differently configured beads on a string.[2031,2043-2045] A crystal structure for the entire urokinase molecule has not been accomplished. However, a crystal structure at a resolution of 2.5 Å has been reported for the catalytic domain. The molecule used was a recombinant, nonglycosylated human u-PA (residues 159-411) with its active site histidine residue derivatized with a peptidyl chloromethylketone.[2046] The catalytic domain of u-PA has the expected overall topography and S1 specificity pocket of a trypsinlike protease, an S2 pocket of hydrophobic character, and a solvent-accessible S3 pocket suitable for binding a wide range of amino acid side chains. The crystal structure of a mutant urokinase catalytic domain (residues 159-404: C122A and N302Q) at a resolution of 1.5 Å has also been reported.[2047]

Activation

Conversion of single-chain urokinase to an active two-chain form occurs principally through hydrolysis of the Lys^{158}-Ile^{159} bond. This molecular form, referred to as *high-molecular-weight tcu-PA,* is composed of NH$_2$-terminal heavy chain (residues 1-158) linked by one disulfide bond to the catalytic domain. In the blood, during fibrinolysis, plasmin is the primary catalyst of this conversion; in addition, both kallikrein and factor XIIa,[2007] products of the intrinsic pathway of coagulation, hydrolyze this bond. A number of other proteases that cleave the Lys^{158}-Ile^{159} bond have also been identified, including several cathepsins,[2048-2051] mast cell tryptase,[2052] nerve growth factor-γ,[2053] human T-cell serine proteinase-1,[2054] and FSAP.[2055] A second, catalytically active form of two-chain urokinase, known as *low-molecular-weight tcu-PA,* is found in plasma when fibrinolysis is stimulated. It is formed by an additional plasmin cleavage at Lys^{135}-Lys^{136}. This yields a truncated heavy chain containing most of the connecting peptide region (residues 136-158) linked to the catalytic domain by the Cys^{148}-Cys^{279} disulfide bond. This cleavage produces a more efficient enzyme, and this low-molecular-weight form is used clinically for thrombolytic therapy. Another low-molecular-weight

form of scu-PA arises from cleavage of the Glu^{143}-Leu^{144} bond by the matrix metalloproteinases Pump 1 and metalloproteinase 3.[2056-2058] This form appears to be a better clot-lysing agent than low-molecular-weight tcu-PA.[2059]

Neutrophil cathepsin G and elastase from granulocytes cleave scu-PA at the Ile^{159}-Ile^{160} bond, yielding a two-chain molecule that is inactive.[2060,2061] Thrombin[2007,2062,2063] and, more efficiently, the thrombin-thrombomodulin complex[2064] cleave scu-PA at Arg^{156}-Phe^{157}, yielding an inactive two-chain urokinase species. The release of the dipeptide Phe^{157}-Lys^{158} from the catalytic domain is catalyzed by cathepsin C[2049] or plasmin.[2065]

Function

t-PA appears to be the primary plasminogen activator in the vasculature, with fibrin-localized scu-PA conversion to tcu-PA acting as an amplifying rather than initiating mechanism for plasmin formation.[2012,2066] Direct scu-PA activation of Glu-plasminogen bound to COOH-terminal lysine residues found in partially proteolyzed fibrin has been proposed as contributing to clot lysis.[2067-2069] This catalytic role of scu-PA, although direct, still depends temporally on t-PA–derived plasmin to create the circumstance (plasmin proteolyzed fibrin) under which it can contribute to overall fibrinolysis.

Extrinsic Activator: Factor VII–Activating Protease

Recently, a novel serine protease in human plasma has been described that can support coagulation by activating factor VII.[491,2055,2070] It was originally described as plasma hyaluronan-binding protein and was isolated by adsorption to immobilized hyaluronic acid as a disulfide-linked heterodimer.[2070] Independently, a thrombin-like amidolytic activity was purified from commercial prothrombin complex concentrates.[2071,2072] Sequencing data indicated that this protease and plasma hyaluronan-binding protein were the same proteins. Subsequently, the protease from prothrombin complex concentrates was shown to be a potent activator of factor VII and termed *FSAP*.[491] The capacity of FSAP to activate factor VII has been challenged.[2073] This protease has also been shown to be an efficient activator of single-chain urokinase and appears to catalyze the inactivating proteolysis of TFPI.[2074] Its single-chain precursor has been purified from plasma.[2075]

Gene Structure and Expression

FSAP has been mapped to chromosome 10 band q25.3.[2076] It spans 35 kb and is composed of 13 exons (*Table 20.10*). Its transcript specifies a protein of 560 amino acids; the first 23 amino acids comprise the signal peptide sequence. Two single nucleotide polymorphisms have been identified. One, called *FSAP Marburg I* (SNP-1), yields a Gly511Glu substitution near the COOH terminus of the protease resulting in impairment of its scu-PA-activating properties.[2077-2079] The second polymorphism, Marburg II, contains a Glu370Gln mutation that does not appear to have an effect on the catalytic properties of FSAP.

Biochemistry and Activation

FSAP is a single-chain glycoprotein containing 537 amino acids with an M_r of 64 kDa (*Figure 20.27*).[2070] It circulates at a concentration of approximately 12 µg/mL (190 nmol/L; *Table 20.10*). It is composed of 5% carbohydrate and is glycosylated at Asn^{31} (NH$_2$-terminal strand) and Asn^{184} (kringle domain).[2075] The structure consists of an aminoterminal strand (residues 1-52) that is followed by three EGF-like domains (residues 53-166), a kringle domain (residues 170-254), and a COOH-terminal serine protease domain (residues 290-537). FSAP has structural regions that are homologous to those found in hepatocyte growth factor activator.[2086] It binds to GAGs such as heparin.

The conversion to the active two-chain form requires cleavage of the Arg^{290}-Ile^{291} bond. This generates a heavy chain (residues 1-290) and a light chain or catalytic domain (residues 291-537). The two chains are linked by a single disulfide bond (Cys^{278}-Cys^{412}). The active site residues of this serine protease are Asp^{382}, His^{339}, and Ser^{486}. Preparations of single-chain FSAP rapidly convert to the two-chain form.

Factor VII activating protease: 78 kDa

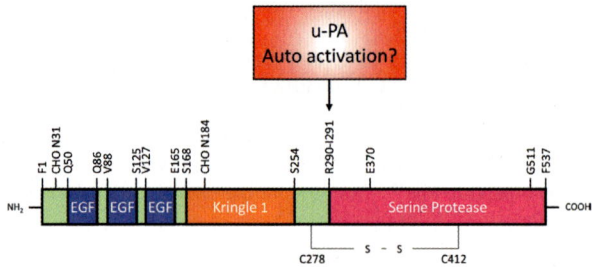

FIGURE 20.27 Schematic of the zymogen precursor of Factor VII activating protease (FSAP). FSAP is a serine protease that circulates as a single chain, catalytically inert molecule. Conversion to the active two-chain form (cleavage at R290-I291) has been reported to occur via several mechanisms including surface-mediated autocatalytic activation, soluble polyanion or polycation-induced autocatalytic activation, and proteolysis by two chain urokinase.[2080-2083] However, the potential for autocatalytic activation differs between plasma-based and purified component assays. Recent studies have reported that surface-mediated activation of FSAP in plasma is restricted to positively charged surfaces[2082] and positively charged molecules like histones.[2084,2085] Two single nucleotide polymorphisms have been identified: G511E (Marburg 1) and G380Q (named Marburg 2). Marburg I FSAP, which shows impaired proteolytic activity, appears to be a risk factor for cardiovascular disease.[2083]

Whether this is due to an intrinsic activity of the single-chain molecule or to trace amounts of the two-chain form in single-chain preparations has not been resolved.[2087] Heparin promotes conversion of single-chain FSAP preparations to the two-chain form,[2088] as do natural RNA[2089] and histones.[2084] The high-molecular-weight form of two-chain urokinase has been shown to convert single-chain FSAP to the two-chain form and may represent a physiologic activator.[2075] The rate of this reaction is affected by heparin. In addition to factor VII and single-chain urokinase, other substrates for FSAP, determined from in vitro assays, include factor V/factor Va, factor VIII/factor VIIIa, fibrinogen, single-chain t-PA, fibronectin, and vitronectin.[2090] Similar to plasmin, two-chain FSAP binds to aprotinin. In vitro assays indicate that it also complexes with serpins such as C1-inhibitor,[2091] α_2-antiplasmin, and antithrombin-heparin.[2055,2092] Stoichiometric inhibitors of FSAP include C1-esterase inhibitor, α_2-antiplasmin, and TFPI.[2093]

Function

The physiologic function of FSAP still is unclear. The ability of two-chain FSAP to convert factor VII to factor VIIa in the absence of tissue factor suggests that it could contribute to the maintenance of normal factor VIIa levels in blood or contribute to the localized production of factor VIIa at the site of vascular injury. In a system of synthetic hemophilia (factor VIII deficiency), two-chain FSAP has been shown to correct the hemostatic defect.[492] Similar results have been found with the addition of exogenous factor VIIa to hemophilia blood.[460] The two-chain form of FSAP appears to be an efficient activator of single-chain urokinase, comparing favorably with plasmin when heparin is present.[2055] It has been suggested[2090] that GAG-binding properties of FSAP may localize it to cell surfaces and extracellular matrix proteins, where it may play a role as an initiator of urokinase-dependent proteolytic cascades. The role of FSAP in inflammatory processes is under investigation.[2080]

INHIBITORS OF THE FIBRINOLYTIC SYSTEM

A wide variety of natural inhibitors of fibrinolysis exist in plasma, blood cells, tissues, and extracellular matrices. These natural inhibitors can act either to inhibit plasmin directly or to block the conversion of plasminogen to plasmin (*Figure 20.23*). In this section,

TAFI, PAI-1, PAI-2, and α_2-antiplasmin inhibitor are reviewed in terms of their gene structure and expression, biochemistry, and function.

Thrombin-Activatable Fibrinolysis Inhibitor

TAFI (E.C.3.4.17.20) (for reviews, see[2094-2098]) is a plasma zymogen with homology to procarboxypeptidases A and B. Its plasma concentration is 75 nmol/L (4.5 µg/mL; *Table 20.10*). TAFI is synthesized in the liver and is thought to circulate in blood in complex with plasminogen. A small pool of TAFI (<1% of plasma concentration) is found in platelets and has been found to enhance the attenuation of fibrinolysis in vitro.[2099,2100] Activation of TAFI yields an exopeptidase (TAFIa) with carboxypeptidase B-like substrate specificity. It catalyzes the removal of basic amino acids (arginines, lysines) from the COOH termini of polypeptides. Its primary physiologic activator appears to be the thrombin-thrombomodulin complex, thus defining TAFIa as a coagulation-dependent activity.[1024] COOH-terminal lysines that appear in fibrin as it degrades have been identified as the primary substrates for TAFIa (*Figure 20.28*). The initial phase of plasmin proteolysis yields products that amplify plasminogen activation by t-PA. These fibrin degradation products thus constitute a positive feedback process, thereby accelerating clot lysis. COOH-terminal lysines that appear in fibrin as it is degraded by plasmin function as additional binding sites where efficient plasminogen activation can occur. Removal of these terminal lysine residues by TAFIa reduces the number of plasminogen-binding sites, thus serving to downregulate the rate of plasmin generation and thereby the rate of clot lysis. Thus, TAFI/TAFIa functions as an antifibrinolytic factor by suppressing the positive feedback pathway of fibrinolysis. The importance in vivo of the TAFI/TAFIa-mediated regulation of fibrinolysis remains to be established. Several studies involving animal models of thrombosis[2036-2039,2101-2103] have provided in vivo evidence consistent with the proposed role of the TAFI/TAFIa system in regulating fibrinolysis. However, TAFI knockout mice develop normally and prove no more sensitive to a wide range of hemostatic challenges than their wild-type littermates.[2104] In humans, TAFI antigen concentration has been correlated with an increase in risk for deep vein thrombosis.[2105,2106]

The nomenclature associated with carboxypeptidase B-type activity in serum reflects the history of its isolation and characterization. The presence of a carboxypeptidase B-type activity in serum that differed from that of carboxypeptidase N, a previously characterized enzyme found in plasma, was first reported by two groups: Hendriks et al[18,2107,2108] named the enzyme *carboxypeptidase unstable* because of its short $t_{1/2}$ compared with carboxypeptidase N; Campbell and Okada[2109] named their activity *carboxypeptidase R* because of its apparent preference for substrates with COOH-terminal arginine residues, again in contrast to carboxypeptidase N, which showed a selectivity for COOH-terminal lysines. Subsequently, Eaton et al[11,2110] purified a novel plasminogen-binding protein from human plasma, which, based on sequence homology and enzymatic properties, proved to be a procarboxypeptidase. They named this *protein plasma procarboxypeptidase B*. Independently, Bajzar et al,[36] using an assay designed to detect the factor responsible for thrombin-dependent inhibition of fibrinolysis, purified a protein from human plasma. Initial characterization of this protein indicated that it was a procarboxypeptidase B-type protein, which converted to an active carboxypeptidase on treatment with thrombin. This group named the protein *TAFI*. Further characterization established that TAFI is identical to protein plasma procarboxypeptidase B.[19,1065] Whether carboxypeptidase R and carboxypeptidase unstable are identical to TAFI has not been resolved because of differences in the reported molecular mass and subunit structure of these proteins.

Gene Structure and Expression

TAFI is a member of a multigene family that includes the pancreatic and mast cell carboxypeptidases but not other carboxypeptidases

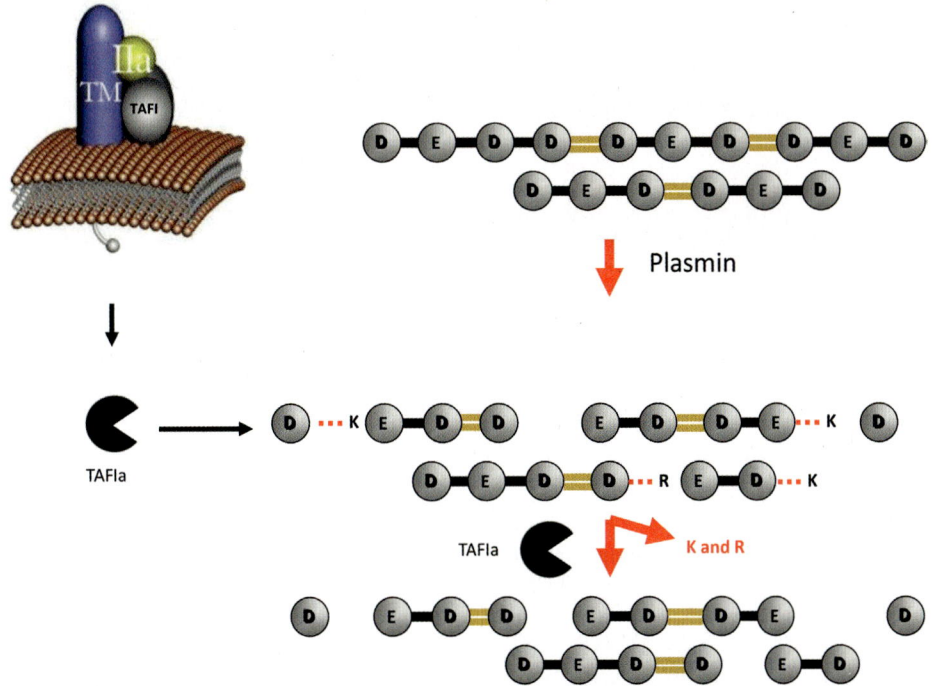

FIGURE 20.28 Mechanism of thrombin-activatable fibrinolysis inhibitor (TAFI) regulation of fibrinolysis. Thrombin-thrombomodulin (IIa•TM) cleaves TAFI to its active carboxypeptidase form TAFIa. TAFIa interferes with fibrinolysis by cleaving COOH-terminal Arg (R) or Lys (K) residues made available as a consequence of partial plasmin digestion of the fibrin clot. Removing these residues attenuates the self-amplifying mechanism of fibrin-based plasmin formation wherein partial plasmin proteolysis of fibrin increases the number of binding sites (COOH-terminal lysines) available for efficient plasminogen activation. (From Mann KG. *Coagulation Explosion.* Vermont Business Graphics; 1997.)

with a specificity for basic amino acids, such as carboxypeptidases N, M, H, and D.[2111,2112] TAFI shares a 34% to 40% amino acid identity with its family members, including exact conservation of cysteine residues and residues critical for catalysis, zinc binding, and substrate binding.

The human gene for TAFI maps to chromosome 13 band q14.13[2113] and is composed of 11 exons within 48 kb of DNA[2111] (*Table 20.9*). When the TAFI gene is compared with the genes from rat pancreatic carboxypeptidases A1, A2, and B and human mast cell carboxypeptidase A, the positions of intron/exon boundaries are conserved, whereas the intron lengths diverge significantly. The TAFI promoter lacks a consensus TATA sequence but does have a 70-bp sequence in the 5′-flanking region of the gene that is required for liver-specific transcription.[2111] Transcription is initiated at multiple sites. Primer extension analysis of human liver Poly (A)+ RNA identified nine major transcription start sites with similar frequencies of usage.[2111] The TAFI transcript is polyadenylated at three different sites.

The TAFI transcript encodes a gene product of 423 amino acids. The first 22 amino acids comprise a signal peptide that is absent in the circulating form of the protein. Three single nucleotide polymorphisms in the coding region of the human TAFI gene have been identified, resulting in two distinct isoforms of TAFI: a base change of C to T at base 678, resulting in a silent mutation; a base change of A to G at base 505, yielding a Thr to Ala substitution at amino acid position 147; and a base change of C to T at base 1057, resulting in an Ile to Thr substitution at TAFI residue 325. No functional difference was observed between purified TAFIa (Ala[147]) and TAFIa (Thr[147]).[2114] However, purified TAFIa (Ile[325]) showed greater activity and stability than TAFIa (Thr[325]).

The plasma concentration of TAFI antigen has been observed to vary approximately 10-fold in the human population. The origin of this variability appears to be primarily genetic.[2115] Polymorphisms in

the TAFI gene that have been shown to be strongly associated with plasma TAFI levels include a number in the 5′-flanking region,[2105,2116] the 3′-untranslated region,[2116] and the coding region.[2117]

Biochemistry

The TAFI transcript specifies a preprotein of 423 amino acids composed of a signal peptide, an activation peptide domain, and a catalytic domain. Removal of the signal peptide yields the circulating zymogen of 401 amino acids (45 kDa); when analyzed by SDS-PAGE, the apparent molecular weight of TAFI is 58 kDa (*Figure 20.29*). The difference in mass derives from a high level of glycosylation involving all four of the potential sites (Asn[22], Asn[51], Asn[63], and Asn[86]) present in the activation peptide domain (residues 1-92). In addition to its structural role in suppressing the catalytic potential of TAFI, the activation peptide domain mediates the association in blood of TAFI with plasminogen.[19] The sequence of the catalytic domain (residues 93-401; 35 kDa) displays exact conservation when compared with pancreatic and mast cell carboxypeptidases of cysteine residues and residues critical for catalysis, Zn[2+] binding, and substrate binding.[19,2111] The activated form of TAFI is a carboxypeptidase that catalyzes the removal of arginine or lysine residues from the COOH termini of polypeptides. TAFIa is inhibited by agents that can chelate Zn[2+], such as o-phenanthroline, and by 2-guanidinoethylmercaptosuccinic acid, a specific inhibitor of pancreatic and mast cell carboxypeptidases.[19,36] TAFIa is an unstable enzyme at physiologic pH and temperature.[18,19,36] At 37 °C, TAFIa has a functional $t_{1/2}$ of approximately 10 minutes; its loss of activity is coincident with a significant change in conformation.[2118]

Activation

The activation of TAFI requires the cleavage of the zymogen at Arg[92], yielding an activation peptide of approximately 15 kDa and an active carboxypeptidase of 35 kDa (*Figure 20.29*). Trypsin,[19] plasmin,[19,2119] plasmin–anionic GAG complex,[2119]

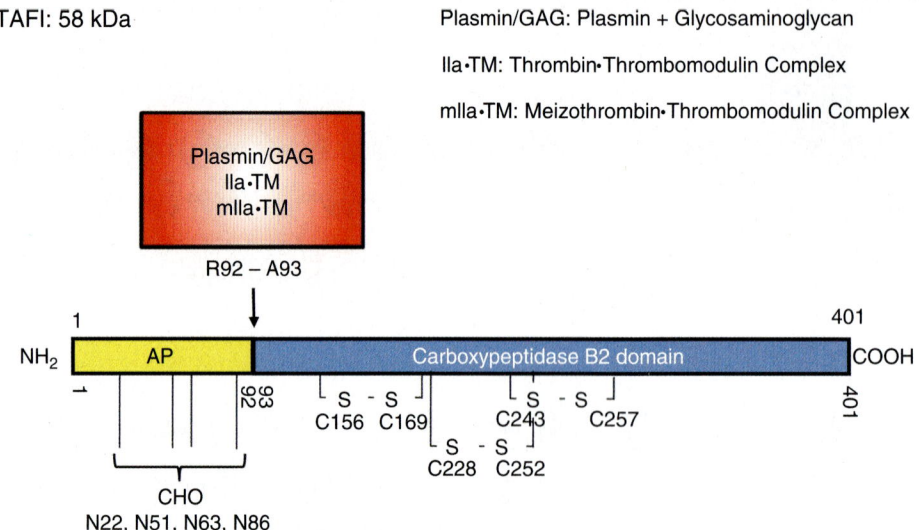

FIGURE 20.29 **Schematic of thrombin-activatable fibrinolysis inhibitor (TAFI).** Activation of TAFI yields an exopeptidase (TAFIa) with carboxypeptidase B–like substrate specificity. It catalyzes the removal of basic amino acids (arginines, lysines) from the COOH termini of polypeptides. TAFI contains four glycosylation sites in its activation peptide region. TAFIa is an unstable enzyme undergoing spontaneous conformational change resulting in a loss of catalytic activity ($t_{1/2}$ = 8-10 min).

thrombin,[19,36] thrombin-thrombomodulin complex,[1024] and meizothrombin-thrombomodulin complex[1153] all catalyze this reaction in vitro. A ranking of these catalysts in terms of relative catalytic efficiency shows the following order: thrombin-thrombomodulin (1.0) > meizothrombin-thrombin (0.1) = plasmin–anionic GAG (0.1) > plasmin (0.006) > thrombin (0.0008). The complement protease MASP-1 also has been shown to activate TAFI.[2120] The relative contributions of thrombin and plasmin to TAFI generation in vivo may be regulated by the availability of their respective cofactors at the site of vascular injury: cell-associated thrombomodulin versus the extent of exposure of subendothelial extracellular matrix. Platelet factor 4 has been reported to inhibit activation of TAFI by the thrombin-thrombomodulin complex.[2121]

Function

Thrombin cleavage of fibrinogen yields insoluble fibrin polymers and soluble fibrinopeptides, all bearing COOH-terminal arginine residues. These COOH-terminal arginines are substrates for TAFIa, and the kinetics of their release in an in vitro clot lysis system[1066] and whole blood system where des-Arg FPB was detected[1068] have been reported. The significance of this removal of arginine residues from these sites is not known. The activation of many of the cofactors and zymogens of the coagulation and fibrinolytic cascades results in the generation of functional proteins with COOH-terminal arginines or lysines. Their status as TAFIa substrates is unknown. Bradykinin and several enkephalins have been shown in vitro to be good TAFIa substrates[2110]; to date, only circumstantial evidence connects TAFIa and bradykinin in vivo.[2122]

Extensive in vitro data[1066,1161,1848,1849,2118,2123,2124] attest to the ability of TAFIa to slow the rate of fibrin degradation by plasmin generated in situ. Proteolysis of insoluble fibrin by plasmin proceeds through repetitive cleavages at lysine residues terminating in the formation of soluble fibrin degradation products. Before solubilization, each cleavage shortens the fibrin molecule and generates a new COOH-terminal lysine residue. COOH-terminal lysines in partially degraded fibrin have been shown to function as potent cofactors for t-PA-catalyzed activation of Glu-plasminogen.[2125-2129] Removal of the COOH-terminal lysines by TAFIa thus reduces the number of sites available for plasminogen binding, thereby reducing the rate of plasmin generation with consequent prolongation of fibrin dissolution[1066,1848,2130] (*Figure 20.28*). TAFIa functions as an attenuator of fibrinolysis,[2131] and thus an adequate rate of TAFIa generation may be critical in the stabilization of the blood clot.

For example, plasmas with specific deficiencies in the coagulation pathway showed reduced rates of thrombin production, decreased levels of TAFIa, and premature clot lysis.[1849,2102,2132]

Regulation

TAFI circulates in plasma bound to plasminogen[19] and is a substrate for factor XIIIa, which catalyzes its covalent attachment to fibrin.[1067] Whether these two mechanisms for concentrating TAFI at the site of fibrin formation contribute to the function of TAFI in vivo is not established. It has been proposed,[2133] because the thrombin-thrombomodulin complex has a K_m 10 to 20 times the plasma concentration of TAFI, that rates of TAFI activation would vary directly with changes in TAFI concentration.

A plasma inhibitor of TAFIa has not been described. Carboxypeptidase inhibitors from potato[2134] and the leech[2135] active against TAFIa have been identified. TAFIa is an unstable enzyme under physiologic conditions.[18,19,36] It undergoes a spontaneous conformational change with a $t_{1/2}$ of 10 minutes at 37 °C.[2118] This appears to be the primary route of inactivation because proteolytic cleavage at Arg[302] by thrombin or plasmin has now been identified as secondary to and dependent on the inactivating conformation change.[2136,2137]

TAFI plasma concentrations vary significantly in the human population. Although genetic factors appear to be the largest contributor to this variation,[2116] a growing number of stimuli have been shown to affect TAFI plasma concentration.[2106,2115,2138-2141] It has been proposed, in light of the intrinsic instability of TAFIa and the absence of a specific inhibitor, that control of the concentration of TAFIa through control of the level of TAFI gene expression is the primary regulator of the TAFI/TAFIa system in vivo.[2142]

Plasminogen Activator Inhibitor-1

PAI-1 is the primary physiologic inhibitor of plasminogen activation in blood, targeting u-PA and t-PA.[2143] It also appears to have a role, independent of its antiproteolytic function, in tissue remodeling by interfering with vitronectin-dependent processes of cell adhesion and migration. Congenital deficiency of PAI-1 is rare, with homozygous individuals displaying abnormal bleeding in response to trauma.[2144-2148] In a normal population, plasma PAI-1 concentration varies over a 15-fold range (6-80 ng/mL; *Table 20.10*)[2149,2150] and exhibits a circadian variation.[2151] Some of this variability stems from polymorphisms in the PAI-1 gene; however, a larger fraction of the variability appears to derive from the responsiveness of PAI-1 gene expression to a wide variety of physiologic effectors and conditions as well as pharmacologic agents.[2152] Higher levels of plasma PAI-1 prolong fibrin removal by shortening the functional lifetime of plasminogen activators, thereby shifting hemostasis to a more thrombotic state.[2153] The $t_{1/2}$ of PAI-1 in blood is <10 minutes. Potential sites of constitutive PAI-1 synthesis in humans include the liver, spleen, adipose tissue, and cells of the vasculature, including endothelial cells, smooth muscle cells, macrophages, and megakaryocytes. The relative contributions from these sources to plasma PAI-1 levels in normal or specific pathologic conditions remain unresolved. The major fraction of PAI-1 in blood is present in platelets, apparently synthesized and stored in the α-granules during the maturation of megakaryocytes.[2154] Although 75% to 80% of platelet PAI-1 is present in the latent form, there appears to be enough active PAI-1 released from platelets at sites of thrombus formation to contribute to the suppression of fibrinolysis.[1995,1996]

PAI-1 is a single-chain protein with an M_r of 50,000 (13% carbohydrate; *Table 20.10*). It is a typical serpin with its reactive site bond, Arg[346]-Met[347], positioned in an exposed loop region[2155] where it is available for complexation with its target proteases. However, this conformation, with the reactive site accessible to proteases, is unstable ($t_{1/2} \leq 90$ minutes), reverting spontaneously to a latent form of the inhibitor in which the reactive loop is buried in β sheet A of the protein core. This positioning of the reactive loop is observed in PAI-1 and other serpins after cleavage of the reactive site bond.[2156] Plasma PAI-1 circulates in noncovalent association with vitronectin[2149,2157] ($K_d \leq 0.05$ nmol/L); in vitro, this association results in a 2-fold increase in its functional $t_{1/2}$ and, in the presence of heparin, increases PAI-1 reactivity with thrombin.[1677]

Gene Structure and Expression

PAI-1 is an inhibitory serpin with significant sequence homology to α_1-antitrypsin, antithrombin, and α_1-antichymotrypsin.[1448,2158-2164] It shares the fundamental structural plan of these serpins: three β sheets, nine α-helices, and a reactive site loop. PAI-1 is distinguished from the other inhibitory serpins in that it lacks cysteine residues.

The human gene for PAI-1 is located on chromosome 7 band q22.1 in close proximity to the loci for erythropoietin, paraoxonase, and cystic fibrosis[2165,2166] (*Table 20.9*). It covers 12.2 kb of DNA with nine exons specifying the 23 amino acids of the signal peptide and 379 amino acids of the mature protein.[2167-2170] Introns, totaling approximately 9000 bp, define boundaries of individual structural subdomains or are found in random coil regions of the protein.[2167,2168] The transcription start site is located 25 bp downstream of a consensus TATA sequence.[2168,2170] The 5′-flanking region of the PAI-1 gene shows an extensive region of nucleotide sequence identity with the 5′-flanking region of the gene encoding t-Pan.[2169,2170] The 3′ region of the human PAI-1 gene contains alternative polyadenylation sites resulting in two mRNA species of different lengths (2.4 and 3.2 kb).[2167]

Normal plasma levels of PAI-1 antigen range between 6 and 80 ng/mL. Polymorphisms in the PAI-1 gene appear to correlate with different plasma levels of PAI-1; thus, genotype-specific regulation of PAI-1 accounts for some of the observed variation in the normal population. Nine polymorphisms have been described, with three of these the subject of human population studies.[2171] A polymorphism located 675 bp upstream of the transcription start site consists of a single guanine insertion/deletion variation (4G/5G) leading to a sequence of four or five guanine nucleotides in the promoter.[2172] Individuals homozygous for the 4G polymorphism have the highest levels of PAI-1; heterozygotes show intermediate levels; those homozygous for the 5G allele have the lowest levels.[2173-2177] The basis of this differential expression of the PAI-1 gene appears to be the specificity of a transcriptional repressor protein that binds the 5G allele and not the 4G allele.[2177] The predictive relationship between the 4G/5G genotype, plasma PAI-1 level, and the risk of thrombosis is controversial.[2178-2180] The two other polymorphisms investigated both in vitro and in human population studies include an eight-allele $(CA)_n$ repeat in intron 3[2181] and

a two-allele Hind III restriction fragment length polymorphism of the 3′-flanking region. Individuals with one of the homozygous genotypes associated with the Hind III site exhibit higher plasma PAI-1 activity than the complementary homozygous individuals.[2181] In vitro studies of the Hind III polymorphism have shown genotype-specific regulation of PAI-1 synthesis by a number of effector molecules.[2182-2185]

Congenital PAI-1 deficiency is a rare disorder, with homozygous PAI-1-deficient individuals showing abnormal bleeding after trauma or surgery.[2144,2145] A study of an extended family with 19 heterozygotes and 7 individuals homozygous for a null mutation in the PAI-1 gene found no significant developmental or other abnormalities in the homozygotes beyond abnormal bleeding episodes.[2147] Homozygous PAI-1-deficient mice display normal fertility, viability, and development, with no identified histologic abnormalities.[2186,2187] A mild hyperfibrinolytic state and greater resistance to venous thrombosis were reported. Mice with combined homozygous deficiency of PAI-1 and α_2-antiplasmin show normal fertility and development while displaying a higher fibrinolytic capacity.[2188] However, this increase appears to depend on the α_2-antiplasmin deficiency alone, suggesting a less critical role for PAI-1 in the regulation of fibrinolysis.

Biochemistry

PAI-1 is a single-chain glycoprotein of 379 amino acids that has no cysteine residues (*Figure 20.30*). It is an inhibitory serpin with a reactive site bond, Arg[346]-Met[347], positioned in a surface-exposed, disordered loop of 20 amino acids.[2155] Reaction with t-PA or u-PA involves rapid formation (second-order rate constant = 10^7 to 10^8 M^{-1} s^{-1}) of a reversible complex; specific interactions between a negatively charged region (amino acids 350-355) of the PAI-1 molecule and positively charged regions in t-PA[2192,2193] or in u-PA[2194] are important to this initial association. Cleavage of the reactive site Arg[346]-Met[347] bond in PAI-1 by the protease triggers a large conformational change in both the inhibitor and the protease that renders the protease unable to efficiently hydrolyze the normally transient ester linkage between its active site serine residue and the carboxyl moiety of the targeted peptide bond. PAI-1 converts to an inactive (latent) form spontaneously; it can be returned to its active conformation by treatment with denaturants.[2195] The crystal structure of latent PAI-1 indicates that the reactive site loop is inserted into the β sheet A of the molecule, making it unavailable to proteases.[2196] The crystal structure of a mutant PAI-1 stabilized in the active conformation by substitutions at four sites (N150→H; K154→T; Q319→L; M354→I) shows the reactive site bond to be located at the apex of a flexible, exterior loop.[2155] The vitronectin binding site of PAI-1 involves five residues located on the exterior of the molecule.[2191] Extensive structural differences have been noted when this region is compared in active and latent conformations of PAI-1.[2155] Stabilization of the conformation of this region of PAI-1 by the PAI-1 vitronectin binding interaction presumably impedes the insertion of the reactive site loop into β sheet A of the molecule.

Function

PAI-1 is the central physiologic inhibitor of the plasminogen activator t-PA in blood. It reacts with both the secreted, single-chain form of t-PA and the two-chain form generated by plasmin during the process of fibrin dissolution. Both PAI-1 and t-PA are characterized by high turnover rates (t-PA, $t_{1/2}$ = 3-4 minutes; PAI-1, $t_{1/2}$ = 10 minutes) with functional PAI-1 circulating concentrations maintained at least at severalfold molar excess over the concentration of functional t-PA (14 pmol/L). From the circulating concentration of PAI-1 and the second-order rate constant for the association of PAI-1 with either form of t-PA (10^7 to 10^8 M^{-1} s^{-1}), the predicted $t_{1/2}$ of t-PA is <1 minute. This is consistent with the observation that approximately 80% of the t-PA antigen in plasma (70 pmol/L) is found complexed with PAI-1. PAI-1-t-PA complexes have a clearance $t_{1/2}$ of approximately 5 minutes.[1927] Although other plasma proteins have been identified in vitro with inhibitory activity toward plasminogen activators (PAI-2, PAI-3, protease nexin), only PAI-1–plasminogen activator complexes have been detected in vivo.[1185,2197]

Plasminogen activator inhibitor-1: 50 kDa

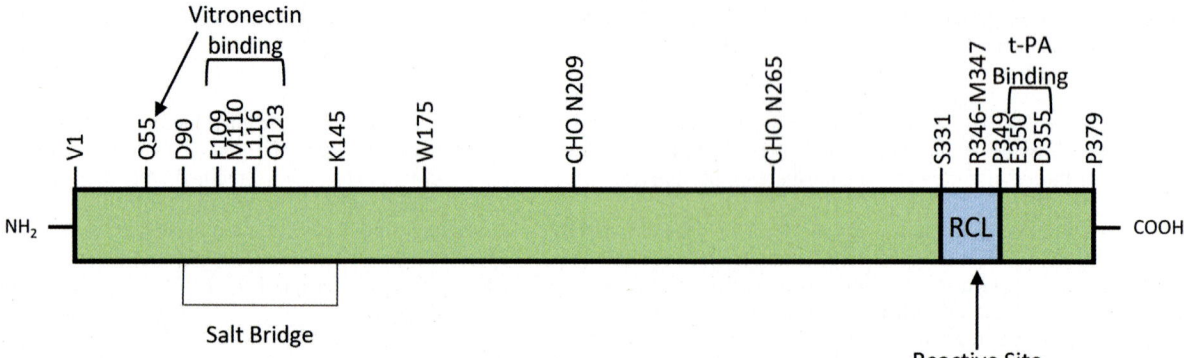

FIGURE 20.30 Schematic of plasminogen activator inhibitor 1 (PAI-1). The protein is a serine protease inhibitor targeting u-PA and t-PA. The protein has no cysteine residues and is unstable, spontaneously converting to an inactive form ($t_{1/2}$ of 1 hour at 37 °C) via insertion of the reactive center loop (RCL) into the core of the protein. Association of PAI-1 with vitronectin stabilizes the active conformation. Two divalent metal ion–binding sites have been identified.[2189] There are three potential N-linked glycosylation sites (N209, N265, and N329), but only two (N209 and N265) are utilized with the glycosylation pattern showing a heterogeneous, tissue-specific variation.[2143] Salt bridges related to the stability of the active form of the inhibitor include between D90 and K145[2189] and D224 and R273.[2190] A key structural feature of the NH₂ terminus of the molecule is the vitronectin-binding site, which appears to bridge two α-helical structures and a ß-strand, thereby blocking insertion of the RCL[2191] and a salt bridge. Key structural features of the COOH terminus of the molecule include the RCL containing the reactive site peptide bond (R346-M347) and the residues involved in its exosite interaction with t-PA.[2192]

PAI-1 is an important inhibitor of u-PA. Unlike t-PA, PAI-1 forms complexes only with the two-chain form of urokinase; it does not complex with the single-chain form of urokinase. The second-order rate constant for the association of PAI-1 and tcu-PA is in the range of 10^8 M^{-1} s^{-1}. Conversion of circulating scu-PA (37-74 pmol/L) to tcu-PA occurs at sites of fibrin lysis. Urokinase is also involved in physiologic and pathologic processes such as embryo development, wound healing, cell migration, inflammation, and metastasis of tumor cells. A large body of in vitro work supports a regulatory role for PAI-1 as a protease inhibitor in u-PA-mediated events outside the vasculature, and as a consequence, its dysregulation has been implicated in the pathogenesis of fibrosis in different organs.[2198]

PAI-1 also appears to be involved in regulating cell adhesion and migration by a mechanism independent of its function as a protease inhibitor. Its high-affinity association with the somatomedin B domain of vitronectin makes it an effective competitor with other ligands such as urokinase-type plasminogen activator receptor (uPAR)[2199-2202] and integrins including $\alpha_V\beta_3$[2203] that also bind to vitronectin at this site. The ability to interfere with the binding of such cell-associated ligands to matrix-associated vitronectin suggests a role for PAI-1 as a regulator of the interaction of cells with the extracellular matrix.

Plasminogen Activator Inhibitor-2

PAI-2 is a member of the serpin subfamily designated the *ovalbumin-related serpins*.[2204] It was initially identified in human placenta as an inhibitor of urokinase.[2205] It has also been referred to as the *placental-type PAI*.[2205-2210] It is not normally detected in plasma, although it has been detected in human thrombi.[2211] During pregnancy, PAI-2 is found in plasma at levels that may exceed those of PAI-1.[2197] PAI-2 appears to have significant functions within the cytoplasm of certain cell types and in the extracellular region outside of the vasculature, where it may regulate urokinase-dependent events. However, its role in hemostasis remains problematic and a definitive intracellular role for PAI-2 is not established.[2212] PAI-2 (–/–) null mice developed normally and did not display any phenotypic abnormalities.[2213]

Gene Structure and Expression

The gene for PAI-2 is located on chromosome 18, bands q21.33–q22.1, and spans 16.5 kb[2214-2219] (*Table 20.9*). Its transcript specifies a protein of 415 amino acids that lacks a cleavable NH₂-terminal signal sequence. PAI-2 is synthesized and secreted by human white blood cells such as monocytes and macrophages and cells of epithelial lineage such as keratinocytes and certain tumor cells.[2220-2223] A large number of agonists have been shown to affect transcription rates of the PAI-2 gene (reviewed in [2204,2224,2225]). For example, the PAI-2 gene has been shown to respond dramatically to TNF[2226] and to lipopolysaccharide.[2227] In human monocytes, exposure to lipopolysaccharide induced approximately a 100-fold increase in PAI-2 mRNA levels.[2228] Posttranscriptional regulation of PAI-2 mRNA levels has also been documented.[2229,2230] Regulation of the stability of PAI-2 mRNA has been shown to derive in part from an AU rich–mRNA destabilizing determinant in the 3′-untranslated region[2230] and from an mRNA instability element identified within exon 4 of the coding region.[2231]

Biochemistry and Function

There are two forms of PAI-2: an intracellular nonglycosylated form (M_r = 47 kDa) and a secreted glycosylated form (M_r = 60 kDa) (*Table 20.10; Figure 20.31*). However, the nonglycosylated form has been observed in the blood of pregnant women.[2197] Glycosylation occurs at Asn[75], Asn[115], and Asn[339]. PAI-2 is structurally distinguished from other serpins by the presence of a unique 33-residue-long loop (CD loop: residues 66-98) positioned between helices C and D. This solvent-exposed loop region has two glutamine residues (Gln[83] and Gln[86]) that have been shown to be sites for factor XIIIa–catalyzed cross-linking of PAI-2 to fibrinogen.[2211,2233] PAI-2 cross-linked to fibrinogen remains functional after its fibrinogen carrier is converted to insoluble fibrin.[2233] The CD loop has also been implicated in the association of intracellular PAI-2 with other cytoplasmic proteins.[2234] The crystal structure of PAI-2 at 2-Å resolution has recently been reported using a PAI-2 mutant lacking the CD loop.[2235] The reactive site bond (Arg[380]-Thr[381]) is located in a highly disordered reactive center loop

PAI-2 secreted glycosylated form: 60 kDa

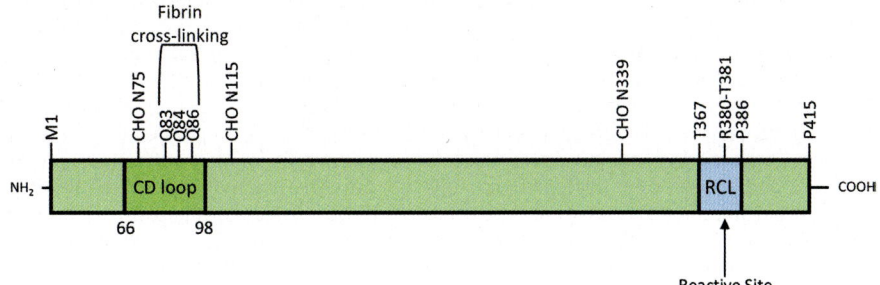

FIGURE 20.31 **Schematic of plasminogen activator 2 (PAI-2).** PAI-2 is a member of the serine protease inhibitor superfamily. Although it shares plasminogen activator inhibitory functions with PAI-1, reacting with both two chain t-PA and two chain u-PA, the two inhibitors are phylogenetically distinct and are classified into different serpin subfamilies.[2204,2212] Unlike PAI-1, PAI-2 does not show binding to heparin, has cysteine residues (C5, C79, C145, C161, C405, ± C413), and does not spontaneously undergo a conformational shift to a functionally inert form. Key structural features of the protein include three N-linked glycosylation sites (N75, N115, and N 339) and a CD loop region, a highly flexible 30-amino-acid structure connecting helices C and D, which contains three transglutamination sites (Q83, Q84, and Q86). Glycosylation at N75 appears to block access to these transglutamination sites[2232]; and a reactive center loop (RCL) containing the reactive site peptide bond (R380-T381). Two forms of PAI-2, differing at residues 120, 404, and 413, have been described. Type A has the composition N120, N404, and S413, while type B shows D120, K404, and C413. Each of these differences reflects a single base change yet all three appear to be linked since they have not been found in isolation.[2204,2212] Functional consequences of these sequence differences have not been identified, but population studies have linked PAI-2 genotype with disease.[2212]

extending from Thr^{367} to Pro^{386}. PAI-2 is a serpin inhibitor that can inhibit plasminogen activators. The second-order rate constants defining its interactions with two-chain urokinase (1×10^6 M^{-1} s^{-1}) and two-chain t-PA (2×10^5 M^{-1} s^{-1}) are approximately 100-fold lower than those characterizing the reaction of PAI-1 with these proteases. Unlike PAI-1, PAI-2 reacts very slowly with the single-chain form of t-PA. Also unlike PAI-1, PAI-2-t-PA or PAI-2-u-PA complexes have not been detected in plasma. Thus, it has been suggested that PAI-2 may not play an important role in regulating intravascular clot lysis. However, fibrin deposition at sites of chronic inflammation within blood vessels may represent an instance in which monocyte-derived PAI-2 could end up cross-linked to fibrin, thereby exerting some effect in the vasculature.[2211,2233] An extravascular role for PAI-2 in aspects of tissue remodeling and wound healing that depend on urokinase catalysis is consistent with the observed induction of PAI-2 production by inflammatory mediators in cell types such as keratinocytes and macrophages.

The nonglycosylated form of PAI-2 is found in the cytosol of a number of cell types. Data supporting a diverse set of roles for intracellular pools of PAI-2 include effects on cellular differentiation,[2234] cell proliferation,[2236] TNF-α-induced apoptosis,[2237,2238] signal transduction,[2239] and, in monocytes, multiple roles in modulating adhesion, proliferation, and differentiation.[2240]

α_2-Antiplasmin (α_2-Plasmin Inhibitor)

α_2-Antiplasmin (or α_2-plasmin inhibitor) is the primary plasmin inhibitor in human plasma[2241-2244] and thus is an important regulator of fibrinolysis.[2245] Congenital deficiency of α_2-antiplasmin is rare, with homozygous individuals displaying a severe to moderate bleeding disorder.[2246] α_2-Antiplasmin is a single-chain glycoprotein with a calculated mass of 58 kDa[2247] and a relative molecular weight of 70 kDa. It is present in plasma at a concentration of 70 mg/L (*Table 20.10*). The primary site of synthesis is the liver, although the kidney may be another contributing source[2248]; its in vivo $t_{1/2}$ is 2.6 days.[2249,2250] Two NH$_2$-terminal variants of α_2-antiplasmin are isolated from human plasma in roughly equivalent amounts: α_2-antiplasmin Met^1, the full-length protein secreted into the blood, and α_2-antiplasmin Asn^1, lacking the first 12 amino acids (Asn^{13} in α_2-antiplasmin Met^1).[2251,2252] α_2-Antiplasmin is a member of the serine protease inhibitor superfamily. It forms a stable 1:1 stoichiometric complex with plasmin that has

no proteolytic or esterase activity.[2242,2243,2253] It is structurally distinct from related serpins in having a 55-amino-acid extension at its COOH terminus.[2254,2255] This region mediates α_2-antiplasmin binding to specific regions (lysine-binding sites) on the kringle domains of plasminogen and plasmin.[2256-2258] Approximately 30% of α_2-antiplasmin in human plasma lacks part of this COOH-terminal region (residues 449-464). This truncated form appears to be functionally inert in plasma,[2258,2259] although it has been shown, when purified, to slowly form complexes with plasmin.[2260,2261]

The α_2-antiplasmin molecule has three domains defining its role in fibrinolysis: the reactive site (Arg^{376}-Met^{377}), the plasminogen-binding site (both of which are critical to its reactivity with plasmin),[2256,2257,2262] and a cross-linking site mediating the attachment of α_2-antiplasmin to the α-chain of fibrin during clotting.[1601] The binding of the plasminogen-binding domain of α_2-antiplasmin to a lysine-binding site of plasmin has been shown to occur more rapidly than the association between the active site of plasmin and the reactive site of α_2-antiplasmin.[2263] Thus, the rate of binding of α_2-antiplasmin depends primarily on the availability of the lysine-binding site(s) of plasmin. This dependence of the rate of inhibition on an exosite interaction between the two molecules results in the differential reactivity of α_2-antiplasmin with its primary targets in clotting blood: plasmin released into the circulating blood ($t_{1/2}$ = 0.1 second) versus plasmin bound through its lysine-binding sites to fibrin or cellular sites at the site of vascular injury ($t_{1/2}$ = 10 seconds).

Gene Structure and Expression

α_2-Antiplasmin is a member of a multigene family of serine protease inhibitors that includes α_1-antitrypsin, antithrombin, PAI-1, and α_1-antichymotrypsin.[1448,2158,2255] These serpins interact with their target proteases at a reactive Arg-X peptide bond positioned in a loop structure located 30 to 40 amino acids from the inhibitor COOH terminus. α_2-Antiplasmin differs from other members of its family in having a 55-amino-acid extension at its COOH terminus.

The human gene for α_2-antiplasmin is located on chromosome 17, band p13.3,[2264] and is composed of 10 exons distributed over 16 kb of DNA[2265] (*Table 20.9*). The 5'-untranslated region and leader sequence are interrupted by three introns; a TATA box sequence is found 17 nucleotides upstream of the transcription initiation site. Exons 4 through 10 code for the protein, with exon 10 specifying both the reactive site and the unique COOH-terminal plasminogen-binding site. One common polymorphism, RGW, has been mechanically linked to differences in the levels of α_2-antiplasmin Met^1 and α_2-antiplasmin Asn^1.[2266,2267]

Congenital α_2-antiplasmin deficiency has been described[2246]; the transmission is autosomal recessive. Bleeding problems vary from severe to moderate in homozygotes. The majority of heterozygotes have no bleeding problems, although exceptions have been described.[2268,2269] One instance of congenital deficiency, α_2-antiplasmin Enschede,[2270] is characterized by dysfunctional full-length α_2-antiplasmin at normal plasma concentrations. All other cases involve quantitative defects with the four characterized instances showing mutations in the coding exons[2271-2273] or an intron splicing donor site[2274] with consequent truncated, nonsecreted peptide products. Homozygous α_2-antiplasmin-deficient mice have been generated.[2275] They display normal fertility, viability, and development, and show no overt bleeding disorder.

Biochemistry

α_2-Antiplasmin is a single-chain glycoprotein of 464 amino acids with an M_r of 70 kDa (13% carbohydrate; *Table 20.10*) (*Figure 20.32*). Glycosylation occurs at Asn^{99}, Asn^{268}, Asn^{282}, and Asn^{289}. α_2-Antiplasmin contains four cysteine residues but only one S–S bridge.[2280] It is a member of the α_1-proteinase inhibitor class of the serine proteinase inhibitor superfamily.[1448,2255]

α_2-Antiplasmin functions as the primary inhibitor of plasmin in blood.[2249] It is synthesized primarily in the liver with a signal peptide of 27 amino acids and circulates at a concentration of 1 µmol/L[2247] with a $t_{1/2}$ of 2.6 days.[2249,2250] Isolation from plasma yields both Met^1-α_2-antiplasmin (464 amino acids) and a truncated form

with an NH$_2$-terminal Asn (Asn^{13}-α_2-antiplasmin)[2251]; the truncated form appears to be generated within circulating blood by a plasma protease.[2275,2279] Plasma α_2-antiplasmin is also found to have two COOH-terminal forms: a slow-reacting, non-plasminogen-binding form (30%) that lacks the terminal 26 amino acids and the fully active molecule with an intact COOH-terminal extension.[2258,2260] Conversion to the non-plasminogen-binding form occurs in the blood.[2259] α_2-Antiplasmin has three functionally important domains: a reactive site, a plasmin/plasminogen-binding site, and a cross-linking site. The reactive site of the inhibitor is the Arg^{376}-Met^{377} peptide bond.[2254] α_2-Antiplasmin reacts with plasmin in a two-step process. First, a rapid (second-order rate constant = $2\text{-}4 \times 10^7$ M^{-1} s^{-1}) reversible interaction yields a 1:1 complex ($K_d = 10^{-10}$ M). Second, a slower first-order ($t_{1/2}$ = 166 seconds) covalent bond forms between the active site seryl residue of plasmin and Arg^{376} of α_2-antiplasmin with subsequent release of a COOH-terminal fragment (residues 377-464) of α_2-antiplasmin. The plasmin/plasminogen-binding domain is located within residues 410 to 464, with Lys^{464} acting as the key residue.[2281-2283] It complexes with lysine-binding site(s) located in the kringle structures of plasminogen and plasmin, exhibiting at least a 10-fold stronger binding to plasmin.[1886] Lysine-binding sites on kringles 1[1886,2284] and 4[2280] have been identified as the points of interaction with α_2-antiplasmin, although their relative importance individually is not resolved.[2280] Maximum rates of α_2-antiplasmin inhibition of plasmin require the unimpeded interaction of both the plasminogen-binding domain and the reactive site of α_2-antiplasmin with their respective target domains in the plasmin molecule.[2263] Cross-linking of α_2-antiplasmin at Gln^{14} to the α-chain of fibrin is catalyzed by activated factor XIII.[2285] In vitro, Asn^{13} α_2-antiplasmin is more efficiently cross-linked to fibrin.[2279,2286]

α_2-antiplasmin (α_2-plasmin inhibitor) – 70 kDa

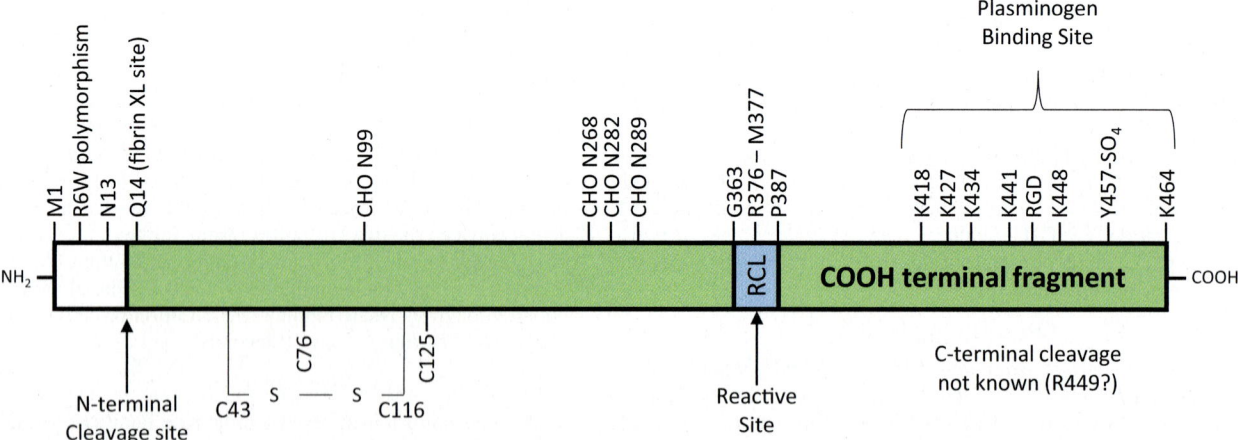

FIGURE 20.32 Schematic of α_2-antiplasmin. α_2-antiplasmin is the primary plasmin inhibitor in plasma and a key suppressor of fibrinolysis. Three important functional regions are depicted: (1) the cross-linking site between α_2-antiplasmin (residue Q14) and fibrin (K303 of the α-chain). Cross-linking of α_2-antiplasmin to fibrin is an important contributor to thrombus stability[1847,2276,2277]; (2) the reactive center loop (RCL) and reactive site bond (R376-M377), the interaction region between the plasmin active site and α_2-antiplasmin; and (3) the C-terminal region (residues 410-464), which interacts with lysine-binding sites on kringles 1 and 4 of plasmin/plasminogen. An RGD sequence is also present in the C-terminal region but its biological role remains to be determined. Once secreted into the blood, α_2-antiplasmin can undergo proteolytic modifications at the C terminus, the N terminus, or both sites, with all four species potentially present in an individual plasma.[2278] Proteolysis at the N terminus is between residue P12 and N13[2251,2252]; the resulting N12 α_2-antiplasmin is cross-linked to fibrin more efficiently than the full-length molecule.[2279] Proteolysis at the C terminus removes ~26 residues; disruption of this exosite on α_2-antiplasmin slows its rate of plasmin inhibition at least 30-fold. The plasma protease responsible for the N-terminal cleavage has been identified,[2279] while the specific cleavage site and enzyme responsible for the C-terminal cleavage in vivo have not. Although clear functional differences have been established between these forms of α_2-antiplasmin and a wide interindividual variation in the distribution of the forms reported, the clinical significance of this heterogeneity remains unclear and is an area of active research.[2278]

Function

α_2-Antiplasmin is the primary plasmin inhibitor in human plasma. Its effective concentration in plasma is in the range of 0.5 μmol/L. Approximately one-third of the circulating pool (1 μmol/L) is poorly reactive,[2258,2260] and another fraction is bound to circulating plasminogen (K_d = 4 μmol/L).[2263] α_2-Antiplasmin stabilizes the fibrin scaffolding of the developing blood clot by attenuating the rate of plasmin-driven fibrinolysis and protects against systemic degradation of fibrinogen and other proteins by plasmin. Fibrin, as the key cofactor for efficient t-PA activation of plasminogen, localizes plasmin generation to the site of fibrin formation. Generated plasmin is partitioned: one fraction is surface associated through binding interactions between its lysine-binding sites and active site and insoluble fibrin; the other fraction mixes with the circulating blood. α_2-Antiplasmin rapidly inhibits solution phase plasmin ($t_{1/2}$ ~ 0.1 second), preventing systemic fibrinogen degradation until more than 50% of its neutralizing capacity has been exhausted.[2249] The in vitro rate of inhibition of fibrin-bound plasmin by α_2-antiplasmin decreases by at least a factor of 100 ($t_{1/2} \geq 10$ seconds).[2287] This decrease in reactivity reflects the dependence of the rate of inhibition on the availability of both the lysine-binding and active sites of plasmin. Offsetting this, α_2-antiplasmin is accumulated on fibrin through a factor XIIIa–catalyzed tethering of the NH_2 terminus of α_2-antiplasmin to the α-chain of fibrin. Approximately 20% of the available α_2-antiplasmin is rapidly bound to fibrin. This process has been shown to play a significant role in stabilizing the fibrin clot against lysis.[1847,2276]

PHYSIOLOGIC REGULATION OF FIBRINOLYSIS

The physiologic regulation of fibrinolysis centers on controlling the rate and location of plasmin formation. Under quiescent conditions, there is little systemic plasmin formation. t-PA is a poor catalyst of the conversion of plasminogen to plasmin in the absence of fibrin. In addition, circulating levels of active t-PA are continually suppressed by reactions with PAI-1, thus further reducing the potential for solution phase plasminogen activation by t-PA. scu-PA has negligible activity toward plasminogen in solution. Furthermore, there is no gradual accumulation of plasmin in the blood because the circulating concentration and efficacy of α_2-antiplasmin limit the $t_{1/2}$ of plasmin formed away from a fibrin surface to 0.1 second. Thus, significant plasmin formation occurs only after the formation of fibrin. t-PA and plasminogen bind to fibrin as the clot forms, localizing plasmin generation to the clot. Initial plasmin degradation of fibrin actually increases the number of plasminogen-binding sites in the fibrin, thus amplifying plasmin formation rates. Plasmin also cleaves scu-PA to generate the active two-chain form of the catalyst, further enhancing rates of plasmin activation. In addition, fibrin-bound plasmin is protected from inactivation by circulating α_2-antiplasmin. These mechanisms ensure that plasmin formation is not premature, that plasmin formation is localized to the clot; the extent of plasmin formation is tied to the amount of fibrin present, thus allowing the process to efficiently dissolve thrombi of different sizes.

Regulation of fibrinolysis is achieved through a dynamic balance between profibrinolytic and antifibrinolytic processes maintained by complex interactions between circulating proteins, clot-based factors, and endothelial cells. Recruitment of the proteins key to fibrinolysis to the site of injury occurs simultaneously with the initiation of fibrin formation. The fibrin clot not only serves as a substrate but also acts in a role similar to the phospholipid surface in coagulation, functioning as a surface for the activation and localization of fibrinolytic proteins. The association of plasminogen and t-PA with fibrin enhances the rate of plasminogen activation by t-PA. Plasmin bound to fibrin is protected from inhibition by α_2-antiplasmin.[2220,2263,2288] These mechanisms both enhance fibrinolysis and serve to limit proteolytic activity to the clot. However, profibrinolytic processes are balanced by antifibrinolytic responses. PAI-1 associates with fibrin and inactivates t-PA and u-PA within the meshwork of the clot.[2289] Factor XIIIa cross-links and stabilizes the fibrin clot and renders it less susceptible to plasmin proteolysis. Factor XIIIa also cross-links α_2-antiplasmin to fibrin; this incorporation has been shown to play an important role in fibrin clot stabilization.[1846,1847,2276] TAFIa removes COOH-terminal lysines from partially proteolyzed fibrin, reducing the number of plasminogen-binding sites and attenuating the rate of plasmin formation. In addition, activated platelets release PAI-1 and α_2-antiplasmin at the fibrin surface, thus supplementing the ongoing downregulation of plasmin levels by the plasma pools of these serpins.[2290-2294]

Cellular Regulation of Fibrinolysis

The fibrin clot and, thus, fibrinolysis are localized to the surface of the blood vessel at sites where the normally nonthrombogenic facade presented by the endothelium is either mechanically removed or altered in its molecular composition. The unperturbed endothelium secretes PAI-1[2295] and is actively antifibrinolytic. Once the endothelial layer is disturbed, α-thrombin is generated and fibrin formation proceeds at that site.[2296] Intact endothelial surfaces in the vicinity of the injury become "activated" via interaction with products of the coagulation cascade, shifting from an antifibrinolytic to a profibrinolytic state. "Activated" endothelial cells express t-PA and u-PA as well as specific receptors for the plasminogen activators.[2297-2299] t-PA is likely the primary activator of plasminogen at the fibrin surface.[1987,2059,2300] u-PA has profibrinolytic activity but appears to be primarily associated with extracellular matrix degradation and initiation of tissue repair and remodeling.[2301-2303]

In addition to receptors for plasminogen activators, receptors for plasminogen[2304,2305] have been identified on a number of cell types including platelets, monocytes, fibroblasts, and endothelial cells, in which they appear to localize and accelerate plasmin formation. Plasmin generated at the cell surface is protected from serpin inhibitors by binding to specific cell receptors. Therefore, the cell surface can serve as a sanctuary for plasmin activity.

Urokinase-Type Plasminogen Activator Receptor

uPAR is synthesized and expressed by normal and malignant cells including monocytes, neutrophils, fibroblasts, platelets, and endothelial cells.[2301,2306-2312] A primary function of uPAR is to localize u-PA-mediated plasmin generation to the cell surface; however, more generally, uPAR mediates cell migration and tissue remodeling during development and wound healing.[2313,2314] Thus, uPAR function appears to be enmeshed with coagulation, fibrinolytic, and inflammatory processes.[2313-2315] uPAR binds both single-chain u-PA and plasminogen via high-affinity interactions, forming a ternary complex that enhances plasminogen activation[2308,2316] and initiates proteolysis of the extracellular matrix.[2317] The receptor is a heterogeneously glycosylated single-chain polypeptide (M_r = 50,000-60,000) of 313 amino acids.[2318] Although uPAR is an integral membrane protein, there is no defined transmembrane sequence. uPAR is instead anchored to the cellular membrane by a glycosyl-phosphatidylinositol moiety.[2319] The glycolipid is most likely attached to Gly^{283}, indicating that the mature protein consists of 283 amino acids.[2319,2320] Because uPAR has no intracellular domain, uPAR-mediated signaling presumably occurs through surface interactions with other components of the plasma membrane. At least 9 stable and 33 membrane-associated binding proteins have been identified.[2321] The neutrophils of individuals experiencing the hematopoietic stem cell disorder paroxysmal nocturnal hemoglobinuria, a disease in which these glycosyl-phosphatidylinositol moieties are lacking, show impaired transendothelial migration.[2310,2322] The absence of the receptor may play a role in the hypercoagulable state associated with this disorder. The crystal structure of uPAR has been reported in its ligand-free form[2323] and complexed with sc-UPA.[2324]

Tissue-Type Plasminogen Activator Receptors

Many structurally unrelated components that bind t-PA have been described. These receptors can be separated into two distinct functional

The Normal Hematologic System

groups: activation receptors and clearance receptors. Activation receptors are described as localizing t-PA onto a cell surface and enhancing the activation of plasminogen by t-PA.[2325] Receptors in the activation category include annexin II (42 kDa),[2326,2327] heparan sulfate and chondroitin sulfate-like proteoglycans,[2328] cytokeratin 8 and 18,[2329,2330] and tubulin.[2331] In patients with promyelocytic leukemia, overexpression of the t-PA receptor annexin II has been associated with a hyperfibrinolytic state resulting in bleeding.[2332] The t-PA receptor(s) on endothelial cells is poorly defined (for descriptions of these receptors, see Bachmann[1861]).

Clearance receptors are responsible for clearing t-PA from the circulation and its subsequent degradation. These receptors control not only the plasma concentration of t-PA but also the levels of inactive t-PA/PAI-1 complexes. t-PA clearance occurs principally in the liver and involves two different receptors: the mannose receptor and the LRP/α_2-macroglobulin receptor. The mannose receptor is a major t-PA receptor and binds t-PA with a high-affinity K_d of 1-4 nmol/L.[2333-2335] Liver endothelial cells and Kupffer cells bind t-PA via the mannose receptor. The other major pathway for t-PA clearance is through the LRP/α_2-macroglobulin receptor. This receptor has a relative molecular weight of 600 kDa.[1861] This receptor mediates the clearance of t-PA, t-PA/PAI-1, and u-PA/PAI-1 complexes; toxins; cytokines; apolipoprotein E-enriched chylomicron remnants; and complexes of α_2-macroglobulin.[2336] Free and PAI-1-complexed t-PA have also been shown to be cleared from the circulation through a glycoprotein 330-kDa LRP receptor and a 130-kDa very-low-density lipoprotein receptor.[2336-2338]

Role of Platelets in the Regulation of Fibrinolysis

Platelets are vital to procoagulant events and contribute to the fibrinolytic process as well. Platelets bind both t-PA and plasminogen and support plasmin generation.[2339-2341] Plasmin bound to the platelet surface is also protected from inhibition by α_2-antiplasmin.[2342] Platelets likewise contribute to the antifibrinolytic mechanism. Activated platelets release PAI-1, α_2-antiplasmin, C1-esterase inhibitor, and α_2-macroglobulin, which function to inhibit plasminogen activators and plasmin. Therefore, platelets, when present at high concentrations, can promote thrombosis and inhibit fibrinolysis.

Several studies have shown that plasmin can directly modify the function of platelets.[2342-2347] When plasmin is present at a low concentration, it can inhibit platelet aggregation by arachidonic acid metabolism or by proteolysis of membrane glycoproteins. At a high plasmin concentration, a proteolytic modification of the platelets occurs that affects fibrinogen binding and platelet aggregation. Plasmin is also able to increase the number of plasminogen-binding sites on the surface of platelets, an alteration that may function as a positive feedback loop for t-PA-mediated plasmin production. Increasing the size of the pool of fibrin-localized, platelet-bound plasminogen would augment the other readily activatable pool (plasminogen bound to fibrin), thereby increasing the amount of plasminogen available for efficient t-PA activation. Plasmin has also been shown to degrade the platelet-binding site for factor XIIIa, decreasing the rate of clot stabilization.[2316]

CONCLUSION

This chapter describes the process of blood coagulation by dividing it into sections based on procoagulant, anticoagulant, and fibrinolytic enzymes, cofactors, and inhibitors in the overall process of fibrin formation and fibrin dissolution. The role of each protein is described as either essential or accessory to hemostasis. The overall process of blood coagulation and fibrinolysis is better described when all the players are considered as contributing to a threshold-limited, complex, intertwined process that together promotes hemostasis.

Our understanding of the coagulation process has ancient historical roots; the accomplishments of numerous clinical and basic investigators have provided a relatively complete description of the inventory, connectivity, and dynamics of the overall process that occurs after vascular injury. Significant progress has been made in achieving a complete set of x-ray crystal structures for all the proteins involved in these processes (*Table 20.5*). The challenge for the future is the use of this knowledge in the development of new technology for the advancement of diagnosis, prophylaxis, and treatment of vascular disease.

ACKNOWLEDGMENTS

We, the authors, would like to thank Matthew Gissel for his assistance in the preparation of this chapter.

References

1. Mann KG. *Normal Hemostasis. Textbook of Internal Medicine*. JB Lippincott & Co.; 1992:1240-1245.
2. Writing GroupMembers, Lloyd-Jones D, Adams RJ, et al. Heart disease and stroke statistics–2010 update: a report from the American Heart Association. *Circulation*. 2010;121(7):e46-e215.
3. Macfarlane RG. An enzyme cascade in the blood clotting mechanism, and its function as a biochemical amplifier. *Nature*. 1964;202:498-499.
4. Davie EW, Ratnoff OD. Waterfall sequence for intrinsic blood clotting. *Science*. 1964;145(3638):1310-1312.
5. Mann KG, Nesheim ME, Church WR, Haley P, Krishnaswamy S. Surface-dependent reactions of the vitamin K-dependent enzyme complexes. *Blood*. 1990;76(1):1-16.
6. Orfeo T, Butenas S, Brummel-Ziedins KE, Mann KG. The tissue factor requirement in blood coagulation. *J Biol Chem*. 2005;280(52):42887-42896.
7. Gailani D, Broze GJ, Jr. Factor XI activation in a revised model of blood coagulation. *Science*. 1991;253(5022):909-912.
8. Radcliffe R, Nemerson Y. Activation and control of factor VII by activated factor X and thrombin. Isolation and characterization of a single chain form of factor VII. *J Biol Chem*. 1975;250(2):388-395.
9. Toole JJ, Knopf JL, Wozney JM, et al. Molecular cloning of a cDNA encoding human antihaemophilic factor. *Biotechnology*. 1984;1992(24):310-315.
10. Hill-Eubanks DC, Parker CG, Lollar P. Differential proteolytic activation of factor VIII-von Willebrand factor complex by thrombin. *Proc Natl Acad Sci U S A*. 1989;86(17):6508-6512.
11. Eaton D, Rodriguez H, Vehar GA. Proteolytic processing of human factor VIII. Correlation of specific cleavages by thrombin, factor Xa, and activated protein C with activation and inactivation of factor VIII coagulant activity. *Biochemistry*. 1986;25(2):505-512.
12. Lollar P, Hill-Eubanks DC, Parker CG. Association of the factor VIII light chain with von Willebrand factor. *J Biol Chem*. 1988;263(21):10451-10455.
13. Nesheim ME, Mann KG. Thrombin-catalyzed activation of single chain bovine factor V. *J Biol Chem*. 1979;254(4):1326-1334.
14. Nesheim ME, Foster WB, Hewick R, Mann KG. Characterization of Factor V activation intermediates. *J Biol Chem*. 1984;259(5):3187-3196.
15. Suzuki K, Dahlback B, Stenflo J. Thrombin-catalyzed activation of human coagulation factor V. *J Biol Chem*. 1982;257(11):6556-6564.
16. Naito K, Fujikawa K. Activation of human blood coagulation factor XI independent of factor XII. Factor XI is activated by thrombin and factor XIa in the presence of negatively charged surfaces. *J Biol Chem*. 1991;266(12):7353-7358.
17. Lorand L, Konishi K. Activation of the fibrin stabilizing factor of plasma by thrombin. *Arch Biochem Biophys*. 1964;105:58-67.
18. Hendriks D, Wang W, Scharpe S, Lommaert MP, van Sande M. Purification and characterization of a new arginine carboxypeptidase in human serum. *Biochim Biophys Acta*. 1990;1034(1):86-92.
19. Eaton DL, Malloy BE, Tsai SP, Henzel W, Drayna D. Isolation, molecular cloning, and partial characterization of a novel carboxypeptidase B from human plasma. *J Biol Chem*. 1991;266(32):21833-21838.
20. Kalafatis M, Swords NA, Rand MD, Mann KG. Membrane-dependent reactions in blood coagulation: role of the vitamin K-dependent enzyme complexes. *Biochim Biophys Acta*. 1994;1227(3):113-129.
21. Collen D, Lijnen HR. Molecular basis of fibrinolysis, as relevant for thrombolytic therapy. *Thromb Haemost*. 1995;74(1):167-171.
22. Henkin J, Marcotte P, Yang HC. The plasminogen-plasmin system. *Prog Cardiovasc Dis*. 1991;34(2):135-164.
23. Mann KG. Thrombin generation in hemorrhage control and vascular occlusion. *Circulation*. 2011;124(2):225-235.
24. Mann KG, Brummel K, Butenas S. What is all that thrombin for? *J Thromb Haemost*. 2003;1(7):1504-1514.
25. Mann KG, Butenas S, Brummel K. The dynamics of thrombin formation. *Arterioscler Thromb Vasc Biol*. 2003;23(1):17-25.
26. Warner ED, BK, Smith HP. A quantitative study of blood clotting. *Am J Physiol*. 1936;114:667-675.
27. Quick AJ. On the constitution of prothrombin. *Arterioscler Thromb Vasc Biol*. 1943;140:212-214.
28. Langdell RD, Wagner RH, Brinkhous KM. Effect of antihemophilic factor on one-stage clotting tests; a presumptive test for hemophilia and a simple one-stage antihemophilic factor assy procedure. *J Lab Clin Med*. 1953;41(4):637-647.
29. Hathaway WE, Belhasen LP, Hathaway HS. Evidence for a new plasma thromboplastin factor. I. Case report, coagulation studies and physicochemical properties. *Blood*. 1965;26(5):521-532.
30. Colman RW, Bagdasarian A, Talamo RC, et al. Williams trait. Human kininogen deficiency with diminished levels of plasminogen proactivator and prekallikrein associated with abnormalities of the Hageman factor-dependent pathways. *J Clin Invest*. 1975;56(6):1650-1662.

31. Hoak JC, Swanson LW, Warner ED, Connor WE. Myocardial infarction associated with severe factor-XII deficiency. *Lancet.* 1966;2(7469):884-886.

32. Telfer TP, Denson KW, Wright DR. A new coagulation defect. *Br J Haematol.* 1956;2(3):308-316.

33. Owen CA, Jr, Cooper T. Parahemophilia. *AMA Arch Intern Med.* 1955;95(2):194-201.

34. Roberts HR, Foster PA. *Inherited Disorders of Prothrombin Conversion.* JB Lippincott Company; 1987.

35. Biggs R, Douglas AS, Macfarlane RG, Dacie JV, Pitney WR. Merskey. Christmas disease: a condition previously mistaken for haemophilia. *Br Med J.* 1952;2(4799):1378-1382.

36. Bajzar L, Manuel R, Nesheim ME. Purification and characterization of TAFI, a thrombin-activable fibrinolysis inhibitor. *J Biol Chem.* 1995;270(24):14477-14484.

37. Lawson JH, Kalafatis M, Stram S, Mann KG. A model for the tissue factor pathway to thrombin. I. An empirical study. *J Biol Chem.* 1994;269(37):23357-23366.

38. Bone B. *Sepsis and Multiple Organ Failure: Consensus or Controversy.* Vol. 16. Springer-Verlag; 1992.

39. Colman RWHJ, Marder VJ, Salzman EW. *Contact Activation Pathway: Inflammatory, Fibrinolytic, Anticoagulant, Antiadhesive, and Antiangiogenic Activities.* Lippincott, Williams & Wilkins; 2001.

40. Renne T, Pozgajova M, Gruner S, et al. Defective thrombus formation in mice lacking coagulation factor XII. *J Exp Med.* 2005;202(2):271-281.

41. Kleinschnitz C, Stoll G, Bendszus M, et al. Targeting coagulation factor XII provides protection from pathological thrombosis in cerebral ischemia without interfering with hemostasis. *J Exp Med.* 2006;203(3):513-518.

42. Nesheim ME, Taswell JB, Mann KG. The contribution of bovine Factor V and Factor Va to the activity of prothrombinase. *J Biol Chem.* 1979;254(21):10952-10962.

43. Krishnaswamy S. Prothrombinase complex assembly. Contributions of protein-protein and protein-membrane interactions toward complex formation. *J Biol Chem.* 1990;265(7):3708-3718.

44. Tracy PB, Nesheim ME, Mann KG. Coordinate binding of factor Va and factor Xa to the unstimulated platelet. *J Biol Chem.* 1981;256(2):743-751.

45. Krishnaswamy S, Field KA, Edgington TS, Morrissey JH, Mann KG. Role of the membrane surface in the activation of human coagulation factor X. *J Biol Chem.* 1992;267(36):26110-26120.

46. Mann KG. Prothrombin. *Methods Enzymol.* 1976;45:123-156.

47. Kalafatis M, Xue J, Lawler CM, Mann KG. Contribution of the heavy and light chains of factor Va to the interaction with factor Xa. *Biochemistry.* 1994;33(21):6538-6545.

48. Walker RK, Krishnaswamy S. The influence of factor Va on the active site of factor Xa. *J Biol Chem.* 1993;268(19):13920-13929.

49. Nemerson Y. Tissue factor and hemostasis. *Blood.* 1988;71(1):1-8.

50. Edgington TS, Mackman N, Brand K, Ruf W. The structural biology of expression and function of tissue factor. *Thromb Haemost.* 1991;66(1):67-79.

51. Nakagaki T, Foster DC, Berkner KL, Kisiel W. Initiation of the extrinsic pathway of blood coagulation: evidence for the tissue factor dependent autoactivation of human coagulation factor VII. *Biochemistry.* 1991;30(45):10819-10824.

52. Morrissey JH, Macik BG, Neuenschwander PF, Comp PC. Quantitation of activated factor VII levels in plasma using a tissue factor mutant selectively deficient in promoting factor VII activation. *Blood.* 1993;81(3):734-744.

53. Drake TA, Morrissey JH, Edgington TS. Selective cellular expression of tissue factor in human tissues. Implications for disorders of hemostasis and thrombosis. *Am J Pathol.* 1989;134(5):1087-1097.

54. Rodgers GM, Greenberg CS, Shuman MA. Characterization of the effects of cultured vascular cells on the activation of blood coagulation. *Blood.* 1983;61(6):1155-1162.

55. Maynard JR, Dreyer BE, Stemerman MB, Pitlick FA. Tissue-factor coagulant activity of cultured human endothelial and smooth muscle cells and fibroblasts. *Blood.* 1977;50(3):387-396.

56. Wilcox JN, Smith KM, Schwartz SM, Gordon D. Localization of tissue factor in the normal vessel wall and in the atherosclerotic plaque. *Proc Natl Acad Sci U S A.* 1989;86(8):2839-2843.

57. Callander NS, Varki N, Rao LV. Immunohistochemical identification of tissue factor in solid tumors. *Cancer.* 1992;70(5):1194-1201.

58. Fleck RA, Rao LV, Rapaport SI, Varki N. Localization of human tissue factor antigen by immunostaining with monospecific, polyclonal anti-human tissue factor antibody. *Thromb Res.* 1990;59(2):421-437.

59. Rodgers GM. Hemostatic properties of normal and perturbed vascular cells. *FASEB J.* 1988;2(2):116-123.

60. Conkling PR, Greenberg CS, Weinberg JB. Tumor necrosis factor induces tissue factor-like activity in human leukemia cell line U937 and peripheral blood monocytes. *Blood.* 1988;72(1):128-133.

61. Lawson JH, Mann KG. Cooperative activation of human factor IX by the human extrinsic pathway of blood coagulation. *J Biol Chem.* 1991;266(17):11317-11327.

62. Mann KG, Krishnaswamy S, Lawson JH. Surface-dependent hemostasis. *Semin Hematol.* 1992;29(3):213-226.

63. Ahmad SS, Rawala-Sheikh R, Walsh PN. Components and assembly of the factor X activating complex. *Semin Thromb Hemost.* 1992;18(3):311-323.

64. Revenko AS, Gao D, Crosby JR, et al. Selective depletion of plasma prekallikrein or coagulation factor XII inhibits thrombosis in mice without increased risk of bleeding. *Blood.* 2011;118(19):5302-5311.

65. Cheng Q, Tucker EI, Pine MS, et al. A role for factor XIIa-mediated factor XI activation in thrombus formation in vivo. *Blood.* 2010;116(19):3981-3989.

66. Gailani D, Renne T. Intrinsic pathway of coagulation and arterial thrombosis. *Arterioscler Thromb Vasc Biol.* 2007;27(12):2507-2513.

67. Nickel KF, Long AT, Fuchs TA, Butler LM, Renne T. Factor XII as a therapeutic target in thromboembolic and inflammatory diseases. *Arterioscler Thromb Vasc Biol.* 2017;37(1):13-20.

68. Kuijpers MJ, van der Meijden PE, Feijge MA, et al. Factor XII regulates the pathological process of thrombus formation on ruptured plaques. *Arterioscler Thromb Vasc Biol.* 2014;34(8):1674-1680.

69. Larsson M, Rayzman V, Nolte MW, et al. A factor XIIa inhibitory antibody provides thromboprotection in extracorporeal circulation without increasing bleeding risk. *Sci Transl Med.* 2014;6(222):222ra217.

70. Visser M, Heitmeier S, Ten Cate H, Spronk HMH. Role of factor XIa and plasma kallikrein in arterial and venous thrombosis. *Thromb Haemost.* 2020;120(6):883-993.

71. Rangaswamy C, Englert H, Deppermann C, Renne T. Polyanions in coagulation and thrombosis: focus on polyphosphate and neutrophils extracellular traps. *Thromb Haemost.* 2021;121(8):1021-1030.

72. Kapoor S, Opneja A, Nayak L. The role of neutrophils in thrombosis. *Thromb Res.* 2018;170:87-96.

73. Doring Y, Libby P, Soehnlein O. Neutrophil extracellular traps participate in cardiovascular diseases: recent experimental and clinical insights. *Circ Res.* 2020;126(9):1228-1241.

74. van der Meijden PE, Munnix IC, Auger JM, et al. Dual role of collagen in factor XII-dependent thrombus formation. *Blood.* 2009;114(4):881-890.

75. Shamanaev A, Emsley J, Gailani D. Proteolytic activity of contact factor zymogens. *J Thromb Haemost.* 2021;19(2):330-341.

76. Revak SD, Cochrane CG, Johnston AR, Hugli TE. Structural changes accompanying enzymatic activation of human Hageman factor. *J Clin Invest.* 1974;54(3):619-627.

77. Saito H, Ratnoff OD, Pensky J. Radioimmunoassay of human Hageman factor (factor XII). *J Lab Clin Med.* 1976;88(2):506-514.

78. Gordon EM, Williams SR, Frenchek B, Mazur CA, Speroff L. Dose-dependent effects of postmenopausal estrogen and progestin on antithrombin III and factor XII. *J Lab Clin Med.* 1988;111(1):52-56.

79. Mitropoulos KA, Martin JC, Burgess AI, et al. The increased rate of activation of factor XII in late pregnancy can contribute to the increased reactivity of factor VII. *Thromb Haemost.* 1990;63(3):349-355.

80. Gordon EM, Johnson TR, Ramos LP, Schmeidler-Sapiro KT. Enhanced expression of factor XII (Hageman factor) in isolated livers of estrogen- and prolactin-treated rats. *J Lab Clin Med.* 1991;117(5):353-358.

81. Stavrou E, Schmaier AH. Factor XII: what does it contribute to our understanding of the physiology and pathophysiology of hemostasis & thrombosis. *Thromb Res.* 2010;125(3):210-215.

82. Woodruff RS, Sullenger B, Becker RC. The many faces of the contact pathway and their role in thrombosis. *J Thromb Thrombolysis.* 2011;32(1):9-20.

83. Ghebrehiwet B, CebadaMora C, Tantral L, Jesty J, Peerschke EI. gC1qR/p33 serves as a molecular bridge between the complement and contact activation systems and is an important catalyst in inflammation. *Adv Exp Med Biol.* 2006;586:95-105.

84. Peerschke EI, Minta JO, Zhou SZ, et al. Expression of gC1q-R/p33 and its major ligands in human atherosclerotic lesions. *Mol Immunol.* 2004;41(8):759-766.

85. Maas C, Govers-Riemslag JW, Bouma B, et al. Misfolded proteins activate factor XII in humans, leading to kallikrein formation without initiating coagulation. *J Clin Invest.* 2008;118(9):3208-3218.

86. Citarella F, Tripodi M, Fantoni A, Bernardi F, Romeo G, Rocchi M. Assignment of human coagulation factor XII (fXII) to chromosome 5 by cDNA hybridization to DNA from somatic cell hybrids. *Hum Genet.* 1988;80(4):397-398.

87. Royle NJ, Nigli N, Cool D, MacGillivray RT, Hamerton JL. Structural gene encoding human factor XII is located at 5q33-qter. *Somat Cell Mol Genet.* 1988;14(2):217-221.

88. Cool DE, MacGillivray RT. Characterization of the human blood coagulation factor XII gene. Intron/exon gene organization and analysis of the 5'-flanking region. *J Biol Chem.* 1987;262(28):13662-13673.

89. Citarella F, Misiti S, Felici A, Aiuti A, La Porta C, Fantoni A. The 5' sequence of human factor XII gene contains transcription regulatory elements typical of liver specific, estrogen-modulated genes. *Biochim Biophys Acta.* 1993;1172(1-2):197-199.

90. Griffin JH, Cochrane CG. Human factor XII (hageman factor). *Methods Enzymol.* 1976;45:56-65.

91. McMullen BA, Fujikawa K, Kisiel W. The occurrence of beta-hydroxyaspartic acid in the vitamin K-dependent blood coagulation zymogens. *Biochem Biophys Res Commun.* 1983;115(1):8-14.

92. Fujikawa K, McMullen BA. Amino acid sequence of human beta-factor XIIa. *J Biol Chem.* 1983;258(18):10924-10933.

93. McMullen BA, Fujikawa K. Amino acid sequence of the heavy chain of human alpha-factor XIIa (activated Hageman factor). *J Biol Chem.* 1985;260(9):5328-5341.

94. Cool DE, Edgell CJ, Louie GV, Zoller MJ, Brayer GD, MacGillivray RT. Characterization of human blood coagulation factor XII cDNA. Prediction of the primary structure of factor XII and the tertiary structure of beta-factor XIIa. *J Biol Chem.* 1985;260(25):13666-13676.

95. Harris RJ, Ling VT, Spellman MW. O-linked fucose is present in the first epidermal growth factor domain of factor XII but not protein C. *J Biol Chem.* 1992;267(8):5102-5107.

96. Pixley RA, Colman RW. Factor XII: hageman factor. *Methods Enzymol.* 1993;222:51-65.

97. Rojkaer R, Schousboe I. Partial identification of the Zn2+-binding sites in factor XII and its activation derivatives. *Eur J Biochem.* 1997;247(2):491-496.

98. Schousboe I. Contact activation in human plasma is triggered by zinc ion modulation of factor XII (Hageman factor). *Blood Coagul Fibrinolysis.* 1993;4(5):671-678.

99. Bernardo MM, Day DE, Olson ST, Shore JD. Surface-independent acceleration of factor XII activation by zinc ions. I. Kinetic characterization of the metal ion rate enhancement. *J Biol Chem.* 1993;268(17):12468-12476.

The Normal Hematologic System

100. Bernardo MM, Day DE, Halvorson HR, Olson ST, Shore JD. Surface-independent acceleration of factor XII activation by zinc ions. II. Direct binding and fluorescence studies. *J Biol Chem.* 1993;268(17):12477-12483.
101. Cochrane CG, Revak SD, Wuepper KD. Activation of Hageman factor in solid and fluid phases. A critical role of kallikrein. *J Exp Med.* 1973;138(6):1564-1583.
102. Revak SD, Cochrane CG, Griffin JH. The binding and cleavage characteristics of human Hageman factor during contact activation. A comparison of normal plasma with plasmas deficient in factor XI, prekallikrein, or high molecular weight kininogen. *J Clin Invest.* 1977;59(6):1167-1175.
103. Griffin JH. Role of surface in surface-dependent activation of Hageman factor (blood coagulation factor XII). *Proc Natl Acad Sci U S A.* 1978;75(4):1998-2002.
104. Kirby EP, McDevitt PJ. The binding of bovine factor XII to kaolin. *Blood.* 1983;61(4):652-659.
105. Wiggins RC, Cochrane CC. The autoactivation of rabbit Hageman factor. *J Exp Med.* 1979;150(5):1122-1133.
106. Miller G, Silverberg M, Kaplan AP. Autoactivatability of human Hageman factor (factor XII). *Biochem Biophys Res Commun.* 1980;92(3):803-810.
107. Silverberg M, Dunn JT, Garen L, Kaplan AP. Autoactivation of human Hageman factor. Demonstration utilizing a synthetic substrate. *J Biol Chem.* 1980;255(15):7281-7286.
108. Dunn JT, Silverberg M, Kaplan AP. The cleavage and formation of activated human Hageman factor by autodigestion and by kallikrein. *J Biol Chem.* 1982;257(4):1779-1784.
109. Espana F, Ratnoff OD. Activation of Hageman factor (factor XII) by sulfatides and other agents in the absence of plasma proteases. *J Lab Clin Med.* 1983;102(1):31-45.
110. Tankersley DL, Finlayson JS. Kinetics of activation and autoactivation of human factor XII. *Biochemistry.* 1984;23(2):273-279.
111. Thorisdottir H, Ratnoff OD, Maniglia AJ. Activation of Hageman factor (factor XII) by bismuth subgallate, a hemostatic agent. *J Lab Clin Med.* 1988;112(4):481-486.
112. Zhuo R, Siedlecki CA, Vogler EA. Autoactivation of blood factor XII at hydrophilic and hydrophobic surfaces. *Biomaterials.* 2006;27(24):4325-4332.
113. Ziats NP, Pankowsky DA, Tierney BP, Ratnoff OD, Anderson JM. Adsorption of Hageman factor (factor XII) and other human plasma proteins to biomedical polymers. *J Lab Clin Med.* 1990;116(5):687-696.
114. Ratnoff OD. Activation of hageman factor by L-homocystine. *Science.* 1968;162(3857):1007-1009.
115. Becker CG, Wagner M, Kaplan AP, et al. Activation of factor XII-dependent pathways in human plasma by hematin and protoporphyrin. *J Clin Invest.* 1985;76(2):413-419.
116. Kurachi K, Fujikawa K, Davie EW. Mechanism of activation of bovine factor XI by factor XII and factor XIIa. *Biochemistry.* 1980;19(7):1330-1338.
117. Fujikawa K, Heimark RL, Kurachi K, Davie EW. Activation of bovine factor XII (Hageman factor) by plasma kallikrein. *Biochemistry.* 1980;19(7):1322-1330.
118. Tans G, Rosing J, Griffin JH. Sulfatide-dependent autoactivation of human blood coagulation Factor XII (Hageman Factor). *J Biol Chem.* 1983;258(13):8215-8222.
119. Hojima Y, Cochrane CG, Wiggins RC, Austen KF, Stevens RL. In vitro activation of the contact (Hageman factor) system of plasma by heparin and chondroitin sulfate E. *Blood.* 1984;63(6):1453-1459.
120. Koenig JM, Chahine A, Ratnoff OD. Inhibition of the activation of Hageman factor (factor XII) by soluble human placental collagens types III, IV, and V. *J Lab Clin Med.* 1991;117(6):523-527.
121. Silverberg M, Diehl SV. The autoactivation of factor XII (Hageman factor) induced by low-Mr heparin and dextran sulphate. The effect of the Mr of the activating polyanion. *Biochem J.* 1987;248(3):715-720.
122. Tans G, Verkleij AJ, Yu J, Griffin JH. Sulfatide bilayers as a surface for contact activation in human plasma. *Biochem Biophys Res Commun.* 1987;149(3):1002-1007.
123. Griep MA, Fujikawa K, Nelsestuen GL. Possible basis for the apparent surface selectivity of the contact activation of human blood coagulation factor XII. *Biochemistry.* 1986;25(21):6688-6694.
124. Johne J, Blume C, Benz PM, et al. Platelets promote coagulation factor XII-mediated proteolytic cascade systems in plasma. *Biol Chem.* 2006;387(2):173-178.
125. Klein S, Spannagl M, Engelmann B. Phosphatidylethanolamine participates in the stimulation of the contact system of coagulation by very-low-density lipoproteins. *Arterioscler Thromb Vasc Biol.* 2001;21(10):1695-1700.
126. Schmaier A. *Contact Activation.* Williams and Wilkins; 1998.
127. Motta G, Rojkjaer R, Hasan AA, Cines DB, Schmaier AH. High molecular weight kininogen regulates prekallikrein assembly and activation on endothelial cells: a novel mechanism for contact activation. *Blood.* 1998;91(2):516-528.
128. Rojkjaer R, Hasan AA, Motta G, Schousboe I, Schmaier AH. Factor XII does not initiate prekallikrein activation on endothelial cells. *Thromb Haemost.* 1998;80(1):74-81.
129. Hovinga JK, Schaller J, Stricker H, Wuillemin WA, Furlan M, Lammle B. Coagulation factor XII Locarno: the functional defect is caused by the amino acid substitution Arg 353-->Pro leading to loss of a kallikrein cleavage site. *Blood.* 1994;84(4):1173-1181.
130. Clarke BJ, Cote HC, Cool DE, et al. Mapping of a putative surface-binding site of human coagulation factor XII. *J Biol Chem.* 1989;264(19):11497-11502.
131. Citarella F, Ravon DM, Pascucci B, Felici A, Fantoni A, Hack CE. Structure/function analysis of human factor XII using recombinant deletion mutants. Evidence for an additional region involved in the binding to negatively charged surfaces. *Eur J Biochem.* 1996;238(1):240-249.
132. Kaplan AP, Austen KF. A pre-albumin activator of prekallikrein. *J Immunol.* 1970;105(4):802-811.
133. Wuepper KD, TEI, Cochrane CG. Plasma kinin system: proenzyme components. *J Immunol.* 1970;105:1307-1311.
134. Cochrane CG, Griffin JH. Molecular assembly in the contact phase of the Hageman factor system. *Am J Med.* 1979;67(4):657-664.
135. Kaplan AP, Austen KF. A prealbumin activator of prekallikrein. II. Derivation of activators of prekallikrein from active Hageman factor by digestion with plasmin. *J Exp Med.* 1971;133(4):696-712.
136. Revak SD, Cochrane CG, Bouma BN, Griffin JH. Surface and fluid phase activities of two forms of activated Hageman factor produced during contact activation of plasma. *J Exp Med.* 1978;147(3):719-729.
137. Revak SD, Cochrane CG. The relationship of structure and function in human Hageman factor. The association of enzymatic and binding activities with separate regions of the molecule. *J Clin Invest.* 1976;57(4):852-860.
138. Gordon EM, Gallagher CA, Johnson TR, Blossey BK, Ilan J. Hepatocytes express blood coagulation factor XII (Hageman factor). *J Lab Clin Med.* 1990;115(4):463-469.
139. Kaplan AP, Silverberg M, Ghebrehiwet B. The intrinsic coagulation/kinin pathway–the classical complement pathway and their interactions. *Adv Exp Med Biol.* 1986;198(pt B):11-25.
140. Chien P, Pixley RA, Stumpo LG, Colman RW, Schreiber AD. Modulation of the human monocyte binding site for monomeric immunoglobulin G by activated Hageman factor. *J Clin Invest.* 1988;82(5):1554-1559.
141. Toossi Z, Sedor JR, Mettler MA, Everson B, Young T, Ratnoff OD. Induction of expression of monocyte interleukin 1 by Hageman factor (factor XII). *Proc Natl Acad Sci U S A.* 1992;89(24):11969-11972.
142. Wachtfogel YT, Pixley RA, Kucich U, et al. Purified plasma factor XIIa aggregates human neutrophils and causes degranulation. *Blood.* 1986;67(6):1731-1737.
143. Schmaier AH. The elusive physiologic role of Factor XII. *J Clin Invest.* 2008;118(9):3006-3009.
144. Mandle R, Jr, Kaplan AP. Hageman factor substrates. Human plasma prekallikrein: mechanism of activation by Hageman factor and participation in hageman factor-dependent fibrinolysis. *J Biol Chem.* 1977;252(17):6097-6104.
145. Forbes CD, Pensky J, Ratnoff OD. Inhibition of activated Hageman factor and activated plasma thromboplastin antecedent by purified serum C1 inactivator. *J Lab Clin Med.* 1970;76(5):809-815.
146. Schreiber AD, Kaplan AP, Austen KF. Inhibition by C1INH of Hagemann factor fragment activation of coagulation, fibrinolysis, and kinin generation. *J Clin Invest.* 1973;52(6):1402-1409.
147. de Agostini A, Lijnen HR, Pixley RA, Colman RW, Schapira M. Inactivation of factor XII active fragment in normal plasma. Predominant role of C-1-inhibitor. *J Clin Invest.* 1984;73(6):1542-1549.
148. Pixley RA, Schapira M, Colman RW. The regulation of human factor XIIa by plasma proteinase inhibitors. *J Biol Chem.* 1985;260(3):1723-1729.
149. Stead N, Kaplan AP, Rosenberg RD. Inhibition of activated factor XII by antithrombin-heparin cofactor. *J Biol Chem.* 1976;251(21):6481-6488.
150. Pixley RA, Schapira M, Colman RW. Effect of heparin on the inactivation rate of human activated factor XII by antithrombin III. *Blood.* 1985;66(1):198-203.
151. Berrettini M, Schleef RR, Espana F, Loskutoff DJ, Griffin JH. Interaction of type 1 plasminogen activator inhibitor with the enzymes of the contact activation system. *J Biol Chem.* 1989;264(20):11738-11743.
152. Kleniewski J, Donaldson VH. Endothelial cells produce a substance that inhibits contact activation of coagulation by blocking the activation of Hageman factor. *Proc Natl Acad Sci U S A.* 1993;90(1):198-202.
153. Ratnoff OD, Everson B, Embury P, et al. Inhibition of the activation of Hageman factor (factor XII) by human vascular endothelial cell culture supernates. *Proc Natl Acad Sci U S A.* 1991;88(23):10740-10743.
154. Ratnoff OD, Gleich GJ, Shurin SB, Kazura J, Everson B, Embury P. Inhibition of the activation of hageman factor (factor XII) by eosinophils and eosinophilic constituents. *Am J Hematol.* 1993;42(1):138-145.
155. Niwano H, Embury PB, Greenberg BD, Ratnoff OD. Inhibitory action of amyloid precursor protein against human Hageman factor (factor XII). *J Lab Clin Med.* 1995;125(2):251-256.
156. Fisher CA, Schmaier AH, Addonizio VP, Colman RW. Assay of prekallikrein in human plasma: comparison of amidolytic, esterolytic, coagulation, and immunochemical assays. *Blood.* 1982;59(5):963-970.
157. McConnell DJ, Mason B. The isolation of human plasma prekallikrein. *Br J Pharmacol.* 1970;38(3):490-502.
158. Mandle RJ, Colman RW, Kaplan AP. Identification of prekallikrein and high-molecular-weight kininogen as a complex in human plasma. *Proc Natl Acad Sci U S A.* 1976;73(11):4179-4183.
159. Scott CF, Colman RW. Function and immunochemistry of prekallikrein-high molecular weight kininogen complex in plasma. *J Clin Invest.* 1980;65(2):413-421.
160. Girolami A, Scarparo P, Candeo N, Lombardi AM. Congenital prekallikrein deficiency. *Expert Rev Hematol.* 2010;3(6):685-695.
161. Bojanini EU, Loaiza-Bonilla A, Pimentel A. Prekallikrein deficiency presenting as recurrent cerebrovascular accident: case report and review of the literature. *Case Rep Hematol.* 2012;2012:723204.
162. Beaubien G, Rosinski-Chupin I, Mattei MG, Mbikay M, Chretien M, Seidah NG. Gene structure and chromosomal localization of plasma kallikrein. *Biochemistry.* 1991;30(6):1628-1635.
163. Yu H, Anderson PJ, Freedman BI, Rich SS, Bowden DW. Genomic structure of the human plasma prekallikrein gene, identification of allelic variants, and analysis in end-stage renal disease. *Genomics.* 2000;69(2):225-234.
164. Veloso D, Shilling J, Shine J, Fitch WM, Colman RW. Recent evolutionary divergence of plasma prekallikrein and factor XI. *Thromb Res.* 1986;43(2):153-160.
165. Chung DW, Fujikawa K, McMullen BA, Davie EW. Human plasma prekallikrein, a zymogen to a serine protease that contains four tandem repeats. *Biochemistry.* 1986;25(9):2410-2417.
166. Ciechanowicz A, Bader M, Wagner J, Ganten D. Extra-hepatic transcription of plasma prekallikrein gene in human and rat tissues. *Biochem Biophys Res Commun.* 1993;197(3):1370-1376.

167. Cerf ME, Raidoo DM. Immunolocalization of plasma kallikrein in human brain. *Metab Brain Dis*. 2000;15(4):315-323.
168. Asakai R, Davie EW, Chung DW. Organization of the gene for human factor XI. *Biochemistry*. 1987;26(23):7221-7228.
169. Scott CF, Liu CY, Colman RW. Human plasma prekallikrein: a rapid high-yield method for purification. *Eur J Biochem*. 1979;100(1):77-83.
170. McMullen BA, Fujikawa K, Davie EW. Location of the disulfide bonds in human coagulation factor XI: the presence of tandem apple domains. *Biochemistry*. 1991;30(8):2056-2060.
171. Page JD, You JL, Harris RB, Colman RW. Localization of the binding site on plasma kallikrein for high-molecular-weight kininogen to both apple 1 and apple 4 domains of the heavy chain. *Arch Biochem Biophys*. 1994;314(1):159-164.
172. Herwald H, Jahnen-Dechent W, Alla SA, Hock J, Bouma BN, Muller-Esterl W. Mapping of the high molecular weight kininogen binding site of prekallikrein. Evidence for a discontinuous epitope formed by distinct segments of the prekallikrein heavy chain. *J Biol Chem*. 1993;268(19):14527-14535.
173. Wuepper KD, Cochrane CG. Plasma prekallikrein: isolation, characterization, and mechanism of activation. *J Exp Med*. 1972;135(1):1-20.
174. Shariat-Madar Z, Mahdi F, Schmaier AH. Identification and characterization of prolylcarboxypeptidase as an endothelial cell prekallikrein activator. *J Biol Chem*. 2002;277(20):17962-17969.
175. Bouma BN, Miles LA, Beretta G, Griffin JH. Human plasma prekallikrein. Studies of its activation by activated factor XII and of its inactivation by diisopropyl phosphofluoridate. *Biochemistry*. 1980;19(6):1151-1160.
176. van der Graaf F, Tans G, Bouma BN, Griffin JH. Isolation and functional properties of the heavy and light chains of human plasma kallikrein. *J Biol Chem*. 1982;257(23):14300-14305.
177. Burger D, Schleuning WD, Schapira M. Human plasma prekallikrein. Immunoaffinity purification and activation to alpha- and beta-kallikrein. *J Biol Chem*. 1986;261(1):324-327.
178. Colman RW, Wachtfogel YT, Kucich U, et al. Effect of cleavage of the heavy chain of human plasma kallikrein on its functional properties. *Blood*. 1985;65(2):311-318.
179. Nagasawa S, Nakayasu T. Human plasma prekallikrein as a protein complex. *J Biochem*. 1973;74(2):401-403.
180. Habal FM, Movat HZ, Burrowes CE. Isolation of two functionally different kininogens from human plasma–separation from proteinase inhibitors and interaction with plasma kallikrein. *Biochem Pharmacol*. 1974;23(16):2291-2303.
181. Toda N, Okamura T. Endothelium-dependent and -independent responses to vasoactive substances of isolated human coronary arteries. *Am J Physiol*. 1989;257(3 pt 2):H988-H995.
182. Hong SL. Effect of bradykinin and thrombin on prostacyclin synthesis in endothelial cells from calf and pig aorta and human umbilical cord vein. *Thromb Res*. 1980;18(6):787-795.
183. Gurewich V, Johnstone M, Loza JP, Pannell R. Pro-urokinase and prekallikrein are both associated with platelets. Implications for the intrinsic pathway of fibrinolysis and for therapeutic thrombolysis. *FEBS Lett*. 1993;318(3):317-321.
184. Loza JP, Gurewich V, Johnstone M, Pannell R. Platelet-bound prekallikrein promotes pro-urokinase-induced clot lysis: a mechanism for targeting the factor XII dependent intrinsic pathway of fibrinolysis. *Thromb Haemost*. 1994;71(3):347-352.
185. Wachtfogel YT, Kucich U, James HL, et al. Human plasma kallikrein releases neutrophil elastase during blood coagulation. *J Clin Invest*. 1983;72(5):1672-1677.
186. Schapira M, Scott CF, Colman RW. Protection of human plasma kallikrein from inactivation by C1 inhibitor and other protease inhibitors. The role of high molecular weight kininogen. *Biochemistry*. 1981;20(10):2738-2743.
187. van der Graaf F, Koedam JA, Bouma BN. Inactivation of kallikrein in human plasma. *J Clin Invest*. 1983;71(1):149-158.
188. Schapira M, Scott CF, Colman RW. Contribution of plasma protease inhibitors to the inactivation of kallikrein in plasma. *J Clin Invest*. 1982;69(2):462-468.
189. van der Graaf F, Koedam JA, Griffin JH, Bouma BN. Interaction of human plasma kallikrein and its light chain with C1 inhibitor. *Biochemistry*. 1983;22(20):4860-4866.
190. Schapira M, Scott CF, James A, et al. High molecular weight kininogen or its light chain protects human plasma kallikrein from inactivation by plasma protease inhibitors. *Biochemistry*. 1982;21(3):567-572.
191. Schmaier AH, Gustafson E, Idell S, Colman RW. Plasma prekallikrein assay: reversible inhibition of C-1 inhibitor by chloroform and its use in measuring prekallikrein in different mammalian species. *J Lab Clin Med*. 1984;104(6):882-892.
192. DeLa Cadena RA, Colman RW. The sequence HGLGHGHEQQHGLGHGH in the light chain of high molecular weight kininogen serves as a primary structural feature for zinc-dependent binding to an anionic surface. *Protein Sci*. 1992;1(1):151-160.
193. Bjork I, Olson ST, Sheffer RG, Shore JD. Binding of heparin to human high molecular weight kininogen. *Biochemistry*. 1989;28(3):1213-1221.
194. Olson ST, Sheffer R, Francis AM. High molecular weight kininogen potentiates the heparin-accelerated inhibition of plasma kallikrein by antithrombin: role for antithrombin in the regulation of kallikrein. *Biochemistry*. 1993;32(45):12136-12147.
195. Meijers JC, Kanters DH, Vlooswijk RA, van Erp HE, Hessing M, Bouma BN. Inactivation of human plasma kallikrein and factor XIa by protein C inhibitor. *Biochemistry*. 1988;27(12):4231-4237.
196. Espana F, Estelles A, Griffin JH, Aznar J. Interaction of plasma kallikrein with protein C inhibitor in purified mixtures and in plasma. *Thromb Haemost*. 1991;65(1):46-51.
197. Koedam JA, Meijers JC, Sixma JJ, Bouma BN. Inactivation of human factor VIII by activated protein C. Cofactor activity of protein S and protective effect of von Willebrand factor. *J Clin Invest*. 1988;82(4):1236-1243.
198. Schmaier AH, Bradford H, Silver LD, et al. High molecular weight kininogen is an inhibitor of platelet calpain. *J Clin Invest*. 1986;77(5):1565-1573.
199. Schmaier AH, Zuckerberg A, Silverman C, Kuchibhotla J, Tuszynski GP, Colman RW. High-molecular weight kininogen. A secreted platelet protein. *J Clin Invest*. 1983;71(5):1477-1489.
200. Scott CF, Shull B, Muller-Esterl W, Colman RW. Rapid direct determination of low and high molecular weight kininogen in human plasma by Particle Concentration Fluorescence Immunoassay (PCFIA). *Thromb Haemost*. 1997;77(1):109-118.
201. Cheung PP, Kunapuli SP, Scott CF, Wachtfogel YT, Colman RW. Genetic basis of total kininogen deficiency in Williams' trait. *J Biol Chem*. 1993;268(31):23361-23365.
202. Kaplan AP, Ghebrehiwet B. The plasma bradykinin-forming pathways and its interrelationships with complement. *Mol Immunol*. 2010;47(13):2161-2169.
203. Takagaki Y, Kitamura N, Nakanishi S. Cloning and sequence analysis of cDNAs for human high molecular weight and low molecular weight prekininogens. Primary structures of two human prekininogens. *J Biol Chem*. 1985;260(14):8601-8609.
204. Kitamura N, Kitagawa H, Fukushima D, Takagaki Y, Miyata T, Nakanishi S. Structural organization of the human kininogen gene and a model for its evolution. *J Biol Chem*. 1985;260(14):8610-8617.
205. Cheung PP, Cannizzaro LA, Colman RW. Chromosomal mapping of human kininogen gene (KNG) to 3q26----qter. *Cytogenet Cell Genet*. 1992;59(1):24-26.
206. Schmaier AH, Kuo A, Lundberg D, Murray S, Cines DB. The expression of high molecular weight kininogen on human umbilical vein endothelial cells. *J Biol Chem*. 1988;263(31):16327-16333.
207. Chen LM, Chung P, Chao S, Chao L, Chao J. Differential regulation of kininogen gene expression by estrogen and progesterone in vivo. *Biochim Biophys Acta*. 1992;1131(2):145-151.
208. Chhibber G, Cohen A, Lane S, Farber A, Meloni FJ, Schmaier AH. Immunoblotting of plasma in a pregnant patient with hereditary angioedema. *J Lab Clin Med*. 1990;115(1):112-121.
209. Takano M, Kondo J, Yayama K, Okamoto H. Expression of low-molecular-weight kininogen mRNA in human fibroblast WI38 cells. *Jpn J Pharmacol*. 1996;71(4):341-343.
210. Higashiyama S, Ohkubo I, Ishiguro H, Sasaki M, Matsuda T, Nakamura R. Heavy chain of human high molecular weight and low molecular weight kininogens binds calcium ion. *Biochemistry*. 1987;26(23):7450-7458.
211. Salvesen G, Parkes C, Abrahamson M, Grubb A, Barrett AJ. Human low-Mr kininogen contains three copies of a cystatin sequence that are divergent in structure and in inhibitory activity for cysteine proteinases. *Biochem J*. 1986;234(2):429-434.
212. Bradford HN, Schmaier AH, Colman RW. Kinetics of inhibition of platelet calpain II by human kininogens. *Biochem J*. 1990;270(1):83-90.
213. Zini JM, Schmaier AH, Cines DB. Bradykinin regulates the expression of kininogen binding sites on endothelial cells. *Blood*. 1993;81(11):2936-2946.
214. Meloni FJ, Schmaier AH. Low molecular weight kininogen binds to platelets to modulate thrombin-induced platelet activation. *J Biol Chem*. 1991;266(11):6786-6794.
215. Meloni FJ, Gustafson EJ, Schmaier AH. High molecular weight kininogen binds to platelets by its heavy and light chains and when bound has altered susceptibility to kallikrein cleavage. *Blood*. 1992;79(5):1233-1244.
216. Jiang YP, Muller-Esterl W, Schmaier AH. Domain 3 of kininogens contains a cell-binding site and a site that modifies thrombin activation of platelets. *J Biol Chem*. 1992;267(6):3712-3717.
217. Wachtfogel YT, DeLa Cadena RA, Kunapuli SP, et al. High molecular weight kininogen binds to Mac-1 on neutrophils by its heavy chain (domain 3) and its light chain (domain 5). *J Biol Chem*. 1994;269(30):19307-19312.
218. Puri RN, Zhou F, Hu CJ, Colman RF, Colman RW. High molecular weight kininogen inhibits thrombin-induced platelet aggregation and cleavage of aggregin by inhibiting binding of thrombin to platelets. *Blood*. 1991;77(3):500-507.
219. Kunapuli SP, Bradford HN, Jameson BA, et al. Thrombin-induced platelet aggregation is inhibited by the heptapeptide Leu271-Ala277 of domain 3 in the heavy chain of high molecular weight kininogen. *J Biol Chem*. 1996;271(19):11228-11235.
220. Hasan AA, Cines DB, Zhang J, Schmaier AH. The carboxyl terminus of bradykinin and amino terminus of the light chain of kininogens comprise an endothelial cell binding domain. *J Biol Chem*. 1994;269(50):31822-31830.
221. Hasan AA, Amenta S, Schmaier AH. Bradykinin and its metabolite, Arg-Pro-Pro-Gly-Phe, are selective inhibitors of alpha-thrombin-induced platelet activation. *Circulation*. 1996;94(3):517-528.
222. Reddigari SR, Kuna P, Miragliotta G, Shibayama Y, Nishikawa K, Kaplan AP. Human high molecular weight kininogen binds to human umbilical vein endothelial cells via its heavy and light chains. *Blood*. 1993;81(5):1306-1311.
223. Hasan AA, Cines DB, Herwald H, Schmaier AH, Muller-Esterl W. Mapping the cell binding site on high molecular weight kininogen domain 5. *J Biol Chem*. 1995;270(33):19256-19261.
224. Retzios AD, Rosenfeld R, Schiffman S. Effects of chemical modifications on the surface- and protein-binding properties of the light chain of human high molecular weight kininogen. *J Biol Chem*. 1987;262(7):3074-3081.
225. Pixley RA, Lin Y, Isordia-Salas I, Colman RW. Fine mapping of the sequences in domain 5 of high molecular weight kininogen (HK) interacting with heparin and zinc. *J Thromb Haemost*. 2003;1(8):1791-1798.
226. Tait JF, Fujikawa K. Identification of the binding site for plasma prekallikrein in human high molecular weight kininogen. A region from residues 185 to 224 of the kininogen light chain retains full binding activity. *J Biol Chem*. 1986;261(33):15396-15401.
227. Tait JF, Fujikawa K. Primary structure requirements for the binding of human high molecular weight kininogen to plasma prekallikrein and factor XI. *J Biol Chem*. 1987;262(24):11651-11656.
228. Vogel R, Kaufmann J, Chung DW, Kellermann J, Muller-Esterl W. Mapping of the prekallikrein-binding site of human H-kininogen by ligand screening of lambda gt11 expression libraries. Mimicking of the predicted binding site by anti-idiotypic antibodies. *J Biol Chem*. 1990;265(21):12494-12502.

229. Kerbiriou DM, Griffin JH. Human high molecular weight kininogen. Studies of structure-function relationships and of proteolysis of the molecule occurring during contact activation of plasma. *J Biol Chem.* 1979;254(23):12020-12027.

230. Bock PE, Shore JD. Protein-protein interactions in contact activation of blood coagulation. Characterization of fluorescein-labeled human high molecular weight kininogen-light chain as a probe. *J Biol Chem.* 1983;258(24):15079-15086.

231. Sun D, McCrae KR. Endothelial-cell apoptosis induced by cleaved high-molecular-weight kininogen (HKa) is matrix dependent and requires the generation of reactive oxygen species. *Blood.* 2006;107(12):4714-4720.

232. Gustafson EJ, Schmaier AH, Wachtfogel YT, Kaufman N, Kucich U, Colman RW. Human neutrophils contain and bind high molecular weight kininogen. *J Clin Invest.* 1989;84(1):28-35.

233. Gustafson EJ, Schutsky D, Knight LC, Schmaier AH. High molecular weight kininogen binds to unstimulated platelets. *J Clin Invest.* 1986;78(1):310-318.

234. Greengard JS, Heeb MJ, Ersdal E, Walsh PN, Griffin JH. Binding of coagulation factor XI to washed human platelets. *Biochemistry.* 1986;25(13):3884-3890.

235. van Iwaarden F, de Groot PG, Sixma JJ, Berrettini M, Bouma BN. High-molecular weight kininogen is present in cultured human endothelial cells: localization, isolation, and characterization. *Blood.* 1988;71(5):1268-1276.

236. Schmaier AH, Smith PM, Purdon AD, White JG, Colman RW. High molecular weight kininogen: localization in the unstimulated and activated platelet and activation by a platelet calpain(s). *Blood.* 1986;67(1):119-130.

237. Greengard JS, Griffin JH. Receptors for high molecular weight kininogen on stimulated washed human platelets. *Biochemistry.* 1984;23(26):6863-6869.

238. Walsh PN, Sinha D, Koshy A, Seaman FS, Bradford H. Functional characterization of platelet-bound factor XIa: retention of factor XIa activity on the platelet surface. *Blood.* 1986;68(1):225-230.

239. Chavakis T, Boeckel N, Santoso S, et al. Inhibition of platelet adhesion and aggregation by a defined region (Gly-486-Lys-502) of high molecular weight kininogen. *J Biol Chem.* 2002;277(26):23157-23164.

240. Chavakis T, Preissner KT. Potential pharmacological applications of the antithrombotic molecule high molecular weight kininogen. *Curr Vasc Pharmacol.* 2003;1(1):59-64.

241. Saito H, Goldsmith GH, Jr. Plasma thromboplastin antecedent (PTA, factor XI): a specific and sensitive radioimmunoassay. *Blood.* 1977;50(3):377-385.

242. Thompson RE, Mandle R, Jr, Kaplan AP. Association of factor XI and high molecular weight kininogen in human plasma. *J Clin Invest.* 1977;60(6):1376-1380.

243. Lipscomb MS, Walsh PN. Human platelets and factor XI. Localization in platelet membranes of factor XI-like activity and its functional distinction from plasma factor XI. *J Clin Invest.* 1979;63(5):1006-1014.

244. Tuszynski GP, Bevacqua SJ, Schmaier AH, Colman RW, Walsh PN. Factor XI antigen and activity in human platelets. *Blood.* 1982;59(6):1148-1156.

245. Schiffman S, Yeh CH. Purification and characterization of platelet factor XI. *Thromb Res.* 1990;60(1):87-97.

246. Walsh PN. The effects of collagen and kaolin on the intrinsic coagulant activity of platelets. Evidence for an alternative pathway in intrinsic coagulation not requiring factor XII. *Br J Haematol.* 1972;22(4):393-405.

247. Schiffman S, Rapaport SI, Chong MM. Platelets and initiation of intrinsic clotting. *Br J Haematol.* 1973;24(5):633-642.

248. Todd T, Perry DJ. A review of long-term prophylaxis in the rare inherited coagulation factor deficiencies. *Haemophilia.* 2010;16(4):569-583.

249. Rapaport SI, Proctor RR, Patch MJ, Yettra M. The mode of inheritance of PTA deficiency: evidence for the existence of major PTA deficiency and minor PTA deficiency. *Blood.* 1961;18:149-165.

250. Asakai R, Chung DW, Ratnoff OD, Davie EW. Factor XI (plasma thromboplastin antecedent) deficiency in Ashkenazi Jews is a bleeding disorder that can result from three types of point mutations. *Proc Natl Acad Sci U S A.* 1989;86(20):7667-7671.

251. Asakai R, Chung DW, Davie EW, Seligsohn U. Factor XI deficiency in Ashkenazi Jews in Israel. *N Engl J Med.* 1991;325(3):153-158.

252. Seligsohn U, Peretz H. Molecular genetics aspects of factor XI deficiency and Glanzmann thrombasthenia. *Haemostasis.* 1994;24(2):81-85.

253. Leiba H, Ramot B, Many A. Heredity and coagulation studies in ten families with factor XI (plasma thromboplastin antecedent) deficiency. *Br J Haematol.* 1965;11(6):654-665.

254. Seligsohn U. Factor XI deficiency. *Thromb Haemost.* 1993;70(1):68-71.

255. Santoro R, Prejano S, Iannaccaro P. Factor XI deficiency: a description of 34 cases and literature review. *Blood Coagul Fibrinolysis.* 2011;22(5):431-435.

256. Sidi A, Seligsohn U, Jonas P, Many M. Factor XI deficiency: detection and management during urological surgery. *J Urol.* 1978;119(4):528-530.

257. Hu CJ, Baglia FA, Mills DC, Konkle BA, Walsh PN. Tissue-specific expression of functional platelet factor XI is independent of plasma factor XI expression. *Blood.* 1998;91(10):3800-3807.

258. Ragni MV, Sinha D, Seaman F, Lewis JH, Spero JA, Walsh PN. Comparison of bleeding tendency, factor XI coagulant activity, and factor XI antigen in 25 factor XI-deficient kindreds. *Blood.* 1985;65(3):719-724.

259. Bolton-Maggs PH, Young Wan-Yin B, McCraw AH, Slack J, Kernoff PB. Inheritance and bleeding in factor XI deficiency. *Br J Haematol.* 1988;69(4):521-528.

260. Baglia FA, Walsh PN. Prothrombin is a cofactor for the binding of factor XI to the platelet surface and for platelet-mediated factor XI activation by thrombin. *Biochemistry.* 1998;37(8):2271-2281.

261. Kato A, Asakai R, Davie EW, Aoki N. Factor XI gene (F11) is located on the distal end of the long arm of human chromosome 4. *Cytogenet Cell Genet.* 1989;52(1-2):77-78.

262. Gailani D, Sun MF, Sun Y. A comparison of murine and human factor XI. *Blood.* 1997;90(3):1055-1064.

263. Clarkson K, Rosenfeld B, Fair J, Klein A, Bell W. Factor XI deficiency acquired by liver transplantation. *Ann Intern Med.* 1991;115(11):877-879.

264. Hsu TC, Shore SK, Seshsmma T, Bagasra O, Walsh PN. Molecular cloning of platelet factor XI, an alternative splicing product of the plasma factor XI gene. *J Biol Chem.* 1998;273(22):13787-13793.

265. Pugh RE, McVey JH, Tuddenham EG, Hancock JF. Six point mutations that cause factor XI deficiency. *Blood.* 1995;85(6):1509-1516.

266. Meijers JC, Davie EW, Chung DW. Expression of human blood coagulation factor XI: characterization of the defect in factor XI type III deficiency. *Blood.* 1992;79(6):1435-1440.

267. Wistinghausen B, Reischer A, Oddoux C, Ostrer H, Nardi M, Karpatkin M. Severe factor XI deficiency in an Arab family associated with a novel mutation in exon 11. *Br J Haematol.* 1997;99(3):575-577.

268. Martincic D, Zimmerman SA, Ware RE, Sun MF, Whitlock JA, Gailani D. Identification of mutations and polymorphisms in the factor XI genes of an African American family by dideoxyfingerprinting. *Blood.* 1998;92(9):3309-3317.

269. Hancock JF, Wieland K, Pugh RE, et al. A molecular genetic study of factor XI deficiency. *Blood.* 1991;77(9):1942-1948.

270. Peretz H, Zivelin A, Usher S, Seligsohn U. A 14-bp deletion (codon 554 del AAGgtaacagagtg) at exon 14/intron N junction of the coagulation factor XI gene disrupts splicing and causes severe factor XI deficiency. *Hum Mutat.* 1996;8(1):77-78.

271. PN W. *Factor XI.* Lippincott, Williams & Wilkins; 2001.

272. Seligsohn U. Factor XI deficiency in humans. *J Thromb Haemost.* 2009;7(suppl 1):84-87.

273. Fujikawa K, Chung DW, Hendrickson LE, Davie EW. Amino acid sequence of human factor XI, a blood coagulation factor with four tandem repeats that are highly homologous with plasma prekallikrein. *Biochemistry.* 1986;25(9):2417-2424.

274. Wiggins RC, Bouma BN, Cochrane CG, Griffin JH. Role of high-molecular-weight kininogen in surface-binding and activation of coagulation Factor XI and prekallikrein. *Proc Natl Acad Sci U S A.* 1977;74(10):4636-4640.

275. Baglia FA, Walsh PN. A binding site for thrombin in the apple 1 domain of factor XI. *J Biol Chem.* 1996;271(7):3652-3658.

276. Baglia FA, Jameson BA, Walsh PN. Identification and chemical synthesis of a substrate-binding site for factor IX on coagulation factor XIa. *J Biol Chem.* 1991;266(35):24190-24197.

277. Sun Y, Gailani D. Identification of a factor IX binding site on the third apple domain of activated factor XI. *J Biol Chem.* 1996;271(46):29023-29028.

278. Sun MF, Zhao M, Gailani D. Identification of amino acids in the factor XI apple 3 domain required for activation of factor IX. *J Biol Chem.* 1999;274(51):36373-36378.

279. Walsh PN, Griffin JH. Contributions of human platelets to the proteolytic activation of blood coagulation factors XII and XI. *Blood.* 1981;57(1):106-118.

280. Baglia FA, Jameson BA, Walsh PN. Identification and characterization of a binding site for platelets in the Apple 3 domain of coagulation factor XI. *J Biol Chem.* 1995;270(12):6734-6740.

281. Baglia FA, Seaman FS, Walsh PN. The Apple 1 and Apple 4 domains of factor XI act synergistically to promote the surface-mediated activation of factor XI by factor XIIa. *Blood.* 1995;85(8):2078-2083.

282. Ho DH, Baglia FA, Walsh PN. Factor XI binding to activated platelets is mediated by residues R(250), K(255), F(260), and Q(263) within the apple 3 domain. *Biochemistry.* 2000;39(2):316-323.

283. Baglia FA, Jameson BA, Walsh PN. Identification and characterization of a binding site for factor XIIa in the Apple 4 domain of coagulation factor XI. *J Biol Chem.* 1993;268(6):3838-3844.

284. Choi SH, Smith SA, Morrissey JH. Polyphosphate is a cofactor for the activation of factor XI by thrombin. *Blood.* 2011;118(26):6963-6970.

285. Morrissey JH, Choi SH, Smith SA. Polyphosphate: an ancient molecule that links platelets, coagulation, and inflammation. *Blood.* 2012;119(25):5972-5979.

286. Bouma BN, Griffin JH. Human blood coagulation factor XI. Purification, properties, and mechanism of activation by activated factor XII. *J Biol Chem.* 1977;252(18):6432-6437.

287. Kurachi K, Davie EW. Activation of human factor XI (plasma thromboplastin antecedent) by factor XIIa (activated Hageman factor). *Biochemistry.* 1977;16(26):5831-5839.

288. Emsley J, McEwan PA, Gailani D. Structure and function of factor XI. *Blood.* 2010;115(13):2569-2577.

289. Broze GJ, Jr, Gailani D. The role of factor XI in coagulation. *Thromb Haemost.* 1993;70(1):72-74.

290. Baglia FA, Walsh PN. Thrombin-mediated feedback activation of factor XI on the activated platelet surface is preferred over contact activation by factor XIIa or factor XIa. *J Biol Chem.* 2000;275(27):20514-20519.

291. Walsh PN. Platelets and factor XI bypass the contact system of blood coagulation. *Thromb Haemost.* 1999;82(2):234-242.

292. Fujikawa K, Legaz ME, Kato H, Davie EW. The mechanism of activation of bovine factor IX (Christmas factor) by bovine factor XIa (activated plasma thromboplastin antecedent). *Biochemistry.* 1974;13(22):4508-4516.

293. Di Scipio RG, Kurachi K, Davie EW. Activation of human factor IX (Christmas factor). *J Clin Invest.* 1978;61(6):1528-1538.

294. Osterud B, Bouma BN, Griffin JH. Human blood coagulation factor IX. Purification, properties, and mechanism of activation by activated factor XI. *J Biol Chem.* 1978;253(17):5946-5951.

295. Smith SB, Gailani D. Update on the physiology and pathology of factor IX activation by factor XIa. *Expert Rev Hematol.* 2008;1(1):87-98.

296. Muller F, Gailani D, Renne T. Factor XI and XII as antithrombotic targets. *Curr Opin Hematol.* 2011;18(5):349-355.

297. Heck LW, Kaplan AP. Substrates of Hageman factor. I. Isolation and characterization of human factor XI (PTA) and inhibition of the activated enzyme by alpha 1-antitrypsin. *J Exp Med.* 1974;140(6):1615-1630.

298. Beeler DL, Marcum JA, Schiffman S, Rosenberg RD. Interaction of factor XIa and antithrombin in the presence and absence of heparin. *Blood*. 1986;67(5):1488-1492.
299. Scott CF, Schapira M, Colman RW. Effect of heparin on the inactivation rate of human factor XIa by antithrombin-III. *Blood*. 1982;60(4):940-947.
300. Scott CF, Schapira M, James HL, Cohen AB, Colman RW. Inactivation of factor XIa by plasma protease inhibitors: predominant role of alpha 1-protease inhibitor and protective effect of high molecular weight kininogen. *J Clin Invest*. 1982;69(4):844-852.
301. Walsh PN, Sinha D, Kueppers F, Seaman FS, Blankstein KB. Regulation of factor XIa activity by platelets and alpha 1-protease inhibitor. *J Clin Invest*. 1987;80(6):1578-1586.
302. Damus PS, Hicks M, Rosenberg RD. Anticoagulant action of heparin. *Nature*. 1973;246(5432):355-357.
303. Soons H, Janssen-Claessen T, Tans G, Hemker HC. Inhibition of factor XIa by antithrombin III. *Biochemistry*. 1987;26(15):4624-4629.
304. Meijers JC, Vlooswijk RA, Bouma BN. Inhibition of human blood coagulation factor XIa by C-1 inhibitor. *Biochemistry*. 1988;27(3):959-963.
305. Saito H, Goldsmith GH, Moroi M, Aoki N. Inhibitory spectrum of alpha 2-plasmin inhibitor. *Proc Natl Acad Sci U S A*. 1979;76(4):2013-2017.
306. Scott CF, Colman RW. Factors influencing the acceleration of human factor XIa inactivation by antithrombin III. *Blood*. 1989;73(7):1873-1879.
307. Rosenberg RD, Damus PS. The purification and mechanism of action of human antithrombin-heparin cofactor. *J Biol Chem*. 1973;248(18):6490-6505.
308. Espana F, Berrettini M, Griffin JH. Purification and characterization of plasma protein C inhibitor. *Thromb Res*. 1989;55(3):369-384.
309. Soons H, Janssen-Claessen T, Hemker HC, Tans G. The effect of platelets in the activation of human blood coagulation factor IX by factor XIa. *Blood*. 1986;68(1):140-148.
310. Cronlund AL, Walsh PN. A low molecular weight platelet inhibitor of factor XIa: purification, characterization, and possible role in blood coagulation. *Biochemistry*. 1992;31(6):1685-1694.
311. Bush AI, Martins RN, Rumble B, et al. The amyloid precursor protein of Alzheimer's disease is released by human platelets. *J Biol Chem*. 1990;265(26):15977-15983.
312. Smith RP, Higuchi DA, Broze GJ, Jr. Platelet coagulation factor XIa-inhibitor, a form of Alzheimer amyloid precursor protein. *Science*. 1990;248(4959):1126-1128.
313. Van Nostrand WE, Schmaier AH, Farrow JS, Cunningham DD. Protease nexin-II (amyloid beta-protein precursor): a platelet alpha-granule protein. *Science*. 1990;248(4956):745-748.
314. Zhang Y, Scandura JM, Van Nostrand WE, Walsh PN. The mechanism by which heparin promotes the inhibition of coagulation factor XIa by protease nexin-2. *J Biol Chem*. 1997;272(42):26139-26144.
315. Dam H. Cholesterinstoffwechsel in Huhnereiern und Hunchen. *Biochemische Zeitschrift*. 1929;215:475-492.
316. Dam H. Cholesterol synthesis in the animal body. *Biochemische Zeitschrift*. 1930;220:158-163.
317. Dam H. Hemmorrhages in chicks reared on artificial diets. A new deficiency disease. *Nature*. 1934;133:909-910.
318. Doisy EA, Binkley SB, Thayer SA. Vitamin K. *Chem Rev*. 1941;28:477-517.
319. Owen CA, Bowie EJ. *The History of the Development of Oral Anticoagulant Drugs*. Arnold; 1996.
320. Magnusson S, Sottrup-Jensen L, Petersen TE, Morris HR, Dell A. Primary structure of the vitamin K-dependent part of prothrombin. *FEBS Lett*. 1974;44(2):189-193.
321. Stenflo J, Fernlund P, Egan W, Roepstorff P. Vitamin K dependent modifications of glutamic acid residues in prothrombin. *Proc Natl Acad Sci U S A*. 1974;71(7):2730-2733.
322. Stenflo J. Vitamin K and the biosynthesis of prothrombin. IV. Isolation of peptides containing prosthetic groups from normal prothrombin and the corresponding peptides from dicoumarol-induced prothrombin. *J Biol Chem*. 1974;249(17):5527-5535.
323. Nelsestuen GL, Zytkovicz TH, Howard JB. The mode of action of vitamin K. Identification of gamma-carboxyglutamic acid as a component of prothrombin. *J Biol Chem*. 1974;249(19):6347-6350.
324. Kulman JD, Harris JE, Haldeman BA, Davie EW. Primary structure and tissue distribution of two novel proline-rich gamma-carboxyglutamic acid proteins. *Proc Natl Acad Sci U S A*. 1997;94(17):9058-9062.
325. Hauschka PV, Lian JB, Cole DE, Gundberg CM. Osteocalcin and matrix Gla protein: vitamin K-dependent proteins in bone. *Physiol Rev*. 1989;69(3):990-1047.
326. Luo G, Ducy P, McKee MD, et al. Spontaneous calcification of arteries and cartilage in mice lacking matrix GLA protein. *Nature*. 1997;386(6620):78-81.
327. Schurgers LJ, Spronk HM, Skepper JN, et al. Post-translational modifications regulate matrix Gla protein function: importance for inhibition of vascular smooth muscle cell calcification. *J Thromb Haemost*. 2007;5(12):2503-2511.
328. Olivera BM. E.E. Just Lecture, 1996. Conus venom peptides, receptor and ion channel targets, and drug design: 50 million years of neuropharmacology. *Mol Biol Cell*. 1997;8(11):2101-2109.
329. Olivera BM, Rivier J, Clark C, et al. Diversity of Conus neuropeptides. *Science*. 1990;249(4966):257-263.
330. Olivera BM, Rivier J, Scott JK, Hillyard DR, Cruz LJ. Conotoxins. *J Biol Chem*. 1991;266(33):22067-22070.
331. Hasanbasic I, Rajotte I, Blostein M. The role of gamma-carboxylation in the anti-apoptotic function of gas6. *J Thromb Haemost*. 2005;3(12):2790-2797.
332. Leytus SP, Foster DC, Kurachi K, Davie EW. Gene for human factor X: a blood coagulation factor whose gene organization is essentially identical with that of factor IX and protein C. *Biochemistry*. 1986;25(18):5098-5102.
333. Patthy L. Evolutionary assembly of blood coagulation proteins. *Semin Thromb Hemost*. 1990;16(3):245-259.
334. Stenberg LM, Brown MA, Nilsson E, Ljungberg O, Stenflo J. A functional prothrombin gene product is synthesized by human kidney cells. *Biochem Biophys Res Commun*. 2001;280(4):1036-1041.
335. Sacchi E, Tagliabue L, Scoglio R, et al. Plasma factor VII levels are influenced by a polymorphism in the promoter region of the FVII gene. *Blood Coagul Fibrinolysis*. 1996;7(2):114-117.
336. Spek CA, Koster T, Rosendaal FR, Bertina RM, Reitsma PH. Genotypic variation in the promoter region of the protein C gene is associated with plasma protein C levels and thrombotic risk. *Arterioscler Thromb Vasc Biol*. 1995;15(2):214-218.
337. Green F, Kelleher C, Wilkes H, Temple A, Meade T, Humphries S. A common genetic polymorphism associated with lower coagulation factor VII levels in healthy individuals. *Arterioscler Thromb*. 1991;11(3):540-546.
338. Burns P, Hoffman CJ, Katz JP, Miller RH, Lawson WE, Hultin MB. Vitamin K-dependent clotting factors are elevated in young adults who have close relatives with ischemic heart disease. *J Lab Clin Med*. 1993;122(6):720-727.
339. Hofmann R, Lehmer A, Buresch M, Hartung R, Ulm K. Clinical relevance of urokinase plasminogen activator, its receptor, and its inhibitor in patients with renal cell carcinoma. *Cancer*. 1996;78(3):487-492.
340. Bladbjerg EM, Tholstrup T, Marckmann P, Sandstrom B, Jespersen J. Dietary changes in fasting levels of factor VII coagulant activity (FVII: C) are accompanied by changes in factor VII protein and other vitamin K-dependent proteins. *Thromb Haemost*. 1995;73(2):239-242.
341. Mukherjee M, Dawson G, Sembhi K, Kakkar VV. Triglyceride dependence of factor VII coagulant activity in deep venous thrombosis. *Thromb Haemost*. 1996;76(4):500-501.
342. Talstad I, Gamst ON. Warfarin resistance due to malabsorption. *J Intern Med*. 1994;236(4):465-467.
343. O'Reilly RA. Warfarin metabolism and drug-drug interactions. *Adv Exp Med Biol*. 1987;214:205-212.
344. Lee CJ, Chandrasekaran V, Wu S, Duke RE, Pedersen LG. Recent estimates of the structure of the factor VIIa (FVIIa)/tissue factor (TF) and factor Xa (FXa) ternary complex. *Thromb Res*. 2010;125(suppl 1):S7-S10.
345. Lee CJ, Lin P, Chandrasekaran V, et al. Proposed structural models of human factor Va and prothrombinase. *J Thromb Haemost*. 2008;6(1):83-89.
346. Bilik R, Superina RA, Poon AO. Coagulation plasma factor levels are early indicators of graft nonfunction following liver transplantation in children. *J Pediatr Surg*. 1992;27(3):302-306.
347. Bilik R, Yellen M, Superina RA. Surgical complications in children after liver transplantation. *J Pediatr Surg*. 1992;27(11):1371-1375.
348. Casella JF, Lewis JH, Bontempo FA, Zitelli BJ, Markel H, Starzl TE. Successful treatment of homozygous protein C deficiency by hepatic transplantation. *Lancet*. 1988;1(8583):435-438.
349. Cransac M, Carles J, Bernard PH, et al. Heterozygous protein C deficiency and dysfibrinogenemia acquired by liver transplantation. *Transpl Int*. 1995;8(4):307-311.
350. Stenflo J, Fernlund P. Beta-hydroxyaspartic acid in vitamin K-dependent plasma proteins from scorbutic and warfarin-treated Guinea pigs. *FEBS Lett*. 1984;168(2):287-292.
351. Gronke RS, VanDusen WJ, Garsky VM, et al. Aspartyl beta-hydroxylase: in vitro hydroxylation of a synthetic peptide based on the structure of the first growth factor-like domain of human factor IX. *Proc Natl Acad Sci U S A*. 1989;86(10):3609-3613.
352. Bristol JA, Ratcliffe JV, Roth DA, Jacobs MA, Furie BC, Furie B. Biosynthesis of prothrombin: intracellular localization of the vitamin K-dependent carboxylase and the sites of gamma-carboxylation. *Blood*. 1996;88(7):2585-2593.
353. Wallin R, Stanton C, Hutson SM. Intracellular maturation of the gamma-carboxyglutamic acid (Gla) region in prothrombin coincides with release of the propeptide. *Biochem J*. 1993;291(pt 3):723-727.
354. Bovill EG, Malhotra OP, Mann KG. Mechanisms of vitamin K antagonism. *Baillieres Clin Haematol*. 1990;3(3):555-581.
355. Wasley LC, Rehemtulla A, Bristol JA, Kaufman RJ. PACE/furin can process the vitamin K-dependent pro-factor IX precursor within the secretory pathway. *J Biol Chem*. 1993;268(12):8458-8465.
356. Drews R, Paleyanda RK, Lee TK, et al. Proteolytic maturation of protein C upon engineering the mouse mammary gland to express furin. *Proc Natl Acad Sci U S A*. 1995;92(23):10462-10466.
357. Foster DC, Holly RD, Sprecher CA, Walker KM, Kumar AA. Endoproteolytic processing of the human protein C precursor by the yeast Kex2 endopeptidase coexpressed in mammalian cells. *Biochemistry*. 1991;30(2):367-372.
358. Wu SM, Cheung WF, Frazier D, Stafford DW. Cloning and expression of the cDNA for human gamma-glutamyl carboxylase. *Science*. 1991;254(5038):1634-1636.
359. Suttie JW. Vitamin K-dependent carboxylase. *Annu Rev Biochem*. 1985;54:459-477.
360. Li T, Chang CY, Jin DY, Lin PJ, Khvorova A, Stafford DW. Identification of the gene for vitamin K epoxide reductase. *Nature*. 2004;427(6974):541-544.
361. Gardill SL, Suttie JW. Vitamin K epoxide and quinone reductase activities. Evidence for reduction by a common enzyme. *Biochem Pharmacol*. 1990;40(5):1055-1061.
362. Furie B, Furie BC. Molecular basis of vitamin K-dependent gamma-carboxylation. *Blood*. 1990;75(9):1753-1762.
363. Cosgriff SW. The effectiveness of an oral vitamin K1 in controlling excessive hypoprothrombinemia during anticoagulant therapy. *Ann Intern Med*. 1956;45(1):14-22.
364. Hirsh J. Optimal intensity and monitoring warfarin. *Am J Cardiol*. 1995;75(6):39B-42B.
365. Hirsh J, Dalen JE, Deykin D, Poller L, Bussey H. Oral anticoagulants. Mechanism of action, clinical effectiveness, and optimal therapeutic range. *Chest*. 1995;108(4 suppl):231S-246S.
366. Danziger J. Vitamin K-dependent proteins, warfarin, and vascular calcification. *Clin J Am Soc Nephrol*. 2008;3(5):1504-1510.
367. Chatrou ML, Winckers K, Hackeng TM, Reutelingsperger CP, Schurgers LJ. Vascular calcification: the price to pay for anticoagulation therapy with vitamin K-antagonists. *Blood Rev*. 2012;26(4):155-166.
368. Drakenberg T, Fernlund P, Roepstorff P, Stenflo J. beta-Hydroxyaspartic acid in vitamin K-dependent protein C. *Proc Natl Acad Sci U S A*. 1983;80(7):1802-1806.

369. McMullen BA, Fujikawa K, Kisiel W, et al. Complete amino acid sequence of the light chain of human blood coagulation factor X: evidence for identification of residue 63 as beta-hydroxyaspartic acid. *Biochemistry*. 1983;22(12):2875-2884.

370. Stenflo J, Lundwall A, Dahlback B. beta-Hydroxyasparagine in domains homologous to the epidermal growth factor precursor in vitamin K-dependent protein S. *Proc Natl Acad Sci U S A*. 1987;84(2):368-372.

371. Stenflo J, Ohlin AK, Owen WG, Schneider WJ. beta-Hydroxyaspartic acid or beta-hydroxyasparagine in bovine low density lipoprotein receptor and in bovine thrombomodulin. *J Biol Chem*. 1988;263(1):21-24.

372. Sunnerhagen MS, Persson E, Dahlqvist I, et al. The effect of aspartate hydroxylation on calcium binding to epidermal growth factor-like modules in coagulation factors IX and X. *J Biol Chem*. 1993;268(31):23339-23344.

373. Derian CK, VanDusen W, Przysiecki CT, et al. Inhibitors of 2-ketoglutarate-dependent dioxygenases block aspartyl beta-hydroxylation of recombinant human factor IX in several mammalian expression systems. *J Biol Chem*. 1989;264(12):6615-6618.

374. Nelson RM, VanDusen WJ, Friedman PA, Long GL. beta-Hydroxyaspartic acid and beta-hydroxyasparagine residues in recombinant human protein S are not required for anticoagulant cofactor activity or for binding to C4b-binding protein. *J Biol Chem*. 1991;266(31):20586-20589.

375. Miletich JP, Broze GJ, Jr. Beta protein C is not glycosylated at asparagine 329. The rate of translation may influence the frequency of usage at asparagine-X-cysteine sites. *J Biol Chem*. 1990;265(19):11397-11404.

376. Grinnell BW, Hermann RB, Yan SB. Human protein C inhibits selectin-mediated cell adhesion: role of unique fucosylated oligosaccharide. *Glycobiology*. 1994;4(2):221-225.

377. Baker ME, French FS, Joseph DR. Vitamin K-dependent protein S is similar to rat androgen-binding protein. *Biochem J*. 1987;243(1):293-296.

378. Fujimaki K, Yamazaki T, Taniwaki M, Ichinose A. The gene for human protein Z is localized to chromosome 13 at band q34 and is coded by eight regular exons and one alternative exon. *Biochemistry*. 1998;37(19):6838-6846.

379. Brenner B, Tavori S, Zivelin A, et al. Hereditary deficiency of all vitamin K-dependent procoagulants and anticoagulants. *Br J Haematol*. 1990;75(4):537-542.

380. Boneh A, Bar-Ziv J. Hereditary deficiency of vitamin K-dependent coagulation factors with skeletal abnormalities. *Am J Med Genet*. 1996;65(3):241-243.

381. Spronk HM, Farah RA, Buchanan GR, Vermeer C, Soute BA. Novel mutation in the gamma-glutamyl carboxylase gene resulting in congenital combined deficiency of all vitamin K-dependent blood coagulation factors. *Blood*. 2000;96(10):3650-3652.

382. Brenner B, Sanchez-Vega B, Wu SM, Lanir N, Stafford DW, Solera J. A missense mutation in gamma-glutamyl carboxylase gene causes combined deficiency of all vitamin K-dependent blood coagulation factors. *Blood*. 1998;92(12):4554-4559.

383. Soriano-Garcia M, Park CH, Tulinsky A, Ravichandran KG, Skrzypczak-Jankun E. Structure of Ca2+ prothrombin fragment 1 including the conformation of the Gla domain. *Biochemistry*. 1989;28(17):6805-6810.

384. Tulinsky A, Park CH, Skrzypczak-Jankun E. Structure of prothrombin fragment 1 refined at 2.8 A resolution. *J Mol Biol*. 1988;202(4):885-901.

385. Park CH, Tulinsky A. Three-dimensional structure of the kringle sequence: structure of prothrombin fragment 1. *Biochemistry*. 1986;25(14):3977-3982.

386. Soriano-Garcia M, Padmanabhan K, de Vos AM, Tulinsky A. The Ca2+ ion and membrane binding structure of the Gla domain of Ca-prothrombin fragment 1. *Biochemistry*. 1992;31(9):2554-2566.

387. Bode W, Mayr I, Baumann U, Huber R, Stone SR, Hofsteenge J. The refined 1.9 A crystal structure of human alpha-thrombin: interaction with D-Phe-Pro-Arg chloromethylketone and significance of the Tyr-Pro-Pro-Trp insertion segment. *EMBO J*. 1989;8(11):3467-3475.

388. Rydel TJ, Ravichandran KG, Tulinsky A, et al. The structure of a complex of recombinant hirudin and human alpha-thrombin. *Science*. 1990;249(4966):277-280.

389. Banner DW, Hadvary P. Crystallographic analysis at 3.0-A resolution of the binding to human thrombin of four active site-directed inhibitors. *J Biol Chem*. 1991;266(30):20085-20093.

390. Martin PD, Robertson W, Turk D, Huber R, Bode W, Edwards BF. The structure of residues 7-16 of the A alpha-chain of human fibrinogen bound to bovine thrombin at 2.3-A resolution. *J Biol Chem*. 1992;267(11):7911-7920.

391. Vitali J, Martin PD, Malkowski MG, et al. The structure of a complex of bovine alpha-thrombin and recombinant hirudin at 2.8-A resolution. *J Biol Chem*. 1992;267(25):17670-17678.

392. Padmanabhan K, Padmanabhan KP, Tulinsky A, et al. Structure of human des(1-45) factor Xa at 2.2 A resolution. *J Mol Biol*. 1993;232(3):947-966.

393. Brandstetter H, Bauer M, Huber R, Lollar P, Bode W. X-ray structure of clotting factor IXa: active site and module structure related to Xase activity and hemophilia B. *Proc Natl Acad Sci U S A*. 1995;92(21):9796-9800.

394. Kemball-Cook G, Johnson DJ, Tuddenham EG, Harlos K. Crystal structure of active site-inhibited human coagulation factor VIIa (des-Gla). *J Struct Biol*. 1999;127(3):213-223.

395. Sichler K, Banner DW, D'Arcy A, et al. Crystal structures of uninhibited factor VIIa link its cofactor and substrate-assisted activation to specific interactions. *J Mol Biol*. 2002;322(3):591-603.

396. Mather T, Oganessyan V, Hof P, et al. The 2.8 A crystal structure of Gla-domainless activated protein C. *EMBO J*. 1996;15(24):6822-6831.

397. Stafford DW. The vitamin K cycle. *J Thromb Haemost*. 2005;3(8):1873-1878.

398. Nelsestuen GL, Shah AM, Harvey SB. Vitamin K-dependent proteins. *Vitam Horm*. 2000;58:355-389.

399. Stenflo J. Contributions of Gla and EGF-like domains to the function of vitamin K-dependent coagulation factors. *Crit Rev Eukaryot Gene Expr*. 1999;9(1):59-88.

400. Sunnerhagen M, Olah GA, Stenflo J, Forsen S, Drakenberg T, Trewhella J. The relative orientation of Gla and EGF domains in coagulation factor X is altered by Ca2+

binding to the first EGF domain. A combined NMR-small angle X-ray scattering study. *Biochemistry*. 1996;35(36):11547-11559.

401. Prendergast FG, Mann KG. Differentiation of metal ion-induced transitions of prothrombin fragment 1. *J Biol Chem*. 1977;252(3):840-850.

402. Gerads I, Govers-Riemslag JW, Tans G, Zwaal RF, Rosing J. Prothrombin activation on membranes with anionic lipids containing phosphate, sulfate, and/or carboxyl groups. *Biochemistry*. 1990;29(34):7967-7974.

403. Pei G, Powers DD, Lentz BR. Specific contribution of different phospholipid surfaces to the activation of prothrombin by the fully assembled prothrombinase. *J Biol Chem*. 1993;268(5):3226-3233.

404. McDonald JF, Shah AM, Schwalbe RA, Kisiel W, Dahlback B, Nelsestuen GL. Comparison of naturally occurring vitamin K-dependent proteins: correlation of amino acid sequences and membrane binding properties suggests a membrane contact site. *Biochemistry*. 1997;36(17):5120-5127.

405. Kung C, Hayes E, Mann KG. A membrane-mediated catalytic event in prothrombin activation. *J Biol Chem*. 1994;269(41):25838-25848.

406. Nelsestuen GL, Kisiel W, Di Scipio RG. Interaction of vitamin K dependent proteins with membranes. *Biochemistry*. 1978;17(11):2134-2138.

407. Schwalbe RA, Ryan J, Stern DM, Kisiel W, Dahlback B, Nelsestuen GL. Protein structural requirements and properties of membrane binding by gamma-carboxyglutamic acid-containing plasma proteins and peptides. *J Biol Chem*. 1989;264(34):20288-20296.

408. Arni RK, Padmanabhan K, Padmanabhan KP, Wu TP, Tulinsky A. Structure of the non-covalent complex of prothrombin kringle 2 with PPACK-thrombin. *Chem Phys Lipids*. 1994;67–68:59-66.

409. Shikamoto Y, Morita T, Fujimoto Z, Mizuno H. Crystal structure of Mg2+- and Ca2+-bound Gla domain of factor IX complexed with binding protein. *J Biol Chem*. 2003;278(26):24090-24094.

410. Huang M, Rigby AC, Morelli X, et al. Structural basis of membrane binding by Gla domains of vitamin K-dependent proteins. *Nat Struct Biol*. 2003;10(9):751-756.

411. Sunnerhagen M, Forsen S, Hoffren AM, Drakenberg T, Teleman O, Stenflo J. Structure of the Ca(2+)-free Gla domain sheds light on membrane binding of blood coagulation proteins. *Nat Struct Biol*. 1995;2(6):504-509.

412. Christiansen WT, Jalbert LR, Robertson RM, Jhingan A, Prorok M, Castellino FJ. Hydrophobic amino acid residues of human anticoagulation protein C that contribute to its functional binding to phospholipid vesicles. *Biochemistry*. 1995;34(33):10376-10382.

413. Jalbert LR, Chan JC, Christiansen WT, Castellino FJ. The hydrophobic nature of residue-5 of human protein C is a major determinant of its functional interactions with acidic phospholipid vesicles. *Biochemistry*. 1996;35(22):7093-7099.

414. Zhang L, Castellino FJ. The binding energy of human coagulation protein C to acidic phospholipid vesicles contains a major contribution from leucine 5 in the gamma-carboxyglutamic acid domain. *J Biol Chem*. 1994;269(5):3590-3595.

415. Doolittle RF, Feng DF, Johnson MS. Computer-based characterization of epidermal growth factor precursor. *Nature*. 1984;307(5951):558-560.

416. Ohlin AK, Landes G, Bourdon P, Oppenheimer C, Wydro R, Stenflo J. Beta-hydroxyaspartic acid in the first epidermal growth factor-like domain of protein C. Its role in Ca2+ binding and biological activity. *J Biol Chem*. 1988;263(35):19240-19248.

417. Sugo T, Bjork I, Holmgren A, Stenflo J. Calcium-binding properties of bovine factor X lacking the gamma-carboxyglutamic acid-containing region. *J Biol Chem*. 1984;259(9):5705-5710.

418. Sugo T, Fernlund P, Stenflo J. erythro-beta-Hydroxyaspartic acid in bovine factor IX and factor X. *FEBS Lett*. 1984;165(1):102-106.

419. Baron M, Norman DG, Harvey TS, et al. The three-dimensional structure of the first EGF-like module of human factor IX: comparison with EGF and TGF-alpha. *Protein Sci*. 1992;1(1):81-90.

420. Ullner M, Selander M, Persson E, Stenflo J, Drakenberg T, Teleman O. Three-dimensional structure of the apo form of the N-terminal EGF-like module of blood coagulation factor X as determined by NMR spectroscopy and simulated folding. *Biochemistry*. 1992;31(26):5974-5983.

421. Montelione GT, Wuthrich K, Burgess AW, et al. Solution structure of murine epidermal growth factor determined by NMR spectroscopy and refined by energy minimization with restraints. *Biochemistry*. 1992;31(1):236-249.

422. Selander-Sunnerhagen M, Ullner M, Persson E, Teleman O, Stenflo J, Drakenberg T. How an epidermal growth factor (EGF)-like domain binds calcium. High resolution NMR structure of the calcium form of the NH2-terminal EGF-like domain in coagulation factor X. *J Biol Chem*. 1992;267(27):19642-19649.

423. Muranyi A, Finn BE, Gippert GP, Forsen S, Stenflo J, Drakenberg T. Solution structure of the N-terminal EGF-like domain from human factor VII. *Biochemistry*. 1998;37(30):10605-10615.

424. Hopfner KP, Lang A, Karcher A, et al. Coagulation factor IXa: the relaxed conformation of Tyr99 blocks substrate binding. *Structure*. 1999;7(8):989-996.

425. Campbell ID, Downing AK. Building protein structure and function from modular units. *Trends Biotechnol*. 1994;12(5):168-172.

426. Stenflo J, Stenberg Y, Muranyi A. Calcium-binding EGF-like modules in coagulation proteinases: function of the calcium ion in module interactions. *Biochim Biophys Acta*. 2000;1477(1-2):51-63.

427. Giannelli F, Green PM, Sommer SS, et al. Haemophilia B: database of point mutations and short additions and deletions–eighth edition. *Nucleic Acids Res*. 1998;26(1):265-268.

428. Husten EJ, Esmon CT, Johnson AE. The active site of blood coagulation factor Xa. Its distance from the phospholipid surface and its conformational sensitivity to components of the prothrombinase complex. *J Biol Chem*. 1987;262(27):12953-12961.

429. Kelly CR, Dickinson CD, Ruf W. Ca2+ binding to the first epidermal growth factor module of coagulation factor VIIa is important for cofactor interaction and proteolytic function. *J Biol Chem*. 1997;272(28):17467-17472.
430. Rand MD, Lindblom A, Carlson J, Villoutreix BO, Stenflo J. Calcium binding to tandem repeats of EGF-like modules. Expression and characterization of the EGF-like modules of human Notch-1 implicated in receptor-ligand interactions. *Protein Sci*. 1997;6(10):2059-2071.
431. Handford P, Downing AK, Rao Z, Hewett DR, Sykes BC, Kielty CM. The calcium binding properties and molecular organization of epidermal growth factor-like domains in human fibrillin-1. *J Biol Chem*. 1995;270(12):6751-6756.
432. Bajaj SP, Rapaport SI, Brown SF. Isolation and characterization of human factor VII. Activation of factor VII by factor Xa. *J Biol Chem*. 1981;256(1):253-259.
433. Fair DS. Quantitation of factor VII in the plasma of normal and warfarin-treated individuals by radioimmunoassay. *Blood*. 1983;62(4):784-791.
434. Rivard GE, Kovac I, Kunschak M, Thone P. Clinical study of recovery and half-life of vapor-heated factor VII concentrate. *Transfusion*. 1994;34(11):975-979.
435. Seligsohn U, Kasper CK, Osterud B, Rapaport SI. Activated factor VII: presence in factor IX concentrates and persistence in the circulation after infusion. *Blood*. 1979;53(5):828-837.
436. Connelly JB, Roderick PJ, Cooper JA, Meade TW, Miller GJ. Positive association between self-reported fatty food consumption and factor VII coagulant activity, a risk factor for coronary heart disease, in 4246 middle-aged men. *Thromb Haemost*. 1993;70(2):250-252.
437. Giansily-Blaizot M, Aguilar-Martinez P, Schved JF. Genotypic heterogeneity may explain phenotypic variations in inherited factor VII deficiency. *Haematologica*. 2002;87(3):328-329.
438. Iannello S, Prestipino M, Belfiore F. Genetic deficiency of factor VII and hemorrhagic diathesis. A case report and literature review. *Panminerva Med*. 1998;40(3):226-238.
439. Ragni MV, Lewis JH, Spero JA, Hasiba U. Factor VII deficiency. *Am J Hematol*. 1981;10(1):79-88.
440. Triplett DA, Brandt JT, Batard MA, Dixon JL, Fair DS. Hereditary factor VII deficiency: heterogeneity defined by combined functional and immunochemical analysis. *Blood*. 1985;66(6):1284-1287.
441. Baribeau G. Congenital hypoproconvertinemia. *Union Med Can*. 1971;100(2):240-247.
442. Carew JA, Pollak ES, High KA, Bauer KA. Severe factor VII deficiency due to a mutation disrupting an Sp1 binding site in the factor VII promoter. *Blood*. 1998;92(5):1639-1645.
443. Boyer C, Wolf M, Rothschild C, et al. An enzyme immunoassay (ELISA) for the quantitation of human factor VII. *Thromb Haemost*. 1986;56(3):250-255.
444. Lechler E. Use of prothrombin complex concentrates for prophylaxis and treatment of bleeding episodes in patients with hereditary deficiency of prothrombin, factor VII, factor X, protein C protein S, or protein Z. *Thromb Res*. 1999;95(4 suppl 1):S39-S50.
445. Cohen LJ, McWilliams NB, Neuberg R, et al. Prophylaxis and therapy with factor VII concentrate (human) immuno, vapor heated in patients with congenital factor VII deficiency: a summary of case reports. *Am J Hematol*. 1995;50(4):269-276.
446. Levi D, Pefkarou A, Fort JA, DeFaria W, Tzakis AG. Liver transplantation for factor VII deficiency. *Transplantation*. 2001;72(11):1836-1837.
447. Berrettini M, Mariani G, Schiavoni M, et al. Pharmacokinetic evaluation of recombinant, activated factor VII in patients with inherited factor VII deficiency. *Haematologica*. 2001;86(6):640-645.
448. Eskandari N, Feldman N, Greenspoon JS. Factor VII deficiency in pregnancy treated with recombinant factor VIIa. *Obstet Gynecol*. 2002;99(5 pt 2):935-937.
449. Hunault M, Bauer KA. Recombinant factor VIIa for the treatment of congenital factor VII deficiency. *Semin Thromb Hemost*. 2000;26(4):401-405.
450. Lusher JM, Roberts HR, Davignon G, et al. A randomized, double-blind comparison of two dosage levels of recombinant factor VIIa in the treatment of joint, muscle and mucocutaneous haemorrhages in persons with haemophilia A and B, with and without inhibitors. rFVIIa Study Group. *Haemophilia*. 1998;4(6):790-798.
451. Shapiro AD, Gilchrist GS, Hoots WK, Cooper HA, Gastineau DA. Prospective, randomised trial of two doses of rFVIIa (NovoSeven) in haemophilia patients with inhibitors undergoing surgery. *Thromb Haemost*. 1998;80(5):773-778.
452. Shapiro AD. Recombinant factor VIIa in the treatment of bleeding in hemophilic children with inhibitors. *Semin Thromb Hemost*. 2000;26(4):413-419.
453. Negrier C, Hay CR. The treatment of bleeding in hemophilic patients with inhibitors with recombinant factor VIIa. *Semin Thromb Hemost*. 2000;26(4):407-412.
454. Ingerslev J. Efficacy and safety of recombinant factor VIIa in the prophylaxis of bleeding in various surgical procedures in hemophilic patients with factor VIII and factor IX inhibitors. *Semin Thromb Hemost*. 2000;26(4):425-432.
455. John M. Eisenberg Center for Clinical Decisions and Communications Science. *Utilization and clinical data on in-hospital, off-label uses of recombinant factor VIIa*. In: *Comparative Effectiveness Review Summary Guides for Clinicians*. Agency for Healthcare Research and Quality (US). 2007.
456. Hedner U. Recombinant activated factor VII as a universal haemostatic agent. *Blood Coagul Fibrinolysis*. 1998;9(suppl 1):S147-S152.
457. van't Veer C, Mann KG. The regulation of the factor VII-dependent coagulation pathway: rationale for the effectiveness of recombinant factor VIIa in refractory bleeding disorders. *Semin Thromb Hemost*. 2000;26(4):367-372.
458. Monroe DM, Hoffman M, Oliver JA, Roberts HR. Platelet activity of high-dose factor VIIa is independent of tissue factor. *Br J Haematol*. 1997;99(3):542-547.
459. Hoffman M, Monroe DM, IIIrd, Roberts HR. Activated factor VII activates factors IX and X on the surface of activated platelets: thoughts on the mechanism of action of high-dose activated factor VII. *Blood Coagul Fibrinolysis*. 1998;9(suppl 1):S61-S65.
460. Butenas S, Brummel KE, Branda RF, Paradis SG, Mann KG. Mechanism of factor VIIa-dependent coagulation in hemophilia blood. *Blood*. 2002;99(3):923-930.
461. Borensztajn K, Chafa O, Alhenc-Gelas M, et al. Characterization of two novel splice site mutations in human factor VII gene causing severe plasma factor VII deficiency and bleeding diathesis. *Br J Haematol*. 2002;117(1):168-171.
462. Carew JA, Pollak ES, Lopaciuk S, Bauer KA. A new mutation in the HNF4 binding region of the factor VII promoter in a patient with severe factor VII deficiency. *Blood*. 2000;96(13):4370-4372.
463. Hunault M, Arbini AA, Carew JA, Peyvandi F, Bauer KA. Characterization of two naturally occurring mutations in the second epidermal growth factor-like domain of factor VII. *Blood*. 1999;93(4):1237-1244.
464. Hunault M, Arbini AA, Carew JA, Bauer KA. Mechanism underlying factor VII deficiency in Jewish populations with the Ala244Val mutation. *Br J Haematol*. 1999;105(4):1101-1108.
465. Takamiya O, Seta M, Tanaka K, Ishida F. Human factor VII deficiency caused by S339C mutation located adjacent to the specificity pocket of the catalytic domain. *Clin Lab Haematol*. 2002;24(4):233-238.
466. McVey JH, Boswell E, Mumford AD, Kemball-Cook G, Tuddenham EG. Factor VII deficiency and the FVII mutation database. *Hum Mutat*. 2001;17(1):3-17.
467. Aasrum M, Prydz H. Gene targeting of tissue factor, factor X, and factor VII in mice: their involvement in embryonic development. *Biochemistry (Mosc)*. 2002;67(1):25-32.
468. Rosen ED, Chan JC, Idusogie E, et al. Mice lacking factor VII develop normally but suffer fatal perinatal bleeding. *Nature*. 1997;390(6657):290-294.
469. de Grouchy J, Dautzenberg MD, Turleau C, Beguin S, Chavin-Colin F. Regional mapping of clotting factors VII and X to 13q34. Expression of factor VII through chromosome 8. *Hum Genet*. 1984;66(2-3):230-233.
470. O'Hara PJ, Grant FJ, Haldeman BA, et al. Nucleotide sequence of the gene coding for human factor VII, a vitamin K-dependent protein participating in blood coagulation. *Proc Natl Acad Sci U S A*. 1987;84(15):5158-5162.
471. Gilgenkrantz S, Briquel ME, Andre E, et al. Structural genes of coagulation factors VII and X located on 13q34. *Ann Genet*. 1986;29(1):32-35.
472. Marder VJ, Shulman NR. Clinical aspects of congenital factor VII deficiency. *Am J Med*. 1964;37:182-194.
473. Greenberg D, Miao CH, Ho WT, Chung DW, Davie EW. Liver-specific expression of the human factor VII gene. *Proc Natl Acad Sci U S A*. 1995;92(26):12347-12351.
474. Pollak ES, Hung HL, Godin W, Overton GC, High KA. Functional characterization of the human factor VII 5'-flanking region. *J Biol Chem*. 1996;271(3):1738-1747.
475. Wilcox JN, Noguchi S, Casanova J. Extrahepatic synthesis of factor VII in human atherosclerotic vessels. *Arterioscler Thromb Vasc Biol*. 2003;23(1):136-141.
476. Erdmann D, Heim J. Orphan nuclear receptor HNF-4 binds to the human coagulation factor VII promoter. *J Biol Chem*. 1995;270(39):22988-22996.
477. Friso S, Lotto V, Choi SW, et al. Promoter methylation in coagulation F7 gene influences plasma FVII concentrations and relates to coronary artery disease. *J Med Genet*. 2012;49(3):192-199.
478. Berkner K, Busby S, Davie E, et al. Isolation and expression of cDNAs encoding human factor VII. *Cold Spring Harb Symp Quant Biol*. 1986;51(pt 1):531-541.
479. Hagen FS, Gray CL, O'Hara P, et al. Characterization of a cDNA coding for human factor VII. *Proc Natl Acad Sci U S A*. 1986;83(8):2412-2416.
480. Sabharwal AK, Birktoft JJ, Gorka J, Wildgoose P, Petersen LC, Bajaj SP. High affinity Ca(2+)-binding site in the serine protease domain of human factor VIIa and its role in tissue factor binding and development of catalytic activity. *J Biol Chem*. 1995;270(26):15523-15530.
481. Higashi S, Nishimura H, Fujii S, Takada K, Iwanaga S. Tissue factor potentiates the factor VIIa-catalyzed hydrolysis of an ester substrate. *J Biol Chem*. 1992;267(25):17990-17996.
482. Toomey JR, Smith KJ, Stafford DW. Localization of the human tissue factor recognition determinant of human factor VIIa. *J Biol Chem*. 1991;266(29):19198-19202.
483. Kumar A, Fair DS. Specific molecular interaction sites on factor VII involved in factor X activation. *Eur J Biochem*. 1993;217(2):509-518.
484. Eigenbrot C, Kirchhofer D, Dennis MS, et al. The factor VII zymogen structure reveals reregistration of beta strands during activation. *Structure*. 2001;9(7):627-636.
485. Banner DW, D'Arcy A, Chene C, et al. The crystal structure of the complex of blood coagulation factor VIIa with soluble tissue factor. *Nature*. 1996;380(6569):41-46.
486. Wildgoose P, Nemerson Y, Hansen LL, Nielsen FE, Glazer S, Hedner U. Measurement of basal levels of factor VIIa in hemophilia A and B patients. *Blood*. 1992;80(1):25-28.
487. Neuenschwander PF, Fiore MM, Morrissey JH. Factor VII autoactivation proceeds via interaction of distinct protease-cofactor and zymogen-cofactor complexes. Implications of a two-dimensional enzyme kinetic mechanism. *J Biol Chem*. 1993;268(29):21489-21492.
488. Lawson JH, Krishnaswamy S, Butenas S, Mann KG. Extrinsic pathway proteolytic activity. *Methods Enzymol*. 1993;222:177-195.
489. Seligsohn U, Osterud B, Brown SF, Griffin JH, Rapaport SI. Activation of human factor VII in plasma and in purified systems: roles of activated factor IX, kallikrein, and activated factor XII. *J Clin Invest*. 1979;64(4):1056-1065.
490. Lawson JH, Butenas S, Mann KG. The evaluation of complex-dependent alterations in human factor VIIa. *J Biol Chem*. 1992;267(7):4834-4843.
491. Kisiel W, Fujikawa K, Davie EW. Activation of bovine factor VII (proconvertin) by factor XIIa (activated Hageman factor). *Biochemistry*. 1977;16(19):4189-4194.
492. Romisch J, Feussner A, Vermohlen S, Stohr HA. A protease isolated from human plasma activating factor VII independent of tissue factor. *Blood Coagul Fibrinolysis*. 1999;10(8):471-479.
493. Puy C, Lopez-Sagaseta J, Hermida J, Montes R. The endothelial cells downregulate the generation of factor VIIa through EPCR binding. *Br J Haematol*. 2010;149(1):111-117.

494. Persson E, Olsen OH. Allosteric activation of coagulation factor VIIa. *Front Biosci (Landmark Ed).* 2011;16:3156-3163.

495. Vadivel K, Bajaj SP. Structural biology of factor VIIa/tissue factor initiated coagulation. *Front Biosci (Landmark Ed).* 2012;17:2476-2494.

496. Osterud B, Rapaport SI. Activation of factor IX by the reaction product of tissue factor and factor VII: additional pathway for initiating blood coagulation. *Proc Natl Acad Sci U S A.* 1977;74(12):5260-5264.

497. Jesty J, Silverberg SA. Kinetics of the tissue factor-dependent activation of coagulation Factors IX and X in a bovine plasma system. *J Biol Chem.* 1979;254(24):12337-12345.

498. Morrison SA, Jesty J. Tissue factor-dependent activation of tritium-labeled factor IX and factor X in human plasma. *Blood.* 1984;63(6):1338-1347.

499. Krishnaswamy S. The interaction of human factor VIIa with tissue factor. *J Biol Chem.* 1992;267(33):23696-23706.

500. Silverberg SA, Nemerson Y, Zur M. Kinetics of the activation of bovine coagulation factor X by components of the extrinsic pathway. Kinetic behavior of two-chain factor VII in the presence and absence of tissue factor. *J Biol Chem.* 1977;252(23):8481-8488.

501. Butenas S, Mann KG. Kinetics of human factor VII activation. *Biochemistry.* 1996;35(6):1904-1910.

502. Osterud B, Miller-Andersson M, Abildgaard U, Prydz H. The effect of antithrombin III on the activity of the coagulation factors VII, IX and X. *Thromb Haemost.* 1976;35(2):295-304.

503. Jesty J. The inhibition of activated bovine coagulation factors X and VII by antithrombin III. *Arch Biochem Biophys.* 1978;185(1):165-173.

504. Rao LV, Nordfang O, Hoang AD, Pendurthi UR. Mechanism of antithrombin III inhibition of factor VIIa/tissue factor activity on cell surfaces. Comparison with tissue factor pathway inhibitor/factor Xa-induced inhibition of factor VIIa/tissue factor activity. *Blood.* 1995;85(1):121-129.

505. Lawson JH, Butenas S, Ribarik N, Mann KG. Complex-dependent inhibition of factor VIIa by antithrombin III and heparin. *J Biol Chem.* 1993;268(2):767-770.

506. Rao LV, Rapaport SI, Hoang AD. Binding of factor VIIa to tissue factor permits rapid antithrombin III/heparin inhibition of factor VIIa. *Blood.* 1993;81(10):2600-2607.

507. Rapaport SI, Rao LV. Initiation and regulation of tissue factor-dependent blood coagulation. *Arterioscler Thromb.* 1992;12(10):1111-1121.

508. Biggs R, Denson KW. The fate of prothrombin and factors Viii, Ix and X Transfused to patients deficient in these factors. *Br J Haematol.* 1963;9:532-547.

509. Thompson AR. Structure, function, and molecular defects of factor IX. *Blood.* 1986;67(3):565-572.

510. Stern DM, Knitter G, Kisiel W, Nawroth PP. In vivo evidence of intravascular binding sites for coagulation factor IX. *Br J Haematol.* 1987;66(2):227-232.

511. Wolberg AS, Stafford DW, Erie DA. Human factor IX binds to specific sites on the collagenous domain of collagen IV. *J Biol Chem.* 1997;272(27):16717-16720.

512. Gui T, Lin HF, Jin DY, et al. Circulating and binding characteristics of wild-type factor IX and certain Gla domain mutants in vivo. *Blood.* 2002;100(1):153-158.

513. Cheung WF, van den Born J, Kuhn K, Kjellen L, Hudson BG, Stafford DW. Identification of the endothelial cell binding site for factor IX. *Proc Natl Acad Sci U S A.* 1996;93(20):11068-11073.

514. van Hylckama Vlieg A, van der Linden IK, Bertina RM, Rosendaal FR. High levels of factor IX increase the risk of venous thrombosis. *Blood.* 2000;95(12):3678-3682.

515. Thompson AR, Chen SH. Characterization of factor IX defects in hemophilia B patients. *Methods Enzymol.* 1993;222:143-169.

516. Shetty S, Ghosh K, Mohanty D. Hemophilia B in a female. *Acta Haematol.* 2001;106(3):115-117.

517. Espinos C, Lorenzo JI, Casana P, Martinez F, Aznar JA. Haemophilia B in a female caused by skewed inactivation of the normal X-chromosome. *Haematologica.* 2000;85(10):1092-1095.

518. Boggio LN, Green D. Acquired hemophilia. *Rev Clin Exp Hematol.* 2001;5(4):389-404. quiz following 431.

519. Giannelli F, Green PM, Sommer SS, et al. Haemophilia B: database of point mutations and short additions and deletions, 7th edition. *Nucleic Acids Res.* 1997;25(1):133-135.

520. Knobe KE, Persson KE, Sjorin E, Villoutreix BO, Stenflo J, Ljung RC. Functional analysis of the EGF-like domain mutations Pro55Ser and Pro55Leu, which cause mild hemophilia B. *J Thromb Haemost.* 2003;1(4):782-790.

521. Krepischi-Santos AC, Carneiro JD, Svartman M, Bendit I, Odone-Filho V, Vianna-Morgante AM. Deletion of the factor IX gene as a result of translocation t(X;1) in a girl affected by haemophilia B. *Br J Haematol.* 2001;113(3):616-620.

522. Vianello F, Belvini D, Dal Bello F, et al. Mild bleeding diathesis in a boy with combined severe haemophilia B (C(10400)-->T) and heterozygous factor V Leiden. *Haemophilia.* 2001;7(5):511-514.

523. Ljung R, Petrini P, Tengborn L, Sjorin E. Haemophilia B mutations in Sweden: a population-based study of mutational heterogeneity. *Br J Haematol.* 2001;113(1):81-86.

524. Ivaskevicius V, Jurgutis R, Rost S, et al. Lithuanian haemophilia A and B registry comprising phenotypic and genotypic data. *Br J Haematol.* 2001;112(4):1062-1070.

525. Chowdhury MR, Kabra M, Menon PS. Factor IX gene polymorphisms in Indian population. *Am J Hematol.* 2001;68(4):246-248.

526. Chan V, Yam I, Yip B, et al. Single nucleotide polymorphisms of the factor IX gene for linkage analysis in the southern Chinese population. *Br J Haematol.* 2000;111(2):540-543.

527. Lefkowitz JB, Nuss R, Haver T, Jacobson L, Thompson AR, Manco-Johnson M. Factor IX Denver, ASN 346-->ASP mutation resulting in a dysfunctional protein with defective factor VIIIa interaction. *Thromb Haemost.* 2001;86(3):862-870.

528. Wu PC, Hamaguchi N, Yu YS, Shen MC, Lin SW. Hemophilia B with mutations at glycine-48 of factor IX exhibited delayed activation by the factor VIIa-tissue factor complex. *Thromb Haemost.* 2000;84(4):626-634.

529. Bowen DJ. Haemophilia A and haemophilia B: molecular insights. *Mol Pathol.* 2002;55(2):127-144.

530. Goodeve AC, Perry DJ, Cumming T, et al. Genetics of haemostasis. *Haemophilia.* 2012;18(suppl 4):73-80.

531. Roth DA, Kessler CM, Pasi KJ, et al. Human recombinant factor IX: safety and efficacy studies in hemophilia B patients previously treated with plasma-derived factor IX concentrates. *Blood.* 2001;98(13):3600-3606.

532. Franchini M, Frattini F, Crestani S, Bonfanti C, Haemophilia B. Current pharmacotherapy and future directions. *Expert Opin Pharmacother.* 2012;13(14):2053-2063.

533. DiMichele DM, Kroner BL. North American immune tolerance study G. The North American immune tolerance registry: practices, outcomes, outcome predictors. *Thromb Haemost.* 2002;87(1):52-57.

534. High K. Gene-based approaches to the treatment of hemophilia. *Ann N Y Acad Sci.* 2002;961:63-64.

535. Herzog RW, Hagstrom JN. Gene therapy for hereditary hematological disorders. *Am J Pharmacogenomics.* 2001;1(2):137-144.

536. Grieger JC, Samulski RJ. Adeno-associated virus as a gene therapy vector: vector development, production and clinical applications. *Adv Biochem Eng Biotechnol.* 2005;99:119-145.

537. Vandendriessche T, Thorrez L, Acosta-Sanchez A, et al. Efficacy and safety of adeno-associated viral vectors based on serotype 8 and 9 vs. lentiviral vectors for hemophilia B gene therapy. *J Thromb Haemost.* 2007;5(1):16-24.

538. Nathwani AC, Davidoff AM, Hanawa H, et al. Sustained high-level expression of human factor IX (hFIX) after liver-targeted delivery of recombinant adeno-associated virus encoding the hFIX gene in rhesus macaques. *Blood.* 2002;100(5):1662-1669.

539. White SJ, Page SM, Margaritis P, Brownlee GG. Long-term expression of human clotting factor IX from retrovirally transduced primary human keratinocytes in vivo. *Hum Gene Ther.* 1998;9(8):1187-1195.

540. Cherington V, Chiang GG, McGrath CA, et al. Retroviral vector-modified bone marrow stromal cells secrete biologically active factor IX in vitro and transiently deliver therapeutic levels of human factor IX to the plasma of dogs after reinfusion. *Hum Gene Ther.* 1998;9(10):1397-1407.

541. Ponder KP. Gene therapy for hemophilia. *Curr Opin Hematol.* 2006;13(5):301-307.

542. High K. Gene transfer for hemophilia: can therapeutic efficacy in large animals be safely translated to patients? *J Thromb Haemost.* 2005;3(8):1682-1691.

543. Nathwani AC, Gray JT, McIntosh J, et al. Safe and efficient transduction of the liver after peripheral vein infusion of self-complementary AAV vector results in stable therapeutic expression of human FIX in nonhuman primates. *Blood.* 2007;109(4):1414-1421.

544. Jiang H, Pierce GF, Ozelo MC, et al. Evidence of multiyear factor IX expression by AAV-mediated gene transfer to skeletal muscle in an individual with severe hemophilia B. *Mol Ther.* 2006;14(3):452-455.

545. Manno CS, Pierce GF, Arruda VR, et al. Successful transduction of liver in hemophilia by AAV-Factor IX and limitations imposed by the host immune response. *Nat Med.* 2006;12(3):342-347.

546. High KA. The gene therapy journey for hemophilia: are we there yet? *Hematology Am Soc Hematol Educ Program.* 2012;2012:375-381.

547. Buckle VCI, Hunter D, Edwards JH. Fine assignment of the coagulation factor IX gene. *Cytogenet Cell Genet.* 1985;40:593-594.

548. Camerino G, Grzeschik KH, Jaye M, et al. Regional localization on the human X chromosome and polymorphism of the coagulation factor IX gene (hemophilia B locus). *Proc Natl Acad Sci U S A.* 1984;81(2):498-502.

549. Chance PF, Dyer KA, Kurachi K, et al. Regional localization of the human factor IX gene by molecular hybridization. *Hum Genet.* 1983;65(2):207-208.

550. Anson DS, Choo KH, Rees DJ, et al. The gene structure of human anti-haemophilic factor IX. *EMBO J.* 1984;3(5):1053-1060.

551. Choo KH, Gould KG, Rees DJ, Brownlee GG. Molecular cloning of the gene for human anti-haemophilic factor IX. *Nature.* 1982;299(5879):178-180.

552. Picketts DJ, Mueller CR, Lillicrap D. Transcriptional control of the factor IX gene: analysis of five cis-acting elements and the deleterious effects of naturally occurring hemophilia B Leyden mutations. *Blood.* 1994;84(9):2992-3000.

553. Naka H, Brownlee GG. Transcriptional regulation of the human factor IX promoter by the orphan receptor superfamily factor, HNF4, ARP1 and COUP/Ear3. *Br J Haematol.* 1996;92(1):231-240.

554. Graves BJ, Johnson PF, McKnight SL. Homologous recognition of a promoter domain common to the MSV LTR and the HSV tk gene. *Cell.* 1986;44(4):565-576.

555. Paonessa G, Gounari F, Frank R, Cortese R. Purification of a NF1-like DNA-binding protein from rat liver and cloning of the corresponding cDNA. *EMBO J.* 1988;7(10):3115-3123.

556. Sladek FM, Zhong WM, Lai E, Darnell JE, Jr. Liver-enriched transcription factor HNF-4 is a novel member of the steroid hormone receptor superfamily. *Genes Dev.* 1990;4(12B):2353-2365.

557. Mueller CR, Maire P, Schibler U. DBP, a liver-enriched transcriptional activator, is expressed late in ontogeny and its tissue specificity is determined posttranscriptionally. *Cell.* 1990;61(2):279-291.

558. Kurachi S, Deyashiki Y, Takeshita J, Kurachi K. Genetic mechanisms of age regulation of human blood coagulation factor IX. *Science.* 1999;285(5428):739-743.

559. Nguyen P, Cornillet P, Potron G. A new case of severe hemophilia B Leyden, associated with a G to C mutation at position -6 of the factor IX promoter. *Am J Hematol.* 1995;49(3):259-260.

560. Reijnen MJ, Peerlinck K, Maasdam D, Bertina RM, Reitsma PH. Hemophilia B Leyden: substitution of thymine for guanine at position -21 results in a disruption of a hepatocyte nuclear factor 4 binding site in the factor IX promoter. *Blood.* 1993;82(1):151-158.

561. Briet E, Bertina RM, van Tilburg NH, Veltkamp JJ. Hemophilia B Leyden: a sex-linked hereditary disorder that improves after puberty. *N Engl J Med.* 1982;306(13):788-790.

562. Briet E, Wijnands MC, Veltkamp JJ. The prophylactic treatment of hemophilia B Leyden with anabolic steroids. *Ann Intern Med.* 1985;103(2):225-226.

563. Brady JN, Notley C, Cameron C, Lillicrap D. Androgen effects on factor IX expression: in-vitro and in-vivo studies in mice. *Br J Haematol.* 1998;101(2):273-279.

564. Kurachi K, Davie EW. Isolation and characterization of a cDNA coding for human factor IX. *Proc Natl Acad Sci U S A.* 1982;79(21):6461-6464.

565. Harris RJ, van Halbeek H, Glushka J, et al. Identification and structural analysis of the tetrasaccharide NeuAc alpha(2-->6)Gal beta(1-->4)GlcNAc beta(1-->3) Fuc alpha 1-->O-linked to serine 61 of human factor IX. *Biochemistry.* 1993;32(26):6539-6547.

566. Agarwala KL, Kawabata S, Takao T, et al. Activation peptide of human factor IX has oligosaccharides O-glycosidically linked to threonine residues at 159 and 169. *Biochemistry.* 1994;33(17):5167-5171.

567. Nishimura H, Takao T, Hase S, Shimonishi Y, Iwanaga S. Human factor IX has a tetrasaccharide O-glycosidically linked to serine 61 through the fucose residue. *J Biol Chem.* 1992;267(25):17520-17525.

568. Kuraya N, Omichi K, Nishimura H, Iwanaga S, Hase S. Structural analysis of O-linked sugar chains in human blood clotting factor IX. *J Biochem.* 1993;114(6):763-765.

569. Rao Z, Handford P, Mayhew M, Knott V, Brownlee GG, Stuart D. The structure of a Ca(2+)-binding epidermal growth factor-like domain: its role in protein-protein interactions. *Cell.* 1995;82(1):131-141.

570. Celie PH, Lenting PJ, Mertens K. Hydrophobic contact between the two epidermal growth factor-like domains of blood coagulation factor IX contributes to enzymatic activity. *J Biol Chem.* 2000;275(1):229-234.

571. Christophe OD, Lenting PJ, Kolkman JA, Brownlee GG, Mertens K. Blood coagulation factor IX residues Glu78 and Arg94 provide a link between both epidermal growth factor-like domains that is crucial in the interaction with factor VIII light chain. *J Biol Chem.* 1998;273(1):222-227.

572. Braunstein KM, Noyes CM, Griffith MJ, Lundblad RL, Roberts HR. Characterization of the defect in activation of factor IX Chapel Hill by human factor XIa. *J Clin Invest.* 1981;68(6):1420-1426.

573. Griffith MJ, Breitkreutz L, Trapp H, et al. Characterization of the clotting activities of structurally different forms of activated factor IX. Enzymatic properties of normal human factor IXa alpha, factor IXa beta, and activated factor IX Chapel Hill. *J Clin Invest.* 1985;75(1):4-10.

574. Jackson CM, Nemerson Y. Blood coagulation. *Annu Rev Biochem.* 1980;49:765-811.

575. Baglia FA, Sinha D, Walsh PN. Functional domains in the heavy-chain region of factor XI: a high molecular weight kininogen-binding site and a substrate-binding site for factor IX. *Blood.* 1989;74(1):244-251.

576. Kurachi K, Fujikawa K, Schmer G, Davie EW. Inhibition of bovine factor IXa and factor Xabeta by antithrombin III. *Biochemistry.* 1976;15(2):373-377.

577. Geng Y, Verhamme IM, Messer A, et al. A sequential mechanism for exosite-mediated factor IX activation by factor XIa. *J Biol Chem.* 2012;287(45):38200-38209.

578. Lenting PJ, ter Maat H, Clijsters PP, Donath MJ, van Mourik JA, Mertens K. Cleavage at arginine 145 in human blood coagulation factor IX converts the zymogen into a factor VIII binding enzyme. *J Biol Chem.* 1995;270(25):14884-14890.

579. Noyes CM, Griffith MJ, Roberts HR, Lundblad RL. Identification of the molecular defect in factor IX Chapel Hill: substitution of histidine for arginine at position 145. *Proc Natl Acad Sci U S A.* 1983;80(14):4200-4202.

580. Giannelli F, Green PM, High KA, et al. Haemophilia B: database of point mutations and short additions and deletions--fourth edition, 1993. *Nucleic Acids Res.* 1993;21(13):3075-3087.

581. Brummel KE, Paradis SG, Butenas S, Mann KG. Thrombin functions during tissue factor-induced blood coagulation. *Blood.* 2002;100(1):148-152.

582. Cawthern KM, van 't Veer C, Lock JB, DiLorenzo ME, Branda RF, Mann KG. Blood coagulation in hemophilia A and hemophilia C. *Blood.* 1998;91(12):4581-4592.

583. Hockin MF, Jones KC, Everse SJ, Mann KG. A model for the stoichiometric regulation of blood coagulation. *J Biol Chem.* 2002;277(21):18322-18333.

584. Rosenberg JS, McKenna PW, Rosenberg RD. Inhibition of human factor IXa by human antithrombin. *J Biol Chem.* 1975;250(23):8883-8888.

585. Schmaier AH, Dahl LD, Hasan AA, Cines DB, Bauer KA, Van Nostrand WE. Factor IXa inhibition by protease nexin-2/amyloid beta-protein precursor on phospholipid vesicles and cell membranes. *Biochemistry.* 1995;34(4):1171-1178.

586. Isawa H, Yuda M, Yoneda K, Chinzei Y. The insect salivary protein, prolixin-S, inhibits factor IXa generation and Xase complex formation in the blood coagulation pathway. *J Biol Chem.* 2000;275(9):6636-6641.

587. Bauer KA. Selective inhibition of coagulation factors: advances in antithrombotic therapy. *Semin Thromb Hemost.* 2002;28(suppl 2):15-24.

588. Nishimura S, Ishida T, Imai K. Monoclonal antibody therapy for disorders of hemostasis and coagulation. *Nihon Rinsho.* 2002;60(3):525-530.

589. Refino CJ, Jeet S, DeGuzman L, Bunting S, Kirchhofer D. A human antibody that inhibits factor IX/IXa function potently inhibits arterial thrombosis without increasing bleeding. *Arterioscler Thromb Vasc Biol.* 2002;22(3):517-522.

590. Sullenger B, Woodruff R, Monroe DM. Potent anticoagulant aptamer directed against factor IXa blocks macromolecular substrate interaction. *J Biol Chem.* 2012;287(16):12779-12786.

591. Roser-Jones C, Chan M, Howard EL, Becker KC, Rusconi CP, Becker RC. Factor IXa as a target for pharmacologic inhibition in acute coronary syndrome. *Cardiovasc Ther.* 2011;29(4):e22-e35.

592. Antman EM. Hirudin in acute myocardial infarction. Safety report from the thrombolysis and thrombin inhibition in myocardial infarction (TIMI) 9A trial. *Circulation.* 1994;90(4):1624-1630.

593. Adams TE, Everse SJ, Mann KG. Predicting the pharmacology of thrombin inhibitors. *J Thromb Haemost.* 2003;1(5):1024-1027.

594. Randomized trial of intravenous heparin versus recombinant hirudin for acute coronary syndromes. The global use of strategies to open Occluded coronary arteries (GUSTO) IIa investigators. *Circulation.* 1994;90(4):1631-1637.

595. Howard EL, Becker KC, Rusconi CP, Becker RC. Factor IXa inhibitors as novel anticoagulants. *Arterioscler Thromb Vasc Biol.* 2007;27(4):722-727.

596. Becker RC, Rusconi C, Sullenger B. Nucleic acid aptamers in therapeutic anticoagulation. Technology, development and clinical application. *Thromb Haemost.* 2005;93(6):1014-1020.

597. Davie EW, Fujikawa K, Kurachi K, Kisiel W. The role of serine proteases in the blood coagulation cascade. *Adv Enzymol Relat Areas Mol Biol.* 1979;48:277-318.

598. Di Scipio RG, Hermodson MA, Yates SG, Davie EW. A comparison of human prothrombin, factor IX (Christmas factor), factor X (Stuart factor), and protein S. *Biochemistry.* 1977;16(4):698-706.

599. Roberts HR, Lechler E, Webster WP, Penick GD. Survival of Transfused factor X in patients with Stuart disease. *Thromb Diath Haemorrh.* 1965;13:305-313.

600. de Visser MC, Poort SR, Vos HL, Rosendaal FR, Bertina RM. Factor X levels, polymorphisms in the promoter region of factor X, and the risk of venous thrombosis. *Thromb Haemost.* 2001;85(6):1011-1017.

601. Uprichard J, Perry DJ. Factor X deficiency. *Blood Rev.* 2002;16(2):97-110.

602. Menegatti M, Peyvandi F. Factor X deficiency. *Semin Thromb Hemost.* 2009;35(4):407-415.

603. Peyvandi F, Menegatti M, Santagostino E, et al. Gene mutations and three-dimensional structural analysis in 13 families with severe factor X deficiency. *Br J Haematol.* 2002;117(3):685-692.

604. Morishita E, Yamaguchi K, Asakura H, et al. One missense mutation in the factor X gene causing factor X deficiency–factor X Kanazawa. *Int J Hematol.* 2001;73(3):390-392.

605. Simioni P, Vianello F, Kalafatis M, et al. A dysfunctional factor X (factor X San Giovanni Rotondo) present at homozygous and double heterozygous level: identification of a novel microdeletion (delC556) and missense mutation (Lys408-->Asn) in the factor X gene. A study of an Italian family. *Thromb Res.* 2001;101(4):219-230.

606. Deam S, Srinivasan N, Westby J, Horn EH, Dolan G. F X Nottingham and F X Taunton. Two novel mutations in factor X resulting in loss of functional activity and an interpretation using molecular modelling. *Thromb Haemost.* 2001;85(2):265-269.

607. Millar DS, Elliston L, Deex P, et al. Molecular analysis of the genotype-phenotype relationship in factor X deficiency. *Hum Genet.* 2000;106(2):249-257.

608. Cooper DN, Millar DS, Wacey A, Pemberton S, Tuddenham EG. Inherited factor X deficiency: molecular genetics and pathophysiology. *Thromb Haemost.* 1997;78(1):161-172.

609. Denson KW, Lurie A, De Cataldo F, Mannucci PM. The factor-X defect: recognition of abnormal forms of factor X. *Br J Haematol.* 1970;18(3):317-327.

610. Vianello F, Lombardi AM, Boldrin C, Luni S, Girolami A. A new factor X defect (factor X Padua 3): a compound heterozygous between true deficiency (Gly(380)->Arg) and an abnormality (Ser(334)-->Pro). *Thromb Res.* 2001;104(3):257-264.

611. Girolami A, Scarparo P, Vettore S, Candeo N, Scandellari R, Lombardi AM. Unexplained discrepancies in the activity–antigen ratio in congenital FX deficiencies with defects in the catalytic domain. *Clin Appl Thromb Hemost.* 2009;15(6):621-627.

612. Choufani EB, Sanchorawala V, Ernst T, et al. Acquired factor X deficiency in patients with amyloid light-chain amyloidosis: incidence, bleeding manifestations, and response to high-dose chemotherapy. *Blood.* 2001;97(6):1885-1887.

613. Beardell FV, Varma M, Martinez J. Normalization of plasma factor X levels in amyloidosis after plasma exchange. *Am J Hematol.* 1997;54(1):68-71.

614. Girmann G, Wilker D, Stadie H, Scheurlen PG. Acquired isolated factor X deficiency associated with systemic amyloidosis. Case report and review of literature. *Klin Wochenschr.* 1980;58(17):859-862.

615. Girolami A, Candeo N, Vettore S, Lombardi AM, Girolami B. The clinical significance of the lack of arterial or venous thrombosis in patients with congenital prothrombin or FX deficiency. *J Thromb Thrombolysis.* 2010;29(3):299-302.

616. Dewerchin M, Liang Z, Moons L, et al. Blood coagulation factor X deficiency causes partial embryonic lethality and fatal neonatal bleeding in mice. *Thromb Haemost.* 2000;83(2):185-190.

617. Miao CH, Leytus SP, Chung DW, Davie EW. Liver-specific expression of the gene coding for human factor X, a blood coagulation factor. *J Biol Chem.* 1992;267(11):7395-7401.

618. Scambler PJ, Williamson R. The structural gene for human coagulation factor X is located on chromosome 13q34. *Cytogenet Cell Genet.* 1985;39(3):231-233.

619. Rocchi M, Roncuzzi L, Santamaria R, Archidiacono N, Dente L, Romeo G. Mapping through somatic cell hybrids and cDNA probes of protein C to chromosome 2, factor X to chromosome 13, and alpha 1-acid glycoprotein to chromosome 9. *Hum Genet.* 1986;74(1):30-33.

620. Huang MN, Hung HL, Stanfield-Oakley SA, High KA. Characterization of the human blood coagulation factor X promoter. *J Biol Chem.* 1992;267(22):15440-15446.

621. Wilberding JA, Castellino FJ. Characterization of the murine coagulation factor X promoter. *Thromb Haemost.* 2000;84(6):1031-1038.

622. Hung HL, High KA. Liver-enriched transcription factor HNF-4 and ubiquitous factor NF-Y are critical for expression of blood coagulation factor X. *J Biol Chem.* 1996;271(4):2323-2331.

623. Hung HL, Pollak ES, Kudaravalli RD, Arruda V, Chu K, High KA. Regulation of human coagulation factor X gene expression by GATA-4 and the Sp family of transcription factors. *Blood.* 2001;97(4):946-951.

624. Di Scipio RG, Hermodson MA, Davie EW. Activation of human factor X (Stuart factor) by a protease from Russell's viper venom. *Biochemistry.* 1977;16(24):5253-5260.

625. Fujikawa K, Davie EW. Bovine factor X (Stuart factor). *Methods Enzymol.* 1976;45:89-95.

626. Nakagawa H, Takahashi N, Fujikawa K, et al. Identification of the oligosaccharide structures of human coagulation factor X activation peptide at each glycosylation site. *Glycoconj J.* 1995;12(2):173-181.

627. Young RJ, Campbell M, Borthwick AD, et al. Structure- and property-based design of factor Xa inhibitors: pyrrolidin-2-ones with acyclic alanyl amides as P4 motifs. *Bioorg Med Chem Lett.* 2006;16(23):5953-5957.

628. Osterud B, Rapaport SI. Synthesis of intrinsic factor X activator. Inhibition of the function of formed activator by antibodies to factor VIII and to factor IX. *Biochemistry.* 1970;9(8):1854-1861.

629. McGee MP, Li LC, Xiong H. Diffusion control in blood coagulation. Activation of factor X by factors IXa/VIIIa assembled on human monocyte membranes. *J Biol Chem.* 1992;267(34):24333-24339.

630. Rand MD, Lock JB, van't Veer C, Gaffney DP, Mann KG. Blood clotting in minimally altered whole blood. *Blood.* 1996;88(9):3432-3445.

631. Butenas S, van 't Veer C, Mann KG. Evaluation of the initiation phase of blood coagulation using ultrasensitive assays for serine proteases. *J Biol Chem.* 1997;272(34):21527-21533.

632. Neuenschwander PF, Morrissey JH. Deletion of the membrane anchoring region of tissue factor abolishes autoactivation of factor VII but not cofactor function. Analysis of a mutant with a selective deficiency in activity. *J Biol Chem.* 1992;267(20):14477-14482.

633. Monkovic DD, Tracy PB. Activation of human factor V by factor Xa and thrombin. *Biochemistry.* 1990;29(5):1118-1128.

634. Gajdusek C, Carbon S, Ross R, Nawroth P, Stern D. Activation of coagulation releases endothelial cell mitogens. *J Cell Biol.* 1986;103(2):419-428.

635. Gasic GP, Arenas CP, Gasic TB, Gasic GJ. Coagulation factors X, Xa, and protein S as potent mitogens of cultured aortic smooth muscle cells. *Proc Natl Acad Sci U S A.* 1992;89(6):2317-2320.

636. Altieri DC, Stamnes SJ. Protease-dependent T cell activation: ligation of effector cell protease receptor-1 (EPR-1) stimulates lymphocyte proliferation. *Cell Immunol.* 1994;155(2):372-383.

637. Bae JS, Yang L, Rezaie AR. Factor X/Xa elicits protective signaling responses in endothelial cells directly via PAR-2 and indirectly via endothelial protein C receptor-dependent recruitment of PAR-1. *J Biol Chem.* 2010;285(45):34803-34812.

638. Altieri DC, Morrissey JH, Edgington TS. Adhesive receptor Mac-1 coordinates the activation of factor X on stimulated cells of monocytic and myeloid differentiation: an alternative initiation of the coagulation protease cascade. *Proc Natl Acad Sci U S A.* 1988;85(20):7462-7466.

639. Altieri DC, Edgington TS. Identification of effector cell protease receptor-1. A leukocyte-distributed receptor for the serine protease factor Xa. *J Immunol.* 1990;145(1):246-253.

640. Tracy PB, Nesheim ME, Mann KG. Platelet factor Xa receptor. *Methods Enzymol.* 1992;215:329-360.

641. Lindhout T, Willems G, Blezer R, Hemker HC. Kinetics of the inhibition of human factor Xa by full-length and truncated recombinant tissue factor pathway inhibitor. *Biochem J.* 1994;297(pt 1):131-136.

642. Huang ZF, Wun TC, Broze GJ, Jr. Kinetics of factor Xa inhibition by tissue factor pathway inhibitor. *J Biol Chem.* 1993;268(36):26950-26955.

643. Iversen N, Lindahl AK, Abildgaard U. Elevated plasma levels of the factor Xa-TFPI complex in cancer patients. *Thromb Res.* 2002;105(1):33-36.

644. Gitel SN, Medina VM, Wessler S. Inhibition of human activated Factor X by antithrombin III and alpha 1-proteinase inhibitor in human plasma. *J Biol Chem.* 1984;259(11):6890-6895.

645. Miletich JP, Jackson CM, Majerus PW. Properties of the factor Xa binding site on human platelets. *J Biol Chem.* 1978;253(19):6908-6916.

646. Marciniak E. Factor-Xa inactivation by antithrombin. 3. Evidence for biological stabilization of factor Xa by factor V-phospholipid complex. *Br J Haematol.* 1973;24(3):391-400.

647. Pinto DJ, Galemmo RA, Jr, Quan ML, et al. Discovery of potent, efficacious, and orally bioavailable inhibitors of blood coagulation factor Xa with neutral P1 moieties. *Bioorg Med Chem Lett.* 2006;16(21):5584-5589.

648. Kakar P, Watson T, Lip GY. Drug evaluation: rivaroxaban, an oral, direct inhibitor of activated factor X. *Curr Opin Investig Drugs.* 2007;8(3):256-265.

649. Kochanny MJ, Adler M, Ewing J, et al. Substituted thiophene-anthranilamides as potent inhibitors of human factor Xa. *Bioorg Med Chem.* 2007;15(5):2127-2146.

650. Eriksson BI, Quinlan DJ, Weitz JI. Comparative pharmacodynamics and pharmacokinetics of oral direct thrombin and factor xa inhibitors in development. *Clin Pharmacokinet.* 2009;48(1):1-22.

651. De Caterina R, Husted S, Wallentin L, et al. New oral anticoagulants in atrial fibrillation and acute coronary syndromes: ESC Working Group on Thrombosis-Task Force on Anticoagulants in Heart Disease position paper. *J Am Coll Cardiol.* 2012;59(16):1413-1425.

652. Weitz JI. New oral anticoagulants: a view from the laboratory. *Am J Hematol.* 2012;87(suppl 1):S133-S136.

653. Augoustides JG. Breakthroughs in anticoagulation: advent of the oral direct factor Xa inhibitors. *J Cardiothorac Vasc Anesth.* 2012;26(4):740-745.

654. Lundblad RL, Kingdon HS, Mann KG. Thrombin. *Methods Enzymol.* 1976;45:156-176.

655. McDuffie FC, Giffin C, Niedringhaus R, et al. Prothrombin, thrombin and prothrombin fragments in plasma of normal individuals and of patients with laboratory evidence of disseminated intravascular coagulation. *Thromb Res.* 1979;16(5-6):759-773.

656. Kisiel W, Hanahan DJ. Purification and characterization of human Factor II. *Biochim Biophys Acta.* 1973;304(1):103-113.

657. Chow BK, Ting V, Tufaro F, MacGillivray RT. Characterization of a novel liver-specific enhancer in the human prothrombin gene. *J Biol Chem.* 1991;266(28):18927-18933.

658. Bancroft JD, McDowell SA, Degen SJ. The human prothrombin gene: transcriptional regulation in HepG2 cells. *Biochemistry.* 1992;31(49):12469-12476.

659. Roberts HR, Lefkowitz JB. *Inherited Disorders of Prothrombin Conversion.* Lippincott; 1994.

660. Rouvier J, Braude R, Altman R. Proceedings: fibrinogenolysis – studies on its degradation products. *Thromb Diath Haemorrh.* 1975;34(1):340.

661. Girolami A, Scandellari R, Scapin M, Vettore S. Congenital bleeding disorders of the vitamin K-dependent clotting factors. *Vitam Horm.* 2008;78:281-374.

662. Sun WY, Degen SJ. Gene targeting in hemostasis. Prothrombin. *Front Biosci.* 2001;6:D222-D238.

663. Xue J, Wu Q, Westfield LA, et al. Incomplete embryonic lethality and fatal neonatal hemorrhage caused by prothrombin deficiency in mice. *Proc Natl Acad Sci U S A.* 1998;95(13):7603-7607.

664. Sun WY, Witte DP, Degen JL, et al. Prothrombin deficiency results in embryonic and neonatal lethality in mice. *Proc Natl Acad Sci U S A.* 1998;95(13):7597-7602.

665. Bancroft JD, Schaefer LA, Degen SJ. Characterization of the Alu-rich 5'-flanking region of the human prothrombin-encoding gene: identification of a positive cis-acting element that regulates liver-specific expression. *Gene.* 1990;95(2):253-260.

666. Degen SJ. The prothrombin gene and its liver-specific expression. *Semin Thromb Hemost.* 1992;18(2):230-242.

667. Degen SJ, Davie EW. Nucleotide sequence of the gene for human prothrombin. *Biochemistry.* 1987;26(19):6165-6177.

668. Degen SJ, MacGillivray RT, Davie EW. Characterization of the complementary deoxyribonucleic acid and gene coding for human prothrombin. *Biochemistry.* 1983;22(9):2087-2097.

669. Poort SR, Rosendaal FR, Reitsma PH, Bertina RM. A common genetic variation in the 3'-untranslated region of the prothrombin gene is associated with elevated plasma prothrombin levels and an increase in venous thrombosis. *Blood.* 1996;88(10):3698-3703.

670. Perez-Ceballos E, Corral J, Alberca I, et al. Prothrombin A19911G and G20210A polymorphisms' role in thrombosis. *Br J Haematol.* 2002;118(2):610-614.

671. Nguyen A. Prothrombin G20210A polymorphism and thrombophilia. *Mayo Clin Proc.* 2000;75(6):595-604.

672. Favaloro EJ, McDonald D, Lippi G. Laboratory investigation of thrombophilia: the good, the bad, and the ugly. *Semin Thromb Hemost.* 2009;35(7):695-710.

673. Coppola A, Tufano A, Cerbone AM, Di Minno G. Inherited thrombophilia: implications for prevention and treatment of venous thromboembolism. *Semin Thromb Hemost.* 2009;35(7):683-694.

674. Butkowski RJ, Elion J, Downing MR, Mann KG. Primary structure of human prethrombin 2 and alpha-thrombin. *J Biol Chem.* 1977;252(14):4942-4957.

675. MacGillivray RT, Davie EW. Characterization of bovine prothrombin mRNA and its translation product. *Biochemistry.* 1984;23(8):1626-1634.

676. Mizuochi T, Fujii J, Kisiel W, Kobata A. Studies on the structures of the carbohydrate moiety of human prothrombin. *J Biochem.* 1981;90(4):1023-1031.

677. Patthy L. Evolution of the proteases of blood coagulation and fibrinolysis by assembly from modules. *Cell.* 1985;41(3):657-663.

678. Castellino FJ, Beals JM. The genetic relationships between the kringle domains of human plasminogen, prothrombin, tissue plasminogen activator, urokinase, and coagulation factor XII. *J Mol Evol.* 1987;26(4):358-369.

679. Deguchi H, Takeya H, Gabazza EC, Nishioka J, Suzuki K. Prothrombin kringle 1 domain interacts with factor Va during the assembly of prothrombinase complex. *Biochem J.* 1997;321(pt 3):729-735.

680. Sugo T, Nakamikawa C, Tanabe S, Matsuda M. Activation of prothrombin by factor Xa bound to the membrane surface of human umbilical vein endothelial cells: its catalytic efficiency is similar to that of prothrombinase complex on platelets. *J Biochem.* 1995;117(2):244-250.

681. Bajaj SP, Butkowski RJ, Mann KG. Prothrombin fragments. Ca2+ binding and activation kinetics. *J Biol Chem.* 1975;250(6):2150-2156.

682. Kotkow KJ, Deitcher SR, Furie B, Furie BC. The second kringle domain of prothrombin promotes factor Va-mediated prothrombin activation by prothrombinase. *J Biol Chem.* 1995;270(9):4551-4557.

683. Krishnaswamy S, Walker RK. Contribution of the prothrombin fragment 2 domain to the function of factor Va in the prothrombinase complex. *Biochemistry.* 1997;36(11):3319-3330.

684. Wood JP, Silveira JR, Maille NM, Haynes LM, Tracy PB. Prothrombin activation on the activated platelet surface optimizes expression of procoagulant activity. *Blood.* 2011;117(5):1710-1718.

685. Whelihan MF, Zachary V, Orfeo T, Mann KG. Prothrombin activation in blood coagulation: the erythrocyte contribution to thrombin generation. *Blood.* 2012;120(18):3837-3845.

686. Krishnaswamy S, Church WR, Nesheim ME, Mann KG. Activation of human prothrombin by human prothrombinase. Influence of factor Va on the reaction mechanism. *J Biol Chem.* 1987;262(7):3291-3299.

687. Kim PY, Nesheim ME. Further evidence for two functional forms of prothrombinase each specific for either of the two prothrombin activation cleavages. *J Biol Chem.* 2007;282(45):32568-32581.

688. Doyle MF, Mann KG. Multiple active forms of thrombin. IV. Relative activities of meizothrombins. *J Biol Chem.* 1990;265(18):10693-10701.

689. Haynes LM, Bouchard BA, Tracy PB, Mann KG. Prothrombin activation by platelet-associated prothrombinase proceeds through the prethrombin-2 pathway via a concerted mechanism. *J Biol Chem.* 2012;287(46):38647-38655.

690. Myrmel KH, Lundblad RL, Mann KG. Characteristics of the association between prothrombin fragment 2 and alpha-thrombin. *Biochemistry.* 1976;15(8):1767-1773.

691. Nesheim ME, Abbott T, Jenny R, Mann KG. Evidence that the thrombin-catalyzed feedback cleavage of fragment 1.2 at Arg154-Ser155 promotes the release of thrombin from the catalytic surface during the activation of bovine prothrombin. *J Biol Chem.* 1988;263(2):1037-1044.

692. Tracy PB, Eide LL, Mann KG. Human prothrombinase complex assembly and function on isolated peripheral blood cell populations. *J Biol Chem.* 1985;260(4):2119-2124.

693. Bovill EG, Tracy RP, Hayes TE, Jenny RJ, Bhushan FH, Mann KG. Evidence that meizothrombin is an intermediate product in the clotting of whole blood. *Arterioscler Thromb Vasc Biol.* 1995;15(6):754-758.

694. Mosesson MW. The roles of fibrinogen and fibrin in hemostasis and thrombosis. *Semin Hematol.* 1992;29(3):177-188.

695. Davey MG, Luscher EF. Actions of thrombin and other coagulant and proteolytic enzymes on blood platelets. *Nature.* 1967;216(5118):857-858.

696. Mann KG, Jenny RJ, Krishnaswamy S. Cofactor proteins in the assembly and expression of blood clotting enzyme complexes. *Annu Rev Biochem.* 1988;57:915-956.

697. Fay PJ. Subunit structure of thrombin-activated human factor VIIIa. *Biochim Biophys Acta.* 1988;952(2):181-190.

698. Kisiel W, Canfield WM, Ericsson LH, Davie EW. Anticoagulant properties of bovine plasma protein C following activation by thrombin. *Biochemistry.* 1977;16(26):5824-5831.

699. Fenton JW,IInd. Regulation of thrombin generation and functions. *Semin Thromb Hemost.* 1988;14(3):234-240.

700. Bar-Shavit R, Benezra M, Eldor A, et al. Thrombin immobilized to extracellular matrix is a potent mitogen for vascular smooth muscle cells: nonenzymatic mode of action. *Cell Regul.* 1990;1(6):453-463.

701. Bar-Shavit R, Kahn AJ, Mann KG, Wilner GD. Identification of a thrombin sequence with growth factor activity on macrophages. *Proc Natl Acad Sci U S A.* 1986;83(4):976-980.

702. McNamara CA, Sarembock IJ, Gimple LW, Fenton JW,IInd, Coughlin SR, Owens GK. Thrombin stimulates proliferation of cultured rat aortic smooth muscle cells by a proteolytically activated receptor. *J Clin Invest.* 1993;91(1):94-98.

703. Sago H, Iinuma K. Cell shape change and cytosolic Ca2+ in human umbilical-vein endothelial cells stimulated with thrombin. *Thromb Haemost.* 1992;67(3):331-334.

704. Tsopanoglou NE, Pipili-Synetos E, Maragoudakis ME. Thrombin promotes angiogenesis by a mechanism independent of fibrin formation. *Am J Physiol.* 1993;264(5 pt 1):C1302-C1307.

705. Folkman J. Tumor angiogenesis. *Adv Cancer Res.* 1985;43:175-203.

706. Tsopanoglou NE, Maragoudakis ME. On the mechanism of thrombin-induced angiogenesis. Potentiation of vascular endothelial growth factor activity on endothelial cells by up-regulation of its receptors. *J Biol Chem.* 1999;274(34):23969-23976.

707. Jenny NSLR, Mann KG. *Thrombin.* Lippincott, Williams & Wilkins; 2006.

708. Bjork I, Lindahl U. Mechanism of the anticoagulant action of heparin. *Mol Cell Biochem.* 1982;48(3):161-182.

709. Rosenberg RD. Chemistry of the hemostatic mechanism and its relationship to the action of heparin. *Fed Proc.* 1977;36(1):10-18.

710. Butenas S, van't Veer C, Mann KG. "Normal" thrombin generation. *Blood.* 1999;94(7):2169-2178.

711. Toomey JR, Kratzer KE, Lasky NM, Stanton JJ, Broze GJ, Jr. Targeted disruption of the murine tissue factor gene results in embryonic lethality. *Blood.* 1996;88(5):1583-1587.

712. Bugge TH, Xiao Q, Kombrinck KW, et al. Fatal embryonic bleeding events in mice lacking tissue factor, the cell-associated initiator of blood coagulation. *Proc Natl Acad Sci U S A.* 1996;93(13):6258-6263.

713. Carmeliet P, Mackman N, Moons L, et al. Role of tissue factor in embryonic blood vessel development. *Nature.* 1996;383(6595):73-75.

714. Carmeliet P, Moons L, Dewerchin M, et al. Insights in vessel development and vascular disorders using targeted inactivation and transfer of vascular endothelial growth factor, the tissue factor receptor, and the plasminogen system. *Ann N Y Acad Sci.* 1997;811:191-206.

715. Scarpati EM, Wen D, Broze GJ, Jr, et al. Human tissue factor: cDNA sequence and chromosome localization of the gene. *Biochemistry.* 1987;26(17):5234-5238.

716. Kao FT, Hartz J, Horton R, Nemerson Y, Carson SD. Regional assignment of human tissue factor gene (F3) to chromosome 1p21-p22. *Somat Cell Mol Genet.* 1988;14(4):407-410.

717. Mackman N, Morrissey JH, Fowler B, Edgington TS. Complete sequence of the human tissue factor gene, a highly regulated cellular receptor that initiates the coagulation protease cascade. *Biochemistry.* 1989;28(4):1755-1762.

718. Mackman N, Fowler BJ, Edgington TS, Morrissey JH. Functional analysis of the human tissue factor promoter and induction by serum. *Proc Natl Acad Sci U S A.* 1990;87(6):2254-2258.

719. Ranganathan G, Blatti SP, Subramaniam M, Fass DN, Maihle NJ, Getz MJ. Cloning of murine tissue factor and regulation of gene expression by transforming growth factor type beta 1. *J Biol Chem.* 1991;266(1):496-501.

720. Geczy CL. Cellular mechanisms for the activation of blood coagulation. *Int Rev Cytol.* 1994;152:49-108.

721. Camerer E, Kolsto AB, Prydz H. Cell biology of tissue factor, the principal initiator of blood coagulation. *Thromb Res.* 1996;81(1):1-41.

722. MCVey JH. *Tissue Factor and Factor VII Initiation of Coagulation.* Lippincott, Williams & Wilkins; 2001.

723. Andoh K, Kubota T, Takada M, Tanaka H, Kobayashi N, Maekawa T. Tissue factor activity in leukemia cells. Special reference to disseminated intravascular coagulation. *Cancer.* 1987;59(4):748-754.

724. Tanaka M, Yamanishi H. The expression of tissue factor antigen and activity on the surface of leukemic cells. *Leuk Res.* 1993;17(2):103-111.

725. Tallman MS, Hakimian D, Kwaan HC, Rickles FR. New insights into the pathogenesis of coagulation dysfunction in acute promyelocytic leukemia. *Leuk Lymphoma.* 1993;11(1-2):27-36.

726. Osterud B, Flaegstad T. Increased tissue thromboplastin activity in monocytes of patients with meningococcal infection: related to an unfavourable prognosis. *Thromb Haemost.* 1983;49(1):5-7.

727. Kadish JL, Wenc KM, Dvorak HF. Tissue factor activity of normal and neoplastic cells: quantitation and species specificity. *J Natl Cancer Inst.* 1983;70(3):551-557.

728. Silberberg JM, Gordon S, Zucker S. Identification of tissue factor in two human pancreatic cancer cell lines. *Cancer Res.* 1989;49(19):5443-5447.

729. Bauer KA, Conway EM, Bach R, Konigsberg WH, Griffin JD, Demetri G. Tissue factor gene expression in acute myeloblastic leukemia. *Thromb Res.* 1989;56(3):425-430.

730. Mueller BM, Reisfeld RA, Edgington TS, Ruf W. Expression of tissue factor by melanoma cells promotes efficient hematogenous metastasis. *Proc Natl Acad Sci U S A.* 1992;89(24):11832-11836.

731. Dvorak HF, Quay SC, Orenstein NS, et al. Tumor shedding and coagulation. *Science.* 1981;212(4497):923-924.

732. Lechner D, Weltermann A. Circulating tissue factor-exposing microparticles. *Thromb Res.* 2008;122(suppl 1):S47-S54.

733. Levi M, van der Poll T, Schultz M. Infection and inflammation as risk factors for thrombosis and atherosclerosis. *Semin Thromb Hemost.* 2012;38(5):506-514.

734. Faulk WP, Labarrere CA, Carson SD. Tissue factor: identification and characterization of cell types in human placentae. *Blood.* 1990;76(1):86-96.

735. Blakely ML, Van der Werf WJ, Berndt MC, Dalmasso AP, Bach FH, Hancock WW. Activation of intragraft endothelial and mononuclear cells during discordant xenograft rejection. *Transplantation.* 1994;58(10):1059-1066.

736. Salom RN, Maguire JA, Hancock WW. Endothelial activation and cytokine expression in human acute cardiac allograft rejection. *Pathology.* 1998;30(1):24-29.

737. Gertler JP, Weibe DA, Ocasio VH, Abbott WM. Hypoxia induces procoagulant activity in cultured human venous endothelium. *J Vasc Surg.* 1991;13(3):428-433.

738. O'Rourke JF, Pugh CW, Bartlett SM, Ratcliffe PJ. Identification of hypoxically inducible mRNAs in HeLa cells using differential-display PCR. Role of hypoxia-inducible factor-1. *Eur J Biochem.* 1996;241(2):403-410.

739. Herbert JM, Corseaux D, Lale A, Bernat A. Hypoxia primes endotoxin-induced tissue factor expression in human monocytes and endothelial cells by a PAF-dependent mechanism. *J Cell Physiol.* 1996;169(2):290-299.

740. Mackman N. Regulation of the tissue factor gene. *Thromb Haemost.* 1997;78(1):747-754.

741. Yan SF, Zou YS, Gao Y, et al. Tissue factor transcription driven by Egr-1 is a critical mechanism of murine pulmonary fibrin deposition in hypoxia. *Proc Natl Acad Sci U S A.* 1998;95(14):8298-8303.

742. Broze GJ, Jr, Leykam JE, Schwartz BD, Miletich JP. Purification of human brain tissue factor. *J Biol Chem.* 1985;260(20):10917-10920.

743. Morrissey JH, Fakhrai H, Edgington TS. Molecular cloning of the cDNA for tissue factor, the cellular receptor for the initiation of the coagulation protease cascade. *Cell.* 1987;50(1):129-135.

744. Spicer EK, Horton R, Bloem L, et al. Isolation of cDNA clones coding for human tissue factor: primary structure of the protein and cDNA. *Proc Natl Acad Sci U S A.* 1987;84(15):5148-5152.

745. Bazan JF. Structural design and molecular evolution of a cytokine receptor superfamily. *Proc Natl Acad Sci U S A.* 1990;87(18):6934-6938.

746. Muller YA, Ultsch MH, de Vos AM. The crystal structure of the extracellular domain of human tissue factor refined to 1.7 A resolution. *J Mol Biol.* 1996;256(1):144-159.

747. Krudysz-Amblo J, Jennings ME,IInd, Mann KG, Butenas S. Carbohydrates and activity of natural and recombinant tissue factor. *J Biol Chem.* 2010;285(5):3371-3382.

748. Krudysz-Amblo J, Jennings ME,IInd, Matthews DE, Mann KG, Butenas S. Differences in the fractional abundances of carbohydrates of natural and recombinant human tissue factor. *Biochim Biophys Acta.* 2011;1810(4):398-405.

749. Paborsky LR, Caras IW, Fisher KL, Gorman CM. Lipid association, but not the transmembrane domain, is required for tissue factor activity. Substitution of the transmembrane domain with a phosphatidylinositol anchor. *J Biol Chem.* 1991;266(32):21911-21916.

750. Paborsky LR, Harris RJ. Post-translational modifications of recombinant human tissue factor. *Thromb Res.* 1990;60(5):367-376.

751. Harlos K, Martin DM, O'Brien DP, et al. Crystal structure of the extracellular region of human tissue factor. *Nature.* 1994;370(6491):662-666.

752. Muller YA, Ultsch MH, Kelley RF, de Vos AM. Structure of the extracellular domain of human tissue factor: location of the factor VIIa binding site. *Biochemistry.* 1994;33(36):10864-10870.

753. Muller YA, Kelley RF, de Vos AM. Hinge bending within the cytokine receptor superfamily revealed by the 2.4 A crystal structure of the extracellular domain of rabbit tissue factor. *Protein Sci.* 1998;7(5):1106-1115.

754. Huang M, Syed R, Stura EA, et al. The mechanism of an inhibitory antibody on TF-initiated blood coagulation revealed by the crystal structures of human tissue factor, Fab 5G9 and TF.G9 complex. *J Mol Biol.* 1998;275(5):873-894.

755. Kahn ML, Zheng YW, Huang W, et al. A dual thrombin receptor system for platelet activation. *Nature.* 1998;394(6694):690-694.

756. Bach R, Konigsberg WH, Nemerson Y. Human tissue factor contains thioester-linked palmitate and stearate on the cytoplasmic half-cystine. *Biochemistry.* 1988;27(12):4227-4231.

The Normal Hematologic System

757. Chen VM, Hogg PJ. Allosteric disulfide bonds in thrombosis and thrombolysis. *J Thromb Haemost.* 2006;4(12):2533-2541.

758. Ahamed J, Versteeg HH, Kerver M, et al. Disulfide isomerization switches tissue factor from coagulation to cell signaling. *Proc Natl Acad Sci U S A.* 2006;103(38):13932-13937.

759. Ruf W, Versteeg HH. Tissue factor mutated at the allosteric Cys186-Cys209 disulfide bond is severely impaired in decrypted procoagulant activity. *Blood.* 2010;116(3):500-501. author reply 502-503.

760. van den Hengel LG, Kocaturk B, Reitsma PH, Ruf W, Versteeg HH. Complete abolishment of coagulant activity in monomeric disulfide-deficient tissue factor. *Blood.* 2011;118(12):3446-3448.

761. Ruf W. Role of thiol pathways in TF procoagulant regulation. *Thromb Res.* 2012;129(suppl 2):S11-S12.

762. Rehemtulla A, Ruf W, Edgington TS. The integrity of the cysteine 186-cysteine 209 bond of the second disulfide loop of tissue factor is required for binding of factor VII. *J Biol Chem.* 1991;266(16):10294-10299.

763. Paborsky LR, Tate KM, Harris RJ, et al. Purification of recombinant human tissue factor. *Biochemistry.* 1989;28(20):8072-8077.

764. Butenas S, Amblo-Krudysz J, Mann KG. Posttranslational modifications of tissue factor. *Front Biosci (Elite Ed).* 2012;4:381-391.

765. Egorina EM, Sovershaev MA, Osterud B. Regulation of tissue factor procoagulant activity by post-translational modifications. *Thromb Res.* 2008;122(6):831-837.

766. Zioncheck TF, Roy S, Vehar GA. The cytoplasmic domain of tissue factor is phosphorylated by a protein kinase C-dependent mechanism. *J Biol Chem.* 1992;267(6):3561-3564.

767. Nemerson Y, Repke D. Tissue factor accelerates the activation of coagulation factor VII: the role of a bifunctional coagulation cofactor. *Thromb Res.* 1985;40(3):351-358.

768. Ruf W, Rehemtulla A, Morrissey JH, Edgington TS. Phospholipid-independent and -dependent interactions required for tissue factor receptor and cofactor function. *J Biol Chem.* 1991;266(4):2158-2166.

769. Pedersen AH, Nordfang O, Norris F, et al. Recombinant human extrinsic pathway inhibitor. Production, isolation, and characterization of its inhibitory activity on tissue factor-initiated coagulation reactions. *J Biol Chem.* 1990;265(28):16786-16793.

770. Neuenschwander PF, Branam DE, Morrissey JH. Importance of substrate composition, pH and other variables on tissue factor enhancement of factor VIIa activity. *Thromb Haemost.* 1993;70(6):970-977.

771. Komiyama Y, Pedersen AH, Kisiel W. Proteolytic activation of human factors IX and X by recombinant human factor VIIa: effects of calcium, phospholipids, and tissue factor. *Biochemistry.* 1990;29(40):9418-9425.

772. Camerer E, Trejo J. Cryptic messages: is noncoagulant tissue factor reserved for cell signaling? *Proc Natl Acad Sci U S A.* 2006;103(39):14259-14260.

773. Morel O, Toti F, Hugel B, et al. Procoagulant microparticles: disrupting the vascular homeostasis equation? *Arterioscler Thromb Vasc Biol.* 2006;26(12):2594-2604.

774. Butenas S, Bouchard BA, Brummel-Ziedins KE, Parhami-Seren B, Mann KG. Tissue factor activity in whole blood. *Blood.* 2005;105(7):2764-2770.

775. Giesen PL, Rauch U, Bohrmann B, et al. Blood-borne tissue factor: another view of thrombosis. *Proc Natl Acad Sci U S A.* 1999;96(5):2311-2315.

776. Butenas S, Orfeo T, Mann KG. Tissue factor in coagulation: which? Where? When? *Arterioscler Thromb Vasc Biol.* 2009;29(12):1989-1996.

777. Date K, Ettelaie C, Maraveyas A. Tissue factor-bearing microparticles and inflammation: a potential mechanism for the development of venous thromboembolism in cancer. *J Thromb Haemost.* 2017;15(12):2289-2299.

778. Krudysz-Amblo J, Jennings ME, 2nd, Knight T, Matthews DE, Mann KG, Butenas S. Disulfide reduction abolishes tissue factor cofactor function. *Biochim Biophys Acta.* 2013;1830(6):3489-3496.

779. Marder VJ, Mannucci PM, Firkin BG, Hoyer LW, Meyer D. Standard nomenclature for factor VIII and von Willebrand factor: a recommendation by the International Committee on Thrombosis and Haemostasis. *Thromb Haemost.* 1985;54(4):871-872.

780. Leyte A, Verbeet MP, Brodniewicz-Proba T, Van Mourik JA, Mertens K. The interaction between human blood-coagulation factor VIII and von Willebrand factor. Characterization of a high-affinity binding site on factor VIII. *Biochem J.* 1989;257(3):679-683.

781. Bendetowicz AV, Morris JA, Wise RJ, Gilbert GE, Kaufman RJ. Binding of factor VIII to von willebrand factor is enabled by cleavage of the von Willebrand factor propeptide and enhanced by formation of disulfide-linked multimers. *Blood.* 1998;92(2):529-538.

782. Mannucci PM. Desmopressin (DDAVP) in the treatment of bleeding disorders: the first 20 years. *Blood.* 1997;90(7):2515-2521.

783. Tuddenham EG, Lane RS, Rotblat F, et al. Response to infusions of polyelectrolyte fractionated human factor VIII concentrate in human haemophilia A and von Willebrand's disease. *Br J Haematol.* 1982;52(2):259-267.

784. Over J, Sixma JJ, Bruine MH, et al. Survival of 125iodine-labeled Factor VIII in normals and patients with classic hemophilia. Observations on the heterogeneity of human factor VIII. *J Clin Invest.* 1978;62(2):223-234.

785. Weiss HJ, Sussman II, Hoyer LW. Stabilization of factor VIII in plasma by the von Willebrand factor. Studies on posttransfusion and dissociated factor VIII and in patients with von Willebrand's disease. *J Clin Invest.* 1977;60(2):390-404.

786. Brinkhous KM, Sandberg H, Garris JB, et al. Purified human factor VIII procoagulant protein: comparative hemostatic response after infusions in hemophilic and von Willebrand disease dogs. *Proc Natl Acad Sci U S A.* 1985;82(24):8752-8756.

787. Hoyer LW. Molecular pathology and immunology of factor VIII (hemophilia A and factor VIII inhibitors). *Hum Pathol.* 1987;18(2):153-161.

788. Rizza CR, Spooner RJ. Treatment of haemophilia and related disorders in Britain and Northern Ireland during 1976-80: report on behalf of the directors of haemophilia centres in the United Kingdom. *Br Med J (Clin Res Ed).* 1983;286(6369):929-933.

789. Kaufman RJ, AS, Fay PJ. *Factor VII and Hemophilia A.* Lippincott, Williams & Wilkins; 2001.

790. Freije D, Schlessinger D. A 1.6-Mb contig of yeast artificial chromosomes around the human factor VIII gene reveals three regions homologous to probes for the DXS115 locus and two for the DXYS64 locus. *Am J Hum Genet.* 1992;51(1):66-80.

791. Migeon BR, McGinniss MJ, Antonarakis SE, et al. Severe hemophilia A in a female by cryptic translocation: order and orientation of factor VIII within Xq28. *Genomics.* 1993;16(1):20-25.

792. Gitschier J, Wood WI, Goralka TM, et al. Characterization of the human factor VIII gene. *Nature.* 1984;312(5992):326-330.

793. Purrello M, Alhadeff B, Esposito D, et al. The human genes for hemophilia A and hemophilia B flank the X chromosome fragile site at Xq27.3. *EMBO J.* 1985;4(3):725-729.

794. Tantravahi U, Murty VV, Jhanwar SC, et al. Physical mapping of the factor VIII gene proximal to two polymorphic DNA probes in human chromosome band Xq28: implications for factor VIII gene segregation analysis. *Cytogenet Cell Genet.* 1986;42(1-2):75-79.

795. Wood WI, Capon DJ, Simonsen CC, et al. Expression of active human factor VIII from recombinant DNA clones. *Nature.* 1984;312(5992):330-337.

796. Webster WP, Zukoski CF, Hutchin P, Reddick RL, Mandel SR, Penick GD. Plasma factor VIII synthesis and control as revealed by canine organ transplantation. *Am J Physiol.* 1971;220(5):1147-1154.

797. Groth CG, Hathaway WE, Gustafsson A, et al. Correction of coagulation in the hemophilic dog by transplantation of lymphatic tissue. *Surgery.* 1974;75(5):725-733.

798. Lewis JH, Bontempo FA, Spero JA, Ragni MV, Starzl TE. Liver transplantation in a hemophiliac. *N Engl J Med.* 1985;312(18):1189-1190.

799. Bontempo FA, Lewis JH, Gorenc TJ, et al. Liver transplantation in hemophilia A. *Blood.* 1987;69(6):1721-1724.

800. Liu L, Xia S, Seifert J. Transplantation of spleen cells in patients with hemophilia A. A report of 20 cases. *Transpl Int.* 1994;7(3):201-206.

801. Kelly DA, Summerfield JA, Tuddenham EG. Localization of factor VIIIC: antigen in Guinea-pig tissues and isolated liver cell fractions. *Br J Haematol.* 1984;56(4):535-543.

802. Wion KL, Kelly D, Summerfield JA, Tuddenham EG, Lawn RM. Distribution of factor VIII mRNA and antigen in human liver and other tissues. *Nature.* 1985;317(6039):726-729.

803. Vehar GA, Keyt B, Eaton D, et al. Structure of human factor VIII. *Nature.* 1984;312(5992):337-342.

804. Jenny RJ, Pittman DD, Toole JJ, et al. Complete cDNA and derived amino acid sequence of human factor V. *Proc Natl Acad Sci U S A.* 1987;84(14):4846-4850.

805. Adams TE, Hockin MF, Mann KG, Everse SJ. The crystal structure of activated protein C-inactivated bovine factor Va: implications for cofactor function. *Proc Natl Acad Sci U S A.* 2004;101(24):8918-8923.

806. Shen BW, Spiegel PC, Chang CH, et al. The tertiary structure and domain organization of coagulation factor VIII. *Blood.* 2008;111(3):1240-1247.

807. Koschinsky ML, Funk WD, van Oost BA, MacGillivray RT. Complete cDNA sequence of human preceruloplasmin. *Proc Natl Acad Sci U S A.* 1986;83(14):5086-5090.

808. Poole S, Firtel RA, Lamar E, Rowekamp W. Sequence and expression of the discoidin I gene family in Dictyostelium discoideum. *J Mol Biol.* 1981;153(2):273-289.

809. Stubbs JD, Lekutis C, Singer KL, et al. cDNA cloning of a mouse mammary epithelial cell surface protein reveals the existence of epidermal growth factor-like domains linked to factor VIII-like sequences. *Proc Natl Acad Sci U S A.* 1990;87(21):8417-8421.

810. Fass DN, Knutson GJ, Katzmann JA. Monoclonal antibodies to porcine factor VIII coagulant and their use in the isolation of active coagulant protein. *Blood.* 1982;59(3):594-600.

811. Andersson LO, Forsman N, Huang K, et al. Isolation and characterization of human factor VIII: molecular forms in commercial factor VIII concentrate, cryoprecipitate, and plasma. *Proc Natl Acad Sci U S A.* 1986;83(9):2979-2983.

812. Fay PJ, Anderson MT, Chavin SI, Marder VJ. The size of human factor VIII heterodimers and the effects produced by thrombin. *Biochim Biophys Acta.* 1986;871(3):268-278.

813. Elder B, Lakich D, Gitschier J. Sequence of the murine factor VIII cDNA. *Genomics.* 1993;16(2):374-379.

814. Bihoreau N, Pin S, de Kersabiec AM, Vidot F, Fontaine-Aupart MP. Copper-atom identification in the active and inactive forms of plasma-derived FVIII and recombinant FVIII-delta II. *Eur J Biochem.* 1994;222(1):41-48.

815. Tagliavacca L, Moon N, Dunham WR, Kaufman RJ. Identification and functional requirement of Cu(I) and its ligands within coagulation factor VIII. *J Biol Chem.* 1997;272(43):27428-27434.

816. Saenko EL, Shima M, Rajalakshmi KJ, Scandella D. A role for the C2 domain of factor VIII in binding to von Willebrand factor. *J Biol Chem.* 1994;269(15):11601-11605.

817. Saenko EL, Scandella D. The acidic region of the factor VIII light chain and the C2 domain together form the high affinity binding site for von willebrand factor. *J Biol Chem.* 1997;272(29):18007-18014.

818. Foster PA, Fulcher CA, Houghten RA, Zimmerman TS. An immunogenic region within residues Val1670-Glu1684 of the factor VIII light chain induces antibodies which inhibit binding of factor VIII to von Willebrand factor. *J Biol Chem.* 1988;263(11):5230-5234.

819. Shima M, Scandella D, Yoshioka A, et al. A factor VIII neutralizing monoclonal antibody and a human inhibitor alloantibody recognizing epitopes in the C2 domain inhibit factor VIII binding to von Willebrand factor and to phosphatidylserine. *Thromb Haemost.* 1993;69(3):240-246.

820. Hsu TC, Pratt KP, Thompson AR. The factor VIII C1 domain contributes to platelet binding. *Blood.* 2008;111(1):200-208.

821. Lenting PJ, Donath MJ, van Mourik JA, Mertens K. Identification of a binding site for blood coagulation factor IXa on the light chain of human factor VIII. *J Biol Chem.* 1994;269(10):7150-7155.
822. Lenting PJ, van de Loo JW, Donath MJ, van Mourik JA, Mertens K. The sequence Glu1811-Lys1818 of human blood coagulation factor VIII comprises a binding site for activated factor IX. *J Biol Chem.* 1996;271(4):1935-1940.
823. Fay PJ, Beattie T, Huggins CF, Regan LM. Factor VIIIa A2 subunit residues 558-565 represent a factor IXa interactive site. *J Biol Chem.* 1994;269(32):20522-20527.
824. O'Brien LM, Medved LV, Fay PJ. Localization of factor IXa and factor VIIIa interactive sites. *J Biol Chem.* 1995;270(45):27087-27092.
825. Fay PJ, Koshibu K. The A2 subunit of factor VIIIa modulates the active site of factor IXa. *J Biol Chem.* 1998;273(30):19049-19054.
826. Payne AB, Miller CH, Kelly FM, Michael Soucie J, Craig Hooper W. The CDC Hemophilia A Mutation Project (CHAMP) mutation list: a new online resource. *Hum Mutat.* 2013;34(2):E2382-E2391.
827. Jenkins PV, Freas J, Schmidt KM, Zhou Q, Fay PJ. Mutations associated with hemophilia A in the 558-565 loop of the factor VIIIa A2 subunit alter the catalytic activity of the factor Xase complex. *Blood.* 2002;100(2):501-508.
828. Ngo JC, Huang M, Roth DA, Furie BC, Furie B. Crystal structure of human factor VIII: implications for the formation of the factor IXa-factor VIIIa complex. *Structure.* 2008;16(4):597-606.
829. Stoilova-McPhie S, Lynch GC, Ludtke S, Pettitt BM. Domain organization of membrane-bound factor VIII. *Biopolymers.* 2013;99(7):448-459.
830. Dalm D, Galaz-Montoya JG, Miller JL, et al. Dimeric organization of blood coagulation factor VIII bound to lipid nanotubes. *Sci Rep.* 2015;5:11212.
831. Autin L, Miteva MA, Lee WH, Mertens K, Radtke KP, Villoutreix BO. Molecular models of the procoagulant factor VIIIa-factor IXa complex. *J Thromb Haemost.* 2005;3(9):2044-2056.
832. Venkateswarlu D. Structural insights into the interaction of blood coagulation co-factor VIIIa with factor IXa: a computational protein-protein docking and molecular dynamics refinement study. *Biochem Biophys Res Commun.* 2014;452(3):408-414.
833. Bajaj SP, Schmidt AE, Mathur A, et al. Factor IXa:factor VIIIa interaction. helix 330-338 of factor ixa interacts with residues 558-565 and spatially adjacent regions of the a2 subunit of factor VIIIa. *J Biol Chem.* 2001;276(19):16302-16309.
834. Griffiths AE, Rydkin I, Fay PJ. Factor VIIIa A2 subunit shows a high affinity interaction with factor IXa: contribution of A2 subunit residues 707-714 to the interaction with factor IXa. *J Biol Chem.* 2013;288(21):15057-15064.
835. Lapan KA, Fay PJ. Localization of a factor X interactive site in the A1 subunit of factor VIIIa. *J Biol Chem.* 1997;272(4):2082-2088.
836. Regan LM, O'Brien LM, Beattie TL, Sudhakar K, Walker FJ, Fay PJ. Activated protein C-catalyzed proteolysis of factor VIIIa alters its interactions within factor Xase. *J Biol Chem.* 1996;271(8):3982-3987.
837. Pittman DD, Wang JH, Kaufman RJ. Identification and functional importance of tyrosine sulfate residues within recombinant factor VIII. *Biochemistry.* 1992;31(13):3315-3325.
838. Michnick DA, Pittman DD, Wise RJ, Kaufman RJ. Identification of individual tyrosine sulfation sites within factor VIII required for optimal activity and efficient thrombin cleavage. *J Biol Chem.* 1994;269(31):20095-20102.
839. Hironaka T, Furukawa K, Esmon PC, et al. Comparative study of the sugar chains of factor VIII purified from human plasma and from the culture media of recombinant baby hamster kidney cells. *J Biol Chem.* 1992;267(12):8012-8020.
840. van Dieijen G, Tans G, Rosing J, Hemker HC. The role of phospholipid and factor VIIIa in the activation of bovine factor X. *J Biol Chem.* 1981;256(7):3433-3442.
841. van Dieijen G, van Rijn JL, Govers-Riemslag JW, Hemker HC, Rosing J. Assembly of the intrinsic factor X activating complex–interactions between factor IXa, factor VIIIa and phospholipid. *Thromb Haemost.* 1985;53(3):396-400.
842. Duffy EJ, Parker ET, Mutucumarana VP, Johnson AE, Lollar P. Binding of factor VIIIa and factor VIII to factor IXa on phospholipid vesicles. *J Biol Chem.* 1992;267(24):17006-17011.
843. Ahmad SS, Rawala-Sheikh R, Walsh PN. Comparative interactions of factor IX and factor IXa with human platelets. *J Biol Chem.* 1989;264(6):3244-3251.
844. Scandura JM, Ahmad SS, Walsh PN. A binding site expressed on the surface of activated human platelets is shared by factor X and prothrombin. *Biochemistry.* 1996;35(27):8890-8902.
845. Ahmad SS, Scandura JM, Walsh PN. Structural and functional characterization of platelet receptor-mediated factor VIII binding. *J Biol Chem.* 2000;275(17):13071-13081.
846. Ahmad SS, London FS, Walsh PN. Binding studies of the enzyme (factor IXa) with the cofactor (factor VIIIa) in the assembly of factor-X activating complex on the activated platelet surface. *J Thromb Haemost.* 2003;1(11):2348-2355.
847. Ahmad SS, Walsh PN. Coordinate binding studies of the substrate (factor X) with the cofactor (factor VIII) in the assembly of the factor X activating complex on the activated platelet surface. *Biochemistry.* 2002;41(37):11269-11276.
848. Lollar P, Knutson GJ, Fass DN. Stabilization of thrombin-activated porcine factor VIII: C by factor IXa phospholipid. *Blood.* 1984;63(6):1303-1308.
849. Lamphear BJ, Fay PJ. Factor IXa enhances reconstitution of factor VIIIa from isolated A2 subunit and A1/A3-C1-C2 dimer. *J Biol Chem.* 1992;267(6):3725-3730.
850. Lamphear BJ, Fay PJ. Proteolytic interactions of factor IXa with human factor VIII and factor VIIIa. *Blood.* 1992;80(12):3120-3126.
851. Fay PJ, Beattie TL, Regan LM, O'Brien LM, Kaufman RJ. Model for the factor VIIIa-dependent decay of the intrinsic factor Xase. Role of subunit dissociation and factor IXa-catalyzed proteolysis. *J Biol Chem.* 1996;271(11):6027-6032.
852. O'Brien DP, Johnson D, Byfield P, Tuddenham EG. Inactivation of factor VIII by factor IXa. *Biochemistry.* 1992;31(10):2805-2812.
853. Fay PJ, Smudzin TM, Walker FJ. Activated protein C-catalyzed inactivation of human factor VIII and factor VIIIa. Identification of cleavage sites and correlation of proteolysis with cofactor activity. *J Biol Chem.* 1991;266(30):20139-20145.
854. Lu D, Kalafatis M, Mann KG, Long GL. Comparison of activated protein C/protein S-mediated inactivation of human factor VIII and factor V. *Blood.* 1996;87(11):4708-4717.
855. Regan LM, Lamphear BJ, Huggins CF, Walker FJ, Fay PJ. Factor IXa protects factor VIIIa from activated protein C. Factor IXa inhibits activated protein C-catalyzed cleavage of factor VIIIa at Arg562. *J Biol Chem.* 1994;269(13):9445-9452.
856. Tracy PB, Giles AR, Mann KG, Eide LL, Hoogendoorn H, Rivard GE. Factor V (Quebec): a bleeding diathesis associated with a qualitative platelet Factor V deficiency. *J Clin Invest.* 1984;74(4):1221-1228.
857. Mann KG, Kalafatis M. Factor V: a combination of Dr Jekyll and Mr Hyde. *Blood.* 2003;101(1):20-30.
858. Kalafatis M. Coagulation factor V: a plethora of anticoagulant molecules. *Curr Opin Hematol.* 2005;12(2):141-148.
859. Camire RM. A new look at blood coagulation factor V. *Curr Opin Hematol.* 2011;18(5):338-342.
860. Dahlback B. Pro- and anticoagulant properties of factor V in pathogenesis of thrombosis and bleeding disorders. *Int J Lab Hematol.* 2016;38(suppl 1):4-11.
861. Cui J, O'Shea KS, Purkayastha A, Saunders TL, Ginsburg D. Fatal haemorrhage and incomplete block to embryogenesis in mice lacking coagulation factor V. *Nature.* 1996;384(6604):66-68.
862. Seligsohn U, Zivelin A, Zwang E. Combined factor V and factor VIII deficiency among non-Ashkenazi Jews. *N Engl J Med.* 1982;307(19):1191-1195.
863. Lippi G, Favaloro EJ, Montagnana M, Manzato F, Guidi GC, Franchini M. Inherited and acquired factor V deficiency. *Blood Coagul Fibrinolysis.* 2011;22(3):160-166.
864. Dansako H, Ishimaru F, Takai Y, et al. Molecular characterization of the ERGIC-53 gene in two Japanese patients with combined factor V-factor VIII deficiency. *Ann Hematol.* 2001;80(5):292-294.
865. Khoriaty R, Vasievich MP, Ginsburg D. The COPII pathway and hematologic disease. *Blood.* 2012;120(1):31-38.
866. Baruch D, Lindhout T, Dupuy E, Caen JP. Thrombin-induced platelet factor Va formation in patients with a gray platelet syndrome. *Thromb Haemost.* 1987;58(2):768-771.
867. Weiss HJ, Lages B. Platelet prothrombinase activity and intracellular calcium responses in patients with storage pool deficiency, glycoprotein IIb-IIIa deficiency, or impaired platelet coagulant activity–a comparison with Scott syndrome. *Blood.* 1997;89(5):1599-1611.
868. Janeway CM, Rivard GE, Tracy PB, Mann KG. Factor V Quebec revisited. *Blood.* 1996;87(9):3571-3578.
869. Fokkema I, Kroon M, Lopez Hernandez JA, et al. The LOVD3 platform: efficient genome-wide sharing of genetic variants. *Eur J Hum Genet.* 2021;29(12):1796-1803.
870. Wang H, Riddell DC, Guinto ER, MacGillivray RT, Hamerton JL. Localization of the gene encoding human factor V to chromosome 1q21-25. *Genomics.* 1988;2(4):324-328.
871. Kane WH, Ichinose A, Hagen FS, Davie EW. Cloning of cDNAs coding for the heavy chain region and connecting region of human factor V, a blood coagulation factor with four types of internal repeats. *Biochemistry.* 1987;26(20):6508-6514.
872. Mazzorana M, Baffet G, Kneip B, Launois B, Guguen-Guillouzo C. Expression of coagulation factor V gene by normal adult human hepatocytes in primary culture. *Br J Haematol.* 1991;78(2):229-235.
873. Gewirtz AM, Shen YM. Effect of phorbol myristate acetate on c-myc, beta-actin, and FV gene expression in morphologically recognizable human megakaryocytes: a kinetic analysis employing in situ hybridization. *Exp Hematol.* 1990;18(8):945-952.
874. Gewirtz AM, Shapiro C, Shen YM, Boyd R, Colman RW. Cellular and molecular regulation of factor V expression in human megakaryocytes. *J Cell Physiol.* 1992;153(2):277-287.
875. Gewirtz AM, Keefer M, Doshi K, Annamalai AE, Chiu HC, Colman RW. Biology of human megakaryocyte factor V. *Blood.* 1986;67(6):1639-1648.
876. Gould WR, Simioni P, Silveira JR, Tormene D, Kalafatis M, Tracy PB. Megakaryocytes endocytose and subsequently modify human factor V in vivo to form the entire pool of a unique platelet-derived cofactor. *J Thromb Haemost.* 2005;3(3):450-456.
877. Bouchard BA, Williams JL, Meisler NT, Long MW, Tracy PB. Endocytosis of plasma-derived factor V by megakaryocytes occurs via a clathrin-dependent, specific membrane binding event. *J Thromb Haemost.* 2005;3(3):541-551.
878. Suehiro Y, Veljkovic DK, Fuller N, et al. Endocytosis and storage of plasma factor V by human megakaryocytes. *Thromb Haemost.* 2005;94(3):585-592.
879. Rowley JW, Oler AJ, Tolley ND, et al. Genome-wide RNA-seq analysis of human and mouse platelet transcriptomes. *Blood.* 2011;118(14):e101-e111.
880. Gertz JM, Bouchard BA. Mechanisms regulating Acquisition of platelet-derived factor V/va by megakaryocytes. *J Cell Biochem.* 2015;116(10):2121-2126.
881. Cerveny TJ, Fass DN, Mann KG. Synthesis of coagulation factor V by cultured aortic endothelium. *Blood.* 1984;63(6):1467-1474.
882. Rodgers GM. Vascular smooth muscle cells synthesize, secrete and express coagulation factor V. *Biochim Biophys Acta.* 1988;968(1):17-23.
883. Kane WH, Majerus PW. Purification and characterization of human coagulation factor V. *J Biol Chem.* 1981;256(2):1002-1007.
884. Nesheim ME, Myrmel KH, Hibbard L, Mann KG. Isolation and characterization of single chain bovine factor V. *J Biol Chem.* 1979;254(2):508-517.
885. Dahlback B. Human coagluation factor V purification and thrombin-catalyzed activation. *J Clin Invest.* 1980;66(3):583-591.
886. Katzmann JA, Nesheim ME, Hibbard LS, Mann KG. Isolation of functional human coagulation factor V by using a hybridoma antibody. *Proc Natl Acad Sci U S A.* 1981;78(1):162-166.
887. Mann KG, Lawler CM, Vehar GA, Church WR. Coagulation Factor V contains copper ion. *J Biol Chem.* 1984;259(21):12949-12951.

888. Undas A, Williams EB, Butenas S, Orfeo T, Mann KG. Homocysteine inhibits inactivation of factor Va by activated protein C. *J Biol Chem.* 2001;276(6):4389-4397.
889. Kalafatis M. Identification and partial characterization of factor Va heavy chain kinase from human platelets. *J Biol Chem.* 1998;273(14):8459-8466.
890. Pittman DD, Tomkinson KN, Michnick D, Selighsohn U, Kaufman RJ. Posttranslational sulfation of factor V is required for efficient thrombin cleavage and activation and for full procoagulant activity. *Biochemistry.* 1994;33(22):6952-6959.
891. Pittman DD, Tomkinson KN, Kaufman RJ. Post-translational requirements for functional factor V and factor VIII secretion in mammalian cells. *J Biol Chem.* 1994;269(25):17329-17337.
892. Fernandez JA, Hackeng TM, Kojima K, Griffin JH. The carbohydrate moiety of factor V modulates inactivation by activated protein C. *Blood.* 1997;89(12):4348-4354.
893. Nicolaes GA, Villoutreix BO, Dahlback B. Partial glycosylation of Asn2181 in human factor V as a cause of molecular and functional heterogeneity. Modulation of glycosylation efficiency by mutagenesis of the consensus sequence for N-linked glycosylation. *Biochemistry.* 1999;38(41):13584-13591.
894. Hoekema L, Nicolaes GA, Hemker HC, Tans G, Rosing J. Human factor Va1 and factor Va2: properties in the procoagulant and anticoagulant pathways. *Biochemistry.* 1997;36(11):3331-3335.
895. Rosing J, Bakker HM, Thomassen MC, Hemker HC, Tans G. Characterization of two forms of human factor Va with different cofactor activities. *J Biol Chem.* 1993;268(28):21130-21136.
896. Kim SW, Ortel TL, Quinn-Allen MA, et al. Partial glycosylation at asparagine-2181 of the second C-type domain of human factor V modulates assembly of the prothrombinase complex. *Biochemistry.* 1999;38(35):11448-11454.
897. Kalafatis M, Rand MD, Mann KG. Factor Va-membrane interaction is mediated by two regions located on the light chain of the cofactor. *Biochemistry.* 1994;33(2):486-493.
898. Villoutreix BO, Dahlback B. Structural investigation of the A domains of human blood coagulation factor V by molecular modeling. *Protein Sci.* 1998;7(6):1317-1325.
899. Pellequer JL, Gale AJ, Getzoff ED, Griffin JH. Three-dimensional model of coagulation factor Va bound to activated protein C. *Thromb Haemost.* 2000;84(5):849-857.
900. Lechtenberg BC, Murray-Rust TA, Johnson DJ, et al. Crystal structure of the prothrombinase complex from the venom of Pseudonaja textilis. *Blood.* 2013;122(16):2777-2783.
901. Saleh M, Peng W, Quinn-Allen MA, et al. The factor V C1 domain is involved in membrane binding: identification of functionally important amino acid residues within the C1 domain of factor V using alanine scanning mutagenesis. *Thromb Haemost.* 2004;91(1):16-27.
902. Peng W, Quinn-Allen MA, Kane WH. Mutation of hydrophobic residues in the factor Va C1 and C2 domains blocks membrane-dependent prothrombin activation. *J Thromb Haemost.* 2005;3(2):351-354.
903. Majumder R, Quinn-Allen MA, Kane WH, Lentz BR. The phosphatidylserine binding site of the factor Va C2 domain accounts for membrane binding but does not contribute to the assembly or activity of a human factor Xa-factor Va complex. *Biochemistry.* 2005;44(2):711-718.
904. Autin L, Steen M, Dahlback B, Villoutreix BO. Proposed structural models of the prothrombinase (FXa-FVa) complex. *Proteins.* 2006;63(3):440-450.
905. Pomowski A, Ustok FI, Huntington JA. Homology model of human prothrombinase based on the crystal structure of Pseutarin C. *Biol Chem.* 2014;395(10):1233-1241.
906. Shim JY, Lee CJ, Wu S, Pedersen LG. A model for the unique role of factor Va A2 domain extension in the human ternary thrombin-generating complex. *Biophys Chem.* 2015;199:46-50.
907. Esmon CT. The subunit structure of thrombin-activated factor V. Isolation of activated factor V, separation of subunits, and reconstitution of biological activity. *J Biol Chem.* 1979;254(3):964-973.
908. Guinto ER, Esmon CT. Formation of a calcium-binding site on bovine activated factor V following recombination of the isolated subunits. *J Biol Chem.* 1982;257(17):10038-10043.
909. Kane WH, Majerus PW. The interaction of human coagulation factor Va with platelets. *J Biol Chem.* 1982;257(7):3963-3969.
910. Laue TM, Johnson AE, Esmon CT, Yphantis DA. Structure of bovine blood coagulation factor Va. Determination of the subunit associations, molecular weights, and asymmetries by analytical ultracentrifugation. *Biochemistry.* 1984;23(7):1339-1348.
911. Thorelli E, Kaufman RJ, Dahlback B. Cleavage requirements for activation of factor V by factor Xa. *Eur J Biochem.* 1997;247(1):12-20.
912. Vicic WJ, Lages B, Weiss HJ. Release of human platelet factor V activity is induced by both collagen and ADP and is inhibited by aspirin. *Blood.* 1980;56(3):448-455.
913. Bradford HN, Annamalai A, Doshi K, Colman RW. Factor V is activated and cleaved by platelet calpain: comparison with thrombin proteolysis. *Blood.* 1988;71(2):388-394.
914. Allen DH, Tracy PB. Human coagulation factor V is activated to the functional cofactor by elastase and cathepsin G expressed at the monocyte surface. *J Biol Chem.* 1995;270(3):1408-1415.
915. Camire RM, Kalafatis M, Tracy PB. Proteolysis of factor V by cathepsin G and elastase indicates that cleavage at Arg1545 optimizes cofactor function by facilitating factor Xa binding. *Biochemistry.* 1998;37(34):11896-11906.
916. Kalafatis M, Mann KG. The role of the membrane in the inactivation of factor va by plasmin. Amino acid region 307-348 of factor V plays a critical role in factor Va cofactor function. *J Biol Chem.* 2001;276(21):18614-18623.
917. Zeibdawi AR, Pryzdial EL. Mechanism of factor Va inactivation by plasmin. Loss of A2 and A3 domains from a Ca2+-dependent complex of fragments bound to phospholipid. *J Biol Chem.* 2001;276(23):19929-19936.
918. Lee CD, Mann KG. Activation/inactivation of human factor V by plasmin. *Blood.* 1989;73(1):185-190.
919. Tracy RP, Rubin DZ, Mann KG, et al. Thrombolytic therapy and proteolysis of factor V. *J Am Coll Cardiol.* 1997;30(3):716-724.
920. Shen L, Dahlback B. Factor V and protein S as synergistic cofactors to activated protein C in degradation of factor VIIIa. *J Biol Chem.* 1994;269(29):18735-18738.
921. Gierula M, Ahnstrom J. Anticoagulant protein S-New insights on interactions and functions. *J Thromb Haemost.* 2020;18(11):2801-2811.
922. Dahlback B. Novel insights into the regulation of coagulation by factor V isoforms, tissue factor pathway inhibitoralpha, and protein S. *J Thromb Haemost.* 2017;15(7):1241-1250.
923. Mast AE, Ruf W. Regulation of coagulation by tissue factor pathway inhibitor: implications for hemophilia therapy. *J Thromb Haemost.* 2022;20(6):1290-1300.
924. Toso R, Camire RM. Removal of B-domain sequences from factor V rather than specific proteolysis underlies the mechanism by which cofactor function is realized. *J Biol Chem.* 2004;279(20):21643-21650.
925. Kane WH, Devore-Carter D, Ortel TL. Expression and characterization of recombinant human factor V and a mutant lacking a major portion of the connecting region. *Biochemistry.* 1990;29(29):6762-6768.
926. Bos MH, Camire RM. A bipartite autoinhibitory region within the B-domain suppresses function in factor V. *J Biol Chem.* 2012;287(31):26342-26351.
927. Kuang SQ, Hasham S, Phillips MD, et al. Characterization of a novel autosomal dominant bleeding disorder in a large kindred from east Texas. *Blood.* 2001;97(6):1549-1554.
928. Vincent LM, Tran S, Livaja R, Bensend TA, Milewicz DM, Dahlback B. Coagulation factor V(A2440G) causes east Texas bleeding disorder via TFPIalpha. *J Clin Invest.* 2013;123(9):3777-3787.
929. Cunha ML, Bakhtiari K, Peter J, Marquart JA, Meijers JC, Middeldorp S. A novel mutation in the F5 gene (factor V Amsterdam) associated with bleeding independent of factor V procoagulant function. *Blood.* 2015;125(11):1822-1825.
930. Zimowski KL, Petrillo T, Ho MD, et al. F5-Atlanta: a novel mutation in F5 associated with enhanced East Texas splicing and FV-short production. *J Thromb Haemost.* 2021;19(7):1653-1665.
931. Peterson JA, Gupta S, Martinez ND, Hardesty B, Maroney SA, Mast AE. Factor V east Texas variant causes bleeding in a three-generation family. *J Thromb Haemost.* 2022;20(3):565-573.
932. Petrillo T, Ayombil F, Van't Veer C, Camire RM. Regulation of factor V and factor V-short by TFPIalpha: relationship between B-domain proteolysis and binding. *J Biol Chem.* 2021;296:100234.
933. Dahlback B, Guo LJ, Livaja-Koshiar R, Tran S. Factor V-short and protein S as synergistic tissue factor pathway inhibitor (TFPIalpha) cofactors. *Res Pract Thromb Haemost.* 2018;2(1):114-124.
934. Dahlback B, Tran S. The preAR2 region (1458-1492) in factor V-Short is crucial for the synergistic TFPIalpha-cofactor activity with protein S and the assembly of a trimolecular factor Xa-inhibitory complex comprising FV-Short, protein S, and TFPIalpha. *J Thromb Haemost.* 2022;20(1):58-68.
935. Mann KG, Hockin MF, Begin KJ, Kalafatis M. Activated protein C cleavage of factor Va leads to dissociation of the A2 domain. *J Biol Chem.* 1997;272(33):20678-20683.
936. Hockin MF, Cawthern KM, Kalafatis M, Mann KG. A model describing the inactivation of factor Va by APC: bond cleavage, fragment dissociation, and product inhibition. *Biochemistry.* 1999;38(21):6918-6934.
937. Bravo MC, Orfeo T, Mann KG, Everse SJ. Modeling of human factor Va inactivation by activated protein C. *BMC Syst Biol.* 2012;6:45.
938. Dahlback B, Carlsson M, Svensson PJ. Familial thrombophilia due to a previously unrecognized mechanism characterized by poor anticoagulant response to activated protein C: prediction of a cofactor to activated protein C. *Proc Natl Acad Sci U S A.* 1993;90(3):1004-1008.
939. Bertina RM, Koeleman BP, Koster T, et al. Mutation in blood coagulation factor V associated with resistance to activated protein C. *Nature.* 1994;369(6475):64-67.
940. Kalafatis M, Bernardi F, Simioni P, Lunghi B, Girolami A, Mann KG. Phenotype and genotype expression in pseudohomozygous factor VLEIDEN: the need for phenotype analysis. *Arterioscler Thromb Vasc Biol.* 1999;19(2):336-342.
941. Ridker PM, Miletich JP, Hennekens CH, Buring JE. Ethnic distribution of factor V Leiden in 4047 men and women. Implications for venous thromboembolism screening. *JAMA.* 1997;277(16):1305-1307.
942. Kalafatis M, Mann KG. Factor VLeiden and thrombophilia. *Arterioscler Thromb Vasc Biol.* 1997;17(4):620-627.
943. Kujovich JL. Factor V Leiden thrombophilia. *Genet Med.* 2011;13(1):1-16.
944. Beauchamp NJ, Daly ME, Hampton KK, Cooper PC, Preston FE, Peake IR. High prevalence of a mutation in the factor V gene within the U.K. population: relationship to activated protein C resistance and familial thrombosis. *Br J Haematol.* 1994;88(1):219-222.
945. Ridker PM, Hennekens CH, Lindpaintner K, Stampfer MJ, Eisenberg PR, Miletich JP. Mutation in the gene coding for coagulation factor V and the risk of myocardial infarction, stroke, and venous thrombosis in apparently healthy men. *N Engl J Med.* 1995;332(14):912-917.
946. Dahlback B. Factor V gene mutation causing inherited resistance to activated protein C as a basis for venous thromboembolism. *J Intern Med.* 1995;237(3):221-227.
947. Abildgaard CF, Suzuki Z, Harrison J, Jefcoat K, Zimmerman TS. Serial studies in von Willebrand's disease: variability versus "variants". *Blood.* 1980;56(4):712-716.
948. Koutts J, Walsh PN, Plow EF, Fenton JW,IInd, Bouma BN, Zimmerman TS. Active release of human platelet factor VIII-related antigen by adenosine diphosphate, collagen, and thrombin. *J Clin Invest.* 1978;62(6):1255-1263.
949. Gill JC, Endres-Brooks J, Bauer PJ, Marks WJ, Jr, Montgomery RR. The effect of ABO blood group on the diagnosis of von Willebrand disease. *Blood.* 1987;69(6):1691-1695.
950. van Schie MC, van Loon JE, de Maat MP, Leebeek FW. Genetic determinants of von Willebrand factor levels and activity in relation to the risk of cardiovascular disease: a review. *J Thromb Haemost.* 2011;9(5):899-908.

951. Moake JL, Olson JD, Troll JH, Jr, Weinger RS, Peterson DM, Cimo PL. Interaction of platelets, von Willebrand factor, and ristocetin during platelet agglutination. *J Lab Clin Med*. 1980;96(1):168-184.

952. Weiss HJ, Rogers J, Brand H. Defective ristocetin-induced platelet aggregation in von Willebrand's disease and its correction by factor VIII. *J Clin Invest*. 1973;52(11):2697-2707.

953. Von Willebrand EA. Hereditary pseudohaemophilia. *Haemophilia*. 1999;5(3):223-231. discussion 222.

954. Jorpes JE. E.A. von WILLEBRAND and von Willebrand's disease. *Nord Med*. 1962;67:729-732.

955. Nilsson IM, Blomback M, Jorpes E, Blomback B, Johansson SA. Von Willebrand's disease and its correction with human plasma fraction 1-0. *Acta Med Scand*. 1957;159(3):179-188.

956. Biggs R, Matthews JM. The treatment of haemorrhage in von Willebrand's disease and the blood level of factor VIII (AHG). *Br J Haematol*. 1963;9:203-214.

957. Rodeghiero F, Castaman G, Dini E. Epidemiological investigation of the prevalence of von Willebrand's disease. *Blood*. 1987;69(2):454-459.

958. Werner EJ, Broxson EH, Tucker EL, Giroux DS, Shults J, Abshire TC. Prevalence of von Willebrand disease in children: a multiethnic study. *J Pediatr*. 1993;123(6):893-898.

959. Berliner SA, Seligsohn U, Zivelin A, Zwang E, Sofferman G. A relatively high frequency of severe (type III) von Willebrand's disease in Israel. *Br J Haematol*. 1986;62(3):535-543.

960. Lenk H, Nilsson IM, Holmberg L, Weissbach G. Frequency of different types of von Willebrand's disease in the GDR. *Acta Med Scand*. 1988;224(3):275-280.

961. Ates E, Bakkaloglu A, Saatci U, Soylemezoglu O. von Willebrand factor antigen compared with other factors in vasculitic syndromes. *Arch Dis Child*. 1994;70(1):40-43.

962. Stevens TR, James JP, Simmonds NJ, et al. Circulating von Willebrand factor in inflammatory bowel disease. *Gut*. 1992;33(4):502-506.

963. Blann AD. von Willebrand factor antigen as an acute phase reactant and marker of endothelial cell injury in connective tissue diseases: a comparison with CRP, rheumatoid factor, and erythrocyte sedimentation rate. *Z Rheumatol*. 1991;50(5):320-322.

964. Pottinger BE, Read RC, Paleolog EM, Higgins PG, Pearson JD. von Willebrand factor is an acute phase reactant in man. *Thromb Res*. 1989;53(4):387-394.

965. Denis CV, Lenting PJ. von Willebrand factor: at the crossroads of bleeding and thrombosis. *Int J Hematol*. 2012;95(4):353-361.

966. Mancuso DJ, Tuley EA, Westfield LA, et al. Structure of the gene for human von Willebrand factor. *J Biol Chem*. 1989;264(33):19514-19527.

967. Mancuso DJ, Tuley EA, Westfield LA, et al. Human von Willebrand factor gene and pseudogene: structural analysis and differentiation by polymerase chain reaction. *Biochemistry*. 1991;30(1):253-269.

968. Shelton-Inloes BB, Chehab FF, Mannucci PM, Federici AB, Sadler JE. Gene deletions correlate with the development of alloantibodies in von Willebrand disease. *J Clin Invest*. 1987;79(5):1459-1465.

969. Jaffe EA, Hoyer LW, Nachman RL. Synthesis of von Willebrand factor by cultured human endothelial cells. *Proc Natl Acad Sci U S A*. 1974;71(5):1906-1909.

970. Sporn LA, Chavin SI, Marder VJ, Wagner DD. Biosynthesis of von Willebrand protein by human megakaryocytes. *J Clin Invest*. 1985;76(3):1102-1106.

971. Wagner DD, Olmsted JB, Marder VJ. Immunolocalization of von Willebrand protein in Weibel-Palade bodies of human endothelial cells. *J Cell Biol*. 1982;95(1):355-360.

972. Schwachtgen JL, Janel N, Barek L, et al. Ets transcription factors bind and transactivate the core promoter of the von Willebrand factor gene. *Oncogene*. 1997;15(25):3091-3102.

973. Slot JW, Bouma BN, Montgomery R, Zimmerman TS. Platelet factor VIII-related antigen: immunofluorescent localization. *Thromb Res*. 1978;13(5):871-881.

974. Coller BS, Hirschman RJ, Gralnick HR. Studies on the Factor VIII/von Willebrand factor antigen on human platelets. *Thromb Res*. 1975;6(6):469-480.

975. Guan J, Guillot PV, Aird WC. Characterization of the mouse von Willebrand factor promoter. *Blood*. 1999;94(10):3405-3412.

976. Jahroudi N, Lynch DC. Endothelial-cell-specific regulation of von Willebrand factor gene expression. *Mol Cell Biol*. 1994;14(2):999-1008.

977. Schwachtgen JL, Remacle JE, Janel N, et al. Oct-1 is involved in the transcriptional repression of the von willebrand factor gene promoter. *Blood*. 1998;92(4):1247-1258.

978. Ardekani AM, Greenberger JS, Jahroudi N. Two repressor elements inhibit expression of the von Willebrand factor gene promoter in vitro. *Thromb Haemost*. 1998;80(3):488-494.

979. Aird WC, Edelberg JM, Weiler-Guettler H, Simmons WW, Smith TW, Rosenberg RD. Vascular bed-specific expression of an endothelial cell gene is programmed by the tissue microenvironment. *J Cell Biol*. 1997;138(5):1117-1124.

980. Edelberg JM, Aird WC, Wu W, et al. PDGF mediates cardiac microvascular communication. *J Clin Invest*. 1998;102(4):837-843.

981. Collins CJ, Underdahl JP, Levene RB, et al. Molecular cloning of the human gene for von Willebrand factor and identification of the transcription initiation site. *Proc Natl Acad Sci U S A*. 1987;84(13):4393-4397.

982. Hamilton KK, Sims PJ. Changes in cytosolic Ca2+ associated with von Willebrand factor release in human endothelial cells exposed to histamine. Study of microcarrier cell monolayers using the fluorescent probe indo-1. *J Clin Invest*. 1987;79(2):600-608.

983. Menon C, Berry EW, Ockelford P. Beneficial effect of D.D.A.V.P. on bleeding-time in von Willebrand's disease. *Lancet*. 1978;2(8092 pt 1):743-744.

984. Takeuchi M, Nagura H, Kaneda T. DDAVP and epinephrine-induced changes in the localization of von Willebrand factor antigen in endothelial cells of human oral mucosa. *Blood*. 1988;72(3):850-854.

985. Denis CV, Christophe OD, Oortwijn BD, Lenting PJ. Clearance of von Willebrand factor. *Thromb Haemost*. 2008;99(2):271-278.

986. Sadler JE, Shelton-Inloes BB, Sorace JM, Harlan JM, Titani K, Davie EW. Cloning and characterization of two cDNAs coding for human von Willebrand factor. *Proc Natl Acad Sci U S A*. 1985;82(19):6394-6398.

987. Lynch DC, Zimmerman TS, Collins CJ, et al. Molecular cloning of cDNA for human von Willebrand factor: authentication by a new method. *Cell*. 1985;41(1):49-56.

988. Shelton-Inloes BB, Titani K, Sadler JE. cDNA sequences for human von Willebrand factor reveal five types of repeated domains and five possible protein sequence polymorphisms. *Biochemistry*. 1986;25(11):3164-3171.

989. Verweij CL, Diergaarde PJ, Hart M, Pannekoek H. Full-length von Willebrand factor (vWF) cDNA encodes a highly repetitive protein considerably larger than the mature vWF subunit. *EMBO J*. 1986;5(8):1839-1847.

990. Titani K, Kumar S, Takio K, et al. Amino acid sequence of human von Willebrand factor. *Biochemistry*. 1986;25(11):3171-3184.

991. Ginsburg D, Handin RI, Bonthron DT, et al. Human von Willebrand factor (vWF): isolation of complementary DNA (cDNA) clones and chromosomal localization. *Science*. 1985;228(4706):1401-1406.

992. Koller E, Winterhalter KH, Trueb B. The globular domains of type VI collagen are related to the collagen-binding domains of cartilage matrix protein and von Willebrand factor. *EMBO J*. 1989;8(4):1073-1077.

993. Sadler JE, Mancuso DJ, Randi AM, Tuley EA, Westfield LA. Molecular biology of von Willebrand factor. *Ann N Y Acad Sci*. 1991;614:114-124.

994. Hunt LT, Barker WC. von Willebrand factor shares a distinctive cysteine-rich domain with thrombospondin and procollagen. *Biochem Biophys Res Commun*. 1987;144(2):876-882.

995. Verweij CL, Hofker M, Quadt R, Briet E, Pannekoek H. RFLP for a human von Willebrand factor (vWF) cDNA clone, pvWF1100. *Nucleic Acids Res*. 1985;13(22):8289.

996. Santoro SA. Adsorption of von Willebrand factor/factor VIII by the genetically distinct interstitial collagens. *Thromb Res*. 1981;21(6):689-691.

997. Cruz MA, Yuan H, Lee JR, Wise RJ, Handin RI. Interaction of the von Willebrand factor (vWF) with collagen. Localization of the primary collagen-binding site by analysis of recombinant vWF a domain polypeptides. *J Biol Chem*. 1995;270(18):10822-10827.

998. Weiss HJ, Turitto VT, Baumgartner HR. Effect of shear rate on platelet interaction with subendothelium in citrated and native blood. I. Shear rate–dependent decrease of adhesion in von Willebrand's disease and the Bernard-Soulier syndrome. *J Lab Clin Med*. 1978;92(5):750-764.

999. Sakariassen KS, Nievelstein PF, Coller BS, Sixma JJ. The role of platelet membrane glycoproteins Ib and IIb-IIIa in platelet adherence to human artery subendothelium. *Br J Haematol*. 1986;63(4):681-691.

1000. Matsushita T, Sadler JE. Identification of amino acid residues essential for von Willebrand factor binding to platelet glycoprotein Ib. Charged-to-alanine scanning mutagenesis of the A1 domain of human von Willebrand factor. *J Biol Chem*. 1995;270(22):13406-13414.

1001. Bockenstedt P, Greenberg JM, Handin RI. Structural basis of von Willebrand factor binding to platelet glycoprotein Ib and collagen. Effects of disulfide reduction and limited proteolysis of polymeric von Willebrand factor. *J Clin Invest*. 1986;77(3):743-749.

1002. Girma JP, Kalafatis M, Pietu G, et al. Mapping of distinct von Willebrand factor domains interacting with platelet GPIb and GPIIb/IIIa and with collagen using monoclonal antibodies. *Blood*. 1986;67(5):1356-1366.

1003. Pareti FI, Fujimura Y, Dent JA, Holland LZ, Zimmerman TS, Ruggeri ZM. Isolation and characterization of a collagen binding domain in human von Willebrand factor. *J Biol Chem*. 1986;261(32):15310-15315.

1004. Ruggeri ZM, De Marco L, Gatti L, Bader R, Montgomery RR. Platelets have more than one binding site for von Willebrand factor. *J Clin Invest*. 1983;72(1):1-12.

1005. Schullek J, Jordan J, Montgomery RR. Interaction of von Willebrand factor with human platelets in the plasma milieu. *J Clin Invest*. 1984;73(2):421-428.

1006. Goto S, Salomon DR, Ikeda Y, Ruggeri ZM. Characterization of the unique mechanism mediating the shear-dependent binding of soluble von Willebrand factor to platelets. *J Biol Chem*. 1995;270(40):23352-23361.

1007. Ruggeri ZM, Bader R, de Marco L. Glanzmann thrombasthenia: deficient binding of von Willebrand factor to thrombin-stimulated platelets. *Proc Natl Acad Sci U S A*. 1982;79(19):6038-6041.

1008. Fujimoto T, Hawiger J. Adenosine diphosphate induces binding of von Willebrand factor to human platelets. *Nature*. 1982;297(5862):154-156.

1009. Fujimoto T, Ohara S, Hawiger J. Thrombin-induced exposure and prostacyclin inhibition of the receptor for factor VIII/von Willebrand factor on human platelets. *J Clin Invest*. 1982;69(6):1212-1222.

1010. Fay PJ, Coumans JV, Walker FJ. von Willebrand factor mediates protection of factor VIII from activated protein C-catalyzed inactivation. *J Biol Chem*. 1991;266(4):2172-2177.

1011. Swords NA, Mann KG. The assembly of the prothrombinase complex on adherent platelets. *Arterioscler Thromb*. 1993;13(11):1602-1612.

1012. Furlan M, Lammle B. Assays of von Willebrand factor-cleaving protease: a test for diagnosis of familial and acquired thrombotic thrombocytopenic purpura. *Semin Thromb Hemost*. 2002;28(2):167-172.

1013. Chung DW, Fujikawa K. Processing of von Willebrand factor by ADAMTS-13. *Biochemistry*. 2002;41(37):11065-11070.

1014. Fujikawa K, Suzuki H, McMullen B, Chung D. Purification of human von Willebrand factor-cleaving protease and its identification as a new member of the metalloproteinase family. *Blood*. 2001;98(5):1662-1666.

1015. Gerritsen HE, Robles R, Lammle B, Furlan M. Partial amino acid sequence of purified von Willebrand factor-cleaving protease. *Blood*. 2001;98(6):1654-1661.

1016. Tsai HM. ADAMTS13 and microvascular thrombosis. *Expert Rev Cardiovasc Ther.* 2006;4(6):813-825.

1017. P M. Die Chemie der Blutgerrinnung. *Ergebnisse der Physiologie.* 1905;4:307.

1018. Fuld E, Spiro K. Der Einfluss einiger gerinnungshemmender Agenzien auf das Vogelplasma. *Beitraege zur chemischen Physiologie und Pathologie, Braunschweig.* 1904;4:171.

1019. Bar-Shavit R, Kahn A, Mudd MS, Wilner GD, Mann KG, Fenton JW,IInd. Localization of a chemotactic domain in human thrombin. *Biochemistry.* 1984;23(3):397-400.

1020. Spraggon G, Everse SJ, Doolittle RF. Crystal structures of fragment D from human fibrinogen and its crosslinked counterpart from fibrin. *Nature.* 1997;389(6650):455-462.

1021. Hantgan R, McDonagh J, Hermans J. Fibrin assembly. *Ann N Y Acad Sci.* 1983;408:344-366.

1022. Lorand L, Jeong JM, Radek JT, Wilson J. Human plasma factor XIII: subunit interactions and activation of zymogen. *Methods Enzymol.* 1993;222:22-35.

1023. Yee VC, Pedersen LC, Le Trong I, Bishop PD, Stenkamp RE, Teller DC. Three-dimensional structure of a transglutaminase: human blood coagulation factor XIII. *Proc Natl Acad Sci U S A.* 1994;91(15):7296-7300.

1024. Bajzar L, Morser J, Nesheim M. TAFI, or plasma procarboxypeptidase B, couples the coagulation and fibrinolytic cascades through the thrombin-thrombomodulin complex. *J Biol Chem.* 1996;271(28):16603-16608.

1025. Lollar P, Parker CG. Subunit structure of thrombin-activated porcine factor VIII. *Biochemistry.* 1989;28(2):666-674.

1026. Berk BC, Taubman MB, Cragoe EJ, Jr, Fenton JW,IInd, Griendling KK. Thrombin signal transduction mechanisms in rat vascular smooth muscle cells. Calcium and protein kinase C-dependent and -independent pathways. *J Biol Chem.* 1990;265(28):17334-17340.

1027. Michel MC, Brass LF, Williams A, Bokoch GM, LaMorte VJ, Motulsky HJ. Alpha 2-adrenergic receptor stimulation mobilizes intracellular Ca2+ in human erythroleukemia cells. *J Biol Chem.* 1989;264(9):4986-4991.

1028. He CJ, Rondeau E, Medcalf RL, Lacave R, Schleuning WD, Sraer JD. Thrombin increases proliferation and decreases fibrinolytic activity of kidney glomerular epithelial cells. *J Cell Physiol.* 1991;146(1):131-140.

1029. Glenn KC, Carney DH, Fenton JW,IInd, Cunningham DD. Thrombin active site regions required for fibroblast receptor binding and initiation of cell division. *J Biol Chem.* 1980;255(14):6609-6616.

1030. Herbert JM, Lamarche I, Dol F. Induction of vascular smooth muscle cell growth by selective activation of the thrombin receptor. Effect of heparin. *FEBS Lett.* 1992;301(2):155-158.

1031. Harlan JM, Thompson PJ, Ross RR, Bowen-Pope DF. Alpha-thrombin induces release of platelet-derived growth factor-like molecule(s) by cultured human endothelial cells. *J Cell Biol.* 1986;103(3):1129-1133.

1032. Vlodavsky I, Folkman J, Sullivan R, et al. Endothelial cell-derived basic fibroblast growth factor: synthesis and deposition into subendothelial extracellular matrix. *Proc Natl Acad Sci U S A.* 1987;84(8):2292-2296.

1033. Ross R, Glomset J, Kariya B, Harker L. A platelet-dependent serum factor that stimulates the proliferation of arterial smooth muscle cells in vitro. *Proc Natl Acad Sci U S A.* 1974;71(4):1207-1210.

1034. Majesky MW, Lindner V, Twardzik DR, Schwartz SM, Reidy MA. Production of transforming growth factor beta 1 during repair of arterial injury. *J Clin Invest.* 1991;88(3):904-910.

1035. Clinton SK, Fleet JC, Loppnow H, et al. Interleukin-1 gene expression in rabbit vascular tissue in vivo. *Am J Pathol.* 1991;138(4):1005-1014.

1036. Douglas SA, Louden C, Vickery-Clark LM, et al. A role for endogenous endothelin-1 in neointimal formation after rat carotid artery balloon angioplasty. Protective effects of the novel nonpeptide endothelin receptor antagonist SB 209670. *Circ Res.* 1994;75(1):190-197.

1037. Sigal SL, Gellman J, Sarembock IJ, et al. Effects of serotonin-receptor blockade on angioplasty-induced vasospasm in an atherosclerotic rabbit model. *Arterioscler Thromb.* 1991;11(3):770-783.

1038. Mugge A, Heistad DD, Densen P, et al. Activation of leukocytes with complement C5a is associated with prostanoid-dependent constriction of large arteries in atherosclerotic monkeys in vivo. *Atherosclerosis.* 1992;95(2-3):211-222.

1039. Seino Y, Ikeda U, Ikeda M, et al. Interleukin 6 gene transcripts are expressed in human atherosclerotic lesions. *Cytokine.* 1994;6(1):87-91.

1040. Malik AB, Fenton JW,IInd. Thrombin-mediated increase in vascular endothelial permeability. *Semin Thromb Hemost.* 1992;18(2):193-199.

1041. Sugama Y, Malik AB. Thrombin receptor 14-amino acid peptide mediates endothelial hyperadhesivity and neutrophil adhesion by P-selectin-dependent mechanism. *Circ Res.* 1992;71(4):1015-1019.

1042. Hollenberg MD, Yang SG, Laniyonu AA, Moore GJ, Saifeddine M. Action of thrombin receptor polypeptide in gastric smooth muscle: identification of a core pentapeptide retaining full thrombin-mimetic intrinsic activity. *Mol Pharmacol.* 1992;42(2):186-191.

1043. Vouret-Craviari V, Van Obberghen-Schilling E, Rasmussen UB, Pavirani A, Lecocq JP, Pouyssegur J. Synthetic alpha-thrombin receptor peptides activate G protein-coupled signaling pathways but are unable to induce mitogenesis. *Mol Biol Cell.* 1992;3(1):95-102.

1044. Vu TK, Hung DT, Wheaton VI, Coughlin SR. Molecular cloning of a functional thrombin receptor reveals a novel proteolytic mechanism of receptor activation. *Cell.* 1991;64(6):1057-1068.

1045. Walker FJ. Regulation of activated protein C by protein S. The role of phospholipid in factor Va inactivation. *J Biol Chem.* 1981;256(21):11128-11131.

1046. Esmon CT. The roles of protein C and thrombomodulin in the regulation of blood coagulation. *J Biol Chem.* 1989;264(9):4743-4746.

1047. Walker FJ, Fay PJ. Regulation of blood coagulation by the protein C system. *FASEB J.* 1992;6(8):2561-2567.

1048. Jenny NS, MK. Thrombin. In: Colman RW, HJ , Marder VJ, Clowes AW, George JN, eds. *Hemostasis and Thrombosis: Basic Principles & Clinical Practice.* Lippincott, Williams & Wilkins; 2001:171-189.

1049. Poort SR, Michiels JJ, Reitsma PH, Bertina RM. Homozygosity for a novel missense mutation in the prothrombin gene causing a severe bleeding disorder. *Thromb Haemost.* 1994;72(6):819-824.

1050. Reuner KH, Ruf A, Grau A, et al. Prothrombin gene G20210-->A transition is a risk factor for cerebral venous thrombosis. *Stroke.* 1998;29(9):1765-1769.

1051. Hillarp A, Zoller B, Svensson PJ, Dahlback B. The 20210 A allele of the prothrombin gene is a common risk factor among Swedish outpatients with verified deep venous thrombosis. *Thromb Haemost.* 1997;78(3):990-992.

1052. Ferraresi P, Marchetti G, Legnani C, et al. The heterozygous 20210 G/A prothrombin genotype is associated with early venous thrombosis in inherited thrombophilias and is not increased in frequency in artery disease. *Arterioscler Thromb Vasc Biol.* 1997;17(11):2418-2422.

1053. Margaglione M, Brancaccio V, Giuliani N, et al. Increased risk for venous thrombosis in carriers of the prothrombin G-->A20210 gene variant. *Ann Intern Med.* 1998;129(2):89-93.

1054. Lundblad RL, Noyes CM, Mann KG, Kingdon HS. The covalent differences between bovine alpha- and beta-thrombin. A structural explanation for the changes in catalytic activity. *J Biol Chem.* 1979;254(17):8524-8528.

1055. Witting JI, Miller TM, Fenton JW,IInd. Human alpha- and gamma-thrombin specificity with tripeptide p-nitroanalide substrates under physiologically relevant conditions. *Thromb Res.* 1987;46(4):567-574.

1056. Stevens WK, Cote HF, MacGillivray RT, Nesheim ME. Calcium ion modulation of meizothrombin autolysis at Arg55-Asp56 and catalytic activity. *J Biol Chem.* 1996;271(14):8062-8067.

1057. Tracy PB, Eide LL, Bowie EJ, Mann KG. Radioimmunoassay of factor V in human plasma and platelets. *Blood.* 1982;60(1):59-63.

1058. Keenan JP, Solum NO. Quantitative studies on the release of platelet fibrinogen by thrombin. *Br J Haematol.* 1972;23(4):461-466.

1059. Niewiarowski S, Thomas DP. Platelet factor 4 and adenosine diphosphate release during human platelet aggregation. *Nature.* 1969;222(5200):1269-1270.

1060. Levine SP, Wohl H. Human platelet factor 4: purification and characterization by affinity chromatography. Purification of human platelet factor 4. *J Biol Chem.* 1976;251(2):324-328.

1061. Lawler JW, Slayter HS, Coligan JE. Isolation and characterization of a high molecular weight glycoprotein from human blood platelets. *J Biol Chem.* 1978;253(23):8609-8616.

1062. Zucker MB, Mosesson MW, Broekman MJ, Kaplan KL. Release of platelet fibronectin (cold-insoluble globulin) from alpha granules induced by thrombin or collagen; lack of requirement for plasma fibronectin in ADP-induced platelet aggregation. *Blood.* 1979;54(1):8-12.

1063. Viskup RW, Tracy PB, Mann KG. The isolation of human platelet factor V. *Blood.* 1987;69(4):1188-1195.

1064. Larsen E, Celi A, Gilbert GE, et al. PADGEM protein: a receptor that mediates the interaction of activated platelets with neutrophils and monocytes. *Cell.* 1989;59(2):305-312.

1065. Hamburger SA, McEver RP. GMP-140 mediates adhesion of stimulated platelets to neutrophils. *Blood.* 1990;75(3):550-554.

1066. Wang W, Boffa MB, Bajzar L, Walker JB, Nesheim ME. A study of the mechanism of inhibition of fibrinolysis by activated thrombin-activable fibrinolysis inhibitor. *J Biol Chem.* 1998;273(42):27176-27181.

1067. Valnickova Z, Enghild JJ. Human procarboxypeptidase U, or thrombin-activable fibrinolysis inhibitor, is a substrate for transglutaminases. Evidence for transglutaminase-catalyzed cross-linking to fibrin. *J Biol Chem.* 1998;273(42):27220-27224.

1068. Brummel KE, Butenas S, Mann KG. An integrated study of fibrinogen during blood coagulation. *J Biol Chem.* 1999;274(32):22862-22870.

1069. von dem Borne PA, Mosnier LO, Tans G, Meijers JC, Bouma BN. Factor XI activation by meizothrombin: stimulation by phospholipid vesicles containing both phosphatidylserine and phosphatidylethanolamine. *Thromb Haemost.* 1997;78(2):834-839.

1070. Tans G, Nicolaes GA, Thomassen MC, et al. Activation of human factor V by meizothrombin. *J Biol Chem.* 1994;269(23):15969-15972.

1071. Di Cera E. Thrombin as an anticoagulant. *Prog Mol Biol Transl Sci.* 2011;99:145-184.

1072. Esmon CT, Owen WG. Identification of an endothelial cell cofactor for thrombin-catalyzed activation of protein C. *Proc Natl Acad Sci U S A.* 1981;78(4):2249-2252.

1073. Bagdasarian A, Colman RW. Subcellular localization and purification of platelet alpha1-antitrypsin. *Blood.* 1978;51(1):139-156.

1074. Schwarz HP, Heeb MJ, Wencel-Drake JD, Griffin JH. Identification and quantitation of protein S in human platelets. *Blood.* 1985;66(6):1452-1455.

1075. Novotny WF, Girard TJ, Miletich JP, Broze GJ, Jr. Platelets secrete a coagulation inhibitor functionally and antigenically similar to the lipoprotein associated coagulation inhibitor. *Blood.* 1988;72(6):2020-2025.

1076. Antoniades HN. Human platelet-derived growth factor (PDGF): purification of PDGF-I and PDGF-II and separation of their reduced subunits. *Proc Natl Acad Sci U S A.* 1981;78(12):7314-7317.

1077. Heldin CH, Westermark B, Wasteson A. Platelet-derived growth factor. Isolation by a large-scale procedure and analysis of subunit composition. *Biochem J.* 1981;193(3):907-913.

1078. Deuel TF, Huang JS, Proffitt RT, Baenziger JU, Chang D, Kennedy BB. Human platelet-derived growth factor. Purification and resolution into two active protein fractions. *J Biol Chem.* 1981;256(17):8896-8899.

1079. Raines EW, Ross R. Platelet-derived growth factor. I. High yield purification and evidence for multiple forms. *J Biol Chem.* 1982;257(9):5154-5160.

1080. Childs CB, Proper JA, Tucker RF, Moses HL. Serum contains a platelet-derived transforming growth factor. *Proc Natl Acad Sci U S A*. 1982;79(17):5312-5316.
1081. Clemmons DR, Isley WL, Brown MT. Dialyzable factor in human serum of platelet origin stimulates endothelial cell replication and growth. *Proc Natl Acad Sci U S A*. 1983;80(6):1641-1645.
1082. King GL, Buchwald S. Characterization and partial purification of an endothelial cell growth factor from human platelets. *J Clin Invest*. 1984;73(2):392-396.
1083. Harrison P, Cramer EM. Platelet alpha-granules. *Blood Rev*. 1993;7(1):52-62.
1084. Hou L, Howells GL, Kapas S, Macey MG. The protease-activated receptors and their cellular expression and function in blood-related cells. *Br J Haematol*. 1998;101(1):1-9.
1085. Vu TK, Wheaton VI, Hung DT, Charo I, Coughlin SR. Domains specifying thrombin-receptor interaction. *Nature*. 1991;353(6345):674-677.
1086. Schmidt VA, Nierman WC, Maglott DR, et al. The human proteinase-activated receptor-3 (PAR-3) gene. Identification within a Par gene cluster and characterization in vascular endothelial cells and platelets. *J Biol Chem*. 1998;273(24):15061-15068.
1087. Estevez B, Kim K, Delaney MK, et al. Signaling-mediated cooperativity between glycoprotein Ib-IX and protease-activated receptors in thrombin-induced platelet activation. *Blood*. 2016;127(5):626-636.
1088. Seegers WH, McCoy L, Kipfer RK, Murano G. Preparation and properties of thrombin. *Arch Biochem Biophys*. 1968;128(1):194-201.
1089. Mann KG, Batt CW. The molecular weights of bovine thrombin and its primary autolysis products. *J Biol Chem*. 1969;244(23):6555-6557.
1090. Rosenberg RD, Waugh DF. Multiple bovine thrombin components. *J Biol Chem*. 1970;245(19):5049-5056.
1091. Boissel JP, Le Bonniec B, Rabiet MJ, Labie D, Elion J. Covalent structures of beta and gamma autolytic derivatives of human alpha-thrombin. *J Biol Chem*. 1984;259(9):5691-5697.
1092. Fenton JWLB, Walz DA, Finlayson JS. Human thrombosis. In: Lundblad RL, FJ , Mann KG, eds. *The Chemistry and Biology of Thrombin*. Ann Arbor Press; 1977:43-70.
1093. Lottenberg R, Hall JA, Fenton JW,IInd, Jackson CM. The action of thrombin on peptide p-nitroanilide substrates: hydrolysis of Tos-Gly-Pro-Arg-pNA and D-Phe-Pip-Arg-pNA by human alpha and gamma and bovine alpha and beta-thrombins. *Thromb Res*. 1982;28(3):313-332.
1094. Lorand L, Credo RB. Thrombin and fibrin stabilization. In: Lundblad RL, FJ , Mann KG, eds. *The Chemistry and Biology of Thrombin*. Ann Arbor Press; 1977:311-323.
1095. Bezeaud A, Denninger MH, Guillin MC. Interaction of human alpha-thrombin and gamma-thrombin with antithrombin III, protein C and thrombomodulin. *Eur J Biochem*. 1985;153(3):491-496.
1096. Seegers WH, McCoy LE, Walz DA, Reuterby J, Andary TJ. Isolation of thrombin-E and the evolution of enzyme activity from prothrombin. *Experientia*. 1974;30(10):1130-1132.
1097. Matafonov A, Sarilla S, Sun MF, et al. Activation of factor XI by products of prothrombin activation. *Blood*. 2011;118(2):437-445.
1098. Lundblad RL, Nesheim ME, Straight DL, et al. Bovine alpha- and beta-thrombin. Reduced fibrinogen-clotting activity of beta-thrombin is not a consequence of reduced affinity for fibrinogen. *J Biol Chem*. 1984;259(11):6991-6995.
1099. Berliner LJ, Shen YY. Physical evidence for an apolar binding site near the catalytic center of human alpha-thrombin. *Biochemistry*. 1977;16(21):4622-4626.
1100. Di Cera E, Guinto ER, Vindigni A, et al. The Na+ binding site of thrombin. *J Biol Chem*. 1995;270(38):22089-22092.
1101. Tulinsky A. Molecular interactions of thrombin. *Semin Thromb Hemost*. 1996;22(2):117-124.
1102. Folkers PJ, Clore GM, Driscoll PC, Dodt J, Kohler S, Gronenborn AM. Solution structure of recombinant hirudin and the Lys-47–Glu mutant: a nuclear magnetic resonance and hybrid distance geometry-dynamical simulated annealing study. *Biochemistry*. 1989;28(6):2601-2617.
1103. Haruyama H, Wuthrich K. Conformation of recombinant desulfatohirudin in aqueous solution determined by nuclear magnetic resonance. *Biochemistry*. 1989;28(10):4301-4312.
1104. Stone SR, Braun PJ, Hofsteenge J. Identification of regions of alpha-thrombin involved in its interaction with hirudin. *Biochemistry*. 1987;26(15):4617-4624.
1105. Braun PJ, Dennis S, Hofsteenge J, Stone SR. Use of site-directed mutagenesis to investigate the basis for the specificity of hirudin. *Biochemistry*. 1988;27(17):6517-6522.
1106. Chang JY, Ngai PK, Rink H, Dennis S, Schlaeppi JM. The structural elements of hirudin which bind to the fibrinogen recognition site of thrombin are exclusively located within its acidic C-terminal tail. *FEBS Lett*. 1990;261(2):287-290.
1107. Stone SR, Hofsteenge J. Kinetics of the inhibition of thrombin by hirudin. *Biochemistry*. 1986;25(16):4622-4628.
1108. Gorman JJ. Inhibition of human thrombin assessed with different substrates and inhibitors. Characterization of fibrinopeptide binding interaction. *Biochim Biophys Acta*. 1975;412(2):273-282.
1109. Olson ST, Bock PE, Kvassman J, et al. Role of the catalytic serine in the interactions of serine proteinases with protein inhibitors of the serpin family. Contribution of a covalent interaction to the binding energy of serpin-proteinase complexes. *J Biol Chem*. 1995;270(50):30007-30017.
1110. Fuchs HE, Shifman MA, Pizzo SV. In vivo catabolism of alpha 1-proteinase inhibitor-trypsin, antithrombin III-thrombin and alpha 2-macroglobulin-methylamine. *Biochim Biophys Acta*. 1982;716(2):151-157.
1111. Ganrot PO. Inhibition of plasmin activity by alpha-2-macroglobulin. *Clin Chim Acta*. 1967;16(2):328-329.
1112. Barrett AJ. Alpha 2-macroglobulin. *Methods Enzymol*. 1981;80(pt C):737-754.
1113. Barrett AJ, Starkey PM. The interaction of alpha 2-macroglobulin with proteinases. Characteristics and specificity of the reaction, and a hypothesis concerning its molecular mechanism. *Biochem J*. 1973;133(4):709-724.
1114. Pizzo SV, Gonias SL. Receptor-mediated protease regulation. In: Conn PM, ed. *The Receptors*. Academic Press; 1984:177-206.
1115. Gonias SL, Pizzo SV. Chemical and structural modifications of alpha 2-macroglobulin: effects on receptor binding and endocytosis studied in an in vivo model. *Ann N Y Acad Sci*. 1983;421:457-471.
1116. Huntington JA. Natural inhibitors of thrombin. *Thromb Haemost*. 2014;111(4):583-589.
1117. Dahlback B, Villoutreix BO. Regulation of blood coagulation by the protein C anticoagulant pathway: novel insights into structure-function relationships and molecular recognition. *Arterioscler Thromb Vasc Biol*. 2005;25(7):1311-1320.
1118. Wildhagen KC, Lutgens E, Loubele ST, ten Cate H, Nicolaes GA. The structure-function relationship of activated protein C. Lessons from natural and engineered mutations. *Thromb Haemost*. 2011;106(6):1034-1045.
1119. Griffin JH, Zlokovic BV, Mosnier LO. Protein C anticoagulant and cytoprotective pathways. *Int J Hematol*. 2012;95(4):333-345.
1120. Mammen EF, Thomas WR, Seegers WH. Activation of purified prothrombin to autoprothrombin I or autoprothrombin II (platelet cofactor II or autoprothrombin II-A). *Thromb Diath Haemorrh*. 1960;5:218-249.
1121. Miletich J, Sherman L, Broze G, Jr. Absence of thrombosis in subjects with heterozygous protein C deficiency. *N Engl J Med*. 1987;317(16):991-996.
1122. Okajima K, Koga S, Kaji M, et al. Effect of protein C and activated protein C on coagulation and fibrinolysis in normal human subjects. *Thromb Haemost*. 1990;63(1):48-53.
1123. Marlar RA, Sills RH, Groncy PK, Montgomery RR, Madden RM. Protein C survival during replacement therapy in homozygous protein C deficiency. *Am J Hematol*. 1992;41(1):24-31.
1124. Bauer KA. Coumarin-induced skin necrosis. *Arch Dermatol*. 1993;129(6):766-768.
1125. Epstein DJ, Bergum PW, Bajaj SP, Rapaport SI. Radioimmunoassays for protein C and factor X. Plasma antigen levels in abnormal hemostatic states. *Am J Clin Pathol*. 1984;82(5):573-581.
1126. McGehee WG, Klotz TA, Epstein DJ, Rapaport SI. Coumarin necrosis associated with hereditary protein C deficiency. *Ann Intern Med*. 1984;101(1):59-60.
1127. Broekmans AW, Bertina RM, Loeliger EA, Hofmann V, Klingemann HG. Protein C and the development of skin necrosis during anticoagulant therapy. *Thromb Haemost*. 1983;49(3):251.
1128. Goldberg SL, Orthner CL, Yalisove BL, Elgart ML, Kessler CM. Skin necrosis following prolonged administration of coumarin in a patient with inherited protein S deficiency. *Am J Hematol*. 1991;38(1):64-66.
1129. Thompson AR. Molecular genetics of hemostatis proteins. In: Colman RW, Hirsh J, Marder VJ, Salzman EW, eds. *Hemostasis and Thrombosis: Basic Principles and Clinical Practice*. Lippincott; 1994:55-80.
1130. Bovill EG, Hasstedt SJ, Leppert MF, Long GL. Hereditary thrombophilia as a model for multigenic disease. *Thromb Haemost*. 1999;82(2):662-666.
1131. Lu D, Bovill EG, Long GL. Molecular mechanism for familial protein C deficiency and thrombosis in protein CVermont (Glu20-->Ala and Val34-->Met). *J Biol Chem*. 1994;269(46):29032-29038.
1132. Hasstedt SJ, Bovill EG, Callas PW, Long GL. An unknown genetic defect increases venous thrombosis risk, through interaction with protein C deficiency. *Am J Hum Genet*. 1998;63(2):569-576.
1133. Plutzky J, Hoskins JA, Long GL, Crabtree GR. Evolution and organization of the human protein C gene. *Proc Natl Acad Sci U S A*. 1986;83(3):546-550.
1134. Kato A, Miura O, Sumi Y, Aoki N. Assignment of the human protein C gene (PROC) to chromosome region 2q14–q21 by in situ hybridization. *Cytogenet Cell Genet*. 1988;47(1-2):46-47.
1135. Spek CA, Greengard JS, Griffin JH, Bertina RM, Reitsma PH. Two mutations in the promoter region of the human protein C gene both cause type I protein C deficiency by disruption of two HNF-3 binding sites. *J Biol Chem*. 1995;270(41):24216-24221.
1136. Miao CH, Ho WT, Greenberg DL, Davie EW. Transcriptional regulation of the gene coding for human protein C. *J Biol Chem*. 1996;271(16):9587-9594.
1137. Furie B, Furie BC. The molecular basis of blood coagulation. *Cell*. 1988;53(4):505-518.
1138. Taylor FB, Jr, Chang A, Hinshaw LB, Esmon CT, Archer LT, Beller BK. A model for thrombin protection against endotoxin. *Thromb Res*. 1984;36(2):177-185.
1139. Comp PC. Hereditary disorders predisposing to thrombosis. *Prog Hemost Thromb*. 1986;8:71-102.
1140. Grinnell BW, WJ, Gerlitz B, et al. Native and modified recombinant human protein C: function, secretion, and posttranslational modifications. In: Bruley DF, DW , eds. *Protein C and Related Anticoagulants*. Gulf Publishing Company; 1991:29-63.
1141. Esmon CT. Protein C. *Prog Hemost Thromb*. 1984;7:25-54.
1142. Stenflo J. Structure and function of protein C. *Semin Thromb Hemost*. 1984;10(2):109-121.
1143. Preissner KT. Biological relevance of the protein C system and laboratory diagnosis of protein C and protein S deficiencies. *Clin Sci (Lond)*. 1990;78(4):351-364.
1144. Ohlin AK, Stenflo J. Calcium-dependent interaction between the epidermal growth factor precursor-like region of human protein C and a monoclonal antibody. *J Biol Chem*. 1987;262(28):13798-13804.
1145. Ohlin AK, Linse S, Stenflo J. Calcium binding to the epidermal growth factor homology region of bovine protein C. *J Biol Chem*. 1988;263(15):7411-7417.
1146. Rezaie AR, Mather T, Sussman F, Esmon CT. Mutation of Glu-80-->Lys results in a protein C mutant that no longer requires Ca2+ for rapid activation by the thrombin-thrombomodulin complex. *J Biol Chem*. 1994;269(5):3151-3154.
1147. Cheng CH, Geng JP, Castellino FJ. The functions of the first epidermal growth factor homology region of human protein C as revealed by a charge-to-alanine scanning mutagenesis investigation. *Biol Chem*. 1997;378(12):1491-1500.
1148. Castellino FJ. Human protein C and activated protein C Components of the human anticoagulation system. *Trends Cardiovasc Med*. 1995;5(2):55-62.

1149. Kisiel W. Human plasma protein C: isolation, characterization, and mechanism of activation by alpha-thrombin. *J Clin Invest.* 1979;64(3):761-769.

1150. Kisiel W, Canfield WM. Snake venom proteases that activate blood-coagulation factor V. *Methods Enzymol.* 1981;80(pt C):275-285.

1151. Weiler-Guettler H, Christie PD, Beeler DL, et al. A targeted point mutation in thrombomodulin generates viable mice with a prethrombotic state. *J Clin Invest.* 1998;101(9):1983-1991.

1152. Varadi K, Philapitsch A, Santa T, Schwarz HP. Activation and inactivation of human protein C by plasmin. *Thromb Haemost.* 1994;71(5):615-621.

1153. Cote HC, Bajzar L, Stevens WK, et al. Functional characterization of recombinant human meizothrombin and Meizothrombin(desF1). Thrombomodulin-dependent activation of protein C and thrombin-activatable fibrinolysis inhibitor (TAFI), platelet aggregation, antithrombin-III inhibition. *J Biol Chem.* 1997;272(10):6194-6200.

1154. Haley PE, Doyle MF, Mann KG. The activation of bovine protein C by factor Xa. *J Biol Chem.* 1989;264(27):16303-16310.

1155. Thompson EA, Salem HH. Factors IXa, Xa, XIa and activated protein C do not have protein C activating ability in the presence of thrombomodulin. *Thromb Haemost.* 1988;59(2):339.

1156. Wu Q, Tsiang M, Lentz SR, Sadler JE. Ligand specificity of human thrombomodulin. Equilibrium binding of human thrombin, meizothrombin, and factor Xa to recombinant thrombomodulin. *J Biol Chem.* 1992;267(10):7083-7088.

1157. McRae SJ, Stafford AR, Fredenburgh JC, Weitz JI. In the presence of phospholipids, glycosaminoglycans potentiate factor Xa-mediated protein C activation by modulating factor Xa activity. *Biochemistry.* 2007;46(13):4195-4203.

1158. Klein JD, Walker FJ. Purification of a protein C activator from the venom of the southern copperhead snake (Agkistrodon contortrix contortrix). *Biochemistry.* 1986;25(15):4175-4179.

1159. Koshiar RL, Somajo S, Norstrom E, Dahlback B. Erythrocyte-derived microparticles supporting activated protein C-mediated regulation of blood coagulation. *PLoS One.* 2014;9(8):e104200.

1160. Norstrom EA, Tran S, Steen M, Dahlback B. Effects of factor Xa and protein S on the individual activated protein C-mediated cleavages of coagulation factor Va. *J Biol Chem.* 2006;281(42):31486-31494.

1161. Bajzar L, Nesheim ME, Tracy PB. The profibrinolytic effect of activated protein C in clots formed from plasma is TAFI-dependent. *Blood.* 1996;88(6):2093-2100.

1162. Bajzar L, Kalafatis M, Simioni P, Tracy PB. An antifibrinolytic mechanism describing the prothrombotic effect associated with factor VLeiden. *J Biol Chem.* 1996;271(38):22949-22952.

1163. Esmon CT. Structure and functions of the endothelial cell protein C receptor. *Crit Care Med.* 2004;32(5 suppl):S298-S301.

1164. Fukudome K, Esmon CT. Identification, cloning, and regulation of a novel endothelial cell protein C/activated protein C receptor. *J Biol Chem.* 1994;269(42):26486-26491.

1165. Montes R, Puy C, Molina E, Hermida J. Is EPCR a multi-ligand receptor? Pros and cons. *Thromb Haemost.* 2012;107(5):815-826.

1166. Hancock WW, Grey ST, Hau L, et al. Binding of activated protein C to a specific receptor on human mononuclear phagocytes inhibits intracellular calcium signaling and monocyte-dependent proliferative responses. *Transplantation.* 1995;60(12):1525-1532.

1167. Ahmad MF, BF, Esmon CT, Hancock WW. Cloning and in vitro analysis of the endothelial protein C receptor (EPCR) on human monocytes show that monocyte EPCR does not mediate the anti-inflammatory effects of activated protein C. *Blood.* 1997;90:32a.

1168. Esmon CT. Inflammation and the activated protein C anticoagulant pathway. *Semin Thromb Hemost.* 2006;32(suppl 1):49-60.

1169. Taylor FB, Jr, Chang A, Esmon CT, D'Angelo A, Vigano-D'Angelo S, Blick KE. Protein C prevents the coagulopathic and lethal effects of Escherichia coli infusion in the baboon. *J Clin Invest.* 1987;79(3):918-925.

1170. Hancock WW, Tsuchida A, Hau H, Thomson NM, Salem HH. The anticoagulants protein C and protein S display potent antiinflammatory and immunosuppressive effects relevant to transplant biology and therapy. *Transplant Proc.* 1992;24(5):2302-2303.

1171. Mosnier LO, Zlokovic BV, Griffin JH. The cytoprotective protein C pathway. *Blood.* 2007;109(8):3161-3172.

1172. Della Valle P, Pavani G, D'Angelo A. The protein C pathway and sepsis. *Thromb Res.* 2012;129(3):296-300.

1173. Sinha RK, Wang Y, Zhao Z, et al. PAR1 biased signaling is required for activated protein C in vivo benefits in sepsis and stroke. *Blood.* 2018;131(11):1163-1171.

1174. Taoka Y, Okajima K, Uchiba M, et al. Activated protein C reduces the severity of compression-induced spinal cord injury in rats by inhibiting activation of leukocytes. *J Neurosci.* 1998;18(4):1393-1398.

1175. Moore KL, Andreoli SP, Esmon NL, Esmon CT, Bang NU. Endotoxin enhances tissue factor and suppresses thrombomodulin expression of human vascular endothelium in vitro. *J Clin Invest.* 1987;79(1):124-130.

1176. Nawroth PP, Handley DA, Esmon CT, Stern DM. Interleukin 1 induces endothelial cell procoagulant while suppressing cell-surface anticoagulant activity. *Proc Natl Acad Sci U S A.* 1986;83(10):3460-3464.

1177. Hirokawa K, Aoki N. Regulatory mechanisms for thrombomodulin expression in human umbilical vein endothelial cells in vitro. *J Cell Physiol.* 1991;147(1):157-165.

1178. Maruyama I, Soejima Y, Osame M, et al. Increased expression of thrombomodulin on the cultured human umbilical vein endothelial cells and mouse hemangioma cells by cyclic AMP. *Thromb Res.* 1991;61(3):301-310.

1179. Ohji T, Urano H, Shirahata A, et al. Transforming growth factor beta 1 and beta 2 induce down-modulation of thrombomodulin in human umbilical vein endothelial cells. *Thromb Haemost.* 1995;73(5):812-818.

1180. Moore KL, Esmon CT, Esmon NL. Tumor necrosis factor leads to the internalization and degradation of thrombomodulin from the surface of bovine aortic endothelial cells in culture. *Blood.* 1989;73(1):159-165.

1181. Conway EM, Rosenberg RD. Tumor necrosis factor suppresses transcription of the thrombomodulin gene in endothelial cells. *Mol Cell Biol.* 1988;8(12):5588-5592.

1182. Lentz SR, Tsiang M, Sadler JE. Regulation of thrombomodulin by tumor necrosis factor-alpha: comparison of transcriptional and posttranscriptional mechanisms. *Blood.* 1991;77(3):542-550.

1183. Ohdama S, Takano S, Ohashi K, Miyake S, Aoki N. Pentoxifylline prevents tumor necrosis factor-induced suppression of endothelial cell surface thrombomodulin. *Thromb Res.* 1991;62(6):745-755.

1184. Yu K, Morioka H, Fritze LM, Beeler DL, Jackman RW, Rosenberg RD. Transcriptional regulation of the thrombomodulin gene. *J Biol Chem.* 1992;267(32):23237-23247.

1185. Heeb MJ, Espana F, Geiger M, Collen D, Stump DC, Griffin JH. Immunological identity of heparin-dependent plasma and urinary protein C inhibitor and plasminogen activator inhibitor-3. *J Biol Chem.* 1987;262(33):15813-15816.

1186. Stief TW, Radtke KP, Heimburger N. Inhibition of urokinase by protein C-inhibitor (PCI). Evidence for identity of PCI and plasminogen activator inhibitor 3. *Biol Chem Hoppe Seyler.* 1987;368(10):1427-1433.

1187. Espana F, GJ. Plasma protein C inhibitor (PCI) inhibits procoagulant and profibrinolytic enzymes. *Blood.* 1987;70:401a.

1188. Dahlback B. Purification of human C4b-binding protein and formation of its complex with vitamin K-dependent protein S. *Biochem J.* 1983;209(3):847-856.

1189. Fair DS, Revak DJ. Quantitation of human protein S in the plasma of normal and warfarin-treated individuals by radioimmunoassay. *Thromb Res.* 1984;36(6):527-535.

1190. Walker FJ. Regulation of activated protein C by a new protein. A possible function for bovine protein S. *J Biol Chem.* 1980;255(12):5521-5524.

1191. Suzuki K, Nishioka J, Matsuda M, Murayama H, Hashimoto S. Protein S is essential for the activated protein C-catalyzed inactivation of platelet-associated factor Va. *J Biochem.* 1984;96(2):455-460.

1192. Walker FJ, Chavin SI, Fay PJ. Inactivation of factor VIII by activated protein C and protein S. *Arch Biochem Biophys.* 1987;252(1):322-328.

1193. Walker FJ. Protein S and the regulation of activated protein C. *Semin Thromb Hemost.* 1984;10(2):131-138.

1194. Walker FJ. Regulation of vitamin K-dependent protein S. Inactivation by thrombin. *J Biol Chem.* 1984;259(16):10335-10339.

1195. Solymoss S, Tucker MM, Tracy PB. Kinetics of inactivation of membrane-bound factor Va by activated protein C. Protein S modulates factor Xa protection. *J Biol Chem.* 1988;263(29):14884-14890.

1196. Marlar RA, Gausman JN. Protein S abnormalities: a diagnostic nightmare. *Am J Hematol.* 2011;86(5):418-421.

1197. Wypasek E, Karpinski M, Alhenc-Gelas M, Undas A. Venous thromboembolism associated with protein S deficiency due to Arg451* mutation in PROS1 gene: a case report and a literature review. *J Genet.* 2017;96(6):1047-1051.

1198. Kang J, Kim HS. Where are the secrets of increased thrombosis and Aneurysm formation with the current Bioresorbable vascular scaffolds hidden? reply. *Circ J.* 2018;82(2):609-610.

1199. Comp PC, Nixon RR, Cooper MR, Esmon CT. Familial protein S deficiency is associated with recurrent thrombosis. *J Clin Invest.* 1984;74(6):2082-2088.

1200. Schwarz HP, Fischer M, Hopmeier P, Batard MA, Griffin JH. Plasma protein S deficiency in familial thrombotic disease. *Blood.* 1984;64(6):1297-1300.

1201. Comp PC, Esmon CT. Recurrent venous thromboembolism in patients with a partial deficiency of protein S. *N Engl J Med.* 1984;311(24):1525-1528.

1202. Broekmans AW, Bertina RM, Reinalda-Poot J, et al. Hereditary protein S deficiency and venous thrombo-embolism. A study in three Dutch families. *Thromb Haemost.* 1985;53(2):273-277.

1203. Kamiya T, Sugihara T, Ogata K, et al. Inherited deficiency of protein S in a Japanese family with recurrent venous thrombosis: a study of three generations. *Blood.* 1986;67(2):406-410.

1204. Mahasandana C, Suvatte V, Chuansumrit A, et al. Homozygous protein S deficiency in an infant with purpura fulminans. *J Pediatr.* 1990;117(5):750-753.

1205. Pegelow CH, Ledford M, Young JN, Zilleruelo G. Severe protein S deficiency in a newborn. *Pediatrics.* 1992;89(4 pt 1):674-676.

1206. Heeb MJ, Mesters RM, Tans G, Rosing J, Griffin JH. Binding of protein S to factor Va associated with inhibition of prothrombinase that is independent of activated protein C. *J Biol Chem.* 1993;268(4):2872-2877.

1207. Heeb MJ, Rosing J, Bakker HM, Fernandez JA, Tans G, Griffin JH. Protein S binds to and inhibits factor Xa. *Proc Natl Acad Sci U S A.* 1994;91(7):2728-2732.

1208. Mitchell CA, Kelemen SM, Salem HH. The anticoagulant properties of a modified form of protein S. *Thromb Haemost.* 1988;60(2):298-304.

1209. Ploos van Amstel HK, Reitsma PH, van der Logt CP, Bertina RM. Intron-exon organization of the active human protein S gene PS alpha and its pseudogene PS beta: duplication and silencing during primate evolution. *Biochemistry.* 1990;29(34):7853-7861.

1210. Watkins PC, Eddy R, Fukushima Y, et al. The gene for protein S maps near the centromere of human chromosome 3. *Blood.* 1988;71(1):238-241.

1211. Schmidel DK, Tatro AV, Phelps LG, Tomczak JA, Long GL. Organization of the human protein S genes. *Biochemistry.* 1990;29(34):7845-7852.

1212. Edenbrandt CM, Lundwall A, Wydro R, Stenflo J. Molecular analysis of the gene for vitamin K dependent protein S and its pseudogene. Cloning and partial gene organization. *Biochemistry.* 1990;29(34):7861-7868.

1213. Ploos van Amstel HK, Reitsma PH, Bertina RM. The human protein S locus: identification of the PS alpha gene as a site of liver protein S messenger RNA synthesis. *Biochem Biophys Res Commun.* 1988;157(3):1033-1038.

1214. Ploos van Amstel HK, Huisman MV, Reitsma PH, Wouter ten Cate J, Bertina RM. Partial protein S gene deletion in a family with hereditary thrombophilia. *Blood.* 1989;73(2):479-483.

1215. Fair DS, Marlar RA. Biosynthesis and secretion of factor VII, protein C, protein S, and the Protein C inhibitor from a human hepatoma cell line. *Blood.* 1986;67(1):64-70.

1216. Hoskins J, Norman DK, Beckmann RJ, Long GL. Cloning and characterization of human liver cDNA encoding a protein S precursor. *Proc Natl Acad Sci U S A.* 1987;84(2):349-353.

1217. Fair DS, Marlar RA, Levin EG. Human endothelial cells synthesize protein S. *Blood.* 1986;67(4):1168-1171.

1218. Stern D, Brett J, Harris K, Nawroth P. Participation of endothelial cells in the protein C-protein S anticoagulant pathway: the synthesis and release of protein S. *J Cell Biol.* 1986;102(5):1971-1978.

1219. Hooper WC, Phillips DJ, Ribeiro MJ, et al. Tumor necrosis factor-alpha downregulates protein S secretion in human microvascular and umbilical vein endothelial cells but not in the HepG-2 hepatoma cell line. *Blood.* 1994;84(2):483-489.

1220. Maillard C, Berruyer M, Serre CM, Dechavanne M, Delmas PD. Protein-S, a vitamin K-dependent protein, is a bone matrix component synthesized and secreted by osteoblasts. *Endocrinology.* 1992;130(3):1599-1604.

1221. Smiley ST, Boyer SN, Heeb MJ, Griffin JH, Grusby MJ. Protein S is inducible by interleukin 4 in T cells and inhibits lymphoid cell procoagulant activity. *Proc Natl Acad Sci U S A.* 1997;94(21):11484-11489.

1222. DiScipio RG, Davie EW. Characterization of protein S, a gamma-carboxyglutamic acid containing protein from bovine and human plasma. *Biochemistry.* 1979;18:899-904.

1223. Lundwall A, Dackowski W, Cohen E, et al. Isolation and sequence of the cDNA for human protein S, a regulator of blood coagulation. *Proc Natl Acad Sci U S A.* 1986;83(18):6716-6720.

1224. Joseph DR, Baker ME. Sex hormone-binding globulin, androgen-binding protein, and vitamin K-dependent protein S are homologous to laminin A, merosin, and Drosophila crumbs protein. *FASEB J.* 1992;6(7):2477-2481.

1225. Gershagen S, Fernlund P, Edenbrandt CM. The genes for SHBG/ABP and the SHBG-like region of vitamin K-dependent protein S have evolved from a common ancestral gene. *J Steroid Biochem Mol Biol.* 1991;40(4-6):763-769.

1226. Stenberg Y, Linse S, Drakenberg T, Stenflo J. The high affinity calcium-binding sites in the epidermal growth factor module region of vitamin K-dependent protein S. *J Biol Chem.* 1997;272(37):23255-23260.

1227. Walker FJ. Properties of chemically modified protein S: effect of the conversion of gamma-carboxyglutamic acid to gamma-methyleneglutamic acid on functional properties. *Biochemistry.* 1986;25(20):6305-6311.

1228. Van Wijnen M, Stam JG, Chang GT, et al. Characterization of mini-protein S, a recombinant variant of protein S that lacks the sex hormone binding globulin-like domain. *Biochem J.* 1998;330(pt 1):389-396.

1229. He X, Shen L, Malmborg AC, Smith KJ, Dahlback B, Linse S. Binding site for C4b-binding protein in vitamin K-dependent protein S fully contained in carboxy-terminal laminin-G-type repeats. A study using recombinant factor IX-protein S chimeras and surface plasmon resonance. *Biochemistry.* 1997;36(12):3745-3754.

1230. Pauls JE, Hockin MF, Long GL, Mann KG. Self-association of human protein S. *Biochemistry.* 2000;39(18):5468-5473.

1231. Ahnstrom J, Andersson HM, Hockey V, et al. Identification of functionally important residues in TFPI Kunitz domain 3 required for the enhancement of its activity by protein S. *Blood.* 2012;120(25):5059-5062.

1232. Ndonwi M, Tuley EA, Broze GJ, Jr. The Kunitz-3 domain of TFPI-alpha is required for protein S-dependent enhancement of factor Xa inhibition. *Blood.* 2010;116(8):1344-1351.

1233. Reglinska-Matveyev N, Andersson HM, Rezende SM, et al. TFPI cofactor function of protein S: essential role of the protein S SHBG-like domain. *Blood.* 2014;123(2):3979-3987.

1234. Somajo S, Ahnstrom J, Fernandez-Recio J, Gierula M, Villoutreix BO, Dahlback B. Amino acid residues in the laminin G domains of protein S involved in tissue factor pathway inhibitor interaction. *Thromb Haemost.* 2015;113(5):976-987.

1235. Yegneswaran S, Wood GM, Esmon CT, Johnson AE. Protein S alters the active site location of activated protein C above the membrane surface. A fluorescence resonance energy transfer study of topography. *J Biol Chem.* 1997;272(40):25013-25021.

1236. Koppelman SJ, Hackeng TM, Sixma JJ, Bouma BN. Inhibition of the intrinsic factor X activating complex by protein S: evidence for a specific binding of protein S to factor VIII. *Blood.* 1995;86(3):1062-1071.

1237. Hackeng TM, Sere KM, Tans G, Rosing J. Protein S stimulates inhibition of the tissue factor pathway by tissue factor pathway inhibitor. *Proc Natl Acad Sci U S A.* 2006;103(9):3106-3111.

1238. Peraramelli S, Rosing J, Hackeng TM. TFPI-dependent activities of protein S. *Thromb Res.* 2012;129(suppl 2):S23-S26.

1239. Peraramelli S, Thomassen S, Heinzmann A, et al. Inhibition of tissue factor:factor VIIa-catalyzed factor IX and factor X activation by TFPI and TFPI constructs. *J Thromb Haemost.* 2014;12(11):1826-1837.

1240. Hackeng TM, Hessing M, van 't Veer C, et al. Protein S binding to human endothelial cells is required for expression of cofactor activity for activated protein C. *J Biol Chem.* 1993;268(6):3993-4000.

1241. Koppelman SJ, van't Veer C, Sixma JJ, Bouma BN. Synergistic inhibition of the intrinsic factor X activation by protein S and C4b-binding protein. *Blood.* 1995;86(7):2653-2660.

1242. Smiley ST, Stitt TN, Grusby MJ. Cross-linking of protein S bound to lymphocytes promotes aggregation and inhibits proliferation. *Cell Immunol.* 1997;181(2):120-126.

1243. Chang GT, Aaldering L, Hackeng TM, Reitsma PH, Bertina RM, Bouma BN. Construction and characterization of thrombin-resistant variants of recombinant human protein S. *Thromb Haemost.* 1994;72(5):693-697.

1244. Dahlback B. Purification of human vitamin K-dependent protein S and its limited proteolysis by thrombin. *Biochem J.* 1983;209(3):837-846.

1245. Suzuki K, Nishioka J, Hashimoto S. Regulation of activated protein C by thrombin-modified protein S. *J Biochem.* 1983;94(3):699-705.

1246. Prowse CV, Esnouf MP. The isolation of a new warfarin-sensitive protein from bovine plasma. *Biochem Soc Trans.* 1977;5(1):255-256.

1247. Broze GJ, Jr, Miletich JP. Human protein Z. *J Clin Invest.* 1984;73(4):933-938.

1248. Broze GJ, Jr. Protein Z-dependent regulation of coagulation. *Thromb Haemost.* 2001;86(1):8-13.

1249. Han X, Fiehler R, Broze GJ, Jr. Isolation of a protein Z-dependent plasma protease inhibitor. *Proc Natl Acad Sci U S A.* 1998;95(16):9250-9255.

1250. Undar L, Karadogan I, Ozturk F. Plasma protein Z levels inversely correlate with plasma interleukin-6 levels in patients with acute leukemia and non-Hodgkin's lymphoma. *Thromb Res.* 1999;94(2):131-134.

1251. Raczkowski CA, RM, Esmon CT, Comp PC. Protein Z is a negatively responding acute phase protein. *Blood.* 1999;70(suppl 1):393a.

1252. Yurdakok M, Gurakan B, Ozbag E, Vigit S, Dundar S, Kirazli S. Plasma protein Z levels in healthy newborn infants. *Am J Hematol.* 1995;48(3):206-207.

1253. Kemkes-Matthes B, Matthes KJ. Protein Z. *Semin Thromb Hemost.* 2001;27(5):551-556.

1254. Bertolino G, Montani N, Lorezutti F, Balduini CL, Gamba G. Behavior of plasma protein Z levels in patients with abnormal hemostasis. *J Thromb Haemost.* 1997;78(suppl 1):235a.

1255. Kemkes-Matthes B, Matthes KJ. Protein Z, a new haemostatic factor, in liver diseases. *Haemostasis.* 1995;25(6):312-316.

1256. Bertolino G, Montani N, Anesi E, Palladini G, Gamba G. Plasma protein Z levels in patients with systemic AL amyloidosis. *Thromb Haemost.* 1999;82(Suppl):136a.

1257. Usalan C, Erdem Y, Altun B, et al. Protein Z levels in haemodialysis patients. *Int Urol Nephrol.* 1999;31(4):541-545.

1258. Miletich JP, Broze GJ, Jr. Human plasma protein Z antigen: range in normal subjects and effect of warfarin therapy. *Blood.* 1987;69(6):1580-1586.

1259. Yin ZF, Huang ZF, Cui J, et al. Prothrombotic phenotype of protein Z deficiency. *Proc Natl Acad Sci U S A.* 2000;97(12):6734-6738.

1260. Corral J, Gonzalez-Conejero R, Hernandez-Espinosa D, Vicente V. Protein Z/Z-dependent protease inhibitor (PZ/ZPI) anticoagulant system and thrombosis. *Br J Haematol.* 2007;137(2):99-108.

1261. Bafunno V, Santacroce R, Margaglione M. The risk of occurrence of venous thrombosis: focus on protein Z. *Thromb Res.* 2011;128(6):508-515.

1262. Vasse M. Protein Z, a protein seeking a pathology. *Thromb Haemost.* 2008;100(4):548-556.

1263. Suzuki K, Nishioka J, Hayashi T, Kosaka Y. Functionally active thrombomodulin is present in human platelets. *J Biochem.* 1988;104(4):628-632.

1264. Kemkes-Matthes B, Matthes KJ. Protein Z deficiency: a new cause of bleeding tendency. *Thromb Res.* 1995;79(1):49-55.

1265. Greten J, Kreis I, Liliensiek B, et al. Localisation of protein Z in vascular lesions of patients with atherosclerosis. *Vasa.* 1998;27(3):144-148.

1266. Almawi WY, Al-Shaikh FS, Melemedjian OK, Almawi AW. Protein Z, an anticoagulant protein with expanding role in reproductive biology. *Reproduction.* 2013;146(2):R73-R80.

1267. Ichinose A, Takeya H, Espling E, Iwanaga S, Kisiel W, Davie EW. Amino acid sequence of human protein Z, a vitamin K-dependent plasma glycoprotein. *Biochem Biophys Res Commun.* 1990;172(3):1139-1144.

1268. Sejima H, Hayashi T, Deyashiki Y, Nishioka J, Suzuki K. Primary structure of vitamin K-dependent human protein Z. *Biochem Biophys Res Commun.* 1990;171(2):661-668.

1269. Heeb MJ, Cabral KM, Ruan L. Down-regulation of factor IXa in the factor Xase complex by protein Z-dependent protease inhibitor. *J Biol Chem.* 2005;280(40):33819-33825.

1270. Yang L, Rezaie AR. Residues of the 39-loop restrict the plasma inhibitor specificity of factor IXa. *J Biol Chem.* 2013;288(18):12692-12698.

1271. Dayer MR, Ghayour O, Dayer MS. Mechanism of protein-z-mediated inhibition of coagulation factor xa by z-protein-dependent inhibitor: a molecular dynamic approach. *ISRN Hematol.* 2012;2012:762728.

1272. Huang X, Dementiev A, Olson ST, Gettins PG. Basis for the specificity and activation of the serpin protein Z-dependent proteinase inhibitor (ZPI) as an inhibitor of membrane-associated factor Xa. *J Biol Chem.* 2010;285(26):20399-20409.

1273. Huang X, Yan Y, Tu Y, et al. Structural basis for catalytic activation of protein Z-dependent protease inhibitor (ZPI) by protein Z. *Blood.* 2012;120(8):1726-1733.

1274. Hogg PJ, Stenflo J. Interaction of human protein Z with thrombin: evaluation of the species difference in the interaction between bovine and human protein Z and thrombin. *Biochem Biophys Res Commun.* 1991;178(3):801-807.

1275. Conway EM. Thrombomodulin and its role in inflammation. *Semin Immunopathol.* 2012;34(1):107-125.

1276. Imada S, Yamaguchi H, Nagumo M, Katayanagi S, Iwasaki H, Imada M. Identification of fetomodulin, a surface marker protein of fetal development, as thrombomodulin by gene cloning and functional assays. *Dev Biol.* 1990;140(1):113-122.

1277. Healy AM, Rayburn HB, Rosenberg RD, Weiler H. Absence of the blood-clotting regulator thrombomodulin causes embryonic lethality in mice before development of a functional cardiovascular system. *Proc Natl Acad Sci U S A.* 1995;92(3):850-854.

1278. Wen DZ, Dittman WA, Deaven LL, Majerus PW, Sadler JE. Human thrombomodulin: complete cDNA sequence and chromosome localization of the gene. *Biochemistry.* 1987;26(14):4350-4357.

1279. Espinosa R,IIIrd, Sadler JE, Le Beau MM. Regional localization of the human thrombomodulin gene to 20p12-cen. *Genomics.* 1989;5(3):649-650.

1280. Jackman RW, Beeler DL, Fritze L, Soff G, Rosenberg RD. Human thrombomodulin gene is intron depleted: nucleic acid sequences of the cDNA and gene predict protein structure and suggest sites of regulatory control. *Proc Natl Acad Sci U S A.* 1987;84(18):6425-6429.

1281. Shirai T, Shiojiri S, Ito H, et al. Gene structure of human thrombomodulin, a cofactor for thrombin-catalyzed activation of protein C. *J Biochem.* 1988;103(2):281-285.

1282. Maruyama I, Bell CE, Majerus PW. Thrombomodulin is found on endothelium of arteries, veins, capillaries, and lymphatics, and on syncytiotrophoblast of human placenta. *J Cell Biol.* 1985;101(2):363-371.

1283. DeBault LE, Esmon NL, Olson JR, Esmon CT. Distribution of the thrombomodulin antigen in the rabbit vasculature. *Lab Invest.* 1986;54(2):172-178.

1284. Conway EM, Nowakowski B, Steiner-Mosonyi M. Human neutrophils synthesize thrombomodulin that does not promote thrombin-dependent protein C activation. *Blood.* 1992;80(5):1254-1263.

1285. Satta N, Freyssinet JM, Toti F. The significance of human monocyte thrombomodulin during membrane vesiculation and after stimulation by lipopolysaccharide. *Br J Haematol.* 1997;96(3):534-542.

1286. McCachren SS, Diggs J, Weinberg JB, Dittman WA. Thrombomodulin expression by human blood monocytes and by human synovial tissue lining macrophages. *Blood.* 1991;78(12):3128-3132.

1287. Conway EM, Nowakowski B. Biologically active thrombomodulin is synthesized by adherent synovial fluid cells and is elevated in synovial fluid of patients with rheumatoid arthritis. *Blood.* 1993;81(3):726-733.

1288. Raife TJ, Lager DJ, Madison KC, et al. Thrombomodulin expression by human keratinocytes. Induction of cofactor activity during epidermal differentiation. *J Clin Invest.* 1994;93(4):1846-1851.

1289. Jackson DE, Mitchell CA, Bird P, Salem HH, Hayman JA. Immunohistochemical localization of thrombomodulin in normal human skin and skin tumours. *J Pathol.* 1995;175(4):421-432.

1290. Lager DJ, Callaghan EJ, Worth SF, Raife TJ, Lentz SR. Cellular localization of thrombomodulin in human epithelium and squamous malignancies. *Am J Pathol.* 1995;146(4):933-943.

1291. Scarpati EM, Sadler JE. Regulation of endothelial cell coagulant properties. Modulation of tissue factor, plasminogen activator inhibitors, and thrombomodulin by phorbol 12-myristate 13-acetate and tumor necrosis factor. *J Biol Chem.* 1989;264(34):20705-20713.

1292. Ishii H, Horie S, Kizaki K, Kazama M. Retinoic acid counteracts both the down-regulation of thrombomodulin and the induction of tissue factor in cultured human endothelial cells exposed to tumor necrosis factor. *Blood.* 1992;80(10):2556-2562.

1293. Hayashi T, Honda G, Suzuki K. An atherogenic stimulus homocysteine inhibits cofactor activity of thrombomodulin and enhances thrombomodulin expression in human umbilical vein endothelial cells. *Blood.* 1992;79(11):2930-2936.

1294. Ogawa S, Gerlach H, Esposito C, Pasagian-Macaulay A, Brett J, Stern D. Hypoxia modulates the barrier and coagulant function of cultured bovine endothelium. Increased monolayer permeability and induction of procoagulant properties. *J Clin Invest.* 1990;85(4):1090-1098.

1295. Esposito C, Gerlach H, Brett J, Stern D, Vlassara H. Endothelial receptor-mediated binding of glucose-modified albumin is associated with increased monolayer permeability and modulation of cell surface coagulant properties. *J Exp Med.* 1989;170(4):1387-1407.

1296. Archipoff G, Beretz A, Bartha K, et al. Role of cyclic AMP in promoting the thromboresistance of human endothelial cells by enhancing thrombomodulin and decreasing tissue factor activities. *Br J Pharmacol.* 1993;109(1):18-28.

1297. Dittman WA, Nelson SC, Greer PK, Horton ET, Palomba ML, McCachren SS. Characterization of thrombomodulin expression in response to retinoic acid and identification of a retinoic acid response element in the human thrombomodulin gene. *J Biol Chem.* 1994;269(24):16925-16932.

1298. Takada Y, Shinkai F, Kondo S, et al. Fluid shear stress increases the expression of thrombomodulin by cultured human endothelial cells. *Biochem Biophys Res Commun.* 1994;205(2):1345-1352.

1299. Malek AM, Jackman R, Rosenberg RD, Izumo S. Endothelial expression of thrombomodulin is reversibly regulated by fluid shear stress. *Circ Res.* 1994;74(5):852-860.

1300. Conway EM, Liu L, Nowakowski B, Steiner-Mosonyi M, Jackman RW. Heat shock of vascular endothelial cells induces an up-regulatory transcriptional response of the thrombomodulin gene that is delayed in onset and does not attenuate. *J Biol Chem.* 1994;269(36):22804-22810.

1301. Tazawa R, Yamamoto K, Suzuki K, Hirokawa K, Hirosawa S, Aoki N. Presence of functional cyclic AMP responsive element in the 3'-untranslated region of the human thrombomodulin gene. *Biochem Biophys Res Commun.* 1994;200(3):1391-1397.

1302. Suzuki K, Kusumoto H, Deyashiki Y, et al. Structure and expression of human thrombomodulin, a thrombin receptor on endothelium acting as a cofactor for protein C activation. *EMBO J.* 1987;6(7):1891-1897.

1303. Petersen TE. The amino-terminal domain of thrombomodulin and pancreatic stone protein are homologous with lectins. *FEBS Lett.* 1988;231(1):51-53.

1304. Kurosawa S, Stearns DJ, Jackson KW, Esmon CT. A 10-kDa cyanogen bromide fragment from the epidermal growth factor homology domain of rabbit thrombomodulin contains the primary thrombin binding site. *J Biol Chem.* 1988;263(13):5993-5996.

1305. Stearns DJ, Kurosawa S, Esmon CT. Microthrombomodulin. Residues 310-486 from the epidermal growth factor precursor homology domain of thrombomodulin will accelerate protein C activation. *J Biol Chem.* 1989;264(6):3352-3356.

1306. Suzuki K, Hayashi T, Nishioka J, et al. A domain composed of epidermal growth factor-like structures of human thrombomodulin is essential for thrombin binding and for protein C activation. *J Biol Chem.* 1989;264(9):4872-4876.

1307. Zushi M, Gomi K, Honda G, et al. Aspartic acid 349 in the fourth epidermal growth factor-like structure of human thrombomodulin plays a role in its Ca(2+)-mediated binding to protein C. *J Biol Chem.* 1991;266(30):19886-19889.

1308. Zushi M, Gomi K, Yamamoto S, Maruyama I, Hayashi T, Suzuki K. The last three consecutive epidermal growth factor-like structures of human thrombomodulin comprise the minimum functional domain for protein C-activating cofactor activity and anticoagulant activity. *J Biol Chem.* 1989;264(18):10351-10353.

1309. Lin JH, McLean K, Morser J, et al. Modulation of glycosaminoglycan addition in naturally expressed and recombinant human thrombomodulin. *J Biol Chem.* 1994;269(40):25021-25030.

1310. Ye J, Rezaie AR, Esmon CT. Glycosaminoglycan contributions to both protein C activation and thrombin inhibition involve a common arginine-rich site in thrombin that includes residues arginine 93, 97, and 101. *J Biol Chem.* 1994;269(27):17965-17970.

1311. Bourin MC, Lindahl U. Glycosaminoglycans and the regulation of blood coagulation. *Biochem J.* 1993;289(pt 2):313-330.

1312. Bourin MC, Ohlin AK, Lane DA, Stenflo J, Lindahl U. Relationship between anticoagulant activities and polyanionic properties of rabbit thrombomodulin. *J Biol Chem.* 1988;263(17):8044-8052.

1313. He X, Ye J, Esmon CT, Rezaie AR. Influence of Arginines 93, 97, and 101 of thrombin to its functional specificity. *Biochemistry.* 1997;36(29):8969-8976.

1314. Tsiang M, Lentz SR, Sadler JE. Functional domains of membrane-bound human thrombomodulin. EGF-like domains four to six and the serine/threonine-rich domain are required for cofactor activity. *J Biol Chem.* 1992;267(9):6164-6170.

1315. Lu RL, Esmon NL, Esmon CT, Johnson AE. The active site of the thrombin-thrombomodulin complex. A fluorescence energy transfer measurement of its distance above the membrane surface. *J Biol Chem.* 1989;264(22):12956-12962.

1316. Conway EM, Boffa MC, Nowakowski B, Steiner-Mosonyi M. An ultrastructural study of thrombomodulin endocytosis: internalization occurs via clathrin-coated and non-coated pits. *J Cell Physiol.* 1992;151(3):604-612.

1317. Conway EM, Pollefeyt S, Collen D, Steiner-Mosonyi M. The amino terminal lectin-like domain of thrombomodulin is required for constitutive endocytosis. *Blood.* 1997;89(2):652-661.

1318. Ye J, Liu LW, Esmon CT, Johnson AE. The fifth and sixth growth factor-like domains of thrombomodulin bind to the anion-binding exosite of thrombin and alter its specificity. *J Biol Chem.* 1992;267(16):11023-11028.

1319. Vindigni A, White CE, Komives EA, Di Cera E. Energetics of thrombin-thrombomodulin interaction. *Biochemistry.* 1997;36(22):6674-6681.

1320. Ye J, Esmon NL, Esmon CT, Johnson AE. The active site of thrombin is altered upon binding to thrombomodulin. Two distinct structural changes are detected by fluorescence, but only one correlates with protein C activation. *J Biol Chem.* 1991;266(34):23016-23021.

1321. Ye J, Esmon CT, Johnson AE. The chondroitin sulfate moiety of thrombomodulin binds a second molecule of thrombin. *J Biol Chem.* 1993;268(4):2373-2379.

1322. Musci G, Berliner LJ, Esmon CT. Evidence for multiple conformational changes in the active center of thrombin induced by complex formation with thrombomodulin: an analysis employing nitroxide spin-labels. *Biochemistry.* 1988;27(2):769-773.

1323. Liu LW, Rezaie AR, Carson CW, Esmon NL, Esmon CT. Occupancy of anion binding exosite 2 on thrombin determines Ca2+ dependence of protein C activation. *J Biol Chem.* 1994;269(16):11807-11812.

1324. Esmon CT, Esmon NL, Harris KW. Complex formation between thrombin and thrombomodulin inhibits both thrombin-catalyzed fibrin formation and factor V activation. *J Biol Chem.* 1982;257(14):7944-7947.

1325. Esmon NL, Carroll RC, Esmon CT. Thrombomodulin blocks the ability of thrombin to activate platelets. *J Biol Chem.* 1983;258(20):12238-12242.

1326. Hofsteenge J, Taguchi H, Stone SR. Effect of thrombomodulin on the kinetics of the interaction of thrombin with substrates and inhibitors. *Biochem J.* 1986;237(1):243-251.

1327. Bourin MC, Boffa MC, Bjork I, Lindahl U. Functional domains of rabbit thrombomodulin. *Proc Natl Acad Sci U S A.* 1986;83(16):5924-5928.

1328. Preissner KT, Delvos U, Muller-Berghaus G. Binding of thrombin to thrombomodulin accelerates inhibition of the enzyme by antithrombin III. Evidence for a heparin-independent mechanism. *Biochemistry.* 1987;26(9):2521-2528.

1329. Lentz SR, Sadler JE. Inhibition of thrombomodulin surface expression and protein C activation by the thrombogenic agent homocysteine. *J Clin Invest.* 1991;88(6):1906-1914.

1330. Maruyama I, Majerus PW. Protein C inhibits endocytosis of thrombin-thrombomodulin complexes in A549 lung cancer cells and human umbilical vein endothelial cells. *Blood.* 1987;69(5):1481-1484.

1331. Maruyama I, Majerus PW. The turnover of thrombin-thrombomodulin complex in cultured human umbilical vein endothelial cells and A549 lung cancer cells. Endocytosis and degradation of thrombin. *J Biol Chem.* 1985;260(29):15432-15438.

1332. Horvat R, Palade GE. Thrombomodulin and thrombin localization on the vascular endothelium; their internalization and transcytosis by plasmalemmal vesicles. *Eur J Cell Biol.* 1993;61(2):299-313.

1333. Beretz A, Freyssinet JM, Gauchy J, et al. Stability of the thrombin-thrombomodulin complex on the surface of endothelial cells from human saphenous vein or from the cell line EA.hy 926. *Biochem J.* 1989;259(1):35-40.

1334. Boehme MW, Deng Y, Raeth U, et al. Release of thrombomodulin from endothelial cells by concerted action of TNF-alpha and neutrophils: in vivo and in vitro studies. *Immunology.* 1996;87(1):134-140.

1335. Takano S, Kimura S, Ohdama S, Aoki N. Plasma thrombomodulin in health and diseases. *Blood.* 1990;76(10):2024-2029.

1336. Glaser CB, Morser J, Clarke JH, et al. Oxidation of a specific methionine in thrombomodulin by activated neutrophil products blocks cofactor activity. A potential rapid mechanism for modulation of coagulation. *J Clin Invest.* 1992;90(6):2565-2573.

1337. Pizzo SV, Wu SM. Alpha-macroglobulins and kunins. In: Colman RW, HJ , Marder VJ, Clowes AW, George JN, eds. *Hemostasis and Thrombosis: Basic Principles & Clinical Practice*. Lippincott, Williams & Wilkins; 2001:367-379.

1338. Sottrup-Jensen L. Alpha 2-macroglobulin and related thiol ester plasma proteins. In: FW P, ed. *The Plasma Proteins*. Academic Press; 1987:191-287.

1339. Travis J, Salvesen GS. Human plasma proteinase inhibitors. *Annu Rev Biochem*. 1983;52:655-709.

1340. Starkey PM, Barrett AJ. Evolution of alpha 2-macroglobulin. The demonstration in a variety of vertebrate species of a protein resembling human alpha 2-macroglobulin. *Biochem J*. 1982;205(1):91-95.

1341. Kruger U. Chronic obstructive lung disease and alpha-2-macroglobulin deficiency in serum–case report. *Pneumologie*. 1993;47(9):531-534.

1342. Kanoh Y, Ohtani H, Koshiba K. Studies on alpha 2 macroglobulin deficiency in association with cancer metastasis. *Nihon Rinsho Meneki Gakkai Kaishi*. 1997;20(1):30-43.

1343. Umans L, Serneels L, Overbergh L, Lorent K, Van Leuven F, Van den Berghe H. Targeted inactivation of the mouse alpha 2-macroglobulin gene. *J Biol Chem*. 1995;270(34):19778-19785.

1344. Webb DJ, Wen J, Lysiak JJ, Umans L, Van Leuven F, Gonias SL. Murine alpha-macroglobulins demonstrate divergent activities as neutralizers of transforming growth factor-beta and as inducers of nitric oxide synthesis. A possible mechanism for the endotoxin insensitivity of the alpha2-macroglobulin gene knock-out mouse. *J Biol Chem*. 1996;271(40):24982-24988.

1345. Matthijs G, Devriendt K, Cassiman JJ, Van den Berghe H, Marynen P. Structure of the human alpha-2 macroglobulin gene and its promotor. *Biochem Biophys Res Commun*. 1992;184(2):596-603.

1346. Kan CC, Solomon E, Belt KT, Chain AC, Hiorns LR, Fey G. Nucleotide sequence of cDNA encoding human alpha 2-macroglobulin and assignment of the chromosomal locus. *Proc Natl Acad Sci U S A*. 1985;82(8):2282-2286.

1347. Fukushima Y, Bell GI, Shows TB. The polymorphic human alpha 2-macroglobulin gene (A2M) is located in chromosome region 12p12.3----p13.3. *Cytogenet Cell Genet*. 1988;48(1):58-59.

1348. Devriendt K, Zhang J, van Leuven F, van den Berghe H, Cassiman JJ, Marynen P. A cluster of alpha 2-macroglobulin-related genes (alpha 2 M) on human chromosome 12p: cloning of the pregnancy-zone protein gene and an alpha 2M pseudogene. *Gene*. 1989;81(2):325-334.

1349. Swenson RP, Howard JB. Structural characterization of human alpha2-macroglobulin subunits. *J Biol Chem*. 1979;254(11):4452-4456.

1350. Sottrup-Jensen L, Stepanik TM, Wierzbicki DM, et al. The primary structure of alpha 2-macroglobulin and localization of a Factor XIIIa cross-linking site. *Ann N Y Acad Sci*. 1983;421:41-60.

1351. Carlsson-Bosted L, Moestrup SK, Gliemann J, Sottrup-Jensen L, Stigbrand T. Three different conformational states of pregnancy zone protein identified by monoclonal antibodies. *J Biol Chem*. 1988;263(14):6738-6741.

1352. Christensen U, Simonsen M, Harrit N, Sottrup-Jensen L. Pregnancy zone protein, a proteinase-binding macroglobulin. Interactions with proteinases and methylamine. *Biochemistry*. 1989;28(24):9324-9331.

1353. Meyer C, Hinrichs W, Hahn U. Human alpha2-macroglobulin–another variation on the venus flytrap. *Angew Chem Int Ed Engl*. 2012;51(21):5045-5047.

1354. Mortensen SB, Sottrup-Jensen L, Hansen HF, Petersen TE, Magnusson S. Primary and secondary cleavage sites in the bait region of alpha 2-macroglobulin. *FEBS Lett*. 1981;135(2):295-300.

1355. Marrero A, Duquerroy S, Trapani S, et al. The crystal structure of human alpha2-macroglobulin reveals a unique molecular cage. *Angew Chem Int Ed Engl*. 2012;51(14):3340-3344.

1356. Sottrup-Jensen L, Petersen TE, Magnusson S. A thiol-ester in alpha 2-macroglobulin cleaved during proteinase complex formation. *FEBS Lett*. 1980;121(2):275-279.

1357. Howard JB. Reactive site in human alpha 2-macroglobulin: circumstantial evidence for a thiolester. *Proc Natl Acad Sci U S A*. 1981;78(4):2235-2239.

1358. Gonias SL, Reynolds JA, Pizzo SV. Physical properties of human alpha 2-macroglobulin following reaction with methylamine and trypsin. *Biochim Biophys Acta*. 1982;705(3):306-314.

1359. Harpel PC. Human plasma alpha 2-macroglobulin. An inhibitor of plasma kallikrein. *J Exp Med*. 1970;132(2):329-352.

1360. Harpel PC. Alpha2-plasmin inhibitor and alpha2-macroglobulin-plasmin complexes in plasma. Quantitation by an enzyme-linked differential antibody immunosorbent assay. *J Clin Invest*. 1981;68(1):46-55.

1361. Mitchell L, Piovella F, Ofosu F, Andrew M. Alpha-2-macroglobulin may provide protection from thromboembolic events in antithrombin III-deficient children. *Blood*. 1991;78(9):2299-2304.

1362. Abbink JJ, Nuijens JH, Eerenberg AJ, et al. Quantification of functional and inactivated alpha 2-macroglobulin in sepsis. *Thromb Haemost*. 1991;65(1):32-39.

1363. Huang SS, O'Grady P, Huang JS. Human transforming growth factor beta.alpha 2-macroglobulin complex is a latent form of transforming growth factor beta. *J Biol Chem*. 1988;263(3):1535-1541.

1364. Borth W, Luger TA. Identification of alpha 2-macroglobulin as a cytokine binding plasma protein. Binding of interleukin-1 beta to "F" alpha 2-macroglobulin. *J Biol Chem*. 1989;264(10):5818-5825.

1365. Matsuda T, Hirano T, Nagasawa S, Kishimoto T. Identification of alpha 2-macroglobulin as a carrier protein for IL-6. *J Immunol*. 1989;142(1):148-152.

1366. Dennis PA, Saksela O, Harpel P, Rifkin DB. Alpha 2-macroglobulin is a binding protein for basic fibroblast growth factor. *J Biol Chem*. 1989;264(13):7210-7216.

1367. Wollenberg GK, LaMarre J, Rosendal S, Gonias SL, Hayes MA. Binding of tumor necrosis factor alpha to activated forms of human plasma alpha 2 macroglobulin. *Am J Pathol*. 1991;138(2):265-272.

1368. Legres LG, Pochon F, Barray M, Gay F, Chouaib S, Delain E. Evidence for the binding of a biologically active interleukin-2 to human alpha 2-macroglobulin. *J Biol Chem*. 1995;270(15):8381-8384.

1369. Kovacs DM. Alpha 2-macroglobulin in late-onset Alzheimer's disease. *Exp Gerontol*. 2000;35(4):473-479.

1370. McGeer PL, McGeer EG. Polymorphisms in inflammatory genes and the risk of Alzheimer disease. *Arch Neurol*. 2001;58(11):1790-1792.

1371. Zappia M, Cittadella R, Manna I, et al. Genetic association of alpha2-macroglobulin polymorphisms with AD in southern Italy. *Neurology*. 2002;59(5):756-758.

1372. Broze GJ, Jr. The role of tissue factor pathway inhibitor in a revised coagulation cascade. *Semin Hematol*. 1992;29(3):159-169.

1373. Broze GJ, Jr, Girard TJ, Novotny WF. Regulation of coagulation by a multivalent Kunitz-type inhibitor. *Biochemistry*. 1990;29(33):7539-7546.

1374. Rapaport SI. The extrinsic pathway inhibitor: a regulator of tissue factor-dependent blood coagulation. *Thromb Haemost*. 1991;66(1):6-15.

1375. Broze GJ. Tissue factor pathway inhibitor and the current concept of blood coagulation. *Blood Coagul Fibrinolysis*. 1995;6(sup 1):S7-S13.

1376. Broze GJ, Jr, Lange GW, Duffin KL, MacPhail L. Heterogeneity of plasma tissue factor pathway inhibitor. *Blood Coagul Fibrinolysis*. 1994;5(4):551-559.

1377. Novotny WF, Girard TJ, Miletich JP, Broze GJ, Jr. Purification and characterization of the lipoprotein-associated coagulation inhibitor from human plasma. *J Biol Chem*. 1989;264(31):18832-18837.

1378. Sanders NL, Bajaj SP, Zivelin A, Rapaport SI. Inhibition of tissue factor/factor VIIa activity in plasma requires factor X and an additional plasma component. *Blood*. 1985;66(1):204-212.

1379. Lesnik P, Vonica A, Guerin M, Moreau M, Chapman MJ. Anticoagulant activity of tissue factor pathway inhibitor in human plasma is preferentially associated with dense subspecies of LDL and HDL and with Lp (a). *Arterioscler Thromb*. 1993;13(7):1066-1075.

1380. Broze GJ, Jr. Tissue factor pathway inhibitor. *Thromb Haemost*. 1995;74(1):90-93.

1381. Broze GJ, Jr. Tissue factor pathway inhibitor: structure-function. *Front Biosci*. 2012;17(1):262.

1382. Maroney SA, Ellery PE, Mast AE. Alternatively spliced isoforms of tissue factor pathway inhibitor. *Thromb Res*. 2010;125:S52-S56.

1383. Maroney SA, Mast AE. Platelet tissue factor pathway inhibitor modulates intravascular coagulation. *Thromb Res*. 2012;129:S21-S22.

1384. Holroyd EW. Tissue factor pathway inhibitor as a multifunctional mediator of vascular structure. *Front Biosci*. 2012;E4(1):392.

1385. Huang ZF, Higuchi D, Lasky N, Broze GJ, Jr. Tissue factor pathway inhibitor gene disruption produces intrauterine lethality in mice. *Blood*. 1997;90(3):944-951.

1386. Chan JCY, Carmeliet P, Moons L, et al. Factor VII deficiency rescues the intrauterine lethality in mice associated with a tissue factor pathway inhibitor deficit. *J Clin Invest*. 1999;103(4):475-482.

1387. Westrick RJ, Bodary PF, Xu Z, Shen YC, Broze GJ, Eitzman DT. Deficiency of tissue factor pathway inhibitor promotes atherosclerosis and thrombosis in mice. *Circulation*. 2001;103(25):3044-3046.

1388. Kato H. Regulation of functions of vascular wall cells by tissue factor pathway inhibitor: basic and clinical aspects. *Arterioscler Thromb*. 2002;22(4):539-548.

1389. LaRosa SP, Opal SM. Tissue factor pathway inhibitor and anitithrombin trial results. *Crit Care Clin*. 2005;21(3):433-448.

1390. Abraham E, Reinhart K, Svoboda P, et al. Assessment of the safety of recombinant tissue factor pathway inhibitor in patients with severe sepsis: a multicenter, randomized, placebo-controlled, single-blind, dose escalation study. *Crit Care Med*. 2001;29(11):2081-2089.

1391. Van der Logt CPE, Kluck PMC, Wiegant J, Landegent JE, Reitsma PH. Refined regional assignment of the human tissue factor pathway inhibitor (TFPI) gene to chromosome band 2q32 by non-isotopic in situ hybridization. *Hum Genet*. 1992;89(5):577-578.

1392. Van der Logt CPE, Reitsma PH, Bertina RM. Intron-exon organization of the human gene coding for the lipoprotein-associated coagulation inhibitor: the factor Xa dependent inhibitor of the extrinsic pathway of coagulation. *Biochemistry*. 1991;30(6):1571-1577.

1393. Girard TJ, Eddy R, Wesselschmidt RL, et al. Structure of the human lipoprotein-associated coagulation inhibitor gene. Intro/exon gene organization and localization of the gene to chromosome 2. *J Biol Chem*. 1991;266(8):5036-5041.

1394. Enjyoji K-i, Emi M, Mukai T, et al. Human tissue factor pathway inhibitor (TFPI) gene: complete genomic structure and localization on the genetic map of chromosome 2q. *Genomics*. 1993;17(2):423-428.

1395. Bajaj MS, Kuppuswamy MN, Saito H, Spitzer SG, Bajaj SP. Cultured normal human hepatocytes do not synthesize lipoprotein-associated coagulation inhibitor: evidence that endothelium is the principal site of its synthesis. *Proc Natl Acad Sci U S A*. 1990;87(22):8869-8873.

1396. Ameri A, Kuppuswamy MN, Basu S, Bajaj SP. Expression of tissue factor pathway inhibitor by cultured endothelial cells in response to inflammatory mediators. *Blood*. 1992;79(12):3219-3226.

1397. Broze GJ, Miletich JP. Isolation of the tissue factor inhibitor produced by HepG2 hepatoma cells. *Proc Natl Acad Sci U S A*. 1987;84(7):1886-1890.

1398. Wun TC, Kretzmer KK, Girard TJ, Miletich JP, Broze GJ, Jr. Cloning and characterization of a cDNA coding for the lipoprotein-associated coagulation inhibitor shows that it consists of three tandem Kunitz-type inhibitory domains. *J Biol Chem*. 1988;263(13):6001-6004.

1399. Novotny WF, Palmier M, Wun TC, Broze GJ, Jr, Miletich JP. Purification and properties of heparin-releasable lipoprotein-associated coagulation inhibitor. *Blood*. 1991;78(2):394-400.

1400. Broze GJ. Tissue factor pathway inhibitor and the revised theory of coagulation. *Annu Rev Med*. 1995;46(1):103-112.

1401. Enjyoji K-i, Miyata T, Kamikubo Yi, Kato II. Effect of heparin on the inhibition of factor xa by tissue factor pathway inhibitor: a segment, Gly212-Phe243, of the third Kunitz domain is a heparin-binding site. *Biochemistry.* 1995;34(17):5725-5735.

1402. Smith PL, Skelton TP, Fiete D, et al. The asparagine-linked oligosaccharides on tissue factor pathway inhibitor terminate with SO4-4GalNAc beta 1, 4GlcNAc beta 1,2 Mana alpha. *J Biol Chem.* 1992;267(27):19140-19146.

1403. Broze GJ, Jr, Warren LA, Novotny WF, Higuchi DA, Girard JJ, Miletich JP. The lipoprotein-associated coagulation inhibitor that inhibits the factor VII-tissue factor complex also inhibits factor Xa: insight into its possible mechanism of action. *Blood.* 1988;71(2):335-343.

1404. Sandset PM, Abildgaard U, Larsen ML. Heparin induces release of extrinsic: coagulation pathway inhibitor (EPI). *Thromb Res.* 1988;50(6):803-813.

1405. Lindahl AK, Abildgaard U, Stokke G. Release of extrinsic pathway inhibitor after heparin injection: increased response in cancer patients. *Thrombosis Res.* 1990;59(3):651-656.

1406. van 't Veer C, Kalafatis M, Bertina RM, Simioni P, Mann KG. Increased tissue factor-initiated prothrombin activation as a result of the Arg506 -> Gln mutation in factor VLEIDEN. *J Biol Chem.* 1997;272(33):20721-20729.

1407. Eitzman DT. Lethal perinatal thrombosis in mice resulting from the interaction of tissue factor pathway inhibitor deficiency and factor V Leiden. *Circulation.* 2002;105(18):2139-2142.

1408. Hamamoto T, Yamamoto M, Nordfang O, Petersen JG, Foster DC, Kisiel W. Inhibitory properties of full-length and truncated recombinant tissue factor pathway inhibitor (TFPI). Evidence that the third Kunitz-type domain of TFPI is not essential for the inhibition of factor VIIa-tissue factor complexes on cell surfaces. *J Biol Chem.* 1993;268(12):8704-8710.

1409. Wesselschmidt R, Likert K, Girard T, Wun TC, Broze GJ, Jr. Tissue factor pathway inhibitor: the carboxy-terminus is required for optimal inhibition of factor Xa. *Blood.* 1992;79(8):2004-2010.

1410. Ndonwi M, Broze G. Protein S enhances the tissue factor pathway inhibitor inhibition of factor Xa but not its inhibition of factor VIIa–tissue factor. *J Thromb Haemost.* 2008;6(6):1044-1046.

1411. van't Veer C, Mann KG. Regulation of tissue factor initiated thrombin generation by the stoichiometric inhibitors tissue factor pathway inhibitor, antithrombin-III, and heparin cofactor-II. *J Biol Chem.* 1997;272(7):4367-4377.

1412. van 't Veer C, Golden NJ, Kalafatis M, Mann KG. Inhibitory mechanism of the protein C pathway on tissue factor-induced thrombin generation: synergistic effect in combination with tissue factor pathway inhibitor. *J Biol Chem.* 1997;272(12):7983-7994.

1413. Warshawsky I, Bu G, Mast A, Saffitz JE, Broze GJ, Schwartz AL. The carboxy terminus of tissue factor pathway inhibitor is required for interacting with hepatoma cells in vitro and in vivo. *J Clin Invest.* 1995;95(4):1773-1781.

1414. Warshawsky I, Broze GJ, Schwartz AL. The low density lipoprotein receptor-related protein mediates the cellular degradation of tissue factor pathway inhibitor. *Proc Natl Acad Sci.* 1994;91(14):6664-6668.

1415. Narita M, Bu G, Olins GM, et al. Two receptor systems are involved in the plasma clearance of tissue factor pathway inhibitor in vivo. *J Biol Chem.* 1995;270(42):24800-24804.

1416. Janciauskiene S. Conformational properties of serine proteinase inhibitors (serpins) confer multiple pathophysiological roles. *Biochim Biophys Acta.* 2001;1535(3):221-235.

1417. Rau JC, Beaulieu LM, Huntington JA, Church FC. Serpins in thrombosis, hemostasis and fibrinolysis. *J Thromb Haemost.* 2007;5:102-115.

1418. Huntington JA. Serpin structure, function and dysfunction. *J Thromb Haemost.* 2011;9:26-34.

1419. Kuhle S, Lane DA, Jochmanns K, et al. Homozygous antithrombin deficiency type II (99 Leu to Phe mutation) and childhood thromboembolism. *Thromb Haemost.* 2001;86(4):1007-1011.

1420. Yamamoto K, Takeshita K, Shimokawa T, et al. Plasminogen activator inhibitor-1 is a major stress-regulated gene: implications for stress-induced thrombosis in aged individuals. *Proc Natl Acad Sci.* 2002;99(2):890-895.

1421. Khan H, Salman KA, Ahmed S. Alpha-1 antitrypsin deficiency in emphysema. *J Assoc Physicians India.* 2002;50:579-582.

1422. Koide M, Shirahama S, Tokura Y, Takigawa M, Hayakawa M, Furukawa F. Lupus erythematosus associated with C1 inhibitor deficiency. *J Dermatol.* 2002;29(8):503-507.

1423. Propst T, Propst A, Dietze O, Judmaier G, Braunsteiner H, Vogel W. Alpha-1-antitrypsin deficiency and liver disease. *Dig Dis.* 1994;12(3):139-149.

1424. Davis RL, Shrimpton AE, Carrell RW, et al. Association between conformational mutations in neuroserpin and onset and severity of dementia. *Lancet.* 2002;359(9325):2242-2247.

1425. Stratikos E, Gettins PG. Formation of the covalent serpin-proteinase complex involves translocation of the proteinase by more than 70 A and full insertion of the reactive center loop into beta-sheet A. *Proc Natl Acad Sci U S A.* 1999;96(9):4808-4813.

1426. Kaslik G, Patthy A, Bálint M, Gráf L. Trypsin complexed with α 1 -proteinase inhibitor has an increased structural flexibility. *FEBS Letts.* 1995;370(3):179-183.

1427. Stavridi ES, O'Malley K, Lukacs CM, et al. Structural change in α-chymotrypsin induced by complexation with α 1 -antichymotrypsin as seen by enhanced sensitivity to proteolysis. *Biochemistry.* 1996;35(33):10608-10615.

1428. Fa M, Bergström F, Karolin J, Johansson LBÅ, Ny T. Conformational studies of plasminogen activator inhibitor type 1 by fluorescence spectroscopy. *Eur J Biochem.* 2000;267(12):3729-3734.

1429. Fa M, Bergström F, Hägglöf P, Wilczynska M, Johansson LBÅ, Ny T. The structure of a serpin–protease complex revealed by intramolecular distance measurements using donor–donor energy migration and mapping of interaction sites. *Structure.* 2000;8(4):397-405.

1430. Hervé M, Ghélis C. Conformational stability of the covalent complex between elastase and α1-proteinase inhibitor. *Arch Biochem Biophys.* 1991;285(1):142-146.

1431. Streusand VJ, Bjork I, Gettins PG, Petitou M, Olson ST. Mechanism of acceleration of antithrombin-proteinase reactions by low affinity heparin. Role of the antithrombin binding pentasaccharide in heparin rate enhancement. *J Biol Chem.* 1995;270(16):9043-9051.

1432. Plotnick MI, Mayne L, Schechter NM, Rubin H. Distortion of the active site of chymotrypsin complexed with a serpin. *Biochemistry.* 1996;35(23):7586-7590.

1433. Baglin TP Carrell RW, Church FC, Esmon CT, Huntington JA. Crystal structures of native and thrombin-complexed heparin cofactor II reveal a multistep allosteric mechanism. *Proc Natl Acad Sci U S A.* 2002;99(17):11079-11084.

1434. Li W, Johnson DJD, Esmon CT, Huntington JA. Structure of the antithrombin–thrombin–heparin ternary complex reveals the antithrombotic mechanism of heparin. *Nat Struct Mol Biol.* 2004;11(9):857-862.

1435. Li W, Adams TE, Nangalia J, Esmon CT, Huntington JA. Molecular basis of thrombin recognition by protein C inhibitor revealed by the 1.6-A structure of the heparin-bridged complex. *Proc Natl Acad Sci.* 2008;105(12):4661-4666.

1436. Li W, Huntington JA. Crystal structures of protease nexin-1 in complex with heparin and thrombin suggest a 2-step recognition mechanism. *Blood.* 2012;120(2):459-467.

1437. Im H, Woo MS, Hwang KY, Yu MH. Interactions causing the kinetic trap in serpin protein folding. *J Biol Chem.* 2002;277(48):46347-46354.

1438. Whisstock J, Skinner R, Lesk AM. An atlas of serpin conformations. *Trends Biochem Sci.* 1998;23(2):63-67.

1439. Huntington JA, Read RJ, Carrell RW. *Nature.* 2000;407(6806):923-926.

1440. Djie MZ, Stone SR, Le Bonniec BF. Intrinsic specificity of the reactive site loop of 1-antitrypsin, 1-antichymotrypsin, antithrombin III, and protease nexin I. *J Biol Chem.* 1997;272(26):16268-16273.

1441. Zhou A, Carrell RW, Huntington JA. The serpin inhibitory mechanism is critically dependent on the length of the reactive center loop. *J Biol Chem.* 2001;276(29):27541-27547.

1442. Lawrence DA. Partitioning of serpin-proteinase reactions between stable inhibition and substrate cleavage is regulated by the rate of serpin reactive center loop insertion into beta -sheet A. *J Biol Chem.* 2000;275(8):5839-5844.

1443. Potempa J, Korzus E, Travis J. The serpin superfamily of proteinase inhibitors: structure, function, and regulation. *J Biol Chem.* 1994;269(23):15957-15960.

1444. Laskowski M, Qasim MA. What can the structures of enzyme-inhibitor complexes tell us about the structures of enzyme substrate complexes? *Biochim Biophys Acta.* 2000;1477(1-2):324-337.

1445. Silverman GA, Bird PI, Carrell RW, et al. The serpins are an expanding superfamily of structurally similar but functionally diverse proteins: evolution, mechanism of inhibition, novel functions, and a revised nomenclature. *J Biol Chem.* 2001;276(36):33293-33296.

1446. Gils A, Declerck PJ. Structure-function relationships in serpins: current concepts and controversies. *Thromb Haemost.* 1998;80(4):531-541.

1447. Wright HT. The structural puzzle of how serpin serine proteinase inhibitors work. *Bioessays.* 1996;18(6):453-464.

1448. Huber R, Carrell RW. Implications of the three-dimensional structure of.alpha.1-antitrypsin for structure and function of serpins. *Biochemistry.* 1989;28(23):8951-8966.

1449. Ye S. Serpins and other covalent protease inhibitors. *Curr Opin Struct Biol.* 2001;11(6):740-745.

1450. Bode W, Huber R. Structural basis of the endoproteinase–protein inhibitor interaction. *Biochim Biophys Acta.* 2000;1477(1-2):241-252.

1451. Collen D, Schetz J, Cock FD, Holmer E, Verstraete M. Metabolism of antithrombin III (heparin cofactor) in man: effects of venous thrombosis and of heparin administration. *Eur J Clin Invest.* 1977;7(1):27-35.

1452. Menache D, O'Malley JP, Schorr JB, et al. Evaluation of the safety, recovery, half-life, and clinical efficacy of antithrombin III (human) in patients with hereditary antithrombin III deficiency. Cooperative Study Group. *Blood.* 1990;75(1):33-39.

1453. Muszbek L, Bereczky Z, Kovács B, Komáromi I. Antithrombin deficiency and its laboratory diagnosis. *Clin Chem Lab Med.* 2010;48:S67-S78.

1454. Harper PL, Luddington RJ, Daly M, et al. The incidence of dysfunctional antithrombin variants: four cases in 210 patients with thromboembolic disease. *Br J Haematol.* 1991;77(3):360-364.

1455. Lane DA, Kunz G, Olds RJ, Thein SL. Molecular genetics of antithrombin deficiency. *Blood Rev.* 1996;10(2):59-74.

1456. Perry DJ, Carrell RW. Molecular genetics of human antithrombin deficiency. *Hum Mutat.* 1996;7(1):7-22.

1457. Picard V, Nowak-Göttl U, Biron-Andreani C, et al. Molecular bases of antithrombin deficiency: twenty-two novel mutations in the antithrombin gene. *Hum Mutat.* 2006;27(6):600-600.

1458. van Boven HH, Lane DA. Antithrombin and its inherited deficiency states. *Semin Hematol.* 1997;34(3):188-204.

1459. Vinazzer H. Hereditary and acquired antithrombin deficiency. *Semin Thromb Hemost.* 1999;25(03):257-263.

1460. White B, Perry D. Acquired antithrombin deficiency in sepsis. *Br J Haematol.* 2001;112(1):26-31.

1461. Wiedermann Ch J, Romisch J. The anti-inflammatory actions of antithrombin–a review. *Acta Med Austriaca.* 2002;29(3):89-92.

1462. Baudo F, Redaelli R, Caimi TM, Mostarda G, Somaini G, de Cataldo F. The continuous infusion of recombinant activated factor VIIa (rFVIIa) in patients with factor VIII inhibitors activates the coagulation and fibrinolytic systems without clinical complications. *Thromb Res.* 2000;99(1):21-24.

1463. Bock SC, Harris JF, Balazs I, Trent JM. Assignment of the human antithrombin III structural gene to chromosome 1q23-25. *Cytogenet Genome Res.* 1985;39(1):67-69.

1464. Olds RJ, Lane DA, Chowdhury V, De Stefano V, Leone G, Thein SL. Complete nucleotide sequence of the antithrombin gene: evidence for homologous recombination causing thrombophilia. *Biochemistry.* 1993;32(16):4216-4224.

1465. Fernandez-Rachubinski FA, Weiner JH, Blajchman MA. Regions flanking exon 1 regulate constitutive expression of the human antithrombin gene. *J Biol Chem.* 1996;271(46):29502-29512.

1466. Murano G, Williams L, Miller-Andersson M, Aronson DL, King C. Some properties of antithrombin-III and its concentration in human plasma. *Thromb Res.* 1980;18(1-2):259-262.

1467. Peterson CB, Blackburn MN. Isolation and characterization of an antithrombin III variant with reduced carbohydrate content and enhanced heparin binding. *J Biol Chem.* 1985;260(1):610-615.

1468. Prochownik EV, Markham AF, Orkin SH. Isolation of a cDNA clone for human antithrombin III. *J Biol Chem.* 1983;258(13):8389-8394.

1469. Bock SC, Wion KL, Vehar GA, Lawn RM. Cloning and expression of the cDNA for human antithrombin III. *Nucleic Acids Res.* 1982;10(24):8113-8125.

1470. Franzen LE, Svensson S, Larm O. Structural studies on the carbohydrate portion of human antithrombin III. *J Biol Chem.* 1980;255(11):5090-5093.

1471. Mizuochi T, Fujii J, Kurachi K, Kobata A. Structural studies of the carbohydrate moiety of human antithrombin III. *Arch Biochem Biophys.* 1980;203(1):458-465.

1472. Turk B, Brieditis I, Bock SC, Olson ST, Björk I. The oligosaccharide side chain on Asn-135 of α-antithrombin, absent in β-antithrombin, decreases the heparin affinity of the inhibitor by affecting the heparin-induced conformational change. *Biochemistry.* 1997;36(22):6682-6691.

1473. Mourey L, Samama J-P, Delarue M, Petitou M, Choay J, Moras D. Crystal structure of cleaved bovine antithrombin III at 3·2 Å resolution. *J Mol Biol.* 1993;232(1):223-241.

1474. Johnson DJD, Langdown J, Li W, Luis SA, Baglin TP, Huntington JA. Crystal structure of monomeric native antithrombin reveals a novel reactive center loop conformation. *J Biol Chem.* 2006;281(46):35478-35486.

1475. Wardell MR, Abrahams JP, Bruce D, Skinner R, Leslie AGW. Crystallization and preliminary X-ray diffraction analysis of two conformations of intact human antithrombin. *J Mol Biol.* 1993;234(4):1253-1258.

1476. Skinner R, Abrahams JP, Whisstock JC, Lesk AM, Carrell RW, Wardell MR. The 2.6 Å structure of antithrombin indicates a conformational change at the heparin binding site. *J Mol Biol.* 1997;266(3):601-609.

1477. Olson ST, Björk I, Shore JD. Kinetic characterization of heparin-catalyzed and uncatalyzed inhibition of blood coagulation proteinases by antithrombin. *Methods Enzymol.* 1993;222:525-559.

1478. Olson ST, Shore JD. Demonstration of a two-step reaction mechanism for inhibition of alpha-thrombin by antithrombin III and identification of the step affected by heparin. *J Biol Chem.* 1982;257(24):14891-14895.

1479. Casu B, Oreste P, Torri G, et al. The structure of heparin oligosaccharide fragments with high anti-(factor Xa) activity containing the minimal antithrombin III-binding sequence Chemical and 13 C nuclear-magnetic-resonance studies. *Biochem J.* 1981;197(3):599-609.

1480. O'Reilly MS. Antiangiogenic activity of the cleaved conformation of the serpin antithrombin. *Science.* 1999;285(5435):1926-1928.

1481. Gray E, Hogwood J, Mulloy B. The anticoagulant and antithrombotic mechanisms of heparin. *Heparin - A Century of Progress.* 2012;207:43-61. Springer Science + Business Media.

1482. Johnson DJD, Li W, Adams TE, Huntington JA. Antithrombin–S195A factor Xa-heparin structure reveals the allosteric mechanism of antithrombin activation. *EMBO J.* 2006;25(9):2029-2037.

1483. Rau J, Mitchell J, Fortenberry Y, Church F. Heparin cofactor II: discovery, properties, and role in controlling vascular homeostasis. *Semin Thromb Hemost.* 2011;37(04):339-348.

1484. Tollefsen DM, Pestka CA, Monafo WJ. Activation of heparin cofactor II by dermatan sulfate. *J Biol Chem.* 1983;258(11):6713-6716.

1485. Tollefsen DM, Majerus DW, Blank MK. Heparin cofactor II. Purification and properties of a heparin-dependent inhibitor of thrombin in human plasma. *J Biol Chem.* 1982;257(5):2162-2169.

1486. Griffith MJ, Carraway T, White GC, Dombrose FA. Heparin cofactor activities in a family with hereditary antithrombin III deficiency: evidence for a second heparin cofactor in human plasma. *Blood.* 1983;61(1):111-118.

1487. Andersson TR, Sie P, Pelzer H, Aamodt LM, Nustad K, Abildgaard U. Elevated levels of thrombin-heparin cofactor II complex in plasma from patients with disseminated intravascular coagulation. *Thromb Res.* 1992;66(5):591-598.

1488. Corral J. Homozygous deficiency of heparin cofactor II: relevance of P17 glutamate residue in serpins, relationship with conformational diseases, and role in thrombosis. *Circulation.* 2004;110(10):1303-1307.

1489. Simioni P, Lazzaro AR, Coser E, Salmistraro G, Girolami A. Hereditary heparin cofactor II deficiency and thrombosis. *Blood Coagul Fibrinolysis.* 1990;1(5):351-556.

1490. Weisdorf DJ, Edson JR. Recurrent venous thrombosis associated with inherited deficiency of heparin cofactor II. *Br J Haematol.* 1991;77(1):125-126.

1491. Andersson TR, Larsen ML, Handeland GF, Abildgaard U. Heparin cofactor II activity in plasma: application of an automated assay method to the study of a normal adult population. *Scand J Haematol.* 1986;36(1):96-102.

1492. Blinder MA, Marasa JC, Reynolds CH, Deaven LL, Tollefsen DM. Heparin cofactor II: cDNA sequence, chromosome localization, restriction fragment length polymorphism, and expression in *Escherichia coli. Biochemistry.* 1988;27(2):752-759.

1493. Herzog R, Lutz S, Blin N, Marasa JC, Blinder MA, Tollefsen DM. Complete nucleotide sequence of the gene for human heparin cofactor II and mapping to chromosomal band 22q11. *Biochemistry.* 1991;30(5):1350-1357.

1494. Ragg H. A new member of the plasma protease inhibitor gene family. *Nucleic Acids Res.* 1986;14(2):1073-1088.

1495. Zhang GS, Mehringer JH, Van Deerlin VMD, Kozak CA, Tollefsen DM. Murine heparin cofactor II: purification, cDNA sequence, expression, and gene structure. *Biochemistry.* 1994;33(12):3632-3642.

1496. Whinna HC, Blinder MA, Szewczyk M, Tollefsen DM, Church FC. Role of lysine 173 in heparin binding to heparin cofactor II. *J Biol Chem.* 1991;266(13):8129-8135.

1497. Blinder MA, Tollefsen DM. Site-directed mutagenesis of arginine 103 and lysine 185 in the proposed glycosaminoglycan-binding site of heparin cofactor II. *J Biol Chem.* 1990;265(1):286-291.

1498. Tollefsen DM. Heparin cofactor II. *Adv Exp Med Biol.* 1997;425:35-44. Springer Science + Business Media.

1499. Ragg H, Ulshofer T, Gerewitz J. On the activation of human leuserpin-2, a thrombin inhibitor, by glycosaminoglycans. *J Biol Chem.* 1990;265(9):5211-5218.

1500. Van Deerlin VM, Tollefsen DM. The N-terminal acidic domain of heparin cofactor II mediates the inhibition of alpha-thrombin in the presence of glycosaminoglycans. *J Biol Chem.* 1991;266(30):20223-20231.

1501. Sheehan JP, Wu Q, Tollefsen DM, Sadler JE. Mutagenesis of thrombin selectively modulates inhibition by serpins heparin cofactor II and antithrombin III. Interaction with the anion-binding exosite determines heparin cofactor II specificity. *J Biol Chem.* 1993;268(5):3639-3645.

1502. Church FC, Pratt CW, Hoffman M. Leukocyte chemoattractant peptides from the serpin heparin cofactor II. *J Biol Chem.* 1991;266(2):704-709.

1503. Joslin G, Wittwer A, Adams S, Tollefsen DM, August A, Perlmutter DH. Cross-competition for binding of alpha 1-antitrypsin (alpha 1 AT)-elastase complexes to the serpin-enzyme complex receptor by other serpin-enzyme complexes and by proteolytically modified alpha 1 AT. *J Biol Chem.* 1993;268(3):1886-1893.

1504. Griffith MJ, Noyes CM, Church FC. Reactive site peptide structural similarity between heparin cofactor II and antithrombin III. *J Biol Chem.* 1985;260(4):2218-2225.

1505. Fortenberry YM, Whinna HC, Gentry HR, Myles T, Leung LLK, Church FC. Molecular mapping of the thrombin-heparin cofactor II complex. *J Biol Chem.* 2004;279(41):43237-43244.

1506. Parker KA, Tollefsen DM. The protease specificity of heparin cofactor II. Inhibition of thrombin generated during coagulation. *J Biol Chem.* 1985;260(6):3501-3505.

1507. Giri TK. Letter to the Editor: heparin cofactor II levels do not predict the development of coronary heart disease – the atherosclerosis risk in Communities (ARIC) study. *Arterioscler Thromb Vasc Biol.* 2005;25(12):2689-2690.

1508. McGuire EA, Tollefsen DM. Activation of heparin cofactor II by fibroblasts and vascular smooth muscle cells. *J Biol Chem.* 1987;262(1):169-175.

1509. Tollefsen DM. Vascular dermatan sulfate and heparin cofactor II. *Prog Mol Biol Transl Sci.* 2010;93:351-372.

1510. Andrew M, Mitchell L, Berry L, et al. An anticoagulant dermatan sulfate proteoglycan circulates in the pregnant woman and her fetus. *J Clin Invest.* 1992;89(1):321-326.

1511. Massouh M, Jatoi A, Gordon EM, Ratnoff OD. Heparin cofactor II activity in plasma during pregnancy and oral contraceptive use. *J Lab Clin Med.* 1989;114(6):697-699.

1512. Liu L, Dewar L, Song Y, et al. Inhibition of thrombin by antithrombin III and heparin cofactor II in vivo. *Thromb Haemost.* 1995;73(3):405-412.

1513. Ikeda Y, Aihara Ki, Yoshida S, et al. Heparin cofactor II, a serine protease inhibitor, promotes angiogenesis via activation of the AMP-activated protein kinase-endothelial nitric-oxide synthase signaling pathway. *J Biol Chem.* 2012;287(41):34256-34263.

1514. Jeppsson JO, Laurell CB, Fagerhol M. Properties of isolated human alpha1-antitrypsins of Pi types M, S and Z. *Eur J Biochem.* 1978;83(1):143-153.

1515. Jeppsson JO, Laurell CB, Nosslin B, Cox DW. Catabolic rate of α 1-antitrypsin of Pi types S, and M malton and of asialylated M-protein in man. *Clin Sci.* 1978;55(1):103-107.

1516. Shalygin VA, Eroshenko LB, Solnyshko AL, Bocharov RV, Shalygin AV. Diagnostic and prognostic significance of study of acute phase proteins in children with appendicular peritonitis. *Klin Lab Diagn.* 2002;2002(7):7-9.

1517. Primhak RA. Alpha-1 antitrypsin deficiency. *Arch Dis Childhood.* 2001;85(1):2-5.

1518. Ekeowa UI, Marciniak SJ, Lomas DA. α 1-antitrypsin deficiency and inflammation. *Exp Rev Clin Immunol.* 2011;7(2):243-252.

1519. Lewis EC. Expanding the clinical indications for alpha(1)-antitrypsin therapy. *Mol Med.* 2012;18:957-970.

1520. Metz R, DiCola M, Kurihara T, et al. Mode of action of RNA/DNA oligonucleotides. *Chest.* 2002;121(3):91S-97S.

1521. Davies J. Prospects for gene therapy in lung disease. *Curr Opin Pharmacol.* 2001;1(3):272-278.

1522. Vadolas J, Williamson R, Ioannou PA. Gene therapy for inherited lung disorders: an insight into pulmonary defence. *Pulm Pharmacol Ther.* 2002;15(1):61-72.

1523. Gooptu B, Lomas DA. Conformational pathology of the serpins: themes, variations, and therapeutic strategies. *Annu Rev Biochem.* 2009;78(1):147-176.

1524. Leicht M, Long GL, Chandra T, et al. Sequence homology and structural comparison between the chromosomal human α1-antitrypsin and chicken ovalbumin genes. *Nature.* 1982;297(5868):655-659.

1525. Rabin M, Watson M, Kidd V, Woo SLC, Breg WR, Ruddle FH. Regional location of α1-antichymotrypsin and α1-antitrypsin genes on human chromosome 14. *Somat Cell Mol Genet.* 1986;12(2):209-214.

1526. Purrello M, Alhadeff B, Whittington E, et al. Comparison of cytologic and genetic distances between long arm subtelomeric markers of human autosome 14 suggests uneven distribution of crossing-over. *Cytogenet Genome Res.* 1987;44(1):32-40.

1527. Darlington GJ, Astrin KH, Muirhead SP, Desnick RJ, Smith M. Assignment of human alpha 1-antitrypsin to chromosome 14 by somatic cell hybrid analysis. *Proc Natl Acad Sci U S A.* 1982;79(3):870-873.

1528. Bao Jj, Reed-Fourquet L, Sifers RN, Kidd VJ, Woo SLC. Molecular structure and sequence homology of a gene related to α1-antitrypsin in the human genome. *Genomics.* 1988;2(2):165-173.

1529. Hofker MH, Nelen M, Klasen EC, et al. Cloning and characterization of an α1-antitrypsin like gene 12 kb downstream of the genuine α1-antitrypsin gene. *Biochem Biophys Res Commun.* 1988;155(2):634-642.

1530. Rollini P. Differential regulation of gene activity and chromatin structure within the human serpin gene cluster at 14q32.1 in macrophage microcell hybrids. *Nucleic Acids Res.* 2000;28(8):1767-1777.

1531. Hu C, Perlmutter DH. Cell-specific involvement of HNF-1β in α1-antitrypsin gene expression in human respiratory epithelial cells. *Am J Physiol Lung Cell Mol Physiol.* 2002;282(4):L757-L765.

1532. Janciauskiene SM, Bals R, Koczulla R, Vogelmeier C, Kohnlein T, Welte T. The discovery of alpha1-antitrypsin and its role in health and disease. *Respir Med.* 2011;105(8):1129-1139.

1533. Brantly M, Nukiwa T, Crystal RG. Molecular basis of alpha-1-antitrypsin deficiency. *Am J Med.* 1988;84(6A):13-31.

1534. Johnson D, Travis J. Structural evidence for methionine at the reactive site of human alpha-1-proteinase inhibitor. *J Biol Chem.* 1978;253(20):7142-7144.

1535. Matheson NR, van Halbeek H, Travis J. Evidence for a tetrahedral intermediate complex during serpin-proteinase interactions. *J Biol Chem.* 1991;266(21):13489-13491.

1536. Loebermann H, Tokuoka R, Deisenhofer J, Huber R. Human alpha 1-proteinase inhibitor. Crystal structure analysis of two crystal modifications, molecular model and preliminary analysis of the implications for function. *J Mol Biol.* 1984;177(3):531-557.

1537. Schulze AJ, Frohnert PW, Engh RA, Huber R. Evidence for the extent of insertion of the active site loop of intact.alpha.1 proteinase inhibitor in.beta.-sheet A. *Biochemistry.* 1992;31(33):7560-7565.

1538. Smith KF, Harrison RA, Perkins SJ. Structural comparisons of the native and reactive-centre-cleaved forms of α 1 -antitrypsin by neutron- and X-ray-scattering in solution. *Biochem J.* 1990;267(1):203-212.

1539. Murakami T, Komiyama Y, Masuda M, Karakawa M, Iwasaka T, Takahashi H. Evaluation of factor XIa 1-antitrypsin in plasma, a contact phase activated coagulation factor inhibitor complex, in patients with coronary artery disease. *Arterioscler Thromb Vasc Biol.* 1995;15(8):1107-1113.

1540. Wuillemin WA, Hack CE, Bleeker WK, Biemond BJ, Levi M, ten Cate H. Inactivation of factor Xia in vivo: studies in chimpanzees and in humans. *Thromb Haemost.* 1996;76(4):549-555.

1541. Scully MF, Toh CH, Hoogendoorn H, et al. Activation of protein C and its distribution between its inhibitors, protein C inhibitor, alpha 1-antitrypsin and alpha 2-macroglobulin, in patients with disseminated intravascular coagulation. *Thromb Haemost.* 1993;69(5):448-453.

1542. Carter PE, Dunbar B, Fothergill JE. Genomic and cDNA cloning of the human C1 inhibitor. Intron-exon junctions and comparison with other serpins. *Eur J Biochem.* 1988;173(1):163-169.

1543. Orfan NA, Kolski GB. Angioedema and C1 inhibitor deficiency. *Ann Allergy.* 1992;69(3):167-172.

1544. Phanish MK. Spontaneous regression of acquired C1 esterase inhibitor deficiency associated with splenic marginal zone lymphoma presenting with recurrent angiooedema. *J Clin Pathol.* 2002;55(10):789-790.

1545. Shiozawa S, Shiozawa K. Angioedema and acquired C1 esterase inhibitor deficiency. *Intern Med.* 2002;41(5):333-334.

1546. Han ED, MacFarlane RC, Mulligan AN, Scafidi J, Davis AE. Increased vascular permeability in C1 inhibitor–deficient mice mediated by the bradykinin type 2 receptor. *J Clin Invest.* 2002;109(8):1057-1063.

1547. Frank MM. Hereditary angioedema: a current state-of-the-art review, VI – novel therapies for hereditary angioedema. *Ann Allergy Asthma Immunol.* 2008;100(1 suppl 2):S23-S29.

1548. Antoniu SA. Therapeutic approaches in hereditary angioedema. *Clin Rev Allergy Immunol.* 2011;41(1):114-122.

1549. Singer MJ, Jones. Hereditary angioedema: a current state-of-the-art review, VI – novel therapies for hereditary angioedema. *Ann Allergy Asthma Immunol.* 2011;100:S23-S29.

1550. Banz Y, Rieben R. Role of complement and perspectives for intervention in ischemia-reperfusion damage. *Ann Med.* 2012;44(3):205-217.

1551. Bock SC, Skriver K, Nielsen E, et al. Human C.hivin.1 inhibitor: primary structure, cDNA cloning, and chromosomal localization. *Biochemistry.* 1986;25(15):4292-4301.

1552. Zahedi K, Prada AE, Davis AE,IIIrd. Structure and regulation of the C1 inhibitor gene. *Behring Inst Mitt.* 1993;1993(93):115-119.

1553. Kang HR, Yim EY, Oh SY, et al. Normal C1 inhibitor mRNA expression level in type I hereditary angioedema patients: newly found C1 inhibitor gene mutations. *Allergy.* 2006;61(2):260-264.

1554. Tosi M. Molecular genetics of C1 inhibitor. *Immunobiology.* 1998;199(2):358-365.

1555. Davis AE,IIIrd, Lu F, Mejia P. C1 inhibitor, a multi-functional serine protease inhibitor. *Thromb Haemost.* 2010;104(5):886-893.

1556. Bos IG, Lubbers YT, Roem D, Abrahams JP, Hack CE, Eldering E. The functional integrity of the serpin domain of C1-inhibitor depends on the unique N-terminal domain, as revealed by a pathological mutant. *J Biol Chem.* 2003;278(32):29463-29470.

1557. Coutinho M, Aulak KS, Davis AE,IIIrd. Functional analysis of the serpin domain of C1 inhibitor. *J Immunol.* 1994;153(8):3648-3654.

1558. Wagenaar-Bos IG, Hack CE. Structure and function of C1-inhibitor. *Immunol Allergy Clin North Am.* 2006;26(4):615-632.

1559. Perkins SJ, Smith KF, Amatayakul S, et al. Two-domain structure of the native and reactive centre cleaved forms of C1 inhibitor of human complement by neutron scattering. *J Mol Biol.* 1990;214(3):751-763.

1560. Perkins SJ, Smith KF, Nealis AS, et al. Secondary structure changes stabilize the reactive-centre cleaved form of SERPINs. *J Mol Biol.* 1992;228(4):1235-1254.

1561. Perkins SJ. Three-dimensional structure and molecular modelling of C1- inhibitor. *Behring Inst Mitt.* 1993;93:63-80.

1562. Laurell AB, Johnson U, Martensson U, Sjoholm AG. Formation of complexes composed of C1r, C1s, and C1 inactivator in human serum on activation of C1. *Acta Pathol Microbiol Scand C.* 1978;86C(6):299-306.

1563. Wuillemin WA, Minnema M, Meijers JC, et al. Inactivation of factor XIa in human plasma assessed by measuring factor XIa-protease inhibitor complexes: major role for C1-inhibitor. *Blood.* 1995;85(6):1517-1526.

1564. Nilsson T. On the interaction between human plasma kallikrein and C1-esterase inhibitor. *Thromb Haemost.* 1983;49(3):193-195.

1565. Geiger M, Zechmeister-Machhart M, Uhrin P, et al. Protein C inhibitor (PCI). *Immunopharmacology.* 1996;32(1-3):53-56.

1566. Seregni E, Botti C, Ballabio G, Bombardieri E. Biochemical characteristics and recent biological knowledge on prostate-specific antigen. *Tumori.* 1996;82(1):72-77.

1567. Suzuki K, Nishioka J, Hashimoto S. Protein C inhibitor. Purification from human plasma and characterization. *J Biol Chem.* 1983;258(1):163-168.

1568. Laurell M, Christensson A, Abrahamsson PA, Stenflo J, Lilja H. Protein C inhibitor in human body fluids. Seminal plasma is rich in inhibitor antigen deriving from cells throughout the male reproductive system. *J Clin Invest.* 1992;89(4):1094-1101.

1569. Laurell M, Stenflo J, Carlson TH. Turnover of *I-protein C inhibitor and *I-alpha 1-antitrypsin and their complexes with activated protein C. *Blood.* 1990;76(11):2290-2295.

1570. Meijers JCM, Marquart JA, Bertina RM, Bouma BN, Rosendaal FR. Protein C inhibitor (plasminogen activator inhibitor-3) and the risk of venous thrombosis. *Br J Haematol.* 2002;118(2):604-609.

1571. Uhrin P, Dewerchin M, Hilpert M, et al. Disruption of the protein C inhibitor gene results in impaired spermatogenesis and male infertility. *J Clin Invest.* 2000;106(12):1531-1539.

1572. Meijers JC, Chung DW. Organization of the gene coding for human protein C inhibitor (plasminogen activator inhibitor-3). Assignment of the gene to chromosome 14. *J Biol Chem.* 1991;266(23):15028-15034.

1573. Billingsley GD, Walter MA, Hammond GL, Cox DW. Physical mapping of four serpin genes: alpha 1-antitrypsin, alpha 1-antichymotrypsin, corticosteroid-binding globulin, and protein C inhibitor, within a 280-kb region on chromosome I4q32.1. *Am J Hum Genet.* 1993;52(2):343-353.

1574. Suzuki K, Deyashiki Y, Nishioka J, et al. Characterization of a cDNA for human protein C inhibitor. A new member of the plasma serine protease inhibitor superfamily. *J Biol Chem.* 1987;262(2):611-616.

1575. Seixas S, Garcia O, Trovoada J, Santos T, Amorim A, Rocha J. Patterns of haplotype diversity within the serpin gene cluster at 14q32.1: insights into the natural history of the α1-antitrypsin polymorphism. *Hum Genet.* 2001;108(1):20-30.

1576. Nishioka J, Ning M, Hayashi T, Suzuki K. Protein C inhibitor secreted from activated platelets efficiently inhibits activated protein C on phosphatidylethanolamine of platelet membrane and microvesicles. *J Biol Chem.* 1998;273(18):11281-11287.

1577. Krebs M, Uhrin P, Vales A, et al. Protein C inhibitor is expressed in human skin. *J Invest Dermatol.* 1999;113(1):32-37.

1578. Radtke KP, Fernández JA, Greengard JS, et al. Protein C inhibitor is expressed in tubular cells of human kidney. *J Clin Invest.* 1994;94(5):2117-2124.

1579. Sun W, Parry S, Ubhayasekera W, Engstrom A, Dell A, Schedin-Weiss S. Further insight into the roles of the glycans attached to human blood protein C inhibitor. *Biochem Biophys Res Commun.* 2010;403(2):198-202.

1580. Fujita M, Izutani W, Takahashi K, Nishizawa K, Shirono H, Koga J. Role of each Asn-linked glycan in the anticoagulant activity of human protein C inhibitor. *Thromb Res.* 2002;105(1):95-102.

1581. Pratt CW, Church FC. General features of the heparin-binding serpins antithrombin, heparin cofactor II and protein C inhibitor. *Blood Coagul Fibrinolysis.* 1993;4(3):479-490.

1582. Neese LL, Wolfe CA, Church FC. Contribution of basic residues of the D and H helices in heparin binding to protein C inhibitor. *Arch Biochem Biophys.* 1998;355(1):101-108.

1583. Li W, Adams TE, Kjellberg M, Stenflo J, Huntington JA. Structure of native protein C inhibitor provides insight into its multiple functions. *J Biol Chem.* 2007;282(18):13759-13768.

1584. España F, Vicente V, Tabernero D, Scharrer I, Griffin JH. Determination of plasma protein C inhibitor and of two activated protein C-inhibitor complexes in normals and in patients with intravascular coagulation and thrombotic disease. *Thromb Res.* 1990;59(3):593-608.

1585. Meijers J, Herwald H. Protein C inhibitor. *Semin Thromb Hemost.* 2011;37(04):349-354.

1586. Suzuki K. The multi-functional serpin, protein C inhibitor: beyond thrombosis and hemostasis. *J Thromb Haemost.* 2008;6(12):2017-2026.

1587. Fortenberry YM, Hlavacek AC, Church FC. Protein C inhibitor inhibits factor VIIa when bound to tissue factor. *J Thromb Haemost.* 2011;9(4):861-863.

1588. Rezaie AR, Cooper ST, Church FC, Esmon CT. Protein C inhibitor is a potent inhibitor of the thrombin-thrombomodulin complex. *J Biol Chem.* 1995;270(43):25336-25339.

1589. Heeb MJ, Espana F, Griffin JH. Inhibition and complexation of activated protein C by two major inhibitors in plasma. *Blood.* 1989;73(2):446-454.

1590. Hoogendoorn H, Nesheim ME, Giles AR. A qualitative and quantitative analysis of the activation and inactivation of protein C in vivo in a primate model. *Blood.* 1990;75(11):2164-2171.

1591. Mosnier LO, Elisen MG, Bouma BN, Meijers JC. Protein C inhibitor regulates the thrombin-thrombomodulin complex in the up- and down regulation of TAFI activation. *Thromb Haemost.* 2001;86(4):1057-1064.

1592. Strandberg K, Astermark J, Bjorgell O, Becker C, Nilsson PE, Stenflo J. Complexes between activated protein C and protein C inhibitor measured with a new method: comparison of performance with other markers of hypercoagulability in the diagnosis of deep vein thrombosis. *Thromb Haemost.* 2001;86(6):1400-1408.

1593. Barkan G, Gaspar A. Zur frage der Reversibilitaet der Fibringerinnung. *Biochemische Zeitschrift.* 1923;139:291-301.

1594. Muszbek L, Ariens RA, Ichinose A. Isth Ssc Subcommittee on factor X. Factor XIII: recommended terms and abbreviations. *J Thromb Haemost.* 2007;5(1):181-183.

1595. KC R. A study on the conversion of fibrin clots. *Am J Physiol.* 1944;142:581-588.

1596. Laki K, Lorand L. On the solubility of fibrin clots. *Science.* 1948;108(2802):280.

1597. Lorand L. A study on the solubility of fibrin clots in urea. *Hung Acta Physiol.* 1948;1(6):192-196.

1598. Muszbek L, Yee VC, Hevessy Z. Blood coagulation factor XIII. *Thromb Res.* 1999;94(5):271-305.

1599. Procyk R, Adamson L, Block M, Blomback B. Factor XIII catalyzed formation of fibrinogen-fibronectin oligomers—a thiol enhanced process. *Thromb Res.* 1985;40(6):833-852.

1600. Procyk R, Blomback B. Factor XIII-induced crosslinking in solutions of fibrinogen and fibronectin. *Biochim Biophys Acta.* 1988;967(2):304-313.

1601. Tamaki T, Aoki N. Cross-linking of alpha 2-plasmin inhibitor to fibrin catalyzed by activated fibrin-stabilizing factor. *J Biol Chem.* 1982;257(24):14767-14772.

1602. Chen R, Doolittle RF. γ-γ Cross-linking sites in human and bovine fibrin. *Biochemistry.* 1971;10(24):4486-4491.

1603. Kanaide H, Shainoff JR. Cross-linking of fibrinogen and fibrin by fibrin-stablizing factor (factor XIIIa). *J Lab Clin Med.* 1975;85(4):574-597.

1604. Mosher DF, Schad PE. Cross-linking of fibronectin to collagen by blood coagulation Factor XIIIa. *J Clin Invest.* 1979;64(3):781-787.

1605. Mosher DF. Cross-linking of fibronectin to collagenous proteins. *Mol Cell Biochem.* 1984;58(1-2):63-68.

1606. Mui PT, Ganguly P. Cross-linking of actin and fibrin by fibrin-stabilizing factor. *Am J Physiol.* 1977;233(3):H346-H349.

1607. Lynch GW, Slayter HS, Miller BE, McDonagh J. Characterization of thrombospondin as a substrate for factor XIII transglutaminase. *J Biol Chem.* 1987;262(4):1772-1778.

1608. Lorand L. Factor XIII and the clotting of fibrinogen: from basic research to medicine. *J Thromb Haemost.* 2005;3(7):1337-1348.

1609. Dardik R, Loscalzo J, Inbal A. Factor XIII (FXIII) and angiogenesis. *J Thromb Haemost.* 2006;4(1):19-25.

1610. Muszbek L, Bereczky Z, Bagoly Z, Komaromi I, Katona E. Factor XIII: a coagulation factor with multiple plasmatic and cellular functions. *Phys Rev.* 2011;91(3):931-972.

1611. Ichinose A. Factor XIII is a key molecule at the intersection of coagulation and fibrinolysis as well as inflammation and infection control. *Int J Hematol.* 2012;95(4):362-370.

1612. Sane DC. Roles of transglutaminases in cardiac and vascular diseases. *Front Biosci.* 2007;12(1):2530.

1613. Weisberg LJ, Shiu DT, Greenberg CS, Kan YW, Shuman MA. Localization of the gene for coagulation factor XIII a-chain to chromosome 6 and identification of sites of synthesis. *J Clin Invest.* 1987;79(2):649-652.

1614. Board PG, Webb GC, McKee J, Ichinose A. Localization of the coagulation factor XIII A subunit gene (F13A) to chromosome bands 6p24→p25. *Cytogenet Genome Res.* 1988;48(1):25-27.

1615. Ichinose A, Davie EW. Characterization of the gene for the a subunit of human factor XIII (plasma transglutaminase), a blood coagulation factor. *Proc Natl Acad Sci.* 1988;85(16):5829-5833.

1616. Webb GC, Coggan M, Ichinose A, Board P. Localization of the coagulation factor XIII B subunit gene (F13B) to chromosome bands 1q31?32.1 and restriction fragment length polymorphism at the locus. *Hum Genet.* 1989;81(2):157-160.

1617. Grundmann U, Nerlich C, Rein T, Zettlmeissl G. Complete cDNA sequence encoding the B subunit of human factor XIII. *Nucl Acids Res.* 1990;18(9):2817-2818.

1618. Ichinose A, McMullen BA, Fujikawa K, Davie EW. Amino acid sequence of the b subunit of human factor XIII, a protein composed of ten repetitive segments. *Biochemistry.* 1986;25(16):4633-4638.

1619. Bottenus RE, Ichinose A, Davie EW. Nucleotide sequence of the gene for the b subunit of human factor XIII. *Biochemistry.* 1990;29(51):11195-11209.

1620. Morley BJ, Campbell RD. Internal homologies of the Ba fragment from human complement component Factor B, a class III MHC antigen. *EMBO J.* 1984;3(1):153-157.

1621. Chung LP, Gagnon J, Reid KBM. Amino acid sequence studies of human C4b-binding protein: N-terminal sequence analysis and alignment of the fragments produced by limited proteolysis with chymotrypsin and the peptides produced by cyanogen bromide treatment. *Mol Immunol.* 1985;22(4):427-435.

1622. Miloszewski KJA, Losowski MS. Fibrin stabilization and factor XIII deficiency. In: Horwood E, ed. *Fibrinogen, Fibrin Stabilization and Finbrinolysis.* L Francis; 1988:175-202.

1623. Kohler HP, Ichinose A, Seitz R, Ariens RAS, Muszbek L. Diagnosis and classification of factor XIII deficiencies. *J Thromb Haemost.* 2011;9(7):1404-1406.

1624. Lowey AG, McDonagh J, Mikkola H, Teller DC, Yee VC. Structure and function of factor XIII. In: Colman RW, HJ , Marder VJ, Clowes AW, George JN, eds. *Hemostasis and Thrombosis.* Lippincott, Williams & Wilkins; 2001:233-247.

1625. Biswas A, Ivaskevicius V, Seitz R, Thomas A, Oldenburg J. An update of the mutation profile of Factor 13 A and B genes. *Blood Rev.* 2011;25(5):193-204.

1626. Ariens RAS. Role of factor XIII in fibrin clot formation and effects of genetic polymorphisms. *Blood.* 2002;100(3):743-754.

1627. Reiner AP, Schwartz SM, Frank MB, et al. Polymorphisms of coagulation factor XIII subunit A and risk of nonfatal hemorrhagic stroke in young white women editorial comment. *Stroke.* 2001;32(11):2580-2587.

1628. Mikkola H, Syrjala M, Rasi V, et al. Deficiency in the A-subunit of coagulation factor XIII: two novel point mutations demonstrate different effects on transcript levels. *Blood.* 1994;84(2):517-525.

1629. Kohler HP, Stickland MH, Ossei-Gerning N, Carter A, Mikkola H, Grant PJ. Association of a common polymorphism in the factor XIII gene with myocardial infarction. *Thromb Haemost.* 1998;79(1):8-13.

1630. Wartiovaara U, Perola M, Mikkola H, et al. Association of FXIII Val34Leu with decreased risk of myocardial infarction in Finnish males. *Atherosclerosis.* 1999;142(2):295-300.

1631. Catto AJ, Kohler HP, Coore J, Mansfield MW, Stickland MH, Grant PJ. Association of a common polymorphism in the factor XIII gene with venous thrombosis. *Blood.* 1999;93(3):906-908.

1632. Franco RF, Reitsma PH, Lourenco D, et al. Factor XIII Val34Leu is a genetic factor involved in the etiology of venous thrombosis. *Thromb Haemost.* 1999;81(5):676-679.

1633. Elbaz A, Poirier O, Canaple S, Chedru F, Cambien F, Amarenco P. The association between the Val34Leu polymorphism in the factor XIII gene and brain infarction. *Blood.* 2000;95(2):586-591.

1634. Renner W, Koppel H, Hoffmann C, et al. Prothrombin G20210A, factor V Leiden, and factor XIII Val34Leu: common mutations of blood coagulation factors and deep vein thrombosis in Austria. *Thromb Res.* 2000;99(1):35-39.

1635. Lorand L. Factor XIII: structure, activation, and interactions with fibrinogen and fibrin. *Ann N Y Acad Sci.* 2001;936:291-311.

1636. Kohler HP, Ariens RA, Whitaker P, Grant PJ. A common coding polymorphism in the FXIII A-subunit gene (FXIIIVal34Leu) affects cross-linking activity. *Thromb Haemost.* 1998;80(4):704.

1637. Kangsadalampai S, Board PG. The Val34Leu polymorphism in the A subunit of coagulation factor XIII contributes to the large normal range in activity and demonstrates that the activation peptide plays a role in catalytic activity. *Blood.* 1998;92(8):2766-2770.

1638. Anwar R, Gallivan L, Edmonds SD, Markham AF. Genotype/phenotype correlations for coagulation factor XIII: specific normal polymorphisms are associated with high or low factor XIII specific activity. *Blood.* 1999;93(3):897-905.

1639. Ariens RA, Philippou H, Nagaswami C, Weisel JW, Lane DA, Grant PJ. The factor XIII V34L polymorphism accelerates thrombin activation of factor XIII and affects cross-linked fibrin structure. *Blood.* 2000;96(3):988-995.

1640. Undas A, Sydor WJ, Brummel K, Musial J, Mann KG, Szczeklik A. Aspirin alters the cardioprotective effects of the factor XIII Val34Leu polymorphism. *Circulation.* 2003;107(1):17-20.

1641. Schwartz ML, Pizzo SV, Hill RL, McKee PA. Human Factor XIII from plasma and platelets. Molecular weights, subunit structures, proteolytic activation, and cross-linking of fibrinogen and fibrin. *J Biol Chem.* 1973;248(4):1395-1407.

1642. Radek JT, Jeong JM, Wilson J, Lorand L. Association of the A subunits of recombinant placental factor XIII with the native carrier B subunits from human plasma. *Biochemistry.* 1993;32(14):3527-3534.

1643. Yorifuji H, Anderson K, Lynch GW, Van de Water L, McDonagh J. B protein of factor XIII: differentiation between free B and complexed B. *Blood.* 1988;72(5):1645-1650.

1644. Katona E, Haramura G, Karpati L, Fachet J, Muszbek L. A simple, quick one-step ELISA assay for the determination of complex plasma factor XIII (A2B2). *Thromb Haemost.* 2000;83(2):268-273.

1645. Takahashi N, Takahashi Y, Putnam FW. Primary structure of blood coagulation factor XIIIa (fibrinoligase, transglutaminase) from human placenta. *Proc Natl Acad Sci.* 1986;83(21):8019-8023.

1646. Ichinose A, Hendrickson LE, Fujikawa K, Davie EW. Amino acid sequence of the a subunit of human factor XIII. *Biochemistry.* 1986;25(22):6900-6906.

1647. Carrell NA, Erickson HP, McDonagh J. Electron microscopy and hydrodynamic properties of factor XIII subunits. *J Biol Chem.* 1989;264(1):551-556.

1648. McDonagh J. Structure and function of factor XIII. In: Colman RW, HJ , Marder VJ, Sandberg H, eds. *Hemostasis and Thrombosis: Basic Principles and Clinical Practice.* Lippincott; 1994:301-313.

1649. Ichinose A, Kaetsu H. Molecular approach to structure-function relationship of human coagulation factor XIII. *Methods Enzymol.* 1993;222:36-51. Elsevier BV.

1650. Pedersen LC, Yee VC, Bishop PD, Trong IL, Teller DC, Stenkamp RE. Transglutaminase factor XIII uses proteinase-like catalytic triad to crosslink macromolecules. *Protein Sci.* 1994;3(7):1131-1135.

1651. Yee VC, Pedersen LC, Bishop PD, Stenkamp RE, Teller DC. Structural evidence that the activation peptide is not released upon thrombin cleavage of factor XIII. *Thromb Res.* 1995;78(5):389-397.

1652. Fox BA, Yee VC, Pedersen LC, et al. Identification of the calcium binding site and a novel Ytterbium site in blood coagulation factor XIII by X-ray crystallography. *J Biol Chem.* 1999;274(8):4917-4923.

1653. Yee V, Le Trong I, Bishop P, Pedersen L, Stenkamp R, Teller D. Structure and function studies of factor XIIIa by x-ray crystallography. *Semin Thromb Hemost.* 1996;22(05):377-384.

1654. Pedersen LC. *X-ray Structure Determination of Factor XIII.* University of Washington; 1994.

1655. Weisberg LJ, Shiu DT, Conkling PR, Shuman MA. Identification of normal human peripheral blood monocytes and liver as sites of synthesis of coagulation factor XIII a-chain. *Blood.* 1987;70(2):579-582.

1656. Wölpl A, Lattke H, Board PG, et al. Coagulation factor XIII a and B subunits in bone marrow and liver transplantation. *Transplantation.* 1987;43(1):151-153.

1657. Poon MC, Russell JA, Low S, et al. Hemopoietic origin of factor XIII A subunits in platelets, monocytes, and plasma. Evidence from bone marrow transplantation studies. *J Clin Invest.* 1989;83(3):787-792.

1658. McDonagh J, McDonagh RP, Del'ge JM, Wagner RH. Factor XIII in human plasma and platelets. *J Clin Invest.* 1969;48(5):940-946.

1659. Henriksson P, Becker S, Lynch G, McDonagh J. Identification of intracellular factor XIII in human monocytes and macrophages. *J Clin Invest.* 1985;76(2):528-534.

1660. Muszbek L, Adány R, Szegedi G, Polgár J, Kávai M. Factor XIII of blood coagulation in human monocytes. *Thromb Res.* 1985;37(3):401-410.

1661. Takagi T, Doolittle RF. Amino acid sequence studies on factor XIII and the peptide released during its activation by thrombin. *Biochemistry.* 1974;13(4):750-756.

1662. Kaetsu H, Hashiguchi T, Foster D, Ichinose A. Expression and release of the a and b subunits from human coagulation factor XIII in baby hamster kidney (BHK) cells. *J Biochem.* 1996;119(5):961-969.

1663. Mignatti P, Morimoto T, Rifkin DB. Basic fibroblast growth factor, a protein devoid of secretory signal sequence, is released by cells via a pathway independent of the endoplasmic reticulum-Golgi complex. *J Cell Physiol.* 1992;151(1):81-93.

1664. Rubartelli A, Cozzolino F, Talio M, Sitia R. A novel secretory pathway for interleukin-1 beta, a protein lacking a signal sequence. *EMBO J.* 1990;9(5):1503-1510.

1665. Kreager JA, Devine DV, Greenberg CS. Cytofluorometric identification of plasmin-sensitive factor XIIIa binding to platelets. *Thromb Haemost.* 1988;60(1):88-93.

1666. Greenberg CS, Shuman MA. Specific binding of blood coagulation factor XIIIa to thrombin-stimulated platelets. *J Biol Chem.* 1984;259(23):14721-14727.

1667. Nagy JA, Kradin RL, McDonagh J. Biosynthesis of factor XIII A and B subunits. *Adv Exp Med Biol.* 1988;231:29-49. Springer Science + Business Media.

1668. Mikuni Y, Iwanaga S, Konishi K. A peptide released from plasma fibrin stabilizing factor in the conversion to the active enzyme by thrombin. *Biochem Biophys Res Commun.* 1973;54(4):1393-1402.

1669. Komaromi I, Bagoly Z, Muszbek L. Factor XIII: novel structural and functional aspects. *J Thromb Haemost.* 2011;9(1):9-20.

1670. Nikolajsen CL, Dyrlund TF, Poulsen ET, Enghild JJ, Scavenius C. Coagulation factor XIIIa substrates in human plasma: identification and incorporation into the clot. *J Biol Chem.* 2014;289(10):6526-6534.

1671. Schroeder V, Kohler HP. Factor XIII: structure and function. *Semin Thromb Hemost.* 2016;42(4):422-428.

1672. Souri M, Ichinose A. Impaired protein folding, dimer formation, and heterotetramer assembly cause intra- and extracellular instability of a Y283C mutant of the A subunit for coagulation factor XIII. *Biochemistry.* 2001;40(45):13413-13420.

1673. Credo RB, Curtis CG, Lorand L. Ca2+-related regulatory function of fibrinogen. *Proc Natl Acad Sci U S A.* 1978;75(9):4234-4237.

1674. Curtis CG, Brown KL, Credo RB, et al. Calcium-dependent unmasking of active center cysteine during activation of fibrin stabilizing factor. *Biochemistry.* 1974;13(18):3774-3780.

1675. Hornyak TJ, Shafer JA. Role of calcium ion in the generation of factor XIII activity. *Biochemistry.* 1991;30(25):6175-6182.

1676. Brummel-Ziedins KE, Branda RF, Butenas S, Mann KG. Discordant fibrin formation in hemophilia. *J Thromb Haemost.* 2009;7(5):825-832.

1677. Naski MC, Lorand L, Shafer JA. Characterization of the kinetic pathway for fibrin promotion of alpha-thrombin-catalyze activation of plasma factor XIII. *Biochemistry.* 1991;30(4):934-941.

1678. Janus TJ, Lewis SD, Lorand L, Shafer JA. Promotion of thrombin-catalyzed activation of factor XIII by fibrinogen. *Biochemistry.* 1983;22(26):6269-6272.

1679. Gorman JJ, Folk JE. Structural features of glutamine substrates for human plasma factor XIIIa (activated blood coagulation factor XIII). *J Biol Chem.* 1980;255(2):419-427.

1680. Chung SI, Folk JE. Kinetic studies with transglutaminases. The human blood enzymes (activated coagulation factor 13 and the Guinea pig hair follicle enzyme. *J Biol Chem.* 1972;247(9):2798-2807.

1681. Lord ST. Fibrinogen and fibrin: scaffold proteins in hemostasis. *Curr Opin Hematol.* 2007;14(3):236-241.

1682. Mosesson MW. Fibrinogen and fibrin structure and functions. *J Thromb Haemost.* 2005;3(8):1894-1904.

1683. Everse SJ. New insights into fibrin (ogen) structure and function. *Vox Sanguinis.* 2002;83:375-382.

1684. Hantgan RR, Simpson-Haidaris PJ, Francis CW, Mader VJ. Fibrinogen structure and physiology. In: Colman RW, Hirsh J, Marder VJ, Clowes AW, George JN, eds. *Hemostasis and Thrombosis: Basic Principles and Clinical Practice.* Lippincott, Williams & Wilkins; 2001:203-232.

1685. Doolittle RF, Yang Z, Mochalkin I. Crystal structure studies on fibrinogen and fibrin. *Ann N Y Acad Sci.* 2001;936:31-43.

1686. Blombäck B. Fibrinogen: evolution of the structure-function concept. *Ann N Y Acad Sci.* 2006;936(1):1-10.

1687. Straub PW. A study of fibrinogen production by human liver slices in vitro by an immunoprecipitin method. *J Clin Invest.* 1963;42(1):130-136.

1688. Takeda Y. Studies of the metabolism and distribution of fibrinogen in healthy men with autologous 125-I-labeled fibrinogen. *J Clin Invest.* 1966;45(1):103-111.

1689. Collen D, Tytgat GN, Claeys H, Piessens R. Metabolism and distribution of fibrinogen. I. Fibrinogen turnover in physiological conditions in humans. *Br J Haematol.* 1972;22(6):681-700.

1690. Rausen AR, Cruchaud A, Mc MC, Gitlin D. A study of fibrinogen turnover in classical hemophilia and congenital afibrinogenemia. *Blood.* 1961;18:710-716.

1691. de Maat MP. Effects of diet, drugs, and genes on plasma fibrinogen levels. *Ann N Y Acad Sci.* 2001;936:509-521.

1692. Blombäck B, Blombäck M, Henschen A, Hessel B, Iwanaga S, Woods KR. N-terminal disulphide knot of human fibrinogen. *Nature.* 1968;218(5137):130-134.

1693. Doolittle RF. Evolution of fibrinogen molecules. *Thromb Diath Haemorrh.* 1970;39:25-42.

1694. Doolittle RF. Differences in the clotting of lamprey fibrinogen by lamprey and bovine thrombins. *Biochem J.* 1965;94(3):735-741.

1695. Doolittle RF. The structure and evolution of vertebrate fibrinogen. *Ann N Y Acad Sci.* 1983;408:13-27.

1696. Takagi T, Doolittle RF. Amino acid sequence studies on the α chain of human fibrinogen. Location of four plasmin attack points and a covalent cross-linking site. *Biochemistry.* 1975;14(23):5149-5156.

1697. Henschen A, Lottspeich F. Sequence homology between γ-chain and β-chain in human fibrin. *Thromb Res.* 1977;11(6):869-880.

1698. Watt KW, Takagi T, Doolittle RF. Amino acid sequence of the beta chain of human fibrinogen: homology with the gamma chain. *Proc Natl Acad Sci.* 1978;75(4):1731-1735.

1699. Doolittle RF. A detailed consideration of a principal domain of vertebrate fibrinogen and its relatives. *Protein Sci.* 1992;1(12):1563-1577.

1700. Kant JA, Fornace AJ, Saxe D, Simon MI, McBride OW, Crabtree GR. Evolution and organization of the fibrinogen locus on chromosome 4: gene duplication accompanied by transposition and inversion. *Proc Natl Acad Sci.* 1985;82(8):2344-2348.

1701. Doolittle RF, Cottrell BA, Riley M. Amino acid compositions of the subunit chains of lamprey fibrinogen. *Biochim Biophys Acta.* 1976;453(2):439-452.

1702. Strong DD, Laudano AP, Hawiger J, Doolittle RF. Isolation, characterization and synthesis of peptides from human fibrinogen that block the staphylococcal clumping reaction and construction of a synthetic clumping particle. *Biochemistry.* 1982;21(6):1414-1420.

1703. Crabtree GR, Kant JA. Coordinate accumulation of the mRNAs for the alpha, beta, and gamma chains of rat fibrinogen following defibrination. *J Biol Chem.* 1982;257(13):7277-7279.

1704. Morgan JG, Holbrook NJ, Crabtree GR. Nucleotide sequence of the gamma chain gene of rat fibrinogen: conserved intronic sequences. *Nucl Acids Res.* 1987;15(6):2774-2776.

1705. Francis CW, Muller E, Henschen A, Simpson PJ, Marder VJ. Carboxyl-terminal amino acid sequences of two variant forms of the gamma chain of human plasma fibrinogen. *Proc Natl Acad Sci.* 1988;85(10):3358-3362.

1706. Pan Y, Doolittle RF. cDNA sequence of a second fibrinogen alpha chain in lamprey: an archetypal version alignable with full-length beta and gamma chains. *Proc Natl Acad Sci.* 1992;89(6):2066-2070.

1707. Weissbach L, Grieninger G. Bipartite mRNA for chicken alpha-fibrinogen potentially encodes an amino acid sequence homologous to beta- and gamma-fibrinogens. *Proc Natl Acad Sci.* 1990;87(13):5198-5202.

1708. Jones FS, Hoffman S, Cunningham BA, Edelman GM. A detailed structural model of cytotactin: protein homologies, alternative RNA splicing, and binding regions. *Proc Natl Acad Sci.* 1989;86(6):1905-1909.

1709. Xu X, Doolittle RF. Presence of a vertebrate fibrinogen-like sequence in an echinoderm. *Proc Natl Acad Sci.* 1990;87(6):2097-2101.

1710. Baker N, Mlodzik M, Rubin G. Spacing differentiation in the developing Drosophila eye: a fibrinogen-related lateral inhibitor encoded by scabrous. *Science.* 1990;250(4986):1370-1377.

1711. Olaisen B, Teisberg P, Gedde-Dahl T. Fibrinogen? chain locus is on chromosome 4 in man. *Hum Genet.* 1982;61(1):24-26.

1712. Henry I, Uzan G, Weil D, et al. The genes coding for A alpha-, B beta-, and gamma-chains of fibrinogen map to 4q2. *Am J Hum Genet.* 1984;36(4):760-768.

1713. Rixon MW, Chan WY, Davie EW, Chung DW. Characterization of a complementary deoxyribonucleic acid coding for the alpha chain of human fibrinogen. *Biochemistry.* 1983;22(13):3237-3244.

1714. Chung DW, Que BG, Rixon MW, Mace M, Davie EW. Characterization of complementary deoxyribonucleic and genomic deoxyribonucleic acid for the beta chain of human fibrinogen. *Biochemistry.* 1983;22(13):3244-3250.

1715. Crabtree GR. The molecular biology of fibrinogen. In: Stamatoyanopolous G, Nienhuis AW, Leder P, Lajerus PW, eds. *The Molecular Basis of Blood Diseases.* Saunders; 1987:631-661.

1716. Fish RJ, Neerman-Arbez M. Fibrinogen gene regulation. *Thromb Haemost.* 2012;108(3):419-426.

1717. Chung DW, Harris JE, Davie EW. Nucleotide sequences of the three genes coding for human fibrinogen. *Adv Exp Med Biol.* 1990;281:39-48. Springer Science + Business Media.

1718. Crabtree GR, Kant JA. Molecular cloning of cDNA for the alpha, beta, and gamma chains of rat fibrinogen. A family of coordinately regulated genes. *J Biol Chem.* 1981;256(18):9718-9723.

1719. Crabtree GR, Kant JA, Fornace AJ, Rauch CA, Fowlkes DM. Regulation and characterization of the mRNAs for the A alpha, B beta and gamma chains of fibrinogen. *Ann N Y Acad Sci.* 1983;408:457-468.

1720. Mizuguchi J, Hu CH, Cao Z, Loeb KR, Chung DW, Davie EW. Characterization of the 5'-flanking region of the gene for the gamma chain of human fibrinogen. *J Biol Chem.* 1995;270(47):28350-28356.

1721. Fowlkes DM, Mullis NT, Comeau CM, Crabtree GR. Potential basis for regulation of the coordinately expressed fibrinogen genes: homology in the 5' flanking regions. *Proc Natl Acad Sci.* 1984;81(8):2313-2316.

1722. Otto JM. The coordinated regulation of fibrinogen gene transcription by hepatocyte-stimulating factor and dexamethasone. *J Cell Biol.* 1987;105(3):1067-1072.

1723. Chung DW, Davie EW. gamma. and.gamma.' chains of human fibrinogen are produced by alternative mRNA processing. *Biochemistry.* 1984;23(18):4232-4236.

1724. Fornace A, Cummings D, Comeau C, Kant J, Crabtree G. Single-copy inverted repeats associated with regional genetic duplications in gamma fibrinogen and immunoglobulin genes. *Science.* 1984;224(4645):161-164.

1725. Fu Y, Grieninger G. Fib420: a normal human variant of fibrinogen with two extended alpha chains. *Proc Natl Acad Sci.* 1994;91(7):2625-2628.

1726. Francis CW, Mosesson MW. Terminology for fibrinogen gamma-chains differing in carboxyl terminal amino acid sequence. *Thromb Haemost.* 1989;62(2):813-814.

1727. Fu Y, Weissbach L, Plant PW, et al. Carboxy-terminal-extended variant of the human fibrinogen alpha subunit: a novel exon conferring marked homology to beta and gamma subunits. *Biochemistry.* 1992;31(48):11968-11972.

1728. Grieninger G. Contribution of the alpha EC domain to the structure and function of fibrinogen-420. *Ann N Y Acad Sci.* 2001;936:44-64.

1729. Green FR. Fibrinogen polymorphisms and atherothrombotic disease. *Ann N Y Acad Sci.* 2006;936(1):549-559.

1730. Vischetti M, Zito F, Donati MB, Iacoviello L. Analysis of gene-environment interaction in coronary heart disease: fibrinogen polymorphisms as an example. *Ital Heart J.* 2002;3(1):18-23.

1731. Iacoviello L, Vischetti M, Zito F, Benedetta Donati M. Genes encoding fibrinogen and cardiovascular risk. *Hypertension.* 2001;38(5):1199-1203.

1732. Martinez J. Congenital dysfibrinogenemia. *Curr Opin Hematol.* 1997;4(5):357-365.

1733. Degen JL. Genetic interactions between the coagulation and fibrinolytic systems. *Thromb Haemost.* 2001;86(1):130-137.

1734. Menart C, Sprunck N, Duhaut P, Pinede L, Demolombe-Rague S, Negrier C. Recurrent spontaneous intracerebral hematoma in a patient with afibrinogenemia. *Thromb Haemost.* 1998;79(1):241-242.

1735. Ehmann WC, Al-Mondhiry H. Splenic rupture in afibrinogenemia: Conservative versus surgical management. *Am J Med.* 1995;99(4):444.

1736. De Marco L, Girolami A, Zimmerman TS, Ruggeri ZM. von Willebrand factor interaction with the glycoprotein IIb/IIa complex. Its role in platelet function as demonstrated in patients with congenital afibrinogenemia. *J Clin Invest.* 1986;77(4):1272-1277.

1737. Ni H, Denis CV, Subbarao S, et al. Persistence of platelet thrombus formation in arterioles of mice lacking both von Willebrand factor and fibrinogen. *J Clin Invest.* 2000;106(3):385-392.

1738. Parameswaran R, Dickinson JP, De Lord S, Keeling DM, Colvin BT. Spontaneous intracranial bleeding in two patients with congenital afibrinogenaemia and the role of replacement therapy. *Haemophilia.* 2000;6(6):705-708.

1739. Suh TT, Holmback K, Jensen NJ, et al. Resolution of spontaneous bleeding events but failure of pregnancy in fibrinogen-deficient mice. *Genes Dev.* 1995;9(16):2020-2033.

1740. Holmback K, Danton MJ, Suh TT, Daugherty CC, Degen JL. Impaired platelet aggregation and sustained bleeding in mice lacking the fibrinogen motif bound by integrin alpha IIb beta 3. *EMBO J.* 1996;15(21):5760-5771.

1741. Phillips DR, Charo IF, Parise LV, Fitzgerald LA. The platelet membrane glycoprotein IIb-IIIa complex. *Blood.* 1988;71(4):831-843.

1742. Bugge TH, Kombrinck KW, Flick MJ, Daugherty CC, Danton MJS, Degen JL. Loss of fibrinogen rescues mice from the pleiotropic effects of plasminogen deficiency. *Cell.* 1996;87(4):709-719.

1743. Drew AF, Kaufman AH, Kombrinck KW, Daugherty CC, Degen JL, Bugge TH. Ligneous conjunctivitis in plasminogen-deficient mice. *Fibrinolysis Proteolysis.* 1997;11:21.

1744. Drew AF, Tucker HL, Kombrinck KW, Simon DI, Bugge TH, Degen JL. Plasminogen is a critical determinant of vascular remodeling in mice. *Circ Res.* 2000;87(2):133-139.

1745. Kao WW, Kao CW, Kaufman AH, et al. Healing of corneal epithelial defects in plasminogen- and fibrinogen-deficient mice. *Invest Ophthalmol Vis Sci.* 1998;39(3):502-508.

1746. Drew AF, Schiman HL, Kombrinck KW, Bugge TH, Degen JL, Kaufman AH. Persistent corneal haze after excimer laser photokeratectomy in plasminogen-deficient mice. *Invest Ophthalmol Vis Sci.* 2000;41(1):67-72.

1747. Degen JL, Drew AF, Palumbo JS, et al. Genetic manipulation of fibrinogen and fibrinolysis in mice. *Ann N Y Acad Sci.* 2001;936:276-290.

1748. Brennan SO, Fellowes AP, George PM. Molecular mechanisms of hypo- and afibrinogenemia. *Ann N Y Acad Sci.* 2001;936:91-100.

1749. Higgins DL, Shafer JA. Fibrinogen Petoskey, a dysfibrinogenemia characterized by replacement of Arg-A alpha 16 by a histidyl residue. Evidence for thrombin-catalyzed hydrolysis at a histidyl residue. *J Biol Chem.* 1981;256(23):12013-12017.

1750. Henschen A, Kehl M, Southan C. Genetically abnormal fibrinogens–strategies for structure elucidation, including fibrinopeptide analysis. *Curr Probl Clin Biochem.* 1984;14:273-320.

1751. Matsuda M. Molecular abnormalities of fibrinogen: the present status of structure elucidation. In: Iwanga S, Takada A, Henschen A, eds. *Fibrinogen 4 Current Basis and Clinical Aspects.* Excerpta Medica; 1990:139-152.

1752. Kaudewitz H, Henschen H, Soria C. The molecular defect of the genetically abnormal fibrinogen Christchurch II. In: Muller , Scheefers-Borchel V, Selmayr E, Henschen A, eds. *BerghausGFibrinogen and its Derivatives.* Elsevier; 1986:31-36.

1753. Ebert RF. *Index of Variant Human Fibrinogen.* CRC Press; 1994.

1754. Hanss M, Biot F. A database for human fibrinogen variants. *Ann N Y Acad Sci.* 2001;936:89-90.

1755. Yu S, Sher B, Kudryk B, Redman CM. Intracellular assembly of human fibrinogen. *J Biol Chem.* 1983;258(22):13407-13410.

1756. Yu S, Sher B, Kudryk B, Redman CM. Fibrinogen precursors. Order of assembly of fibrinogen chains. *J Biol Chem.* 1984;259(16):10574-10581.

1757. Hirose S, Oda K, Ikehara Y. Biosynthesis, assembly and secretion of fibrinogen in cultured rat hepatocytes. *Biochem J.* 1988;251(2):373-377.

1758. Lee SY, Lee KP, Lim JW. Identification and biosynthesis of fibrinogen in human uterine cervix carcinoma cells. *Thromb Haemost.* 1996;75(3):466-470.

1759. Haidaris PJ. Induction of fibrinogen biosynthesis and secretion from cultured pulmonary epithelial cells. *Blood.* 1997;89:873-882.

1760. Haidaris PJ, Courtney MA. Tissue-specific and ubiquitous expression of fibrinogen gamma-chain mRNA. *Blood Coagul Fibrinolysis.* 1990;1(4-5):433-437.

1761. Haidaris PJ, Courtney MA. Liver-specific RNA processing of the ubiquitously transcribed rat fibrinogen gamma-chain gene. *Blood.* 1992;79(5):1218-1224.

1762. Nickerson JM, Fuller GM. Modification of fibrinogen chains during synthesis: glycosylation of B.beta. and.gamma. chains. *Biochemistry.* 1981;20(10):2818-2821.

1763. Nickerson JM, Fuller GM. In vitro synthesis of rat fibrinogen: identification of preA alpha, preB beta, and pre gamma polypeptides. *Proc Natl Acad Sci.* 1981;78(1):303-307.

1764. Townsend RR, Hilliker E, Li YT, Laine RA, Bell WR, Lee YC. Carbohydrate structure of human fibrinogen. Use of 300-MHz 1H-NMR to characterize glycosidase-treated glycopeptides. *J Biol Chem.* 1982;257(16):9704-9710.

1765. Köttgen E, Hell B, Müller C, Tauber R. Demonstration of glycosylation variants of human fibrinogen, using the new technique of glycoprotein lectin immunosorbent assay (GLIA). *Biol Chem Hoppe-Seyler.* 1988;369(2):1157-1166.

1766. Langer BG, Hong SK, Schmelzer CH, Bell WR. Deglycosylation of a native, protease-sensitive glycoprotein by peptide N-glycosidase F without protease inhibitors. *Anal Biochem.* 1987;166(1):212-217.

1767. Seydewitz HH, Kaiser C, Rothweiler H, Witt I. The location of a second in vivo phosphorylation site in the Aα-chain of human fibrinogen. *Thromb Res.* 1984;33(5):487-498.

1768. Blombäck B, Hessel B, Hogg D. Disulfide bridges in NH2-terminal part of human fibrinogen. *Thromb Res.* 1976;8(5):639-658.

1769. Zhang JZ, Kudryk B, Redman CM. Symmetrical disulfide bonds are not necessary for assembly and secretion of human fibrinogen. *J Biol Chem.* 1993;268(15):11278-11282.

1770. Zhang JZ, Redman C. Fibrinogen assembly and secretion: role of intrachain disulfide loops. *J Biol Chem.* 1996;271(47):30083-30088.

1771. Zhang JZ, Redman CM. Identification of B beta chain domains involved in human fibrinogen assembly. *J Biol Chem.* 1992;267(30):21727-21732.

1772. Zhang JZ, Redman CM. Role of interchain disulfide bonds on the assembly and secretion of human fibrinogen. *J Biol Chem.* 1994;269(1):652-658.

1773. Zhang JZ, Redman CM. Assembly and secretion of fibrinogen. Involvement of amino-terminal domains in dimer formation. *J Biol Chem.* 1996;271(21):12674-12680.

1774. Jenkins GR, Seiffert D, Parmer RJ, Miles LA. Regulation of plasminogen gene expression by interleukin-6. *Blood.* 1997;89(7):2394-2403.

1775. Nieuwenhuizen W. Sites in fibrin involved in the acceleration of plasminogen activation by t-PA. Possible role of fibrin polymerisation. *Thromb Res.* 1994;75(3):343-347.

1776. Bailey K, Astbury WT, Rudall KM. Fibrinogen and fibrin as members of the keratin-myosin group. *Nature.* 1943;151(3843):716-717.

1777. Crick FHC, Kendrew JC. X-ray analysis and protein structure. *Adv Protein Chem.* 1957;12:133-214. Elsevier BV.

1778. Scheraga HA, Laskowski M. The fibrinogen-fibrin conversion. *Adv Protein Chem.* 1957;12:1-131. Elsevier BV.

1779. Shulman S. The size and shape of bovine fibrinogen. Studies of sedimentation, diffusion and viscosity 1. *J Am Chem Soc.* 1953;75(23):5846-5852.

1780. Caspary EA, Kekwick RA. Some physicochemical properties of human fibrinogen. *Biochem J.* 1957;67(1):41-48.

1781. Hall CE. The fibrinogen molecule: its size, shape, and mode of polymerization. *J Cell Biol.* 1959;5(1):11-27.

1782. Cohen C. Invited discussion at 1960 symposium on protein structure. *J Polym Sci.* 1961;49:144-145.

1783. Nussenzweig V, Seligmann M, Pelmont J, Grabar P. The products of degradation of human fibrinogen by plasmin. I. Separation and physicochemical properties. *Ann Inst Pasteur (Paris).* 1961;100:377-389.

1784. Marder VJ, Shulman NR, Carroll WR. High molecular weight derivatives of human fibrinogen produced by plasmin. I. Physicochemical and immunological characterization. *J Biol Chem.* 1969;244(8):2111-2119.

1785. Rao SP, Poojary MD, Elliott BW, Jr, Melanson LA, Oriel B, Cohen C. Fibrinogen structure in projection at 18 A resolution. Electron density by co-ordinated cryo-electron microscopy and X-ray crystallography. *J Mol Biol.* 1991;222(1):89-98.

1786. Brown JH, Volkmann N, Jun G, Henschen-Edman AH, Cohen C. The crystal structure of modified fibrinogen. *Proc Natl Acad Sci USA.* 2000;97(1):85-90.

1787. Yang Z, Mochalkin I, Veerapandian L, Riley M, Doolittle RF. Crystal structure of native chicken fibrinogen at 5.5-A resolution. *Proc Natl Acad Sci.* 2000;97(8):3907-3912.

1788. Yang Z, Kollman JM, Pandi L, Doolittle RF. Crystal structure of native chicken fibrinogen at 2.7 Å resolution. *Biochemistry.* 2001;40(42):12515-12523.

1789. Doolittle RF, Watt KWK, Cottrell BA, Strong DD, Riley M. The amino acid sequence of the α-chain of human fibrinogen. *Nature.* 1979;280(5722):464-468.

1790. Murakawa M, Okamura T, Kamura T, Shibuya T, Harada M, Niho Y. Diversity of primary structures of the carboxy-terminal regions of mammalian fibrinogen A alpha-chains. Characterization of the partial nucleotide and deduced amino acid sequences in five mammalian species; rhesus monkey, pig, dog, mouse and Syrian hamster. *Thromb Haemost.* 1993;69(4):351-360.

1791. Kollman JM, Pandi L, Sawaya MR, Riley M, Doolittle RF. Crystal structure of human fibrinogen. *Biochemistry.* 2009;48(18):3877-3886.

1792. Madrazo J, Brown JH, Litvinovich S, et al. Crystal structure of the central region of bovine fibrinogen (E5 fragment) at 1.4-A resolution. *Proc Natl Acad Sci.* 2001;98(21):11967-11972.

1793. Yee VC, Pratt KP, Côté HCF, et al. Crystal structure of a 30 kDa C-terminal fragment from the γ chain of human fibrinogen. *Structure.* 1997;5(1):125-138.

1794. Doolittle RF, Everse SJ, Spraggon G, Veerapandian L. Crystal structures of fragments D and double-D from fibrinogen and fibrin. *Blood Coagul Fibrinolysis.* 1998;9(7):670.

1795. Pratt KP, Cote HCF, Chung DW, Stenkamp RE, Davie EW. The primary fibrin polymerization pocket: three-dimensional structure of a 30-kDa C-terminal chain fragment complexed with the peptide Gly-Pro-Arg-Pro. *Proc Natl Acad Sci USA.* 1997;94(14):7176-7181.

1796. Yang Z, Spraggon G, Pandi L, Everse SJ, Riley M, Doolittle RF. Crystal structure of fragment D from lamprey fibrinogen complexed with the peptide Gly-his-Arg-pro-amide. *Biochemistry.* 2002;41(32):10218-10224.

1797. Kostelansky MS, Betts L, Gorkun OV, Lord ST. 2.8 Å crystal structures of recombinant fibrinogen fragment D with and without two peptide ligands: GHRP binding to the "b" site disrupts its Nearby calcium-binding site. *Biochemistry.* 2002;41(40):12124-12132.

1798. Kostelansky MS, Lounes KC, Ping LF, Dickerson SK, Gorkun OV, Lord ST. Probing the γ2 calcium-binding site: studies with γD298,301A fibrinogen reveal changes in the γ294-301 loop that alter the integrity of the "a" polymerization site. *Biochemistry.* 2007;46(17):5114-5123.

1799. Carr ME, Hermans J. Size and density of fibrin fibers from Turbidity. *Macromolecules.* 1978;11(1):46-50.

1800. Ferry JD. The mechanism of polymerization of fibrinogen. *Proc Natl Acad Sci U S A.* 1952;38(7):566-569.

1801. Laudano AP, Doolittle RF. Synthetic peptide derivatives that bind to fibrinogen and prevent the polymerization of fibrin monomers. *Proc Natl Acad Sci.* 1978;75(7):3085-3089.

1802. Litvinov RI. Polymerization of fibrin: specificity, strength, and stability of knob-hole interactions studied at the single-molecule level. *Blood.* 2005;106(9):2944-2951.

1803. Everse SJ, Spraggon G, Veerapandian L, Riley M, Doolittle RF. Crystal structure of fragment double-D from human fibrin with two different bound ligands. *Biochemistry.* 1998;37(24):8637-8642.

1804. Everse SJ, Spraggon G, Veerapandian L, Doolittle RF. Conformational changes in fragments D and double-D from human fibrin(ogen) upon binding the peptide ligand Gly-his-Arg-pro-amide. *Biochemistry.* 1999;38(10):2941-2946.

1805. Doolittle RF, Chen A, Pandi L. Differences in binding specificity for the homologous γ- and β-chain "holes" on fibrinogen: exclusive binding of Ala-his-Arg-pro-amide by the β-chain hole. *Biochemistry.* 2006;45(47):13962-13969.

1806. Betts L, Merenbloom BK, Lord ST. The structure of fibrinogen fragment D with the 'A' knob peptide GPRVVE. *J Thromb Haemost.* 2006;4(5):1139-1141.

1807. Mihályi E, Högfeldt E, Sillén LG, Kinell P-O. Electrophoretic investigation of fibrin and fibrinogen dissolved in urea solutions. *Acta Chem Scand.* 1950;4:351-358.

1808. Bailey K, Bettelheim FR, Lorand L, Middlebrook WR. Action of thrombin in the clotting of fibrinogen. *Nature.* 1951;167(4241):233-234.

1809. Blomback B. Studies on the action of thrombotic enzymes on bovine fibrinogen as measured by N-terminal analysis. *Arkiv För Kemi Mineralogi Och Geologi.* 2003;12:321.

1810. Doolittle RF. Structural aspects of the fibrinogen to fibrin conversion. *Adv Protein Chem.* 1973;27:1-109.

1811. Blomback B, Hessel B, Hogg D, Therkildsen L. A two-step fibrinogen–fibrin transition in blood coagulation. *Nature.* 1978;275(5680):501-505.

1812. Blomback B. Isolation of fibrinopeptides by chromatography. *Arkiv För Kemi Mineralogi Och Geologi.* 1958;12:173.

1813. Shainoff JR, Page IH. Cofibrins and fibrin intermediates as indicators of thrombin activity in vivo. *Circ Res.* 1960;8:1013-1022.

1814. Hanna LS, Scheraga HA, Francis CW, Marder VJ. Comparison of structures of various human fibrinogens and a derivative thereof by a study of the kinetics of release of fibrinopeptides. *Biochemistry.* 1984;23(20):4681-4687.

1815. Lewis SD, Shields PP, Shafer JA. Characterization of the kinetic pathway for liberation of fibrinopeptides during assembly of fibrin. *J Biol Chem.* 1985;260(18):10192-10199.

1816. Mihalyi E. Clotting of bovine fibrinogen. Kinetic analysis of the release of fibrinopeptides by thrombin and of the calcium uptake upon clotting at high fibrinogen concentrations. *Biochemistry.* 1988;27(3):976-982.

1817. Vindigni A, Di Cera E. Release of fibrinopeptides by the slow and fast forms of thrombin. *Biochemistry.* 1996;35(14):4417-4426.

1818. Pechik I, Yakovlev S, Mosesson MW, Gilliland GL, Medved L. Structural basis for sequential cleavage of fibrinopeptides upon fibrin assembly. *Biochemistry.* 2006;45(11):3588-3597.

1819. Bettelheim FR, Bailey K. The products of the action of thrombin on fibrinogen. *Biochim Biophys Acta.* 1952;9(5):578-579.

1820. Barlow GH, Holleman WH, Lorand L. The action of Arvin on fibrin stabilizing factor (factor 13). *Res Commun Chem Pathol Pharmacol.* 1970;1(1):39-42.

1821. Edgar W, Prentice CRM. The proteolytic actions of ancrod on human fibrinogen and polypeptide chains. *Thromb Res.* 1973;2:85-96.

1822. Dyr JE, Blomback B, Hessel B, Kornalik F. Conversion of fibrinogen to fibrin induced by preferential release of fibrinopeptide B. *Biochim Biophys Acta.* 1989;990(1):18-24.

1823. Mosesson MW, DiOrio JP, Muller MF, et al. Studies on the ultrastructure of fibrin lacking fibrinopeptide B (beta-fibrin). *Blood.* 1987;69(4):1073-1081.

1824. Shainoff JR, Dardik BN. Fibrinopeptide B and aggregation of fibrinogen. *Science.* 1979;204(4389):200-202.

1825. Doolittle RF. Fibrinogen and fibrin. In: Bloom AL, Thomas DP, eds. *Hemostasis and Thrombosis.* Churchill Livingstone; 1981:163-191.

1826. Hantgan RR, Hermans J. Assembly of fibrin. A light scattering study. *J Biol Chem.* 1979;254(22):11272-11281.

1827. Hantgan R, Fowler W, Erickson H, Hermans J. Fibrin assembly: a comparison of electron microscopic and light scattering results. *Thromb Haemost.* 1980;44(3):119-124.

1828. Weisel JW, Phillips GN, Cohen C. The structure of fibrinogen and fibrin: II. Architecture of the fibrin clot. *Ann N Y Acad Sci.* 1983;408:367-379.

1829. Fowler WE, Hantgan RR, Hermans J, Erickson HP. Structure of the fibrin protofibril. *Proc Natl Acad Sci.* 1981;78(8):4872-4876.

1830. Mosesson MW, Siebenlist KR, Amrani DL, DiOrio JP. Identification of covalently linked trimeric and tetrameric D domains in crosslinked fibrin. *Proc Natl Acad Sci.* 1989;86(3):1113-1117.

1831. Kudryk B, Okada M, Redman CM, Blomback B. Biosynthesis of dog fibrinogen. Characterization of nascent fibrinogen in the rough endoplasmic reticulum. *Eur J Biochem.* 1982;125(3):673-682.

1832. Gorkun OV, Veklich YI, Medved LV, Henschen AH, Weisel JW. Role of the .alpha.C domains of fibrin in clot formation. *Biochemistry.* 1994;33(22):6986-6997.

1833. Weisel JW, Papsun DM. Involvement of the cooh-terminal portion of the alpha-chain of fibrin in the branching of fibers to form a clot. *Thromb Res.* 1987;47(2):155-163.

1834. Doolittle RF, Pandi L. Binding of synthetic B knobs to fibrinogen changes the character of fibrin and inhibits its ability to activate tissue plasminogen activator and its Destruction by plasmin. *Biochemistry.* 2006;45(8):2657-2667.

1835. Folk JE, Finlayson JS. The ε-(γ-Glutamyl)Lysine crosslink and the catalytic role of transglutaminases. *Adv Protein Chem.* 1977;31:1-133. Elsevier BV.

1836. Pisano JJ, Finlayson JS, Peyton MP. Cross-link in fibrin polymerized by factor XIII: egr-(ggr-Glutamyl)lysine. *Science.* 1968;160(3830):892-893.

1837. Shen LL, Hermans J, McDonagh J, McDonagh RP, Carr M. Effects of calcium ion and covalent crosslinking on formation and elasticity of fibrin gels. *Thromb Res.* 1975;6(3):255-265.

1838. Gerth C, Roberts WW, Ferry JD. Rheology of fibrin clots II. *Biophys Chem.* 1974;2(3):208-217.

1839. McDonagh RP, McDonagh J, Duckert F. The influence of fibrin crosslinking on the kinetics of urokinase-induced clot lysis. *Br J Haematol.* 1971;21(3):323-332.

1840. Shen LL, McDonagh RP, McDonagh J, Hermans J. Early events in the plasmin digestion of fibrin and fibrinogen. Effects of plasmin on fibrin polymerization. *J Biol Chem.* 1977;252(17):6184-6189.

1841. Francis CW, Marder VJ. Increased resistance to plasmic degradation of fibrin with highly crosslinked alpha-polymer chains formed at high factor XIII concentrations. *Blood.* 1988;71(5):1361-1365.

1842. Chen R, Doolittle RF. Identification of the polypeptide chains involved in the cross-linking of fibrin. *Proc Natl Acad Sci U S A.* 1969;63(2):420-427.

1843. McKee PA, Mattock P, Hill RL. Subunit structure of human fibrinogen, soluble fibrin, and cross-linked insoluble fibrin. *Proc Natl Acad Sci.* 1970;66(3):738-744.

1844. Cottrell BA, Strong DD, Watt KWK, Doolittle RF. Amino acid sequence studies on the .alpha. chain of human fibrinogen. Exact location of crosslinking acceptor sites. *Biochemistry.* 1979;18(24):5405-5410.

1845. Gaffney PJ, Whitaker AN. Fibrin crosslinks and lysis rates. *Thromb Res.* 1979;14(1):85-94.

1846. Sakata Y, Aoki N. Cross-linking of alpha 2-plasmin inhibitor to fibrin by fibrin-stabilizing factor. *J Clin Invest.* 1980;65(2):290-297.

1847. Sakata Y, Aoki N. Significance of cross-linking of α2-plasmin inhibitor to fibrin in inhibition of fibrinolysis and in hemostasis. *J Clin Invest.* 1982;69(3):536-542.

1848. Sakharov DV, Plow EF, Rijken DC. On the mechanism of the antifibrinolytic activity of plasma carboxypeptidase B. *J Biol Chem.* 1997;272(22):14477-14482.

1849. Broze GJ, Jr, Higuchi DA. Coagulation-dependent inhibition of fibrinolysis: role of carboxypeptidase-U and the premature lysis of clots from hemophilic plasma. *Blood.* 1996;88(10):3815-3823.

1850. Marder VJ. Immunologic structure of finbrinogen and its plasmin degradation products. Theoretical and clinical considerations. In: Laki K, ed. *Fibrinogen.* Marcel Dekker Inc. Edward Arnold (Publishers Ltd.); 1968:339-358.

1851. Marder VJ. Physiochemical studies of intermediate and final products of plasmin digestion of human fibrinogen. *Thromb Diath Haemorr.* 1970;80:187-195.

1852. Larrieu MJ, Marder VJ, Inceman S. Effects of fibrinogen degradation products on platelets and coagulation. *Thromb Diath Haemorrh Suppl.* 1966;20:215-226.

1853. Marder VJ, Shulman NR, Carroll WR. The importance of intermediate degradation products of fibrinogen in fibrinolytic hemorrhage. *Trans Assoc Am Physicians.* 1967;80:156-167.

1854. Francis CW, Marder VJ, Barlow GH. Plasmic degradation of crosslinked fibrin. *J Clin Invest.* 1980;66(5):1033-1043.

1855. Pizzo SV, Taylor LM, Jr, Schwartz ML, Hill RL, McKee PA. Subunit structure of fragment D from fibrinogen and cross-linked fibrin. *J Biol Chem.* 1973;248(13):4584-4590.

1856. Marder VJ, Francis CW. Plasmin degradation of cross-linked fibrin. *Ann N Y Acad Sci.* 1983;408:397-406.

1857. Francis C, Marder V. A molecular model of plasmic degradation of crosslinked fibrin. *Semin Thromb Hemost.* 1982;8(01):25-35.

1858. Gaffney PJ, Brasher M. Subunit structure of the plasmin-induced degradation products of crosslinked fibrin. *Biochim Biophys Acta.* 1973;295(1):308-313.

1859. Hudry-Clergeon G, Paturel L, Suscillon M. Identification of a (D-D)...E complex in degradation products of bovine fibrin stabilized by factor XIII. *Pathol Biol (Paris).* 1974;22:47-52.

1860. Gaffney PJ, Lane DA, Kakkar VV, Brasher M. Characterisation of a soluble D dimer-E complex in crosslinked fibrin digests. *Thromb Res.* 1975;7(1):89-99.

1861. Bachmann F. Plasminogen-plasmin enzyme system. In: Colman RW, Hirsh J, Marder VJ, Clowes AW, George JN, eds. *Hemostasis and Thrombosis: Basic Principles and Clinical Practice.* Lippencott Williams & Wilkins; 2001:275-320.

1862. Bugge TH, Flick MJ, Daugherty CC, Degen JL. Plasminogen deficiency causes severe thrombosis but is compatible with development and reproduction. *Genes Dev.* 1995;9(7):794-807.

1863. Ploplis VA, Carmeliet P, Vazirzadeh S, et al. Effects of disruption of the plasminogen gene on thrombosis, growth, and health in mice. *Circulation.* 1995;92(9):2585-2593.

1864. Murray JC, Buetow KH, Donovan M, et al. Linkage disequilibrium of plasminogen polymorphisms and assignment of the gene to human chromosome 6q26-6q27. *Am J Hum Genet.* 1987;40(4):338-350.

1865. Petersen TE, Martzen MR, Ichinose A, Davie EW. Characterization of the gene for human plasminogen, a key proenzyme in the fibrinolytic system. *J Biol Chem.* 1990;265(11):6104-6111.

1866. Ichinose A. Multiple members of the plasminogen-apolipoprotein(a) gene family associated with thrombosis. *Biochemistry.* 1992;31(12):3113-3118.

1867. Magnaghi P, Citterio E, Malgaretti N, Acquati F, Ottolenghi S, Taramelli R. Molecular characterisation of the human apo(a) -plasminogen gene family clustered on the telomeric region of chromosome 6 (6q26-27). *Hum Mol Genet.* 1994;3(3):437-442.

1868. Kida M, Wakabayashi S, Ichinose A. Characterization of the 5'-flanking regions of plasminogen-related genes A and B. *FEBS Lett.* 1997;404(1):95-99.

1869. Raum D, Marcus D, Alper C, Levey R, Taylor P, Starzl T. Synthesis of human plasminogen by the liver. *Science.* 1980;208(4447):1036-1037.

1870. Collen D, Tytgat G, Claeys H, Verstraete M, Wallén P. Metabolism of plasminogen in healthy subjects: effect of tranexamic acid. *J Clin Invest.* 1972;51(6):1310-1318.

1871. Wallen P, Wiman B. Characterization of human plasminogen. I. On the relationship between different molecular forms of plasminogen demonstrated in plasma and found in purified preparations. *Biochim Biophys Acta.* 1970;221(1):20-30.

1872. Wallen P, Wiman B. Characterization of human plasminogen. II. Separation and partial characterization of different molecular forms of human plasminogen. *Biochim Biophys Acta.* 1972;257(1):122-134.

1873. Summaria L, Arzadon L, Bernabe P, Robbins KC. Studies on the isolation of the multiple molecular forms of human plasminogen and plasmin by isoelectric focusing methods. *J Biol Chem.* 1972;247(14):4691-4702.

1874. Pirie-Shepherd SR, Jett EA, Andon NL, Pizzo SV. Sialic acid content of plasminogen 2 glycoforms as a regulator of fibrinolytic activity. Isolation, carbohydrate analysis, and kinetic characterization of six glycoforms of plasminogen. *J Biol Chem.* 1995;270(11):5877-5881.

1875. Takada A, Takada Y. Physiology of plasminogen: with special reference to activation and degradation. *Pathophysiol Haemost Thromb.* 1988;18(1):25-35.

1876. Gonzalez-Gronow M, Grenett HE, Fuller GM, Pizzo SV. The role of carbohydrate in the function of human plasminogen: comparison of the protein obtained from molecular cloning and expression in *Escherichia coli* and COS cells. *Biochim Biophys Acta.* 1990;1039(3):269-276.

1877. Hatton MWC, Southward S, Ross-Ouellet B. Catabolism of plasminogen glycoforms I and II in rabbits: relationship to plasminogen synthesis by the rabbit liver in vitro. *Metabolism.* 1994;43(11):1430-1437.

1878. Mølgaard L, Ponting CP, Christensen U. Glycosylation at Asn-289 facilitates the ligand-induced conformational changes of human Glu-plasminogen. *FEBS Letts.* 1997;405(3):363-368.

1879. Hatton MWC, Day S, Ross B, Southward SMR, Dereske M, Richardson M. Plasminogen II accumulates five times faster than plasminogen I at the site of a balloon de-endothelializing injury in vivo to the rabbit aorta: comparison with other hemostatic proteins. *J Lab Clin Med.* 1999;134(3):260-266.

1880. Pirie-Shepherd SR, Stevens RD, Andon NL, Enghild JJ, Pizzo SV. Evidence for a novel O-linked sialylated trisaccharide on Ser-248 of human plasminogen 2. *J Biol Chem.* 1997;272(11):7408-7411.

1881. Forsgren M, Råden B, Israelsson M, Larsson K, Hedén LO. Molecular cloning and characterization of a full-length cDNA clone for human plasminogen. *FEBS Lett.* 1987;213(2):254-260.

1882. Malinowski DP, Sadler JE, Davie EW. Characterization of a complementary deoxyribonucleic acid coding for human and bovine plasminogen. *Biochemistry.* 1984;23(18):4243-4250.

1883. Rakoczi I, Wiman B, Collen D. On the biological significance of the specific interaction between fibrin, plasminogen and antiplasmin. *Biochim Biophys Acta.* 1978;540(2):295-300.

1884. Wiman B, Wallén P. The specific interaction between plasminogen and fibrin. A physiological role of the lysine binding site in plasminogen. *Thromb Res.* 1977;10(2):213-222.

1885. Thorsen S, Clemmensen I, Sottrup-Jensen L, Magnusson S. Adsorption to fibrin of native fragments of known primary structure from human plasminogen. *Biochim Biophy Acta.* 1981;668(3):377-387.

1886. Wiman B, Lijnen HR, Collen D. On the specific interaction between the lysine-binding sites in plasmin and complementary sites in alpha2-antiplasmin and in fibrinogen. *Biochim Biophys Acta.* 1979;579(1):142-154.

1887. Lijnen HR, Hoylaerts M, Collen D. Isolation and characterization of a human plasma protein with affinity for the lysine binding sites in plasminogen. Role in the regulation of fibrinolysis and identification as histidine-rich glycoprotein. *J Biol Chem.* 1980;255(21):10214-10222.

1888. Selim TE, Ghoneim HR, Uknis AB, Colman RW, DeLa Cadena RA. High-molecular-mass and low-molecular-mass kininogens block plasmin-induced platelet aggregation by forming a complex with kringle 5 of plasminogen/plasmin. *Eur J Biochem.* 1997;250(2):532-538.

1889. Silverstein RL, Leung LL, Harpel PC, Nachman RL. Complex formation of platelet thrombospondin with plasminogen. Modulation of activation by tissue activator. *J Clin Invest.* 1984;74(5):1625-1633.

1890. Thorsen S, Astrup T. Substrate composition and the effect of epsilon-aminocaproic acid on tissue plasminogen activator and urokinase-induced fibrinolysis. *Thromb Diath Haemorrh.* 1974;32(2-3):306-324.

1891. Violand BN, Byrne R, Castellino FJ. The effect of alpha-,omega-amino acids on human plasminogen structure and activation. *J Biol Chem.* 1978;253(15):5395-5401.

1892. Sjoholm I, Wiman B, Wallean P. Studies on the conformational changes of plasminogen induced during activation to plasmin and by 6-Aminohexanoic acid. *Eur J Biochem.* 1973;39(2):471-479.

1893. Castellino F. Biochemistry of human plasminogen. *Semin Thromb Hemost.* 1984;10(01):18-23.

1894. Mangel W, Lin B, Ramakrishnan V. Characterization of an extremely large, ligand-induced conformational change in plasminogen. *Science.* 1990;248(4951):69-73.

1895. Ramakrishnan V, Patthy L, Mangel WF. Conformation of Lys-plasminogen and the kringle 1-3 fragment of plasminogen analyzed by small-angle neutron scattering. *Biochemistry.* 1991;30(16):3963-3969.

1896. O'Reilly M. Angiostatin: a novel angiogenesis inhibitor that mediates the suppression of metastases by a lewis lung carcinoma. *Cell.* 1994;79(2):315-328.

1897. Peisach E, Wang J, de los Santos T, Reich E, Ringe D. Crystal structure of the proenzyme domain of plasminogen. *Biochemistry.* 1999;38(34):11180-11188.

1898. Violand BN, Castellino FJ. Mechanism of the urokinase-catalyzed activation of human plasminogen. *J Biol Chem.* 1976;251(13):3906-3912.

1899. Claeys H, Vermylen J. Physico-chemical and proenzyme properties of NH2-terminal glutamic acid and NH2-terminal lysine human plasminogen. *Biochim Biophys Acta.* 1974;342(2):351-359.

1900. Kluft C, Dooijewaard G, Emeis JJ. Role of the contact system in fibrinolysis. *Semin Thromb Hemost.* 1987;13(1):50-68.

1901. Colman RW. Activation of plasminogen by human plasma kallikrein. *Biochem Biophys Res Commun.* 1969;35(2):273-279.

1902. Mandle RJ, Jr, Kaplan AP. Hageman-factor-dependent fibrinolysis: generation of fibrinolytic activity by the interaction of human activated factor XI and plasminogen. *Blood.* 1979;54(4):850-862.

1903. Goldsmith GH, Saito H, Ratnoff OS. The activation of plasminogen by Hageman factor (Factor XII) and Hageman factor fragments. *J Clin Invest.* 1978;62(1):54-60.

1904. Schousboe I, Feddersen K, Rojkjaer R. Factor XIIa is a kinetically favorable plasminogen activator. *Thromb Haemost.* 1999;82(3):1041-1046.

1905. Booyse FM, Scheinbuks J, Radek J, Osikowicz G, Feder S, Quarfoot AJ. Immunological identification and comparison of plasminogen activator forms in cultured normal human endothelial cells and smooth muscle cells. *Thromb Res.* 1981;24(5-6):495-504.

1906. Goldsmith GH, Ziats NP, Robertson AL. Studies on plasminogen activator and other proteases in subcultured human vascular cells. *Exp Mol Pathol.* 1981;35(2):257-264.

1907. Levin EG. Cultured bovine endothelial cells produce both urokinase and tissue-type plasminogen activators. *J Cell Biol.* 1982;94(3):631-636.

1908. Levin EG. Latent tissue plasminogen activator produced by human endothelial cells in culture: evidence for an enzyme-inhibitor complex. *Proc Natl Acad Sci.* 1983;80(22):6804-6808.

1909. Allen RA, Pepper DS. Isolation and properties of human vascular plasminogen activator. *Thromb Haemost.* 1981;45(1):43-50.

1910. Papadaki M, Ruef J, Nguyen KT, et al. Differential regulation of protease activated receptor-1 and tissue plasminogen activator expression by shear stress in vascular smooth muscle cells. *Circ Res.* 1998;83(10):1027-1034.

1911. Wang Y, Hand AR, Wang YH, et al. Functional and morphologic evidence of the presence of tissue-plasminogen activator in vascular nerves: implications for a neurologic control of vessel wall fibrinolysis and rigidity. *J Neurosci Res.* 1998;53(4):443-453.

1912. Brisson-Jeanneau C, Solberg LA, Sultan Y. Presence of functionally active tissue plasminogen activator in human CFU-M derived megakaryocytes in vitro. *Fibrinolysis.* 1990;4(2):107-115.

1913. Brisson-Jeanneau C, Nelles L, Rouer E, Sultan Y, Benarous R. Tissue-plasminogen activator RNA detected in megakaryocytes by in situ hybridization and biotinylated probe. *Histochemistry.* 1990;95(1):23-26.

1914. Bankl HC, Grobschmidt K, Pikula B, Bankl H, Lechner K, Valent P. Mast cells are augmented in deep vein thrombosis and express a profibrinolytic phenotype. *Human Pathology.* 1999;30(2):188-194.

1915. Sillaber C, Baghestanian M, Bevec D, et al. The mast cell as site of tissue-type plasminogen activator expression and fibrinolysis. *J Immunol.* 1999;162(2):1032-1041.

1916. Hart PH. Human monocytes can produce tissue-type plasminogen activator. *J Exp Med.* 1989;169(4):1509-1514.

1917. Tyagi SC, Lewis K, Pikes D, et al. Stretch-induced membrane type matrix metalloproteinase and tissue plasminogen activator in cardiac fibroblast cells. *J Cell Physiol.* 1998;176(2):374-382.

1918. Collen D, Lijnen HR, Todd PA, Goa KL. Tissue-type plasminogen activator. *Drugs.* 1989;38(3):346-388.

1919. Lucas FV, Miller ML. The fibrinolytic system: recent advances. *Cleve Clin J Med.* 1988;55(6):531-541.

1920. Rijken DC, Juhan-Vague I, de Cock F, Collen D. Measurement of human tissue-type plasminogen activator by a two-site immunoradiometric assay. *J Lab Clin Med.* 1983;101(2):274-284.

1921. Stalder M, Hauert J, Kruithof EKO, Bachmann F. Release of vascular plasminogen activator (v-PA) after venous stasis: electrophoretic—zymographic analysis of free and complexed v-PA. *Br J Haematol.* 1985;61(1):169-176.

1922. Holvoet P, Cleemput H, Collen D. Assay of human tissue-type plasminogen activator (t-PA) with an enzyme-linked immunosorbent assay (ELISA) based on three murine monoclonal antibodies to t-PA. *Thromb Haemost.* 1985;54(3):684-687.

1923. Nicoloso G, Hauert J, Kruithof EK, Van Melle G, Bachmann F. Fibrinolysis in normal subjects--comparison between plasminogen activator inhibitor and other components of the fibrinolytic system. *Thromb Haemost.* 1988;59(2):299-303.

1924. Takada Y, Takada A. Plasma levels of t-pa, free pai-1 and a complex of t-pa with pai-1 in human males and females at various ages. *Thromb Res.* 1989;55(5):601-609.

1925. Booth NA, Walker E, Maughan R, Bennett B. Plasminogen activator in normal subjects after exercise and venous occlusion: t-PA circulates as complexes with C1-inhibitor and PAI-1. *Blood.* 1987;69(6):1600-1604.

1926. Eitzman DT, Fay WP, Ginsburg D. Plasminogen activator inhibitor-1. In: Becker RC, ed. *Textbook of Coronary Thrombosis and Thrombolysis.* Kluwer Academic Publishers; 1997:65-78.

1927. Chandler WL, Alessi MC, Aillaud MF, Henderson P, Vague P, Juhan-Vague I. Clearance of tissue plasminogen activator (TPA) and TPA/plasminogen activator inhibitor type 1 (PAI-1) complex: relationship to elevated TPA antigen in patients with high PAI-1 activity levels. *Circulation.* 1997;96(3):761-768.

The Normal Hematologic System

1928. Garabedian HD, Gold HK, Leinbach RC, Yasuda T, Johns JA, Collen D. Dose-dependent thrombolysis, pharmacokinetics and hemostatic effects of recombinant human tissue-type plasminogen activator for coronary thrombosis. *Am J Cardiol.* 1986;58(9):673-679.
1929. Camani C, Kruithof EK. Clearance receptors for tissue-type plasminogen activator. *Int J Hematol.* 1994;60(2):97-109.
1930. Emeis JJ, van den Hoogen CM, Jense D. Hepatic clearance of tissue-type plasminogen activator in rats. *Thromb Haemost.* 1985;54(3):661-664.
1931. Bakhit C, Lewis D, Billings R, Malfroy B. Cellular catabolism of recombinant tissue-type plasminogen activator. Identification and characterization of a novel high affinity uptake system on rat hepatocytes. *J Biol Chem.* 1987;262(18):8716-8720.
1932. Benham FJ, Spurr N, Povey S, et al. Assignment of tissue-type plasminogen activator to chromosome 8 in man and identification of a common restriction length polymorphism within the gene. *Mol Biol Med.* 1984;2(4):251-259.
1933. Browne MJ, Tyrrell AWR, Chapman CG, et al. Isolation of a human tissue-type plasminogen-activator genomic DNA clone and its expression in mouse L cells. *Gene.* 1985;33(3):279-284.
1934. Fisher R, Waller EK, Grossi G, Thompson D, Tizard R, Schleuning WD. Isolation and characterization of the human tissue-type plasminogen activator structural gene including its 5' flanking region. *J Biol Chem.* 1985;260(20):11223-11230.
1935. Degen SJ, Rajput B, Reich E. The human tissue plasminogen activator gene. *J Biol Chem.* 1986;261(15):6972-6985.
1936. Bulens F, Ibanez-Tallon I, Van Acker P, et al. Retinoic acid induction of human tissue-type plasminogen activator gene expression via a direct repeat element (DR5) located at -7 kilobases. *J Biol Chem.* 1995;270(13):7167-7175.
1937. Merchiers P. Identification of a multihormone responsive enhancer far upstream from the human tissue-type plasminogen activator gene. *J Biol Chem.* 1997;272(1):663-671.
1938. Merchiers P, Bulens F, Stockmans I, et al. 1,25-Dihydroxyvitamin D 3 induction of the tissue-type plasminogen activator gene is mediated through its multihormone-responsive enhancer. *FEBS Lett.* 1999;460(2):289-296.
1939. Merchiers P, Bulens F, De Vriese A, Collen D, Belayew A. Involvement of Sp1 in basal and retinoic acid induced transcription of the human tissue-type plasminogen activator gene. *FEBS Lett.* 1999;456(1):149-154.
1940. Henderson BR, Sleigh MJ. TATA box-independent transcription of the human tissue plasminogen activator gene initiates within a sequence conserved in related genes. *FEBS Lett.* 1992;309(2):130-134.
1941. Costa M, Shen Y, Maurer F, Medcalf RL. Transcriptional regulation of the tissue-type plasminogen-activator gene in human endothelial cells: identification of nuclear factors that recognise functional elements in the tissue-type plasminogen-activator gene promoter. *Eur J Biochem.* 1998;258(1):123-131.
1942. Ouyang Y, HP, Huang C. Influence of 5'-untranslated region (UTR) sequence on the regulation of tissue plasminogran activator (t-PA) mRNA expression. *Sci China Series B.* 1995;40:1378-1383.
1943. Huarte J, Belin D, Vassalli A, Strickland S, Vassalli JD. Meiotic maturation of mouse oocytes triggers the translation and polyadenylation of dormant tissue-type plasminogen activator mRNA. *Genes Dev.* 1987;1(10):1201-1211.
1944. Ouyang Y, HP, Huang C. Inhibitory effect of 3'-untranslated region (3'-UTR) of human-tissue plasminogen activator (ht-PA) mRNA on its expression. *Science China Ser B.* 1995;38:1253-1260.
1945. van der Bom JG, de Knijff P, Haverkate F, et al. Tissue plasminogen activator and risk of myocardial infarction: the Rotterdam study. *Circulation.* 1997;95(12):2623-2627.
1946. Tishkoff SA, Ruano G, Kidd JR, Kidd KK. Distribution and frequency of a polymorphic Alu insertion at the plasminogen activator locus in humans. *Hum Genet.* 1996;97(6):759-764.
1947. Iacoviello L, Di Castelnuovo A, de Knijff P, et al. Alu-repeat polymorphism in the tissue-type plasminogen activator (t-PA) gene, t-PA levels and risk of familial myocardial infarction (MI). *Fibrinolysis.* 1996;10:13-16.
1948. Ridker PM, Baker MT, Hennekens CH, Stampfer MJ, Vaughan DE. Alu-repeat polymorphism in the gene coding for tissue-type plasminogen activator (t-PA) and risks of myocardial infarction among middle-aged men. *Arterioscler Thromb Vasc Biol.* 1997;17(9):1687-1690.
1949. Steeds R, Adams M, Smith P, Channer K, Samani NJ. Distribution of tissue plasminogen activator insertion/deletion polymorphism in myocardial infarction and control subjects. *Thromb Haemost.* 1998;79(5):980-984.
1950. Ludwig M, Wohn KD, Schleuning WD, Olek K. Allelic dimorphism in the human tissue-type plasminogen activator (TPA) gene as a result of an Alu insertion/deletion event. *Hum Genet.* 1992;88(4):388-392.
1951. Rigat B, Hubert C, Alhenc-Gelas F, Cambien F, Corvol P, Soubrier F. An insertion/deletion polymorphism in the angiotensin I-converting enzyme gene accounting for half the variance of serum enzyme levels. *J Clin Invest.* 1990;86(4):1343-1346.
1952. Ladenvall P, Wall U, Jern S, Jern C. Identification of eight novel single-nucleotide polymorphisms at human tissue-type plasminogen activator (t-PA) locus: association with vascular t-PA release in vivo. *Thromb Haemost.* 2000;84(2):150-155.
1953. Ladenvall P, Johansson L, Jansson JH, et al. Tissue-type plasminogen activator -7,351C/T enhancer polymorphism is associated with a first myocardial infarction. *Thromb Haemost.* 2002;87(1):105-109.
1954. Carmeliet P, Schoonjans L, Kieckens L, et al. Physiological consequences of loss of plasminogen activator gene function in mice. *Nature.* 1994;368(6470):419-424.
1955. Carmeliet P, Collen D. Targeted gene manipulation and transfer of the plasminogen and coagulation systems in mice. *Fibrinolysis.* 1996;10(4):195-213.
1956. Pohl G, Kaellstroem M, Bergsdorf N, Wallen P, Joernvall H. Tissue plasminogen activator: peptide analyses confirm an indirectly derived amino acid sequence, identify the active site serine residue, establish glycosylation sites, and localize variant differences. *Biochemistry.* 1984;23(16):3701-3707.
1957. Pennica D, Holmes WE, Kohr WJ, et al. Cloning and expression of human tissue-type plasminogen activator cDNA in *E. coli. Nature.* 1983;301(5897):214-221.
1958. Wallen P, Pohl PG, Bergsdorf N, et al. Structural characterization of tissue plasminogen activator purified by immunosorbent chromatography. In: Davidson JF, BF , Bouvier CA, et al. eds. *Progress in Fibrinolysis.* Churchill-Livingstone; 1983:338-343.
1959. Berg DT, Grinnell BW. Signal and propeptide processing of human tissue plasminogen activator: activity of a pro-tPA derivative. *Biochem Biophys Res Commun.* 1991;179(3):1289-1296.
1960. Jörnvall H, Pohl G, Bergsdorf N, Wallén P. Differential proteolysis and evidence for a residue exchange in tissue plasminogen activator suggest possible association between two types of protein microheterogeneity. *FEBS Lett.* 1983;156(1):47-50.
1961. Boose JA, Kuismanen E, Gerard R, Sambrook J, Gething MJ. The single-chain form of tissue-type plasminogen activator has catalytic activity: studies with a mutant enzyme that lacks the cleavage site. *Biochemistry.* 1989;28(2):635-643.
1962. Rijken DC, Hoylaerts M, Collen D. Fibrinolytic properties of one-chain and two-chain human extrinsic (tissue-type) plasminogen activator. *J Biol Chem.* 1982;257(6):2920-2925.
1963. Rijken DC, Groeneveld E. Isolation and functional characterization of the heavy and light chains of human tissue-type plasminogen activator. *J Biol Chem.* 1986;261(7):3098-3102.
1964. Rånby M, Bergsdorf N, Nilsson T. Enzymatic properties of the one-and two-chain form of tissue plasminogen activator. *Thromb Res.* 1982;27(2):175-183.
1965. Ny T, Elgh F, Lund B. The structure of the human tissue-type plasminogen activator gene: correlation of intron and exon structures to functional and structural domains. *Proc Natl Acad Sci.* 1984;81(17):5355-5359.
1966. Bányai L, Váradi A, Patthy L. Common evolutionary origin of the fibrin-binding structures of fibronectin and tissue-type plasminogen activator. *FEBS Lett.* 1983;163(1):37-41.
1967. Verde P, Stoppelli MP, Galeffi P, Di Nocera P, Blasi F. Identification and primary sequence of an unspliced human urokinase poly(A)+ RNA. *Proc Natl Acad Sci.* 1984;81(15):4727-4731.
1968. Holland SK, Harlos K, Blake CC. Deriving the generic structure of the fibronectin type II domain from the prothrombin Kringle 1 crystal structure. *EMBO J.* 1987;6(7):1875-1880.
1969. van Zonneveld AJ, Veerman H, Pannekoek H. On the interaction of the finger and the kringle-2 domain of tissue-type plasminogen activator with fibrin. Inhibition of kringle-2 binding to fibrin by epsilon-amino caproic acid. *J Biol Chem.* 1986;261(30):14214-14218.
1970. Verheijen JH, Caspers MP, Chang GT, de Munk GA, Pouwels PH, Enger-Valk BE. Involvement of finger domain and kringle 2 domain of tissue-type plasminogen activator in fibrin binding and stimulation of activity by fibrin. *EMBO J.* 1986;5(13):3525-3530.
1971. De Munk GAW, Caspers MPM, Chang GTG, Pouwels PH, Enger-Valk BE, Verheijen JH. Binding of tissue-type plasminogen activator to lysine, lysine analogs, and fibrin fragments. *Biochemistry.* 1989;28(18):7318-7325.
1972. Downing AK, Driscoll PC, Harvey TS, et al. Solution structure of the fibrin binding finger domain of tissue-type plasminogen activator determined by 1H nuclear magnetic resonance. *J Mol Biol.* 1992;225(3):821-833.
1973. Lijnen HR, Collen D. Strategies for the improvement of thrombolytic agents. *Thromb Haemost.* 1991;66(1):88-110.
1974. Madison EL. Probing structure-function relationships of tissue-type plasminogen activator by site-specific mutagenesis. *Fibrinolysis.* 2002;8(suppl 1):221.
1975. De Vos AM, Ultsch MH, Kelley RF, et al. Crystal structure of the kringle 2 domain of tissue plasminogen activator at 2.4-.ANG. resolution. *Biochemistry.* 1992;31(1):270-279.
1976. De Serrano VS, Sehl LC, Castellino FJ. Direct identification of lysine-33 as the principal cationic center of the ω-amino acid binding site of the recombinant kringle 2 domain of tissue-type plasminogen activator. *Arch Biochem Biophys.* 1992;292(1):206-212.
1977. Chang Y, Zajicek J, Castellino FJ. Role of tryptophan-63 of the kringle 2 domain of tissue-type plasminogen activator in its thermal stability, folding, and ligand binding properties. *Biochemistry.* 1997;36(25):7652-7663.
1978. Chang Y, Nilsen SL, Castellino FJ. Functional and structural consequences of aromatic residue substitutions within the kringle-2 domain of tissue-type plasminogen activator. *J Pept Res.* 1999;53(6):656-664.
1979. Davie EW, Ichinose A, Leytus SP. Structural features of the proteins participating in blood coagulation and fibrinolysis. *Cold Spring Harb Symp Quant Biol.* 1986;51(pt 1):509-514.
1980. Andreasen PA, Petersen LC. Diversity in catalytic properties of single chain and two chain tissue-type plasminogen activator. *Fibrinolysis.* 1991;5:207-215.
1981. Lamba D, Bauer M, Huber R, et al. The 2.3 Å crystal structure of the catalytic domain of recombinant two-chain human tissue-type plasminogen activator. *J Mol Biol.* 1996;258(1):117-135.
1982. Renatus M. Lysine 156promotes the anomalous proenzyme activity of tPA: X-ray crystal structure of single-chain human tPA. *EMBO J.* 1997;16(16):4797-4805.
1983. Harris RJ, Leonard CK, Guzzetta AW, Spellman MW. Tissue plasminogen activator has an O-linked fucose attached to threonine-61 in the epidermal growth factor domain. *Biochemistry.* 1991;30(9):2311-2314.
1984. Hajjar KA, Reynolds CM. alpha-Fucose-mediated binding and degradation of tissue-type plasminogen activator by HepG2 cells. *J Clin Invest.* 1994;93(2):703-710.
1985. Parekh RB, Dwek RA, Thomas JR, et al. Cell-type-specific and site-specific N-glycosylation of type I and type II human tissue plasminogen activator. *Biochemistry.* 1989;28(19):7644-7662.
1986. Spellman MW, Basa LJ, Leonard CK, et al. Carbohydrate structures of human tissue plasminogen activator expressed in Chinese hamster ovary cells. *J Biol Chem.* 1989;264(24):14100-14111.
1987. Hoylaerts M, Rijken DC, Lijnen HR, Collen D. Kinetics of the activation of plasminogen by human tissue plasminogen activator. Role of fibrin. *J Biol Chem.* 1982;257(6):2912-2919.

1988. Zamarron C, Lijnen HR, Collen D. Kinetics of the activation of plasminogen by natural and recombinant tissue-type plasminogen activator. *J Biol Chem.* 1984;259(4):2080-2083.

1989. Loscalzo J. Structural and kinetic comparison of recombinant human single- and two-chain tissue plasminogen activator. *J Clin Invest.* 1988;82(4):1391-1397.

1990. Dichek D, Quertermous T. Thrombin regulation of mRNA levels of tissue plasminogen activator and plasminogen activator inhibitor-1 in cultured human umbilical vein endothelial cells. *Blood.* 1989;74(1):222-228.

1991. Diamond S, Eskin S, McIntire L. Fluid flow stimulates tissue plasminogen activator secretion by cultured human endothelial cells. *Science.* 1989;243(4897):1483-1485.

1992. Emeis JJ. Regulation of the acute release of tissue-type plasminogen activator from the endothelium by coagulation activation products. *Ann N Y Acad Sci.* 1992;667(1 Plasminogen A):249-258.

1993. van den Eijnden-Schrauwen Y, Kooistra T, de Vries RE, Emeis JJ. Studies on the acute release of tissue-type plasminogen activator from human endothelial cells in vitro and in rats in vivo: evidence for a dynamic storage pool. *Blood.* 1995;85(12):3510-3517.

1994. Fay WP, Eitzman DT, Shapiro AD, Madison EL, Ginsburg D. Platelets inhibit fibrinolysis in vitro by both plasminogen activator inhibitor-1-dependent and -independent mechanisms. *Blood.* 1994;83(2):351-356.

1995. Levi M, Biemond BJ, van Zonneveld AJ, ten Cate JW, Pannekoek H. Inhibition of plasminogen activator inhibitor-1 activity results in promotion of endogenous thrombolysis and inhibition of thrombus extension in models of experimental thrombosis. *Circulation.* 1992;85(1):305-312.

1996. Braaten JV, Handt S, Jerome WG, Kirkpatrick J, Lewis JC, Hantgan RR. Regulation of fibrinolysis by platelet-released plasminogen activator inhibitor 1: light scattering and ultrastructural examination of lysis of a model platelet-fibrin thrombus. *Blood.* 1993;81(5):1290-1299.

1997. Steffens GJ, Günzler WA, Ötting F, Frankus E, Flohé L. The complete amino acid sequence of low molecular mass urokinase from human urine. *Hoppe Seylers Z Physiol Chem.* 1982;363(2):1043-1058.

1998. Günzler WA, Steffens GJ, Ötting F, Kim S-MA, Frankus E, Flohé L. The primary structure of high molecular mass urokinase from human urine. The complete amino arid sequence of the A chain. *Hoppe Seylers Z Physiol Chem.* 1982;363(2):1155-1166.

1999. Husain SS, Gurewich V, Lipinski B. Purification and partial characterization of a single-chain high-molecular-weight form of urokinase from human urine. *Arch Biochem Biophys.* 1983;220(1):31-38.

2000. Stump DC, Thienpont M, Collen D. Urokinase-related proteins in human urine. Isolation and characterization of single-chain urokinase (pro-urokinase) and urokinase-inhibitor complex. *J Biol Chem.* 1986;261(3):1267-1273.

2001. Shatos MA, Orfeo T, Doherty JM, Penar PL, Collen D, Mann KG. Thrombin stimulates urokinase production and DNA synthesis in cultured human cerebral microvascular endothelial cells. *Arterioscler Thromb Vasc Biol.* 1995;15(7):903-911.

2002. van Hinsbergh VWM. Regulation of the synthesis and secretion of plasminogen activators by endothelial cells. *Pathophysiol Haemost Thromb.* 1988;18(4-6):307-327.

2003. Wun TC, Schleuning WD, Reich E. Isolation and characterization of urokinase from human plasma. *J Biol Chem.* 1982;257(6):3276-3283.

2004. Stump DC, Lijnen HR, Collen D. Purification and characterization of single-chain urokinase-type plasminogen activator from human cell cultures. *J Biol Chem.* 1986;261(3):1274-1278.

2005. Darras V, Thienpont M, Stump DC, Collen D. Measurement of urokinase-type plasminogen activator (u-PA) with an enzyme-linked immunosorbent assay (ELISA) based on three murine monoclonal antibodies. *Thromb Haemost.* 1986;56(3):411-414.

2006. Collen D, Zamarron C, Lijnen HR, Hoylaerts M. Activation of plasminogen by pro-urokinase. II. Kinetics. *J Biol Chem.* 1986;261(3):1259-1266.

2007. Ichinose A, Fujikawa K, Suyama T. The activation of pro-urokinase by plasma kallikrein and its inactivation by thrombin. *J Biol Chem.* 1986;261(8):3486-3489.

2008. Kasai S, Arimura H, Nishida M, Suyama T. Primary structure of single-chain pro-urokinase. *J Biol Chem.* 1985;260(22):12382-12389.

2009. Stump DC, Lijnen HR, Collen D. Purification and characterization of a novel low molecular weight form of single-chain urokinase-type plasminogen activator. *J Biol Chem.* 1986;261(36):17120-17126.

2010. Gurewich V, Pannell R, Broeze RJ, Mao J. Characterization of the intrinsic fibrinolytic properties of pro-urokinase through a study of plasmin-resistant mutant forms produced by site-specific mutagenesis of lysine(158). *J Clin Invest.* 1988;82(6):1956-1962.

2011. Gurewich V, Pannell R. Fibrin binding and zymogenic properties of single-chain urokinase (Pro-urokinase). *Semin Thromb Hemost.* 1987;13(02):146-151.

2012. Pannell R, Gurewich V. Activation of plasminogen by single-chain urokinase or by two-chain urokinase--a demonstration that single-chain urokinase has a low catalytic activity (pro-urokinase). *Blood.* 1987;69(1):22-26.

2013. Lijnen HR. Elements of the fibrinolytic system. *Ann N Y Acad Sci.* 2001;936:226-236.

2014. Han B, Nakamura M, Mori I, Nakamura Y, Kakudo K. Urokinase-type plasminogen activator system and breast cancer (Review). *Oncol Rep.* 2005;14(1):105-112.

2015. Blasi F. Proteolysis, cell adhesion, chemotaxis, and invasiveness are regulated by the u-PA-u-PAR-PAI-1 system. *Thromb Haemost.* 1999;82(2):298-304.

2016. Quax PH, van Leeuwen RT, Verspaget HW, Verheijen JH. Protein and messenger RNA levels of plasminogen activators and inhibitors analyzed in 22 human tumor cell lines. *Cancer Res.* 1990;50(5):1488-1494.

2017. Evans DM, Sloan-Stakleff K, Arvan M, Guyton DP. Time and dose dependency of the suppression of pulmonary metastases of rat mammary cancer by amiloride. *Clin Exp Metastasis.* 1998;16(4):353-357.

2018. Banerji A, Fernandes A, Bane S, Ahire S. The field bean protease inhibitor has the potential to suppress B16F10 melanoma cell lung metastasis in mice. *Cancer Lett.* 1998;129(1):15-20.

2019. Kobayashi H, Gotoh J, Fujie M, Shinohara H, Moniwa N, Terao T. Inhibition of metastasis of lewis lung carcinoma by a synthetic peptide within growth factor-like domain of urokinase in the experimental and spontaneous metastasis model. *Int J Cancer.* 1994;57(5):727-733.

2020. Xiao G, Liu YE, Gentz R, et al. Suppression of breast cancer growth and metastasis by a serpin myoepithelium-derived serine proteinase inhibitor expressed in the mammary myoepithelial cells. *Proc Natl Acad Sci.* 1999;96(7):3700-3705.

2021. Rabbani S, Harakidas P, Davidson DJ, Henkin J, Mazar AP. Prevention of prostate-cancer metastasisin vivo by a novel synthetic inhibitor of urokinase-type plasminogen activator (uPA). *Int J Cancer.* 1995;63(6):840-845.

2022. Alonso DF, Farias EF, Ladeda V, Davel L, Puricelli L, Bal de Kier Joffe E. Effects of synthetic urokinase inhibitors on local invasion and metastasis in a murine mammary tumor model. *Breast Cancer Res Treat.* 1996;40(3):209-223.

2023. Jankun J, Keck RW, Skrzypczak-Jankun E, Swiercz R. Inhibitors of urokinase reduce size of prostate cancer xenografts in severe combined immunodeficient mice. *Cancer Res.* 1997;57(4):559-563.

2024. Riccio A, Grimaldi G, Verde P, Sebastio G, Boast S, Blasi F. The human urokinase-plasminogen activator gene and its promoter. *Nucl Acids Res.* 1985;13(8):2759-2771.

2025. Tripputi P, Blasi F, Verde P, Cannizzaro LA, Emanuel BS, Croce CM. Human urokinase gene is located on the long arm of chromosome 10. *Proc Natl Acad Sci.* 1985;82(13):4448-4452.

2026. Günzler WA, Steffens GJ, Ötting F, Buse G, Flohé L. Structural relationship between human high and low molecular mass urokinase. *Hoppe Seylers Z Physiol Chem.* 1982;363(1):133-142.

2027. Holmes WE, Pennica D, Blaber M, et al. Cloning and expression of the gene for pro-urokinase in Escherichia coli. *Bio/Technology.* 1985;3(10):923-929.

2028. Gyetko MR, Chen GH, McDonald RA, et al. Urokinase is required for the pulmonary inflammatory response to Cryptococcus neoformans. A murine transgenic model. *J Clin Invest.* 1996;97(8):1818-1826.

2029. Shapiro RL, Duquette JG, Nunes I, et al. Urokinase-type plasminogen activator-deficient mice are predisposed to staphylococcal botryomycosis, pleuritis, and effacement of lymphoid follicles. *Am J Pathol.* 1997;150(1):359-369.

2030. Beck JM, Preston AM, Gyetko MR. Urokinase-type plasminogen activator in inflammatory cell recruitment and host defense against Pneumocystis carinii in mice. *Infect Immun.* 1999;67(2):879-884.

2031. Li X, Bokman AM, Llinás M, Smith RAG, Dobson CM. Solution structure of the kringle domain from urokinase-type plasminogen activator. *J Mol Biol.* 1994;235(5):1548-1559.

2032. Franco P, Iaccarino C, Chiaradonna F, et al. Phosphorylation of human pro-urokinase on ser 138/303 impairs its receptor-dependent ability to promote myelomonocytic adherence and motility. *J Cell Biol.* 1997;137(3):779-791.

2033. Mazar AP, Buko A, Petros AM, et al. Domain analysis of urokinase plasminogen activator (u-PA): preparation and characterization of intact A-chain molecules. *Fibrinolysis.* 2003;6(suppl 1):49-55.

2034. He CJ, Rebibou JM, Peraldi MN, Meulders Q, Rondeau E. Growth factor-like effect of urokinase type plasminogen activator in human renal cells. *Biochem Biophys Res Commun.* 1991;176(3):1408-1416.

2035. Koopman JL. Mitogenic effects of urokinase on melanoma cells are independent of high affinity binding to the urokinase receptor. *J Biol Chem.* 1998;273(50):33267-33272.

2036. Rabbani SA, Gladu J, Mazar AP, Henkin J, Goltzman D. Induction in human osteoblastic cells (SaOS2) of the early response genesfos, jun, andmyc by the amino terminal fragment (ATF) of urokinase. *J Cell Physiol.* 1997;172(2):137-145.

2037. Goncharova EA, Vorotnikov AV, Gracheva EO, et al. Activation of p38 MAP-kinase and Caldesmon phosphorylation are essential for urokinase-induced human smooth muscle cell migration. *Biol Chem.* 2002;383(1):115-126.

2038. Lee KN, Jackson KW, McKee PA. Effect of a synthetic carboxy-terminal peptide of α2-antiplasmin on urokinase-induced fibrinolysis. *Thromb Res.* 2002;105(3):263-270.

2039. Mukhina S. The chemotactic action of urokinase on smooth muscle cells is dependent on its kringle domain. Characterization of interactions and contribution to chemotaxis. *J Biol Chem.* 2000;275(22):16450-16458.

2040. Gurewich V, Pannell R, Louie S, Kelley P, Suddith RL, Greenlee R. Effective and fibrin-specific clot lysis by a zymogen precursor form of urokinase (pro-urokinase). A study in vitro and in two animal species. *J Clin Invest.* 1984;73(6):1731-1739.

2041. Pannell R, Gurewich V. Pro-urokinase: a study of its stability in plasma and of a mechanism for its selective fibrinolytic effect. *Blood.* 1986;67(5):1215-1223.

2042. Ellis V, Scully MF, Kakkar VV. Plasminogen activation by single-chain urokinase in functional isolation. A kinetic study. *J Biol Chem.* 1987;262(31):14998-15003.

2043. Nowak UK, Li X, Teuten AJ, Smith RAG, Dobson CM. NMR studies of the dynamics of the multidomain protein urokinase-type plasminogen activator. *Biochemistry.* 1993;32(1):298-309.

2044. Hansen AP, Petros AM, Meadows RP, Fesik SW. Backbone dynamics of a two-domain protein: 15N relaxation studies of the amino-terminal fragment of urokinase-type plasminogen activator. *Biochemistry.* 1994;33(51):15418-15424.

2045. Hansen AP, Petros AM, Meadows RP, et al. Solution structure of the amino-terminal fragment of urokinase-type plasminogen activator. *Biochemistry.* 1994;33(16):4847-4864.

2046. Spraggon G, Phillips C, Nowak UK, et al. The crystal structure of the catalytic domain of human urokinase-type plasminogen activator. *Structure.* 1995;3(7):681-691.

2047. Nienaber V, Wang J, Davidson D, Henkin J. Re-Engineering of human urokinase provides a system for structure-based drug design at high resolution and reveals a novel structural subsite. *J Biol Chem.* 2000;275(10):7239-7248.

2048. Kobayashi H, Schmitt M, Goretzki L, et al. Cathepsin B efficiently activates the soluble and the tumor cell receptor-bound form of the proenzyme urokinase-type plasminogen activator (Pro-uPA). *J Biol Chem.* 1991;266(8):5147-5152.

2049. Nauland U, Rijken DC. Activation of thrombin-inactivated single-chain urokinase-type plasminogen activator by dipeptidyl peptidase I (cathepsin C). *Eur J Biochem.* 1994;223(2):497-501.
2050. Goretzki L, Schmitt M, Mann K, et al. Effective activation of the proenzyme form of the urokinase-type plasminogen activator (pro-uPA) by the cysteine protease cathepsin L. *FEBS Lett.* 1992;297(1-2):112-118.
2051. Drag B, Petersen LC. Activation of pro-urokinase by cathepsin G in the presence of glucosaminoglycans. *Fibrinolysis.* 1994;8(3):192-199.
2052. Stack MS, Johnson DA. Human mast cell tryptase activates single-chain urinary-type plasminogen activator (pro-urokinase). *J Biol Chem.* 1994;269(13):9416-9419.
2053. Wolf BB, Vasudevan J, Henkin J, Gonias SL. Nerve growth factor-gamma activates soluble and receptor-bound single chain urokinase-type plasminogen activator. *J Biol Chem.* 1993;268(22):16327-16331.
2054. Brunner G, Simon MM, Kramer MD. Activation of pro-urokinase by the human T cell-associated serine proteinase HuTSP-1. *FEBS Lett.* 1990;260(1):141-144.
2055. Römisch J, Vermöhlen S, Feussner A, Stöhr HA. The FVII activating protease cleaves single-chain plasminogen activators. *Pathophysiol Haemost Thromb.* 2000;29(5):292-299.
2056. Marcotte PA, Kozan IM, Dorwin SA, Ryan JM. The matrix metalloproteinase pump-1 catalyzes formation of low molecular weight (pro)urokinase in cultures of normal human kidney cells. *J Biol Chem.* 1992;267(20):13803-13806.
2057. Ugwu F, Van Hoef B, Bini A, Collen D, Lijnen HR. Proteolytic cleavage of urokinase-type plasminogen activator by Stromelysin-1 (MMP-3). *Biochemistry.* 1998;37(20):7231-7236.
2058. Orgel D, Schröder W, Hecker-Kia A, Weithmann KU, Kolkenbrock H, Ulbrich N. The cleavage of pro-urokinase type plasminogen activator by Stromelysin-1. *Clin Chem Lab Med.* 1998;36(9):697-702.
2059. Collen D, Lijnen HR. Basic and clinical aspects of fibrinolysis and thrombolysis. *Blood.* 1991;78(12):3114-3124.
2060. Schmitt M, Kanayama N, Henschen A, et al. Elastase released from human granulocytes stimulated with N-formyl-chemotactic peptide prevents activation of tumor cell prourokinase (pro-uPA). *FEBS Lett.* 1989;255(1):83-88.
2061. Learmonth MP, Li W, Namiranian S. Modulation of the cell binding property of single chain urokinase-type plasminogen activator by neutrophil cathepsin G. *Fibrinolysis.* 1992;6(suppl 4):113-116.
2062. Braat EAM, Levi M, Bos R, et al. Inactivation of single-chain urokinase-type plasminogen activator by thrombin in human subjects. *J Lab Clin Med.* 1999;134(2):161-167.
2063. Braat EA, Rijken DC. The inactivation of single-chain urokinase-type plasminogen activator by thrombin may provide an additional explanation for the antifibrinolytic effect of factor XI. *Thromb Haemost.* 1999;81(4):657.
2064. de Munk GAW, Parkinson JF, Groeneveld E, Bang NU, Rijken DC. Role of the glycosaminoglycan component of thrombomodulin in its acceleration of the inactivation of single-chain urokinase-type plasminogen activator by thrombin. *Biochem. J.* 1993;290(3):655-659.
2065. Lijnen HR, Hoef B, Collen D. Activation with plasmin of two-chain urokinase-type plasminogen activator derived from single-chain urokinase-type plasminogen activator by treatment with thrombin. *Eur J Biochem.* 1987;169(2):359-364.
2066. Robbins KC, Summaria L, Hsieh B, Shah RJ. The peptide chains of human plasmin. Mechanism of activation of human plasminogen to plasmin. *J Biol Chem.* 1967;242(10):2333-2342.
2067. Fleury V, Lijnen HR, Angles-Cano E. Mechanism of the enhanced intrinsic activity of single-chain urokinase-type plasminogen activator during ongoing fibrinolysis. *J Biol Chem.* 1993;268(25):18554-18559.
2068. Longstaff C, Clough AM, Gaffney PJ. Kinetics of plasmin activation of single chain urinary-type plasminogen activator (scu-PA) and demonstration of a high affinity interaction between scu-PA and plasminogen. *J Biol Chem.* 1992;267(1):173-179.
2069. Lenich C, Pannell R, Gurewich V. The effect of the carboxy-terminal lysine of urokinase on the catalysis of plasminogen activation. *Thromb Res.* 1991;64(1):69-80.
2070. Choi-Miura NH, Tobe T, Sumiya J., et al. Purification and characterization of a novel hyaluronan-binding protein (PHBP) from human plasma: it has three EGF, a kringle and a serine protease domain, similar to hepatocyte growth factor Activator. *J Biochem.* 1996;119(6):1157-1165.
2071. Hunfeld A, Etscheid M, Koenig H, Seitz R, Dodt J. Identification of the thrombin-like activity of PCC's. *Ann Hematol.* 1998;76:A101.
2072. Hunfeld A, Etscheid M, König H, Seitz R, Dodt J. Detection of a novel plasma serine protease during purification of vitamin K-dependent coagulation factors. *FEBS Lett.* 1999;456(2):290-294.
2073. Stavenuiter F, Dienava-Verdoold I, Boon-Spijker MG, Brinkman HJM, Meijer AB, Mertens K. Factor seven activating protease (FSAP): does it activate factor VII? *J Thromb Haemost.* 2012;10(5):859-866.
2074. Kanse SM, Declerck PJ, Ruf W, Broze G, Etscheid M. Factor VII-activating protease promotes the proteolysis and inhibition of tissue factor pathway inhibitor. *Arterioscler Thromb Vasc Biol.* 2011;32(2):427-433.
2075. Kannemeier C, Feussner A, Stöhr H-A, Weisse J, Preissner KT, Römisch J. Factor VII and single-chain plasminogen activator-activating protease. *Eur J Biochem.* 2001;268(13):3789-3796.
2076. Sumiya J, Asakawa S, Tobe T, et al. Isolation and characterization of the plasma hyaluronan-binding protein (PHBP) gene (HABP2). *J Biochem.* 1997;122(5):983-990.
2077. Roemisch J, Feussner A, Nerlich C, Stoehr HA, Weimer T. The frequent Marburg I polymorphism impairs the pro-urokinase activating potency of the factor VII activating protease (FSAP). *Blood Coagul Fibrinolysis.* 2002;13(5):433-441.
2078. Gulesserian T, Hron G, Endler G, Eichinger S, Wagner O, Kyrle PA. Marburg I polymorphism of factor VII-activating protease and risk of recurrent venous thromboembolism. *Thromb Haemost.* 2005;95(1):65-67.
2079. Sedding D, Daniel JM, Muhl L, et al. The G534E polymorphism of the gene encoding the factor VII–activating protease is associated with cardiovascular risk due to increased neointima formation. *J Exp Med.* 2006;203(13):2801-2807.
2080. Stephan F, Aarden LA, Zeerleder S. FSAP, a new player in inflammation? *Hämostaseologie.* 2012;32(1):51-55.
2081. Kanse SM, Etscheid M. Factor VII activating protease (FSAP): caught in the crossfire between polycations and polyanions. *J Thromb Haemost.* 2010;8(3):556-558.
2082. Sperling C, Maitz MF, Grasso S, Werner C, Kanse SM. A positively charged surface triggers coagulation activation through factor VII activating protease (FSAP). *ACS Appl Mater Interf.* 2017;9(46):40107-40116.
2083. Zeerleder S. Factor VII-activating protease: hemostatic protein or immune regulator? *Semin Thromb Hemost.* 2018;44(2):151-158.
2084. Yamamichi S, Fujiwara Y, Kikuchi T, Nishitani M, Matsushita Y, Hasumi K. Extracellular histone induces plasma hyaluronan-binding protein (factor VII activating protease) activation in vivo. *Biochem Biophys Res Commun.* 2011;409(3):483-488.
2085. Grasso S, Neumann A, Lang IM, Etscheid M, von Kockritz-Blickwede M, Kanse SM. Interaction of factor VII activating protease (FSAP) with neutrophil extracellular traps (NETs). *Thromb Res.* 2018;161:36-42.
2086. Miyazawa K, Shimomura T, Kitamura A, Kondo J, Morimoto Y, Kitamura N. Molecular cloning and sequence analysis of the cDNA for a human serine protease reponsible for activation of hepatocyte growth factor. Structural similarity of the protease precursor to blood coagulation factor XII. *J Biol Chem.* 1993;268(14):10024-10028.
2087. Etscheid M, Hunfeld A, Konig H, Seitz R, Dodt J. Activation of proPHBSP, the zymogen of a plasma hyaluronan binding serine protease, by an intermolecular autocatalytic mechanism. *Biol Chem.* 2000;381(12):1223-1231.
2088. Choi-Miura NH, Takahashi K, Yoda M, Saito K, Mazda T, Tomita M. Proteolytic activation and inactivation of the serine protease activity of plasma hyaluronan binding protein. *Biol Pharm Bull.* 2001;24(5):448-452.
2089. Nakazawa F, Kannemeier C, Shibamiya A, et al. Extracellular RNA is a natural cofactor for the (auto-)activation of Factor VII-activating protease (FSAP). *Biochem J.* 2005;385(pt 3):831-838.
2090. Romisch J. Factor VII activating protease (FSAP): a novel protease in hemostasis. *Biol Chem.* 2002;383(7-8):1119-1124.
2091. Choi-Miura NH, Saito K, Takahashi K, Yoda M, Tomita M. Regulation mechanism of the serine protease activity of plasma hyaluronan binding protein. *Biol Pharm Bull.* 2001;24(3):221-225.
2092. Etscheid M, Beer N, Seitz R, Dodt J. Regulation of the plasma hyaluronan-binding seine protease. *Ann Hematol.* 2002;81:A16.
2093. Stephan F, Dienava-Verdoold I, Bulder I, et al. Tissue factor pathway inhibitor is an inhibitor of factor VII-activating protease. *J Thromb Haemost.* 2012;10(6):1165-1171.
2094. Nesheim M, Bajzar L. The discovery of TAFI. *J Thromb Haemost.* 2005;3(10):2139-2146.
2095. Mosnier LO, Bouma BN. Regulation of fibrinolysis by thrombin activatable fibrinolysis inhibitor, an unstable carboxypeptidase B that unites the pathways of coagulation and fibrinolysis. *Arterioscle Thromb Vasc Biol.* 2006;26(11):2445-2453.
2096. Boffa MB, Koschinsky ML. Curiouser and curiouser: recent advances in measurement of thrombin-activatable fibrinolysis inhibitor (TAFI) and in understanding its molecular genetics, gene regulation, and biological roles. *Clin Biochem.* 2007;40(7):431-442.
2097. Heylen E. An update on the role of carboxypeptidase U (TAFIa) in fibrinolysis. *Front Biosci.* 2011;16(1):2427.
2098. Declerck PJ. Thrombin activatable fibrinolysis inhibitor. *Hämostaseologie.* 2011;31(3):165-173.
2099. Mosnier LO. Identification of thrombin activatable fibrinolysis inhibitor (TAFI) in human platelets. *Blood.* 2003;101(12):4844-4846.
2100. Schadinger SL, Lin JHH, Garand M, Boffa MB. Secretion and antifibrinolytic function of thrombin-activatable fibrinolysis inhibitor from human platelets. *J Thromb Haemost.* 2010;8(11):2523-2529.
2101. Redlitz A, Nicolini FA, Malycky JL, Topol EJ, Plow EF. Inducible carboxypeptidase activity: a role in clot lysis in vivo. *Circulation.* 1996;93(7):1328-1330.
2102. Minnema MC, Friederich PW, Levi M, et al. Enhancement of rabbit jugular vein thrombolysis by neutralization of factor XI. In vivo evidence for a role of factor XI as an anti-fibrinolytic factor. *J Clin Invest.* 1998;101(1):10-14.
2103. Gresele P, Momi S, Berrettini M, et al. Activated human protein C prevents thrombin-induced thromboembolism in mice. Evidence that activated protein c reduces intravascular fibrin accumulation through the inhibition of additional thrombin generation. *J Clin Invest.* 1998;101(3):667-676.
2104. Nagashima M. Thrombin-activatable fibrinolysis inhibitor (TAFI) deficient mice. *Front Biosci.* 2002;7(1-3):d556.
2105. Franco RF, Fagundes MG, Meijers JC, et al. Identification of polymorphisms in the 5'-untranslated region of the TAFI gene: relationship with plasma TAFI levels and risk of venous thrombosis. *Haematologica.* 2001;86(5):510-517.
2106. van Tilburg NH, Rosendaal FR, Bertina RM. Thrombin activatable fibrinolysis inhibitor and the risk for deep vein thrombosis. *Blood.* 2000;95(9):2855-2859.
2107. Hendriks D, Wang W, Scharpe S. Carboxypeptidase U: a novel plasma carboxypeptidase with affinity for plasminogen. *Fibrinolysis.* 1994;8:24.
2108. Hendriks D, Scharpé S, Sande M, Lommaert MP. Characterisation of a carboxypeptidase in human serum distinct from carboxypeptidase N. *Clin Chem Lab Med.* 1989;27(5):277-286.
2109. Campbell W, Okada H. An arginine specific carboxypeptidase generated in blood during coagulation or inflammation which is unrelated to carboxypeptidase N or its subunits. *Biochem Biophys Res Commun* 1989;162(3):933-939.
2110. Tan AK, Eaton DL. Activation and characterization of procarboxypeptidase B from human plasma. *Biochemistry.* 1995;34(17):5811-5816.

2111. Boffa MB, Reid TS, Joo E, Nesheim ME, Koschinsky ML. Characterization of the gene encoding human TAFI (Thrombin-Activable fibrinolysis inhibitor; plasma pro-carboxypeptidase B). *Biochemistry.* 1999;38(20):6547-6558.

2112. Skidgel RA. Basic carboxypeptidases: regulators of peptide hormone activity. *Trends Pharmacol Sci.* 1988;9(8):299-304.

2113. Vanhoof G, Wauters J, Schatteman K, et al. The gene for human carboxypeptidase U (CPU)—a proposed novel regulator of plasminogen activation—maps to 13q14.11. *Genomics.* 1996;38(3):454-455.

2114. Zhao L, Morser J, Bajzar L, Nesheim M, Nagashima M. Identification and characterization of two thrombin-activatable fibrinolysis inhibitor isoforms. *Thromb Haemost.* 1998;80(6):949-955.

2115. Juhan-Vague I, Renucci JF, Grimaux M, et al. Thrombin-activatable fibrinolysis inhibitor antigen levels and cardiovascular risk factors. *Arterioscler Thromb Vascu Biol.* 2000;20(9):2156-2161.

2116. Henry M. Identification of polymorphisms in the promoter and the 3' region of the TAFI gene: evidence that plasma TAFI antigen levels are strongly genetically controlled. *Blood.* 2001;97(7):2053-2058.

2117. Brouwers GJ. A novel, possibly functional, single nucleotide polymorphism in the coding region of the thrombin-activatable fibrinolysis inhibitor (TAFI) gene is also associated with TAFI levels. *Blood.* 2001;98(6):1992-1993.

2118. Boffa MB, Wang W, Bajzar L, Nesheim ME. Plasma and recombinant thrombin-activable fibrinolysis inhibitor (TAFI) and activated TAFI compared with respect to glycosylation, thrombin/thrombomodulin-dependent activation, thermal stability, and enzymatic properties. *J Biol Chem.* 1998;273(4):2127-2135.

2119. Mao SS, Cooper CM, Wood T, Shafer JA, Gardell SJ. Characterization of plasmin-mediated activation of plasma procarboxypeptidase B: modulation by glycosaminoglycans. *J Biol Chem.* 1999;274(49):35046-35052.

2120. Hess K, Ajjan R, Phoenix F, Dobó J, Gál P, Schroeder V. Effects of MASP-1 of the complement system on activation of coagulation factors and plasma clot formation. *PLoS One.* 2012;7(4):e35690.

2121. Mosnier LO. Platelet factor 4 inhibits thrombomodulin-dependent activation of thrombin-activatable fibrinolysis inhibitor (TAFI) by thrombin. *J Biol Chem.* 2010;286(1):502-510.

2122. Koschinsky ML, Boffa MB, Nesheim ME, et al. Association of a single nucleotide polymorphism in CPB2 encoding the thrombin-activable fibrinolysis inhibitor (TAFI) with blood pressure. *Clin Genet.* 2002;60(5):345-349.

2123. Von dem Borne PA, Bajzar L, Meijers JC, Nesheim ME, Bouma BN. Thrombin-mediated activation of factor XI results in a thrombin-activatable fibrinolysis inhibitor-dependent inhibition of fibrinolysis. *J Clin Invest.* 1997;99(10):2323-2327.

2124. Plow EF, Herren T, Redlitz A, Miles LA, Hoover-Plow JL. The cell biology of the plasminogen system. *FASEB J.* 1995;9(10):939-945.

2125. Suenson E, Lutzen O, Thorsen S. Initial plasmin-degradation of fibrin as the basis of a positive feed-back mechanism in fibrinolysis. *Eur J Biochem.* 1984;140(3):513-522.

2126. Pannell R, Black J, Gurewich V. Complementary modes of action of tissue-type plasminogen activator and pro-urokinase by which their synergistic effect on clot lysis may be explained. *J Clin Investig.* 1988;81(3):853-859.

2127. Norrman B, Wallen P, Ranby M. Fibrinolysis mediated by tissue plasminogen activator. Disclosure of a kinetic transition. *Eur J Biochem.* 1985;149(1):193-200.

2128. Fleury V, Angles-Cano E. Characterization of the binding of plasminogen to fibrin surfaces: the role of carboxy-terminal lysines. *Biochemistry.* 1991;30(30):7630-7638.

2129. Sakharov DV, Rijken DC. Superficial accumulation of plasminogen during plasma clot lysis. *Circulation.* 1995;92(7):1883-1890.

2130. Foley JH, Cook PF, Nesheim ME. Kinetics of activated thrombin-activatable fibrinolysis inhibitor (TAFIa)-catalyzed cleavage of C-terminal lysine residues of fibrin degradation products and removal of plasminogen-binding sites. *J Biol Chem.* 2011;286(22):19280-19286.

2131. Nesheim M. Fibrinolysis and the plasma carboxypeptidase. *Curr Opin Hematol.* 1998;5(5):309-313.

2132. Bouma BN, Mosnier LO, Meijers JC, Griffin JH. Factor XI dependent and independent activation of thrombin activatable fibrinolysis inhibitor (TAFI) in plasma associated with clot formation. *Thromb Haemost.* 1999;82(6):1703-1708.

2133. Bajzar L. Thrombin activatable fibrinolysis inhibitor and an antifibrinolytic pathway. *Arterioscler Thromb Vasc Biol.* 2000;20(12):2511-2518.

2134. Ryan CA, Hass GM, Kuhn RW. Purification and properties of a carboxypeptidase inhibitor from potatoes. *J Biol Chem.* 1974;249(17):5495-5499.

2135. Reverter D. A carboxypeptidase inhibitor from the medical leech Hirudo medicinalis. ISOLATION, sequence analysis, cDNA cloning, recombinant expression, and characterization. *J Biol Chem.* 1998;273(49):32927-32933.

2136. Boffa MB. Roles of thermal instability and proteolytic cleavage in regulation of activated thrombin-activable fibrinolysis inhibitor. *J Biol Chem.* 2000;275(17):12868-12878.

2137. Marx PF. Inactivation of active thrombin-activable fibrinolysis inhibitor takes place by a process that involves conformational instability rather than proteolytic cleavage. *J Biol Chem.* 2000;275(17):12410-12415.

2138. Sato T, Miwa T, Akatsu H, et al. Pro-carboxypeptidase R is an acute phase protein in the mouse, whereas carboxypeptidase N is not. *J Immunol.* 2000;165(2):1053-1058.

2139. Silveira A, Schatteman K, Goossens F, et al. Plasma procarboxypeptidase U in men with symptomatic coronary artery disease. *Thromb Haemost.* 2000;84(3):364-368.

2140. Schatteman KA, Goossens FJ, Scharpe SS, Neels HM, Hendriks DF. Assay of procarboxypeptidase U, a novel determinant of the fibrinolytic cascade, in human plasma. *Clin Chem.* 1999;45(6 pt 1):807-813.

2141. Chetaille P, Alessi MC, Kouassi D, Morange PE, Juhan-Vague I. Plasma TAFI antigen variations in healthy subjects. *Thromb Haemost.* 2000;83(6):902-905.

2142. Boffa MB. A role for CCAAT/Enhancer-binding protein in hepatic expression of thrombin-activable fibrinolysis inhibitor. *J Biol Chem.* 2002;277(28):25329-25336.

2143. Van De Craen B, Declerck PJ, Gils A. The biochemistry, physiology and pathological roles of PAI-1 and the requirements for PAI-1 inhibition in vivo. *Thromb Res.* 2012;130(4):576-585.

2144. Dieval J, Nguyen G, Gross S, Delobel J, Kruithof EK. A lifelong bleeding disorder associated with a deficiency of plasminogen activator inhibitor type 1. *Blood.* 1991;77(3):528-532.

2145. Fay WP, Shapiro AD, Shih JL, Schleef RR, Ginsburg D. Complete deficiency of plasminogen-activator inhibitor type 1 due to a frame-shift mutation. *New Engl J Med.* 1992;327(24):1729-1733.

2146. Lee MH, Vosburgh E, Anderson K, McDonagh J. Deficiency of plasma plasminogen activator inhibitor 1 results in hyperfibrinolytic bleeding. *Blood.* 1993;81(9):2357-2362.

2147. Fay WP, Parker AC, Condrey LR, Shapiro AD. Human plasminogen activator inhibitor-1 (PAI-1) deficiency: characterization of a large kindred with a null mutation in the PAI-1 gene. *Blood.* 1997;90(1):204-208.

2148. Minowa H, Takahashi Y, Tanaka T, et al. Four cases of bleeding diathesis in children due to congenital plasminogen activator inhibitor-1 deficiency. *Pathophysiol Haemost Thromb.* 2000;29(5):286-291.

2149. Declerck PJ, De Mol M, Alessi MC, et al. Purification and characterization of a plasminogen activator inhibitor 1 binding protein from human plasma. Identification as a multimeric form of S protein (vitronectin). *J Biol Chem.* 1988;263(30):15454-15461.

2150. Declerck PJ, Alessi MC, Verstreken M, Kruithof EK, Juhan-Vague I, Collen D. Measurement of plasminogen activator inhibitor 1 in biologic fluids with a murine monoclonal antibody-based enzyme-linked immunosorbent assay. *Blood.* 1988;71(1):220-225.

2151. Wiman B, Hamsten A. The fibrinolytic enzyme system and its role in the etiology of thromboembolic disease. *Semin Thromb Hemost.* 1990;16(03):207-216.

2152. Stiko A, Hervio L, Loskutoff DJ. Plasminogen activator inhibitors. In: Colman RW, HJ , Marder VJ, Clowes AW, George JN, eds. *Hemostasis and Thrombosis: Basic Principles and Clinical Practice.* Lippincott Williams & Wilkins; 2002:355-365.

2153. Huber K. Plasminogen activator inhibitor type-1 (part two): role for failure of thrombolytic therapy. PAI-1 resistance as a potential benefit for new fibrinolytic agents. *J Thromb.* 2001;11(3):195-202.

2154. Alessi MC, Chomiki N, Fossat C, Berthier R, Juhan-Vague I. Plasminogen activator inhibitor 1 (PAI-1) gene expression in human megacaryocytes. *Fibrinolysis.* 1994;8:28.

2155. Sharp AM, Stein PE, Pannu NS, et al. The active conformation of plasminogen activator inhibitor 1, a target for drugs to control fibrinolysis and cell adhesion. *Structure.* 1999;7(2):111-118.

2156. Aertgeerts K, De Bondt HL, De Ranter CJ, Declerck PJ. Mechanisms contributing to the conformational and functional flexibility of plasminogen activator inhibitor-1. *Nat Struct Mol Biol.* 1995;2(10):891-897.

2157. Wiman B, Almquist Å, Sigurdardottir O, Lindahl T. Plasminogen activator inhibitor 1 (PAI) is bound to vitronectin in plasma. *FEBS Lett.* 1988;242(1):125-128.

2158. Schulze AJ, Huber R, Bode W, Engh RA. Structural aspects of serpin inhibition. *FEBS Lett.* 1994;344(2-3):117-124.

2159. Ginsburg D, Zeheb R, Yang AY, et al. cDNA cloning of human plasminogen activator-inhibitor from endothelial cells. *J Clin Investig.* 1986;78(6):1673-1680.

2160. Ny T, Sawdey M, Lawrence D, Millan JL, Loskutoff DJ. Cloning and sequence of a cDNA coding for the human beta-migrating endothelial-cell-type plasminogen activator inhibitor. *Proc Natl Acad Sci.* 1986;83(18):6776-6780.

2161. Sawdey M, Ny T, Loskutoff DJ. Messenger RNA for plasminogen activator inhibitor. *Thromb Res.* 1986;41(2):151-160.

2162. Pannekoek H, Veerman H, Lambers H, et al. Endothelial plasminogen activator inhibitor: a new member of the serpin gene family. *Thromb Res.* 1986;41:20.

2163. Andreasen PA, Riccio A, Welinder KG, et al. Plasminogen activator inhibitor type-1: reactive center and amino-terminal heterogeneity determined by protein and cDNA sequencing. *FEBS Letts.* 1986;209(2):213-218.

2164. Wun TC, Kretzmer KK. cDNA cloning and expression in *E. coli* of a plasminogen activator inhibitor (PAI) related to a PAI produced by Hep G2 hepatoma cell. *FEBS Lett.* 1987;210(1):11-16.

2165. Klinger KW, Winqvist R, Riccio A, et al. Plasminogen activator inhibitor type 1 gene is located at region q21.3-q22 of chromosome 7 and genetically linked with cystic fibrosis. *Proc Natl Acad Sci.* 1987;84(23):8548-8552.

2166. Schwartz CE, Stanislovitis P, Phelan MC, Klinger K, Taylor HA, Stevenson RE. Deletion mapping of plasminogen activator inhibitor, type I (PLANH1) and β-glucuronidase (GUSB) in 7q21→q22. *Cytogenet Genome Res.* 1991;56(3-4):152-153.

2167. Loskutoff DJ, Linders M, Keijer J, Veerman H, Van Heerikhuizen H, Pannekoek H. Structure of the human plasminogen activator inhibitor 1 gene: nonrandom distribution of introns. *Biochemistry.* 1987;26(13):3763-3768.

2168. Strandberg L, Lawrence D, Ny T. The organization of the human-plasminogen-activator-inhibitor-1 gene. Implications on the evolution of the serine-protease inhibitor family. *Eur J Biochem.* 1988;176(3):609-616.

2169. Bosnia PJ, Kooistra T, Siemieniak DR, Slightom JL. Further characterization of the 5'-flanking DNA of the gene encoding human plasminogen activator inhibitor-1. *Gene.* 1991;100:261-266.

2170. Bosma PJ, van den Berg EA, Kooistra T, Siemieniak D, Slightom JL. 238 Promotor and structural gene nucleotide sequences of the human plasminogen activator inhibitor 1 (PAI-1) gene. *Fibrinolysis.* 1988;2:103.

2171. Nordt TK, Lohrmann J, Bode C. Regulation of PAI-1 expression by genetic polymorphisms. *Thromb Res.* 2001;103:S1-S5.

2172. Dawson SJ, Wiman B, Hamsten A, Green F, Humphries S, Henney AM. The two allele sequences of a common polymorphism in the promoter of the plasminogen activator inhibitor-1 (PAI-1) gene respond differently to interleukin-1 in HepG2 cells. *J Biol Chem.* 1993;268(15):10739-10745.

2173. Nordenhem A, Wiman B. Plasminogen activator inhibitor-1 (PAI-1) content in platelets from healthy individuals genotyped for the 4G/5G polymorphism in the PAI-1 gene. *Scand J Clin Lab Invest.* 1997;57(5):453-461.
2174. Ye S, Green FR, Scarabin PY, et al. The 4G/5G genetic polymorphism in the promoter of the plasminogen activator inhibitor-1 (PAI-1) gene is associated with differences in plasma PAI-1 activity but not with risk of myocardial infarction in the ECTIM study. Etude CasTemoins de I'nfarctus du Mycocarde. *Thromb Haemost.* 1995;74(3):837-841.
2175. Margaglione M, Cappucci G, Colaizzo D, et al. The PAI-1 gene locus 4G/5G polymorphism is associated with a family history of coronary artery disease. *Arterioscler Thromb Vasc Biol.* 1998;18(2):152-156.
2176. Margaglione M, Cappucci G, d'Addedda M, et al. PAI-1 plasma levels in a general population without clinical evidence of atherosclerosis: relation to environmental and genetic determinants. *Arterioscler Thromb Vasc Biol.* 1998;18(4):562-567.
2177. Eriksson P, Kallin B, van 't Hooft FM, Bavenholm P, Hamsten A. Allele-specific increase in basal transcription of the plasminogen-activator inhibitor 1 gene is associated with myocardial infarction. *Proc Natl Acad Sci U S A.* 1995;92(6):1851-1855.
2178. Ridker PM, Hennekens CH, Lindpaintner K, Stampfer MJ, Miletich JP. Arterial and venous thrombosis is not associated with the 4G/5G polymorphism in the promoter of the plasminogen activator inhibitor gene in a large cohort of US men. *Circulation.* 1997;95(1):59-62.
2179. Huber K, Christ G, Wojta J, Gulba D. Plasminogen activator inhibitor type-1 in cardiovascular disease. *Thromb Res.* 2001;103:S7-S19.
2180. Tsantes AE, Nikolopoulos GK, Bagos PG, Bonovas S, Kopterides P, Vaiopoulos G. The effect of the plasminogen activator inhibitor-1 4G/5G polymorphism on the thrombotic risk. *Thromb Res.* 2008;122(6):736-742.
2181. Dawson S, Hamsten A, Wiman B, Henney A, Humphries S. Genetic variation at the plasminogen activator inhibitor-1 locus is associated with altered levels of plasma plasminogen activator inhibitor-1 activity. *Arterioscler Thromb Vasc Biol.* 1991;11(1):183-190.
2182. Grenett HE, Benza RL, Li XN, et al. Expression of plasminogen activator inhibitor type I in genotyped human endothelial cell cultures: genotype-specific regulation by insulin. *Thromb Haemost.* 1999;82(5):1504-1509.
2183. Booyse FM, Aikens ML, Grenett HE. Endothelial cell fibrinolysis: transcriptional regulation of fibrinolytic protein gene expression (t-PA, u-PA, and PAI-1) by low alcohol. *Alcohol Clin Exp Res.* 1999;23(6):1119-1124.
2184. Li XN, Grenett HE, Benza RL, et al. Genotype-specific transcriptional regulation of PAI-1 expression by Hypertriglyceridemic VLDL and Lp(a) in cultured human endothelial cells. *Arterioscler Thromb Vasc Biol.* 1997;17(11):3215-3223.
2185. Grenett HE, Benza RL, Fless GM, Li XN, Davis GC, Booyse FM. Genotype-specific transcriptional regulation of PAI-1 gene by insulin, Hypertriglyceridemic VLDL, and Lp(a) in Transfected, cultured human endothelial cells. *Arterioscler Thromb Vasc Biol.* 1998;18(11):1803-1809.
2186. Carmeliet P, Kieckens L, Schoonjans L, et al. Plasminogen activator inhibitor-1 gene-deficient mice. I. Generation by homologous recombination and characterization. *J Clin Investig.* 1993;92(6):2746-2755.
2187. Carmeliet P, Stassen JM, Schoonjans L, et al. Plasminogen activator inhibitor-1 gene-deficient mice. II. Effects on hemostasis, thrombosis, and thrombolysis. *J Clin Investig.* 1993;92(6):2756-2760.
2188. Dewerchin M, Collen D, Lijnen HR. Enhanced fibrinolytic potential in mice with combined homozygous deficiency of alpha2-antiplasmin and PAI-1. *Thromb Haemost.* 2001;86(2):640-646.
2189. Jensen JK, Thompson LC, Bucci JC, et al. Crystal structure of plasminogen activator inhibitor-1 in an active conformation with normal thermodynamic stability. *J Biol Chem.* 2011;286(34):29709-29717.
2190. Dupont DM, Blouse GE, Hansen M, et al. Evidence for a pre-latent form of the serpin plasminogen activator inhibitor-1 with a detached beta-strand 1C. *J Biol Chem.* 2006;281(47):36071-36081.
2191. Lawrence DA, Berkenpas MB, Palaniappan S, Ginsburg D. Localization of vitronectin binding domain in plasminogen activator inhibitor-1. *J Biol Chem.* 1994;269(21):15223-15228.
2192. Madison EL, Goldsmith EJ, Gerard RD, Gething MJH, Sambrook JF. Serpin-resistant mutants of human tissue-type plasminogen activator. *Nature.* 1989;339(6227):721-724.
2193. Madison EL, Goldsmith EJ, Gething MJ, Sambrook JF, Gerard RD. Restoration of serine protease-inhibitor interaction by protein engineering. *J Biol Chem.* 1990;265(35):21423-21426.
2194. Adams DS, Griffin LA, Nachajko WR, Reddy VB, Wei CM. A synthetic DNA encoding a modified human urokinase resistant to inhibition by serum plasminogen activator inhibitor. *J Biol Chem.* 1991;266(13):8476-8482.
2195. Hekman CM, Loskutoff DJ. Endothelial cells produce a latent inhibitor of plasminogen activators that can be activated by denaturants. *J Biol Chem.* 1985;260(21):11581-11587.
2196. Mottonen J, Strand A, Symersky J, et al. Structural basis of latency in plasminogen activator inhibitor-1. *Nature.* 1992;355(6357):270-273.
2197. Kruithof EK, Tran-Thang C, Gudinchet A, et al. Fibrinolysis in pregnancy: a study of plasminogen activator inhibitors. *Blood.* 1987;69(2):460-466.
2198. Ghosh AK, Vaughan DE. PAI-1 in tissue fibrosis. *J Cell Physiol.* 2012;227(2):493-507.
2199. Kjoller L, Kanse SM, Kirkegaard T, et al. Plasminogen activator inhibitor-1 represses integrin- and vitronectin-mediated cell migration independently of its function as an inhibitor of plasminogen activation. *Exp Cell Res.* 1997;232(2):420-429.
2200. Waltz DA, Natkin LR, Fujita RM, Wei Y, Chapman HA. Plasmin and plasminogen activator inhibitor type 1 promote cellular motility by regulating the interaction between the urokinase receptor and vitronectin. *J Clin Invest.* 1997;100(1):58-67.
2201. Kanse SM, Kost C, Wilhelm OG, Andreasen PA, Preissner KT. The urokinase receptor is a major vitronectin-binding protein on endothelial cells. *Exp Cell Res.* 1996;224(2):344-353.
2202. Deng G, Curriden SA, Wang S, Rosenberg S, Loskutoff DJ. Is plasminogen activator inhibitor-1 the molecular switch that governs urokinase receptor-mediated cell adhesion and release? *J Cell Biol.* 1996;134(6):1563-1571.
2203. Stefansson S, Lawrence DA. The serpin PAI-1 inhibits cell migration by blocking integrin alpha V beta 3 binding to vitronectin. *Nature.* 1996;383(6599):441-443.
2204. Kruithof EK, Baker MS, Bunn CL. Biological and clinical aspects of plasminogen activator inhibitor type 2. *Blood.* 1995;86(11):4007-4024.
2205. Kawano T, Morimoto K, Uemura Y. Partial purification and properties of urokinase inhibitor from human placenta. *J Biochem.* 1970;67(3):333-342.
2206. Kawano T, Uemura Y. Inhibition of tissue activator by urokinase inhibitor. *Thromb Diath Haemorrh.* 1971;25(1):129-133.
2207. Kawano T, Morimoto K, Uemura Y. Urokinase inhibitor in human placenta. *Nature.* 1968;217(5125):253-254.
2208. Astedt B, Hagerstrand I, Lecander I. Cellular localisation in placenta of placental type plasminogen activator inhibitor. *Thromb Haemost.* 1986;56(1):63-65.
2209. Holmberg L, Lecander I, Persson B, Astedt B. An inhibitor from placenta specifically binds urokinase and inhibits plasminogen activator released from ovarian carcinoma in tissue culture. *Biochim Biophys Acta.* 1978;544(1):128-137.
2210. Astedt B, Lecander I, Brodin T, Lundblad A, Low K. Purification of a specific placental plasminogen activator inhibitor by monoclonal antibody and its complex formation with plasminogen activator. *Thromb Haemost.* 1985;53(1):122-125.
2211. Ritchie H, Robbie LA, Kinghorn S, Exley R, Booth NA. Monocyte plasminogen activator inhibitor 2 (PAI-2) inhibits u-PA-mediated fibrin clot lysis and is cross-linked to fibrin. *Thromb Haemost.* 1999;81(1):96-103.
2212. Lee JA, Cochran BJ, Lobov S, Ranson M. Forty years later and the role of plasminogen activator inhibitor type 2/SERPINB2 is still an enigma. *Semin Thromb Hemost.* 2011;37(4):395-407.
2213. Dougherty KM, Pearson JM, Yang AY, Westrick RJ, Baker MS, Ginsburg D. The plasminogen activator inhibitor-2 gene is not required for normal murine development or survival. *Proc Natl Acad Sci U S A.* 1999;96(2):686-691.
2214. Webb AC, Collins KL, Snyder SE, et al. Human monocyte Arg-Serpin cDNA. Sequence, chromosomal assignment, and homology to plasminogen activator-inhibitor. *J Exp Med.* 1987;166(1):77-94.
2215. Samia JA, Alexander SJ, Horton KW, et al. Chromosomal organization and localization of the human urokinase inhibitor gene: perfect structural conservation with ovalbumin. *Genomics.* 1990;6(1):159-167.
2216. Schleuning WD, Medcalf RL, Hession C, Rothenbuhler R, Shaw A, Kruithof EK. Plasminogen activator inhibitor 2: regulation of gene transcription during phorbol ester-mediated differentiation of U-937 human histiocytic lymphoma cells. *Mol Cell Biol.* 1987;7(12):4564-4567.
2217. Wun TC, Reich E. An inhibitor of plasminogen activation from human placenta. Purification and characterization. *J Biol Chem.* 1987;262(8):3646-3653.
2218. Ye RD, Wun TC, Sadler JE. cDNA cloning and expression in *Escherichia coli* of a plasminogen activator inhibitor from human placenta. *J Biol Chem.* 1987;262(8):3718-3725.
2219. Ye RD, Ahern SM, Le Beau MM, Lebo RV, Sadler JE. Structure of the gene for human plasminogen activator inhibitor-2. The nearest mammalian homologue of chicken ovalbumin. *J Biol Chem.* 1989;264(10):5495-5502.
2220. Kruithof EK. Plasminogen activator inhibitors: a review. *Enzyme.* 1988;40(2-3):113-121.
2221. Chapman HA, Jr, Stone OL. A fibrinolytic inhibitor of human alveolar macrophages. Induction with endotoxin. *Am Rev Respir Dis.* 1985;132(3):569-575.
2222. Saksela O, Hovi T, Vaheri A. Urokinase-type plasminogen activator and its inhibitor secreted by cultured human monocyte-macrophages. *J Cell Physiol.* 1985;122(1):125-132.
2223. Wohlwend A, Belin D, Vassalli JD. Plasminogen activator-specific inhibitors produced by human monocytes/macrophages. *J Exp Med.* 1987;165(2):320-339.
2224. Bachmann F. The enigma PAI-2. Gene expression, evolutionary and functional aspects. *Thromb Haemost.* 1995;74(1):172-179.
2225. Dear AE, MR. The cellular and molecular biology of plasminogen activator inhibitor type-2. *Fibrinolysis.* 1995;9:321-330.
2226. Medcalf RL, Kruithof EK, Schleuning WD. Plasminogen activator inhibitor 1 and 2 are tumor necrosis factor/cachectin-responsive genes. *J Exp Med.* 1988;168(2):751-759.
2227. Schwartz BS, Monroe MC, Levin EG. Increased release of plasminogen activator inhibitor type 2 accompanies the human mononuclear cell tissue factor response to lipopolysaccharide. *Blood.* 1988;71(3):734-741.
2228. Suzuki T, Hashimoto S, Toyoda N, et al. Comprehensive gene expression profile of LPS-stimulated human monocytes by SAGE. *Blood.* 2000;96(7):2584-2591.
2229. Maurer F, Tierney M, Medcalf RL. An AU-rich sequence in the 3'-UTR of plasminogen activator inhibitor type 2 (PAI-2) mRNA promotes PAI-2 mRNA decay and provides a binding site for nuclear HuR. *Nucleic Acids Res.* 1999;27(7):1664-1673.
2230. Maurer F, Medcalf RL. Plasminogen activator inhibitor type 2 gene induction by tumor necrosis factor and phorbol ester involves transcriptional and post-transcriptional events. Identification of a functional nonameric AU-rich motif in the 3'-untranslated region. *J Biol Chem.* 1996;271(42):26074-26080.
2231. Tierney MJ, Medcalf RL. Plasminogen activator inhibitor type 2 contains mRNA instability elements within exon 4 of the coding region. Sequence homology to coding region instability determinants in other mRNAs. *J Biol Chem.* 2001;276(17):13675-13684.
2232. Jensen PH, Schuler E, Woodrow G, et al. A unique interhelical insertion in plasminogen activator inhibitor-2 contains three glutamines, Gln83, Gln84, Gln86, essential for transglutaminase-mediated cross-linking. *J Biol Chem.* 1994;269(21):15394-15398.

2233. Ritchie H, Lawrie LC, Crombie PW, Mosesson MW, Booth NA. Cross-linking of plasminogen activator inhibitor 2 and alpha 2-antiplasmin to fibrin(ogen). *J Biol Chem.* 2000;275(32):24915-24920.

2234. Jensen PJ, Wu Q, Janowitz P, Ando Y, Schechter NM. Plasminogen activator inhibitor type 2: an intracellular keratinocyte differentiation product that is incorporated into the cornified envelope. *Exp Cell Res.* 1995;217(1):65-71.

2235. Harrop SJ, Jankova L, Coles M, et al. The crystal structure of plasminogen activator inhibitor 2 at 2.0 A resolution: implications for serpin function. *Structure.* 1999;7(1):43-54.

2236. Hibino T, Matsuda Y, Takahashi T, Goetinck PF. Suppression of keratinocyte proliferation by plasminogen activator inhibitor-2. *J Invest Dermatol.* 1999;112(1):85-90.

2237. Dickinson JL, Bates EJ, Ferrante A, Antalis TM. Plasminogen activator inhibitor type 2 inhibits tumor necrosis factor alpha-induced apoptosis. Evidence for an alternate biological function. *J Biol Chem.* 1995;270(46):27894-27904.

2238. Dickinson JL, Norris BJ, Jensen PH, Antalis TM. The C-D interhelical domain of the serpin plasminogen activator inhibitor-type 2 is required for protection from TNF-alpha induced apoptosis. *Cell Death Differ.* 1998;5(2):163-171.

2239. Shafren DR, Gardner J, Mann VH, Antalis TM, Suhrbier A. Picornavirus receptor down-regulation by plasminogen activator inhibitor type 2. *J Virol.* 1999;73(9):7193-7198.

2240. Yu H, Maurer F, Medcalf RL. Plasminogen activator inhibitor type 2: a regulator of monocyte proliferation and differentiation. *Blood.* 2002;99(8):2810-2818.

2241. Collen D. Identification and some properties of a new fast-reacting plasmin inhibitor in human plasma. *Eur J Biochem.* 1976;69(1):209-216.

2242. Mullertz S, Clemmensen I. The primary inhibitor of plasmin in human plasma. *Biochem J.* 1976;159(3):545-553.

2243. Moroi M, Aoki N. Isolation and characterization of alpha2-plasmin inhibitor from human plasma. A novel proteinase inhibitor which inhibits activator-induced clot lysis. *J Biol Chem.* 1976;251(19):5956-5965.

2244. Collen D, De C, Verstraete M. Immunochemical distinction between antiplasmin and alpha-antitrypsin. *Thromb Res.* 1975;7(1):245-249.

2245. Schaller J, Gerber SS. The plasmin-antiplasmin system: structural and functional aspects. *Cell Mol Life Sci.* 2011;68(5):785-801.

2246. Favier R, Aoki N, de Moerloose P. Congenital alpha(2)-plasmin inhibitor deficiencies: a review. *Br J Haematol.* 2001;114(1):4-10.

2247. Aoki N, Sumi Y, Miura O, Hirosawa S. Human alpha 2-plasmin inhibitor. *Methods Enzymol.* 1993;223:185-197.

2248. Menoud PA, Sappino N, Boudal-Khoshbeen M, Vassalli JD, Sappino AP. The kidney is a major site of alpha(2)-antiplasmin production. *J Clin Invest.* 1996;97(11):2478-2484.

2249. Collen D, Wiman B. Turnover of antiplasmin, the fast-acting plasmin inhibitor of plasma. *Blood.* 1979;53(2):313-324.

2250. Mast AE, Enghild JJ, Pizzo SV, Salvesen G. Analysis of the plasma elimination kinetics and conformational stabilities of native, proteinase-complexed, and reactive site cleaved serpins: comparison of alpha 1-proteinase inhibitor, alpha 1-antichymotrypsin, antithrombin III, alpha 2-antiplasmin, angiotensinogen, and ovalbumin. *Biochemistry.* 1991;30(6):1723-1730.

2251. Bangert K, Johnsen AH, Christensen U, Thorsen S. Different N-terminal forms of alpha 2-plasmin inhibitor in human plasma. *Biochem J.* 1993;291(pt 2):623-625.

2252. Koyama T, Koike Y, Toyota S, Miyagi F, Suzuki N, Aoki N. Different NH2-terminal form with 12 additional residues of alpha 2-plasmin inhibitor from human plasma and culture media of Hep G2 cells. *Biochem Biophys Res Commun.* 1994;200(1):417-422.

2253. Wiman B, Collen D. Purification and characterization of human antiplasmin, the fast-acting plasmin inhibitor in plasma. *Eur J Biochem.* 1977;78(1):19-26.

2254. Holmes WE, Nelles L, Lijnen HR, Collen D. Primary structure of human alpha 2-antiplasmin, a serine protease inhibitor (serpin). *J Biol Chem.* 1987;262(4):1659-1664.

2255. Lijnen HR, Holmes WE, Hoef B, Wiman B, Rodriguez H, Collen D. Amino-acid sequence of human alpha2-antiplasmin. *Eur J Biochem.* 1987;166(3):565-574.

2256. Hortin GL, Gibson BL, Fok KF. Alpha 2-antiplasmin's carboxy-terminal lysine residue is a major site of interaction with plasmin. *Biochem Biophys Res Commun.* 1988;155(2):591-596.

2257. Wiman B, Almquist A, Ranby M. The non-covalent interaction between plasmin and alpha 2-antiplasmin. *Fibrinolysis.* 1989;3:231-235.

2258. Sugiyama N, Sasaki T, Iwamoto M, Abiko Y. Binding site of alpha 2-plasmin inhibitor to plasminogen. *Biochim Biophys Acta.* 1988;952(1):1-7.

2259. Wiman B, Nilsson T, Cedergren B. Studies on a form of alpha 2-antiplasmin in plasma which does not interact with the lysine-binding sites in plasminogen. *Thromb Res.* 1982;28(1):193-199.

2260. Christensen U, Clemmensen I. Purification and reaction mechanisms of the primary inhibitor of plasmin from human plasma. *Biochem J.* 1978;175(2):635-641.

2261. Clemmensen I, Thorsen S, Mullertz S, Petersen LC. Properties of three different molecular forms of the alpha 2 plasmin inhibitor. *Eur J Biochem.* 1981;120(1):105-112.

2262. Hortin GL, Trimpe BL, Fok KF. Plasmin's peptide-binding specificity: characterization of ligand sites in alpha 2-antiplasmin. *Thromb Res.* 1989;54(6):621-632.

2263. Wiman B, Collen D. On the kinetics of the reaction between human antiplasmin and plasmin. *Eur J Biochem.* 1978;84(2):573-578.

2264. Kato A, Hirosawa S, Toyota S, et al. Localization of the human alpha 2-plasmin inhibitor gene (PLI) to 17p13. *Cytogenet Cell Genet.* 1993;62(4):190-191.

2265. Hirosawa S, Nakamura Y, Miura O, Sumi Y, Aoki N. Organization of the human alpha 2-plasmin inhibitor gene. *Proc Natl Acad Sci U S A.* 1988;85(18):6836-6840.

2266. Christiansen VJ, Jackson KW, Lee KN, McKee PA. The effect of a single nucleotide polymorphism on human alpha 2-antiplasmin activity. *Blood.* 2007;109(12):5286-5292.

2267. Lee KN, Jackson KW, Christiansen VJ, Lee CS, Chun JG, McKee PA. Why alpha-antiplasmin must be converted to a derivative form for optimal function. *J Thromb Haemost.* 2007;5(10):2095-2104.

2268. Kordich L, Feldman L, Porterie P, Lago O. Severe hemorrhagic tendency in heterozygous alpha 2-antiplasmin deficiency. *Thromb Res.* 1985;40(5):645-651.

2269. Griffin GC, Mammen EF, Sokol RJ, Perrotta AL, Stoyanovich A, Abildgaard CF. Alpha 2-antiplasmin deficiency. An overlooked cause of hemorrhage. *Am J Pediatr Hematol Oncol.* 1993;15(3):328-330.

2270. Holmes WE, Lijnen HR, Nelles L, et al. Alpha 2-antiplasmin Enschede: alanine insertion and abolition of plasmin inhibitory activity. *Science.* 1987;238(4824):209-211.

2271. Miura O, Sugahara Y, Aoki N. Hereditary alpha 2-plasmin inhibitor deficiency caused by a transport-deficient mutation (alpha 2-PI-Okinawa). Deletion of Glu137 by a trinucleotide deletion blocks intracellular transport. *J Biol Chem.* 1989;264(30):18213-18219.

2272. Miura O, Hirosawa S, Kato A, Aoki N. Molecular basis for congenital deficiency of alpha 2-plasmin inhibitor. A frameshift mutation leading to elongation of the deduced amino acid sequence. *J Clin Invest.* 1989;83(5):1598-1604.

2273. Yoshinaga H, Nakahara M, Koyama T, et al. A single thymine nucleotide deletion responsible for congenital deficiency of plasmin inhibitor. *Thromb Haemost.* 2002;88(1):144-148.

2274. Yoshinaga H, Hirosawa S, Chung DH, Miyasaka N, Aoki N, Favier R. A novel point mutation of the splicing donor site in the intron 2 of the plasmin inhibitor gene. *Thromb Haemost.* 2000;84(2):307-311.

2275. Lijnen HR. Gene targeting in hemostasis. Alpha2-antiplasmin. *Front Biosci.* 2001;6:D239-D247.

2276. Fraser SR, Booth NA, Mutch NJ. The antifibrinolytic function of factor XIII is exclusively expressed through alpha(2)-antiplasmin cross-linking. *Blood.* 2011;117(23):6371-6374.

2277. Jansen JW, Haverkate F, Koopman J, Nieuwenhuis HK, Kluft C, Boschman TA. Influence of factor XIIIa activity on human whole blood clot lysis in vitro. *Thromb Haemost.* 1987;57(2):171-175.

2278. Abdul S, Leebeek FW, Rijken DC, Uitte de Willige S. Natural heterogeneity of alpha2-antiplasmin: functional and clinical consequences. *Blood.* 2016;127(5):538-545.

2279. Lee KN, Jackson KW, Christiansen VJ, Chung KH, McKee PA. A novel plasma proteinase potentiates alpha2-antiplasmin inhibition of fibrin digestion. *Blood.* 2004;103(10):3783-3788.

2280. Christensen U, Bangert K, Thorsen S. Reaction of human alpha2-antiplasmin and plasmin stopped-flow fluorescence kinetics. *FEBS Lett.* 1996;387(1):58-62.

2281. Frank PS, Douglas JT, Locher M, Llinas M, Schaller J. Structural/functional characterization of the alpha 2-plasmin inhibitor C-terminal peptide. *Biochemistry.* 2003;42(4):1078-1085.

2282. Gerber SS, Lejon S, Locher M, Schaller J. The human alpha(2)-plasmin inhibitor: functional characterization of the unique plasmin(ogen)-binding region. *Cell Mol Life Sci.* 2010;67(9):1505-1518.

2283. Lu BG, Sofian T, Law RH, Coughlin PB, Horvath AJ. Contribution of conserved lysine residues in the alpha2-antiplasmin C terminus to plasmin binding and inhibition. *J Biol Chem.* 2011;286(28):24544-24552.

2284. Mimuro J, Koike Y, Sumi Y, Aoki N. Monoclonal antibodies to discrete regions in alpha 2-plasmin inhibitor. *Blood.* 1987;69(2):446-453.

2285. Reed GL, Matsueda GR, Haber E. Platelet factor XIII increases the fibrinolytic resistance of platelet-rich clots by accelerating the crosslinking of alpha 2-antiplasmin to fibrin. *Thromb Haemost.* 1992;68(3):315-320.

2286. Sumi Y, Ichikawa Y, Nakamura Y, Miura O, Aoki N. Expression and characterization of pro alpha 2-plasmin inhibitor. *J Biochem.* 1989;106(4):703-707.

2287. Wiman B, Collen D. On the role of alpha 2-antiplasmin in the regulation of fibrinolysis. In: Collen D, Wiman B, Verstraete M, eds. *The Physiological Inhibitors of Coagulation and Fibrinolysis.* Elsevier; 1979:177-185.

2288. Sprengers ED, Kluft C. Plasminogen activator inhibitors. *Blood.* 1987;69(2):381-387.

2289. Reilly CF, Hutzelmann JE. Plasminogen activator inhibitor-1 binds to fibrin and inhibits tissue-type plasminogen activator-mediated fibrin dissolution. *J Biol Chem.* 1992;267(24):17128-17135.

2290. Plow EF, Miles LA, Collen D. Platelet α2-antiplasmin. *Methods in Enzymology.* Elsevier BV; 1989:296-300.

2291. Plow EF, Collen D. The presence and release of alpha 2-antiplasmin from human platelets. *Blood.* 1981;58(6):1069-1074.

2292. Gogstad GO, Stormorken H, Solum NO. Platelet α2-antiplasmin is located in the platelet α-granules. *Thromb Res.* 1983;31(2):387-390.

2293. Erickson LA, Hekman CM, Loskutoff DJ. The primary plasminogen-activator inhibitors in endothelial cells, platelets, serum, and plasma are immunologically related. *Proc Natl Acad Sci U S A.* 1985;82(24):8710-8714.

2294. Kruithof EK, Tran-Thang C, Bachmann F. Studies on the release of a plasminogen activator inhibitor by human platelets. *Thromb Haemost.* 1986;55(2):201-205.

2295. Philips M, Juul A-G, Thorsen S. Human endothelial cells produce a plasminogen activator inhibitor and a tissue-type plasminogen activator-inhibitor complex. *Biochim Biophys Acta.* 1984;802(1):99-110.

2296. Stern D, Nawroth P, Handley D, Kisiel W. An endothelial cell-dependent pathway of coagulation. *Proc Natl Acad Sci.* 1985;82(8):2523-2527.

2297. Levin EG, Santell L, Osborn KG. The expression of endothelial tissue plasminogen activator in vivo: a function defined by vessel size and anatomic location. *J Cell Sci.* 1997;110(pt 2):139-148.

2298. Grant PJ, Medcalf RL. Hormonal regulation of haemostasis and the molecular biology of the fibrinolytic system. *Clin Sci.* 1990;78(1):3-11.

2299. Hajjar KA, Hamel NM, Harpel PC, Nachman RL. Binding of tissue plasminogen activator to cultured human endothelial cells. *J Clin Invest.* 1987;80(6):1712-1719.

The Normal Hematologic System

2300. Bachmann F, Kruithof IE. Tissue plasminogen activator: chemical and physiological aspects. *Semin Thromb Hemost.* 1984;10(01):6-17.

2301. Blasi F. Urokinase-type plasminogen activator: proenzyme, receptor, and inhibitors. *J Cell Biol.* 1987;104(4):801-804.

2302. Danø K, Andreasen PA, Grøndahl-Hansen J, Kristensen P, Nielsen LS, Skriver L. *Plasminogen activators, tissue degradation, and cancer. Advances in Cancer Research.* Elsevier BV; 1985:139-266.

2303. Blasi F. Surface receptors for urokinase plasminogen activator. *Fibrinolysis.* 1988;2(2):73-84.

2304. Kwon M, MacLeod TJ, Zhang Y, Waisman DM. S100A10, annexin A2, and annexin a2 heterotetramer as candidate plasminogen receptors. *Front Biosci.* 2005;10:300-325.

2305. Das R, Pluskota E, Plow EF. Plasminogen and its receptors as regulators of cardiovascular inflammatory responses. *Trends Cardiovasc Med.* 2010;20(4):120-124.

2306. Miles LA, Levin EG, Plescia J, Collen D, Plow EF. Plasminogen receptors, urokinase receptors, and their modulation on human endothelial cells. *Blood.* 1988;72(2):628-635.

2307. Miles LA, Plow EF. Receptor mediated binding of the fibrinolytic components, plasminogen and urokinase, to peripheral blood cells. *Thromb Haemost.* 1987;58(3):936-942.

2308. Cubellis MV, Nolli ML, Cassani G, Blasi F. Binding of single-chain pro-urokinase to the urokinase receptor of human U937 cells. *J Biol Chem.* 1986;261(34):15819-15822.

2309. Vassalli JD. A cellular binding site for the Mr 55,000 form of the human plasminogen activator, urokinase. *J Cell Biol.* 1985;100(1):86-92.

2310. Ploug M, Plesner T, Ronne E, et al. The receptor for urokinase-type plasminogen activator is deficient on peripheral blood leukocytes in patients with paroxysmal nocturnal hemoglobinuria. *Blood.* 1992;79(6):1447-1455.

2311. Romer J, Lund LR, Eriksen J, Pyke C, Kristensen P, Dano K. The receptor for urokinase-type plasminogen activator is expressed by keratinocytes at the leading edge during re-epithelialization of mouse skin wounds. *J Invest Dermatol.* 1994;102(4):519-522.

2312. Pyke C, Kristensen P, Ralfkiaer E, et al. Urokinase-type plasminogen activator is expressed in stromal cells and its receptor in cancer cells at invasive foci in human colon adenocarcinomas. *Am J Pathol.* 1991;138(5):1059-1067.

2313. Rosso MD, Margheri F, Serrati S, Chilla A, Laurenzana A, Fibbi G. The urokinase receptor system, A key regulator at the intersection between inflammation, Immunity, and coagulation. *CPD.* 2011;17(19):1924-1943.

2314. Mazar AP, Ahn RW, O'Halloran TV. Development of novel therapeutics targeting the urokinase plasminogen activator receptor (uPAR) and their translation toward the clinic. *CPD.* 2011;17(19):1970-1978.

2315. Fuhrman B. The urokinase system in the pathogenesis of atherosclerosis. *Atherosclerosis.* 2012;222(1):8-14.

2316. Ellis V, Dano K. Potentiation of plasminogen activation by an anti-urokinase monoclonal antibody due to ternary complex formation. A mechanistic model for receptor-mediated plasminogen activation. *J Biol Chem.* 1993;268(7):4806-4813.

2317. Ellis V, Pluog M, Plesner T, Dano K. *Gene Expression and Function of the Cellular Receptor for uPA (uPAR).* CRC Prss; 1995.

2318. Roldan AL, Cubellis MV, Masucci MT, et al. Cloning and expression of the receptor for human urokinase plasminogen activator, a central molecule in cell surface, plasmin dependent proteolysis. *EMBO J.* 1990;9(2):467-474.

2319. Ploug M, Ronne E, Behrendt N, Jensen AL, Blasi F, Dano K. Cellular receptor for urokinase plasminogen activator. Carboxyl-terminal processing and membrane anchoring by glycosyl-phosphatidylinositol. *J Biol Chem.* 1991;266(3):1926-1933.

2320. Moller LB, Ploug M, Blasi F. Structural requirements for glycosyl-phosphatidylinositol-anchor attachment in the cellular receptor for urokinase plasminogen activator. *Eur J Biochem.* 1992;208(2):493-500.

2321. Eden G, Archinti M, Furlan F, Murphy R, Degryse B. The urokinase receptor interactome. *CPD.* 2011;17(19):1874-1889.

2322. Ploug M, Eriksen J, Plesner T, Hansen NE, Dano K. A soluble form of the glycolipid-anchored receptor for urokinase-type plasminogen activator is secreted from peripheral blood leukocytes from patients with paroxysmal nocturnal hemoglobinuria. *Eur J Biochem.* 1992;208(2):397-404.

2323. Xu X, Gårdsvoll H, Yuan C, Lin L, Ploug M, Huang M. Crystal structure of the urokinase receptor in a ligand-free form. *J Mol Biol.* 2012;416(5):629-641.

2324. Barinka C, Parry G, Callahan J, et al. Structural basis of interaction between urokinase-type plasminogen activator and its receptor. *J Mol Biol.* 2006;363(2):482-495.

2325. Hajjar KA. Cellular receptors in the regulation of plasmin generation. *Thromb Haemost.* 1995;74(1):294-301.

2326. Dudani AK, Ganz PR. Endothelial cell surface actin serves as a binding site for plasminogen, tissue plasminogen activator and lipoprotein(a). *Br J Haematol.* 1996;95(1):168-178.

2327. Flood EC, Hajjar KA. The annexin A2 system and vascular homeostasis. *Vasc Pharmacol.* 2011;54(3-6):59-67.

2328. Bohm T, Geiger M, Binder BR. Isolation and characterization of tissue-type plasminogen activator binding proteoglycans from human umbilical vein endothelial cells. *Arterioscler Thromb Vasc Biol.* 1996;16(5):665-672.

2329. Kralovich KR, Li L, Hembrough TA, Webb DJ, Karns LR, Gonias SL. *J Protein Chem.* 1998;17(8):845-854.

2330. Hembrough TA, Kralovich KR, Li L, Gonias SL. Cytokeratin 8 released by breast carcinoma cells in vitro binds plasminogen and tissue-type plasminogen activator and promotes plasminogen activation. *Biochem J.* 1996;317(3):763-769.

2331. Beebe DP, Wood LL, Moos M. Characterization of tissue plasminogen activator binding proteins isolated from endothelial cells and other cell types. *Thromb Res.* 1990;59(2):339-350.

2332. Menell JS, Cesarman GM, Jacovina AT, McLaughlin MA, Lev EA, Hajjar KA. Annexin II and bleeding in acute promyelocytic leukemia. *N Engl J Med.* 1999;340(13):994-1004.

2333. Taylor ME, Conary JT, Lennartz MR, Stahl PD, Drickamer K. Primary structure of the mannose receptor contains multiple motifs resembling carbohydrate-recognition domains. *J Biol Chem.* 1990;265(21):12156-12162.

2334. Otter M, Barrett-Bergshoeff MM, Rijken DC. Binding of tissue-type plasminogen activator by the mannose receptor. *J Biol Chem.* 1991;266(21):13931-13935.

2335. Noorman F, Barrett-Bergshoeff MM, Rijken DC. Role of carbohydrate and protein in the binding of tissue-type plasminogen activator to the human mannose receptor. *Eur J Biochem.* 1998;251(1-2):107-113.

2336. Andreasen PA, Sottrup-Jensen L, Kjøller L, et al. Receptor-mediated endocytosis of plasminogen activators and activator/inhibitor complexes. *FEBS Lett.* 1994;338(3):239-245.

2337. Moestrup SK. The α2-macroglobulin receptor and epithelial glycoprotein-330: two giant receptors mediating endocytosis of multiple ligands. *Biochim Biophys Acta.* 1994;1197(2):197-213.

2338. Kasza A, Petersen HH, Heegaard CW, et al. Specificity of serine proteinase/serpin complex binding to very-low-density lipoprotein receptor and alpha2-macroglobulin receptor/low-density-lipoprotein-receptor-related protein. *Eur J Biochem.* 1997;248(2):270-281.

2339. Miles LA, Plow EF. Binding and activation of plasminogen on the platelet surface. *J Biol Chem.* 1985;260(7):4303-4311.

2340. Miles LA, Ginsberg MH, White JG, Plow EF. Plasminogen interacts with human platelets through two distinct mechanisms. *J Clin Investig.* 1986;77(6):2001-2009.

2341. Adelman B, Rizk A, Hanners E. Plasminogen interactions with platelets in plasma. *Blood.* 1988;72(5):1530-1535.

2342. Redlitz A, Fowler BJ, Plow EF, Miles LA. The role of an Enolase-related molecule in plasminogen binding to cells. *Eur J Biochem.* 1995;227(1-2):407-415.

2343. Schafer AI, Adelman B. Plasmin inhibition of platelet function and of arachidonic acid metabolism. *J Clin Invest.* 1985;75(2):456-461.

2344. Schafer AI, Zavoico GB, Loscalzo J, Maas AK. Synergistic inhibition of platelet activation by plasmin and prostaglandin I2. *Blood.* 1987;69(5):1504-1507.

2345. Niewiarowski S, Senyi AF, Gillies P. Plasmin-induced platelet aggregation and platelet release reaction. Effects on hemostasis. *J Clin Invest.* 1973;52(7):1647-1659.

2346. Miller JL, Katz AJ, Feinstein MB. Plasmin inhibition of thrombin-induced platelet aggregation. *Thromb Diath Haemorrh.* 1975;33(2):286-309.

Chapter 21 ■ Endothelium: Angiogenesis and the Regulation of Hemostasis

GEORGE M. RODGERS

NORMAL ANGIOGENESIS

Blood circulation requires the production and maintenance of a vast network of vessels that have specialized functions depending on their organ location. The vascular network involves a complex interaction between endothelial cells (ECs), specialized cells such as smooth muscle cells and pericytes, and the extracellular matrix (ECM). *Vasculogenesis* is the de novo development of vessels.[1] It is seen mainly at the embryonic stage of development with the differentiation of a common pluripotent precursor, the hemangioblast, into endothelial and hematopoietic cells. *Angiogenesis* is the development of new vessels from preexisting vessels.[1] It is an essential process for wound healing and the maintenance of the integrity of the vascular network. Pathologic angiogenesis is seen in disease states including cancer and retinal and autoimmune diseases.[2]

As outlined by Conway, Collen, and Carmeliet,[1] physiologic angiogenesis is a well-organized stepwise process that involves dilation and increased permeability of the parent vessel, dissolution of the ECM, division and migration of EC, cord formation and the development of lumina, and, finally, the maintenance of new vessel integrity. The entire process involves the complex and choreographed effects of multiple inducers and inhibitors (*Table 21.1*).

The first step in angiogenesis is vasodilation. This is mediated through the activation of the soluble guanylate cyclase by nitric oxide (NO).[3] NO also upregulates vascular endothelial growth factor (VEGF) production.[4] By causing intercellular adhesion molecules to redistribute (platelet-EC adhesion molecule-1 and VE-cadherin, among others), VEGF induces an increase in vascular permeability.[5,6] The VEGF-induced increase in vascular permeability is negatively controlled by angiopoietin-1 (Ang1) through its receptor, Tie2.[7] The next key step to vascular development is the dissolution of the ECM, which is accomplished by proteases belonging to the matrix metalloproteinase family.[8,9] These proteases also induce the liberation of EC growth factors from the ECM, including VEGF and basic fibroblast growth factor. The action of matrix metalloproteinases is negatively controlled by a family of protease inhibitors, including the tissue inhibitors of metalloproteinases.[10]

Degradation of the extravascular matrix allows the development of the key element of the angiogenesis process, namely, EC division and migration. The list of factors that stimulate this process is extensive (*Table 21.1*), but a key role is played by VEGF in concert with Ang1.[6,11-16] Angiopoietin-2 (Ang2) could have angiogenic effects in the presence of VEGF, whereas it is antiangiogenic in the absence of VEGF.[14-17] Other factors that stimulate angiogenesis include basic fibroblast growth factor and platelet-derived growth factor.[18,19] EC growth is negatively controlled by endogenous angiogenesis inhibitors that include angiostatin, endostatin, interferons, and antithrombin.[20-22] ECs then migrate in large part through the action of integrins ($\alpha_v\beta_3$ and $\alpha_v\beta_1$).[23] The end result of EC division and migration is sprouting and the formation of cords.[1] This is followed by lumen formation, which is controlled by different VEGF isoforms, Ang1, and integrins.[1,15] Thrombospondin-1 acts as an endogenous inhibitor of lumen development.[1]

Once formed, new vessels survive for years.[1] This prolonged survival is maintained by the interaction of VEGF with its receptor VEGFR-2, phosphoinositide 3-kinase, β-catenin, and VE-cadherin.[1,24] The angiopoietins also play a role in maintaining vessel survival through their receptors Tie1 and Tie2. Ang1 stabilizes the vessel, whereas Ang2 has an opposite effect[14,15,25] (see Angiopoietins and their Receptors). An essential element in the maintenance of the integrity of vessels is their "coating" with smooth muscle cells and pericytes.[26] Evidence suggests that vascular smooth muscle cells and ECs have a common precursor.[27] On stimulation with platelet-derived growth factor-BB, these precursor cells differentiate into smooth muscle cells, whereas VEGF stimulation drives them to differentiate into EC.[27] Besides providing physical support for endothelial vessels, smooth muscle cells and pericytes are a source of factors that are important for the maintenance and control of vascular integrity and function.[1,26] The ECM plays a key role in that respect by being a dynamic storage site for growth factors and proenzymes that are important in vessel function and angiogenesis.[1]

Vascular Endothelial Growth Factor and Its Receptors

VEGF is the pivotal factor controlling angiogenesis. As such, it is the best-studied angiogenic factor. Several proteins belong to the VEGF family and include VEGF (also known as *VEGF-A*), VEGF-B, VEGF-C, VEGF-D, and placental growth factor.[14] Although VEGF-A is the main angiogenic factor discussed here, VEGF-B seems to play an important role in coronary vascular development.[28] VEGF-C and VEGF-D are likely important in lymphangiogenesis.[29]

Being the major regulator of angiogenesis, VEGF is a mitogen and survival factor for EC.[11,14] As mentioned earlier, it is also a potent inducer of vascular permeability, an essential step in the angiogenic process.[1,11,14] It has two well-characterized receptors, VEGFR-1 and VEGFR-2 (also known as *Flt-1* and *Flk-1/kinase domain receptor*, respectively).[14] They are both tyrosine kinases. VEGFR-2 is the main effector of a VEGF-induced chemotactic and mitogenic response in EC. VEGFR-2 also mediates the ECs' permeability effects.[14] VEGFR-1 seems to negatively control the VEGF effects by acting as a decoy.[14,30,31] Indeed, mice that have been engineered not to express VEGFR-1 have evidence of excess and disorganized angiogenesis.[30]

Angiopoietins and Their Receptors

Angiopoietins and Tie receptors play an important role in angiogenesis.[32] At least four angiopoietins have been identified.[14] However, only Ang1 and Ang2 have been fully characterized. They interact with the Tie tyrosine kinase receptors, mainly Tie2. Ang1 plays an important role in stabilizing the vasculature.[14] Supportive cells express Ang1 and interact with EC through the Tie2 receptor. Genetically engineered mouse embryos that lack Ang1 develop a normal primary vasculature. However, they do not undergo further vascular remodeling.[16] Transgenic mice that overexpress Ang1 have evidence of vascularization characterized by larger vessels rather than a greater number of vessels.[15] In addition, those vessels are resistant to leak, further supporting the role of Ang1 as a stabilizing factor.

The function of Ang2 has been more difficult to characterize.[14,17] It too binds with high affinity to the Tie2 receptor. Transgenic overexpression of Ang2 in mice is embryonically lethal and induces a phenotype that is similar to Ang1 or Tie2 knockout experiments. Thus, it has been suggested that Ang2, by acting as an antagonist of Tie2, negates the stabilizing effects of Ang1 on the vasculature. As such, Ang2 may be a destabilizing factor that helps initiate angiogenesis and vascular remodeling.[14]

NOTCH Signaling

Carmeliet and Jain[33] and Welti et al[34] have proposed models for vessel development whereby in the angiogenesis process ECs can be divided into two categories, namely, tip cells and stalk cells. Tip cells migrate and lead vessel development, whereas stalk cells divide. The process is controlled by the NOTCH signaling pathway. VEGF activation of VEGFR-2 leads to upregulation of DLL4 in tip cells. DLL4 then activates NOTCH in stalk cells. NOTCH downregulates VEGFR-2

Table 21.1. Activators and Inhibitors of Angiogenesis

Activators	Function	Inhibitors	Function
VEGF, VEGF-C, PlGF, and homologues	Stimulate angiogenesis, permeability; stimulate lymphangiogenesis, pathologic angiogenesis	VEGFR-1, soluble VEGFR-1, and NP-1	Sink for VEGF, VEGF-B, PlGF (VEGFR-1), and $VEGFR_{165}$ (NP-1)
VEGFR	VEGFR-2: angiogenic signaling; VEGFR-3: (lymph) angiogenic signaling	Ang2	Ang1 antagonist; induces vessel regression in the absence of angiogenic signals
Ang1 and Tie2 receptor	Ang1: stabilizes vessels, inhibits permeability	TSP-1	ECM proteins; inhibits EC migration, growth, and adhesion
	Ang2: destabilizes vessels before sprouting	TSP-2	Inhibits angiogenesis
Platelet-derived growth factor-BB and receptors	Recruit smooth muscle cells	Meth-1, Meth-2	Contains metalloprotease, thrombospondin, and disintegrin domains
TGF-β_1, endoglin, TGF-β receptors	Stabilize vessels by stimulating ECM production	Angiostatin and related plasminogen kringles	Inhibits EC survival and migration
Fibroblast growth factor, hepatocyte growth factor, monocyte chemotactic protein-1	Stimulate angiogenesis, stimulate arteriogenesis	Endostatin	Inhibits EC survival and migration
Integrins $\alpha_v \beta_3$, $\alpha_v \beta_5$	MMP receptors	Vasostatin, calreticulin	Inhibits EC growth
VE-cadherin, platelet-EC adhesion molecule	EC junctional molecules, promote EC survival	Platelet factor-4	Heparin-binding molecule; inhibits binding of bFGF and VEGF
Ephrins	Regulate arterial/venous specifications	Tissue inhibitors of metalloproteinases, MMP inhibitors	Suppresses pathologic angiogenesis
		Proteolytic fragment of MMP	Inhibits binding of MMP2 to $\alpha_v \beta_3$
Plasminogen activators, MMPs	Cell migration and matrix remodeling; liberate bFGF/VEFG from ECM; activate TGF-β_1; generate angiostatin		
Plasminogen activator inhibitor-1	Stabilizes nascent vessels (prevents ECM dissolution)	IFN-α, -β, -γ; IL-4, -12, -18	Inhibits EC migration, IFN-α downregulates bFGF
Nitric oxide synthase, cyclooxygenase-2	Nitric oxide/prostaglandins stimulate angiogenesis and vasodilation	Prothrombin kringle 2 antithrombin fragment	Suppresses EC growth
AC133	Angioblast differentiation	Prolactin fragment; secreted protein (acidic and rich in cysteine) fragment	Inhibits bFGF and VEGF; inhibits EC binding and activity of VEGF
ADAMTS13	Proangiogenic	von Willebrand factor	Antiangiogenic

Abbreviations: ADAMTS13, a disintegrin and metalloproteinase with a thrombospondin type 1 motif, member 13; Ang, angiopoietin; bFGF, basic fibroblast growth factor; EC, endothelial cell; ECM, extracellular matrix; IFN, interferon; IL, interleukin; Meth, metalloproteinase and thrombospondin; MMP, matrix metalloproteinase; NP, neuropilin; PlGF, placental growth factor; TGF, transforming growth factor; TSP, thrombospondin; VE-cadherin, vascular endothelial cadherin; VEGF, vascular endothelial growth factor; VEGFR, vascular endothelial growth.
Adapted from Conway EM, Collen D, Carmeliet P. Molecular mechanisms of blood vessel growth. *Cardiovasc Res.* 2001;49:507-521. Reproduced by permission of European Society of Cardiology.

and upregulates VEGFR-1 in stalk cells, making them less sensitive to VEGF-stimulated sprouting. The end result is to maintain the lead of tip cells in vessel development.[35] However, NOTCH stimulates stalk cell proliferation in vivo through activation of WNT signaling.[36] NOTCH upregulates its own inhibitor Nrarp in stalk cells.[37] It has been observed that the tip cell position is dynamic with stalk cells moving into the tip position depending on modulation of VEGFR-1 and VEGFR-2 expression.[33,37]

Role of ADAMTS13 and von Willebrand Factor

ADAMTS13 is primarily known as the von Willebrand factor (vWF) cleaving protease. However, emerging data indicate that these two proteins are also involved in angiogenesis. For example, ADAMTS13 is proangiogenic.[38] Knockdown of endogenous ADAMT13 inhibits angiogenesis.[39] Loss of vWF results in enhanced angiogenesis, and this is classically seen in patients with von Willebrand disease and gastrointestinal bleeding associated with angiodysplasia.[40]

Origin of Endothelium

Asahara et al have shown that human buffy coat cells can differentiate into cells expressing endothelial markers, including VEGFR-1, VEGFR-2, and CD31.[41] This raises the possibility that circulating endothelial stem cells can be recruited to sites of angiogenesis. This may be particularly relevant for tumor angiogenesis, whereby tumors can develop their vasculature both from recruitment of local endothelium and circulating endothelial stem cells.[42] Factors involved in the recruitment of endothelial stem cells may include stromal cell–derived factor-1, thrombopoietin, and soluble kit ligand.[2]

Angiogenesis in Normal and Malignant Hematopoiesis

There is mounting evidence suggesting the presence of a common precursor for ECs and hematopoietic cells.[43] This hemangioblast gives rise to both ECs and hematopoietic cells in embryonic development. Embryonic stem cells express VEGFR-2 and can give rise, depending on culture conditions, to hematopoietic progenitor cells and angioblasts.[43] Stimulation of hematopoietic stem cells with growth factors,

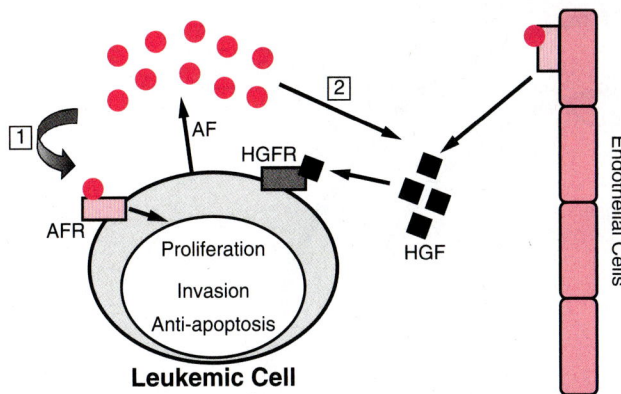

FIGURE 21.1 Hypothesis for the role of angiogenesis in leukemia. 1, Angiogenic factors (AFs) produced by leukemic cells can stimulate cell growth and invasion, or inhibit apoptosis (autocrine mechanism). 2, AFs produced by leukemic cells can also stimulate endothelial cell (EC) proliferation and the production of EC hematopoietic growth factors (HGFs) (paracrine mechanism). AFR, angiogenic factor receptor; HGFR, hematopoietic growth factor receptor. (From Dickson DJ, Shami PJ.Angiogenesis in acute and chronic leukemias. *Leuk Lymphoma.* 2001;42(5):847-853. Reprinted by permission of Taylor & Francis Ltd. http://www.tandfonline.com)

including kit ligand, interleukin-3, granulocyte-macrophage colony-stimulating factor, and granulocyte colony-stimulating factor, induces the release by those cells of VEGF, which then induces the release of hematopoietic growth factors by bone marrow ECs.[43] Thus, there is a dynamic interaction between hematopoietic and endothelial elements in the bone marrow.

Several studies have shown evidence of increased angiogenesis in hematopoietic malignancies.[44] Such evidence has been demonstrated in multiple myeloma and lymphomas, as well as in acute and chronic leukemias.[45-52] Malignant hematopoietic cells have been shown to produce angiogenic factors, including VEGF.[44] Similar to the effect observed in normal hematopoiesis, VEGF stimulates the production of hematopoietic growth factors by ECs.[44] Consequently, malignant cells exploit their environment to their advantage by developing a synergistic relationship with ECs (*Figure 21.1*). This has led to the active investigation of antiangiogenic agents as a novel therapeutic strategy for hematologic malignancies.

In addition to the effects of the vascular endothelium in modulating and responding to angiogenic stimuli, the vascular endothelium also influences other functions,[53,54] including vasoconstriction, selective permeability, hemostasis, antigen presentation, and the inflammatory response. The EC surface is a dynamic interface between soluble and cellular constituents of the blood and the remainder of the body.[55] A brief discussion of ECs structure and regulation of hemostasis follows.

ENDOTHELIAL CELL STRUCTURE

Individual ECs measure approximately 20 to 50 μm^2 in surface area. The total vascular surface area in a normal adult is estimated to be at least 4000 m^2.[55] However, the geometry of the vascular system is not static. The surface area facing a unit volume of blood differs, depending on the vascular bed being considered. For example, the surface area-to-volume ratio is approximately 1000 times greater in capillaries than in large blood vessels.[56] This vascular geometry has implications for regulation of hemostasis and is discussed later.

ECs are anchored to the vessel wall by the basement membrane secreted by ECs and smooth muscle cells. The basement membrane contains a large number of connective tissue components, including collagen, microfibrils, glycosaminoglycans (GAGs), fibronectin, and thrombospondin. These components may serve as ligands for a number of cell adhesion processes that are important in angiogenesis, hemostasis, vascular repair, and inflammation.[54,57]

ECs typically exist as a cell monolayer, exhibiting contact inhibition and a cobblestone appearance. Two types of cell-cell junctional

structures have been reported: adherens junctions and tight junctions. These structures regulate permeability and maintain polarity.[58]

ECs contain unique intracellular structures called *Weibel-Palade bodies*[59]; these organelles contain the adhesion protein vWF, which is secreted constitutively and also in response to cell stimulation.[60] The Weibel-Palade body membrane contains P-selectin, which is expressed on the EC surface after EC activation. When expressed on the vascular surface, P-selectin mediates neutrophil and monocyte adhesion to the vessel wall.[61] Selectin-independent platelet adhesion to endothelium has also been reported.[62] Integrins mediating platelet-EC and leukocyte-EC interactions are discussed in Chapters 19 and 7, respectively. Additional EC proteins have been reported to undergo regulated release or cell-surface expression, including tissue plasminogen activator (TPA), interleukin-8, endothelin-1, and multimerin.[63] These and other proteins may be contained in Weibel-Palade bodies or other distinct organelles.

Endothelial Cell Phenotypes: Resting vs Activated

The concept of differing EC phenotypes (e.g., resting [constitutive] vs activated) has been applied to numerous EC functions,[64] including the inflammatory response, regulation of coagulation, and angiogenesis. This chapter focuses on EC phenotypes as related to the functions of angiogenesis, and hemostasis and thrombosis. Other EC functions have been reviewed elsewhere.[54,64]

THE VESSEL WALL AND HEMOSTASIS: GENERAL CONCEPTS

The three major cell types of the normal vessel wall are ECs (intima), smooth muscle cells (media), and connective tissue elements, such as fibroblasts (adventitia). The circulating coagulation proteins contained in the blood are in immediate contact with quiescent vascular endothelium that normally presents a thromboresistant surface in that ECs are unable to initiate coagulation[65,66] or promote platelet adhesion and activation.[67-70] Thus, in the absence of vascular trauma or perturbation (activation), blood remains fluid as a result of antithrombotic activities expressed by ECs. However, after traumatic vascular injury, exposure of blood to cells within the vessel wall, especially fibroblasts, or to the ECM (subendothelium) results in rapid initiation of coagulation because fibroblasts[65] and subendothelium contain EC remnants[71] that constitutively express tissue factor (TF) procoagulant activity. Alternatively, perturbation (activation) of EC by stimuli, such as cytokines,[72] may induce altered EC hemostatic function (in the absence of vascular injury), resulting in net EC expression of thrombotic activity. These hemostatic properties of unperturbed and perturbed EC are critical in determining the coagulant balance of the vessel wall and the extent of activation of coagulation.

A cell-based model of hemostasis has been presented in which fibroblasts or perturbed EC express TF to initiate coagulation; amplification and propagation of coagulation then occur on the platelet surface. Modulation of coagulation occurs via EC antithrombotic activities and plasma protease inhibitors.[73]

ANTITHROMBOTIC PROPERTIES OF UNPERTURBED ENDOTHELIUM

Antithrombotic mechanisms responsible for unperturbed (native) EC thromboresistance are illustrated in *Figure 21.2*. Major antithrombotic properties can be classified as antiplatelet activities, anticoagulant activities, and fibrinolytic activities.

Antiplatelet Activities

The vascular endothelium inhibits platelet function by several mechanisms. The EC plasma membrane does not permit adherence of resting platelets.[74] In addition, ECs synthesize and secrete three potent antiplatelet agents: prostacyclin (PGI_2), NO, and certain adenine nucleotides. PGI_2 is constitutively synthesized by EC cyclooxygenase (prostaglandin H synthase) and phospholipase A_2 in response to

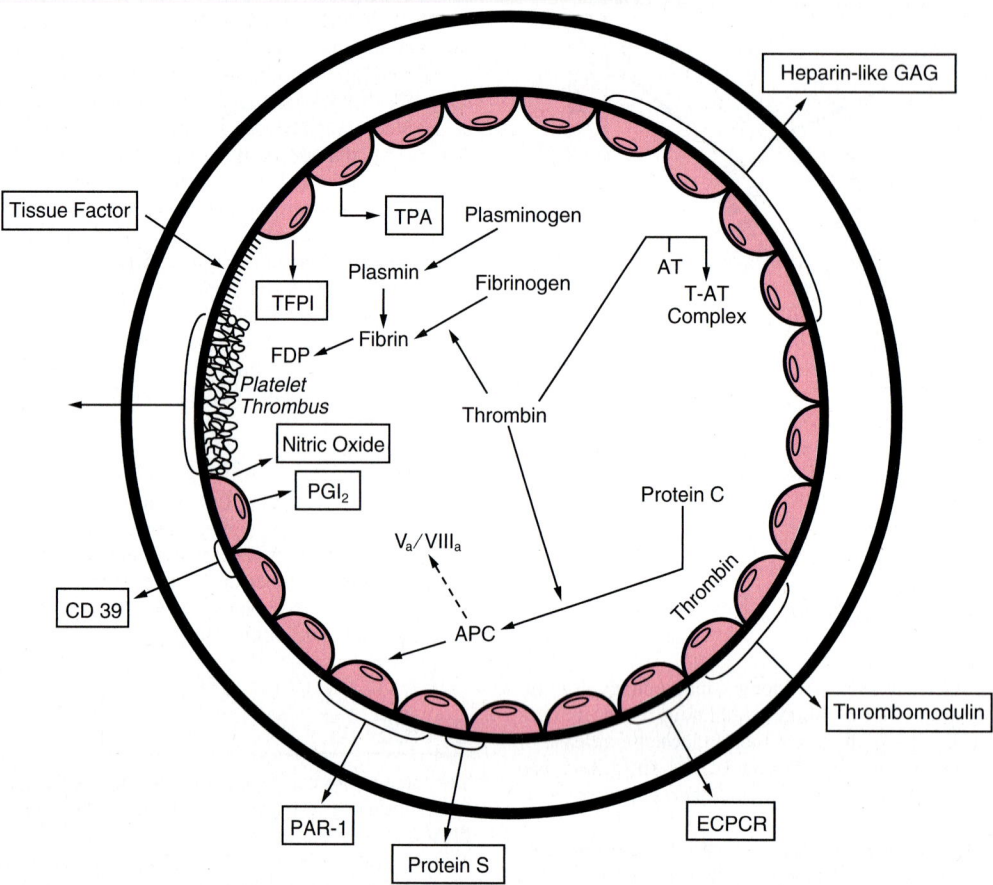

FIGURE 21.2 Vessel wall antithrombotic properties. The major antithrombotic properties are depicted in boxes. Heparin-like glycosaminoglycans (GAG), such as heparan sulfate, catalyze inactivation of serine proteases, such as thrombin (T) and factor Xa, by antithrombin (AT). Formation of the T-thrombomodulin complex activates protein C to activated protein C (APC). The endothelial cell (EC) protein C receptor (ECPCR) promotes protein C activation. Binding of APC to EC-bound protein S (and factor V) promotes proteolysis of factors Va and VIIIa (dashed line), inhibiting coagulation. APC also possesses anti-inflammatory properties that are mediated by EC protease-activated receptor (PAR)-1. This APC activity requires ECPCR (data not shown). Secretion of vessel wall prostacyclin (PGI2) and nitric oxide and expression of CD39 limit platelet thrombus formation at sites of vascular injury. Tissue plasminogen activator (TPA) is secreted and bound to EC to initiate fibrinolysis. Secretion of tissue factor pathway inhibitor (TFPI) by EC suppresses tissue factor-mediated initiation of coagulation. Dermatan sulfate–catalyzed activation of heparin cofactor II and an inhibitor to contact activation are not illustrated in the figure. FDP, fibrin degradation products. (Modified from Rodgers GM. Hemostatic properties of normal and perturbed vascular cells. *FASEB J.* 1988;2(2):116-123. Copyright © FASEB. Reprinted by permission of John Wiley & Sons, Inc.)

thrombin[75] and other vasoactive agonists.[76] In addition to its ability to prevent adhesion of activated platelets to EC, PGI2 also possesses potent vasodilating properties.[68] PGI2 inhibits platelet function by increasing the levels of platelet cyclic adenosine monophosphate. Aspirin inhibits the synthesis of PGI2 by irreversibly acetylating and inactivating EC cyclooxygenase.[77] Recovery of PGI2 production by EC occurs with subsequent EC synthesis of cyclooxygenase.

A second inducible form of cyclooxygenase, called *cyclooxygenase-2*, has been identified in a variety of cells, including ECs.[78] Both cyclooxygenase proteins are homologous, with similar molecular weights and structural features. Investigators believe that cyclooxygenase-2 mediates the vascular response to injury and inflammation.

Although thought to be important primarily in regulating vascular tone,[79,80] NO is also a potent inhibitor of platelet adhesion to the vascular endothelium.[69] Constitutive and inducible pathways generate NO from the terminal guanidino nitrogen of arginine in a reaction catalyzed by NO synthetase.[79,81] The constitutive mechanism generates small amounts of NO and mediates physiologic responses. Increased synthesis of NO occurs in response to cytokines (inducible pathway), such as tumor necrosis factor, to mediate inflammatory events.[80] Both the constitutive and inducible forms of NO synthetase are present in ECs. Other stimuli to NO generation include adenosine diphosphate (ADP), thrombin, shear stress, and bradykinin. EC-derived NO also inhibits leukocyte adhesion, as well as vascular smooth muscle cell proliferation. Elevated levels of cyclic guanosine monophosphate

result from NO stimulation and mediate the biologic activities of this antiplatelet agent. Synthesis of NO is insensitive to the effects of aspirin.

A third EC antiplatelet property is ectoenzymes that rapidly metabolize ADP and adenosine triphosphate to adenosine monophosphate and adenosine, respectively.[82] ADP is a potent platelet agonist, and adenosine is a potent inhibitor of platelet function. Thus, ECs can convert a platelet agonist to an antiplatelet agent by this mechanism. EC ectoenzymes are insensitive to the effects of aspirin. This ectoenzyme antiplatelet property of EC may explain earlier reports of EC thromboresistance to platelet adhesion. The EC ecto-ADPase responsible for inhibition of platelet function is CD39.[83] Deletion of this EC receptor in mice results in a prothrombotic state and platelet dysfunction.[84]

Anticoagulant Activities

Vascular ECs synthesize and express heparin-like GAG, such as heparan sulfate and dermatan sulfate, on their luminal surface.[85] These GAGs catalyze the inactivation of serine proteases, such as thrombin and factor Xa, by protease inhibitors, such as antithrombin and heparin cofactor II, respectively, via formation of a covalent protease-antiprotease complex. Of these two protease inhibitors, antithrombin is considered to be more important.[86] The molecular basis for the effect of heparin in promoting antithrombin neutralization of serine proteases involves interaction of a specific pentasaccharide sequence of the EC heparin-like molecule with an allosteric site on the antithrombin molecule.[85,86] This interaction results in conformational changes in antithrombin that permit more efficient binding to, and inhibition of, protease molecules. In vivo, antithrombin molecules are associated with EC GAG,[85] providing a mechanism for instantaneous control over activation of coagulation.

Another key vascular anticoagulant activity is the protein C pathway that consists of two plasma proteins, protein C and protein S, and an EC receptor, thrombomodulin (*Figure 21.2*). ECs synthesize and express protein S[87] and thrombomodulin,[88] whereas protein C is synthesized by the liver. Thrombin generation leads to thrombin's binding to thrombomodulin; the thrombin-thrombomodulin complex then activates protein C to generate activated protein C (APC).[89] APC binds to protein S, resulting in inhibition of coagulation by proteolysis of two coagulation cofactor proteins, factors Va and VIIIa. Inactivation of factors Va and VIIIa prevents further thrombin formation. It appears that APC downregulation of coagulation (proteolysis of factors Va and VIIIa) occurs more efficiently on the vascular endothelium rather than on platelets.[90]

An additional component of the protein C pathway exists: the EC protein C receptor (ECPCR). This protein binds protein C to enhance protein C activation by the thrombin-thrombomodulin complex.[91] ECPCR is found primarily on large-vessel endothelium[92] and is induced by thrombin stimulation. Blocking ECPCR with a monoclonal antibody in a primate model indicates that ECPCR plays a major role in in vivo protein C activation.[93]

APC possesses activities other than those associated with anticoagulant activity. In gene-expression studies using microarray techniques, APC was found to modulate anti-inflammatory and cell-survival pathways. APC suppressed adhesion molecule expression, decreased activity of the nuclear factor-κB transcription pathway, and inhibited apoptosis.[94] Recent information suggests that APC uses the ECPCR to signal EC via the protease-activated receptor (PAR)-1 pathway (see Hemostatic Properties of Perturbed Endothelium).[95]

Regulation of TF procoagulant activity by a plasma protein called TFPI has been described.[96,97] This protein is synthesized primarily by EC[98] and is an important regulator of TF–factor VIIa activation of factor X (discussed in Chapter 20). In addition, TFPI can inhibit vascular cell proliferation.[99] Heparin or low-molecular-weight heparin releases TFPI from EC storage sites.[100]

Fibrinolytic Activities

ECs synthesize and secrete plasminogen activators, primarily TPA, in response to stimulation by thrombin or vasoactive stimuli, such as histamine and vasopressin.[101] TPA has been localized to the Weibel-Palade organelles in EC.[102] Specific EC receptors for TPA exist.[103] In response to inflammatory mediators, ECs synthesize another plasminogen activator, urokinase,[104] which activates plasminogen in the fluid phase or bound to fibrin. Activation of plasminogen by TPA generates plasmin; localization of TPA and plasminogen to the fibrin clot leads to physiologic fibrinolysis and release of soluble fibrin degradation products (*Figure 21.2*). Fibrin degradation products possess potent antiplatelet and antithrombin activities and contribute to the anticoagulant effect of fibrinolysis. Activation of plasminogen is regulated by PAIs. The major inhibitor of TPA is PAI-1; PAI-1 is secreted by vascular EC.[105] This inhibitor also regulates urokinase activity. Details of the fibrinolytic mechanism and its regulation are discussed in Chapter 20.

PROTHROMBOTIC PROPERTIES OF UNPERTURBED ENDOTHELIUM

Unperturbed ECs possess procoagulant activities that promote coagulation after vascular injury or perturbation.[72] However, in the absence of initiating stimuli, these activities remain latent and do not contribute to thrombosis. Major prothrombotic activities of resting EC include binding sites (receptors) for coagulation zymogens or proteases (factor XII,[106] factor XI,[107] factors X and Xa,[108-110] factors IX and IXa,[108,111] thrombin,[112] cofactor proteins [high-molecular-weight kininogen,[113]

factor VIIIa, and factor Va[114]]) and synthesis and expression of factor V[115,116] and vWF.[117] Resting ECs can also activate bound factor XII and promote functional cleavage of prekallikrein.[106] Investigators have reported a factor XII–independent pathway for prekallikrein activation on EC; this activation is mediated by an EC-associated thiol protease.[113] In addition, when high-molecular-weight kininogen is bound to EC, factor XI (XIa) can associate with EC to promote factor IX activation.[118] However, ECs also secrete an inhibitor to contact activation.[119] These prothrombotic activities are illustrated in *Figure 21.3*.

EC receptors for coagulation proteases permit assembly of complexes consisting of cofactor proteins, proteases, and zymogen substrates that result in optimal activation and localization of coagulation.[120] Factor V is secreted primarily into the fluid phase,[115] whereas vWF is secreted both in the plasma and in the subendothelium, providing a source of adhesive protein for the platelet response to vascular injury.[121]

HEMOSTATIC PROPERTIES OF PERTURBED ENDOTHELIUM

In this discussion, the term *EC perturbation* means exposure of EC to diverse stimuli, such as traumatic vascular injury, certain cytokines, atherogenic stimuli (homocysteine, modified low-density lipoprotein [LDL]), lipopolysaccharide (endotoxin), immune complexes, and certain infectious organisms. From this list, it is obvious that a variety of inflammatory, infectious, or malignant disorders, as well as metabolic defects, may be associated with hemostatic dysfunction resulting from altered EC hemostatic properties. The major hemostatic properties reviewed in this section include TF activity, thrombomodulin activity (protein C pathway), factor V activation, and fibrinolytic activities (TPA, PAI-1). In general, these activities are concordantly regulated, with stimuli that induce TF expression also suppressing protein C activation and fibrinolysis. The net result of these events is that the perturbed EC surface is converted from an antithrombotic surface to a prothrombotic surface.

The key hemostatic activity induced by EC perturbants is TF expression, the major initiator of coagulation.[122] Stimuli reported to induce EC TF activity include cytokines, lipopolysaccharide, oxidized LDL, homocysteine, and certain infectious organisms. Expression of EC TF antigen in pathologic human and primate tissues using immunohistochemical methods has been reported,[123-125] including vascular tissue from patients with sickle cell anemia[126] and skin biopsies from patients treated with intradermal cytokines.[127] The importance of vessel wall TF activity in arterial and venous thrombosis has been confirmed,[128] and a mouse model of arterial thrombosis suggested that activated endothelium, not platelets, primarily supported prothrombinase activity.[129] Studies with human arterial vascular tissue indicate that vascular tissue alone (in the absence of platelets) can generate large amounts of thrombin.[130]

EC TF procoagulant activity may be modulated by a novel EC protease, PAR-2. PARs represent a group of G protein–coupled receptors present in ECs and other tissues.[131] Thrombin or other proteases cleave the amino terminus of the receptor exodomain; the amino-terminus fragment then binds to the cell-associated domain of the receptor to activate the protease.[132]

There are four members of the PAR family.[131] Human PAR-1, PAR-3, and PAR-4 can be activated by thrombin, and it is proposed that their in vivo role is to sense thrombin generation.[131] ECs contain both PAR-1 and PAR-2,[131,133] but thrombin does not activate PAR-2. Rather, data indicate that PAR-2 may be activated directly by TF–factor VIIa and indirectly by TF–factor VIIa-generated factor Xa.[134] It has been proposed that PAR-2 may function as a coagulation protease "sensor" and thereby contribute to EC activation by pathologic stimuli.[134] EC PAR-2 may mediate additional thrombin-induced vascular functions, including leukocyte adhesion[135] and mitogenesis.[136] PAR-1 also mediates the EC response to APC; APC and ECPCR cleave PAR-1 to initiate signaling events.[95] The role of PARs in vascular biology and disease has been reviewed.[137,138]

The Normal Hematologic System

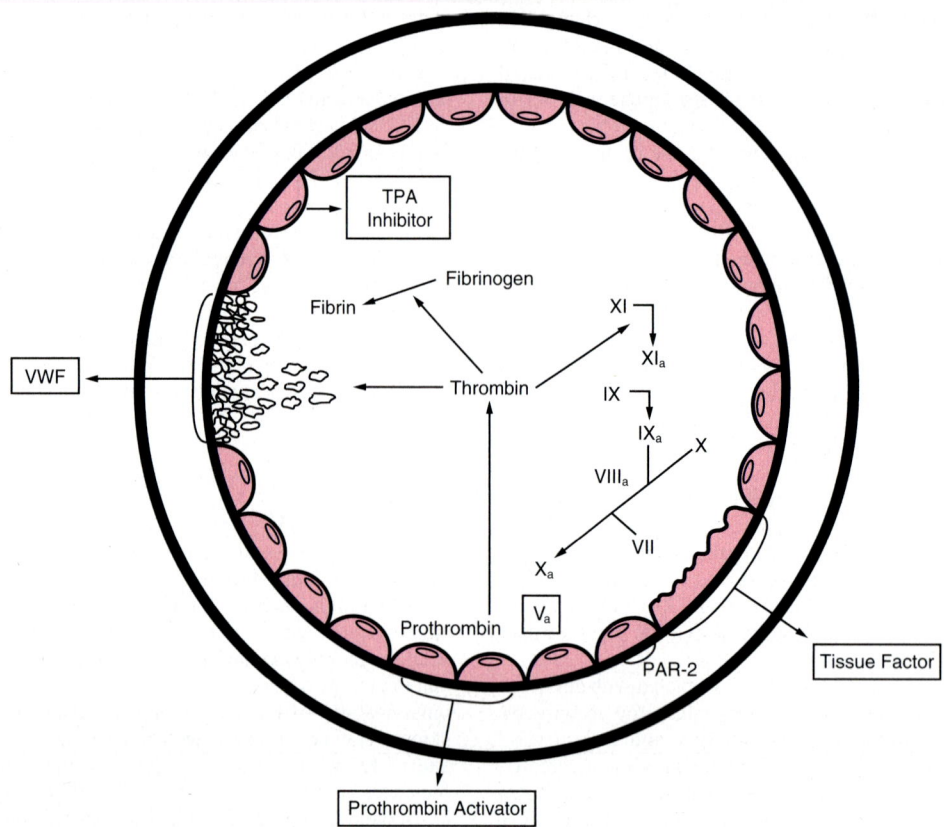

FIGURE 21.3 Vessel wall prothrombotic properties. The major prothrombotic properties are depicted in boxes. Expression of tissue factor activity initiates coagulation, and endothelial cell (EC) synthesis of factor V promotes thrombin formation. Thrombin formation is enhanced by feedback activation of factor XI. Vessel wall injury also promotes platelet adhesion and thrombus formation by exposure of subendothelial von Willebrand factor (vWF). An inducible EC prothrombin activator may directly generate thrombin. EC can be induced to express an activator of factor V (Va). Thrombin exerts multiple procoagulant activities, including platelet activation and cleavage of fibrinogen, resulting in the fibrin clot. Thrombin binding to thrombomodulin activates thrombin-activatable fibrinolysis inhibitor to downregulate fibrinolysis (data not shown). EC secretion of tissue plasminogen activator (TPA) inhibitor further stabilizes the fibrin clot by preventing fibrinolysis. Also not shown are EC-binding sites for coagulation zymogens or proteases. Protease-activated receptor (PAR)-2 is activated by the tissue factor–factor VIIa complex and factor Xa to contribute to EC activation by pathologic stimuli. (Modified from Rodgers GM. Hemostatic properties of normal and perturbed vascular cells. *FASEB J.* 1988;2:116-123. Copyright © FASEB. Reprinted by permission of John Wiley & Sons, Inc.)

An additional mechanism for EC generation of thrombin has been reported. Perturbed ECs express a prothrombin activator that can generate thrombin independent of the intrinsic and extrinsic coagulation pathways.[139] The description of trypsin expression by cultured EC and by vascular EC in situ suggests that a variety of EC-derived proteases may also regulate blood coagulation.[140]

Regulation of the anticoagulant protein C pathway by EC perturbants has also been a subject of interest because of the recurrent thrombotic disorders associated with deficiency of protein C pathway components (proteins C and S).[88,89] Downregulation of the protein C pathway has focused on thrombomodulin, the EC membrane protein that activates protein C after complexing with thrombin. The effects of tumor necrosis factor on the protein C pathway appear to result from enhanced endocytosis and subsequent degradation of thrombomodulin.[141] In addition, tumor necrosis factor, a cytokine that reduces protein C activation, has been reported to inhibit transcription of thrombomodulin RNA.[142]

Another important EC hemostatic property regulated by relevant perturbing stimuli is secretion of PAI-1 and TPA. Treatment of cultured EC with interleukin-1 results in both diminished TPA secretion and increased PAI-1 secretion.[143] Increased amounts of PAI-1 relative to TPA diminish vascular fibrinolytic activity, resulting in enhanced thrombotic potential because of failure to lyse fibrin thrombi.

In addition to the humoral and biochemical stimuli discussed earlier, biomechanical forces (shear stress) can regulate EC gene expression and phenotype.[144] For example, either laminar or turbulent shear stress has been reported to regulate a large number of EC genes differentially, including adhesion molecules and growth factors, as well as

hemostasis proteins.[145] Shear stress also attenuates cytokine-induced EC TF expression.[146] These data indicate that vascular endothelium is responsive to biomechanical stimuli.

Diversity of Endothelial Cell Hemostatic Properties

There is significant heterogeneity in arterial, venous, and capillary EC with regard to expression of hemostatic and other functional activities.[147] For example, aortic ECs express more factor V activity than do venous ECs,[109] and PGI$_2$, a major metabolite secreted by human venous EC, is not substantially produced by human capillary cells.[148] Increases in blood flow lead to upregulation of NO synthase messenger RNA in aortic, but not pulmonary, arterial EC.[149] Vascular anticoagulant activity in the microcirculation is reinforced by geometric aspects of the vessel wall.[56] For example, the thrombomodulin concentration in the microcirculation would increase more than a 1000-fold[56] compared with a large vessel. Consequently, in large vessels, thrombin circulates freely to catalyze coagulation, whereas in the microcirculation, thrombin exists mostly bound to thrombomodulin, promoting anticoagulation.[89]

The differential concentration of thrombomodulin in large versus small vessels may also affect vascular fibrinolysis in specific vascular beds. Thrombin-activatable fibrinolysis inhibitor is stimulated by low thrombomodulin concentrations but decreased at high concentrations of thrombomodulin.[150] This implies that enhanced fibrinolysis would be seen in the microcirculation that contains high levels of thrombomodulin activity.

These data suggest a vascular model in which procoagulant activities are dominant in the arterial circulation and anticoagulant activities are dominant in the microcirculation. This distribution of vascular hemostatic properties is consistent with the necessity for rapid thrombin generation and fibrin clot formation after arterial injury, while providing the venous and microcirculation with anticoagulant mechanisms to protect against thrombosis.[72] The concept of EC diversity is also supported by gene-expression profile studies that have identified characteristic expression patterns of arterial versus venous EC, as well as large versus microvascular EC.[151]

References

1. Conway EM, Collen D, Carmeliet P. Molecular mechanisms of blood vessel growth. *Cardiovasc Res.* 2001;49:507-521.
2. Carmeliet P, Jain RK. Angiogenesis in cancer and other diseases. *Nature.* 2000;407:249-257.
3. Nathan C. Nitric oxide as a secretory product of mammalian cells. *FASEB J.* 1992;6:3051-3064.
4. Kimura H, Weisz A, Kurashima Y, et al. Hypoxia response element of the human vascular endothelial growth factor gene mediates transcriptional regulation by nitric oxide: control of hypoxia-inducible factor-1 activity by nitric oxide. *Blood.* 2000;95:189-197.
5. Eliceiri BP, Paul R, Schwartzberg PL, et al. Selective requirement for Src kinases during VEGF-induced angiogenesis and vascular permeability. *Mol Cell.* 1999;4:915-924.
6. Gale NW, Yancopoulos GD. Growth factors acting via endothelial cell-specific receptor tyrosine kinases: VEGFs, angiopoietins, and ephrins in vascular development. *Genes Dev.* 1999;13:1055-1066.
7. Thurston G, Rudge JS, Ioffe E, et al. Angiopoietin-1 protects the adult vasculature against plasma leakage. *Nat Med.* 2000;6:460-463.
8. Nelson AR, Fingleton B, Rothenberg ML, Matrisian LM. Matrix metalloproteinases: biologic activity and clinical implications. *J Clin Oncol.* 2000;18:1135-1149.
9. Stetler-Stevenson WG. Matrix metalloproteinases in angiogenesis: a moving target for therapeutic intervention. *J Clin Invest.* 1999;103:1237-1241.
10. Brew K, Dinakarpandian D, Nagase H. Tissue inhibitors of metalloproteinases: evolution, structure and function. *Biochim Biophys Acta.* 2000;1477:267-283.
11. Ferrara N, Gerber HP. The role of vascular endothelial growth factor in angiogenesis. *Acta Haematol.* 2001;106:148-156.
12. Veikkola T, Karkkainen M, Claesson-Welsh L, Alitalo K. Regulation of angiogenesis via vascular endothelial growth factor receptors. *Cancer Res.* 2000;60:203-212.
13. Singh H, Tahir TA, Alawo DO, et al. Molecular control of angiopoietin signaling. *Biochem Soc Trans.* 2011;39:1592-1596.
14. Yancopoulos GD, Davis S, Gale NW, et al. Vascular-specific growth factors and blood vessel formation. *Nature.* 2000;407:242-248.
15. Suri C, McClain J, Thurston G, et al. Increased vascularization in mice overexpressing angiopoietin-1. *Science.* 1998;282:468-471.
16. Suri C, Jones PF, Patan S, et al. Requisite role of angiopoietin-1, a ligand for the TIE2 receptor, during embryonic angiogenesis. *Cell.* 1996;87:1171-1180.
17. Maisonpierre PC, Suri C, Jones PF, et al. Angiopoietin-2, a natural antagonist for Tie2 that disrupts in vivo angiogenesis. *Science.* 1997;277:55-60.
18. Fernandez B, Buehler A, Wolfram S, et al. Transgenic myocardial overexpression of fibroblast growth factor-1 increases coronary artery density and branching. *Circ Res.* 2000;87:207-213.
19. Carmeliet P. Fibroblast growth factor-1 stimulates branching and survival of myocardial arteries: a goal for therapeutic angiogenesis? *Circ Res.* 2000;87:176-178.
20. O'Reilly MS, Holmgren L, Shing Y, et al. Angiostatin: a novel angiogenesis inhibitor that mediates the suppression of metastases by a Lewis lung carcinoma. *Cell.* 1994;79:315-328.
21. O'Reilly MS, Boehm T, Shing Y, et al. Endostatin: an endogenous inhibitor of angiogenesis and tumor growth. *Cell.* 1997;88(2):277-285.
22. Carmeliet P. Mechanisms of angiogenesis and arteriogenesis. *Nat Med.* 2000;6:389-395.
23. Eliceiri BP, Cheresh DA. The role of alphav integrins during angiogenesis: insights into potential mechanisms of action and clinical development. *J Clin Invest.* 1999;103:1227-1230.
24. Carmeliet P, Lampugnani MG, Moons L, et al. Targeted deficiency or cytosolic truncation of the VE-cadherin gene in mice impairs VEGF-mediated endothelial survival and angiogenesis. *Cell.* 1999;98:147-157.
25. Holash J, Maisonpierre PC, Compton D, et al. Vessel cooption, regression, and growth in tumors mediated by angiopoietins and VEGF. *Science.* 1999;284:1994-1998.
26. Hirschi KK, D'Amore PA. Pericytes in the microvasculature. *Cardiovasc Res.* 1996;32:687-698.
27. Yamashita J, Itoh H, Hirashima M, et al. Flk1-positive cells derived from embryonic stem cells serve as vascular progenitors. *Nature.* 2000;408(6808):92-96.
28. Bellomo D, Headrick JP, Silins GU, et al. Mice lacking the vascular endothelial growth factor-B gene (Vegfb) have smaller hearts, dysfunctional coronary vasculature, and impaired recovery from cardiac ischemia. *Circ Res.* 2000;86:E29-E35.
29. Olofsson B, Jeltsch M, Eriksson U, Alitalo K. Current biology of VEGF-B and VEGF-C. *Curr Opin Biotechnol.* 1999;10:528-535.
30. Fong GH, Rossant J, Gertsenstein M, Breitman ML. Role of the Flt-1 receptor tyrosine kinase in regulating the assembly of vascular endothelium. *Nature.* 1995;376:66-70.
31. Hiratsuka S, Minowa O, Kuno J, et al. Flt-1 lacking the tyrosine kinase domain is sufficient for normal development and angiogenesis in mice. *Proc Natl Acad Sci U S A.* 1998;95:9349-9354.
32. Saharinen P, Eklund L, Alitalo K. Therapeutic targeting of the angiopoietin—TIE pathway. *Nat Rev Drug Discov.* 2017;16(9):635-661.
33. Carmeliet P, Jain RK. Molecular mechanisms and clinical applications of angiogenesis. *Nature.* 2011;473:298-307.
34. Welti J, Loges S, Dimmeler S, Carmeliet P. Recent molecular discoveries in angiogenesis and antiangiogenic therapies in cancer. *J Clin Invest.* 2013;123:3190-3200.
35. Phng LK, Potente M, Leslie JD, et al. Nrarp coordinates endothelial Notch and Wnt signaling to control vessel density in angiogenesis. *Dev Cell.* 2009;16:70-82.
36. Phng LK, Gerhardt H. Angiogenesis: a team effort coordinated by notch. *Dev Cell.* 2009;16:196-208.
37. Jakobsson L, Franco CA, Bentley K, et al. Endothelial cells dynamically compete for the tip cell position during angiogenic sprouting. *Nat Cell Biol.* 2010;12:943-953.
38. Lee M, Keener J, Xiao J, Long Zheng X, Rodgers GM. ADAMTS13 and its variants promote angiogenesis via upregulation of VEGF and VEGFR2. *Cell Mol Life Sci.* 2015;72:349-356.
39. Tang H, Lee M, Kim EH, Bishop D, Rodgers GM. siRNA-Knockdown of ADAMTS-13 modulates endothelial cell angiogenesis. *Microvasc Res.* 2017;113:65-70.
40. Randi AM. Endothelial dysfunction in von Willebrand disease: angiogenesis and angiodysplasia. *Thromb Res.* 2016;141(suppl 2):S55-S58.
41. Asahara T, Murohara T, Sullivan A, et al. Isolation of putative progenitor endothelial cells for angiogenesis. *Science.* 1997;275:964-967.
42. Perry BN, Arbiser JL. The duality of angiogenesis: implications for therapy of human disease. *J Invest Dermatol.* 2006;126:2160-2166.
43. Ribatti D, Vacca A, De Falco G, et al. Role of hematopoietic growth factors in angiogenesis. *Acta Haematol.* 2001;106:157-161.
44. Dickson DJ, Shami PJ. Angiogenesis in acute and chronic leukemias. *Leuk Lymphoma.* 2001;42:847-853.
45. Tosi P, Tura S. Antiangiogenic therapy in multiple myeloma. *Acta Haematol.* 2001;106:208-213.
46. Salven P. Angiogenesis in lymphoproliferative disorders. *Acta Haematol.* 2001;106:184-189.
47. Hussong JW, Rodgers GM, Shami PJ. Evidence of increased angiogenesis in patients with acute myeloid leukemia. *Blood.* 2000;95:309-313.
48. Padro T, Ruiz S, Bieker R, et al. Increased angiogenesis in the bone marrow of patients with acute myeloid leukemia. *Blood.* 2000;95:2637-2645.
49. Aguayo A, Kantarjian H, Manshouri T, et al. Angiogenesis in acute and chronic leukemias and myelodysplastic syndromes. *Blood.* 2000;96:2240-2245.
50. Kini AR, Kay NE, Peterson LC. Increased bone marrow angiogenesis in B cell chronic lymphocytic leukemia. *Leukemia.* 2000;14:1414-1418.
51. Albitar M. Angiogenesis in acute myeloid leukemia and myelodysplastic syndrome. *Acta Haematol.* 2001;106:170-176.
52. Di Raimondo F, Palumbo GA, Molica S, Giustolisi R. Angiogenesis in chronic myeloproliferative disorders. *Acta Haematol.* 2001;106:177-183.
53. Petty RG, Pearson JD. Endothelium—the axis of vascular health and disease. *J R Coll Physicians Lond.* 1989;23:92-102.
54. Cines DB, Pollak ES, Buck CA, et al. Endothelial cells in physiology and in the pathophysiology of vascular disorders. *Blood.* 1998;91:3527-3561.
55. Aird WC. Spatial and temporal dynamics of the endothelium. *J Thromb Haemost.* 2005;3:1392-1406.
56. Busch C, Cancilla PA, DeBault LE, et al. Use of endothelium cultured on microcarriers as a model for the microcirculation. *Lab Invest.* 1982;47:498-504.
57. Carlos TM, Harlan JM. Leukocyte-endothelial adhesion molecules. *Blood.* 1994;84:2068-2101.
58. Dejana E, Corada M, Lampugnani MG. Endothelial cell-to-cell junctions. *FASEB J.* 1995;9:910-918.
59. Weibel ER, Palade GE. New cytoplasmic components in arterial endothelia. *J Cell Biol.* 1964;23:101-113.
60. Wagner DD, Olmstead JB, Marder VJ. Immunolocalization of von Willebrand protein in Weibel–Palade bodies of human endothelial cells. *J Cell Biol.* 1982;95:355-360.
61. McEver RP, Beckstead JH, Moore KL, et al. GMP-140, a platelet membrane alpha-granule protein, is also synthesized by vascular endothelial cells and is localized in Weibel–Palade bodies. *J Clin Invest.* 1989;84:92-99.
62. André P, Denis CV, Ware J, et al. Platelets adhere to and translocate on von Willebrand factor presented by endothelium in stimulated veins. *Blood.* 2000;96:3322-3328.
63. Rondaij MG, Bierings R, Kragt A, van Mourik JA, Voorberg J. Dynamics and plasticity of Weibel–Palade bodies in endothelial cells. *Arterioscler Thromb Vasc Biol.* 2006;26:1002-1007.
64. Augustin HG, Kozian DH, Johnson RC. Differentiation of endothelial cells: analysis of the constitutive and activated endothelial cell phenotypes. *Bioessays.* 1994;16:901-906.
65. Rodgers GM, Greenberg CS, Shuman MA. Characterization of the effects of cultured vascular cells on the activation of blood coagulation. *Blood.* 1983;61:1155-1162.
66. Rosenberg RD, Rosenberg JS. Natural anticoagulant mechanisms. *J Clin Invest.* 1984;74:1-6.
67. Jaffe EA. Physiologic functions of normal endothelial cells. *Ann N Y Acad Sci.* 1985;454:279-291.
68. Moncada S. Prostacyclin and arterial wall biology. *Arteriosclerosis.* 1982;2:193-207.
69. Radomski MW, Palmer RMJ, Moncada S. Endogenous nitric oxide inhibits human platelet adhesion to vascular endothelium. *Lancet.* 1987;2:1057-1058.
70. Zimmermann H. Nucleotides and CD39: principal modulatory players in hemostasis and thrombosis. *Nat Med.* 1999;5:987-988.
71. Mulder AB, Hegge-Paping KS, Magielse CP, et al. Tumor necrosis factor alpha-induced endothelial tissue factor is located on the cell surface rather than in the subendothelial matrix. *Blood.* 1994;84:1559-1566.

72. Rodgers GM. Hemostatic properties of normal and perturbed vascular cells. *FASEB J.* 1988;2:116-123.

73. Monroe DM, Hoffman M. What does it take to make the perfect clot? *Arterioscler Thromb Vasc Biol.* 2006;26:41-48.

74. Czervionke RL, Hoak JC, Fry GL. Effect of aspirin on thrombin-induced adherence of platelets to cultured cells from the blood vessel wall. *J Clin Invest.* 1978;62:847-856.

75. Weksler BB, Marcus AJ, Jaffe EA. Synthesis of prostaglandin I$_2$ (prostacyclin) by cultured human and bovine endothelial cells. *Proc Natl Acad Sci U S A.* 1977;74:3922-3926.

76. Jaffe EA. Endothelial cell structure and function. In: Hoffman R, Benz EJ, Shattil SJ, et al, eds. *Hematology: Basic Principles and Practice.* Churchill Livingstone; 1991:1198-1213.

77. Roth GJ, Siok CJ. Acetylation of the NH$_2$-terminal serine of prostaglandin synthetase by aspirin. *J Biol Chem.* 1978;253:3782-3784.

78. Hla T, Neilson K. Human cyclooxygenase-2 cDNA. *Proc Natl Acad Sci U S A.* 1992;89:7384-7388.

79. Moncada S, Palmer RM, Higgs EA. Nitric oxide: physiology, pathophysiology, and pharmacology. *Pharmacol Rev.* 1991;43:109-142.

80. Lowenstein CJ, Dinerman JL, Snyder SH. Nitric oxide: a physiologic messenger. *Ann Intern Med.* 1994;120:227-237.

81. Palmer RM, Ashton DS, Moncada S. Vascular endothelial cells synthesize nitric oxide from l-arginine. *Nature.* 1988;333:664-666.

82. Pearson JD, Gordon JL. Nucleotide metabolism by endothelium. *Annu Rev Physiol.* 1985;47:617-627.

83. Marcus AJ, Broekman MJ, Drosopoulos JH, et al. The endothelial cell ecto-ADPase responsible for inhibition of platelet function is CD39. *J Clin Invest.* 1997;99:1351-1360.

84. Enjyoji K, Sevigny J, Lin Y, et al. Targeted disruption of CD39/ATP diphosphohydrolase results in disordered hemostasis and thromboregulation. *Nat Med.* 1999;5:1010-1017.

85. Bourin MC, Lindahl U. Glycosaminoglycans and the regulation of blood coagulation. *Biochem J.* 1993;289:313-330.

86. Bock SC. Antithrombin III and heparin cofactor II. In: Colman RW, Hirsh J, Marder VJ, et al, eds. *Hemostasis and Thrombosis: Basic Principles and Clinical Practice.* 4th ed. Lippincott Williams & Wilkins; 2001:321-333.

87. Stern D, Brett J, Harris K, Nawroth P. Participation of endothelial cells in the protein C-protein S anticoagulant pathway: the synthesis and release of protein S. *J Cell Biol.* 1986;102:1971-1978.

88. Esmon CT. The regulation of natural anticoagulant pathways. *Science.* 1987;235:1348-1352.

89. Esmon CT. The roles of protein C and thrombomodulin in the regulation of blood coagulation. *J Biol Chem.* 1989;264:4743-4746.

90. Oliver JA, Monroe DM, Church FC, et al. Activated protein C cleaves factor V$_a$ more efficiently on endothelium than on platelet surfaces. *Blood.* 2002;100:539-546.

91. Esmon CT. The endothelial cell protein C receptor. *Thromb Haemost.* 2000;83:639-643.

92. Laszik Z, Mitro A, Taylor FB, et al. Human protein C receptor is present primarily on endothelium of large blood vessels: implications for control of the protein C pathway. *Circulation.* 1997;96:3633-3640.

93. Taylor FB, Peer GT, Lockhart MS, et al. Endothelial cell protein C receptor plays an important role in protein C activation in vivo. *Blood.* 2001;97:1685-1688.

94. Joyce DE, Gelbert L, Ciaccia A, et al. Gene expression profile of antithrombotic protein C defines new mechanisms modulating inflammation and apoptosis. *J Biol Chem.* 2001;276:11199-11203.

95. Reiwald M, Petrovan RJ, Donner A, et al. Activation of endothelial cell protease activated receptor 1 by the protein C pathway. *Science.* 2002;296:1880-1882.

96. Wun T-C, Kretzmer KK, Girard TJ, et al. Cloning and characterization of a cDNA coding for the lipoprotein-associated coagulation inhibitor shows that it consists of three tandem Kunitz-type inhibitory domains. *J Biol Chem.* 1988;263:6001-6004.

97. Rapaport SI. Inhibition of factor VII$_a$/tissue factor-induced blood coagulation: with particular emphasis upon a factor X$_a$-dependent inhibitory mechanism. *Blood.* 1989;73:359-365.

98. Bajaj MS, Kuppuswamy MN, Saito H, et al. Cultured normal human hepatocytes do not synthesize lipoprotein-associated coagulation inhibitor: evidence that endothelium is the principal site of its synthesis. *Proc Natl Acad Sci U S A.* 1990;87:8869-8873.

99. Kato H. Regulation of functions of vascular wall cells by tissue factor pathway inhibitor: basic and clinical aspects. *Arterioscler Thromb Vasc Biol.* 2002;22:535-548.

100. Sandset PM, Abildgaard U, Larsen ML. Heparin induces release of extrinsic coagulation pathway inhibitor (EPI). *Thromb Res.* 1988;50:803-813.

101. Grant PJ, Medcalf RL. Hormonal regulation of haemostasis and the molecular biology of the fibrinolytic system. *Clin Sci (Lond).* 1990;78:3-11.

102. Huber D, Cramer EM, Kaufmann JE, et al. Tissue-type plasminogen activator (t-PA) is stored in Weibel–Palade bodies in human endothelial cells both in vitro and in vivo. *Blood.* 2002;15:3637-3645.

103. Hajjar KA, Hamel NM, Harpel PC, Nachman RL. Binding of tissue plasminogen activator to cultured human endothelial cells. *J Clin Invest.* 1987;80:1712-1719.

104. Levin EG, Loskutoff DJ. Cultured bovine endothelial cells produce both urokinase and tissue type plasminogen activators. *J Cell Biol.* 1982;94:631-636.

105. Philips M, Juul AG, Thorsen S. Human endothelial cells produce a plasminogen activator inhibitor and a tissue-type plasminogen activator-inhibitor complex. *Biochim Biophys Acta.* 1984;802:99-110.

106. Reddigari SR, Shibayama Y, Brunnee T, Kaplan AP. Human Hageman factor (Factor XII) and high molecular weight kininogen compete for the same binding site on human umbilical vein endothelial cells. *J Biol Chem.* 1993;268:11982-11987.

107. Shariat-Mader Z, Mahdi F, Schmaier AH. Factor XI assembly and activation on human umbilical vein endothelial cells in culture. *Thromb Haemost.* 2001;85:544-551.

108. Heimark RL, Schwartz SM. Binding of coagulation factors IX and X to the endothelial cell surface. *Biochem Biophys Res Commun.* 1983;111:723-731.

109. Rodgers GM, Shuman MA. Characterization of the interaction between factor X$_a$ and bovine aortic endothelial cells. *Biochim Biophys Acta.* 1985;844:320-329.

110. Stern DM, Nawroth PP, Kisiel W, et al. A coagulation pathway on bovine aortic segments leading to generation of factor X$_a$ and thrombin. *J Clin Invest.* 1984;74:1910-1921.

111. Stern DM, Drillings M, Nossel HL, et al. Binding of factors IX and IX$_a$ to cultured vascular endothelial cells. *Proc Natl Acad Sci U S A.* 1983;80:4119-4123.

112. Shuman MA. Thrombin-cellular interactions. *Ann N Y Acad Sci.* 1986;485:228-239.

113. Motta G, Rojkjaer R, Hasan AAK, et al. High molecular weight kininogen regulates prekallikrein assembly and activation on endothelial cells: a novel mechanism for contact activation. *Blood.* 1998;91:516-528.

114. Maruyama I, Salem HH, Majerus PW. Coagulation factor V$_a$ binds to human umbilical vein endothelial cells and accelerates protein C activation. *J Clin Invest.* 1984;74:224-230.

115. Cerveny TJ, Fass DN, Mann KG. Synthesis of coagulation factor V by cultured aortic endothelium. *Blood.* 1984;63:1467-1474.

116. Rodgers GM, Shuman MA. Prothrombin is activated on vascular endothelial cells by factor X$_a$ and calcium. *Proc Natl Acad Sci U S A.* 1983;80:7001-7005.

117. Jaffe EA, Hoyer LW, Nachman RL. Synthesis of antihemophilic factor antigen by cultured human endothelial cells. *J Clin Invest.* 1973;52:2757-2764.

118. Berrettini M, Schleef RR, Heeb MJ, et al. Assembly and expression of an intrinsic factor IX activator complex on the surface of cultured human endothelial cells. *J Biol Chem.* 1992;267:19833-19839.

119. Ratnoff OD, Everson B, Embury P, et al. Inhibition of the activation of Hageman factor (factor XII) by human vascular endothelial cell supernates. *Proc Natl Acad Sci U S A.* 1991;88:10740-10743.

120. Mann KG, Lawson JH. The role of the membrane in the expression of the vitamin K-dependent enzymes. *Arch Pathol Lab Med.* 1992;116:1330-1336.

121. Houdijk WP, deGroot PG, Nievelstein PF, Sakariassen KS, Sixma JJ. Subendothelial proteins and platelet adhesion: von Willebrand factor and fibronectin, not thrombospondin, are involved in platelet adhesion to extracellular matrix of human vascular endothelial cells. *Arteriosclerosis.* 1986;6:24-33.

122. Nemerson Y. Tissue factor and hemostasis. *Blood.* 1988;71:1-8.

123. Courtney MA, Haidaris PJ, Marder VJ, Sporn LA. Tissue factor mRNA expression in the endothelium of an intact umbilical vein. *Blood.* 1996;87:174-179.

124. Drake TA, Cheng J, Chang A, Taylor FB. Expression of tissue factor, thrombomodulin, and E-selectin in baboons with lethal *Escherichia coli* sepsis. *Am J Pathol.* 1993;142:1458-1470.

125. More L, Sim R, Hudson M, et al. Immunohistochemical study of tissue factor expression in normal intestine and idiopathic inflammatory bowel disease. *J Clin Pathol.* 1993;46:703-708.

126. Hammerschmidt DE. Tissue factor expression in sickle cell anemia. *J Lab Clin Med.* 2001;137:440.

127. Speiser W, Kapiotis S, Kopp CW, et al. Effect of intradermal tumor necrosis factor-alpha-induced inflammation on coagulation factors in dermal vessel endothelium: an in vivo study of human skin biopsies. *Thromb Haemost.* 2001;85:362-367.

128. Day SM, Reeve JL, Pedersen B, et al. Macrovascular thrombosis is driven by tissue factor derived primarily from the blood vessel wall. *Blood.* 2005;105:192-198.

129. Ivanciu L, Krishnaswamy S, Camire RM. New insights into the spatiotemporal localization of prothrombinase in vivo. *Blood.* 2014;124:1705-1714.

130. Pathak A, Zhao R, Monroe DM, et al. Thrombin generation in vascular tissue. *J Thromb Haemost.* 2006;4:60-67.

131. Coughlin SR. How the protease thrombin talks to cells. *Proc Natl Acad Sci U S A.* 1999;96:11023-11027.

132. Vu TK, Hung DT, Wheaton VI, Coughlin SR. Molecular cloning of a functional thrombin receptor reveals a novel proteolytic mechanism of receptor activation. *Cell.* 1991;64:1057-1068.

133. Alm AK, Norstrom E, Sundelin J, Nystedt S. Stimulation of proteinase activated receptor-2 causes endothelial cells to promote blood coagulation in vitro. *Thromb Haemost.* 1999;81:984-988.

134. Camerer E, Huang W, Coughlin SR. Tissue factor- and factor X-dependent activation of protease-activated receptor-2 by factor VII$_a$. *Proc Natl Acad Sci U S A.* 2000;97:5255-5260.

135. Hattori R, Hamilton KK, Fugate RD, McEver RP, Sims PJ. Stimulated secretion of von Willebrand factor is accompanied by rapid redistribution to the cell surface of the intracellular granule membrane protein GMP-140. *J Biol Chem.* 1989;264:7768-7771.

136. Mirza H, Yatsula V, Bahou WF. The proteinase activated receptor-2 (PAR-2) mediates mitogenic responses in human vascular endothelial cells. *J Clin Invest.* 1996;97:1705-1714.

137. Hirano K. The roles of proteinase-activated receptors in the vascular physiology and pathophysiology. *Arterioscler Thromb Vasc Biol.* 2007;27:27-36.

138. Nieman MT. Protease-activated receptors in hemostasis. *Blood.* 2016;128:169-177.

139. Liu L, Rodgers GM. Characterization of an inducible endothelial cell prothrombin activator. *Blood.* 1996;88:2989-2994.

140. Koshikawa N, Nagashima Y, Miyagi Y, et al. Expression of trypsin in vascular endothelial cells. *FEBS Lett.* 1997;409:442-448.

141. Moore KL, Esmon CT, Esmon NL. Tumor necrosis factor leads to the internalization and degradation of thrombomodulin from the surface of bovine aortic endothelial cells in culture. *Blood.* 1989;73:159-165.

142. Dittman WA, Majerus PW. Structure and function of thrombomodulin: a natural anticoagulant. *Blood.* 1990;75:329-336.

143. Bevilacqua MP, Schleef RR, Gimbrone MA, Loskutoff DJ. Regulation of the fibrinolytic system of cultured human vascular endothelium by interleukin 1. *J Clin Invest.* 1986;78:587-591.

144. Hathcock JJ. Flow effects on coagulation and thrombosis. *Arterioscler Thromb Vasc Biol.* 2006;26:1729-1737.

145. Garcia-Cardena G, Comander J, Anderson KR, Blackman BR, Gimbrone MA, Jr. Biomechanical activation of vascular endothelium as a determinant of its functional phenotype. *Proc Natl Acad Sci U S A.* 2001;98:4478-4485.

146. Matsumoto Y, Kawai Y, Watanabe K, et al. Fluid shear stress attenuates tumor necrosis factor-alpha-induced tissue factor expression in cultured human endothelial cells. *Blood.* 1998;91:4164-4172.

147. Aird WC, Edelberg JM, Weiler-Guettler H, Simmons WW, Smith TW, Rosenberg RD. Vascular bed-specific expression of an endothelial cell gene is programmed by the tissue microenvironment. *J Cell Biol.* 1997;138:1117-1124.

148. Charo IF, Shak S, Karasek MA, Davison PM, Goldstein IM. Prostaglandin I_2 is not a major metabolite of arachidonic acid in cultured endothelial cells from human foreskin microvessels. *J Clin Invest.* 1984;74:914-919.

149. Everett AD, Le Cras TD, Xue C, Johns RA. eNOS expression is not altered in pulmonary vascular remodeling due to increased pulmonary blood flow. *Am J Physiol.* 1998;274:L1058-L1065.

150. Mosnier LO, Meijers JC, Bouma BN. Regulation of fibrinolysis in plasma by TAFI and protein C is dependent on the concentration of thrombomodulin. *Thromb Haemost.* 2001;85:5-11.

151. Chi JT, Chang HY, Haraldsen G, et al. Endothelial cell diversity revealed by global expression profiling. *Proc Natl Acad Sci U S A.* 2003;100:10623-10628.

The Normal Hematologic System

Part 3

TRANSFUSION MEDICINE

Chapter 22 ■ Red Cell, Platelet, and White Cell Antigens

ERIC A. GEHRIE • HEATHER M. SMETANA • PAUL M. NESS

INTRODUCTION

The most common reason for a transfusion medicine physician to be contacted by a hematology service is for assistance with procuring an optimal blood component for infusion. In the posttransfusion period, transfusion services are most frequently queried for advice on the management of an adverse event, such as a suspected transfusion reaction or a disappointing response to transfusion. In both situations, the primary responsibility of the transfusion service is to interpret laboratory data relating to the transfused red blood cells (RBCs), platelets (PLTs), and (rarely) white blood cells and to determine the most likely clinical implications of these data in the context of the transfusion recipient. In this chapter, we aim to review the RBC, white blood cell, and PLT antigens that are most relevant to the practice of hematology. The emphasis of this chapter is on the clinical aspects of these topics that would be of interest to the practicing hematologist. For a detailed accounting of the biochemistry and genetics of blood group antigen systems, we refer the readers to previously published treatises.[1-4]

RBC ANTIGENS AND ANTIBODIES

The surface of the human erythrocyte is covered with hundreds of distinct antigens, which have been studied by immunohematologists for over 100 years. Some of these antigens are only expressed on RBCs, but others are found on organs, tissues, and fluids throughout the body. Transfusion of RBCs requires assessment of antibodies to RBC antigens that are circulating in the recipient's blood. Some of these antibodies, such as anti-A and anti-B (also known as isohemagglutinins), are naturally occurring. But, for individuals who have been previously exposed to allogeneic RBCs (eg, previous RBC transfusion or pregnancy), consideration must be given to the possibility that antibodies to allogeneic RBC antigens have been formed (alloimmunization). Importantly, transfusion of plasma containing blood components, including platelets, can also induce hemolysis if the transfused plasma contains antibodies that cross-react with antigens expressed on the recipient's RBCs (such as anti-A or anti-B). Herein, we highlight clinical considerations relating to RBC antigens, as well as antibodies that interact with them.

Major RBC Antigens

Of the many hundreds of antigens described in the blood banking literature, no group is more clinically important than the ABO blood group antigens. The A and B antigens are defined by immunodominant sugars: N-acetyl-D-galactosamine (A antigen) and D-galactose (B antigen). The A and B antigens are expressed on a precursor antigen called H. In blood group O individuals, H is the only expressed antigen (ie, there is no "O" antigen). The biochemistry of the ABO blood group is depicted in *Figure 22.1*. Among individuals of blood group A, B, or AB, expression of the A and B antigens on RBCs is weak at birth, but full expression occurs within the first few years of life.[5] Naturally occurring antibodies to the A and B antigens are generally present 3 to 6 months after birth and reach adult levels by early childhood.[6,7]

The purpose of blood group typing (the "type" portion of the "type and screen" test) is to determine whether the patient expresses one, both, or neither of the A or B antigens on their endogenous RBCs. This analysis is critical, as the assignment of an incorrect blood type to a patient could result in the provision of incompatible RBCs, which may induce an acute, life-threatening, intravascular hemolytic transfusion reaction.[8,9] Owing to the severity of this type of reaction, both donor and recipient are required to undergo two separately performed blood typing tests prior to the routine issuance of RBCs for transfusion.[10] In addition, blood banks are required to enforce strict rules regarding patient sample identification, as retrospective analysis has shown that patient identification errors are the most frequent cause of incompatible blood erroneously administered to a recipient.[11-14] RBCs (group O are required for patients without a blood type on file in the blood bank),[10] plasma, and platelets may be released by the blood bank without performing compatibility testing in emergency situations.

Serology

The expression (or lack thereof) of A and B antigens on RBCs is determined using monoclonal reagents. These reagents are derived from a single B-cell clone or a mixture of several clones, are highly reliable, and routinely subjected to quality control procedures in the blood bank. Typical results for ABO blood grouping of red cells (forward grouping) and plasma (reverse grouping) are depicted in *Table 22.1*.

Occasionally, weak expression of A (or, less commonly B) antigens can require further workup before type-specific RBCs can be issued for transfusion. The causes for unexpected serologic reactions during blood groupings are discussed in detail in the blood banking literature.[7] Some of the more common subtypes of A or B antigen are listed in *Table 22.2*.

In general, patients who are blood group A fall into two distinct categories: those whose RBCs agglutinate in the presence of the lectin *Dolichos biflorus* and those that do not. Blood from patients who are blood group A_1 agglutinates in the presence of this lectin; subgroups of A (such as A_2, etc.) do not. In the European population, the A_2 blood group is by far the most common subtype of A, as it is found in approximately 20% of blood group A population.[7] However, the A_2 subtype is far less common in other ethnicities, such as in Japan, where it is rare.[15] The A_2 subtype is rarely clinically relevant, but sometimes these patients form anti-A_1, which can interfere with blood grouping and, in rare instances, mediate a hemolytic transfusion reaction. Some blood banks may issue blood group A RBCs to patients with known anti-A_1 if there is no clinical history of hemolysis (which is rare), while others may always provide group O RBCs (out of an abundance of caution).

Expression of Major RBC Antigens on Organs and Tissues

In addition to being expressed on RBCs, the A and B antigens are also expressed on vascular endothelium, lung, heart, liver, kidney, and bone tissue.[16] Because genes controlling ABO and human leukocyte antigen (HLA) are inherited independently, major blood group antigens need to be taken into account in stem cell as well as solid

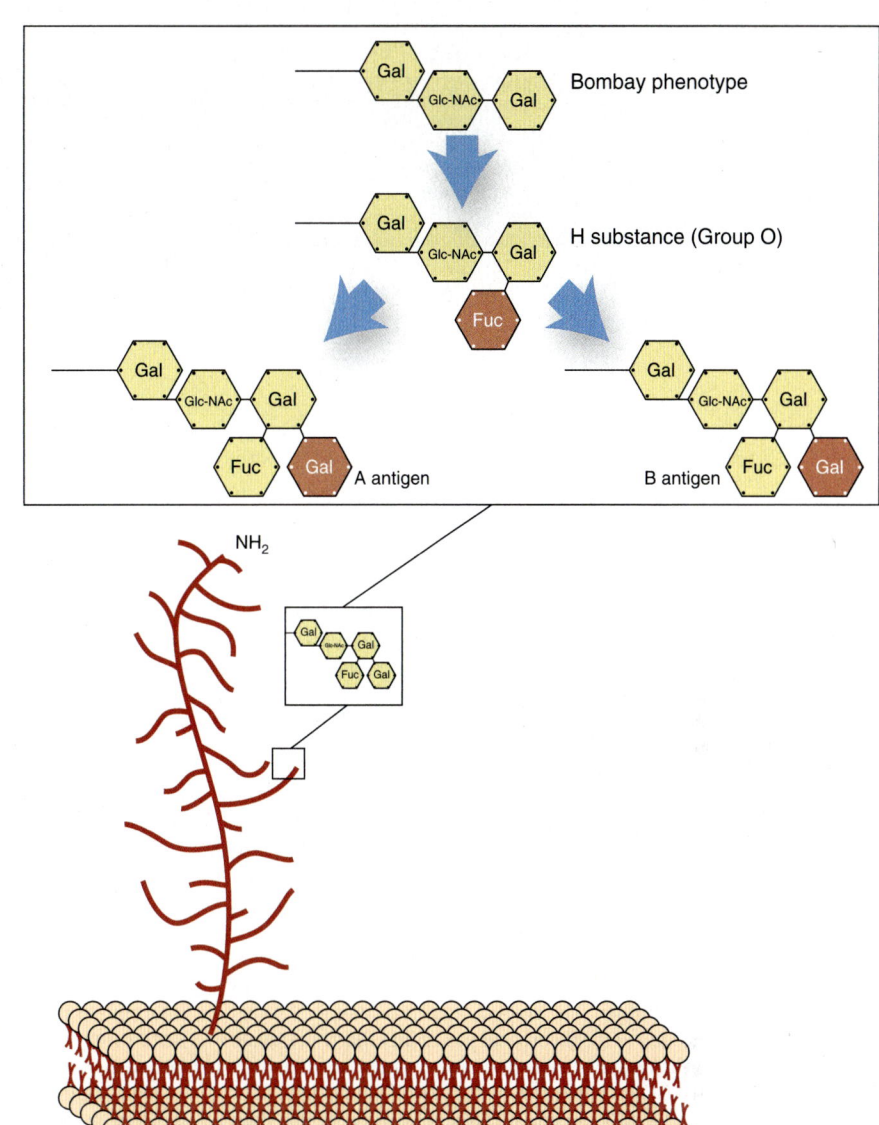

FIGURE 22.1 Biosynthesis of ABO blood group antigens. The antigens of the ABO system are located on the carbohydrate of type II oligosaccharides. H transferase is required to add fucose to the oligosaccharide chain and form H substance. Without the presence of H substance, A transferase and B transferase are not able to add terminal sugar moieties to the oligosaccharide chain. Fuc, l-fucose; Gal, d-galactose; Glc-Nac, d-N-acetyl-glucosamine.

Transfusion Medicine

Table 22.1. Expected Serologic Reactions for the Major ABO Blood Groups

Blood Group (Frequency in US Blood Donors)	Reaction of Patient Cells with Anti-A	Reaction of Patient Cells with Anti-B	Reaction of Group A Cells with Patient Plasma	Reaction of Group B Cells with Patient Plasma	Interpretation
O (45%-49%)	0	0	4+	4+	No A or B antigen on RBCs; anti-A and anti-B in plasma
A (27%-40%)	4+	0	0	2+	A antigen on RBCs; anti-B in plasma
B (11%-20%)	0	4+	3+	0	B antigen on RBCs; anti-A in plasma
AB (4%)	3+	3+	0	0	A and B antigen on RBCs; no anti-A or anti-B in plasma

Adapted from Harmening DM, Firestone D. The ABO blood group system. In: Harmening DM, ed. *Modern Blood Banking and Transfusion Practices.* 5th ed. FA Davis; 2005:110; Fung MK, ed. Chapter 12: *ABO, H, and Lewis blood groups and structurally related antigens.* In: *AABB Technical Manual.* 18th ed. AABB Press; 2014:292, Table 12.1.

Table 22.2. Some Important Subtypes of Blood Group A and Blood Group B

	Group A Subtypes				Group B Subtypes		
	Expected Reaction of Patient RBCs with Reagent anti-A	Anti-B Detectable in Patient Serum?	Associated with Hemolysis in Response to transfusion with Group A RBCs?		Expected Reaction of Patient RBCs with Reagent anti-B	Anti-A Detectable in Patient Serum	Associated with Hemolysis in Response to transfusion with Group B RBCs?
A_2	Normal	Yes	<3%	B_3	Weak	Yes	Almost never
A_3	Weak	Yes	Almost never	B_x	Weak	Yes	Almost never
A_x	Weak	Yes	Almost never	B_m	Weak	Yes	Almost never
A_{end}	Weak	Yes	Almost never	B_{el}	None	Yes	Almost never
A_m	Weak	Yes	Almost never				
A_y	None	Yes	Almost never				
A_{el}	None	Yes	Almost never				

Adapted from Harmening DM, Firestone D. The ABO blood group system. In: Harmening DM, ed. *Modern Blood Banking and Transfusion Practices.* 5th ed. FA Davis; 2005:120-121.

organ transplantation, as there is no guarantee that an HLA-matched donor will be ABO compatible (or vice versa). While modern medical advancements have permitted the transplantation of hematopoietic stem cells and some solid organs with protocols to reduce incompatible antibody titers (eg, liver, kidney), ABO incompatibility between donor and recipient remains a major impediment to adult cardiac transplantation. Note is made that, unlike solid organs, stem cell grafts can be modified in the laboratory to reduce the quantity of incompatible RBCs or plasma.[17]

Secretors

Approximately 80% of the population express the major blood group antigens in their saliva, free floating in their plasma, and in their other body fluids. These individuals have inherited a gene (Se (FUT2) or secretor genotype) that results in the production of an enzyme (alpha-2-L-fucosyltransferase) that allows the H antigen to be expressed in body fluids. In blood group A, B, or AB individuals, the H antigen on both RBCs and free floating in body fluids is further modified to express the A and/or B antigen. The clinical significance of this observation is generally limited to the theoretical possibility that individuals with free floating antigens are less likely to demonstrate hemolysis as a consequence of an ABO incompatible plasma or platelet transfusion. It is also notable that secretors express different Lewis antigens than nonsecretors. This concept is depicted in *Figure 22.2* and is discussed in more detail in the section discussing the Lewis antigens below.

Bombay and Para-Bombay

In rare instances, patients can have a genetic absence (Bombay nonsecretor) or deficiency (Para-Bombay or Bombay secretor) of the H antigen. These individuals appear to be blood group O during routine blood typing, because the H antigen is required for expression of the A or B antigen. Importantly, these patients develop anti-H in addition to anti-A and anti-B, and the anti-H is usually detected by antibody screening tests. In a patient with Bombay or Para-Bombay phenotype, anti-H can mediate severe intravascular hemolysis. If alerted, the blood bank or reference laboratory can differentiate a blood group O individual from an H-deficient or H-absent individual using a protein (lectin) derived from the *Ulex europaeus* plant, which will react with (agglutinate) blood group O RBCs but not with RBCs from patients with Bombay phenotype. Note that, in most cases, it is very difficult to procure compatible RBCs for patients with the Bombay phenotype, as the only acceptable RBC donor is a donor who is also of the Bombay blood type.

Minor RBC Antigens and Antibodies

In addition to the A, B, and H antigens, there are hundreds of additional RBC antigens that are referred to as "minor" antigens. Many of the minor RBC antigens are clinically significant, capable of causing hemolysis in transfusion recipients, hemolytic disease of the fetus and newborn (HDFN), and complications during stem cell (or rarely solid organ) transplantation. The minor RBC antigens are summarized in *Table 22.3.* We emphasize that the salient difference between uncrossmatched RBCs provided during an emergency and routine crossmatched RBCs is only crossmatched RBCs are required to account for these antigens. Emergency release units have no such requirement, as they are only required to account for the recipient's ABO type (or to use group O donor cells).

It is well known that most antibodies to minor RBC fade to the point of becoming undetectable by routine laboratory testing over a period of months to years after formation.[20] This tendency, referred to as antibody evanescence in the transfusion literature, frustrates the study of alloimmunization and can confuse clinicians because the current antibody screening test can appear to be negative yet the blood bank will insist that the patient has a history of antibodies. In addition, because antibodies can quickly reemerge after transfusion with RBCs that express the cognate antigen, the risk of a hemolytic transfusion reaction is believed to be higher among patients who have a history of intermittent transfusion without follow-up or of transfusion at unaffiliated hospitals or clinics. The timeframe for antibody evanescence is believed to be antibody specific.

Antibody evanescence is perhaps the most common reason for a delayed hemolytic transfusion reaction. The most common scenario is a patient presenting to a hospital for the first time, with a history of blood transfusion at an outside hospital, which they may or may not recall. If the blood bank is not informed of the patient's transfusion history, and/or previously formed antibodies have evanesced to a level below the lower limit of detection for the antibody screen, then the antibody will not be accounted for in the crossmatch. Transfusion reactions may be precipitated by the resulting anamnestic response and can range from severe (eg, intravascular hemolysis with associated disseminated intravascular coagulation and renal injury) to mild (eg, mild, but clinically significant extravascular hemolysis) to clinically silent (eg, asymptomatic patient with mildly elevated indirect bilirubin and lactate dehydrogenase).[21] The silent reactions are described as delayed *serologic* transfusion reactions; although these have no immediate clinical sequelae, subsequent transfusions may produce a hemolytic transfusion reaction and the antibodies that persist may delay blood availability.[22] The development of antibody registries, which would ideally contain blood bank records for transfused patients, would be a tremendous resource toward the goal of preventing these reactions, particularly for patients with cancer or sickle cell disease who are at higher risk of being transfused at more than one hospital.

Rh Antigens and Antibodies

The Rh (historically referred to as the Rhesus) antigens are perhaps the most frequently encountered minor RBC antigens in the blood bank. While there are 56 Rh antigens identified to date, the blood bank is mainly concerned with the D antigen, as antibodies to the D antigen

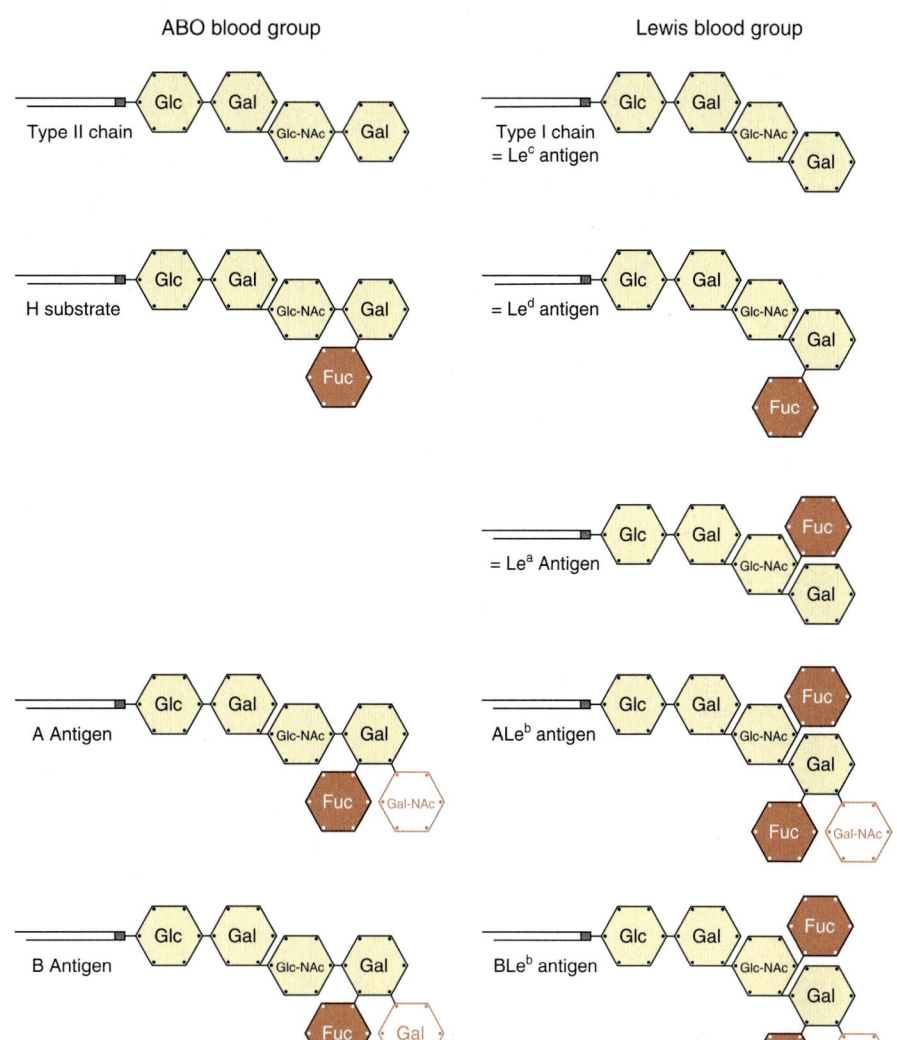

ABO blood group

Lewis blood group

FIGURE 22.2 Differences between ABO (A) and Lewis (B) blood groups. ABO blood group antigens are synthesized in the red cells on type II oligosaccharides, but Lewis blood group antigens are produced in the plasma on type I oligosaccharides and then adsorbed onto the red cell surface. Type II oligosaccharide chains differ from type I chains in the linking position of the terminal galactose moiety. The Le (FUT3) gene encodes type III H transferase, which adds a fucose group (red-colored fucose group) to the second-last sugar moiety of the type I oligosaccharide chain. Synthesis of the Lec and Led antigens does not depend on the activity of the Le gene. Fuc, l-fucose; Gal, d-galactose; Gal-Nac, d-N-acetyl-galactosamine; Glc, d-glucosamine; Glc-Nac, d-N-acetyl-glucosamine.

Transfusion Medicine

(anti-D) can mediate severe hemolytic transfusion reactions, as well as HDFN. Individuals who express the D antigen are referred to as being RhD positive, while individuals who do not express the D antigen are referred to as RhD negative. Other clinically significant Rh antigens include C, c, E, and e antigens.

The Rh antigens are expressed by two closely linked genes, *RHD* and *RHCE*, that have inverted gene orientation and share significant sequence homology. The *RHD* gene codes for the presence or absence of the D antigen, while the *RHCE* gene codes for any of the four combinations of C/c and E/e antigens (CE, Ce, cE, ce).

The blood bank uses specialized terminology to simplify the communication of patterns of expression of these antigens (*Table 22.4*). Note that the "d" antigen is not an Rh antigen; the use of "d" in Rh nomenclature only signifies the absence of the D antigen. In order to prevent formation of anti-D, RhD-negative individuals are generally transfused with RhD-negative RBCs; this is especially true among females of childbearing potential given the risk of HDFN posed by anti-D.

Although RhD is a highly immunogenic antigen, it is generally possible to prevent alloimmunization to the D antigen, when exposed, in an RhD-negative individual by administering an adequate dose of RhIG within 72 hours of exposure to RhD-positive RBCs.[23-25] Without administration of RhIG, the probability of alloimmunization may be as high as 90% in certain patient populations.[26] RhIG is a concentrate of anti-D that is manufactured from individuals who are sensitized to the RhD antigen.[25] It is not recombinant. The mechanism of action of RhIG is not specifically known, although it is believed that administered RhIG binds to enough D antigen sites on RBCs to result in removal from circulation, reduction in immunogenicity, and some degree of suppression of the maternal immune response to the antigen. The risk of alloimmunization to the D antigen is quite heterogeneous depending on the type of exposure and the overall clinical scenario. For example, injection of just a few milliliters of RBCs into a healthy volunteer would be expected to induce alloimmunization in >90% of individuals, while hospitalized patients and oncology patients are at far lower risk.[27]

In the hematology population, there has traditionally been concern that RhD-negative patients with cancer could form anti-D via exposure to platelets collected from RhD-positive blood donors. Although Rh antigens such as D are not expressed on platelets, each platelet concentrate contains a small number (generally <0.1 mL if collected by apheresis) of RBCs, due to incomplete separation of RBCs from platelets during collection. Exposure to these RhD-positive RBCs could lead to alloimmunization to the D antigen (historically, this incidence was reported to be up to 19%[27-29]; however, modern platelet manufacturing techniques have greatly diminished the volume of RBCs that are contained within a unit of platelets. Accordingly, the incidence of alloimmunization to the D antigen as a result of platelet transfusion has greatly decreased, with a large, multicenter clinical trial reporting an alloimmunization rate of 1.4%, even without RhIG prophylaxis.[30] As a result, RhIG is generally not administered to RhD-negative patients receiving platelets from RhD-positive donors unless

Table 22.3. International Society for Blood Transfusion Schematic of Blood Group Systems

ISBT No.	System Name (symbol)	No. of Antigens	Antigen(s)	Gene Name by HUGO Gene Nomenclature	Gene Product(s)	Chromosomal Location
001	ABO (ABO)	4	A, B, A,B, A1	ABO	A = α-3-N-acetylgalactosaminyltransferase B = α-3-D galactosyltransferase	9q34.2
002	MNS (MNS)	50	M, N, S, s, U, He, Mi^a, M^c, Vw, Mur, M^g, Vr, M^e, Mt^a, St^a, Ri^a, Cl^a, Ny^a, Hut, Hil, M^v, Far, s^D, Mit, Dantu, Hop, Nob, En^a, ENKT, N, Or, DANE, TSEN, MINY, MUT, SAT, ERIK, Os^a, ENEP, ENEH, HAG, ENAV, MARS, ENDA, ENEV, MNTD, SARA, KIPP, JENU, SUMI	GYPA GYPB (GYPE)	Glycophorin A (GYPA; CD235a) Glycophorin B (GYPB; CD235b) Glycophorin E (GYPE)	4q31.21
003	P1PK	3	P1, P^k, NOR	A4GALT	CD77	22q13.2
004	Rh (RH)	56	D, C, E, c, e, f, Ce, C^w, C^x, V, E^w, G, Hr$_o$, Hr, hr^s, VS, C^G, CE, D^w, c-like, cE, hr^H, Rh29, Go^a, hr^B, Rh32, Rh33, Hr^B, Rh35, Be^a, Evans, Rh39, Tar, Rh41, Rh42, Crawford, Nou, Riv, Sec, Dav, JAL, STEM, FPTT, MAR, BARC, JAHK, DAK, LOCR, CENR, CEST, CELO, CEAG, PARG, CEVF, CEWA, CETW	RHD RHCE	Acetylated RhD protein Acetylated RhCE protein (CD240)	1p36.11
005	Lutheran (LU)	27	Lu^a, Lu^b, Lu3, Lu4, Lu5, Lu6, Lu7, Lu8, Lu9, Lu11, Lu12, Lu13, Lu14, Lu16, Lu17, Au^a, Au^b, Lu20, Lu21, LURC, LUIT, LUGA, LUAC, LUBI, LUYA, LUNU, LURA	BCAM	B-cell adhesion molecule (CD239)	19q13.2
006	Kell (KEL)	36	K, k, Kp^a, Kp^b, Ku, Js^a, Js^b, Ul^a, K11, K12, K13, K14, K16, K17, K18, K19, Km, Kp^c, K22, K23, K24, VLAN, TOU, RAZ, VONG, KALT, KTIM, KYO, KUCI, KANT, KASH, KELP, KETI, KHUL, KYOR, KEAL	KEL	Zinc endopeptidase (CD238)	7q33
007	Lewis (LE)	6	Le^a, Le^b, Le^{ab}, Le^{bH}, Ale^b, Ble^b	FUT3	α-1,3/1,4-L-Fucosyltransferase	19p13.3
008	Duffy (FY)	5	Fy^a, Fy^b, Fy3, Fy5, Fy6	ACKR1	Duffy antigen receptor for chemokines (CD234)	1q21-q22
009	Kidd (JK)	3	Jk^a, Jk^b, Jk3	SLC14A1	Urea transporter	18q11-q12
010	Diego (DI)	23	Di^a, Di^b, Wr^a, Wr^b, Wd^a, Rb^a, WARR, ELO, Wu, Bp^a, Mo^a, Hg^a, Vg^a, Sw^a, BOW, NFLD, Jn^a, KREP, Tr^a, Fr^a, SW1, DISK, DIST	SLC4A1	Anion exchanger 1, solute carrier family 4/band 3 (CD233)	17q21.31
011	Yt (YT)	5	Yt^a, Yt^b, YTEG, YTLI, YTOT	ACHE	Acetylcholinesterase	7q22
012	Xg (XG)	2	Xg^a, CD99	XG MIC2	Xg^a glycoprotein (CD99)	Xp22.32
013	Scianna (SC)	9	Sc1, Sc2, Sc3, Rd, STAR, SCER, SCAN, SCAR, SCAC	ERMAP	Erythrocyte membrane-associated protein (ERMAP)	1p34.2
014	Dombrock (DO)	10	Do^a, Do^b, Gy^a, Hy, Jo^a, DOYA, DOMR, DOLG, DOLC, DODE	ART4	ADP-ribosyltransferase 4 (CD297)	12p13-p12
015	Colton (CO)	4	Co^a, Co^b, Co3, Co4	AQP1	Aquaporin-1 (AQP1)	7p14
016	Landsteiner-Wiener (LW)	3	LW^a, LW^{ab}, LW^b	ICAM4	Intracellular adhesion molecule 4 (ICAM4) (CD242)	19p13.2
017	Chido/Rodgers (CH/RG)	9	Chapter 1, Chapter 2, Chapter 3, Chapter 4, Chapter 5, Chapter 6, WH, Rg1, Rg2	C4A C4B	Complement component 4A protein Complement component 4B protein	6p21.3
018	H (H)	1	H	FUT1	Galactoside 2-α-L-fucosyltransferase 1 (CD173)	19q13.33
019	Kx (XK)	1	Kx	XK	Membrane transport protein XK	Xp21.1

(Continued)

Table 22.3. International Society for Blood Transfusion Schematic of Blood Group Systems (Continued)

ISBT No.	System Name (symbol)	No. of Antigens	Antigen(s)	Gene Name by HUGO Gene Nomenclature	Gene Product(s)	Chromosomal Location
020	Gerbich (GE)	13	Ge2, Ge3, Ge4, Wb, Ls^a, An^a, Dh^a, GEIS, GEPL, GEAT, GETI, GECT, GEAR	GYPC	Glycophorin C (GPC; CD236) and GPD (glycophorin C precursor)	2q14-q21
021	Cromer (CROM)	20	Cr^a, Tc^a, Tc^b, Tc^c, Dr^a, Es^a, IFC, WES^a, WES^b, UMC, GUTI, SERF, ZENA, CROV, CRAM, CROZ, CRUE, CRAG, CROK, CORS	CD55	CD55/decay accelerating factor (DAF)	1q32
022	Knops (KN)	12	Kn^a, Kn^b, McC^a, Sl1, Yk^a, McC^b, Sl2, Sl3, KCAM, KDAS, DACY, YCAD	CR1	CD35	1q32.2
023	Indian (IN)	6	In^a, In^b, INFI, INJA, INRA, INSL	CD44	CD44	11p13
024	Ok (OK)	3	Ok^a, OKGV, OKVM	BSG	Basigin (CD147)	19p13.3
025	Raph (RAPH)	1	MER2	CD151	CD151	11p15.5
026	John Milton Hagen (JMH)	8	JMH, JMHK, JMHL, JMHG, JMHM, JMHQ, JMHN, JMHA	SEMA7A	Semaphorin 7A (CD108)	15q22.3-q23
027	I (I)	1	I	GCNT2	I-α-1, 6-N-acetylglucosaminyltransferase A	6p24.2
028	Globoside (GLOB)	2	P, PX2	B3GALNT1	UDP-N-acetyl-galactosamineglobotriaosylceramide 3-α-N-acetylgalactosaminyl-transferase	3q25
029	Gill (GIL)	1	GIL	AQP3	Aquaporin-3 (AQP3)	9p13
030	Rh-associated glycoprotein (RHAG)	4	Duclos, Ol^a, DSLK, Kg	RHAG	CD241	6p12.3
031	Forssman (FOR)	1	FORS1	GBGT1	Globoside alpha-1,3-N-acetylgalactosaminyltransferase 1	9q34.13-q34.3
032	JR	1	Jr^a	ABCG2	ATP-binding cassette, subfamily G (WHITE), member 2 (CD338)	4q22.1
033	LAN	1	Lan	ABCB6	ATP-binding cassette, subfamily B (MDR/TAP), member 6	2q36
034	VEL	1	Vel	SMIM1	SMIM1	1p36.32
035	CD59	1	CD59.1	CD59	CD59	11p13
036	Augustine	4	AUG1, At^a, ATML, ATAM	SLC29A1	Equilibrative nucleoside transporter 1 (ENT1)	6p21.1
037	KANNO	1	KANNO1	PRNP	CD230	20p13
038	SID	1	Sd^a	B4GALNT2	B4GALNT2-encoded transferase	17q21.32
039	CTL2	2	RIF, VER	SLC44A2		19p13.2
040	PEL	1	PEL	ABCC4		13q32.1
041	MAM	1	MAM	EMP3		19q13.33
042	EMM	1	Emm	PIGG		4p16.3
043	ABCC1	1	WLF	ABCC1		16p13.11

HUGO Gene Nomenclature Committee (www.genenames.org)[18]; ISBT, International Society of Blood Transfusion[19]; No, number.

Data from Daniels GL, Fletcher A, Garratty G, et al. International Society of Blood Transfusion Working Party on terminology for red cell surface antigens. *Vox Sang.* 2004;87:304-316; Denomme GA, Rios M, Reid ME. *Molecular Protocols in Transfusion Medicine.* Academic Press, 2000; Logdberg L, Reid MA, Lamont RE, et al. Human blood group genes 2004: chromosomal locations and cloning strategies. *Transfus Med Rev.* 2005;19:45-57; Costa FP, Hue-Roye K, Sausais L, et al. Absence of DOMR, a new antigen in the Dombrock blood group system that weakens expression of Do(b), Gy(a), Hy, Jo(a), and DOYA antigens. *Transfusion.* 2010;50:2026-2031; Smart EA, Storry JR. The OK blood group system: a review. *Immunohematology.* 2010:26:124-126; Walker PS, Reid ME. The Gerbich blood group system: a review. *Immunohematology.* 2010:26:124-126; International Society of Blood Transfusion Working Party on terminology for red cell antigens web site. http://www.isbtweb.org. Accessed January 25, 2017; and HUGO Gene Nomenclature Committee (HGNC) web site. www.genenames.org. Accessed January 25, 2017.

Transfusion Medicine

Table 22.4. Terminology Used to Describe Rh Blood Group Antigens

Weiner Terminology	Fisher-Race Terminology	Haplotype Frequency in Various Racial Groups			
		African American	Asian	Native American	Caucasian
r	Dce	26%	3%	11%	37%
r'	dCe	2%	2%	2%	2%
r''	dcE	<1%	<1%	6%	1%
r^y	dCE	<1%	1%	<1%	<1%
R_0	Dce	44%	3%	2%	4%
R_1	DCe	17%	70%	44%	42%
R_2	DcE	11%	21%	34%	14%
R_z	DCE	<1%	1%	6%	<1%

Adapted from Harmening DM, Firestone D. The ABO blood group system. In: Harmening DM, ed. *Modern Blood Banking and Transfusion Practices*, 5th ed. FA Davis; 2005:136.

the patient is of childbearing potential, although prescribing patterns are highly heterogenous.

Individuals of different racial backgrounds typically express Rh antigens at different frequencies. For example, individuals of Asian or Native American descent are much less likely to be RhD negative, compared with individuals of Caucasian or African American background. In addition, African Americans are much less likely to express the C or E antigens compared with Caucasians. Some of these expression patterns could explain the frequency of the development of antibodies to these antigens in various ethnic groups.

Blood banks employ a number of techniques in order to identify patients with unusually low expression of D antigen on their RBCs. The reason for this is that patients with lower expression of the D antigen may be at risk of developing anti-D if they are exposed to RhD-positive RBCs. It is not generally possible to reliably determine which patients with low expression of the D antigen are at risk of alloimmunization to the D antigen as a result of transfusion based on serologic tests alone. Consequently, many experts recommend performing *RHD* genotyping on patients with weak serologic testing results, especially if alloimmunization to the D antigen would be of significant clinical impact (eg, for women of childbearing potential).[31] For a discussion of this approach, see the section "*Determining the Rh status of patients with low serologic expression of RhD*".

Kell Antigens and Antibodies

Similar to Rh, the Kell antigens are clinically significant and frequently taken into consideration during the crossmatch. The Kell antigens are believed to be nearly as immunogenic as the D antigen.[32] Although there are 36 antigens in the Kell blood group system, the only antibody that is routinely clinically encountered is the K antigen. The remaining antigens are generally either relatively common (expressed by >90% of individuals) or infrequently encountered (expressed by <5% of individuals), making them far less likely to result in alloimmunization.[33]

Alloantibodies to K antigens are frequently IgG class and are capable of mediating both hemolytic transfusion reaction as well as HDFN. Unfortunately, anti-K has been reported to mediate severe hemolytic disease of the fetus and newborn, even at relatively low titers, compared with anti-D. The ability of anti-K to mediate HDFN at low titers is believed to be due to the expression of the K antigen on erythroid precursors, allowing anti-K to suppress erythropoiesis.[34] On rare occasions, an IgM class anti-K can be produced in response to infection, although, in contrast to the more typically encountered IgG class anti-K, the clinical significance of IgM class anti-K is uncertain.[35]

In addition, the introduction of daratumumab (anti-CD38) therapy into the medical mainstream for multiple myeloma has increased demand for K antigen–negative RBCs for transfusion. The reason for this growing concern is that many blood banks use a chemical technique to remove CD38 from the surface of reagent RBCs used to

perform antibody screening on patients receiving daratumumab therapy. Unfortunately, the Kell antigens (as well as several families of antigens that are generally not clinically important) are also susceptible to this chemical treatment (usually dithiothreitol), and thus, unless the patient is definitively known to express K antigen on their native RBCs, they are generally transfused with RBCs from donors whose cells do not express the K antigen.[36,37] Some blood banks ask that a blood sample is sent to the blood bank for a complete workup prior to the initiation of daratumumab therapy. Fortunately, more than 90% of blood donors in the United States are K antigen negative, making the procurement of these cells relatively routine for most transfusion services. For additional information regarding the impact of monoclonal antineoplastic agents on the blood compatibility testing process please see the section "*Impact of Novel Cancer Drugs on Transfusion Compatibility Testing.*"

It is important to note that the Kell antigen is linked to the Xk protein by a disulfide bond. The Xk protein is not a member of the Kell antigen system; it is a separate blood group system encoded by a separate gene (*XK*), which is located on the X chromosome (see *Table 22.3*).

Patients with the X-linked McLeod syndrome suffer from neurologic, psychiatric, and muscular complications and are sometimes identified by the presence of acanthocytes on their peripheral blood smear. Patients with McLeod syndrome also can have a diminished expression of Kell antigens on their RBCs (McLeod phenotype), and one particular Kell antigen (K_m) is completely absent from RBCs of patients with McLeod phenotype. Patients with McLeod phenotype are therefore at risk for developing anti-K_m if they are transfused with RBCs. Developing anti-K_m would make a transfusion recipient incompatible with almost all blood donors. Even more dramatically, people who have both McLeod phenotype and X-linked chronic granulomatous disease can develop anti-K_m as well as anti-Kx, which would make finding compatible blood essentially impossible. As a result, it is recommended to seek the advice of a transfusion medicine expert prior to transfusing a patient with McLeod syndrome, particularly if they also have chronic granulomatous disease.[33]

Kidd Antigens and Antibodies

There are three antigens in the Kidd system (Jk^a, Jk^b, and JK3). These antigens are anchored to Human Urea Transporter 11 (HUT11). It is believed that HUT11 helps to protect RBCs from being damaged while traversing the urea-rich environment of the renal medulla. The RBCs of individuals who lack expression of both the Jk^a and the Jk^b antigen are susceptible to in vitro hemolysis by concentrated urea; however, RBCs from these individuals have normal lifespan and normal function in vivo. Outside of RBCs, Kidd antigens are also expressed on renal endothelium.

Because JK3 is expressed essentially universally, the only two antigens that are generally relevant to the blood bank are Jk^a and Jk^b.

Approximately 70% to 80% of individuals of Caucasian or Asian descent express each of these antigens on their RBCs. However, among African Americans, Jk^a expression is more frequent (approximately 90%) but Jk^b expression is less frequent (approximately 40%). Jk^a and Jk^b antigens are expressed during the first trimester of fetal life.[4]

Antibodies to Jk^a and Jk^b are generally clinically significant, complement fixing, IgG class antibodies that are capable of mediating severe intravascular hemolysis and HDFN. These antibodies are particularly troublesome for blood banks because they tend to remain detectable for only a short period of time before evanescence. As a result, they are a relatively common cause of delayed hemolytic transfusion reactions.

Duffy Antigens and Antibodies

There are five antigens in the Duffy blood group system, each of which is expressed on a chemokine receptor (the Duffy antigen receptor for chemokines, or DARC). Of these antigens, only two are generally clinically important: Fy^a and Fy^b. The remaining antigens (Fy3, Fy5, and Fy6) rarely complicate compatibility testing. Duffy antigens are expressed throughout the body on various organ endothelium, including in the brain and the kidney.[16]

Antigen expression patterns of Fy^a and Fy^b are highly variable among different ethnic groups. Most striking is that approximately 68% of African Americans (and up to 100% of Africans) do not express either antigen on their RBCs.[33] In contrast, nearly 100% of Caucasians and 76% of Chinese individuals express at least one of these two antigens on their RBCs.[38] This observation is likely explained by the fact that individuals who express neither Fy^a nor Fy^b on their RBCs are resistant to infection by *Plasmodium vivax* and *Plasmodium knowlesi*.[33] The mutation (GATA) that is responsible for the lack of Duffy antigen expression on the RBCs of African-descended populations is erythroid specific. As a result, many African-descended individuals are incapable of forming anti-Fy^b in response to transfusion owing to expression of Duffy antigens on tissues other than RBCs.[33] As a result, prophylactic antigen matching programs for sickle cell disease populations generally do not require provision of Fy^b-negative RBCs.[39]

Antibodies to Fy^a and Fy^b are both generally clinically significant, warm-reacting, IgG antibodies that can mediate both hemolytic transfusion reactions as well as HDFN.

MNS Antigens and Antibodies

The MNS blood group system consists of 50 antigens. Of these, only five—M, N, S, s, and U—are likely to cause complications in clinical practice; the remaining antigens are mostly either too high or too low in incidence to be encountered, except in rare circumstances.[40] The M and N antigens are expressed on glycophorin A (CD235a), while the S, s, and U antigens are expressed on glycophorin B (CD235b). Both of these glycophorins are receptors for *Plasmodium falciparum*. Glycophorin A and the M and N antigens are present on renal tissues.[41] There are not major differences in M, N, S, s, or U expression in different ethnic groups, with the exception of the rare S-s-U- phenotype, which is found in approximately 2% of individuals of African descent.

Anti-M is frequently encountered in the blood bank. Generally, these antibodies are cold-reacting, IgM class entities that can complicate the blood bank crossmatching process, but they are clinically insignificant. However, warm-reacting, IgG class anti-M can mediate hemolytic transfusion reactions and HDFN.[42] As with anti-M, antibodies to the N antigen are generally not clinically significant.

In contrast to anti-M and anti-N, antibodies to S and s are generally IgG class, warm-reacting, clinically significant entities. Anti-S and anti-s can mediate hemolytic transfusion reactions and HDFN.[43-45]

Anti-U is occasionally encountered by transfusion services. This clinically significant antibody is capable of mediating hemolysis as well as fetal anemia. Patients with anti-U do not express S or s and thus are at risk of forming all three antibodies. Because the U antigen (which is an abbreviation for Universal) is extremely high incidence, it can be very difficult to procure U antigen negative units of RBCs for transfusion, although these units often can be obtained within a week or two from rare donor networks.[33] In cases where RBC transfusion is pursued for patients with an anti-U, it is important to obtain RBCs from a donor who is truly U negative, not U variant, as patients with anti-U can have hemolytic transfusion reactions in response to transfusion with RBCs from U variant donors, who may type as U negative by serologic methods.

Lewis Antigens and Antibodies

Unlike the other antigens discussed in this chapter, the Lewis antigens are not produced by the RBC; rather, they are produced in the plasma and secretions and are then adsorbed onto the surface of the RBC. There are two principal antigens in the Lewis system, Le^a and Le^b; the other Lewis antigens are amalgams of the Le^a or Le^b antigens with the A and/or B antigens. Expression of Le^a is controlled by a fucosyltransferase (FUT3), while expression of Le^b requires the underlying presence of the secretor (Se) gene. Because the antigens are adsorbed, transfused RBCs eventually come to express the same Lewis antigen pattern as the patient's native RBCs. The physiology of pregnancy frequently results in a transient reduction of Lewis antigen expression on RBCs. In addition, the Lewis antigens adsorb onto cells other than RBCs, including gastrointestinal, renal, and genitourinary tissues, and platelets. Lewis antigens are not well expressed at birth and are not fully developed until age 5 years.[35] Le^b is a receptor for norovirus and *Helicobacter pylori*. The genetics of the Lewis system are of great interest to serologists, and are discussed in detail in blood bank reference textbooks, but are of limited importance to the practicing hematologist.[7,46]

Lewis antibodies are almost always cold-reactive, IgM antibodies that are not clinically significant. These antibodies are most frequently identified among pregnant women with (frequently transient) reduction in Lewis antigen expression. In that context, Lewis antibodies are almost never clinically significant. On occasion, however, a pathologic Lewis antibody can be identified.[47,48] In these rare occasions, the blood bank may insist on providing antigen-negative, crossmatch-compatible RBCs for transfusion. *Figure 22.3* depicts the biochemistry of the GLOB (which houses the P antigen), I, and ABO blood groups.

P Antigens and Antibodies

Historically, blood bankers referred to the P1PK blood group system as consisting of four antigens: P, P_1, P^k, and Luke (LKE). More recently, these antigens have been subdivided into different antigen systems, with P_1, P^k, and NOR in the P1PK blood group system and P and PX2 in the GLOB blood group system. Anti-PP_1P_k and anti-P have been reported to mediate repeated spontaneous abortion.[49,50] Approximately 21% of Europeans and 6% of Africans lack expression of the P_1 antigen on their RBCs. Approximately one-quarter of these individuals have circulating anti-P_1, which is almost always a clinically insignificant, cold-reacting, IgM class antibody.[7] However, when alloanti-P_1 does react at body temperature, hemolytic transfusion reactions can result.[51] Hemolytic disease of the fetus and newborn is thought not to be mediated by alloanti-P_1, mainly due to the inability of IgM to cross the placenta and the limited expression of P_1 antigen on fetal RBCs.[40] Antibodies to P^k are quite rare but can sometimes mediate severe hemolysis.

Autoantibodies with specificity for the P antigen are believed to mediate paroxysmal cold hemoglobinuria. Unlike the antibodies mentioned above, these autoantibodies (frequently referred to as Donath-Landsteiner antibodies) bind at low temperatures and then mediate hemolysis at 37°C. Interestingly, these antibodies typically result in a negative direct antiglobulin test (DAT) for IgG, owing to the tendency for these antibodies to dissociate from RBCs at 37°C. The DAT is generally positive for complement only.[52] In the modern era, these antibodies are almost always observed in pediatric patients.[53] Note is made that the P antigen is also the target for parvovirus B19, which is associated with aplastic crisis in hematology patients.[54]

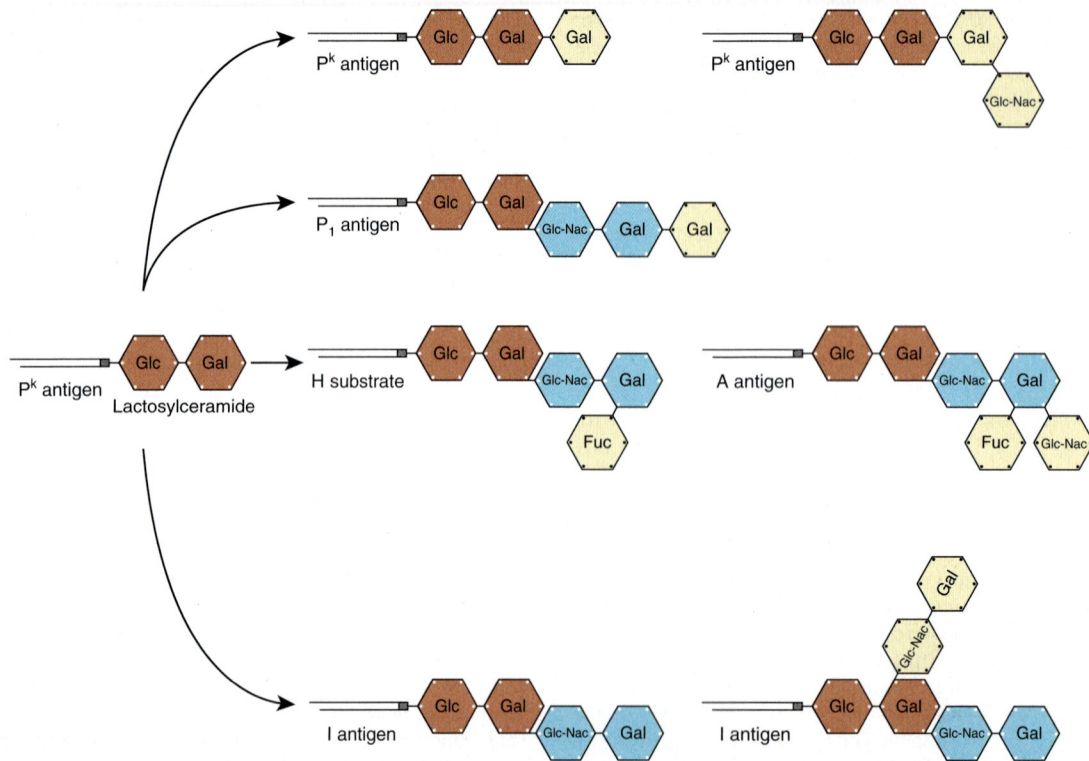

FIGURE 22.3 The relationship among ABO, P, and Ii blood group systems. These antigens are located on terminal oligosaccharides. Among these blood groups, the structure in common is lactosylceramide (red sugar moieties). Lewis group antigens also share similar structures, but they are not synthesized in red cells. Fuc, l-fucose; Gal, d-galactose; Gal-Nac, d-N-acetyl-galactosamine; Glc, d-glucosamine; Glc-Nac, d-N-acetyl-glucosamine.

I and i Antigens and Antibodies

The I and i antigens are high-incidence antigens expressed on RBC N-linked glycoproteins and glycolipids.[7,38] The i antigen is highly expressed at birth, but the amount of i antigen reduces over the first 2 years of life, in favor of increasing expression of the I antigen.[40]

Anti-I is almost always an IgM class autoagglutinin. Every adult would be expected to have at least some circulating anti-I, although special techniques (such as 4°C testing) may be needed to detect this antibody in some situations. Rarely, a pathologic variant of anti-I can be produced, usually as a result of an underlying malignancy or *Mycoplasma pneumoniae* infection. These pathologic forms of anti-I can attach to RBCs and mediate hemolysis at body temperature (cold agglutinin syndrome).[40,52] Anti-i is rare and is associated with Epstein-Barr virus infection (infectious mononucleosis). Since anti-I is found in low titer in all adults, it is important to recognize that its detection in a workup for a hemolytic anemia probably does not indicate a cause of immune hemolysis.

Other Antigen Systems

There are numerous other RBC antigen systems that are beyond the scope of this chapter and are reviewed in detail elsewhere.[1-4] The names and characteristics of these antigens are reviewed in *Table 22.3*.

Prophylactic Antigen Matching in Chronically Transfused Populations

Among chronically transfused patients with sickle cell disease, alloimmunization to minor RBC antigens has been shown to be associated with worse clinical outcomes.[55-57] For this reason, expert opinion has favored prophylactic provision of C-, E-, and K-negative RBCs for many years.[39,58] However, there is significant controversy in this area, because not all studies have shown that provision of prophylactically matched RBCs, particularly matched to the C and E antigens, have actually prevented alloimmunization in all cases. This is due to the high degree of *RHCE* genetic diversity among the African American population, which accounts for 90% of the sickle cell disease population in the United States. While prevention of alloimmunization is clearly an important clinical priority, opponents of the prophylactic antigen matching strategy point out that the standard approach employed by most blood banks increases costs, and increases the number of patients requiring a limited resource (antigen-negative RBCs), but may not prevent alloimmunization due to *RHCE* variants.[59-62] As discussed below, the theoretical solution to this problem is to perform *RHCE* genotyping of both transfusion donors and recipients, with high enough resolution to make it possible to account for *RHCE* variants among both donors and recipients in the crossmatch. However, at present, this approach is not feasible, and unfortunately, little progress has been made in this regard in the last 5 years. An area of emerging interest is the impact of alloimmunization on clinical and economic outcomes in patients with myelodysplastic syndromes, beta thalassemia, hereditary hemorrhagic telangiectasia, as well as other types of anemia.[63,64]

Owing to the high rate of alloimmunization among individuals with sickle cell disease, the low incidence of the K antigen expression on RBCs among blood donors, and the infrequency of *KEL* variants in the African American population, many groups recommend transfusing patients with sickle cell anemia whose RBCs do not express the K antigen with RBCs from donors that also are K antigen negative.[65-70] Owing to the infrequency of *KEL* variants in the sickle cell disease population, this approach would likely be highly effective at preventing alloimmunization to the K antigen.

Autoantibodies

In the blood bank, warm- or cold-reacting autoantibodies are often detected during blood typing or antibody screening. It is uncommon for these antibodies to be clinically significant, and most blood banks regard their presence as a nuisance. However, if autoantibodies are suspected during a blood bank workup, most transfusion services will perform a DAT to confirm the presence of autoantibodies. It is important to note, however, that the positive predictive value for clinically significant hemolysis is extremely low (<2%).[52] Autoimmune hemolytic anemias are covered in more detail in Chapter 31, but for the purposes of this chapter, it is important to emphasize that most warm-reacting, IgG class autoantibodies show specificity for all common Rh phenotype test cells. In contrast, many cold-reacting, IgM class autoantibodies show specificity for the I antigen (auto anti-I).

The Use of Genetic Testing in the Blood Bank

While serological testing remains the corner stone of immunohematologic methodologies to issue compatible blood products, there are several situations in which serology cannot be relied upon to determine the antigen status of an individual. In the postgenomic era, molecular immunohematology (MIH) or genotyping is increasingly used in the blood donor centers and hospital-based blood banks. The practical application of MIH in blood banking is afforded by the knowledge of the molecular basis for the presence or absence of an antigen on the red cell surface (ie, genotype-phenotype correlation). Therefore, in certain situations, one can type the genetic region controlling the antigen(s) of interest to predict the patient's red cell phenotype with confidence. The majority of blood group antigens are single nucleotide polymorphisms, which are easy to detect using simple molecular methods. Some practical applications of genotyping in the blood bank include:

To predict the red cell phenotype of a recently transfused patient, or a patient with a positive DAT.

In a recently transfused patient (transfused within the last 3 months), the presence of donor red cells in the patient's blood can interfere with determining the patient's native red cell phenotype by serology. Extracting the DNA from the patient's white blood cells and performing genotyping offers an alternative approach to predict the patient's native red cell phenotype in these situations.

Differentiating Between an Alloantibody and an Autoantibody

Whether reactivity identified during an antibody screening test is due to an allo- or autoantibody can be an important determinant of whether antigen-negative RBCs must be provided for future transfusions.[71] Genotyping can be used to predict the patient's native red cell phenotype in situations where a patient has antibodies to an antigen that their own red cells appear to express based on serologic testing. This can be particularly useful in situations where there is concern that the patient may have a variant antigen, such as in patients with sickle cell disease, although caution is advised in the interpretation of commercially available genotype kits, which at present do not detect all of the variants required to make a holistic assessment of *RHD* or *RHCE* gene variants.

Determining the Rh Status of Patients With Low Serologic Expression of RhD

Weak serological reactivity to the D antigen can be attributed to genetic changes that cause either a partial D expression or weak D expression. Partial D is the result of amino acid changes on the surface of the transmembrane protein, which results in absence of some of the D antigen epitopes. In contrast, amino acid changes in weak D are clustered in the transmembrane portion of the protein, which result in reduced density of the antigen on the surface but expression of all D antigen epitopes. If genotyping reveals that an individual is weak D types 1, 2, 3, or 4.1, then they should generally be regarded as RhD positive. In contrast, genotyping data consistent with partial D or other variants of weak D other than types 1, 2, 3 or 4.1 is associated with a much higher risk of alloimmunization.[72,73] Patients with weak D types other than 1, 2, 3 or 4.1 are thus regarded as RhD negative for the purposes of transfusion and RhIG prophylaxis during pregnancy.[73] However, all weak D or partial D blood donors are regarded as RhD positive for the purposes of blood donation, even if they only type very weakly for the D antigen.[10] This is a protective step to prevent alloimmunization in the transfusion recipient.

Prenatal Testing to Determine Risk of Hemolytic Disease of the Fetus and Newborn

When a pregnant woman has a positive antibody screening test, the determination of whether or not the cognate antigen is expressed on fetal erythrocytes informs the obstetrician as to whether or not the pregnancy may be affected by HDFN. Generally, the workup begins by determining whether or not the father of the fetus expresses the corresponding antigen on his RBCs. If he does not, then the workup is generally complete. However, if the father's RBCs do express the corresponding antigen serologically, then a molecular test may be indicated to determine whether he is heterozygous or homozygous for the gene that encodes the antigen. If the father is a homozygote, then the fetus is an obligate carrier of one copy of the gene and is at risk for HDFN. However, if the father is a heterozygote, then the fetus has a 50% chance of inheriting the gene that would confer risk for HDFN. Therefore, if the father is found to be a heterozygote, molecular testing may be pursued to determine which gene the fetus inherited. Molecular testing of fetal cells may also be pursued in circumstances where the paternity of the fetus is unknown or if the father is not amenable to testing.

Provision of Genotype-Matched RBCs for Transfusion

In groups of patients who are at high risk of alloimmunization, such as patients with sickle cell disease or transfusion-dependent thalassemia, there is significant interest in using genetically matched RBCs for transfusion in order to prevent alloimmunization and delayed hemolytic transfusion reactions.[74] Although there has never been a clinical trial comparing the efficacy of genetically matched RBCs to serologically matched RBCs for the prevention of alloimmunization, only genetically matched RBCs would take *RHD* and *RHCE* gene variants into account and theoretically would prevent alloimmunization events that cannot be prevented with serologic approaches.[59,62] As a result, genetically matched RBCs are considered to be theoretically advantageous compared with serologically matched RBCs.[75] At present, it seems that the patients who would most clearly benefit from the availability of genetically matched RBCs are those who already have formed an alloantibody to a variant RHCE antigen. Unfortunately, those cells are in such short supply that they are frequently unavailable even for this limited population as genetically matched RBCs are only available in limited supply in much of the world.[76]

Limitations and Challenges of Molecular Typing

The field of molecular immunohematology and its applications in transfusion medicine are rapidly increasing. However, the interpretation of molecular typing can be complicated for several reasons, including several alleles of a gene can code for the same antigen (eg, ABO antigens); molecular events in other parts of the gene may lead to nonexpression of apparently normal antigens (eg, GATA promoter mutation in Fy gene results in nonexpression of Fy antigens on RBCs but does not affect expression on tissues); presence of hybrid alleles (eg, Rh system); large deletions and presence of pseudogenes (eg, Rh system); and mutations in modifying or interacting genes that can control the expression of antigen on the red cell surface (eg, interaction of RHAG with Rh; interaction of Kx with Kell). The knowledge of the molecular basis of many antigens is evolving, and it is likely that not all of the molecular changes that can affect the phenotypic expression of antigens in every ethnicity are known. Finally, molecular typing requires more time than routine immunohematology, which may not be practical in cases when immediate intervention is needed. Given the growth of molecular testing in all areas of laboratory medicine, it is anticipated that molecular typing of blood antigens will play an increasing role in the hospitals and donor centers of the future.

RBC Antigens in Hematopoietic Stem Cell Transplantation

Because HLA and ABO antigens are inherited independently, up to half of stem cell grafts are not fully ABO compatible with their recipients.[17] In situations where the recipient has circulating anti-A and/or anti-B that cross-reacts with A or B antigens expressed on the graft (eg, a group A donor for a group O recipient), the incompatibility is referred to as "major." Major incompatibility is associated with an increased risk for acute hemolytic events as well as delayed RBC, granulocyte, and PLT engraftment. In some situations, pure RBC aplasia may result (see Chapter 40). All of these effects are believed to be primarily mediated by the presence of circulating anti-A or anti-B in the recipient. Many stem cell laboratories will deplete the content of RBCs in these grafts in an effort to reduce the severity of acute hemolysis. It is uncommon to attempt to reduce the titer of anti-A or anti-B in a recipient prior to transplant via apheresis or another means.

A minor ABO mismatch occurs when the stem cell graft contains plasma that is incompatible with the ABO type of the recipient's RBCs (eg, a group O donor for a group A recipient). This scenario can be associated with acute hemolysis (mediated by anti-A and/or anti-B present in the stem cell infusion) or with delayed hemolysis (mediated by anti-A and/or anti-B produced by B lymphocytes that are present in the graft). Acute hemolysis can be mitigated by reducing the volume of incompatible plasma present in the graft; the delayed hemolysis generally presents between 5 and 15 days post infusion.

Bidirectional mismatch occurs when major and minor ABO incompatibilities are both present (eg, a group A donor for a group B recipient). Bidirectional mismatch is associated with all of the complications of both major and minor ABO incompatibilities. There are conflicting reports of the implications of ABO incompatibility on clinical outcomes (such as survival and graft-versus-host disease), but studies in the literature to date report either equivalent or worse outcomes in ABO incompatible transplants.[77-83]

Transfusion support during ABO incompatible transplantation must account for both donor and recipient blood types. The first choice is to provide RBCs, PLTs, and plasma that are ABO compatible with both donor and recipient blood types. Depending on the blood types involved, this protocol can put substantial pressure on the need to transfuse group O RBCs and group AB platelets and plasma, all of which are generally in short supply. The blood bank may substitute out of group plasma products in this situation, generally utilizing a decision tree that is designed to limit the amount of incompatible anti-A, which is generally higher titer and more pathological than anti-B (see *Table 22.5*).

Antibodies to minor blood group antigens (such as anti-D, anti-K) may also complicate stem cell transplant.[17] Similar to ABO incompatibility, immediate hemolysis can result if minor RBC antibodies are circulating at the same time that RBCs expressing the cognate antigen are infused (or vice versa). This problem can theoretically be addressed by modifying the graft to limit the volume of incompatible RBCs or plasma, although this intervention is rarely pursued. More problematically, chronic hemolysis can result if recipient B cells that produce minor blood group antibodies survive conditioning and donor-derived RBCs expressing the corresponding antigen are produced by the engrafted marrow (passenger lymphocyte syndrome). If incompatible RBCs are unwittingly transfused, exchange transfusion may be required to remove them.[84] The oncology and blood bank teams should maintain open lines of communication regarding transplant scheduling so that the blood bank can have sufficient time to procure the best possible RBCs, which would involve accounting for both ABO type and any minor RBC antibodies, for transfusion in the transplant period.

Red Blood Cell Antigens and Solid Organ Transplantation

Both major and minor RBC antigens are relevant to solid organ transplantation. Renal transplantation across ABO is of particular importance. Patients receiving a transplant have approximately twice the life expectancy as patients on hemodialysis.[85] In addition, it has been estimated that 1500 additional renal transplants could occur annually in the United States if ABO compatibility between donor and recipient was not an impediment to transplant.[85] However, renal tissue extensively expresses A and B antigens, and outcomes in renal transplantation are believed to be particularly sensitive to ABO incompatibility between donor and recipient.

Prior to the late 1980s, very few ABO incompatible renal transplantations were attempted and graft survival for more than 1 year was rare.[86] Beginning in the late 1980s, ABO incompatible renal transplantation using kidneys from blood group A donors with less than full expression of A antigen (A_2 subtype) was attempted, with improved outcomes. However, more recently, experience has shown that ABO incompatibility can be overcome using intravenous immune globulin (IVIG) and plasmapheresis therapy, with patient survival at least equal to patients receiving ABO compatible grafts.

There are several case reports in the literature attributing episodes of humoral renal allograft rejection to Kidd antibodies. In these reports, the transplant recipient, who was sensitized to Jk^a or Jk^b, received an allograft from a donor who expressed the corresponding antigen. In most cases, rejection was reported to occur when the recipients were noncompliant with their antirejection medication.[87-89] In one case, rejection may have been precipitated by a hemolytic transfusion reaction mediated by anti-Jk^a.[90] Grafts were able to be salvaged with medical therapy in half of the cases. The recent literature has not added much information to the evaluation of this scenario. Generally speaking, the impact of minor RBC antibodies on renal transplantation outcomes remains largely theoretical and there are no specific protocols or guidelines that define a standard of care.

Although liver transplantation is generally regarded as less sensitive to ABO incompatibility than renal transplantation, early experience (mainly in the 1980s) with ABO incompatible liver transplantation was associated with a less than 50% success rate.[91] In the 1990s, Japanese studies found that ABO incompatible liver transplant was more likely to be successful in infants, compared with older children or adults, theoretically due to the limited expression of A and B antigens on size-matched grafts, as well as the paucity of anti-A and anti-B in infant plasma. More recently, with the advent of rituximab, the success rate of ABO incompatible liver transplantation substantially increased.[92,93]

Cardiac transplant is believed to be exquisitely sensitive to ABO compatibility. In adults, ABO incompatibility is generally regarded as an absolute contraindication to cardiac transplantation. While there are instances where ABO incompatible transplant is reported in the medical literature, these cases are generally due to a medical error that led to a lack of recognition that there was ABO incompatibility between donor and recipient. Approximately half of such patients died within 2 months of transplantation.[94] In pediatric patients, however, ABO incompatible cardiac transplantation is established medical practice that has been shown to reduce mortality of children awaiting cardiac transplant.[95,96] The differences between adult and pediatric outcomes is likely due to the fact that infants may not exhibit much anti-A or anti-B in their plasma until they reach their first birthday.[97]

IVIG-Mediated Hemolysis

Although there is no known therapeutic benefit to the inclusion of antibodies to the A and B blood group antigens in IVIG, it is known that IVIG contains these antibodies. Hundreds of hemolytic reactions to IVIG have been reported in the medical literature, mostly in patients of blood group A or AB.[98-100] The risk of hemolysis is higher when the dose of IVIG is 2 g/kg or greater or when the IVIG contains antibodies to A or B antigens of 1:32 or greater titer.[98] While the frequency of this complication has subsided in recent years, mainly due to efforts within the manufacturing of IVIG to limit the quantity of anti-A and anti-B, clinically, it remains reasonable to carefully monitor patients receiving high-dose IVIG infusions for signs or symptoms of hemolysis. For patients with a known history of a hemolytic reaction, it may be necessary to divide doses of IVIG and to administer therapy during a hospital admission.[101] If RBC transfusion is needed as a result of IVIG-induced hemolysis, transfusion with group O RBCs is generally recommended.

Impact of Novel Cancer Drugs on Transfusion Compatibility Testing

In the past several years, clinical use of antibodies targeting CD38 have become exceedingly common and additional antibodies targeting CD47 are in advanced clinical development (see *Table 22.6*). While CD38 and CD47 are important markers of hematologic malignancies, they also happen to be expressed on the surface of erythrocytes. Thus, treatment

Table 22.5. Transfusion Support During ABO Incompatible Stem Cell Transplantation

| Diagnosis to Infusion | | | Infusion to RBC Engraftment | | | | | From RBC Engraftment Onward | | | | |
| | | | | Platelets | | Plasma | | | Platelets | | Plasma | |
Recipient	Donor	All Products	RBCs	First Choice	Second Choices	First Choice	Second Choices	RBCs	First Choice	Second Choices	First Choice	Second Choices
O	A	Recipient	O	A	AB, B, O	A	AB	Donor	A	AB, B, O	A	AB
O	B	Recipient	O	B	AB, A, O	B	AB	Donor	B	AB, A, O	B	AB
O	AB	Recipient	O	AB	A, B, O	AB	NA	Donor	AB	A, B, O	AB	NA
A	AB	Recipient	A	AB	A, B, O	AB	NA	Donor	AB	A, B, O	AB	NA
B	AB	Recipient	B	AB	B, A, O	AB	NA	Donor	AB	B, A, O	AB	NA
A	O	Recipient	O	A	AB, B, O	A	AB	Donor	A	AB, B, O	A	AB
B	O	Recipient	O	B	AB, A, O	B	AB	Donor	B	AB, A, O	B	AB
AB	O	Recipient	O	AB	A, B, O	AB	NA	Donor	AB	A, B, O	AB	NA
AB	A	Recipient	A	AB	A, B, O	AB	NA	Donor	AB	A, B, O	AB	NA
AB	B	Recipient	B	AB	B, A, O	AB	NA	Donor	AB	B, A, O	AB	NA
A	B	Recipient	O	AB	B, A, O	AB	NA	Donor	AB	B, A, O	AB	NA
B	A	Recipient	O	AB	O, A, B	AB	NA	Donor	AB	A, B, O	AB	NA

Reprinted from Booth GS, Gehrie EA, Bolan CD, et al. Clinical guide to ABO-incompatible allogeneic stem cell transplantation. *Biol Blood Marrow Transplant.* 2013;19(8):1152-1158. Copyright © 2013 American Society for Blood and Marrow Transplantation. With permission.

Transfusion Medicine

Table 22.6. Therapeutic Monoclonal Antibodies Associated With Interference With the Blood Bank Workup

Specificity	Drug Names
Anti-CD38	• Daratumumab • Isatuximab • Daratumumab/hyaluronidase
Anti-CD47	• Magrolimab[a] • DSP107[b] • CC-90002[c]

[a]Not FDA approved. Currently in phase 3 trials for higher risk myelodysplastic syndrome and acute myeloid leukemia and phase 2 trials for head and neck squamous cell carcinoma and solid tumors, and a phase Ib/2 trial for diffuse large B-cell lymphoma.
[b]Not FDA approved as of January 2022. Currently in phase 1b trial for acute myeloid leukemia and myelodysplastic syndromes and a phase 1/2 trial for advanced solid tumors.
[c]Phase 1 trial discontinued due to efficacy and development of drug antibodies.[102]

Table 22.7. Properties of HLA Class I, Class II, and Class III

HLA	Antigens Encoded	Purpose
HLA class I	A, B, C, E, F, and G	Adaptive immunity
HLA class II	DP, DQ, DR, DN, and DO	Adaptive immunity
HLA class III	TNFα, TNFβ, 21-hydroxylase, C2, C4A, C4B, Bf	Innate immunity

Abbreviations: HLA, human leukocyte antigen; TNF, tumor necrosis factor.

with CD38 or CD47 antibodies can result in agglutination of RBCs, frustrating blood bank testing as well as potentially causing hemolysis (particularly with anti-CD47).[36,103,104] Patients being considered for either therapy should ideally have a blood bank workup performed prior to initiation of the therapy, so that the patient's blood type can be established with certainty. Blood banks should strongly consider phenotyping the patient's pretreatment RBCs so that future test results can be interpreted in the context of the patient's pretreatment sample, which can help to differentiate off-target drug effect from alloimmunization. As mentioned above, in some situations the blood bank may determine that patients treated with anti-CD38 should be provided with RBCs from donors who are negative for the K antigen, which modestly increases the complexity of the blood procurement process. Overall, the blood bank can only determine that a specialized pretransfusion strategy (such as phenotyping or provision of K antigen–negative cells) is needed if it is aware that the patient is being treated with anti-CD38 or anti-CD47. Thus, proactive communication with the blood bank about these patients can help to reduce the probability of an adverse event and reduce the time required to complete pretransfusion testing.

WHITE BLOOD CELL ANTIGENS AND ANTIBODIES

In humans, white blood cell antigens include HLAs and human neutrophil antigens (HNAs). Several diseases, hematologic entities, or adverse reactions to transfusion are associated with antibodies to these antigens, including neonatal alloimmune neutropenia (NAIN), chronic benign autoimmune neutropenia of infancy (AIN), allograft rejection, transfusion-related acute lung injury (TRALI), post-stem cell transplant immune neutropenia, and granulocyte transfusion refractoriness.[105]

It is important to emphasize that RBC and platelet transfusions today contain far fewer "contaminating" leukocytes than in the past. Nearly all RBCs and platelet components in the United States are leukoreduced prior to transfusion, and a whole blood filter also exists for whole blood, which is gaining traction as a trauma resuscitation product. Importantly, there is more than a 99% reduction in a unit of RBCs or apheresis platelets as a result of leukofiltration.[10] Leukoreduction has been credited with a reduction in the incidence of febrile, nonhemolytic transfusion reactions,[106] as well as with a reduction in HLA alloimmunization and platelet refractoriness[107,108] in transfusion recipients.

HLA Antigens and Antibodies

HLA is the term used to describe the major histocompatibility complex molecules in humans. These genes, which encode HLAs, are found on chromosome 6, are highly polymorphic, and are expressed in a codominant fashion. HLA antigens are divided into class I, ~57,000-Dalton proteins that are expressed on all nucleated cells, and class II, 63,000-Dalton proteins that are only expressed on dedicated antigen-presenting cells such as macrophages, dendritic cells, and B lymphocytes. Class III HLA antigens encode aspects of the innate immune system (see *Table 22.7*).

HLA antigens are the primary means of determining a "match" for stem cell or solid organ transplantation and are also applicable to platelet transfusion as platelets express class I HLA (mainly HLA-A and HLA-B). In general, HLA matching between a donor and a recipient is based on at least HLA-A, HLA-B, HLA-C, HLA-DR, and HLA-DQ for stem cell transplant and at least HLA-A, HLA-B, and HLA-DR for renal transplantation. Owing to the codominant expression of HLA antigens, there are two possible matches at each locus. Assuming that a patient's mother and father usually express different HLA antigens over these loci, the probability of a full match between a parent and a child is very small. However, the probability that any given sibling is a full match is 25%. HLA matching is associated with improved graft survival in renal transplant and a reduced probability of graft versus host disease in stem cell transplantation.[109,110] Liver, heart, and lung transplantation, in contrast, may be performed without regard to the degree of HLA match between donor and recipient.[111] HLA antigen expression is also associated with susceptibility to various diseases, including systemic lupus erythematosus, celiac disease, ankylosing spondylitis, dermatitis herpetiformis, and narcolepsy.[112-114]

In transfusion practice, HLA antigens are most frequently discussed with reference to refractoriness to platelet transfusion. HLA antigens are variably expressed on red cells so they do not present problems in red cell transfusion practice. Granulocytes can be transfused for neutropenic patients, but the efficacy of providing HLA compatible granulocytes has not been rigorously demonstrated and the heterogeneity of HLA types in donors and the requirements to administer granulocytes at least daily would make HLA matching of granulocytes for transfusion very difficult.[115]

Platelets are known to express HLA antigens. Generally, in clinical practice, platelets for patients with refractoriness are matched for HLA-A and HLA-B antigens, although HLA-C antigen matching may be considered in some special clinical situations.[116] Platelet matching does not include consideration of HLA class II antigens. HLA matching is graded according to a four-antigen matching system, depicted in *Table 22.8*.

This grading schematic is of limited utility for some platelet refractory patients, because it does not take into account the degree of ABO match between donor and recipient (platelets express ABO antigens in addition to HLA antigens). In addition, the availability of an acceptable match (usually described as grade B or better) can be very limited.[117] In response to these limitations, many transfusion services will attempt to improve response to platelet transfusion by giving the freshest possible ABO-matched or ABO-identical units prior to pursuing an HLA-matched platelet. This strategy is rationalized because platelets also express ABO antigens, and thus ABO-matched platelets avoid immune clearance mediated by incompatible ABO antibodies. If there is a high index of suspicion that HLA antibodies are mediating refractoriness, another strategy is to perform a test for HLA antibodies or platelet-specific antibodies in the plasma of the transfusion recipient and seeking out platelet units that do not react with their known antibodies (so-called antigen avoidance). Compared with a search for antigen-matched platelets, this approach can greatly increase the availability of a product that will provide acceptable transfusion support for alloimmunized, refractory patients. In addition, this approach may produce equivalent results for refractory transfusion recipients.[118] However, this platelet matching procedure does not prevent further alloimmunization to HLA-mismatched antigens. None of these

Table 22.8. Grading Schematic for HLA-Matched Platelets

Grade	Description
A	All 4 antigens match
B1U	3 antigens match, remaining antigen unknown or blank[a]
B1X	3 antigens match, fourth antigen from a cross-reactive group
B2U	2 antigens match, third antigen blank,[a] fourth antigen from a cross-reactive group
C	3 antigens match, fourth antigen mismatched
D	At least two mismatched antigens
R	Random

[a]A blank antigen is most likely caused by homozygosity for a particular HLA antigen.
Abbreviation: HLA, human leukocyte antigen.
Adapted with permission from Fung MK, Grossman BJ, Hillyer CD, Westhoff CM. *Technical Manual.* 18th ed. American Association of Blood Banks; 2014. Table 18.4. Copyright © 2014 by AABB.

strategies would be expected to improve response to platelet transfusion if the refractoriness is mediated by a nonimmune condition, such as splenic sequestration, disseminated intravascular coagulation, uncontrolled hemorrhage, or other clinical events that can produce nonimmune refractoriness.

In addition to complicating platelet transfusion, HLA antibodies have also been implicated in the pathogenesis of febrile nonhemolytic transfusion reactions and TRALI. To diminish these transfusion complications, there are now guidelines to limit the incidence of HLA-sensitized donors in the plasma and platelet supply. These steps have mainly been accomplished by excluding female donors from the donor pool and testing apheresis platelet donors for HLA antibodies.[119]

HNA Antigens and Antibodies

The central cells in the body that express HNAs are those of the granulocyte lineage, although some of these antigens (principally HNA-3) are also expressed on other important cells such as lung endothelium, which explains the association between antibodies to these entities and some proposed etiologies of TRALI.[120-122] There are a total of 14 HNA alleles described to date, which are expressed on five glycoproteins,[122] which are summarized in the following paragraphs.[105] In addition to TRALI, antibodies to HNA antigens are associated with several important pathological entities, such as NAIN, AIN, febrile nonhemolytic transfusion reactions, transfusion-related alloimmune neutropenia, failure to engraft after stem cell transplantation, and kidney transplant rejection—but testing is not routine in hospital-based blood banks and these antigens play no role in routine pretransfusion compatibility testing.[122] Many of the clinical entities are described in detail in other chapters of this text. For a detailed explanation of modern techniques to HNA typing and antibody detection please see Browne et al.[122]

HNA-1 is found only on neutrophils and basophils and consists of five alleles, including HNA-1a (previously NA1), HNA-1b (previously NA2), and HNA-1c (previously SH).[123] These antigens are expressed on FCγ receptor IIIb, which is also referred to as CD16b.[123,124] Almost all individuals of European, Asian, Native American, and African ancestry express HNA-1 antigens, but the allele frequency of HNA-1a versus -1b or -1c varies by ethnicity.[122,123] Most individuals express at least one, and up to 4, HNA-1 alleles, but lack of expression of HNA-1 (HNA-1 null) does not appear to be associated with infection or autoimmune disease.[122,125] Individuals who lack expression of these antigens can become alloimmunized if they are exposed to the antigens, usually in the context of blood transfusion or pregnancy. Antibodies to HNA-1a, 1b, and 2 have the strongest association with NAIN, although other antibodies have also been implicated in case reports.[122,126-130]

HNA-2 (CD177) is a high-incidence antigen expressed on neutrophils.[123] Interestingly, antibodies that appear to have HNA-2

specificity do not seem to bind directly to HNA-2, and thus, they are technically classified as isoantibodies rather than alloantibodies.[120,131] Nonetheless, anti-HNA-2 has been associated with TRALI, AIN, post–stem cell transplant neutropenia.[105,122,132-135]

The HNA-3 (previously referred to as 5b and 5a) system is expressed on the choline transporter-like protein 2 (CTL2) molecule, which is also expressed on platelets, lymphocytes, and other cells including those found in the colon, lung, and liver.[105,120,122,123] Antibodies to HNA-3a are far more frequent than antibodies to HNA-3b.[105] Anti-HNA-3a has been associated with at least six fatal cases of TRALI and, along with antibodies to HNA-2, are the most important causes of HNA-induced TRALI cases.[122,136] These antibodies may also mediate kidney allograft rejection.[122,137,138]

HNA-4 (previously Mart) is expressed on CD11b.[123] It has been identified on neutrophils, lymphocytes, and other cells.[105,122] Antibodies to HNA-4a (and also possibly antibodies to HNA-4b) are associated with AIN, and autoantibodies to CD11b are associated with autoimmune neutropenia and may impair neutrophil function.[122,139,140]

The HNA-5 (previously Ond) system only consists of one allele, HNA-5a.[122,123] The HNA-5a molecule is carried on CD11a.[122] Anti-HNA-5a has been described in a patient with hypoplastic anemia; in that patient, survival of his skin graft was attributed in part due to anti-HNA-5a, although his serum also contained anti-HNA-1b.[141,142] More recently, anti-HNA-5a has also been associated with NAIN, although these reports are not frequent.[122,143]

Platelet Antigens and Antibodies

In addition to the previously discussed HLA and ABO antigens, both of which are expressed on platelets, there are clinically important antigens that are mainly known due to their expression on platelets. These antigens include human platelet antigens (HPAs; which are expressed on platelets as well as endothelial cells and leukocytes), which are an ever-expanding category of (currently) 41 antigens, the last of which was first described in 2019.[105,144] For a current listing of HPA antigens as well as relevant citations relating to their discovery and clinical characteristics, see *The Human Platelet Antigen Database.*[145] The "w" designation refers to antigens where antibodies to both antithetical antigens have yet to be discovered.[105]

The first platelet alloantigen to be discovered was HPA-1a (previously referred to as Zwᵃ or Plᴬ¹). The HPA-1a antigen is bound to the β-subunit of the platelet fibrinogen receptor (GPIIb/IIIa). Antibodies to HPA-1a can be formed by the approximately 2% of the population that is homozygous for HPA-1b. Among Caucasians, anti-HPA-1a is the most common cause of neonatal alloimmune thrombocytopenia (NAIT) and is also the most frequent HPA antibody specificity associated with posttransfusion purpura (PTP; although anti-HPA-1b and anti-HPA-5b are also relatively common). PTP can cause a dramatic reduction in platelet count approximately 1 week after transfusion,[146,147] and additional information can be found in the section of this textbook on transfusion complications.

With respect to NAIT, anti-HPA-1a was traditionally considered the most important antibody. However, there are several reasons why the contribution of antibodies besides anti-HPA-1a to the incidence of NAIT may be underappreciated. First, there are significant differences in HPA allele frequencies between different ethnicities. For example, while virtually 100% of individuals of European, African, or Brazilian ancestry are homozygous for HPA-4a, a small percentage (still <1%) of individuals of Asian descent express the HPA-4b allele.[148] As a result, anti-HPA-4b has been linked to immune-mediated platelet transfusion refractoriness, NAIT, and posttransfusion purpura in Asian descended populations.[105,149] Similar to anti-HPA-4b, HPA 21-bw also has a higher allele frequency among individuals of Asian descent and is associated with severe NAIT.[149-152] Overall, a large number of antibodies, including anti-HPA-6bw, anti-HPA-8-bw, anti-HPA-9-bw, anti-HPA-11bw, and anti-HPA-13-bw, and, most recently, anti-HPA-35bw, have all been associated with NAIT.[144,153-158] Therefore, it is becoming clearer that a second cause of underdetection of NAIT mediated by HPAs other than HPA-1a is the lack of sophisticated testing laboratories with available specific reagents.

In addition to forming antibodies to HPA, individuals lacking other platelet antigens—defects that in and of themselves lead to defects in platelet aggregation—can form additional clinically significant allo-antibodies if they are sensitized by platelet transfusion or pregnancy. For example, patients with Glanzmann thrombasthenia, an inherited bleeding disorder due to a deleted or an abnormal platelet fibrinogen receptor resulting in absent aggregation, can form antibodies to the highly immunogenic GPIIb/IIIa antigen in response to platelet transfusion.[105] Patients with Bernard-Soulier syndrome, who lack the von Willebrand receptor on platelets and in whom aggregation is normal in response to agonists except for ristocetin, can produce anti-GPIb/IX/V if they are exposed to the antigen. Both anti-GPIIb/IIIa and anti-GPIb/IX/V can mediate immune refractoriness to platelet transfusion and can also cross the placenta resulting in neonatal thrombocytopenia.[159,160] In addition, among patients with these congenital platelet disorders, these antibodies may be confused with HLA antibodies (and vice versa) as a cause of transfusion refractoriness. Regarding collagen receptor defects, patients who do not express CD36 (glycoprotein IV) on platelets (who are generally of Asian or African ancestry) can become sensitized to CD36 by transfusion or pregnancy.[161] Anti-CD36 may mediate platelet refractoriness, posttransfusion purpura, or NAIT.[162-164] In addition, some cases of thrombocytopenia appear to be caused by the development of antibodies to the primary platelet collagen receptor, GPVI.[105,165,166] It is believed that GPVI autoantibodies can cause bleeding by effectively removing GPVI molecules from the platelet surface, depriving the platelet of the capability to bind collagen.[105]

As discussed previously, platelets express both ABO and HLA antigens on their surface. Because antibodies to A and B antigens are naturally occurring, all transfusion recipients have the immune capacity to clear platelets expressing incompatible ABO antigens, even if they have never been transfused before.[167,168] Interestingly, individuals who are blood group A_2, a subset of blood group A that is identified in approximately 20% of Caucasians, are believed to express quite small amounts of the A antigen on their platelets. Transfusion of platelets from A_2 donors has been used as a strategy to overcome platelet refractoriness in patients with high-titer anti-A.[169] Unfortunately, this strategy is not viable as a routine practice because the hospital blood bank is generally unable to determine which of their platelet donors are blood group A_1 versus A_2.

CONCLUSION

RBC, white blood cell, and platelet antigens and antibodies are all relevant to the practice of clinical hematology. The technologists and physicians in the blood bank can be an expert resource to determine the clinical significance of these antigens, as well as antibodies that are formed as a result of sensitization to these antigens. These issues can be important in patients with difficult transfusion problems or in the diagnosis and management of patients with suspected autoimmune hematologic diseases. In the future, molecular methodologies will likely play a larger role in the assessment of these antigens and their disease and transfusion practice implications.

ACKNOWLEDGMENT

We wish to acknowledge the authors of the previous version of this chapter, with special consideration to R. Sue Shirey and Dr. Karen King, who have both passed away in the interim between editions.

References

1. Harmening D. *Modern Blood Banking and Transfusion Medicine.* 7th ed. FA Davis; 2018.
2. Cohn C. *Technical Manual.* 20th ed. AABB Press; 2020.
3. Reid M. *Blood Group Antigen Factsbook.* 3rd ed. Elsevier; 2012.
4. Daniels G. *Human Blood Groups.* 3rd ed. Wiley; 2013.
5. Denise M, Firestone D. The ABO blood group system. In: Harmening DM, ed. *Modern Blood Banking and Transfusion Practices.* ed. 5th ed. FA Davis; 2005:108-111.
6. Auf der Maur C, Hodel M, Nydegger UE, Rieben R. Age dependency of ABO histo-blood group antibodies: reexamination of an old dogma. *Transfusion.* 1993;33(11):915-918. PubMed PMID: 8259597

7. Cooling I. ABO, H, and Lewis blood groups and structurally related antigens. In: Fung M, *AABB Technical Manual.* ed. 18th ed. AABB Press; 2014.
8. Janatpour KA, Kalmin ND, Jensen HM, Holland PV. Clinical outcomes of ABO-incompatible RBC transfusions. *Am J Clin Pathol.* 2008;129(2):276-281.PubMed PMID: 18208808. doi:10.1309/VXY1ULAFUY6E6JT3.
9. Gehrie EA, Savani BN, Booth GS. Risk factors for hemolytic transfusion reactions resulting from ABO and minor red cell antigen incompatibility: from mislabeled samples to stem cell transplant and sickle cell disease. *Blood Rev.* 2021;45:100719. PubMed PMID: 32561028,doi:10.1016/j.blre.2020.100719.
10. AABB. *Standards for Blood Banks and Transfusion Services.* 32nd ed. AABB; 2020.
11. Linden JV, Wagner K, Voytovich AE, Sheehan J. Transfusion errors in New York State: an analysis of 10 years' experience. *Transfusion.* 2000;40(10):1207-1213. PubMed PMID: 11061857
12. Kaufman RM, Dinh A, Cohn CS, et al. Electronic patient identification for sample labeling reduces wrong blood in tube errors. *Transfusion.* 2019;59(3):972-980. Epub 20181214. PubMed PMID: 30549289. doi:10.1111/trf.15102.
13. Callum J, Etchells E, Shojania K. Addressing the identity crisis in healthcare: positive patient identification technology reduces wrong patient events. *Transfusion.* 2019;59(3):899-902. PubMed PMID: 30840332. doi:10.1111/trf.15160.
14. Lumadue JA, Boyd JS, Ness PM. Adherence to a strict specimen-labeling policy decreases the incidence of erroneous blood grouping of blood bank specimens. *Transfusion.* 1997;37(11-12):1169-1172. PubMed PMID: 9426641. doi:10.1046/j.1537-2995.1997.37111298088047.x.
15. Yoshida A, Dave V, Hamilton HB. Imbalance of blood group A subtypes and the existence of superactive B gene in Japanese in Hiroshima and Nagasaki. *Am J Hum Genet.* 1988;43(4):422-428. PubMed PMID: 3177385; PMCID: PMC1715517.
16. Flegel WA. Pathogenesis and mechanisms of antibody-mediated hemolysis. *Transfusion.* 2015;55(suppl 2):S47-S58. doi: 10.1111/trf.13147. PubMed PMID: 26174897; PMCID: PMC4503931.
17. Booth GS, Gehrie EA, Bolan CD, Savani BN. Clinical guide to ABO-incompatible allogeneic stem cell transplantation. *Biol Blood Marrow Transpl.* 2013;19(8):1152-1158. PubMed PMID: 23571461. doi:10.1016/j.bbmt.2013.03.018.
18. HUGO Gene Nomenclature Committee [Internet] [cited 11/28/2021]http://www.genenames.org .
19. International Society of Blood Transfusion Working Party on Terminology for Red Cell Antigens [Internet] [cited 11/28/2021]http://www.isbtweb.org .
20. Tormey CA, Stack G. The persistence and evanescence of blood group alloantibodies in men. *Transfusion.* 2009;49(3):505-512. PubMed PMID: 19040411. doi:10.1111/j.1537-2995.2008.02014.x.
21. Mazzei CA, Kopko PM. Noninfectious complications of blood transfusion. In: Fung MK, Grossman BJ, Hillyer CD, Westhoff CM, eds. *Technical Manual.* ed. 18th ed. AABB; 2014:665-696.
22. Ness PM, Shirey RS, Thoman SK, Buck SA. The differentiation of delayed serologic and delayed hemolytic transfusion reactions: incidence, long-term serologic findings, and clinical significance. *Transfusion.* 1990;30(8):688-693. PubMed PMID: 2219254
23. Thornton JG, Page C, Foote G, Arthur GR, Tovey LA, Scott JS. Efficacy and long term effects of antenatal prophylaxis with anti-D immunoglobulin. *BMJ.* 1989;298(6689):1671-1673. PubMed PMID: 2547468; PMCID: PMC1836780.
24. Pollack W, Ascari WQ, Kochesky RJ, O'Connor RR, Tripodi D. Studies on Rh prophylaxis. 1. Relationship between doses of anti-Rh and size of antigenic stimulus. *Transfusion.* 1971;11(6):333-339. PubMed PMID: 5002765
25. Behring C. *RhO(D) Immune Globulin Intravenous (Human).* Package Insert; 2016.
26. Urbaniak SJ, Robertson AE. A successful program of immunizing Rh-negative male volunteers for anti-D production using frozen/thawed blood. *Transfusion.* 1981;21(1):64-69. PubMed PMID: 6781108
27. Goldfinger D, McGinniss MH. Rh-incompatible platelet transfusions--risks and consequences of sensitizing immunosuppressed patients. *N Engl J Med.* 1971;284(17):942-944. PubMed PMID: 4994614. doi:10.1056/NEJM197104292841704.
28. Baldwin ML, Ness PM, Scott D, Braine H, Kickler TS. Alloimmunization to D antigen and HLA in D-negative immunosuppressed oncology patients. *Transfusion.* 1988;28(4):330-333.PubMed PMID: 3133844
29. McLeod BC, Piehl MR, Sassetti RJ. Alloimmunization to RhD by platelet transfusions in autologous bone marrow transplant recipients. *Vox Sang.* 1990;59(3):185-189.PubMed PMID: 2124754
30. Cid J, Lozano M, Ziman A, et al. Biomedical Excellence for Safer Transfusion c. Low frequency of anti-D alloimmunization following D+ platelet transfusion: the Anti-D Alloimmunization after D-incompatible Platelet Transfusions (ADAPT) study. *Br J Haematol.* 2015;168(4):598-603. PubMed PMID: 25283094; PMCID: PMC4314459. doi:10.1111/bjh.13158.
31. Kacker S, Vassallo R, Keller MA, et al. Financial implications of RHD genotyping of pregnant women with a serologic weak D phenotype. *Transfusion.* 2015;55(9):2095-2103. PubMed PMID: 25808011; PMCID: PMC4739823. doi:10.1111/trf.13074.
32. Stack G, Tormey CA. Estimating the immunogenicity of blood group antigens: a modified calculation that corrects for transfusion exposures. *Br J Haematol.* 2016;175(1):154-160. PubMed PMID: 27340943. doi:10.1111/bjh.14175.
33. Storry J. Other blood group systems and antigens. In: Fung M, *AABB Technical Manual.* ed. 18th ed. AABB Press; 2014:337-366.
34. *Human Blood Groups.* 3rd ed: Wiley-Blackwell; 2013.
35. Klein HG, AD ABO, H Le. In: Klein HGAD, *P1PK, GLOB, I and FORS Blood Group Systems.* ed. Wiley-Blackwell; 2014..
36. Chapuy CI, Aguad MD, Nicholson RT, et al. International validation of a dithiothreitol (DTT)-based method to resolve the daratumumab interference with blood compatibility testing. *Transfusion.* 2016. PubMed PMID: 27600566. doi:10.1111/trf.13789.

37. Chapuy CI, Nicholson RT, Aguad MD, et al. Resolving the daratumumab interference with blood compatibility testing. *Transfusion*. 2015;55(6 Pt 2):1545-1554. PubMed PMID: 25764134. doi:10.1111/trf.13069.

38. Beattie K. The Duffy blood group system: distribution, serology and genetics. In: Pierce SRMC, *Blood Group Systems: Duffy, Kidd and Lutheran*. ed. AABB; 1988.

39. Chou ST, Alsawas M, Fasano RM, et al. American Society of Hematology 2020 guidelines for sickle cell disease: transfusion support. *Blood Adv*. 2020;4(2):327-355. PubMed PMID: 31985807; PMCID: PMC6988392. doi:10.1182/bloodadvances.2019001143.

40. Leger RM, Calhoun L. Other major blood group systems. In: Harmening DM, ed. *Modern Blood Banking & Transfusion Practices*. ed. 5th ed.. FA Davis; 2005:162-192.

41. Hawkins P, Anderson SE, McKenzie JL, McLoughlin K, Beard ME, Hart DN. Localization of MN blood group antigens in kidney. *Transpl Proc*. 1985;17(2):1697-1700. PubMed PMID: 3984026

42. Yasuda H, Ohto H, Nollet KE, et al. Hemolytic disease of the fetus and newborn with late-onset anemia due to anti-M: a case report and review of the Japanese literature. *Transfus Med Rev*. 2014;28(1):1-6. PubMed PMID: 24262303. doi:10.1016/j.tmrv.2013.10.002.

43. Reddy VS, Kohan R. Severe hemolytic disease of fetus and newborn due to anti-s antibodies. *J Clin Neonatol*. 2014;3(2):128-129. PubMed PMID: 25024987; PMCID: PMC4089131. doi:10.4103/2249-4847.134719.

44. Yousuf R, Abdul Aziz S, Yusof N, Leong CF. Hemolytic disease of the fetus and newborn caused by anti-D and anti-S alloantibodies: a case report. *J Med Case Rep*. 2012;6:71. PubMed PMID: 22348809; PMCID: PMC3299637. doi:10.1186/1752-1947-6-71.

45. Adam S, Lombaard H. *Autologous Intrauterine Transfusion in a Case of Anti-U*. *Transfusion*; 2016. PubMed PMID: 27664105. doi:10.1111/trf.13806.

46. Taghizadeh M, Harmening DM. The Lewis system and the biological significance. In: Harmening DM, ed. *Modern Blood Banking & Transfusion Practices*. ed. 5th ed. FA Davis; 2005:148-161.

47. Irani MS, Figueroa D, Savage G. Acute hemolytic transfusion reaction due to anti-Le(b). *Transfusion*. 2015;55(10):2486-2488. PubMed PMID: 26018602. doi:10.1111/trf.13178.

48. Duncan V, Pham HP, Williams LAIII. A possible case of a haemolytic transfusion reaction caused by anti-Le(a) antibody. *Blood Transfus*. 2015;13(3):535-536. PubMed PMID: 26057494; PMCID: PMC4614310. doi:10.2450/2015.0286-14.

49. Yoshida H, Ito K, Kusakari T, et al. Removal of maternal antibodies from a woman with repeated fetal loss due to P blood group incompatibility. *Transfusion*. 1994;34(8):702-705. PubMed PMID: 8073488.

50. Shirey RS, Ness PM, Kickler TS, et al. The association of anti-P and early abortion. *Transfusion*. 1987;27(2):189-191. PubMed PMID: 3824479.

51. Arndt PA, Garratty G, Marfoe RA, Zeger GD. An acute hemolytic transfusion reaction caused by an anti-P1 that reacted at 37 degrees C. *Transfusion*. 1998;38(4):373-377. PubMed PMID: 9595020.

52. PLaG G. *Immune Hemolytic Anemias*. 2nd ed. Churchill Livingstone; 2004.

53. Zeller MP, Arnold DM, Al Habsi K, et al. Paroxysmal cold hemoglobinuria: a difficult diagnosis in adult patients. *Transfusion*. 2016. PubMed PMID: 27807852. doi:10.1111/trf.13888.

54. Mallouh AA, Qudah A. An epidemic of aplastic crisis caused by human parvovirus B19. *Pediatr Infect Dis J*. 1995;14(1):31-34. PubMed PMID: 7715986

55. Telen MJ, Afenyi-Annan A, Garrett ME, Combs MR, Orringer EP, Ashley-Koch AE. Alloimmunization in sickle cell disease: changing antibody specificities and association with chronic pain and decreased survival. *Transfusion*. 2015;55(6 Pt 2):1378-1387. Epub 20141201. PubMed PMID: 25444611; PMCID: PMC4451450. doi:10.1111/trf.12940.

56. Nickel RS, Hendrickson JE, Fasano RM, et al. Impact of red blood cell alloimmunization on sickle cell disease mortality: a case series. *Transfusion*. 2016;56(1):107-114. Epub 20151028. PubMed PMID: 26509333. doi:10.1111/trf.13379.

57. Tormey CA, Hendrickson JE. Transfusion-related red blood cell alloantibodies: induction and consequences. *Blood*. 2019;133(17):1821-1830. Epub 20190226. PubMed PMID: 30808636; PMCID: PMC6484385. doi:10.1182/blood-2018-08-833962.

58. Services USDoHaH. *Evidence-Based Management of Sickle Cell Disease: Expert Panel Report, 2014*; 2014.

59. Gehrie EA, Ness PM, Bloch EM, Kacker S, Tobian AAR. Medical and economic implications of strategies to prevent alloimmunization in sickle cell disease. *Transfusion*. 2017;57(9):2267-2276. Epub 20170626. PubMed PMID: 28653325; PMCID: PMC5695925. doi:10.1111/trf.14212.

60. Kacker S, Ness PM, Savage WJ, et al. Economic evaluation of a hypothetical screening assay for alloimmunization risk among transfused patients with sickle cell disease. *Transfusion*. 2014;54(8):2034-2044. PubMed PMID: 24571485; PMCID: PMC4138280. doi:10.1111/trf.12585.

61. Kacker S, Ness PM, Savage WJ, et al. Cost-effectiveness of prospective red blood cell antigen matching to prevent alloimmunization among sickle cell patients. *Transfusion*. 2014;54(1):86-97. PubMed PMID: 23692415; PMCID: PMC3758770. doi: 10.1111/trf.12250.

62. Chou ST, Jackson T, Vege S, Smith-Whitley K, Friedman DF, Westhoff CM. High prevalence of red blood cell alloimmunization in sickle cell disease despite transfusion from Rh-matched minority donors. *Blood*. 2013;122(6):1062-1071. PubMed PMID: 23723452. doi: 10.1182/blood-2013-03-490623.

63. Zheng J, Pollak J, Henderson K, Hendrickson JE, Tormey CA. A novel association between high red blood cell alloimmunization rates and hereditary hemorrhagic telangiectasia. *Transfusion*. 2018;58(3):775-780. PubMed PMID: 29210083. doi: 10.1111/trf.14451.

64. Singhal D, Kutyna MM, Chhetri R, et al. Red cell alloimmunization is associated with development of autoantibodies and increased red cell transfusion requirements

65. Tahhan HR, Holbrook CT, Braddy LR, Brewer LD, Christie JD. Antigen-matched donor blood in the transfusion management of patients with sickle cell disease. *Transfusion*. 1994;34(7):562-569. PubMed PMID: 8053036

66. Castro O, Sandler SG, Houston-Yu P, Rana S. Predicting the effect of transfusing only phenotype-matched RBCs to patients with sickle cell disease: theoretical and practical implications. *Transfusion*. 2002;42(6):684-690. PubMed PMID: 12147019.

67. Ambruso DR, Githens JH, Alcorn R, et al. Experience with donors matched for minor blood group antigens in patients with sickle cell anemia who are receiving chronic transfusion therapy. *Transfusion*. 1987;27(1):94-98. PubMed PMID: 3810834

68. Sakhalkar VS, Roberts K, Hawthorne LM, et al. Allosensitization in patients receiving multiple blood transfusions. *Ann N Y Acad Sci*. 2005;1054:495-499. PubMed PMID: 16339705. doi: 10.1196/annals.1345.072.

69. Adams RJ, McKie VC, Hsu L, et al. Prevention of a first stroke by transfusions in children with sickle cell anemia and abnormal results on transcranial Doppler ultrasonography. *N Engl J Med*. 1998;339(1):5-11. PubMed PMID: 9647873. doi: 10.1056/NEJM199807023390102.

70. Vichinsky EP, Luban NL, Wright E, et al. Prospective RBC phenotype matching in a stroke-prevention trial in sickle cell anemia: a multicenter transfusion trial. *Transfusion*. 2001;41(9):1086-1092. PubMed PMID: 11552063

71. Ipe TS, Wilkes JJ, Hartung HD, Chou ST, Friedman DF. Severe hemolytic transfusion reaction due to anti-D in a D+ patient with sickle cell disease. *J Pediatr Hematol Oncol*. 2015;37(2):e135-37. PubMed PMID: 25171447; PMCID: PMC4333075. doi: 10.1097/MPH.0000000000000241.

72. Flegel WA, Denomme GA, Queenan JT, et al. It's time to phase out "serologic weak D phenotype" and resolve D types with RHD genotyping including weak D type 4. *Transfusion*. 2020;60(4):855-859. PubMed PMID: 32163599. doi: 10.1111/trf.15741.

73. Sandler SG, Flegel WA, Westhoff CM, et al. It's time to phase in RHD genotyping for patients with a serologic weak D phenotype. College of American Pathologists Transfusion Medicine Resource Committee Work Group. *Transfusion*. 2015;55(3):680-689. PubMed PMID: 25438646; PMCID: PMC4357540. doi: 10.1111/trf.12941.

74. Putzulu RPN, Orlando N, Massini G, et al. The role of molecular typing and perfect match transfusion in sickle cell disease and thalassaemia: an innovative transfusion strategy. *Transfus Apher Sci*. 2017. doi: j.transci.2017.01.003.

75. Matteocci A, Pierelli L. Red blood cell alloimmunization in sickle cell disease and in thalassaemia: current status, future perspectives and potential role of molecular typing. *Vox Sang*. 2014;106(3):197-208. PubMed PMID: 24117723. doi: 10.1111/vox.12086.

76. Karafin MS, Field JJ, Gottschall JL, Denomme GA. Barriers to using molecularly typed minority red blood cell donors in support of chronically transfused adult patients with sickle cell disease. *Transfusion*. 2015;55(6 Pt 2):1399-1406. PubMed PMID: 25757390. doi: 10.1111/trf.13037.

77. Sieff C, Bicknell D, Caine G, Robinson J, Lam G, Greaves MF. Changes in cell surface antigen expression during hemopoietic differentiation. *Blood*. 1982;60(3):703-713. PubMed PMID: 6286014.

78. Kim JG, Sohn SK, Kim DH, et al. Impact of ABO incompatibility on outcome after allogeneic peripheral blood stem cell transplantation. *Bone Marrow Transplant*. 2005;35(5):489-495. PubMed PMID: 15654350. doi: 10.1038/sj.bmt.1704816.

79. Helming AM, Brand A, Wolterbeek R, van Tol MJ, Egeler RM, Ball LM. ABO incompatible stem cell transplantation in children does not influence outcome. *Pediatr Blood Cancer*. 2007;49(3):313-317. PubMed PMID: 16960869. doi: 10.1002/pbc.21025.

80. Stussi G, Muntwyler J, Passweg JR, et al. Consequences of ABO incompatibility in allogeneic hematopoietic stem cell transplantation. *Bone Marrow Transpl*. 2002;30(2):87-93. PubMed PMID: 12132047. doi: 10.1038/sj.bmt.1703621.

81. Buckner CD, Clift RA, Sanders JE, et al. ABO-incompatible marrow transplants. *Transplantation*. 1978;26(4):233-238. PubMed PMID: 30194.

82. Bacigalupo A, Van Lint MT, Occhini D, et al.. ABO compatibility and acute graft-versus-host disease following allogeneic bone marrow transplantation. *Transplantation*. 1988;45(6):1091-1094. PubMed PMID: 3289150.

83. Sora F, De Matteis S, Piccirillo N, et al. Rituximab for pure red cell aplasia after ABO-mismatched allogeneic peripheral blood progenitor cell transplantation. *Transfusion*. 2005;45(4):643-645. PubMed PMID: 15819690. doi: 10.1111/j.0041-1132.2005.00445.x.

84. Young PP, Goodnough LT, Westervelt P, Diersio JF. Immune hemolysis involving non-ABO/RhD alloantibodies following hematopoietic stem cell transplantation. *Bone Marrow Transplant*. 2001;27(12):1305-1310. PubMed PMID: 11548850.

85. Montgomery RA, Locke JE, King KE, et al. ABO incompatible renal transplantation: a paradigm ready for broad implementation. *Transplantat*. 2009;87(8):1246-1255. PubMed PMID: 19384174. doi: 10.1097/TP.0b013e31819f2024.

86. Rydberg L. ABO-incompatibility in solid organ transplantation. *Transfus Med*. 2001;11(4):325-342. PubMed PMID: 11532188.

87. Hamilton MS, Singh V, Warady BA. Additional case of acute cellular kidney rejection associated with the presence of antibodies to the red blood cell Kidd antigen. *Pediatr Transplant*. 2008;12(8):918-919. PubMed PMID: 18433406. doi: 10.1111/j.1399-3046.2008.00954.x.

88. Hamilton MS, Singh V, Warady BA. Plasma cell-rich acute cellular rejection of a transplanted kidney associated with antibody to the red cell Kidd antigen. *Pediatr Transplant*. 2006;10(8):974-977. PubMed PMID: 17096770. doi: 10.1111/j.1399-3046.2006.00608.x.

in myelodysplastic syndrome. *Haematologica*. 2017;102(12):2021-2029. Epub 20171005. PubMed PMID: 28983058; PMCID: PMC5709101. doi: 10.3324/haematol.2017.175752.

89. Rourk ASJ. Implications of the Kidd blood group system in renal transplantation. *Immunohematol.* 2012;28:91-94.

90. Holt S, Donaldson H, Hazlehurst G, et al. Acute transplant rejection induced by blood transfusion reaction to the Kidd blood group system. *Nephrol Dial Transplant.* 2004;19(9):2403-2406. PubMed PMID: 15299103. doi: 10.1093/ndt/gfh333.

91. Gordon RD, IS, Esquivel CO, et al. Experience with primary liver transplantation across ABO blood groups. *Transplant Proc.* 1987;19(6):4575-4579.

92. Ikegami T, Shirabe K, Soejima Y, Taketomi A, Maehara Y. Feasibility of ABO-incompatible living donor liver transplantation in the rituximab era. *Liver Transplant.* 2010;16(11):1332-1333; author reply 4-5. doi: 10.1002/lt.22160. PubMed PMID: 21031550

93. Shirakawa H, Ishida H, Shimizu T, et al. The low dose of rituximab in ABO-incompatible kidney transplantation without a splenectomy: a single-center experience. *Clin Transplant.* 2011;25(6):878-884. PubMed PMID: 21175849 doi:10.1111/j.1399-0012.2010.01384.x.

94. Cooper DK. Clinical survey of heart transplantation between ABO blood group-incompatible recipients and donors. *J Heart Transplant.* 1990;9(4):376-381. PubMed PMID: 2398432

95. West LJ, Karamlou T, Dipchand AI, Pollock-BarZiv SM, Coles JG, McCrindle BW. Impact on outcomes after listing and transplantation, of a strategy to accept ABO blood group-incompatible donor hearts for neonates and infants. *J Thorac Cardiovasc Surg.* 2006;131(2):455-461. PubMed PMID: 16434278. doi: 10.1016/j.jtcvs.2005.09.048.

96. Roche SL, Burch M, O'Sullivan J, et al. Multicenter experience of ABO-incompatible pediatric cardiac transplantation. *Am J Transplant.* 2008;8(1):208-215. PubMed PMID: 18021280. doi: 10.1111/j.1600-6143.2007.02040.x.

97. West LJ, Pollock-Barziv SM, Dipchand AI, et al. ABO-incompatible heart transplantation in infants. *N Engl J Med.* 2001;344(11):793-800. PubMed PMID: 11248154. doi: 10.1056/NEJM200103153441102.

98. Bellac CL, Hottiger T, Jutzi MP, et al. The role of isoagglutinins in intravenous immunoglobulin-related hemolysis. *Transfusion.* 2015;55(suppl 2):S13-S22. PubMed PMID: 26174892. doi: 10.1111/trf.13113.

99. Taylor E, Vu D, Legare C, Keene D. Intravenous immune globulin-related hemolysis: comparing two different methods for case assessment. *Transfusion.* 2015;55(suppl 2):S23-S27. PubMed PMID: 26174894. doi:doi: 10.1111/trf.13096.

100. Berg R, Shebl A, Kimber MC, Abraham M, Schreiber GB. Hemolytic events associated with intravenous immune globulin therapy: a qualitative analysis of 263 cases reported to four manufacturers between 2003 and 2012. *Transfusion.* 2015;55(suppl 2):S36-S46. PubMed PMID: 26174896. doi: 10.1111/trf.13198.

101. Rubin TLA, Gehrie E, Hsu FI. Hemolysis associated with IVIG therapy (abstract). *J Allergy.* 2016;137(suppl 2):AB257.

102. Zeidan AM, DeAngelo DJ, Palmer J, et al. Phase 1 study of anti-CD47 monoclonal antibody CC-90002 in patients with relapsed/refractory acute myeloid leukemia and high-risk myelodysplastic syndromes. *Ann Hematol.* 2022. PubMed PMID: 34981142. doi: 10.1007/s00277-021-04734-2.

103. Jones AD, Moayeri M, Nambiar A. Impact of new myeloma agents on the transfusion laboratory. *Pathology.* 2021;53(3):427-437. PubMed PMID: 33707006. doi: 10.1016/j.pathol.2021.01.001.

104. Brierley CK, Staves J, Roberts C, et al. The effects of monoclonal anti-CD47 on RBCs, compatibility testing, and transfusion requirements in refractory acute myeloid leukemia. *Transfusion.* 2019;59(7):2248-2254. PubMed PMID: 31183877, doi:doi: 10.1111/trf.15397.

105. Curtis BR. Platelet and granulocyte antigens and antibodies. In: Fung MK, ed. *Technical Manual.* ed. 18th ed. AABB; 2014:453-474.

106. King KE, Shirey RS, Thoman SK, Bensen-Kennedy D, Tanz WS, Ness PM. Universal leukoreduction decreases the incidence of febrile nonhemolytic transfusion reactions to RBCs. *Transfusion.* 2004;44(1):25-29. PubMed PMID: 14692963.

107. The Trial to Reduce Alloimmunization to Platelets Study Group. Leukocyte reduction and ultraviolet B irradiation of platelets to prevent alloimmunization and refractoriness to platelet transfusions. *N Engl J Med.* 1997;337(26):1861-1869. PubMed PMID: 9417523. doi: 10.1056/NEJM199712253372601.

108. Cardillo A, Heal JM, Henrichs K, et al. Reducing the need for HLA-matched platelet transfusion. *N Engl J Med.* 2021;384(25):2451-2452. PubMed PMID: 34161713. doi: 10.1056/NEJMc2034764.

109. Opelz G, Wujciak T, Dohler B, Scherer S, Mytilineos J. HLA compatibility and organ transplant survival. Collaborative Transplant Study. *Rev Immunogenet.* 1999;1(3):334-342. PubMed PMID: 11256424.

110. Hansen JA, Yamamoto K, Petersdorf E, Sasazuki T. The role of HLA matching in hematopoietic cell transplantation. *Rev Immunogenet.* 1999;1(3):359-373. PubMed PMID: 11256427.

111. Ketheesan N, Tay GK, Witt CS, Christiansen FT, Taylor RR, Dawkins RL. The significance of HLA matching in cardiac transplantation. *J Heart Lung Transplant.* 1999;18(3):226-230. PubMed PMID: 10328148.

112. Pile KD. Broadsheet number 51: HLA and disease associations. *Pathology.* 1999;31(3):202-212. PubMed PMID: 10503262.

113. Thorsby E. Invited anniversary review: HLA associated diseases. *Hum Immunol.* 1997;53(1):1-11. PubMed PMID: 9127141. doi: 10.1016/S0198-8859(97)00024-4.

114. Klein J, Sato A. The HLA system. Second of two parts. *N Engl J Med.* 2000;343(11):782-786. PubMed PMID: 10984567. doi: 10.1056/NEJM200009143431106.

115. TH P. The ring study: a randomized controlled trial of GCSF-stimulated granulocytes in granulocytopenic patients. *Blood.* 2014;124:SCI-16.

116. Saito S, Ota S, Seshimo H, et al. Platelet transfusion refractoriness caused by a mismatch in HLA-C antigens. *Transfusion.* 2002;42(3):302-308. PubMed PMID: 11961234.

117. Bolgiano DC, LE, Slichter SJ. A model to determine required pool size for HLA-typed community donor apheresis programs. *Transfusion.* 1989;29:306-310.

118. Petz LD, Garratty G, Calhoun L, et al. Selecting donors of platelets for refractory patients on the basis of HLA antibody specificity. *Transfusion.* 2000;40(12):1446-1456. PubMed PMID: 11134563.

119. Toy P, Gajic O, Bacchetti P, et al. Transfusion-related acute lung injury: incidence and risk factors. *Blood.* 2012;119(7):1757-1767. PubMed PMID: 22117051; PMCID: PMC3286351. doi: 10.1182/blood-2011-08-370932.

120. KEWebert, SJames, DMArnold, HWChan, NMHeddle, JGKelton. Red cell, platelet, and white cell antigens. In: Greer JP Daniel A, Glader B, List AF, Means RT, Paraskevas F, et al., eds. Wintrobe's Clinical Hematology. 13th ed. Lippincott Williams & Wilkins.

121. Storch EK, Hillyer CD, Shaz BH. Spotlight on pathogenesis of TRALI: HNA-3a (CTL2) antibodies. *Blood.* 2014;124(12):1868-1872. PubMed PMID: 25006121. doi: 10.1182/blood-2014-05-538181.

122. Browne T, Dearman RJ, Poles A. Human neutrophil antigens: nature, clinical significance and detection. *Int J Immunogenet.* 2021;48(2):145-156. Epub 20200924. PubMed PMID: 32970372. doi: 10.1111/iji.12514.

123. Bux J. Human neutrophil alloantigens. *Vox Sang.* 2008;94(4):277-285. PubMed PMID: 18208407. doi: 10.1111/j.1423-0410.2007.01031.x.

124. Bux J, Stein EL, Bierling P, et al. Characterization of a new alloantigen (SH) on the human neutrophil Fc gamma receptor IIIb. *Blood.* 1997;89(3):1027-1034. PubMed PMID: 9028335.

125. Flesch BK, Reil A. Molecular genetics of the human neutrophil antigens. *Transfus Med Hemother.* 2018;45(5):300-309. Epub 20180817PubMed PMID: 30498408; PMCID: PMC6257083. doi: 10.1159/000491031.

126. Curtis BR, Reno C, Aster RH. Neonatal alloimmune neutropenia attributed to maternal immunoglobulin G antibodies against the neutrophil alloantigen HNA-1c (SH): a report of five cases. *Transfusion.* 2005;45(8):1308-1313. PubMed PMID: 16078917. doi: 10.1111/j.1537-2995.2005.00199.x.

127. Reil A, Sachs UJ, Siahanidou T, Flesch BK, Bux J. HNA-1d: a new human neutrophil antigen located on Fcgamma receptor IIIb associated with neonatal immune neutropenia. *Transfusion.* 2013;53(10):2145-2151. PubMed PMID: 23347194. doi: 10.1111/trf.12086.

128. Stroncek DF, Skubitz KM, Plachta LB, et al. Alloimmune neonatal neutropenia due to an antibody to the neutrophil Fc-gamma receptor III with maternal deficiency of CD16 antigen. *Blood.* 1991;77(7):1572-1580. PubMed PMID: 1826224.

129. Huizinga TW, Kuijpers RW, Kleijer M, et al. Maternal genomic neutrophil FcRIII deficiency leading to neonatal isoimmune neutropenia. *Blood.* 1990;76(10):1927-1932. PubMed PMID: 1978690.

130. Mraz GA, Crighton GL, Christie DJ. Antibodies to human neutrophil antigen HNA-4b implicated in a case of neonatal alloimmune neutropenia. *Transfusion.* 2016;56(5):1161-1165. PubMed PMID: 26749553. doi: 10.1111/trf.13463.

131. Kissel K, Scheffler S, Kerowgan M, Bux J. Molecular basis of NB1 (HNA-2a, CD177) deficiency. *Blood.* 2002;99(11):4231-4233. PubMed PMID: 12010833

132. Bux J, Becker F, Seeger W, Kilpatrick D, Chapman J, Waters A. Transfusion-related acute lung injury due to HLA-A2-specific antibodies in recipient and NB1-specific antibodies in donor blood. *Br J Haematol.* 1996;93(3):707-713. PubMed PMID: 8652399

133. Leger R, Palm S, Wulf H, Vosberg A, Neppert J. Transfusion-related lung injury with leukopenic reaction caused by fresh frozen plasma containing anti-NB1. *Anesthesiology.* 1999;91(5):1529-1532. PubMed PMID: 10551607

134. Stroncek DF, Shapiro RS, Filipovich AH, Plachta LB, Clay ME. Prolonged neutropenia resulting from antibodies to neutrophil-specific antigen NB1 following marrow transplantation. *Transfusion.* 1993;33(2):158-163. PubMed PMID: 8430456

135. Yomtovian R, Kline W, Press C, et al. Severe pulmonary hypersensitivity associated with passive transfusion of a neutrophil-specific antibody. *Lancet.* 1984;1(8371):244-246. PubMed PMID: 6142994

136. Reil A, Keller-Stanislawski B, Gunay S, Bux J. Specificities of leucocyte alloantibodies in transfusion-related acute lung injury and results of leucocyte antibody screening of blood donors. *Vox Sang.* 2008;95(4):313-317. PubMed PMID: 19138261. doi: 10.1111/j.1423-0410.2008.01092.x.

137. Key TCV, Day S, Goodwin J, et al. Human neutrophil antibodies associated with early and chronic antibody mediated rejection in kidney transplant recipients. *J Ren Transplant Sci.* 2019;2:81-84.

138. Key TCV, Day S, Goodwin P, et al. Human neutrophil antibodies are associated with severe early rejection in kidney transplant recipients. *Transplantation.* 2018;102:S214.

139. Fung YL, Pitcher LA, Willett JE, et al. Alloimmune neonatal neutropenia linked to anti-HNA-4a. *Transfus Med.* 2003;13(1):49-52. PubMed PMID: 12581454

140. Hartman KR, Wright DG. Identification of autoantibodies specific for the neutrophil adhesion glycoproteins CD11b/CD18 in patients with autoimmune neutropenia. *Blood.* 1991;78(4):1096-1104. PubMed PMID: 1678288.

141. Simsek S, van der Schoot CE, Daams M, et al. Molecular characterization of antigenic polymorphisms (Ond(a) and Mart(a)) of the beta 2 family recognized by human leukocyte alloantisera. *Blood.* 1996;88(4):1350-1358. PubMed PMID: 8695853.

142. Pegels JG, Bruynes EC, Korthals Altes HR, Engelfriet CP, von dem Borne AE. Immune Unresponsiveness to platelets. A case study. *Vox Sang.* 1982;42(4):211-216. PubMed PMID: 7046248.

143. Porcelijn L, Abbink F, Terraneo L, Onderwater-vd Hoogen L, Huiskes E, de Haas M. Neonatal alloimmune neutropenia due to immunoglobulin G antibodies against human neutrophil antigen-5a. *Transfusion.* 2011;51(3):574-577. PubMed PMID: 20735765. doi: 10.1111/j.1537-2995.2010.02858.x.

144. Bertrand G, Danger Y, Croisille L, et al. A new platelet alloantigen (Efs(a) , HPA-35bw) on glycoprotein IIIa leading to neonatal alloimmune thrombocytopenia. *Transfusion.* 2019;59(7):2463-2464. PubMed PMID: 30942487. doi: 10.1111/trf.15283.

145. Platelet Antigen Database [Internet] [cited 12/6/2021]https://www.versiti.org/medical-professionals/precision-medicine-expertise/platelet-antigen-database#hpadatabase .

146. Woelke C, Eichler P, Washington G, Flesch BK. Post-transfusion purpura in a patient with HPA-1a and GPIa/IIa antibodies. *Transfus Med.* 2006;16(1):69-72. PubMed PMID: 16480442. doi: 10.1111/j.1365-3148.2005.00633.x.

147. Hawkins J, Aster RH, Curtis BR. Post-transfusion purpura: current perspectives. *J Blood Med.* 2019;10:405-415. PubMed PMID: 31849555; PMCID: PMC6910090. doi: 10.2147/JBM.S189176.

148. Immuno Polymorphism Database [cited 2022 1/21]https://www.ebi.ac.uk/ipd/imgt/hla/.

149. Peterson JA, Pechauer SM, Gitter ML, Szabo A, Curtis BR, Aster RH. The human platelet polymorphisms associated with neonatal alloimmune thrombocytopenia. *Transfusion.* 2012;52(4):915-916. PubMed PMID: 22490273; PMCID: PMC4427891. doi: 10.1111/j.1537-2995.2011.03508.x.

150. Peterson JA, Gitter ML, Kanack A, et al. New low-frequency platelet glycoprotein polymorphisms associated with neonatal alloimmune thrombocytopenia. *Transfusion.* 2010;50(2):324-333. PubMed PMID: 19821948; PMCID: PMC3568744. doi: 10.1111/j.1537-2995.2009.02438.x.

151. Shibata Y, Matsuda I, Miyaji T, Ichikawa Y. Yuka, a new platelet antigen involved in two cases of neonatal alloimmune thrombocytopenia. *Vox Sang.* 1986;50(3):177-180. PubMed PMID: 3716290.

152. Morel-Kopp MC, Blanchard B, Kiefel V, Joly C, Mueller-Eckhardt C, Kaplan C. Anti-HPA-4b (anti-Yuk(a)) neonatal alloimmune thrombocytopenia: first report in a Caucasian family. *Transfus Med.* 1992;2(4):273-276. PubMed PMID: 1339581.

153. Kroll H, Kiefel V, Santoso S, Mueller-Eckhardt C. Sra, a private platelet antigen on glycoprotein IIIa associated with neonatal alloimmune thrombocytopenia. *Blood.* 1990;76(11):2296-2302. PubMed PMID: 2257303.

154. Kroll H, Yates J, Santoso S. Immunization against a low-frequency human platelet alloantigen in fetal alloimmune thrombocytopenia is not a single event: characterization by the combined use of reference DNA and novel allele-specific cell lines expressing recombinant antigens. *Transfusion.* 2005;45(3):353-358. PubMed PMID: 15752152. doi: 10.1111/j.1537-2995.2005.04218.x.

155. Simsek S, Vlekke AB, Kuijpers RW, Goldschmeding R, von dem Borne AE. A new private platelet antigen, Groa, localized on glycoprotein IIIa, involved in neonatal alloimmune thrombocytopenia. *Vox Sang.* 1994;67(3):302-306. PubMed PMID: 7863631.

156. Santoso S, Amrhein J, Hofmann HA, et al. A point mutation Thr(799)Met on the alpha(2) integrin leads to the formation of new human platelet alloantigen Sit(a) and affects collagen-induced aggregation. *Blood.* 1999;94(12):4103-4111. PubMed PMID: 10590055.

157. McFarland JG, Blanchette V, Collins J, Newman PJ, Wang R, Aster RH. Neonatal alloimmune thrombocytopenia due to a new platelet-specific alloantibody. *Blood.* 1993;81(12):3318-3323. PubMed PMID: 8507868.

158. Kekomaki R, Jouhikainen T, Ollikainen J, Westman P, Laes M. A new platelet alloantigen, Tua, on glycoprotein IIIa associated with neonatal alloimmune thrombocytopenia in two families. *Br J Haematol.* 1993;83(2):306-310. PubMed PMID: 8457479.

159. Poon MC, d'Oiron R. Alloimmunization in congenital deficiencies of platelet surface glycoproteins: focus on glanzmann's thrombasthenia and bernard-soulier's syndrome. *Semin Thromb Hemost.* 2018;44(6):604-614. PubMed PMID: 29879742. doi: 10.1055/s-0038-1648233.

160. Nurden AT. Glanzmann thrombasthenia. *Orphanet J Rare Dis.* 2006;1:10. Epub 20060406. PubMed PMID: 16722529; PMCID: PMC1475837. doi: 10.1186/1750-1172-1-10.

161. Peterson JA, McFarland JG, Curtis BR, Aster RH. Neonatal alloimmune thrombocytopenia: pathogenesis, diagnosis and management. *Br J Haematol.* 2013;161(1):3-14. PubMed PMID: 23384054; PMCID: PMC3895911. doi: 10.1111/bjh.12235.

162. Curtis BR, Ali S, Glazier AM, Ebert DD, Aitman TJ, Aster RH. Isoimmunization against CD36 (glycoprotein IV): description of four cases of neonatal isoimmune thrombocytopenia and brief review of the literature. *Transfusion.* 2002;42(9):1173-1179. PubMed PMID: 12430674.

163. Bierling P, Godeau B, Fromont P, et al. Posttransfusion purpura-like syndrome associated with CD36 (Naka) isoimmunization. *Transfusion.* 1995;35(9):777-782. PubMed PMID: 7570941.

164. Ikeda H, Mitani T, Ohnuma M, et al. A new platelet-specific antigen, Naka, involved in the refractoriness of HLA-matched platelet transfusion. *Vox Sang.* 1989;57(3):213-217. PubMed PMID: 2617957.

165. Boylan B, Chen H, Rathore V, et al. Anti-GPVI-associated ITP: an acquired platelet disorder caused by autoantibody-mediated clearance of the GPVI/FcRgamma-chain complex from the human platelet surface. *Blood.* 2004;104(5):1350-1355. PubMed PMID: 15150079. doi: 10.1182/blood-2004-03-0896.

166. Akiyama M, Kashiwagi H, Todo K, et al. Presence of platelet-associated anti-glycoprotein (GP)VI autoantibodies and restoration of GPVI expression in patients with GPVI deficiency. *J Thromb Haemostasis.* 2009;7(8):1373-1383. PubMed PMID: 19522742. doi: 10.1111/j.1538-7836.2009.03510.x.

167. Slichter SJ, Davis K, Enright H, et al. Factors affecting posttransfusion platelet increments, platelet refractoriness, and platelet transfusion intervals in thrombocytopenic patients. *Blood.* 2005;105(10):4106-4114. PubMed PMID: 15692069; PMCID: PMC1895076. doi: 10.1182/blood-2003-08-2724.

168. Julmy F, Ammann RA, Taleghani BM, Fontana S, Hirt A, Leibundgut K. Transfusion efficacy of ABO major-mismatched platelets (PLTs) in children is inferior to that of ABO-identical PLTs. *Transfusion.* 2009;49(1):21-33. PubMed PMID: 18774963. doi: 10.1111/j.1537-2995.2008.01914.x.

169. Skogen B, Rossebo Hansen B, Husebekk A, Havnes T, Hannestad K. Minimal expression of blood group A antigen on thrombocytes from A2 individuals. *Transfusion.* 1988;28(5):456-459. PubMed PMID: 3138793.

Transfusion Medicine

MRIGENDER SINGH VIRK • SUCHITRA PANDEY • JENNIFER ANDREWS

INTRODUCTION

The first documented transfusion of blood in humans occurred in 1667, but it was not until almost 300 years later that transfusion became a therapeutic practicality after Landsteiner's landmark discovery in the early 1900s of blood groups and agglutinating antibodies. The development of anticoagulants, blood preservatives, and sterile collection sets in the middle of the 20th century made blood banking possible by enabling the collection and preservation of donor blood for later use.

In the past few decades, the complexity of transfusion medicine has exploded. Both infectious and noninfectious complications of transfusion have led to practice changes involving blood donor screening, component production and modification, compatibility testing, and blood utilization. The menu of blood component options and therapeutic services has progressively expanded, along with efforts to establish evidence-based guidelines for their optimal use. Specialized recommendations have been developed for supporting specific patient populations, such as immunosuppressed patients, chronic transfusion recipients, hematopoietic cell transplant recipients, and neonates.[1] In the United States, Food and Drug Administration (FDA) regulations govern all aspects of blood collection, component processing, storage, compatibility testing, and administration. The FDA requires blood establishments to comply with stringent quality assurance standards that ensure control of processes and restrict variability. The AABB (Association for the Advancement of Blood & Biotherapies, formerly known as the American Association of Blood Banks) and the College of American Pathologists issue accreditations and standards that further establish best practices in the United States.[2]

Today, transfusion medicine/blood banking is itself a Board-recognized clinical specialty. In addition to overseeing the complex donor center and transfusion service operations, transfusion medicine physicians are increasingly important participants in the clinical care team. Transfusion medicine specialists guide the selection of therapeutic options to best support a patient's medical needs and coordinate the supply and delivery of these blood components and therapeutic services.[3] This chapter serves as a review of the current state of transfusion medicine.

BLOOD DONOR EVALUATION

Donor Selection

Donor selection is undertaken with two goals in mind: to ensure the safety of the donor giving blood and to provide safe blood components for patients. During donor qualification, a series of overlapping safeguards is utilized including positive donor identification, maintenance of donor records, predonation educational materials, a health history questionnaire, a limited physical examination, and sophisticated donor testing. With implementation of rigorous donor screening criteria, it is estimated that approximately 41% to 63% of the US population is eligible to donate blood, but only approximately 5% of the currently eligible donor population annually donate.[4,5]

In the United States, blood components (i.e., red blood cells [RBCs], plasma, platelets, cryoprecipitate, and granulocytes) are collected and prepared from unpaid volunteer donors. These donors have a decreased risk of transmitting infectious agents, especially in the "window period" (infection to detection) when screening tests fail to detect infection. Paying donors for transfusion products was discontinued in the 1970s after studies showed that paid donors had a much higher prevalence of hepatitis.[6] Commercial manufacturers of plasma-derived medicines (e.g., albumin, intravenous immunoglobulin [IVIG], coagulation factor concentrates) still use paid donors,

but comply with FDA-approved donor eligibility criteria and employ pathogen reduction processes during manufacturing that reduce infectious risks, as discussed later in this chapter.

Prior to donation, the donor reviews educational materials as a part of donor qualification. This includes an explanation of the donation process, a list of medications that require temporary or indefinite donor deferral, an explanation of the testing process, and a discussion of specific high-risk behaviors that preclude donor eligibility. The donor must be informed that testing may not detect all infections and that they should not donate blood to obtain infectious disease results.

The donor completes a medical questionnaire developed by the FDA and AABB intended to ensure both donor and patient safety. This includes a review of the donor's current health, questions about specific infectious disease risk factors (e.g., travel history, high-risk behaviors), recent immunizations and medication use, and several general health history questions (e.g., cancer history, heart or lung problems, bleeding conditions). Responses are reviewed with the donor by qualified staff. The donor must meet hemoglobin (Hb), minimum weight, temperature, blood pressure, pulse, and arm visual inspection criteria prior to donation. Male donors must have a Hb value of at least 13.0 g/dL and females at least 12.5 g/dL.[7] Donors must weigh a minimum of 50 kg (110 pounds) and must be deemed to be in good health with a normal temperature (less than or equal to 99.5 °F) and a blood pressure and pulse within acceptable limits (blood pressure systolic between 90 and 180 mm Hg and diastolic between 50 and 100 mm Hg; pulse must be regular and between 50 and 100 beats per minute).[7] The phlebotomy site must be inspected and not have evidence of infection, inflammation, or lesions that may indicate parenteral drug abuse.[7]

The donor must sign the health history form, verifying that all questions were answered truthfully, that the donation process is understood, and that they consent to testing for infectious agents transmitted by transfusion, including human immunodeficiency virus (HIV) and hepatitis. Donors are additionally provided instructions to call the blood center subsequent to the donation if they develop illness or if they have concerns related to the safety of their blood.

BLOOD COLLECTION AND PROCESSING

Modern transfusion practices rely primarily upon component therapy (e.g., RBCs, platelets, cryoprecipitate, and plasma) rather than whole blood transfusions (*Table 23.1*). Component potency can be maintained with storage of each product type under its ideal conditions. Maximum efficiency of resources can also be achieved, as a single blood donation can provide component therapy to multiple patients.

Blood (Manual) Donation

The majority of RBC and plasma products transfused in the United States are prepared from whole blood donations. Blood is collected through a large-bore phlebotomy needle that allows rapid blood flow and mixing with an anticoagulant solution present in the primary collection bag. The volume drawn is standardized for the collection bag used and results in either a 450 milliliter (mL) (±10%) or a 500 mL (±10%) whole blood collection.[8]

Automated Blood Collection and Separation Devices: Apheresis

The term *apheresis* is derived from a Greek word that means to separate or to take away. In modern blood banking and transfusion medicine, this refers to a process in which whole blood is collected through a closed circuit, separated into its constituent elements (often through centrifugation), and specific blood components are retained in

Table 23.1. Blood Components and Indications for Use

Component	Composition	Volume	Indications and Expected Benefit
Whole blood	RBC and plasma (approx. Hct, 40%); WBCs; platelets[a]	500 mL	To increase red cell mass and plasma volume (plasma deficient in labile clotting factors V and VIII); for hypovolemic anemia, massive transfusion, or exchange transfusion in neonates
Packed RBCs	RBC and 25-75 mL plasma (approx. Hct, 75%); WBCs; platelets[a]	250 mL	To increase red cell mass in symptomatic anemia; 10 mL/kg raises Hct by 10%
RBCs, adenine-saline added	RBC and 100 mL of additive solution (approx. Hct, 60%); WBCs; platelets[a]; little plasma	330 mL	To increase red cell mass in symptomatic anemia; 10 mL/kg raises Hct by 8%
RBCs, leukocytes reduced (prepared by filtration)	>85% original volume of RBCs; $<5 \times 10^6$ WBCs	>85% of original volume	To increase red cell mass; $<5 \times 10^6$ WBCs to decrease the likelihood of febrile reactions, immunization to platelets (HLA antigens), or CMV transmission
RBCs, washed	RBCs (approx. Hct, 75%); reduced WBCs; no plasma	225 mL	To increase red cell mass; and reduce risk of allergic reactions to plasma proteins; or reduce free potassium dose
RBCs, frozen	RBCs (approx. Hct, 75%)	225 mL	To increase red cell mass; minimize febrile or allergic transfusion reactions; use for prolonged RBC blood storage
RBCs, deglycerolized	$<5 \times 10^6$ WBCs; no platelets; no plasma		
Granulocytes, pheresis	Granulocytes ($>1.0 \times 10^{10}$ polymorphonuclear cells/U); lymphocytes; platelets ($>2.0 \times 10^{11}$/U); some RBCs	220 mL	To provide granulocytes for selected patients with sepsis and severe neutropenia ($<0.5 \times 10^9$/L)
Platelet concentrates	Platelets ($>5.5 \times 10^{10}$/U); RBCs; WBCs; plasma	50 mL	Bleeding owing to thrombocytopenia or thrombocytopathy; 1 U/10 kg raises platelet count by $17-50 \times 10^9$/L
Platelets, pheresis	Platelets ($>3 \times 10^{11}$/U); RBCs; WBCs; plasma	300 mL	Same as platelets; sometimes HLA matched; benefit is equivalent to six platelet concentrates
Platelets, leukocytes reduced	Platelets (as above); $<5 \times 10^6$ WBCs/final dose of pooled or pheresis platelets	300 mL	Same as platelets; $<5 \times 10^6$ WBCs to decrease the likelihood of febrile reactions, alloimmunization to leukocytes (HLA antigens), or CMV transmission
FFP; thawed plasma; liquid plasma	FFP: all coagulation factors; thawed and liquid plasma: reduced factors V and VIII	200 mL	Treatment of some coagulation disorders; 10 mL/kg of FFP raises factor levels by approximately 10%
Cryoprecipitate	Fibrinogen; factors VIII and XIII; von Willebrand factor	15 mL	Deficiency of fibrinogen, 1 U/5 kg raises fibrinogen 70 mg/dL; also used for factor XIII replacement; not first-choice therapy for hemophilia A, von Willebrand disease, topical fibrin sealant

[a]WBCs and platelets are nonfunctional.
Abbreviations: approx., approximate; CMV, cytomegalovirus; FFP, fresh frozen plasma; Hct, hematocrit; HLA, human leukocyte antigen; RBC, red blood cell; WBC, white blood cell.
Modified with permission from King KE, ed. *Blood Transfusion Therapy: A Physician's Handbook*. 11th ed. American Association of Blood Banks; 2014. Table 1. Copyright © 2014 by AABB.

collection bags while the remaining blood is returned to the donor or patient. Apheresis technology has become a routine collection method for transfusable blood components and the majority of platelets transfused in the United States are collected via apheresis.[9]

In blood banking, the major advantage of apheresis donations is that only the desired blood component or components are collected, while the remaining blood is returned to the donor. This makes it possible to obtain multiple unit-equivalent doses of platelets, plasma, or RBCs from a single donation. Because there is limited loss of RBCs during an apheresis donation, plasma and platelet apheresis donors can donate more frequently than whole blood donors. The specific components collected during an apheresis donation may be based upon individual donor characteristics (e.g., ABO/Rh type, gender, Hb level), as well as inventory management needs.

Complications of Donation

Whole blood and apheresis collections are very safe; however, a small number of donors experience adverse reactions during, or shortly after, donation. Approximately 2% to 3% of all presenting donors experience a complication, the most common being a vasovagal reaction with or without loss of consciousness followed by local injury related to the needle, such as a hematoma.[10] Individual reaction rates vary widely based upon donor age, gender, donation type, and donation history. First-time donors and young donors (16-22 years old) have higher reaction rates than repeat donors and older donors, respectively. During apheresis collections, blood that is anticoagulated with citrate is returned to the donor. Although citrate is rapidly metabolized, a citrate reaction can occur due to transient hypocalcemia. Symptoms are usually mild, such as paresthesias and tingling, and are managed by slowing the rate of return of citrated blood and/or giving oral calcium.[1] Importantly, the majority of donor reactions are mild and resolve quickly without requiring medical attention. To better understand donor reactions and improve donor safety, implementation of standardized reaction definitions is needed along with widespread hemovigilance reporting.[11,12] Hemovigilance is currently largely voluntary in the United States but mandatory in other countries.

Recently, there has been an increased focus on iron deficiency in blood donors. Certain donor populations, such as young donors, frequent donors, and premenopausal women, are at increased risk of developing iron deficiency with blood donation.[13] AABB standards require that donors be given educational materials about the risks of postdonation iron deficiency and mitigation strategies.[2] Strategies include increasing the interdonation interval in high-risk donors, ferritin testing, and postdonation iron supplementation. One study showed that a minimum of 18 mg of elemental iron daily for 60 days can replace the iron lost in a whole blood donation.[13]

Transfusion Medicine

DONOR TESTING

Every blood donation undergoes a series of tests to determine its suitability for transfusion. In the United States, as of late 2016, the following tests must be performed on every unit collected: ABO group and Rh(D) type; red cell antibody screen; serologic tests for infectious disease markers including hepatitis B surface antigen (HBsAg), antibodies to hepatitis B core (HBc) antigen, hepatitis C, HIV-1 and -2, human T-cell lymphotropic virus I and II, and syphilis; and nucleic acid tests for HIV-1 RNA, hepatitis C virus (HCV) RNA, hepatitis B virus (HBV) DNA, and West Nile virus (WNV) RNA (*Table 23.2*).[2] In 2010, the FDA recommended one-time testing of allogeneic donors for antibodies to *Trypanosoma cruzi* (the causative agent of Chagas disease).[14] In 2016, FDA required that all blood donations be tested for Zika virus (ZIKV) RNA, but in 2021 FDA allowed discontinuation of ZIKV testing, since ZIKV no longer had sufficient incidence or prevalence to affect the potential donor population.[15] Finally, in 2019, FDA recommended that nucleic acid testing (NTA) for *Babesia microti* be performed on all donations collected in 14 high-risk states and Washington D.C.[16]

Beyond the required donor tests, additional tests may be performed on a portion of collections based upon inventory management needs, patient order requests, specific donor attributes (e.g., gender, pregnancy history), donation type, and other factors. For plasma, apheresis platelets, and whole blood products, AABB standards require that HLA antibody testing be negative for female donors with pregnancy history in order to mitigate the risk of transfusion-related acute lung injury (TRALI). Other tests performed on blood donations include cytomegalovirus (CMV) serology and phenotyping for minor RBC antigens. These may be utilized as part of a broad strategy to support overall transfusion safety or may be used to help support specific patient clinical needs.

Table 23.2. Infectious Disease Screening Tests Performed on US Blood Donations

Infection	Tests Designed to Detect
HBV	Hepatitis B surface antigen
	IgG antibody to hepatitis B core antigen
	HBV DNA by NAT[a]
HCV	IgG antibody to hepatitis C peptides
	HCV RNA by NAT[a]
HIV-1/-2	IgG antibody to HIV-1/-2
	HIV-1 RNA by NAT[a]
HTLV-I/-II	IgG antibody to HTLV-I/-II
Syphilis	IgG antibody to treponemal antigens
	Or nontreponemal serologic reactivity (e.g., rapid plasma reagin)
WNV	WNV RNA[a,b]
Trypanosoma cruzi	IgG antibody to *T. cruzi*[c]
Babesia microti	*Babesia microti* DNA by NAT[d]

[a]For donor screening, NAT is usually performed on minipools of 6 to 16 donor samples.
[b]Transition to individual sample NAT testing when there is increased WNV activity in blood collection region.
[c]*T. cruzi* antibody testing may be limited to one-time testing of each donor.
[d]Individual sample NAT for donations collected in the following high-risk states/areas: Connecticut, Delaware, Maine, Maryland, Minnesota, Massachusetts, New Hampshire, New Jersey, New York, Pennsylvania, Rhode Island, Vermont, Virginia, Wisconsin, and Washington, D.C.
Abbreviations: NAT, nucleic acid testing; HBV, hepatitis B virus; HCV, hepatitis C virus; HIV, human immunodeficiency virus; HTLV, human T-cell lymphotropic virus; Ig, immunoglobulin; WNV, West Nile virus; ZIKV, Zika virus.

RED BLOOD CELL PRESERVATION AND STORAGE

Anticoagulant/Preservative Solutions

Citrate-based anticoagulants are used for both manual whole blood and automated apheresis collections. Citrate chelates ionized calcium in blood, blocking calcium-dependent coagulation in the collection bag and stored component. After transfusion, the recipient's liver readily metabolizes the infused citrate, limiting any adverse patient effects. Several additional preservatives are included in RBC anticoagulant solutions to help maintain RBC viability. These include dextrose for cell maintenance and phosphate buffers to help retain a stable pH during storage.

A citrate-phosphate-dextrose (CPD) solution fortified with adenine, citrate-phosphate-dextrose-adenine (CPDA-1) became available in the United States in 1978. The addition of adenine allows for improved maintenance of adenosine triphosphate (ATP) content and RBC viability during storage. Initial concerns about potential toxicity of adenine proved to be unfounded. CPDA-1 remains a commonly used RBC anticoagulant-preservative and permits RBC storage for up to 35 days.[8]

Whole Blood

Whole blood (WB) is usually separated into components for transfusion therapy, but recently whole blood transfusions have increased in certain settings such as trauma including prehospital transfusions. Whole blood is stored at 1 °C to 6 °C and has a shelf life of 35 days in CPDA-1 and 21 days in CPD/citrate-phosphate-double dextrose.[2] WB can be leukocyte reduced via a platelet-sparing leukoreduction filter or can remain non–leukocyte reduced. WB contains cold-stored platelets, which may provide an improved hemostatic effect in a bleeding patient. WB can provide RBCs, plasma, and platelets with a single transfusion providing massive transfusion.

Packed Red Cells vs Red Cells in Additive Solutions

During the manufacture of RBC components, whole blood is centrifuged and red cells ("packed RBCs") are separated from most of the "platelet-rich plasma." Approximately 100 mL of anticoagulant-containing plasma must remain with the RBCs to provide a metabolic substrate during storage. CPDA-1 RBC components have a final hematocrit (Hct) of 65% to 80% and a volume between 225 and 350 mL.[8] An alternative approach to red cell preservation involves more complete removal of the anticoagulated plasma from the red cells ("dry pack"), with only approximately 20 to 30 mL of residual plasma remaining.[8] An additive solution (AS) is then added to resuspend the red cells (100 mL AS/450 mL collection; 110 mL AS/500 mL collection). AS-RBCs have a final Hct of 55% to 65% and a volume between 300 and 400 mL.[8] Licensed ASs contain some combination of dextrose, adenine, sodium chloride, and are with or without mannitol. ASs better maintain stored red cell viability and allow for RBC storage for up to 42 days.[8] RBCs in AS are now the most common preparations for transfusion in the United States.

Changes in Red Cells During Storage

RBC components must be stored at 1 °C to 6 °C to maintain optimal functionality and to prevent growth of bacteria. Stored liquid RBCs undergo a variety of changes that may have major influences on their viability and function after transfusion.[17] The RBC "storage lesion" refers to the series of structural, biochemical, and metabolic changes that occur when RBCs are stored ex vivo.

Structural Changes

A number of red cell structural changes contribute to decreased cell survival after storage.[17] RBCs are normally disc shaped; however, soon after storage, they become spherical with surface projections (sphero-echinocytosis). Later defects include loss of membrane lipids and protein, as well as alterations in structural proteins. Loss of membrane deformability correlates with cellular viability after infusion. The more severe membrane changes are irreversible and likely contribute to decreased posttransfusion RBC survival.[17]

Biochemical Changes

Red cells lack mitochondria and depend solely on glycolysis for ATP generation. During component storage, red cells metabolize the limited glucose available, producing lactic and pyruvic acids, and resulting in a lowered pH. As glycolysis slows, RBC ATP content falls. Because human RBCs contain no enzymes to synthesize adenine or other purines de novo, the nucleotide pool gradually becomes exhausted. The presence of adenine and inorganic phosphate in anticoagulant-preservative (CPDA-1) and ASs improves the cells' ability to regenerate ATP. This helps sustain the energy-requiring process that preserves cell membrane integrity and cellular function.

Plasma potassium concentrations in stored RBCs increase because of passive leakage of intracellular potassium from the cells. This is because the major membrane Na^+-K^+ ATPase that normally maintains the K^+ gradient does not function well at 1 °C to 6 °C. Plasma potassium increases approximately 1 mEq/L/d during RBC storage and peaks at approximately 60 to 70 mEq/L depending on the storage media used and RBC Hct.[1] Gamma irradiation of red cells to prevent transfusion-associated graft-vs-host disease (TA-GVHD; see section on TA-GVHD) doubles the rate of potassium leakage.[18] Stored RBCs reabsorb potassium after transfusion.

The accumulation of potassium in stored blood increases the risk of hyperkalemia-induced cardiac arrhythmia or cardiac arrest in select patients.[19] Care must be taken in situations in which large volumes of older, higher-potassium RBCs are used for at-risk vulnerable patients. This includes large-volume transfusions to infants and neonates, to prime cardiopulmonary bypass, dialysis or apheresis circuits, and high-flow administration into central venous circulation.

Red Cell 2,3-Diphosphoglycerate

Another significant change in stored RBCs is 2,3-diphosphoglycerate (DPG) depletion and a resulting leftward shift in the oxygen-Hb dissociation curve. This shift results in increased affinity of Hb for oxygen and less oxygen delivered peripherally to the tissue.[20,21] In CPD, CPDA-1, and AS-stored red cells, 2,3-DPG is depleted after about 2 weeks. 2,3-DPG levels improve rapidly within the first 6 hours after transfusion, and return to near-normal levels within 24 hours.[22] The clinical implication of blood transfusions with decreased 2,3-DPG content is controversial.[20-23]

Clinical Implications of Stored Blood

Whether the age of transfused blood affects clinical outcomes is highly controversial, with many studies coming to different conclusions.[24] For methodologic reasons, the ability of even well-designed, randomized controlled trials to demonstrate significant clinical differences based on the age of transfused blood has been questioned[25]; and to date, a number of prospective, randomized clinical trials in adults[25-27] and one in pediatrics[28,29] have found no difference in clinical outcomes for patients receiving older vs younger blood.

Frozen Red Cells

RBC components may undergo further processing to allow for long-term frozen storage. The most common method uses "high-concentration" glycerol (40%, wt/vol) to cryopreserve RBCs for up to 10 years with storage at −65 °C or colder.[8] After thawing, glycerol is removed by washing the RBCs in successively lower concentrations of sodium chloride. This process should retain 80% or more of the RBCs present in the original blood product. In most cases, postthaw storage is limited to 24 hours because an open system is used to process the thawed red cells.

The cost of processing and storing frozen RBCs, as well as a shortened postthaw outdate, has limited the utility of frozen RBC components. The current primary indication for freezing RBCs is the storage of rare RBC products with uncommon blood types to support hard-to-match patients. Prolonged frozen storage of autologous red cells in the event of a planned or postponed surgery may also be performed.

In Vivo Recovery of Stored Red Cells

After transfusion of stored blood, red cells that have developed lethal degrees of damage are removed promptly from the circulation of the recipient. Red cells that survive the first 24 hours after transfusion have normal survival thereafter.[30] Therefore, a common criterion by which the adequacy for transfusion of banked blood is assessed is the proportion of transfused red cells that remain in circulation at 24 hours after transfusion. Generally, at least 75% survival at 24 hours is considered evidence of adequate stored RBC viability; however, the ability of RBCs to consistently meet this threshold has been questioned.[31] Compared with refrigerated units, frozen deglycerolized RBCs appear to be equally safe and efficacious with regard to transfusion response, adverse reactions, and clinical outcomes.[32]

PLATELET PREPARATION AND STORAGE

Platelets, like erythrocytes, are actively metabolizing cells that require specific conditions during their preparation and storage to optimally maintain viability and function. Platelet components may be prepared from whole blood or apheresis collections.

Preparation of Platelet Concentrates

In a minority of centers in the United States, and more commonly in other countries, whole blood collections undergo further processing to produce a 40 to 70 mL *platelet concentrate* component. Four to six ABO identical platelet concentrate units may be pooled before storage, or just prior to transfusion, to result in a therapeutic adult dose. Whole blood intended for further platelet manufacture is collected into CPD or CPDA-1 bags, transported in conditions that support cooling toward room temperature (20 °C-24 °C), and must be processed within 8 hours of collection.

In the American production method, supernatant platelet–rich plasma is separated from whole blood RBCs at low-speed centrifugation and is expressed into a satellite bag (*Figure 23.1*). The platelet-rich plasma is then centrifuged a second time to concentrate the platelets and express off the majority of the platelet-poor plasma into another transfer bag. After 1 hour, the platelets are gently resuspended in the remaining plasma (40-70 mL) to produce a platelet concentrate component. Approximately 60% to 75% of the donor platelets, or a minimum of 5.5×10^{10} platelets/U, are recovered in the final unit.[33]

In Europe and Canada, whole blood platelet concentrates are prepared by the buffy coat method. Briefly, the whole blood unit is centrifuged at high speed, and the platelet-poor plasma and the buffy coat are withdrawn, each into its own satellite bag. The buffy coat is then centrifuged at low speed to separate the platelets from the red and white cells. The functional quality of these platelets is comparable to those prepared by the American method.[33] Platelet concentrates prepared by the buffy coat method contain fewer white cells than those prepared from platelet-rich plasma, although filtration is still necessary to meet the European standards for leukoreduced products.

Apheresis (Pheresis) Platelets

Apheresis platelets must contain at least 3×10^{11} platelets in approximately 300 mL of plasma by AABB standards.[2] This is equivalent to four to six whole blood–derived platelet concentrates.[8] Apheresis platelets are leukoreduced by the collection technology and do not require further filtration.

The primary clinical advantage of apheresis platelets is that a single donor can provide a therapeutic patient dose from one blood donor. This minimizes recipient exposure to possible infectious agents and in addition allows for the provision of HLA-matched or antigen-negative units to support platelet refractory patients.

Platelet Storage and Functional Integrity

Platelet components prepared from both whole blood and apheresis collections are stored under the same conditions. Platelet survival and function are optimized by storage at room temperature (20 °C-24 °C) with gentle agitation to help support gas exchange.[34] Platelet bags are gas permeable, allowing oxygen to enter and CO_2 to leave the component. This supports continued platelet oxidative metabolism and limits acidosis. Although platelet viability is maintained for up to 7 days of storage, room temperature shelf life was previously only approved for

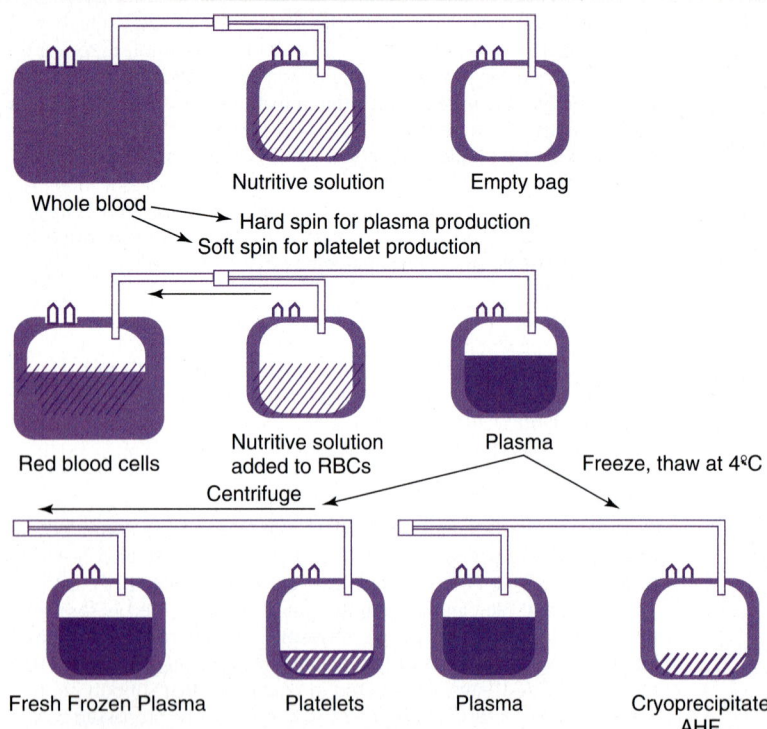

Whole blood → Hard spin for plasma production
Soft spin for platelet production

Nutritive solution

Empty bag

Red blood cells

Nutritive solution added to RBCs

Plasma

Freeze, thaw at 4ºC

Centrifuge

Fresh Frozen Plasma

Platelets

Plasma

Cryoprecipitate AHF

FIGURE 23.1 Preparation of components from a whole blood donation. AHF, antihemophilic factor; RBC, red blood cell. (Reprinted with permission from Jeter EK, Spivey MA. Blood components and their use. In: *Introduction to Transfusion Medicine: A Case Study Approach*. American Association of Blood Banks Press; 1996:5, Figures 1-2. Copyright © 1996 by AABB.)

5 days in the United States because of the risk of bacterial growth. However, guidance from the FDA in the fall of 2021 does allow extension of apheresis platelet shelf life to 7 days if large-volume delayed sampling for bacterial cultures is performed to increase sensitivity of the platelet culture.[35] Further discussion of platelet bacterial contamination and mitigation occurs later in this chapter.

Even under optimal storage conditions, platelets, like red cells, develop changes related to component storage. The mechanisms responsible for platelet storage lesion changes are not fully understood but appear to be multifactorial. Platelet storage lesion changes may be associated with loss of platelet recovery, decreased survival, and impaired hemostatic activity after transfusion.

Platelets with good viability have a discoid morphology that reflects light and produces a "swirling" visual effect within the component. During storage, platelets may become activated and become spherical in shape. Activated platelets lack a "swirling" appearance, as the resulting change in shape does not readily diffract light. Platelet activation may occur following exposure to foreign surfaces, vigorous handling, exposure to low pH, cold temperatures, and a variety of other factors. Platelet activation is accompanied by surface expression of sequestered granular membrane proteins (P-selectin and CD63), conformational changes of the glycoprotein IIb/IIIa fibrinogen receptor, and release of platelet granule contents (e.g., β-thromboglobulin, platelet factor 4, etc.). Responsiveness to single agonists (e.g., adenosine phosphate) rapidly declines during storage but can recover after transfusion within the recipient.[36] Lactic acid produced during platelet metabolism ultimately results in pH changes that may further impact platelet function. Studies have shown that platelets begin to suffer deleterious effects below a pH of 6.5 to 6.8 and are irreversibly damaged with a sustained pH < 6.2.[37]

Platelet Additive Solutions

Platelet additive solutions (PASs) have been developed to ameliorate platelet storage lesion changes and improve platelet quality. These are isotonic solutions designed to replace approximately 65% of the plasma used in the storage of platelets.[38] Compounds such as citrate, acetate, phosphate, potassium, magnesium, and glucose have proved to be important constituents of PAS. In vitro evaluation of platelet morphology and function has shown platelets to be better preserved in

PAS compared with traditional plasma. Additionally, platelets stored in PAS appear to have equivalent clinical efficacy for controlling bleeding compared with traditional platelet components.[39] Removal of plasma has additional potential advantages including decreased patient reactions (e.g., allergic, febrile, ABO-incompatible hemolysis, TRALI), use in pathogen inactivation, and utilization of the plasma removed for fractionation or transfusion.

Cold-Stored Platelets

There are numerous benefits to storing platelets at 1 °C to 6 °C including the increase in hemostatic activity of the platelets, reduction of bacterial contamination risk, extension of the platelet's shelf life, and improvement of logistics relating to platelet transport and storage.[40] Cold storage of platelets can increase platelet activation and hemostatic function, which offers an advantage in patients with bleeding.[41] However, cold storage can reduce in vivo survival compared to platelets stored at room temperature.[42] In the United States, regulations allow apheresis platelets to be stored at 1 °C to 6 °C without agitation for up to 3 days for use in patients with active bleeding. Of note, some blood collection establishments have now obtained a variance from the FDA to allow storage for up to 14 days, which improves inventory management.

PREPARATION OF PLASMA COMPONENTS

Plasma can be obtained from whole blood or apheresis collections. Plasma may be used directly for transfusion (e.g., fresh frozen plasma [FFP], plasma frozen within 24 hours [PF24], liquid plasma), further processed into cryoprecipitate, or sent to commercial facilities to be manufactured into plasma-derived products.

Plasma Components for Transfusion

There are a variety of different transfusable plasma components that may be produced, briefly described here.

Fresh Frozen Plasma, Plasma Frozen Within 24 Hours

FFP and PF24 are generally considered clinically interchangeable (i.e., equivalent efficacy), and in practice, physicians will place an order for "plasma" or FFP and the transfusion service will fill the order with

FFP or PF24 according to inventory availability. Both whole blood and apheresis collections may be used to prepare a standard 200 to 250 mL FFP or PF24 component. Apheresis-derived 400 to 600 mL "jumbo" units may also be available. FFP and PF24 are stored at −18 °C or below for up to 1 year. These units are thawed in a water bath at 30 °C to 37 °C or in an FDA-cleared device (e.g., microwave defroster).[8] After thawing, FFP and PF24 may be stored refrigerated at 1 °C to 6 °C for up to 24 hours before use. The distinguishing feature between FFP and PF24 is when freezing is initiated after donor collection.

FFP is prepared by centrifuge separation of citrated plasma from whole blood and frozen within 8 hours of collection. Alternatively, FFP may also be prepared by freezing citrated apheresis plasma within 6 hours of collection. Under these conditions, there is minimal loss of activity of the labile coagulation factors V and VIII. One milliliter of FFP contains approximately 1 IU of each coagulation factor activity.

PF24 (previously known as FP24) has largely replaced FFP production in the United States. PF24 must be separated and frozen within 24 hours of collection. This allows blood centers to make transfusable plasma out of donations collected in locations that are not able to be processed within 8 hours of collection. The content of PF24 is identical to that of FFP except that the factor VIII content may be reduced to 80% that of FFP.[43] Protein C levels are also reduced. The factor VIII content of PF24 is more than sufficient for support of clinical coagulation, especially in light of the fact that the reference interval of factor VIII is 50% to 150% of normal.

Liquid Plasma, Thawed Plasma

Liquid plasma is a term for plasma that is separated from whole blood and stored at 1 °C to 6 °C without freezing. Liquid plasma must be separated and infused no later than 5 days after the expiration date of the whole blood from which it was prepared. Therefore, a CPD whole blood collection (21-day shelf life) would enable preparation of up to a 26-day shelf-life liquid plasma unit. The labile coagulation proteins, factor V and factor VIII, significantly decrease during liquid plasma storage to 39% and 60% of their respective mean initial activity.[44] The primary utilization of liquid plasma is in the immediate support of trauma patients, however, and these levels are sufficient to support clinical hemostasis in bleeding patients (i.e., 30% of normal). With implementation of thawed plasma, liquid plasma is not as commonly used by hospitals.

Thawed plasma is a term for FFP or PF24 that is thawed and stored refrigerated at 1 °C to 6 °C for up to 5 days after thawing. The only significant difference between these products and FFP/PF24 is the content of the labile coagulation factors (V and VIII). After 5 days of refrigerated storage, factor VIII and V levels are at about 65% to 75% of their original levels. Other coagulation factors, including fibrinogen, ADAMTS13, and factors II, VII, IX, X, and XIII, are generally stable under refrigerated storage conditions.[45] Thawed plasma can be made immediately available to support massive transfusions as well as limit unnecessary waste when FFP or PF24 is thawed and then not used by a patient. *Thawed plasma* represents approximately 53% of plasma issued by hospitals. For most clinical indications, thawed plasma is considered clinically equivalent to FFP or PF24 and is used interchangeably within the transfusion service based upon inventory management needs.

Plasma, Cryoprecipitate Reduced

Cryoprecipitate-reduced plasma is the transfusable plasma prepared from whole blood–derived FFP after thawing, centrifugation, and removal of cryoprecipitate (see "Cryoprecipitated Antihemophilic Factor"). This product is also referred to as "cryo-poor plasma." After removal of cryoprecipitate, the supernatant plasma is refrozen within 24 hours of thawing and has the same storage conditions as FFP/PF24. Cryo-poor plasma is deficient in fibrinogen, factor VIII, von Willebrand factor (vWF), and factor XIII. This plasma was initially thought to be superior to FFP for treatment of thrombotic thrombocytopenic purpura (TTP) because of its lower vWF content. Randomized studies have verified that this component is therapeutically effective for TTP; however, it is not superior to FFP.[46]

Cryoprecipitated Antihemophilic Factor

Cryoprecipitated antihemophilic factor or *cryoprecipitate* is an extract of FFP that is enriched in high-molecular-weight plasma proteins. It is prepared by thawing one unit of whole blood–derived FFP at 1 °C to 6 °C and recovering the high-molecular-weight proteins that form as a cold-insoluble precipitate. Precipitated protein is concentrated by centrifugation, and all except approximately 15 mL of supernatant plasma is removed. The resulting 5 to 20 mL cryoprecipitate component may be stored at −18 °C or below for up to 1 year.[8] Each unit of cryoprecipitate contains approximately 80 to 120 U of factor VIII and at least 150 mg of fibrinogen. It also contains factor XIII, fibronectin, and the high-molecular-weight multimers of vWF. Multiple units of cryoprecipitate may be pooled before administration to result in a therapeutic patient dose.

Cryoprecipitate was originally developed for the treatment of hemophilia A (factor VIII deficiency). However, in the United States, it is no longer used for this indication, as safer pathogen-inactivated factor concentrates or recombinant alternatives exist. At the present time, cryoprecipitate is most often used for correction of hypofibrinogenemia in bleeding patients. Cryoprecipitate has also been used topically, along with thrombin and calcium, as a "fibrin glue." However, commercial products that are much more effective as topical hemostatic or sealant agents are now available. Plasma-derived fibrinogen concentrates for intravenous infusion exist, however, and are currently approved in the United States for treatment of congenital fibrinogen deficiency.

Plasma-Derived Therapeutics

Plasma derivatives are made from plasma pooled from thousands of donors. Paid plasmapheresis donors provide the majority of plasma for further fractionation (~70%), with the remainder coming from excess ("recovered") plasma from volunteer whole blood donations.[47] Donor plasma is generally pooled into 2000 to 4000 L batches and specific proteins of interest are separated, purified, and concentrated on the basis of differing protein solubility characteristics. The most commonly used fractionation method is based on Cohn's cold ethanol fractionation process, developed in the 1940s.[48] As the temperature, ionic strength, pH, and ethanol concentration are varied, plasma can be separated into various fractions. Fraction I contains factor VIII and fibrinogen, fraction II contains the immunoglobulins, and fraction V contains albumin. Fractions III and IV contain a number of other coagulation factors and proteins. Although other approaches such as ion exchange chromatography have been applied to the preparation of certain plasma products, Cohn's method remains the standard.

Because the plasma pools used for the production of plasma derivatives involve collections from many donors, the major risk of these products is related to the transmission of blood-borne infectious agents. Therefore, beyond routine donor screening and testing, additional safety measures are required to mitigate infectious disease risk of fractionated products. Bacteria, intracellular viruses, and parasites are not readily transmitted by plasma derivatives because they are destroyed by the freeze-thaw steps or removed by filtration during processing. The fractionation process itself additionally includes several dedicated steps of pathogen removal/inactivation intended to address both known infectious disease agents (e.g., HIV, HCV, HBV) and emerging or unrecognized infectious disease risks. Use of prolonged heating or treatment with organic solvents and detergents (S/D) inactivates enveloped viruses. Pooled plasma products, however, could still transmit infectious agents that lack a lipid envelope and that are resistant to heat. Human parvovirus B19 and hepatitis A are two such agents. The FDA requires screening for, and exclusion of, donations that contain high titers of the B19 virus, which may be associated with infectious risk in the final prepared product. Many plasma derivatives undergo additional purification steps such as affinity chromatography, precipitation, or nanofiltration that would further reduce their contamination by infectious agents.[48] No documented transmission of HIV, HBV, or HCV by products subjected to dedicated viral inactivation treatments has been reported since the 1980s.[49]

There are many commercial plasma derivatives available. Some examples are described in the following.

Solvent/Detergent-Treated Plasma

Because plasma is essentially acellular, it can be virally inactivated using agents that would otherwise destroy cellular blood components. Solvent/detergent-treated plasma (S/D plasma) is made from hundreds or thousands of units of FFP that have been thawed, pooled, subjected to treatment with organic S/D, filtered, and refrozen.[50] S/D plasma was developed to reduce the risk of transmitting enveloped viruses, such as HIV, HCV, and HBV. Nonenveloped viruses (e.g., hepatitis A virus [HAV], parvovirus B19) are not inactivated by this process, nor are prions. A version of this product introduced in the United States in the late 1990s was withdrawn after reports of thromboembolic complications. A new S/D plasma was licensed in the United States in 2013 and is related to a version that has been used extensively in Europe with an established safety record. The current available S/D plasma does not appear to have any thromboembolic complication. S/D plasma has similar levels to FFP for most clotting factors, and clinical study supports that S/D plasma is therapeutically equivalent to, and has the same general indications of, FFP.[50] In contrast to individual donor plasma units (i.e., FFP, PF24), S/D plasma has not been associated with TRALI, presumably because of the dilution of antibodies from individual donors during plasma pooling.

Coagulation Factor Concentrates

Various coagulation factor concentrates are available and include both plasma-derived and recombinant formulations. These are discussed in detail elsewhere as part of the management of inherited or acquired coagulation disorders (Chapters 53 and 54). Notable coagulation factor derivatives include concentrates of fibrinogen, purified factor IX, factor VIII/vWF, and plasma complex concentrates containing vitamin-K-dependent coagulation factors.

Immunoglobulins

Intramuscular, intravenous, and subcutaneous immunoglobulin preparations may all be prepared through pooled human plasma fractionation. Intramuscular immunoglobulin preparations contain dimeric and polymeric IgG as a result of the fractionation procedure, which are capable of nonspecifically activating complement by both the classic and alternative pathways. This mechanism probably explains the major adverse effects that occur if these products are administered intravenously.[48] Products labeled for intramuscular use must therefore not be given intravenously.

IVIGs are produced by additional chemical modifications designed to decrease the aggregation of IgG. Nonspecific complement activation is reduced, whereas the ability of IgG to interact with pathogenic organisms and complement is retained. Many of these products may also be administered subcutaneously.

Nonspecific immunoglobulin preparations contain a broad spectrum of antibodies naturally present in the donor population. They are most often used for treatment of primary immunodeficiency or as immune modulators.[51] Hyperimmune globulins are made by selecting plasma with high titers of a specific antibody or by specifically immunizing donors to produce such antibodies. Such preparations are primarily for intramuscular use; however, in some instances, they may also be made into intravenous formulations. Examples of hyperimmune preparations include Rh immune globulin to prevent Rh(D) alloimmunization and hepatitis B, varicella zoster, and tetanus immunoglobulin preparations to provide temporary passive protection against infections.

BLOOD COMPONENT MODIFICATION

"Closed" vs "Open" Systems

Blood components may undergo further modification within the blood bank or the hospital transfusion service to meet specific patient transfusion needs. If component manipulation is done without opening the system to the outside environment (i.e., closed system), the component may be stored to the limit of its original shelf life. If the bag or tubing is entered, however, the system is considered potentially open to air/bacteria, and the product outdates in 4 hours if stored at room temperature or 24 hours if refrigerated. Devices using high-temperature welds can sterilely attach additional containers or tubing to the original unit in a way that prevents entry of bacteria. With these "sterile connection devices," blood components may be split into aliquots, filtered, or otherwise manipulated without loss of shelf life.

Leukocyte Reduction

When whole blood collections are separated by centrifugation, white blood cells (WBCs) sediment at the interface between red cells and platelet-rich plasma. Therefore, WBCs typically contaminate both red cell and platelet concentrate components, with concentrations of approximately 10^9 WBCs per product. WBCs in blood components can mediate febrile transfusion reactions, stimulate HLA alloimmunization in transfusion recipients, and transmit some cell-associated pathogens such as CMV.[20] Therefore, it is desirable to remove WBCs from transfusable blood components.

Selective leukoreduction filters have been developed capable of at least a 3-log reduction of WBCs in blood components. These synthetic fiber filters remove WBCs by a combination of mesh density, chemical attraction, and active adhesion. To meet FDA criteria for leukocyte reduction, all RBC units must have less than 5×10^6 WBCs/U and at least 85% of the original red cell content.[52]

Leukocyte reduction of RBC components is most often performed by blood collection centers within the first few days after collection using an integral or sterilely connected filtration system. Filtration prior to storage reduces WBC breakdown products in the blood component. The vast majority of RBC units collected, prepared, or modified in the United States are leukocyte reduced.

Apheresis platelets contain very few WBCs and usually qualify as leukoreduced ($<5 \times 10^6$ WBCs), without the need for additional filtration. In contrast, whole blood–derived platelet concentrates contain large numbers of WBCs. Many of the febrile transfusion reactions related to these products appear to be due to cytokines produced by contaminating WBCs during storage.[53,54] Therefore, removal of WBCs from whole blood–derived platelet concentrates before storage is beneficial. One system that is approved in the United States allows prestorage leukocyte reduction and pooling of whole blood platelets.

Washed Products

Saline washing with automated cell washers can be used to reduce the amount of plasma and acellular elements present in cellular blood products. Although cell washing was previously used for leukocyte reduction, it is no longer used for this purpose. Today, washing is primarily used to remove glycerol from previously frozen RBC units and to reduce unwanted plasma proteins. Washers are capable of removing approximately 99% of plasma proteins from red cell and platelet products. Therefore, washing may be used to remove ABO antibodies for plasma-incompatible platelet transfusions or remove constituents that predispose rare patients to develop significant or repeated allergic/anaphylactic reactions (e.g., removal of IgA-containing plasma for an IgA-deficient patient with a significant reaction history). Washing is also used to reduce RBC supernatant potassium, which may be required prior to massive or rapid infusion of stored RBCs to neonates.

Washing on an automated cell processor takes approximately 30 to 45 min/U. Because the washing procedure is usually performed in an "open" system, red cells have only a 24-hour shelf-life after washing. A closed processing system has been developed that may permit longer storage of washed cells. Washing results in up to a 20% loss of RBCs from the original component.[1] Although many facilities perform red cell washing, fewer offer washed platelets. Because they are stored at room temperature, platelets have only a 4-hour shelf life after washing. Washing additionally results in up to a 33% loss of platelets from the original component and loss of platelet function through activation.[55]

Irradiation of Blood Products

Gamma irradiation of cellular blood components is used to prevent TA-GVHD by impairing the proliferative capacity of T lymphocytes in the blood component. The recommended dose for the irradiation of blood and blood products is 2500 cGy at the center of the irradiation field, with a minimum dose of 1500 cGy at any point in the field.[2,56] This dose of radiation has no significant adverse effect on red cell, platelet, or granulocyte function. However, there are changes in the red cell membrane that result in an increased loss of potassium from the cell, limiting the storage time of red cell components to 28 days.[18] The amount of accumulated free potassium in the supernatant of irradiated red cells may be clinically important in massive transfusion, especially in neonates.[57] It may be desirable to irradiate proximate to transfusion, or wash stored irradiated RBCs if massive transfusion of irradiated products is required for a patient at risk for hyperkalemia. The dose of irradiation used for cellular blood components is not sufficient to inactivate pathogens.[58] Leukocyte reduction is not a substitute for irradiation in the prevention of TA-GVHD.

ADDITIONAL BLOOD CENTER ACTIVITIES

Beyond the collection, manufacture, testing, and distribution of blood components, blood centers often participate in a number of additional activities in the support of clinical transfusion medicine. The blood service provider often functions as the primary transfusion medicine specialty resource available to support community hospitals. Blood center–based transfusion medicine physicians may provide clinical case consultation and educational training and participate on hospital-based transfusion committees. A blood center reference lab may be available to provide primary or referral patient transfusion testing. Some blood centers provide actual patient care through therapeutic apheresis or therapeutic phlebotomy services. Finally, the blood service provider may support hospital blood utilization review and implementation of patient blood management (PBM) practices. Close collaboration between the blood center and transfusing facilities can not only ensure a safe and available supply of blood but also support best transfusion medicine practices.

ALTERNATIVES TO ALLOGENEIC DONOR BLOOD

Directed and Autologous Donations

A *directed* donation (DD) is a donation in which an individual directs their donated blood product to a specific designated patient. The donor is often a family member or friend of a patient who has a current or anticipated need for blood. Directed donors must meet all routine donation criteria; however, medical exceptions can be made if a clinical situation warrants it. Data show that DDs are no safer than regular community donations from an infectious disease perspective. Directed donors are more likely to be first-time donors, who also have a higher incidence of HIV and HCV than do repeat blood donors.[59] Parents donating blood for their children have an even higher incidence of positive infectious disease testing than nonrelated DDs.[60] DDs from blood relatives should be irradiated to prevent TA-GVHD. DDs are useful in rare circumstances to support specific patient transfusion needs when allogeneic blood is not available (e.g., rare HLA or RBC phenotypes obtained from family members) but are generally discouraged.

An *autologous* donation is where a patient donates for their own use, typically prior to a planned surgery. Autologous donations have declined dramatically in the United States with implementation of improved transfusion safety standards. In a recent AABB survey, autologous donations represented only 0.5% of total collections in the United States.[61] Candidates for autologous donation are individuals who can tolerate, and compensate for, the acute loss of blood associated with donation and who are scheduled for a procedure likely to require a transfusion. Like DDs, autologous donations have the greatest medical benefit when used for a patient who has specific transfusion needs that render them incompatible with most allogeneic donors (e.g., the presence of multiple or high-frequency RBC antibodies).

The use of a patient's own (autologous) blood can reduce or eliminate the need for allogeneic blood. There are three types of autologous blood collection procedures. In preoperative autologous donation (PAD), patients donate one or more units of blood to a blood bank during the weeks preceding an elective procedure. In acute normovolemic hemodilution (ANH), blood units are collected in the operating room immediately prior to surgery. In autologous blood cell salvage, blood lost during or after a surgical procedure is salvaged for reinfusion.

Preoperative Autologous Donation

PAD is mainly used in patients for whom crossmatch-compatible blood cannot otherwise be made available, as in patients with rare blood groups or with multiple alloantibodies. For autologous collections, the donor eligibility criteria are not as stringent as those for allogeneic donors. The key consideration is whether the patient can tolerate the acute withdrawal of a unit of whole blood representing 10% to 15% of their blood volume. Patients with significant cerebral or cardiac disease should be evaluated before they are enrolled in a PAD program. Adolescents are also eligible for autologous blood donation in certain states in the United States, but the volume of blood collected and anticoagulant used must be adjusted to body weight.

An autologous donor may donate blood every 3 days as long as the donor's Hb remains at or above 11 g/dL. An "aggressive" donation schedule stimulates a more substantial endogenous erythropoietin response and compensatory erythropoiesis to the "iatrogenic" blood loss (donation), with the potential for more autologous units collected or a higher patient Hb at surgery.[62] In most instances, the units of blood are stored in the liquid state for up to 35 to 42 days. They may be frozen for patients with multiple alloantibodies, but this significantly increases the cost and is not routinely recommended.[63]

Autologous collections must be tested for ABO group and Rh type, and labeled *For Autologous Use Only*. If autologous blood is to be transfused at an institution that is not the collecting facility, the blood unit must be tested for transfusion-transmitted infectious diseases.[64] Units with reactive infectious disease tests must be labeled with biohazard labels. Regulators permit the use of autologous units with positive infectious disease tests. However, some hospital transfusion services or committees do not accept such units because of concerns related to the risk of accidental transfusion of the unit into the wrong patient.

Transfusion complications, such as bacterial contamination, febrile nonhemolytic transfusion reactions (FNHTRs), allergic reactions, and volume overload can occur with autologous transfusion. The possibility of an accident or error such as the transfusion of the wrong unit or an allogeneic unit into the autologous donor/patient has been reported to be 1.2%.[64] The frequency of PAD has significantly declined in recent decades, given its high cost, risks, and currently very low risks from allogeneic blood.[65]

Acute Normovolemic Hemodilution

The second approach to autologous blood procurement involves the withdrawal of blood immediately before the surgical procedure and replacing the blood with crystalloid, colloid, or both, thereby acutely lowering the patient's Hb.[66,67] The blood lost during surgery is therefore relatively dilute, reducing total red cell loss. The higher Hct blood withdrawn immediately prior to surgery is used for transfusion. Patients most likely to benefit from this maneuver are those with anticipated large surgical blood losses who can tolerate low intraoperative Hbs.[68]

Units collected by ANH can be stored at room temperature for up to 8 hours or at 1 °C to 6 °C for up to 24 hours.[69] The first unit collected is typically transfused last (since it's the most hemoconcentrated), though the order of units transfused may be modified if the first unit is nearing expiration or the surgery is ending. The relative efficacy of ANH in comparison to other blood conservation techniques has been debated.[70,71] The cost of ANH is less than that of PAD because of less incremental cost associated with collecting the blood and no required testing, though familiarity and experience with this technique vary among anesthesiologists.[71]

Intraoperative and Postoperative Salvage and Reinfusion

A third approach to autologous transfusion is the collection and retransfusion of blood lost during or after surgery.[72] Perioperative salvage has been shown to be effective in reducing the need for allogenic blood in a variety of surgical procedures. The AABB publishes *Standards for Perioperative Autologous Blood Collection and Administration*, which provides guidance for use of these blood-conservation options.[69]

There are two basic techniques available. Intraoperatively, an anti-coagulated vacuum suction device can be used to collect blood from the surgical field and deliver it to a centrifuge-like device that washes the shed blood with saline before it is reinfused. Only red cells are salvaged by this method (platelets and plasma are lost). There has been concern about the safety of reinfusing materials suctioned from obstetric, cancerous, or contaminated surgical fields. Published experience to date, however, suggests that reinfusion of salvaged and washed cells after processing with leukoreduction filters may be safe in these settings.[73,74] Postoperatively, blood shed into joints or body cavities can be collected into sterile containers. The salvaged material must be filtered to remove fat and particles, and may then be reinfused either directly or after washing. The shed fluid contains red cell stroma, free Hb, activated clotting factors, and fibrin degradation products. It appears that there is not an increased risk associated with infusion of unwashed shed blood if the volume reinfused is limited to approximately 1 L. There is little value to salvaging shed blood in settings where the volume of fluid drained from the surgical site is small or has a low Hct. Because these devices are expensive, patient selection is important.[75]

Erythropoiesis Stimulating Agents

Erythropoiesis stimulating agents (ESAs) have been used to stimulate red cell production in advance of perioperative blood loss to increase preoperative red cell mass[76] and to facilitate the number of autologous units that can be collected preoperatively.[62,77,78] The use of epoetin alfa has been approved to facilitate autologous blood donation in the European Union, Canada, and Japan, but not in the United States.[79] Epoetin alfa has also been approved for use in patients undergoing major, noncardiac surgery who are anemic preoperatively (males with Hb ≤ 13 g/dL, females <12 g/dL) in the United States and Canada.

Artificial Oxygen Carriers

Hb-based oxygen carriers (HBOCs) increase the oxygen delivery by increasing total Hb. Some aspects that make artificial oxygen carriers particularly appealing include prospect of being free of most or all of the infectious risks of allogeneic blood, no need to perform blood typing or crossmatch, extended shelf-life and possibility of storage at room temperature, fewer inventory constraints, and possibility of development of homogeneous and standardized products with controlled characteristics optimized to achieve the goal of oxygen delivery without raising all other complexities of allogeneic blood.[80-83]

Despite being an effective oxygen carrier, vasoconstriction (initially attributed to extravasation of the HBOC into interstitial space and scavenging nitric oxide),[84] hypertension, and renal, pancreatic, and liver injury have been described as complications. A meta-analysis of 16 trials for 5 different HBOCs indicated that regardless of the individual product or indication studied, HBOCs are associated with significantly higher risk of death (relative risk [RR] of 1.30) and myocardial infarction (MI; RR of 2.71) compared with the controls.[85] Approaches such as purification, polymerization, cross-linking, conjugating with other macromolecules, and encapsulating in vesicles or other nanoparticles have been pursued to minimize toxicity and associated complications in subsequent generations of HBOCs. A new generation of products is in development to serve as an "oxygen bridge," in which anemia management with the use of ESA and intravenous iron therapy to promote compensatory erythropoiesis of cellular Hb can be achieved. To date, no artificial oxygen carrier has been approved by the FDA for human use in the United States.

USE OF BLOOD COMPONENTS

Table 23.1 lists the blood components available for clinical use and briefly summarizes the indications for use of each. The use of each component is discussed in detail in the following sections.

Patient Informed Consent

Since 2015, despite approximately 11 million units of RBCs being transfused in the United States annually, the benefit of blood has never been demonstrated with well-designed trials. For purposes of obtaining the patient's informed consent, the treating physician and patient must understand the relative risks and benefits of blood transfusion.

The elements of transfusion consent comprise a discussion of blood transfusion risks and benefits, alternatives to blood, an opportunity to ask questions, and patient consent.[86] Consent should occur as far in advance of transfusion as possible so that alternatives to allogeneic blood, such as autologous blood, can be made available. Some states in the United States have legislated that alternatives to allogeneic blood be available to patients who request them. It should also be noted that blood transfusion has been legislated to be a medical service not subject to commerce and trade laws, thus excluding the principle of implied warranty and granting blood banks and physicians immunity from product liability.[87]

Patient Blood Management

Increased awareness of the costs associated with blood transfusion[88] and recognition of the potential adverse patient outcomes[89] have stimulated the development of initiatives in blood management, defined as the appropriate use of blood and blood components with a goal of minimizing their use. This goal has been motivated historically by (1) known blood risks, (2) unknown blood risks, (3) preservation of the national blood inventory, and (4) constraints from escalating costs.[90]

PBM is an evidence-based approach that is patient-focused, proactive, multidisciplinary (transfusion medicine specialists, surgeons, anesthesiologists, and critical care specialists), and multiprofessional (physicians, nurses, pump technologists, and pharmacists).[90] Preventative strategies are emphasized to identify, evaluate, and manage anemia[91] (e.g., preadmission testing, pharmacologic therapy,[66,92] and reduced iatrogenic blood losses from diagnostic testing)[93]; to optimize hemostasis (e.g., point-of-care testing)[94]; and to establish decision thresholds (e.g., guidelines) for the appropriate administration of blood therapy (the role of these activities in reducing the need for blood transfusion is illustrated in *Figure 23.2*).[90,91]

PBM strategies in a variety of settings including patients undergoing cardiac surgery have been shown to be safe and effective in reducing transfusion, while at the same time delivering high-quality patient outcomes. One institution reported that only 11% of patients undergoing cardiac surgeries received blood transfusions; this program ranked first in their state in the United States for lowest risk-adjusted mortality in patients undergoing open heart surgery.[95]

RED BLOOD CELL TRANSFUSION

The transfusion of RBCs is a balance between the benefits of maintaining oxygen delivery and the inherent risks from blood. Chronic anemia is generally well tolerated because of the compensatory expansion of intravascular plasma volume, increased cardiac output, vasodilatation, increased blood flow owing to decreased viscosity, and, not least, increased RBC 2,3-DPG, with a right shift of the oxygen dissociation curve, so that oxygen is unloaded to the peripheral tissues more readily.[96] Moreover, blood transfusion has been identified as one of the most overused (and inappropriate) therapeutic interventions by national accreditation organizations (The Joint Commission) and medical societies such as the American Board of Internal Medicine in the United States.[97] Guidelines for RBC transfusion therapy have been published by a number of medical societies.[91,98]

The therapeutic goal of an RBC transfusion is to improve oxygen delivery so as to maintain maximal oxygen consumption. The compensatory response to an acute anemia is to increase cardiac output to maintain adequate oxygen delivery.[96] In a normal heart, increased lactate production and an oxygen-extraction ratio of 50% occur at a Hb of approximately 3.5 to 4 g/dL,[99] whereas in a model of coronary stenosis, the anaerobic state occurs at a Hb of approximately 6 to 7 g/dL.[100] No single, universal Hb level can serve as an absolute need for transfusion. However, the use of a laboratory value in conjunction with

Patient Blood Management

	Optimize erythropoiesis	Minimize blood loss	Manage anemia
Preoperative	• Identify, evaluate, and treat underlying anemia • Preoperative autologous blood donation • Consider erythropoiesis stimulating agents (ESA) if nutritional anemias ruled out/treated • Refer for further evaluation if necessary	• Identify and manage bleeding risk (past/family history) • Review medications (antiplatelet, anticoagulation therapy) • Minimize iatrogenic blood loss • Procedure planning and rehearsal	• Compare estimated blood loss with patient-specific tolerable blood loss • Assess/optimize patient's physiological reserve (eg, pulmonary and cardiac function) • Formulate patient-specific management plan using appropriate blood conservation modalities to manage anemia
Intraoperative	• Time surgery with optimization of red blood cell mass (note: unmanaged anemia is a contraindication for elective surgery)	• Meticulous hemostasis and surgical techniques • Blood-sparing surgical techniques • Anesthetic blood-conserving strategies • Acute normovolemic hemodilution • Cell salvage/reinfusion • Pharmacological/hemostatic agents	• Optimize cardiac output • Optimize ventilation and oxygenation • Evidence-based transfusion strategies
Postoperative	• Manage nutritional/correctable anemia (eg, avoid folate deficiency, iron-restricted erythropoiesis) • ESA therapy if appropriate • Be aware of drug interactions that can cause anemia (eg, ACE inhibitor)	• Monitor and manage bleeding • Maintain normothermia (unless hypothermia indicated) • Autologous blood salvage • Minimize iatrogenic blood loss • Hemostasis/anticoagulation management • Be aware of adverse effects of medications (eg, acquired Vit K deficiency)	• Maximize oxygen delivery • Minimize oxygen consumption • Avoid/treat infections promptly • Evidence-based transfusion strategies

FIGURE 23.2 Patient blood management. These principles applied in the perisurgical period enable treating physicians to have the time and tools to provide patient-centered, evidenced-based patient blood management in order to minimize allogeneic blood transfusions. ACE, angiotensin-converting enzyme. (Reprinted with permission from Goodnough LT, Shander A. Patient blood management. *Anesthesiology.* 2012;116(6):1367-1376. Copyright © 2012 the American Society of Anesthesiologists, Inc.)

clinical assessment of the patient status would permit a rational decision regarding the appropriateness of transfusion before the onset of hypoxia or ischemia.[101]

Experience in surgical patients refusing transfusion provides insight into the circumstances in which transfusion may be of benefit. In a review of 16 reports of the surgical outcomes in Jehovah's Witness patients who underwent major surgery without blood transfusion, mortality associated with anemia occurred in only 1.4% of the 1404 operations.[102] A more detailed analysis of 61 studies of Jehovah's Witness patients found that, with the exception of three patients who died after cardiac surgery, all deaths attributed to anemia occurred in patients with Hb ≤ 5 g/dL.[103] In one large study of surgical patients refusing transfusion, the risk of death was found to be higher in patients with cardiovascular disease (CVD) than in those without.[104] A subsequent analysis[105] found that although the risk of death was low in patients with postoperative Hb levels of 7.1 to 8.0 g/dL, morbidity occurred in 9.4%; the odds of death in patients with a postoperative Hb level ≤8 g/dL increased 2.5 times for each gram decrease in Hb level.[105]

Indications for RBC Transfusion

Pediatric Patients

The first randomized, prospective, multicenter trial (the TRIPICU study) to evaluate a Hb "trigger" in children was published in 2007.[106] In this study, over 600 children admitted to pediatric intensive care units (PICUs) were randomized to either a restrictive-strategy group where the Hb threshold for transfusion was 7 g/dL or a liberal-strategy transfusion group where the Hb threshold was 9.5 g/dL. The restrictive strategy resulted in a 44% decrease in the number of RBC transfusions without increasing rates of new or progressive multiorgan dysfunction,

the primary outcome of the study. A number of secondary outcomes, including sepsis, transfusion reactions, nosocomial respiratory infections, catheter-related infections, adverse events, length of stay in the ICU and hospital, and mortality, were no different between the groups. The authors recommended a restrictive RBC transfusion strategy in pediatric patients who are stable in the PICU.[106,107]

Additionally, the Tissue Oxygenation by Transfusion in Severe Anemia With Lactic Acidosis (TOTAL) trial involving children aged 6 to 60 months presenting with severe anemia owing to malaria or sickle cell disease revealed significant improvements in signs and symptoms of anemia after RBC transfusion to raise Hb concentrations from 3.7 to 7.1 g/dL.[108] Serum lactate levels decreased from 9.1 to ≤3 mmol/L 6 hours after transfusion in 59% of the children. Similarly, cerebral tissue oxygen saturation, as measured by near-infrared spectrometry, increased by over 5% at the completion of transfusion. Furthermore, rates of stupor or coma were reduced by half, whereas respiratory distress decreased by 60%. These findings suggest that tissue perfusion with Hb concentrations of 7 g/dL may be sufficient in very young children. Recent clinical guidelines, based in part on this study and the TRIPICU study as well as expert consensus when evidence was lacking, were published by the Transfusion and Anemia Expertise Initiative (TAXI) in an effort to avoid unnecessary transfusions in children with Hb values above 7 g/dL and/or in children with other diagnoses such as nonhemorrhagic shock or congenital heart disease.[107]

Other randomized trials investigating Hb thresholds have been completed in neonates.[109-111] The Premature Infants in Need of Transfusion (PINT) study published in 2006[109] suggested that liberal RBC transfusions were beneficial to neurocognitive outcomes of premature infants at 18 to 22 months, in contrast to a randomized clinical trial published in 2005 that showed poorer neurologic outcomes at

7- to 10-year follow-up for those premature infants who were transfused liberally.[110] The Transfusion of Prematures (TOP) trial, an open, multicenter trial randomizing more than 1800 extremely low–birth-weight neonates to a higher or lower Hb threshold across neonatal ICUs in the United States, and the Effects of Transfusion Thresholds on Neurocognitive Outcomes of Extremely Low-Birth-Weight Infants (ETTNO) trial, a multicenter parallel-group randomized superiority trial of liberal vs restrictive RBC transfusion strategies in >1000 neonates at 36 centers in Europe, both recently showed that a higher Hb threshold did not improve survival or neurocognitive outcome.[111,112]

The notable exception in which liberal RBC transfusions have been found to be superior for improved clinical outcomes is in children with sickle cell anemia, who have overt stroke or abnormal transcranial Doppler (TCD) ultrasonography and who are managed with chronic blood transfusions to keep the percentage of Hb sickle (HbS) less than 30% and the total Hb level at approximately 10 g/dL.[113,114] Interruption of such aggressive transfusion therapy when children reach the age of 18 to 20 years during transition of care to adult medical services has been associated with increased mortality and overt stroke events.[115]

Adult Patients

Symptomatic manifestations of medical anemias generally occur when the Hb is below two-thirds of normal (i.e., <9-10 g/dL), as basal cardiac output increases and is manifested by symptoms of increased cardiac work.[96] The historical practice was to correct mild-to-moderate anemia with RBC transfusions in order to ablate these signs and symptoms by transfusing blood prophylactically. This historical view was reflected in one publication that stated "when the concentration of hemoglobin is less than 8 to 10 g/dL, it is wise to give a blood transfusion before operation."[116]

A readjustment of the transfusion trigger from a Hb of 10 g/dL to a lower threshold was triggered by concern over blood risks, particularly HIV, accompanied by the realization in populations such as Jehovah's Witness patients, who decline blood transfusions because of religious beliefs, that morbidity and mortality related to anemia do not increase until the Hb is very low.[105] Data from this population indicate that the critical level of hemodilution, as defined as the point at which oxygen consumption starts to decrease because of insufficient oxygen delivery, occurs at a Hb level of approximately 4 g/dL,[117] which was corroborated in a recent study of RBC transfusions in Ugandan children with sickle cell anemia or malaria infection.[108]

For anemic patients known to have CVD, perioperative mortality has been reported to be increased significantly when compared with patients not known to have CVD.[104] Management of anemia and the Hb threshold for RBC therapy should therefore be different for these patients. A post hoc analysis of one study[118] was accompanied by an editorial observing that "survival tended to decrease for patients with preexisting heart disease in the restrictive transfusion strategy group, suggesting that critically ill patients with heart and vascular disease may benefit from higher Hb."[119] One previously published clinical practice guideline concluded, "the presence of coronary artery disease likely constitutes an important factor in determining a patient's tolerance to low Hb."[120] A retrospective analysis of 79,000 elderly patients (>65 years of age) hospitalized with acute MI in the United States found that blood transfusion in patients whose admission Hct values were less than 33% was associated with significantly lower mortality rates.[121] A more aggressive use of blood transfusion in the management of anemia in elderly patients who have cardiac disease might well be warranted.[122-124]

There are an increasing number of controlled, randomized trials in adults providing Level I evidence for restrictive blood transfusion practices. A previous systematic review of the literature up to the year 2000 identified 10 trials.[125] The authors concluded at that time that the existing evidence supported the use of restrictive transfusion triggers in patients who were free of serious cardiac disease. A Cochrane systematic review of prospective randomized trials to 2016[126] compared "high" vs "low" Hb thresholds of 31 trials involving a total of 12,587 patients. The authors found that (1) "low" Hb thresholds were well tolerated and (2) RBC transfusions were reduced by 43% (confidence interval [CI] 49%-65%) in patients randomized to the "low" Hb cohorts. A meta-analysis found that a restrictive RBC transfusion strategy aiming to allow a Hb concentration as low as 7 g/dL reduced cardiac events, rebleeding, bacterial infections, and mortality.[127]

There are seven key randomized, clinical trials in adult patients that compare "restrictive" vs "liberal" RBC transfusion strategies in various clinical settings (*Table 23.3*). The Transfusion Requirements in Critical Care (TRICC) trial[128] found that intensive care patients could tolerate a restrictive transfusion strategy (Hb range 7-9 g/dL, 8.2 g/dL on average) as well as patients transfused more liberally (Hb range 10-12 g/dL, 10.5 g/dL on average), with no differences in 30-day mortality rates. Similarly, in the Transfusion Requirements in Septic Shock (TRISS) trial[133] of lower (<7 g/dL) vs higher (<9 g/dL) Hb thresholds for transfusion in patients with septic shock, equivalent 90-day

Table 23.3. Seven Key Clinical Trials of Blood Transfusion in Adults

Clinical Setting (References)	Hemoglobin Threshold (g/dL)	Age (Years)	Patients Transfused (%)	Deviation (%) From Transfusion Protocol	Mean Hemoglobin[a] at Transfusion (g/dL)	Participation (%) of Eligible Patients
Intensive care[128]	7 vs 10	57 58	67 99	1.4 4.3	8.5 10.7	41
CT surgery[129]	8 vs 10	59 vs 61	47 78	1.6 0.0	9.1 10.5	75
Hip fracture repair[130]	8 vs 10	82 vs 82	41 97	9.0 5.6	7.9 9.2	56
Acute upper GI bleeding[131]	7 vs 9	NA NA	49 86	9.0 3.0	7.3 8.0	93
Symptomatic coronary artery disease[132]	8 vs 10	74 vs 67	28.3 NA[b]	1.8 9.1	7.9 9.3	12.2
Sepsis trial[133]	7 vs 9	67 vs 67	64 vs 99	5.9 vs 2.2	7.7 vs 9.3	82
TITR[134]	7.5 vs 9	70 vs 71	53.4 92.2	30 vs 45	8-9 9.2-9.8	98

[a]Average daily hemoglobin.
[b]NA: not available.
Abbreviations: CT, computed tomography; GI, gastrointestinal; TITR, transfusion indication threshold reduction.
From Goodnough LT, Schrier SL. Evaluation and management of anemia in the elderly. *Am J Hematol*. 2014;89(1):88-96. Copyright © 2013 Wiley Periodicals, Inc. Reprinted by permission of John Wiley & Sons, Inc.

mortalities (43% vs 45%, respectively) were found for patients in the two cohorts. However, a retrospective study of 2393 patients[135] consecutively admitted to the ICU found that an admission Hct <25%, in the absence of transfusion, was associated with long-term mortality so that there may be Hct levels below which the risk-to-benefit imbalance for transfusion reverses.

The Transfusion Requirements After Cardiac Surgery (TRACS) trial[129] was a large, single-center study of patients randomized to receive either restrictive (Hct >24%) or liberal (Hct >30%) RBC transfusions postoperatively. Thirty-day all-cause mortality was not different (10% vs 11%, respectively) between the two cohorts. The Transfusion Requirements in Cardiac Surgery (TRICS) III trial was an international noninferiority trial that compared restrictive and liberal RBC transfusion strategies in adults undergoing cardiac surgery with cardiopulmonary bypass that found no differences in the primary outcomes between the two groups.[136] The Functional Outcomes in Cardiovascular Patients Undergoing Surgical Hip Fracture Repair (FOCUS) trial found that elderly (mean > 80 years of age) patients who underwent repair of hip fracture surgery tolerated a Hb trigger without RBC transfusions postoperatively to as low as 8 g/dL (or higher with transfusions, if symptomatic).[130] Subsequently, a single-center prospective study[131] of patients with upper gastrointestinal bleeding demonstrated that patients randomized to a restrictive (Hb < 7 g/dL) vs a liberal (Hb < 9 g/dL) Hb threshold for blood transfusions had significantly improved outcomes, including mortality at 45 days and rates of rebleeding.

The Myocardial Ischemia and Transfusion (MINT) trial[132] was a pilot feasibility study of liberal (Hb ≥ 10 g/dL) vs restrictive (Hb < 8 g/dL) transfusion thresholds in patients with symptomatic coronary artery disease (acute coronary syndrome or stable angina undergoing cardiac catheterization) that was terminated after enrollment of 110 patients; of eligible screened patients, only 12% were enrolled. The primary, composite outcome (death, MI, or revascularization) occurred in 10.9% of the liberal transfusion cohort, compared with 25.9% of the restrictive cohort ($P = .054$); and mortality occurred in 1.8% and 13.0%, respectively ($P = .032$). Additionally, the Transfusion Indication Threshold Reduction (TITRe2) trial,[134] which focused on postoperative coronary artery bypass graft surgery and valve surgery patients, found no difference in primary outcomes of ischemic events (MI, stroke, bowel infarction, acute kidney injury) or infection (sepsis or wound infection) between restrictive (Hb < 7.5 g/dL) and liberal (Hb < 9 g/dL) transfusion triggers (35.1% vs 33.0%, $P = .30$). However, they observed more 30-day deaths in the restrictive group as compared with the liberal group (4.2% vs 2.6%, $P = .045$). Furthermore, a recent meta-analysis stratifying study patients into "context-specific" risk groups based upon patient characteristics and clinical setting found increased risk of inadequate oxygen delivery and mortality among patients with CVD undergoing cardiac or vascular surgery, as well as elderly patients undergoing orthopedic surgery.[124,137] A meta-analysis of 11 trials in 3011 patients with CVD, who were randomized to restrictive vs liberal transfusion triggers, found no 30-day mortality risk between thresholds (1.15, 0.88-1.50), but the risk of acute coronary syndrome managed with restrictive (7-8 g/dL) compared with liberal (9-10 g/dL) transfusions increased (risk ratio 1.78-1.18-2.70, $P = .01$).[124] These trials provide evidence that a more liberal transfusion practice to maintain higher Hb thresholds may represent prudent management of high-risk patients with coronary artery disease or who are undergoing cardiac surgery.

Clinical Practice Guidelines

The number of published clinical practice guidelines[91] for RBC transfusions attests to the increasing interest and importance of appropriate blood utilization by professional societies and health care institutions.[138] The guidelines generally acknowledge the necessity of considering patient covariables or other patient-specific criteria for making transfusion decisions. Among published guidelines, it is generally agreed that transfusion is not of benefit when Hb is greater than 10 g/dL, but may be beneficial when Hb is less than 6 to 7 g/dL, or less than 8 g/dL for patients at risk for acute coronary syndromes.[139]

However, any approach that would use only a Hb value for RBC transfusion rather than the overall assessment of the patient risks over-interpreting available evidence for a "transfusion trigger" and risks underestimating both the heterogeneity of anemias (e.g., acute vs chronic) and the heterogeneity of patients (i.e., comorbidities). Given the increasing evidence that shows blood transfusions are poorly effective and possibly harmful, the guiding principle for transfusion therapy should be that "Less is More." The AABB[140] and American Society of Hematology[141] have published recommendations from the American Board of Internal Medicine's Choosing Wisely campaign advocating single-unit RBC transfusions for nonbleeding hospitalized patients, which had previously been recommended by the American College of Physicians nearly 25 years ago.[142] Additional RBC units should be prescribed only after reassessment of the patient between transfusion decisions.

Red Cell Transfusion in Specific Settings

Trauma

One of the most important indications for blood transfusion is the restoration of circulating blood elements after the loss of large amounts of blood. In general, adults who lose <20% of their blood volume (or ~1 L) do well without red cell transfusion, provided that fluid resuscitation is adequate to maintain the circulating blood volume and that further blood loss is avoided. Young healthy patients can sustain losses of up to 30% to 40% of blood volume as long as intravascular blood volume is adequately maintained.

Massive hemorrhage is generally defined as transfusion of more than 10 U of RBC (one complete blood volume replacement) within 24 hours. In traumatic injury, hemorrhage is a major cause of morbidity and is responsible for almost 50% of deaths occurring within 24 hours of injury. In addition, postpartum hemorrhage can complicate labor and delivery because of uterine atony or abnormal placentation.[143,144]

An estimated 10% of military trauma patients and 3% to 5% of civilian trauma patients receive massive transfusion support.[145-147] There appears to be an important subset of patients with rapid bleeding who may benefit from blood components in addition to RBCs. Both Moore et al.[148] and Holcomb et al.[145] demonstrated that patients receiving 10 U of RBCs in the first 6 hours after injury had a higher rate of mortality than those receiving the same quantity of RBCs over a 24-hour period. Early identification of this patient population and specific massive transfusion support protocols involving multiple blood components at fixed ratios have been associated with improved survival.[149] In response, transfusion services have implemented protocols to quickly and efficiently provide packages of blood products to patients with massive hemorrhage. One review highlights some of the limitations of the available evidence and identifies areas in need of additional study.[150]

Trauma studies have evaluated the impact of more aggressive ratios of plasma to RBC units and noted an association with improved survival with use of massive transfusion protocols.[151] Such studies support using a more aggressive plasma/RBC ratio, reporting a significant reduction (41% vs 62%) in 30-day mortality as compared with those that received less plasma.[152] The Pragmatic, Randomized Optimal Platelet and Plasma Ratios (PROPPR) trial compared 24-hour and 30-day mortality associated with severe trauma using plasma, platelets, and RBCs in a 1:1:1 ratio compared with a 1:1:2 ratio and found no difference in all-cause mortality.[153] Death due to exsanguination was found to be decreased in the 1:1:1 group, and a subgroup analysis found that early platelet transfusion resulted in improved hemostasis and reduced mortality.[154]

Elective Surgery

In preparation for surgery, preoperative requests for typed and crossmatched blood should be based on the predetermined likelihood of a procedure requiring a blood transfusion. "Maximum surgical blood order schedules" or "standard blood orders" specify the number of units that should be crossmatched for a variety of procedures and include guidelines for pretransfusion assessment. A pretransfusion request for type and crossmatch should be sent to the blood bank if it is likely (≥10% probability) that blood will be required for a specific surgical procedure. The request should be for a type and screen if it is unlikely (<10%) that the patient will require blood. As discussed previously under PBM, preoperative evaluation and management of anemia to correct deficits in red cell mass (anemia) is the single most important determinant in likelihood of perioperative blood transfusions.[90,155]

Nutritional Deficiencies

Patients who are anemic solely because of deficiency of iron, folate, or B_{12} rarely require transfusion. In chronic anemias, physiologic adaptations to anemia, including elevated red cell 2,3-DPG content and increased cardiac output, compensate to preserve oxygen transport and delivery. Transfusion is rarely indicated in these patients when there is time to manage and correct anemia.

Hemolytic Anemias

Patients with acute or chronic hemolytic anemias may require red cell transfusion; often, this need arises at the time of a hemolytic or aplastic crisis. Such patients are often critically ill, and safe transfusion requires careful clinical attention. In warm autoimmune hemolytic anemia,[156] the clinician may be faced with a severely anemic patient for whom crossmatch-compatible blood cannot be obtained. These patients produce an antibody that reacts with all RBCs including their own, and the transfusion of serologically incompatible red cells may be necessary. At Hb < 6 g/dL, most patients require transfusion. In these cases, withholding transfusion in the absence of "compatible" RBCs places the patient at needless risk. Although "incompatible" cells will have a shorter-than-normal life span, transfusion reactions are infrequent. The risk of complications is increased if the patient has an undetected alloantibody in addition to the autoantibody. If time allows, special techniques should be used to evaluate these patients for alloantibodies prior to transfusion (see "Red Cell Autoantibodies"). Consultation with a transfusion medicine specialist is recommended in these cases.

Hereditary Red Cell Disorders

In children with thalassemia (Chapter 35), bone marrow hyperplasia with its undesirable effects on the skeleton may be ameliorated, and iron absorption decreased, by regular transfusions to maintain a near-normal Hb concentration.[157] Such a program is possible only in conjunction with an aggressive iron chelation program, as the iron load otherwise leads to fatal hemosiderosis. In patients with sickle cell disease and vaso-occlusive crises (Chapter 34), the adverse microvascular effects of sickle cells can be relieved temporarily by hydration with crystalloid therapy to restore intravascular volume, rather than with RBC transfusions (to avoid unnecessary risks of alloimmunization and iron overload). Transfusion or red cell exchange may be indicated when impaired oxygenation leads to <90% O_2 saturation in acute chest syndrome. The multicenter Stroke Prevention Trial in Sickle Cell Anemia (STOP) showed a significant decrease in the incidence of stroke in patients with abnormal TCD studies who were treated with simple or exchange transfusions to maintain their HbS concentrations <30%, compared with patients who remained on standard supportive care with transfusion only when clinically indicated.[158] A recent prospective trial also showed prevention of silent infarction with chronic transfusion therapy.[159]

Pretransfusion Testing of Red Cells
Compatibility Testing Process

The process of selecting red cells for transfusion involves three stages—blood typing, antibody screening, and crossmatching. Blood typing involves determination of the ABO group and Rh type of both the recipient and donor specimens. The recipient's serum or plasma is screened for the presence of unexpected red cell antibodies. Crossmatching, either serologically or electronically, after selection of a donor unit of the appropriate type determines whether the donor cells are compatible with the recipient's plasma.

Properly selected blood products will be compatible with the recipient, indicating that transfusion should not result in hemolysis of donor red cells. Because only the ABO and Rh(D) red cell antigens are matched in routine transfusion practice, there are always significant antigenic differences between donors and recipients, both for red cells and for the accompanying leukocytes, platelets, and plasma. Repeated exposure to foreign antigens with chronic transfusion or from pregnancy may result in antibody formation in the recipient.

There is no room for error in the provision of blood for transfusion. If clerical or laboratory error results in the donor and recipient being mismatched for the ABO group, transfusion of even a few milliliters of red cells may lead to a life-threatening acute hemolytic transfusion reaction (AHTR) with shock, intravascular coagulation, and acute renal failure. Such reactions are uncommon because of rigid adherence to a routine designed to maximize safety at all levels of the transfusion process; however, with the decrease in the risk of transfusion-transmitted infections, such reactions are becoming one of the leading risks of transfusion.[160] Careful identification of the patient for whom the blood is ordered, including complete labeling of the blood type and antibody screen specimen at the bedside of that patient, is essential. Careful ABO blood typing along with comparing the results with historical records for each patient adds to the level of safety. Ensuring positive identification of crossmatched units of blood and verifying that the information identifying the unit with the intended recipient is reviewed in the presence of that recipient before the administration of the blood are crucial.[1,2]

Blood Typing

The presence of ABO antigens is determined by testing patient RBCs with anti-A and anti-B reagent sera by one of a variety of methods including slide, tube, gel, or microplate tests.[1] Identifying which ABO antigens are on the surface of an individual's RBCs is called the *forward typing* or *forward grouping*. Cells agglutinated only with anti-A serum are group A; those reacting only with anti-B are group B. Those reacting with both antisera are group AB, and red cells that fail to agglutinate with either anti-A or anti-B are group O.

"Reverse typing" or "reverse grouping" should be performed to confirm the reaction obtained by the forward typing test. This involves testing patient serum or plasma with reagent red cells of known A1 and B type. Agglutination of the red cells indicates the presence of anti-A or anti-B in the individual's serum. The conclusions of forward and reverse tests should agree, as shown in *Table 23.4*.

The Rh(D) type of red cells is determined by examining the cells' reaction with anti-D serum from commercial sources. Commercial antisera may be modified by the manufacturer with the addition of high concentrations of protein or by chemically altering the IgG molecules in such a way that they perform as direct agglutinins in the laboratory. This permits rapid, reliable testing to determine the D antigen status of the cells. However, these high-protein reagents may cause false-positive reactions because of spontaneous aggregation of some red cells in their presence. If this happens, an Rh-negative patient could be typed as Rh positive if the recommended Rh control is not tested simultaneously. This problem has led to the development of low-protein, saline-reactive monoclonal reagents. Monoclonal anti-D

Table 23.4. ABO Grouping

| Patient Blood Group | Expected Reactions of | | | |
| | Patient's Cells With | | Patient's Serum With | |
	Anti-A	Anti-B	A Cells	B Cells
O	None	None	+	+
A	+	None	None	+
B	None	+	+	None
AB	+	+	None	None

reagents contain both human IgM and polyclonal IgG antibodies and are currently most widely used. They can also be used in the antiglobulin test for weak D. As with all reagents, manufacturers' instructions must be followed.[1]

Red cells reacting weakly with anti-D reagents are called weak D. If donor blood is being tested, the absence of D must be confirmed. If the initial test for D is negative, a second, more sensitive test must be performed using a method that detects weak D. If D is detected by either method, the unit is labeled RhD positive.[1,2] In patients, testing for weak D is not required. Patients who are typed as RhD negative, but who are really weak D positive will not be adversely affected by the transfusion of RhD-negative products.[161] An exception to this rule is for newborns who demonstrate an RhD-negative blood type and are born to RhD-negative mothers. Weak D testing must be done in this scenario to verify the infant's RhD type and determine the mother's need for anti-D immunoprophylaxis. Before concluding that a patient is weak D positive, care must be taken to ensure that the patient has not recently been transfused with RhD-positive red cells or experienced a large fetal-maternal hemorrhage.

Testing for Red Cell Antibodies

Antibodies in potential blood transfusion recipients fall into several categories. The most common blood group antibodies that are clinically significant and may be implicated in hemolytic transfusion reactions or hemolytic disease of the fetus and newborn are shown in *Table 23.5*.

All human plasmas contain naturally occurring antibodies that react with the complementary antigens of the ABO system. These are of great importance in transfusion, as they are complement-fixing IgM antibodies and transfusion of incompatible red cells can lead to acute hemolytic reactions. Many people also have naturally occurring antibodies (usually low-titer IgM antibodies reacting at or below room temperature) that react with some antigens of the Lewis, P1PK, Ii, MN, or other systems. These are rarely active above room temperature and are only occasionally clinically significant. Finally, people exposed to foreign red cells by prior transfusion or pregnancy may produce IgG antibodies to antigens of certain other systems, primarily Rh (C, c, D, E, e), Kell, Duffy, Kidd, and Ss, but many less common possibilities exist. These red cell antibodies are clinically significant.[162] They do not often lead to intravascular hemolytic reactions, but transfused incompatible red cells may exhibit decreased survival caused by increased clearance in the reticuloendothelial system (RES). Many of these IgG antibodies can also cause hemolytic disease of the fetus and newborn.

There are two major classes of antibodies that react with red cells. Complete or saline antibodies agglutinate red cells suspended in saline solution; these are usually IgM. Antibodies that do not react visibly in saline and are capable of producing agglutination reactions only with special techniques to make their interaction with red cells detectable are called *incomplete agglutinins*; these are generally IgG antibodies.

The best example of a room temperature saline agglutination test is that used in ABO typing. Other red cell antibodies that are readily detected in saline suspension are those belonging to the Lewis, MN, P1PK, and Ii blood group systems. With the important exception of ABO system antibodies, many of the others detected with this test are of no clinical significance, as they are not reactive at 37 °C.

The best examples of incomplete agglutinins, or IgG antibodies, are those that react with antigens of the Rh system. If such antibodies are not detected in the recipient, immediate hemolysis of transfused, incompatible red cells is extremely rare. However, their presence may lead to a significantly decreased survival of transfused cells and the development of an extravascular hemolytic syndrome (delayed hemolytic transfusion reaction [DHTR]).

Table 23.5. Significance of Certain Blood Group Antibodies

Blood Group System	Antibody	Relative Frequency in Antibody Screening	Hemolytic Transfusion Reaction	Hemolytic Disease of the Fetus and Newborn
ABO	Anti-A	All group B and O	Yes	Yes
	Anti-B	All group A and O	Yes	Yes
Rhesus	Anti-D	Common	Yes	Yes
	Anti-c	Common	Yes	Yes
	Anti-E	Common	Yes	Yes
	Anti-C	Common	Yes	Yes
	Anti-e	Uncommon	Yes	Yes
Kell	Anti-K	Common	Yes	Yes
	Anti-k	Rare	Yes	Yes
Kidd	Anti-Jk[a]	Common	Yes	Yes
	Anti-Jk[b]	Rare	Yes	Yes
Duffy	Anti-Fy[a]	Common	Yes	Yes
	Anti-Fy[b]	Uncommon	Yes	Yes
MNS	Anti-M	Common	Rare	Rare
	Anti-N	Rare	Rare	Rare
	Anti-S	Uncommon	Yes	Yes
	Anti-s	Rare	Yes	Yes
Lewis	Anti-Le[a]	Common	Yes	No
	Anti-Le[b]	Uncommon	No	No
P	Anti-P$_1$	Common	Rare	No
Ii	Anti-I	Uncommon	No	No

Antiglobulin Test

The antiglobulin (Coombs) test (*Figures 23.3* and *23.4*) is based on the reaction between an antihuman globulin (AHG) reagent and antibody- or complement-coated red cells. AHG reagents are commercially available and are prepared either by the injection of an animal with human globulin or through hybridoma technology. AHG reagents may be polyspecific or monospecific. The polyspecific reagents contain antibodies with both antihuman IgG and anticomplement activity. Monospecific AHG reagents, anti-IgG, anti-C3b, and anti-C3d, are used to determine which protein is responsible for a positive *direct antiglobulin test (DAT)*.[1]

The DAT is performed by washing the patient's cells with saline, adding polyspecific AHG, and observing for agglutination (*Figure 23.3*). Positive reactions (agglutination) suggest the presence of IgG antibodies or complement bound to the red cell.[1] The *indirect* antiglobulin test is used to determine the presence of red cell antibodies in serum or plasma (*Figure 23.4*). Reagent red cells are incubated with the patient's serum or plasma, washed to remove unbound immunoglobulins, mixed with AHG (usually monospecific anti-IgG), and then centrifuged briefly. The cell button is gently resuspended and examined for agglutination. A positive reaction suggests that IgG antibodies in the patient's plasma have bound to the reagent cells. A positive indirect antiglobulin test therefore indicates the presence of antibodies capable of reacting with red cells and possibly capable of hemolyzing such cells if they were transfused.

Direct and indirect antiglobulin tests are the simplest approaches to the detection of IgG anti–red cell antibodies. Because many of these serologic reactions are rather weak, the addition of various media has been used to enhance the agglutination reaction. These tests involve procedures that diminish the mutually repulsive electrostatic forces between red cells, permitting visible agglutination by IgG antibodies. Antigens that often require such enhancing tests include those of the Kidd (Jk^a and Jk^b), Rh (D, C, E, c, e), Kell, and Duffy (Fy^a and Fy^b) systems.

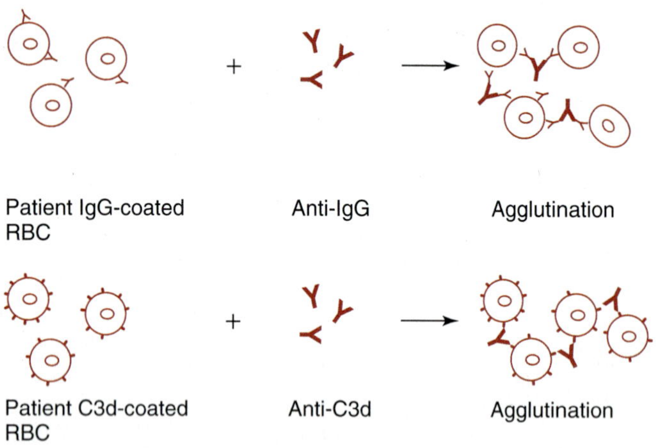

![Direct antiglobulin test diagram showing Patient IgG-coated RBC plus Anti-IgG yielding Agglutination, and Patient C3d-coated RBC plus Anti-C3d yielding Agglutination]

Patient IgG-coated RBC   Anti-IgG   Agglutination

Patient C3d-coated RBC   Anti-C3d   Agglutination

FIGURE 23.3 Direct antiglobulin test with anti-immunoglobulin G (IgG) and anti-C3d. RBC, red blood cell. (Reprinted with permission from Jeter EK, Spivey MA. Blood components and their use. In: *Introduction to Transfusion Medicine: A Case Study Approach.* American Association of Blood Banks Press; 1996:56. Figure 3-4. Copyright © 1996 by AABB.)

Media That Enhance Agglutination

Adding albumin, low–ionic strength saline, or polyethylene glycol solutions to antibody identification tests can enhance the sensitivity of the test system.[163] These solutions augment the antibody-antigen interaction in a variety of ways, enhancing the detection of weak or otherwise undetectable antibodies. Treating reagent red cells with proteolytic enzymes such as papain or ficin also increases the sensitivity for some antibodies such as those reacting with Rh and Kidd system antigens. These enzyme reagents weaken or destroy other red cell antigens (M, N, Fy^a, Fy^b, and, in some cases, S, s), a trait that can be helpful in the identification of multiple red cell antibodies in a single serum sample.[1]

Other Antibody Identification Tests

Sera containing several antibodies may be analyzed by adsorbing with one or more selected red cells.[1] Antibodies so adsorbed may be eluted from the cells, and their specificity may be determined. Alternatively, the specificity of antibodies not adsorbed and remaining in the supernatant can be identified. When necessary, the identity of certain antibodies may be confirmed by their inhibition by soluble antigens, such as A, B, and Lewis substances, present in the saliva of secretors.[164] Neonatal (cord) red cells exhibit a number of antigens very weakly and may be used to investigate antibody specificity.

Selection of Red Cells for Transfusion

A series of serologic tests is used to select donor blood for patients. Although individual transfusion services prefer different specific methods, the general principles of compatibility testing are the same.

A properly labeled, fresh sample of patient blood must be provided. If the patient has been transfused or has been pregnant within the preceding 3 months, the specimen must be obtained within 3 days of the anticipated transfusion.

Donor

The ABO group of the donor unit must be confirmed. The donor unit RhD typing must also be repeated if the unit is labeled as RhD negative. These tests are performed to confirm the blood type and to ensure that the unit has not been mislabeled.

Recipient

The recipient's ABO group and RhD type must be determined. The recipient's serum is screened for the presence of antibodies that may have been induced by prior pregnancy or transfusion. A set of commercially prepared group O red cells, expressing 18 clinically relevant antigens (D, C, E, c, e, M, N, S, s, P_1, Le^a, Le^b, K, k, Fy^a, Fy^b, Jk^a, and Jk^b), is used in this test in accordance with FDA rules. The use of group O reagent red cells avoids agglutination by anti-A or anti-B. These reagent cells are incubated with the patient's serum and tested with the indirect antiglobulin test for reactions indicating the presence of antibody in the serum.[1]

If such screening reactions are positive, antibody specificity can be determined by reaction of the serum with a commercially prepared panel of reagent red cells of known antigenic composition. If an antibody has been found on the screen and the patient's clinical status allows, it is best to withhold transfusion until identification is complete. The incidence of unexpected RBC antibodies in patients requiring transfusion is low.[165,166]

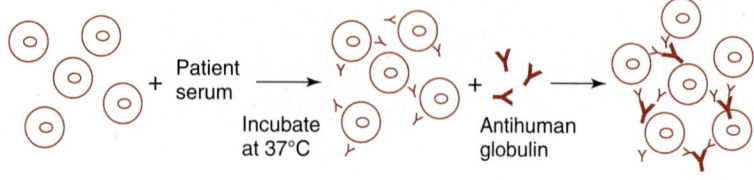

Test RBCs   + Patient serum → Incubate at 37°C → IgG bound to test RBCs   + Antihuman globulin → Agglutination

FIGURE 23.4 Indirect antiglobulin test. IgG, immunoglobulin G; RBC, red blood cell. (Reprinted with permission from Jeter EK, Spivey MA. Blood components and their use. In: *Introduction to Transfusion Medicine: A Case Study Approach.* American Association of Blood Banks Press; 1996:56. Figure 3-3. Copyright © 1996 by AABB.)

Type and Screen

If it is unlikely that blood will be required, for example, for a surgical procedure with <10% likelihood of transfusion, a "type and screen" rather than a crossmatch should be requested. In this instance, the blood bank types the patient's blood and screens for unexpected antibodies; if antibodies are not found, the blood bank ensures that blood of the appropriate group is available for transfusion if necessary. In such an event, a telephone call or electronic "call slip" can trigger a rapid crossmatch test, and blood will be available with minimal delay. The appropriate use of type and screen improves the efficiency of the blood bank. It assists in inventory control by not segregating blood for patients who are unlikely to require it and is therefore more cost-effective.

Crossmatch

If no antibody has been detected on the screen and there is no record of the previous presence of a clinically significant antibody, only verification of ABO compatibility between the donor unit and recipient is required before transfusion. This can be done either by an immediate spin crossmatch or a computer crossmatch.

The immediate spin crossmatch consists of mixing the patient's serum with donor saline–suspended red cells at room temperature, spinning the tube, and reading the results immediately. The purpose of this test is to detect ABO incompatibility because of the presence of anti-A, anti-B, or both, in the patient's serum.

The conditions for computer or "electronic" crossmatch are outlined in the AABB Standards.[2] Briefly, the computer system must be validated to prevent release of ABO-incompatible blood. This computer crossmatch can be used only for patients who do not have a record of clinically significant antibodies. The recipient's ABO blood group must have been determined on at least two separate tests. The system must contain complete information on the donor unit and the recipient, including ABO group and RhD type. Data entered must be verified as correct before the release of blood. The system must contain logic to alert the user to discrepancies for either the donor unit or the recipient, including unit labeling, blood typing, and ABO incompatibilities.

If a clinically significant red cell antibody has been found when a patient's plasma or serum is screened for unexpected antibodies, antibody identification should be performed. Once the antibody specificity has been identified, donor units that lack the corresponding antigen should be selected, and a crossmatch using an indirect antiglobulin test should be performed on each unit to ensure compatibility. The physician should also be advised about the nature of the problem, as well as the potential for delays if further units are required.

Once a unit of blood is crossmatched for a patient, there must be positive identification of the patient and the blood product both in the laboratory before release of a blood product to the bedside as well as at the patient's bedside by the transfusionist. Before every transfusion, the requisition, the label on the blood product, and the patient's identification must be checked. These aspects of patient and blood product identification are critical safety steps and must be documented.[2]

Uncrossmatched Blood for Emergency Transfusion

For patients in hemorrhagic shock, it is necessary to transfuse blood immediately, and no blood bank testing should be attempted before emergency transfusion. The risk of transfusing group O "uncrossmatched" red cells is extremely low and is certainly much lower than the risk of the patient's death if blood transfusion is delayed. If a patient is to be given uncrossmatched blood, a specimen of the patient's blood should be obtained prior to transfusion so that typing and screening can be performed while the transfusion is proceeding.

Once the patient's blood type has been determined, ABO-compatible uncrossmatched blood may be used.[2] Until the patient's RhD type is determined, uncrossmatched blood should be Rh(D) negative when used in women of childbearing age, in whom sensitization to D would be undesirable. As RhD-negative blood is often in limited supply, RhD-positive blood is often used for emergency transfusion

of older females and of males of unknown blood type. In such cases, sensitization may occur, but the risk of an immediate hemolytic reaction is low.[167]

Despite the lack of a crossmatch, transfusion of type-specific blood under emergency situations is safe. The incidence of red cell alloantibodies in healthy people is low, and most such antibodies do not cause dangerous acute intravascular hemolytic transfusion reactions. However, the decision to use uncrossmatched blood is the responsibility of the patient's attending physician, who must weigh the risks against the expected benefits and document in the patient's record the need for the uncrossmatched blood.

Table 23.6 outlines the selection of blood and plasma by ABO type. If the blood type is known, ABO-compatible red cells and plasma can be selected. If the blood type is not known, group O red cells should be used. If plasma is required, group AB plasma should be used because it contains no anti-A or anti-B.[168] Group A plasma has also been demonstrated to be safe for trauma resuscitation in patients of unknown blood type when group AB plasma is unavailable or in limited supply.[169]

Crossmatching Problems

Standard serologic techniques often depend on agglutination as an end point. There are several agglutinating phenomena that can interfere with the correct interpretation of these serologic tests and may delay antibody identification and crossmatching. *Pseudoagglutination* refers to red cell clumping (rouleaux formation) that typically occurs in the presence of dysproteinemias, or after the administration of dextran or hydroxyethyl starch. Dilution in saline abolishes the reaction.[1] *Autoagglutination* refers to red cell agglutination by the patient's own serum or plasma and often indicates the presence of a cold agglutinin. Washing patient red cells with warm saline can often remove enough of the antibodies so that testing can be completed. *Polyagglutination* is the phenomenon in which a patient's red cells are agglutinated by most or all group-compatible sera. During bacterial or viral infections, enzymes of the infecting organism can cause alteration of antigenic structures on the red cell membrane, exposing previously hidden antigens such as T, or more rarely Tn.[170] Most adult sera contain naturally acquired antibodies capable of reacting with these cryptantigens. The situation may be elucidated by testing the patient's red cells with cord serum, which lacks the antibodies necessary for this reaction, and by examining for reactions with plant lectins that have specific activity with the antigens involved in polyagglutination.[171]

Red Cell Autoantibodies

A positive indirect antiglobulin test against all screening and donor red cells often indicates the presence of an IgG, warm-reacting autoantibody. The patient's DAT is also positive. Such autoantibodies

Table 23.6. Selection of Blood and Plasma by ABO Type

Component	Recipient ABO Type	Selection of Blood Component	
		Preferred	Alternate
Red blood cells	O	O	None
	A	A	O
	B	B	O
	AB	AB	A, B, O
Fresh frozen plasma	O	O	A, B, AB
	A	A	AB
	B	B	AB
	AB	AB	None

Modified with permission from Jeter EK, Spivey MA. *Introduction to Transfusion Medicine: A Case Study Approach.* American Association of Blood Banks Press; 1996. Table 1-2. Copyright © 1996 by AABB.

may preclude the identification of any serologically compatible donor units. If red cells are transfused, it is essential that ABO compatibility be ensured. The patient's serum should be screened for alloantibodies that might be masked by the autoantibody.[172] Such screening requires the removal of the autoantibody from the patient's serum so that any alloantibodies present can be identified. If the patient has not been transfused within the last 3 to 4 months, this can be done by absorbing autoantibody from the serum with autologous red cells, from which already attached antibody has been removed by enzyme or chemical treatment.[1] Alternatively, the autoantibody may be removed by adsorption with a panel of cells selected to lack the antigens to which the patient may become alloimmunized. This process is referred to as an alloadsorption or differential adsorption. The autoantibody-depleted serum can then be examined for the presence of residual alloantibodies, and a serologic crossmatch can be done. If only the autoreactive antibody is present, transfusion of red cells is generally well tolerated.

Alloantibody to High-Incidence Antigens

Occasionally, a patient may have a red cell antibody that does not react with the patient's own cells but reacts with all donor red cells. Identification of these antibodies is particularly challenging, requiring rare cells that lack common red cell antigens. Assistance of specialized laboratories may be needed both to identify the antibody to a *high-incidence* antigen and to locate compatible blood. In some of these cases, it is not clear whether the antibody is likely to cause significant hemolysis. The utilization of DNA-based methodologies to identify donors with rare blood types is a useful tool in these challenging situations.[173]

Drugs

Some drugs may stimulate an autoantibody in the patient that reacts with all reagent cells tested as well as with donor red cell units crossmatched.[174] Drug-induced immune hemolytic anemia is classified by four mechanisms—immune complex formation, drug adsorption (hapten), autoantibody production, and nonimmunologic protein adsorption. Drugs implicated include α-methyldopa, levodopa, fludarabine, and procainamide.[1] In some cases, the in vitro findings may be identical to those found in autoimmune hemolytic anemias. The presence of these antibodies may or may not be clinically significant but may result in a delay if a transfusion is required. In most cases, however, drug-induced antibodies are associated with a positive DAT that is not part of the standard pretransfusion or crossmatch testing, and the indirect antiglobulin test is negative. An emerging class of monoclonal antibodies used as biologic therapies in patients with refractory malignancies such as daratumumab can also interfere with compatibility testing.

Red Cell Genotyping

The use of DNA-based methods for red cell antigen identification can assist in securing the optimal blood products for transfusion. The molecular bases for many of the major blood group antigens have been identified and DNA-based methods for their detection developed. Because these methods do not directly detect the presence of red cell antigens, challenges with widespread application still exist.[175] When used with standard serologic testing, however, such methods are useful in identifying donors for patients with multiple red cell antibodies or blood donors with rare antigen types. Additionally, these methods are helpful in determining a patient's red cell antigen makeup when chronically or recently transfused or when access to a blood specimen increases patient risk (e.g., fetus).

Special Considerations in Neonatal Transfusion
Pretransfusion Testing

The so-called naturally occurring IgM ABO antibodies do not begin to appear until approximately 3 to 6 months of age. However, IgG antibodies of maternal origin, including maternal anti-A, anti-B or anti-A, B, may be passively transferred to the fetus. Thus, pretransfusion testing in the newborn consists of ABO and RhD typing of the

infant's cells and an antibody screen for passively transferred maternal IgG antibodies, including anti-A or anti-B if applicable. If the initial antibody screen is negative, the infant may be transfused with products compatible with the infant's ABO/RhD type, and no further compatibility testing is required for the first 4 months of life during hospitalization. If a clinically significant antibody of maternal origin is detected, units that are antigen negative or crossmatch compatible must be issued until the antibody is no longer detectable in the infant's serum.[2]

Selection of Products for Neonatal Transfusion

Preterm infants may require multiple transfusions in the first weeks to months of life. It has become common practice to limit donor exposure by reserving one unit or one-half unit for a single preterm infant.[176] Serial aliquots may be obtained using a sterile connection device for the life of the unit.[177-179] Blood products for low-birth-weight infants should be irradiated to prevent TA-GVHD and should be CMV safe (i.e., CMV antibody negative or leukoreduced; Chapter 44). Red cells stored in either CPDA-1 or ASs may be used for standard dose aliquot transfusions (i.e., 10-15 mL/kilogram [kg]). However, the safety of ASs has not been demonstrated in the setting of massive transfusion of infants (i.e., more than 15-20 mL/kg in a neonate). The amount of free potassium in the supernatant of the irradiated blood may also become clinically important in the setting of massive transfusion, given the potential risk of transfusion-associated hyperkalemic cardiac arrest.[57,180] For massively transfused infants at an increased risk of hyperkalemia, the dose of free potassium in the red cell product may be decreased by delaying irradiation of a fresh unit until just before issue or by washing older RBCs.

Exchange Transfusion

Historically the most common indication for exchange transfusion in the neonate was hyperbilirubinemia that had not responded adequately to phototherapy, particularly that associated with hemolytic disease of the fetus and newborn. However, the frequency of this procedure has decreased significantly over the past few decades such that it should only be undertaken at a center with appropriate expertise.[176,181]

Red cells collected in CPD or CPDA-1 that are less than 1 week old are preferred.[165] Because several clotting factors in newborns are at the low end of hemostatic levels, some centers perform exchanges using whole blood, or red cells reconstituted with plasma, to prevent further lowering of factor levels by the exchange. RBCs used for the exchange transfusion should be irradiated to prevent TA-GVHD.[1]

Administration of Blood

The first step before the administration of blood or of a blood product is to obtain consent for the transfusion from the patient. Every hospital should set its own policy for obtaining this consent. A note in the chart indicating that the risks of transfusion as well as the indications and alternatives have been discussed with the patient and that the patient has accepted this form of therapy may be adequate depending on applicable laws and regulations. There must be a written order for the administration of the product.[2]

All blood products should be given through an appropriate blood administration set containing a filter, and careful aseptic technique should be practiced at all times. There must be confirmation and documentation that the information identifying the blood product with the patient has been verified in the presence of the patient.[2]

Vital signs should be documented before and after transfusion and as clinically required. For the first 15 minutes after the infusion has begun, the patient should be kept under close observation to detect any signs of a serious transfusion reaction. If none is observed, the infusion rate may be increased. One unit of red cells is often given in 1 to 4 hours, depending on the amount to be transfused and the patient's cardiovascular status. Infusion of a unit for longer than 4 hours is not recommended, as there is a risk of bacterial proliferation because the opened unit is at room temperature. Normal (0.9%) saline, 5% albumin, or ABO-compatible plasma may be added. No other solution and no medication should be added to or infused through the same tubing as a blood product, unless there is documentation of compatibility or FDA approval.[2] Dextrose causes red cells to agglutinate or hemolyze, and hypotonic saline causes hemolysis. Ringer's lactate or other solutions containing calcium must never be added to a blood product because the calcium present in them leads to coagulation. After the transfusion has been completed, the transfusion tag or record should become part of the patient's chart.

When the patient being transfused is in severe congestive heart failure, additional measures should be taken. The indications for transfusion should be carefully considered, weighing them against the potential risks of transfusion, and unnecessary transfusions should be avoided by adhering to restrictive thresholds for hemodynamically stable patients.[140] Administration of diuretics before or during the transfusion may be necessary to prevent aggravation of heart failure by volume overload. In the presence of heart failure, transfusion should proceed slowly (e.g., 1 mL/kg/h), with careful observation and additional diuretics given if clinically indicated. If slower rates than this are needed, the blood component may be divided by the blood bank into two or more parts and each part transfused over 4 hours. The unused portions should be kept in the blood bank until needed for transfusion.

PLATELET TRANSFUSION

Modern treatment for hematologic malignancies would not be possible without the ability to prevent or treat thrombocytopenic bleeding. Similarly, many surgical procedures would not be feasible without platelet transfusions.

Administration of Platelets

The preparation of platelet concentrates is described in the section "Platelet Preparation and Storage." Platelet transfusions must be administered within 4 hours once the blood bag is opened by puncturing one of the sealed ports,[2] but the infusion time is usually about 30 minutes. Platelets should be examined for abnormal appearance before they are transfused, and must be administered through a filter approved for platelet use; a standard blood set with a 170- or 260 μm filter is acceptable.

Dosage and Expected Response

The typical adult dose, whether prepared from whole blood or by apheresis, is 3 to 6×10^{11} platelets. Only two-thirds of transfused platelets are expected to remain in the circulation of the recipient because of pooling of platelets, particularly in the spleen. The maximum expected increase in circulating platelet count can be estimated after transfusion of a platelet product containing the minimum of 3×10^{11} platelets into a 70 kg adult with a blood volume of 5 L as follows: maximum increase in platelet count = $\frac{2}{3} \times 3 \times 10^{11}$ platelets distributed in 5 L blood volume = 40×10^9/L. In practice, the observed posttransfusion platelet recovery in patients is often much lower than expected from the calculation in this example. Hematology patients typically achieve an increment of approximately 20×10^9/L after infusion of 3×10^{11} platelets, about 50% of expected.[182] A recovery as low as 30% of expected is generally considered "acceptable." This would correspond to an increase in platelet count of approximately 13×10^9/L after transfusion of one apheresis platelet product to a 70 kg adult. The expected and "acceptable" increases in platelet count would be proportionately lower in a larger adult and higher with transfusion of a larger dose of platelets.

Many investigators have assessed the acceptability of a posttransfusion platelet increment by calculating a corrected count increment (CCI). With CCI, the measured increment in circulating platelet count is corrected for the patient's size and for the dose of platelets given as follows:

$$CCI = \left(\text{posttransfusion count} - \text{pretransfusion count} \right)$$
$$\times \text{body surface area} \left(m^2 \right) / \text{number of platelets administered} \left(10^{11} \right)$$

The maximum achievable CCI is approximately 25×10^9/L. The typical CCI in patients is approximately one-half of this, and the lowest "acceptable" CCI is considered to be 7.5×10^9/L at 1 hour and 4.5×10^9/L at 20 to 24 hours. Patients with in vivo recoveries or CCIs lower than acceptable values should be evaluated for causes of platelet refractoriness such as an enlarged spleen or alloimmunization (as discussed in the section "Platelet Refractoriness and Alloimmunization").

In healthy adults, the half-life of transfused platelets is 3 to 5 days.[34] In thrombocytopenic patients, however, platelet survival is reduced. A fixed rate of platelet consumption of 7.1×10^9/L/d has been measured in otherwise stable patients with severe thrombocytopenia.[183] It is assumed that this platelet consumption is associated with maintenance of vascular integrity. The rate of platelet consumption may be higher in critically ill patients.

Given the limited absolute increase in platelet count achieved with the standard dose of platelets and the presence of ongoing platelet consumption, many patients return to their baseline platelet count within 1 to 2 days of platelet transfusion. In stable patients, the transfusion-free interval may be increased by administering larger doses of platelets with each transfusion.[184,185] However, this strategy can result in an increase in the total number of platelets transfused.[182] A recent randomized controlled trial[186] demonstrated that "low-dose" prophylactic platelet transfusions are not associated with greater bleeding than with "standard" or "high-dose" platelet transfusions.

Indications for Platelet Transfusion

The risks of posttraumatic and spontaneous bleeding increase as the platelet count falls. In general, assuming that platelet function is normal, there is minimal risk of spontaneous bleeding because of thrombocytopenia at platelet counts >50×10^9/L, and this level is usually sufficient to permit surgical procedures. As the count falls below this level, there is an increasing risk of microvascular bleeding, characterized by petechiae, ecchymoses, oozing at venipuncture and incision sites, epistaxis, menorrhagia, gastrointestinal bleeding, or intracranial hemorrhage.

The precise degree of bleeding risk at any given platelet count is difficult to determine, as many other clinical variables have important effects. These include the cause of thrombocytopenia, the duration of thrombocytopenia, the nature of concurrent disease processes including sepsis, uremia, vasculitis, or malignant processes invading blood vessels or other organs; the coexistence of coagulopathies, such as liver disease, vitamin K deficiency, intravascular coagulation, or heparin treatment; and the presence of drugs such as acetylsalicylic acid or semisynthetic penicillins that interfere with platelet function.[187]

In general, the risk of significant spontaneous hemorrhage increases gradually as the platelet count drops to <70×10^9/L and further increases at counts <5×10^9/L.[186]

For therapeutic platelet transfusions, algorithms for platelet transfusions based on point-of-care testing have demonstrated promise in patients who have platelet-derived bleeding such as those in cardiothoracic surgery[94] and in trauma.[153,188,189] Additional evidence-based studies in platelet transfusion are needed.[190]

Prophylactic Platelet Transfusion

The indications for prophylactic transfusion remain controversial. Historically, it was common practice to transfuse platelets when the count was <20×10^9/L. Current guidelines from the United States and the United Kingdom recommend a transfusion trigger of a platelet count of 10×10^9/L for platelets transfused prophylactically.[191,192] These guidelines are based on outcomes from randomized clinical trials that compared prophylactic triggers of 10×10^9/L vs 20×10^9/L in patients with acute leukemia and in autologous and allogeneic hematopoietic stem cell transplant recipients.[193-196] The transfusion trigger of a platelet count of 10×10^9/L resulted in a decreased number of platelet transfusions without an increased frequency of significant hemorrhage. In these studies, however, the trigger for transfusion was liberalized in the presence of clinical factors suspected to increase the risk of hemorrhage, such as fever, an increased WBC count, coagulopathy, bleeding, or invasive procedures. When significant hemorrhagic events occurred, they were often in patients with morning platelet counts $>20 \times 10^9$/L. Infection, vascular lesions, or prolonged duration of thrombocytopenia may contribute to the risk of significant hemorrhage.[194] Thus, it appears that a prophylactic transfusion trigger of 10×10^9/L is as safe as one of 20×10^9 in most patients with acute leukemia or after myeloablative hematopoietic cell transplant, but an assessment of individual clinical risk factors is appropriate.

Two recent large randomized controlled trials have addressed the question of whether prophylactic platelet transfusions should be used in patients with hematologic malignancies.[197,198] Both showed that prophylactic platelet transfusions reduced the risk of bleeding. However, this effect was less marked in patients receiving autologous hematopoietic stem cell transplants.

Very limited data are available to guide the use of prophylactic platelet transfusion before invasive procedures. A platelet count $>50 \times 10^9$/L is usually recommended before major surgical procedures.[191,199,200] The safety of performing surgical procedures at counts below this level has not been formally evaluated in clinical trials. Some procedures such as bone marrow aspirations and biopsies may be safely performed in patients with very low platelet counts of $<20 \times 10^9$/L without platelet transfusion, but recent recommendations from the AABB are that patients undergoing elective central venous catheter placement should receive a platelet transfusion if the platelet count is $<20 \times 10^9$/L and that patients undergoing elective diagnostic lumbar puncture should receive a platelet transfusion if the platelet count is $<50 \times 10^9$/L.[191] However, the minimum safe platelet level for other invasive procedures remains to be defined.

Prophylactic transfusion of platelets is generally *not* recommended in patients with platelet consumption disorders, such as immune thrombocytopenic purpura (ITP) and TTP. In ITP, there is reduced recovery and survival of transfused platelets; platelet transfusion used as prophylaxis to prevent bleeding does not usually produce a sustained increase in platelet count. Platelets are activated in TTP, leading to a hypercoagulable state. However, platelet transfusion may be used to treat life-threatening bleeding in patients with these disorders.

Therapeutic Platelet Transfusion

Rapid massive bleeding is unlikely to be solely owing to thrombocytopenia and suggests the presence of a vascular injury. Rapid massive bleeding in the postoperative setting is usually surgical in nature and therefore not correctable by platelet transfusion. However, bypass-induced platelet dysfunction may contribute to bleeding after cardiac surgery,[201] and platelet transfusion may improve hemostasis in such situations. Platelet transfusion is most useful in thrombocytopenic patients with microvascular bleeding (e.g., oozing or mucous membrane or gastrointestinal bleeding). Transfusion to achieve a platelet count of 50×10^9/L is generally recommended for bleeding patients.[191,199,200] However, hemostasis may be achieved through repeated platelet transfusion even in the absence of a demonstrable rise in platelet count.

Dilutional thrombocytopenia may occur after massive transfusion of red cells and plasma volume expanders. In the absence of platelet consumption, a platelet count of $<50 \times 10^9$/L is not generally seen, unless more than two blood volumes (20 red cell units in an adult) have been replaced.[202-204] However, in settings such as trauma where there is activation of coagulation and consumption of platelets in addition to blood loss, there is some evidence that preemptive use of platelets in the resuscitation support may be of benefit.[154,189,205]

In all situations, the clinical decision regarding platelet transfusions requires consideration of several variables, including an estimation of platelet count and function, the cause of thrombocytopenia, and assessment of coagulation; the presence or likelihood of bleeding (the development of petechiae, spontaneous mucous membrane oozing, and retinal hemorrhages may be danger signals indicating hemostatic incompetence); and the hazards of transfusion.

Platelet Refractoriness and Alloimmunization

Refractoriness to platelet transfusions is a clinical state that can be defined as an unacceptably low recovery of transfused platelets on two or more occasions. As noted previously, a CCI of $<7.5 \times 10^9$/L at 1 hour and $<4.5 \times 10^9$/L at 20 to 24 hours after the transfusion is a commonly used definition of an unacceptable response. Clinical factors reported to be associated with refractoriness to platelet transfusion are listed in *Table 23.7*.[206-208]

Immune Causes of Refractoriness and the Prevention of HLA Alloimmunization

The major immune cause of refractoriness is the presence of HLA antibodies. These antibodies are stimulated by pregnancy or by transfusion of WBC-containing blood products. Platelets bear HLA class I antigens on their surface. Transfusion of platelets that are serologically incompatible with a preexisting HLA antibody typically results in no increase in platelet counts.[209]

The TRAP (Trial to Reduce Alloimmunization to Platelets) found that in patients with acute myelogenous leukemia receiving non–leukocyte-reduced blood components, the incidence of HLA alloimmunization was 33% in those who had never been pregnant and 62% in those who had been pregnant; in patients receiving leukocyte-reduced blood components, it was 9% and 32%, respectively.[210]

The incidence of clinically significant alloantibodies to human platelet antigens (HPAs) in transfusion recipients is unclear. Antibodies to HPAs have been detected almost exclusively in patients who also have broadly reactive HLA antibodies. Using the sensitive monoclonal antibody immobilization of platelet antigen assays, investigators have reported detection of antibodies to HPAs in as many as 25% of HLA-alloimmunized transfusion recipients.[211] A significant proportion of the antibodies detected have ill-defined specificity, and the contribution of such antibodies to platelet refractoriness is unclear. The presence of HPA antibodies in patients who are broadly sensitized to HLA presents an enormous transfusion support challenge. Although many blood centers maintain HLA-typed donor registries, at present, very few of these donors are typed for HPAs.

Nonimmune Causes of Refractoriness

Of the nonimmune factors implicated in refractoriness, underlying infection is the most important.[212] Transfused platelets pool in the enlarged spleen and increasing the dose of platelets does not necessarily improve the posttransfusion increment. Each of the other nonimmune factors listed in *Table 23.7* has been reported to be associated

Table 23.7. Factors Reported to Be Associated With Platelet Refractoriness

Immune Factors
Alloantibodies
Anti–human leukocyte antigen
Antiplatelet glycoprotein
ABO
Autoantibodies
Immune thrombocytopenic purpura
Drug-related
Nonimmune Factors
Splenomegaly
Fever, infection
Disseminated intravascular coagulation
Immune complexes
Bone marrow transplantation
Amphotericin

with refractoriness, although the importance of each factor has not been demonstrated consistently.[208]

Diagnosis and Management of Alloimmunization

The appropriate investigation and management of platelet refractoriness require consideration of information from a clinical assessment of the patient as well as laboratory investigations. The first step is a clinical evaluation for possible nonimmune clinical causes and is frequently omitted. Any significant clinical factors such as infection should be treated if possible.

If poor responses to platelet transfusions persist, the patient should be tested for HLA antibodies, and, if present, platelet transfusions matched for the HLA-A and -B antigens of the patient can be used.[209] The provision of HLA-matched platelets is enabled by the establishment of panels of HLA-typed platelet donors who can be asked to donate platelets by apheresis. This requires logistic coordination and may result in a time lag before the product is available. There are a number of ways to select HLA-matched platelet transfusions. Traditionally, recipient and donor are matched for HLA-A and -B antigens as the most important antibodies in causing platelet refractoriness. Refinements to HLA matching have been made including grading of the quality of HLA match and its revision to include "permissive" mismatches,[213] the identification of the specificity of HLA antibodies and the issue of HLA-matched platelets based on their specificity,[214] and, more recently, the use of software tools such as "HLA matchmaker" to predict HLA compatibility by identifying immunogenic epitopes in antibody-accessible regions of HLA molecules.[215] A recent systematic review found that HLA-matched platelet transfusions improved 1 hour posttransfusion platelet increments but did not consistently improve the 24-hour increments, and failed to demonstrate any reduction in mortality or bleeding, as the studies were inadequately powered for these outcomes.[216] Alternatively, HLA-compatible platelets may be identified by selecting donors with HLA-A and HLA-B antigens that do not correspond with the HLA antibody profile of the patient. This process provides patients with a larger compatible donor pool compared to finding an exact HLA match and improves 1-hour CCI relative to random donor platelets but can result in exposure to new HLA antigens and further alloimmunization.

It is important to monitor patients' responses to platelet transfusion and to reevaluate them serologically if they do not respond to products that were previously acceptable. It should also be noted that HLA antibodies may appear or disappear over the course of a patient's treatment.[212]

Platelet Transfusions for Patients Refractory to HLA-Matched Platelet Transfusions

Responses to HLA-matched platelet transfusions should be carefully monitored. If there are improved responses, HLA-matched platelet transfusions should be continued. If there are poor responses to HLA-matched platelet transfusions, the reasons should be sought, including HLA incompatibility, which is most likely to occur in patients with unusual HLA types with few well-matched donors, nonimmune platelet consumption, and HPA and ABO incompatibility.

Platelet crossmatching of the patient's plasma against the lymphocytes and platelets of donors of HLA-matched platelet transfusions that have failed to produce satisfactory responses may be very helpful in identifying the cause of the poor responses.[217] Platelet crossmatching can also be used as an alternative approach for the management of refractory patients with HLA-matched platelet transfusions.[218] Typically, the patient's plasma is tested against platelet samples of ABO-compatible apheresis platelet donors. Donor platelets lacking reactivity are considered to be "crossmatch compatible" and the associated platelet concentrates selected for transfusion in preference to those from random donors. An advantage of platelet crossmatching over a strategy of HLA-matched platelet transfusions is its timeliness where the HLA types of platelet-refractory patients are not yet known. A disadvantage is the need to carry out testing each time a platelet transfusion is required.

The management of patients with HLA or HPA alloimmunization with no compatible donors may be very difficult. There is no evidence that alloimmunized patients benefit from prophylactic transfusions of incompatible platelets that do not produce an increase in the platelet count, and prophylactic platelet support should be discontinued. If bleeding occurs, platelet transfusions from random donors or the best-matched donors, despite being incompatible, may reduce the severity of hemorrhage, although large doses of platelets may be required. Other management approaches for severe alloimmune refractoriness such as the use of high-dose IVIG,[219] splenectomy, and plasma exchange have not been shown to be effective.

The management of patients with nonimmune platelet consumption is similarly problematic. Treatment of the underlying illness is indicated. Common practice is to continue with daily platelet transfusions as prophylactic platelet support, but it is not known whether this approach is effective, or whether platelet transfusions should be discontinued or the dose of platelets increased. IVIG is also ineffective in this scenario. Antifibrinolytic drugs, such as aminocaproic acid and tranexamic acid, may be beneficial in controlling bleeding in thrombocytopenic patients,[220,221] but the A-TREAT (American Trial Using Tranexamic Acid in Thrombocytopenia) suggests that these therapies are not effective for bleeding prophylaxis.[222]

Selection of Platelet Products

ABO Group

The clinical importance of ABO compatibility in platelet transfusion is controversial. Platelets bear both intrinsic[223] and adsorbed[224] antigens of the ABO system. Transfusion of ABO-incompatible platelets may be associated with decreased posttransfusion platelet recovery and normal survival.[225] The reduction in recovery is variable and may be related to the isohemagglutinin titer of the recipient. Rarely, a high titer (>1:256) of anti-A or anti-B may cause frank refractoriness to ABO-incompatible platelets.[226]

Platelet products contain a significant amount of donor plasma. Rarely, high-titer donor isohemagglutinins in platelet products may cause intravascular hemolysis of recipient red cells,[227] especially platelets from group O donors.[228] Although ABO-identical platelets may result in increased platelet recovery, this strategy has not been shown to provide a benefit in terms of morbidity and survival.[229,230] In addition, the strict use of ABO-identical platelets may result in increased outdating of products and waste.[231]

RhD Type

Platelets do not carry Rh antigens, and the donor's RhD type is important only because the red cells present in the platelet concentrate may immunize RhD-negative recipients. The reported frequency of D alloimmunization in D-negative recipients after transfusion of D-positive platelets has varied in studies. It is possible that the difference in observations is related both to an increase in intensity of chemotherapy and to a substantial reduction in the red cell content of platelet products. Most platelet products transfused in the United States are apheresis derived, and these products contain a significantly smaller volume of red cells compared to whole blood derived platelet concentrates.[232] A study of 485 D-negative recipients of D-positive platelets in 11 centers between 2010 and 2012 found that only 7 of 485 (1.44%) recipients had a primary anti-D response.[232] There were no statistically significant differences between the primary anti-D formers and the other patients in terms of gender, age, receipt of immunosuppressive therapy, proportion of patients with hematologic/oncologic diseases, transfusion of whole blood–derived or apheresis platelets or both, and total number of transfused platelet products. A single-institution retrospective analysis of RhD-negative patients receiving RhD-positive platelets found that none of the 130 patients who received apheresis platelets were alloimmunized and formed anti-D. The use of RhD immunoprophylaxis may be considered when transfusing RhD-negative females of childbearing age with RhD-positive platelets, and institution-specific policies should be developed based on the method of platelet collection.[233]

Transfusion Medicine

Cold-Stored Platelets

Platelet transfusions have most frequently been used for the prophylactic treatment of thrombocytopenia in patients with malignancies, and a key determinant of their quality has been the length of survival in circulation. Platelets stored at room temperature have demonstrated a longer half-life in circulation relative to refrigerated platelets and have therefore been the most widely available platelet product in hospital blood banks.[234] However, more recent literature has suggested that the hemostatic potential of cold-stored platelets may be superior to room temperature platelets for actively bleeding patients. These studies showed that cold-stored platelets were less susceptible to storage lesion due to reduced metabolic activity, which resulted in improved aggregation, clot strength, and bleeding times.[235] A safety and feasibility pilot trial comparing cold-stored platelets stored up to 14 days and room temperature platelets stored for the conventional 5 days in cardiothoracic surgery found no significant differences in total blood use, chest drainage, adverse events, length of stay, and mortality.[236] This new data, along with the increased use of therapeutic platelet transfusions in settings with active bleeding (surgery, trauma, and massive transfusions) and reduced need for prophylactic transfusions due to lower thresholds, has renewed interest in cold-stored platelets. In addition, the potential for a significantly longer shelf life and reduced concerns of bacterial contamination may cause a shift in blood bank inventories after considering the effects on transfusion safety and waste.

PLASMA TRANSFUSION

Use of Plasma Components

Plasma is utilized in patients who are deficient in coagulation factors and who can benefit from an increase in levels. Plasma can be used for replacement of clotting factors consumed during massive hemorrhage, for reversal of warfarin (if a prothrombin complex concentrate is unavailable), and as the replacement fluid for plasma-exchange procedures in patients with TTP and some other disorders (see Therapeutic Apheresis).[8,237,238] Plasma should not be used as volume expanders or for all therapeutic plasma exchange (TPE) procedures because alternative fluids with lower risks of infectious diseases, allergic reactions, and TRALI are available for these purposes (e.g., crystalloid, albumin, starch). The appropriate dose of plasma is a minimum of 15 mL/kg, to provide approximately a 30% increase in coagulation factor levels.[239,240] The expected rise in coagulation factor activity for a 70 kg adult is approximately 7% for each plasma unit.

Efficacy of Plasma Transfusions

In an evidence-based review, the AABB recommended plasma therapy for only a few clinical indications, based on the available Level 1 evidence in the literature (which was assessed to be of "weak quality")[241]: trauma patients with substantial hemorrhage, patients undergoing complex cardiovascular surgery, patients with TTP, emergency reversal of warfarin-associated coagulopathy, and management of patients with coagulation factor deficiencies for which no concentrates are available.[242] Patients with mild prolongations of the international normalized ratio (INR < 1.7) are not at risk of bleeding and do not need plasma therapy for minor procedures,[239] but these patients make up the majority of patients receiving plasma transfusions. However, logistical/technical barriers that prevent effective and timely plasma therapy (possibly resulting in plasma therapies that are "too little, too late"), along with very few randomized, controlled clinical trials, have probably contributed to the paucity of evidence demonstrating a clinical benefit for plasma therapy.[92,243] One of the few such clinical trials compared plasma therapy vs a 4-factor prothrombin concentrate in patients with major bleeding who were on vitamin K antagonists.[244] The 4-factor concentrate corrected INRs to less than 1.3 within 30 minutes in 62% of patients, compared with only 9.6% of patients receiving plasma.

One of the largest prospective studies of plasma transfusions and their effect on INR and bleeding included both medical and surgical patients with pretransfusion INR of between 1.1 and 1.85.[245] The authors reported that <1% of patients had normalization of their INR and only 15% had at least 50% correction. The median dose of plasma was 2 U (only 5-7 mL/kg), and there was no correlation between plasma dose and change in INR. This study had many of the limitations common in this clinical arena: lack of control groups, only modest prolongation in coagulation tests, poorly defined clinical end points (e.g., change in Hb or need for transfusion), or an inadequate dose of plasma therapy.[246]

The paucity of evidence for benefit of plasma transfusion therapy has been accompanied by growing evidence that risks of plasma have been underrecognized. In a prospective study, 8% of transfused patients developed transfusion-associated cardiac overload.[247] TRALI[248] is a significant cause of morbidity/mortality from blood transfusions, whose incidence has declined subsequently with use of plasma from male donors or female donors who have no history of pregnancy.[249]

WHOLE BLOOD TRANSFUSION

Component therapy has been central to transfusion medicine practice for decades, but with the increased recognition of trauma patients requiring early administration of fixed ratio transfusions (1 RBC:1 FFP:1 PLT), there has been increased interest in the use of whole blood. Whole blood has been frequently utilized in military trauma and several civilian institutions now carry this product in their inventories. The AABB allows for the use of whole blood that is ABO-identical, unless there are policies that address the upper limits of isohemagglutinins (anti-A and anti-B), specify indications for its use, and define a maximum volume that can be transfused out of group. This has popularized the use of low-titer type O whole blood (LTOWB) for the initial resuscitation of trauma. The benefits of LTOWB over component therapy include a more concentrated blood product that contains a lower volume of preservative solution and cold-stored platelets that may provide superior hemostasis in bleeding patients.[235,250] Seheult et al. demonstrated that there was no measurable difference in hemolysis markers when comparing LTOWB for type O patients to out-of-group transfusions and the use of whole blood for trauma resulted in similar mortality rates when compared to component therapy (18.5% vs 24.4%, $P = .24$).[251-253] The hospital lengths of stay and median number of transfusions also did not differ between the groups. Although literature on whole blood use in civilian settings in limited, early evidence points to a safe and efficacious product that will likely increase in utilization for trauma, prehospital transfusion, and massive transfusions.

GRANULOCYTE TRANSFUSIONS

Severe bacterial and fungal infections in the setting of prolonged chemotherapy-associated neutropenia are common causes of morbidity and mortality in the treatment of malignancy. Risk of serious bacterial infection appears as the neutrophil count falls below 1.0×10^9/L and increases rapidly below 0.5×10^9/L. Fungal infections occur with much higher frequency as the neutrophil count falls below 0.2×10^9/L.[254] Other risk factors include the duration of neutropenia and the rate of fall of the neutrophil count. The use of growth factors (e.g., granulocyte colony–stimulating factor [G-CSF]) has reduced the severity and duration of neutropenia, but many patients still have long periods of poor granulocyte production, lasting 2 to 3 weeks or longer.[255] Prophylactic antibiotics and anti-fungal therapies are sometimes prescribed to mitigate risks of serious bacterial and fungal infections in select patient populations, such as those with hematologic malignancies.[256,257] Although the idea of enhancing host defenses with granulocyte infusions dates back 60 years, difficulty obtaining adequate granulocyte yields as well as safety concerns stifled the initial interest generated after early clinical successes in the 1970s.[258] Modern apheresis techniques, growth factors that increased yields, and positive results from clinical trials led to renewed interest in applying granulocyte therapy to a wider range of patients and the completion of a randomized clinical controlled trial to evaluate their effectiveness.[259]

Clinical Indications and Efficacy

The most recent Cochrane review of all 10 randomized clinical trials performed between 1975 and 2015, including the Resolving Infection in Neutropenia with Granulocytes (RING) trial, concluded that there is insufficient evidence to support or refute the use of granulocyte transfusions in neutropenic patients.[260] In 321 participants in six studies eligible for quantitative analysis, there was no difference in all-cause mortality up to 30 days comparing participants receiving granulocyte transfusions vs those who did not (RR 0.75, 95% CI 0.54-1.04). Some older studies were likely limited by the apheresis techniques used and the low cell yields obtained, as most donors were pretreated with corticosteroids only. However, further analysis showed no difference in mortality in patients receiving higher vs lower doses of granulocytes. Though in the five trials published before 2000 there may have been a reduction in overall mortality in those patients who received granulocytes vs those who did not (RR 0.53, 95% CI 0.33-0.85), supportive care including antibiotics and antifungal medications, including prophylactic use, has changed substantially. Based on this information, granulocyte therapy may warrant consideration in severely neutropenic patients with bacterial infections unresponsive to typical antimicrobial therapy, but should be considered experimental and ideally should be conducted within the context of an ongoing clinical trial.

The RING multicenter, randomized controlled trial was undertaken to definitively assess the efficacy of granulocyte transfusions in the modern era.[259] However, the study was terminated early because of low accrual and thus was not powered to detect a true benefit to this therapy. There was no difference in overall survival or microbial response in 56 patients who received granulocytes vs 54 patients who did not (P = .64). Post hoc analysis showed that patients who received higher-dose granulocyte infusions did better than those who received lower doses. However, the authors caution that there is likely no real clinical difference between these groups.

The effect of the prophylactic use of granulocyte transfusions to diminish the risk of serious infections in severely neutropenic patients during therapy of hematologic malignancies and after bone marrow transplantation has been investigated.[261] Although prophylactic granulocyte transfusion may decrease the risk of septicemia, the increased incidence of adverse effects observed with this therapy, including HLA sensitization, may outweigh the beneficial effects.[262-268] The use of prophylactic granulocyte transfusions should be carefully considered and viewed as experimental.

Donor Preparation/Selection

High granulocyte yields were initially obtained using preparations from donors with chronic myelogenous leukemia.[269] Subsequently, methods were developed to collect sufficient granulocytes from normal donors. Apheresis became the standard method for collection of granulocyte concentrates.[270] The quantity and quality of granulocytes obtained depend on the apheresis collection technique as well as the number of circulating donor neutrophils. Infusion of hydroxyethyl starch or dextran to improve the sedimentation of donor red cells during centrifugation improves the efficiency of apheresis, but the granulocyte yield remains low. Data suggested a daily granulocyte dose of about 10×10^{10} cells would be needed to achieve benefit.[271] Oral corticosteroids produce a transient donor neutrophilia, but the collection yield remains in the range of 2 to 3×10^{10}.[272] Studies have shown the ability of G-CSF to increase the dose/collection. Donors treated with G-CSF with or without corticosteroids produce yields ranging from 2.4 to 9.9×10^{10} granulocytes. Although adverse effects are common, most are mild and consist of bone pain, headache, myalgias, and/or fatigue. Data from the bone marrow transplant literature support the short-term safety of G-CSF use in healthy donors, although rare serious adverse events have been reported.[273] Based on available evidence, donor pretreatment with a single dose of G-CSF (300-600 μg

subcutaneously) with dexamethasone (8 mg orally) 12 hours before collection gives reliable yields in a well-tolerated and cost-effective manner. Although repeated daily G-CSF stimulation and granulocyte collection have been reported,[274] standard practice is to perform only one collection per donor.

Prospective granulocyte donors should meet all FDA and AABB standards for donation. Because granulocyte products must be transfused before completion of donor infectious disease testing, donors who have been previously tested within 30 days are strongly preferred. Donors should also be free of disorders that might be exacerbated by dexamethasone (e.g., diabetes) or G-CSF (e.g., arthritis, vasculitis, splenomegaly, gout, thrombocytopenia). Donor-recipient pairs should be ABO compatible because of the RBC content in the product. RBC compatibility must be verified for each granulocyte product. CMV infections are a significant risk when seropositive donors are used for immunocompromised CMV-seronegative patients; therefore, these patients should receive granulocytes from CMV-negative donors since this product cannot be leukoreduced.[269]

Granulocyte Collection/Storage

Once an appropriate donor has been selected and prepared, granulocytes are typically collected by leukapheresis during which 7 to 10 L of blood is processed over 3 to 4 hours. Hydroxyethyl starch is often used to reduce RBC contamination by sedimentation. According to AABB Standards, at least 1×10^{10} granulocytes/apheresis is collected.[2] Current techniques achieve mean yields of 4 to 8×10^{10}/leukapheresis in 200 to 400 mL of plasma, with 10 to 30 mL of RBCs, and 1 to 6×10^{11} platelets. Although granulocytes can be stored for up to 24 hours at room temperature, transfusion within 8 hours of collection is recommended.

Administration of Granulocytes

Granulocytes should be administered on a daily basis until the patient's endogenous neutrophil count rises to 0.5×10^9/L or until the infection clears. Granulocyte concentrates should be given through a standard filter set to ensure that aggregates are not administered. The concentrate should be given slowly (over 1-2 hours), with the patient under constant observation, including the use of pulse oximetry. Transfusion reactions occur in 10% to 50% of patients but are usually mild, consisting of fever and chills. Premedication with antihistamines, acetaminophen, or steroids is common practice before infusion. More severe reactions occur in 1% to 5% of patients and tend to be pulmonary in nature. A serious potential interaction between granulocyte transfusions and amphotericin B has been reported,[275] but this association has not been substantiated by others.[276,277] Nevertheless, many physicians administer granulocytes and amphotericin at least 8 to 12 hours apart to limit the potential for increased pulmonary toxicity. If there are any signs or symptoms of respiratory distress, the transfusion should be discontinued immediately, the recipient should be examined for hypoxemia or pulmonary edema, and a chest radiograph should be done to assess for pulmonary infiltrates. If major adverse effects do occur, the recipient should be studied for the presence of antibodies that react with neutrophils. Granulocyte products contain lymphocytes and are capable of causing TA-GVHD. Thus, all granulocyte products should be irradiated to prevent TA-GVHD without significantly impairing granulocyte function.[278] Pre- and posttransfusion neutrophil counts should be determined to guide therapy. With large doses (>8×10^{10}), neutrophil increments may exceed 2×10^9/L immediately after infusion and may last for 24 to 48 hours.

ADVERSE EFFECTS OF BLOOD TRANSFUSION

The potential complications of blood transfusion therapy are many, but most present problems only in patients requiring repeated or large numbers of transfusions. The risks associated with the transfusion of any specific unit of blood are low. However, the risks must be weighed against the benefits at the time each transfusion is ordered.

Transfusion complications can be classified as immunologic and nonimmunologic (*Table 23.8*). Many of the immune reactions are caused by the stimulation of antibody production by foreign antigens present on transfused red cells, leukocytes, platelets, or plasma proteins. Such alloimmunization may lead to immunologically mediated reactions when transfusions carrying these antigens are administered in the future. These include hemolytic reactions caused by incompatibility for red cell antigens; febrile or pulmonary reactions caused by leukocyte and HLA antigens; allergic or anaphylactic reactions caused by soluble antigens, usually plasma proteins, in the transfused material; and TA-GVHD caused by engraftment of transfused lymphocytes in immunosuppressed recipients. The rates of transfusion reactions are shown in *Table 23.9*.[279]

The nonimmune reactions are caused by the physical or chemical properties of the transfused blood products, as well as contaminating infectious agents. Nonimmune reactions include circulatory overload and certain adverse effects encountered specifically during massive transfusions.

Table 23.8. Adverse Effects of Transfusion

Immunologic
Alloimmunization to:
Red cell antigens
Human leukocyte antigen antigens
Platelet-specific antigens
Neutrophil-specific antigens
Hemolytic transfusion reactions
Acute
Delayed
Febrile nonhemolytic transfusion reactions
Transfusion-related acute lung injury
Allergic transfusion reactions
Posttransfusion purpura
Transfusion-associated graft-vs-host disease
Nonimmunologic
Transfusion-associated circulatory overload
Massive transfusion
Metabolic (hyperkalemia, hypocalcemia)
Hypothermia
Transfusion hemosiderosis
Infectious
Hepatitis: A, B, C, D, other
Human immunodeficiency virus-1/-2
Human T-lymphotropic virus-I/-II
Syphilis
Cytomegalovirus
Arboviruses: West Nile virus, Zika virus
Parasites: malaria, *Babesia*, trypanosomes
Variant Creutzfeldt-Jakob disease
Bacterial contamination
Emerging pathogens
Unknown
Transfusion-related immunomodulatory effects
Red blood cell storage lesions

Immunologic Transfusion Reactions
Alloimmunization to Transfused Antigens
Alloantibodies Reacting With Red Cell Antigens

Although the antigenic composition of donor red cells differs from that of the recipient, only a minority of multitransfused recipients develop red cell alloantibodies. Antibodies to Rh-system antigens and to Kell (K) are most often detected, though transfusion-induced antibodies to other minor red cell antigens such as Fy and Jk are also commonly found.[280]

The production of such antibodies is a property of both the recipient's immune response and the immunogenicity of the different red cell antigens. The risk of red cell alloimmunization has been estimated at 2% in sporadically transfused patients.[280] The reported incidence of RBC alloimmunization for patients with thalassemias is 5% to 10%[281] vs 7% to 59% for those with sickle cell anemia.[282] The increased incidence of alloimmunization in sickle cell patients has been attributed to the difference in race between the blood donor pool and the patient population.[283] As a result, there is a greater likelihood of minor antigen incompatibility between donor and recipient. The differing immunogenicity of various red cell antigens also plays a role. For patients with sickle cell anemia, red cells phenotypically matched for Rh (including C, c, E, and e) and Kell (K, k) antigens are recommended. This measure was shown to reduce the alloimmunization rate in this population from 3% to 0.3% per unit transfused.[284]

Alloantibodies Reacting With Leukocyte Antigens

Alloimmunization to HLA and other leukocyte-associated antigens has been discussed earlier with respect to problems encountered in platelet transfusion. These antibodies occur mainly in multiparous women[285] and multitransfused patients. In patients receiving nonleukoreduced transfusion support for aplastic anemia or acute leukemia, 20% to 70% become immunized to HLA antigens.[286] Interestingly, HLA alloimmunization is significantly increased in male patients with preexisting RBC antibodies compared with multiple transfused

Table 23.9. Rates of Transfusion Reactions

	Prevalence (per 100,000 U Transfused)
Allergic transfusion reaction	112.2
Anaphylactic transfusion reaction	8
Acute hemolytic transfusion reaction	2.5-7.9
Delayed hemolytic transfusion reaction	40
Delayed serologic transfusion reaction	48.9-75.7
Febrile nonhemolytic transfusion reaction	1000-3000
Hyperhemolytic transfusion reaction	Unknown
Hypotensive transfusion reaction	1.8-9.0
Massive transfusion-associated reactions (citrate, potassium, cold toxicity)	Unknown
Posttransfusion purpura	Unknown
Septic transfusion reaction	0.03-3.3 (product dependent)
Transfusion-associated circulatory overload	10.9
Transfusion-associated graft-vs-host disease	Extremely rare (near 0%) with irradiation or pathogen reduction methods
Transfusion-related acute lung injury	0.4-1.0 with mitigation (varies by component and postimplementation of risk mitigation strategies)

Reprinted from Delaney M, Wendel S, Bercovitz RS, et al. Transfusion reactions: prevention, diagnosis, and treatment. *Lancet.* 2016;388(10061):2825-2836. Copyright © 2016 Elsevier. With permission.

male patients without such antibodies.[287] As discussed in the section "Platelet Transfusion," the prophylactic use of leukocyte-reduced blood products significantly reduces the incidence of HLA alloimmunization in patients with no prior exposure to these antigens.

Alloantibodies Reacting With Plasma Proteins

Although antibodies to soluble plasma proteins such as lipoproteins and to Gm and Inv determinants on IgG are often detectable in multitransfused patients, transfusion reactions have rarely been attributed to such antibodies.[288] Some anaphylactic reactions are attributed to anti-IgA antibodies,[289] especially in patients who are IgA-deficient, although the presence of antibodies that react with IgA is not always clearly correlated with the occurrence of this type of transfusion reaction.[290]

Hemolytic Transfusion Reactions

The development of antibodies capable of reacting with red cell antigens may lead to destruction of transfused red cells. The clinical significance of such reactions ranges from life-threatening to trivial. Whether hemolysis occurs immediately within the circulation, more slowly within the RES, or not at all depends on the antigen and antibody involved.[291]

The incidence of such reactions is variably reported. A review of fatal hemolytic reactions in the 1970s and 1980s reported to the US Bureau of Biologics (now the FDA's Center for Biologics Evaluation and Research or CBER) found that 86% were caused by ABO incompatibility, and of these, 89% were caused by simple clerical error.[292] More recent FDA data have shown a decrease in deaths because of ABO incompatibility, although hemolytic transfusion reactions still represent a leading cause of transfusion-related mortality.[293]

Acute (Intravascular) Hemolytic Transfusion Reactions

Acute hemolytic transfusion reactions are most typically associated with ABO incompatibility. Anti-A and anti-B antibodies are predominantly IgM and are capable of binding complement and causing immediate intravascular destruction of red cells. An AHTR caused by ABO incompatibility is usually related to human error (see "Compatibility Testing Process"). Other red cell antigens such as Jk^a and Fy^a (which may bind complement) may also lead to such reactions.

Infrequently, hemolytic transfusion reactions may be caused by destruction of recipient red cells after the transfusion of plasma-containing antibodies.[294] For example, anti-A_1 occurring naturally in group A donors of subgroup A_2 has been reported to cause hemolytic transfusion reactions.[295] Hemolytic transfusion reactions have also been reported in association with apheresis platelets containing abnormally high titer (>1:256) anti-A or anti-B antibodies in the plasma. Plasma volume reduction is recommended for such products if the plasma is incompatible with the recipient.[296] Hemolytic reactions caused by the transfusion of plasma containing other antibodies are extremely rare, as blood donors are screened for red cell antibodies other than ABO.

Signs and Symptoms. AHTRs occur soon after the incompatible transfusion has begun. Fever with or without chills is one of the most common manifestations of such reactions. More severe signs and symptoms include anxiety, chest or back pain, flushing, dyspnea, tachycardia, hypotension, and disseminated intravascular coagulation (DIC).[1] If the patient is under general anesthesia or unconscious, these symptoms may not be recognized immediately; only severe hypotension and evidence of oozing or hemoglobinuria serve as clues to the presence of a hemolytic reaction.

AHTRs may be life-threatening especially if unrecognized, since severity of complications including acute renal failure, shock, DIC, and ultimately death is related to the amount of incompatible blood transfused. It has been estimated that a fatal acute hemolytic reaction occurs in ~0.4 of 1,000,000 red cell transfusions. The mortality of a severe AHTR increases with the amount of blood transfused.

Pathophysiology. The primary event in AHTRs is the interaction between the antibody and the red cell membrane, resulting in the development of immune complexes, activation of complement leading to the release of C3a and C5a with anaphylatoxic activity, and the coagulation mechanism via cytokines and factor XII (leading to both consumptive coagulopathy and generation of bradykinin). Vasomotor mediators implicated in the transfusion reaction include histamine, serotonin, and cytokines. Shock results from release of such vasoactive substances.[291]

The renal failure that may occur in this setting is of complex and poorly understood etiology but appears to be primarily ischemic, caused by a combination of hypotension, vasoconstriction (via nitric oxide inactivation by Hb), and intravascular coagulation.

Management. On any suspicion of a hemolytic transfusion reaction, the transfusion must be discontinued immediately, as the severity of the reaction is related to the volume of red cells infused. A recheck of the patient's identity with the information on the discontinued blood unit (a "clerical check") is necessary to rule out patient identification errors. The reaction must be reported to the blood bank without delay; a posttransfusion blood sample and the discontinued bag of blood should be sent to the blood bank for investigation of the cause of the reaction. Hydration must be begun immediately to prevent renal failure. An infusion of normal saline is given to maintain the blood pressure and increase the urine flow rate to 100 mL/h. Diuretics may be needed to maintain urine output. Once renal failure is established, the usual supportive measures, including fluid restriction, management of electrolyte balance, and dialysis, are required. Consultation with nephrology, hematology, and critical care specialists may be required.

Additional interventions may be needed depending on the severity of the reaction. The patient may require support of the defective hemostatic mechanisms with platelets and cryoprecipitate or plasma.

Investigation of AHTRs. The following steps must be carried out in the investigation of patients with all transfusion reactions. The patient's identity must be confirmed, and all the records on the patient and the donor blood label must be checked for clerical errors. A new sample of blood must be drawn from the patient and sent to the blood bank with the discontinued unit of blood. The posttransfusion sample must be visually checked for hemolysis. In intravascular reactions, free plasma Hb can be detected most quickly by centrifuging a tube of blood anticoagulated with ethylenediaminetetraacetic acid (EDTA) or heparin; pink to red plasma indicates intravascular hemolysis. A DAT must be performed on the specimen submitted at the time of the reaction. If the test is positive, the pretransfusion sample should also be tested, because the patient may have had a positive DAT before transfusion.

Red cell typing should be repeated on all specimens. If the posttransfusion ABO and Rh types do not agree with pretransfusion results, there has been an error in patient identification or typing. Antibody detection tests may be repeated on the pre- and postreaction samples. In a minority of patients in whom there is a high clinical suspicion of a hemolytic transfusion reaction, no immunologic abnormality may be identified. In some, repeated examination for antibodies over a prolonged period of time may eventually reveal the cause; in others, results may be persistently negative. Blood bank physicians may request additional studies or tests, including other markers of hemolysis.

Prevention. Most AHTRs are preventable. The most likely cause is human error, such as mislabeling of the patient sample, drawing the sample from the wrong patient, transcription errors, and transfusion of the wrong unit with the recipient. Mechanisms to ensure positive identification of the patient (recipient), the blood sample, and the transfusion component must be in place to prevent AHTRs.[2]

Delayed Hemolytic Transfusion Reactions

DHTRs generally are much milder than those occurring immediately, and red cell destruction is predominantly extravascular.[297] The transfused red cells are destroyed between 2 and 10 days after a transfusion. Investigation may reveal the presence of a red cell antibody not detected in the pretransfusion blood sample. The DAT is often positive. The positivity is transient and may be missed if it is performed too late. The DAT reverts to negative as the incompatible red cells are removed from the circulation.

Transfusion Medicine

DHTRs almost always represent secondary, or anamnestic, antibody responses. On first exposure to an immunogenic red cell antigen, a primary antibody response generally is delayed in onset and slow to reach its peak. The antibody level gradually declines, and antibody screening and crossmatch tests may be negative by the time the patient needs a transfusion. After a subsequent transfusion, the previously sensitized recipient manifests a much more brisk (secondary) immune response, with high concentrations of IgG antibody developing within days. Donor cells remaining in the circulation may become coated with antibody and removed by the RES. Only rarely does primary immunization after transfusion lead to a DHTR.[298]

In DHTRs, destruction of the sensitized red cells is predominantly extravascular, that is, the IgG-coated red cells are removed by the RES. Often, there are no symptoms, with a new red cell antibody and positive DAT detected incidentally (termed a delayed serologic transfusion reaction).[299] If present, symptoms and signs may include fever, falling Hb, jaundice, and, infrequently, hemoglobinemia and hemoglobinuria. Rarely, the reactions may be dramatic; renal failure is uncommon, but fatalities have been reported. Antibodies to Kidd (Jk) antigens and to antigens of the Rh system are the major causes of DHTRs, with anti-Kell and anti-Duffy (Fy) implicated in most other delayed reactions. Anti-Kidd antibodies are particularly troublesome because the plasma concentration of these antibodies declines more rapidly than others, so pretransfusion tests are more commonly negative in patients who are in fact sensitized.[167]

Investigation of DHTRs

If a DHTR is suspected, a fresh blood sample should be obtained from the patient. This sample should be screened for the presence of previously undetectable red cell antibodies. A DAT should be done. If it is positive, the antibodies should be eluted from the red cells and identified. If the transfused cells have already been destroyed, the DAT will not be positive, but an antibody should be detectable in the patient's serum. The treating physician must be advised and the patient given a card or record indicating the presence of the antibody to be presented to all future physicians and other transfusing facilities. The blood bank must retain a permanent record of clinically significant antibodies because the antibody may again become undetectable.

Management of DHTRs

In most instances, no specific therapy is necessary. The few patients who experience severe reactions should be treated with adequate hydration. The physician and patient should be informed about the antibody so that crossmatch-compatible blood negative for the offending antigen(s) is administered in the future, especially if the patient transfers to other institutions where blood bank records are not shared (such as at most hospitals in the United States).

Pseudohemolytic Transfusion Reactions

In patients manifesting a clinical syndrome consistent with intravascular hemolysis, but in whom no blood group incompatibility can be identified, explanations other than AHTRs and DHTRs should be considered. Conditions that mimic hemolytic transfusion reactions are called *pseudohemolytic transfusion reactions*.[291] These include bacterial contamination with organisms such as *Yersinia*, resorption of large hematomas, and hemolysis caused by drug reactions or vascular prostheses. Pretransfusion hemolysis of donor blood caused by mechanical trauma, freezing, heat, or hypotonic solutions should always be considered a potential cause of such a reaction.[291]

Febrile Nonhemolytic Transfusion Reactions

FNHTRs have been reported in a variable proportion of patients receiving transfusions, ranging between 1.0% and 3.0% (*Table 23.9*); they are more common in multitransfused patients. The typical reaction consists of a fever of 1 °C or greater, usually during or within a few hours of the transfusion. Rigors, chills, headache, or tachypnea may occur.[300] Occasionally, the reaction may be severe, but usually these reactions are mild. Whatever their degree, febrile transfusion reactions usually run their course within a few hours.

Alloimmunization to antigens on leukocytes and platelets is one of the most common causes of FNHTRs. HLA antibodies are most commonly found, followed by platelet-specific antibodies and granulocyte-specific antibodies.[301]

Another cause of FNHTRs is the transfusion of cytokines that have developed during product storage, especially in nonleukoreduced whole blood–derived platelet concentrates stored at room temperature.[302] During storage, leukocytes in platelet concentrates release cytokines that appear to be responsible for the febrile reaction.[53] The incidence of FNHTRs to nonleukoreduced platelet concentrates increases with the age of the platelet concentrate and the leukocyte concentration in the product. The concentration of cytokines in platelet concentrates and incidence of FNHTRs can be decreased by leukoreducing the products soon after collection; see the section "Platelet Preparation and Storage."

Management of Febrile Reactions

The approach to management of febrile transfusion reactions must be based on an understanding of all the possible causes (*Figure 23.5*). Although many such reactions are caused by WBC alloimmunization or cytokines, fever may also be an indication of an unsuspected hemolytic transfusion reaction or contamination of the donor blood by bacteria or endotoxin. For these reasons, every transfusion complicated by a febrile transfusion reaction should be discontinued until the patient has been carefully assessed by a physician and the blood bank alerted. The physician, depending on the clinical condition of the patient and the institution's policies regarding such steps, may elect to restart the transfusion if a hemolytic or bacterially contaminated transfusion has been ruled out.

The possibility of a hemolytic reaction should be considered when fever occurs. If suspected, the donor unit, along with a patient blood specimen, should be returned to the blood bank for investigation. The donor unit and patient blood should be cultured if there is any suspicion of bacterial contamination.

The symptoms of FNHTRs may be ameliorated with an antipyretic such as acetaminophen or hydrocortisone in patients who develop severe reactions. Meperidine may be used to decrease or stop severe shaking chills. Antihistamines are indicated only if the patient also has allergic symptoms such as hives.

Prevention of Febrile Transfusion Reactions

Febrile transfusion reactions to red cells occur most commonly in patients who have been sensitized to WBC antigens by previous transfusions or pregnancies. In such patients, the risk of a febrile transfusion reaction varies with the leukocyte content of the donor unit. The use of leukoreduced red cells decreases the incidence of FNHTRs.[300]

Transfusion-Related Acute Lung Injury

TRALI most commonly presents as severe respiratory distress of sudden onset, caused by a syndrome of noncardiogenic pulmonary edema resembling the adult respiratory distress syndrome. Chills, fever, chest pain, hypotension, and cyanosis, as well as the usual manifestations of pulmonary edema, may be seen. TRALI is reported by the FDA as the second most common cause of transfusion-associated fatality.[293]

It is hypothesized that TRALI reactions may be the result of two cumulative events: the first event is linked to the patient (i.e., underlying sepsis, hematologic disease, or postsurgical status), and the second event is related to the transfusion of potential granulocyte primers such as inflammatory cytokines, active lipids, or alloantibodies.[303] The diagnosis of a TRALI reaction is based on the onset of acute lung injury within 6 hours of transfusion,[304] characterized by an acute onset of hypoxemia (oxygen saturation <90% by pulse oximetry for a patient breathing room air or a $PaO_2/FiO_2 \leq 300$ mm Hg), bilateral infiltrates on frontal chest radiograph, and no evidence of circulatory overload.

Management involves supportive measures for the pulmonary edema and hypoxia, including ventilatory support if required.[305] The AABB requires evaluation of donors implicated in TRALI.[2] Donors whose blood is implicated in such reactions should be examined for the presence of granulocyte-specific and HLA antibodies that react

All transfusions must be stopped when a patient is experiencing a reaction and assessed by a provider
Provide supportive therapy to support vital organ function (cardiac, pulmonary, renal)
for questions regarding transfusion reaction diagnosis or management, call the transfusion service, or other appropriate physician

Reaction	Symptoms	Interventions

Increase in temperature

| Possible febrile nonhaemolytic reaction | Incremental increase <1°C above baseline and no other new symptoms | • Close observation, frequent vital signs
• If stable and no other new symptoms, then continue with transfusion |
| Possible bacterial contamination

Possible hemolysis | Incremental increase ≥1°C above baseline, or incremental increase <1°C with any other new symptoms (chills or rigors, hypotension, nausea, or vomiting) | • Stop transfusion, keep intravenous line open, assess patient, check patient ID and unit ID and compatibility.
• Antipyretic drug.
• Consider blood cultures (patient); empirical antibiotics if neutropenic.
• Do not resume transfusion.
• Strongly consider culturing blood product if ≥2°C increase in temperature or if high clinical suspicion of sepsis.
• Notify blood transfusion laboratory; return unit (with administration set) plus posttransfusion patient sample to blood transfusion laboratory. |

For consistently febrile patient due to underlying disease or treatment, when possible:
• Avoid starting transfusion if patient's temperature is increasing.
• Treat fever with antipyretic drug before starting transfusion.
• If incremental increase in temperature ≥1°C above baseline treat as mentioned earlier (stop and do not resume transfusion, cultures if indicated)
• Notify blood transfusion laboratory, return unit (with administration set) plus posttransfusion patient sample to blood transfusion laboratory.

Allergic symptoms

| Urticaria | Mild hives, rash, or skin itching only | • Stop transfusion, keep intravenous line open, and assess patient.
• Antihistamines.
• Notify patient clinician and blood transfusion laboratory; sample not required.
• If symptoms resolve, then can resume transfusion.
• If symptoms do not improve or worsen or recur then discontinue transfusion; return unit (with administration set) to blood transfusion laboratory. |
| Possible allergic reaction | Hives, rash, itching, and/or any other new symptoms (throat, eye and tongue swelling, etc.) | • Stop transfusion, keep intravenous line open, assess patient, check patient ID and unit ID and compatibility.
• Antihistamines.
• Do not resume transfusion.
• Notify blood transfusion laboratory; return unit (with administration set) plus posttransfusion patient sample to blood transfusion laboratory. |

Respiratory symptoms

| Possible anaphylaxis, transfusion-associated circulatory overload, septic transfusion reaction, or transfusion-related acute lung injury | Bronchospasm, dyspnea, tachypnea, and hypoxemia, copious frothy pink-tinged fluid (from endotrachel tube) | • Stop transfusion, keep intravenous line open, assess patient, check patient ID and unit ID and patient compatibility.
• Treat symptoms as indicated (adrenaline, antihistamines, steroids; oxygen and respiratory support, diuretics; fluid, blood pressure, and renal support).
• Chest radiograph for presence of bilateral interstitial infiltrate, if suggestive of transfusion-related acute lung injury.
• Blood cultures (patient and product), if high clinical suspicion of sepsis.
• Do not resume transfusion.
• Notify blood transfusion laboratory; return unit with administration set, plus posttransfusion patient sample. Associated products can be quaratined. |

All other symptoms

| Possible anaphylaxis, hemolytic transfusion reaction, fluid overload, or transfusion-related acute lung injury | Chills, rigors, hypotension, nausea or vomiting, feeling of impending doom, back or chest pain, intravenous site pain, cough, dyspnea, hypoxia | • Stop transfusion, keep intravenous line open, assess unit, check patient ID and unit ID and patient compatibility.
• Treat symptoms as indicated (adrenaline, antihistamines, steroids; oxygen and respiratory support, diuretics; fluid, blood pressure, and renal support).
• Blood cultures (patient and product) if high clinical suspicion of sepsis.
• Do not resume transfusion.
• Notify blood transfusion laboratory; return unit with administration set, plus posttransfusion patient sample. Associated products can be quaratined. |

FIGURE 23.5 Transfusion reaction decision tree. Algorithm to guide assessment and actions to take when a transfusion reaction is initially identified. Actions should go from left to right. (From Delaney M, Wendel S, Bercovitz RS, et al. Transfusion reactions: prevention, diagnosis, and treatment. *Lancet*. 2016;388(10061):2825-2836.)

Transfusion Medicine

with recipient leukocytes. It is recommended to avoid further transfusion of plasma-containing products from implicated donors found to have anti-HLA or anti-granulocyte antibodies.

Strategies such as the use of male donors only for plasma and plasma used for suspension of buffy coat–derived platelet pools, and screening of female apheresis donors have resulted in a substantial reduction in cases of TRALI.[249,306] The rate of TRALI after full implementation of mitigation strategies declined from 2.88 per 100,000 components in 2007 to 0.60 per 100,000 components in 2017 (*Table 23.9*).[307]

Allergic Reactions

Allergic reactions are common in transfusion recipients, particularly with platelet transfusions with an estimated incidence of up to 3% for platelet transfusions, but their actual incidence may be higher because they are often not reported.[279] They range in severity from urticarial lesions (hives), other skin rashes, bronchospasm, and angioedema to anaphylactic shock. Minor reactions are dose related, with an incidence related to the volume of plasma transfused. Whole blood and plasma are more likely than red cells to cause such reactions; washed red cells are rarely implicated. Minor urticarial reactions are the only transfusion reactions that do not necessitate immediate discontinuation of the transfusion or reporting of a suspected transfusion reaction. Fortunately, the incidence of severe anaphylactic transfusion reactions is very low, as such reactions can be life-threatening.

Most allergic reactions are thought to be mediated by recipient IgE to proteins or other soluble substances in donor plasma. The interaction between the antigen and IgE stimulates the release of histamine from mast cells and basophils. Most patients do not have repeated allergic reactions, but those with a history of atopy are at higher risk for additional reactions. For patients with repeated moderate-to-severe allergic reactions, premedication with a H_1-blocking antihistamine is usually sufficient for prevention, though evidence is lacking for use of premedication in patients with a history of mild allergic reactions.[308] If maximal premedication (e.g., adding an H_2-blocking antihistamine and corticosteroids) fails to control the allergic response, reducing the plasma content of the transfused blood product is another option, either by centrifuging the product and removing almost all the plasma by washing or by transfusing platelets stored in PAS.

In patients with severe anaphylactoid or anaphylactic reactions, antibodies reacting with IgA in donor plasma should be considered.[279] The incidence of genetically determined IgA deficiency in the otherwise normal population is high, ranging from 1 in 400 to 1 in 500.[309] Without necessarily having prior transfusion exposure, approximately 20% to 25% of such patients produce antibodies to IgA, generally class-specific (i.e., reacting with all IgA molecules). Such patients should be transfused, when necessary, with washed red cells[310] or with IgA-deficient blood products. In addition, many patients with normal IgA levels have antibodies that react with some, but not all, IgA molecules; the incidence of such limited-specificity antibodies has been reported at 2% of normal adults.[311] The concentration of such limited-specificity antibodies generally is low, and the resulting reactions are usually milder, but the possibility of a major reaction exists.[289]

Posttransfusion Purpura

Posttransfusion purpura[312,313] is the development of life-threatening thrombocytopenia 5 to 10 days after transfusion. This rare complication is caused by the development of alloantibodies directed against platelet-specific antigens; anti-HPA-1a is often implicated, although antibodies with other specificities have also been reported (Chapter 48). Posttransfusion purpura is thought to occur as a result of a secondary immunologic response to the platelet-specific antigen, most patients having been sensitized by prior pregnancy or transfusion. However, the mechanism of destruction of the patient's own platelets is uncertain. Management includes high-dose IVIG[314]; other therapies such as corticosteroids or plasma exchange are ineffective.

Posttransfusion thrombocytopenia may also be associated with the passive administration of a platelet-specific antibody.[315] Both anti-HPA-1a and anti-HPA-5a have been implicated; these cases can be considered as passive posttransfusion purpura. The resulting thrombocytopenia occurs within hours of the transfusion. It is important to identify the donors of these blood products to prevent further infusion of plasma-containing products from such donors.

Transfusion-Related Immunomodulation

Allogeneic blood transfusion results in the transfer of not only RBCs but also significant amounts of potential immune effector cells, their products (e.g., cytokines), and various substances that may be seen by the host immune system as foreign antigens. A large body of literature exists that substantiates the modulation of host immune systems by transfused allogeneic blood, raising the possibility of the development of clinical syndromes generally referred to as *transfusion-related immunomodulation* (TRIM).[316] Beneficial transfusion-related immunomodulatory effects have been reported in renal transplant patients, women with recurrent spontaneous abortions, and patients with Crohn disease.[317]

A large number of clinical studies have been performed, specifically addressing two potential harmful TRIM-associated effects: cancer recurrence and postoperative bacterial infections. The aim of the studies has been to document TRIM and to ascertain the potential benefit of leukoreduction or use of autologous blood. Despite some reported observations of a transfusion-associated increased risk of cancer recurrence or postoperative infections, many studies include potential confounders or sources of bias. Meta-analyses have concluded that a deleterious clinical effect of transfusion immunomodulation remains controversial.[318,319]

Transfusion-Associated Graft-vs-Host Disease

Most cellular blood products, including red cell, platelet, and granulocyte products, contain viable, immunocompetent T lymphocytes. When transfused into immunocompromised recipients, such as patients undergoing hematopoietic stem cell transplantation and patients with congenital or acquired immunodeficiency and Hodgkin lymphoma, and fetuses, these donor lymphocytes may proliferate in the patient and lead to the clinical syndrome of transfusion-associated GVHD.[320,321] TA-GVHD has also been reported in immunocompetent patients, especially those who receive transfusions from family members or from random donors who share HLA antigens, as is the case when the donor is homozygous for a shared HLA haplotype.[322,323] In fact, a recent international review reported that over half of patients with TA-GVHD were immunocompetent as opposed to the traditional notion that immunocompromised patients are most at risk.[324] In these cases, the recipient does not recognize the donor cells as foreign, allowing the transfused lymphocytes to proliferate and cause TA-GVHD. A higher incidence has been reported in countries such as Japan, whose populations are genetically similar.

Transfusion of leukocyte or platelet concentrates or fresh blood has been responsible for most cases of TA-GVHD. Frozen-thawed plasma products (FFP, cryoprecipitate) have not been definitively associated with TA-GVHD, though fresh, never-frozen plasma (which contains viable lymphocytes) has been implicated.[324] TA-GVHD occurs earlier than that seen after bone marrow transplantation, usually within 1 to 2 weeks, but is otherwise similar.[325] Fever is the most common symptom, followed by a typical erythematous, maculopapular skin rash that begins centrally and spreads peripherally to the hands and feet. Abnormalities of hepatic function, nausea, and bloody diarrhea often occur as the process progresses. Leukopenia followed by pancytopenia because of marrow failure is quite common in TA-GVHD and is seen most often 2 to 3 weeks after the onset of symptoms. The diagnosis is based on the clinical picture and can be confirmed histologically with a skin biopsy. Laboratory confirmation that the GVHD is transfusion induced can be obtained by demonstrating the presence of donor lymphocytes in the patient. This can be done by HLA typing of patient and donor cells by DNA methods for class I and II antigens, by cytogenetic analysis, or by analysis of DNA microsatellite polymorphisms or variable number tandem repeats. Severe systemic infections are the most common cause of death, which often occurs within 3 to 4 weeks from the time of the implicated transfusion. Despite aggressive treatment, the fatality rate in TA-GVHD is significantly higher than that associated with bone marrow transplantation and has been reported to be >90%.[324,325]

Corticosteroids, antithymocyte globulin, cyclosporine, growth factors, and stem cell transplant have all been used with minimal success in the treatment of TA-GVHD. Rather, the focus has been on the prevention of TA-GVHD by pretransfusion irradiation of all cellular blood products administered to patients at risk. Irradiation inhibits proliferation of donor lymphocytes, with little significant adverse effect on red cell, platelet, or granulocyte function. Although data from Serious Hazards of Transfusion (SHOT) have indicated a reduction in cases of TA-GVHD since universal leukoreduction of blood components was implemented in the United Kingdom,[326] leukoreduction alone is insufficient to prevent TA-GVHD.[324]

Based primarily on case reports and reviews, a number of immunosuppressed and immunocompetent patient groups can be stratified according to risk for developing TA-GVHD[325] (*Table 23.10*).

Nonimmunologic Adverse Effects of Blood Transfusion
Transfusion-Associated Circulatory Overload

Transfusion of red cell preparations or plasma products may result in transfusion-associated circulatory load (TACO) in 1% to 8% of transfusions.[247,327] It is the number one cause of mortality and major morbidity in reports from SHOT and the FDA.[293,326] Risk factors include older age or infanthood, renal failure, preexisting fluid overload, cardiac dysfunction, and rapid administration of large volumes of blood components. Diagnostic criteria include symptom onset within 1 to 2 hours of transfusion, increased central venous pressure, left heart failure, positive fluid balance, pulmonary edema, raised brain natriuretic peptide, and widened cardiothoracic ratio on chest radiograph.[1,279]

Treatment of TACO involves stopping the transfusion and administering oxygen and diuretics, which may be both therapeutic and diagnostic. Prevention of TACO is preferable by identifying patients at risk, giving small volumes of transfusions slowly, and careful monitoring of patients.[279]

Massive Transfusion

Clinical effects associated with massive transfusion are multifactorial and associated with patient factors such as the causative event itself, for example, trauma and shock, and with factors associated with transfusion of large volumes of stored donor blood.[279]

Metabolic Effects and Hypothermia

Stored blood differs in its composition from that circulating in the body. The elevated K^+ content in the supernatant surrounding stored red cells rarely leads to hyperkalemia, but it is a risk in massive transfusion of infants, or in patients with renal failure. It can lead to cardiac complications and can be detected by measurement of the potassium and electrocardiogram changes. Longer storage of blood and irradiation are risk factors. Transfusion-associated hyperkalemia has been frequently associated with rapid transfusion of large volumes of blood to neonates, which can be minimized by the use of fresh RBC units irradiated at the time of issue for large-volume transfusions.

Plasma contains a significant amount of citrate as anticoagulant; recipients with normal circulatory status promptly metabolize this in the liver, but during plasma exchange or in patients in shock or severe liver failure, citrate excess may lead to hypocalcemia and result in changes in cardiac function. Hypocalcemic reactions caused by citrate may be treated by intravenous calcium infusion.

Hypothermia may occur if a large volume of cold blood is infused rapidly. Hypothermia is one of the most common complications of massive transfusion and contributes to the associated coagulopathy. Blood-warming devices are available that can adequately warm the

Table 23.10. Patients at Increased Risk for Transfusion-Associated Graft-vs-Host Disease

High Risk
Stem cell transplant (allogeneic and autologous)
Intrauterine transfusions
Granulocyte transfusions
Transfusions from blood relatives
Congenital immunodeficiencies
Hodgkin disease
Moderate Risk
Hematologic malignancy (acute myelogenous leukemia/acute lymphocytic leukemia/non-Hodgkin lymphoma, multiple myeloma)
Patients treated with purine-analog drugs (e.g., chronic lymphocytic leukemia)
Malignancies treated with intensive chemo-/radiotherapy (i.e., neuroblastoma, sarcoma)
Solid-organ transplant recipients
Preterm infants
Newborns receiving exchange transfusion
Low/Theoretical Risk
Human immunodeficiency virus/acquired immunodeficiency syndrome
Healthy term newborns

Modified from Schroeder ML. Transfusion-associated graft-versus-host disease. *Br J Haematol.* 2002;117:275-287. Copyright © 2002 Blackwell Science Ltd. Reprinted by permission of John Wiley & Sons, Inc.

blood administered, even during a rapid and massive transfusion. All patients who are receiving large amounts of red cells and plasma should have those products administered through blood-warming devices. Blood warmers must be checked regularly to ensure that they maintain their temperature. If the blood is overheated, hemolysis and the associated complications of transfusing hemolyzed blood may result.

Any one of these potential problems alone is rarely significant. However, in the critically ill patient who requires massive transfusion, acidosis, hypoxemia, hypothermia, hypocalcemia, and hypo- or hyperkalemia often coexist, with a consequent risk of cardiac arrhythmias. Neonates receiving exchange transfusions are particularly susceptible to such physical and metabolic effects.[57,328]

Massively transfused patients are often affected by sepsis, shock, and intravascular coagulation, which may aggravate the dilutional hemostatic defects. Transfusion therapy of such patients is best guided by laboratory measurements, but clinical assessment is most important because conventional coagulation tests take time to obtain. As discussed earlier in this chapter in the section "Red Cell Transfusion in Specific Settings: Trauma," for patients undergoing rapid massive transfusion, the first line of treatment (with regard to hemostatic blood products) should include plasma to correct the levels of coagulation factors, as well as platelet products.[143,145,146,151,153,329]

Iron Overload: Transfusion Hemosiderosis

Iron overload is a major problem in patients who require long-term red cell transfusion support for chronic anemias because of bone marrow failure or chronic hemolysis. Each unit of red cells contains approximately 0.20 g of iron. After a large number of red cell transfusions, in the absence of blood loss, the recipient develops the stigmata of transfusion hemosiderosis: impaired growth, failure of sexual maturation, myocardial and hepatic dysfunction, hyperpigmentation, and, often, diabetes. Patients such as those with thalassemia or sickle cell anemia who are at risk of this complication should receive prophylactic aggressive iron chelation therapy.

INFECTIOUS COMPLICATIONS OF BLOOD TRANSFUSION

Overview of Blood Donor Screening for Infectious Diseases

Over the past 30 years, there have been significant advances in the safety of the blood supply, as demonstrated by decreased rates of the major viral infectious disease risks (*Table 23.11*). This has resulted from improved donor selection/deferral policies, advances in donor testing, and broad improvements in public health care.[330] Consequently, transfusions are safer now than ever before from an infectious disease standpoint.

A number of conditions must be met for an infectious disease to be transmitted by blood transfusion. The disease must have an asymptomatic phase during which it is present in the donor blood, survive component processing and storage, be infective via an intravenous route, and be able to manifest a disease in a susceptible patient population. A variety of different infectious disease agents have been identified that may be transmitted through blood. For some of these agents, donor testing is required on each and every donation, whereas for others, testing may be performed on only a subset of donations or may not be performed at all. In the absence of donor testing, screening questions may exist to defer donors with a risk of infection. The infections discussed in this chapter represent some of the most important transfusion-related infectious disease risks.

Testing Strategy

Current donor testing relies upon serologic, antigen, or NAT technologies. These are selected based upon the characteristics of the individual infectious disease risk (e.g., chronic or self-limited infections) and the performance of the individual tests (i.e., sensitivity and specificity). For logistic and cost reasons, many of the viral NATs are performed on pooled samples from 6 to 16 donors using automated methods. If a pool is positive, further testing is done to identify the individual donor of the positive result. All donor screening tests have a "window period" after donor exposure when the infectious agent may circulate in the blood but be below the limit of detection by the test method. Advances in testing technology have progressively decreased the window period for donor testing significantly, contributing to transfusion safety. Several infectious agents (i.e., HBV, HCV, HIV) are additionally subject to multiple redundant tests which reduces the overall risk that may be associated with an individual test failure, which is very rare.

Residual Risks of Infection

Table 23.2 lists the tests currently performed on volunteer blood donations in the United States. It is thought that the residual risk of transmitting HIV and hepatitis by transfusion is related mainly to window period donations. The probability that a donation was made during the window period can be calculated from the observed incidence of new infections in blood donors and the length of the window period.[59,331] The implementation of NAT for HIV, HCV, and HBV has permitted direct detection of donors with newly acquired infections (i.e., donors who are NAT positive, antibody negative). New HIV, HCV, and HBV infections in repeat blood donors are very rare. However, studies indicate that first-time donors are two to three times more likely than repeat donors to have newly acquired infection.[59] Thus, current estimates of transfusion risk include an adjustment for a two- to threefold higher probability that a first-time donor is in the window period compared with a repeat donor.[331-333] *Table 23.11* shows the current risk estimates for transfusion-transmitted HIV, HCV, and HBV based on the length of the window period and the estimated frequency of window period donations.

Because the current risks of transmitting HIV, HCV, and HBV are low, the absolute benefit gained from further incremental improvements in blood donor testing for these infections would be very small. The implementation of individual-unit NAT for HIV, HCV, and HBV, for example, would be associated with extremely high cost, with very little incremental improvement in blood safety in the United States.[334]

Transfusion-Associated Hepatitis

Before the development of serologic tests capable of determining the cause of transfusion-associated hepatitis (TAH), all TAH infections were thought to be owing to hepatitis B (the "serum hepatitis" agent). After the HBsAg test became available, however, it was discovered that hepatitis B accounted for only about 25% to 30% of TAH cases.[335] Subsequent studies excluded HAV, CMV, and the Epstein-Barr virus as common causes of TAH. The designation non-A, non-B (NANB) hepatitis was created to describe the majority of TAH cases.[336] In 1989, the major causative agent of NANB hepatitis was identified as HCV.[337,338] Widespread testing of all blood donations for this virus was implemented in 1990. An improved test for hepatitis C became available in 1992. Since NAT, TAH has become rare (*Table 23.11*).

Hepatitis B

Donor screening for HBV includes detection of the virus through NAT (HBV DNA), antigen testing (HBsAg), and testing for antibodies against the hepatitis B core antigen (anti-HBc). The HBV pooled NAT window period is estimated to be 21.2 to 29.2 days, an 8.8-day reduction from HBsAg testing.[339] The residual risk of HBV transmission by blood is now estimated to be 1 per 765,000 to 1 per 1,006,000 transfusions (*Table 23.11*).[332]

Hepatitis C

Donor screening for HCV includes NAT for HCV RNA as well as HCV antibody testing. It is estimated that the donor RNA test detects infection an average of 7.4 days after exposure. Based on the window period/incidence modeling, the risk of HCV transmission by transfusion of blood products is now estimated to be approximately 1 in 1,149,000 (*Table 23.11*).[332]

Hepatitis A Virus

Transfusion-related transmission of HAV by transfusable blood products is rare.[340] However, transmission of HAV has been associated with pooled plasma products.[341] Because HAV is not lipid enveloped, infectivity is not eliminated by solvent/detergent treatment. Therefore, immunization to HAV is recommended for patients who are expected to receive pooled plasma products, such as patients with clotting disorders.[341] The FDA does not require donor screening for this agent; however, some plasma-derivative manufacturers test plasma pools for HAV nucleic acid in an effort to reduce the risk of transmitting this agent. In addition, during a common source outbreak of HAV, blood collection facilities may elicit information and defer donors who report possible exposure.

Human Immunodeficiency Virus Type 1 and Type 2

Current donor screening for HIV includes NAT for HIV-1 RNA and testing for antibodies to HIV-1 and HIV-2. The window period for HIV, based on time to detection of RNA via minipool nucleic acid screening, is currently estimated at 9 days.[332] The current estimated risk of HIV transmission by transfusion is approximately 1:1,467,000 U (*Table 23.11*). Donor questioning regarding HIV risk behavior and the temporary exclusion of individuals at increased risk of being in the HIV window period are critical and essential elements of this safety level.[1] Whether certain deferral periods could be shortened without compromising blood transfusion safety has been the topic of intense public discussion.[342] In April 2020, the FDA recommended that the deferral period related to HIV risk factors, such as men who have sex with men (MSM), can be decreased from 12 months (or indefinite deferrals for some risk factors) to 3 months.[343]

Infections Transmitted by Arthropods

Over the past 2 decades, significant attention has been focused on infectious agents that can be transmitted to donors by insects and

Table 23.11. Transfusion-Associated Adverse Events

I. Infectious Agents

Transfusion-transmitted disease routinely tested	
Hepatitis B virus (1970 [surface antigen]; 1986-1987 [core antibody]; 2009 [Nucleic Acid])	1:765,000-1:1,106,000
Human immunodeficiency virus (1985 [antibody]; 2000 [nucleic acid])	1:1,467,000
Hepatitis C virus (1986-1987 [alanine aminotransferase]; 1990 [antibody]; 1999 [nucleic acid])	1:1,149,000
Human T-cell lymphotropic virus (1988 [antibody])	Very rare
West Nile virus (2003 [nucleic acid])	Very rare
Bacteria (in platelets only; 2004)	1:20,000
Trypanosoma cruzi (2007 [antibody])	Very rare
Syphilis	Very rare
Cytomegalovirus (for patients at risk)	Rare
Transfusion-transmitted disease not currently, routinely tested	Very rare or unknown
Hepatitis A virus	
Parvovirus B19	
Dengue fever virus	
Malaria	
Hepatitis E	
Babesia sp.	
Plasmodium sp.	
Leishmania sp.	
Brucella sp.	
New variant Creutzfeldt-Jakob disease prions	
Zika virus	
Unknown pathogens	

II. Transfusion-Associated Adverse Reaction Events

Estimated risk per unit infused

ABO incompatible blood transfusions	1 in 60,000
Symptoms	40%
Fatalities	1 in 600,000
Delayed serologic reactions	1 in 1600
Delayed hemolytic reactions	1 in 6700
Transfusion-related acute lung injury	1 in 20,000
Graft-vs-host disease	Very rare
Posttransfusion purpura	Very rare
Febrile, nonhemolytic transfusion reactions	
Red blood cells	1 in 200
Platelets	1 in 5-20
Allergic reactions	1 in 30-100
Transfusion-associated circulatory overload	1 in 12
Anaphylactic reactions (IgA deficiency)	1 in 150,000
Iron overload	Estimated 80-100 U for adults
Transfusion-related immunosuppression	Unestablished
Storage lesions	Unestablished

Modified from Goodnough LT. Blood management: transfusion medicine comes of age. *Lancet*. 2013;381:1791-1792; Stramer SL, Notari EP, Krysztof DE, Dodd RY. Hepatitis B virus testing by minipool nucleic acid testing: does it improve blood safety? *Transfusion*. 2013;53:2449-2458; Zou S, Dorsey KA, Notari, EP et al. Prevalence, incidence, and residual risk of human immunodeficiency virus and hepatitis C virus infections among United States blood donors since the introduction of nucleic acid testing. *Transfusion*. 2010;50:1495-1504.

further transmitted to patients via transfusion. This category of pathogens includes WNV, *Trypanosoma cruzi* (*T. cruzi*), *Babesia*, malaria, ZIKV, and other potential emerging infections.

West Nile Virus

WNV is a *Flavivirus* maintained in nature in a mosquito-bird-mosquito transmission cycle. *Culex* mosquitoes are generally considered the principal vectors of WNV. Humans are "dead-end" hosts, meaning that once they become infected, they do not spread the infection. WNV was first detected in the United States in 1999 and has since spread through the North American continent in annual epidemics. Eighty percent of infected individuals are asymptomatic, 20% have a relatively nonspecific febrile illness, and <1% develop neuroinvasive disease (meningitis, encephalitis, or flaccid paralysis), which can lead to chronic disability or death.

WNV was first demonstrated to be transmissible by transfusion in 2002, when infection in 23 recipients was linked to blood components later found to contain WNV RNA but no WNV antibody.[344] In 2003, minipool NAT screening of blood donations for WNV RNA was implemented throughout the United States using investigational assays. WNV NAT assays are now FDA licensed. WNV transmissions despite minipool donor testing led to the discovery that 20% to 30% of donors with WNV infection may be missed by minipool testing because of low levels of circulating virus.[345] Therefore, at times of high WNV activity, donor WNV RNA screening must be performed on individual donations.

Zika Virus

ZIKV is also a *Flavivirus*; however, unlike WNV, it does not currently have a known natural nonhuman primate animal reservoir that can serve as an amplifying host. Instead, ZIKV is primarily transmitted through a mosquito-human-mosquito transmission cycle. The *Aedes aegypti* mosquito is thought to be the principal vector of ZIKV, and it also may be transmitted by *Aedes albopictus*. Sexual transmission of ZIKV has also been reported. ZIKV infection is asymptomatic in approximately 80% of individuals; however, infection during pregnancy is a cause of microcephaly, miscarriage/stillbirth, and other significant developmental abnormalities.[346] ZIKV infection has also been associated with increased incidence of Guillain-Barré syndrome.

In 2015 to 2016, an explosive ZIKV epidemic expanded from Brazil to involve most of the Americas. During this time period, four cases of transfusion-transmitted ZIKV were identified in Brazil. In July 2016, the first cases of local transmission of ZIKV occurring in the continental United States were reported from southern Florida. The FDA, shortly thereafter, recommended universal donor testing for ZIKV using an investigational individual donor nucleic acid test (ID-NAT).[347] In 2018, the FDA updated their recommendation to allow minipool testing for ZIKV with conversion to individual donations testing when there was evidence of local mosquito-borne transmission. However, in May 2021, the FDA determined that ZIKV no longer had sufficient incidence or prevalence in the US donor population and allowed blood collection facilities to discontinue testing for ZIKV. ZIKV epidemiology in the United States will continue to be monitored, and if needed, ZIKV donor screening may be reinstated.[348]

Malaria

Malaria is a common infection globally. Transfusion-transmitted malaria is rare in the United States with zero to three cases reported yearly.[349] This degree of safety is remarkable considering that screening is accomplished entirely by donor questioning, rather than testing. According to current FDA guidelines, individuals are deferred from blood donation for 3 months after travel to a malaria-endemic area and for 3 years after living in a malaria-endemic area.[350] Of the donors implicated in the cases of transfusion-transmitted malaria in the United States, approximately 60% (including the majority of *Plasmodium falciparum* infections) should have been excluded by donor deferral criteria. The remaining cases are largely related to chronic asymptomatic infections in donors who are beyond the deferral period.[349]

Babesiosis

Babesiosis is caused by a protozoan parasite that infects human RBCs. It is transmitted by the *Ixodes* tick, the same vector that transmits the causative agents of Lyme disease. The majority of US *Babesia* cases are caused by *Babesia microti*, which is endemic to the Northeast and upper Midwest. Less commonly infections are caused by *Babesia duncani* mainly in Western states, and babesiosis caused by a *Babesia divergens*-like organism has been reported in multiple states.

Incubation ranges from 1 to 6 weeks or longer. Symptoms range from none to mild flulike to a malaria-type illness with hemolytic anemia. The parasitemic period is reported to last from 2 to 7 months but may persist for more than 2 years.[351,352] Although *Babesia* transmission is seasonal and coincides with tick activity (typically May-September), tick-borne and transfusion-transmitted infections are reported year-round. Since 1980, more than 200 transfusion-transmitted *Babesia* (TTB) cases have been reported.[353,354] The majority of TTB cases are associated with *Babesia microti*, but three reported cases have been caused by *Babesia duncani* and 1 possible case from *Babesia divergens*. RBC transfusions are most commonly implicated but a few cases have been reported with platelet transfusion. Symptoms in transfusion recipients usually occur 1 to 9 weeks (and as long as 6 months) after transfusion, and asplenic, immunocompromised, elderly, and neonatal patients are at increased risk for severe infection.

Approximately 95% of TTB cases are reported from 14 US states and Washington, D.C., and since 2019, based on FDA recommendations, blood donations collected in these high-risk regions have been tested for *Babesia microti* by a licensed nucleic acid test.[354] Donors with a positive test are deferred for at least 2 years. Approved pathogen reduction technology effective against *Babesia* can also be used as an alternative to testing to mitigate the risk of TTB.

Trypanosoma cruzi

T. cruzi, the protozoan parasite that causes Chagas disease, is endemic to portions of Mexico, Central America, and South America. It is transmitted to humans by the reduviid bug. Acute infection is usually self limited, although rarely it may involve myocarditis or meningoencephalitis and may be fatal, particularly in immunocompromised patients. In most cases, however, the acute infection goes undiagnosed, and the infection becomes chronic. After decades, 20% to 30% of chronically infected individuals develop cardiac or intestinal dysfunction that can be fatal. The transmission of *T. cruzi* by transfusion is well documented in endemic areas.[355] A blood donor screening assay for *T. cruzi* antibody became available in the United States in 2007. The vast majority of the infected donors detected have been immigrants from endemic areas; US-acquired *T. cruzi* appears to be rare. Therefore, in 2010, the FDA endorsed a strategy of testing each US donor only once for this infection.[14] Only five cases of transfusion-transmitted *T. cruzi* were reported in the United States between 1987 and 2011, and recipient tracing after implementation of routine donor testing has identified another two definite and one possible case.[356] All have involved the transfusion of a platelet component and have predominantly involved highly immunocompromised recipients.

Transmissible Spongiform Encephalopathies: Creutzfeldt-Jakob Disease and Variant Creutzfeldt-Jakob Disease

Both classical Creutzfeldt-Jakob disease (CJD) and variant Creutzfeldt-Jakob disease (vCJD) are rapidly progressive fatal infections of the nervous system caused by prions. Individuals at increased risk for classic CJD are currently excluded from blood donation in the United States, despite evidence that this disease is not transmissible by transfusion.

In contrast, vCJD does appear to be transmissible by transfusion. Human vCJD is caused by the same prion that causes bovine spongiform encephalopathy (BSE), or "mad cow disease." As of April 2012, four cases of apparent transfusion-transmitted vCJD had been identified in the United Kingdom, where a BSE epidemic occurred between 1980 and 1996. In addition, one case of vCJD had been identified postmortem in a hemophilia patient in the United Kingdom who died

of other causes. Worldwide, steps have been taken in an effort to minimize the risk of vCJD transmission by blood products in the absence of a donor screening test for the infection. In the United States, individuals are currently excluded from donating blood if they lived in the United Kingdom for 3 months or more between 1980 and 1996, if they lived in France or Ireland for 5 years or more between 1980 and 2001, or if they have received a transfusion in the United Kingdom, France, or Ireland since 1980.[357] Because prions lack lipid coats and nucleic acid, the causative agent of vCJD or CJD would not be inactivated by any of the pathogen-inactivation processes currently in use or under development.

Potential Emerging Infections

The emergence of new or novel pathogens that could impact the blood supply has proven to be unpredictable. With the expansion of global travel and trade, continued close evaluation of nonendemic pathogens that could impact the US blood supply is essential. This requires up-to-date epidemiologic data and should be evaluated in a risk-based decision framework based on the National AABB Hemovigilance Database. This analysis is available online and is updated periodically. The goal of these evaluations is to develop a systematic approach to risk assessment and provide timely education and recommendations toward possible mitigation interventions. Over 70 emerging infectious disease agents with the potential to impact blood safety have been identified to date. For each infectious agent, a supplemental fact sheet is maintained that provides background information on the disease along with information on the priority level, likelihood of blood transmission, potential impact on blood safety, possible safety measures, and other general disease characteristics.[358,359] Example agents that have been included in this analysis include ZIKV, chikungunya virus, dengue virus, hepatitis E virus, and yellow fever virus. If an emerging disease is deemed to be a relevant transfusion transmitted infection, FDA provides recommendations to mitigate risk and maintain blood safety, such as additional donor history questions and/or testing.

COVID-19

In December 2019, a novel coronavirus (SARS-CoV-2) was discovered in Wuhan, China and since then has quickly spread resulting in a global pandemic. COVID-19 is the infection caused by SARS-CoV-2 and although the majority of people infected are asymptomatic or have mild symptoms, COVID-19 can cause severe respiratory illness and death. As of this writing, there have been over 340 million cases reported in the United States with approximately 610,000 deaths.[360] With regard to blood safety, respiratory viruses are not known to be transfusion transmitted, and there have been no reported cases of transfusion-transmitted SARS-CoV-2 worldwide. Nevertheless, to ensure blood safety and also the safety of donors and blood center staff, the FDA has recommended that individuals diagnosed with COVID-19 should wait 14 days after symptom resolution (or after a positive test if asymptomatic) before donating blood. However, screening blood donors with a COVID-19 test is not recommended. Donors who have been vaccinated with a nonreplicating, inactivated, or mRNA-based vaccine (which currently includes all vaccines being administered in the United States) are eligible.[361]

Notably early in the pandemic, COVID-19 convalescent plasma (CCP) was introduced as an investigational passive antibody therapy for SARS-CoV-2 infection. CCP is collected from donors who have recovered from a confirmed COVID-19 infection and are symptom free for at least 14 days, have evidence of high-titer antibodies against SARS-CoV-2 using an FDA-approved assay, and meet all other criteria for blood donation.[362] Data from an expanded access protocol (more than 90,000 units transfused in the United States) indicate that CCP transfusion is safe.[363] Although there are still questions regarding CCP's efficacy, since some clinical trials did not show benefit, based on the available data, the FDA has provided Emergency Use Authorization (EUA) for use of high-titer CCP in hospitalized patients with COVID-19 early in their disease course or with impaired humoral immunity.[364-368] Studies have shown that transfusion of CCP in patients with moderate-to-severe disease (e.g., respiratory failure requiring mechanical ventilation) is not associated with clinical benefit.[369,370] However, one study showed that transfusion of high-titer CCP in older patients with mild disease and within 72 hours of symptom onset reduced the risk of progression to severe respiratory disease.[371] At this time, outpatient transfusion of CCP is not included under the current EUA, but CCP can be administered in this setting in a clinical trial. Numerous clinical trials with CCP are still underway, and findings from these studies might help to resolve some of the uncertainties around this investigational treatment.

Bacterial Contamination

Bacterial contamination of blood components is the most prevalent transfusion-associated infectious risk in North America and Europe. This is in part owing to the significant safety gains seen with implementation of sophisticated viral infectious disease screening and the continued limitations of current bacterial testing and mitigation strategies. The consequence of transfusing bacterially contaminated blood ranges in severity from being clinically asymptomatic to resulting in a self-limited infection, fulminant septic shock, or even death. A total of 20 fatalities attributed to blood products contaminated with bacteria were reported to the FDA from 2015 to 2019, representing 10% of reported transfusion-related deaths.[293]

Platelet components are at highest risk of bacterial contamination and proliferation due to room temperature storage, while contamination of refrigerated RBCs and frozen plasma products is uncommon. However, certain organisms such as *Yersinia enterocolitica* proliferate in red cells at storage temperatures of 1 °C to 6 °C. Potential sources of bacteria include asymptomatic donor bacteremia, bacteria from the donor's skin, and, rarely, environmental contamination.

Prevention

Recognition of morbidity and mortality from transfusion of bacterially contaminated platelets has prompted the FDA and AABB to implement specific mitigation measures related to the collection and testing of these components. Bacteria in the deeper layers of skin cannot be addressed by surface disinfectants; thus, a diversion pouch is required for any collections intended to prepare a platelet product.[2] In this system, the first few milliliters of donor blood that may contain bacteria from the phlebotomy skin plug are diverted into a sample pouch to reduce contamination of the final component. Since 2004, the AABB has also required bacterial testing of platelet components. The quantity of bacteria in blood components just after collection is too low to detect by current diagnostic assays; therefore, there is a 24-hour hold after collection to allow potentially contaminating bacteria to multiply to detectable levels. Then, a sample is taken from each product and inoculated into a blood culture bottle. If the culture is negative after at least 12 hours, the product can be released for transfusion, but the culture is continued for the shelf life of the unit.[372]

About 1 in 5000 apheresis platelets are found by bacterial culture screening to be bacterially contaminated.[373] This screening process is imperfect, however, and fails to detect more than 50% of bacterially contaminated platelets.[374] The residual risk of contamination per transfused unit on the day of transfusion is estimated to be 1 in 2500.[375] Despite this limitation, reported rates of septic transfusion reactions and patient fatalities have significantly decreased after implementation of primary platelet culture testing.[293,376] This is presumably owing to culture testing's ability to detect high bacterial contamination most concerning for severe, life-threatening reactions.[377]

An additional bacterial mitigation strategy involves the use of a rapid bacterial detection test performed on the platelet unit typically in the hospital just prior to transfusion. Two rapid diagnostic tests are currently approved for this use to detect contaminated units missed by primary culture methods. Utilization of one of these methods was reported to find bacteria in approximately 1 in 3000 apheresis platelets that had been negative on their culture screen.[378] These alternative tests are associated with false positives and logistical challenges, however, and still fail to detect some contaminated products.[379]

Given the residual risk that remains for bacterial contamination of platelets, the FDA has released a series of additional mitigation recommendations set to implement by October 2021. Surveillance data on platelets stored up to 5 days have shown that 95% to 100% of septic reactions related to platelets have occurred with transfusion of day 4 and day 5 stored platelets. Thus, for a 5 day platelet after the primary culture is performed at 24 hours, the FDA recommends that either a secondary culture is performed no earlier than day 3 or the platelet is tested with a rapid test prior to transfusion. Alternatively, a larger sample can be taken for the primary culture after at least 36 hours of incubation to increase sensitivity. The FDA has also provided options to extend the shelf life of the platelet to 7 days, for example if the large volume sampling for primary culture is performed after at least 48 hours of incubation. Finally, treating platelets with an approved pathogen reduction technology is an acceptable alternative to bacterial cultures. These strategies will decrease the residual risk of bacterial contamination in platelets and increase blood safety.[372]

Septic Transfusion Reactions

Septic transfusion reactions are far less common than the rates of bacterial contamination previously described. This may be owing to a variety of factors including insufficient inoculums to cause clinical manifestations, contamination with nonpathogenic species, bacterial death or inhibition during refrigerated storage, and the patient already being on antibiotic medication. For clinically apparent reactions, bacterial infections are reported to occur in at least 1:75,000 platelet transfusions and at least 1:500,000 red cell transfusions.[380] It has been suggested, however, that septic transfusion reactions are underrecognized and that the patient risk is 10- to 40-fold higher than what passive hemovigilance incidence data suggest.[375]

Possible clinical manifestations of transfusion-transmitted bacterial infections include a fever ≥38 °C (100.4 °F) with a rise ≥1 °C (1.8 °F), chills, rigors, tachycardia, dyspnea, hypotension, nausea/vomiting, and shock. The vast majority of septic transfusion reactions become symptomatic during or within 4 hours after completion of the transfusion. However, more delayed reactions may be seen depending upon the specific bacterial contaminant and the underlying patient clinical condition. In general, contamination with gram-negative bacteria results in a more rapid appearance of symptoms because of high levels of endotoxins that may build up in the component during storage.

If a septic transfusion reaction is suspected, the transfusion should be immediately stopped and supportive therapy should be provided. Patient blood cultures should be performed prior to initiation of antibiotic therapy and the blood product or products should be returned to the transfusion service. The transfusion service may perform a Gram stain and culture on the returned component per facility policies. A definitive diagnosis of transfusion-transmitted bacterial infection requires identification of the same organism from the blood product and patient, but can be presumed in a culture-negative patient with clinical sepsis if bacteria are isolated from the transfused unit.[381]

Cytomegalovirus

CMV is a DNA virus in the herpesvirus family.[382] Like other herpesviruses, it remains latent after acute infection, with the potential for reactivation.[383] In immunologically normal adults, CMV disease manifestations range from none to a mononucleosis-like syndrome. In immunosuppressed or immunodeficient patients, however, both primary CMV and CMV reactivation may be associated with significant clinical manifestations including thrombocytopenia, hemolytic anemia, pneumonitis, colitis, hepatitis, meningoencephalitis, and even death. The incidence of severe disease can be reduced by prophylactic treatment of high-risk patients with antiviral drugs or by careful monitoring/screening of such patients and initiation of therapy with the first evidence of infection.[382] At least 60% of the US population has been exposed to CMV with a seroprevalence of 90% in those aged >80 years.[384]

WBCs of the monocyte lineage are the most likely to carry latent CMV in the blood of previously infected donors. CMV, therefore, may be transmitted through the transfusion of cellular blood components (i.e., RBCs, platelets, liquid never-frozen plasma). The incidence of transmission of CMV by transfusion appears to be low

(<1%) in immunologically normal recipients.[385] Immunodeficient patients, however, are at increased risk of acquiring CMV from transfusion. CMV transmission to these patients can be greatly reduced by restricting their cellular components to products obtained from CMV-seronegative donors or by use of leukoreduced blood components.[382]

Most studies have detected no transmission of CMV by leukoreduced blood components. Some transmissions were detected, however, in a large randomized study that evaluated the incidence of CMV infection and CMV disease in 502 bone marrow transplant recipients randomized to receive either leukoreduced (i.e., leukofiltered) or CMV antibody–negative blood components.[386] CMV infection was observed in 1.3% of recipients of seronegative components and in 2.4% of recipients of leukoreduced components, a difference that was not statistically significant. However, in the leukoreduced arm, all CMV-infected patients developed disease, and five out of six died; in the serologically screened arm, there were no cases of CMV-related disease or death. A meta-analysis estimated that the risk of transfusion-transmitted CMV is approximately 1.5% with use of CMV antibody–screened components, compared to 2.5% with leukoreduced, antibody-unscreened, components.[387] Most of the cellular components in the United States are leukoreduced. Whether it is clinically beneficial to perform CMV antibody screening in addition to leukoreduction remains controversial.[382]

It is generally recommended that cellular products with a reduced risk of transmitting CMV (leukoreduced or CMV antibody negative) be used for patients at increased risk of severe primary CMV disease, including unborn babies (i.e., intrauterine transfusion), low-birth-weight infants of seronegative mothers, seronegative recipients of seronegative solid-organ or hematopoietic stem cell transplants, and seronegative patients with severe cellular immunodeficiency (e.g., severe combined immunodeficiency patients). Products with reduced CMV risk also are often provided for seronegative patients who are likely to require transplantation in the future, to reduce their future risk of CMV-reactivation disease.[382]

There is no clinical benefit of providing products of reduced CMV risk to patients who are already seropositive. Although second-strain infections may occur, these have not been shown to be clinically important, given the high risk of reactivation disease these patients face. In CMV-positive recipients of allogeneic hematopoietic stem cell transplants, the use of CMV-positive stem cell donors has no detectable adverse effect on patient outcomes.[388] Therefore, it seems that CMV-seropositive blood components would also be acceptable in this setting.

Seronegative recipients of seropositive organ and stem cell transplants are at high risk of CMV disease[389] and are likely to be monitored closely, treated prophylactically, or both. It is unclear whether providing blood products with reduced CMV risk to such patients is of clinical benefit.

Pathogen-Reduction Technologies

Donor screening and testing cannot completely eliminate the possibility of transfusion-transmitted infection or blood-product contamination. Additionally, there exists a period of time after a new or emerging infectious disease threat has been identified until screening or testing can be implemented to protect the blood supply. Pathogen reduction of blood components represents a proactive means to address these limitations and prevent transfusion-transmitted disease. In principle, pathogen-reduction technology (PRT) has the potential to broadly reduce or eliminate infectious disease risk without the need to screen for or test specific pathogens.

The ideal PRT would effectively inactivate residual pathogens without adversely affecting the function, toxicity, or immunogenicity of the blood component. The two major approaches to pathogen inactivation involve methods to disrupt viral lipid envelopes and methods to damage nucleic acids and prevent pathogen replication. Early PRT focused on plasma components, as these do not contain cells that may be disrupted by a harsh inactivation preprocess. Most commercial plasma derivatives are treated with heat or organic S/D. S/D treatment inactivates lipid-coated agents. Cellular blood components, however, cannot withstand this treatment.

Most PRTs for cellular products consist of blood product additives that bind to and damage DNA or RNA and thereby prevent residual pathogens from proliferating in the blood component or in the recipient. This method is especially appealing for cellular blood components because RBCs and platelets lack nuclei and do not require functional nucleic acids. Inactivation of nucleic acids in the lymphocytes of a blood product is an additional PRT benefit because this is able to prevent WBC replication and TA-GVHD. The efficacy of PRT is dependent on the technology used and characteristics of individual specific infectious disease agents. In general, current technologies are able to result in at least a 4 to 5 log reduction of pathogens in model testing.[390] Because of concern that nucleic acid–altering agents could cause long-term toxicity in transfusion recipients, many of the PRT systems include processes that remove the DNA-binding agent or inactivate it.

PRTs can reduce the residual risk related to window period transmissions of HIV, HCV, and HBV, but these residual risks are small. The primary benefit of PRTs, therefore, is to reduce transmission of agents for which there are currently no tests.[391] Pathogen reduction treatments are costly; however, incremental costs of PRT can be offset if they are approved by regulators as eliminating the need for irradiation, CMV antibody screening, and bacterial testing. Elimination of platelet bacterial testing would also expedite release of these products.

As of summer 2021, PRT currently available in the United States includes a pooled S/D plasma derivative and PRT treatments of platelets, individual transfusable plasma components, and cryoprecipitate. Examples of pathogen reduction technologies are listed in *Table 23.12*.[392] PRT platelet treatments appear to be associated with some loss of platelet product potency.[393,394] Additional work continues on the development of PRT for treatment of whole blood and RBCs.

THERAPEUTIC APHERESIS

Therapeutic apheresis is an important modality of therapy in the management of a number of diseases. The term *plasmapheresis* refers to the selective removal of plasma. This includes the collection of plasma from normal donors. A *TPE*, on the other hand, refers to the removal of a large proportion of a patient's plasma and replacement with crystalloid or colloid fluids or plasma product. These terms are often used interchangeably. Therapeutic cytapheresis, the removal of red cells, leukocytes, or platelets, is used in the management of patients with hemoglobinopathies, leukostasis, or thrombocytosis, respectively.

Guidelines for clinical practice have been developed by the American Society for Apheresis and are regularly updated every 3 to 7 years with a systematic review of the medical literature. The current guidelines published in 2019[395] review the therapeutic apheresis procedures most commonly performed, that is, TPE, RBC exchange, erythrocytapheresis, thrombocytapheresis, leukocytapheresis, extracorporeal photopheresis, immunoadsorption, selective removal methods, adsorptive cytapheresis, and membrane differential filtration. Additionally, the guidelines contain 84 specific disease fact sheets listing the type of apheresis procedure indicated and the rationale for it, the recommended blood volume to be exchanged, and the duration of the treatment.

The disorders for which therapeutic apheresis has been used are divided into four categories: category I, for which apheresis is the accepted first line of therapy; category II, for which apheresis is considered a second-line therapy, after a patient has failed or is unable to undergo the first-line therapy; category III, for which the optimum role of apheresis therapy is not established and decision-making should be individualized; and category IV disorders, in which published evidence demonstrates or suggests apheresis to be ineffective or harmful.[395] The indications for TPE (category I) are listed in *Table 23.13*.

Table 23.12. Pathogen Reduction Technologies for Transfusable Blood Components

Component	Technology	Manufacturer
Plasma: commercially prepared pools	Solvent/detergent treatment[a]	Octapharma
Plasma: individual units	• Amotosalen (psoralen) + UV light[a] • Riboflavin (vitamin B$_2$) + UV light • Methylene blue + light	Cerus Terumo BCT MacoPharma
Platelets	• Amotosalen (psoralen) + UV light[a] • Riboflavin (vitamin B$_2$) + UV light • UV light	Cerus Terumo BCT MacoPharma
Red blood cells	• Amustaline and glutathione	Cerus
Whole blood	• Riboflavin (vitamin B$_2$) + UV light	Terumo BCT
Cryoprecipitate (Pathogen Reduced Cryoprecipitated Fibrinogen Complex)	• Amotosalen (psoralen) + UV light[a]	Cerus

[a]Approved by the FDA for use in the United States.
Abbreviation: UV, ultraviolet.
Modified with permission from Cohn CS, Delaney M, Johnson ST, Katz LM, eds. *Technical Manual.* 20th ed. AABB Press; 2020. Copyright © 2020 by AABB; INTERCEPT® Blood System for Cryoprecipitation Package Insert For the manufacturing of Pathogen Reduced Cryoprecipitated Fibrinogen Complex. Accessed July 19, 2021. https://www.fda.gov/media/143996/download

Table 23.13. Category and Grade Recommendations for TPE Category I Indications

Disease Name	Indication	Category	Grade
Acute inflammatory demyelinating polyradiculoneuropathy/Guillain-Barré syndrome	Primary	I	1A
Acute liver failure	TPE-high volume	I	1A
Antiglomerular basement membrane disease (Goodpasture syndrome) Catastrophic antiphospholipid antibody syndrome[a]	DAH Dialysis independence	I I I	1C 1B 2C
Chronic inflammatory demyelinating polyradiculoneuropathy		I	1B
Focal segmental glomerulosclerosis	Recurrent in transplanted kidney	I	1B
Hyperviscosity in monoclonal gammopathies	Symptomatic Prophylaxis for rituximab	I I	1B 1C
Liver transplantation	Desensitization, ABO incompatible LD	I	1C
Myasthenia gravis	Acute, short-term treatment	I	1B
N-methyl D-aspartate receptor antibody encephalitis		I	1C
Paraproteinemic demyelinating neuropathies/chronic acquired demyelinating polyneuropathies	IgG/IgA IgM	I I	1B 1C
Renal transplantation, ABO compatible	Antibody-mediated rejection Desensitization, LD	I I	1B 1B
Renal transplantation, ABO incompatible	Desensitization, LD	I	1B
Thrombotic microangiopathy, complement mediated[b]	Factor H autoantibodies	I	2C
Thrombotic microangiopathy, drug associated	Ticlopidine	I	2B
Thrombotic thrombocytopenic purpura Vasculitis, ANCA-associated	MPA/GPA/RLV: RPGN, Cr ≥ 5.7 MPA/GPA/RLV: DAH	I I I	1A 1A 1C
Wilson disease	Fulminant	I	1C

[a]New fact sheets in 2019 edition.
[b]TMA-specific fact sheets.
Abbreviations: TPE, therapeutic plasma exchange; DAH, diffuse alveolar hemorrhage; LD, living donor; MPA, microscopic polyangiitis; GPA, granulomatosis with polyangiitis; RLV, renal-limited vasculitis; RPGN, rapidly progressive glomerulonephritis.
Modified from Padmanabhan A, Connelly-Smith L, Aqui N, et al. Guidelines on the use of therapeutic apheresis in clinical practice—evidence-based approach from the Writing Committee of the American Society for Apheresis: the eighth special issue. *J Clin Apher.* 2019;34(3):171-354. Copyright © 2019 Wiley Periodicals, Inc. Reprinted by permission of John Wiley & Sons, Inc.

Therapeutic Plasma Exchange

Indications

The therapeutic goal of TPE is to remove plasma components such as monoclonal proteins and cryoglobulins, immune complexes, lipoproteins, or toxins responsible for physical or metabolic problems. These may include removal of autoantibodies, as in myasthenia gravis and Goodpasture syndrome, or alloantibodies, as in posttransfusion purpura.

The existence and pathogenic role of antibodies or immune complexes are presumed in several situations often treated with TPE, including neurologic disorders such as Guillain-Barré syndrome,[396,397] polyneuropathy,[398] and various nephritides.[399] In TTP, TPE using cryoprecipitate-reduced plasma[400] or frozen plasma as the replacement fluid serves to either replace the missing vWF-cleaving metalloprotease or to remove autoantibodies to this protein.[46,401] TPE or plasma transfusion[402-404] may be life-saving in this disease, as it controls the microangiopathy.

Technical Considerations

The amount of plasma to be removed from the patient is determined by the physician, depending on the clinical situation. A patient's plasma volume may be estimated at 40 mL/kg, determined from a nomogram based on the patient's sex, height, weight, and Hct, or estimated according to the weight and Hct by the following formula:

$$\text{Circulating blood volume} = \text{patient weight}\,(\text{kg}) \times 70 \text{ mL/kg}$$

$$\text{Circulating plasma volume} = \text{circulating blood volume}$$
$$\times \left(1 - \text{Hct}\left[\text{expressed as a decimal}\right]\right)$$

TPE is typically performed with 1.0 to 1.5 plasma volume exchanges or approximately 3000 to 4500 mL in an adult. If < 1000 mL is removed from an adult, it may be possible to replace the loss with crystalloid alone; if a more extensive plasma exchange is performed, use of a colloid is necessary. Albumin (5%) is the replacement fluid most commonly used in the United States. FFP or PF24 is indicated in certain instances, such as TTP or as a component of the replacement fluid in the setting of a coagulopathy.

After exchange of 1 or 1.5 plasma volume exchange, approximately 62% or 88%, respectively, of the original plasma has been removed. The efficiency of plasma exchange decreases with further exchange.

In practice, measurement of plasma protein concentrations after exchange has confirmed the approximate validity of these estimates. However, efficacy varies with the plasma factor to be removed. IgM, which is largely confined to the intravascular space, is removed most efficiently.[405,406] IgG is removed less efficiently by plasma exchange because only one-third of the body's IgG is located in the intravascular space, although IgG levels can be reduced by repeated TPE. Patients receiving plasma exchange for immunologic diseases generally have 1.0 to 1.5 plasma volumes exchanged at each procedure; this is often repeated, for a total of five exchanges over a period of 7 to 10 days. Such plasma exchange schedules have been determined empirically based on calculations that a 1-log (90%) reduction of IgG is achieved after five TPE sessions.

Therapeutic Cytapheresis

Therapeutic leukapheresis is used in the treatment of patients with leukostasis as a result of extremely high circulating concentrations of leukemia cells.[407,408] At myeloid blast counts >100 × 10⁹/L, there is an increasing risk of cerebral and pulmonary leukostasis, resulting in impaired capillary blood flow resulting from obstruction of small vessels. This situation may be encountered in acute leukemias but rarely in chronic lymphocytic leukemia or chronic myelogenous leukemia. Therapeutic leukapheresis decreases the circulating blast count more rapidly than chemotherapy alone; chemotherapy must be instituted promptly once the patient is stabilized, to prevent rebound leukocytosis. The only exception is in pregnancy, in which leukapheresis may be indicated until after the delivery of the fetus, thereby protecting the fetus from the teratogenic effects of chemotherapy. Collection of leukocytes by apheresis, followed by ex vivo exposure of the leukocytes to UV light in the presence of a psoralen, and reinfusion of the treated leukocytes ("photopheresis") has become standard therapy for cutaneous T-cell lymphoma. This procedure may be useful in the treatment of other disorders such as GVHD.

Therapeutic plateletpheresis[409] is performed very rarely and is not considered to be first-line therapy. It is indicated in patients with very high platelet counts, usually >1.0 to 1.5 × 10¹²/L, in whom the high count is directly responsible for serious thrombotic or hemorrhagic problems, or in whom other urgent clinical situations necessitate immediate lowering of the platelet count. Therapeutic plateletpheresis must be followed by cytotoxic therapy to prevent rebound after the procedure, or its effect is very short-lived.

Erythrocytapheresis (red cell exchange) is used in sickle cell disease to replace sickled cells with normal erythrocytes and thereby prevent thromboses and improve capillary circulation.[407] Stroke prevention by maintaining HbS level below 30% and acute chest syndrome are the two major indications for red cell exchange in patients with sickle disease.[395]

Therapeutic Adsorption of Plasma Constituents

Apheresis technology may be used to selectively remove constituents of plasma implicated in disease processes. In these procedures, a patient's plasma is withdrawn and separated by apheresis technology, passed over a selective adsorption column, and reinfused into the patient. This technique has been used to selectively remove IgG (staphylococcal protein A columns) or low-density lipoprotein (LDL) cholesterol. Selective apheresis may specifically treat diseases such as LDL-hypercholesterolemia. Patients with LDL-hypercholesterolemia are at risk of developing severe coronary artery disease despite a low-fat diet and cholesterol-lowering agents. Selective LDL apheresis involves separation of the patient's plasma, followed by selective removal of apoB-containing atherogenic lipoproteins, preserving the cardioprotective high-density lipoprotein cholesterol, after which the cleansed plasma is recombined with the cellular portion of the blood and returned to the patient. This procedure was shown to be safe and efficacious in controlling patients with familial hypercholesterolemia.[410]

Adverse Effects

Adverse reactions to therapeutic apheresis are common but usually mild.[411] In a survey of 18 centers with 125 to 500 therapeutic apheresis procedures performed per center, 4.75% of procedures were complicated by mostly reversible adverse effects in 3429 responses.[411] They included vasovagal reactions, fluid imbalance with hypovolemia or overload, fever, chills, and hypocalcemic citrate reactions ranging from paresthesias to arrhythmias. If plasma is used as the replacement fluid, urticarial reactions may be encountered. Mild dilutional coagulopathy and thrombocytopenia occur but are rarely significant.[412] Problems related to venous access are common. Infections related to indwelling venous lines are not uncommon. Deaths, though very rare, have also been reported with therapeutic apheresis.[413] It is important that patients be carefully assessed and the indications reviewed before implementing this form of therapy.

SUMMARY

Blood transfusion is an important option for therapy in a wide variety of disorders. Collaboration between transfusion medicine professionals and patient care teams is essential to ensure the effective application of strategies for PBM so that blood transfusion is only used when necessary and so that transfusion practice is both safe and appropriate.

ACKNOWLEDGMENTS

The authors wish to thank Jonathan Hughes, Michael Murphy, and Lawrence T. Goodnough for their very thorough chapter on transfusion medicine in the previous edition, which provided an excellent template for our update on this chapter.

References

1. Cohn CSDM, Johnson ST, Katz LM. *Technical Manual*. 20th ed. Bethesda, MD: AABB Press; 2020.
2. *32nd Edition Standards for Blood Banks and Transfusion Services*. vol. 32: AABB Press; 2020.
3. Goodnough LT. What is a transfusion medicine specialist? *Transfusion*. 1999;39(9):1031-1033.
4. James AB, Hillyer CD, Shaz BH. Demographic differences in estimated blood donor eligibility prevalence in the United States. *Transfusion*. 2012;52(5):1050-1061.
5. Riley W, Schwei M, McCullough J. The United States' potential blood donor pool: estimating the prevalence of donor-exclusion factors on the pool of potential donors. *Transfusion*. 2007;47(7):1180-1188.
6. Domen RE. Paid-versus-volunteer blood donation in the United States: a historical review. *Transfus Med Rev*. 1995;9(1):53-59.
7. Food and Drug Adminstration. Requirements for blood and blood components intended for transfusion or for further manufacturing use. Final Rule. *Fed Regist*. 2015;29841-29906.
8. An acceptable circular of information for the use of human blood and blood components. Accessed January 12, 2018. http://www.fda.gov/downloads/BiologicsBloodVaccines/GuidanceComplianceRegulatoryInformation/Guidances/Blood/UCM364593.pdf. November 2013.

9. Jones JM, Sapiano MRP, Mowla S, Bota D, Berger JJ, Basavaraju SV. Has the trend of declining blood transfusions in the United States ended? Findings of the 2019 National Blood Collection and Utilization Survey. *Transfusion*. 2021:61.
10. Land KWB. *2012 AABB United States Donor Hemovigilance Report*. Accessed January 12, 2018. https://www.aabb.org/research/hemovigilance/Documents/aabb-donor-hemovigilance-report-2012.pdf. 2012.
11. International Society of Blood Transfusion. *Standards for Surveillance of Complications Related to Blood Donation*. Accessed December 11, 2014 http://wwww.isbtweb.org/fileadmin/user_upload/2_Donor-Standard-Definitions.pdf.
12. Townsend M, Kamel H, Van Buren N, et al. Development and validation of donor adverse reaction severity grading tool: enhancing objective grade assignment to donor adverse events. *Transfusion*. 2020;60(6):1231-1242.
13. Szczepiorkowski ZHT. *AABB Association Bulletin #17-02. Updated Strategies to Limit or Prevent Iron Deficiency in Blood Donors*. Accessed June 29, 2021. https://www.aabb.org/docs/default-source/default-document-library/resources/association-bulletins/ab17-02.pdf. 2017.
14. Food and Drug Adminstration. *Guidance for Industry: Use of Serological Tests to Reduce the Transmission of Trypanosoma cruzi Infection in Whole Blood and Blood Components Intended for Transfusion*. FDA Guidance. Accessed December 2010http://www.fda.gov/BiologicsBloodVaccines/GuidanceComplianceRegulatoryInformation/Guidances/Blood/ucm528600.pdf.
15. *Information for blood establishments regarding FDA's determination that Zika virus is no longer a relevant transfusion-transmitted infection. Withdrawal of Guidance Titled "Revised Recommendations for Reducing the Risk of Zika Virus Transmission by Blood and Blood Components."* May 2021. Accessed 29, 2021. https://www.fda.gov/vaccines-blood-biologics/blood-blood-products/information-blood-establishments-regarding-fdas-determination-zika-virus-no-longer-relevant.
16. Recommendations for reducing the risk of transfusion-transmitted babesiosis. *Guidance for Industry*. May 2019. Accessed 29, 2021. https://www.fda.gov/regulatory-information/search-fda-guidance-documents/recommendations-reducing-risk-transfusion-transmitted-babesiosis.
17. Glynn SA, Klein HG, Ness PM. The red blood cell storage lesion: the end of the beginning. *Transfusion*. 2016;56(6):1462-1468.
18. Davey RJ, McCoy NC, Yu M, Sullivan JA, Spiegel DM, Leitman SF. The effect of prestorage irradiation on posttransfusion red cell survival. *Transfusion*. 1992;32(6):525-528.
19. Vraets A, Lin Y, Callum JL. Transfusion-associated hyperkalemia. *Transfus Med Rev*. 2011;25(3):184-196.
20. Simon TL, McCullough J, Snyder EL, Solheim BG, Strauss RG. *Rossi's Principles of Transfusion Medicine*. 5th ed. Chichester, West Sussex; Hoboken, NJ: John Wiley & Sons Inc.; 2016.
21. Sohmer PR, Dawson RB. The significance of 2,3-DPG in red blood cell transfusions. *CRC Crit Rev Clin Lab Sci*. 1979;11(2):107-174.
22. Beutler E, Wood L. The in vivo regeneration of red cell 2,3 diphosphoglyceric acid (DPG) after transfusion of stored blood. *J Lab Clin Med*. 1969;74(2):300-304.
23. What is the clinical importance of alterations of the hemoglobin oxygen affinity in preserved blood—especially as produced by variations of red cell 2,3 DPG content? *Vox Sang*. 1978;34(2):111-127.
24. Koch CG, Li L, Sessler DI, et al. Duration of red-cell storage and complications after cardiac surgery. *N Engl J Med*. 2008;358(12):1229-1239.
25. Pereira A. Will clinical studies elucidate the connection between the length of storage of transfused red blood cells and clinical outcomes? An analysis based on the simulation of randomized controlled trials. *Transfusion*. 2013;53(1):34-40.
26. Steiner ME, Ness PM, Assmann SF, et al. Effects of red-cell storage duration on patients undergoing cardiac surgery. *N Engl J Med*. 2015;372(15):1419-1429.
27. Lacroix J, Hebert PC, Fergusson DA, et al. Age of transfused blood in critically ill adults. *N Engl J Med*. 2015;372(15):1410-1418.
28. Heddle NM, Cook RJ, Arnold DM, et al. Effect of short-term vs. long-term blood storage on mortality after transfusion. *N Engl J Med*. 2016;375(20):1937-1945.
29. Fergusson DA, Hebert P, Hogan DL, et al. Effect of fresh red blood cell transfusions on clinical outcomes in premature, very low-birth-weight infants: the ARIPI randomized trial. *JAMA*. 2012;308(14):1443-1451.
30. Moroff G, Sohmer PR, Button LN. Proposed standardization of methods for determining the 24-hour survival of stored red cells. *Transfusion*. 1984;24(2):109-114.
31. Dumont LJ, AuBuchon JP. Evaluation of proposed FDA criteria for the evaluation of radiolabeled red cell recovery trials. *Transfusion*. 2008;48(6):1053-1060.
32. Fabricant L, Kiraly L, Wiles C, et al. Cryopreserved deglycerolized blood is safe and achieves superior tissue oxygenation compared with refrigerated red blood cells: a prospective randomized pilot study. *J Trauma Acute Care Surg*. 2013;74(2):371-376. Discussion 376-377.
33. Murphy S, Heaton WA, Rebulla P. Platelet production in the old world—and the new. *Transfusion*. 1996;36(8):751-754.
34. Murphy S. Platelet storage for transfusion. *Semin Hematol*. 1985;22(3):165-177.
35. *FDA Guidance for Industry*. December 2020. Accessed 29, 2021. https://www.fda.gov/regulatory-information/search-fda-guidance-documents/bacterial-risk-control-strategies-blood-collection-establishments-and-transfusion-services-enhance.
36. Rinder HM, Snyder EL, Tracey JB, et al. Reversibility of severe metabolic stress in stored platelets after in vitro plasma rescue or in vivo transfusion: restoration of secretory function and maintenance of platelet survival. *Transfusion*. 2003;43(9):1230-1237.
37. Murphy S, Munoz S, Parry-Billings M, Newsholme E. Amino acid metabolism during platelet storage for transfusion. *Br J Haematol*. 1992;81(4):585-590.
38. Vassallo RR, Adamson JW, Gottschall JL, et al. In vitro and in vivo evaluation of apheresis platelets stored for 5 days in 65% platelet additive solution/35% plasma. *Transfusion*. 2010;50(11):2376-2385.
39. Kerkhoffs JL, Eikenboom JC, Schipperus MS, et al. A multicenter randomized study of the efficacy of transfusions with platelets stored in platelet additive solution II versus plasma. *Blood*. 2006;108(9):3210-3215.
40. Waters L, Cameron M, Padula MP, Marks DC, Johnson L. Refrigeration, cryopreservation and pathogen inactivation: an updated perspective on platelet storage conditions. *Vox Sang*. 2018;113(4):317-328.
41. Reddoch-Cardenas KM, Bynum JA, Meledeo MA, et al. Cold-stored platelets: a product with function optimized for hemorrhage control. *Transfus Apher Sci*. 2019;58(1):16-22.
42. Stolla M, Fitzpatrick L, Gettinger I, et al. In vivo viability of extended 4 degrees C-stored autologous apheresis platelets. *Transfusion*. 2018;58(10):2407-2413.
43. Cardigan R, Lawrie AS, Mackie IJ, Williamson LM. The quality of fresh-frozen plasma produced from whole blood stored at 4 degrees C overnight. *Transfusion*. 2005;45(8):1342-1348.
44. Matijevic N, Wang YW, Cotton BA, et al. Better hemostatic profiles of never-frozen liquid plasma compared with thawed fresh frozen plasma. *J Trauma Acute Care Surg*. 2013;74(1):84-90. Discussion 90-91.
45. Yazer MH, Cortese-Hassett A, Triulzi DJ. Coagulation factor levels in plasma frozen within 24 hours of phlebotomy over 5 days of storage at 1 to 6 degrees C. *Transfusion*. 2008;48(12):2525-2530.
46. Raife TJ, Friedman KD, Dwyre DM. The pathogenicity of von Willebrand factor in thrombotic thrombocytopenic purpura: reconsideration of treatment with cryopoor plasma. *Transfusion*. 2006;46(1):74-79.
47. Laub R, Baurin S, Timmerman D, Branckaert T, Strengers P. Specific protein content of pools of plasma for fractionation from different sources: impact of frequency of donations. *Vox Sang*. 2010;99(3):220-231.
48. Ofosu FA, Freedman J, Semple JW. Plasma-derived biological medicines used to promote haemostasis. *Thromb Haemost*. 2008;99(5):851-862.
49. Tabor E. The epidemiology of virus transmission by plasma derivatives: clinical studies verifying the lack of transmission of hepatitis B and C viruses and HIV type 1. *Transfusion*. 1999;39(11-12):1160-1168.
50. Hellstern P, Solheim BG. The use of solvent/detergent treatment in pathogen reduction of plasma. *Transfus Med Hemother*. 2011;38(1):65-70.
51. Darabi K, Abdel-Wahab O, Dzik WH. Current usage of intravenous immune globulin and the rationale behind it: the Massachusetts General Hospital data and a review of the literature. *Transfusion*. 2006;46(5):741-753.
52. Guidance for Industry: *Pre-storage Leukocyte Reduction of Whole Blood and Blood Components Intended for Transfusion*. FDA CBER. September 2012. Accessed January 12, 2018 http://www.fda.gov/downloads/BiologicsBloodVaccines/GuidanceComplianceRegulatoryInformation/Guidances/Blood/UCM320641.pdf.
53. Heddle NM, Klama L, Singer J, et al. The role of the plasma from platelet concentrates in transfusion reactions. *N Engl J Med*. 1994;331(10):625-628.
54. Heddle NM, Klama LN, Griffith L, Roberts R, Shukla G, Kelton JG. A prospective study to identify the risk factors associated with acute reactions to platelet and red cell transfusions. *Transfusion*. 1993;33(10):794-797.
55. Veeraputhiran M, Ware J, Dent J, et al. A comparison of washed and volume-reduced platelets with respect to platelet activation, aggregation, and plasma protein removal. *Transfusion*. 2011;51(5):1030-1036.
56. Groner A. Pathogen safety of plasma-derived products—Haemate P/Humate-P. *Haemophilia*. 2008;14 (suppl 5):54-71.
57. Holman P, Blajchman MA, Heddle N. Noninfectious adverse effects of blood transfusion in the neonate. *Transfus Med Rev*. 1995;9(3):277-287.
58. Hiemstra H, Tersmette M, Vos AH, Over J, van Berkel MP, de Bree H. Inactivation of human immunodeficiency virus by gamma radiation and its effect on plasma and coagulation factors. *Transfusion*. 1991;31(1):32-39.
59. Dorsey KA, Moritz ED, Steele WR, Eder AF, Stramer SL. A comparison of human immunodeficiency virus, hepatitis C virus, hepatitis B virus, and human T-lymphotropic virus marker rates for directed versus volunteer blood donations to the American Red Cross during 2005 to 2010. *Transfusion*. 2013;53(6):1250-1256.
60. Jacquot C, Seo A, Miller PM, et al. Parental versus non-parental-directed donation: an 11-year experience of infectious disease testing at a pediatric tertiary care blood donor center. *Transfusion*. 2017;57(11):2799-2803.
61. Whitaker B, Rajbhandary S, Kleinman S, Harris A, Kamani N. Trends in United States blood collection and transfusion: results from the 2013 AABB Blood Collection, Utilization, and Patient Blood Management Survey. *Transfusion*. 2016;56(9):2173-2183.
62. Goodnough LT, Skikne B, Brugnara C. Erythropoietin, iron, and erythropoiesis. *Blood*. 2000;96(3):823-833.
63. Birkmeyer JD, Goodnough LT, AuBuchon JP, Noordsij PG, Littenberg B. The cost-effectiveness of preoperative autologous blood donation for total hip and knee replacement. *Transfusion*. 1993;33(7):544-551.
64. Mackey JLK. *AABB Position on Testing of Autologous Units. Association Bulletin 95-4*. Bethesda, MD: American Association of Blood Banks; 1995.
65. Vassallo R, Goldman M, Germain M, Lozano M, Collaborative B. Preoperative autologous blood donation: waning indications in an era of improved blood safety. *Transfus Med Rev*. 2015;29(4):268-275.
66. Goodnough LT, Brecher ME, Kanter MH, AuBuchon JP. Transfusion medicine. Second of two parts—blood conservation. *N Engl J Med*. 1999;340(7):525-533.
67. Monk TG, Goodnough LT, Brecher ME, et al. Acute normovolemic hemodilution can replace preoperative autologous blood donation as a standard of care for autologous blood procurement in radical prostatectomy. *Anesth Analg*. 1997;85(5):953-958.
68. Goodnough LT, Monk TG, Brecher ME. Acute normovolemic hemodilution should replace the preoperative donation of autologous blood as a method of autologous-blood procurement. *Transfusion*. 1998;38(5):473-476.
69. *9th Edition Standards for Perioperative Autologous Blood Collection and Administration*. vol. 9. Bethesda, MD: AABB Press; 2021.

70. Segal JB, Blasco-Colmenares E, Norris EJ, Guallar E. Preoperative acute normovolemic hemodilution: a meta-analysis. *Transfusion.* 2004;44(5):632-644.

71. Monk TG, Goodnough LT, Brecher ME, Colberg JW, Andriole GL, Catalona WJ. A prospective randomized comparison of three blood conservation strategies for radical prostatectomy. *Anesthesiology.* 1999;91(1):24-33.

72. Williamson KR, Taswell HF. Intraoperative blood salvage: a review. *Transfusion.* 1991;31(7):662-675.

73. Ashworth A, Klein AA. Cell salvage as part of a blood conservation strategy in anaesthesia. *Br J Anaesth.* 2010;105(4):401-416.

74. Sikorski RA, Rizkalla NA, Yang WW, Frank SM. Autologous blood salvage in the era of patient blood management. *Vox Sang.* 2017;112(6):499-510.

75. Ritter MA, Keating EM, Faris PM. Closed wound drainage in total hip or total knee replacement. A prospective, randomized study. *J Bone Joint Surg Am.* 1994;76(1):35-38.

76. Effectiveness of perioperative recombinant human erythropoietin in elective hip replacement. Canadian Orthopedic Perioperative Erythropoietin Study Group. *Lancet.* 1993;341(8855):1227-1232.

77. Goodnough LT, Rudnick S, Price TH, et al. Increased preoperative collection of autologous blood with recombinant human erythropoietin therapy. *N Engl J Med.* 1989;321(17):1163-1168.

78. Goodnough LT, Price TH, Friedman KD, et al. A phase III trial of recombinant human erythropoietin therapy in nonanemic orthopedic patients subjected to aggressive removal of blood for autologous use: dose, response, toxicity, and efficacy. *Transfusion.* 1994;34(1):66-71.

79. Goodnough LT, Monk TG, Andriole GL. Erythropoietin therapy. *N Engl J Med.* 1997;336(13):933-938.

80. Kocian R, Spahn DR. Haemoglobin, oxygen carriers and perioperative organ perfusion. *Best Pract Res Clin Anaesthesiol.* 2008;22(1):63-80.

81. Shander A, Goodnough LT. Why an alternative to blood transfusion? *Crit Care Clin.* 2009;25(2):261-277. Table of Contents.

82. Goodnough LT, Shander A. Blood management. *Arch Pathol Lab Med.* 2007;131(5):695-701.

83. Goodnough LT, Shander A. Evolution in alternatives to blood transfusion. *Hematol J.* 2003;4(2):87-91.

84. Hai CM. Systems biology of HBOC-induced vasoconstriction. *Curr Drug Discov Technol.* 2012;9(3):204-211.

85. Natanson C, Kern SJ, Lurie P, Banks SM, Wolfe SM. Cell-free hemoglobin-based blood substitutes and risk of myocardial infarction and death: a meta-analysis. *JAMA.* 2008;299(19):2304-2312.

86. Welch HG, Meehan KR, Goodnough LT. Prudent strategies for elective red blood cell transfusion. *Ann Intern Med.* 1992;116(5):393-402.

87. Starr DP. *Blood: An Epic History of Medicine and Commerce.* 1st ed. New York: Alfred A. Knopf; 1998.

88. Shander A, Hofmann A, Ozawa S, Theusinger OM, Gombotz H, Spahn DR. Activity-based costs of blood transfusions in surgical patients at four hospitals. *Transfusion.* 2010;50(4):753-765.

89. Goodnough LT. Blood management: transfusion medicine comes of age. *Lancet.* 2013;381(9880):1791-1792.

90. Goodnough LT, Shander A. Patient blood management. *Anesthesiology.* 2012;116(6):1367-1376.

91. Goodnough LT, Levy JH, Murphy MF. Concepts of blood transfusion in adults. *Lancet.* 2013;381(9880):1845-1854.

92. Goodnough LT, Shander A. Current status of pharmacologic therapies in patient blood management. *Anesth Analg.* 2013;116(1):15-34.

93. Salisbury AC, Reid KJ, Alexander KP, et al. Diagnostic blood loss from phlebotomy and hospital-acquired anemia during acute myocardial infarction. *Arch Intern Med.* 2011;171(18):1646-1653.

94. Despotis GJ, Joist JH, Goodnough LT. Monitoring of hemostasis in cardiac surgical patients: impact of point-of-care testing on blood loss and transfusion outcomes. *Clin Chem.* 1997;43(9):1684-1696.

95. Moskowitz DM, McCullough JN, Shander A, et al. The impact of blood conservation on outcomes in cardiac surgery: is it safe and effective? *Ann Thorac Surg.* 2010;90(2):451-458.

96. Finch CA, Lenfant C. Oxygen transport in man. *N Engl J Med.* 1972;286(8):407-415.

97. Bulger J, Nickel W, Messler J, et al. Choosing wisely in adult hospital medicine: five opportunities for improved healthcare value. *J Hosp Med.* 2013;8(9):486-492.

98. Goodnough LT, Panigrahi AK. Blood transfusion therapy. *Med Clin North Am.* 2017;101(2):431-447.

99. Levy PS, Chavez RP, Crystal GJ, et al. Oxygen extraction ratio: a valid indicator of transfusion need in limited coronary vascular reserve? *J Trauma.* 1992;32(6):769-773. Discussion 773-764.

100. Levy PS, Kim SJ, Eckel PK, et al. Limit to cardiac compensation during acute isovolemic hemodilution: influence of coronary stenosis. *Am J Physiol.* 1993;265(1 Pt 2):H340-H349.

101. Goodnough LT, Despotis GJ, Hogue CW, Jr, Ferguson TB, Jr. On the need for improved transfusion indicators in cardiac surgery. *Ann Thorac Surg.* 1995;60(2):473-480.

102. Kitchens CS. Are transfusions overrated? Surgical outcome of Jehovah's Witnesses. *Am J Med.* 1993;94(2):117-119.

103. Viele MK, Weiskopf RB. What can we learn about the need for transfusion from patients who refuse blood? The experience with Jehovah's Witnesses. *Transfusion.* 1994;34(5):396-401.

104. Carson JL, Duff A, Poses RM, et al. Effect of anaemia and cardiovascular disease on surgical mortality and morbidity. *Lancet.* 1996;348(9034):1055-1060.

105. Carson JL, Noveck H, Berlin JA, Gould SA. Mortality and morbidity in patients with very low postoperative Hb levels who decline blood transfusion. *Transfusion.* 2002;42(7):812-818.

106. Lacroix J, Hebert PC, Hutchison JS, et al. Transfusion strategies for patients in pediatric intensive care units. *N Engl J Med.* 2007;356(16):1609-1619.

107. Valentine SL, Bembea MM, Muszynski JA, et al. Consensus recommendations for RBC transfusion practice in critically ill children from the pediatric critical care transfusion and anemia expertise initiative. *Pediatr Crit Care Med.* 2018;19(9):884-898.

108. Dhabangi A, Ainomugisha B, Cserti-Gazdewich C, et al. Effect of transfusion of red blood cells with longer vs shorter storage duration on elevated blood lactate levels in children with severe anemia: the TOTAL randomized clinical trial. *JAMA.* 2015;314(23):2514-2523.

109. Kirpalani H, Whyte RK, Andersen C, et al. The Premature Infants in Need of Transfusion (PINT) study: a randomized, controlled trial of a restrictive (low) versus liberal (high) transfusion threshold for extremely low birth weight infants. *J Pediatr.* 2006;149(3):301-307.

110. Bell EF, Strauss RG, Widness JA, et al. Randomized trial of liberal versus restrictive guidelines for red blood cell transfusion in preterm infants. *Pediatrics.* 2005;115(6):1685-1691.

111. Kirpalani H, Bell EF, Hintz SR, et al. Higher or lower hemoglobin transfusion thresholds for preterm infants. *N Engl J Med.* 2020;383(27):2639-2651.

112. Franz AR, Engel C, Bassler D, et al. Effects of liberal vs restrictive transfusion thresholds on survival and neurocognitive outcomes in extremely low-birth-weight infants: the ETTNO randomized clinical trial. *JAMA.* 2020;324(6):560-570.

113. Adams RJ, McKie VC, Hsu L, et al. Prevention of a first stroke by transfusions in children with sickle cell anemia and abnormal results on transcranial Doppler ultrasonography. *N Engl J Med.* 1998;339(1):5-11.

114. Adams RJ, Brambilla D; Optimizing Primary Stroke Prevention in Sickle Cell Anemia Trial I. Discontinuing prophylactic transfusions used to prevent stroke in sickle cell disease. *N Engl J Med.* 2005;353(26):2769-2778.

115. McLaughlin JF, Ballas SK. High mortality among children with sickle cell anemia and overt stroke who discontinue blood transfusion after transition to an adult program. *Transfusion.* 2016;56(5):1014-1021.

116. Adams RCLJ. Anesthesia in cases of poor surgical risk: some suggestions for decreasing the risk. *Anesthesiology.* 1942;3:603-607.

117. van Woerkens EC, Trouwborst A, van Lanschot JJ. Profound hemodilution: what is the critical level of hemodilution at which oxygen delivery-dependent oxygen consumption starts in an anesthetized human? *Anesth Analg.* 1992;75(5):818-821.

118. Hebert PC, Yetisir E, Martin C, et al. Is a low transfusion threshold safe in critically ill patients with cardiovascular diseases? *Crit Care Med.* 2001;29(2):227-234.

119. Parrillo JE. Journal supplements, anemia management, and evidence-based critical care medicine. *Crit Care Med.* 2001;29(9):S139-S140.

120. Guidelines for red blood cell and plasma transfusion for adults and children. *Int J Risk Saf Med.* 1997;10(4):255-271.

121. Wu WC, Rathore SS, Wang Y, Radford MJ, Krumholz HM. Blood transfusion in elderly patients with acute myocardial infarction. *N Engl J Med.* 2001;345(17):1230-1236.

122. Goodnough LT, Bach RG. Anemia, transfusion, and mortality. *N Engl J Med.* 2001;345(17):1272-1274.

123. Goodnough LT, Schrier SL. Evaluation and management of anemia in the elderly. *Am J Hematol.* 2014;89(1):88-96.

124. Docherty AB, O'Donnell R, Brunskill S, et al. Effect of restrictive versus liberal transfusion strategies on outcomes in patients with cardiovascular disease in a non-cardiac surgery setting: systematic review and meta-analysis. *BMJ.* 2016;352:i1351.

125. Carson JL, Hill S, Carless P, Hebert P, Henry D. Transfusion triggers: a systematic review of the literature. *Transfus Med Rev.* 2002;16(3):187-199.

126. Carson JL, Stanworth SJ, Roubinian N, et al. Transfusion thresholds and other strategies for guiding allogeneic red blood cell transfusion. *Cochrane Database Syst Rev.* 2016;10:CD002042.

127. Salpeter SR, Buckley JS, Chatterjee S. Impact of more restrictive blood transfusion strategies on clinical outcomes: a meta-analysis and systematic review. *Am J Med.* 2014;127(2):124-131 e123.

128. Hebert PC, Wells G, Blajchman MA, et al. A multicenter, randomized, controlled clinical trial of transfusion requirements in critical care. Transfusion Requirements in Critical Care Investigators, Canadian Critical Care Trials Group. *N Engl J Med.* 1999;340(6):409-417.

129. Hajjar LA, Vincent JL, Galas FR, et al. Transfusion requirements after cardiac surgery: the TRACS randomized controlled trial. *JAMA.* 2010;304(14):1559-1567.

130. Carson JL, Terrin ML, Noveck H, et al. Liberal or restrictive transfusion in high-risk patients after hip surgery. *N Engl J Med.* 2011;365(26):2453-2462.

131. Villanueva C, Colomo A, Bosch A, et al. Transfusion strategies for acute upper gastrointestinal bleeding. *N Engl J Med.* 2013;368(1):11-21.

132. Carson JL, Brooks MM, Abbott JD, et al. Liberal versus restrictive transfusion thresholds for patients with symptomatic coronary artery disease. *Am Heart J.* 2013;165(6):964-971 e961.

133. Holst LB, Haase N, Wetterslev J, et al. Lower versus higher hemoglobin threshold for transfusion in septic shock. *N Engl J Med.* 2014;371(15):1381-1391.

134. Murphy GJ, Pike K, Rogers CA, et al. Liberal or restrictive transfusion after cardiac surgery. *N Engl J Med.* 2015;372(11):997-1008.

135. Mudumbai SC, Cronkite R, Hu KU, et al. Association of admission hematocrit with 6-month and 1-year mortality in intensive care unit patients. *Transfusion.* 2011;51(10):2148-2159.

136. Mazer CD, Whitlock RP, Fergusson DA, et al. Restrictive or liberal red-cell transfusion for cardiac surgery. *N Engl J Med.* 2017;377(22):2133-2144.

137. Hovaguimian F, Myles PS. Restrictive versus liberal transfusion strategy in the perioperative and acute care settings: a context-specific systematic review and meta-analysis of randomized controlled trials. *Anesthesiology*. 2016;125(1):46-61.
138. Goodnough LT, Shah N. Is there a "magic" hemoglobin number? Clinical decision support promoting restrictive blood transfusion practices. *Am J Hematol*. 2015;90(10):927-933.
139. Carson JL, Guyatt G, Heddle NM, et al. Clinical practice guidelines from the AABB: red blood cell transfusion thresholds and storage. *JAMA*. 2016;316(19):2025-2035.
140. Callum JL, Waters JH, Shaz BH, Sloan SR, Murphy MF. The AABB recommendations for the Choosing Wisely campaign of the American Board of Internal Medicine. *Transfusion*. 2014;54(9):2344-2352.
141. Hicks LK, Bering H, Carson KR, et al. The ASH Choosing Wisely(R) campaign: five hematologic tests and treatments to question. *Blood*. 2013;122(24):3879-3883.
142. Audet AM, GL. American College of Physicians Position Paper: strategies for elective red blood cell transfusion. *Ann Intern Med*. 1992;116:403-406.
143. Burtelow M, Riley E, Druzin M, Fontaine M, Viele M, Goodnough LT. How we treat: management of life-threatening primary postpartum hemorrhage with a standardized massive transfusion protocol. *Transfusion*. 2007;47(9):1564-1572.
144. Butwick AJ, Goodnough LT. Transfusion and coagulation management in major obstetric hemorrhage. *Curr Opin Anaesthesiol*. 2015;28(3):275-284.
145. Holcomb JB, Jenkins D, Rhee P, et al. Damage control resuscitation: directly addressing the early coagulopathy of trauma. *J Trauma*. 2007;62(2):307-310.
146. Borgman MA, Spinella PC, Perkins JG, et al. The ratio of blood products transfused affects mortality in patients receiving massive transfusions at a combat support hospital. *J Trauma*. 2007;63(4):805-813.
147. Como JJ, Dutton RP, Scalea TM, Edelman BB, Hess JR. Blood transfusion rates in the care of acute trauma. *Transfusion*. 2004;44(6):809-813.
148. Moore FA, Nelson T, McKinley BA, et al. Massive transfusion in trauma patients: tissue hemoglobin oxygen saturation predicts poor outcome. *J Trauma*. 2008;64(4):1010-1023.
149. Cotton BA, Dossett LA, Au BK, Nunez TC, Robertson AM, Young PP. Room for (performance) improvement: provider-related factors associated with poor outcomes in massive transfusion. *J Trauma*. 2009;67(5):1004-1012.
150. Goodnough LT, Spain DA, Maggio P. Logistics of transfusion support for patients with massive hemorrhage. *Curr Opin Anaesthesiol*. 2013;26(2):208-214.
151. Shaz BH, Dente CJ, Nicholas J, et al. Increased number of coagulation products in relationship to red blood cell products transfused improves mortality in trauma patients. *Transfusion*. 2010;50(2):493-500.
152. Gunter OL, Jr, Au BK, Isbell JM, Mowery NT, Young PP, Cotton BA. Optimizing outcomes in damage control resuscitation: identifying blood product ratios associated with improved survival. *J Trauma*. 2008;65(3):527-534.
153. Holcomb JB, Tilley BC, Baraniuk S, et al. Transfusion of plasma, platelets, and red blood cells in a 1:1:1 vs a 1:1:2 ratio and mortality in patients with severe trauma: the PROPPR randomized clinical trial. *JAMA*. 2015;313(5):471-482.
154. Cardenas JC, Zhang X, Fox EE, et al. Platelet transfusions improve hemostasis and survival in a substudy of the prospective, randomized PROPPR trial. *Blood Adv*. 2018;2(14):1696-1704.
155. Goodnough LT, Maniatis A, Earnshaw P, et al. Detection, evaluation, and management of preoperative anaemia in the elective orthopaedic surgical patient: NATA guidelines. *Br J Anaesth*. 2011;106(1):13-22.
156. Petz LD, Garratty G, *Immune Hemolytic Anemias*. 2nd ed. Philadelphia, PA: Churchill Livingstone/Elsevier Science; 2004.
157. Greenwalt TJ, Zelenski KR. Transfusion support for haemoglobinopathies. *Clin Haematol*. 1984;13(1):151-165.
158. Lee MT, Piomelli S, Granger S, et al. Stroke prevention trial in sickle cell anemia (STOP): extended follow-up and final results. *Blood*. 2006;108(3):847-852.
159. DeBaun MR, Gordon M, McKinstry RC, et al. Controlled trial of transfusions for silent cerebral infarcts in sickle cell anemia. *N Engl J Med*. 2014;371(8):699-710.
160. Stainsby D, Russell J, Cohen H, Lilleyman J. Reducing adverse events in blood transfusion. *Br J Haematol*. 2005;131(1):8-12.
161. Sandler SG, Flegel WA, Westhoff CM, et al. It's time to phase in RHD genotyping for patients with a serologic weak D phenotype. College of American Pathologists Transfusion Medicine Resource Committee Work Group. *Transfusion*. 2015;55(3):680-689.
162. Garratty G. What is a clinically significant antibody? *ISBT Sci Ser*. 2012;7:54-57.
163. Shirey RS, Boyd JS, Ness PM. Polyethylene glycol versus low-ionic-strength solution in pretransfusion testing: a blinded comparison study. *Transfusion*. 1994;34(5):368-370.
164. Byrne KM, Mercado CMC, Nnabue TN, Paige TD, Flegel WA. Inhibition of blood group antibodies by soluble substances. *Immunohematology*. 2019;35(1):19-22.
165. Winters JL, Pineda AA, Gorden LD, et al. RBC alloantibody specificity and antigen potency in Olmsted County, Minnesota. *Transfusion*. 2001;41(11):1413-1420.
166. Hoeltge GA, Domen RE, Rybicki LA, Schaffer PA. Multiple red cell transfusions and alloimmunization. Experience with 6996 antibodies detected in a total of 159,262 patients from 1985 to 1993. *Arch Pathol Lab Med*. 1995;119(1):42-45.
167. Klein HG, Anstee DJ. *Mollison's Blood Transfusion in Clinical Medicine*. 12th ed. Chichester, West Sussex, UK: Wiley-Blackwell; 2014.
168. Novak DJ, Bai Y, Cooke RK, et al. Making thawed universal donor plasma available rapidly for massively bleeding trauma patients: experience from the Pragmatic, Randomized Optimal Platelets and Plasma Ratios (PROPPR) trial. *Transfusion*. 2015;55(6):1331-1339.
169. Dunbar NM, Yazer MH, Biomedical Excellence for Safer Transfusion Collaborative. A possible new paradigm? A survey-based assessment of the use of thawed group A plasma for trauma resuscitation in the United States. *Transfusion*. 2016;56(1):125-129.
170. Ramasethu J, Luban N. T activation. *Br J Haematol*. 2001;112(2):259-263.
171. Levene C, Levene NA, Buskila D, Manny N. Red cell polyagglutination. *Transfus Med Rev*. 1988;2(3):176-185.
172. Wallhermfechtel MA, Pohl BA, Chaplin H. Alloimmunization in patients with warm autoantibodies. A retrospective study employing three donor alloabsorptions to aid in antibody detection. *Transfusion*. 1984;24(6):482-485.
173. Anstee DJ. Red cell genotyping and the future of pretransfusion testing. *Blood*. 2009;114(2):248-256.
174. Arndt PA. Drug-induced immune hemolytic anemia: the last 30 years of changes. *Immunohematology*. 2014;30(2):44-54.
175. Flegel WA, Gottschall JL, Denomme GA. Integration of red cell genotyping into the blood supply chain: a population-based study. *Lancet Haematol*. 2015;2(7):e282-289.
176. Reece JT, Sesok-Pizzini D. Inventory management and product selection in pediatric blood banking. *Clin Lab Med*. 2021;41(1):69-81.
177. Hume H, Bard H. Small volume red blood cell transfusions for neonatal patients. *Transfus Med Rev*. 1995;9(3):187-199.
178. Luban NL, Strauss RG, Hume HA. Commentary on the safety of red cells preserved in extended-storage media for neonatal transfusions. *Transfusion*. 1991;31(3):229-235.
179. Wang-Rodriguez J, Mannino FL, Liu E, Lane TA. A novel strategy to limit blood donor exposure and blood waste in multiply transfused premature infants. *Transfusion*. 1996;36(1):64-70.
180. Lee AC, Reduque LL, Luban NL, Ness PM, Anton B, Heitmiller ES. Transfusion-associated hyperkalemic cardiac arrest in pediatric patients receiving massive transfusion. *Transfusion*. 2014;54(1):244-254.
181. Wolf MF, Childers J, Gray KD, et al. Exchange transfusion safety and outcomes in neonatal hyperbilirubinemia. *J Perinatol*. 2020;40(10):1506-1512.
182. Tinmouth AT, Freedman J. Prophylactic platelet transfusions: which dose is the best dose? A review of the literature. *Transfus Med Rev*. 2003;17(3):181-193.
183. Hanson SR, Slichter SJ. Platelet kinetics in patients with bone marrow hypoplasia: evidence for a fixed platelet requirement. *Blood*. 1985;66(5):1105-1109.
184. Norol F, Bierling P, Roudot-Thoraval F, et al. Platelet transfusion: a dose-response study. *Blood*. 1998;92(4):1448-1453.
185. Klumpp TR, Herman JH, Gaughan JP, et al. Clinical consequences of alterations in platelet transfusion dose: a prospective, randomized, double-blind trial. *Transfusion*. 1999;39(7):674-681.
186. Slichter SJ, Kaufman RM, Assmann SF, et al. Dose of prophylactic platelet transfusions and prevention of hemorrhage. *N Engl J Med*. 2010;362(7):600-613.
187. Beutler E. Platelet transfusions: the 20,000/microL trigger. *Blood*. 1993;81(6):1411-1413.
188. Lal DS, Shaz BH. Massive transfusion: blood component ratios. *Curr Opin Hematol*. 2013;20(6):521-525.
189. Young PP, Cotton BA, Goodnough LT. Massive transfusion protocols for patients with substantial hemorrhage. *Transfus Med Rev*. 2011;25(4):293-303.
190. Delaney M, Meyer E, Cserti-Gazdewich C, et al. A systematic assessment of the quality of reporting for platelet transfusion studies. *Transfusion*. 2010;50(10):2135-2144.
191. Kaufman RM, Djulbegovic B, Gernsheimer T, et al. Platelet transfusion: a clinical practice guideline from the AABB. *Ann Intern Med*. 2015;162(3):205-213.
192. Estcourt LJ, Birchall J, Allard S, et al. Guidelines for the use of platelet transfusions. *Br J Haematol*. 2017;176(3):365-394.
193. Rebulla P, Finazzi G, Marangoni F, et al. The threshold for prophylactic platelet transfusions in adults with acute myeloid leukemia. Gruppo Italiano Malattie Ematologiche Maligne dell'Adulto. *N Engl J Med*. 1997;337(26):1870-1875.
194. Wandt H, Frank M, Ehninger G, et al. Safety and cost effectiveness of a 10 x 10(9)/L trigger for prophylactic platelet transfusions compared with the traditional 20 x 10(9)/L trigger: a prospective comparative trial in 105 patients with acute myeloid leukemia. *Blood*. 1998;91(10):3601-3606.
195. Heckman KD, Weiner GJ, Davis CS, Strauss RG, Jones MP, Burns CP. Randomized study of prophylactic platelet transfusion threshold during induction therapy for adult acute leukemia: 10,000/microL versus 20,000/microL. *J Clin Oncol*. 1997;15(3):1143-1149.
196. Zumberg MS, del Rosario ML, Nejame CF, et al. A prospective randomized trial of prophylactic platelet transfusion and bleeding incidence in hematopoietic stem cell transplant recipients: 10,000/L versus 20,000/microL trigger. *Biol Blood Marrow Transplant*. 2002;8(10):569-576.
197. Stanworth SJ, Estcourt LJ, Powter G, et al. A no-prophylaxis platelet-transfusion strategy for hematologic cancers. *N Engl J Med*. 2013;368(19):1771-1780.
198. Wandt H, Schaefer-Eckart K, Wendelin K, et al. Therapeutic platelet transfusion versus routine prophylactic transfusion in patients with haematological malignancies: an open-label, multicentre, randomised study. *Lancet*. 2012;380(9850):1309-1316.
199. Practice guidelines for blood component therapy: a report by the American Society of Anesthesiologists Task Force on blood component therapy. *Anesthesiology*. 1996;84(3):732-747.
200. Goodnough LT, Grishaber JE, Monk TG, Catalona WJ. Acute preoperative hemodilution in patients undergoing radical prostatectomy: a case study analysis of efficacy. *Anesth Analg*. 1994;78(5):932-937.
201. Harker LA, Malpass TW, Branson HE, Hessel EA,II, Slichter SJ. Mechanism of abnormal bleeding in patients undergoing cardiopulmonary bypass: acquired transient platelet dysfunction associated with selective alpha-granule release. *Blood*. 1980;56(5):824-834.
202. Counts RB, Haisch C, Simon TL, Maxwell NG, Heimbach DM, Carrico CJ. Hemostasis in massively transfused trauma patients. *Ann Surg*. 1979;190(1):91-99.
203. Miller RD, Robbins TO, Tong MJ, Barton SL. Coagulation defects associated with massive blood transfusions. *Ann Surg*. 1971;174(5):794-801.

204. Ketchum L, Hess JR, Hiippala S. Indications for early fresh frozen plasma, cryoprecipitate, and platelet transfusion in trauma. *J Trauma.* 2006;60(suppl 6):S51-S58.

205. Callum JL, Nascimento B, Tien H, Rizoli S. Editorial: "formula-driven" versus "lab-driven" massive transfusion protocols—at a state of clinical equipoise. *Transfus Med Rev.* 2009;23(4):247-254.

206. Nance ST, Slichter S, American Association of Blood Banks; International Society of Blood Transfusion. *Transfusion Medicine in the 1990's.* Arlington, VA: American Association of Blood Banks; 1990.

207. Bishop JF, McGrath K, Wolf MM, et al. Clinical factors influencing the efficacy of pooled platelet transfusions. *Blood.* 1988;71(2):383-387.

208. Novotny VM. Prevention and management of platelet transfusion refractoriness. *Vox Sang.* 1999;76(1):1-13.

209. Yankee RA, Graff KS, Dowling R, Henderson ES. Selection of unrelated compatible platelet donors by lymphocyte HL-A matching. *N Engl J Med.* 1973;288(15):760-764.

210. Trial to Reduce Alloimmunization to Platelets Study Group. Leukocyte reduction and ultraviolet B irradiation of platelets to prevent alloimmunization and refractoriness to platelet transfusions. *N Engl J Med.* 1997;337(26):1861-1869.

211. Schnaidt M, Northoff H, Wernet D. Frequency and specificity of platelet-specific alloantibodies in HLA-immunized haematologic-oncologic patients. *Transfus Med.* 1996;6(2):111-114.

212. Doughty HA, Murphy MF, Metcalfe P, Rohatiner AZ, Lister TA, Waters AH. Relative importance of immune and non-immune causes of platelet refractoriness. *Vox Sang.* 1994;66(3):200-205.

213. Duquesnoy RJ, Filip DJ, Aster RH. Influence of HLA-A2 on the effectiveness of platelet transfusions in alloimmunized thrombocytopenic patients. *Blood.* 1977;50(3):407-412.

214. Petz LD, Garratty G, Calhoun L, et al. Selecting donors of platelets for refractory patients on the basis of HLA antibody specificity. *Transfusion.* 2000;40(12):1446-1456.

215. Nambiar A, Duquesnoy RJ, Adams S, et al. HLAMatchmaker-driven analysis of responses to HLA-typed platelet transfusions in alloimmunized thrombocytopenic patients. *Blood.* 2006;107(4):1680-1687.

216. Pavenski K, Rebulla P, Duquesnoy R, et al. Efficacy of HLA-matched platelet transfusions for patients with hypoproliferative thrombocytopenia: a systematic review. *Transfusion.* 2013;53(10):2230-2242.

217. Waters AH, Minchinton RM, Bell R, Ford JM, Lister TA. A cross-matching procedure for the selection of platelet donors for alloimmunized patients. *Br J Haematol.* 1981;48(1):59-68.

218. Wiita AP, Nambiar A. Longitudinal management with crossmatch-compatible platelets for refractory patients: alloimmunization, response to transfusion, and clinical outcomes (CME). *Transfusion.* 2012;52(10):2146-2154.

219. Kickler T, Braine HG, Piantadosi S, Ness PM, Herman JH, Rothko K. A randomized, placebo-controlled trial of intravenous gammaglobulin in alloimmunized thrombocytopenic patients. *Blood.* 1990;75(1):313-316.

220. Gardner FH, Helmer RE,III. Aminocaproic acid. Use in control of hemorrhage in patients with amegakaryocytic thrombocytopenia. *JAMA.* 1980;243(1):35-37.

221. Kalmadi S, Tiu R, Lowe C, Jin T, Kalaycio M. Epsilon aminocaproic acid reduces transfusion requirements in patients with thrombocytopenic hemorrhage. *Cancer.* 2006;107(1):136-140.

222. Gernsheimer TBBS, Triulzi DJ, Key NS, El Kassar N, Herren H, May S. Effects of tranexamic acid prophylaxis on bleeding outcomes in hematologic malignancy: the a-TREAT trial. *Blood.* 2020;136:1-2.

223. Dunstan RA, Simpson MB, Knowles RW, Rosse WF. The origin of ABH antigens on human platelets. *Blood.* 1985;65(3):615-619.

224. Kelton JG, Hamid C, Aker S, Blajchman MA. The amount of blood group A substance on platelets is proportional to the amount in the plasma. *Blood.* 1982;59(5):980-985.

225. Aster RH. New approaches to an old problem. Refractoriness to platelet transfusions. *Transfusion.* 1988;28(2):95-96.

226. Lee EJ, Schiffer CA. ABO compatibility can influence the results of platelet transfusion. Results of a randomized trial. *Transfusion.* 1989;29(5):384-389.

227. McManigal S, Sims KL. Intravascular hemolysis secondary to ABO incompatible platelet products. An underrecognized transfusion reaction. *Am J Clin Pathol.* 1999;111(2):202-206.

228. Josephson CD, Mullis NC, Van Demark C, Hillyer CD. Significant numbers of apheresis-derived group O platelet units have "high-titer" anti-A/A,B: implications for transfusion policy. *Transfusion.* 2004;44(6):805-808.

229. Shehata N, Tinmouth A, Naglie G, Freedman J, Wilson K. ABO-identical versus nonidentical platelet transfusion: a systematic review. *Transfusion.* 2009;49(11):2442-2453.

230. Solves P, Carpio N, Balaguer A, et al. Transfusion of ABO non-identical platelets does not influence the clinical outcome of patients undergoing autologous haematopoietic stem cell transplantation. *Blood Transfus.* 2015;13(3):411-416.

231. Henrichs KF, Howk N, Masel DS, et al. Providing ABO-identical platelets and cryoprecipitate to (almost) all patients: approach, logistics, and associated decreases in transfusion reaction and red cell alloimmunization incidence. *Transfusion.* 2012;52(3):635-640.

232. Cid J, Lozano M, Ziman A, et al. Low frequency of anti-D alloimmunization following D+ platelet transfusion: the Anti-D Alloimmunization after D-incompatible Platelet Transfusions (ADAPT) study. *Br J Haematol.* 2015;168(4):598-603.

233. O'Brien KL, Haspel RL, Uhl L. Anti-D alloimmunization after D-incompatible platelet transfusions: a 14-year single-institution retrospective review. *Transfusion.* 2014;54(3):650-654.

234. Murphy S, Gardner FH. Effect of storage temperature on maintenance of platelet viability--deleterious effect of refrigerated storage. *N Engl J Med.* 1969;280(20):1094-1098.

235. Reddoch KM, Pidcoke HF, Montgomery RK, et al. Hemostatic function of apheresis platelets stored at 4 degrees C and 22 degrees C. *Shock.* 2014;41 (suppl 1):54-61.

236. Strandenes G, Sivertsen J, Bjerkvig CK, et al. A pilot trial of platelets stored cold versus at room temperature for complex cardiothoracic surgery. *Anesthesiology.* 2020;133(6):1173-1183.

237. *Blood Transfusion Therapy: A Physician's Handbook,* 13th ed. AABB Press; 2020.

238. Wiviott SD, Trenk D, Frelinger AL, et al. Prasugrel compared with high loading- and maintenance-dose clopidogrel in patients with planned percutaneous coronary intervention: the Prasugrel in Comparison to Clopidogrel for Inhibition of Platelet Activation and Aggregation-Thrombolysis in Myocardial Infarction 44 trial. *Circulation.* 2007;116(25):2923-2932.

239. Holland LL, Brooks JP. Toward rational fresh frozen plasma transfusion: the effect of plasma transfusion on coagulation test results. *Am J Clin Pathol.* 2006;126(1):133-139.

240. Chowdary P, Saayman AG, Paulus U, Findlay GP, Collins PW. Efficacy of standard dose and 30 ml/kg fresh frozen plasma in correcting laboratory parameters of haemostasis in critically ill patients. *Br J Haematol.* 2004;125(1):69-73.

241. Murad MH, Stubbs JR, Gandhi MJ, et al. The effect of plasma transfusion on morbidity and mortality: a systematic review and meta-analysis. *Transfusion.* 2010;50(6):1370-1383.

242. Roback JD, Caldwell S, Carson J, et al. Evidence-based practice guidelines for plasma transfusion. *Transfusion.* 2010;50(6):1227-1239.

243. Goodnough LT, Shander A. How I treat warfarin-associated coagulopathy in patients with intracerebral hemorrhage. *Blood.* 2011;117(23):6091-6099.

244. Sarode R, Milling TJ, Jr, Refaai MA, et al. Efficacy and safety of a 4-factor prothrombin complex concentrate in patients on vitamin K antagonists presenting with major bleeding: a randomized, plasma-controlled, phase IIIb study. *Circulation.* 2013;128(11):1234-1243.

245. Abdel-Wahab OI, Healy B, Dzik WH. Effect of fresh-frozen plasma transfusion on prothrombin time and bleeding in patients with mild coagulation abnormalities. *Transfusion.* 2006;46(8):1279-1285.

246. Goodnough LT. Does plasma transfusion therapy have a role in clinical medicine? *Crit Care Med.* 2013;41(8):2041-2042.

247. Li G, Rachmale S, Kojicic M, et al. Incidence and transfusion risk factors for transfusion-associated circulatory overload among medical intensive care unit patients. *Transfusion.* 2011;51(2):338-343.

248. Shaz BH, Stowell SR, Hillyer CD. Transfusion-related acute lung injury: from bedside to bench and back. *Blood.* 2011;117(5):1463-1471.

249. Lin Y, Saw CL, Hannach B, Goldman M. Transfusion-related acute lung injury prevention measures and their impact at Canadian Blood Services. *Transfusion.* 2012;52(3):567-574.

250. Armand R, Hess JR. Treating coagulopathy in trauma patients. *Transfus Med Rev.* 2003;17(3):223-231.

251. Seheult JN, Triulzi DJ, Alarcon LH, Sperry JL, Murdock A, Yazer MH. Measurement of haemolysis markers following transfusion of uncrossmatched, low-titre, group O+ whole blood in civilian trauma patients: initial experience at a level 1 trauma centre. *Transfus Med.* 2017;27(1):30-35.

252. Seheult JN, Bahr M, Anto V, et al. Safety profile of uncrossmatched, cold-stored, low-titer, group O+ whole blood in civilian trauma patients. *Transfusion.* 2018;58(10):2280-2288.

253. Seheult JN, Anto V, Alarcon LH, Sperry JL, Triulzi DJ, Yazer MH. Clinical outcomes among low-titer group O whole blood recipients compared to recipients of conventional components in civilian trauma resuscitation. *Transfusion.* 2018;58(8):1838-1845.

254. Bodey GP, Buckley M, Sathe YS, Freireich EJ. Quantitative relationships between circulating leukocytes and infection in patients with acute leukemia. *Ann Intern Med.* 1966;64(2):328-340.

255. Crawford J, Ozer H, Stoller R, et al. Reduction by granulocyte colony-stimulating factor of fever and neutropenia induced by chemotherapy in patients with small-cell lung cancer. *N Engl J Med.* 1991;325(3):164-170.

256. Mikulska M, Averbuch D, Tissot F, et al. Fluoroquinolone prophylaxis in haematological cancer patients with neutropenia: ECIL critical appraisal of previous guidelines. *J Infect.* 2018;76(1):20-37.

257. Flowers CR, Seidenfeld J, Bow EJ, et al. Antimicrobial prophylaxis and outpatient management of fever and neutropenia in adults treated for malignancy: American Society of Clinical Oncology clinical practice guideline. *J Clin Oncol.* 2013;31(6):794-810.

258. Dale DC, Liles WC, Price TH. Renewed interest in granulocyte transfusion therapy. *Br J Haematol.* 1997;98(3):497-501.

259. Price TH, Boeckh M, Harrison RW, et al. Efficacy of transfusion with granulocytes from G-CSF/dexamethasone-treated donors in neutropenic patients with infection. *Blood.* 2015;126(18):2153-2161.

260. Estcourt LJ, Stanworth SJ, Hopewell S, Doree C, Trivella M, Massey E. Granulocyte transfusions for treating infections in people with neutropenia or neutrophil dysfunction. *Cochrane Database Syst Rev.* 2016;4:CD005339.

261. Mousset S, Hermann S, Klein SA, et al. Prophylactic and interventional granulocyte transfusions in patients with haematological malignancies and life-threatening infections during neutropenia. *Ann Hematol.* 2005;84(11):734-741.

262. Winston DJ, Ho WG, Howell CL, et al. Cytomegalovirus infections associated with leukocyte transfusions. *Ann Intern Med.* 1980;93(5):671-675.

263. Clift RA, Sanders JE, Thomas ED, Williams B, Buckner CD. Granulocyte transfusions for the prevention of infection in patients receiving bone-marrow transplants. *N Engl J Med.* 1978;298(19):1052-1057.

264. Ford JM, Cullen MH, Roberts MM, Brown LM, Oliver RT, Lister TA. Prophylactic granulocyte transfusions: results of a randomized controlled trial in patients with acute myelogenous leukemia. *Transfusion.* 1982;22(4):311-316.

265. Schiffer CA, Aisner J, Daly PA, Schimpff SC, Wiernik PH. Alloimmunization following prophylactic granulocyte transfusion. *Blood*. 1979;54(4):766-774.

266. Strauss RG, Connett JE, Gale RP, et al. A controlled trial of prophylactic granulocyte transfusions during initial induction chemotherapy for acute myelogenous leukemia. *N Engl J Med*. 1981;305(11):597-603.

267. Winston DJ, Ho WG, Young LS, Gale RP. Prophylactic granulocyte transfusions during human bone marrow transplantation. *Am J Med*. 1980;68(6):893-897.

268. Winston DJ, Ho WG, Gale RP. Prophylactic granulocyte transfusions during chemotherapy of acute nonlymphocytic leukemia. *Ann Intern Med*. 1981;94(5):616-622.

269. Atallah E, Schiffer CA. Granulocyte transfusion. *Curr Opin Hematol*. 2006;13(1):45-49.

270. Menitove JE, Abrams RA. Granulocyte transfusions in neutropenic patients. *Crit Rev Oncol Hematol*. 1987;7(1):89-113.

271. Bodey GP. Infection in cancer patients. A continuing association. *Am J Med*. 1986;81(1A):11-26.

272. Dale DC, Fauci AS, Guerry DI, Wolff SM. Comparison of agents producing a neutrophilic leukocytosis in man. Hydrocortisone, prednisone, endotoxin, and etiocholanolone. *J Clin Invest*. 1975;56(4):808-813.

273. Martino M, Fedele R, Massara E, Recchia AG, Irrera G, Morabito F. Long-term safety of granulocyte colony-stimulating factor in normal donors: is it all clear? *Expert Opin Biol Ther*. 2012;12(5):609-621.

274. Ikemoto J, Yoshihara S, Fujioka T, et al. Impact of the mobilization regimen and the harvesting technique on the granulocyte yield in healthy donors for granulocyte transfusion therapy. *Transfusion*. 2012;52(12):2646-2652.

275. Wright DG, Robichaud KJ, Pizzo PA, Deisseroth AB. Lethal pulmonary reactions associated with the combined use of amphotericin B and leukocyte transfusions. *N Engl J Med*. 1981;304(20):1185-1189.

276. Karp DD, Ervin TJ, Tuttle S, Gorgone BC, Lavin P, Yunis EJ. Pulmonary complications during granulocyte transfusions: incidence and clinical features. *Vox Sang*. 1982;42(2):57-61.

277. Dana BW, Durie BG, White RF, Huestis DW. Concomitant administration of granulocyte transfusions and amphotericin B in neutropenic patients: absence of significant pulmonary toxicity. *Blood*. 1981;57(1):90-94.

278. Hubel K, Dale DC, Liles WC. Granulocyte transfusion therapy: update on potential clinical applications. *Curr Opin Hematol*. 2001;8(3):161-164.

279. Delaney M, Wendel S, Bercovitz RS, et al. Transfusion reactions: prevention, diagnosis, and treatment. *Lancet*. 2016;388(10061):2825-2836.

280. Evers D, Middelburg RA, de Haas M, et al. Red-blood-cell alloimmunisation in relation to antigens' exposure and their immunogenicity: a cohort study. *Lancet Haematol*. 2016;3(6):e284-e292.

281. Vichinsky E, Neumayr L, Trimble S, et al. Transfusion complications in thalassemia patients: a report from the centers for disease control and prevention (CME). *Transfusion*. 2014;54(4):972-981. Quiz 971.

282. Yazdanbakhsh K, Ware RE, Noizat-Pirenne F. Red blood cell alloimmunization in sickle cell disease: pathophysiology, risk factors, and transfusion management. *Blood*. 2012;120(3):528-537.

283. Vichinsky EP, Earles A, Johnson RA, Hoag MS, Williams A, Lubin B. Alloimmunization in sickle cell anemia and transfusion of racially unmatched blood. *N Engl J Med*. 1990;322(23):1617-1621.

284. Vichinsky EP, Luban NL, Wright E, et al. Prospective RBC phenotype matching in a stroke-prevention trial in sickle cell anemia: a multicenter transfusion trial. *Transfusion*. 2001;41(9):1086-1092.

285. Overweg J, Engelfriet CP. Cytotoxic leucocyte iso-antibodies formed during the first pregnancy. *Vox Sang*. 1969;16(2):97-104.

286. Dutcher JP, Schiffer CA, Aisner J, Wiernik PH. Alloimmunization following platelet transfusion: the absence of a dose-response relationship. *Blood*. 1981;57(3):395-398.

287. Buetens O, Shirey RS, Goble-Lee M, et al. Prevalence of HLA antibodies in transfused patients with and without red cell antibodies. *Transfusion*. 2006;46(5):754-756.

288. McVerry BA, Machin SJ. Incidence of allo-immunization and allergic reactions to cryoprecipitate in haemophilia. *Vox Sang*. 1979;36(2):77-80.

289. Sandler SG, Mallory D, Malamut D, Eckrich R. IgA anaphylactic transfusion reactions. *Transfus Med Rev*. 1995;9(1):1-8.

290. Rivat L, Rivat C, Daveau M, Ropartz C. Comparative frequencies of anti-IgA antibodies among patients with anaphylactic transfusion reactions and among normal blood donors. *Clin Immunol Immunopathol*. 1977;7(3):340-348.

291. Beauregard P, Blajchman MA. Hemolytic and pseudo-hemolytic transfusion reactions: an overview of the hemolytic transfusion reactions and the clinical conditions that mimic them. *Transfus Med Rev*. 1994;8(3):184-199.

292. Sazama K. Reports of 355 transfusion-associated deaths: 1976 through 1985. *Transfusion*. 1990;30(7):583-590.

293. FDA. *Fatalities Reported to FDA Following Blood Collection and Transfusion Annual Summary for Fiscal Year* 2019. Accessed June 8, 2021. https://www.fda.gov/media/147628/download.

294. Pierce RN, Reich LM, Mayer K. Hemolysis following platelet transfusions from ABO-incompatible donors. *Transfusion*. 1985;25(1):60-62.

295. Lundberg WB, McGinniss MH. Hemolytic transfusion reaction due to anti-A. *Transfusion*. 1975;15(1):1-9.

296. Fontaine MJ, Mills AM, Weiss S, Hong WJ, Viele M, Goodnough LT. How we treat: risk mitigation for ABO-incompatible plasma in plateletpheresis products. *Transfusion*. 2012;52(10):2081-2085.

297. Chaplin H, Jr. The implication of red cell-bound complement in delayed hemolytic transfusion reaction. *Transfusion*. 1984;24(3):185-187.

298. Patten E, Reddi CR, Riglin H, Edwards J. Delayed hemolytic transfusion reaction caused by a primary immune response. *Transfusion*. 1982;22(3):248-250.

299. Ness PM, Shirey RS, Thoman SK, Buck SA. The differentiation of delayed serologic and delayed hemolytic transfusion reactions: incidence, long-term serologic findings, and clinical significance. *Transfusion*. 1990;30(8):688-693.

300. Goel R, Tobian AAR, Shaz BH. Noninfectious transfusion-associated adverse events and their mitigation strategies. *Blood*. 2019;133(17):1831-1839.

301. Brubaker DB. Clinical significance of white cell antibodies in febrile nonhemolytic transfusion reactions. *Transfusion*. 1990;30(8):733-737.

302. Davenport RD, Kunkel SL. Cytokine roles in hemolytic and nonhemolytic transfusion reactions. *Transfus Med Rev*. 1994;8(3):157-168.

303. Silliman CC, Ambruso DR, Boshkov LK. Transfusion-related acute lung injury. *Blood*. 2005;105(6):2266-2273.

304. Kleinman S, Caulfield T, Chan P, et al. Toward an understanding of transfusion-related acute lung injury: statement of a consensus panel. *Transfusion*. 2004;44(12):1774-1789.

305. Vlaar AP, Juffermans NP. Transfusion-related acute lung injury: a clinical review. *Lancet*. 2013;382(9896):984-994.

306. Chapman CE, Stainsby D, Jones H, et al. Ten years of hemovigilance reports of transfusion-related acute lung injury in the United Kingdom and the impact of preferential use of male donor plasma. *Transfusion*. 2009;49(3):440-452.

307. Vossoughi S, Gorlin J, Kessler DA, et al. Ten years of TRALI mitigation: measuring our progress. *Transfusion*. 2019;59(8):2567-2574.

308. Tobian AA, King KE, Ness PM. Transfusion premedications: a growing practice not based on evidence. *Transfusion*. 2007;47(6):1089-1096.

309. Oen K, Petty RE, Schroeder ML. Immunoglobulin A deficiency: genetic studies. *Tissue Antigens*. 1982;19(3):174-182.

310. Yap PL, Pryde EA, McClelland DB. IgA content of frozen-thawed-washed red blood cells and blood products measured by radioimmunoassay. *Transfusion*. 1982;22(1):36-38.

311. Vyas GN, Perkins HA. Letter: anti-IgA in blood donors. *Transfusion*. 1976;16(3):289-290.

312. Abramson N, Eisenberg PD, Aster RH. Post-transfusion purpura: immunologic aspects and therapy. *N Engl J Med*. 1974;291(22):1163-1166.

313. Pegels JG, Bruynes EC, Engelfriet CP, von dem Borne AE. Post-transfusion purpura: a serological and immunochemical study. *Br J Haematol*. 1981;49(4):521-530.

314. Hamblin TJ, Naorose Abidi SM, Nee PA, Copplestone A, Mufti GJ, Oscier DG. Successful treatment of post-transfusion purpura with high dose immunoglobulins after lack of response to plasma exchange. *Vox Sang*. 1985;49(2):164-167.

315. Scott EP, Moilan-Bergeland J, Dalmasso AP. Posttransfusion thrombocytopenia associated with passive transfusion of a platelet-specific antibody. *Transfusion*. 1988;28(1):73-76.

316. Vamvakas EC, Blajchman MA. Deleterious clinical effects of transfusion-associated immunomodulation: fact or fiction? *Blood*. 2001;97(5):1180-1195.

317. Vamvakas EC, Blajchman MA. Transfusion-related immunomodulation (TRIM): an update. *Blood Rev*. 2007;21(6):327-348.

318. Vamvakas EC. Meta-analysis of randomized controlled trials investigating the risk of postoperative infection in association with white blood cell-containing allogeneic blood transfusion: the effects of the type of transfused red blood cell product and surgical setting. *Transfus Med Rev*. 2002;16(4):304-314.

319. Vamvakas EC. Deleterious clinical effects of transfusion immunomodulation: proven beyond a reasonable doubt. *Transfusion*. 2006;46(3):492-494. Author reply 494-495.

320. Brubaker DB. Human posttransfusion graft-versus-host disease. *Vox Sang*. 1983;45(6):401-420.

321. Anderson KC, Weinstein HJ. Transfusion-associated graft-versus-host disease. *N Engl J Med*. 1990;323(5):315-321.

322. Petz LD, Calhoun L, Yam P, et al. Transfusion-associated graft-versus-host disease in immunocompetent patients: report of a fatal case associated with transfusion of blood from a second-degree relative, and a survey of predisposing factors. *Transfusion*. 1993;33(9):742-750.

323. Triulzi D, Duquesnoy R, Nichols L, et al. Fatal transfusion-associated graft-versus-host disease in an immunocompetent recipient of a volunteer unit of red cells. *Transfusion*. 2006;46(6):885-888.

324. Kopolovic I, Ostro J, Tsubota H, et al. A systematic review of transfusion-associated graft-versus-host disease. *Blood*. 2015;126(3):406-414.

325. Schroeder ML. Transfusion-associated graft-versus-host disease. *Br J Haematol*. 2002;117(2):275-287.

326. Bolton-Maggs PPD, Watt A, eds. *On Behalf of the Serious Hazards of Transfusion (SHOT) Steering Group. The 2015 Annual SHOT Report*. 2016. Accessed September 9, 2016 http://www.shotuk.org/wp-content/uploads/SHOT-2015-Annual-Report-Web-Edition-Final-bookmarked-1.pdf.

327. Lieberman L, Maskens C, Cserti-Gazdewich C, et al. A retrospective review of patient factors, transfusion practices, and outcomes in patients with transfusion-associated circulatory overload. *Transfus Med Rev*. 2013;27(4):206-212.

328. Luban NL. Massive transfusion in the neonate. *Transfus Med Rev*. 1995;9(3):200-214.

329. Cotton BA, Gunter OL, Isbell J, et al. Damage control hematology: the impact of a trauma exsanguination protocol on survival and blood product utilization. *J Trauma*. 2008;64(5):1177-1182. Discussion 1182-1173.

330. Zou S, Stramer SL, Dodd RY. Donor testing and risk: current prevalence, incidence, and residual risk of transfusion-transmissible agents in US allogeneic donations. *Transfus Med Rev*. 2012;26(2):119-128.

331. Glynn SA, Kleinman SH, Wright DJ, Busch MP, Study NRED. International application of the incidence rate/window period model. *Transfusion*. 2002;42(8):966-972.

332. Zou S, Dorsey KA, Notari EP, et al. Prevalence, incidence, and residual risk of human immunodeficiency virus and hepatitis C virus infections among United States blood donors since the introduction of nucleic acid testing. *Transfusion*. 2010;50(7):1495-1504.

Transfusion Medicine

333. Stramer SL, Glynn SA, Kleinman SH, et al. Detection of HIV-1 and HCV infections among antibody-negative blood donors by nucleic acid-amplification testing. *N Engl J Med.* 2004;351(8):760-768.

334. Busch MP, Glynn SA, Stramer SL, et al. A new strategy for estimating risks of transfusion-transmitted viral infections based on rates of detection of recently infected donors. *Transfusion.* 2005;45(2):254-264.

335. Aach RD, Kahn RA. Post-transfusion hepatitis: current perspectives. *Ann Intern Med.* 1980;92(4):539-546.

336. Prince AM, Brotman B, Grady GF, et al. Long-incubation post-transfusion hepatitis without serological evidence of exposure to hepatitis-B virus. *Lancet.* 1974;2(7875):241-246.

337. Choo QL, Kuo G, Weiner AJ, Overby LR, Bradley DW, Houghton M. Isolation of a cDNA clone derived from a blood-borne non-A, non-B viral hepatitis genome. *Science.* 1989;244(4902):359-362.

338. Kuo G, Choo QL, Alter HJ, et al. An assay for circulating antibodies to a major etiologic virus of human non-A, non-B hepatitis. *Science.* 1989;244(4902):362-364.

339. Stramer SL, Notari EP, Krysztof DE, Dodd RY. Hepatitis B virus testing by minipool nucleic acid testing: does it improve blood safety? *Transfusion.* 2013;53(10 Pt 2):2449-2458.

340. Hughes JA, Fontaine MJ, Gonzalez CL, Layon AG, Goodnough LT, Galel SA. Case report of a transfusion-associated hepatitis A infection. *Transfusion.* 2014;54(9):2202-2206.

341. Advisory Committee on Immunization P, Fiore AE, Wasley A, Bell BP. Prevention of hepatitis A through active or passive immunization: recommendations of the Advisory Committee on Immunization Practices (ACIP). *MMWR Recomm Rep.* 2006;55(RR-7):1-23.

342. *UDoHaHSHACoBSaA. Committee Recommendations.* June 2010. Washington, DC: HHS. Accessed January 12, 2018. https://www.hhs.gov/ohaidp/initiatives/blood-tissue-safety/advisory-committee/recommendations/index.html. In.

343. FDA Guidance for Industry. *Revised Recommendations for Reducing the Risk of Human Immunodeficiency Virus Transmission by Blood and Blood Products.* April 2020. Accessed July 2021. https://www.fda.gov/regulatory-information/search-fda-guidance-documents/revised-recommendations-reducing-risk-human-immunodeficiency-virus-transmission-blood-and-blood.

344. Pealer LN, Marfin AA, Petersen LR, et al. Transmission of West Nile virus through blood transfusion in the United States in 2002. *N Engl J Med.* 2003;349(13):1236-1245.

345. Busch MP, Caglioti S, Robertson EF, et al. Screening the blood supply for West Nile virus RNA by nucleic acid amplification testing. *N Engl J Med.* 2005;353(5):460-467.

346. Petersen LR, Jamieson DJ, Powers AM, Honein MA. Zika virus. *N Engl J Med.* 2016;374(16):1552-1563.

347. Goodnough LT, Marques MB. Zika virus and patient blood management. *Anesth Analg.* 2017;124(1):282-289.

348. *Information for blood establishments regarding FDA's determination that Zika virus is no longer a relevant transfusion-transmitted infection. Withdrawal of Guidance Titled "Revised Recommendations for Reducing the Risk of Zika Virus Transmission by Blood and Blood Components."* May 2021. Accessed July 2021. https://www.fda.gov/vaccines-blood-biologics/blood-blood-products/information-blood-establishments-regarding-fdas-determination-zika-virus-no-longer-relevant.

349. Mungai M, Tegtmeier G, Chamberland M, Parise M. Transfusion-transmitted malaria in the United States from 1963 through 1999. *N Engl J Med.* 2001;344(26):1973-1978.

350. FDA. *Revised Recommendations to Reduce the Risk of Transfusion-Transmitted Malaria.* Accessed July 2021. https://www.fda.gov/regulatory-information/search-fda-guidance-documents/revised-recommendations-reduce-risk-transfusion-transmitted-malaria. April 2020.

351. Moritz ED, Winton CS, Tonnetti L, et al. Screening for *Babesia microti* in the U.S. Blood supply. *N Engl J Med.* 2016;375(23):2236-2245.

352. Krause PJ, Spielman A, Telford SR,III, et al. Persistent parasitemia after acute babesiosis. *N Engl J Med.* 1998;339(3):160-165.

353. Herwaldt BL, Linden JV, Bosserman E, Young C, Olkowska D, Wilson M. Transfusion-associated babesiosis in the United States: a description of cases. *Ann Intern Med.* 2011;155(8):509-519.

354. Guidance For Industry. *Recommendations for Reducing the Risk of Transfusion-Transmitted Babesiosis;* May 2019. https://www.fda.gov/regulatory-information/search-fda-guidance-documents/recommendations-reducing-risk-transfusion-transmitted-babesiosis.

355. Kalina U, Bickhard H, Schulte S. Biochemical comparison of seven commercially available prothrombin complex concentrates. *Int J Clin Pract.* 2008;62(10):1614-1622.

356. Benjamin RJ, Stramer SL, Leiby DA, Dodd RY, Fearon M, Castro E. *Trypanosoma cruzi* infection in North America and Spain: evidence in support of transfusion transmission. *Transfusion.* 2012;52(9):1913-1921. quiz 1912.

357. Food and Drug Adminstration. *Guidance for Industry: Recommendations to Reduce the Possible Risk of Transmission of Creutzfeldt-Jakob Disease (CJD) and Variant Creutzfeldt-Jakob Disease (vCJD) by Blood and Blood Components.* August 2020. Accessed 18, 2021. https://www.fda.gov/regulatory-information/search-fda-guidance-documents/recommendations-reduce-possible-risk-transmission-creutzfeldt-jakob-disease-and-variant-creutzfeldt.

358. Stramer SL, Hollinger FB, Katz LM, et al. Emerging infectious disease agents and their potential threat to transfusion safety. *Transfusion.* 2009;49 (suppl 2):1S-29S.

359. AABB. *Fact Sheets Created or Update Post Publication of the Transfusion August 2009 Supplement.* Accessed July 18, 2021. https://www.aabb.org/regulatory-and-advocacy/regulatory-affairs/infectious-diseases/emerging-infectious-disease-agents/fact-sheets-created-or-updated-post-publication-of-the-transfusion-august-2009-supplement.

360. *CDC. COVID-19.* Accessed 23, 2021. https://www.cdc.gov/coronavirus/2019-ncov/index.html.

361. *Updated information for blood establishments regarding the COVID-19 pandemic and blood donation.* FDA. January 2021. Accessed 23, 2021. https://www.fda.gov/vaccines-blood-biologics/safety-availability-biologics/updated-information-blood-establishments-regarding-covid-19-pandemic-and-blood-donation.

362. Guidance For Industry. *Investigational COVID-19 Convalescent Plasma.* Accessed 23, 2021. https://www.fda.gov/regulatory-information/search-fda-guidance-documents/investigational-covid-19-convalescent-plasma. February 2021.

363. Joyner MJ, Bruno KA, Klassen SA, et al. Safety update: COVID-19 convalescent plasma in 20,000 hospitalized patients. *Mayo Clin Proc.* 2020;95(9):1888-1897.

364. Thompson MA, Henderson JP, Shah PK, et al. Association of convalescent plasma therapy with survival in patients with hematologic cancers and COVID-19. *JAMA Oncol.* 2021.

365. Group RC. Convalescent plasma in patients admitted to hospital with COVID-19 (RECOVERY): a randomised controlled, open-label, platform trial. *Lancet.* 2021;397(10289):2049-2059.

366. FDA. *In Brief: FDA Updates Emergency Use Authorization for COVID-19 Convalescent Plasma to Reflect New Data.* February 2021 Accessed 23, 2021. https://www.fda.gov/news-events/fda-brief/fda-brief-fda-updates-emergency-use-authorization-covid-19-convalescent-plasma-reflect-new-data.

367. Joyner MJ, Carter RE, Senefeld JW, et al. Convalescent plasma antibody levels and the risk of death from Covid-19. *N Engl J Med.* 2021;384(11):1015-1027.

368. Salazar E, Christensen PA, Graviss EA, et al. Treatment of coronavirus disease 2019 patients with convalescent plasma reveals a signal of significantly decreased mortality. *Am J Pathol.* 2020;190(11):2290-2303.

369. Simonovich VA, Burgos Pratx LD, Scibona P, et al. A randomized trial of convalescent plasma in Covid-19 severe pneumonia. *N Engl J Med.* 2021;384(7):619-629.

370. Piechotta V, Iannizzi C, Chai KL, et al. Convalescent plasma or hyperimmune immunoglobulin for people with COVID-19: a living systematic review. *Cochrane Database Syst Rev.* 2021;5:CD013600.

371. Libster R, Perez Marc G, Wappner D, et al. Early high-titer plasma therapy to prevent severe Covid-19 in older adults. *N Engl J Med.* 2021;384(7):610-618.

372. Guidance For Industry. Bacterial risk control strategies for blood collection establishments and transfusion services to enhance the safety and availability of platelets for transfusion. Accessed 19, 2021. https://www.fda.gov/regulatory-information/search-fda-guidance-documents/bacterial-risk-control-strategies-blood-collection-establishments-and-transfusion-services-enhance. December 2020.

373. Eder AF, Kennedy JM, Dy BA, et al. Limiting and detecting bacterial contamination of apheresis platelets: inlet-line diversion and increased culture volume improve component safety. *Transfusion.* 2009;49(8):1554-1563.

374. Dumont LJ, Kleinman S, Murphy JR, et al. Screening of single-donor apheresis platelets for bacterial contamination: the PASSPORT study results. *Transfusion.* 2010;50(3):589-599.

375. Hong H, Xiao W, Lazarus HM, Good CE, Maitta RW, Jacobs MR. Detection of septic transfusion reactions to platelet transfusions by active and passive surveillance. *Blood.* 2016;127(4):496-502.

376. Vamvakas EC, Blajchman MA. Transfusion-related mortality: the ongoing risks of allogeneic blood transfusion and the available strategies for their prevention. *Blood.* 2009;113(15):3406-3417.

377. Jacobs MR, Good CE, Lazarus HM, Yomtovian RA. Relationship between bacterial load, species virulence, and transfusion reaction with transfusion of bacterially contaminated platelets. *Clin Infect Dis.* 2008;46(8):1214-1220.

378. Jacobs MR, Smith D, Heaton WA, Zantek ND, Good CE, Group PGDS. Detection of bacterial contamination in prestorage culture-negative apheresis platelets on day of issue with the Pan Genera Detection test. *Transfusion.* 2011;51(12):2573-2582.

379. Tomasulo P, Su L. Is it time for new initiatives in the blood center and/or the hospital to reduce bacterial risk of platelets? *Transfusion.* 2011;51(12):2527-2533.

380. Eder AF, Kennedy JM, Dy BA, et al. Bacterial screening of apheresis platelets and the residual risk of septic transfusion reactions: the American Red Cross experience (2004-2006). *Transfusion.* 2007;47(7):1134-1142.

381. Eder AF, Goldman M. How do I investigate septic transfusion reactions and blood donors with culture-positive platelet donations? *Transfusion.* 2011;51(8):1662-1668.

382. Blajchman MA, Goldman M, Freedman JJ, Sher GD. Proceedings of a consensus conference: prevention of post-transfusion CMV in the era of universal leukoreduction. *Transfus Med Rev.* 2001;15(1):1-20.

383. Hahn G, Jores R, Mocarski ES. Cytomegalovirus remains latent in a common precursor of dendritic and myeloid cells. *Proc Natl Acad Sci U S A.* 1998;95(7):3937-3942.

384. Staras SA, Dollard SC, Radford KW, Flanders WD, Pass RF, Cannon MJ. Seroprevalence of cytomegalovirus infection in the United States, 1988-1994. *Clin Infect Dis.* 2006;43(9):1143-1151.

385. Preiksaitis JK, Brown L, McKenzie M. The risk of cytomegalovirus infection in seronegative transfusion recipients not receiving exogenous immunosuppression. *J Infect Dis.* 1988;157(3):523-529.

386. Bowden RA, Slichter SJ, Sayers M, et al. A comparison of filtered leukocyte-reduced and cytomegalovirus (CMV) seronegative blood products for the prevention of transfusion-associated CMV infection after marrow transplant. *Blood.* 1995;86(9):3598-3603.

387. Vamvakas EC. Is white blood cell reduction equivalent to antibody screening in preventing transmission of cytomegalovirus by transfusion? A review of the literature and meta-analysis. *Transfus Med Rev.* 2005;19(3):181-199.

388. Boeckh M, Nichols WG. The impact of cytomegalovirus serostatus of donor and recipient before hematopoietic stem cell transplantation in the era of antiviral prophylaxis and preemptive therapy. *Blood.* 2004;103(6):2003-2008.

389. Preiksaitis JK, Sandhu J, Strautman M. The risk of transfusion-acquired CMV infection in seronegative solid-organ transplant recipients receiving non-WBC-reduced blood components not screened for CMV antibody (1984 to 1996): experience at a single Canadian center. *Transfusion.* 2002;42(4):396-402.

390. Kaiser-Guignard J, Canellini G, Lion N, Abonnenc M, Osselaer JC, Tissot JD. The clinical and biological impact of new pathogen inactivation technologies on platelet concentrates. *Blood Rev.* 2014;28(6):235-241.

391. McCullough J. Pathogen inactivation: a new paradigm for preventing transfusion-transmitted infections. *Am J Clin Pathol.* 2007;128(6):945-955.

392. Dunbar NM, Beth B. Indications for therapeutic plasma exchange in thrombotic microangiopathies. *Hematol Am Soc Hematol Educ Program.* 2016;13(6):4-5.

393. Irsch J, Lin L. Pathogen inactivation of platelet and plasma blood components for transfusion using the INTERCEPT blood system. *Transfus Med Hemother.* 2011;38(1):19-31.

394. Marschner S, Goodrich R. Pathogen reduction technology treatment of platelets, plasma and whole blood using Riboflavin and UV light. *Transfus Med Hemother.* 2011;38(1):8-18.

395. Padmanabhan A, Connelly-Smith L, Aqui N, et al. Guidelines on the use of therapeutic apheresis in clinical practice—evidence-based approach from the writing committee of the American Society for Apheresis: the eighth special issue. *J Clin Apher.* 2019;34(3):171-354.

396. Plasma Exchange/Sandoglobulin Guillain-Barre Syndrome Trial Group. Randomised trial of plasma exchange, intravenous immunoglobulin, and combined treatments in Guillain-Barre syndrome. *Lancet.* 1997;349(9047):225-230.

397. Cheng BC, Chang WN, Chen JB, et al. Long-term prognosis for Guillain-Barre syndrome: evaluation of prognostic factors and clinical experience of automated double filtration plasmapheresis. *J Clin Apher.* 2003;18(4):175-180.

398. Weinstein R. Therapeutic apheresis in neurological disorders. *J Clin Apher.* 2000;15(1-2):74-128.

399. Levy JB, Pusey CD. Still a role for plasma exchange in rapidly progressive glomerulonephritis? *J Nephrol.* 1997;10(1):7-13.

400. Rock G, Shumak KH, Sutton DM, Buskard NA, Nair RC. Cryosupernatant as replacement fluid for plasma exchange in thrombotic thrombocytopenic purpura. Members of the Canadian Apheresis Group. *Br J Haematol.* 1996;94(2):383-386.

401. Moake JL. Thrombotic thrombocytopenic purpura and the hemolytic uremic syndrome. *Arch Pathol Lab Med.* 2002;126(11):1430-1433.

402. Rock GA, Shumak KH, Buskard NA, et al. Comparison of plasma exchange with plasma infusion in the treatment of thrombotic thrombocytopenic purpura. Canadian Apheresis Study Group. *N Engl J Med.* 1991;325(6):393-397.

403. Bukowski RM, King JW, Hewlett JS. Plasmapheresis in the treatment of thrombotic thrombocytopenic purpura. *Blood.* 1977;50(3):413-417.

404. Matzdorff AC. Thrombotic thrombocytopenic purpura. *N Engl J Med.* 2006;355(6):630. Author reply 630.

405. Derksen RH, Schuurman HJ, Meyling FH, Struyvenberg A, Kater L. The efficacy of plasma exchange in the removal of plasma components. *J Lab Clin Med.* 1984;104(3):346-354.

406. Volkin RL, Starz TW, Winkelstein A, et al. Changes in coagulation factors, complement, immunoglobulins, and immune complex concentrations with plasma exchange. *Transfusion.* 1982;22(1):54-58.

407. Grima KM. Therapeutic apheresis in hematological and oncological diseases. *J Clin Apher.* 2000;15(1-2):28-52.

408. Lichtman MA, Rowe JM. Hyperleukocytic leukemias: rheological, clinical, and therapeutic considerations. *Blood.* 1982;60(2):279-283.

409. Goldfinger D, Thompson R, Lowe C, Kurz L, Belkin G. Long-term plateletpheresis in the management of primary thrombocytosis. *Transfusion.* 1979;19(3):336-338.

410. Sachais BS, Katz J, Ross J, Rader DJ. Long-term effects of LDL apheresis in patients with severe hypercholesterolemia. *J Clin Apher.* 2005;20(4):252-255.

411. McLeod BC, Sniecinski I, Ciavarella D, et al. Frequency of immediate adverse effects associated with therapeutic apheresis. *Transfusion.* 1999;39(3):282-288.

412. Chirnside A, Urbaniak SJ, Prowse CV, Keller AJ. Coagulation abnormalities following intensive plasma exchange on the cell separator. II. Effects on factors I, II, V, VII, VIII, IX, X and antithrombin III. *Br J Haematol.* 1981;48(4):627-634.

413. Huestis DW. Mortality in therapeutic haemapheresis. *Lancet.* 1983;1(8332):1043.

Section 1 ▪ INTRODUCTION

Chapter 24 ▪ Anemia: General Considerations

ROBERT T. MEANS JR. • BERTIL GLADER

INTRODUCTION

This introductory chapter focuses on the general concepts of anemia, the classification of the most common types of anemia, the approach to patients with hemolysis, and the assessment of posthemorrhagic anemia. Anemia, one of the most common findings in clinical medicine, rarely is a disease by itself. Most commonly, it is a sign of an acquired or a genetic abnormality. The various medical conditions that lead to anemia encompass the full spectrum of human disease.

DEFINITION OF ANEMIA

Red blood cells (RBCs) circulate in the peripheral blood for 100 to 120 days, and approximately 1% of the body's RBCs are removed and replaced each day. Senescent RBCs are removed from the circulation by macrophages in the spleen, liver, and bone marrow (Chapter 6). An erythropoietic feedback loop ensures that the total red cell mass remains constant. Reduced RBC mass results from loss of RBCs from the circulation at a rate greater than their production: this may reflect increased RBC destruction, decreased RBC production, or both.

Anemia is functionally defined as an insufficient RBC mass to deliver optimal oxygen to peripheral tissues. For practical purposes, any of the three concentration measurements performed on whole blood can be used to establish the presence of anemia: the hemoglobin (Hb) concentration, typically expressed as grams Hb per deciliter (g/dL) or as grams per liter in Systeme Internationale (SI) units; the hematocrit (Hct; also called the *packed cell volume [PCV]* or *volume of packed red blood cells [vPRC]*), which represents the proportion of blood volume comprising RBCs and expressed as a percentage or as a decimal (SI); and the RBC concentration in cells per microliter (10^6/μL) or per liter (10^{12}/L; SI).

In the past, these parameters were measured using manual physical and chemical techniques. The term "hematocrit" originally referred to the graduated tube in which the vPRC was measured following centrifugation. Both the term and the parameter came into general usage after Maxwell Wintrobe designed a novel tube that allowed highly reproducible results.[1,2] Now these parameters are determined by electronic cell counters and Hb analyzers (Chapter 1). In most of the current analyzers, RBC concentration, Hb concentration, and mean corpuscular volume (MCV in fL) are directly measured. These measured values are used to calculate the Hct, mean corpuscular hemoglobin (MCH), and mean corpuscular hemoglobin concentration (MCHC):

$$MCV = Hct(L/L) \times 1000/\text{red cell count}(10^{12}/L)$$

Many physicians prefer to define anemia using the Hb concentration, although for practical purposes the Hct is comparably reliable. The electronic counters also generate an index of red cell size, the red cell distribution width (RDW; *Figure 24.1*). The RDW is a quantitative measure of the variation in red cell size, and the higher the values, the more heterogeneous the RBC population size. The mean normal Hb and Hct values and the lower limits of the normal ranges of these parameters depend on the age and gender of subjects, as well as their altitude of residence.

Anemia in Adults

Normal values for Hb and Hct are based on population surveys. The 37,489-person sample studied during the third National Health and Nutrition Examination Survey (NHANES III), 1988 to 1994, was selected statistically as representative of the entire population of the United States.[3] Age, gender, and race as well as geographic and socioeconomic factors were factored into the selection process. In adult subjects (age 15-59 years), the lower limit of normal (defined by the range representing 95% of the standard population) was 13.2 g/dL in men and 11.7 g/dL in women (*Figure 24.2*). Values for African-American subjects were approximately 0.5 to 1.0 g/dL lower than those of Caucasian subjects. Consistent with these observations, the World Health Organization (WHO) defines the lower limit of normal for Hb concentration at sea level to be 12.0 g/dL in women and 13.0 g/dL in men.[4]

Hemoglobin Values in the Elderly

Anemia is a common condition in the older population. In a community-dwelling American population of individuals over 65 years, 8.5% have a hemoglobin concentration meeting the WHO definition of anemia.[5] Other investigators have confirmed that the prevalence of anemia rises steadily with age, increasing from approximately 10% in individuals 65 years and older to 20% in individuals over 85 years.[6] It is a significant predictor of morbidity, mortality, and performance status in the elderly, whether considered as a general risk factor or in the setting of a specific clinical circumstance, such as heart failure.[7] Although a majority of cases reflect clinical conditions such as iron deficiency and B_{12} or folate deficiency, the decline in testosterone production in male aging,[8] and the impact on erythropoietin (Epo) production of the routine decline in creatinine clearance with advancing age,[7] the etiology of a significant proportion of these anemias cannot be readily explained.[6] Studies of mechanisms of the development of otherwise unexplained anemia in the aging population have suggested the involvement of a number of possible mechanisms, from an increased incidence of underlying diseases that may be associated with cytokine activation and the anemia of chronic disease[9,10] to changes in the hematopoietic reserve,[11,12] or even in the characteristics of hematopoietic progenitors themselves.[13] Taken together, slightly lower limits of normal Hb concentration may be applicable in evaluating the elderly. **However, the too-easy acceptance of mild anemia as a physiologic phenomenon in the elderly runs the risk of ignoring a potentially valuable, early clue to an important underlying disorder.**

Hemoglobin Values in Infants and Children

At the other extreme of life, the definition of anemia in infancy and childhood is different from that in adults. The lower limit of normal

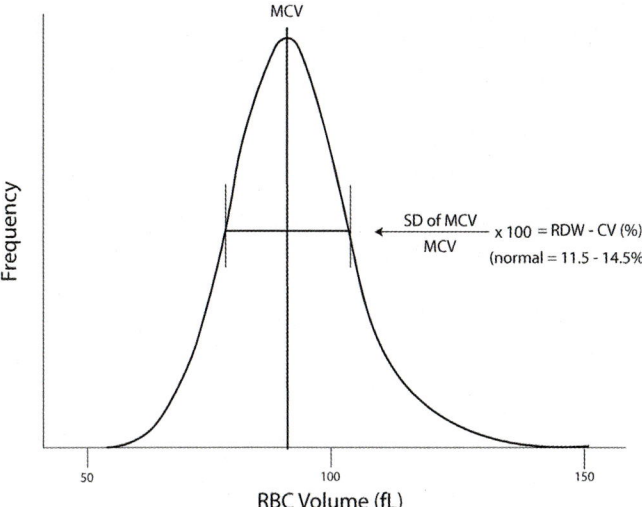

FIGURE 24.1 Frequency distribution curve of erythrocyte volume. Red blood cells (RBCs) are normally distributed about a mean cell volume (MCV) of 90 fL. Red blood cell distribution width (RDW-CV) is a measure of the range of variation of RBC volume that is reported as part of a standard complete blood count. Normal reference range of RDW-CV in human RBCs is 11.5% to 14.5%. A change in RDW is useful in evaluating the cause of different anemias.

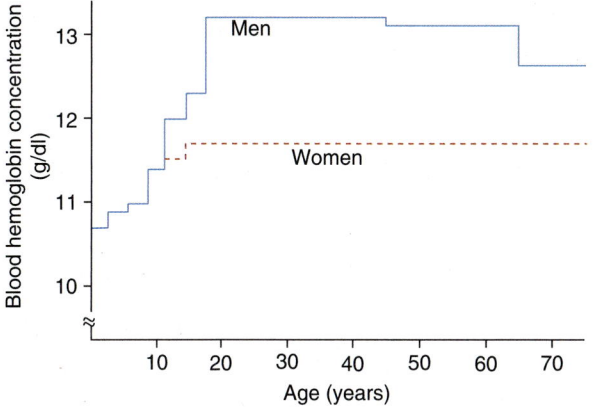

FIGURE 24.2 The lower limit of normal blood hemoglobin concentration in men and women of various ages. Values were calculated from a sample of 11,547 subjects selected to represent the population of the United States. Subjects with iron deficiency, those who were pregnant, or those who had an abnormal hemoglobin value were excluded from the sample. (Data from Dallman PR, Yip R, Johnson C. Prevalence and causes of anemia in the United States, 1976 to 1980. *Am J Clin Nutr.* 1984;39(3):437-445.)

Hb concentration at birth is 14 g/dL, and this decreases to 11 g/dL by 1 year of age. This Hb decrement, referred to as the *physiologic anemia of infancy*, occurs as part of the normal physiologic adaptation from the relatively hypoxic intrauterine existence to the well-oxygenated extrauterine environment (Chapter 45). Also, as fetal erythropoiesis is replaced, the MCV decreases from birth (100-130 fL) to 1 year of age (70-85 fL).

Even after the first year of life, normal childhood Hb and MCV values remain considerably lower than those occurring in adolescents and adults (*Table 24.1*). From the NHANES II study, the lower limit of normal Hb concentration in both male and female children, aged 1 to 2 years, was 10.7 g/dL, and the value rose with advancing age until adult levels were reached at age 15 to 18 years.

There has been no completely satisfactory explanation for these differences in normal Hb values of children and adults, but it is not due to nutritional deficiencies. It has been demonstrated that serum inorganic phosphate is 50% higher in children than in adults, and this

Table 24.1. Red Blood Cell Characteristics in Childhood

Age	Lowest Normal Hb (g/dL)	Normal Red Blood Cell Size Mean Corpuscular Volume (fL)	Fetal Hb (%)
Birth	14.0	100-130	55-90
1 mo	12.0	90-110	50-80
2 mo	10.5	80-100	30-55
3-6 mo	10.5	75-90	5-25
6 mo-1 y	11.0	70-85	<5
1-4 y	11.0	70-85	<1
4 y-puberty	11.5	75-100	<1
Adult female	12.0	80-100	<1
Adult male	13.0	80-100	<1

Abbreviation: Hb, hemoglobin.

hyperphosphatemia is associated with elevated erythrocyte adenosine triphosphate and 2,3-diphosphoglycerate content. As a result of these changes in erythrocyte organic phosphates, hemoglobin oxygen affinity is decreased in children compared with that in adults. On this basis, it has been postulated that lower Hb values in children may be due to altered Hb-oxygen affinity and thereby represent a *physiologic anemia of childhood*.[14] At puberty, the Hb concentration in children reaches the same levels seen in adults. The higher Hb levels in males presumably are a reflection of the effects of androgens on erythropoiesis.

Limitations in the Use of Hb Concentration, Hct, and RBC Measurements in Defining Anemia

For practical purposes, the blood Hb and Hct determinations are equally useful in assessing for anemia in most patients, but there are limitations that must be recognized:

1. Hb and Hct changes may reflect altered plasma volume, not a change in RBC mass (*Table 24.2*). In pregnancy, for example, the plasma volume increases, thereby decreasing the Hb concentration, although, in fact, total RBC mass actually is increased, but to a lesser degree than the plasma volume (Chapter 43). Similarly, individuals with massive splenomegaly may have some anemia because of hypersplenism, but the degree of anemia may appear more severe because of an increased plasma volume. Conversely, burn patients lose plasma through the injured skin, leaving Hb and Hct concentrated at a higher level. Other causes of dehydration with depletion of intravascular space also produce a spuriously high Hb concentration. In chronically ill patients with a reduced red cell mass, the magnitude of anemia may be masked by an associated contraction of the plasma volume.[15]

2. Another consideration is that Hb and Hct changes may reflect underlying physiologic conditions with different oxygen needs. For example, chronically hypoxemic subjects, such as individuals who live at high altitudes or patients with a right-to-left cardiac shunt, typically have erythrocytosis with elevated Hb/Hct levels. A normal Hb/Hct level in such a patient actually may represent anemia by the functional criterion of not meeting tissue oxygen requirements adequately.

3. Some abnormal Hb variants have an altered ability to bind and release oxygen, and this can be associated with changes in Hb concentration (Chapter 36).

4. Acute blood loss is another example of the problem of denoting anemia by the Hb concentration or Hct. Immediately after loss of a liter of blood, the Hb concentration/Hct is unchanged, because the initial response to acute hemorrhage is vasoconstriction. The shift of fluid from extravascular to intravascular space, and thus the

Table 24.2. Conditions Associated With Discordance Between Hemoglobin Concentration and Red Cell Mass

Increase in plasma volume relative to RBC mass (Hb disproportionately low)
Hydremia of pregnancy
Congestive splenomegaly
Recumbency (vs. upright)
Decrease in plasma volume relative to RBC mass (Hb high, normal, or low; but high relative to RBC mass)
Dehydration
Protracted diarrhea (especially in infants)
Peritoneal dialysis with hypertonic solutions
Diabetic acidosis
Diabetes insipidus with restricted fluid intake
Burn patients
Stress erythrocytosis, spurious polycythemia
Decrease in plasma volume and RBC mass (Hb normal, RBC mass low)
Acute blood loss
Chronic disease

Abbreviations: Hb, hemoglobin; RBC, red blood cell.

decrease in Hb concentration and Hct, does not begin for 6 h, and can continue for 48 to 72 h. Reticulocytosis occurs after 24 to 48 h.

5. Impaired partial synthesis of one globin chain, as in thalassemia trait, may be reflected in a low Hb (10 g/dL) and a high RBC count (6.5 million/μL), thus giving anemia by one measure (Hb) and erythrocytosis by another (RBC). This demonstrates why the RBC count is the least reliable and least commonly used indicator of anemia.

In addition to the issues listed, changes in posture also have effects on red cell concentration that can influence Hb and Hct measurements. When normal individuals assume a recumbent position, the Hct falls an average 7% (range, 4%-10%) within 1 h.[16] When the upright position is resumed, the Hct increases by a similar amount within 15 min. These changes have been attributed to alterations in plasma volume as fluid moves between the circulation and the extravascular spaces in the lower limbs because of hydrostatic forces. Hb concentrations and Hct exhibit diurnal variation and are highest in the morning, decreasing slightly (usually <0.5 Hb g/dL) over the course of the day. This is attributed to overnight volume depletion and not to alterations in erythropoiesis.[17]

CLINICAL EFFECTS OF ANEMIA

Patients with anemia usually seek medical attention because of decreased work or exercise tolerance, shortness of breath, palpitations, or other signs of cardiorespiratory adjustments to anemia. They may be asymptomatic, but their friends or family may note pallor. It is not uncommon that anemia in a child is first recognized by a visiting relative, the process sometimes occurring so slowly as to not be noted by parents or other immediate family members.

Cardiovascular and Pulmonary Features of Anemia

The clinical manifestations of anemia depend on the magnitude and rate of reduction in the oxygen-carrying capacity of the blood, the ability of the cardiovascular and pulmonary systems to compensate for the anemia, and the associated features of the underlying disorder that resulted in the development of anemia. The Hb concentration is not the only determinant of observed symptoms. Coexistent cardiovascular or pulmonary disease, particularly in older individuals, may exaggerate

the symptoms associated with a degree of anemia that would be well tolerated under other circumstances.

If the anemia has been insidious in onset and there is no cardiopulmonary disease, the patient's adjustment may be so effective that the blood Hb concentration may fall to 8 g/dL or even lower before the patient experiences enough symptoms to appreciate the situation.[18] In cases of iron deficiency anemia, pernicious anemia, or other types of slowly developing anemia, Hb concentrations may reach levels of 6 g/dL or lower before patients are motivated to seek medical attention.[19] This is particularly true in children where no limitations of physical activity may be apparent despite the existence of very severe anemia.[20] The physiologic adjustments that take place with a slowly falling red cell mass chiefly involve the cardiovascular system and changes in the Hb-oxygen dissociation curve.

In many patients, respiratory and circulatory symptoms are noticeable only after exertion. However, when anemia is sufficiently severe, dyspnea and awareness of vigorous or rapid heart action may be noted even at rest. When anemia develops rapidly, shortness of breath, tachycardia, dizziness or faintness (particularly upon arising from a sitting or recumbent posture), and extreme fatigue are prominent. In chronic anemia, only moderate dyspnea or palpitation may occur; but in some patients, congestive heart failure associated with high cardiac output,[21] angina pectoris,[22] or intermittent claudication can be the presenting manifestation. In patients with severe chronic anemia, tachycardia and postural hypotension may not be present because the total blood volume actually may be increased due to an expanded plasma volume. In the elderly particularly, cardiovascular adaptation to anemia is predominantly by increasing stroke volume rather than by heart rate.[23] In these cases, blood transfusion may precipitate congestive heart failure by aggravating an already expanded blood volume. Concern about this possibility should not preclude expansion of the blood's oxygen-carrying capacity by transfusion if necessary; but the judicious use of diuretics in the peritransfusion period should be considered in patients with clinical signs of volume overload.

Heart murmurs are a common cardiac sign associated with anemia. They usually are systolic and best heard in the pulmonic area.[24] Often, they are moderate in intensity, and at times may be rough in quality and raise suspicion of organic valvular heart disease. In a study from Bosnia, 25% of the heart murmurs investigated in a pediatric cardiology clinic were attributable to anemia and resolved with its correction.[25]

Pallor

Pallor is a sign of anemia, but many factors other than Hb concentration affect skin color. These include the degree of dilation of peripheral vessels, the extent of pigmentation, and the fluid content of the subcutaneous tissues. Some people routinely have pale-appearing skin without being anemic. Patients with myxedema may manifest pallor without anemia. In simple vasovagal syncope, pallor results from cutaneous vasoconstriction and is not a sign of anemia. Jaundice, cyanosis, individual skin pigmentation, and dilation of the peripheral vessels all can mask the pallor of anemia.

The pallor associated with anemia is best detected in the mucous membranes of the mouth and pharynx, the conjunctivae, the lips, and the nail beds. In the hands, the skin of the palms first becomes pale, but the creases may retain their usual pink color until the Hb concentration is less than 7 g/dL.

A distinctly sallow color implies chronic anemia. A lemon-yellow pallor suggests pernicious anemia, but it is observed only when the condition is well advanced. Definite pallor associated with mild scleral and cutaneous icterus suggests hemolytic anemia. Marked pallor associated with petechiae or ecchymoses suggests more generalized bone marrow failure due to acute leukemia, aplasia, or myelodysplastic syndromes (MDSs).

Skin and Mucosal Changes

Other changes in the integument occur with anemia. Thinning, loss of luster, and early graying of the hair may occur, the last especially in patients with pernicious anemia, in whom it may precede the development of anemia. Alopecia in patients with pernicious anemia may be autoimmune in origin.[26] The nails may lose their luster, become brittle, and break easily. This finding is especially noticeable in chronic iron deficiency anemia,[27] in which the nails may actually become concave instead of convex. Chronic leg ulcers may occur, especially in patients with sickle cell anemia but occasionally in patients with other hemolytic anemias. Glossitis occurs in association with pernicious anemia. When nutritional deficiency is associated with anemia, symmetric dermatitis may develop, fissures may be present at the angles of the mouth, glossitis may occur, and erythematous lesions on the face, neck, hands, or elbows may be found.

Neuromuscular Features

Headache, vertigo, tinnitus, faintness, scotomata, lack of mental concentration, drowsiness, restlessness, and muscular weakness are common symptoms of severe anemia. Paresthesias are common in pernicious anemia and may be associated with other symptoms and signs of peripheral neuropathy, and more especially with combined system disease.

Ophthalmologic Findings

A variety of ophthalmologic findings have been observed in anemic patients.[28] Approximately 20% of such patients have flame-shaped hemorrhages, hard exudates, cottonwool spots, or tortuous retinal veins. The hemorrhages occur even in the absence of coexisting thrombocytopenia. Papilledema related solely to anemia has been described,[29] and it clears when the anemia disappears.

Gastrointestinal Changes

Gastrointestinal symptoms are common in anemic patients. Some are manifestations of the underlying disorder (e.g., hiatal hernia, duodenal ulcer, gastric carcinoma, or inflammatory bowel disease); others may be a consequence of the anemic condition, whatever its cause. Glossitis and atrophy of tongue papillae commonly occur in pernicious anemia and less often in iron deficiency anemia. Painful, ulcerative, and necrotic lesions in the mouth and pharynx occur in aplastic anemia and in acute leukemia, usually reflecting the neutropenia accompanying these conditions. Dysphagia may occur in chronic iron deficiency anemia.

EVALUATION AND CLASSIFICATION OF ANEMIA

History and Physical Examination

All aspects of the history and clinical examination are important. The duration of the symptoms and their onset, whether insidious or acute, should be established. **It is very helpful to know the most recent date at which a routine hematologic examination was normal**.

The family history is most useful for increasing suspicion of hereditary hemolytic diseases, hereditary bleeding disorders, and congenital vascular abnormalities such as hereditary hemorrhagic telangiectasias. Key clues are histories of bleeding, jaundice, gallstones at an early age, and splenectomy not related to trauma (see "Approach to Hemolysis").

The patient's occupation, household customs, and hobbies must be ascertained because certain drugs, solvents, and other chemicals may produce hemolytic anemia or aplastic anemia, as well as granulocytopenia and thrombocytopenia. Also, social habits (alcohol use), travel history (to areas endemic for malaria or other high-risk infections), and drug history are each important in ascertaining the underlying etiology.

The dietary history is critical to the analysis, and questions regarding the diet must be specific in the hope of obtaining quantitative information. Very young children, those who obtain the bulk of their nutrition from cow's milk (very low in iron), are at risk for iron deficiency anemia. Changes in weight are important in both adults and children. Formerly obese individuals who have undergone bariatric surgery and other individuals who have undergone gastric resection are at risk for anemia from iron, copper, and other nutrient deficiencies.[30]

The patient should be questioned about early graying of the hair, burning sensations of the tongue, skin changes, sores about the angles of the mouth, and discomfort and brittleness of the fingernails, which are symptoms of anemias caused by deficiency of specific nutrients.

Change in stool habits may be an important clue to neoplasms of the colon and rectum underlying the anemia. The significance of tarry stools often is not appreciated by patients, and specific inquiry is necessary. The amount of blood lost from hemorrhoids may be overlooked or overestimated. In men, occult blood loss most often is from the gastrointestinal tract.

In women, additional important information includes an appraisal of the amount of blood lost during menstruation. Data about number of pads or tampons used and the presence or absence of clots should be obtained. The average amount of blood normally lost per period is approximately 50 mL, representing roughly 25 mg of elemental iron. Menstrual flow is considered excessive if more than 12 pads are used each period, if there are more than 2 days of heavy bleeding per period, if clots are passed after the first day, or if the period duration exceeds 7 days. The number of pregnancies and abortions and the interval since the most recent of these are also important, for each represents significant iron loss.

The presence or absence of fever must be noted; its presence suggests infection, lymphoma, and other neoplasm or collagen vascular disease. Paresthesias and difficulty in walking suggest pernicious anemia. Abnormal color of the urine, suggesting blood or Hb, may signify urinary tract disease or hematologic problems. Bilirubin is not detected in the urine of people with uncomplicated hemolytic anemia ("acholuric jaundice"), but a darker than normal color may result from the increased excretion of urobilinogen and its conversion to urobilin.

Bruises, ecchymoses, and petechiae are other important points in the history. Their presence indicates that the disorder-producing anemia may also involve platelets or the liver. Alternatively, the anemia itself may be the consequence of blood loss resulting from a disorder of hemostasis.

In all instances, the presence or absence of symptoms suggestive of an underlying disease such as chronic renal disease, liver disease, chronic infection, endocrinopathy, or malignancy must be explored. Anemia can be the presenting feature of many of these disorders.

The physical examination can provide further clues to the cause of anemia. Scleral icterus suggests the presence of hemolytic anemia or ineffective erythropoiesis. Sternal tenderness near the middle or lower third of the sternum, of which the patient may have been unaware, may represent acute expansion of hematopoietic marrow. Palpation of the liver and spleen and a systematic check for lymphadenopathy can provide clues to infection, lymphoma, leukemia, or metastatic carcinoma.

In the absence of a strongly suspected etiology (iron deficiency in an otherwise healthy young woman, for example), the initial patient evaluation should include a urinalysis. Even when the color of the urine does not suggest blood, the routine urinalysis should be tested for occult blood. A positive reaction may be due to hematuria, hemoglobinuria, or even myoglobinuria. Hematuria may be differentiated from the other conditions by finding RBCs on microscopic examination of the urine, or by centrifuging a fresh urine specimen, thereby clearing the bloody color from the supernatant and depositing the RBCs in the bottom of the tube. Hematuria reflects disease of the kidneys or urinary tract. Sickle cell trait may be accompanied by microscopic hematuria. Hemoglobinuria implies intravascular hemolysis.

Evaluation of Basic Hematology Laboratory Data

To identify the cause of anemia, information from the medical history and physical examination must be integrated with some key laboratory tests. There is no one simple classification of anemia. A useful approach entails asking several questions, outlined in the following sections (*Figure 24.3*).

Disorders of Red Blood Cells

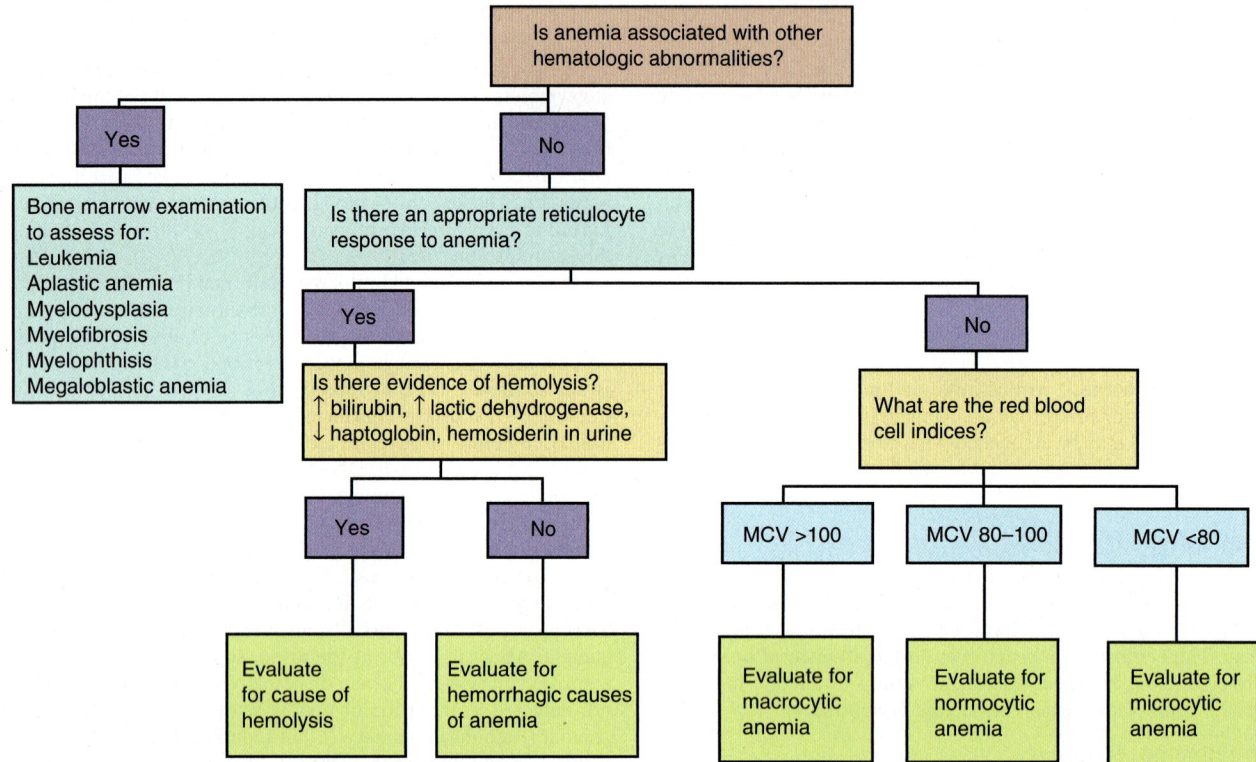

FIGURE 24.3 **Questions to ask in the initial evaluation of anemia.** ↑, increased; ↓, decreased; MCV, mean corpuscular volume (fL).

Is Anemia Associated With Other Hematologic Abnormalities?

Specifically, is the anemia associated with thrombocytopenia or abnormalities in white blood cell numbers or the presence of abnormal leukocytes? If the answer to this question is yes, consideration must be given to the possibility of bone marrow failure due to aplastic anemia, leukemia, or other malignant marrow disease. Alternatively, pancytopenia can be secondary to peripheral destruction or sequestration of cells as in hypersplenism. In most cases, these disorders can be differentiated by careful review of screening hematologic studies and close attention to the medical history and physical examination.

Is There an Appropriate Reticulocyte Response to Anemia?

The number of erythrocytes in the circulation at a given time is the result of a dynamic equilibrium between the delivery of red cells into the circulation on the one hand and their destruction or loss from the circulation on the other. Each day, approximately 1% of the RBC pool is replaced by young erythrocytes released from the marrow. The homeostatic mechanisms of the body bring about recovery from anemia by accelerating erythropoiesis, and this response of the normal marrow is brought about through the release of Epo. At maximum stimulation, the bone marrow is capable of producing erythrocytes at six to eight times the normal rate.

The reticulocyte count provides an initial assessment of whether the cause of anemia is due to impaired RBC production or due to increased loss in the peripheral circulation (e.g., blood loss, hemolysis) (*Figure 24.3*). Previously, the reticulocyte count was measured by microscopic examination of a smear prepared from fresh blood stained with a supravital stain, such as new methylene blue. The normal reticulocyte count by light microscopy is 0.5% to 1.5% of the total red cells. Nowadays, automated methods based on flow cytometry have become widely utilized to measure the reticulocyte count. Automated methods count a larger number of cells and exhibit a greater degree of reproducibility.[31]

In the presence of anemia, the reticulocyte count must be corrected because of the reduced number of RBCs in an anemic patient. An

Table 24.3. Methods of Correcting the Reticulocyte Count for the Degree of Anemia

Reticulocyte count = % reticulocytes in RBC population
Corrected reticulocyte count = % reticulocytes × (patient Hct/45)
Reticulocyte production index = Corrected reticulocyte count ÷ maturation time in peripheral blood in days[a]
(Normal values of all the above-mentioned 0.5% – 1.5%)
Absolute reticulocyte count = % reticulocytes × RBC count/L(^{3})
(Normal values for the absolute reticulocyte count are from 25 to 75 × 10^9/L; values <100 × 10^9/L indicate an inappropriately low erythropoietic response to anemia)

[a]Reticulocyte maturation time = 1 day for Hct ≥40%; 1.5 days for Hct 30%-40%; 2.0 days for Hct 20%-30%; 2.5 days for Hct <20%.
Data from Hillman RS, Finch CA. *Red Cell Manual.* 5th ed. F. A. Davis; 1985.

additional correction of this parameter needs to be made because reticulocytes released under intense Epo stimulation remain in the peripheral blood for more than the usual 1-day survival time of reticulocytes produced in steady state. There are a number of ways to adjust the reticulocyte count for the degree of anemia (*Table 24.3*). Although all of these methods have value, the absolute reticulocyte count is traditionally the easiest to estimate. The normal absolute reticulocyte count is 25 to 75 × 10^3/μL.

Automated reticulocyte counting also allows the evaluation of other parameters, such as reticulocyte hemoglobin content (CHr) and the proportion of immature reticulocytes (immature reticulocyte fraction, IRF). Whether not these parameters are available in a clinic or hospital depends on the automated hematology analyzer in use there. Terminology used to describe these parameters also varies depending on precise methodology and laboratory equipment, for example, CHr, reticulocyte hemoglobin equivalent (RET-He), and reticulocyte hemoglobin cellular content (RHCc) are different methods of assessing the same functional parameter.[32] These parameters can provide information in a number of clinical settings. A reduced IRF is an early sign of red cell underproduction, and an increase in IRF may be an early marker of marrow engraftment in posttransplant patients or of response to therapy in patients receiving B_{12}, iron, or Epo. A low CHr (<28 pg) suggests iron deficiency and predicts response to iron replacement. Similar to IRF, an increase in CHr is an early sign of response to iron. A decreased CHr is a strong indicator of ineffective erythropoiesis, particularly in dialysis patients.[32] A more detailed discussion of newer reticulocyte indices can be found in various reviews.[32–34]

If Anemia Is Associated With Reticulocytosis, Is There Any Evidence for Hemolysis?

The most characteristic presentation of hemolysis is reticulocytosis with some degree of hyperbilirubinemia as a marker of increased heme catabolism. Other markers reflect direct red cell injury (e.g., increased serum lactic dehydrogenase) or increased production and clearance of free Hb (e.g., low serum haptoglobin, hemoglobinemia, hemoglobinuria, and increased urinary hemosiderin). The evaluation and diagnostic considerations related to hemolytic anemia are complex and are considered separately elsewhere in this chapter (see "Approach to Hemolysis").

If Anemia Is Associated With a Lower-Than-Appropriate Reticulocyte Response, What Are the Red Cell Indices?

Anemia with low reticulocytes usually reflects some impairment of normal erythropoiesis, and this can be due to two kinds of defects. Erythropoiesis may be impaired because of a reduction in red cell precursors (hypogenerative). Alternatively, red cell production may be ineffective, a condition characterized by erythroid hyperplasia in the bone marrow, but with the production of essentially nonviable red cells, most of which do not reach circulation.

There are numerous causes of anemia with low reticulocyte counts, and it is in this group that analysis of RBCs indices is most helpful. Of these, the MCV tends to be the single most useful measurement,[33] although some clinicians prefer to use the MCH.[35] The MCV and MCH almost always correlate closely.[36]

An initial step in the classification of anemias with low reticulocyte counts separates them into three groups on the basis of average cell size: the macrocytic, microcytic, and normocytic anemias (*Figure 24.3*). Anemia is classified as macrocytic if the MCV exceeds 100 fL. Usually, the MCH is also increased, whereas the MCHC remains within normal limits (*Figure 24.4*). Microcytic anemia is identified when the MCV is less than 80 fL in adults. The anemia is normocytic when the indices are within normal limits, with an MCV between 80 and 100 fL. In children, MCV values vary as a function of age, and, correspondingly, the definition of microcytic, normocytic, and macrocytic differ accordingly (*Table 24.1*). As a practical matter for those who take care of children, it is important to know the age-related differences in RBC size, because many laboratory reports only contain adult normal values, often signaling the child's age-appropriate hematologic values as abnormal.

The MCHC is useful in detecting severe hypochromia, but it is rarely abnormal when the MCV is normal.[37,38] A reduced value for MCHC is observed most often in association with iron deficiency, and this index tends to be the last to fall as iron deficiency worsens.[39] The changes in MCHC with iron deficiency were seen more frequently in the past when centrifugal methods were used to determine the Hct before the availability of electronic cell counting. Because of plasma trapping, centrifugal Hct methods overestimate the volume of packed red cells and, therefore, underestimate MCHC.

Is the Anemia Associated With a Low Reticulocyte Response and Microcytic Red Blood Cells?

The large majority of patients in this category have defects in cellular Hb synthesis because of iron deficiency, thalassemia trait, or Hb E syndromes (see "Approach to Microcytic Anemia").

Is the Anemia Associated With a Low Reticulocyte Response and Macrocytic Red Blood Cells?

In these patients, the anemia is characterized by reticulocytopenia with red cells having an increased MCV. Many of these disorders are due to megaloblastic anemia resulting in impaired nuclear development, and the formation of other blood cells is also affected (see "Approach to Macrocytic Anemia").

Is the Anemia Associated With a Low Reticulocyte Response and Normocytic Red Blood Cells?

Normocytic anemia, low reticulocyte count, and normal bilirubin levels are seen in a large number of patients with anemia. The anemia of inflammation (AI), formerly called anemia of chronic disease (ACD), usually is normocytic, although occasionally may be slightly microcytic. Microcytic AI is more common when the anemia is long-standing. The anemia of renal failure is normocytic and largely is due to reduced Epo production. Acquired pure red cell aplasia (PRCA) is a normocytic anemia, which occurs in adults and children (see "Approach to Normocytic Anemia").

Is the Anemia Associated With Populations of Red Cells of Different Size?

The red cell indices represent mean values and do not reveal any variation that may exist within a population of cells. The MCV can be normal if there are combined abnormalities, such as when iron deficiency (decreased MCV) is accompanied by a megaloblastic anemia (increased MCV). For these reasons, it is important to examine the peripheral blood smear. The electronically derived RDW allows for recognition of these phenomena because it quantifies RBC size heterogeneity (anisocytosis) in a population of cells, and this has proved to be of value.[33] An increased RDW value usually, but not always, is an early and pronounced finding in iron deficiency and most megaloblastic anemias. RDW in heterozygous thalassemia is usually normal. In iron deficiency, the RDW value may become abnormal even before the MCV falls below the lower limits of normal.

Is the Anemia Associated With Abnormalities Seen on the Blood Smear?

Despite the technical advances provided by current electronic complete blood cell count (CBC) measurements, review of the peripheral blood smear remains a critical aspect of the diagnostic evaluation for anemia. It confirms the electronically determined classification of RBC size. Most importantly, it also allows for recognition of the many

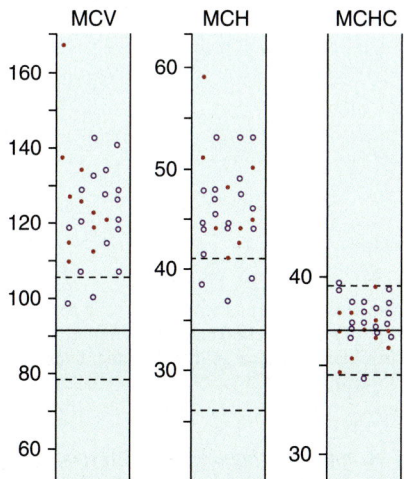

FIGURE 24.4 Erythrocyte indices in 28 patients with untreated or relapsed pernicious anemia. Dashed lines enclose the 95% confidence limits in normal subjects. Solid dots indicate males; open circles indicate females. MCH, mean corpuscular hemoglobin; MCHC, mean corpuscular hemoglobin concentration; MCV, mean corpuscular volume. (From Hallberg L. Blood volume, hemolysis and regeneration of blood in pernicious anemia. *Scand J Clin Lab Invest.* 1955;7(suppl 16). Copyright © Medisinsk Fysiologisk Forenings Forlag (MFFF), reprinted by permission of Taylor & Francis Ltd, http://www.tandfonline.com on behalf of Medisinsk Fysiologisk Forenings Forlag (MFFF).)

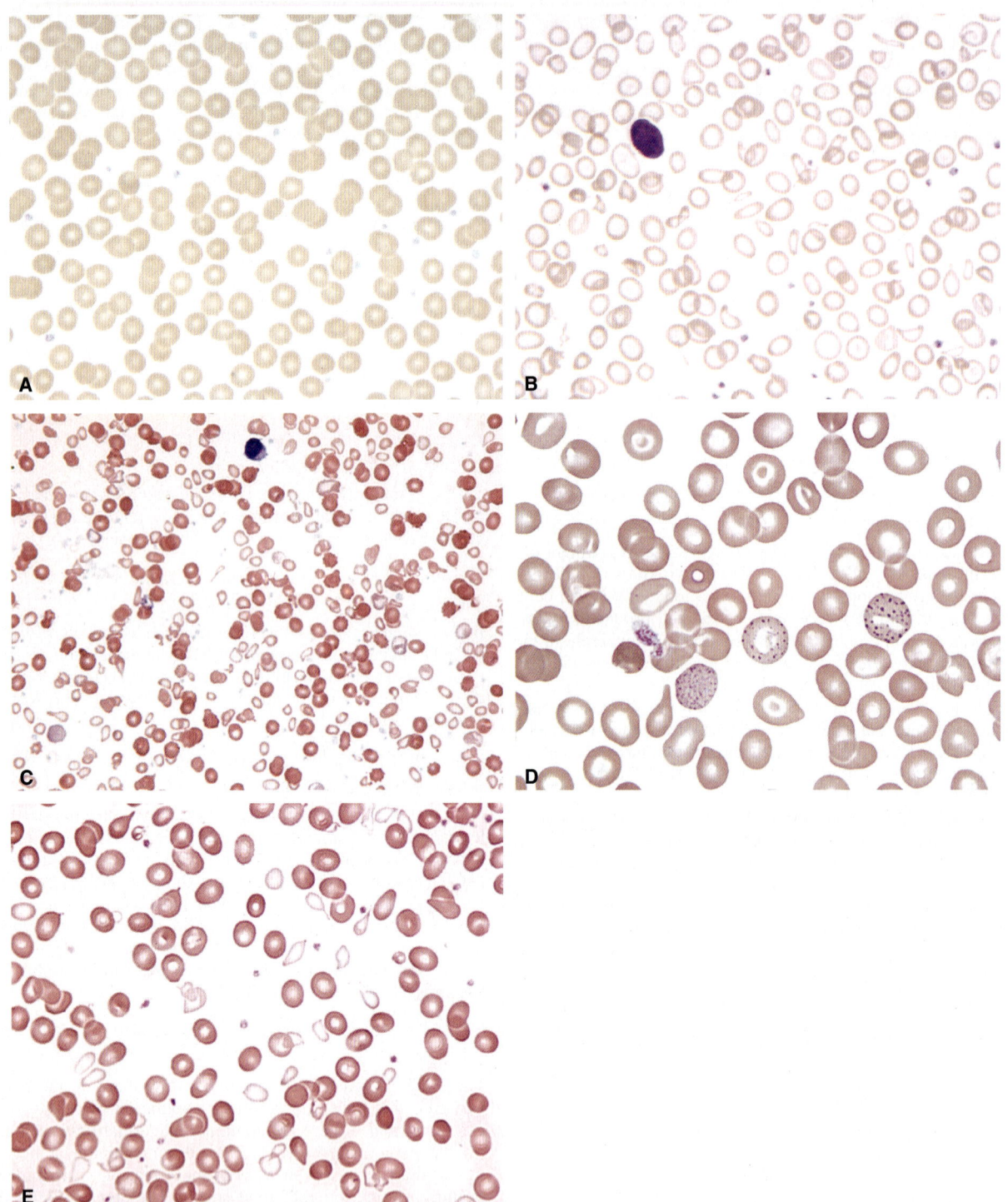

FIGURE 24.5 **Peripheral blood smear of erythrocytes in a variety of hypochromic, microcytic anemia. A.** Normal red cells. **B.** Iron deficiency anemia. Note the large area of central pallor. **C.** Dimorphic population of cells in iron deficiency anemia responding to treatment. **D.** Thalassemia minor. The cells are thin and appear pale but are nearly normal in diameter. Note the basophilic stippling in several RBCs. **E.** Sideroblastic anemia. A hypochromic, microcytic population of cells is mixed with relatively normocytic red blood cell.

variations in RBC size and shape that frequently are seen in patients with hemolysis.

Microcytes and macrocytes can be detected on the blood smear on the basis of a change in red cell diameter. Normal red cells approximate the size of the nucleus of a small lymphocyte, and the area of central pallor is one-third to one-half of the diameter of the red cell (*Figure 24.5A*). An increase in the area of central pallor of erythrocytes on the blood smear is indicative of hypochromia, and when the change is pronounced, little more than a faint ring of color in the

periphery may be apparent (*Figure 24.5B*). Hypochromia and microcytosis almost always occur together.

The automated analysis of the blood has made the erythrocyte indices more accurate and reproducible.[33] However, the evaluation of the blood smear remains important because it may reveal abnormal cell populations too small to affect the erythrocyte indices. For example, as iron deficiency develops, some microcytic cells are produced while the RBC indices are still normal. Furthermore, as B_{12} deficiency progresses, some characteristic oval macrocytes and hypersegmented

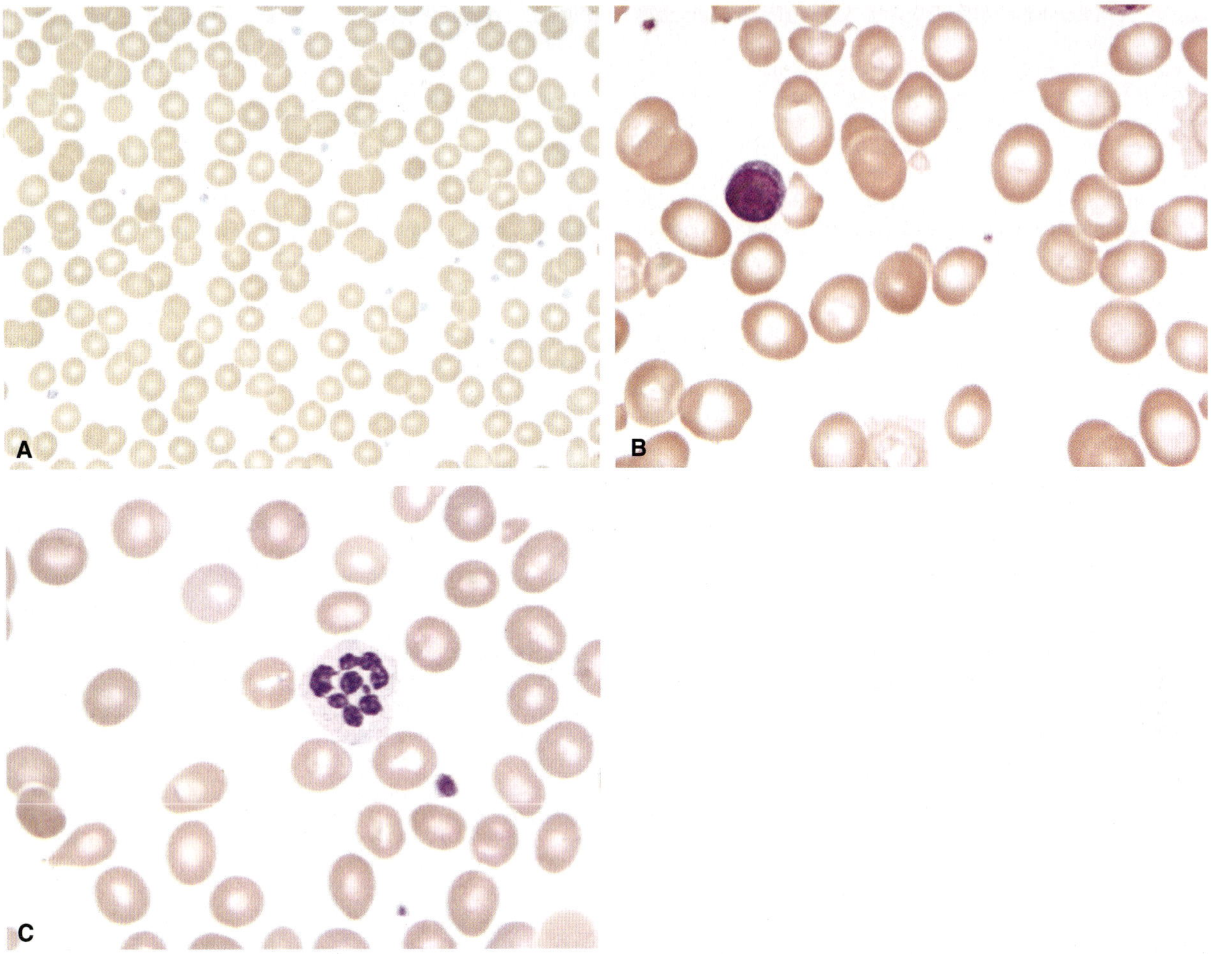

FIGURE 24.6 **Megaloblastic anemia. A.** Normal red cells. **B.** Macro-ovalocytes in pernicious anemia. **C.** Hypersegmented neutrophils seen in a patient with megaloblastic anemia.

neutrophils may appear long before there are MCV or Hb changes (*Figure 24.6B* and *C*). Moreover, examination of the smear is important for detecting conditions characterized by two populations of cells, only one of which is of abnormal size. This dimorphic anemia is particularly characteristic of sideroblastic anemias (*Figure 24.5E*). It is also seen in iron deficiency after iron therapy is started (*Figure 24.5C*) and in iron-deficient individuals who have been transfused.

Review of the blood smear may reveal underlying causes of the anemia. A leukoerythroblastic picture (teardrop RBC, nucleated RBC, early white blood cell precursors, or abnormalities in platelet size) suggests marrow infiltration by malignant cells, granulomas, or lipid deposits (*Figure 24.7*). The marked elevation in serum proteins in multiple myeloma may result in a stacking of RBCs in rouleaux formation. The appearance of RBC in agglutinates (as opposed to their stacking into rouleaux) is seen with cold agglutinin disease. One of the most valuable outcomes of reviewing the blood smear is that it often reveals abnormal red cell shapes characteristic of certain hemolytic anemias, like hereditary spherocytosis.

Is a Bone Marrow Examination Needed to Clarify the Cause of Anemia?

Examination of the bone marrow is most useful in reticulocytopenic anemias, particularly when there is more than one hematopoietic cell line affected. Both hypoplasia and marrow infiltrative disease due to leukemia, tumor, or granulomas (myelophthisic anemia) may readily be demonstrated in the bone marrow aspirate and biopsy. Myelofibrosis can be recognized as a component of myeloid metaplasia. If the marrow is normocellular except for reduced erythropoiesis, the underlying cause may be red cell aplasia, renal disease, or endocrinopathy.

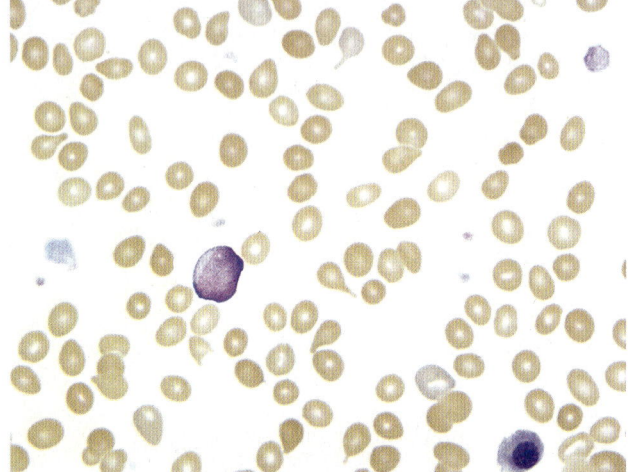

FIGURE 24.7 **Peripheral blood smear.** A leukoerythroblastic response seen in a patient with metastatic breast cancer.

Examination of iron in bone marrow macrophages traditionally was considered the definitive way to demonstrate decreased iron stores. Nowadays, the diagnosis of iron deficiency can be made by simple blood tests in most cases, thus obviating the need for an iron stain of the bone marrow. On the other hand, to make the diagnosis of sideroblastic anemia, a bone marrow examination is necessary to identify ringed sideroblasts. Megaloblastic anemias usually can be recognized by peripheral blood findings, but a marrow examination will confirm the diagnosis.

In some anemias with low reticulocyte counts, marrow erythropoiesis surprisingly is quite active. This is referred to as *ineffective erythropoiesis*, and it occurs when developing red cells are defective and are destroyed before they leave the marrow or shortly thereafter. In healthy individuals, a very small fraction of erythropoiesis is ineffective; however, in certain conditions, especially megaloblastic anemias, thalassemias, sideroblastic anemias, and congenital dyserythropoietic anemias, ineffective erythropoiesis becomes greatly exaggerated. The increased intramedullary destruction of erythroblasts in these conditions is associated with accelerated heme catabolism, resulting in an elevated unconjugated bilirubin level in the plasma. The serum lactate dehydrogenase level, a marker of cell destruction, also can be markedly elevated. Ineffective erythropoiesis can be confused with hemolytic anemia because signs of excessive red cell destruction and erythroid hyperplasia of the bone marrow are found in both conditions. However, the two conditions are distinguished from one another by the degree of reticulocytosis, which is increased in hemolytic anemia and usually low in ineffective erythropoiesis.

APPROACH TO MACROCYTIC ANEMIA

The MCV is increased in 1.7% to 3.6% of cases involving patients seeking medical care, often in the absence of anemia.[40,41] Mild macrocytosis (MCV of 100-110 fL) is particularly common and often remains unexplained, even after careful study.[40,41] Nevertheless, this finding should not be ignored, because it can be an important early clue to reversible disease. In pernicious anemia, macrocytosis and/or neuropsychiatric symptoms may precede anemia development.[42,43]

Morphologic and biochemical criteria allow macrocytic anemias to be divided into two groups: megaloblastic anemias and nonmegaloblastic macrocytic anemias. The types of macrocytic anemias that clinicians encounter vary considerably depending on the population served. If alcoholism is common in the population, it is likely to be the most common cause. In patients with cancer, high MCVs are most likely due to chemotherapy. In hospitals largely serving the elderly, pernicious anemia and other nutritional anemias may predominate.[43]

When confronted with a diagnostic problem involving macrocytic anemia, the physician should first distinguish between megaloblastic and nonmegaloblastic anemia (*Figure 24.8*). Morphologic examination is helpful in making this distinction.

Megaloblastic Anemias

The term *megaloblast* is a designation that was first applied by Ehrlich to the abnormal erythrocyte precursors found in the bone marrow of patients with pernicious anemia. Megaloblasts are characterized by their large size and by specific alterations in the appearance of their nuclear chromatin (*Figure 24.9*). These distinctive cells are now known to be the morphologic expression of a biochemical abnormality: retarded DNA synthesis.[44] RNA synthesis remains unimpaired while cell division is restricted.[45] As a result, cytoplasmic components, especially Hb, are synthesized in excessive amounts during the delay between cell divisions. An enlarged cell is the product of such a process. Megaloblastic anemias are defined by the presence of these cells or by other evidence of defective DNA synthesis.

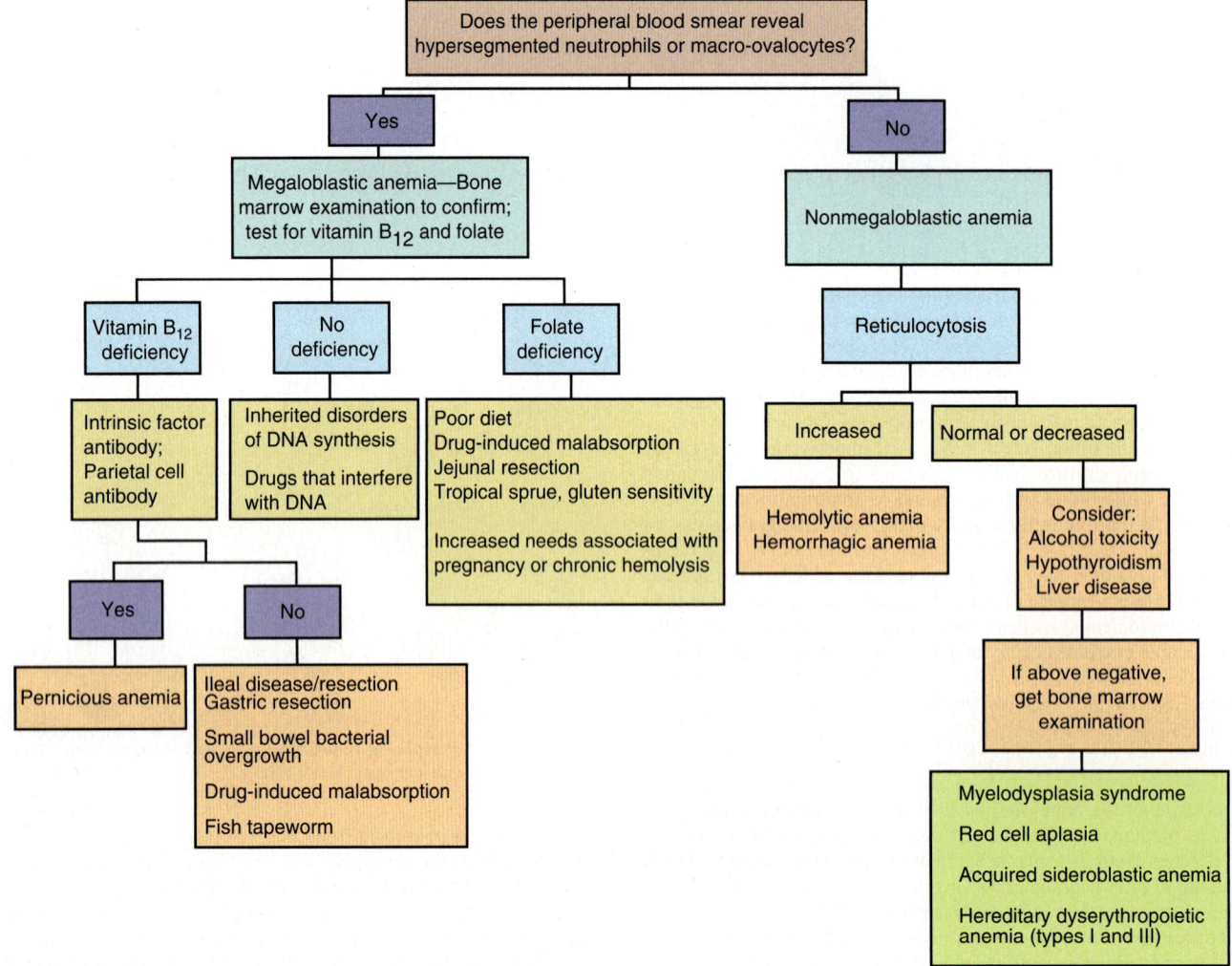

FIGURE 24.8 **Diagnostic approach to a patient with macrocytic anemia.**

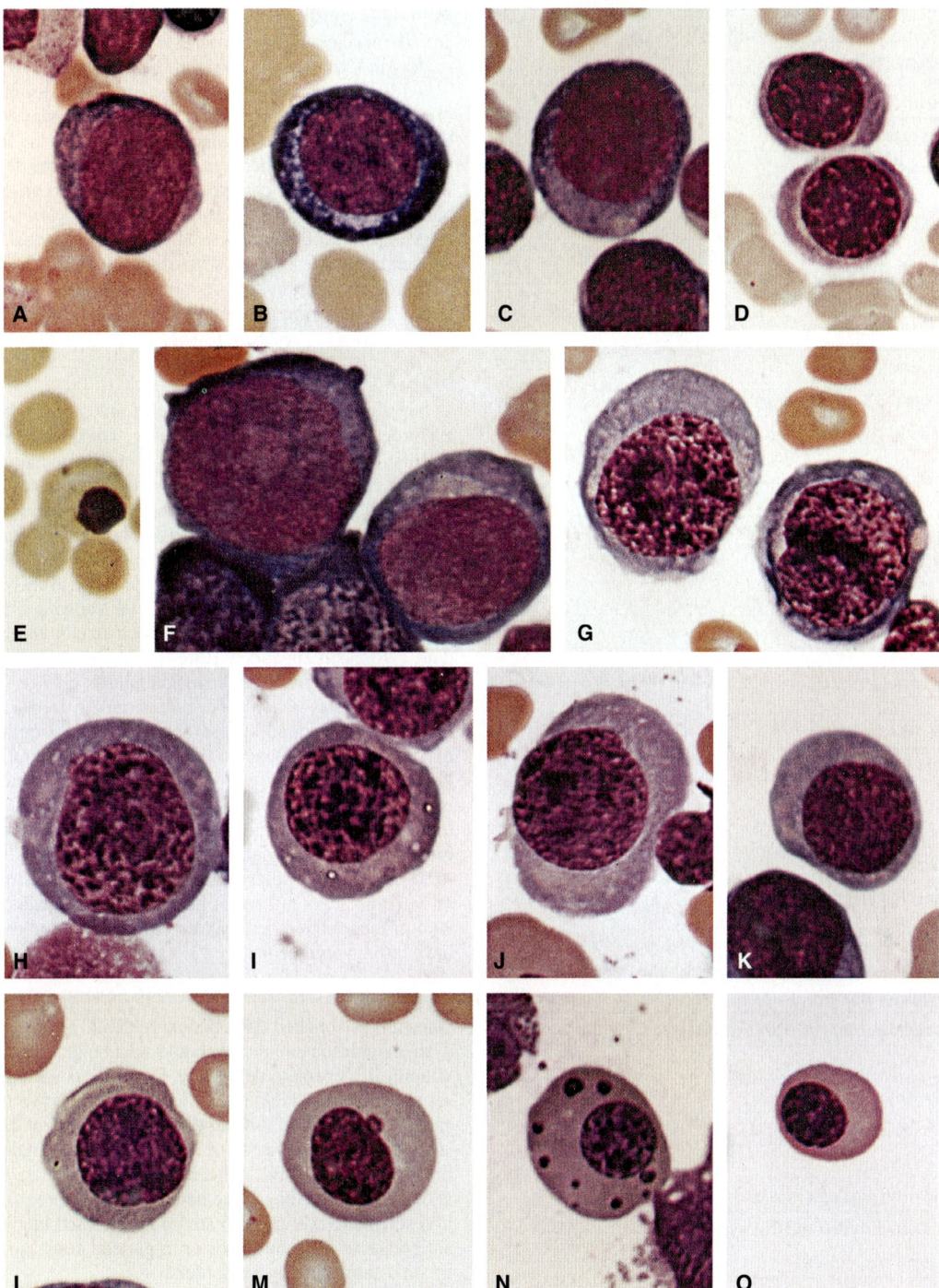

FIGURE 24.9 Normoblasts and megaloblasts contrasted (Wright stain × 1000). A-E. Normoblast. **A.** Pronormoblast. **B.** Basophilic normoblast. **C.** Early polychromatophilic normoblast. **D.** Late polychromatophilic normoblast. **E.** Orthochromatic normoblast with stippling. **F-O.** Megaloblasts. **F.** Promegaloblast (*left*) and basophilic megaloblast (*right*). **G-K.** Polychromatophilic megaloblasts. **L-O.** Orthochromatic megaloblasts.

A pathogenetic classification of the causes of megaloblastic anemias is presented in *Table 24.4.* Most often, megaloblastic anemia is the consequence of deficiency of vitamin B_{12}. Folate deficiency, formerly a major cause of megaloblastic anemia, has become far less frequent due to food fortification. Less commonly, megaloblastic anemia results from inherited or drug-induced disorders of DNA synthesis.

Hematologic Features of Megaloblastic Anemia

Examination of the blood smear often reveals the two most valuable findings for differentiating megaloblastic from nonmegaloblastic anemia: neutrophil hypersegmentation and oval macrocytes.

Neutrophil hypersegmentation is one of the most sensitive and specific signs of megaloblastic anemia (*Figure 24.6C*). Normally, the nuclei of circulating, segmented neutrophils have fewer than five lobes. In megaloblastic anemia, neutrophils with six or more lobes may be detected. In a large study, more than 98% of patients with megaloblastic anemia had at least one six-lobed neutrophil out of 100 cells examined, as compared with only 2% of normal control subjects.[46] Hypersegmentation is among the first hematologic abnormalities to appear as the megaloblastic state develops.[47] It persists for an average of 14 days after institution of specific therapy.[48]

Table 24.4. Pathogenetic Classification of Megaloblastic Anemia

Vitamin B$_{12}$ deficiency
Dietary deficiency (vegan diet)
Lack of intrinsic factor
Pernicious anemia
Gastric surgery
Ingestion of caustic materials
Biologic competition for vitamin B$_{12}$:
Small-bowel bacterial overgrowth
Fish tapeworm disease
Familial selective vitamin B$_{12}$ malabsorption (Imerslund-Gräsbeck syndrome)
Drug-induced vitamin B$_{12}$ malabsorption
Chronic pancreatic disease
Zollinger-Ellison syndrome
Diseases of the ileum
Previous ileal resection
Regional enteritis
Folate deficiency
Dietary deficiency
Increased requirements:
Pregnancy
Chronic hemolytic anemia
Alcoholism
Congenital folate malabsorption
Drug-induced folate deficiency
Extensive intestinal (jejuna) resection
Combined folate and vitamin B$_{12}$ deficiency
Tropical sprue
Gluten-sensitive enteropathy
Inherited or acquired disorders of DNA synthesis
Orotic aciduria
Lesch-Nyhan syndrome
Thiamine-responsive megaloblastic anemia
Transcobalamin II deficiency
Homocystinuria and methylmalonic aciduria
Drug- and toxin-induced disorders of DNA synthesis
Folate antagonists (e.g., methotrexate)
Purine antagonists (e.g., 6-mercaptopurine)
Pyrimidine antagonists (e.g., cytosine arabinoside)
Alkylating agents (e.g., cyclophosphamide)
Zidovudine (AZT, Retrovir)
Trimethoprim
Oral contraceptives
Nitrous oxide
Arsenic

The main products of megaloblastic erythropoiesis are macrocytic erythrocytes with a distinctly oval shape. Such cells are well filled with Hb, and often central pallor is reduced or absent (*Figure 24.6B*). The oval shape may be useful in distinguishing megaloblastic anemias from other causes of macrocytosis: the macroreticulocytes that characterize accelerated erythropoiesis tend to be round and distinctly blue or gray in Romanowsky/Wright-Giemsa dyes.

Although oval macrocytes are prominent in megaloblastic anemia, the size and shape of the erythrocytes may vary considerably. Quantitative measures of anisocytosis, such as the RDW, are substantially increased, and the increase may precede the development of anemia.[49] Morphologic changes on the blood smear, however, are most conspicuous when anemia is pronounced.

Megaloblastic anemias usually develop gradually, and the degree of anemia is often severe when first detected. Hb values less than 7 or 8 g/dL are not unusual. As noted earlier, macrocytosis characteristically precedes the development of anemia, sometimes by very prolonged periods. The MCV usually is between 110 and 130 fL.

Bone Marrow

A megaloblastic marrow is cellular and usually hyperplastic, with erythrocyte precursors predominating. The characteristic megaloblasts are distinguished by their large size and especially by their delicate nuclear chromatin. The chromatin has been described as particulate or sieve-like, as distinguished from the normal denser chromatin of normoblasts (*Figure 24.9*). This morphologic change may be detected at all stages of erythrocyte development; however, the identification of orthochromatic megaloblasts is particularly useful in the recognition of megaloblastic anemia because they differ so markedly from any cell found in normal marrow. In the orthochromatic megaloblast, the abundant cytoplasm appears mature (pink), whereas the nucleus appears immature as the result of the megaloblastic change.

Leukopoiesis is also abnormal; extremely large (up to 20 or 30 μm) leukocytes are found. These abnormalities of cellular development may occur at any stage in the myeloid series, but they are particularly common among the metamyelocytes. The nuclei of these giant metamyelocytes are enlarged, both absolutely and in relation to the total cell size. Nuclear shape and chromatin structure or staining properties may also be abnormal.

In general, megakaryopoiesis is less disturbed than that of either of the other two cell lines; however, when megaloblastic change is severe, megakaryocytes may be reduced in number and patients may have thrombocytopenia.

Vitamin B$_{12}$ and Folate Levels in Serum and Erythrocytes

Once it is established that a patient has CBC and morphologic evidence of megaloblastic anemia, it should next be determined if this is due to vitamin B$_{12}$ or folate deficiency. Useful tests include measurement of serum folate and vitamin B$_{12}$ levels. The relative merits of different assays are discussed in Chapter 37. Measurement of other parameters such as serum homocysteine and serum methylmalonic acid can confirm a diagnosis of B$_{12}$ deficiency, particularly when initial assays are at odds with the clinical and hematologic picture. Vitamin B$_{12}$ absorption studies (Schilling test) are no longer used in clinical practice, but antibodies to intrinsic factor or to parietal cells can further define the specific causes of these disorders.

Nonmegaloblastic Macrocytic Anemias

Nonmegaloblastic macrocytic anemias are not united by any common pathogenetic mechanism. They simply represent macrocytic anemias in which the RBC precursors appear normal without the characteristic nuclear and cytoplasmic findings of megaloblastosis. When macrocytosis is found, it tends to be mild; the MCV usually ranges from 100 to 110 fL and rarely exceeds 120 fL.[40] Several causes of nonmegaloblastic macrocytosis are recognized (*Table 24.5*).

Accelerated Erythropoiesis

Mild to moderate macrocytosis often follows Epo-mediated acceleration of red cell production, as may be induced by blood loss or hemolysis. In part, this increased cell size occurs because reticulocytes are approximately 25% larger than mature red cells.[50] In addition, under conditions of accelerated red cell production, a premature release of bone marrow reticulocytes (shift reticulocytes) occurs, and these cells are even larger and contain more RNA than normal circulating reticulocytes.[32] Lastly, an erythroblast cell division may be skipped under this erythropoietic stress, a phenomenon that results in a macroreticulocyte that is approximately twice the normal size.[32]

Chronic Alcohol Use

Macrocytosis, usually mild, has been reported in more than two-thirds of steady users of alcohol, many of whom have no anemia.[51] The finding is so characteristic of the condition that macrocytosis has been used as part of the screening procedure for the detection of chronic alcohol use. It may be present in both heavy and moderate drinkers.[52] Macrocytosis and anemia in alcoholic individuals have several causes. Folate deficiency from poor nutrition can lead to megaloblastic anemia, and alcoholic cirrhosis may be associated with spur-cell hemolytic anemia. Most commonly, however, alcoholic macrocytosis is associated with none of these factors and instead results from poorly defined direct effects of alcohol on the bone marrow. There are no morphologic findings such as those that occur in megaloblastic anemia. Serum and erythrocyte folate levels are usually normal, and the macrocytosis does not respond to folate treatment. If the patient abstains from alcohol, the MCV returns to normal levels after 2 to 4 months.

Liver Disease

The causes of anemia in liver disease are multifactorial, resulting from intravascular dilution due to hypervolemia, impaired ability of the marrow to respond optimally to the anemia, and, in some patients, a severe hemolytic anemia associated with morphologically abnormal erythrocytes (spur cells; Chapters 33 and 42). The anemia is usually mild to moderate. In patients with cirrhosis, the Hb level averages approximately 12 g/dL and remains above 10 g/dL in the absence of bleeding or severe hemolysis. The anemia of liver disease is mildly macrocytic: the MCV rarely exceeds 115 fL in the absence of megaloblastic changes in the bone marrow. Macrocytosis in liver disease typically reflects changes in RBC membrane lipid composition and is discussed in Chapter 42.

Miscellaneous Anemias

Macrocytosis may accompany various anemias with low reticulocyte counts including MDS (Chapter 80), congenital bone marrow failure disorders such as Diamond-Blackfan anemia (Chapter 40), and Fanconi anemia (Chapter 38). Less commonly, macrocytosis can be a feature of certain congenital dyserythropoietic anemias (CDAs) (Chapter 41) and myelophthisic conditions. The reason for macrocytosis in these disorders is not well understood.

Spurious macrocytosis can result from laboratory artifacts. Cold agglutinins, marked leukocytosis, or other acute-phase reactants can lead to an incorrect high MCV value.[53] Care is needed so that these situations do not lead to a fruitless search for a disorder known to cause macrocytic anemia. Because reticulocytes are larger than mature

RBCs, significant reticulocytosis can increase the MCV. This is not a spurious macrocytosis, but it is misleading.

APPROACH TO MICROCYTIC ANEMIA

Most microcytic anemias are due to deficient Hb synthesis, often associated with iron deficiency or impaired iron use (*Table 24.6*). The differentiation of iron deficiency from the ACD and the differentiation of iron deficiency from thalassemia trait syndromes are both common clinical issues. Significant microcytosis is detected in nearly 3% of all patients who require admission to the hospital.[54,55]

The typical Hb level seen in adults with a variety of microcytic anemias is presented in *Table 24.7*. The laboratory evaluation of microcytic anemias focuses on screening hematologic studies, followed by more definitive tests to distinguish iron deficiency anemia, the ACD, hemoglobinopathies, or sideroblastic anemias (*Figure 24.10*). A few commonly used studies are described subsequently; others are described elsewhere in this text.

Table 24.6. Pathogenic Classification of Microcytic Anemias

Disorders of iron metabolism
Iron deficiency anemia
Anemia of inflammation/anemia of chronic disease
Disorders of globin synthesis
Alpha and beta thalassemias
Hemoglobin E syndromes (AE, EE, E-β-thalassemia)
Hemoglobin C syndromes (AC, CC)
Sideroblastic anemias
Hereditary sideroblastic anemia
Acquired sideroblastic anemia
Refractory anemia with ringed sideroblasts
Malignancies
Myeloproliferative disorders
Lead intoxication (usually normocytic)

Table 24.5. Nonmegaloblastic Macrocytic Anemias

Hemolytic anemia/reticulocytosis
Posthemorrhagic anemia
Chronic alcohol abuse
Liver disease
Myelodysplastic syndrome
Myelophthisic anemias
Aplastic anemia
Acquired sideroblastic anemia
Congenital dyserythropoietic anemia (CDA) types I and III
Diamond-Blackfan anemia
Hypothyroidism
Spurious macrocytosis (paraproteinemia, inflammation)

Table 24.7. Typical Hemoglobin and Mean Corpuscular Volume Values in Adults With Certain Anemias

Condition	Hb Concentration (g/dL)	MCV (fL)
Normal men	16 (14-18)	89 (80-100)
Normal women	14 (12-16)	89 (80-100)
Iron deficiency anemia	8 (4-12)	74 (55-85)
Anemia of chronic diseases	10 (8-13)	85 (75-95)
β-Thalassemias minor	12 (9-14)	68 (55-75)
β-Thalassemias major	(2-7)	(48-72)
Hemoglobin H disease	9 (7-11)	70 (53-88)
Hemoglobin E trait (AE)	14 (12-17)	73 (71-78)
Homozygous hemoglobin E (EE)	12 (11-15)	64 (58-76)
Hemoglobin C disease (CC)	10 (7-14)	77 (55-93)
Congenital sideroblastic anemia	6 (4-10)	77 (49-104)
Acquired sideroblastic anemia	10 (7-12)	104 (83-118)

Values are means, with approximate range in parentheses.
Abbreviations: Hb, hemoglobin; MCV, mean corpuscular volume.

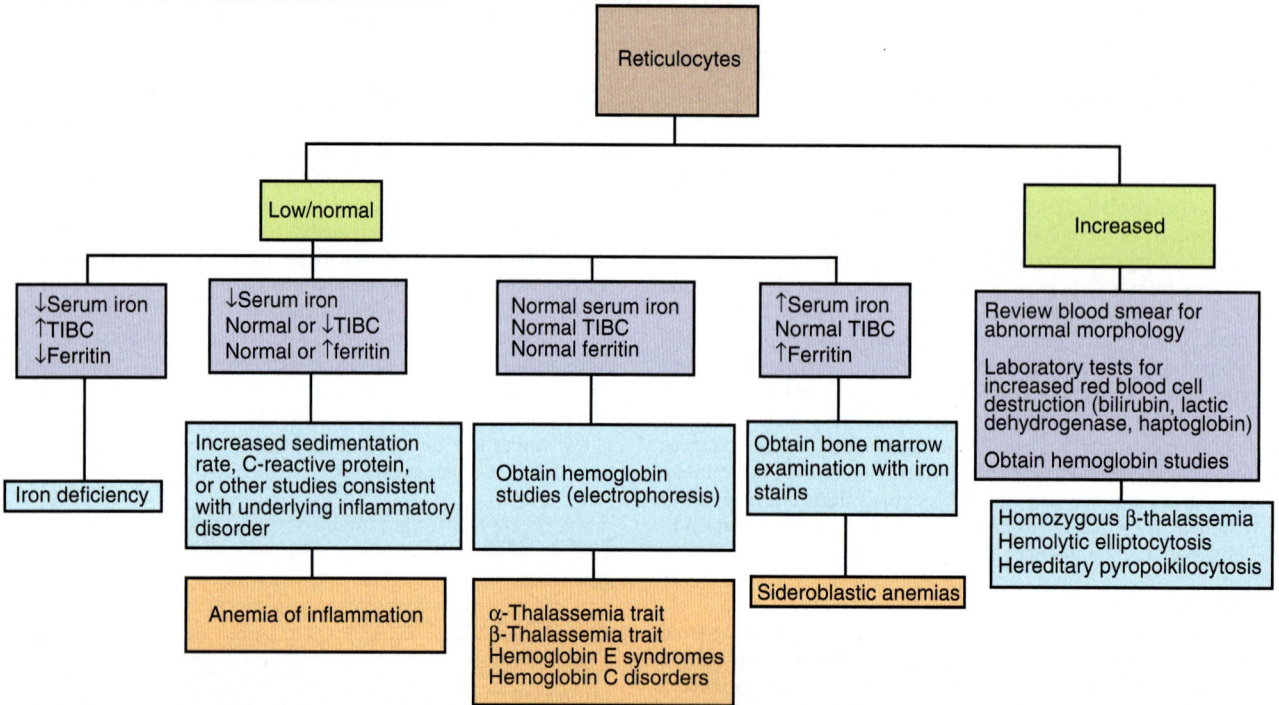

FIGURE 24.10 **Diagnostic approach to a patient with microcytic anemia.** ↑, increased; ↓, decreased; TIBC, total iron-binding capacity.

Iron Pathway Disorders

The principal source of iron for Hb production is transferrin, the iron-transport protein in plasma. Under normal circumstances, plasma iron levels are not rate limiting in erythropoiesis, and transferrin is able to supply all the iron required for normal or accelerated production rates. However, in iron deficiency anemia, the storage sites in macrophages are depleted of iron and the plasma iron concentration falls. When transferrin saturation with iron is less than 16%, the red cell production rate decreases, and hypochromic, microcytic cells are manufactured. This state is known as *iron-deficient erythropoiesis.*

In AI (Chapter 42), the macrophage iron level is normal or increased, but export of iron from macrophages is downregulated.[56] Thus, iron accumulates in the macrophage, while plasma iron level falls, and the marrow is deprived of adequate supplies.

Together, iron deficiency anemia and AI are among the most common causes of anemia. Iron deficiency predominates in children and young women, but it also occurs in older individuals in whom it may reflect occult bleeding because of underlying pathology. AI is more common among elderly people,[57] but it also can occur in younger individuals affected by certain chronic inflammatory states.

Distinguishing typical iron deficiency anemia from AI is usually not difficult. Anemia, hypochromia, and microcytosis are typically more pronounced in iron deficiency, as are the degrees of anisocytosis and poikilocytosis. AI is usually normocytic. However, when iron deficiency is early and mild, the morphologic findings in the two conditions may be similar.

Tests to distinguish iron deficiency anemia and AI are discussed in detail in Chapters 25 and 42. Some general comments follow.

Measurement of Serum Iron and Iron-Binding Capacity

Serum iron levels are a measure of the amount of iron bound to transferrin. Total iron-binding capacity (TIBC) is an indirect measurement of transferrin in terms of the amount of iron it will bind. Transferrin can also be measured directly by immunologic techniques that are available in most laboratories.

A limitation in the use of serum iron determinations is the considerable variability in values.[58] Serum iron values in an individual can vary from 10% to 40% within a single day or from day to day,[59,60]

and many normal subjects demonstrate a predictable diurnal variation, with the highest values in the morning and lowest values in the evening.[61] The iron regulatory protein hepcidin has a diurnal pattern also, and this provides a potential mechanism for the diurnal serum iron variation.[62] In contrast to serum iron, TIBC (or transferrin) values show less significant diurnal variation.[63,64] It is also important to recognize that serum iron levels are influenced by the recent ingestion and absorption of iron medication or of food iron. In one report, tea (containing phytates that may bind iron) decreased serum iron 50% while consumption of orange juice (containing ascorbic acid that may improve absorption) increased iron 2-fold.[65] Fasting serum iron concentrations more accurately reflect iron stores.[66]

TIBC saturation is calculated with the following formula: TIBC saturation (%) = (serum iron × 100)/TIBC. The normal value is 20% to 45%. Values below 16% are noted in association with both iron deficiency and AI. The degree of reduction tends to be greater in iron deficiency than in chronic disorders, but considerable overlap exists between these two conditions. In both children and adults, however, a value of less than 5% is almost certainly due to iron deficiency anemia. In sideroblastic anemias, and in transfused thalassemic patients, the TIBC saturation invariably is increased and often approaches 100%. In laboratories that measure transferrin directly, an iron transferrin saturation index that provides the same information as the TIBC saturation is calculated.

The absolute value for TIBC may be helpful in distinguishing between iron deficiency and the anemia of chronic disorders. The TIBC often is increased in iron deficiency and decreased in AI, and some consider this to be the best test to distinguish these two disorders.[67] However, in hospitalized patients, elevated TIBC is an insensitive marker of iron deficiency.[68]

Serum Ferritin

Determination of serum ferritin concentration also is used for evaluating iron stores in patients with iron deficiency.[69] Ferritin is chiefly an intracellular iron storage protein, but trace amounts also are secreted into plasma. In most clinical circumstances, the serum ferritin concentration is proportional to total body iron stores. In contrast to serum iron measurements, ferritin values are not influenced by recent iron therapy.[69]

Serum ferritin values in men tend to rise steadily with age. These levels show little or no diurnal variation. The serum ferritin level in patients with AI (also called anemia of chronic disease) may increase disproportionately relative to the increase in iron stores, probably because ferritin is an acute-phase reactant. This phenomenon complicates the diagnosis of iron deficiency when it coexists with inflammatory disease. In some other illnesses, the serum ferritin level increases because of factors other than augmented iron stores. One such condition is liver disease, in which damage to the hepatic cell can cause the release of intracellular ferritin (nonglycosylated and iron-rich).[70] Serum ferritin values also may be inappropriately increased in association with various malignancies, especially hematologic malignancies.[71]

Evaluation of Bone Marrow Iron Stores

In bone marrow aspirates, hemosiderin appears as golden-yellow refractile granules. More often, the specimen is stained by the Prussian blue method, in which hemosiderin is blue.[72] Experienced observers can grade the marrow hemosiderin stores from 0 to 6+.[73] In iron deficiency, marrow hemosiderin is absent (grade 0) compared with normal (grade 1+ to 3+). Iron is always present in AI (grade 2+ to 5+) and is greatly increased in sideroblastic anemia, thalassemia major, and other iron-loading anemias (grade 5+ to 6+). Nowadays the marrow assessment of iron is used much less, because serum ferritin and soluble transferrin receptor (TfR) provide simpler measurements that correlate with clinical iron states in AI and other iron deficiency states.

Soluble Transferrin Receptors

TfRs are disulfide-linked transmembrane proteins that facilitate the entry of transferrin-bound iron into cells (Chapter 25). A soluble, truncated form of the protein can be detected in plasma, and its immunologic quantification can be useful in detecting iron deficiency and distinguishing it from AI. Values in iron-deficient subjects are clearly increased and are typically not increased in uncomplicated ACD.[74] Therefore, TfR determination may be useful in distinguishing iron deficiency from AI, but it must be interpreted in association with the ferritin concentration.[68] It has been proposed that the ratio of serum TfR concentration to the logarithm of the serum ferritin concentration has better capacity to distinguish iron deficiency from ACD than does the unadjusted serum TfR concentration.[75] Serum TfR levels also vary with the total mass of red cell precursors and serves as a marker of the degree of erythropoiesis. Therefore, the value increases in hemolytic anemia, thalassemia, and polycythemia and decreases in hypoplastic anemia and renal failure.[76]

Other Tests to Assess Iron Metabolism

Erythrocyte Zinc Protoporphyrin

Red cell precursors normally synthesize slightly more protoporphyrin than is needed for heme synthesis. The excess remains with the cell throughout its lifespan and has been called free erythrocyte protoporphyrin. When iron is not available for heme synthesis, protoporphyrin accumulates in excess as zinc protoporphyrin (ZPP). ZPP increases dramatically in iron deficiency and is an effective population screening test for iron deficiency, particularly in children and in resource-poor environments. The erythrocyte ZPP content is also greatly increased in lead poisoning, but it is normal in thalassemia.[77,78]

Liver Iron Stores

Iron stores can also be evaluated by liver biopsy using both histochemical and chemical methods of analysis. Measurement of hepatic iron stores has been used mainly to assess iron overload states and is not generally helpful in assessing iron stores for erythropoiesis. Currently, however, magnetic resonance imaging using T2* technology is replacing liver biopsy as a noninvasive way to measure liver iron content.[79,80]

Disorders of Hemoglobin Synthesis

The Hb disorders associated with microcytosis include the thalassemias and certain structural Hb variants.

The thalassemias are a group of inherited disorders in which synthesis of one of the normal polypeptide chains of globin is deficient (Chapter 35). In mild forms of the disease (thalassemia minor), hypochromia and microcytosis are prominent, whereas anemia is absent or mild. In other thalassemic disorders, including homozygous β-thalassemia (β-thalassemia major) and Hb E β-thalassemia, hypochromic microcytic anemia is usually quite severe.

Some structurally abnormal Hb may also be associated with moderate microcytosis. This is particularly characteristic of patients carrying an Hb E gene. Heterozygotes for this hemoglobinopathy typically have normochromic microcytosis without anemia. Homozygotes have a greater degree of microcytosis and either mild or no anemia. As with thalassemia, Hb E diseases are characterized by reduced β-chain synthesis.[81] Normochromic microcytosis also occurs in homozygous Hb C disease.[82] Target cells are also common in these disorders.

The possibility of thalassemia minor often is raised by a finding that the microcytosis is more severe than might be expected for the mild degree of anemia. In addition, basophilic stippling and target cells tend to be more prominent in thalassemia than in iron deficiency. An important feature of thalassemia trait–like conditions (which include the Hb E syndromes) is that microcytosis often is associated with very high-normal to elevated RBC counts despite having little or no anemia. This characteristic has allowed several different measures for differentiating iron deficiency from thalassemia trait and Hb E disorders. One of the most useful is a modification of the Mentzer index,[83] which is based on the MCV and RBC count:

MCV/RBC (10^6) > 14 (suggestive of iron deficiency)
MCV/RBC (10^6) 12 to 14 (indeterminate)
MCV/RBC (10^6) <12 (suggestive of thalassemia trait disorders)

RDW, a measure of anisocytosis derived from erythrocyte volume distribution, has been proposed to distinguish iron deficiency from thalassemia minor in patients with microcytosis.[84,85] Anisocytosis is an early and prominent finding in iron deficiency, often detectable before significant microcytosis, hypochromia, or even anemia is apparent. The normal value for RDW is 13.4% ± 1.2% (mean, 2 SD), and the upper limit of normal is 14.6%. In iron deficiency, the RDW is increased above normal, sometimes greater than 20%, a reflection of the anisocytosis associated with iron-deficient erythropoiesis. In contrast to iron deficiency, anisocytosis tends to be absent or mild in thalassemia minor, and consequently the RDW usually is normal, although occasionally it is slightly increased.[61] Overall an increased RDW appears to be 90% to 100% sensitive for iron deficiency but only 50% to 70% specific.[86] An increased value for RDW in an otherwise normal CBC most often represents early iron deficiency, but other nutritional deficiencies are also possible causes.

Distinguishing homozygous β-thalassemia (β-thalassemia major) from β-thalassemia minor is rarely a problem, because the former is accompanied by signs of hemolysis and ineffective erythropoiesis; there are also characteristic findings on the blood smear, including nucleated red cells, extreme anisocytosis and poikilocytosis, and target cells (Chapter 35). However, it is a common diagnostic problem to distinguish patients with the β-thalassemia trait from those with iron deficiency. In almost all cases of β-thalassemia trait, the fraction of Hb A_2 is increased, whereas the value for Hb A_2 is normal or decreased in iron deficiency.[87] It was previously thought that, if a patient with β-thalassemia trait is iron deficient at the time of evaluation, the Hb A_2 might be normal. A number of recent studies contradict this observation.[83,88]

α-Thalassemia syndromes result from decreased α-globin chain synthesis that is directed by four structural genes on chromosome 16. Four different α-thalassemia syndromes have been recognized. Silent carrier state individuals lack one α globin gene; the α,β-globin chain synthetic ratio is less than 1, but these individuals are hematologically normal and have no clinical problems. α-Thalassemia trait individuals lack two α-globin genes, α-globin synthesis is impaired, and there is a mild hypochromic microcytic anemia. α-Thalassemia trait can occur in two genotypes: type 1 or *cis* deletion (--/αα) or type 2 or *trans* deletion (-α/-α). Hb H disease is caused by the deletion of three α-globin genes, and the consequence of this is a mild to moderate hemolytic anemia. Beyond the neonatal period, the unbalanced chain synthesis leads to an excess in β-globin chains that form Hb H (β₄ tetramers). Hb H is mildly unstable, particularly in the presence of oxidant stress, and can cause intermittent hemolysis. Homozygous α-thalassemia (hydrops) is due to a deletion of all four α-globin genes, resulting in severe anemia due to the complete absence of α-globin chains. This disorder is incompatible with life, and fetuses are aborted early, are stillborn, or die within the first few hours of life.

A common clinical problem is to identify the α-thalassemia trait, which has a presentation similar to that of the β-thalassemia trait and to iron deficiency. The diagnosis often has been a presumptive one, made after excluding iron deficiency, β-thalassemia trait, and any other abnormal Hb. The α-thalassemia syndromes occur primarily in those of Asian and African descent, and it is of interest that in Africans with α-thalassemia trait, the globin gene deletions occur on different chromosomes (type 2, *trans* deletions), whereas in Asians with α-thalassemia trait, the gene deletions occur on the same chromosome (type 1, *cis* deletion). As a consequence of these racial differences, Hb H disease and homozygous α-thalassemia occurs only in Asians. Moreover, virtually all Africans with α-thalassemia have the α-thalassemia trait (Chapter 35).

GENERAL DIAGNOSTIC APPROACH TO HEMOGLOBINOPATHIES AND THALASSEMIAS

The clinical and laboratory features of specific thalassemia and hemoglobinopathy disorders are discussed in the chapters addressing those conditions. Thalassemia and hemoglobinopathy syndromes are suspected in patients with microcytosis, in patients with unexplained hemolytic anemia, and in patients with the red cell abnormalities suggestive of hemoglobinopathies, such as sickle cells or the characteristic inclusions of Hb C disease. The general approach to identification of these disorders is quantitative hemoglobin analysis, and in the past the principal tool was hemoglobin electrophoresis. Hb C, Hb E, Hb S, and Hb H can be detected by electrophoresis. The presence of increased amounts of Hb A₂ and/or Hb F indicates β-thalassemia variants. The most common approach to hemoglobin electrophoresis uses cellulose acetate at alkaline pH (usually pH 8.2-8.6); however, Hb A₂ and Hb C migrate to the same position and must be distinguished by electrophoresis at an acidic pH on citrate agar. Specific quantitative tests using alkali denaturation for Hb F or ion-exchange microcolumns for Hb A₂ are widely available. Techniques have been developed to separate a number of Hb types not clearly distinguished in cellulose acetate or citrate agar. These new methods utilizing high-performance liquid chromatography and capillary zone electrophoresis have replaced electrophoretic methods as the primary testing platforms for hemoglobin identification in most reference laboratories.[89,90] DNA sequencing is often employed in the analysis of rare or novel Hb variants.

α-Thalassemia syndromes are not associated with increases in Hb A₂ and Hb F and thus not detectable by hemoglobin quantitation studies unless three α genes are deleted, resulting in Hb H disease. For this reason, the diagnosis of the α-thalassemia trait was traditionally presumptive, based on family studies and exclusion of iron deficiency and β-thalassemia. Specific DNA-based testing that can quantify the number of alleles is readily available and can confirm a diagnosis of alpha thalassemia trait. It is particularly useful in prenatal diagnosis and the counseling of potential parents at risk for having children with homozygous α-thalassemia. Unstable Hbs are detected by the isopropanol stability test.

Sideroblastic Anemias

The sideroblastic anemias are due to acquired and hereditary disorders of heme synthesis (Chapter 26). A classic morphologic feature of this type of anemia, as seen in the peripheral blood smear, is the presence of erythrocyte dimorphism (*Figure 24.5E*), with a microcytic population of cells mixed with a normal red cell population and the presence of occasional heavily stippled hypochromic cells. In

hereditary (X-linked) sideroblastic anemia, the anemia and microcytosis are pronounced (*Table 24.7*), and these changes are accompanied by considerable anisocytosis and poikilocytosis. The serum iron concentration usually is elevated, and the TIBC is increased. In all cases of sideroblastic anemia, regardless of the specific etiology, impaired heme synthesis leads to retention of iron within the mitochondria. Morphologically, this is seen in marrow aspirates, which reveal many nucleated red cells with iron granules (i.e., aggregates of iron in mitochondria) that have a perinuclear distribution.[91,92] These distinctive cells, known as *ring sideroblasts*, are found only in pathologic states and are distinct from the sideroblasts (erythroblasts with diffuse cytoplasmic ferritin granules) seen in 30% to 50% of normal RBCs precursors in marrow. Most common sideroblastic anemias occur in middle age and later life, and these acquired disorders can be idiopathic or secondary to drugs, alcohol, or myeloproliferative disorders (*Table 24.6*). In addition, there are rare congenital sideroblastic anemias that conform to an X-linked pattern of inheritance, usually occurring in males, although skewed lyonization has resulted in females being affected. Autosomal-dominant and sporadic cases also occur. Several different genetic mutations have been identified in these congenital sideroblastic anemias (Chapter 26). Severe anemias are recognized in infancy or in early childhood, whereas milder cases may not become apparent until early adulthood or later. Patients may present with pallor, icterus, moderate splenomegaly, or hepatomegaly. Iron overload is a major complication of this disorder. In some cases in which there is little or no anemia, there still may be clinical evidence of iron overload (i.e., diabetes mellitus and liver dysfunction).

APPROACH TO NORMOCYTIC ANEMIA

Normocytic anemias are those in which the values for MCV are within normal limits, between 80 and 100 fL in adults. At times, however, the anemias that fall into this category may also present as macrocytic or microcytic. For example, the anemia associated with hypothyroidism or with liver disease may be either normocytic or slightly macrocytic. In addition, because of reticulocytosis, the anemia associated with acute hemorrhage or chronic hemolysis may be normocytic or slightly macrocytic. AI, although most often normocytic, is sometimes microcytic, and its pathogenesis is best understood in the context of microcytic anemias, as described earlier. Lastly, iron deficiency early in the course of anemia may be normocytic before becoming microcytic.

The normocytic anemias are not related to one another by common pathogenetic mechanisms. In many instances, anemia is only of incidental importance, a manifestation of a systemic disease with other, more serious consequences. Importantly, however, sometimes anemia is the first evidence of disease and the sign leading to discovery of the underlying disorder.

Despite the varied etiologies and the often-incidental nature of normocytic anemias, they can be classified in a way that forms a basis for diagnostic investigation (*Figure 24.11*). As a first step, it should be determined whether the erythropoietic response is appropriate to the degree of anemia. When bone marrow function is unimpaired and the iron supply is ample, erythropoiesis can increase many-fold. In most cases, marrow examination is not necessary to determine that the erythropoietic response is adequate, because reticulocytosis may be prominent, and polychromatophilic macrocytes may be detected on routinely stained blood smears. These manifestations of appropriate marrow response are typical of hemolytic anemia and posthemorrhagic anemia. The history, physical examination, and signs of excessive erythrocyte destruction (e.g., hyperbilirubinemia) provide the information necessary to differentiate these two conditions. The diagnostic approaches to anemias due to hemolysis and after acute hemorrhage are discussed separately.

When anemia is apparent but the erythropoietic response is less than appropriate, most likely the underlying disorder directly or indirectly affects the bone marrow. Indirect effects should be investigated first, because often a diagnosis can be made without resorting to marrow aspiration and biopsy. For example, several disorders are associated with reduced secretion of Epo (*Table 24.8*). In these conditions, screening tests

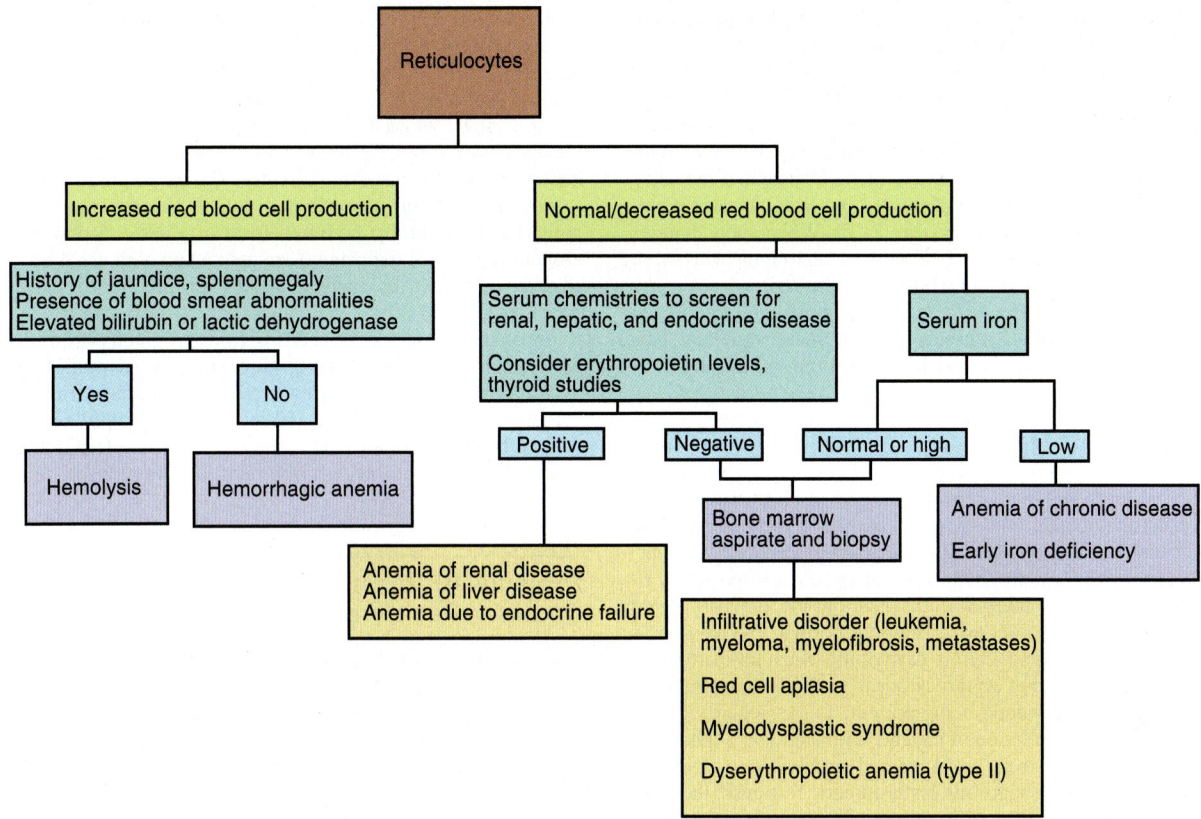

FIGURE 24.11 Diagnostic approach to a patient with normocytic anemia.

Table 24.8. Classification of the Normocytic Anemias

Anemia associated with appropriately increased erythrocyte production

Posthemorrhagic anemia

Hemolytic anemia

Anemia of systemic diseases

Anemia of renal insufficiency

Anemia of liver disease

Anemia of inflammation

Anemia of endocrine deficiency

Protein-calorie malnutrition

Anemia with impaired marrow response

Red blood cell aplasia

Acquired pure red cell aplasia in adults

Transient erythroblastopenia of childhood

Transient aplastic crises associated with hemolysis

Aplastic anemia (pancytopenia)

Bone marrow infiltrative disorders

Leukemia

Myeloma

Other myelophthisic anemias

Myelodysplastic anemias

Congenital dyserythropoietic anemia (CDA) type II

usually uncover an underlying systemic disease, and for this purpose, renal function, liver function, and thyroid status should be assessed using appropriate biochemical tests. Although severe protein-calorie malnutrition is accompanied by reduced Epo secretion and a mild normocytic anemia, such undernutrition is rare in developed countries and thus is not likely to be confused with other systemic disorders. AI typically presents as a normocytic anemia with low reticulocytes. This can be recognized by the underlying inflammatory state and the previously described iron studies. One of the elements of AI is a blunted Epo response due to the presence of inflammatory cytokines (Chapter 42).

Normocytic anemia with marked reticulocytopenia is also a characteristic of several disorders not caused by Epo deficiency such as the PRCA syndromes. Acquired PRCA in adults represents a relatively rare group of disorders usually occurring in the fifth to seventh decades of life (Chapter 40). The anemia can occur as a primary disorder or as secondary to some other disease. Early studies suggested an association with thymoma, but more recent data indicate this is much less common. Most cases of PRCA are seen with a variety of hematologic malignancies (in particular, chronic lymphocytic leukemia) and also with nonhematologic malignancies (primarily thymoma) and inflammatory disorders like rheumatoid arthritis or systemic lupus erythematous, and in association with a variety of drugs and chemicals. Laboratory data reveal isolated anemia, reticulocytopenia, and a bone marrow almost completely devoid of erythroblasts. The remainder of the CBC is normal.

Transient erythroblastopenia of childhood (TEC) is a form of PRCA occurring in young children, caused by transient antibody-mediated suppression of normal erythropoiesis that frequently follows a viral infection (Chapter 41). In contrast to Diamond-Blackfan syndrome, there are no congenital abnormalities and no abnormal RBC features. The natural history of TEC is one of spontaneous recovery over a few weeks.

Aplastic crises with hemolytic anemia are a self-limiting form of red cell aplasia seen in patients with chronic hemolytic anemia. It is

Disorders of Red Blood Cells

characterized by a rapid decrease in the steady-state Hb concentration and a very low reticulocyte count (see "Approach to Hemolysis").

When normocytic anemia with reticulocytopenia is associated with leukopenia and thrombocytopenia, there should be suspicion for intrinsic marrow disease due to aplastic anemia, leukemia, myelofibrosis, or myelophthisis. Morphologic abnormalities suggestive of marrow infiltration found on the blood smear include nucleated red cells, teardrop poikilocytes, immature leukocytes, and large, bizarre platelets or megakaryocyte fragments (*Figure 24.7*). When such changes are detected, as well as in any patient with anemia along with other cytopenias, marrow aspiration and biopsy are indicated.

Of the different CDAs, type II CDA is the most common, and it is the one that almost always presents as a normocytic anemia. This disorder is recognized by distinct multinuclearity of the marrow normoblasts (Chapter 41).

APPROACH TO HEMOLYSIS

Hemolytic disorders are characterized by signs of accelerated erythrocyte destruction together with those of vigorous blood regeneration. Under maximal stimulation, the normal marrow is capable of undergoing hyperplasia until its production rate increases approximately 6- to 8-fold.[32] With optimal marrow compensation, the survival of red cells in the circulation can decrease from the normal 120 days to as few as 15 to 20 days without anemia developing. Such an increase in destruction and production of erythrocytes can result in a compensated hemolytic state without anemia being present. In this regard, it is of interest that a significant fraction of patients with hereditary spherocytosis are not anemic. However, when red cell survival is so short that anemia develops despite a vigorous erythropoietic response, the term *hemolytic anemia* is appropriate.

Pathogenesis and Classification

Disorders associated with hemolytic anemia have been classified in various ways, none of which is entirely satisfactory. On clinical grounds, hemolytic anemias have been divided into acute and chronic forms, but such a division is of limited usefulness because acute exacerbations may develop during the course of chronic hemolytic disorders. Of somewhat greater use is a classification based on the site of hemolysis, whether it is predominantly within the circulation (intravascular) or within tissue macrophages (extravascular). Most hemolytic diseases are characterized by extravascular red cell destruction. The intravascular hemolytic disorders are accompanied by unique manifestations, such as hemoglobinemia, hemoglobinuria, and hemosiderinuria, and this type of hemolysis is easily recognized (*Table 24.9*).[93]

Hemolytic disorders may also be considered to be caused by an intrinsic defect of the red cell itself or caused by extrinsic agents acting on otherwise normal red cells. It is this classification that generally is most useful to the clinician (*Table 24.10*). Most intrinsic defects are inherited, whereas the extrinsic ones are typically acquired. Exceptions to this generalization are few; these include paroxysmal nocturnal hemoglobinuria (Chapter 32), an acquired disorder characterized by an intrinsic red cell defect. Certain inherited intrinsic defects (e.g., the most common form of glucose-6-phosphate dehydrogenase [G6PD] deficiency) are associated with no ill effects in the absence of an extrinsic agent, usually an infection or exposure to a drug (see Chapter 30).

Intrinsic and extrinsic abnormalities originally were defined by performing cross-transfusion erythrocyte survival studies. When normal erythrocytes are transfused to patients with an extrinsic cause for hemolysis, the donated cells are destroyed as rapidly as the patient's own cells. On the other hand, when the patient's RBCs are removed from their unfavorable environment and transfused to a normal

Table 24.9. Hemolytic Anemias Characterized by Significant Intravascular Red Cell Destruction

Paroxysmal nocturnal hemoglobinuria (PNH)
Erythrocyte fragmentation disorders
Transfusion reactions resulting from ABO isoantibodies
Paroxysmal cold hemoglobinuria
Acquired autoimmune hemolytic anemia (AIHA)
Associated with certain infections
Blackwater fever in falciparum malaria
Clostridial sepsis
Caused by certain chemical agents
Arsine poisoning
Snake and spider venoms
Drug reactions with G6PD deficiency
Intravenous administration of distilled water
Thermal injury

Table 24.10. Classification of the Most Common Causes of Hemolysis

Acquired Hemolytic Disorders
Immunohemolytic anemias
Autoimmune hemolytic anemia
Hemolytic disease of the newborn
Transfusion of incompatible blood
Mechanical hemolytic anemia
Prosthetic valves and other cardiac abnormalities
Hemolytic uremic syndrome
Thrombotic thrombocytopenic purpura
March hemoglobinuria
Disseminated intravascular coagulation
Infection
Protozoa (malaria, toxoplasmosis, leishmaniasis, babesiosis)
Bacteria (clostridial infection, cholera, bartonellosis, typhoid, etc.)
Other causes
Paroxysmal nocturnal hemoglobinuria
Spur-cell anemia in liver disease
Associated with hemodialysis and uremia
Thermal RBC injury
Hypophosphatemia
Snake venoms
Inherited Hemolytic Disorders
RBC membrane abnormalities
Hereditary spherocytosis
Hereditary elliptocytosis syndromes
Hereditary stomatocytosis; xerocytosis
RBC enzyme disorders
Glucose-6-phosphate dehydrogenase deficiency
Pyruvate kinase deficiency
RBC hemoglobin disorders
Sickle cell anemia syndromes
Thalassemia syndromes
Unstable hemoglobin disorders

recipient, their survival time is normal. In contrast, when the disorder is due to an intrinsic red cell defect, the RBCs of the patient, when given to a normal recipient, are removed from the circulation more rapidly than those of the recipient; the normal erythrocytes, if transfused into the patient, maintain a normal lifespan. Although such cross-transfusion experiments were important in clarifying the pathogenesis of various hemolytic disorders, obviously they have no current role in the evaluation of patients.

The intrinsic disorders of the erythrocyte are due to defects affecting the red cell membrane (Chapter 29), disorders of red cell metabolism (Chapter 30), or various Hb abnormalities (Chapters 35 and 36) (*Table 24.10*).

The acquired hemolytic anemias are further subclassified on the basis of the extrinsic factors causing hemolysis. These include antibodies and other immune mechanisms (Chapter 31) and other non-immune causes (Chapter 33) including physical trauma, infectious agents, physical agents, chemical agents, hypophosphatemia, and liver disease (spur-cell anemia). A separate category is needed for paroxysmal nocturnal hemoglobinuria, which is unique among the acquired hemolytic anemias in that it is related to an intrinsic abnormality of the red cell (Chapter 32).

Each of these different hemolytic anemias is discussed in detail elsewhere in this book. The remainder of this section focuses on the general clinical and laboratory features that are common to most congenital and acquired hemolytic anemias.

Clinical Features of Congenital Hemolytic Anemia
Degree of Anemia

The severity of anemia varies greatly, even among patients with the same congenital disorder. Most commonly, the anemia with congenital hemolytic disorders is mild to moderate because the shortened erythrocyte survival is partially offset by increased erythropoietic activity of the bone marrow. Often, patients accommodate remarkably well to the anemia and may exhibit few signs or symptoms. Consequently, detection can be delayed until later in childhood and discovered incidentally. Moreover, some patients have no anemia at all. The disease may then remain unsuspected until late in adult life unless jaundice, an acute hemolytic or aplastic episode ("crisis"), or complications of chronic hemolysis like cholelithiasis from bilirubin gallstones draw attention to the condition. Sometimes, such cases are discovered only when another family member receives a diagnosis.

In some congenital hemolytic disorders, such as β-thalassemia major, the rate of red cell destruction far exceeds the erythropoietic capacity of the marrow, and these individuals usually have a very severe anemia requiring lifelong red cell transfusions.

Jaundice

Jaundice often is first noted in the neonatal period,[94] and phototherapy frequently is used to reduce the hyperbilirubinemia; sometimes, exchange transfusions are required. In some older children and adults with congenital hemolytic anemia, icterus is absent or mild enough to pass unnoticed. Careful inquiry often elicits a history of episodes of jaundice or the passing of dark urine associated with minor infections. In other cases, jaundice is persistent but never becomes intense. Often, slight scleral icterus is the only sign of hemolytic disease. As noted earlier, the jaundice of hemolytic disease is typically acholuric; the bilirubin, being unconjugated, is not excreted in the urine. Furthermore, pruritus is absent. These features help distinguish the icterus of hemolytic disease from that found with disorders of the hepatobiliary system.

Aplastic Crises

Aplastic crises result from transient failure of red cell production (*Figure 24.12*) caused by infection with the type B19 human parvovirus.[95,96] The same virus also causes erythema infectiosum (fifth disease, a common childhood exanthem).[97] In adults, it may cause an acute polyarthropathy syndrome as well as aseptic meningitis.[98]

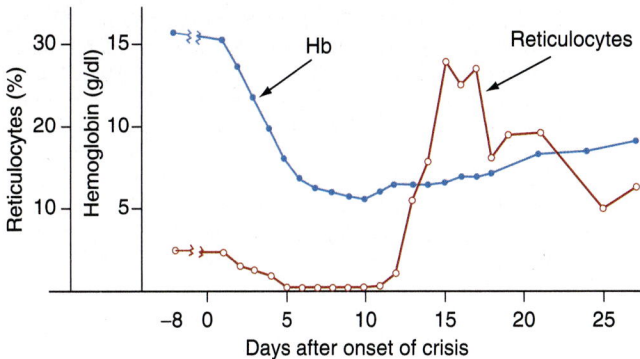

FIGURE 24.12 **Severe aplastic crisis in a patient with hereditary spherocytosis who previously had well-compensated hemolysis.** Note the profound reticulocytopenia during the early phases of the reaction, followed by reticulocytosis. Hb, hemoglobin. (Data plotted from Owren P. Congenital hemolytic jaundice. The pathogenesis of the "hemolytic crisis. *Blood.* 1948;3:231-248.)

In utero, it can cause fetal death with hydrops fetalis.[99] Parvovirus infection may occur sporadically, but most often it is an epidemic disease that can affect several family members simultaneously or multiple people in a large geographic area. School-age children (age 5-10 years) are most at risk for parvovirus infection, but cases have been reported in young adults.[100] Any patient with moderately severe chronic hemolytic disease who becomes infected with parvovirus is at risk for an aplastic crisis. Blood Hb concentrations fall several grams/dL, sometimes to life-threatening levels, and the reticulocyte count falls abruptly to less than 1%.[95,96] The magnitude of the crisis depends on the severity of the underlying hemolytic process. In most cases, leukocyte and platelet counts are unaffected, but neutropenia and thrombocytopenia can occur and, rarely, may be severe. The bone marrow is cellular, but erythroid hypoplasia is the characteristic finding; in particular, the more mature erythrocyte precursors tend to disappear. Giant pronormoblasts may be observed. Recovery is heralded by reticulocytosis. The entire episode, from onset of symptoms to reappearance of reticulocytes, lasts approximately 10 to 12 days in subjects with normal immunologic responses but may persist much longer in patients with defective or suppressed immune systems.[101] Parvovirus infection also produces erythroid aplasia in normal subjects, but the decrease in Hb concentration is minimal when erythrocyte survival is normal, and such small changes go undetected.[102] During the acute phase of aplastic crisis, parvovirus DNA can be detected in the serum by polymerase chain reaction assays.[103] The appearance of a specific immunoglobulin (Ig) M (IgM) antibody in serum is a marker of recent infection. It is replaced by an IgG antibody that persists for years and is found in 60% of normal subjects.[103] A single infection apparently confers lifelong immunity. However, parvovirus antibody titers are only helpful for diagnosis in immunocompetent patients.

Splenomegaly

The spleen commonly is enlarged in patients with congenital hemolytic anemias, except for individuals with sickle cell anemia (HbSS) older than 5 years of age, in whom the spleen has undergone autoinfarction. Most often, the degree of enlargement is mild to moderate. At times, detection of splenomegaly is the first clue to the underlying hematologic disease. It is not uncommon for children with hereditary spherocytosis to be recognized initially by the finding of splenomegaly during a routine physical examination in an otherwise healthy child.

Cholelithiasis

Gallstones and its complications play a significant role in the clinical manifestations of congenital hemolytic anemias. Symptoms of gallbladder disease rarely may be the initial manifestations of a hemolytic process and the ones that bring the illness to the attention of a physician. Gallstones typical of hemolytic anemia are so-called pigment stones and are typically black or very dark brown in color.[104,105] They differ from mineral-based stones (calcium, etc.) and cholesterol stones, neither of which are associated with hemolysis. The hepatic bile of patients with hemolytic anemia contains greatly increased amounts and concentrations of unconjugated bilirubin, decreased concentrations of bile acids, and increased concentrations of ionized calcium.[106]

The prevalence of cholelithiasis in patients with hemolytic anemia increases with age and with the intensity of the hemolytic process. In a large study series involving Jamaican patients with sickle cell anemia, the prevalence ranged from 8% among patients 16 to 25 years old to 55% in patients older than age 35 years with reticulocyte counts greater than 15%.[107]

Leg Ulcers

Chronic ulcerations in the legs are uncommon complications of chronic hemolytic disease. They are particularly characteristic of sickle cell anemia (Chapter 34)[108] and also occur in association with other hemolytic disorders such as hereditary spherocytosis or beta thalassemia[109,110] (Chapters 29 and 35). The ulcers often are bilateral and tend to involve the areas overlying or proximal to the medial or lateral malleoli. They tend to be chronic or recurrent and, upon healing, leave the skin indurated and pigmented. Hydroxyurea, which is extensively prescribed in sickle cell patients, can also produce malleolar skin ulcers.[108]

Skeletal Abnormalities

When hemolytic anemia is severe during active phases of growth and development, the pronounced expansion of erythroid bone marrow may lead to a tower-shaped skull, thickening and striation of frontal and parietal bones ("frontal bossing"), maxillary and dental abnormalities, and other distortions of bony structures. Such abnormalities are particularly characteristic of severe thalassemia major, the so-called thalassemic facies (Chapter 36). It is much less common to see these skeletal malformations than it was 30 years ago, because now patients with severe β-thalassemia syndromes are transfused aggressively with red cells to maintain a higher Hb level, and this suppresses expansion of the erythroid marrow and its subsequent effects on bone structure. However, in patients with thalassemia intermedia, a slightly milder clinical variant not necessitating RBC transfusions, the characteristic bone changes may occur because of the expanded size of the erythroid marrow. The skeletal changes may also occur in patients with sickle cell anemia and rarely in patients with other forms of congenital hemolytic anemia.[111]

Clinical Features of Acquired Hemolytic Anemia

Hemolytic anemia sometimes develops acutely, such as after the transfusion of incompatible blood, or following the ingestion of an oxidant drug or fava beans by patients with G6PD deficiency, or in association with an acute febrile illness. Some instances of autoimmune hemolytic anemia, thrombotic thrombocytopenic purpura, and other hemolytic disorders may also begin abruptly. Fever and chills are the most common symptoms and may be accompanied by aching pains in the back and abdomen, headaches, malaise, and vomiting.[112] Abdominal pain may be severe, and the accompanying muscular spasm and rigidity may simulate the signs of an acute abdominal condition requiring surgical evaluation. Pallor, jaundice, tachycardia, and other symptoms of severe anemia may be prominent.

Acquired hemolytic anemia can also begin insidiously, developing gradually over a period of weeks or months. Cardiovascular adjustments to the anemia may be adequate, and patients may have few symptoms. Pallor, scleral icterus, or a jaundiced complexion may be the first evidence of illness, and, often, these signs are noticed by friends or associates before they are appreciated by the patient or the family. As in congenital hemolytic anemia, the course may be interrupted by aplastic crises.[113]

In other instances, the clinical setting may be dominated by the manifestations of an underlying disease of which the hemolytic anemia is one manifestation. For example, signs and symptoms of lymphoma, systemic lupus erythematosus, or mycoplasma pneumonia may overshadow those of the associated hemolytic process.

Laboratory Features of Hemolysis

The laboratory studies used to identify a hemolytic process include those related to the increase in erythrocyte destruction and those related to the compensatory increase in the rate of erythropoiesis (*Table 24.11*).

Signs of Increased Red Blood Cell Destruction

Serum Bilirubin

The amount of bilirubin in the circulation depends in part on the rate at which the bilirubin is formed and in part on the efficiency with which it is excreted by the liver. Hyperbilirubinemia is a hallmark of hemolytic anemia (*Figure 24.13*), although occasionally the serum bilirubin is within the normal range despite brisk hemolytic disease.[114] The increased serum bilirubin level in hemolysis almost always consists of the unconjugated (indirect-reacting) pigment. The conjugated fraction typically remains within or near normal limits, and no bilirubin is evident in the urine. Except for during the neonatal period, values greater than 5 mg/dL are unusual in patients with hemolytic anemia and suggest coexisting hepatic dysfunction.

Serum Lactate Dehydrogenase

Serum lactate dehydrogenase (LDH) often is increased in patients with hemolytic anemia, although not to as great an extent as in megaloblastic anemia. The increase in LDH probably results from release of the erythrocyte enzyme into the plasma during hemolysis.[115] Increased serum LDH is a nonspecific finding, because it also is elevated in other medical conditions associated with tissue injury.

Serum Haptoglobin

When Hb enters the plasma, it binds to haptoglobin, and the complex is removed by hepatocytes. As a result, serum haptoglobin decreases in individuals with hemolytic disease. Moreover, despite the intravascular site of haptoglobin function, this protein becomes depleted in association with both intravascular and extravascular hemolysis. Haptoglobin also decreases in megaloblastic anemia and other

Table 24.11. Laboratory Signs of Hemolysis

Accelerated red cell destruction
Increased serum unconjugated bilirubin level
Increased serum lactate dehydrogenase
Increased carbon monoxide production
Decreased serum haptoglobin
Hemoglobinemia
Hemoglobinuria
Hemosiderinuria
Methemalbuminemia
Decreased serum hemopexin
Accelerated erythropoiesis
Reticulocytosis
Macrocytosis
Blood smear findings
Polychromatophilia
Basophilic, stippling
Erythroblastosis
Abnormal red blood cell shapes
Bone marrow (erythroid hyperplasia)

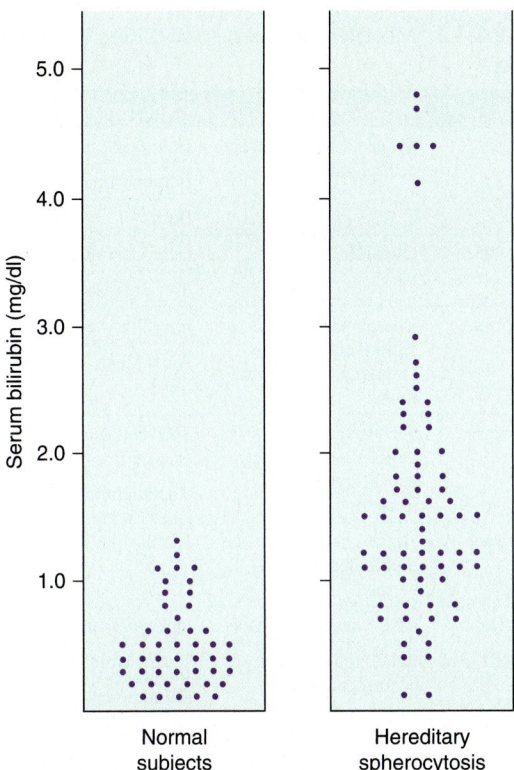

FIGURE 24.13 **Total serum bilirubin values in 48 normal subjects and 72 patients with hereditary spherocytosis.** (Data from Mackinney A, Norton NE, Kosower NS. Ascertaining genetic carriers of hereditary spherocytosis by statistical analysis of multiple laboratory tests. *J Clin Invest*. 1962;41:554-555.)

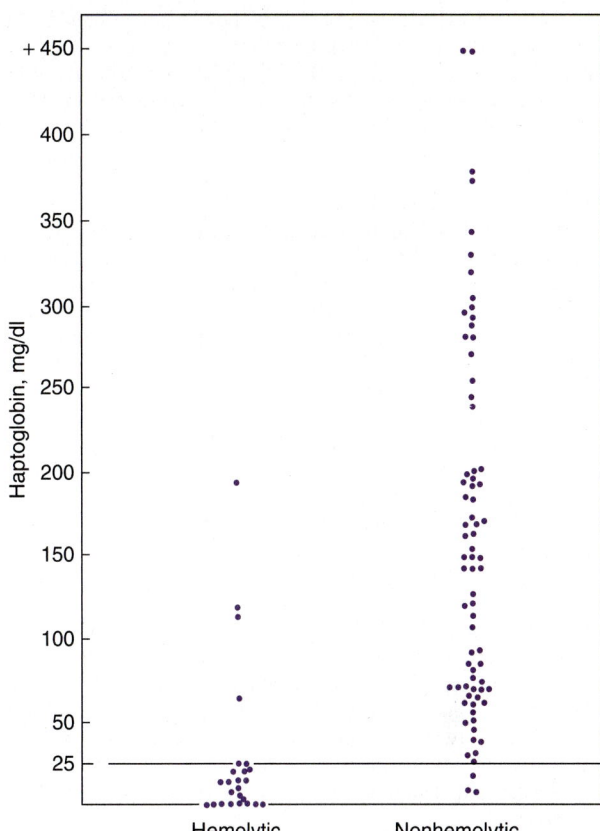

FIGURE 24.14 **Serum haptoglobin in hemolytic and nonhemolytic disease.** (Reproduced with permission from Marchand A, Galen RS, Van Lente F. The predictive value of serum haptoglobin in hemolytic disease. *JAMA*. 1980;243(19):1909-1911. Copyright © 1980 American Medical Association. All rights reserved.)

conditions with intramedullary hemolysis (ineffective erythropoiesis) (*Figure 24.14*). In microangiopathic hemolytic anemias with intravascular hemolysis, low haptoglobin levels are the most sensitive marker of red cell destruction and may be seen in the absence of anemia or hemoglobinemia.[116]

The interpretation of haptoglobin levels sometimes is complicated by the fact that haptoglobin is an acute-phase reactant, the synthesis of which increases in response to inflammatory, infectious, or malignant disease. Haptoglobin values may also fall in association with liver disease because of impaired synthesis and or may be decreased because of hereditary deficiency of the protein.

Erythrocyte Survival

The strictest definition of hemolysis requires demonstration that the red cell lifespan is reduced. From a practical perspective, however, erythrocyte lifespan determinations are rarely necessary, because they provide little additional information beyond what can be assessed by more easily obtained data, such as serial observations of the degree of anemia, reticulocytosis, and jaundice. For these reasons, determination of red cell survival is rarely performed.

Rate of Carbon Monoxide Production

Determinations of the rate of endogenous carbon monoxide production provide accurate assessments of the rate of heme catabolism. With these methods, values of approximately 2 to 10 times the normal rate have been detected in small groups of patients with hemolytic disease. However, these methods are not available for routine clinical use.[117]

Signs of Intravascular Hemolysis

When erythrocytes are destroyed within the circulation, and also when extravascular destruction is so rapid that it exceeds the capacity of the macrophage system, Hb is released into the plasma. The disposal of Hb and its heme group occurs by several mechanisms

(Chapter 6), and characteristic laboratory abnormalities are found (*Table 24.11*).

Hemoglobinemia

At low concentrations, plasma Hb may be measured by means of the benzidine reaction, which allows detection not only of Hb but also of any other heme pigments that may be present. If special precautions are observed to avoid artifactual hemolysis during collection of blood, normal values of less than 1 mg/dL of plasma are found. Plasma usually appears visibly red when Hb exceeds 50 mg/dL. At levels greater than 100 mg/dL, Hb can be measured directly by the cyanomethemoglobin method.

Detectable plasma Hb levels are normal in most patients with hereditary hemolytic anemias, including hereditary spherocytosis, but can be markedly increased in severe, acquired, and immunohemolytic anemia, at times reaching 100 mg/dL. Particularly high values, up to 1000 mg/dL, are found only in patients with disorders associated with intravascular hemolysis.[118]

Hemoglobinuria

When plasma Hb exceeds the haptoglobin binding capacity, Hb dimers are excreted into the urine, resulting in hemoglobinuria. Urine that contains Hb ranges from faint pink to deeper red, or even to almost black, similar to a cola beverage.

Hemoglobinuria can be distinguished from hematuria (whole RBCs in the urine) by microscopic examination of a freshly voided urine specimen. Urine also may appear red because of ingestion of certain drugs (pyridium) or food (beets), or because of porphyrinuria (Chapter 28) or myoglobinuria. Of these various red urinary pigments, only Hb and myoglobin produce a positive reaction in the commonly available tests for occult blood.

Hemoglobinuria must be distinguished from myoglobinuria, which occurs as the result of massive muscle injury. Myoglobin is a heme pigment of low molecular weight (17,000 Da); it is not bound by haptoglobin and therefore does not accumulate to an appreciable extent in plasma. Thus, inspection of the plasma can help distinguish myoglobinuria from hemoglobinuria, the presence of a red color in the plasma favoring the latter. More precise identification is accomplished by spectroscopic analysis.

Urine Hemosiderin and Urinary Iron Excretion

Hb in the glomerular filtrate is partially reabsorbed by the proximal tubular cells, and the Hb iron is incorporated into ferritin and hemosiderin. Subsequently, the iron-containing tubular cells are sloughed into the urine. Hemosiderinuria, therefore, constitutes reliable evidence that hemoglobinemia has occurred in the recent past. After an acute episode of intravascular hemolysis, however, several days may pass before increased iron excretion can be detected. Moreover, the abnormality may persist for some time after the episode has terminated. In most conditions associated with chronic intravascular hemolysis, such as in some of the fragmentation hemolysis syndromes, increased iron excretion is a constant finding, whereas hemoglobinuria occurs only intermittently. Hemosiderinuria may be detected by means of a qualitative test based on the Prussian blue reaction.[119]

Methemalbumin and Hemopexin

Hb in plasma is readily oxidized to methemoglobin, from which the heme group easily detaches. The liberated heme binds to hemopexin and also to albumin, forming methemalbumin. Hemopexin-heme and methemalbumin impart a coffee-brown color to plasma. Low hemopexin values are seen in thalassemia major, sickle cell anemia, and the fragmentation hemolytic anemia that follows cardiac surgical procedures. The measurement of hemopexin is seldom used to assess hemolytic anemia.

Signs of Accelerated Erythropoiesis

Laboratory signs of increased erythropoiesis are almost always present in patients with chronic hemolytic disease. In patients who have had an acute hemolytic episode, signs of increased red cell production appear after 3 to 6 days (*Table 24.11*). These same signs of increased RBC production also occur after hemorrhage and after specific therapy for anemia caused by iron, folate, or vitamin B_{12} deficiency.

Reticulocytosis

An increased number of reticulocytes continues to be the most readily available and most often used index of accelerated erythropoiesis. In cases of hemolytic anemia, the erythrocyte production rate and the absolute reticulocyte count is usually greatly increased when hemolysis is severe enough to produce anemia. In most types of hemolytic anemia, the reticulocyte count consistently increases to levels that correlate fairly well with the severity of the process. Exceptions occur during aplastic crises. In addition, some patients with acquired autoimmune hemolytic anemia may have normal or decreased reticulocyte counts. In one report of 308 cases, 18% had a reticulocyte count less than $100 \times 10^6/\text{mL}$.[120] In these cases, it is thought that the autoantibodies are directed against marrow erythroid precursors as well as against circulating erythrocytes.

Morphologic Findings in the Blood

When reticulocytes are increased, polychromatophilia and fine basophilic stippling are apparent on routinely stained smears of blood. Macrocytosis is found in association with most hemolytic disorders because of Epo-mediated stimulation of Hb synthesis and because prematurely released ("shift") reticulocytes are significantly larger than normal erythrocytes. Exceptions occur in hereditary spherocytosis and sickle cell anemia, diseases in which the intrinsic defect of the cell tends to decrease its size.

When hemolysis is brisk, nucleated erythrocytes may be found in the blood (erythroblastosis), usually in numbers below 1% of all the nucleated cells. In infants, however, erythroblastosis may be more striking, especially in hemolytic disease of the newborn.

Table 24.12. Morphologic Abnormalities in Hemolytic Anemia

Cell	Description	Clinical Disorders
Spherocyte	Spheroid RBC with no central pallor	Hereditary spherocytosis
		Immunohemolytic anemia
		Burns
Elliptocytes	Oval RBC	Hereditary elliptocytosis
		Megaloblastic anemia
Stomatocytes	Uniconcave red cell; slitlike rather than circular area of central pallor	Hereditary stomatocytosis
		Alcoholism
Acanthocytes	5-10 spicules of various lengths, irregular in spacing and thickness	Spur-cell anemia with liver disease
		Abetalipoproteinemia
Echinocytes	10-30 spicules evenly distributed over cell surface	Uremia
Sickle cells	RBC with sickle shape	Sickle cell anemia
Target cells	Solid area in center of central pallor	Thalassemia
		Hemoglobin C disorders
		Liver disease
		Lecithin-cholesterol acyl-transferase deficiency
		Postsplenectomy
Schistocytes	Triangular, helmet-shaped, fragmented, or greatly distorted cell; small	Microangiopathic anemia
		Turbulent blood flow
		Hemolytic uremic syndrome

Neutrophilic leukocytosis and thrombocytosis may accompany hemolytic anemia. These findings tend to be most common and most pronounced in patients with acute hemolytic anemias. Platelets are not only numerous but also large. The changes are less pronounced in chronic hemolytic processes.

Bone Marrow

The major alteration in the bone marrow in hemolytic anemia is erythroid hyperplasia, as manifested by a reduction in the myeloid to erythroid ratio.

Laboratory Tests Useful in the Differential Diagnosis of Hemolysis

Specific Morphologic Abnormalities

Detection of certain distortions of red cell shape is of particular diagnostic use because their presence suggests only one or a few entities. Descriptive features of certain such abnormal red cells are presented in *Table 24.12* and illustrated in *Figures 24.15* and *24.16.* .

Spherocytes, erythrocytes that lack an area of central pallor (*Fig. 24.15B*), are the hallmark of hereditary spherocytosis. They are also found in most patients with acquired immunohemolytic anemias (*Fig. 24.15C*), thermal injury, hypophosphatemia, or certain kinds of chemical poisoning. They typically have a smaller diameter than normal red blood cells.

Oval cells or elliptocytes (*Figure 24.15D*) are the sine qua non of common hereditary elliptocytosis that usually is a morphologic curiosity and not associated with significant hemolysis. However, some hereditary elliptocytosis variants are also associated with marked poikilocytosis (*Figure 24.15E* and *F*), and these individuals have significant hemolytic anemia.

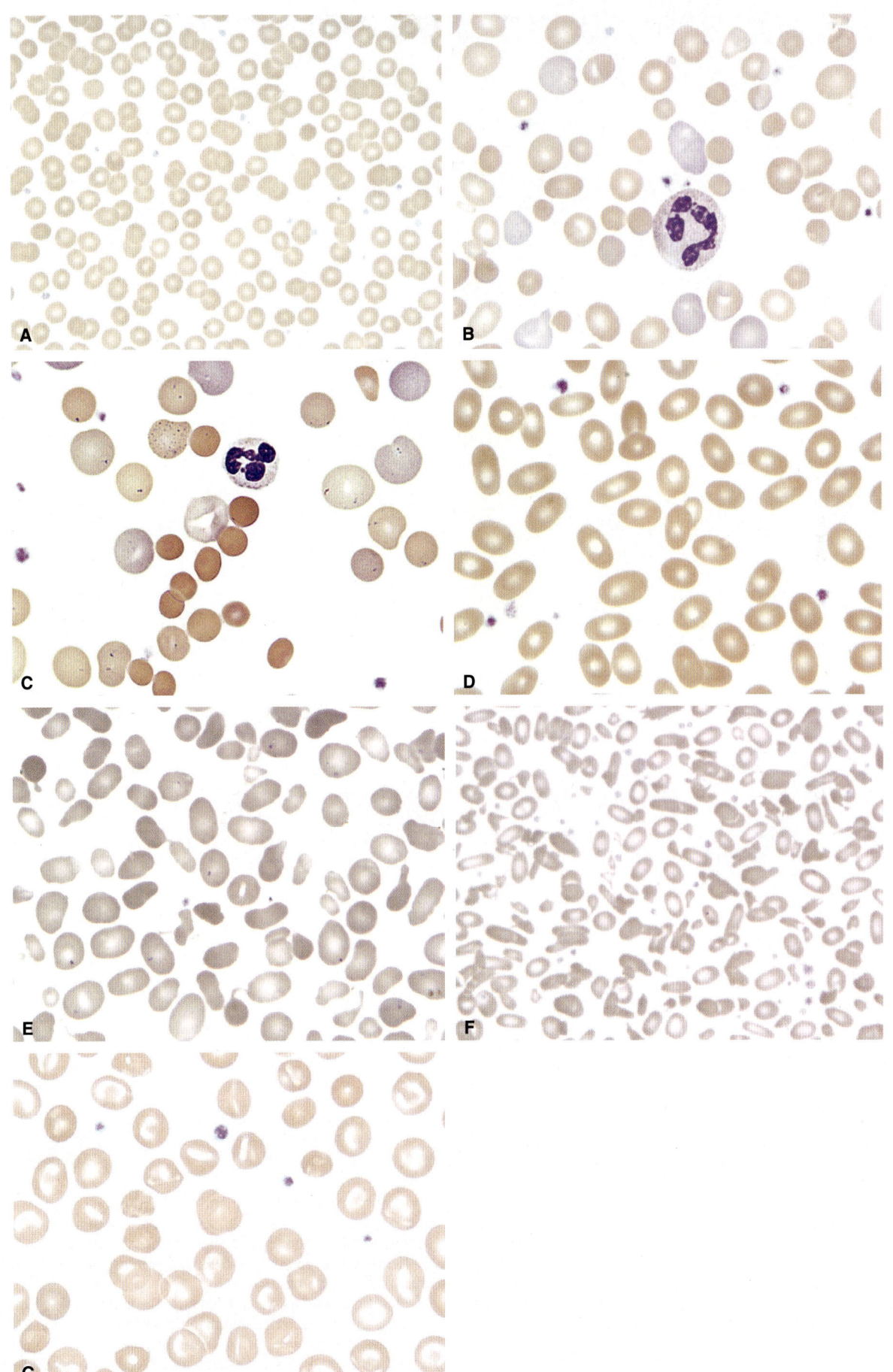

FIGURE 24.15 Red blood cell abnormalities associated with hemolysis. A. Normal red blood cells for comparison. **B.** Microspherocytes from patient with hereditary spherocytosis. **C.** Spherocytes from patient with autoimmune hemolytic anemia **D.** Hereditary elliptocytosis—common variant with minimal or no hemolysis. **E.** Hereditary elliptocytosis—hemolytic variant. **F.** Hereditary elliptocytosis—pyropoikilocytosis variant. **G.** Hereditary stomatocytosis.

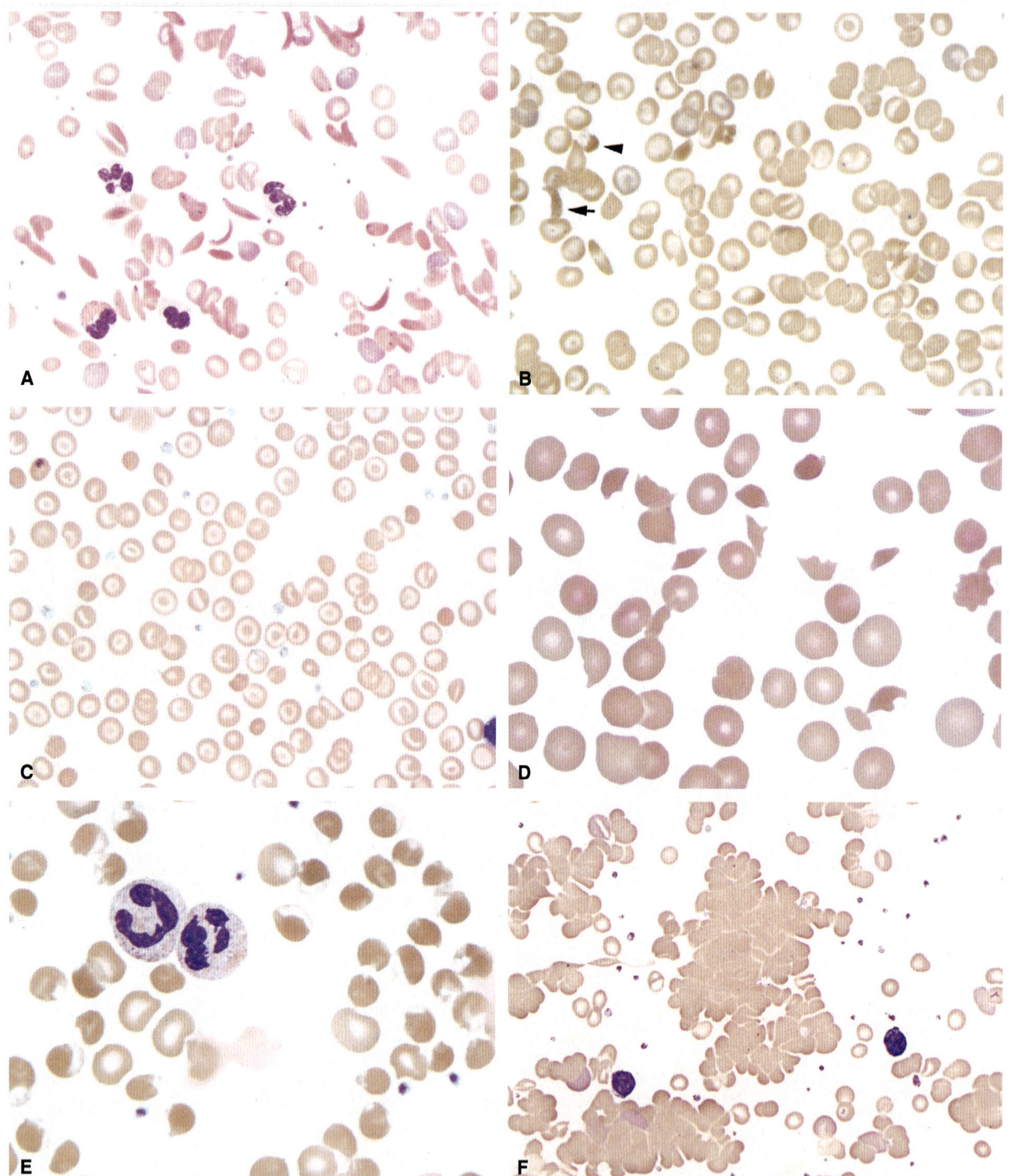

FIGURE 24.16 **A.** Sickle cell (HbSS) anemia. **B.** Sickle hemoglobin SC disease. **C.,** Target cells in hemoglobin EE. **D.** Schistocytes in patient with thrombotic thrombocytopenic purpura. **E.** Blister cell from oxidative assault in patient with glucose-6-phosphate dehydrogenase deficiency. **F.** Autoagglutination in cold agglutinin disease.

Stomatocytes (*Figure 24.15G*) are erythrocytes with a central slit or mouth-shaped (stoma) area of central pallor when examined on dried smears. In wet preparations, they are uniconcave rather than biconcave, giving them a bowl-like appearance. A few stomatocytes may be observed in blood smears prepared from normal individuals. Acquired stomatocytosis has been associated with hepatobiliary disease, vinca alkaloid administration, and neoplasms. Stomatocytes are also associated with rare hereditary disorders of red cell cation permeability, sitosterolemia, and familial deficiency of high-density lipoproteins (Chapter 29).

Acanthocytes indicate disturbed erythrocyte lipid composition; they occur in association with abetalipoproteinemia and the spur-cell anemia that occasionally accompanies hepatic cirrhosis.

Echinocytes (sea urchin cells) are a nonspecific abnormality and are also found in uremia.

Sickle cell anemia was named after the unmistakable sickle-shaped red cells that characterize that disorder (*Figure 24.16A* and *B*).

Target cells (*Figure 24.16C*) are characteristic of thalassemia, Hb E syndromes, and Hb C disorders. Target cells also occur in nonhemolytic states, such as obstructive jaundice and after splenectomy.

Schistocytes, helmet cells, or other fragmented red cells (*Figure 24.16D*) suggest hemolysis associated with physical trauma to the erythrocyte or with diseases affecting small blood vessels.

Bite cells are erythrocytes that look as if a semicircular bite has been taken from one edge. Hemighosts are red cells that look as if the Hb has shifted to one side of the cell, leaving the other side clear. These hemighosts also are referred to as *blister cells* and may appear to contain a coagulum of Hb that has separated from the membrane (*Figure 24.16E*). These cells are seen in patients with oxidant-induced injury such as in G6PD deficiency.

Autoagglutination may be apparent in blood smears (*Figure 24.16F*) or may even be visible to the naked eye when the blood is allowed to flow along the side of a glass container. The phenomenon is particularly characteristic of immunohemolytic disease caused by cold agglutinins. Autoagglutination must be distinguished from rouleaux formation, a manifestation of multiple myeloma and related diseases and the phenomenon responsible for accelerated rates of erythrocyte sedimentation.

Direct Antiglobulin Test

The test used for detection of immunohemolytic anemia is the direct antiglobulin or Coombs test (see discussion in Chapter 31). Positive test results indicate that the red cells are coated with IgG or complement components, especially C3. However, 3% to 11% of patients with autoimmune hemolytic disease have negative test results because the amount of globulin on the cell surface is below the detection limits. IgA-induced hemolytic anemia or IgM associated hemolytic anemia that does not fix complement may also have a negative direct antiglobulin test.[121] Occasionally, patients have weakly positive test results and no clinical evidence of hemolysis. Positive tests are found in as many as 36% of patients with AIDS without evidence of hemolysis.[122]

Osmotic Fragility Test

The osmotic fragility test is a measure of the resistance of erythrocytes to hemolysis by osmotic stress. The test consists of exposing red cells to decreasing strengths of hypotonic saline solutions and measuring the degree of hemolysis. A symmetric, sigmoidal curve is obtained in most subjects (*Figure 24.17*). Increased fragility is indicated by a shift of the curve to the left, whereas osmotic resistance (reduced fragility) is signified by a rightward shift of the curve. Increased osmotic fragility is observed in conditions associated with spherocytosis. With prior incubation of sterile blood for 24 h, the increased osmotic fragility of spherocytes is greatly accentuated, whereas normal cells become only slightly more fragile. Determination of osmotic fragility is of value chiefly in confirming important morphologic findings, especially the

presence of spherocytes. In most cases, however, the osmotic fragility test does not provide information that was not already available from an expert examination of a well-prepared, stained blood smear. Eosin-5-maleimide (EMA) binding to erythrocytes, a flow cytometry–based method reflecting relative amounts of band 3 protein, is now considered to be one of the most sensitive tests for detecting HS and has largely replaced osmotic fragility testing.[123] Osmotic gradient ektacytometry also is more sensitive and specific than the osmotic fragility test for the diagnosis of hereditary spherocytosis, but it is not widely available.[124]

Tests for Hemolytic Disorders Associated With Heinz Body Formation

In certain disorders, the hemolytic process involves precipitation of Hb, with the formation of inclusions known as *Heinz bodies*. These inclusions are rapidly removed by the spleen. Heinz body formation is the principal mechanism of hemolysis in G6PD deficiency and related disorders (Chapter 30), in unstable Hb disease (Chapter 36), in the thalassemias (Chapter 35), and in certain kinds of chemical injury (Chapter 33). Heinz bodies are not observed when ordinary staining procedures are used but require the use of special supravital stains (*Figure 24.18*). Cells containing these inclusions may be found in the blood during an acute hemolytic episode in subjects with G6PD deficiency and in splenectomized individuals with unstable Hb disease. When the spleen is intact, however, the inclusions are removed with such efficiency that the inclusion-containing cells often are not seen.

Diagnostic Strategy in the Patient With Hemolytic Anemia
Establishing the Presence of Hemolytic Anemia

The most common manifestations of chronic hemolytic anemia include anemia and reticulocytosis, often associated with various signs of excessive blood destruction. In contrast, an acute hemolytic anemia may not be accompanied initially by signs of accelerated red cell production. Such a diagnosis may be suspected because of the abrupt onset of hemoglobinuria or other signs of intravascular hemolysis or because of a rapid fall in blood Hb concentration from previously stable levels.

Conditions Sometimes Mistaken for Hemolytic Anemia

Anemias associated with acute hemorrhage and those with partially treated nutritional deficiency states are characterized by transient anemia and reticulocytosis (*Table 24.13*). They usually can be distinguished from hemolytic disease by the absence of icterus and by a rising Hct on subsequent determinations.

Anemias caused by ineffective erythropoiesis often are accompanied by jaundice and erythroid marrow hyperplasia; however, the reticulocyte count usually is not increased.

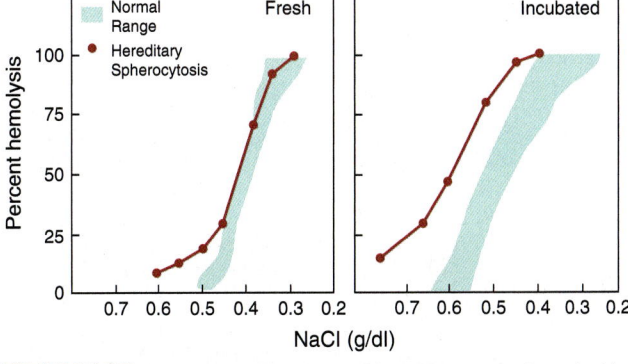

FIGURE 24.17 Osmotic fragility (as manifested by percent hemolysis) of normal and hereditary spherocytosis (HS) erythrocytes after incubation in salt solutions of varying tonicity. In fresh HS erythrocytes, note the "tail" of cells with increased sensitivity as a result of splenic conditioning (*left*). In the incubated red blood cell (RBC), note that the entire HS population of RBCs is more osmotically sensitive (*right*). (Reprinted from Glader BE, Naumovski L. Hereditary red blood cell disorders. In: Rimoin DL, Connor JM, Pyeritz RE, Emery AE, eds. *Principles and Practice of Medical Genetics*. 3rd ed. Churchill Livingstone; 1996 Copyright © 1996 Elsevier. With permission.)

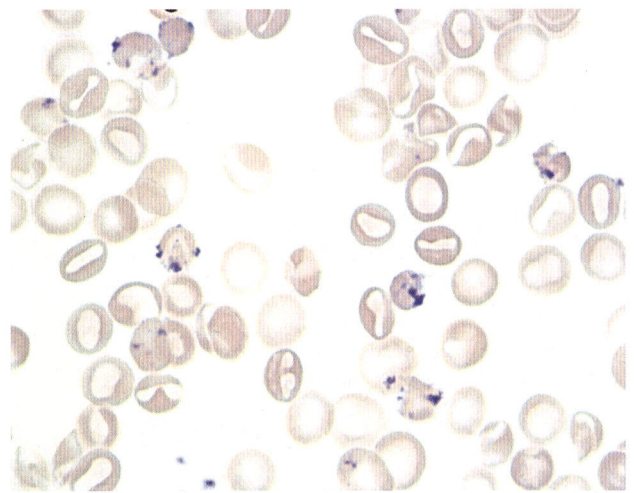

FIGURE 24.18 Heinz bodies (seen with brilliant cresyl blue supravital stains of blood) during hemolytic episodes in patient with G6PD deficiency.

A particularly confusing situation may arise after occult hemorrhage into the retroperitoneal space or other tissue compartments; anemia develops rapidly, and reticulocytosis follows. Furthermore, indirect hyperbilirubinemia may occur as the result of reabsorption of the products of Hb breakdown at the site of hemorrhage. Thus, the picture of hemolytic anemia may be simulated in several ways. Diagnosis depends on detecting signs of the hemorrhage itself or the disease process leading to it. If occult hemorrhage is suspected, serial observations usually clarify the situation; once the hemorrhage ceases, the Hct, reticulocyte count, and bilirubin values return to normal.

In individuals with acholuric jaundice but without anemia, the differential diagnosis lies between a compensated hemolytic state and Gilbert syndrome or other disorders of bilirubin catabolism. Reticulocytosis or morphologic abnormalities of erythrocytes are typical findings in the former. In mild compensated hemolytic disease, however, one cannot always be certain that the hematologic values will be abnormal. Fasting induces an exaggerated increase in bilirubin levels in patients with Gilbert syndrome,[125] and this phenomenon may be useful in distinguishing Gilbert syndrome from hemolytic anemia.

Anemia associated with marrow invasion may be accompanied by erythroblastosis and abnormalities of erythrocyte shape. Mild reticulocytosis may develop because of premature release of cells from the marrow. Usually, however, patients do not have jaundice, and evidence of the invasive disease may be detected by examination of the bone marrow.

Determining the Specific Cause of Hemolysis

Information from the medical history and physical examination, careful review of the CBC and peripheral blood smear, and results from the direct antiglobulin test, taken together, form the basis of the initial diagnosis assessment of hemolysis. From these data, five groups of patients can be distinguished.

1. *Those patients in whom the diagnosis is clear because of medical history such as obvious exposure to infectious, chemical, or physical agents.* Some infections, such as malaria, can cause hemolysis directly, whereas in other cases it is more indirect, associated with an underlying G6PD deficiency or an unstable Hb, such as Hb H.
2. *Those patients with a positive direct antiglobulin test.* Such individuals may be presumed to have immunohemolytic anemia. The subsequent investigation requires a search for an underlying disease as well as a serologic study of the nature of the antibody.
3. *Those patients with antiglobulin-negative, spherocytic hemolytic anemia.* Such patients probably have hereditary spherocytosis. It is appropriate to confirm the presence of spherocytes by flow cytometry to measure EMA binding to erythrocytes and also to attempt to establish the familial nature of the illness by studying family members. Immunohemolytic anemia may be associated with spherocytosis and is occasionally associated with a negative antiglobulin reaction. Exposure to chemical or infectious agents producing spherocytosis may not always be easy to establish.
4. *Those patients with other specific morphologic abnormalities of erythrocytes.* The significance of various types of abnormally shaped red cells was discussed previously. Some poikilocytes, such as elliptocytes and sickle cells, are virtually pathognomonic findings.
5. *Those with no specific morphologic abnormalities and a negative reaction to the antiglobulin test.* These patients warrant a battery of screening tests, including quantitative hemoglobin studies, the isopropanol stability test for unstable Hb disease, tests for common red cell enzymes such as G6PD and pyruvate kinase, and a screening test for paroxysmal nocturnal hemoglobinuria.

If all of these procedures yield normal results, making the diagnosis is likely to be difficult. Some of the possibilities include one of the rarer erythrocyte enzyme deficiencies or an unusual variant of CDA. To help facilitate making these diagnoses, there are now a number of molecular panels commercially available to help identify red cell membrane protein and enzyme mutations.

APPROACH TO ACUTE POSTHEMORRHAGIC ANEMIA

When blood loss occurs in small amounts over a prolonged period, no anemia develops until iron stores are depleted. In such circumstances, the hematologic findings are those of iron deficiency anemia. On the other hand, when larger amounts of blood are lost over shorter periods of time, anemia may develop, although iron stores remain adequate. This latter condition is called *acute posthemorrhagic anemia.*

The patient may be symptomatic and appear to be in shock, or the entire situation might be confused with an acute hemolytic process.

The physiologic changes that occur with acute blood loss in otherwise healthy individuals are summarized in *Table 24.14.* The immediate effects of acute hemorrhage are primarily cardiovascular. The plasma volume and red cell mass are reduced in proportional amounts; consequently, no decrease is observed in the Hct.[126] Because of the time required for extracellular fluid to restore the blood volume, the amount of blood loss tends to be underestimated by the degree of anemia, especially early in the disease course. The platelet count may increase, often reaching levels above normal within 1 h, and values greater than 1 million platelets/μL can be observed. There also can be a neutrophilic leukocytosis over 2 to 5 h. Typically, the leukocyte

Table 24.13. Conditions Sometimes Mistaken for Hemolytic Anemia

Associated with anemia and reticulocytosis
Hemorrhage
Recovery from iron, folate, or vitamin B_{12} deficiency
Recovery from marrow failure
Associated with jaundice and anemia
Ineffective erythropoiesis (intramedullary hemolysis)
Bleeding into a body cavity or tissue
Associated with jaundice without anemia
Defective bilirubin conjugation
Crigler-Najjar syndrome
Gilbert syndrome
Marrow invasion (myelofibrosis, metastatic disease)
Myoglobinuria

Table 24.14. Clinical Features of Acute Hemorrhage in Healthy Young Adults

Volume of Blood Loss (mL)	Blood Volume (%)	Symptoms
500-1000	10-20	Few if any symptoms
1000-1500	20-30	Asymptomatic while at rest in a recumbent position; light-headedness and hypotension when upright; tachycardia
1500-2000	30-40	Symptoms present when subject is recumbent; thirst, shortness of breath, clouding or loss of consciousness; blood pressure, cardiac output, venous pressure decrease; pulse usually becomes rapid; extremities become cold, clammy, and pale
2000-2500	40-50	Lactic acidosis, shock; irreversible shock, death

count is 10 to 20 × 10^4/μL. The leukocytosis is explained in part by the effect of epinephrine on granulocyte demargination and release from the marrow granulocyte reserve.

When first detected, the anemia following acute hemorrhage is normocytic with few signs of erythrocyte regeneration. The Hct or Hb may not reach the minimum value until 3 days or more after the hemorrhage ceases.

Some increase in the number of reticulocytes is usually detected within 3 to 5 days, and maximal values are reached at 6 to 11 days.[32] The degree of reticulocytosis is related to the magnitude of hemorrhage but rarely exceeds 15%. Other signs of erythrocyte regeneration include polychromatophilia and macrocytosis, and the MCV may transiently increase. If the patient is seen for the first time during this stage, the findings may be mistaken for those of hemolytic anemia; however, signs of increased bilirubin production are conspicuously absent, unless there has been bleeding into a body cavity or tissue space.

An external hemorrhage of a magnitude sufficient to cause significant anemia is usually evident. Similarly, substantial bleeding from the gastrointestinal or female reproductive tract is likely to be a dramatic event with readily detected signs and symptoms. Internal bleeding, as from a ruptured aneurysm, may be less apparent but should be suspected when there is the abrupt onset of shock or unexplained hypotension and tachycardia. Often, these manifestations are accompanied by symptoms referable to the site of bleeding. Hemorrhage into the retroperitoneal space, a body cavity, or a cyst, or in association with a hip or pelvic fracture, sometimes presents a diagnostic problem. There may be a rapid onset of anemia accompanied by hyperbilirubinemia arising from the breakdown and absorption of RBCs. Under such circumstances, the picture may be transiently confused with acute hemolytic anemia. In all cases, the onset of a sudden, unexplained anemia should lead to the suspicion of covert bleeding. The suspicion is strengthened if signs of regeneration, such as reticulocytosis, appear and no evidence of excessive blood destruction is found.

Surgery is a special circumstance in which hemorrhage is predictable. Surgical mortality is clearly increased when patients are severely anemic. An older guideline requiring preoperative transfusion if the Hb is less than 10 g/dL has been replaced by a lower trigger point, 7 g/dL, in otherwise healthy, younger patients.[127] In patients at increased cardiovascular risk who undergo major general or vascular surgery procedures, a less restrictive transfusion threshold may be appropriate.[128] Surgeons and anesthesiologists use several techniques to avoid the need for allogeneic transfusions. These techniques include the use of autotransfusion of cells harvested during surgery and or hypervolemic hemodilution.[129] The preoperative or postoperative use of Epo injection with concurrent intravenous iron has proved disappointing because of a relatively slow correction but may have a role in severely anemic patients who refuse transfusion.[129,130]

References

1. Means RTJ. It all started in New Orleans: Wintrobe, the hematocrit and the definition of normal. *Am J Med Sci.* 2011;341(1):64-65.
2. Koepke JA. *Practical Laboratory Hematology.* Churchill Livingstone; 1991:587.
3. Hollowell JG, van Assendelft OW, Gunter EW, Lewis BG, Najjar M, Pfeiffer C. Hematological and iron-related analytes—reference data for persons aged 1 year and over: United States, 1988-94. *Vital and health statistics series 11, Data from the national health survey.* 2005;247:1-156.
4. Khusun H, Yip R, Schultink W, Dillon DH. World Health Organization hemoglobin cut-off points for the detection of anemia are valid for an Indonesian population. *J Nutr.* 1999;129(9):1669-1674.
5. Zakai NA, Katz R, Hirsch C, et al. A prospective study of anemia status, hemoglobin concentration, and mortality in an elderly cohort: the Cardiovascular Health Study. *Arch Intern Med.* 2005;165(19):2214-2220.
6. Guralnik JM, Eisenstaedt RS, Ferrucci L, Klein HG, Woodman RC. Prevalence of anemia in persons 65 years and older in the United States: evidence for a high rate of unexplained anemia. *Blood.* 2004;104(8):2263-2268.
7. Ble A, Fink JC, Woodman RC, et al. Renal function, erythropoietin, and anemia of older persons: the InCHIANTI study. *Arch Intern Med.* 2005;165(19):2222-2227.
8. Spivak JL. Anemia in the elderly: time for new blood in old vessels. *Arch Intern Med.* 2005;165(19):2187-2189.
9. Daly MP, Sobal J. Anemia in the elderly. A survey of physicians' approaches to diagnosis and workup. *J FamPract.* 1989;28(5):524-528.
10. Stander PE. Anemia in the elderly. Symptoms, causes, and therapies. *Postgrad Med.* 1989;85(2):85-90.
11. Morra L, Moccia F, Mazzarello GP, Bessone G, Del NE, Ponassi GA. Defective burst-promoting activity of T lymphocytes from anemic and nonanemic elderly people. *Ann Hematol.* 1994;68(2):67-71.
12. Morra L, Moccia F, Mazzarello GP, Bessone G, Mela GS, Ponassi GA. Defective in vitro growth of BFU-E of elderly subjects revealed by hydrocortisone. *Biomed Pharmacother.* 1993;47(4):167-171.
13. Lipschitz DA, Udupa KB, Milton KY, Thompson CO. Effect of age on hematopoiesis in man. *Blood.* 1984;63(3):502-509.
14. Card RT, Brain MC. The "anemia" of childhood: evidence for a physiologic response to hyperphosphatemia. *N Engl J Med.* 1973;288(8):388-392.
15. Caregaro L, Di Pascoli L, Favaro A, Nardi M, Santonastaso P. Sodium depletion and hemoconcentration: overlooked complications in patients with anorexia nervosa?. *Nutrition.* 2005;21(4):438-445.
16. Fawcett J Wynn V. Effects of posture on plasma volume and some blood constituents. *J Clin Pathol.* 1960;13:304-310.
17. Jones AR, Twedt D, Swaim W, Gottfried E. Diurnal change of blood count analytes in normal subjects. *Am J Clin Pathol.* 1996;106(6):723-727.
18. Dawson AA, Ogston D, Fullerton HW. Evaluation of diagnostic significance of certain symptoms and physical signs in anaemic patients. *Br Med J.* 1969;3(668):436-439.
19. Desforges JF. Anemia in uremia. *Arch Intern Med.* 1970;126(5):808-811.
20. Cropp GJ. Cardiovascular function in children with severe anemia. *Circulation.* 1969;39(6):775-784.
21. Anand IS. Pathophysiology of anemia in heart failure. *Heart Fail Clin.* 2010;6(3):279-288.
22. Zeidman A, Fradin Z, Blecher A, Oster HS, Avrahami Y, Mittelman M. Anemia as a risk factor for ischemic heart disease. *Isr Med Assoc J.* 2004;6(1):16-18.
23. Aessopos A, Deftereos S, Farmakis D, et al. Cardiovascular adaptation to chronic anemia in the elderly: an echocardiographic study. *Clin Invest Med.* 2004;27(5):265-273.
24. Muhe L, Oljira B, Degefu H, Jaffar S, Weber MW. Evaluation of clinical pallor in the identification and treatment of children with moderate and severe anaemia. *Trop Med Int Health : TM & IH.* 2000;5(11):805-810.
25. Mesihovic-Dinarevic S, Ibrahimovic J, Hasanbegovic E, Icindic-Nakas E, Smajic A. Heart murmur and anaemia in the pediatric population. *Bosn J Basic Med Sci/ Udruzenje basicnih medicinskih znanosti = Association of Basic Medical Sciences.* 2005;5(3):39-45.
26. MacLean KJ, Tidman MJ. Alopecia areata: more than skin deep. *Practitioner.* 2013;257(1764):29-32.
27. Jacobsen E, Blenning C, Judkins D. Clinical inquiry: what nutritional deficiencies and toxic exposures are associated with nail changes? *J Fam Pract.* 2012;61(3):164-165.
28. Turco CD, La Spina C, Mantovani E, Gagliardi M, Lattanzio R, Pierro L. Natural history of premacular hemorrhage due to severe acute anemia: clinical and anatomical features in two untreated patients. *Ophthalmic Surg Lasers Imaging Retina.* 2014;45. Online:E5-7.
29. Haider BA, Yakoob MY, Bhutta ZA. Effect of multiple micronutrient supplementation during pregnancy on maternal and birth outcomes. *BMC Publ Health.* 2011;11(Suppl 3):S19.
30. Wu J Ricker M, Meunch J. Copper deficiency as a cause of unexplained hematologic and neurologic deficits in patient with prior gastrointestional surgery. *J Am Board Fam Med.* 2006;19:191-194.
31. Preloznik-Zupan I, Cernelc P, Zontar D. Reticulocyte analysis using light microscopy and two different flow cytometric procedures. *Pflugers Archiv Eur J Phy.* 2000;440(5 Suppl):R185-R187.
32. Piva E, Brugnara C, Spolaore F, Plebani M. Clinical utility of reticulocyte parameters. *Clin Lab Med.* 2015;35(1):133-163.
33. Buttarello M. Laboratory diagnosis of anemia: are the old and new red cell parameters useful in classification and treatment, how? *Int J Lab Hematol.* 2016;38(Suppl 1):123-132.
34. Joosten E, Lioen P, Brusselmans C, Indevuyst C, Boeckx N. Is analysis of the reticulocyte haemoglobin equivalent a useful test for the diagnosis of iron deficiency anaemia in geriatric patients? *Eur J Intern Med.* 2013;24(1):63-66.
35. Hershko C, Bar-Or D, Gaziel Y, et al. Diagnosis of iron deficiency anemia in a rural population of children. Relative usefulness of serum ferritin, red cell protoporphyrin, red cell indices, and transferrin saturation determinations. *Am J Clin Nutr.* 1981;34(8):1600-1610.
36. Mohammed Mujib AS, Mohammad Mahmud AS, Halder M, Monirul Hasan CM. Study of hematological parameters in children suffering from iron deficiency anaemia in Chattagram Maa-o-Shishu General Hospital, Chittagong, Bangladesh. *Anemia.* 2014;2014:503981.
37. Marsh WL, Jr., Koenig HM. The laboratory evaluation of microcytic red blood cells. *Crit Rev Clin Lab Sci.* 1982;16(3):195-254.
38. Gottfried EL. Erythrocyte indexes with the electronic counter. *N Engl J Med.* 1979;300(22):1277.
39. Patton WN, Cave RJ, Harris RI. A study of changes in red cell volume and haemoglobin concentration during phlebotomy induced iron deficiency and iron repletion using the Technicon H1. *Clin Lab Haematol.* 1991;13(2):153-161.
40. Takahashi N, Kameoka J, Takahashi N, et al. Causes of macrocytic anemia among 628 patients: mean corpuscular volumes of 114 and 130 fL as critical markers for categorization. *Int J Hematol.* 2016;104(3):344-357.
41. Savage DG, Ogundipe A, Allen RH, Stabler SP, Lindenbaum J. Etiology and diagnostic evaluation of macrocytosis. *Am J Med Sci.* 2000;319(6):343-352.

42. Lachner C, Steinle NI, Regenold WT. The neuropsychiatry of vitamin B12 deficiency in elderly patients. *J Neuropsychiatry Clin Neurosci.* 2012;24(1):5-15.

43. Wong CW, Ip CY, Leung CP, Leung CS, Cheng JN, Siu CY. Vitamin B12 deficiency in the institutionalized elderly: a regional study. *Exp Gerontol.* 2015;69:221-225.

44. Wickramasinghe SN. Kinetics and morphology of haemopoiesis in pernicious anaemia. *Br J Haematol.* 1972;22(2):111-115.

45. Ganzoni A, Hillman RS, Finch CA. Maturation of the macroreticulocyte. *Br J Haematol.* 1969;16(1):119-135.

46. Lindenbaum J, Nath BJ. Megaloblastic anaemia and neutrophil hypersegmentation. *Br J Haematol.* 1980;44(3):511-513.

47. Neogi SS, Thomas M, Sharma A, Kumar J, Khanduri U. Early markers of occult megaloblastosis for low-cost detection of hyperhomocysteinemia in patients with ischaemic stroke: preventive approach for primary health care. *Can J Physiol Pharmacol.* 2014;92(9):713-716.

48. Nath BJ, Lindenbaum J. Persistence of neutrophil hypersegmentation during recovery from megaloblastic granulopoiesis. *Ann Intern Med.* 1979;90(5):757-760.

49. Beguin Y, Clemons GK, Pootrakul P, Fillet G. Quantitative assessment of erythropoiesis and functional classification of anemia based on measurements of serum transferrin receptor and erythropoietin. *Blood.* 1993;81(4):1067-1076.

50. D'Onofrio G, Chirillo R, Zini G, Caenaro G, Tommasi M, Micciulli G. Simultaneous measurement of reticulocyte and red blood cell indices in healthy subjects and patients with microcytic and macrocytic anemia. *Blood.* 1995;85(3):818-823.

51. Latvala J, Parkkila S, Niemela O. Excess alcohol consumption is common in patients with cytopenia: studies in blood and bone marrow cells. *Alcohol Clin Exp Res.* 2004;28(4):619-624.

52. Koivisto H, Hietala J, Anttila P, Parkkila S, Niemela O. Long-term ethanol consumption and macrocytosis: diagnostic and pathogenic implications. *J Lab Clin Med.* 2006;147(4):191-196.

53. Lindenbaum J. Status of laboratory testing in the diagnosis of megaloblastic anemia. *Blood.* 1983;61(4):624-627.

54. Okuno T, Chou A. The significance of small erythrocytes. *Am J Clin Pathol.* 1975;64(1):48-52.

55. Cunningham LO, Rising JA. Erythrocyte microcytosis: clinical implications in 100 patients. *Am J Med Sci.* 1977;273(2):149-155.

56. Artz AS, Xue QL, Wickrema A, et al. Unexplained anaemia in the elderly is characterised by features of low grade inflammation. *Br J Haematol.* 2014;167(2):286-289.

57. Yip R, Dallman PR. The roles of inflammation and iron deficiency as causes of anemia. *Am J Clin Nutr.* 1988;48(5):1295-1300.

58. Tietz NW, Rinker AD, Morrison SR. When is a serum iron really a serum iron? A follow-up study on the status of iron measurements in serum. *Clin Chem.* 1996;42(1):109-111.

59. Statland B, Winkel P, Bokelund H. Variation of serum iron concentration in young healthy men: within day-and day-to-day changes. *Clin Biochem.* 1976;9:26-29.

60. Werkman HP, Trijbels JM, Schretlen ED. The "short-term" iron rhythm. *Clin Chim Acta.* 1974;53(1):65-68.

61. Archer NM, Brugnara C. Diagnosis of iron-deficient states. *Crit Rev Clin Lab Sci.* 2015;52(5):256-272.

62. Schaap CC, Hendriks JC, Kortman GA, et al. Diurnal rhythm rather than dietary iron mediates daily hepcidin variations. *Clin Chem.* 2013;59(3):527-535.

63. Dale JC, Burritt MF, Zinsmeister AR. Diurnal variation of serum iron, iron-binding capacity, transferrin saturation, and ferritin levels. *Am J Clin Pathol.* 2002;117(5):802-808.

64. Sennels HP, Jorgensen HL, Hansen AL, Goetze JP, Fahrenkrug J. Diurnal variation of hematology parameters in healthy young males: the Bispebjerg study of diurnal variations. *Scand J Clin Lab Invest.* 2011;71(7):532-541.

65. Rossander L, Hallberg L, Björn-Rasmussen E. Absorption of iron from breakfast meals. *Am J Clin Nutr.* 1979;32(12):2484-2489.

66. Nguyen LT, Buse JD, Baskin L, Sadrzadeh SMH, Naugler C. Influence of diurnal variation and fasting on serum iron concentrations in a community-based population. *Clin Biochem.* 2017;50(18):1237-1242.

67. Wians FH,Jr., Urban JE, Keffer JH, Kroft SH. Discriminating between iron deficiency anemia and anemia of chronic disease using traditional indices of iron status vs transferrin receptor concentration. *Am J Clin Pathol.* 2001;115(1):112-118.

68. Means RT, Allen J, Sears DA, Schuster SJ. Serum soluble transferrin receptor and the prediction of marrow aspirate results in a heterogeneous group of patients. *Clin Lab Haematol.* 1999;21:161-167.

69. Daru J, Colman K, Stanworth SJ, De La Salle B, Wood EM, Pasricha SR. Serum ferritin as an indicator of iron status: what do we need to know? *Am J Clin Nutr.* 2017;106:1634S-1639S.

70. Moirand R, Lescoat G, Delamaire D, et al. Increase in glycolsylated and nonglycosylated serum ferritin in chronic alcoholism and their evolution during alcohol withdrawal. *Alcohol Clin Exp Res.* 1991;15:963-969.

71. Sackett K, Cunderlik M, Sahni N, Killeen AA, Olson AP. Extreme hyperferritinemia: causes and impact on diagnostic reasoning. *Am J Clin Pathol.* 2016;145(5):646-650.

72. Rath CE, Finch CA. Sternal marrow hemosiderin; a method for the determination of available iron stores in man. *J Lab Clin Med.* 1948;33(1):81-86.

73. Gale E, Torrance J, Bothwell T. The quantitative estimation of total iron stores in human bone marrow. *J Clin Invest.* 1963;42:1076-1082.

74. Speeckaert MM, Speeckaert R, Delanghe JR. Biological and clinical aspects of soluble transferrin receptor. *Crit Rev Clin Lab Sci.* 2010;47(5–6):213-228.

75. Skikne BS, Punnonen K, Caldron PH, et al. Improved differential diagnosis of anemia of chronic disease and iron deficiency anemia: A prospective multicenter evaluation of soluble transferrin receptor (sTfR) and the sTfR/log ferritin index (sTfR Index). *Am J Hematol.* 2011;86:923-927.

76. Beguin Y. Soluble transferrin receptor for the evaluation of erythropoiesis and iron status. *Clin Chim Acta.* 2003;329(1–2):9-22.

77. Marsh WL, Jr., Nelson DP, Koenig HM. Free erythrocyte protoporphyrin (FEP) II. The FEP test is clinically useful in classifying microcytic RBC disorders in adults. *Am J Clin Pathol.* 1983;79(6):661-666.

78. Stockman JA,III, Weiner LS, Simon GE, Stuart MJ, Oski FA. The measurement of free erythrocyte porphyrin (FEP) as a simple means of distinguishing iron deficiency from beta-thalassemia trait in subjects with microcytosis. *J Lab Clin Med.* 1975;85(1):113-119.

79. Wood JC. Magnetic resonance imaging measurement of iron overload. *Curr Opin Hematol.* 2007;14(3):183-190.

80. Wood JC, Enriquez C, Ghugre N, et al. MRI R2 and R2* mapping accurately estimates hepatic iron concentration in transfusion-dependent thalassemia and sickle cell disease patients. *Blood.* 2005;106(4):1460-1465.

81. Vichinsky E. Hemoglobin E Syndromes. Hematology/the Education Program of the American Society of Hematology American Society of Hematology Education Program; 2007:79-83.

82. Bain BJ. Hemoglobin C disease. *Am J Hematol.* 2015;90(2):174.

83. Amid A, Haghi-Ashtiani B, Kirby-Allen M, Haghi-Ashtiani MT. Screening for thalassemia carriers in populations with a high rate of iron deficiency: revisiting the applicability of the Mentzer Index and the effect of iron deficiency on Hb A2 levels. *Hemoglobin.* 2015;39(2):141-143.

84. Urrechaga E, Borque L, Escanero JF. The role of automated measurement of RBC subpopulations in differential diagnosis of microcytic anemia and beta-thalassemia screening. *Am J Clin Pathol.* 2011;135(3):374-379.

85. Urrechaga E, Hoffmann J. Critical appraisal of discriminant formulas for distinguishing thalassemia from iron deficiency in patients with microcytic anemia. *Clin Chem Lab Med.* 2017;55(10):1582-1591.

86. McClure S, Custer E, Bessman JD. Improved detection of early iron deficiency in nonanemic subjects. *JAMA.* 1985;253:1021-1023.

87. Urrechaga E, Hoffmann JJ, Izquierdo S, Escanero JF. Differential diagnosis of microcytic anemia: the role of microcytic and hypochromic erythrocytes. *Int J Lab Hematol.* 2015;37:334-340.

88. Sharma P, Das R, Trehan A, et al. Impact of iron deficiency on hemoglobin A2% in obligate beta-thalassemia heterozygotes. *Int J Lab Hematol.* 2015;37(1):105-111.

89. Ryan K, Bain BJ, Worthington D, et al. Significant haemoglobinopathies: guidelines for screening and diagnosis. *Br J Haematol.* 2010;149(1):35-49.

90. Kutlar F. Diagnostic approach to hemoglobinopathies. *Hemoglobin.* 2007;31(2):243-250.

91. Mollin D. Sideroblasts and sideroblastic aneamia. *Br J Haematol.* 1965;11:41-48.

92. Bessis M, Jensen WN. Sideroblastic anaemia, mitochondria and erythroblast iron. *Br J Haematol.* 1965;11:49-51.

93. Barcellini W, Fattizzo B. Clinical applications of hemolytic markers in the differential diagnosis and management of hemolytic anemia. *Dis Markers.* 2015;2015:635670.

94. Olusanya BO, Emokpae AA, Zamora TG, Slusher TM. Addressing the burden of neonatal hyperbilirubinaemia in countries with significant glucose-6-phosphate dehydrogenase deficiency. *Acta Paediat.* 2014;103(11):1102-1109.

95. Kobayashi Y, Hatta Y, Ishiwatari Y, Kanno H, Takei M. Human parvovirus B19-induced aplastic crisis in an adult patient with hereditary spherocytosis: a case report and review of the literature. *BMC Res Notes.* 2014;7:137.

96. Slavov SN, Kashima S, Pinto AC, Covas DT. Human parvovirus B19: general considerations and impact on patients with sickle-cell disease and thalassemia and on blood transfusions. *FEMS Immunol Med Microbiol.* 2011;62(3):247-262.

97. Valentin MN, Cohen PJ. Pediatric parvovirus B19: spectrum of clinical manifestations. *Cutis.* 2013;92(4):179-184.

98. Oiwa H, Shimada T, Hashimoto M, et al. Clinical findings in parvovirus B19 infection in 30 adult patients in Kyoto. *Mod Rheumatol/The Jpn Rheum Assoc.* 2011;21(1):24-31.

99. Ornoy A, Ergaz Z. Parvovirus B19 infection during pregnancy and risks to the fetus. *Birth Defects Res.* 2017;109(5):311-323.

100. Young N, Mortimer P. Viruses and bone marrow failure. *Blood.* 1984;63(4):729-737.

101. Kurtzman GJ, Cohen BJ, Field AM, Oseas R, Blaese RM, Young NS. Immune response to B19 parvovirus and an antibody defect in persistent viral infection. *J Clin Invest.* 1989;84(4):1114-1123.

102. Potter CG, Potter AC, Hatton CS, et al. Variation of erythroid and myeloid precursors in the marrow and peripheral blood of volunteer subjects infected with human parvovirus (B19). *J Clin Invest.* 1987;79(5):1486-1492.

103. Heegaard ED, Brown KE. Human parvovirus B19. *Clin Microbiol Rev.* 2002;15(3):485-505.

104. Lammert F, Gurusamy K, Ko CW, et al. Gallstones. *Nat Rev Dis Prim.* 2016;2:16024.

105. Qiao T, Ma RH, Luo XB, Yang LQ, Luo ZL, Zheng PM. The systematic classification of gallbladder stones. *PLoS One.* 2013;8(10):e74887.

106. Trotman BW. Pigment gallstone disease. *Gastroenterol Clin North Am.* 1991;20(1):111-126.

107. McCall IW, Desai P, Serjeant BE, Serjeant GR. Cholelithiasis in Jamaican patients with homozygous sickle cell disease. *Am J Hematol.* 1977;3:15-21.

108. Minniti CP, Kato GJ. Critical Reviews: How we treat sickle cell patients with leg ulcers. *Am J Hematol.* 2016;91(1):22-30.

109. Giraldi S, Abbage KT, Marinoni LP, et al. Leg ulcer in hereditary spherocytosis. *Pediatr Dermatol.* 2003;20(5):427-428.

110. Saad GS, Musallam KM, Taher AT. The surgeon and the patient with beta-thalassaemia intermedia. *Br J Surg.* 2011;98(6):751-760.

111. Bedair EM, Helmy AN, Yakout K, Soliman AT. Review of radiologic skeletal changes in thalassemia. *Pediatr Endocrinol Rev.* 2008;6(Suppl 1):123-126.

112. Savage WJ. Transfusion reactions. *Hematol Oncol Clin North Am.* 2016;30(3):619-634.

113. Kudoh T, Yoto Y, Suzuki N, et al. Human parvovirus B19-induced aplastic crisis in iron deficiency anemia. *Acta Paediatr Jpn.* 1994;36(4):448-449.

114. Berlin NI, Berk PD. Quantitative aspects of bilirubin metabolism for hematologists. *Blood.* 1981;57(6):983-999.

115. Van Lente F, Marchand A, Galen RS. Diagnosis of hemolytic disease by electrophoresis of erythrocyte lactate dehydrogenase isoenzymes on cellulose acetate or Agarose. *Clin Chem.* 1981;27(8):1453-1455.

116. Shih AW, McFarlane A, Verhovsek M. Haptoglobin testing in hemolysis: measurement and interpretation. *Am J Hematol.* 2014;89(4):443-447.

117. Franco RS. The measurement and importance of red cell survival. *Am J Hematol.* 2009;84(2):109-114.

118. Ham T. Hemoglobinuria. *Am J Med.* 1955;18:990-1006.

119. Sears DA, Anderson PR, Foy AL, Williams HL, Crosby WH. Urinary iron excretion and renal metabolism of hemoglobin in hemolytic diseases. *Blood.* 1966;28(5):708-725.

120. Barcellini W, Fattizzo B, Zaninoni A, et al. Clinical heterogeneity and predictors of outcome in primary autoimmune hemolytic anemia: a GIMEMA study of 308 patients. *Blood.* 2014;124(19):2930-2936.

121. Segel GB, Lichtman MA. Direct antiglobulin ("Coombs") test-negative autoimmune hemolytic anemia: a review. *Blood Cells Mol Dis.* 2014;52(4):152-160.

122. Chetty T, Bouwer N, Wan YO, Mahlangu J. Immunoglobulin subtyping and quantification in direct antiglobulin test: positive haemolysis in an HIV-prevalent setting. *J Clin Pathol.* 2022;75:117-120.

123. Bianchi P, Fermo E, Vercellati C, et al. Diagnostic power of laboratory tests for hereditary spherocytosis: a comparison study in 150 patients grouped according to molecular and clinical characteristics. *Haematologica.* 2012;97(4):516-523.

124. Llaudet-Planas E, Vives-Corrons JL, Rizzuto V, et al. Osmotic gradient ektacytometry: A valuable screening test for hereditary spherocytosis and other red blood cell membrane disorders. *Int J Lab Hematol.* 2018;40(1):94-102.

125. Strassburg CP. Hyperbilirubinemia syndromes (Gilbert-Meulengracht, Crigler-Najjar, Dubin-Johnson, and Rotor syndrome). *Best Pract Res Clin Gastroenterol.* 2010;24(5):555-571.

126. Riddez L, Hahn RG, Brismar B, Strandberg A, Svensen C, Hedenstierna G. Central and regional hemodynamics during acute hypovolemia and volume substitution in volunteers. *Crit Care Med.* 1997;25(4):635-640.

127. Carson JL, Guyatt G, Heddle NM, et al. Clinical practice guidelines from the AABB: red blood cell transfusion thresholds and storage. *JAMA.* 2016;316(19):2025-2035.

128. Kougias P, Sharath S, Mi Z, Biswas K, Mills JL. Effect of postoperative permissive Anemia and cardiovascular risk status on outcomes after major general and vascular surgery operative interventions. *Ann Surg.* 2019;270(4):602-611.

129. Scharman CD, Burger D, Shatzel JJ, Kim E, DeLoughery TG. Treatment of individuals who cannot receive blood products for religious or other reasons. *Am J Hematol.* 2017;92(12):1370-1381.

130. Posluszny JA, Jr., Napolitano LM. How do we treat life-threatening anemia in a Jehovah's Witness patient?. *Transfusion.* 2014;54(12):3026-3034.

Disorders of Red Blood Cells

Chapter 25 ■ Iron Deficiency and Related Disorders

ELIZABETA NEMETH • MARIE HOLLENHORST • LAWRENCE T. GOODNOUGH

INTRODUCTION

Iron deficiency has been recognized since medieval times. Chlorosis, a term derived from the Greek word meaning green, was applied by Varandaeus to a disorder that was later described in 1554 as "De morbo virgineo."[1] The disease became well known as the "green-sickness," due to a greenish pallor occurring almost exclusively in teenaged girls,[2] depicted in paintings by the Dutch masters and was alluded to by Shakespeare. Other clinical features were breathlessness, palpitations, slight ankle edema, and gastrointestinal complaints. Emotional disturbances, depression, irritability, and moodiness were common.

Chlorosis became especially common in the last decade of the 19th century and then declined in incidence. Today, most believe that chlorosis resulted from a combination of factors affecting adolescent girls: the demands of growth and the onset of menses, an inadequate diet, and a legacy of poor iron stores from early childhood. In the 1830s, anemia, hypochromia, and lack of iron in the blood were linked to this disorder. In 1832, Pierre Blaud described the response of chlorosis to his deservedly famous pills (ferrous sulfate plus potassium carbonate). Many observers, including Niemeyer and Osler, confirmed his findings.[3] Ferrous sulfate remains a cornerstone of modern treatment of iron deficiency.

In the late 1920s and early 1930s, a distinct hypochromic anemia was described. Like chlorosis, chronic hypochromic anemia chiefly affected women. It differed from chlorosis in that it was detected later in life, especially in the fourth and fifth decades.[4] Other distinguishing clinical features were epithelial changes involving the tongue and nails, and achlorhydria. The anemia most often affected women with poor diets, multiple pregnancies, or menstrual irregularities. Today, menstruating women continue to be among the most likely individuals to develop iron deficiency, along with young children whose growth outpaces their iron supply. An understanding of normal iron physiology is essential to best appreciate the pathophysiology of iron deficiency anemia (IDA).

NORMAL IRON PHYSIOLOGY

Total Body Iron

Iron endowment varies with age and sex. Full-term infants begin life with approximately 75 mg/kg body weight of iron, primarily acquired from their mothers during the third trimester of gestation. These abundant stores are rapidly depleted over the first few months of life, and most young children have tenuous iron balance, as their intake must keep pace with rapid growth. Requirements decrease after adolescence, and men have a small, gradual increase in iron stores throughout life. The body iron content of normal adult men is 50 mg/kg body weight or greater. In contrast, postpubertal women have increased losses of iron due to menstruation, pregnancy, and childbirth, resulting in a body iron endowment averaging 35 mg/kg. After menopause, women accumulate iron linearly in parallel with adult men.

Most of the body iron is found in hemoglobin and myoglobin, the heme-containing oxygen transport and storage proteins (*Table 25.1*). Smaller amounts of iron are incorporated into enzymes with active sites containing heme, iron-sulfur clusters, or iron coordinated by protein side chains. These include enzymes of electron transport chain, peroxidases, catalases, and ribonucleotide reductase. Most nonheme iron (approximately 1 g in adult men or 200-500 mg in adult women)

is stored as ferritin in macrophages and hepatocytes. Only a tiny fraction of iron (~0.1%) is in transit in the plasma, bound to the carrier protein, transferrin.

Iron Balance

Iron is not actively excreted from the body; it is eliminated only through the loss of epithelial cells from the gastrointestinal tract, epidermal cells of the skin, and, in menstruating women, red blood cells (RBCs). On the basis of long-term studies of body iron turnover, the total average daily loss of iron has been estimated at ~1 to 2 mg in normal adult men and nonmenstruating women.[5] Although iron is a physiologic component of sweat, only a tiny amount of iron (22.5 µg/L) is lost by this route.[6] Urinary iron excretion amounts to <0.05 mg/d and is largely accounted for by sloughed cells. Menstruating women lose an additional, highly variable amount over each menstrual cycle, from 0.006 (average) to more than 0.025 mg/kg/d.[7]

These iron losses are normally balanced by an equivalent amount of iron absorbed from the diet (1-2 mg/d). Only a fraction of dietary iron is absorbed: the bioavailability of iron from mixed diets in industrialized countries is estimated at 14% to 18%, although less may be absorbed if iron stores are replete.[8] The iron bioavailability for vegetarian diets is lower, ranging from 5% to 12%. Fractional absorption of dietary iron can increase up to 3- to 5-fold (3-5 mg/d) if iron stores are depleted. Thus, iron balance is primarily, if not exclusively, achieved by control of absorption rather than by control of excretion.

Intestinal Absorption

Iron is absorbed in the duodenum, and humans and other omnivorous mammals have at least two distinct pathways for iron absorption: one for uptake of heme iron and another for ferrous (Fe^{2+}) iron. Heme iron is derived from hemoglobin, myoglobin, and other heme proteins in foods of animal origin, representing approximately 10% to 15% of iron content in the typical Western diet. However, because it is more easily absorbed than nonheme iron, heme-derived iron accounts for two-thirds of *absorbed* iron in meat-eating humans. Exposure to acid and proteases present in gastric juices frees the heme from its apoprotein. Heme is taken up by mucosal cells, but the specific transporter is still unknown. Once heme iron enters the cell, the porphyrin ring is enzymatically cleaved by heme oxygenase.[9] The liberated iron then probably follows the same pathways as those used by nonheme iron. Although enterocytes express the heme exporter protein feline leukemia virus, subgroup C receptor 1 (FLVCR1), this protein does not export intact dietary heme into plasma.[10] Absorption of heme iron is relatively unaffected by the overall composition of the diet.

Dietary nonheme iron is largely in the form of ferric hydroxide or loosely bound to organic molecules such as phytates, oxalate, sugars, citrate, lactate, and amino acids. Low gastric pH is thought to be important for the solubility of inorganic iron. Dietary constituents may also have profound effects on the absorption of nonheme iron, making the bioavailability of food iron highly variable. Ascorbate enhances inorganic iron absorption, whereas calcium inhibits it.[11] Depending on various combinations of enhancing and inhibitory factors, dietary iron assimilation can vary as much as 10-fold.

Molecular Mechanisms of Iron Absorption

Absorption of nonheme iron occurs in the duodenum, where ferrous iron is imported into enterocytes by divalent metal ion transporter 1

Table 25.1. Iron Distribution in Humans[a]

Protein	Function	Fe amount
Hemoglobin	Erythrocyte oxygen transport	2.6 g
Ferritin	Intracellular iron storage	1 g
Transferrin	Plasma iron transport	3 mg
Myoglobin	Muscle oxygen storage	130 mg
Enzymes and other proteins	Electron transport, oxygen sensing, DNA synthesis and other processes	150 mg

[a]Amounts estimated for a 70 kg adult male; adult females generally have lower iron stores (100-400 mg).

(DMT1, also known as Nramp2, DCT1, SLC11A2). DMT1 is a protein with 12 predicted transmembrane segments, which is expressed on the apical surface of absorptive enterocytes. Levels of DMT1 are markedly increased in iron-deficient animals.[12] DMT1 may also contribute to the absorption of other nutritionally important metals (e.g., Mn^{2+}) in addition to iron.[13] Evidence in vitro demonstrates that DMT1 is a proton-coupled symporter.[14] The Na^+/H^+ exchanger-3 (NHE3) in the duodenum is the primary determinant of the acidic microclimate in the intestine, providing the proton electrochemical gradient as the driving force for iron uptake.[15]

DMT1 does not transport the Fe^{3+} form of iron, but most dietary nonheme iron arrives at the brush border as Fe^{3+} ion. A duodenal cytochrome b–like ferrireductase enzyme, Dcytb (also called CYBRD1), likely reduces dietary Fe^{3+} to make it a substrate for transport by DMT1. Dcytb is induced in response to stimuli that increase iron absorption; however, because knockout mice appear to have normal metabolism, Dcytb may not be the only ferrireductase enzyme involved in absorption of nonheme iron.[16]

A variable fraction of iron taken into the mucosal cell is delivered to the plasma. The remainder is used by the cell or incorporated into ferritin,[17] an intracellular iron storage protein discussed in a later section. Iron retained in mucosal ferritin is not absorbed; rather, it is lost from the body when the senescent mucosal cells are sloughed into the intestine at the end of their 3- to 4-day lifespan (10^{11} cells/d).[18]

Iron not stored in the absorptive enterocytes is transferred across the basolateral membrane of the cell to the lamina propria and ultimately to the plasma. This is accomplished, at least in part, by the iron exporter ferroportin (also known as FPN1, IREG1, MTP1, SLC40A1), a multitransmembrane segment protein expressed on the basolateral surface of enterocytes.[19] Ferroportin is also expressed in other tissues involved in handling large iron fluxes including macrophages recycling iron from senescent RBCs, hepatocytes storing iron, and placental trophoblast delivering iron from mother to fetus. Complete ablation of ferroportin in mice, including extraembryonic tissues, resulted in embryonic death, whereas selective inactivation that preserved placental ferroportin expression resulted in live births, demonstrating the essential function of ferroportin in maternofetal iron transfer.[20] Ferroportin is also essential for systemic iron homeostasis, as inactivation of ferroportin in all tissues in mice other than placenta led to the development of severe anemia resembling iron deficiency and stemmed from the inability to mobilize iron from enterocytes, macrophages, and hepatocytes.

Similar to apical iron uptake, basolateral iron efflux is aided by an enzyme that changes the oxidation state of iron. Ferroportin exports Fe^{2+}, and this iron must be oxidized to its Fe^{3+} form to bind to transferrin. A membrane-bound multicopper oxidase, hephaestin, has been implicated in this process. Mice with intestine-specific knockout of hephaestin have decreased intestinal iron absorption and develop systemic iron deficiency,[21] although not severe enough to cause anemia in adult animals. This suggests that additional ferroxidases may contribute or that ferroxidase activity

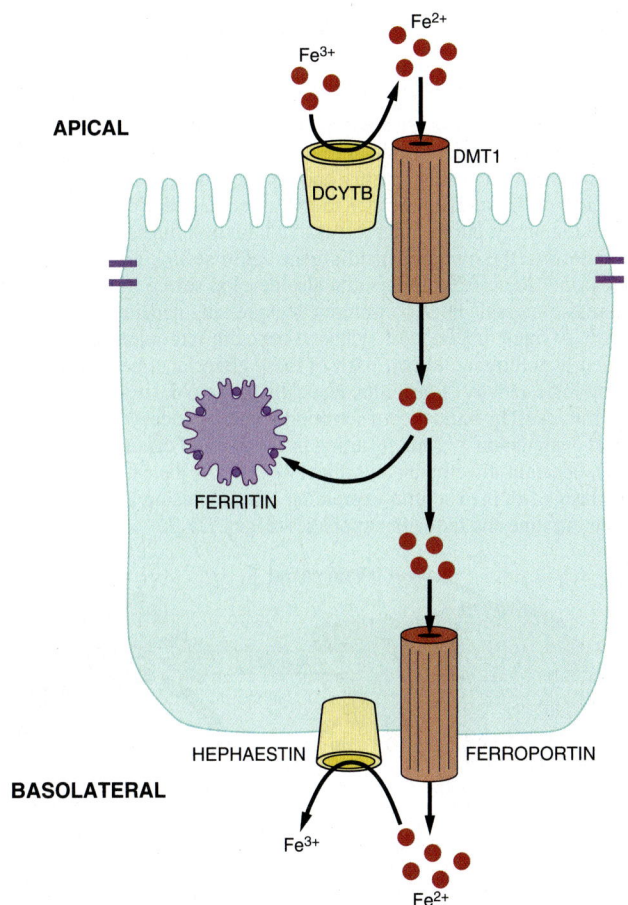

FIGURE 25.1 Nonheme iron absorption in the intestine. This figure shows a drawing of an absorptive enterocyte from the proximal duodenum. The apical brush border is at the top. Dietary nonheme iron enters the gut as the ferric (Fe^{3+}) ion and is converted to the ferrous (Fe^{2+}) ion by a surface reductase activity, probably mediated by the duodenal cytochrome b–like (DCYTB) protein. The Fe^{2+} iron enters the cell through the action of divalent metal ion transporter 1 (DMT1). Within the cell, some iron is stored, and some is transported across the basolateral membrane. Ferroportin functions as a basolateral Fe^{2+} iron transporter. Ferroxidase hephaestin facilitates basolateral iron export, by oxidizing iron to the Fe^{3+} form to bind to plasma apotransferrin.

is not absolutely required for iron absorption. Ceruloplasmin, the ferroxidase involved in efflux of iron from hepatocytes and macrophages, may also contribute to enterocyte iron export.[22] A model incorporating current knowledge of nonheme iron transport is shown in *Figure 25.1*.

Regulation of Iron Absorption

Because the total body iron content is largely determined by the efficiency of absorption of iron, the regulation of absorption has long been of great interest. Both systemic mechanisms as well as local mechanisms within enterocytes (discussed later in the chapter) regulate dietary iron uptake. The systemic signals that are of prime importance in determining absorptive rate are the amount of storage iron in the body and the erythropoietic activity. When storage iron is depleted, iron absorption is increased; when it is excessive, iron absorption is decreased.[23] Intestinal iron absorption also increases when the red cell production rate is increased. This is observed in effective as well as in ineffective erythropoiesis in which erythroid precursors are destroyed relatively close to their site of origin in the bone marrow (as seen in thalassemia syndromes, congenital dyserythropoietic anemias, and sideroblastic anemias). Hormone hepcidin controls iron absorption in response to both changing iron stores and erythropoietic activity.

Hepcidin and Systemic Regulation of Iron Metabolism

Hormone hepcidin has emerged as the key systemic regulator of iron homeostasis. Hepcidin is a small peptide of 25 amino acids, produced in the liver, secreted into the plasma, and excreted through the kidneys.[24,25] Hepcidin is structurally similar to antimicrobial peptides involved in innate immunity, but its main role is to inhibit iron fluxes into plasma.[26] Mutations in the human hepcidin gene cause severe, early-onset iron overload.[27] Mice lacking hepcidin also develop severe iron overload,[28] whereas transgenic mice constitutively expressing hepcidin have severe IDA.[29] A single injection of synthetic hepcidin into mice exerts a prolonged hypoferremic effect.[30] All of these effects can be explained by the biologic activity of hepcidin. Hepcidin binds to the iron exporter ferroportin, causing occlusion of ferroportin and its endocytosis and lysosomal degradation[31,32] and resulting in cessation of cellular iron export. Thus, hepcidin directly and coordinately controls the entry of iron into the plasma from ferroportin-expressing cells, including absorptive cells of the intestine and tissue macrophages (*Figure 25.2*).

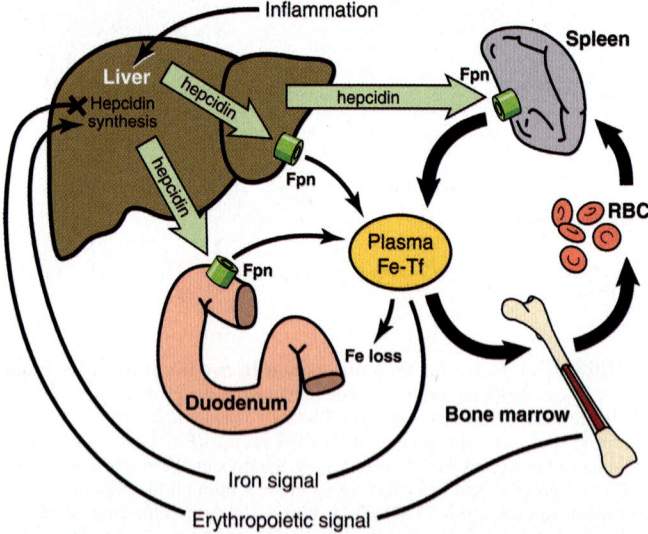

FIGURE 25.2 Regulation of systemic iron homeostasis by hepcidin. Hepcidin controls the entry of iron into plasma by causing degradation of its receptor, the iron exporter ferroportin. The major iron flows that are regulated by hepcidin-ferroportin interactions include the release of iron from macrophages that recycle iron in the spleen and liver, dietary iron absorption in the duodenum, and, at least in part, the release of iron from storage in hepatocytes. The feedback stimulation of hepcidin by plasma holotransferrin and iron stores ensures that extracellular iron concentration and iron stores stay within normal limits. Hepcidin synthesis is suppressed by erythropoietic activity, ensuring a sufficient supply of iron to the bone marrow when demand for hemoglobin synthesis is high. During inflammation, hepcidin production is stimulated and iron entry into plasma is inhibited, causing the hypoferremia and anemia of inflammation. Fpn, ferroportin; RBC, red blood cell. (Reprinted with permission from Ganz T. Molecular control of iron transport. *J Am Soc Nephrol.* 2007;18(2):394-400.)

Alterations in hepcidin production lead to changes in iron absorption and recycling. Multiple signals are known to regulate hepcidin expression, including iron, erythropoiesis, inflammation, and growth factors. Like other hormones that are feedback regulated by the substances whose concentration they control, hepcidin expression is regulated by iron. When iron is deficient, hepatocytes produce less hepcidin, allowing more iron to enter plasma. When iron is abundant, hepcidin production increases, limiting further iron absorption and release from stores. In human volunteers ingesting a single dose of oral iron, hepcidin concentrations in serum or urine increased within several hours and were proportional to the increase in transferrin saturation (Tsat).[33] Serum hepcidin concentrations in healthy subjects also correlate with body iron stores as reflected by serum ferritin. The specific forms of iron that increase hepcidin synthesis include diferric plasma transferrin and iron stores in the liver, and the transduction pathways that regulate hepcidin synthesis in response to these iron forms are still being elucidated.

The bone morphogenetic protein (BMP) pathway with its canonical signaling via Smad proteins has a central role in the regulation of hepcidin transcription. BMP receptors are tetramers of serine/threonine kinase receptors, with two type I and two type II subunits. Recent data indicate that type I subunits ALK2 and ALK3 and type II subunits ActRIIA and BMPRII are specific BMP receptors involved in iron regulation.[34,35] Binding of BMP ligands to the receptors triggers phosphorylation of Smads1/5/8, which then form a complex with Smad4, translocate into the nucleus and activate transcription of the hepcidin gene. In the liver, BMP pathway signaling to hepcidin is modulated by the BMP coreceptor hemojuvelin expressed on hepatocytes and by the ligands BMP6 and 2 produced by the liver endothelial cells.[36-38] Hepatic ablation of any of these regulators in mice (HJV, BMP receptors, BMP ligands, Smad1/5/8 or Smad 4) decreases hepcidin expression, resulting in the development of iron overload.[39,40] In humans, HJV mutations result in severe hepcidin deficiency and cause juvenile hemochromatosis,[41] whereas heterozygous missense mutations in the BMP6 propeptide have been linked to mild to moderate iron loading.[42]

How BMP receptors and HJV interact with iron-sensing molecules is still not understood. The two transferrin receptors TfR1 and TfR2, and HFE, a major histocompatibility complex (MHC) class I–like membrane protein, may serve as holotransferrin sensors.[26] TfR1 and TfR2 bind holotransferrin. Because holotransferrin-binding site on TfR1 overlaps with that of HFE, increasing concentrations of holotransferrin result in displacement of HFE from TfR1, and free HFE then interacts with TfR2.[43,44] In addition, TfR2 protein itself is stabilized by binding of holotransferrin.[45] The formation of the HFE/TfR2 complex is thus proportional to holotransferrin concentration. How the complex stimulates hepcidin expression is not well understood, but it seems to potentiate the BMP pathway signaling. The role of HFE or TfR2 in hepcidin regulation by iron is supported by genetic evidence: HFE and TfR2 mutations in humans or mice cause hepcidin deficiency and an adult form of hemochromatosis.[26] HFE may also regulate hepcidin expression without complexing with TfR2.[46] HFE was shown to interact with the BMP receptor type I ALK3,[47] one of the critical regulators of hepcidin expression. HFE prevents ubiquitination and proteasomal degradation of ALK3 protein, thus increasing ALK3 expression at the cell surface, which again results in greater Smad signaling to increase hepcidin transcription. Two other membrane proteins, a serine protease matriptase-2 (MT-2, also called transmembrane protease serine 6, TMPRSS6), and the receptor neogenin also influence hepcidin synthesis, likely by modulating hemojuvelin concentration on the cell membrane.[48,49] The concentration of hepatic MT-2 is acutely increased by iron deficiency,[50,51] suggesting that MT-2 may also function as an iron sensor, although the mechanism is unknown. Mutations in MT-2 in humans and mice lead to increased hepcidin expression and development of iron-restricted anemia, discussed later in this chapter.

As already mentioned, hepcidin synthesis also increases in response to increased liver iron stores. Although the underlying mechanism is still not fully elucidated, increase in hepatic iron concentrations stimulates liver endothelial BMP6 and BMP2 synthesis.[38,39,52,53]

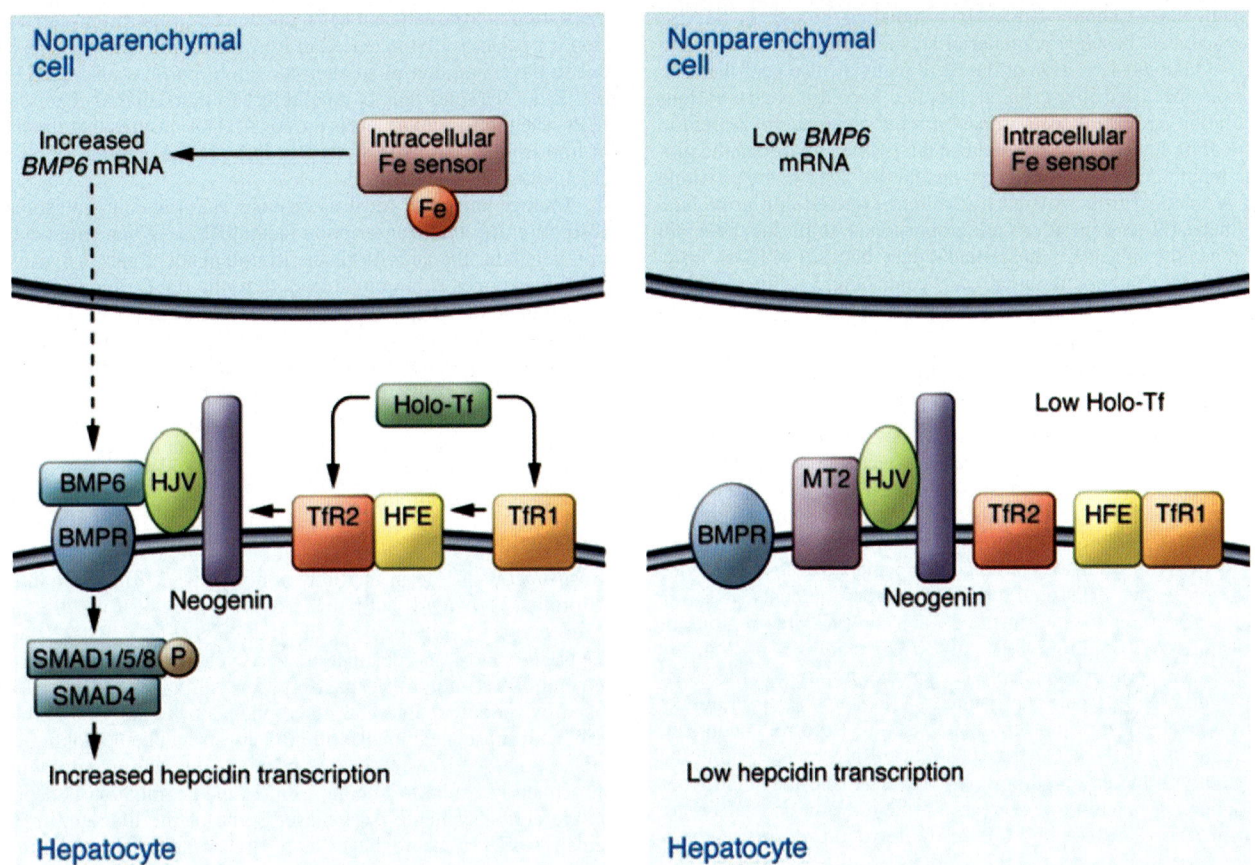

FIGURE 25.3 Molecular mechanisms of hepcidin regulation by iron. Left panel: high-iron conditions. Extracellular iron in the form of holotransferrin (HoloTf) is sensed by the two transferrin receptors (TfR1 and TfR2). Binding of HoloTf to its receptors promotes hemochromatosis protein (HFE) interaction with TfR2 instead of TfR1, and the HFE/TfR2 complex then sensitizes the bone morphogenetic protein receptor (BMPR) to its ligands such as BMP6 or 2. HFE may also directly stabilize BMPR (ALK3) by preventing its ubiquitination. Hemojuvelin (HJV), a membrane-linked BMP coreceptor also potentiates the BMPR activation. Once activated, BMPRs initiate SMAD signaling, which increases hepcidin transcription. High intracellular iron in parenchymal and/or endothelial cells of the liver enhances BMP6 and 2 production, eventually leading to activation of the BMPR on hepatocytes. Right panel: low-iron conditions. Low HoloTf concentrations and low intracellular iron both lead to decreased BMP pathway signaling and decreased hepcidin mRNA expression. Furthermore, matriptase-2 (MT-2) protease is stabilized in low-iron conditions and cleaves HJV, thus further decreasing the signaling through the BMP pathway. (Adapted with permission of American Society for Clinical Investigation from Zhao N, Zhang AS, Enns CA. Iron regulation by hepcidin. *J Clin Invest.* 2013;123(6):2337-2343; permission conveyed through Copyright Clearance Center, Inc.)

BMP6 and BMP2 then act on hepatocytes to increase hepcidin mRNA proportionally to iron loading of the liver.[54] *Figure 25.3*[55] summarizes our current understanding of the molecular mechanisms involved in hepcidin regulation by iron.

Hepcidin synthesis, and consequently absorption of iron and its availability for erythropoiesis, is regulated by erythropoiesis itself. Increased erythropoietic activity due to bleeding, hemolysis, or administration of erythropoietin in humans or mice causes hepcidin suppression.[56-58] Very low hepcidin concentrations are observed in patients with absolute IDA, or anemias with high erythropoietic activity.[59] In turn, low hepcidin allows increased absorption of dietary iron and release of iron from stores, thus increasing iron supply to the bone marrow for hemoglobin synthesis. The mechanism by which erythropoiesis regulates hepcidin production is becoming better understood and depends on the production of a hepcidin-suppressive factor by the erythroid precursors in the bone marrow.[57,60] Erythroferrone (ERFE), a member of the tumor necrosis factor (TNF)-α superfamily of cytokines, is a mediator of hepcidin suppression during stress erythropoiesis.[61,62] ERFE baseline levels are very low, but its production by erythroid precursors rapidly increases when these cells are stimulated by erythropoietin (EPO). Erythroid precursors secrete ERFE into circulation, and the hormone then acts on hepatocytes to reduce hepcidin expression. ERFE is thought to function as a BMP trap, sequestering BMP2, 6 and 2/6 heterodimers away from their cell surface receptors, specifically ALK3.[63-65] ERFE-deficient mice fail to suppress hepcidin

acutely after phlebotomy or EPO injections, demonstrating the essential role of ERFE in linking erythropoietic activity to iron homeostasis. Because hepcidin suppression is impaired, ERFE-deficient mice have a delay in recovery from anemia caused by hemorrhage or severe inflammation.[62,66] Nevertheless, chronic administration of EPO in mice suppresses hepcidin even in the absence of ERFE,[67] indicating that additional mechanisms exist to lower hepcidin production when erythropoietic activity is chronically increased.

The suppressive effect of erythropoiesis on hepcidin is particularly prominent in diseases with ineffective erythropoiesis such as β-thalassemia,[68-70] where erythrocyte precursors massively expand but undergo apoptosis rather than maturing into erythrocytes. The severe suppression of hepcidin, particularly in untransfused β-thalassemia, leads to increased iron absorption and the development of lethal iron overload. ERFE is now thought to contribute to the pathological suppression of hepcidin in anemias with ineffective erythropoiesis. Deletion of ERFE in β-thalassemia mice restored hepcidin expression to normal levels and partially improved their iron overload phenotype.[71] ERFE serum levels are greatly elevated in patients with β-thalassemia,[72] both as a result of increased number of erythroid precursors and because of EPO-dependent induction of ERFE expression in these precursors. Elevated ERFE was also reported in sickle cell disease and myelodysplastic syndrome.[73,74]

Hepcidin gene expression is induced in response to inflammatory cytokines,[75] accounting for iron sequestration in the anemia of inflammation (see Chapter 42).[56,76] IL-6 signaling through the STAT-3 pathway seems to be a key regulator of hepcidin expression in inflammation,[77,78] but the activation of the BMP pathway also contributes.[79] Apart from increased transcription, elevated hepcidin concentrations in circulation can result from impaired renal clearance of hepcidin. Because of its small size (2.7 kD), hepcidin is filtered through the glomerular membrane and is then taken up and degraded in the proximal tubule. A fraction of the filtered hepcidin is excreted into urine, and urinary hepcidin concentrations are proportionate to plasma hepcidin levels in healthy subjects.[59] In chronic kidney diseases (CKDs), however, hepcidin clearance is impaired,[80] contributing to the hormone accumulation in plasma.

Regulation of Iron Absorption by Intracellular Mechanisms

In addition to being regulated by systemic signals, iron absorption is subject to local regulation by intracellular mechanisms in duodenal enterocytes. At least two mechanisms have been described: one related to enterocyte iron levels and the other to the hypoxia pathway.

Intracellular iron levels in enterocytes (and most other cells) are sensed by two iron regulatory proteins (IRP1 and IRP2).[81] When cytoplasmic iron is low, IRPs bind to iron regulatory elements (IREs),[82] stem-loop structures located in the 5′ or 3′ untranslated regions of different mRNAs. Binding of IRPs to 3′IREs stabilizes mRNAs by protecting them from endonucleolytic cleavage, resulting in increased protein synthesis. mRNAs that contain 3′ IREs encode iron uptake proteins such as transferrin receptor and a DMT1 isoform. In contrast, IRP binding to 5′IREs blocks translation of mRNA by preventing the interaction with the cap-binding complex eIF4F and the small ribosomal subunit,[83] resulting in decreased protein synthesis. 5′IREs are present in ferritin mRNA and one of the ferroportin transcripts. In iron-replete cells, IRPs do not bind to IREs, resulting in greater degradation of 3′IRE-containing transcripts (e.g., TfR1), and increased translation of 5′IRE-containing transcripts (e.g., ferritin or ferroportin), thus shifting the cellular phenotype from an iron-importing to an iron-storing or iron-exporting one.

How does intracellular iron concentration modulate IRP binding to IREs? IRP1 contains a 4Fe-4S iron-sulfur cluster that, when saturated with iron, converts IRP1 to a cytosolic aconitase that catalyzes the conversion of citrate to isocitrate.[84-86] In this enzyme form, IRP1 has low affinity for IREs in mRNAs. When iron-poor, IRP1 loses its aconitase activity and greatly increases its affinity for IREs. In the case of IRP2, intracellular iron levels control its degradation.[87,88] In iron-replete cells, IRP2 is ubiquitinated by an iron-sensitive E3 ubiquitin ligase complex containing FBXL5 protein,[89] and ubiquitinated IRP2 is degraded by proteasomes.

Targeted inactivation of the genes encoding murine IRPs has shed light on the roles of IRP1 and IRP2 in vivo. The specific roles of each IRPs are not entirely clear, but they may respond differently over the physiologically relevant range of oxygen tensions.[90] Loss of both IRP proteins is incompatible with life,[91] whereas deficiency of either yields viable and fertile animals indicating that IRP1 and IRP2 are, at least in part, functionally redundant. Nevertheless, deficiency of each IRP alone does have phenotypic consequences. Loss of IRP1 resulted in polycythemia, pulmonary hypertension, and cardiac hypertrophy in mice,[92] and this was related to inappropriately increased hypoxia-inducible factor (HIF)-2α levels in several tissues. HIF2α mRNA contains 5′IRE that is controlled by IRP1. Thus, IRP1 plays an important role in erythropoiesis and pulmonary and cardiovascular systems. Loss of IRP2 in mice resulted in microcytic anemia, erythropoietic protoporphyria, and neurological problems, indicating that IRP2 plays an important role in erythropoiesis and the nervous system.[92] Tissue-specific knockout of both IRPs in the intestine of mice resulted in dysregulation of multiple iron transporters, confirming the role of IRPs in the regulation of iron transport in enterocytes. The knockout mice also had impaired intestinal function and died within 4 weeks of birth.[93]

Even though IRPs regulate translation of ferroportin mRNA through the 5′ IRE and thus would be expected to prevent ferroportin translation in iron-deficient cells, duodenal ferroportin protein expression is paradoxically increased in iron deficiency. This may be in part due to the expression of an alternative ferroportin transcript (FPN1B) that lacks IRE and thus is not subject to translational repression by IRPs when intracellular levels are low.[94] This ensures that the transfer of iron from absorptive enterocytes into plasma continues even when enterocytes are iron deficient.

Another important local mechanism that regulates intestinal iron absorption involves transcription factor HIF2α. When enterocytes are iron deficient, the activity of the iron-dependent prolyl hydroxylase domain enzymes is inhibited, leading to the stabilization of HIF2α in the duodenum.[95] HIF2α in turn increases the expression of DcytB, DMT1, and ferroportin mRNAs, resulting in an increase in iron uptake.[96] Thus, duodenal HIF-2α is a critical local regulator of iron absorption by coordinating the increase in both apical and basolateral iron transport during iron deficiency. Prolyl hydroxylase inhibitors, the new class of agents for treatment of anemia in CKD, exert beneficial effects likely in part by potentiating the duodenal HIF2α activity to increase iron absorption.

Iron Cycle

Most functional iron in the body is not derived from daily intestinal absorption (1-2 mg/d) but rather from recycling of iron (20-25 mg/d) from senescent erythrocytes and other cells (*Figure 25.4*). The most important source and destination of recycled iron is the erythron. At the end of a 4-month lifespan, effete erythrocytes are engulfed and lysed by reticuloendothelial macrophages or hemolysed extracellularly with subsequent uptake of RBC ghosts and hemoglobin by macrophages.[97] In either case, macrophages degrade hemoglobin, and subsequently heme, to liberate iron. Heme degradation is dependent on the action of heme oxygenase. Some of the liberated iron may remain stored in macrophages as ferritin or hemosiderin, but most is delivered to the plasma through ferroportin, and the rate of iron export is determined by the hepcidin-ferroportin interaction. In plasma, iron becomes bound to transferrin, completing the cycle. A small amount of iron, probably <2 mg, leaves the plasma each day to enter hepatic parenchymal cells and other tissues. Here, the iron is stored or used for synthesis of cellular heme proteins, such as myoglobin and the cytochromes.

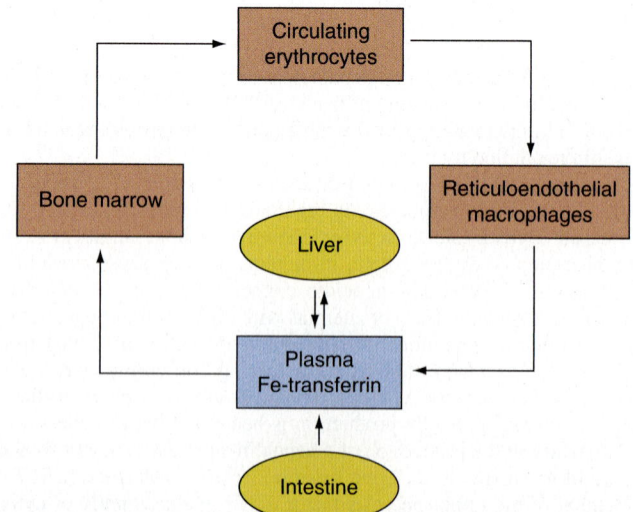

FIGURE 25.4 Iron cycle in humans. Iron (Fe) enters the body through the small intestine and travels in the plasma bound to transferrin. It is delivered to the erythroid bone marrow, where it is incorporated into hemoglobin and released into the circulation in mature erythrocytes. After a life span of approximately 120 days, erythrocytes are engulfed by macrophages in the reticuloendothelial system. There the Fe is extracted from hemoglobin and returned to plasma, where it becomes bound to transferrin, completing the cycle. Fe in excess of tissue needs is stored in the liver.

Plasma Transport

The plasma iron-binding protein, transferrin, is a glycoprotein with a molecular weight of approximately 80 kDa.[98] Transferrin is synthesized chiefly in the liver and actively secreted by hepatocytes. Transferrin keeps iron nonreactive in the circulation and extravascular fluid, delivering it to cells bearing TFR1. The rate of transferrin synthesis shows an inverse relationship to iron in stores; when iron stores are depleted, more transferrin is synthesized, and when iron stores are overfilled, the level of transferrin decreases. The biological role of this regulation is still unclear, but transferrin levels are considered a biomarker of body iron stores.

The normal concentration of transferrin in plasma is approximately 2 to 3 g/L. It can be measured immunologically or can be quantified in terms of the amount of iron it will bind, a measure called the total iron-binding capacity (TIBC). Transferrin has two homologous iron-binding domains, each of which binds an atom of trivalent (ferric) iron.[91] In the average subject, the plasma iron concentration is ~18 μmol/L (100 μg/dL) and TIBC is ~56 μmol/L (300 μg/dL). Transferrin saturation (TSAT) is also a useful metric for assessing iron status; it is calculated as (iron/TIBC)*100. Only about one-third of the available transferrin-binding sites are occupied in an iron-replete individual, leaving a large capacity to buffer variations in ingested and recycled iron. Plasma iron concentration varies over the course of the day, with the highest values in the morning and the lowest in the evening. Levels of serum transferrin are more constant, and there is no apparent diurnal variation in TIBC.

Iron Delivery to Erythroid Precursors

The biologic importance of transferrin in erythropoiesis is illustrated by abnormalities observed in patients and mice with congenital atransferrinemia.[99-103] When transferrin is severely deficient, red cells display the morphologic stigmata of iron deficiency. This occurs despite the fact that intestinal iron absorption is markedly increased, in response to a perceived need for iron for erythropoiesis. Nonhematopoietic tissues avidly assimilate the non-transferrin-bound metal. Similarly, mutant mice lacking tissue receptors for transferrin die during embryonic development from severe anemia, apparently resulting from ineffective iron delivery to erythroid precursor cells.[103]

Transferrin delivers its iron to developing erythroblasts and other cells by binding to specific cell-surface receptors. The transferrin receptor (TFRC, TfR1) is a disulfide-linked homodimer of a glycoprotein with a single membrane-spanning segment and a short cytoplasmic segment. It is a type II membrane protein, with its N terminus located within the cell. The native molecular weight of TfR1 is ~180 kDa. Each TfR1 homodimer can bind two transferrin molecules. Diferric transferrin is bound with higher affinity (dissociation constant $2-7 \times 10^{-9}$ M) than monoferric transferrin. As a result, diferric transferrin has a competitive advantage in delivering iron to the erythroid precursors.[104] Apotransferrin has little affinity for the receptor at physiologic pH but considerable affinity at lower pH, an important factor in intracellular iron release.

Transferrin receptor 2 (TfR2), which shares ~45% homology with TfR1 in its large extracellular domain,[105] binds transferrin with lower affinity, and its role in cellular iron uptake is unclear. TfR2 is highly expressed in the liver and, as discussed earlier in this chapter, acts as an iron sensor that regulates hepcidin expression.[26] TfR2 is also expressed in erythroid precursor cells, where it interacts with the EPO receptor (EpoR) and enhances the delivery of EpoR to cell surface when extracellular iron availability is high.[106]

The role of TfR1 is relatively well understood. TfR1 numbers are modulated during erythroid cell maturation, reaching their peak in intermediate basophilic erythroblasts. Very few TfR1 molecules are found on burst-forming-unit erythroid cells, and only slightly greater numbers are found on colony-forming-unit erythroid cells. The rate of iron uptake is directly related to the number of receptors. The number decreases as reticulocytes mature, and late in maturation, erythroid cells shed all remaining receptors by exocytosis and by proteolytic cleavage.[107] The shed receptors (referred to as soluble

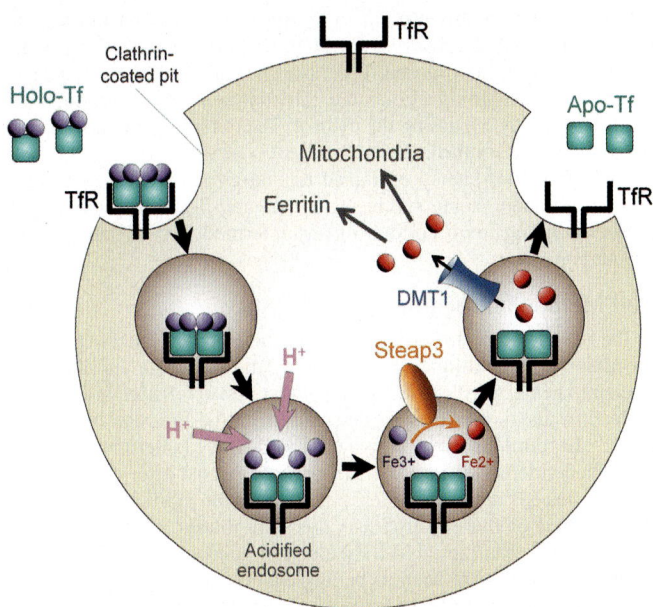

FIGURE 25.5 Cellular uptake of iron-transferrin. Iron bound to plasma Tf (holo-Tf) is delivered to the cell by binding to cell-surface transferrin receptor 1 (TfR). The ligand-receptor complex enters the cell through invagination of clathrin-coated pits to form specialized endosomes. The endosomes become acidified through the entry of protons, releasing Fe^{3+} iron from Tf and strengthening the apo-Tf/TfR complex at low pH. The released iron is reduced to Fe^{2+} by STEAP3 ferrireductase and exits the endosome through the divalent metal ion transporter 1 (DMT1) to go to sites of storage and use within the cell (ferritin, mitochondria). The apo-Tf/TFR complex then returns to the cell surface, where apo-Tf is released. Both Tf and TFR participate in multiple rounds of iron delivery.

transferrin receptors, sTfR) can be found in plasma in a concentration that correlates with the rate of erythropoiesis.[108] An increase in plasma sTfR is a sensitive indicator of erythroid mass and erythroid iron deficiency.[109,110]

After ligand and receptors interact, iron-loaded transferrin undergoes receptor-mediated endocytosis (*Figure 25.5*). Specialized endocytic vesicles form, which are acidified to a pH of 5 to 6 by the influx of protons. The low pH facilitates release of iron from transferrin and strengthens the apotransferrin-receptor interaction. Released iron is reduced by an endosomal ferrireductase, STEAP3,[111] and transferred to the cytosol by DMT1.[112] Because DMT1 must cotransport protons with iron atoms, vesicle acidification is also important for the function of this transporter. After iron enters the cytosol, the protein components of the endosome return to the membrane surface, where neutral pH promotes the release of apotransferrin to the plasma. Both transferrin and TfR1 participate in multiple rounds of iron delivery.

Mutations in DMT1 can have profound effect on erythroid development. Although rare, DMT1 mutations have been described in several patients with congenital IDA.[113,114] The patients suffer from severe microcytic, hypochromic anemia, due to the inability to transport iron out of Tf/TfR1 endocytic vesicles, thus preventing iron delivery for heme synthesis. Although DMT1 is also involved in duodenal iron absorption, most of these patients develop hepatic overload at a young age, suggesting that iron absorption is at least partially intact, probably due to dietary heme absorption. Blood transfusions to correct the anemia also contribute to patients iron overload.

Once inside the cell, erythroid iron must be shuttled to the mitochondrion, where it will be incorporated into protoporphyrin IX by ferrochelatase, the final enzyme of heme biosynthesis. How iron that is exported from endosome reaches the mitochondrion and is transported across the outer mitochondrial membrane is not well understood. Iron transport across the inner mitochondrial membrane seems to be mediated by mitoferrin-1, a transmembrane iron transporter. Inactivation of the mitoferrin-1 gene in mice prevents RBC production, underscoring the importance of this protein in erythroid biology. An alternative mechanism for iron delivery from Tf/TfR endosome to the mitochondrion has also been proposed. The "kiss and run" hypothesis suggests that the Tf-containing endosome directly contacts the mitochondrion,[115] thereby bypassing the cytosol. The details of the mechanism remain to be determined.

A highly coordinated erythroid regulatory system exists to balance iron uptake, heme synthesis, and α- and β-globin protein synthesis, avoiding toxic buildup of any intermediates of hemoglobin production.[116]

Iron Metabolism Within Erythroblasts

In the normal subject, ~80% to 90% of the iron that enters erythroid precursor cells is ultimately taken up by mitochondria and incorporated into heme. Most of the remainder is stored in ferritin.[117] Granules of ferritin may sometimes be detected using the Prussian blue reaction.[118] Erythroblasts with Prussian blue–positive (siderotic) granules are called sideroblasts, and, if the granules persist after enucleation, the mature cells are called siderocytes. In normal individuals, approximately half of the erythroblasts are sideroblasts, each containing less than five small granules. By electron microscopy, these normal siderotic granules are seen to be aggregations of ferritin, often surrounded by a membrane (siderosomes). Another kind of sideroblast, the ringed sideroblast, is found only under pathologic circumstances (sideroblastic anemias; see Chapter 26). In the ringed sideroblast, siderotic granules form a full or partial ring around the nucleus, and electron microscopy reveals that the iron is deposited in mitochondria.

Intriguingly, even though erythroid precursors require large amounts of iron and heme for hemoglobin synthesis, they have been found to express the heme exporter FLVCR and the iron exporter ferroportin. FLVCR, initially identified as the receptor for feline leukemia virus subgroup C that causes erythroid aplasia in cats, is highly expressed in early erythroid precursors. Of the two isoforms, FLVCR1a localizes to the plasma membrane, and FLVCR1b localizes to mitochondria. The loss of both FLVCR isoforms in mice caused embryonic lethality due to the lack of definitive erythropoiesis.[119] When FLVCR was ablated postnatally, the mice developed a hyperchromic macrocytic anemia with proerythroblast maturation arrest. It appears that expression of Flvcr1a and 1b has to be coordinated to ensure the optimal size of the cytosolic heme pool, which is required to sustain proliferation and differentiation of committed erythroid progenitors.[120]

Erythroid precursors as well as mature RBCs also express ferroportin,[94,121] and this is thought to function as a safety valve to remove excess iron, protecting cells from oxidative stress. Interestingly, erythroid cells preferentially express non-IRE ferroportin transcript during the stages of rapid iron uptake, thus avoiding any iron-induced increase in ferroportin translation dependent on the IRE/IRP system.

Macrophage Iron Recycling

Although there are many types of tissue macrophages, those that participate in the catabolism of RBCs can be subdivided into two categories. One type, exemplified by pulmonary alveolar macrophages, is able to phagocytose erythrocytes or other cells and convert the iron they contain into storage forms but lacks the ability to return the iron to the circulation. This type of macrophage appears to retain the iron throughout its life span. The second type of macrophage, comprising the reticuloendothelial system, acquires iron in a similar fashion but is able to return it to the plasma. The latter macrophages, found especially in the sinuses of the spleen and liver, play a primary role in the normal reutilization of iron from aged red cells, allowing completion of the iron cycle shown in *Figure 25.4*.

Aged red cells may be phagocytosed by the reticuloendothelial macrophages, or may be retained within the splenic extracellular matrix through specific adhesion molecules, and undergo hemolysis.[97] The remnant erythrocyte ghosts and released hemoglobin are then taken up by the splenic macrophages. Once hemoglobin is taken up by macrophages, it undergoes proteolytic degradation in the phagolysosome, and heme is exported from phagolysosomes by the heme transporter HRG1[122] and is degraded in the cytosol by heme oxygenase

to yield biliverdin, carbon monoxide, and iron.[123] Iron can then be stored in ferritin or exported from macrophages through ferroportin, the iron exporter that is also found on the basolateral surface of absorptive enterocytes. Some iron is immediately released as erythrophagocytosis causes both induction of ferroportin mRNA expression by heme released from hemoglobin, as well as induction of ferroportin protein translation by heme-derived iron acting via the IRE/IRP system.[124] Iron stored in ferritin can be mobilized later in response to iron demand. This mobilization is likely achieved by modulating expression of hepcidin, the iron-regulatory hormone that causes degradation of macrophage ferroportin. Expression of hepcidin decreases when erythroid iron needs increase, allowing more ferroportin molecules to remain on the membrane of recycling macrophages.[125] Iron exported through ferroportin must be oxidized to be bound to transferrin. The ferroxidase reaction is catalyzed by the plasma copper protein, ceruloplasmin. When the gene encoding ceruloplasmin was disrupted in mice, macrophages failed to release their iron at a normal rate, resulting in hypoferremia despite the presence of normal iron stores. A similar phenomenon was noted in aceruloplasminemic human subjects.[126] Ceruloplasmin acts by catalyzing the oxidation of ferrous iron to the ferric form, which is a prerequisite for iron binding by apotransferrin.

Because of the large daily iron flux through erythrophagocytosing macrophages (20-25 mg), iron release from macrophages is a critical determinant of the availability of iron for plasma transferrin and, consequently, for erythropoiesis. The anemia of inflammation,[127] also called the anemia of chronic disease,[128] characterized by macrophage iron retention, illustrates the deleterious effects of perturbing the delicate balance between macrophage iron storage and release (see Chapter 42).

Intracellular iron in macrophages is stored in ferritin. Ferritin is the protein shell constructed of 24 molecules of two distinct ferritin subunits, designated H (for heavy or heart) and L (for light or liver), and these proteins are ubiquitously expressed. H and L ferritins have distinct functions: the H subunit catalyzes oxidation of Fe^{2+} to Fe^{3+} necessary for iron deposition in the cavity, whereas the L subunit binds Fe^{3+} ions to function as a nucleation site for the formation of the iron core.[129] Deletion of ferritin H in mice causes early embryonic lethality indicating that there is no functional redundancy between the two ferritin subunits.[130] The role of ferritin is to store iron and release it in a controlled manner; this provides cellular protection against oxidative damage that would be caused by highly reactive free iron[131] and allows rapid iron availability in times of cellular need.

At least 20 distinct ferritin heteropolymers, with varying proportions of L and H chains, have been isolated from human tissue.[132] Fully assembled, iron-free apoferritin has a molecular weight of approximately 400 to 500 kDa. Apoferritin is formed first, and iron is added later. A cytosolic iron chaperone, poly (rC)-binding protein 1 (PCBP1), delivers iron in the form of Fe^{2+} to ferritin.[133] Iron then enters ferritin through one of the six penetrating channels. As it passes into the core, it is oxidized to the Fe^{3+} form by molecular oxygen, with ferritin H catalyzing the oxidative process.[134] Theoretically, a single ferritin molecule could hold up to ~4500 iron atoms. More often, molecules with 2000 or fewer iron atoms are found. The iron is stored as a trivalent polymer of ferric hydroxide and phosphate.

In a wide variety of cell types, the synthesis of apoferritin is stimulated by exposure to iron.[135] This effect is due to the presence of 5′IRE in ferritin mRNA,[136] so that translation of ferritin is regulated by the IRE/IRP system described earlier in the chapter.

Mobilization of iron from ferritin is a regulated process that utilizes autophagy mechanisms. Autophagic turnover of ferritin is dependent on the selective cargo receptor NCOA4.[137] The levels of NCOA4 change according to intracellular iron levels. When intracellular iron levels are low, NCOA4 is abundant and recruits ferritin into autophagosomes, resulting in degradation of ferritin and liberation of iron. In contrast, when intracellular iron levels are high, NCOA4 itself is targeted for degradation by HERC2 ubiquitin ligase, thus preventing ferritin degradation.[138] Accordingly, NCOA4-deficient mice had altered baseline iron homeostasis, with mild impairment in erythropoiesis and iron accumulation in the liver and spleen. Furthermore, the mice had highly inappropriate response to iron deficiency; iron could not be mobilized from ferritin, and mice developed severe microcytic hypochromic anemia and ineffective erythropoiesis.[139] Therefore, ferritinophagy is an essential process that ensures efficient utilization of iron.

Ferritin is also found in plasma in small amounts (12-300 µg/L), and in the absence of inflammation,[140] the circulating ferritin concentration correlates closely with the amount of iron in stores. Plasma ferritin appears to be actively secreted into plasma, primarily by macrophages but is iron-poor compared with tissue ferritin.[141] The biological role of plasma ferritin is not known. It has been proposed that plasma ferritin represents residual ferritin after iron-rich ferritin secreted from cells is selectively taken up by neighboring cells via TFR1 and other ferritin receptors.[142] This mechanism could serve to redistribute iron within tissues.

Iron Metabolism in Other Tissues

Iron is required in small amounts by *all* tissues for the synthesis of iron-containing enzymes and proteins, including cytochromes, catalase, ribonucleotide reductase, ferrochelatase, aconitase, and prolyl hydroxylases. Cells are generally thought to acquire their iron from transferrin through binding to cell-surface transferrin receptor 1, although some cells can also take up non-transferrin-bound iron (NTBI) via specific NTBI transporters. Nevertheless, under normal conditions, all the iron in circulation is bound to transferrin, and TfR1-mediated iron uptake is essential for normal function of most tissues. For example, tissue-specific knockout of TfR1 in cardiomyocytes, skeletal muscle, or dopaminergic neurons caused severe organ dysfunction and early death in each of these models.[143-145] Human missense mutation in TfR1 that was associated with impaired internalization of TfR1 and iron deficiency in lymphocytes caused combined immunodeficiency due to severe impairment in the function of T and B cells.[146] Proliferating cells in many tissues have increased numbers of TFR1 compared with their quiescent counterparts, reflecting their need for iron.

The placenta also accepts iron from transferrin and may do so even at relatively low plasma iron levels, thus effectively competing with the maternal erythroid bone marrow. The export of iron from placental trophoblast into fetal circulation occurs through ferroportin.

IRON DEFICIENCY ANEMIA

Pathogenesis of Iron Deficiency Anemia

Although its handling is frequently termed "iron metabolism," iron itself is not metabolized; iron disorders are the result of iron imbalance or maldistribution. IDA, hemochromatosis, and the anemia of chronic disease/inflammation are each examples of this principle.

Three pathogenic factors are implicated in the anemia of iron deficiency. First, hemoglobin synthesis is impaired as a consequence of reduced iron supply. Second, there is a generalized defect in cellular proliferation. Third, survival of erythroid precursors and erythrocytes is reduced, particularly when the anemia is severe.

When Tsat falls below ~15%, the supply of iron to the marrow is inadequate to meet basal requirements for hemoglobin production (generally ~25 mg of iron daily in average adults). As a result, the amount of free erythrocyte protoporphyrin increases, reflecting the excess of protoporphyrin over iron in heme synthesis. Globin protein synthesis is reduced and each cell that is produced contains less hemoglobin, resulting in microcytosis and hypochromia. This is the normal adaptive response to iron deficiency in humans and mice. If globin synthesis was not decreased in heme deficiency, misfolding and precipitation of excess globin chains would lead to apoptosis. Globin synthesis is controlled by heme availability at both transcriptional and translational levels. Heme regulates globin gene expression by its ability to bind a transcription suppressor Bach1. When heme is deficient, Bach1 associates with small Maf proteins (sMaf) and causes transcriptional repression of globin genes.[147] When heme is abundant, heme binding to Bach1 causes its dissociation from sMafs and Bach1 degradation,[148] permitting sMaf interaction with transcriptional activators to increase expression of globin genes.

On the translational level, heme regulates globin synthesis by binding to and controlling the activity of heme-regulated eIF2α kinase (HRI).[149] HRI functions by phosphorylating the α subunit of a key regulatory translation initiation factor eIF2 and preventing its participation in the initiation of translation. With high intracellular heme concentrations, heme binds to HRI and renders it inactive, but in heme deficiency, heme dissociates from HRI and the kinase is activated by autophosphorylation. HRI then phosphorylates eIF2α, preventing the recycling of eIF2 for another round of protein synthesis initiation, resulting in reduced globin protein synthesis and preventing formation of toxic globin precipitates in the absence of heme. In $Hri^{-/-}$ mice, the adaptive hypochromic and microcytic response to iron deficiency was absent.[116] Iron deficiency and consequently decreased heme levels instead resulted in aggregation of globins within the erythrocytes and their precursors, causing increased apoptosis of erythroid precursors in the bone marrow and spleen and accelerated destruction of mature RBCs, which were hyperchromic and normocytic.

Cellular proliferation is also restricted in iron deficiency, resulting in decreased number of RBCs. Although there is relative erythroid hyperplasia in the bone marrow, both the degree of erythroid hyperplasia and the reticulocyte count are low for the degree of anemia. There is a significant component of "ineffective erythropoiesis" in iron deficiency, and a proportion of immature erythroid cells in iron-deficient subjects are so defective that they are rapidly destroyed.

Genetic Forms of Iron Deficiency Anemia

Genes involved in hereditary IDA are listed in *Table 25.2.*[90,102,150-153] The main biological and clinical difference in genetic forms of IDA are outlined in *Table 25.3.*

Several forms of genetic IDA are associated with hypochromic, microcytic anemia and iron overload outside of the erythron. These are caused by autosomal recessive mutations in several genes and are exceedingly rare. DMT1 (SLC*11A2*) encodes an iron transporter

Table 25.2. Genes Involved in Hereditary Iron Deficiency Anemia

Protein (Gene Symbol)	Chromosome	Protein Function	Disease Caused by Mutations
DMT1 (SLC11A2)	12	Transmembrane iron transporter	Hypochromic, microcytic anemia, usually with hepatic iron overload[113,114]
Glutaredoxin 5 (GLRX5)	14	Participates in iron-sulfur cluster biogenesis	Anemia with iron overload and sideroblasts[150]
Transferrin (TF)	3	Plasma iron-binding protein; ligand for TfR1 and TfR2	Atransferrinemia, iron deficiency anemia with tissue iron overload[99,100,102]
Ceruloplasmin (CP)	3	Plasma ferroxidase	Aceruloplasminemia, mild iron deficiency anemia associated with iron accumulation in the liver and brain[151]
Matriptase-2 (TMPRSS6)	22	Hepcidin suppressor, acts by cleaving membrane hemojuvelin	Iron-refractory iron deficiency anemia[152-154]

Abbreviations: DMT1, divalent metal ion transporter 1; TfR1 and 2, transferrin receptors 1 and 2.
Modified from Andrews NC. Forging a field: the golden age of iron biology. *Blood.* 2008;112(2):219-230. Copyright © 2008 American Society of Hematology. With permission.

Table 25.3. Main Biologic and Clinical Differences in Genetic Forms of Iron Deficiency Anemia

	DMT1	Glutaredoxin 5	Atransferrinemia	Aceruloplasminemia	TMPRSS6
Age at diagnosis	At birth	Usually midlife	Late onset provided some Tf is present	Late onset with moderate anemia	18-24 mo
Liver iron overload	Yes	Yes	Yes	Yes	No
Brain damage	No	No	No	Yes	No
Serum iron	High	High	Low	Low	Low
Transferrin saturation	High	High	High or nonmeasurable	Low	Low
Ringed sideroblasts	No	Yes	No	No	No
Hepcidin levels	Low to normal	Not yet measured	Low	Low	High for anemia
Ferritin	Low to mildly elevated	High	High	High	Low to normal

Abbreviations: DMT1, divalent metal ion transporter 1; Tf, transferrin; TMPRSS6, matriptase-2.
Provided courtesy of Photis Beris.

involved in dietary iron absorption and in iron transfer from Tf/TfR1 endosomes into the cytosol of erythroid precursors. Glutaredoxin 5 (GLRX5) is an enzyme involved in mitochondrial iron-sulfur cluster biogenesis. Human patients carrying these mutations have similar blood films and erythrocyte abnormalities, but they also have hepatic iron overload that is not fully explained by their transfusion histories.[113,114,155-157] Deficiency of serum transferrin, called hypotransferrinemia or atransferrinemia, is due to mutations in the transferrin gene itself.[102,158] This interrupts iron delivery to erythroid precursors, triggering an increase in intestinal iron absorption and deposition of excess iron in tissues. Deficiency of another major plasma protein, ceruloplasmin, also causes mild IDA associated with iron accumulation in the liver and brain.[151] Iron deficiency results from lack of ferroxidase activity needed to mobilize iron from storage.[151,159]

Some patients have congenital, iron-refractory iron deficiency anemia (IRIDA) without iron overload.[153,154,160-162] The disease is caused by recessive mutations in *Tmprss6* gene, which encodes serine protease matriptase-2. Matriptase-2 is highly expressed in the liver and acts by cleaving HJV, a BMP coreceptor and a key regulator of hepcidin expression.[49,153] Measurement of serum hepcidin concentrations in patients with IRIDA confirmed that hepcidin levels were much higher than would be expected for the degree of iron deficiency and anemia, where hepcidin is usually undetectable.[153,154] How TMPRSS6 expression or activity is regulated is still unknown, but hepatocyte iron deficiency was shown to stabilize matriptase-2 protein,[51] which dampens BMP signaling and decreases hepcidin expression. Further studies will be needed to evaluate the possibility that less severe or heterozygous mutations increase susceptibility to common, acquired IDA. In genome-wide association studies, common variants of TMPRSS6 were associated with alterations in hemoglobin levels, serum iron, or erythrocyte volume,[163-165] suggesting that TMPRSS6 has a critical role in maintenance of iron homeostasis and normal erythropoiesis.

CLINICAL FEATURES OF IRON DEFICIENCY

Stages in the Development of Iron Deficiency

When it is not a result of acute blood loss, iron deficiency is the end result of a long period of negative iron balance. As the total body iron level begins to fall, a characteristic sequence of events ensues. First, the iron stores in the hepatocytes and the macrophages of the liver, spleen, and bone marrow are depleted. Once stores are gone, plasma iron content decreases and the supply of iron to marrow becomes inadequate for normal hemoglobin production. Consequently, the amount of free erythrocyte protoporphyrin increases, production of microcytic erythrocytes begins, and the blood hemoglobin level decreases, eventually reaching abnormal levels.

This progression corresponds to three recognized stages. The first stage, also called prelatent iron deficiency or iron depletion, represents a reduction in iron stores without reduced serum iron levels.[166] This

Table 25.4. Stages in the Development of Iron Deficiency

	Stage 1 (Prelatent)	Stage 2 (Latent)	Stage 3 (Anemia)
Bone marrow iron	Reduced	Absent	Absent
Serum ferritin	Reduced	<30 µg/L	<30 µg/L
Transferrin saturation	Normal	<16%	<16%
Free erythrocyte protoporphyrin, zinc protoporphyrin	Normal	↑	↑
Serum transferrin receptor	Normal	↑	↑
Reticulocyte hemoglobin content	Normal	↓	↓
Hemoglobin	Normal	Normal	Reduced
Mean corpuscular volume	Normal	Normal	Reduced
Symptoms	Rare	Fatigue, malaise in some patients	Pallor, pica, epithelial changes

↑, increased; ↓, decreased.

stage is usually detected by a low serum ferritin measurement, unless inflammation is present in which case serum ferritin does not reflect storage iron.[140] Latent iron deficiency is said to exist when iron stores are exhausted but the blood hemoglobin level remains higher than the lower limit of normal.[167] In this second stage, certain biochemical abnormalities of iron-limited erythropoiesis may be detected, including reduced transferrin saturation, increased TIBC,[168] increased free erythrocyte protoporphyrin,[169] increased zinc protoporphyrin,[170] and increased serum transferrin receptor (sTfR).[171] The mean corpuscular volume usually remains within normal limits, but a few microcytes may be detected on a blood smear. Patients report generalized fatigue or malaise, even though they are not yet anemic.

Finally, in the third stage, the blood hemoglobin concentration falls below the lower limit of normal and IDA is apparent. Iron-containing enzymes, such as the cytochromes, also reach abnormally low levels during this period. Clinical manifestations include a constellation of constitutional symptoms: fatigue, decreased exercise tolerance with tachycardia, dermatologic manifestations, decreased intellectual performance, dysphagia, depression, and restless legs syndrome.[172] This progression forms the basis for the stages of iron deficiency outlined in *Table 25.4*. It has been confirmed by experiments in which normal volunteers were gradually depleted of iron by phlebotomy.[173]

Prevalence

Iron deficiency is the most common nutritional deficiency in both developing and developed countries. Anemia may be defined by cutoff hemoglobin values of 12.1 g/dL in women and 13.7 g/dL in men.[174] IDA is defined as anemia resulting from iron deficiency. In the United States, the most comprehensive surveys for IDA have been the National Health and Nutrition Examination Surveys (NHANES). According to data from NHANES III, covering the years 1988 to 1994, the prevalence of hypoferremia in the United States was <1% in adult men <50 years of age, 2% to 4% in adult men >50 years of age, 9% to 11% in menstruating teenagers and women, and 5% to 7% in postmenopausal women. Because serum ferritin is an acute phase reactant regulated by inflammation, these data may underestimate the prevalence of IDA in some populations, particularly the elderly. Recent analyses have estimated prevalence of IDA in the elderly (>65 years of age) and extreme elderly (>75 years of age) ranging from 10% to 36%.[175-177] The prevalence of IDA is higher in low- to middle-income countries, and it is estimated that globally ~1.2 billion people are affected with IDA.[178]

There are several other large and important patient populations in which anemia has been recognized as an independent risk factor for a number of adverse clinical outcomes, including patients with CKD, malignancies, and congestive heart failure. Iron deficiency is highly prevalent in each of these settings, for which treatment guidelines have been published.[179-181]

Iron deficiency is particularly common in young children and pregnant women and has been associated with increased risk for adverse maternal and neonatal outcomes.[182] Iron deficiency was detected in 9% of infants and toddlers, with anemia in approximately one-third of those children.[183] In infancy, the occurrence of iron deficiency was equal in both sexes. It is usually detected between the ages of 6 and 20 months. The peak incidence was at a younger age in infants born prematurely than in those born at term, because premature infants do not have full opportunity to acquire maternal iron during the third trimester. The prevalence of iron deficiency was also higher among people living in chronic poverty.[184] Iron deficiency tends to run in families, possibly as a result of economic factors. If an iron-deficient child is identified, the mother and siblings of that child are frequently also deficient. Definitive data regarding the benefits and harms of screening children and pregnant women for iron deficiency is lacking. The United States Preventative Services Task Force (USPSTF) previously recommended screening pregnant women and 1-year-old children for iron deficiency but currently concludes that the balance of benefits versus harms of screening in unselected children ages 6 to 24 months and pregnant women cannot be determined based on the available evidence.[185,186] In contrast, the American Academy of Pediatrics recommends universal screening for anemia at approximately 1 year of age.[187] In addition, the Academy recommends testing for iron deficiency in infants with anemia and/or iron deficiency risk factors.[187]

Iron deficiency occurs as a late manifestation of prolonged negative iron balance (e.g., chronic blood loss), as a result of acute blood loss, or because of failure to meet an increased physiologic need for iron. The normal mechanisms for maintaining iron balance were discussed earlier in this chapter. Factors leading to negative iron balance, increased requirements, or inadequate iron for erythropoiesis are listed in *Table 25.5*. In many instances, multiple etiologic factors are involved. The association of a marginal diet with some source of blood loss, such as that associated with menstruation, is a common combination. Another example is hookworm infestation, which produces anemia primarily in those people whose diets are marginally adequate.

Diet

The total amount of iron in the diet roughly correlates with caloric content; in the United States, the average diet contains ~6 mg of iron per 1000 kcal. The bioavailability of dietary iron in specific foods was described earlier in this chapter.

The early stages of human evolution were characterized by hunter-gatherer food patterns and by diets rich in meat. In evolutionary terms,

Table 25.5. Etiologic Factors in Iron-Deficiency Anemia

Negative Iron Balance
Decreased Iron Intake
Inadequate diet
Impaired absorption
Achlorhydria
Gastric surgery
Celiac disease
Helicobacter pylori infection
Duodenal bypass
Drugs that increase gastric pH
Tannins, phytates, bran
Competing metals
Inflammation, ↑ hepcidin
Increased Iron Loss
Blood donation
Iatrogenic: diagnostic phlebotomy for testing
Gastrointestinal bleeding
Intestinal parasites
Anatomic lesions: hemorrhoids, gastritis, diverticulosis, varices, hiatal hernia, Meckel diverticulum, arteriovenous malformation, peptic ulcer
Neoplasm
Inflammatory bowel disease
Cow's milk protein allergy (infants and children)
Use of salicylate or nonsteroidal anti-inflammatory agents
Excessive menstrual flow
Gynecologic neoplasm
Bladder neoplasm
Epistaxis
Hemoglobinuria
Self-induced bleeding (autophlebotomy)
Pulmonary hemosiderosis
Tuberculosis
Bronchiectasis
Hereditary hemorrhagic telangiectasia
Anticoagulant, antiplatelet therapies
Chronic hemodialysis
Runner anemia
Increased Requirements
Infancy
Pregnancy
Lactation
Genetic Forms of Iron Deficiency Anemia
See *Tables 25.2* and *25.3*

agriculture is a recent development to which humans have not fully adapted. Thus, individuals whose diets are rich in meat, a source of heme iron, usually absorb more iron from their diets than vegetarians. The increased prevalence of iron deficiency among the economically deprived and people in developing countries is explained in part by the fact that heme iron is less abundant in their diets.

Disorders of Red Blood Cells

Because many factors influence the bioavailability of iron, it is difficult to make recommendations about the optimal amount of iron in the diet. In the usual mixed diets of Western countries, adult men should consume 5 to 10 mg/d and adult women should consume 7 to 20 mg/d.[166] Because women are usually smaller and consume less food than men, and because their requirements are greater, their daily iron intake may be marginal. Iron deficiency is rarely seen in American men, in the absence of occult RBC losses, as a result of diet alone. Exceptions to this rule are sufficiently unusual to justify case reports.[188]

In many countries, foods are fortified to compensate for the insufficient amounts of iron in the diet.[189] For infants, fortified milk- or soy-based formulas and dry cereals are important sources of iron in the diet.

Impaired Absorption

Achlorhydria is common in iron-deficient subjects, both as a result of the deficiency and as a factor in its development.[190] Gastric acid facilitates absorption of nonheme iron,[191] by increasing its solubility rather than affecting the activity of the proton-symporter DMT1, and absorption of inorganic iron is profoundly impaired in patients with atrophic gastritis. Therapeutic measures used to reduce gastric acidity, such as the administration of antacids and drugs that block acid production, also impair iron absorption but usually not to a clinically significant degree. Gastric infection with *Helicobacter pylori* is recognized as an important cause of otherwise unexplained IDA, which responds to eradication of the bacterial infection.[192]

IDA is a common complication of gastric surgeries, including Roux-en-Y gastric bypass, total gastrectomy,[193] partial gastrectomy,[194] and vagotomy with gastroenterostomy.[195] Reduction in gastric acidity is only one factor in the impaired iron absorption that follows such operations. Other gastric secretions that aid in iron absorption may also be lost.[196] Also, because most iron absorption takes place in the proximal duodenum, the rapid intestinal transit that follows loss of the reservoir function of the stomach may lead to decreased absorption. For the same reason, iron deficiency is more common when the duodenum is surgically bypassed.[195] Finally, recurrent bleeding, as well as increased sloughing of iron-containing epithelial cells, may contribute to the development of postgastrectomy anemia.[196]

In addition to gastrectomy, other defects in the gastrointestinal tract may lead to malabsorption of iron, contributing to the development of iron deficiency. The anemia associated with celiac disease (gluten sensitivity, sprue, idiopathic steatorrhea) is often hypochromic rather than megaloblastic[197,198]; in fact, IDA may be the initial and dominant manifestation of celiac disease, with steatorrhea detectable only by laboratory test analysis.[197] Both malabsorption and intestinal blood loss are factors in the development of iron deficiency.[198] Most patients with tropical sprue are deficient in iron.[199]

Copper Deficiency

It has long been known that copper deficiency is associated with abnormalities in iron metabolism and IDA. In recent years, it has become clear that this is due, at least in part, to the importance of the copper-containing ferroxidases ceruloplasmin and hephaestin. As mentioned earlier in this chapter, these enzymes are required for the optimal mobilization of iron from cells to plasma. They oxidize Fe^{2+} exported by ferroportin into the Fe^{3+} form, which can then bind to apotransferrin.

Blood Loss

Blood loss is a significant cause of IDA. It is important not only because of its prevalence but also because the accurate detection, precise diagnosis, and proper management of the bleeding lesion may be of far greater importance to the ultimate well-being of the patient than repletion of iron stores. Each 1 mL of RBC contains ~1 mg of iron. Thus, assuming the consumption of an average diet, chronic RBC loss of as little as 1 to 2 mL/d can result in a negative iron balance.

Gastrointestinal Bleeding

Gastrointestinal bleeding is the most common cause of iron deficiency in adult men and is second only to menstrual blood loss as a cause in women. Any hemorrhagic lesion of the alimentary tract may cause iron deficiency. Most commonly, the lesions cause occult bleeding or the chronic loss of small amounts of blood. They may go unnoticed or may be tolerated until the symptoms of anemia supervene. The list of etiologies presented here is not meant to be comprehensive; many other, less common lesions have been reported to occur in association with isolated cases of IDA.

Two-thirds of patients with hemorrhoids experience rectal bleeding, which is usually obvious to the patient. Nevertheless, a large majority of patients allow at least 1 year to elapse before seeking medical attention, and perhaps one-third wait for more than 10 years. Nevertheless, although hemorrhoids are frequently associated with IDA, the clinician should be reluctant to accept them as the only bleeding lesions; a careful investigation is warranted because hemorrhoids may divert attention from another, less obvious lesion elsewhere in the alimentary tract.

Upper gastrointestinal bleeding is typically due to duodenal or gastric ulcers or gastritis, all of which can cause sufficient blood loss to result in iron deficiency. Certain drugs are associated with gastrointestinal bleeding. Of these, nonsteroidal anti-inflammatory drugs (NSAIDs), including aspirin, are the most important. NSAID administration causes mucosal damage manifested by petechial hemorrhage, erosions, and ulcers. The problem is more likely to occur in elderly patients and women and with higher ("anti-inflammatory") doses than with lower ("analgesic") ones.[200]

Low-dose aspirin (81 mg/d in the United States) was previously recommended for routine use in primary prevention of atherosclerotic cardiovascular disease (ASCVD) leading to widespread use of this medication. However, more recent analyses have shown that low-dose aspirin lacks a net benefit in this context, as the net benefit in terms of prevention of ASCVD is balanced by an increased risk of bleeding. Recent guidelines recommend against use of aspirin for primary prevention in adults >70 years or those of any age with increased bleeding risk.[201] Other drugs associated with gastrointestinal bleeding include stanozolol, anticoagulants, antiplatelet agent therapy for coronary artery disease, corticosteroids, and ethacrynic acid.

IDA occurs in ~15% of patients with esophageal hiatal hernia.[202] Anemia is particularly common (30%) with the paraesophageal variety of lesion and in large hernias.[203] Reasons for the bleeding include reflux esophagitis and trauma to the gastric mucosa at the neck of the hernial sac.[202]

Colonic diverticuli can also bleed in patients with diverticulosis and diverticulitis. Usually, the blood loss is small and intermittent and may resemble the pattern of hemorrhoidal bleeding. Intestinal bleeding can also result from the presence of adenomatous polyps. In a survey of 32 patients with ulcerative colitis, 26 (81%) had IDA.[204] Average fecal blood loss of 6 to 25 mL/d was noted in five patients who were moderately anemic with relatively mild symptoms of colitis.

A careful investigation for other sources of intestinal blood loss is warranted to exclude the possibility of a neoplasm. IDA may be the first sign of a malignant neoplasm of the gastrointestinal tract, especially in men and postmenopausal women.[140,205] Carcinoma of the cecum is often clinically silent until anemia occurs. Less often, in carcinomas of other parts of the colon, as well as of the stomach and the ampulla of Vater, IDA may be the only initial symptom.

An important cause of gastrointestinal blood loss in tropical areas is infection with intestinal and genitourinary parasites,[206] including whipworm, *Trichuris trichiura*[207]; hookworm, *Necator americanus* or *Ancylostoma duodenale*[208]; and schisotosomes.[209] Hookworm is particularly important, affecting some 20% of the world's population.[199] It is endemic in a zone extending from the southern United States to northern Argentina in the Western hemisphere, as well as in Mediterranean countries, South Asia, and Africa. The worms attach to the upper small intestine and suck blood from the host. The amount of blood lost is proportional to the number of worms harbored, which can be estimated by the fecal excretion of hookworm eggs. Female subjects harboring >100 worms (5 mL/d of blood loss) and male subjects harboring >250 worms (12.5 mL/d of blood loss) tend to become anemic.[208] Other factors affecting iron balance including an iron-deficient diet, repeated pregnancies, and achlorhydria are contributory factors in development of hookworm anemia. The anemia may be improved with iron therapy, whether or not the worms are removed. Conversely, removal of worms with an effective antihelminthic agent does not correct the anemia unless iron stores are replenished.

Schistosomiasis and trichuriasis are other parasitic infections associated with iron deficiency.[206] With *Schistosoma mansoni,* blood loss is from the intestine, whereas with *Schistosoma haematobium* the loss is from the urinary tract.[209] *Trichuris* (whipworm) is known to cause iron deficiency in inhabitants of Central America.[207]

Menstruation

Menstrual blood loss is the most common cause of iron deficiency in women.[7,210,211] In healthy, normal women, menstrual blood flow averages ~35 mL per menstrual period and the upper limit of normal is ~80 mL per period. Although flow varies considerably among different women, it is remarkably constant from one period to the next in the same person. In Swedish women with a dietary intake of ~10 mg of iron per day, 67% of women with menstrual blood loss >80 mL per period were anemic.[211] In another study, British women with IDA lost an average of 85 mL per period.[210] In contrast, a Canadian population with flows >80 mL per period had no overt anemia or hypoferremia.[212]

Menstrual blood flow is increased by the use of certain intrauterine contraceptive devices[213] and is reduced by the use of oral contraceptives. Estimating menstrual blood loss from information obtained in interviews is difficult because few women have a basis for determining the normality of their flow. It is important to elicit a history including a detailed description of the events during each menstrual period. Any of the following findings are indications of excessive menstrual flow: (a) need to change pad or tampon more frequently than every 3 hours; (b) use of more than 21 pads or tampons per cycle; (c) passage of clots greater than 1 cm in diameter; (d) frequent need to change the pad/tampon during the night.

Blood Donation

Regular blood donation is an important cause of iron deficiency.[214] Each unit of blood donated contains 200 mL RBC[215] equaling ~200 mg of iron. In most blood centers, a hemoglobin concentration, which is an insensitive determination for iron status, is the only indicator for IDA. In an analysis of the RISE (Retrovirus Epidemiology Donor Iron Status Evaluation) study[216] of frequent blood donors, two-thirds of women and almost half the men were iron deficient: the true prevalence is even higher, since the RISE study enrolled only frequent donors who had been accepted for donation and excluded those deferred because of anemia. The unavoidable conclusion is that presently, blood collection practices fail to protect committed blood donors from iron deficiency.[217] Increasing evidence of the potential adverse consequences of iron deficiency on blood donor health prompted the AABB to issue a bulletin in 2017 recommending that blood collection establishments take actions to monitor and/or mitigate the risk of iron deficiency associated with blood donation. Suggested approaches include iron supplementation, ferritin measurements, and/or lengthening of the interdonation interval.[218]

Alveolar Hemorrhage

Acute hemorrhage into the pulmonary alveoli may be severe enough to cause the blood hemoglobin level to fall 1.5 to 3.0 g/dL in 24 hours.[219] Reticulocytosis and hyperbilirubinemia often accompany such episodes, leading to an incorrect diagnosis of hemolytic anemia. Iron in the shed blood is converted to hemosiderin by pulmonary macrophages, but it cannot be used for hemoglobin synthesis. Thus, repeated hemorrhages can lead to iron deficiency despite a normal total amount of body iron. Hemoptysis and alveolar infiltrates are the other prominent manifestations. However, if the hemorrhages are small, the hemoptysis may be unnoticed, making the diagnosis difficult without

a chest x-ray examination. Patients may swallow the blood-containing sputum, rendering the stools positive for occult blood and resulting in further diagnostic confusion.

Idiopathic pulmonary hemosiderosis, an illness of children and young adults, is characterized by alveolar hemorrhage that is not due to another form of lung disease.[220,221] IDA almost invariably accompanies the disease and may be the initial and only symptom. Hemoptysis and alveolar infiltrates, however, are common manifestations. Interstitial fibrosis may develop after repeated episodes, with dyspnea, clubbing, and even cor pulmonale.

Anemia is also a common finding in antiglomerular basement membrane antibody disease (Goodpasture syndrome).[221] The presence of renal disease distinguishes this illness from other forms of pulmonary hemosiderosis, but kidney involvement may not be evident early in the course of the disease or the degree of proteinuria or microscopic hematuria may be modest. Eventually, however, most patients develop azotemia. Focal or diffuse glomerulonephritis is evident from renal biopsy, and linear deposits of immunoglobulins are characteristic of, although not completely specific for, the disease. Detection of antibasement membrane antibodies in serum is ~80% to 85% sensitive and 98% specific for the diagnosis.[219]

Other illnesses associated with pulmonary alveolar hemorrhage include rapidly progressive glomerulonephritis, systemic lupus erythematosus, and certain other collagen vascular diseases and systemic vasculitides. The presence of antineutrophil cytoplasm antibodies or other autoantibodies is considered a particularly poor prognostic sign in patients with pulmonary hemosiderosis. Alveolar hemorrhage is also observed as a toxic reaction to trimellitic anhydride, d-penicillamine, or lymphangiography.

Hemoglobinuria

Paroxysmal nocturnal hemoglobinuria can result in urinary iron losses averaging 1.8 to 7.8 mg/d.[222] Consequently, this rare disorder often is complicated by hypoferremia and hypochromic anemia.[223] Hemoglobinuria in other disorders, such as the erythrocyte fragmentation syndromes associated with prosthetic cardiac valves, also may be complicated by iron deficiency.[224]

Factitious Anemia

Self-induced blood-letting (autophlebotomy) is an unusual cause of iron deficiency.[225] In almost all reported instances, such anemia occurred in unmarried women in paramedical occupations. Blood was removed by venipuncture or injuring preexisting hemorrhoids, by laceration of the gastrointestinal tract with such instruments as knitting needles, or by means that remained obscure. At least one case was reported in which an infant apparently developed severe iron deficiency as a result of deliberate parental action in which all iron from the child's diet was removed.[220]

Hereditary Hemorrhagic Telangiectasia

Hereditary hemorrhagic telangiectasia is an uncommon disorder characterized by recurrent hemorrhages from the nose, gastrointestinal tract, and other sites. IDA, sometimes very difficult to manage, is an important complication of the illness (see Chapter 51).[226]

Iatrogenic Blood Loss

Diagnostic phlebotomy can result in substantial iron losses in patients with chronic disorders, particularly in hospitalized patients.[227] A study at the Cleveland Clinic Health System[228] evaluated nearly 190,000 hospitalizations of patients not anemic at admission and found that 74% developed hospital-acquired anemia. Although hospital-acquired anemia is clearly multifactorial in etiology, diagnostic phlebotomy is a significant contributor. A large European study reported that intensive care unit (ICU) patients were phlebotomized on average 41 ± 40 mL/d.[229] A different ICU study reported that median contribution of diagnostic blood loss to total blood loss was 17% (range 10%-28%).[230] Phlebotomy was shown to not only precipitate or aggravate IDA but also increase the need for allogeneic blood transfusion in critical care patients.[231]

Disorders of Red Blood Cells

Chronic Renal Failure Treated With Hemodialysis

Iron deficiency affects a significant fraction of patients treated with hemodialysis now that the anemia related to CKD is treated with pharmacologic agents and blood transfusions are restricted.[232] Absolute iron deficiency results from the loss of blood associated with the dialysis process and diagnostic tests. Gastrointestinal blood losses may also be substantial, averaging 6.27 mL/d in one study.[233] Telangiectasias are among the most common bleeding gastrointestinal lesions in patients with renal failure. Other factors contributing to negative iron balance include reduced dietary iron intake and malabsorption of iron caused by elevated hepcidin.[234]

Administration of erythropoiesis stimulating agents (ESAs) results in a "functional iron deficiency" even when body iron stores are replete.[235] The intense, periodic erythropoietic stimulus due to ESA therapy exceeds the mobilization of iron from macrophages, so that adequate transferrin-bound iron is not available to RBC precursors.[235,236] For this reason, parenteral iron supplementation is often provided as an adjunct to ESA therapy in patients with end stage kidney disease.[140,235]

Runner Anemia

IDA can occur in long-distance runners.[237] Over 50% of regular joggers and competitive runners become iron deficient. Mild mechanical hemolysis accompanies strenuous exercise, resulting in hemoglobinemia and hemoglobinuria (also called march hemoglobinuria). Gastrointestinal bleeding also contributes to blood loss and iron deficiency.[238] Fecal blood excretion increases substantially after a race or an intense training exercise and may reach 5 to 7 mL/d. Stress, intestinal ischemia, and the jarring effect of running have been advanced as possible explanations for the gastrointestinal blood loss. Reduced iron absorption due to subclinical inflammation and inappropriately high hepcidin may also contribute to the development of IDA in athletes.[239]

Decreased Total Body Iron at Birth

Body iron concentration in normal neonates averages ~75 to 100 mg/kg weight. Similar concentrations are found throughout fetal development, resulting in a linear relationship between body iron and body weight. Newborn babies in the upper range of normal birth weights have more iron than those in the lower range. Premature infants are at higher risk of iron deficiency during the first year of life, because they have not had the full opportunity to accumulate iron stores during the third trimester of gestation.

Newborn iron levels can be influenced by the technique that the obstetrician uses to clamp the umbilical cord at delivery.[240] As much as 100 mL of fetal blood may remain in the placenta with early clamping of the cord. Cord clamping delayed for only 3 minutes can result in a 58% increase in red cell volume. If delayed clamping is impractical, as in cesarean section procedures, a similar effect can be achieved by clamping the cord at the placental end, raising the clamp, and allowing gravity to drain the cord.[241] Although the newborn has no immediate need for these erythrocytes, the iron they contain can be used later to meet the demands of growth.

Maternal iron status during pregnancy affects infant's iron endowment because maternal iron deficiency compromises fetal iron acquisition.[242] Suboptimal iron supply to the fetus can have detrimental effects on the fetal development.[243] Decreased iron stores at birth are also associated with long-term cognitive deficits in infancy and childhood.[244] The iron endowment at birth is important because those stores are utilized until 6 to 9 months of age.[243] Iron supplementation of iron-deficient mothers during pregnancy was shown to have positive effects on both maternal and neonatal outcomes.[243]

Growth

In the absence of disease, iron requirements of an adult man are relatively low and vary little. In contrast, in infancy, childhood, and adolescence, the requirements for iron are relatively great because of the increased needs of rapidly growing tissues. The most rapid relative growth rates in human development occur in the first year of life. Body weight and blood volume approximately triple, and the circulating hemoglobin mass nearly doubles. Still greater relative growth occurs in premature and low-birth-weight infants. Premature infants weighing 1.5 kg may increase their weight and blood volume 6-fold and may triple the circulating hemoglobin mass in 1 year. To meet the demands imposed by growth, the normal-term infant must acquire 135 to 200 mg of iron during the first year of life. A premature infant may require as much as 350 mg in the same period.[245]

The relatively slower rates of growth in children through the remainder of the first decade require a positive iron balance of ~0.2 to 0.3 mg/d. The growth spurt that occurs in the early teens requires a positive balance of ~0.5 mg/d in girls and 0.6 mg/d in boys.[166] Toward the end of this period, the onset of menstruation occurs in girls, and their requirements then equal those of adult women.

Diet in Infancy and Childhood

Iron stores in the infant are typically depleted by 4 to 6 months of age as a result of the demands of growth. During this critical period, a normal full-term infant must absorb ~0.4 to 0.6 mg of iron daily from the diet. To achieve this level of absorption, an iron intake of 1 mg/kg/d is recommended for full-term infants, 2 to 4 mg/kg/d for preterm infants, and at least 6 mg (to a maximum of 15 mg) for preterm infants receiving EPO therapy.[246] These amounts may be difficult to achieve without supplementation.

Both human milk and cow's milk contain relatively small amounts of iron, but the infant more readily absorbs the iron in human milk. In one study, 49% of the iron in human breast milk was absorbed, compared with 10% of the iron in cow's milk.[247] As a result, iron deficiency is relatively uncommon in the first 6 months of life in infants exclusively fed breast milk.

Formula-fed infants are likely to become iron-deficient unless iron-supplemented formulas are used. In the United States, such formulas are often supplemented with iron (10-12 mg/L) as ferrous sulfate, of which a variable proportion is absorbed.[246] Approximately 7% to 12% of the iron in cow's milk–based formulas is absorbed, with the lower percentage seen when formulas with higher iron content are given.[248] Less iron is absorbed from soy-based formulas, but soy formulas containing 12 mg/L of iron appear to be adequate.[249] Fortified dry cereals for infants are another important source of iron in the diet of both breast-fed and formula-fed infants. Currently, infant cereals are fortified with small-particle elemental iron at a concentration of 0.45 mg/g, from which ~4% is absorbed.[250] Two servings per day will supply the needs of most infants.

Excessive intake of cow's milk is an important cause of iron deficiency in the first 2 years of life.[245,251] Not only is cow's milk a poor source of iron, but it may also cause gastrointestinal blood loss (see Blood Loss in Infancy section). In general, cow's milk should not be given to infants <1 year of age, although it may be tolerated if the remainder of the diet is iron rich.[252] A unique disorder termed Bahima disease, described in Uganda, was attributed to the practice of feeding children a diet of cow's milk almost exclusively.[253]

Blood Loss in Infancy

Occult hemorrhage, often without obvious anatomic lesions, may be observed in some iron-deficient infants.[250,254] The process is often accompanied by diffuse disease of the bowel with protein-losing enteropathy and impaired absorption of other nutrients.[255] It probably results from hypersensitivity to a heat-labile protein in cow's milk.[256] The daily loss of 1 to 4 mL of blood, along with increased serum albumin turnover, was observed while fresh cow's milk was consumed, and these abnormalities ceased abruptly with the substitution of heat-treated or soybean-protein feeding formulas.

Pregnancy and Lactation

Pregnancy is a major drain on the limited iron reserves of young women. Each pregnancy results in an average loss to the mother of 740 mg of iron, the equivalent of ~700 mL of RBC, or 1700 mL of blood. An additional 450 mg of iron must be available to support the expanded blood volume during pregnancy. The latter amount of iron does not represent a net loss after delivery because the iron is returned to stores; it must be available, however, during the pregnancy or iron deficiency will supervene.

Prorated over the full term of pregnancy, the iron requirement amounts to ~2.5 mg/d (*Table 25.6*). Because most of the loss occurs during the third trimester, the requirement is small early in pregnancy and rises to as much as 3.0 to 7.5 mg/d in the third trimester.[257] These amounts are greater than those that can be absorbed from even the best of diets, and stores may be insufficient to meet them. Nevertheless, the USPSTF concludes that the current evidence is insufficient to assess the balance of benefits and harms of routine iron supplementation for pregnant women to prevent adverse maternal health and birth outcomes.[186] While strong data to support a benefit are lacking, most experts recommend that pregnant women take prenatal vitamins that provide 15 to 30 mg of iron per day. In the absence of supplements, maternal iron deficiency may occur, usually manifesting in the third trimester.

Lactation results in a daily iron loss of ~0.5 to 1.0 mg. The iron content of human breast milk is probably not affected by the maternal iron stores.[258] Because normal menstruation is usually inhibited while breastfeeding continues, iron requirements in the lactating mother approximate those of the menstruating woman.

Signs and Symptoms of Iron Deficiency

The onset of IDA is usually insidious, and the progression of symptoms is gradual. As a result, patients accommodate remarkably well to advancing anemia and may delay a visit to their physicians for prolonged periods.

Fatigue and Other Nonspecific Symptoms

IDA can be associated with irritability, palpitations, dizziness, breathlessness, headache, and fatigue. Fatigue is a particularly common complaint among patients. Even latent iron deficiency (i.e., iron deficiency without any anemia at all) has been described to result in fatigue.[259] Iron therapy has been shown to ameliorate fatigue. In a randomized clinical trial of intravenous (IV) iron therapy in 90 premenopausal nonanemic women presenting with fatigue, serum ferritin ≤50 ng/mL, and Hgb ≥ 12 g/dL, fatigue scopes decreased significantly within 6 weeks of IV iron therapy compared with placebo, particularly in women with baseline serum ferritin ≤15 ng/mL.[260]

Neuromuscular System

Despite the lack of symptoms at rest, investigators have demonstrated that even mild degrees of IDA impair muscular performance, as measured by standardized exercise tests.[261] Total exercise time, maximal workload, heart rate, and serum lactate levels after exercise are all affected adversely in proportion to the degree of anemia. Furthermore, work performance and productivity at tasks requiring sustained or prolonged activity are impaired in iron-deficient subjects and improve when iron is administered.[262] As a result, measures directed toward iron nutrition of a workforce can produce important economic dividends, more than offsetting the costs of the treatment program.

Abnormalities in muscle metabolism are noted even when iron deficiency is mild. Animal studies demonstrate that muscle function is disturbed in iron deficiency. The spontaneous activity level of iron-deficient rats decreased,[263] and short-term exercise tolerance in treadmill running tests was reduced, even at mild degrees of deficiency.[264] These abnormalities could not be explained by anemia alone, because they persisted after anemia was corrected by exchange transfusion.[265] Cellular and animal studies showed that iron deficiency impairs skeletal muscle energetics, leading to shift toward anaerobic metabolism, shift to glycolysis, impaired oxidative metabolism, and derangements in mitochondrial morphology.[266]

A variety of behavioral disturbances have been observed in iron-deficient children.[267-270] These children have been reported to be irritable and disruptive, with short attention spans and a lack of interest in their surroundings. Neurologic development in infants[271] and scholastic performance in older children[272] may be impaired. Cognitive performance is defective in iron-deficient rats.[273] All of these behavioral abnormalities are ameliorated with the initiation of iron therapy.

The ability to maintain body temperature on exposure to cold is impaired in iron-deficient patients.[274] Occasional patients experience neuralgia pains, vasomotor disturbances, or numbness and tingling. In children, iron deficiency has been associated with neurologic sequelae, including developmental delay, ischemic stroke, increased intracranial pressure, papilledema, and the clinical picture of pseudotumor cerebri.[275] The pathogenesis is probably complex, involving severe anemia, thrombocytosis, and reduced levels of tissue iron enzymes.

Epithelial Tissues

Patients with long-standing iron deficiency may develop a constellation of symptoms characterized by defective structure or function of epithelial tissues. Especially affected are the nails, the tongue and mouth, the hypopharynx, and the stomach. These epithelial lesions tend to occur together in the same patients at the same time,[276] but they may also occur as isolated findings.

In iron-deficient subjects, the fingernails may become brittle, fragile, or longitudinally ridged, but these findings are quite nonspecific. Alterations more typical of iron deficiency are nail thinning, flattening, and ultimately the development of koilonychia, concave or "spoon-shaped" nails (*Figure 25.6*). Koilonychia is now rarely seen in clinical practice, but of 400 babies attending a well-baby clinic in West Virginia before 1970, 5.5% had koilonychia and nearly all of these infants appeared to be iron deficient.[277] Koilonychia is a relatively nonspecific finding, which can also result from prolonged, repeated exposure to hot soapsuds and other caustic agents.

Oral abnormalities, including atrophy of the lingual papillae, are the most common of iron deficiency–induced epithelial changes (*Figure 25.7, Table 25.7*). These may present as soreness or burning of the tongue, either spontaneously or stimulated by food or drink, and by varying degrees of redness.[276] The filiform papillae over the anterior two-thirds of the tongue are the first to atrophy and may disappear completely. In severe cases, fungiform papillae also may be affected, leaving the tongue completely smooth and waxy or glistening.[278] These changes are generally reversed after 1 to 2 weeks of iron

Table 25.6. Iron Balance in Pregnancy

Iron Fate	Mean Amount (mg)
Lost to fetus	−270
Lost to placenta	−90
Expansion of maternal RBC mass	−450
Baseline maternal body iron loss	−230
Total iron needs during pregnancy	**−1040**
RBC mass contraction after delivery	+450
Iron lost with bleeding at delivery	−150
Net pregnancy iron loss to the mother	**−740**

Abbreviation: RBC, red blood cell.

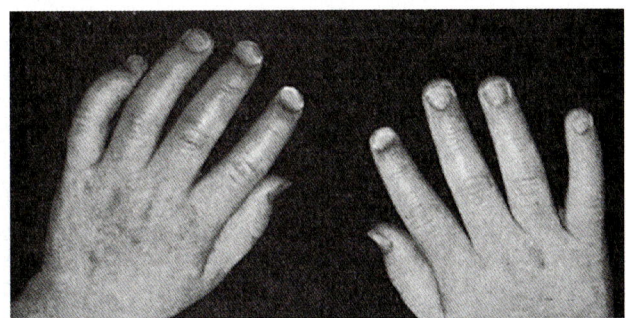

FIGURE 25.6 Koilonychia in a 1½-year-old child with iron-deficiency anemia.

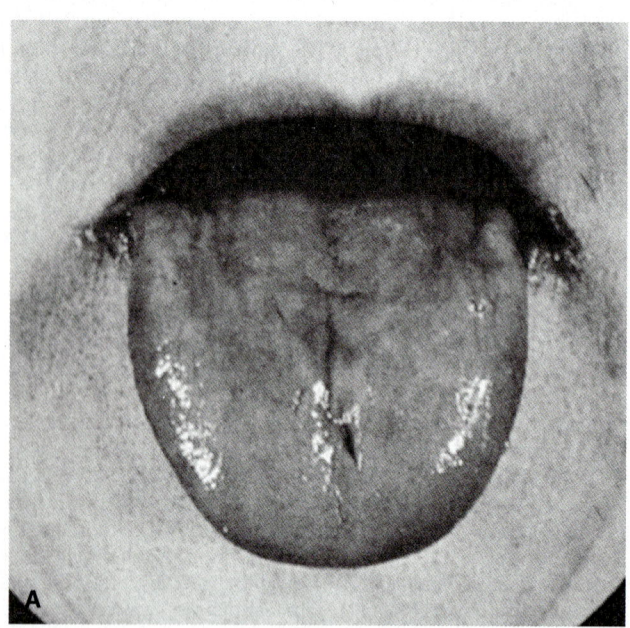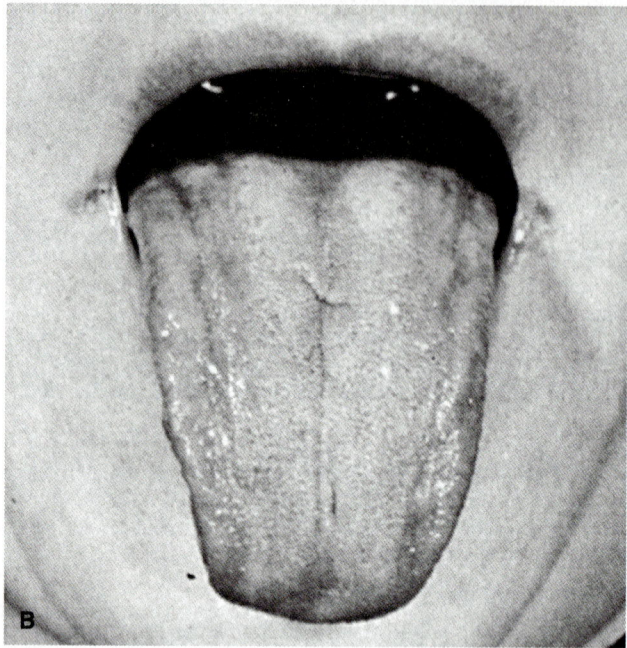

FIGURE 25.7 **Tongue of a patient with iron-deficiency anemia.** Moderately severe papillary atrophy evident before therapy (A) and restoration after iron repletion (B). (Courtesy of R. W. Monto, Detroit, MI.)

Table 25.7. Epithelial Lesions Associated With Iron Deficiency

Site	Finding
Nails	Flattening Koilonychia
Tongue	Soreness Mild papillary atrophy Absence of filiform papillae
Mouth	Angular stomatitis
Hypopharynx	Dysphagia Esophageal webs
Stomach	Achlorhydria Gastritis

therapy. Angular stomatitis, characterized by ulcerations or fissures at the corners of the mouth, is a less specific sign of iron deficiency, and it also occurs in riboflavin and pyridoxine deficiencies.

The association of dysphagia, angular stomatitis, and lingual abnormalities with hypochromic anemia was reported as early as the beginning of the 20th century. Patients with sideropenic dysphagia (also known as Paterson-Kelly syndrome in the United Kingdom and Plummer-Vinson syndrome in the United States) note a gradual onset of difficulty swallowing and describe discomfort localized to the area of the neck near the cricoid cartilage. They experience dysphagia with solid foods but have little problem with liquids. If not treated, the dysphagia worsens, and ultimately the diet is so restricted that it interferes with the maintenance of balanced nutrition.

The most common anatomic lesion is a "web" of mucosa at the juncture between the hypopharynx and the esophagus.[279] These webs, which may be multiple, usually extend from the anterior wall into the lumen of the esophagus, but they may encircle the lumen completely, forming a cuff-like structure. In some patients, a benign stricture is noted, and the opening into the esophagus at the cricoid area may be reduced to the size of a pinhole or slit. Both webs and strictures may be demonstrated by radiographic examination after barium swallow.

At biopsy, the webs appear to be constructed of normal epithelium with underlying loose connective tissue, sometimes showing a chronic inflammatory reaction. In a small percentage, hyperchromatic nuclei and increased mitotic activity are observed in the basal cell layer. Biopsy of the strictures demonstrates chronic, nonspecific inflammation and degeneration of striated muscle. Carcinoma in the postcricoid area has been noted as a late complication of the syndrome in 4% to 16% of patients.[276] For relief of the dysphagia, clinicians often must rupture the webs, dilate the stenosis, or both, although treatment with iron supplements relieves dysphagia in mild cases if the associated webs are small.[280,281]

Immunity and Infection

The relationship between iron deficiency and infection is complex.[282] Iron deficiency clearly results in at least two abnormalities in the immune response: defective lymphocyte-mediated immunity and impaired bacterial killing by phagocytes. Evidence of defective cellular immunity includes as much as a 35% reduction in the number of circulating T cells. Lymphocyte iron deficiency caused by impaired iron uptake due to a mutation in TfR1 was shown to lead to combined immunodeficiency. The patients had impaired proliferation of T and B cells and impaired antibody production, highlighting the importance of iron in the function of immune cells.[146] In a study of infants, IDA at time of vaccination predicted decreased response to diphtheria, pertussis, and pneumococcal vaccines[283] and iron supplementation at time of vaccination increased humoral vaccine response.

The nitroblue tetrazolium dye test of phagocyte function yielded abnormal results in iron-deficient children, and the abnormality could be corrected by iron administration.[284] Furthermore, a decrease in the magnitude of the "oxidative burst" accompanying phagocytosis was observed.[285] Finally, killing of several types of pathogenic bacteria by neutrophils is defective.[286]

In experiments in an iron-deficient mouse model, lack of hepcidin was responsible for the high inflammatory response to lipopolysaccharide treatment.[287] Taken together, these abnormalities provide a basis for an expectation that resistance to infection may be impaired in iron deficiency. However, a clinically relevant relationship between states of iron deficiency and susceptibility to infections remains controversial.[288] Conversely, considerable data suggest that iron deficiency and iron sequestration by binding proteins protect against infection by depriving the invading organisms of the metal.[289] Thus, optimal immune function is highly dependent on iron balance; both iron-deficient and iron-overloaded hosts may be at higher risk for infection.

Pica

Pica is a striking symptom of iron deficiency. Hippocrates wrote that a "craving to eat earth" was associated with "corruption of the blood." Abnormal eating patterns were also a prominent manifestation of chlorosis. Pagophagia, defined as the purposeful eating of at least one tray of ice daily for 2 months, is a common form of pica. In one study, the ingestion of ice averaged nearly 2 kg/d, and some patients ate an astounding 4 to 9 kg/d.[290] This dramatic symptom was relieved within 1 to 14 days after iron was administered. Another study found that pagophagia was a symptom of iron deficiency in 23 of 38 consecutive adult patients, and iron therapy was curative.[291] Pica is especially striking when the patient consumes bizarre, nonfood substances.[292]

Crosby estimated the incidence of pica in his iron-deficient patients to be 50%.[293] Approximately half of them ate ice; the rest experienced "food pica." The latter consists of compulsively eating one food, often something that is brittle and makes a crunching sound when chewed.[294] Because patients may be ashamed of this compulsive habit, they often do not volunteer the information during the medical interview. Direct, tactful inquiry is necessary to elicit the history of pica.

Genitourinary System

Disturbances in menstruation are common in iron deficiency, and not infrequently, iron deficiency results from, or is exacerbated by, excessive menstrual blood loss.

There may be evidence that iron deficiency decreases fertility. The Nurses' Health Study II suggested that the consumption of iron supplements and nonheme iron from foods may decrease the risk of ovulatory infertility.[295] A study in female rats reported a delay in conception and lower conception rate in iron-deficient animals.[296]

Skeletal System

Changes in the skull similar to those found in association with thalassemia or chronic hemolytic anemia have been reported in children with IDA of long duration.[297] The diploic spaces may be widened and the outer tables thinned, at times with vertical striations producing a hair-on-end appearance. In addition, abnormalities of the long bones are noted, especially the metacarpals and phalanges, with expansion of the medulla and thinning of the cortices.[298] These changes likely result from expansion of the erythroid marrow during bone growth and development.

LABORATORY EVALUATION

Complete Blood Count and Peripheral Smear

The severity of anemia depends on the presenting circumstances of iron deficiency. If discovered when the patient is being evaluated for preadmission testing for elective surgery, or for an underlying or unrelated disease (*Figure 25.8*),[175,298] the anemia can be mild to moderate (Hgb 8 g/dL to 12 g/dL). If symptoms of anemia are the presenting complaint, the blood hemoglobin level may be 8 g/dL or lower.

Anisocytosis is an important early sign in iron deficiency and one that has differential diagnostic value when quantified.[299] The red cell distribution width (RDW) is increased in iron deficiency, and this often is useful in distinguishing iron deficiency from thalassemia trait conditions in which the RDW is normal. Both the percentage and the absolute number of reticulocytes may be normal or slightly increased. In experimentally induced iron deficiency in certain animal species, including rats, mice, and pigs, reticulocytosis is pronounced. The chief finding on blood smear is hypochromia, observed as an increase in the size of the region of central pallor (*Figure 25.9*). The more severe the anemia, the more severe the hypochromia and the greater the percentage of erythrocytes affected. When hypochromia is extreme, most of the RBCs appear as mere rings. Tiny microcytes and a moderate number of poikilocytes, particularly tailed and elongated elliptical forms (pencil cells), are also found. In almost all instances, however, a variable number of well-filled red corpuscles are present, and some macrocytes, often polychromatophilic, can be distinguished. The mean corpuscular volume and mean corpuscular hemoglobin values are reduced in most patients, and the mean corpuscular hemoglobin concentration is reduced in long-standing or severe disease. The degree of change in the red cell indices is related in part to the duration and in part to the severity of the anemia. In mild iron deficiency of short duration, the indices may be within normal ranges.

Iron-Related Indices

The laboratory diagnosis of absolute iron deficiency has traditionally been based on low serum iron, low percent Tsat, and low ferritin.[140] However, it has long been known that inflammation can mimic some aspects of iron deficiency by impairing the utilization of existing iron stores for red cell production and inducing an iron-sequestration syndrome and hypoferremia.[300] The molecular mechanisms that underlie the redistribution of iron during inflammation are discussed in Chapter 45; they may center on cytokine-stimulated overproduction of hepcidin, particularly IL-6.[26]

Serum ferritin has the potential to differentiate true iron deficiency from inflammatory iron sequestration. However, both inflammation and intracellular iron accumulation stimulate the production of the iron storage protein ferritin whose soluble form is detectable in circulation. Therefore, interpretation of serum ferritin in patients with inflammation due to comorbidities is more challenging. The generally accepted cutoff level for serum ferritin to indicate absolute iron deficiency has been ≤12 ng/mL.[301] However, studies correlating the presence or absence of stainable iron with serum ferritin in patients and in normal individuals, and also patients with anemia responsive to iron therapy, indicate that this threshold level of ferritin had only a sensitivity of 25% for detecting iron deficiency.[302] The sensitivity could be improved to 92%, with a positive predictive value of 83%, by using a diagnostic cutoff value of ≤30 ng/mL.

The differentiation among absolute iron deficiency, functional iron deficiency, and iron-sequestration syndromes (*Figure 25.10*) is important for patient management.[235] Functional iron deficiency is manifest by a fall in iron saturation either during endogenous erythropoietin–stimulated erythropoiesis[235,303] or with initiation of ESA therapy even in normal volunteers with adequate iron stores.[235,304] The manifestation of functional iron deficiency is reduced transferrin saturation in the presence of normal ferritin levels, as illustrated in *Figure 25.11*.[305] Absolute iron deficiency may be the presenting sign of occult blood loss from gastrointestinal lesions including malignancy.[205] An iron sequestration phenotype is indicative of an underlying inflammatory disorder, in which commonly used laboratory tests such as serum iron, total iron-binding capacity, mean corpuscular volume, transferrin saturation, and ferritin provide limited diagnostic value.[128,306]

Increased soluble transferrin receptor (sTfR) has been reported to be an indicator of iron deficiency,[307] since sTfR is released by erythropoietic precursors in proportion to their expansion and degree of their iron deficiency and is not increased by inflammation. However, this assay was found to have a specificity of 84% and a positive predictive value of only 58% in a population of patients likely to be typical of the most difficult diagnostic environments for assessing iron status.[302] Interpretation of increased sTfR therefore may be challenging, even in the absence of known causes of increased erythropoiesis other than iron deficiency. Similarly, attempts to combine ferritin and sTfR results (sTfR/log ferritin)[308] still fall short when analyzed for diagnostic sensitivity and specificity and must be corrected for acute phase reactant changes in the setting of inflammation.[306]

The development of sensitive, accurate, and reproducible immunoassays[59,309] and mass-spectrometric assays[310] for human hepcidin has allowed detailed definition of physiologic and pathologic changes of hepcidin in healthy volunteers and in patients. In contrast to ferritin, changes in hepcidin concentrations are frequently the cause of, rather than the result of, iron disorders. Measurements of hepcidin may be useful for diagnosing absolute iron deficiency or differentiating it from iron sequestration syndromes.[235] In absolute iron deficiency, serum hepcidin concentrations are very low.[59] Low hepcidin would also identify patients most likely to respond to iron therapy. In iron sequestration syndromes, on the other hand, hepcidin would be expected to be high as the pathogenic mediator of iron restriction in

Disorders of Red Blood Cells

EVALUATION OF ANEMIA

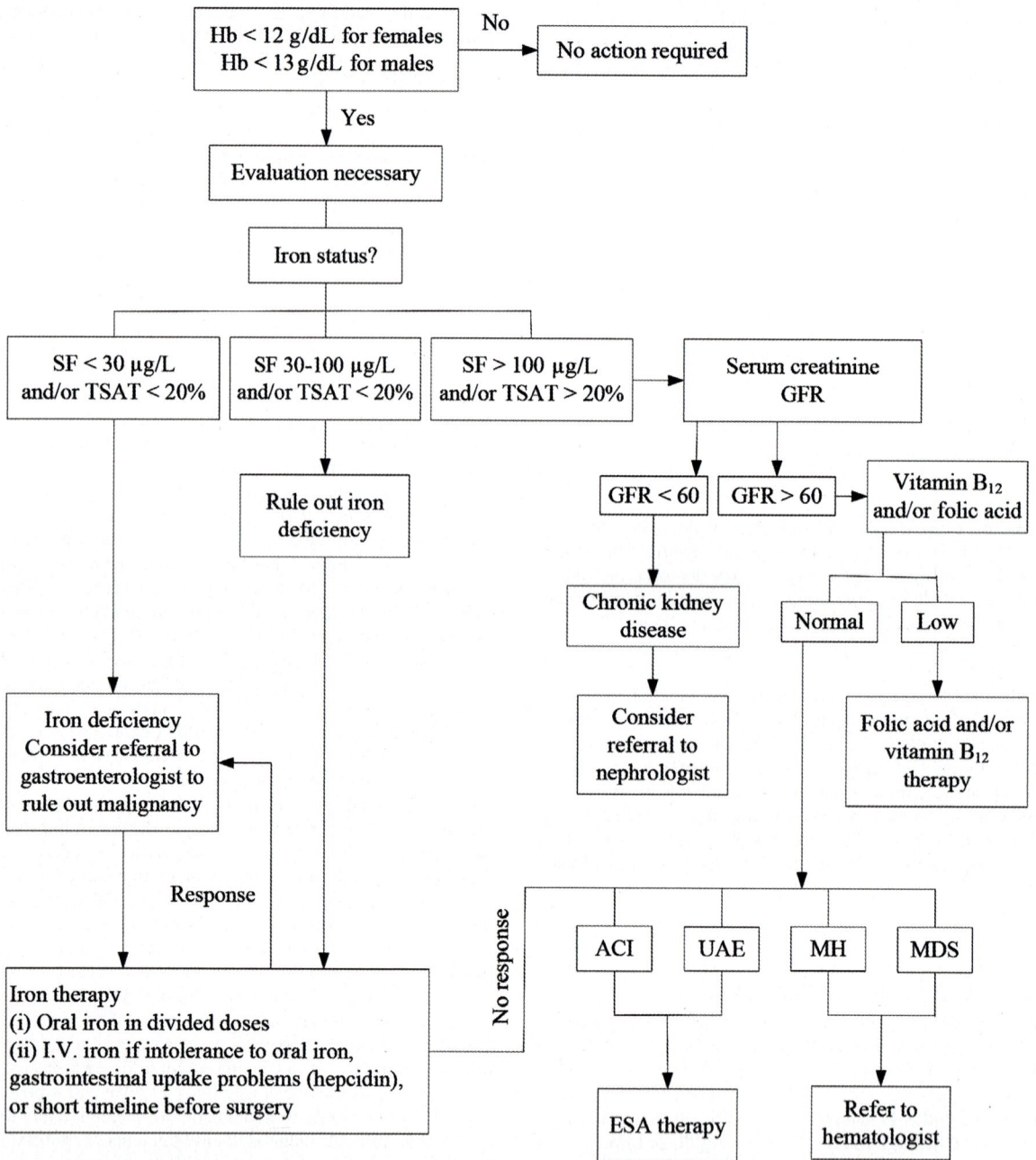

FIGURE 25.8 **Screening, evaluation, and management of anemia.** Algorithm for the detection, evaluation, and management of anemia. ACI, anemia of inflammation; ESA, erythropoiesis stimulating agent; GFR, glomerular filtration rate; Hb, hemoglobin; I.V., intravenous; MDS, myelodysplastic syndrome; MH, malignant hematology; SF, serum ferritin; Tsat, transferrin saturation; UFA, undifferentiated anemia. (From Goodnough LT, Schrier SL. Evaluation and management of anemia in the elderly. *Am J Hematol.* 2014;89:88-96. Copyright © 2013 Wiley Periodicals, Inc. Reprinted by permission of John Wiley & Sons, Inc.)

inflammation. In patients with mixed presentations, hepcidin may be regulated by opposing stimuli and its levels tend to be variable.[311] For example, in conditions with mixed iron deficiency and inflammation, hepcidin may be low, normal, or elevated depending on the degree of iron deficiency or inflammation. In resistance to ESA therapy due to CKD, hepcidin levels may be high because of decreased hepcidin renal clearance and possibly inflammation. In the absence of inflammation, in conditions of accelerated erythropoiesis due to endogenous EPO or ESA stimulation, hepcidin levels will be low. Thus, in patients with mixed conditions, hepcidin levels may not help treating physicians arrive at a definitive diagnosis but may give guidance in identifying patients who are likely to respond to iron (oral vs IV) therapy

(i.e., hepcidin levels are low with marginal storage iron or accelerated erythropoiesis). More complex algorithms will need to be developed and tested to provide optimal guidance in the evaluation and management of anemia.[312] Expected changes in hepcidin levels and iron parameters in various clinical conditions, in iron therapy strategies, and in the potential use of hepcidin-targeted therapies in patients with various forms of anemia are summarized in *Table 25.8.*

Clinically, it would be helpful to detect the earliest changes in red cell indices that reflect iron-restricted erythropoiesis. One approach would be to identify newly formed iron-deficient cells when they are released from the bone marrow as reticulocytes. Flow cytometric analysis of reticulocytes allows determination of reticulocyte hemoglobin

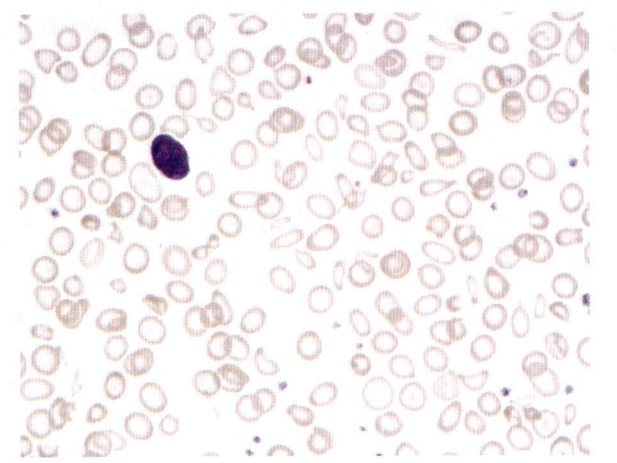

FIGURE 25.9 Blood smear from a patient with microcytic anemia due to iron deficiency. (Courtesy of Irma Pereira MT [ASCP] SH.)

content (CHr)[313] or percentage of hypochromic reticulocytes (% HYPO).[314] The CHr measure may be a useful measurement as it is a real-time parameter (reflecting iron-restricted erythropoiesis over the last 48 hours).[314] Many existing laboratory analyzers are capable of measuring CHr but may require modification with software patches.

Leukocytes and Platelets

The leukocytes are usually normal in number, but mild granulocytopenia may occur in long-standing cases of iron deficiency. Recent large-volume hemorrhage may cause a slight neutrophilic leukocytosis, and occasional myelocyte may be found in peripheral blood. In iron deficiency due to parasitic infestation, eosinophilia may be present.

Thrombocytosis commonly accompanies iron deficiency.[315] The platelet count often increases to approximately twice the normal level, and values return to normal after iron therapy. Recent work suggests that the thrombocytosis in iron deficiency is driven by an iron-related switch in the lineage commitment of megakaryocyte-erythroid progenitor cells (MEPs). Low bone marrow iron biases MEPs toward megakaryocyte commitment at the expense of erythroid commitment.[316]

Bone Marrow

Macrophage iron is absent or severely reduced in the marrow, spleen, and liver of iron-deficient subjects. Fewer than 10% of the marrow erythroblasts are sideroblasts. In addition, the iron-deficient bone marrow is characterized by mild to moderate erythroid hyperplasia. There may be striking nuclear distortions, resembling those found in

Iron Deficiency States

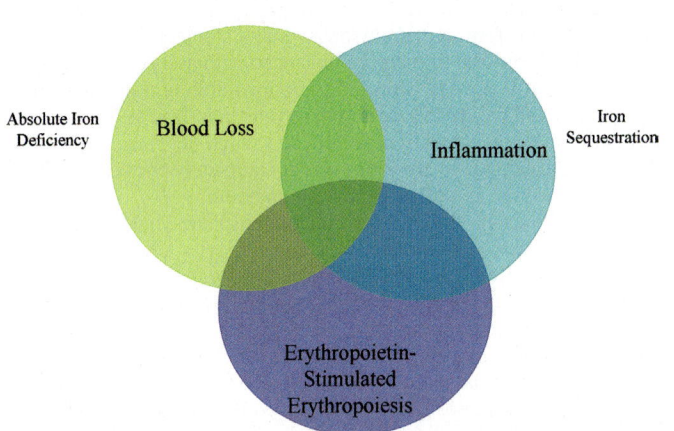

FIGURE 25.10 Iron deficiency states. The relationships between absolute iron deficiency, iron sequestration, and functional iron deficiency are illustrated. Patients can have one or more combinations that all result in iron-restricted erythropoiesis. (From Goodnough LT. Iron deficiency syndromes and iron-restricted erythropoiesis. *Transfusion.* 2012;52:1584-1592. Copyright © 2011 American Association of Blood Banks. Reprinted by permission of John Wiley & Sons, Inc.)

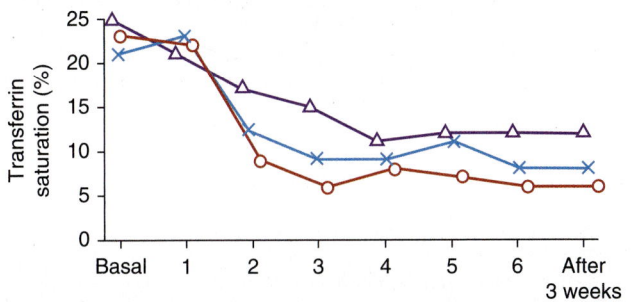

FIGURE 25.11 The impact of endogenous erythropoietin-mediated erythropoiesis or erythropoiesis-stimulating agent (ESA)–mediated erythropoiesis on iron saturation. Patients undergoing autologous blood donation prior to elective orthopedic surgery are shown at baseline and after treatment with placebo or one of two doses of recombinant human erythropoietin (rHuEPO) at each visit during the donation period. All patients received supplemental oral iron. Mean transferrin saturation in 24 patients receiving placebo (△), 300 U/kg rHuEPO (×), or 600 U per rHuEPO (é). (From Mercuriali F, Zanella A, Barosi G, et al. Use of erythropoietin to increase the volume of autologous blood donated by orthopedic patients. *Transfusion.* 1993;33(1):55-60. Copyright © 1993 AABB. Reprinted by permission of John Wiley & Sons, Inc.)

Table 25.8. Potential Role of Hepcidin in Diagnosis and Management of Patients With Iron-Restricted Erythropoiesis

Condition	Expected Hepcidin Levels	Iron Parameters	Iron Therapy Strategies	Potential Hepcidin Therapy
Absolute iron deficiency anemia	Low	Low Tsat and ferritin	PO or IV if poorly tolerated or malabsorbed	No
Functional iron deficiency (ESA therapy, CKD)	Variable, depending on ±CKD	Low Tsat, variable ferritin	IV	Antagonist (if hepcidin levels not low)
Iron sequestration (anemia of inflammation)	High	Low Tsat, normal to elevated ferritin	IV	Antagonist
Mixed anemia (AI/IDA) or (AI/functional iron deficiency)	Variable	Low Tsat, low to normal ferritin	IV[a]	Antagonist (if hepcidin levels not low)

[a]Mixed anemia is a diagnosis of exclusion without a therapeutic trial of iron.
Abbreviations: CKD, chronic kidney disease; ESA, erythropoiesis-stimulating agent; IV, intravenous; PO, oral; Tsat, transferrin saturation.
From Goodnough LT. Iron deficiency syndromes and iron-restricted erythropoiesis. *Transfusion.* 2012;52(7):1584-1592. Copyright © 2011 American Association of Blood Banks. Reprinted by permission of John Wiley & Sons, Inc.

Disorders of Red Blood Cells

dyserythropoietic anemias.[317] Karyorrhexis and nuclear budding are particularly common, but multinuclearity, nuclear fragmentation, and even intranuclear bridging may be observed. The individual erythroblasts appear small and may have scanty cytoplasm, often with irregular, ragged borders. When therapy is given, erythroid hyperplasia initially increases, but as erythropoiesis is restored to normal, the cellularity of the marrow likewise becomes normal.

MANAGEMENT OF IRON DEFICIENCY

Management is primarily focused on repletion of iron stores. Most of the time, this therapy is straightforward, simple, and inexpensive. The response to treatment is predictable and gratifying. There is, however, an important caveat: correction of the iron deficiency is only part of the task confronting the clinician. Particularly in older adults, iron deficiency may be an early sign of a serious illness, such as an occult gastrointestinal malignancy. Clearly, correction of the anemia without recognition and treatment of a possible underlying disease is poorly practiced medicine. The cause of IDA should be and must be identified in the great majority of cases.

Iron can be administered orally or intravenously. The oral route is the least expensive. Importantly, therapeutic doses are quite different for oral and IV preparations. Most iron-deficient patients respond well to oral therapy, but IV administration of iron may sometimes be required. A treatment algorithm is illustrated in *Figure 25.12*.[318]

Oral Iron Therapy

The most common preparation used orally is ferrous sulfate, which has been a mainstay of treatment for iron deficiency since it was first introduced by the French physician Pierre Blaud in the 19th century. In addition to ferrous sulfate, there are a number of other oral iron preparations, including ferrous gluconate and ferrous fumarate. There

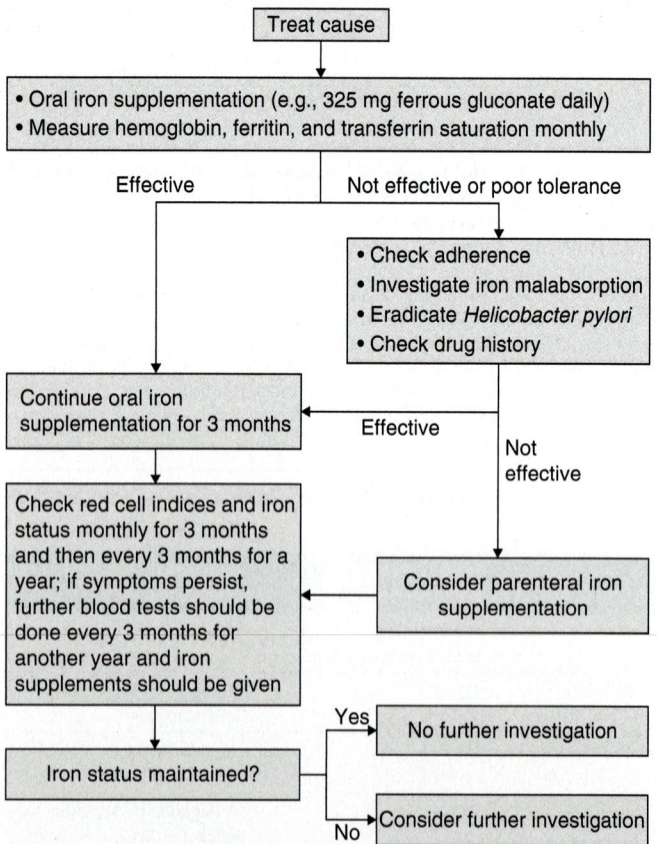

FIGURE 25.12 **Algorithm for treatment of iron deficiency.** ESA, erythropoiesis-stimulating agent. (Reprinted from Lopez A, Cacoub P, Macdougall IC, et al. Iron deficiency anemia. *Lancet.* 2016;387(10021):907-916. Copyright © 2016 Elsevier. With permission.)

are no data to suggest superiority of one preparation over another, and most are inexpensive. Although iron deficiency clearly promotes increased absorption, individual variations are great and absorption may be vastly different at varying degrees of anemia and in the presence of complicating illnesses.[319,320]

Recent evidence suggests that alternate-day dosing is at least as effective and may be more effective than daily or more frequent dosing and results in fewer adverse effects. A typical regimen would be one ferrous sulfate tablet every other day; each 325 mg tablet contains 65 mg elemental iron. Iron is absorbed more when the stomach is empty; when iron ingestion occurs after or with a meal, absorption decreases substantially.[321] However, since gastrointestinal irritation is common when the stomach is empty, patients are frequently advised to take oral iron immediately after or even with a meal. The gain in patient acceptance may be more important than the reduced absorption of iron. However, it is important to remember that absorption is enhanced by the presence of orange juice, meat, poultry, and fish, whereas other substances such as cereals, tea, and milk inhibit it. This is particularly important in toddlers, because administration of oral iron with milk often compromises therapy.

For iron-deficient children, the optimal dosage is 3 mg elemental iron per kilogram of body weight given orally once daily. Palatable elixirs and syrups are the most satisfactory pediatric preparations, although they can stain the teeth if not given carefully. Children usually tolerate this form of therapy on an empty stomach.

Absorption of oral iron can be enhanced with ascorbate by at least 30%, because it prevents formation of insoluble and unabsorbable compounds and reduces ferric iron to ferrous iron. Iron absorption and release from stores may be impaired due to high hepcidin levels from diminished clearance by the kidneys, not completely corrected by routine hemodialysis, as well as from inflammation.

Ferric citrate, an oral iron-containing phosphate binder, is proving to be an effective iron supplement in patients with CKD. In addition to decreasing serum phosphate, ferric citrate was shown to increase hemoglobin, serum ferritin, and Tsat and reduce the use of IV iron and ESA in patients on hemodialysis and in non-dialysis-dependent CKD.[322] The effectiveness may, at least in part, be related to the ability to administer very large doses of iron without gastrointestinal irritation. The mechanism of ferric citrate absorption in the gut remains to be demonstrated.

Another ferric iron preparation, ferric maltol, was reported to have improved tolerance in patients with previous intolerance to other oral iron formulations.[323]

Regardless of the form of oral therapy used, treatment should be continued for at least 1 month after the anemia is relieved to replete iron stores.

Side Effects of Oral Iron Therapy

Some patients given oral iron report gastrointestinal symptoms, including heartburn, nausea, abdominal cramps, and diarrhea. In one double-blind study, ferrous sulfate, ferrous gluconate, ferrous fumarate, and placebo were administered in identically appearing tablets.[324] No significant differences were found among the three iron salts. Approximately 12% of subjects had symptoms that could reasonably be ascribed to iron ingestion. Often, tolerance of iron salts improves when a small dose is given at first and increased over the course of several days to the full dose.

Enteric-coated preparations are designed to reduce side effects by retarding dissolution of the iron. However, this effect may markedly decrease absorption, especially in achlorhydric individuals, whose gastric juice cannot dissolve the coating. Sustained-release preparations also reduce side effects by retarding dissolution, but in so doing, the most actively absorbing regions of the intestine are bypassed and absorption is therefore reduced.[325]

Failure of Oral Iron Therapy

Clinicians often encounter patients said to have IDA unresponsive to oral therapy. The most common explanations for failure to respond to oral iron include (1) incorrect diagnosis, (2) complicating illness, (3) medication nonadherence, (4) inadequate prescription (dose or form), (5) continuing iron loss in excess of intake, and (6) malabsorption of iron.

In managing a problem of alleged failure to respond to iron, it is important to review the data on which the diagnosis of IDA was based and to take note of any laboratory procedures that might have yielded erroneous information. At times, even though iron deficiency is present, a coexisting cause for anemia may impair response. Examples are iron deficiency as a complication of the anemia of inflammation in rheumatoid arthritis, chronic gastrointestinal blood loss such as *H. pylori* infection, as well as so-called dimorphic anemia, in which iron deficiency and pernicious anemia coexist.

In some patients, ongoing RBC losses exceed the capacity of oral iron therapy to effectively treat iron deficiency. If this situation is not correctable (e.g., in the case of hereditary hemorrhagic telangiectasia), parenteral iron therapy must be given. Finally, some patients may be unable to tolerate or absorb oral iron. Patients with IRIDA have a mutation in the protease TMPRSS6 causing increased hepcidin production[152-154] and are refractory to oral iron therapy but partially responsive to IV iron therapy.

In individuals who are compliant with oral therapy and not actively bleeding, but still poorly responsive to treatment, addition of ascorbic acid (usually 500 mg twice a day) may improve iron absorption and the hemoglobin response.[326,327] Subclinical ascorbic acid deficiency has been suggested as an etiology of refractory IDA.[328]

Even under the best of circumstances, oral iron supplementation is poorly tolerated and patients may be nonadherent, not only from side effects of oral iron but because of their diagnosis or the therapy they are undergoing for their disease. Nevertheless, in stable patients with mild to moderate anemia in which there is some time for management strategies, and particularly in those patients in whom diagnostic laboratory testing has not definitively ruled out iron-restricted erythropoiesis, a therapeutic trial of oral or parenteral iron therapy can be recommended.[329] In general, absorption of oral iron inversely correlates with hepcidin levels.[330] Thus, hepcidin measurements may help to determine a priori which patients are good candidates for oral iron therapy.[312] Exceptions may be patients who malabsorb iron because of damage to the intestinal lining such as in celiac disease and in patients undergoing treatment with proton-pump inhibitors.

In a study of patients with anemia,[302] 5 of 54 who had bone marrow examinations had absent iron stores indicating absolute iron deficiency. There were an additional eight patients who were categorized as iron deficient because of their response to oral iron therapy; half of these had serum ferritins ≥12 ng/mL and one of the patients had a serum ferritin >100 ng/mL. This analysis suggests that, in the absence of a diagnostic bone marrow examination, it is difficult to confidently rule out iron deficiency and an empiric trial of oral iron therapy over 14 days duration[331] is desirable in order to identify patients who have absolute iron deficiency. Subsequent management would include evaluating patients for serious underlying illness, including malignancy.[205]

Failure to respond to a trial of oral iron therapy does not rule out iron-restricted erythropoiesis or even true iron deficiency in the setting of inflammation, as inflammatory hepcidin elevation would cause impaired iron absorption.[26] Furthermore, ongoing blood (and iron) losses may exceed even maximal gastrointestinal absorption of iron.[332] Clinical situations are often complex, and blood loss, iron-restricted erythropoiesis, and high hepcidin levels can coexist in patients in whom absorption of dietary iron or oral iron supplements is impaired. In these instances and in circumstances of ongoing blood loss,[332] IV iron therapy may be needed either as a diagnostic trial or as definitive therapy.[333]

Intravenous Iron Therapy

IV iron administration is recommended in renal dialysis patients undergoing ESA therapy.[334] Patients treated with IV iron (100 mg twice weekly) achieved a 46% reduction in ESA dosage required to maintain hematocrit (Hct) levels between 30% and 34%, compared with patients supplemented with oral iron.[335] To further address the management of iron-restricted erythropoiesis in patients with CKD

undergoing dialysis, a randomized controlled trial evaluated the efficacy of IV iron supplementation in patients with ferritin between 500 and 1200 ng/mL.[336] The administration of IV iron (and increasing the dose of ESA by 25%) resulted in a greater correction of anemia compared with increasing the dose of ESA alone. After the end of the trial, there was greater success in reducing the dose of ESA in the patients receiving IV iron, compared with the non-iron-treated arm.

IV iron therapy also improves responses to ESA therapy in patients with inflammatory bowel disease[337] compared with responses in a similar patient group who receive oral iron supplementation.[338] Decreased CHr is an indicator of functional iron deficiency in the face of increased iron demand stimulated by ESA therapy.[307] The requirement for a kinetic balance between iron delivery and level of erythropoietin stimulation may explain the need for IV iron supplemental therapy in ESA-treated patients, even those with replete iron stores.[334] The clinical response to the combination of IV iron and ESA therapy may be attributed to the ability of the parenteral route to circumvent the inflammation-induced block to intestinal iron absorption and deliver a large dose of iron to the reticuloendothelial system, which could increase iron efflux from macrophages, perhaps by increasing the translation of ferroportin mRNA.

Currently approved intravenous iron preparations are listed in *Table 25.9*.[339] The risk-benefit profile of IV iron continues to undergo evaluation in renal dialysis patients,[334,340] as well as in patients with anemia of chronic diseases.[128] IV iron can allow up to a 5-fold greater erythropoietic response to significant blood loss anemia in normal individuals.[341] One potential limitation to IV iron therapy may be that much of the administered iron ends up in the reticuloendothelial system as storage iron, from where it may not be readily available for erythropoiesis, particularly if hepcidin concentrations are elevated. However, in patients with iron deficiency, 50% of IV iron was incorporated into hemoglobin within 3 to 4 weeks.[342] For patients with anemia of chronic disease or renal failure, IV iron is mobilized less rapidly from the reticuloendothelial system.[343] Nevertheless, when IV iron was given to patients with the anemia of rheumatoid arthritis, cellular hemoglobin concentrations increased significantly.[344] In a systemic review and meta-analysis of 15 randomized trials of oral versus IV iron therapy in postpartum patients with IDA, Hb concentrations were almost 1 g/dL higher after 6 weeks in women who received IV iron.[345]

In patients with malignancy and chemotherapy-induced anemia, a number of trials have studied IV iron in the setting of therapy with ESAs. In one study[346] of patients undergoing chemotherapy, 155 patients were treated with ESA and randomized to receive no iron, oral iron as 325 mg of ferrous sulfate twice daily, 100-mg boluses of IV iron dextran weekly until the total calculated iron deficit was administered, or a single dose of IV iron dextran to the same calculated dose. There were significant improvements in hemoglobin levels and hematopoietic responses in both patient groups treated with IV iron, compared with those receiving oral iron or no iron therapy.

Another study[347] assigned 189 patients to receive ESA weekly plus no iron, oral iron as 325 mg of ferrous sulfate thrice daily, or IV ferrous gluconate as 125 mg weekly boluses. The cohort treated with IV iron had improved hemoglobin and hematopoietic responses compared with the other cohorts. A third study[348] randomly assigned 67 patients with lymphoproliferative malignancies not receiving chemotherapy with IV or no iron. Again, IV iron resulted in improved hemoglobin and hematopoietic responses. A fourth study of 398 patients with chemotherapy-induced anemia who were treated with ESA therapy found significant improvement in hemoglobin levels and hematopoietic responses in the patient cohort treated with IV iron,[349] further confirmed by a fifth study.[350]

Iron-restricted erythropoiesis has been shown to be a consideration at time of cancer diagnosis even before ESA therapy: 17% of carefully screened patients were found to have serum ferritins <100 ng/mL and 59% had Tsat less than 20% at diagnosis.[351] In addition, renewed attention has been placed on the dose-response relationship between ESA dosage and red cell production responses in ESA-treated patients. Once ESA therapy is administered, even subjects with normal baseline levels develop Tsat and ferritin decreases to levels

Table 25.9. Currently Available Intravenous Iron Preparations

Generic Name	Iron Dextran, Low Molecular Weight	Ferric Gluconate	Iron Sucrose	Ferumoxytol	Ferric Carboxymaltose	Ferric Derisomaltose
Trade Name	INFeD (US) CosmoFer (UK)	Ferrlecit	Venofer	Feraheme	Injectafer (US) Ferinject (UK)	Monofer
Carbohydrate	Low-molecular-weight dextran	Gluconate	Sucrose	Carboxymethyl dextran	Carboxymaltose	Isomaltoside 1000
Molecular weight measured by manufacturer (Da)	165,000	289,000-440,000	34,000-60,000	750,000	150,000	150,000
Total-dose or >500-mg infusion	Yes	No	No	Yes	Yes	Yes
Premedication	TDI only	No	No	No	No	No
Test dose required	Yes	No	No	No	No	No
Iron concentration (mg/mL)	50	12.5	20	30	50	100
Vial volume (mL)	2	5	5	17	2 or 10	1, 2, 5, or 10
Black box warning	Yes	No	No	Yes	No	No
Preservative	None	Benzyl alcohol	None	None	None	None

Ferric gluconate and iron sucrose are also referred to as iron salts.
Abbreviation: TDI, total dose infusion.
Adapted with permission from Goodnough LT, Shander A. Current status of pharmacologic therapies in patient blood management. *Anesth Analg.* 2013;116(1):15-34. Copyright © 2013 International Anesthesia Research Society.

indicating iron-restricted erythropoiesis.[304] Accordingly, guidelines by the National Comprehensive Cancer Network have recommended that iron studies be obtained at baseline to identify patients who are candidates for supplemental iron therapy and that if subsequent hemoglobin levels after 4 weeks of ESA therapy indicate no response (<1 g/dL increase in hemoglobin), then IV iron supplemental therapy should be considered, along with an increase in ESA dose.[352]

On the one hand, the hypoferremia and anemia of inflammation can be viewed as a mechanism of defense against providing iron to unwanted pathogens, and therefore adaptive. On the other hand, others are not convinced that iron deficiency or iron-restrictive anemia should be regarded as a desirable condition that benefits patients with infection or inflammation. Although more evidence is clearly needed, in patients who show symptoms attributable to moderate or severe anemia of inflammation, and who do not suffer from overwhelming or difficult-to-control infection, iron-restricted erythropoiesis can and should be treated, an argument that is not new.[353] In iron-restricted anemias other than absolute iron deficiency, the optimal treatment is still evolving and may be improved by the ongoing development of hepcidin-targeted therapies.[354]

Important clinical subjects for further study in this area should include improving the diagnosis of various forms of iron-restricted anemia in complex clinical settings, testing optimal combinations of ESA and IV iron treatments, analysis of the relative risk-benefits of ESA and IV iron therapy, and the appropriate use of adjuncts such as anti-inflammatory therapy or frequent dialysis. Basic scientific insights that could facilitate the progress in this area include understanding the molecular nature of the erythropoietic iron regulator and suppressor of hepcidin, details of the mechanisms by which circulating and stored iron regulates hepcidin, the contribution of hepcidin-independent mechanisms to anemia of inflammation, and the role of genetics in sporadic iron deficiency.

Side Effects of Parenteral Iron Therapy

Side effects may be local or systemic. With IV injection, rates of administration greater than 100 mg/min are associated with pain in the vein injected, flushing, and a metallic taste.[355] Such reactions are brief in duration and relieved immediately by slowing the injection. Systemic reactions may be either immediate or delayed. Immediate side effects include hypotension, headache, malaise, urticaria, nausea, and rare anaphylactoid reactions.[356,357] Delayed reactions include lymphadenopathy, myalgia, arthralgia, and fever. Most of the reactions are mild and transient, but the anaphylactoid reactions due to some iron dextran preparations may be life-threatening,[355] although high-molecular-weight iron dextran, which was associated with most severe adverse reactions, is no longer commercially available.[358] For iron dextran therapy, the clinician should be prepared for the possibility of anaphylaxis by having epinephrine, oxygen, and facilities for resuscitation available. Sodium ferric gluconate, iron sucrose, and iron saccharate are much better tolerated than iron-dextran formulas, as long as the recommended dosages are not exceeded.[140,333,359] Long-term effects of the IV iron preparations, including phosphorus homeostasis, will require careful study in relevant clinical settings.[360]

Response to Therapy

When specific iron therapy is given, patients often show rapid subjective improvement, with disappearance or marked diminution of fatigue, lassitude, and other nonspecific symptoms. This response may occur before any improvement in anemia is observed. For example, pica has been reported to be relieved within 1 week of therapy.[290]

The earliest hematologic evidence of response to treatment is an increase in the percentage of reticulocytes and their hemoglobin content. The reticulocytes attain a maximal value on the fifth to tenth day after institution of therapy and thereafter gradually return to normal. The maximal value usually ranges from 5% to 10% and is inversely related to the level of hemoglobin. The reticulocyte response may not be detectable in mild IDA.

The blood hemoglobin level is the most accurate measure of the degree of anemia in iron deficiency. During the response to therapy, the red cell count may increase temporarily to normal range, but the hemoglobin value lags behind. The red cell indices may remain abnormal for some time after the normal hemoglobin level is restored. As recovery occurs, a normocytic cell population gradually replaces the microcytic cell population, and one of the early signs of response to therapy is an increase in the RDW from pretreatment levels. When treatment is fully effective, hemoglobin reaches normal levels by 2 months after therapy is initiated.

Of the epithelial lesions in iron deficiency, those affecting the tongue and nails are the most responsive to treatment. After 1 to 2 weeks, small regenerating filiform papillae are observed. After 3 months, the tongue has usually returned to normal; however, in patients with severe anemia, some atrophy may persist. Koilonychia usually disappears in 3 to 6 months, with the concavity moving toward the end of the nail as the nail grows. Gastritis and the associated defects in gastric secretion often do not respond to therapy, especially in older adults. In patients younger than 30 years, gastric acid secretion and normal epithelial architecture may be restored.[190]

Dysphagia may be relieved by iron therapy if the associated post-cricoid webs are small or medium sized.[280] The webs themselves are not altered, however, and relapse of the anemia is associated with recurring dysphagia. With more severe lesions, dilatation of the esophagus is required for relief.

Relapse occurs in a significant fraction of patients who respond to iron treatment, in part because of nonadherence with the full course of therapy and in part because of recurrence (or continuation) of the predisposing condition or illness.

Preventive Treatment

Certain people are at such high risk for developing iron deficiency that prophylactic measures may be considered. These include infants, pregnant women, regular blood donors, and women with menorrhagia. Iron supplementation has been recommended for pregnant women for almost half a century. However, the advantages of iron supplementation in pregnant women without a diagnosis of iron deficiency have not been definitively established,[361,362] and the USPSTF determined that there was insufficient evidence to clarify the benefits and harms of routine iron supplementation for pregnant women.[363]

The American Academy of Pediatrics made recommendations for iron supplementation in infants.[187,246] They recommend that exclusively or partially breast-fed infants receive supplemental iron at 1 mg/kg/d until appropriate iron-containing foods are introduced to the diet. Formula-fed infants should be given formula supplemented with 12 mg/L of iron through the first year of life. Iron-fortified cereal should be given at the time that a solid diet is begun.

Acute Iron Intoxication

The accidental ingestion of iron compounds by children who have mistaken the tablets for candy is a worrisome problem, particularly with toddlers whose mothers are taking iron-containing prenatal vitamin supplements.[364] A few such cases have also been reported in adults.[365] Those persons who died had swallowed 3 to 10 g or more.

Symptoms of iron intoxication have been classified in four stages. In stage 1, gastrointestinal symptoms predominate (vomiting, diarrhea, and melena). Shock may ensue, followed by dyspnea, lethargy, and coma. These events occur in the first 6 hours after ingestion. In stage 2, lasting from 6 to 24 hours after ingestion, transient improvement occurs and may continue to recovery. In stage 3, metabolic acidosis is present. Death may take place 12 to 48 hours after ingestion. Stage 4 consists of intestinal obstruction as a late complication caused by scarring of the intestine.

These ill effects are the consequence of the local irritative action of the iron, resulting in mucosal ulceration and bleeding. Capillary dilatation and diapedesis of red cells may occur. Many factors cause the shock, including the absorption of iron in amounts far above the binding capacity of the plasma. Serum iron values as high as 3000 µg/dL have been observed. Late coma is the result of hypoxia, metabolic disturbances, and hepatic damage.

The introduction of deferoxamine as a therapeutic agent has greatly modified the outlook.[366] In the setting of acute iron poisoning, this hexadentate chelator, which has a high specific affinity for iron, can be given orally and intravenously. The molecular complex is small and is excreted quickly by the kidneys. Nonetheless, it is prudent to manage iron poisoning in consultation with an experienced toxicologist.

ACKNOWLEDGMENTS

Portions of this chapter were adapted from previous editions written by G. Richard Lee and Nancy Andrews.

References

1. WHO, CDC. *Assessing the Iron Status of Populations: Including Literature Reviews. Report of a Joint World Health Organization/Centers for Disease Control and Prevention Technical Consultation on the Assessment of Iron Status at the Population Level, Geneva, Switzerland.* World Health Organization/Centers for Disease Control and Prevention; 2007. 6-8 April 2004.
2. Witte DL, Angstadt DS, Davis SH, Schrantz RD. Predicting bone marrow iron stores in anemic patients in a community hospital using ferritin and erythrocyte sedimentation rate. *Am J Clin Pathol.* 1988;90(1):85-87.
3. World Health Organization. *Global Nutrition Targets 2025: Anaemia Policy Brief.* World Health Organization; 2014. WHO/NMH/NHD/14.4.
4. Yip R, Parvanta I, Cogswell ME, et al. Recommendations to prevent and control iron deficiency in the United States. *MMWR Morb Mortal Wkly Rep.* 1998;47:1-29.
5. Green R, Charlton R, Seftel H, et al. Body iron excretion in man: a collaborative study. *Am J Med.* 1968;45(3):336-353. (In eng).
6. Brune M, Magnusson B, Persson H, Hallberg L. Iron losses in sweat. *Am J Clin Nutr.* 1986;43(3):438-443. (In eng).
7. Hallberg L, Rossander-Hulten L. Iron requirements in menstruating women. *Am J Clin Nutr.* 1991;54(6):1047-1058. (In eng).
8. Hurrell R, Egli I. Iron bioavailability and dietary reference values. *Am J Clin Nutr.* 2010;91(5):1461s-1467s. (In eng). doi: 10.3945/ajcn.2010.28674F
9. Raffin SB, Woo CH, Roost KT, Price DC, Schmid R. Intestinal absorption of hemoglobin iron-heme cleavage by mucosal heme oxygenase. *J Clin Invest.* 1974;54(6):1344-1352. (In eng). doi: 10.1172/jci107881
10. Fiorito V, Forni M, Silengo L, Altruda F, Tolosano E. Crucial role of FLVCR1a in the maintenance of intestinal heme homeostasis. *Antioxidants Redox Signal.* 2015;23(18):1410-1423. (In eng). doi: 10.1089/ars.2014.6216
11. Lopez MA, Martos FC. Iron availability: an updated review. *Int J Food Sci Nutr.* 2004;55(8):597-606. (In eng). doi: 10.1080/09637480500085820
12. Gunshin H, Mackenzie B, Berger UV, et al. Cloning and characterization of a mammalian proton-coupled metal-ion transporter. *Nature.* 1997;388(6641):482-488. (In eng). doi: 10.1038/41343
13. Illing AC, Shawki A, Cunningham CL, Mackenzie B. Substrate profile and metal-ion selectivity of human divalent metal-ion transporter-1. *J Biol Chem.* 2012 (In eng). doi: 10.1074/jbc.M112.364208
14. Mackenzie B, Ujwal ML, Chang MH, Romero MF, Hediger MA. Divalent metal-ion transporter DMT1 mediates both H+-coupled Fe2+ transport and uncoupled fluxes. *Pflügers Archiv* 2006;451(4):544-558. (In eng). doi: 10.1007/s00424-005-1494-3
15. Shawki A, Engevik MA, Kim RS, et al. Intestinal brush-border Na+/H+ exchanger-3 drives H+-coupled iron absorption in the mouse. *Am J Physiol Gastrointest Liver Physiol.* 311(3):G423-G430. 2016:ajpgi.00167.2016. (In eng). doi: 10.1152/ajpgi.00167.2016
16. McKie AT. The role of Dcytb in iron metabolism: an update. *Biochem Soc Trans.* 2008;36(pt 6):1239-1241. (In eng). doi: 10.1042/bst0361239
17. Sheehan RG, Frenkel EP. The control of iron absorption by the gastrointestinal mucosal cell. *J Clin Invest* 1972;51(2):224-231. (In eng). doi: 10.1172/jci106807
18. Potten CS, Loeffler M. Stem cells: attributes, cycles, spirals, pitfalls and uncertainties. Lessons for and from the crypt. *Development.* 1990;110(4):1001-1020. (In eng).
19. Donovan A, Brownlie A, Zhou Y, et al. Positional cloning of zebrafish ferroportin1 identifies a conserved vertebrate iron exporter. *Nature.* 2000;403(6771):776-781. (In eng). doi: 10.1038/35001596
20. Donovan A, Lima CA, Pinkus JL, et al. The iron exporter ferroportin/Slc40a1 is essential for iron homeostasis. *Cell Metabol.* 2005;1(3):191-200. (In eng). doi: 10.1016/j.cmet.2005.01.003
21. Fuqua BK, Lu Y, Darshan D, et al. The multicopper ferroxidase hephaestin enhances intestinal iron absorption in mice. *PLoS One.* 2014;9(6):e98792. (In eng). doi: 10.1371/journal.pone.0098792
22. Cherukuri S, Potla R, Sarkar J, Nurko S, Harris ZL, Fox PL. Unexpected role of ceruloplasmin in intestinal iron absorption. *Cell Metabol.* 2005;2(5):309-319. (In eng). doi: 10.1016/j.cmet.2005.10.003
23. Finch C. Regulators of iron balance in humans. *Blood.* 1994;84(6):1697-1702.
24. Krause A, Neitz S, Magert HJ, et al. LEAP-1, a novel highly disulfide-bonded human peptide, exhibits antimicrobial activity. *FEBS Lett.* 2000;480(2-3):147-150. (In eng).
25. Park CH, Valore EV, Waring AJ, Ganz T. Hepcidin, a urinary antimicrobial peptide synthesized in the liver. *J Biol Chem.* 2001;276(11):7806-7810. (In eng). doi: 10.1074/jbc.M008922200
26. Ganz T, Nemeth E. Hepcidin and disorders of iron metabolism. *Annu Rev Med.* 2011;62:347-360. (In eng). doi: 10.1146/annurev-med-050109-142444
27. Roetto A, Papanikolaou G, Politou M, et al. Mutant antimicrobial peptide hepcidin is associated with severe juvenile hemochromatosis. *Nat Genet.* 2003;33(1):21-22. (In eng). doi: 10.1038/ng1053
28. Viatte L, Lesbordes-Brion JC, Lou DQ, et al. Deregulation of proteins involved in iron metabolism in hepcidin-deficient mice. *Blood.* 2005;105(12):4861-4864. (In eng). doi: 10.1182/blood-2004-12-4608
29. Nicolas G, Bennoun M, Porteu A, et al. Severe iron deficiency anemia in transgenic mice expressing liver hepcidin. *Proc Natl Acad Sci U S A.* 2002;99(7):4596-4601. (In eng). doi: 10.1073/pnas.072632499

30. Rivera S, Nemeth E, Gabayan V, Lopez MA, Farshidi D, Ganz T. Synthetic hepcidin causes rapid dose-dependent hypoferremia and is concentrated in ferroportin-containing organs. *Blood*. 2005;106(6):2196-2199. (In eng). doi: 10.1182/blood-2005-04-1766
31. Nemeth E, Tuttle MS, Powelson J, et al. Hepcidin regulates cellular iron efflux by binding to ferroportin and inducing its internalization. *Science*. 2004;306(5704):2090-2093. (In eng). doi: 10.1126/science.1104742
32. Aschemeyer S, Qiao B, Stefanova D, et al. Structure-function analysis of ferroportin defines the binding site and an alternative mechanism of action of hepcidin. *Blood*. 2018;131(8):899-910. doi: 10.1182/blood-2017-05-786590
33. Lin L, Valore EV, Nemeth E, Goodnough JB, Gabayan V, Ganz T. Iron transferrin regulates hepcidin synthesis in primary hepatocyte culture through hemojuvelin and BMP2/4. *Blood*. 2007;110(6):2182-2189. (In eng). doi: 10.1182/blood-2007-04-087593. blood-2007-04-087593 [pii].
34. Steinbicker AU, Bartnikas TB, Lohmeyer LK, et al. Perturbation of hepcidin expression by BMP type I receptor deletion induces iron overload in mice. *Blood*. 2011;118(15):4224-4230. (In eng). doi: 10.1182/blood-2011-03-339952
35. Xia Y, Babitt JL, Sidis Y, Chung RT, Lin HY. Hemojuvelin regulates hepcidin expression via a selective subset of BMP ligands and receptors independently of neogenin. *Blood* 2008;111(10):5195-5204. (In eng). doi: 10.1182/blood-2007-09-111567
36. Andriopoulos B, Jr, Corradini E, Xia Y, et al. BMP6 is a key endogenous regulator of hepcidin expression and iron metabolism. *Nat Genet*. 2009;41(4):482-487. (In eng). doi: 10.1038/ng.335
37. Meynard D, Kautz L, Darnaud V, Canonne-Hergaux F, Coppin H, Roth MP. Lack of the bone morphogenetic protein BMP6 induces massive iron overload. *Nat Genet*. 2009;41(4):478-481. (In eng). doi: 10.1038/ng.320
38. Canali S, Wang CY, Zumbrennen-Bullough KB, Bayer A, Babitt JL. Bone morphogenetic protein 2 controls iron homeostasis in mice independent of Bmp6. *Am J Hematol*. 2017;92(11):1204-1213. doi: 10.1002/ajh.24888
39. Fisher AL, Babitt JL. Coordination of iron homeostasis by bone morphogenetic proteins: current understanding and unanswered questions. *Dev Dyn*. 2021;251(1):26-46. doi: 10.1002/dvdy.372
40. Ramos E, Kautz L, Rodriguez R, et al. Evidence for distinct pathways of hepcidin regulation by acute and chronic iron loading in mice. *Hepatology*. 2011;53(4):1333-1341. (In eng). doi: 10.1002/hep.24178
41. Papanikolaou G, Samuels ME, Ludwig EH, et al. Mutations in HFE2 cause iron overload in chromosome 1q-linked juvenile hemochromatosis. *Nat Genet*. 2004;36(1):77-82. (In eng). doi: 10.1038/ng1274
42. Daher R, Kannengiesser C, Houamel D, et al. Heterozygous mutations in BMP6 pro-peptide lead to inappropriate hepcidin synthesis and moderate iron overload in humans. *Gastroenterology*. 2016;150(3):672-683.e4. (In eng). doi: 10.1053/j.gastro.2015.10.049
43. Schmidt PJ, Toran PT, Giannetti AM, Bjorkman PJ, Andrews NC. The transferrin receptor modulates Hfe-dependent regulation of hepcidin expression. *Cell Metabol*. 2008;7(3):205-214. (In eng). doi: 10.1016/j.cmet.2007.11.016
44. Gao J, Chen J, Kramer M, Tsukamoto H, Zhang AS, Enns CA. Interaction of the hereditary hemochromatosis protein HFE with transferrin receptor 2 is required for transferrin-induced hepcidin expression. *Cell Metabol*. 2009;9(3):217-227. (In eng). doi: 10.1016/j.cmet.2009.01.010
45. Johnson MB, Enns CA. Diferric transferrin regulates transferrin receptor 2 protein stability. *Blood*. 2004;104(13):4287-4293. (In eng). doi: 10.1182/blood-2004-06-2477
46. Schmidt PJ, Fleming MD. Transgenic HFE-dependent induction of hepcidin in mice does not require transferrin receptor-2. *Am J Hematol* 2012;87(6):588-595. (In eng). doi: 10.1002/ajh.23173
47. Wu XG, Wang Y, Wu Q, et al. HFE interacts with the BMP type I receptor ALK3 to regulate hepcidin expression. *Blood*. 2014;124(8):1335-1343. (In eng). doi: 10.1182/blood-2014-01-552281
48. Lee DH, Zhou LJ, Zhou Z, et al. Neogenin inhibits HJV secretion and regulates BMP-induced hepcidin expression and iron homeostasis. *Blood*. 2010;115(15):3136-3145. (In eng). doi: 10.1182/blood-2009-11-251199
49. Silvestri L, Pagani A, Nai A, De Domenico I, Kaplan J, Camaschella C. The serine protease matriptase-2 (TMPRSS6) inhibits hepcidin activation by cleaving membrane hemojuvelin. *Cell Metab*. 2008;8(6):502-511. doi: 10.1016/j.cmet.2008.09.012
50. Zhang AS, Anderson SA, Wang J, et al. Suppression of hepatic hepcidin expression in response to acute iron deprivation is associated with an increase of matriptase-2 protein. *Blood*. 2011;117(5):1687-1699. (In eng). doi: 10.1182/blood-2010-06-287292
51. Zhao N, Nizzi CP, Anderson SA, et al. Low intracellular iron increases the stability of matriptase-2. *J Biol Chem*. 2015;290(7):4432-4446. (In eng). doi: 10.1074/jbc.M114.611913
52. Enns CA, Ahmed R, Wang J, et al. Increased iron loading induces Bmp6 expression in the non-parenchymal cells of the liver independent of the BMP-signaling pathway. *PLoS One*. 2013;8(4):e60534. (In eng). doi: 10.1371/journal.pone.0060534
53. Rausa M, Pagani A, Nai A, et al. Bmp6 expression in murine liver non parenchymal cells: a mechanism to control their high iron exporter activity and protect hepatocytes from iron overload? *PLoS One*. 2015;10(4):e0122696, doi: 10.1371/journal.pone.0122696
54. Kautz L, Meynard D, Monnier A, et al. Iron regulates phosphorylation of Smad1/5/8 and gene expression of Bmp6, Smad7, Id1, and Atoh8 in the mouse liver. *Blood*. 2008;112(4):1503-1509. (In eng). doi: 10.1182/blood-2008-03-143354
55. Camaschella C, Nai A, Silvestri L. Iron metabolism and iron disorders revisited in the hepcidin era. *Haematologica*. 2020;105(2):260-272. doi: 10.3324/haematol.2019.232124
56. Nicolas G, Chauvet C, Viatte L, et al. The gene encoding the iron regulatory peptide hepcidin is regulated by anemia, hypoxia, and inflammation. *J Clin Invest*. 2002;110(7):1037-1044. (In eng). doi: 10.1172/jci15686
57. Pak M, Lopez MA, Gabayan V, Ganz T, Rivera S. Suppression of hepcidin during anemia requires erythropoietic activity. *Blood*. 2006;108(12):3730-3735. (In eng). doi: 10.1182/blood-2006-06-028787
58. Ashby DR, Gale DP, Busbridge M, et al. Erythropoietin administration in humans causes a marked and prolonged reduction in circulating hepcidin. *Haematologica*. 2010;95(3):505-508. (In eng). doi: 10.3324/haematol.2009.013136
59. Ganz T, Olbina G, Girelli D, Nemeth E, Westerman M. Immunoassay for human serum hepcidin. *Blood*. 2008;112(10):4292-4297.
60. Kautz L, Nemeth E. Molecular liaisons between erythropoiesis and iron metabolism. *Blood*. 2014;124(4):479-482, doi: 10.1182/blood-2014-05-516252
61. Srole DN, Ganz T. Erythroferrone structure, function, and physiology: iron homeostasis and beyond. *J Cell Physiol*. 2021;236(7):4888-4901. doi: 10.1002/jcp.30247
62. Kautz L, Jung G, Valore EV, Rivella S, Nemeth E, Ganz T. Identification of erythroferrone as an erythroid regulator of iron metabolism. *Nat Genet*. 2014;46(7):678-684. doi: 10.1038/ng.2996
63. Arezes J, Foy N, McHugh K, et al. Erythroferrone inhibits the induction of hepcidin by BMP6. *Blood*. 2018;132(14):1473-1477. doi: 10.1182/blood-2018-06-857995
64. Arezes J, Foy NJ, McHugh K, et al. Antibodies against the erythroferrone N-terminal domain prevent hepcidin suppression and ameliorate murine thalassemia. *Blood*. 2020;135(8):547-557. doi: 10.1182/blood.2019003140
65. Wang CY, Xu Y, Traeger L, et al. Erythroferrone lowers hepcidin by sequestering BMP2/6 heterodimer from binding to the BMP type I receptor ALK3. *Blood*. 2020;135(6):453-456. doi: 10.1182/blood.2019002620
66. Kautz L, Jung G, Nemeth E, Ganz T. Erythroferrone contributes to recovery from anemia of inflammation. *Blood*. 2014;124(16):2569-2574. (In eng). doi: 10.1182/blood-2014-06-584607
67. Coffey R, Sardo U, Kautz L, Gabayan V, Nemeth E, Ganz T. Erythroferrone is not required for the glucoregulatory and hematologic effects of chronic erythropoietin treatment in mice. *Physiol Rep*. 2018;6(19):e13890. doi: 10.14814/phy2.13890
68. Origa R, Galanello R, Ganz T, et al. Liver iron concentrations and urinary hepcidin in beta-thalassemia. *Haematologica*. 2007;92(5):583-588.
69. Kearney SL, Nemeth E, Neufeld EJ, et al. Urinary hepcidin in congenital chronic anemias. *Pediatr Blood Cancer*. 2007;48(1):57-63. (In eng). doi: 10.1002/pbc.20616
70. Jones E, Pasricha SR, Allen A, et al. Hepcidin is suppressed by erythropoiesis in hemoglobin E beta-thalassemia and beta-thalassemia trait. *Blood*. 2015;125(5):873-880. (In eng). doi: 10.1182/blood-2014-10-606491
71. Kautz L, Jung G, Du X, et al. Erythroferrone contributes to hepcidin suppression and iron overload in a mouse model of beta-thalassemia. *Blood*. 2015;126(17):2031-2037. doi: 10.1182/blood-2015-07-658419
72. Ganz T, Jung G, Naeim A, et al. Immunoassay for human serum erythroferrone. *Blood*. 2017;130(10):1243-1246. doi: 10.1182/blood-2017-04-777987
73. Mangaonkar AA, Thawer F, Son J, et al. Regulation of iron homeostasis through the erythroferrone-hepcidin axis in sickle cell disease. *Br J Haematol*. 2020;189(6):1204-1209. doi: 10.1111/bjh.16498
74. Bondu S, Alary AS, Lefevre C, et al. A variant erythroferrone disrupts iron homeostasis in SF3B1-mutated myelodysplastic syndrome. *Sci Transl Med*. 2019;11(500):eaav5467. doi: 10.1126/scitranslmed.aav5467
75. Nemeth E, Valore EV, Territo M, Schiller G, Lichtenstein A, Ganz T. Hepcidin, a putative mediator of anemia of inflammation, is a type II acute-phase protein. *Blood*. 2003;101(7):2461-2463. (In eng). doi: 10.1182/blood-2002-10-3235
76. Weinstein DA, Roy CN, Fleming MD, Loda MF, Wolfsdorf JI, Andrews NC. Inappropriate expression of hepcidin is associated with iron refractory anemia: implications for the anemia of chronic disease. *Blood*. 2002;100(10):3776-3781. (In eng). doi: 10.1182/blood-2002-04-1260
77. Nemeth E, Rivera S, Gabayan V, et al. IL-6 mediates hypoferremia of inflammation by inducing the synthesis of the iron regulatory hormone hepcidin. *J Clin Invest*. 2004;113(9):1271-1276. (In eng). doi: 10.1172/jci20945
78. Wrighting DM, Andrews NC. Interleukin-6 induces hepcidin expression through STAT3. *Blood*. 2006;108(9):3204-3209. (In eng). doi: 10.1182/blood-2006-06-027631
79. Steinbicker AU, Sachidanandan C, Vonner AJ, et al. Inhibition of bone morphogenetic protein signaling attenuates anemia associated with inflammation. *Blood*. 2011;117(18):4915-4923. (In eng). doi: 10.1182/blood-2010-10-313064
80. Zaritsky J, Young B, Wang HJ, et al. Hepcidin—potential novel biomarker for iron status in chronic kidney disease. *Clin J Am Soc Nephrol*. 2009;4(6):1051-1056. (In eng). doi: 10.2215/cjn.05931108
81. Hentze MW, Muckenthaler MU, Andrews NC. Balancing acts: molecular control of mammalian iron metabolism. *Cell*. 2004;117(3):285-297. (In eng).
82. Eisenstein RS. Iron regulatory proteins and the molecular control of mammalian iron metabolism. *Annu Rev Nutr*. 2000;20:627-662. (In eng). doi: 10.1146/annurev.nutr.20.1.627
83. Muckenthaler M, Gray NK, Hentze MW. IRP-1 binding to ferritin mRNA prevents the recruitment of the small ribosomal subunit by the cap-binding complex eIF4F. *Mol Cell*. 1998;2(3):383-388. (In eng).
84. Kaptain S, Downey WE, Tang C, et al. A regulated RNA binding protein also possesses aconitase activity. *Proc Natl Acad Sci U S A*. 1991;88(22):10109-10113. (In eng).
85. Constable A, Quick S, Gray NK, Hentze MW. Modulation of the RNA-binding activity of a regulatory protein by iron in vitro: switching between enzymatic and genetic function? *Proc Natl Acad Sci U S A*. 1992;89(10):4554-4558. (In eng).
86. Haile DJ, Rouault TA, Tang CK, Chin J, Harford JB, Klausner RD. Reciprocal control of RNA-binding and aconitase activity in the regulation of the iron-responsive element binding protein: role of the iron-sulfur cluster. *Proc Natl Acad Sci U S A*. 1992;89(16):7536-7540. (In eng).
87. Guo B, Phillips JD, Yu Y, Leibold EA. Iron regulates the intracellular degradation of iron regulatory protein 2 by the proteasome. *J Biol Chem*. 1995;270(37):21645-21651. (In eng).

88. Samaniego F, Chin J, Iwai K, Rouault TA, Klausner RD. Molecular characterization of a second iron-responsive element binding protein, iron regulatory protein 2. Structure, function, and post-translational regulation. J Biol Chem. 1994;269(49):30904-30910. (In eng).

89. Salahudeen AA, Thompson JW, Ruiz JC, et al. An E3 ligase possessing an iron-responsive hemerythrin domain is a regulator of iron homeostasis. Science. 2009;326(5953):722-726. (In eng). doi: 10.1126/science.1176326

90. Meyron-Holtz EG, Ghosh MC, Rouault TA. Mammalian tissue oxygen levels modulate iron-regulatory protein activities in vivo. Science 2004;306(5704):2087-2090. (In eng). doi: 10.1126/science.1103786

91. Smith SR, Ghosh MC, Ollivierre-Wilson H, Hang Tong W, Rouault TA. Complete loss of iron regulatory proteins 1 and 2 prevents viability of murine zygotes beyond the blastocyst stage of embryonic development. Blood Cells Mol Dis. 2006;36(2):283-287. (In eng). doi: 10.1016/j.bcmd.2005.12.006

92. Ghosh MC, Zhang DL, Rouault TA. Iron misregulation and neurodegenerative disease in mouse models that lack iron regulatory proteins. Neurobiol Dis. 2015;81:66-75. doi: 10.1016/j.nbd.2015.02.026

93. Galy B, Ferring-Appel D, Kaden S, Grone HJ, Hentze MW. Iron regulatory proteins are essential for intestinal function and control key iron absorption molecules in the duodenum. Cell Metabol. 2008;7(1):79-85. (In eng). doi: 10.1016/j.cmet.2007.10.006

94. Zhang DL, Hughes RM, Ollivierre-Wilson H, Ghosh MC, Rouault TA. A ferroportin transcript that lacks an iron-responsive element enables duodenal and erythroid precursor cells to evade translational repression. Cell Metab. 2009;9(5):461-473. doi: 10.1016/j.cmet.2009.03.006

95. Schwartz AJ, Das NK, Ramakrishnan SK, et al. Hepatic hepcidin/intestinal HIF-2alpha axis maintains iron absorption during iron deficiency and overload. J Clin Invest. 2018;129(1):336-348. doi: 10.1172/JCI122359

96. Taylor M, Qu A, Anderson ER, et al. Hypoxia-inducible factor-2alpha mediates the adaptive increase of intestinal ferroportin during iron deficiency in mice. Gastroenterology. 2011;140(7):2044-2055. doi: 10.1053/j.gastro.2011.03.007

97. Klei TRL, Dalimot J, Nota B, et al. Hemolysis in the spleen drives erythrocyte turnover. Blood. 2020;136(14):1579-1589. doi: 10.1182/blood.2020005351

98. Aisen P. Transferrin receptor 1. Int J Biochem Cell Biol. 2004;36(11):2137-2143. (In eng). doi: 10.1016/j.biocel.2004.02.007

99. Goya N, Miyazaki S, Kodate S, Ushio B. A family of congenital atransferrinemia. Blood 1972;40(2):239-245. (In eng).

100. Heilmeyer L, Keller W, Vivell O, et al. Congenital atransferrinemia in a 7-year-old girl. Dtsch Med Wochenschr. 1961;86:1745-1751. (In ger). doi: 10.1055/s-0028-1113001

101. Kaplan J, Craven C, Alexander J, Kushner J, Lamb J, Bernstein S. Regulation of the distribution of tissue iron. Lessons learned from the hypotransferrinemic mouse. Ann N Y Acad Sci. 1988;526:124-135. (In eng).

102. Beutler E, Gelbart T, Lee P, Trevino R, Fernandez MA, Fairbanks VF. Molecular characterization of a case of atransferrinemia. Blood. 2000;96(13):4071-4074. (In eng).

103. Levy JE, Jin O, Fujiwara Y, Kuo F, Andrews NC. Transferrin receptor is necessary for development of erythrocytes and the nervous system. Nat Genet. 1999;21(4):396-399. (In eng). doi: 10.1038/7727

104. Huebers HA, Csiba E, Huebers E, Finch CA. Molecular advantage of diferric transferrin in delivering iron to reticulocytes: a comparative study. Proc Soc Exp Biol Med. 1985;179(2):222-226. (In eng).

105. Kawabata H, Nakamaki T, Ikonomi P, Smith RD, Germain RS, Koeffler HP. Expression of transferrin receptor 2 in normal and neoplastic hematopoietic cells. Blood. 2001;98(9):2714-2719. (In eng).

106. Forejtnikova H, Vieillevoye M, Zermati Y, et al. Transferrin receptor 2 is a component of the erythropoietin receptor complex and is required for efficient erythropoiesis. Blood. 2010;116(24):5357-5367. (In eng). doi: 10.1182/blood-2010-04-281360

107. Ahn J, Johnstone RM. Origin of a soluble truncated transferrin receptor. Blood. 1993;81(9):2442-2451. (In eng).

108. Beguin Y. Soluble transferrin receptor for the evaluation of erythropoiesis and iron status. Clin Chim Acta. 2003;329(1-2):9-22. (In eng).

109. Huebers HA, Beguin Y, Pootrakul P, Einspahr D, Finch CA. Intact transferrin receptors in human plasma and their relation to erythropoiesis. Blood. 1990;75(1):102-107. (In eng).

110. R'Zik S, Beguin Y. Serum soluble transferrin receptor concentration is an accurate estimate of the mass of tissue receptors. Exp Hematol. 2001;29(6):677-685. (In eng).

111. Ohgami RS, Campagna DR, Greer EL, et al. Identification of a ferrireductase required for efficient transferrin-dependent iron uptake in erythroid cells. Nat Genet. 2005;37(11):1264-1269. (In eng). doi: 10.1038/ng1658

112. Fleming MD, Romano MA, Su MA, Garrick LM, Garrick MD, Andrews NC. Nramp2 is mutated in the anemic Belgrade (b) rat: evidence of a role for Nramp2 in endosomal iron transport. Proc Natl Acad Sci U S A. 1998;95(3):1148-1153. (In eng).

113. Iolascon A, d'Apolito M, Servedio V, Cimmino F, Piga A, Camaschella C. Microcytic anemia and hepatic iron overload in a child with compound heterozygous mutations in DMT1 (SCL11A2). Blood. 2006;107(1):349-354. (In eng). doi: 10.1182/blood-2005-06-2477

114. Beaumont C, Delaunay J, Hetet G, Grandchamp B, de Montalembert M, Tchernia G. Two new human DMT1 gene mutations in a patient with microcytic anemia, low ferritinemia, and liver iron overload. Blood. 2006;107(10):4168-4170. (In eng). doi: 10.1182/blood-2005-10-4269

115. Sheftel AD, Zhang AS, Brown C, Shirihai OS, Ponka P. Direct interorganellar transfer of iron from endosome to mitochondrion. Blood. 2007;110(1):125-132. (In eng). doi: 10.1182/blood-2007-01-068148

116. Han AP, Yu C, Lu L, et al. Heme-regulated eIF2alpha kinase (HRI) is required for translational regulation and survival of erythroid precursors in iron deficiency. EMBO J. 2001;20(23):6909-6918. (In eng). doi: 10.1093/emboj/20.23.6909

117. Primosigh JV, Thomas ED. Studies on the partition of iron in bone marrow cells. J Clin Invest. 1968;47(7):1473-1482. (In eng). doi: 10.1172/jci105841

118. Douglas AS, Dacie JV. The incidence and significance of iron-containing granules in human erythrocytes and their precursors. J Clin Pathol. 1953;6(4):307-313. (In eng).

119. Keel SB, Doty RT, Yang Z, et al. A heme export protein is required for red blood cell differentiation and iron homeostasis. Science. 2008;319(5864):825-828. (In eng). doi: 10.1126/science.1151133

120. Mercurio S, Petrillo S, Chiabrando D, et al. The heme exporter Flvcr1 regulates expansion and differentiation of committed erythroid progenitors by controlling intracellular heme accumulation. Haematologica. 2015;100(6):720-729. (In eng). doi: 10.3324/haematol.2014.114488

121. Zhang DL, Ghosh MC, Ollivierre H, Li Y, Rouault TA. Ferroportin deficiency in erythroid cells causes serum iron deficiency and promotes hemolysis due to oxidative stress. Blood. 2018. doi: 10.1182/blood-2018-04-842997

122. White C, Yuan X, Schmidt PJ, et al. HRG1 is essential for heme transport from the phagolysosome of macrophages during erythrophagocytosis. Cell Metabol. 2013;17(2):261-270. (In eng). doi: 10.1016/j.cmet.2013.01.005

123. Maines MD. The heme oxygenase system: a regulator of second messenger gases. Annu Rev Pharmacol Toxicol. 1997;37:517-554. (In eng). doi: 10.1146/annurev.pharmtox.37.1.517

124. Delaby C, Pilard N, Puy H, Canonne-Hergaux F. Sequential regulation of ferroportin expression after erythrophagocytosis in murine macrophages: early mRNA induction by haem, followed by iron-dependent protein expression. Biochem J. 2008;411(1):123-131. (In eng). doi: 10.1042/bj20071474

125. Ganz T. Hepcidin and iron regulation, 10 years later. Blood. 2011;117(17):4425-4433.

126. Harris ED. The iron-copper connection: the link to ceruloplasmin grows stronger. Nutr Rev. 1995;53(6):170-173. (In eng).

127. Weiss G, Ganz T, Goodnough LT. Anemia of inflammation. Blood. 2019;133(1):40-50. doi: 10.1182/blood-2018-06-856500

128. Weiss G, Goodnough LT. Anemia of chronic disease. N Engl J Med. 2005;352(10):1011-1023. (In eng). doi: 10.1056/NEJMra041809. 352/10/1011 [pii].

129. Finazzi D, Arosio P. Biology of ferritin in mammals: an update on iron storage, oxidative damage and neurodegeneration. Arch Toxicol. 2014;88(10):1787-1802. (In eng). doi: 10.1007/s00204-014-1329-0

130. Ferreira C, Santambrogio P, Martin ME, et al. H ferritin knockout mice: a model of hyperferritinemia in the absence of iron overload. Blood. 2001;98(3):525-532. (In eng).

131. Arosio P, Levi S. Cytosolic and mitochondrial ferritins in the regulation of cellular iron homeostasis and oxidative damage. Biochim Biophys Acta. 2010;1800(8):783-792. (In eng). doi: 10.1016/j.bbagen.2010.02.005

132. Drysdale JW, Adelman TG, Arosio P, et al. Human isoferritins in normal and disease states. Semin Hematol. 1977;14(1):71-88. (In eng).

133. Shi H, Bencze KZ, Stemmler TL, Philpott CC. A cytosolic iron chaperone that delivers iron to ferritin. Science. 2008;320(5880):1207-1210. (In eng). doi: 10.1126/science.1157643

134. ACOG Practice Bulletin No. 95: anemia in pregnancy. Obstet Gynecol. 2008;112(1):201-207.

135. Munro H. The ferritin genes: their response to iron status. Nutr Rev. 1993;51(3):65-73. (In eng).

136. Hentze MW, Caughman SW, Rouault TA, et al. Identification of the iron-responsive element for the translational regulation of human ferritin mRNA. Science. 1987;238(4833):1570-1573. (In eng).

137. Mancias JD, Wang X, Gygi SP, Harper JW, Kimmelman AC. Quantitative proteomics identifies NCOA4 as the cargo receptor mediating ferritinophagy. Nature. 2014;509(7498):105-109. (In eng). doi: 10.1038/nature13148

138. Mancias JD, Pontano Vaites L, Nissim S, et al. Ferritinophagy via NCOA4 is required for erythropoiesis and is regulated by iron dependent HERC2-mediated proteolysis. Elife. 2015;4:e10308. (In eng). DOI: 10.7554/eLife.10308.

139. Bellelli R, Federico G, Matte A, et al. NCOA4 deficiency impairs systemic iron homeostasis. Cell Rep. 2016;14(3):411-421. (In eng). doi: 10.1016/j.celrep.2015.12.065

140. Goodnough LT, Nemeth E, Ganz T. Detection, evaluation, and management of iron-restricted erythropoiesis. Blood. 2010;116(23):4754-4761. (In eng). doi: 10.1182/blood-2010-05-286260. blood-2010-05-286260 [pii].

141. Cohen LA, Gutierrez L, Weiss A, et al. Serum ferritin is derived primarily from macrophages through a nonclassical secretory pathway. Blood. 2010;116(9):1574-1584. (In eng). doi: 10.1182/blood-2009-11-253815

142. Truman-Rosentsvit M, Berenbaum D, Spektor L, et al. Ferritin is secreted via 2 distinct nonclassical vesicular pathways. Blood. 2018;131(3):342-352. doi: 10.1182/blood-2017-02-768580

143. Barrientos T, Laothamatas I, Koves TR, et al. Metabolic catastrophe in mice lacking transferrin receptor in muscle. EBioMedicine. 2015;2(11):1705-1717. (In eng). doi: 10.1016/j.ebiom.2015.09.041

144. Xu W, Barrientos T, Mao L, Rockman HA, Sauve AA, Andrews NC. Lethal cardiomyopathy in mice lacking transferrin receptor in the heart. Cell Rep. 2015;13(3):533-545. doi: 10.1016/j.celrep.2015.09.023

145. Matak P, Matak A, Moustafa S, et al. Disrupted iron homeostasis causes dopaminergic neurodegeneration in mice. Proc Natl Acad Sci U S A. 2016;113(13):3428-3435. (In eng). doi: 10.1073/pnas.1519473113

146. Jabara HH, Boyden SE, Chou J, et al. A missense mutation in TFRC, encoding transferrin receptor 1, causes combined immunodeficiency. Nat Genet. 2016;48(1):74-78. doi: 10.1038/ng.3465

Disorders of Red Blood Cells

147. Tahara T, Sun J, Nakanishi K, et al. Heme positively regulates the expression of beta-globin at the locus control region via the transcriptional factor Bach1 in erythroid cells. *J Biol Chem.* 2004;279(7):5480-5487. (In eng). doi: 10.1074/jbc.M302733200

148. Zenke-Kawasaki Y, Dohi Y, Katoh Y, et al. Heme induces ubiquitination and degradation of the transcription factor Bach1. *Mol Cell Biol.* 2007;27(19):6962-6971. (In eng). doi: 10.1128/mcb.02415-06

149. Chen JJ. Regulation of protein synthesis by the heme-regulated eIF2alpha kinase: relevance to anemias. *Blood.* 2007;109(7):2693-2699. (In eng). doi: 10.1182/blood-2006-08-041830

150. Camaschella C, Campanella A, De Falco L, et al. The human counterpart of zebrafish shiraz shows sideroblastic-like microcytic anemia and iron overload. *Blood.* 2007;110(4):1353-1358. (In eng). doi: 10.1182/blood-2007-02-072520

151. Harris ZL, Takahashi Y, Miyajima H, Serizawa M, MacGillivray RT, Gitlin JD. Aceruloplasminemia: molecular characterization of this disorder of iron metabolism. *Proc Natl Acad Sci U S A.* 1995;92(7):2539-2543. (In eng).

152. Folgueras AR, de Lara FM, Pendas AM, et al. Membrane-bound serine protease matriptase-2 (Tmprss6) is an essential regulator of iron homeostasis. *Blood.* 2008;112(6):2539-2545. (In eng). doi: 10.1182/blood-2008-04-149773

153. Finberg KE, Heeney MM, Campagna DR, et al. Mutations in TMPRSS6 cause iron-refractory iron deficiency anemia (IRIDA). *Nat Genet.* 2008;40(5):569-571. (In eng). doi: 10.1038/ng.130

154. Guillem F, Lawson S, Kannengiesser C, Westerman M, Beaumont C, Grandchamp B. Two nonsense mutations in the TMPRSS6 gene in a patient with microcytic anemia and iron deficiency. *Blood.* 2008;112(5):2089-2091. (In eng). doi: 10.1182/blood-2008-05-154740

155. Mims MP, Guan Y, Pospisilova D, et al. Identification of a human mutation of DMT1 in a patient with microcytic anemia and iron overload. *Blood.* 2005;105(3):1337-1342. (In eng). doi: 10.1182/blood-2004-07-2966

156. Priwitzerova M, Nie G, Sheftel AD, Pospisilova D, Divoky V, Ponka P. Functional consequences of the human DMT1 (SLC11A2) mutation on protein expression and iron uptake. *Blood.* 2005;106(12):3985-3987. (In eng). doi: 10.1182/blood-2005-04-1550

157. Lam-Yuk-Tseung S, Camaschella C, Iolascon A, Gros P. A novel R416C mutation in human DMT1 (SLC11A2) displays pleiotropic effects on function and causes microcytic anemia and hepatic iron overload. *Blood Cells Mol Dis.* 2006;36(3):347-354. (In eng). doi: 10.1016/j.bcmd.2006.01.011

158. Trenor CC,IIIrd, Campagna DR, Sellers VM, Andrews NC, Fleming MD. The molecular defect in hypotransferrinemic mice. *Blood.* 2000;96(3):1113-1118. (In eng).

159. Di Raimondo D, Pinto A, Tuttolomondo A, Fernandez P, Camaschella C, Licata G. Aceruloplasminemia: a case report. *Intern Emerg Med.* 2008;3(4):395-399. (In eng). doi: 10.1007/s11739-008-0150-2

160. Hartman KR, Barker JA. Microcytic anemia with iron malabsorption: an inherited disorder of iron metabolism. *Am J Hematol.* 1996;51(4):269-275. (In eng). doi: 10.1002/(sici)1096-8652(199604)51:4<269::aid-ajh4>3.0.co;2-u

161. Lappas M. Markers of endothelial cell dysfunction are increased in human omental adipose tissue from women with pre-existing maternal obesity and gestational diabetes. *Metabolism.* 2014;63(6):860-873. (Research Support, Non-U.S. Gov't) (In Eng). doi: 10.1016/j.metabol.2014.03.007

162. Pearson HA, Lukens JN. Ferrokinetics in the syndrome of familial hypoferremic microcytic anemia with iron malabsorption. *J Pediatr Hematol Oncol.* 1999;21(5):412-417. (In eng).

163. Benyamin B, Ferreira MA, Willemsen G, et al. Common variants in TMPRSS6 are associated with iron status and erythrocyte volume. *Nat Genet.* 2009;41(11):1173-1175. (In eng). doi: 10.1038/ng.456

164. Chambers JC, Zhang W, Li Y, et al. Genome-wide association study identifies variants in TMPRSS6 associated with hemoglobin levels. *Nat Genet.* 2009;41(11):1170-1172. (In eng). doi: 10.1038/ng.462

165. Ganesh SK, Zakai NA, van Rooij FJ, et al. Multiple loci influence erythrocyte phenotypes in the CHARGE Consortium. *Nat Genet.* 2009;41(11):1191-1198. (In eng). doi: 10.1038/ng.466

166. Heinrich HC. Iron deficiency without anemia. *Lancet.* 1968;2(7565):460. (In eng).

167. Verloop MC. Iron depletion without anemia: a controversial subject. *Blood.* 1970;36(5):657-671. (In eng).

168. Ballas SK. Normal serum iron and elevated total iron-binding capacity in iron-deficiency states. *Am J Clin Pathol.* 1979;71(4):401-403. (In eng).

169. Koller ME, Romslo I, Finne PH, Brockmeier F, Tyssebotn I. The diagnosis of iron deficiency by erythrocyte protoporphyrin and serum ferritin analyses. *Acta Paediatr Scand.* 1978;67(3):361-366. (In eng).

170. Labbe RF, Vreman HJ, Stevenson DK. Zinc protoporphyrin: a metabolite with a mission. *Clin Chem.* 1999;45(12):2060-2072. (In eng).

171. Cook JD. The measurement of serum transferrin receptor. *Am J Med Sci.* 1999;318(4):269-276. (In eng).

172. Trost LB, Bergfeld WF, Calogeras E. The diagnosis and treatment of iron deficiency and its potential relationship to hair loss. *J Am Acad Dermatol.* 2006;54(5):824-844. (In eng). doi: 10.1016/j.jaad.2005.11.1104

173. Conrad ME, Crosby WH. The natural history of iron deficiency induced by phlebotomy. *Blood.* 1962;20:173-185. (In eng).

174. Beutler E, Waalen J. The definition of anemia: what is the lower limit of normal of the blood hemoglobin concentration? *Blood.* 2006;107(5):1747-1750. (In eng). doi: 10.1182/blood-2005-07-3046

175. Goodnough LT, Schrier SL. Evaluation and management of anemia in the elderly. *Am J Hematol.* 2014;89(1):88-96. (In eng). doi: 10.1002/ajh.23598

176. Guralnik JM, Eisenstaedt RS, Ferrucci L, Klein HG, Woodman RC. Prevalence of anemia in persons 65 years and older in the United States: evidence for a high rate of unexplained anemia. *Blood.* 2004;104(8):2263-2268. (In eng). doi: 10.1182/blood-2004-05-1812

177. Ferrucci L, Semba RD, Guralnik JM, et al. Proinflammatory state, hepcidin, and anemia in older persons. *Blood.* 2010;115(18):3810-3816. (In eng). doi: 10.1182/blood-2009-02-201087

178. Disease GBD, Injury I, Prevalence C. Global, regional, and national incidence, prevalence, and years lived with disability for 328 diseases and injuries for 195 countries, 1990-2016: a systematic analysis for the Global Burden of Disease Study 2016. *Lancet.* 2017;390(10100):1211-1259. doi: 10.1016/S0140-6736(17)32154-2

179. Onken JE, Bregman DB, Harrington RA, et al. Ferric carboxymaltose in patients with iron-deficiency anemia and impaired renal function: the REPAIR-IDA trial. *Nephrol Dial Transplant.* 2014;29(4):833-842. (In eng). doi: 10.1093/ndt/gft251

180. Onken JE, Bregman DB, Harrington RA, et al. A multicenter, randomized, active-controlled study to investigate the efficacy and safety of intravenous ferric carboxymaltose in patients with iron deficiency anemia. *Transfusion.* 2014;54(2):306-315. (In eng). doi: 10.1111/trf.12289

181. Tim Goodnough L, Comin-Colet J, Leal-Noval S, et al. Management of anemia in patients with congestive heart failure. *Am J Hematol.* 2017;92(1):88-93. doi: 10.1002/ajh.24595

182. Drukker L, Hants Y, Farkash R, Ruchlemer R, Samueloff A, Grisaru-Granovsky S. Iron deficiency anemia at admission for labor and delivery is associated with an increased risk for Cesarean section and adverse maternal and neonatal outcomes. *Transfusion.* 2015;55(12):2799-2806. (In eng). doi: 10.1111/trf.13252

183. Looker AC, Dallman PR, Carroll MD, Gunter EW, Johnson CL. Prevalence of iron deficiency in the United States. *JAMA.* 1997;277(12):973-976. (In eng).

184. Karp RJ, Haaz WS, Starko K, Gorman JM. Iron deficiency in families of iron-deficient inner-city school children. *Am J Dis Child.* 1974;128(1):18-20. (In eng).

185. Siu AL, USPST Force. Screening for iron deficiency anemia in young children: USPSTF recommendation statement. *Pediatrics.* 2015;136(4):746-752. doi: 10.1542/peds.2015-2567

186. Siu AL, Force USPST. Screening for iron deficiency anemia and iron supplementation in pregnant women to improve maternal health and birth outcomes: U.S. Preventive Services task force recommendation statement. *Ann Intern Med.* 2015;163(7):529-536. (In eng). doi: 10.7326/M15-1707

187. Baker RD, Greer FR, Pediatrics CoNAAo. Diagnosis and prevention of iron deficiency and iron-deficiency anemia in infants and young children (0-3 years of age). *Pediatrics.* 2010;126(5):1040-1050. (In eng). doi: 10.1542/peds.2010-2576

188. Rosenbaum E, Leonard JW. Nurtritional iron deficiency anemia in an adult male. Report of a case. *Ann Intern Med.* 1964;60:683-688. (In eng).

189. Hurrell RF. Fortification: overcoming technical and practical barriers. *J Nutr.* 2002;132(4 suppl):806S-812S. (In eng).

190. Jacobs A, Lawrie JH, Entwistle CC, Campbell H. Gastric acid secretion in chronic iron-deficiency anaemia. *Lancet.* 1966;2(7456):190-192. (In eng).

191. Skikne BS, Lynch SR, Cook JD. Role of gastric acid in food iron absorption. *Gastroenterology.* 1981;81(6):1068-1071. (In eng).

192. Hershko C, Lahad A, Kereth D. Gastropathic sideropenia. *Best Pract Res Clin Haematol.* 2005;18(2):363-380. (In eng). doi: 10.1016/j.beha.2004.10.002

193. Adams JF. The clinical and metabolic consequences of total gastrectomy. II. Anaemia. Metabolism of iron, vitamin B12 and folic acid. *Scand J Gastroenterol.* 1968;3(2):145-151. (In eng).

194. Hines JD, Hoffbrand AV, Mollin DL. The hematologic complications following partial gastrectomy. A study of 292 patients. *Am J Med.* 1967;43(4):555-569. (In eng).

195. Magnusson BE. Iron absorption after antrectomy with gastroduodenostomy. Studies on the absorption from food and from iron salt using a double radioiron isotope technique and whole-body counting. *Scand J Haematol Suppl.* 1976;26:1-111. (In eng).

196. Sutton DR, Stewart JS, Baird IM, Coghill NF. "Free" iron loss in atrophic gastritis, post-gastrectomy states, and adult coeliac disease. *Lancet.* 1970;2(7669):387-389. (In eng).

197. Kilpatrick ZM, Katz J. Occult celiac disease as a cause of iron deficiency anemia. *JAMA.* 1969;208(6):999-1001. (In eng).

198. Kosnai I, Kuitunen P, Siimes MA. Iron deficiency in children with coeliac disease on treatment with gluten-free diet. Role of intestinal blood loss. *Arch Dis Child.* 1979;54(5):375-378. (In eng).

199. Fleming AF. Iron deficiency in the tropics. *Clin Haematol.* 1982;11(2):365-388. (In eng).

200. Graham DY, Smith JL. Gastroduodenal complications of chronic NSAID therapy. *Am J Gastroenterol.* 1988;83(10):1081-1084. (In eng).

201. Arnett DK, Blumenthal RS, Albert MA, et al. 2019 ACC/AHA guideline on the primary prevention of cardiovascular disease: a report of the American college of cardiology/American heart association task force on clinical practice guidelines. *J Am Coll Cardiol.* 2019;74(10):e177-e232. doi: 10.1016/j.jacc.2019.03.010

202. Windsor CW, Collis JL. Anaemia and hiatus hernia: experience in 450 patients. *Thorax.* 1967;22(1):73-78. (In eng).

203. Cameron AJ. Incidence of iron deficiency anemia in patients with large diaphragmatic hernia. A controlled study. *Mayo Clin Proc.* 1976;51(12):767-769. (In eng).

204. Beal RW, Skyring AP, McRae J, Firkin BG. The anemia of ulcerative colitis. *Gastroenterology.* 1963;45:589-603. (In eng).

205. Raje D, Mukhtar H, Oshowo A, Ingham Clark C. What proportion of patients referred to secondary care with iron deficiency anemia have colon cancer? *Dis Colon Rectum.* 2007;50(8):1211-1214. (In eng). doi: 10.1007/s10350-007-0249-y

206. Stephenson LS, Latham MC, Ottesen EA. Malnutrition and parasitic helminth infections. *Parasitology.* 2000;121(suppl):S23-S38. (In eng).

207. Stephenson LS, Holland CV, Cooper ES. The public health significance of Trichuris trichiura. *Parasitology.* 2000;121(suppl):S73-S95. (In eng).

208. Roche M, Layrisse M. The nature and causes of "hookworm anemia". *Am J Trop Med Hyg.* 1966;15(6):1029-1102. (In eng).

209. Stephenson L. The impact of schistosomiasis on human nutrition. *Parasitology.* 1993;107(suppl):S107-S123. (In eng).

210. Jacobs A, Butler EB. Menstrual blood-loss in iron-deficiency anaemia. *Lancet.* 1965;2(7409):407-409. (In eng).

211. Hallberg L, Hogdahl AM, Nilsson L, Rybo G. Menstrual blood loss—a population study. Variation at different ages and attempts to define normality. *Acta Obstet Gynecol Scand* 1966;45(3):320-351. (In eng).

212. Beaton GH, Thein M, Milne H, Veen MJ. Iron requirements of menstruating women. *Am J Clin Nutr.* 1970;23(3):275-283. (In eng).

213. Hefnawi F, Askalani H, Zaki K. Menstrual blood loss with copper intrauterine devices. *Contraception.* 1974;9(2):133-139. (In eng).

214. Simon TL, Garry PJ, Hooper EM. Iron stores in blood donors. *JAMA.* 1981;245(20):2038-2043. (In eng).

215. Goodnough LT, Bravo JR, Hsueh YS, Keating LJ, Brittenham GM. Red blood cell mass in autologous and homologous blood units. Implications for risk/benefit assessment of autologous blood crossover and directed blood transfusion. *Transfusion.* 1989;29(9):821-822. (In eng).

216. Cable RG, Glynn SA, Kiss JE, et al. Iron deficiency in blood donors: analysis of enrollment data from the REDS-II Donor Iron Status Evaluation (RISE) study. *Transfusion.* 2011;51(3):511-522. (In eng). doi: 10.1111/j.1537-2995.2010.02865.x

217. Brittenham GM. Iron deficiency in whole blood donors. *Transfusion.* 2011;51(3):458-461. (In eng). doi: 10.1111/j.1537-2995.2011.03062.x

218. AABB. Updated strategies to limit or prevent iron deficiency in blood donors. *Association Bulletin.* 1984;100:843-845.

219. Leatherman JW, Davies SF, Hoidal JR. Alveolar hemorrhage syndromes: diffuse microvascular lung hemorrhage in immune and idiopathic disorders. *Medicine (Baltim)* 1984;63(6):343-361. (In eng).

220. Ernst TN, Philp M. Severe iron deficiency anemia. An example of covert child abuse (Munchausen by proxy). *West J Med.* 1986;144(3):358-359. (In eng).

221. Specks U. Diffuse alveolar hemorrhage syndromes. *Curr Opin Rheumatol.* 2001;13(1):12-17. (In eng).

222. Hartmann RC, Jenkins DE, Jr, McKee LC, Heyssel RM. Paroxysmal nocturnal hemoglobinuria: clinical and laboratory studies relating to iron metabolism and therapy with androgen and iron. *Medicine (Baltim).* 1966;45(5):331-363. (In eng).

223. Kann HE, Jr, Mengel CE, Wall RL. Paroxysmal nocturnal hemoglobinuria "obscured" by the presence of iron deficiency. *Ann Intern Med.* 1967;67(3):593-596. (In eng).

224. Roeser HP, Powell LW. Urinary iron excretion in valvular heart disease and after heart valve replacement. *Blood.* 1970;36(6):785-792. (In eng).

225. Stone DR, Duran A, Fine KC. Lab-fraud anemia. *N Engl J Med.* 1988;319(11):727-728. (In eng). doi: 10.1056/nejm198809153191119

226. Peery WH. Clinical spectrum of hereditary hemorrhagic telangiectasia (Osler-Weber-Rendu disease). *Am J Med.* 1987;82(5):989-997. (In eng).

227. Koch CG, Li L, Sun Z, et al. Hospital-acquired anemia: prevalence, outcomes, and healthcare implications. *J Hosp Med.* 2013;8(9):506-512. (In eng). doi: 10.1002/jhm.2061

228. Salisbury AC, Reid KJ, Alexander KP, et al. Diagnostic blood loss from phlebotomy and hospital-acquired anemia during acute myocardial infarction. *Arch Intern Med.* 2011;171(18):1646-1653. (In eng). doi: 10.1001/archinternmed.2011.361

229. Vincent JL, Baron JF, Reinhart K, et al. Anemia and blood transfusion in critically ill patients. *JAMA.* 2002;288(12):1499-1507. (In eng).

230. von Ahsen N, Muller C, Serke S, Frei U, Eckardt KU. Important role of nondiagnostic blood loss and blunted erythropoietic response in the anemia of medical intensive care patients. *Crit Care Med.* 1999;27(12):2630-2639. (In eng).

231. Napolitano LM. Scope of the problem: epidemiology of anemia and use of blood transfusions in critical care. *Crit Care.* 2004;8(suppl 2):S1-S8. (In eng). doi: 10.1186/cc2832

232. Goodnough LT, Strasburg D, Riddell J, Verbrugge D, Wish J. Has recombinant human erythropoietin therapy minimized red-cell transfusions in hemodialysis patients? *Clin Nephrol* 1994;41(5):303-307. (In eng).

233. Rosenblatt SG, Drake S, Fadem S, Welch R, Lifschitz MD. Gastrointestinal blood loss in patients with chronic renal failure. *Am J Kidney Dis.* 1982;1(4):232-236. (In eng).

234. Ganz T, Nemeth E. Iron balance and the role of hepcidin in chronic kidney disease. *Semin Nephrol.* 2016;36(2):87-93. (In eng). doi: 10.1016/j.semnephrol.2016.02.001

235. Goodnough LT. Iron deficiency syndromes and iron-restricted erythropoiesis. *Transfusion.* 2012;52(7):1584-1592. (In eng). doi: 10.1111/j.1537-2995.2011.03495.x

236. Goodnough LT, Skikne B, Brugnara C. Erythropoietin, iron, and erythropoiesis. *Blood.* 2000;96(3):823-833. (In eng).

237. Dang CV. Runner's anemia. *JAMA* 2001;286(6):714-716. (In eng).

238. Stewart JG, Ahlquist DA, McGill DB, Ilstrup DM, Schwartz S, Owen RA. Gastrointestinal blood loss and anemia in runners. *Ann Intern Med.* 1984;100(6):843-845. (In eng).

239. McClung JP. Iron status and the female athlete. *J Trace Elem Med Biol.* 2012;26(2-3):124-126. (In eng). doi: 10.1016/j.jtemb.2012.03.006

240. Pisacane A. Neonatal prevention of iron deficiency. *BMJ.* 1996;312(7024):136-137. (In eng).

241. Daniel DG, Weerakkody AN. Neonatal prevention of iron deficiency. Blood can be transfused from cord clamped at placental end. *BMJ.* 1996;312(7038):1102-1103. (In eng).

242. Scholl TO. Maternal iron status: relation to fetal growth, length of gestation, and iron endowment of the neonate. *Nutr Rev.* 2011;69(suppl 1):S23-S29. (In eng). doi: 10.1111/j.1753-4887.2011.00429.x

243. Cao C, O'Brien KO. Pregnancy and iron homeostasis: an update. *Nutr Rev.* 2013;71(1):35-51. (In eng). doi: 10.1111/j.1753-4887.2012.00550.x

244. Lozoff B, Beard J, Connor J, Barbara F, Georgieff M, Schallert T. Long-lasting neural and behavioral effects of iron deficiency in infancy. *Nutr Rev.* 2006;64(5 pt 2):S34-S43; discussion S72-91. (In eng)

245. Oski FA, Stockman JA,IIIrd. Anemia due to inadequate iron sources or poor iron utilization. *Pediatr Clin North Am.* 1980;27(2):237-253. (In eng).

246. Garcia-Ramos Estarriol L, Gonzalez Diaz JP, Duque Hernandez J. Dietetic ingestion and feeding habits during the first year of life. *Anales Espanoles de Pediatria.* 2000;52:523-529.

247. Saarinen UM, Siimes MA, Dallman PR. Iron absorption in infants: high bioavailability of breast milk iron as indicated by the extrinsic tag method of iron absorption and by the concentration of serum ferritin. *J Pediatr.* 1977;91(1):36-39. (In eng).

248. Saarinen UM, Siimes MA. Iron absorption from infant milk formula and the optimal level of iron supplementation. *Acta Paediatr Scand.* 1977;66(6):719-722. (In eng).

249. Hertrampf E, Cayazzo M, Pizarro F, Stekel A. Bioavailability of iron in soy-based formula and its effect on iron nutriture in infancy. *Pediatrics.* 1986;78(4):640-645. (In eng).

250. Rios E, Hunter RE, Cook JD, Smith NJ, Finch CA. The absorption of iron as supplements in infant cereal and infant formulas. *Pediatrics.* 1975;55(5):686-693. (In eng).

251. Sandoval C, Berger E, Ozkaynak MF, Tugal O, Jayabose S. Severe iron deficiency anemia in 42 pediatric patients. *Pediatr Hematol Oncol.* 2002;19(3):157-161. (In eng). doi: 10.1080/088800102753541305

252. Yeung GS, Zlotkin SH. Efficacy of meat and iron-fortified commercial cereal to prevent iron depletion in cow milk-fed infants 6 to 12 months of age: a randomized controlled trial. *Can J Public Health.* 2000;91(4):263-267. (In eng).

253. Jelliffe DB, Blackman V. Bahima disease. Possible "milk anemia" in late childhood. *J Pediatr.* 1962;61:774-779. (In eng).

254. Wilson JF, Lahey ME, Heiner DC. Studies on iron metabolism. V. Further observations on cow's milk-induced gastrointestinal bleeding in infants with iron-deficiency anemia. *J Pediatr.* 1974;84(3):335-344. (In eng).

255. Guha DK, Walia BN, Tandon BN, Deo MG, Ghai OP. Small bowel changes in iron-deficiency anaemia of childhood. *Arch Dis Child.* 1968;43(228):239-244. (In eng).

256. Woodruff CW, Wright SW, Wright RP. The role of fresh cow's milk in iron deficiency. II. Comparison of fresh cow's milk with a prepared formula. *Am J Dis Child.* 1972;124(1):26-30. (In eng).

257. Bothwell TH. Iron requirements in pregnancy and strategies to meet them. *Am J Clin Nutr.* 2000;72(1 suppl):257s-264s. (In eng).

258. Celada A, Busset R, Gutierrez J, Herreros V. No correlation between iron concentration in breast milk and maternal iron stores. *Helv Paediatr Acta.* 1982;37(1):11-16. (In eng).

259. Beutler E, Larsh SE, Gurney CW. Iron therapy in chronically fatigued, nonanemic women: a double-blind study. *Ann Intern Med.* 1960;52:378-394. (In eng).

260. Krayenbuehl PA, Battegay E, Breymann C, Furrer J, Schulthess G. Intravenous iron for the treatment of fatigue in nonanemic, premenopausal women with low serum ferritin concentration. *Blood.* 2011;118(12):3222-3227. (In eng). doi: 10.1182/blood-2011-04-346304

261. Gardner GW, Edgerton VR, Senewiratne B, Barnard RJ, Ohira Y. Physical work capacity and metabolic stress in subjects with iron deficiency anemia. *Am J Clin Nutr.* 1977;30(6):910-917. (In eng).

262. Edgerton VR, Gardner GW, Ohira Y, Gunawardena KA, Senewiratne B. Iron-deficiency anaemia and its effect on worker productivity and activity patterns. *Br Med J.* 1979;2(6204):1546-1549. (In eng).

263. Glover J, Jacobs A. Activity pattern of iron-deficient rats. *Br Med J.* 1972;2(5814):627-628. (In eng).

264. Koziol BJ, Ohira Y, Edgerton VR, Simpson DR. Changes in work tolerance associated with metabolic and physiological adjustment to moderate and severe iron deficiency anemia. *Am J Clin Nutr.* 1982;36(5):830-839. (In eng).

265. Finch CA, Gollnick PD, Hlastala MP, Miller LR, Dillmann E, Mackler B. Lactic acidosis as a result of iron deficiency. *J Clin Invest.* 1979;64(1):129-137. (In eng). doi: 10.1172/jci109431

266. Stugiewicz M, Tkaczyszyn M, Kasztura M, Banasiak W, Ponikowski P, Jankowska EA. The influence of iron deficiency on the functioning of skeletal muscles: experimental evidence and clinical implications. *Eur J Heart Fail.* 2016;18(7):762-773, doi: 10.1002/ejhf.467

267. Oski FA. The nonhematologic manifestations of iron deficiency. *Am J Dis Child.* 1979;133(3):315-322. (In eng).

268. Lozoff B. Iron deficiency and infant development. *J Pediatr.* 1994;125(4):577-578. (In eng).

269. Lozoff B, Klein NK, Nelson EC, McClish DK, Manuel M, Chacon ME. Behavior of infants with iron-deficiency anemia. *Child Dev.* 1998;69(1):24-36. (In eng).

270. Oski FA, Honig AS, Helu B, Howanitz P. Effect of iron therapy on behavior performance in nonanemic, iron-deficient infants. *Pediatrics.* 1983;71(6):877-880. (In eng).

271. Lozoff B. Perinatal iron deficiency and the developing brain. *Pediatr Res.* 2000;48(2):137-139. (In eng).

272. Grantham-McGregor S, Ani C. A review of studies on the effect of iron deficiency on cognitive development in children. *J Nutr.* 2001;131(2s-2):649S-666S; discussion 666S-668S. (In Eng).

273. Massaro TF, Widmayer P. The effect of iron deficiency on cognitive performance in the rat. *Am J Clin Nutr* 1981;34(5):864-870. (In eng).

274. Martinez-Torres C, Cubeddu L, Dillmann E, et al. Effect of exposure to low temperature on normal and iron-deficient subjects. *Am J Physiol.* 1984;246(3 pt 2):R380-R383. (In eng).

275. Yager JY, Hartfield DS. Neurologic manifestations of iron deficiency in childhood. *Pediatr Neurol.* 2002;27(2):85-92. (In eng).

276. Butte NF, Lopez-Alarcon MG, Garza C. *Nutrient Adequacy of Exclusive Breastfeeding for the Term Infant during the First Six Months of Life.* WHO; 2001.

277. Hogan GR, Jones B. The relationship of koilonychia and iron deficiency in infants. *J Pediatr.* 1970;77(6):1054-1057. (In eng).

278. Jacobs A, Cavill I. The oral lesions of iron deficiency anaemia: pyridoxine and ribo-flavin status. *Br J Haematol.* 1968;14(3):291-295. (In eng).

279. Ekberg O, Malmquist J, Lindgren S. Pharyngo-oesophageal webs in dyspha-geal patients. A radiologic and clinical investigation in 1134 patients. *Röfo.* 1986;145(1):75-80. (In eng). doi: 10.1055/s-2008-1048889

280. Chisholm M, Ardran GM, Callender ST, Wright R. A follow-up study of patients with post-cricoid webs. *Q J Med.* 1971;40(159):409-420. (In eng).

281. Khosla SN. Cricoid webs--incidence and follow-up study in Indian patients. *Postgrad Med J.* 1984;60(703):346-348. (In eng).

282. Theurl I, Fritsche G, Ludwiczek S, Garimorth K, Bellmann-Weiler R, Weiss G. The macrophage: a cellular factory at the interphase between iron and immunity for the control of infections. *Biometals.* 2005;18(4):359-367. (In eng). doi: 10.1007/s10534-005-3710-1

283. Stoffel NU, Uyoga MA, Mutuku FM, et al. Iron deficiency anemia at time of vac-cination predicts decreased vaccine response and iron supplementation at time of vaccination increases humoral vaccine response: a birth cohort study and a random-ized trial follow-up study in Kenyan infants. *Front Immunol.* 2020;11:1313. doi: 10.3389/fimmu.2020.01313

284. Chandra RK, Saraya AK. Impaired immunocompetence associated with iron defi-ciency. *J Pediatr.* 1975;86(6):899-902. (In eng).

285. Yetgin S, Altay C, Ciliv G, Laleli Y. Myeloperoxidase activity and bactericidal func-tion of PMN in iron deficiency. *Acta Haematol.* 1979;61(1):10-14. (In eng).

286. Dallman PR. Iron deficiency and the immune response. *Am J Clin Nutr.* 1987;46(2):329-334. (In eng).

287. Pagani A, Nai A, Corna G, et al. Low hepcidin accounts for the proinflammatory status associated with iron deficiency. *Blood.* 2011;118(3):736-746. doi: 10.1182/blood-2011-02-337212

288. Oppenheimer SJ. Iron and its relation to immunity and infectious disease. *J Nutr.* 2001;131(2S-2):616S-633S; discussion 633S-635S. (In eng).

289. Ganz T, Aronoff GR, Gaillard C, et al. Iron administration, infection, and ane-mia management in CKD: untangling the effects of intravenous iron therapy on immunity and infection risk. *Kidney Med.* 2020;2(3):341-353. doi: 10.1016/j.xkme.2020.01.006

290. Coltman CA, Jr. Pagophagia and iron lack. *JAMA.* 1969;207(3):513-516. (In eng).

291. Reynolds RD, Binder HJ, Miller MB, Chang WW, Horan S. Pagophagia and iron deficiency anemia. *Ann Intern Med.* 1968;69(3):435-440. (In eng).

292. Moore DF, Jr, Sears DA. Pica, iron deficiency, and the medical history. *Am J Med.* 1994;97(4):390-393. (In eng).

293. Crosby WH. Pica. *JAMA.* 1976;235(25):2765. (In eng).

294. Crosby WH. Food pica and iron deficiency. *Arch Intern Med.* 1971;127(5):960-961. (In eng).

295. Chavarro JE, Rich-Edwards JW, Rosner BA, Willett WC. Iron intake and risk of ovulatory infertility. *Obstet Gynecol.* 2006;108(5):1145-1152. (In eng). doi: 10.1097/01.AOG.0000238333.37423.ab

296. Li YQ, Cao XX, Bai B, Zhang JN, Wang MQ, Zhang YH. Severe iron deficiency is associated with a reduced conception rate in female rats. *Gynecol Obstet Invest.* 2014;77(1):19-23. (In eng). doi: 10.1159/000355112

297. Lanzkowsky P. Radiological features of iron-deficiency anemia. *Am J Dis Child.* 1968;116(1):16-29. (In eng).

298. Goodnough LT, Maniatis A, Earnshaw P, et al. Detection, evaluation, and manage-ment of preoperative anaemia in the elective orthopaedic surgical patient: NATA guidelines. *Br J Anaesth.* 2011;106(1):13-22. (In eng). doi: 10.1093/bja/aeq361. aeq361 [pii].

299. Bessman JD, Gilmer PR, Jr, Gardner FH. Improved classification of anemias by MCV and RDW. *Am J Clin Pathol.* 1983;80(3):322-326. (In eng).

300. Freireich EJ, Miller A, Emerson CP, Ross JF. The effect of inflammation on the utili-zation of erythrocyte and transferrin bound radioiron for red cell production. *Blood.* 1957;12(11):972-983. (In eng).

301. Ali MA, Luxton AW, Walker WH. Serum ferritin concentration and bone marrow iron stores: a prospective study. *Can Med Assoc J.* 1978;118(8):945-946. (In eng).

302. Mast AE, Blinder MA, Gronowski AM, Chumley C, Scott MG. Clinical utility of the soluble transferrin receptor and comparison with serum ferritin in several popu-lations. *Clin Chem.* 1998;44(1):45-51. (In eng).

303. Goodnough LT, Price TH, Rudnick S. Iron-restricted erythropoiesis as a limitation to autologous blood donation in the erythropoietin-stimulated bone marrow. *J Lab Clin Med.* 1991;118(3):289-296. (In eng). doi: 0022-2143(91)90073-G [pii]

304. Eschbach JW, Haley NR, Egrie JC, Adamson JW. A comparison of the responses to recombinant human erythropoietin in normal and uremic subjects. *Kidney Int.* 1992;42(2):407-416. (In eng).

305. Mercuriali F, Zanella A, Barosi G, et al. Use of erythropoietin to increase the volume of autologous blood donated by orthopedic patients. *Transfusion.* 1993;33(1):55-60. (In eng).

306. Thomas C, Thomas L. Anemia of chronic disease: pathophysiology and laboratory diagnosis. *Lab Hematol.* 2005;11(1):14-23. (In eng). doi: 10.1532/lh96.04049

307. Ferguson BJ, Skikne BS, Simpson KM, Baynes RD, Cook JD. Serum transferrin receptor distinguishes the anemia of chronic disease from iron deficiency anemia. *J Lab Clin Med.* 1992;119(4):385-390. (In eng).

308. Punnonen K, Irjala K, Rajamaki A. Serum transferrin receptor and its ratio to serum ferritin in the diagnosis of iron deficiency. *Blood.* 1997;89(3):1052-1057. (In eng).

309. Girelli D, Nemeth E, Swinkels DW. Hepcidin in the diagnosis of iron disorders. *Blood.* 2016;127(23):2809-2813. (In eng). doi: 10.1182/blood-2015-12-639112.

310. Castagna A, Campostrini N, Zaninotto F, Girelli D. Hepcidin assay in serum by SELDI-TOF-MS and other approaches. *J Proteomics.* 2010;73(3):527-536. (In eng). doi: 10.1016/j.jprot.2009.08.003

311. Pasricha SR. Is it time for hepcidin to join the diagnostic toolkit for iron deficiency? *Expert Rev Hematol.* 2012;5(2):153-155. (In eng). doi: 10.1586/ehm.12.2

312. Bregman DB, Morris D, Koch TA, He A, Goodnough LT. Hepcidin levels predict nonresponsiveness to oral iron therapy in patients with iron deficiency anemia. *Am J Hematol.* 2013;88(2):97-101. (In eng). doi: 10.1002/ajh.23354

313. Brugnara C, Zurakowski D, DiCanzio J, Boyd T, Platt O. Reticulocyte hemoglobin content to diagnose iron deficiency in children. *JAMA.* 1999;281(23):2225-2230. (In eng).

314. Macdougall IC. What is the most appropriate strategy to monitor functional iron deficiency in the dialysed patient on rhEPO therapy? Merits of percentage hypo-chromic red cells as a marker of functional iron deficiency. *Nephrol Dial Transplant.* 1998;13(4):847-849. (In eng).

315. Hicsonmez G, Suzer K, Suloglu G, Donmez S. Platelet counts in children with iron deficiency anemia. *Acta Haematol.* 1978;60(2):85-89. (In eng).

316. Xavier-Ferrucio J, Scanlon V, Li X, et al. Low iron promotes megakaryocytic com-mitment of megakaryocytic-erythroid progenitors in humans and mice. *Blood.* 2019;134(18):1547-1557, doi: 10.1182/blood.2019002039

317. Hill RS, Pettit JE, Tattersall MH, Kiley N, Lewis SM. Iron deficiency and dyseryth-ropoiesis. *Br J Haematol.* 1972;23(4):507-512. (In eng).

318. Lopez A, Cacoub P, Macdougall IC, Peyrin-Biroulet L. Iron deficiency anaemia. *Lancet.* 2016;387(10021):907-916. doi: 10.1016/S0140-6736(15)60865-0

319. Moretti D, Goede JS, Zeder C, et al. Oral iron supplements increase hepcidin and decrease iron absorption from daily or twice-daily doses in iron-depleted young women. *Blood.* 2015;126(17):1981-1989.

320. Stoffel NU, Cercamondi CI, Brittenham G, et al. Iron absorption from oral iron supplements given on consecutive versus alternate days and as single morning doses versus twice-daily split dosing in iron-depleted women: two open-label, ran-domised controlled trials. *Lancet Haematol.* 2017;4(11):e524-e533. doi: 10.1016/S2352-3026(17)30182-5

321. Grebe G, Martinez-Torres C, Layrisse M. Effect of meals and ascorbic acid on the absorption of a therapeutic dose of iron as ferrous and ferric salts. *Curr Ther Res Clin Exp.* 1975;17(4):382-397. (In eng).

322. Ganz T, Bino A, Salusky IB. Mechanism of action and clinical attributes of auryxia((R)) (ferric citrate). *Drugs.* 2019;79(9):957-968. doi: 10.1007/s40265-019-01125-w

323. Khoury A, Pagan KA, Farland MZ. Ferric maltol: a new oral iron formulation for the treatment of iron deficiency in adults. *Ann Pharmacother.* 2021;55(2):222-229. doi: 10.1177/1060028020941014

324. Hallberg L, Ryttinger L, Solvell L. Side-effects of oral iron therapy. A double-blind study of different iron compounds in tablet form. *Acta Med Scand Suppl.* 1966;459:3-10. (In eng).

325. Callender ST. Quick- and slow-release iron: a double-blind trial with a single daily dose regimen. *Br Med J.* 1969;4(5682):531-532. (In eng).

326. Baird IM, Walters RL, Sutton DR. Absorption of slow-release iron and effects of ascorbic acid in normal subjects and after partial gastrectomy. *Br Med J.* 1974;4(5943):505-508. (In eng).

327. Israels MC, Simmons AV. Ferrous sulphate with ascorbic acid in iron-deficiency anaemia. *Lancet.* 1967;1(7503):1297-1299. (In eng).

328. Cacciola E, Consoli U, Giustolisi R. Ascorbic acid deficiency may be a cause of refractoriness to iron-therapy in the treatment of iron-deficiency anemia. *Haematologica.* 1994;79(1):96-97. (In eng).

329. Goodnough LT. The new age of iron: evaluation and management of iron-restricted erythropoiesis. *Semin Hematol.* 2009;46(4):325-327. (In eng). doi: 10.1053/j.semin-hematol.2009.07.002. S0037-1963(09)00105-X [pii]

330. Ruivard M, Laine F, Ganz T, et al. Iron absorption in dysmetabolic iron overload syndrome is decreased and correlates with increased plasma hepcidin. *J Hepatol.* 2009;50(6):1219-1225. (In eng). doi: 10.1016/j.jhep.2009.01.029

331. Koch TA, Myers J, Goodnough LT. Intravenous iron therapy in patients with iron deficiency anemia: dosing considerations. *Anemia.* 2015;2015:763576. (In eng). doi: 10.1155/2015/763576

332. Van Wyck DB, Mangione A, Morrison J, Hadley PE, Jehle JA, Goodnough LT. Large-dose intravenous ferric carboxymaltose injection for iron deficiency anemia in heavy uterine bleeding: a randomized, controlled trial. *Transfusion.* 2009;49(12):2719-2728. (In eng). doi: 10.1111/j.1537-2995.2009.02327.x. TRF2327 [pii].

333. Auerbach M, Goodnough LT, Picard D, Maniatis A. The role of intravenous iron in anemia management and transfusion avoidance. *Transfusion.* 2008;48(5):988-1000. (In eng). doi: 10.1111/j.1537-2995.2007.01633.x. TRF01633 [pii].

334. Inker LA, Astor BC, Fox CH, et al. KDOQI US commentary on the 2012 KDIGO clinical practice guideline for the evaluation and management of CKD. *Am J Kidney Dis.* 2014;63(5):713-735. (In eng). doi: 10.1053/j.ajkd.2014.01.416

335. Silverberg DS, Iaina A, Peer G, et al. Intravenous iron supplementation for the treat-ment of the anemia of moderate to severe chronic renal failure patients not receiving dialysis. *Am J Kidney Dis.* 1996;27(2):234-238. (In eng).

336. Coyne DW, Kapoian T, Suki W, et al. Ferric gluconate is highly efficacious in anemic hemodialysis patients with high serum ferritin and low transferrin satura-tion: results of the Dialysis Patients' Response to IV Iron with Elevated Ferritin (DRIVE) Study. *J Am Soc Nephrol.* 2007;18(3):975-984. (In eng). doi: 10.1681/asn.2006091034

337. Gasche C, Dejaco C, Waldhoer T, et al. Intravenous iron and erythropoietin for ane-mia associated with Crohn disease. A randomized, controlled trial. *Ann Intern Med.* 1997;126(10):782-787. (In eng).

338. Schreiber S, Howaldt S, Schnoor M, et al. Recombinant erythropoietin for the treat-ment of anemia in inflammatory bowel disease. *N Engl J Med.* 1996;334(10):619-623. (In eng). doi: 10.1056/nejm199603073341002

339. Auerbach M. Ferumoxytol as a new, safer, easier-to-administer intravenous iron: yes or no? *Am J Kidney Dis.* 2008;52(5):826-829. (In eng). doi: 10.1053/j.ajkd.2008.09.006

340. Thurnham DI. Interactions between nutrition and immune function: using inflammation biomarkers to interpret micronutrient status. *Proc Nutr Soc.* 2014;73(1):1-8.

341. Hillman RS, Henderson PA. Control of marrow production by the level of iron supply. *J Clin Invest.* 1969;48(3):454-460. (In eng). doi: 10.1172/jci106002

342. Wood JK, Milner PF, Pathak UN. The metabolism of iron-dextran given as a total-dose infusion to iron deficient Jamaican subjects. *Br J Haematol.* 1968;14(2):119-129. (In eng).

343. Beamish MR, Davies AG, Eakins JD, Jacobs A, Trevett D. The measurement of reticuloendothelial iron release using iron-dextran. *Br J Haematol.* 1971;21(6):617-622. (In eng).

344. Bentley DP, Williams P. Parenteral iron therapy in the anaemia of rheumatoid arthritis. *Rheumatol Rehabil.* 1982;21(2):88-92. (In eng).

345. Sultan P, Bampoe S, Shah R, et al. Oral vs intravenous iron therapy for postpartum anemia: a systematic review and meta-analysis. *Am J Obstet Gynecol.* 2019;221(1):19-29 e3. doi: 10.1016/j.ajog.2018.12.016

346. Auerbach M, Ballard H, Trout JR, et al. Intravenous iron optimizes the response to recombinant human erythropoietin in cancer patients with chemotherapy-related anemia: a multicenter, open-label, randomized trial. *J Clin Oncol.* 2004;22(7):1301-1307. (In eng). doi: 10.1200/jco.2004.08.119

347. Henry DH, Dahl NV, Auerbach M, Tchekmedyian S, Laufman LR. Intravenous ferric gluconate significantly improves response to epoetin alfa versus oral iron or no iron in anemic patients with cancer receiving chemotherapy. *Oncologist.* 2007;12(2):231-242. (In eng). doi: 10.1634/theoncologist.12-2-231

348. Hedenus M, Birgegard G, Nasman P, et al. Addition of intravenous iron to epoetin beta increases hemoglobin response and decreases epoetin dose requirement in anemic patients with lymphoproliferative malignancies: a randomized multicenter study. *Leukemia.* 2007;21(4):627-632. (In eng). doi: 10.1038/sj.leu.2404562

349. Bastit L, Vandebroek A, Altintas S, et al. Randomized, multicenter, controlled trial comparing the efficacy and safety of darbepoetin alpha administered every 3 weeks with or without intravenous iron in patients with chemotherapy-induced anemia. *J Clin Oncol.* 2008;26(10):1611-1618. (In eng). doi: 10.1200/jco.2006.10.4620

350. Auerbach M, Silberstein PT, Webb RT, et al. Darbepoetin alfa 300 or 500 mg once every 3 weeks with or without intravenous iron in patients with chemotherapy-induced anemia. *Am J Hematol.* 2010;85(9):655-663. (In eng). doi: 10.1002/ajh.21779

351. Warnecke C, Zaborowska Z, Kurreck J, et al. Differentiating the functional role of hypoxia-inducible factor (HIF)-1alpha and HIF-2alpha (EPAS-1) by the use of RNA interference: erythropoietin is a HIF-2alpha target gene in Hep3B and Kelly cells. *FASEB J.* 2004;18(12):1462-1464.

352. Weinberg ED. Iron withholding: a defense against infection and neoplasia. *Physiol Rev.* 1984;64(1):65-102.

353. Crosby WH. The rationale for treating iron deficiency anemia. *Arch Intern Med.* 1984;144(3):471-472. (In eng).

354. Ruchala P, Nemeth E. The pathophysiology and pharmacology of hepcidin. *Trends Pharmacol Sci.* 2014;35(3):155-161. (In eng). doi: 10.1016/j.tips.2014.01.004

355. Hamstra RD, Block MH, Schocket AL. Intravenous iron dextran in clinical medicine. *JAMA.* 1980;243(17):1726-1731. (In eng).

356. Wang C, Graham DJ, Kane RC, et al. Comparative risk of anaphylactic reactions associated with intravenous iron products. *JAMA.* 2015;314(19):2062-2068. (In eng). doi: 10.1001/jama.2015.15572

357. Macdougall IC, Bircher AJ, Eckardt KU, et al. Iron management in chronic kidney disease—conclusions from a "kidney disease: improving global outcomes" (KDIGO) controversies conference. *Kidney Int.* 2016;89(1):28-39. (In eng). doi: 10.1016/j.kint.2015.10.002

358. Auerbach M, Adamson J, Bircher A, et al. On the safety of intravenous iron, evidence trumps conjecture. *Haematologica.* 2015;100(5):e214-5. (In eng). doi: 10.3324/haematol.2014.121004

359. Trumbo H, Kaluza K, Numan S, Goodnough LT. Frequency and associated costs of anaphylaxis-and hypersensitivity-related adverse events for intravenous iron products in the USA: an analysis using the US food and drug administration adverse event reporting system. *Drug Saf.* 2021;44(1):107-119. doi: 10.1007/s40264-020-01022-2

360. Kalantar-Zadeh K, Ganz T, Trumbo H, Seid MH, Goodnough LT, Levine MA. Parenteral iron therapy and phosphorus homeostasis: a review. *Am J Hematol.* 2021;96(5):606-616. doi: 10.1002/ajh.26100

361. Beaton GH. Iron needs during pregnancy: do we need to rethink our targets? *Am J Clin Nutr.* 2000;72(1 suppl):265S-271S.

362. Haram K, Nilsen ST, Ulvik RJ. Iron supplementation in pregnancy--evidence and controversies. *Acta Obstet Gynecol Scand.* 2001;80(8):683-688. (In eng).

363. U.S. Preventive Services. *Iron Deficiency Anemia in Pregnant Women: Screening and Supplementation.* Accessed August 29, 2016 http://www.uspreventiveservicestaskforce.org/Page/Document/UpdateSummaryFinal/iron-deficiency-anemia-in-pregnant-women-screening-and-supplementation

364. Morris CC. Recent trends in pediatric iron poisonings. *South Med J.* 2000;93(12):1229. (In eng).

365. Wallack MK, Winkelstein A. Acute iron intoxication in an adult. *JAMA.* 1974;229(10):1333-1334. (In eng).

366. Mills KC, Curry SC. Acute iron poisoning. *Emerg Med Clin North Am.* 1994;12(2):397-413. (In eng).

Disorders of Red Blood Cells

Chapter 26 ▪ Sideroblastic Anemias

MARK D. FLEMING

INTRODUCTION

The sideroblastic anemias (SAs) are a heterogeneous group of bone marrow disorders uniquely characterized by pathologic iron deposits in erythroblast mitochondria (*Figure 26.1A*).[1-4] Iron-encrusted mitochondria account for the so-called ring sideroblast, an erythroblast in which numerous Prussian blue–positive granules appear in a perinuclear distribution on bone marrow aspirate preparations (*Figure 26.1B*); definitive mitochondrial localization requires transmission electron microscopy, which is not typically performed on clinical samples.

When known, the basis for the mitochondrial iron accumulation in the SAs is a consequence of primary defects in heme biosynthesis, iron-sulfur (Fe-S) cluster biogenesis, or mitochondrial protein synthesis and/or oxidative phosphorylation, creating an imbalance between mitochondrial iron import and utilization. Iron delivery to the erythroid cell does not appear to be downregulated in the face of these alterations, and iron continues to be transported normally to mitochondria, where it accumulates.[5,6] In some cases, particularly those situations wherein heme synthesis is impaired, globin synthesis is also secondarily reduced.[7,8]

Similar to other erythroid disorders with defective cytoplasmic or nuclear maturation, the SAs are characterized by variable degrees of ineffective erythropoiesis.[9,10] Erythroid hyperplasia of the bone marrow may be accompanied by a reduced, normal, or only slightly increased reticulocyte count, depending on the contribution of a coexisting reduction in red blood cell (RBC) survival. The plasma iron turnover rate is increased, but iron incorporation into circulating red cells is reduced. A slight hyperbilirubinemia as well as an increase in urobilinogen excretion may be noted as a result of a raised erythropoietic component of the "early-label" bilirubin peak.[11] Thus, it can be inferred that a substantial proportion of the developing ring sideroblasts are nonviable and their apoptosis within the marrow accounts for the kinetic abnormalities.[12-14]

The mean corpuscular volume (MCV) varies considerably from one form of SA to another. Often, RBC dimorphism is conspicuous, with a hypochromic/microcytic population of cells existing side by side with a normal or macrocytic one (*Figure 26.1C* and *D*). In most cases, the red cell distribution width (RDW) is increased. The siderotic mitochondria of the developing cell may be retained in some circulating erythrocytes—Pappenheimer bodies on the Wright-stained blood smear—and are regularly found with concurrent hypofunction or absence of the spleen; these cells are the nearly pathognomonic siderocytes that are also demonstrable on iron-stained peripheral smears (*Figure 26.1E* and *F*).[15] While historical classifications, particularly of the myelodysplastic syndromes with ring sideroblasts, often emphasized a minimum fraction of erythroblasts being ring sideroblasts required to support the diagnosis of SA, it is increasingly evident that even an occasional definitive ring sideroblast can be an important clue to making a molecular diagnosis. Conversely, some congenital anemias not regarded as sideroblastic per se, particularly β-thalassemia and congenital dyserythropoietic anemia type I, may have moderate number of cells that are indistinguishable from ring sideroblasts on iron-stained aspirate smears.

A common feature of many irreversible SAs is an excess of total body iron. The serum iron concentration is increased, even in the absence of transfusion, often to the point of complete saturation of transferrin, and the level of serum ferritin roughly reflects the degree of iron overload. The ineffective erythropoiesis mediates increased intestinal absorption of iron by suppressing hepcidin production by a mechanism that involves the erythroid factor erythroferrone, which sequesters bone morphogenetic proteins that ordinarily stimulates hepcidin production in the liver.[16-20] The consequent iron overloaded state is called erythropoietic hemochromatosis, a form of secondary iron overload, and its clinical and pathologic features and course can rival those of hereditary hemochromatosis (see Chapter 27).[21,22] Concomitant genetic hemochromatosis may accentuate the iron overload,[23-25] but its prevalence in patients with SA does not appear to be greater than that in the general population.[26-28]

The causes of SA are diverse (*Table 26.1*). Within the congenital group, the nonsyndromic forms appear as isolated anemia; X-linked SA (XLSA) and an autosomal recessive type caused by defects in SLC25A38 occur most frequently. Less common are a number of syndromically diverse forms involving multiple organ systems. Acquired SA is much more common than the congenital types and occurs in middle-aged and older individuals as a clonal disorder, manifesting only anemia or multilineage dysplasia or myeloproliferative features. Diverse environmental factors, such as ethanol, certain drugs, copper deficiency, and hypothermia, produce a sideroblastic phenotype that is fully reversible.

HISTORICAL ASPECTS

The history of SAs can be said to have begun in 1945 with Cooley's report of a family with X-linked microcytic hypochromic anemia.[29] Nearly synchronously, iron-containing granules in erythroblasts, including their peculiar perinuclear distribution, were described separately[30,31] and 10 years later were demonstrated to represent iron-laden mitochondria.[2] Over the next 2 decades, these ring sideroblasts were recognized in pyridoxine-responsive anemia and in numerous patients with "refractory anemia" of unknown cause, hereditary or acquired, forming the basis for a 1965 symposium and adoption of the term SA.[3] By then, concurrent iron overload was also fully appreciated.[32,33] With the advent of modern genetic techniques such as DNA mutation analysis, positional cloning, and whole exome sequencing, beginning in 1992 the genetic causes of SAs and their pathogenesis progressively succumbed to discovery, such that now a great majority can be attributed to germline or somatic mutations in specific genes.[34]

HEME SYNTHESIS IN ERYTHROID CELLS

Developing erythroid cells have the greatest requirement of any cell type for heme; more than 70% of the body heme is in the form of hemoglobin. The expression and regulation of erythroid heme synthesis are unique in that they are linked to (a) the differentiation events occurring in response to erythropoietin signaling on erythroid precursors that induces the machinery for porphyrin synthesis, (b) the availability of iron, and (c) the production of globin during the development of the red cell. As in hepatocytes, 5-aminolevulinate (ALA) synthase (ALAS) and hydroxymethylbilane synthase (HMBS, also known as porphobilinogen [PBG] deaminase), have considerably lower relative activities than the remaining enzymes in the heme biosynthetic pathway (see Chapter 6) and are sites of pathway regulation.[35] In contrast to the liver, the relative activity of ferrochelatase, the terminal enzyme in the pathway, also appears to be low in erythroid cells. Furthermore, developing red cells express erythroid-specific isozymes or, alternatively spliced messenger RNA (mRNA) transcripts of the first four enzymes of heme synthesis, namely, ALAS, ALA dehydratase, HMBS, and uroporphyrinogen III synthase.

ALAS, the first and rate-controlling enzyme of heme synthesis, is translated in the cytosol as a precursor protein with an N-terminal signal sequence that is proteolytically cleaved and processed upon

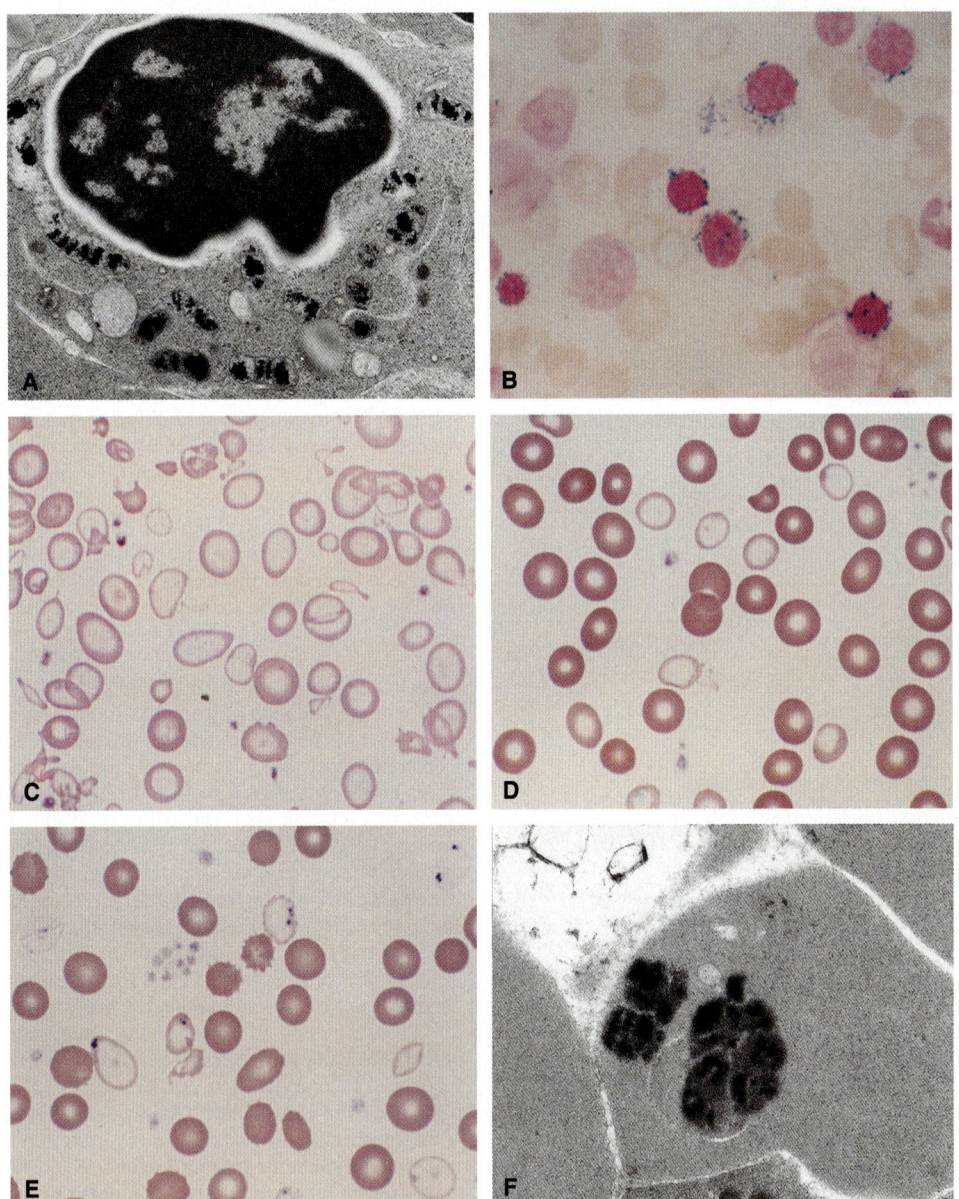

FIGURE 26.1 Morphologic features of sideroblastic anemia. A, Electron micrograph of an erythroblast with iron-laden mitochondria. B, Bone marrow smear (Prussian blue stain) with ring sideroblasts. C and D, Blood smears (Wright stain) of severe and mild sideroblastic anemia. E, Siderocytes (Wright stain). F, Electron micrograph of a Pappenheimer body in a peripheral red blood cell.

transport into the mitochondrial matrix.[36,37] The mature mitochondrial protein catalyzes the formation of ALA from glycine and succinyl coenzyme A (CoA) and requires pyridoxal 5′-phosphate (PLP) as a cofactor. The erythroid-specific mitochondrial carrier family protein SLC25A38 transports glycine from the cytosol across the mitochondrial inner membrane to meet the high requirement of ALAS for this substrate.[38,39] Two distinct genes encode ALAS isoenzymes.[40,41] The housekeeping gene, *ALAS1*, located on chromosome 3,[41,42] is expressed ubiquitously,[43] whereas the erythroid-specific gene, *ALAS2*, is on the X chromosome.[40,41,44,45] Expression of the housekeeping gene, at least in hepatocytes, is controlled by glucose levels and is increased by certain steroids, drugs, and chemicals, playing a role in the development of the acute hepatic porphyrias (see Chapter 28). ALAS1 protein is negatively regulated by heme, the end product of the pathway, so that heme levels tightly regulate ALAS1 activity in a feedback manner.[43] Expression of the erythroid isoform is essential for hemoglobin production in erythroblasts, and ALAS1 cannot compensate for a lack of ALAS2.[46] *ALAS2* is transcribed in concert with other erythroid genes through the action of

erythropoietin[36,43] (*Figure 26.2*); it is not repressed by heme but is upregulated by hypoxia.[47] Cellular iron supply also controls *ALAS2* mRNA levels,[48] whereas exogenous heme inhibits translation of *ALAS2* mRNA.[49] Translation of *ALAS2* mRNA is regulated by interaction of its cis-acting iron-responsive element (IRE)[50,51] with iron regulatory proteins (IRP1 and IRP2; also called IRE binding proteins 1 and 2)[52-54] that are modulated through Fe-S clusters or heme generated in mitochondria in response to cellular iron status (*Figure 26.2*) (see Chapter 25).[55,56] In this manner, regulation of protoporphyrin production is linked to iron availability and mitochondrial function. The low ALAS activity observed in erythroid cells in iron deficiency is consistent with such a control mechanism.[57] Although the signal sequences of the ALAS1 and ALAS2 precursor proteins contain two heme-binding motifs implicated in regulating translocation of the enzyme into mitochondria by interaction of heme with these motifs (*Figure 26.2*),[58,59] mitochondrial import of ALAS2 does not appear to be affected by heme.[60] It had been suggested that ALAS2 uniquely associates with the succinyl-CoA synthetase βA subunit to stabilize the ALAS2, to control the generation of its substrate succinyl-CoA,

Table 26.1. Classification of the Sideroblastic Anemias

Congenital SA
Nonsyndromic
X-linked sideroblastic anemia
SLC25A38 deficiency
Iron-sulfur cluster biogenesis deficiency (HSPA9, HSCB, and GLRX5 deficiency)
Associated with erythropoietic protoporphyria
Syndromic
X-linked sideroblastic anemia with ataxia
Congenital sideroblastic anemia and B-cell immunodeficiency (SIFD)
Pearson marrow-pancreas syndrome
Myopathy, lactic acidosis, and sideroblastic anemia and related disorders
Thiamine-responsive megaloblastic anemia
Acquired clonal SA
Refractory anemia with ring sideroblasts (MDS-RS-SLD)
Refractory cytopenia with multilineage dysplasia and ring sideroblasts
Refractory anemia with ring sideroblasts and thrombocytosis
Reversible SA: associated with
Alcoholism
Certain drugs (isoniazid, chloramphenicol, linezolid)
Copper deficiency (nutritional, malabsorption, zinc ingestion, copper chelation)
Hypothermia

Abbreviations: MDS, myelodysplastic syndrome; MDS-RS-SLD, MDS with ring sideroblasts and single lineage dysplasia; SA, sideroblastic anemia; SIFD, sideroblastic anemia with B-cell immunodeficiency, periodic fevers, and developmental delay.

or both.[61] However, recent metabolomic data indicate that the majority of succinyl-CoA required for heme synthesis derives from deamination of glutamate to α-ketoglutarate and subsequent conversion to succinyl-CoA by α-ketoglutarate dehydrogenase (KDH). This apparently occurs *without* equilibrating through the tricarboxylic acid cycle and may be facilitated by a direct interaction between ALAS2 and KDH.[62]

ALA dehydratase (ALAD), a cytosolic Fe-S enzyme,[63] catalyzes the formation of the pyrrole PBG from two molecules of ALA. Two tissue-specific isozymes are produced by a single gene, which contains two promoter regions, generating housekeeping and erythroid-specific transcripts with alternative noncoding first exons.[64,65] Although both transcripts encode identical polypeptides, the erythroid-regulated form provides for the production of the large amounts of heme for hemoglobin. ALAD is not a rate-limiting enzyme for heme biosynthesis, as it is present in many fold excess amounts.[35]

HMBS, which forms the linear tetrapyrrole hydroxymethylbilane from four molecules of PBG in the cytosol (see Chapter 6), is also expressed as two tissue-specific isozymes from a single gene,[66] owing to the presence of two overlapping transcriptional units, each with its own promoter: an upstream ubiquitous promoter and a downstream promoter active only in erythroid cells. Alternative splicing generates two mRNAs. One encodes the ubiquitous HMBS enzyme, and the other encodes the erythroid-specific isozyme. To what extent the erythroid-specific enzyme has a regulatory role in the overall production of heme in erythroid cells is not known. In response to erythropoietin or hypoxia, bone marrow HMBS activity increases 3.5-fold, apparently by de novo synthesis.[67]

The gene for uroporphyrinogen III synthase, likewise, has two promoters that result in housekeeping and erythroid-specific transcripts with unique 5′-untranslated sequences.[68] As for ALAD and HMBS,

the erythroid-promoter activity is increased during erythroid differentiation. Uroporphyrinogen decarboxylase, the fifth enzyme of the pathway, located in the cytosol, is not known to have distinctive regulation in erythroid cells; however, its mRNA is markedly increased in erythroid tissue[69] and the enzyme activity is higher in erythroid cells than in the liver.[35]

After translation, the three terminal enzymes of heme biosynthesis (coproporphyrinogen oxidase, protoporphyrinogen oxidase, and ferrochelatase), such as ALAS, are transported to their mitochondrial site of action. Single genes encode these enzymes, and erythroid-specific transcription products are not known for them. However, erythroid-specific regulation of their expression is accommodated by the presence of promoter sequences in their genes for binding of erythroid transcription factors (e.g., GATA binding factor 1 [GATA1] and nuclear factor erythroid 2 [NFE2])[70-72] to enhance production of these enzymes during erythropoiesis.[73] Ferrochelatase, the last enzyme of the heme synthetic pathway, catalyzes the insertion of iron into protoporphyrin to form heme. Relative to the activity of ALAS, ferrochelatase is in considerable excess,[35,74] but the enzyme becomes rate limiting as a defective protein in erythropoietic protoporphyria (see Chapter 28). Because it contains an Fe-S cluster, its expression and stability are also dependent on cellular iron levels and Fe-S cluster biogenesis.[75,76] Its activity is further regulated by an essential mitochondrial ATPase inhibitory factor 1 (ATPIF1) through modulation of mitochondrial pH and redox potential.[77]

The large amounts of iron required for erythroid heme synthesis are delivered through transferrin receptor–mediated endocytosis of iron transferrin (see Chapter 25), and iron availability ultimately limits heme synthesis in erythroid cells.[78] High expression of transferrin receptors is also linked to erythropoietin-induced differentiation.[43,78] With erythroid maturation and the accumulation of cellular hemoglobin, the transferrin receptor number progressively decreases.[78] While surface transferrin receptors and iron uptake are increased in iron-deficient erythroblasts,[79,80] they are not altered in states of impaired heme synthesis, such as in the presence of succinylacetone[81] or in erythroid cells from patients with SA.[5] Transport of iron out of the endosome by the divalent metal transporter DMT1 requires an endosomal ferrireductase (Steap3) in erythroid cells.[82] How the further transfer of iron to mitochondria and to apoferritin is accomplished is not understood. It may be facilitated by a cytoplasmic chaperone[83] or through direct interaction of endosomes with mitochondria.[84] Iron is imported across the mitochondrial inner membrane by mitoferrin 1 (SLC25A37), which is highly expressed in erythroid cells and stabilized by interacting with the ATP-binding cassette protein ABCB10.[85,86] An oligomeric complex of mitoferrin 1, ABCB10, and ferrochelatase appears to facilitate the incorporation of iron into protoporphyrin to form heme.[87] Iron imported into the mitochondrion is also used for the generation of Fe-S clusters, which in part are exported to the cytosol by an ABCB7-dependent process for their addition to IRP1 and other cytosolic Fe-S proteins[56] required for the regulation of the translation of *ALAS2* mRNA,[88] and for the expression and stabilization of ferrochelatase and ALAD.[63,75,76]

The export of heme out of the mitochondrion into the cytosol for its pairing with globins of hemoglobin and other cytosolic heme proteins is mediated at least in the mouse by an isoform of the feline leukemia virus C receptor (FLVCR1), named FLVCR1b.[89]

The events coordinating the production of globin chains with the rate of heme synthesis are well understood. Beyond the orchestration of the erythroid differentiation program by erythroid-specific transcription factors, heme controls globin gene expression at the transcriptional level.[90,91] Heme is also required for initiation of globin mRNA translation, and it acts by inhibiting a protein kinase called heme-regulated inhibitor (HRI), which inactivates the translational initiation factor 2-α (eIF2α) in the absence of heme (Figure 26.2).[92] Moreover, the absence of this kinase adversely modifies the phenotype of disorders of heme synthesis (iron deficiency, protoporphyria) and of globin production (β-thalassemia).[92]

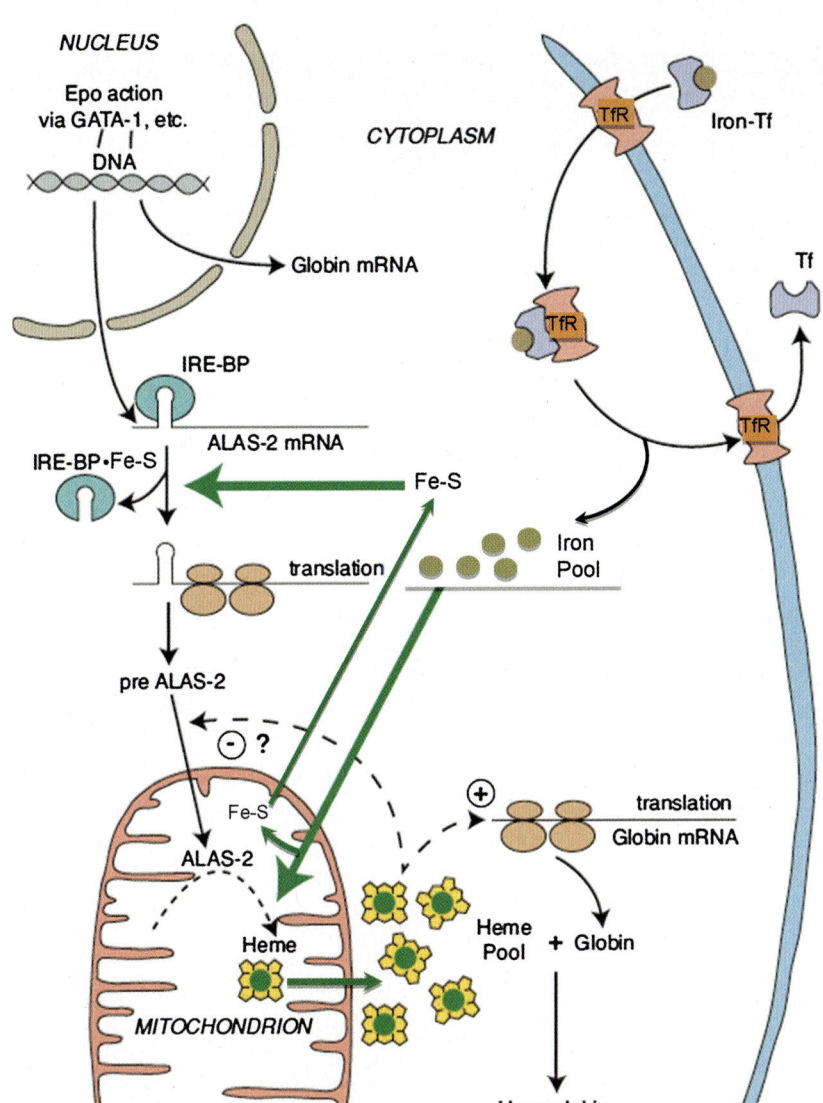

FIGURE 26.2 Pathways of regulation of erythroid 5-aminolevulinate synthase (ALAS2). Epo, erythropoietin; Fe-S, iron-sulfur cluster; IRE-BP, iron-responsive element binding protein; mRNA, messenger RNA; Tf, transferrin; TfR, transferrin receptor; −, inhibition; +, stimulation. (Modified from May BK, Dogra SC, Sadlon TJ, et al. Molecular regulation of heme biosynthesis in higher vertebrates. *Prog Nucleic Acid Res Mol Biol.* 1995;51:1-51. Copyright © 1995 Academic Press Inc. With permission.)

CONGENITAL SIDEROBLASTIC ANEMIAS

The congenital SAs are not uncommon. They are clinically and genetically heterogeneous, with diverse underlying causes, inheritance patterns, RBC phenotypes, and other associated features (*Table 26.2*). The severity of anemia is highly variable even within a specific diagnosis, and clinical features are often overlapping between diagnoses. Many are nonsyndromic, appearing as isolated anemia without other hematologic or systemic effects. The syndromic forms also have nonhematologic manifestations that may be the predominant clinical phenotype. Genetic analysis has revealed a spectrum of specific abnormalities. At present, the defined underlying defects fall into three general and interconnected pathways: heme biosynthesis, Fe-S cluster biogenesis, and mitochondrial protein synthesis or respiration. However, in about one-third of cases, a genetic cause remains undiscovered.[34]

Nonsyndromic Congenital Sideroblastic Anemias
Inheritance Patterns, Molecular Basis, and Pathogenesis

X-Linked Sideroblastic Anemia
This form of SA is by far the most common cause of congenital disease and is due to mutations in ALAS2. Although it is not the only form of XLSA, as the name would suggest, the inheritance follows an X-linked pattern, with the anemia occurring most commonly in males. A clue to the diagnosis is often coexistence of anemia in a patient's maternal uncles or male cousins.[29,93-99] Minimal expression of the erythroid abnormality may be seen in carrier females, which is consistent with stochastic X-chromosome. However, in many kindreds, the anemia has occurred only in females[100-104]; in these cases the genetic defect is typically lethal in hemizygous male conceptions.[105]

Early observations implicated defects in ALAS as underlying the impaired heme biosynthesis in this form of SA. In patients who responded to pyridoxine supplementation, the incorporation of glycine, but not of ALA, into heme was reduced in reticulocytes.[106] ALAS activity in bone marrow was low before pyridoxine administration and returned to normal or supranormal levels after an erythropoietic response.[98,107,108] It was presumed that the residual activity or stability of a defective erythroid ALAS was enhanced by additional supply of its coenzyme PLP through a mass action effect (e.g., if the enzyme had a reduced affinity for the coenzyme[108] or was abnormally sensitive to proteolysis).[109] Pharmacologic amounts of pyridoxine are typically required to induce an erythropoietic response, but the response is variable and rarely is the hemoglobin completely normalized. Individuals may present with profound anemia only in adulthood or even very late in life,[98,110-112] suggesting that the disorder can progress with time. In some cases, prior additional dietary or medicinal intake of pyridoxine,[113] possible changes in pyridoxine metabolism with advancing age,[114] or initiation of hemodialysis[115,116] can be factors in unmasking milder phenotypes that were not symptomatic at a younger age.

Table 26.2. Genetic and Hematologic Features of the Congenital Sideroblastic Anemias

	Mode of Inheritance	Defective Enzyme/ Protein	Gene/ Chromosomal Location of Gene	Erythrocyte		Severity of Anemia
				Mean Corpuscular Volume	Protoporphyrin	
X-linked Sideroblastic Anemia	X-linked	ALAS2	*ALAS2*/Xp11.21	Decreased[a]	Decreased	Mild to severe
Mitochondrial Glycine Carrier Deficiency	Autosomal recessive	SLC25A38	*SLC25A38*/3p22.1	Decreased	Decreased	Severe
Iron-Sulfur Cluster Biogenesis Deficiency	Autosomal recessive	HSPA9, HSCB, Glutaredoxin 5	*HSPA9*/5q31.1, *HSCB*/22q12.1, *GLRX5*/14q32.13	Decreased Decreased Decreased	Not reported Not reported	Moderate Moderate Severe
Erythropoietic Protoporphyria	Autosomal recessive	Ferrochelatase	*FECH*/18q21.3	Decreased	Markedly increased	Mild
X-linked Sideroblastic Anemia with Ataxia	X-linked	ABCB7 mitochondrial transporter	*ABCB7*/Xq13.3	Decreased	Increased	Mild
CSA and B-cell Immunodeficiency (SIFD)	Autosomal recessive	tRNA nucleotidyl transferase	*TRNT1*/3p25.1	Decreased	Not reported	Severe
Myopathy, Lactic Acidosis, and Sideroblastic Anemia (MLASA) Variants	Autosomal recessive	Pseudouridine synthase 1 Mitochondrial tyrosyl tRNA synthetase 2 NADH dehydrogenase Mitochondrial leucyl-tRNA synthetase	*PUS1*/12q24.33 *YARS2*/12p11.21 *NDUFB11*/Xp11.23 *LARS2*/3p21.3	Normal/ increased Normal/ increased Normal/ increased Not reported	Not reported Not reported Not reported Not reported	Severe Moderate to severe Moderate Severe
	Maternal	ATP synthase 6	*MT-ATP6*/mitochondrial	Decreased/ normal	Not reported	Moderate to Severe
Pearson Syndrome	Maternal	Respiratory chain components	*Multiple*/mitochondrial	Increased	Increased	Severe
Thiamine-Responsive Megaloblastic Anemia	Autosomal recessive	Thiamine transporter	*SLC19A2*/1q23.3	Increased	Normal/increased	Mild to severe

[a]Often normal or increased in females expressing the disorder.
Abbreviations: ATP, adenosine triphosphate; CSA, congenital sideroblastic anemia; tRNA, transfer RNA.

In female patients expressing the disease, skewed X-chromosome inactivation in hematopoietic tissue that occurs with advancing age,[117] or, in certain cases, a familial predisposition to X-chromosome skewing, involving progressive inactivation of the X chromosome bearing the normal allele, has been the explanation as the anemia usually evolved in adulthood[103,104] or late in life.[118] Constitutive skewed X inactivation to account for disease expression in females in childhood is uncommon, but reported.

After the cloning and characterization of *ALAS2*,[50,119] and its localization to the X chromosome, linkage of the disorder to the locus was established,[98,120] and many heterogeneous missense mutations involving invariant or highly conserved amino acid residues in the catalytic domain of the enzyme have been found to cause the disorder (*Figure 26.2*).[121] The underlying molecular defect in ALAS2 has even been defined[25,122-124] in several of the index families described in the 1940s.[29,94,97,125] Nonsense mutations, splicing alleles, and mutations in the promoter region of the *ALAS2* gene have been the exceptions; null mutations are seen only in heterozygous females. A small minority of families have a mutation in a GATA1 transcription factor binding site in an enhancer element located in intron 1 of the gene.[126,127] A majority of the mutations reside in exons 5 and 9; the latter contains the PLP-binding lysine (Lys391) of the enzyme (*Figure 26.3*).[128]

Among over 90 distinct mutations so far encountered, only about 20% have occurred in more than one unrelated family or proband, and close to one-third of the probands are female. An apparent somatic mutation in the *ALAS2* gene was found in an older male patient with acquired SA.[129]

To some extent, the sites of ALAS2 mutations and the severity of anemia or the degree of its responsiveness to pyridoxine supplements can be correlated; many mutations are predictably pyridoxine responsive, whereas others are predictably unresponsive. The activity of the recombinant enzyme is reduced for many, but not all, ALAS2 mutants so far examined and is variably enhanced by PLP.[98,99,112,122,130-132] Some mutants have altered substrate kinetics[132,133] or fail to bind to the β-subunit of succinyl-CoA synthetase.[61,133] A three-dimensional structure model of the human enzyme[134] and the crystal structures of the significantly homologous ALAS of *Rhodobacter capsulatus*[135] and *Saccharomyces cerevisiae*[136] have made it possible to explain how altered structure by many of the naturally occurring mutations that give rise to XLSA affects the function of the enzyme. For example, mutations changing an amino acid located in the vicinity of the PLP-binding site often exhibit a response to pyridoxine, whereas mutations involving sites of substrate binding, enzyme stability, or folding are refractory to pyridoxine.[135,137] However, while clinical severity can be

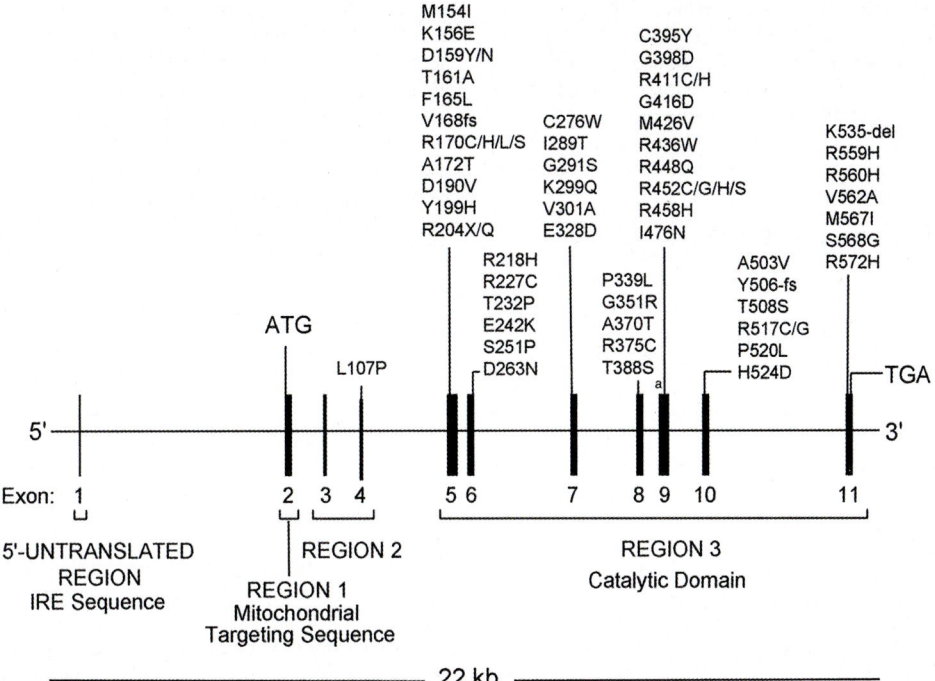

FIGURE 26.3 Diagram of the structure of the human erythroid 5-aminolevulinate synthase gene (*ALAS2*) and the location of a majority of mutations identified in X-linked sideroblastic anemia. Two mutations in the promoter region and mutations disrupting the intron 1 enhancer of ALAS2 are not indicated. ^aCodon 391, the pyridoxal 5′-phosphate binding lysine. ATG, methionine translational start codon; IRE, iron-responsive element; kb, kilobases; TGA, translational stop codon. (Data from Reference 121 and unpublished material.)

related at least in part to the effect of a specific mutation on enzyme function, marked variation in severity of anemia has been observed between some kindreds bearing the same mutation as well as within a few kinships,[98,99,138,139] implicating undefined genetic differences or environmental factors for the apparent variable penetrance.

Mitochondrial Carrier Protein SLC25A38 Deficiency

A significant proportion of congenital SA (~15%), and most of the nonsyndromic, hypochromic microcytic cases without ALAS2 mutations, are due to biallelic mutations in the gene encoding the erythroid-specific mitochondrial inner membrane carrier protein SLC25A38.[38,140] The SLC25A38 protein has an amino terminal mitochondrial targeting signal and three mitochondrial carrier family protein domains that encode six transmembrane helices. From its structural features, the protein is predicated to function as an amino acid transporter. Data obtained in the yeast *S. cerevisiae* deficient in the protein indicated a heme biosynthetic defect and suggested that it serves as a glycine importer across the inner mitochondrial membrane.[38] Glycine transport activity was later confirmed by expression of the protein in proteoliposomes.[39]

Heterogeneous mutations spread throughout the SLC25A38 protein have been reported in more than 90 families, including multiple sibling pairs.[38,121,140-143] Presumptive null alleles, including nonsense, frameshift, and splicing mutations, are most common; however, approximately one-third of mutations are missense variants occurring in conserved amino acids and nearly exclusively in transmembrane domains. Two-thirds of patients are homozygous and one-third are compound heterozygotes for specific mutations, reflecting the increased frequency of rare recessive diseases such as in consanguineous pedigrees. That many patients are complete nulls suggests that there is some, but insufficient, redundancy in the supply of mitochondrial glycine for heme synthesis in erythroid cells, possibly through mechanisms that involve the interconversion of glycine and serine.

Iron-Sulfur Cluster Biogenesis Deficiency

The human counterpart of a zebrafish mutant (*shiraz*) deficient in glutaredoxin 5,[55] which is essential for the synthesis of Fe-S clusters such

as for IRP1 and thus influences ALAS2 translation, has been identified in two patients. In the first, a homozygous mutation in the *GLRX5* gene that affects intron 1 splicing and markedly reduces GLRX5 RNA production was associated with microcytic SA.[144] The anemia was detected in the fifth decade, became severe by age 60 years, and improved with iron chelation therapy for the associated iron overload. Studies in cell lines derived from the patient demonstrated severe impairment of Fe-S cluster biogenesis and revealed markedly reduced levels of ferrochelatase.[145] Biallelic GLRX5 mutations in a second case were also associated with severe microcytic anemia that was improved by iron chelation.[146]

Heterogeneous mutations in *HSPA9*, which encodes the mitochondrial heat shock protein 70 homologue A9 (HSPA9) that serves as a chaperone protein in Fe-S cluster biogenesis, were described in 11 families or isolated cases with normocytic or slightly microcytic SA,[147] including a large family described 30 years earlier.[148] In some cases, a single severe HSPA9 loss-of-function allele is associated with a common synonymous nucleotide polymorphism in the other *HSPA9* allele that is underexpressed; this is a pathogenetic theme also typically true in patients with erythropoietic protoporphyria who have a common intronic variant that reduces protein expression (see Chapter 28). A single patient with compound heterozygous mutations in the HSPA9 cochaperone, HSCB, has been described.[149] These defects likely also lead to repressed *ALAS2* translation, similar to glutaredoxin 5 deficiency.

Sideroblastic Anemia in Erythropoietic Protoporphyria

Marked deficiency of ferrochelatase underlies erythropoietic protoporphyria as a result of a large variety of mutations in the gene encoding the enzyme (see Chapter 28). The defect is expressed in erythroid cells and leads to marked accumulation of metal-free protoporphyrin, the substrate of the enzyme, during the final stages of erythroid maturation when the defective ferrochelatase becomes rate limiting for heme production.[150] Erythroid heme synthesis appears to be sufficiently compromised in most patients to cause a mild microcytic hypochromic anemia.[151] In 10 patients, marrow ring sideroblasts with typical mitochondrial iron deposits were observed,[152,153] but not in one sibling pair with mild microcytosis without anemia.[150] Bone marrow examination has generally not been performed in this disorder, so the incidence of ring sideroblasts is not known. The genetic heterogeneity in protoporphyria likely accounts for the phenotypic variation of the hematologic features; most patients are compound heterozygotes for a common deep intronic variant that is associated with reduced *FECH* mRNA expression and a protein coding variant with markedly reduced ferrochelatase activity, the latter of which are very diverse.[154,155]

Clinical and Laboratory Features of XLSA and SLC25A38 Deficiency

If severe, XLSA is recognized in infancy or early childhood. However, not infrequently, the disorder is mild or even asymptomatic and may be discovered only in young adulthood or even in later life. Because the severity of anemia can also vary within kindreds,[98,99,139] diagnosis in family members may be delayed or overlooked unless complete pedigree studies or DNA analyses for an ALAS2 mutation identified in the proband are performed. In contrast, patients with SLC25A38 genetic defects typically present at birth or in early childhood with severe anemia, requiring transfusion.[143]

In time, nearly all patients develop iron overload. Mild to moderate enlargement of the liver and spleen is common, but liver function is usually normal or only mildly disturbed at presentation. Liver biopsy reveals iron deposition that is indistinguishable from hereditary hemochromatosis (*Figure 26.4*).[33] In the X-linked form, the iron burden does not correlate with the severity of anemia, and, not infrequently, well-established but asymptomatic micronodular cirrhosis is discovered in the third or fourth decade in patients with only mild anemia.[156] Hepatocellular carcinoma developed in two reported cases.[138,157] Clinical diabetes or abnormal glucose tolerance may or may not be related to iron overload. Skin hyperpigmentation is uncommon. The most dangerous manifestations of the iron overload are cardiac arrhythmias and congestive heart failure, which usually occur late in the disease course. In severely affected infants or young children, growth and development tend to be impaired.[96]

The hallmark is a hypochromic microcytic anemia. In severe cases, microcytosis and hypochromia are extreme (mean corpuscular volume [MCV], 50-60 fl), and striking anisocytosis, poikilocytosis, target cells, and occasional siderocytes are prominent findings on blood smear (*Figure 26.1C*). The RDW is usually abnormally wide and, notably, dimorphism is seen in males with the X-linked form as well as in autosomal forms of the disease.[93,140,148] Some female carriers of the X-linked trait have a biphasic red cell volume histogram (*Figure 26.5*) or only a very small microcytic erythrocyte population.[25,97] However, most women who are anemic (i.e., HGB <11 g/dL) because of XLSA exhibit RBC macrocytosis, although dimorphism may be evident (*Figure 26.1D*). Leukocyte and platelet values usually are normal; they may be reduced in the presence of splenomegaly (hypersplenism). Erythroid hyperplasia is found on marrow examination, and maturation is usually normoblastic with poorly hemoglobinized, "ragged" cytoplasm. Megaloblastic changes may be observed if coexisting folate deficiency is present. Marrow macrophage iron is increased, and the telltale ring sideroblast is most prominent among late, nondividing erythroblasts.[158,159] Transferrin saturation is increased, as is the serum ferritin level, and transferrin levels tend to be decreased. Ferrokinetic studies reflect ineffective erythropoiesis. A reduced serum haptoglobin level is consistent with the ineffective erythropoiesis.

The erythrocyte protoporphyrin level is usually low or normal.[9] In one female patient, the low protoporphyrin level was shown to be restricted to the microcytic red cells.[100] Kindreds in which the erythrocyte protoporphyrin is increased[148] can be considered to represent disorders other than XLSA or SLC25A38 deficiency.

Treatment and Prognosis

Approximately two-thirds of patients with SA caused by ALAS2 mutations, but not other forms of the condition, can be expected to respond to pyridoxine administration. Doses of 50 to 100 mg/day are large compared with the estimated adult daily requirement for vitamin B_6 of 1.5 to 2.0 mg and are sufficient for a maximal response, although in some cases a supplement of only 2 to 4 mg/day was found to be effective.[98] Higher doses may be toxic, resulting in neurologic symptoms. No convincing evidence is available that the parenteral route or PLP, the active coenzyme form, is more effective than oral administration. However, the response to pyridoxine is quite variable. With an optimal response, reticulocytosis is observed, blood hemoglobin concentration returns to normal or near-normal levels in 1 to 2 months, and low erythrocyte protoporphyrin levels increase to normal.[9,160] The morphologic red cell abnormalities then diminish but very rarely completely resolve, even when ALAS activity and the hemoglobin level are restored with pyridoxine supplementation. Approximately two-thirds of responding patients experience a distinct but suboptimal improvement with pyridoxine administration, and the hemoglobin concentration stabilizes at less than normal levels. When an effect of pyridoxine is achieved, continued maintenance treatment is necessary because relapses follow within several months after discontinuance of the vitamin. In a few instances, subsequent remissions with resumed treatment were less complete.[9] In the occasional case with accompanying megaloblastic changes or documented folate deficiency, folic acid should be given, which should lead to normoblastic maturation, suboptimal reticulocytosis, and some increase in the hemoglobin level.

Patients with SLC25A38-associated congenital SA nearly invariably require chronic transfusion and are most commonly managed similarly to patients with β-thalassemia major. In severely anemic individuals with ALAS2 mutations who do not respond to pyridoxine, periodic red cell transfusions are necessary to relieve symptoms and to allow normal growth and development of children. However, in most cases, save occasional patients with very severe mutations, such as mutations in the intron 1 GATA1-binding site, chronic transfusion is typically not required.

Depending on the assessed extent of iron overload, by liver biopsy or by hepatic and cardiac magnetic resonance imaging, an iron depletion program should be instituted to prevent or stabilize already established organ damage.[102,161-163] In many patients with mild to moderate XLSA, therapeutic phlebotomy is well tolerated and even preferred in the absence of contraindications such as heart disease.[102,156,164-166] After the initial removal of all storage iron, maintenance phlebotomies should be continued indefinitely. For patients with severe anemia, or for those who depend on regular transfusions and thus become massively iron loaded, an iron-chelating agent is administered.[167,168] As recommended for thalassemia, deferoxamine is infused over 12 hours subcutaneously or intravenously, at 40 mg/kg/day, and for at least 5 days each week.[168] Although iron removal with deferoxamine is enhanced by ascorbate, large supplements can cause acute cardiac toxicity by facilitating excessive mobilization of ferritin iron, and any intake of the vitamin should be limited to 200 mg daily.[169] The risks of deferoxamine treatment are minimal.[162,170] Occasional local reactions can be controlled with the inclusion of small amounts of hydrocortisone in the infusate. Rare hypersensitivity is amenable to desensitization.[171] Reported visual and auditory neurotoxicity is unlikely without excessive doses of the drug. The newer, orally active tridentate iron chelator deferasirox (Exjade) has an efficacy similar to deferoxamine or better[163,172]; the recommended initial daily dose is 20 mg/kg and can be increased to 30 mg/kg. Although the long-term safety profile of this agent is not fully known, it has emerged as a preferred iron chelator. The goal of iron chelation therapy is to maintain the serum ferritin concentration below 500 µg/L. The increased risk of infection with *Yersinia* (and perhaps other organisms) in iron overload, although uncommon, increases further with deferoxamine treatment.[162,173] Removal of the excess iron has occasionally reduced the severity of the anemia[5,25,165,166] by improving erythroblast mitochondrial function, such as restoration of secondary ferrochelatase deficiency[166]; by enhancing pyridoxine responsiveness[25]; and by diminishing the ineffective erythropoiesis.[165]

Splenectomy in congenital SA appears to be nearly invariably complicated by thromboembolic complications and, often, a fatal outcome.[110,111,122,143,174,175] Factors other than persistent thrombocytosis seem to play a role. Control of the platelet count and anticoagulant therapy usually are not effective, so splenectomy is contraindicated

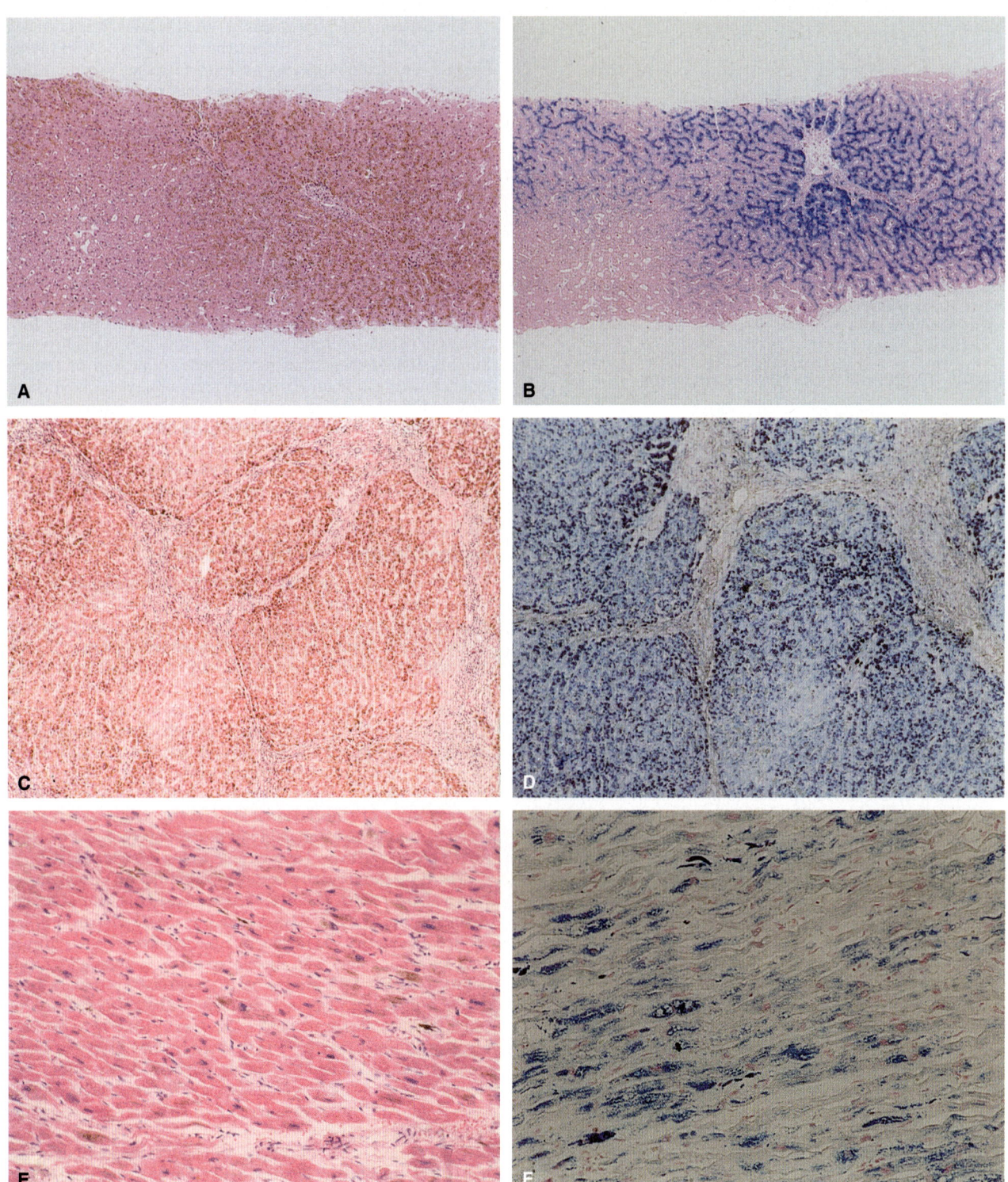

FIGURE 26.4 Histopathology of the iron overload in congenital sideroblastic anemia. A and B, Liver biopsy section of a 26-year-old man with SLC25A38 deficiency and moderate hemochromatosis. C and D, Autopsy liver section of a 45-year-old man with X-linked sideroblastic anemia, micronodular cirrhosis, and hemochromatosis. E and F, Section from the heart of the latter patient with marked hemosiderosis. A, C, and E, Hematoxylin stain; B, D, and F, Prussian blue stain.

save for a case of clinical urgency such as traumatic splenic rupture or otherwise untreatable splenic abscess.

These supportive measures provide for a favorable prognosis and often for normal survival. Curative bone marrow transplantation was achieved in seven reported patients without known molecular defects,[176-180] including recovery from chronic graft-versus-host disease after subsequent orthotopic liver transplantation in one of these cases[181];

one patient succumbed to graft-versus-host disease and prior iron overload.[179] Hematopoietic stem cell transplantation has also been successful in multiple cases with SLC25A38 deficiency[143,182]; pre-implantation diagnosis resulted in unaffected twin offspring in one family.[183]

In contrast to acquired clonal SA, transformation to acute leukemia has not been observed.

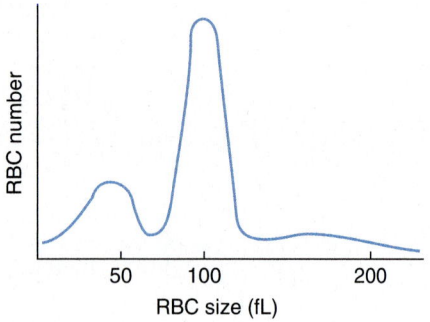

FIGURE 26.5 Dimorphic red cell distribution in a female patient with mild X-linked sideroblastic anemia. RBC, red blood cell. (Redrawn from the output of a Coulter analyzer.)

Syndromic Congenital Sideroblastic Anemias

X-Linked Sideroblastic Anemia With Ataxia

In a large kindred with XLSA associated with nonprogressive ataxia (XLSA/A),[184] linkage to the phosphoglycerate kinase locus at Xq13 was demonstrated[185] and linkage to *ALAS2* was excluded.[45] Cloning and chromosomal mapping to Xq13.1-q13.3 of the human *ABCB7* gene,[186,187] the ortholog of the *ATM1* gene in yeast that encodes a transporter protein required for mitochondrial iron homeostasis and the maturation of cytosolic Fe-S cluster proteins,[188] led to identification of a mutation in this gene as the underlying defect in the kindred.[189] Distinct mutations in the ABCB7 have been identified in four additional families.[190-192] All the mutations result in substitutions of conserved amino acids and affect a region of the protein involved in binding and transport of a substrate. It is postulated that ABCB7 participates in the export of a component, possibly Fe-S complexed with glutathione, from mitochondria required for assembly of cytosolic Fe-S clusters.[193,194] Expression of wild-type ABCB7, but not mutant ABCB7, in Atm1p-deficient yeast restores phenotypic defects as well as the production of cytosolic Fe-S proteins.[190] As in humans with ABCB7 mutations, loss of Atm1p leads to mitochondrial siderosis in the yeast.[193] How heme synthesis becomes impaired in erythroid cells has not been elucidated and may be a consequence of reduced Fe-S cluster biogenesis impacting the translation of ALAS2.[55,145] Because free protoporphyrin, as well as zinc protoporphyrin, accumulates in erythrocytes,[184,190-192] the maturation of ferrochelatase,[76,195] an Fe-S–containing protein, is probably also affected. Neither ALAS nor ferrochelatase has been examined in erythroid cells with the XLSA/A defects. The mechanism for the neural dysfunction in this disorder remains elusive.

Among five kindreds so far encountered, the neurologic features predominate and include delayed motor and cognitive development, incoordination, and nonprogressive cerebellar hypoplasia or atrophy with or without atrophy of the pons and medulla.[184,190-192,196] The anemia is mild to moderate, and morphologic features are indistinguishable from other heritable forms of SA, including variable abnormalities in female carriers, as observed in XLSA. Both free and zinc protoporphyrin are increased. Iron overload has not been evident.

Congenital Sideroblastic Anemia With B-Cell Immunodeficiency, Fevers, and Developmental Delay

This syndrome of severe microcytic SA with B-cell immunodeficiency, periodic fevers, and developmental delay is caused by autosomal recessive biallelic mutations in TRNT1.[197,198] This gene encodes an essential template-independent nucleotidyl transferase that adds the trinucleotide cytosine-cytosine-adenosine (CCA) to the 3′ end of all nuclear and mitochondrial transfer RNAs before they can engage in the polypeptide assembly on ribosomes. The defects lead to metabolic dysfunction in multiple body systems, but their pathogenesis is not defined. At the cellular level, formation of respiratory chain complexes is impaired in patient-derived fibroblasts.[199]

The presentation of the disease is often in infancy and can be quite variable, with a subset of the patients having predominantly immunologic, ophthalmologic, or neurologic, rather than hematologic, compromise.[200,201] Milder phenotypes may present in adulthood. The anemia, unlike most of the other syndromic congenital SAs, tends to be markedly microcytic (MCV 50-70) and hypochromic, likely because of effects on globin protein translation, and often requires chronic transfusion. Neurodegeneration, seizures, cerebellar abnormalities, sensorineural deafness, cardiomyopathy, hepatopathy, and other multisystem derangements are variably present. Many patients have recurrent aseptic febrile episodes, similar to those seen in periodic fever syndromes, which can lead to life-threatening metabolic crises. Early death is commonly attributed to cardiac or multiorgan failure.

Based on the associated immunologic and inflammatory features in this syndrome, anti–tumor necrosis factor (TNF) therapy has been administered in multiple patients, resulting in clinical benefit.[201] Suppression of the inflammatory state, reduction of transfusion requirements, and improved growth were observed. The therapy was most beneficial if initiated early in life. Several patients have undergone successful bone marrow transplantation, whereas others have succumbed in the peri- and posttransplant setting because of exacerbation of inflammatory or metabolic abnormalities. Consequently, stem cell transplantation should be approached with extreme care in these patients.

Pearson Marrow-Pancreas Syndrome

This progressive, congenital multisystem mitochondrial disorder is associated with sporadic large deletions of mitochondrial DNA, leading to the loss of multiple proteins encoded by the mitochondrial genome.[202,203] About one-half of cases are heteroplasmic for a 4977-bp deletion that involves mitochondrially encoded subunits of respiratory complex I (NADH dehydrogenase), complex IV (cytochrome c oxidase), and complex V (ATP synthase) as well as several mitochondrial *tRNA* genes.[202] The spectrum of mitochondrial genomic deletions is nonoverlapping, but all cases involve deletion of at least one of the 22 mitochondrially encoded mitochondrial tRNAs. Thus, translation of mitochondrially encoded proteins would be affected. The heteroplasmic nature of mitochondrial DNA at the cellular and organ levels accounts for the high variability of tissues involved and the potential for the phenotype to evolve over time within one individual.

The disorder generally presents within the first 6 months of life with anemia, failure to thrive, metabolic acidosis, and exocrine pancreatic insufficiency.[204] Also common is the development of hepatic and renal failure. Some infants lack the metabolic derangements, initially presenting only with anemia, resulting in oversight of this syndrome. Typically, 25% are anemic in the neonatal period; by 6 months of age, anemia is evident in 75% of cases. Any associated neutropenia and thrombocytopenia are milder. The anemia tends to be severe and is normocytic or macrocytic.[205] In the bone marrow, erythroid precursors are often reduced in number, and occasionally nearly absent, but ring sideroblasts are usually prominent.[206] A feature shared with several other syndromic SAs is the presence of striking vacuoles in myeloid and erythroid precursors.[207]

Approximately half of patients succumb to the metabolic derangements. The anemia may improve or remit in up to one-third of cases by 10 years of age. Survivors often develop the Kearns-Sayre syndrome (chronic progressive external ophthalmoplegia with myopathy).[203,208] Treatment is supportive, with RBC transfusions required, as necessary for anemia. Owing to multisystem involvement, hematopoietic stem cell transplantation is generally not indicated.

Mitochondrial Myopathy, Lactic Acidosis, and Sideroblastic Anemia and Related Phenotypes

Mitochondrial myopathy, lactic acidosis, and SA (MLASA) was first defined as an autosomal recessive oxidative phosphorylation disorder caused by mutations in pseudouridylate synthase 1 (PUS1).[209,210] Missense and nonsense mutations have been described.[211-213] PUS1 posttranscriptionally modifies uridine to pseudouridine on mitochondrial and cytoplasmic tRNAs, rendering them more stable[214]; decreased PUS1 activity likely causes faulty translation of mitochondrial mRNAs encoding components of respiratory complexes. The disorder is characterized by muscle weakness, resting lactic acidemia, and normocytic SA with clinical onset in childhood or adolescence.[210] Some cases have exhibited intellectual impairment and/or craniofacial abnormalities. Diminished oxidative phosphorylation is reflected in decreased activity of mitochondrial enzymes of the respiratory chain as well as in the raised blood lactic acid level. The myopathy and the anemia are variably progressive, and transfusions are usually required by the third decade of life if not earlier.

Mutations in mitochondrial tyrosyl tRNA synthetase 2 (YARS2) lead to a very similar clinical phenotype (MLASA2), reduce levels of the enzyme, and result in decreased mitochondrial protein synthesis and respiratory chain dysfunction.[215] More than 30 distinct mutations have been reported and are associated with heterogeneous phenotypes.[215-217] Patients of Lebanese Christian descent are particularly common because of a founder mutation present in that population. Clinical onset ranges from infancy to adolescence. Generalized muscle weakness and cardiomyopathy are prominent features. Patients with biallelic YARS2 mutations may not have SA; in one-third of 17 cases in one report, SA was not evident or it resolved.[218] Blood lactate levels are elevated in the presence of myopathy. When examined, deficiencies of muscle cytochrome c oxidase and respiratory chain complex activities were found.

A recurring mutation in the respiratory complex I protein NDUFB11 underlies a third disorder reminiscent of MLASA that has been reported in six male patients, appropriate to the gene location on the X chromosome.[219,220] All of the patients have the same, recurrent mutation, p.Phe93del, which results in respiratory insufficiency caused by loss of complex I stability and activity.[219] In vitro studies suggested primarily a proliferation defect in erythropoiesis. The anemia is normocytic and moderately severe. Associated features have been variable among patients and have included short stature, developmental delay, or myopathy.

Mutations in leucyl-tRNA synthetase (LARS2), which, like YARS2, ligates leucine to its cognate mitochondrial tRNA, caused reduced enzyme activity and complex I protein levels in one reported patient.[221] The associated clinical features consisted of hydrops, lactic acidosis, SA, and multisystem failure.

A heteroplasmic missense mutation in mitochondrial ATPase 6 (MT-ATP6), a subunit of complex V (ATP synthase of the oxidative phosphorylation system) that is encoded by the mitochondrial gene MT-ATP6, was associated with severe mitochondrial respiratory impairment and an "MLASA-plus" phenotype in one patient.[222] Three additional cases subsequently described with the same mutation, p.Ser148Asn, included one severely affected individual similar to the first reported patient, and two patients with a much milder phenotype, presumably attributable to variable tissue heteroplasmy.[223] Consequently, this disorder may be better considered within the rubric of mitochondrial heteroplasmy disorders such as Pearson syndrome.

Thiamine-Responsive Megaloblastic Anemia

This autosomal recessive syndrome, also known as Rogers syndrome,[224] is caused by mutations in the *SLC19A2* gene, which encodes a high-affinity thiamine transporter.[225-227] About 50 distinct mutations have been reported.[121,228] Most are nonsense or frameshift mutations; missense mutations result in proteins that are not properly targeted to the cell membrane.[229,230] The megaloblastic features of the anemia are considered to be due to defective nucleic acid synthesis owing to limited intracellular thiamine, which impairs the pentose phosphate pathway and de novo synthesis of ribose-5-P.[231] The unique additional feature of marrow ring sideroblasts, which are an inconstant feature, may relate to the role of thiamine in the generation of succinyl-CoA, a substrate of ALAS2.[232]

The cardinal clinical characteristic of the syndrome is the triad of megaloblastic anemia, non–type I diabetes mellitus, and sensorineural deafness. Other clinical features have been described in some cases.[228] The disorder has typically manifested between infancy and adolescence.[228,233] Some patients have a milder phenotype, and a few have presented as adults.

Hematologic findings are macrocytic anemia, variable degrees of neutropenia and thrombocytopenia with megaloblastic changes, and fewer marrow ring sideroblasts than in other congenital SAs.[233] Thiamine (vitamin B_1) in pharmacologic doses (25 mg/d) usually improves the anemia and the diabetes initially, but it has become ineffective in adulthood.[234]

Undefined Congenital Sideroblastic Anemia(s)

Up to one-third of cases of congenital SA are currently molecularly unexplained.[235] These may have autosomal or X-linked defects in previously identified genes causing the phenotype that may be detected with other approaches of mutational analysis (e.g., methods that detect large deletions or chromosomal rearrangements). Novel genetic defects are also possible in some previously described kindreds. For example, in one family, SA occurred in a vertical distribution including father-to-son transmission and consistent with a dominant trait.[236] In another family manifesting the anemia in both genders, a defect in mitochondrial DNA was postulated[237]; the mild anemia was characterized by erythrocyte dimorphism and macrocytosis.

Animal Models of Congenital Sideroblastic Anemia

The first genetically designed animal model of SA was developed in zebrafish (the *sau* mutant, *sauternes*), in which hematopoiesis resembles that of higher vertebrates also at the molecular level, as hematopoietic gene expression and function are conserved.[238] The chemically induced mutant gene encodes the zebrafish ortholog of human ALAS2 and expresses embryonic hypochromic anemia with severe heme deficiency. The two mutations, p.Val249Asp and p.Leu305Gln, are in exon 6 and exon 7, respectively, and are in phylogenetically conserved amino acids. However, the mutants' blood cells did not reveal ring sideroblasts, perhaps because of species differences in cellular iron metabolism.

A second congenital SA model in zebrafish (the *sir* mutant, *shiraz*) has a deficiency of glutaredoxin 5, an essential component of Fe-S cluster assembly, and expresses hypochromic anemia.[55] In the absence of the Fe-S cluster, IRP1 blocks *ALAS2* translation by binding to the IRE of the ALAS2 mRNA. As in the ALAS2 zebrafish mutant, ring sideroblasts were not observed and may reflect species differences.

In a transgenic mouse model with homozygous deficiency of Alas2, erythroid differentiation is arrested, and embryos die by day 11.5,[46] and animals lacking the GATA1-binding site in intron 1 also die of anemia in utero.[239] Mice chimeric for *Alas2*-null mutant cells or transgenic mice generated with partial ALAS2 expression exhibit the phenotype of human XLSA, with severe anemia and typical ring sideroblasts in the marrow.[240]

In another mouse model, deletion of the *Abcb7* gene led to fatal neonatal bone marrow failure, demonstrating that Abcb7 is essential for hematopoiesis.[241] While marrow ring sideroblasts were not observed in these animals or in animals chimeric for the mouse ortholog of the human Abcb7 p.Glu433Lys mutation, siderocytes were detected in the peripheral blood. Conditional deletion of HSCB in the bone marrow leads to a similar, lethal phenotype with a transient population of siderocytes.[149]

A mouse null allele in the *Pus1* gene results in mitochondrial myopathy, but with no evidence of anemia or sideroblasts.[242]

The combination of isoniazid (INH) and cycloserine administered to guinea pigs produces SA in a few weeks.[243,244] Blood PLP concentrations become reduced, and bone marrow ALAS as well as ferrochelatase activity is diminished.[244] The latter may be secondary to mitochondrial damage by the iron deposits.

The *flexed-tail* (*f/f*) mouse has a transient embryonic and neonatal anemia associated with siderotic granules (iron-laden mitochondria) in erythrocytes and reduced heme synthesis, which coincides with the physiologic cessation of hepatic erythropoiesis.[245,246] The defect is a frameshift mutation in sideroflexin 1 (*Sfxn1*) that encodes a high-affinity mitochondrial serine importer that contributes to mitochondrial one-carbon metabolism, supports heme synthesis, and helps to maintain respiratory complex III function.[247-249]

ACQUIRED CLONAL SIDEROBLASTIC ANEMIA

Since the initial description of acquired idiopathic SA by Bjorkman,[250] a considerable spectrum of its manifestations has been recognized. The anemia is a component of certain subsets of stem cell disorders, namely, the myelodysplastic syndromes (MDSs)[251-253] and the myeloproliferative neoplasms.[254,255] Uncommonly, the ring sideroblast abnormality has been observed in acute leukemia and in erythroleukemia at the time of diagnosis.[256,257] The disorder arises in conjunction with the clonal overgrowth of a somatic mutant hematopoietic progenitor cell that has a proliferative advantage over the normal cell population and was thus included among the MDS.[251] Three variants with ring sideroblasts are distinguished and were recently renamed[253]: refractory anemia with ring sideroblasts as MDS with ring sideroblasts and single lineage dysplasia (RARS//MDS-RS-SLD), refractory cytopenia with multilineage dysplasia and ring sideroblasts as MDS with ring sideroblasts and multilineage dysplasia (RCMD-RS//MDS-RS-MLD), and RARS with thrombocytosis as MDS/MPN with ring sideroblasts and thrombocytosis (RARS-T//MDS/MPN-RS-T) (*Table 26.1*).

Etiology and Pathogenesis
Clonality

The clonal nature of the disorder was first suggested by the morphologic and kinetic findings of two populations of red cells, the short-lived cell population being the product of the abnormal clone that bears the characteristic ring sideroblasts.[258-260] This hypothesis was confirmed by identifying a single glucose-6-phosphate dehydrogenase isozyme in hematopoietic cells, but not in fibroblasts, of an individual who was also heterozygous for a glucose-6-phosphate dehydrogenase polymorphism.[261] Further evidence was provided by cytogenetic studies, which corroborated the clonality of the abnormal hematopoiesis.[262-264] Chromosomal abnormalities are detectable in bone marrow cells of up to 50% of patients, and deletions in chromosomes 5, 11, and 20 as well as trisomy 8 and loss of Y occur most frequently.[265,266] Although structurally abnormal X chromosomes are uncommon in general in MDS, Xq13 breakpoints are particularly associated with MDS with RS.[267] A unique recurring cytogenetic abnormality is an isodicentric chromosome Xq13.1 (idicXq13.1), which is seen only in females.[268]

The strongest molecular correlate of ring sideroblasts in MDS-RS-SLD, MDS-RS-MLD, and MDS/MPN-RS-T (collectively MDS with RS) is specific somatic mutations in splicing factor SF3B1, a core component of the splicing machinery (spliceosome) that recognizes the 3′ splice acceptor site in nascent mRNAs; heterozygous clonal *SF3B1* mutations can be identified in 70% to 90% of such cases,[269-272] and, in most, it is the sole detectable clonal abnormality. Thus, mutant SF3B1 appears not only to be a driver of the MDS phenotype but also to initiate the production of the ring sideroblast.[269,273] Patients with MDS/MPN-RS-T, on the other hand, characteristically bear somatic SF3B1 mutations as well as gain-of-function hematopoietic receptor tyrosine kinase signaling pathway mutations, most commonly JAK2 p.Val617Phe (~60%)[274-276] and less commonly other JAK2, or MPL, or CALR variants.[277] Regardless of the specific phenotype, the observed SF3B1 mutations are restricted to missense variants in the C-terminal HEAT domains (residues 622-781), with the most common, p.Val700Glu, accounting for approximately 60% of alleles.[278] These mutations appear to be neomorphic variants that result in aberrant 3′ splice site selection and abnormally spliced mRNAs, many of which are degraded by nonsense-mediated decay, resulting in gene downregulation.[279] Mutations in several other 3′ spliceosome components, including SRSF2, ZRSR2, and PRPF8, are also seen in MDS with RS, but it is unclear if these variants are enriched beyond the MDS population as a whole.[269,280]

Pathogenesis of Ring Sideroblasts in Myelodysplastic Syndromes

Considerable effort has been expended to try to unify the genetics and pathogenesis of the congenital and acquired clonal SAs. This was particularly true prior to the discovery of mutations in the spliceosome machinery in the acquired forms. In the light of current knowledge that the genes mutated in each case are mutually exclusive and that aberrant splicing has the potential to misregulate a diverse set of target genes, it is certain that the pathogenesis of acquired ring sideroblasts is multifactorial.

Various studies of MDS with RS indicated that the biosynthesis of heme is impaired at the levels of ALAS and ferrochelatase. Reduced activity of ALAS in marrow cells was the most consistent abnormality in earlier series of patients[108,109,281,282] and was particularly demonstrable in the youngest erythroblast fraction.[283] In occasional patients, the addition of PLP enhanced the low enzyme activity in vitro, but reported erythropoietic responses to pyridoxine or to PLP administration,[284] as well as restoration of low ALAS activity to normal,[281,285] were unusual and may have reflected an inherited defect of ALAS2.[103,112] In a later study, the activity of detergent-solubilized ALAS in bone marrow cells was actually somewhat increased,[286] suggesting enhanced translation of the enzyme in response to raised cellular iron levels.

A constant feature is mild to moderate elevation of the erythrocyte protoporphyrin,[258] rarely reaching values encountered in protoporphyria (see Chapter 28).[35,258,260,287] The latter cases may now be explained by a likely acquired deletion of a ferrochelatase allele caused by a cytogenetic abnormality of the clonal disorder.[288] The erythrocyte protoporphyrin increases further after pyridoxine administration but without improvement of the anemia,[258,281,289] suggesting a block at the ferrochelatase step. Impaired activity of this enzyme was found in approximately half of patients studied,[108,282] likely representing a secondary effect of the mitochondrial iron deposition. Studies of iron metabolism in erythroid cells revealed increased accumulation of nonheme iron into membrane or mitochondrial fractions and reduced incorporation of iron into heme.[5,6] Thus, impaired iron utilization for heme biosynthesis remains the common denominator in the pathogenesis.

Subsequently, a defect(s) intrinsic to mitochondria, causing diminished heme production in the abnormal clone as well as accounting for the decreased activity of several other mitochondrial enzymes (i.e., cytochrome oxidase, oligomycin-sensitive ATP, and mitochondrial serine protease) in granulocytes and erythroblasts,[290] was sought. Diverse heteroplasmic point mutations of conserved nucleotides in mitochondrial DNA, as well as in transfer RNAs and mitochondrial ribosomal RNAs, were found in hematopoietic cells of patients with clonal SA.[291] Many of these affect cytochrome c oxidase and may be implicated in impaired reduction of iron for its incorporation into protoporphyrin by ferrochelatase. Such mitochondrial defects are consistent with the heterogeneity of hemoglobin content found between individual erythroblasts by scanning microspectrophotometry,[292] as well as with the variable size of erythrocyte and ring sideroblast cell populations. A gradual accumulation of affected erythroid precursors and the known higher mutation rate in mitochondrial DNA than in nuclear DNA would provide a basis for the slowly progressive nature of the anemia and its expression in later life, respectively.

The description of SF3B1 mutations in a majority of cases of MDS with RS has stimulated substantial work to identify genes, particularly those encoding proteins involved in congenital SA and other mitochondrial pathways that are aberrantly spliced and/or misregulated in the MDS with RS progenitor population. Gene expression studies have shown that a number of genes implicated in congenital SA and mitochondrial iron metabolism, including *ALAS2*, *GLRX5*, and *SLC25A37*,[293] are upregulated, whereas the transcript encoding ABCB7 is reduced due to nonsense-mediated decay of a misspliced mRNA.[294-296] In addition to *ABCB7*, mRNAs for the heme synthesis protein protoporpyrinogen oxidase (PPOX), TMEM14C, which is a mitochondrial inner membrane protein that is essential for heme synthesis and erythropoiesis, and thought to transport protoporphyrinogen IX into the mitochondrial matrix, and MAP37K1, involved in transforming growth factor b (TGFb) and BMP signaling, are consistently misregulated in many human models.[297-299] Very recently, it has been demonstrated that the ring sideroblast phenotype is partially complemented by the forced overexpression of either ABCB7 or TMEM14C, and their combined expression nearly completely abolishes RS formation,[299] providing evidence that the ontogeny of the RS is almost certainly largely related to coordinate misregulation of these two genes. Nonetheless, while these observations explain the morphologic phenotype, they do not explain the neoplastic phenotype, which appears to be related to the missplicing of BRD9 (Bromodomain Containing 9), a member of the noncanonical mammalian SWI/SNF chromatin remodeling complex. Mutant SF3B1 appears to recognize an aberrant, deep intronic branchpoint within BRD9, causing the inclusion of an exon that is derived from an endogenous retroviral element, and leading to degradation of BRD9 mRNA.[300,301] This species-specific pathogenesis indicates why hematopoietic-specific Sf3b1mutant knockin mouse models develop macrocytosis and functional abnormalities in hematopoietic precursors, but not a neoplastic phenotype.[302,303]

Clinical and Laboratory Features

The disorder occurs in middle-aged and older individuals. It is extraordinarily uncommon in individuals younger than 30 years; in such cases, a late presentation of a congenital SA should be considered. The anemia frequently develops insidiously and may be discovered during a routine examination or in association with an unrelated complaint. The older individual more often experiences symptoms of fatigue and angina if there is coexisting coronary artery disease. Physical examination may reveal no abnormality except for pallor. Hepatosplenomegaly is found in one-third to half of patients.

The anemia is usually moderate and may be normocytic but more often is macrocytic (*Figure 26.6*). The mean corpuscular hemoglobin concentration is normal or slightly reduced, and a variable population of hypochromic cells may also be found on blood smear. A particularly characteristic finding is the presence of basophilic stippling that stains for iron in occasional hypochromic cells.[23,258] Typical Pappenheimer bodies are uncommon unless there is associated hyposplenism. Leukocyte and platelet values are usually within the normal range.

Characteristically, the erythrocyte protoporphyrin is moderately increased, up to 300 µg/dL (normal is 20-80 µg/dL). Values ranged from 1055 to 10,514 µg/dL in patients with acquired loss of a ferrochelatase allele in the hematopoietic clone, and some had associated dermal photosensitivity.[35,260,287]

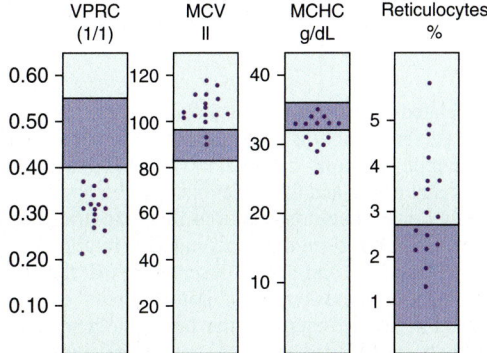

FIGURE 26.6 Characteristics of the anemia in 17 patients with acquired clonal sideroblastic anemia. Shaded areas, normal range (mean ± 2 SD). MCHC, mean corpuscular hemoglobin concentration; MCV, mean corpuscular volume; VPRC, volume of packed red cells. (Reprinted with permission from Kushner JP, Lee GR, Wintrobe MM, et al. Idiopathic refractory sideroblastic anemia. Clinical and laboratory investigation of 17 patients and review of the literature. *Medicine (Baltimore).* 1971;50(3):139-159.)

Serum transferrin saturation is increased in most patients and exceeds 90% in approximately one-third.[258] Substantially increased deposition of iron is found in the liver, but hepatic dysfunction is rare at presentation. Serum ferritin levels are elevated.

Erythroid hyperplasia is found on bone marrow examination. Mild megaloblastic changes are common and may or may not be related to accompanying folate deficiency. Marrow hemosiderin content is increased, and ring sideroblasts constitute up to 100% of the erythroblasts unless masked by concomitant iron deficiency.[258,304,305] In contrast to the microcytic congenital SAs, where they are most prominent in later stages, ring sideroblasts are evident at all stages of erythroid maturation.[158] Because the hematologic phenotype is usually indistinguishable from XLSA in women,[103,104] analysis of DNA for an ALAS2 mutation should be strongly considered in those patients who lack an SF3B1 mutation, other spliceosome mutation, or a variant not commonly associated with clonal hematopoiesis of indeterminate potential.

The presence of erythroid abnormalities in isolation on bone marrow examination constitutes the MDS-RS-SLD subtype of the disorder in the World Health Organization (WHO) classification of MDS (see Chapter 74).[253] Associated moderate leukopenia, thrombocytopenia, or both tend to be accompanied by other myelodysplastic features, such as morphologically abnormal leukocytes (e.g., the pseudo-Pelger anomaly) or immature forms in the peripheral blood,[265] and define the WHO category MDS-RS-MLD.[253] The presence of leukocytosis, thrombocytosis, or both is indicative of a mixed myelodysplastic-myeloproliferative neoplasm, MDS/MPN-RS-T.[254,255]

Natural History

The natural history of acquired SA is commonly characterized by a chronic, stable anemia and, uncommonly, by a progressive marrow failure state or leukemic evolution.[265,306] Many patients are not significantly incapacitated by the anemia. In patients without abnormalities of the other hematopoietic cell lines and with minimal iron overload, often no progression occurs for many years.[265] Such individuals frequently succumb to other concurrent diseases. Nevertheless, continued medical follow-up is indicated.

Excessive absorption of dietary iron occurs over time in many, if not all, patients with stable disease and can be attributed to the ineffective erythropoiesis, as in congenital SAs and other disorders with long-standing ineffective erythropoiesis.[18] The consequent iron accumulation closely resembles that of hereditary hemochromatosis. Inadvertent administration of iron for the anemia and red cell transfusions add predictably to the parenchymal iron deposition.[167,306,307]

Iron overload, particularly when accentuated by repeated transfusions, can be a significant cause of morbidity and mortality, particularly liver or heart failure,[306,308] and is improved with iron chelation therapy.[309,310] When the serum ferritin level is 500 µg/L or higher, along with the increased transferrin saturation, it should be countered. Histologic and chemical determination of iron in the liver biopsy or liver iron quantitation by magnetic resonance imaging provides the optimal assessment of the degree of iron overload. In mildly or moderately anemic individuals, iron removal can be accomplished with graded phlebotomies. Patients with more severe anemia or who are transfusion dependent require iron chelation as described for congenital SAs. Because each unit of blood deposits ~200 mg of iron, iron overload develops fairly rapidly with regular transfusions, and it is controlled more easily if treatment with an iron chelator is begun after approximately 20 units of blood have been given. In some cases, anemia was improved after iron removal[5,311-313]; an independent effect of deferoxamine on erythropoiesis was also implicated.[312,313]

The survival of patients with isolated anemia who are stable and not transfusion dependent may not differ from that of healthy individuals. A prospective study of 232 patients, which validated the proposal of the two types of the disorder, provided prognostic information.[265] In pure SA, with the marrow failure restricted to the erythroid cell lineage and now called MDS-RS-SLD, overall survival was the same as in age-matched controls, and leukemic transformation was not observed. In MDS-RS-MLD, having features of impaired

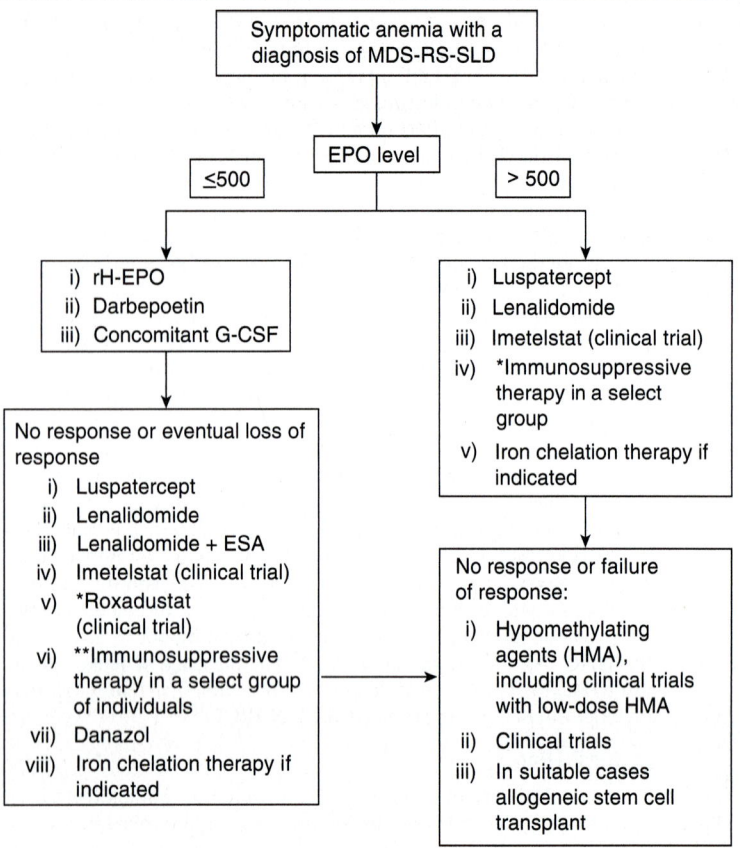

FIGURE 26.7 Schematic approach for the management of myelodysplastic syndrome with ring sideroblasts and single lineage dysplasia. EPO, erythropoietin; ESA, erythropoiesis stimulating agents; G-CSF, granulocyte colony-stimulating factor; MDS-RS, myelodysplastic syndrome with ring sideroblasts; rH, recombinant human. *Roxadustat acts as a hypoxia inducible factor prolyl hydroxylase inhibitor and increases the endogenous production of erythropoietin. **Immunosuppressive therapy could be considered in patients with hypoplastic bone marrows, presence of oligoclonal T-cell large granular lymphocyte leukemia and HLA DR-15 genotype. (From Patnaik MM, Tefferi A. Myelodysplastic syndromes with ring sideroblasts (MDS-RS) and MDS/myeloproliferative neoplasm with RS and thrombocytosis (MDS/MPN-RS-T)—"2021 update on diagnosis, risk-stratification, and management." *Am J Hematol.* 2021;96:379-394. Copyright © 2021 Wiley Periodicals LLC. Reprinted by permission of John Wiley & Sons, Inc.)

granulopoiesis, megakaryopoiesis, or both, survival was reduced to 56% at 3 years, and, in approximately 5% of cases, evolution to acute leukemia occurred. Other factors associated with the development of leukemia are the presence of few ring sideroblasts, more severe ineffective erythropoiesis, and impaired bone marrow colony formation.[265,306] Additional mutations appear to be necessary for leukemic evolution[314] that can be reversed with chemotherapy, but the initial manifested defect expressed in the sideroblastic state persists.[315,316] The probability of leukemic transformation is also increased in the presence of certain bone marrow karyotype abnormalities (eg, monosomy 7, deletion 20q, or complex defects).[306,317] When SA followed therapy for various malignant disorders, leukemic evolution tended to be the rule.[318,319]

Treatment

Treatment has historically consisted largely of supportive measures; however, there are an increasing number of nontargeted and targeted therapies available or in clinical trials. Transfusion of packed red cells is necessary for patients with symptomatic anemia, but it should be kept to a minimum because it accelerates the iron overload. Pyridoxine administration cannot be expected to be beneficial because ALAS2 defects are not involved in the pathogenesis. The effectiveness of erythropoietin has been examined in patients with MDS, including the subtypes with ring sideroblasts. Most, if not all, patients with uncomplicated SA have high levels of endogenous erythropoietin, and it would appear unlikely that additional administration of the hormone would be beneficial. However, prolonged administration of recombinant erythropoietin, with or without granulocyte colony-stimulating factor, can lead to gratifying improvement or even correction of the anemia in around 40% of patients,[320,321] in particular in individuals who have a low or intermediate-1 International Prognostic Scoring System (IPSS) score.[322] A response is more likely to occur if the endogenous serum erythropoietin level is not commensurate with the degree of the anemia,[323] and large doses may be required.

Many studies evaluating various drug regimens for myelodysplasia, generally speaking, have included the subtypes with ring sideroblasts. The drugs used have included the hypomethylating agents 5-azacytidine and decitabine, anti-TNF fusion protein (etanercept), antithymocyte globulin, thalidomide and its derivative lenalidomide, and valproic acid.[324-326] On average, major responses with improved erythropoiesis or hematopoiesis have been less than 50% (see Chapter 80). The activin receptor ligand trap, Luspatercept, which blocks a number of growth factors in the transforming growth factor beta (TGF-β) family that are overexpressed in ineffective erythropoiesis, has recently been approved for the treatment of patients with lower-risk MDS, including those with RA.[327,328] A phase I study of an SF3B1 inhibitor targeting the spliceosome has been initiated as a strategy to counter the molecular basis of the disorders.[329,330] Based on these recent advancements, a multitiered approach to the treatment of the patient with low-grade MDS with RS has been developed (*Figure 26.7*).

REVERSIBLE SIDEROBLASTIC ANEMIAS

Alcoholism

Anemia associated with alcoholism usually has numerous causes.[331] A ring sideroblast abnormality is never the sole cause but occurs in 25% to 30% of anemic alcoholic patients[332,333] and probably only in the presence of malnutrition and folate deficiency.[333,334]

The production of heme is impaired by ethanol, as indicated by the ability of heme to restore the concomitantly inhibited globin synthesis in reticulocytes[335] and by the observation that the HRI activity of globin translation increases.[336] Inhibitory effects of alcohol have been observed at several steps of the heme biosynthetic pathway. Reduced activity of erythrocyte ALAD may be related to zinc depletion.[337,338] Activity levels of erythrocyte uroporphyrinogen decarboxylase, leukocyte coproporphyrinogen oxidase, and ferrochelatase are also decreased in alcoholic patients; those of ALAS and HMBS are increased.[337,338] Abnormalities of vitamin B_6 metabolism have also been observed. Serum levels of PLP are low in chronically ill alcoholic persons[339] but do not correlate with the presence or absence of ring sideroblasts.[333] Acetaldehyde enhanced the degradation of

PLP,[339,340] and, in one study, alcohol-induced SA responded to PLP but not to the combination of folic acid and pyridoxine.[341] The colony formation of early (burst-forming unit–erythroid) and late (colony-forming unit–erythroid) human erythroid progenitor cells is preferentially suppressed by ethanol and acetaldehyde over that of myeloid cell progenitors at concentrations found in vivo and is partially reversed by folinic acid and pyridoxine.[342] Thus, a direct role of vitamin B_6 deficiency in the sideroblastic change is uncertain. Important in the pathogenesis may be the direct effects of ethanol, acetaldehyde, or both on the heme biosynthetic steps or on mitochondrial metabolism because these agents also inhibit hepatic mitochondrial protein synthesis.[343]

Blood hemoglobin values range from 6 to 10 g/dL, and the MCV is normal or increased. The transient sideroblastic change is commonly evident in dimorphic circulating erythrocytes. Siderocytes, present in approximately one-third of patients, are a specific finding[331] and provide the most persistent clue for the ethanol-associated ring sideroblast defect. Megaloblastic hematopoiesis resulting from folate deficiency is frequent but not always present.[331] Vacuolization of pronormoblasts may be observed. The percentage of marrow ring sideroblasts ranges up to 70%, and they typically represent later stage normoblasts.[334] Marrow iron stores are usually increased, as are the serum transferrin saturation and the serum ferritin level.

Withdrawal of alcohol is followed by the disappearance of ring sideroblasts within a few days to 2 weeks (*Figure 26.8*).[332] Recovery from the anemia may occur over several weeks and also depends on the presence of other erythroid defects induced by alcohol,[332] as well as any associated medical illness that affects erythropoiesis (see Chapter 42). A prompt recovery phase may exhibit reticulocytosis and erythroid hyperplasia in the bone marrow resembling hemolytic anemia.[332]

Drugs
Antituberculosis Agents

Reversible SA occurs in association with the treatment of tuberculosis with INH; pyrazinamide and cycloserine have also been implicated.[344] These drugs interfere with vitamin B_6 metabolism, and deprivation of PLP reduces ALA synthesis and thus heme production.[344] INH reacts with pyridoxal to form a hydrazone and inhibits pyridoxal phosphokinase. Bone marrow ALAS activity is also inhibited by INH in a dose-dependent manner in vitro and is restored by PLP.[108] Cycloserine inhibits PLP-requiring enzyme reactions and directly inactivates pyridoxal.[344] Pyrazinamide appears to have anti–vitamin B_6 properties, but a specific mechanism has not been determined.

The relative incidence of anemia in relation to the extensive use of these drugs appears to be low, perhaps because of the regular concomitant administration of pyridoxine. Unknown contributory

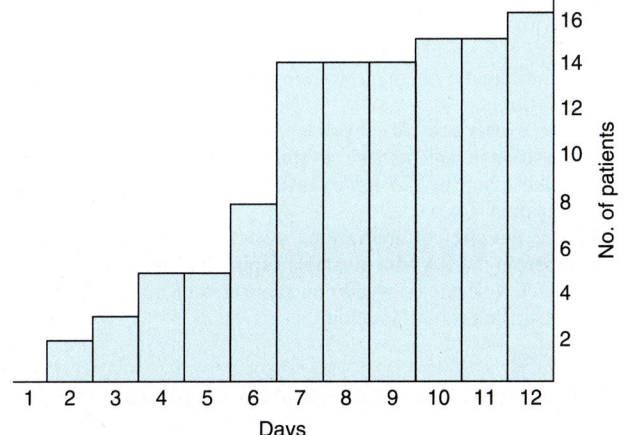

FIGURE 26.8 The rate of clearance in days of ring sideroblasts in 16 alcoholic patients after alcohol intake ceased. (From Eichner ER, Hillman RS. The evolution of anemia in alcoholic patients. *Am J Med.* 1971;50:218-232. Copyright © 1971 Elsevier. With permission.)

factors or another hematologic disorder may render certain individuals more susceptible to the antipyridoxine effects of the drugs.[344] In one study, ring sideroblasts or increased erythroblast iron was found in 58% of all patients treated for tuberculosis.[345] Anemia has occurred from 1 to 10 months after institution of INH treatment. It is moderately severe (volume of packed red cells, 0.20-0.26 L/L), the red cell indices are usually reduced, and the erythrocytes show dimorphic morphologic features with prominent hypochromia and microcytosis.[346] Ring sideroblasts are invariably present in the bone marrow. Serum pyridoxal concentrations were subnormal in most patients studied.[347] Transferrin saturation tends to be increased. The anemia is usually promptly and fully reversed on withdrawal of the drug or by administering large doses of pyridoxine while continuing use of the drug.

Chloramphenicol and Linezolid

In contrast to the sporadic or idiosyncratic and usually fatal aplastic anemia occurring within weeks or months of chloramphenicol use, the dose-dependent and reversible hematologic toxicity of the drug is predictable and characterized by suppression of erythropoiesis[348] and by the ring sideroblast abnormality.[349] A primary mitochondrial injury by the agent impairs heme synthesis as well as erythroid differentiation and proliferation. Therapeutic concentrations of chloramphenicol (10 μg/mL) inhibit the synthesis of mitochondrially encoded proteins, such as cytochrome a + a_3 and b, and thus mitochondrial respiration.[350,351] Impaired heme synthesis is evident in reduced activities of ferrochelatase[352] and ALAS,[353] which appear to be secondary effects as these enzymes are synthesized in the cytosol. The greater sensitivity of erythroid cells to chloramphenicol has been demonstrated in vitro, in that therapeutic concentrations of the drug inhibit erythroid colony growth but not granulocyte colony growth.[354]

The anemia may reach moderately severe levels. Bone marrow study reveals variable degrees of hypocellularity and ring sideroblasts as well as prominent vacuolization of early erythroid precursors. Erythrokinetic parameters reflect a hypoproliferative state. Reticulocytopenia, increased serum iron values, and prolonged plasma iron clearance are characteristic.[348] These abnormalities, as well as the ring sideroblasts and anemia, disappear on withdrawal of the drug.

Linezolid causes reversible myelosuppression, and the ring sideroblast abnormality has also been observed.[355] Its toxicity resembles that of chloramphenicol in that it inhibits mitochondrial protein synthesis (mRNA translation), although it blocks assembly of the initiation complex, while chloramphenicol inhibits peptidyl transferases and thus peptide elongation.[356] Vacuolization of erythroid precursors is common, and the hematologic abnormalities disappear when the drug is discontinued.

Other Drugs

Several miscellaneous drugs have been implicated in producing SA in a few patients. These include fusidic acid, busulfan, melphalan, penicillamine, and the copper-chelating agent triethylene tetramine dihydrochloride.

Copper Deficiency

Deficiency of copper generally does not occur in humans because requirements are low relative to its wide distribution in food.[357] However, copper deficiency anemia is encountered in various clinical settings and typically leads to SA and neutropenia. It has developed after prolonged parenteral nutrition[358-361] and forced enteral feeding[362,363] if copper was not included in the formulations and in association with intestinal malabsorption[363]; some patients have had prior gastrointestinal operations, for example, gastrectomy, bariatric surgery.[364,365] Copper deficiency also occurs with the use of copper-chelating agents[366] and after prolonged ingestion of zinc, such as in the form of zinc supplements[367] and with the chronic use of denture cream containing zinc.[368,369] In seven

Disorders of Red Blood Cells

instances, the deficiency developed from prolonged ingestion of coins associated with psychiatric illness and was attributed to their zinc content.[370-374]

A novel syndrome of severe SA with the neurologic manifestations of central nervous system demyelination, or peripheral neuropathy with optic neuritis, or myelopathy and profound copper deficiency was recognized only recently[375-377] and was proposed to represent another combined system disorder resembling vitamin B$_{12}$ deficiency.[378] Subsequently, numerous cases with this syndrome were reported.[364] In some, excess zinc ingestion was present and remote prior gastric resection was noted frequently.[364] Myeloneuropathy has been the most frequent neurologic abnormality.

The pathogenesis of copper deficiency–induced SA is understood in part from extensive studies of the severe anemia that develops late in the course of dietary copper deficiency in swine.[379] In these animals, the anemia is microcytic and hypochromic and is associated with several defects of iron metabolism. Intestinal absorption and mobilization of iron from reticuloendothelial cells and hepatocytes to transferrin are impaired because of the associated lack of ceruloplasmin (ferroxidase). In reticulocytes of deficient animals, protoporphyrin production from glycine and ALA and ferrochelatase activity are not reduced,[379] but iron metabolism in erythroid mitochondria is impaired in that heme synthesis from ferric iron and protoporphyrin is decreased.[357] It was postulated that the reduction of ferric iron to ferrous iron is defective, being somehow linked to the diminished levels of cytochrome oxidase also observed. Low levels of intracellular copper enzymes, such as cytochrome oxidase, may interfere with hematopoiesis in other ways and also account for the neutropenia as well as the neuropathology in humans. The cause of copper deficiency after ingestion of excess zinc has been attributed to induction of the intestinal protein metallothionein by zinc,[380] which preferentially binds copper,[381] prevents its absorption, and enhances its excretion.[382]

The anemia of copper deficiency is progressive and may be profound if untreated. The MCV usually is normal or slightly increased at presentation; hypochromic microcytic erythrocytes may be detectable on the blood smear. The granulocytes are commonly less than 1000/mm^3; the platelet count is usually normal. The bone marrow tends to be hypoplastic, with impaired myeloid maturation.[358,359] Vacuolization of early erythroid and granulocytic precursors is a prominent finding, as are large iron-positive cytoplasmic inclusions in plasma cells.[358,377] In most instances, moderate numbers of ring sideroblasts are observed, particularly if the anemia is sufficiently severe. The hematologic features occasionally led to the erroneous diagnosis of an MDS before the copper deficiency was recognized.[377,383,384]

Serum iron levels and transferrin saturation are normal. The serum copper and ceruloplasmin levels are uniformly low. In cases of zinc-induced copper deficiency, serum zinc levels are increased from 2- to 3-fold above the mean normal value.

With correction of the copper deficit, recovery of the hematologic abnormalities is uniformly prompt and complete. In some cases, recovery followed discontinuation of the excess zinc intake alone. Zinc, as a therapeutic agent, should thus be prescribed with caution, and its use as a stimulus for general well-being should be discouraged. Moreover, the zinc content has been removed from denture cream products. The neurologic abnormalities may improve or only stabilize with continued copper supplementation.[364,376,377] The usual dose of copper (2 mg of elemental copper/d) may not be sufficient for all patients as relapse has occurred,[385] and long-term follow-up is advised for all patients.

Hypothermia

In 1982, O'Brien et al described three patients who, during episodic hypothermia, exhibited erythroid hypoplasia and ring sideroblasts as well as thrombocytopenia in the presence of a normal number of megakaryocytes.[386] As the body temperature returned to normal, these changes slowly reversed. The ring sideroblast abnormality might be explained by the well-known inhibition of the translocation of proteins into mitochondria by reduced temperature.[386,387] Heme synthesis[388] and iron incorporation into hemoglobin by reticulocytes[389] have also been shown to be diminished at lowered temperatures.

KEY CLINICAL SUMMARY POINTS

- **General definition of SA**

  SA comprises a wide spectrum of heritable or acquired erythropoietic disorders. Regardless of clinical and peripheral blood abnormalities, the unifying feature of all forms of SA is the presence of bone marrow ring sideroblasts.

- **Prompt diagnosis of a SA**

  Consider in all adults and children/infants with unexplained anemia of any severity from history, clinical examination, and basic laboratory data. Certain features are suggestive: history of chronic anemia; exposure to factors causing reversible SA (*Table 26.1*); family history of anemia; presence of neurologic abnormalities, myopathy, lactic acidosis, and immunodeficiency in children or young adults.

  Suspect a congenital SA in the presence of microcytosis without evidence of iron deficiency or thalassemia; the MCV and erythrocyte morphology are most accurate before any red cell transfusion (*Figure 26.9*).

  Establish the diagnosis of SA by performing a Prussian blue stain on the bone marrow aspirate smear.

- **Differential diagnosis**

  If ring sideroblasts are evident in the marrow, review the patient's constellation of clinical findings to narrow the differential diagnosis (*Table 26.1* and *Figure 26.9*).

  Where the causative gene is known, mutation analysis provides definitive diagnosis of a congenital SA, allowing anticipation of associated syndromic features and initiation of treatment prior to the evolution of complications; some molecular genetic tests are available in several clinical laboratories listed on the www.genetests.org website, and others may be available in certain research laboratories.

  Evaluate for iron overload with serum iron profile and ferritin; assess parenchymal organ involvement as indicated.

- **Treatment**

  Withdraw an identified reversible cause.

  Recommend a therapeutic trial of pyridoxine (adult dose 50-100 mg/d) in patients with microcytic SA until the genetic cause can be determined; the vitamin is effective only in some cases with XLSA. Females with normocytic or macrocytic XLSA tend not to respond to pyridoxine.

  For symptomatic anemia, provide supportive treatment with red cell transfusion.

  Remove excess body iron by phlebotomy if anemia is mild, by use of iron chelation in patients with severe/transfusion-dependent anemia.

  Prescribe thiamine (25 mg/d) in the thiamine-responsive megaloblastic anemia syndrome.

  Manage the clinical aberrations associated with the syndromic forms of congenital SA with available supportive measures.

  For selected, severe nonsyndromic congenital SAs, consider hematopoietic stem cell transplantation.

- **Follow-up**

  Educate the patient and family about the disease and relevant inheritance.

  Encourage patients to keep records of diagnostic studies and recommended therapy.

  In cases with congenital SA, provide for examination of family members and for their genetic testing as indicated.

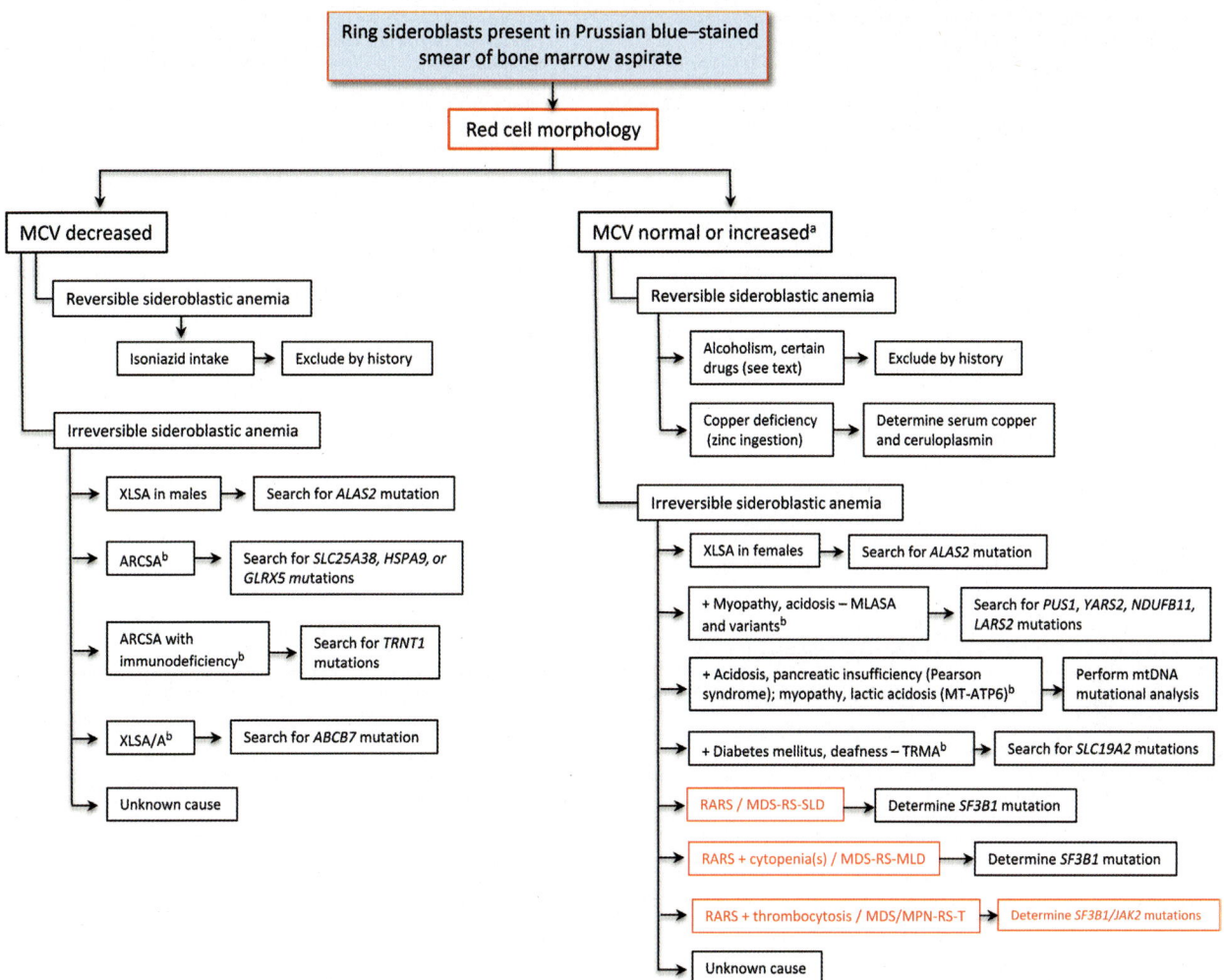

FIGURE 26.9 Schema for diagnostic evaluation of patients with a sideroblastic anemia. ARCSA, autosomal recessive sideroblastic anemia; MCV, mean corpuscular volume; MLASA, myopathy, lactic acidosis, and sideroblastic anemia; MPN, myeloproliferative neoplasm; MT-ATP6, mitochondrial ATPase 6; mtDNA, mitochondrial DNA; RARS//MDS-RS-SLD, refractory anemia with ring sideroblasts as MDS with ring sideroblasts and single lineage dysplasia; RS-MLD, ring sideroblasts and multilineage dysplasia; TRMA, thiamine-responsive megaloblastic anemia; XLSA, X-linked sideroblastic anemia; XLSA/A, X-linked sideroblastic anemia with ataxia. [a]Microcytic hypochromic red cells may be present in the blood smear in many, but not all, of these disorders. [b]Typically present in infancy or childhood.

Website Resource

The website www.uptodate.com contains two sections on SAs: causes and pathophysiology; diagnosis and treatment.

ACKNOWLEDGMENT

The editors acknowledge the contributions of Dr. Sylvia Bottomley, who was the sole author or lead author of this chapter over several previous editions.

References

1. Bottomley SS, Fleming MD. Sideroblastic anemia: diagnosis and management. *Hematol Oncol Clin North Am.* 2014;28(4):653-670. v.
2. Caroli J, Bernard J, Bessis M, Combrisson A, Malassenet R, Breton J. Hemochromatose avec anemie hypochrome et absence d'hemoglobine anormale. *Presse Med.* 1957;65(88):1991-1996.
3. Mollin DL. Sideroblasts and sideroblastic anaemia. *Br J Haematol.* 1965;11:41-48.
4. Sorenson GD. Electron microscopic observations of bone marrow from patients with sideroblastic anemia. *Am J Pathol.* 1962;40:297-314.
5. Bottomley SS. The spectrum and role of iron overload in sideroblastic anemia. *Ann NY Acad Sci.* 1988;526(1):331-332.
6. May A, de Souza P, Barnes K, Kaaba S, Jacobs A. Erythroblast iron metabolism in sideroblastic marrows. *Br J Haematol.* 1982;52(4):611-621.
7. White JM, Brain MC, Ali MA. Globin synthesis in sideroblastic anaemia. I. Alpha and beta peptide chain synthesis. *Br J Haematol.* 1971;20(3):263-275.
8. White JM, Ali MA. Globin synthesis in sideroblastic anaemia. II. The effect of pyridoxine,-aminolaevulinic acid and haem, in vitro. *Br J Haematol.* 1973;24(4):481-489.
9. Harris JW, Horrigan DL. Pyridoxine-responsive anemia—prototype and variations on the theme. *Vitam Horm.* 1964;22:721-753.
10. Singh AK, Shinton NK, Williams JD. Ferrokinetic abnormalities and their significance in patients with sideroblastic anaemia. *Br J Haematol.* 1970;18(1):67-77.
11. Barrett PV, Cline MJ, Berlin NI. The association of the urobilin "early peak" and erythropoiesis in man. *J Clin Invest.* 1966;45(11):1657-1667.
12. Muta K, Krantz SB. Inhibition of heme synthesis induces apoptosis in human erythroid progenitor cells. *J Cell Physiol.* 1995;163(1):38-50.
13. Matthes TW, Meyer G, Samii K, Beris P. Increased apoptosis in acquired sideroblastic anaemia. *Br J Haematol.* 2000;111(3):843-852.
14. Hellstrom-Lindberg E, Schmidt-Mende J, Forsblom AM, Christensson B, Fadeel B, Zhivotovsky B. Apoptosis in refractory anaemia with ringed sideroblasts is initiated at the stem cell level and associated with increased activation of caspases. *Br J Haematol.* 2001;112(3):714-726.
15. Cartwright GE, Deiss A. Sideroblasts, siderocytes, and sideroblastic anemia. *N Engl J Med.* 1975;292(4):185-193.
16. Pippard MJ, Weatherall DJ. Iron absorption in non-transfused iron loading anaemias: prediction of risk for iron loading, and response to iron chelation treatment, in beta thalassaemia intermedia and congenital sideroblastic anaemias. *Haematologia.* 1984;17(1):17-24.
17. Tanno T, Bhanu NV, Oneal PA, et al. High levels of GDF15 in thalassemia suppress expression of the iron regulatory protein hepcidin. *Nat Med.* 2007;13(9):1096-1101.
18. Tanno T, Miller JL. Iron loading and overloading due to ineffective erythropoiesis. *Adv Hematol.* 2010;2010:358283.
19. Kautz L, Jung G, Valore EV, Rivella S, Nemeth E, Ganz T. Identification of erythroferrone as an erythroid regulator of iron metabolism. *Nat Genet.* 2014;46(7):678-684.

20. Arezes J, Foy N, McHugh K, et al. Erythroferrone inhibits the induction of hepcidin by BMP6. *Blood*. 2018;132(14):1473-1477.

21. Bottomley SS. Secondary iron overload disorders. *Semin Hematol*. 1998;35(1):77-86.

22. Bottomley SS. Iron overload in sideroblastic and other non-thalassemic anemias. In: Barton JC, Edwards CQ, eds. *Hemochromatosis: Genetics, Pathophysiology, Diagnosis and Treatment*. Cambridge University Press; 2000:442-452.

23. Cartwright GE, Edwards CQ, Skolnick MH, Amos DB. Association of HLA-linked hemochromatosis with idiopathic refractory sideroblastic anemia. *J Clin Invest*. 1980;65(5):989-992.

24. Yaouanq J, Grosbois B, Jouanolle AM, Goasguen J, Leblay R. Haemochromatosis Cys282Tyr mutation in pyridoxine-responsive sideroblastic anaemia. *Lancet*. 1997;349(9063):1475-1476.

25. Cotter PD, May A, Li L, et al. Four new mutations in the erythroid-specific 5-aminolevulinate synthase (ALAS2) gene causing X-linked sideroblastic anemia: increased pyridoxine responsiveness after removal of iron overload by phlebotomy and coinheritance of hereditary hemochromatosis. *Blood*. 1999;93(5):1757-1769.

26. Bottomley SS, Wasson EG, Wise PD. Role of the hemochromatosis HFE gene mutation(s) in the iron overload of hereditary sideroblastic anemia *Blood*. 1997;90(suppl 1):11b.

27. Beris P, Samii K, Darbellay R, et al. Iron overload in patients with sideroblastic anaemia is not related to the presence of the haemochromatosis Cys282Tyr and His63Asp mutations. *Br J Haematol*. 1999;104(1):97-99.

28. Grosbois B, Bibes B, Jouanolle AM, et al. Haemochromatosis mutations and idiopathic acquired sideroblastic anemia (IASA). *Blood*. 1999;94(suppl 1):15b.

29. Cooley TB. A severe type of hereditary anemia with elliptocytosis. Interesting sequence of splenectomy. *Am J Med Sci*. 1945;209:561-568.

30. McFadzean A, Davis LJ. Iron-staining erythrocytic inclusions with especial reference to acquired haemolytic anaemia. *Glasgow Med J*. 1947;28(9):237-279.

31. Dacie JV, Doniach I. The basophilic property of the iron-containing granules in siderocytes. *J Pathol Bacteriol*. 1947;59(4):684-686.

32. Brain MC, Herdan A. Tissue iron stores in sideroblastic anaemia. *Br J Haematol*. 1965;11:107-113.

33. Hathway D, Harris JW, Stenger RJ. Histopathology of the liver in pyridoxine-responsive anemia. *Arch Pathol*. 1967;83(2):175-179.

34. Ducamp S, Fleming MD. The molecular genetics of sideroblastic anemia. *Blood*. 2019;133(1):59-69.

35. Bottomley SS, Muller-Eberhard U. Pathophysiology of heme synthesis. *Semin Hematol*. 1988;25(4):282-302.

36. Sadlon TJ, Dell'Oso T, Surinya KH, May BK. Regulation of erythroid 5-aminolevulinate synthase expression during erythropoiesis. *Int J Biochem Cell Biol*. 1999;31(10):1153-1167.

37. Dzikaite V, Kanopka A, Brock JH, Kazlauskas A, Melefors O. A novel endoproteolytic processing activity in mitochondria of erythroid cells and the role in heme synthesis. *Blood*. 2000;96(2):740-746.

38. Guernsey DL, Jiang H, Campagna DR, et al. Mutations in mitochondrial carrier family gene SLC25A38 cause nonsyndromic autosomal recessive congenital sideroblastic anemia. *Nat Genet*. 2009;41(6):651-653.

39. Lunetti P, Damiano F, De Benedetto G, et al. Characterization of human and yeast mitochondrial glycine carriers with implications for heme biosynthesis and anemia. *J Biol Chem*. 2016;291(38):19746-19759.

40. Cox TC, Bawden MJ, Abraham NG, et al. Erythroid 5-aminolevulinate synthase is located on the X chromosome. *Am J Hum Genet*. 1990;46(1):107-111.

41. Bishop DF, Henderson AS, Astrin KH. Human delta-aminolevulinate synthase: assignment of the housekeeping gene to 3p21 and the erythroid-specific gene to the X chromosome. *Genomics*. 1990;7(2):207-214.

42. Cotter PD, Drabkin HA, Varkony T, Smith DI, Bishop DF. Assignment of the human housekeeping delta-aminolevulinate synthase gene (ALAS1) to chromosome band 3p21.1 by PCR analysis of somatic cell hybrids. *Cytogenet Cell Genet*. 1995;69(3–4):207-208.

43. May B, Dogra SC, Sadlon TJ, Bhasker CR, Cox TC, Bottomley SS. Molecular regulation of heme biosynthesis in higher vertebrates. *Prog Nucleic Acid Res Mol Biol*. 1995;51:1-51.

44. Cotter PD, Willard HF, Gorski JL, Bishop DF. Assignment of human erythroid delta-aminolevulinate synthase (ALAS2) to a distal subregion of band Xp11.21 by PCR analysis of somatic cell hybrids containing X; autosome translocations. *Genomics*. 1992;13(1):211-212.

45. Cox TC, Kozman HM, Raskind WH, May BK, Mulley JC. Identification of a highly polymorphic marker within intron 7 of the ALAS2 gene and suggestion of at least two loci for X-linked sideroblastic anemia. *Hum Mol Genet*. 1992;1(8):639-641.

46. Nakajima O, Takahashi S, Harigae H, et al. Heme deficiency in erythroid lineage causes differentiation arrest and cytoplasmic iron overload. *EMBO J*. 1999;18(22):6282-6289.

47. Hofer T, Wenger RH, Kramer MF, Ferreira GC, Gassmann M. Hypoxic up-regulation of erythroid 5-aminolevulinate synthase. *Blood*. 2003;101(1):348-350.

48. Fuchs O, Ponka P. The role of iron supply in the regulation of 5-aminolevulinate synthase mRNA levels in murine erythroleukemia cells. *Neoplasma*. 1996;43(1):31-36.

49. Smith SJ, Cox TM. Translational control of erythroid delta-aminolevulinate synthase in immature human erythroid cells by heme. *Cell Mol Biol (Noisy-le-grand)*. 1997;43(1):103-114.

50. Cox TC, Bawden MJ, Martin A, May BK. Human erythroid 5-aminolevulinate synthase: promoter analysis and identification of an iron-responsive element in the mRNA. *EMBO J*. 1991;10(7):1891-1902.

51. Dandekar T, Stripecke R, Gray NK, et al. Identification of a novel iron-responsive element in murine and human erythroid delta-aminolevulinic acid synthase mRNA. *EMBO J*. 1991;10(7):1903-1909.

52. Melefors O, Goossen B, Johansson HE, Stripecke R, Gray NK, Hentze MW. Translational control of 5-aminolevulinate synthase mRNA by iron-responsive elements in erythroid cells. *J Biol Chem*. 1993;268(8):5974-5978.

53. Bhasker CR, Burgiel G, Neupert B, Emery-Goodman A, Kuhn LC, May BK. The putative iron-responsive element in the human erythroid 5-aminolevulinate synthase mRNA mediates translational control. *J Biol Chem*. 1993;268(17):12699-12705.

54. Gray NK, Hentze MW. Iron regulatory protein prevents binding of the 43S translation pre-initiation complex to ferritin and eALAS mRNAs. *EMBO J*. 1994;13(16):3882-3891.

55. Wingert RA, Galloway JL, Barut B, et al. Deficiency of glutaredoxin 5 reveals Fe-S clusters are required for vertebrate haem synthesis. *Nature*. 2005;436(7053):1035-1039.

56. Rouault TA. The role of iron regulatory proteins in mammalian iron homeostasis and disease. *Nat Chem Biol*. 2006;2(8):406-414.

57. Houston T, Moore MR, McColl KE, Fitzsimons E. Erythroid 5-aminolaevulinate synthase activity during normal and iron deficient erythropoiesis. *Br J Haematol*. 1991;78(4):561-564.

58. Lathrop JT, Timko MP. Regulation by heme of mitochondrial protein transport through a conserved amino acid motif. *Science*. 1993;259(5094):522-525.

59. Goodfellow BJ, Dias JS, Ferreira GC, Henklein P, Wray V, Macedo AL. The solution structure and heme binding of the presequence of murine 5-aminolevulinate synthase. *FEBS Lett*. 2001;505(2):325-331.

60. Munakata H, Sun JY, Yoshida K, et al. Role of the heme regulatory motif in the heme-mediated inhibition of mitochondrial import of 5-aminolevulinate synthase. *J Biochem*. 2004;136(2):233-238.

61. Furuyama K, Sassa S. Interaction between succinyl CoA synthetase and the heme-biosynthetic enzyme ALAS-E is disrupted in sideroblastic anemia. *J Clin Invest*. 2000;105(6):757-764.

62. Burch JS, Marcero JR, Maschek JA, et al. Glutamine via α-ketoglutarate dehydrogenase provides succinyl-CoA for heme synthesis during erythropoiesis. *Blood*. 2018;132(10):987-998.

63. Liu G, Sil D, Maio N, et al. Heme biosynthesis depends on previously unrecognized acquisition of iron-sulfur cofactors in human amino-levulinic acid dehydratase. *Nat Commun*. 2020;11(1):6310.

64. Kaya AH, Plewinska M, Wong DM, Desnick RJ, Wetmur JG. Human delta-aminolevulinate dehydratase (ALAD) gene: structure and alternative splicing of the erythroid and housekeeping mRNAs. *Genomics*. 1994;19(2):242-248.

65. Bishop TR, Miller MW, Beall J, Zon LI, Dierks P. Genetic regulation of delta-aminolevulinate dehydratase during erythropoiesis. *Nucleic Acids Res*. 1996;24(13):2511-2518.

66. Chretien S, Dubart A, Beaupain D, et al. Alternative transcription and splicing of the human porphobilinogen deaminase gene result either in tissue-specific or in house-keeping expression. *Proc Natl Acad Sci U S A*. 1988;85(1):6-10.

67. Beru N, Goldwasser E. Studies of the effect of erythropoietin on heme synthesis. *Adv Exp Med Biol*. 1989;271:87-94.

68. Aizencang G, Solis C, Bishop DF, Warner C, Desnick RJ. Human uroporphyrinogen-III synthase: genomic organization, alternative promoters, and erythroid-specific expression. *Genomics*. 2000;70(2):223-231.

69. Romeo PH, Raich N, Dubart A, et al. Molecular cloning and nucleotide sequence of a complete human uroporphyrinogen decarboxylase cDNA. *J Biol Chem*. 1986;261(21):9825-9831.

70. Takahashi S, Taketani S, Akasaka JE, et al. Differential regulation of copro-porphyrinogen oxidase gene between erythroid and nonerythroid cells. *Blood*. 1998;92(9):3436-3444.

71. Taketani S, Inazawa J, Abe T, et al. The human protoporphyrinogen oxidase gene (PPOX): organization and location to chromosome 1. *Genomics*. 1995;29(3):698-703.

72. Magness ST, Tugores A, Diala ES, Brenner DA. Analysis of the human ferrochelatase promoter in transgenic mice. *Blood*. 1998;92(1):320-328.

73. Busfield SJ, Riches KJ, Sainsbury AJ, Rossi E, Garcia-Webb P, Klinken SP. Retrovirally-produced erythropoietin effectively induces differentiation and proliferation of J2E erythroid cells. *Growth Factors*. 1993;9(2):87-97.

74. Houston T, Moore MR, McColl KE, Fitzsimons EJ. Regulation of haem biosynthesis in normoblastic erythropoiesis: role of 5-aminolaevulinic acid synthase and ferrochelatase. *Biochim Biophys Acta*. 1994;1201(1):85-93.

75. Taketani S, Adachi Y, Nakahashi Y. Regulation of the expression of human ferrochelatase by intracellular iron levels. *Eur J Biochem*. 2000;267(15):4685-4692.

76. Crooks DR, Ghosh MC, Haller RG, Tong WH, Rouault TA. Posttranslational stability of the heme biosynthetic enzyme ferrochelatase is dependent on iron availability and intact iron-sulfur cluster assembly machinery. *Blood*. 2010;115(4):860-869.

77. Shah DI, Takahashi-Makise N, Cooney JD, et al. Mitochondrial ATPIF1 regulates haem synthesis in developing erythroblasts. *Nature*. 2012;491(7425):608-612.

78. Ponka P. Tissue-specific regulation of iron metabolism and heme synthesis: distinct control mechanisms in erythroid cells. *Blood*. 1997;89(1):1-25.

79. Bottomley SS, Moore MZ. Regulation of iron metabolism in erythroblasts. *Blood*. 1985;66:43a.

80. Muta K, Nishimura J, Ideguchi H, Umemura T, Ibayashi H. Erythroblast transferrin receptors and transferrin kinetics in iron deficiency and various anemias. *Am J Hematol*. 1987;25(2):155-163.

81. Bottomley SS, Wolfe LC, Bridges KR. Iron metabolism in K562 erythroleukemic cells. *J Biol Chem*. 1985;260(11):6811-6815.

82. Ohgami RS, Campagna DR, Greer EL, et al. Identification of a ferrireductase required for efficient transferrin-dependent iron uptake in erythroid cells. *Nat Genet*. 2005;37(11):1264-1269.

83. Shi H, Bencze KZ, Stemmler TL, Philpott CC. A cytosolic iron chaperone that delivers iron to ferritin. *Science*. 2008;320(5880):1207-1210.

84. Sheftel AD, Zhang AS, Brown C, Shirihai OS, Ponka P. Direct interorganellar transfer of iron from endosome to mitochondrion. *Blood.* 2007;110(1):125-132.

85. Shaw GC, Cope JJ, Li L, et al. Mitoferrin is essential for erythroid iron assimilation. *Nature.* 2006;440(7080):96-100.

86. Chen W, Paradkar PN, Li L, et al. Abcb10 physically interacts with mitoferrin-1 (Slc25a37) to enhance its stability and function in the erythroid mitochondria. *Proc Natl Acad Sci U S A.* 2009;106(38):16263-16268.

87. Chen W, Dailey HA, Paw BH. Ferrochelatase forms an oligomeric complex with mitoferrin-1 and Abcb10 for erythroid heme biosynthesis. *Blood.* 2010;116(4):628-630.

88. Rouault TA. Linking physiological functions of iron. *Nat Chem Biol.* 2005;1(4):193-194.

89. Chiabrando D, Marro S, Mercurio S, et al. The mitochondrial heme exporter FLVCR1b mediates erythroid differentiation. *J Clin Invest.* 2012;122(12):4569-4579.

90. Charnay P, Maniatis T. Transcriptional regulation of globin gene expression in the human erythroid cell line K562. *Science.* 1983;220(4603):1281-1283.

91. Tahara T, Sun J, Nakanishi K, et al. Heme positively regulates the expression of beta-globin at the locus control region via the transcriptional factor Bach1 in erythroid cells. *J Biol Chem.* 2004;279(7):5480-5487.

92. Chen JJ. Regulation of protein synthesis by the heme-regulated eIF2alpha kinase: relevance to anemias. *Blood.* 2007;109(7):2693-2699.

93. Rundles RW, Falls HF. Hereditary (sex-linked?) anemia. *Am J Med Sci.* 1946;211:641-658.

94. Losowsky MS, Hall R. Hereditary sideroblastic anaemia. *Br J Haematol.* 1965;11:70-85.

95. Elves MW, Bourne MS, Israels MC. Pyridoxine-responsive anaemia determined by an X-linked gene. *J Med Genet.* 1966;3(1):1-4.

96. Prasad AS, Tranchida L, Konno ET, et al. Hereditary sideroblastic anemia and glucose-6-phosphate dehydrogenase deficiency in a Negro family. *J Clin Invest.* 1968;47(6):1415-1424.

97. Holmes J, May A, Geddes D, Jacobs A. A family study of congenital X linked sideroblastic anaemia. *J Med Genet.* 1990;27(1):26-28.

98. Cox TC, Bottomley SS, Wiley JS, Bawden MJ, Matthews CS, May BK. X-linked pyridoxine-responsive sideroblastic anemia due to a Thr388-to-Ser substitution in erythroid 5-aminolevulinate synthase. *N Engl J Med.* 1994;330(10):675-679.

99. Prades E, Chambon C, Dailey TA, Dailey HA, Briere J, Grandchamp B. A new mutation of the ALAS2 gene in a large family with X-linked sideroblastic anemia. *Hum Genet.* 1995;95(4):424-428.

100. Lee GR, MacDiarmid WD, Cartwright GE, Wintrobe MM. Hereditary, X-linked, sideroachrestic anemia. The isolation of two erythrocyte populations differing in Xga blood type and porphyrin content. *Blood.* 1968;32(1):59-70.

101. Weatherall DJ, Pembrey ME, Hall EG, Sanger R, Tippett P, Gavin J. Familial sideroblastic anaemia: problem of Xg and X chromosome inactivation. *Lancet.* 1970;2(7676):744-748.

102. Peto TE, Pippard MJ, Weatherall DJ. Iron overload in mild sideroblastic anaemias. *Lancet.* 1983;1(8321):375-378.

103. Bottomley SS, Wise PD, Wasson EG, et al. X-linked sideroblastic anemia in ten female probands due to ALAS2 mutations and skewed X chromosome inactivation. *Am J Hum Genet.* 1998;63(suppl):A352.

104. Aivado M, Gattermann N, Rong A, et al. X-linked sideroblastic anemia associated with a novel ALAS2 mutation and unfortunate skewed X-chromosome inactivation patterns. *Blood Cells Mol Dis.* 2006;37(1):40-45.

105. Rose C, Callebaut I, Pascal L, et al. Lethal ALAS2 mutation in males X-linked sideroblastic anaemia. *Br J Haematol.* 2017;178(4):648-651.

106. Vogler WR, Mingioli ES. Heme synthesis in pyridoxine-responsive anemia. *N Engl J Med.* 1965;273(7):347-353.

107. Aoki Y, Urata G, Wada O, Takaku F. Measurement of delta-aminolevulinic acid synthetase activity in human erythroblasts. *J Clin Invest.* 1974;53(5):1326-1334.

108. Konopka L, Hoffbrand AV. Haem synthesis in sideroblastic anaemia. *Br J Haematol.* 1979;42(1):73-83.

109. Aoki Y, Muranaka S, Nakabayashi K, Ueda Y. Delta-Aminolevulinic acid synthetase in erythroblasts of patients with pyridoxine-responsive anemia. Hypercatabolism caused by the increased susceptibility to the controlling protease. *J Clin Invest.* 1979;64(5):1196-1203.

110. Byrd RB, Cooper T. Hereditary iron-loading anemia with secondary hemochromatosis. *Ann Intern Med.* 1961;55:103-123.

111. Bottomley SS. Sideroblastic anemia: death from iron overload. *Hosp Pract.* 1991;26(suppl 3):55-56.

112. Cotter PD, May A, Fitzsimons EJ, et al. Late-onset X-linked sideroblastic anemia. Missense mutations in the erythroid delta-aminolevulinate synthase (ALAS2) gene in two pyridoxine-responsive patients initially diagnosed with acquired refractory anemia and ringed sideroblasts. *J Clin Invest.* 1995;96(4):2090-2096.

113. Rosenberg SJ, Bennett JM. Pyridoxine-responsive anemia. *N Y State J Med.* 1969;69(11):1430-1433.

114. Joosten E, van den Berg A, Riezler R, et al. Metabolic evidence that deficiencies of vitamin B-12 (cobalamin), folate, and vitamin B-6 occur commonly in elderly people. *Am J Clin Nutr.* 1993;58(4):468-476.

115. Nankivell BJ. Vitamin B$_6$ deficiency on hemodialysis causing sideroblastic anemia. *Nephron.* 1991;59(4):674-675.

116. Furuyama K, Harigae H, Kinoshita C, et al. Late-onset X-linked sideroblastic anemia following hemodialysis. *Blood.* 2003;101(11):4623-4624.

117. Busque L, Mio R, Mattioli J, et al. Nonrandom X-inactivation patterns in normal females: lyonization ratios vary with age. *Blood.* 1996;88(1):59-65.

118. Cazzola M, May A, Bergamaschi G, Cerani P, Rosti V, Bishop DF. Familial-skewed X-chromosome inactivation as a predisposing factor for late-onset X-linked sideroblastic anemia in carrier females. *Blood.* 2000;96(13):4363-4365.

119. Conboy JG, Cox TC, Bottomley SS, Bawden MJ, May BK. Human erythroid 5-aminolevulinate synthase. Gene structure and species-specific differences in alternative RNA splicing. *J Biol Chem.* 1992;267(26):18753-18758.

120. Noble JS, Taylor GR, Losowsky MS, et al. Linkage analysis of a large pedigree with hereditary sideroblastic anaemia. *J Med Genet.* 1995;32(5):389-392.

121. The Human Gene Mutation Database (HGMD®). http://www.hgmd.cf.ac.uk/ac/index.php.

122. Cotter PD, Rucknagel DL, Bishop DF. X-linked sideroblastic anemia: identification of the mutation in the erythroid-specific delta-aminolevulinate synthase gene (ALAS2) in the original family described by Cooley. *Blood.* 1994;84(11):3915-3924.

123. Edgar AJ, Losowsky MS, Noble JS, Wickramasinghe SN. Identification of an arginine452 to histidine substitution in the erythroid 5-aminolaevulinate synthetase gene in a large pedigree with X-linked hereditary sideroblastic anaemia. *Eur J Haematol.* 1997;58(1):1-4.

124. Koc S, Bishop DF, Li L, et al. Iron overload in pyridoxine-responsive X-linked sideroblastic anemia: greater severity in a heterozygote than in her hemizygous brother. *Blood.* 1997;90(suppl):16b.

125. Cotton HB, Harris JW. Familial pyridoxine-responsive anemia. *J Clin Invest.* 1962;31:1352.

126. Campagna DR, de Bie CI, Schmitz-Abe K, et al. X-linked sideroblastic anemia due to ALAS2 intron 1 enhancer element GATA-binding site mutations. *Am J Hematol.* 2014;89(3):315-319.

127. Kaneko K, Furuyama K, Fujiwara T, et al. Identification of a novel erythroid-specific enhancer for the ALAS2 gene and its loss-of-function mutation which is associated with congenital sideroblastic anemia. *Haematologica.* 2014;99(2):252-261.

128. Ferreira GC, Neame PJ, Dailey HA. Heme biosynthesis in mammalian systems: evidence of a Schiff base linkage between the pyridoxal 5′-phosphate cofactor and a lysine residue in 5-aminolevulinate synthase. *Protein Sci.* 1993;2(11):1959-1965.

129. May A, Al-Sabah AI, Lawless SL. Acquired sideroblastic anemia unresponsive to pyridoxine caused by a somatic mutation in ALAS 2. *Blood.* 2005;106:988a-989a.

130. Cotter PD, Baumann M, Bishop DF. Enzymatic defect in "X-linked" sideroblastic anemia: molecular evidence for erythroid delta-aminolevulinate synthase deficiency. *Proc Natl Acad Sci U S A.* 1992;89(9):4028-4032.

131. Furuyama K, Harigae H, Heller T, et al. Arg452 substitution of the erythroid-specific 5-aminolaevulinate synthase, a hot spot mutation in X-linked sideroblastic anaemia, does not itself affect enzyme activity. *Eur J Haematol.* 2006;76(1):33-41.

132. Bottomley SS, Wise PD, Wasson EG, et al. The spectrum of molecular defects in the erythroid 5-aminolevulinate synthase gene in hereditary sideroblastic anemia *Blood.* 1998;92(suppl 1):669a.

133. Bishop DF, Tchaikovskii V, Hoffbrand AV, Fraser ME, Margolis S. X-linked sideroblastic anemia due to carboxyl-terminal ALAS2 mutations that cause loss of binding to the beta-subunit of succinyl-CoA synthetase (SUCLA2). *J Biol Chem.* 2012;287(34):28943-28955.

134. Shoolingin-Jordan PM, Al-Daihan S, Alexeev D, et al. 5-Aminolevulinic acid synthase: mechanism, mutations and medicine. *Biochim Biophys Acta.* 2003;1647(1–2):361-366.

135. Astner I, Schulze JO, van den Heuvel J, Jahn D, Schubert WD, Heinz DW. Crystal structure of 5-aminolevulinate synthase, the first enzyme of heme biosynthesis, and its link to XLSA in humans. *EMBO J.* 2005;24(18):3166-3177.

136. Brown BL, Kardon JR, Sauer RT, Baker TA. Structure of the mitochondrial aminolevulinic acid synthase, a key heme biosynthetic enzyme. *Structure.* 2018;26(4):580-589.e584.

137. Bottomley SS, Fleming MD. Sideroblastic anemias: molecular basis, pathophysiology and clinical aspects. In: Kadish KM, Smith KM, Guilard R, eds. *Handbook of Porphyrin Science with Applications to Chemistry, Physics, Materials Science, Engineering Biology and Medicine.* Vol. 29. World Scientific Publishing; 2013:43-87.

138. Barton JC, Lee PL. Disparate phenotypic expression of ALAS2 R452H (nt 1407 G → A) in two brothers, one with severe sideroblastic anemia and iron overload, hepatic cirrhosis, and hepatocellular carcinoma. *Blood Cells Mol Dis.* 2006;36(3):342-346.

139. Cazzola M, May A, Bergamaschi G, Cerani P, Ferrillo S, Bishop DF. Absent phenotypic expression of X-linked sideroblastic anemia in one of 2 brothers with a novel ALAS2 mutation. *Blood.* 2002;100(12):4236-4238.

140. Kannengiesser C, Sanchez M, Sweeney M, et al. Missense SLC25A38 variations play an important role in autosomal recessive inherited sideroblastic anemia. *Haematologica.* 2011;96(6):808-813.

141. Liu G, Guo S, Kang H, et al. Mutation spectrum in Chinese patients affected by congenital sideroblastic anemia and a search for a genotype-phenotype relationship. *Haematologica.* 2013;98(12):e158-e160.

142. Mehri M, Zarin M, Ardalani F, Najmabadi H, Azarkeivan A, Neishabury M. Novel mutations in mitochondrial carrier family gene SLC25A38, causing congenital sideroblastic anemia in Iranian families, identified by whole exome sequencing. *Blood Cells Mol Dis.* 2018;71:39-44.

143. Heeney MM, Berhe S, Campagna DR, et al. SLC25A38 congenital sideroblastic anemia: phenotypes and genotypes of 31 individuals from 24 families, including 11 novel mutations, and a review of the literature. *Hum Mutat.* 2021;42(11):1367-1383.

144. Camaschella C, Campanella A, De Falco L, et al. The human counterpart of zebrafish shiraz shows sideroblastic-like microcytic anemia and iron overload. *Blood.* 2007;110(1):1353-1358.

145. Ye H, Jeong SY, Ghosh MC, et al. Glutaredoxin 5 deficiency causes sideroblastic anemia by specifically impairing heme biosynthesis and depleting cytosolic iron in human erythroblasts. *J Clin Invest.* 2010;120(5):1749-1761.

146. Liu G, Guo S, Anderson GJ, Camaschella C, Han B, Nie G. Heterozygous missense mutations in the GLRX5 gene cause sideroblastic anemia in a Chinese patient. *Blood.* 2014;124(17):2750-2751.

147. Schmitz-Abe K, Ciesielski SJ, Schmidt PJ, et al. Congenital sideroblastic anemia due to mutations in the mitochondrial HSP70 homologue HSPA9. *Blood.* 2015;126(25):2734-2738.

148. van Waveren Hogervorst GD, van Roermund HP, Snijders PJ. Hereditary sideroblastic anaemia and autosomal inheritance of erythrocyte dimorphism in a Dutch family. *Eur J Haematol.* 1987;38(5):405-409.

149. Crispin A, Guo C, Chen C, et al. Mutations in the iron-sulfur cluster biogenesis protein HSCB cause congenital sideroblastic anemia. *J Clin Invest.* 2020;130(10):5245-5256.

150. Bottomley SS, Tanaka M, Everett MA. Diminished erythroid ferrochelatase activity in protoporphyria. *J Lab Clin Med.* 1975;86(1):126-131.

151. Holme SA, Worwood M, Anstey AV, Elder GH, Badminton MN. Erythropoiesis and iron metabolism in dominant erythropoietic protoporphyria. *Blood.* 2007;110(12):4108-4110.

152. Scott AJ, Ansford AJ, Webster BH, Stringer HC. Erythropoietic protoporphyria with features of a sideroblastic anaemia terminating in liver failure. *Am J Med.* 1973;54(2):251-259.

153. Rademakers LH, Koningsberger JC, Sorber CW, et al. Accumulation of iron in erythroblasts of patients with erythropoietic protoporphyria. *Eur J Clin Invest.* 1993;23(2):130-138.

154. Gouya L, Puy H, Lamoril J, et al. Inheritance in erythropoietic protoporphyria: a common wild-type ferrochelatase allelic variant with low expression accounts for clinical manifestation. *Blood.* 1999;93(6):2105-2110.

155. Gouya L, Deybach JC, Lamoril J, et al. Modulation of the phenotype in dominant erythropoietic protoporphyria by a low expression of the normal ferrochelatase allele. *Am J Hum Genet.* 1996;58(2):292-299.

156. Fairbanks VF, Dickson ER, Thompson ME. Hereditary sideroblastic anemia. *Hosp Pract.* 1991;26(suppl 3):53-55.

157. Cuijpers MLH, van Spronsen DJ, Muus P, Hamel BCJ, Swinkels DW. Need for early recognition and therapeutic guidelines of congenital sideroblastic anaemia. *Int J Hematol.* 2011;94(1):97-100.

158. Hall R, Losowsky MS. The distribution of erythroblast iron in sideroblastic anaemias. *Br J Haematol.* 1966;12(3):334-340.

159. Wickramasinghe SN, Fulker MJ, Losowsky MS, Hall R. Microspectrophotometric and electron microscopic studies of bone marrow in hereditary sideroblastic anaemia. *Acta Haematol.* 1971;45(4):236-244.

160. Raab SO, Haut A, Cartwright GE, Wintrobe MM. Pyridoxine-responsive anemia. *Blood.* 1961;18:285-302.

161. Schafer AI, Rabinowe S, Le Boff MS, Bridges K, Cheron RG, Dluhy R. Long-term efficacy of deferoxamine iron chelation therapy in adults with acquired transfusional iron overload. *Arch Intern Med.* 1985;145(7):1217-1221.

162. Porter JB. Practical management of iron overload. *Br J Haematol.* 2001;115(2):239-252.

163. Porter JB. Concepts and goals in the management of transfusional iron overload. *Am J Hematol.* 2007;82(12 suppl):1136-1139.

164. Harris JW, Danish EH, Brittenham GM, McLaren CE. Pyridoxine responsive hereditary sideroblastic erythropoiesis and iron overload: two microcytic subpopulations in the affected male, one normocytic and one microcytic subpopulation in the obligate female carrier. *Am J Hematol.* 1993;42(4):400-401.

165. Hines JD. Effect of pyridoxine plus chronic phlebotomy on the function and morphology of bone marrow and liver in pyridoxine-responsive sideroblastic anemia. *Semin Hematol.* 1976;13(2):133-140.

166. Vogler WR, Mingioli ES. Porphyrin synthesis and heme synthetase activity in pyridoxine-responsive anemia. *Blood.* 1968;32(6):979-988.

167. Marcus RE, Huehns ER. Transfusional iron overload. *Clin Lab Haematol.* 1985;7(3):195-212.

168. Olivieri NF, Brittenham GM. Iron-chelating therapy and the treatment of thalassemia. *Blood.* 1997;89(3):739-761.

169. Nienhuis AW, Benz EJ, Jr, Propper R, et al. Thalassemia major: molecular and clinical aspects. NIH conference. *Ann Intern Med.* 1979;91(6):883-897.

170. Kushner JP, Porter JP, Olivieri NF. Secondary iron overload. *Hematology Am Soc Hematol Educ Program.* 2001;2001:47-61.

171. Miller KB, Rosenwasser LJ, Bessette JA, Beer DJ, Rocklin RE. Rapid desensitisation for desferrioxamine anaphylactic reaction. *Lancet.* 1981;1(8228):1059.

172. Cappellini MD, Cohen A, Piga A, et al. A phase 3 study of deferasirox (ICL670), a once-daily oral iron chelator, in patients with beta-thalassemia. *Blood.* 2006;107(9):3455-3462.

173. Robins-Browne RM, Prpic JK. Effects of iron and desferrioxamine on infections with *Yersinia enterocolitica. Infect Immun.* 1985;47(3):774-779.

174. Aleali SH, Castro O, Spencer RP, Finch SC. Sideroblastic anemia with splenic abscess and fatal thromboemboli after splenectomy. *Ann Intern Med.* 1975;83(5):661-663.

175. Byrne MT, Bergman AK, Ruiz AI, Silver BJ, Maciejewski JP, Tiu RV. Postsplenectomy thrombembolic disease in congenital sideroblastic anaemia. *BMJ Case Rep.* 2010;2010.

176. Gonzalez MI, Caballero D, Vazquez L, et al. Allogeneic peripheral stem cell transplantation in a case of hereditary sideroblastic anaemia. *Br J Haematol.* 2000;109(3):658-660.

177. Urban C, Binder B, Hauer C, Lanzer G. Congenital sideroblastic anemia successfully treated by allogeneic bone marrow transplantation. *Bone Marrow Transpl.* 1992;10(4):373-375.

178. Ayas M, Al-Jefri A, Mustafa MM, Al-Mahr M, Shalaby L, Solh H. Congenital sideroblastic anaemia successfully treated using allogeneic stem cell transplantation. *Br J Haematol.* 2001;113(4):938-939.

179. Medeiros BC, Kolhouse JF, Cagnoni PJ, et al. Nonmyeloablative allogeneic hematopoietic stem cell transplantation for congenital sideroblastic anemia. *Bone Marrow Transpl.* 2003;31(11):1053-1055.

180. Meo A, Ruggeri A, La Rosa MA, Zanghi L, Morabito N, Duca L. Iron burden and liver fibrosis decrease during a long-term phlebotomy program and iron chelating treatment after bone marrow transplantation. *Hemoglobin.* 2006;30(1):131-137.

181. Urban CH, Deutschmann A, Kerbl R, et al. Organ tolerance following cadaveric liver transplantation for chronic graft-versus-host disease after allogeneic bone marrow transplantation. *Bone Marrow Transpl.* 2002;30(8):535-537.

182. Kim MH, Shah S, Bottomley SS, Shah NC. Reduced-toxicity allogeneic hematopoietic stem cell transplantation in congenital sideroblastic anemia. *Clin Case Rep.* 2018;6(9):1841-1844.

183. Kakourou G, Vrettou C, Kattamis A, et al. Complex preimplantation genetic diagnosis for beta-thalassaemia, sideroblastic anaemia, and human leukocyte antigen (HLA)-typing. *Syst Biol Reprod Med.* 2016;62(1):69-76.

184. Pagon RA, Bird TD, Detter JC, Pierce I. Hereditary sideroblastic anaemia and ataxia: an X linked recessive disorder. *J Med Genet.* 1985;22(4):267-273.

185. Raskind WH, Wijsman E, Pagon RA, et al. X-linked sideroblastic anemia and ataxia: linkage to phosphoglycerate kinase at Xq13. *Am J Hum Genet.* 1991;48(2):335-341.

186. Savary S, Allikmets R, Denizot F, et al. Isolation and chromosomal mapping of a novel ATP-binding cassette transporter conserved in mouse and human. *Genomics.* 1997;41(2):275-278.

187. Shimada Y, Okuno S, Kawai A, et al. Cloning and chromosomal mapping of a novel ABC transporter gene (hABC7), a candidate for X-linked sideroblastic anemia with spinocerebellar ataxia. *J Hum Genet.* 1998;43(2):115-122.

188. Kispal G, Csere P, Prohl C, Lill R. The mitochondrial proteins Atm1p and Nfs1p are essential for biogenesis of cytosolic Fe/S proteins. *EMBO J.* 1999;18(14):3981-3989.

189. Allikmets R, Raskind WH, Hutchinson A, Schueck ND, Dean M, Koeller DM. Mutation of a putative mitochondrial iron transporter gene (ABC7) in X-linked sideroblastic anemia and ataxia (XLSA/A). *Hum Mol Genet.* 1999;8(5):743-749.

190. Bekri S, Kispal G, Lange H, et al. Human ABC7 transporter: gene structure and mutation causing X-linked sideroblastic anemia with ataxia with disruption of cytosolic iron-sulfur protein maturation. *Blood.* 2000;96(9):3256-3264.

191. Maguire A, Hellier K, Hammans S, May A. X-linked cerebellar ataxia and sideroblastic anaemia associated with a missense mutation in the ABC7 gene predicting V411L. *Br J Haematol.* 2001;115(4):910-917.

192. D'Hooghe M, Selleslag D, Mortier G, et al. X-linked sideroblastic anemia and ataxia: a new family with identification of a fourth ABCB7 gene mutation. *Eur J Paediatr Neurol.* 2012;16(6):730-735.

193. Lill R. Function and biogenesis of iron-sulphur proteins. *Nature.* 2009;460(7257):831-838.

194. Srinivasan V, Pierik AJ, Lill R. Crystal structures of nucleotide-free and glutathione-bound mitochondrial ABC transporter Atm1. *Science.* 2014;343(6175):1137-1140.

195. Taketani S, Kakimoto K, Ueta H, Masaki R, Furukawa T. Involvement of ABC7 in the biosynthesis of heme in erythroid cells: interaction of ABC7 with ferrochelatase. *Blood.* 2003;101(8):3274-3280.

196. Hellier KD, Hatchwell E, Duncombe AS, Kew J, Hammans SR. X-linked sideroblastic anaemia with ataxia: another mitochondrial disease? *J Neurol Neurosurg Psychiatry.* 2001;70(1):65-69.

197. Wiseman DH, May A, Jolles S, et al. A novel syndrome of congenital sideroblastic anemia, B-cell immunodeficiency, periodic fevers, and developmental delay (SIFD). *Blood.* 2013;122(1):112-123.

198. Chakraborty PK, Schmitz-Abe K, Kennedy EK, et al. Mutations in TRNT1 cause congenital sideroblastic anemia with immunodeficiency, fevers, and developmental delay (SIFD). *Blood.* 2014;124(18):2867-2871.

199. Liwak-Muir U, Mamady H, Naas T, et al. Impaired activity of CCA-adding enzyme TRNT1 impacts OXPHOS complexes and cellular respiration in SIFD patient-derived fibroblasts. *Orphanet J Rare Dis.* 2016;11(1):79.

200. DeLuca AP, Whitmore SS, Barnes J, et al. Hypomorphic mutations in TRNT1 cause retinitis pigmentosa with erythrocytic microcytosis. *Hum Mol Genet.* 2016;25(1):44-56.

201. Giannelou A, Wang H, Zhou Q, et al. Aberrant tRNA processing causes an autoinflammatory syndrome responsive to TNF inhibitors. *Ann Rheum Dis.* 2018;77(4):612-619.

202. Rotig A, Bourgeron T, Chretien D, Rustin P, Munnich A. Spectrum of mitochondrial DNA rearrangements in the Pearson marrow-pancreas syndrome. *Hum Mol Genet.* 1995;4(8):1327-1330.

203. Rotig A, Cormier V, Blanche S, et al. Pearson's marrow-pancreas syndrome. A multisystem mitochondrial disorder in infancy. *J Clin Invest.* 1990;86(5):1601-1608.

204. Farruggia P, Di Marco F, Dufour C. Pearson syndrome. *Expert Rev Hematol.* 2018;11(3):239-246.

205. Smith OP, Hann IM, Woodward CE, Brockington M. Pearson's marrow/pancreas syndrome: haematological features associated with deletion and duplication of mitochondrial DNA. *Br J Haematol.* 1995;90(2):469-472.

206. Bader-Meunier B, Mielot F, Breton-Gorius J, et al. Hematologic involvement in mitochondrial cytopathies in childhood: a retrospective study of bone marrow smears. *Pediatr Res.* 1999;46(2):158-162.

207. Pearson HA, Lobel JS, Kocoshis SA, et al. A new syndrome of refractory sideroblastic anemia with vacuolization of marrow precursors and exocrine pancreatic dysfunction. *J Pediatr.* 1979;95(6):976-984.

208. Simonsz HJ, Barlocher K, Rotig A. Kearns-Sayre's syndrome developing in a boy who survived Pearson's syndrome caused by mitochondrial DNA deletion. *Doc Ophthalmol.* 1992;82(1–2):73-79.

209. Bykhovskaya Y, Casas K, Mengesha E, Inbal A, Fischel-Ghodsian N. Missense mutation in pseudouridine synthase 1 (PUS1) causes mitochondrial myopathy and sideroblastic anemia (MLASA). *Am J Hum Genet.* 2004;74(6):1303-1308.

210. Casas KA, Fischel-Ghodsian N. Mitochondrial myopathy and sideroblastic anemia. *Am J Med Genet.* 2004;125A(2):201-204.

211. Zeharia A, Fischel-Ghodsian N, Casas K, et al. Mitochondrial myopathy, sideroblastic anemia, and lactic acidosis: an autosomal recessive syndrome in Persian Jews caused by a mutation in the PUS1 gene. *J Child Neurol.* 2005;20(5):449-452.

212. Fernandez-Vizarra E, Berardinelli A, Valente L, Tiranti V, Zeviani M. Nonsense mutation in pseudouridylate synthase 1 (PUS1) in two brothers affected by myopathy, lactic acidosis and sideroblastic anaemia (MLASA). *J Med Genet.* 2007;44(3):173-180.

213. Sasarman F, Nishimura T, Thiffault I, Shoubridge EA. A novel mutation in YARS2 causes myopathy with lactic acidosis and sideroblastic anemia. *Hum Mutat.* 2012;33(8):1201-1206.

214. Patton JR, Bykhovskaya Y, Mengesha E, Bertolotto C, Fischel-Ghodsian N. Mitochondrial myopathy and sideroblastic anemia (MLASA): missense mutation in the pseudouridine synthase 1 (PUS1) gene is associated with the loss of tRNA pseudouridylation. *J Biol Chem.* 2005;280(20):19823-19828.

215. Riley LG, Cooper S, Hickey P, et al. Mutation of the mitochondrial tyrosyl-tRNA synthetase gene, YARS2, causes myopathy, lactic acidosis, and sideroblastic anemia—MLASA syndrome. *Am J Hum Genet.* 2010;87(1):52-59.

216. Riley LG, Menezes MJ, Rudinger-Thirion J, et al. Phenotypic variability and identification of novel YARS2 mutations in YARS2 mitochondrial myopathy, lactic acidosis and sideroblastic anaemia. *Orphanet J Rare Dis.* 2013;8:193.

217. Riley LG, Heeney MM, Rudinger-Thirion J, et al. The phenotypic spectrum of germline *YARS2* variants: from isolated sideroblastic anemia to mitochondrial myopathy, lactic acidosis and sideroblastic anemia 2. *Haematologica.* 2018;103(12):2008-2015.

218. Sommerville EW, Ng YS, Alston CL, et al. Clinical features, molecular heterogeneity, and prognostic implications in YARS2-related mitochondrial myopathy. *JAMA Neurol.* 2017;74(6):686-694.

219. Lichtenstein DA, Crispin AW, Sendamarai AK, et al. A recurring mutation in the respiratory complex 1 protein NDUFB11 is responsible for a novel form of X-linked sideroblastic anemia. *Blood.* 2016;128(15):1913-1917.

220. Torraco A, Bianchi M, Verrigni D, et al. A novel mutation in NDUFB11 unveils a new clinical phenotype associated with lactic acidosis and sideroblastic anemia. *Clin Genet.* 2017;91(3):441-447.

221. Riley LG, Rudinger-Thirion J, Schmitz-Abe K, et al. LARS2 variants associated with hydrops, lactic acidosis, sideroblastic anemia, and multisystem failure. *JIMD Rep.* 2016;28:49-57.

222. Burrage LC, Tang S, Wang J, et al. Mitochondrial myopathy, lactic acidosis, and sideroblastic anemia (MLASA) plus associated with a novel de novo mutation (m.8969G>A) in the mitochondrial encoded ATP6 gene. *Mol Genet Metab.* 2014;113(3):207-212.

223. Berhe S, Heeney MM, Campagna DR, et al. Recurrent heteroplasmy for the MT-ATP6 p.Ser148Asn (m.8969G>A) mutation in patients with syndromic congenital sideroblastic anemia of variable clinical severity. *Haematologica.* 2018;103(12):e561-e563.

224. Porter FS, Rogers LE, Sidbury JB, Jr. Thiamine-responsive megaloblastic anemia. *J Pediatr.* 1969;74(4):494-504.

225. Labay V, Raz T, Baron D, et al. Mutations in SLC19A2 cause thiamine-responsive megaloblastic anaemia associated with diabetes mellitus and deafness. *Nat Genet.* 1999;22(3):300-304.

226. Fleming JC, Tartaglini E, Steinkamp MP, Schorderet DF, Cohen N, Neufeld EJ. The gene mutated in thiamine-responsive anaemia with diabetes and deafness (TRMA) encodes a functional thiamine transporter. *Nat Genet.* 1999;22(3):305-308.

227. Diaz GA, Banikazemi M, Oishi K, Desnick RJ, Gelb BD. Mutations in a new gene encoding a thiamine transporter cause thiamine-responsive megaloblastic anaemia syndrome. *Nat Genet.* 1999;22(3):309-312.

228. Bergmann AK, Sahai I, Falcone JF, et al. Thiamine-responsive megaloblastic anemia: identification of novel compound heterozygotes and mutation update. *J Pediatr.* 2009;155(6):888-892.e881.

229. Baron D, Assaraf YG, Cohen N, Aronheim A. Lack of plasma membrane targeting of a G172D mutant thiamine transporter derived from Rogers syndrome family. *Mol Med.* 2002;8(8):462-474.

230. Subramanian VS, Marchant JS, Parker I, Said HM. Cell biology of the human thiamine transporter-1 (hTHTR1). Intracellular trafficking and membrane targeting mechanisms. *J Biol Chem.* 2003;278(6):3976-3984.

231. Boros LG, Steinkamp MP, Fleming JC, Lee WN, Cascante M, Neufeld EJ. Defective RNA ribose synthesis in fibroblasts from patients with thiamine-responsive megaloblastic anemia (TRMA). *Blood.* 2003;102(10):3556-3561.

232. Abboud MR, Alexander D, Najjar SS. Diabetes mellitus, thiamine-dependent megaloblastic anemia, and sensorineural deafness associated with deficient alpha-ketoglutarate dehydrogenase activity. *J Pediatr.* 1985;107(4):537-541.

233. Neufeld EJ, Fleming JC, Tartaglini E, Steinkamp MP. Thiamine-responsive megaloblastic anemia syndrome: a disorder of high-affinity thiamine transport. *Blood Cells Mol Dis.* 2001;27(1):135-138.

234. Ricketts CJ, Minton JA, Samuel J, et al. Thiamine-responsive megaloblastic anaemia syndrome: long-term follow-up and mutation analysis of seven families. *Acta Paediatr.* 2006;95(1):99-104.

235. Bergmann AK, Campagna DR, McLoughlin EM, et al. Systematic molecular genetic analysis of congenital sideroblastic anemia: evidence for genetic heterogeneity and identification of novel mutations. *Pediatr Blood Cancer.* 2010;54(2):273-278.

236. Amos RJ, Miller AL, Amess JA. Autosomal inheritance of sideroblastic anaemia. *Clin Lab Haematol.* 1988;10(3):347-353.

237. Tuckfield A, Ratnaike S, Hussein S, Metz J. A novel form of hereditary sideroblastic anaemia with macrocytosis. *Br J Haematol.* 1997;97(2):279-285.

238. Brownlie A, Donovan A, Pratt SJ, et al. Positional cloning of the zebrafish sauternes gene: a model for congenital sideroblastic anaemia. *Nat Genet.* 1998;20(3):244-250.

239. Zhang Y, Zhang J, An W, et al. Intron 1 GATA site enhances ALAS2 expression indispensably during erythroid differentiation. *Nucleic Acids Res.* 2017;45(2):657-671.

240. Harigae H, Nakajima O, Suwabe N, et al. Aberrant iron accumulation and oxidized status of erythroid-specific delta-aminolevulinate synthase (ALAS2)-deficient definitive erythroblasts. *Blood.* 2003;101(3):1188-1193.

241. Pondarre C, Campagna DR, Antiochos B, Sikorski L, Mulhern H, Fleming MD. Abcb7, the gene responsible for X-linked sideroblastic anemia with ataxia, is essential for hematopoiesis. *Blood.* 2007;109(8):3567-3569.

242. Mangum JE, Hardee JP, Fix DK, et al. Pseudouridine synthase 1 deficient mice, a model for mitochondrial myopathy with sideroblastic anemia, exhibit muscle morphology and physiology alterations. *Sci Rep.* 2016;6:26202.

243. Harriss EB, Macgibbon BH, Mollin DL. Experimental sideroblastic anaemia. *Br J Haematol.* 1965;11:99-106.

244. Tanaka M, Bottomley SS. Bone marrow delta-aminolevulinic acid synthetase activity in experimental sideroblastic anemia. *J Lab Clin Med.* 1974;84(1):92-98.

245. Gruneberg H. The anaemia of flexed-tail mice (Mus musculus). II. Siderocytes. *J Genet.* 1942;44:246-271.

246. Chui DH, Sweeney GD, Patterson M, Russell ES. Hemoglobin synthesis in siderocytes of flexed-tailed mutant (f/f) fetal mice. *Blood.* 1977;50(1):165-177.

247. Fleming MD, Campagna DR, Haslett JN, Trenor CC,III, Andrews NC. A mutation in a mitochondrial transmembrane protein is responsible for the pleiotropic hematological and skeletal phenotype of flexed-tail (f/f) mice. *Genes Dev.* 2001;15(6):652-657.

248. Kory N, Wyant GA, Prakash G, et al. SFXN1 is a mitochondrial serine transporter required for one-carbon metabolism. *Science.* 2018;362(6416):eaat9528.

249. Acoba MG, Alpergin ESS, Renuse S, et al. The mitochondrial carrier SFXN1 is critical for complex III integrity and cellular metabolism. *Cell Rep.* 2021;34(11):108869.

250. Bjorkman SE. Chronic refractory anemia with sideroblastic bone marrow; a study of four cases. *Blood.* 1956;11(3):250-259.

251. Bennett JM. Classification of the myelodysplastic syndromes. *Clin Haematol.* 1986;15(4):909-923.

252. Juneja SK, Imbert M, Sigaux F, Jouault H, Sultan C. Prevalence and distribution of ringed sideroblasts in primary myelodysplastic syndromes. *J Clin Pathol.* 1983;36(5):566-569.

253. Arber DA, Orazi A, Hasserjian R, et al. The 2016 revision to the World Health Organization classification of myeloid neoplasms and acute leukemia. *Blood.* 2016;127(20):2391-2405.

254. Streeter RR, Presant CA, Reinhard E. Prognostic significance of thrombocytosis in idiopathic sideroblastic anemia. *Blood.* 1977;50(3):427-432.

255. Broseus J, Florensa L, Zipperer E, et al. Clinical features and course of refractory anemia with ring sideroblasts associated with marked thrombocytosis. *Haematologica.* 2012;97(7):1036-1041.

256. Catovsky D, Shaw MT, Hoffbrand AV, Dacie JV. Sideroblastic anaemia and its association with leukaemia and myelomatosis: a report of five cases. *Br J Haematol.* 1971;20(4):385-393.

257. Eastman PM, Schwartz R, Schrier SL. Distinctions between idiopathic ineffective erythropoiesis and di Guglielmo's disease: clinical and biochemical differences. *Blood.* 1972;40(4):487-499.

258. Kushner JP, Lee GR, Wintrobe MM, Cartwright GE. Idiopathic refractory sideroblastic anemia: clinical and laboratory investigation of 17 patients and review of the literature. *Medicine (Baltim).* 1971;50(3):139-159.

259. Dacie JV, Smith MD, White JC, Mollin DL. Refractory normoblastic anaemia: a clinical and haematological study of seven cases. *Br J Haematol.* 1959;5(1):56-82.

260. Riedler GF, Straub PW. Abnormal iron incorporation, survival protoporphyrin content and fluorescence of one red cell population in preleukemic sideroblastic anemia. *Blood.* 1972;40(3):345-352.

261. Prchal JT, Throckmorton DW, Carroll AJ,III, Fuson EW, Gams RA, Prchal JF. A common progenitor for human myeloid and lymphoid cells. *Nature.* 1978;274(5671):590-591.

262. Amenomori T, Tomonaga M, Jinnai I, et al. Cytogenetic and cytochemical studies on progenitor cells of primary acquired sideroblastic anemia (PASA): involvement of multipotent myeloid stem cells in PASA clone and mosaicism with normal clone. *Blood.* 1987;70(5):1367-1372.

263. Lawrence HJ, Broudy VC, Magenis RE, et al. Cytogenetic evidence for involvement of B lymphocytes in acquired idiopathic sideroblastic anemias. *Blood.* 1987;70(4):1003-1005.

264. Suzuki H, Asano H, Ohashi H, et al. Clonality analysis of refractory anemia with ring sideroblasts: simultaneous study of clonality and cytochemistry of bone marrow progenitors. *Leukemia.* 1999;13(1):130-134.

265. Germing U, Gattermann N, Aivado M, Hildebrandt B, Aul C. Two types of acquired idiopathic sideroblastic anaemia (AISA): a time-tested distinction. *Br J Haematol.* 2000;108(4):724-728.

266. Heim S, Mitelman F. Chromosome abnormalities in the myelodysplastic syndromes. *Clin Haematol.* 1986;15(4):1003-1021.

267. Dewald GW, Brecher M, Travis LB, Stupca PJ. Twenty-six patients with hematologic disorders and X chromosome abnormalities. Frequent idic(X)(q13) chromosomes and Xq13 anomalies associated with pathologic ringed sideroblasts. *Cancer Genet Cytogenet.* 1989;42(2):173-185.

268. Dierlamm J, Michaux L, Criel A, et al. Isodicentric (X)(q13) in haematological malignancies: presentation of five new cases, application of fluorescence in situ hybridization (FISH) and review of the literature. *Br J Haematol.* 1995;91(4):885-891.

269. Yoshida K, Sanada M, Shiraishi Y, et al. Frequent pathway mutations of splicing machinery in myelodysplasia. *Nature.* 2011;478(7367):64-69.

270. Papaemmanuil E, Cazzola M, Boultwood J, et al. Somatic SF3B1 mutation in myelodysplasia with ring sideroblasts. *N Engl J Med.* 2011;365(15):1384-1395.

271. Visconte V, Makishima H, Jankowska A, et al. SF3B1, a splicing factor is frequently mutated in refractory anemia with ring sideroblasts. *Leukemia.* 2012;26(3):542-545.
272. Patnaik MM, Lasho TL, Hodnefield JM, et al. SF3B1 mutations are prevalent in myelodysplastic syndromes with ring sideroblasts but do not hold independent prognostic value. *Blood.* 2012;119(2):569-572.
273. Malcovati L, Cazzola M. Recent advances in the understanding of myelodysplastic syndromes with ring sideroblasts. *Br J Haematol.* 2016;174(6):847-858.
274. Szpurka H, Tiu R, Murugesan G, et al. Refractory anemia with ringed sideroblasts associated with marked thrombocytosis (RARS-T), another myeloproliferative condition characterized by JAK2 V617F mutation. *Blood.* 2006;108(7):2173-2181.
275. Gattermann N, Billiet J, Kronenwett R, et al. High frequency of the JAK2 V617F mutation in patients with thrombocytosis (platelet count > 600 × 109/L) and ringed sideroblasts more than 15% considered as MDS/MPD, unclassifiable. *Blood.* 2007;109(3):1334-1335.
276. Schmitt-Graeff AH, Teo SS, Olschewski M, et al. JAK2V617F mutation status identifies subtypes of refractory anemia with ringed sideroblasts associated with marked thrombocytosis. *Haematologica.* 2008;93(1):34-40.
277. Patnaik MM, Tefferi A. Refractory anemia with ring sideroblasts (RARS) and RARS with thrombocytosis (RARS-T): 2017 update on diagnosis, risk-stratification, and management. *Am J Hematol.* 2017;92(3):297-310.
278. Janusz K, Del Rey M, Abaigar M, et al. A two-step approach for sequencing spliceosome-related genes as a complementary diagnostic assay in MDS patients with ringed sideroblasts. *Leuk Res.* 2017;56:82-87.
279. Darman RB, Seiler M, Agrawal AA, et al. Cancer-associated SF3B1 hotspot mutations induce cryptic 3′ splice site selection through use of a different branch point. *Cell Rep.* 2015;13(5):1033-1045.
280. Kurtovic-Kozaric A, Przychodzen B, Singh J, et al. PRPF8 defects cause missplicing in myeloid malignancies. *Leukemia.* 2015;29(1):126-136.
281. Bottomley SS, Tanaka M, Self J. Delta-aminolevulinic acid synthetase activity in normal human bone marrow and in patients with idiopathic sideroblastic anemia. *Enzyme.* 1973;16(1):138-145.
282. Bottomley SS. Porphyrin and iron metabolism in sideroblastic anemia. *Semin Hematol.* 1977;14(2):169-185.
283. Fitzsimons EJ, May A, Elder GH, Jacobs A. 5-Aminolaevulinic acid synthase activity in developing human erythroblasts. *Br J Haematol.* 1988;69(2):281-285.
284. Mason DY, Emerson PM. Primary acquired sideroblastic anaemia: response to treatment with pyridoxal-5-phosphate. *Br Med J.* 1973;1(5850):389-390.
285. Meier PJ, Fehr J, Meyer UA. Pyridoxine-responsive primary acquired sideroblastic anaemia. In vitro and in vivo effects of vitamin B6 on decreased 5-aminolaevulinate synthase activity. *Scand J Haematol.* 1982;29(5):421-424.
286. Bottomley SS, Healy HM, Brandenburg MA, May BK. 5-Aminolevulinate synthase in sideroblastic anemias: mRNA and enzyme activity levels in bone marrow cells. *Am J Hematol.* 1992;41(2):76-83.
287. Lim HW, Cooper D, Sassa S, Dosik H, Buchness MR, Soter NA. Photosensitivity, abnormal porphyrin profile, and sideroblastic anemia. *J Am Acad Dermatol.* 1992;27(2, Pt 2):287-292.
288. Sarkany RP, Ross G, Willis F. Acquired erythropoietic protoporphyria as a result of myelodysplasia causing loss of chromosome 18. *Br J Dermatol.* 2006;155(2):464-466.
289. Bottomley SS. Observations on free erythrocyte protoporphyrin in sideroachrestic anemia. *Clin Chim Acta.* 1965;12:543-545.
290. Aoki Y. Multiple enzymatic defects in mitochondria in hematological cells of patients with primary sideroblastic anemia. *J Clin Invest.* 1980;66(1):43-49.
291. Wulfert M, Kupper AC, Tapprich C, et al. Analysis of mitochondrial DNA in 104 patients with myelodysplastic syndromes. *Exp Hematol.* 2008;36(5):577-586.
292. Coulombel L, Tchernia G, Mielot F, Mohandas N. Hemoglobin content of individual erythroblasts in hematopoietic dysplasia: marked heterogeneity at late stages of maturation. *Exp Hematol.* 1984;12(7):587-593.
293. Dolatshad H, Pellagatti A, Liberante FG, et al. Cryptic splicing events in the iron transporter ABCB7 and other key target genes in SF3B1-mutant myelodysplastic syndromes. *Leukemia.* 2016;30(12):2322-2331.
294. Nikpour M, Scharenberg C, Liu A, et al. The transporter ABCB7 is a mediator of the phenotype of acquired refractory anemia with ring sideroblasts. *Leukemia.* 2013;27(4):889-896.
295. Boultwood J, Pellagatti A, Nikpour M, et al. The role of the iron transporter ABCB7 in refractory anemia with ring sideroblasts. *PLoS One.* 2008;3(4):e1970.
296. Dolatshad H, Pellagatti A, Fernandez-Mercado M, et al. Disruption of SF3B1 results in deregulated expression and splicing of key genes and pathways in myelodysplastic syndrome hematopoietic stem and progenitor cells. *Leukemia.* 2015;29(5):1092-1103.
297. del Rey M, Benito R, Fontanillo C, et al. Deregulation of genes related to iron and mitochondrial metabolism in refractory anemia with ring sideroblasts. *PLoS One.* 2015;10(5):e0126555.
298. Yien YY, Robledo RF, Schultz IJ, et al. TMEM14C is required for erythroid mitochondrial heme metabolism. *J Clin Invest.* 2014;124(10):4294-4304.
299. Clough CA, Pangallo J, Sarchi M, et al. Coordinated missplicing of TMEM14C and ABCB7 causes ring sideroblast formation in SF3B1-mutant myelodysplastic syndrome. *Blood.* 2022;139(13):2038-2049.
300. Yoshimi A, Lin KT, Wiseman DH, et al. Coordinated alterations in RNA splicing and epigenetic regulation drive leukaemogenesis. *Nature.* 2019;574(7777):273-277.
301. Inoue D, Chew GL, Liu B, et al. Spliceosomal disruption of the non-canonical BAF complex in cancer. *Nature.* 2019;574(7778):432-436.
302. Obeng EA, Chappell RJ, Seiler M, et al. Physiologic expression of Sf3b1(K700E) causes impaired erythropoiesis, aberrant splicing, and sensitivity to therapeutic spliceosome modulation. *Cancer Cell.* 2016;30(3):404-417.
303. Mupo A, Seiler M, Sathiaseelan V, et al. Hemopoietic-specific Sf3b1-K700E knock-in mice display the splicing defect seen in human MDS but develop anemia without ring sideroblasts. *Leukemia.* 2017;31(3):720-727.
304. Stavem P, Rorvik TO, Rootwelt K, Josefsen JO. Severe iron deficiency causing loss of ring sideroblasts. *Scand J Haematol.* 1983;31(4):389-391.
305. Minuk LA, Hsia CC. Refractory anemia with ring sideroblasts masked by iron deficiency anemia. *Blood.* 2011;117(22):5793.
306. Cazzola M, Barosi G, Gobbi PG, Invernizzi R, Riccardi A, Ascari E. Natural history of idiopathic refractory sideroblastic anemia. *Blood.* 1988;71(2):305-312.
307. Schafer AI, Cheron RG, Dluhy R, et al. Clinical consequences of acquired transfusional iron overload in adults. *N Engl J Med.* 1981;304(6):319-324.
308. Malcovati L. Impact of transfusion dependency and secondary iron overload on the survival of patients with myelodysplastic syndromes. *Leuk Res.* 2007;31(suppl 3):S2-S6.
309. Leitch HA, Leger CS, Goodman TA, et al. Improved survival in patients with myelodysplastic syndrome receiving iron chelation therapy. *Clin Leuk.* 2008;2:205-211.
310. Neukirchen J, Fox F, Kundgen A, et al. Improved survival in MDS patients receiving iron chelation therapy-a matched pair analysis of 188 patients from the Dusseldorf MDS registry. *Leuk Res.* 2012;36(8):1067-1070.
311. French TJ, Jacobs P. Sideroblastic anaemia associated with iron overload treated by repeated phlebotomy. *S Afr Med J.* 1976;50(15):594-596.
312. Jensen PD, Heickendorff L, Pedersen B, et al. The effect of iron chelation on haemopoiesis in MDS patients with transfusional iron overload. *Br J Haematol.* 1996;94(2):288-299.
313. Del Rio Garma J, Fernandez Lago C, Batlle Fonrodona FJ. Desferrioxamine in the treatment of myelodysplastic syndromes. *Haematologica.* 1997;82(5):639-640.
314. Raskind WH, Tirumali N, Jacobson R, Singer J, Fialkow PJ. Evidence for a multistep pathogenesis of a myelodysplastic syndrome. *Blood.* 1984;63(6):1318-1323.
315. Barton JC, Conrad ME, Parmley RT. Acute lymphoblastic leukemia in idiopathic refractory sideroblastic anemia: evidence for a common lymphoid and myeloid progenitor cell. *Am J Hematol.* 1980;9(1):109-115.
316. Hussein KK, Salem Z, Bottomley SS, Livingston RB. Acute leukemia in idiopathic sideroblastic anemia: response to combination chemotherapy. *Blood.* 1982;59(3):652-656.
317. Yunis JJ, Lobell M, Arnesen MA, et al. Refined chromosome study helps define prognostic subgroups in most patients with primary myelodysplastic syndrome and acute myelogenous leukaemia. *Br J Haematol.* 1988;68(2):189-194.
318. Khaleeli M, Keane WM, Lee GR. Sideroblastic anemia in multiple myeloma: a preleukemic change. *Blood.* 1973;41(1):17-25.
319. Kitahara M, Cosgriff TM, Eyre HJ. Sideroblastic anemia as a preleukemic event in patients treated for Hodgkin's disease. *Ann Intern Med.* 1980;92(5):625-627.
320. Mantovani L, Lentini G, Hentschel B, et al. Treatment of anaemia in myelodysplastic syndromes with prolonged administration of recombinant human granulocyte colony-stimulating factor and erythropoietin. *Br J Haematol.* 2000;109(2):367-375.
321. Terpos E, Mougiou A, Kouraklis A, et al. Prolonged administration of erythropoietin increases erythroid response rate in myelodysplastic syndromes: a phase II trial in 281 patients. *Br J Haematol.* 2002;118(1):174-180.
322. Jadersten M, Montgomery SM, Dybedal I, Porwit-MacDonald A, Hellstrom-Lindberg E. Long-term outcome of treatment of anemia in MDS with erythropoietin and G-CSF. *Blood.* 2005;106(3):803-811.
323. Wallvik J, Stenke L, Bernell P, Nordahl G, Hippe E, Hast R. Serum erythropoietin (EPO) levels correlate with survival and independently predict response to EPO treatment in patients with myelodysplastic syndromes. *Eur J Haematol.* 2002;68(3):180-185.
324. Santini V. Treatment of low-risk myelodysplastic syndromes. *Hematology Am Soc Hematol Educ Program.* 2016;2016(1):462-469.
325. Giagounidis A. Current treatment algorithm for the management of lower-risk MDS. *Hematology Am Soc Hematol Educ Program.* 2017;2017(1):453-459.
326. Greenberg PL, Stone RM, Al-Kala A, et al. Myelodysplastic syndromes, version 2.2017, NCCN clinical practice guidelines in oncology. *J Natl Compr Canc Netw.* 2017;15:60-87.
327. Mies A, Hermine O, Platzbecker U. Activin receptor II ligand traps and their therapeutic potential in myelodysplastic syndromes with ring sideroblasts. *Curr Hematol Malig Rep.* 2016;11(6):416-424.
328. Fenaux P, Platzbecker U, Mufti GJ, et al. Luspatercept in patients with lower-risk myelodysplastic syndromes. *N Engl J Med.* 2020;382(2):140-151.
329. Brierley CK, Steensma DP. Targeting splicing in the treatment of myelodysplastic syndromes and other myeloid neoplasms. *Curr Hematol Malig Rep.* 2016;11(6):408-415.
330. Steensma DP, Wermke M, Klimek VM, et al. Phase I first-in-human dose escalation study of the oral SF3B1 modulator H3B-8800 in myeloid neoplasms. *Leukemia.* 2021;35(12):3542-3550.
331. Savage D, Lindenbaum J. Anemia in alcoholics. *Medicine (Baltim).* 1986;65(5):322-338.
332. Eichner ER, Hillman RS. The evolution of anemia in alcoholic patients. *Am J Med.* 1971;50(2):218-232.
333. Pierce HI, McGuffin RG, Hillman RS. Clinical studies in alcoholic sideroblastosis. *Arch Intern Med.* 1976;136(3):283-289.
334. Hines JD. Reversible megaloblastic and sideroblastic marrow abnormalities in alcoholic patients. *Br J Haematol.* 1969;16(1):87-101.
335. Freedman ML, Cohen HS, Rosman J, Forte FJ. Ethanol inhibition of reticulocyte protein synthesis: the role of haem. *Br J Haematol.* 1975;30(3):351-363.
336. Freedman ML, Rosman J. A rabbit reticulocyte model for the role of hemin-controlled repressor in hypochromic anemias. *J Clin Invest.* 1976;57(3):594-603.
337. McColl KE, Thompson GG, Moore MR, Goldberg A. Acute ethanol ingestion and haem biosynthesis in healthy subjects. *Eur J Clin Invest.* 1980;10(2, pt. 1):107-112.

338. Abdulla M, Svensson S. Effect of oral zinc intake on delta-aminolaevulinic acid dehydratase in red blood cells. *Scand J Clin Lab Invest.* 1979;39(1):31-36.

339. Lumeng L. The role of acetaldehyde in mediating the deleterious effect of ethanol on pyridoxal 5'-phosphate metabolism. *J Clin Invest.* 1978;62(2):286-293.

340. Lumeng L, Li TK. Vitamin B_6 metabolism in chronic alcohol abuse. Pyridoxal phosphate levels in plasma and the effects of acetaldehyde on pyridoxal phosphate synthesis and degradation in human erythrocytes. *J Clin Invest.* 1974;53(3):693-704.

341. Hines JD, Cowan DH. Studies on the pathogenesis of alcohol-induced sideroblastic bone-marrow abnormalities. *N Engl J Med.* 1970;283(9):441-446.

342. Meagher RC, Sieber F, Spivak JL. Suppression of hematopoietic-progenitor-cell proliferation by ethanol and acetaldehyde. *N Engl J Med.* 1982;307(14):845-849.

343. Burke JP, Rubin E. The effects of ethanol and acetaldehyde on the products of protein synthesis by liver mitochondria. *Lab Invest.* 1979;41(5):393-400.

344. Bottomley SS. Sideroblastic anaemia. In: Jacobs A, Worwood M, eds. *Iron in Biochemistry and Medicine II.* Academic Press; 1980:363-392.

345. Roberts PD, Hoffbrand AV, Mollin DL. Iron and folate metabolism in tuberculosis. *Br Med J.* 1966;2(5507):198-202.

346. Haden HT. Pyridoxine-responsive sideroblastic anemia due to antituberculous drugs. *Arch Intern Med.* 1967;120(5):602-606.

347. Standal BR, Kao-Chen SM, Yang GY, Char DF. Early changes in pyridoxine status of patients receiving isoniazid therapy. *Am J Clin Nutr.* 1974;27(5):479-484.

348. Scott JL, Finegold SM, Belkin GA, Lawrence JS. A controlled double-blind study of the hematologic toxicity of chloramphenicol. *N Engl J Med.* 1965;272:1137-1142.

349. Skinnider LF, Ghadially FN. Chloramphenicol-induced mitochondrial and ultrastructural changes in hemopoietic cells. *Arch Pathol Lab Med.* 1976;100(11):601-605.

350. Martelo OJ, Manyan DR, Smith US, Yunis AA. Chloramphenicol and bone marrow mitochondria. *J Lab Clin Med.* 1969;74(6):927-940.

351. Firkin FC. Mitochondrial lesions in reversible erythropoietic depression due to chloramphenicol. *J Clin Invest.* 1972;51(8):2085-2092.

352. Manyan DR, Arimura GK, Yunis AA. Chloramphenicol-induced erythroid suppression and bone marrow ferrochelatase activity in dogs. *J Lab Clin Med.* 1972;79(1):137-144.

353. Rosenberg A, Marcus O. Effect of chloramphenicol on reticulocyte delta-aminolaevulinic acid synthetase in rabbits. *Br J Haematol.* 1974;26(1):79-83.

354. Yunis AA, Adamson JW. Differential in vitro sensitivity of marrow erythroid and granulocytic colony forming cells to chloramphenicol. *Am J Hematol.* 1977;2(4):355-363.

355. Saini N, Jacobson JO, Jha S, Saini V, Weinger R. The perils of not digging deep enough—uncovering a rare cause of acquired anemia. *Am J Hematol.* 2012;87(4):413-416.

356. Kloss P, Xiong L, Shinabarger DL, Mankin AS. Resistance mutations in 23 S rRNA identify the site of action of the protein synthesis inhibitor linezolid in the ribosomal peptidyl transferase center. *J Mol Biol.* 1999;294(1):93-101.

357. Williams DM. Copper deficiency in humans. *Semin Hematol.* 1983;20(2):118-128.

358. Dunlap WM, James GW,III, Hume DM. Anemia and neutropenia caused by copper deficiency. *Ann Intern Med.* 1974;80(4):470-476.

359. Vilter RW, Bozian RC, Hess EV, Zellner DC, Petering HG. Manifestations of copper deficiency in a patient with systemic sclerosis on intravenous hyperalimentation. *N Engl J Med.* 1974;291(4):188-191.

360. Hirase N, Abe Y, Sadamura S, et al. Anemia and neutropenia in a case of copper deficiency: role of copper in normal hematopoiesis. *Acta Haematol.* 1992;87(4):195-197.

361. Saitoh T, Matsushima T, Toyama K, et al. Copper deficiency pancytopenia with infectious complications after hemolytic anemia. *Ann Hematol.* 2006;85(12):881-882.

362. Nagano T, Toyoda T, Tanabe H, et al. Clinical features of hematological disorders caused by copper deficiency during long-term enteral nutrition. *Intern Med.* 2005;44(6):554-559.

363. Halfdanarson TR, Kumar N, Hogan WJ, Murray JA. Copper deficiency in celiac disease. *J Clin Gastroenterol.* 2009;43(2):162-164.

364. Kumar N. Copper deficiency myelopathy (human swayback). *Mayo Clin Proc.* 2006;81(10):1371-1384.

365. Choi EH, Strum W. Hypocupremia-related myeloneuropathy following gastrojejunal bypass surgery. *Ann Nutr Metab.* 2010;57(3–4):190-192.

366. Perry AR, Pagliuca A, Fitzsimons EJ, Mufti GJ, Williams R. Acquired sideroblastic anaemia induced by a copper-chelating agent. *Int J Hematol.* 1996;64(1):69-72.

367. Fiske DN, McCoy HE,III, Kitchens CS. Zinc-induced sideroblastic anemia: report of a case, review of the literature, and description of the hematologic syndrome. *Am J Hematol.* 1994;46(2):147-150.

368. Nations SP, Boyer PJ, Love LA, et al. Denture cream: an unusual source of excess zinc, leading to hypocupremia and neurologic disease. *Neurology.* 2008;71(9):639-643.

369. Hedera P, Peltier A, Fink JK, Wilcock S, London Z, Brewer GJ. Myelopolyneuropathy and pancytopenia due to copper deficiency and high zinc levels of unknown origin II. The denture cream is a primary source of excessive zinc. *Neurotoxicology.* 2009;30(6):996-999.

370. Broun ER, Greist A, Tricot G, Hoffman R. Excessive zinc ingestion. A reversible cause of sideroblastic anemia and bone marrow depression. *JAMA.* 1990;264(11):1441-1443.

371. Bennett DR, Baird CJ, Chan KM, et al. Zinc toxicity following massive coin ingestion. *Am J Forensic Med Pathol.* 1997;18(2):148-153.

372. Hassan HA, Netchvolodoff C, Raufman JP. Zinc-induced copper deficiency in a coin swallower. *Am J Gastroenterol.* 2000;95(10):2975-2977.

373. Kumar A, Jazieh AR. Case report of sideroblastic anemia caused by ingestion of coins. *Am J Hematol.* 2001;66(2):126-129.

374. Pawa S, Khalifa AJ, Ehrinpreis MN, Schiffer CA, Siddiqui FA. Zinc toxicity from massive and prolonged coin ingestion in an adult. *Am J Med Sci.* 2008;336(5):430-433.

375. Schleper B, Stuerenburg HJ. Copper deficiency-associated myelopathy in a 46-year-old woman. *J Neurol.* 2001;248(8):705-706.

376. Prodan CI, Holland NR, Wisdom PJ, Burstein SA, Bottomley SS. CNS demyelination associated with copper deficiency and hyperzincemia. *Neurology.* 2002;59(9):1453-1456.

377. Gregg XT, Reddy V, Prchal JT. Copper deficiency masquerading as myelodysplastic syndrome. *Blood.* 2002;100(4):1493-1495.

378. Prodan CI, Holland NR, Wisdom PJ, Bottomley SS. Myelopathy due to copper deficiency. *Neurology.* 2004;62(9):1655-1656. author reply 1656.

379. Lee GR, Cartwright GE, Wintrobe MM. Heme biosynthesis in copper deficient swine. *Proc Soc Exp Biol Med.* 1968;127(4):977-981.

380. Cousins RJ. Absorption, transport, and hepatic metabolism of copper and zinc: special reference to metallothionein and ceruloplasmin. *Physiol Rev.* 1985;65(2):238-309.

381. Day FA, Panemangalore M, Brady FO. In vivo and ex vivo effects of copper on rat liver metallothionein. *Proc Soc Exp Biol Med.* 1981;168(3):306-310.

382. Brewer GJ, Hill GM, Prasad AS, Cossack ZT, Rabbani P. Oral zinc therapy for Wilson's disease. *Ann Intern Med.* 1983;99(3):314-319.

383. Kumar N, Elliott MA, Hoyer JD, Harper CM, Jr, Ahlskog JE, Phyliky RL. Myelodysplasia," myeloneuropathy, and copper deficiency. *Mayo Clin Proc.* 2005;80(7):943-946.

384. Weihl CC, Lopate G. Motor neuron disease associated with copper deficiency. *Muscle Nerve.* 2006;34(6):789-793.

385. Prodan CI, Bottomley SS, Holland NR, Lind SE. Relapsing hypocupraemic myelopathy requiring high-dose oral copper replacement. *J Neurol Neurosurg Psychiatry.* 2006;77(9):1092-1093.

386. O'Brien H, Amess JA, Mollin DL. Recurrent thrombocytopenia, erythroid hypoplasia and sideroblastic anaemia associated with hypothermia. *Br J Haematol.* 1982;51(3):451-456.

387. Pfanner N, Hartl FU, Neupert W. Import of proteins into mitochondria: a multi-step process. *Eur J Biochem.* 1988;175(2):205-212.

388. Morell H, Savoie JC, London IM. The biosynthesis of heme and the incorporation of glycine into globin in rabbit bone marrow in vitro. *J Biol Chem.* 1958;233(4):923-929.

389. Jandl JH, Inman JK, Simmons RL, Allen DW. Transfer of iron from serum iron-binding protein to human reticulocytes. *J Clin Invest.* 1959;38(1, pt 1):161-185.

Disorders of Red Blood Cells

Chapter 27 ■ Hemochromatosis

JAMES C. BARTON • CHARLES J. PARKER

IRON OVERLOAD

Iron overload is the consequence of iron accumulation that exceeds iron loss. Examples include (1) absorption of excessive amounts of normal dietary iron (hemochromatosis, disorders of ineffective erythropoiesis), (2) absorption of excessive amounts due to consumption of high quantities of iron (eg, African iron overload, medicinal iron overload), and (3) iatrogenic iron overload due to requirement for chronic transfusion (eg, aplastic anemia, myelodysplastic syndrome). The definition of iron overload typically includes a description of an individual's iron phenotype, such as (1) an elevated serum ferritin concentration without other explanation, (2) abnormally high transferrin saturation, (3) excessive iron in the liver or myocardium, and (4) a greater than normal number of phlebotomies to induce iron-limited erythropoiesis.

HISTORY

In 1865, Trousseau reported a 28-year-old Parisian man whose autopsy revealed hepatomegaly and hypertrophic cirrhosis. In 1871, Troisier described a 51-year-old Parisian man who had bronzing of the skin. The patient's autopsy revealed an enlarged, chocolate-colored liver. Microscopy showed pigmented granules within and outside of the hepatocytes. In 1886, the term *cirrhose pigmentaire* was used to describe the triad of skin bronzing, diabetes mellitus, and hepatic cirrhosis. von Recklinghausen introduced the term *hämochromatose* in his 1889 description of 12 patients evaluated at autopsy who had iron pigmentation involving multiple organs. Sheldon described 311 cases of hemochromatosis in his 1935 monograph.[1]

DIFFERENTIAL DIAGNOSIS OF IRON OVERLOAD

Both heritable and acquired disorders are associated with increased body iron stores (*Table 27.1*).

HEMOCHROMATOSIS

Ferroportin (p.SLC40A1), a transmembrane protein, is the tissue exporter of iron and is expressed primarily on the surface of duodenal enterocytes, hepatocytes, and reticuloendothelial cells (see Chapter 25 for a detailed description of iron homeostasis). Ferroportin is the only known receptor of hepcidin (a word derived from hepatic bactericidal protein). After hepcidin binding, the hepcidin-ferroportin complex is internalized and degraded. Therefore, hepcidin expression is the ultimate regulator of iron homeostasis due to its effects on ferroportin. When plasma hepcidin concentration is high, ferroportin density is low, limiting duodenal absorption of iron and availability of iron recycled from senescent erythrocytes by the reticuloendothelial system. When plasma hepcidin concentration is low, expression of cellular ferroportin is high, resulting both in an increase of gastrointestinal absorption of iron and availability of recycled iron. Consequently, proteins that control expression of *HAMP* (the gene that encodes hepcidin, an acronym for hepatic antimicrobial peptide) indirectly control cell surface expression of ferroportin (see Chapter 25 for a detailed description of the proteins involved in regulation of *HAMP* expression). Polymorphisms and mutations in genes that encode proteins involved in the hepcidin-ferroportin axis underlie the pathophysiology of hemochromatosis.[a]

---

[a]While this Chapter was in press, "*Hemochromatosis classification: update and recommendations by the BIOIRON Society*" was published (*Blood.* 2022; 139:3018-29). Although the nomenclatures used differ from those in this Chapter, the disease entities can be cross-referenced based on the molecular pattern shown in Table 4 of the *Blood* paper.

HFE Hemochromatosis

The mutant gene that causes most cases of hemochromatosis in non-Hispanic Western European whites was found to be linked to the human leukocyte antigen (HLA) locus on the short arm of chromosome 6. In 1996, the gene was isolated by positional cloning and named *HFE* (homeostatic iron regulator).[2] Consistent with diagnoses of hemochromatosis previously obtained by HLA-A and -B typing, *HFE* is located at 6p21.3, ~4 mB telomeric to the HLA locus. The structure of *HFE* is similar to that of other HLA class I–like genes. Two common *HFE* missense mutations (p.C282Y and p.H63D) account for most cases of *HFE* hemochromatosis.[2] Most patients with *HFE* hemochromatosis are homozygous for p.C282Y (exon 4; c.845G→A; rs1800562). A small proportion of patients with *HFE* hemochromatosis are compound heterozygotes (p.C282Y/p.H63D). HFE protein is a component of the complex that senses the status of circulating iron in combination with transferrin receptor 1 (TfR1) and transferrin receptor 2 (TfR2) and effects hepcidin transcription through interaction of components of the complex (HFE and TfR2) with receptors (bone morphogenic receptors type I and II) for bone morphogenic protein 2 (BMP-2) and bone morphogenic protein 6 (BMP-6) (discussed in more detail below and in Chapter 25).

HFE Mutations

At least 97 mutations of the *HFE* gene have been reported.[3] The most common genotype of persons with *HFE* hemochromatosis is p.C282Y homozygosity.[2] The second most common *HFE* mutation in patients with hemochromatosis is p.H63D (exon 2; 187C→G; rs1799945) in a compound heterozygous genotype with p.C282Y (*Table 27.2*).[2] Of the reported pathogenic *HFE* mutations, most are missense or nonsense mutations. Some mutations involve a nucleotide change that does not result in an amino acid substitution (synonymous mutations). Other mutations occur in noncoding regions of *HFE*.[3] It is expected that other rare *HFE* mutations will be discovered in adults with hemochromatosis phenotypes.

HFE Mutations and Iron Loading

Pathogenic mutations typically cause iron overload when they occur in homozygosity or in compound heterozygosity. At least 37 *HFE* mutations are associated with clinically significant iron loading, including p.C282Y, p.R330M, IVS3 (+1) G→T, p.E168X, p.C282S, p.R74X, and p.G93fs.[3] About 25 mutations have a modest or moderate effect on iron accumulation, including p.H63D, p.S65C, p.G93R, p.I105T, and p.E168Q. Approximately 36 *HFE* mutations have been identified in individuals without iron overload or in whom the effect of the mutation on iron accumulation could not be determined.[3] Synonymous mutations do not affect iron absorption.[3]

Juvenile Hemochromatosis

Juvenile hemochromatosis is characterized by nontransfusion iron overload, often severe, that typically occurs in children or young adults. Patients with juvenile hemochromatosis have pathogenic *HJV*, *HAMP*, or *TFR2* genotypes.

Hemojuvelin (*HJV*) Hemochromatosis

HJV hemochromatosis is an autosomal recessive disorder due to inheritance of two pathogenic mutations (either homozygosity or compound heterozygosity) in the hemojuvelin gene (*HJV*; chromosome 1q21.1).[7-9] The iron overload phenotype is more severe at the same age than that of typical patients with *HFE* hemochromatosis. Penetrance of *HJV* hemochromatosis genotypes to cause iron overload is also greater. *HJV* hemochromatosis often causes abdominal pain

Table 27.1. Heritable and Acquired Disorders Associated With Iron Overload: Differential Diagnosis

Heritable Disorder	Chromosome	Pattern of Inheritance	Cause of Iron Loading
HFE hemochromatosis	6p21.3	Autosomal recessive	Mutations of *HFE*, excess consumption of dietary or supplemental iron
HJV hemochromatosis	1q21	Autosomal recessive	Mutations of hemojuvelin
HAMP hemochromatosis	19q13	Autosomal recessive	Hepcidin antimicrobial peptide gene mutations
TFR2 hemochromatosis	7q22	Autosomal recessive	Inactivation of transferrin receptor 2
SLC40A1 hemochromatosis	2q32	Autosomal dominant	Ferroportin gene mutations
H-ferritin hemochromatosis	11q12-q13	Autosomal dominant	H-ferritin gene mutations
Porphyria cutanea tarda	1p34	Autosomal dominant or sporadic	Heterogeneous
Atransferrinemia	3q21	Autosomal recessive	Transferrin gene mutations and red cell transfusions
Aceruloplasminemia	3q23-q24	Autosomal recessive	Ceruloplasmin gene mutations
Hereditary hyperferritinemia and cataract syndrome	19q13.1-q13.3.3	Autosomal dominant	L-ferritin gene mutations
Friedreich ataxia	9p23-p11,9q13	Autosomal recessive	Frataxin gene mutations
Panthothenate kinase-associated neurodegeneration	20p13-p12.3	Autosomal recessive	Panthothenate kinase gene mutations
β-Thalassemia major	11p15.5	Autosomal recessive	β-Globin gene mutations, chronic hemolysis, red cell transfusions
Other Chronic Hemolytic Anemias			
Hereditary X-linked sideroblastic anemia	Xp11.21; Xp11.3	X-Linked	δ-Aminolevulinic acid synthase gene mutations; respiratory complex 1 protein gene (*NDUFB11*) mutation (p.F93del)
X-Linked sideroblastic anemia with ataxia	Xq13.1-q13.3	X-Linked	*ABCB7* mutations
MLASA syndrome	12q24.33	Autosomal recessive	Pseudouridine synthase-1 mutations
GLRX5 sideroblastic anemia	14q32.13	Autosomal recessive	Glutaredoxin-5 mutations
DMT1 iron overload	12q13	Autosomal recessive	*SLC11A2* mutations
Pyruvate kinase deficiency	1q21	Autosomal recessive	Pyruvate kinase gene mutations
G6PD deficiency	Xq28	X-Linked	G6PD gene mutations
Congenital dyserythropoietic anemias	Type I 15q15.1-q15.3	Autosomal recessive	Ineffective erythropoiesis
	Type II 20q11.2	Autosomal recessive	Ineffective erythropoiesis
	Type III 15q21	Autosomal dominant	Ineffective erythropoiesis
Acquired Disorder	**Cause of Iron Loading**	**Heritability**	
Transfusion iron overload	Erythrocyte infusions		
African iron overload	Consumption of traditional beer containing iron	Multiple family members sometimes affected	
Neonatal hemochromatosis	Alloimmunity, increased in utero iron transfer and liver injury	Multiple siblings sometimes affected	
Medicinal iron overload	Excessive supplemental iron ingestion, parenteral iron injections		
Myelodysplasia with ringed sideroblasts	Excessive iron absorption; erythrocyte transfusion	Increased prevalence of *HFE* p.C282Y heterozygosity	
Portacaval shunt	Excessive iron absorption		
Hemodialysis	Excessive iron infusions		
Nonalcoholic fatty liver disease	Excessive iron absorption		

Abbreviations: ABCB7, ATP-binding cassette, subfamily B, member 7; DMT1, divalent metal transporter-1; G6PD, glucose-6-phosphate dehydrogenase; MLASA, myopathy with lactic acidosis and sideroblastic anemia; SLC11A2, solute carrier family 11, member 2.
Modified from Edwards CQ, Barton JC. Hemochromatosis. In: Greer JP, Arber DA, Glader B, et al, eds. *Wintrobe's Clinical Hematology.* 13th ed. Philadelphia, PA: Lippincott Williams & Wilkins; 2014:662–681.

Disorders of Red Blood Cells

Table 27.2. Prevalence of *HFE* Genotypes in the United States[a]

Race/Ethnicity	N	p.C282Y/p.C282Y, %	p.C282Y/p.H63D, %	p.H63D/p.H63D, %	p.C282Y/wt, %	p.H63D/wt, %	Wt/Wt, %
Non-Hispanic White							
Kaiser	32,820	0.44	1.75	2.35	9.58	23.18	62.69
NHANES III	2016	0.30	2.33	2.38	9.82	23.66	61.51
HEIRS Study	44,082	0.64	2.06	2.33	10.32	23.90	60.75
Non-Hispanic Black/African American							
Kaiser	1501	0	0.27	0.19	3.53	8.39	87.61
NHANES III	1600	0.06	0.06	0.31	2.38	5.63	91.56
HEIRS Study	27,124	0.015	0.13	0.11	2.23	5.60	91.91
Mexican American/Hispanic							
Kaiser	2986	0.17	0.70	1.34	3.05	20.09	74.65
NHANES III	1555	0.03	0.39	0.90	2.64	20.58	75.43
HEIRS Study	12,459	0.056	0.39	1.23	2.82	17.65	77.86
Native American							
HEIRS Study	648	0.15	1.08	1.08	5.40	19.75	72.53
Pacific Islander							
HEIRS Study	698	0	0	0	2.15	8.88	89.97
Asian							
Kaiser	1814	0	0	0.28	0.22	6.84	92.67
HEIRS Study	12,772	0	0	0.23	0.13	8.38	91.27
Other/multiple/unknown							
Kaiser	2581	0.23	1.16	1.51	6.35	17.05	73.69
HEIRS Study	1928	0.31	0.99	1.09	5.76	16.23	75.62

[a]Approximately 20% of HEIRS Study participants were enrolled in Hamilton, Ontario, Canada. wt, wild type indicates absence of *HFE* p.C282Y or p.H63D except in the Kaiser study wherein a very small percentage of "wt" chromosomes in participants with p.C282Y/wt were p.S65C.[4] These are unadjusted prevalence rates. Weighted prevalence estimates[5] or prevalence estimates from Hardy-Weinberg proportions[6] may differ slightly. NHANES, National Health and Nutrition Examination Survey. Data were tabulated from these sources: Kaiser,[4] NHANES III,[5] and HEIRS Study.[6]

and hepatomegaly in children, hypogonadotrophic hypogonadism in teenagers, and arthropathy, osteoporosis, heart failure, cardiac arrhythmias, and cirrhosis before the age of 30 years.[10,11] Estimated daily iron absorption was 3.2 to 3.9 mg in some patients (whereas absorption of ~1 mg of iron daily is normal for men).[12]

The most common mutation (p.G320V) has been detected in patients of diverse European ethnicities.[13,14] More than 30 pathogenic *HJV* mutations have been reported. Many mutations are confined to specific kinships.[13,14] Some patients with *HJV* hemochromatosis also have an abnormal *HFE* genotype, although such a coexisting abnormality does not account for or exacerbate iron overload.[15]

Through interactions with BMP receptors, hemojuvelin participates in transcriptional regulation of *HAMP* (see Chapter 25). Mutations that underlie *HJV* hemochromatosis decrease hemojuvelin activity, resulting in decreased hepcidin transcription, thereby decreasing hepcidin available for binding and inactivation of ferroportin. Consequently, iron export from absorptive enterocytes via ferroportin into the plasma is increased and transferrin saturation is increased due to more efficient recycling of iron from senescent erythrocytes by the reticuloendothelial system.

Hepcidin (*HAMP*) Hemochromatosis

HAMP hemochromatosis, a rare disorder inherited as an autosomal recessive trait, is associated with iron overload phenotypes of variable severity and age at diagnosis.[16] *HAMP* hemochromatosis is due to mutations in the hepcidin gene (*HAMP*, chromosome 19q13.12). Mutations that limit *HAMP* transcription cause hemochromatosis by altering the balance of the hepcidin-ferroportin axis as described above for *HJV* hemochromatosis.

C70R was the first reported pathogenic *HAMP* mutation.[17] Approximately 12 other pathogenic *HAMP* mutations have been described. Some patients, usually those heterozygous for pathogenic promoter or coding region mutations, also have *HFE* mutations that may contribute to the development of iron overload ("digenic" hemochromatosis).

Transferrin Receptor-2 (*TFR2*) Hemochromatosis

Hemochromatosis *TFR2* is a rare autosomal recessive disorder of Europeans, Asians, and blacks of sub-Saharan African descent caused by mutations of the transferrin receptor-2 gene (*TFR2*; chromosome 7q22.1).[18,19] The clinical phenotype is variable, although penetrance is high. Some patients present in the second decade with multiorgan iron overload typical of juvenile hemochromatosis. Iron overload and its clinical manifestations in other patients are mild and may not progress, even without therapy.

TFR2 p.Y250X and p.R455Q have been detected in individuals or kindreds who were not closely related. Consanguinity has been identified in some affected families. More than 20 pathogenic *TFR2* mutations have been reported.[20] Single-nucleotide polymorphism (SNP) analysis for the four most common variants identifies mutations in less than one-half of persons known or suspected to have *TFR2* hemochromatosis, whereas almost all variants are detected by direct gene sequencing. TfR2 is a component of the complex that senses the status of circulating iron in combination with transferrin receptor 1 and HFE and effects hepcidin transcription through interaction of components of the complex with the receptor for BMP receptors (see Chapter 25). Pathogenic *TFR2* mutations result in decreased transcription of hepcidin[21] and thereby increase iron absorption by altering the balance of the hepcidin-ferroportin axis.

Ferroportin (*SLC40A1*) Hemochromatosis

Ferroportin hemochromatosis, an uncommon heterogeneous disorder transmitted as an autosomal dominant trait, is caused by mutations of the gene encoding the hepcidin receptor ferroportin (*SLC40A1*, chromosome 2q32.2).[22-24] There are two distinct ferroportin hemochromatosis phenotypes. Loss-of-function mutations encode ferroportin that either is not presented normally on the cell surface or has defective iron transport activity. Such mutations decrease iron export from the intestine and inhibit iron egress from macrophages. Phenotypes include normal or low transferrin saturation, mild anemia, predominance of iron retention in macrophages, and decreased tolerance to phlebotomy therapy. Increased iron absorption, often mild, is attributed to compensatory mechanisms responsive to anemia. Gain-of-function mutations encode ferroportin that cannot bind hepcidin normally or be internalized after hepcidin binding ("hepcidin resistance"). Consequently, iron absorption via enterocytes and iron export by macrophages are increased. Phenotypes include high transferrin saturation, normal hemoglobin concentrations, predominance of iron deposition in hepatocytes, and tolerance of phlebotomy therapy that is similar to that of patients with *HFE* hemochromatosis.

Ferroportin mutations are cosmopolitan. Most reported mutations are restricted to single families, although *SLC40A1* p.V162del has been reported in patients with iron overload from Australia, Europe, and Asia. p.A77D has been reported in patients with iron overload in Italy, Australia, and India, and p.Q248H (exon 6; c.744G → T; rs11568350) is a polymorphism found in native blacks in sub-Saharan Africa and in African Americans. Serum ferritin concentrations are higher in some native sub-Saharan Africans and African Americans with p.Q248H, especially men, although p.Q248H alone does not appear to cause clinically significant iron overload.[25-27]

Interaction of *HFE* and Non-*HFE* Iron-Related Mutations

Iron overload has been reported in patients who inherited one or more *HFE* mutations and a mutation of a non-*HFE* gene that is also involved in iron metabolism ("digenic" hemochromatosis). An example is the development of hemochromatosis in patients who inherited one or more *HFE* mutations and a mutation of the hepcidin gene (*HAMP*).[28] Iron loading has also occurred in patients who inherited an *HFE* mutation in the heterozygous state and either a mutation of the hemojuvelin gene (*HJV*)[26] or the transferrin receptor-2 gene (*TFR2*) in the heterozygous state.[29] In such patients, iron loading is often interpreted to be a synergistic effect of digenic inheritance because it seems unlikely that either mutation alone would cause iron overload.

More severe iron phenotypes have been reported in cohorts of unrelated patients with hemochromatosis who inherited the common hemochromatosis ancestral haplotype on chromosome 6p (HLA-B*07, HLA-A*03, D6S105(8), *HFE* p.C282Y).[30] Iron phenotypes of greater severity in p.C282Y homozygotes are also associated with a microhaplotype on chromosome 6p.[31] To date, a candidate modifier gene on chromosome 6p that would account for these observations has not been identified.

Alleles of non-*HFE* iron-related genes reported to be modifiers of iron phenotypes of unrelated *HFE* p.C282Y homozygotes are controversial.[3,32] These include common alleles of *TF*; *BMP2* (rs235756); SNPs in *ARNTL*, *TFR2*, *CYBRD*, and *GNPAT* p.D519G (rs11558492). In some studies, *GNPAT* p.D519G was associated with greater iron overload in p.C282Y homozygotes[33-35] and p.C282Y/p.H63D compound heterozygotes.[36] Other studies reported no significant association of p.D519G with iron overload severity.[37-40] Heterozygosity for the *HAMP* promoter mutation nc.-153C→T was associated with massive iron overload in one p.C282Y homozygote,[41] but the frequency of this mutation was too low to account for transferrin saturation and serum ferritin phenotype heterogeneity in 785 Hemochromatosis and Iron Overload Screening (HEIRS) Study participants, regardless of *HFE* genotype or race/ethnicity.[42] A variant in the D-loop of mitochondrial DNA at nucleotide 16189 (mtDNA 16189T→C) was associated with more severe iron phenotypes in patients with hemochromatosis in one study but not in another report.

Effects of Hepcidin

Hepcidin, encoded by *HAMP*, is the central regulator of iron absorption. It is a low-molecular-weight (20-25 amino acids), thionin-like, defensin-like peptide with eight cysteine residues linked as four disulfide bridges. Hepcidin has antimicrobial activity against bacteria and fungi, is present in plasma, and is excreted in urine. Hepcidin is synthesized in hepatocytes in response to anemia, hypoxia, and inflammatory stimuli mediated by interleukin-6 and in the presence of adequate or increased amounts of plasma iron. Hepcidin concentrations are inversely related to iron absorption. Hepcidin is also involved in the abnormalities of iron metabolism that occur in the anemia of chronic disease.

Ferroportin, the hepcidin receptor, occurs as a multimer on the surfaces of cells that bind and recycle iron: enterocytes (basolateral surfaces), macrophages, hepatocytes, and placental syncytiotrophoblasts. Hepcidin binding to cell-surface ferroportin induces ferroportin tyrosine phosphorylation, dephosphorylation, and proteosomal degradation through the ubiquitin pathway. Thus, hepcidin regulates plasma iron concentrations and tissue iron distribution by its impact on ferroportin expression.

Hepcidin Function in Hemochromatosis

Dysregulation of hepcidin production and hepcidin deficiency underlie the pathophysiology of *HFE*, *HJV*, *HAMP*, and *TFR2* hemochromatosis. For example, hepcidin expression by the liver is inappropriately low in patients with *HFE* hemochromatosis and iron overload,[43] and thus iron absorption continues despite increased iron stores. Macrophages display increased cell-surface ferroportin and thus export more iron, causing elevation of serum iron concentration, transferrin saturation, and plasma non-transferrin-bound iron (NTBI). Preferential deposition of iron in hepatocytes occurs because their avidity for NTBI is great.

In patients with "classic" (loss-of-function) ferroportin hemochromatosis, iron overload is caused by a mutation in the ferroportin gene (*SLC40A1*) that results in diminished quantities or absence of normally functional ferroportin ("hepcidin resistance").[44] Hepcidin production and regulation are not decreased. Because iron export by macrophages is decreased, serum iron concentration and transferrin saturation are normal or decreased, and excess iron in the liver is deposited predominantly in Kupffer cells.

Expression of *HFE* Protein

Small amounts of HFE occur in almost all normal cells and tissues. HFE protein expression is prominent in gastric epithelial cells, tissue macrophages, blood monocytes and granulocytes, and the syncytiotrophoblast.[3] HFE immunoreactivity in crypt enterocytes appears in a decreasing gradient from villous crypts to villous tips and from duodenum to ileum. In mice, intestinal knockout of *Hfe* results in no obvious iron phenotype, whereas hepatocyte-specific *Hfe* knockout recapitulates the iron phenotype of a whole-body knockout.

HFE protein is one of several upstream regulators of hepcidin transcription[45] (see Chapter 25). Compared with wild-type *HFE* control subjects, hepcidin concentration is significantly lower in untreated patients with hemochromatosis and *HFE* p.C282Y homozygosity. There is a significant inverse correlation between the expression of hepcidin and hepatic iron concentration in untreated patients with *HFE* hemochromatosis.[43] These observations indicate that *HFE* protein participates in regulating hepcidin expression in response to iron concentration and that the liver is important in the pathophysiology of *HFE* hemochromatosis.[43] Thus, p.C282Y homozygosity results in decreased hepcidin responsiveness to iron, causing a relative or absolute hepcidin deficiency (and consequently greater expression of ferroportin).[45] Hemojuvelin and TfR2 also contribute to regulation of *HAMP* transcription. Alterations of these proteins as consequences of pathogenic mutations in their corresponding genes, as with HFE protein and *HFE* mutations, lead to iron overload through perturbation of the hepcidin-ferroportin axis (see Chapter 25).

Disorders of Red Blood Cells

Protein Effects of *HFE* Gene Mutations

An extracellular portion of *HFE* protein (HFE) binds β_2-microglobulin at a site that includes two disulfide bridges. The most common mutation of *HFE* associated with iron overload (p.C282Y) is caused by a mutation of one nucleotide (exon 4; c.845G→A) of *HFE*.[2] In HFE C282Y protein, a cysteine is replaced by a tyrosine residue at amino acid position 282. Thus, β_2-microglobulin does not bind to cell surfaces normally in p.C282Y homozygotes because a disulfide bridge is absent. C282Y protein that does not reach the cell surface may sequester bone morphogenic receptor type I (Alk3), thereby preventing Alk3 from trafficking to the surface[46] (*Figure 27.1*). The affinity of C282Y protein for transferrin receptor is also decreased, although the significance of this to iron absorption has not been determined.[3] The increase in iron absorption associated with HFE *H63D* may be a consequence of failure of the mutant protein to protect Alk3 from ubiquitin-mediated degradation[46] (*Figure 27.1*). Other pathogenic *HFE* mutations cause splicing errors, alter transferrin receptor binding, or cause premature termination of translation.[3]

Intestinal Mucosal Iron Uptake in *HFE* Hemochromatosis

Duodenal cytochrome b, a plasma membrane protein encoded by *CYBRD1*, functions as a ferric reductase. In one study of patients with untreated *HFE* hemochromatosis, but not another, there was a post-translational increase in *CYBRD1* expression in relation to body iron stores.[48,49] Divalent metal transporter-1 on the apical microvillous membranes of absorptive enterocytes transports iron (and other divalent cations) from the intestinal lumen into enterocytes by an H+-coupled mechanism. Untreated p.C282Y homozygotes have inappropriate upregulation of both divalent metal transporter-1 and ferroportin mRNA expression in proportion to their serum ferritin concentrations.[49,50] Hephaestin, a transmembrane copper-dependent ferroxidase, transports iron from enterocytes into the plasma. Duodenal hephaestin is not upregulated in *HFE* hemochromatosis.[49] Duodenal cytochrome b, divalent metal transporter-1, ferroportin, and hephaestin mRNA expression are positively related in *HFE* hemochromatosis.[48]

IRON ABSORPTION AND TOXICITY IN *HFE* HEMOCHROMATOSIS

Abnormal Iron Absorption

Normal adults absorb an amount of iron each day that precisely balances daily losses (men ~1 mg, premenopausal women 1 to 3 mg). In some adults with hemochromatosis, the daily absorption of dietary iron is inappropriately great, but is usually ≤2 mg.[51,52] The absorption of heme iron in patients with hemochromatosis was greater than predicted in normal volunteers.[53] In juvenile hemochromatosis, average daily iron absorption may exceed 3 mg. Phlebotomy therapy of some patients with *HFE* hemochromatosis may increase daily iron absorption to 10 mg. Iron absorption may remain inappropriately elevated long after iron deficiency resolves. Iron loading in hemochromatosis, regardless of genetic subtype, is caused either by an abnormality in hepcidin synthesis or a decrease of its activity via decreased inhibition of ferroportin.

Organ and Cellular Injury due to Iron Overload

Iron bound to transferrin or stored in normal amounts in ferritin is not toxic. Iron storage sites, especially hepatocytes and Kupffer cells, become overloaded after years of excessive iron absorption. In the presence of excessive iron stores and increased release of iron from macrophages and other sites caused by absolute or relative hepcidin deficiency, the iron-binding capacity of transferrin is exceeded and plasma nonferritin, NTBI occurs. Plasma NTBI in adults with

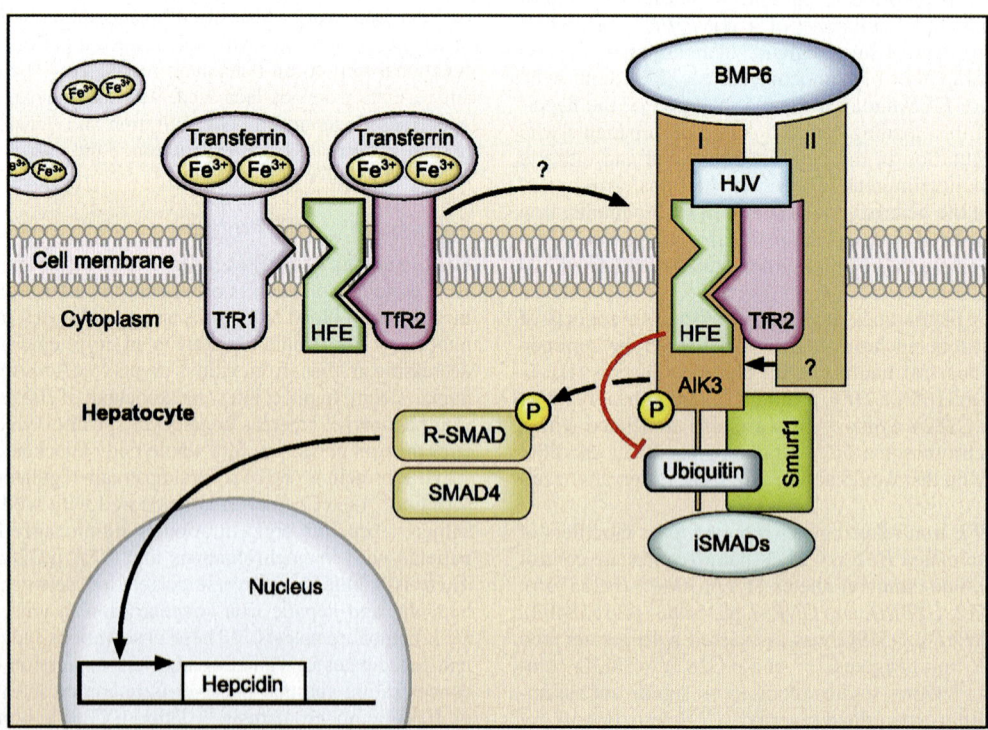

FIGURE 27.1 **Protein-protein interactions that control hepcidin expression in hepatocytes.** Regulated protein-protein interactions among HFE, TfR2, HJV (proteins altered in subtypes of hemochromatosis), BMP receptors, and BMP ligands play a critical role in sensing transferrin-bound Fe to control hepcidin expression in hepatocytes. HFE binds to BMP receptor type I (Alk3) to prevent its ubiquitination and proteosomal degradation. As a result, expression of Alk3 is increased on the cell surface, activating BMP/SMAD signaling and hepcidin transcription. Both *HFE* p.C282Y and p.H63D protein variants are able to interact with Alk3 but failed to increase Alk3 protein levels as detected on the cell surface of hepatocytes in both cultured hepatocytes and mouse liver. The respective underlying mechanisms differ. Although the p.H63D variant did not inhibit Alk3 ubiquitination, the *HFE* p.C282Y protein protected Alk3 from ubiquitination, similar to wild-type HFE. The authors speculated that HFE p.C282Y protein, which does not reach the cell membrane, sequesters Alk3 inside cells, thereby preventing Alk3 from trafficking to the cell surface.[47]

hemochromatosis is detectable at transferrin saturation ~35% and increases in parallel with progressively greater transferrin saturation.[54,55] In untreated Utah hemochromatosis homozygotes, transferrin saturation values were 82% to 87% (men) and 69% to 81% (women).[56]

NTBI readily enters cells. Hepatocytes, cardiac myocytes, β-cells of the pancreatic islets, pancreatic exocrine cells, and gonadotroph cells of the anterior pituitary have high affinity for NTBI. Iron-induced injury to these and other organs and tissues contributes to the defining clinical characteristics of patients with untreated hemochromatosis. Iron overload of the spleen in *HFE* hemochromatosis is relatively less than in some types of non-*HFE* hemochromatosis iron overload.

Free iron generates reactive oxygen species (oxyradicals). Hydroxyl radicals are thought to be involved in iron-related damage of enzymes, proteins, nucleic acids, and polysaccharides. It is likely that hydroxyl, alkoxyl, and peroxyl radicals are involved in lipid peroxidation that disrupts membrane-dependent functions of lysosomes, mitochondria, endoplasmic reticulum, cell membranes, and DNA. Excess iron and iron-induced oxyradicals activate hepatic stellate cells that undergo transformation to fibroblasts. Excess iron and iron-induced oxyradicals are also carcinogens in hepatocytes and possibly in extrahepatic parenchymal cells. Ferroptosis is an iron-dependent type of nonapoptotic cell death.[57] In mouse models of hemochromatosis, a ferroptosis inhibitor reduced iron overload-induced liver injury,[58] although ferroptosis-mediated hepatocellular injury or death in *HFE* hemochromatosis, if any, has not been reported.

Prevalence of *HFE* p.C282Y Homozygosity in Different Populations

The prevalence of *HFE* p.C282Y is relatively high in non-Hispanic whites native to Central, Western, and Northern Europe. In a study of 65,238 Norwegians, 0.68% were p.C282Y homozygotes.[59] The prevalence of *HFE* p.C282Y is also relatively high in non-Hispanic whites of derivative countries, including Canada, Australia, and the United States.[60] Among 29,676 subjects of northern European ancestry in the Australian HealthIron Study, 203 were homozygous for p.C282Y (0.65% [95% confidence interval: 0.59, 0.78]).[61] In three large population-based screening studies in the United States,[4-6] the prevalence of *HFE* p.C282Y homozygosity was 0.30% to 0.44% in non-Hispanic whites, 0% to 0.015% in non-Hispanic blacks/African Americans, and 0.03% to 0.17% in Mexican Americans/Hispanics (*Table 27.2*). Among non-Hispanic whites, p.H63D/p.H63D and p.C282Y/p.H63D genotypes were about 4 and 3.5 times more common, respectively, than p.C282Y/p.C282Y genotypes (*Table 27.2*).[4-6]

The prevalence of *HFE* mutations is relatively low in regions or population subgroups with little or no ancestry from Western and Central Europe, including sub-Saharan Africa (black Native Africans), the Middle East, and Asia, and in Native Americans in North, Central, and South America.[3,60] In one study, the prevalence of *HFE* p.C282Y in Native Americans was one-half of that in non-Hispanic whites (*Table 27.2*).[6] p.C282Y is uncommon in Pacific Islanders and rare in Asians (*Table 27.2*).[4,6] There are extensive *HFE* mutation and genotype frequency data in different countries and in different regions within countries.[3,62-64]

Proportions of *HFE* p.C282Y Homozygotes in Hemochromatosis Cohorts

In the first report of the *HFE* gene, 83% of subjects with hemochromatosis were *HFE* p.C282Y homozygotes.[2] The prevalence of p.C282Y homozygosity in patients with hemochromatosis in France, Germany, United Kingdom, Norway, Denmark, Belgium, Austria, Spain, and Portugal is 57% to 100%.[65] The prevalence of p.C282Y homozygosity in patients with hemochromatosis in Italy is 33% to 69% and in Greece is 50%.[65] In the United States, Canada, and Australia, the prevalence of p.C282Y homozygosity in patients with hemochromatosis is 59% to 100%.[65] In Argentina, Brazil, and Ecuador, the prevalence of p.C282Y homozygosity in patients with hemochromatosis is 4%, 28%, and 0%, respectively.[65] In patients with hemochromatosis in Austria,

Italy, Spain, Greece, Russia, United States, and Brazil, the prevalence of *HFE* genotypes that do not include p.C282Y, p.H63D, or p.S65C is ≥10%.[65] Variability in these prevalence estimates is due in part to differences in clinical or screening venues or diagnostic criteria and inclusion (or exclusion) of family members with hemochromatosis.

Postscreening Evaluation of *HFE* p.C282Y Homozygotes in the HEIRS Study

HEIRS Study participants were invited for postscreening evaluation if they were *HFE* p.C282Y homozygotes or if they had elevated transferrin saturation (>50% men, >45% women) or elevated serum ferritin (>300 μg/L men, >200 μg/L women). Age- and sex-matched control participants without p.C282Y or p.H63D who had transferrin saturation and serum ferritin concentrations in the middle 50th percentile for the respective five enrollment centers were also invited for comprehensive postscreening evaluations. The prevalence of chronic fatigue, hyperpigmentation, and reports of joint stiffness, swelling, or tenderness of the second and third metacarpophalangeal (MCP) joints were significantly greater in p.C282Y homozygotes with elevated serum ferritin concentrations than control participants.[66] The sex- and age-adjusted prevalences of self-reported symptoms and signs of liver disease, heart disease, diabetes, and other major clinical manifestations of hemochromatosis were similar in p.C282Y homozygotes and control participants.[66] The prevalence of biopsy-proven hepatic fibrosis (stage 3 or 4) in 302 p.C282Y homozygotes was 0.66%.[67] Screening for iron overload with serum ferritin and transferrin saturation also detected participants with viral hepatitis and other noniron liver diseases.[67]

In *HFE* p.C282Y homozygotes, diabetes was associated with greater age, male sex, MCP joint hypertrophy, greater blood neutrophil counts, and metabolic syndrome.[68] The prevalence of hypothyroidism and hyperthyroidism was similar in p.C282Y homozygotes identified by screening and control subjects.[69] The average mean corpuscular volume (MCV) was greater in p.C282Y homozygotes (men and women) and reflects increased mean transferrin saturation and mean serum ferritin. An additional effect of p.C282Y homozygosity on MCV and hemoglobin concentrations was detected in women.[70] The major histocompatibility complex is linked to white blood cell and lymphocyte counts in adults unselected for *HFE* genotypes. p.C282Y homozygosity is significantly associated with blood lymphocyte and basophil counts.[71]

CLINICAL FEATURES OF HEMOCHROMATOSIS

Prevalence of Hemochromatosis in Men and Women

Hemochromatosis is transmitted as an autosomal recessive condition. Therefore, it is predicted that the proportions of male and female *HFE* p.C282Y homozygotes in specific populations are approximately equal, although men with hemochromatosis have more overt iron overload, organ injury, and related illness than women.[72] In addition, men with hemochromatosis have ~2.5-fold more mobilizable storage iron than women. Iron absorption in men may be stimulated by hepcidin suppression induced by testosterone.[73] Women are partially protected from severe iron overload by the obligatory iron costs of menses, pregnancy, and lactation. Regardless, some men never develop iron overload and some women develop severe iron overload. Thus, other acquired or heritable factors influence the expression of iron phenotypes in patients with *HFE* p.C282Y homozygosity.

Symptoms

The presence or absence of symptoms in patients with hemochromatosis is related to the severity and duration of iron overload at diagnosis. Individuals diagnosed during a routine office visit are expected to have no organ injury and many little or no overload. This phenotype is common among women, young men, children, and the healthy siblings who undergo family screening after a proband is diagnosed. Other patients have symptoms and seek medical evaluation that leads to the diagnosis of hemochromatosis (*Table 27.3*).[1,56,72,74-80] These patients usually have clinically significant iron overload with evidence

Table 27.3. Observations in 97 Utah Hemochromatosis Probands

	59 Symptomatic Probands (%)	38 Screening Probands (%)	P value[a]
Symptoms			
Asymptomatic	0	90	0.0001
Abdominal pain	48	5	0.0001
Weakness, lethargy	54	5	0.0001
Palpitations	37	5	0.0010
Impotence (men)	25	3	0.0080
Weight loss	17	5	0.0160
Clinical Findings			
Skin pigmentation	71	19	0.0001
Arthropathy	48	10	0.0001
Hepatomegaly	56	3	0.0001
Liver enzyme elevation	68	8	0.0001
Liver iron stain grade 3-4[b]	98	21	0.0001
Hepatic cirrhosis	42	0	0.0001
Diabetes mellitus	27	0	0.0010
Cardiomegaly	14	0	0.0370
Documented hypogonadism	16	0	0.0260

[a]$P < .05$ is defined as significant.
[b]Scale of 0 to 4; normal grade 0 to 1.
Data summarized from Witte DL, Crosby WH, Edwards CQ, et al. Practice guideline development Task Force of the College of American Pathologists. Hereditary hemochromatosis. *Clin Chim Acta.* 1996;245:139–200. Modified from Edwards CQ, Griffen LM, Bulaj ZJ, et al. *Hemochromatosis: Genetics, Pathophysiology, Diagnosis and Treatment.* Cambridge, UK: Cambridge University Press, 2000; 314.

of organ injury. The prevalence of symptoms, physical signs, and laboratory abnormalities in patients with hemochromatosis (symptomatic probands), that of probands identified during screening, and that of their homozygous relatives identified during family evaluation (clinically unselected homozygotes) are displayed in *Table 27.4.*[81] Among persons who are diagnosed with hemochromatosis or discovered to have *HFE* p.C282Y homozygosity during screening, 90% to 98% are asymptomatic.

The most common symptom in nonscreening patients with hemochromatosis at diagnosis is arthralgias (~40% of homozygotes).[56]

MCP joints, especially the second and third, are most commonly involved with typical hemochromatosis arthropathy.[82] Pain or other manifestations can also occur in knees, hips, shoulders, and other diarthrodial joints. Weakness, fatigue, and lethargy are common but nonspecific symptoms. Weight loss, abdominal pain, loss of libido in men, and palpitations also occur in some iron-loaded homozygotes.

Physical Examination Abnormalities

Gray or bronze pigmentation is the most common physical examination abnormality in hemochromatosis homozygotes diagnosed in nonscreening settings (35%-84%). Other common findings include arthropathy (13%-68%), hepatomegaly (54%-93%), splenomegaly (10%-55%), irregular heartbeat, congestive heart failure, telangiectasias, loss of midline body hair, and testicular atrophy. The frequency of physical abnormalities in 10 nonscreening hemochromatosis cohorts is shown in *Table 27.5.* The prevalence of self-reported illness according to *HFE* genotype in a large California population screening study is displayed in *Table 27.6.*

Laboratory Abnormalities

The most common laboratory abnormalities in adults with untreated hemochromatosis are elevated values of serum iron concentration, transferrin saturation, and serum ferritin concentration.[83] Transferrin saturation may also be elevated in children, teenagers, and iron-depleted adult homozygotes. This finding is due not to iron overload but to increased export of iron by macrophages via deregulated ferroportin expression caused by hepcidin deficiency. Therefore, elevated transferrin saturation may also occur in hemochromatosis homozygotes without physical or laboratory manifestations of iron overload.

The specificity of transferrin saturation and serum ferritin values for diagnosis of *HFE* hemochromatosis is low. In the HEIRS Study, 10% to 12% of participants with an elevated serum ferritin concentration (200-1000 μg/L) were *HFE* p.C282Y homozygotes.[84] Transferrin saturation values and serum ferritin concentrations by *HFE* genotype in adult participants in a large California screening study are shown in *Table 27.7.*[85]

Elevated serum concentrations of alanine and aspartate aminotransferases occur in untreated patients with hemochromatosis diagnosed in nonscreening venues (8%-92%). The prevalence of this abnormality varies markedly according to the method of case ascertainment (*Tables 27.3* and *27.5*). Usually, concentrations of these enzymes are two to five times the upper reference limit in nonscreening subjects. If hepatic failure is present, serum transaminase and bilirubin concentrations may be markedly elevated. In patients with hemochromatosis, there is a strong positive correlation between elevated serum concentrations of collagen type IV with hepatic fibrosis or cirrhosis.[86] In a retrospective study of 181 subjects with hemochromatosis, the aspartate aminotransferase:platelet ratio index

Table 27.4. Transferrin Saturation and Serum Ferritin Values of 505 Utah Hemochromatosis Homozygotes[a]

	Symptomatic Probands		Screening Probands Identified by Elevated Transferrin Saturation		Clinically Unselected Homozygous Relatives of Probands	
	Men (136)	Women (48)	Men (66)	Women (41)	Men (113)	Women (101)
Mean age, y	51	51	37	45	41	44
Mean percent transferrin saturation	87	81	82	79	82	69
Median serum ferritin, μg/L (10th, 90th percentiles)	1300 (518, 3164)	657 (242, 2682)	421 (99, 1274)	319 (69, 1023)	552 (147, 1495)	170 (28, 580)

[a]P values calculated by the Kruskal-Wallis test for comparison of serum ferritin concentrations were: symptomatic probands versus screening probands: <0.001 for men, 0.002 for women; symptomatic probands versus clinically unselected homozygous relatives: <0.001 for men, <0.001 for women; screening probands identified versus clinically unselected homozygous relatives: 0.37 for men, 0.004 for women.
Modified from Bulaj ZJ, Ajioka RS, Phillips JD, et al. Disease-related conditions in relatives of patients with hemochromatosis. *N Engl J Med.* 2000;343(21):1529-1535.

Table 27.5. Clinical Observations (%) in Patients With Hemochromatosis[a]

Author	Sheldon[1]	Finch[74]	Milman[75]	Fargion[76]	Niederau[77]	Adams[78]	Moirand[72]	Bell[79]	Bulaj[56]	Aleman[80]
Year published	1935	1955	1991	1992	1996	1996	1997	2000	2000	2011
Patients, n	311	787	179	212	251	194	352	120	505	373
Men	295	711	140	181	224	141	176	55	315	266
Women	16	76	39	31	27	53	176	65	190	107
Symptoms										
Weakness	13	70	79	—	82	64	54	40	—	29
Weight loss	—	44	69	—	—	—	—	—	—	—
Arthralgias	—	—	44	—	44	—	40	24	—	37
Abdominal pain	26	29	34	—	56	—	—	—	—	—
Loss of libido and/or impotence	6	14	41	—	36	—	—	—	—	—
Amenorrhea	—	—	10	—	15	—	—	—	—	—
Cardiac complaints	—	33	—	—	—	—	—	—	—	—
Asymptomatic	—	—	—	—	—	—	—	55	—	—
Physical and Laboratory Findings										
Skin pigmentation	84	85	70	35	72	38	52	—	—	—
Hepatomegaly	92	93	84	75	81	41	—	—	—	—
Abnormal hepatic function tests	—	—	92	—	—	30	—	32	10	—
Cirrhosis	92	92	84	69	57	—	20	5	17	15
Hepatoma	6	14	—	12	—	4	—	—	3	—
Splenomegaly	55	50	12	—	10	—	—	—	8	—
Diabetes	79	82	47	30	—	24	12	4	10	13
Testicular atrophy	—	16	—	24[b]	—	18	—	—	—	—
Hypogonadism, documented	—	—	—	—	—	—	—	—	—	—
Hypogonadotrophic hypogonadism	—	—	—	—	—	—	—	—	5	—
Arthropathy	—	—	—	13	—	37	—	24	—	—
Cardiac arrhythmia	—	35	—	20	35	14	14	—	8	—
Congestive heart failure	—	33	15	—	—	14	—	—	—	—

[a]From eight countries.
[b]Findings in men only; not all men were studied.
Modified with permission from Edwards CQ, Griffen LM, Bulaj ZJ, et al. Estimate of the frequency of morbid complications of hemochromatosis. In: Barton JC, Edwards CQ, eds. *Hemochromatosis: Genetics, Pathophysiology, Diagnosis and Treatment.* Cambridge University Press; 2000:312-317. Copyright © 2000 Cambridge University Press.

Disorders of Red Blood Cells

Table 27.6. Self-Reported Health Problems and *HFE* Genotypes in a California Screening Study

	Men, % (n)	Women, % (n)
Arthropathy		
p.C282Y/p.C282Y	28.6 (16/56)	42.6 (29/68)
p.C282Y/p.H63D	38.4 (112/292)	47.5 (143/301)
wt/wt[a]	36.5 (3975/10,889)	46.5 (5324/11,458)
Diabetes		
p.C282Y/p.C282Y	1.8 (1/56)	8.8 (6/68)
p.C282Y/p.H63D	9.9 (29/292)	5.0 (15/301)
wt/wt[a]	9.6 (1045/10,889)	7.4 (843/11,458)
Liver Problems		
p.C282Y/p.C282Y	7.1 (4/56)	7.1 (6/68)
p.C282Y/p.H63D	3.8 (11/292)	3.8 (11/301)
wt/wt[a]	4.5 (534/11,889)	4.5 (392/11,458)
Arrhythmias		
p.C282Y/p.C282Y)	14.3 (8/56)	33.8 (23/68)
p.C282Y/p.H63D)	18.2 (53/292)	34.2 (103/301)
wt/wt[a]	17.2 (1868/10,889)	32.6 (3730/11,458)
Impotence		
p.C282Y/p.C282Y	26.8 (15/56)	—
p.C282Y/p.H63D	40.4 (118/292)	—
wt/wt[a]	35.9 (3904/10,889)	—

[a]wt, wild type (absence of *HFE* p.C282Y or p.H63D).[4]
Modified from Beutler E, Felitti VJ, Koziol JA, et al. Penetrance of 845G→A (C282Y) *HFE* hereditary haemochromatosis mutation in the USA. *Lancet.* 2002;359(9302):211-218. Copyright © 2002 Elsevier. With permission.

and fibrosis-4 index scores identified patients with advanced hepatic fibrosis with 81% accuracy.[87]

The significance of elevated serum concentrations of hepatic transaminases is often different in *HFE* p.C282Y homozygotes detected in screening programs than in nonscreening patients. In the HEIRS Study participants with hyperferritinemia, mean serum concentrations of transaminase activities were significantly lower in p.C282Y homozygotes than in nonhomozygotes. The probability of being a p.C282Y homozygote increased as the transaminase activities decreased. Thus, HEIRS Study participants with hyperferritinemia detected in screening were more likely to be p.C282Y homozygotes if they had normal liver transaminase activities.[81]

Serum concentrations of ceruloplasmin, a copper-containing ferroxidase, are significantly lower in patients with hemochromatosis than in control subjects or patients with nonhemochromatosis iron overload. In persons with hemochromatosis, achieving iron depletion with phlebotomy therapy does not change serum ceruloplasmin concentrations.[88]

The average hemoglobin concentration is greater in untreated *HFE* p.C282Y homozygotes than in control subjects without common *HFE* mutations.[70,89] Likewise, the MCV of many untreated p.C282Y homozygotes is greater than the upper reference limit, even in patients without liver disease.[89] The mean red blood cell (RBC) count and mean coefficient of variation of MCV (RBC distribution width) are lower in p.C282Y homozygotes.[89] These erythrocyte-associated characteristics, usually more pronounced in men than in women, are attributed to the ample amounts of iron available to marrow erythroblasts via transferrin. In patients with *HFE* hemochromatosis, the soluble transferrin receptor concentration begins to rise at higher values of transferrin saturation than in control subjects, suggesting that recognition of iron available for erythropoiesis is also altered in *HFE* hemochromatosis. Genome-wide linkage analyses confirm that a locus/loci on chromosome 6p21 is/are significantly associated with hemoglobin concentration.[90] This locus is presumed to be *HFE*. In 23,681 Caucasian adults who attended a California health maintenance clinic, mean hemoglobin and MCV were also significantly greater in those with northern than southern European ancestry.[91] In 119 referred patients with hemochromatosis and p.C282Y homozygosity in Australia, MCV >97.9 fL was associated with a likelihood ratio of 2.2 for development of arthritis.[92] Lymphocyte and basophil counts are positively associated with p.C282Y homozygosity, after adjustment for other factors.[71]

Common endocrine-related laboratory abnormalities include the following: elevation of fasting serum glucose concentration; elevated or subnormal serum thyroid-stimulating hormone concentrations[69]; and blood test evidence of hypogonadism, usually hypogonadotrophic hypogonadism, with decreased serum concentrations of testosterone, dihydrotestosterone, luteinizing hormone, and follicle-stimulating hormone.[93] In *HFE* hemochromatosis, hypogonadotrophic or idiopathic hypogonadism occurs almost exclusively in men. In juvenile-onset hemochromatosis, the prevalence of hypogonadotrophic hypogonadism at diagnosis is similar in males and females.

Radiography

Approximately 50% of untreated homozygotes have radiographic changes typical of hemochromatosis hand arthropathy.[9,94,95] Such patients are usually older and have serum ferritin concentrations >1000 μg/L.[95] Plain radiographs reveal narrowing of the metacarpophalangeal joint spaces (especially those of the second and third metacarpophalangeal joints), hook osteophytes, subperiosteal bone resorption, and periarticular demineralization. Patients with typical metacarpophalangeal changes often have similar changes in interphalangeal, intercarpal, and radiocarpal joints. Shoulders, elbows, knees, ankles, and toes are affected in some patients. In some cases, plain radiographs of knees or other diarthrodial joints reveal chondrocalcinosis.[95,96] Bone mineral

Table 27.7. Transferrin Saturation and Serum Ferritin in a California Screening Study

HFE Genotype	Wt/Wt[a]	p.C282Y/Wt[a]	p.C282Y/p.H63D	p.C282Y/p.C282Y
Men, n	12,601	1603	300	73
Mean percent transferrin saturation	27	31	40	64
Mean serum ferritin, μg/L[b]	118	122	191	395
Women, n	13,674	1690	305	79
Mean percent transferrin saturation	23	27	32	46
Mean serum ferritin, μg/L[b]	52	56	70	159

[a]wt, wild type (absence of *HFE* p.C282Y and p.H63D) except that a very small percentage of "wt" chromosomes in participants with p.C282Y/wt were p.S65C.[4]
[b]Geometric mean.
Modified from Beutler E, Felitti VJ, Koziol JA, et al. Penetrance of 845G→A (C282Y) *HFE* hereditary haemochromatosis mutation in the USA. *Lancet.* 2002;359(9302):211-218. Copyright © 2002 Elsevier. With permission.

loss unexplained by hypogonadism or cirrhosis is common in patients with hemochromatosis and severe iron overload, especially men.[97,98]

In 49 patients with iron-loaded hemochromatosis, four sequences of low-field magnetic resonance (MR) images (0.2 T) identified degenerative or inflammatory joint abnormalities in 84% of symptomatic and 42% of asymptomatic individuals.[99] Investigators in Austria and Germany performed physical examinations, functional evaluations, and two-view hand radiographs to assess differences in hand osteoarthritis among 141 individuals with hemochromatosis and 158 non–iron-loaded subjects with idiopathic osteoarthritis of the hands. Hemochromatosis hand osteoarthritis was more prevalent, but functionally less severe, than idiopathic hand osteoarthritis.[100]

Dual-energy computerized tomography (CT) scanning can distinguish hepatic iron from fat. In a dual-energy CT scan, an iron-loaded liver appears brighter than paraspinous muscles. MR imaging has largely replaced CT scanning in the evaluation of livers that are presumed to be cirrhotic. Advantages of MR scanning include superior contrast resolution, multiplanar capability, greater sensitivity and specificity in the detection and characterization of abnormalities, and no use of ionizing radiation. MR imaging can be used to identify hepatic cirrhosis, regenerating nodules, increased iron, and hepatocellular carcinoma in patients with hemochromatosis.

Where appropriate hardware and software are available, MR can be used to quantify hepatic iron content (milligrams of iron per gram of liver tissue).[101] Storage iron quantified by MR imaging is correlated with iron chemically measured in a liver biopsy sample. Thus, MR scanning can provide credible estimation of the hepatic iron concentration in patients who do not undergo liver biopsy. Using the same method, semiquantitative assessment of myocardial iron can be determined. MR imaging quantification of hepatic and myocardial iron can be repeated as indicated by the patient's clinical condition. Such analysis is sensitive and noninvasive and does not involve ionizing radiation.[102-104]

Liver Abnormalities

Liver morphology by microscopy is usually normal in homozygotes whose serum ferritin concentrations are not elevated. In patients whose serum ferritin concentrations are elevated, the hepatic parenchymal cell stainable iron and measured hepatic iron concentration are usually increased. Cirrhosis is not expected to occur until the hepatic iron concentration is ~22 mg of iron per gram of liver dry weight (normal, ~1 mg of iron per gram dry weight).[105] Many nonscreening male homozygotes have hepatic fibrosis or cirrhosis when hemochromatosis is diagnosed (Tables 27.3, 27.5, and 27.8).[56] Most women with hemochromatosis do not have fibrosis or cirrhosis at diagnosis. HFE p.C282Y homozygotes who are identified only because they participated in screening studies rarely have heavy liver iron overload or hepatic fibrosis (Table 27.8).[56,67,81]

Cirrhosis risk in hemochromatosis is influenced by multiple factors. In 368 HFE p.C282Y homozygotes with biopsy-proven cirrhosis, cirrhosis risk was significantly associated with age, diabetes, daily alcohol intake, and iron removed by phlebotomy, taking into account the effect of other variables.[106] Chronic infection by hepatitis

C virus may contribute to cirrhosis risk in some patients with hemochromatosis, although the prevalence of anti-hepatitis C antibody in postscreening participants with p.C282Y homozygosity (0.3%) and chronic hepatitis C virus infection in referred adults with p.C282Y homozygosity (1.0%) in North America was similar to that of control participants with HFE wt/wt and normal screening transferrin saturation and serum ferritin concentrations.[107] Cirrhosis risk is increased in p.C282Y homozygotes who also have the rs23619C allele of the PCSK7 gene (proprotein convertase subtilisin/kexin type 7 gene; chromosome 11q23.3).[108] This allele occurs in ~5% of Europeans. In two studies, GNPAT p.D519G was not a risk factor for cirrhosis in p.C282Y homozygotes.[40,106] The prevalence of hepatic fibrosis, cirrhosis, and hepatocellular carcinoma in patients with hemochromatosis is presented in Tables 27.3, 27.5, and 27.8.

The prevalence of nonalcoholic fatty liver disease was significantly greater in 54 patients with hemochromatosis and HFE p.C282Y homozygosity than 20 control subjects.[109] Patients with hemochromatosis had significantly lower serum phosphatidylcholine and significantly higher phosphatidylethanolamine and triglyceride concentrations than healthy control subjects. PNPLA3 polymorphism (CC vs CG/GG) was not significantly associated with iron and lipid measures.[109] In 214 Australian patients with hemochromatosis and p.C282Y homozygosity, steatosis was independently associated with fibrosis, male sex, excess alcohol consumption, and hepatic iron content.[110] Both higher body mass index and alcohol consumption were independently associated with the presence of steatosis.[110] The risk of nonalcoholic fatty liver disease is also increased in p.C282Y heterozygotes[111] and p.C282Y/p.H63D compound heterozygotes.[112]

In 36 men in Massachusetts who had nonalcoholic steatohepatitis, 2.8% were HFE p.C282Y homozygotes, 17.0% were p.C282Y heterozygotes, 5.6% were p.H63D homozygotes, and 44.0% were p.H63D heterozygotes.[113] In 348 control subjects, none was a p.C282Y homozygote, 11.0% were p.C282Y heterozygotes, 2.9% were p.H63D homozygotes, and 26.0% were p.H63D heterozygotes. Individuals with nonalcoholic steatohepatitis who had an HFE mutation had higher concentrations of transferrin saturation and serum ferritin, and those with p.C282Y had significantly higher concentrations of alanine aminotransferase and a greater degree of hepatic fibrosis than those without p.C282Y.[113] Insulin resistance syndrome is common in people who have nonalcoholic steatohepatitis, with or without mutations of HFE.

HFE MUTATIONS AND OTHER CONDITIONS

Arthropathy

Arthropathy is common in patients diagnosed with hemochromatosis in nonscreening settings and is a major cause of morbidity in some individuals. The proportion of nonscreening patients who have severe iron overload is relatively high and the prevalence of hemochromatosis arthropathy is significantly greater in patients whose serum ferritin is > 1000 μg/L at diagnosis,[114,115] although one HFE p.C282Y homozygote without iron overload at diagnosis had typical arthropathy.[116]

Table 27.8. Liver Biopsy Findings in 372 Utah Hemochromatosis Homozygotes

| Liver histology | Symptomatic Probands | | Screening probands[a] | | Clinically Unselected Homozygous Relatives of Probands | |
	Men (n = 123)	Women (n = 44)	Men (n = 54)	Women (n = 33)	Men (n = 78)	Women (n = 40)
Cirrhosis, % (n)	44.7 (55)	22.7 (10)	5.6 (3)	6.3 (2)	17.9 (14)	5.0 (2)
Fibrosis, % (n)	26.0 (32)	20.5 (9)	11.1 (6)	6.3 (2)	16.7 (13)	10.0 (4)
Hepatocellular carcinoma, % (n)	11.4 (14)	0	0	0	2.6 (2)	0

[a]Identified by elevated transferrin saturation.
Modified from Bulaj ZJ, Ajioka RS, Phillips JD, et al. Disease-related conditions in relatives of patients with hemochromatosis. N Engl J Med. 2000;343(21):1529-1535.

Disorders of Red Blood Cells

p.C282Y homozygosity, male sex, and older age are significant independent risk factors for hand arthropathy.[117]

Hemochromatosis homozygotes with hand arthropathy usually experience symmetrical arthralgias in the second and third MCP and proximal interphalangeal joints.[118] MCP joint swelling, decreased range of motion, and decreased ability to make a fist are typical physical examination findings. Persons with hemochromatosis and iron overload phenotypes have increased utilization of hip arthroplasty procedures.[98,119-121] Utilization of knee arthroplasty was increased in persons with hemochromatosis phenotypes in one study[120] but not in another study.[121] In a meta-analysis, persons with hemochromatosis had risk for ankle replacement surgery.[122]

Typical hemochromatosis arthropathy is uncommon in persons diagnosed to have hemochromatosis in screening programs because the proportion of persons identified with hemochromatosis who have severe iron overload is low. Among the 98,529 participants in the HEIRS Study (36,474 men and 62,055 women), there was no significant difference in the prevalence of self-reported arthritis between groups of HFE p.C282Y homozygotes and age- and sex-matched participants without HFE mutations.[6] In another large questionnaire study, the prevalence of arthropathy in 45 p.C282Y homozygotes identified by screening and 9299 control subjects did not differ significantly.[85] The results of another screening study confirmed these results.[123]

The prevalence of common HFE mutations did not differ significantly in 1000 patients who had inflammatory arthritis and in 1000 normal control subjects.[124] In another study of patients without a diagnosis of hemochromatosis, the prevalence of p.C282Y was greater in those with radiographic evidence of hand osteoarthritis than in control subjects. Serum ferritin concentrations were similar in patients with and without hand osteoarthritis.[125] Some p.C282Y homozygotes develop rheumatoid factor–positive rheumatoid arthritis,[126,127] ankylosing spondylitis,[127] psoriatic arthritis, gouty arthritis, or other types of arthropathy not due to iron overload. Osteoporosis defined by decreased bone mineral density was present in 34% of 38 p.C282Y homozygotes and p.C282Y/p.H63D compound heterozygotes who had not undergone iron depletion therapy. Osteopenia was present in 79%.[97] Serum vitamin D and parathyroid hormone concentrations were normal. Hypogonadism was present in 13%.[97] Arthralgias often respond to nonsteroidal anti-inflammatory drugs (NSAIDs). Two patients whose arthralgias did not improve with NSAIDs and tramadol were treated with five daily subcutaneous injections of anakinra (receptor antagonist of IL-1α and IL-1β). Relief of arthralgias was transient.[128]

Diabetes Mellitus

Diabetes was reported in early accounts of hemochromatosis, and its occurrence was essential for the diagnosis of hemochromatosis for many years. Diabetes remains especially common among patients with hemochromatosis who also have severe iron overload and cirrhosis, although such cases are uncommon. Iron is deposited preferentially in the β cells of the pancreatic islets.[129] Diabetes and hemochromatosis segregate independently as genetic traits.[130]

Iron-associated injury of pancreatic β cells and consequent decreased insulin secretion would account for diabetes in some patients with hemochromatosis. Some patients have low insulin concentrations.[131] Some patients with impaired glucose tolerance and cirrhosis without diabetes diagnoses have decreased insulin response to glucose and decreased sensitivity to insulin.[132] In one study of patients with hemochromatosis who also had impaired glucose tolerance (86% of whom were obese) without insulin resistance, acute insulin responses to glucose were 68% lower than those of control subjects.[133]

After the discovery of HFE in 1996, hemochromatosis case definition changed from that of a rare, severe iron overload phenotype to a relatively common, mild or asymptomatic disorder defined primarily by p.C282Y homozygosity. The prevalence of diabetes in nonscreening case series of patients with hemochromatosis with p.C282Y homozygosity has decreased to rates similar to those of age- and sex-matched members of the general population.[134,135] Among 98,529 HEIRS Study participants, there was no significant difference in the prevalence of

self-reported diabetes between groups of p.C282Y homozygotes and age- and sex-matched participants with normal HFE genotypes.[6] In a study of 22,347 control subjects without HFE mutations, 8.4% reported having diabetes, whereas 5.6% of 124 p.C282Y homozygotes reported having diabetes. Similarly, 7.0% of p.C282Y/p.H63D compound heterozygotes had diabetes.[85] Earlier diagnosis of hemochromatosis due to iron phenotyping and HFE genotyping in probands and family members and subsequent phlebotomy therapy could account partly for the decreasing prevalence of diabetes associated with hemochromatosis.

Transferrin receptors and divalent metal transporter-1 in the normal human pancreas are expressed predominantly in the islets and are presumed to be physiologic means by which iron enters islet cells. In HFE hemochromatosis, iron loading of parenchymal cells is also due to uptake of NTBI from plasma. In human pancreas, hepcidin is localized exclusively to β-cell secretory granules that store insulin.[136] Hepcidin expression in pancreatic β cells is regulated by iron in vitro.[136] Thus, hepcidin in pancreatic β cells, in addition to that in hepatocytes, may contribute to iron homeostasis and blood glucose regulation.

Cirrhosis contributes to insulin resistance, hyperglucagonemia, and diabetogenesis in some patients with hemochromatosis. In 368 HFE p.C282Y homozygotes with biopsy-proven cirrhosis, the odds ratio for diabetes was significantly increased (3.3; [1.1, 9.7]), taking into account the effect of other variables.[106] In another study of nonscreening hemochromatosis probands with p.C282Y homozygosity, diabetes was not independently associated with either biopsy-proven cirrhosis or the aggregate variable "liver disorders."[135] In men with p.C282Y homozygosity, the prevalence of diabetes in those with markedly increased iron stores (50% cirrhosis) and those with normal or mildly increased iron stores (no cirrhosis) did not differ significantly (14% diabetes vs 15% diabetes, respectively).[33]

Type 2 diabetes is the most common type of diabetes in patients with hemochromatosis and HFE p.C282Y homozygosity. A history of diabetes in first-degree family members is a major predictor of diabetes in hemochromatosis probands.[135] Thus, a genetic factor(s) increases diabetes risk in persons with and without HFE hemochromatosis.[135,137] Obesity or increased body mass index is also associated with decreased insulin secretory capacity and increased diabetes risk in patients with HFE hemochromatosis.[68,134,135,138-140] Similar abnormalities occur in mouse models of hemochromatosis.[141] In p.C282Y homozygotes identified in screening, there were significant positive associations of serum ferritin concentrations with homeostatic model assessment of insulin resistance fourth quartile, metabolic syndrome, and diabetes.[68] In genome-wide association studies, type 2 diabetes has not been significantly associated with HLA region genes. Although autoimmune diabetes is associated with loci on chromosome 6p, autoimmune diabetes was not diagnosed in 235 nonscreening p.C282Y homozygotes.[127]

Screening patients with type 2 diabetes for hemochromatosis is not justified unless they also have other manifestations typical of hemochromatosis or iron overload. Nonscreening patients with hemochromatosis, HFE p.C282Y homozygosity, and diabetes had decreased survival after hemochromatosis diagnosis, although a high proportion also had cirrhosis and severe iron overload.[142] In an analysis of 84,865 Danes in the general population, persons with increased transferrin saturation or p.C282Y homozygosity had 2- to 6-fold greater risks of death due to diabetes than persons without common HFE mutations.[143] Complications and management of diabetes in patients with and without hemochromatosis are similar.[144] There are no substantial longitudinal observations of p.C282Y homozygotes and their posthemochromatosis diagnoses of diabetes or impaired fasting glucose.

Other Endocrinopathy

Hypogonadism, typically hypogonadotrophic hypogonadism,[93] is common in men with HFE hemochromatosis and severe iron overload (Tables 27.3 and 27.5). This complication is usually due to selective deposition of iron in gonadotroph cells of the anterior pituitary.[1,93,145] In 141 iron-loaded hemochromatosis patients, 9 (6%) had subnormal testosterone concentrations. Eight of these nine (89%) also had low values of luteinizing hormone and follicle-stimulating hormone, consistent with hypogonadotrophic hypogonadism.[93] Hypothalamic dysfunction occurs in some patients. It is reasonable to evaluate men with hypopituitarism of unknown cause for hemochromatosis.[146] In 13 nonscreening hemochromatosis patients whose first symptoms occurred before the age of 30 years, 77% had hypogonadotrophic hypogonadism.[14] Some patients with hemochromatosis have hypogonadotrophic hypogonadism due to noniron causes or primary gonadal failure unrelated to iron overload.

Abnormal thyroid function occurs in some patients with *HFE* hemochromatosis. In 49 nonscreening adults with homozygous hemochromatosis, 3 of 34 men (8.8%) had hypothyroidism and elevated titers of antithyroid antibodies.[147] Fifteen women with homozygous hemochromatosis had normal thyroid function.[147] In 235 nonscreening hemochromatosis probands with p.C282Y homozygosity, autoimmune (Hashimoto) thyroiditis was diagnosed in 19 probands (8.1%).[127] The prevalence of autoimmune thyroiditis was greater in women than in men (14.4% vs 3.6%, respectively; odds ratio 4.6 [95% confidence interval: 1.6, 13.1]).[127] Although autoimmune thyroiditis risk is linked in part to the *AITD-1* locus on chromosome 6p,[148] positivity for HLA-A*03 or HLA-A and -B haplotypes did not differ significantly between 19 hemochromatosis probands with and 216 probands without autoimmune thyroiditis.[127] In the HEIRS Study, hypothyroidism was detected in 1.7% of 176 screening p.C282Y homozygotes and 1.3% of 312 control participants without common *HFE* mutations.[69] Autoimmune thyroiditis was diagnosed in two of four siblings with juvenile hemochromatosis and severe iron overload.[9,149] Autoimmune thyroiditis did not segregate with *HJV* alleles on Ch1q in this kinship.[9,149]

In a study of 49 nonscreening adults with HLA-linked hemochromatosis, one man (2.9%) had hyperthyroidism.[147] In 235 nonscreening hemochromatosis probands, 1 (0.4%) had Graves disease.[127] In the HEIRS Study, 0.6% of 176 p.C282Y homozygotes and 1% of 312 control participants without p.C282Y or p.H63D had hyperthyroidism. These differences were not statistically significant.[69]

The greater prevalence of autoimmune thyroid disorders in nonscreening than screening patients with *HFE* hemochromatosis and the occurrence of autoimmune thyroiditis in *HJV* hemochromatosis suggest that iron overload contributes to the pathogenesis of thyroid conditions. Histologic examination of thyroid glands at autopsy of men who died of hemochromatosis revealed that siderosis, fibrosis, and lymphocytic infiltration are common.[1] It has been postulated that iron deposition causes thyroid injury, leading to the development of antithyroid antibodies and hypothyroidism.[147] In nonscreening probands with hemochromatosis, multivariable analyses revealed that female sex and family history of autoimmune condition(s) were significantly associated with autoimmune thyroiditis.[127]

Iron is deposited in the adrenal cortex and parathyroid glands of patients with advanced hemochromatosis.[1] In 19 patients with hemochromatosis and iron overload, including 7 with cirrhosis, no functional abnormality of the pituitary-adrenal axis or mineralocorticoid status was detected.[150] A 25-year-old man who presented with adrenocortical insufficiency, hypogonadotrophic hypogonadism, cardiomyopathy, and non-*HFE* hemochromatosis had no common, noniron cause of adrenocortical insufficiency.[151] Primary aldosterone deficiency was not observed in patients with hemochromatosis and severe iron overload.[152] One patient with hemochromatosis also had hypoparathyroidism.[153] The function of pancreatic α-cells is preserved in persons with hemochromatosis.[154]

Polycystic ovary syndrome affects ~5% of white women and is often associated with decreased serum hepcidin concentrations. In a case-control study of women with polycystic ovarian syndrome unselected for hemochromatosis followed by a randomized clinical trial, the imbalance between increased iron stores and reduced hepcidin concentrations was related to characteristic insulin resistance and androgen excess.[155] Homozygosity for the *HFE* p.C282Y mutation is also associated with decreased serum hepcidin. In a study of 107 unrelated women with p.C282Y homozygosity, a 13- and a 16-year-old (1.9%) had polycystic ovary syndrome. Each had elevated serum ferritin concentration and grade 3 or 4 hepatic parenchymal stainable iron.[156]

Low serum hepcidin concentration due to both polycystic ovary syndrome with amenorrhea at a young age and *HFE* hemochromatosis may contribute to early age-of-onset iron overload.

HEMOCHROMATOSIS, IRON, AND CANCER RISK

Mechanisms by which *HFE* p.C282Y and iron could increase risks for premalignant lesions and invasive cancer include iron overload with consequential DNA damage,[157] perturbed iron metabolism at the tissue or cellular level that facilitates tumor cell growth and modifies immune responses,[158] and linkage of p.C282Y with cancer-associated alleles on chromosome 6p.[159] Age; sex; smoking; alcohol use; consumption of greater quantities of iron; exposure to carcinogens in food, drinks, and workplaces; elevated body mass index; family histories of malignancy; and other heritable and acquired factors could also increase cancer risk.

Hepatocellular Carcinoma

The relative risk of hepatocellular carcinoma in patients with hemochromatosis is 219-fold higher in those with than in those without cirrhosis.[160,161] Among patients who have both end-stage hemochromatosis and cirrhosis, 10% to 29% develop hepatoma.[160,162-165] About 3% to 4% of patients with hemochromatosis complicated by cirrhosis develop hepatocellular carcinoma per year.[166] The risk of hepatocellular carcinoma is greater in men than in women with hemochromatosis phenotypes[167-169] or *HFE* p.C282Y homozygosity.[169,170] In a study of Swiss patients with hemochromatosis phenotypes, only higher age at diagnosis was significantly associated with development of hepatocellular carcinoma, after adjustment for other variables.[169] There are also reports of hepatocellular carcinoma in patients with hemochromatosis who did not have cirrhosis.[171-174]

Hepatocellular carcinoma in hemochromatosis may be multifocal and may not cause the marked elevation of serum α-fetoprotein concentrations that are common in patients with a large nodular hepatocellular carcinoma. Multifocal hepatocellular carcinoma may not be visible by ultrasonography until the diameter of the nodules is ≥ 1 cm. The histology of primary liver cancer in hemochromatosis is heterogeneous. Although the majority of primary liver cancers in hemochromatosis are of the hepatocellular type, biliary cancers also occur, including cholangiocarcinoma and combined hepatocellular and cholangiocarcinoma.[164,174]

In some reports, the proportion of patients with hepatocellular carcinoma who also have *HFE* p.C282Y homozygosity[175,176] or p.C282Y heterozygosity is significantly increased.[175,177,178] In another report, the prevalence of *HFE* mutations was similar in patients with hepatocellular carcinoma and in control subjects.[179] In a prospective evaluation of 234 French patients with cirrhosis, 12 (5.1%) were p.C282Y homozygotes and 3 (1.3%) were p.C282Y/p.H63D compound heterozygotes.[180] Positive associations of *HFE* mutations, chronic viral hepatitis, and hepatocellular carcinoma have been reported.[176,178] Guidelines have been published about the evaluation and management of patients who have hepatocellular carcinoma.[181-183]

Surveillance for Hepatocellular Carcinoma

The recommendations in three guidelines about surveillance for hepatocellular carcinoma among persons who have cirrhosis of any cause have been summarized. All guidelines recommended surveillance at 6-month intervals using hepatic ultrasonography. One guideline recommended measurement of serum α-fetoprotein at the time of hepatic ultrasonography.[184]

Colorectal Polyps and Colorectal Cancer

The risk for colorectal cancer was increased 2-fold in *HFE* p.C282Y homozygotes in a cohort of 28,509 screening participants in Australia.[185] In 6849 Swiss patients with hemochromatosis, the standardized incidence ratio for colon adenocarcinoma was increased 40%.[186] In screening study participants in Australia, p.C282Y/p.H63D compound heterozygotes and p.C282Y heterozygotes did not have increased risks for colorectal cancer.[185] In 475 case patients and

833 control subjects in the United States, the prevalence of p.C282Y and p.H63D mutations was greater in patients with colorectal cancer.[187] When controlled for age, race, sex, red meat consumption, use of NSAIDs, and total iron intake, subjects with any *HFE* mutation were more likely to have colon cancer than subjects without *HFE* mutations. Colon cancer risk associated with an *HFE* gene mutation was similar in those with and without a family history of colon cancer.[187]

Cancer risk increases with increasing age and total iron intake among subjects with mutations.[187] In a study of 362 individuals from Australia and Poland with confirmed causative DNA mismatch repair gene mutations, those with p.H63D homozygosity had a 3-fold greater risk of developing colorectal cancer than *HFE* wild-type homozygotes and p.H63D heterozygotes combined.[188] In 327 patients with colorectal cancer with a family history of colorectal cancer and 322 randomly selected controls in the United Kingdom, p.C282Y heterozygosity, p.H63D heterozygosity, or compound heterozygosity for p.C282Y/p.H63D was not associated with significantly increased colorectal cancer risk.[189] In a study of 226 cases of colorectal cancer and 437 matched referents in Sweden, neither serum ferritin concentrations nor *HFE* mutations were associated with colorectal cancer risk.[190] The risk of advanced distal adenomatous colorectal polyps is not significantly related to p.C282Y or p.H63D or dietary iron intake.[191]

Gastrins, peptide hormones synthesized mainly by G cells of the gastric antrum, induce proliferation of the colonic epithelium. Increased plasma concentrations of gastrins could account in part for the greater risk of colorectal cancer in *HFE* p.C282Y homozygotes observed in some studies. Increased concentrations of circulating amidated and nonamidated gastrins are typical of p.C282Y homozygotes (and C57BL/6J *Hfe*$^{-/-}$ mice).[192] In a study of 128,992 subscribers to a health maintenance program, a supranormal serum gastrin level was associated with a nearly 4-fold greater risk for colorectal malignancy a mean interval of 15.3 years later.[193] Gastrin-17 promotes in vitro growth of human colon cancer HT-29 cells via their gastrin receptors (CCK-2).[194]

Other Types of Cancer

The risk of breast cancer in women with *HFE* p.C282Y homozygosity was increased 2-fold in a cohort study of 28,509 screening participants in Australia, whereas p.C282Y/p.H63D compound heterozygotes and p.C282Y heterozygotes did not have increased risks of breast cancer.[185] In Canadian women, p.C282Y was associated with a 5-fold increased risk of ovarian cancer and decreased survival after diagnosis of ovarian cancer.[195] The risk of prostate cancer in men in Australia with p.C282Y homozygosity or p.C282Y/p.H63D compound heterozygosity was not increased.[185] In Finland, the allele frequency of p.C282Y and p.H63D in 843 consecutive men with prostate cancer and 118 men with breast cancer and population-based controls did not differ significantly.[196]

The standardized incidence ratio for squamous cell carcinoma of the esophagus was increased 3-fold in Swedish patients with hemochromatosis.[186] Neither *HFE* p.C282Y nor p.H63D was associated with increased risk for pancreatic cancer in 958 patients with diverse preexisting pancreatic abnormalities.[197] In a study of Swiss patients with hemochromatosis diagnosed in the interval 1965 to 2013, standardized incidence ratios for esophageal adenocarcinoma and gastric, small bowel, and rectal cancer were not increased.[186] In a meta-analysis, the risk of developing cancers other than hepatocellular carcinoma in 66,263 people with *HFE* mutations and in 226,515 control subjects without *HFE* mutations did not differ significantly.[198]

PORPHYRIA CUTANEA TARDA

The most common type of porphyria is sporadic porphyria cutanea tarda (PCT). An elevated amount of storage iron is characteristic of this disorder. The presence of one or two *HFE* p.C282Y or p.H63D mutations is common in subjects with sporadic PCT and increased storage iron. Some patients with PCT (either sporadic or familial) and heavy iron loading are homozygous for *HFE* mutations.[199-201]

PCT occurs in individuals who have decreased activity of uroporphyrinogen decarboxylase that results in the accumulation of uroporphyrinogen I. In the presence of excess iron, accumulated uroporphyrinogen undergoes iron-mediated oxidation, resulting in the production of uroporphomethene. Uroporphomethene further inhibits the already decreased activity of uroporphyrinogen decarboxylase.[202,203] An association of the uroporphyrinogen decarboxylase gene on chromosome 1q and hemochromatosis alleles on chromosome 6p was first reported in 1989[199] and substantiated after *HFE* was cloned and common *HFE* mutations were identified.[200,204,205] In a study of 108 subjects in Utah with PCT, 19% were p.C282Y homozygotes and 7% were p.C282Y/p.H63D compound heterozygotes.[200] The *HFE* mutation(s) cause increased iron absorption that further suppresses uroporphyrinogen decarboxylase activity resulting in the accumulation of uroporphyrin I in organs. Deposition of porphyrin in skin causes photosensitivity, blistering, and scarring.

Risk factors for the expression of PCT include common *HFE* mutations,[206-211] hepatitis C, alcohol abuse, oral estrogen therapy (but possibly not transdermal estrogen),[200,212] vaginal contraceptive ring,[211] and tamoxifen.[213] Hepatitis C infection, a potent risk factor, occurs in 28% to 74% of individuals with PCT. In a 2002 study of 39 consecutive patients with PCT in Galveston, Texas, 9% had *HFE* genotype p.C282Y/p.C282Y, 9% had p.C282Y/wt, 12% had p.C282Y/p.H63D, 9% had p.H63D/p.H63D, and 26% had p.H63D/wt.[207] Among these patients, 79% drank alcohol, 73% of 11 women took estrogens, 86% were smokers, and 74% were positive for hepatitis C antibody. Thus, *HFE* mutations were common and PCT expression was multifactorial. Three or more risk factors for expression of PCT were detected in 92% of the 39 patients.[207]

In France, 17% of patients with PCT had *HFE* p.C282Y (4% of controls). There was no significant difference in the prevalence of the p.H63D and p.S65C or compound p.C282Y/p.H63D heterozygosity between groups. Hepatitis C antibodies were detected in 28% of patients with PCT.[208] In a study of 190 German patients with sporadic PCT and 115 age-matched healthy blood donors, 39% of patients with porphyria had *HFE* p.C282Y (vs 3% of controls) and 12% were p.C282Y homozygotes (vs 0% of controls).[206] The p.H63D mutation was present in 45% of patients with porphyria (10% of controls). Nine percent of patients with porphyria were p.C282Y/p.H63D compound heterozygotes. Among Basques, patients with PCT did not have increased prevalence of *HFE* p.C282Y, p.H63D, or p.S65C, although 35% had hepatitis C.[209]

ANEMIAS, HEMOCHROMATOSIS, AND IRON OVERLOAD

Erythropoietic activity has a greater influence on hepcidin expression than body iron status.[214] Hepcidin expression is decreased when erythropoiesis is increased (eg, post phlebotomy, hemolysis, and administration of erythropoietin). The signal that induces this process appears to be mediated by molecules released by erythroid precursors. In 2014, Kautz and colleagues isolated erythroferrone (ERFE), a hormone produced by erythroblasts that mediates hepcidin suppression during stress erythropoiesis.[215] Subsequently, ERFE was shown to contribute to hepcidin suppression and iron overload in murine models of β-thalassemia and recovery from inflammation.[216,217] It has been suggested that ERFE is involved in inherited anemias with ineffective erythropoiesis, anemia of chronic kidney disease, and iron-refractory iron deficiency anemia.[215,218] ERFE is produced by marrow erythroblasts, and its biosynthesis is regulated by erythropoietin. ERFE inhibits hepcidin synthesis by binding bone morphogenetic proteins and thereby inhibiting the bone morphogenetic protein receptor pathway that controls hepcidin transcription (Chapter 25).[215,219,220] Therefore, ERFE regulates iron metabolism through the hepcidin-ferroportin axis. Other candidate signaling molecules, at least in the context of ineffective erythropoiesis, include growth differentiation factor 15 (GDF15) and twisted gastrulation protein homolog 1 (TWSG1).[221-224]

Hereditary Spherocytosis

Individuals who have hereditary spherocytosis may develop severe iron overload and hepatic cirrhosis if they are *HFE* p.C282Y homozygotes or heterozygotes.[225] Iron overload can also occur in patients with hereditary spherocytosis who do not have common *HFE* mutations.[226] In a Utah family, for example, two brothers with p.C282Y homozygosity had iron overload.[225] Iron overload in the propositus with both hemochromatosis and hereditary spherocytosis was much more severe than that of his brother who had hemochromatosis without hereditary spherocytosis. The son of the propositus was a p.C282Y heterozygote who also had hereditary spherocytosis. His serum ferritin concentration and liver iron stores were modestly elevated. A man with hereditary spherocytosis without common *HFE* mutations developed iron overload in association with daily consumption of iron supplements for 15 years.[225] A woman with hereditary stomatocytosis and *HFE* p.S65C heterozygosity developed severe iron overload.[227] Conceivably, ERFE production in response to the chronic hemolysis of hereditary spherocytosis could contribute to an iron-loading phenotype.

β-Thalassemia

β-Thalassemia minor and hemochromatosis sometimes occur in the same person. In one family, three persons had both β-thalassemia minor and hemochromatosis and four others had hemochromatosis alone.[228] A man who consumed large quantities of daily iron supplements developed severe iron overload. He was diagnosed to have both *HFE* p.C282Y homozygosity and β-thalassemia minor.[226] In a study of 22 iron-loaded Italian patients with β-thalassemia minor and 62 of their relatives, the severity of iron-related complications in p.C282Y homozygotes who also had β-thalassemia trait was increased.[229] Among 152 Italian men with β-thalassemia minor, the four with p.H63D homozygosity had higher mean serum ferritin concentrations than those without p.H63D.[230] Among 71 Italian patients with transfusion-dependent β-thalassemia major, the most severe iron overload was observed in the only patient who had p.H63D homozygosity.[231] The development of iron overload in persons with β-thalassemia minor without p.C282Y or p.H63D homozygosity is uncommon. Ineffective erythropoiesis due to β-thalassemia minor could enhance iron absorption in some p.C282Y or p.H63D homozygotes.[229-231] It is plausible that mutations in non-*HFE* iron-related genes or acquired factors increase iron absorption in some persons with β-thalassemia minor. ERFE likely contributes to iron loading in thalassemia, including transfusion-independent β-thalassemia intermedia.[216]

The risk of coinheritance of β-thalassemia minor and common *HFE* mutations varies across populations because there are significant regional differences in the prevalence of these respective traits.[60,232] In several European populations, the prevalence of p.C282Y and p.H63D in patients with β-thalassemia minor does not differ significantly from that of corresponding control subjects.[229,231] In Sardinia, an area not reached by Celtic migrations, the prevalence of β-thalassemia is relatively high (12%).[232] The prevalence of p.H63D is similar to that of other European populations but p.C282Y is rare.[60] There are small cohorts of patients with β-thalassemia in Egypt, Turkey, Iraq, and northern India, but their prevalence of p.H63D did not differ significantly from that of control populations and p.C282Y was not detected.

X-Linked Sideroblastic Anemia

Some men with X-linked sideroblastic anemia (hemizygotes for pathogenic mutations of the aminolevulinate synthase gene, *ALAS2*), ringed sideroblasts, and iron overload also have *HFE* mutations. This pattern of "digenic" iron overload was first described in a 59-year-old French man who had X-linked sideroblastic anemia, hepatic iron overload, and p.C282Y/p.H63D compound heterozygosity. His iron overload was much more severe than that of his 61-year-old brother who had X-linked sideroblastic anemia but no *HFE* mutation.[233] By increasing ERFE production, the ineffective erythropoiesis of X-linked sideroblastic anemia may contribute to an iron-loading phenotype.[234]

Among 18 unrelated patients with X-linked sideroblastic anemia, 17.0% had *HFE* p.C282Y (5.5% in white controls) and 23.0% had p.H63D (15.0% in controls).[235] Prevalence of the p.C282Y mutation was significantly greater in patients with sideroblastic anemia than in controls, but the prevalence of p.H63D was similar in both groups. After iron depletion, the responsiveness of anemia to pyridoxine supplementation increased in some patients. Coinheritance of one or more *HFE* mutations and an otherwise mild *ALAS2* mutation was associated with heavy iron overload.[236] The iron status of patients with mutations of *ALAS2*, with or without *HFE* mutations, has been reviewed.[237]

Refractory Anemia With Ringed Sideroblasts

Iron accumulation varies in this myelodysplastic disorder.[238] In 40 patients from Switzerland, Greece, and France who had refractory anemia with ringed sideroblasts and nontransfusion iron overload, 1.3% had *HFE* p.C282Y. This prevalence was similar to that in 200 normal control subjects (2.5%). The prevalence of the p.H63D mutation was also similar in patients and controls (19% and 13%, respectively).[239] The investigators suggested that ineffective erythropoiesis alone could account for the increased intestinal absorption of iron in most nontransfused patients. In a report from Cleveland of 140 patients with myelodysplastic syndrome, 21.4% of 42 patients with refractory anemia with ringed sideroblasts were p.C282Y heterozygotes, compared with 9.8% of 198 healthy race-matched controls.[240] ERFE likely contributes to the iron-loading phenotype of myelodysplastic syndromes.[234,241]

Infections in Hemochromatosis Patients

Individuals with hemochromatosis, especially those with cirrhosis, are susceptible to severe infection by organisms that rarely cause illness in people with normal body iron stores. Analyses of US Multiple-Cause Mortality Data (1979-1992) revealed that decedents with hemochromatosis were 15.3, 2.2, 1.5, and 1.4 times more likely to have chronic liver disease or cirrhosis, bacteremia, septicemia, and (unspecified) bacterial infection, respectively, than decedents without hemochromatosis.[242]

Vibrio vulnificus can cause fatal primary septicemia[243,244] and serious wound infections[245] in persons with hemochromatosis. Invasive organisms thrive in blood that has elevated iron content[244] and can also derive iron from erythrocytes or hemoglobin. Mortality of *V. vulnificus* infection in hepcidin knockout mice with iron overload was greater than that of wild-type control mice.[246] Dietary iron depletion or administration of a hepcidin agonist decreased mortality.[246] In two respective persons with hemochromatosis, non-01 *Vibrio cholerae* caused hemorrhagic bullous skin lesions and bacteremia[247] and a skin lesion and an intracerebral abscess.[248]

Yersinia enterocolitica can cause bacteremia and multiple hepatic abscesses in persons with hemochromatosis.[249,250] In hepcidin knockout mice, mortality of "siderophilic" *Y. enterocolitica* O9 *infection was 100%, whereas no iron-depleted* hepcidin knockout mice *died of infection.*[251] *Yersinia pseudotuberculosis* can cause septicemia[252] and multiple hepatic abscesses in persons with hemochromatosis.[253] *Hjv* (−/−) and *HFE* (p.C282Y/p.C282Y) mice developed colonization of deep tissues by *Y. pseudotuberculosis* after oral inoculation.[254] A laboratory strain of *Y. pestis* caused the death of a man with *HFE* p.C28Y homozygosity and hepatic iron overload.[255,256]

Serious or fatal infections due to *Escherichia coli* in patients with hemochromatosis include spontaneous bacterial peritonitis,[257-259] nonnosocomial pneumonia,[260] and nonnosocomial meningitis.[261] Iron overload from a normal diet in hepcidin knockout mice and intravenous iron overload in wild-type mice potentiated infection and death due to intraperitoneal injection of pathogenic *E. coli*.[262] Iron depletion of hepcidin knockout mice prevented mortality due to infection.[262]

In a 2020 multinational study, *HFE* p.C282Y was not a risk factor for SARS-CoV-2 infection (COVID-19), after adjustment for other variables.[263]

Subnormal Immunoglobulins

Approximately 30% of hemochromatosis probands with *HFE* p.C282Y homozygosity had subnormal IgG isotypes, especially subclasses IgG1 or IgG3.[264] Phlebotomy therapy did not affect serum IgG or IgG subclass concentrations.[264] There was concordance of Ig and hemochromatosis phenotypes in probands and respective HLA-identical siblings and a significant positive association of selective IgG deficiency with p.C282Y-bearing chromosome 6p HLA haplotypes that included HLA-A*03, B*07. In another study, subnormal serum IgG3 concentrations were linked to chromosome 6p SNP microhaplotypes in hemochromatosis probands with p.C282Y homozygosity.[265] Patients with hemochromatosis who have subnormal IgG subclass isotypes and frequent or severe respiratory tract infections may benefit from IgG replacement therapy. Protein-losing enteropathy or nephrotic syndrome can also cause severe Ig deficiency in p.C282Y homozygotes.

Cardiomyopathy

Heart-related abnormalities include arrhythmia detected by electrocardiography, cardiomegaly on chest radiography, and decreased ejection fraction on echocardiography. In *HFE* hemochromatosis, these abnormalities are often due to noniron causes. In juvenile-onset hemochromatosis, cardiac abnormalities are usually caused by siderosis of cardiac myocytes and Purkinje fibers.

Hemochromatosis can cause cardiac arrhythmias or congestive heart failure due to siderosis of conducting fibers and cardiac myocytes. This complication is much more prevalent in juvenile hemochromatosis than *HFE* hemochromatosis. It was estimated that German adults with hemochromatosis had a 300-fold increased risk of developing cardiomyopathy.[160] In a study of US Multiple-Cause Mortality Files (1979-1992), the association of cardiomyopathy and hemochromatosis was 4.8-fold higher than the expected ratio.[242] In a Swedish study of nationwide, population-based health and census registers, the risk of cardiomyopathy in persons with hemochromatosis was significantly elevated (hazard ratio 3.2 [95% confidence interval: 2.15, 4.81]).[266]

Atherosclerosis

The prevalence of coronary atherosclerosis in a large autopsy study was lower in decedents with iron overload than control subjects.[267] In a study of US Multiple-Cause Mortality Files, manifestations of ischemic heart disease tended to be lower in patients who died with hemochromatosis.[242] In 300 Canadian subjects with coronary atherosclerosis, higher serum ferritin concentrations in those with coronary atherosclerosis diagnosed before age 50 y was not related to *HFE* p.C282Y or p.H63D[268] In 265 Puerto Rican patients with premature (age <50 y) coronary and/or peripheral atherosclerosis, p.C282Y prevalence was lower and that of p.H63D was similar to those of 272 healthy control subjects.[269] In a study of 30,916 white adults aged 25 to 98 years, there was no consistent association of the prevalence of coronary heart disease and either serum iron indicators or *HFE* mutations.[270] Total mean serum cholesterol and low-density lipoprotein concentrations were lower in *HFE* p.C282Y homozygotes than *HFE* wild-type participants.[271] Low macrophage expression of hepcidin in persons with hemochromatosis could contribute to their decreased risk of coronary atherosclerosis.[272] Hemochromatosis or iron overload is not significantly related to risk of carotid atherosclerosis or stroke.[273-276] Peripheral artery atherosclerosis is uncommon in patients with hemochromatosis and insulin-dependent diabetes.[267,277] The hazard ratio of ischemic heart disease was not increased in first-degree relatives of persons with hemochromatosis.[266] Together, "There is overwhelming evidence that atherosclerosis, coronary artery disease, stroke, and peripheral artery disease are neither prominent clinical features nor frequent causes of death in genetic hemochromatosis."[186]

DIAGNOSIS

History and Physical Examination Findings

Recent guidelines and reviews have been published about screening, evaluation and management of individuals suspected to have hemochromatosis, and evaluation of relatives of a person who has *HFE* hemochromatosis.[166,278-280] A large percentage of *HFE* p.C282Y homozygotes who are identified during screening studies do not have symptoms or persistently elevated serum ferritin concentrations.[6,66,85] Currently, screening of the general population for hemochromatosis is not recommended.[281]

Hemochromatosis with iron overload should be suspected in an individual who has some combination of the following: arthralgias, right upper quadrant abdominal pain, impotence, palpitations, unexplained fatigue or weight loss, gray-bronze skin, hepatomegaly, stigmata of portal hypertension, diabetes, or hypogonadism. People in whom the diagnosis is established after seeking evaluation due to illness usually have several of the symptoms and physical examination abnormalities stated above. Only heavily iron-loaded patients with far-advanced organ injury have all of the above symptoms and physical examination abnormalities. Most hemochromatosis homozygotes do not have these findings. Individuals in whom the diagnosis is established during routine screening are nearly always asymptomatic and have no physical examination abnormalities. The wide variation in the frequency of symptoms and signs of hemochromatosis from 10 nonscreening cohorts is displayed in *Table 27.5*.

Laboratory Findings

Transferrin saturation, the first blood test to become elevated in hemochromatosis homozygotes, is typically >60% in symptomatic men and >50% in symptomatic women.[56,81,282] Total serum iron-binding capacity is often mildly reduced and unbound iron-binding capacity is usually decreased in untreated homozygotes.[283] In iron-loaded patients, serum ferritin concentration is elevated. The sensitivity of elevated transferrin saturation to identify a patient with hemochromatosis is 94% to 98%, and its specificity is 70% to 98%.[81,282] Typical results of transferrin saturation and serum ferritin concentration in different groups of hemochromatosis homozygotes are displayed in *Tables 27.4* and *27.7*. Liver stainable iron and the hepatic iron index are also elevated in iron-loaded homozygotes. Recommendations about obtaining liver specimens by biopsy are available.[106,284] SNP analyses of *HFE* p.C282Y, p.H63D, and p.S65C are widely available. p.C282Y homozygosity was present in 89% of patients with hemochromatosis in the Utah studies, regardless of the presence or absence of iron overload.[56]

Evaluation of Relatives

It is important to study the siblings of hemochromatosis probands. Test selection is the same as for the index patient: transferrin saturation; serum ferritin concentration; and *HFE* mutation analysis to identify p.C282Y, p.H63D, and p.S65C alleles. Young homozygous siblings of a hemochromatosis proband may have a normal serum ferritin concentration.[56] Serum ferritin concentrations should be measured at 2- or 3-year intervals. When the serum ferritin concentration becomes elevated, it is reasonable to begin intermittent phlebotomy therapy to prevent accumulation of excess iron in the liver and other organs.

Relatives homozygous for hemochromatosis who have serum ferritin >700 µg/L[285] or >1000 µg/L[283,286] and elevated serum concentrations of hepatic transaminases should undergo liver biopsy to determine the presence or absence of hepatic fibrosis or cirrhosis and permit measurement of hepatic iron stores. A liver biopsy typical of iron-loaded homozygotes appears in *Figure 27.2*. Most relatives homozygous for hemochromatosis identified during family screening are less iron-loaded and have fewer complications than their corresponding probands. Where available and validated, MRI can be used to quantify hepatic iron content and assess liver anatomy.

Heterozygous Relatives

HFE p.C282Y heterozygotes do not become iron-loaded unless they have an additional disorder that increases iron accumulation.[287] There was no difference in the amount of heme iron or nonheme iron absorption in p.C282Y heterozygotes and normal control subjects. Similarly, NTBI concentrations, transferrin saturation, or serum ferritin concentrations did not differ significantly between p.C282Y heterozygotes and normal controls.[288] Transferrin

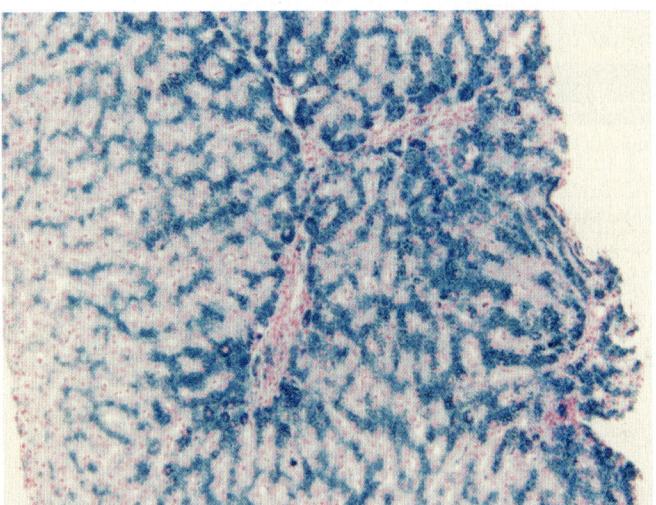

FIGURE 27.2 Grade 4 hepatic parenchymal cell stainable iron in a 30-year-old asymptomatic woman with *HFE* p.C282Y homozygosity who was evaluated after her symptomatic brother was diagnosed to have hemochromatosis (TIFF image × 200 original magnification).

saturation and serum ferritin concentration measurements in p.C282Y heterozygotes and normal individuals are displayed in *Table 27.7*.[85]

Because ~10% of whites of Central, Western, and Northern European ancestry are *HFE* p.C282Y heterozygotes, the occurrence of hemochromatosis in consecutive generations of whites is common. Transferrin saturation or unbound iron-binding capacity should be measured in all siblings of the proband and in the interested parents and adult children of homozygotes.

Homozygous Relatives

In a study of the relatives of 291 hemochromatosis probands, 214 homozygous relatives were identified.[56] Stratification of these 214 clinically unselected individuals by age and sex revealed that 90% of the homozygous male relatives were iron-loaded by age 40 years and that 52% of them had iron-related organ injury. Clinically unselected female homozygous relatives became iron-loaded approximately 1 decade later than men. After age 50 years, 88% of clinically unselected female homozygous relatives became iron-loaded and 16% of them had iron-related organ injury.[56] The results of transferrin saturation and serum ferritin concentration tests in 291 probands and their 214 clinically unselected homozygous relatives in the Utah studies are displayed in *Table 27.4*.

Hemochromatosis in African Americans

In 1950, Krainin and Kahn described a black man in New York who had hemochromatosis and hepatic iron overload.[289] In 1995 to 1996, nontransfusion iron overload was described in African Americans in two case series.[290,291] Nontransfusion iron overload was identified in African Americans in two hospital autopsy studies,[292,293] a coroner autopsy series,[294] and a liver biopsy series.[295]

In 2001, it was reported that two unrelated African American men had hemochromatosis phenotypes and hemochromatosis-associated *HFE* genotypes.[296] The prevalence of p.C282Y homozygosity in African Americans in two large US population studies was 0 to 0.0001.[83,297] Five African American participants in screening programs had *HFE* p.C282Y homozygosity.[83,271,298] The occurrence of p.C282Y in African Americans is consistent with European American ancestry.[299] Hemochromatosis phenotypes in African Americans also occur in association with pathogenic mutations in *HJV*[19] and *SLC40A1* p.D270V.[300] X-linked sideroblastic anemia and iron overload occur in African American men with *ALAS2* p.R452S, an allele that probably arose in Africa.[301-303]

Hyperferritinemia in African Americans is strongly associated with chronic hepatitis C viral infection.[304] Persistent hyperferritinemia in African Americans without evidence of hepatitis C is positively associated with male sex, age, transferrin saturation, serum GGT concentrations, and number of units of erythrocyte transfusion, after adjustment for other variables.[304]

SLC40A1 p.Q248H, a polymorphism in sub-Saharan African blacks and African Americans, is also associated with hyperferritinemia, especially in men,[305-307] although p.Q248H probably does not cause iron overload in the absence of other factors. The prevalence of p.Q248H in African Americans with elevated or normal transferrin saturations and serum ferritin concentrations did not differ significantly[26] and the odds ratio estimate of p.Q248H in African Americans with iron overload who lacked *HFE* p.C282Y was not significantly increased.[25] The ferroportin 248 amino acid is not highly conserved, and the mutation does not affect a portion of the ferroportin molecule critical to hepcidin binding or iron transport.[27]

H-Ferritin Hemochromatosis

Four members of a Japanese family had a single point mutation (A49U) in the iron-responsive element motif of H-ferritin mRNA that accounted for a novel subtype of autosomal dominant iron overload.[308] Laboratory features in affected family members included elevated transferrin saturations, elevated serum ferritin concentrations, increased hepatocyte iron, and iron deposition in Kupffer cells and splenic macrophages. In vitro studies suggested that iron abnormalities were due to impaired ferroxidase activity generated by H-ferritin subunits.[308] Although it is presumed that members of this family with iron overload absorbed supranormal quantities of iron, there is no report of iron absorption or blood or urine hepcidin concentrations in this kinship.

MANAGEMENT

Phlebotomy Therapy

There are detailed discussions of phlebotomy therapy for patients with *HFE* hemochromatosis.[81,309] There is objective evidence of benefit of normalizing serum ferritin concentrations by therapeutic phlebotomy in patients with hemochromatosis, even in those who present with mild or moderate elevation of serum ferritin (300-1000 μg/L).[310] Overall, men require approximately twice as many units of phlebotomy to induce iron depletion as women.[72,81,311] Manifestations of hemochromatosis and associated iron overload that respond to and those that do not improve after phlebotomy therapy are displayed in *Table 27.9*. All siblings of index patients with juvenile hemochromatosis should be evaluated for hemochromatosis. Sibling(s) with hemochromatosis should be treated promptly to achieve iron depletion.

Initial Weekly Phlebotomy Schedule

The main treatment of patients with hemochromatosis with iron overload is phlebotomy.[81,309,311] It is important to begin phlebotomy promptly after the diagnosis of iron overload is established. In a phlebotomy of 500 mL of blood with a hematocrit of 40%, 200 mL of packed RBCs are removed. Because 1 mL of packed erythrocytes contains ~1 mg of iron, each 500-mL phlebotomy removes ~200 mg of iron. Serum ferritin concentrations, not serum iron concentrations or transferrin saturations, should be used to monitor relative amounts of storage iron during phlebotomy.[314]

Most iron-loaded homozygotes tolerate removal of 500 mL of blood each week. Some women, small individuals, or elderly patients may only tolerate removal of 250 mL of blood each week. In patients with heavy iron overload who have cardiac arrhythmias or hepatic failure, twice-weekly phlebotomy with or without iron chelation therapy may improve cardiac and hepatic function quickly. Phlebotomy therapy should be continued until hemoglobin drops by 1 to 2 g/dL below baseline, the MCV drops by 3 to 5 fL below baseline, and serum ferritin concentration drops to 20 to 50 μg/L. These findings provide evidence of iron-limited erythropoiesis, which concludes the initial phase of phlebotomy therapy. The patient then enters the lifelong maintenance phase of phlebotomy therapy.[81,309,311,314,315]

Table 27.9. Changes Expected After Phlebotomy Therapy

Manifestations Attributed to Hemochromatosis or Iron Overload	Expected treatment Outcome(s)
No complications	Prevention of complications of iron overload; normal life expectancy
Weakness, fatigue, lethargy	May resolve
Abdominal pain	Resolution usual
Elevated serum hepatic transaminase concentration(s)	Improvement or resolution
Hepatomegaly	Resolution often occurs
Hepatic cirrhosis[a]	Usually no change
Increased risk for primary liver cancer[b]	May persist in patients with cirrhosis
Right upper quadrant pain[c]	Resolution if due only to iron overload
Arthropathy	Arthralgias may improve; joint deformity unlikely to resolve; worsening sometimes occurs
Hypogonadotrophic hypogonadism	May resolve if pituitary injury is not extensive
Diabetes mellitus	Occasional improvement, often temporary
Hyperthyroidism, hypothyroidism	Resolution rare
Cardiomyopathy	Resolution sometimes
Hyperpigmentation	Resolution usual
Hyperferritinemia	Resolution
Hyperferremia[d]	Usually decreases
Elevated ceruloplasmin concentration	Little or no change
Elevated mean corpuscular volume	Decrease or resolution
Excess absorption and storage of nonferrous metals[e]	Little or no change
Increased risk of infection with *Vibrio vulnificus,* other bacteria	Little or no change
Subnormal immunoglobulin concentration(s)	Little or no change

[a]Regression was reported in some patients.[312]
[b]Increased risk is usually only in those who have hepatic cirrhosis.
[c]Right upper quadrant pain that is only due to iron overload usually decreases, whereas pain due to hepatocellular carcinoma, portal vein thrombosis, gallbladder disease, or other noniron causes usually does not decrease.
[d]Serum iron concentrations may be normal or subnormal in persons with hemochromatosis due to severe iron deficiency, chronic inflammatory or infectious disease, vitamin C deficiency, or prolonged fasting.
[e]Cobalt, manganese, zinc, and lead. In one study of *HFE* p.C282Y homozygotes, there was a positive association of blood cadmium concentrations and duration/units of phlebotomy.[313]
Modified from Barton JC, McDonnell SM, Adams PC, et al. Management of hemochromatosis. *Ann Intern Med.* 1998;129(11):932-939. Copyright © 1998 American College of Physicians. All Rights Reserved. Reprinted with the permission of American College of Physicians, Inc.

Erythrocytapheresis is an alternative to phlebotomy therapy. In a large randomized trial that compared these two treatment modalities, erythrocytapheresis achieved iron depletion in patients with *HFE* hemochromatosis at about the same rate as traditional weekly phlebotomy but the former was more expensive for hospitals and probably more time-consuming for technicians.[316] Erythrocytapheresis is not available at every facility. These results do not support a general recommendation of erythrocytapheresis use to achieve iron depletion in patients with *HFE* hemochromatosis.

Deferasirox, an oral iron chelator, was evaluated as a means of achieving iron depletion in *HFE* p.C282Y homozygotes without cirrhosis whose pretreatment serum ferritin concentrations were 300 to 2000 μg/L. Adverse events, reported in <10% of patients, were generally dose related and included diarrhea, nausea, abdominal pain, and elevated serum alanine transaminase or creatinine concentrations. Decrements of serum ferritin concentrations were dose dependent.[317] Deferoxamine is also US Food and Drug Administration (FDA) approved for treatment iron overload in patients with hemochromatosis. Another oral iron chelator, deferiprone, has been approved by the FDA to treat transfusion iron overload in patients with thalassemia syndromes in whom current chelation therapy is inadequate.

Lifelong Maintenance Phlebotomy

After iron depletion is accomplished, lifelong maintenance of normal iron stores by phlebotomy therapy begins. Removal of 500 mL of blood every 2 to 4 months (every 3-6 months in women) prevents reaccumulation of excessive organ storage iron. The goals of lifelong maintenance phlebotomy therapy include maintenance of a normal hemoglobin concentration and maintenance of serum ferritin <300 μg/L in men and <200 μg/L in women.[318] A very low serum ferritin concentration and the presence of anemia indicate that the frequency of phlebotomy therapy can be decreased to 4- or 6-month intervals.

Patients and physicians often want to estimate the duration of weekly phlebotomy therapy to achieve iron depletion. Based on a study of the correlation of serum ferritin concentrations with the number of grams of iron removed by phlebotomy therapy, 1 μg/L of pretreatment serum ferritin concentration corresponded to ~8 mg of mobilizable iron.[285] A person whose pretreatment serum ferritin concentration is 600 μg/L is likely to have ~4800 mg of mobilizable storage iron. Each milliliter of centrifuged RBCs contains about 1 mg of iron and each 500-mL unit of blood with a hematocrit of 40% contains ~200 mg of iron. Therefore, a patient whose serum ferritin is 600 μg/L is predicted to undergo ~24 units of phlebotomy to achieve iron depletion ((8 × 600) = 4800; (4800 mg/200 mg iron/unit) = 24 units). This estimate holds reasonably well except in patients whose serum ferritin concentration is elevated out of proportion to storage iron due to hepatic necrosis or another source of inflammation that causes hyperferritinemia. In some cases, measuring serum ferritin concentration every few phlebotomies is comforting to patients and physicians. After patients achieve iron depletion by phlebotomy, the number of units of blood removed, multiplied by 200 mg iron per phlebotomy, provides an estimate of the amount of iron that was removed (quantitative phlebotomy). Hemochromatosis patients who take proton pump inhibitor therapy for nonhemochromatosis indications may require fewer annual maintenance phlebotomies.[319]

Hemochromatosis Homozygotes as Blood Donors

Experts at the US National Institutes of Health studied patients with hemochromatosis as blood donors.[320] They evaluated 1402 units of blood from hemochromatosis donors and concluded that, if such individuals do not have serologic results necessitating deferral, their blood units do not pose a health risk for recipients and could significantly augment the blood supply at the Institutes. After 27 months of study, blood from donors with hemochromatosis represented 14% of all blood donations. In another report, an ethicist concluded that patients with hemochromatosis can be free, voluntary, altruistic blood donors if they do not request any benefit other than blood removal.[321]

In a retrospective assessment of 3 years of transfusion-transmissible infections in Australia from hemochromatosis (therapeutic) and volunteer whole-blood donors, the rate of infection was lower among donors with hemochromatosis (8.4 infections/100,000 donations) than volunteer donors (21.6 infections/100,000 donations). Thus, blood from therapeutic donors posed less risk for recipients than that of first-time volunteer blood donors.[322] It has been estimated that blood from healthy patients with hemochromatosis could add millions of units to the US blood supply,[323] although most US blood banks do not provide medical services needed by many persons with hemochromatosis. When phlebotomy therapy is performed in a setting other than a blood bank, blood cannot be collected and processed properly for future transfusion.

Thirty-five blood services from 33 countries on five continents responded to an internet-based questionnaire about how blood services use blood from individuals with hemochromatosis. Blood services in the United States did not participate. Some blood centers (31%) do not accept blood from either hemochromatosis homozygotes or heterozygotes. The remaining 69% accept blood donations from some heterozygotes and homozygotes, whether asymptomatic or symptomatic. Some centers allow heterozygotes and homozygotes to donate blood more often (frequency not stated) than those who have not been discovered to have a hemochromatosis gene mutation. There were diverse reasons that some centers do not accept donations from hemochromatosis homozygotes or heterozygotes, such as legislation, legal regulations, internal regulations, personal opinion or preference, or expert consensus. Donation policies varied between countries and within some countries. Among the centers that accepted hemochromatosis blood for transfusion, 1% to 5% of the total number of blood donations were made by donors known to have one or more hemochromatosis gene mutations.[324]

Clinical Changes After Iron Depletion

Phlebotomy-related changes related to manifestations attributed to iron overload are displayed in *Table 27.9*.[309] Malaise and asthenia are common, nonspecific presenting manifestations in nonscreening patients that resolve in some patients after they achieve iron depletion. Regression of hepatic fibrosis was studied in 36 patients with hemochromatosis who underwent two liver biopsies, the first one before and the second after iron depletion, with an interval of at least 2 years between biopsies.[312] Regression of fibrosis occurred in 9 of 13 patients whose initial fibrosis was far advanced (grade 3) and in 8 of 23 whose initial biopsy showed cirrhosis (grade 4). Iron depletion with phlebotomy results in increased insulin secretory capacity in some persons with hemochromatosis and diabetes, but insulin resistance may persist.[325] In patients with arthropathy typical of hemochromatosis, joint pain and swelling may decrease and joint mobility may increase after iron depletion, although degenerative changes rarely improve. In unusual cases, thyroid function returns to normal in adults with hemochromatosis after iron depletion with phlebotomy. Impotence and other abnormalities caused by hypogonadotrophic hypogonadism are common in men with HLA-linked hemochromatosis. Phlebotomy rarely alleviates these manifestations in men younger than 40 years and has not been documented to have benefit in men 40 years or older.

Women with juvenile-onset hemochromatosis and hypogonadotrophic hypogonadism due to iron overload rarely if ever experience return of menses or fertility after iron depletion alone. In patients with hemochromatosis without hepatic cirrhosis or typical arthropathy at diagnosis, iron depletion and subsequent lifelong maintenance phlebotomy therapy may prevent the development of these conditions.

Dietary Recommendations

Much more iron can be removed in each 500-mL phlebotomy each week than can be absorbed during that week. For this reason, it is not necessary to impose dietary restrictions in an attempt to avoid foods that contain iron. Regardless, heme iron of meat, especially that of red meat, is readily absorbed. It is reasonable to advise patients to eat red meat in moderation to decrease dietary intake of saturated fat and animal protein, and to increase consumption of fresh vegetables and fruit, as for anyone else who follows a prudent cardiovascular diet.[309] Persons with hemochromatosis have increased risk of developing life-threatening infections with *V. vulnificus* from raw shellfish (see Infections in Hemochromatosis Patients). It is prudent to advise these individuals not to consume raw shellfish, although consumption of cooked shellfish is safe.

Alcohol Intake

Cirrhosis in *HFE* p.C282Y homozygotes is significantly associated with daily alcohol intake.[106] A study of 368 p.C282Y homozygotes revealed that daily intake of each 14 g of alcohol increases risk of cirrhosis 1.5-fold, after adjustment of other variables.[106] In other studies, it was estimated that consumption of 30 g[164,326] or >60 g[327,328] of alcohol per day can worsen iron-related liver damage. Consumption of alcohol by persons with cirrhosis may increase the risk of hepatocellular carcinoma.[164,328] Individuals with hepatic damage due to iron overload may benefit by avoiding consumption of alcohol.

Vitamins

It is reasonable to advise patients with hemochromatosis to avoid medicinal intake of vitamin C (ascorbic acid) because it can increase the absorption of dietary iron, mobilization of storage iron, or production of free radicals. Vitamin C also may cause oxidative damage of the myocardium and cardiac conduction system, resulting in rare fatal arrhythmias in iron-loaded patients who have hemochromatosis or thalassemia major.[329-331] It is also reasonable to advise patients with hemochromatosis not take multiple vitamins that contain iron.

PROGNOSIS

Cirrhosis and diabetes mellitus present at diagnosis of hemochromatosis with iron overload are major causes of decreased survival in older patients. Early studies revealed that the survival in patients treated with phlebotomy was greater than that of untreated patients.[162] Therapy also reduced deaths due to cardiac and hepatic failure.[162] In a study of 111 patients with hemochromatosis in England, the average survival of 85 people who underwent phlebotomy therapy was 63 months, compared with 18 months in the 26 subjects who did not become iron depleted.[162] In a study of 251 patients with hemochromatosis in Germany, survival of those who became iron depleted was similar to that of the background population.[77] Patients with hemochromatosis with diabetes had a 10-year survival of 65%. In patients without diabetes, the survival was 90%.[77] The 10-year survival of patients with hemochromatosis with cirrhosis was 72%, whereas survival of patients without cirrhosis was 82%. Patients who could not be iron depleted within 18 months after the onset of phlebotomy therapy also had decreased survival.[77] Survival of patients with hemochromatosis was similar in another report.[62] In 422 hemochromatosis probands homozygous for *HFE* p.C282Y, serum ferritin >1000 μg/L at diagnosis was positively associated with male sex and cirrhosis. Even with phlebotomy treatment, the relative risk of death from iron overload was 5-fold greater in probands with serum ferritin >1000 μg/L.[332] Patients with hemochromatosis had lower post–liver transplant survival than patients without iron storage disease, mostly due to extrahepatic causes.[333] Absolute telomere length, a factor directly associated with survival in some studies, was shorter in patients with hemochromatosis and iron overload than in patients with hemochromatosis without iron overload or normal control subjects.[334]

Cardiomyopathy due to cardiac siderosis is the predominant cause of premature death in persons with juvenile-onset hemochromatosis. Initiating therapy is urgent. Combined phlebotomy and deferoxamine or deferasirox along with supportive cardiac care may improve or restore cardiac function.[335] In other cases, combination chelation therapy with deferiprone and deferoxamine removed excessive cardiac iron.[336,337]

References

1. Sheldon JH. *Haemochromatosis*. London: Oxford University Press; 1935.
2. Feder JN, Gnirke A, Thomas W, et al. A novel MHC class I-like gene is mutated in patients with hereditary haemochromatosis. *Nat Genet*. 1996;13(4):399-408.
3. Barton JC, Edwards CQ, Acton RT. *HFE* gene: structure, function, mutations, and associated iron abnormalities. *Gene*. 2015;574(2):179-192.
4. Waalen J, Felitti V, Gelbart T, Ho NJ, Beutler E. Penetrance of hemochromatosis. *Blood Cells Mol Dis*. 2002;29(3):418-432.
5. Steinberg KK, Cogswell ME, Chang JC, et al. Prevalence of C282Y and H63D mutations in the hemochromatosis (*HFE*) gene in the United States. *JAMA*. 2001;285(17):2216-2222.
6. Adams PC, Reboussin DM, Barton JC, et al. Hemochromatosis and iron-overload screening in a racially diverse population. *N Engl J Med*. 2005;352(17):1769-1778.
7. Roetto A, Totaro A, Cazzola M, et al. Juvenile hemochromatosis locus maps to chromosome 1q. *Am J Hum Genet*. 1999;64(5):1388-1393.
8. Rivard SR, Lanzara C, Grimard D, et al. Juvenile hemochromatosis locus maps to chromosome 1q in a French Canadian population. *Eur J Hum Genet*. 2003;11(8):585-589.
9. Murugan RC, Lee PL, Kalavar MR, Barton JC. Early age-of-onset iron overload and homozygosity for the novel hemojuvelin mutation HJV R54X (exon 3; c.160A-->T) in an African American male of West Indies descent. *Clin Genet*. 2008;74(1):88-92.
10. Cazzola M, Cerani P, Rovati A, Iannone A, Claudiani G, Bergamaschi G. Juvenile genetic hemochromatosis is clinically and genetically distinct from the classical HLA-related disorder. *Blood*. 1998;92(8):2979-2981.
11. Janosi A, Andrikovics H, Vas K, et al. Homozygosity for a novel nonsense mutation (G66X) of the *HJV* gene causes severe juvenile hemochromatosis with fatal cardiomyopathy. *Blood*. 2005;105(1):432.
12. Barton JC, Rao SV, Pereira NM, et al. Juvenile hemochromatosis in the southeastern United States: a report of seven cases in two kinships. *Blood Cells Mol Dis*. 2002;29(1):104-115.
13. Lanzara C, Roetto A, Daraio F, et al. Spectrum of hemojuvelin gene mutations in 1q-linked juvenile hemochromatosis. *Blood*. 2004;103(11):4317-4321.
14. Papanikolaou G, Samuels ME, Ludwig EH, et al. Mutations in *HFE2* cause iron overload in chromosome 1q-linked juvenile hemochromatosis. *Nat Genet*. 2004;36(1):77-82.
15. Rivard SR, Mura C, Simard H, et al. Clinical and molecular aspects of juvenile hemochromatosis in Saguenay-Lac-Saint-Jean (Quebec, Canada). *Blood Cells Mol Dis*. 2000;26(1):10-14.
16. Roetto A, Papanikolaou G, Politou M, et al. Mutant antimicrobial peptide hepcidin is associated with severe juvenile hemochromatosis. *Nat Genet*. 2003;33(1):21-22.
17. Roetto A, Daraio F, Porporato P, et al. Screening hepcidin for mutations in juvenile hemochromatosis: identification of a new mutation (C70R). *Blood*. 2004;103(6):2407-2409.
18. Camaschella C, Roetto A, Cali A, et al. The gene *TFR2* is mutated in a new type of haemochromatosis mapping to 7q22. *Nat Genet*. 2000;25(1):14-15.
19. Majore S, Ricerca BM, Radio FC, et al. Type 3 hereditary hemochromatosis in a patient from sub-Saharan Africa: is there a link between African iron overload and TFR2 dysfunction?. *Blood Cells Mol Dis*. 2013;50(1):31-32.
20. Joshi R, Shvartsman M, Moran E, et al. Functional consequences of transferrin receptor-2 mutations causing hereditary hemochromatosis type 3. *Mol Genet Genomic Med*. 2015;3(3):221-232.
21. Nemeth E, Roetto A, Garozzo G, Ganz T, Camaschella C. Hepcidin is decreased in *TFR2* hemochromatosis. *Blood*. 2005;105(4):1803-1806.
22. Montosi G, Donovan A, Totaro A, et al. Autosomal-dominant hemochromatosis is associated with a mutation in the ferroportin (*SLC11A3*) gene. *J Clin Invest*. 2001;108(4):619-623.
23. Cremonesi L, Forni GL, Soriani N, et al. Genetic and clinical heterogeneity of ferroportin disease. *Br J Haematol*. 2005;131(5):663-670.
24. De Domenico I, Ward DM, Nemeth E, et al. The molecular basis of ferroportin-linked hemochromatosis. *Proc Natl Acad Sci USA*. 2005;102(25):8955-8960.
25. Barton JC, Acton RT, Lee PL, West C. *SLC40A1* Q248H allele frequencies and Q248H-associated risk of non-*HFE* iron overload in persons of sub-Saharan African descent. *Blood Cells Mol Dis*. 2007;39(2):206-211.
26. Barton JC, Lafreniere SA, Leiendecker-Foster C, et al. *HFE, SLC40A1, HAMP, HJV, TFR2*, and *FTL* mutations detected by denaturing high-performance liquid chromatography after iron phenotyping and *HFE* C282Y and H63D genotyping in 785 HEIRS Study participants. *Am J Hematol*. 2009;84(11):710-714.
27. Schimanski LM, Drakesmith H, Merryweather-Clarke AT, et al. In vitro functional analysis of human ferroportin (FPN) and hemochromatosis-associated *FPN* mutations. *Blood*. 2005;105(10):4096-4102.
28. Merryweather-Clarke AT, Cadet E, Bomford A, et al. Digenic inheritance of mutations in *HAMP* and *HFE* results in different types of haemochromatosis. *Hum Mol Genet*. 2003;12(17):2241-2247.
29. Pietrangelo A, Caleffi A, Henrion J, et al. Juvenile hemochromatosis associated with pathogenic mutations of adult hemochromatosis genes. *Gastroenterology*. 2005;128(2):470-479.
30. Barton JC, Harmon L, Rivers C, Acton RT. Hemochromatosis: association of severity of iron overload with genetic markers. *Blood Cells Mol Dis*. 1996;22(3):195-204.
31. Costa M, Cruz E, Barton JC, et al. Effects of highly conserved major histocompatibility complex (MHC) extended haplotypes on iron and low CD8+ T lymphocyte phenotypes in *HFE* C282Y homozygous hemochromatosis patients from three geographically distant areas. *PLoS One*. 2013;8(11):e79990.
32. Radio FC, Majore S, Aurizi C, et al. Hereditary hemochromatosis type 1 phenotype modifiers in Italian patients. The controversial role of variants in *HAMP, BMP2, FTL* and *SLC40A1* genes. *Blood Cells Mol Dis*. 2015;55(1):71-75.
33. McLaren CE, Emond MJ, Subramaniam VN, et al. Exome sequencing in *HFE* C282Y homozygous men with extreme phenotypes identifies a *GNPAT* variant associated with severe iron overload. *Hepatology*. 2015;62(2):429-439.
34. Barton JC, Chen WP, Emond MJ, et al. *GNPAT* p.D519G is independently associated with markedly increased iron stores in *HFE* p.C282Y homozygotes. *Blood Cells Mol Dis*. 2017:6315-6320.
35. Besson-Fournier C, Martinez M, Vinel JP, Aguilar-Martinez P, Coppin H, Roth MP. Further support for the association of *GNPAT* variant rs11558492 with severe iron overload in hemochromatosis. *Hepatology*. 2016;63(6):2054-2055.
36. Secondes ES, Wallace DF, Rishi G, et al. Increased frequency of *GNPAT* p.D519G in compound *HFE* p.C282Y/p.H63D heterozygotes with elevated serum ferritin levels. *Blood Cells Mol Dis*. 2020;85:102463.
37. Ryan E, Russell J, Ryan JD, Crowe J, Stewart S. *GNPAT* variant is not associated with severe iron overload in Irish C282Y homozygotes. *Hepatology*. 2016;63(6):2055-2056.
38. Tchernitchko D, Scotet V, Lefebvre T, et al. GNPAT polymorphism rs11558492 is not associated with increased severity in a large cohort of *HFE* p.Cys282Tyr homozygous patients. *Hepatology*. 2017;65(3):1069-1071.
39. Levstik A, Stuart A, Adams PC. *GNPAT* variant (D519G) is not associated with an elevated serum ferritin or iron removed by phlebotomy in patients referred for C282Y-linked hemochromatosis. *Ann Hepatol*. 2016;15(6):907-910.
40. Greni F, Valenti L, Mariani R, et al. *GNPAT* rs11558492 is not a major modifier of iron status: study of Italian hemochromatosis patients and blood donors. *Ann Hepatol*. 2017;16(3):451-456.
41. Aguilar-Martinez P, Giansily-Blaizot M, Bismuth M, Cunat S, Igual H, Schved JF. *HAMP* promoter mutation nc.-153C>T in non p.C282Y homozygous patients with iron overload. *Haematologica*. 2010;95(4):687-688.
42. Barton JC, Leiendecker-Foster C, Li H, DelRio-LaFreniere S, Acton RT, Eckfeldt JH. *HAMP* promoter mutation nc.-153C>T in 785 HEIRS Study participants. *Haematologica*. 2009;94(10):1465-1466.
43. Bridle KR, Frazer DM, Wilkins SJ, et al. Disrupted hepcidin regulation in *HFE*-associated haemochromatosis and the liver as a regulator of body iron homoeostasis. *Lancet*. 2003;361(9358):669-673.
44. Papanikolaou G, Tzilianos M, Christakis JI, et al. Hepcidin in iron overload disorders. *Blood*. 2005;105(10):4103-4105.
45. Ganz T. Hepcidin and iron regulation, 10 years later. *Blood*. 2011;117(17):4425-4433.
46. Wu XG, Wang Y, Wu Q, et al. HFE interacts with the BMP type I receptor ALK3 to regulate hepcidin expression. *Blood*. 2014;124(8):1335-1343.
47. Muckenthaler MU. How mutant *HFE* causes hereditary hemochromatosis. *Blood*. 2014;124(8):1212-1213.
48. Zoller H, Theurl I, Koch RO, McKie AT, Vogel W, Weiss G. Duodenal cytochrome b and hephaestin expression in patients with iron deficiency and hemochromatosis. *Gastroenterology*. 2003;125(3):746-754.
49. Stuart KA, Anderson GJ, Frazer DM, et al. Duodenal expression of iron transport molecules in untreated haemochromatosis subjects. *Gut*. 2003;52(7):953-959.
50. Zoller H, Koch RO, Theurl I, et al. Expression of the duodenal iron transporters divalent-metal transporter 1 and ferroportin 1 in iron deficiency and iron overload. *Gastroenterology*. 2001;120(6):1412-1419.
51. Bezwoda WR, Disler PB, Lynch SR, et al. Patterns of food iron absorption in iron-deficient white and indian subjects and in venesected haemochromatotic patients. *Br J Haematol*. 1976;33(3):425-436.
52. Milder MS, Cook JD, Finch CA. Influence of food iron absorption on the plasma iron level in idiopathic hemochromatosis. *Acta Haematol*. 1978;60(2):65-75.
53. Lynch SR, Skikne BS, Cook JD. Food iron absorption in idiopathic hemochromatosis. *Blood*. 1989;74(6):2187-2193.
54. Aruoma OI, Bomford A, Polson RJ, Halliwell B. Nontransferrin-bound iron in plasma from hemochromatosis patients: effect of phlebotomy therapy. *Blood*. 1988;72(4):1416-1419.
55. Loreal O, Gosriwatana I, Guyader D, Porter J, Brissot P, Hider RC. Determination of non-transferrin-bound iron in genetic hemochromatosis using a new HPLC-based method. *J Hepatol*. 2000;32(5):727-733.
56. Bulaj ZJ, Ajioka RS, Phillips JD, et al. Disease-related conditions in relatives of patients with hemochromatosis. *N Engl J Med*. 2000;343(21):1529-1535.
57. Dixon SJ, Lemberg KM, Lamprecht MR, et al. Ferroptosis: an iron-dependent form of nonapoptotic cell death. *Cell*. 2012;149(5):1060-1072.
58. Wang H, An P, Xie E, et al. Characterization of ferroptosis in murine models of hemochromatosis. *Hepatology*. 2017;66(2):449-465.
59. Asberg A, Hveem K, Thorstensen K, et al. Screening for hemochromatosis: high prevalence and low morbidity in an unselected population of 65,238 persons. *Scand J Gastroenterol*. 2001;36(10):1108-1115.
60. Merryweather-Clarke AT, Pointon JJ, Jouanolle AM, Rochette J, Robson KJ. Geography of *HFE* C282Y and H63D mutations. *Genet Test*. 2000;4(2):183-198.

61. Allen KJ, Gurrin LC, Constantine CC, et al. Iron-overload-related disease in *HFE* hereditary hemochromatosis. *N Engl J Med.* 2008;358(3):221-230.

62. Edwards CQ, Barton JC. Hemochromatosis. In: Greer JP, Foerster J, Rodgers GM, Paraskevas F, Glader B, eds. *Wintrobe's Clinical Hematology.* 13th ed. Philadelphia: Lippincott Williams & Wilkins; 2014:662-681.

63. Heath KM, Axton JH, McCullough JM, Harris N. The evolutionary adaptation of the C282Y mutation to culture and climate during the European Neolithic. *Am J Phys Anthropol.* 2016;160(1):86-101.

64. Wallace DF, Subramaniam VN. The global prevalence of *HFE* and non-*HFE* hemochromatosis estimated from analysis of next-generation sequencing data. *Genet Med.* 2016;18(6):618-626.

65. Edwards CQ, Barton JC. Hemochromatosis. In: Greer JP, Rodgers GM, Glader B, et al., eds. *Wintrobe's Clinical Hematology.* 14th ed. Philadelphia: Wolters Kluwer; 2019:665-690.

66. McLaren GD, McLaren CE, Adams PC, et al. Clinical manifestations of hemochromatosis in *HFE* C282Y homozygotes identified by screening. *Can J Gastroenterol.* 2008;22(11):923-930.

67. Adams PC, Passmore L, Chakrabarti S, et al. Liver diseases in the Hemochromatosis and Iron Overload Screening Study. *Clin Gastroenterol Hepatol.* 2006;4(7):918-923.

68. Barton JC, Barton JC, Adams PC, Acton RT. Risk factors for insulin resistance, metabolic syndrome, and diabetes in 248 *HFE* C282Y homozygotes identified by population screening in the HEIRS Study. *Metab Syndr Relat Disord.* 2016;14(2):94-101.

69. Barton JC, Leiendecker-Foster C, Reboussin DM, Adams PC, Acton RT, Eckfeldt JH. Thyroid-stimulating hormone and free thyroxine levels in persons with *HFE* C282Y homozygosity, a common hemochromatosis genotype: the HEIRS Study. *Thyroid.* 2008;18(8):831-838.

70. McLaren CE, Barton JC, Gordeuk VR, et al. Determinants and characteristics of mean corpuscular volume and hemoglobin concentration in white *HFE* C282Y homozygotes in the Hemochromatosis and Iron Overload Screening Study. *Am J Hematol.* 2007;82(10):898-905.

71. Barton JC, Barton JC, Acton RT. White blood cells and subtypes in *HFE* p.C282Y and wild-type homozygotes in the Hemochromatosis and Iron Overload Screening Study. *Blood Cells Mol Dis.* 2017:639-714.

72. Moirand R, Adams PC, Bicheler V, Brissot P, Deugnier Y. Clinical features of genetic hemochromatosis in women compared with men. *Ann Intern Med.* 1997;127(2):105-110.

73. Bachman E, Feng R, Travison T, et al. Testosterone suppresses hepcidin in men: a potential mechanism for testosterone-induced erythrocytosis. *J Clin Endocrinol Metab.* 2010;95(10):4743-4747.

74. Finch SC, Finch CA. Idiopathic hemochromatosis, an iron storage disease. A. Iron metabolism in hemochromatosis. *Medicine (Baltim).* 1955;34(4):381-430.

75. Milman N. Hereditary haemochromatosis in Denmark 1950-1985. Clinical, biochemical and histological features in 179 patients and 13 preclinical cases. *Dan Med Bull.* 1991;38(4):385-393.

76. Fargion S, Mandelli C, Piperno A, et al. Survival and prognostic factors in 212 Italian patients with genetic hemochromatosis. *Hepatology.* 1992;15(4):655-659.

77. Niederau C, Fischer R, Purschel A, Stremmel W, Haussinger D, Strohmeyer G. Long-term survival in patients with hereditary hemochromatosis. *Gastroenterology.* 1996;110(4):1107-1119.

78. Adams PC, Valberg LS. Evolving expression of hereditary hemochromatosis. *Semin Liver Dis.* 1996;16(1):47-54.

79. Bell H, Berg JP, Undlien DE, et al. The clinical expression of hemochromatosis in Oslo, Norway. Excessive oral iron intake may lead to secondary hemochromatosis even in *HFE* C282Y mutation negative subjects. *Scand J Gastroenterol.* 2000;35(12):1301-1307.

80. Aleman S, Endalib S, Stal P, et al. Health check-ups and family screening allow detection of hereditary hemochromatosis with less advanced liver fibrosis and survival comparable with the general population. *Scand J Gastroenterol.* 2011;46(9):1118-1126.

81. Witte DL, Crosby WH, Edwards CQ, Fairbanks VF, Mitros FA. Practice guideline development task force of the College of American Pathologists. Hereditary hemochromatosis. *Clin Chim Acta.* 1996;245(2):139-200.

82. Schumacher HR, Straka PC, Krikker MA, Dudley AT. The arthropathy of hemochromatosis. Recent studies. *Ann N Y Acad Sci.* 1988:526224-526233.

83. Barton JC, Acton RT, Dawkins FW, et al. Initial screening transferrin saturation values, serum ferritin concentrations, and *HFE* genotypes in whites and blacks in the Hemochromatosis and Iron Overload Screening Study. *Genet Test.* 2005;9(3):231-241.

84. Adams PC, Speechley M, Barton JC, McLaren CE, McLaren GD, Eckfeldt JH. Probability of C282Y homozygosity decreases as liver transaminase activities increase in participants with hyperferritinemia in the hemochromatosis and iron overload screening study. *Hepatology.* 2012;55(6):1722-1726.

85. Beutler E, Felitti VJ, Koziol JA, Ho NJ, Gelbart T. Penetrance of 845G→A (C282Y) *HFE* hereditary haemochromatosis mutation in the USA. *Lancet.* 2002;359(9302):211-218.

86. George DK, Ramm GA, Walker NI, Powell LW, Crawford DH. Elevated serum type IV collagen: a sensitive indicator of the presence of cirrhosis in haemochromatosis. *J Hepatol.* 1999;31(1):47-52.

87. Chin J, Powell LW, Ramm LE, Hartel GF, Olynyk JK, Ramm GA. Utility of serum biomarker indices for staging of hepatic fibrosis before and after venesection in patients with hemochromatosis caused by variants in *HFE. Clin Gastroenterol Hepatol.* 2020;19(7):1459-1468e5.

88. Cairo G, Conte D, Bianchi L, Fraquelli M, Recalcati S. Reduced serum ceruloplasmin levels in hereditary haemochromatosis. *Br J Haematol.* 2001;114(1):226-229.

89. Barton JC, Bertoli LF, Rothenberg BE. Peripheral blood erythrocyte parameters in hemochromatosis: evidence for increased erythrocyte hemoglobin content. *J Lab Clin Med.* 2000;135(1):96-104.

90. Iliadou A, Evans DM, Zhu G, et al. Genomewide scans of red cell indices suggest linkage on chromosome 6q23. *J Med Genet.* 2007;44(1):24-30.

91. Beutler E, Felitti V, Gelbart T, Waalen J. Haematological effects of the C282Y *HFE* mutation in homozygous and heterozygous states among subjects of northern and southern European ancestry. *Br J Haematol.* 2003;120(5):887-893.

92. Rehman A, Carroll GJ, Powell LW, Ramm LE, Ramm GA, Olynyk JK. Arthropathy in hereditary haemochromatosis segregates with elevated erythrocyte mean corpuscular volume. *Scand J Rheumatol.* 2021;50(2):139-142.

93. McDermott JH, Walsh CH. Hypogonadism in hereditary hemochromatosis. *J Clin Endocrinol Metab.* 2005;90(4):2451-2455.

94. Stevens SM, Edwards CQ. Hemnochromaotsis arthropathy: clinical features and management. *J Muscoskel Med.* 2009:2615-2624.

95. Carroll GJ, Breidahl WH, Olynyk JK. Characteristics of the arthropathy described in hereditary hemochromatosis. *Arthritis Care Res.* 2012;64(1):9-14.

96. Axford JS, Bomford A, Revell P, Watt I, Williams R, Hamilton EB. Hip arthropathy in genetic hemochromatosis. Radiographic and histologic features. *Arthritis Rheum.* 1991;34(3):357-361.

97. Guggenbuhl P, Deugnier Y, Boisdet JF, et al. Bone mineral density in men with genetic hemochromatosis and *HFE* gene mutation. *Osteoporos Int.* 2005;16(12):1809-1814.

98. Richette P, Ottaviani S, Vicaut E, Bardin T. Musculoskeletal complications of hereditary hemochromatosis: a case-control study. *J Rheumatol.* 2010;37(10):2145-2150.

99. Frenzen K, Schafer C, Keysser G. Erosive and inflammatory joint changes in hereditary hemochromatosis arthropathy detected by low-field magnetic resonance imaging. *Rheumatol Int.* 2013;33(8):2061-2067.

100. Dallos T, Sahinbegovic E, Stamm T, et al. Idiopathic hand osteoarthritis vs haemochromatosis arthropathy—a clinical, functional and radiographic study. *Rheumatology.* 2013;52(5):910-915.

101. Wood JC. Impact of iron assessment by MRI. *Hematology Am Soc Hematol Educ Program.* 2011:443-450.

102. Anderson LJ. Assessment of iron overload with T2* magnetic resonance imaging. *Prog Cardiovasc Dis.* 2011;54(3):287-294.

103. Gulati V, Harikrishnan P, Palaniswamy C, Aronow WS, Jain D, Frishman WH. Cardiac involvement in hemochromatosis. *Cardiol Rev.* 2014;22(2):56-68.

104. Mavrogeni S, Markousis-Mavrogenis G, Markussis V, Kolovou G. The emerging role of cardiovascular magnetic resonance imaging in the evaluation of metabolic cardiomyopathies. *Horm Metab Res.* 2015;47(9):623-632.

105. Bassett ML, Halliday JW, Powell LW. Value of hepatic iron measurements in early hemochromatosis and determination of the critical iron level associated with fibrosis. *Hepatology.* 1986;6(1):24-29.

106. Barton JC, McLaren CE, Chen WP, et al. Cirrhosis in hemochromatosis: independent risk factors in 368 *HFE* p.C282Y homozygotes. *Ann Hepatol.* 2018;17(5):871-879.

107. Barton JC, Barton JC, Adams PC. Prevalence and characteristics of anti-HCV positivity and chronic hepatitis C virus infection in *HFE* p.C282Y homozygotes. *Ann Hepatol.* 2019;18(2):354-359.

108. Stickel F, Buch S, Zoller H, et al. Evaluation of genome-wide loci of iron metabolism in hereditary hemochromatosis identifies *PCSK7* as a host risk factor of liver cirrhosis. *Hum Mol Genet.* 2014;23(14):3883-3890.

109. Seessle J, Gan-Schreier H, Kirchner M, Stremmel W, Chamulitrat W, Merle U. Plasma lipidome, *PNPLA3* polymorphism and hepatic steatosis in hereditary hemochromatosis. *BMC Gastroenterol.* 2020;20(1):230.

110. Powell EE, Ali A, Clouston AD, et al. Steatosis is a cofactor in liver injury in hemochromatosis. *Gastroenterology.* 2005;129(6):1937-1943.

111. Valenti L, Dongiovanni P, Fracanzani AL, et al. Increased susceptibility to nonalcoholic fatty liver disease in heterozygotes for the mutation responsible for hereditary hemochromatosis. *Dig Liver Dis.* 2003;35(3):172-178.

112. Ye Q, Qian BX, Yin WL, Wang FM, Han T. Association between the HFE C282Y, H63D polymorphisms and the risks of non-alcoholic fatty liver disease, liver cirrhosis and hepatocellular carcinoma: an updated systematic review and meta-analysis of 5,758 cases and 14,741 controls. *PLoS One.* 2016;11(9):e0163423.

113. Bonkovsky HL, Jawaid Q, Tortorelli K, et al. Non-alcoholic steatohepatitis and iron: increased prevalence of mutations of the *HFE* gene in non-alcoholic steatohepatitis. *J Hepatol.* 1999;31(3):421-429.

114. Valenti L, Fracanzani AL, Rossi V, et al. The hand arthropathy of hereditary hemochromatosis is strongly associated with iron overload. *J Rheumatol.* 2008;35(1):153-158.

115. Carroll GJ, Breidahl WH, Bulsara MK, Olynyk JK. Hereditary hemochromatosis is characterized by a clinically definable arthropathy that correlates with iron load. *Arthritis Rheum.* 2011;63(1):286-294.

116. Chehade S, Adams PC. Severe hemochromatosis arthropathy in the absence of iron overload. *Hepatology.* 2019;70(3):1064-1065.

117. Nguyen CD, Morel V, Pierache A, et al. Bone and joint complications in patients with hereditary hemochromatosis: a cross-sectional study of 93 patients. *Ther Adv Musculoskelet Dis.* 2020. 12:17597320X20939405.

118. Schumacher HR, Jr. Hemochromatosis and arthritis. *Arthritis Rheum.* 1964;7:741-750.

119. Kroner PT, Mareth KF, Wijarnpreecha K, Palmer WC. Hereditary hemochromatosis is associated with increased use of joint replacement surgery: results of a nationwide analysis. *Semin Arthritis Rheum.* 2020;50(2):360-365.

120. Elmberg M, Hultcrantz R, Simard JF, Carlsson A, Askling J. Increased risk of arthropathies and joint replacement surgery in patients with genetic hemochromatosis: a study of 3,531 patients and their 11,794 first-degree relatives. *Arthritis Care Res.* 2013;65(5):678-685.

121. Wang Y, Gurrin LC, Wluka AE, et al. *HFE* C282Y homozygosity is associated with an increased risk of total hip replacement for osteoarthritis. *Semin Arthritis Rheum.* 2012;41(6):872-878.

Disorders of Red Blood Cells

122. Wijarnpreecha K, Aby ES, Panjawatanan P, et al. Hereditary hemochromatosis and risk of joint replacement surgery: a systematic review and meta-analysis. *Eur J Gastroenterol Hepatol.* 2021;33(1):96-101.

123. Sherrington CA, Knuiman MW, Divitini ML, Bartholomew HC, Cullen DJ, Olynyk JK. Population-based study of the relationship between mutations in the hemochromatosis (*HFE*) gene and arthritis. *J Gastroenterol Hepatol.* 2006;21(3):595-598.

124. Willis G, Scott DG, Jennings BA, Smith K, Bukhari M, Wimperis JZ. *HFE* mutations in an inflammatory arthritis population. *Rheumatology.* 2002;41(2):176-179.

125. Ross JM, Kowalchuk RM, Shaulinsky J, Ross L, Daniel R, Phatak PD. Association of heterozygous hemochromatosis C282Y gene mutation with hand osteoarthritis. *J Rheumatol.* 2003;30(1):121-125.

126. Lonardo A, Neri P, Mascia MT, Pietrangelo A. Hereditary hemochromatosis masquerading as rheumatoid arthritis. *Ann Ital Med Int.* 2001;16(1):46-49.

127. Barton JC, Barton JC. Autoimmune conditions in 235 hemochromatosis probands with *HFE* C282Y homozygosity and their first-degree relatives. *J Immunol Res.* 2015;453046.

128. Latourte A, Frazier A, Briere C, Ea HK, Richette P. Interleukin-1 receptor antagonist in refractory haemochromatosis-related arthritis of the hands. *Ann Rheum Dis.* 2013;72(5):783-784.

129. Hartroft WS. Islet pathology in diabetes. *Diabetes.* 1956;5(2):98-104.

130. Saddi R, Feingold J. Idiopathic haemochromatosis: an autosomal recessive disease. *Clin Genet.* 1974;5(3):234-241.

131. Hramiak IM, Finegood DT, Adams PC. Factors affecting glucose tolerance in hereditary hemochromatosis. *Clin Invest Med.* 1997;20(2):110-118.

132. Dymock IW, Cassar J, Pyke DA, Oakley WG, Williams R. Observations on the pathogenesis, complications and treatment of diabetes in 115 cases of haemochromatosis. *Am J Med.* 1972;52(2):203-210.

133. McClain DA, Abraham D, Rogers J, et al. High prevalence of abnormal glucose homeostasis secondary to decreased insulin secretion in individuals with hereditary haemochromatosis. *Diabetologia.* 2006;49(7):1661-1669.

134. O'Sullivan EP, McDermott JH, Murphy MS, Sen S, Walsh CH. Declining prevalence of diabetes mellitus in hereditary haemochromatosis–the result of earlier diagnosis. *Diabetes Res Clin Pract.* 2008;81(3):316-320.

135. Barton JC, Barton JC, Acton RT. Diabetes in first-degree family members: a predictor of type 2 diabetes in 159 nonscreening Alabama hemochromatosis probands with *HFE* C282Y homozygosity. *Diabetes Care.* 2014;37(1):259-266.

136. Kulaksiz H, Fein E, Redecker P, Stremmel W, Adler G, Cetin Y. Pancreatic beta-cells express hepcidin, an iron-uptake regulatory peptide. *J Endocrinol.* 2008;197(2):241-249.

137. Weires MB, Tausch B, Haug PJ, Edwards CQ, Wetter T, Cannon-Albright LA. Familiality of diabetes mellitus. *Exp Clin Endocrinol Diabetes.* 2007;115(10):634-640.

138. Wilson JG. Iron and glucose homeostasis: new lessons from hereditary haemochromatosis. *Diabetologia.* 2006;49(7):1459-1461.

139. Abbas MA, Abraham D, Kushner JP, McClain DA. Anti-obesity and pro-diabetic effects of hemochromatosis. *Obesity.* 2014;22(10):2120-2122.

140. Acton RT, Barton JC, Barton JC. Serum ferritin, insulin resistance, and metabolic syndrome: clinical and laboratory associations in 769 non-hispanic whites without diabetes mellitus in the HEIRS Study. *Metab Syndr Relat Disord.* 2015;13(2):57-63.

141. Cooksey RC, Jouihan HA, Ajioka RS, et al. Oxidative stress, beta-cell apoptosis, and decreased insulin secretory capacity in mouse models of hemochromatosis. *Endocrinology.* 2004;145(11):5305-5312.

142. Barton JC, Barton JC, Acton RT. Longer survival associated with HLA-A*03, B*14 among 212 hemochromatosis probands with *HFE* C282Y homozygosity and HLA-A and -B typing and haplotyping. *Eur J Haematol.* 2010;85(5):439-447.

143. Ellervik C, Mandrup-Poulsen T, Tybjaerg-Hansen A, Nordestgaard BG. Total and cause-specific mortality by elevated transferrin saturation and hemochromatosis genotype in individuals with diabetes: two general population studies. *Diabetes Care.* 2014;37(2):444-452.

144. Barton JC, Acton RT. Diabetes in *HFE* hemochromatosis. *J Diabetes Res.* 2017;9826930.

145. Kelly TM, Edwards CQ, Meikle AW, Kushner JP. Hypogonadism in hemochromatosis: reversal with iron depletion. *Ann Intern Med.* 1984;101(5):629-632.

146. Lewis AS, Courtney CH, Atkinson AB. All patients with 'idiopathic' hypopituitarism should be screened for hemochromatosis. *Pituitary.* 2009;12(3):273-275.

147. Edwards CQ, Kelly TM, Ellwein G, Kushner JP. Thyroid disease in hemochromatosis. Increased incidence in homozygous men. *Arch Intern Med.* 1983;143(10):1890-1893.

148. Ban Y, Greenberg DA, Davies TF, Jacobson E, Concepcion E, Tomer Y. Linkage analysis of thyroid antibody production: evidence for shared susceptibility to clinical autoimmune thyroid disease. *J Clin Endocrinol Metab.* 2008;93(9):3589-3596.

149. Lee PL, Beutler E, Rao SV, Barton JC. Genetic abnormalities and juvenile hemochromatosis: mutations of the *HJV* gene encoding hemojuvelin. *Blood.* 2004;103(12):4669-4671.

150. Walsh CH, Murphy AL, Cunningham S, McKenna TJ. Mineralocorticoid and glucocorticoid status in idiopathic haemochromatosis. *Clin Endocrinol.* 1994;41(4):439-443.

151. Varkonyi J, Kaltwasser JP, Seidl C, Kollai G, Andrikovics H, Tordai A. A case of non-*HFE* juvenile haemochromatosis presenting with adrenocortical insufficiency. *Br J Haematol.* 2000;109(1):252-253.

152. Hempenius LM, Van Dam PS, Marx JJ, Koppeschaar HP. Mineralocorticoid status and endocrine dysfunction in severe hemochromatosis. *J Endocrinol Invest.* 1999;22(5):369-376.

153. Krysiak R, Okopien B. Hypoparathyroidism and hypogonadism as a clinical manifestation of hemochromatosis. *Przegl Lek.* 2013;70(1):35-37.

154. Nelson RL, Baldus WP, Rubenstein AH, Go VL, Service FJ. Pancreatic alpha-cell function in diabetic hemochromatotic subjects. *J Clin Endocrinol Metab.* 1979;49(3):412-416.

155. Luque-Ramirez M, Alvarez-Blasco F, Alpanes M, Escobar-Morreale HF. Role of decreased circulating hepcidin concentrations in the iron excess of women with the polycystic ovary syndrome. *J Clin Endocrinol Metab.* 2011;96(3): 846-852.

156. Barton JC, Barton JC. Hemochromatosis, *HFE* C282Y homozygosity, and polycystic ovary syndrome: report of two cases and possible effects of androgens and hepcidin. *Acta Haematol.* 2011;126(3):138-140.

157. Meneghini R. Iron homeostasis, oxidative stress, and DNA damage. *Free Radic Biol Med.* 1997;23(5):783-792.

158. Deugnier Y, Turlin B, Loreal O. Iron and neoplasia. *J Hepatol.* 1998;28:121-125.

159. Santos GC, Zielenska M, Prasad M, Squire JA. Chromosome 6p amplification and cancer progression. *J Clin Pathol.* 2007;60(1):1-7.

160. Niederau C, Fischer R, Sonnenberg A, Stremmel W, Trampisch HJ, Strohmeyer G. Survival and causes of death in cirrhotic and in noncirrhotic patients with primary hemochromatosis. *N Engl J Med.* 1985;313(20):1256-1262.

161. Bruix J, Sherman M. Management of hepatocellular carcinoma. *Hepatology.* 2005;42(5):1208-1236.

162. Bomford A, Williams R. Long term results of venesection therapy in idiopathic haemochromatosis. *Q J Med.* 1976;45(180):611-623.

163. Tiniakos G, Williams R. Cirrhotic process, liver cell carcinoma and extrahepatic malignant tumors in idiopathic haemochromatosis. Study of 71 patients treated with venesection therapy. *Appl Pathol.* 1988;6(2):128-138.

164. Deugnier YM, Guyader D, Crantock L, et al. Primary liver cancer in genetic hemochromatosis: a clinical, pathological, and pathogenetic study of 54 cases. *Gastroenterology.* 1993;104(1):228-234.

165. Beaton MD, Adams PC. Prognostic factors and survival in patients with hereditary hemochromatosis and cirrhosis. *Can J Gastroenterol.* 2006;20(4):257-260.

166. Bacon BR, Adams PC, Kowdley KV, Powell LW, Tavill AS. Diagnosis and management of hemochromatosis: 2011 practice guideline by the American association for the study of liver diseases. *Hepatology.* 2011;54(1):328-343.

167. Elmberg M, Hultcrantz R, Ekbom A, et al. Cancer risk in patients with hereditary hemochromatosis and in their first-degree relatives. *Gastroenterology.* 2003;125(6):1733-1741.

168. Haddow JE, Palomaki GE, McClain M, Craig W. Hereditary hemochromatosis and hepatocellular carcinoma in males: a strategy for estimating the potential for primary prevention. *J Med Screen.* 2003;10(1):11-13.

169. Nowak A, Giger RS, Krayenbuehl PA. Higher age at diagnosis of hemochromatosis is the strongest predictor of the occurrence of hepatocellular carcinoma in the Swiss hemochromatosis cohort: a prospective longitudinal observational study. *Medicine (Baltim).* 2018;97(42):e12886.

170. Atkins JL, Pilling LC, Masoli JAH, et al. Association of hemochromatosis *HFE* p.C282Y homozygosity with hepatic malignancy. *JAMA.* 2020;324(20):2048-2057.

171. von DS, Lersch C, Schulte-Frohlinde E, et al. Hepatocellular carcinoma associated with hereditary hemochromatosis occurring in non-cirrhotic liver. *Z Gastroenterol.* 2006;44(1):39-42.

172. Goh J, Callagy G, McEntee G, O'Keane JC, Bomford A, Crowe J. Hepatocellular carcinoma arising in the absence of cirrhosis in genetic haemochromatosis: three case reports and review of literature. *Eur J Gastroenterol Hepatol.* 1999;11(8): 915-919.

173. Pellise M, Gonzalez-Abraldes J, Navasa M, Miquel R, Bruguera M. Hepatocellular carcinoma in a patient with hereditary hemochromatosis without cirrhosis. *Gastroenterol Hepatol.* 2001;24(3):132-134.

174. Morcos M, Dubois S, Bralet MP, Belghiti J, Degott C, Terris B. Primary liver carcinoma in genetic hemochromatosis reveals a broad histologic spectrum. *Am J Clin Pathol.* 2001;116(5):738-743.

175. Pirisi M, Toniutto P, Uzzau A, et al. Carriage of *HFE* mutations and outcome of surgical resection for hepatocellular carcinoma in cirrhotic patients. *Cancer.* 2000;89(2):297-302.

176. Fargion S, Stazi MA, Fracanzani AL, et al. Mutations in the *HFE* gene and their interaction with exogenous risk factors in hepatocellular carcinoma. *Blood Cells Mol Dis.* 2001;27(2):505-511.

177. Hellerbrand C, Poppl A, Hartmann A, Scholmerich J, Lock G. *HFE* C282Y heterozygosity in hepatocellular carcinoma: evidence for an increased prevalence. *Clin Gastroenterol Hepatol.* 2003;1(4):279-284.

178. Fracanzani AL, Fargion S, Stazi MA, et al. Association between heterozygosity for *HFE* gene mutations and hepatitis viruses in hepatocellular carcinoma. *Blood Cells Mol Dis.* 2005;35(1):27-32.

179. Racchi O, Mangerini R, Rapezzi D, et al. Mutations of the *HFE* gene and the risk of hepatocellular carcinoma. *Blood Cells Mol Dis.* 1999;25(5–6):350-353.

180. Funakoshi N, Chaze I, Alary AS, et al. The role of genetic factors in patients with hepatocellular carcinoma and iron overload–a prospective series of 234 patients. *Liver Int.* 2016;36(5):746-754.

181. Bruix J, Sherman M. Management of hepatocellular carcinoma: an update. *Hepatology.* 2011;53(3):1020-1022.

182. Kudo M, Izumi N, Kokudo N, et al. Management of hepatocellular carcinoma in Japan: consensus-based clinical practice guidelines proposed by the Japan society of hepatology (JSH) 2010 updated version. *Dig Dis.* 2011;29(3):339-364.

183. European Association for the Study of the Liver. EASL-EORTC clinical practice guidelines: management of hepatocellular carcinoma. *J Hepatol.* 2012;56(4):908-943.

184. van Meer MS, de Man RA, Siersema PD, van Erpecum KJ. Surveillance for hepatocellular carcinoma in chronic liver disease: evidence and controversies. *World J Gastroenterol.* 2013;19(40):6744-6756.

185. Osborne NJ, Gurrin LC, Allen KJ, et al. *HFE* C282Y homozygotes are at increased risk of breast and colorectal cancer. *Hepatology.* 2010;51(4):1311-1318.

186. Niederau C. Iron overload and atherosclerosis. *Hepatology.* 2000;32(3):672-674.

187. Shaheen NJ, Silverman LM, Keku T, et al. Association between hemochromatosis (*HFE*) gene mutation carrier status and the risk of colon cancer. *J Natl Cancer Inst.* 2003;95(2):154-159.

188. Shi Z, Johnstone D, Talseth-Palmer BA, et al. Haemochromatosis *HFE* gene polymorphisms as potential modifiers of hereditary nonpolyposis colorectal cancer risk and onset age. *Int J Cancer.* 2009;125(1):78-83.

189. Robinson JP, Johnson VL, Rogers PA, et al. Evidence for an association between compound heterozygosity for germ line mutations in the hemochromatosis (*HFE*) gene and increased risk of colorectal cancer. *Cancer Epidemiol Biomarkers Prev.* 2005;14(6):1460-1463.

190. Ekblom K, Marklund SL, Palmqvist R, et al. Iron biomarkers in plasma, *HFE* genotypes, and the risk for colorectal cancer in a prospective setting. *Dis Colon Rectum.* 2012;55(3):337-344.

191. McGlynn KA, Sakoda LC, Hu Y, et al. Hemochromatosis gene mutations and distal adenomatous colorectal polyps. *Cancer Epidemiol Biomarkers Prev.* 2005;14(1):158-163.

192. Smith KA, Kovac S, Anderson GJ, Shulkes A, Baldwin GS. Circulating gastrin is increased in hemochromatosis. *FEBS Lett.* 2006;580(26):6195-6198.

193. Thorburn CM, Friedman GD, Dickinson CJ, Vogelman JH, Orentreich N, Parsonnet J. Gastrin and colorectal cancer: a prospective study. *Gastroenterology.* 1998;115(2):275-280.

194. Colucci R, Blandizzi C, Tanini M, Vassalle C, Breschi MC, Del TM. Gastrin promotes human colon cancer cell growth via CCK-2 receptor-mediated cyclooxygenase-2 induction and prostaglandin E2 production. *Br J Pharmacol.* 2005;144(3):338-348.

195. Gannon PO, Medelci S, Le PC, et al. Impact of hemochromatosis gene (*HFE*) mutations on epithelial ovarian cancer risk and prognosis. *Int J Cancer.* 2011;128(10):2326-2334.

196. Syrjakoski K, Fredriksson H, Ikonen T, et al. Hemochromatosis gene mutations among Finnish male breast and prostate cancer patients. *Int J Cancer.* 2006;118(2):518-520.

197. Hucl T, Kylanpaa-Back ML, Witt H, et al. *HFE* genotypes in patients with chronic pancreatitis and pancreatic adenocarcinoma. *Genet Med.* 2007;9(7):479-483.

198. Ellervik C, Birgens H, Tybjaerg-Hansen A, Nordestgaard BG. Hemochromatosis genotypes and risk of 31 disease endpoints: meta-analyses including 66,000 cases and 226,000 controls. *Hepatology.* 2007;46(4):1071-1080.

199. Edwards CQ, Griffen LM, Goldgar DE, Skolnick MH, Kushner JP. HLA-linked hemochromatosis alleles in sporadic porphyria cutanea tarda. *Gastroenterology.* 1989;97(4):972-981.

200. Bulaj ZJ, Phillips JD, Ajioka RS, et al. Hemochromatosis genes and other factors contributing to the pathogenesis of porphyria cutanea tarda. *Blood.* 2000;95(5):1565-1571.

201. Olsson KS, Ritter B, Hansson N. The HLA-A1-B8 haplotype hitchhiking with the hemochromatosis mutation: does it affect the phenotype?. *Eur J Haematol.* 2007;79(5):429-434.

202. Danton M, Lim CK. Porphomethene inhibitor of uroporphyrinogen decarboxylase: analysis by high-performance liquid chromatography/electrospray ionization tandem mass spectrometry. *Biomed Chromatogr.* 2007;21(7):661-663.

203. Phillips JD, Bergonia HA, Reilly CA, Franklin MR, Kushner JP. A porphomethene inhibitor of uroporphyrinogen decarboxylase causes porphyria cutanea tarda. *Proc Natl Acad Sci U S A.* 2007;104(12):5079-5084.

204. Roberts AG, Whatley SD, Morgan RR, Worwood M, Elder GH. Increased frequency of the haemochromatosis Cys282Tyr mutation in sporadic porphyria cutanea tarda. *Lancet.* 1997;349(9048):321-323.

205. Bonkovsky HL, Poh-Fitzpatrick M, Pimstone N, et al. Porphyria cutanea tarda, hepatitis C, and *HFE* gene mutations in North America. *Hepatology.* 1998;27(6):1661-1669.

206. Tannapfel A, Stolzel U, Kostler E, et al. C282Y and H63D mutation of the hemochromatosis gene in German porphyria cutanea tarda patients. *Virchows Arch.* 2001;439(1):1-5.

207. Egger NG, Goeger DE, Payne DA, Miskovsky EP, Weinman SA, Anderson KE. Porphyria cutanea tarda: multiplicity of risk factors including *HFE* mutations, hepatitis C, and inherited uroporphyrinogen decarboxylase deficiency. *Dig Dis Sci.* 2002;47(2):419-426.

208. Lamoril J, Andant C, Gouya L, et al. Hemochromatosis (*HFE*) and transferrin receptor-1 (*TFRC1*) genes in sporadic porphyria cutanea tarda (sPCT). *Cell Mol Biol (Noisy-Le-Grand).* 2002;48(1):33-41.

209. Castiella A, Zapata E, de Juan MD, et al. Porphyria cutanea tarda. An analysis of *HFE* gene mutations, hepatitis viruses, alcohol intake, and other risk factors in 54 patients from Guipuzcoa, Basque Country, Spain. *Rev Esp Enferm Dig.* 2008;100(12):774-778.

210. Munoz-Santos C, Guilabert A, Moreno N, et al. Familial and sporadic porphyria cutanea tarda: clinical and biochemical features and risk factors in 152 patients. *Medicine (Baltim).* 2010;89(2):69-74.

211. Barton JC, Edwards CQ. Porphyria cutanea tarda associated with *HFE* C282Y homozygosity, iron overload, and use of a contraceptive vaginal ring. *J Community Hosp Intern Med Perspect.* 2016;6(1):30380.

212. Ryan CF, Sendi H, BonkovskyHepatitis HLC. Porphyria cutanea tarda and liver iron: an update. *Liver Int.* 2012;32(6):880-893.

213. Bertoli LF, Barton JC. Remission of porphyria cutanea tarda after anastrozole treatment against breast cancer. *Clin Breast Cancer.* 2007;7(9):716-718.

214. Fleming RE, Ponka P. Iron overload in human disease. *N Engl J Med.* 2012;366(4):348-359.

215. Kautz L, Jung G, Valore EV, Rivella S, Nemeth E, Ganz T. Identification of erythroferrone as an erythroid regulator of iron metabolism. *Nat Genet.* 2014;46(7):678-684.

216. Kautz L, Jung G, Du X, et al. Erythroferrone contributes to hepcidin suppression and iron overload in a mouse model of beta-thalassemia. *Blood.* 2015;126(17):2031-2037.

217. Kautz L, Jung G, Nemeth E, Ganz T. Erythroferrone contributes to recovery from anemia of inflammation. *Blood.* 2014;124(16):2569-2574.

218. Pasricha SR, McHugh K, Drakesmith H. Regulation of hepcidin by erythropoiesis: the story so far. *Annu Rev Nutr.* 2016:36417-36434.

219. Arezes J, Foy N, McHugh K, et al. Erythroferrone inhibits the induction of hepcidin by BMP6. *Blood.* 2018;132(14):1473-1477.

220. Arezes J, Foy N, McHugh K, et al. Antibodies against the erythroferrone N-terminal domain prevent hepcidin suppression and ameliorate murine thalassemia. *Blood.* 2020;135(8):547-557.

221. Tanno T, Porayette P, Sripichai O, et al. Identification of TWSG1 as a second novel erythroid regulator of hepcidin expression in murine and human cells. *Blood.* 2009;114(1):181-186.

222. Tanno T, Bhanu NV, Oneal PA, et al. High levels of GDF15 in thalassemia suppress expression of the iron regulatory protein hepcidin. *Nat Med.* 2007;13(9):1096-1101.

223. Tamary H, Shalev H, Perez-Avraham G, et al. Elevated growth differentiation factor 15 expression in patients with congenital dyserythropoietic anemia type I. *Blood.* 2008;112(13):5241-5244.

224. Casanovas G, Swinkels DW, Altamura S, et al. Growth differentiation factor 15 in patients with congenital dyserythropoietic anaemia (CDA) type II. *J Mol Med (Berl).* 2011;89(8):811-816.

225. Edwards CQ, Skolnick MH, Dadone MM, Kushner JP. Iron overload in hereditary spherocytosis: association with HLA-linked hemochromatosis. *Am J Hematol.* 1982;13(2):101-109.

226. Barton JC, Lee PL, West C, Bottomley SS. Iron overload and prolonged ingestion of iron supplements: clinical features and mutation analysis of hemochromatosis-associated genes in four cases. *Am J Hematol.* 2006;81(10):760-767.

227. Barton JC, Sawada-Hirai R, Rothenberg BE, Acton RT. Two novel missense mutations of the *HFE* gene (I105T and G93R) and identification of the S65C mutation in Alabama hemochromatosis probands. *Blood Cells Mol Dis.* 1999;25(3-4):147-155.

228. Edwards CQ, Skolnick MH, Kushner JP. Coincidental nontransfusional iron overload and thalassemia minor: association with HLA-linked hemochromatosis. *Blood.* 1981;58(4):844-848.

229. Piperno A, Mariani R, Arosio C, et al. Haemochromatosis in patients with beta-thalassaemia trait. *Br J Haematol.* 2000;111(3):908-914.

230. Melis MA, Cau M, Deidda F, Barella S, Cao A, Galanello R. H63D mutation in the *HFE* gene increases iron overload in beta-thalassemia carriers. *Haematologica.* 2002;87(3):242-245.

231. Longo F, Zecchina G, Sbaiz L, Fischer R, Piga A, Camaschella C. The influence of hemochromatosis mutations on iron overload of thalassemia major. *Haematologica.* 1999;84(9):799-803.

232. Weatherall DJ, Clegg JB. *Frontmatter. The Thalassaemia Syndromes.* London: Blackwell Science Ltd.; 2008:i-xiv.

233. Yaouanq J, Grosbois B, Jouanolle AM, Goasguen J, Leblay R. Haemochromatosis Cys282Tyr mutation in pyridoxine-responsive sideroblastic anaemia. *Lancet.* 1997;349(9063):1475-1476.

234. Ganz T. Erythropoietic regulators of iron metabolism. *Free Radic Biol Med.* 2019:13369-13374.

235. Cotter PD, May A, Li L, et al. Four new mutations in the erythroid-specific 5-aminolevulinate synthase (*ALAS2*) gene causing X-linked sideroblastic anemia: increased pyridoxine responsiveness after removal of iron overload by phlebotomy and coinheritance of hereditary hemochromatosis. *Blood.* 1999;93(5):1757-1769.

236. Lee PL, Barton JC, Rao SV, Acton RT, Adler BK, Beutler E. Three kinships with ALAS2 P520L (c. 1559 C→T) mutation, two in association with severe iron overload, and one with sideroblastic anemia and severe iron overload. *Blood Cells Mol Dis.* 2006;36(2):292-297.

237. Bottomley SS. Sideroblastic anemias. In: Greer JP, Arber DA, Glader B, et al., eds. *Wintrobe's Clinical Hematology.* 13th ed. Philadelphia: Lippincott Williams & Wilkins; 2014:643-661.

238. Cazzola M, Barosi G, Gobbi PG, Invernizzi R, Riccardi A, Ascari E. Natural history of idiopathic refractory sideroblastic anemia. *Blood.* 1988;71(2):305-312.

239. Beris P, Samii K, Darbellay R, et al. Iron overload in patients with sideroblastic anaemia is not related to the presence of the haemochromatosis Cys282Tyr and His63Asp mutations. *Br J Haematol.* 1999;104(1):97-99.

240. Nearman ZP, Szpurka H, Serio B, et al. Hemochromatosis-associated gene mutations in patients with myelodysplastic syndromes with refractory anemia with ringed sideroblasts. *Am J Hematol.* 2007;82(12):1076-1079.

241. Srole DN, Ganz T. Erythroferrone structure, function, and physiology: iron homeostasis and beyond. *J Cell Physiol.* 2021;236(7):4888-4901.

242. Yang Q, McDonnell SM, Khoury MJ, Cono J, Parrish RG. Hemochromatosis-associated mortality in the United States from 1979 to 1992: an analysis of multiple-cause mortality data. *Ann Intern Med.* 1998;129(11):946-953.

243. Hlady WG, Klontz KC. The epidemiology of *Vibrio* infections in Florida, 1981-1993. *J Infect Dis.* 1996;173(5):1176-1183.

244. Bullen JJ, Spalding PB, Ward CG, Gutteridge JM. Hemochromatosis, iron and septicemia caused by *Vibrio vulnificus. Arch Intern Med.* 1991;151(8):1606-1609.

245. Barton JC, Acton RT. Hemochromatosis and *Vibrio vulnificus* wound infections. *J Clin Gastroenterol.* 2009;43(9):890-893.

246. Arezes J, Jung G, Gabayan V, et al. Hepcidin-induced hypoferremia is a critical host defense mechanism against the siderophilic bacterium *Vibrio vulnificus. Cell Host Microbe.* 2015;17(1):47-57.

247. Fernandez JM, Serrano M, De Arriba JJ, Sanchez MV, Escribano E, Ferreras P. Bacteremic cellulitis caused by Non-01, Non-0139 *Vibrio cholerae*: report of a case in a patient with hemochromatosis. *Diagn Microbiol Infect Dis.* 2000;37(1):77-80.

248. Torp-Pedersen T, Nielsen XC, Olsen KE, Barfod TS. Intracerebral abscess after infection with non-toxigenic *Vibrio cholerae. Ugeskr Laeger.* 2012;174(8):498-499.

249. Collazos J, Guerra E, Fernandez A, Mayo J, Martinez E. Miliary liver abscesses and skin infection due to *Yersinia enterocolitica* in a patient with unsuspected hemochromatosis. *Clin Infect Dis.* 1995;21(1):223-224.

250. Benbrika S, Boukari L, Stirnemann J, et al. A case of yersiniasis with multiple liver abscesses. *Rev Med Interne.* 2005;26(2):151-152.

251. Stefanova D, Raychev A, Arezes J, et al. Endogenous hepcidin and its agonist mediate resistance to selected infections by clearing non-transferrin-bound iron. *Blood.* 2017;130(3):245-257.

252. Conway SP, Dudley N, Sheridan P, Ross H. Haemochromatosis and aldosterone deficiency presenting with *Yersinia pseudotuberculosis* septicaemia. *Postgrad Med.* 1989;65(761):174-176.

253. Mennecier D, Lapprand M, Hernandez E, et al. Liver abscesses due to *Yersinia pseudotuberculosis* discloses a genetic hemochromatosis. *Gastroenterol Clin Biol.* 2001;25(12):1113-1115.

254. Miller HK, Schwiesow L, Au-Yeung W, Auerbuch V. Hereditary hemochromatosis predisposes mice to *Yersinia pseudotuberculosis* infection even in the absence of the type III secretion system. *Front Cell Infect Microbiol.* 2016:669.

255. Centers for Disease Control and Prevention (CDC). Fatal laboratory-acquired infection with an attenuated *Yersinia pestis* Strain–Chicago, Illinois, 2009. *MMWR Morb Mortal Wkly Rep.* 2011;60(7):201-205.

256. Frank KM, Schneewind O, Shieh WJ. Investigation of a researcher's death due to septicemic plague. *N Engl J Med.* 2011;364(26):2563-2564.

257. McClatchie S, Taylor HE, Henry AT. Acute abdominal pain and shock associated with haemochromatosis. *Can Med Assoc J.* 1950;63(5):485-488.

258. Finlayson DC, Brooks JR, Vandam LD. Hemochromatosis, abdominal pain, shock and death. *Ann Surg.* 1963:158256-158259.

259. Sydow M, Crozier TA, Schauer A, Burchardi H. Septic shock with acute abdomen in idiopathic hemochromatosis. *Anasthesiol Intensivmed Notfallmed Schmerzther.* 1993;28(4):258-260.

260. Corke PJ, McLean AS, Stewart D, Adams S. Overwhelming Gram-negative septic shock in haemochromatosis. *Anaesth Intensive Care.* 1995;23(3):346-349.

261. Christopher GW. *Escherichia coli* bacteremia, meningitis, and hemochromatosis. *Arch Intern Med.* 1985;145(10):1908.

262. Stefanova D, Raychev A, Deville J, et al. Hepcidin protects against lethal *Escherichia coli* sepsis in mice inoculated with isolates from septic patients. *Infect Immun.* 2018;86(7).

263. Delanghe JR, Speeckaert MM, De Buyzere ML. COVID-19 infections are also affected by human *ACE1* D/I polymorphism. *Clin Chem Lab Med.* 2020;58(7):1125-1126.

264. Barton JC, Bertoli LF, Acton RT. Common variable immunodeficiency and IgG subclass deficiency in central Alabama hemochromatosis probands homozygous for *HFE* C282Y. *Blood Cells Mol Dis.* 2003;31(1):102-111.

265. Barton JC, Barton JC, Cruz E, Teles MJ, Guimaraes JT, Porto G. Chromosome 6p SNP microhaplotypes and IgG3 levels in hemochromatosis probands with *HFE* p.C282Y homozygosity. *Blood Cells Mol Dis.* 2020;85:102461.

266. Elmberg M, Hultcrantz R, Simard JF, Stal P, Pehrsson K, Askling J. Risk of ischaemic heart disease and cardiomyopathy in patients with haemochromatosis and in their first-degree relatives: a nationwide, population-based study. *J Intern Med.* 2012;272(1):45-54.

267. Miller M, Hutchins GM. Hemochromatosis, multiorgan hemosiderosis, and coronary artery disease. *JAMA.* 1994;272(3):231-233.

268. Nassar BA, Zayed EM, Title LM, et al. Relation of *HFE* gene mutations, high iron stores and early onset coronary artery disease. *Can J Cardiol.* 1998;14(2):215-220.

269. Franco RF, Zago MA, Trip MD, et al. Prevalence of hereditary haemochromatosis in premature atherosclerotic vascular disease. *Br J Haematol.* 1998;102(5):1172-1175.

270. Waalen J, Felitti V, Gelbart T, Ho NJ, Beutler E. Prevalence of coronary heart disease associated with *HFE* mutations in adults attending a health appraisal center. *Am J Med.* 2002;113(6):472-479.

271. Pankow JS, Boerwinkle E, Adams PC, et al. *HFE* C282Y homozygotes have reduced low-density lipoprotein cholesterol: the Atherosclerosis Risk in Communities (ARIC) Study. *Transl Res.* 2008;152(1):3-10.

272. Kraml P. The role of iron in the pathogenesis of atherosclerosis. *Physiol Res.* 2017;66(Suppl 1):S55-S67.

273. Rossi E, McQuillan BM, Hung J, Thompson PL, Kuek C, Beilby JP. Serum ferritin and C282Y mutation of the hemochromatosis gene as predictors of asymptomatic carotid atherosclerosis in a community population. *Stroke.* 2000;31(12):3015-3020.

274. Njajou OT, Hollander M, Koudstaal PJ, et al. Mutations in the hemochromatosis gene (*HFE*) and stroke. *Stroke.* 2002;33(10):2363-2366.

275. Yunker LM, Parboosingh JS, Conradson HE, et al. The effect of iron status on vascular health. *Vasc Med.* 2006;11(2):85-91.

276. Ellervik C, Tybjaerg-Hansen A, Appleyard M, Sillesen H, Boysen G, Nordestgaard BG. Hereditary hemochromatosis genotypes and risk of ischemic stroke. *Neurology.* 2007;68(13):1025-1031.

277. Passa P, Rousselie F, Gauville C, Canivet J. Retinopathy and plasma growth hormone levels in idiopathic hemochromatosis with diabetes. *Diabetes.* 1977;26(2):113-120.

278. Barton JC, Adams PC. Clinical guidelines: *HFE* hemochromatosis-screening, diagnosis and management. *Nat Rev Gastroenterol Hepatol.* 2010;7(9):482-484.

279. Pietrangelo A. Hereditary hemochromatosis: pathogenesis, diagnosis, and treatment. *Gastroenterology.* 2010;139(2):393-408.

280. Gan EK, Powell LW, Olynyk JK. Natural history and management of *HFE*-hemochromatosis. *Semin Liver Dis.* 2011;31(3):293-301.

281. Nadakkavukaran IM, Gan EK, Olynyk JK. Screening for hereditary haemochromatosis. *Pathology.* 2012;44(2):148-152.

282. Powell LW, George DK, McDonnell SM, Kowdley KV. Diagnosis of hemochromatosis. *Ann Intern Med.* 1998;129(11):925-931.

283. Allen KJ, Bertalli NA, Osborne NJ, et al. *HFE* Cys282Tyr homozygotes with serum ferritin concentrations below 1000 microg/L are at low risk of hemochromatosis. *Hepatology.* 2010;52(3):925-933.

284. Bassett ML, Hickman PE, Dahlstrom JE. The changing role of liver biopsy in diagnosis and management of haemochromatosis. *Pathology.* 2011;43(5):433-439.

285. Bassett ML, Halliday JW, Ferris RA, Powell LW. Diagnosis of hemochromatosis in young subjects: predictive accuracy of biochemical screening tests. *Gastroenterology.* 1984;87(3):628-633.

286. Morrison ED, Brandhagen DJ, Phatak PD, et al. Serum ferritin level predicts advanced hepatic fibrosis among U.S. patients with phenotypic hemochromatosis. *Ann Intern Med.* 2003;138(8):627-633.

287. Bulaj ZJ, Griffen LM, Jorde LB, Edwards CQ, Kushner JP. Clinical and biochemical abnormalities in people heterozygous for hemochromatosis. *N Engl J Med.* 1996;335(24):1799-1805.

288. Hunt JR, Zeng H. Iron absorption by heterozygous carriers of the *HFE* C282Y mutation associated with hemochromatosis. *Am J Clin Nutr.* 2004;80(4):924-931.

289. Krainin P, Kahn BS. Hemochromatosis: report of a case in a Negro; discussion of iron metabolism. *Ann Intern Med.* 1950;33(452):462.

290. Barton JC, Edwards CQ, Bertoli LF, Shroyer TW, Hudson SL. Iron overload in African Americans. *Am J Med.* 1995;99(6):616-623.

291. Wurapa RK, Gordeuk VR, Brittenham GM, Khiyami A, Schechter GP, Edwards CQ. Primary iron overload in African Americans. *Am J Med.* 1996;101(1):9-18.

292. Brown KE, Khan CM, Zimmerman MB, Brunt EM. Hepatic iron overload in blacks and whites: a comparative autopsy study. *Am J Gastroenterol.* 2003;98(7):1594-1598.

293. Barton JC, Acton RT, Anderson LE, Alexander CB. A comparison between whites and blacks with severe multi-organ iron overload identified in 16,152 autopsies. *Clin Gastroenterol Hepatol.* 2009;7(7):781-785.

294. Barton JC, Acton RT, Richardson AK, Brissie RM. Stainable hepatic iron in 341 African American adults at coroner/medical examiner autopsy. *BMC Clin Pathol.* 2005;5:1-8.

295. Barton JC, Bertoli LF, Alford TJ, Barton JC, Edwards CQ. Hepatic iron in African Americans who underwent liver biopsy. *Am J Med Sci.* 2015;349(1):50-55.

296. Barton JC, Acton RT. Inheritance of two *HFE* mutations in African Americans: cases with hemochromatosis phenotypes and estimates of hemochromatosis phenotype frequency. *Genet Med.* 2001;3(4):294-300.

297. Beutler E, Felitti V, Gelbart T, Ho N. The effect of *HFE* genotypes on measurements of iron overload in patients attending a health appraisal clinic. *Ann Intern Med.* 2000;133(5):329-337.

298. MacClenahan K, Moran R, McDermott S, Longshore JW. Prevalence of hereditary hemochromatosis mutations in the upper savannah region of South Carolina. *Proc Greenwood Genet Center.* 2000:1945-1950.

299. Acton RT, Wiener HW, Barton JC. Estimates of European American ancestry in African Americans using *HFE* p.C282Y. *Genet Test Mol Biomarkers.* 2020;24(9):578-583.

300. Lee PL, Gaasterland T, Barton JC. Mild iron overload in an African American man with *SLC40A1* D270V. *Acta Haematol.* 2012;128(1):28-32.

301. Collins TS, Arcasoy MO. Iron overload due to X-linked sideroblastic anemia in an African American man. *Am J Med.* 2004;116(7):501-502.

302. Sussman NL, Lee PL, Dries AM, Schwartz MR, Barton JC. Multi-organ iron overload in an African-American man with *ALAS2* R452S and *SLC40A1* R561G. *Acta Haematol.* 2008;120(3):168-173.

303. Lee PL, Reid TJ,III, Bottomley SS, Barton JC. Sideroblastic anemia, iron overload, and *ALAS2* R452S in African-American males: phenotype and genotype features of five unrelated patients. *Am J Hematol.* 2011;86(9):787-789.

304. Barton JC, Barton JC, Adams PC. Clinical and laboratory associations with persistent hyperferritinemia in 373 black Hemochromatosis and Iron Overload Screening Study participants. *Ann Hepatol.* 2017;16(5):802-811.

305. Beutler E, Barton JC, Felitti VJ, et al. Ferroportin 1 (*SCL40A1*) variant associated with iron overload in African-Americans. *Blood Cells Mol Dis.* 2003;31(3):305-309.

306. Gordeuk VR, Caleffi A, Corradini E, et al. Iron overload in Africans and African-Americans and a common mutation in the *SCL40A1* (ferroportin 1) gene. *Blood Cells Mol Dis.* 2003;31(3):299-304.

307. Rivers CA, Barton JC, Gordeuk VR, et al. Association of ferroportin Q248H polymorphism with elevated levels of serum ferritin in African Americans in the hemochromatosis and iron overload screening (HEIRS) study. *Blood Cells Mol Dis.* 2007;38(3):247-252.

308. Kato J, Fujikawa K, Kanda M, et al. A mutation, in the iron-responsive element of H ferritin mRNA, causing autosomal dominant iron overload. *Am J Hum Genet.* 2001;69(1):191-197.

309. Barton JC, McDonnell SM, Adams PC, et al. Management of hemochromatosis. Hemochromatosis management working group. *Ann Intern Med.* 1998;129(11):932-939.

310. Ong SY, Gurrin LC, Dolling L, et al. Reduction of body iron in *HFE*-related haemochromatosis and moderate iron overload (Mi-Iron): a multicentre, participant-blinded, randomised controlled trial.. *Lancet Haematol.* 2017;4(12):e607-e614.

311. Edwards CQ, Dadone MM, Skolnick MH, Kushner JP. Hereditary haemochromatosis. *Clin Haematol.* 1982;11(2):411-435.

312. Falize L, Guillygomarc'h A, Perrin M, et al. Reversibility of hepatic fibrosis in treated genetic hemochromatosis: a study of 36 cases. *Hepatology.* 2006;44(2):472-477.

313. Akesson A, Stal P, Vahter M. Phlebotomy increases cadmium uptake in hemochromatosis. *Environ Health Perspect.* 2000;108(4):289-291.

314. Barton JC, Bottomley SS. Iron deficiency due to excessive therapeutic phlebotomy in hemochromatosis. *Am J Hematol.* 2000;65(3):223-226.

315. Barton JC, Bertoli LF, Rothenberg BE. Screening for hemochromatosis in routine medical care: an evaluation of mean corpuscular volume and mean corpuscular hemoglobin. *Genet Test.* 2000;4(2):103-110.

316. Sundic T, Hervig T, Hannisdal S, et al. Erythrocytapheresis compared with whole blood phlebotomy for the treatment of hereditary haemochromatosis. *Blood Transfus.* 2014;12(Suppl 1):s84-s89.

317. Phatak P, Brissot P, Wurster M, et al. A phase 1/2, dose-escalation trial of deferasirox for the treatment of iron overload in *HFE*-related hereditary hemochromatosis. *Hepatology.* 2010;52(5):1671-1779.

318. Adams PC, Barton JC. How I treat hemochromatosis. *Blood.* 2010;116(3):317-325.

319. Dirweesh A, Anugwom CM, Li Y, Vaughn BP, Lake J. Proton pump inhibitors reduce phlebotomy burden in patients with *HFE*-related hemochromatosis: a systematic review and meta-analysis. *Eur J Gastroenterol Hepatol.* 2020;10:1327-1331.

320. Leitman SF, Browning JN, Yau YY, et al. Hemochromatosis subjects as allogeneic blood donors: a prospective study. *Transfusion.* 2003;43(11):1538-1544.

321. Pennings G. Demanding pure motives for donation: the moral acceptability of blood donations by haemochromatosis patients. *J Med Ethics.* 2005;31(2):69-72.

322. Hoad V, Bentley P, Bell B, Pathak P, Chan HT, Keller A. The infectious disease blood safety risk of Australian hemochromatosis donations. *Transfusion.* 2016;56(12):2934-2940.

323. Leitman SF. Hemochromatosis: the new blood donor. *Hematology Am Soc Hematol Educ Program.* 2013:645-650.

324. Pauwels NS, De BE, Compernolle V, Vandekerckhove P. Worldwide policies on haemochromatosis and blood donation: a survey among blood services. *Vox Sang.* 2013;105(2):121-128.

325. Abraham D, Rogers J, Gault P, Kushner JP, McClain DA. Increased insulin secretory capacity but decreased insulin sensitivity after correction of iron overload by phlebotomy in hereditary haemochromatosis. *Diabetologia.* 2006;49(11):2546-2551.

326. LeSage GD, Baldus WP, Fairbanks VF, et al. Hemochromatosis: genetic or alcohol-induced?. *Gastroenterology.* 1983;84(6):1471-1477.

327. Fletcher LM, Dixon JL, Purdie DM, Powell LW, Crawford DH. Excess alcohol greatly increases the prevalence of cirrhosis in hereditary hemochromatosis. *Gastroenterology.* 2002;122(2):281-289.

328. Fletcher LM, Powell LW. Hemochromatosis and alcoholic liver disease. *Alcohol.* 2003;30(2):131-136.

329. O'Brien RT. Ascorbic acid enhancement of desferrioxamine-induced urinary iron excretion in thalassemia major. *Ann N Y Acad Sci* 1974;232(0):221-225.

330. Herbert V, Shaw S, Jayatilleke E. Vitamin C-driven free radical generation from iron. *J Nutr.* 1996;126(4 Suppl):1213S-1220S.

331. McLaran CJ, Bett JH, Nye JA, Halliday JW. Congestive cardiomyopathy and haemochromatosis—rapid progression possibly accelerated by excessive ingestion of ascorbic acid. *Aust N Z J Med.* 1982;12(2):187-188.

332. Barton JC, Barton JC, Acton RT, So J, Chan S, Adams PC. Increased risk of death from iron overload among 422 treated probands with *HFE* hemochromatosis and serum levels of ferritin greater than 1000 µg/L at diagnosis. *Clin Gastroenterol Hepatol.* 2012;10(4):412-416.

333. Dobrindt EM, Keshi E, Neulichedl J, et al. Long-term outcome of orthotopic liver transplantation in patients with hemochromatosis: a summary of a 30-year transplant program. *Transplant Direct.* 2020;6(6):e560.

334. Martin M, Millan A, Ferraro F, et al. Leukocyte telomere length is associated with iron overload in male adults with hereditary hemochromatosis. *Biosci Rep.* 2020;40(10):1916.

335. Kelly AL, Rhodes DA, Roland JM, Schofield P, Cox TM. Hereditary juvenile haemochromatosis: a genetically heterogeneous life-threatening iron-storage disease. *QJM.* 1998;91(9):607-618.

336. Blank R, Wolber T, Maeder M, Rickli H. Reversible cardiomyopathy in a patient with juvenile hemochromatosis. *Int J Cardiol.* 2006;111(1):161-162.

337. Fabio G, Minonzio F, Delbini P, Bianchi A, Cappellini MD. Reversal of cardiac complications by deferiprone and deferoxamine combination therapy in a patient affected by a severe type of juvenile hemochromatosis (JH). *Blood.* 2007;109(1):362-364.

Disorders of Red Blood Cells

Chapter 28 ■ Porphyrias

MAKIKO YASUDA • JOHN D. PHILLIPS • ROBERT J. DESNICK

INTRODUCTION

The *porphyrias* are inborn errors of heme biosynthesis, each resulting from a different defective enzyme in the heme biosynthetic pathway (*Figure 28.1*). There are eight major porphyrias, which are inherited as autosomal dominant, autosomal recessive, or X-linked traits. Seven of them are caused by dominant or biallelic recessive loss-of-function mutations in their respective heme biosynthetic genes, and one, X-linked protoporphyria (XLP), results from gain-of-function mutations in erythroid-specific 5-aminolevulinic acid synthase (*ALAS2*). The genes encoding these enzymes have been cloned, their chromosomal locations identified, and DNA analyses have revealed >1000 pathogenic mutations causing all the porphyrias. The metabolic blocks resulting from the defective enzymes are expressed either in the liver or in the bone marrow, the sites where most of the body heme is produced. The porphyrias can be classified into three major groups based on their presenting symptoms and site of pathology: (1) the acute hepatic porphyrias (AHPs), for which there are four; (2) the hepatocutaneous porphyria, porphyria cutanea tarda (PCT); and (3) the three erythropoietic cutaneous porphyrias (*Table 28.1*). PCT can occur as an inherited or acquired form, both primarily influenced by certain metabolic and environmental factors. Some "late-onset porphyrias" result from acquired clonal hematopoietic disorders such as myelodysplasias, due to the clonal expansion of a somatic mutation in a heme biosynthetic enzyme, which leads to expression of the porphyria.

Although the pathophysiologic mechanisms that result in the clinical manifestations of the porphyrias are only partly understood, two cardinal features prevail: life-threatening episodic acute neurological symptoms in the AHPs and cutaneous photosensitivity in the hepatocutaneous and erythropoietic cutaneous porphyrias. The neurologic manifestations are associated with increased production of the putative neurotoxic porphyrin precursors, 5-aminolevulinic acid

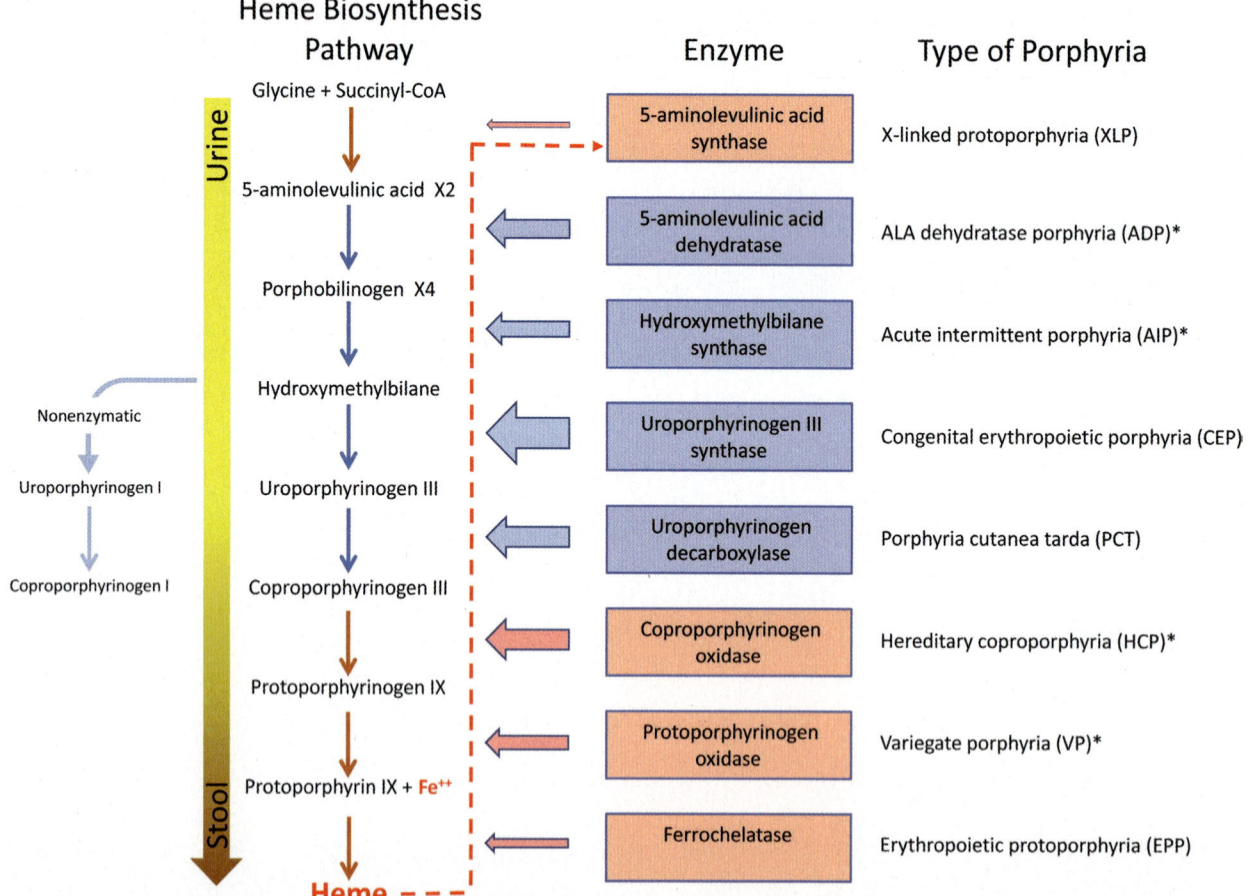

FIGURE 28.1 **The heme biosynthetic pathway, its enzymes, and the eight forms of human porphyria associated with genetic defects of these enzymes.** The enzymes are located in mitochondria (peach boxes) or in the cytosol (blue boxes); the sizes of boxed arrows indicate the relative enzymatic activities in erythroid cells. The major compound accumulated and excreted in excess in the seven porphyrias beyond the 5-aminolevulinate (ALA) synthase step is the substrate of the respective deficient enzyme; increased activity of the erythroid ALA synthase (ALAS2) in X-linked protoporphyria leads to increased flux of intermediates through the pathway and accumulation of protoporphyrin. In the acute or inducible porphyrias (asterisk), reduced hepatic heme synthesis causes increased ALA production through release of the normal negative feedback on the rate-limiting ALA synthase step exerted by heme,[1] indicated by the red dashed line. The broad downward arrow (in yellow) reflects the decreasing water solubility of the biosynthetic intermediates and their excretion in urine or stool. Nonenzymatic closure of the linear tetrapyrrole hydroxymethylbilane when uroporphyrinogen III synthase is deficient yields the dead-end isomers uroporphyrinogen I and coproporphyrinogen I. Fe^{2+}, ferrous iron.

Table 28.1. Classification of Major Porphyrias

I. Acute Hepatic Porphyrias
Without Cutaneous Manifestations:
Acute intermittent porphyria (AIP)
ALA dehydratase–deficient porphyria (ADP)
With Cutaneous Manifestations:
Variegate porphyria (VP)
Hereditary coproporphyria (HCP)

II. Hepatocutaneous Porphyria
Porphyria cutanea tarda (PCT)

III. Erythropoietic Cutaneous Porphyrias
Congenital erythropoietic porphyria (CEP)
Erythropoietic protoporphyria (EPP)
X-linked protoporphyria (XLP)

(ALA) and porphobilinogen (PBG), which characterize the AHPs. The cutaneous photosensitivity is a manifestation of the unique photoactive properties of porphyrins (the oxidized forms of the natural porphyrinogens in the heme synthesis pathway) in those porphyrias in which the enzyme defects cause porphyrin accumulation (*Figure 28.1*). These distinguishing clinical manifestations of the porphyrias form the basis for their classification in *Table 28.1*. Clinical and biochemical diagnoses can be made by its characteristic profile of accumulated and excreted heme biosynthetic metabolic intermediates (*Table 28.2*). Diagnoses can be confirmed by identification of the

pathogenic mutation(s) causing the porphyria. Approved treatments are available for the AHPs and hepatocutaneous and erythropoietic cutaneous porphyrias.

MAMMALIAN HEME BIOSYNTHESIS AND ITS REGULATION

Heme is an iron-containing cofactor and signaling molecule that is essential to virtually all aerobic organisms and is involved in a wide variety of biological processes, including oxygen transport, drug metabolism, electron transfer, circadian rhythm, and micro-RNA processing.[1-7] Heme is synthesized from glycine and succinyl coenzyme A through the action of eight enzymatic reactions (*Figure 28.1*).[8] These eight enzymes are encoded by nine genes, as the first and rate-limiting enzyme in the pathway, ALAS, has two genes that encode unique housekeeping (ALAS1) and erythroid-specific (ALAS2) isozymes.[9,10] The first and last three reactions occur in the mitochondria, whereas the intermediate four steps take place in the cytosol. The first three heme biosynthetic enzymes successively convert glycine and succinyl to the porphyrin precursors ALA, PBG, and then to hydroxymethylbilane (HMB), a linear tetrapyrrole (*Figure 28.1*). The next four enzymes convert HMB to various PBGs or porphyrins, which are cyclic tetrapyrroles, and finally, ferrochelatase (FECH), the last enzyme in the pathway, inserts iron into protoporphyrin IX to form heme. A complete and ubiquitous lack of heme biosynthesis is not compatible with human life. Thus, all living porphyria patients have at least a small amount of residual activity of their respective heme biosynthetic enzymes.

Table 28.2. Genetic and Key Metabolic Features of the Porphyrias

	Inheritance	Defective Enzyme	Gene (Symbol/Location[a])	Enzyme Activity (%)[b] Heterozygote	Enzyme Activity (%)[b] Homozygote[c]	Heme Precursor(s) Accumulated/Excreted[d]	Route of Excretion	Tissue Source
X-linked protoporphyria	X-linked	Erythroid 5-aminolevulinate synthase	*ALAS2*/Xp11.21	2 to 3 × normal	–	**Metal-free (50%-85%) and Zn-proto IX** (15%-50%)	Feces	Bone marrow
ALA dehydratase	Autosomal recessive	ALA dehydratase	*ALAD*/9q32	–	<10	**ALA[f]**, Copro III	Urine	Liver
Acute intermittent	Autosomal dominant	HMB Synthase (PBG deaminase)	*HMBS*/11q23.3	50	1-18	**PBG[f], ALA[f]**	Urine	Liver
Congenital erythropoietic	Autosomal recessive	Uroporphyrinogen III synthase	*UROS*/10q26.2	–	1-20	**Uro I,** Copro I	Urine	Bone marrow
Porphyria Cutanea tarda	Autosomal dominant or acquired	Uroporphyrinogen decarboxylase	*UROD*/1p34.1	50	3-27	**Uro I + III, 7-COOH porphyrin**	Urine	Liver
Hereditary coproporphyria	Autosomal dominant	Coproporphyrinogen oxidase	*CPOX*/3q11.2	50	2-10[e]	**Copro III** PBG[f], ALA[f]	Feces Urine	Liver
Variegate	Autosomal dominant	Protoporphyrinogen oxidase	*PPOX*/1q22	50	<20	**Proto IX, Copro III** PBG[f], ALA[f], Copro III[f]	Feces Urine Urine	Liver
Protoporphyria	Autosomal recessive	Ferrochelatase	*FECH*/18q21.3	–	<10	**>85% metal-free protoporphyrin**	Feces	Bone marrow
Protoporphyria[g] (most common)	Autosomal recessive	Ferrochelatase	*FECH*/18q21.3 + *IVS3-48C* allele[g]	–	20-30[g]	**>85% metal-free proto IX**	Feces	Bone marrow

Abbreviations: ALA, 5-aminolevulinic acid; copro, coproporphyrin; HMB, hydroxymethylbilane; PBG, porphobilinogen; proto, protoporphyrin; uro, uroporphyrin; Zn, zinc.
[a]Gene symbol and chromosomal location as listed in the Human Gene Mutation Database, located at http://www.hgmd.org.
[b]Percentage of normal.
[c]Often a compound heterozygote.
[d]The major metabolite(s) and route are shown in boldface. The route of porphyrin excretion is determined by the number of carboxyl groups on the porphyrin and hence by its water solubility.
[e]In harderoporphyria, the activity is 18% to 24% of normal (see text).
[f]Increased in urine during acute attack; in variegate porphyria urine coproporphyrin is increased when symptoms are only cutaneous.
[g]In this case, one allele has a pathogenic mutation and the other has the *FECH* "low expression" allele (*IVS3-48C*) (see text).

While heme is synthesized in essentially all nucleated cells, the predominant sites of synthesis are the bone marrow (~80% of total body heme), for hemoglobin synthesis, and the liver (~15%), mainly for synthesis of drug-metabolizing and mitochondrial cytochrome enzymes.[11] Due to their differences in heme demand, the liver and erythron have distinct mechanisms of regulating heme biosynthesis.[9,10] Tight regulation is crucial, as heme deficiency leads to insufficient amounts of critical hemoproteins or heme signaling, whereas excessive amounts are cytotoxic. In the erythron, heme biosynthesis is controlled by the availability of iron, which regulates ALAS2 at the translational level.[12-19] In the liver, where the metabolic demand for heme is constantly fluctuating, for example due to ingestion of cytochrome P450-inducing drugs or hormonal changes, heme synthesis is controlled by the "free" or labile heme pool, via ALAS1. Under heme-replete conditions, heme represses ALAS1 expression, primarily by (1) inhibiting *ALAS1* mRNA synthesis; (2) blocking transport of the enzyme's precursor into the mitochondria where it is processed into the mature and active protein; and (3) stimulating ALAS protein degradation via Ion peptidase 1 (LONP1), a mitochondrial protease.[20-25] When hepatic heme pools decrease, the negative feedback is lost and ALAS1 synthesis is induced.

Heme degradation is controlled by heme oxygenase (HO), which includes the inducible (HO-1) and constitutive HO-2 isoforms.[26-30] HO-1 is induced by heme, its natural substrate, as well as oxidative stress. Both HO isozymes break down heme into equimolar amounts of carbon monoxide, iron, and biliverdin, which is subsequently metabolized to bilirubin through the action of biliverdin reductase.[31-33]

ACUTE HEPATIC PORPHYRIAS

Four porphyrias manifest with clinically indistinguishable episodic acute neurovisceral symptoms and are classified as AHPs (*Table 28.1*). These include acute intermittent porphyria (AIP), variegate porphyria (VP), hereditary coproporphyria (HCP), and the ultrarare ALA dehydratase (ALAD)-deficient porphyria (ADP), which are associated with deficiencies of hydroxymethylbilane synthase (HMBS), protoporphyrinogen oxidase (PPOX), coproporphyrinogen oxidase (CPOX), and ALAD, respectively.[34] The life-threatening acute attacks typically begin with severe abdominal pain and may progress to include a myriad of symptoms associated with dysfunction of the autonomic, peripheral, and central nervous systems.

The attacks are precipitated by "porphyrinogenic" factors that directly or indirectly induce hepatic ALAS1 activity. Well-established precipitating factors include certain drugs, particularly those that induce hepatic cytochrome P450 enzymes, and hormonal fluctuation, the main culprit likely being progesterone, as female AIP heterozygotes often experience attacks during the luteal phase of their menstrual cycles.[35-37] Other precipitating factors include fasting or low-carbohydrate diets, stress, and infections.[9,38] When hepatic ALAS1 activity is induced, the respective deficiencies in downstream heme biosynthetic enzymes likely become rate-limiting, leading to insufficient heme production and depletion of the "free" heme pool in the liver. This leads to de-repression of ALAS1[20-25] and its further induction. Under these circumstances, HMBS, which is normally the second least abundant heme biosynthetic enzyme next to ALAS1,[11] becomes rate-limiting, resulting in the massive accumulation of the porphyrin precursors, ALA and PBG, in the liver. One exception is ADP, in which only ALA accumulates, as the defective enzyme, ALAD, is upstream of PBG. The ALA and PBG that are overproduced in the liver are released into the blood and excreted through the urine.

Precipitating factors induce hepatic *ALAS1* expression by increasing the demand for heme and/or by stimulating its transcription.[9] Prototypic porphyrinogenic drugs and steroid hormones increase heme demand because their metabolism is mediated by cytochrome P450 enzymes, which are hemoproteins. Such drugs and steroids also induce xenobiotic-sensing nuclear receptors such as pregnane X receptor and constitutive androstane receptor, which have been shown to bind to drug response enhancer motifs located upstream of the *ALAS1* coding region and induce gene transcription.[39] Fasting or extreme carbohydrate restriction, on the other hand, induces the transcriptional co-activator, peroxisome proliferator-activated receptor gamma coactivator 1alpha, which promotes direct binding of transcription factors to the promoter region of *ALAS1*, activating its transcription.[38] Infection and stress induce the heme catabolizing enzyme, HO-1, and thereby deplete hepatic heme pools and induce *ALAS1* expression.[9]

Diagnosis is often missed or delayed in patients with AHPs because the acute neurovisceral symptoms are nonspecific and mimic those that are caused by more common etiologies. In fact, a US study found that the mean lag time from disease onset to AHP diagnosis is approximately 15 years.[40] In patients who are exhibiting symptoms, first-line testing involves assessment of PBG levels in a spot urine sample that was collected during symptoms.[41] Elevated levels (>4 times upper normal) establish a diagnosis of an AHP (i.e., AIP, VP, or HCP), as PBG is not associated with any other known condition in human. Normal levels effectively rule out AHPs, with the exception of ADP, which is extremely rare with <10 verified cases to date.[42] Once the diagnosis of an AHP is established, second-line tests performed in urine, fecal, and blood samples will identify the specific type of porphyria based on their unique biochemical characteristics, which are described for each of the AHPs in their respective "Laboratory Findings" sections. Identification of the pathogenic AHP mutation by molecular testing confirms the diagnosis and permits detection of other positive family members so that they too can be counseled to avoid precipitating factors. Molecular testing is highly effective for the AHPs, as it successfully detects >96% of mutations causing AIP, HCP, and VP.[43] Importantly, treatment for acute attacks is the same for all four AHPs. Thus, treatment should be initiated immediately once a biochemical diagnosis of an AHP is established, even if the specific porphyria type has yet to be determined.

Acute Intermittent Porphyria

AIP (also known as Swedish porphyria), the most common AHP, is an autosomal dominant disorder due to the approximately half-normal activity of HMBS (also known as porphobilinogen deaminase [PBGD]), the third enzyme in the heme biosynthetic pathway (*Figure 28.1*).[21] The prevalence of symptomatic AIP is estimated to be 5.4 per 1,000,000 in Europe[44] and is likely similar elsewhere in the world. An exception is northern Scandinavia, which has a notably higher prevalence (~1 per 10,000 in Sweden) due to founder effects.[44,45] The vast majority of AIP heterozygotes are clinically latent their entire lives, never experiencing an acute attack. In fact, recent studies have estimated that as few as 0.5% to 1% of AIP heterozygotes who carry a pathogenic *HMBS* mutation exhibit symptoms.[46,47]

Clinical Description

Acute attacks typically begin at or after puberty and predominantly affect women (80%-90%) of child-bearing age.[48] Although rare, childhood onset of attacks has been reported, and interestingly, occurred mostly in males.[49] The acute symptoms usually last for several days but may continue for several months and are separated by symptomless intervals varying from months to decades. Most symptomatic AIP heterozygotes have one or few attacks in their lifetime, while a small number of them, estimated to be 3% to 5% in Europe,[44,50] experience frequent recurring attacks (>4 per year).

The most common and typically the first symptom of an acute attack is a crippling abdominal pain that is usually generalized and is often accompanied by nausea, vomiting, constipation, and/or diarrhea (*Table 28.3*). The abdomen is usually soft, with no rebound tenderness or other signs of peritoneal irritation. X-ray may show mild ileus of the bowel, in which case dilated bowel loops may be palpable. Tachycardia and systemic arterial hypertension, which reflect increased sympathetic activity, are reported to occur in 40% to 50% of attacks.[40] In patients with recurrent attacks, prodromal symptoms, including "brain fog," irritability, and fatigue, may be recognized days prior to onset of acute and severe pain.[51]

With prolonged or more severe attacks, a motor-dominant peripheral axonal neuropathy may also occur.[52] It can be manifested as pain in the extremities, back, buttocks, or chest or weakness in one or more

Table 28.3. Signs and Symptoms of Acute Intermittent Porphyria

Signs and Symptoms	Incidence (%)
Abdominal pain	85-95
Vomiting	43-88
Constipation	48-84
Tachycardia	28-80
Muscle weakness	42-68
Mental changes	40-58
Hypertension	36-54
Extra-abdominal pains	50-52
Sensory deficit	9-38
Fever	9-37
Convulsions	9-20
Respiratory paralysis	9-14

Data from four reports, 525 patients: Stein JA, Tschudy DP. Acute intermittent porphyria. A clinical and biochemical study of 46 patients. *Medicine (Baltimore)*. 1970;49:1-16; Waldenström J. The porphyrias as inborn errors of metabolism. *Am J Med*. 1957;22:758-773; Goldberg A. Acute intermittent porphyria: a study of 50 cases. *Q J Med*. 1959;28:183-209; Bonkovsky HL, Maddukuri VC, Yazici C, et al. Acute intermittent porphyria in the USA: Features of 108 subjects from Porphyrias Consortium. *Am J Med*. 2014;127:1233-1241.

extremities, especially the upper extremities and proximal musculature that may progress to quadriparesis.[53,54] Bulbar and respiratory muscle paralysis can be life-threatening. If peripheral nerve deficits develop, they may clear slowly, over months or years, or never completely. Sensory neuropathy is rare. Blindness may result from both occipital lobe and optic nerve involvement.[55-57] Other CNS disturbances may include acute anxiety and irritability with progression to confusion, frank psychosis, and coma, which occasionally dominate the clinical presentation.[54,58,59] Major seizures occur in 10% to 20% of attacks and are commonly accompanied by marked hyponatremia that is attributed to inappropriate secretion of antidiuretic hormone (ADH).[40,60]

In recent years, it has become increasingly appreciated that many symptomatic AIP patients also experience persistent chronic symptoms even during their attack-free phase. A recent natural history study in a cohort of 110 AHP patients with recurrent attacks, mostly consisting of female AIP heterozygotes, showed that ~65% of them experienced ongoing pain, nausea, fatigue, insomnia, and anxiety that significantly reduced quality of life (QOL).[61] Depression, including suicidal tendencies, may occur with frequent attacks or with chronic symptoms.

In older reports, the mortality rate from neurologic involvement was approximately 30%,[62] which has since decreased dramatically due to improved diagnosis, avoidance of porphyrinogenic drugs, and the development of hemin therapy. The overall prognosis of AIP is good, particularly if diagnosis is made in a timely manner and treatment is initiated early, before serious nerve damage occurs.[63]

Long-Term Complications

Symptomatic AIP patients, particularly those with continuous elevation of ALA and PBG concentrations, are at increased risk of developing late complications, including chronic kidney disease (CKD), chronic hypertension, and primary liver cancers (PLCs). ~60% of symptomatic AIP patients develop hypertension and a CKD characterized by chronic tubulointerstitial nephropathy that is rarely associated with proteinuria.[64,65] The hypertension may predispose to CKD, although recent studies suggest that porphyrin precursors are directly nephrotoxic and are likely the culprit of AHP-associated CKD[64] (see "Pathogenesis of Long-term Complications" section). In rare cases, AIP patients with end-stage renal disease (ESRD) develop blistering skin lesions resembling those of PCT due to impaired excretion and the consequential accumulation of photoreactive porphyrins.[66]

The risk of developing PLCs, which consists predominantly of hepatocellular carcinoma (HCC) and, to a much lesser extent, cholangiocarcinoma, are elevated by as much as 60-fold in symptomatic AHP patients, particularly those who are >60 years old and have persistent porphyrin precursor elevation.[67,68] Although some studies indicate that symptomatic AIP women are more prone to developing PLCs compared to their male counterparts,[63,69] a recent large-scale (>1000 AIP patients) prospective study showed that gender does not impact risk.[68] Of interest, only 20% to 30% of HCC cases in AIP were associated with cirrhosis, whereas HCC that occurs in the general population almost always (80%-90%) coexists with cirrhosis.

Molecular Basis and Pathogenesis

AIP is due to pathogenic mutations in the gene encoding HMBS, which catalyzes the deamination and condensation of four PBG molecules to form HMB (*Figure 28.1*).[8] There are two HMBS isozymes encoded by a single *HMBS* gene (located at chromosomal region 11q23.3)[70] through the activity of independently regulated housekeeping and erythroid-specific promoters and alternative splicing (*Figure 28.2*).[71-73] The mRNA encoding the housekeeping form of *HMBS* has exon 1 spliced to exon 3, with translation initiation in exon 1. In erythroid cells, exon 1 is excluded from the transcript and translation begins in exon 3, thereby resulting in a protein lacking the first 17 amino acids of the housekeeping isozyme. Therefore, mutations within exon 1 or at the exon 1/intron 1 junction restrict the HMBS enzymatic defect to nonerythroid tissues and account for the normal enzymatic activity in erythrocytes.[10]

To date, >520 *HMBS* mutations have been reported.[74] Most mutations are identified in single or a small number of pedigrees, although certain mutations that occur at CpG dinucleotides (e.g., p.Arg173Trp and p.Arg167Gln), which are mutational hotspots, are more common.[10,75] Founder mutations occur in restricted geographic areas; for example, the p.Trp198Ter mutation is a founder mutation in Sweden and Norway.[76] It is estimated that approximately 3% of all index cases with AIP have de novo mutations.[77] Roughly 40% of reported mutations are missense or nonsense mutations, while the remaining consist of splice site mutations, insertions or deletions, and a much smaller number of promoter region mutations.[74] In general, no correlation between the genotypes and phenotypes has been found, although some prevalent mutations (e.g., p.Trp198Ter, p.Arg173Trp) have been reported to exhibit higher penetrance.[78,79] The structure of HMBS has been solved and functional outcomes of the mutations can be predicted.[80-82]

Recent studies have shown that pathogenic *HMBS* mutations are rather common, occurring at a frequency of 1 per ~1300 to 1700 Caucasians.[46,47] Why only ~1% of these heterozygotes develop symptoms is not understood. Notably, the penetrance of AIP is considerably higher within families that have a symptomatic heterozygote, ranging between 20% and 35%,[47,83] compared to the 1% in the general population. This suggests that modifier genes and/or environmental factors modulate the susceptibility to developing symptomatic disease. Thus far, such genetic modifiers have not been identified.

Pathogenesis of Acute Attacks

While two major hypotheses regarding the pathogenesis of the acute attacks have been proposed, including (1) neurotoxicity of the porphyrin precursors and (2) cellular heme deficiency in neuronal tissues, recent evidence strongly supports the former. First, orthotopic liver transplantation completely prevented attacks in AIP heterozygotes who, prior to transplantation, had uncontrollable frequently recurring attacks.[84-86] In the reverse scenario, two unrelated nonporphyric males were transplanted livers isolated from AIP heterozygotes with severe recurring attacks in a domino liver transplantation and developed acute attack symptoms with elevated ALA and PBG.[87] Together, these findings strongly indicate that the liver is the main site of pathology, giving rise to two major possibilities: (1) that neurotoxic molecules are released from the liver; or (2) that hepatic heme deficiency leads to

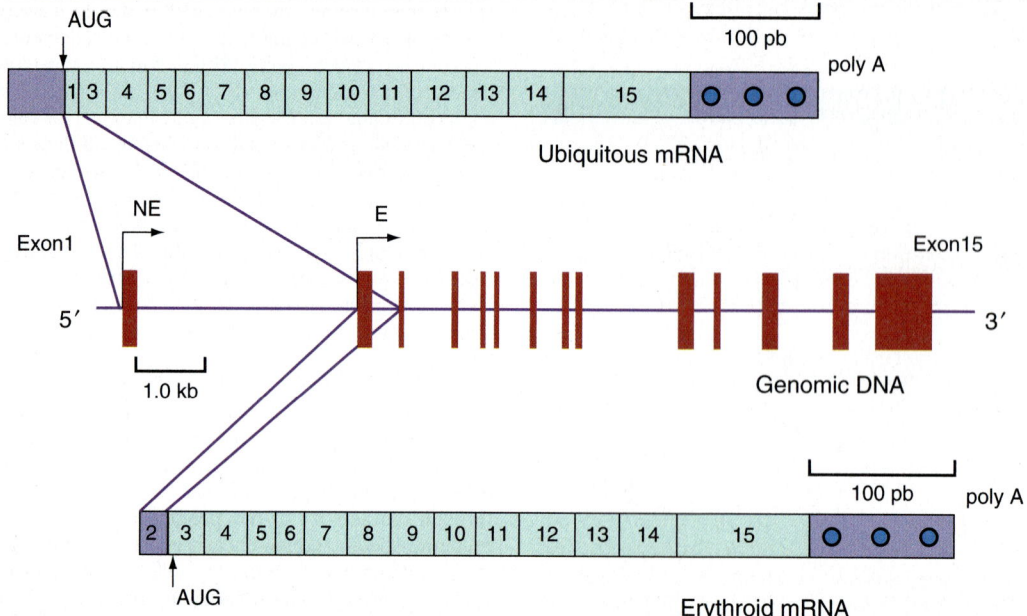

FIGURE 28.2 Structure of the human porphobilinogen deaminase gene and its two transcripts produced by alternative splicing. AUG, methionine translational start site; E, erythroid promoter; mRNA, messenger ribonucleic acid; NE, nonerythroid promoter. (Reprinted from Deybach JC, Puy H. Acute intermittent porphyria: from clinical to molecular aspects. In: Kadish KM, Smith KM, Guilard R, eds. *The Porphyrin Handbook: Medical Aspects of Porphyrins*. Vol 14. Academic Press; 2003;14:23-41. Copyright © 2003 Elsevier. With permission.)

acute attack symptomology. The recent observation that a RNA interference (RNAi) therapeutic (i.e., givosiran) against hepatocyte *ALAS1* effectively protects AHP patients from developing acute attacks[88,89] strongly supports the former hypothesis, as this therapeutic inhibits the production of porphyrin precursors but is not expected to increase hepatic heme pools.

The main neurotoxic culprit is thought to be ALA, as it is markedly elevated in the plasma in all four AHPs, whereas PBG is not increased in ADP. Further, plasma ALA is increased in other conditions, including lead poisoning and hereditary tyrosinemia type 1 (HT1), which are also associated with neurological dysfunction that has a strikingly similar presentation to porphyric attacks. *In vivo* studies in animal models also support the neurotoxicity of ALA. For example, injection of ALA into cerebral ventricles of rats induced seizures.[90] Additionally, disruption of peptide transporter 2 (PEPT2), which acts as an efflux transporter of ALA at the choroid plexus, led to elevated ALA in the cerebrospinal fluid (CSF), impaired neuromotor function, and decreased survival rates in mice that were systemically administered ALA.[91] It has been proposed that ALA may exert neurotoxicity by modulating GABA activity in neuronal tissues, as ALA is structurally very similar to GABA and displays agonist-like effects in vitro.[92-94] Alternatively, ALA may be neurotoxic due to its pro-oxidative properties, as demonstrated in vitro.[95,96] The neurotoxicity of PBG remains to be investigated, although injection of PBG into rat cerebral ventricles induced seizures as potently as did ALA.[90]

However, it should be noted that increases in plasma ALA and/or PBG alone do not fully explain the pathogenic mechanism of acute attacks. First, there are AIP heterozygotes classified as asymptomatic high excretors who have continuous and considerable elevation of plasma ALA and PBG concentrations but do not exhibit overt symptoms. Additionally, symptomatic patients often have markedly elevated plasma and urinary ALA and PBG levels that are only slightly lower compared to peak levels during attacks, even when they are asymptomatic.[61] These observations suggest that while porphyrin precursor accumulation is a prerequisite, that alone is not sufficient to express the disease. Another unresolved issue is how ALA and PBG, which do not readily permeate the blood-brain barrier,[91,97] cause CNS disturbances. One possible explanation is that additional pathological mechanisms, such as neuronal heme deficiency[11] or mitochondrial insufficiency,[98-100] are also involved in the development of CNS

dysfunction. Further studies are needed to fully understand the pathogenic mechanism(s) underlying the acute attacks.

Pathogenesis of Late Complications

ALA and/or PBG are also implicated in the pathogenesis of CKD that frequently develops as a late complication in AHP patients with active disease. In the kidney, PEPT2 is involved in the reabsorption of ALA in proximal tubules. Recent studies have shown that the prevalence of CKD is significantly higher in AIP heterozygotes carrying a *PETP2* variant (PEPT2*1*1) associated with increased renal ALA reabsorption compared to those with the other common *PEPT2* genotypes (PEPT2*2*2 or PEPT2*1*2).[101] Furthermore, co-incubation of cultured human renal epithelial cells with ALA and PBG increased expression of proinflammatory and profibrogenic factors and induced apoptosis.[64]

The pathogenesis of AIP-related chronic hypertension and PLCs is poorly understood. For the latter, several mechanisms have been proposed, including (1) direct hepatotoxicity of ALA[96,102]; (2) decreased HO-1-mediated antioxidative effects due to reduced hepatic heme levels[103]; and (3) that biallelic inactivation of heme biosynthetic genes, which has been reported in few cases of AHP-associated HCC, interferes with tumor suppressor activity.[104,105]

Laboratory Findings

Results of routine hematologic tests are typically within normal limits even during attacks, although occasionally a leukocytosis is observed and may lead to an erroneous impression of an abdominal condition requiring emergency operation (e.g., appendicitis). Serum transaminases are increased during attacks in some patients and may be chronically elevated in patients with recurrent attacks. The urine is often red or brown in color, especially on standing in light, due to oxidation of PBG into porphobilin and spontaneous polymerization into porphyrins. For this reason, urinary samples collected from individuals with suspicion of an AHP needs to be protected from light, either by wrapping in foil or by placing the specimen in an amber bag. The discoloration of urine has often led to the suspicion and eventual diagnosis of an AHP.

The telltale sign of an AIP attack is urinary overexcretion of ALA and PBG. Normally, there are only trace amounts of ALA and PBG in the plasma, and 24-hour urinary excretion levels of ALA and PBG are

<7 and <4 mg, respectively. During acute attacks, the urinary excretion of PBG generally ranges from 20 to 200 mg daily, while urinary ALA excretion is roughly half of that of PBG.[55] Plasma ALA and PBG may be increased as high as 300 µg/dL.[41] The elevated plasma and urinary ALA and PBG decrease during remission and may return to normal, although they frequently remain elevated for prolonged periods, especially in AIP.[106]

As outlined earlier, the first step in diagnosing AIP is establishing markedly increased urinary PBG levels.[41] Quantitation of PBG in a spot urine that has been normalized for creatinine is sufficient; 24-hour urine collection is unnecessary. ALA and PBG are typically quantitated simultaneously using liquid chromatography with tandem mass spectrometry (LC-MS/MS[107]). While this method is highly sensitive and specific, in the United States, the average turnaround time for receiving results is 4 to 7 days, meaning a substantial delay in diagnosis. Rapid qualitative screening tests for PBG such as the Watson-Schwartz test[108] may be useful in establishing a diagnosis, if they are available in-house. However, results of qualitative tests must always be confirmed by quantitative tests.

Total fecal porphyrin concentrations and coproporphyrin I/III isomer ratios are essentially normal in AIP, which distinguish it from VP and HCP. Demonstration of approximately half-normal HMBS enzymatic activity in erythrocytes is diagnostic, but there are two major limitations to this test: (1) *HMBS* mutations that are in exon 1 or at the exon 1/intron 1 junction, estimated to be present in ~5% of AIP patients, will be missed (see AIP "Molecular Basis and Pathogenesis" section[109]); and (2) there is significant overlap between the ranges of activity in affected and normal individuals,[110] making it difficult to interpret the results in some cases.

Hyponatremia (serum $Na^+ < 130$ mEq/L) is often observed during acute attacks in the presence of elevated ADH. For this reason, the hyponatremia is often attributed to syndrome of inappropriate ADH (SIADH). However, it should be noted that most AHP patients have decreased blood volume,[55] rather than increased circulating volume, which is characteristic of SIADH. Thus, the hyponatremia that occurs in AHP may be a result of vomiting, and the increased ADH may reflect appropriate response to the decreased blood volume. Hypomagnesemia associated with tetany has also been reported.[111]

In the presence of encephalopathy, magnetic resonance imaging (MRI) studies often show reversible contrast-enhancing cerebral subcortical white matter lesions of variable size with normal diffusion-weighted MR images, interpreted to represent vasogenic edema.[112] These transient lesions have been documented in a large number of AIP cases, most of them occurring in the posterior lobes although frontal and parietal changed have also been reported.[112] In some cases with cortical blindness, similar lesions were limited to the occipital lobes.[113] The CSF is usually normal. Electrophysiologic studies and microscopic examination of nervous tissue indicate that the acute attack affects primarily neuronal bodies, leading to an acute axonal degeneration of peripheral and autonomic nerves and to neuronal loss and gliosis in the CNS.[114-116]

Treatment

Treatment of Ongoing Attack

When an acute attack occurs, patients usually require hospitalization because the clinical course is difficult to predict and causes for the symptoms other than porphyria must be excluded. Precipitating factors, especially drugs that are porphyrinogenic, or likely porphyrinogenic, should be removed whenever possible. Pain should be treated with nonporphyrinogenic analgesics and narcotics such as morphine. Fluid, electrolyte, and caloric deficits should be restored. Carbohydrate is administered orally or intravenously (as 10% dextrose in 0.45% saline), so that the equivalent of 300 to 500 g of glucose is given daily.[41] Propranolol has been effective in reducing tachycardia and hypertension in some patients[117] but must be used very cautiously if at all in patients with hypovolemia.[118]

Carbohydrate loading may suffice for mild attacks, particularly if the attack was precipitated by fasting or a low-carbohydrate diet. However, for most acute attacks, therapy with intravenous hemin is

necessary. Hemin acts by restoring the depleted hepatic heme pool and suppressing *ALAS1* expression in the liver, thereby decreasing production of the putative neurotoxic heme precursors, ALA and PBG.[119] There are two approved hemin formulations, including Panhematin (Recordati Rare Diseases), a lyophilized hematin preparation available in the United States, and heme arginate (Normosang, Orphan Europe), a heme-arginine complex in solution that is used in Europe and other parts of the world, including South Africa, Japan, and South America. Of note, Panhematin was the first drug to be approved under the US Orphan Drug Act.

The standard treatment for acute attacks is administration of hemin at a dose of 3 to 4 mg/kg body weight via a large vein or central line once daily for 3 to 5 days. After infusion of hemin, dramatic reductions in ALA and PBG concentrations in plasma and urine are usually observed, and clinical symptoms often improve within 48 to 72 hours. In some cases, particularly if treatment is delayed, response to hemin might be slow, in which case treatment can be extended. It is recommended and common practice for hemin to be reconstituted in 25% human serum albumin rather than sterile water, which is indicated by the product label. This is because the albumin stabilizes the hemin in solution, which otherwise rapidly degrades and may lead to a transient coagulopathy or infusion site phlebitis due to pro-coagulant effects of the heme degradation products.[120,121] Other less common side effects of hemin include fever, aching, malaise, and hemolysis.[41] As hemin contains 9% iron by weight, long-term repeated heme treatment can lead to iron overload and hepatic fibrosis.[122] This is prevented by monitoring the serum ferritin and by phlebotomy or iron chelation therapy as indicated.

The management of seizures is a considerable challenge. If they are related to hyponatremia and/or hypomagnesemia, correction of these derangements may control them. However, if seizures are related to the porphyric diathesis or are a chronic associated problem, their management may be difficult because most anticonvulsants are porphyrinogenic and contraindicated.[123] Several antiepileptic drugs (e.g., gabapentin, vigabatrin, and levetiracetam) are not metabolized by the liver and are the treatment of choice for epilepsy in AHPs.[124,125]

Orthotopic liver transplantation has become established as a treatment option for severe refractory AIP in carefully selected patients as it leads to phenotypic cure.[68,84] A recent follow-up study on 38 European AIP patients showed that all 37 patients who received an orthotopic liver transplantation remained attack free for up to 19 years.[68] On the contrary, one patient who received an auxiliary transplantation without removal of the native liver continued to have recurring attacks post-transplantation, suggesting that removal of the AIP liver may be critical for effective treatment. An increased incidence of hepatic artery thrombosis associated with the procedure was reported, with the recommendation to use antiplatelet therapy after transplantation.[126]

Prevention of Acute Attacks

Prevention of acute attacks by avoiding potential precipitating factors, such as porphyrinogenic drugs and caloric restriction, is the cornerstone of treating the patient in whom the diagnosis has been established. Latent heterozygous relatives should also be counseled to avoid factors that may precipitate an attack. The most extensive and up-to-date drug database that classifies drugs based on their relative risk of inducing a porphyric attack can be found at the website: www.drugs-porphyria.org. Patients should be warned that fasting may induce attacks; they should regularly take in sufficient calories to maintain a normal body weight and promptly consult a physician whenever adequate oral intake is interrupted by intercurrent illness.

In women whose recurrent and frequent attacks are related to the menstrual cycle, prevention may be achieved by suppression of ovulation with gonadotropin-releasing hormone (GnRH) analogs.[127,128] Improvement in severity and frequency of attacks following treatment has been reported in up to 80% of female AIP heterozygotes.[129] Prolonged administration of GnRH analogs is associated with decreased bone mineral density, and therefore, addition of low-dose estradiol or bisphosphonate should be considered in patients who continue treatment beyond 6 months. After 1 to 2 years, GnRH analogs should bc discontinued and the need for continued oral contraceptive treatment should be re-evaluated.[41]

Patients with recurrent attacks may also be treated with prophylactic hemin infusions, typically once or twice a week, to prevent the attacks. This approach may be particular effective for AIP heterozygotes whose attacks are recurrent but noncyclic.[41] Frequent hemin administration often requires insertion of a central venous access port and may lead to hepatic iron overload, necessitating periodic phlebotomies or iron-chelator therapy, as noted earlier. After 1 to 2 years, prophylactic hemin should be discontinued to assess whether continued therapy is necessary.[41]

More recently, Givosiran (Givlaari; Alnylam Pharmaceuticals), a subcutaneously administered RNAi therapeutic that silences the induced expression of hepatocyte *ALAS1* mRNA, and thereby decreases plasma ALA and PBG concentrations, has been approved in the United States and several other countries for treatment of AHPs. The *ALAS1*-targeted siRNA is conjugated to N-acetylgalactosamine (GalNAc), which permits nearly exclusive uptake by hepatocytes via asialoglycoprotein receptor–mediated endocytosis.[130] In a phase III clinical trial, monthly subcutaneous administration of Givosiran reduced annual attacks by ~74% and markedly improved QOL in AHP patients with recurring attacks.[88] Currently, Givosiran is administered once monthly at a dose of 2.5 mg/kg body weight as a prophylactic treatment against recurrent acute attacks. In the United States, it is indicated for adult patients, whereas in European countries, it is approved for patients 12 years and older. Renal and liver function should be monitored periodically, as increases in alanine transferase and decreased glomerular filtration rate have been reported.[88] Homocysteine levels should also be assessed prior to and periodically during treatment, as clinically and biochemically active AIP heterozygotes are prone to developing hyperhomocysteinemia (HHcy) that may be further exacerbated by Givosiran administration.[131-133] While the mechanism of Givosiran-related HHcy remains to be elucidated, the condition is rapidly reversed by supplementation of pyridoxine or a multivitamin formulation.[132]

Emerging Therapies

Several novel therapeutic approaches for AIP are currently under development, including (1) enzyme replacement therapy; (2) gene therapy; and (3) molecular chaperone approaches. Early attempts to develop recombinant HMBS enzyme replacement therapy failed to show efficacy in a clinical trial.[134] Recent preclinical studies have demonstrated that conjugation of the HMBS enzyme to apolipoprotein A1 (ApoA1), the major protein component of high-density lipoprotein that mediates its uptake by hepatocytes, provides durable protection against induced acute attacks when administered intravenously or subcutaneously into a well-established mouse model of AIP.[135,136] While adeno-associated virus (AAV)-mediated delivery of a therapeutic *HMBS* gene to hepatocytes effectively prevented and treated biochemically induced acute attacks in the AIP mice,[137,138] a phase I/II clinical trial of AAV2/5-gene therapy did not improve ALA and PBG levels in AIP patients, presumably due to insufficient hepatocyte transduction.[139] Therefore, more recent efforts have been directed toward modifying the therapeutic vector to improve transduction efficiency.[140,141] Preclinical studies have also shown that lipid nanoparticle (LNP)-mediated delivery of the normal human *HMBS* mRNA to hepatocytes effectively prevented and treated the biochemically induced acute attacks in the AIP mice.[142] Efforts are also being directed to apply molecular chaperones to stabilize and enhance the activity of wild-type HMBS, encoded by the intact *HMBS* allele, as a treatment for AIP.[143]

Long-Term Management

Pregnancy is generally well-tolerated in women with AIP, although occasionally, hormonal fluctuation early in the process may induce or exacerbate acute attack symptoms.[144,145] Women with inadequate caloric intake and hyperemesis gravidarum are most at risk of developing acute attacks[146] and need to be monitored and treated accordingly to prevent the attacks. If an acute attack occurs and hemin therapy is indicated, it can be administered to the pregnant patient, as there is no evidence of adverse effects in the mother or fetus.[147]

As symptomatic AIP patients are at increased risk of developing hypertension and CKD, blood pressure should be controlled using nonporphyrinogenic drugs and kidney function should be carefully monitored. AIP patients who develop ESRD benefit from kidney transplantation.[66]

While clinically and biochemically active patients >60 years are considered to be at most risk of developing PLCs, latent individuals may also be at increased risk compared to the general population. For this reason, some porphyria experts recommended that all AIP heterozygotes be screened at least annually by liver imaging starting at 50 years old to facilitate early tumor detection.[148]

At-risk family members of the proband should be encouraged to undergo genetic testing for the pathogenic *HMBS* mutation. Latent heterozygotes should be counseled to avoid factors that are potentially porphyrinogenic.

Homozygous Dominant AIP

Rarely, individuals have biallelic pathogenic *HMBS* mutations that result in markedly reduced (<4%) HMBS enzymatic activity. These patients typically present with infancy onset of severe psychomotor retardation and constitutively elevated plasma and urinary ALA and PBG and may also develop ataxia, nystagmus, and dystonia.[149-151] Most patients die in early childhood, although some with higher residual HMBS activity (13%-18%) survive to adulthood and present with a milder, slowly progressive neuropathy.[152] While mild neurovisceral symptoms were reported in a female homozygous dominant AIP (HD-AIP) adult,[152] acute attacks were absent in the remaining six HD-AIP children reported to date. It has been proposed that the marked CNS dysfunction in HD-AIP is due to ALA and/or PBG that is overproduced and accumulates within the CNS tissues, distinct from the AHPs, in which porphyrin precursor overproduction is limited to the liver.[97] This suggests that effective therapies for HD-AIP likely need to target the CNS and that liver-targeted therapies for the AHPs are ineffective for HD-AIP. In line with this, orthotopic liver transplantation in two HD-AIP patients, a 1.5-year-old child and a 46-year-old woman, did not halt neurological decline.[60,152]

Variegate Porphyria

VP is an autosomal dominant disorder with low penetrance caused by loss-of-function mutations in the gene encoding PPOX, the enzyme that catalyzes the penultimate step of heme biosynthesis (*Figure 28.1*). The disease is termed "variegate" as it may be manifested by acute attacks, cutaneous photosensitivity, or both. It is also referred to as the "South African genetic porphyria" because of its remarkably highly prevalence in this country due to a founder effect traceable to a single Dutch couple that arrived in Cape Town in 1688.[153,154] Although much less prevalent elsewhere, patients have been identified around the world and the estimated prevalence of symptomatic VP in Europe is 3.2 per 1,000,000.[44]

Clinical Description

Similar to AIP, VP patients rarely express disease manifestation before puberty, and symptoms are more common in women than men.[155] Of the symptomatic VP patients, ~60% are reported to present with only cutaneous symptoms, while ~20% exhibit only neurovisceral symptoms, and the remaining display both.[156,157] These proportions were strikingly similar between large VP patient cohorts from South African and Europe (France and the United Kingdom).[156,157]

The typical cutaneous presentation is adult-onset chronic blistering lesions, including subepidermal vesicles and bullae with erosions that are limited to sun-exposed areas, especially the backs of the hands (*Figure 28.3*). These lesions result from the severe mechanical fragility of the skin induced by phototoxic porphyrin accumulation, which leave the skin prone to blister formation.[155] The subepidermal vesicles, bullae, and erosions crust over and heal slowly. If the blisters rupture, they may become infected. These skin lesions are clinically and histologically indistinguishable from those that occur in PCT. Other chronic skin findings include scarring, thickening, milia (small, 1- to 2-mm, firm, whitish papules), and focal hyperpigmentation or

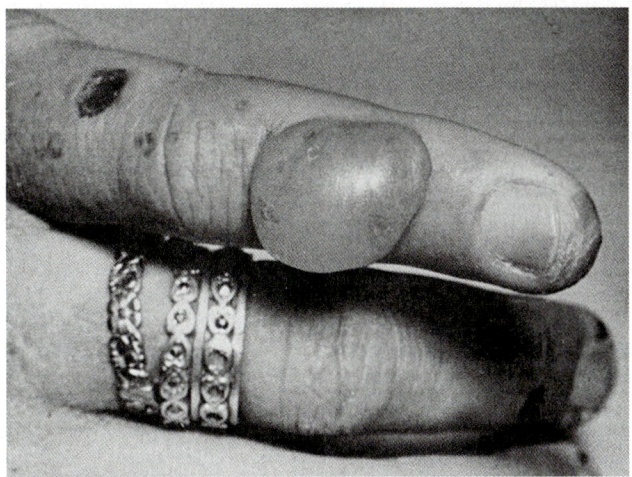

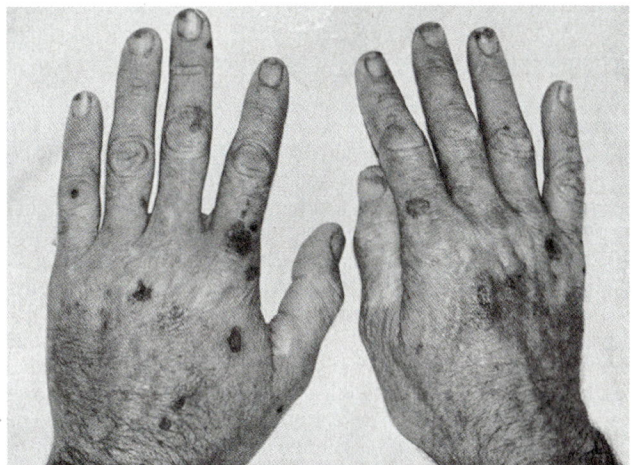

FIGURE 28.3 Cutaneous manifestations of variegate porphyria. A, Bulla on index finger, pigmented scars, and collapsed blisters at the fingertips of a 27-year-old woman. B, Hands of a 36-year-old man. Note erosions on the back of hands, depigmented scars of past lesions, and subungual involvement. (Courtesy of Dr Lennox Eales, University of Cape Town, South Africa.)

hypopigmentation. Facial hypertrichosis and hyperpigmentation may also be present.[155]

The neurovisceral attacks of VP do not differ in any important respect from those of AIP, although they are generally less frequent and less severe compared to the latter.[153] Notably, the proportion of VP heterozygotes who have acute attacks has decreased over the years, from 30% to 40% in the 1980s, to <10% as of 2005,[153] presumably due to more sensitive diagnostic testing, physician and patient education, and less use of drugs that precipitate symptoms. As with AIP, the risk of developing chronic renal disease and HCC is increased in patients with VP, especially in those who are over 50 years old and have persistent elevation of ALA and PBG.[158,159]

Molecular Basis and Pathogenesis

VP results from the deficiency of PPOX, which oxidizes the fully reduced protoporphyrinogen IX to protoporphyrin IX.[8] PPOX activity is approximately half-normal in all tissues[160,161] and accounts for the observed pattern of porphyrin excretion (*Table 28.2*). The gene that encodes the enzyme was the last of the heme synthesis genes to be cloned and characterized,[162,163] and it has been mapped to chromosome 1 (1q23.3).[164]

Over 200 distinct *PPOX* mutations have been identified in patients with VP throughout the world, with roughly half of them being missense or nonsense mutations, the others consisting of insertions, deletions, and splice site and promoter mutations.[74] Most mutations occur in single or few pedigrees,[157] whereas the exon 3 *PPOX*

founder mutation, p.Arg59Trp, is found in 95% of VP patients in South Africa.[154] Studies indicate that as many as 3 per 1000 South Africans are heterozygous for this mutation.[153,154] When expressed in *Escherichia coli*, the p.Arg59Trp mutant protein had an almost undetectable catalytic activity, presumably related to its location in the binding motif of flavin adenine dinucleotide, an essential cofactor for the enzyme.[165] In general, pathogenic *PPOX* mutations that cause VP are severe and result in very little, if any, enzymatic activity.[157] Analyses of 104 unrelated VP families from France and the United Kingdom showed no clear correlation between the type of mutation (e.g., missense, nonsense, etc.) and presenting symptoms.[157]

Pathogenesis

The cutaneous damage produced by the accumulated porphyrins in plasma and capillaries of the skin is the consequence of the photoactive porphyrins. Porphyrins absorb light at ~400 to 410 nm (Soret band) and release the energy at ~620 nm, as fluorescence. It is the high energy photon emission in an aerobic environment of tissues that produces reactive oxygen species (superoxide anion and other reactive metabolites)[166] that are damaging to cells. The complement system is light-activated in vivo in the skin of porphyric patients, promoting release of proteases from dermal mast cells. Chemotactic cytokines also are generated, and the peroxides produced by high-energy photons activate polymorphonuclear leukocytes, in turn activating the complement system that may act synergistically to form the bullous cutaneous lesions. As a consequence of these events, the dermal-epidermal junction becomes disrupted and leads to skin fragility and the formation of vesicles and bullae that easily rupture.

The accumulation of plasma ALA and PBG and the consequential neurovisceral symptoms in VP are attributed to an associated relative deficiency of hepatic HMBS activity,[11,167] as described earlier (see "Acute Hepatic Porphyrias" section). In support of this, LNP-mediated delivery of wild-type *HMBS* mRNA into a chemically induced VP rabbit model with approximately half-normal hepatic PPOX activity (and normal HMBS activity) completely corrected the accumulation of porphyrin precursors and the attack-like symptoms, including hypertension and neuromotor impairment.[168] *In vitro* studies have shown that the porphyrinogens that accumulate in VP, coproporphyrinogen and protoporphyrinogen, act as allosteric inhibitors of HMBS, and therefore, may further exacerbate the relative HMBS deficiency.[169]

Laboratory Findings

The most distinguishing laboratory abnormality in VP is the excretion of large and roughly equal amounts of coproporphyrin III and protoporphyrin in the feces, particularly in patients with active disease.[41,155,156] In South African patients, fecal protoporphyrin excretion reached 1500 μg/g dry weight, and fecal coproporphyrin excretion reached 1300 μg/g dry weight during the symptomatic phase (normal total fecal porphyrin excretion is less than 200 μg/g).[156] The diagnosis of VP can be established by fecal analysis during an acute attack, during periods when only cutaneous manifestations are present, or during a clinically latent period. However, up to 30% of asymptomatic VP heterozygotes have normal fecal porphyrin profiles.[170]

Another distinctive finding in VP is the fluorescence emission maximum at wavelength 626 to 628 nm on plasma fluorescence scanning, which is performed by exposing a saline-diluted patient plasma sample to light (excitation 405 nm) to excite the porphyrins and identifying peak fluorescence emission.[171] Importantly, this qualitative test distinguishes VP from the other two AHPs associated with elevated PBG (i.e., AIP and HCP) as well as PCT, which all display a peak between 618 and 620 nm.[11,171] As this test is highly specific and sensitive, rapid, and easy to administer, it is often the first test performed in patients with elevated PBG levels to screen for VP.[11] Although plasma fluorescence scanning is the most sensitive biochemical test to establish a diagnosis of VP in asymptomatic patients, it only detects ~50% of such heterozygotes, and therefore is not sufficiently sensitive compared to DNA analysis.[156,172,173]

During acute attacks, ALA and PBG are markedly elevated in the plasma and urine, although typically less prominent compared to attacks associated with AIP.[41] In contrast to AIP, plasma and urinary ALA and PBG generally return to normal after an acute attack[156,170] and are usually normal or only slightly increased in patients in whom the only clinical manifestations are cutaneous. During latent periods, urinary porphyrin excretion is usually normal. However, during acute attacks, nonenzymatic conversion of PBG to uroporphyrin I may occur, giving rise to artificially elevated urinary porphyrin excretion.[34,156,170] When cutaneous symptoms alone are present, coproporphyrin is the major urinary porphyrin, but uroporphyrin excretion may also be increased.[156]

Treatment

Acute attacks should be prevented and treated as outlined for AIP. Hemin is used for severe attacks and is most effective if administered early in the course of the attack.[174] Glucose may be of benefit for mild attacks.[156] Givosiran is indicated for adult patients (or patients 12 years and older in Europe) with recurrent neurovisceral attacks. Its effectiveness to prevent cutaneous symptoms has yet to be tested. Protection against sun exposure, including protective clothing (e.g., wide-brimmed hats, gloves) and the use of tinted glass for windows and cars, is the only practical way to deal with the photosensitivity. Despite the skin lesions being clinically and histologically similar to that of PCT, effective treatments for PCT, including low-dose hydroxychloroquine or phlebotomy, are not therapeutic for the cutaneous lesions in VP. Kidney function and screening for PLCs should be performed as outlined in the "Long-term Management" section for AIP.

One VP patient with progressive disease underwent orthotopic liver transplantation due to alcohol-induced cirrhosis and had complete resolution of persistent symptoms and biochemical abnormalities.[175] Thus, liver transplantation may be considered for VP patients with severe and frequent attacks for whom all other treatment options have been exhausted.

Identifying asymptomatic VP heterozygotes in families is important because, as in AIP, acute attacks can often be prevented by avoiding precipitating drugs or other precipitating factors. Biochemical studies apart from assay of the PPOX enzyme, which is not readily available, are often inconclusive in asymptomatic individuals, and therefore, molecular analysis is the definitive approach for detection of carriers.

Homozygous Dominant VP

At least 14 unrelated homozygous dominant VP (HD-VP) patients with biallelic compound heterozygous or homozygous *PPOX* mutations and PPOX activities ranging between 5% and 25% of normal have been reported to date.[10,170] The major clinical features are infancy-onset severe cutaneous photosensitivity and photomutilation, which may be accompanied by skeletal deformities of the hand, especially shortening of the fingers, psychomotor delay, seizures, nystagmus, sensory neuropathy, and retarded growth. Mild acute attacks were reported in a 26-year-old female patient[176] but were absent in the other case reports. Biochemical findings are consistent with those of autosomal dominant VP, but in addition, patients have elevated erythrocyte protoporphyrin, predominantly zinc protoporphyrin.[177] Of note, HD-VP patients homozygous for the common South African mutation, p.Arg59Trp, have not been identified to date, presumably because this mutation is severe and nearly abolishes PPOX activity and is, therefore, incompatible with life.[154]

Hereditary Coproporphyria

HCP is transmitted as an autosomal dominant trait with reduced penetrance. It is caused by pathogenic mutations in the gene encoding CPOX (*Figure 28.1*), the sixth enzyme in the heme biosynthetic pathway. The prevalence of symptomatic HCP is estimated to be 1 to 2 in 1,000,000[44,178]; it is the third most prevalent AHP, behind AIP and VP. Similar to VP, patients can manifest with acute neurovisceral attack, chronic cutaneous photosensitivity, or both, although cutaneous symptoms are less frequent compared to VP.

Clinical Description

As with AIP and VP, this disease is generally latent before puberty and most of those who manifest are women.[11,34] Most symptomatic HCP patients (80%-90%) present with acute neurovisceral attacks that are similar to those of AIP and VP but are generally less frequent and less severe.[34,179] Photosensitivity is much less common compared to VP, reported to occur in only 5% to 13% of patients, and unlike in the latter, it tends to occur mainly in the presence of neurovisceral episodes.[11,179,180] Rarely, intermittent episodes of cutaneous symptoms that are similar to those described for VP may be the only clinical manifestation of the disease.[11] Cutaneous symptoms may be more pronounced in HCP patients who have chronic liver disease that impair biliary excretion of coproporphyrin, as this results in retention and accumulation of the photoreactive porphyrin in the plasma.[181] Few cases of HCC associated with HCP have been reported.[182,183] Like AIP and VP patients, HCP patients who are clinically and biochemically active are considered to be at heightened risk of developing long-term complications, including PLCs and CKD and chronic hypertension.

Molecular Basis and Pathogenesis

HCP is caused by the deficient activity of CPOX, which catalyzes the two-step decarboxylation of coproporphyrinogen III to protoporphyrinogen IX.[8] CPOX activity is reduced to half-normal in the liver[184] and all tissues examined, including cultured skin fibroblasts,[185] lymphocytes,[186] and kidney.[187] The cloning and characterization of the *CPOX* gene,[188-190] located on chromosome 3 (3q12),[191] led to the identification of numerous mutations in the gene. Over 90 different *CPOX* mutations have been reported to date, and almost all have been restricted to single families.[74,192] Approximately 40% of mutations are missense, ~14% are small deletions, and ~10% are nonsense, while the remainder of mutations include splice site mutations, gross deletion, and small insertions and duplications.[74] These mutations are spread throughout the *CPOX* gene. Despite the marked allelic heterogeneity at the molecular level and a wide range of residual enzyme activities of mutant proteins, clinical features are similar.[193]

The pathogenesis of the clinical features can be viewed as the same as in VP, with induction of ALAS1 during attacks.[194] The photosensitivity occurs mainly during periods of a neurovisceral attack, presumably because plasma levels of the photosensitizing coproporphyrin become sufficiently elevated.

Laboratory Findings

As in VP, urinary ALA and PBG are typically increased only during attacks and concentrations are usually lower compared to attacks associated with AIP.[41] A characteristic biochemical finding in HCP is the marked elevation of fecal coproporphyrin, which is usually increased after puberty and may approach or exceed 10,000 µg/g dry weight during an attack (10-220 times normal).[195] Another distinguishing feature is increased fecal coproporphyrin isomer III-to-isomer I ratio to >2 (normal is <0.5),[11,195] which is often present even in latent cases in whom fecal coproporphyrin concentrations may be normal.[180,192] Urinary coproporphyrin excretion may be profoundly increased during an attack but is usually normal during remissions and is not diagnostic.

Treatment

HCP should be treated and managed as described under AIP and VP. Intravenous hemin is effective for acute attacks[196,197] as well as for needed maintenance therapy with regular infusions.[198] Givosiran is effective in preventing acute porphyric attacks and is indicated for adult (≥12 years in Europe) HCP patients with recurrent attacks.[88,199] To date, liver transplantation has not been performed in a patient with HCP, but given its effectiveness to treat AIP-associated attacks, it may be considered as a last resort therapeutic option for HCP that is refractory to other treatments. Cutaneous symptoms are managed as described for VP.

Homozygous Dominant HCP

To date, there have been several reported cases of homozygous dominant HCP (HD-HCP) with biallelic *CPOX* mutations. The majority of these patients have a clinically distinct form of HD-HCP called harderoporphyria, which is associated with accumulation of a tricarboxylic coproporphyrin, harderoporphyrin,[200,201] an intermediate metabolite in the conversion of coproporphyrin to protoporphyrin IX. Nine confirmed cases of harderoporphyria have been reported thus far,[202] all presenting with neonatal-onset hemolytic anemia and jaundice that typically improve after early childhood. One child was reported to also develop acute attacks and died from its complications at the age of 5 years.[203] Patients also exhibit variable photosensitivity in adulthood.

Biochemically, these patients have elevation of fecal porphyrins, with the predominant porphyrin being harderoporphyrin. Urinary coproporphyrin and harderoporphyrin combined are increased about 20-fold relative to normal. CPOX enzyme activity ranged between 18% and 24% of normal.[204]

With the exception of two patients, one of whom was homozygous for the *CPOX* mutation encoding p.His327Arg[203] and another whom was compound heterozygous for p.Asp233Gly and c.1207-1218del12,[202] all patients were either homozygous for the exon 6 p.Lys404Glu mutation or carried this mutation in trans with a splicing defect that deleted exon 6.[202,204] Studies have indicated that the CPOX amino acid residues D400 to K405 are in the enzyme active site and are directly involved in the enzyme's second step decarboxylation of harderoporphyrinogen to protoporphyrinogen IX.[204]

Two young HD-HCP females, both with <10% of normal CPOX activity, were confirmed to have marked elevation of fecal porphyrins, predominantly coproporphyrin III, thereby ruling out the diagnosis of harderoporphyria.[205,206] One presented with skin pigmentation, hypertrichosis, and episodic acute neurovisceral attacks accompanied by ALA and PBG elevations, while the other had CEP-like symptoms, including skin fragility and erythrodontia. Interestingly, one of these patients was compound heterozygous for the *CPOX* mutations p.His-327Arg, which caused harderoporphyria at homozygosity, in combination with p.His307Arg.

ALAD Deficiency Porphyria

ADP (also referred to as "plumbo porphyria" or "Doss porphyria") is by far the rarest of the eight major inherited porphyrias, and to date, has been documented in only eight cases worldwide. Unlike the other three AHPs, it is an autosomal recessive disorder caused by biallelic pathogenic *ALAD* mutations. This is likely related to the fact that in human liver, ALAD is vastly abundant relative to the heme biosynthetic enzymes that are associated with the three autosomal dominant AHPs (i.e., HMBS, CPOX, and PPOX).[8] Patients present with acute neurovisceral crises that are similar to the other AHPs, although disease onset is typically much younger and symptoms are generally more severe. Cutaneous symptoms are absent. Due to the small case numbers to date, it is the least understood porphyria, and the natural history and treatment experience with this disease are extremely limited.

Clinical Description

Of interest, all documented ADP cases to date have been male patients, contrary to the other three AHPs, in which manifesting patients are mostly women. The clinical findings vary among the small number of cases with ADP. Of the eight documented cases, two had disease onset at birth, five experienced their first acute attack between 7 and 15 years old, while one patient developed mild ADP at 63 years in conjunction with a myeloproliferative disorder (i.e., polycythemia vera [PV]).[42] Similar to the other AHPs, the neurovisceral symptoms were episodic and included severe pain in the abdomen and/or extremities, nausea and/or vomiting, hypertension, peripheral neuropathy, and in some cases, paralysis.

Molecular Basis and Pathogenesis

ALAD (also known as PBG synthase) is the second enzyme in the heme biosynthetic pathway (*Figure 28.1*) that catalyzes the condensation of two ALA molecules to form PBG.[8] It is encoded by the *ALAD* gene, located on chromosome 9 (9q34).[207] The gene contains two promoter regions that generate housekeeping and erythroid-specific transcripts by alternative splicing of a separate noncoding exon 1 (i.e., exons 1A or 1B) to exon 2; both transcripts encode identical ALAD polypeptides.[208]

All eight documented ADP cases were compound heterozygotes, with the exception of the 63-year-old patient with PV, who was heterozygous for the germline pathogenic *ALAD* mutation, p.Gly133Arg. The ADP in this patient presumably developed as a result of clonal expansion of a cell lineage carrying the *ALAD* mutation.[42] The 13 pathogenic *ALAD* mutations reported to date consist of 9 missense, 3 splice site mutations, and a small deletion. When expressed individually in vitro, the missense mutations displayed 0% to 41% of wild-type ALAD activity.[209] These activities generally correlate with disease severity, although in vitro enzyme activity was available for both *ALAD* mutations in only four ADP patients.[209] It has been proposed that the deficient ALAD enzymatic activity is due to conformational changes in the enzyme. Human ALAD is maximally active as a homooctomer, but pathogenic *ALAD* missense mutations associated with ADP were shown to favor the less catalytically active hexamer formation.[210] More recently, human ALAD was shown to be an iron-sulfur protein, and one reported mutation (p.Cys132Arg) is expected to disrupt coordination of an iron-sulfur cluster that is critical for maximal enzymatic activity.[42]

The mechanism for the dominating neurologic features present in ADP appears to be similar to that discussed for AIP, and the large accumulation of ALA caused by the biosynthetic block supports its implicated importance as a neurotoxin in the pathogenesis, as aforementioned. However, unlike the other three AHPs in which porphyrin precursor overproduction is limited to the liver, it is not entirely clear whether the ALA that is overproduced in ADP is contributed solely by the liver, or if there is added contribution by the bone marrow. The latter is supported by the observations that (1) liver transplantation in a severely affected ADP child did not correct the biochemical abnormalities, although it did improve clinical symptoms[211]; (2) a patient with infantile onset of disease who was unresponsive to hemin went into clinical remission following suppression of heme biosynthesis in bone marrow with blood transfusion and hydroxyurea[212]; and (3) ADP patients have substantial elevation of erythrocyte zinc protoporphyrin. Contrary to these findings, it was recently documented that hepatic *ALAS1* mRNA in plasma and urinary exosomes of an ADP patient was elevated to levels comparable to those in AIP patients during attacks,[42] suggesting that the liver is a major source of ALA overproduction in ADP. Further studies are needed to fully elucidate the pathogenesis of this ultrarare porphyria.

Laboratory Findings

The characteristic laboratory findings in ADP are markedly increased plasma and urinary ALA that are ~10-fold and 8- to 80-fold over the normal values, respectively.[213] In general, the amount of ALA excreted in urine correlates with disease severity.[42] As aforementioned, ALA is also elevated in lead poisoning and HT1. The former can be excluded from the diagnosis by quantifying blood lead levels, while the latter can be differentiated by assessing plasma or urinary concentrations of succinyl acetone, a structural analog and potent inhibitor of ALAD that forms in HT-1 due to deficiency of the fumarylacetoacetate hydrolase enzyme.

In the eight documented ADP probands, erythrocyte ALAD activities were less than 15% of normal[42] and did not show a clear correlation with disease severity. Erythrocyte zinc protoporphyrin is increased, from 3 to 30 times normal. Urinary coproporphyrin III is also typically raised 10- to 70-fold and may result from conversion of ALA to porphyrinogens in tissues other than those that accumulate ALA (i.e., the liver and perhaps also bone marrow).[8] Fecal porphyrins are normal in most cases. Despite the defects in both alleles, erythropoiesis does not appear to be compromised, although hemoglobin values were often not reported. Heterozygotes for an ALAD defect have no biochemical abnormalities except for the reduced levels of ALAD activity.[214]

Treatment

Supportive measures as outlined for AIP are generally helpful for acute episodes of ADP as well. Roughly half of the ADP patients who were administered hemin showed good clinical response, while oral or intravenous glucose was sufficient to treat symptoms and correct the biochemical abnormalities in the patient who developed mild ADP in conjunction with PV.[42] One child with infantile onset was treated with orthotopic liver transplantation at 6 years old, following unsuccessful treatment with hemin infusions.[211] While the high basal urinary excretion of ALA and porphyrin remained unchanged, the patient no longer exhibited increased urinary ALA and PBG when challenged with porphyrinogenic drugs or with intercurrent illnesses and no longer experienced pain 1 year following transplantation.[211] Givosiran is indicated for adult patients (>12 years in Europe) with ADP, but to date, there have not been reports of ADP patients being treated with the RNAi therapeutic.

HEPATOCUTANEOUS PORPHYRIA

PCT is considered to be a hepatocutaneous porphyria, as it is characterized by blistering skin lesions due to porphyrin accumulation in the liver and release into the plasma. It is unique among the porphyrias in that it occurs both as a sporadic form, in the absence of a uroporphyrinogen decarboxylase (*UROD*) mutation, as well as a familial form that is inherited as an autosomal dominant trait.

Porphyria Cutanea Tarda

Clinically, PCT has been considered the most frequently encountered porphyric disorder. A primary comorbidity in sporadic PCT is the presence of hepatitis C virus (HCV) infection; however, the current treatment of HCV infections (genotypes 1-6) with the antivirals, sofosbuvir and velpatasvir, has effectively reduced this confounding factor in sporadic PCT. There are now studies that show a reversal of the PCT cutaneous lesions and elevated porphyrin abnormalities when HCV was eliminated.[215] Since most sporadic PCT patients have HCV infections as a precipitating factor, the antiviral treatment has become widely accepted for PCT and has markedly reduced the PCT prevalence.

There are both genetic and environmental factors that cause the reduced hepatic activity of UROD (*Figure 28.1*), resulting in the accumulation of uroporphyrins (oxidized uroporphyrinogens), their release into the plasma, and excretion in the urine.[34] Clinically, PCT manifests as a photosensitive bullous dermatosis as a consequence of the circulating accumulated photoactive porphyrins. Neurovisceral symptoms do not occur. Symptoms typically arise in adult life (hence the name *tarda*) and are brought on by conditions driving hepatic siderosis, and/or environmental factors such as alcohol abuse, HCV or HIV infections, or oral estrogen therapy. Three subtypes of the disease have been recognized: familial, sporadic, and toxic.

Clinical Description

Skin lesions very similar to those in VP are found predominantly on light-exposed areas such as the face and hands, and in women, on the legs and feet as well. There is little discomfort with sun exposure per se; however, blue (visible) light triggers an insidious cutaneous damage. The most common complaint is marked skin fragility in areas subjected to repeated minor trauma, such as the hands and forearms (*Figure 28.4*). Vesicles and bullae form primarily on the dorsa of the hands and may erode, leaving atrophic scars that often display zones of both hyperpigmentation and hypopigmentation. Milia are commonly noted on the hands and, at times, on the face.

Facial hypertrichosis occurs in most patients, is generally more noticeable in women, and may be an isolated presenting feature. Hypertrichosis, sometimes striking, is occasionally observed on areas of the skin that are rarely exposed to the sun, such as the trunk and legs. Other findings include hyperpigmentation of facial skin, alopecia, and scleroderma-like changes on the skin of the face, neck, and hands. The histologic appearance of the scleroderma-like lesions is identical to

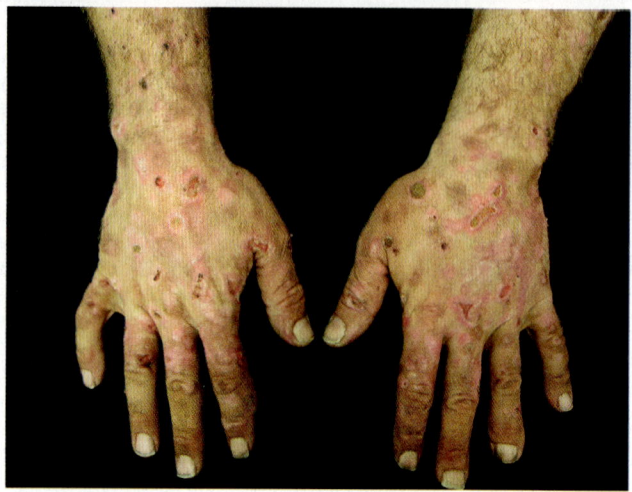

FIGURE 28.4 Porphyria cutanea tarda in a 56-year-old man. Note many erosions and denuded skin areas from ruptured blisters over the hands and forearms and an occasional blister.

that seen in patients with systemic scleroderma. Occasionally, patients have overt signs and symptoms of underlying liver disease, but no good correlation exists between the degree of liver disease and the occurrence or severity of the porphyria.

Molecular Basis and Pathogenesis

Familial PCT (type II), an autosomal dominant subtype that accounts for ~20% of PCT cases,[216,217] results from pathogenetic mutations in the *UROD* gene that reduce the enzymatic activity to half-normal in all tissues. UROD catalyzes the fifth heme biosynthetic step, in which uroporphyrinogen III is converted to coproporphyrinogen III (*Figure 28.1*). The human *UROD* cDNA and gene have localized to chromosome 1 (1p34)[218] and have been sequenced. Over 140 mutations have been reported in the *UROD* gene,[74,219] which usually encode unstable or inactive enzyme. The UROD crystal structure[220,221] has been determined.

Sporadic PCT (type I) results from reduced UROD activity restricted to the liver.[222-224] The catalytic activity and the immunoreactivity of UROD are normal in erythrocytes,[224] while the hepatic catalytic activity is decreased, but immunoreactive enzyme is present in normal or increased amounts.[224] After treatment (see below), both catalytic activity and immunoreactivity become normal.[225] These findings, and the lack of a family history of sporadic PCT, implied that this subtype is acquired and not inherited. At the molecular level, no mutations are present in the *UROD* gene or its promoter region.[226] However, in a few families, clinically manifest PCT was associated with decreased UROD activity in the liver and normal activity in erythrocytes and other tissues.[219] These cases have been called *type III PCT* because molecular studies have not identified *UROD* mutations, and yet multiple family members were affected.[227]

The photosensitivity symptoms result from the accumulating porphyrins, which are released into plasma and exert the photochemical reactions in the skin, as described for VP. Sclerodermoid changes in skin result from a light-independent effect (the "dark effect") of the porphyrin on collagen synthesis by skin fibroblasts.[228] The pathogenesis of the hyperpigmentation, hypopigmentation, and hypertrichosis is poorly understood.

Clinical expression of both familial and sporadic PCT is nearly always associated with prevalent confounding factors that cause hepatic injury, so the disorder remains silent without these. In large PCT studies, most patients had more than one of four cardinal hepatotoxic risk factors, namely excess hepatic iron, excessive alcohol use, viral infection (HCV and/or HIV), or oral medicinal estrogen use. Each of these risk factors is far more common than the previously estimated frequency of PCT (approximately 1 per 25,000).[34]

Mechanism of Hepatic Iron Pathogenesis

The central role of iron in the clinical expression of PCT has been recognized since 1961.[229,230] Numerous studies have documented hepatocellular siderosis in most patients with significant uroporphyrinuria. The iron deposits are generally moderate in amount, 1.5 to 4 times normal, but are usually greater with coinheritance of mutations in the *HFE* gene that lead to hemochromatosis.[231] On average, ~35% of PCT patients are heterozygous for the p.Cys282Tyr mutation in *HFE*, and 15% are homozygous or double heterozygotes for the p.His63Asp mutation in *HFE*. The cause of excess hepatic iron in the remaining cases appears to result from downregulation of hepcidin expression regardless of iron status and consequent to the oxidative stress associated with the other risk factors for PCT. Transfusional iron overload also promotes clinical expression of PCT.[232]

Depletion of iron by repetitive phlebotomy[233] or by administration of deferoxamine[234] uniformly induces both clinical and biochemical remissions. Replenishment of iron stores promptly reignites symptoms in patients in whom a remission has been induced by phlebotomy. An inhibitor of UROD was found in liver cytosol of a mouse model and PCT patients. The inhibitor is a partially oxidized uroporphyrinogen, a porphomethene, that is generated by iron or uncoupling of cytochrome P450s.[235,236] This is consistent with the diminished hepatic UROD activity without reduction in enzyme protein in symptomatic PCT patients and the restoration of hepatic UROD activity to its genetically determined level after iron depletion. The mechanism for the generation of sufficient porphomethene in patients with sporadic PCT that does not occur in iron overload states in general remains to be defined. The oxidative environment in the hepatocyte generated by the common environmental risk factors accompanying clinical expression of the disorder, as well as other traits such as the allele variants of CYP1A2 and G51M1A,[237] probably plays an important role.[238]

Precipitating Factors

Ethanol exacerbates PCT. Heavy alcohol intake was found in 25% to 100% of patients in many studies, and hepatic cirrhosis is not uncommon. The association of clinically expressed PCT with alcoholism would relate to its hepatotoxicity and its effect of stimulating iron absorption.[239]

A striking association between symptomatic PCT, familial and sporadic, and HCV is well recognized. Although most patients with HCV do not develop PCT, as many as 80% of PCT patients are chronically infected with the virus. This infection elicits oxidative stress in hepatocytes as well as downregulation of hepcidin expression and explains, in part, the liver damage in PCT. Association of PCT with HIV infection also occurs, and such patients may be infected with both HIV and HCV. Dual infection causes more severe hepatic disease; whether the HIV virus per se plays a role in the expression of PCT is not known. Thus, patients should be evaluated for the presence of HCV and HIV at the time of diagnosis.

The association of estrogen ingestion and expression of PCT occurs only in a very small percentage of patients who ingest estrogens, consistent with an underlying predisposition to the disease. The cutaneous symptoms have occurred with the use of estrogen as a postmenopausal supplement, for contraception, and for prostatic carcinoma. The mechanism of the estrogen effect is thought to relate to its adverse effects on the liver such as steatosis and steatohepatitis. It is generally a lesser factor because venesection alone has brought about full recovery. For women needing estrogen supplements at the usual dose, transdermal preparations have been shown to be safe, provided that storage iron is removed and maintained at a low level.

Additional susceptibility factors that are positively associated with PCT are smoking, allele variants of CYP1A2 and GSTM, and ascorbic acid deficiency. Several diverse drugs and radiation have also been implicated in precipitating PCT in a few cases.

Renal Dialysis

Patients with renal failure undergoing hemodialysis may develop PCT. Iron overload is not uncommon in these patients, and intravenous iron used in conjunction with erythropoietin for the anemia may precipitate clinical PCT. Hemodialysis or peritoneal dialysis does not effectively clear circulating plasma uroporphyrins, presumably because porphyrins are bound to proteins and can form polymers too large to cross the dialysis membrane.

Laboratory Findings

Patients with symptomatic PCT have markedly increased amounts of porphyrins in the urine. Uroporphyrin and heptacarboxylic porphyrin predominate, with lesser amounts of coproporphyrin and small amounts of 5- and 6-carboxylate porphyrins. Typically, the daily urinary excretion of uroporphyrin is approximately 3000 µg (normal, <50 µg), but considerably higher values may be found. Uroporphyrin in the urine is predominantly isomer I, whereas the heptacarboxylic porphyrin is predominantly isomer III. Photosensitive cutaneous symptoms rarely occur when the daily urinary excretion of uroporphyrin is <1000 µg. Urinary coproporphyrin rarely exceeds 600 µg daily.[240] An unusual and distinctive tetracarboxylic porphyrin, isocoproporphyrin, is excreted in feces,[241] and a slight increase may be noted in total fecal porphyrin excretion.[34] Plasma porphyrins are typically increased, with a fluorescence peak at neutral pH near 619 nm. Erythrocyte protoporphyrin may be moderately increased and is primarily zinc protoporphyrin.

Treatment

Exposure to alcohol and oral estrogen supplements in women, as well as smoking, should be avoided. Abstinence from alcohol can lead to remissions in some patients, especially if the PCT is associated with alcoholic liver disease, but removal of iron by phlebotomy can induce remissions even if alcohol intake continues.[233,242] In patients with PCT where HCV is the primary risk factor, antiviral treatment is effective as a single-agent therapy.[243] With the advent of markedly improved treatment of HCV with direct-acting antiviral agents (simeprevir, sofosbuvir, etc), they have become the treatment of choice for patients with PCT.[244,245] Transdermal administration of estrogen was found to be safe in a small number of patients,[246] and this avoids any possible first-pass effects of the hormone on the liver.

Previously, effective treatment of both sporadic and familial PCT was the removal of iron stores by phlebotomy, which leads to clinical and biochemical remission in virtually every case and may improve concomitant HCV infection. Phlebotomy should be initiated if there are no contraindications, with 500 mL removed every 1 to 2 weeks. Initial serum transferrin saturation and ferritin values are obtained to estimate the iron burden. Liver biopsy should be considered to assess the disease status of associated viral hepatitis and hemochromatosis and cirrhosis. Clinical remissions often occur after the removal of approximately 3 L of blood[233,240]; patients who also have hemochromatosis may require more frequent phlebotomies, including regular maintenance phlebotomies. The optimal approach is to achieve mild iron deficiency, defined by an onset of iron-limited erythropoiesis in which the mean corpuscular volume is decreased to low normal, the serum transferrin saturation is low normal, and the serum ferritin is near 20 µg/L or lower. Although further overproduction of uroporphyrin is minimized, the slow release of chronically accumulated, relatively hydrophobic porphyrins may take months to return to baseline. Patients should be advised that formation of new skin lesions ceases gradually, and full recovery often extends over several months to a year or more.[240] Remissions for years are the rule[233,240] and are permanent when the known precipitating factors are avoided or removed; any clinical and biochemical relapse responds to another course of phlebotomies.[233,240] It is expected that in patients with effectively treated HCV sustained remission will be maintained unless the patient again becomes infected with the virus.

Hydroxychloroquine and chloroquine have also been used in the treatment of PCT. After administration of chloroquine (0.5-1.0 g/d) for several days, a large amount of the porphyrins stored in the liver is mobilized and excreted in the urine. This purging effect results from the formation of an easily excreted water-soluble complex between uroporphyrin and the drug. The chloroquine effect was often accompanied by malaise, anorexia, fever, and signs of hepatocellular

Disorders of Red Blood Cells

damage. Subsequent use of lower doses made it possible to avoid the toxic response without impairing efficacy,[247] but this maneuver does not always preclude toxicity.[240] Low-dose hydroxychloroquine is as effective as phlebotomy.[248] Despite the potential hepatic reaction to this antimalarial and its needed readministration in time, this agent provides an alternative treatment particularly for patients for whom phlebotomy is unsuitable. Patients with associated *HFE* hemochromatosis appear not to respond to this therapy unless iron removal is initiated.[249]

The use of sunscreen agents effective in the Soret band of the spectrum and avoidance of sunlight through protective clothing can be useful until the beneficial effects of phlebotomy, low-dose chloroquine, or antiviral removal of the HCV are achieved.

Treatment of PCT patients with renal failure presents special challenges. The disorder may be particularly severe because such patients lack the renal excretory pathway for porphyrins, leading to higher porphyrin levels in plasma and tissues. Chloroquine-porphyrin complexes are not filtered out by standard hemodialysis. High-flux hemodialysis appears to remove porphyrins from plasma better and may be of some benefit. The treatment of choice is the administration of recombinant erythropoietin to mobilize stored iron and relieve the anemia so that phlebotomies can be performed as necessary to induce remission. This method is preferable to depleting iron stores by iron chelation. In patients refractory to these treatment methods, the porphyria fully resolved after renal transplantation.[250]

Hepatocellular Carcinoma

An increased frequency of HCCs is recognized in patients with PCT,[251] and such tumors are associated with a long symptomatic period before the start of treatment as well as with the presence of cirrhosis or chronic active hepatitis. Iron overload may also play a role. Thus, in the presence of hepatitis or cirrhosis, surveillance for HCC with regular hepatic imaging is indicated. In contrast, documented evidence supports a PCT-like illness as a manifestation of porphyrin-producing hepatoma in an otherwise normal liver (paraneoplastic PCT) in several cases.[252] When the tumor could be surgically removed, the cutaneous symptoms and biochemical abnormalities remitted.[252]

Toxic Porphyria Cutanea Tarda

In Turkey between 1956 and 1961, an epidemic of acquired porphyria affecting more than 3000 people occurred as a result of exposure to flour made from seed-wheat that had been treated with the fungicide, hexachlorobenzene.[253,254] Members of both sexes were affected, and many of the subjects were children. Affected people developed hepatomegaly, hypertrichosis, hyperpigmentation, uroporphyrinuria, and a photosensitive dermatosis. Uroporphyrinuria and a variety of other signs and symptoms persisted in some individuals for more than 25 years, and no effective therapy has been devised for this toxic porphyria. Animal models demonstrated that hexachlorobenzene leads to the formation of the porphomethene inhibitor of hepatic UROD. Iron magnifies this inhibitory effect, and clear genetic susceptibility to this type of acquired porphyria has been shown in mice.[255]

Other polyhalogenated aromatic hydrocarbons have also produced a toxic porphyria in humans. 2,3,7,8-Tetrachlorodibenzo-*p*-dioxin, a by-product in the manufacture of the herbicides 2,4-dichlorophenoxyacetic acid, 2,4,5-trichlorophenoxyacetic acid, and some polychlorinated biphenyls have proved porphyrinogenic for humans; all of these compounds are very strong inducers of cytochrome P450 enzymes that require heme. As in the case of hexachlorobenzene-induced porphyria, iron magnifies the inhibition of UROD, and iron depletion minimizes the inhibitory effect of these agents. The parallel between the permissive effects of iron in these toxic porphyria models and the role of iron in the pathogenesis of both familial and sporadic PCT is striking.

Hepatoerythropoietic Porphyria

In the rare homozygous form of familial PCT, hepatoerythropoietic porphyria (HEP), the skin changes described for PCT usually occur before the age of 5 years, and photosensitivity may be severe, resembling CEP and including disfigurement. Mild anemia, developmental delay, and seizures also have been reported. Other features are pink urine, dental fluorescence, and occasionally hepatosplenomegaly. These patients have residual UROD enzyme activity ranging from 3% to 20% of normal.[34,256,257] To date, over 40 *UROD* mutations causing HEP (homozygous or compound heterozygous) have been reported. Treatment for HEP is the same as for PCT. Severe anemia and cutaneous symptoms may respond to erythropoietin.[258] Preclinical efforts toward somatic gene therapy for HEP patients were initiated by demonstrating correction of the enzyme defect with retroviral gene transfer in transformed B-cell lines[259] and may become a prospect in vivo in the future. Prenatal exclusion of HEP has been performed.[260]

ERYTHROPOIETIC CUTANEOUS PORPHYRIAS

Three disorders, congenital erythropoietic porphyria (CEP), erythropoietic protoporphyria (EPP), and X-linked protoporphyria (XLP), a genetic variant of EPP, are classified as erythropoietic cutaneous porphyrias (*Table 28.1*). Recently, another genetic variant of EPP, CLPX protoporphyria, was identified but thus far only in one family. These disorders present with cutaneous photosensitivity that results from the marked accumulation of photoreactive porphyrins in the bone marrow and circulating erythrocytes. Unlike the other porphyrias, XLP is caused by gain-of-function of a heme biosynthetic enzyme.

Congenital Erythropoietic Porphyria

CEP (also known as Günther disease) is an ultrarare (~300 reported cases), panethnic, autosomal recessive disorder due to loss-of-function mutations in the uroporphyrinogen synthase (*UROS*) gene, which lead to the markedly deficient or absent activity of UROS, the fourth enzyme in the pathway (*Figure 28.1*). The enzymatic defect leads to the erythroid accumulation of uroporphyrin I and coproporphyrin I isomers, which are released into the circulation, gain access to tissues, and are primarily excreted in the urine. The accumulation of these photoactive metabolites, particularly in the skin, leads to the intense photosensitivity of CEP patients. Clinically, the disease is first detected in infancy, but it may not become apparent until later in life, dependent on the amount of residual UROS activity.

Clinical Description

Typically, the first sign of CEP is the reddish or pink urine discoloration of the infant's diapers, which fluoresces under Wood's light.[261] Particular attention to the discoloration should lead to the diagnosis of CEP prior to phototherapy for neonatal icterus, which can result in whole-body third-degree burns. Exposure to visible light is followed by the development of vesicular or bullous lesions containing a porphyrin-rich, fluorescent fluid. The lesions tend to heal slowly, leaving pigmented scars (*Figure 28.5A*). Often, they become infected, ulcerated, and necrotic. Over a period of years, patients develop progressive mutilation and disfigurement with loss of portions of the fingers, nose, eyelids, or ears (*Figure 28.5B*). Ocular effects include thinning and necrosis of the sclera; corneal scarring can lead to blindness.[262,263] Skin not exposed to light is unaffected. Hypertrichosis is prominent and fine hair growth may cover much of the face and extremities. Patients adopt extreme precautions to avoid the sun. Deposition of porphyrins in the dentin of the teeth causes them to appear red (erythrodontia), brown, or yellowish. Even if discoloration is not apparent in ordinary light, the teeth exhibit red fluorescence in UV light. At necropsy, the entire skeleton has this red fluorescence. Osteopenia and osteolytic lesions can occur. Anemia is detected in most patients, usually the spleen is enlarged. The most severe phenotypes are transfusion-dependent.

Molecular Basis and Pathogenesis

The accumulating porphyrins in CEP reflect a defect in the conversion of HMB to the III isomer of uroporphyrinogen. Cyclization of the linear tetrapyrrole to the biologically active III isomer requires UROS (*Figure 28.1*). Affected individuals are homozygotes or compound heterozygotes for *UROS* mutations that reduce the enzyme's activity

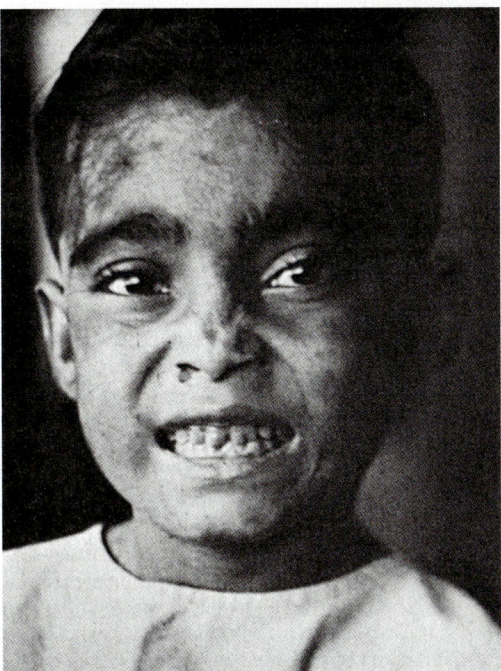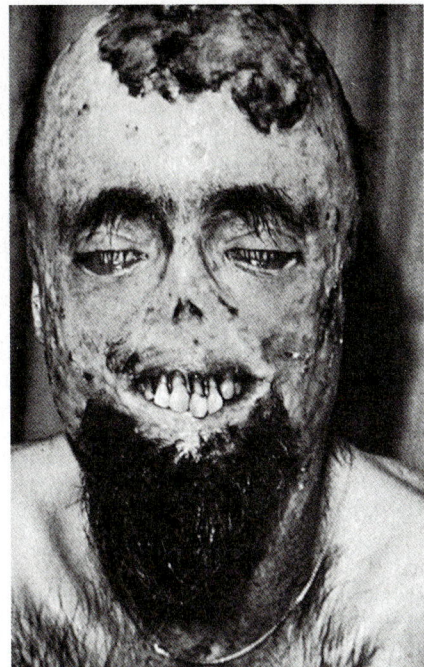

FIGURE 28.5 Congenital erythropoietic porphyria. A, In an Indian boy. Note facial hypertrichosis, scarring, and discoloration of the teeth. B, In a 50-year-old Caucasian man. Note the severe photomutilation. (Courtesy of Dr Neville Pimstone, University of California, Davis, CA.)

to 1%-20% of normal. Nonenzymatic cyclization of HMB produces uroporphyrinogen I, an isomer that can be converted to coproporphyrinogen I, but no further so both accumulate.

The *UROS* gene resides on chromosome 10 (10q25.2-q26.3) and has alternative promoters that generate identical housekeeping and erythroid-specific transcripts. Over 55 different *UROS* mutations have been reported,[74] the most common being p.Cys73Arg, which occurs in about one-third of patients and causes the most severe phenotype of nonimmune hydrops fetalis, transfusion-dependent anemia from birth, or both, particularly in homoallelic cases. Less clinically severe patients have been heteroallelic. The mutant proteins expressed in prokaryotic systems, or gene promoter-reporter activities for promoter mutations, have provided more precise genotype/phenotype correlations. However, there may be a marked divergence of phenotypic expression among siblings, suggesting undefined modifying factors.[264]

Variant CEP patients with mutations in the X-linked erythroid transcription factor GATA-binding protein 1 have been reported.[265,266] CEP also occurred with a milder phenotype in adults associated with a myelodysplastic syndrome (MDS); the pattern of excess porphyrin accumulation was similar to the childhood-onset CEP, but at lower concentrations.[267]

Although large quantities of porphyrin I isomers are released from erythroid cells in CEP patients, they are deposited in multiple tissues.[268] However, the clinical damage occurs in the skin and subcutaneous regions through oxygen-dependent phototoxic reactions on excitation by light. This relentless process leads in varying degrees to the formation of subepidermal bullae, secondary infection, scarring, epidermal atrophy, and resorption of acral structures. Anemia results from both hemolysis and ineffective erythropoiesis. Associated splenic sequestration leads to splenomegaly and variable leukopenia and thrombocytopenia.

Laboratory Findings

The anemia is normocytic, normochromic, and of variable severity. Detailed morphologic descriptions of the blood and bone marrow have been reported. Anisocytosis, poikilocytosis, polychromasia, basophilic stippling, and nucleated erythrocytes are fairly common features of the peripheral blood.[269] Following splenectomy, needle-like fluorescent red cell inclusions that may represent precipitated porphyrin have been observed.[269] Morphologic abnormalities of the bone marrow range

from erythroid hyperplasia to striking dyserythropoiesis. Nuclear inclusions containing hemoglobin may be present. Results of studies of the marrow with light and fluorescence microscopy reflect the coexistence of normal and abnormal erythropoietic cells.[270,271] Fluorescence is restricted to the morphologically abnormal cells and is most marked in cell nuclei. Kinetically, the anemia is characterized by both a shortened red cell survival and ineffective erythropoiesis.[272] Its morphologic and kinetic features closely resemble those of congenital dyserythropoietic anemia type I.

The characteristic metabolic abnormalities are the greatly increased urinary excretion of uroporphyrin and coproporphyrin I isomers. Total urinary porphyrin excretion may exceed 100 mg daily (normal is <300 μg), and the urine usually fluoresces on exposure to UV light. Fecal excretion of the more hydrophobic porphyrins, especially coproporphyrin I, is greatly increased.[34] The concentration of uroporphyrin I is increased in erythrocytes and plasma; the marrow porphyrin content exceeds that of the peripheral blood or other tissues.[34]

Treatment

Patients rely on avoidance of sunlight exposure and should be instructed to wear photoprotective clothing, including gloves and broad-brimmed hats. Conventional sunscreen agents are ineffective because they do not screen out the wavelengths in the Soret band of the visible spectrum (around 400 nm) that are responsible for inducing porphyrin-mediated photosensitivity.[166] Reflective sunblocks, such as zinc oxide and titanium oxide, are useful, but not often used.[273]

Accumulation of the porphyrins in erythroid tissue can be reduced by suppression of erythropoiesis with chronic hypertransfusion and concomitant iron chelation therapy,[274,275] or with hydroxyurea.[276] Most recently, treatment with the iron chelator, deferasirox, to inhibit *ALAS2* mRNA translation in a CEP patient resulted in a marked decrease of porphyrin accumulation, amelioration of hemolysis, and reduced photosensitivity.[277]

Hematopoietic stem cell transplantation (HSCT) remains the only curative treatment and has been successful in most of 22 patients.[263,278] Given the potential severe complications of HSCT, only severely affected, transfusion-dependent patients should be considered. Prenatal diagnosis can be made by demonstrating the fetal diagnosis by enzyme assay or mutation analysis of cultured amniotic fluid cells or chorionic villi.[279,280]

Disorders of Red Blood Cells

Erythropoietic Protoporphyria and X-Linked Protoporphyria

EPP is an autosomal recessive cutaneous disorder due to loss-of-function mutations in the *FECH* gene, which markedly reduce FECH enzymatic activity, resulting in the erythroid accumulation of its photoactive substrate, protoporphyrin IX (*Figure 28.1; Table 28.2*). EPP is likely the most common porphyria with an estimated prevalence of 1 per 75,000 to 200,000, particularly since the recent and curative antiviral treatment of HCV in PCT patients has reduced its frequency, which underlie most PCT cases. In addition, there are two recently described genetic variants of EPP, XLP, and CLPX porphyria. Both EPP variants have the same biochemical and clinical manifestations as EPP[281] (*Table 28.2*). XLP is caused by gain-of-function mutations in the last exon of *ALAS2*, while CLPX porphyria is due to mutations in the *CLPX* mitochondrial protein unfoldase gene that result in increased stability of ALAS2.[282] Both variants are characterized by accumulation of large amounts of metal-free protoporphyrin in erythroid tissue that is readily released into the plasma and taken up into dermal endothelial cells, leading to the acute photosensitivity.

Clinical Description

EPP typically manifests as photosensitivity in childhood. However, the cutaneous features of the photosensitivity are unlike those in patients with other porphyrias, which include bullae, scarring, sensitivity to trauma, hypertrichosis, and hyperpigmentation. EPP and XLP patients experience a prodrome when first exposed to sunlight in a few minutes to an hour or longer. These cutaneous sensations on the sun-exposed skin include stinging, prickling, itching, or burning (photoparesthesias) sensations. These are the warning signals to exit the sun immediately. About 25% of patients experience the prodromal sensations by 10 minutes and another 35% experience the sensations by 30 minutes of sun exposure. Continued sun exposure induces severe excruciating pain followed by erythema, urticaria, and edema, which can last 2 to 7 days.[283,284] Chronic skin changes may include shallow pitted scars or pseudovesicles over the cheeks and nose and thickened leathery skin (pachydermia) over the dorsa of the hands (*Figure 28.6A and B*).[283,285,286]

A number of EPP patients have been identified with palmar keratoderma.[287] They represent a subtype of EPP, which is characterized by seasonal palmar keratoderma, relatively low erythrocyte protoporphyrin concentrations, and biallelic pathogenic *FECH* mutations. These individuals appear to carry a lower risk of liver disease than other patients with EPP.[288]

Cholelithiasis tends to develop early in life[283] and ultimately occurs in approximately 10% of patients. The gallstones fluoresce and consist, in part, of precipitated protoporphyrin.[289] Vitamin D deficiency is common as a result of sun avoidance and is associated with a high prevalence of osteoporosis and osteopenia.[290] Pregnancy and breastfeeding may be associated with reduced photosensitivity and erythrocyte protoporphyrin levels.[291]

Although EPP is generally a disorder with variable clinical manifestations limited to the skin, a small subset of patients (less than 5%) develop progressive liver disease, leading to cirrhosis in the second to fourth decades of life and requiring liver transplantation. At autopsy, massive hepatic deposits of protoporphyrin are found.[292,293] Associated with the liver failure are rising blood protoporphyrin levels with progressive cholestasis, hemolysis, increasing photosensitivity, and neurologic crises resembling those of the acute porphyrias. The neurologic dysfunction was best correlated with a markedly increased level of plasma protoporphyrin and was believed to cause neurotoxicity, leading to axonal degeneration.[294]

Molecular Basis and Pathogenesis

In patients with EPP, decreased FECH activity (10%-30% of normal) is found in bone marrow, reticulocytes, liver, cultured skin fibroblasts, and lymphocytes. However, the protoporphyrin accumulates principally, if not entirely, in erythroid cells, whose contribution to heme production far exceeds that of all other tissues. Patients often exhibit a mild hypochromic-microcytic anemia as a consequence of the FECH deficiency and are frequently iron deficient. Protoporphyrin accumulates in bone marrow erythroblasts just before the nucleus is lost. Reticulocytes and young erythrocytes are the major source of protoporphyrin in plasma once released from these cells. The hydrophobic structure and low-water solubility necessitate protoporphyrin excretion exclusively through the biliary tract rather than urine.

The inheritance of EPP was first described as autosomal dominant with incomplete penetrance, or autosomal recessive in a few families. However, FECH activity in tissue lysates from patients with EPP symptoms was 20% to 30% of normal, and not the 50% expected for an autosomal dominant trait. Moreover, most obligate carriers of the disorder have no symptoms and their erythrocyte and fecal protoporphyrin levels are normal with tissue FECH activity of about 50% of normal.

Since the cloning and characterization of the human *FECH* gene,[295] located on chromosome 18 (18q21.3), over 215 different mutations have been identified.[74] Subsequently, it was found that over 95% of EPP patients had also inherited a "low-expression" *FECH* allele *trans* to a deleterious mutant allele.[296,297] The "low-expression" allele in the third intron of the *FECH* gene (*IVS3-48 T/C*) directs the use of an aberrant acceptor splice site in the gene.[297] The aberrantly spliced mRNA fraction is degraded, decreasing the steady-state level of normal *FECH* mRNA from this allele by more than 20% and explaining the observed FECH activity of less than 30% in this subset of EPP patients. The frequency of the hypomorphic *IVS3-48C* allele differs widely between ethnic groups, ranging from ~34% in Japanese to less than 1% in West Africans, and in general correlates with the prevalence of clinical EPP among individuals with a mutant *FECH* allele in the different populations.[298] Because the structure of FECH is a homodimer,[299] some mutations may lead to nonfunctional homodimers, resulting in a residual enzyme activity of less than 50% in the absence of the low-expression allele. Once the combination of *FECH* mutations leads to an enzyme activity of 30% or less of mean normal, the disease phenotype is expressed.

XLP accounts for ~2% and 10% of patients with an EPP phenotype in the United Kingdom and the United States, respectively.[300] In XLP patients, the FECH enzyme activity is normal, but erythrocyte protoporphyrin concentrations may be higher than in EPP, especially in males, whereas the levels in female heterozygotes can range from normal to levels as high as in their affected male relatives. This variability in females results from random X-chromosome inactivation.[301] Up to 50% of the accumulated protoporphyrin is zinc-protoporphyrin, indicating that the supply of the iron substrate as well as FECH activity becomes rate limiting. At least five mutations have been identified in the last exon (exon 11) of the *ALAS2* gene that lead to the deletion or elongation of C-terminal amino acids of the enzyme. Enzymatic activity of recombinant mutants is increased two- to threefold[302] as a result of altered protein conformation.[303] These gain-of-function mutations explain the increase in protoporphyrin and contrasts with other previously described *ALAS2* mutations that decrease enzyme activity and cause X-linked sideroblastic anemia (see Chapter 26).

CLPX protoporphyria, an autosomal dominant disorder, has only been described in one family to date, with affected individuals having markedly increased levels of zinc and free protoporphyrin as in XLP. There was a missense mutation in the *CLPX* gene[282] that reduced the ATPase activity of the CLPX protein, thereby decreasing the turnover of the ALAS2 enzyme and leading to increased ALA production. The body iron status may account for the variable severity among the family members.

The pathophysiology of EPP is mediated by accumulated metal-free protoporphyrin. As it leaks out of erythroid cells into the plasma, it gains entry into tissues. It is extracted solely by the liver and secreted unchanged into the bile. The liver is capable of clearing large amounts of protoporphyrin, but its secretion across the canalicular membrane and into the bile appears to be rate limiting.[284] Yet, despite microscopic evidence of hepatobiliary changes in many EPP patients, cholestasis leads to cirrhosis and hepatic failure in only a few (less than 5%).

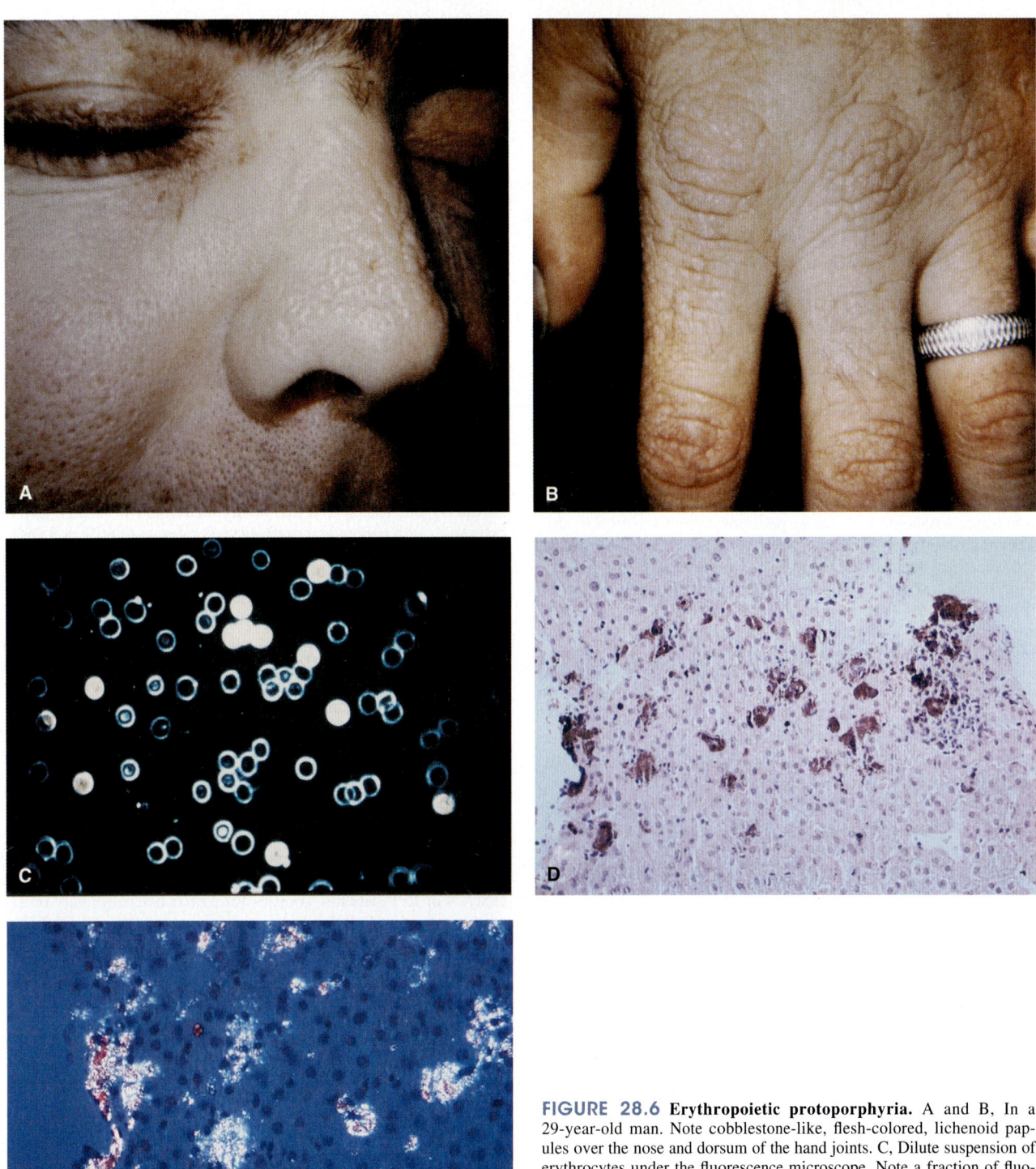

FIGURE 28.6 Erythropoietic protoporphyria. A and B, In a 29-year-old man. Note cobblestone-like, flesh-colored, lichenoid papules over the nose and dorsum of the hand joints. C, Dilute suspension of erythrocytes under the fluorescence microscope. Note a fraction of fluorescing cells. D and E, Needle biopsy section of the liver. Note deposits of protoporphyrin pigment in the parenchyma and a portal triad (D), and birefringence of the deposits, including a dark Maltese cross figure near the left center (E). (C, Courtesy of Dr Maureen Poh-Fitzpatrick, Columbia University, New York.)

In the skin, the hydrophobic protoporphyrin transfers readily from erythrocytes into the plasma and is taken up by the endothelial cells of the superficial capillaries in the upper dermis. When the photons penetrate these capillaries, the photoactive protoporphyrin triggers the light-induced skin symptoms.[285,304] Porphyrin-sensitized, oxygen-dependent histochemical reactions and the activation of complement eliciting an inflammatory response are involved in the light-induced pathogenesis.[305,306] The conjugated double-bond structure of protoporphyrin renders it highly photoactive, resulting in the unique acute epidermal phototoxicity,[307] in contrast to the porphyrins that accumulate in the other porphyrias with cutaneous photosensitivity. The activated porphyrin also stimulates fibroblast proliferation, accounting for a characteristic waxy appearance of the sun-exposed skin.[306]

Laboratory Findings

The defining laboratory manifestation of a protoporphyria is a greatly increased total erythrocyte protoporphyrin concentration. In EPP, reported values range from 600 to 4500 µg/dL (normal, less than 80 µg/dL).[34,283] It is essential to fractionate the total protoporphyrin for the relative proportions of metal-free protoporphyrin and zinc protoporphyrin, because in EPP, the metal-free form is more than 85% and zinc protoporphyrin is less than 15%.[308-310] In the XLP and CLPX variants, the proportion of zinc protoporphyrin ranges from 15% to 50% and its greater abundance can almost always differentiate them from EPP; total erythrocyte protoporphyrin values range from 1130 to 11,000 µg/dL in XLP, the higher values in males. Increased levels of erythrocyte protoporphyrin are observed in other conditions, including iron deficiency, lead poisoning, anemia of chronic inflammation, and hemolytic disorders, but only rarely do they exceed 300 µg/dL, and the protoporphyrin is the zinc chelate. In protoporphyria, plasma protoporphyrin is usually increased as well, and a normal plasma porphyrin in a patient with increased erythrocyte protoporphyrin may exclude EPP. The life-threatening liver disease may be predicted by increasing erythrocyte and plasma protoporphyrin levels along with altered liver function tests. In patients with severe protoporphyric liver disease, the erythrocyte protoporphyrin concentration generally exceeds 2000 µg/dL, and values greater than 8000 µg/dL have been reported.

Fluorescence microscopy of a dilute suspension of freshly obtained blood reveals fluorescence in a variable proportion of erythrocytes (*Figure 28.6C*).[307] Protoporphyrin is increased chiefly in young erythrocytes. In asymptomatic carriers, a small population of such fluorocytes may be detected even when the erythrocyte protoporphyrin concentration is normal.[311]

Fecal protoporphyrin excretion is often increased in symptomatic patients.[283] Values may be as high as 1400 µg/g of dry weight (normally less than 100 µg/g) and vary widely from patient to patient. An increasing ratio of erythrocyte to fecal protoporphyrin and an increasing ratio of biliary protoporphyrin to biliary bile acids may also suggest impending hepatic decompensation.[292,312,313] Urinary porphyrin and porphyrin precursor concentrations are normal.

Although most patients with EPP have mild microcytic/hypochromic anemia and reduced iron stores, intestinal absorption of iron does not appear to be impaired, yet hepcidin levels are unaltered.[314] Limited assimilation of iron appears to be an adaptive feature of the disorder. Studies of red cell survival and iron kinetics failed to detect a characteristic abnormality, but hemolysis has been occasionally reported. Some cases exhibit ring sideroblasts in erythroblasts (see Chapter 26), but others do not.

The majority of patients with EPP have no clinical evidence of liver disease, although 20% to 30% have slight elevations of liver enzymes. In eight families with XLP, a higher percentage of liver dysfunction was noted. However, in most if not in all cases, the liver contains dark brown pigment deposits in hepatocytes, Kupffer cells, and portal macrophages as well as within the lumens of ductules and interlobular ducts that exhibit the characteristic red fluorescence of protoporphyrin when transilluminated with wavelengths 380 to 500 nm (*Figure 28.6D*). These deposits are crystalline in nature on electron microscopy. They also exhibit a distinctive type of birefringence, not shared by any other pigment known to occur in the liver, that is demonstrable in routinely fixed and hematoxylin and eosin–stained paraffin-embedded sections (*Figure 28.6E*). Not infrequently, the pigmentation is accompanied by bile stasis and varying degrees of portal inflammation, fibrosis, and ductular proliferation. In patients who have developed liver failure, liver histology shows micronodular or macronodular cirrhosis and massive deposits of the pigment throughout.

Targeted DNA sequencing of *FECH* or *ALAS2* identified mutations in about 95% of patients. Because large intragenic deletions in *FECH* are not uncommon, their identification requires the use of a gene dosage analyses.

Treatment

The use of protective clothing, gloves, hats, etc is essential when outdoors. Topical sunscreens are not effective. The only readily available effective topical preparations are opaque formulations containing oxidates of zinc or titanium. Indoors or in a vehicle, window glass is not protective if not tinted, and operating room lights without yellow filters during prolonged surgical or dental procedures may cause phototoxic reactions.

Afamelanotide (brand name Scenesse, manufactured by Clinuvel, Melbourne, Australia), a synthetic analog of α-melanocyte-stimulating hormone, improves sun tolerance in EPP and XLP by increasing skin pigmentation by promoting melanin production and reduces free radical formation and cytokine production.[315] It is available in Europe and the United States for adults. The preparation is a 16 mg sustained-release resorbable implant formulation of afamelanotide that is inserted subcutaneously every other month. Two randomized trials (74 patients in Europe, 94 patients in the United States)[315] and a retrospective study of 115 EPP patients[316] demonstrated that this prophylactic treatment increased sunlight tolerance and improved QOL. The agent does not affect porphyrin production or alter the underlying disease process. Once severe liver damage has occurred, no form of medical therapy is currently effective. Thus, liver transplantation should be undertaken as a life-saving measure. The results have been favorable, with patient and graft survival rates up to 66% at 5 years.[317] However, the protoporphyrin burden from erythroid tissue remains and recurrence of protoporphyrin hepatopathy is common, supporting the need for bone marrow transplantation in these patients. HSCT has been performed in several EPP patients with a prior liver transplant to treat or prevent disease recurrence in the graft.[318] In a small child with XLP and severe hepatic fibrosis, HSCT was successful with marked improvement of the fibrosis.[319] Identification of patients at risk of severe liver disease remains a challenge.

The most definitive treatment for the disease would be replacement of the defective gene in affected tissues. *In vitro* studies have demonstrated effective transfer of the normal *FECH* cDNA into cultured fibroblasts from patients with EPP that corrected the biochemical defect.[320,321] In another in vitro approach, antisense oligonucleotide treatment of erythroid cells from an EPP patient abrogated the aberrant splicing of the common polymorphic IVS3-48C allele, reducing protoporphyrin accumulation to an asymptomatic level.[322] Genetic analysis of EPP patients' spouses for *FECH* heterozygosity or a low-expression *FECH* allele allows assessment for the risk EPP in their offspring as well as an indication for prenatal testing or preimplantation genetic diagnosis.

Long-Term Management

It is advisable to monitor erythrocyte and plasma protoporphyrin levels as well as liver function tests annually for early detection of protoporphyric hepatopathy. Reversible causes of liver dysfunction should be identified and treated. Patients should avoid excess exposure to alcohol and hepatotoxic drugs as well as drugs or hormone preparations that impair hepatic excretory function. Preventive hepatitis A and B vaccinations are recommended. Annual complete blood count and ferritin are advised to detect development of significant iron deficiency that may increase protoporphyrin levels and accentuate photosensitivity. Vitamin D deficiency is prevented by monitoring serum 25-hydroxy vitamin D levels and by providing vitamin supplementation.

Late-Onset Protoporphyria

EPP that is clinically indistinguishable from the inherited forms may develop later in life in the setting of an MDS[323] or a myeloproliferative disorder.[324] In these cases, a clone with mutated *FECH* alleles expands to dominate erythropoiesis. Over 15 such patients have been described[325]; most have loss of a *FECH* allele as from a complete or partial deletion of chromosome 18, and the presence of the sideroblastic anemia MDS subtype is common (see Chapter 26).[326,327]

DUAL PORPHYRIAS

On the basis of clinical and biochemical studies, approximately 15 patients and their families have been described to have dual porphyrias, resulting from simultaneous deficiency of two heme biosynthetic enzymes. To date, eight different combinations have been reported, including UROD and PPOX; UROD and HMBS; UORD and UROS; UROD and CPOX; HMBS and PPOX; PPOX and CPOX; CPOX and UROS; and CPOX and ALAD.[328] In some cases, the disease manifestations were severe or even fatal. Although these cases were reported as early as the 1980s, it was not until 2006 that DNA sequencing confirmed the presence of molecular defects in two heme biosynthetic genes in two patients. One patient had a mutation in their *CPOX* and *ALAD* genes[329] while the other had *UROD* and *HMBS* mutations[330] that were confirmed to be pathogenic by in vitro expression assays.[330] Thus, these studies identified the first bona fide dual porphyria patient.

The most well-known report of a dual porphyria is "Chester porphyria," which was described in a large kindred residing in Chester, UK. Affected family members exhibited acute neurovisceral attacks and biochemical characteristics consistent with co-existence of AIP and VP, most notably, deficient HMBS and PPOX activities in peripheral blood leukocytes.[331] However, DNA analyses of this family revealed only a nonsense mutation in the *HMBS* gene and did not detect a defect in *PPOX*.[332] Given the rarity of *PPOX* mutations that are undetectable by standard DNA sequencing (e.g., mutations deep in the intron, large deletions, etc.), it is highly likely that these individuals have AIP, rather than a dual porphyria. These findings highlight the importance of confirming the diagnosis of dual porphyrias with molecular testing.

KEY CLINICAL SUMMARY POINTS

Broad Definitions of the Eight Major Porphyrias

The porphyrias comprise a group of distinct genetic disorders, each resulting from the partial deficiency (with one exception) of a specific enzyme in the eight-step heme biosynthetic pathway (*Figure 28.1*) with its root cause known at the molecular level. The pathophysiology of clinical manifestations rests on the toxicity profile of the accumulated pathway intermediate(s) (*Table 28.2*) caused by the enzyme deficiency, much like roadwork causing a traffic jam in front of the roadwork. Additionally, although heme synthesis is essential in all cells, the metabolic block of a defective enzyme in porphyrias is expressed either in the liver or in the erythroid tissue, the principal sites of body heme production.

Acute hepatic porphyrias (AIP, VP, HCP, ADP) are clinically expressed when the impaired heme pathway in the liver is taxed further through its marked induction by factors such as drugs (P450 inducers), progesterone, and dietary restrictions, so that the putatively neurotoxic ALA and/or PBG accumulate, leading exclusively to neurovisceral manifestations. The sites of the primary biosynthetic block in VP and HCP account for porphyrin accumulations also causing cutaneous photosensitivity.

Porphyria cutanea tarda (PCT), or *chronic hepatic porphyria,* is expressed in the liver and is linked to deficient UROD in combination with various hepatotoxins (iron, alcohol, viral hepatitis, estrogen), causing insidious, protracted skin fragility and a bullous photodermatosis due to uroporphyrin accumulation. Although familial PCT (type II), associated with inherited UROD deficiency, is less common than the sporadic (type I) form, a genetic basis for the latter has not been identified.

Erythropoietic protoporphyria (EPP) is expressed in erythroid cells where the deficient FECH activity becomes rate limiting for heme synthesis. The nature of the accumulated metal-free protoporphyrin uniquely elicits acute cutaneous photosensitivity without blistering or skin fragility. Fulminant protoporphyric liver disease occurs unpredictably in less than 5% of patients.

X-linked protoporphyria (XLP), like EPP, is expressed in erythroid tissue but is much less common. It is unique among the porphyrias in that it is caused by gain-of-function mutations in the erythroid ALAS (ALAS2). The two- to threefold increase of ALA synthase in erythroid tissue drives the pathway excessively, so that FECH and iron become rate limiting. Protoporphyrin accumulates in greater amounts, and protoporphyric liver disease is more frequent than in EPP.

Congenital erythropoietic porphyria (CEP) is expressed in erythroid cells where the roadblock caused by marked UROS deficiency coupled to the site of 85% of body heme production results in massive uroporphyrin and coproporphyrin accumulation, causing the most severe photodermatosis of the cutaneous porphyrias with usual onset in early life.

In the presence of clinical manifestations, accurate diagnosis of each porphyria can be established with characteristic laboratory test abnormalities.

Diagnosis and Treatment of Acute Hepatic Porphyrias (AIP, VP, HCP)
Diagnosis

Consider an acute porphyria attack in all adults with unexplained symptoms seen in acute porphyria (*Table 28.3*). Suggestive features are as follows: abdominal pain, muscle weakness, CNS disturbance, seizures, hyponatremia, dark or orange-red urine.

Test for *increased urine PBG* in single-voided sample, which is singularly specific for diagnosis of an acute attack in AIP, VP, and HCP. Then save same urine sample to establish the porphyria type by quantitation of ALA, PBG, and porphyrin levels together with measurements of plasma porphyrin, fecal porphyrins, and erythrocyte PBGD (*Table 28.2*).

During remission, these quantitative tests can usually but not always establish the diagnosis. Suggestive but inconclusive results can be confirmed by mutational analysis.

Treatment

For a biochemically documented *acute attack*: (1) Usually hospitalize patient for control of acute symptoms: withdraw unsafe medications, correct dehydration/electrolyte imbalance; provide nutritional support and narcotic analgesics for pain, phenothiazine for nausea/vomiting, β-adrenergic blockers for hypertension; consider seizure precautions. (2) Begin hemin (3-4 mg/kg/d for at least 4 days) as soon as possible; give intravenous glucose (10%, 300 g/d) for mild attacks or while awaiting hemin delivery. (3) Monitor patient closely for respiratory and neurologic status; serum electrolytes, magnesium, and renal function; bladder distention.

Follow-Up

(1) Educate patient and family about the disease, its inheritance, precipitating factors, and important preventive measures. (2) Encourage patient to wear medical alert bracelet and to keep records of diagnostic studies and recommended therapy. (3) Treat chronic manifestations such as pain and depression, and disability. (4) Provide access to genetic testing for patient and family members. (5) Monitor for renal function and HCC with hepatic imaging. (6) For severe recurrent attacks unresponsive to supportive therapy, consider curative liver transplantation as a last resort. For up-to-date information regarding treatment and long-term management of AHPs, see References 41, 130, and 333.

Diagnosis and Treatment of Porphyria Cutanea Tarda
Diagnosis

Consider in all patients with symptoms of cutaneous fragility, blister formation, poorly healing ulcerations.

Plasma porphyrin is increased. Urine uroporphyrin with 7-carboxylate porphyrin is usually greater than 1000 µg/24 hours. In type II PCT, erythrocyte UROD activity is approximately 50% of normal and is normal in type I PCT.

Assess for factors precipitating clinical disease: iron overload with serum transferrin saturation, serum ferritin, and DNA analysis for genetic hemochromatosis; hepatitis C, HIV; alcohol excess; estrogen use; chronic renal disease.

Treatment

(1) Discontinue any risk agents. (2) Perform one unit (500 mL) phlebotomy every 2 weeks to a serum ferritin level of 20; if phlebotomy is contraindicated or not tolerated, use oral hydroxychloroquine (100 mg twice a week) or chloroquine (125 mg twice a week). (3) In the presence of chronic renal disease, facilitate phlebotomy with erythropoietin. (4) Provide sunscreen agent against the 400 to 420 nm light spectrum until primary therapy is effective. (5) Treat any concomitant hepatitis after the patient is deironed.

Follow-Up

(1) Educate patient about the disease and preventive measures. (2) Monitor plasma porphyrin yearly for potential symptom recurrence. (3) In the presence of hepatitis or cirrhosis, monitor yearly for HCC with hepatic imaging. (4) Consider mutation analysis if type II PCT is likely, and then genetic testing of family members.

Diagnosis and Treatment of Protoporphyrias (EPP, XLP, CLPX)

Diagnosis

Consider in infants/children with cutaneous symptoms of intense burning pain often within minutes of sun/light exposure, with or without redness or swelling. Chronic changes of sun-exposed skin include shallow facial scars and/or leathery skin over dorsal hands. Very rarely advanced liver disease may be the predominant presenting feature. In adults, the clinical phenotype suggests late-onset disease associated with a clonal hematopoietic disorder.

In EPP, erythrocyte protoporphyrin is greater than 600 µg/dL, greater than 85% as metal-free; plasma porphyrin is usually increased. In XLP and CLPX defect, 50% to 85% of erythrocyte protoporphyrin is metal-free and 15% to 50% is zinc-protoporphyrin. Fecal porphyrins may be increased or normal.

Assess hepatic function.

Treatment

(1) Avoid sunlight (including long-wave UV light that passes through windows) with protective clothing. (2) Suggest a tanning product that increases pigmentation. (3) Advise a trial of synthetic β-carotene (Lumitene, Tishcon Corporation, Westbury, New York) to improve sunlight tolerance. (4) Prescribe the α-melanocyte-stimulating hormone analog afamelanotide (Scenesse; Clinuvel, Melbourne, Australia); it is available in Europe and the United States. (5) Prevent vitamin D insufficiency with supplementation if blood levels are low. (6) Avoid cholestatic agents (e.g., estrogens).

For severe liver disease: cholestyramine and other porphyrin absorbents, plasmapheresis and intravenous hemin may be helpful; liver transplantation and/or HSCT may be required.

Follow-Up

(1) Educate patient and family about the disease. (2) Provide patient and family members access to genetic testing. (3) Monitor erythrocyte protoporphyrin(s) and hepatic function yearly; if cholelithiasis is suspected, monitor with imaging.

Diagnosis and Treatment of Congenital Erythropoietic Porphyria

Diagnosis

Consider in infants/children with symptoms of marked skin fragility, bullous photodermatosis prone to infection, disfigurement of face and hands in time; red, fluorescent diaper may be an initial clue for the disorder. Beginning in adults, the cutaneous symptoms most likely reflect late-onset disease associated with a clonal hematopoietic disorder.

Measurement of erythrocyte, plasma, urine, and fecal porphyrins reveals massively increased levels of uroporphyrin I and coproporphyrin I.

Evaluate for hemolytic anemia and test for dental fluorescence.

Treatment

(1) Rigorously protect from sunlight and treat infected skin lesions. (2) Give red cell transfusions for symptomatic anemia; splenectomy may be necessary for marked hypersplenism. (3) Consider inducing iron restriction with deferasirox for disease manifestations. (4) Erythrocyte hypertransfusion reduces porphyrin accumulation and requires management of attendant iron overload. (5) Porphyrin binders (e.g., oral charcoal) may reduce the porphyrin burden. (6) Consider HSCT for severe progressive disease; it has been successful and curative in a majority of patients so treated.

Follow-Up

See Reference 280.

Mutation Analysis

After biochemical studies have defined the type of porphyria, DNA analysis to identify the disease-causing mutation(s) is recommended, permitting rapid and accurate detection of asymptomatic at-risk family members. Mutation analysis is available for each porphyria at **Sema4** (www.sema4.com). For the AHPs, genetic testing is offered free of charge to those who are eligible through **Invitae** (www.invitae.com/en/alnylam-act-ahp/).

Website Resources

www.rarediseasesnetwork.org
www.porphyria.org (Porphyria patient advocacy organization)
www.uptodate.com
www.drugs-porphyria.org (Drug database for AHPs)
www.porphyria.com
www.panhematin.com

ACKNOWLEDGMENT

The authors and editor acknowledge the contribution of Dr. Sylvia Bottomley as author of this chapter in the previous several editions of Wintrobe.

References

1. Chiabrando D, Vinchi F, Fiorito V, et al. Heme in pathophysiology: a matter of scavenging, metabolism and trafficking across cell membranes. *Front Pharmacol.* 2014;5:61.
2. Mense SM, Zhang L. Heme: a versatile signaling molecule controlling the activities of diverse regulators ranging from transcription factors to MAP kinases. *Cell Res.* 2006;16:681-692.
3. Ogawa K, Sun J, Taketani S, et al. Heme mediates derepression of Maf recognition element through direct binding to transcription repressor Bach1. *EMBO J.* 2001;20:2835-2843.
4. Poulos TL. Heme enzyme structure and function. *Chem Rev.* 2014;114:3919-3962.
5. Reedy CJ, Gibney BR. Heme protein assemblies. *Chem Rev.* 2004;104:617-649.
6. Shimizu T, Lengalova A, Martinek V, et al. Heme: emergent roles of heme in signal transduction, functional regulation and as catalytic centres. *Chem Soc Rev.* 2019;48:5624-5657.
7. Wu N, Yin L, Hanniman EA, et al. Negative feedback maintenance of heme homeostasis by its receptor, Rev-erbalpha. *Genes Dev.* 2009;23:2201-2209.
8. Phillips JD. Heme biosynthesis and the porphyrias. *Mol Genet Metab.* 2019;128:164-177.
9. Peoc'h K, Nicolas G, Schmitt C, et al. Regulation and tissue-specific expression of delta-aminolevulinic acid synthases in non-syndromic sideroblastic anemias and porphyrias. *Mol Genet Metab.* 2019;128:190-197.
10. Yasuda M, Chen B, Desnick RJ. Recent advances on porphyria genetics: inheritance, penetrance & molecular heterogeneity, including new modifying/causative genes. *Mol Genet Metab.* 2019;128:320-331.
11. Puy H, Gouya L, Deybach JC. Porphyrias. *Lancet.* 2010;375:924-937.
12. Galy B, Ferring-Appel D, Sauer SW, et al. Iron regulatory proteins secure mitochondrial iron sufficiency and function. *Cell Metab.* 2010;12:194-201.
13. Harigae H, Suwabe N, Weinstock PH, et al. Deficient heme and globin synthesis in embryonic stem cells lacking the erythroid-specific delta-aminolevulinate synthase gene. *Blood.* 1998;91:798-805.
14. Hentze MW, Muckenthaler MU, Andrews NC. Balancing acts: molecular control of mammalian iron metabolism. *Cell.* 2004;117:285-297.
15. Ishikawa H, Kato M, Hori H, et al. Involvement of heme regulatory motif in heme-mediated ubiquitination and degradation of IRP2. *Mol Cell.* 2005;19:171-181.
16. Kaldy P, Menotti E, Moret R, et al. Identification of RNA-binding surfaces in iron regulatory protein-1. *EMBO J.* 1999;18:6073-6083.
17. Reichard JF, Motz GT, Puga A. Heme oxygenase-1 induction by NRF2 requires inactivation of the transcriptional repressor BACH1. *Nucleic Acids Res.* 2007;35:7074-7086.

18. Sadlon TJ, Dell'Oso T, Surinya KH, et al. Regulation of erythroid 5-aminolevulinate synthase expression during erythropoiesis. *Int J Biochem Cell Biol.* 1999;31:1153-1167.

19. Sanchez M, Galy B, Schwanhaeusser B, et al. Iron regulatory protein-1 and -2: transcriptome-wide definition of binding mRNAs and shaping of the cellular proteome by iron regulatory proteins. *Blood.* 2011;118:e168-e179.

20. Ades IZ, Stevens TM, Drew PD. Biogenesis of embryonic chick liver delta-aminolevulinate synthase: regulation of the level of mRNA by hemin. *Arch Biochem Biophys.* 1987;253:297-304.

21. Cable EE, Miller TG, Isom HC. Regulation of heme metabolism in rat hepatocytes and hepatocyte cell lines: delta-aminolevulinic acid synthase and heme oxygenase are regulated by different heme-dependent mechanisms. *Arch Biochem Biophys.* 2000;384:280-295.

22. Hayashi N, Watanabe N, Kikuchi G. Inhibition by hemin of in vitro translocation of chicken liver delta-aminolevulinate synthase into mitochondria. *Biochem Biophys Res Commun.* 1983;115:700-706.

23. Lathrop JT, Timko MP. Regulation by heme of mitochondrial protein transport through a conserved amino acid motif. *Science.* 1993;259:522-525.

24. Yamamoto M, Kure S, Engel JD, et al. Structure, turnover, and heme-mediated suppression of the level of mRNA encoding rat liver delta-aminolevulinate synthase. *J Biol Chem.* 1988;263:15973-15979.

25. Tian Q, Li T, Hou W, et al. Lon peptidase 1 (LONP1)-dependent breakdown of mitochondrial 5-aminolevulinic acid synthase protein by heme in human liver cells. *J Biol Chem.* 2011;286:26424-26430.

26. Trakshel GM, Kutty RK, Maines MD. Cadmium-mediated inhibition of testicular heme oxygenase activity: the role of NADPH-cytochrome c (P-450) reductase. *Arch Biochem Biophys.* 1986;251:175-187.

27. Maines MD, Trakshel GM, Kutty RK. Characterization of two constitutive forms of rat liver microsomal heme oxygenase. Only one molecular species of the enzyme is inducible. *J Biol Chem.* 1986;261:411-419.

28. Yoshida T, Kikuchi G. Purification and properties of heme oxygenase from pig spleen microsomes. *J Biol Chem.* 1978;253:4224-4229.

29. Yoshida T, Kikuchi G. Purification and properties of heme oxygenase from rat liver microsomes. *J Biol Chem.* 1979;254:4487-4491.

30. Maines MD, Ibrahim NG, Kappas A. Solubilization and partial purification of heme oxygenase from rat liver. *J Biol Chem.* 1977;252:5900-5903.

31. Singleton JW, Laster L. Biliverdin reductase of Guinea pig liver. *J Biol Chem.* 1965;240:4780-4789.

32. Yamaguchi T, Komoda Y, Nakajima H. Biliverdin-IX alpha reductase and biliverdin-IX beta reductase from human liver. Purification and characterization. *J Biol Chem.* 1994;269:24343-24348.

33. Tenhunen R, Marver HS, Schmid R. The enzymatic conversion of heme to bilirubin by microsomal heme oxygenase. *Proc Natl Acad Sci U S A.* 1968;61:748-755.

34. Anderson KE, Sassa S, Bishop DF. Disorders of heme Biosynthesis: X-linked sideroblastic anemia and the porphyrias. In: Scriver CS, Beaudet AI, Sly WS, eds. *The Molecular and Metabolic Bases of Inherited Disease.* 8th ed. McGraw-Hill; 2001:2961-3062.

35. de Matteis F. Disturbances of liver porphyrin metabolism caused by drugs. *Pharmacol Rev.* 1967;19:523-557.

36. Miller LK, Kappas A. The effect of progesterone on activities of delta-aminolevulinic acid synthetase and delta-aminolevulinic acid dehydratase in estrogen-primed avian oviduct. *Gen Comp Endocrinol.* 1974;22:238-244.

37. Sassa S, Bradlow HL, Kappas A. Steroid induction of delta-aminolevulinic acid synthase and porphyrins in liver. Structure-activity studies and the permissive effects of hormones on the induction process. *J Biol Chem.* 1979;254:10011-10020.

38. Handschin C, Lin J, Rhee J, et al. Nutritional regulation of hepatic heme biosynthesis and porphyria through PGC-1alpha. *Cell.* 2005;122:505-515.

39. Podvinec M, Handschin C, Looser R, et al. Identification of the xenosensors regulating human 5-aminolevulinate synthase. *Proc Natl Acad Sci U S A.* 2004;101:9127-9132.

40. Bonkovsky HL, Maddukuri VC, Yazici C, et al. Acute porphyrias in the USA: features of 108 subjects from porphyrias consortium. *Am J Med.* 2014;127:1233-1241.

41. Anderson KE. Acute hepatic porphyrias: current diagnosis & management. *Mol Genet Metab.* 2019;128:219-227.

42. Lahiji AP, Anderson KE, Chan A, et al. 5-Aminolevulinate dehydratase porphyria: update on hepatic 5-aminolevulinic acid synthase induction and long-term response to hemin. *Mol Genet Metab.* 2020;131:418-423.

43. Whatley SD, Mason NG, Woolf JR, et al. Diagnostic strategies for autosomal dominant acute porphyrias: retrospective analysis of 467 unrelated patients referred for mutational analysis of the HMBS, CPOX, or PPOX gene. *Clin Chem.* 2009;55:1406-1414.

44. Elder G, Harper P, Badminton M, et al. The incidence of inherited porphyrias in Europe. *J Inherit Metab Dis.* 2013;36:849-857.

45. Floderus Y, Shoolingin-Jordan PM, Harper P. Acute intermittent porphyria in Sweden. Molecular, functional and clinical consequences of some new mutations found in the porphobilinogen deaminase gene. *Clin Genet.* 2002;62:288-297.

46. Chen B, Solis-Villa C, Hakenberg J, et al. Acute intermittent porphyria: predicted pathogenicity of HMBS variants indicates extremely low penetrance of the autosomal dominant disease. *Hum Mutat.* 2016;37:1215-1222.

47. Lenglet H, Schmitt C, Grange T, et al. From a dominant to an oligogenic model of inheritance with environmental modifiers in acute intermittent porphyria. *Hum Mol Genet.* 2018;27:1164-1173.

48. Innala E, Backstrom T, Bixo M, et al. Evaluation of gonadotropin-releasing hormone agonist treatment for prevention of menstrual-related attacks in acute porphyria. *Acta Obstet Gynecol Scand.* 2010;89:95-100.

49. Balwani M, Singh P, Seth A, et al. Acute intermittent porphyria in children: a case report and review of the literature. *Mol Genet Metab.* 2016;119:295-299.

50. Andersson C, Innala E, Backstrom T. Acute intermittent porphyria in women: clinical expression, use and experience of exogenous sex hormones. A population-based study in Northern Sweden. *J Intern Med.* 2003;254:176-183.

51. Naik H, Stoecker M, Sanderson SC, et al. Experiences and concerns of patients with recurrent attacks of acute hepatic porphyria: a qualitative study. *Mol Genet Metab.* 2016;119:278-283.

52. Albers SY, Fink JK. Porphyric neuropathy. *Muscle Nerve.* 2004;30:410-422.

53. Pischik E, Kauppinen R. Neurological manifestations of acute intermittent porphyria. *Cell Mol Biol.* 2009;55:72-83.

54. Gurses C, Durukan A, Sencer S, et al. A severe neurological sequela in acute intermittent porphyria: presentation of a case from encephalopathy to quadriparesis. *Br J Radiol.* 2008;81:e135-e140.

55. Stein JA, Tschudy DP. Acute intermittent porphyria. A clinical and biochemical study of 46 patients. *Medicine (Baltimore).* 1970;49:1-16.

56. Kang SY, Kang JH, Choi JC, et al. Posterior reversible encephalopathy syndrome in a patient with acute intermittent porphyria. *J Neurol.* 2010;257:663-664.

57. DeFrancisco M, Savino PJ, Schatz NJ. Optic atrophy in acute intermittent porphyria. *Am J Ophthalmol.* 1979;87:221-224.

58. Carney MW. Hepatic porphyria with mental symptoms. Four missed cases. *Lancet.* 1972;2:100-101.

59. Crimlisk HL. The little imitator—porphyria: a neuropsychiatric disorder. *J Neurol Neurosurg Psychiatry.* 1997;62:319-328.

60. Bonkovsky HL, Dixon N, Rudnick S. Pathogenesis and clinical features of the acute hepatic porphyrias (AHPs). *Mol Genet Metab.* 2019;128:213-218.

61. Gouya L, Ventura P, Balwani M, et al. EXPLORE: a prospective, multinational, natural history study of patients with acute hepatic porphyria with recurrent attacks. *Hepatology.* 2020;71:1546-1558.

62. Beattie AD, Goldberg A. Acute intermittent porphyria. Natural history and prognosis. In: Doss M, ed. *Porphyrins in Human Diseases.* Karger; 1976:245-250.

63. Baravelli CM, Aarsand AK, Sandberg S, et al. Sick leave, disability, and mortality in acute hepatic porphyria: a nationwide cohort study. *Orphanet J Rare Dis.* 2020;15:56.

64. Pallet N, Mami I, Schmitt C, et al. High prevalence of and potential mechanisms for chronic kidney disease in patients with acute intermittent porphyria. *Kidney Int.* 2015;88:386-395.

65. Andersson C, Lithner F. Hypertension and renal disease in patients with acute intermittent porphyria. *J Intern Med.* 1994;236:169-175.

66. Lazareth H, Talbi N, Kamar N, et al. Kidney transplantation improves the clinical outcomes of Acute Intermittent Porphyria. *Mol Genet Metab.* 2020;131:259-266.

67. Kauppinen R, Mustajoki P. Acute hepatic porphyria and hepatocellular carcinoma. *Br J Cancer.* 1988;57:117-120.

68. Lissing M, Vassiliou D, Floderus Y, et al. Risk of primary liver cancer in acute hepatic porphyria patients: a matched cohort study of 1244 individuals. *J Intern Med.* 2022;291:824-836.

69. Sardh E, Wahlin S, Bjornstedt M, et al. High risk of primary liver cancer in a cohort of 179 patients with Acute Hepatic Porphyria. *J Inherit Metab Dis.* 2013;36:1063-1071.

70. Namba H, Narahara K, Tsuji K, et al. Assignment of human porphobilinogen deaminase to 11q24.1→q24.2 by in situ hybridization and gene dosage studies. *Cytogenet Cell Genet.* 1991;57:105-108.

71. Yoo HW, Warner CA, Chen CH, et al. Hydroxymethylbilane synthase: complete genomic sequence and amplifiable polymorphisms in the human gene. *Genomics.* 1993;15:21-29.

72. Grandchamp B, De Verneuil H, Beaumont C, et al. Tissue-specific expression of porphobilinogen deaminase. Two isoenzymes from a single gene. *Eur J Biochem.* 1987;162:105-110.

73. Chretien S, Dubart A, Beaupain D, et al. Alternative transcription and splicing of the human porphobilinogen deaminase gene result either in tissue-specific or in housekeeping expression. *Proc Natl Acad Sci U S A.* 1988;85:6-10.

74. Human Gene Mutation Database. *HGMD®Professional 2022.* Accessed June 1, 2022. www.hgmd.org

75. Cooper DN, Youssoufian H. The CpG dinucleotide and human genetic disease. *Hum Genet.* 1988;78:151-155.

76. Tjensvoll K, Bruland O, Floderus Y, et al. Haplotype analysis of Norwegian and Swedish patients with acute intermittent porphyria (AIP): extreme haplotype heterogeneity for the mutation R116W. *Dis Markers.* 2003;19:41-46.

77. Whatley SD, Roberts AG, Elder GH. De-novo mutation and sporadic presentation of acute intermittent porphyria. *Lancet.* 1995;346:1007-1008.

78. Andersson C, Floderus Y, Wikberg A, et al. The W198X and R173W mutations in the porphobilinogen deaminase gene in acute intermittent porphyria have higher clinical penetrance than R167W. A population-based study. *Scand J Clin Lab Invest.* 2000;60:643-648.

79. Fraunberg M, Pischik E, Udd L, et al. Clinical and biochemical characteristics and genotype-phenotype correlation in 143 Finnish and Russian patients with acute intermittent porphyria. *Medicine (Baltimore).* 2005;84:35-47.

80. Gill R, Kolstoe SE, Mohammed F, et al. Structure of human porphobilinogen deaminase at 2.8 A: the molecular basis of acute intermittent porphyria. *Biochem J.* 2009;420:17-25.

81. Brownlie PD, Lambert R, Louie GV, et al. The three-dimensional structures of mutants of porphobilinogen deaminase: toward an understanding of the structural basis of acute intermittent porphyria. *Protein Sci.* 1994;3:1644-1650.

82. Chen B, Solis-Villa C, Erwin AL, et al. Identification and characterization of 40 novel hydroxymethylbilane synthase mutations that cause acute intermittent porphyria. *J Inherit Metab Dis.* 2019;42:186-194.

Disorders of Red Blood Cells

83. Baumann K, Kauppinen R. Penetrance and predictive value of genetic screening in acute porphyria. *Mol Genet Metab.* 2020;130:87-99.

84. Soonawalla ZF, Orug T, Badminton MN, et al. Liver transplantation as a cure for acute intermittent porphyria. *Lancet.* 2004;363:705-706.

85. Yasuda M, Erwin AL, Liu LU, et al. Liver transplantation for acute intermittent porphyria: biochemical and pathologic studies of the explanted liver. *Mol Med.* 2015;21:487-495.

86. Lissing M, Nowak G, Adam R, et al. Liver transplantation for acute intermittent porphyria. *Liver Transpl.* 2021;27:491-501.

87. Dowman JK, Gunson BK, Bramhall S, et al. Liver transplantation from donors with acute intermittent porphyria. *Ann Intern Med.* 2011;154:571-572.

88. Balwani M, Sardh E, Ventura P, et al. Phase 3 trial of RNAi therapeutic givosiran for acute intermittent porphyria. *N Engl J Med.* 2020;382:2289-2301.

89. Sardh E, Harper P. RNAi therapy with givosiran significantly reduces attack rates in acute intermittent porphyria. *J Intern Med.* 2022;291:593-610.

90. Pierach CA, Edwards PS. Neurotoxicity of delta-aminolevulinic acid and porphobilinogen. *Exp Neurol.* 1978;62:810-814.

91. Hu Y, Shen H, Keep RF, et al. Peptide transporter 2 (PEPT2) expression in brain protects against 5-aminolevulinic acid neurotoxicity. *J Neurochem.* 2007;103:2058-2065.

92. Brennan MJ, Cantrill RC. Delta-aminolaevulinic acid is a potent agonist for GABA autoreceptors. *Nature.* 1979;280:514-515.

93. Muller WE, Snyder SH. delta-Aminolevulinic acid: influences on synaptic GABA receptor binding may explain CNS symptoms of porphyria. *Ann Neurol.* 1977;2:340-342.

94. Puy H, Deybach JC, Bogdan A, et al. Increased delta aminolevulinic acid and decreased pineal melatonin production. A common event in acute porphyria studies in the rat. *J Clin Invest.* 1996;97:104-110.

95. Felitsyn N, McLeod C, Shroads AL, et al. The heme precursor delta-aminolevulinate blocks peripheral myelin formation. *J Neurochem.* 2008;106:2068-2079.

96. Onuki J, Chen Y, Teixeira PC, et al. Mitochondrial and nuclear DNA damage induced by 5-aminolevulinic acid. *Arch Biochem Biophys.* 2004;432:178-187.

97. Yasuda M, Gan L, Chen B, et al. Homozygous hydroxymethylbilane synthase knock-in mice provide pathogenic insights into the severe neurological impairments present in human homozygous dominant acute intermittent porphyria. *Hum Mol Genet.* 2019;28:1755-1767.

98. Dixon N, Li T, Marion B, et al. Pilot study of mitochondrial bioenergetics in subjects with acute porphyria. *Mol Genet Metab.* 2019;128:228-235.

99. Homedan C, Laafi J, Schmitt C, et al. Acute intermittent porphyria causes hepatic mitochondrial energetic failure in a mouse model. *Int J Biochem Cell Biol.* 2014;51:93-101.

100. Homedan C, Schmitt C, Laafi J, et al. Mitochondrial energetic defects in muscle and brain of a Hmbs−/− mouse model of acute intermittent porphyria. *Hum Mol Genet.* 2015;24:5015-5023.

101. Tchernitchko D, Tavernier Q, Lamoril J, et al. A variant of peptide transporter 2 predicts the severity of porphyria-associated kidney disease. *J Am Soc Nephrol.* 2017;28:1924-1932.

102. Onuki J, Teixeira PC, Medeiros MH, et al. Is 5-aminolevulinic acid involved in the hepatocellular carcinogenesis of acute intermittent porphyria? *Cell Mol Biol.* 2002;48:17-26.

103. Peoc'h K, Manceau H, Karim Z, et al. Hepatocellular carcinoma in acute hepatic porphyrias: a Damocles Sword. *Mol Genet Metab.* 2019;128:236-241.

104. Molina L, Zhu J, Trepo E, et al. Biallelic hydroxymethylbilane synthase inactivation defines a homogenous clinico-molecular subtype of hepatocellular carcinoma. *J Hepatol.* 2022;77(4):1038-1046.

105. Schneider-Yin X, van Tuyll van Serooskerken AM, Siegesmund M, et al. Biallelic inactivation of protoporphyrinogen oxidase and hydroxymethylbilane synthase is associated with liver cancer in acute porphyrias. *J Hepatol.* 2015;62:734-738.

106. Marsden JT, Rees DC. Urinary excretion of porphyrins, porphobilinogen and delta-aminolaevulinic acid following an attack of acute intermittent porphyria. *J Clin Pathol.* 2014;67:60-65.

107. Zhang J, Yasuda M, Desnick RJ, et al. A LC-MS/MS method for the specific, sensitive, and simultaneous quantification of 5-aminolevulinic acid and porphobilinogen. *J Chromatogr B Analyt Technol Biomed Life Sci.* 2011;879:2389-2396.

108. Pierach CA, Cardinal R, Bossenmaier I, et al. Comparison of the Hoesch and the Watson-Schwartz tests for urinary porphobilinogen. *Clin Chem.* 1977;23:1666-1668.

109. Whatley SD, Roberts AG, Llewellyn DH, et al. Non-erythroid form of acute intermittent porphyria caused by promoter and frameshift mutations distant from the coding sequence of exon 1 of the HMBS gene. *Hum Genet.* 2000;107:243-248.

110. Sassa S, Granick S, Bickers DR, et al. A microassay for uroporphyrinogen I synthase, one of three abnormal enzyme activities in acute intermittent porphyria, and its application to the study of the genetics of this disease. *Proc Natl Acad Sci U S A.* 1974;71:732-736.

111. Tschudy DP, Valsamis M, Magnussen CR. Acute intermittent porphyria: clinical and selected research aspects. *Ann Intern Med.* 1975;83:851-864.

112. Jaramillo-Calle DA, Solano JM, Rabinstein AA, et al. Porphyria-induced posterior reversible encephalopathy syndrome and central nervous system dysfunction. *Mol Genet Metab.* 2019;128:242-253.

113. Kupferschmidt H, Bont A, Schnorf H, et al. Transient cortical blindness and bioccipital brain lesions in two patients with acute intermittent porphyria. *Ann Intern Med.* 1995;123:598-600.

114. Albers JW, Robertson WC Jr, Daube JR. Electrodiagnostic findings in acute porphyric neuropathy. *Muscle Nerve.* 1978;1:292-296.

115. Ten Eyck FW, Martin WJ, Kernohan JW. Acute porphyria: necropsy studies in nine cases. *Proc Staff Meet Mayo Clin.* 1961;36:409-422.

116. Thorner PS, Bilbao JM, Sima AA, et al. Porphyric neuropathy: an ultrastructural and quantitative case study. *Can J Neurol Sci.* 1981;8:281-287.

117. Douer D, Weinberger A, Pinkhas J, et al. Treatment of acute intermittent porphyria with large doses of propranolol. *J Am Med Assoc.* 1978;240:766-768.

118. Bonkowsky HL, Tschudy DP. Letter: hazard of propranolol in treatment of acute porphyria. *Br Med J.* 1974;4:47-48.

119. Bonkowsky HL, Tschudy DP, Collins A, et al. Repression of the overproduction of porphyrin precursors in acute intermittent porphyria by intravenous infusions of hematin. *Proc Natl Acad Sci U S A.* 1971;68:2725-2729.

120. Goetsch CA, Bissell DM. Instability of hematin used in the treatment of acute hepatic porphyria. *N Engl J Med.* 1986;315:235-238.

121. Green D, Ts'ao CH. Hematin: effects on hemostasis. *J Lab Clin Med.* 1990;115:144-147.

122. Willandt B, Langendonk JG, Biermann K, et al. Liver fibrosis associated with iron accumulation due to long-term heme-arginate treatment in acute intermittent porphyria: a case series. *JIMD Rep.* 2016;25:77-81.

123. Winkler AS, Peters TJ, Elwes RD. Neuropsychiatric porphyria in patients with refractory epilepsy: report of three cases. *J Neurol Neurosurg Psychiatry.* 2005;76:380-383.

124. Hahn M, Gildemeister OS, Krauss GL, et al. Effects of new anticonvulsant medications on porphyrin synthesis in cultured liver cells: potential implications for patients with acute porphyria. *Neurology.* 1997;49:97-106.

125. Zaatreh MM. Levetiracetam in porphyric status epilepticus: a case report. *Clin Neuropharmacol.* 2005;28:243-244.

126. Dowman JK, Gunson BK, Mirza DF, et al. Liver transplantation for acute intermittent porphyria is complicated by a high rate of hepatic artery thrombosis. *Liver Transpl.* 2012;18:195-200.

127. Schulenburg-Brand D, Gardiner T, Guppy S, et al. An audit of the use of gonadorelin analogues to prevent recurrent acute symptoms in patients with acute porphyria in the United Kingdom. *JIMD Rep.* 2017;36:99-107.

128. Stein P, Badminton M, Barth J, et al. Best practice guidelines on clinical management of acute attacks of porphyria and their complications. *Ann Clin Biochem.* 2013;50:217-223.

129. Pischik E, Kauppinen R. An update of clinical management of acute intermittent porphyria. *Appl Clin Genet.* 2015;8:201-214.

130. Nair JK, Willoughby JL, Chan A, et al. Multivalent N-acetylgalactosamine-conjugated siRNA localizes in hepatocytes and elicits robust RNAi-mediated gene silencing. *J Am Chem Soc.* 2014;136:16958-16961.

131. To-Figueras J, Wijngaard R, Garcia-Villoria J, et al. Dysregulation of homocysteine homeostasis in acute intermittent porphyria patients receiving heme arginate or givosiran. *J Inherit Metab Dis.* 2021;44:961-971.

132. Vassiliou D, Sardh E. Homocysteine elevation in givosiran treatment: suggested ALAS1 siRNA effect on cystathionine beta-synthase. *J Intern Med.* 2021;290:928-930.

133. Ventura P, Corradini E, Di Pierro E, et al. Hyperhomocysteinemia in patients with acute porphyrias: a potentially dangerous metabolic crossroad?. *Eur J Intern Med.* 2020;79:101-107.

134. Andersson C, Peterson J, Anderson KE, et al. Randomized clinical trial of recombinant human porphobilinogen deaminase (rhPBGD) in acute attacks of porphyria. Porphyrins and Porphyrias International Meeting. 2007:152-216.

135. Cordoba KM, Serrano-Mendioroz I, Jerico D, et al. Recombinant porphobilinogen deaminase targeted to the liver corrects enzymopenia in a mouse model of acute intermittent porphyria. *Sci Transl Med.* 2022;14:eabc0700.

136. Lindberg RL, Porcher C, Grandchamp B, et al. Porphobilinogen deaminase deficiency in mice causes a neuropathy resembling that of human hepatic porphyria. *Nat Genet.* 1996;12:195-199.

137. Yasuda M, Bishop DF, Fowkes M, et al. AAV8-mediated gene therapy prevents induced biochemical attacks of acute intermittent porphyria and improves neuromotor function. *Mol Ther.* 2010;18:17-22.

138. Unzu C, Sampedro A, Mauleon I, et al. Sustained enzymatic correction by rAAV-mediated liver gene therapy protects against induced motor neuropathy in acute porphyria mice. *Mol Ther.* 2011;19:243-250.

139. D'Avola D, Lopez-Franco E, Sangro B, et al. Phase I open label liver-directed gene therapy clinical trial for acute intermittent porphyria. *J Hepatol.* 2016;65:776-783.

140. Serrano-Mendioroz I, Sampedro A, Alegre M, et al. An inducible promoter responsive to different porphyrinogenic stimuli improves gene therapy vectors for acute intermittent porphyria. *Hum Gene Ther.* 2018;29:480-491.

141. Serrano-Mendioroz I, Sampedro A, Serna N, et al. Bioengineered PBGD variant improves the therapeutic index of gene therapy vectors for acute intermittent porphyria. *Hum Mol Genet.* 2018;27:3688-3696.

142. Jiang L, Berraondo P, Jerico D, et al. Systemic messenger RNA as an etiological treatment for acute intermittent porphyria. *Nat Med.* 2018;24:1899-1909.

143. Bustad HJ, Toska K, Schmitt C, et al. A pharmacological chaperone therapy for acute intermittent porphyria. *Mol Ther.* 2020;28:677-689.

144. Marsden JT, Rees DC. A retrospective analysis of outcome of pregnancy in patients with acute porphyria. *J Inherit Metab Dis.* 2010;33:591-596.

145. Tollanes MC, Aarsand AK, Sandberg S. Excess risk of adverse pregnancy outcomes in women with porphyria: a population-based cohort study. *J Inherit Metab Dis.* 2011;34:217-223.

146. Aggarwal N, Bagga R, Sawhney H, et al. Pregnancy with acute intermittent porphyria: a case report and review of literature. *J Obstet Gynaecol Res.* 2002;28:160-162.

147. Wenger S, Meisinger V, Brucke T, et al. Acute porphyric neuropathy during pregnancy – effect of haematin therapy. *Eur Neurol.* 1998;39:187-188.

148. Innala E, Andersson C. Screening for hepatocellular carcinoma in acute intermittent porphyria: a 15-year follow-up in northern Sweden. *J Intern Med.* 2011;269:538-545.

149. Solis C, Martinez-Bermejo A, Naidich TP, et al. Acute intermittent porphyria: studies of the severe homozygous dominant disease provides insights into the neurologic attacks in acute porphyrias. *Arch Neurol.* 2004;61:1764-1770.

150. Llewellyn DH, Smyth SJ, Elder GH, et al. Homozygous acute intermittent porphyria: compound heterozygosity for adjacent base transitions in the same codon of the porphobilinogen deaminase gene. *Hum Genet.* 1992;89:97-98.

151. Beukeveld GJ, Wolthers BG, Nordmann Y, et al. A retrospective study of a patient with homozygous form of acute intermittent porphyria. *J Inherit Metab Dis.* 1990;13:673-683.

152. Stutterd CA, Kidd A, Florkowski C, et al. Expanding the clinical and radiological phenotypes of leukoencephalopathy due to biallelic HMBS mutations. *Am J Med Genet A.* 2021;185:2941-2950.

153. Hift RJ, Meissner PN. An analysis of 112 acute porphyric attacks in Cape Town, South Africa: evidence that acute intermittent porphyria and variegate porphyria differ in susceptibility and severity. *Medicine (Baltimore).* 2005;84:48-60.

154. Meissner PN, Dailey TA, Hift RJ, et al. A R59W mutation in human protoporphyrinogen oxidase results in decreased enzyme activity and is prevalent in South Africans with variegate porphyria. *Nat Genet.* 1996;13:95-97.

155. Singal AK, Anderson KE. Variegate porphyria. In: Adam MP, Mirzaa GM, Pagon RA, et al, eds. *GeneReviews®.* 1993.

156. Eales L, Day RS, Blekkenhorst GH. The clinical and biochemical features of variegate porphyria: an analysis of 300 cases studied at Groote Schuur Hospital, Cape Town. *Int J Biochem.* 1980;12:837-853.

157. Whatley SD, Puy H, Morgan RR, et al. Variegate porphyria in Western Europe: identification of PPOX gene mutations in 104 families, extent of allelic heterogeneity, and absence of correlation between phenotype and type of mutation. *Am J Hum Genet.* 1999;65:984-994.

158. Luvai A, Mbagaya W, Narayanan D, et al. Hepatocellular carcinoma in variegate porphyria: a case report and literature review. *Ann Clin Biochem.* 2015;52:407-412.

159. Schneider-Yin X, van Tuyll van Serooskerken AM, Went P, et al. Hepatocellular carcinoma in variegate porphyria: a serious complication. *Acta Derm Venereol.* 2010;90:512-515.

160. Brenner DA, Bloomer JR. The enzymatic defect in variegate porphyria. Studies with human cultured skin fibroblasts. *N Engl J Med.* 1980;302:765-769.

161. Deybach JC, de Verneuil H, Nordmann Y. The inherited enzymatic defect in porphyria variegata. *Hum Genet.* 1981;58:425-428.

162. Puy H, Robreau AM, Rosipal R, et al. Protoporphyrinogen oxidase: complete genomic sequence and polymorphisms in the human gene. *Biochem Biophys Res Commun.* 1996;226:226-230.

163. Taketani S, Inazawa J, Abe T, et al. The human protoporphyrinogen oxidase gene (PPOX): organization and location to chromosome 1. *Genomics.* 1995;29:698-703.

164. Roberts AG, Whatley SD, Daniels J, et al. Partial characterization and assignment of the gene for protoporphyrinogen oxidase and variegate porphyria to human chromosome 1q23. *Hum Mol Genet.* 1995;4:2387-2390.

165. Dailey HA, Dailey TA. Characteristics of human protoporphyrinogen oxidase in controls and variegate porphyrias. *Cell Mol Biol.* 1997;43:67-73.

166. Spikes JD. Photobiology of porphyrins. *Prog Clin Biol Res.* 1984;170:19-39.

167. Meissner PN, Day RS, Moore MR, et al. Protoporphyrinogen oxidase and porphobilinogen deaminase in variegate porphyria. *Eur J Clin Invest.* 1986;16:257-261.

168. Jerico D, Cordoba KM, Jiang L, et al. mRNA-based therapy in a rabbit model of variegate porphyria offers new insights into the pathogenesis of acute attacks. *Mol Ther Nucleic Acids.* 2021;25:207-219.

169. Meissner P, Adams P, Kirsch R. Allosteric inhibition of human lymphoblast and purified porphobilinogen deaminase by protoporphyrinogen and coproporphyrinogen. A possible mechanism for the acute attack of variegate porphyria. *J Clin Invest.* 1993;91:1436-1444.

170. Meissner P, Hift RJ, Corrigal A. Variegate porphyria. In: Kadish KM, Smith KM, Guilard R, eds. *The Porphyrin Handbook-Medical Aspects of Porphyrias.* Academic Press; 2003:89-120.

171. Poh-Fitzpatrick MB. A plasma porphyrin fluorescence marker for variegate porphyria. *Arch Dermatol.* 1980;116:543-547.

172. Da Silva V, Simonin S, Deybach JC, et al. Variegate porphyria: diagnostic value of fluorometric scanning of plasma porphyrins. *Clin Chim Acta.* 1995;238:163-168.

173. Sies CW, Davidson JS, Florkowski CM, et al. Plasma fluorescence scanning did not detect latent variegate porphyria in nine patients with non-p.R59W mutations. *Pathology.* 2005;37:324-326.

174. Mustajoki P, Nordmann Y. Early administration of heme arginate for acute porphyric attacks. *Arch Intern Med.* 1993;153:2004-2008.

175. Stojeba N, Meyer C, Jeanpierre C, et al. Recovery from a variegate porphyria by a liver transplantation. *Liver Transpl.* 2004;10:935-938.

176. Corrigall AV, Hift RJ, Davids LM, et al. Homozygous variegate porphyria in South Africa: genotypic analysis in two cases. *Mol Genet Metab.* 2000;69:323-330.

177. Kordac V, Martasek P, Zeman J, et al. Increased erythrocyte protoporphyrin in homozygous variegate porphyria. *Photo Dermatol.* 1985;2:257-259.

178. With TK. Hereditary coproporphyria and variegate porphyria in Denmark. *Dan Med Bull.* 1983;30:106-112.

179. Kaftory R, Edel Y, Snast I, et al. Greater disease burden of variegate porphyria than hereditary coproporphyria: an Israeli nationwide study of neurocutaneous porphyrias. *Mol Genet Metab Rep.* 2021;26:100707.

180. Kuhnel A, Gross U, Doss MO. Hereditary coproporphyria in Germany: clinical-biochemical studies in 53 patients. *Clin Biochem.* 2000;33:465-473.

181. Wang B, Bissell DM. Hereditary coproporphyria. In: Adam MP, Mirzaa GM, Pagon RA, et al, eds. *GeneReviews®.* 1993.

182. Andant C, Puy H, Faivre J, et al. Acute hepatic porphyrias and primary liver cancer. *N Engl J Med.* 1998;338:1853-1854.

183. Andant C, Puy H, Bogard C, et al. Hepatocellular carcinoma in patients with acute hepatic porphyria: frequency of occurrence and related factors. *J Hepatol.* 2000;32:933-939.

184. Hawk JL, Magnus IA, Parkes A, et al. Deficiency of hepatic coproporphyrinogen oxidase in hereditary coproporphyria. *J R Soc Med.* 1978;71:775-777.

185. Elder GH, Evans JO, Thomas N. The primary enzyme defect in hereditary coproporphyria. *Lancet.* 1976;2:1217-1219.

186. Grandchamp B, Nordmann Y. Decreased lymphocyte coproporphyrinogen III oxidase activity in hereditary coproporphyria. *Biochem Biophys Res Commun.* 1977;74:1089-1095.

187. Doss M, von Tiepermann R, Pfluger KH. Coexistence of hereditary coproporphyria and epilepsy: coproporphyrinogen oxidase deficiency in liver and kidney. *J Neurol.* 1981;226:25-33.

188. Delfau-Larue MH, Martasek P, Grandchamp B. Coproporphyrinogen oxidase: gene organization and description of a mutation leading to exon 6 skipping. *Hum Mol Genet.* 1994;3:1325-1330.

189. Martasek P, Camadro JM, Delfau-Larue MH, et al. Molecular cloning, sequencing, and functional expression of a cDNA encoding human coproporphyrinogen oxidase. *Proc Natl Acad Sci U S A.* 1994;91:3024-3028.

190. Taketani S, Kohno H, Furukawa T, et al. Molecular cloning, sequencing and expression of cDNA encoding human coproporphyrinogen oxidase. *Biochim Biophys Acta.* 1994;1183:547-549.

191. Cacheux V, Martasek P, Fougerousse F, et al. Localization of the human coproporphyrinogen oxidase gene to chromosome band 3q12. *Hum Genet.* 1994;94:557-559.

192. Allen KR, Whatley SD, Degg TJ, et al. Hereditary coproporphyria: comparison of molecular and biochemical investigations in a large family. *J Inherit Metab Dis.* 2005;28:779-785.

193. Lamoril J, Puy H, Whatley SD, et al. Characterization of mutations in the CPO gene in British patients demonstrates absence of genotype-phenotype correlation and identifies relationship between hereditary coproporphyria and harderoporphyria. *Am J Hum Genet.* 2001;68:1130-1138.

194. McIntyre N, Pearson AJ, Allan DJ, et al. Hepatic delta-aminolaevulinic acid synthetase in an attack of hereditary coproporphyria and during remission. *Lancet.* 1971;1:560-564.

195. Martasek P. Hereditary coproporphyria. *Semin Liver Dis.* 1998;18:25-32.

196. Schoenfeld N, Mamet R, Dotan I, et al. Relation between uroporphyrin excretion, acute attacks of hereditary coproporphyria and successful treatment with haem arginate. *Clin Sci (Lond).* 1995;88:365-369.

197. Manning DJ, Gray TA. Haem arginate in acute hereditary coproporphyria. *Arch Dis Child.* 1991;66:730-731.

198. Ma E, Mar V, Varigos G, et al. Haem arginate as effective maintenance therapy for hereditary coproporphyria. *Australas J Dermatol.* 2011;52:135-138.

199. Upchurch M, Donnelly JP, Deremiah E, et al. Hereditary coproporphyria mimicking guillain-barre syndrome after COVID-19 infection. *Cureus.* 2022;14:e21586.

200. Lamoril J, Martasek P, Deybach JC, et al. A molecular defect in coproporphyrinogen oxidase gene causing harderoporphyria, a variant form of hereditary coproporphyria. *Hum Mol Genet.* 1995;4:275-278.

201. Lamoril J, Puy H, Gouya L, et al. Neonatal hemolytic anemia due to inherited harderoporphyria: clinical characteristics and molecular basis. *Blood.* 1998;91:1453-1457.

202. Moghe A, Ramanujam VMS, Phillips JD, et al. Harderoporphyria: case of lifelong photosensitivity associated with compound heterozygous coproporphyrinogen oxidase (CPOX) mutations. *Mol Genet Metab Rep.* 2019;19:100457.

203. Hasanoglu A, Balwani M, Kasapkara CS, et al. Harderoporphyria due to homozygosity for coproporphyrinogen oxidase missense mutation H327R. *J Inherit Metab Dis.* 2011;34:225-231.

204. Schmitt C, Gouya L, Malonova E, et al. Mutations in human CPO gene predict clinical expression of either hepatic hereditary coproporphyria or erythropoietic harderoporphyria. *Hum Mol Genet.* 2005;14:3089-3098.

205. Doss MO, Gross U, Lamoril J, et al. Compound heterozygous hereditary coproporphyria with fluorescing teeth. *Ann Clin Biochem.* 1999;36(pt 5):680-682.

206. Grandchamp B, Phung N, Nordmann Y. Homozygous case of hereditary coproporphyria. *Lancet.* 1977;2:1348-1349.

207. Potluri VR, Astrin KH, Wetmur JG, et al. Human delta-aminolevulinate dehydratase: chromosomal localization to 9q34 by in situ hybridization. *Hum Genet.* 1987;76:236-239.

208. Kaya AH, Plewinska M, Wong DM, et al. Human delta-aminolevulinate dehydratase (ALAD) gene: structure and alternative splicing of the erythroid and housekeeping mRNAs. *Genomics.* 1994;19:242-248.

209. Maruno M, Furuyama K, Akagi R, et al. Highly heterogeneous nature of delta-aminolevulinate dehydratase (ALAD) deficiencies in ALAD porphyria. *Blood.* 2001;97:2972-2978.

210. Jaffe EK, Stith L. ALAD porphyria is a conformational disease. *Am J Hum Genet.* 2007;80:329-337.

211. Thunell S, Henrichson A, Floderus Y, et al. Liver transplantation in a boy with acute porphyria due to aminolaevulinate dehydratase deficiency. *Eur J Clin Chem Clin Biochem.* 1992;30:599-606.

212. Neeleman RA, van Beers EJ, Friesema EC, et al. Clinical remission of delta-aminolevulinic acid dehydratase deficiency through suppression of erythroid heme synthesis. *Hepatology.* 2019;70:434-436.

213. Sassa S. ALAD porphyria. *Semin Liver Dis.* 1998;18:95-101.

214. Bird TD, Hamernyik P, Nutter JY, et al. Inherited deficiency of delta-aminolevulinic acid dehydratase. *Am J Hum Genet.* 1979;31:662-668.

215. Tong Y, Song YK, Tyring S. Resolution of porphyria cutanea tarda in patients with hepatitis C following ledipasvir-sofosbuvir combination therapy. *JAMA Dermatol.* 2016;152:1393-1395.

Disorders of Red Blood Cells

216. Elder GH, Roberts AG, de Salamanca RE. Genetics and pathogenesis of human uroporphyrinogen decarboxylase defects. *Clin Biochem.* 1989;22:163-168.

217. Kushner JP, Barbuto AJ, Lee GR. An inherited enzymatic defect in porphyria cutanea tarda: decreased uroporphyrinogen decarboxylase activity. *J Clin Invest.* 1976;58:1089-1097.

218. Dubart A, Mattei MG, Raich N, et al. Assignment of human uroporphyrinogen decarboxylase (URO-D) to the p34 band of chromosome 1. *Hum Genet.* 1986;73:277-279.

219. Singal AK, Philips JD. Porphyria cutanea tarda. In: Kadish KM, Smith KM, Guillard R, eds. *Handbook of Porphyrin Science With Application to Chemistry, Physics, Materials Science, Engineering Biology and Medicine.* World Scientific Publishing; 2014:219-261.

220. Phillips JD, Parker TL, Schubert HL, et al. Functional consequences of naturally occurring mutations in human uroporphyrinogen decarboxylase. *Blood.* 2001;98:3179-3185.

221. Badenas C, To-Figueras J, Phillips JD, et al. Identification and characterization of novel uroporphyrinogen decarboxylase gene mutations in a large series of porphyria cutanea tarda patients and relatives. *Clin Genet.* 2009;75:346-353.

222. de Verneuil H, Aitken G, Nordmann Y. Familial and sporadic porphyria cutanea: two different diseases. *Hum Genet.* 1978;44:145-151.

223. Felsher BF, Carpio NM, Engleking DW, et al. Decreased hepatic uroporphyrinogen decarboxylase activity in porphyria cutanea tarda. *N Engl J Med.* 1982;306:766-769.

224. Elder GH, Lee GB, Tovey JA. Decreased activity of hepatic uroporphyrinogen decarboxylase in sporadic porphyria cutanea tarda. *N Engl J Med.* 1978;299:274-278.

225. Elder GH, Urquhart AJ, De Salamanca RE, et al. Immunoreactive uroporphyrinogen decarboxylase in the liver in porphyria cutanea tarda. *Lancet.* 1985;2:229-233.

226. Garey JR, Franklin KF, Brown DA, et al. Analysis of uroporphyrinogen decarboxylase complementary DNAs in sporadic porphyria cutanea tarda. *Gastroenterology.* 1993;105:165-169.

227. Mendez M, Poblete-Gutierrez P, Garcia-Bravo M, et al. Molecular heterogeneity of familial porphyria cutanea tarda in Spain: characterization of 10 novel mutations in the UROD gene. *Br J Dermatol.* 2007;157:501-507.

228. Varigos G, Schiltz JR, Bickers DR. Uroporphyrin I stimulation of collagen biosynthesis in human skin fibroblasts. A unique dark effect of porphyrin. *J Clin Invest.* 1982;69:129-135.

229. Ippen H. General symptoms of late skin porphyria (porphyria cutanea tarda) as an indication for its treatment. Article in German. *Dtsch Med Wochenschr.* 1961;86:127-133.

230. Lamont NM, Hathorn M, Joubert SM. Porphyria in the African: a study of 100 cases. *Q J Med.* 1961;30:373-392.

231. Felsher BF, Jones ML, Redeker AG. Iron and hepatic uroporphyrin synthesis. Relation in porphyria cutanea tarda. *J Am Med Assoc.* 1973;226:663-665.

232. Goulding JM, Purohit G, Borg A, et al. Porphyria cutanea tarda complicating transfusion-dependent myelodysplastic syndrome. *Br J Haematol.* 2007;136:2.

233. Ippen H. Treatment of porphyria cutanea tarda by phlebotomy. *Semin Hematol.* 1977;14:253-259.

234. Rocchi E, Gibertini P, Cassanelli M, et al. Iron removal therapy in porphyria cutanea tarda: phlebotomy versus slow subcutaneous desferrioxamine infusion. *Br J Dermatol.* 1986;114:621-629.

235. Phillips JD, Bergonia HA, Reilly CA, et al. A porphomethene inhibitor of uroporphyrinogen decarboxylase causes porphyria cutanea tarda. *Proc Natl Acad Sci U S A.* 2007;104:5079-5084.

236. Phillips JD, Kushner JP, Bergonia HA, et al. Uroporphyria in the Cyp1a2−/− mouse. *Blood Cells Mol Dis.* 2011;47:249-254.

237. Wickliffe JK, Abdel-Rahman SZ, Lee C, et al. CYP1A2*1F and GSTM1 alleles are associated with susceptibility to porphyria cutanea tarda. *Mol Med.* 2011;17:241-247.

238. Ryan Caballes F, Sendi H, Bonkovsky HL. Hepatitis C, porphyria cutanea tarda and liver iron: an update. *Liver Int.* 2012;32:880-893.

239. Felsher BF, Kushner JP. Hepatic siderosis and porphyria cutanea tarda: relation of iron excess to the metabolic defect. *Semin Hematol.* 1977;14:243-251.

240. Grossman ME, Bickers DR, Poh-Fitzpatrick MB, et al. Porphyria cutanea tarda. Clinical features and laboratory findings in 40 patients. *Am J Med.* 1979;67:277-286.

241. Elder GH. Differentiation of porphyria cutanea tarda symptomatica from other types of porphyria by measurement of isocoproporphyrin in faeces. *J Clin Pathol.* 1975;28:601-607.

242. Topi GC, Amantea A, Griso D. Recovery from porphyria cutanea tarda with no specific therapy other than avoidance of hepatic toxins. *Br J Dermatol.* 1984;111:75-82.

243. Rich JD, Mylonakis E, Nossa R, et al. Highly active antiretroviral therapy leading to resolution of porphyria cutanea tarda in a patient with AIDS and hepatitis C. *Dig Dis Sci.* 1999;44:1034-1037.

244. Singal AK, Venkata KVR, Jampana S, et al. Hepatitis C treatment in patients with porphyria cutanea tarda. *Am J Med Sci.* 2017;353:523-528.

245. Combalia A, To-Figueras J, Laguno M, et al. Direct-acting antivirals for hepatitis C virus induce a rapid clinical and biochemical remission of porphyria cutanea tarda. *Br J Dermatol.* 2017;177:e183-e184.

246. Bulaj ZJ, Franklin MR, Phillips JD, et al. Transdermal estrogen replacement therapy in postmenopausal women previously treated for porphyria cutanea tarda. *J Lab Clin Med.* 2000;136:482-488.

247. Ashton RE, Hawk JL, Magnus IA. Low-dose oral chloroquine in the treatment of porphyria cutanea tarda. *Br J Dermatol.* 1984;111:609-613.

248. Singal AK, Kormos-Hallberg C, Lee C, et al. Low-dose hydroxychloroquine is as effective as phlebotomy in treatment of patients with porphyria cutanea tarda. *Clin Gastroenterol Hepatol.* 2012;10:1402-1409.

249. Stolzel U, Kostler E, Schuppan D, et al. Hemochromatosis (HFE) gene mutations and response to chloroquine in porphyria cutanea tarda. *Arch Dermatol.* 2003;139:309-313.

250. Ewing S, Crosby DL. Renal transplantation for porphyria cutanea tarda. *N Engl J Med.* 1997;336:811.

251. Fracanzani AL, Taioli E, Sampietro M, et al. Liver cancer risk is increased in patients with porphyria cutanea tarda in comparison to matched control patients with chronic liver disease. *J Hepatol.* 2001;35:498-503.

252. Ochiai T, Morishima T, Kondo M. Symptomatic porphyria secondary to hepatocellular carcinoma. *Br J Dermatol.* 1997;136:129-131.

253. Schmid R. Cutaneous porphyria in Turkey. *N Engl J Med.* 1960;263:397-398.

254. Can C, Nigogosyan G. Acquired toxic porphyria cutanea tarda due to hexachlorobenzene. Report of 348 cases caused by this fungicide. *J Am Med Assoc.* 1963;183:88-91.

255. Smith AG, Francis JE. Genetic variation of iron-induced uroporphyria in mice. *Biochem J.* 1993;291(pt 1):29-35.

256. de Verneuil H, Beaumont C, Deybach JC, et al. Enzymatic and immunological studies of uroporphyrinogen decarboxylase in familial porphyria cutanea tarda and hepatoerythropoietic porphyria. *Am J Hum Genet.* 1984;36:613-622.

257. Toback AC, Sassa S, Poh-Fitzpatrick MB, et al. Hepatoerythropoietic porphyria: clinical, biochemical, and enzymatic studies in a three-generation family lineage. *N Engl J Med.* 1987;316:645-650.

258. Horina JH, Wolf P. Epoetin for severe anemia in hepatoerythropoietic porphyria. *N Engl J Med.* 2000;342:1294-1295.

259. Fontanellas A, Mazurier F, Moreau-Gaudry F, et al. Correction of uroporphyrinogen decarboxylase deficiency (hepatoerythropoietic porphyria) in Epstein-Barr virus-transformed B-cell lines by retrovirus-mediated gene transfer: fluorescence-based selection of transduced cells. *Blood.* 1999;94:465-474.

260. Ged C, Ozalla D, Herrero C, et al. Description of a new mutation in hepatoerythropoietic porphyria and prenatal exclusion of a homozygous fetus. *Arch Dermatol.* 2002;138:957-960.

261. Pollack SS, Rosenthal MS. Images in clinical medicine. Diaper diagnosis of porphyria. *N Engl J Med.* 1994;330:114.

262. Di Pierro E, Brancaleoni V, Granata F. Advances in understanding the pathogenesis of congenital erythropoietic porphyria. *Br J Haematol.* 2016;173:365-379.

263. To-Figueras J, Millet O, Herrero C. Congenital erythropoietic porphyria. In: Kadish KM, Smith KM, Guillard R, eds. *Handbook of Porphyrin Science With Application to Chemistry, Physics, Materials Sience, Engineering Biology and Medicine.* World Scientific Publishing; 2014:151-217.

264. To-Figueras J, Ducamp S, Clayton J, et al. ALAS2 acts as a modifier gene in patients with congenital erythropoietic porphyria. *Blood.* 2011;118:1443-1451.

265. Phillips JD, Steensma DP, Pulsipher MA, et al. Congenital erythropoietic porphyria due to a mutation in GATA1: the first trans-acting mutation causative for a human porphyria. *Blood.* 2007;109:2618-2621.

266. Di Pierro E, Russo R, Karakas Z, et al. Congenital erythropoietic porphyria linked to GATA1-R216W mutation: challenges for diagnosis. *Eur J Haematol.* 2015;94:491-497.

267. Sarkany RP, Ibbotson SH, Whatley SD, et al. Erythropoietic uroporphyria associated with myeloid malignancy is likely distinct from autosomal recessive congenital erythropoietic porphyria. *J Invest Dermatol.* 2011;131:1172-1175.

268. Bhutani LK, Sood SK, Das PK, et al. Congenital erythropoietic porphyria. An autopsy report. *Arch Dermatol.* 1974;110:427-431.

269. Haining RG, Cowger ML, Shurtleff DB, et al. Congenital erythropoietic porphyria. I. Case report, special studies and therapy. *Am J Med.* 1968;45:624-637.

270. Kushner JP, Pimstone NR, Kjeldsberg CR, et al. Congenital erythropoietic porphyria, diminished activity of uroporphyrinogen decarboxylase and dyserythropoiesis. *Blood.* 1982;59:725-737.

271. Varadi S. Haematological aspects in a case of erythropoietic porphyria. *Br J Haematol.* 1958;4:270-280.

272. London IM, West R, Shemin D, et al. Porphyrin formation and hemoglobin metabolism in congenital porphyria. *J Biol Chem.* 1950;184:365-371.

273. Magnus IA. The cutaneous porphyrias. *Semin Hematol.* 1968;5:380-408.

274. Haining RG, Cowger ML, Labbe RF, et al. Congenital erythropoietic porphyria. II. The effects of induced polycythemia. *Blood.* 1970;36:297-309.

275. Piomelli S, Poh-Fitzpatrick MB, Seaman C, et al. Complete suppression of the symptoms of congenital erythropoietic porphyria by long-term treatment with high-level transfusions. *N Engl J Med.* 1986;314:1029-1031.

276. Guarini L, Piomelli S, Poh-Fitzpatrick MB. Hydroxyurea in congenital erythropoietic porphyria. *N Engl J Med.* 1994;330:1091-1092.

277. Egan DN, Yang Z, Phillips J, et al. Inducing iron deficiency improves erythropoiesis and photosensitivity in congenital erythropoietic porphyria. *Blood.* 2015;126:257-261.

278. Katugampola RP, Anstey AV, Finlay AY, et al. A management algorithm for congenital erythropoietic porphyria derived from a study of 29 cases. *Br J Dermatol.* 2012;167:888-900.

279. Ged C, Moreau-Gaudry F, Taine L, et al. Prenatal diagnosis in congenital erythropoietic porphyria by metabolic measurement and DNA mutation analysis. *Prenat Diagn.* 1996;16:83-86.

280. Deybach JC, Grandchamp B, Grelier M, et al. Prenatal exclusion of congenital erythropoietic porphyria (Gunther's disease) in a fetus at risk. *Hum Genet.* 1980;53:217-221.

281. Whatley SD, Ducamp S, Gouya L, et al. C-terminal deletions in the ALAS2 gene lead to gain of function and cause X-linked dominant protoporphyria without anemia or iron overload. *Am J Hum Genet.* 2008;83:408-414.

282. Yien YY, Ducamp S, van der Vorm LN, et al. Mutation in human CLPX elevates levels of delta-aminolevulinate synthase and protoporphyrin IX to promote erythropoietic protoporphyria. *Proc Natl Acad Sci U S A.* 2017;114:E8045-E8052.

283. DeLeo VA, Poh-Fitzpatrick M, Mathews-Roth M, et al. Erythropoietic protoporphyria. 10 years experience. *Am J Med.* 1976;60:8-22.
284. Avner DL, Berenson MM. Hepatic clearance and biliary secretion of protoporphyrin in the isolated, in situ-perfused rat liver. *J Lab Clin Med.* 1982;99:885-894.
285. Baart de la Faille H, Bijlmer-Iest JC, van Hattum J, et al. Erythropoietic protoporphyria: clinical aspects with emphasis on the skin. *Curr Probl Dermatol.* 1991;20:123-134.
286. Berke M, Redeker AG. Erythropoietic protoporporphyria with eczema solare: report of 3 cases. *Arch Dermatol.* 1963;87:507-511.
287. Holme SA, Anstey AV, Finlay AY, et al. Erythropoietic protoporphyria in the U.K.: clinical features and effect on quality of life. *Br J Dermatol.* 2006;155:574-581.
288. Holme SA, Whatley SD, Roberts AG, et al. Seasonal palmar keratoderma in erythropoietic protoporphyria indicates autosomal recessive inheritance. *J Invest Dermatol.* 2009;129:599-605.
289. Goerz G, Krieg T, Bolsen K, et al. Erythropoietic protoporphyria: porphyrin content of a gall-stone (author's transl). Article in German. *Arch Dermatol Res (1975).* 1976;256:283-289.
290. Biewenga M, Matawlie RHS, Friesema ECH, et al. Osteoporosis in patients with erythropoietic protoporphyria. *Br J Dermatol.* 2017;177:1693-1698.
291. Heerfordt IM, Wulf HC. Patients with erythropoietic protoporphyria have reduced erythrocyte protoporphyrin IX from early in pregnancy. *Br J Dermatol.* 2017;177:e38-e40.
292. Meerman L. Erythropoietic protoporphyria. An overview with emphasis on the liver. *Scand J Gastroenterol Suppl.* 2000;(232):79-85.
293. Bloomer JR, Enriquez R. Evidence that hepatic crystalline deposits in a patient with protoporphyria are composed of protoporphyrin. *Gastroenterology.* 1982;82:569-573.
294. Lock G, Holstege A, Mueller AR, et al. Liver failure in erythropoietic protoporphyria associated with choledocholithiasis and severe post-transplantation polyneuropathy. *Liver.* 1996;16:211-217.
295. Nakahashi Y, Taketani S, Okuda M, et al. Molecular cloning and sequence analysis of cDNA encoding human ferrochelatase. *Biochem Biophys Res Commun.* 1990;173:748-755.
296. Gouya L, Deybach JC, Lamoril J, et al. Modulation of the phenotype in dominant erythropoietic protoporphyria by a low expression of the normal ferrochelatase allele. *Am J Hum Genet.* 1996;58:292-299.
297. Gouya L, Puy H, Robreau AM, et al. The penetrance of dominant erythropoietic protoporphyria is modulated by expression of wildtype FECH. *Nat Genet.* 2002;30:27-28.
298. Gouya L, Martin-Schmitt C, Robreau AM, et al. Contribution of a common single-nucleotide polymorphism to the genetic predisposition for erythropoietic protoporphyria. *Am J Hum Genet.* 2006;78:2-14.
299. Burden AE, Wu C, Dailey TA, et al. Human ferrochelatase: crystallization, characterization of the [2Fe-2S] cluster and determination that the enzyme is a homodimer. *Biochim Biophys Acta.* 1999;1435:191-197.
300. Whatley SD, Mason NG, Holme SA, et al. Molecular epidemiology of erythropoietic protoporphyria in the U.K. *Br J Dermatol.* 2010;162:642-646.
301. Brancaleoni V, Balwani M, Granata F, et al. X-chromosomal inactivation directly influences the phenotypic manifestation of X-linked protoporphyria. *Clin Genet.* 2016;89:20-26.
302. Bishop DF, Tchaikovskii V, Nazarenko I, et al. Molecular expression and characterization of erythroid-specific 5-aminolevulinate synthase gain-of-function mutations causing X-linked protoporphyria. *Mol Med.* 2013;19:18-25.
303. Fratz EJ, Clayton J, Hunter GA, et al. Human erythroid 5-aminolevulinate synthase mutations associated with X-linked protoporphyria disrupt the conformational equilibrium and enhance product release. *Biochemistry.* 2015;54:5617-5631.
304. Brun A, Western A, Malik Z, et al. Erythropoietic protoporphyria: photodynamic transfer of protoporphyrin from intact erythrocytes to other cells. *Photochem Photobiol.* 1990;51:573-577.
305. Poh-Fitzpatrick MB. Molecular and cellular mechanisms of porphyrin photosensitization. *Photo Dermatol.* 1986;3:148-157.
306. Lim HW. Pathophysiology of cutaneous lesions in porphyrias. *Semin Hematol.* 1989;26:114-119.
307. Magnus IA, Jarrett A, Prankerd TA, et al. Erythropoietic protoporphyria. A new porphyria syndrome with solar urticaria due to protoporphyrinaemia. *Lancet.* 1961;2:448-451.
308. Bottomley SS, Tanaka M, Everett MA. Diminished erythroid ferrochelatase activity in protoporphyria. *J Lab Clin Med.* 1975;86:126-131.
309. Balwani M, Naik H, Anderson KE, et al. Clinical, biochemical, and genetic characterization of north American patients with erythropoietic protoporphyria and X-linked protoporphyria. *JAMA Dermatol.* 2017;153:789-796.
310. Gou EW, Balwani M, Bissell DM, et al. Pitfalls in erythrocyte protoporphyrin measurement for diagnosis and monitoring of protoporphyrias. *Clin Chem.* 2015;61:1453-1456.
311. Went LN, Klasen EC. Genetic aspects of erythropoietic protoporphyria. *Ann Hum Genet.* 1984;48:105-117.
312. Poh-Fitzpatrick MB. Protoporphyrin metabolic balance in human protoporphyria. *Gastroenterology.* 1985;88:1239-1242.
313. Morton KO, Schneider F, Weimer MK, et al. Hepatic and bile porphyrins in patients with protoporphyria and liver failure. *Gastroenterology.* 1988;94:1488-1492.
314. Bossi K, Lee J, Schmeltzer P, et al. Homeostasis of iron and hepcidin in erythropoietic protoporphyria. *Eur J Clin Invest.* 2015;45:1032-1041.
315. Langendonk JG, Balwani M, Anderson KE, et al. Afamelanotide for erythropoietic protoporphyria. *N Engl J Med.* 2015;373:48-59.
316. Biolcati G, Marchesini E, Sorge F, et al. Long-term observational study of afamelanotide in 115 patients with erythropoietic protoporphyria. *Br J Dermatol.* 2015;172:1601-1612.
317. Poh-Fitzpatrick MB, Wang X, Anderson KE, et al. Erythropoietic protoporphyria: altered phenotype after bone marrow transplantation for myelogenous leukemia in a patient heteroallelic for ferrochelatase gene mutations. *J Am Acad Dermatol.* 2002;46:861-866.
318. Windon AL, Tondon R, Singh N, et al. Erythropoietic protoporphyria in an adult with sequential liver and hematopoietic stem cell transplantation: a case report. *Am J Transplant.* 2018;18:745-749.
319. Butler DF, Ginn KF, Daniel JF, et al. Bone marrow transplant for X-linked protoporphyria with severe hepatic fibrosis. *Pediatr Transplant.* 2015;19:E106-E110.
320. Mathews-Roth MM, Michel JL, Wise RJ. Amelioration of the metabolic defect in erythropoietic protoporphyria by expression of human ferrochelatase in cultured cells. *J Invest Dermatol.* 1995;104:497-499.
321. Magness ST, Brenner DA. Ferrochelatase cDNA delivered by adenoviral vector corrects biochemical defect in protoporphyric cells. *Hum Gene Ther.* 1995;6:1285-1290.
322. Oustric V, Manceau H, Ducamp S, et al. Antisense oligonucleotide-based therapy in human erythropoietic protoporphyria. *Am J Hum Genet.* 2014;94:611-617.
323. Sarkany RP, Ross G, Willis F. Acquired erythropoietic protoporphyria as a result of myelodysplasia causing loss of chromosome 18. *Br J Dermatol.* 2006;155:464-466.
324. Goodwin RG, Kell WJ, Laidler P, et al. Photosensitivity and acute liver injury in myeloproliferative disorder secondary to late-onset protoporphyria caused by deletion of a ferrochelatase gene in hematopoietic cells. *Blood.* 2006;107:60-62.
325. Yoshioka A, Fujiwara S, Kawano H, et al. Late-onset erythropoietic protoporphyria associated with myelodysplastic syndrome treated with azacitidine. *Acta Derm Venereol.* 2018;98:275-277.
326. Bottomley SS, Muller-Eberhard U. Pathophysiology of heme synthesis. *Semin Hematol.* 1988;25:282-302.
327. Lim HW, Cooper D, Sassa S, et al. Photosensitivity, abnormal porphyrin profile, and sideroblastic anemia. *J Am Acad Dermatol.* 1992;27:287-292.
328. Poblete-Gutierrez P, Badeloe S, Wiederholt T, et al. Dual porphyrias revisited. *Exp Dermatol.* 2006;15:685-691.
329. Harraway JR, Florkowski CM, Sies C, et al. Dual porphyria with mutations in both the UROD and HMBS genes. *Ann Clin Biochem.* 2006;43:80-82.
330. Akagi R, Inoue R, Muranaka S, et al. Dual gene defects involving delta-aminolaevulinate dehydratase and coproporphyrinogen oxidase in a porphyria patient. *Br J Haematol.* 2006;132:237-243.
331. McColl KE, Thompson GG, Moore MR, et al. Chester porphyria: biochemical studies of a new form of acute porphyria. *Lancet.* 1985;2:796-799.
332. Poblete-Gutierrez P, Wiederholt T, Martinez-Mir A, et al. Demystification of Chester porphyria: a nonsense mutation in the Porphobilinogen Deaminase gene. *Physiol Res.* 2006;55(suppl 2):S137-S144.
333. Balwani M, Wang B, Anderson K, et al. Acute hepatic porphyrias: recommendations for evaluation and long-term management. *Hepatology.* 2017;66:1314-1322.

Chapter 29 ■ Hereditary Spherocytosis, Hereditary Elliptocytosis, and Other Disorders Associated With Abnormalities of the Erythrocyte Membrane

PATRICK G. GALLAGHER • BERTIL GLADER

This chapter focuses on hemolytic disorders and abnormalities of red blood cell shape resulting from alterations of the erythrocyte membrane. The major emphasis is on the hereditary spherocytosis (HS) and hereditary elliptocytosis (HE) syndromes because these are most commonly encountered by clinicians.[1] The traditional classification of these disorders has been based on red blood cell (RBC) shape changes, retained in this chapter because of its clinical applicability (*Figure 29.1*). There has been an explosion of knowledge regarding the biology of the erythrocyte membrane, providing a better understanding of membrane structure and function as well as revealing the heterogeneous and diverse pathobiology of these disorders. Readers should consult prior editions of this text for detailed references for previously cited primary references.

THE ERYTHROCYTE MEMBRANE

The erythrocyte membrane, because of its easy accessibility, is the most studied biologic membrane. Composed of a lipid bilayer and an underlying cortical membrane skeleton (*Figure 29.2*), the erythrocyte membrane provides the red cell with the deformability and stability required to withstand its travels through the circulation. The erythrocyte is subjected to high sheer stress in the arterial system, dramatic changes in size in the microcirculation with capillary diameters as small as 7.5 microns, and marked fluctuations in tonicity, pH, and pO_2 as it travels through the body.[2]

The lipid bilayer is composed primarily of phospholipids intercalated with unesterified cholesterol and glycolipids. Phospholipids are asymmetrically organized, with the choline phospholipids, phosphatidylcholine (PC) and sphingomyelin, primarily in the outer half of the bilayer, and the amino phospholipids, phosphatidylethanolamine and phosphatidylserine (PS), in the inner half of the bilayer.[3] In pathologic states, such as thalassemia, sickle cell disease, and diabetes, loss of phospholipid asymmetry with externalization of PS leads to activation of blood clotting via conversion of prothrombin to thrombin and facilitates macrophage attachment to erythrocytes, marking them for destruction.[4]

Lipids are arranged in domains within the bilayers, as large, lipid-rich macroscopic domains, protein-bound microscopic domains, or domains associated with the detergent-resistant fraction of the membrane (called DRM or lipid rafts).[5,6] The role(s) of these domains has yet to be elucidated, but DRM domains may facilitate malarial invasion of the erythrocyte.[7,8]

The erythrocyte membrane contains about 15 major proteins and hundreds of minor ones.[9,10] Typically, membrane proteins are classified as *integral*, penetrating or crossing the lipid bilayer and interacting with the hydrophobic lipid core, or *peripheral*, interacting with integral proteins or lipids at the membrane surface but not penetrating into the bilayer core. The integral membrane proteins include the glycophorins, the Rh proteins, Kell and Duffy antigens, and transport proteins such as band 3 (AE1, anion exchanger 1), Na^+, K^+-ATPase, Ca^{2+}-ATPase, and Mg^{2+}-ATPase. An assortment of membrane receptors and antigens are present on various integral membrane proteins. Peripheral membrane proteins include the structural proteins of the spectrin-actin based membrane skeleton.[11]

The membrane skeleton, composed of an intricately interwoven meshwork of proteins, interacts with both integral membrane proteins and the lipid bilayer.[11] The major proteins of the membrane skeleton include spectrin, actin, ankyrin, protein 4.1R, and protein 4.2 (*Figure 29.2* and *Table 29.1*).

Spectrin is the principal structural component of the membrane skeleton, as well as its most abundant protein, comprising 25% to 30% of membrane protein. Spectrin functions include provision of structural support for the lipid bilayer, maintenance of cellular shape, and regulation of lateral movement of integral membrane proteins.[13] Spectrin is composed of α and ß chains, which despite a number of similarities, including both containing 106 amino acid α-helical "spectrin repeats" composed of triple-helices linked by short connecting regions, are distinct proteins encoded by separate genes. αß-Spectrin chains intertwine in an antiparallel manner to form 100-nm-long heterodimers. These αß-spectrin heterodimers self-associate with other αß-spectrin heterodimers to form $(\alpha\beta)_2$ heterotetramers, the functional spectrin subunit in the erythrocyte.[14] Tetramers provide significant flexibility and structural support for the lipid bilayer, helping maintain cellular shape.[12,13] Spectrin heterodimer-tetramer interconversion is governed by a simple thermodynamic equilibrium that favors tetramer formation.[15]

The primary linkage of spectrin to the plasma membrane is via binding of spectrin tetramers to ankyrin, which in turn binds to the integral protein band 3.[16] Protein 4.2 binds to band 3 and probably to ankyrin, presumably promoting their interactions.[17]

A second linkage of spectrin to the plasma membrane is mediated by its association with the "junctional complex," a multiprotein complex that includes spectrin, actin, adducin, and protein 4.1R.[18] Protein 4.1R directly interacts with both spectrin and actin, as well as other proteins of the junctional complex and the plasma membrane including band 3, glycophorin C (GPC), p55, calmodulin, CD44, pIC1n, CASK, mature parasite-infected antigen, and phosphatidylserine. Other important junctional complex proteins include the ß subtype of actin, tropomyosin, tropomodulin, p55, and adducin.[13] Adducin is a heterodimer of structurally related proteins, α-, ß-, or γ-adducin, which functions in the early assembly of the spectrin/actin complex by capping the ends of fast-growing actin filaments and by recruiting spectrin to the ends of actin filaments.[18,19]

Another membrane skeleton linkage to the plasma membrane is mediated via binding of a multiprotein complex containing the Rh proteins, the RH-associated glycoproteins, CD47, LW, glycophorin B, and protein 4.2 to ankyrin.

Erythrocyte membrane disorders result from alterations in the quantity or quality (or both) of individual proteins and their dynamic interactions with each other.[2,20] Disruption of the vertical protein-protein interactions of the membrane, that is, the spectrin-ankyrin-band 3 linkage or the band 3–protein 4.2 interaction, leads to uncoupling of the membrane skeleton from the lipid bilayer. This leads to membrane instability with loss of lipids and some integral membrane proteins, resulting in loss of membrane surface area and the phenotype of spherocytosis (*Figure 29.2*). Disruption of the horizontal interactions of membrane skeleton proteins, including perturbation of spectrin self-association or junctional complex protein-protein interactions, leads to membrane instability, altered membrane deformability and mechanical properties, and the phenotype of elliptocytosis (*Figure 29.2*).[21]

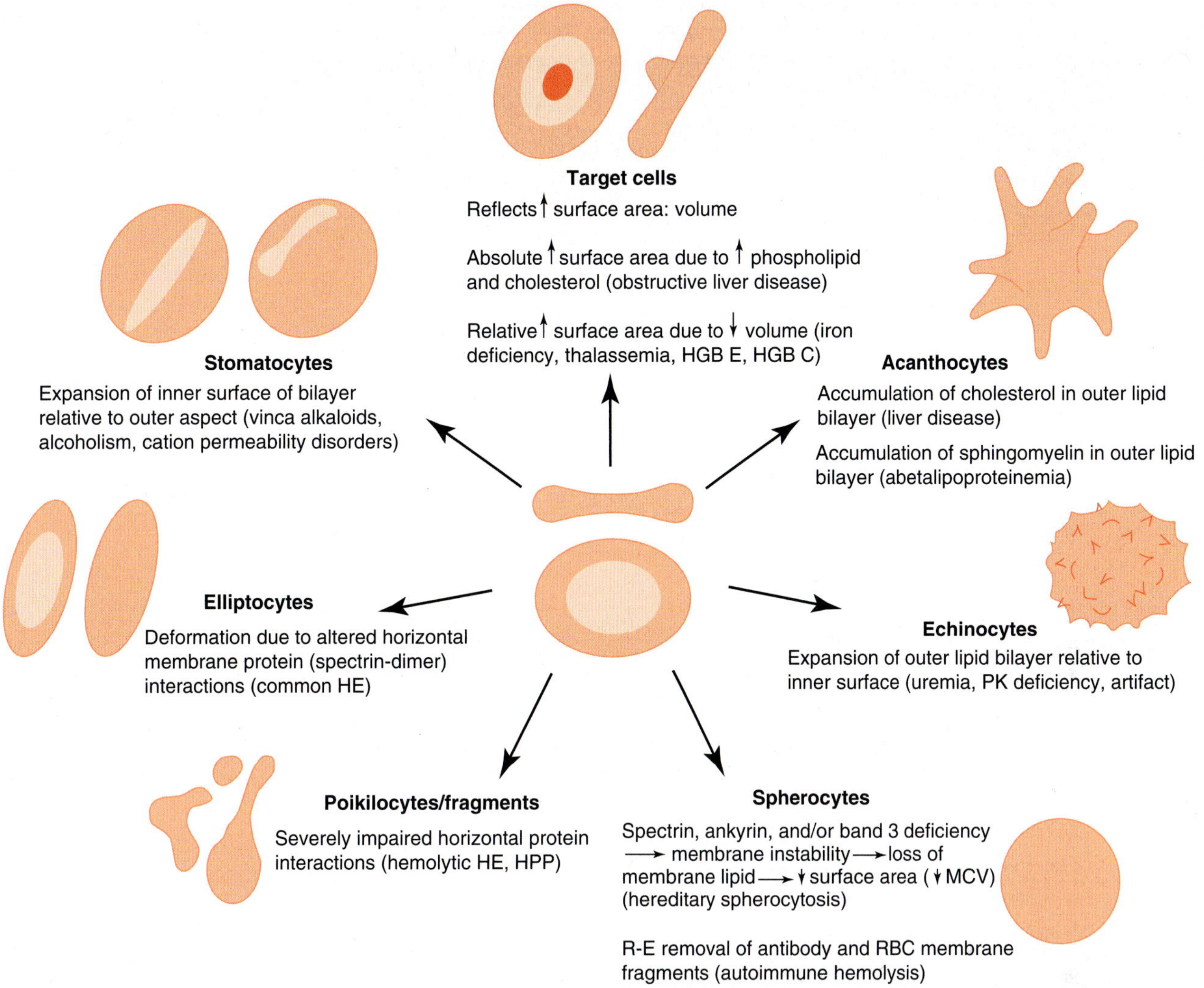
Target cells
Reflects ↑ surface area: volume
Absolute ↑ surface area due to ↑ phospholipid and cholesterol (obstructive liver disease)
Relative ↑ surface area due to ↓ volume (iron deficiency, thalassemia, HGB E, HGB C)
Stomatocytes
Expansion of inner surface of bilayer relative to outer aspect (vinca alkaloids, alcoholism, cation permeability disorders)
Acanthocytes
Accumulation of cholesterol in outer lipid bilayer (liver disease)
Accumulation of sphingomyelin in outer lipid bilayer (abetalipoproteinemia)
Elliptocytes
Deformation due to altered horizontal membrane protein (spectrin-dimer) interactions (common HE)
Echinocytes
Expansion of outer lipid bilayer relative to inner surface (uremia, PK deficiency, artifact)
Poikilocytes/fragments
Severely impaired horizontal protein interactions (hemolytic HE, HPP)
Spherocytes
Spectrin, ankyrin, and/or band 3 deficiency ⟶ membrane instability ⟶ loss of membrane lipid ⟶ ↓ surface area (↓ MCV) (hereditary spherocytosis)
R-E removal of antibody and RBC membrane fragments (autoimmune hemolysis)

FIGURE 29.1 Diagrammatic representation of abnormal cells associated with alterations in the erythrocyte membrane. HE, hereditary elliptocytosis; HGB, hemoglobin; HPP, hereditary pyropoikilocytosis; MCV, mean corpuscular volume; PK, pyruvate kinase; R-E, reticuloendothelial.

Glycophorin A
Glycophorin C
Band 3
Band 3
Band 3
Band 3
p55
Adducin
4.2
Ankyrin
4.9
Actin
Tropomyosin
β-Spectrin
α-Spectrin
Tropomodulin
Vertical Interaction
Horizontal Interaction

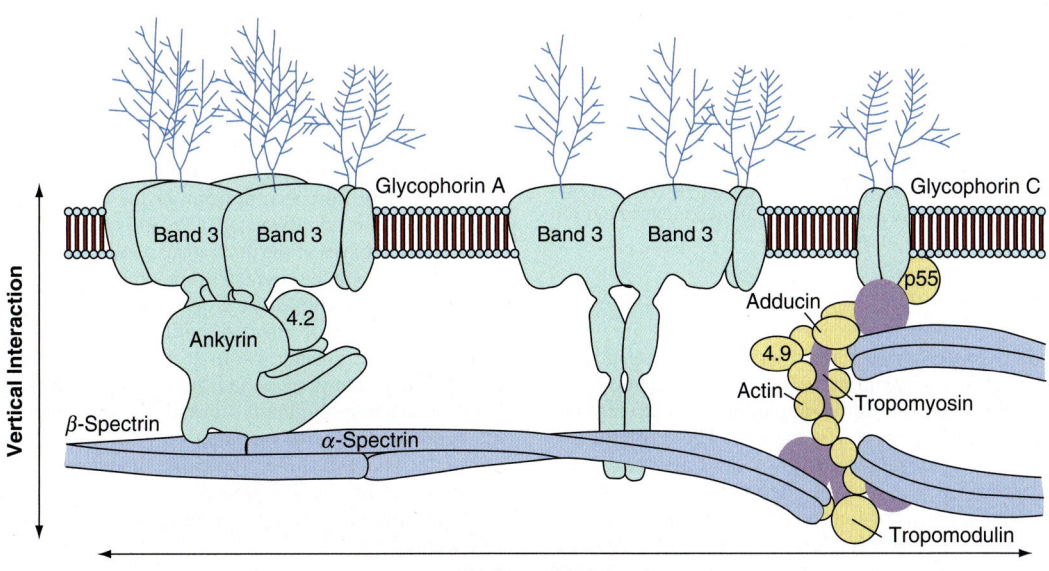

FIGURE 29.2 The erythrocyte membrane. A model of the major proteins of the erythrocyte membrane is shown: α- and ß-spectrin, ankyrin, band 3 (the anion exchanger), 4.1R (protein 4.1R) and 4.2 (protein 4.2), Rh (Rhesus polypeptide), RhAG (Rh-associated glycoprotein), LW (Landsteiner-Weiner glycoprotein), actin and glycophorin. Membrane protein-protein and protein-lipid interactions are often divided into two categories: (1) *vertical interactions*, which are perpendicular to the plane of the membrane and involve spectrin-ankyrin-band 3protein 4.2 interactions and weak interactions between spectrin and the negatively charged lipids of the inner half of the membrane lipid bilayer, and (2) *horizontal interactions*, which are parallel to the plane of the membrane and include interactions between junctional complex proteins and spectrin or other membrane proteins. (Adapted from Perrotta S, Gallagher PG, Mohandas N. Hereditary spherocytosis. *Lancet*. 2008;372(9647):1411-1426. Copyright © 2008 Elsevier. With permission.)

Table 29.1. Major Human Erythrocyte Membrane Proteins, Their Genes, and Associated Disorders

SDS-Page band	Protein	Amino Acids (#)	Molecular Weight × 10³ (Gel/ Calculated)	Oligomeric State	Gene Symbol	Chromosomal Location	Exons (#)	Associated Disorders
1	α-Spectrin	2429	240/281	Heterodimer/ tetramer	SPTA1	1q22-q23	52	HE, HPP, HS
2	β-Spectrin	2137	220/246	Heterodimer/ tetramer	SPTB	14q23-q24.1	32	HE, HPP, HS
2.1ᵃ	Ankyrin-1	1880	210/206	Monomer	ANK1	8p11.2	42	HS
2.9	α-Adducin	—	97/80	Heterodimer/ tetramer	ADD1	4p16.3	16	—
2.9	β-Adducin	726	97/80	Heterodimer/ tetramer	ADD2	2p13.3	17	—
3	Band 3 (AE1), anion exchanger1	911	90-100/102	Dimer or tetramer	SLC4A1	17q21	20	HS, HAc, SAO, HSt
4.1ᵇ	Protein 4.1R	588	80 + 78/66	Monomer	EPB41	1p33-p34.2	>23	HE
4.2	Protein 4.2	691	2/77	Dimer or trimer	EPB42	15q15-q21	13	HS[12]
4.9	Dematin	383	48-52/43-46	Trimer	EPB49	8p21.1	15	—
4.9	p55	466	55/53	Dimer	MPP1	Xq28	12	—
5	β-Actin	375	43/42	Oligomer	ACTB	7pter-q22	6	—
5	Tropomodulin	359	43/41	Monomer	TMOD	9q22	9	—
6	G3PD	335	35/36	Tetramer	GAPD	12p13	9	—
7	Stomatin	288	31/32	Oligomer	STOM	9q33.2	7	HSt
7	Tropomyosin	239	27 + 29/28	Heterodimer	TPM3	1q31	13	—
PAS-1ᶜ	Glycophorin A	131	36/14	Dimer	GYPA	4q31.21	7	—
PAS-2ᶜ	Glycophorin C	128	32/14	—	GYPC	2q14-q21	4	HE
PAS-3ᶜ	Glycophorin B	72	20/8	Dimer	GYPB	4q31.21	5	—
PAS-3ᶜ	Glycophorin D	107	23/11	—	GYPD	2q14 q21	4	HE

ᵃMultiple ankyrin isoforms are seen on SDS-PAGE gels numbered 2.1, 2.1, 0.23, etc.
ᵇProtein 4.1R is a doublet (4.1a and 4.1b) on SDS-PAGE gels, with 4.1a derived from 4.1b by deamidation.
ᶜGlycophorins are visible only on PAS-stained gels.
Abbreviations: G3PD, glucose 3-phosphate dehydrogenase; HAc, hereditary acanthocytosis; HE, hereditary elliptocytosis; HPP, hereditary pyropoikilocytosis; HS, hereditary spherocytosis; HSt, hereditary stomatocytosis; PAS, periodic acid Schiff stain; SAO, Southeast Asian ovalocytosis; SDS-PAGE, sodium dodecyl sulfate-polyacrylamide gel electrophoresis.
Modified from Gallagher PG, Lux SE. Disorders of the erythrocyte membrane. In: Nathan DG, Orkin SH, Ginsburg D, et al., eds. *Nathan and Oski's Hematology of Infancy and Childhood.* 6th ed. WB Saunders; 2003:567-568. Copyright © 2003 Elsevier. With permission.

Development of biochemical techniques has allowed the separation and quantification of membrane proteins (*Figure 29.3*) and the detection of membrane protein abnormalities in many hereditary red cell disorders. Advances in molecular biology have allowed determination of the precise genetic defects in many cases.

HEREDITARY SPHEROCYTOSIS

HS is a hemolytic disorder characterized by anemia, intermittent jaundice, splenomegaly, and responsiveness to splenectomy.[22,23] There is marked clinical heterogeneity, ranging from an asymptomatic condition to a fulminant hemolytic anemia. The morphologic hallmark of HS is the spherocyte, created by loss of membrane surface area and characterized by abnormal erythrocyte osmotic fragility in vitro. The interesting history of HS is recounted in detail by Dacie[24] and Packman.[25] The earliest clinical account of the disorder is probably the 1871 report of Vanlair and Masius,[26] and the 1934 studies of Haden drew attention to a probable structural abnormality of the membrane as the basis for hemolysis.[27] Subsequent investigation of HS afforded important insights into the structure and function of cell membranes and the role of the spleen in maintaining erythrocyte integrity.

Prevalence and Genetics

HS is the most common of the hereditary hemolytic anemias among people of Northern European descent. In the United States, the incidence of the disorder is approximately 1 in 3000 to 5000.[22,23] When mild and asymptomatic forms of the disease are considered, the incidence is closer to 1:2000.[28,29] The disease is encountered worldwide, but its incidence and prevalence in other ethnic groups are not clearly established.

In the majority of affected families, HS is transmitted in an autosomal dominant manner. Up to 25% of patients with HS demonstrate nondominant inheritance, and the parents of these patients are clinically and hematologically normal.[30,31] In many of these patients, HS is due to a de novo mutation. In others, it is inherited in an autosomal recessive fashion, typically linked to abnormalities in the α-spectrin or protein 4.2 genes.[32,33] A few cases of severe, homozygous HS have been reported, usually in cases where there is parental consanguinity.[34,35]

Pathogenesis

The pathogenesis of HS involves the interplay between an intrinsic erythrocyte membrane protein defect and an intact spleen that selectively retains, damages, and eventually destroys abnormal HS erythrocytes.

Membrane Protein Defects

The primary lesion in HS erythrocytes is caused by membrane protein defects that result in membrane instability. The first biochemical defect recognized in patients with HS was spectrin deficiency, and the

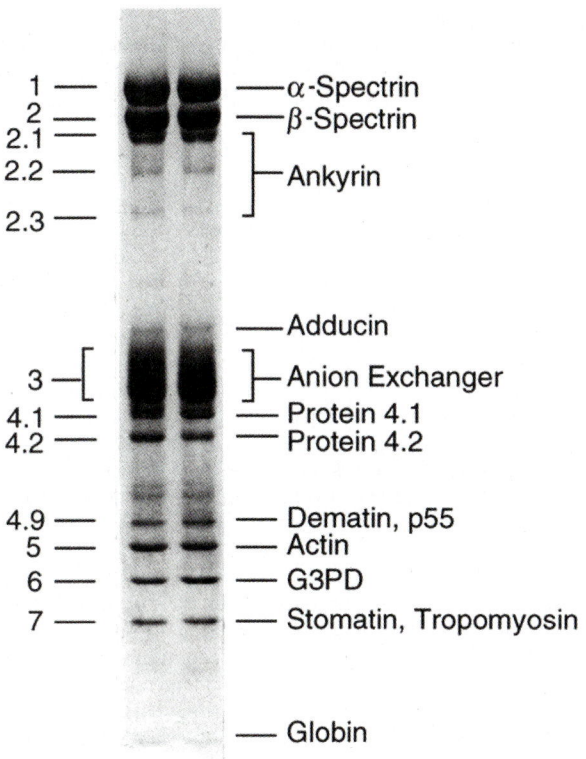

FIGURE 29.3 Protein composition of the red blood cell membrane skeleton. The major components of the erythrocyte membrane as separated by sodium dodecyl sulfate–polyacrylamide gel electrophoresis and revealed by. Coomassie blue staining. G3PD, glucose 3-phosphate dehydrogenase. (Reprinted from Gallagher PG, Tse WT, Forget BG. Clinical and molecular aspects of disorders of the erythrocyte membrane skeleton. *Semin Perinatol.* 1990;14(5):351-367. Copyright © 1990 Elsevier. With permission.)

degree of spectrin deficiency was found to correlate with the extent of spherocytosis, the degree of abnormality of the osmotic fragility test, and severity of hemolysis.[30,31,36-38] In some cases, spectrin deficiency is the result of impaired synthesis, whereas in other instances, it is caused by quantitative or qualitative deficiencies of other proteins that integrate spectrin into the cell membrane, especially ankyrin.[32] In the latter case, free spectrin is degraded, thereby leading to spectrin deficiency. Analysis of red cell membrane proteins in patients with HS has identified several major abnormal patterns: spectrin deficiency alone, combined spectrin and ankyrin deficiency, band 3 deficiency, protein 4.2 deficiency, or no obvious biochemical abnormality. Each of the variant subsets is associated with mutations that result in different protein abnormalities, laboratory findings, and varied clinical expression (*Table 29.2*).[39,40]

Spectrin Deficiency

In the erythrocyte, α-spectrin is synthesized in 3- to 4-fold excess with β-spectrin synthesis rate limiting for membrane assembly of αβ-spectrin heterotetramers.[41,42] Excess α-chains normally are degraded. Clinical abnormalities caused by α-spectrin deficiency are found only in the homozygous or compound heterozygous state, as heterozygotes produce sufficient normal α-spectrin to balance ß-spectrin production and maintain a normal phenotype. In contrast, defects of ß-spectrin are clinically apparent in the heterozygous state because synthesis of ß-spectrin is rate limiting. Red cell membranes from patients with autosomal recessive HS due to α-spectrin deficiency have only 40% to 50% the normal amount of spectrin, whereas spectrin levels range from 60% to 80% in patients with autosomal dominant HS due to ß-spectrin defects.[22,23]

Determination of the precise genetic defects in α-spectrin-linked HS has identified a number of associated mutations. Several variant alleles have been associated with α-spectrin-deficient, nondominant HS.[43,44] These include spectrin[Bug Hill], an alanine to aspartic acid substitution in the αII domain, and spectrin[LEPRA], low expression Prague, a C to T substitution associated with increased utilization of an alternative acceptor splice site in intron 30. As series of laboratory, biochemical, and genetic studies revealed, spectrin[LEPRA] is the primary cause of severe, nondominant HS due to perturbed α-spectrin mRNA splicing.[32]

Mutations of ß-spectrin mutations impair ß-spectrin synthesis or produce truncated ß-spectrin chains that are unstable or do not bind to ankyrin and, thus, are not assembled onto the membrane skeleton.[45,46] One HS-associated ß-spectrin variant, ß-Spectrin[Kissimmee], is a point

Disorders of Red Blood Cells

Table 29.2. Classification of Hereditary Spherocytosis (HS)

	Carrier	Mild Spherocytosis	Moderate Spherocytosis	Moderately Severe Spherocytosis[a]	Severe Spherocytosis[b]
Hemoglobin (g/dL)	Normal	11-15	8-12	6-8	<6
Reticulocytes (%)	1-3	3-8	8	10	10
Bilirubin (mg/dL)	0-1	1-2	2	2-3	3
Spectrin content (% of normal)[c]	100	80-100	50-80	40-80[d]	20-50
Peripheral smear	Normal	Mild spherocytosis	Spherocytosis	Spherocytosis	Spherocytosis and poikilocytosis
Osmotic fragility fresh blood	Normal	Normal or slightly increased	Distinctly increased	Distinctly increased	Distinctly increased
Incubated blood	Slightly increased	Distinctly increased	Distinctly increased	Distinctly increased	Markedly increased

[a]Values in untransfused patients.
[b]By definition, patients with severe spherocytosis are transfusion dependent.
[c]Normal (±SD) = 245 ± 27 × 10⁵ spectrin dimers per erythrocyte. In most patients, ankyrin content is decreased to a comparable degree. A minority of patients with HS lack band 3 or protein 4.2 and may have mild to moderate spherocytosis with normal amounts of spectrin and ankyrin.
[d]The spectrin content is variable in this group of patients, presumably reflecting heterogeneity of the underlying pathophysiology.
From Walensky LD, Narla M, Lux SE. Disorders of the red blood cell membrane. In: Handin RI, Lux SE, Stossel TO, eds. *Blood: Principles and Practice of Hematology.* 2nd ed. Lippincott Williams & Wilkins; 2003:1753. Reprinted with permission from Dr. Robert I. Handin.

mutation that leads to defective binding of spectrin to protein 4.1R.[47] Occasionally, cases of ß-spectrin-linked HS arise de novo.[48]

Ankyrin Defects

Combined spectrin and ankyrin deficiency is the most common biochemical abnormality found in the red cell membrane in cases of typical, autosomal dominant HS.[49] Ankyrin is the principal binding site for spectrin on the red cell membrane, and studies of membrane skeleton assembly indicate that ankyrin deficiency leads to decreased incorporation of spectrin on the membrane despite normal spectrin synthesis. As expected, there is proportional deficiency of spectrin and ankyrin in these erythrocytes (*Figure 29.4*).

Ankyrin gene mutations are the most common defect associated with dominant HS. The majority of ankyrin defects are private point mutations in the coding region of the ankyrin gene associated with reduced or absent expression of the mutant allele.[34] Around 15% to 20% of these mutations arise de novo.[50] A few cases of spectrin/ankyrin-deficient HS are associated with mutations in the ankyrin gene erythroid promoter.[51-53]

HS has been associated with karyotypic abnormalities involving deletions or translocations of the ankyrin-1 gene locus on chromosome 8p. Ankyrin deletions may be part of a contiguous gene syndrome associated with HS, mental retardation, typical facies, and hypogonadism.[54,55]

Band 3 Deficiency

Heterozygous band 3 mutations are found in 10% to 25% of patients with autosomal-dominant HS.[56,57] Erythrocyte membranes demonstrate a 20% to 40% decrease of band 3 content and decreased or absent protein 4.2. Red cell anion transport is decreased proportional to the band 3 deficiency. Numerous band 3 gene mutations spread throughout the regions encoding both the cytoplasmic and membrane-spanning domains have been described. Many of these are null mutations associated with markedly reduced or absent band 3 mRNA. Others are missense mutations that disrupt band 3–membrane protein

interactions or disrupt normal band 3 cellular trafficking from the endoplasmic reticulum to the plasma membrane.[57,58]

Affected patients typically exhibit mild to moderate HS.[22,23] Mushroom-shaped or "pincered" red cells on peripheral smear have been associated with band 3–deficient HS. Homozygotes or compound heterozygotes for band 3 mutations usually exhibit more severe HS. Band 3 alleles that influence band 3 expression have been reported that, when inherited *in trans* to a band 3 mutation, aggravate band 3 deficiency and worsen the clinical phenotype.[59-61] Although band 3 is expressed in the distal tubules of the kidney, only a few patients with band 3–associated HS exhibit defects in urinary acidification.[62,63]

Protein 4.2 Deficiency

Autosomal recessive HS has been described in a subset of patients, primarily those of Japanese ancestry, whose erythrocyte membranes demonstrate marked deficiency of protein 4.2.[64] In some cases, there is coexisting deficiency of band 3 and ankyrin. Clinical severity and red cell morphology are variable, with spherocytes, elliptocytes, or sphero-ovalocytes on peripheral smear. A few mutations of the protein 4.2 gene have been described in these patients, primarily null or missense mutations. One missense mutation, Protein 4.2[Nippon], associated with a spherocytic, ovalocytic, and elliptocytic hemolytic anemia, is relatively common in Japan.[65] Protein 4.2 deficiency also occurs in association with HS-associated mutations in the cytoplasmic domain of band 3, likely due to disruption of band 3–protein 4.2 interactions.

Erythrocyte Abnormalities

The molecular basis of HS is heterogeneous; thus, it is likely that the loss of membrane surface area is a consequence of several molecular mechanisms (*Figure 29.5*). The common denominator is a weakening of protein-protein interactions that link the membrane skeleton to the lipid bilayer, leading to microvesiculation, loss of membrane surface area, decreased surface to volume ratio, and spherocytosis. In cases associated with spectrin deficiency, the membrane skeleton is unable to provide adequate support for the lipid bilayer, causing destabilization of the lipid bilayer with the resultant loss of band 3–containing membrane microvesicles. In cases associated with band 3 deficiency, the lipid-stabilizing effect of band 3 is lost, releasing band 3–free microvesicles from the membrane. The loss of membrane surface area transforms red cells from biconcave discs to spherocytes with decreased cellular deformability, limiting their ability to pass through the sinusoids of the spleen and predisposing them to splenic entrapment, conditioning, and destruction.

The membrane defect in HS leads to a variety of secondary metabolic changes. These include increased sodium and potassium flux across the HS membrane, which leads to increased membrane sodium-potassium adenosine triphosphatase activation; accelerated adenosine triphosphate (ATP) breakdown; increased glycolytic rate; decreased 2,3-diphosphoglycerate (2,3-DPG) concentration, and lower intracellular pH. HS erythrocytes are slightly dehydrated, although the reason for decreased RBC water content is not known. Possibilities include activation of K-Cl cotransport, a pathway that leads to dehydration and is activated by acid pH, possibly in the acid environment of the splenic cords, or increased Na^+/K^+ pump activity stimulated in response to increased passive cation leaks, leading to decreased total cation content, water efflux from the red cell, and cellular dehydration. Dehydration of HS red cells is important because it can further impair their deformability.

Role of the Spleen

The spleen plays a critical role in the pathobiology of HS, as destruction of spherocytes in the spleen is the primary cause of hemolysis in patients with HS.[66] The survival of HS red cells infused into normal recipients is reduced, whereas the survival of normal red cells in subjects with HS is normal. Despite the persistence of spherocytosis after splenectomy, red cell survival is normal or only slightly reduced.

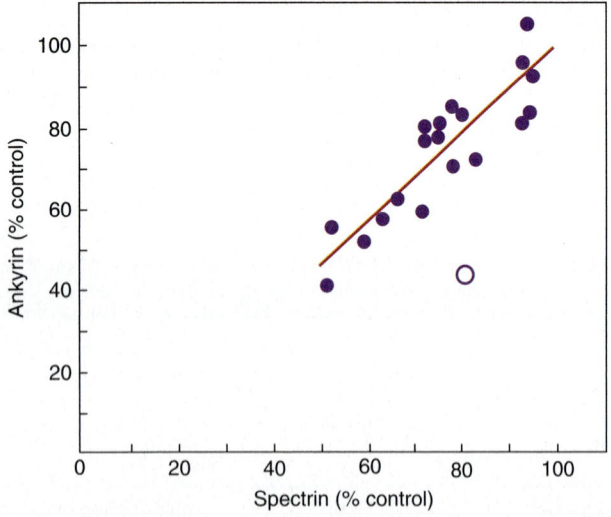

FIGURE 29.4 Role of spectrin and ankyrin in hereditary spherocytosis. The relationship between spectrin and ankyrin content in erythrocytes of patients with dominant hereditary spherocytosis. Each point, expressed as a percentage of control (100%), represents the mean value for a kindred for both spectrin and ankyrin levels. The line represents a computer-generated fitting of the data for 19 of the 20 kindreds. The degree of spectrin and ankyrin deficiencies is essentially identical in these kindreds with one exception (*open circle*), an otherwise typical family in which erythrocytes are primarily ankyrin deficient. (Reprinted from Savvides P, Shalev O, John KM, et al. Combined spectrin and ankyrin deficiency is common in autosomal dominant hereditary spherocytosis. *Blood.* 1993;82(10):2953-2960. Copyright © 1993 American Society of Hematology. With permission.)

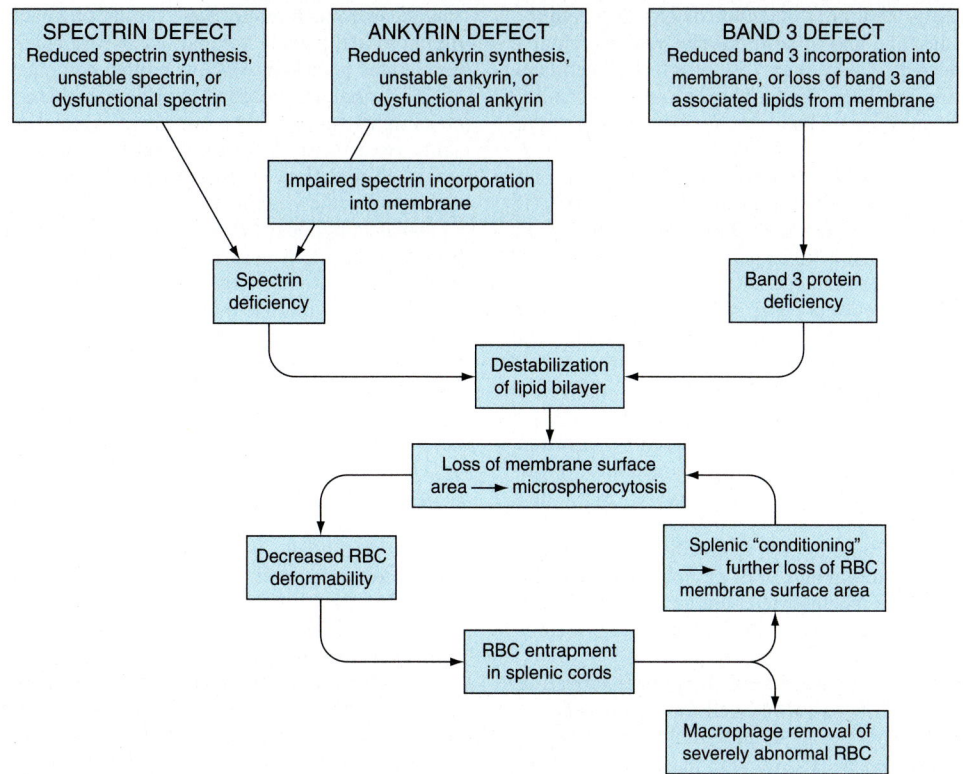

FIGURE 29.5 Pathophysiology of hereditary spherocytosis (HS). The primary defect in HS is a deficiency of membrane surface area, leading to the formation of spherocytes. Decreased surface area may be produced by different mechanisms: Defects of spectrin and ankyrin lead to reduced density of the spectrin-actin membrane skeleton, destabilizing the overlying lipid bilayer and releasing band 3–containing microvesicles, or defects of band 3 and protein 4.2 lead to band 3 deficiency and loss of its lipid-stabilizing effect, resulting in the loss of band 3–free microvesicles. Both pathways result in loss of membrane surface area, spherocyte formation, and decreased deformability. These deformed erythrocytes become trapped in the hostile environment of the spleen cords, where splenic conditioning inflicts further membrane damage or they are removed by splenic macrophages.

Taken together, these observations demonstrate that an intrinsic red cell defect leads to RBC destruction, but only in the presence of an extrinsic factor—an intact spleen.

Splenic Entrapment

The unique anatomy of the splenic vasculature leads to sequestration of spherocytes selectively in the spleen. Arterial blood enters directly into the splenic cords, a network of channels formed by reticulum cells and lined by macrophages. Most of the blood that enters the splenic cords passes rapidly through direct channels, which reenter the venous system after traversing fenestrations between the lining endothelial cells. A small fraction of blood in the splenic cords percolates more slowly through this maze before reaching the venous sinuses. The hematocrit of blood from the splenic cords is high, the environment is acidic, and red cells are exposed to macrophages that line these channels. The size of fenestrations in the venous sinuses is small relative to the RBC size, and to pass through requires significant deformability of the red cell and its membrane.[67] This, however, is a major problem for spherocytes, which have lost surface area and are dehydrated. Spleens removed from patients with HS reveal congested cords, relatively empty venous sinuses, and few spherocytes traversing sinus walls. The most severely damaged spherocytes, cells unable to negotiate the fenestrations in the venous sinus, are removed from the circulation by macrophages. However, impaired deformability of HS red cells is only significant for the passage of these cells through the spleen. After splenectomy, red cell survival normalizes, even though spherocytes persist and sometimes are increased. Splenectomy has no effect on surface area loss by HS reticulocytes or mature red cells, because surface area loss is due to the intrinsic membrane lesion in these cells, an independent event that continues even after splenectomy.

Splenic Conditioning

In addition to trapping HS red cells, the spleen also "conditions" these cells in a way that accelerates membrane loss and spherocyte formation. Some conditioned red cells reenter the systemic circulation, gradually shifting from osmotically normal to osmotically fragile cells during their circulation. Osmotically fragile microspherocytes are concentrated in and emanate from the splenic pulp. The more conditioned or spheroidal cells are responsible for the most fragile portion, or "the tail" of the fresh osmotic fragility curve. The conditioning effect of the spleen is a cumulative injury, thought to result from several passages through the organ. The mechanism(s) of splenic conditioning is not clear. It may be the result of hemoconcentration and erythrostasis with macrophage-induced membrane injury, possibly related to the lower pH in the spleen. The calculated transit time for spherocytes is short relative to the time required for severe metabolic compromise; thus, it is unlikely that metabolic depletion is important, and the ATP content of HS cells in the spleen is normal.

Clinical Features

Anemia, jaundice, and splenomegaly are the clinical features of HS most commonly encountered. However, signs and symptoms are highly variable, both with respect to age of onset and severity.[22,23] for example, anemia or hyperbilirubinemia may be of such magnitude as to require exchange transfusion in the neonatal period or cases may escape clinical recognition altogether, presenting very late in life.[68] Anemia usually is mild to moderate, but it may be absent, mild, moderate, or severe requiring transfusion. Beyond the neonatal period, jaundice is intermittent and is associated with fatigue, cold exposure, emotional distress, or pregnancy. An increase in scleral icterus and a darker urine color is commonly seen in children with nonspecific viral infections. Even when patients have no detectable jaundice, there is usually laboratory evidence of ongoing hemolysis. Splenomegaly is the rule, and in large family studies, palpable spleens have been detected in more than 75% of affected members. No apparent correlation has been shown between spleen size and disease severity, but it may exist. The liver is normal in size and function.

From a clinical perspective, it has been useful to classify HS according to the severity of disease (*Table 29.2*).[22,23] Moderate HS is the most common presentation, recognized as a chronic hemolytic disorder with characteristic spherocytes on peripheral blood smear and an autosomal dominant pattern of inheritance.

Mild HS occurs in 20% to 30% of cases of HS. Anemia is absent, as the bone marrow is able to fully compensate for the persistent destruction of red cells, and there is little or no splenomegaly.[69,70] Because patients in this group usually are asymptomatic, they often are not diagnosed until later in life. Sometimes, they are identified as a result of hemolytic or aplastic episodes triggered by infection. Occasionally, the condition is identified through family surveys performed to document the hereditary nature of hemolytic disease in a relative.

Moderate HS accounts for 60% to 75% of all HS cases. It is associated with mild to moderate anemia, modest splenomegaly, and intermittent jaundice.[69,70] The reticulocyte count and serum bilirubin levels are elevated. Patients may require transfusion during intercurrent illness.

Severe HS occurs in ~5% of cases of HS. It is characterized by severe hemolytic anemia, the need for red cell transfusion particularly during infancy and early childhood, and usually an incomplete response to splenectomy. The pattern of inheritance is frequently nondominant.[30,31,35]

The silent carrier of HS exists in families with autosomal recessive HS. In most cases, carriers have no signs of HS or minimal signs of HS, for example, a slightly increased reticulocyte count, a few spherocytes on peripheral blood smear, a minimally abnormal incubated osmotic fragility, or abnormal erythrocyte spectrin content detected when using sensitive techniques.[30] Using a conservative estimate of 1:5000 HS incidence in the United States, combined with the observation that ~25% of cases are autosomal recessive, it has been calculated that the HS silent carrier state might exist in 1.4% of the US population.

HS in Infancy

In the neonatal period, jaundice is likely to be the most prominent feature of HS. About 30 to 50% of adult patients with HS report a history of neonatal jaundice and the diagnosis of HS is prominent in etiologic studies of severe neonatal hyperbilirubinemia.[71,72] The magnitude of hyperbilirubinemia may be severe, requiring phototherapy or exchange transfusion.[73] Virtually all infants with HS who are homozygous for the mutation responsible for Gilbert syndrome are jaundiced enough to require phototherapy.[73] Most newborns with HS are not anemic, in contrast to having jaundice, sometimes making diagnosis difficult.[74] Spherocytosis on the peripheral blood smear and reticulocytosis are frequently minimal or absent. However, anemia develops rapidly over the first few weeks of life in many infants and may require transfusion.[73] Maturation of splenic filtering and development of the splenic circulation appear to increase the rate of hemolysis after birth; at the same time, the erythropoietic response to anemia is blunted. Within a few months, erythropoiesis increases, anemia improves, and the need for red cell transfusions disappears in all but the most severely affected infants.

Complications

The two major complications seen in HS are episodes of worsening anemia and the development of gall bladder disease.

Exacerbations of anemia occur in almost all patients with HS, even in most patients with HS who have mild or clinically silent disease, associated with various stresses such as infection, major surgery, trauma, and pregnancy. For example, previously mild anemia

can become much more severe during pregnancy, usually because of the increased plasma volume but occasionally as a consequence of accelerated hemolysis.[75] As with other chronic hemolytic states, some anemic crises are preceded by a febrile illness and may be observed concurrently in more than one affected member of a single family. In some cases, there may be increased hemolysis (decreased hemoglobin, increased reticulocytes, increased bilirubin concentration) associated with nonspecific viral infections.[76]

Aplastic/hypoplastic crises resulting from parvovirus B19 infection may occur, just as is seen in individuals with other chronic hemolytic disorders.[77] Parvovirus B19 selectively infects erythroid precursors and inhibits their growth. Erythropoietic arrest leads to a sudden decrease in hemoglobin concentration and reticulocytopenia. Recovery occurs within 7 to 10 days and is heralded by reticulocytosis and thrombocytosis. Parvovirus infection may be the first manifestation of HS, and multiple HS family members infected with parvovirus have developed aplastic crises at the same time, leading to descriptions of "epidemics" of HS.[78] Infection with parvovirus is a particular threat to susceptible pregnant women, because it can infect the fetus, leading to severe anemia, hydrops fetalis, and fetal death.

Less commonly, exaggeration of anemia is the result of exhaustion of folate reserves by the sustained increase in net DNA synthesis.[79] Megaloblastic arrest of erythropoiesis has been observed most commonly during pregnancy, in association with liver disease, or in patients recovering from an aplastic crisis.

Cholelithiasis is common in HS just as in other chronic hemolytic disorders. Bilirubin pigment gallstones may be found in infants and young children,[80] but the incidence of gallstones increases markedly with age, and they are present in 40% to 80% of adults. The history of family members with cholelithiasis in the second or third decade of life is a clue to the possibility of HS or another inherited hemolytic disorder. In patients with mild HS, cholelithiasis may be the initial presentation of the disease. The development of gallstones is increased approximately 5-fold in patients with HS who are homozygotes for the uridine diphosphate-glucuronosyltransferase mutation responsible for Gilbert syndrome.[81,82] Because of their high incidence, patients with HS should be periodically examined by ultrasound for the presence of gallstones, beginning early in childhood.

A few other unusual complications have been noted in patients with HS. Heterotopia of the bone marrow has been noted rarely in the renal pelvis or along the vertebral column.[83] These extramedullary masses of marrow may be mistaken for malignant tumors. After the spleen is removed, they undergo fatty metamorphosis. Hemosiderosis and multiple endocrine disorders resulting from transfusion-induced iron overload have been described. Interestingly, symptomatic iron overload also has been reported in some nontransfused patients with HS who are heterozygous for the hemochromatosis gene. Cases of HS and hematologic malignancy, including multiple myeloma, leukemia, and myeloproliferative disorders, have been reported, suggested to be linked to the persistent hematopoietic stress of HS, but the relationship with HS, if more than coincidental, remains to be determined. Gout and chronic leg ulcers/dermatitis are unusual complications in adults with HS.[84,85] Other rare complications include thrombosis, spinocerebellar degenerative syndromes, movement disorder with myopathy, and hypertrophic cardiomyopathy.[86]

Laboratory Features

The classic laboratory features of HS include anemia, reticulocytosis, increased mean corpuscular hemoglobin concentration (MCHC), spherocytes on the peripheral blood smear, hyperbilirubinemia, and an abnormal osmotic fragility test.

Anemia is typically mild, accompanied by reticulocytosis with values of 5% to 20%. This compensation is associated with increased erythropoiesis and elevated levels of erythropoietin.[69,70] Erythrocyte indices demonstrate a normal or borderline low mean corpuscular volume (MCV) despite increased numbers of reticulocytes, reflecting the membrane loss and dehydration. The MCHC is usually increased (>35%) due to mild cellular dehydration.[87,88] Examination of indices obtained by automated cell counters can be used as a screening test for HS. In unsplenectomized children, an MCHC >35.4 g/dL and a red cell distribution width (RDW) >14 had a sensitivity of 63% and a specificity of 100%[88] for the diagnosis of HS. Histograms of hyperdense erythrocytes (MCHC > 40 g/dL) obtained from laser-based cell counters have been used as a screening tests for HS, and when combined with an elevated MCHC, have been claimed to identify nearly all cases of HS.

RBC morphology is distinctive but not diagnostic. Patients with typical HS have obvious spherocytes on peripheral blood smear. Spherocytes lack central pallor, their mean cell diameter is decreased, and they appear more intensely hemoglobinized. Spherocytes are a feature of many hemolytic anemias; thus, their identification alone does not establish a diagnosis of HS. The number of spherocytes and microspherocytes varies considerably from patient to patient, as few as 1 to 3/hpf in mild HS to as many as 20 to 30/hpf in moderate HS (*Figure 29.6*). In severe HS, many poikilocytes are also present in addition to the spherocytosis. Unlike the spherocytes associated with immune hemolytic disease and thermal injury, most HS spherocytes are fairly uniform in size and density. Varying degrees of polychromatophilia and anisocytosis are noted. Because the degree of spherocytosis or "conditioning" is a function of cell age, reticulocytes and young red cells are morphologically normal. Specific morphologic findings, including pincered erythrocytes (band 3), spherocytic acanthocytes (ß-spectrin), or spherostomatocytes (protein 4.2) have been correlated with specific membrane defects.[22,23]

Osmotic Fragility

Red cells behave as perfect osmometers when suspended in varying concentrations of hypotonic salt solutions, and osmotic fragility (OF) of red cells is a measure of their spheroidicity. With a decreased membrane surface area relative to volume, spherocytes are unable to withstand the introduction of small amounts of free water that occurs when they are placed in progressively more hypotonic solutions. Consequently, spherocytes hemolyze more than discoid RBCs at any salt concentration (*Figure 29.7*). Hemolysis is determined by measuring the fraction of total hemoglobin released from red cells into the extracellular fluid at progressively more dilute salt concentrations. The fresh osmotic fragility test detects circulating spherocytes, cells that have been conditioned by the spleen. This appears as a "tail" produced by a small population of abnormal cells that undergo hemolysis at salt concentrations that do not affect normal red cells. The most sensitive test to detect spherocytes is the incubated OF test performed after

incubating RBCs 18 to 24 hours under sterile conditions at 37 °C. This procedure takes advantage of the observation that all erythrocytes lose membrane under these incubation conditions; however, the process is markedly accelerated in HS red cells. Hemolysis of HS cells may be complete at solute concentrations that cause little or no lysis of normal cells. HS individuals may have a normal fresh OF if reduced surface area is balanced by a reduction in volume (due to cell dehydration), but the OF after prolonged incubation at 37 °C is usually abnormal. Although OF correlates well with the magnitude of spherocytosis, no correlation is observed between OF and hemoglobin concentration. The sensitivity of the incubated OF test may be outweighed by a loss of its specificity, that is, spherocytes due to any cause exhibit abnormal incubated OF. A normal OF does not exclude the diagnosis of HS, as 10% to 20% of patients with HS, that is, those with mild HS, lack circulating spherocytes.

Eosin-5-Maleimide Binding

Eosin-5-maleimide (EMA) binding to erythrocytes, a flow cytometry-based method reflecting relative amounts of band 3 and Rh-related proteins, has been utilized as a screening test for HS.[89] It is claimed to have a higher predictive value than osmotic fragility testing based on the observation that there have been no reports of positive results in immune-mediated or non-membrane-associated hemolytic disease. However, these tests are not specific, detecting other erythrocyte

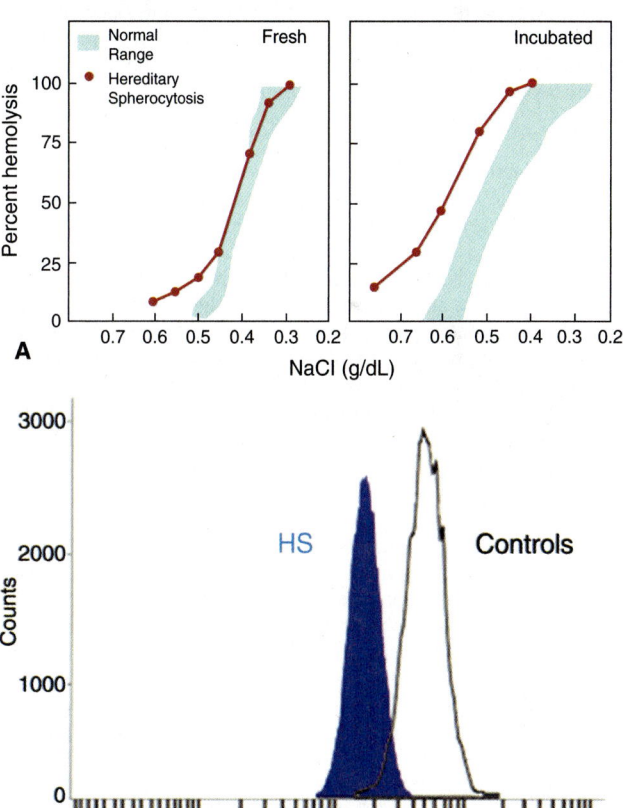

FIGURE 29.7 Osmotic fragility curves in hereditary spherocytosis. Diagrams of the osmotic fragility (OF) test, as manifested by percent hemolysis, of normal and hereditary spherocytosis (HS) erythrocytes after dilution in salt solutions of varying tonicity. *(Left)* In the fresh OF, a "tail" of osmotically sensitive HS erythrocytes produced by splenic conditioning is seen prior to splenectomy. *(Right)* In the incubated OF, the entire population of HS erythrocytes is more osmotically sensitive. (Reprinted from Glader BE, Naumovski L. Hereditary red blood cell disorders. In: Rimoin DL, Connor JM, Pyeritz RE, Korf BR, eds. *Emery and Rimoin's Principles and Practice of Medical Genetics.* 5th ed. Churchill Livingstone; 2006. Copyright © 2006 Elsevier. With permission.)

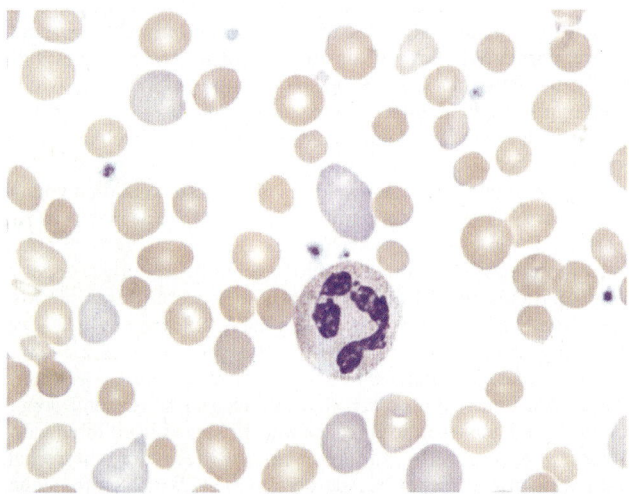

FIGURE 29.6 Hereditary spherocytosis. A typical Wright-stained peripheral blood smear from a patient with autosomal dominant hereditary spherocytosis is shown. Small, dense, round, conditioned spherocytes that lack central pallor are visible throughout.

Disorders of Red Blood Cells

abnormalities, especially those associated with abnormal band 3, including congenital dyserythropoietic anemia and abnormalities of erythrocyte hydration and viscosity, including sickle cell disease and cryohydrocytosis.[90,91] In addition, normal EMA binding has been reported in some cases of spectrin-deficient HS. The EMA binding test has gained wide popularity due to its ease in execution and relatively low cost of performance. Similar to osmotic fragility testing, its predictive value is enhanced if family history, clinical information, and additional laboratory data are also available.[91]

Osmotic gradient ektacytometry is more sensitive and specific than the osmotic fragility or EMA binding tests for the diagnosis of HS, but it is not widely available.

Other laboratory tests used to diagnose HS include the autohemolysis test, the spontaneous hemolysis of red cells incubated under sterile conditions without glucose, the glycerol lysis test, and the pink test, but these are rarely used nowadays and they offer no advantage over the osmotic fragility test. The cryohemolysis test has also been used as a screening test in HS.[89]

In the past, doubt existed whether HS could be diagnosed in the newborn period because many infants with HS have few circulating spherocytes. Moreover, fresh red cells from normal neonates are relatively resistant to osmotic lysis, whereas incubated infant erythrocytes are osmotically more fragile. However, OF and EMA binding detect HS in many but not all infants if appropriate normal neonatal RBC controls are used.

The bone marrow is characterized by erythroid hyperplasia. Normoblasts may constitute 25% to 60% of all nucleated cells. When complicated by folate deficiency, megaloblastic features of both myeloid and erythroid precursors are prominent. Examination of the bone marrow is not needed to diagnose HS.

Molecular Studies

Once the diagnosis of HS is made, it is possible to further characterize the specific membrane lesion. Studies using polyacrylamide gel electrophoresis separation or specific radioimmunoassays allow quantification of major membrane proteins, looking for abnormalities in spectrin, ankyrin, band 3, protein 4.2, or other proteins. Detection of the specific genetic abnormality is accomplished via mutation screening or direct DNA sequence analyses. However, these studies are cumbersome, expensive, and available only in select research laboratories. Detailed molecular studies, which have proven to be highly informative for understanding of both the pathogenesis of HS and normal membrane structure and function, are utilized for studying difficult or particularly interesting and informative cases.

Diagnosis

The diagnosis of HS generally is straightforward. Often, there is a family history of HS or a family history of anemia, splenectomy, or cholecystectomy. The signs and symptoms of HS are nonspecific and associated with many chronic hemolytic states (mild pallor, intermittent jaundice, and splenomegaly). Typical laboratory features include mild anemia, reticulocytosis, increased MCHC and RDW, normal MCV despite reticulocytosis, spherocytes on the peripheral blood smear, hyperbilirubinemia, and an abnormal incubated osmotic fragility test. Other disorders, such as immune hemolytic disease, glucose-6-phosphate dehydrogenase deficiency, certain syndromes of red cell fragmentation, and thermal and chemical injury of red cells, also are associated with spherocytosis. In most of these conditions, spherocytes are but one of several types of abnormal RBCs present, whereas in HS, there are few abnormal forms other than spherocytes. Additional historical data, such as onset later in life, temporal relationship to prescription of various medications such as methyldopa, or symptoms attributable to malignancy or connective tissue disease, as well as additional laboratory data, such as a positive direct antiglobulin reaction in immune hemolytic disease, may help differentiate other disorders from HS.

Use of genetic testing for diagnosis is becoming more common.[92] Some practitioners perform genetic testing prior to

splenectomy (see below) to ensure the correct diagnosis, especially to exclude the diagnosis of hereditary xerocytosis (HX), a condition that may mimic HS where splenectomy is contraindicated due to the occurrence of post splenectomy thrombotic complications. Molecular testing has its pitfalls including detection of variants of uncertain significance, making genetic diagnosis uncertain, and failure of detection of mutations outside gene coding regions and intron/exon boundaries such as deep intronic mutations, distal regulatory elements, and intragenic deletions and rearrangements.

Treatment

For practical purposes, the treatment of HS revolves around supportive care, splenectomy, and management of postsplenectomy complications.[93,94]

Neonates with severe hyperbilirubinemia caused by HS are at risk for kernicterus,[72] and such infants should be treated with phototherapy or exchange transfusion, or both, as clinically indicated.[95] Red cell transfusions are sometimes needed during hemolytic or aplastic crises. Erythropoietin therapy for the first few months of life has been suggested to diminish the need for red cell transfusions until erythropoiesis reaches its full postnatal expression,[96,97] but this therapy is not well studied.

Folic acid is required to sustain erythropoiesis, and normal dietary folate may be inadequate for children and some adults with chronic hemolytic anemia. For this reason, patients with HS are instructed to take supplementary folic acid to prevent the rare megaloblastic crises, although in mild cases, this is probably unnecessary.

HS is unique among the congenital hemolytic anemias in that splenectomy is permanently curative except in some severe, autosomal recessive cases,[98,99] and even these severe cases exhibit significant clinical improvement.[66,100] Within days of splenectomy, jaundice fades, the hemoglobin concentration rises, and red cell survival is dramatically improved. Transfusion requirements are decreased or eliminated, and the risk of cholelithiasis is reduced. Spherocytosis and increased osmotic fragility persist, but the tail of the fresh osmotic fragility curve, created by splenic conditioning, disappears. The MCV may fall but the MCHC does not change significantly.

For many years splenectomy was recommended for all patients with HS without regard to clinical severity. The rationale was that splenectomy eliminated the need for transfusion therapy, ensured freedom from aplastic crises, and minimized the risk of gall bladder disease. This position has been tempered in recent years because it is now known that the spleen has a critical immunologic role in protecting against certain types of infections and overwhelming postsplenectomy infection with encapsulated bacteria, especially *Streptococcus pneumonia,* may occur. The emergence of penicillin-resistant pneumococci has heightened concerns, as has growing recognition of increased risk of postsplenectomy cardiovascular disease, particularly thrombosis and pulmonary hypertension.[101-105] Finally, the important role of the spleen in protection of individuals living in geographic regions where parasitic diseases such as malaria or babesiosis occur has reemerged as international travel has become more common.

The risk of postsplenectomy sepsis is greatest in children younger than 5 years, but even older children and adults are at increased risk. Death from sepsis may occur decades after splenectomy.[106,107] In one comprehensive review, postsplenectomy infection was assessed in 850 patients with HS, 786 of whom were children.[108] Most patients had undergone surgery during the first 5 years of life. A total of 30 cases of septicemia (3.52%) and 19 septic deaths (2.23%) were identified. The estimated rate of mortality from sepsis was approximately 200 times greater than that expected in the general population. Although most septic episodes were observed in children whose spleens were removed in the first years of life, older children and adults were also susceptible. Another report of 226 patients splenectomized for HS estimated the mortality from overwhelming sepsis to be 0.73/1000 years. Mortality rates for 35 children who underwent splenectomy prior to 6 years of age and for 191 individuals who were older than 6 at the time of splenectomy were 1.12/1000 and 0.66/1000 years of life post splenectomy, respectively, far beyond that of the general population. Rates for both these studies may overestimate the postsplenectomy risk, as some of the participants underwent splenectomy prior to introduction of the pneumococcal vaccine.

The rationale that splenectomy prevents development of gallstones and symptomatic biliary tract disease, as well as obviates the need for major gallbladder surgery, is not as valid today as in the past. Development of laparoscopic cholecystectomy has had a significant impact on the management of nonanemic patients with mild HS who have gallstones. In these patients, if they have no signs or symptoms related to their hemolytic anemia, it is reasonable to follow them without splenectomy. If surveillance ultrasound examinations reveal gallstones, laparoscopic cholecystectomy can be performed, preventing biliary tract disease.

The benefits of splenectomy must be balanced against the immediate and long-term risks of the procedure.[109,110] Recently published HS management guidelines recognize these concerns and recommend discussion between health care providers, patient, and family when splenectomy is entertained.[93] It seems reasonable to splenectomize patients with HS with severe hemolytic anemia, patients with significant complications of anemia including growth failure, skeletal changes, extramedullary hematopoietic tumors, and leg ulcers/dermatitis. Splenectomy for patients with moderate HS and compensated, asymptomatic anemia is controversial and should be undertaken on a case-by-case basis. Patients with mild HS and compensated hemolysis can be managed expectantly and referred for splenectomy if clinically indicated. The higher risk of overwhelming sepsis in young children who undergo splenectomy makes it important to defer the operation until at least age 6 years in all but the most severe patients. Before splenectomy, patients should receive immunization with pneumococcal, *Haemophilus influenzae*, and meningococcal vaccines. Based on these considerations, rates of splenectomy in HS are decreasing.[111]

Laparoscopic splenectomy, associated with less postoperative discomfort, quicker recovery, shorter hospitalization, and decreased cost, is now the preferred method for splenectomy.[112,113] Operative complications of splenectomy, which include local infection, bleeding, and pancreatitis, are uncommon.[114] Partial splenectomy has initially been explored for infants and very young children with severe HS.[115-119] The purpose of partial splenectomy is to preserve splenic immunologic function, reducing splenic destruction of spherocytes and thereby palliating hemolysis and anemia. Follow-up demonstrates that there is sustained and clinically significant laboratory parameters and clinical signs and symptoms in many patients, but regrowth of the spleen remnant leading to increased clinical severity of HS necessitating total splenectomy may occur in up to one-third of cases.[120] The role of radiologic imaging as part of the preoperative evaluation prior to partial splenectomy has been emphasized.[121] Proponents of this procedure note that splenic function is preserved in young children when the risk of overwhelming sepsis is highest and that chronic transfusions and iron overload are decreased. Opponents of partial splenectomy note that patients who can be well managed with judicious transfusion therapy may be subjected to two operative procedures with general anesthesia.

Post splenectomy care includes counseling of patients or parents to seek prompt medical care during febrile illness. Use of early antibiotic therapy for splenectomized febrile children has led to a decrease in the incidence of severe postsplenectomy infection, leading some to propose having antibiotics available at home for immediate treatment of febrile illness. The emergence of penicillin-resistant pneumococci requires consideration when selecting antibiotic therapy in splenectomized patients.

The role of prophylactic antibiotics post splenectomy is a matter of current controversy, and few data exist to provide recommendations. Some recommend that all splenectomized children (and adults) receive penicillin prophylactically for life. Others recommend prophylaxis up to 6 years of age, while others prescribe antibiotics for 10 years post

splenectomy. There are even fewer data regarding the prescription of prophylactic antibiotics in adults post splenectomy.

There have been several reports of major thrombotic events post splenectomy for HS.[101,102,122] Some of these cases have actually been variants of stomatocytosis, where post splenectomy risk of thrombosis is well known. Anticoagulants have not been evaluated in this setting.

HEREDITARY ELLIPTOCYTOSIS SYNDROMES

The HE syndromes are a family of genetically determined erythrocyte disorders characterized by elliptical red cells on the peripheral blood smear (*Figure 29.8*).[123] Some HE syndromes are associated with symptomatic hemolytic disease, although most are clinically silent and are discovered incidentally when a blood smear is reviewed. The varied clinical and hematologic manifestations of HE are an expression of the numerous molecular defects that give rise to an elliptocytic-shaped erythrocyte.

The HE syndromes are classified into several groups (*Table 29.3*).[124] *Common HE* is a dominantly inherited condition characterized by many elliptocytes in the peripheral blood smear. The clinical severity of common HE is extremely variable, ranging from an incidental asymptomatic condition, most commonly observed, to a mild to moderate hemolytic anemia. The clinical expression of *hemolytic HE* ranges from a moderate hemolytic anemia to severe, near fatal or fatal hemolytic anemia. *Hereditary pyropoikilocytosis* (HPP) is a severe hemolytic anemia, with red cell fragments, poikilocytes, and microspherocytes seen on peripheral blood smear. From a clinical perspective, it is difficult to distinguish severe hemolytic HE from HPP. Once regarded as a separate condition, HPP is now recognized to be a variant of the HE disorders. *Spherocytic HE* is a rare condition in which both ovalocytes and spherocytes are present on the blood smear. *Southeast Asian ovalocytosis* (SAO), also known as stomatocytic elliptocytosis, is an HE variant prevalent in the malaria-infested belt of Southeast Asia and the South Pacific, and it is characterized by rigid spoon-shaped cells that have either a longitudinal slit or a transverse ridge.

Prevalence of Hereditary Elliptocytosis Variants

When considered together, the HE variants occur with an estimated frequency of 1:1000 to 5000. The distribution of HE is worldwide, and no racial or ethnic group appears to be spared.[124] In the US population, the prevalence of HE is approximately 3 to 5/10,000, and it appears to be much more common among patients of African ancestry. In areas where malaria is endemic, HE occurs considerably more frequently. In one study from equatorial Africa, common HE had a prevalence of 0.6%. Resistance of hereditary elliptocytes to invasion by malaria parasites may explain the high prevalence.[125]

Pathogenesis of Hereditary Elliptocytosis Disorders

The HE disorders are caused by intrinsic membrane protein abnormalities, which lead to an alteration in RBC membrane function, changes in RBC shape, and, in some cases, hemolysis.

Membrane Protein Defects

The primary defect of the membrane skeleton leading to the HE phenotype was suggested by the retention of an elliptical shape by membrane ghosts and skeletons prepared from hereditary elliptocytes, uniform instability of HE membrane ghosts and skeletons to mechanical stress, and abnormal heat sensitivity of spectrin prepared from the red cells of some patients with HE. Subsequent studies have shown that the principle defect in HE is mechanical weakness or fragility of the erythrocyte membrane skeleton, due to qualitative and/or quantitative defects in several membrane skeleton proteins, α- and ß-spectrin, protein 4.1R, or GPC.[124]

The majority of HE-associated defects occur in spectrin, the principal structural protein of the membrane skeleton. Spectrin is composed of α- and ß-spectrin, two structurally similar, nonidentical proteins encoded by separate genes. The majority of spectrin is

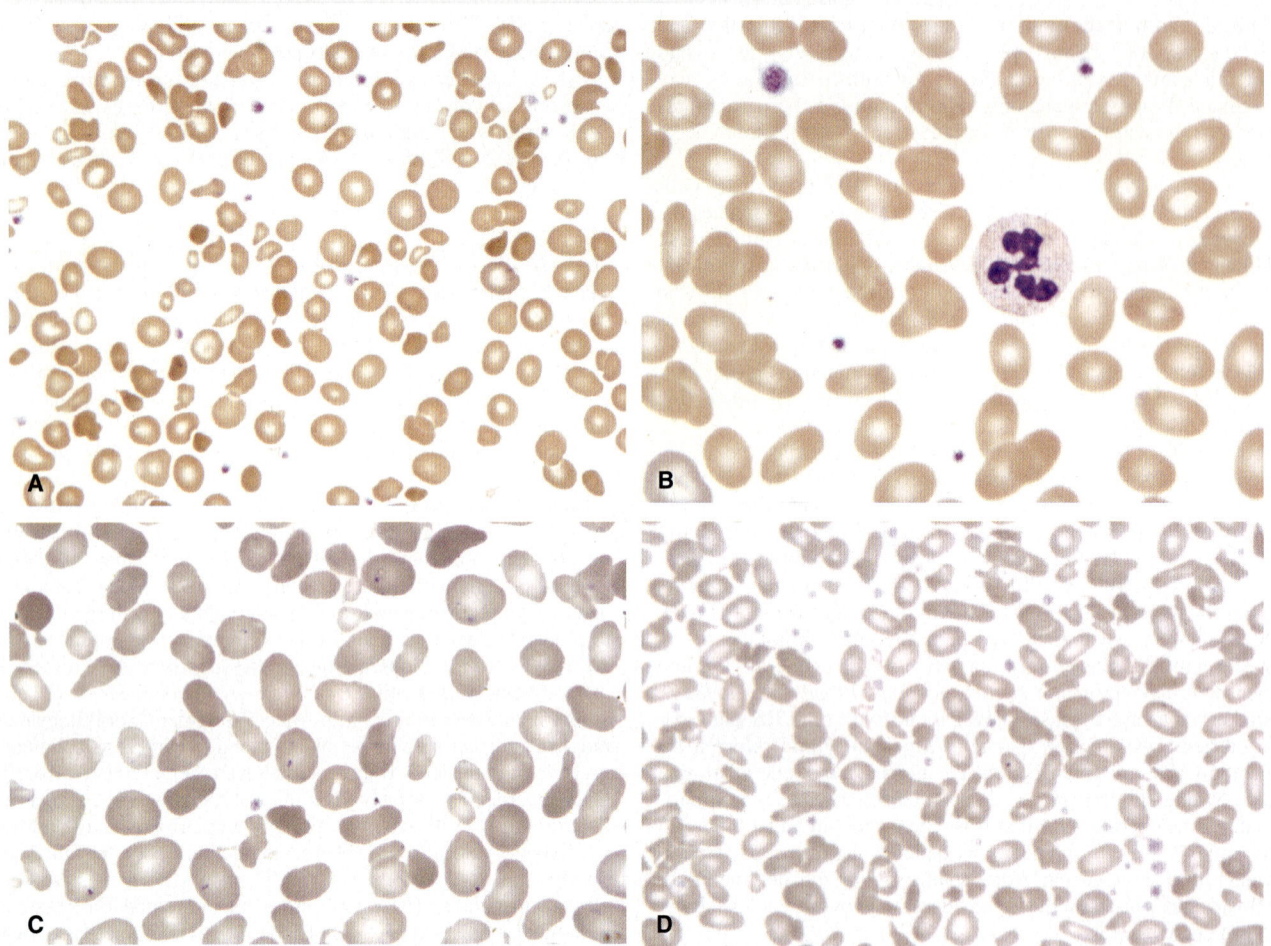

FIGURE 29.8 **Hereditary elliptocytosis.** Peripheral blood smears representative of different hereditary elliptocytosis syndromes are shown. A, Micropoikilocytes and elliptocytes in a neonate with transient poikilocytosis and an α-spectrin gene mutation. B, Same child at 7 months of age, now exhibiting morphology of common hereditary elliptocytosis. C, Compound heterozygous hereditary elliptocytosis due to two α-spectrin self-association–site structural mutations. Note distorted red cell shapes, elliptocytes, and fragments. D, Hereditary pyropoikilocytosis. Red cell abnormalities are similar to those in (A) and (C) with prominent budding and fragmentation. (Courtesy of Irma Pereira MT [ASCP]SH.)

Table 29.3. Classification of Hereditary Elliptocytosis (HE) Syndromes

	Common HE	Hemolytic HE	Hereditary Pyropoikilocytosis	Spherocytic Elliptocytes	Southeast Asian Ovalocytosis
Anemia	None	Moderate-severe	Severe	Mild to moderate	None
Hemolysis	None-mild	Moderate-severe	Severe	Mild to moderate	None
Splenomegaly	None	Present	Present	Present	None
Peripheral blood smear	15%-90% elliptocytes	Elliptocytes; poikilo-cytes; fragments	Poikilocytosis; RBC budding with frag-ments; elliptocytes; microspherocytes	Rounded elliptocytes; spherocytes	Rounded elliptocytes, some having a trans-verse bar dividing cell
Osmotic fragility	Normal	Normal/increased	Increased	Increased	Normal to decreased
Inheritance	Dominant	Recessive	Recessive	Dominant	Dominant
Other	Poikilocytosis with severe hemolysis, seen transiently in some infants	Normal/low mean cor-puscular volume	Low/very low mean corpuscular volume		Rigid erythrocytes

triple helical repeats connected by nonhelical segments. The "spectrin repeat," originally defined in erythroid cells, is a conserved triple helical, coiled-coil bundle of amino acids found in a diverse array of proteins that participate in protein-protein interactions and complex formation with functions as diverse as membrane assembly and signal transduction.[11,13] In the erythrocyte, α- and ß-spectrin assemble side to side in an antiparallel position, forming a flexible rod in which the NH$_2$ terminus of α-spectrin and the COOH terminus of ß-spectrin form an α-ß heterodimer. These heterodimers self-associate to form an atypical triple helical repeat in which one helix is contributed

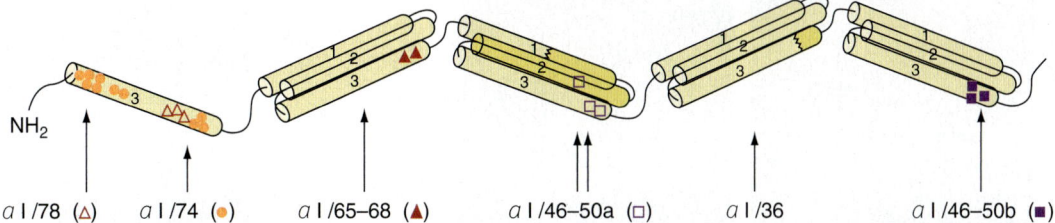

FIGURE 29.9 **Defects of the αβ-spectrin self-association site in hereditary elliptocytosis (HE) and hereditary pyropoikilocytosis (HPP).** A model of the triple-helical spectrin repeats that constitute the αβ-spectrin self-association site is shown. Limited tryptic digestion of spectrin, followed by two-dimensional gel electrophoresis, identifies abnormal cleavage sites (*arrows*) in spectrin associated with various mutations. Symbols denote positions of various genetic defects identified in patients with HE or HPP. In most cases, the mutation found is adjacent to the abnormal cleavage site, either in the same helical coil or in helical coils juxtaposed next to each other in the triple-helical model. The hashed lines denote the location of spectrin chain truncations. (Reprinted and modified from Gallagher PG, Tse WT, Forget BG. Clinical and molecular aspects of disorders of the erythrocyte membrane skeleton. *Semin Perinatol.* 1990;14(5):351-367. Copyright © 1990 Elsevier. With permission.)

by the NH_2 terminus of α-spectrin and two helices are contributed by the COOH terminus of ß-spectrin to form tetramers, the form of spectrin critical for membrane stability as well as erythrocyte shape and function. Spectrin tetramers are connected into a highly ordered two-dimensional lattice through binding, at their tail ends, to actin oligomers at the junctional complex, facilitated by protein 4.1R, into a uniform hexagonal lattice.[12,18] Studies have shown that local dissociation of tetramers and reassociation of dimers provide the membrane the ability to accommodate the distortions required for passage through the microvasculature.[15]

Disruption of erythrocyte membrane skeleton protein interactions by mutations that alter protein structure, function, or amount leads to diminished membrane mechanical stability and, in severe cases, to hemolysis. Most cases of HE are caused by spectrin mutations that perturb the interactions between αß-spectrin heterodimers, impairing spectrin tetramer formation, and, consequently, disrupting the integrity and mechanical stability of the membrane skeleton.[14] Mutation of protein 4.1R likely perturbs formation of the spectrin-actin-protein 4.1R-GPC junctional complex and attachment of this complex to the membrane. In 4.1R-deficient erythrocytes, abnormalities in membrane stability and cellular deformability are proportional to levels of protein 4.1R.

Spectrin Abnormalities

Most elliptogenic spectrin mutations are located in the region of spectrin self-association, impairing tetramer formation (*Figure 29.9*). These mutations create abnormal proteolytic cleavage sites that typically reside in the third helix of a repetitive segment and give rise to abnormal tryptic peptides on two-dimensional tryptic peptide maps of spectrin. Abnormal tryptic digests of spectrin extracted from HE erythrocytes were first used to identify HE mutations, followed by identification of the precise genetic defects after cloning of the α- and ß-spectrin genes. In α-spectrin, most reported mutations are amino acid substitutions. In ß-spectrin, mutations are amino acid substitutions and truncations of the COOH terminus of the ß-spectrin chain. When inherited in the heterozygous state, these mutations lead to typical HE. When inherited in *trans* to modifier alleles that worsen clinical severity, mild to moderate hemolytic HE is seen. Homozygosity and compound heterozygosity are associated with hemolytic HE and/or HPP. Several cases of homozygous ß-spectrin self-association site mutations have been associated with fatal or near-fatal fetal and neonatal anemia.[126]

Although most HE mutations are in the region of spectrin self-association site, a few spectrin mutations distant from this region have been described. In the heterozygous state, these mutations are asymptomatic, but they may be associated with hemolytic HE or HPP in the homozygous state.

Functionally, HE-associated self-association contact site missense mutations likely disrupt predicted conformational rearrangements in the predicted protein structure (*Figure 29.10*).[127] Mutations outside the self-association region likely disrupt long-range protein-protein

interactions, disrupting positively coupled, cooperative interactions of spectrin self-association, spectrin-ankyrin binding, and ankyrin-band 3 binding.[21] Thus these mutations may act to block repeat-to-repeat transfer of conformational information, decrease the ability of spectrin to *trans*-regulate ankyrin binding, and disrupt the register of spectrin repeats and perturb binding of other proteins, for example, ankyrin, to spectrin.[21,128]

Clinically, the most severe clinical phenotypes are associated with mutation of the αß-spectrin self-association contact site, the atypical hybrid repeat created by two helices of ß-spectrin and one of α-spectrin. Modifier alleles also influence clinical severity.[129] The most common of these is the low-expression allele, spectrin α[LELY] (LELY: low-expression allele from Lyon).[130,131] In α[LELY], a mutation in intron 45 leads to variable splicing and loss of exon 46 in about half of the α-spectrin mRNA synthesized. Spectrin proteins lacking exon 46 have a reduced ability to participate in dimer and tetramer assembly and are degraded. When α[LELY] is present as the only variant, it is clinically silent because normal α-spectrin is synthesized in large excess. However, when α[LELY] is present in *trans* to an α-spectrin HE mutant, incorporation of the latter into heterodimers is favored, thereby leading to increased proportion of the elliptocytogenic spectrin in red cells and worsening clinical severity. Conversely, when coinherited in *cis* to an HE α-spectrin mutation, it reduces the amount of the mutation incorporated into heterodimers and ameliorates clinical severity. α[LELY] is a common allele, affecting ~30% of α-spectrin alleles of Europeans and 20% of Japanese and West Africans.[132]

Protein 4.1R Defects

Protein 4.1R abnormalities associated with HE are much less common than spectrin mutations. One site on protein 4.1R binds to the distal end of the spectrin αß-heterodimer increasing the binding of spectrin to oligomeric actin. The NH_2-terminal domain of 4.1R interacts with GPC, phosphatidylinositol, and phosphatidylserine, facilitating the attachment of the distal end of spectrin to the membrane. Complex patterns of alternate splicing lead to the production of various tissue- and developmental stage–specific isoforms of 4.1R, including an erythropoiesis stage-specific splicing event that generates the 80-kDa mature erythroid protein 4.1R isoform.[133]

Deficiency of protein 4.1R has been described in several kindreds from southern France and northern Africa.[124] Partial deficiency of protein 4.1R is associated with mild dominantly inherited HE. Heterozygotes have approximately 50% of the normal amount of protein 4.1R and have mild hemolytic anemia. Homozygotes have no detectable protein 4.1R and a severe transfusion-dependent hemolytic anemia with prominent elliptocytosis and spherocytosis. Homozygous 4.1R-deficient erythrocytes are deficient in p55 and GPC, fragment more rapidly than normal at moderate sheer stresses, and display a dramatically disrupted skeletal network.

Structural abnormalities of protein 4.1R associated with HE have also been found including deletions and duplications of the exons encoding the spectrin-binding domain.[134,135]

Disorders of Red Blood Cells

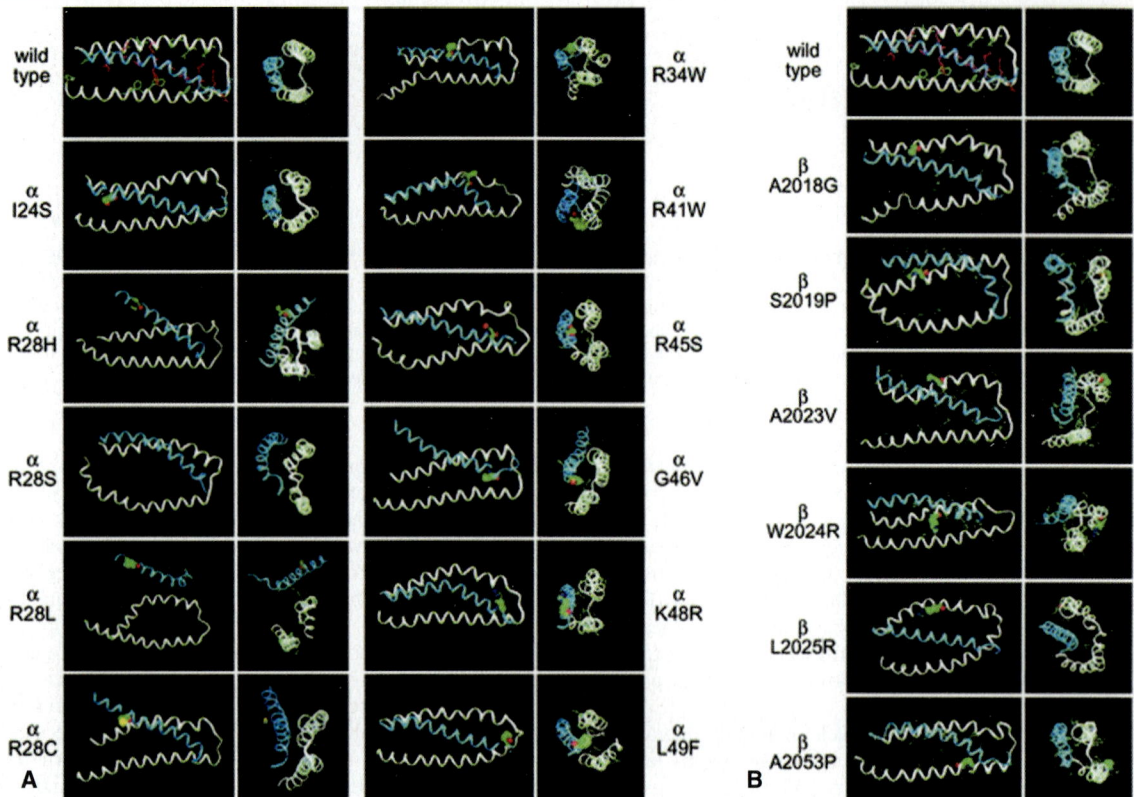

FIGURE 29.10 Molecular modeling of mutations of the αβ-spectrin self-association site. Using dynamic modeling and energy minimization, the three-dimensional structure of the αβ-self-association contact site was determined and the structural consequences of elliptocytosis-associated mutations were determined. A, Mutations involving α-spectrin. B, Mutations involving β-spectrin. Longitudinal and end-on views are shown for each mutation. The mutated residue is depicted using a solid-filled representation. Every pathologic point mutation, including seemingly conservative substitutions such as G for A, A for V, or K for R (single-letter amino acid codes), led to conformational rearrangements in the predicted structure. The degree of structural disruption, as measured by root-mean-square deviation of the predicted backbone structure, correlated strongly with the severity of clinical disease associated with each mutation. (Reprinted from Zhang Z, Weed SA, Gallagher PG, et al. Dynamic molecular modeling of pathogenic mutations in the spectrin self-association domain. *Blood.* 2001;98(6):1645-1653. Copyright © 2001 American Society of Hematology. With permission.)

Glycophorin C Deficiency

The Leach phenotype, typically associated with a 7-kb deletion of genomic DNA that removes exons 3 and 4 from the GPC/GPD locus, is characterized by GPC deficiency with elliptocytosis. GPC-deficient erythrocytes are also partially deficient in 4.1R, speculated to be the basis for the elliptocytosis, and lack p55. These abnormalities are presumed to be caused by disruption of a multiprotein complex that recruits, assembles, or stabilizes each other on the membrane. In contrast to other forms of HE, heterozygous carriers of GPC deficiency are asymptomatic with normal RBC morphology. Homozygous-deficient individuals have mild elliptocytosis but no anemia.

Membrane Abnormalities Leading to Elliptocyte Formation

Disruption of erythrocyte membrane skeleton protein interactions by mutations that alter protein structure, function, or amount leads to diminished membrane mechanical stability and, in severe cases, to hemolysis. The mechanism by which these protein defects result in elliptocyte formation is not clear. Elliptocytes acquire their shape after release from the marrow and as they age in vivo. Normal erythrocytes assume an elliptical shape in capillaries and in vitro when exposed to shear stress. They resume a normal biconcave shape after passage through the microcirculation and in vitro after removal of shear stress. If mechanical distortion is maintained for long periods, even normal red cells remain misshapen, suggesting that the membrane skeleton is altered because of sustained shape change. In HE, it is possible that altered membrane protein interactions lead to skeletal reorganization after less extensive deformation or shear stress. With repeated distortions imposed by passage through small capillaries, cells with unstable membrane skeletons gradually elongate to form irreversible elliptocytes. Erythrocytes with more severe skeletal defects presumably are unable to withstand normal circulatory shear stress and undergo fragmentation. This may explain the poikilocytosis seen in homozygous HE and HPP. In all hemolytic HE and HPP syndromes, more severely distorted cells are retained in splenic cords, thus splenectomy markedly ameliorates the associated anemia. Despite alterations in membrane mechanical fragility and stability, intravascular hemolysis has little role in the destruction of HE erythrocytes as hemoglobinuria, hemoglobinemia, or hemosiderinuria are not features of the hemolytic HE syndromes.

Clinical Features

The HE syndrome variants are clinically and hematologically heterogeneous, sharing the feature of elliptocytes on peripheral smear (*Table 29.3*). There is much overlap when these disorders are classified on a clinical, biochemical, or molecular basis.

Common Hereditary Elliptocytosis

Individuals with common HE are typically discovered accidently when elliptocytes are identified during routine evaluation of the peripheral blood film.[124] These individuals usually are not anemic, their red cell survival is normal, and there is no splenomegaly. In contrast to the clinical picture, the peripheral blood smear is striking, containing 15% to 100% elliptocytes (*Figure 29.7*). Episodic hemolytic anemia may occur during acute or chronic illnesses. Other common HE cases involve mild compensated hemolysis without anemia.

Hemolytic anemia with prominent elliptocytosis and poikilocytosis, termed by some as infantile poikilocytosis or infantile pyknocytosis, may be observed in the first few months of life. It is most common in patients of African ancestry. Affected infants have moderately severe hemolytic anemia and hyperbilirubinemia in the newborn period, the latter often necessitating exchange transfusion. The blood smear is characterized by elliptocytosis, marked red cell fragmentation, and poikilocytosis (*Figure 29.8B*). These morphologic changes are indistinguishable from those noted in patients with HPP. In contrast to HPP, the hemolysis and anemia abate, evolving to asymptomatic typical common HE throughout childhood (*Figure 29.8C*). The basis for this phenomenon is unknown, but increased concentrations of free 2,3-DPG observed in the neonatal period may contribute to membrane instability by perturbing protein 4.1R-actin interactions.[136]

Hemolytic Hereditary Elliptocytosis

In some cases of HE, the hemolytic process is incompletely compensated and patients have a chronic hemolytic anemia of variable severity.[124] Morphologic characteristics may include poikilocytosis, microelliptocytosis, and red cell fragmentation. The spleen may be enlarged, and gallstones occur with increased frequency. As in other hemolytic states, abrupt episodes of more severe anemia may occur in association with viral infection or other intercurrent illnesses and hemolytic, aplastic, and megaloblastic crises may occur. There is overlap between the findings in patients with hemolytic HE and HPP (see below).

In some families, hemolytic HE has been transmitted through several generations. In other families, not all individuals with HE manifest chronic hemolysis, but instead exhibit asymptomatic common HE or, at the other end of the spectrum, severe HPP. This variation reflects the genetic heterogeneity of the HE syndromes. Some α-spectrin mutations, such as mutations of codon 28, disrupt numerous critical protein-protein interactions leading to severe membrane dysfunction and are associated with greater clinical severity. Thus homozygous or compound heterozygous patients with different spectrin mutations manifest variable clinical severity.[137] In some cases, inheritance of modifier alleles, such as the common α^{LELY} allele, that alter α-spectrin expression may worsen or ameliorate the clinical course. Even patients with mutations of different HE genes, such as patients with both α and ß-spectrin self-association site mutations, have been described. Given the vast combination of mutant alleles and modifier alleles, it is not surprising that there is great clinical, laboratory, and biochemical variability in the HE syndromes.

Hereditary Pyropoikilocytosis

This severe congenital hemolytic anemia, which overlaps with severe hemolytic HE, is characterized by a peripheral blood smear that resembles those seen in patients with thermal burns.[138] Affected individuals, typically of African ancestry, present in infancy or early childhood with moderate to severe hemolytic anemia and unlike common HE, the hemolytic anemia is life-long rather than transient. Complications of chronic hemolysis, including splenomegaly, cholelithiasis, and growth retardation, have been described. Intermittent transfusions may be required. Splenectomy improves or ameliorates the anemia. Most impressive are changes in red cell morphology, which include extreme poikilocytosis, microspherocytosis, microelliptocytosis, membrane budding, and cell fragments. The MCV may be extremely low, 30 to 50 fl, the MCHC is normal, and osmotic fragility is increased. Thermal instability of HPP erythrocytes, susceptibility to budding and fragmentation upon heating to 46 °C, once thought to be diagnostic of HPP, is not unique as it is also found in some HE erythrocytes. Unlike HE red cells, HPP erythrocytes are also partially deficient in spectrin.

Studies of the genetics of HPP have revealed that many HPP probands have inherited structural mutations on both α-spectrin alleles from HE parents in a homozygous or compound heterozygous manner. In others, the HPP proband has inherited a structural mutation of spectrin from an HE parent on one allele and a null allele of α-spectrin

from an asymptomatic parent whose red cells have no detectable biochemical abnormality.[139] This null or "thalassemia-like" allele, which synthesizes little or no normal spectrin, enhancing the relative expression of the structural spectrin mutant and contributing to a superimposed spectrin deficiency, is most often due to inheritance of the spectrin^{LEPRA} allele.[32]

Spherocytic Elliptocytosis

This syndrome is characterized morphologically by two populations of cells: red cells that are more rounded than typical hereditary elliptocytes and a variable number of microspherocytes.[124] In contrast to other HE syndromes with hemolysis, no poikilocytes or fragments are seen. The disorder has been seen primarily in families of European descent and may account for as many as 15% to 25% of cases of HE in whites. Affected individuals have an incompletely compensated hemolytic process with mild anemia and predisposition to aplastic crises. The relative numbers of spherocytes and elliptocytes vary considerably, even within families. As in HS, the osmotic fragility and mechanical fragility may be increased. Splenectomy is curative.

Southeast Asian Ovalocytosis

This interesting variant, also known as *stomatocytic elliptocytosis,* is characterized morphologically by plump, rounded elliptocytes (ovalocytes), many of which have one or two transverse ridges. These red cells are found in people from Malaysia, New Guinea, Indonesia, and the Philippines. Outside the neonatal period, their presence is not associated with shortened RBC life span, anemia, or hemolysis.[140,141] SAO RBCs demonstrate increased red cell rigidity, increased thermal stability, and decreased osmotic fragility.[142]

The molecular defect in SAO results from an abnormal band 3 protein lacking codons 400 to 408 at the cytoplasmic and membrane-spanning domains.[143] All individuals with the SAO phenotype are heterozygotes, with one normal band 3 allele and one mutant band 3 allele. The homozygous state has never been observed and is thought to be lethal in utero.[144] There is tight binding of band 3 protein to ankyrin in SAO red cells, restricting the lateral mobility of band 3. Because band 3 protein is a receptor for malarial parasites, its reduced mobility may limit invagination and penetration by the parasite. *In vitro,* SAO erythrocytes are resistant to invasion by several strains of malaria. Studies of children in Papua New Guinea indicate that SAO does not actually reduce the incidence of infection with *Plasmodium falciparum,* but it does provide remarkable protection against cerebral malaria. This effect is likely due to reduced cytoadherence of SAO red cells to the cerebral vasculature, but the exact mechanism is not yet known.[124] In populations in which SAO is prevalent, its frequency is increased in older individuals, suggesting a favorable effect on longevity.

Laboratory Evaluation

Initial laboratory studies in a patient with a suspected HE syndrome should assess whether the patient is anemic (hemoglobin concentration/hematocrit), whether the anemia is well compensated (reticulocyte count), and whether the anemia is caused by accelerated RBC destruction (increased serum lactate dehydrogenase and bilirubin concentration). The mean cell volume (MCV) also is important because some hemolytic HE and HPP variants with RBC fragmentation often demonstrate severe microcytosis as a result of RBC fragmentation.

Careful evaluation of the blood smear is essential both for the diagnosis of HE and the classification of the disorder into major subtypes. At least 15% and often as many as 50% to 90% of red cells are elliptical, whereas smears from normal subjects contain fewer than 15% elliptocytes. In patients in whom elliptocytosis is the only morphologic abnormality, hemolysis is usually minimal or absent with the exception of spherocytic elliptocytosis, in which the presence of "fat" ovalocytes is associated with accelerated red cell destruction. In other patients with hemolytic forms of HE, poikilocytosis almost always is seen on the blood film, and in HPP, many red cells circulate as cell fragments and microspherocytes, producing a marked decrease in mean cell volume. Osmotic fragility is normal in nonhemolytic HE but is increased in hemolytic HE variants with poikilocytosis, HPP, and spherocytic elliptocytosis.

The finding of more than 30% oval red cells on the peripheral blood film, some containing a central slit or a transverse ridge, together with an absence of clinical and laboratory evidence of hemolysis in an individual from Southeast Asia or the South Pacific is highly suggestive of SAO. A screening test for SAO is the failure of ovalocytes to undergo membrane changes (form spicules) after metabolic depletion or when suspended in hypertonic salt solutions. The mechanism of this resistance to change in shape presumably is because of the extreme rigidity of the red cell membrane. The osmotic fragility is decreased (i.e., resistant to hemolysis) in SAO red cells.

Acquired elliptocytosis is sometimes observed in patients with myelodysplasia syndromes.[145,146]

Once the diagnosis of an HE syndrome is established, it is possible to further characterize the specific membrane lesion. Biochemical studies including studies of membrane protein quality and quantity; functional studies of spectrin, such as analyses of spectrin self-association; and tryptic mapping of spectrin digests to detect mutant spectrin peptides can be performed. Genetic studies to identify specific mutations and associated modifier alleles can also be performed. Like HS, these studies, available in specialized research laboratories, are indicated for studying difficult or particularly interesting and informative cases.

Treatment

In view of the benign nature of typical HE, therapeutic intervention is not indicated in most individuals. Patients with HE variants associated with severe hemolytic anemia should be provided supportive care comparable with that in HS, for example, supplemental folic acid,

periodic screening for cholelithiasis, and transfusion during hemolytic or aplastic crisis. Splenectomy is followed by dramatic improvement or normalization of the hemoglobin concentration and decrease in the reticulocyte count, despite persistence of elliptocytes on peripheral smear.

No therapeutic interventions are required for individuals with SAO.

STOMATOCYTIC DISORDERS

Stomatocytes are erythrocytes with a central slit or mouth-shaped (stoma) area of central pallor when examined on dried smears. In wet preparations, they are uniconcave rather than biconcave, giving them a bowl-like appearance. *In vitro,* stomatocytes are produced by drugs that intercalate into the inner half of the lipid bilayer, thereby expanding the inner lipid surface area relative to that of the outer half of the bilayer. In contrast, echinocytes (RBCs with numerous fine spicules) are thought to be the result of preferential expansion of the outer lipid bilayer relative to the inner layer. A few stomatocytes may be observed in blood smears prepared from normal individuals.[147] Acquired stomatocytosis has been associated with acute alcoholism and hepatobiliary disease, vinca alkaloid administration, neoplasms, and cardiovascular disease. Stomatocytosis is also sometimes observed as a processing artifact. Stomatocytes are associated with rare hereditary disorders of red cell cation permeability known as the hereditary stomatocytosis syndromes,[148] aberrant Rh blood group antigen expression, sitosterolemia, and familial deficiency of high-density lipoproteins. Each of these stomatocytic disorders is associated with mild to moderate hemolysis.

To appreciate the pathophysiology of the hereditary stomatocytosis syndromes (*Table 29.4*), an understanding of normal red cell cation and water transport is essential.[149] The RBC membrane, which is

Table 29.4. Features of Hereditary Stomatocytosis Syndromes

| | Stomatocytosis (hydrocytosis) | | | Intermediate Syndromes | | Xerocytosis |
	Severe Hemolysis	Mild Hemolysis	Cryohydrocytosis	Stomatocytic Xerocytosis	Xerocytosis with High PC	Xerocytosis
Hemolysis	Severe	Mild to moderate	Moderate	Mild	Moderate	Moderate
Anemia	Severe	Mild to moderate	Mild to moderate	None	Mild	Moderate
Blood smear	Stomatocytes	Stomatocytes	Stomatocytes or normal	Stomatocytes	Targets	Targets, echinocytes
MCV (80-100 μ^3)[a]	110-150	95-130	90-105	91-98	84-92	100-110
MCHC (32%-36%)	24-30	26-29	34-40	33-39	34-38	34-38
Unincubated osmotic fragility	Very increased	Increased	Normal	Decreased	Very decreased	Very decreased
RBC Na$^+$ (5-12 mEq/LRBC)	60-100	30-60	40-50	10-20	10-15	10-20
RBC K$^+$ (90-103 mEq/LRBC)	20-55	40-85	55-65	75-85	75-90	60-80
RBC Na$^+$ +K$^+$ (95-110 mEq/LRBC)	110-140	115-145	100-105	87-103	93-99	75-90
Phosphatidylcholine content	Normal	±Increased	Normal	Normal	Increased	Normal
Cold autohemolysis	No	No	Yes	No	No	?
Effect of splenectomy	Good	Good	Fair	?	?	?Poor
Genetics	AD, ?AR	AD	AD	AD	AD	AD

[a]Values in parentheses are the normal range.
Abbreviations: AD, autosomal dominant; AR, autosomal recessive; LRBC, liter of red blood cells.
Modified from Walensky LD, Narla M, Lux SE. Disorders of the red blood cell membrane. In: Handin RI, Lux SE, Stossel TP, eds. *Blood: Principles and Practice of Hematology.* 2nd ed. Lippincott Williams & Wilkins; 2003:1753. Reprinted with permission from Dr. Robert I. Handin.

freely permeable to water, controls its volume primarily through regulation of the monovalent cation content. Small passive cation leaks (Na$^+$ in, K$^+$ out) are normally balanced by the active outward transport of sodium (3 mEq/red cell/hour) and inward transport of potassium (2 mEq/red cell/hour). These cation pumps are linked, require ATP, and are dependent on the membrane enzyme Na$^+$-K$^+$-adenosine triphosphatase. If the membrane permeability leak to monovalent cations increases, cation pumps have limited compensatory ability, and, if this capacity is exceeded, the red cell volume changes in parallel with the total cation change. Red cells swell when the inward sodium leak exceeds the potassium leak out; red cells shrink when the potassium leak out exceeds the inward sodium leak. These membrane permeability abnormalities are recognized by observing altered RBC hydration (decreased or increased MCHC) and altered red cell sodium, potassium, and total monovalent cation content.

Hereditary Stomatocytosis

Hereditary stomatocytosis (also known as hereditary hydrocytosis, or overhydrated stomatocytosis) refers to a heterogeneous group of autosomal dominant hemolytic anemias caused by altered sodium permeability of the red cell membrane (*Table 29.4*).[150,151] The major pathophysiologic abnormality is the result of a marked increase in sodium permeability (15-40 times normal) leading to increased RBC sodium, a lesser decrease in intracellular potassium, an increase in total monovalent cation content, and, thereby, an increase in cell water. Despite a marked compensatory increase of active sodium and potassium transport, increased pump activity is unable to compensate for the markedly increased inward sodium leak. Treatment of these cells with dimethyl adipimidate (a bifunctional imidoester that cross-links proteins) normalizes membrane permeability, corrects cell cation and water content, improves membrane deformability, and corrects the abnormal RBC morphology. Moreover, these treated RBCs have an improved survival in vivo. In most patients, excess cation permeability is associated with an absence of red cell membrane protein band 7 on sodium dodecyl sulfate gels. This protein is referred to as band 7.2b or stomatin,[152-154] and its function is currently unknown. No abnormalities in the stomatin gene, which has been isolated and cloned, have been identified in stomatin-deficient individuals with hereditary stomatocytosis. Homozygous knock-out mice that completely lack the murine analog of erythrocyte stomatin exhibit no features of the hereditary stomatocytosis syndrome seen in humans, suggesting that stomatin deficiency is not the proximate cause of the disease in humans, although it may be a marker for another membrane defect that is responsible.[155]

The severity of hemolytic disease is diverse, both between different families and among affected members of the same family. In most patients, symptoms related to intermittent anemia and jaundice are so mild that no therapy is required. Rarely, the anemia is of sufficient severity to require transfusion therapy. Exchange transfusion for severe neonatal hyperbilirubinemia was required in one case. Splenomegaly is an expected corollary of severe anemia. Approximately 10% to 50% of circulating red cells are stomatocytes (*Figure 29.11*). The MCV is elevated, often strikingly; the MCHC is normal or low (because of increased cell water content); and osmotic fragility is increased. Red cell sodium content is increased, and potassium content is decreased. In most patients, hemolytic anemia is improved after splenectomy, but splenectomy is considered contraindicated in most cases because there is a high risk of postsplenectomy thromboembolic disease and chronic pulmonary hypertension. This has been attributed to increased erythrocyte-endothelial cell adhesion due to increased phosphatidylserine exposure of overhydrated erythrocytes.[156] Fortunately, most patients have compensated hemolysis and splenectomy is not required.

Hereditary Xerocytosis

Hereditary xerocytosis (also known as dessicocytosis or dehydrated stomatocytosis) is a rare autosomal dominant hemolytic anemia characterized by red cell dehydration due to net potassium loss from cells that is not accompanied by a proportional gain of sodium (*Table*

29.4).[150,157] Measurement of RBC cations reveals a slight increase in cell sodium content, a greater decrease in potassium concentration, and, thus, a decrease in the net intracellular cation content and cell dehydration. In some cases, reduced red cell 2,3-DPG has been noted. In several families, an increase in erythrocyte PC content has been observed. Although the total red cell membrane protein content may be elevated, specific abnormalities of stomatin or other membrane proteins have not been observed. The red cells in HX are sensitive to shear stress and readily undergo membrane fragmentation.

Patients with xerocytosis characteristically have mild to moderate hemolysis. The MCHC is increased, reflecting cellular dehydration. The MCV also is slightly increased, reflecting both increased reticulocyte count and artifact from electronic cell counters, which due to alterations in cellular stiffness, estimate the MCV about 10% too high.[158] The peripheral blood film reveals stomatocytes, target cells, spiculated cells, and some cells in which hemoglobin is concentrated ("puddled") in discrete areas on the cell periphery (*Figure 29.11*). Peripheral blood smears from mildly affected patients are nearly normal. The osmotic fragility is decreased. Splenectomy has minimal effect on the hemolytic anemia and increases the risk of thrombosis,[159,160] and is, therefore, to be avoided. A subset of patients with HX also exhibit transient in utero ascites, nonimmune hydrops fetalis, and/or pseudohyperkalemia, which are unrelated to the degree of anemia.[161-163] The basis for the transient ascites and hydrops is unknown.

Most cases of HX are due to mutations in the mechanotransduction protein PIEZO1.[164-166] PIEZO1 is encoded by the FAM38A gene on chromosome 16, located in the region previously linked to both

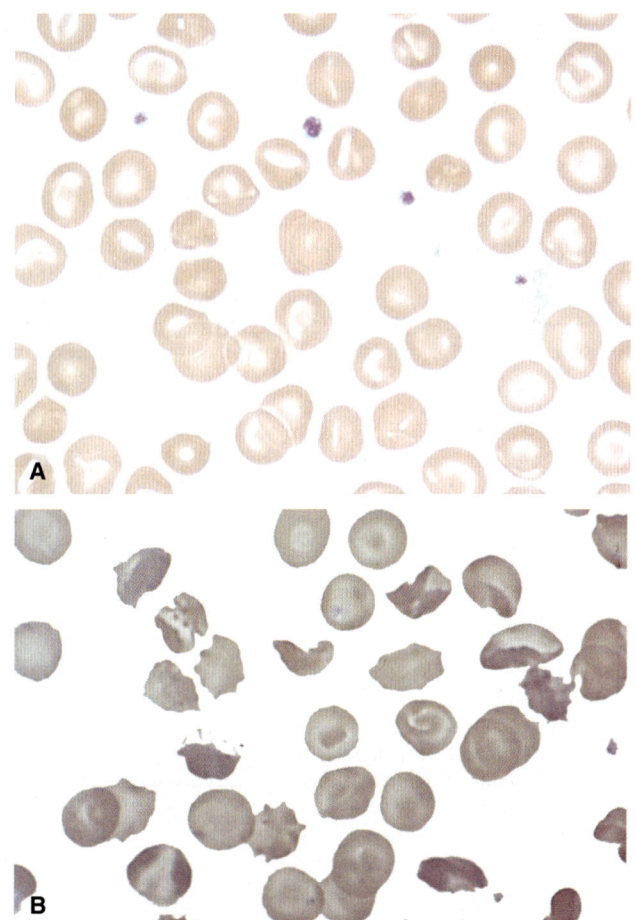

FIGURE 29.11 Hereditary stomatocytosis. A, Wright-stained peripheral blood smear from a patient with hereditary hydrocytosis. Instead of central pallor, characteristic erythrocytes have a central mouthlike or "stoma" appearance, hence the term *stomatocytosis*. B, Wright-stained peripheral blood smear from a patient with hereditary xerocytosis, showing dense, abnormal erythrocyte forms where hemoglobin appears puddled at the periphery.

hereditary xerocytosis and pseudohyperkalemia (see Intermediate Stomatocytic Syndromes).[167-169] Studies indicate that PIEZO1-mutant erythrocytes exhibit increased cation permeability associated with alterations in channel kinetics.[170,171] Thus PIEZO proteins play a previously unrecognized role in erythrocyte volume regulation, with PIEZO1-mutant erythrocytes gradually becoming dehydrated during their repeated cycles of travel through the microcirculation, associated with changes in oxygenation/deoxygenation. Extending these observations, PIEZO proteins may participate in the initial calcium-permeable cation conductance pathways involved in sickle cell dehydration.[164,172,173] A common PIEZO1 allele has been identified in African populations associated with erythrocyte dehydration and attenuates *Plasmodium* infection.[174] Finally, when PIEZO1 mutations are coinherited with other inherited anemias with erythrocyte dehydration, such as sickle cell disease, significant erythrocyte dehydration worsens clinical severity.[175]

In a subset of patients with HX, defects of the Gardos channel encoded by the *KCNN4* gene have been described.[176-178]

Intermediate Stomatocytic Syndromes

Some cases of hereditary RBC cation permeability abnormalities share features of both hereditary stomatocytosis and xerocytosis including cryohydrocytosis, stomatocytic xerocytosis, and xerocytosis with high PC (*Table 29.4*).[150,179] Affected individuals have stomatocytes and target cells on the peripheral blood smear. The osmotic fragility of red cells is either normal or slightly increased. The sodium and potassium permeabilities are somewhat increased, but the intracellular cation concentration and the red cell volume usually are normal or slightly reduced.

Cryohydrocytosis is a variant of hydrocytosis with abnormal cation transport and overhydrated red cells (*Table 29.4*). Cryohydrocytosis cells exhibit a profound increase in cation permeability in vitro at low temperatures (5 °C) compared with 37 °C. A similar susceptibility to cold-induced cation permeability in which potassium and water loss predominates and xerocytes instead of hydrocytes are present has also been described. Blood samples left at room temperature for a few hours may manifest pseudohyperkalemia as a result of potassium efflux from red cells into the plasma. Despite the mildly dehydrated red cells, no anemia or hemolysis is associated with this defect. Careful analysis of potassium loss at low temperatures is an excellent way to distinguish between cryohydrocytosis, pseudohyperkalemia, and intermediate forms; at least five different phenotypes can be distinguished. In a group of patients with cryohydrocytosis, two different mutations in the Rh-associated glycoprotein (RhAG), Ile61Arg or Phe65Ser, were found.[180] Additional studies support the role of Rh proteins as an ammonia channel in erythrocytes, with the cryohydrocytosis-associated mutations leading to increased cation conductance/permeability.[181,182]

A subgroup of stomatin-deficient patients with cryohydrocytosis with hepatosplenomegaly, cataracts, seizures, and movement disorders has been described. In two affected kindreds, mutations in the glucose transporter 1 (GLUT1), encoded by the SLC2A1 gene, have been found.[183]

Study of a group of patients with stomatocytosis, spherocytosis, and spherostomatocytosis with large cation leaks at 0 °C revealed varying patterns of cation loss over a range of temperatures. Erythrocyte membranes from some of these patients demonstrated band 3 deficiency. Several missense mutations in exon 17, encoding an intramembrane domain of band 3, were discovered in these patients.[122] *In vitro* studies suggested that these mutations convert band 3 from an anion exchanger to a nonselective cation leak channel.[184]

Rh-Null Disease

Most hematologists are familiar with the Rh antigen because of the immune sensitization that occurs in Rh-negative individuals exposed to Rh-positive red cells. The Rh locus (*RH30*) is composed of two closely linked genes, one encoding the D polypeptide and the other encoding the CE protein.[185] The importance of the Rh locus for membrane integrity was recognized through the discovery of rare

individuals whose red cells have absent (Rh_{null}) or markedly decreased (Rh_{mod}) Rh antigen expression.[186] Rh proteins are part of a multiprotein complex that includes two Rh proteins and two RhAGs.[187] Other proteins that associate with this complex include CD47, LW, glycophorin B, and protein 4.2. The Rh-RhAG complex interacts with ankyrin to link the membrane skeleton to the lipid bilayer.[188]

Rh_{null} and Rh_{mod} disease are characterized by mild to moderate normocytic, normochromic hemolytic anemia with stomatocytes and occasional spherocytes on peripheral blood smear. Although the clinical syndromes are the same, the genetic basis of the Rh deficiency syndrome is heterogeneous, with at least two groups defined. The "amorph type" is due to defects involving the *RH30* locus encoding the RhD and RhCE polypeptides. The "regulatory type" of Rh_{null} and Rh_{mod} phenotypes results from suppressor or "modifier" mutations at the *RH50* locus encoding the Rh-associated glycoproteins. When one chain of the Rh-RhAG complex is absent, the entire Rh multiprotein complex is either not transported to or assembled at the membrane.

Sitosterolemia

Sitosterolemia, also known as phytosterolemia, is a recessively inherited disorder associated with elevated plasma levels of plant sterols.[189] Affected patients exhibit early-onset xanthomatosis and premature coronary artery disease.[190] Hematologic manifestations include macrothrombocytopenia and stomatocytic hemolytic anemia.[191,192] Mutations in the transporters ABCG5 or ABCG8 lead to gastrointestinal hyperabsorption and decreased biliary elimination of plant sterols as well as altered cholesterol metabolism.[193] Plant sterols are not synthesized endogenously in humans but are passively absorbed in the intestine.[194] ABCG5 and ABCG8 actively pump plant sterols out of the intestinal cells back into the intestine and out of liver cells into bile ducts. It has been suggested that the stomatocytic phenotype is due to intercalation of plant sterols into the inner leaflet of the lipid bilayer.[191]

Familial Deficiency of High-Density Lipoproteins

Familial deficiency of high-density lipoproteins (Tangier disease) is a rare autosomal recessive disorder associated with accumulation of cholesterol esters in many tissues.[195] Affected patients exhibit markedly reduced high-density lipoproteins and mild hypertriglyceridemia. Accretion of cholesterol leads to enlarged yellow or orange-colored tonsils, hepatosplenomegaly, cloudy corneas, neuropathy, and premature atherosclerosis. Hematologic manifestations include a mild to moderate hemolytic anemia with stomatocytosis. Erythrocyte membranes have low free cholesterol content, leading to a decreased cholesterol to phospholipid ratio and a relative increase in PC. Patients with Tangier disease have mutations in ABCA1, a protein involved in the cellular export of cholesterol.

ACANTHOCYTIC DISORDERS

Acanthocytes are dense, contracted red cells with several irregularly spaced "thorny" projections on the surface. Acanthocytes differ from echinocytes in that there are fewer projections, and the width and length of these projections vary considerably. No central pallor is evident. By contrast, echinocytic spicules are similar in dimension and evenly distributed around the cell periphery. Acquired acanthocytosis is encountered in patients with severe liver disease, in malnourished states such as anorexia nervosa,[13] in hypothyroidism, and after splenectomy. Acanthocytosis also is seen in hereditary disorders such as abetalipoproteinemia, the McLeod phenotype, and the neuroacanthocytosis syndromes.

Spur Cell Anemia

Acanthocytosis in liver disease (hepatocellular injury) is attributable to a marked increase in the cholesterol content and the cholesterol to phospholipid ratio of red cell membranes (*Figure 29.12*).[196] This red cell lipid profile is in contrast to the equal increase in both cholesterol and phospholipid seen in obstructive liver disease. In cirrhotic liver disease, abnormal lipoproteins produced by the liver are loaded

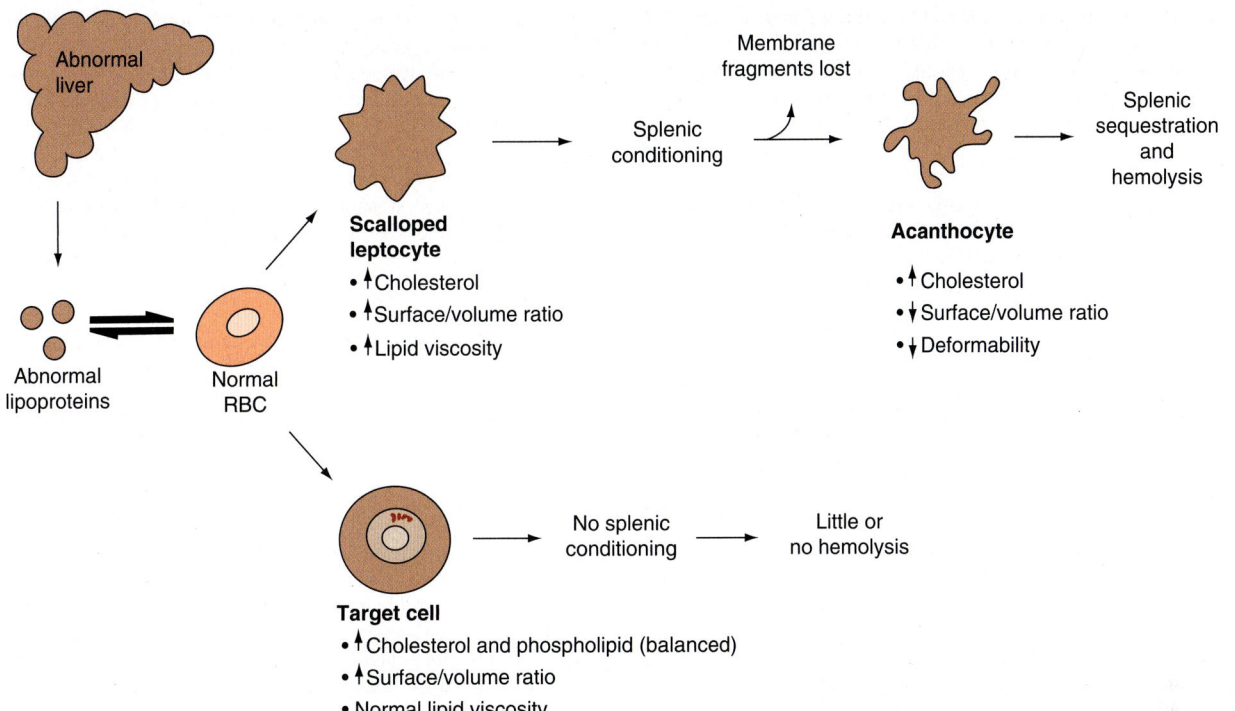

FIGURE 29.12 Alterations of erythrocyte shape in liver disease. Schematic illustration of the pathophysiology of acanthocyte ("spur cell") and target cell formation in liver disease. RBC, red blood cell. (Reprinted from Gallagher PG, Lux SE. Disorders of the erythrocyte membrane. In: Nathan DG, Orkin SH, Ginsburg D, et al., eds. *Nathan and Oski's Hematology of Infancy and Childhood.* 6th ed. WB Saunders; 2003:645. Copyright © 2003 Elsevier. With permission.)

with cholesterol; this excess cholesterol is readily transferred to RBCs, resulting in the formation of flat, scalloped cells.[197] These cells, however, are further conditioned by the spleen, resulting in membrane fragmentation, and the evolution of acanthocytes that look like "spurs."

These spur RBCs are cholesterol loaded, with a decreased surface area to volume ratio, and their cellular deformability is decreased. Once formed, spur cells are destroyed over time by the spleen, accounting for the hemolytic anemia associated with severe liver disease. Such patients usually have moderate to severe hemolysis, hyperbilirubinemia, splenomegaly, as well as clinical and laboratory evidence of liver disease. This acanthocytic, spur cell anemia, typically associated with alcoholism, can occur in any condition associated with severe hepatocyte injury.[198]

Abetalipoproteinemia

Abetalipoproteinemia is a rare, autosomal recessive disorder characterized by acanthocytosis, malabsorption of fat, hypolipidemia, retinitis pigmentosa, and progressive ataxia.[199] Although affected infants ostensibly are normal at birth, steatorrhea, abdominal distention, and growth failure develop in the first months of life. Retinitis pigmentosa and progressive ataxia are first noted in children between 5 and 10 years of age. Without treatment, neurologic disability is progressive, with death usually occurring during the second or third decade. In some cases, cardiac arrhythmias and heart failure precede death. Many of the clinical abnormalities have been attributed to fat-soluble vitamin deficiency, especially vitamin E, but this has not been well studied. Retinal and neuromuscular abnormalities may be stabilized by the administration of vitamin E.

The primary biochemical defect is failure to synthesize or secrete lipoprotein-containing products of the apolipoprotein B gene, the B apoproteins B100 and B48, or defects in the multifunctional microsomal triglyceride transfer protein (MTP),[200] required for production of apoprotein B–containing beta-lipoproteins.[201] Absorption of lipids through the intestine is defective, serum cholesterol levels are extremely low, and serum beta lipoprotein is absent. Secondary alterations in CD1 lead to immune defects.[202] The serum appears

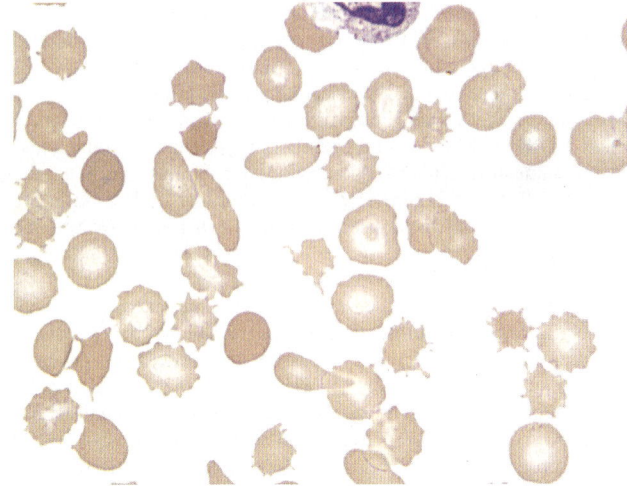

FIGURE 29.13 Acanthocytes. Blood smear from patient with liver disease. Note the numerous erythrocytes with thorny projections, or acanthocytes. (Courtesy of Irma Pereira MT [ASCP]SH.)

transparent. Clinical manifestations are variable depending upon the extent to which apolipoprotein B–mediated metabolic processes are affected.

Acanthocyte formation is thought to reflect an increase in the surface area of the outer lipid bilayer relative to the inner bilayer, attributed to increased sphingomyelin in the outer bilayer mirroring the altered plasma lipid profile of these patients presumably due to lipid exchange. Normal red cells become acanthocytic when infused into individuals with abetalipoproteinemia. In affected patients, red cell precursors and young erythrocytes are of normal shape, with acanthocyte formation increasing with erythrocyte aging, reaching up to 50% to 90% of erythrocytes on peripheral smear (*Figure 29.13*). For unknown reasons, the anemia in abetalipoproteinemia (increased sphingomyelin) is minimal to mild, whereas in spur cell anemia (increased cholesterol) there is moderate to severe hemolysis. Occasionally, severe anemia is observed in patients with abetalipoproteinemia. This is usually the result of broad nutritional deficiencies, including folate deficiency, related to malabsorption.

McLeod Phenotype

The McLeod phenotype, named after the first patient described, is an X-linked abnormality of the Kell blood group system.[203,204] Red cells, leukocytes, or both from affected patients react poorly with Kell antisera. Associated findings in affected males include acanthocytosis ranging from 8% to 85%, a mild, well-compensated hemolytic anemia, and susceptibility to alloimmunization by Kell antigens. Elevated serum creatine phosphokinase levels are seen, often accompanied by myopathy and peripheral neuropathy. Central nervous system abnormalities may appear, particularly after the fourth decade of life.[205] Females have only occasional acanthocytes and minimal to no hemolysis. Because of the susceptibility to alloimmunization, it is important to diagnose affected patients because, if they are transfused, they may develop antibodies compatible only with McLeod red cells.

The McLeod phenotype is the result of mutation in the XK gene located on the X chromosome, which encodes a membrane protein necessary for Kell antigen expression. XK is linked to Kell, a zinc endopeptidase that carries the Kell antigens, by a disulfide bond. McLeod erythrocytes lack XK and Kell proteins. Contiguous X-chromosome gene deletions including the XK gene have led to McLeod individuals with coinherited chronic granulomatous disease, Duchenne muscular dystrophy, and/or retinitis pigmentosa.[206]

Neuroacanthocytosis Syndromes

The neuroacanthocytoses are a group of degenerative neurologic disorders marked by great phenotypic and genetic heterogeneity that share the feature of acanthocytes on peripheral blood smear.[207,208] These disorders include the X-linked McLeod syndrome described above, chorea-acanthocytosis (ChAc), and other neurodegenerative disorders including Huntington Disease-Like 2 (HDL2) due to mutations in the junctophilin-3 gene and pantothenate kinase–associated neurodegeneration (formerly known as Hallervorden-Spatz syndrome and its allelic variant HARP syndrome—hypobetalipoproteinemia, acanthocytosis, retinitis pigmentosa, pallidal degeneration) due to mutations in pantothenate kinase 2 (PANK2) gene.[205,209-211] The etiology of the acanthocytic erythroid phenotype in these disorders is unknown. Further investigation of the pathobiology in erythroid cells may provide important insights into the neurodegenerative processes affecting the brain.

ChAc is an autosomal recessive disorder characterized by acanthocytes, normolipoproteinemia, and progressive neurologic disease beginning in adolescence or adult life. Neurologic manifestations are variable and may include limb chorea, progressive orofacial dyskinesia, tongue biting, muscle wasting, and hypotonia. Mutations have been identified in the chorein gene (also known as *CHAC* or VPS13A-vacuolar protein sorting 13 homolog A) in patients with ChAC.[212-216] The role of chorein is unknown, either in erythrocytes or in the brain. In yeast, its homologue is involved in protein sorting and transport. Abnormalities in erythrocyte membrane phosphorylation have been identified, and perturbations in a network of interconnected kinases suggested to play a role in acanthocyte formation.[217,218]

ECHINOCYTIC DISORDERS

Echinocytes are RBCs with numerous fine uniform spicules equally throughout the cell surface. These cells differ morphologically from acanthocytes, which have fewer projections, and the spicules vary in size. It is thought that echinocytes are the result of preferential expansion of the outer lipid bilayer relative to the inner layer. As mentioned previously, stomatocytes, in contrast, are produced by agents that expand the inner lipid surface area relative to the outer half of the bilayer. The presence of echinocytes on the peripheral blood film often is an artifact caused by interactions of red cells with glass. However, echinocytes also are seen in association with hemolytic anemias in patients with hypophosphatemia,

pyruvate kinase deficiency, uremia, and in some long-distance runners. The mechanism of echinocytosis in these diverse disorders is not clear. *In vitro,* a variety of factors, such as exposure of red cells to certain drugs, calcium loading, or ATP depletion, can induce echinocyte formation. In echinocytes produced by ATP depletion or calcium loading, it has been suggested that altered phospholipid distribution is a consequence of decreased aminophospholipid translocase activity, an ATP-dependent enzyme that actively translocates aminophospholipids from the outer half of the bilayer to the inner half echinocytes.

TARGET CELL DISORDERS

Target cells are discoid RBCs with a centralized hemoglobinized area in the clear center, resembling a bull's eye or target. Target cells are the morphologic expression of an increase in the ratio of the cell surface area to cell volume. This ratio is influenced by increases in surface area as well as decreases in cell volume. An absolute increase in cell surface area due to net membrane accumulation of phospholipids and cholesterol is the basis of target cell formation in obstructive liver disease and disorders of intrahepatic cholestasis (*Figure 29.12*). This accumulation is caused by abnormal low-density lipoproteins that occur in obstructive jaundice. These low-density lipoproteins are laden with cholesterol and lecithin, which is readily transferable to red cell membrane, thereby leading to an expansion of the cell membrane surface. This process explains why patients with HS who develop sudden obstructive jaundice due to cholelithiasis have a decrease in hemolysis and normalization of osmotic fragility, that is, the increased membrane surface area temporarily normalizes the previously abnormal surface area: volume ratio of spherocytes. Decreased cell volume leading to target cell formation is associated with decreased hemoglobin synthesis (thalassemia or iron deficiency), several structural mutations of hemoglobin (S, C, D, E), or some primary disorders of cell hydration.

Target cells have decreased osmotic fragility, as the excess of membrane surface area leads to an increase of the critical hemolytic volume. Typically, an increase in cell surface area does not affect red cell survival; decreased cell volume associated with cellular dehydration or reduced hemoglobin synthesis may.

Immediately post splenectomy, target cells appear, reaching levels of 2% to 10%. Like other target cells, membrane lipids are increased, osmotic fragility is decreased, and the cell surface area to volume ratio is increased.[219] As discussed above, splenic conditioning normally removes excess membrane from erythrocytes. The exact mechanism responsible is not defined, although the reduction in red cell lipid content suggests that lipases may be involved. Post splenectomy, red cells may eventually lose their excess lipid by conditioning in nonsplenic sites, leading to a gradual decrease in target cells.

Familial Lecithin-Cholesterol Acyltransferase Deficiency

Target cells are also observed on peripheral smears of patients with lecithin-cholesterol acyltransferase (LCAT) deficiency. Familial LCAT deficiency is a rare, autosomal recessive disorder due to mutations in LCAT, an enzyme that catalyzes the transfer of fatty acids from PC to cholesterol.[220-222] Manifestations include mild anemia, corneal opacities, hyperlipidemia, renal disease, and premature atherosclerosis.[221,223,224] In the circulation, LCAT is complexed with high-density lipoproteins. Deficient plasma LCAT activity is responsible for a marked decrease in plasma levels of unesterified cholesterol and an increase in the amount of free cholesterol. The red cell membrane may contain twice the normal amounts of unesterified cholesterol, but PC also is increased, whereas sphingomyelin and phosphatidylethanolamine are reduced. These RBC lipid changes are reversible when the target cells are incubated with normal plasma. Typically, the anemia of LCAT deficiency is mild with both hemolysis and decreased erythropoiesis due to renal disease implicated in its etiology. Foam cells and "sea-blue histiocytes" laden with unesterified cholesterol and PC are found in the bone marrow and the spleen of affected patients. A variety of therapeutic strategies are being pursued to improve plasma lipid metabolism by increasing LCAT activity to treat LCAT deficiency and the related disorder fish-eye disease.[225]

Website Resources

http://www.ncbi.nlm.nih.gov/pubmedhealth/PMH0001557/
http://ghr.nlm.nih.gov/condition/hereditary-spherocytosis
http://ghr.nlm.nih.gov/condition/hereditary-spherocytosis/show/OMIM
http://emedicine.medscape.com/article/206107-overview

References

1. Delaunay J. The molecular basis of hereditary red cell membrane disorders. *Blood Rev.* 2007;21:1-20.

2. Mohandas N, Chasis JA, Shohet SB. The influence of membrane skeleton on red cell deformability, membrane material properties, and shape. *Semin Hematol.* 1983;20:225-242.

3. Balasubramanian K, Schroit AJ. Aminophospholipid asymmetry: a matter of life and death. *Annu Rev Physiol.* 2003;65:701-734.

4. Kuypers FA, de Jong K. The role of phosphatidylserine in recognition and removal of erythrocytes. *Cell Mol Biol (Noisy-le-grand).* 2004;50:147-158.

5. Holthuis JC, van Meer G, Huitema K. Lipid microdomains, lipid translocation and the organization of intracellular membrane transport (Review). *Mol Membr Biol.* 2003;20:231-241.

6. Salzer U, Prohaska R. Stomatin, flotillin-1, and flotillin-2 are major integral proteins of erythrocyte lipid rafts. *Blood.* 2001;97:1141-1143.

7. Hiller NL, Akompong T, Morrow JS, Holder AA, Haldar K. Identification of a stomatin orthologue in vacuoles induced in human erythrocytes by malaria parasites. A role for microbial raft proteins in apicomplexan vacuole biogenesis. *J Biol Chem.* 2003;278:48413-48421.

8. Murphy SC, Samuel BU, Harrison T, et al. Erythrocyte detergent-resistant membrane proteins: their characterization and selective uptake during malarial infection. *Blood.* 2004;103:1920-1928.

9. Gautier EF, Leduc M, Ladli M, et al. Comprehensive proteomic analysis of murine terminal erythroid differentiation. *Blood Adv.* 2020;4:1464-1477.

10. Gautier EF, Leduc M, Cochet S, et al. Absolute proteome quantification of highly purified populations of circulating reticulocytes and mature erythrocytes. *Blood Adv.* 2018;2:2646-2657.

11. Bennett V, Baines AJ. Spectrin and ankyrin-based pathways: metazoan inventions for integrating cells into tissues. *Physiol Rev.* 2001;81:1353-1392.

12. Discher DE. New insights into erythrocyte membrane organization and microelasticity. *Curr Opin Hematol.* 2000;7:117-122.

13. Morrow JS, Rimm DL, Kennedy SP, Cianci CD, Sinard JH, Weed SA. Of membrane stability and mosaics: the spectrin cytoskeleton. In: Hoffman J, Jamieson J, eds. *Handbook of Physiology.* Oxford; 1997:485-540.

14. Ipsaro JJ, Harper SL, Messick TE, Marmorstein R, Mondragon A, Speicher DW. Crystal structure and functional interpretation of the erythrocyte spectrin tetramerization domain complex. *Blood.* 2010;115:4843-4852.

15. An X, Lecomte MC, Chasis JA, Mohandas N, Gratzer W. Shear-response of the spectrin dimer-tetramer equilibrium in the red blood cell membrane. *J Biol Chem.* 2002;277:31796-31800.

16. Mohler PJ, Bennett V. Defects in ankyrin-based cellular pathways in metazoan physiology. *Front Biosci.* 2005;10:2832-2840.

17. Cohen CM, Dotimas E, Korsgren C. Human erythrocyte membrane protein band 4.2 (pallidin). *Semin Hematol.* 1993;30:119-137.

18. Gilligan DM, Bennett V. The junctional complex of the membrane skeleton. *Semin Hematol.* 1993;30:74-83.

19. Franco T, Low PS. Erythrocyte adducin: a structural regulator of the red blood cell membrane. *Transfus Clin Biol.* 2010;17:87-94.

20. Mohandas N, Chasis JA. Red blood cell deformability, membrane material properties and shape: regulation by transmembrane, skeletal and cytosolic proteins and lipids. *Semin Hematol.* 1993;30:171-192.

21. Giorgi M, Cianci CD, Gallagher PG, Morrow JS. Spectrin oligomerization is cooperatively coupled to membrane assembly: a linkage targeted by many hereditary hemolytic anemias? *Exp Mol Pathol.* 2001;70:215-230.

22. Eber S, Lux SE. Hereditary spherocytosis—defects in proteins that connect the membrane skeleton to the lipid bilayer. *Semin Hematol.* 2004;41:118-141.

23. Perrotta S, Gallagher PG, Mohandas N. Hereditary spherocytosis. *Lancet.* 2008;372:1411-1426.

24. Dacie J. *The Haemolytic Anaemias.* Churchill Livingstone; 1985.

25. Packman CH. The spherocytic haemolytic anaemias. *Br J Haematol.* 2001;112:888-899.

26. Vanlair CF, Masius JB. De la microythemie. *Bull R Acad Med Belg.* 1871;5:515.

27. Haclen RL. The mechanism of the increased fragility of the erythrocytes in congenital hemolytic jaundice. *Am J Med Sci.* 1934;188:441-449.

28. Eber SW, Pekrun A, Neufeldt A, Schroter W. Prevalence of increased osmotic fragility of erythrocytes in German blood donors: screening using a modified glycerol lysis test. *Ann Hematol.* 1992;64:88-92.

29. Godal HC, Heisto H. High prevalence of increased osmotic fragility of red blood cells among Norwegian blood donors. *Scand J Haematol.* 1981;27:30-34.

30. Agre P, Asimos A, Casella JF, McMillan C. Inheritance pattern and clinical response to splenectomy as a reflection of erythrocyte spectrin deficiency in hereditary spherocytosis. *N Engl J Med.* 1986;315:1579-1583.

31. Agre P, Orringer EP, Bennett V. Deficient red-cell spectrin in severe, recessively inherited spherocytosis. *N Engl J Med.* 1982;306:1155-1161.

32. Gallagher PG, Maksimova Y, Lezon-Geyda K, et al. Aberrant splicing contributes to severe α-spectrin-linked congenital hemolytic anemia. *J Clin Invest.* 2019;129:2878-2887.

33. Chonat S, Risinger M, Sakthivel H, et al. The spectrum of SPTA1-associated hereditary spherocytosis. *Front Physiol.* 2019;10:815.

34. Edelman EJ, Maksimova Y, Duru F, Altay C, Gallagher PG. A complex splicing defect associated with homozygous ankyrin-deficient hereditary spherocytosis. *Blood.* 2007;109:5491-5493.

35. Yetgin S, Aytac S, Gurakan F, Yurdakok M. Nonimmune hydrops fetalis in two cases of consanguineous parents and associated with hereditary spherocytosis and hemophagocytic hystiocytosis. *J Perinatol.* 2007;27:252-254.

36. Coetzer TL, Lawler J, Liu SC, et al. Partial ankyrin and spectrin deficiency in severe, atypical hereditary spherocytosis. *N Engl J Med.* 1988;318:230-234.

37. Eber SW, Armbrust R, Schroter W. Variable clinical severity of hereditary spherocytosis: relation to erythrocytic spectrin concentration, osmotic fragility, and autohemolysis. *J Pediatr.* 1990;117:409-416.

38. Hanspal M, Yoon SH, Yu H, et al. Molecular basis of spectrin and ankyrin deficiencies in severe hereditary spherocytosis: evidence implicating a primary defect of ankyrin. *Blood.* 1991;77:165-173.

39. Gallagher PG. Update on the clinical spectrum and genetics of red blood cell membrane disorders. *Curr Hematol Rep.* 2004;3:85-91.

40. Huisjes R, Makhro A, Llaudet-Planas E, et al. Density, heterogeneity and deformability of red cells as markers of clinical severity in hereditary spherocytosis. *Haematologica.* 2020;105:338-347.

41. Hanspal M, Hanspal JS, Kalraiya R, et al. Asynchronous synthesis of membrane skeletal proteins during terminal maturation of murine erythroblasts. *Blood.* 1992;80:530-539.

42. Moon RT, Lazarides E. beta-Spectrin limits alpha-spectrin assembly on membranes following synthesis in a chicken erythroid cell lysate. *Nature.* 1983;305:62-65.

43. Tse WT, Gallagher PG, Jenkins PB, et al. Amino-acid substitution in alpha-spectrin commonly coinherited with nondominant hereditary spherocytosis. *Am J Hematol.* 1997;54:233-241.

44. Wichterle H, Hanspal M, Palek J, Jarolim P. Combination of two mutant alpha spectrin alleles underlies a severe spherocytic hemolytic anemia. *J Clin Invest.* 1996;98:2300-2307.

45. Hassoun H, Vassiliadis JN, Murray J, et al. Characterization of the underlying molecular defect in hereditary spherocytosis associated with spectrin deficiency. *Blood.* 1997;90:398-406.

46. Hassoun H, Vassiliadis JN, Murray J, et al. Hereditary spherocytosis with spectrin deficiency due to an unstable truncated beta spectrin. *Blood.* 1996;87:2538-2545.

47. Becker PS, Tse WT, Lux SE, Forget BG. Beta spectrin kissimmee: a spectrin variant associated with autosomal dominant hereditary spherocytosis and defective binding to protein 4.1. *J Clin Invest.* 1993;92:612-616.

48. Miraglia del Giudice E, Lombardi C, Francese M, et al. Frequent de novo monoallelic expression of beta-spectrin gene (SPTB) in children with hereditary spherocytosis and isolated spectrin deficiency. *Br J Haematol.* 1998;101:251-254.

49. Savvides P, Shalev O, John KM, Lux SE. Combined spectrin and ankyrin deficiency is common in autosomal dominant hereditary spherocytosis. *Blood.* 1993;82:2953-2960.

50. Miraglia del Giudice E, Francese M, Nobili B, et al. High frequency of de novo mutations in ankyrin gene (ANK1) in children with hereditary spherocytosis. *J Pediatr.* 1998;132:117-120.

51. Raskind CH, Dembry LM, Gallagher PG. Vancomycin-resistant enterococcal bacteremia and necrotizing enterocolitis in a preterm neonate. *Pediatr Infect Dis J.* 2005;24:943-944.

52. Gallagher PG, Sabatino DE, Basseres DS, et al. Erythrocyte ankyrin promoter mutations associated with recessive hereditary spherocytosis cause significant abnormalities in ankyrin expression. *J Biol Chem.* 2001;276:41683-41689.

53. Gallagher PG, Steiner LA, Liem RI, et al. Mutation of a barrier insulator in the human ankyrin-1 gene is associated with hereditary spherocytosis. *J Clin Invest.* 2010;120:4453-4465.

54. Lux SE, Tse WT, Menninger JC, et al. Hereditary spherocytosis associated with deletion of human erythrocyte ankyrin gene on chromosome 8. *Nature.* 1990;345:736-739.

55. Miya K, Shimojima K, Sugawara M, et al. A de novo interstitial deletion of 8p11.2 including ANK1 identified in a patient with spherocytosis, psychomotor developmental delay, and distinctive facial features. *Gene.* 2012;506:146-149.

56. Jarolim P, Murray JL, Rubin HL, et al. Characterization of 13 novel band 3 gene defects in hereditary spherocytosis with band 3 deficiency. *Blood.* 1996;88:4366-4374.

57. Jarolim P, Rubin HL, Brabec V, et al. Mutations of conserved arginines in the membrane domain of erythroid band 3 lead to a decrease in membrane-associated band 3 and to the phenotype of hereditary spherocytosis. *Blood.* 1995;85:634-640.

58. Quilty JA, Reithmeier RA. Trafficking and folding defects in hereditary spherocytosis mutants of the human red cell anion exchanger. *Traffic.* 2000;1:987-998.

59. Alloisio N, Maillet P, Carre G, et al. Hereditary spherocytosis with band 3 deficiency. Association with a nonsense mutation of the band 3 gene (allele Lyon), and aggravation by a low-expression allele occurring in trans (allele Genas). *Blood.* 1996;88:1062-1069.

60. Alloisio N, Texier P, Vallier A, et al. Modulation of clinical expression and band 3 deficiency in hereditary spherocytosis. *Blood.* 1997;90:414-420.

61. Bracher NA, Lyons CA, Wessels G, Mansvelt E, Coetzer TL. Band 3 Cape Town (E90K) causes severe hereditary spherocytosis in combination with band 3 Prague III. *Br J Haematol.* 2001;113:689-693.

62. Ribeiro ML, Alloisio N, Almeida H, et al. Severe hereditary spherocytosis and distal renal tubular acidosis associated with the total absence of band 3. *Blood.* 2000;96:1602-1604.

63. Wrong O, Bruce LJ, Unwin RJ, Toye AM, Tanner MJ. Band 3 mutations, distal renal tubular acidosis, and Southeast Asian ovalocytosis. *Kidney Int.* 2002;62:10-19.

64. Yawata Y, Kanzaki A, Yawata A, Doerfler W, Ozcan R, Eber SW. Characteristic features of the genotype and phenotype of hereditary spherocytosis in the Japanese population. *Int J Hematol.* 2000;71:118-135.

65. Bouhassira EE, Schwartz RS, Yawata Y, et al. An alanine-to-threonine substitution in protein 4.2 cDNA is associated with a Japanese form of hereditary hemolytic anemia (protein 4.2NIPPON). *Blood.* 1992;79:1846-1854.

66. Lusher JM, Barnhart MI. The role of the spleen in the pathoophysiology of hereditary spherocytosis and hereditary elliptocytosis. *Am J Pediatr Hematol Oncol.* 1980;2:31-39.

67. Park Y, Best CA, Badizadegan K, et al. Measurement of red blood cell mechanics during morphological changes. *Proc Natl Acad Sci U S A.* 2010;107:6731-6736.

68. Mendelbaum H. Congenital hemolytic jaundice: initial hemolytic crisis occurring at the age of 75. *Ann Intern Med.* 1939;13:872-883.

69. Guarnone R, Centenara E, Zappa M, Zanella A, Barosi G. Erythropoietin production and erythropoiesis in compensated and anaemic states of hereditary spherocytosis. *Br J Haematol.* 1996;92:150-154.

70. Rocha S, Costa E, Catarino C, et al. Erythropoietin levels in the different clinical forms of hereditary spherocytosis. *Br J Haematol.* 2005;131:534-542.

71. Saada V, Cynober T, Brossard Y, et al. Incidence of hereditary spherocytosis in a population of jaundiced neonates. *Pediatr Hematol Oncol.* 2006;23:387-397.

72. Sgro M, Campbell D, Shah V. Incidence and causes of severe neonatal hyperbilirubinemia in Canada. *CMAJ (Can Med Assoc J).* 2006;175:587-590.

73. Berardi A, Lugli L, Ferrari F, et al. Kernicterus associated with hereditary spherocytosis and UGT1A1 promoter polymorphism. *Biol Neonate.* 2006;90:243-246.

74. Gallagher PG. Difficulty in diagnosis of hereditary spherocytosis in the neonate. *Pediatrics.* 2021;148:e2021051100.

75. Pajor A, Lehoczky D, Szakacs Z. Pregnancy and hereditary spherocytosis. Report of 8 patients and a review. *Arch Gynecol Obstet.* 1993;253:37-42.

76. Gehlbach SH, Cooper BA. Haemolytic anaemia in infectious mononucleosis due to inapparent congenital spherocytosis. *Scand J Haematol.* 1970;7:141-144.

77. Young NS. Hematologic manifestations and diagnosis of parvovirus B19 infections. *Clin Adv Hematol Oncol.* 2006;4:908-910.

78. Lefrere JJ, Courouce AM, Girot R, Bertrand Y, Soulier JP. Six cases of hereditary spherocytosis revealed by human parvovirus infection. *Br J Haematol.* 1986;62:653-658.

79. Delamore IW, Richmond J, Davies SH. Megaloblastic anaemia in congenital spherocytosis. *Br Med J.* 1961;1:543-545.

80. Tamary H, Aviner S, Freud E, et al. High incidence of early cholelithiasis detected by ultrasonography in children and young adults with hereditary spherocytosis. *J Pediatr Hematol Oncol.* 2003;25:952-954.

81. Economou M, Tsatra I, Athanassiou-Metaxa M. Simultaneous presence of Gilbert syndrome and hereditary spherocytosis: interaction in the pathogenesis of hyperbilirubinemia and gallstone formation. *Pediatr Hematol Oncol.* 2003;20:493-495.

82. Iolascon A, Faienza MF, Moretti A, Perrotta S, Miraglia del Giudice E. UGT1 promoter polymorphism accounts for increased neonatal appearance of hereditary spherocytosis. *Blood.* 1998;91:1093.

83. Kugler D, Jager D, Barth J. A patient with pancreatitis, anaemia and an intrathoracic tumour. Diagnosis: tumour-simulating asymptomatic intrathoracic extramedullary haematopoiesis (EMH) in a patient with hereditary spherocytosis. *Eur Respir J.* 2006;27:856-859.

84. Giraldi S, Abbage KT, Marinoni LP, et al. Leg ulcer in hereditary spherocytosis. *Pediatr Dermatol.* 2003;20:427-428.

85. Rabhi S, Benjelloune H, Meziane M, et al. Hereditary spherocytosis with leg ulcers healing after splenectomy. *South Med J.* 2011;104:150-152.

86. Alter P, Maisch B. Non-compaction cardiomyopathy in an adult with hereditary spherocytosis. *Eur J Heart Fail.* 2007;9:98-99.

87. Cynober T, Mohandas N, Tchernia G. Red cell abnormalities in hereditary spherocytosis: relevance to diagnosis and understanding of the variable expression of clinical severity. *J Lab Clin Med.* 1996;128:259-269.

88. Michaels LA, Cohen AR, Zhao H, Raphael RI, Manno CS. Screening for hereditary spherocytosis by use of automated erythrocyte indexes. *J Pediatr.* 1997;130:957-960.

89. King MJ, Smythe JS, Mushens R. Eosin-5-maleimide binding to band 3 and Rh-related proteins forms the basis of a screening test for hereditary spherocytosis. *Br J Haematol.* 2004;124:106-113.

90. Bianchi P, Fermo E, Vercellati C, et al. Diagnostic power of laboratory tests for hereditary spherocytosis: a comparison study in 150 patients grouped according to molecular and clinical characteristics. *Haematologica.* 2012;97:516-523.

91. D'Alcamo E, Agrigento V, Sclafani S, et al. Reliability of EMA binding test in the diagnosis of hereditary spherocytosis in Italian patients. *Acta Haematol.* 2011;125:136-140.

92. Fermo E, Vercellati C, Marcello AP, et al. Targeted next generation sequencing and diagnosis of congenital hemolytic anemias: a three years experience monocentric study. *Front Physiol.* 2021;12:684569.

93. Bolton-Maggs PH, Stevens RF, Dodd NJ, et al. Guidelines for the diagnosis and management of hereditary spherocytosis. *Br J Haematol.* 2004;126:455-474.

94. Bolton-Maggs PH, Langer JC, Iolascon A, Tittensor P, King MJ; General Haematology Task Force of the British Committee for Standards in, H. Guidelines for the diagnosis and management of hereditary spherocytosis--2011 update. *Br J Haematol.* 2012;156:37-49.

95. Christensen RD, Henry E. Hereditary spherocytosis in neonates with hyperbilirubinemia. *Pediatrics.* 2010;125:120-125.

96. Hosono S, Hosono A, Mugishima H, et al. Successful recombinant erythropoietin therapy for a developing anemic newborn with hereditary spherocytosis. *Pediatr Int.* 2006;48:178-180.

97. Tchernia G, Delhommeau F, Perrotta S, et al. Recombinant erythropoietin therapy as an alternative to blood transfusions in infants with hereditary spherocytosis. *Hematol J.* 2000;1:146-152.

98. Baird RN, Macpherson AI, Richmond J. Red-blood-cell survival after splenectomy in congenital spherocytosis. *Lancet.* 1971;2:1060-1061.

99. Chapman RG, McDonald LL. Red cell life span after splenectomy in hereditary spherocytosis. *J Clin Invest.* 1968;47:2263-2267.

100. Reliene R, Mariani M, Zanella A, et al. Splenectomy prolongs in vivo survival of erythrocytes differently in spectrin/ankyrin- and band 3-deficient hereditary spherocytosis. *Blood.* 2002;100:2208-2215.

101. Bonderman D, Jakowitsch J, Adlbrecht C, et al. Medical conditions increasing the risk of chronic thromboembolic pulmonary hypertension. *Thromb Haemost.* 2005;93:512-516.

102. Hayag-Barin JE, Smith RE, Tucker FC, Jr. Hereditary spherocytosis, thrombocytosis, and chronic pulmonary emboli: a case report and review of the literature. *Am J Hematol.* 1998;57:82-84.

103. Jardine DL, Laing AD. Delayed pulmonary hypertension following splenectomy for congenital spherocytosis. *Intern Med J.* 2004;34:214-216.

104. Smedema JP, Louw VJ. Pulmonary arterial hypertension after splenectomy for hereditary spherocytosis. *Cardiovasc J S Afr.* 2007;18:84-89.

105. Wandersee NJ, Olson SC, Holzhauer SL, Hoffmann RG, Barker JE, Hillery CA. Increased erythrocyte adhesion in mice and humans with hereditary spherocytosis and hereditary elliptocytosis. *Blood.* 2004;103:710-716.

106. Hansen K, Singer DB. Asplenic-hyposplenic overwhelming sepsis: postsplenectomy sepsis revisited. *Pediatr Dev Pathol.* 2001;4:105-121.

107. Schilling RF. Estimating the risk for sepsis after splenectomy in hereditary spherocytosis. *Ann Intern Med.* 1995;122:187-188.

108. Singer DB. Postsplenectomy sepsis. *Perspect Pediatr Pathol.* 1973;1:285-311.

109. Casale M, Perrotta S. Splenectomy for hereditary spherocytosis: complete, partial or not at all?. *Expert Rev Hematol.* 2011;4:627-635.

110. Schilling RF. Risks and benefits of splenectomy versus no splenectomy for hereditary spherocytosis - a personal view. *Br J Haematol.* 2009;145:728-732.

111. Vercellati C, Zaninoni A, Marcello AP, et al. Changing trends of splenectomy in hereditary spherocytosis: the experience of a reference Centre in the last 40 years. *Br J Haematol.* 2022;198(5):912-915.

112. Balague C, Targarona EM, Cerdan G, et al. Long-term outcome after laparoscopic splenectomy related to hematologic diagnosis. *Surg Endosc.* 2004;18:1283-1287.

113. Rescorla FJ, Engum SA, West KW, Tres Scherer LR,IIIrd, Rouse TM, Grosfeld JL. Laparoscopic splenectomy has become the gold standard in children. *Am Surg.* 2002;68:297-301. discussion 301-292.

114. Abdullah F, Zhang Y, Camp M, et al. Splenectomy in hereditary spherocytosis: review of 1,657 patients and application of the pediatric quality indicators. *Pediatr Blood Cancer.* 2009;52:834-837.

115. Dutta S, Price VE, Blanchette V, Langer JC. A laparoscopic approach to partial splenectomy for children with hereditary spherocytosis. *Surg Endosc.* 2006;20:1719-1724.

116. Rice HE, Oldham KT, Hillery CA, Skinner MA, O'Hara SM, Ware RE. Clinical and hematologic benefits of partial splenectomy for congenital hemolytic anemias in children. *Ann Surg.* 2003;237:281-288.

117. Stoehr GA, Stauffer UG, Eber SW. Near-total splenectomy: a new technique for the management of hereditary spherocytosis. *Ann Surg.* 2005;241:40-47.

118. Tchernia G, Gauthier F, Mielot F, et al. Initial assessment of the beneficial effect of partial splenectomy in hereditary spherocytosis. *Blood.* 1993;81:2014-2020.

119. Yoshimoto A, Fujimura M, Nakao S. Pulmonary hypertension after splenectomy in hereditary stomatocytosis. *Am J Med Sci.* 2005;330:195-197.

120. Buesing KL, Tracy ET, Kiernan C, et al. Partial splenectomy for hereditary spherocytosis: a multi-institutional review. *J Pediatr Surg.* 2011;46:178-183.

121. Hollingsworth CL, Rice HE. Hereditary spherocytosis and partial splenectomy in children: review of surgical technique and the role of imaging. *Pediatr Radiol.* 2010;40:1177-1183.

122. Bruce LJ, Robinson HC, Guizouarn H, et al. Monovalent cation leaks in human red cells caused by single amino-acid substitutions in the transport domain of the band 3 chloride-bicarbonate exchanger, AE1. *Nat Genet.* 2005;37:1258-1263.

123. Dhermy D, Garbarz M, Lecomte MC, et al. Hereditary elliptocytosis: clinical, morphological and biochemical studies of 38 cases. *Nouv Rev Fr Hematol.* 1986;28:129-140.

124. Gallagher PG. Hereditary elliptocytosis: spectrin and protein 4.1R. *Semin Hematol.* 2004;41:142-164.

125. Dhermy D, Schrevel J, Lecomte MC. Spectrin-based skeleton in red blood cells and malaria. *Curr Opin Hematol.* 2007;14:198-202.

126. Gallagher PG, Weed SA, Tse WT, et al. Recurrent fatal hydrops fetalis associated with a nucleotide substitution in the erythrocyte beta-spectrin gene. *J Clin Invest.* 1995;95:1174-1182.

127. Zhang Z, Weed SA, Gallagher PG, Morrow JS. Dynamic molecular modeling of pathogenic mutations in the spectrin self-association domain. *Blood.* 2001;98:1645-1653.

128. Johnson CP, Gaetani M, Ortiz V, et al. Pathogenic proline mutation in the linker between spectrin repeats: disease caused by spectrin unfolding. *Blood.* 2007;109:3538-3543.

129. Delaunay J, Nouyrigat V, Proust A, et al. Different impacts of alleles alphaLEPRA and alphaLELY as assessed versus a novel, virtually null allele of the SPTA1 gene in trans. *Br J Haematol.* 2004;127:118-122.

130. Alloisio N, Morle L, Marechal J, et al. Sp alpha V/41: a common spectrin polymorphism at the alpha IV-alpha V domain junction. Relevance to the expression level of hereditary elliptocytosis due to alpha-spectrin variants located in trans. *J Clin Invest.* 1991;87:2169-2177.

131. Wilmotte R, Marechal J, Morle L, et al. Low expression allele alpha LELY of red cell spectrin is associated with mutations in exon 40 (alpha V/41 polymorphism) and intron 45 and with partial skipping of exon 46. *J Clin Invest.* 1993;91:2091-2096.

132. Marechal J, Wilmotte R, Kanzaki A, et al. Ethnic distribution of allele alpha LELY, a low-expression allele of red-cell spectrin alpha-gene. *Br J Haematol.* 1995;90:553-556.

133. Chasis JA, Coulombel L, McGee S, et al. Differential use of protein 4.1 translation initiation sites during erythropoiesis: implications for a mutation-induced stage-specific deficiency of protein 4.1 during erythroid development. *Blood.* 1996;87:5324-5331.

134. Conboy J, Marchesi S, Kim R, Agre P, Kan YW, Mohandas N. Molecular analysis of insertion/deletion mutations in protein 4.1 in elliptocytosis. II. Determination of molecular genetic origins of rearrangements. *J Clin Invest.* 1990;86:524-530.

135. Conboy J, Mohandas N, Tchernia G, Kan YW. Molecular basis of hereditary elliptocytosis due to protein 4.1 deficiency. *N Engl J Med.* 1986;315:680-685.

136. Mentzer WC, Jr, Iarocci TA, Mohandas N, et al. Modulation of erythrocyte membrane mechanical stability by 2,3-diphosphoglycerate in the neonatal poikilocytosis/elliptocytosis syndrome. *J Clin Invest.* 1987;79:943-949.

137. Iarocci TA, Wagner GM, Mohandas N, Lane PA, Mentzer WC. Hereditary poikilocytic anemia associated with the co-inheritance of two alpha spectrin abnormalities. *Blood.* 1988;71:1390-1396.

138. Zarkowsky HS, Mohandas N, Speaker CB, Shohet SB. A congenital haemolytic anaemia with thermal sensitivity of the erythrocyte membrane. *Br J Haematol.* 1975;29:537-543.

139. Costa DB, Lozovatsky L, Gallagher PG, Forget BG. A novel splicing mutation of the {alpha}-spectrin gene in the original hereditary pyropoikilocytosis kindred. *Blood.* 2005;106:4367-4369.

140. Laosombat V, Dissaneevate S, Peerapittayamongkol C, Matsuo M. Neonatal hyperbilirubinemia associated with Southeast Asian ovalocytosis. *Am J Hematol.* 1999;60:136-139.

141. Laosombat V, Viprakasit V, Dissaneevate S, et al. Natural history of Southeast Asian ovalocytosis during the first 3 years of life. *Blood Cells Mol Dis.* 2010;45:29-32.

142. Mohandas N, Winardi R, Knowles D, et al. Molecular basis for membrane rigidity of hereditary ovalocytosis. A novel mechanism involving the cytoplasmic domain of band 3. *J Clin Invest.* 1992;89:686-692.

143. Liu SC, Palek J, Yi SJ, et al. Molecular basis of altered red blood cell membrane properties in Southeast Asian ovalocytosis: role of the mutant band 3 protein in band 3 oligomerization and retention by the membrane skeleton. *Blood.* 1995;86:349-358.

144. Liu SC, Jarolim P, Rubin HL, et al. The homozygous state for the band 3 protein mutation in Southeast Asian Ovalocytosis may be lethal. *Blood.* 1994;84:3590-3591.

145. Manabe M, Hagiwara Y, Asada R, Tanizawa N, Nanno S, Koh KR. Acquired elliptocytosis in a patient with myelodysplastic syndrome harbouring a novel unbalanced whole-arm translocation, der(14;20)(q10;p10). *Br J Haematol.* 2022;196:7.

146. Quiroz-Cervantes KS, Juárez-Salcedo LM, Nuevo I, Guillén H, Arbeteta J, Golbano N. Acquired elliptocytosis in a patient with a myelodysplastic syndrome associated with 20q deletion. *Br J Haematol.* 2019;185:206.

147. Davidson RJ, How J, Lessels S. Acquired stomatocytosis: its prevalence of significance in routine haematology. *Scand J Haematol.* 1977;19:47-53.

148. Mentzer WC, Jr, Smith WB, Goldstone J, Shohet SB. Hereditary stomatocytosis: membrane and metabolism studies. *Blood.* 1975;46:659-669.

149. Stewart GW, Turner EJ. The hereditary stomatocytoses and allied disorders: congenital disorders of erythrocyte membrane permeability to Na and K. *Baillieres Best Pract Res Clin Haematol.* 1999;12:707-727.

150. Delaunay J. The hereditary stomatocytoses: genetic disorders of the red cell membrane permeability to monovalent cations. *Semin Hematol.* 2004;41:165-172.

151. Bruce LJ. Hereditary stomatocytosis and cation leaky red cells--recent developments. *Blood Cells Mol Dis.* 2009;42:216-222.

152. Fricke B, Argent AC, Chetty MC, et al. The "stomatin" gene and protein in overhydrated hereditary stomatocytosis. *Blood.* 2003;102:2268-2277.

153. Fricke B, Parsons SF, Knopfle G, von During M, Stewart GW. Stomatin is mistrafficked in the erythrocytes of overhydrated hereditary stomatocytosis, and is absent from normal primitive yolk sac-derived erythrocytes. *Br J Haematol.* 2005;131:265-277.

154. Lande WM, Thiemann PV, Mentzer WC, Jr. Missing band 7 membrane protein in two patients with high Na, low K erythrocytes. *J Clin Invest.* 1982;70:1273-1280.

155. Zhu Y, Paszty C, Turetsky T, et al. Stomatocytosis is absent in "stomatin"-deficient murine red blood cells. *Blood.* 1999;93:2404-2410.

156. Gallagher PG, Chang SH, Rettig MP, et al. Altered erythrocyte endothelial adherence and membrane phospholipid asymmetry in hereditary hydrocytosis. *Blood.* 2003;101:4625-4627.

157. Glader BE, Fortier N, Albala MM, Nathan DG. Congenital hemolytic anemia associated with dehydrated erythrocytes and increased potassium loss. *N Engl J Med.* 1974;291:491-496.

158. Sauberman N, Fairbanks G, Lutz HU, Fortier NL, Snyder LM. Altered red blood cell surface area in hereditary xerocytosis. *Clin Chim Acta.* 1981;114:149-161.

159. Schroter W, Ungefehr K, Tillmann W. Role of the spleen in congenital stomatocytosis associated with high sodium-low potassium erythrocytes. *Klin Wochenschr.* 1981;59:173-179.

160. Smith BD, Segel GB. Abnormal erythrocyte endothelial adherence in hereditary stomatocytosis. *Blood.* 1997;89:3451-3456.

161. Basu AP, Carey P, Cynober T, et al. Dehydrated hereditary stomatocytosis with transient perinatal ascites. *Arch Dis Child Fetal Neonatal Ed.* 2003;88:F438-F439.

162. Grootenboer S, Schischmanoff PO, Cynober T, et al. A genetic syndrome associating dehydrated hereditary stomatocytosis, pseudohyperkalaemia and perinatal oedema. *Br J Haematol.* 1998;103:383-386.

163. Grootenboer-Mignot S, Cretien A, Laurendeau I, et al. Sub-lethal hydrops as a manifestation of dehydrated hereditary stomatocytosis in two consecutive pregnancies. *Prenat Diagn.* 2003;23:380-384.

164. Zarychanski R, Schulz VP, Houston BL, et al. Mutations in the mechanotransduction protein PIEZO1 are associated with hereditary xerocytosis. *Blood.* 2012;120(9):1908-1915.

165. Jankovsky N, Caulier A, Demagny J, et al. Recent advances in the pathophysiology of PIEZO1-related hereditary xerocytosis. *Am J Hematol.* 2021;96:1017-1026.

166. Andolfo I, Russo R, Rosato BE, et al. Genotype-phenotype correlation and risk stratification in a cohort of 123 hereditary stomatocytosis patients. *Am J Hematol.* 2018;93:1509-1517.

167. Carella M, Stewart G, Ajetunmobi JF, et al. Genomewide search for dehydrated hereditary stomatocytosis (hereditary xerocytosis): mapping of locus to chromosome 16 (16q23-qter). *Am J Hum Genet.* 1998;63:810-816.

168. Iolascon A, Stewart GW, Ajetunmobi JF, et al. Familial pseudohyperkalemia maps to the same locus as dehydrated hereditary stomatocytosis (hereditary xerocytosis). *Blood.* 1999;93:3120-3123.

169. Houston BL, Zelinski T, Israels SJ, et al. Refinement of the hereditary xerocytosis locus on chromosome 16q in a large Canadian kindred. *Blood Cells Mol Dis.* 2011;47(4):226-231.

170. Glogowska E, Schneider ER, Maksimova Y, et al. Novel mechanisms of PIEZO1 dysfunction in hereditary xerocytosis. *Blood.* 2017;130:1845-1856.

171. Cahalan SM, Lukacs V, Ranade SS, Chien S, Bandell M, Patapoutian A. Piezo1 links mechanical forces to red blood cell volume. *Elife.* 2015;4:e07370.

172. Vandorpe DH, Xu C, Shmukler BE, et al. Hypoxia activates a Ca2+-permeable cation conductance sensitive to carbon monoxide and to GsMTx-4 in human and mouse sickle erythrocytes. *PLoS One.* 2010;5:e8732.

173. Ma YL, Rees DC, Gibson JS, Ellory JC. The conductance of red blood cells from sickle cell patients: ion selectivity and inhibitors. *J Physiol.* 2012;590:2095-2105.

174. Ma S, Cahalan S, LaMonte G, et al. Common PIEZO1 allele in African populations causes RBC dehydration and attenuates Plasmodium infection. *Cell.* 2018;173:443-455 e412.

175. Yang E, Voelkel EB, Lezon-Geyda K, Schulz VP, Gallagher PG. Hemoglobin C trait accentuates erythrocyte dehydration in hereditary xerocytosis. *Pediatr Blood Cancer.* 2017;64:10.1002/pbc.26444.

176. Rapetti-Mauss R, Lacoste C, Picard V, et al. A mutation in the Gardos channel is associated with hereditary xerocytosis. *Blood.* 2015;126:1273-1280.

177. Glogowska E, Lezon-Geyda K, Maksimova Y, Schulz VP, Gallagher PG. Mutations in the Gardos channel (KCNN4) are associated with hereditary xerocytosis. *Blood.* 2015;126:1281-1284.

178. Fermo E, Bogdanova A, Petkova-Kirova P, et al. Gardos Channelopathy': a variant of hereditary Stomatocytosis with complex molecular regulation. *Sci Rep.* 2017;7:1744.

179. Clark MR, Shohet SB, Gottfried EL. Hereditary hemolytic disease with increased red blood cell phosphatidylcholine and dehydration: one, two, or many disorders? *Am J Hematol.* 1993;42:25-30.

180. Bruce LJ, Guizouarn H, Burton NM, et al. The monovalent cation leak in overhydrated stomatocytic red blood cells results from amino acid substitutions in the Rh-associated glycoprotein. *Blood.* 2009;113:1350-1357.

181. Genetet S, Ripoche P, Picot J, et al. Human RhAG ammonia channel is impaired by the Phe65Ser mutation in overhydrated stomatocytic red cells. *Am J Physiol Cell Physiol.* 2012;302:C419-C428.

182. Stewart AK, Shmukler BE, Vandorpe DH, et al. Loss-of-function and gain-of-function phenotypes of stomatocytosis mutant RhAG F65S. *Am J Physiol Cell Physiol.* 2011;301:C1325-C1343.

183. Flatt JF, Guizouarn H, Burton NM, et al. Stomatin-deficient cryohydrocytosis results from mutations in SLC2A1: a novel form of GLUT1 deficiency syndrome. *Blood.* 2011;118:5267-5277.

184. Guizouarn H, Martial S, Gabillat N, Borgese F. Point mutations involved in red cell stomatocytosis convert the electroneutral anion exchanger 1 to a non-selective cation conductance. *Blood.* 2007;110:2158-2165.

185. Van Kim CL, Colin Y, Cartron JP. Rh proteins: key structural and functional components of the red cell membrane. *Blood Rev.* 2005;20:93-110.

186. Sturgeon P. Hematological observations on the anemia associated with blood type Rhnull. *Blood.* 1970;36:310-320.

187. Nicolas V, Le Van Kim C, Gane P, et al. Rh-RhAG/ankyrin-R, a new interaction site between the membrane bilayer and the red cell skeleton, is impaired by Rh(null)-associated mutation. *J Biol Chem.* 2003;278:25526-25533.

188. Nicolas V, Mouro-Chanteloup I, Lopez C, et al. Functional interaction between Rh proteins and the spectrin-based skeleton in erythroid and epithelial cells. *Transfus Clin Biol.* 2006;13:23-28.

189. Tada H, Nomura A, Ogura M, et al. Diagnosis and management of sitosterolemia 2021. *J Atheroscler Thromb.* 2021;28:791-801.

190. Niu DM, Chong KW, Hsu JH, et al. Clinical observations, molecular genetic analysis, and treatment of sitosterolemia in infants and children. *J Inherit Metab Dis.* 2010;33:437-443.

191. Rees DC, Iolascon A, Carella M, et al. Stomatocytic haemolysis and macrothrombocytopenia (Mediterranean stomatocytosis/macrothrombocytopenia) is the haematological presentation of phytosterolaemia. *Br J Haematol.* 2005;130:297-309.

192. Wang G, Wang Z, Liang J, Cao L, Bai X, Ruan C. A phytosterolemia patient presenting exclusively with macrothrombocytopenia and stomatocytic hemolysis. *Acta Haematol.* 2011;126:95-98.

193. Stefkova J, Poledne R, Hubacek JA. ATP-binding cassette (ABC) transporters in human metabolism and diseases. *Physiol Res.* 2004;53:235-243.

194. Wang DQ. Regulation of intestinal cholesterol absorption. *Annu Rev Physiol.* 2007;69:221-248.

195. Koseki M, Yamashita S, Ogura M, et al. Current diagnosis and management of Tangier disease. *J Atheroscler Thromb.* 2021;28:802-810.

Disorders of Red Blood Cells

196. Cooper RA. Anemia with spur cells: a red cell defect acquired in serum and modified in the circulation. *J Clin Invest*. 1969;48:1820-1831.

197. Cooper RA. Hemolytic syndromes and red cell membrane abnormalities in liver disease. *Semin Hematol*. 1980;17:103-112.

198. Raffa GA, Byrnes DM, Byrnes JJ. The diagnosis is in the smear: a case and review of spur cell anemia in Cirrhosis. *Case Rep Hematol*. 2021;2021:8883335.

199. Takahashi M, Okazaki H, Ohashi K, et al. Current diagnosis and management of abetalipoproteinemia. *J Atheroscler Thromb*. 2021;28:1009-1019.

200. Hussain MM, Rava P, Walsh M, Rana M, Iqbal J. Multiple functions of microsomal triglyceride transfer protein. *Nutr Metab*. 2012;9:14.

201. Tarugi P, Averna M, Di Leo E, et al. Molecular diagnosis of hypobetalipoproteinemia: an ENID review. *Atherosclerosis*. 2007;195:e19-e27.

202. Zeissig S, Dougan SK, Barral DC, et al. Primary deficiency of microsomal triglyceride transfer protein in human abetalipoproteinemia is associated with loss of CD1 function. *J Clin Invest*. 2010;120:2889-2899.

203. Danek A, Rubio JP, Rampoldi L, et al. McLeod neuroacanthocytosis: genotype and phenotype. *Ann Neurol*. 2001;50:755-764.

204. Reid ME, Mohandas N. Red blood cell blood group antigens: structure and function. *Semin Hematol*. 2004;41:93-117.

205. Roulis E, Hyland C, Flower R, Gassner C, Jung HH, Frey BM. Molecular basis and clinical overview of McLeod syndrome compared with other neuroacanthocytosis syndromes: a review. *JAMA Neurol*. 2018;75:1554-1562.

206. Lhomme F, Peyrard T, Babinet J, et al. Chronic granulomatous disease with the McLeod phenotype: a french national retrospective case series. *J Clin Immunol*. 2020;40:752-762.

207. Walker RH, Jung HH, Dobson-Stone C, et al. Neurologic phenotypes associated with acanthocytosis. *Neurology*. 2007;68:92-98.

208. Jung HH, Danek A, Walker RH. Neuroacanthocytosis syndromes. *Orphanet J Rare Dis*. 2011;6:68.

209. Hayflick SJ, Westaway SK, Levinson B, et al. Genetic, clinical, and radiographic delineation of Hallervorden-Spatz syndrome. *N Engl J Med*. 2003;348:33-40.

210. Pellecchia MT, Valente EM, Cif L, et al. The diverse phenotype and genotype of pantothenate kinase-associated neurodegeneration. *Neurology*. 2005;64:1810-1812.

211. Peikert K, Danek A, Hermann A. Current state of knowledge in Chorea-Acanthocytosis as core Neuroacanthocytosis syndrome. *Eur J Med Genet*. 2018;61:699-705.

212. Dobson-Stone C, Velayos-Baeza A, Filippone LA, et al. Chorein detection for the diagnosis of chorea-acanthocytosis. *Ann Neurol*. 2004;56:299-302.

213. Rampoldi L, Dobson-Stone C, Rubio JP, et al. A conserved sorting-associated protein is mutant in chorea-acanthocytosis. *Nat Genet*. 2001;28:119-120.

214. Ueno S, Maruki Y, Nakamura M, et al. The gene encoding a newly discovered protein, chorein, is mutated in chorea-acanthocytosis. *Nat Genet*. 2001;28:121-122.

215. Tomiyasu A, Nakamura M, Ichiba M, et al. Novel pathogenic mutations and copy number variations in the VPS13A gene in patients with chorea-acanthocytosis. *Am J Med Genet B Neuropsychiatr Genet*. 2011;156B:620-631.

216. Walker RH, Schulz VP, Tikhonova IR, et al. Genetic diagnosis of neuroacanthocytosis disorders using exome sequencing. *Mov Disord*. 2012;27:539-543.

217. De Franceschi L, Scardoni G, Tomelleri C, et al. Computational identification of phospho-tyrosine sub-networks related to acanthocyte generation in neuroacanthocytosis. *PLoS One*. 2012;7:e31015.

218. De Franceschi L, Tomelleri C, Matte A, et al. Erythrocyte membrane changes of chorea-acanthocytosis are the result of altered Lyn kinase activity. *Blood*. 2011;118:5652-5663.

219. de Haan LD, Werre JM, Ruben AM, Huls HA, de Gier J, Staal GE. Alterations in size, shape and osmotic behaviour of red cells after splenectomy: a study of their age dependence. *Br J Haematol*. 1988;69:71-80.

220. Hovingh GK, de Groot E, van der Steeg W, et al. Inherited disorders of HDL metabolism and atherosclerosis. *Curr Opin Lipidol*. 2005;16:139-145.

221. Roshan B, Ganda OP, Desilva R, et al. Homozygous lecithin:cholesterol acyltransferase (LCAT) deficiency due to a new loss of function mutation and review of the literature. *J Clin Lipidol*. 2011;5:493-499.

222. Mehta R, Elías-López D, Martagón AJ, et al. LCAT deficiency: a systematic review with the clinical and genetic description of Mexican kindred. *Lipids Health Dis*. 2021;20:70.

223. Argyropoulos G, Jenkins A, Klein RL, et al. Transmission of two novel mutations in a pedigree with familial lecithin:cholesterol acyltransferase deficiency: structure-function relationships and studies in a compound heterozygous proband. *J Lipid Res*. 1998;39:1870-1876.

224. Asztalos BF, Schaefer EJ, Horvath KV, et al. Role of LCAT in HDL remodeling: investigation of LCAT deficiency states. *J Lipid Res*. 2007;48:592-599.

225. Yang K, Wang J, Xiang H, Ding P, Wu T, Ji G. LCAT- targeted therapies: progress, failures and future. *Biomed Pharmacother*. 2022;147:112677.

Chapter 30 ■ Hereditary Hemolytic Anemias Due to Red Blood Cell Enzyme Disorders

RACHAEL F. GRACE • BERTIL GLADER

OVERVIEW OF ERYTHROCYTE METABOLISM

Mature red blood cells (RBCs) are anucleate (thereby incapable of cell division), are devoid of ribosomes (thereby incapable of protein synthesis), and lack mitochondria (thereby incapable of oxidative phosphorylation). Despite these limitations, RBCs survive 100 to 120 days in the circulation and effectively deliver oxygen to peripheral tissues. Glucose is the main metabolic substrate of RBCs, and it is metabolized by two major pathways: the glycolytic or "energy producing" pathway and the hexose monophosphate (HMP) shunt or "protective" pathway. Under normal conditions, approximately 90% of glucose flows through glycolysis, with a much smaller fraction channeled through the HMP pathway. However, the fraction of glucose entering the pentose phosphate pathway can increase significantly under conditions of increased oxidative stress. The major products of glycolysis are ATP (a source of energy for numerous RBC membrane and metabolic reactions), NADH (a necessary cofactor for methemoglobin reduction by cytochrome b5 reductase), and 2,3-diphosphoglycerate (2,3-DPG) or 2,3-biphosphoglycerate (2,3-BPG), an important intermediate that modulates hemoglobin-oxygen affinity) (*Figure 30.1*). Mature RBCs are incapable of de novo purine or pyrimidine synthesis, although many enzymes of nucleotide metabolism are present in erythrocytes. The later are known to be important for RBC preservation in vitro; it is also recognized that abnormalities in purine and pyrimidine metabolism are associated with inherited hemolytic disease.

The consequences of red cell enzymopathies are diverse. Some enzyme variants cause hemolytic disease with anemia being the sole expression of the enzymopathy. In other enzyme disorders, hemolysis is one feature of a multisystem disease affecting many tissues. Also, in some cases, erythrocyte enzyme abnormalities have no adverse effects on RBC function, and, if they occur in patients with hemolytic anemia, it is not always clear that the enzyme deficiency and hemolysis are causally related. This chapter focuses on the varied enzyme defects associated with hemolysis. These RBC enzyme disorders are due to abnormalities in the HMP shunt and glutathione metabolism, glycolytic enzyme deficiencies, and abnormalities in purine and pyrimidine metabolism.

DISORDERS OF HEXOSE MONOPHOSPHATE SHUNT AND GLUTATHIONE METABOLISM

The HMP shunt pathway metabolizes 5% to 10% of glucose utilized by RBCs, and this is critical for protecting red cells against oxidant injury (*Figure 30.2*). The HMP pathway is the only RBC source of reduced nicotinamide adenine dinucleotide phosphate (NADPH), a cofactor important in glutathione metabolism. RBCs contain relatively high concentrations of reduced glutathione (GSH), a sulfhydryl containing tripeptide (glutamylcysteinylglycine), which functions as an intracellular reducing agent that protects cells against oxidant injury. Oxidants, such as superoxide anion (O_2^-) and hydrogen peroxide (H_2O_2), are produced by exogenous factors (i.e., drugs, infection) and also are formed within red cells as a consequence of reactions of hemoglobin with oxygen. However, when these oxidants accumulate within red cells, hemoglobin and other proteins are oxidized, leading to loss of function and RBC death. Under normal circumstances this does not occur, since GSH, in conjunction with the enzyme glutathione peroxidase (GPx), rapidly inactivates these compounds. During the oxidant detoxification process, however, GSH is converted to oxidized glutathione (GSSG) and GSH levels fall. In order to sustain protection against persistent oxidant injury, GSH levels must be maintained, and this is accomplished by glutathione reductase (GSR), which catalyzes reduction of GSSG to GSH. This reaction requires the NADPH generated by glucose-6-phosphate dehydrogenase (G6PD), the first enzymatic reaction of the HMP shunt. Thus, it is the tight coupling of the HMP shunt and glutathione metabolism that is responsible for protecting intracellular proteins from oxidative assault. Almost all hemolytic episodes related to altered HMP shunt and glutathione metabolism are due to G6PD deficiency, and this enzyme deficiency affects millions of people throughout the world.[1-6] Rare cases of hemolysis associated with decreased GSR activity, GPx deficiency, and deficiencies of GSH synthetic enzymes also have been described.

GLUCOSE-6-PHOSPHATE DEHYDROGENASE DEFICIENCY

The importance of this enzyme for red cell integrity was first recognized following the observation that some African American soldiers taking the antimalarial drug primaquine would develop acute hemolytic anemia with hemoglobinuria (*Figure 30.3*). Initially it was observed that GSH was decreased in the RBC of susceptible individuals during acute hemolytic episodes. Subsequently, the activity of G6PD, one of the enzymes needed to keep adequate GSH levels, was found to be deficient in affected red cells.[7,8] Soon thereafter, the worldwide distribution of G6PD deficiency became apparent and the variation of clinical expression of enzyme deficiency was discovered. In most individuals with G6PD deficiency, there is no anemia in the steady state, reticulocyte counts are normal, but RBC survival may be slightly decreased. However, episodic exacerbations of hemolysis accompanied by anemia occur in association with the administration of certain drugs, with some infections, and with the eating of fava

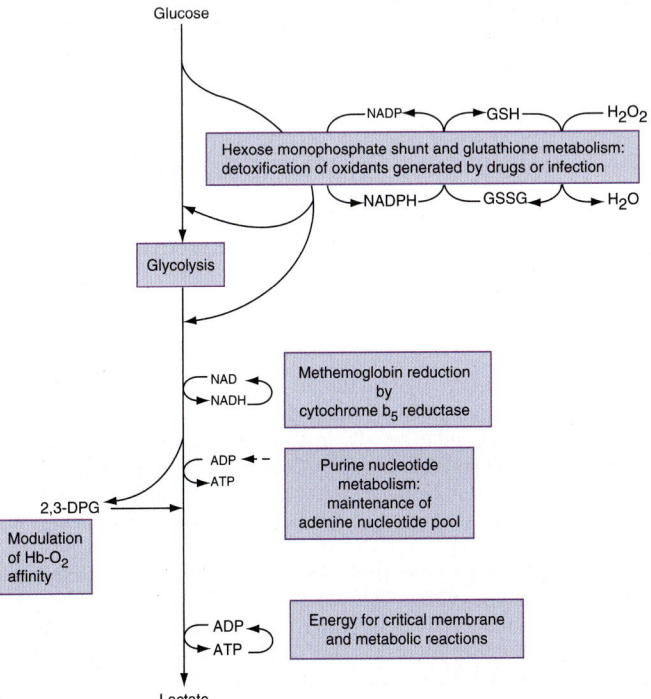

FIGURE 30.1 Summary of overall glycolysis, hexose monophosphate shunt, glutathione metabolism, and RBC nucleotide metabolism.

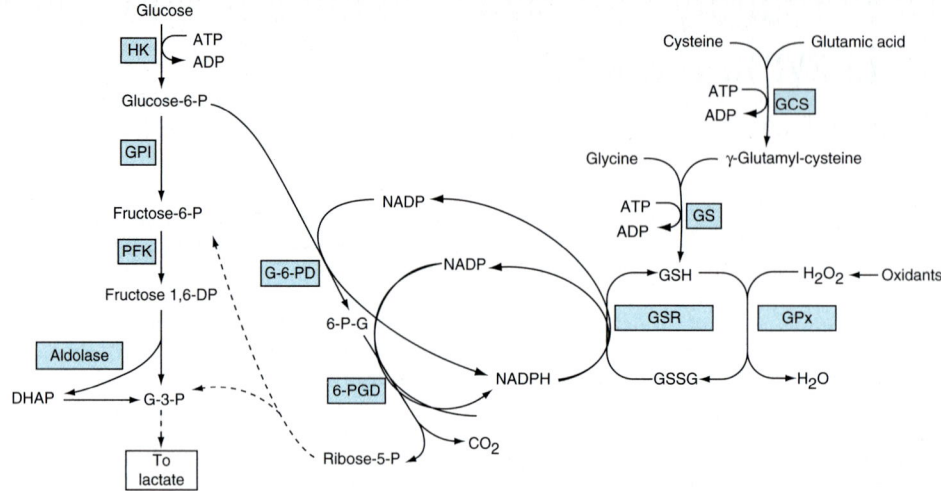

FIGURE 30.2 Hexose monophosphate shunt, enzymes of glutathione metabolism, protection from oxidant assault, and relationship to glycolytic metabolism. Enzyme abbreviations: 6-PGD, 6-phosphogluconate dehydrogenase; G-6-PD, glucose-6-phosphate dehydrogenase; GCS, γ-glutamyl-cysteine-synthetase; GPI, glucose phosphate isomerase; GPx, glutathione peroxidase; GS, glutathione synthetase; GSR, glutathione reductase; HK, hexokinase; PFK, phosphofructokinase. Substrate abbreviations: 6-P-G, 6-phosphogluconate; DHAP, dihydroxyacetone phosphate; G-3-P, glyceraldehyde 3-phosphate; GSH, reduced glutathione, GSSG, oxidized glutathione; R-5-P, ribose 5-phosphate.

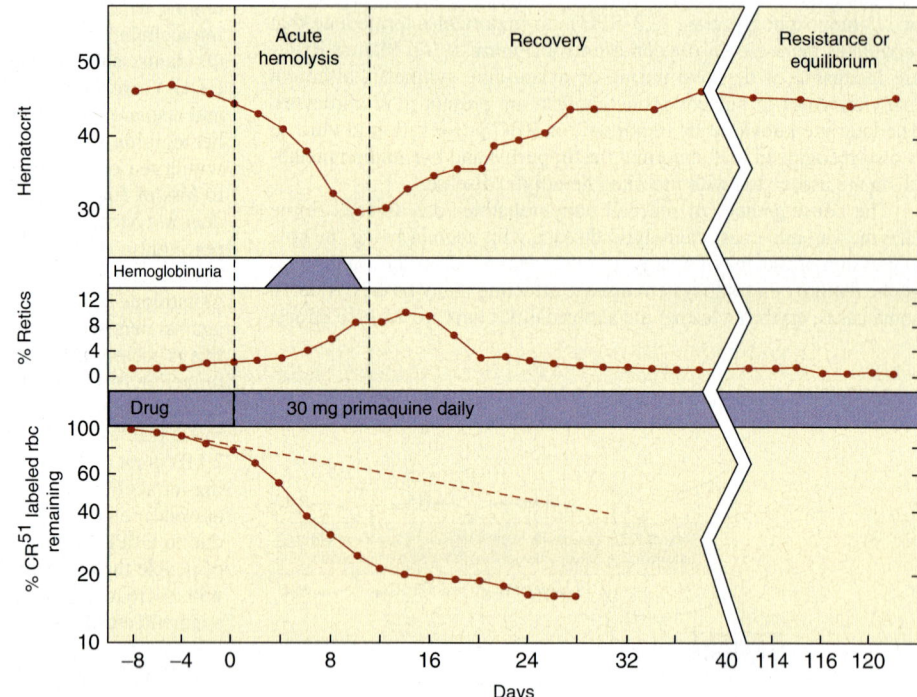

FIGURE 30.3 The course of primaquine-induced hemolysis in the G6PD A- variant. (Reprinted with permission from Alving AS, Johnson CF, Tarlov AR, et al. Mitigation of the haemolytic effect of primaquine and enhancement of its action against exoerythrocytic forms of the Chesson strain of *Plasmodium vivax* by intermittent regimens of drug administration. *Bull World Health Organ.* 1960;22(6):621-631.)

beans. In a minority of cases, G6PD deficiency is associated with a chronic hemolytic process. To date, over 200 G6PD variants with known mutations have been recognized.[5]

Prevalence and Geographic Distribution

Deficiency of G6PD is the most common metabolic disorder of RBCs and has been estimated to affect over 400 million people worldwide.[2,3,9] Although global in its distribution, G6PD deficiency is encountered with the greatest frequency in the tropical and subtropical zones of the Eastern Hemisphere. The incidence of the deficiency state is approximately 12% in African American men and 8% in Brazilians of African ancestry. As many as 20% of female African Americans may be heterozygous for G6PD mutations, and as many as 1% are homozygous. In Sardinia, the incidence varies from 35% at low altitudes to 3% in areas above 600 m. The deficiency state has been reported from

most areas of Greece, again with the greatest frequency (20%-32%) in the lowlands. In the male Asian population, the incidence of G6PD deficiency is estimated to be 14% in Cambodia, 2.6% in India, 2.1% in China, and less than 0.1% in Japan. Given that ancestry is often both diverse and unknown, G6PD testing should be evaluated in all individuals before administration of medications known to trigger hemolysis in deficient individuals.

Because of its high incidence among populations in which malaria was once endemic, G6PD deficiency is thought to have conferred a selective advantage against infection by falciparum malaria.[10] Partial indirect support for this is that G6PD deficiency in Sardinia is more common at sea level compared with higher elevations, and this also parallels the endemicity of malaria. In addition, it has been observed that parasitized female heterozygotes for G6PD deficiency (who therefore have normal and G6PD-deficient RBC) have more malarial parasites in normal erythrocytes compared with their own G6PD-deficient cells.[11] Moreover, it has been demonstrated that the in vitro growth of malarial parasites is inhibited in G6PD-deficient red cells.[12] The precise reasons for the observed inhibition of parasite growth in G6PD-deficient red cells are not known. One possibility is that the oxidant stress that causes GSH instability, and destroys the host RBC, also kills the parasite.[2]

The Enzyme and Its Variants

The monomeric form of G6PD contains 515 amino acids and has a molecular weight of 59 kD.[13,14] The active form of G6PD in vivo is a dimer that requires NADP for its stability.[15] The G6PD gene contains 13 exons and is over 18 kb in length.[14,16,17]

The normal or wild-type enzyme is G6PD B, although many variant enzymes have been identified. By international agreement, standardized methods have been used to characterize these enzyme variants, which differ on the basis of biochemical properties such as kinetic activity, electrophoretic mobility, the Michaelis constant for its substrate glucose 6-phosphate and cofactor NADP, the ability to utilize different substrate analogues, heat stability, and pH optima. Throughout the years the published list of recognized G6PD biochemical variants has been periodically updated, and over 400 biochemical variant forms of G6PD are recognized.[3] However, differences between some variants are subtle and most likely reflect minor technical differences between laboratories rather than true enzyme differences. Moreover, the advances in molecular biology have revealed that many biochemical G6PD variants, in fact, have the same DNA defect (see below).

The World Health Organization (WHO) has classified G6PD variants on the magnitude of the enzyme deficiency and also the severity of hemolysis.[18] **Class I variants** have very severe enzyme deficiency (less than 10%-20% of normal) and have chronic hemolytic anemia. **Class II variants** also have severe enzyme deficiency (less than 10% of normal), but there is usually only intermittent hemolysis. **Class III variants** have moderate enzyme deficiency (10%-60% of normal) with intermittent hemolysis usually associated with infection or drugs. **Class IV variants** have no enzyme deficiency or hemolysis. **Class V variants** are those in which enzyme activity is increased. Variants in the last two groups, although of much interest to biologists, geneticists, and anthropologists, are of no major clinical significance.

The normal wild-type enzyme, G6PD B, has normal catalytic activity and is not associated with hemolysis (class IV). A commonly encountered variant is G6PD A+, which is found in 20% to 30% of individuals of African descent.[19] It has normal catalytic properties and does not cause hemolysis (class IV). It differs from G6PD B in that it has a much faster electrophoretic mobility (the letters A and B refer to relative electrophoretic mobilities). The structure of G6PD A+ differs from that of G6PD B by the substitution of a single amino acid, an asparagine for aspartate at the 126th position of the protein.[20] Another common variant, G6PD A−, is the enzyme responsible for primaquine sensitivity in individuals of African descent, and it is the most common variant associated with mild to moderate hemolysis (class III). This G6PD variant is found in 10% to 15% of African Americans, and with similar frequencies in western and central Africa.[21] It has an electrophoretic mobility identical to that of G6PD A+. However, this is an unstable enzyme and its catalytic activity, although nearly normal in bone marrow cells and reticulocytes,[22] decreases markedly in older RBC.[23] Hence, this variant is designated G6PD A− compared with G6PD A+ (the + and − denote enzyme activity). G6PD Mediterranean is a common abnormal variant found in people whose origins are in the Mediterranean area. However, this same variant also is found in the Mideast and India.[2] The electrophoretic mobility of G6PD Mediterranean is identical to that of G6PD B, but its catalytic activity is markedly reduced, and hemolysis can be severe (class II).[22]

Genetics

The gene for G6PD is located on the X chromosome (band X q28). The fact that healthy males and females have the same enzyme activity in their red cells is explained by the Lyon hypothesis.[1,24] This hypothesis maintains that one of two X chromosomes in each cell of the female embryo is inactivated and remains inactive throughout subsequent cell divisions for the duration of life. In fact, it was studies by Beutler on females with G6PD deficiency that were used in proof of the Lyon hypothesis.[25] Enzyme deficiency is expressed in males carrying a variant gene, whereas heterozygous females usually are clinically normal. However, dependent upon the degree of lyonization, and the degree to which the abnormal G6PD variant is expressed, the mean RBC enzyme activity in females may be normal, moderately reduced, or grossly deficient. A female with 50% normal G6PD activity has 50% normal red cells and 50% G6PD-deficient red cells. The G6PD-deficient cells in females, however, are as vulnerable to hemolysis as are enzyme-deficient RBCs in males.

Advances in molecular biology have further enhanced our understanding of G6PD deficiency, and now more than 200 different gene mutations have been identified.[2,5,26,27] Almost all these DNA changes are missense mutations leading to single amino acid substitutions in the enzyme. Large deletions have not been identified, suggesting that complete absence of G6PD might be lethal.[3] The mutations are located throughout the entire coding region of the gene.[28] However, in class I variants associated with chronic hemolysis, mutations are clustered around exon 10, an area that governs the formation of the active G6PD dimer.[28,29] The correlation between the different biochemical variants, the site of genetic mutation, and the extent of hemolysis is a matter of current investigation.[2]

An interesting example of how molecular biology has enhanced our understanding relates to G6PD A−, once thought to be a single unstable variant found in Blacks throughout the world. However, molecular analysis now has demonstrated that G6PD A− may have more than one genotype (*Table 30.1*). In all cases there is a (376A > G) mutation, which is also the nucleotide substitution characteristic of G6PD A+. In addition, the G6PD A− variants have a second mutation, and in the majority of cases it is (202G > A).[3,30] A smaller fraction of G6PD A-subjects have the second substitution, (680G > T) or (968T > C).[31] Thus, the G6PD A− variant, once thought to be a single homogeneous mutation in Africans, now turns out to represent at least three different genotypes.[3] Also, a number of G6PD variants originally described in non-Africans are now found to have one of the known G6PD A−mutations (*Table 30.1*). For example, G6PD Betica,[32] a Spanish variant, and G6PD Matera,[33] an Italian variant, have demonstrated base substitutions at nucleotides 202 and 376, identical to the common G6PD A− variant. They are examples, therefore, of G6PD A−. One subject with G6PD Betica had base substitutions at nucleotides 376 and 968, identical to the less common G6PD A− variant.[32]

There are several other variants that appear clinically and biochemically heterogeneous but have been found to be genetically uniform. For example, G6PD Mediterranean involves many different ethnic groups, although most individuals have the same genetic defect, a single base substitution (563C > T). Moreover, just as in the case of G6PD A-, many of the different biochemical variants have turned out to have the same molecular defect as G6PD Mediterranean (*Table 30.1*).

In China, there are at least 21 variants causing G6PD deficiency. The three most common are G6PD Canton (1376G > T), G6PD Kaiping (1388G > A), and G6PD Gaohe (95A > G).[34] G6PD Canton and G6PD Gaohe are mainly regarded as WHO class II variants, while G6PD Kaiping is considered a WHO class III variant. These three variants account for over 70% of G6PD deficiency cases in China. The most common G6PD mutation in Southeast Asia is G6PD Mahidol (487G > A), a class III variant. Of interest, while India borders China, none of the Chinese G6PD variants are found in India where the most common type is G6PD Mediterranean (563C > T).

Because leukocyte G6PD is regulated by the same gene as that of red cells, documentation of decreased enzyme activity in the white blood cells of deficient individuals is not surprising.[35,36] Because of the normally short survival of leukocytes, however, most individuals with G6PD deficiency do not manifest impairment of phagocytosis or bactericidal activity of granulocytes.[36,37] The exception to this occurs with class I G6PD deficiency where some affected individuals may have neutrophil dysfunction and increased susceptibility to bacterial infection[38].

Table 30.1. Biochemical, Epidemiological, and Clinical Features of Select G6PD Variants

G6PD variant Classification	Nucleotide Substitution	Amino Acid Substitution	Population	WHO Classification
A- Alabama Betica Ferrara Septic	202 G > A 376 A > G	68 Val > Met 126 Asn > Asp	Africa, Italy, Spain Canary Islands, Mexico	3
A+	376 A > >G	126 Asn > Asp	Africa	4
A-	376 A > G 680 G > T	126 Asn > Asp 227 Asn > Asp	Africa, Spain Canary Islands	3
A- Betica Selma	376 A > G 968 T > C	126 Asn > Asp 387 Arg > Cys		3
Mahidol	487 G > A	163 Gly > Asp	Southeast Asia, China, Twain	3
Mediterranean Birmingham Cagili Dallas Panama Sassari	563 C > T	188 Ser > Phe	Italy, Greece, Saudi Arabia, Iran, Iraq, Israel, Egypt	2
Walter Reed Iowa Iowa City Springfield	1156 A > G	386 Lys > Glu		1
Union	1360 C > T	454 Arg > Cys	Philippians, Spain, Italy	2
Canton Maewo	1376 G > T	459 Arg > Leu	China, Twain	3
Kaiping Anant Dhon Petrich-like Sapporo-like	1388 G > A	463 Arg > His		2

Data modified from Beutler E. Glucose-6-phosphate dehydrogenase deficiency. *N Engl J Med.* 1991;324(3):169-74; Beutler E. G6PD deficiency. *Blood.* 1994;84(11):3613-36; and Miwa S, Fujii H. Molecular basis of erythroenzymopathies associated with hereditary hemolytic anemia: tabulation of mutant enzymes. *Am J Hematol.* 1996;51(2):122-132.

Pathophysiology

As red cells age, the activity of G6PD declines. The normal enzyme (G6PD B) has an in vivo half-life of 62 days.[22] Despite this loss of enzyme activity, normal old RBCs contain sufficient G6PD activity to generate NADPH and thereby sustain GSH levels in the face of oxidant stress. In contrast, the G6PD variants associated with hemolysis are unstable and have much shorter half-lives. The activity of G6PD A- in reticulocytes is normal, but it declines rapidly thereafter with a half-life of only 13 days.[22,39] The instability of G6PD Mediterranean is even more pronounced, with a half-life measured in hours.[22] The clinical correlate of this age-related enzyme instability is that hemolysis in patients with G6PDA- generally is mild and limited to older deficient erythrocytes. In contrast, the enzymatic defect in G6PD Mediterranean is due to much greater enzyme instability, and RBC of all ages are grossly deficient. Consequently, the entire RBC population of individuals with G6PD Mediterranean is susceptible to oxidant-induced injury, and this can lead to severe hemolytic anemia.

G6PD-deficient erythrocytes exposed to oxidants (infection, drugs, fava beans) become depleted of GSH. This reaction is central to the cell injury in this disorder since once GSH is depleted there is further oxidation of other RBC sulfhydryl-containing proteins. Oxidation of the sulfhydryl groups on hemoglobin leads to the formation of denatured globin or sulfhemoglobin. The latter form insoluble masses, which attach to the red cell membrane by disulfide bridges, and these

are known as Heinz bodies. Also, with some class I variants the oxidation of membrane sulfhydryl groups leads to the accumulation of membrane polypeptide aggregates, presumably due to disulfide bond formation between spectrin dimers and other membrane proteins. The end result of these changes is the production of rigid, nondeformable erythrocytes that are susceptible to stagnation and destruction by reticuloendothelial macrophages in the spleen and liver. Both extravascular and intravascular hemolysis occurs in G6PD-deficient individuals, the latter giving rise to hemoglobinemia and hemoglobinuria.

Clinical and Hematologic Features

The clinical expression of G6PD variants encompasses a continuous spectrum of hemolytic syndromes. In most affected individuals, the deficiency state goes unrecognized, while in some it causes episodic or chronic anemia. The common clinical entities encountered are acute hemolytic anemia, favism, and neonatal hyperbilirubinemia. Congenital chronic nonspherocytic hemolytic anemia due to G6PD deficiency is rare.

Acute Hemolytic Anemia

With most G6PD variants, hemolysis occurs only after exposure to oxidant stresses. In the steady state, there is no anemia, evidence of increased red cell destruction, or alteration in blood morphology. Sudden destruction of enzyme-deficient erythrocytes is triggered by drugs having a high redox potential, by ingestion of fava beans, and by selected infectious or metabolic perturbations. The clinical and laboratory features of an acute hemolytic episode are best illustrated in a figure from a classic study with primaquine-induced hemolysis in individuals with G6PD A⁻ (*Figure 30.3*).[8] After 2 to 4 days of primaquine ingestion, all the signs, symptoms, and laboratory results characteristic of an acute hemolytic episode are observed. Jaundice, pallor, and dark urine, with or without abdominal and back pain, are sudden in onset. An abrupt decrement of 3 to 4 g/dL in hemoglobin concentration occurs. The peripheral blood smear contains spherocytes and eccentrocytes or "blister" cells. In response to anemia, red cell production increases; an increase in reticulocytes is apparent within 5 days and is maximal by 7 to 10 days after onset of hemolysis. Despite continued drug exposure, the acute hemolytic process ends spontaneously after about 1 week, and the hemoglobin concentration thereafter returns to normal levels. The anemia is self-limited because the old susceptible population of erythrocytes is replaced by younger RBC with sufficient G6PD activity to withstand an oxidative assault. Although red cell survival remains shortened as long as use of the drug continues, compensation by the erythroid marrow effectively abolishes the anemia in subjects with G6PD A⁻. In contrast, hemolysis occurring with the G6PD Mediterranean variant is much more severe because a larger population of circulating erythrocytes is vulnerable to injury.[40] Hemolytic crises occur in heterozygous female subjects, as well as in hemizygous male patients. Of interest, the incidence of clinically significant G6PD deficiency in elderly women reportedly is increased, and this is thought to reflect skewed lionization that occurs with aging. In a fascinating study from Hong Kong, the incidence of G6PD deficiency in elderly females (80-107 years) was increased (1.73%) compared with newborn girls (0.27%)[41] In virtually all cases, acute hemolytic episodes are due to administration of drugs, associated with infection, or due to fava bean exposure.

Drug-Induced Hemolysis

Primaquine is but one of several drugs that can precipitate hemolysis. The common denominator of these drugs is their interaction with hemoglobin and oxygen, thus accelerating the intracellular formation of H_2O_2 and other oxidizing radicals. The published lists of suspect drugs are lengthy; however, many of the putative hemolytic agents were incriminated before it was recognized that infections often mimic the adverse effects of drugs. Consequently, many hemolytic events previously ascribed to drugs may, in fact, have resulted from infections for which drugs were given. Aspirin is such a drug, and it now is recognized that it can safely be given to individuals with class II and III G6PD variants. Some common drugs and chemicals, however, are predictably injurious for all G6PD-deficient individuals,[3,42] and these agents, including primaquine and rasburicase, are listed in *Table 30.2*. Other drugs, although producing a modest shortening of survival of G6PD-deficient red cells, can be given safely in usual therapeutic doses to individuals with class II and III G6PD variants (*Table 30.2*).[43] Ascorbic acid is safe in usual therapeutic doses, although large amounts may pose problems. Similarly, acetaminophen (Tylenol), aminoptyrine, sulfisoxazole (Gantrisin), sulfamethoxazole, and vitamin K can be given safely in usual therapeutic doses.[42] It should be noted that other agents that are not drugs also can cause hemolysis in G6PD-deficient individuals. Examples of these include naphthalene (moth balls), henna compounds (used for hair dyes, tattoos), and some Chinese herbs.[44] The sexual enhancement drug "RUSH," which may contain amyl or isobutyl nitrite, has also been reported to cause hemolysis in G6PD-deficient individuals.[45] Notably, drugs that can induce methemoglobinemia, such as lidocaine and dapsone, can be additionally problematic for G6PD-deficient individuals due to the contraindication to use of methylene blue.

Infection-Induced Hemolysis

Infection is one of the most common factors inciting hemolysis.[46,47] About 20% of G6PD-deficient individuals with pneumonia experience an abrupt drop in hemoglobin concentration.[46] A variety of infectious agents has been implicated: salmonella, *Escherichia coli*, beta-hemolytic streptococci, and rickettsiae. Hemolysis is particularly prominent in G6PD-deficient individuals with viral hepatitis. The accelerated destruction of red cells imposes a bilirubin load on an already damaged liver, resulting in an exaggerated increase in serum bilirubin level. Despite the magnitude of bilirubin retention, however, convalescence is generally complete and uneventful. Although hemolysis triggered by infection characteristically is mild, on rare occasion acute renal failure secondary to massive intravascular hemolysis can occur.[48,49] The mechanism for destruction of G6PD-deficient red cells during infection is not known. One possible explanation for this relationship is that oxidants generated by phagocytosing macrophages may diffuse into the extracellular medium where they pose an oxidative threat to G6PD-deficient erythrocytes.[50]

Table 30.2. Common Drugs and Chemicals Associated With Hemolysis in G6PD Deficiency

Drugs	Chemicals
Unsafe (Class I, II, and III G6PD Variants)	
Diaminodiphenyl sulfone (Dapsone)	Henna (Lawsone)
Methylene blue	Naphthalene (Mothballs)
Nalidixic acid (Neg—Gram)	Phenylhydrazine
Niridazole (Ambilhar)	Trinitrotoluene (TNT)
Nitrofurantoin (Furadantin)	
Phenazopyridine (Pyridium)	
Primaquine	
"RUSH" (isobutyl nitrate, amyl nitrate)	
Urate oxidase (Rasburicase)	
Medicines previously considered unsafe, but PROBABLY SAFE given in usual therapeutic doses to individuals with Class II and III G6PD deficiency*	
Acetaminophen (Tylenol)	Phenylbutazone
Acetylsalicylic acid (Aspirin)	Phenytoin
Antazoline (Antistine)	Probenecid (Benemid)
Antipyrine	Procainamide hydrochloride (Pronestyl)
Ascorbic acid	Pyrimethamine (Daraprim)
Benzhexol (Artane)	Quinine
Chloramphenicol	Streptomycin
Chlorguanidine (Proguanil, Paludrine)	Sulfacytine
Chloroquine	Sulfacetamide
Colchicine	Sulfadiazine
Cotrimoxazole	Sulfamethoxazole (Gantanol)
Diphenhydramine (Benadryl)	Sulfamethoxazole/trimethoprim
Glyburide	Sulfamethoxypyridazine (Kynex)
Isoniazid	Sulfanilamide
L-Dopa	Sulfisoxazole (Gantrisin)
Nalidixic acid (Neg—Gram)	Tiaprofenic acid
p-Aminobenzoic acid	Trimethoprim
p-Aminosalicylic acid	Tripelennamine (Pyribenzamine)
Trimethoprim	Vitamin K

*Safety for WHO class I G6PD deficiency is generally not known.
Data modified from Beutler E. Glucose-6-phosphate dehydrogenase deficiency: a historical perspective. *Blood*. 2008;111(1):16-24.

Hemolysis Associated With Diabetic Acidosis

Diabetic ketoacidosis rarely is associated with triggering destruction of G6PD-deficient red cells.[51] Correction of acidosis and restoration of glucose homeostasis reverses the hemolytic process. Changes in blood pH, glucose,[52] and pyruvate[53] have been proposed as possible mechanisms for hemolysis. Also, occult infection may be a common trigger for inducing both acute hemolysis and diabetic acidosis.

Favism

Exposure to the fava bean (*Vicia fava*, broad bean) is toxic and potentially fatal for some individuals with G6PD deficiency, and this has been known, allegedly, since the time of Pythagoras.[1,54] Unlike other agents capable of inducing hemolysis, the fava bean is toxic for only some G6PD-deficient individuals. Class II variants, such as G6PD Mediterranean, most usually are implicated, and as a result, favism is encountered commonly in Italy, Greece, and the Middle East, areas where fava beans are a dietary staple.[3,55,56] It also occurs in some of the Asian G6PD variants. Africans and African Americans with G6PD A⁻ are much less susceptible, although hemolytic episodes have been reported.[57]

Most cases of favism result from ingestion of fresh beans. Consequently, the peak seasonal incidence of this disorder in the Mediterranean is in the spring and coincides with harvesting of the bean.[58] Hemolysis of comparable severity can follow consumption of fried fava beans, a popular Chinese snack. Favism has been observed in nursing infants of mothers who have eaten the beans,[58] as well as in a newborn infant whose mother had eaten fava beans 5 days before delivery.[59] Enzyme deficiency was held responsible for fatal hydrops fetalis in a male infant of a hematologically normal Chinese woman who ingested fava beans during the final month of pregnancy.[60]

Favism occurs most commonly in children between the ages of 1 and 5 years. As with other clinical manifestations of G6PD deficiency syndromes, it is seen primarily in males, although it can also occur in females with severe enzyme deficiency. Symptoms of acute intravascular hemolysis occur within 5 to 24 hours of ingestion of the bean. Headache, nausea, back pain, chills, and fever are followed by hemoglobinuria, anemia, and jaundice. The drop in hemoglobin concentration is precipitous and often severe and may require a red cell transfusion.

Favism does not occur in all susceptible G6PD individuals, and it is thought that additional genetic factors are involved, presumably related to how fava bean oxidants are metabolized. Furthermore, the reaction to the fava bean by the same individual at different times may not be consistent.[54] Clearly, a factor other than enzyme deficiency is operative. Two pyrimidine aglycones, divicine and isouramil, have been implicated as the toxic components of fava beans.[61] Both compounds rapidly overwhelm the GSH-generating capacity of G6PD-deficient cells and reproduce many of the metabolic derangements noted during hemolytic episodes. To date, however, there are no convincing data to explain the erratic hemolytic episodes seen in favism. The more common occurrence of favism in children in comparison with adults may relate to the ratio of fava beans consumed to the child's body weight.[54]

Neonatal Hyperbilirubinemia

Hyperbilirubinemia associated with G6PD deficiency is well documented in the newborn period, rarely noted at the time of birth with a peak incidence of clinical onset between days 2 and 3.[62-64] In most cases, there is more jaundice than anemia. Close monitoring of serum bilirubin levels in infants known to be G6PD deficient is warranted.[65-67] Neonatal hyperbilirubinemia is seen with G6PD Mediterranean (class II) variants. An increase in the incidence of neonatal hyperbilirubinemia is also seen in Southeast Asia and China, and a significant fraction of the latter is associated with G6PD Canton.[68] African American infants with G6PD A⁻ (class III) once were considered to be at minimal risk, but this is no longer held, and significant hyperbilirubinemia can occur in these neonates.[62,69,70] Untreated hyperbilirubinemia can lead to kernicterus with severe neurologic injury or death.[71,72] It is of interest that data from the USA Kernicterus Registry from 1992 to 2004 indicate that over 30% of kernicterus cases are associated with G6PD deficiency.[73]

The observation that the incidence of hyperbilirubinemia in G6PD-deficient infants born in Australia to Greek immigrants is lower than that noted in deficient infants in Greece suggests that local environmental variables are probably important.[74] Herbs used in traditional Chinese medicine and clothing impregnated with naphthalene also are examples of covert oxidants to which susceptible infants may be exposed. Lastly, certain drugs and fava bean ingestion by mothers in late gestation have been implicated as the inciting stimulus of hemolysis in newborns.[60,70]

Although the cause of hyperbilirubinemia in G6PD-deficient infants sometimes reflects accelerated red cell breakdown, usually there is no obvious RBC destruction or oxidant exposure. It has been suggested that hyperbilirubinemia may have another etiology, possibly related to impaired liver clearance of bilirubin. In support of this hypothesis are the observations that carboxyhemoglobin production, a marker of hemolysis or RBC breakdown, is the same in neonates with G6PD Mediterranean, with and without hyperbilirubinemia.[75] It is now thought that the variable degree of hyperbilirubinemia in G6PD-deficient neonates reflects the presence or absence of the variant form of uridine-diphosphoglucuronyl-transferase responsible for Gilbert syndrome.[67] The relative importance of the latter is underscored by the observation that most jaundiced G6PD-deficient neonates are not anemic and that evidence for increased bilirubin production secondary to hemolysis often is lacking.[76]

Congenital Nonspherocytic Hemolytic Anemia

A small fraction of G6PD-deficient individuals have chronic lifelong hemolysis in the absence of infection or drug exposure. These rare class I G6PD variants are extremely heterogeneous with respect to biochemical kinetics but have in common very low in vitro activity and/or marked enzyme instability.[29] Most of these variants have DNA mutations at exon 10, an area that affects monomer-dimer interactions and thereby enzyme activity.[29] The hemolytic anemia associated with class I variants is indistinguishable from the congenital nonspherocytic hemolytic syndromes related to glycolytic enzyme deficiencies.

Anemia and jaundice often are noted first in the newborn period. Hyperbilirubinemia often necessitates exchange transfusion. Typically, hemolysis occurs in the absence of a recognized triggering factor, although exposure to drugs or chemicals with oxidant potential exaggerates an already established hemolytic process. Beyond infancy, signs and symptoms of the hemolytic disorder are subtle and inconstant. Exaggeration of anemia occurs after exposure to drugs with oxidant properties, even those that are safe for individuals with class II and III G6PD variants.

No hematologic alterations of the class I variants are distinctive. The hemolytic process may be fully compensated, although mild to moderate anemia is the rule (hemoglobin 8-10 g/dL). Under basal conditions the usual reticulocyte count is 10% to 15%.

In a few instances, leukocyte dysfunction associated with class I variant G6PD deficiency has been described.[38] The abnormality is characterized functionally by defective bactericidal activity (but normal chemotaxis and phagocytosis) and clinically by recurrent infections with catalase-positive organisms. Overall, however, clinical infections are not a major problem in G6PD deficiency.

Diagnosis

Because of its prevalence and worldwide distribution, G6PD deficiency should be given serious consideration in the differential diagnosis of any nonimmune hemolytic anemia. Most commonly, anemia is first recognized during or after an infectious illness, after exposure to one of several suspect drugs or chemicals, or following exposure to fava beans. Also, G6PD deficiency should be considered in neonates with excessive and unexplained hyperbilirubinemia. Clinical and hematologic features reflect the severity of hemolysis but are not themselves specifically from G6PD deficiency. Irregularly contracted erythrocytes (eccentrocytes with hemoglobin puddled to one side of the RBC) and "bite" cells are seen in the Wright-stained peripheral blood smear. Previously, these bite cells were considered a consequence of splenic removal of Heinz bodies. Now, however, it is recognized that these

RBCs contain a coagulum of hemoglobin that has separated from the membrane, often leaving an unstained non-hemoglobin-containing cell membrane (i.e., having the appearance of a bite removed from the cell).[77] These morphologic alterations are a consequence of the oxidative assault on hemoglobin. Brilliant cresyl blue supravital stains of the peripheral blood may reveal Heinz bodies during hemolytic episodes.

The specific diagnosis of G6PD deficiency is made by adding a measured amount of hemolysate to an assay mixture containing substrate (glucose 6-phosphate) and cofactor (NADP) and then spectrophotometrically measuring the rate of NADPH generation. Alternatively, a variety of screening tests that utilize hemolysate as a source of enzyme also can be used. The fluorescent spot test is the simplest, most reliable, and most sensitive of the screening methods.[78] This test is based on the fluorescence of NADPH, after glucose 6-phosphate and NADP are added to a hemolysate of test cells. Other screening methods detect NADPH generation indirectly by measuring the transfer of hydrogen ions from NADPH to an acceptor. In the methemoglobin reduction test,[79] methylene blue is the acceptor used for the transfer of hydrogen from NADPH to methemoglobin, thereby facilitating its reduction. It is important to mention this test because, when combined with a technique for the elution of methemoglobin from intact cells, it can be used to detect relative G6PD sufficiency of individual RBCs,[80] thereby detecting the carrier state with approximately 75% reliability. Regardless of the screening test used to detect G6PD deficiency, it should be recognized that false-negative results can occur if the most severe enzyme-deficient RBCs have been removed by hemolysis. This can be a problem in diagnosing females and individuals with G6PD A-, especially during the reticulocytosis following acute hemolysis. In these cases, family members can be studied. An alternative approach to diagnosis is to wait until the hemolytic crisis is over and reevaluate the patient after the RBC mass is repopulated with cells of all ages (approximately 2 to 3 months). False-negative tests are less of a problem in diagnosing G6PD deficiency when quantitative spectrophotometric enzyme assays are utilized.

Treatment

Management of the patient with G6PD deficiency is determined by the clinical syndrome with which it is associated. Individuals having variants associated with acute hemolysis may have a significant fall in hemoglobin concentration requiring an RBC transfusion. This is the case more commonly in G6PD Mediterranean (class II) than in G6PD A⁻ (class III). All affected individuals should avoid exposure to fava beans and drugs known to trigger hemolysis. Pregnant and nursing women known to be heterozygous for the deficiency also should avoid ingestion of drugs with oxidant potential, because some gain access to the fetal circulation and to breast milk. If the indication for its use is critical, however, an offending drug justifiably may be given despite modest shortening of red cell survival. For example, primaquine is safely given to individuals with the G6PD A⁻ variant, provided it is started cautiously (15 mg/d or 45 mg once or twice weekly) and the blood count is monitored closely.[81] The mild anemia caused by its administration is rapidly corrected by a compensatory erythropoietic effort and does not recur unless the dose of drug is escalated. In addition, the risk/benefit profile of rasburicase must also be considered in patients with tumor lysis syndrome.

Chronic nonspherocytic hemolytic anemia due to class I G6PD variants may require more active intervention. Exchange transfusion during the first week of life often is required to prevent bilirubin encephalopathy. Beyond the newborn period, anemia rarely is of such severity as to require regular blood transfusions. During aplastic crises, however, transfusions may be lifesaving, and transfusions can also be needed in the setting of increased hemolysis induced by viral triggers. As with other syndromes resulting from G6PD deficiency, drugs capable of exaggerating hemolysis should be avoided. Splenectomy, although occasionally bringing about a modest improvement in hemoglobin concentration,[82] is generally without benefit. Because of its antioxidant properties, vitamin E had been proposed as a therapeutic agent, but subsequent evaluation of large doses of the vitamin failed to demonstrate an ameliorative effect on anemia.[83]

Therapy for hyperbilirubinemia and neonatal hemolysis resulting from G6PD deficiency includes the following: phototherapy or exchange transfusion to prevent kernicterus, RBC transfusion for symptomatic anemia, removal of potential oxidants that may be contributing to hemolysis, and treatment of associated infections. In infants known to be G6PD deficient, prevention of severe hyperbilirubinemia by administration of a single intramuscular dose of Sn-mesoporphyrin, an inhibitor of heme oxygenase, is highly effective and appears safe, but this therapy is not yet clinically available.[84] A study from Nigeria has reported a much poorer outcome for G6PD-deficient infants born at home, presumably a reflection of delayed identification and treatment of hyperbilirubinemia in these neonates.[72] In the United States, guidelines have been established for following hyperbilirubinemia in babies after discharge from the hospital.[62]

Screening

Aside from the District of Columbia and Pennsylvania, there is no generalized neonatal screening program for G6PD deficiency in the United States. The approach in the United States has been to recognize that neonatal hyperbilirubinemia may be caused by G6PD deficiency and these infants should be tested and monitored closely. In some countries where the predominant G6PD variants are class II mutations, screening programs have been instituted. Neonatal screening for G6PD deficiency has been very effective in reducing the incidence of favism later in life in Sardinia[85] and other regions where this potentially fatal complication is common.[63]

Routine blood bank screening has been considered unwarranted, and G6PD deficiency is not considered a problem in transfusion medicine. Even in areas where G6PD deficiency is endemic, screening of blood donors is not required. One careful evaluation of the recipients of G6PD-deficient blood uncovered no deleterious consequences.[86] However, patients receiving G6PD Mediterranean blood may have an increased serum bilirubin and lactate dehydrogenase (LDH) concentration following transfusion, and this can be confused with a transfusion reaction.[87] In premature infants, simple transfusions with G6PD-deficient red cells have been associated with hemolysis and severe hyperbilirubinemia requiring exchange transfusion.[88] Also, massive intravascular hemolysis has occurred in an Indian neonate following an exchange transfusion with G6PD-deficient blood.[89] In view of these occurrences, it has been recommended that, in areas where G6PD deficiency (presumably class II variants) is common, donor blood should be screened for the enzyme before transfusing premature infants[88] or using the blood for a neonatal exchange transfusion.[89] This recommendation currently is not standard blood banking practice.

RELATED DISORDERS OF HMP SHUNT AND GLUTATHIONE METABOLISM

In addition to G6PD, other enzymes of the HMP shunt pathway (6-phosphogluconate dehydrogenase [6PGD]), the closely linked reactions of glutathione metabolism (GSR, GPx), and the glutathione synthetic pathway are important in protecting RBCs against oxidant injury. Rare abnormalities in these enzymes have been reported, and, in some cases, they are associated with hemolysis.

6-Phosphogluconate Dehydrogenase Deficiency

The enzyme 6PGD catalyzes the conversion of 6-phosphogluconate to pentose 5-phosphate (*Figure 30.2*), and, in the process, NADPH is generated from NADP. Deficiency of 6PGD is well documented, although it appears to have little or no significance for red cell viability. Presumably this reflects the fact that NADPH is generated by the proximal enzyme, G6PD, suggesting that the second dehydrogenase may not be necessary for cell integrity.

Glutathione Reductase Deficiency

GSSG is reduced in the presence of NADPH by GSR (*Figure 30.2*). The enzyme contains flavin adenine dinucleotide (FAD) as a prosthetic component, and as a result, normal enzyme activity is dependent on the dietary availability of riboflavin. Not surprisingly, partial GSR deficiency is a relatively common feature of disorders that are compounded by suboptimal nutrition. GSR levels are restored within days by the administration of physiologic quantities of riboflavin.[90] The association between riboflavin-induced GSR deficiency and various disease states is of no hematologic consequence.[91]

Genetically determined GSR deficiency has been documented in three siblings who were offspring of consanguineous parents.[92] Enzyme activity was not enhanced by incubation of hemolysates with FAD. Despite near absence of erythrocyte GSR activity, the siblings were hematologically normal, except for episodes of hemolysis after the ingestion of fava beans. All three of the siblings acquired cataracts at an early age (24-32 years).[93] Since this report, there have been no new reported cases of hereditary GSR deficiency associated with hemolysis.

Glutathione Peroxidase Deficiency

GPx catalyzes the oxidation of GSH by peroxides, including hydrogen peroxide and organic hydroperoxides (*Figure 30.2*). Rare cases of hemolysis in association with moderate deficiency of erythrocyte GPx activity have been described in adults and children.[94] Of all the reported cases suggesting a relationship between hemolysis and GPx deficiency, one of the most persuasive was that of a 9-month-old Japanese girl with chronic nonspherocytic hemolytic anemia.[95] This patient's erythrocyte GPx activity was 17% of control activity, while her hematologically normal parents had 51% to 66% control enzyme activity. However, it is not known whether this specific enzyme defect was responsible for the patient's chronic hemolytic anemia. The general consensus today is that GPx deficiency is probably not a cause of hemolysis or other hematologic problems as many healthy individuals, particularly those of Jewish or Mediterranean ancestry, have reduced GPx activity without evidence of hemolysis.[96] Moreover, low GPx activity, in the absence of hemolysis, also is observed in healthy people from New Zealand with Selenium (Se) deficiency (Se being an integral part of GPx).[97] In view of these observations, the role of GPx deficiency as a cause of hemolysis is questioned. Some argue that GPx is only one of the cellular mechanisms available to detoxify peroxides. Under physiologic conditions, catalase and nonenzymatic reduction of oxidants by GSH also may be important factors regulating the rate of H_2O_2 detoxification. From a clinical perspective, because of the questionable role of GPx, any patient with hemolytic anemia and reduced GPx activity should be extensively evaluated for other causes of hemolysis.

Defects in Glutathione Synthesis

Glutathione is actively synthesized in RBC and has an intracellular half-life of only 4 days, in part due to cellular efflux of GSSG. RBCs are capable of de novo GSH synthesis, and this requires two critical enzymes (*Figure 30.2*). Gamma-glutamyl-cysteine synthetase (GCS) catalyzes the first step in GSH synthesis, the formation of gamma-glutamyl-cysteine from glutamic acid and cysteine. Glutathione synthetase (GS) catalyzes the formation of GSH from glutamyl-cysteine and glycine. In many tissues, but not RBC, these two enzymes are part of the gamma glutamyl cycle, which is involved with the synthesis and degradation of GSH and also thought to have a role in amino acid transport across cell membranes. Hereditary hemolytic anemia, characterized by reduced GSH content, has been reported in patients with deficiencies of both GCS and GS activity. The clinical effects of these disorders depends on the severity of enzyme deficiency and whether the gamma glutamyl cycle also is affected in nonerythroid tissues.[98]

GCS deficiency, also called gamma-glutamyl-cysteine ligase (GCL) deficiency, is a rare hemolytic anemia[98] that was first described in two adult siblings (Konrad et al)[111]. Both had a life-long history of mild hemolytic anemia, intermittent jaundice, cholelithiasis, and splenomegaly. They also manifested severe neurologic dysfunction and generalized aminoaciduria.[99] This disorder is an autosomal recessive condition and, in the family studied, presumed carriers had reduced GCS activity, although erythrocyte GSH levels were normal. Hemolytic anemia was seen only in the homozygous state where

erythrocyte GSH levels were approximately 5% of normal, and there was markedly reduced GCS activity. A third patient with GCS deficiency, unrelated to the first cases, was a 22-year-old woman with markedly reduced RBC GCS activity, severely reduced erythrocyte GSH concentration, and chronic hemolytic anemia.[100] Family members of this patient had 50% reduced enzyme activity but no decrease in RBC-glutathione content or evidence of hemolysis. Of particular interest, in contrast to the first patients described with GCS deficiency, this patient had no neurologic disease. To date there have been a total of 10 probands reported with GCS deficiency and hemolysis, and 4 of these have also had severe neurological disease.[101-104] The molecular defect in these cases has been associated with different missense mutations in the *GCLC* and *GCLM* genes, which encode the two GCS subunits. There is no specific therapy for GCS deficiency. Supportive care for this chronic hemolytic anemia should be similar to that of other congenital hemolytic disorders, including management of neonatal hyperbilirubinemia, transfusion support for aplastic crisis, consideration of periodic gallbladder ultrasound for bilirubin gallstones, and monitoring for iron loading.

GS deficiency has been incriminated as the cause of chronic hemolytic anemia alone (due to isolated RBC enzyme deficiency) and as the cause of a generalized syndrome (due to enzyme deficiency in many tissues), characterized by mild hemolytic disease, severe metabolic acidosis, and neurologic deterioration. The first syndrome, mild hemolytic anemia, has been described in several families.[105-109] Exposure to oxidant drugs and to fava beans has occasioned temporary acceleration of hemolysis. Splenomegaly has been noted in approximately half of the reported cases. A concurrent deficiency of glutathione-S-transferase is thought to be caused by the instability of this enzyme in the absence of adequate intracellular GSH.[106] The second more generalized syndrome is characterized by mild hemolytic anemia, persistent metabolic acidosis presenting in the newborn period, and progressive cerebral and cerebellar degeneration.[110] Acidosis is caused by the accumulation of 5-oxoproline, a metabolic product of γ-glutamyl-cysteine. Abnormally large quantities of the dipeptide are produced because of the loss of feedback inhibition of γ-glutamyl-cysteine synthetase by GSH. This disorder is suspected in patients with hemolytic anemia and markedly reduced RBC GSH content. Virtually no GS activity is detected in homozygous-deficient individuals.[111] Rarely, therapy is required for the hematologic consequences of GS deficiency. Exposure to drugs and chemicals with oxidant potential should be avoided by those individuals with chronic hemolytic anemia, and acetaminophen should additionally be avoided in those with associated oxoprolinemia.[112] In some cases, splenectomy has been efficacious in modifying the anemia, although hemolysis may continue as manifested by persistent reticulocytosis.[108] In those individuals with GS deficiency and oxoprolinemia, administration of oral sodium bicarbonate or citrate is necessary to control acidosis, and some clinicians have suggested vitamins C and E to be beneficial as well.[113]

GLYCOLYTIC ENZYMES ABNORMALITIES— GENERAL CONSIDERATIONS

Hemolytic anemias due to glycolytic enzymopathies are relatively rare, affecting a few thousand individuals. This is in contrast to G6PD deficiency, which affects millions throughout the world. Abnormalities in virtually every glycolytic enzyme have been described, although over 90% of cases associated with hemolysis are due to pyruvate kinase (PK) deficiency (*Figure 30.4*). Most glycolytic enzymopathies manifest an autosomal recessive pattern of inheritance. Heterozygotes almost always are hematologically normal, although their RBCs contain less than normal levels of enzyme activity. It once was thought that hemolysis occurred only in those individuals who were homozygous for the enzyme deficiency. However, true homozygosity for a given mutant enzyme now is known to be less common and usually restricted to consanguineous kindred. The vast majority of cases of hemolytic anemia due to glycolytic enzyme deficiencies are a consequence of double heterozygosity for two different enzyme variants,

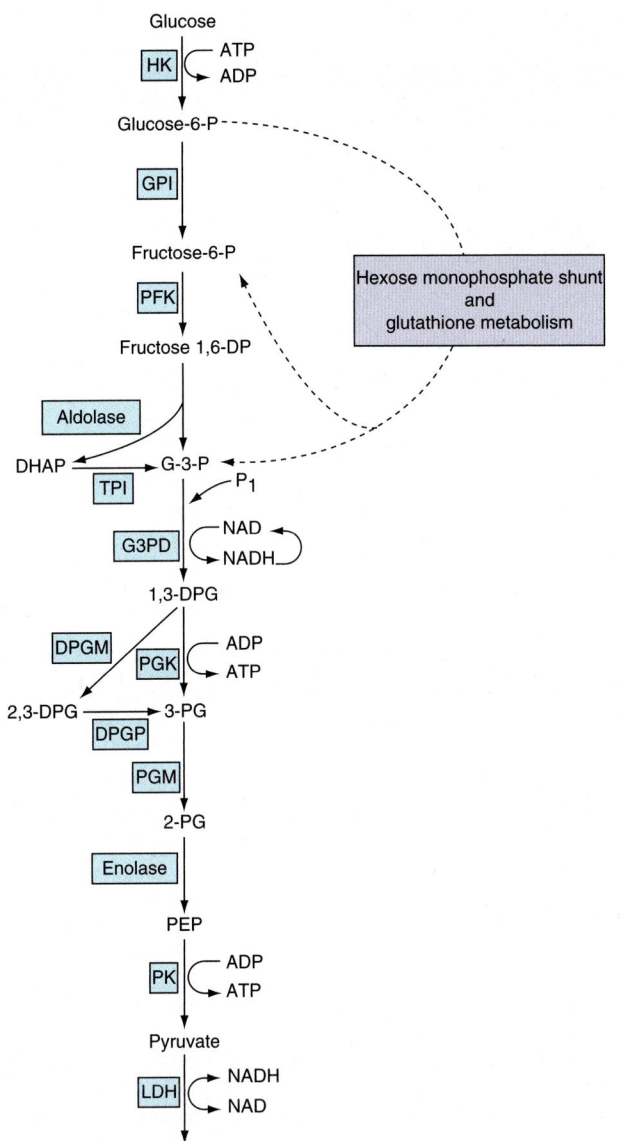

FIGURE 30.4 Overall metabolic pathway of glycolysis in the erythrocyte.
Enzyme abbreviations: 2,3 DPGM, 2,3 diphosphoglycerate mutase; 2,3-DPGP, 2,3-diphosphoglycerate phosphatase; G3PD, glyceraldehyde-3-phosphate dehydrogenase; GPI, glucose phosphate isomerase; HK, hexokinase; LDH, lactate dehydrogenase; PFK, phosphofructokinase; PGK, phosphoglycerate kinase; PGM, phosphoglycerate mutase; PK, pyruvate kinase; TPI, triose phosphate isomerase. Substrate abbreviations: 1,3-DPG, 1,3-diphosphoglycerate; 2-PG, 2-phosphoglycerate; 3-PG, 3-phosphoglycerate; DHAP, dihydroxyacetone phosphate; G-3-P, glyceraldehyde 3-phosphate; PEP, phosphoenolpyruvate.

and this accounts for the diverse biochemical and clinical heterogeneity of the red cell glycolytic enzymopathies. The one exception to this autosomal mode of inheritance for glycolytic enzymopathies is phosphoglycerate kinase (PGK) deficiency, which is an X-linked disorder.

Clinical manifestations of hemolysis due to glycolytic enzymopathies include chronic anemia, reticulocytosis, and some degree of indirect hyperbilirubinemia. Although the hemolytic process is often recognized and diagnosed in childhood, diagnosis in adolescents and adults is not uncommon. Frequently, there is a history of neonatal jaundice, often requiring an exchange transfusion, and rarely causing kernicterus. The magnitude of chronic anemia varies; there may be accelerated hemolysis with some nonspecific infections or transient aplastic crises associated with parvovirus infection. In some enzymopathies, such as PK deficiency, the manifestations of enzyme deficiency are isolated to the erythrocyte. In other cases, such as in

phosphofructokinase (PFK), aldolase, triose phosphate isomerase (TPI), and PGK deficiencies, the enzyme deficiency affects multiple cell types, and therefore, hemolytic anemia is but one feature of multisystem disease (see *Table 30.3*).

The possibility of a glycolytic defect is considered when chronic hemolytic anemia cannot be explained by the more common causes (i.e., hereditary spherocytosis or hemoglobinopathies). There are no specific morphologic abnormalities, although anisocytosis and poikilocytosis are common. In virtually all cases, a specific assay of RBC enzyme activity and/or genetic testing are necessary to make the diagnosis.

GENETIC TESTING IN EVALUATING DISORDERS OF GLYCOLYSIS

Diagnosis in patients with glycolytic enzyme abnormalities can be complex, particularly in patients managed with regular transfusions.[114] Transfused blood and/or reticulocytosis confounds enzyme testing. Mutant erythrocytes can also be so unstable that they are rapidly hemolyzed, and the remaining cells may be biochemically less abnormal. Consequently, "false negative" assays can obscure the correct diagnosis. Diagnosis is important with regard to monitoring and supportive care, the role of splenectomy, hematopoietic stem cell transplantation, and as newer disease-targeted therapies evolve.

In regularly transfused children, after a careful family history, laboratory studies of the parents often yield important clues to the diagnosis. Initial screening of parents typically consists of blood counts with erythrocyte indices, peripheral blood smear, and a reticulocyte count. When the parents are hematologically normal, this suggests an autosomal recessive disorder or a new dominant mutation. Historically, direct enzyme assays have been considered the gold standard for the diagnosis of disorders of erythrocyte metabolism. Enzyme analyses in transfusion-dependent patients are problematic, as results are confounded by transfused erythrocytes. The availability of clinical molecular testing has grown for disorders of glycolysis. There are advantages and disadvantages of molecular testing compared with direct enzyme assay. Molecular testing can be performed in transfused patients, it can be utilized for prenatal diagnosis, and sample shipping and preparation are less complicated than for direct enzyme assay. However, unless the patient is homozygous for a known variant, parent DNA samples are needed to ascertain if the variants detected are in *cis* or *trans* for diagnosis. Variants of uncertain significance create an additional diagnostic dilemma as it is not clear whether these variants are pathogenic and related to disease. Furthermore, patients have also been found to have low enzyme activity with nonconfirmatory genetic testing, suggesting that either molecular testing may miss variants outside the coding region. For these patients, diagnostic classification is challenging.

For disorders of red cell glycolysis, enzyme assays and molecular studies are complementary techniques. In many patients, direct enzyme analysis is adequate for initial diagnosis, with molecular testing serving as a confirmatory test. The complementary aspects of functional and molecular testing are especially useful in difficult cases, in which enzyme assays demonstrate only relatively low levels of activity compared with other red cell age-dependent enzymes or in which molecular testing shows only one mutation or a variant of unknown significance. This complementary diagnostic approach to patients can lead to the specific diagnosis in chronic hemolytic anemias, which is critical for specific monitoring and treatment strategies. This diagnostic precision is key given the availability of approved disease-directed treatments and other therapies in clinical development.

Supportive care for RBC glycolytic defects is similar to that of other chronic hemolytic anemias. RBC transfusions often are needed. Splenectomy usually is beneficial in severely anemic patients since the spleen (along with the liver) participates in the destruction of enzymatically abnormal cells. In most cases, however, the response to splenectomy is only partial, although RBC transfusion requirements may decrease. Cholelithiasis is a common problem, and periodic gallbladder ultrasound examinations are necessary in all patients with

Table 30.3. Features of Glycolytic and Nucleotide Enzymopathies

Enzymopathy	Approximate Fraction of Enzymopathies[a]	Mode of Inheritance	Effects of Enzymopathy
Hexokinase	<1%	AR	Mild/severe CNSHA
Glucose phosphate isomerase	3%-5%	AR	Mod/severe CNSHA; ±neurologic deficits
Phosphofructokinase	<1%	AR	Mild CNSHA; ±myopathy
Aldolase	<1%	AR	Mild/mod CNSHA; ±myopathy
Triose phosphate isomerase	<1%	AR	Mod/severe CNSHA; neurologic deficits
Phosphoglycerate kinase	<1%	X-linked	Mild/severe CNSHA; ±neurologic deficits; ±myopathy
Pyruvate kinase	80%-90%	AR	Mod/severe CNSHA
Pyrimidine 5'nucleotidase	2%-3%	AR	Moderate CNSHA
Adenosine deaminase excess	<1%	AD	Mild CNSHA
Adenylate kinase	<1%	AR	CNSHA ±neurologic deficits

Abbreviations: AD, autosomal dominant; CNSHA, chronic nonspherocytic hemolytic anemia; R, autosomal recessive.
[a]Approximate estimates derived from several sources: Beutler E. Red cell enzyme defects as nondiseases and as diseases. *Blood.* 1979;54(1):1-7; Tanaka KR, Zerez CR, Red cell enzymopathies of the glycolytic pathway. *Semin Hematol.* 1990;27(2):165-185; Eber SW. Disorders of erythrocyte glycolysis and nucleotide metabolism. In: Handin R, Lux S, Stossel T, eds. *Blood: Principles and Practice of Hematology.* Lippincott, Williams & Wilkins; 2003:1887-1920; and Mentzer W. *Pyruvate Kinase Deficiency and Disorders of Glycolysis.* WB Saunders; 2003.

glycolytic enzymopathies, even following splenectomy. Transfusion-independent iron loading is a frequent complication in RBC glycolytic disorders; thus, routine monitoring is indicated, with ferritin and/or magnetic resonance imaging (MRI) once a child or young adult can cooperate. The biologic and clinical features of specific glycolytic disorders are summarized in the following paragraphs.

PYRUVATE KINASE DEFICIENCY

Of the enzymatic deficiencies involving glycolysis, PK deficiency is the most common, and the most extensively studied cases have been reported.[115-117] The actual number of cases worldwide is unknown because patients historically were not reported unless there were unusual associated findings. The development of patient registries for PK deficiency has helped to better characterize the spectrum of symptoms and complications in patients with this anemia.

Geographic Distribution

Most cases of PK deficiency have been reported from Europe, the United States, and Japan; however, the disorder occurs worldwide.[118-120] The frequency of the heterozygote state has been estimated on the basis of studies that screened various populations for low enzyme activity. In Germany and in the United States, the prevalence of apparent heterozygosity for PK deficiency has been estimated to be about 1%.[119] A particularly high frequency exists among both the Pennsylvania Amish, in whom the disorder can be traced to a single immigrant couple causing a founder effect, and in the Romany population.[121,122] In studies looking at the most common PK mutations found in a Caucasian population, a prevalence of PK deficiency has been estimated to be 1 per 20,000 population.[123] A more recent meta-analysis estimates a prevalence of 3.2 to 8.5 per million in Western populations.[124]

Biochemical Genetics

PK catalyzes the conversion of phosphoenolpyruvate to pyruvate; this is one of the two glycolytic reactions resulting in net ATP production (*Figure 30.4*). PK is a tetrameric protein with a molecular weight of 230 kDa. There are two different PK genes (*PKM2* and *PKLR*), which encode for four distinct PK isozymes.

The *PKM2* gene is on chromosome 15 (15q22),[125] and it encodes for two isozymes (PK-M2 and PK-M1). PK-M2 is the isozyme present in all tissues during fetal life. As fetal maturation proceeds, other tissue-specific PK isozymes begin to appear. PK-M2 persists as the predominant isoenzyme in mature leukocytes and certain other tissues (platelets, lung, kidney spleen, adipose tissue). In addition, PK-M2 is the major isozyme in erythroid precursors.[126] PK-M1, which differs from PK-M2 as a result of alternative splicing, is the PK isozyme present in mature muscle and brain tissue.[127]

The *PKLR* gene is on chromosome 1(1q21)[128]; it also encodes for two isozymes (PK-L and PK-R). PK-L is the predominant isozyme in hepatocytes. PK-R is the isozyme present in mature erythrocytes.[116] The hemolytic anemia associated with PK deficiency is due to mutations of the *PKLR* gene. In some patients with hemolytic anemia, a decrease in the liver PK-L isozyme has also been observed, but this is typically of no clinical significance since the liver also has residual PK-M2 activity. During normal erythroid differentiation, the PK isozyme switches from the M2 to the R-type.[126] Of interest, in one severe form of PK deficiency (PK Beppu), PK-M2-type persists in mature erythrocytes, and it has been proposed that this compensatory PK-M2 production allows affected red cells to survive, analogous to the beneficial effect of persistent fetal hemoglobin production in homozygous beta thalassemia.[126]

Over 300 different mutations of the *PKLR* gene have been identified as causes of chronic hemolytic anemia. Most of these are missense mutations (approximately 70%), and the others are either nonsense or insertional mutations, deletions, or splicing abnormalities.[116,129,130] Most PK mutations are very rare, occurring only once, and, at this time, approximately 25% of patients diagnosed appear to have a newly described pathogenic variant. The variable phenotypic expression of PK deficiency undoubtedly reflects the heterogeneity of these different PK mutants and that most patients have compound heterozygous variants. A few mutations are seen with some frequency. The mutation in a significant fraction of affected individuals from norther Northern Europe and the United States (30%-40%) is 1529G > A (510Arg > Gln).[131,132] This particular mutation is common in the United States and in northern Europe, and homozygosity for this mutation was seen in children from a polygamist community in the western United States.[133] A second common mutation, 1456C > T (484Arg > Trp), is observed in Spain, Portugal, and Italy where it accounts for approximately 30% of all cases. A third common mutation, 1468C > T (Arg490 > Trp), is found predominantly in Japan. The mutation seen in the Amish population with PK deficiency is 1436G > A (479Arg > His).[134] The PK deficiency in the Romany (Gypsy) population is due to a deletion of 1149 bp, resulting in the deletion of exon 11.[122]

At one time, PK deficiency was thought to be a consequence of decreased production of a structurally normal enzyme, but it is now recognized that most PK variants are abnormal proteins that differ with respect to their biochemical kinetics and physical properties.[135,136] The heterozygous state for a PK variant is clinically silent with no hemolysis or anemia.

There is little or no relationship between red cell PK activity in vitro and severity of hemolysis.[119,126,137] In part, this reflects the fact that in vitro assay conditions are very different from what exists in vivo. In addition, the presence of young RBC, or reticulocytes, with elevated enzyme activity can mask the presence of a very unstable PK variant, or there can be persistence of PK-M2 in mature RBC.[126,138,139] Furthermore, the erythrocytes most deficient in PK can be so unstable that they are rapidly hemolyzed, with the remaining cells being overrepresented in the enzyme assay. Since most individuals with PK deficiency are compound heterozygotes for two different *PKLR* mutants,[126] the study of RBC from affected patients characterizes the mixture of PK variants without providing specific information about the individual enzymes. In those minority of individuals with homozygous disease, a relationship between defective PK enzymes and severity of hemolysis occasionally is apparent.[135,136,140] Initial studies suggest that PK protein levels may be a better correlate with severity of hemolysis and the need for transfusion.[137]

Ongoing molecular biology studies are focused on determining the relationship of specific mutations (genotype) with hemolysis (phenotype).[116,129] Given the number of different mutations and frequency of compound heterozygotes, analyses of genotype-phenotype relationships have focused on grouping variants by the types of mutations (two missense mutations, one missense/one drastic mutation, or two drastic mutations). Although there are limitations to this type of categorization, these analyses have found that patients with more severe mutations have a lower hemoglobin post splenectomy, a higher number of lifetime transfusions and total volume, a higher rate of splenectomy, and a higher frequency of iron overload.[141] Despite these findings the same degree of phenotypic similarity exists within siblings as between nonsiblings with PK deficiency. In addition, within cohorts with the same homozygous mutation, for example, 1592 G > A (510 Arg > Gln), there is significant variability in the severity of disease.

Pathophysiology

PK deficiency results in impaired glucose utilization and, thereby, decreased pyruvate and lactate production. In addition, glycolytic intermediates proximal to the block accumulate in red cells, and, of particular interest, the levels of 2,3-DPG may increase up to 3-fold.[142] The major impairment due to PK deficiency is a diminished capacity to generate ATP.[143] Paradoxically, however, PK-deficient patients with high reticulocyte counts may have normal or even elevated levels of ATP.[143] This occurs because PK-deficient reticulocytes generate ATP through mitochondrial oxidative phosphorylation, and this is associated with a 6- to 7-fold increase in oxygen consumption compared with normal reticulocytes.[143,144] The advantage of oxidative phosphorylation for PK-deficient reticulocytes is that ATP can be generated without relying on glycolysis. When reticulocytes mature, however, mitochondria disappear, oxidative phosphorylation ceases, and ATP levels fall. The effects of this will vary because there are marked cellular differences in the PK activity of PK-deficient red cells. In severely PK-deficient RBCs, the fall in ATP leads to cell injury, although the precise ATP-dependent reactions leading to irreversible membrane injury are not known. The end result is a loss of membrane plasticity and the formation of rigid RBC marked for premature destruction in the spleen.[145]

The reticulocytes most deficient in PK are doomed to almost immediate extinction once they lose their mitochondria. Less severely

deficient cells survive to a nearly normal age, their ATP needs satisfied despite marginal metabolic resources.[144] This vulnerability of enzyme-deficient reticulocytes is seen in erythroid kinetic studies that demonstrate that reticulocyte-rich fractions of blood from PK-deficient subjects have a shorter survival than do reticulocyte-poor fractions.[144,145] Given the unique metabolic abnormalities of the PK-deficient reticulocyte, it is understandable why the spleen poses a problem for them. Because of their greater adhesive tendencies, reticulocytes endure a longer sojourn in the spleen, where limited oxygen and glucose restrict effective oxidative phosphorylation.[144] Impaired ATP production then leads to RBC destruction in the spleen or in the liver after escape from the spleen.[145,146] Because severely deficient reticulocytes are metabolically more stable in the absence of the spleen, a paradoxical, sustained robust reticulocytosis follows splenectomy.[119]

As noted previously, the concentration of 2,3-DPG may be up to three times normal.[147] This increase is responsible for a rightward shift in the oxygen dissociation curve of hemoglobin. As a result, it is hypothesized that patients with PK deficiency have greater exercise tolerance than would be expected from the degree of anemia.[142] In clinical practice, however, tolerance and symptoms of low hemoglobin levels vary substantially among patients with PK deficiency.[148]

Clinical Features

The clinical symptoms of PK deficiency are quite variable, ranging from hydrops fetalis to pronounced neonatal jaundice requiring multiple exchange transfusions, and occasionally complicated by kernicterus, to a fully compensated hemolytic process detected as an incidental finding in adults.[149,150] Unlike the hyperbilirubinemia associated with G6PD deficiency, the jaundice noted in PK-deficient infants invariably is associated with anemia and often with splenomegaly. Approximately one-quarter of patients with PK deficiency will have complications in utero or at the time of birth, including intrauterine growth retardation, perinatal anemia requiring transfusions, hydrops, and preterm birth.[117] After birth, most newborns will develop severe jaundice and hemolysis requiring phototherapy and/or simple or exchange transfusions. Fulminant neonatal presentations have been described with hypoglycemia, hyperferritinemia, hepatosplenomegaly, and respiratory distress.[151,152] Severe hepatic disease with evolution to liver failure has been reported in several neonates.[153,154]

Beyond the neonatal period, anemia of varying degree, jaundice, and splenomegaly characterize erythrocyte PK deficiency. There are no specific or distinguishing clinical characteristics of this disorder; no tissues are affected besides the red cells. Notably, some patients with PK deficiency have no jaundice at birth and only a mild, chronic hemolytic anemia. These patients often are diagnosed later in childhood or adulthood; thus, PK deficiency should be suspected in individuals of any age with a chronic hemolytic anemia without evidence of an immune-mediated process, membranopathy, or hemoglobinopathy.

The burden of RBC transfusions in PK deficiency is quite variable and is dependent on both patient- and provider-specific factors. Young children are more often reliant on frequent transfusions to decrease symptoms and improve growth.[155] For some young children, decreasing the frequency of transfusions to permit a lower hemoglobin nadir will allow assessment of the reticulocyte response. The reticulocyte response may be adequate to transition to transfusion independence over time, even without a splenectomy. However, for many children and adolescents, transfusion needs decrease after splenectomy. Approximately one-fifth of patients with PK deficiency have never been transfused. Most commonly, patients receive intermittent transfusions in the setting of periodic hemolytic triggers, such as viral infections. Erythrocytopheresis has been reported as a treatment to improve symptoms.[156] Anemia in PK deficiency may be better tolerated than similarly low hemoglobin levels in other anemias because of the increased red cell 2,3-DPG content, which is responsible for a rightward shift in the hemoglobin-oxygen dissociation curve. Fatigue and symptoms of anemia are quite variable between patients with similar hemoglobin levels and in individual patients as they age.[117,148,157] Patients can develop difficulty with concentration. It is important to

Disorders of Red Blood Cells

assess symptoms on a regular basis and over time when determining patient management and need for intervention including transfusions.

Similar to other chronic hemolytic anemias, the clinical course may be complicated by aplastic crises, characterized by an abrupt but temporary arrest of erythropoiesis and a precipitous drop in hemoglobin concentration and reticulocyte count. These crises usually are related to infection with parvovirus B19, which is cytotoxic for erythroid progenitors. Gallstones are a frequent complication with many children and adolescents requiring cholecystectomy. The risk of gallstones is lifelong, occurs in 70% of adults, and continues even after splenectomy due to ongoing hemolysis. Nearly half of patients who had a splenectomy without simultaneous cholecystectomy will go on to have a cholecystectomy later in life; thus, cholecystectomy should be considered at the time of splenectomy, even in patients without evidence of concurrent gallstones.

Iron overload is a predictable complication of chronic transfusion therapy, but iron loading frequently also occurs in patients with PK deficiency in the absence of transfusions.[158-160] Transfusion-independent iron loading in PK deficiency is underrecognized, occurring at all ages and in patients with both mild and more severe anemia. In one cohort of patients who were not regularly transfused and had an MRI for liver iron assessment, 82% had iron overload.[159] Approximately 50% of children with PK deficiency younger than 18 years have iron overload.[155] Since iron loading is common in PK deficiency, patients should have iron monitoring at least annually with ferritin measurements and, when patients are able to have a nonsedated assessment, with MRI assessment in those with ferritin >500 ng/mL. Depending on the degree of iron burden, iron chelation and/or phlebotomy may be periodically prescribed in nontransfused patients through their lifetime. The pathophysiology of transfusion-independent iron loading in these patients is not well understood; however, both ineffective erythropoiesis and coinheritance of hereditary hemochromatosis may contribute to iron loading in the more minimally transfused patients.[161]

Bone changes associated with hyperplastic bone marrow, such as those seen in thalassemia, occasionally may result in frontal bossing. Patients with PK deficiency are also at risk for osteopenia; in a cohort of 159 patients, 75% had osteopenia or osteoporosis by dual-energy x-ray absorptiometry (DXA) Thus, close attention to vitamin D and calcium intake may be beneficial with consideration of monitoring with DXA scans for baseline assessment in late adolescence or early adulthood. Chronic leg ulcers, pulmonary hypertension, and extramedullary hematopoiesis occur rarely.[117] Screening echocardiograms should be considered in those older than 30 years, prior to pregnancy, and in patients with concerning symptoms.[150] Pregnancy has been associated with good maternal and fetal outcomes.[162] However, the degree of hemolysis often worsens during the pregnancy, and most women will be transfused during the pregnancy or after the delivery.[161] Multidisciplinary care with a hematologist and high-risk obstetrician is recommended with close attention to fetal growth to determine transfusion frequency. Pregnant women with PK deficiency should be careful to avoid prenatal vitamins containing iron.

Diagnosis

Anemia due to PK deficiency is mild to severe in degree. The hemoglobin concentration characteristically is 6 to 12 g/dL.[119] The peripheral blood smear reveals all the morphologic hallmarks of accelerated erythropoiesis: polychromatophilia, anisocytosis, poikilocytosis, and variable numbers of nucleated red cells. Irregularly contracted erythrocytes with surface spicules, ecchinocytes,[163] poikilocytes,[143] and acanthocytes[164] have been observed in the blood smears of some affected individuals. Before splenectomy, the reticulocyte count may be increased (5%-15%), but after splenectomy, reticulocyte counts paradoxically increase and can be as high as 50% to 70%.[119,136] The robust reticulocytosis is due to the longer survival of PK-deficient reticulocytes following splenectomy.

The hematologic features of PK deficiency are not distinctive. Current diagnostic algorithms recommend both RBC enzyme testing and *PKLR* genotyping to confirm PK diagnosis in most patients. In cases where PK deficiency is suspected, a direct quantitative assay of the enzyme is essential. Leukocytes must be excluded from the system, because the leukocyte *PKM2* gene is not affected in hemolytic variants to PK deficiency and the PK activity of white blood cells is 300 times that of normal red cells.[165] Most deficient individuals have 5% to 25% of the normal mean activity. However, the diagnosis of PK deficiency should be suspected when the PK enzyme activity is normal but relatively low in comparison with other age-dependent RBC enzymes. Thus, PK activity should always be measured along with another RBC age-dependent enzyme such as hexokinase (HK) or G6PD. The PK:HK ratio has a 98% sensitivity for the diagnosis of PK deficiency in nontransfused patients.[137]

Heterozygous carriers of a PK variant have approximately half normal activity, although there is considerable overlap with normal.

In families with a child with PK deficiency, the issue of prenatal diagnosis in subsequent pregnancies is a matter of concern. Molecular diagnostic techniques for the prenatal diagnosis of PK deficiency have proven to be useful.[166] In addition, in patients who are transfused before the enzyme disorder is recognized, the dilution of enzyme-deficient RBC with transfused cells often makes it difficult to make the diagnosis based on chemical enzyme analysis. The increased availability of genetic testing for PK deficiency allows for molecular diagnosis in patients in whom enzyme analysis is challenging and for confirmation of enzyme deficiency.[114] This is particularly important as disease-modifying therapies are becoming available.[157,167]

Treatment

During the first years of life, symptomatic anemia, often manifested as poor growth, is managed with red cell transfusions. The decision for transfusion therapy throughout childhood and adulthood must relate to patients' tolerance of anemia rather than an arbitrary level of hemoglobin. Because of increased red cell 2,3-DPG content, there is variability in patient tolerance to anemia.[142,150]

Splenectomy partially ameliorates the anemia in many patients and can be beneficial in decreasing the transfusion burden. However, because of the well-known risk of postsplenectomy sepsis due to encapsulated organism bacteremia in young children, surgery should be delayed until 5 years of age whenever possible. In determining the timing of splenectomy, one must weigh the risk of postsplenectomy sepsis with the risks of RBC transfusions and iron loading. Also, there is a postsplenectomy thrombosis risk, estimated to be 10% for splenectomized patients with PK deficiency.[117] Preoperative assessment of red cell survival, splenic sequestration, and/or spleen size is of no value in selecting patients for splenectomy, and this in part reflects the importance of the liver as another site of red cell destruction. Splenectomy most commonly improves the anemia but does not completely correct the hemolysis.[119,143,145] Transfusion requirements, if present before splenectomy, almost always decrease or are eliminated. In most patients, an incompletely compensated hemolytic process persists with reticulocytosis and indirect hyperbilirubinemia.

A severe hemolytic anemia associated with PK deficiency in Basenji dogs has been corrected by hemopoietic stem cell transplant (HSCT).[168] Similarly, marrow transplantation has been shown to be effective in mutant mice with splenomegaly and chronic hemolytic anemia due to PK deficiency.[169] These successes in animal studies clearly indicate a possible role for HSCT in humans. In one report, 16 patients with PK deficiency have undergone HSCT in Europe and Asia with a range of conditioning regimens and management strategies.[170] In this cohort, there was a 74% cumulative survival and a high rate of graft-vs-host disease, particularly in patients transplanted at age greater than 10 years. Despite the report of success with stem cell transplant in several patients, in almost all cases of hemolytic anemia due to PK deficiency, the risk-benefit ratio of red cell transfusions and/or splenectomy over HSCT currently remains weighted in favor of splenectomy over stem cell transplantation. This is particularly true now in light of new disease-targeted treatment approaches available for adults.[157]

Since PK deficiency is due to a single gene defect, affecting primarily one cell line, it is considered a candidate disease for gene therapy.[171,172] A preclinical model of gene therapy in PK-deficient mice using a lentiviral vector has shown success with an increase in PK activity and hemoglobin and a decrease in reticulocyte count and spleen size.[173,174] Metabolic studies in these corrected mice are consistent with improved flow through the glycolytic pathway. Based on these data, a lentivirus gene therapy for PK deficiency is currently in clinical trials with reported initial normalization of hemoglobin and hemolytic markers in two adult patients.[175]

Several activators of red cell PK are in clinical development. Mitapivat (AG-348) is an allosteric small-molecule PK activator that has been studied in a phase 2 and two phase 3 clinical trials in adults with PK deficiency. This drug activates wild-type PK in vitro as well as mutant PK across a wide spectrum of variants. In preclinical studies, the drug activates PK and enhances glycolytic flux in mice.[176,177] In healthy volunteers, the drug induces PK activity in vivo and increases RBC ATP and decreases 2,3-DPG. In a global phase 2 clinical trial of 52 adults with PK deficiency, 50% of patients had a median hemoglobin increase of >1 g/dL (median 3.4 g/dL).[167] Improvement in markers of hemolysis was correlated with the increase in hemoglobin. Responses in hemoglobin occurred soon after drug was administered (median of 10 days) and were sustained with ongoing treatment. Of note, the hemoglobin response related to the *PKLR* genotype and PK protein level. Patients with at least one missense mutation and higher PK protein levels had an increased probability of a hemoglobin response. Phase 3 trials in both transfused and nontransfused adults with PK deficiency have shown similar safety and efficacy.[157] Since the majority of individuals with PK deficiency are compound heterozygotes with at least one missense *PKLR* mutation, mitapivat has the potential to raise the hemoglobin and decrease hemolysis in a substantial proportion of affected adults. In the United States, mitapivat recently has been approved by the US Food and Drug Administration for use in adults with PK deficiency.

Future studies will determine whether this activator is an effective and safe potential treatment for patients with PK deficiency.

OTHER GLYCOLYTIC ENZYMOPATHIES

Hexokinase Deficiency

HK catalyzes the conversion of glucose to glucose 6-phosphate (*Figure 30.4*). As the first enzyme in the glycolytic pathway, HK has a strategic role in the regulation of glucose consumption. The activity of HK declines rapidly as red cells age, and, in older cells, HK activity is lower than that of any other glycolytic enzyme.

There are four HK isozymes, and each one is coded for by a different gene (HK1, HK2, HK3, HK4). The HK1 gene codes for the HK found in erythrocytes, and this gene maps to chromosome 10.[178] Type I HK isozyme also is present in lymphocytes and platelets. However, deficiency of type I HK isozyme in lymphocytes is offset by an increase in the amount of type III isozyme.[179] The inheritance pattern of HK deficiency is autosomal recessive. As with PK deficiency, deficient HK activity may result from quantitative deficiency of an apparently normal enzyme,[180,181] abnormalities that affect substrate affinity, or heat stability. Because clinical genetic testing has become more widely available, the molecular defect has been identified in an increasing number of cases of HK deficiency.[182-184]

At least 30 patients with HK deficiency have been described in families of European, Mediterranean, Scandinavian, and Asian background.[178,180,184] This low number of reported patients may be due to a high number of cases that lead to fetal demise due to severe anemia or underdiagnoses because of underrecognition or diagnostic challenges. Moreover, as new patients are diagnosed, they are unlikely to be reported in the literature in the absence of unusual clinical or molecular features.

There are no unique RBC features associated with HK deficiency. The diagnosis rests on the assay of red cell HK activity. Because HK is among the most age dependent of red cell enzymes, its activity must be considered in relation to the reticulocyte count or the activity of other age-dependent enzymes, such as PK.[181] Given the rarity of this diagnosis, if a patient is found to have low enzyme activity, this should be confirmed with molecular testing.

Symptoms may be out of proportion to expected based on the degree of anemia due to low levels of erythrocyte 2,3-DPG, which reduce oxygen release to tissues at any given oxygen tension.[142] Since the diagnosis is rare, the clinical complications are not clear but are likely to be similar to other congenital hemolytic anemias. Monitoring may be needed for complications such as gallstones and transfusion-independent iron loading.

Disease severity is variable, ranging from fully compensated hemolysis to anemia requiring regular RBC transfusions. In about 25% of reported cases, neonatal hyperbilirubinemia can occur and may require exchange transfusion. In many affected individuals, mild anemia or recurrent episodes of jaundice are not noted until after the first decade of life. Splenomegaly is common. Regular RBC transfusions may be required in severely affected patients. Splenectomy ameliorates but does not cure the hemolytic process.[181] Treatment with hemopoietic stem cell transplant has been described in a single patient.[185]

Glucose phosphate Isomerase Deficiency

Glucose phosphate isomerase (GPI) catalyzes the interconversion of fructose 6-phosphate and glucose 6-phosphate (*Figure 30.4*). GPI deficiency is the second most common glycolytic enzymatic defect associated with hemolytic disease.[186] Since the first description of the disorder in 1968, less than 100 cases have been reported.[187] Similarly to the other glycolytic enzyme disorders, many more cases probably exist but are not published or listed in any rare disease registry. It is estimated that 0.2% of North Americans are heterozygous for a GPI mutant.[188]

The gene for GPI is located on chromosome 19. GPI deficiency is autosomal recessive, caused by homozygous or compound heterozygous mutant alleles.[126,189] Multiple pathogenic gene mutations associated with hemolysis have been identified.[55,126,187] A single form of GPI is synthesized by all cells of the body; consequently, structural mutations of the enzyme are expressed in all tissues. However, because most mutations result in enzyme instability,[190] the defect imposes functional compromise mainly in older mature erythrocytes. Both missense mutations and gene deletions have been described.[187,189] Heterozygotes for mutant alleles have reduced red cell GPI activity but are hematologically normal without hemolysis.

Red cell morphology is characterized by anisocytosis, poikilocytosis, polychromatophilia, and often the presence of nucleated red cells. Definitive diagnosis requires specific enzyme assay of an RBC hemolysate. Prenatal diagnosis of GPI by enzymatic assay of amniotic fluid cells has been demonstrated in a kindred with unusually severe hemolytic disease.[191] Multiple GPI mutations have been identified, and molecular testing for confirmation is available.[192]

The severity of hemolytic disease is quite variable. Hydrops fetalis with death in neonates has been reported,[191,193] and anemia and hyperbilirubinemia complicate the postnatal course in many patients.[194] Chronic transfusion therapy may be required. As with other congenital hemolytic anemias, the clinical course may be complicated by aplastic and hyperhemolytic episodes with infectious illness. Developmental delay and excessive stores of hepatic glycogen were noted in a single patient.[195] Neuromuscular impairment (hypotonia, ataxia, dysarthria, mental retardation) occasionally has been seen, but only in certain variants.[187,196] Splenectomy has eliminated or dramatically reduced the transfusion requirement in most patients. Postsplenectomy hemoglobin concentrations are 8 to 10 g/dL. Similar to PK deficiency, reticulocyte counts may increase dramatically (50%-75%) post splenectomy.[188] Transfusion-independent iron loading has been reported,[197] and patients are at a lifetime risk for gallstones.

Phosphofructokinase Deficiency

PFK catalyzes the phosphorylation of fructose 6-phosphate to fructose 1,6-diphosphate, and this is one of the rate-limiting reactions of glycolysis (*Figure 30.4*). The PFK enzyme in RBC is a tetrameric protein made up of varying combinations of muscle or M type subunits, liver or L type subunits, and platelet or P type subunits.[198-200] Three different structural loci encode for these M, L, or P subunits of PFK. The M type subunit is encoded for a gene on chromosome 1.[201,202] The L type

PFK subunit is encoded by a gene located on chromosome 21.[203] The gene encoding for the P subunits of PFK is located on chromosome 10.[204] The subunits are variably expressed in different tissues. Muscle and liver PFK are composed exclusively of M4 and L4 tetramers, respectively. RBC contains equal amounts of M and L subtypes and all possible tetrameric variations are present (L_4; $L_3 M_1$; $L_2 M_2$; $L_1 M_3$; M_4).[200] Neutrophil PFK is composed primarily of L4 homotetramers, and platelet PFK consists of both P and L subunits. The variable structure of PFK in different tissues provides an explanation for the diversity of syndromes associated with deficiency states. These syndromes include chronic hemolytic disease with myopathy, hemolytic disease alone, and myopathy alone.[205]

The first PFK deficiency syndrome described was characterized by congenital nonspherocytic hemolytic disease and myopathy (Tarui disease, glycogenosis type VII).[206] At least 40 unrelated families have been identified with this very rare deficiency.[207] PFK deficiency is inherited as an autosomal recessive disorder. The myopathy is characterized by muscle fatigue and cramping with exercise and pathologically increased muscle glycogen.[208] There is a mild compensated hemolytic anemia. The hemoglobin concentration can be normal, or even increased. Both myopathy and hemolytic disease result from the total lack of M subunit expression. Biopsies of muscle reveal that PFK activity is completely lacking, while erythrocyte PFK activity is about 50% of normal. The red cell PFK in these patients is composed exclusively of L4 subunits.[200,208] Glycolytic intermediates proximal to PFK are increased in concentration, and those distal to the block are decreased. Of particular interest, 2,3-DPG is decreased,[209] and this presumably leads an unfavorable shift of the hemoglobin-oxygen affinity, thereby accounting for the mild erythrocytosis in some patients and absence of anemia despite shortened red cell survival in others.

PFK deficiency also has been implicated as the cause of hemolytic disease in the absence of myopathy.[210,211] Some individuals manifest mild myopathic symptoms during ischemic exercise tolerance tests.[211] This syndrome is attributed to the synthesis of an unstable but catalytically active M subunit. Muscle cells are protected because of continued synthesis of the enzyme, whereas anucleate erythrocytes, incapable of protein synthesis, sustain early loss of enzyme activity.[210] A ketogenic diet has been reported to improve the myopathy symptoms in several patients.[212,213] Although myopathy without hemolysis has also been attributed to PFK deficiency, hemolytic disease may have been dismissed because of the absence of anemia related to the shift in hemoglobin-oxygen affinity.[211] Heterozygosity for deficiency in the L subunit is associated with about 50% red cell PFK activity but with no myopathic or hemolytic features.[211,214,215]

Aldolase Deficiency

Aldolase catalyzes the conversion of fructose 1,6-diphosphate to dihydroxyacetone and glyceraldehyde 3-phosphate (*Figure 30.4*). Aldolase is a tetrameric protein, and three tissue isozymes (A, B, C) have been identified. Type A aldolase, the main isozyme in RBCs and muscle, has been characterized and cloned. The gene that encodes aldolase A is located on chromosome 16.

Aldolase deficiency is a very rare cause of hemolytic anemia and has been identified in only seven kindred. The first case was documented in a consanguineous family with a child with mild hemolytic anemia as well as hepatomegaly associated with increased glycogen deposition and psychomotor retardation.[216] A second report of aldolase deficiency in a Japanese family described more severe hemolytic anemia (hemoglobin 6 g/dL; 7%-8% reticulocytes) without attendant hepatomegaly or developmental delay.[217] In a third case, a 4-year-old boy in Germany was identified with aldolase deficiency.[218] He had a history of neonatal jaundice, recurrent episodes of jaundice beyond the newborn period, and anemia requiring red cell transfusions in the first year of life. In addition, however, he had a myopathy characterized by severe muscle weakness, exercise intolerance, and laboratory evidence of rhabdomyolysis in association with fever and an upper respiratory infection. In a fourth reported case, a young girl of Sicilian extraction had a transfusion-dependent hemolytic anemia requiring splenectomy at age 3 years.[219] She also had a myopathy with recurrent and

progressive episodes of rhabdomyolysis. She died due to hyperkalemia and rhabdomyolysis during a febrile illness associated with gastrointestinal hemorrhage at age 4 years. Three siblings have been reported to have a homozygous mutation in the aldolase A gene associated with episodic rhabdomyolysis without hemolytic anemia despite low RBC aldolase activity.[220] Another case report includes a 24-year-old male, diagnosed in adulthood, who had recurrent myalgia and dark urine following exercise or fever and chronic hemolytic anemia associated with hyperferritinemia.[221] Molecular analysis in each of the above cases has identified several different missense or nonsense mutations, each resulting in a thermolabile unstable enzyme.[218,219,222,223] The mechanism of hemolysis in these cases is uncertain; however, deficient red cells accumulate proximal glycolytic intermediates, especially fructose 1,6-diphosphate.

Triose Phosphate Isomerase Deficiency

TPI catalyzes the reversible isomerization of glyceraldehyde 3-phosphate and dihydroxyacetone phosphate (*Figure 30.4*). TPI is a dimeric enzyme composed of identical subunits. Several electrophoretically distinct bands result from posttranslational modification of a single protein[224] that is encoded by a single structural gene located on the short arm of chromosome 12.[225] Only one isozyme of TPI is produced, and, thus, enzyme deficiency involves all body tissues. Enzyme activity is greatly reduced in red cells, as well as leukocytes, muscle, and skin fibroblasts. TPI is autosomal recessive, and the majority of reported cases are homozygous. Several different point mutations in the TPI gene have been identified and reviewed.[226,227] The majority of the mutants result in heat-labile enzymes with residual catalytic activity. The enzyme abnormality in almost all cases is due to a single amino acid substitution that results in an unstable enzyme, and this variant is due to a 315G → C mutation that results in an amino acid substitution (104 Glu → Asp).[226] Heterozygotes, with 50% RBC TPI activity, are clinically normal. Of interest, the frequency of the heterozygous state for TPI deficiency is relatively high (0.1%-0.5% in Caucasians, 5.5% in African Americans).[228] Despite this estimate, less than 40 individuals with symptomatic disease have been identified.[226] The very low incidence of clinically significant homozygous TPI deficiency suggests incompatibility with fetal life.

The diagnosis of TPI deficiency is suspected in young children with chronic hemolytic disease not due to the more common causes of hemolysis. Associated motor neurologic symptoms should further raise the index of suspicion for TPI deficiency. There are no specific RBC abnormalities. In suspected cases, it is necessary to assay for TPI activity in an RBC hemolysate. Since the majority of cases are associated with the codon 104 mutation, chorionic villous biopsy samples and molecular techniques have been used for prenatal diagnosis.[229]

Hemolysis due to TPI deficiency is one aspect of a multiple system disease. This enzymopathy is associated with severe neurologic features characterized by spasticity, motor retardation, and hypotonia.[226] TPI deficiency is a progressive, ultimately fatal disease. In most cases, anemia and hyperbilirubinemia have been noted at birth or during the first weeks of life.[226,230,231] The degree of anemia is variable, but most affected infants and children require periodic blood transfusions. Death from hemolytic anemia in the first week of life occurred in a sibling and a cousin of the patient described in the first reported case.[230] Splenectomy appears to have no discernible benefit.[230] Late in the first year of life, spasticity and a delay in the acquisition of motor skills are noted. Neurologic involvement generally is progressive, giving rise to paraparesis, weakness, and hypotonia. Recurrent systemic infections are a problem in most affected children, but it is not known whether these are related to impaired TPI activity in phagocytes. Death, probably from cardiac arrhythmias, usually occurs before the fifth birthday. In the only adult thus far identified as having TPI deficiency,[232] neurologic dysfunction, although profound, was stable. An interesting report of TPI deficiency with chronic hemolytic anemia has been described in a 13-year-old boy and his 23-year-old brother. Noteworthy was the observation that the 13-year-old boy had hyperkinetic torsion dyskinesia but his 23-year-old brother had no neurological abnormalities.[233-235]

Phosphoglycerate Kinase Deficiency

PGK catalyzes the conversion of 1,3-diphosphoglycerate (1,3-DPG) to 3-phosphoglycerate. This is one of two glycolytic reactions resulting in net ATP generation from ADP (*Figure 30.1*). An alternative fate of 1,3-DPG is the formation of 2,3-DPG, a reaction catalyzed by 2,3-diphosphoglyceromutase (2,3-DPGM). The product of the later reaction is 2,3-DPG, an important intermediate that is known to enhance oxygen release from hemoglobin. Hereditary deficiency of PGK activity has been recognized as a rare cause of chronic hemolytic anemia for 50 years.[236] Red cells severely deficient in PGK predictably accumulate DHAP, have higher than normal concentrations of 2,3-DPG, and have decreased concentrations of ATP. The altered intermediate profile in PGK-deficient RBC thus reflects an increased flow of triose phosphates through the DPG pathway at the expense of ATP generation.

The genetics of this disorder are unique among glycolytic enzymopathies in that it is X-linked.[236] PGK is known to be encoded by a single structural gene on the X-chromosome q13.[237] Biochemical variants of PGK with abnormal kinetics and/or enzyme instability have been reported in 26 separate families,[238] and several different variants have been described, most of which are due to missense mutations.[238,239]

Male hemizygotes with little or no enzyme activity are symptomatic with chronic hemolysis that can be severe, often requiring RBC transfusions.[236,240,241] In contrast, females, who are mosaics, have normal and PGK-deficient red cells, and there may be variable degrees of hemolysis.[236,242] Clinical exacerbations of hemolysis, most of which appear to be triggered by intercurrent infections, are responsible for recurrent episodes of jaundice. Splenectomy obviates transfusion in most patients but does not fully correct the hemolytic process. In deficient male patients, PGK activity is decreased in leukocytes,[236] platelets, muscle, liver, and brain, as well as in red cells. Although leukocyte PGK activity may also be low, there is no evidence that affected individuals have leukocyte dysfunction or increased infections. Of far greater consequence than the hemolysis is progressive neurologic deterioration. Some deficient males experience apparent normal development until 3 to 4 years of age, when motor regression, expressive aphasia, and emotional liability become apparent. Seizures and progressive extrapyramidal disease follow late in the first decade.[236,240,243,244] Most PGK variants cause symptoms of both hemolysis and neurologic disease (PGK-Uppsala, PGK-Tokyo, PGK-Matsue, PGK-Michigan); however, there are exceptions. PGK-Shizuoka is characterized by hemolysis and muscle disease,[245] while PGK-San Francisco has only hemolysis without other symptoms.[246] Another variant is characterized by neurologic and muscle disease with no hemolysis.[247] At the other extreme, recurrent exertional rhabdomyolysis producing renal failure but without associated neurologic or hematologic disease has been observed in PGK-Creteil.[248] The absence of hemolysis in this variant is most intriguing since red cell PGK activity was less than 3% of normal. Molecular studies demonstrate that patients with both hemolysis and neurologic symptoms have unstable molecular variants, whereas those with myopathy without hemolytic or neurological symptoms have variants that affect the stability of the enzyme and its catalytic properties. Thus, molecular testing may help to predict later clinical findings in patients with PGK deficiency.[239]

Glycolytic Enzymopathies of Doubtful Clinical Significance

Hemolysis has been associated with deficiencies of other glycolytic enzymes, but the causal relationship between enzymopathy and reported hematologic disturbances is far from clear.[186] These include glyceraldehyde-3-phosphate dehydrogenase deficiency, 2,3-DPGM deficiency, enolase deficiency, and LDH deficiency. For more details regarding these enzymopathies, the reader is referred to Wintrobe, 13th edition.

While DPGM deficiency does not cause hemolysis, very reduced levels of this enzyme are associated with a low 2,3-DPG concentration in RBC, a left shifted oxygen dissociation curve, and a compensatory erythrocytosis.[249] In most cases this is an autosomal recessive inheritance (see Chapter 45).

ABNORMALITIES OF PURINE AND PYRIMIDINE NUCLEOTIDE METABOLISM

Mature RBCs are incapable of de novo purine or pyrimidine synthesis, although many enzymes of nucleotide metabolism are present in erythrocytes (*Figure 30.5*). The latter are now known to be important for RBC preservation in vitro, and it also is recognized that abnormalities in purine and pyrimidine metabolism are associated with inherited hemolytic disease.

Initial interest in RBC nucleotide metabolism was stimulated by blood bank concerns related to ATP and 2,3-DPG loss during storage of RBCs. Several studies demonstrated that inosine, adenosine, and adenine each could minimize loss of organic phosphates and thereby improve viability of stored blood. These studies defined an important role for purine nucleoside metabolism in maintaining energy pools of stored RBC, and this has had a major impact on the science of transfusion medicine.

In certain immune and metabolic disorders due to inborn errors of purine metabolism, erythrocytes share the same enzymatic deficiency, without any adverse effect on RBC function or viability. The RBC enzyme abnormalities in these cases can serve as a marker of disease in other tissues, and in some cases assay of red cell enzyme activity is used for diagnostic purposes.[250] The two most common disorders in which the red cell is used as this type of diagnostic tool are adenosine deaminase (ADA) deficiency associated with severe combined immune deficiency[251] and purine nucleoside phosphorylase deficiency associated with impaired T-cell immunity.[252]

Red cell purine and pyrimidine enzyme disorders also have been associated with inherited hemolytic syndromes, and these cases have further identified the important role of nucleotide metabolism in mature erythrocytes. The remainder of this section focuses on the pyrimidine and purine enzyme disorders associated with hemolysis: pyrimidine 5′ nucleotidase deficiency, ADA excess, and adenylate kinase (AK) deficiency.

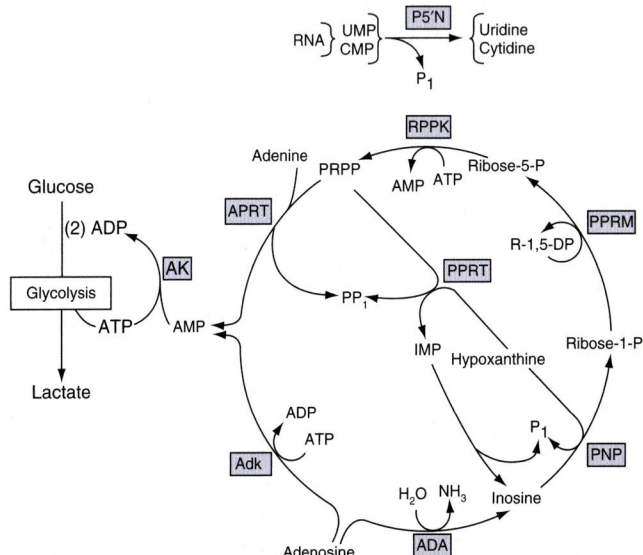

FIGURE 30.5 Schema of purine and pyrimidine metabolism in mature erythrocytes. Enzyme abbreviations: ADA, adenosine deaminase; AdK, adenosine kinase; AK, adenylate kinase; APRT, adenine phosphoribosyltransferase; P5′N, pyrimidine 5′ nucleotidase; PNP, purine nucleoside phosphorylase; PPRM, pyrophosphoribosyl mutase; PPRT, pyrophosphoribosyl transferase; RPPK, ribopyrophosphoryl kinase. Substrate abbreviations: AMP, adenosine monophosphate; IMP, inosine monophosphate.

Pyrimidine 5′nucleotidase Deficiency

Ribosomal RNA in normal reticulocytes is degraded to 5′ nucleotides. The enzyme pyrimidine 5′nucleotidase (P5′N) further catalyzes the degradation of cytidine and uridine mononucleotides to inorganic phosphate and the corresponding nucleoside. Although the mononucleotides are impermeable to the RBC membrane, after P5′N exposure, the nucleosides can passively diffuse from the cell. P5′N thus rids maturing reticulocytes of pyrimidine degradation products of RNA without compromising the purine (adenine) nucleotide pool necessary for energy-dependent reactions. Another enzyme, thymidylate nucleotidase, is thought to catalyze the degradation of thymidine monophosphate in a similar manner. This is supported by the observation that P5′N-deficient cells exhibit brisk nucleotidase activity when thymidine and deoxyuridine monophosphates are used as substrates.[253-255]

Reticulocytes deficient in P5′N accumulate large quantities of cytidine and uridine compounds, increasing the total nucleotide pool to more than five times that present in normal red cells.[254,256] Cases of P5′N deficiency formerly were classified as "high ATP syndromes" owing to the erroneous assumption that the large amount of nucleotide was adenine phosphate rather than pyrimidine phosphate.[257,258] In addition to the increased nucleotide pool content, elevated levels of GSH[259] and decreased activity of ribose phosphate pyrophosphate (PRPP) synthetase are consistent but there are unexplained findings of P5′N deficiency.[257,258] As a consequence of impaired ribosomal degradation, intracellular aggregates form in P5′N-deficient cells, and these appear as basophilic stippling on Wright-stained peripheral blood smears.

The gene encoding P5′N is located on chromosome 7p15-p14. Over 20 different mutations of P5′N have been reported in 30 different families with this enzyme deficiency.[260]

Pyrimidine 5′N deficiency is a rare RBC defect, yet it is the most common enzyme abnormality affecting nucleotide metabolism.[186,255,260] Over 60 patients representing a wide geographic distribution have been reported with a predisposition for people of Mediterranean, Jewish, and African ancestry.[260,261] In all families studied, the disorder follows an autosomal recessive mode of transmission. Family members who are biochemical heterozygotes are hematologically normal, whereas homozygotes with <5%-10% of normal P5′N activity have lifelong hemolytic anemia associated with splenomegaly and intermittent jaundice. The disorder is characterized by mild to moderate anemia, reticulocytosis, and hyperbilirubinemia. Transfusions usually are not required. Splenectomy is followed by a modest increase in hemoglobin concentration but affords no significant benefit.[258,262,263] There are no associated P5′N abnormalities in platelets or leukocytes. Developmental delay has been noted.[264]

The possibility of P5′N deficiency as the cause of hemolysis is suggested by the presence of marked basophilic stippling, a unique RBC morphologic feature characteristic of this hemolytic disorder. Definitive diagnosis requires demonstration of decreased RBC nucleotidase activity[262] or increased pyrimidine nucleotides in erythrocytes. Normally, RBC nucleotides are almost entirely adenine nucleotides. However, in P5′N deficiency, up to 80% of the nucleotide pool may be pyrimidine nucleotides. The latter is the basis for a simple screening test that utilizes ultraviolet spectroscopy to demonstrate a shift in the absorption spectrum of red cell lysates.[263]

The mechanism by which P5′N deficiency leads to hemolytic anemia is not known, although there have been a variety of proposed mechanisms.[265,266]

P5′N enzyme is readily inactivated by heavy metals such as lead, and it has been proposed that the basophilic stippling in lead poisoning is secondary to acquired P5′N deficiency.[267] As blood lead levels approach 200 μg/dL packed red cells, P5′N activity decreases to levels comparable with those associated with the homozygous deficiency state, intracellular pyrimidine nucleotides accumulate, and basophilic stippling can be demonstrated.[254,268]

Adenosine Deaminase Excess

Adenosine is a common substrate for two different enzymes, adenosine kinase (ADK) and ADA. The Km (adenosine) is much lower for ADK than for ADA, and, thus, normally metabolism proceeds through ADK with phosphorylation of adenosine to form AMP (*Figure 30.5*). In the presence of plasma adenosine, ADK thereby helps maintain the red cell adenine nucleotide pool.[269,270] The enzyme ADA catalyzes the deamination of adenosine to form inosine.

Hereditary deficiency of ADA is associated with severe combined immunodeficiency,[251] and since the enzyme deficiency also exists in erythrocytes, assay of red cell ADA can be used to diagnose this immune disorder. Red cell adenine nucleotide content is increased in severe ADA deficiency, but this has no adverse effects on RBC and there is no anemia.

Surprisingly, hereditary hemolytic anemia occurs in association with a 60- to 100-fold excess of normal ADA activity,[271] and this has been described in a few families including a large kindred of English-Irish ancestry and in a Japanese family.[272] In these patients with hemolysis and increased RBC-ADA activity, erythrocyte ATP content is reduced.[271,272] The decrease in adenine nucleotides presumably occurs because although elevated ADA activity, despite the higher Km for adenosine, effectively competes with normal levels of ADK, thereby producing a "relative" deficiency of the later enzyme.[262,270]

In patients with hemolytic anemia and marked ADA excess, the purified enzyme exhibits normal biochemical properties and the defect appears to be due to excess production of a structurally normal enzyme.[273,274] The synthesis of this enzyme is directed by a gene on chromosome 20, and posttranslational modifications result in different tissue isozymes. No specific DNA mutation has been identified to account for increased ADA production in patients with hemolytic anemia.

This rare hemolytic enzymopathy is unique because it is associated with an enzyme excess and also because it is inherited in an autosomal dominant pattern.[271,275] Clinical features include mild to moderate anemia, reticulocytosis, and hyperbilirubinemia. No other tissues share in enzyme excess, and there are no other systemic effects. There are no distinguishing clinical, hematologic, or morphologic features to aid in the diagnosis of this condition. The specific diagnosis can be suspected if red cell ATP levels are low and confirmed by demonstrating increased ADA activity in a hemolysate. Usually no specific therapy is indicated since most patients have very mild anemia. In contrast to these rare patients with a marked excess of enzyme activity and hemolytic anemia, a much smaller increase in enzyme activity (2- to 4-fold) has been observed in most patients with congenital hypoplastic anemia (Diamond-Blackfan syndrome)[276,277] (see Chapter 43).

Adenylate Kinase Deficiency

AK catalyzes the interconversion of adenine nucleotides (AMP + ATP → 2 ADP) (*Figure 30.5*). This is thought to be the only enzyme reaction in mature RBC that can lead to ADP synthesis from AMP, and thus AK would appear to have a critical role in salvaging AMP and protecting the erythrocyte adenine nucleotide pool.[278] In erythrocytes, AMP is formed in two reactions: the ADK-mediated phosphorylation of adenosine and the APRT-mediated phosphorylation of PRPP. There are three isozymes: AK1, AK2, and AK3.[279] AK1 is the isozyme in red cells, muscle, and brain.

Hereditary nonspherocytic hemolytic anemia in association with AK deficiency has been described in nine different kindred distributed worldwide.[278,280-286] AK deficiency is autosomal recessive; heterozygotes are hematologically normal. Molecular analysis has revealed the gene defect in six of the known kindred with chronic hemolysis and AK deficiency, including missense mutations, nonsense mutations, and deletions.[126,279,284-286]

A moderate to severe chronic nonspherocytic hemolytic anemia has been reported in almost all affected individuals. Splenectomy sometimes is beneficial.[283,287] Developmental delay has been reported in some cases with severe erythrocyte AK deficiency,[281,283-285] and this may reflect that AK1 is the isozyme in both RBC and brain.

The causal relationship of this enzyme abnormality to hemolysis is not entirely clear because some individuals with profound AK deficiency have no evidence of hemolysis.[278] In two siblings, there was congenital hemolytic anemia and less than 1% normal erythrocyte AK activity in an 8-year-old girl while her brother also had no detectable AK activity but was hematologically normal.[278] In another family with AK deficiency, a 4-year-old girl had chronic hemolysis with occasional exacerbations during infections.[282] Her RBC had no detectable AK activity while her parents had half-normal activity. In this patient, decreased activity of other phosphotransferases was noted; in particular, PRPP synthetase activity was reduced, just as in P5′N deficiency. The authors proposed that defects in multiple phosphotransferases may be responsible for the shortened lifespan of AK-deficient RBC.[282] The significance of these observations is unknown.

References

1. Beutler E. Glucose-6-phosphate dehydrogenase deficiency: a historical perspective. *Blood.* 2008;111(1):16-24.
2. Mason PJ, Bautista JM, Gilsanz F. G6PD deficiency: the genotype-phenotype association. *Blood Rev.* 2007;21(5):267-283.
3. Beutler E. G6PD deficiency. *Blood.* 1994;84(11):3613-3636.
4. Luzzatto L. Glucose 6-phosphate dehydrogenase deficiency: from genotype to phenotype. *Haematologica.* 2006;91(10):1303-1306.
5. Luzzatto L, Ally M, Notaro R. Glucose-6-phosphate dehydrogenase deficiency. *Blood.* 2020;136(11):1225-1240.
6. Luzzatto L, Nannelli C, Notaro R. Glucose-6-Phosphate dehydrogenase deficiency. *Hematol Oncol Clin North Am.* 2016;30(2):373-393.
7. Carson PE, Flanagan CL, Ickes CE, Alving A. S.. Enzymatic deficiency in primaquine sensitive erythrocytes. *Science.* 1956;124:484-485.
8. Alving A, Johnson CF, Tarlov AR, Brewer GJ, Kellermeyer RW, Carson PE. Mitigation of the haemolytic effect of primaquine and enhancement of its action against exoerythrocytic forms of the Chesson strain of Plasmodium vivax by intermittent regimens of drug administration. *Bull WHO.* 1960;22:621-631.
9. Nkhoma ET, Nkhoma ET, Poole C, Vannappagari V, Hall SA, Beutler E. The global prevalence of glucose-6-phosphate dehydrogenase deficiency: a systematic review and meta-analysis. *Blood Cells Mol Dis.* 2009;42(3):267-278.
10. Luzzatto L. Genetics of red cells and susceptibility to malaria. *Blood.* 1979;54(5):961-976.
11. Luzzatto L, Usanga FA, Reddy S. Glucose-6-phosphate dehydrogenase deficient red cells: resistance to infection by malarial parasites. *Science.* 1969;164(881):839-842.
12. Luzzatto L, Sodeinde O, Martini G. Genetic variation in the host and adaptive phenomena in Plasmodium falciparum infection. *Ciba Found Symp.* 1983;94:159-173.
13. Cohen P, Rosemeyer MA. Human glucose-6-phosphate dehydrogenase: purification of the erythrocyte enzyme and the influence of ions on its activity. *Eur J Biochem.* 1969;8(1):1-7.
14. Persico MG, Viglietto G, Martini G, et al. Isolation of human glucose-6-phosphate dehydrogenase (G6PD) cDNA clones: primary structure of the protein and unusual 5' non-coding region. *Nucleic Acids Res.* 1986;14(6):2511-2522.
15. Mason P. New insights into G6PD deficiency. *Br J Haematol.* 1996;94:585-591.
16. Martini G, Toniolo D, Vulliamy T, et al. Structural analysis of the X-linked gene encoding human glucose 6-phosphate dehydrogenase. *EMBO J.* 1986;5(8):1849-1855.
17. Takizawa T, Huang IY, Ikuta T, Yoshida A. Human glucose-6-phosphate dehydrogenase: primary structure and cDNA cloning. *Proc Natl Acad Sci U S A.* 1986;83(12):4157-4161.
18. Beutler E. The molecular biology of enzymes of erythrocyte metabolism. In: Stamatoyannopoulos G, Majerus PW, Varmus H, eds. *The Molecular Basis of Blood Disease.* W B Saunders; 1993.
19. Boyer S, Porter IH, Weilbacher RG. Electrophoretic heterogeneity fo glucose-6-phosphate dehydrogenase and its relationship to enzyme deficiency in man. *Proc Natl Acad Sci USA.* 1962;48:1868-1876.
20. Yoshida A. A single amino acid substitution (asparagine to aspartic acid) between normal (B+) and the common Negro variant (A+) of human glucose-6-phosphate dehydrogenase. *Proc Natl Acad Sci USA.* 1967;57:835-840.
21. Reys L, Manso C, Stamatoyannopoulos G. Genetic studies on southeastern Bantu of Mozambique. I. Variants of glucose-6-phosphate dehydrogenase. *Am J Hum Genet.* 1970;22(2):203-215.
22. Piomelli S, Corash LM, Davenport DD, Miraglia J, Amorosi EL. In vivo lability of glucose-6-phosphate dehydrogenase in GdA- and GdMediterranean deficiency. *J Clin Invest.* 1968;47(4):940-948.
23. Morelli A, Benatti U, Gaetani GF, De Flora A. Biochemical mechanisms of glucose-6-phosphate dehydrogenase deficiency. *Proc Natl Acad Sci U S A.* 1978;75(4):1979-1983.
24. Lyon MF. Gene action in the X-chromosome of the mouse (mus musculus L). *Nature.* 1961;190:372.
25. Beutler Ee.a, Yeh M Fairbanks VF. The normal human female as a mosaic of X-chromosome activity: studies using the gene for G-6-PD deficiency as a marker. *Proc Natl Acad Sci U S A.* 1962;48:9-16.
26. Luzzatto L, Mehta A, Vulliamy T, et al. Glucose-6-Phosphate dehydrogenase deficiency. In: Scriver C, ed. *The Metabolic and Molecular Bases of Inherited Disease.* McGraw Hill; 2001:4517-4553.
27. Beutler E, Vulliamy TJ. Hematologically important mutations: glucose-6-phosphate dehydrogenase. *Blood Cells Mol Dis.* 2002;28(2):93-103.
28. Mehta A, Mason PJ, Vulliamy TJ. Glucose-6-phosphate dehydrogenase deficiency. *Baillieres Best Pract Res Clin Haematol.* 2000;13(1):21-38.
29. Fiorelli G, Martinez di Montemuros F, Cappellini MD. Chronic non-spherocytic haemolytic disorders associated with glucose-6-phosphate dehydrogenase variants. *Baillieres Best Pract Res Clin Haematol.* 2000;13(1):39-55.
30. Hirono A, Beutler E. Molecular cloning and nucleotide sequence of cDNA for human glucose-6-phosphate dehydrogenase variant A(-). *Proc Natl Acad Sci U S A.* 1988;85(11):3951-3954.
31. Beutler E, Kuhl W, Vives-Corrons J, Prchal J. Molecular heterogeneity of glucose-6-phosphate dehydrogenase A. *Blood.* 1989;74(7):2550-2555.
32. Beutler E. Glucose-6-phosphate dehydrogenase: new perspectives. *Blood.* 1989;73(6):1397-1401.
33. Vulliamy TJ, D'Urso M, Battistuzzi G, et al. Diverse point mutations in the human glucose-6-phosphate dehydrogenase gene cause enzyme deficiency and mild or severe hemolytic anemia. *Proc Natl Acad Sci U S A.* 1988;85(14):5171-5175.
34. Jiang W, Yu G, Liu P, et al. Structure and function of glucose-6-phosphate dehydrogenase-deficient variants in Chinese population. *Hum Genet.* 2006;119(5):463-478.
35. Cooper MR, DeChatelet LR, McCall CE, La Via MF, Spurr CL, Baehner RL. Complete deficiency of leukocyte glucose-6-phosphate dehydrogenase with defective bactericidal activity. *J Clin Invest.* 1972;51(4):769-778.
36. Schiliro G, Russo A, Mauro L, Pizzarelli G, Marino S. Leukocyte function and characterization of leukocyte glucose-6-phosphate dehydrogenase in Sicilian mutants. *Pediatr Res.* 1976;10(8):739-742.
37. Miller DR, Wollman MR. A new variant of glucose-6-phosphate dehydrogenase deficiency hereditary hemolytic anemia, G6PD Cornell: erythrocyte, leukocyte, and platelet studies. *Blood.* 1974;44(3):323-331.
38. Costa E, Vasconcelos J, Santos E, Laranjeira A, Melo JC, Barbot J. Neutrophil dysfunction in a case of glucose-6-phosphate dehydrogenase deficiency. *J Pediatr Hematol Oncol.* 2002;24(2):164-165.
39. Yoshida A, Stamatoyannopoulos G, Motulsky AG. Negro variant of glucose-6-phosphate dehydrogenase deficiency (A-) in man. *Science.* 1967;155(758):97-99.
40. Pannacciulli I, Salvidio E, Tizianello A, Parravidino G. Hemolytic effects of standard single dosages of primaquine and chloroquine on G-6-PD-deficient caucasians. *J Lab Clin Med.* 1969;74(4):653-661.
41. Au WY, Lam V, Pang A, et al. Glucose-6-phosphate dehydrogenase deficiency in female octogenarians, nanogenarians, and centenarians. *J Gerontol A Biol Sci Med Sci.* 2006;61(10):1086-1089.
42. Beutler E. Glucose-6-phosphate dehydrogenase deficiency. *N Engl J Med.* 1991;324(3):169-174.
43. Youngster I, Arcavi L, Schechmaster R, et al. Medications and glucose-6-phosphate dehydrogenase deficiency: an evidence-based review. *Drug Saf.* 2010;33(9):713-726.
44. Raupp P, Hassan JA, Varughese P, Kristiansson B. Henna causes life threatening haemolysis in glucose-6-phosphate dehydrogenase deficiency. *Arch Dis Child.* 2001;85(5):411-412.
45. Beaupre SR, Schiffman FJ. Rush hemolysis. A "bite-cell" hemolytic anemia associated with volatile liquid nitrite use. *Arch Fam Med.* 1994;3(6):545-548.
46. Burka E, Weaver Z,III, Marks P. Clinical spectrum of hemolytic anemia associated with glucose-6-phosphate dehydrogenase deficiency. *Ann Intern Med.* 1966;64:817-825.
47. Shannon K, Buchanan GR. Severe hemolytic anemia in black children with glucose-6-phosphate dehydrogenase deficiency. *Pediatrics.* 1982;70(3):364-369.
48. Phillips SM, Silvers NP. Glucose-6 phosphate dehydrogenase deficiency, infectious hepatitis, acute hemolysis, and renal failure. *Ann Intern Med.* 1969;70(1):99-104.
49. Whelton A, Donadio JV, Jr, Elisberg BL. Acute renal failure complicating rickettsial infections in glucose-6-phosphate dehydrogenase-deficient individuals. *Ann Intern Med.* 1968;69(2):323-328.
50. Baehner RL, Nathan DG, Castle WB. Oxidant injury of caucasian glucose-6-phosphate dehydrogenase-deficient red blood cells by phagocytosing leukocytes during infection. *J Clin Invest.* 1971;50(12):2466-2473.
51. Gellady AM, Greenwood RD. G-6-PD hemolytic anemia complicating diabetic ketoacidosis. *J Pediatr.* 1972;80(6):1037-1038.
52. Glader BE. Role of elevated glucose concentrations in the hemolysis of glucose-6-phosphate dehydrogenase deficient erythroycytes (38474). *Proc Soc Exp Biol Med.* 1975;148(1):50-53.
53. Beutler E, Guinto E. Mechanism of stimulation of the hexose monophosphate shunt of erythrocytes by pyruvate. *Enzyme.* 1974;18(1):7-18.
54. Luzzatto L, Arese P. Favism and glucose-6-phosphate dehydrogenase deficiency. *N Engl J Med.* 2018;378(11):1068-1069.
55. Xu W, Beutler E. The characterization of gene mutations for human glucose phosphate isomerase deficiency associated with chronic hemolytic anemia. *J Clin Invest.* 1994;94(6):2326-2329.
56. Vulliamy T, Luzzatto L. Glucose-6-Phosphate dehydrogenase deficiency and related disorders. In: Handin R, Lux S, Stossel T, eds. *Blood: Principles and Practice of Hematology.* Lippincott, Williams & Wilkins; 2003:1921-1950.
57. Galiano S, Gaetani GF, Barabino A, et al. Favism in the African type of glucose-6-phosphate dehydrogenase deficiency (A-). *BMJ.* 1990;300(6719):236.
58. Kattamis CA, Kyriazakou M, Chaidas S. Favism: clinical and biochemical data. *J Med Genet.* 1969;6(1):34-41.
59. Corchia C, , Balata A, Meloni GF, Meloni T. Favism in a female newborn infant whose mother ingested fava beans before delivery. *J Pediatr.* 1995;127(5):807-808.
60. Mentzer WC, Collier E. Hydrops fetalis associated with erythrocyte G-6-PD deficiency and maternal ingestion of fava beans and ascorbic acid. *J Pediatr.* 1975;86(4):565-567.
61. Chevion M, Navok T, Glaser G, Mager J. The chemistry of favism-inducing compounds. The properties of isouramil and divicine and their reaction with glutathione. *Eur J Biochem.* 1982;127(2):405-409.
62. Maisels MJ. Neonatal jaundice. *Pediatr Rev.* 2006;27(12):443-454.
63. Valaes T. Severe neonatal jaundice associated with glucose-6-phosphate dehydrogenase deficiency: pathogenesis and global epidemiology. *Acta Paediatr Suppl.* 1994;394:58-76.

64. Kaplan M, Hammerman C. Glucose-6-phosphate dehydrogenase deficiency: a hidden risk for kernicterus. *Semin Perinatol*. 2004;28(5):356-364.
65. Kaplan M, Hammerman C, Feldman R, Brisk R. Predischarge bilirubin screening in glucose-6-phosphate dehydrogenase-deficient neonates. *Pediatrics*. 2000;105(3 pt 1):533-537.
66. Kaplan M, Hammerman C, Beutler E. Hyperbilibubinaemia, glucose-6-phosphate dehydrogenase deficiency and Gilbert syndrome. *Eur J Pediatr*. 2001;160:195.
67. Kaplan M, Algur N, Hammerman C. Onset of jaundice in glucose-6-phosphate dehydrogenase-deficient neonates. *Pediatrics*. 2001;108(4):956-959.
68. Huang CS, Hung KL, Huang MJ, Li YC, Liu TH, Tang TK. Neonatal jaundice and molecular mutations in glucose-6-phosphate dehydrogenase deficient newborn infants. *Am J Hematol*. 1996;51(1):19-25.
69. Kaplan M, Hammerman C. Glucose-6-phosphate dehydrogenase-deficient neonates: a potential cause for concern in North America. *Pediatrics*. 2000;106(6):1478-1479.
70. Kaplan M, Hoyer JD, Herschel M, Hammerman C, Stevenson DK. Glucose-6-phosphate dehydrogenase activity in term and near-term, male African American neonates. *Clin Chim Acta*. 2005;355(1-2):113-117.
71. Oyebola DD. Care of the neonate and management of neonatal jaundice as practised by Yoruba traditional healers of Nigeria. *J Trop Pediatr*. 1983;29(1):18-22.
72. Slusher TM, Vreman HJ, McLaren DW, Lewison LJ, Brown AK, Stevenson DK. Glucose-6-phosphate dehydrogenase deficiency and carboxyhemoglobin concentrations associated with bilirubin-related morbidity and death in Nigerian infants. *J Pediatr*. 1995;126(1):102-108.
73. Johnson L, Bhutani VK, Karp K, Sivieri EM, Shapiro SM. Clinical report from the pilot USA kernicterus Registry (1992 to 2004). *J Perinatol*. 2009;29(suppl 1):S25-S45.
74. Drew JH, Kitchen WH. Jaundice in infants of Greek parentage: the unknown factor may be environmental. *J Pediatr*. 1976;89(2):248-252.
75. Kaplan M, Vreman HJ, Hammerman C, Leiter C, Abramov A, Stevenson DK. Contribution of haemolysis to jaundice in Sephardic Jewish glucose-6-phosphate dehydrogenase deficient neonates. *Br J Haematol*. 1996;93(4):822-827.
76. Kaplan M, Beutler E, Vreman HJ, et al. Neonatal hyperbilirubinemia in glucose-6-phosphate dehydrogenase-deficient heterozygotes. *Pediatrics*. 1999;104(1 pt 1):68-74.
77. Arese P, De Flora A. Pathophysiology of hemolysis in glucose-6-phosphate dehydrogenase deficiency. *Semin Hematol*. 1990;27(1):1-40.
78. Fairbanks V, Beutler E. A simple method for detection of erythrocyte glucose-6-phosphate dehydrogenase (G-6-PD spot test). *Blood*. 1962;20:591-601.
79. Brewer G, Tarlov AR, Alving AS. The methemoglobin reduction test for primaquine-type sensitivity of erythrocytes. *JAMA*. 1962;180:386-388.
80. Gall J. Studies of glucose-6-phosphate dehydrogenase activity of individual erythrocytes: the methemoglobin elution test for identification of females heterozygous for G6PD deficiency. *Am J Hum Genet*. 1965;17:359-368.
81. Brewer G, Zarafonetis CJD. The haemolytic effect of various regimens of primaquine with chloroquine in American negroes with G6PD deficiency and the lack of an effect of various antimalarial suppressive agents on erythrocyte metabolism. *Bull World Health Organ*. 1976;36:303-308.
82. Balinsky D, Gomperts E, Cayanis E, et al. Glucose-6-phosphate dehydrogenase Johannesburg: a new variant with reduced activity in a patient with congenital nonspherocytic haemolytic anaemia. *Br J Haematol*. 1973;25(3):385-392.
83. Johnson GJ, Vatassery GT, Finkel B, Allen DW. High-dose vitamin E does not decrease the rate of chronic hemolysis in glucose-6-phosphate dehydrogenase deficiency. *N Engl J Med*. 1983;308(17):1014-1017.
84. DeSandre GH, Wong RJ, Morioka I, Contag CH, Stevenson DK. The effectiveness of oral tin mesoporphyrin prophylaxis in reducing bilirubin production after an oral heme load in a transgenic mouse model. *Biol Neonate*. 2006;89(3):139-146.
85. Meloni T, Forteleoni G, Meloni GF. Marked decline of favism after neonatal glucose-6-phosphate dehydrogenase screening and health education: the northern Sardinian experience. *Acta Haematol*. 1992;87(1-2):29-31.
86. McCurdy PR, Morse EE. Glucose-6-phosphate dehydrogenase deficiency and blood transfusion. *Vox Sang*. 1975;28(3):230-237.
87. Shalev O, Manny N, Sharon R. Posttransfusional hemolysis in recipients of glucose-6-phosphate dehydrogenase-deficient erythrocytes. *Vox Sang*. 1993;64(2):94-98.
88. Mimouni F, Shohat S, Reisner SH. G6PD-deficient donor blood as a cause of hemolysis in two preterm infants. *Isr J Med Sci*. 1986;22(2):120-122.
89. Kumar P, Sarkar S, Narang A. Acute intravascular haemolysis following exchange transfusion with G-6-PD deficient blood. *Eur J Pediatr*. 1994;153(2):98-99.
90. Beutler E. Effect of flavin compounds on glutathione reductase activity: in vivo and in vitro studies. *J Clin Invest*. 1969;48(10):1957-1966.
91. Beutler E, Srivastava SK. Relationship between glutathione reductase activity and drug-induced haemolytic anaemia. *Nature*. 1970;226(247):759-760.
92. Loos H, Roos D, Weening R, Houwerzijl J. Familial deficiency of glutathione reductase in human blood cells. *Blood*. 1976;48(1):53-62.
93. Kamerbeek NM, van Zwieten R, de Boer M, et al. Molecular basis of glutathione reductase deficiency in human blood cells. *Blood*. 2007;109(8):3560-3566.
94. Necheles TF, Steinberg MH, Cameron D. Erythrocyte glutathione-peroxidase deficiency. *Br J Haematol*. 1970;19(5):605-612.
95. Nishimura Y, Chida N, Hayashi T, Arakawa T. Homozygous glutathione-peroxidase deficiency of erythrocytes and leukocytes. *Tohoku J Exp Med*. 1972;108(3):207-217.
96. Beutler E, Matsumoto F. Ethnic variation in red cell glutathione peroxidase activity. *Blood*. 1975;46(1):103-110.
97. Perona G, Guidi GC, Piga A, Cellerino R, Menna R, Zatti M. In vivo and in vitro variations of human erythrocyte glutathione peroxidase activity as result of cells ageing, selenium availability and peroxide activation. *Br J Haematol*. 1978;39(3):399-408.
98. Ristoff E, Larsson A. Inborn errors in the metabolism of glutathione. *Orphanet J Rare Dis*. 2007;2:16.
99. Prins H, Oort M, Loos JA, et al. Congenital Nonspherocytic hemolytic anemia, associated with glutathione deficiency of the erythrocytes. *Blood*. 1966;27:145-166.
100. Beutler E, Moroose R, Kramer L, Gelbart T, Forman L. Gamma-glutamylcysteine synthetase deficiency and hemolytic anemia. *Blood*. 1990;75(1):271-273.
101. Beutler E, Gelbart T, Kondo T, Matsunaga AT. The molecular basis of a case of gamma-glutamylcysteine synthetase deficiency. *Blood*. 1999;94(8):2890-2894.
102. Ristoff E, Augustson C, Geissler J, et al. A missense mutation in the heavy subunit of gamma-glutamylcysteine synthetase gene causes hemolytic anemia. *Blood*. 2000;95(7):2193-2196.
103. Manu Pereira M, Gelbart T, Ristoff E, et al. Chronic non-spherocytic hemolytic anemia associated with severe neurological disease due to gamma-glutamylcysteine synthetase deficiency in a patient of Moroccan origin. *Haematologica*. 2007;92(11):e102-e105.
104. Almusafri F, Elamin HE, Khalaf TE, Ali A, Ben-Omran T, El-Hattab AW. Clinical and molecular characterization of 6 children with glutamate-cysteine ligase deficiency causing hemolytic anemia. *Blood Cells Mol Dis*. 2017;65:73-77.
105. Mohler DN, Majerus PW, Minnich V, Hess CE, Garrick MD. Glutathione synthetase deficiency as a cause of hereditary hemolytic disease. *N Engl J Med*. 1970;283(23):1253-1257.
106. Beutler E, Gelbart T, Pegelow C. Erythrocyte glutathione synthetase deficiency leads not only to glutathione but also to glutathione-S-transferase deficiency. *J Clin Invest*. 1986;77(1):38-41.
107. Hirono A, Iyori H, Sekine I, et al. Three cases of hereditary nonspherocytic hemolytic anemia associated with red blood cell glutathione deficiency. *Blood*. 1996;87(5):2071-2074.
108. Corrons JL, Alvarez R, Pujades A, et al. Hereditary non-spherocytic haemolytic anaemia due to red blood cell glutathione synthetase deficiency in four unrelated patients from Spain: clinical and molecular studies. *Br J Haematol*. 2001;112(2):475-482.
109. AMA drug evaluations. *JAMA*, 1968;203(8):702-710.
110. Skullerud K, Marstein S, Schrader H, Brundelet PJ, Jellum E. The cerebral lesions in a patient with generalized glutathione deficiency and pyroglutamic aciduria (5-oxoprolinuria). *Acta Neuropathol*. 1980;52(3):235-238.
111. Konrad PN, Richards F, Valentine WN, Paglia DE. -Glutamyl-cysteine synthetase deficiency. A cause of hereditary hemolytic anemia. *N Engl J Med*. 1972;286(11):557-561.
112. Signolet I, Chenouard R, Oca F, et al. Recurrent isolated neonatal hemolytic anemia: think about glutathione synthetase deficiency. *Pediatrics*. 2016:138(3):e20154324.
113. Atwal PS, Medina CR, Burrage LC, Sutton VR. Nineteen-year follow-up of a patient with severe glutathione synthetase deficiency. *J Hum Genet*. 2016;61(7):669-672.
114. Gallagher PG, Glader B. Diagnosis of pyruvate kinase deficiency. *Pediatr Blood Cancer*. 2016;63(5):771-772.
115. Zanella A, Bianchi P, Fermo E. Pyruvate kinase deficiency. *Haematologica*. 2007;92(6):721-723.
116. Zanella A, Fermo E, Bianchi P, Chiarelli LR, Valentini G. Pyruvate kinase deficiency: the genotype-phenotype association. *Blood Rev*. 2007;21(4):217-231.
117. Grace RF, Bianchi P, van Beers EJ, et al. Clinical spectrum of pyruvate kinase deficiency: data from the pyruvate kinase deficiency natural history study. *Blood*. 2018;131(20):2183-2192.
118. Tanaka KR, Zerez CR. Red cell enzymopathies of the glycolytic pathway. *Semin Hematol*. 1990;27(2):165-185.
119. Tanaka KR, Paglia DE. Pyruvate kinase deficiency. *Semin Hematol*. 1971;8(4):367-396.
120. Zanella A, Bianchi P. Red cell pyruvate kinase deficiency: from genetics to clinical manifestations. *Baillieres Best Pract Res Clin Haematol*. 2000;13(1):57-81.
121. Bowman H. Pyruvate kinase deficient hemolytic anemia in an Amish isolate. *Am J Hum Genet*. 1965;17:1-8.
122. Baronciani L, Beutler E. Molecular study of pyruvate kinase deficient patients with hereditary nonspherocytic hemolytic anemia. *J Clin Invest*. 1995;95(4):1702-1709.
123. Beutler E, Gelbart T. Estimating the prevalence of pyruvate kinase deficiency from the gene frequency in the general white population. *Blood*. 2000;95(11):3585-3588.
124. Secrest MH, Storm M, Carrington C, et al. Prevalence of pyruvate kinase deficiency: a systematic literature review. *Eur J Haematol*. 2020;105(2):173-184.
125. Tani K, Yoshida MC, Satoh H, et al. Human M2-type pyruvate kinase: cDNA cloning, chromosomal assignment and expression in hepatoma. *Gene*. 1988;73(2):509-516.
126. Miwa S, Fujii H. Molecular basis of erythroenzymopathies associated with hereditary hemolytic anemia: tabulation of mutant enzymes. *Am J Hematol*. 1996;51(2):122-132.
127. Noguchi T, Inoue H, Tanaka T. The M1- and M2-type isozymes of rat pyruvate kinase are produced from the same gene by alternative RNA splicing. *J Biol Chem*. 1986;261(29):13807-13812.
128. Tani K, Fujii H, Tsutsumi H, et al. Human liver type pyruvate kinase: cDNA cloning and chromosomal assignment. *Biochem Biophys Res Commun*. 1987;143(2):431-438.
129. Zanella A, Fermo E, Bianchi P, Valentini G. Red cell pyruvate kinase deficiency: molecular and clinical aspects. *Br J Haematol*. 2005;130(1):11-25.
130. Bianchi P, Fermo E. Molecular heterogeneity of pyruvate kinase deficiency. *Haematologica*. 2020;105(9):2218-2228.
131. Baronciani L, Beutler E. Analysis of pyruvate kinase-deficiency mutations that produce nonspherocytic hemolytic anemia. *Proc Natl Acad Sci U S A*. 1993;90(9):4324-4327.
132. Lenzner C, Nurnberg P, Thiele B, et al. Mutations in the pyruvate kinase L gene in patients with hereditary hemolytic anemia. *Blood*. 1994;83(10):2817-2822.
133. Christensen RD, Yaish HM, Johnson CB, Bianchi P, Zanella A. Six children with pyruvate kinase deficiency from one small town: molecular characterization of the PK-LR gene. *J Pediatr*. 2011;159(4):695-697.

134. Kanno H, Ballas S, Miwa S, Fujii H, Bowman H. Molecular abnormality of erythrocyte pyruvate kinase deficiency in the Amish. *Blood*. 1994;83(8):2311-2316.

135. Miwa S. Pyruvate kinase variants characterized by the methods recommended by the International Committee for Standardization in Haematology. *Hemoglobin*. 1980;4(5-6):627-633.

136. Miwa S, Fujii H, Takegawa S, et al. Seven pyruvate kinase variants characterized by the ICSH recommended methods. *Br J Haematol*. 1980;45(4):575-583.

137. Al-Samkari H, Addonizio K, Glader B, et al. The pyruvate kinase (PK) to hexokinase enzyme activity ratio and erythrocyte PK protein level in the diagnosis and phenotype of PK deficiency. *Br J Haematol*. 2021;192(6):1092-1096.

138. Baronciani L, Magalhães IQ, Mahoney Jr. DH, et al. Study of the molecular defects in pyruvate kinase deficient patients affected by nonspherocytic hemolytic anemia. *Blood Cells Mol Dis*. 1995;21(1):49-55.

139. Beutler E, Forman L, Rios-Larrain E. Elevated pyruvate kinase activity in patients with hemolytic anemia due to red cell pyruvate kinase "deficiency." *Am J Med*. 1987;83(5):899-904.

140. Shinohara K, Tanaka KR. Pyruvate kinase deficiency hemolytic anemia: enzymatic characterization studies in twelve patients. *Hemoglobin*. 1980;4(5-6):611-625.

141. Bianchi P, Fermo E, Lezon-Geyda K, et al. Genotype-phenotype correlation and molecular heterogeneity in pyruvate kinase deficiency. *Am J Hematol*. 2020;95(5):472-482.

142. Oski FA, Marshall BE, Cohen PJ, Sugerman HJ, Miller LD. The role of the left-shifted or right-shifted oxygen-hemoglobin equilibrium curve. *Ann Intern Med*. 1971;74(1):44-46.

143. Keitt AS. Pyruvate kinase deficiency and related disorders of red cell glycolysis. *Am J Med*. 1966;41(5):762-785.

144. Mentzer WC, Jr, Baehner RL, Schmidt-Schönbein H, Robinson SH, Nathan DG. Selective reticulocyte destruction in erythrocyte pyruvate kinase deficiency. *J Clin Invest*. 1971;50(3):688-699.

145. Nathan DG, Oski FA, Miller DR, Gardner FH. Life-span and organ sequestration of the red cells in pyruvate kinase deficiency. *N Engl J Med*. 1968;278(2):73-81.

146. Nathan D, Oski FA, Sidel VW, et al. Extreme hemolysis and red-cell distortion in erythrocyte pyruvate kinase deficiency. *N Engl J Med*. 1965;272:118-123.

147. Grimes A, Meisler A, Dacie JV. Hereditary non-spherocytic haemolytic anaemia. A study of red-cell carbohydrate metabolism in twelve cases of pyruvate-kinase deficiency. *Br J Haematol*. 1964;10:403-411.

148. Al-Samkari H, Van Beers EJ, Kuo KHM, et al. The variable manifestations of disease in pyruvate kinase deficiency and their management. *Haematologica*. 2020;105(9):2229-2239.

149. Grace RF, Zanella A, Neufeld EJ, et al. Erythrocyte pyruvate kinase deficiency: 2015 status report. *Am J Hematol*. 2015;90(9):825-830.

150. Grace RF, Barcellini W. Management of pyruvate kinase deficiency in children and adults. *Blood*. 2020;136(11):1241-1249.

151. Cotton F, Bianchi P, Zanella A, et al. A novel mutation causing pyruvate kinase deficiency responsible for a severe neonatal respiratory distress syndrome and jaundice. *Eur J Pediatr*. 2001;160(8):523-524.

152. Pissard S, de Montalembert M, Bachir D, et al. Pyruvate kinase (PK) deficiency in newborns: the pitfalls of diagnosis. *J Pediatr*. 2007;150(4):443-445.

153. Olivier F, Wieckowska A, Piedboeuf B, Alvarez F. Cholestasis and hepatic failure in a neonate: a case report of severe pyruvate kinase deficiency. *Pediatrics*. 2015;136(5):e1366-e1368.().

154. Raphael MF, Van Wijk R, Schweizer JJ, et al. Pyruvate kinase deficiency associated with severe liver dysfunction in the newborn. *Am J Hematol*. 2007;82(11):1025-1028.

155. Chonat S, Eber SW, Holzhauer S, et al. Pyruvate kinase deficiency in children. *Pediatr Blood Cancer*. 2021;68(9):e29148.

156. Jensen RFG, Dziegiel MH, Rieneck K, Birgens H, Glenthøj A. Erythrocytapheresis as a novel treatment option for adult patients with pyruvate kinase deficiency. *Haematologica*. 2020;105(7):e373-e375.

157. Al-Samkari H, Galactéros F, Glenthøj A, et al. Mitapivat versus placebo for pyruvate kinase deficiency. *N Engl J Med*. 2022;386(15):1432-1442.

158. Salem HH, Van Der Weyden MB, Firkin BG. Iron overload in congenital erythrocyte pyruvate kinase deficiency. *Med J Aust*. 1980;1(11):531-532.

159. van Beers EJ, van Straaten S, Morton DH, et al. Prevalence and management of iron overload in pyruvate kinase deficiency: report from the Pyruvate Kinase Deficiency Natural History Study. *Haematologica*. 2019;104(2):e51-e53.

160. Boscoe AN, Yan Y, Hedgeman E, et al. Comorbidities and complications in adults with pyruvate kinase deficiency. *Eur J Haematol*. 2021;106(4):484-492.

161. Rider NL, Strauss KA, Brown K, et al. Erythrocyte pyruvate kinase deficiency in an old-order Amish cohort: longitudinal risk and disease management. *Am J Hematol*. 2011;86(10):827-834.

162. Wax JR, Pinette MG, Cartin A, Blackstone J. Pyruvate kinase deficiency complicating pregnancy. *Obstet Gynecol*. 2007;109(2 pt 2):553-555.

163. Nathan DG, Oski FA, Sidel VW, Gardner FH, Diamond LK. Studies of erythrocyte spicule formation in haemolytic anaemia. *Br J Haematol*. 1966;12(4):385-395.

164. Oski F, Nathan DG, Sidel VW. Extreme hemolysis and red-cell distortion in erythrocyte pyruvate kinase deficiency. *N Engl J Med*. 1964;270:1023-1030.

165. Hanel HK. Pyruvate kinase in human erythrocytes. *Scand J Haematol*. 1969;6(3):173-174.

166. Baronciani L, Beutler E. Prenatal diagnosis of pyruvate kinase deficiency. *Blood*. 1994;84(7):2354-2356.

167. Grace RF, Rose C, Layton DM, et al. Safety and efficacy of mitapivat in pyruvate kinase deficiency. *N Engl J Med*. 2019;381(10):933-944.

168. Weiden PL, Storb R, Graham TC, Schroeder ML. Severe hereditary haemolytic anaemia in dogs treated by marrow transplantation. *Br J Haematol*. 1976;33(3):357-362.

169. Morimoto M, Kanno H, Asai H, et al. Pyruvate kinase deficiency of mice associated with nonspherocytic hemolytic anemia and cure of the anemia by marrow transplantation without host irradiation. *Blood*. 1995;86(11):4323-4330.

170. van Straaten S, Bierings M, Bianchi P, et al. Worldwide study of hematopoietic allogeneic stem cell transplantation in pyruvate kinase deficiency. *Haematologica*. 2018;103(2):e82-e86.

171. Kanno H, Utsugisawa T, Aizawa S, et al. Transgenic rescue of hemolytic anemia due to red blood cell pyruvate kinase deficiency. *Haematologica*. 2007;92(6):731-737.

172. Meza NW, Alonso-Ferrero ME, Navarro S, et al. Rescue of pyruvate kinase deficiency in mice by gene therapy using the human isoenzyme. *Mol Ther*. 2009;17(12):2000-2009.

173. Garcia-Gomez M, Calabria A, Garcia-Bravo M, et al. Safe and efficient gene therapy for pyruvate kinase deficiency. *Mol Ther*. 2016;24(7):1187-1198.

174. Garate Z, Quintana-Bustamante O, Crane AM, et al. Generation of a high number of healthy erythroid cells from gene-edited pyruvate kinase deficiency patient-specific induced pluripotent stem cells. *Stem Cell Rep*. 2015;5(6):1053-1066.

175. Shah A, López Lorenzo JL, Navarro S, et al. Lentiviral mediated gene therapy for pyruvate kinase deficiency: interim results of a global phase 1 study for adult and pediatric patients. *Blood*. 2021;138:563.

176. Kung C, Hixon J, Kosinski PA, et al. AG-348 enhances pyruvate kinase activity in red blood cells from patients with pyruvate kinase deficiency. *Blood*. 2017;130(11):1347-1356.

177. Kung C, Hill C., Chen Y, et al. AD-348 Activation of pyruvate Kinase in vivo enhances red cell Glycolysis in mice. *Blood*. 2014;124:4010.

178. Kanno H. Hexokinase: gene structure and mutations. *Baillieres Best Pract Res Clin Haematol*. 2000;13(1):83-88.

179. Rijksen G, Akkerman J, van den Wall Bake A, Hofstede D, Staal G. Generalized hexokinase deficiency in the blood cells of a patient with nonspherocytic hemolytic anemia. *Blood*. 1983;61(1):12-18.

180. Beutler E, Dyment PG, Matsumoto F. Hereditary nonspherocytic hemolytic anemia and hexokinase deficiency. *Blood*. 1978;51(5):935-940.

181. Valentine WN, Oski FA, Paglia DE, Baughan MA, Schneider AS, Naiman JL. Hereditary hemolytic anemia with hexokinase deficiency. Role of hexokinase in erythrocyte aging. *N Engl J Med*. 1967;276(1):1-11.

182. Bianchi M, Magnani M. Hexokinase mutations that produce nonspherocytic hemolytic anemia. *Blood Cells Mol Dis*. 1995;21(1):2-8.

183. van Wijk R, Rijksen G, Huizinga EG, Nieuwenhuis HK, van Solinge WW. HK Utrecht: missense mutation in the active site of human hexokinase associated with hexokinase deficiency and severe nonspherocytic hemolytic anemia. *Blood*. 2003;101(1):345-347.

184. Koralkova P, Mojzikova R, van Oirschot B, et al. Molecular characterization of six new cases of red blood cell hexokinase deficiency yields four novel mutations in HK1. *Blood Cells Mol Dis*. 2016;59:71-76.

185. Khazal S, Polishchuk V, Manwani D, Gallagher PG, Prinzing S, Mahadeo KM. Allogeneic bone marrow transplantation for treatment of severe hemolytic anemia attributable to hexokinase deficiency. *Blood*. 2016;128(5):735-737.

186. Beutler E. Red cell enzyme defects as nondiseases and as diseases. *Blood*. 1979;54(1):1-7.

187. Kugler W, Lakomek M. Glucose-6-phosphate isomerase deficiency. *Baillieres Best Pract Res Clin Haematol*, 2000;13(1):89-101.

188. Paglia DE, Holland P, Baughan MA, Valentine WN. Occurrence of defective hexosephosphate isomerization in human erythrocytes and leukocytes. *N Engl J Med*. 1969;280(2):66-71.

189. Baronciani L, Zanella A, Bianchi P, et al. Study of the molecular defects in glucose phosphate isomerase-deficient patients affected by chronic hemolytic anemia. *Blood*. 1996;88(6):2306-2310.

190. Zanella A, Izzo C, Rebulla P, et al. The first stable variant of erythrocyte glucose-phosphate isomerase associated with severe hemolytic anemia. *Am J Hematol*. 1980;9(1):1-11.

191. Whitelaw AG, Rogers PA, Hopkinson DA, et al. Congenital haemolytic anaemia resulting from glucose phosphate isomerase deficiency: genetics, clinical picture, and prenatal diagnosis. *J Med Genet*. 1979;16(3):189-196.

192. Fermo E, Vercellati C, Marcello AP, et al. Clinical and molecular spectrum of glucose-6-phosphate isomerase deficiency. Report of 12 new cases. *Front Physiol*. 2019;10:467.

193. Ravindranath Y, Paglia DE, Warrier I, et al. Glucose phosphate isomerase deficiency as a cause of hydrops fetalis. *N Engl J Med*. 1987;316:258-261.

194. Hutton JJ, Chilcote RR. Glucose phosphate isomerase deficiency with hereditary nonspherocytic hemolytic anemia. *J Pediatr*. 1974;85(4):494-497.

195. Van Biervliet JP, Vlug A, Bartstra H, Rotteveel JJ, Vaan GAM, Staal GEJ. A new variant of glucosephosphate isomerase deficiency. *Humangenetik*. 1975;30(1):35-40.

196. Kedar PS, Dongerdiye R, Chilwirwar P, et al. Glucose phosphate isomerase deficiency: high prevalence of p.Arg347His mutation in Indian population associated with severe hereditary non-spherocytic hemolytic anemia coupled with neurological dysfunction. *Indian J Pediatr*. 2019;86(8):692-699.

197. Manco L, Bento C, Victor BL, et al. Hereditary nonspherocytic hemolytic anemia caused by red cell glucose-6-phosphate isomerase (GPI) deficiency in two Portuguese patients: clinical features and molecular study. *Blood Cells Mol Dis*. 2016;60:18-23.

198. Kahn A, Meienhofer MC, Cottreau D, Lagrange JLo, Dreyfus JC. Phosphofructokinase (PFK) isozymes in man. I. Studies of adult human tissues. *Hum Genet*. 1979;48(1):93-108.

199. Meienhofer MC, Lagrange J, Cottreau D, Lenoir G, Dreyfus J, Kahn A. Phosphofructokinase in human blood cells. *Blood*. 1979;54(2):389-400.

Disorders of Red Blood Cells

200. Vora S, Seaman C, Durham S, Piomelli S. Isozymes of human phosphofructokinase: identification and subunit structural characterization of a new system. *Proc Natl Acad Sci U S A.* 1980;77(1):62-66.
201. Vora S, Durham S, de Martinville B, George DL, Francke U. Assignment of the human gene for muscle-type phosphofructokinase (PFKM) to chromosome 1 (region cen leads to q32) using somatic cell hybrids and monoclonal anti-M antibody. *Somat Cell Genet.* 1982;8(1):95-104.
202. Vaisanen PA, Reddy GR, Sharma PM, et al. Cloning and characterization of the human muscle phosphofructokinase gene. *DNA Cell Biol.* 1992;11(6):461-470.
203. Van Keuren M, Drabkin H, Hart I, Harker D, Patterson D, Vora S. Regional assignment of human liver-type 6-phosphofructokinase to chromosome 21q22.3 by using somatic cell hybrids and a monoclonal anti-L antibody. *Hum Genet.* 1986;74(1):34-40.
204. Vora S, Miranda AF, Hernandez E, Francke U. Regional assignment of the human gene for platelet-type phosphofructokinase (PFKP) to chromosome 10p: novel use of polyspecific rodent antisera to localize human enzyme genes. *Hum Genet.* 1983;63(4):374-379.
205. Valentine WN, Paglia DE. Erythrocyte enzymopathies, hemolytic anemia, and multisystem disease: an annotated review. *Blood.* 1984;64(3):583-591.
206. Tarui S, Kono N, Nasu T, Nishikawa M. Enzymatic basis for the coexistence of myopathy and hemolytic disease in inherited muscle phosphofructokinase deficiency. *Biochem Biophys Res Commun.* 1969;34(1):77-83.
207. Fujii H, Miwa S. Other erythrocyte enzyme deficiencies associated with non-haematological symptoms: phosphoglycerate kinase and phosphofructokinase deficiency. *Baillieres Best Pract Res Clin Haematol.* 2000;13(1):141-148.
208. Layzer RB, Rowland LP, Ranney H. Muscle phosphofructokinase deficiency. *Trans Am Neurol Assoc.* 1967;92:99-101.
209. Tarui S, Kono N, Kuwajima M, Kitani T. Hereditary and acquired abnormalities in erythrocyte phosphofructokinase activity: the close association with altered 2,3-diphosphoglycerate levels. *Hemoglobin.* 1980;4(5-6):581-592.
210. Kahn A, Etiemble J, Meienhofer MC, Bovin P. Erythrocyte phosphofructokinase deficiency associated with an unstable variant of muscle phosphofructokinase. *Clin Chim Acta.* 1975;61(3):415-419.
211. Vora S, Davidson M, Seaman C, et al. Heterogeneity of the molecular lesions in inherited phosphofructokinase deficiency. *J Clin Invest.* 1983;72(6):1995-2006.
212. Simila ME, Auranen M, Piirila PL. Beneficial effects of ketogenic diet on phosphofructokinase deficiency (glycogen storage disease type VII). *Front Neurol.* 2020;11:57.
213. Reason SL, Godfrey RJ. The potential of a ketogenic diet to minimize effects of the metabolic fault in glycogen storage disease V and VII. *Curr Opin Endocrinol Diabetes Obes.* 2020;27(5):283-290.
214. Etiemble J, Simeon J, Buc HA, Picat C, Boulard M, Boivin P. A liver-type mutation in a case of pronounced erythrocyte phosphofructokinase deficiency without clinical expression. *Biochim Biophys Acta.* 1983;759(3):236-242.
215. Etiemble J, Picat C, Siméon J, Blatrix C, Boivin P. Inherited erythrocyte phosphofructokinase deficiency: molecular mechanism. *Hum Genet.* 1980;55(3):383-390.
216. Beutler E, Scott S, Bishop A, Margolis N, Matsumo F, Kuhl W. Red cell aldolase deficiency and hemolytic anemia: a new syndrome. *Trans Assoc Am Phys.* 1973;86:154-166.
217. Miwa S, Fujii H, Tani K, et al. Two cases of red cell aldolase deficiency associated with hereditary hemolytic anemia in a Japanese family. *Am J Hematol.* 1981;11(4):425-437.
218. Kreuder J, Borkhardt A, Repp R, et al. Brief report: inherited metabolic myopathy and hemolysis due to a mutation in aldolase A. *N Engl J Med.* 1996;334(17):1100-1104.
219. Neufeld N, Tolan DR, Murray MF, et al. Hemolytic anemia and severe rhabdomyolysis due to compound heterozygous mutations of the gene for erythrocyte/muscle Isozyme of Aldolase: ALDOA(Arg303X/Cys338Tyr). *Blood.* 2002;100:225(a).
220. Mamoune A, Bahuau M, Hamel Y, et al. A thermolabile aldolase A mutant causes fever-induced recurrent rhabdomyolysis without hemolytic anemia. *PLoS Genet.* 2014;10(11):e1004711.
221. Papadopoulos C, Svingou M, Kekou K, et al. Aldolase A deficiency: Report of new cases and literature review. *Mol Genet Metab Rep.* 2021;27:100730.
222. Kishi H, Mukai T, Hirono A, Fujii H, Miwa S, Hori K. Human aldolase A deficiency associated with a hemolytic anemia: thermolabile aldolase due to a single base mutation. *Proc Natl Acad Sci U S A.* 1987;84(23):8623-8627.
223. Takasaki Y, Takasaki I, Mukai T, Hori K. Human aldolase A of a hemolytic anemia patient with Asp-128—Gly substitution: characteristics of an enzyme generated in E. coli transfected with the expression plasmid pHAAD128G. *J Biochem (Tokyo).* 1990;108(2):153-157.
224. Yuan PM, Talent JM, Gracy RW. Molecular basis for the accumulation of acidic isozymes of triosephosphate isomerase on aging. *Mech Ageing Dev.* 1981;17(2):151-162.
225. McKusick VA. The anatomy of the human genome. *Am J Med.* 1980;69(2):267-276.
226. Schneider AS. Triosephosphate isomerase deficiency: historical perspectives and molecular aspects. *Baillieres Best Pract Res Clin Haematol.* 2000;13(1):119-140.
227. Aissa K, Kamoun F, Sfaihi L, et al. Hemolytic anemia and progressive neurologic impairment: think about triosephosphate isomerase deficiency. *Fetal Pediatr Pathol.* 2014;33(4):234-238.
228. Mohrenweiser HW, Fielek S. Elevated frequency of carriers for triosephosphate isomerase deficiency in newborn infants. *Pediatr Res.* 1982;16(11):960-963.
229. Arya R, Lalloz MR, Nicolaides KH, Bellingham AJ, Layton DM. Prenatal diagnosis of triosephosphate isomerase deficiency. *Blood.* 1996;87(11):4507-4509.
230. Schneider A, Valentine WN, Hattori M, et al. Hereditary hemolytic anemia with triosephosphate ismerase deficiency. *N Engl J Med.* 1965;272:229-235.
231. Valentine W, Schneider A, Baughan MA, et al. Hereditary hemolytic anemia with triosephosphate isomerase deficiency. *Am J Med.* 1966;41:27-41.
232. Harris S, Paglia DE, Jaffe ER, et al. Triosephosphate isomerase deficiency in an adult. *Clin Res.* 1970;18:529-530.
233. Hollan S, Fujii H, Hirono K, et al. Hereditary triosephosphate isomerase (TPI) deficiency: two severely affected brothers one with and one without neurological symptoms. *Hum Genet.* 1993;92(5):486-490.
234. Hollan S, Magócsi M, Fodor E, Horányi M, Harsányi V, Farkas T. Search for the pathogenesis of the differing phenotype in two compound heterozygote Hungarian brothers with the same genotypic triosephosphate isomerase deficiency. *Proc Natl Acad Sci U S A.* 1997;94(19):10362-10366.
235. Harris C, Nelson B, Farber D, et al. Child neurology: triosephosphate isomerase deficiency. *Neurology.* 2020;95(24):e3448-e3451.
236. Valentine WN, Hsieh HS, Paglia DE, et al. Hereditary hemolytic anemia associated with phosphoglycerate kinase deficiency in erythrocytes and leukocytes. A probable X-chromosome-linked syndrome. *N Engl J Med.* 1969;280(10):528-534.
237. Chen SH, Malcom LA, Yoshida A, Giblett ER. Phosphoglycerate kinase: an X-linked polymorphism in man. *Am J Hum Genet.* 1971;23(1):87-91.
238. Beutler E. *PGK deficiency. Br J Haematol.* 2007;136(1):3-11.
239. Chiarelli LR, Morera SM, Bianchi P, et al. Molecular insights on pathogenic effects of mutations causing phosphoglycerate kinase deficiency. *PLoS One.* 2012;7(2):e32065.
240. Dodgson SJ, Lee CS, Holland RA, O'Sullivan WJ, Vowels MR. Erythrocyte phosphoglycerate kinase deficiency: enzymatic and oxygen binding studies. *Aust N Z J Med.* 1980;10(6):614-621.
241. Hjelm M, Wadam B, Yoshida A. A phosphoglycerate kinase variant, PGK Uppsala, associated with hemolytic anemia. *J Lab Clin Med.* 1980;96(6):1015-1021.
242. Kraus AP, Langston MF, Jr, Lynch BL. Red cell phosphoglycerate kinase deficiency. A new cause of non-spherocytic hemolytic anemia. *Biochem Biophys Res Commun.* 1968;30(2):173-177.
243. Konrad PN, McCarthy DJ, Mauer AM, Valentine WN, Paglia DE. Erythrocyte and leukocyte phosphoglycerate kinase deficiency with neurologic disease. *J Pediatr.* 1973;82(3):456-460.
244. Miwa S, Nakashima K, Oda S, Ogawa H, Nagafuji H. Phosphoglycerate kinase (PKG) deficiency hereditary nonspherocytic hemolytic anemia: report of a case found in a Japanese family. *Nippon Ketsueki Gakkai Zasshi.* 1972;35(4):511-514.
245. Fujii H, Kanno H, Hirono A, Shiomura T, Miwa S. A single amino acid substitution (157 Gly---Val) in a phosphoglycerate kinase variant (PGK Shizuoka) associated with chronic hemolysis and myoglobinuria. *Blood.* 1992;79(6):1582-1585.
246. Guis MS, Karadsheh N, Mentzer WC. Phosphoglycerate kinase San Francisco: a new variant associated with hemolytic anemia but not with neuromuscular manifestations. *Am J Hematol.* 1987;25(2):175-182.
247. Coppens S, Koralkova P, Aeby A, et al. Recurrent episodes of myoglobinuria, mental retardation and seizures but no hemolysis in two brothers with phosphoglycerate kinase deficiency. *Neuromuscul Disord.* 2016;26(3):207-210.
248. Rosa R, George C, Fardeau M, Calvin M, Rapin M, Rosa J. A new case of phosphoglycerate kinase deficiency: PGK Creteil associated with rhabdomyolysis and lacking hemolytic anemia. *Blood.* 1982;60(1):84-91.
249. Hoyer JD, Allen SL, Beutler E, Kubik K, West C, Fairbanks VF. Erythrocytosis due to bisphosphoglycerate mutase deficiency with concurrent glucose-6-phosphate dehydrogenase (G-6-PD) deficiency. *Am J Hematol.* 2004;75(4):205-208.
250. Glader BE, Sullivan DW. The red blood cell as a biopsy tool. *Clin Haematol.* 1981;10(1):209-222.
251. Giblett ER, Anderson J, Cohen F, Pollara B, Meuwissen H. Adenosine-deaminase deficiency in two patients with severely impaired cellular immunity. *Lancet.* 1972;2(7786):1067-1069.
252. Giblett ER, Ammann A, Sandman R, Wara D, Diamond L. Nucleoside-phosphorylase deficiency in a child with severely defective T-cell immunity and normal B-cell immunity. *Lancet.* 1975;1(7914):1010-1013.
253. Paglia DE, Valentine WN, Brockway RA. Identification of thymidine nucleotidase and deoxyribonucleotidase activities among normal isozymes of 5'-nucleotidase in human erythrocytes. *Proc Natl Acad Sci U S A.* 1984;81(2):588-592.
254. Paglia DE, Valentine W, Keitt A, Brockway R, Nakatani M. Pyrimidine nucleotidase deficiency with active dephosphorylation of dTMP: evidence for existence of thymidine nucleotidase in human erythrocytes. *Blood.* 1983;62(5):1147-1149.
255. Vives-Corrons JL. Chronic non-spherocytic haemolytic anaemia due to congenital pyrimidine 5' nucleotidase deficiency: 25 years later. *Baillieres Best Pract Res Clin Haematol.* 2000;13(1):103-118.
256. Swanson MS, Angle CR, Stohs SJ, et al. 31P NMR study of erythrocytes from a patient with hereditary pyrimidine-5'-nucleotidase deficiency. *Proc Natl Acad Sci U S A.* 1983;80(1):169-172.
257. Valentine WN, Anderson HM, Paglia DE, et al. Studies on human erythrocyte nucleotide metabolism. II. Nonspherocytic hemolytic anemia, high red cell ATP, and ribosephosphate pyrophosphokinase (RPK, E.C.2.7.6.1) deficiency. *Blood.* 1972;39(5):674-684.
258. Valentine WN, Bennett JM, Krivit W, et al. Nonspherocytic haemolytic anaemia with increased red cell adenine nucleotides, glutathione and basophilic stippling and ribosephosphate pyrophosphokinase (RPK) deficiency: studies on two new kindreds. *Br J Haematol.* 1973;24(2):157-167.
259. Ben-Bassat I, Brok-Simoni F, Kende G, Holtzmann F, Ramot B. A family with red cell pyrimidine 5'-nucleotidase deficiency. *Blood.* 1976;47(6):919-922.
260. Zanella A, Bianchi P, Fermo E, Valentini G. Hereditary pyrimidine 5'-nucleotidase deficiency: from genetics to clinical manifestations. *Br J Haematol.* 2006;133(2):113-123.
261. Chiarelli LR, , Fermo E, Zanella A, Valentini G. Hereditary erythrocyte pyrimidine 5'-nucleotidase deficiency: a biochemical, genetic and clinical overview. *Hematology.* 2006;11(1):67-72.

262. Paglia DE, Valentine WN. Hereditary and acquired defects in the pyrimidine nucleotidase of human erythrocytes. *Curr Top Hematol.* 1980;3:75-109.

263. Valentine WN, Fink K, Paglia DE, Harris SR, Adams WS. Hereditary hemolytic anemia with human erythrocyte pyrimidine 5'-nucleotidase deficiency. *J Clin Invest.* 1974;54(4):866-879.

264. Beutler E, Baranko P, Feagler J, et al. Hemolytic anemia due to pyrimidine-5'-nucleotidase deficiency: report of eight cases in six families. *Blood.* 1980;56(2):251-255.

265. Paglia DE, Valentine WN, Nakatani M, Rauth BJ. Selective accumulation of cytosol CDP-choline as an isolated erythrocyte defect in chronic hemolysis. *Proc Natl Acad Sci U S A.* 1983;80(10):3081-3085.

266. Swanson MS, , Markin R, Stohs S, Angle C. Identification of cytidine diphosphodiesters in erythrocytes from a patient with pyrimidine nucleotidase deficiency. *Blood.* 1984;63(3):665-670.

267. Paglia DE, Valentine WN, Dahlgren JG. Effects of low-level lead exposure on pyrimidine 5'-nucleotidase and other erythrocyte enzymes. Possible role of pyrimidine 5'-nucleotidase in the pathogenesis of lead-induced anemia. *J Clin Invest.* 1975;56(5):1164-1169.

268. Valentine WN, Paglia DE, Fink K, Madokoro G. Lead poisoning: association with hemolytic anemia, basophilic stippling, erythrocyte pyrimidine 5'-nucleotidase deficiency, and intraerythrocytic accumulation of pyrimidines. *J Clin Invest.* 1976;58(4):926-932.

269. Paglia DE, Valentine WN. Red cell nucleotide abnormalities. *Prog Clin Biol Res.* 1984;165:213-225.

270. Paglia DE, Valentine WN. Haemolytic anaemia associated with disorders of the purine and pyrimidine salvage pathways. *Clin Haematol.* 1981;10(1):81-98.

271. Valentine WN, Paglia DE, Tartaglia AP, Gilsanz F. Hereditary hemolytic anemia with increased red cell adenosine deaminase (45- to 70-fold) and decreased adenosine triphosphate. *Science.* 1977;195(4280):783-785.

272. Miwa S, Fujii H, Matsumoto N, et al. A case of red-cell adenosine deaminase overproduction associated with hereditary hemolytic anemia found in Japan. *Am J Hematol.* 1978;5(2):107-115.

273. Chottiner EG, , Ginsburg D, Tartaglia A, Mitchell B. Erythrocyte adenosine deaminase overproduction in hereditary hemolytic anemia. *Blood.* 1989;74(1):448-453.

274. Fujii H, Miwa S, Tani K, Fujinami N, Asano H. Overproduction of structurally normal enzyme in man: hereditary haemolytic anaemia with increased red cell adenosine deaminase activity. *Br J Haematol.* 1982;51(3):427-430.

275. Paglia D, Valentine WN, Tartaglia AP, et al. Perturbations in erythrocyte adenine nucleotide metabolism: a dominantly inherited hemolytic disorder with implications regarding normal mechanisms of adenine nucleotide preservation. *Blood.* 1976;48:959.

276. Glader BE, Backer K, Diamond LK. Elevated erythrocyte adenosine deaminase activity in congenital hypoplastic anemia. *N Engl J Med.* 1983;309(24):1486-1490.

277. Fargo JH, Kratz CP, Giri N, et al. Erythrocyte adenosine deaminase: diagnostic value for Diamond-Blackfan anaemia. *Br J Haematol.* 2013;160(4):547-554.

278. Beutler E, Carson D, Dannawi H, et al. Metabolic compensation for profound erythrocyte adenylate kinase deficiency. A hereditary enzyme defect without hemolytic anemia. *J Clin Invest.* 1983;72(2):648-655.

279. Matsuura S, Igarashi M, Tanizawa Y, et al. Human adenylate kinase deficiency associated with hemolytic anemia. A single base substitution affecting solubility and catalytic activity of the cytosolic adenylate kinase. *J Biol Chem.* 1989;264(17):10148-10155.

280. Szeinberg A, Kahana D, Gavendo S, Zaidman J, Ben-Ezzer J. Hereditary deficiency of adenylate kinase in red blood cell. *Acta Haematol.* 1969;42(2):111-126.

281. Boivin P, Galand C, Hakim J, Simony D, Seligman M. A new erythroenzymopathy: congenital non-spherocytic hemolytic anemia and hereditary erythrocytic adenylate kinase deficiency. [Article in French]. *Presse Med.* 1971;79(6):215-218.

282. Lachant NA, Zerez C, Barredo J, Lee D, Savely S, Tanaka K. Hereditary erythrocyte adenylate kinase deficiency: a defect of multiple phosphotransferases? *Blood.* 1991;77(12):2774-2784.

283. Toren A, Brok-Simoni F, Ben-Bassat I, et al. Congenital haemolytic anaemia associated with adenylate kinase deficiency. *Br J Haematol.* 1994;87(2):376-380.

284. Bianchi P, Zappa M, Bredi E, et al. A case of complete adenylate kinase deficiency due to a nonsense mutation in AK-1 gene (Arg 107--> Stop, CGA--> TGA) associated with chronic haemolytic anaemia. *Br J Haematol.* 1999;105(1):75-79.

285. Qualtieri A, Pedace V, Bisconte MG, et al. Severe erythrocyte adenylate kinase deficiency due to homozygous A-->G substitution at codon 164 of human AK1 gene associated with chronic haemolytic anaemia. *Br J Haematol.* 1997;99(4):770-776.

286. Vives-Corrons JL, Garcia E, Tussel JJ, Varughese KI, West C, Beutler E. Red cell adenylate kinase deficiency. Molecular study of three new mutations (118 G{Rightarrow}A,190 G{Rightarrow}A, and GAC deletion) associated with non-spherocytic hemolytic anemia. *Blood.* 2003;102(1):353-356.

287. Niizuma H, Kanno H, Sato A, Ogura H, Imaizumi M. Splenectomy resolves hemolytic anemia caused by adenylate kinase deficiency. *Pediatr Int.* 2017;59(2):228-230.

Disorders of Red Blood Cells

Chapter 31 ■ Autoimmune Hemolytic Anemia

RICHARD C. FRIEDBERG • CLARA LO

CLASSIFICATION

In autoimmune hemolytic anemia (AIHA), pathologic antibodies (autoantibodies) attach to and lead to the destruction (hemolysis) of endogenous erythrocytes (red blood cells, RBCs) resulting in anemia. By definition, both autoantibodies and associated RBC consumption must be identified. AIHA is readily subclassified according to the characteristic temperature activity of the responsible antibodies (*Table 31.1*). Cold-active antibodies typically have little, if any, activity at body temperature but have greater affinity for RBCs as the temperature decreases toward 0 °C. Conversely, warm-active antibodies have their greatest affinity at 37 °C. Generally speaking, cold-active antibodies are typically immunoglobulin (Ig) M, fix complement, and lead to immediate intravascular RBC destruction or hepatic-mediated clearance. In contrast, warm-active antibodies are typically IgG, may or may not fix complement, and primarily lead to RBC loss by splenic-mediated clearance of sensitized cells. Patients who express both (mixed) cold- and warm-active antibodies are particularly troublesome clinically because of the dual impact from severe RBC destruction and often present a diagnostic and therapeutic challenge.[1] Drug-induced immune hemolytic anemia (DI-IHA) is caused by warm-active antibodies that may be clinically and serologically indistinguishable from the idiopathic warm autoimmune type (α-methyldopa type) or may be dependent on the presence of the drug in serologic studies

Table 31.1. Classification of Immune Hemolytic Anemias

Cold-Active Antibodies
Cold agglutinin disease
Primary or idiopathic
Secondary
Lymphoproliferative diseases
Autoimmune disorders
Infections
Mycoplasma pneumoniae
Infectious mononucleosis
Other viruses
Paroxysmal cold hemoglobinuria
Syphilis
Measles, mumps, other viruses
Mixed cold- and warm-active antibodies
Warm-active antibodies
Idiopathic autoimmune hemolytic anemia
Secondary autoimmune hemolytic anemia
Lymphoproliferative disorders
Autoimmune and immunodeficiency disorders
Malignancy
Viral infections
Drug-induced immune hemolytic anemia
Drug adsorption type (penicillin)
Neoantigen type (quinidine/stibophen)
Autoimmune type (α-methyldopa)
Nonimmune type (first-generation cephalosporins)
Transplant-associated hemolytic anemia
Hematopoietic stem cell transplant
Minor ABO group mismatch
Major ABO group mismatch
Passive antibody transfer
Solid organ transplant
Passenger lymphocyte syndrome
Passive antibody transfer

to demonstrate attachment of the antibody to the RBC. The clinical spectrum of drug-induced antibody attachment to RBCs ranges from asymptomatic positive serologic studies to life-threatening massive hemolysis.[2] Finally, a different type of immune-mediated hemolytic anemia can occur as a complication of organ transplantation. Because the antibodies are generated from donor-derived lymphocytes, the disorder is not truly of "auto" immune origin but can be thought of as a graft-vs-host disorder.

Etiology of the Immune Response in Autoimmune Hemolytic Anemia

Immunologic tolerance is a state in which the individual is incapable of developing an immune response to a specific antigen. Self-tolerance refers to lack of responsiveness to an individual's own (self) antigens, which is the normal state. Autoimmunity results from a loss of self-tolerance, leading to T cells or antibodies reacting against self-antigens and the consequent tissue injury. In AIHA, autoantibodies are directed against targets on the individual's own RBCs ("self-antigens"), leading to their enhanced clearance through Fc-receptor-mediated phagocytosis ("extravascular hemolysis") or complement-mediated breakdown ("intravascular hemolysis"). AIHA may be in large part due to self-reactive antibodies against erythrocyte band 3, an anion transporter found in the RBC membrane that is involved in RBC senescence.[3,4]

Central Tolerance

Central tolerance refers to the normal deletion of self-reactive T- and B-lymphocyte clones during their maturation in the central lymphoid organs (thymus for T cells; bone marrow for B cells).[5] Central tolerance prevents widespread autoimmunity by preferentially selecting nonautoreactive (ie, "normal") T cells for circulation into the periphery ("intrathymic negative selection"). Central tolerance is not complete, and a population of T cells with intermediate avidity for self-antigens invariably escapes into the circulation. Under certain conditions these cells can become activated and lead to organ-specific or systemic autoimmune disease.[6,7]

Peripheral Tolerance

The mechanisms by which self-reactive T cells that escape intrathymic negative selection and are deleted in the peripheral tissues constitute peripheral tolerance, including anergy, suppression by regulatory T cells, and clonal deletion by activation-induced cell death (see *Figure 31.1*).

Anergy refers to prolonged or irreversible functional inactivation of lymphocytes. Activation of antigen-specific T cells requires two signals: (1) recognition of peptide antigen in association with self-major histocompatibility complex (MHC) molecules on the surface of antigen-presenting cells and (2) a set of costimulatory signals provided by antigen-presenting cells (the costimulators B7-1 and B7-2). In the absence of costimulators, a negative signal is delivered, and the T lymphocyte becomes anergic. Anergic lymphocytes cannot be activated even if the relevant antigen is presented by antigen-presenting cells (eg, dendritic cells) that can deliver costimulation. Anergy also affects B cells because they encounter antigen in the absence of specific helper T cells. They become unable to respond to subsequent antigenic stimulation and may be excluded from lymphoid follicles.[6]

Suppression by regulatory T cells involves CD4+ cells that coexpress CD25, the α chain of the interleukin-2 (IL-2) receptor, but some CD4+ cells that lack CD25 may also induce peripheral tolerance by suppression. These T cells can suppress (inhibit) lymphocyte

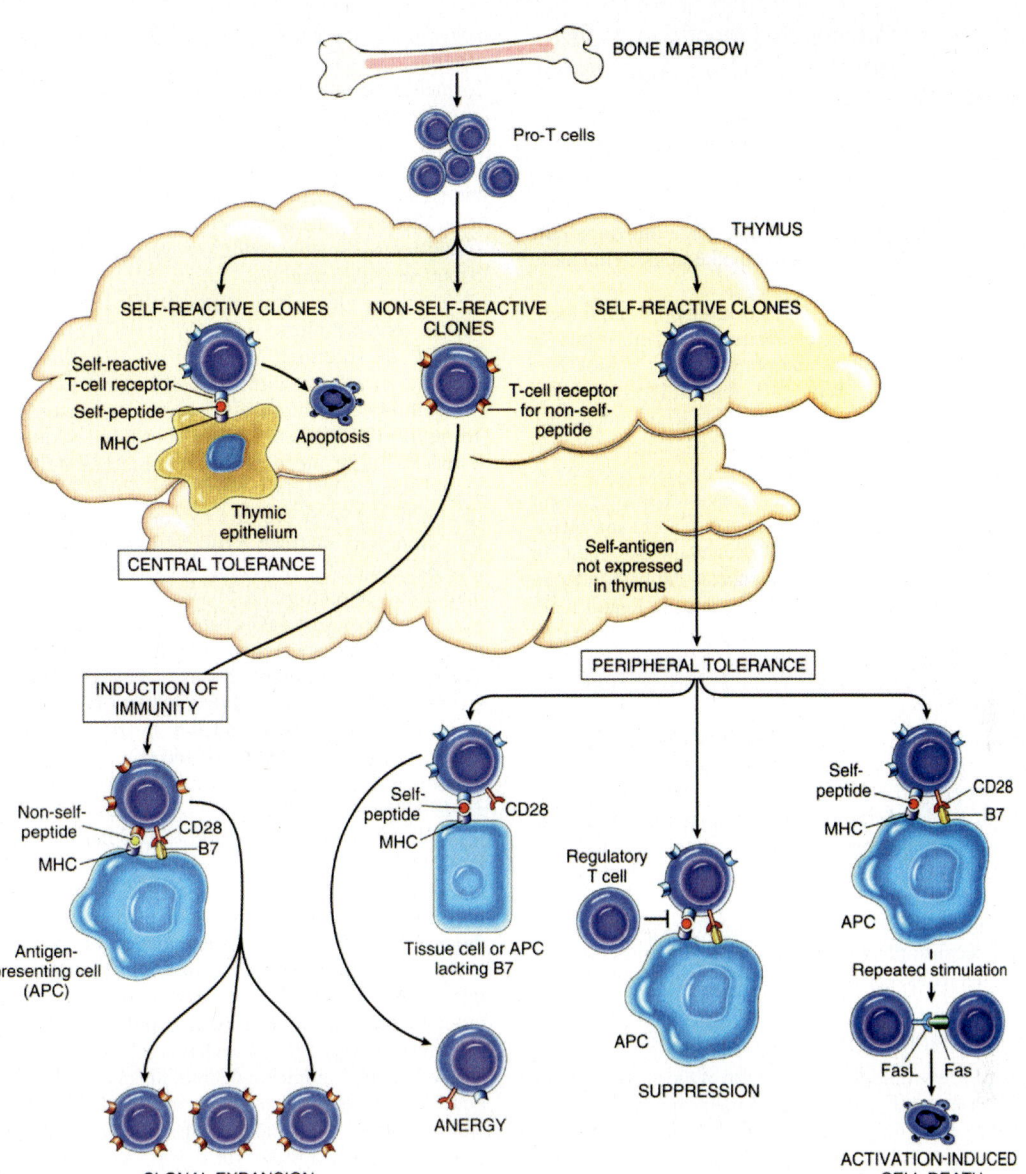

FIGURE 31.1 Schematic illustration of the mechanisms involved in central and peripheral tolerance. The principal mechanisms of tolerance in CD4+ T cells are shown. MHC, major histocompatibility complex. (Reprinted from Abbas AK, Diseases of immunity. In: Kumar V, Abbas AK, Fausto N, eds. *Robbins and Cotran Pathologic Basis of Disease.* 7th ed. Saunders; 2005:223-225. Copyright © 2005 Elsevier. With permission.)

activation and effector functions in part by the secretion of cytokines such as IL-10 and transforming growth factor-β. However, the precise mechanism of their action is unknown.

Clonal deletion by activation-induced cell death refers to the process by which CD4+ T cells that are activated by self-antigens may receive signals that cause apoptosis. Lymphocytes express Fas (CD95), a member of the tumor necrosis factor (TNF) receptor family, and activated lymphocytes express FasL, a membrane protein that is structurally homologous to the cytokine TNF. The engagement of Fas by FasL induces apoptosis of activated autoreactive T cells. Self-antigens that are abundant in peripheral tissues cause repeated and persistent stimulation of self-antigen–specific T cells, leading eventually to their elimination via Fas-mediated apoptosis. FasL on T cells engaging Fas on the B cells may also delete self-reactive B cells.[6]

Factors Affecting Initiation of Autoimmunity

Autoimmunity can be affected by a number of different factors, including the nature of the autoantigens, genetic associations, and environmental factors. In AIHA, autoantigenic T-cell epitopes have been mapped for the RhD autoantigen.[8] Although these autoantigenic sites may be a potential target for novel therapeutic interventions, the precise mechanism of disease initiation remains unclear. In addition, MHC class I and class II genes may predispose individuals to certain types of autoimmune disease. For example, the human leukocyte antigen (HLA)-DQ-6 molecule has been associated with AIHA. However, the genetic association is multifactorial as with most other autoimmune diseases. Finally, inflammatory stimuli such as viral and bacterial infections have been implicated as environmental triggers of autoimmunity, possibly because of antigenic mimicry leading to tolerance breakdown, that is, environmental or infectious agents may have molecular structures similar to self-antigens. Other possible mechanisms involve production of interferon γ during viral infection that causes upregulation of FcRI. Alternatively, viral infection may cause a change in the expression pattern of Fc receptors as a result of transcriptional activation or other mechanisms (discussed further under section Immunoglobulin G–mediated Red Blood Cell Destruction).[9]

Mechanism of Immune-Mediated Red Blood Cell Lysis

The most important features of RBC destruction by IgM and IgG antibodies are summarized in *Table 31.2*.

Immunoglobulin M–Mediated Red Blood Cell Destruction

Destruction of erythrocytes sensitized with IgM antibodies is mediated by the complement system, either directly by cytolysis or indirectly via interaction of RBC-bound activation and degradation fragments of C3 with specific receptors on reticuloendothelial cells, principally liver macrophages (Kupffer cells).

The pentameric structure of IgM enables efficient complement activation. High-titer IgM antibodies can cause direct intravascular hemolysis by generating the cytolytic membrane attack complex of complement on the RBC surface. With sufficient antibody density, complement activation may be robust enough to overwhelm the inhibitory activity of the complement-regulatory proteins DAF (CD55) and MIRL (CD59) on the RBC surface and result in hemolysis.[10] However, in most clinical situations, IgM antierythrocyte antibodies are present in sublytic quantities. Under these conditions, DAF (CD55) and MIRL (CD59) are able to prevent direct RBC lysis. Nonetheless, some C3b is deposited on the RBC surface as a consequence of the IgM-induced complement activation, and interactions of C3b and its ligand iC3b with their specific complement receptors (CRs) on liver macrophages (Kupffer cells) are ultimately responsible for the immune destruction of RBCs under sublytic conditions. *Table 31.3* summarizes the characteristics of various CRs.[10-12]

Although ligation of erythrocyte-bound C3b to CR1 on Kupffer cells may mediate some of the clearance, interaction between RBC-bound iC3b and macrophage CR3 is probably the principal mediator of extravascular destruction of complement-sensitized erythrocytes. Clearance of the complement-sensitized RBCs is likely mediated by phagocytosis, because the liver lacks the unique anatomy of the spleen and is thus unable to sequester cells. Once RBC-bound iC3b has been converted to C3dg (ligand for CR2), the RBCs are no longer subject to immune destruction because phagocytic cells do not express the specific receptor for C3dg. Thus, erythrocytes bearing only C3dg have a normal lifespan.[13,14]

Immunoglobulin G–Mediated Red Blood Cell Destruction

IgG is a relatively ineffective initiator of activation of the classical complement pathway. Consequently, direct complement-mediated cytolysis of RBCs induced by IgG antibodies is unusual (a notable exception is the Donath-Landsteiner (D-L) antibody of paroxysmal cold hemoglobinuria [PCH]). In the absence of complement activation, clearance of IgG-sensitized erythrocytes is primarily splenic. Two distinct processes appear to be involved. First, binding to Fc receptors expressed by tissue macrophages in the red pulp of the spleen can mediate direct and complete phagocytosis. Second, partial phagocytosis, in which the phagocytes remove a portion of the membrane, results in a decrease in the surface area to volume ratio and the consequent generation of spherocytes, the classic morphologic hallmark of immune hemolytic anemia. The loss of deformability as a consequence of spherocyte formation results in sequestration of the abnormal RBCs in the red pulp because the consequent rigidity limits their ability to traverse the splenic cords into the sinuses. The trapped spherocytes are vulnerable to phagocytosis by macrophages that are found in abundance in the splenic cords. In addition, the life span of the sequestered RBCs is shortened by the unfavorable metabolic environment found in the splenic cords (splenic conditioning). Once trapped, RBC destruction is complete within minutes.

The liver clears IgG-coated RBCs less efficiently than does the spleen. Nevertheless, the liver plays a clinically significant role in RBC destruction. The quantity of antibody fixed to the RBC roughly correlates with the site of destruction (smaller amounts of antibody lead mainly to splenic sequestration, whereas larger amounts of antibody lead to increased sequestration within the liver).[15,16] The more rapid clearance of RBCs sensitized with a higher density of IgG antibodies and the shift in clearance from the spleen to the liver are due to complement activation.[16] Although IgG alone can mediate RBC clearance, the concomitant presence of RBC-bound C3 fragments greatly enhances the rate of immune-mediated destruction.

Phagocytosis of IgG-coated RBCs occurs in the spleen and is mediated by surface receptors for the Fcγ region of the IgG molecule. There are three different classes of Fcγ receptors. FcγRI mediates in vitro cytotoxic activity. FcγRII inhibits B-lymphocyte and mast-cell activation. FcγRIII is responsible for phagocytosis, endocytosis, and antibody-dependent cell-mediated cytotoxicity and therefore plays a key role in hemolysis. The characteristics of FcγR are summarized in *Table 31.4*.

Of the four subclasses of IgG, IgG3 has the highest affinity for the FcγR and therefore is most efficient at causing extravascular hemolysis (IgG3 > IgG1 > IgG4 >>> IgG2).[17,18] The critical role of Fcγ receptors in immune destruction in vivo is further demonstrated by the therapeutic approach to management of AIHA and immune thrombocytopenic purpura (ITP). Treatment with corticosteroids, intravenous immunoglobulin G (IVIG), anti-D, and/or splenectomy is aimed at reducing the capacity of reticuloendothelial cells to mediate immune clearance of IgG-sensitized RBCs.[19] Administration of monoclonal antibody 2.4G2 in mice, which binds to and blocks mouse FcγRII and FcγRIII, allows rapid recovery after induction of AIHA, suggesting that alteration of the balance of stimulatory to inhibitory Fcγ receptors has a marked effect on disease progression and susceptibility. Understanding the detailed structure of the Fcγ receptors may lead to the development of novel therapeutic strategies. For example, molecules that inhibit the binding of the FcγR to an IgG-coated RBC or those that might inhibit the Fcγ receptor signaling at the different steps leading to phagocytosis may be useful therapeutic tools. Treatments that decrease expression of the activating Fcγ receptor or increase expression of the inhibitory Fcγ receptor may also be effective.[9]

Table 31.2. Red Cell Destruction by IgM and IgG Antibodies

Antibody	Intravascular Clearance	Extravascular Clearance Liver	Extravascular Clearance Spleen	Complement Dependency	Hemoglobinuria	Bilirubinemia	Specificity of Antiglobulin Test
IgM low titer[a]	+	+	−	+	±	+	Complement
IgM high titer[a]	+	−	−	+	+	+	Complement
IgG low titer[b]	−	−	+	−	−	+	Immunoglobulin
IgG high titer[b]	−	±	+	−	±	+	Immunoglobulin

[a]Anti-A or anti-B blood group antibodies are examples of IgM antibodies that can be present at low or high concentrations.
[b]Anti-Rh$_0$(D) is an example of an IgG antibody that can be present at low or high concentrations.

Table 31.3. Characteristics of Complement Receptors

Receptor	Characteristics	Complement Ligand	Cellular Distribution	Function
CR1 (CD35)	210-330 kDa Four allotypes Single-chain glycoprotein 30 SCRs	C3b (high affinity) C4b iC3b (weak affinity)	RBCs; neutrophils; mono-cytes; macrophages; B cells and some T cells, follicular dendritic cells; Langerhans cells; Kupfer cells	Regulates C3, C4, and C5 convertase of classic and alternative pathways of complements; factor 1 cofactor, RBC CR1, phago-cyte CR1
CR2 (CD21)	145 kDa; integral membrane glycoprotein 15 SCRs	C3dg, C3d	B cells, follicular dendritic cells	Immune modulation, cellu-lar receptor for the Epstein-Barr virus
CR3 (CD11b/CD18)	165 kDa (CD11b); 95 kDa (CD18); heterodimer	iC3b	Neutrophils, monocytes, macrophages, NK cells, cytotoxic T cells	Adherence and phagocytosis of opsonized RBCs
CR4 (CD11c/CD18)	150 kDa (CD11c); 95 kDa (CD18); heterodimer	iC3b	Neutrophils, monocytes, macrophages, NK cells, cytotoxic T cells	Undefined

NK, natural killer; RBC, red blood cell; SCR, short consensus repeat.

Table 31.4. Characteristics of Fcγ Receptors

Receptor	Characteristics	Affinity for IgG	Cellular Distribution	Function
FcγRI (CD64)	72 kDa; integral membrane gly-coprotein IgG	High ($1\text{-}3 \times 10^{-8}$ L/M)	Monocytes, tissue macro-phages, neutrophils	Binds monomeric IgG interfer-on-γ stimulated ADCC and reset-ting of IgG-coated RBCs; not essential for phagocytosis
FcγRII (CDw32)	40 kDa; integral membrane glycoprotein	Low (2×10^{-5} L/M)	Monocytes, tissue macro-phages, neutrophils, platelets, B cells	Binds aggregated IgG, mediates ADCC, weak mediator of reset-ting, important for phagocytosis
FcγRIII (CD16)	50-80 kDa; both integral mem-brane (FcγRIIIa) and glycosyl phosphatidylinositol-anchored (FcγRIIIb) forms	Low (5×10^{-5} L/M)	Neutrophils (FcγRIIIb), tissue macrophages, NK cells (FcγIIIa)	Binds aggregated IgG, important for clearance of IgG-sensitized RBCs

ADCC, antibody-dependent cell-mediated cytotoxicity; NK, natural killer; RBC, red blood cell.

Disorders of Red Blood Cells

Laboratory Diagnosis

Two criteria must be met to diagnose AIHA: clinical or laboratory evi-dence of hemolysis and serologic evidence of an autoantibody.

Common Laboratory Features

The basic tests to evaluate hemolysis include a complete blood count (CBC) with peripheral smear, bilirubin, lactate dehydro-genase (LDH, particularly isoenzyme 1), haptoglobin, and urine hemoglobin or hemosiderin. Universal signs of hemolysis include decreased serum hemoglobin and hematocrit, increased serum LDH and unconjugated bilirubin, and polychromasia and reticu-locytosis given adequate hematopoietic reserve. Haptoglobin is typically reduced, although sequential levels should be assessed because the protein is an acute-phase reactant and thereby depen-dent on both hepatic function and systemic stress. Intravascular hemolysis further manifests with increased free hemoglobinemia, increased hemoglobinuria, hemosiderinuria, methemalbumin-emia, and decreased serum haptoglobin. Hemoglobinemia is usu-ally evident in the specimen collection tube as a distinctly red- or pink-tinged serum or plasma. Hemolysis in AIHA can be either intravascular or extravascular. Typically, intravascular hemolysis is rapid and aggressive, whereas extravascular hemolysis is milder. The peripheral blood smear may reveal spherocytes in warm AIHA or RBC agglutination in cold AIHA.

Serologic Investigation

The demonstration of RBC surface-bound immunoglobulin or evidence of complement fixation supports the diagnosis of immune-mediated RBC destruction. IgM-coated RBCs may spontaneously agglutinate because the pentameric antibody can directly cross-link RBCs. The capability of IgM antibodies to agglutinate saline-suspended RBCs without additional reagents led to the traditional terminology of "com-plete" antibodies. In contrast, IgG antibodies typically require anti-human globulin (AHG) as a cofactor to agglutinate saline-suspended RBCs and are thus termed "incomplete" antibodies.

The explanation for this serologic difference lies in the physi-cal properties of the RBCs and the antibody molecules involved. Erythrocytes have a strong net negative surface charge ("zeta poten-tial") produced by the sialoglycoprotein coat, such that the shortest separation attainable between two RBCs is approximately 18 nm. Other factors may also play a role in maintaining the separation dis-tance, such as water that is tightly bound to the surface of the RBCs. IgM molecules, with their large pentameric structure, create a 30-nm distance between adjacent binding sites and can therefore bridge two RBCs. The smaller IgG can accommodate a span of only 12 nm between antigen-recognition sites and thus usually cannot lead to agglutination alone.[20] Exogenous AHG can bridge IgG molecules, which explains the term "incomplete." However, some IgG antibod-ies can indeed agglutinate RBCs (eg, anti-A, anti-B, and anti-M), revealing the influence on agglutination of the number of antigen sites per RBC[21] and how far the antigenic determinants project from the surface of the RBC. The blood group–defining A and B oligosaccharides extend well beyond the lipid bilayer membrane.[22] In addition to their relative abundance, they are also close together on the RBC surface, potentiating agglutination. The critical number of IgG molecules required to agglutinate RBCs is ~7000 to 20,000 per RBC, whereas the requisite number of IgM molecules is only 25 to 50 per RBC.[23,24] Although serologic tricks such as enzyme treatment, centrifugation, and addition of substances such as albumin, polyvinylpyrrolidone (PVP), and dextran have been used to enhance agglutination by IgG antibodies, the most common way to determine the presence of immune system components on RBCs is with the direct antiglobulin test (DAT, direct Coombs).

Direct Antiglobulin Test (Direct Coombs Test)

In 1908, Moreschi described antiglobulin reactions as an aid to RBC agglutination.[25] This work remained largely unnoticed until 1945, when the investigation of anti-RBC antibodies was revolutionized with the development of the antiglobulin test by Coombs et al[26] and its role in the identification of maternal IgG on fetal RBCs in hemolytic disease of the newborn in 1946.[27] The principle of the DAT is quite simple. To ascertain whether RBCs carry surface-bound immunoglobulin and/or complement, antisera with reactivity to human immunoglobulin and/or complement molecules is added to a suspension of the RBCs in question, providing the necessary cross-link to elicit agglutination. *Figure 31.2* illustrates the principle of the test.[28] An ethylenediaminetetra-acetic acid–collected sample from the patient is used to prevent subsequent complement adherence to the RBC membrane in vitro. The test is performed by first washing the RBCs to remove nonspecifically adhered proteins. Following the addition of AHG, the mixture is centrifuged to enhance agglutination. The result is interpreted by resuspending the RBCs gently and observing carefully for clumps. Magnifying mirrors or low-power microscopy may aid in discerning weak reactions. Negative reactions are further incubated at room temperature, centrifuged, and read again, because this additional incubation promotes positive reactions in the presence of the complement.[29] Initial testing is done with polyspecific AHG (antisera), which contain anti-IgG, anti-C3d, and, occasionally, some anti-light-chain activity. Monospecific reagents differentiate between IgG and C3d to further define the specificity. Other monospecific antisera are available for C3b, C4b, C4d, and IgG heavy chain.[30] Specific antiserum for IgM or IgA is rarely used, because IgM is not usually found attached to the RBC surface ex vivo and IgA is very rarely a cause of immunoglobulin coating by itself.[31,32] The US Food and Drug Administration has licensed monoclonal reagents, the most common of which is anti-C3d, which do not cross-react with other complement components.[30]

Early DAT methodology suffered from relative insensitivity. More recent developments have improved the sensitivity for RBC-bound immunoglobulin and complement. The traditional tube method described earlier detects a lower limit of 150 to 200 IgG molecules per RBC.[33] With PVP enhancement and an autoanalyzer, the detection limit decreases to as few as eight IgG per RBC producing 5% agglutination. If bromelin is added as well, the sensitivity increases even further, with one IgG per RBC producing 5% agglutination and three IgG per RBC producing 50% agglutination.[34] Additional acceptable techniques include flow cytometry, enzyme-linked antiglobulin tests (enzyme-linked immunosorbent assay), radioimmunoassays using ^{125}I-labeled anti-IgG or staphylococcal protein A, solid-phase techniques using microtiter plates, and gel testing.[35] However, only the tube test, solid-phase test, and gel tests are in common use. Of these, the solid-phase and gel tests are the most standardized and have largely replaced older tube testing technology.

A positive DAT does not always mean decreased RBC survival. Most patients with a positive DAT have no obvious clinical signs of hemolytic anemia. DAT interpretation must consider the context of clinical history and other laboratory findings. Outside of AIHA, a positive DAT may also be seen with (a) alloantibodies in a recipient of

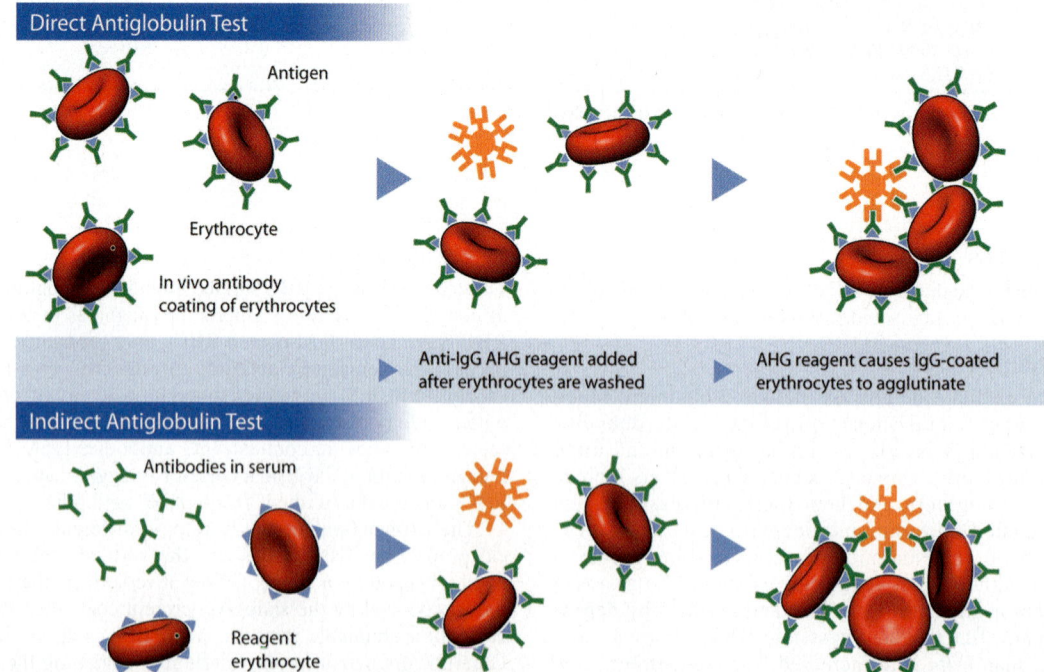

FIGURE 31.2 Direct antiglobulin test (DAT) and indirect antiglobulin test (IAT). The DAT reflects in vivo antibody sensitization of RBCs. Erythrocytes are washed to remove any unbound antibodies, and anti-IgG antihuman globulin (AHG) reagent is then added. IgG antibodies cannot cause direct RBC agglutination, but IgG-coated RBCs will agglutinate in the presence of AHG-containing anti-IgG. This test can also be performed using anticomplement AHG reagent. If it is present, RBC-bound IgG can be eluted for specificity determination. The IAT is used to detect the presence of IgG antibodies in serum (in vitro sensitization). Reagent RBCs are incubated in the presence of serum that may contain antibodies. If they are present, antibodies bind to their target antigens on the reagent RBCs. After incubation, the RBCs are washed to remove unbound antibodies. Anti-IgG AHG reagent is added and will cause IgG-coated erythrocytes to agglutinate. (From Zarandona JM, Yazer MH. Teaching case report. The role of the Coombs test in evaluating hemolysis in adults. *Can Med Assoc J.* 2006;174(3):305-307. Copyright © 2006 CMA Media Inc. or its licensors.)

RBC or plasma transfusion, (b) antibodies from maternal circulation that cross the placenta and coat the fetal RBCs, (c) antibodies directed against certain drugs that bind to the RBC membrane (eg, penicillin), (d) nonspecifically adsorbed proteins including immunoglobulins and Wharton jelly, (e) RBC-bound complement, and (f) antibodies produced by passenger lymphocytes in transplanted organs or hematopoietic components. Further evaluation of a positive DAT in a patient with clinical and laboratory evidence of hemolysis includes testing for clinically significant antibodies to RBC antigens and testing the eluate. *Figure 31.3* illustrates an approach to the evaluation of a positive DAT.[29] A negative DAT, on the other hand, does not exclude AIHA. Possible causes of a negative DAT with clinical evidence of hemolysis include an IgA or IgM autoantibody, insufficient antibody molecules for detection, and low-affinity autoantibodies.[35] Repeat testing, enhancement techniques, and the use of nonroutine reagents may be required when the clinical suspicion is strong.[29]

Indirect Antiglobulin Test (Indirect Coombs Test)

Approximately 80% of patients with AIHA have autoantibodies in their serum as well as on their RBCs.[36] The antibodies in their serum or plasma and the antibodies eluted from their RBCs (the "eluate") are detected by the indirect antiglobulin test (IAT; more commonly known as the antibody screen). Unlike the DAT, which uses patient RBCs with reagent serum, the IAT tests patient serum against reagent RBCs. Immunoglobulin from the patient serum attaches to the reagent RBCs and is detected with antiglobulin sera, which cross-link the RBCs together and produce agglutination, as in the DAT (see *Figure 31.2*).[28]

Warm autoantibodies are typically panagglutinins, reacting with all cells in the diagnostic RBC panel (ie, panreactive). Formerly, panagglutinins were believed to react with a basic determinant of the Rh antigen system because they do not react with the very rare Rh_{null} RBCs, which do not express Rh antigens.[37] However, as more eluates are studied with a broader population of rare null phenotypes, it has been shown that, in addition to Rh, autoantibodies react to LW antigens, glycophorins A, B, C, and D, and, very rarely, Kidd or Kell blood group system antigens.[38] A small number of case reports describing AIHA associated with ABO antigens exist.[39,40]

Daratumumab, a monoclonal antibody used to treat relapsed/refractory multiple myeloma, can interfere with the IAT.[41] The drug works by targeting the CD38 portion of malignant cells. However, RBCs show variable expression of CD38 and cause the drug to attach to the RBC reagent cells used in the IAT, causing the appearance of a panreactive antibody that can mimic a warm-reactive autoantibody. The AABB issued a memorandum on how blood banks can effectively address panreactivity caused by daratumumab. Dithiothreitol (DTT), a common reagent in blood banks, can be used as an inexpensive and practical way to dissolve panreactivity caused by daratumumab. However, DTT is known to destroy the Kell antigen blood group and other less frequently encountered blood group antigens, causing anti-Kell antibodies to be missed. As a precaution, blood banks may issue Kell phenotype matched or Kell negative units to circumvent this problem. Other promising alternative solutions, such as umbilical cord RBC screening cells and neutralization, are not widely available yet.

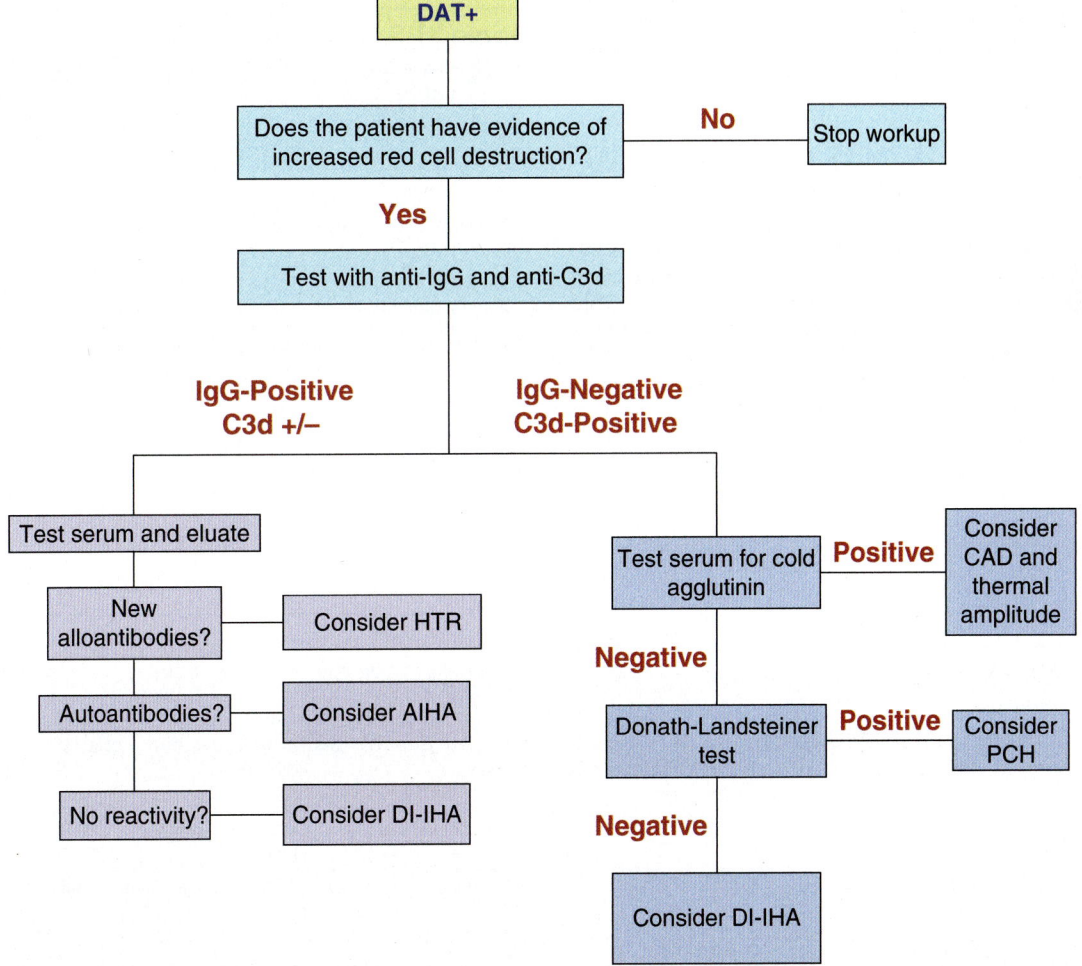

FIGURE 31.3 Flowchart suggesting a rational clinical laboratory approach for investigating a positive direct antiglobulin test (DAT). AIHA, autoimmune hemolytic anemia; CAD, cold agglutinin disease; DI-IHA, drug-induced immune hemolytic anemia; HTR, hemolytic transfusion reaction; PCH, paroxysmal cold hemoglobinuria. (Modified with permission from Brecher ME, ed. *Technical Manual.* 15th ed. American Association of Blood Banks; 2005:480. Appendix 20-1. Copyright © 2005 by AABB.)

Disorders of Red Blood Cells

Elution

If the DAT is positive for RBC-bound antibody, that antibody can be eluted (removed) from the RBC with the aid of acid or xylene, and any binding specificities can be further investigated with a reagent red cell panel. Elutions are not typically performed on DAT specimens positive only for complement, because these molecules do not exhibit antigen specificity. Occasionally, however, when antibody presence is suspected but perhaps at too low a concentration to be detected on the RBCs, eluates may show reactivity. Elution tends to produce a more concentrated antibody solution, so reactions are often stronger. Once the antibody is in solution, indirect antiglobulin techniques may help define the antibody characteristics.[29]

Other Serologic Techniques

Generally, autoantibodies are panreactive, whereas alloantibodies exhibit antigen specificity, reacting only with specific antigen-positive RBCs. In certain situations, an autoantibody may mimic an alloantibody. For example, an alloantibody to a high-incidence antigen in a posttransfusion setting can mimic an autoantibody with a positive DAT (mixed field) and reactions with all panel cells. In addition, autoantibodies may exhibit apparent specificity. Autoadsorption and antigenic phenotyping can help differentiate autoantibodies and alloantibodies, especially if the patient has not been transfused recently. Autoadsorption uses autologous RBCs to adsorb autoantibodies before repeating serum testing for alloantibodies. If an antibody exhibits specificity, demonstration that autologous RBCs are negative for the corresponding antigen confirms the alloantibody; in the absence of a recent transfusion, a positive result suggests that it is an autoantibody. Autoadsorption can also be used to crossmatch donor RBC units for patients with warm autoantibodies who have not been recently transfused.[29]

IMMUNE HEMOLYTIC ANEMIAS CAUSED BY COLD-ACTIVE ANTIBODIES

Cold-active antibodies exhibit greater titer and RBC-binding activity as the temperature decreases toward 0 °C. Two different clinical syndromes are manifested from cold autoimmune antibodies. Cold agglutinin disease (CAD) is associated with IgM antibodies usually directed at the RBC *I* antigen. CAD typically occurs in adult patients and may be primary or secondary to another disease process, usually infectious. In contrast, PCH is caused by an IgG hemolysin, the D-L antibody.[42] Both PCH and CAD are less common than warm AIHA and make up approximately 20% or less of AIHAs (see *Tables 31.5* and *31.6*).

Cold Agglutinin Disease

Although Landsteiner first described cold agglutinins in 1903,[43] it was not until the late 1940s and early 1950s that the connection between cold autoantibodies and RBC destruction was firmly made. In the 1950s, Schubothe coined the term "CAD," and the disorder became recognized as a separate entity from other acquired hemolytic processes.[44] The responsible pathologic IgM antibodies are distinguished from naturally occurring cold autoantibodies by their titer and *thermal amplitude,* a term describing the range of temperatures over which the antibody is reactive. Natural cold autoantibodies occur with titers less than 1:64 at 4 °C and have little to no activity at higher temperatures. However, pathologic cold agglutinins typically have titers well over 1:512 and may react at 28 to 31 °C (peripheral body temperature) or even up to 37 °C[31] (see *Table 31.6* and *Figure 31.4*).

Primary vs Secondary Cold Agglutinin Disease

Primary or idiopathic CAD is typically an affliction of older adults, with a peak incidence around age 70 years.[44] Both sexes are affected, but women predominate.[45] A monoclonal IgMκ antibody is the usual culprit, and, as with other monoclonal gammopathies of unknown significance, may be a harbinger of future B-cell neoplasms. Most commonly, patients tolerate a relatively benign, waxing and waning hemolytic anemia.

Patients with Waldenström macroglobulinemia or other B-cell neoplasms may produce monoclonal anti-RBC antibodies with cold reactivity. As in primary CAD, they are nearly always IgMκ. This type of secondary CAD may be effectively treated with antineoplastic

Table 31.5. Cold Autoantibodies

	Primary Cold Agglutinin Disease	Secondary Cold Autoantibodies	Paroxysmal Cold Hemoglobinuria
Immunoglobulin	IgM	IgM	IgG
Clonality	Monoclonal	Monoclonal or polyclonal	Polyclonal
Direct antiglobulin test	C3	C3	C3
Hemolysis	Chronic, mild	Self-limited, mild to severe	Episodic, self-limited, mild to severe
Target RBC antigen	*I*	*I, i*	*P*

RBC, red blood cell.

Table 31.6. Serologic Overview of Hemolytic Anemias

	Cold Agglutinin Disease	Paroxysmal Cold Hemoglobinuria	Mixed Warm and Cold Autoimmune Hemolytic Anemia	Warm Autoimmune Hemolytic Anemia	Drug-Induced Hemolytic Anemia
Percentage of cases	16%-32%	32% (children); rare in adults	7%-8%	40%-70%	12%-18%
Direct antiglobulin test	C3	C3	IgG ± complement	IgG ± C3; rarely C3 alone	IgG or C3; occasionally IgG ± C3
Ig	IgM	IgG	IgG, IgM	IgG, occasionally with IgA or IgM	IgG
RBC eluate	Nonreactive	Nonreactive	IgG	IgG	IgG or nonreactive
Antibody specificity	*I > i >> Pr*	*P*	Panreactive	Panagglutinin	Rh related
			Unclear > I > others	Rarely Rh	Drug dependent

RBC, red blood cell.

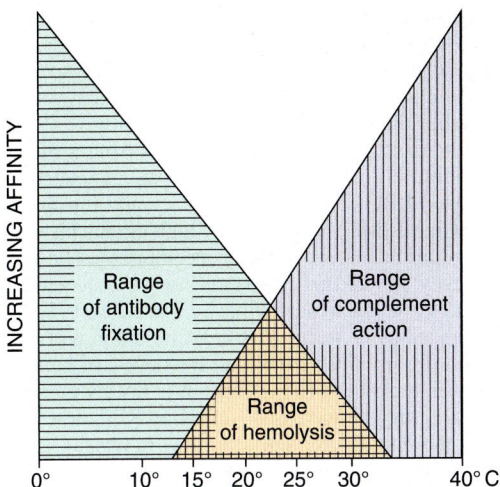

FIGURE 31.4 Temperature ranges for cold agglutinin fixation and lytic complement action. (Reprinted from Schubothe H. The cold hemagglutinin disease. *Semin Hematol.* 1966;3(1):27-47. Copyright © 1966 Elsevier. With permission.)

Table 31.7. **Secondary Cold Agglutinin Disease**

Neoplasms
Waldenström macroglobulinemia
Angioimmunoblastic lymphoma
Other lymphomas
Chronic lymphocytic leukemia
Kaposi sarcoma
Myeloma
Nonhematologic malignancy (rare)
Infections
Mycoplasma pneumoniae
Mononucleosis (Epstein-Barr virus)
Adenovirus
Cytomegalovirus
Encephalitis
Influenza viruses
Rubella
Varicella
Human immunodeficiency virus
Mumps
Ornithosis
Legionnaires disease
Escherichia coli
Subacute bacterial endocarditis
Listeriosis
Syphilis
Trypanosomiasis
Malaria
Other
Autoimmune diseases
Tropical eosinophilia

chemotherapy. A return of hemolysis may herald a tumor relapse. Other non-B-cell tumors reported in association with cold antibody production include squamous cell carcinoma of the lung, metastatic adrenal adenocarcinoma, metastatic adenocarcinoma of the colon, basal cell carcinoma, and a mixed parotid tumor.[46]

Another scenario of secondary cold autoantibody hemolysis occurs after *Mycoplasma pneumoniae* infection or infectious mononucleosis and is more commonly seen in younger adults. This transient, self-limited process is mediated by polyclonal IgM (κ or γ), lasts a few weeks, and seldom requires more than supportive care. In rare cases, massive intravascular hemolysis and acute renal failure may be seen (see *Table 31.7*).

The novel severe acute respiratory syndrome coronavirus 2 (SARS-CoV-2) responsible for coronavirus disease 2019 (COVID-19) has also been associated with CAD.[47,48] Cases have been seen more commonly in adults and more rarely in children.[49] The pathophysiology is postulated to be related to SARS-CoV-2 associated immunologic and inflammation activation. The degree of hemolytic anemia can be severe, requiring several RBC transfusions.[49,50]

Antibody Characteristics

Immunochemistry and Origin

As stated earlier, nearly all cold agglutinins are IgM. A few reports of IgG or IgA agglutinins are recorded, and a mixed IgM-IgG has been seen in infectious mononucleosis and angioimmunoblastic lymphadenopathy.[51] Those patients with non-IgM antibodies are more likely to have cold autoantibody hemolysis secondary to another disease and are less likely to display specificity for the *I* antigen.[45,52]

Anti-idiotypic antibodies and direct nucleotide sequencing of the rearranged immunoglobulin variable-region genes have revealed significant cross-reactivity and homologies among cold autoantibodies with similar specificity.[53,54] For instance, the monoclonal anti-idiotypic antibody 9G4 recognizes an idiotypic determinant present on the heavy chains of both anti-*I* and anti-*i* cold agglutinins as well as the responsible neoplastic B cells.[55] Essentially all pathologic anti-*I* and anti-*i* cold agglutinins are derived from a distinct subset of heavy-chain variable-region genes called V_H4 family genes, specifically V_H4-21.[56] In 40% of the patients, a circulating B-cell clone can be identified with a distinctive karyotypic marker (trisomy 3q11-q29; trisomy 12; or 48XX+3+12). The chromosomal abnormalities were associated with chronic idiopathic cold agglutinin syndrome as well as with monoclonal cold agglutinins secondary to a neoplasm.[57-59] In addition, the cold agglutinins have the same serologic specificity and isoelectric focusing spectrotype and are therefore likely derived from a preneoplastic or neoplastic B-cell clone.[7]

I/i Blood Group System Specificity

More than 90% of cold-active antibodies have the *I* antigen as their target on the RBC, and the *i* antigen is the binding site for a significant portion of the remaining 10%.[31] The closely related *I/i* antigens are high-frequency carbohydrates similar to the ABO antigens. The RBC surface densities of *I* and *i* are inversely proportional, with neonatal RBCs exclusively expressing large amounts of *i* antigen, usually converting to exclusively *I* antigen by 18 months of age. Consequently, adult RBCs are used to detect anti-*I* agglutinins and cord RBCs are needed to detect anti-*i* agglutinins. Extremely rare cases have been described of adults who never express *I* antigen on the RBCs. Other uncommon but reported antigen targets include *Pr*. Anti-Pr cold agglutinins tend to be high titer, with a wide thermal range, and cause symptomatic anemia.[60,61] Other infrequent targets are *Gd, Fl, Vo, Li, Sa, Lud, M, N, Me, Om, D, Sd*ᵃ, and *P*.[38,45,62] The fact that *M. pneumoniae* induces anti-*I* antibodies in the majority of patients is potentially related to the finding that sialylated *I/i* antigens serve as specific *Mycoplasma* receptors.[63] Minor modification of this antigen may incite autoantibodies. Another theory suggests that an *I*-like antigen appears on the organism itself, and cross-reacting antibodies lead to RBC lysis.[64] Despite the high rate of antibody production, clinically significant hemolysis occurs in very few patients.[65] Infectious mononucleosis is also associated with CAD, but to a much lesser degree than *Mycoplasma*. Only 0.1% to 3.0% of patients with mononucleosis have clinical hemolysis,[66] although anti-i is present in 8% to 69% of sera postinfection.[67,68] Therefore, the majority of patients with antibodies are asymptomatic. Anti-I activity is usually noted as well but not to the same degree. Also, anti-Pr and anti-N have been reported.[69] Both IgM and IgG antibodies as well as IgM rheumatoid-like factors reacting with IgG may act as cold agglutinins after infectious mononucleosis.[70,71] See *Table 31.7* for a list of other infectious diseases associated with cold agglutinins, most of which are anti-I, although anti-i has been seen in cytomegalovirus infections and in lymphomas.[72]

Functional Characteristics

Cold agglutinins attach to the RBC in the cooler peripheral circulation. As the blood returns to the warmer core circulation, the antibody dissociates from the RBC. Antibodies that attach, fix complement, and then dissociate are free to attack another erythrocyte and begin the process again.[73] Complement fixation and activation, which are responsible for the destruction of the RBCs, are far more efficient at the warmer core temperatures. However, with a high antibody titer and wide thermal amplitude, there may be sufficient temperature overlap to produce hemolysis at 22 ± 10 °C[44] (see *Figure 31.4*). Because of this diversity of temperature requirements for optimal activity of the antibody and complement, RBC destruction is usually not particularly severe with cold autoantibodies. Quite impressive exceptions occur, and these are typically the antibodies with either high titers (>1:1000) or activity up to 37 °C even in the face of modest titers. Thermal amplitude is a better predictor of hemolysis than titer.[51,74] High-titer cold agglutinins with a narrow thermal amplitude may produce a clinical picture with bursts of hemolysis associated with exposure to cold, often manifested as intermittent hemoglobinuria between quiescent periods.[73]

A frequent misconception about cold agglutinins is the assumption that they are cryoglobulins, whereas in fact they are two distinct disease processes. Both may cause cyanosis and Raynaud phenomenon in cooler temperatures. However, cryoglobulins do not fix complement on the RBCs or lead to hemolysis.

Clinical Manifestations

Mild, chronic hemolytic anemia with exacerbations in the winter is the general rule for CAD. Rarely does the hemoglobin drop below 7 g/dL.[75] Pallor and jaundice may occur if the rate of hemolysis is greater than the endogenous capability to metabolize bilirubin.[45] Some patients have intermittent bursts of hemolysis associated with hemoglobinemia and hemoglobinuria on exposure to cold and may be forced to move to warmer climates to minimize attacks. Acrocyanosis can occur from agglutination of RBCs in the cooler vessels of the hands, ears, nose, and feet.[31,45] Digits may become cold, stiff, painful, or numb and may turn purplish. Limbs may manifest *livedo reticularis*, a mottled appearance that is readily reversible upon warming of the affected area. Only rarely does actual gangrene of the digits develop, and nearly all of these cases have an associated cryoglobulin.[76] A minority of patients with chronic CAD have mild splenomegaly or hepatomegaly. The spleen may be enlarged or more frequently palpable in secondary cold agglutinins because of lymphoma or infectious mononucleosis.[45]

If hemolysis does occur after *Mycoplasma* infections, it typically begins during the postpneumonia recovery period when cold autoantibody titers are peaking. The process, even if severe, resolves spontaneously within 1 to 3 weeks.[31] Hemolytic anemia after infectious mononucleosis may begin with the onset of illness or within the next 3 weeks.[45] The self-limited, postinfectious CAD tends to affect younger patients, whereas the chronic idiopathic form is a disease of the elderly, with peak incidence at age 70 years.[44]

Laboratory Features

Mild chronic anemia is the rule, but the hemoglobin may fall to 5 to 6 g/dL, especially in the winter months in cold climates. The peripheral smear, if not obtained from a carefully collected prewarmed specimen properly maintained warm until spread on a warm slide, may show significant agglutination and RBC clumping under magnification. Occasionally, clumping is so extensive as to be grossly visible without magnification and may even preclude an adequate smear examination. Agglutinates are frequently visible in the specimen tube and can appear to be a large clot. Dissolution with warming demonstrates that the clumped and clotted appearance is the result of a cold agglutinin rather than Rouleaux formation or fibrin strands. Often, the first suspicion of a cold agglutinin comes from a failed attempt to obtain a valid RBC count and indices on an automated CBC. The initially reported RBC count is often artifactually low and the mean corpuscular volume (MCV) artifactually high, producing a spuriously high mean corpuscular hemoglobin concentration. The reticulocyte count is modestly elevated except in rare cases of concomitant marrow failure, such as those due to parvovirus B19 infection.[77] Spherocytosis is not pronounced as in warm AIHA. White blood cell (WBC) and platelet counts are usually normal, but low levels of both have been reported,[45] as has leukocytosis.[45] Bilirubin is mildly elevated, rarely >3 mg/dL. LDH may be increased (reflecting RBC destruction), and complement and haptoglobin are often low or absent. During brisk hemolysis, hemoglobinuria and hemoglobinemia are manifest. The DAT is positive, with polyspecific and anticomplement antisera. As above, IgM has dissociated and is not detectable. In extremely rare cases, the antibody involved is IgG or IgA, either alone or in addition to IgM.[31,45] Mixed warm and cold autoantibodies are not rare (discussed later). Titers measured at 4 °C may range from 1:1000 to 1:1,000,000, although typical values are between 1:1000 and 1:500,000. Much lower levels can be clinically significant if activity is measurable at 37 °C. Postinfectious CAD titers are lower (<1:4000) than the chronic idiopathic or lymphoma-associated varieties. In patients with monoclonal IgM, evaluation of serum proteins frequently reveals an M spike, shown by serial observations to be stable in the chronic idiopathic disease.[78]

Management

Primary Cold Agglutinin Disease

Because of the generally mild chronic nature of the anemia, the majority of patients need no specific therapy other than the general principle of avoiding temperatures below those at which their antibody shows activity. In some cases, this may necessitate a move to a warmer climate. For patients with more severe anemia and cardiovascular compromise, aggressive therapy is indicated.

B Cell–Directed Regimens

Rituximab, a chimeric human/murine monoclonal CD20 antibody, has emerged as the first-line therapy success in CAD in several case reports and series.[79,80] The proposed mechanism of action involves complement-dependent cytotoxicity, antibody-dependent cellular cytotoxicity, direct apoptotic effects, and inhibition of B-cell proliferation. The most effective and best-evaluated treatment is rituximab in standard lymphoma dose (375 mg/m² each week for 4 weeks). Berentsen et al, in an open, uncontrolled prospective phase 2 study of rituximab in CAD showed that 20 of 27 patients responded with a median duration of response of 11 months.[81] Most patients who relapsed responded to retreatment with rituximab. Similar results were obtained by other studies.[82] In some pediatric patients, success was achieved with just two infusions.[83]

Therapy with fludarabine and rituximab has been evaluated in a limited number of patients refractory to rituximab with variable response.[84] However, fludarabine has been associated with grade 3 and 4 neutropenia, along with frequent infections.[80,84] Combination bendamustine and rituximab has also been studied, also with variable responses; there are also reports of grade 3 and 4 neutropenia, although with fewer infections.[85,86] In summary, rituximab is an efficacious, well-tolerated treatment that is associated with high response rates, although complete and sustained remissions are uncommon. In refractory patients, combination with fludarabine or bendamustine is an option.

Immunosuppressive and Steroid Therapy

Previous therapies aimed to suppress production of aberrant IgM protein. Treatments included corticosteroids, alkylating agents, and purine nucleoside analogs. Case series of corticosteroid therapy in CAD report response rates no greater than 14%. The need for high doses of corticosteroids limits their viability as a long-term treatment.[85,87] Several small series have documented a poor clinical response to alkylating agents and have also noted the need for long-term exposure, with clinically significant adverse effects in those who respond.

Plasmapheresis. Given the predominantly intravascular distribution of IgM, a logical conclusion would be that plasmapheresis or plasma exchange should provide rapid relief from hemolysis due to cold autoantibodies. Unfortunately, the results have been somewhat disappointing.[88,89] Simply removing the circulating antibody does not diminish ongoing endogenous antibody production, so improvements are transient at best. In patients with chronic CAD, plasmapheresis should probably be combined with immunosuppressive therapy in an attempt to decrease antibody production.[90] Successful use of plasmapheresis to temporarily decrease cold agglutinin titers to permit safe coronary artery bypass surgery has been reported.[91] Other reports of successful cardiac surgery involving warm cardioplegia have circumvented the need for cold exposure and thus the risk of hemolysis.[92,93] Cryofiltration apheresis has been used for acute exacerbations and for surgical procedures requiring hypothermia, such as coronary artery bypass surgery with cardioplegia. In one small study, two of five such patients who received cryofiltration apheresis had a favorable response with a reduction in titer.[94]

Blood Transfusion. Although most patients with CAD have mild anemia and do not need transfusion, RBC support may be required in patients who are clinically symptomatic or severely anemic.[95] Patients with high-titer or wide-thermal-amplitude antibodies can pose extremely difficult serologic problems for the blood bank laboratory. Testing needs to be performed carefully at 37 °C to minimize the effects of the cold agglutinin so that a search for alloantibodies may be properly performed.[31] This still does not eliminate interference from some particularly pesky autoantibodies. Time-consuming and technically challenging cold autoadsorptions may be necessary to rule out the presence of underlying alloantibodies. Occasionally, incompatible units may need to be issued because of residual agglutination from the cold autoantibody. Most cold agglutinins are directed at the *I* antigen, which is present on nearly all adult donor RBCs. Locating *i* adult RBCs (ie, *I*-negative) is not practical because of their extreme rarity. Reports have documented *i* adult RBCs effectiveness and lack thereof.[96,97] If transfusion is necessary to treat significant cardiovascular compromise, RBC infusion through an in-line blood warmer at 37 °C is recommended.[97] Uncontrolled heating of RBC products is quite dangerous because of the damaging effects of excessive heat and should be avoided. If blood warmers are not available, transfusion may still be accomplished by the slow infusion of room temperature RBCs into a large vein while keeping the patient warm.[31,45]

Splenectomy. Given that most CAD-induced RBC destruction is hepatic, it should be no surprise that splenectomy has been quite ineffective in treating CAD and is therefore not advised. In the rare patient who has the unusual serologic characteristic of hemolysins reactive at 37 °C as well as agglutinating activity at cooler temperatures, splenectomy may be of some benefit.[31]

Complement Inhibition. Because the hemolytic anemia of cold reactive antibodies is mediated by complement, the use of anti-C5 reagents (eg, eculizumab) and other complement-modifying agents may be of benefit.[80,85,98] Eculizumab is a monoclonal antibody used to treat paroxysmal nocturnal hemoglobinuria; it binds to complement protein C5, inhibiting formation of the terminal complement complex. Roth et al described eculizumab use in 12 patients with transfusion-dependent CAD that was refractory to rituximab.[99] However, as C-5 blockade does not affect the C3b-induced extravascular hemolysis, most patients in the study only had a small hemoglobin improvement.[99]

Shi et al published a study demonstrating that a mouse monoclonal anti-C1s antibody (TNT003) effectively blocked classical complement pathway activation in an in vitro system.[100] This led to the development of the humanized monoclonal antibody sutimlimab (TNT009). A small clinical trial using sutimlimab in patients with CAD demonstrated rapid hemoglobin increases of >2 g/dL and normalization of

bilirubin.[101,102] Patients in the sutimlimab study were vaccinated against encapsulated organisms, and there were no reported meningococcal infections.[102]

Complement inhibition does have its limitations. The ischemic symptoms reported in CAD are not complement mediated and therefore are not alleviated. Furthermore, complement inhibitors are not curative and therefore will have to be continued indefinitely. In some situations, complement inhibition may be useful as a bridge to B cell–directed treatment.[103]

Secondary Cold Agglutinin Disease

Hemolysis from infection-associated cold agglutinins lasts for 2 to 3 weeks, and therapy is typically not required. The exception has been seen in CAD associated with SARS-CoV-2 infection, in which patients have been reported to have severe anemia requiring multiple transfusions.[49,50] Given the transient nature of the antibody, even in the rare patient with significant hemolysis, supportive measures such as transfusion and plasmapheresis should suffice. Attempts to alter antibody production with immunosuppressives are generally not indicated. Patients with cold agglutinins and malignancies should have their treatment regimens directed at their underlying disease, with addition of supportive measures as the clinical situation dictates.

Paroxysmal Cold Hemoglobinuria

PCH was the first hemolytic anemia to be described because of its dramatic presentation of intermittent attacks of pain, fever, and hemoglobinuria following exposure to cold. In their classic 1904 paper, Donath and Landsteiner[42] described an antibody that produces the characteristic syndrome. The D-L antibody is a hemolysin that binds to RBCs at low temperatures in the periphery and fixes complement. When the RBCs return to the warm central body core, they are destroyed by complement lysis. The D-L antibody occurs in three clinical syndromes: (a) chronic PCH associated with late-stage or congenital syphilis, (b) acute transient PCH occurring after an infectious illness, and (c) chronic idiopathic PCH. The first type was formerly the most common; but with effective treatments for syphilis, it is now quite rare. Chronic idiopathic PCH has always been uncommon. The acute transient variety is believed to be one of the most common causes of acute hemolytic anemia of children[104,105] (see *Table 31.6*).

Antibody Characteristics

Immunochemistry and Origin

Typically, PCH antibodies are polyclonal IgG.[106] Originally described in patients with advanced or congenital syphilis, the antibody is not cross-reactive in syphilis serology tests in patients with syphilis or in those who manifest the acute transient variety of PCH.[107,108] PCH has been reported in family members, suggesting a genetic predisposition.[45] The origin or stimulus for antibody production is likely microorganism antigen(s) that induce antibodies that cross-react with the *P* blood group system.[109]

P Antigen Specificity

The antibody in PCH is directed against the *P* antigen, which is a glycosphingolipid globoside found on the RBCs of most individuals.[110,111] The *P* antigen is similar to the Forssman glycolipids present in many microorganisms.[109] This similarity suggests that infectious agents may elicit D-L antibodies as a result of cross-reactivity.

Functional Characteristics

The D-L IgG antibody is a potent hemolysin, causing significant RBC destruction even in low titers. The D-L antibody is classically described as a "biphasic" hemolysin. This is based on the test for the antibody originally described by Donath and Landsteiner, whereby the patient's serum is incubated with RBCs at 0 to 4 °C and then warmed to 37 °C to produce lysis. The antibody requires the cooler temperatures to bind to the RBC, but complement-mediated lysis does not proceed until the temperature is raised. For optimal lysis, complement C1 should be available when the antibody initially binds.[107,108] Upon warming, C4, C2, and the remainder of the complement cascade bind and disrupt the membrane, producing lysis. Some D-L antibodies have a wider thermal amplitude and bind to the RBC at temperatures compatible with complement activity. These seem to be "monophasic" hemolysins, in that cooling is not necessary to produce binding activity. Some believe that the distinction between biphasic and monophasic activity is unwarranted, representing only differences in thermal amplitude.[45] Also, other cold-active antibodies that vigorously fix complement may produce in vitro hemolysis biphasically but yet not have the distinguishing characteristics (IgG, anti-*P* specificity) that qualify them as true D-L antibodies.

Clinical Manifestations

Although uncommon, PCH may not be as rare as initial reports suggested. In a series of all hemolytic anemias, the incidence has ranged from 1.7% to 10.0%.[31,66,112] PCH may account for more than 40% of immune hemolytic anemias in children <5 years of age.[113] The sudden onset of fever, back or leg pain, and hemoglobinuria after exposure to cold are the hallmarks of PCH. Cold exposure may be only a few minutes, and symptoms may follow shortly or several hours later. Fever to 40 °C is not unusual. Other symptoms may include pain or an ache in the back, legs, or abdomen; cramps; headache; nausea; vomiting; and diarrhea. The first urine voided after the onset is dark red to black and typically clears in a few hours. Rarely, this condition persists for a few days. The spleen may be palpable during an attack and shortly thereafter, and mild jaundice may appear.[45] Vasomotor phenomena manifest as cold urticaria, tingling of hands and feet, cyanosis, and Raynaud phenomenon; even gangrene has been reported.[114,115] Systemic symptoms may appear without the hemoglobinuria and vice versa.

There does not appear to be any racial or gender predilection in PCH. Children are almost exclusively affected by the acute transient syndrome.[31,45] An antecedent upper respiratory infection in children is usually identified, although the responsible organism may not be determined. Attacks have been associated with measles, measles vaccinations, mumps, *M. pneumonia*, influenza A, adenovirus, varicella, cytomegalovirus, *Haemophilus influenzae*, and infectious mononucleosis.[116-122] Although episodes are typically self-limited and nonrecurring, they can be quite severe and even life-threatening without supportive care.

The original chronic PCH associated with syphilis has all but disappeared. The diagnosis of chronic PCH now should prompt an investigation for occult syphilis infection and, in its absence, should be considered the idiopathic variety.

Laboratory Features

Hematologic findings in PCH are typical for acute, severe intravascular hemolysis. Hemoglobin levels <5 g/dL can be seen.[113,116,117,121] The peripheral smears may show spherocytes, nucleated RBCs, polychromatophilia, anisocytosis, poikilocytosis,[31] and erythrophagocytosis by neutrophils.[117-120] The WBC count may be depressed very early in the attack, but is usually normal or high. Platelet counts are usually normal. Reticulocytopenia is quite common early in the episode, and reticulocytosis appears in the recovery phase.[45] Once haptoglobin is exhausted, hemoglobinuria results. The plasma is frequently tinged red, reflecting the free hemoglobin. As in other instances of hemolysis, the LDH and bilirubin (mostly unconjugated) are elevated. Complement levels are depressed.

Urine tests are positive for hemoglobin and methemoglobin, giving it its dark red-to-black appearance. Occasionally, RBCs are found in the sediment, but the discoloration is primarily pigment. Renal insufficiency with elevated blood urea nitrogen and creatinine is rare.[122] Hemosiderinuria is found in patients with the chronic variety.

The D-L test is a simple procedure involving incubating patient serum in melting ice with washed group O, *P*-positive RBCs, and fresh normal serum as a source of complement. Later, the tube is transferred to 37 °C for a second incubation. Lysis visible to the naked eye after the warm incubation is a positive test.[29] Appropriate controls should be run simultaneously. Other serologic testing in the blood bank should reveal a positive DAT with anticomplement antisera. The anti-IgG DAT is rarely positive, because of dissociation of the antibody

from the RBC at warmer temperatures. If the blood specimen is processed at cold temperatures, RBC surface-bound IgG can occasionally be demonstrated.[31] The D-L antibody may be demonstrated using the IAT. The method of using an ice-cold saline wash to avoid elution of the antibody and then testing with monospecific antisera for IgG is a sensitive indicator for antibody presence.[31] Differentiation between cold agglutinins and the D-L antibody can be made by careful characterization of the antibody involved, including specificity and immunoglobulin class. The classic age discrepancy and the rare occurrence of cold agglutinins in children may lend clinical support to the diagnosis.

Management of Paroxysmal Cold Hemoglobinuria

Treatment of acute attacks is essentially supportive. Given the transient nature of the syndrome, little else is indicated. In severely anemic children, steroids (prednisone 1 mg/kg/d) are usually given, although their benefit has not been documented.[113,118] Blood transfusion may be safely accomplished with standard banked blood, even though essentially all donor units are *P*-antigen positive. Delaying a needed transfusion to locate the rare unit of *pp* blood (ie, *P* negative) among 200,000 U[29] may put the patient in far more danger than transfusing readily available units. Warming both the patient and the blood is advisable. The hemoglobin rises to the expected amount in most situations. In the rare patient in whom the hemoglobin does not rise, rare-donor files may be able to locate *pp* or Tj(a−) units. When this *pp* unit is available, transfusion results have been excellent.[123] As with other immune hemolytic anemias, critical situations may be ameliorated by plasmapheresis.[124] Chronic PCH is best treated by the avoidance of cold and rarely requires any other therapy. Patients who have documented syphilis should be appropriately treated, and most show response.[125]

IMMUNE HEMOLYTIC ANEMIAS CAUSED BY MIXED COLD- AND WARM-ACTIVE ANTIBODIES

Some patients with warm AIHA also possess a cold agglutinin. Although the majority of these cold agglutinins are not clinically significant, they may occasionally demonstrate sufficient thermal amplitude (>30 °C) or high titer (>1:1000 at 0-4 °C) to indicate CAD. Similar to the separate entities, mixed-type AIHA can be either idiopathic or secondary to lymphoproliferative disorders or systemic lupus erythematosus (SLE). Patients usually have a chronic course interrupted by severe exacerbations, which can result in a hemoglobin level <5 g/dL. These exacerbations do not appear to be associated with cold exposure, and they do not result in acrocyanosis or Raynaud phenomenon.[126]

The laboratory workup demonstrates a DAT that is positive for both IgG and C3. As with the separate diseases, the mixed-type AIHA produces difficulties with the antibody screen and the cross-match. The RBC eluate typically indicates a panreactive warm IgG autoantibody. The cold autoantibody usually exhibits specificity against the *I* antigen, but reactivity against *i* has been reported.[126,127] Because of technical difficulties associated with performing the cross-match, due to the autoantibody interference, cross-match-incompatible units may have to be transfused in situations where patients are severely symptomatic or severely anemic.[94] Mixed-type AIHA appears to respond to treatment in a manner similar to warm AIHA. Patients generally respond to steroids, and immunosuppressive agents and splenectomy have been employed successfully as well. Associated diseases, if present, also need to be treated to optimize recovery[126] (see *Table 31.6*).

IMMUNE HEMOLYTIC ANEMIAS CAUSED BY WARM-ACTIVE ANTIBODIES

Autoantibodies with greatest activity at 37 °C are responsible for the majority of patients with AIHA. Excluding drug-induced autoantibodies, ~70% of all patients with AIHA have the warm-antibody type.[31,66] In general, these autoantibodies are IgG, may or may not fix complement, and typically destroy RBCs by extravascular hemolysis in the spleen (exceptions do occur). They may be secondary to an underlying disease, or in some cases, no underlying process is ever identified, and they are labeled *idiopathic*. Certain drugs may induce development of warm-active antibodies, even generating a true autoantibody in the absence of a distinct autoimmune disorder (see *Table 31.6*).

Primary vs Secondary Autoimmune Hemolytic Anemia

Warm autoantibodies are responsible for 48% to 70% of AIHA cases.[31,128] Primary or idiopathic warm AIHA accounts for less than half of the cases. It can occur in any age group, and females predominate (2:1) in most series.[66,106,129] There is no racial predilection, but a genetic predisposition is suggested by intrafamilial occurrences.[45] No blood group has been consistently shown to be selectively affected. HLA-A1, -B7, and -B8 recur in the literature as being overrepresented in this population, although not all series have reached this conclusion.[130-133] The incidence of AIHA has been reported to be in the range of 1:50,000 to 75,000,[87,128] rising with age, but most of the increase is in the secondary hemolytic anemias as opposed to idiopathic. The immune system abnormality that leads to the production of the pathologic antibody in either primary or secondary hemolytic anemia is still not completely understood.

With an aggressive search and long follow-up, most patients with warm autoantibodies are found to have an underlying associated condition. Lymphoproliferative disorders such as chronic lymphocytic leukemia (CLL) and other, non-Hodgkin lymphoma are the leading causes of secondary cases.[134] Other secondary causes include autoimmune disorders (eg, SLE, rheumatoid arthritis, scleroderma, and ulcerative colitis), nonlymphoid neoplasms (eg, ovarian dermoid cysts, teratomas, and carcinomas), immunodeficiency disorders (eg, acquired immunodeficiency syndrome, dysglobulinemia, and hypogammaglobulinemia), and childhood viral illnesses.[134] Warm AIHA has also been reported in association with both pediatric and adult cases of COVID-19 infection.[47,135] As a result of these secondary causes, the incidence of warm AIHA increases starting around 40 years of age. Children have a peak incidence in the first 4 years of life (see *Table 31.8*).

Antibody Characteristics

Immunochemistry and Origin

Most antibodies are IgG with a preponderance of IgG1 and, to a lesser extent, of IgG3.[136] The subtypes vary in their efficiency at causing hemolysis because of the higher affinities of the macrophage Fc receptors for the IgG1 and IgG3 subclasses.[137,138] Various combinations of IgG subclasses may occur together. Although it is uncommon for IgA or IgM to occur in concert with IgG, it is even less common for them to occur singly[31,32] (see *Tables 31.4* and *31.6*).

Blood Group Specificity

Warm autoantibodies are panagglutinins, reacting with all the RBCs in the diagnostic panel. Of the reported specificities, Rh is by far the most common (70%), including all but the Rh$_{null}$ erythrocytes. Occasionally, the IAT identifies an antibody with relative Rh specificity for a particular Rh antigen such as *e*. It is extremely rare for antibodies of true specificity to occur in the absence of those of broader specificity. Thus, little is to be gained by transfusing antigen-negative blood to these patients. Other blood group specificities that have been reported include Wright (Wr^b), En^a, Duffy (Fy^b), Gerbich (Ge), Kidd (Jk^a), Kell (K), Lutheran (Lu), LW, M, N, S, Pr, A, B, I^T, Sc3, U, Vel, and Xg^a.[38,45]

Clinical Manifestations

Warm AIHA has a highly variable clinical presentation. Typically, patients insidiously develop anemic symptoms such as weakness, dizziness, fatigue, and dyspnea on exertion. Other, less specific symptoms include fever, bleeding, coughing, abdominal pain, and weight loss.[139] Cases with insidious onset generally follow a chronic

Table 31.8. Diseases or Conditions Associated With Warm Autoimmune Antibodies

Autoimmune disorders
Systemic lupus erythematosus
Rheumatoid arthritis
Scleroderma
Ulcerative colitis
Antiphospholipid antibodies
Lymphoproliferative disorders
Chronic lymphocytic leukemia
Acute myelocytic leukemia
Hodgkin lymphoma
Non-Hodgkin lymphoma
Waldenström macroglobulinemia
Other lymphoproliferative disorders
Multiple myeloma
Other neoplastic disorders
Thymoma
Ovarian dermoid cyst
Teratoma
Kaposi sarcoma
Carcinoma
Viral infections
Epstein-Barr virus
Hepatitis C virus
HIV/AIDS
Other
Diphtheria-pertussis-tetanus vaccinations
Pregnancy
Bone marrow transplantation
Congenital immune deficiency states
Hypogammaglobulinemia
Dysglobulinemia

AIDS, acquired immunodeficiency syndrome; HIV, human immunodeficiency virus.

waxing and waning course. In patients with fulminant hemolysis, the anemic symptoms can be accompanied by jaundice, pallor, edema, and dark urine (hemoglobinuria). Splenomegaly, hepatomegaly, and lymphadenopathy may accompany the anemia. This more acute, potentially life-threatening presentation is usually associated with viral infections, especially in children. Postinfectious acute-onset hemolysis tends to be short lived.[45] In cases of secondary disease, the symptoms of AIHA may precede the recognition of the underlying illness by months to years, but ultimately the symptoms of the underlying disorder predominate. When presentation includes massive splenomegaly or lymphadenopathy, an underlying lymphoproliferative disorder should be considered. Symptoms can be precipitated by trauma, surgery, infection, pregnancy, and psychologic stress (see *Table 31.9*).

Pregnancy

The rate of autoantibody formation in pregnant women has been reported at 1:50,000, 5-fold greater than in an age-comparable control population.[140] Hemolysis tends to increase during the pregnancy and may remit after delivery. Maternal hemoglobin levels <5 g/dL have

Table 31.9. Warm Autoimmune Hemolytic Anemia: Presenting Signs and Symptoms

Sign	Frequency (%)	Symptom	Frequency (%)
Splenomegaly	82	Weakness	88
Hepatomegaly	45	Dizziness	50
Lymphadenopathy	34	Fever	37
Jaundice	21	Bleeding	10
Thyromegaly	10	Dyspnea	9
Edema	6	Cough	6
Cardiac failure	5	Weight loss	5
Pallor	4	Gastrointestinal disturbance	5
		Anorexia	4
		Dark urine	3
		Angina	2
		Confusion	2

Modified from Pirofsky B. Clinical aspects of autoimmune hemolytic anemia. *Semin Hematol.* 1976;13(4):251-265. Copyright © 1976 Elsevier. With permission.

been reported.[141] Infants born to mothers with hemolytic anemia may or may not suffer any hemolysis. Fetal and neonatal IgG are of maternal origin and diminish postpartum naturally with clearance. Maternal antibody-producing lymphocytes do not typically cross the placenta. Even if difficulties are encountered initially, the infant should normalize in a matter of weeks, because there is no endogenous ongoing neonatal production of pathologic antibodies.[142,143]

Infancy and Childhood

AIHA in infancy and childhood can be quite different from that in adults. The disease onset is more likely to be sudden and severe, usually preceded by a viral prodrome. There is a slight male predominance, and the prognosis is relatively good for a complete and lasting remission within several weeks of the onset. Most children respond well to steroids, and rarely is splenectomy considered.[45] A particular association of childhood vaccines and hemolytic anemia has been documented.[144,145]

Evans Syndrome

Children can have very severe Evans syndrome, the concomitant occurrence of warm AIHA and ITP described in 1949.[146-148] The thrombocytopenia may precede, coincide with, or follow the AIHA.[120] This is more common in children and is less likely to respond well to therapy.[149,150] Steroids is generally the first-line therapy, with approximately 80% success rate.[151] Multiagent protocols have shown some success.[152,153] Rituximab also has demonstrated clinical utility in patients with relapsed, refractory, or steroid-depending Evans syndrome, with the exception of those who have underlying autoimmune lymphoproliferative syndrome so may benefit from other therapies such as mycophenolate mofetil or sirolimus (see section Management).[151]

Laboratory Features

Hemoglobin and hematocrit values at presentation can vary from essentially normal in the compensated hemolyzing patient to extremely low in the rare patient with fulminant RBC destruction. The MCV is usually elevated, reflecting the increased proportion of young RBCs and perhaps a relative folate deficiency in patients with chronic hemolysis. Reticulocyte counts are usually elevated as well, sometimes remarkably so, but may be depressed early in the course.[154] Reticulocytopenia may have myriad causes, including marrow shutdown from intervening infection, malignancy myelophthisis, parvovirus B19 infection, or

the possibility of the autoimmune antibody being directed at antigens in great concentration on the reticulocytes themselves.[45,155-157] The bone marrow is usually hyperplastic even in the face of reticulocytopenia.[154] The peripheral smear typically reflects the reticulocytosis with polychromatophilia and macrocytosis, as well as nucleated RBCs. Spontaneous agglutination is uncommon with warm autoantibodies but may occur if the RBCs are strongly sensitized with immunoglobulin. Spherocytes are produced in varying quantity. Albeit unusual, the presence of erythrophagocytosis by monocytes, or rarely neutrophils, on the peripheral smear is an indication of AIHA.[158]

WBC counts are usually slightly elevated, but they may also be depressed. Thrombocytopenia should raise the consideration of Evans syndrome.[154] Both leukopenia and thrombocytopenia may be immune mediated, as shown in some cases by the presence of antileukocyte and antiplatelet antibodies.[159] Platelet dysfunction may occur as well.[160] Serum bilirubin is elevated but rarely >5 mg/dL in the absence of concomitant liver disease, with the major fraction unconjugated.[161] Hemoglobinemia and depressed or absent haptoglobin can be seen in rapid hemolysis, even if extravascular. Urobilinogens are increased, and hemoglobinuria and hemosiderinuria may follow severe hemolysis. Resultant renal failure has been reported.[162] Stercobilinogens may turn the stool dark. Biologic false-positive syphilis test results are common, and other abnormal antibodies have been reported, including antithyroid antibodies, rheumatoid factors, and anticardiolipin antibodies. Serum immunoglobulin abnormalities have been reported with elevated or depressed levels, but with no consistent pattern.[163,164]

The hallmark of immune-mediated hemolytic anemia is the presence of immunoglobulin, complement, or both on the surface of the RBCs. In >95% of warm AIHA cases, the DAT is positive. Series vary in their DAT results. Between 20% and 66% have only IgG on the surface, 24% to 63% have IgG and C3, 7% to 14% have only C3, and 1% to 4% are DAT negative.[31,128,165] Patients with SLE are particularly prone to positive tests for complement on their RBCs. IgG1 predominates, either alone or in combination with other subclasses, and IgG4 is uncommon. In rare cases of warm hemolysins, IgM antibodies that fix complement and are associated with severe, life-threatening hemolysis have been reported.[166] It is even more uncommon for IgG antibodies to act as hemolysins.[167] The severity of hemolysis is loosely correlated with the quantity of antibody bound to the RBC and the strength of the DAT.[168,169] However, other factors play a large role in the significance of the clinical picture, such as the immunoglobulin subclass, with IgG3 being the most efficient at binding to Fc receptors.

Still other characteristics remain undefined to explain why immune hemolysis occurs in patients with a negative DAT and why some other patients with RBC-bound immunoglobulin have no increase in RBC turnover. If standard techniques do not demonstrate a positive DAT, other, more sensitive techniques may be successful. The antibody screen reveals the presence of the panagglutinin in the serum in 80% of cases. Specificity for other antigens can be sought as described earlier but is difficult to obtain accurately without a large selection of rare, antigen-negative RBCs and is of marginal clinical benefit.

Management of Warm AIHA

General principles of treatment are guided by the severity of hemolysis. Those patients with a positive DAT, mild reticulocytosis, and normal hematocrit are not routinely subjected to steroid therapy. Folate deficiency can be prevented with daily supplements, which probably should be given to any patient with hemolysis. When the RBC life span shortens beyond the point of marrow compensation and a consequent anemia appears, intervention is indicated. Given the high proportion of secondary hemolytic anemias, a search for an underlying disorder that requires specific therapy, such as a lymphoproliferative disorder, is indicated (see *Table 31.8*). Treatment of the secondary disorder may also bring the AIHA under control. However, in some situations, each disorder must be addressed separately. Many treatment options exist for these patients, who can have vast differences in the severity of their disease.[170-172]

First-line Treatment

Glucocorticoids are the initial therapy of choice for warm AIHA, usually on the order of 1.0 to 1.5 mg/kg or 40 mg/m^2/d of prednisone or its equivalent.[85] Higher daily doses or high-dose pulsed therapy may be efficacious.[171,173] Response may not be evident for 3 to 4 days but should be noticeable by 7 days. Reticulocyte counts may increase, and the hemoglobin should rise 2 to 3 g/dL/wk. Once the hemoglobin reaches 10 g/dL, weaning of the steroid can begin, at a rate to parallel the response. Rapid responders can reduce their dose by 50% over 4 to 6 weeks. Beyond this point, tapering should proceed more slowly over 3 to 4 months. Some even continue a low dose for prolonged periods thereafter to prevent relapse, although no data exist to support this practice fully. This schedule should be adjusted for the individual response to the treatment and for any significant side effects that result. Side effects include increased susceptibility to infection, hypertension, fluid retention, diabetes, myopathy, peptic ulceration, osteoporosis, and even reversible facial cosmetic changes and may be intolerable. Alternate-day steroid therapy decreases some of the side effects and may still be effective. Consideration should be given to concomitant prophylactic antacids, bisphosphonates, vitamin D, and calcium according to the recommendation of the American College of Rheumatology. Careful monitoring of blood glucose and aggressive treatment of diabetes is recommended because diabetes is a major risk factor for treatment-related deaths from infections.[174]

The mechanism of action of steroids is multifactorial. Initially, steroids act through tissue macrophages, delaying the reticuloendothelial clearance of IgG- and C3-coated RBCs.[175] Steroids may act by reducing antibody avidity[176] and eventually may actually decrease antibody production.[177] Initial responses to steroids are generally excellent, with ~80% of patients having a prompt reduction in hemolysis. In one series, only 7% took longer than 2 weeks, and even fewer more than 3 weeks. Therefore, if there has been no improvement after 3 weeks of therapy, the patient may be considered a steroid treatment failure. Recurrence of hemolysis after remission is usually gradual, especially if the steroids were weaned over a prolonged period.

Relapse of warm AIHA occurs in the vast majority of patients. Approximately 40% to 50% of patients require maintenance doses of prednisone (5-20 mg/d).[178] If the maintenance prednisone dose is >15 mg/d, other measures should be considered. Free autoantibody in the serum (positive IAT or antibody screen) may disappear, but the DAT remains positive in most patients, although perhaps weaker.[45] Complete and lasting remission rates from steroids alone are reported as occurring in only 16% to 35% of patients,[177,179] so the majority of patients with warm AIHA require additional therapy.

Second-Line Treatment

Second-line treatment is a strong consideration in patients who are refractory to initial steroids, in those who need more than 15 mg/d prednisone as a maintenance dose, in those with intolerable side effects, or in those where compliance is a concern.[85] Splenectomy and rituximab are the only second-line treatments with a proven short-term efficacy.[180]

Splenectomy. Splenectomy may be considered in all patients without contraindications because the short-term efficacy is high. So far, splenectomy is the only treatment that may provide freedom from treatment in a substantial number of patients for more than 2 years and possibly cure in ~20%.[180]

The rationale for splenectomy is 2-fold. The spleen is the major site of RBC sequestration and destruction in warm AIHA, resulting from the interaction of IgG antibodies with the macrophage Fc receptors. Splenectomy has little effect on the clearance of IgM-coated RBCs and therefore would not be indicated in the unusual patient with a warm-active IgM antibody. The spleen is also believed to be a major producer of IgG antibodies.[31,32] Overall responses are probably 60% to 75%, but many of these patients relapse or remain on steroids, albeit at lower, more tolerable doses.[31,181,182] The likelihood of response to splenectomy may be higher in idiopathic AIHA than in secondary AIHA.[183] The perioperative risk of splenectomy is low. Splenectomy can safely be performed laparoscopically in almost all

cases of primary AIHA, because the spleen is usually of normal size. The mortality of laparoscopic splenectomy (all indications) was 0.5% in a large national study. All patients should receive postoperative thromboprophylaxis with low-molecular-weight heparin, probably even beyond hospital discharge. They should also be informed about the higher risk of venous thromboembolism. The withdrawal of steroids after splenectomy should be done slowly (as described for primary treatment) to prevent hemolytic crises in case of recurrence.

The major relevant long-term risk is a lifelong persisting higher rate of infections (the most feared is overwhelming pneumococcal septicemia). Splenectomy rates have gradually declined to <10% of cases due to increased infection risk, especially in the first year post splenectomy.[184] There is a 3% to 5% risk of sepsis due to encapsulated bacteria, with a mortality rate up to 50%.[184] If splenectomy is performed, all measures must be taken to prevent complications. All patients must have preoperative vaccination against pneumococci, meningococci, and haemophilus, and vaccinations should be repeated every 5 years. Patients must be informed about the risk of infections and should be advised to take antibiotics in case of fever. Conditions for which splenectomy may be inadvisable include age >65 years, previous history of or significant risk for thromboembolism, immunodeficiency, lymphoproliferative disorder, or autoimmune conditions.[184]

Rituximab. Rituximab is becoming the preferred second-line treatment for patients with warm AIHA, as it has an ~80% overall response rate and sustained response of ~60% at 3 years.[85,185] Rituximab is a chimeric human/murine monoclonal anti-CD20 antibody approved for use in lymphoma. Successful rituximab use in refractory warm AIHA and Evans syndrome has been documented in several case reports and series.[186-190] Regimens identical to the lymphoma treatment (375 mg/m^2/wk for 4 weeks) have produced remissions in some patients who were refractory to other therapeutic regimens. A response rate of 87% was reported for one series of refractory pediatric patients. Twenty-three percent of the responders relapsed, but subsequent courses of rituximab induced additional remissions.[190] Thus far, few side effects have been reported, but rare reactions to the infusion have been documented.[191] B-cell counts remain low for months after treatment, raising the risk of infections due to poor immune response.[192] The efficacy and toxicity of rituximab monotherapy was tested in additional retrospective studies in a mixed population of refractory primary or secondary AIHA. These studies have been summarized in a review by Lechner et al.[180] The overall response rate was 82%. Safety data available are limited, and adverse events include two patients with severe infections and one patient with myocardial infarction.[193] The most severe potential long-term complication of rituximab treatment was progressive multifocal leukoencephalopathy, which, however, has been observed in only two patients with AIHA.[180] If remissions remain durable and potential side effects are less harmful than other treatments for warm AIHA, such as prolonged steroid use or splenectomy, rituximab may become accepted second-line therapy.

Immunosuppressive Therapy

Immunosuppressive therapy is indicated for patients who have failed to respond to splenectomy and/or rituximab therapy.[180] Most of the evidence for the use of the agents dates from the pre-rituximab era, and recent evidence is limited. Cyclophosphamide is an effective immunosuppressive agent with capability to suppress the immune response, even if administered after antigen presentation.[194] This is particularly desirable for administration after the onset of immune hemolysis. Beneficial effects of cyclophosphamide therapy are reported in reviews.[177,178,181] Blood counts should be followed up closely. Other significant side effects from the antimetabolites and cyclophosphamide include hemorrhagic cystitis, bladder fibrosis, secondary malignancies, sterility, and alopecia.[31,178,195,196] No properly controlled trial exists from which to draw conclusions, but the reviews and case reports suggest a response rate of approximately 40% to 60% in those patients who did not respond to steroids and splenectomy.[180,182] A reasonable immunosuppressive regimen might include cyclophosphamide (60 mg/m^2/d), concomitantly with prednisone (40 mg/m^2/d). Prednisone may be tapered over 3 months or so and the cytotoxic agent continued for 6 months before reducing the dose gradually.[182] Bone marrow suppression may dictate minor dose adjustments. Rapid withdrawal has led to rebound immune response.[197] Alternatively, high-dose cyclophosphamide (50 mg/kg/d for 4 days) has produced a complete remission in 66% of patients who were refractory to other therapies. Severe myelotoxicity and its attendant potential for complications are expected.[198]

Mycophenolate mofetil, an inhibitor of inosine 5'-monophosphate dehydrogenase, is an immunosuppressant initially employed to treat allograft rejection. It has been shown to induce complete or partial remission of hemolysis in case reports. Doses begin at 1 g/d and are then increased to 2 g/d. In cases of partial remission, reduction in doses of other immunosuppressives was possible without sacrificing efficacy. Mycophenolate mofetil has also been shown to be a viable second-line agent therapy for children with refractory AIHA.[199] Long-term side effects are not fully established. Short-term side effects consist primarily of headache, gastrointestinal intolerance, and mild myelosuppression.[188,189,200,201]

Cyclosporine A has been used both successfully and unsuccessfully in patients with refractory hemolytic anemia, as were many of the other immunosuppressive medications previously described. Doses of 3 mg/kg/d with target serum levels of 200 to 400 ng/mL produced remissions.[190,202] It has also been used in combination with other remedies with some success, including danazol and prednisone.[153,192,193,203,204]

Sirolimus has also garnered attention for the treatment of relapsed and refractory AIHA.[204,205] It has also been effectively used as a monotherapy, steroid-sparing agent in refractory cases. It is particularly effective for patients who have AIHA associated with autoimmune lymphoproliferative syndrome (ALPS).[204] Bride et al demonstrated in their case series that children with AIHA associated with ALPS achieved complete response within 1 to 3 months.[205] In this series, sirolimus was given at a dose of 2 to 2.5 mg/m^2/d. Few side effects were reported, including most commonly grade 1 to 2 mucositis, typically within the first 3 months of therapy. Other potential side effects include hypercholesterolemia and hypertriglyceridemia, sun sensitivity, and gastroesophageal reflux.

Transfusion

As with CAD, red cell transfusion support may be required in patients who are clinically symptomatic or severely anemic. Patients with warm AIHA should be tested for the presence of coexisting alloantibodies, which may have developed following pregnancies or prior transfusions. Alloantibodies, rather than autoantibodies, may cause major transfusion reactions in such patients if not discovered. However, identifying an alloantibody in the presence of an autoantibody takes additional time. Thus, if the patient needs to be transfused emergently, transfusion should be given before the availability of the results. Most patients will tolerate even serologically incompatible blood. Blood bank personnel should be involved early in the decision to transfuse to minimize delays and possible confusion.[206]

Other Therapies

IVIG has not enjoyed the success in AIHA that it has in ITP. Case reports of success[207-209] and failure[210,211] have appeared. Escalating the dose from the standard 0.4 to 1.0 g/kg/d (for 5 days) may be helpful. In one refractory patient, weekly maintenance infusions of 800 mg/kg/wk helped control transfusion requirements.[212] The mechanism of action of IVIG is not completely clear. Recent evidence suggests that IVIG exerts inhibitory effects on dendritic cells by downregulating costimulatory molecules, blocking maturation, and modifying their interactions with lipopolysaccharide and cytokines.[213] Other postulated mechanisms include modulating expression and function of Fc receptors, interfering with the activation of complement, modulating immune response through anti-idiotype antibodies, and effects on B and T cells.[214]

Plasmapheresis has been used with limited success in attempts to remove the antibody.[31,215,216] However, in some patients, fulminant hemolysis proceeds unchecked and plasmapheresis may serve as a temporizing measure until other immunosuppressive therapies can take effect. Selective removal of IgG with staphylococcal protein A columns has also been reported with some benefit.[217]

Stem cell transplantation (SCT) has been described for many severe, life-threatening autoimmune syndromes, including hemolytic anemia and Evans syndrome. Sources of the stem cells have been autologous, HLA-matched sibling, and cord blood.[218,219] Relapses and the expected range of complications, including death, have occurred. For very severe and refractory cases of Evans syndrome, SCT offers the only chance of long-term cure. Available data suggest that allogeneic SCT may be superior to autologous SCT, but both carry risks of severe morbidity and of transplant-related mortality. As more refractory patients are seen, stem cell reconstitution after high-dose immune suppressive regimens will no doubt expand. Cure of Evans syndrome following reduced-intensity conditioning has been reported and should be considered for younger patients in the context of controlled clinical trials.[220]

Alemtuzumab is a humanized anti-CD52 monoclonal antibody that is an effective therapy for B-CLL, mycosis fungoides, and T-cell prolymphocytic leukemia. There have been recent case reports that suggest alemtuzumab may be useful for the treatment of AIHA in patients with B-CLL who have failed other treatments.[221,222]

Bortezomib is a 26S proteasome inhibitor that has had some reported successes in patients who had AIHA post bone marrow transplant.[223] Khandelwal et al also reported some success in treating seven children with AIHA with bortezomib.[224] The mechanism of action is through targeting plasma cells, based on the theory that plasma cells not targetable by other therapies might be the etiology of disease refractoriness.

Complications

Hoffmann suggests that venous thromboembolism is an underrecognized complication of AIHA and may, in some instances, be related to coexistent antiphospholipid antibodies.[225] Although it is premature to recommend anticoagulant prophylaxis in general for patients with AIHA hemolytic episodes, consideration might be given to those at particularly high risk, such as those with evidence of coexisting antiphospholipid antibodies.

DRUG-INDUCED IMMUNE HEMOLYTIC ANEMIA

Drugs can produce hemolysis by both immune and nonimmune mechanisms. In the 1970s and 1980s, α-methyldopa and high-dose penicillin were responsible for the majority of cases of DI-IHA. In recent years, there has been a significant decline in DI-IHA due to α-methyldopa and high-dose penicillin because of declining use of those medications. More recent estimates of the incidence of DI-IHA are approximately 1 per million.[226] Second- and third-generation cephalosporins, especially cefotetan and ceftriaxone, have been associated increasingly with cases of immune hemolytic anemia, accounting for ~80% of the DI-IHA.[227] Rarely, these cases of cephalosporin-induced immune hemolytic anemia are fatal. Other antibiotic agents associated with immune hemolytic anemia include β-lactamase inhibitors (clavulanate, sulbactam, and tazobactam) found in combination with β-lactam antibiotics in Timentin (ticarcillin/clavulanate), Unasyn (ampicillin/sulbactam), Zosyn (piperacillin/tazobactam), and piperacillin.[227] AIHA has been noted with increased incidence in patients receiving purine nucleoside analogs such as fludarabine, cladribine, and pentostatin for hematologic malignancies.[225] The mechanism by which these drugs cause AIHA is unclear (see *Figure 31.4, Tables 31.6* and *31.10*).

Mechanisms

Drug-induced antibodies can be divided into two main groupings based on the requirement for the drug in detection. Drug-dependent antibodies (penicillin type or immune complex type) require the presence of the drug in the test system, whereas drug-independent antibodies (autoantibodies) do not (see *Table 31.11* and *Figure 31.5*).

Drug-dependent antibodies may be true autoantibodies with serology that is identical to warm AIHA. There are three major

Table 31.10. Drugs Associated With Immune Hemolysis or Autoantibodies

Acetaminophen	Doxepin	Omeprazole
Aminopyrine	"Ecstasy"	Oxaliplatin
Amphotericin B	Elliptinium acetate	p-Aminosalicylic acid
Ampicillin	Erythromycin	Penicillin G
Antazoline	Etodolac	Phenacetin
Apazone (azapropazone)	Fenfluramine	Podophyllotoxin
Buthiazide (butazide)	Fenoprofen	Probenecid
Carbenicillin	Fludarabine	Procainamide
Carbimazole	Fluorescein	Propyphenazone
Carboplatin	5-Fluorouracil	Pyramidon
Catergen	Glafenine	Quinidine
Cefotaxime	Hydralazine	Quinine
Cefotetan	Hydrochlorothiazide	Ranitidine
Cefoxitin	Ibuprofen	Rifampin (rifampicin)
Ceftazidime	Insecticides	Sodium pentothal
Ceftriaxone	Insulin	Stibophen
Cephaloridine	Interferon-α	Streptomycin
Cephalothin	Intravenous contrast media	Sulfonamides
Chaparral	Isoniazid	Sulfonylurea derivative
Chlorambucil	Latamoxef	Sulindac
Chlorinated hydrocarbons	Levodopa	Suprofen
2-Chlorodeoxyadenosine	Mefenamic acid	Suramin
Chlorpromazine	Mefloquine	Teniposide
Chlorpropamide	Melphalan	Tetracycline
Cianidanol	6-Mercaptopurine	Thiazides
Ciproflaxin	Mephenytoin	Thiopental
Cisplatin	Methadone	Thioridazine
Cladribine	Methicillin	Tolbutamide
Cyclofenil	Methotrexate	Tolmetin
Diclofenac	Methyldopa	Triamterene
Diethylstilbestrol	Nafcillin	Trimellitic anhydride
Diglycoaldehyde	Nalidixic acid	Zomepirac
Dipyrone	Nomifensine	

Modified from Arndt PA, Garratty G. The changing spectrum of drug-induced immune hemolytic anemia. *Semin Hematol.* 2005;42(3):137-144. Copyright © 2005 Elsevier. With permission.

mechanisms by which drugs can cause immune hemolysis in vivo[228] (see *Figure 31.5*):

1. The drug adsorption mechanism, in which the antibody reacts with a drug tightly bound to the RBC membrane
2. The neoantigen or immune complex mechanism, in which the drug combines loosely with the RBC membrane and the antibody reacts with new antigenic site(s) created by the combination of drug and membrane
3. The autoimmune mechanism, which is indistinguishable from true AIHA without drug exposure

Some medications may produce hemolysis by more than one mechanism, and differentiating among them is not always possible.

Nonimmunologic adsorption of proteins to the RBC membrane can also cause a positive DAT but is not associated with increased RBC destruction.

Drug Adsorption Mechanism (Penicillin Type)

In a penicillin-type drug absorption mechanism, the drug binds tightly to the RBC membrane and the antibody attaches to the drug without direct interaction with the erythrocyte. Penicillin binds to the RBC membrane covalently and can be demonstrated on the RBC in most patients receiving high doses of the drug, even in the absence of antibody.[229] Attachment of only the drug does not harm the erythrocyte. However, when the drug is given in large doses (>10 million U/d), it can induce production of IgG antibody, which attaches to the membrane-bound drug, thus producing a positive DAT with AHG sera.[229] Eluates from these RBCs do not react with RBC panels, in contrast to the previously discussed true autoimmune antibodies, which display panagglutinin activity. The explanation lies in the fact that penicillin-induced antibodies are attached to the drug alone and not to membrane components of the erythrocyte. If reagent cell suspensions are first coated with penicillin, agglutination occurs with all RBCs, thus providing a diagnostic testing strategy when drug-induced hemolysis is suspected.[31]

The benzylpenicilloyl determinant is the primary antigen-binding site. High-titered IgG antibenzylpenicilloyl antibodies are responsible for the positive DAT and appear in ~3% of patients receiving high doses of the drug.[230] Only some of these patients develop hemolysis.[31] Rare exceptions of complement fixation to the RBCs exist in patients on penicillin. These have been associated with IgG attachment, and the DAT is positive with both anti-IgG and anti-C3 sera.[231,232]

RBC destruction in the drug adsorption mechanism of hemolysis is through sequestration by splenic macrophages of the IgG-coated RBCs.[233,234] Rarely, when associated with complement fixation, the RBCs may be lysed (intravascular hemolysis).[235] Anemia develops gradually over 7 to 10 days and can be life-threatening if not recognized and the drug discontinued. Once the medication is stopped, the hemolysis resolves over the ensuing couple of weeks. However, the DAT may remain positive for several weeks. Of clinical importance is the observation that other signs of penicillin hypersensitivity, such as urticaria and airway reactivity, are usually absent.[31]

Other drugs can also cause hemolysis by this mechanism. Cephalosporins,[236-240] tetracycline,[241,242] tolbutamide,[243] and semisynthetic penicillins[244,245] can cause DI-IHA by this mechanism.

Neoantigen Mechanism (Quinidine/Stibophen Type)

The neoantigen mechanism is also known as the immune complex mechanism. The antibody is specific for a combination antigen, or neoantigen, created jointly by the drug and RBCs. Investigations with rare antigen-negative RBCs revealed that two antibodies have specific sites on the RBC membrane to which they attach along with the drug.[246,247]

The neoantigen mechanism differs from the drug adsorption mechanism in a few key areas. Unlike the penicillin model, these drugs bind very loosely to the RBC membrane. Only a small dose of the medication is required for hemolysis to occur, as opposed to the very large doses of penicillin required. Hemolysis is usually sudden, severe, and accompanied by hemoglobinuria[2] instead of the subacute anemia typically seen with the drug adsorption type. Renal failure is a frequent occurrence in the neoantigen mechanism.[248,249] The effector phase is mediated predominantly by complement fixation and subsequent intravascular hemolysis. Some sequestration of RBCs occurs in splenic macrophages or the liver via CRs. The DAT is positive only for the presence of complement, and IgM or IgG is rarely still attached to the RBC.[31] Therefore, eluates are nonreactive primarily because there is no immunoglobulin to elute. In vitro, serum reacts with RBCs only in the presence of the drug or a reactive metabolite.[31] These drugs may also induce thrombocytopenia by similar mechanisms.[250,251]

Table 31.11. Mechanisms of Drug-Induced Hemolysis or Positive Direct Antiglobulin Test

	Drug Adsorption	Neoantigen	Autoimmune	Nonimmune Adsorption
Prototype drug	Penicillin	Quinidine/stibophen	α-Methyldopa	First-generation cephalosporins
Role of drug	Cell-bound hapten	Antibody binds drug + RBC	Induces drug-independent RBC antibody	Modifies RBC membrane; adsorbs proteins nonspecifically
Typical direct antiglobulin test	IgG	Complement	IgG	Non-Ig
Antibody reactions	Reacts only with drug-coated cells	Reacts only with drug present	Drug-independent panagglutinin	No antibody present
Typical clinical presentation	Subacute onset; mild to severe hemolysis	Acute onset; severe hemolysis	Insidious onset; chronic mild hemolysis	No hemolysis

RBC, red blood cell.

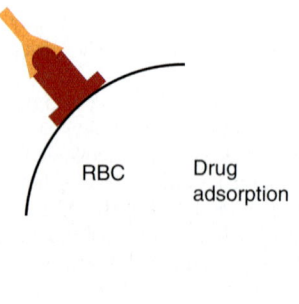

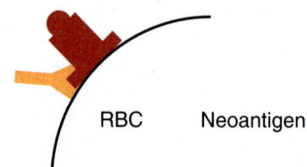

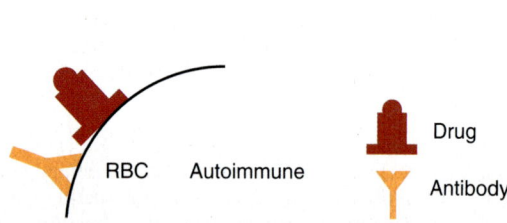

FIGURE 31.5 **A proposed theory of drug-induced antibody reactions.** A, The antibody attaches only to the drug, which is tightly bound to the red blood cell (RBC) membrane (penicillin type). B, The antibody attaches to a neoantigen created by components of both the drug and the RBC membrane (quinidine/stibophen type). C, The antibody attaches mainly to the membrane, not requiring the presence of the drug (α-methyldopa type). (Adapted from Habibi B. Drug induced red blood cell autoantibodies co-developed with drug specific antibodies causing haemolytic anaemias. *Br J Haematol.* 1985;61(1):139-143. Copyright © 1985 British Society for Haematology. Reprinted by permission of John Wiley & Sons, Inc.)

Autoimmune Mechanism (α-Methyldopa Type)

Unlike the previous two mechanisms, which require the presence of the offending drug for antibody reaction with the RBC membrane, hemolysis induced by α-methyldopa is truly autoimmune in nature. Antibodies bind to erythrocyte membrane antigens in a manner indistinguishable from the sporadic AIHA discussed earlier. With declining use of α-methyldopa, these antibodies are now seen in association with cladribine, fludarabine, levodopa, mefenamic acid, and procainamide.[227] The etiology of these antibodies is unknown, but the drugs

likely directly stimulate the immune system to mimic an autoimmune disease. The DAT is positive with anti-IgG and is usually negative with anti-C3. The eluate shows a panreactive antibody. The characteristics of the IgG antibody eluted from the RBCs are strikingly similar to those in idiopathic warm AIHA. They are polyclonal[252] and bind as a panagglutinin to reagent cells even in the absence of the drug. As in warm AIHA, these antibodies have a predilection for Rh antigens, with some specific anti-c and anti-e documented.[252,253]

Despite a high incidence of immunoglobulin coating of RBCs, only a minority of patients actually develop clinical hemolysis.[2] Explanations of this phenomenon have been unsatisfactory. The amount of antibody on the RBC correlates poorly with in vivo hemolysis, and no threshold has been well established.[66,254]

Nonimmunologic Protein Adsorption Mechanism

Proteins other than immunoglobulins may attach nonspecifically to the RBC membrane and cause positive antiglobulin reactions. These do not cause increased RBC destruction and are of importance only because of the need to differentiate them from those of clinical significance. This is most commonly seen in patients on cephalosporins, which produce a positive DAT in ~3% of patients.[255,256] Other drugs that have been associated with this mechanism include cefotetan, cisplatin, diglycoaldehyde, oxaliplatin, suramin, and the β-lactamase inhibitors clavulanate, sulbactam, and tazobactam.[227] Many different RBC-bound proteins have been detected within a few days of instituting the medication, including fibrinogen, albumin, complement, immunoglobulins, and α_2-macroglobulin.[256] Clinical distinction between this benign finding and other, potentially significant ones involves the demonstration of a nonreactive eluate with cephalosporin-treated RBCs and the absence or low titer of antidrug antibodies in the serum.[31] In the absence of hemolysis, a positive DAT is not a cause for discontinuing the medication.

Multiple Mechanisms-Unifying Hypothesis

Many medications have been implicated in producing hemolysis by more than one mechanism, sometimes simultaneously in the same patient. Arndt and Garratty have referred to a unifying hypothesis in their review.[227] The drug or its metabolites interact with the constituents of the RBC membrane, resulting in production of different populations of antibodies. Of these antibodies, some react with drug epitopes alone (drug adsorption). Other antibodies may react with drug and membrane components (neoantigen mechanism), and others with RBC membrane components (autoantibody mimickers) (see *Figure 31.6*).

Clinical Manifestations

The clinical features of DI-IHA are similar to those found in idiopathic AIHA, including pallor, jaundice, and easy fatigability. Splenomegaly is common, but lymphadenopathy and hepatomegaly should not be attributed to drug-related hemolysis.[257] The severity of these symptoms depends on the rate of hemolysis, which is, in part, dependent on the mechanism involved. Those patients with the neoantigen mechanism are at the greatest risk for plummeting hemoglobins, hemoglobinuria, and renal failure.[2,248,258] Cefotetan has been implicated in many severe hemolytic reactions.[259-261] Fatal reactions are rare but may occur.[240,262] Cefotetan, ceftriaxone, and fludarabine have been associated with fatalities.[227,263] The drug adsorption and autoimmune varieties are typically characterized by insidious onset of hemolysis over days to weeks. A careful medication history is necessary to evaluate the possibility of a culprit drug in all patients with AIHA.

Laboratory Features

Just as with idiopathic AIHA, anemia with reticulocytosis and a positive DAT are hallmarks of the condition. Elevated indirect bilirubin and LDH are common findings. Rampant RBC destruction leads to hemoglobinemia, hemoglobinuria, and elevated creatinine levels. Distinguishing the mechanisms involved can be accomplished by the serologic results. One can differentiate the neoantigen mechanism from cold autoantibodies by the absence of high-titer cold agglutinins or D-L antibodies in the drug-induced cases. Drug-induced antibodies also do not react in the absence of the drug or a metabolite in IATs. Only a careful history and resolution of the hemolysis after discontinuation of the drug can differentiate the α-methyldopa variety from true autoimmune antibodies. Antibodies to cefotetan react to very high titers against drug-treated RBCs and at lower titers with untreated RBCs with or without drug present. Antibodies to ceftriaxone are the immune complex type.[227] The positive DAT may persist for a few weeks to months after stopping the medication responsible, especially with the autoimmune mechanism.[31]

Management

A careful drug history, including over-the-counter medications, nutritional or dietary supplements, and illicit drugs, is imperative. Discontinuing the implicated medication is usually all that is necessary in the management of drug-induced hemolytic anemia. Problems may arise when a positive DAT occurs, and uncertainty exists as to whether significant RBC destruction is occurring. As previously described, many medications may be associated with a positive DAT test and yet not cause hemolysis. The drug need not be stopped in these patients.

In cases of brisk hemolysis associated with the neoantigen mechanism, stopping the offending agent can be life-saving. Although the helpfulness of prednisone therapy is questionable,[264] it has been used with some success in fludarabine-associated DI-IHA.[263] Transfusion can be accomplished, usually without difficulty in cross-matching, because the

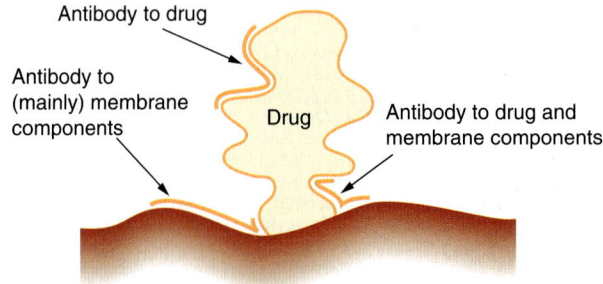

FIGURE 31.6 Proposed unifying hypothesis for drug-induced antibody reactions. The thicker darker lines represent antigen-binding sites on the F_{ab} region of the drug-induced antibody. Drugs (haptens) bind loosely (or firmly) to cell membranes, and antibodies can be made to (A) the drug (producing in vitro reactions typical of a drug adsorption [penicillin-type] reaction); (B) membrane components, or mainly membrane components (producing in vitro reactions typical of autoantibody); or (C) part-drug, part-membrane components (producing an in vitro reaction typical of the so-called immune complex mechanism). (Reprinted with permission from Garratty G. Target antigens for red-cell bound autoantibodies. In: Nance SJ, ed. *Clinical and Basic Science Aspects of Immunohematology.* American Association of Blood Banks; 1991:33-72. Figure 3-1. Copyright © 1991 by AABB.)

antibodies in the drug adsorption and neoantigen mechanisms are drug dependent. However, patients with the autoimmune mechanism may encounter the same difficulties as previously discussed in the section on warm AIHA. It is important to keep in mind that transfused RBCs may be destroyed at the same rate as endogenous RBCs if drug or active metabolites are still circulating. Prognosis is typically excellent for these patients after discontinuation of the drug. With the variety of choices of pharmaceuticals available, alternative therapies are nearly always accessible to treat the underlying condition adequately.

TRANSPLANT-ASSOCIATED IMMUNE HEMOLYTIC ANEMIAS

Although it is not technically an autoimmune hemolytic process, the immune hemolysis associated with transplantation is analogous in many ways. In both cases, antibodies are generated against endogenous self-antigens; the key distinction lies in the source of the antibody-producing lymphocytes. That source can be either the lymphocytes and their precursors contained in a stem cell product being utilized for hematopoietic reconstitution or they can be lymphocytes that are merely passengers contained in the vascular and perivascular regions of a solid organ being transplanted[265] (see *Table 31.12*).

Hematopoietic Stem Cell Transplants

Hematopoietic stem cell transplants can be ABO compatible or ABO mismatched. The mismatch can include major, minor, or both major and minor ABO incompatibilities.[266] ABO-compatible stem cell transplants have the same ABO type for the donor and recipient. A *major ABO mismatch* implies the introduction of a foreign ABO antigen, as would be seen with a group O recipient of a group A, B, or AB donor stem cell product. A *minor ABO mismatch* implies the introduction of a foreign ABO antibody (isohemagglutinin), as would be seen with a group A, B, or AB recipient of a group O donor stem cell product. Both major and minor incompatibilities would be seen with a group A recipient of a group B donor product or a group B recipient of a group A donor product. Appropriate selection of RBC- and plasma-containing blood products can help minimize the complications of passive antibody transfer.[266] The acute impact of a minor incompatible stem cell transplant is ameliorated with a simple washing of the donor product to prevent passive transfer of preexisting antibodies. However, when

Table 31.12. Timing of Posttransplant Immune Hemolytic Anemia

Immediate	Days-Weeks-Months
Hemolysis of original RBCs due to ABO antibodies in the donor stem cell product (minor ABO group mismatch)	Passenger lymphocyte syndrome
Passive transfer of ABO antibodies: infusion of plasma, platelets, IVIG, intravenous anti-D, and anti-lymphocyte globulin	Passive transfer of ABO antibodies: infusion of plasma, platelets, IVIG, intravenous anti-D, and anti-lymphocyte globulin
Hemolysis of donor RBCs contained in stem cell product by original preexisting ABO antibodies (major ABO group mismatch)	Hemolysis of donor RBCs produced by the newly engrafted marrow caused by residual ABO antibodies (major ABO group mismatch)
	Alloantibodies produced by residual cells of the original immune system
	Alloantibodies produced by engrafted cells of the donor's immune system (week-months)
Autoimmune hemolytic anemia	Autoimmune hemolytic anemia

IVIG, intravenous immunoglobulin; RBC, red blood cell.

there is a minor incompatibility, the novel hematopoietic stem cells will eventually produce lymphocytes that generate antibodies against the recipient's original remaining RBCs. This immune hemolysis may begin 7 to 10 days post transplant and can be abrupt and severe. As the patient's original but now incompatible RBCs are destroyed, they are replaced by a combination of transfused cells and postengraftment novel donor-type RBCs. Consequently, the immune-mediated RBC destruction is limited by the residual original-type RBCs remaining.

Solid Organ Transplants and the Passenger Lymphocyte Syndrome

The immune hemolysis associated with solid organ transplantation is typically due to a *passenger lymphocyte syndrome*. This situation can be seen with just about any solid organ being transplanted, as long as the donor and recipient share an RBC incompatibility. The classic example involves a group O organ transplanted into a group A recipient. Donor lymphocytes that are merely passengers in the transplanted organ react to recipient (endogenous) RBCs and generate antirecipient RBC antibodies. The consequent hemolytic anemia is more frequent, with transplanted organs containing significant lymphoid mass. The incidence is lowest in kidney transplant recipients (9%-17%), intermediate among liver transplant recipients (29%-40%), and highest in heart-lung transplant recipients (70%).[266-269] Extensive perfusion of transplanted organs does not necessarily prevent this passenger lymphocyte syndrome, implying extravascular lymphocyte sequestration. Unlike the hemolysis associated with minor ABO-incompatible hematopoietic stem cell transplants, the target RBCs are not replaced by transfusion and a novel engrafted marrow. Consequently, the immune-mediated RBC destruction is limited only by the survival of the passenger lymphocytes.

References

1. Sokol RG, Hewitt S, Stamps BK. Autoimmune haemolysis. Mixed warm and cold antibody type. *Acta Haematol.* 1983;69:266-274.
2. Worlledge SM. Immune drug-induced hemolytic anemias. *Semin Hematol.* 1969;6:181-200.
3. De Angelis, De Matteis MC, Cozzi MR, et al. Abnormalities of membrane protein composition in patients with autoimmune hemolytic anemia. *Br J Haematol.* 1996;95:273-277.
4. Shen CR, Youssef AR, Devine A. Peptides containing a dominant T-cell epitope from red cell band 3 have in vivo immunomodulatory properties in NZB mice with autoimmune hemolytic anemia. *Blood.* 2003;102:3800-3806.
5. Shlomchik MJ. Mechanisms of immune self-tolerance and how they fail in autoimmune disease. In: Silberstein L, ed. *Autoimmune Disorders of Blood.* American Association of Blood Banks; 1996:1-34.
6. Abbas AK. Diseases of immunity. In: Kumar V, Abbas A, Fausto N, eds. *Robbins and Cotran Pathologic Basis of Disease.* 7th ed. Elsevier Saunders; 2005:223-225.
7. Semple JW, Freedman J. Autoimmune pathogenesis and autoimmune hemolytic anemia. *Semin Hematol.* 2005;42:122-130.
8. Hall AM, Ward FJ, Vickers MA, Stott LM, Urbaniak SJ, Barker RN. Interleukin mediated regulatory T-cell responses to epitopes on a human red blood cell autoantigen. *Blood.* 2002;100:4529-4536.
9. Worth GR, Jones BA, Schreiber AD. Fc receptor structure/function and role in immune complex-mediated autoimmune disease. *Hematology Am Soc Hematol Educ Program.* 2004;2004:54-58.
10. Brown EJ. Complement receptors, adhesion, and phagocytosis. *Infect Agents Dis.* 1992;2:63-70.
11. Cooper NR, Moore MD, Nemerow GR. Immunobiology of CR2, the B lymphocyte receptor for Epstein-Barr virus and the C3d complement fragment. *Annu Rev Immunol.* 1988;6:85-113.
12. Ross GD, Medof ME. Membrane complement receptors specific for bound fragments of C3. *Adv Immunol.* 1985;37:217-267.
13. Frank MM, Fries LF. The role of complement in inflammation and phagocytosis. *Immunol Today.* 1991;12:322-326.
14. Lachmann PJ, Voak D, Oldroyd RG, Downie DM, Bevan PC. Use of monoclonal anti-C3 antibodies to characterize the fragments of C3 that are found on erythrocytes. *Vox Sang.* 1983;45:367-372.
15. Logue G, Rosse WF. Immunologic mechanisms in autoimmune hemolytic disease. *Semin Hematol.* 1976;13:277-289.
16. Frank MM, Schreiber AD, Atkinson JP. NIH conference. Pathophysiology of immune hemolytic anemia. *Ann Intern Med.* 1977;87:210-222.
17. Unkless JC. Function and heterogeneity of human Fc receptors for immunoglobulin G. *J Clin Invest.* 1989;83:355-361.
18. van de Winkel JG, Anderson CL. Biology of human immunoglobulin G Fc receptors. *J Leukoc Biol.* 1991;49:511-524.
19. Anderson DR, Kelton JG. Mechanisms of intravascular and extravascular cell destruction. In: Nance SJ, ed. *Immune Destruction of Red Cells.* American Association of Blood Banks; 1989:1-52.
20. van Oss CJ, Absolom DR. Hemagglutination and the closest distance approach of normal, neuraminidase, and papain-treated erythrocytes. *Vox Sang.* 1983;47:250-256.
21. Leikola J, Pasanen VJ. Influence of antigen receptor density on agglutination of red blood cells. *Int Arch Allergy Appl Immunol.* 1970;39:352-360.
22. Fukuda M, Fukuda MV, Hakomori SI. Developmental change and genetic defect in the carbohydrate structure of band 3 glycoprotein of human erythrocyte membrane. *J Biol Chem.* 1979;254:3700-3703.
23. Economidou J, Hughes-Jones NC, Gardner B. The functional activities of IgG and IgM anti-A and anti-B. *Immunology.* 1967;13:227-234.
24. Greenbury CL, Moore D, Nunn LAC. Reaction of 7S and 19S components of immune rabbit antisera with human group A and AB red cells. *Immunology.* 1963;6:421.
25. Moreschi C. Neue Tatsachen über die Blut Körpenchenagglutination. *Zentralbl Bakteriol.* 1908;46:49-51.
26. Coombs RRA, Mourant AE, Race RR. A new test for the detection of weak and "incomplete" Rh agglutinins. *Br J Exp Pathol.* 1945;26:255-266.
27. Coombs RRA, Mourant AE, Race RR. In vivo isosensitization of red cells in babies with haemolytic disease. *Lancet.* 1946;1:264-266.
28. Zarandona JM, Yazer MH. Teaching case report. The role of the Coombs test in evaluating hemolysis in adults. *Can Med Assoc J.* 2006;174:305-307.
29. Brecher ME, ed. *Technical Manual.* 15th ed. American Association of Blood Banks; 2005.
30. South SF. Use of the direct antiglobulin test in routine testing. In: Wallace M, Levitt J, eds. *Current Applications and Interpretations of the Direct Antiglobulin Test.* American Association of Blood Banks; 1988:25-45.
31. Petz LD, Garratty G. *Acquired Immune Hemolytic Anemias.* Churchill Livingstone; 1980.
32. Sokol RJ, Booker DJ, Stamps R, Booth JR, Hook V. IgA red cell autoantibodies and autoimmune hemolysis. *Transfusion.* 1997;37:175-181.
33. Garratty G. Novel mechanisms for immune destruction of circulating autologous cells. In: Silberstein L, ed. *Autoimmune Disorders of Blood.* American Association of Blood Banks; 1996:79-114.
34. Burkhart P, Rosenfield RE, Hsu TC. Instrumental PVP-augmented antiglobulin tests I. Detection of allogeneic antibodies coating otherwise normal erythrocytes. *Vox Sang.* 1974;26:289-304.
35. Garratty G. Immune hemolytic anemia associated with negative routine serology. *Semin Hematol.* 2005;42:156-164.
36. Issitt PD, Pavone BG, Goldfinger D, et al. Anti Wrb and other autoantibodies responsible for positive direct antiglobulin tests in 150 individuals. *Br J Haematol.* 1976;34:5-18.
37. Weiner W, Vox GH. Serology of acquired hemolytic anemias. *Blood.* 1963;22:606-613.
38. Garratty G. Target antigens for red-cell-bound autoantibodies. In: Nance SJ, ed. *Clinical and Basic Science Aspects of Immunohematology.* American Association of Blood Banks; 1991:33-72.
39. Szymanski IO, Roberts PL, Rosenfield RE. Anti-A autoantibody with severe intravascular hemolysis. *N Engl J Med.* 1976;294:995-996.
40. Sokol RJ, Hewitt S, Booker DJ, Morris BM. Patients with red cell autoantibodies: selection of blood for transfusion. *Clin Lab Haematol.* 1988;10:257-264.
41. Dizon MF. The challenges of daratumumab in transfusion medicine. *Lab Med.* 2017;48(1):6-9.
42. Donath J, Landsteiner K. Ueber paroxysmal hämoglobinurie. *München Med Wochenschr.* 1904;51:1590-1593.
43. Landsteiner K. Uber Besiehungen zwischen den Blutserum und den Kürper Kürperzeller. *München Med Wochenschr.* 1903;50:1812.
44. Schubothe H. The cold hemagglutinin disease. *Semin Hematol.* 1966;3:27-47.
45. Dacie J. *The Auto-Immune Haemolytic Anaemias.* 3rd ed. Churchill Livingstone; 1992.
46. Wortman J, Rosse W, Logue G. Cold agglutinin autoimmune hemolytic anemia in nonhematologic malignancies. *Am J Hematol.* 1979;6:275-283.
47. Lazarian G, Quinquenel A, Bellal M, et al. Autoimmune haemolytic anaemia associated with COVID-19 infection. *Br J Haematol.* 2020;190(1):29-31.
48. Brazel D, Eid T, Harding C. Warm and cold autoimmune hemolytic anemia in the setting of COVID-19 disease. *Cureus.* 2021;13(9):e18127.
49. Zama D, Pancaldi L, Baccelli F, et al. Autoimmune hemolytic anemia in children with COVID-19. *Pediatr Blood Cancer.* 2021;69(2):e29330.
50. Jacobs J, Eichbaum Q. COVID-19 associated with severe autoimmune hemolytic anemia. *Transfusion.* 2021;61:635-640.
51. Pruzanski W, Shumak KH. Biologic activity of cold reactive autoantibodies. *N Engl J Med.* 1977;297:538-542.
52. Roelcke D, Hack H, Kreft H, MacDonald B, Pereira A, Habibi B. IgA cold agglutinins recognize Pr and Sa antigens expressed on glycophorins. *Transfusion.* 1993;33:472-475.
53. Williams R, Kunkel H, Capra J. Antigenic specificities related to the cold agglutinin activity of gamma M globulins. *Science.* 1968;161:379.
54. Silberstein LE, Jefferies LC, Goldman J, et al. Variable region gene analysis of pathologic human auto-antibodies to the related i and I red blood cell antigens. *Blood.* 1991;73:2372-2386.
55. Stevenson F, Smith G, North J, Hamblin TJ, Glennie MJ. Identification of normal B-cell counterparts of neoplastic CLLs which secrete cold agglutinins of anti-I and anti-I specificity. *Br J Haematol.* 1989;72:9-15.
56. Pascual V, Victor K, Spellerberg M, Hamblin TJ, Stevenson FK, Capra JD. VH restriction among human cold agglutinins. The VH4-21 gene segment is required to encode anti-I and anti-i specificities. *J Immunol.* 1992;149:2337-2344.

57. Michaux L, Dierlamm J, Wlodarska L, et al. Trisomy 3q11-q29 is recurrently observed in B-cell non-Hodgkin's lymphomas associated with cold agglutinin syndrome. *Ann Hematol.* 1998;76:201-204.

58. Silberstein LE, Robertson GA, Harris AC, Moreau L, Besa E, Nowell PC. Etiologic aspects of cold agglutinin disease: evidence for cytogenetically defined clones of lymphoid cells and the demonstration that an anti-Pr cold autoantibody is derived from a chromosomally aberrant B-cell clone. *Blood.* 1986;67:1705-1709.

59. Silberstein LE, Goldman J, Kant JA, Spitalnik SL. Comparative biochemical and genetic characterization of clonally related human B-cell lines secreting pathogenic anti-Pr2 cold agglutinins. *Arch Biochem Biophys.* 1988;264:244-252.

60. Roelcke D. Cold agglutination. *Transfus Med Rev.* 1989;3:140-166.

61. Konig AL, Schabel A, Sugg U, Brand U, Roelcke D. Autoimmune hemolytic anemia caused by IgG lambda-monotypic cold agglutinins of anti-Pr specificity after rubella infection. *Transfusion.* 2001;41:488-492.

62. von dem Borne AE, Mol JJ, Joustra-Maas N, Pegels JG, Langenhuijsen MM, Engelfriet CP. Autoimmune haemolytic anaemia with monoclonal IgM(k) anti-P cold autohaemolysins. *Br J Haematol.* 1982;50:345-350.

63. Loomes LM, Uemure KI, Childs RA, et al. Erythrocyte receptors for Mycoplasma pneumonia are sialylated oligosaccharides of Ii antigen type. *Nature.* 1984;307:560-563.

64. Costea N, Yakulis V, Heller P. Inhibition of cold agglutinins (anti-I) by M. pneumoniae antigens. *Proc Soc Exp Biol Med.* 1972;139:476-479.

65. Tanowitz HB, Robbins N, Leidich N. Hemolytic anemia associated with severe Mycoplasma pneumoniae pneumonia. *N Y State J Med.* 1978;78:2231-2232.

66. Dacie JV, Worlledge SM. Autoimmune hemolytic anemias. In: Brown EB, Moore CV, eds. *Progress in Hematology.* Vol 6. Grune & Stratton; 1969:82-120.

67. Jenkins WJ, Koster HG, Marsh WL, Carter RL. Infectious mononucleosis: an unsuspected source of anti-I. *Br J Haematol.* 1965;11:480-483.

68. Horwitz CA, Moulds J, Henle W, et al. Cold agglutinins in infectious mononucleosis and heterophil-antibody-negative mononucleosis-like syndromes. *Blood.* 1977;50:195-200.

69. Bowman HS, Marsh WL, Schumacher HR, Oyen R, Reihart J. Auto anti-N immunohemolytic anemia in infectious mononucleosis. *Am J Clin Pathol.* 1974;61:465-472.

70. Goldberg L, Barnett E. Mixed IgG-IgM cold agglutinin. *J Immunol.* 1967;99:803-809.

71. Gronemeyer P, Chaplin H, Ghazarian V, Tuscany F, Wilner GD. Hemolytic anemia complicating infectious mononucleosis due to the interaction of an IgG cold anti-I and an IgM cold rheumatoid factor. *Transfusion.* 1981;21:715-718.

72. Horwitz CA, Skradski K, Reece E, et al. Haemolytic anaemia in previously healthy adult patients with CMV infections: report of two cases and an evaluation of subclinical haemolysis in CMV mononucleosis. *Scand J Haematol.* 1984;33:35-42.

73. Evans RS, Turner E, Bingham M. Studies with radioiodinated cold agglutinins of ten patients. *Am J Med.* 1965;38:378.

74. Rosse WF, Adams JP. The variability of hemolysis in the cold agglutinin syndrome. *Blood.* 1980;56:409-416.

75. Evans RS, Bingham M, Turner E. Autoimmune hemolytic disease: observations of serological reactions and disease activity. *Ann N Y Acad Sci.* 1965;124:422-440.

76. Ferriman DG, Dacie JV, Kelle KD, Fullerton JM. The association of Raynaud's phenomena, chronic haemolytic anaemia, and the formation of cold antibodies. *Q J Med.* 1951;20:275-292.

77. Chitnavis VN, Patou G, Makar YF, Kendra JR. B19 parvovirus-induced red cell aplasia complicating acute cold antibody-mediated haemolytic anaemia. *Br J Haematol.* 1990;76:433-434.

78. Harboe M, Torvisk H. Protein abnormalities in the cold haemagglutinin syndrome. *Scand J Haematol.* 1969;6:416-426.

79. Swiecicki P. Cold agglutinin disease. *Blood.* 2013;122(7):1114-1121.

80. Berentsen S. How I treat cold agglutinin disease. *Blood.* 2021;137(10):1295-1303.

81. Berentsen S, Ulvestad E, Gjertsen BT, et al. Rituximab for primary chronic cold agglutinin disease: a prospective study of 37 courses of therapy in 27 patients. *Blood.* 2004;103(8):2925-2928.

82. Schollkopf C, Kjeldsen L, Bjerrum OW, et al. Rituximab in chronic cold agglutinin disease: a prospective study of 20 patients. *Leuk Lymphoma.* 2006;47(2):253-260.

83. Hongeng S, Tardtong P, Worapongpaiboon S, Ungkanont A, Jootar S. Successful treatment of refractory autoimmune haemolytic anaemia in a post-unrelated bone marrow transplant paediatric patient with rituximab. *Bone Marrow Transplant.* 2002;29:871-872.

84. Berentsen S, Randen U, Vagan AM, et al. High response rate and durable remissions following fludarabine and rituximab combination therapy for chronic cold agglutinin disease. *Blood.* 2010;116(17):3180-3184.

85. Berentsen S, Barcellini W. Autoimmune hemolytic anemias. *N Engl J Med.* 2021;385(15):1407-1419.

86. Berentsen S, Randen U, Oksman M, et al. Bendamustine plus rituximab for chronic cold agglutinin disease: results of a Nordic prospective multicenter trial. *Blood.* 2017;130(4):537-541.

87. Schreiber AD, Herskovitz BS, Goldwein M. Low-titer cold-hemagglutinin disease. *N Engl J Med.* 1977;296:1490-1494.

88. Taft EG, Propp RP, Sullivan SA. Plasma exchange for cold agglutinin hemolytic anemia. *Transfusion.* 1977;17:173-176.

89. Rodenhuis S, Maas A, Hazenberg CA, Das PC, Nieweg HO. Inefficacy of plasma exchange in cold agglutinin hemolytic anemia 舒 a case study. *Vox Sang.* 1985;49:20-25.

90. Nydegger UE, Kazatchkine MD, Miescher PA. Immunopathologic and clinical features of hemolytic anemia due to cold agglutinins. *Semin Hematol.* 1991;28:66-77.

91. Zoppi M, Oppliger R, Althaus U, Nydegger U. Reduction of plasma cold agglutinin titers by means of plasmapheresis to prepare a patient for coronary bypass surgery. *Infusionsther Transfusionsmed.* 1993;20:19-22.

92. Innet LM, Lester JL,III, Tait N. Cold agglutinins: preoperative diagnosis leads to an uneventful perfusion. *Perfusion.* 1995;10:343-345.

93. Agarwal SK, Ghosh PK, Gupta D. Cardiac surgery and cold-reactive proteins. *Ann Thorac Surg.* 1995;60:1143-1150.

94. Siami FS, Siami GA. A last resort modality using cryofiltration apheresis for the treatment of cold hemagglutinin disease in a Veterans Administration hospital. *Ther Apher Dial.* 2004;8:398-403.

95. McCullough J. *Transfusion Medicine.* 2nd ed. Elsevier; 2005:341.

96. Woll JE, Smith CM, Nusbacher J. Treatment of acute cold agglutinin hemolytic anemia with transfusion of adult i RBCs. *JAMA.* 1974;229:1779-1780.

97. Bell CA, Zwicker H, Sacks HJ. Autoimmune hemolytic anemia: routine serologic evaluation in a general hospital population. *Am J Clin Pathol.* 1973;60:903-911.

98. Hillmen P, Hall C, Marsh JC, et al. Effect of eculizumab on hemolysis and transfusion requirements in patients with paroxysmal nocturnal hemoglobinuria. *N Engl J Med.* 2004;350:552-559.

99. Roth A, Huttmann A, Rother RP, Duhrsen U, Philipp T. Long-term efficacy of the complement inhibitor eculizumab in cold agglutinin disease. *Blood.* 2009;113(16):3885-3886.

100. Shi J, Rose EL, Singh A, et al. TNT003, an inhibitor of the serine protease C1s, prevents complement activation induced by cold agglutinins. *Blood.* 2014;123(26):4015-4022.

101. Jager U, D'Sa S, Schorgenhofer C, et al. Inhibition of complement C1s improves severe hemolytic anemia in cold agglutinin disease: a first-in-human trial. *Blood.* 2019;133(9):893-901.

102. Roth A, Barcellini W, D'Sa S, et al. Sutimlimab in cold agglutinin disease. *N Engl J Med.* 2021;384(14):1323-1334.

103. Berentsen S. Cold agglutinins: fending off the attack. *Blood.* 2019;133(9):885-886.

104. Heddle NM. Acute paroxysmal cold hemoglobinuria. *Transfus Med Rev.* 1989;3:219-229.

105. Göttsche B, Salama A, Mueller-Eckhardt C. Donath-Landsteiner autoimmune hemolytic anemia in children. A study of 22 cases. *Vox Sang.* 1990;58:281-286.

106. Gelfand EW, Abramson N, Segel GB, Nathan DG. Buffy-coat observations and red cell antibodies in acquired hemolytic anemia. *N Engl J Med.* 1971;284:1250-1252.

107. Hinz CB, Jr, Picken ME, Lepow IH. Studies on immune human hemolysis. I. The kinetics of the Donath-Landsteiner reaction and the requirement for complement in the reaction. *J Exp Med.* 1961;113:177-192.

108. Hinz CF, Jr. Serologic and physicochemical characterization of Donath-Landsteiner antibodies from six patients. *Blood.* 1963;22:600-605.

109. Schwarting GA, Kundu SK, Marcus DM. Reaction of antibodies that cause paroxysmal cold hemoglobinuria (PCH) with globoside and Forssman glycosphingolipids. *Blood.* 1979;53:186-192.

110. Levine P, Celano MJ, Falkowski F. The specificity of the antibody in paroxysmal cold hemoglobinuria. *Transfusion.* 1963;3:278-280.

111. Levine P, Celano MJ, Falkowski F. The specificity of the antibody in paroxysmal cold hemoglobinuria (P.C.H.). *Ann N Y Acad Sci.* 1966;124:456-461.

112. van Loghem JJ, van der Hart M, Dorfmeier H. *Serological studies in acquired hemolytic anemia. Sixth International Congress of the International Society of Hematology.* Grune & Stratton; 1958.

113. Sokol RJ, Hewitt S, Stamps BK. Autoimmune haemolysis associated with Donath-Landsteiner antibodies. *Acta Haematol.* 1982;68:268-277.

114. Hernandez JA, Steane SM. Erythrophagocytosis by segmented neutrophils in paroxysmal cold hemoglobinuria. *Am J Clin Pathol.* 1984;81:787-789.

115. Hunt JH. The Raynaud phenomena: a critical review. *Q J Med.* 1936;5:399-444.

116. O'Neill BJ, Marshall WC. Paroxysmal cold haemoglobinuria and measles. *Arch Dis Child.* 1967;42:183-186.

117. Bunch DF, Schwarz DM, Bird GW. Paroxysmal cold haemoglobinuria following measles immunization. *Arch Dis Child.* 1972;47:299-300.

118. Colley EW. Paroxysmal cold haemoglobinuria after mumps. *Br Med J.* 1964;1:1552-1553.

119. Boccardi V, D'Annibali S, DiNatale G, Girelli G, Summonti D. Mycoplasma pneumoniae infection complicated by paroxysmal cold hemoglobinuria with anti-P specificity of biphasic hemolysin. *Blut.* 1977;34:211-214.

120. Sokol RJ, Hewitt S, Stamps BK. Autoimmune haemolysis in childhood and adolescence. *Acta Haematol.* 1984;72:245-257.

121. Wolach B, Heddle N, Barr RD, Pai KR, Blajchman MA. Transient Donath-Landsteiner haemolytic anaemia. *Br J Haematol.* 1981;48:425-434.

122. Mohler DH, Farris BL, Pearre AA. Paroxysmal cold hemoglobinuria with acute renal failure. *Arch Intern Med.* 1963;112:36-40.

123. Rausen AR, LeVine R, Hsu TC, Rosenfield RE. Compatible transfusion therapy for paroxysmal cold hemoglobinuria. *Pediatrics.* 1975;55:275-278.

124. Roy-Burman A, Glader BE. Resolution of severe Donath-Landsteiner autoimmune hemolytic anemia temporally associated with institution of plasmapheresis. *Crit Care Med.* 2002;30:931-934.

125. Nelson MG, Nicholl B. Paroxysmal cold haemoglobinuria. *Ir J Med Sci.* 1960;410:49-57.

126. Shulman IA, Branch DR, Nelson JM, Thompson JC, Saxena S, Petz LD. Autoimmune hemolytic anemia with both cold and warm autoantibodies. *JAMA.* 1985;253:1746-1748.

127. Kajii E, Miura Y, Ikemoto S. Characterization of autoantibodies in mixed type autoimmune hemolytic anemia. *Vox Sang.* 1991;60:45-52.

128. Sokol R, Hewitt S, Stamps BK. Autoimmune haemolysis: an 18-year study of 865 cases referred to a regional transfusion centre. *Br Med J (Clin Res Ed).* 1981;282:2023-2027.

129. Dausset J, Colombani J. The serology and the prognosis of 128 cases of autoimmune hemolytic anemia. *Blood.* 1959;14:1280-1301.

Disorders of Red Blood Cells

130. Da Costa JAG, White AG, Parker AC, et al. Increased incidence of HL-A1 and 8 in patients showing IgG or complement coating on their red cells. *J Clin Pathol.* 1974;27:353-355.

131. Clauvel JP, Marcelli-Barge A, Gautier Coggia I, Poirier JC, Benajam A, Dausset J. HLA antigens and idiopathic autoimmune hemolytic anemias. *Transplant Proc.* 1974;6:447-448.

132. Abdel-Khalik A, Paton L, White AG, Urbaniak SJ. Human leucocyte antigens A, B, C and DRW in idiopathic "warm" autoimmune haemolytic anaemia. *Br Med J.* 1980;280:760-761.

133. Toolis F, Parker AC, White A, Urbaniak S. Familial autoimmune hemolytic anaemia. *Br Med J.* 1977;1:1392.

134. Dacie J. *Secondary or Symptomatic Haemolytic Anaemias.* 3rd ed. Churchill Livingstone; 1995.

135. Lopez C, Kim J, Pandey A, et al. Simultaneous onset of COVID-19 and autoimmune haemolytic anaemia. *Br J Haematol.* 2020;190(1):31-32.

136. Engelfriet CP, Overbeeke MA, von dem Borne AE. Autoimmune hemolytic anemia. *Semin Hematol.* 1992;29:3-12.

137. Ravetch J, Kinet JP. Fc receptors. *Annu Rev Immunol.* 1991;9:457-492.

138. Anderson CL, Looney RJ. Human leukocyte IgG Fc receptors. *Immunol Today.* 1986;7:264.

139. Pirofsky B. Clinical aspects of autoimmune hemolytic anemia. *Semin Hematol.* 1976;13:251-265.

140. Sokol RJ, Hewitt S, Stamps B. Erythrocyte autoantibodies, autoimmune haemolysis and pregnancy. *Vox Sang.* 1982;43:169-176.

141. Chaplin H, Jr, Cohen R, Bloomberg G, Kaplan HJ, Moore JA, Dorner I. Pregnancy and idiopathic autoimmune haemolytic anaemia: a prospective study during 6 months gestation and 3 months post-partum. *Br J Haematol.* 1973;24:219-229.

142. Starksen NF, Bell WE, Kickler TS. Unexplained hemolytic anemia associated with pregnancy. *Am J Obstet Gynecol.* 1983;146:617-622.

143. Burt RL, Prichard RW. Acquired hemolytic anaemia in pregnancy: report of a case. *Obstet Gynecol.* 1957;10:444-450.

144. Johnson ST, McFarland JG, Kelly KJ, Casper JT, Gottschall JL. Transfusion support with RBCs from an Mk homozygote in a case of autoimmune hemolytic anemia following diphtheria-pertussis-tetanus vaccination. *Transfusion.* 2002;42:567-571.

145. Downes KA, Domen RE, McCarron KF, Bringelsen KA. Acute autoimmune hemolytic anemia following DTP vaccination: report of a fatal case and review of the literature. *Clin Pediatr.* 2001;40:355-358.

146. Muwakkit S, Rachid R, Bazarbachi A, Araysi T, Dbaibo GS. Treatment-resistant infantile Evans syndrome. *Pediatr Int.* 2001;43:502-504.

147. Evans RS, Duane RT. Acquired hemolytic anaemia: I. The relation of antibody activity to activity of the disease. II. The significance of thrombocytopenia and leukopenia. *Blood.* 1949;4:1196-1213.

148. Evans RS, Takahashi K, Duane RT, Payne R, Liu C. Primary thrombocytopenic purpura and acquired hemolytic anaemia. Evidence for a common etiology. *Arch Intern Med.* 1951;87:48-65.

149. Crosby WH, Rappaport H. Autoimmune hemolytic anaemia. I. Analysis of hematologic observations with particular reference to their prognostic value. A survey of 57 cases. *Blood.* 1957;12:42-55.

150. Wang WC. Evans syndrome in childhood: pathophysiology, clinical course, and treatment. *Am J Pediatr Hematol Oncol.* 1988;10:330-338.

151. Miano M. How I manage Evans syndrome and AIHA cases in children. *Br J Haematol.* 2016;172(4):524-534.

152. Scaradavou A, Bussel J. Evans syndrome results of a pilot study utilizing a multiagent treatment protocol. *J Pediatr Hematol Oncol.* 1995;17:290-295.

153. Ucar B, Akgun N, Aydogdu SD, Kirel B, Idem S. Treatment of refractory Evans' syndrome with cyclosporine and prednisone. *Pediatr Int.* 1999;41:104-107.

154. Liesveld JL, Rowe JM, Lichtman MA. Variability of the erythropoietic response in autoimmune hemolytic anemia: analysis of 189 cases. *Blood.* 1987;69:820-826.

155. Mangan KF, Besa EC, Shadduck RK, Tedrow H, Ray PK. Demonstration of two distinct antibodies in autoimmune hemolytic anemia with reticulocytopenia and red cell aplasia. *Exp Hematol.* 1984;12:788-793.

156. Hauke G, Fauser AA, Weber S, Maas D. Reticulocytopenia in severe autoimmune hemolytic anemia (AIHA) of the warm antibody type. *Blut.* 1983;46:321-327.

157. Lefrère JJ, Courouce AM, Bertrand Y, Girot R, Soulier JP. Human parvovirus and aplastic crisis in chronic hemolytic anemias: a study of 24 observations. *Am J Hematol.* 1986;23:271-275.

158. Zinkham WH, Diamond LK. In vitro erythrophagocytosis in acquired hemolytic anemia. *Blood.* 1952;7:592-601.

159. Fagiolo E. Platelet and leukocyte antibodies in autoimmune hemolytic anemia. *Acta Haematol.* 1976;56:97-106.

160. Russell NH, Keenan JP, Frais MA. Thrombocytopathy associated with autoimmune hemolytic anemia. *Br Med J.* 1978;2:604.

161. Tisdale WA, Klatskin G, Kinsella ED. Significance of the indirect-reacting fraction of serum bilirubin in hemolytic jaundice. *Am J Med.* 1959;26:214-227.

162. Payne R, Spaet TH, Aggeler PM. An unusual antibody pattern in a case of idiopathic acquired hemolytic anemia. *J Lab Clin Med.* 1955;46:245-254.

163. Kretschmer V, Mueller-Eckhardt C. Autoimmune hemolytic anemias. II. Immunoglobulins and b1-globulin in the serum with special regard to the immunochemical type of autoantibodies and the course of the disease. *Blut.* 1972;25:159-168.

164. Mueller-Eckhardt C, Möhring F, Kretschmer V, Höbel W, Löffler H. Reappraisal of the clinical and etiologic significance of immunoglobulin deviations in autoimmune hemolytic anemia ("warm type"). *Blut.* 1977;34:39-47.

165. Chaplin H, Jr. Clinical usefulness of specific antiglobulin reagents in autoimmune hemolytic anemias. *Prog Hematol.* 1973;7:25-49.

166. Araguás C, Martín-Vega C, Massagué I, de Latorre FJ. "Complete" warm hemolysins producing an autoimmune hemolytic anemia. *Vox Sang.* 1990;59:125-126.

167. Wolf MW, Roelcke D. Incomplete warm hemolysins. *Clin Immunol Immunopathol.* 1989;51:68-76.

168. Lalezari P. Serologic profile in autoimmune hemolytic disease: pathophysiologic and clinical interpretations. *Semin Hematol.* 1976;13:291-310.

169. van der Meulen FW, de Bruin HG, Goosen PC, et al. Quantitative aspects of the destruction of red cells sensitized with IgG1 autoantibodies: an application of flow cytofluorometry. *Br J Haematol.* 1980;46:47-56.

170. Gehrs BC, Friedberg RC. Autoimmune hemolytic anemia. *Am J Hematol.* 2002;69:258-271.

171. Petz LD. Treatment of autoimmune hemolytic anemias. *Curr Opin Hematol.* 2001;8:411-416.

172. Dacie SJ. The immune haemolytic anaemias: a century of exciting progress in understanding. *Br J Haematol.* 2001;114:770-785.

173. Meyer O, Stahl D, Beckhove P, Huhn D, Salama A. Pulsed high-dose dexamethasone in chronic autoimmune haemolytic anaemia of warm type. *Br J Haematol.* 1997;98:860-862.

174. Nakasone H, Kako S, Endo H, et al. Diabetes mellitus is associated with high early-mortality and poor prognosis in patients with autoimmune hemolytic anemia. *Hematology.* 2009;14(6):361-365.

175. King KE, Ness PM. Treatment of autoimmune hemolytic anemia. *Semin Hematol.* 2005;42:131-136.

176. Rosse WF. Quantitative immunology of immune hemolytic anemia. II. The relationship of cell bound antibody of hemolysis and the effect of treatment. *J Clin Invest.* 1971;50:734-743.

177. Zupanska B, Sylwestrowicz T, Pawelsi S. The results of prolonged treatment of autoimmune hemolytic anemia. *Hematologia.* 1971;4:425-433.

178. Murphy S, LoBuglio AF. Drug therapy in autoimmune hemolytic anemia. *Semin Hematol.* 1976;13:323-334.

179. Allgood JW, Chaplin H. Idiopathic acquired autoimmune hemolytic anemia: a review of forty-seven cases treated from 1955 through 1965. *Am J Med.* 1967;43:254-273.

180. Lechner K, Jager U. How I treat autoimmune hemolytic anemias in adults *Blood.* 2010;116(11):1831-1838.

181. Gibson J. Autoimmune hemolytic anemia: current concepts. *Aust N Z J Med.* 1988;18:625-637.

182. Pirofsky B, Bardana EJ, Jr. Autoimmune hemolytic anemia: II. Therapeutic aspects. *Haematol.* 1974;7:376-385.

183. Akpek G, McAneny D, Weintraub L. Comparative response to splenectomy in Coombs-positive autoimmune hemolytic anemia with or without associated disease. *Am J Hematol.* 1999;61:98-102.

184. Barcellini W, Fattizzo B. How I treat warm autoimmune hemolytic anemia. *Blood.* 2021;137(10):1283-1294.

185. Reynaud Q, Durieu I, Dutertre M, et al. Efficacy and safety of rituximab in autoimmune hemolytic anemia: a meta-analysis of 21 studies. *Autoimmune Rev.* 2015;14(4):304-313.

186. Ahrens N, Kingreen D, Seltsam A, Salama A. Treatment of refractory autoimmune haemolytic anaemia with anti-CD20 (rituximab). *Br J Haematol.* 2001;114:244-245.

187. Quartier P, Brethon B, Philippet P, Landman-Parker J, Le Deist F, Fischer A. Treatment of childhood autoimmune haemolytic anaemia with rituximab. *Lancet.* 2001;358:1511-1513.

188. Perrotta S, Locatelli F, La Manna A, Cennamo L, De Stefano P, Nobili B. Anti-CD20 monoclonal antibody (rituximab) for life-threatening autoimmune haemolytic anaemia in a patient with systemic lupus erythematosus. *Br J Haematol.* 2002;116:465-467.

189. McMahon C, Babu L, Hodgson A, Hayat A, Connell NO, Smith OP. Childhood refractory autoimmune haemolytic anaemia: is there a role for anti-CD20 therapy (rituximab)? *Br J Haematol.* 2002;117:480-483.

190. Zecca M, Nobili B, Ramenghi U, et al. Rituximab for the treatment of refractory autoimmune hemolytic anemia in children. *Blood.* 2003;101:3857-3861.

191. Kunkel L, Wong A, Maneatis T, et al. Optimizing the use of rituximab for treatment of B-cell non-Hodgkin's lymphoma: a benefit-risk update. *Semin Oncol.* 2000;27(suppl 12):53-61.

192. van der Kolk LE, Baars JW, Prins MH, van Oers MH. Rituximab treatment results in impaired secondary humoral immune responsiveness. *Blood.* 2002;100:2257-2259.

193. Bussone G, Ribeiro E, Dechartres A, et al. Safety of rituximab in adults with warm antibody autoimmune haemolytic anemia: retrospective analysis of 27 cases. *Am J Hematol.* 2009;84(3):153-157.

194. Floersheim GL. A comparative study of the effects of anti-tumor and immunosuppressive drugs on antibody forming and erythropoietic cells. *Clin Exp Immunol.* 1970;6:861-870.

195. Johnson WW, Meadows DC. Urinary bladder fibrosis and telangiectasia associated with long-term cyclophosphamide therapy. *N Engl J Med.* 1971;284:290-294.

196. Kumar R, Biggart JD, McEvoy J, McGeown MG. Cyclophosphamide and reproductive function. *Lancet.* 1972;1:1212-1214.

197. Cheema AR, Hersh EM. Patient survival after chemotherapy and its relationship to in vitro lymphocyte blastogenesis. *Cancer.* 1971;28:851-855.

198. Moyo VM, Smith D, Brodsky I, Crilley P, Jones RJ, Brodsky RA. High-dose cyclophosphamide for refractory autoimmune hemolytic anemia. *Blood.* 2002;100:704-706.

199. Howard J, Hoffbrand AV, Prentice HG, Mehta A. Mycophenolate mofetil for the treatment of refractory auto-immune haemolytic anaemia and auto-immune thrombocytopenia purpura. *Br J Haematol.* 2002;117:712-715.

200. Zimmer-Molsberger B, Knauf W, Thiel E. Mycophenolate mofetil for severe autoimmune haemolytic anemia. *Lancet.* 1997;350:1003-1004.

201. Emilia G, Messora C, Longo G, Bertesi M. Long-term salvage treatment by cyclosporin in refractory autoimmune haematological disorders. *Br J Haematol.* 1996;93:341-344.

202. Chemlal K, Wyplosz B, Grange MJ, Lassoued K, Clauvel JP. Salvage therapy and long-term remission with danazol and cyclosporine in refractory Evan's syndrome. *Am J Hematol.* 1999;62:200.

203. Rackoff WR, Manno CS. Treatment of refractory Evans syndrome with alternate-day cyclosporine and prednisone. *Am J Pediatr Hematol Oncol.* 1994;16:156-159.

204. Miano M, Scalzone M, Perri K, et al. Mycophenolate mofetil and Sirolimus as second or further line treatment in children with chronic refractory primitive or secondary autoimmune cytopenias: a single centre experience. *Br J Hematology.* 2015;171(2):247-253.

205. Bride KL, Vincent T, Smith-Whitley K, et al. Sirolimus is effective in relapsed/refractory autoimmune cytopenias: results of a prospective multi-institutional trial. *Blood.* 2016;127(1):17-28.

206. Garratty G, Petz LD. Approaches to selecting blood for transfusion to patients with autoimmune hemolytic anemia. *Transfusion.* 2002;42(11):1390.

207. Bussell JB, Cunningham-Rundles C, Abraham C. Intravenous treatment of autoimmune hemolytic anemia with very high dose gammaglobulin. *Vox Sang.* 1986;51:264-269.

208. Leickly FE, Buckley RH. Successful treatment of auto-immune hemolytic anemia in common variable immunodeficiency with high-dose intravenous gamma globulin. *Am J Med.* 1987;82:159-162.

209. Majer RV, Hyde RD. High-dose intravenous immunoglobulin in the treatment of autoimmune haemolytic anaemia. *Clin Lab Haematol.* 1988;10:391-395.

210. Salama A, Mahn I, Neuzner J, Graubner M, Mueller-Eckhardt C. IgG therapy in autoimmune haemolytic anaemia of warm type. *Blut.* 1984;48:391-392.

211. Weinblatt ME. Treatment of immune hemolytic anemia with gammaglobulin [letter]. *J Pediatr.* 1987;110:817.

212. Vandenberghe P, Zachee P, Verstraete S, Demuynck H, Boogaerts MA, Verhoef GE. Successful control of refractory and life-threatening autoimmune hemolytic anemia with intravenous immunoglobulins in a man with the primary antiphospholipid syndrome. *Ann Hematol.* 1996;73:253-256.

213. Bayry J, Lacroix-Desmazes S, Carbonneil C, et al. Inhibition of maturation and function of dendritic cells by intravenous immunoglobulin. *Blood.* 2003;101:758-765.

214. Mackay IR, Rosen FS. Immunomodulation of autoimmune and inflammatory diseases with intravenous immune globulin. *N Engl J Med.* 2001;345:747-755.

215. Anderson O, Taaning E, Rosenkvist J, Møller NE, Mogensen HH. Autoimmune haemolytic anaemia treated with multiple transfusion, immunosuppressive therapy, plasma exchange, and desferrioxamine. *Acta Paediatr Scand.* 1984;73:145-148.

216. Kutti J, Wadenvik H, Safai-Kutti S, et al. Successful treatment of refractory autoimmune haemolytic anaemia by plasmapheresis. *Scand J Haematol.* 1984;32:149-152.

217. Jaweed M, Nifong TP, Domen RE, Rybka WB. Durable response to combination therapy including staphylococcal protein A immunoadsorption in life threatening refractory autoimmune hemolysis. *Transfusion.* 2002;42:1217-1220.

218. Seeliger S, Baumann M, Mohr M, Jürgens H, Frosch M, Vormoor J. Autologous peripheral blood stem cell transplantation and anti-B-cell directed immunotherapy for refractory auto-immune haemolytic anaemia. *Eur J Pediatr.* 2001;160:492-496.

219. Raetz E, Beatty PG, Adams RH. Treatment of severe Evans syndrome with an allogeneic cord blood transplant. *Bone Marrow Transplant.* 1997;20:427-429.

220. Norton A, Roberts I. Management of Evans syndrome. *Br J Haematol.* 2006;132:125-137.

221. Lundin J, Karlsson C. Alemtuzumab therapy for severe autoimmune hemolysis in a patient with B-cell chronic lymphocytic leukemia. *Med Oncol.* 2006;23:137-139.

222. Cheung WW, Hwang GY. Alemtuzumab induced complete remission of autoimmune hemolytic anemia refractory to corticosteroids, splenectomy and rituximab. *Haematologica.* 2006;91(suppl 5):ECR13.

223. Waespe N, Zeilhofer U, Gungor T. Treatment-refractory multi-lineage autoimmune cytopenia after unrelated cord blood transplantation: remission after combined bortezomib and vincristine treatment. *Pediatr Blood Cancer.* 2014;61(11):2112-2114.

224. Khandelwal P, Davies SM, Grimley MS, et al. Bortezomib for refractory autoimmunity in pediatrics. *Biol Blood Marrow Transplant.* 2014;20(10):1654-1659.

225. Hoffmann P. Immune hemolytic anemia 舒 selected topics. *Hematology Am Soc Hematol Educ Program.* 2006;2006:13-18.

226. Petz LD, Garratty G. *Immune Hemolytic Anemias.* 2nd ed. Churchill Livingstone; 2004.

227. Arndt PA, Garratty G. The changing spectrum of drug-induced hemolytic anemia. *Semin Hematol.* 2005;42:137-144.

228. Habibi B. Drug-induced red blood cell autoantibodies co-developed with drug specific antibodies causing haemolytic anaemias. *Br J Haematol.* 1985;61:139-143.

229. Levine BB, Redmond A. Immunochemical mechanisms of penicillin induced Coombs positivity and hemolytic anemia in man. *Int Arch Allergy Appl Immunol.* 1967;31:594-606.

230. Petz LD. Immunologic cross-reactivity between penicillins and cephalosporins: a review. *J Infect Dis.* 1978;137S:S74-S79.

231. Kerr RO, Caramone J, Dalmasso AP, Kaplan ME. Two mechanisms of erythrocyte destruction in penicillin-induced hemolytic anemia. *N Engl J Med.* 1972;287:1322-1325.

232. Ries CA, Rosenbaum TJ, Garratty G, Petz LD, Fudenberg HH. Penicillin-induced immune hemolytic anemia. *JAMA.* 1975;233:432-435.

233. Swanson MA, Chanmougan D, Schwartz RS. Immunohemolytic anemia due to anti-penicillin antibodies. *N Engl J Med.* 1966;274:178-181.

234. Nesmith LW, Davis JW. Hemolytic anemia caused by penicillin. *JAMA.* 1968;203:27-30.

235. Funicella T, Weinger RS, Moake JL, Spruell M, Rossen RD. Penicillin-induced immunohemolytic anemia associated with circulating immune complexes. *Am J Hematol.* 1977;3:219-223.

236. Gralnick HR, Wright LD, McGinniss MH. Coombs' positive reactions associated with sodium cephalothin therapy. *JAMA.* 1967;199:725-726.

237. Gralnick HR, McGinniss MH, Elton W, McCurdy P. Hemolytic anemia associated with cephalothin. *JAMA.* 1971;217:1193-1197.

238. Branch DR, Berkowitz LR, Becker RL, et al. Extravascular hemolysis following the administration of cefamandole. *Am J Hematol.* 1985;18:213-219.

239. Chambers LA, Donovan BA, Kruskall MS. Ceftazidime-induced hemolysis patient with drug-dependent antibodies reactive by immune complex and drug adsorption mechanisms. *Am J Clin Pathol.* 1991;95:393-396.

240. Garratty G, Nance S, Lloyd M, Domen R. Fatal immune hemolytic anemia due to cefotetan. *Transfusion.* 1992;32:269-271.

241. Simpson MB, Pryzbylik J, Innis B, Denham MA. Hemolytic anemia after tetracycline therapy. *N Engl J Med.* 1985;312:840-842.

242. Wenz B, Klein RL, Lalezari P. Tetracycline-induced immune hemolytic anemia. *Transfusion.* 1974;14:265-269.

243. Malacarne P, Castaldi G, Bertusi M, Zavagli G. Tolbutamide-induced hemolytic anemia. *Diabetes.* 1977;26:156-158.

244. Tuffs L, Manoharan A. Flucloxacillin-induced haemolytic anaemia. *Med J Aust.* 1986;144:559-560.

245. Seldon MR, Bain B, Johnson CA, Lennox CS. Ticarcillin-induced immune haemolytic anaemia. *Scand J Haematol.* 1982;28:459-460.

246. Habibi B, Bretagne Y. Blood group antigens may be the receptors for specific drug-antibody complexes reacting with red blood cells. [Article in French]. *C R Seances Acad Sci III.* 1983;296:693-696.

247. Salama A, Mueller-Eckhardt C. On the mechanisms of sensitization and attachment of antibodies to RBC in drug-induced immune hemolytic anemia. *Blood.* 1987;69:1006-1010.

248. Muirhead EE, Halden ER, Groves M. Drug-dependent Coombs' (antiglobulin) test and anemia. *Arch Intern Med.* 1958;101:87.

249. Muirhead EF, Groves M, Guy R, Halden ER, Bass RK. Acquired hemolytic anemia, exposures to insecticides and positive Coombs' test dependent on insecticide preparations. *Vox Sang.* 1959;4:277.

250. Christie DJ, Mullen PC, Aster RH. Fab-mediated binding of drug-dependent antibodies to platelets in quinidine- and quinine-induced thrombocytopenia. *J Clin Invest.* 1985;75:310-314.

251. Smith ME, Reid DM, Jones CE, Jordan JV, Kautz CA, Shulman NR. Binding of quinine- and quinidine dependent drug antibodies to platelets is mediated by the Fab domain of immunoglobulin G and is not Fc dependent. *J Clin Invest.* 1987;79:912-917.

252. Bakemeier RF, Leddy JP. Erythrocyte autoantibody associated with alpha methyldopa: heterogeneity of structure and specificity. *Blood.* 1968;32:1-14.

253. LoBuglio AF, Jandl JH. The nature of the alpha-methyldopa red-cell antibody. *N Engl J Med.* 1967;276:658-665.

254. Garratty G, Nance SJ. Correlation between in vivo hemolysis and the amount of red cell-bound IgG measured by flow cytometry. *Transfusion.* 1990;30:617-631.

255. Abraham GN, Petz LD, Fudenberg HH. Immunohaematological cross-allergenicity between penicillin and cephalothin in humans. *Clin Exp Immunol.* 1968;3:343-357.

256. Spath P, Garratty G, Petz LD. Studies on the immune response to penicillin and cephalothin in humans. II. Immunohematologic reactions to cephalothin administration. *J Immunol.* 1971;107:860-869.

257. Worlledge SM, Carstairs KC, Dacie JV. Autoimmune haemolytic anaemia associated with alpha-methyldopa therapy. *Lancet.* 1966;2:135-139.

258. MacGibbon BH, Loughridge LW, Hourihane DO, Boyd DW. Autoimmune haemolytic anaemia with acute renal failure due to phenacetin and p-aminosalicylic acid. *Lancet.* 1960;1:7.

259. Garratty G, Leger RM, Arndt PA. Severe immune hemolytic anemia associated with prophylactic use of cefotetan in obstetric and gynecologic procedures. *Am J Obstet Gynecol.* 1999;181:103-104.

260. Naylor CS, Steele L, Hsi R, Margolin M, Goldfinger D. Cefotetan-induced hemolysis associated with antibiotic prophylaxis for cesarean delivery. *Am J Obstet Gynecol.* 2000;182:1427-1428.

261. Ray EK, Warkentin TE, O'Hoski PL, Gregor P. Delayed onset of life-threatening immune hemolysis after perioperative antimicrobial prophylaxis with cefotetan. *Can J Surg.* 2000;43:461-462.

262. Garratty G, Postoway N, Schwellenbach J, McMahill PC. A fatal case of ceftriaxone (Rocephin)-induced hemolytic anemia associated with intravascular immune hemolysis. *Transfusion.* 1991;31:176-179.

263. Borthakur G, O'Brien S, Wierda WG, et al. Immune anemias in patients with chronic lymphocytic leukaemia treated with fludarabine, cyclophosphamide and rituximab-incidence and predictors. *Br J Haematol.* 2007;136(6):800-805.

264. Petz LD. Drug-induced autoimmune hemolytic anemia. *Transfus Med Rev.* 1993;7:242-254.

265. Petz LD. Immune hemolysis associated with transplantation. *Semin Hematol.* 2005;42:145-155.

266. Friedberg RC. Transfusion therapy in the patient undergoing hematopoietic stem cell transplantation. *Hematol Oncol Clin North Am.* 1994;8:1105-1116.

267. Ramsey G. Red cell antibodies arising from solid organ transplants. *Transfusion.* 1991;31:76-86.

268. Magrin GT, Street AM, Williams TJ, Esmore DS. Clinically significant anti-A derived from B lymphocytes after single lung transplantation. *Transplantation.* 1993;56:466-467.

269. Ramsey GE, Sherman LA. Transfusion therapy in solid organ transplantation. *Hematol Oncol Clin North Am.* 1994;8:1117-1129.

Disorders of Red Blood Cells

Chapter 32 ■ Paroxysmal Nocturnal Hemoglobinuria

CHARLES J. PARKER • RUSSELL E. WARE

ABBREVIATIONS

APC   alternative pathway of complement
BMF   bone marrow failure
DAF   decay accelerating factor (CD55)
FLAER   fluorescent aerolysin
GlcNAc-PI   N-acetylglucosaminyl-phosphatidylinositol
GPI   glycosyl phosphatidylinositol
GPI-AP glycosyl phosphatidylinositol–anchored protein
GPI-AP⁻ glycosyl phosphatidylinositol–anchored protein deficient
GPI-AP⁺ glycosyl phosphatidylinositol–anchored protein sufficient
LDH   lactate dehydrogenase
MIRL   membrane inhibitor of reactive lysis (CD59)
MDS   myelodysplastic syndrome
PNH   paroxysmal nocturnal hemoglobinuria
PNH-sc subclinical PNH

DEFINITION

Paroxysmal nocturnal hemoglobinuria (PNH) is a disease of the hematopoietic stem cell, although it is usually classified as a hemolytic anemia. PNH arises as a result of *nonmalignant* clonal expansion of one or *several* hematopoietic stem cells that have acquired a somatic mutation of *PIGA*.[1,2] The *PIGA* gene is located on the X chromosome, and it encodes an enzyme that is an essential component of the complex biosynthetic pathway that generates glycosyl phosphatidylinositol (GPI). The GPI moiety serves as a membrane anchor for >25 proteins of diverse function that are normally expressed on hematopoietic cells. As a consequence of somatic mutation of *PIGA*, progeny of affected stem cells are deficient in all GPI-anchored proteins (GPI-APs). Among the GPI-APs normally expressed on hematopoietic cells are the complement regulatory proteins CD55 (decay accelerating factor, DAF) and CD59 (membrane inhibitor of reactive lysis, MIRL), and it is deficiency of these two proteins that accounts for the complement-mediated intravascular hemolysis that is the hallmark clinical manifestation of the disease. In addition to complement-mediated intravascular hemolysis, an element of bone marrow failure (BMF) is present in all patients, and PNH frequently arises in association with a defined BMF process, particularly aplastic anemia, and to a lesser extent, low-grade myelodysplastic syndrome (MDS). Thrombophilia is a major cause of morbidity and mortality in PNH.[3]

PNH is characterized, in the classic case, by macroscopic hemoglobinuria. When intravascular hemolysis occurs at night, while the patient is asleep, hemoglobin accumulates in the bladder, and the patient becomes alarmed the following morning by the startlingly abnormal appearance of the first voided urine. The hemoglobinuria is painless and ranges in color from red to brown to black. Typically, the gross hemoglobinuria resolves during the course of the day. In most patients, however, the classic pattern is absent at diagnosis. In these patients, the disease is characterized by symptoms of lethargy, malaise, and asthenia, and by laboratory evidence of chronic, low-grade intravascular hemolysis that may or may not be punctuated by episodes of macroscopic hemoglobinuria, usually occurring in association with infection or unusual stress such as trauma or surgery. Thrombocytopenia, leukopenia, and thrombosis involving unusual sites are other notable clinical characteristics of PNH. As cited above, a close association exists between PNH and certain BMF syndromes, but the basis of this association is incompletely understood.

The history of PNH has been chronicled.[4-8] Strübing published a remarkable paper on PNH in 1882, clearly recognizing the uniqueness of the disease and providing laboratory support for his prescient hypothesis on the etiology of the nocturnal hemoglobinuria (positing that it was caused by the acidosis that resulted from carbon dioxide accumulation associated with sleep-related hypoventilation). Marchiafava and Nazari (1911) and Micheli (1931) subsequently detailed the clinical characteristics of the disease (in some older literature, PNH is called Marchiafava-Micheli syndrome). By 1953, at least 162 cases had been collected. Although the advent of flow cytometry has greatly improved diagnostic sensitivity and specificity, undoubtedly some cases go undiagnosed as the classical signs and symptoms are often absent at presentation. Even today there may be a significant time lapse between the onset of clinical symptoms and the correct diagnosis. Failure to distinguish hemoglobinuria (when present) from hematuria, the rarity of the disease that limits familiarity with its protean clinical manifestation, and the absence of gross hemoglobinuria at presentation in many cases are the primary factors that account for the delay in diagnosis.

It can be argued that the term paroxysmal nocturnal hemoglobinuria is imprecise because it describes only one feature of the illness, a feature, moreover, that is found in only one-quarter of affected individuals at presentation. Nonetheless, the term has been established through long, popular use and consequently is part of the essence of the disease.

ETIOLOGY AND PATHOGENESIS

Sensitivity to Complement-Mediated Lysis

The chronic intravascular hemolysis that is the clinical hallmark of PNH is due to the abnormal sensitivity of the erythrocytes to complement-mediated lysis.[9] From 1937 to 1939, Ham and Dingle made the seminal observations that connected the hemolysis to complement.[7] Those studies demonstrated that the abnormal cells are hemolyzed when incubated in acidified serum and that the hemolysis is complement dependent. The lysis of the defective cells in acidified serum (a process that activates the alternative pathway of complement [APC]) became the standard technique for the diagnosis of PNH, and appropriately, the assay was called Ham test. Approximately 10 years after the studies of Ham and Dingle, cross-transfusion studies confirmed that hemolysis in PNH results from an intrinsic abnormality of the red blood cell (RBC). In those studies, Dacie reported that normal erythrocytes survive normally in patients with PNH, whereas the life span of PNH erythrocytes is shortened both in the patient and in a normal recipient. Not all PNH red cells are equally sensitive to complement-mediated lysis, however, and cohorts of relatively long-lived and very short-lived cells can be distinguished in red cell survival studies. Moreover, the proportions of complement-sensitive and complement-insensitive cells vary greatly among patients. Generally, the percentage of abnormal cells remains stable in an individual patient, although there are clearly exceptions. The percentage of markedly complement-sensitive cells correlates with the clinical course of each patient with respect to the hemolytic component of the disease and perhaps to thrombotic propensity.

A defining feature of PNH is *phenotypic mosaicism* based on sensitivity of the erythrocytes to complement-mediated lysis. This remarkable characteristic was first clearly elucidated by Rosse and Dacie in 1966,[10] and Rosse further refined the analysis in 1973.[11] Using an in vitro test that quantitates the sensitivity of erythrocytes to complement-mediated lysis (the complement lysis sensitivity assay), three phenotypes of PNH erythrocytes were identified (*Table 32.1; Figures 32.1* and *32.2*). One of the phenotypes (designated PNH I) was characterized by normal or near-normal sensitivity to complement,

Table 32.1. PNH Phenotypes

Phenotypic Designation	Complement Sensitivity[a]	GPI-AP Expression by Flow Cytometry[b]	Type of *PIG-A* Mutation
PNH I	Normal	Normal	None
PNH II	Moderately sensitive (3-4 times greater than normal)	Dim positive	Missense (partial *PIGA* inactivation)
PNH III	Markedly sensitive (15-25 times greater than normal)	Negative	Nonsense, frameshifts, deletions, insertions (complete inactivation of *PIGA*)

Abbreviations: GPI-AP, glycosyl phosphatidylinositol–anchored proteins; PNH, paroxysmal nocturnal hemoglobinuria.
[a]Based on the complement lysis sensitivity assay of Rosse and Dacie.
[b]Based on flow cytometric analysis of GPI-AP expression of erythrocytes.

whereas another phenotype (designated PNH III) was 15 to 25 times more susceptible to lysis. A third phenotype (PNH II) was of intermediate sensitivity, about 3 to 5 times more susceptible than normal cells. Most patients have a mixture of type I and type III cells, but mosaics of type I, type II, and type III as well as type I and type II are also observed.

As noted above, the proportion of complement-sensitive and -insensitive cells varies greatly among patients. For example, the erythrocytes of one patient (hypothetical patient A) may comprise 10% PNH III cells and 90% PNH I cells, whereas another patient (hypothetical patient B) may have 75% PNH III cells and 25% PNH I cells. The intensity of the hemolytic component of the disease is related to the size of the PNH III population.[12] The proportions of sensitive and insensitive cells usually remain stable for long periods (years to decades), but population shifts may be observed during the course of the disease, and in some patients, the abnormal clone remits spontaneously.[13,14] The threshold for biochemical evidence of intravascular hemolysis is crossed when the population of GPI-deficient neutrophils (as a measure of the PNH clone size) is 20% to 25% or greater.[15] Patients with a clone size of 20% to 25% usually have 3% to 5% PNH erythrocytes (the population of PNH III cells is smaller than

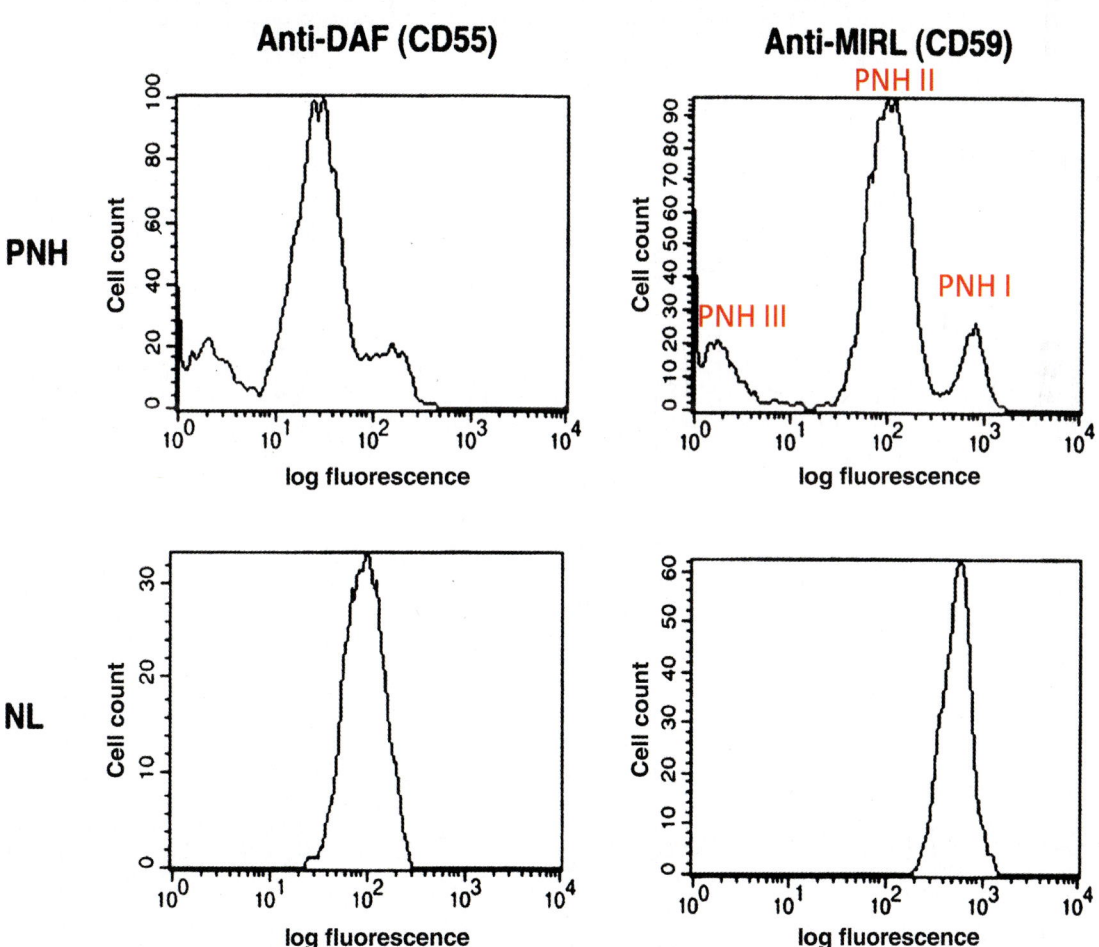

FIGURE 32.1 Phenotypic mosaicism in PNH. Erythrocytes from a patient with PNH and from a normal volunteer donor (NL) were analyzed by flow cytometry using anti-DAF (CD55) and anti-MIRL (CD59) as primary antibodies. The histogram of the erythrocytes from the normal donor shows uniformly positive staining with both antibodies. In contrast, the patient's histogram (PNH) suggests three discrete populations of cells (a negative population [called PNH III], a population with partial expression of CD55 and CD59 [called PNH II], and a population with normal expression [called PNH I]). Statistical analysis of the three groups of cells from the patient showed that the negative population contributed 14% to the total, the intermediate population contributed 75%, and the normal population contributed 11%. DAF, decay accelerating factor; MIRL, membrane inhibitor of reactive lysis. (Modified from Endo M, Ware RE, Vreeke TM, et al. Molecular basis of the heterogeneity of expression of glycosyl phosphatidylinositol-anchored proteins in paroxysmal nocturnal hemoglobinuria. *Blood.* 1996;87(6):2546-2557. Copyright © 1996 American Society of Hematology. With permission.)

Disorders of Red Blood Cells

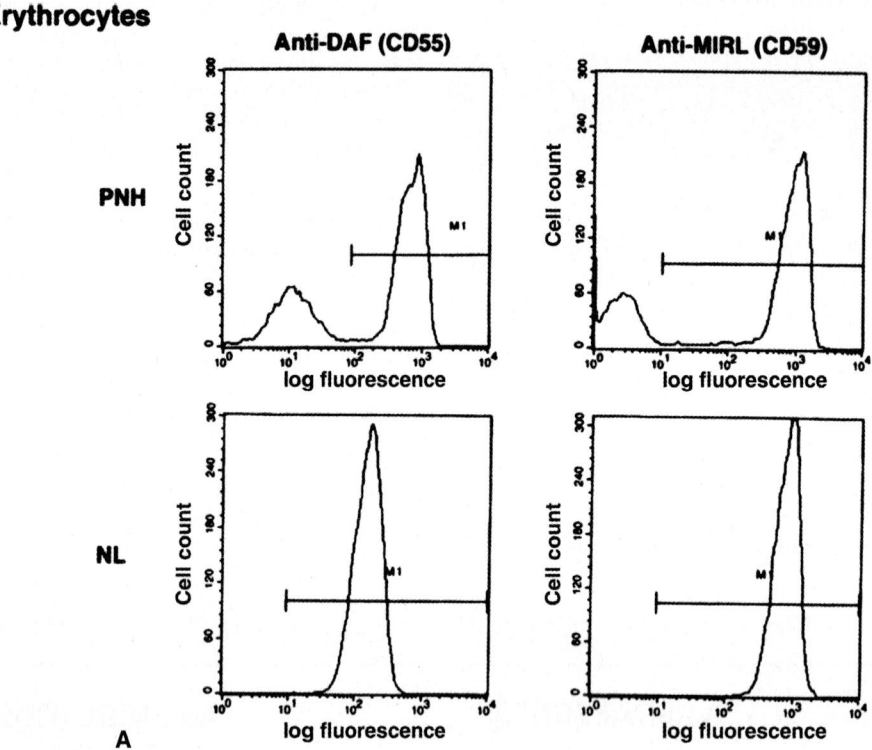

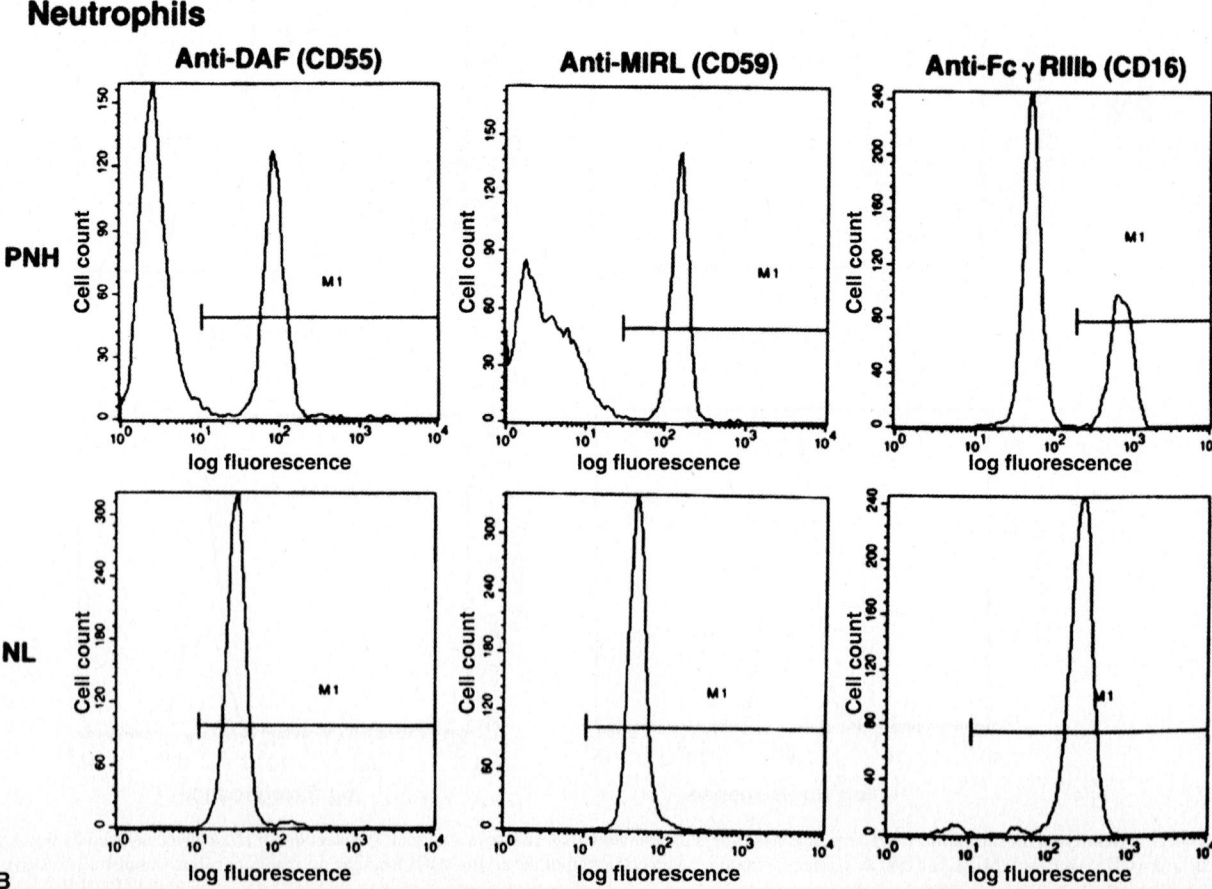

FIGURE 32.2 Analysis of glycosyl phosphatidylinositol-anchored proteins (GPI-AP) on erythrocytes (A) and granulocytes (B) from a patient with PNH.
Erythrocytes and isolated granulocytes from a patient with PNH and from a normal volunteer donor (NL) were analyzed by flow cytometry using anti-DAF (CD55), anti-MIRL (CD59), or anti-FcγRIIIb (CD16b) (granulocytes only) as primary antibodies. The histograms of the cells from the normal donor show uniformly positive staining with both antibodies. In contrast, the patient's histograms (PNH) demonstrate two discrete populations of cells. In the case of the erythrocytes (A), 30% of the cells are negative for DAF and MIRL expression, and 70% show normal expression. In the case of the granulocytes (B), 65% are negative for DAF and MIRL expression. The same population of cells shows abnormal expression of FcγRIIIb, but the deficiency is partial rather than absolute. Together, these results demonstrate three characteristic features of PNH: (1) The hematopoietic cells are a mosaic of normal and GPI-AP-deficient cells; (2) the proportion of abnormal granulocytes is greater than the proportion of abnormal erythrocytes; (3) the deficiency of FcγRIIIb is partial rather than absolute. DAF, decay accelerating factor; MIRL, membrane inhibitor of reactive lysis.

the clone size, because the complement-sensitive red cells are quickly and selectively destroyed intravascularly). As a rule, visibly hemoglobinuria is absent when PNH III erythrocytes constitute less than 20% of the red cell population (corresponding to a PNH clone size of 40%-60%).[12] Paroxysms of gross hemoglobinuria occur when the PNH III population ranges from 20% to 50% of the population (corresponding to a PNH clone size of 60%-90%), and constant hemoglobinuria is associated with greater than 50% PNH III erythrocytes (PNH clone size >90%). PNH II cells (the erythrocytes with intermediate sensitivity to complement), even when present in high proportions, are associated with no visible hemoglobinuria unless an intervening factor such as stress, infection, surgery, or trauma that activates complement supervenes.

The proportion of abnormal cells is greater in the marrow than in the blood and, among circulating erythrocytes, is greatest in young cell populations (the percentage of GPI-deficient reticulocytes is similar to the percentage of GPI-deficient neutrophils).

PNH is not an immune-mediated hemolytic anemia that arises as a consequence of the development of autoantibodies. Rather, failure to regulate APC activation on the erythrocyte surface underlies the hemolysis of PNH (*Figure 32.3*).[9] Under physiological conditions, the alternative pathway is in a state of continuous, low-grade activation. Normal erythrocytes are not hemolyzed as a result of this low-grade alternative pathway activation because specific cell-surface proteins have evolved that inhibit the activity of complement (*Figure 32.3*). In contrast, PNH erythrocytes are deficient in the two most important erythrocyte membrane regulators of complement (CD55 and CD59), and consequently, they are subject to chronic, spontaneous hemolysis in vivo (*Figure 32.3*). Failure to inhibit alternative pathway activation has a profound effect on red cell survival, as studies have shown that the half-life of complement-sensitive PNH cells is approximately 6 days (compared with 60 days for normal erythrocytes).

Rosse and colleagues reported the first clear evidence of the nature of the aberrant interactions of PNH erythrocytes with complement in 1973 and 1974.[16,17] Those investigators showed that, when complement is activated in vitro by either the classical or the alternative pathway, PNH erythrocytes bind much greater amounts of activated complement C3 than normal erythrocytes. The difference in C3

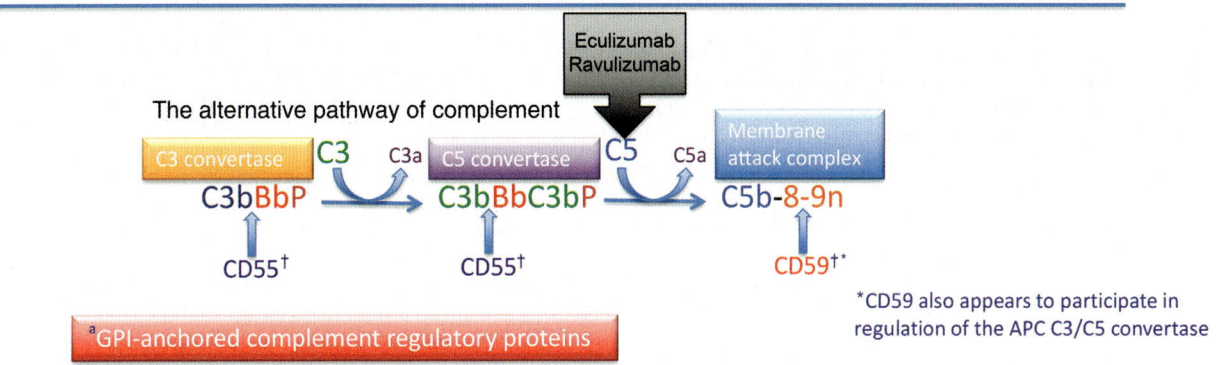

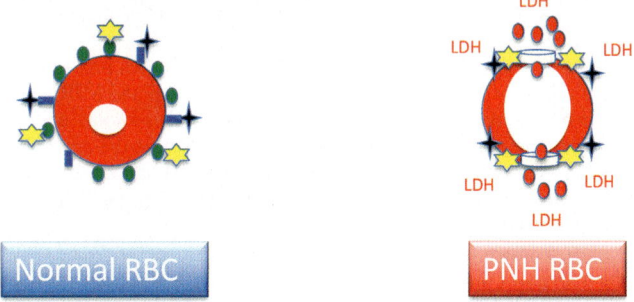

FIGURE 32.3 **Complement-mediated lysis of PNH erythrocytes.** The hemolysis of PNH is due to aberrant regulation of the alternative pathway of complement (APC). The APC is a component of the innate immune system. Unlike the classical pathway of complement that requires a recognition factor such as antibody to activate the pathway, the APC is continuously active. Therefore, safeguards have evolved to protect host cells against APC-mediated injury. In the case of erythrocytes, two GPI-APs, CD55 and CD59, serve this function. Two enzymatic convertases amplify the activity of the APC (top panel). The C3 convertase consists of activated C3 (C3b), activated factor B (Bb, the enzymatic subunit of the complexes that is proteolytically activated by factor D, a trace plasma protein that may be activated by one of the mannose-binding lectin-associated serine proteases), and factor P (formerly called properdin). Factor P stabilizes the C3 convertase, allowing each convertase to activate many molecules of C3 and, in the process, generate the weak anaphylatoxin, C3a. The C5 convertase is similar in structure to the C3 convertase except that two molecules of C3b are required to position C5 for cleavage by activated factor B (Bb). Many molecules of C5 are cleaved by the C5 convertase, and this process generates many molecules of the potent anaphylatoxin and neutrophil chemoattractant, C5a. Activated C5 (C5b) is the nidus for formation of the membrane attack complex (MAC) of complement consisting of C5b, C6, C7, C8, and multiple molecules of C9. The MAC inserts into the lipid bilayer of the cell, forming a transmembrane torus that results in osmotic lysis. CD55 (DAF) blocks the formation and stability of both the C3 and C5 convertases, while CD59 (MIRL) blocks the formation of the cytolytic MAC, primarily by inhibiting binding and multiplicity of C9. There is also evidence that CD59 participates in regulation of the C3/C5 convertase. Eculizumab is a humanized monoclonal anti-C5 antibody that prevents activation of C5 by the C5 convertase. Consequently the MAC cannot form (and C5a is not generated), accounting for the inhibition of the intravascular hemolysis of PNH. However, eculizumab does not inhibit formation of the C3 convertase, accounting for the opsonization by activation and degradation products of C3 observed in patients with PNH treated with eculizumab. Normal RBCs are protected against APC-mediated injury (black crosses represent APC C3 and C5 convertase formation and yellow stars represent MAC formation) by CD55 (blue ovals) and CD59 (green ovals) (bottom panel). PNH cells lacking the complement inhibitory proteins CD55 and CD59 undergo complement-mediated lysis, releasing cellular contents including hemoglobin (red circles) and LDH into the plasma.

Disorders of Red Blood Cells

deposition was particularly striking when acidified serum was used to activate the alternative pathway. Subsequent studies showed that PNH red cells lacked the capacity to regulate the formation and stability of the amplification C3 convertases of complement,[18,19] thus accounting for the greater binding of activated C3. A second defect was suggested by experiments demonstrating that PNH erythrocytes also failed to regulate the activity of the cytolytic membrane attack complex (MAC) of complement.[20,21] Collectively these observations indicated that PNH erythrocytes had two complement regulatory defects, one that affected regulation of the C3 convertases and a second that affected regulation of the MAC (*Figure 32.3*).

Erythrocyte Membrane Protein Deficiencies

Acetylcholinesterase

While Beck and Valentine reported in 1951 that neutrophils from patients with PNH were deficient in leukocyte alkaline phosphatase,[22] the first *erythrocyte* membrane protein that was found to be deficient in PNH was acetylcholinesterase.[23] In 1959, Auditore and Hartmann[23] presented evidence that the extent of the acetylcholinesterase deficiency correlated with the severity of the hemolysis. More detailed studies by others[24] showed that PNH I red cells had a relatively normal amount of acetylcholinesterase, while PNH III erythrocytes were profoundly deficient. Although the deficiency of acetylcholinesterase plays no role in the abnormal susceptibility of PNH red cells to complement-mediated lysis, ultimately the observations that the red cells lack acetylcholinesterase and that the neutrophils lack alkaline phosphatase provided important insights into the fundamental defect that underlies the pathophysiology of the hemolysis of PNH.

Decay Accelerating Factor (CD55)

In 1983, two groups reported that PNH erythrocytes were deficient in DAF (CD55).[25,26] DAF, first identified by Hoffman[27,28] in 1969 and subsequently purified to homogeneity by Nicholson-Weller and colleagues in 1982,[29] is a 70-kD protein that inhibits the formation and stability of the C3 convertases of complement (*Figure 32.3*). Thus, the absence of DAF provided a plausible explanation for the greater binding of activated C3 to PNH erythrocytes. Detailed studies, however, demonstrated that DAF does not regulate the activity of the MAC of complement. Those results implied that PNH erythrocytes were deficient in a second complement regulatory protein that was functionally distinct from DAF.

Membrane Inhibitor of Reactive Lysis (CD59)

In 1989, Holguin et al[30] reported the isolation from normal erythrocytes of an 18-kD protein called membrane inhibitor of reactive lysis (MIRL, CD59) that protected PNH III red cells against complement-mediated lysis (*Figure 32.3*). As anticipated, PNH cells were found to be deficient in MIRL, and additional studies by those investigators and others demonstrated that MIRL inhibits complement-mediated lysis by blocking the assembly of the MAC [30-33] (*Figure 32.3*). Subsequently, evidence was also presented that MIRL inhibits the activity of the C3/C5 convertase of the APC, although the mechanism that underlies this inhibition is incompletely understood.[34-36]

By comparing expression of DAF and MIRL on PNH I, PNH II, and PNH III erythrocytes, the functional basis of the different complement-sensitivity phenotypes was determined.[37] Those studies showed that PNH III cells are completely deficient in both DAF and MIRL, whereas PNH II cells are partially deficient in the two complement-regulatory proteins and PNH I cells have normal expression. Thus, the variability in sensitivity to lysis among the different phenotypes is explained by quantitative differences in expression of DAF and MIRL. Additional experiments demonstrated that the combined deficiency of DAF and MIRL was sufficient to explain the enhanced susceptibility of PNH erythrocytes to hemolysis in acidified serum.[36]

Of the two complement regulatory proteins, MIRL is more important than DAF in protecting cells from complement-mediated lysis in vivo. Antigens of the Cromer-related blood group complex are located on DAF, and rare cases of a null phenotype called Inab have been reported.[38] Like PNH cells, Inab erythrocytes are deficient in DAF, but unlike PNH erythrocytes, MIRL expression is normal on Inab red cells.[35] Although Inab erythrocytes bind more activated C3 when exposed to acidified serum in vitro,[35] they undergo little or no hemolysis. Furthermore, subjects with the Inab phenotype have no known hematological abnormalities, and in particular, they have no clinical evidence of hemolysis.[32,38] These observations show that isolated deficiency of DAF does not produce the PNH syndrome. In contrast, a patient with an inherited, isolated deficiency of MIRL (CD59) had a syndrome that was indistinguishable from PNH.[39,40] Clinically, the patient experienced recurrent episodes of hemoglobinuria, suggesting that MIRL is essential for protecting erythrocytes against complement-mediated lysis in vivo. Recurrent thromboembolic events were also observed in this patient. That patient had normal DAF expression, but in vitro, his cells were susceptible to hemolysis in acidified serum, implying that MIRL deficiency accounts primarily for the positive Ham test in PNH.[36]

Nevo and colleagues reported on five patients, from four unrelated families, who presented in infancy with symmetric muscle weakness accompanied by hypotonia and absent deep tendon reflexes involving the legs more than the arms.[41] The neurological disease was classified as chronic inflammatory demyelinating polyneuropathy. Symptomatic episodes were accompanied by hemolytic anemia characterized by reticulocytosis, negative direct antiglobulin tests, elevated serum lactate dehydrogenase concentration, and low haptoglobin concentration. Leukopenia and anemia were not observed. There was no report of thrombotic complications, although the oldest of the patients in the study was 5 years old. Whole exome sequencing of DNA from one of the patients identified a homozygous missense mutation in the gene that encodes CD59 (p.Cys89Tyr). Subsequent studies identified the same mutation in the other four patients. The mutation segregated with the disease in the families and had a carrier rate of 1:66 among Jewish persons of North-African origin. Cell surface expression of CD59 was absent from the erythrocytes of patients while expression of CD55 was normal. A patient from Germany with a discrete homozygous mutation of CD59 has also been reported.[42] Together, these studies confirm the importance of CD59 in the pathophysiology of the complement-mediated hemolysis of PNH and further suggest an important pathological role for aberrant regulation of the cytolytic MAC of complement in chronic inflammatory demyelinating polyneuropathy, and perhaps other diseases characterized by loss of myelin and axonal integrity.

While the above studies provide interesting insights into the individual functions of DAF and MIRL in vivo, it is important to remember that, in PNH, both proteins are deficient (because both are GPI anchored). Therefore, it is the *combined deficiency of DAF and MIRL that results in the markedly abnormal susceptibility of the red cells of PNH to complement-mediated lysis.*

Basis of the Protein Deficiencies in PNH

If only DAF or only MIRL were deficient in PNH, it would have been logical to hypothesize that the disease was due to mutations affecting the gene that encodes the particular protein. That PNH cells were deficient in multiple proteins (MIRL, DAF, and acetylcholinesterase on red cells and leukocyte alkaline phosphatase on neutrophils), however, eliminated the possibility that the gene for each protein was mutant. Rather, a more plausible hypothesis was that the PNH defect involved a posttranslational modification common to all of the proteins that are deficient in PNH. In 1984, Medof and colleagues[43] reported that isolated DAF spontaneously reincorporated into erythrocyte membranes. This property of DAF had been appreciated by Hoffman in 1969.[27,28] Working with the butanol-saturated aqueous phase of a crude extract prepared from normal human erythrocyte stroma, he showed that the sample contained a factor capable of inhibiting complement-mediated lysis by accelerating the decay of the C3 convertase. He further showed that this substance (that he called decay accelerating factor of stroma, DAF-S) had the capacity to reincorporate into red cells and remain functionally active. In 1980, Low and Zilversmit[44] demonstrated that alkaline phosphatase that had been solubilized from cells by butanol extraction exhibited the capacity to bind to phospholipid vesicles. In this case, the incorporation was thought to be due to the attachment of a phosphatidylinositol moiety to the enzyme. Subsequent experiments demonstrated that isolated acetylcholinesterase also spontaneously reincorporated into cell membranes. Previous studies had shown that alkaline phosphatase, acetylcholinesterase, and 5'-ectonucleotidase (another protein that is deficient in PNH) were released from the cell surface by treatment with phosphatidylinositol-specific phospholipase C. The cumulative work of a number of investigators showed that both the capacity to reincorporate into membranes and susceptibility to cleavage by phosphatidylinositol-specific phospholipase C were characteristic of a group of amphipathic membrane proteins that shared the common structural feature of being anchored to the cell surface through the GPI moiety. The structural link between DAF and acetylcholinesterase, alkaline phosphatase, and 5'-ectonucleotidase was made in 1986 by Davitz et al[45] and Medof et al[46] when those investigators presented evidence that DAF is a GPI-AP. Subsequent studies confirmed that MIRL is also an GPI-AP.[47] The results of those studies suggested the following paradigm: *all proteins that are deficient in PNH are GPI anchored, and all GPI-anchored proteins that are expressed by hematopoietic cells are deficient in PNH.* All data to date are consistent with this postulate.

GPI-APs are functionally diverse. In addition to the complement regulatory proteins (DAF [CD55] and MIRL [CD59]) and enzymes (acetylcholinesterase, alkaline phosphatase, and 5'-ectonucleotidase [CD73]) discussed above, proteins with a variety of receptor, adhesion, and immune modulatory functions (e.g., FcγRIIIb [CD16b], urokinase receptor [CD87], endotoxin binding protein receptor [CD14], and LFA-3 [CD58]) are also GPI anchored. Furthermore, a number of proteins whose function is unknown are GPI anchored. Over 130 human proteins have been shown to be GPI anchored.[1] A partial list of the GPI-APs that have been shown to be deficient on the hematopoietic cells of patients with PNH is shown (*Table 32.2*). This number is less than the total number of GPI-anchored human proteins because PNH is an acquired disease that affects only hematopoietic cells. Thus, GPI-APs that are present on somatic tissues other than hematopoietic cells are expressed normally in patients with PNH. Although PNH cells lack a number of functionally diverse membrane constituents, the only pathological component of the disease that is unequivocally causally related to GPI-AP deficiency is the abnormal susceptibility of the erythrocytes to complement-mediated lysis (*Table 32.2*).

Molecular Basis of PNH

The observation that, based on sensitivity to complement, the peripheral blood of patients with PNH is a mosaic comprising both normal and abnormal cells suggested that the abnormal cells were the progeny of a mutant clone and that they coexisted with the progeny of residual normal stem cells. Furthermore, that PNH is an acquired rather than an inherited disease implied that the abnormal clone arises as a consequence of a somatic mutation. In 1970, Oni et al[48] analyzed G6PD isoforms in both the complement-sensitive and complement-insensitive erythrocytes of a female patient with PNH who was heterozygous at the G6PD locus. The complement-insensitive cells expressed both G6PD isoforms, indicating a polyclonal origin for this cohort. In contrast, the complement-sensitive cells expressed only one isoform, a finding consistent with clonality. These studies provided the first experimental evidence in support of the clonal hypothesis of PNH. In 1969, Aster and Enright[49] reported that a portion of both the platelet and granulocyte populations from patients with PNH was abnormally sensitive to complement-mediated cytolysis. This publication represented another watershed event in the understanding of the origins of PNH, because it indicated that the mutation arose in a primitive hematopoietic stem cell that has the capacity to differentiate along myeloid lines. Subsequent studies showed that monocytes are also affected, and, in most patients, affected lymphocytes can be demonstrated. Together with the observation that all proteins that are deficient in PNH are GPI anchored, these studies suggested that PNH

Table 32.2. Glycosyl Phosphatidylinositol–Anchored Proteins Deficient in PNH[a]

Protein
Complement Regulatory Proteins[b]
• CD55 (decay accelerating factor, DAF)
• CD59 (membrane inhibitor of reactive lysis, MIRL)
Proteins with Immunological Significance
• CD58 (lymphocyte function antigen-3, LFA-3)
• CD16b (Fc receptor gamma IIIb, FcRgIIIb, CD16b)
• CD14 (endotoxin-binding protein)
Receptors
• CD87 (urokinase plasminogen activator receptor, uPAR)
• Folate receptor
• Cellular prion protein (on resting platelets)[c]
Enzymes
• Leukocyte alkaline phosphatase
• Acetylcholinesterase
• 5'-Ectonucleotidase
Miscellaneous Proteins
• CD24
• CD48
• CD52 (Campath-1)
• CD66c
• CD66b (formerly CD67)
• CD90 (Thy-1)
• CD108 (JMH-bearing protein)
• p50-80, GP109, GP157, GP175, GP500

[a]Partial list.
[b]Deficiency of complement regulatory proteins underlies the hemolytic anemia of PNH.
[c]Deficient on resting platelets, but putative transmembrane form expressed on activated platelets.

arises as a result of a somatic mutation affecting a pluripotent hematopoietic stem/progenitor cell and that the gene that is mutant is essential for the normal biosynthesis of the GPI anchor.

The GPI anchor is a complex structure with at least 25 proteins being essential for assembly of the moiety[1,50,51] (*Figure 32.4*). Hypothetically, the PNH phenotype would result if any of these proteins were nonfunctional because if the GPI anchor is not synthesized, GPI-APs are not expressed. Accordingly, it seemed probable that PNH would be found to be heterogeneous at the molecular level as mutations affecting any one of several genes that encode elements critical for GPI anchor assembly would produce the disease phenotype. In 1992[52] and 1993,[53] however, two groups published the surprising finding that GPI-protein-deficient lymphocyte cell lines derived from different patients with PNH all belonged to the same complementation class (class A) of GPI-AP-deficient cell lines. Additional experiments confirmed that the PNH cell lines had the same biochemical defect as the complementation class A mutants. Like the class A mutants, the PNH cell lines failed to synthesize N-acetylglucosaminyl-phosphatidylinositol (GlcNAc-PI), the first intermediate in the pathway of GPI anchor assembly (*Figures 32.4* and *32.5*).

A gene that restores normal expression of GPI-APs in the complementation class A PNH cell lines was identified by Kinoshita and colleagues in 1993.[54,55] As predicted by the studies cited above, the gene, called *PIGA* (for phosphatidylinositol glycan-class A), encodes a protein that is essential for the normal synthesis of GlcNAc-PI.[54] Subsequently, Takeda et al[55] showed that *PIGA* complements the

Disorders of Red Blood Cells

Deficiency of glycosyl phosphatidylinosito anchored proteins is a defining characteristic of PNH

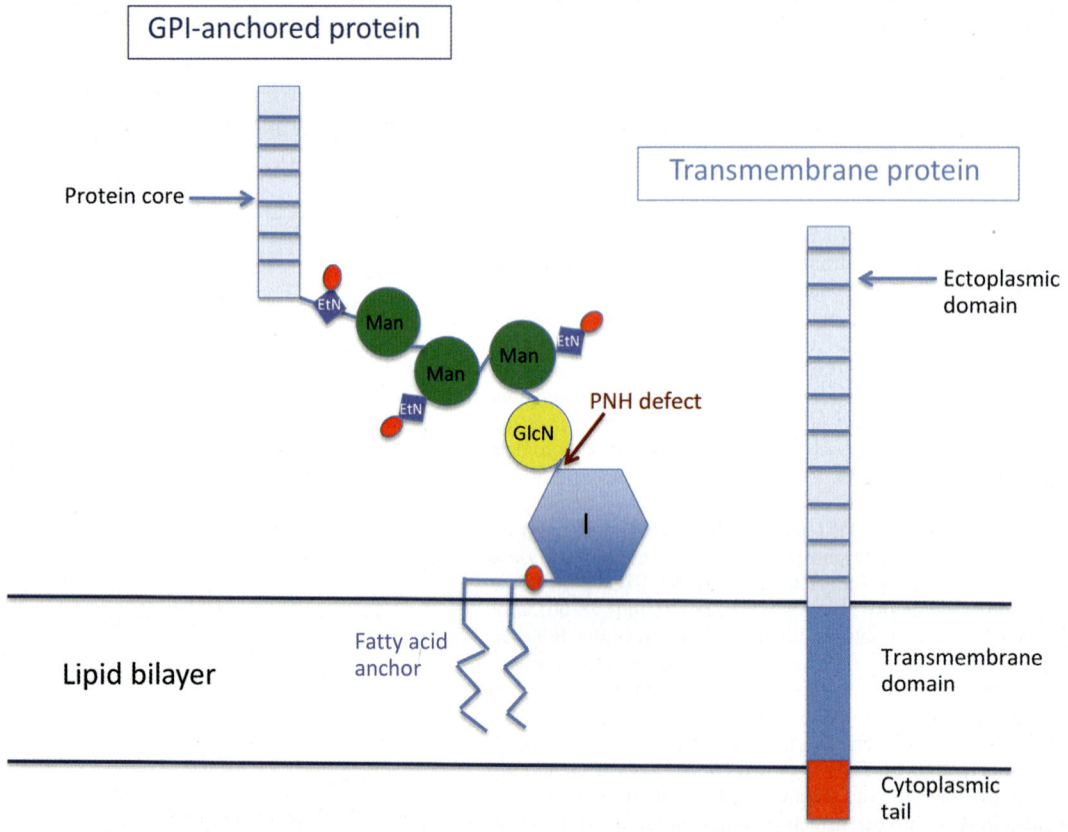

FIGURE 32.4 Structure of glycosyl phosphatidylinositol–anchored proteins. Transmembrane proteins have three domains: an ectoplasmic domain (rectangle with horizontal lines), a transmembrane domain (blue rectangle), and a cytoplasmic domain (red rectangle). In contrast, glycosyl phosphatidylinositol (GPI)-anchored proteins lack the cytoplasmic and transmembrane domains. This class of proteins is anchored to the cell by a GPI moiety consisting of phosphatidylinositol (blue hexagon), glucosamine (yellow circle), and three mannose residues (green circles). The GPI moiety is linked to the COOH terminus of the protein portion of the molecule by ethanolamine phosphate. The *PIGA* gene product is essential for the transfer of the nucleotide sugar uridine diphosphate-N-acetylglucosamine (UDP-GlcNAc) to phosphatidylinositol (PI) to form GlcNAc-PI, the first intermediate in the synthesis of the GPI anchor. Hematopoietic cells in PNH are deficient in all proteins that are GPI anchored because a somatic mutation in a hematopoietic stem cell partially or completely inactivates the *PIGA* gene product. Consequently, the GPI moiety is not synthesized. The arrow indicates the step in GPI synthesis that is defective in PNH.

deficient expression of GPI-APs in PNH lymphoblastoid cell lines and that those cell lines harbored somatic mutations in *PIGA*. Together, those studies defined both the biochemical and the molecular basis of the deficiency of GPI-APs in PNH (*Figure 32.5*).

In addition, Takeda and colleagues observed that a heterozygous mutation was sufficient to produce the PNH phenotype.[55] As presaged by the studies of Hyman et al,[56] the dominant expression of the somatic mutation was explained when *PIGA* was mapped to chromosome Xp22.1 (*Figure 32.5*). As males have a single X chromosome, any functionally significant mutation affecting PIGA is expressed. Females are functionally haploid due to X inactivation in somatic tissues. Therefore, somatic mutations in *PIGA* appear dominant when they occur on the active X chromosome. With rare exception,[57,58] somatic mutations affecting *PIGA* account for the PNH phenotype in all patients in whom the genetic basis has been identified.

More than 25 proteins are involved in the synthesis of the GPI anchor moiety.[1] Hypothetically, somatic mutation of any of the genes that encode these proteins would produce the PNH phenotype (i.e., deficiency of GPI-APs). Why then is PNH essentially always due to mutation of PIGA? The commonly agreed upon answer to this question is based on mathematical probability. Among the genes involved in GPI-AP synthesis, *PIGA* alone is located on the X chromosome.[1] Therefore, only one mutational event is required to produce the PNH

phenotype as males have one X chromosome, and in females, only one of the two X chromosomes is active in somatic tissues (*Figure 32.5*). Because all other genes involved in GPI-AP synthesis are autosomal, two somatic mutational events in the same gene would be required to eliminate synthesis of the GPI anchor and produce the PNH phenotype. Thus, based on mutational frequency (~1.1×10^{-8} per nucleotide position per haploid genome), the probability that deficiency of GPI-APs in PNH would be due to somatically mutated *PIGA* is many orders of magnitude greater than the probability that the deficiency would be due to somatic mutation of both of the alleles of any of the more than 25 autosomal genes involved in GPI anchor synthesis.

Hypothetically, germline mutation of one of the alleles of an autosomal gene involved in GPI-AP synthesis could predispose an individual to develop an autosomal form of PNH, and a case report supports this mechanism as a rare cause of the disease.[57] In this case, the gene involved was *PIGT*, which is located on chromosome 20. The germline mutation was a single-base substitution in the splice acceptor site of intron 10, whereas the somatic mutation was an 8.2-Mb deletion that included the entire *PIGT* gene. In addition to hemolysis, this patient had a history of urticaria before the onset of PNH and developed ulcerative colitis after the onset of PNH, and all symptoms, including hemolysis, responded to treatment with eculizumab, indicating a role of complement activation in their etiology. Three additional patients (two

Pathophysiology of PNH

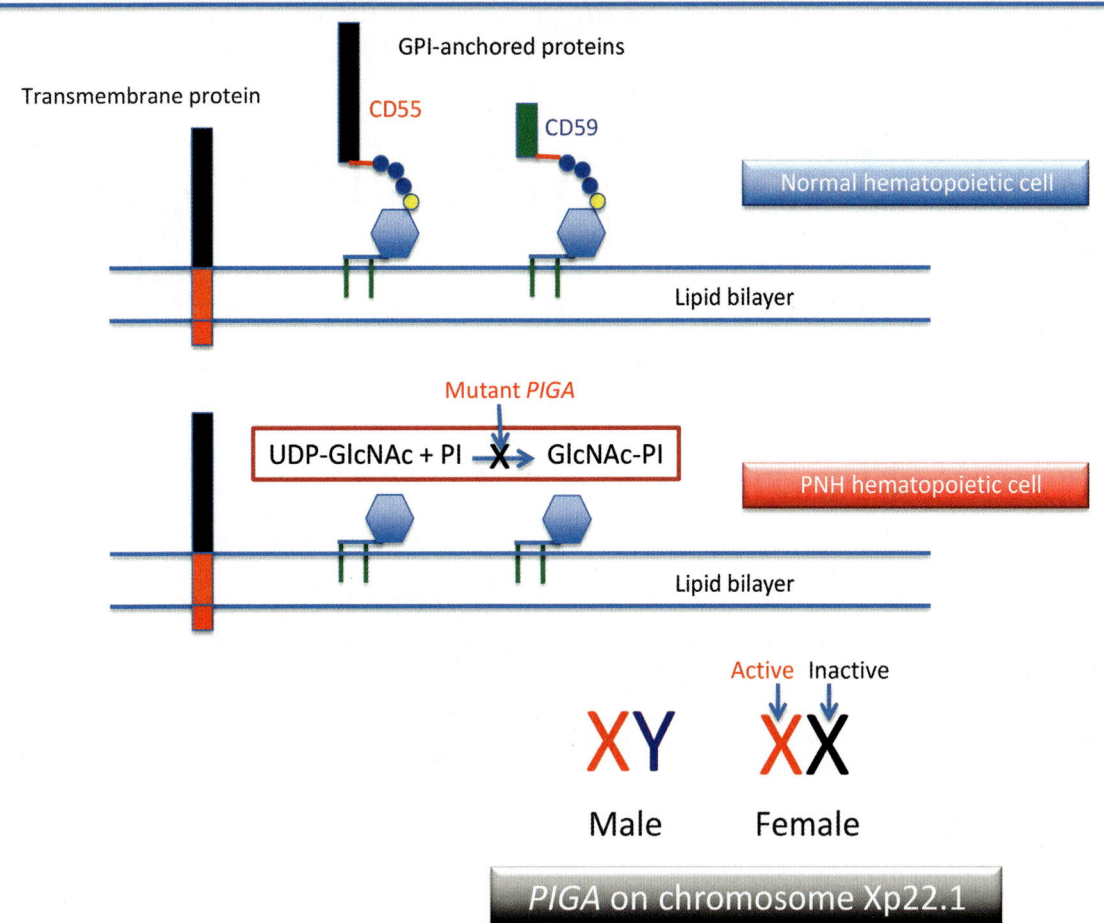

FIGURE 32.5 The molecular basis of PNH. Normal hematopoietic stem cells express both transmembrane and GPI-anchored proteins (top panel). PNH stem cells express transmembrane proteins normally but fail to express GPI-APs because the first step in the synthesis of the anchor is inactivated because the gene (*PIGA*) that encodes the enzyme that is required for transfer of the nucleotide sugar, uridine diphosphate-N-acetylglucosamine (UDP-GlcNAc), to phosphatidy-linositol (PI) is mutant (middle panel). Of the more than 25 genes involved in the synthesis of the GPI anchor, only *PIGA* is located on the X chromosome (all others are autosomal). Location on the X chromosome accounts for the observation that essentially all cases of PNH are due to somatic mutation of *PIGA* because inactivation of only one allele is required to produce the PNH phenotype as males have one X chromosome and in females only one of the two X chromosomes is active in somatic tissues (bottom panel).

from Japan and one from Germany) with a combination of germline and somatic mutations in *PIGT* have been identified, and in each case, hemolysis was accompanied by inflammatory conditions not observed in patients with *PIGA* mutations. The basis of the inflammatory conditions observed in the three patients with atypical PNH is speculative, but it may be due to accumulation of free GPI, which does not occur when *PIGA* is mutant.[59] Recently, a patient with PNH due to copy number neutral loss of heterozygosity of a region on chromosome 15 in which there was a germline mutation of PIGB was described.[58]

Congenital abnormalities of genes involved in GPI-AP synthesis. Germline mutations in at least 12 genes (including *PIGA*) involved in biosynthesis of the GPI anchor moiety have been reported.[1] In these individuals, mutations are hypomorphic and consequently GPI deficiency is partial. Furthermore, expression of GPI-AP on blood cells from these patients is subnormal only on granulocytes, with expression on erythrocytes being nearly normal. Therefore, hemolysis is not observed. The phenotype of patients with germline mutation of genes involved in GPI-AP assembly varies but often involves neurological abnormalities, including mental retardation and seizures, and hyperphosphatasia.

Analysis of *PIGA* has revealed that the same mutation can be identified in isolated neutrophils, monocytes, and lymphocytes from

individual patients with PNH, confirming that the disease involves a hematopoietic stem/progenitor cell.[55,60] More than 170 *PIGA* mutations have been identified in affected cells of patients with PNH. Only three large deletions have been observed[61-63] (*Figure 32.6*). The remaining mutations consist of nucleotide substitutions of the missense or nonsense types or small deletions or insertions that cause frame-shifts and introduce premature termination codons (*Figure 32.6*). The mutations are distributed randomly over the entire coding region and at splice junctions (*Figure 32.6*). At least 19 mutations have been observed in more than one patient. Absence of repetitive mutations indicates that *PIGA* lacks molecular hot spots. The simplest explanation for these observations is that clonal selection and expansion depends on complete or nearly complete inactivation of PIGA such that expression of GPI-AP proteins is below a critical threshold. Therefore, all *PIGA* mutations in PNH are loss-of-function mutations.

Studies of *PIGA* mutations have also provided insights into the molecular basis of the phenotypic mosaicism of PNH.[60] Cloned lymphocyte cell lines were established from the peripheral blood of a patient whose erythrocytes were a mixture of PNH I, PNH II, and PNH III cells (*Figure 32.7*). Based on expression of GPI-APs, lymphocyte clones with four different phenotypes were observed. Analysis of clones with normal expression of GPI-AP revealed no

Mutations in PNH Cause Partial or Complete Loss-of-Function of *PIGA*

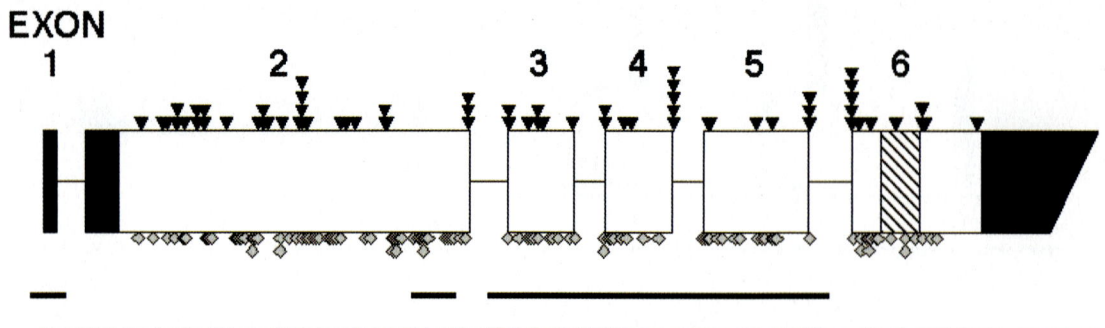

▼ : Base Substitution

◇ : Deletion / Insertion

— : Large Deletion / Insertion

FIGURE 32.6 Diagram of the human *PIGA* gene and the locations of somatic mutations reported in patients with PNH. The boxes represent exons within the *PIGA* gene, and the blackened areas denote noncoding regions. Lines connecting the exons represent introns. The hatched region within exon 6 indicates the putative *PIGA* transmembrane domain. Single nucleotide substitutions are indicated above the gene as inverted triangles, while small nucleotide deletions and insertions are identified beneath the gene by diamonds. Large DNA deletions and insertions are denoted by horizontal lines below the gene. (From Nishimura J, Murakami Y, Kinoshita T. Paroxysmal nocturnal hemoglobinuria: An acquired genetic disease. *Am J Hematol.* 1999;62(3):175-182. Copyright © 1999 Wiley-Liss, Inc. Reprinted by permission of John Wiley & Sons, Inc.)

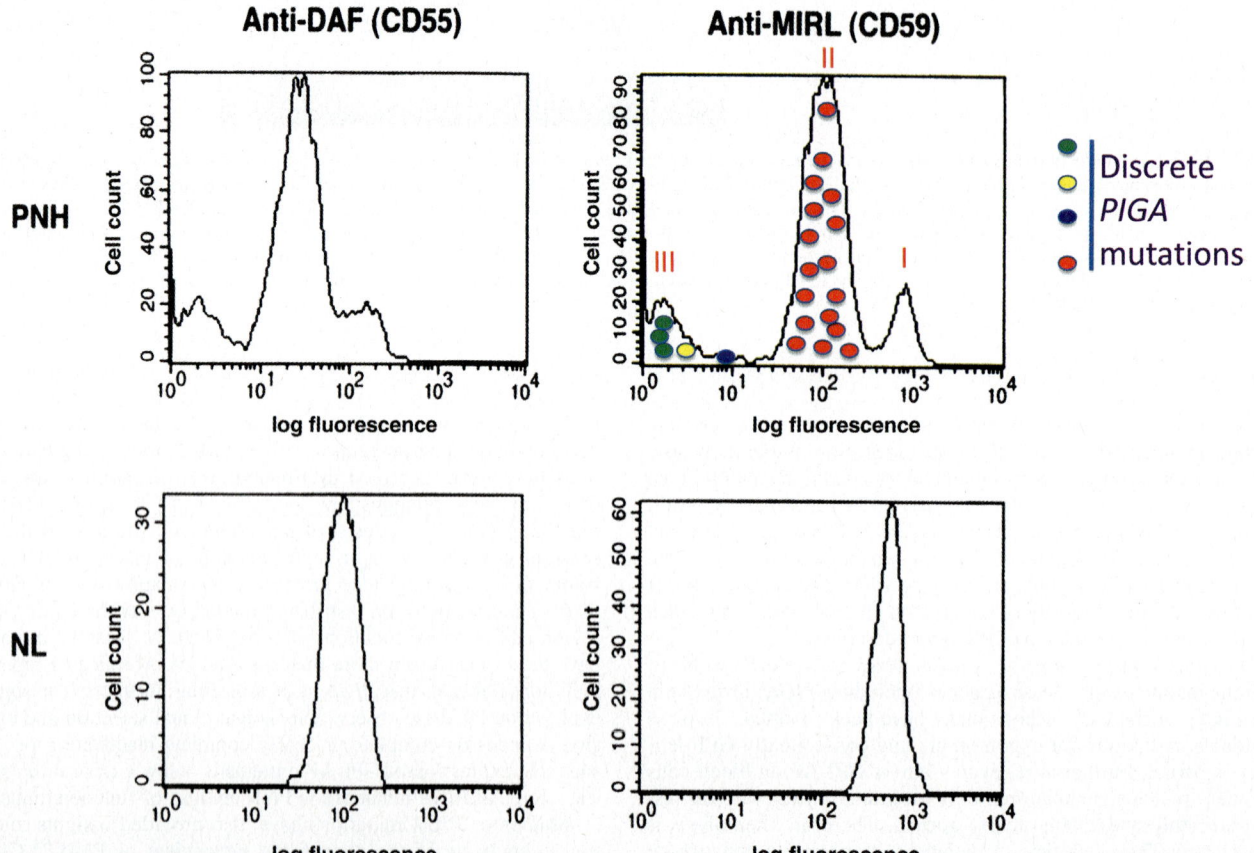

FIGURE 32.7 ***PIGA* genotype determines PNH phenotype. A flow cytometry histogram modeled after that of the patient with PNH shown in** *Figure 32.1* **is illustrated.** In this case, approximately 75% of the patient's hematopoiesis was derived from a clone (upper right panel, red filled circles) with a *PIGA* missense mutation that produced the PNH II phenotype. Three discrete *PIGA* mutations that produced a null phenotype were found among the PNH III cells (green, yellow, and blue filled circles). These three clones together contributed 11% of the patient's hematopoiesis. In this case, the PNH II clone has expanded more than any of the PNH III clones. DAF, decay accelerating factor; MIRL, membrane inhibitor of reactive lysis; NL, normal volunteer donor.

somatic *PIGA* mutations. In contrast, among the four phenotypically distinct lymphocyte clones with abnormal GPI-AP expression, four discrete *PIGA* mutations were identified (*Figure 32.7*). In the lymphocyte clones with the PNH II phenotype, a missense mutation that changed a highly conserved amino acid was found. This observation suggests that cells with partial expression of GPI-APs (PNH II) are derived from stem cells with mutations that incompletely inactivate PIGA. In the case of the lymphocyte clones with the PNH III phenotype, three separate mutations were identified, each of which was expected to inactivate completely the *PIGA* gene product (*Figure 32.7*). Collectively, these experiments demonstrate that the phenotypic mosaicism that is characteristic of PNH is a consequence of genotypic mosaicism. Furthermore, because any mutation that completely inactivates PIGA results in PNH III cells, phenotypically identical cells can have different *PIGA* genotypes (*Figure 32.7*).

Studies of the pattern of X-chromosomal inactivation indicated that, in the female patient with four different *PIGA* mutations, the abnormal clones were not derived from a common ancestor.[60] Furthermore, that each of the mutations was discrete demonstrated that the mutational events occurred independently rather than by clonal evolution. These results demonstrate that PNH is not strictly a monoclonal process and have important implications for the origins of the disease.

Studies of mutational frequency in PNH have produced conflicting results. Some of the disparity is almost certainly due to differences in experimental design and interpretation of data. While an abnormally high mutational rate may contribute to generation of multiple *PIGA*-mutant clones, a selective advantage for GPI-AP-deficient stem/progenitor cells and variable extent of expansion of the mutant clones appears to be necessary to explain the outgrowth of multiple PNH clones, some of which dominate hematopoiesis and some of which persist subclinically.

The Pathophysiology of PNH Is Unique

Despite the progress that has been made in determining the basis of the abnormal sensitivity of the erythrocytes to complement-mediated lysis and the global absence of GPI-APs from hematopoietic cells, an issue that is fundamental to a more complete understanding of PNH remains largely enigmatic. In order for PNH to become clinically evident, the hematopoietic stem cells bearing the mutant *PIGA* must expand so that progeny sufficient to produce symptoms and signs of the disease are generated. In many instances, GPI-AP-deficient (GPI-AP⁻) cells dominate hematopoiesis in patients with PNH, suggesting that the mutant stem cell has either a greater proliferative capacity or a survival advantage relative to GPI-AP-sufficient (GPI-AP⁺) stem cells. That *PIGA* mutations are necessary for the development of PNH is incontrovertible. At issue is whether *PIGA* mutations are both necessary and *sufficient* to account for the PNH syndrome and whether the *PIGA* mutation provides an absolute or a conditional growth/survival advantage.

PNH differs from monoclonal hematopoietic stem cell disorders such as chronic myelogenous leukemia in which the t(9;21) that generates the fusion protein BCR-ABL is sufficient to account for the proliferative and survival advantage of the mutant cell, and in which all normal hematopoiesis is progressively and invariably displaced as a consequence of the uncontrolled proliferation of a transformed clone. In PNH, the peripheral blood is a mosaic of normal and abnormal cells and the proportion of GPI-AP⁻:GPI-AP⁺ cells varies greatly among patients, and that ratio tends to remain fixed over long periods of observations. Therefore, although PNH is a clonal disease, it is more aptly categorized as a disease in which the mutant cells have a conditional cellular survival/growth advantage, rather than as a malignant disease.

The oligoclonal nature of PNH[60] suggests that a powerful selection process that is most likely based on phenotype is at work in the bone marrow. According to this hypothesis, stem cells with mutant *PIGA* have an advantage because of some pathological process (likely immune mediated) that involves a GPI-AP. For example, an autoimmune process could arise in which the target antigen is a GPI-AP expressed on hematopoietic stem cells. Under those circumstances,

PIGA-mutant stem cells (lacking GPI-AP) would escape immune-mediated destruction because the target antigen is absent (*Figure 32.8*). In this case, the *PIGA*-mutant stem cells would have a survival advantage rather than an intrinsic growth advantage, which would account for their greater contribution to hematopoiesis.

Hematopoietic cells express a relatively large number of functionally diverse GPI-AP (*Table 32.2*). Thus, absence of all GPI-AP is probably not required for the clonal selection of the mutant stem cells. Rather, the selective advantage may be dependent on the absence of a single protein that is GPI anchored, and the reason for the global deficiency of GPI-AP is that *PIGA* is located on the X chromosome. According to this supposition, an autosomal gene encodes the GPI-AP that is conditionally detrimental (e.g., an antigen targeted for immune destruction or a receptor for a negative growth regulator). Inasmuch as two alleles rather than one must be mutated, the probability of inactivating an autosomal gene through somatic mutagenesis is remote compared with the probability of inactivating an X-linked gene. Therefore, stem cells with a deficiency of the detrimental GPI-AP are most likely to arise as a consequence of *PIGA* mutations, as is the case in patients with CLL treated with Campath1H (antibody to CD52, an autosomal GPI-AP).[64] Assuming that the GPI-AP complement regulatory proteins are not the targets of the underlying pathological process, the hemolytic anemia that is the clinical hallmark of PNH may represent an epiphenomenon related to the chromosomal location of *PIGA*.

Although a compelling case can be made in support of the paradigm that the *PIGA* mutation bestows a conditional growth advantage upon the affected stem cell, the hypothesis that the mutant stem cells have an absolute growth or survival advantage must also be considered. Data that both support and challenge this hypothesis can be found.[65-67] The most compelling argument against an intrinsic growth or survival advantage for *PIGA*-mutant cells is made by the results of studies using transgenic mice.[68] By using homologous recombination, Kawagoe et al[69] disrupted *Piga* (the murine homologue of *PIGA*). Only mice with a low degree of chimerism survived. Among those animals, the percentage of GPI-AP⁻ erythrocytes ranged from ~1% to 5%. During 10 months of observation, the ratio of GPI-AP⁻:GPI-AP⁺ peripheral blood cells did not increase. Studies by others using conditional knockout technology have confirmed these observations.[68,70]

What Is the Origin of the PIGA-Mutant Stem Cells?

Patients with PNH often have more than one *PIGA*-mutant clone.[60,71] A tenet of the Darwinian selection hypothesis, as it applies to PNH, is that *PIGA*-mutant hematopoietic stem cells are present during the time when the selection pressure is applied to the bone marrow. *PIGA*-mutant hematopoietic elements have been identified in the peripheral blood and bone marrow of normal volunteers, providing experimental support for this concept, although whether the GPI-AP-deficient cells identified in normal individuals originate from a hematopoietic stem cells with mutant *PIGA* has been questioned.[72] While there are experimental data that suggest that the mutational frequency of the gene is abnormally high,[72] that *PIGA* is located on the X chromosome (so that only one allele need be mutated for the phenotype to become apparent) likely accounts for the existence of multiple discrete clones in many patients with PNH.

A Two-Step Model of PNH Pathogenesis

Studies by Inoue and colleagues suggest that a two-step mechanism may account for the unique pathophysiology of PNH[73] (*Figure 32.8*). Those investigators identified two patients whose *PIGA*-mutant cells had a concurrent, acquired rearrangement of chromosome 12. Detailed analysis showed that, in both cases, the chromosome 12 rearrangement resulted in disruption of the 3′ translated region of *HMGA2*. As a consequence, a negative regulatory region of the locus was disrupted, resulting in ectopic expression of the gene. *HMGA2* is a member of the high mobility group of proteins (*HMGA1a, HMGA1b, HMGA2*) that function as architectural transcription factors. HMG members possess no intrinsic transcriptional activity. Instead, these nonhistone phosphoproteins orchestrate assembly of stereospecific transcriptional

Hypothetical Model for Selection and Expansion of *PIGA*-Mutant, GPI-AP Deficient
Hematopoietic Stem/Progenitor Cells in Classic PNH

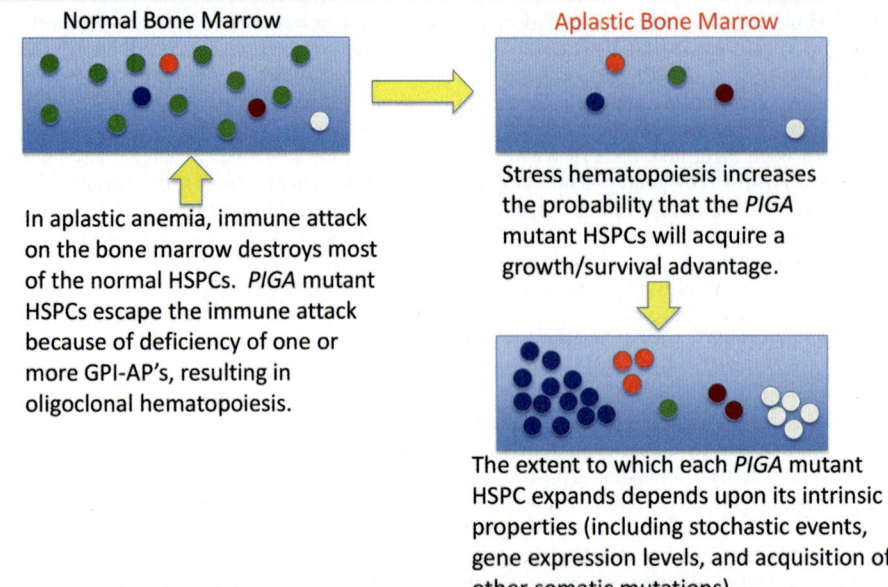

FIGURE 32.8 **Hypothetical model for the etiology of PNH in the setting of immune-mediated bone marrow failure.** The green circles indicated normal stem/progenitor cells while the blue, red, brown, and white circles represent quiescent *PIGA*-mutant stem/progenitor cells (top left panel). Under immune attack, the *PIGA*-mutant cells survive, while most of the normal cells are destroyed (top right panel). The extent to which the surviving *PIGA*-mutant stem/progenitor cells expand depends upon the intrinsic properties of the mutant cells. GPI-AP, glycosyl phosphatidylinositol-anchored protein; HSPC, hematopoietic stem and progenitor cell.

regulatory proteins into enhanceosomes. The cellular targets of *HMGA2* are incompletely defined but appear to include cyclin A and E2F1.

Molecular studies established a causal role for *HMGA2* in benign mesenchymal tumors. Rearrangement of 12q13-15 is observed in these neoplasms, but tumorigenesis does not depend on generation of chimeric proteins derived from fusion of *HMGA2* with specific translocation partners. Rather, clonal expansion induced by *HMGA2* appears to result from deregulated expression of the protein. For the two patients with PNH, ectopic expression was a consequence of gain-of-function mutational events caused by disruption of the 3′ untranslated region (UTR) shown to contain elements that negatively regulate *HMGA2* mRNA stability including the mircoRNA let-7a.[74,75] Additional studies will be required to determine whether aberrant expression of *HMGA2* underlies clonal expansion in patients with PNH without structural abnormalities of 12q13-15, but subsequent studies support this concept by showing that *HMGA2* was aberrantly expressed in the peripheral blood cells of patients with PNH without chromosomal rearrangements,[76] that aberrant expression of *HMGA2* as a consequence of vector integration that disrupts the 3′ UTR during gene therapy for thalassemia results in clonal expansion of hematopoiesis,[75] that truncation of the 3′ UTR of *HMGA2* in murine HSCs results in myeloproliferative-like hematopoiesis,[74] and that *HMGA2* promotes long-term engraftment and myeloerythroid differentiation of human HS/PCs.[77] Together, these observations support the hypothesis that expression of level of *HMGA2* is an important determinant of the extent of clonal expansion of *PIGA*-mutant hematopoietic stem/progenitor cells in PNH.

Clonal expansion of *PIGA*-mutant cells has also been reported in association with mutation of JAK2V617F and BCR-ABL.[78] Whole exome sequencing has been used to identify somatic mutations in GPI-AP⁺ and GPI-AP⁻ cells from the same patient and in patients with aplastic anemia, some of whom had a population of GPI-AP-deficient cells.[79,80] While those studies identified genes known to be involved in clonal expansion including *TET2, DNMT3A,* and *ASXL1,* the contribution of these mutated genes to clonal expansion in PNH remains speculative as somatic mutations of these genes are found in 2% of healthy volunteers and 5% to 6% of individuals over 70 years of age.

In contrast to a disorder characterized by cellular transformation and malignant cellular growth, PNH manifests many of the characteristics of a benign tumor as there is limited expansion of *PIGA*-mutant clones (the peripheral blood of patients is a relatively stable mosaic of normal and abnormal cells), *PIGA*-mutant cells respect tissue boundaries (there is no invasion of nonhematopoietic tissues), *PIGA*-mutant cells respond appropriately to signals that normally regulate hematopoiesis (function is not autonomous), and transformation into acute leukemia occurs rarely (PNH is not a premalignant condition).[81] The studies of Inoue and colleagues[73] suggest the concept of PNH as a benign tumor of the bone marrow with aberrant expression of *HMGA2* producing the proliferative phenotype that underlies clonal expansion.[82]

The findings of Inoue et al provide new insights into the etiology of the nonmalignant clonal hematopoiesis of PNH.[82] These studies support a two-step process consisting of (i) clonal selection based on phenotype (i.e., GPI-AP deficiency resulting from mutant *PIGA*)[83] and (ii) clonal expansion as a consequence of aberrant expression of a gene that bestows a growth/survival advantage (*Figure 32.8*). Clonal selection may induce exit of *PIGA*-mutant stem cells from a dormant state, thereby favoring acquisition of growth/survival properties (through somatic mutation or aberrant gene expression) that result in clonal expansion. The variable expansion of *PIGA*-mutant clones among patients and among mutant clones in the same patient could be explained by heterogeneity involving the expansion-causing event (nature of second somatic mutation or the degree of gene overexpression) that occurs in the *PIGA*-mutant hematopoietic stem/progenitor cell. According to this hypothesis, mutant *PIGA* is promiscuous with respect to the expansion-causing event. But the benign nature of PNH suggests that the process involved in clonal expansion of *PIGA*-mutant stem/progenitor cells is different from those that underlie malignant clonal diseases such as acute leukemia.

In summary, the basis of the clonal dominance in PNH is incompletely understood; however, available evidence supports a two-step model of pathogenesis (*Figure 32.8*). Step 1 of this model is *clonal selection.* In this case, a loss-of-function mutation affecting *PIGA* causes deficiency of GPI-APs on affected stem cells. These mutant stem cells have a relative growth or survival advantage that is enhanced in the setting of BMF (e.g., aplastic anemia).[83] Thus, principles of Darwinian evolution may apply to development of PNH. Strong support for the hypothesis that the clonal selection process is immune mediated comes from studies of HLA patterns in patients with acquired aplastic anemia.[84] Approximately 10% of patients with acquired aplastic anemia have a population of hematopoietic cells that are homozygous for HLA alleles. In most cases, homozygosity is acquired through homologous recombination resulting in copy number neutral loss of heterozygosity, although somatic mutations that inactivate one allele may cause functional loss of heterozygosity.[85] A patient with aplastic anemia may have oligoclonal hematopoiesis due to coexistence of separate clones with mutation of *PIGA* or loss of heterozygosity of HLA.[86] *Clonal expansion*, step 2 of the PNH pathogenesis model, is envisioned as a consequence of clonal evolution in which aberrant gene expression (as a result of somatic mutation or gene overexpression) bestows upon the *PIGA*-mutant stem cell/progenitor cell an absolute proliferative/survival advantage.[73,82] The extent of expansion of a particular clone and the dominance of one *PIGA*-mutant clone in the presence of other *PIGA* mutants may be mediated by the nature of the second event that may be molecularly heterogeneous, or may be determined by the extent of gene overexpression. Alternatively, a limited number of second mutations may partner with mutant *PIGA*, and the extent of clonal expansion may be determined by how the second mutation affects gene function. Together, these steps suggest that *PIGA* mutations are necessary but *not* sufficient for the development of clinical PNH.

Aplastic Anemia and PNH

An association between aplastic anemia and PNH has been recognized for more than 60 years, and numerous studies have confirmed the association. The probability is negligible that these two rare diseases would occur together so frequently by chance. Therefore, a pathophysiological link between PNH and aplastic anemia must exist. Modern studies using high-sensitivity flow cytometry and involving large numbers of patients diagnosed with PNH, aplastic anemia, MDS, or unclassified BMF have shown that approximately 50% of those patients diagnosed with aplastic anemia have detectable PNH cells (i.e., GPI-AP-deficient red cells and granulocytes). In general, the percentage of PNH cells is small with the median being approximately 0.2%. Therefore, the vast majority of patients with aplastic anemia with concurrent PNH have subclinical disease (i.e., no clinical or biochemical evidence of hemolysis). In the study by Sugimori and colleagues involving 749 patients with aplastic anemia, those who were at or above the 90th percentile for percentage of PNH cells had approximately 23% GPI-AP-deficient granulocytes.[87] Clinical evidence of PNH is observed when the percentage of GPI-AP-deficient granulocytes is approximately 25%. Therefore, approximately 10% of patients with PNH and aplastic anemia have clinically significant PNH at the time of diagnosis. Although the number of patients studied was relatively small (29 and 37, respectively),[88,89] for patients with aplastic anemia treated with immunosuppressive therapy who are followed longitudinally for up to 20 years, approximately 35% developed clinically apparent PNH. Hillmen et al.[81] reported that 23 of 80 patients (29%) with clinically significant PNH had an antecedent history of aplastic anemia, and in a series of 220 French patients with PNH, Socié and colleagues identified 65 (30%) in whom the diagnosis of aplastic anemia preceded that of clinical PNH.[90] Together, these results suggest that the selective pressure that favors the survival of *PIGA*-mutant cells occurs frequently in the setting of aplastic anemia but that the clinical syndrome of PNH is apparent at a significantly lower frequency.

Aplastic anemia can also develop in patients with PNH with no antecedent history of BMF. In the French group of 220 patients, approximately 10% of patients with PNH with no prior history of aplastic anemia developed pancytopenia during the relatively short period of observation covered by the study (median follow-up of 2 years).[90] The estimated cumulative incidence of pancytopenia was 8.2% (±2.4%, SE) at 2 years and 14.2% (±3.3%, SE) at 4 years.[90] This incidence of subsequent development of pancytopenia appears to

be somewhat higher than that observed in a longer study reported by Hillmen et al in which 5 of 80 (6%) patients with PNH subsequently developed aplasia.[81] The time between the diagnosis of aplastic anemia and the development of clinical PNH varies from a few months to several years. In the series reported by Socié et al,[90] the median time between diagnosis of aplastic anemia and laboratory evidence of PNH was 3.1 years (range 0.17-15 years).

In summary, while approximately 50% of patients with aplastic anemia have a detectable population of GPI-AP-hematopoietic cells at diagnosis,[91] 10% to 30% (depending on the duration of observation) have or subsequently develop clinically apparent PNH.[92,93] In the remainder, GPI-AP- cells persist subclinically or disappear,[87,91] suggesting that mutant *PIGA* (and the consequent deficiency of GPI-APs) is necessary for clonal selection but is insufficient to account for the clonal expansion required for clinical manifestations of PNH to become apparent. The simplest interpretation of these observations is that factors in addition to mutant *PIGA* contribute to the development of clinical signs and symptoms of PNH by affecting the extent to which the *PIGA*-mutant stem cells expand.

As expansion of the mutant clones occurs later in the course of aplastic anemia, the process could be influenced directly or indirectly by therapy. Although many patients with aplastic anemia who develop PNH are treated with immunosuppressive therapy (e.g., anti-thymocyte globulin and cyclosporin), there is no evidence that immunosuppression causes PNH.[93] Patients with aplastic anemia who respond to androgens appear equally likely to develop PNH.[90]

The basis of the relationship between PNH and aplastic anemia is speculative. Essentially all patients with PNH have some evidence of BMF (e.g., thrombocytopenia, leukopenia, or both) during the course of their disease. Therefore, the immune-mediated bone marrow injury that underlies aplastic anemia appears to play a central role in the development of PNH by providing the conditions that favor the growth/survival of *PIGA*-mutant, GPI-AP-deficient stem cells. Currently, there is no evidence that the types of *PIGA* mutations that occur in PNH/aplastic anemia are different from those observed in classic PNH.[94] Furthermore, a distinction between classic PNH and PNH/aplastic anemia may be artificial, as the underlying pathophysiological process could be the same. According to this hypothesis, in classic PNH, the aplastic or hypoplastic component is subclinical and short-lived, with disease noted only after the *PIGA*-mutant clone(s) have expanded sufficiently to dominate hematopoiesis.

Myelodysplastic Syndrome and PNH

In the study by Sugimori and colleagues that used high-sensitivity flow cytometry to identify GPI-AP- granulocytes, 514 patients with MDS were analyzed and 87 (17%) were found to have a detectable population of PNH granulocytes. As was the case with aplastic anemia, the median percentage of abnormal cells was low (in the range of 0.2%) with approximately 10% of the patients having clinically significant PNH. Notably, the PNH granulocytes were observed only in patients with low-risk MDS (in this case, refractory anemia and refractory cytopenias with multilineage dysplasia). PNH granulocytes were not observed in patients with higher-risk MDS, including those with refractory anemia with excess blasts and refractory anemia with ring sideroblasts. In a prospective multicenter study from Japan (called OPTIMA), 822 patients with MDS were analyzed and 132 (16.1%) had GPI-AP- granulocytes.[95] Approximately 20% of patients with refractory cytopenia with unilineage dysplasia, refractory cytopenias with multilineage dysplasia, MDS-unclassified, and 5q- MDS had detectable PNH granulocytes while no patients with refractory anemia ring sideroblasts, refractory anemia with excess blasts-1, or refractory anemia with excess blasts-2 had GPI-AP- granulocytes. These studies suggest that the conditions that favor selection of GPI-AP- cells are present is some patients with low-risk forms of MDS but not in patients with higher-risk disease. The basis for this difference is speculative but may reflect an immune-mediated contribution to disease pathology, as there is clinical evidence that patients with low-risk MDS who have detectable PNH cells are more likely to respond to immunosuppression.[96,97] The OPTIMA study also included 512 patients who were classified as indistinguishable BMF, and 141 (27.5%) were found to have a population of GPI-AP⁻ granulocytes.[95] Additional analysis will be required to determine the clinical significance of this observation, but based on findings in patients with aplastic anemia and low-risk MDS, these patients may have an immune-mediated form of BMF that responds to immunosuppressive therapy.[98]

Patients with BMF (categorized as either MDS-unclassified or aplastic anemia) with del13q in particular have a high probability of responding to immunosuppressive therapy, and the vast majority of these patients have a detectable PNH clone.[99] In samples analyzed, the GPI-AP- cells were del13q negative, indicating that the PNH cells and the del13q cells were derived from separate clones.[99] This finding suggests that the mechanism that protects PNH cells from immune attack shares features with the mechanism that protects the del13q cells from immune-mediated destruction.

Leukocytes and Platelets

Deficiency of GPI-APs on neutrophils, monocytes, platelet, and lymphocytes has been demonstrated in the peripheral blood of patients with PNH, and identical *PIGA* mutations have been identified in neutrophils, monocytes, and lymphocytes from the same patient.[55,60] Together, these studies indicate that the somatic mutation that gives rise to PNH affects a hematopoietic stem cell/progenitor cell. Most patients with PNH have pancytopenia, or either neutropenia or thrombocytopenia in combination with anemia, at some point during the course of their illness. The neutropenia and thrombocytopenia, however, are due to abnormal hematopoiesis rather than to increased peripheral, complement-mediated destruction, as in vivo studies have demonstrated normal survival of neutrophils and platelets in patients with PNH. That absence of GPI-anchored complement regulatory proteins from PNH neutrophils and platelets does not affect their survival implies that these cell types (unlike erythrocytes) have mechanisms in addition to those provided by CD55 and CD59 that protect them from complement-mediated destruction in vivo.

In vitro studies have shown functional abnormalities of PNH leukocytes and platelets. Furthermore, deficiency of some of the GPI-APs from PNH leukocytes and platelets would seem to have important functional consequences (e.g., deficiency of FcγRIIIb from neutrophils, deficiency of urokinase-type plasminogen activator receptor from monocytes and neutrophils, deficiency of LFA-3 from lymphocytes, deficiency of the folate receptor from hematopoietic stem cells) (*Table 32.2*). However, evidence that deficiency of GPI-APs other than erythrocyte CD55 and CD59 contribute to the pathophysiological manifestations of PNH is largely anecdotal. At least in some cases, functional redundancy appears to account for the lack of untoward consequences associated with deficiency of GPI-APs.

Hematopoietic Stem Cells

The PNH defect can be demonstrated in erythroid and granulocytic precursors grown in vitro (i.e., CFU-E, BFU-E, and CFU-GM).[72] Two populations of colonies can be identified in such studies, and they differ from one another in complement sensitivity and expression of acetylcholinesterase.[100] These latter observations support the concept of a clonal process originating from a mutant hematopoietic stem cell.

Cytogenetic studies on hematopoietic cells of patients with PNH have yielded mixed results. The issue is complicated because patients with aplastic anemia can have karyotypic abnormalities. Araten and colleagues reported karyotypic abnormalities in 11 of 46 (24%) patients with PNH examined in a retrospective study.[101] In seven of those patients, there was evidence of clonal regression, and none of the patients developed excess of blasts or transformed into acute leukemia. These findings suggest that karyotypic abnormalities in PNH do not predict progression into a malignant phenotype. To date, the only nonrandom chromosomal abnormality specific for PNH involves rearrangement of 12q13-15 that results in ectopic expression of *HMGA2*.[102] A systematic study of a large number of patients is needed to determine if other nonrandom karyotypic abnormalities that contribute to the clonal expansion of *PIGA*-mutant cells exist.

Uncommonly (~1%), patients with PNH develop acute leukemia.[81,90] In some cases, the leukemic clone arises from the PNH clone because the blasts are GPI-AP deficient.[103] Similar observations have been made in MDS arising in the setting of PNH.[104] However, in other cases, PNH cells disappear following the onset of the leukemia[105] or myelodysplasia.[106] While transformation into acute leukemia or other clonal myelopathies is uncommon in PNH, the incidence is probably higher than in the general population. Therefore, an element of genetic instability perhaps due to stress hematopoiesis may be associated with PNH or the process that underlies PNH.

CLINICAL MANIFESTATIONS

PNH usually begins insidiously with the abrupt onset of clinically apparent hemoglobinuria being the presenting symptom in only 25% of cases.[107,108] The course is chronic with a generally stable clinical pattern in a given individual. The illness ranges in severity from a mild, clinically benign process to a chronically debilitating, potentially lethal disease. The diagnosis is made most frequently in the fourth to fifth decades of life,[81,90,108] but PNH is also encountered in childhood[109] and in old age (age range 16-75 years[81] and 6-82 years[90] in two large series). Both genders are affected with perhaps a slight female predominance, and PNH has been described in many racial groups. The disease has no familial tendency. As noted above (*Congenital abnormalities of genes involved in GPI-AP synthesis*) the clinical phenotype of patients with inherited mutations of genes involved in GPI-AP synthesis (including *PIGA*) is different from that of patients with PNH due to somatic mutation of PIGA affecting bone marrow stem/progenitor cell. As previously noted (see *Membrane Inhibitor of Reactive Lysis [CD59]*), patients with an inherited deficiency of MIRL (CD59) have a hemolytic component similar to that of PNH, with some patients also having chronic inflammatory demyelinating polyneuropathy. Flow cytometry would differentiate these patients from those with PNH due to somatic mutation of *PIGA*, as GPI-AP other than CD59 would be expressed normally.

Most commonly, patients with classic PNH complain initially of malaise, lethargy, and asthenia. Yellowish discoloration of the skin (jaundice) and sclera (icterus) may be observed by astute family members.

Hemoglobinuria

Although essentially all patients with classic PNH have episodes of hemoglobinuria at some time during their illness, this defining symptom is reported as part of the initial evaluation in only one-quarter of all patients (*Table 32.3*). Nocturnal hemoglobinuria appears to result from an increase in the rate of hemolysis that occurs during sleep. It is not related to time of day, however, because the pattern can be reversed if the patient is kept awake at night and allowed to sleep during the

Table 32.3. Presenting Features in 80 Patients With PNH

Signs and Symptoms	Number of Patients (%)
Symptoms of anemia	28 (35)
Hemoglobinuria	21 (26)
Hemorrhagic signs and symptoms	14 (18)
Aplastic anemia	10 (13)
Gastrointestinal symptoms	8 (10)
Hemolytic anemia and jaundice	7 (9)
Iron-deficiency anemia	5 (6)
Thrombosis or embolism	5 (6)
Infections	4 (5)
Neurological signs and symptoms	3 (4)

Used with permission of John Wiley & Sons from Dacie JV, Lewis SM. Paroxysmal nocturnal haemoglobinuria: clinical manifestations, haematology, and nature of the disease. *Ser Haematol.* 1972;5(3):3-23; permission conveyed through Copyright Clearance Center, Inc.

day. In patients with nocturnal hemoglobinuria, the urine is usually darkly discolored in the morning and clears gradually over the course of the day. When hemolysis is intense, however, macroscopic hemoglobinuria persists throughout the day.

The cause of the nocturnal exacerbation is poorly understood. Retention of CO_2 causing a slight fall in plasma pH sufficient to activate the APC is a possible explanation, but this hypothesis has been challenged. Hemoglobinuria is sometimes mistaken for hematuria, which can lead to delay in the proper diagnosis.

Episodic Hemolysis

In addition to the sleep-related pattern, most patients with classic PNH experience irregular but recurrent exacerbations of intravascular hemolysis and hemoglobinuria. Paroxysms may be precipitated by a variety of events including infections (even minor ones), surgery, transfusions, iron supplementation, vaccinations, and menstruation. Attacks of hemoglobinuria are unrelated to cold exposure, thus distinguishing PNH clinically from paroxysmal cold hemoglobinuria. Mild hemolytic episodes often pass without significant symptoms, but more severe attacks may be associated with substernal, lumbar, or abdominal pain together with drowsiness, malaise, fever, and headaches. The abdominal pain may be colicky and may last for 1 to 2 days. The abdomen may be tender, especially in the left upper quadrant, with guarding and rebound tenderness. The back pain resembles that noted in patients with other types of intravascular hemolysis (such as in an ABO incompatible transfusion reaction) and is most severe in the lumbar region. Headaches may be excruciating and sometimes last for days.

Marrow Hypoplasia

As noted above, there is a close association between PNH and BMF syndromes (see *Aplastic Anemia and PNH*). We recommend screening for PNH in all patients with aplastic anemia, low-risk MDS (*see Myelodysplastic Syndrome and PNH*), and uncategorized BMF with marrow hypoplasia. Because many patients with PNH/aplastic anemia, PNH/low-risk MDS, and PNH/BMF have only a small proportion of complement-sensitive cells, biochemical markers associated with hemolytic anemia are often absent. Identifying even a small, subclinical PNH (PNH-sc) clone in patients with BMF is clinically important as a growing body of evidence suggests that a PNH clone is a surrogate marker for immune pathology, and consequently patients with a PNH have a higher probability of responding to immunosuppressive therapy.[95,98]

Thromboembolic Complications

PNH is associated with a striking predisposition toward intravascular thrombosis, especially within the venous circulation.[81,90,110,111] Intra-abdominal veins are the most commonly affected. Cerebral vein and superficial dermal vein thrombosis also appear to be represented disproportionately. Thrombotic disease accounts for about 50% of all deaths in patients with PNH. Fatal thrombosis usually involves the portal system or the brain.

Recurrent abdominal pain is the dominant clinical manifestation in some patients with PNH (*Table 32.3*). The cause of the pain is often obscure but may be severe enough to suggest an acute abdomen warranting emergency surgery. The possibility that thrombosis in the portal or mesenteric veins is the cause of the pain should be considered in this setting. Both transient intestinal ischemia and intestinal infarction due to thrombosis involving the microcirculation are other possible causes.

Hepatic venous thrombosis (Budd-Chiari syndrome) is a serious, potentially fatal complication of PNH.[112,113] In various series, 15% to 30% of patients with PNH had hepatic venous thrombosis, and this complication might be even more common because affected individuals can be asymptomatic when Budd-Chiari syndrome is in its early stage.[114] The clinical manifestations include nausea, abdominal pain, variable degrees of ascites, variceal bleeding, and signs of liver failure. Often the liver increases abruptly in size, but hepatomegaly is not always noted. Three pathophysiologic stages of hepatic venous

thrombosis have been defined.[114] In the early or mildest stage, only venules or small hepatic veins are involved. Patients may be asymptomatic, and therefore, the condition may go unrecognized. Mild, easily controlled ascites is detected in some patients. In the second stage, larger hepatic veins are partially occluded. Ascites is noted in most patients with such abnormalities. Some individuals develop variceal bleeding, and a few become jaundiced. The third or advanced stage is characterized by complete occlusion of large hepatic veins. Ascites is almost always present, jaundice is common, and variceal bleeding occurs in a few patients. This stage is often fatal.

An increase in the concentration of serum lactate dehydrogenase (LDH), alanine aminotransferase, and aspartate aminotransferase may be an early clue to the presence of hepatic vein thrombosis. Serum concentration of conjugated bilirubin also may increase, but other biochemical tests of liver function are of limited value. Ultrasonography is the most effective noninvasive method for early detection of hepatic vein thrombosis with a sensitivity and specificity of 85% or more.[115,116] Computed tomographic and magnetic resonance imaging (MRI) scans are more sensitive than ultrasound. MRI is better for visualizing the whole length of the vena cava and may permit differentiation of the acute form from the subacute form of the disease.[116] Radioactive isotope scanning demonstrates patchy uptake in most of the liver, except for a normal functioning, hypertrophied caudate lobe that is spared because of its separate venous drainage. Hepatic venography is definitive, but this procedure carries more risk than noninvasive techniques. Biopsy may demonstrate congestion and liver cell loss, but the procedure is hazardous and not always informative.

Small-vessel thrombosis may cause severe and refractory headaches or presage progressive cerebrovascular thrombosis.[117] Isotopic brain scanning and electroencephalography usually are of little help in monitoring patients with PNH with headaches.

Renal Abnormalities

Both acute and chronic renal insufficiency occurs in patients with PNH.[118,119] Acute renal insufficiency is associated with hemoglobinuric crises and may resolve without residual damage. In one series of 19 patients with PNH, however, 12 individuals had reduced values for creatinine clearance while their underlying disease was stable. Furthermore, at least three of these patients had progressive renal insufficiency. Patients with PNH may, over time, also develop hematuria, proteinuria, hypertension, subnormal capacity to concentrate urine, or some combination of these abnormalities. The kidneys usually are enlarged when examined radiographically, and MRI may reveal hemosiderin deposition. The renal abnormalities probably result from repeated thrombotic episodes involving small venules.

Dysphagia and Male Impotence

When closely questioned, many patients with PNH complain of painful or difficult swallowing. This symptom is often worse in the morning and appears to be exacerbated during hemolytic episodes. Studies of peristalsis have shown that the esophageal contractions that occur in this setting have 9 to 10 times the normal force. The pathogenesis of these esophageal complaints is speculative. Inasmuch as hemoglobin binds nitric oxide, it has been proposed that the plasma free hemoglobin that is a consequence of the chronic intravascular hemolysis characteristic of PNH acts as a sump for nitric oxide.[120,121] Esophageal (and intestinal) spasm may ensue due to consumption by plasma free hemoglobin of the smooth muscle relaxing activity of nitric oxide. This hypothesis is supported by observations that patients receiving artificial hemoglobin also experience dysphagia and odynophagia.[122]

Male impotence is common in patients with PNH and is worse during hemolytic exacerbations.[121] As is the case with dysphagia, nitric oxide deficiency that is a consequence of the sump effect of plasma-free hemoglobin may underlie the erectile dysfunction.

Infections

The apparent increased incidence of infections in patients with PNH may be attributable to leukopenia, treatment with corticosteroids, or functional defects in leukocytes (although compelling empirical

Disorders of Red Blood Cells

support is lacking). Even mild infections may constitute a serious hazard because they may precipitate a hemolytic exacerbation.

Physical Examination

Findings are largely nonspecific (related to anemia, thrombocytopenia, or neutropenia). Icterus and jaundice may be observed in patients with brisk hemolysis. Moderate splenomegaly and mild to moderate hepatomegaly are sometimes observed and should raise concerns about hepatic or splenic vein thrombosis.

LABORATORY FINDINGS

Blood

Essentially all patients with PNH are anemic, and in many, the anemia is severe. The red cells are usually macrocytic, as observed in other BMF syndromes, but the MCV varies considerably among patients. Occasionally, the red cells may appear hypochromic and microcytic due to iron deficiency resulting from chronic and acute hemoglobinuria with consequent urinary loss of hemoglobin iron. Moderate anisocytosis and poikilocytosis are common, but spherocytes and schistocytes are not observed in the peripheral blood film. Polychromatophilia, reflecting reticulocytosis, is observed unless BMF is severe. Relative reticulocytosis may be marked, but the absolute reticulocyte count is often lower than that found in association with other hemolytic disorders at comparable degrees of anemia. This discrepancy reflects underlying marrow dysfunction that is invariably a component of the disease. Normoblasts (nucleated RBCs) may also be found in the peripheral blood film. The osmotic and mechanical fragility of the erythrocytes is normal, and the reaction to the direct antiglobulin (Coombs) test is negative (although it may become positive in patients treated with eculizumab; see below).

Leukopenia is often observed and may be marked, especially in the setting of PNH/aplastic anemia. The leukopenia is a consequence of bone marrow rather than complement-mediated destruction.[123] Neutrophil alkaline phosphatase (a GPI-AP) expression is low or absent. Functional leukocyte defects have been demonstrated, but their clinical relevance is conjectural.

Thrombocytopenia of moderate to severe degree is common, but platelet life span and function are normal.[124] Thus, like the leukopenia, the thrombocytopenia of PNH is a consequence of BMF. Bleeding due to severe thrombocytopenia may contribute to the morbidity and mortality of the disease.

Plasma

The plasma may be golden brown, reflecting the presence of increased levels of unconjugated bilirubin, hemoglobin, and methemalbumin. Predictably, serum haptoglobin concentration is low or absent and the serum LDH concentration is markedly elevated, reflecting intravascular hemolysis.

Urine

When the rate of blood destruction is increased, the urine contains increased amounts of urobilinogen. In addition, intravascular hemolysis leads to depletion of serum haptoglobin, which results in the continuous presence of hemoglobin in the glomerular filtrate of the kidney. The cells of the proximal convoluted tubules that reabsorb much of the hemoglobin become heavily laden with iron. The excretion of this iron in the form of granules gives rise to hemosiderinuria. In addition, spectroscopic examination may reveal variable amounts of free hemoglobin. The continuous loss of relatively large amounts of iron as a consequence of hemoglobinuria can result in iron deficiency. Average daily losses of up to 16 mg have been observed, and as much as 4 mg of iron excreted in 24 hours has been demonstrated even in the absence of gross hemoglobinuria. Albuminuria has been detected immediately before and after an episode of hemoglobinuria, and long-term study of patients with PNH has shown an unexpectedly high incidence of functional renal abnormalities, such as hematuria, hyposthenuria, tubular malfunction, and declining creatinine clearance.[118,119]

Bone Marrow

In patients with classic PNH, normoblastic hyperplasia is a characteristic finding. As many as 50% of the nucleated cells may be normoblasts, but only occasionally are megaloblastic changes evident. The absence of morphological changes consistent with megaloblastic anemia suggests that deficiency of the GPI-anchored form of the folate receptor (Table 32.2) does not result in abnormalities in folate metabolism that are clinically significant. The number of megakaryocytes may be decreased. When pancytopenia is evident, a hypoplastic marrow is usually observed, although in some patients, pancytopenia is associated with a cellular marrow, a feature that is more consistent with the ineffective hematopoiesis associated with a myelodysplastic process.

Cytogenetic Studies

Although a number of karyotypic abnormalities have been reported in PNH,[101] the only nonrandom chromosomal aberrations specific for PNH involves rearrangement of the *HMGA2* locus on 12q13-15.[73] Apparently, the presence of karyotypically abnormal bone marrow cells is not a negative prognostic factor in PNH.[101]

Diagnostic Tests

Until the early 1990s, the diagnosis of PNH was based on the results of special tests that exploited the abnormal sensitivity of PNH red cells to lysis by complement. Among the available assays, Ham test (acidified serum lysis) and the sucrose lysis test (sugar water test of Hartmann) were most commonly used for the clinical diagnosis of PNH. While those tests are sensitive and specific when properly performed, and relatively simple in both theory and practice, their accuracy is strongly operator dependent. Therefore, in the hands of an inexperienced technician, results are not always reliable. This problem is compounded by the fact that the tests are usually performed on a sporadic basis in most clinical laboratories because the diagnosis of PNH is entertained relatively uncommonly.

The recognition that deficiency of GPI-AP underlies PNH has resulted in the development of a simple, reliable method for diagnosing the disease.[125] By analyzing expression of GPI-AP on hematopoietic cells using monoclonal antibodies and flow cytometry, the abnormal cells can be readily identified (Figures 32.1 and 32.2). The simplest method is to analyze expression of MIRL (CD59) on erythrocytes (Figure 32.1). Because it is normally present in relatively high density, red cells with either complete or partial deficiency of MIRL are easily distinguished from normal (Figure 32.1). Therefore, PNH I (normal expression), PNH II (partial expression), and PNH III (negative expression) erythrocytes can be identified by analyzing the flow cytometry histogram (Figure 32.1). Analysis of erythrocyte DAF (CD55) expression is also informative. Because erythrocytes express ~6- to 8-fold less DAF (CD55) than MIRL (CD59), however, separation into discrete populations may be less obvious when anti-DAF is used as the primary antibody. By using both antibodies, the diagnosis can be confirmed (Figures 32.1 and 32.2A).

The size of the PNH clone is best determined by analysis of GPI-AP expression on granulocytes. Unlike the life span of peripheral blood RBCs that is markedly shortened as a consequence of deficiency of the GPI-anchored complement regulatory proteins CD55 and CD59, the life span of *PIGA*-mutant, GPI-AP-deficient polymorphonuclear neutrophils (PMNs) is normal.[123] Therefore, the percentage of GPI-AP-deficient PMNs is believed to be an accurate reflection of the contribution of the mutant clone(s) to hematopoiesis. The value of determining the size of the PNH clone is that some of the clinical manifestations of the disease, particularly the risk of thromboembolic complications, appear to be proportional to clone size.[126,127] Analysis of GPI-AP on granulocytes is technically more challenging than on erythrocytes, due to the difficulties associated with shipping, processing, and analyzing these fragile cells. Furthermore, granulocyte expression must be analyzed within 24 to 48 hours after the blood sample is acquired, whereas erythrocytes can be analyzed 1 to 2 weeks after the blood is obtained if the sample is properly stored at 4 °C.

GPI-AP-deficient populations that comprise >1%-3% of the red cells can be identified by standard flow cytometry. Concern that recent red cell transfusion might result in a false-negative result seems unfounded. Because the assay is very sensitive and because the proportion of GPI-AP-deficient cells is greater in the reticulocyte population than in the peripheral blood as a whole, massive transfusion that both replaces essentially all of the patient's blood volume and also completely suppresses erythropoiesis would be required to produce a false-negative result. Transfusion will have an impact on the percentage of GPI-AP-deficient red cells that are observed, but the possibility that the diagnosis would be obscured by transfusion is remote. Conversely, it is unlikely that a recent hemolytic episode would result in a false-negative result because all the abnormal cells are destroyed. However, when documenting the proportion of affected cells and determining the precise erythrocyte phenotype, the analysis is best done when the patient has not been recently transfused, as well as when the patient is not experiencing a hemolytic crisis.

By careful gating and by using triple antibody staining techniques, the sensitivity of flow cytometry can be enhanced by about 3 orders of magnitude, such that as few as 0.003% GPI-AP-deficient cells (RBCs and white blood cells) can be consistently and reproducibly detected[91] (*Figure 32.9*). This high-resolution analysis is used to identify patients with PNH-sc (*Figure 32.9B*). Patients with PNH-sc in the setting of aplastic anemia or low-risk variants of myelodysplastic syndrome appear to have a more benign clinical course than patients without PNH-sc.[91,97,128] In addition, some[91,97,128] but not all[129] studies suggest that patients with PNH-sc respond more favorably to immunosuppressive therapy.[95,98]

A diagnostic assay for PNH using fluorescent aerolysin (FLAER) that exploits the unique properties of the bacterial toxin aerolysin has been developed.[130] This channel-forming protein binds directly to the GPI anchor. By fluorochrome labeling of a modified recombinant form of the protein that does not cause lysis, this reagent can be used to detect leukocytes with the PNH phenotype.[130] The primary advantage of this assay is that, because it detects all GPI-APs, it is specific for PNH. The primary disadvantage is that the FLAER reagent does not bind well to the GPI anchor on RBCs. Thus FLAER cannot be used to characterize GPI-AP expression on erythrocytes.

Analysis of expression of GPI-AP on erythrocytes is a highly specific test for PNH. There is no other known disease in which the

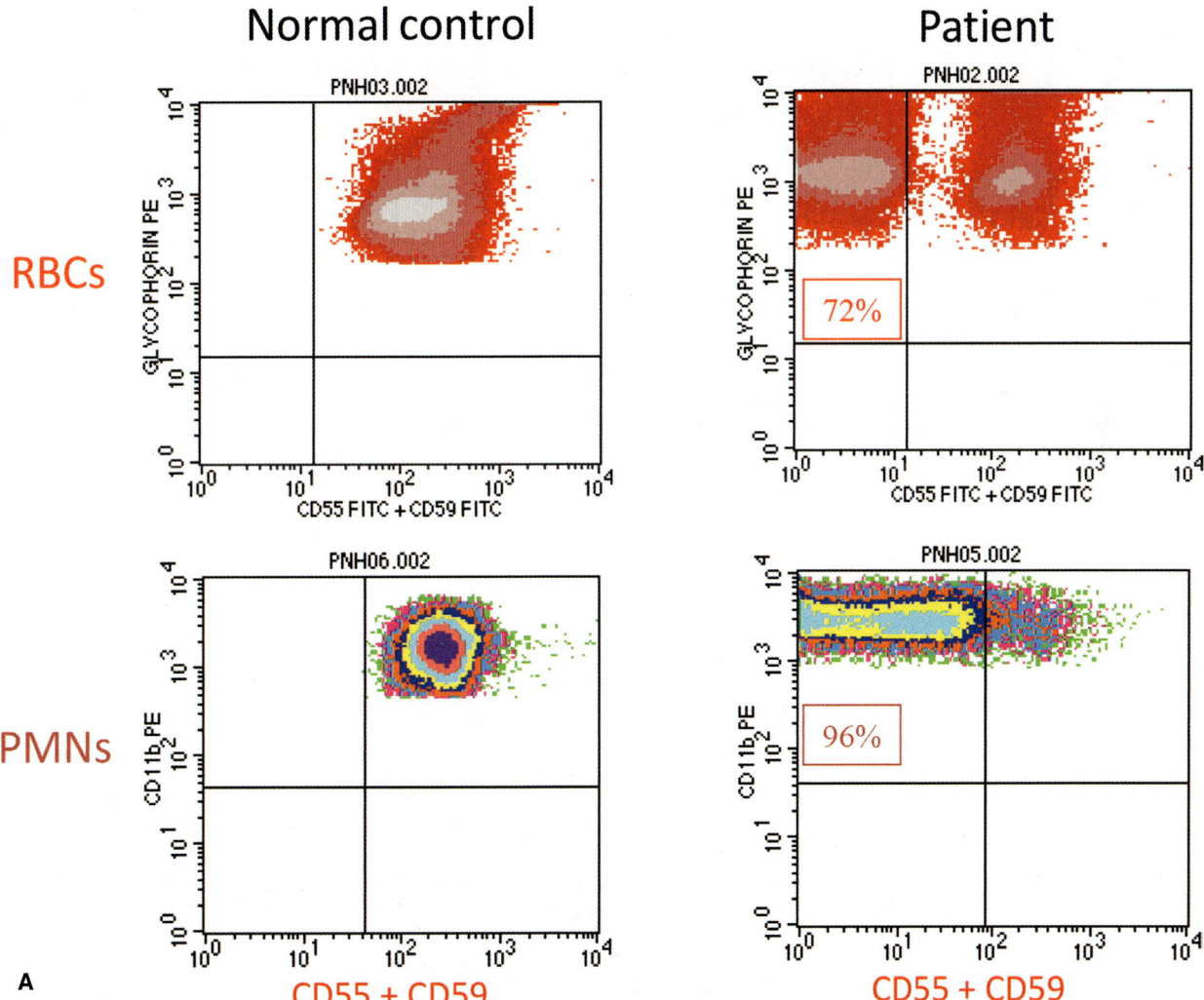

FIGURE 32.9 High-sensitivity flow cytometry for diagnosis of PNH. A, Two-color flow cytometry histogram of erythrocytes (upper panels) and neutrophils (lower panels) from a normal volunteer (left) and from a patient with classic PNH (right). Erythrocytes were stained with phycoerythrin (PE)-labeled anti-glycophorin A (vertical axis) and a combination of fluorescein isothiocyanate (FITC)-labeled anti-CD55 and anti-CD59 (horizontal axis). Neutrophils were stained with PE-labeled CD11b (vertical axis) and FITC-labeled anti-CD55 and anti-CD59 (horizontal axis). No GPI-AP-deficient erythrocytes or neutrophils were among ~100,000 cells counted in this analysis for the normal control, whereas the patient had 72% GPI-AP-deficient erythrocytes and 96% GPI-AP-deficient neutrophils. B, Two-color flow cytometry histogram of erythrocytes and neutrophils from two patients with aplastic anemia but with no clinical evidence of PNH. In the example on the left, approximately 0.077% of the erythrocytes and 0.74% of the neutrophils failed to express CD55 and CD59. In the example on the right, 3% of the erythrocytes and 21% of the neutrophils failed to express CD55 and CD59. PMNs, polymorphonuclear neutrophils; RBCs, red blood cells.

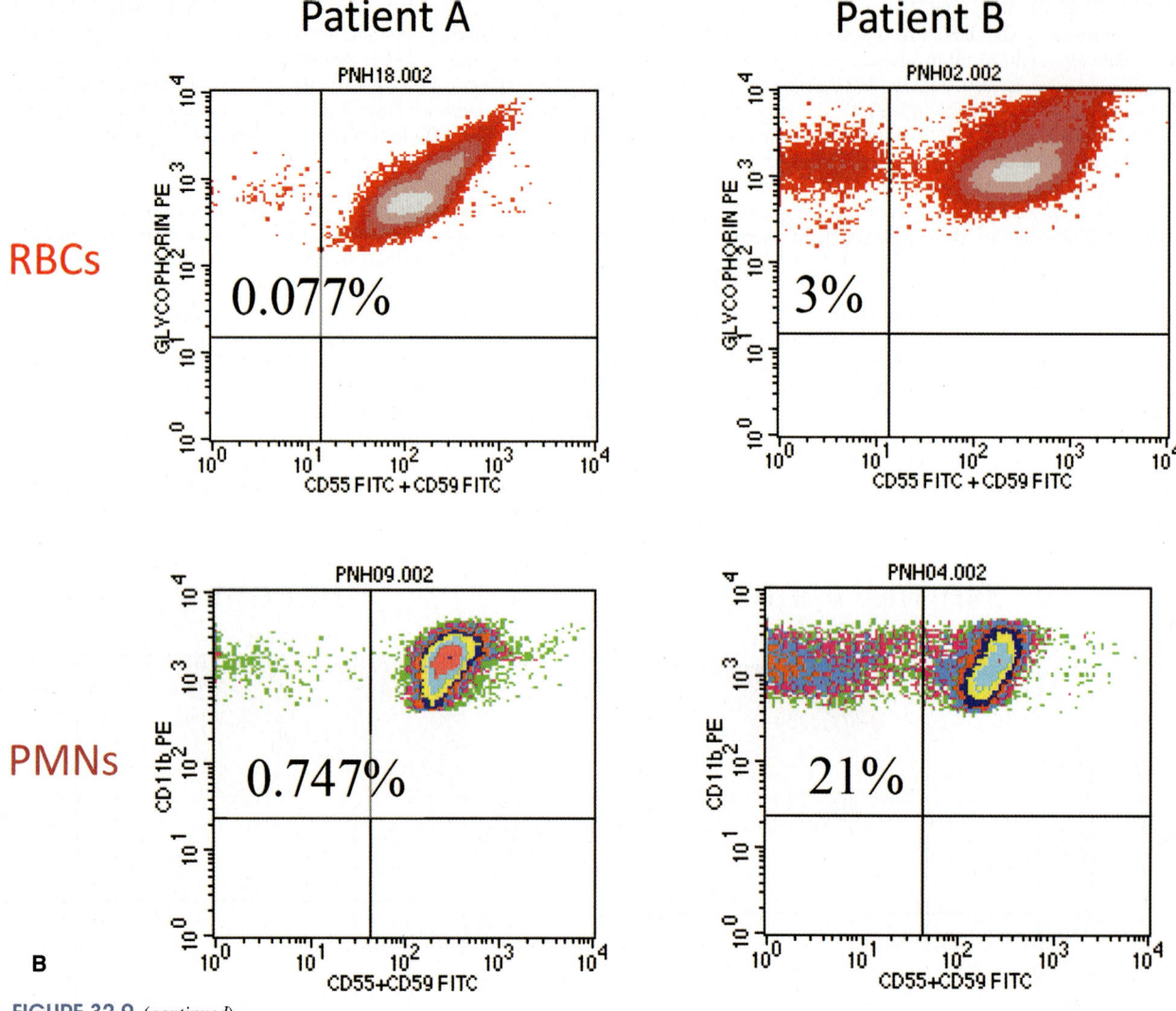

FIGURE 32.9 (*continued*)

erythrocytes include a mosaic of both GPI-AP$^+$ and GPI-AP$^-$ cells. Subjects with isolated deficiency of either DAF (the Inab phenotype) or MIRL (CD59) will be identified by this method (assuming that anti-DAF and anti-MIRL antibodies are used). Such patients are extremely rare, however, and their flow cytometry histograms are readily distinguishable from patients with PNH because 100% of the cells are abnormal (not a mosaic as in PNH) and expression of only one GPI-AP is deficient.

DIFFERENTIAL DIAGNOSIS

The diagnosis of PNH must be considered in any patient who has the following: (1) signs and symptoms of intravascular hemolysis (manifested by an abnormally high LDH) of undefined cause (i.e., Coombs negative), with or without macroscopic hemoglobinuria often accompanied by iron deficiency; (2) pancytopenia in association with hemolysis; (3) venous thrombosis affecting unusual sites, especially intra-abdominal, cerebral, or dermal locations accompanied by evidence of hemolysis; (4) unexplained recurrent bouts of abdominal pain, low backache, or headache in the presence of chronic hemolysis; and (5) Budd-Chiari syndrome.

It is important to document evidence of hemolysis before proceeding with tests more specific for clinical PNH. As discussed above, a history of gross hemoglobinuria (nocturnal or otherwise) is not part of the initial clinical presentation in approximately three-fourths of

patients with PNH (*Table 32.3*). However, except for patients with PNH-sc, *laboratory* evidence of hemolysis is a constant feature of the disease. Quantitation of serum LDH is particularly informative because intravascular hemolysis results in markedly elevated values. If LDH concentrations are difficult to interpret because of other comorbid conditions (e.g., liver disease), then alternative evidence for chronic intravascular hemolysis should be sought (e.g., low serum haptoglobin, urine hemosiderin, elevated indirect bilirubin). Without evidence of hemolysis, more specific tests for *clinical* PNH are generally unwarranted. PNH must be differentiated from antibody-mediated hemolytic anemias, especially paroxysmal cold hemoglobinuria and the cold agglutinin syndrome, and from HEMPAS (hereditary erythroblastic multinuclearity with a positive acidified serum lysis test or congenital dyserythropoietic anemia type II). The mechanism that underlies the abnormal susceptibility of HEMPAS erythrocytes to acidified serum lysis is different from that of PNH.[131] By using flow cytometry, there is no difficulty distinguishing PNH from other hemolytic diseases because deficiency of GPI-APs affecting a portion of the erythrocytes is diagnostic of PNH.

By definition, patients with PNH-sc have no clinical or laboratory evidence of hemolysis. PNH-sc is diagnosed by using high-resolution flow cytometry. Patients with aplastic anemia and low-risk variants of MDS should undergo screening for PNH-sc at diagnosis and yearly thereafter. Finding PNH-sc appears to have important prognostic and therapeutic implications, as patients with PNH-sc/aplastic anemia or

PNH-sc/low-risk MDS may have a more benign clinical course and a higher rate of response to immunosuppressive therapy than those without PNH-sc.[91,95,97,98,128]

TREATMENT

The size of the PNH clone and the type and severity of the BMF component of the disease are the main factors that determine the clinical course. Some patients have a relatively benign clinical course with only a moderate degree of anemia and minimal hemolysis, and for such patients, no PNH-specific treatment is required. Other patients have severe anemia punctuated by hemolytic crises and thromboembolic complications; in such patients, treatment of the complement-mediated hemolytic anemia is clearly warranted and can be transformative. In other patients, the disease is dominated by BMF rather than by hemolysis, and in those patients, the focus of treatment should be on the underlying marrow failure process. By taking into account the size of the PNH clone and the type and severity of the BMF component of the disease, a classification has been developed that provides a rational basis for management.

Clinical Classification

The basic approach to classifying PNH is straightforward. Flow cytometric analysis of peripheral blood erythrocytes and granulocytes is needed to determine the phenotype of the red cells and the size of the PNH clone (based on the percentage of GPI-AP-deficient granulocytes). CBC, reticulocyte count, serum concentration of LDH, bilirubin (fractionated), haptoglobin, and iron stores are needed to assess the degree of marrow failure and hemolysis, and whether iron deficiency is present. Bone marrow aspirate and biopsy and cytogenetic analysis are needed to characterize the status of the bone marrow. Once the basic evaluation is complete, patients should be classified based on the categories developed by the International PNH Interest Group.[3]

The three categories are as follows (*Figure 32.10*):

Classic PNH. Patients with Classic PNH have clinical evidence of intravascular hemolysis (reticulocytosis, abnormally high concentration of serum LDH and indirect bilirubin, and abnormally low concentration of serum haptoglobin) but have no evidence of another defined bone marrow abnormality. A cellular marrow with erythroid hyperplasia and normal or near-normal morphology, but without nonrandom karyotypic abnormalities, is consistent with classic PNH. The PNH clone is large (>50% and often >90%). Patients with even a large population of PNH II erythrocytes, however, will have minimal hemolysis unless they experience a process such as trauma, infection, or surgery that significantly enhances complement activation.

PNH in the setting of another specified bone marrow disorder. This subcategory of patients have at least laboratory evidence of hemolysis and also have concomitantly a defined underlying marrow abnormality. Bone marrow analysis and cytogenetics are used to determine if PNH arose in association with aplastic anemia or MDS. Standard criteria are used for diagnosis of the bone marrow abnormality (e.g., aplastic anemia, low-risk MDS). Finding nonrandom karyotypic abnormalities that are associated with a specific bone marrow abnormality may contribute diagnostically (e.g., abnormalities of chromosomes 5q, 7, and 20q are associated with MDS). The large majority of patients with PNH/AA and PNH/MDS has relatively small PNH clones (25%-50%) and require no specific PNH therapy, and in these cases, treatment should focus on the underlying BMF syndrome.[93] Approximately half of the patients with clinical PNH in the setting of BMF, however, will require therapy (anticomplement treatment for hemolysis or anticoagulation for thrombosis) during the course of their illness.[93]

Subclinical PNH (PNH-sc). Patients with PNH-sc have no clinical or laboratory evidence of hemolysis. Small populations of GPI-AP-deficient hematopoietic cells (peripheral blood erythrocytes, granulocytes, or both) are detected by sensitive flow cytometric analysis.[87] PNH-sc is observed in association with BMF syndromes, particularly aplastic anemia, low-risk MDS, and unclassified hypoplastic marrow failure. In approximately 90% of these cases, the proportion of GPI-AP-deficient cells is <25%.[87] These patients require no PNH-specific therapy; however, as noted above, finding a population of GPI-AP-deficient erythrocytes in patients with aplastic anemia may be clinically relevant, as some[91,97,128] but not all[129] studies suggest that these patients have a particularly high probability of responding to immunosuppressive therapy with a more rapid rate of onset of response compared with patients with aplastic anemia without a population of GPI-AP-deficient erythrocytes.[95,98] Treatment with immunosuppressive therapy appears to have no influence on the size of the PNH clone.[93]

An algorithmic approach to management of PNH based on the above disease classification is shown (*Figure 32.11*).

Management of the Anemia of PNH

Coombs-negative hemolytic anemia is the clinical hallmark of PNH, but because the disease usually arises in the setting of an underlying

Disorders of Red Blood Cells

Classification of PNH Guides Management

Classification of PNH*

	Category	Rate of Intravascular Hemolysis†	Bone Marrow Characteristics	Flow Cytometry	Benefit from Eculizumab
Clinical PNH	Classic	Florid (markedly abnormal LDH, often with episodic macroscopic hemoglobinuria)	Cellular marrow due to erythroid hyperplasia and normal or near-normal morphology	Large population (>50%) of GPI-AP deficient PMNs	Yes
	PNH in the setting of another bone marrow failure syndrome§	Usually mild (often with minimal to modest abnormalities of biochemical markers of hemolysis)	Evidence of a concomitant bone marrow failure syndrome§	Although variable, the percentage of GPI-AP deficient PMNs is usually relatively small (25-50%)	Variable. Some patients have clinically significant hemolysis and benefit from treatment
	Subclinical	No clinical or biochemical evidence of intravascular hemolysis	Evidence of a concomitant bone marrow failure syndrome§	Small (usually <1%) population of GPI-AP deficient PMNs detected by high-resolution flow cytometry	No

* Based on recommendations of the International PNH Interest Group (*Blood* 2005;106:3699-3709)
† Based on episodes of macroscopic hemoglobinuria, serum LDH concentration, and reticulocyte count
§ Aplastic anemia or low risk myelodysplastic syndrome

FIGURE 32.10 Classification of PNH. This classification is modified based on the recommendations of the International PNH Interest Group.

abnormality of the bone marrow, hemolysis may account for only part of a patient's anemia. Furthermore, the erythrocytes of PNH are a mosaic of normal and abnormal cells and the portion of GPI-AP-deficient RBCs varies among patients (*Figures 32.1* and *32.2*). For example, in hypothetical patient A, 15% of the circulating RBCs may be GPI-AP deficient, while, in hypothetical patient B, 75% GPI-AP-deficient erythrocytes may be observed (*Figure 32.12*). In the former,

hemolysis would contribute modestly to an observed anemia, while in the latter, a significant hemolytic component would be expected (*Figure 32.12*). Another complicating factor is that deficiency of GPI-AP may be partial rather than complete (*Figures 32.1* and *32.12*), and partial expression of CD55 and CD59 is sufficient to protect PNH II cells from spontaneous complement-mediated lysis in vivo.[37] Therefore, even if a patient has a high proportion of PNH II cells,

Management of PNH Based on Disease Classification

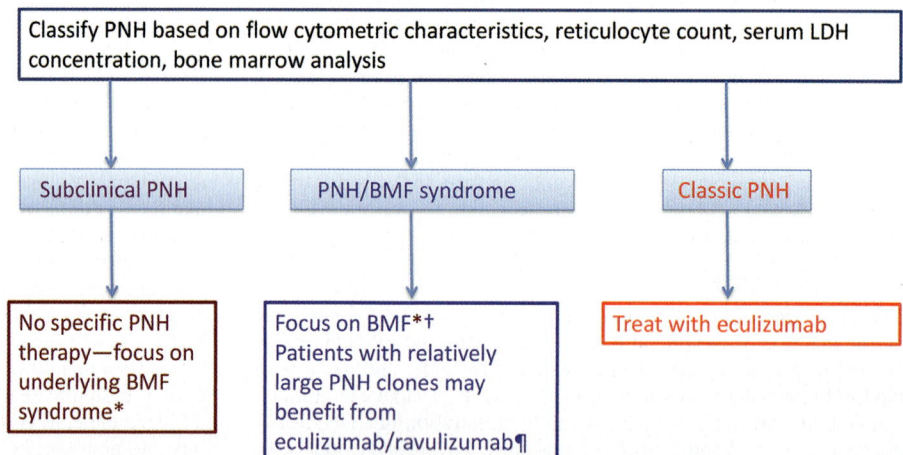

FIGURE 32.11 Algorithm for management of PNH based on disease classification. Disease classification is based on the recommendations of the International PNH Interest Group (*Figure 32.10*). (Used with permission of American Society of Hematology from Parker CJ. Update on the diagnosis and management of paroxysmal nocturnal hemoglobinuria. *Hematology Am Soc Hematol Educ Program.* 2016;2016(1):208-216; permission conveyed through Copyright Clearance Center, Inc.)

BMF, bone marrow failure (aplastic anemia and low-risk MDS)
*Some, but not all, studies suggest a favorable response to immunosuppressive therapy (IST). Treatment with IST does not affect PNH clone size
†Hematopoietic stem cell transplant eradicates the PNH clone
¶Approximately 50% of patients with PNH/BMF require treatment for hemolysis or thrombosis

Clone Size and Phenotype Are Clinically Relevant

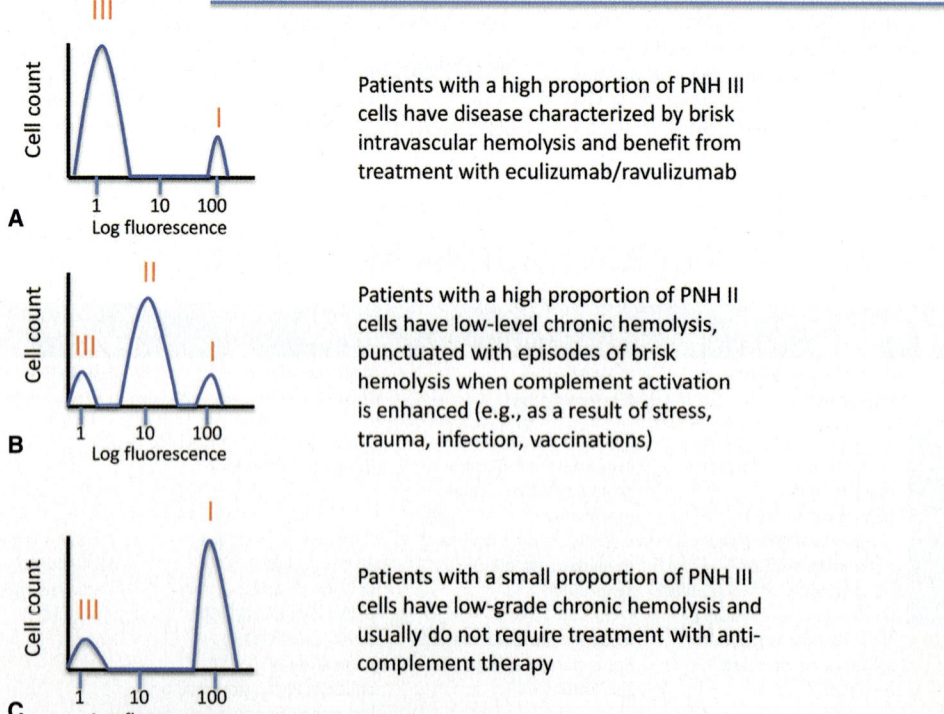

FIGURE 32.12 Impact of phenotype and degree of mosaicism on the hemolytic anemia of PNH. Mock histograms of erythrocytes from patients with PNH stained with anti-CD59 are illustrated. The proportion and type of abnormal erythrocytes varies greatly among patients with PNH, and these characteristics are important determinants of clinical manifestations. In general, patients with a high percentage of type III erythrocytes have clinically apparent hemolysis (A). If the erythrocytes are partially deficient in GPI-AP, hemolysis may be modest even if the percentage of the affected cells is high (B). A patient may have a diagnosis of PNH, but if the proportion of type III cells is low, only biochemical evidence of hemolysis may be observed (C).

only modest evidence of spontaneous hemolysis is usually observed (*Figure 32.12*). But brisk hemolysis can occur in patients with predominantly PNH II erythrocytes in situation where complement activation is enhanced (e.g., by infection, trauma, surgery, vaccination, pregnancy, unusual stress).

Prior to initiating therapy, an effort should be made to determine how much of the anemia is a consequence of hemolysis and how much is due to impaired erythropoiesis (*Table 32.4*). Review of the complete blood count is informative because evidence of thrombocytopenia, leukopenia, or both suggests ineffective hematopoiesis or bone marrow hypoplasia. The capacity of the marrow to respond to the anemia can be inferred from the reticulocyte count. An element of marrow failure is likely a contributing factor in a patient with PNH who has anemia with an inappropriately low reticulocyte count.

Biochemical parameters of hemolysis should be assessed (*Table 32.4*). Normal or minimal elevation of LDH argues against hemolysis as a major contributing factor to the anemia. The presence of urine hemosiderin suggests chronic intravascular hemolysis, but provides no quantitative information, while gross hemoglobinuria indicates clinically significant intravascular hemolysis.

The concentration of erythropoietin should be determined, as renal dysfunction may complicate PNH.[118] Iron deficiency due to hemosiderinuria/hemoglobinuria is common.

Treatment of anemia that is primarily a consequence of BMF should be aimed at the underlying disease (e.g., aplastic anemia, MDS). Patients with PNH/aplastic anemia or PNH/low-risk MDS appear to have a favorable response to immunosuppressive therapy.[91,97,98,128] If absolute or relative erythropoietin deficiency is thought to contribute to the anemia, replacement with the recombinant protein is warranted, but patients should be closely monitored as erythropoietin supplementation could exacerbate hemolysis by increasing production of GPI-AP-deficient erythrocytes (patients treated with eculizumab would be protected against such a hemolytic exacerbation). There are also anecdotal reports of patients responding to pharmacological doses of erythropoietin even when the endogenous concentration is high.[132] Androgens may also be beneficial in patients with PNH who have a hypoproliferative component to their anemia.[133] Complement inhibitory therapy (e.g., eculizumab) would not be expected to have efficacy in the treatment of anemia due to marrow failure.

Complement Inhibitory Therapy

Patients with evidence of clinically significant intravascular hemolysis (markedly elevated LDH, macroscopic hemoglobinuria, reticulocytosis, transfusion dependence) are candidates for treatment with eculizumab or ravulizumab (Soliris, Ultomris, respectively, Alexion Pharmaceuticals Inc). However, patients need not be transfusion dependent to benefit from eculizumab/ravulizumab as the debilitating

---

Table 32.4. Information Useful for Managing Anemia in Patients With PNH

- Complete blood count
- Reticulocyte count
- Serum concentration of lactate dehydrogenase (LDH), bilirubin (total and direct fractions), haptoglobin
- Urine hemosiderin[a]
- Flow cytometric analysis of erythrocytes and granulocytes for expression of GPI-AP
- Serum concentration of blood urea nitrogen and creatinine
- Serum erythropoietin concentration
- Serum iron studies (iron concentration, total iron binding capacity, transferrin saturation, serum ferritin concentration)

[a]Indicative of chronic hemolysis but provides no quantitative information.
Modified from Parker C, Omine M, Richards S, et al. Diagnosis and management of paroxysmal nocturnal hemoglobinuria. *Blood*. 2005;106(12):3699-3709. Copyright © 2005 American Society of Hematology. With permission.

---

symptoms of lethargy, malaise, and asthenia that accompany the chronic, complement-mediated intravascular of PNH are ameliorated by treatment with eculizumab/ravulizumab.

Eculizumab is a humanized monoclonal antibody that binds complement C5, preventing its activation to C5b by the APC C5 convertase and thereby inhibiting MAC formation (*Figure 32.1*).[134] In 2007, eculizumab was approved by both the US Food and Drug Administration (FDA) and the European Medicines Agency for treatment of the hemolysis of PNH. The drug is now available in countries outside of North American and Europe. Treatment of patients who have classic PNH with eculizumab reduces transfusion requirements, ameliorates the anemia of PNH, and improves quality of life.[14,135,136] Following treatment, serum LDH concentration returns to normal or near normal, with approximately two-thirds achieving transfusion independence,[108] but mild to moderate anemia, hyperbilirubinemia, and reticulocytosis persist in essentially all treated patients.

Eculizumab also appears to reduce the risk of thromboembolic complications.[137] For patients being treated with eculizumab who have no prior history of thromboembolic complications, prophylactic anticoagulation may be unnecessary, while it is recommended that anticoagulation continue for those patients who experienced a thromboembolic event prior to initiating therapy with eculizumab.[108] Eculizumab is expensive (~$650,000/y in the United States), and it has no effect either on the underlying stem cell abnormality or on the associated BMF. Consequently, treatment must continue indefinitely and leukopenia, thrombocytopenia, and reticulocytopenia, if present, persist. Patients treated with eculizumab are at risk for infection with *Neisseria* organisms, and vaccination against *Neisseria meningitidis* is required prior to initiation of therapy. Nonetheless, deaths from meningococcal sepsis have been observed in patients being treated with eculizumab. Some advocate the use of prophylactic penicillin in patients treated with eculizumab, as the currently available vaccine does not protect against some species of meningococcus.[108] Treatment with eculizumab appears to have a favorable impact on survival, as a study of 79 patients treated between 2002 and 2010 showed the same survival as that of age- and sex-matched controls from the general population.[108] However, the contribution of eculizumab to survival in this study cannot be quantified accurately as a control patient group was not included.

In December 2018, the FDA-approved ravulizumab for treatment of patients with PNH. Like eculizumab, ravulizumab is a humanized, monoclonal antibody that binds to complement C5, thereby preventing enzymatic cleavage by the C5 convertase and subsequent MAC formation. Ravulizumab was engineered to take advantage of immunoglobulin recycling by the neonatal Fc receptor. This modification extended the half-life of ravulizumab, allowing for dosing every 8 weeks (vs every 2 weeks for eculizumab). Clinical trials showed that ravulizumab is noninferior to eculizumab both in the treatment of patients whose disease was well controlled with eculizumab and in patients who were naïve to anticomplement therapy.[138,139] The incidence of breakthrough hemolysis may be lower in patients treated with ravulizumab compared with those treated with eculizumab.[140] The cost of 1 year of treatment with ravulizumab is approximately 10% less than that of eculizumab.

Reasons for Eculizumab/Ravulizumab Failure

The recommended maintenance dose of eculizumab is fixed (900 mg every 2 weeks ± 2 days) rather than being based on weight or body surface area. Owing to differences in the rate of drug metabolism, some patients may show evidence of breakthrough intravascular hemolysis (e.g., a rise in LDH and development of constitutional symptoms) near the end of a treatment cycle. This process (breakthrough hemolysis) is usually a pharmacokinetics issue, because in some patients, toward the end of the treatment cycle, the concentration of eculizumab falls below that required for complete inhibition of C5. This type of breakthrough hemolysis can be diagnosed by monitoring the CH_{50} or the concentration of free eculizumab.[73] Detectable levels of CH_{50} ($\geq 10\%$ of normal) and concentrations of eculizumab lower than 50 µg/mL suggest suboptimal dosing of eculizumab. This issue can be addressed by increasing the dose of eculizumab from 900 mg every 2 weeks to 1200 mg every 2 weeks or by shorting the dosing interval from 14 to 12 days. Breakthrough hemolysis can also occur when a patient has a complication, such as an intercurrent infection (including COVID-19), that causes brisk complement activation (pharmacodynamic breakthrough hemolysis). These patients may require additional eculizumab to control hemolysis until the inciting event has resolved as the risk of thrombosis increases in this setting.

All patients with PNH have an element of BMF, and patients treated with eculizumab who have higher degrees of relative reticulocytopenia may remain anemic or even transfusion dependent despite excellent control of intravascular hemolysis. Iron stores and serum erythropoietin concentration should be quantified in these patients, and if iron stores are adequate, and serum erythropoietin concentration is inappropriately low, a trial of recombinant erythropoietin is warranted in patients who have symptomatic anemia or who are transfusion dependent. Following treatment with eculizumab, serum LDH returns to normal or near normal, but mild to moderate anemia and laboratory evidence of hemolysis persist in essentially all treated patients.[135]

A subgroup of eculizumab-treated patients experience only modest improvement in anemia, and some remain transfusion dependent.[141] In these patients, hemolysis is mediated by opsonization of the PNH erythrocytes by activation and degradation products of complement C3, and when tested, they are found to be Coombs positive for C3 but not IgG.[142-145] The known pathophysiology of the PNH predicts that CD55 deficiency would result in ongoing extravascular hemolysis of PNH erythrocytes as a consequence of C3 opsonization (*Figure 32.3*), as eculizumab does not block the activity of the APC C3 convertase that is unregulated because of DAF deficiency (*Figure 32.3*). In addition, CD59 appears to have inhibitory activity against the APC C3/C5 convertase, and therefore its deficiency may contribute to the C3 opsonization observed in patients with PNH treated with eculizumab.[34-36] Support for the hypothesis that C3 opsonization can lead to extravascular hemolysis in patients treated with eculizumab is provided by the studies of Risitano and colleagues[145] who showed that, in patients treated with eculizumab, a portion of the PNH erythrocytes (i.e., the CD59-deficient population) had complement C3 bound. Those studies also confirmed the Coombs-negative designation of PNH, as no C3 was found bound to PNH erythrocytes prior to initiation of treatment with eculizumab, implying that PNH erythrocytes upon which complement has been activated are destroyed directly as a consequence of MAC-mediated cytolysis. Therefore, those studies provide a plausible explanation for the persistent hemolytic anemia observed in patients with PNH treated with eculizumab.[146] By inhibiting formation of the MAC, eculizumab prevents direct cytolysis of PNH erythrocytes, allowing the manifestations of CD55 and CD59 deficiency to become apparent in the form of aberrant regulation of the APC C3 convertase and the consequent deposition of activated C3 on the cell surface (*Figure 32.3*).[147] Covalently bound activation and degradation products of C3 then serve as opsonins that are recognized by specific receptors on reticuloendothelial cells resulting in extravascular

hemolysis. The extravascular hemolysis of patients with PNH receiving eculizumab does not require treatment in the absence of constitutional symptoms, symptoms of anemia, or transfusion dependence. As the process is extravascular, splenectomy or corticosteroids may ameliorate the hemolysis in symptomatic or transfusion-dependent patients by removing or inhibiting the function of phagocytic cells. Long-term use of corticosteroids is associated with significant toxicity, however, and concerns about both postoperative and late complications temper enthusiasm for splenectomy. It is also conceivable that the primary site of phagocytosis is hepatic rather than splenic. In such cases, response to splenectomy would likely be inadequate. Based on experience in the treatment of refractory autoimmune hemolytic anemia, a trial of danazol can be considered; however, rituximab is not indicated as the process is mediated by C3 opsonization rather than opsonization by IgG antibodies.

Because some patients have a suboptimal response to eculizumab/ravulizumab due to extravascular hemolysis due to C3 opsonization, there is interest in developing therapeutic products that block formation of the C3 convertase so as to prevent both extravascular hemolysis due to C3 opsonization and intravascular hemolysis mediated by the MAC (*Figure 32.13*). A small peptide inhibitor of complement C3 (pegcetacoplan) was shown to significantly increase hemoglobin concentrations in patients with PNH who remained anemic (hemoglobin concentration <10.5 gm/dL) while on treatment with eculizumab.[148] Transfusion requirements were also reduced among the patients treated with pegcetacoplan compared with those who remained on treatment with eculizumab. Pegcetacoplan requires twice weekly subcutaneous infusion (compared with an every-8-week infusion of ravulizumab). In May 2021, pegcetacoplan (Empaveli) received FDA approval for treatment of adult patients with PNH. Several of the newer C3 convertase inhibitors are small molecules that are active orally (*Figure 32.13*).[149] Additional studies are needed to define more clearly the safety and efficacy of C3 convertase inhibitors and to determine their role in the management of PNH.

Nishimura and colleagues identified a polymorphism of C5 in 11 Japanese patients with PNH who had a poor response to treatment with eculizumab.[150,151] An anti-C5 antibody directed against an epitope different from that recognized by eculizumab completely blocked the hemolytic activity in the sera of the patients with this C5 polymorphism. The prevalence of the polymorphism in the Japanese population appears to be in the range of 3.5%. The polymorphism was also identified in the Han Chinese population.

Androgenic Steroids, Cortical Steroids, and Immunosuppressive Therapy

Although efficacy is controversial,[3] some patients with PNH respond to treatment with androgenic steroids and prednisone.[133]

Approximately one-third of patients appear to respond to androgen therapy with an increase in hemoglobin concentration, a reduction in transfusion requirement, or both; however, attempting to identify the responders in advance is problematic. The mechanism by which androgenic steroids ameliorate the anemia of PNH is not understood,

Inhibition of APC C3 Convertase Formation by Blocking Complement Factor D or Complement C3

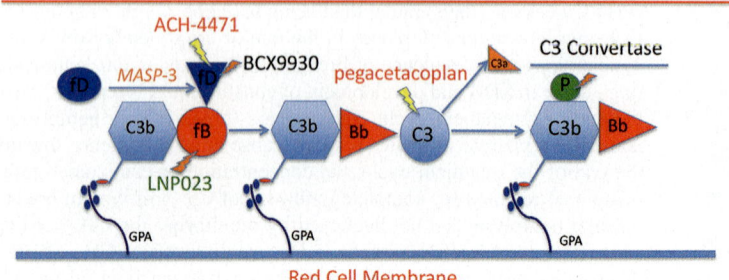

Red Cell Membrane

FIGURE 32.13 Pharmacologic inhibition of C3 convertase formation. Because some patients treated with C5 inhibitors, eculizumab and ravulizumab, have a suboptimal response due to extravascular hemolysis mediated by C3 opsonization, development of therapeutic agents that block the formation of C3 convertase of the alternative pathway of complement are under development with several drugs in trial in human. Lightning bolts indicate targets for pharmacologic intervention. ACH-4471, an oral factor D inhibitor is being developed by Achillion Pharmaceuticals; BCX9930, an oral factor D inhibitor is being developed by Biocryst; LNP023 (iptacopan), an oral factor B inhibitor is being developed by Roche. Pegcetacoplan, an infusible, small molecule inhibitor of C3, developed by Apellis Pharmaceuticals, was approved by the FDA in May 2021 for treatment of adult patients with PNH. Properdin (factor P) is a hypothetical target for pharmacologic inhibition. GPA, glycophorin-alpha.

although the rapid onset of action is consistent with complement inhibition.[152] The adverse effects of androgen therapy can be substantial, ranging from virilization in women and acne and hypercholesterolemia in both sexes to serious liver disease, including peliosis hepatitis and hepatocellular carcinoma. Although neither of the last two complications has been reported in androgen-treated patients with PNH, some suggest androgens might predispose to an insidious form of hepatic vein thrombosis.[133] These considerations make prudent the institution of androgen therapy for only 6 to 8 weeks, with discontinuation if no clear response is observed. Oral preparations such as fluoxymesterone (5-30 mg/d) or oxymetholone (10-50 mg/d) have been used most commonly. Because of fewer virilizing adverse effects, the synthetic androgen danazol (400-800 mg/d in two divided doses) is an attractive alternative to anabolic steroids. Once hemolysis is controlled, a dose of 200 to 400 mg/d may be sufficient to sustain the response. Monitoring of plasma lipids and liver function studies is mandatory.

Corticosteroids have been used as treatment for both chronic hemolysis and acute hemolytic exacerbations. As is the case with androgenic steroids, treatment is not based on compelling empiric data, and there is no experimental evidence that provides a plausible explanation for why steroids should ameliorate the hemolysis of PNH. Nonetheless, some patients appear to respond rapidly and dramatically to glucocorticoids (given in the dosage range of 0.25-1.0 mg/kg/d of prednisone). The rapid response (often within 24 hours of initiating therapy) suggests that complement inhibition accounts for the antihemolytic activity of glucocorticoid therapy. Such an effect could be direct (the result of inhibition of the activity of some component of the APC) or indirect (the result of dampening a process, such as inflammation, that stimulates activation of complement).

The main value of corticosteroids may be in attenuating acute hemolytic exacerbations.[3] Under these circumstances, brief pulses of prednisone may reduce the severity and duration of the crisis while avoiding the untoward consequences associated with long-term use. The value of steroids in treating chronic hemolysis is limited by toxicity, however, and the harm that can accrue from long-term use cannot be overemphasized. An every-other-day schedule may attenuate some of the adverse effects of chronic steroid use, but patients may note worsening of symptoms on the off day. Careful follow-up is essential, and both bacterial prophylaxis and prophylaxis against steroid-induced osteopenia are recommended. Awareness of the potentially debilitating effects of steroid myopathy and sensitivity to the disfiguring consequences of iatrogenic Cushing syndrome are essential for proper management.

Responses to immunosuppressive therapy with cyclosporin and anti-thymocyte globulin have been reported.[153-155] This approach to management has been applied primarily to patients with PNH/aplastic anemia, and as noted above, immunosuppressive therapy appears to have no effect on the size of the PNH clone.[93] Use of high-dose cyclophosphamide for treatment of PNH and PNH/aplastic anemia has been investigated.[15]

Transfusions

Blood transfusions may be required for treatment of anemia. The recommendation that the blood be given in the form of saline-washed or frozen-thawed, deglycerolized red cells in order to avert a hemolytic episode due to complement within the accompanying plasma has been questioned.[156] But hemofiltration is recommended to prevent transfusion reactions resulting from interaction between donor leukocytes and recipient antibodies. Transfused red cells survive normally in patients with PNH, and transfusion to nearly normal hemoglobin levels can produce short-lived "remissions." Clinical improvement may result from a temporary decrease in the production of abnormal cells with a consequent reduction of hemolysis and other disease-associated epiphenomena. Iatrogenic hemochromatosis can occur from chronic transfusions, but this process will be delayed due to iron loss from hemoglobinuria and hemosiderinuria. In fact, iron overload in patients with classic PNH is rare. But iron overload remains a concern in patients who require chronic transfusion when the anemia is primarily a consequence of marrow failure rather than hemolysis.

Iron

As a result of chronic hemoglobinuria and hemosiderinuria, iron deficiency eventually develops in most patients (even in heavily transfused patients).[157] The amount of iron lost should be replaced, since iron-limited erythropoiesis may contribute to the anemia and hemolysis appears to be exacerbated by iron deficiency. Most patients tolerate oral iron therapy well, but hemolytic episodes have been precipitated by such treatment. This phenomenon probably results from the outpouring of a cohort of young erythrocytes, a larger proportion of which is complement sensitive. Parenteral iron repletion is generally safe. If hemoglobinuria after iron therapy is troublesome, hematopoiesis can be suppressed by a brief period of transfusion during which iron stores are repleted. Alternatively, a short course of high doses of prednisone given during the early phases of iron replacement therapy may ameliorate the hemolytic exacerbation. For patients treated with eculizumab, a hemolytic exacerbation would not be induced by iron replacement, and iron deficiency should not develop in patients on eculizumab as inhibition of hemolysis eliminates hemoglobinuria and the consequent iron loss.

Splenectomy

Reports of amelioration of hemolysis and improvement in cytopenias following splenectomy are anecdotal. Concerns about lack of proven efficacy and the potential for postoperative complications, particularly thrombosis, limit enthusiasm for splenectomy in the management of PNH.[3]

Folate

Although most normal Western diets supply adequate folate, supplemental folate (1-5 mg/d) is recommended to ensure compensation for increased utilization associated with heightened erythropoiesis that is a consequence of hemolysis.

Bone Marrow Transplantation

Bone marrow or other forms of stem cell transplantation has been used in the treatment of PNH for nearly 40 years.[158] The unique pathophysiology of PNH should be taken into account when planning a transplant strategy. PNH is a nonmalignant clonal disease, and observations of a patient who underwent a syngeneic stem cell transplant[159] underscore two important differences in response to transplant for PNH, compared with transplant for malignant clonal myelopathies such as acute leukemia. First, cytoreduction of the "tumor" cell burden prior to transplant conditioning is not required, whereas the success of transplant for acute leukemia (and other malignant clonal disorders) is dependent on maximum pretransplant tumor debulking. Second, graft-vs.-tumor effect is not essential for eradication of the PNH clone, whereas graft-vs.-tumor effect plays a critical role in the outcome of transplant for malignant disorders.

The optimal transplant conditioning regimen for PNH should be decided on a case-by-case basis.[3] Clearly some conditioning is essential as infusion of syngeneic donor marrow without conditioning has limited, transient efficacy due to reemergence of the PNH clone.[160] Using a nonmyeloablative regimen, Childs and colleagues reported that eradication of the PNH clone was incomplete without any graft-vs.-tumor effect,[161] but as noted above, a myeloablative regimen can completely eradicate the PNH clone without graft-vs.-tumor effect.[159] Together, these observations can be used in planning a transplant strategy for patients with PNH, depending upon the anticipated or desired role of graft-vs.-tumor effect in the therapeutic process.

While allogeneic BMT is potentially curative, the benefits must be weighed against the significant morbidity and mortality associated with the procedure. As an example, the experience of the International Bone Marrow Transplant Registry was reviewed.[162] A total of 57 patients were included in that study with 48 receiving HLA-identical sibling transplants. The 2-year probability of survival for this group was 56%. Only one of seven patients who underwent unrelated donor transplant was alive after 5 years of follow-up. However, improvements in HLA matching using molecular techniques may improve outcomes with unrelated donors. Successful treatment of patients with PNH using nonmyeloablative stem cell transplantation has also been reported.[161,163,164]

When BMT is used to treat patients with PNH/aplastic anemia or PNH-sc/aplastic anemia, the decision for transplantation should be guided primarily by recommendations for management of that particular marrow failure syndrome, typically based on the degree of aplasia and transfusion dependence. For patients with classic PNH, both recurrent life-threatening thrombosis and refractory, transfusion-dependent hemolytic anemia are indications for transplantation. In the pre-eculizumab era, patients with PNH who had thrombosis at presentation had only a 40% survival rate at 4 years.[90] Progression to pancytopenia was also a risk factor that negatively affects survival[90] as did development of myelodysplastic syndrome or acute leukemia, age over 55 years at diagnosis, and thrombocytopenia at diagnosis (*Table 32.5*). Perhaps surprisingly, however, an antecedent history of aplastic anemia has been reported to influence favorably survival in a multivariate analysis (*Table 32.5*).[90] That rarely some patients with PNH undergo spontaneous remission must also be taken into account when deciding on the appropriateness of allogeneic BMT as treatment for PNH.[81,165]

In the unusual circumstance in which the patient has a syngeneic twin, bone marrow transplantation is the most appropriate therapy for classic PNH because absence of graft-vs.-host disease greatly reduces transplant-associated morbidity and mortality, while graft-vs.-tumor effect is not necessary for eradiation of the *PIGA*-mutant clone.[159,166] Syngeneic transplantation without preconditioning has been unsuccessful because abnormal hematopoiesis usually returns, suggesting that the residual *PIGA*-mutant stem cells have a survival or proliferative advantage relative to the transplanted GPI-AP+ cells.[160] This same phenomenon may limit the efficacy of gene therapy, as transducing *PIGA*-mutant stem cells with normal *PIGA* would hypothetically eliminate the conditional growth or survival advantage. An attractive alternative approach to gene therapy would take advantage of the fact that the hematopoietic stem cells of patients with PNH are a mosaic. Conceivably, the GPI-AP+ cells can be selected and used for marrow rescue following myeloablation. The success of this approach depends upon developing a method for separating uniformly and efficiently the GPI-AP+ population from the GPI-AP− population and acquiring GPI-AP+ stem cells sufficient to repopulate the ablated marrow. Fluorescence-activated cell sorting may be useful for this purpose as CD34+, CD38− hematopoietic stem cells express both CD55 and CD59.[167]

The question now arises regarding when and how best to perform transplant in the eculizumab era.[168,169] Short-term treatment with eculizumab may provide an opportunity to reduce hemolysis and stabilize the blood counts, serving as a bridge to a planned transplant. In one recent report, with good success, eculizumab was used until 2 weeks before a highly lymphoablative conditioning regimen.[170]

Before the availability of eculizumab, the primary indications for transplantation for PNH were BMF, recurrent life-threatening thrombosis, and uncontrollable hemolysis.[3,168] The latter process can be eliminated by treatment with eculizumab, and the thrombophilia of PNH is also reduced following inhibition of intravascular hemolysis by eculizumab.[171] Nonetheless, transplantation is the only curative therapy for PNH, and the availability of molecularly defined, matched unrelated donors; less toxic conditioning regimens; reductions in transplantation-related morbidity and mortality; and improvements in posttransplantation supportive care make this option a viable alternative to medical management.[168,171] The decisions of who should receive transplantation and when it should be performed are complex, however, and require an understanding of the unique pathobiology of PNH and the input of physicians experienced in transplantation and medical management of PNH.[168,172] The recent studies of Kelly et al[108] showing normal survival for patients with PNH treated with eculizumab, notwithstanding the extreme cost of long-term therapy, make the decision concerning medical management versus transplantation challenging.

Prevention and Treatment of Thrombosis

In contrast to our thorough understanding of the basis of the hemolysis, much less is known about the mechanisms that underlie the thrombophilia of PNH[110,111,173] (*Table 32.6*).

A recent review of 13 retrospective studies of PNH in nonpregnant patients revealed considerable variation in the reported rate of thromboembolic disease; however, overall 14.4% (95% confidence interval 7.6-25.5) of the patients included in these studies were affected.[174] Thromboembolic complications of PNH appear to be more common among patients from Western countries (with the exception of Mexico[175]), with intra-abdominal (hepatic and mesenteric veins) and cerebral veins being the most commonly involved sites (*Table 32.6*). Nine of these studies described cause of death with 22% of the mortality being due to venous thrombosis (higher among Westerners).

Clinicians should be particularly alert for thrombotic disease in patients with indwelling catheters, after surgical procedures, during prolonged sedentary periods, and during the puerperium period (pregnancy and PNH are discussed below). Female patients should avoid the use of estrogen-containing oral contraceptives because these agents increase the risk of serious thrombotic disease.

Treatment of thromboembolic complications of PNH. Anticoagulation is required for treatment of venous thrombosis (including cerebral vein thrombosis) associated with PNH, with thrombolytic therapy being advocated for extensive acute or life-threatening hepatic vein thrombosis (see below). Mild to moderate thrombocytopenia (platelet count between 50,000 and 100,000/μL) is not a contraindication to anticoagulation; however, platelet transfusion may be required for patients with counts <50,000/μL. Occasional episodes of hemolysis coincident with the administration of heparin have been reported,[133] and this phenomenon has been attributed to activation of the APC by heparin. This complication is rare, however, and concern for exacerbation of hemolysis by heparin should not deter its use in standard pharmacological doses in situations where anticoagulation is warranted. Once adequately anticoagulated with heparin, coumadin therapy should be initiated with a goal of maintaining the international normalized ratio between 2.0 and 3.0. Although data on recurrence rates have not been generated, patients with PNH who experience a thromboembolic episode probably warrant indefinite anticoagulation.

For hepatic vein thrombosis or other life-threatening thromboembolic complications, prompt treatment with heparin or thrombolytic agents is recommended.[113,176] Even with heparin therapy, extensive hepatic vein thrombosis is associated with a poor prognosis.[117,176] Experience with thrombolytic therapy in this setting is limited, but success has been reported with the use of streptokinase, urokinase, and tissue plasminogen activator.[176,177] A recent review of 9 patients receiving intravenous tissue plasminogen activator on 15 occasions reported serious hemorrhagic complications in 3 patients.[178]

Table 32.5. Risk Factors Affecting Survival Before the Availability of Eculizumab

Factor	Relative Risk of Disease-Related Mortality (95% Confidence Interval)	P value
Development of thrombosis	10.2 (6.0-17)	<.0001
Progression to pancytopenia	5.5 (2.8-11)	<.0001
Myelodysplastic disease or acute leukemia	19.1 (7.3-50)	<.001
Age over 55 y	4.0 (2.4-6.9)	<.0001
More than one treatment	2.1 (1.3-3.6)	<.003
Thrombocytopenia at diagnosis	2.2 (1.3-3.8)	<.003
Aplastic anemia antedating PNH	0.32 (0.14-0.72)	<.023

Abbreviation: PNH, paroxysmal nocturnal hemoglobinuria.
Modified from Socié G, Mary JY, de Gramont A, et al. Paroxysmal nocturnal hemoglobinuria: long-term follow-up and prognostic factors. *Lancet.* 1996;348(9027):573-577. Copyright © 1996 Elsevier. With permission.

Table 32.6. Thrombosis and PNH

- The pathogenesis of the thrombophilia of PNH is incompletely understood
- Sites of thrombosis that are disproportionately represented in PNH
  - Hepatic vein (Budd-Chiari syndrome)
  - Mesenteric veins
  - Portal vein
  - Cerebral veins
  - Dermal veins
- Propensity toward thrombosis appears roughly proportional to the size of the PNH clone[a]
- The risk of thromboembolic disease appears higher in Caucasian and African American patients than in patients of Asian/Pacific Island or Hispanic ancestry even when adjusted for clone size
- Caucasian and African American patients with >50% GPI-AP-deficient granulocytes who have no contraindications are candidates for prophylactic anticoagulation with warfarin if they are not being treated with eculizumab or ravulizumab[b]
- Patients with PNH who have experienced a thromboembolic event should remain anticoagulated indefinitely, even if under treatment with eculizumab

Abbreviations: GPI-AP, glycosyl phosphatidylinositol–anchored protein; INR, international normalized ratio; PNH, paroxysmal nocturnal hemoglobinuria.
[a]The size of the PNH clone is determined by flow cytometric analysis of expression of GPI-AP on peripheral blood granulocytes. Patients with a clone size >50%, who are not on complement-inhibitory therapy, are candidates for primary prophylactic anticoagulation.
[b]Standard intensity warfarin therapy (INR 2.0-3.0) is recommended for chronic therapy.
Modified from Parker C, Omine M, Richards S, et al. Diagnosis and management of paroxysmal nocturnal hemoglobinuria. *Blood.* 2005;106:3699-3709. Copyright © 2005 American Society of Hematology. With permission.

Accordingly, thrombolysis must be considered a high-risk intervention. One young patient with PNH with chronic hepatic vein thrombosis and Budd-Chiari syndrome markedly improved his hepatic blood flow following successful bone marrow transplantation.[166]

Prophylactic anticoagulation. In the study of Socié et al. that antedated the use of eculizumab,[90] 30% of French patients experienced an episode of thrombosis within 8 years of the diagnosis of PNH, and based on Kaplan-Meier estimates, approximately 50% of patients were predicted to have this complication by 15 years. Because of the relatively high incidence of thrombosis (particularly among Westerners) and its associated morbidity and mortality, an argument can be made for prophylactic anticoagulation in patients without contraindications such as severe thrombocytopenia.[127] A nonrandomized study with a relatively short follow-up period suggested a significant reduction in thrombotic events when patients with PNH with >50% GPI-AP-deficient granulocytes received prophylactic anticoagulation with coumadin[127] (*Table 32.6*). A second, retrospective study supports the use of prophylactic anticoagulation for patients with large PNH clones (>50%-60%).[126] The benefits of prophylactic anticoagulation, however, must be weighed against potential adverse effects of long-term anticoagulation. Patients at risk for cerebral vein thrombosis and portal/hepatic vein thrombosis would likely derive the greatest benefit from prophylactic anticoagulation. A method for identifying that subgroup of patients, however, has not been developed.

Eculizumab appears to reduce the risk of thromboembolic complications.[137] For patients being treated with eculizumab who have no prior history of thromboembolic complications, prophylactic anticoagulation may be unnecessary.[108] Because patients with PNH with prior thrombosis are at higher risk for recurrent thrombosis, anticoagulation for eculizumab-treated patients who experienced a prior thromboembolic event should be continued indefinitely.[108,171]

Pregnancy and PNH

Pregnancy is often hazardous in PNH,[179-181] by adding stressors to the anemia and thrombophilia that affect all pregnant women; however, patients with PNH can have successful, uncomplicated pregnancies.[181-184] In the pre-eculizumab era, De Gramont and colleagues[181] reported that approximately one-third of 38 pregnancies observed in 28 patients with PNH were uncomplicated and that life-threatening complications in mothers were uncommon. Complications experienced by mothers in that series were mainly hemorrhage and acute hemolysis. However, 45% of the pregnancies resulted in either spontaneous miscarriage or elective termination. Other studies[179] have reported a maternal mortality of ~6% with the major complications being related to thrombosis (particularly Budd-Chiari syndrome). Fetal wastage and prematurity were also reported to be relatively common. Based upon a review of 20 published reports that described the outcome of 33 pregnant women with PNH from the pre-eculizumab era, Ray and colleagues[174] calculated an all-cause maternal mortality rate of 20.8% (95% confidence intervals 7.3-39.0). Approximately half of all infants were delivered preterm. Three deaths were reported among 34 live births (perinatal mortality of 8.8% with 95% confidence intervals of 1.9-23.7).

When possible, patients with PNH who are contemplating pregnancy should be counseled about the potential for both maternal and fetal complications. However, in approximately 25% of cases of PNH and pregnancy, PNH is first diagnosed during pregnancy.[174] Whether this is due simply to the increased likelihood of obtaining blood counts during pregnancy, or potentially a more causal association, remains undetermined. What is clear, however, is that optimal care of a pregnant patient with PNH requires the combined expertise of an experienced team of medical providers who are familiar with PNH. Early labor induction or elective C-section may be warranted to reduce the risks of extended gestation for both the mother and baby.[185]

Patients who do not have access to complement inhibitory therapy should receive therapeutic doses of subcutaneous heparin during pregnancy. Low-molecular-weight heparin may be advantageous because it is associated with a lower incidence of drug-induced thrombocytopenia compared with unfractionated heparin. Nonetheless, the platelet count should be monitored weekly, as thrombocytopenia frequently complicates PNH during pregnancy. Patients should undergo hepatic ultrasound monthly to monitor the patency of hepatic veins. Anticoagulation should be initiated as soon as the pregnancy is documented and continue 3 months into the postpartum period.[174] Coumadin has teratogenic effects, so it should be used for anticoagulation only during the postpartum period.

Available evidence to guide treatment of pregnant patients with PNH who have access to eculizumab was initially limited. Because eculizumab is a hybrid of IgG2 and IgG4, little antibody is believed to cross the placenta. Two 2010 reports documented the safety of treatment throughout gestation for both mother and baby.[186,187] Since then, numerous successful pregnancy outcomes in patients with PNH treated with eculizumab have been reported and eculizumab appears to be safe for use during pregnancy.[188,189] A survey involving members of the International PNH Interest Group and physicians participating in an International PNH Registry (75 pregnancies in patients treated with eculizumab) found that 8% (6 cases) of the 75 pregnancies included in the study resulted in a first-trimester miscarriage, stillbirths were reported in 4% (including one case in a set of twins), 54% experienced breakthrough hemolysis and required a higher dose of eculizumab or a decrease in the dosing interval, and 9% required transfusions during pregnancy.[188] The survey reported a 29% rate of premature birth, with no apparent trend for cause of premature delivery. There were no reported thrombotic episodes during pregnancy, but two thrombotic events occurred early in the postpartum period. Low-molecular-weight heparin was used in 88% of pregnancies, with 10 hemorrhagic events reported. Twenty cord-blood samples were assayed for eculizumab; the drug was detected in seven of the samples. A total of 25 infants were breastfed, and in 10 of these cases, breast milk was examined for the presence of eculizumab; the drug was not detected in any of the 10 breast milk samples. The drug does not affect the complement system of the newborn.[190] Therefore, for patients who are being treated with eculizumab and become pregnant, eculizumab can be continued, although dose adjustment may be required. Addition of low-molecular-weight heparin should be considered if the patient has a history of thromboembolic complications. If there is no history of thromboembolic events, low-molecular-weight heparin may not be necessary if D-dimer levels remain normal.[189] Data on use of ravulizumab during pregnancy are not available. Because ravulizumab binds to the neonatal Fc receptor that is expressed on the placenta, a hypothetical concern exists that inhibition of fetal complement could result. For this reason, during pregnancy, consideration should be given to replacing ravulizumab with eculizumab through the postdelivery period.

For patients with PNH and a history of thromboembolism who become pregnant but are not being treated with eculizumab, low-molecular-weight heparin should be started early in pregnancy with consideration given to addition of eculizumab beginning in the second trimester. If there is no history of thrombosis, treatment with eculizumab beginning in the second trimester is a reasonable option with low-molecular-weight heparin added if the D-dimer levels become abnormal.[189]

Pediatric PNH

PNH can occur in the young (about 10% of patients are younger than 21 years),[3,81,90,165] but it is often misdiagnosed and mismanaged.[109,191] A retrospective analysis of 26 cases[109] underscored the many similarities between childhood and adult PNH. Signs and symptoms of hemolysis, BMF, and thrombosis dominate the clinical picture, with hemoglobinuria occurring less often in young patients. A generally good response to immunosuppressive therapy (six of nine patients) was observed. However, based on the lack of spontaneous remissions and poor long-term survival (80% at 5 years, 60% at 10 years, and 28% at 20 years), sibling-matched stem cell transplantation is the recommended treatment for childhood PNH. A Dutch study confirmed the common presentation of BMF in 11 children with PNH[191] and reported that 5 patients eventually received BMT (3 matched unrelated donors and 2 matched family donors) of whom 4 were alive. A recent cohort of 12 children with PNH documented 5 with myelodysplastic features without excess blasts or malignant transformation.[192] Mortality appears high in young patients with PNH treated with transplantation using unrelated donors, although surviving cases have been reported.[164,191] In the eculizumab era, the urgency for stem cell transplantation may be lessened.

Owing to the ease of diagnostic testing for PNH via flow cytometry, and a heightened index of suspicion among pediatric hematologists, the number of cases identified in the pediatric and adolescent age range is increasing. Eculizumab appears to be a safe and effective therapy for pediatric PNH,[193] and its long-term use should be recommended over unrelated transplantation in most cases. Ravulizumab is not FDA approved for children with PNH (although it is approved for children with atypical hemolytic uremic syndrome).

Dysphagia, Male Impotence, Abdominal Pain

Many patients with PNH are troubled by dysphagia and odynophagia, especially during hemolytic exacerbations.[3] These symptoms appear to be a consequence of esophageal spasm. The cause of the spasm is unproven, but it may be due to acquired deficiency of nitric oxide (NO), a bioactive molecule that mediates smooth muscle relaxation.[121,122] Males with PNH may experience episodes of impotence, particularly during hemolytic exacerbations. The cause of the impotence may also be a consequence of decreased bioavailability of NO. Sildenafil citrate has shown efficacy in the treatment of hypercontractile motility disorders of the esophagus, including idiopathic achalasia, where the mechanism of disease appears to be impaired NO production similar to that reported for erectile dysfunction.[194-196] Therefore, sildenafil citrate and pharmacologically related compounds are candidate therapies for both the dysphagia/odynophagia and male impotence of PNH. Agents such as oral or dermal nitroglycerine that supply NO pharmacologically have also shown efficacy.

Some patients with PNH are debilitated by recurrent episodes of colicky abdominal pain.[3] The etiology of the abdominal pain is largely speculative, but thrombosis of mesenteric vessels appears to play a role in some cases. Vascular spasm may also contribute to this process. Vigorous hydration and pain control are the mainstays of management, but mesenteric vein thrombosis can result in intestinal infarction necessitating surgical intervention. Still to be determined are the roles of anticoagulation, complement inhibition, and NO supplementation in the management of abdominal pain of PNH.

Geographic/Ethnic Differences

The natural history of PNH appears different for Americans and Europeans compared with Asian/Pacific Islanders and Hispanics.[165,175,197-199] In general, the manifestations of BMF are more common in Asians/Pacific Islanders and Hispanics. In contrast, thrombosis and infection appear more common in American and European patients (*Table 32.6*). The basis of these phenotypic differences is unknown, but the relationship of ethnicity and geography to the natural history of PNH should be considered when formulating a management plan.

PNH and COVID-19

The complement system is activated in patients with SARS-CoV-2 infection, but the contribution of complement activation to the pathophysiology of COVID-19 is incompletely understood.[200] Anecdotal reports and small case series suggest that the clinical course of patients with PNH treated with complement C5 inhibitory therapy (eculizumab/ravulizumab) who develop COVID-19 is heterogeneous.[201-203] Accordingly, randomized, prospective studies are needed to determine the effects of complement inhibitory therapy on the clinical course of COVID-19 in the general population.

Treatment with eculizumab/ravulizumab in patients with PNH who develop COVID-19 infection should continue uninterrupted. Given the high risk of thromboembolic complications associated with SARS-CoV-2 infection, additional doses of eculizumab/ravulizumab may be warranted in patients with PNH who develop breakthrough hemolysis while infected with the virus (see section Reasons for Eculizumab/Ravulizumab Failure). Although not unique to SARS-CoV-2 vaccines, adverse reactions, including breakthrough hemolysis, may occur in patients with PNH.[204] Whether treatment is warranted depends on the severity of the vaccine associated adverse event, particularly the presence of clinically significant hemolysis. Although patients should be alerted to the risk of complications, PNH is not a contraindication to vaccination.

DISEASE COURSE AND PROGNOSIS

PNH is a chronic disease. Retrospective studies that antedated the use of eculizumab suggested a median survival of 10 to 15 years.[81,90] Approximately 25% of patients survive for 25 years or longer after diagnosis.[81] The major causes of morbidity and mortality are thrombosis, bleeding, and infections. The latter two complications are due to thrombocytopenia and neutropenia, respectively, which are consequences of the abnormal hematopoiesis that underlies this stem cell disorder and marrow hypoplasia.

Eculizumab is changing the natural history of PNH, as a study of 79 patients with mostly classic PNH who were treated with eculizumab for up to 9 years had a cumulative percent survival that was equal to that of an age- and sex-matched normal population. The precise contribution of eculizumab to survival, however, could not be determined as there was no control patient group.[108]

Reports from the pre-eculizumab era noted that the severity of the illness lessens with time, and in one series, approximately one-third of patients who survive 10 years experienced a spontaneous clinical remission.[81] These cases suggest that, in time, the abnormal clone can gradually lose its relative proliferative or survival advantage. That the disease spontaneously remits in some instances provides a basis for hope for both patient and physician. In addition, this feature of the disease should enter into management decisions, particularly when the patient is a candidate for allogeneic bone marrow transplantation.[81] Spontaneous remission, however, appears to occur primarily in patients with PNH/aplastic anemia with small clones with such remission being unlikely in patients with classic PNH.

Development of other clonal myelopathies including myelodysplastic disease and acute leukemia adversely affects prognosis.[90] The incidence of acute leukemia in association with PNH appears to be in the range of 1%,[90] although higher (7.7% in a study of Japanese patients[197]) and lower (0 of 80 patients in a study from England[81]) incidences have been reported. The rate of myelodysplastic disease in association with PNH is on the order of 5%.[90] Other clonal myelopathies that have been reported in association with PNH include myelofibrosis, chronic lymphocytic leukemia, chronic myelocytic leukemia, polycythemia vera, and erythroleukemia. In some instances, the clonal myelopathy arises in the PNH clone,[103,104] whereas in other instances it arises in a GPI-AP+ clone.[105,106] The association of PNH with other stem cell disorders particularly myelodysplasia and acute leukemia suggests that genetic instability is a component of the disease.[205] This process may be a consequence of the as yet undefined bone marrow injury that underlies PNH.

Future Directions for Clinical and Basic Research

Because of the rarity of PNH, prospective randomized studies are challenging. Consequently, most treatment recommendations are based on low-quality retrospective data or expert opinion. Among the important issues that need to be addressed through careful clinical studies are the following:

a. Guidelines for management of the thrombophilia of PNH
b. Guidelines for stem cell transplantation
c. Guidelines for the use of eculizumab/ravulizumab
d. Development of additional anticomplement therapy
e. Guidelines for management of pregnancy and PNH

Basic research into the mechanism of the thrombophilia of PNH and the basis of clonal selection and clonal dominance will likely produce new insights into the pathobiology of PNH and the physiology of benign and malignant clonal hematopoiesis, and development of new complement inhibitory drugs will provide additional therapeutic options.[206]

References

1. Maeda K, Murakami Y, Kinoshita T. Synthesis, genetics, and congenital diseases of GPI-anchored proteins. In: Kanakura Y, Kinoshita T, Nishimura J, eds. *Paroxysmal Nocturnal Hemoglobinuria: From Bench to Bedside.* Springer; 2017:11-54.
2. Parker CJ. Update on the diagnosis and management of paroxysmal nocturnal hemoglobinuria. *Hematology Am Soc Hematol Educ Program.* 2016;2016:208-216.
3. Parker C, Omine M, Richards S, et al. Diagnosis and management of paroxysmal nocturnal hemoglobinuria. *Blood.* 2005;106:3699-3709.
4. Crosby WH. Paroxysmal nocturnal hemoglobinuria; a classic description by Paul Strubling in 1882, and a bibliography of the disease. *Blood.* 1951;6:270-284.
5. Rosse W. *A Brief History of PNH. PNH and the GPI-Linked Proteins.* Academic Press; 2000:1-20.
6. Parker CJ. Historical aspects of paroxysmal nocturnal haemoglobinuria: "defining the disease." *Br J Haematol.* 2002;117:3-22.
7. Parker CJ. Paroxysmal nocturnal hemoglobinuria: an historical overview. *Hematology Am Soc Hematol Educ Program.* 2008:93-103.
8. Rosse WF. A history of research of PNH: defining a disease. In: Kanakura Y, Kinoshita T, Nishimura J, eds. *Paroxysmal Nocturnal Hemoglobinuria: From Bench to Bedside.* Springer; 2017:1-10.
9. Parker CJ. Complement and PNH. In: Kanakura Y, Kinoshita T, Nishimura J, eds. *Paroxysmal Nocturnal Hemoglobinuria: From Bench to Bedside.* Springer; 2017:67-95.
10. Rosse WF, Dacie JV. Immune lysis of normal human and paroxysmal nocturnal hemoglobinuria (PNH) red blood cells. II. The role of complement components in the increased sensitivity of PNH red cells to immune lysis. *J Clin Invest.* 1966;45:749-757.
11. Rosse WF. Variations in the red cells in paroxysmal nocturnal haemoglobinuria. *Br J Haematol.* 1973;24:327-342.
12. Rosse WF. Paroxysmal nocturnal hemoglobinuria--present status and future prospects. *West J Med.* 1980;132:219-228.
13. Nishimura J, Hirota T, Kanakura Y, et al. Long-term support of hematopoiesis by a single stem cell clone in patients with paroxysmal nocturnal hemoglobinuria. *Blood.* 2002;99:2748-2751.
14. Hillmen P, Young NS, Schubert J, et al. The complement inhibitor eculizumab in paroxysmal nocturnal hemoglobinuria. *N Engl J Med.* 2006;355:1233-1243.
15. Pu JJ, Mukhina G, Wang H, Savage WJ, Brodsky RA. Natural history of paroxysmal nocturnal hemoglobinuria clones in patients presenting as aplastic anemia. *Eur J Haematol.* 2011;87(1):37-45.
16. Logue GL, Rosse WF, Adams JP. Mechanisms of immune lysis of red blood cells in vitro. I. Paroxysmal nocturnal hemoglobinuria cells. *J Clin Invest.* 1973;52:1129-1137.
17. Rosse WF, Logue GL, Adams J, Crookston JH. Mechanisms of immune lysis of the red cells in hereditary erythroblastic multinuclearity with a positive acidified serum test and paroxysmal nocturnal hemoglobinuria. *J Clin Invest.* 1974;53:31-43.
18. Pangburn MK, Schreiber RD, Trombold JS, Muller-Eberhard HJ. Paroxysmal nocturnal hemoglobinuria: deficiency in factor H-like functions of the abnormal erythrocytes. *J Exp Med.* 1983;157:1971-1980.
19. Parker CJ, Baker PJ, Rosse WF. Increased enzymatic activity of the alternative pathway convertase when bound to the erythrocytes of paroxysmal nocturnal hemoglobinuria. *J Clin Invest.* 1982;69:337-346.
20. Packman CH, Rosenfeld SI, Jenkins DE, Jr, Thiem PA, Leddy JP. Complement lysis of human erythrocytes. Differeing susceptibility of two types of paroxysmal nocturnal hemoglobinuria cells to C5b-9. *J Clin Invest.* 1979;64:428-433.
21. Parker CJ, Wiedmer T, Sims PJ, Rosse WF. Characterization of the complement sensitivity of paroxysmal nocturnal hemoglobinuria erythrocytes. *J Clin Invest.* 1985;75:2074-2084.
22. Beck WS, Valentine WN. Biochemical studies on leucocytes. II. Phosphatase activity in chronic lymphatic leukemia, acute leukemia, and miscellaneous hematologic condidtions. *J Lab Clin Med.* 1951;38:245-253.
23. Auditore JV, Hartmann RC. Paroxysmal nocturnal hemoglobinuria II. erythrocyte acetylcholinesterase defect. *Am J Med.* 1959;27:401-410.
24. Kunstling TR, Rosse WF. Erythrocyte acetylcholinesterase deficiency in paroxysmal nocturnal hemoglobinuria (PNH). A comparison of the complement-sensitive and insensitive populations. *Blood.* 1969;33:607-616.
25. Nicholson-Weller A, March JP, Rosenfeld SI, Austen KF. Affected erythrocytes of patients with paroxysmal nocturnal hemoglobinuria are deficient in the complement regulatory protein, decay accelerating factor. *Proc Natl Acad Sci U S A.* 1983;80:5066-5070.
26. Pangburn MK, Schreiber RD, Muller-Eberhard HJ. Deficiency of an erythrocyte membrane protein with complement regulatory activity in paroxysmal nocturnal hemoglobinuria. *Proc Natl Acad Sci U S A.* 1983;80:5430-5434.
27. Hoffmann EM. Inhibition of complement by a substance isolated from human erythrocytes. II. Studies on the site and mechanism of action. *Immunochemistry.* 1969;6:405-419.
28. Hoffmann EM. Inhibition of complement by a substrate isolated from human erythroctes: I. Extraction from human erythrocyte stromta. *Immunochemistry.* 1969;6:391-403.
29. Nicholson-Weller A, Burge J, Fearon DT, Weller PF, Austen KF. Isolation of a human erythrocyte membrane glycoprotein with decay-accelerating activity for C3 convertases of the complement system. *J Immunol.* 1982;129:184-189.
30. Holguin MH, Fredrick LR, Bernshaw NJ, Wilcox LA, Parker CJ. Isolation and characterization of a membrane protein from normal human erythrocytes that inhibits reactive lysis of the erythrocytes of paroxysmal nocturnal hemoglobinuria. *J Clin Invest.* 1989;84:7-17.
31. Lehto T, Meri S. Interactions of soluble CD59 with the terminal complement complexes. CD59 and C9 compete for a nascent epitope on C8. *J Immunol.* 1993;151:4941-4949.
32. Merry AH, Rawlinson VI, Uchikawa M, Daha MR, Sim RB. Studies on the sensitivity to complement-mediated lysis of erythrocytes (Inab phenotype) with a deficiency of DAF (decay accelerating factor). *Br J Haematol.* 1989;73:248-253.
33. Rollins SA, Zhao J, Ninomiya H, Sims PJ. Inhibition of homologous complement by CD59 is mediated by a species-selective recognition conferred through binding to C8 within C5b-8 or C9 within C5b-9. *J Immunol.* 1991;146:2345-2351.
34. Ezzell JL, Wilcox LA, Bernshaw NJ, Parker CJ. Induction of the paroxysmal nocturnal hemoglobinuria phenotype in normal human erythrocytes: effects of 2-aminoethylisothiouronium bromide on membrane proteins that regulate complement. *Blood.* 1991;77:2764-2773.
35. Holguin MH, Martin CB, Bernshaw NJ, Parker CJ. Analysis of the effects of activation of the alternative pathway of complement on erythrocytes with an isolated deficiency of decay accelerating factor. *J Immunol.* 1992;148:498-502.

Disorders of Red Blood Cells

36. Wilcox LA, Ezzell JL, Bernshaw NJ, Parker CJ. Molecular basis of the enhanced susceptibility of the erythrocytes of paroxysmal nocturnal hemoglobinuria to hemolysis in acidified serum. *Blood*. 1991;78:820-829.

37. Holguin MH, Wilcox LA, Bernshaw NJ, Rosse WF, Parker CJ. Relationship between the membrane inhibitor of reactive lysis and the erythrocyte phenotypes of paroxysmal nocturnal hemoglobinuria. *J Clin Invest*. 1989;84:1387-1394.

38. Telen MJ, Green AM. The Inab phenotype: characterization of the membrane protein and complement regulatory defect. *Blood*. 1989;74:437-441.

39. Motoyama N, Okada N, Yamashina M, Okada H. Paroxysmal nocturnal hemoglobinuria due to hereditary nucleotide deletion in the HRF20 (CD59) gene. *Eur J Immunol*. 1992;22:2669-2673.

40. Yamashina M, Ueda E, Kinoshita T, et al. Inherited complete deficiency of 20-kilodalton homologous restriction factor (CD59) as a cause of paroxysmal nocturnal hemoglobinuria. *N Engl J Med*. 1990;323:1184-1189.

41. Nevo Y, Ben-Zeev B, Tabib A, et al. CD59 deficiency is associated with chronic hemolysis and childhood relapsing immune-mediated polyneuropathy. *Blood*. 2013;121:129-135.

42. Hochsmann B, Dohna-Schwake C, Kyrieleis HA, Pannicke U, Schrezenmeier H. Targeted therapy with eculizumab for inherited CD59 deficiency. *N Engl J Med*. 2014;370:90-92.

43. Medof ME, Kinoshita T, Nussenzweig V. Inhibition of complement activation on the surface of cells after incorporation of decay-accelerating factor (DAF) into their membranes. *J Exp Med*. 1984;160:1558-1578.

44. Low MG, Zilversmit DB. Role of phosphatidylinositol in attachment of alkaline phosphatase to membranes. *Biochemistry*. 1980;19:3913-3918.

45. Davitz MA, Low MG, Nussenzweig V. Release of decay-accelerating factor (DAF) from the cell membrane by phosphatidylinositol-specific phospholipase C (PIPLC). Selective modification of a complement regulatory protein. *J Exp Med*. 1986;163:1150-1161.

46. Medof ME, Walter EI, Roberts WL, Haas R, Rosenberry TL. Decay accelerating factor of complement is anchored to cells by a C-terminal glycolipid. *Biochemistry*. 1986;25:6740-6747.

47. Holguin MH, Wilcox LA, Bernshaw NJ, Rosse WF, Parker CJ. Erythrocyte membrane inhibitor of reactive lysis: effects of phosphatidylinositol-specific phospholipase C on the isolated and cell-associated protein. *Blood*. 1990;75:284-289.

48. Oni SB, Osunkoya BO, Luzzatto L. Paroxysmal nocturnal hemoglobinuria: evidence for monoclonal origin of abnormal red cells. *Blood*. 1970;36:145-152.

49. Aster RH, Enright SE. A platelet and granulocyte membrane defect in paroxysmal nocturnal hemoglobinuria: usefulness for the detection of platelet antibodies. *J Clin Invest*. 1969;48:1199-1210.

50. Murakami Y, Siripanyaphinyo U, Hong Y, Tashima Y, Maeda Y, Kinoshita T. The initial enzyme for glycosylphosphatidylinositol biosynthesis requires PIG-Y, a seventh component. *Mol Biol Cell*. 2005;16:5236-5246.

51. Kinoshita T, Inoue N, Takeda J. Defective glycosyl phosphatidylinositol anchor synthesis and paroxysmal nocturnal hemoglobinuria. *Adv Immunol*. 1995;60:57-103.

52. Armstrong C, Schubert J, Ueda E, et al. Affected paroxysmal nocturnal hemoglobinuria T lymphocytes harbor a common defect in assembly of N-acetyl-D-glucosamine inositol phospholipid corresponding to that in class A Thy-1- murine lymphoma mutants. *J Biol Chem*. 1992;267:25347-25351.

53. Takahashi M, Takeda J, Hirose S, et al. Deficient biosynthesis of N-acetylglucosaminyl-phosphatidylinositol, the first intermediate of glycosyl phosphatidylinositol anchor biosynthesis, in cell lines established from patients with paroxysmal nocturnal hemoglobinuria. *J Exp Med*. 1993;177:517-521.

54. Miyata T, Takeda J, Iida Y, et al. The cloning of PIG-A, a component in the early step of GPI-anchor biosynthesis. *Science*. 1993;259:1318-1320.

55. Takeda J, Miyata T, Kawagoe K, et al. Deficiency of the GPI anchor caused by a somatic mutation of the PIG-A gene in paroxysmal nocturnal hemoglobinuria. *Cell*. 1993;73:703-711.

56. Hyman R, Cunningham K, Stallings V. Evidence for a genetic basis for the class A Thy-1-defect. *Immunogenetics*. 1980;10:261-271.

57. Krawitz PM, Hochsmann B, Murakami Y, et al. A case of paroxysmal nocturnal hemoglobinuria caused by a germline mutation and a somatic mutation in PIGT. *Blood*. 2013;122:1312-1315.

58. Langemeijer S, Schaap C, Preijers F, et al. Paroxysmal nocturnal hemoglobinuria caused by CN-LOH of constitutional PIGB mutation and 70-kbp microdeletion on 15q. *Blood Adv*. 2020;4:5755-5761.

59. Hochsmann B, Murakami Y, Osato M, et al. Complement and inflammasome overactivation mediates paroxysmal nocturnal hemoglobinuria with autoinflammation. *J Clin Invest*. 2019;129:5123-5136.

60. Endo M, Ware RE, Vreeke TM, et al. Molecular basis of the heterogeneity of expression of glycosyl phosphatidylinositol anchored proteins in paroxysmal nocturnal hemoglobinuria. *Blood*. 1996;87:2546-2557.

61. Luzzatto L, Nafa K. Genetics of PNH. In: Young NS, Moss J, eds. *Paroxysmal Nocturnal Hemoglobinuria and the Glycosylphosphatidylinositol-Linked Proteins*. Academic Press; 2000:21-47.

62. Nishimura J, Murakami Y, Kinoshita T. Paroxysmal nocturnal hemoglobinuria: an acquired genetic disease. *Am J Hematol*. 1999;62:175-182.

63. Nafa K, Bessler M, Castro-Malaspina H, Jhanwar S, Luzzatto L. The spectrum of somatic mutations in the PIG-A gene in paroxysmal nocturnal hemoglobinuria includes large deletions and small duplications. *Blood Cells Mol Dis*. 1998;24:370-384.

64. Hertenstein B, Wagner B, Bunjes D, et al. Emergence of CD52-, phosphatidylinositolglycan-anchor-deficient T lymphocytes after in vivo application of Campath-1H for refractory B-cell non-Hodgkin lymphoma. *Blood*. 1995;86:1487-1492.

65. Iwamoto N, Kawaguchi T, Horikawa K, et al. Preferential hematopoiesis by paroxysmal nocturnal hemoglobinuria clone engrafted in SCID mice. *Blood*. 1996;87:4944-4948.

66. Brodsky RA, Vala MS, Barber JP, Medof ME, Jones RJ. Resistance to apoptosis caused by PIG-A gene mutations in paroxysmal nocturnal hemoglobinuria. *Proc Natl Acad Sci U S A*. 1997;94:8756-8760.

67. Chen R, Nagarajan S, Prince GM, et al. Impaired growth and elevated fas receptor expression in PIGA(+) stem cells in primary paroxysmal nocturnal hemoglobinuria. *J Clin Invest*. 2000;106:689-696.

68. Kinoshita T, Bessler M, Takeda J. Animal models of PNH. In: Young NS, Moss J, eds. *Paroxysmal Nocturnal Hemoglobinuria and the Glycosylphosphatidylinositol-Linked Proteins*. Academic Press; 2000:139-158.

69. Kawagoe K, Kitamura D, Okabe M, et al. Glycosylphosphatidylinositol-anchor-deficient mice: implications for clonal dominance of mutant cells in paroxysmal nocturnal hemoglobinuria. *Blood*. 1996;87:3600-3606.

70. Murakami Y, Kinoshita T. Animal models of paroxysmal nocturnal hemoglobinuria. In: Kanakura Y, Kinoshita T, Nishimura J, eds. *Paroxysmal Nocturnal Hemoglobinuria: From Bench to Bedside*. Springer; 2017:55-66.

71. Mortazavi Y, Merk B, McIntosh J, Marsh JC, Schrezenmeier H, Rutherford TR. The spectrum of PIG-A gene mutations in aplastic anemia/paroxysmal nocturnal hemoglobinuria (AA/PNH): a high incidence of multiple mutations and evidence of a mutational hot spot. *Blood*. 2003;109:2833-2841.

72. Hu R, Mukhina GL, Piantadosi S, Barber JP, Jones RJ, Brodsky RA. PIG-A mutations in normal hematopoiesis. *Blood*. 2005;105:3848-3854.

73. Inoue N, Izui-Sarumaru T, Murakami Y, et al. Molecular basis of clonal expansion of hematopoiesis in 2 patients with paroxysmal nocturnal hemoglobinuria (PNH). *Blood*. 2006;108:4232-4236.

74. Ikeda K, Mason PJ, Bessler M. 3′UTR-truncated Hmga2 cDNA causes MPN-like hematopoiesis by conferring a clonal growth advantage at the level of HSC in mice. *Blood*. 2011;117:5860-5869.

75. Cavazzana-Calvo M, Payen E, Negre O, et al. Transfusion independence and HMGA2 activation after gene therapy of human beta-thalassaemia. *Nature*. 2010;467:318-322.

76. Murakami Y, Inoue N, Shichishima T, et al. Deregulated expression of HMGA2 is implicated in clonal expansion of PIGA deficient cells in paroxysmal nocturnal haemoglobinuria. *Br J Haematol*. 2012;156:383-387.

77. Kumar P, Beck D, Galeev R, et al. HMGA2 promotes long-term engraftment and myeloerythroid differentiation of human hematopoietic stem and progenitor cells. *Blood Adv*. 2019;3:681-691.

78. Sugimori C, Padron E, Caceres G, et al. Paroxysmal nocturnal hemoglobinuria and concurrent JAK2(V617F) mutation. *Blood Cancer J*. 2012;2:e63.

79. Shen W, Clemente MJ, Hosono N, et al. Deep sequencing reveals stepwise mutation acquisition in paroxysmal nocturnal hemoglobinuria. *J Clin Invest*. 2014;124:4529-4538.

80. Yoshizato T, Dumitriu B, Hosokawa K, et al. Somatic mutations and clonal hematopoiesis in aplastic anemia. *N Engl J Med*. 2015;373:35-47.

81. Hillmen P, Lewis SM, Bessler M, Luzzatto L, Dacie JV. Natural history of paroxysmal nocturnal hemoglobinuria. *N Engl J Med*. 1995;333:1253-1258.

82. Inoue N, Kinoshita T. Pathogenesis of clonal dominance in PNH: growth advantage in PNH. In: Kanakura Y, Kinoshita T, Nishimura J, eds. *Paroxysmal Nocturnal Hemoglobinuria: From Bench to Bedside*. Springer; 2017:229-252.

83. Kawaguchi T, Nakakuma H. Pathogenesis of clonal dominance in PNH: selection mechanisms in PNH. In: Kanakura Y, Kinoshita T, Nishimura J, eds. *Paroxysmal Nocturnal Hemoglobinuria: From Bench to Bedside*. Springer; 2017: 215-228.

84. Katagiri T, Sato-Otsubo A, Kashiwase K, et al. Frequent loss of HLA alleles associated with copy number-neutral 6pLOH in acquired aplastic anemia. *Blood*. 2011;118:6601-6609.

85. Ueda T, Hayakawa J, Yamanishi M, Maeda M, Fukunaga Y. Efficacy of eculizumab in a patient with paroxysmal nocturnal hemoglobinuria requiring transfusions 14 years after a diagnosis in childhood. *J Nippon Med Sch*. 2013;80:155-159.

86. Babushok DV, Duke JL, Xie HM, et al. Somatic HLA mutations expose the role of class I-mediated autoimmunity in aplastic anemia and its clonal complications. *Blood Adv*. 2017;1:1900-1910.

87. Sugimori C, Mochizuki K, Qi Z, et al. Origin and fate of blood cells deficient in glycosylphosphatidylinositol-anchored protein among patients with bone marrow failure. *Br J Haematol*. 2009;147:102-112.

88. Schubert J, Vogt HG, Zielinska-Skowronek M, et al. Development of the glycosylphosphatidylinositol-anchoring defect characteristic for paroxysmal nocturnal hemoglobinuria in patients with aplastic anemia. *Blood*. 1994;83: 2323-2328.

89. Griscelli-Bennaceur A, Gluckman E, Scrobohaci ML, et al. Aplastic anemia and paroxysmal nocturnal hemoglobinuria: search for a pathogenetic link. *Blood*. 1995;85:1354-1363.

90. Socie G, Mary JY, de Gramont A, et al. Paroxysmal nocturnal haemoglobinuria: long-term follow-up and prognostic factors. French Society of Haematology. *Lancet*. 1996;348:573-577.

91. Sugimori C, Chuhjo T, Feng X, et al. Minor population of CD55-CD59- blood cells predicts response to immunosuppressive therapy and prognosis in patients with aplastic anemia. *Blood*. 2006;107:1308-1314.

92. Frickhofen N, Heimpel H, Kaltwasser JP, Schrezenmeier H. Antithymocyte globulin with or without cyclosporin A: 11-year follow-up of a randomized trial comparing treatments of aplastic anemia. *Blood*. 2003;101:1236-1242.

93. Scheinberg P, Marte M, Nunez O, Young NS. Paroxysmal nocturnal hemoglobinuria clones in severe aplastic anemia patients treated with horse anti-thymocyte globulin plus cyclosporine. *Haematologica*. 2010;95:1075-1080.

94. Nagarajan S, Brodsky RA, Young NS, Medof ME. Genetic defects underlying paroxysmal nocturnal hemoglobinuria that arises out of aplastic anemia. *Blood.* 1995;86:4656-4661.

95. Nakao S. Clinical significance of a small population of glycosylphosphatidylinositol-anchored proteins membrane proteins (GPI-APs)-deficient cells in the management of bone marrow failure. In: Kanakura Y, Kinoshita T, Nishimura J, eds. *Paroxysmal Nocturnal Hemoglobinuria:From Bench to Bedside.* Springer; 2017:185-195.

96. Dunn DE, Tanawattanacharoen P, Boccuni P, et al. Paroxysmal nocturnal hemoglobinuria cells in patients with bone marrow failure syndromes. *Ann Intern Med.* 1999;131:401-408.

97. Wang H, Chuhjo T, Yasue S, Omine M, Nakao S. Clinical significance of a minor population of paroxysmal nocturnal hemoglobinuria-type cells in bone marrow failure syndrome. *Blood.* 2002;100:3897-3902.

98. Wang B, He B, Zhu YD, Wu W. The predictive value of pre-treatment paroxysmal nocturnal hemoglobinuria clone on response to immunosuppressive therapy in patients with aplastic anemia: a meta-analysis. *Hematology.* 2020;25:464-472.

99. Hosokawa K, Katagiri T, Sugimori N, et al. Favorable outcome of patients who have 13q deletion: a suggestion for revision of the WHO "MDS-U" designation. *Haematologica.* 2012;97:1845-1849.

100. Rotoli B, Robledo R, Scarpato N, Luzzatto L. Two populations of erythroid cell progenitors in paroxysmal nocturnal hemoglobinuria. *Blood.* 1984;64:847-851.

101. Araten DJ, Swirsky D, Karadimitris A, et al. Cytogenetic and morphological abnormalities in paroxysmal nocturnal haemoglobinuria. *Br J Haematol.* 2001;115:360-368.

102. Inoue N, Murakami Y, Kinoshita T. Molecular genetics of paroxysmal nocturnal hemoglobinuria. *Int J Hematol.* 2003;77:107-112.

103. Devine DV, Gluck WL, Rosse WF, Weinberg JB. Acute myeloblastic leukemia in paroxysmal nocturnal hemoglobinuria. Evidence of evolution from the abnormal paroxysmal nocturnal hemoglobinuria clone. *J Clin Invest.* 1987;79:314-317.

104. Longo L, Bessler M, Beris P, Swirsky D, Luzzatto L. Myelodysplasia in a patient with pre-existing paroxysmal nocturnal haemoglobinuria: a clonal disease originating from within a clonal disease. *Br J Haematol.* 1994;87:401-403.

105. Krause JR. Paroxysmal nocturnal hemoglobinuria and acute non-lymphocytic leukemia. A report of three cases exhibiting different cytologic types. *Cancer.* 1983;51:2078-2082.

106. van Kamp H, Smit JW, van den Berg E, Ruud Halie M, Vellenga E. Myelodysplasia following paroxysmal nocturnal haemoglobinuria: evidence for the emergence of a separate clone. *Br J Haematol.* 1994;87:399-400.

107. Dacie JV, Lewis SM. Paroxysmal nocturnal haemoglobinuria: clinical manifestations, haematology, and nature of the disease. *Ser Haematol.* 1972;5:3-23.

108. Kelly RJ, Hill A, Arnold LM, et al. Long-term treatment with eculizumab in paroxysmal nocturnal hemoglobinuria: sustained efficacy and improved survival. *Blood.* 2011;117:6786-6792.

109. Ware RE, Hall SE, Rosse WF. Paroxysmal nocturnal hemoglobinuria with onset in childhood and adolescence. *N Engl J Med.* 1991;325:991-996.

110. Sloand EM, Young NS. Thrombotic complications in PNH. In: Young NS, Moss J, eds. *Paroxysmal Nocturnal Hemoglobinuria and the Glycosylphosphatidylinositol-Linked Proteins.* Academic Press; 2000:101-112.

111. Ninomiya H, Hill A. Thrombophilia in PNH. In: Kanakura Y, Kinoshita T, Nishimura J, eds. *Paroxysmal Nocturnal Hemoglobinuria: From Bench to Bedside.* Springer; 2017:153-172.

112. Hartmann RC, Luther AB, Jenkins DE, Jr, Tenorio LE, Saba HI. Fulminant hepatic venous thrombosis (Budd-Chiari syndrome) in paroxysmal nocturnal hemoglobinuria: definition of a medical emergency. *Johns Hopkins Med J.* 1980;146:247-254.

113. Leibowitz AI, Hartmann RC. The Budd-Chiari syndrome in paroxysmal nocturnal haemoglobinuria--revisited. *Br J Haematol.* 1981;49:659-660.

114. Valla D, Dhumeaux D, Babany G, et al. Hepatic vein thrombosis in paroxysmal nocturnal haemoglobinuria. A spectrum from asymptomatic occlusion of hepatic venules to fatal Budd-Chiari syndrome. *Gastroenterology.* 1987;93:569-575.

115. Birgens HS, Hancke S, Rosenklint A, Hansen NE. Ultrasonic demonstration of clinical and subclinical hepatic venous thrombosis in paroxysmal nocturnal haemoglobinuria. *Br J Haematol.* 1986;64:737-743.

116. Menon KV, Shah V, Kamath PS. The Budd-Chiari syndrome. *N Engl J Med.* 2004;350:578-585.

117. Peytremann R, Rhodes RS, Hartmann RC. Thrombosis in paroxysmal nocturnal hemoglobinuria (PNH) with particular reference to progressive, diffuse hepatic venous thrombosis. *Ser Haematol.* 1972;5:115-136.

118. Hillmen P, Elebute M, Kelly R, et al. Long-term effect of the complement inhibitor eculizumab on kidney function in patients with paroxysmal nocturnal hemoglobinuria. *Am J Hematol.* 2010;85:553-559.

119. Clark DA, Butler SA, Braren V, Hartmann RC, Jenkins DE, Jr. The kidneys in paroxysmal nocturnal hemoglobinuria. *Blood.* 1981;57:83-89.

120. Hill A, Sapsford RJ, Scally A, et al. Under-recognized complications in patients with paroxysmal nocturnal haemoglobinuria: raised pulmonary pressure and reduced right ventricular function. *Br J Haematol.* 2012;158(3):409-414.

121. Hill A. Hemolysis in PNH: depletion of nitric oxide. In: Kanakura Y, Kinoshita T, Nishimura J, eds. *Paroxysmal Nocturnal Hemoglobinuria: From Bench to Bedside.* Springer; 2017:121-136.

122. Murray JA, Ledlow A, Launspach J, Evans D, Loveday M, Conklin JL. The effects of recombinant human hemoglobin on esophageal motor functions in humans. *Gastroenterology.* 1995;109:1241-1248.

123. Brubaker LH, Essig LJ, Mengel CE. Neutrophil life span in paroxysmal nocturnal hemoglobinuria. *Blood.* 1977;50:657-662.

124. Devine DV, Siegel RS, Rosse WF. Interactions of the platelets in paroxysmal nocturnal hemoglobinuria with complement. Relationship to defects in the regulation of complement and to platelet survival in vivo. *J Clin Invest.* 1987;79:131-137.

125. Borowitz MJ, Craig FE, Digiuseppe JA, et al. Guidelines for the diagnosis and monitoring of paroxysmal nocturnal hemoglobinuria and related disorders by flow cytometry. *Cytometry B Clin Cytom.* 2010;78:211-230.

126. Moyo VM, Mukina GL, Barrett ES, Brodsky RA. Natural history of paroxysmal nocturnal haemoglobinuria using modern diagnostic assays. *Br J Haematol.* 2004;126:133-138.

127. Hall C, Richards S, Hillmen P. Primary prophylaxis with warfarin prevents thrombosis in paroxysmal nocturnal hemoglobinuria (PNH). *Blood.* 2003;102:3587-3591.

128. Ishiyama K, Chuhjo T, Wang H, Yachie A, Omine M, Nakao S. Polyclonal hematopoiesis maintained in patients with bone marrow failure harboring a minor population of paroxysmal nocturnal hemoglobinuria-type cells. *Blood.* 2003;102:1211-1216.

129. Scheinberg P, Wu CO, Nunez O, Young NS. Predicting response to immunosuppressive therapy and survival in severe aplastic anaemia. *Br J Haematol.* 2009;144:206-216.

130. Brodsky RA, Mukhina GL, Li S, et al. Improved detection and characterization of paroxysmal nocturnal hemoglobinuria using fluorescent aerolysin. *Am J Clin Pathol.* 2000;114:459-466.

131. Tomita A, Parker CJ. Aberrant regulation of complement by the erythrocytes of hereditary erythroblastic multinuclearity with a positive acidified serum lysis test (HEMPAS). *Blood.* 1994;83:250-259.

132. Balleari E, Gatti AM, Mareni C, Massa G, Marmont AM, Ghio R. Recombinant human erythropoietin for long-term treatment of anemia in paroxysmal nocturnal hemoglobinuria. *Haematologica.* 1996;81:143-147.

133. Rosse WF. Treatment of paroxysmal nocturnal hemoglobinuria. *Blood.* 1982;60:20-23.

134. Parker C. Eculizumab for paroxysmal nocturnal haemoglobinuria. *Lancet.* 2009;373:759-767.

135. Hillmen P, Hall C, Marsh JC, et al. Effect of eculizumab on hemolysis and transfusion requirements in patients with paroxysmal nocturnal hemoglobinuria. *N Engl J Med.* 2004;350:552-559.

136. Brodsky RA, Young NS, Antonioli E, et al. Multicenter phase 3 study of the complement inhibitor eculizumab for the treatment of patients with paroxysmal nocturnal hemoglobinuria. *Blood.* 2008;111:1840-1847.

137. Hillmen P, Muus P, Duhrsen U, et al. Effect of the complement inhibitor eculizumab on thromboembolism in patients with paroxysmal nocturnal hemoglobinuria. *Blood.* 2007;110:4123-4128.

138. Kulasekararaj AG, Hill A, Rottinghaus ST, et al. Ravulizumab (ALXN1210) vs eculizumab in C5-inhibitor-experienced adult patients with PNH: the 302 study. *Blood.* 2019;133:540-549.

139. Lee JW, Peffault de Latour R, Brodsky RA, et al. Effectiveness of eculizumab in patients with paroxysmal nocturnal hemoglobinuria (PNH) with or without aplastic anemia in the International PNH Registry. *Am J Hematol.* 2019;94:E37-E41.

140. Brodsky RA, Peffault de Latour R, Rottinghaus ST, et al. Characterization of breakthrough hemolysis events observed in the phase 3 randomized studies of ravulizumab versus eculizumab in adults with paroxysmal nocturnal hemoglobinuria. *Haematologica.* 2021;106:230-237.

141. Risitano AM, Marotta S, Ricci P, et al. Anti-complement treatment for paroxysmal nocturnal hemoglobinuria: time for proximal complement inhibition? A position paper from the SAAWP of the EBMT. *Front Immunol.* 2019;10:1157.

142. Berzuini A, Montanelli F, Prati D. Hemolytic anemia after eculizumab in paroxysmal nocturnal hemoglobinuria. *N Engl J Med.* 2010;363:993-994.

143. Risitano AM, Notaro R, Luzzatto L, Hill A, Kelly R, Hillmen P. Paroxysmal nocturnal hemoglobinuria--hemolysis before and after eculizumab. *N Engl J Med.* 2010;363:2270-2272.

144. Risitano AM, Notaro R, Luzzatto L, Hill A, Kelly R, Hillmen P. Paroxysmal nocturnal hemoglobinuria--hemolysis before and after eculizumab. *N Engl J Med.* 2011;363:2270-2272.

145. Risitano AM, Notaro R, Marando L, et al. Complement fraction 3 binding on erythrocytes as additional mechanism of disease in paroxysmal nocturnal hemoglobinuria patients treated by eculizumab. *Blood.* 2009;113:4094-4100.

146. Notaro R, Risitano A. Clinical effects of eculizumab in PNH: extravascular hemolysis after eculizumab treatment. In: Kanakura Y, Kinoshita T, Nishimura J, eds. *Paroxysmal Nocturnal Hemoglobinuria: From Bench to Bedside.* Springer; 2017:283-296.

147. Lindorfer MA, Pawluczkowycz AW, Peek EM, Hickman K, Taylor RP, Parker CJ. A novel approach to preventing the hemolysis of paroxysmal nocturnal hemoglobinuria: both complement-mediated cytolysis and C3 deposition are blocked by a monoclonal antibody specific for the alternative pathway of complement. *Blood.* 2010;115:2283-2291.

148. Hillmen P, Szer J, Weitz I, et al. Pegcetacoplan versus eculizumab in paroxysmal nocturnal hemoglobinuria. *N Engl J Med.* 2021;384:1028-1037.

149. Kulesekararaj A, Risitano AM, Maciejewski JP, et al. Phase 2 study of danicopan in paroxysmal nocturnal hemoglobinuria patients with an inadequate response to eculizumab. *Blood.* 2021;138(20):1928-1938.

150. Nishimura J, Kinoshita T, Kanakura Y. Clinical effects of eculizumab in PNH: poor responders to eculizumab. In: Kanakura Y, Kinoshita T, Nishimura J, eds. *Paroxysmal Nocturnal Hemoglobinuria: From Bench to Bedside.* Springer; 2017:297-306.

151. Nishimura J, Yamamoto M, Hayashi S, et al. Genetic variants in C5 and poor response to eculizumab. *N Engl J Med.* 2014;370:632-639.

152. Hartmann RC, Jenkins DE, Jr, McKee LC, Heyssel RM. Paroxysmal nocturnal hemoglobinuria: clinical and laboratory studies relating to iron metabolism and therapy with androgen and iron. *Medicine (Baltim).* 1966;45:331-363.

153. Schubert J, Scholz C, Geissler RG, Ganser A, Schmidt RE. G-CSF and cyclosporin induce an increase of normal cells in hypoplastic paroxysmal nocturnal hemoglobinuria. *Ann Hematol.* 1997;74:225-230.

Disorders of Red Blood Cells

154. Stoppa AM, Vey N, Sainty D, et al. Correction of aplastic anaemia complicating paroxysmal nocturnal haemoglobinuria: absence of eradication of the PNH clone and dependence of response on cyclosporin A administration. *Br J Haematol.* 1996;93:42-44.

155. van Kamp H, van Imhoff GW, de Wolf JT, Smit JW, Halie MR, Vellenga E. The effect of cyclosporine on haematological parameters in patients with paroxysmal nocturnal haemoglobinuria. *Br J Haematol.* 1995;89:79-82.

156. Rosse WF. Transfusion in paroxysmal nocturnal hemoglobinuria: to wash or not to wash. *Transfusion.* 1989;29:663-664.

157. Hartmann RC, Kolhouse JF. Viewpoints on the management of paroxysmal nocturnal hemoglobinuria (PNH). *Ser Haematol.* 1972;5:42-60.

158. Antin JH, Ginsburg D, Smith BR, Nathan DG, Orkin SH, Rappeport JM. Bone marrow transplantation for paroxysmal nocturnal hemoglobinuria: eradication of the PNH clone and documentation of complete lymphohematopoietic engraftment. *Blood.* 1985;66:1247-1250.

159. Frei-Lahr D, Inoue N, Wittwer C, et al. Molecular complete remission of clonal hemaotpoiesis in a patient with paroxysmal nocturnal hemologinuria (PNH) after syngeneic stem cell transplant (SCT). *Blood.* 2006;108:5362.

160. Endo M, Beatty PG, Vreeke TM, Wittwer CT, Singh SP, Parker CJ. Syngeneic bone marrow transplantation without conditioning in a patient with paroxysmal nocturnal hemoglobinuria: in vivo evidence that the mutant stem cells have a survival advantage. *Blood.* 1996;88:742-750.

161. Takahashi Y, McCoy JP, Jr, Carvallo C, et al. In vitro and in vivo evidence of PNH cell sensitivity to immune attack after nonmyeloablative allogeneic hematopoietic cell transplantation. *Blood.* 2004;103:1383-1390.

162. Saso R, Marsh J, Cevreska L, et al. Bone marrow transplants for paroxysmal nocturnal haemoglobinuria. *Br J Haematol.* 1999;104:392-396.

163. Suenaga K, Kanda Y, Niiya H, et al. Successful application of nonmyeloablative transplantation for paroxysmal nocturnal hemoglobinuria. *Exp Hematol.* 2001;29:639-642.

164. Woodard P, Wang W, Pitts N, et al. Successful unrelated donor bone marrow transplantation for paroxysmal nocturnal hemoglobinuria. *Bone Marrow Transplant.* 2001;27:589-592.

165. Nishimura JI, Kanakura Y, Ware RE, et al. Clinical course and flow cytometric analysis of paroxysmal nocturnal hemoglobinuria in the United States and Japan. *Medicine (Baltim).* 2004;83:193-207.

166. Graham ML, Rosse WF, Halperin EC, Miller CR, Ware RE. Resolution of Budd-Chiari syndrome following bone marrow transplantation for paroxysmal nocturnal haemoglobinuria. *Br J Haematol.* 1996;92:707-710.

167. Prince GM, Nguyen M, Lazarus HM, Brodsky RA, Terstappen LW, Medof ME. Peripheral blood harvest of unaffected CD34+ CD38- hematopoietic precursors in paroxysmal nocturnal hemoglobinuria. *Blood.* 1995;86:3381-3386.

168. Peffault de Latour R. Transplantation for bone marrow failure: current issues. *Hematology Am Soc Hematol Educ Program.* 2016;2016:90-98.

169. Socie G, Peffault de Latour R. Hematopoietic stem cell transplant in PNH. In: Kanakura Y, Kinoshita T, Nishimura J, eds. *Paroxysmal Nocturnal Hemoglobinuria: From Bench to Bedside.* Springer; 2017:307-318.

170. Taniguchi K, Okada M, Yoshihara S, et al. Strategy for bone marrow transplantation in eculizumab-treated paroxysmal nocturnal hemoglobinuria. *Int J Hematol.* 2011;94:403-407.

171. Parker CJ. Management of paroxysmal nocturnal hemoglobinuria in the era of complement inhibitory therapy. *Hematology Am Soc Hematol Educ Program.* 2011;2011:21-29.

172. Parker CJ. Bone marrow failure syndromes: paroxysmal nocturnal hemoglobinuria. *Hematol Oncol Clin North Am.* 2009;23:333-346.

173. Hill A, Kelly RJ, Hillmen P. Thrombosis in paroxysmal nocturnal hemoglobinuria. *Blood.* 2013;121:4985-4996. quiz 5105.

174. Ray JG, Burows RF, Ginsberg JS, Burrows EA. Paroxysmal nocturnal hemoglobinuria and the risk of venous thrombosis: review and recommendations for management of the pregnant and nonpregnant patient. *Haemostasis.* 2000;30:103-117.

175. Gongora Bianchi RA. Paroxysmal nocturnal hemoglobinuria: the Mexican experience. *Rev Invest Clin.* 1997;49:85S-88S.

176. McMullin MF, Hillmen P, Jackson J, Ganly P, Luzzatto L. Tissue plasminogen activator for hepatic vein thrombosis in paroxysmal nocturnal haemoglobinuria. *J Intern Med.* 1994;235:85-89.

177. Sholar PW, Bell WR. Thrombolytic therapy for inferior vena cava thrombosis in paroxysmal nocturnal hemoglobinuria. *Ann Intern Med.* 1985;103:539-541.

178. Araten DJ, Notaro R, Thaler HT, et al. Thrombolytic therapy is effective in paroxysmal nocturnal hemoglobinuria: a series of nine patients and a review of the literature. *Haematologica.* 2012;97:344-352.

179. Bais J, Pel M, von dem Borne A, van der Lelie H. Pregnancy and paroxysmal nocturnal hemoglobinuria. *Eur J Obstet Gynecol Reprod Biol.* 1994;53:211-214.

180. Bais JM, Pel M. Late maternal mortality due to paroxysmal nocturnal hemoglobinuria and pregnancy. *Eur J Obstet Gynecol Reprod Biol.* 1995;58:211.

181. De Gramont A, Krulik M, Debray J. Paroxysmal nocturnal haemoglobinuria and pregnancy. *Lancet.* 1987;1:868.

182. Beresford CH, Gudex DJ, Symmans WA. Paroxysmal nocturnal haemoglobinuria and pregnancy. *Lancet.* 1986;2:1396-1397.

183. Jacobs P, Wood L. Paroxysmal nocturnal haemoglobinuria and pregnancy. *Lancet.* 1986;2:1099.

184. Svigos JM, Norman J. Paroxysmal nocturnal haemoglobinuria and pregnancy. *Aust N Z J Obstet Gynaecol.* 1994;34:104-106.

185. Melo A, Gorgal-Carvalho R, Amaral J, et al. Clinical management of paroxysmal nocturnal haemoglobinuria in pregnancy: three case reports. *Blood transfusion = Trasfusione del sangue.* 2011;9:99-103.

186. Kelly R, Arnold L, Richards S, et al. The management of pregnancy in paroxysmal nocturnal haemoglobinuria on long-term eculizumab. *Br J Haematol.* 2010;149:446-450.

187. Marasca R, Coluccio V, Santachiara R, et al. Pregnancy in PNH: another eculizumab baby. *Br J Haematol.* 2010;150:707-708.

188. Kelly RJ, Hochsmann B, Szer J, et al. Eculizumab in pregnant patients with paroxysmal nocturnal hemoglobinuria. *N Engl J Med.* 2015;373:1032-1039.

189. Miyasaka N, Miura O. Pregancy in paroxsymal hemoglobinuria. In: Kanakura Y, Kinoshita T, Nishimura J, eds. *Paroxysmal Nocturnal Hemoglobinuira: From Bench to Bedside.* Springer; 2017:347-358.

190. Hallstensen RF, Bergseth G, Foss S, et al. Eculizumab treatment during pregnancy does not affect the complement system activity of the newborn. *Immunobiology.* 2015;220:452-459.

191. van den Heuvel-Eibrink MM, Bredius RG, te Winkel ML, et al. Childhood paroxysmal nocturnal haemoglobinuria (PNH), a report of 11 cases in the Netherlands. *Br J Haematol.* 2005;128:571-577.

192. Curran KJ, Kernan NA, Prockop SE, et al. Paroxysmal nocturnal hemoglobinuria in pediatric patients. *Pediatr Blood Cancer.* 2012;59:525-529.

193. Reiss UM, Schwartz J, Sakamoto KM, et al. Efficacy and safety of eculizumab in children and adolescents with paroxysmal nocturnal hemoglobinuria. *Pediatr Blood Cancer.* 2014;61:1544-1550.

194. Bortolotti M, Mari C, Lopilato C, Porrazzo G, Miglioli M. Effects of sildenafil on esophageal motility of patients with idiopathic achalasia. *Gastroenterology.* 2000;118:253-257.

195. Bortolotti M, Pandolfo N, Giovannini M, Mari C, Miglioli M. Effect of Sildenafil on hypertensive lower oesophageal sphincter. *Eur J Clin Invest.* 2002;32:682-685.

196. Eherer AJ, Schwetz I, Hammer HF, et al. Effect of sildenafil on oesophageal motor function in healthy subjects and patients with oesophageal motor disorders. *Gut.* 2002;50:758-764.

197. Fujioka S, Takayoshi T. Prognostic features of paroxysmal nocturnal hemoglobinuria in Japan. *Acta Haematol Japan.* 1989;52:1386-1394.

198. Kruatrachue M, Wasi P, Na-Nakorn S. Paroxysmal nocturnal haemoglobinuria in Thailand with special reference to as association with aplastic anaemia. *Br J Haematol.* 1978;39:267-276.

199. Araten DJ, Thaler HT, Luzzatto L. High incidence of thrombosis in african-American and Latin-American patients with paroxysmal nocturnal haemoglobinuria. *Thromb Haemost.* 2005;93:88-91.

200. Java A, Apicelli AJ, Liszewski MK, et al. The complement system in COVID-19: friend and foe? *JCI Insight.* 2020;5(15):e140711.

201. Araten DJ, Belmont HM, Schaefer-Cutillo J, Iyengar A, Mattoo A, Reddy R. Mild clinical course of COVID-19 in 3 patients receiving therapeutic monoclonal antibodies targeting C5 complement for hematologic disorders. *Am J Case Rep.* 2020;21:e927418.

202. Kulasekararaj AG, Lazana I, Large J, et al. Terminal complement inhibition dampens the inflammation during COVID-19. *Br J Haematol.* 2020;190:e141-e143.

203. Pike A, Muus P, Munir T, et al. COVID-19 infection in patients on anti-complement therapy: the Leeds National Paroxysmal Nocturnal Haemoglobinuria service experience. *Br J Haematol.* 2020;191:e1-e4.

204. Gerber GF, Yuan X, Yu J, et al. COVID-19 vaccines induce severe hemolysis in paroxysmal nocturnal hemoglobinuria. *Blood.* 2021;137:3670-3673.

205. Horikawa K, Kawaguchi T, Ishihara S, et al. Frequent detection of T cells with mutations of the hypoxanthine-guanine phosphoribosyl transferase gene in patients with paroxysmal nocturnal hemoglobinuria. *Blood.* 2002;99:24-29.

206. Risitano A. Future strategies of complement inhibition in paroxysmal nocturnal hemoglobinuria. In: Kanakura Y, Kinoshita T, Nishimura J, eds. *Paroxysmal Nocturnal Hemoglobinuria: From Bench to Bedside.* Springer; 2017:319-346.

Chapter 33 ■ Acquired Nonimmune Hemolytic Disorders

ROBERT T. MEANS JR. • BERTIL GLADER

INTRODUCTION

In some cases, hemolysis is antibody mediated (see Chapters 31 and 44). In other patients, such as those with glucose-6-phosphate dehydrogenase (G6PD) deficiency (see Chapter 30) or those with unstable hemoglobins (see Chapter 36), there is an underlying propensity of the red blood cell (RBC) to be more susceptible to injury. In still other cases, such as paroxysmal nocturnal hemoglobinuria, hemolysis occurs as a consequence of an acquired clonal abnormality in the RBC membrane (see Chapter 32). Hemolytic anemia also occurs when otherwise normal red cells are injured directly by infectious agents, chemicals, thermal injury, mechanical stresses, or altered metabolites. These etiologies of hemolysis are the focus of this chapter.

HEMOLYSIS DUE TO INFECTION

A variety of infectious processes can lead to hemolytic destruction of normal RBCs. In some cases, such as in *Mycoplasma pneumoniae* infection or with infections related to paroxysmal cold hemoglobinuria, hemolysis is related to antibody-mediated cell destruction (see Chapter 31). With the infections described in this section, hemolysis is largely the result of direct nonimmune effects on erythrocytes. Some of the infections discussed here are not major problems in North America or Europe; however, to the extent that there is significant international travel to and from endemic areas, recognition of these infections is important for health care providers worldwide.

Malaria

Malaria can be an acute, chronic, or recurrent febrile disease caused in humans by four species of *Plasmodium*: *Plasmodium vivax, Plasmodium falciparum, Plasmodium malariae,* and *Plasmodium ovale*. Infections with *P. falciparum* are the major form of malaria in Africa and Southeast Asia, whereas *P. vivax* is most common in Central America and India. These protozoan microorganisms are capable of parasitizing erythrocytes and other body tissues. Malaria is spread by female mosquitoes of the genus *Anopheles* (*Figure 33.1*). The sexual phase of the *Plasmodium* life cycle takes place within the mosquito. The semitropical and tropical endemic distribution of malaria corresponds to the distribution of the vector.

On a worldwide basis, malaria is the most prevalent of all serious diseases; it has been estimated that approximately 2.5 billion people are at risk for malaria and that approximately 500 million people are infected with *P. falciparum*.[1,2] Malarial deaths have been declining, with 435,000 deaths reported worldwide in 2017. The majority of deaths are reported to occur in African children.[3] Malaria has not been endemic in the United States since the 1940s, and the overwhelming majority of US cases reflect exposure from travel or residence in endemic areas. However, there has been a steady increase in US incidence since the 1970s, with more than 2000 reported cases in 2017.[4] Malaria can also be transmitted by blood transfusions[5] or by sharing needles among intravenous drug abusers.[6]

Clinical Manifestations

The clinical features of malaria have been reviewed extensively.[7,8] Of the various malarial species, *P. falciparum* infection causes the most morbidity and mortality. It can be associated with respiratory distress, renal failure, impaired consciousness, hypotension, malignant hyperthermia, or even death in its acute stage.

Anemia is common in malaria. It is particularly characteristic of *P. falciparum*. However, severe anemia alone does not affect prognosis.[9] In tropical areas, anemia tends to be most prevalent and most severe in children aged 1 to 5 years,[10] whereas only moderate anemia is usually noted in adolescents and adults.

In children, the circulating parasite count is inversely proportional to the hematocrit.[11] Leukocyte numbers may be normal, but patients often have leukopenia. Thrombocytopenia has been observed in more than 80% of patients with *P. falciparum* or *P. vivax* malaria,[12] often associated with splenomegaly.[9,13]

The most serious hematologic complication of malaria is acute intravascular hemolytic anemia (blackwater fever), which occurs as a rare event in the course of infection by *P. falciparum*. The clinical manifestations are fulminating, the intravascular hemolysis being associated with prostration, vomiting, chills, and fever. Hemoglobinemia, hemoglobinuria, and hyperbilirubinemia are consistent features, and in the most severe episodes, acute oliguric renal failure supervenes.

Pathogenesis

After a bite from the female *Anopheles* mosquito, sporozoites introduced into the circulation go to the liver parenchyma where they proliferate into thousands of merozoites (*Figure 33.1*). The duration of this liver development stage varies between species. The infected hepatocytes next release merozoites into the bloodstream where they invade erythrocytes.

The ability of various *Plasmodia* to infect red cells is related to their attachment to specific membrane receptors. Of the species that infect humans, *P. vivax* and *P. ovale* invade only reticulocytes. *P. malariae* invades mature red cells, and *P. falciparum* invades erythrocytes of all ages. As a result, the proportion of cells parasitized in *P. vivax* malaria rarely exceeds 1%, whereas as many as 50% of cells may be affected in *P. falciparum* malaria. *P. vivax* invades only Duffy blood group–positive red cells; in West Africa where the Duffy antigen is missing on red cells, *P. vivax* malaria is almost nonexistent.[14] *P. vivax* also has an increased avidity for blood type O erythrocytes.[15] *P. falciparum* apparently has two classes of receptors: erythrocyte-binding ligand, which binds to sialic acid groups on the erythrocyte membrane protein glycophorin (type A, B, or C), and *P. falciparum* reticulocyte binding homolog (PfRh), which binds to neuraminidase-resistant, nonsialated ligands like complement receptor 1, CD147, and semaphorin 7a.[16]

Further development of the parasite within red cells is along one of two pathways, either asexual or sexual differentiation (*Figure 33.1*). Sexual forms, or gametocytes, continue their development within mosquitoes. The asexual differentiation of parasites in red cells proceeds from young ring forms through trophozoites to produce schizonts containing 6 to 32 merozoites (*Figure 33.2*). In the process, parasites use 25% to 75% of the hemoglobin of the cell.[17] The intraerythrocytic phase lasts 24 to 72 hours, depending on the species. The schizonts then lyse, the cell ruptures, and the merozoites are released to invade other cells, thereby continuing the erythrocyte cycle. The simultaneous rupture of billions of schizonts from red cells is associated with the classic paroxysms of malarial fever.

Erythrocytes parasitized by certain strains of *P. falciparum* develop electron-dense knobs that mediate the attachment of the infected red cells to venules.[18] Such sequestration of parasite-infected RBC creates an obstruction to tissue perfusion. In addition, the sequestration in venules prevents parasitized cells from entering the splenic circulation, thereby evading destruction and enhancing merozoite development; this phenomenon may be a factor in the rapid development of anemia in severe infections.[19]

The anemia in malaria is caused by a combination of factors that include parasite-mediated RBC destruction, splenic removal of infected RBCs, and decreased red cell production (*Table 33.1*). Hemoglobin digestion and cell disruption by the parasite are clearly

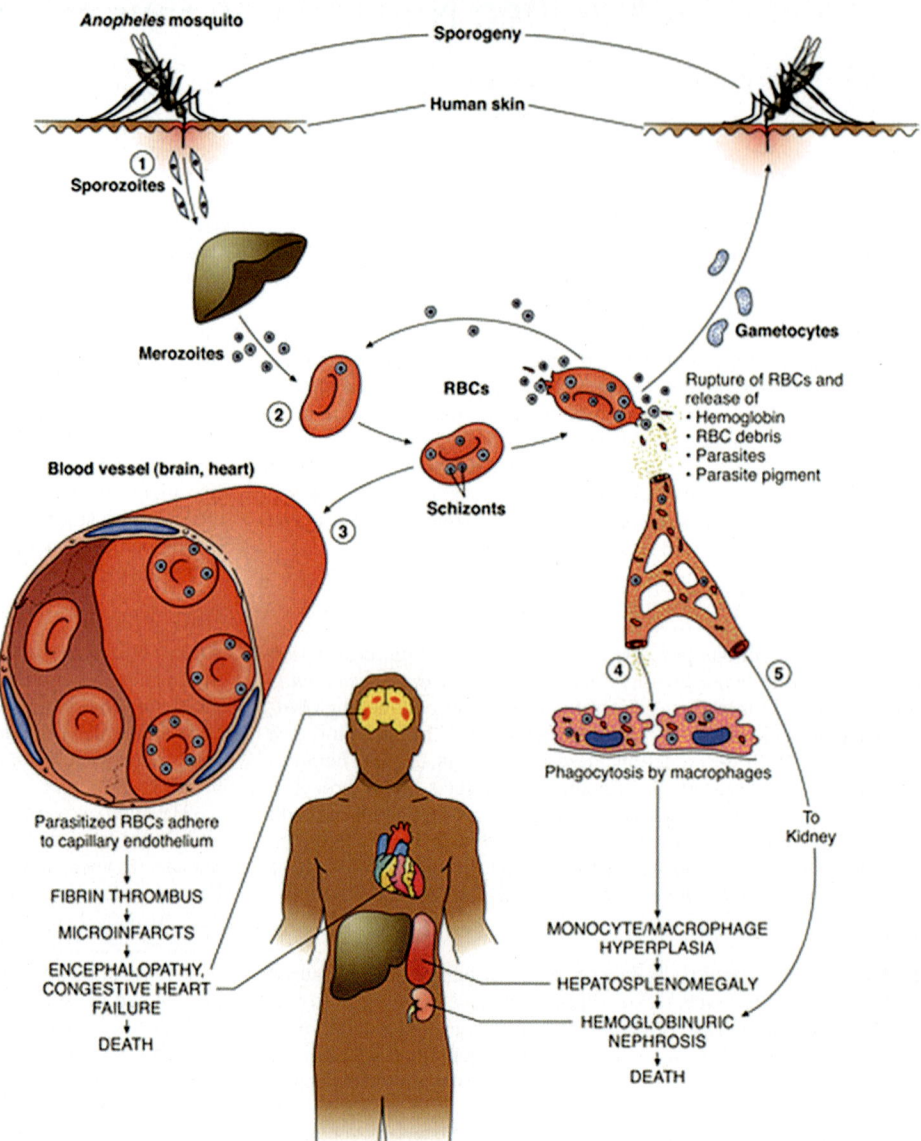

FIGURE 33.1 Life cycle of malaria. An *Anopheles* mosquito bites an infected person, taking blood that contains microgametocytes and macrogametocytes (sexual forms). In the mosquito, sexual multiplication ("sporogony") produces infective sporozoites in the salivary glands. (*1*) During the mosquito bite, sporozoites are inoculated into the bloodstream of the vertebrate host. Some sporozoites leave the blood and enter the hepatocytes, where they multiply asexually (exoerythrocytic schizogony) and form thousands of uninucleated merozoites. (*2*) Rupture of hepatocytes releases merozoites, which penetrate erythrocytes and become trophozoites, which then divide to form numerous schizonts (intraerythrocytic schizogony). Schizonts divide to form more merozoites, which are released on the rupture of erythrocytes and reenter other erythrocytes to begin a new cycle. After several cycles, subpopulations of merozoites develop into microgametocytes and macrogametocytes, which are taken up by another mosquito to complete the cycle. (*3*) Parasitized erythrocytes obstruct capillaries of the brain, heart, kidney, and other deep organs. Adherence of parasitized erythrocytes to capillary endothelial cells causes fibrin thrombi, which produce microinfarcts. These result in encephalopathy, congestive heart failure, pulmonary edema, and frequent death. Ruptured erythrocytes release hemoglobin, erythrocyte debris, and malarial pigment. (*4*) Phagocytosis leads to monocyte/macrophage hyperplasia and hepatosplenomegaly. (*5*) Released hemoglobin produces hemoglobinuric nephrosis, which may be fatal. (Reprinted with permission from Rubin E, Farber JL. *Pathology.* 3rd ed. Lippincott-Raven; 1999.)

the major causes of hemolysis.[9] Anemia often persists for weeks following treatment of malaria, and this results in part from relative marrow failure, as occurs in association with other forms of infection. These effects may be mediated by inflammation[20] (see Chapter 42). Serum erythropoietin levels are often inadequate for the degree of anemia. The bone marrow response to erythropoietin also appears to be impaired.[21] Circulating concentration of the iron-regulatory peptide hepcidin, a key mediator of the anemia of inflammation/chronic disease, is elevated early in the course of malaria. This results in impaired iron mobilization.[22] The malarial pigment hemozoin, a product of hemoglobin degradation, can inhibit erythropoiesis.[23] Dyserythropoiesis with characteristic morphologic findings may occur in malaria. It is thought that this contributes to the slow recovery seen after a single malarial attack and also to the persistence of anemia in individuals with chronic parasitemia.[24]

Even after complete clearance of the parasites, hemolysis may persist for 4 to 5 weeks.[9] A complement-mediated process may be responsible in part, and the direct antiglobulin test is often positive.[25]

The percentage of reticulocytes tends to be low during active infection and increases transiently after effective treatment. In *P. vivax* malaria, however, the low reticulocyte count may be explained in part by the increased affinity of the organism for immature erythroid precursors and reticulocytes.[26]

The pathogenesis of acute intravascular hemolysis (blackwater fever) remains uncertain, and currently this complication is rare, although it still occurs.[27] Blackwater fever does not reflect an unusual degree of parasitemia. In many historic cases, the acute intravascular hemolysis appears to have been precipitated by therapeutic quinine acting as a hapten (*Table 33.1*), although cases involving untreated individuals have also been reported. Some episodes thought to represent blackwater fever may have resulted from the use of primaquine-like drugs in G6PD-deficient patients.[28]

Certain inherited red cell disorders appear to confer resistance to malaria, either by inhibiting parasitic invasion or by slowing intracellular growth. It is thought that these phenomena may contribute to increased prevalence of such inherited diseases because of their effects on survival (balanced polymorphism). These disorders include sickle cell trait, G6PD deficiency, thalassemia,[29] hemoglobin E variants, hemoglobin C variants,[30] ovalocytosis of the Melanesian (Malayan) type,[31] and lack of the Duffy blood group antigen.[29]

Diagnosis

Diagnosis of malaria outside endemic areas is often delayed because it is not suspected.[32] Such delays are dangerous because the early mortality rate from *P. falciparum* malaria approaches 10%, and these deaths can be prevented with adequate treatment. Malaria should be

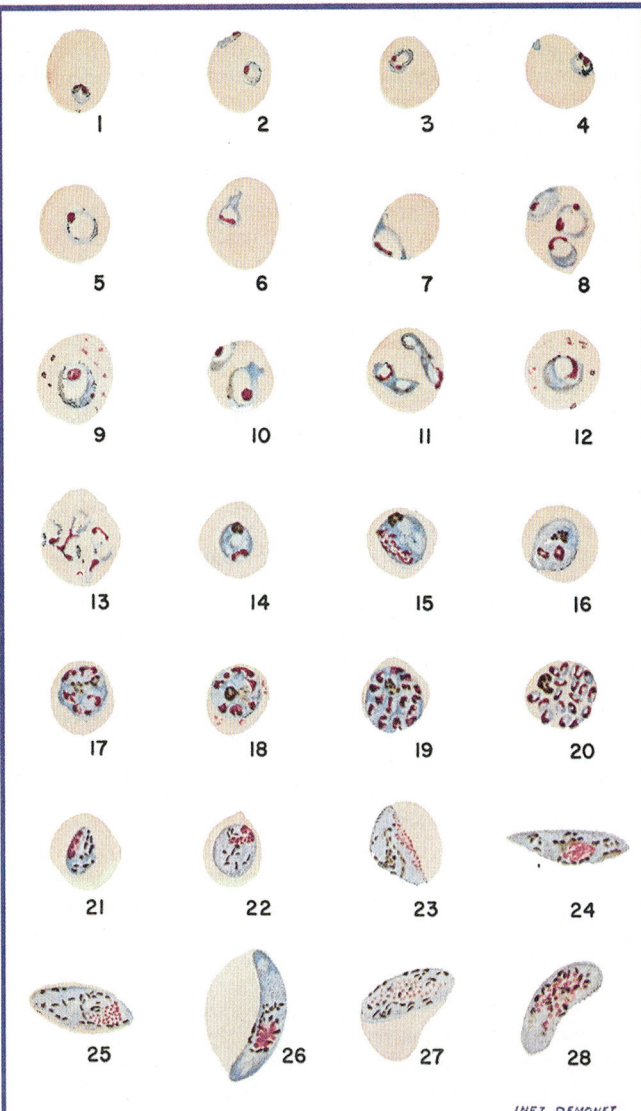

FIGURE 33.2 *Plasmodium falciparum.* (*1*) Very young ring form trophozoite. (*2*) Double infection of single cell with young trophozoites, one a marginal form, the other a signet ring form. (*3,4*) Young trophozoites showing double chromatin dots. (*5-7*) Developing trophozoites. (*8*) Three medium trophozoites in one cell. (*9*) Trophozoite showing pigment in a cell containing Maurer spots. (*10,11*) Two trophozoites in each of two cells showing variation of forms that parasites may assume. (*12*) Almost mature trophozoite showing haze of pigment throughout cytoplasm. (*13*) Aestivoautumnal slender forms. (*14*) Mature trophozoite showing clumped pigment. (*15*) Parasite in the process of initial chromatin division. (*16-19*) Various phases of the development of the schizont. (*20*) Mature schizont. (*21-24*) Successive forms in the development of the gametocyte, usually not found in the circulation. (*25*) Immature macrogametocyte. (*26*) Mature macrogametocyte. (*27*) Immature microgametocyte. (*28*) Mature microgametocyte. (Reproduced from Wilcox A. *Manual for the Microscopical Diagnosis of Malaria in Man. National Institutes of Health Bulletin No. 180.* U.S. Public Health Service; 1951.)

considered in the differential diagnosis of any febrile patient returning from an endemic zone.

Diagnosis traditionally has required identification of parasites on the blood smear (*Figure 33.2*). They can be recognized on ordinary Wright-stained smears, but the chances for detection and identification of species are enhanced by the use of thick smears. Single negative smears do not exclude the disease with certainty in patients with low-grade infections. Parasites may be detected in blood during any phase of the illness, but the chances of detection are greatest during afebrile periods. *P. falciparum* disease is distinguished from that caused by

Table 33.1. Factors Contributing to Anemia in Malaria

Accelerated Red Blood Cell (RBC) Destruction
Direct parasite destruction of red cells
Decreased deformability of parasitized RBCs and destruction by splenic macrophages
Erythrocyte retention in the spleen
Macrophage-mediated destruction of parasitized RBCs in marrow and liver sinusoids
Destruction of nonparasitized cells by immune mechanisms
Destruction of nonparasitized cells by hypersplenism and hyperactive macrophages
Hapten (quinine)-induced intravascular hemolysis (blackwater fever)
Decreased RBC Production
Bone marrow suppression as a result of inflammatory cytokines
Inadequate erythropoietin production
Impaired iron mobilization mediated by hepcidin
Dyserythropoiesis
Suppression of erythropoiesis by hemozocin

Modified from Menendez C, Fleming AF, Alonso PL. Malaria-related anemia. *Parasitol Today.* 2000;16(11):469-476.

other strains by heavy parasitemia involving all ages of erythrocytes and by the lack of trophozoites and schizonts; usually, only ring forms and the distinctive, banana-shaped gametocytes are apparent.

Simple test strips that take 10 to 15 minutes are available for diagnosis of malaria from a drop of fingerstick blood. The sensitivity of these tests is probably as good as microscopy. Diagnosis by rapid polymerase chain reaction is also available.[33] Regardless of the method used, it is important to distinguish *P. falciparum* malaria from other malarial species because of therapeutic considerations and because only *P. falciparum* infection has the potential for being rapidly fatal.

Management

Therapeutic considerations for malaria include supportive medical care for anemia and other complications. Administration of folate to patients with malaria is controversial because its use is associated with higher hematocrits and it may also prolong parasitemia.[34] Chemoprophylaxis should be recommended to all people traveling to an endemic area.[35] Because of the spread of drug-resistant strains of *P. falciparum*, no single regimen is completely effective. Knowledge of the characteristics of the malarial strains in the sites to be visited is essential. Because of changes in drug resistance and the development of new agents, physicians should become familiar with current guidelines from the US Centers for Disease Control and Prevention (http://www.cdc.gov/travel/malinfo.htm) before recommending a regimen to a prospective traveler.

Babesiosis

Infection by tick-borne protozoans of the genus *Babesia* is rare in humans.[36] The infection has been reported in Nantucket and other islands off the northeastern US shore, as well as in neighboring coastal areas of New England. It is also found in north central states, Washington, and California. In the United States, *Babesia microti* is the causative agent, whereas *Babesia divergens* is the species identified in Europe. *Babesia divergens* cases are usually more severe and mostly occur in asplenic patients.[36] Babesiosis can also be transmitted by blood transfusion.[37]

Babesiosis is characterized by an acute febrile illness and hemolytic anemia, very similar to malaria. In most cases, it is a mild self-limited disorder that goes undiagnosed and thus is not reported. It is likely that the true incidence of babesiosis in healthy hosts is underrecognized. However, in asplenic individuals, it can produce serious, often-fatal illness with hemolytic anemia, renal failure, or pulmonary edema.[38]

Laboratory features include hemoglobinuria, hyperbilirubinemia, normocytic anemia, thrombocytopenia, and sometimes leukopenia. Bone marrow examination may show hemophagocytosis, with the overall clinical picture resembling hemophagocytic lymphohistiocytosis.[39] Both *B. microti* and *B. divergens* can be seen in RBCs on the peripheral blood smear, and this can be confused with malaria.[38] Serologic antibody tests and polymerase chain reaction–based assays are available to aid in diagnosis.[36]

In mild cases of babesiosis, no treatment may be necessary. In more severe cases, antibiotics may be required.[39] Red cell exchange transfusions have been used as well.[36]

Trypanosomiasis

Moderate to severe hemolytic anemia is a regular feature of African trypanosomiasis (sleeping sickness).[40] This often-fatal illness is caused by *Trypanosoma brucei gambiense* or *Trypanosoma brucei rhodesiense*. The diseases induced by these two subspecies are similar, except that *T. brucei gambiense* infection follows a more chronic course. The organisms are transmitted to humans and domestic animals by the bite of the tsetse fly.

Normocytic anemia with reticulocytosis is prominent. Red cell survival is shortened, and autoagglutination of erythrocytes with accelerated erythrocyte sedimentation is characteristically observed. The results of the direct antiglobulin test may be positive. Erythrophagocytosis by macrophages is seen throughout the reticuloendothelial system.[41]

The toxic effects of the parasite and immunologic mechanisms both are implicated in the destruction of red cells. The intensity of the hemolytic anemia may fluctuate with the degree of parasitemia. Transient hepatosplenomegaly and decreased serum complement levels accompany the episodes. Marrow failure often supervenes during the terminal phases of the illness. Diagnosis depends on serologic tests or demonstration of the parasite in the blood.[40]

Chagas disease (American trypanosomiasis; *Trypanosoma cruzi*) is commonly associated with a mild degree of anemia, in many cases resembling the anemia of inflammation/chronic disease.[40]

Visceral Leishmaniasis (Kala-Azar)

Leishmaniasis is an infection caused by intracellular protozoan parasites transmitted by sandflies. There are three main forms of *Leishmania* infections in humans: cutaneous, mucocutaneous, and visceral. The major hematologic problems occur with the visceral infection (kala-azar) and involve the lymph nodes, liver, spleen, and bone marrow. The disorder is caused by *Leishmania donovani* and is found throughout Asia and Africa, affecting individuals of all ages. A variant parasite, *Leishmania donovani infantum* is the form that causes kala-azar in southern Europe and North Africa, and it primarily affects young children and infants. Visceral and cutaneous leishmaniasis mainly occur in local endemic areas; however, they may be contracted on visits to endemic areas.[42]

Following an incubation period of 1 to 3 months, there is the insidious onset of fever, sweating, malaise, and anorexia, but these acute symptoms gradually abate. Next, hepatosplenomegaly gradually evolves, and this stage of illness is associated with anemia, neutropenia, and thrombocytopenia. In young children with acute visceral leishmaniasis, particularly in Mediterranean populations, the clinical and hematologic features may be more aggressive with a rapid onset of severe hemolytic anemia.[43]

The bone marrow is hyperplastic with dyserythropoietic changes, and the diagnosis can usually be made by finding macrophages containing intracellular parasites (Leishman-Donovan bodies). The overall hematologic picture is typical of hypersplenism. Hemolysis is the major cause of anemia in leishmaniasis.[44]

In most cases, there is no evidence of immune hemolysis, although both immunoglobulin G and complement are occasionally found on the red cells. Similar to what is seen in malaria, nonsensitized red cells are destroyed by macrophages recruited to the spleen and liver as part of the inflammatory response to the parasite.

Bartonellosis (Carrion Disease)

A severe, acute hemolytic anemia is produced in humans by *Bartonella bacilliformis*, a flagellated bacillus.[45] The infection is limited to South America, particularly in the Andean valleys of Peru, Ecuador, and Columbia, at elevations of 500 to 3000 m.[46] The bacillus is transmitted by the sand fly (*Phlebotomus*) and probably by other arthropods. After a 2- to 3-week incubation period, the acute phase of the illness, known as Oroya fever, begins. It is marked by malaise, headache, muscle pains, remittent fever, chills, and rapid onset of severe anemia. The highest rates of infection are in children.[46]

The findings in the blood are characteristic of acute extravascular blood destruction. On Wright- or Giemsa-stained blood smears, numerous *Bartonella* organisms are apparent in the erythrocyte.[45] The organisms are rod shaped (1-2 m in length and 0.2-0.5 m in width) or round (0.3-1.0 m in diameter).

In patients who recover from the acute phase, a quiescent period ensues during which the organisms disappear from the blood. A chronic, eruptive stage follows: verruca peruviana, a benign condition characterized by hemangioma-like lesions of the skin but without hematologic manifestations.[47]

Bartonella infection can be treated by antibiotic combinations containing chloramphenicol and other antibiotics, often a β-lactam. Verruca peruviana is typically treated with streptomycin-containing regimens.[48]

Clostridial Sepsis

Clostridium perfringens septicemia occurs after septic abortion or in association with a diseased biliary tree, traumatic wound infections, cancer, leukemia, endocarditis, gastrointestinal arteriovenous malformations, or necrotizing enterocolitis of newborns. Sometimes no underlying disease is identified.[49] Profound, often life-threatening acute hemolytic anemia is a regular feature of clostridial sepsis. Signs of intravascular red cell destruction are prominent, and many microspherocytes are found in the blood. The hemolysis can be rapid and massive, with hematocrit values falling to very low levels in a matter of hours. High levels of circulating free hemoglobin may interfere with results from laboratory analyzers.[50] Hemolysis is thought to result from the elaboration of a clostridial toxin, a phospholipase that attacks erythrocyte membrane lipids to form highly lytic lysolecithins.[51] The diagnosis should be suspected when fever, jaundice, and intravascular hemolysis occur together in a patient with a history of previous gastrointestinal or genitourinary surgery, a recent wound, cancer, or other disease. Clostridial infections respond to antibiotic therapy, but in order to affect outcome, treatment must be started quickly, usually before culture results are available.[52]

Other Bacterial Infections

Acute hemolytic anemia with bacterial infection is common, especially in childhood. A wide array of organisms and mechanisms has been implicated (*Table 33.2*).

HEMOLYSIS DUE TO DRUGS AND CHEMICALS

Many drugs and chemicals injure normal red cells to cause hemolytic anemia. Some of the more common occurrences are summarized below. (Drug-induced immune hemolysis is discussed in Chapter 31.)

Oxidant Drugs and Chemicals

Certain chemical agents can bring about the oxidative denaturation of hemoglobin, leading to the sequential formation of methemoglobin, sulfhemoglobin, and Heinz bodies. In some cases, the chemical itself acts as an oxidizing agent; more often, however, it interacts with oxygen to form free radicals or peroxides. These free radicals or peroxides, if produced in quantities too great to be detoxified by the glutathione-dependent reduction system, denature hemoglobin and damage other cellular structures, such as the cell membrane.[53] Individuals deficient in G6PD or other components of glutathione-dependent detoxification processes are particularly sensitive to the hemolytic effects of oxidant

Table 33.2. Other Infectious Agents and Mechanisms Associated With Hemolytic Anemia

Intravascular Hemolysis

Vibrio cholera
Salmonella typhi (typhoid fever)
Bacterial endocarditis (various organisms)

Erythrophagocytosis

Hemophilus influenza (mediated by capsular polysaccharide absorption)
Borrelia recurrentis

Neuraminidase Release (red cell sialic acid cleavage and exposure of T antigen)

Clostridium perfringens
Streptococcus pneumoniae
Vibrio (various species)
Bacteroides (various species)
Escherichia coli (various subspecies)
Actinomyces (various species)

Splenic Sequestration/Other Mechanical

Borrelia recurrentis
Bacterial endocarditis (various organisms)

Unknown

Staphylococcus (various species)
Streptococcus (various species)
Mycobacterium tuberculosis (military tuberculosis)
Leptospira interrogans (leptospirosis)

Particular infectious agents may be associated with more than one mechanism.

compounds. These agents may also unmask otherwise insignificant defects in the metabolic pathways that defend the erythrocyte against oxidative stress.[54] However, some of these agents are powerful enough to overcome the defense mechanisms of otherwise normal erythrocytes and can cause hemolysis if given to healthy subjects in higher-than-usual doses or if renal failure leads to unusually high blood levels.

Hemolytic anemia caused by oxidant drugs varies considerably in severity. Usually, the anemia is noted within 1 to 2 weeks after drug therapy is initiated with laboratory findings of low hemoglobin, reticulocytosis, hyperbilirubinemia, and low serum haptoglobin. In some cases, hemoglobinemia and hemoglobinuria may be apparent. Cyanosis with methemoglobinemia or sulfhemoglobinemia is sometimes noted. The hemolytic process usually disappears within 1 to 3 weeks after the use of the offending drug has been discontinued.

Morphologic findings characteristic of hemolytic anemia caused by oxidant drugs and chemicals are shown in *Figure 33.3* and include the following: Heinz bodies (seen with brilliant cresyl blue supravital stains of blood during hemolytic episodes; *Figure 33.3A*); "bite cells" (seen in routine Wright-stained blood smear; *Figure 33.3B*); and hemighosts, also called "blister cells" or eccentrocytes (*Figure 33.3C*). These hemighosts appear to contain a large vacuole. Hemighosts appear only when hemolysis is brisk[55] and probably indicate a particularly severe degree of oxidant damage. All of these morphologic alterations are consequences of oxidative assault on hemoglobin.

Although the treatment of drug-induced nonimmune hemolysis is largely supportive, erythropoietin has been used in cases associated with a blunted erythropoietic response, particularly in the hemolytic anemia that is observed in patients with hepatitis C treated with ribavirin (see Chapter 42).

Heavy Metal Toxicity

Arsine Arsine (AsH_3) is the most acutely toxic form of arsenic. It is a colorless, nonirritating, highly toxic gas that is produced by the action of water or acid on a metallic arsenide. Exposure to arsine is most common in the chemical, metallurgical, and microelectronics industries.[56]

Manifestations of poisoning appear 2 to 24 hours after exposure and include abdominal pain, nausea, and vomiting; the passage of dark red urine; jaundice; anemia; reticulocytosis; leukocytosis; and other signs of acute hemolytic anemia. Hemoglobinemia and hemoglobinuria are found, and acute, oliguric renal failure may ensue as a result. The antiglobulin test result is negative. Although fatalities can occur, with rapid treatment eventual recovery is common. Proposed mechanisms of red cell damage include oxidative formation of hemoglobin adducts and damage to the red cell membrane sodium/potassium pump.[56]

The treatment of choice for acute toxicity is red cell and plasma exchange transfusion to remove the arsenic-containing erythrocytes and toxic intermediates in the plasma and to restore the blood hemoglobin levels.[57,58]

Lead Risk factors for lead toxicity are related to occupational hazards in adults and to environmental exposure in children.[59,60] Acute toxicity occurs when lead accidently gets into a food or water source. Such acute poisoning leads to lead encephalopathy (headache, confusion, stupor, coma, and seizures), and in addition, there is abdominal colic, hypertension, and hemolytic anemia. Chronic exposure over time is also associated with a variety of neurologic, gastrointestinal, reproductive, and hematologic complications.

The peripheral smear shows extensive coarse basophilic stippling and reticulocytosis. Red cell morphology is not otherwise characteristic. The diagnosis of lead-related hemolysis can be suspected from a history of lead exposure, the physical finding of the gingival lead sulfide line, and coarse basophilic stippling of red cells. The diagnosis is confirmed by measuring of blood and urine lead levels.

Lead inhibits two steps in heme synthesis: *d*-aminolevulinic acid dehydratase and heme synthetase (or ferrochelatase). The latter enzyme catalyzes the insertion of iron into protoporphyrin IX to form heme. The lead-induced inhibition of ferrochelatase is responsible for the increase in free erythrocyte protoporphyrin seen in this disorder and is also the basis of a simple screening test for lead toxicity.

Proposed mechanisms for hemolysis in lead toxicity include lead-induced lipid peroxidation, inhibition of the enzyme pyrimidine 5′-nucleotidase, and phosphoribosyltransferase inhibition.[61,62] Chelation, with or without antioxidant agents, is the established treatment for lead poisoning.[63]

Copper Hemolytic episodes as a result of copper toxicity have been noted in humans after exposure to toxic amounts of copper sulfate.[64] Copper appears to induce hemolysis through hemoglobin oxidation and consequent lipid peroxidation.[65]

Excess copper accumulation since birth produces the clinical manifestations of Wilson disease (hepatolenticular degeneration), which include hemolysis. Wilson disease is caused by defects in the copper-transporting intracellular ATPase ATP7B. This leads to a deficiency of ceruloplasmin, the plasma copper transport protein. It usually becomes symptomatic in the teens or early 20s. Hemolytic anemia can be associated with the early stages of Wilson disease and may be the first manifestation of the disorder, or it may be associated with hepatic decompensation.[66] However, it may appear late in the course of the disease if chelation therapy is discontinued. The hemolytic episodes in Wilson disease are usually transient and self-limited, but they may be severe and recurrent. The incidence of hemolysis at diagnosis is 5% to 20%.[66] The usual treatment for Wilson disease is chelation, but severe hemolysis may require plasmapheresis.[67]

Water (Osmotic Hemolysis)

There are anecdotal reports of hemolysis following inadvertent injection of water and other hypotonic fluids under circumstances like dialysis, irrigation of an operative field, or even fresh water drowning.[68,69] The entry of more than 0.6 L of water into the circulation causes hemoglobinemia and hemoglobinuria as a result of osmotic hemolysis.

HEMOLYSIS WITH VENOMS

Spider Bites

Certain spider bites produce severe, necrotic, gangrenous lesions ("necrotic arachnidism") that may be associated with hemolytic anemia or disseminated intravascular coagulation, and occasionally

Disorders of Red Blood Cells

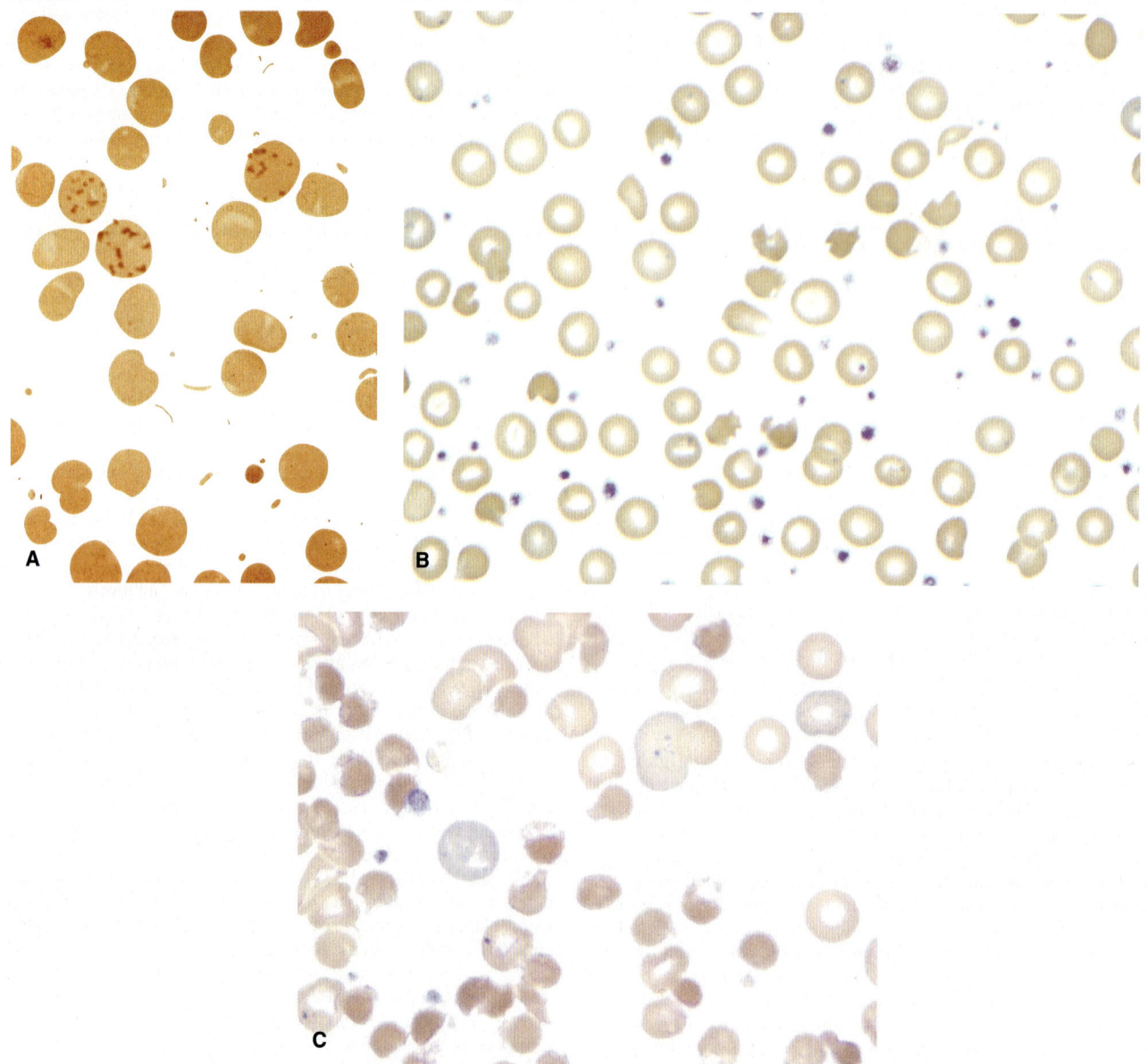

FIGURE 33.3 Morphologic findings characteristic of hemolytic anemia caused by oxidant drugs and chemicals. A. Heinz bodies (seen with brilliant cresyl blue supravital stains of blood during hemolytic episodes). B. "Bite cells" (seen in routine Wright-stained blood smear) as erythrocytes that look as if a semicircular bite has been taken from one edge. C. "Blister cells" or hemighosts (seen in routine Wright-stained blood smear) appear as if hemoglobin has shifted to one side of the cell, leaving the other side clear. These blister red blood cells contain a coagulum of hemoglobin that has separated from the membrane, leaving an unstained non-hemoglobin-containing cell membrane.[124] This image is from a patient receiving Pyridium. (Courtesy of Irma Pereira, MT [ASCP] SH.)

with renal failure.[70] In South America and the southwestern part of the United States, the spiders implicated are the brown recluse spider (*Loxosceles reclusa*) and other *Loxosceles* species.[71,72] In the north-western United States, a similar picture follows the bite of the hobo spider, *Tegenaria agrestis*.[73]

Although most spider bites result in only local complications, systemic manifestations, including intravascular hemolytic anemia, may develop within several hours to 5 days later. Hemoglobinuria and severe anemia are characteristic findings; spherocytes and leukocytosis are found in the blood. Thrombocytopenia has also been observed, sometimes associated with diffuse intravascular coagulation. In many cases, red cells are coated with complement and nonspecific antibodies and the direct antiglobulin test is positive.[70,72] Most often, the hemolytic episode subsides spontaneously in about 1 week, but occasionally, severe reactions occur with renal failure and death.

Described mechanisms of hemolysis include direct vascular toxicity and fibrinogenolysis, complement-dependent intravascular hemolysis associated with cleavage of glycophorin from the red cell membrane, and effects of phospholipase and sphingomyelinase activity found in venom.[72,74-76]

Treatment of spider bite–induced hemolysis is largely supportive. There are some in vitro data suggesting that eculizumab or other complement inhibitors might be beneficial in severe cases.[72]

Snake Bites

Snake bites are a significant health problem worldwide, especially in parts of Asia where thousands of people die from them annually.[77] Snake venoms vary in composition based on species, location, and even time of year. The hematologic problems from snake venom include a venom-induced consumptive coagulopathy clinically resembling disseminated intravascular coagulation and intravascular hemolysis.[78] Hemolysis can be seen following envenomation with most poisonous snakes, including cobras, Australian king brown snakes, Tunisian saw-scaled (carpet) vipers, North American rattlesnakes, habu snakes, and the several species of Russell viper (*Daboia russelli*) found throughout India and the rest of Asia.

The clinical presentation of intravascular hemolysis from snake bites can be acute and fulminant, or the effects can be delayed for a few hours to days. Hemoglobinemia and hemoglobinuria are present, the severity of which varies with the degree of envenomation and species of snake. Proteomic studies show a vast array of bioactive substances in snake venom,[79] many of which may be contributing to hemolysis. The best studied of these is phospholipase A_2, which has direct toxicity for many tissues, including the red cell membrane.[80] Venom from the habu snake contains enzymes that activate complement and cleaves CD55 and CD59 from the red cell membrane, thus leaving the red cell susceptible to complement-induced lysis.[81] Other snake venoms contain protein kinase C inhibitors implicated in hemolysis.[82]

Bee Stings

The effects of bee stings can be immediate or delayed. "Immediate" reactions are related to anaphylaxis. "Delayed" reactions refer to patients who are asymptomatic after massive bee envenomation but 12 to 24 hours later may have evidence of hemolysis, disseminated intravascular coagulation, thrombocytopenia, rhabdomyolysis, liver dysfunction, or renal failure.[83] The delayed effects are related to the degree of envenomation and require attack by large numbers of bees. Although the definition of massive envenomation is more than 50 stings,[84] adults may be able to tolerate a significantly larger number (>100) before severe problems occur.[85] The venom contains melittin and phospholipase A_2, which together disrupt the red cell membrane and cause hemolysis.[86] Hemolytic reactions to bee stings are rare. Renal failure is a much more significant problem than hemolytic anemia.

HEMOLYSIS WITH THERMAL INJURY

Burns

Acute hemolytic anemia has been observed after extensive thermal burns. Signs of intravascular hemolysis are associated with schistocytes, spherocytes, and echinocytes in the blood along with increased osmotic and mechanical fragility of the erythrocytes.[87] The severity of anemia is related to the area of body surface affected, with >20% surface area severely burned being the major determinant.[88] In a series of 130 consecutive severely burned patients admitted to a critical care unit, 39 (30%) had undetectable plasma haptoglobin (an indicator of intravascular hemolysis) at the time of admission. All but one of the patients (97%) had >20% surface area burned.[89]

Hemolysis occurs, and fragmented red cells appear, during the first 24 to 48 hours after the burn and may be miscounted as platelets by electronic counting methods.[90] Up to 30% of the circulating red cell mass may be destroyed in the first 48 hours after the burn.[91] After the acute hemolytic episode, anemia develops and may last for many weeks, although signs of hemolysis disappear. This later stage of the anemia of thermal injury is probably a form of the anemia of inflammation.[92]

The acute hemolytic reaction in burned patients results from the direct effects of heat on erythrocytes. When red cells are heated to temperatures >47 °C, irreversible morphologic and functional abnormalities occur, the severity of which is related to the temperature and the duration of exposure.[93] The major alterations are fragmentation of the cells and the development of spherocytes, accompanied by an increase in osmotic and mechanical fragility. These changes result from irreversible denaturation of the cytoskeletal protein spectrin and the red cell anion exchanger.[94] Mildly heat-damaged erythrocytes are removed predominantly by the spleen.[95]

Heated Fluids and Blood

Overheating of biologic fluids is another clinical circumstance resulting in thermal red cell damage. Typically, it occurs as a result of failure of safety devices or protocols, although hemolysis has been reported after placing a microwave-warmed towel over an intravenous infusion site.[96] Transfused blood does not exhibit significant hemolysis unless warmed to greater than 47 °C.[93] Use of US Food and Drug Administration–approved inline blood warmers equipped with thermometers and alarms, and close adherence to the manufacturer's specific directions, should provide a safety level that prevents the accidental overheating of blood.

FRAGMENTATION HEMOLYSIS

When red cells are subjected to intravascular trauma, they may undergo premature fragmentation and intravascular hemolysis, thereby resulting in hemoglobinemia, hemoglobinuria, decreased haptoglobin, and hemosiderinuria. The hallmark of this type of hemolysis is the fragmented red cell or schistocyte, and these cells take the form of crescents, helmets, triangles, and/or microspherocytes (*Figure 33.4*). Hemolytic anemias resulting from red cell fragmentation are associated with abnormalities of the heart and great vessels, diseases of small vessels, disseminated intravascular coagulation, and hypertension (*Table 33.3*). In most of these conditions, hemolysis is one of many clinical findings and is usually not the major problem.

Cardiac and Large Vessel Abnormalities
Etiology

Soon after the advent of open-heart surgery came the realization that the postoperative course of some patients was complicated by the development of anemia of varying severity. The discovery of fragmented red cells as a characteristic feature of this type of anemia was made in 1961, when Sayed et al described these morphologic alterations in a patient who developed severe and persistent intravascular hemolysis after repair of an ostium primum defect with Teflon.[97] It is now well recognized that fragmented erythrocytes with intravascular hemolysis are commonly associated with a wide variety of structural defects of the heart or great vessels (*Table 33.3*). The pathogenetic mechanism involved in this process is turbulent flow across the particular anatomic lesion or prosthetic device.[98,99] Surgically inserted prosthetic devices, particularly heart valves, furnish the most striking examples of red cell fragmentation. Most of the prosthetic valves associated with hemolytic anemia involve the aortic valve, but cases of hemolysis caused by mitral valve replacement or repair and by repair

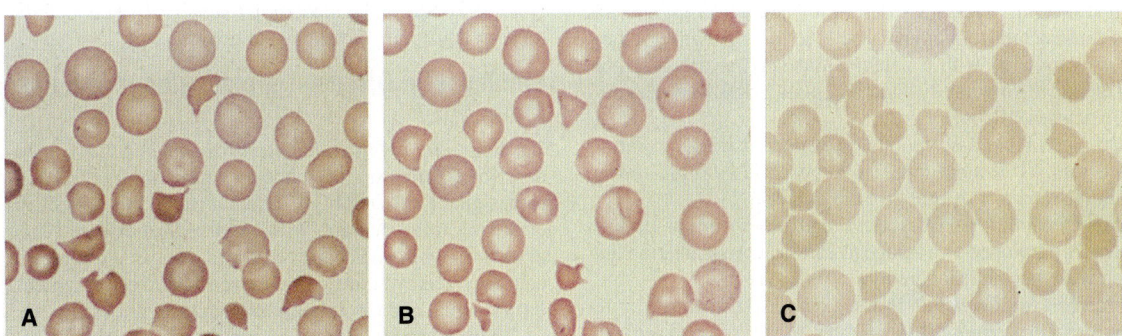

FIGURE 33.4 Schistocytes in patients with (A) thrombotic thrombocytopenic purpura, (B) disseminated intravascular coagulation, and (C) aortic valve replacement.

Table 33.3. Causes of Red Cell Fragmentation

Associated With Abnormalities of the Heart and Great Vessels
Synthetic valvular prostheses
Valve homografts
Valve xenografts and xenobioprostheses
Autograft valvoplasties
Ruptured chordae tendineae
Intracardiac patch repairs
Unoperated valve disease (especially aortic stenosis)
Coarctation of the aorta
Associated With Small Vessel Disease Microangiopathic Hemolytic Anemia
Thrombotic thrombocytopenic purpura (TTP)
Hemolytic uremic syndrome (HUS)
HUS/TTP-related disorders
Disseminated carcinoma
Chemotherapy/drugs
Transplant-associated microangiopathy
Pregnancy and postpartum period
HELLP syndrome
TTP/HUS
Malignant hypertension
Disseminated intravascular coagulation
Immune mechanisms
Lupus erythematosus
Acute glomerulonephritis
Scleroderma
Wegener granulomatosis
Associated with vascular malformations
Hemangiomas
Giant hemangioma (Kasabach-Merritt syndrome)
Hemangioendothelioma of the liver
Plexiform lesions in pulmonary hypertension
Pathogenesis unclear
March hemoglobinuria

HELLP, hemolysis, elevated liver enzymes, and low platelet counts.

of ruptured chordae tendineae have also been reported. The use of bioprostheses has reduced the risk of hemolysis greatly, although red cell fragmentation still occurs after the insertion of porcine xenografts or bioprostheses constructed from bovine tissue. In these patients, hemolysis is usually associated with a paravalvular leak, a torn cusp, or other manifestations of valvular dysfunction, including infective endocarditis or calcification.[100]

Intracardiac patch repairs of various types may also lead to intravascular hemolysis.[101] Typical cases involve patients with Teflon patches used in the repair of ostium primum defects.

Mechanical ventricular assist devices and other similar pump-based technologies employed as a bridge to cardiac transplantation are also associated with mechanical hemolysis.[102]

Although red cell fragmentation is associated most strikingly with intracardiac surgical procedures, intravascular hemolysis with red cell fragmentation also occurs in many patients with valvular heart disease who have not had surgery. Most often, this is noted in patients

who have severe aortic valve disease, especially aortic stenosis.[103] Hemolysis can also be seen in some patients with other defects, including mitral valve disease, ruptured aneurysm of the sinus of Valsalva, coarctation of the aorta, ventricular septal defect, and patent ductus arteriosus. The hemolysis accompanying native valvular heart disease is usually minor and rarely severe.

Incidence

If highly sensitive tests capable of identifying subclinical hemolysis such as haptoglobin or erythrocyte creatine are used, evidence of hemolysis is present in a majority of aortic valves prostheses and is common in other locations. The incidence with transcatheter aortic valve replacement is less than 30%.[98,103,104] Clinically significant hemolytic disease with detectable red cell fragments is much less common. The hemoglobin concentrations of groups of patients with prosthetic valves generally do not differ from matched controls.[98] An incidence of clinically significant hemolysis of 3% to 5% is probably a reasonable estimate for contemporary series.[105]

Clinical Manifestations

No distinctive clinical features are noted, other than those related to preexistent heart disease or cardiac surgery. The development of hemolysis sometimes coincides with severe deterioration of cardiac function because of the tear of a valve cusp or the loosening of valve attachments. When the hemolysis is clinically significant, jaundice may be present.

Laboratory Findings

The blood findings of these patients vary widely, depending on the severity of the hemolytic process. The hemoglobin level may be normal if the hemolysis is compensated, but it may be extremely low. Most cells are normocytic and normochromic, but there are also variable numbers of fragmented erythrocytes identical to the schistocytes seen in patients with microangiopathic hemolytic anemia (*Figure 33.4*). The number of fragmented cells apparent in the blood smear directly reflects the severity of the hemolytic process and the degree of turbulent flow. In patients with long-standing hemolysis, iron stores may be depleted because of hemoglobinuria and hemosiderinuria and the red cells may appear hypochromic because of iron deficiency. Hemosiderinuria is present in many patients when hemoglobinuria is not detectable. The serum bilirubin level is slightly or moderately raised. Serum haptoglobin is reduced or absent. Lactic dehydrogenase levels are usually elevated. The reaction to the antiglobulin test is usually, but not always, negative. On rare occasions, a positive direct antiglobulin test is observed in patients with valve disease.[106] Mechanical damage may expose subsurface antigens, which then elicit the production of autoantibodies.

Treatment

Primary management is directed toward resolving the problem of turbulent flow. Hematologic management is essentially supportive. When iron deficiency develops because of prolonged hemosiderinuria, iron therapy is indicated. Erythropoietin has been used to reduce the need for blood transfusion in the rare patients with severe sustained hemolysis.[106] Folate supplementation may also assist in maintaining an adequate erythropoietic response to hemolysis.

Small Vessel Disease (Microangiopathic Hemolytic Anemia)

The term *microangiopathic hemolytic anemia* was coined originally to describe thrombotic thrombocytopenic purpura (TTP). It is now used to designate any hemolytic anemia related to red cell fragmentation occurring in association with small vessel disease (*Table 33.3*). The term *thrombotic microangiopathy* is also used to describe syndromes characterized by hemolytic anemia with red cell fragmentation, thrombocytopenia, and thrombotic lesions in small blood vessels.

TTP and the hemolytic uremic syndrome (HUS) are similar disorders included in this category. They share many laboratory and clinical features, and the clinical distinction between TTP and HUS is not always clear. There are also TTP/HUS-related conditions seen with pregnancy, cancer, collagen vascular disease, drug therapy, tissue transplantation, and other disorders (*Table 33.3*). A detailed discussion of TTP, HUS, and related disorders can be found in Chapter 49, and TTP related to pregnancy is discussed in Chapter 43.

Hemolysis Due to Malignant Hypertension

An association between red cell fragmentation and malignant hypertension was first recorded in 1954 and has since been confirmed in many other studies.[107] The pathogenesis of microangiopathic hemolytic anemia in malignant hypertension is attributed to the presence of fibrinoid necrosis within the arterioles, which, in turn, appears to depend on the presence of hypertension.

Hemolysis Due to Disseminated Intravascular Coagulation

Microangiopathic hemolytic anemia is associated with a variety of disorders characterized by disseminated intravascular coagulation, including sepsis, purpura fulminans, heat stroke, and abruptio placentae. In all of these clinical conditions, red cell fragmentation is thought to result from the deposition of fibrin within the microvasculature. Fortunately, hemolysis is often not severe and may not contribute significantly to the morbidity of the disease. Because the underlying disease comes under control with appropriate therapy, the fragmentation of red cells also ceases.[108,109]

Fragmentation Hemolysis With Immune Disorders

Microangiopathic hemolytic anemia may be a feature of diseases in which the microvasculature is damaged by immune mechanisms. Connective tissue diseases characterized by vasculitis, which occasionally lead to red cell fragmentation, include lupus erythematosus,[110] rheumatoid arthritis, Sjögren syndrome, polyarteritis nodosa, polymyositis, scleroderma, Wegener granulomatosis, giant cell arteritis, and Still disease.[111-113] The diverse symptomatology of vasculitic disorders, along with the presence of microangiopathic hemolysis, may lead to these disorders being confused with TTP. ADAMTS13 activity levels, although often lower in vasculitic disorders than in healthy patients, are rarely as low as is typical for TTP (discussed in Chapter 49).[114] Microangiopathic hemolysis in vasculitic disorders is attributed to immune complex mechanisms.

Giant Hemangiomas and Hemangioendotheliomas

Microangiopathic hemolytic anemia has been identified in patients with giant hemangiomas (Kasabach-Merritt syndrome and similar disorders) and in patients with hemangioendotheliomas of the liver.[115,116] It is thought that local coagulation in the abnormal blood vessels plays a role in red cell fragmentation.[117] Management of the hemangioma by surgery or chemotherapy resolves the microangiopathic hemolytic anemia and consumption coagulopathy.

March Hemoglobinuria

March hemoglobinuria is an unusual hemolytic disorder in which transient hemoglobinemia and hemoglobinuria develop in susceptible individuals after strenuous exercise that involves forceful contact of the body with a hard surface. Although red cell fragmentation is not always evident, the condition carries all the hallmarks of acute intravascular hemolysis, which presumably results from the mechanical disruption of circulating red cells. Relatively few cases have been reported since Fleischer described the first case in 1881. Clinically inapparent hemoglobinemia may be more common.

March hemoglobinuria primarily affects young persons. Although apparently more common in males, it is also reported in women. Hemoglobinuria is precipitated by prolonged marches or competitive running, but the syndrome has also been noted with repetitive hand strikes, as in karate practitioners or conga drum players.[118] Passage of red or dark urine after physical exertion is often the only complaint. Occasionally, symptoms include nausea; vague abdominal, back, or thigh pain; or a burning feeling in the soles of the feet. Renal failure from hemoglobin toxicity has been reported.[119] Hemoglobinuria

characteristically occurs immediately after exercise and lasts for only a few hours. March hemoglobinuria most commonly affects athletes at the beginning of a running career or on resumption of road training.[120]

Laboratory studies show evidence of intravascular hemolysis, specifically hemoglobinemia and a decreased serum haptoglobin concentration. Significant anemia is uncommon. The bilirubin concentration rarely exceeds 2 mg/dL. Serum lactic dehydrogenase levels may be elevated. The urine contains hemoglobin; after recurrences, it may also contain hemosiderin. Long-distance runners may develop iron deficiency attributable to hemosiderinuria, although the possibility of exercise-associated gastrointestinal bleeding in long-distance runners must also be considered.[121] Swimmers, who do not sustain comparable trauma, can have a similar clinical scenario.[122,123]

Hemoglobinuria can be prevented by the use of shoes with thicker and more resilient soles than those usually worn. There is some experimental data (using tubes of blood placed in the shoe soles of susceptible individuals and controls) suggesting that gait or running technique plays a role.[124]

No specific therapy is usually needed for individuals with march hemoglobinuria. Attacks may be prevented by wearing shoes with more resilient soles and by changing to a less traumatic running style. Banfi and colleagues have reported that immersion of the legs in cold water for several minutes, either before or after training, prevents hemolysis and hemoglobinuria in rugby players.[125]

OTHER CAUSES OF HEMOLYSIS

Hemolytic anemia is also seen in association with a number of nonhematologic systemic disorders, and in most cases, there are several etiologies to the anemia.

Hypersplenism

Normal functions of the spleen include the monitoring and processing of "old" and "damaged" red cells. These functions are executed by macrophages that line reticuloendothelial sinuses of the spleen, and also the liver and bone marrow (see Chapter 66). Macrophages have receptors that recognize immunoglobulin and complement molecules on the RBC surface and, possibly, receptors that detect alterations in the outer portion of the phospholipid bilayer. The spleen is the most stringent of the reticuloendothelial filters, and this is aided by the slow rate of blood flow through the splenic red pulp.

Broadly defined, the term *hypersplenism* refers to sequestration and/or destruction of blood cells occurring in an enlarged spleen, associated with peripheral anemia, neutropenia, and/or thrombocytopenia. In humans, it is generally held that splenomegaly from any cause can be associated with increased filtering, extended macrophage attack, and increased erythrocyte destruction.[126] Rarely does hypersplenism cause significant hemolysis. However, under conditions where macrophages are activated, there may be increased red cell destruction, and this may explain the accelerated hemolysis commonly seen with splenomegaly in infections, in particular with malaria.[13]

Massive splenomegaly is often associated with an increased plasma volume, and in these cases, the low hemoglobin or hematocrit gives a falsely low estimate of the true red cell mass.

Liver Disease

Anemia in liver disease has many causes, including hemolysis. Etiologies of hemolysis in liver disease include portal hypertension and associated splenomegaly, spur cell anemia, and other less obvious red cell membrane changes associated with an altered pattern of lipid deposition in liver disease. These are discussed in Chapter 42.

The hemolysis from portal hypertension and splenomegaly is generally mild, with varying degrees of compensatory increase in red cell production. Attempts to correct portal hypertension have utilized angiographic techniques to create a communication between the intrahepatic portal vein and the hepatic vein. The placement of these transjugular intrahepatic portosystemic shunts avoids the anesthetic and surgical risks of other shunting procedures; however, some 10% of patients develop mild intravascular hemolysis.[127] The hemolysis is usually self-limited and rarely requires intervention.

Renal Disease

Hemolytic anemia and renal failure together can occur with the thrombotic microangiopathies (see Chapter 49). Anemia is also a frequent complication of primary renal disease, the most common cause being as a result of impaired erythropoietin production (see Chapter 42). However, in some cases, there is also a hemolytic component to the anemia of renal failure. In part, it may reflect effects of metabolites that accumulate in uremia and that correct with more aggressive dialysis, and, in part, it may reflect abnormal red cell membrane phospholipid expression, analogous to that seen in liver disease.[128,129] These are discussed in Chapter 42.

Hypophosphatemia

Severe hypophosphatemia can occur in patients undergoing prolonged antacid therapy, in those receiving intravenous hyperalimentation without phosphorus supplementation, in debilitated and starved people, and in alcoholics. In addition to confusion, weakness, anorexia, malaise, paresthesias, and electroencephalographic and electromyographic changes, hypophosphatemia can cause hemolytic anemia.[130] Microspherocytosis can be a feature of this syndrome.

POSTPERFUSION SYNDROME

Cardiopulmonary bypass can be associated with several adverse reactions, including acute intravascular hemolysis, leukopenia, a hemostatic deficit, and nonspecific systemic inflammatory reactions, collectively referred to as the postperfusion syndrome.

After cardiopulmonary bypass, intravascular hemolysis can occur with hemoglobinemia.[131] The mechanism of hemolysis associated in these patients is not damage from mechanical forces during bypass but is rather complement activation with resultant deposition of C5b-9 on red cells and immediate intravascular hemolysis.[132]

The hemolytic process is transient. Hematologic treatment is directed toward RBC support as needed until spontaneous resolution occurs.

References

1. Hay SI, Guerra CA, Gething PW, et al. A world malaria map: plasmodium falciparum endemicity in 2007. *PLoS Med.* 2009;6(3):e1000048.
2. Guerra CA, Snow RW, Hay SI. Mapping the global extent of malaria in 2005. *Trends Parasitol.* 2006;22(8):353-358.
3. Gelband H, Bogoch II, Rodriguez PS, et al. Is malaria an important cause of death among adults? *Am J Trop Med Hyg.* 2020;103(1):41-47.
4. Mace KE, Lucchi NW, Tan KR. Malaria surveillance - United States, 2017. *MMWR Surveill Summ.* 2021;70(2):1-35.
5. Allain JP. Malaria and transfusion: a neglected subject coming back to the forefront. *Clin Infect Dis.* 2010;51(10):1199-1200.
6. Alavi SM, Alavi L, Jaafari F. Outbreak investigation of needle sharing-induced malaria, Ahvaz, Iran. *Int J Infect Dis.* 2010;14(3):e240-e242.
7. Sypniewska P, Duda JF, Locatelli I, Althaus CR, Althaus F, Genton B. Clinical and laboratory predictors of death in African children with features of severe malaria: a systematic review and meta-analysis. *BMC Med.* 2017;15(1):147.
8. White NJ, Pukrittayakamee S, Hien TT, Faiz MA, Mokuolu OA, Dondorp AM. Malaria. *Lancet.* 2014;383(9918):723-735.
9. White NJ. Anaemia and malaria. *Malar J.* 2018;17(1):371.
10. Perrin LH, Mackey LJ, Miescher PA. The hematology of malaria in man. *Semin Hematol.* 1982;19(2):70-82.
11. Okafor HU, Nwaiwu O. Anemia of persistent malarial parasitemia in Nigerian children. *J Trop Pediatr.* 2001;47(5):271-275.
12. Saravu K, Docherla M, Vasudev A, Shastry BA. Thrombocytopenia in vivax and falciparum malaria: an observational study of 131 patients in Karnataka, India. *Ann Trop Med Parasitol.* 2011;105(8):593-598.
13. Leoni S, Buonfrate D, Angheben A, Gobbi F, Bisoffi Z. The hyper-reactive malarial splenomegaly: a systematic review of the literature. *Malar J.* 2015;14:185.
14. Langhi DM, Jr, Bordin JO. Duffy blood group and malaria. *Hematology.* 2006;11(5):389-398.
15. Resende SS, Milagres VG, Chaves DG, et al. Increased susceptibility of blood type O individuals to develop anemia in Plasmodium vivax infection. *Infect Genet Evol.* 2017;50:87-92.
16. Satchwell TJ. Erythrocyte invasion receptors for Plasmodium falciparum: new and old. *Transfus Med.* 2016;26(2):77-88.
17. Tham WH, Schmidt CQ, Hauhart RE, et al. Plasmodium falciparum uses a key functional site in complement receptor type-1 for invasion of human erythrocytes. *Blood.* 2011;118(7):1923-1933.
18. Gritzmacher CA, Reese RT. Reversal of knob formation on Plasmodium falciparum-infected erythrocytes. *Science.* 1984;226(4670):65-67.
19. Davis TM, Krishna S, Looareesuwan S, et al. Erythrocyte sequestration and anemia in severe falciparum malaria. Analysis of acute changes in venous hematocrit using a simple mathematical model. *J Clin Invest.* 1990;86(3):793-800.
20. Ong'echa JM, Davenport GC, Vulule JM, Hittner JB, Perkins DJ. Identification of inflammatory biomarkers for pediatric malarial anemia severity using novel statistical methods. *Infect Immun.* 2011;79(11):4674-4680. IAI.
21. Leowattana W, Krudsood S, Tangpukdee N, Brittenham G, Looareesuwan S. Defective erythropoietin production and reticulocyte response in acute Plasmodium falciparum malaria-associated anemia. *Southeast Asian J Trop Med Public Health.* 2008;39(4):581-588.
22. Casals-Pascual C, Huang H, Lakhal-Littleton S, et al. Hepcidin demonstrates a biphasic association with anemia in acute Plasmodium falciparum malaria. *Haematologica.* 2012;97(11):1695-1698.
23. Awandare GA, Kempaiah P, Ochiel DO, Piazza P, Keller CC, Perkins DJ. Mechanisms of erythropoiesis inhibition by malarial pigment and malaria-induced proinflammatory mediators in an in vitro model. *Am J Hematol.* 2011;86(2):155-162.
24. Wickramasinghe SN, Looareesuwan S, Nagachinta B, White NJ. Dyserythropoiesis and ineffective erythropoiesis in Plasmodium vivax malaria. *Br J Haematol.* 1989;72(1):91-99.
25. Abdalla S, Weatherall DJ. The direct antiglobulin test in P. falciparum malaria. *Br J Haematol.* 1982;51(3):415-425.
26. Tamez PA, Liu H, Fernandez-Pol S, Haldar K, Wickrema A. Stage-specific susceptibility of human erythroblasts to Plasmodium falciparum malaria infection. *Blood.* 2009;114(17):3652-3655.
27. Bruneel F, Gachot B, Wolff M, et al. Resurgence of blackwater fever in long-term European expatriates in Africa: report of 21 cases and review. *Clin Infect Dis.* 2001;32(8):1133-1140.
28. Lon C, Spring M, Sok S, et al. Blackwater fever in an uncomplicated Plasmodium falciparum patient treated with dihydroartemisinin-piperaquine. *Malar J.* 2014;13:96.
29. Kariuki SN, Williams TN. Human genetics and malaria resistance. *Hum Genet.* 2020;139(6-7):801-811.
30. Roberts DJ, Williams TN. Haemoglobinopathies and resistance to malaria. *Redox Rep.* 2003;8(5):304-310.
31. Husain-Chishti A, Ruff P. Malaria and ovalocytosis--molecular mimicry? *Biochim Biophys Acta.* 1991;1096(3):263-264.
32. Bronzan RN, McMorrow ML, Kachur SP. Diagnosis of malaria: challenges for clinicians in endemic and non-endemic regions. *Mol Diagn Ther.* 2008;12(5):299-306.
33. Runsewe-Abiodun IT, Efunsile M, Ghebremedhin B, et al. Malaria diagnostics: a comparative study of blood microscopy, a rapid diagnostic test and polymerase chain reaction in the diagnosis of malaria. *J Trop Pediatr.* 2012;58(2):163-164.
34. Mulenga M, Malunga P, Bennett S, et al. Folic acid treatment of Zambian children with moderate to severe malaria anemia. *Am J Trop Med Hyg.* 2006;74(6):986-990.
35. Lalloo DG, Shingadia D, Bell DJ, Beeching NJ, Whitty CJM, Chiodini PL. UK malaria treatment guidelines 2016. *J Infect.* 2016;72(6):635-649.
36. Krause PJ. Human babesiosis. *Int J Parasitol.* 2019;49(2):165-174.
37. Cable RG, Leiby DA. Risk and prevention of transfusion-transmitted babesiosis and other tick-borne diseases. *Curr Opin Hematol.* 2003;10(6):405-411.
38. Homer MJ, Aguilar-Delfin I, Telford SR,IIIrd, Krause PJ, Persing DH. Babesiosis. *Clin Microbiol Rev.* 2000;13(3):451-469.
39. Gibbons MD, Mendoza DP, Waheed A, Barshak MB, Villalba JA. Case 14-2021: a 64-year-old woman with fever and pancytopenia. *N Engl J Med.* 2021;384(19):1849-1857.
40. Roberts DJ. Hematologic changes asociated with specific infections in the tropics. *Hematol Oncol Clin North Am.* 2016;30(2):395-415.
41. Fleming AF. Haematological manifestations of malaria and other parasitic diseases. *Clin Haematol.* 1981;10(3):983-1011.
42. Buonomano R, Brinkmann F, Leupin N, et al. Holiday souvenirs from the Mediterranean: three instructive cases of visceral leishmaniasis. *Scand J Infect Dis.* 2009;41(10):777-781.
43. Li Volti S, Fischer A, Musumeci S. Hematological and serological aspects of Mediterranean kala-azar in infancy and childhood. *Acta Trop.* 1980;37(4):351-365.
44. Saha Roy S, Chowdhury KD, Sen G, Biswas T. Oxidation of hemoglobin and redistribution of band 3 promote erythrophagocytosis in visceral leishmaniasis. *Mol Cell Biochem.* 2009;321(1-2):53-63.
45. Gomes C, Ruiz J. Carrion's disease: the sound of silence. *Clin Microbiol Rev.* 2018;31(1):e00056-17.
46. Chamberlin J, Laughlin LW, Romero S, et al. Epidemiology of endemic Bartonella bacilliformis: a prospective cohort study in a Peruvian mountain valley community. *J Infect Dis.* 2002;186(7):983-990.
47. Maguina C, Garcia PJ, Gotuzzo E, Cordero L, Spach DH. Bartonellosis (Carrión's disease) in the modern era. *Clin Infect Dis.* 2001;33(6):772-779.
48. Angelakis E, Raoult D. Pathogenicity and treatment of Bartonella infections. *Int J Antimicrob Agents.* 2014;44(1):16-25.
49. Fujita H, Nishimura S, Kurosawa S, Akiya I, Nakamura-Uchiyama F, Ohnishi K. Clinical and epidemiological features of *Clostridium perfringens* bacteremia: a review of 18 cases over 8 year-period in a tertiary care center in metropolitan Tokyo area in Japan. *Intern Med.* 2010;49(22):2433-2437.
50. Smit B, van der Helm MW, Bosma M, Hudig F, Russcher H. Massive hemolysis due to *Clostridium perfringens*: a laboratory's perspective. *Clin Chem Lab Med.* 2020;58(11):e295-e297.
51. Hubl W, Mostbeck B, Hartleb H, Pointner H, Kofler K, Bayer PM. Investigation of the pathogenesis of massive hemolysis in a case of *Clostridium perfringens* septicemia. *Ann Hematol.* 1993;67(3):145-147.
52. Watt J, Amini A, Mosier J, et al. Treatment of severe hemolytic anemia caused by *Clostridium perfringens* sepsis in a liver transplant recipient. *Surg Infect.* 2012;13(1):60-62.

53. De Franceschi L, Fattovich G, Turrini F, et al. Hemolytic anemia induced by riba-virin therapy in patients with chronic hepatitis C virus infection: role of membrane oxidative damage. *Hepatology*. 2000;31(4):997-1004.

54. Grattagliano I, Russmann S, Palmieri VO, Portincasa P, Palasciano G, Lauterburg BH. Glutathione peroxidase, thioredoxin, and membrane protein changes in erythro-cytes predict ribavirin-induced anemia. *Clin Pharmacol Ther*. 2005;78(4):422-432.

55. Chan TK, Chan WC, Weed RI. Erythrocyte hemighosts: a hallmark of severe oxida-tive injury in vivo. *Br J Haematol*. 1982;50(4):575-582.

56. Pakulska D, Czerczak S. Hazardous effects of arsine: a short review. *Int J Occup Med Environ Health*. 2006;19(1):36-44.

57. Song Y, Wang D, Li H, Hao F, Ma J, Xia Y. Severe acute arsine poisoning treated by plasma exchange. *Clin Toxicol*. 2007;45(6):721-727.

58. Danielson C, Houseworth J, Skipworth E, Smith D, McCarthy L, Nanagas K. Arsine toxicity treated with red blood cell and plasma exchanges. *Transfusion*. 2006;46(9):1576-1579.

59. Schwartz BS, Hu H. Adult lead exposure: time for change. *Environ Health Perspect*. 2007;115(3):451-454.

60. Chandran L, Cataldo R. Lead poisoning: basics and new developments. *Pediatr Rev*. 2010;31(10):399-405. quiz 406.

61. Baranowska-Bosiacka I, Dziedziejko V, Safranow K, et al. Inhibition of erythrocyte phosphoribosyltransferases (APRT and HPRT) by Pb2+: a potential mechanism of lead toxicity. *Toxicology*. 2009;259(1-2):77-83.

62. Casado MF, Cecchini AL, Simao AN, Oliveira RD, Cecchini R. Free radical-mediated pre-hemolytic injury in human red blood cells subjected to lead acetate as evaluated by chemiluminescence. *Food Chem Toxicol*. 2007;45(6):945-952.

63. Kim JJ, Kim YS, Kumar V. Heavy metal toxicity: an update of chelating therapeutic strategies. *J Trace Elem Med Biol*. 2019;54:226-231.

64. Franchitto N, Gandia-Mailly P, Georges B, et al. Acute copper sulphate poisoning: a case report and literature review. *Resuscitation*. 2008;78(1):92-96.

65. Fernandes A, Mira ML, Azevedo MS, Manso C. Mechanisms of hemolysis induced by copper. *Free Radic Res Commun*. 1988;4(5):291-298.

66. Patil M, Sheth KA, Krishnamurthy AC, Devarbhavi H. A review and current per-spective on Wilson disease. *J Clin Exp Hepatol*. 2013;3(4):321-336.

67. Asfaha S, Almansori M, Qarni U, Gutfreund KS. Plasmapheresis for hemo-lytic crisis and impending acute liver failure in Wilson disease. *J Clin Apher*. 2007;22(5):295-298.

68. Zatopkova L, Hejna P, Janik M. Hemolytic staining of the endocardium of the left heart chambers: a new sign for autopsy diagnosis of freshwater drowning. *Forensic Sci Med Pathol*. 2015;11(1):65-68.

69. Pendergrast JM, Hladunewich MA, Richardson RM. Hemolysis due to inadvertent hemodialysis against distilled water: perils of bedside dialysate preparation. *Crit Care Med*. 2006;34(10):2666-2673.

70. Robinson JR, Kennedy VE, Doss Y, Bastarache L, Denny J, Warner JL. Defining the complex phenotype of severe systemic loxoscelism using a large electronic health record cohort. *PLoS One*. 2017;12(4):e0174941.

71. Murray LM, Seger DL. Hemolytic anemia following a presumptive brown recluse spider bite. *J Toxicol Clin Toxicol*. 1994;32(4):451-456.

72. Gehrie EA, Nian H, Young PP. Brown Recluse spider bite mediated hemolysis: clin-ical features, a possible role for complement inhibitor therapy, and reduced RBC surface glycophorin A as a potential biomarker of venom exposure. *PLoS One*. 2013;8(9):e76558.

73. Prevention CDC. Necrotic arachnidism—pacific northwest, 1988-1996. *MMWR Morb Mortal Wkly Rep*. 1996;45(21):433-436.

74. Tambourgi DV, Morgan BP, de Andrade RM, Magnoli FC, van Den Berg CW. Loxosceles intermedia spider envenomation induces activation of an endogenous metalloproteinase, resulting in cleavage of glycophorins from the erythrocyte sur-face and facilitating complement-mediated lysis. *Blood*. 2000;95(2):683-691.

75. Van Den Berg CW, De Andrade RM, Magnoli FC, Marchbank KJ, Tambourgi DV. Loxosceles spider venom induces metalloproteinase mediated cleavage of MCP/CD46 and MHCI and induces protection against C-mediated lysis. *Immunology*. 2002;107(1):102-110.

76. Chaves-Moreira D, Chaim OM, Sade YB, et al. Identification of a direct hemolytic effect dependent on the catalytic activity induced by phospholipase-D (dermone-crotic toxin) from brown spider venom. *J Cell Biochem*. 2009;107(4):655-666.

77. Longbottom J, Shearer FM, Devine M, et al. Vulnerability to snakebite envenoming: a global mapping of hotspots. *Lancet*. 2018;392(10148):673-684.

78. Isbister GK. Snakebite doesn't cause disseminated intravascular coagulation: coag-ulopathy and thrombotic microangiopathy in snake envenoming. *Semin Thromb Hemost*. 2010;36(4):444-451.

79. Oliveira IS., Cardoso IA, Bordon K.CF, et al. Global proteomic and functional anal-ysis of *Crotalus durissus* collineatus individual venom variation and its impact on envenoming. *J Proteonomics*. 2019;191:153-165.

80. Mukherje AK, Ghosal SK, Maity CR. Some biochemical properties of Russell's viper (*Daboia russelli*) venom from Eastern India: correlation with clinico-pathological manifestation in Russell's viper bite. *Toxicon*. 2000;38(2):163-175.

81. Yamamoto C, Tsuru D, Oda-Ueda N, Ohno M, Hattori S, Kim ST. Trimeresurus flavoviridis (habu snake) venom induces human erythrocyte lysis through enzymatic lipolysis, complement activation and decreased membrane expression of CD55 and CD59. *Pharmacol Toxicol*. 2001;89(4):188-194.

82. Chiou SH, Chuang MH, Hung CC, et al. Inhibition of protein kinase C by snake venom toxins: comparison of enzyme inhibition, lethality and hemolysis among dif-ferent cardiotoxin isoforms. *Biochem Mol Biol Int*. 1995;35(5):1103-1112.

83. Kolecki P. Delayed toxic reaction following massive bee envenomation. *Ann Emerg Med*. 1999;33(1):114-116.

84. Rahimian R, Shirazi FM, Schmidt JO, Klotz SA. Honeybee stings in the era of killer bees: anaphylaxis and toxic envenomation. *Am J Med*. 2020;133(5):621-626.

85. Bresolin NL, Carvalho LC, Goes EC, Fernandes R, Barotto AM. Acute renal failure following massive attack by Africanized bee stings. *Pediatr Nephrol*. 2002;17(8):625-627.

86. Munoz-Arizpe R, Valencia-Espinoza L, Velasquez-Jones L, Abarca-Franco C, Gamboa-Marrufo J, Valencia-Mayoral P. Africanized bee stings and pathogenesis of acute renal failure. *Nephron*. 1992;61(4):478.

87. Lawrence C, Atac B. Hematologic changes in massive burn injury. *Crit Care Med*. 1992;20(9):1284-1288.

88. Kilyewala C, Alenyo R, Ssentongo R. Determinants and time to blood transfu-sion among thermal burn patients admitted to Mulago Hospital. *BMC Res Notes*. 2017;10(1):258.

89. Dépret F, Dunyach C, De Tymowski C, et al. Undetectable haptoglobin is asso-ciated with major adverse kidney events in critically ill burn patients. *Crit Care*. 2017;21(1):245.

90. Dinsdale RJ, Devi A, Hampson P, et al. Changes in novel haematological param-eters following thermal injury: a prospective observational cohort study. *Sci Rep*. 2017;7:3211.

91. Davies JW, Topley E. The disappearance of red cells in patients with burns. *Clin Sci*. 1956;15(1):135-148.

92. Posluszny JA, Muthumalaiappan K, Kini A, et al. Burn injury dampens erythroid cell production through reprioritizing bone marrow hematopoietic response. *J Trauma*. 2011;71(5):1288-1296.

93. Poder TG, Nonkani WG, Tsakeu Leponkouo E. Blood warming and hemolysis: a systematic review with meta-analysis. *Transfus Med Rev*. 2015;29(3):172-180.

94. Ivanov IT, Zheleva A, Zlatanov I. Anion exchanger and the resistance against ther-mal haemolysis. *Int J Hyperther*. 2011;27(3):286-296.

95. Dimitriou PA, Depascouale AK, Germenis AE, Antipas SE. Kinetics of heat-damaged homologous erythrocytes. A five-compartmental analysis. *Eur J Nucl Med*. 1990;17(1-2):49-54.

96. Wu N, Foung S, Hoopes P, Lizak G, Smith S. Microwave heat-induced hemolysis. *Clin Pediatr*. 1985;24(11):645-645.

97. Sayed HM, Dacie JV, Handley DA, Lewis SM, Cleland WP. Haemolytic anaemia of mechanical origin after open heart surgery. *Thorax*. 1961;16:356-360.

98. Okumiya T, Ishikawa-Nishi M, Doi T, et al. Evaluation of intravascular hemoly-sis with erythrocyte creatine in patients with cardiac valve prostheses. *Chest*. 2004;125(6):2115-2120.

99. Dasi LP, Simon HA, Sucosky P, Yoganathan AP. Fluid mechanics of artificial heart valves. *Clin Exp Pharmacol Physiol*. 2009;36(2):225-237.

100. Shapira Y, Vaturi M, Sagie A. Hemolysis associated with prosthetic heart valves: a review. *Cardiol Rev*. 2009;17(3):121-124.

101. Sideris EB, Leung M, Yoon JH, et al. Occlusion of large atrial septal defects with a centering buttoned device: early clinical experience. *Am Heart J*. 1996;131(2):356-359.

102. Gopalan RS, Arabia FA, Noel P, Chandrasekaran K. Hemolysis from aortic regurgi-tation mimicking pump thrombosis in a patient with a HeartMate II left ventricular assist device: a case report. *ASAIO J*. 2012;58(3):278-280.

103. Sugiura T, Okumiya T, Kubo T, Takeuchi H, Matsumura Y. Evaluation of intravas-cular hemolysis with erythrocyte creatine in patients with aortic stenosis. *Int Heart J*. 2016;57(4):430-433.

104. Širáková A, Toušek P, Bednář F, et al. Intravascular haemolysis after transcatheter aortic valve implantation with self-expandable prosthesis: incidence, severity, and impact on long-term mortality. *Eur Heart J Suppl*. 2020;22(suppl F):F44-f50.

105. Demirsoy E, Yilmaz O, Sirin G, et al. Hemolysis after mitral valve repair: a report of five cases and literature review. *J Heart Valve Dis*. 2008;17(1):24-30.

106. Huang HL, Lin FC, Hung KC, Wang PN, Wu D. Hemolytic anemia in native valve infective endocarditis: a case report and literature review. *Jpn Circ J*. 1999;63(5):400-403.

107. Mitaka H, Yamada Y, Hamada O, Kosaka S, Fujiwara N, Miyakawa Y. Malignant hypertension with thrombotic microangiopathy. *Intern Med*. 2016;55(16):2277-2280.

108. Kurosawa S, Stearns-Kurosawa DJ. Complement, thrombotic microangiopathy and disseminated intravascular coagulation. *J Intensive care*. 2014;2(1):65.

109. Boral BM, Williams DJ, Boral LI. Disseminated intravascular coagulation. *Am J Clin Pathol*. 2016;146(6):670-680.

110. Lansigan F, Isufi I, Tagoe CE. Microangiopathic haemolytic anaemia resembling thrombotic thrombocytopenic purpura in systemic lupus erythematosus: the role of ADAMTS13. *Rheumatology (Oxford)*. 2011;50(5):824-829.

111. Shenkman B, Einav Y. Thrombotic thrombocytopenic purpura and other thrombotic microangiopathic hemolytic anemias: diagnosis and classification. *Autoimmun Rev*. 2014;13(4-5):584-586.

112. Quemeneur T, Noel LH, Kyndt X, et al. Thrombotic microangiopathy in adult Still's disease. *Scand J Rheumatol*. 2005;34(5):399-403.

113. George JN, Charania RS. Evaluation of patients with microangiopathic hemolytic anemia and thrombocytopenia. *Semin Thromb Hemost*. 2013;39(2):153-160.

114. Liu F, Feys HB, Dong N, Zhao Y, Ruan C. Alteration of ADAMTS13 antigen lev-els in patients with idiopathic thrombotic thrombocytopenic purpura, idiopathic thrombocytopenic purpura and systemic lupus erythematosus. *Thromb Haemost*. 2006;95(4):749-750.

115. O'Rafferty C, O'Regan GM, Irvine AD, Smith OP. Recent advances in the patho-biology and management of Kasabach-Merritt phenomenon. *Br J Haematol*. 2015;171(1):38-51.

116. Banton KL, D'Cunha J, Laudi N, et al. Postoperative severe microangiopathic hemo-lytic anemia associated with a giant hepatic cavernous hemangioma. *J Gastrointest Surg*. 2005;9(5):679-685.

117. Inceman S, Tangun Y. Chronic defibrination syndrome due to a giant heman-gioma associated with microangiopathic hemolytic anemia. *Am J Med*. 1969;46(6):997-1002.

118. Vasudev M, Bresnahan BA, Cohen EP, Hari PN, Hariharan S, Vasudev BS. Percussion hemoglobinuria—a novel term for hand trauma-induced mechanical hemolysis: a case report. *J Med Case Rep.* 2011;5:508.

119. Khalighi MA, Henriksen KJ, Chang A, Meehan SM. March hemoglobinuria-associated acute tubular injury. *Clin Kidney J.* 2014;7(5):488-489.

120. Eichner ER. Runner's macrocytosis: a clue to footstrike hemolysis. Runner's anemia as a benefit versus runner's hemolysis as a detriment. *Am J Med.* 1985;78(2):321-325.

121. Thalmann M, Sodeck GH, Kavouras S, et al. Proton pump inhibition prevents gastrointestinal bleeding in ultramarathon runners: a randomised, double blinded, placebo controlled study. *Br J Sports Med.* 2006;40(4):359-362. discussion 362.

122. Pelliccia A, Di Nucci GB. Anemia in swimmers: fact or fiction? Study of hematologic and iron status in male and female top-level swimmers. *Int J Sports Med.* 1987;8(3):227-230.

123. Selby GB, Eichner ER. Endurance swimming, intravascular hemolysis, anemia, and iron depletion. New perspective on athlete's anemia. *Am J Med.* 1986;81(5):791-794.

124. Davidson RJ. March or exertional haemoglobinuria. *Semin Hematol.* 1969;6(2):150-161.

125. Banfi G, Melegati G. Effect on sport hemolysis of cold water leg immersion in athletes after training sessions. *Lab Hematol.* 2008;14(2):15-18.

126. Rosse WF. The spleen as a filter. *N Engl J Med.* 1987;317(11):704-706.

127. Sanyal AJ, Freedman AM, Purdum PP, Shiffman ML, Luketic VA. The hematologic consequences of transjugular intrahepatic portosystemic shunts. *Hepatology.* 1996;23(1):32-39.

128. Bonomini M, Sirolli V. Uremic toxicity and anemia. *J Nephrol.* 2003;16(1):21-28.

129. Bonomini M, Sirolli V, Reale M, Arduini A. Involvement of phosphatidylserine exposure in the recognition and phagocytosis of uremic erythrocytes. *Am J Kidney Dis.* 2001;37(4):807-814.

130. Bacchetta J, Salusky IB. Evaluation of hypophosphatemia: lessons from patients with genetic disorders. *Am J Kidney Dis.* 2012;59(1):152-159.

131. Rezoagli E, Ichinose F, Strelow S, et al. Pulmonary and systemic vascular resistances after cardiopulmonary bypass: role of hemolysis. *J Cardiothorac Vasc Anesth.* 2017;31(2):505-515.

132. Salama A, Hugo F, Heinrich D, et al. Deposition of terminal C5b-9 complement complexes on erythrocytes and leukocytes during cardiopulmonary bypass. *N Engl J Med.* 1988;318(7):408-414.

Chapter 34 ■ Sickle Cell Anemia and Other Sickling Syndromes

PARUL RAI • JANE SILVA HANKINS • JEREMIE E. ESTEPP

INTRODUCTION

This chapter discusses hemoglobin (Hb) variants that cause alterations in erythrocyte morphology and rheology. Sickle Hb (Hb S) is a variant Hb of great clinical importance due to high prevalence and worldwide distribution. There is no reliable assessment of the global burden of Hb S, but more than 100 million individuals are estimated to have a sickle cell trait (Hb S) and the estimated number of newborns born with homozygous Hb SS (sickle cell anemia [SCA]) globally was approximately 300,000 in 2010 and will increase to 400,000 in 2040,[1] making SCA one the most common heritable hematologic diseases affecting humans.

Long before they were recognized in the western hemisphere, sickling disorders were known in Africa by onomatopoeic names denoting the recurrent, unrelenting, and painful nature of the crises. Although symptoms of SCA could be traced in one Ghanaian family to the year 1670,[2] disorders of Hb synthesis went unrecognized by the scientific community until 1910, when James Herrick, a Chicago cardiologist, recorded observations made during investigation of anemia in a 20-year-old West Indian student.[3] Herrick's report led not only to the recognition of hundreds of abnormalities of Hb synthesis but also to a series of remarkable scientific advances involving protein chemistry, molecular biology, physiology, and genetics. The term *sickle cell anemia* was first used in 1922, when it was recognized that a common African ancestry was present in all initial cases described.[4] In 1949, Linus Pauling and collaborators demonstrated for the first time that an abnormal protein was causally linked to a disease, giving rise to the "era of molecular medicine."

Each major hemoglobinopathy occurs in both a heterozygous and a homozygous form. In the heterozygous state, red cells contain both normal adult Hb (Hb A) and the variant Hb. Because they rarely have phenotypic expressions of clinical significance, heterozygotes are said to have the trait for that abnormality, for example, sickle cell trait. In the homozygous state, Hb A is totally lacking, and clinical manifestations are of variable severity; individuals so affected have SCA (Hb SS). In addition, disease may result from the combination of two variant Hbs or from a variant Hb and an interacting thalassemia gene. These double heterozygous states are designated by both aberrant gene products, such as Hb SC disease or Hb S/β-thalassemia. The term *sickle cell disease* is used as an umbrella term to refer to all the sickling syndromes, although the compound heterozygous Hb S/β⁰-thalassemia is commonly grouped with HbSS and referred to as SCA, because of phenotypic similarity to Hb SS.

EPIDEMIOLOGY

Hb S, so called because of the sickle shape it imparts to deoxygenated red cells, is responsible for a wide spectrum of disorders that vary with respect to the degree of anemia, frequency of crises, extent of organ injury, and duration of survival. Some of the sickling syndromes lack significant pathologic potential, but they are easily confused with clinically aggressive disorders based on laboratory evaluation; consequently, precision in diagnosis is essential both to proper clinical management and to meaningful genetic counseling.

The highest prevalence of Hb S in the world is in sub-Saharan Africa, followed by the Arabian and Indian subcontinents. It occurs with lower frequency in the rest of the world as the result of voluntary or forced population migration from high-prevalence areas.[5] Results of studies of deoxyribonucleic acid (DNA) polymorphisms linked to the β^S gene suggest that it arose from three independent mutations in tropical Africa.[6,7] The most common β^S chromosome haplotype is found in Benin and central West Africa. A second haplotype is prevalent in Senegal and the African West Coast, and a third is seen in the Central African Republic (Bantu-speaking Africa). The same three haplotypes are associated with the β^S gene in black Americans and Jamaicans.[8] The Hb S gene in the eastern province of Saudi Arabia and in Central India is associated with a different DNA structure that is not encountered in Africa and probably represents a fourth independent occurrence of the sickle cell mutation.[7] Only the Benin and Senegal haplotypes are prevalent among North Africans, Greeks, and Italians, suggesting that the β^S mutation spread to the Mediterranean basin from West Africa.[7,9] In some parts of Africa, as many as 25% of the population have sickle cell trait, whereas in the United States (among African Americans), Latin America, and the Caribbean, the prevalence of the sickle gene varies from approximately 2% to 8% (*Table 34.1*). In the United States, the expected incidence of SCD at birth among African Americans varies by geographic location. Contemporary data from the Centers for Disease Control (CDC) Registry and Surveillance System for Hemoglobinopathies and recent literature reported variable prevalence by state, ranging from 1 in 260 to 1 in 467 live African American births.[37,38] Taking into account trends in decreased mortality among children, approximately 100,000 cases of SCD would be expected in the United States.[39]

Recognition that sickle cell trait has its highest prevalence in areas that are hyperendemic for malaria suggested that Hb S afforded selective protection against lethal forms of malaria (*Figure 34.1*)[40] and subsequently geographical links between highest HbS allele frequencies and malaria endemicity have been reported on a global scale.[41] In the blood of children with sickle cell trait and malaria, preferential sickling of parasitized cells has been observed, which leads to faster clearance of these infected red cells and impaired parasite growth.[42] An independent mechanism of protection against malaria appears to be mediated by a selective expression of two species of micro-ribonucleic acid (RNA) in sickle trait red blood cells (RBCs), which integrate into *Plasmodium falciparum* mRNAs and inhibit translation and parasite growth.[43,44]

PATHOPHYSIOLOGY

Hb is a tetramer composed of two alpha globin and two beta globin chains. The sickle mutation substitutes thymine for adenine in the sixth codon of the β globin gene (GAG → GTG), thereby encoding valine instead of glutamic acid (p.Glu6Val) in that position. This ostensibly minor change in structure is responsible for profound changes in molecular stability and solubility of the Hb molecule.

Molecular Basis of Sickling

The root cause of sickle cell pathobiology is polymerization of Hb S,[45] resulting in the classically sickled erythrocyte (also known as a

Table 34.1. Worldwide Prevalence of Sickle Cell Trait and Disease

Region	Trait Prevalence (%)	Disease Prevalence (%)	References
Africa			
Nigeria	24.5	2	10-12
Republic of Congo	23.3	0.96	13
Tanzania	13.0		14
Burkina Faso		1.75	15
Uganda	13.3	0.7	16
Europe			
Belgium		0.07	17
France	0.7	0.06	18,19
England		0.05	20
Spain		0.001-0.03	21
South America			
Brazil	4-9.8	0.08-0.3	22-24
Venezuela	2.5		25
North America			
United States (African Americans)	8.0	0.16	26
United States (Hispanics)	0.03-0.06	0.04	23
Central America			
Jamaica	10.0		27
Asia			
India	5.0-7.0	0.4-1.0	28-33
Oman	6.0		34
Saudi Arabia	2.0-27.0	0.2-1.4	35,36

drepanocyte) that may be observed directly with either light or scanning electron microscopy (*Figure 34.2*).

Mammalian Hb transitions between two classic states, known as the relaxed (R) and tense (T) states, which have a high and low affinity for oxygen, respectively. The R state of Hb is normally bound to oxygen, while the T state of Hb is the unbound form.[46] Hb S polymer fibers consist of deoxygenated Hb S in the T state, while HbS in the oxygenated R state is excluded from fibers due to steric hindrance.[45] In individuals with SCD, HbS may polymerize following delivery of oxygen to peripheral tissues while deoxygenated, giving rise to the classic stiff and rigid "sickle-shaped" erythrocyte. This phenomenon then precipitates the complex downstream cascade of events that characterize the disease, including hemolysis, ischemia, vascular-endothelial damage, inflammation, hypercoagulability, increased neutrophil adhesiveness, and platelet activation.[47,48] Upon reoxygenation, these Hb S polymers dissolve or "melt," and the sickle erythrocyte loses most of those pathologic properties.

Structure of Hemoglobin S Polymer

The structure of the deoxygenated Hb S polymer has been deduced from studies involving the use of electron microscopy (*Figure 34.3*) and X-ray diffraction. The polymerized Hb fiber is a helical structure with 14 Hb tetramers in each layer; these form a central core of four strands and an outer sheath of 10 additional strands with an overall diameter of about 21 nm. Only one of the two β6 Val residues appears to participate in the intermolecular contact; it fits into a hydrophobic

pocket formed by a β85 Phe and a β88 Leu residue on a β chain of a nearby Hb S tetramer. Bonds between contact points include both hydrophobic and electrostatic forces.

Physiologic Determinants of Polymerization

The equilibrium between the liquid and solid phases of Hb S is determined by four variables: oxygen tension, Hb S concentration, temperature, and the intraerythocyte concentration of other Hb molecules other than Hb S (e.g., Hb A, Hb A_2, Hb F). Polymerization occurs only with deoxygenation, which results in a fall in oxygen affinity, thereby stabilizing the deoxy state. An increase in 2,3-diphosphoglycerate (DPG) decreases the affinity of Hb S for oxygen and enhances gelation. Likewise, a decrease in pH decreases oxygen affinity via the Bohr effect, thereby increasing the amount of deoxy Hb S at any given oxygen tension. There is a positive correlation between Hb S concentration and gelation. Under standard laboratory conditions, gelation occurs as the concentration of deoxy Hb S is raised above 20.8 g/dL. Because the mean Hb concentration of the red cell is normally >30 g/dL, intracellular gelation of Hb S is a predictable consequence of deoxygenation.

The influence of other Hbs on Hb S polymerization is variable. Both Hb A and Hb F have an inhibitory effect on gelation. When these Hbs are deoxygenated, they enter the sickle polymer less readily than does deoxy Hb S, thereby retarding gelation by a dilutional effect. Other Hbs interfere with polymer formation less well. By measuring the minimum gelling concentration of various mixtures of Hbs, the extent of interaction can be quantitated. Deoxy Hb S molecules copolymerize most effectively with other Hb S molecules and, in decreasing order, with Hb C, D, O-Arab, A, J, and F. In contrast, the doubly heterozygous state for Hb S and hereditary persistence of fetal Hb (HPFH), in which red cells contain approximately 70% Hb S and 30% Hb F, is not associated with clinical disease. Based on Hb F concentration from benign sickle variants such as Hb S/HPFH, an Hb F concentration >10 pg/cell is a threshold above which Hb S polymerization is prevented.[49]

Kinetics of Sickling

Sickling is not an instantaneous phenomenon; the kinetics of sickling suggest that molecular polymerization occurs in stages. The delay period between deoxygenation and polymerization is attributed to nucleation processes, in which Hb S tetramers form small aggregates without modification of internal viscosity. When these aggregates reach a critical mass, a rapid addition of free Hb units occurs to form fibers that then undergo alignment to form a tactoid. A red cell spends <1 to 2 seconds in the arterial circulation and 1 second in the microcirculation; it then takes <15 seconds returning to the lungs. If the delay time is >15 seconds, the cell can return to the lungs and be reoxygenated before any significant polymerization has begun, but if the delay time is between 1 and 15 seconds, gelation occurs while the cell is in the venous circulation. Sickling in the large veins does not produce vaso-occlusion, but the cell membrane may be damaged, resulting in a loss of water and a shorter delay time in subsequent trips through the circulation. If the delay time is less than 1 second, gelation can occur while the cell is in one of the narrow vessels of the microcirculation. Because the cell is much less deformable, it may not be able to "squeeze" through and may become transiently or permanently stuck. Under physiologic conditions, the delay between complete deoxygenation and erythrocyte sickling is <2 seconds. Small increments in deoxyhemoglobin concentration (e.g., those that occur with loss of cell water) profoundly shorten the delay time, thereby potentiating sickling. The delay time, however, is strongly influenced by changes in Hb concentration, the presence of Hbs other than Hb S, temperature, pH, and DPG. Increased intracellular DPG decreases the oxygen-binding affinity of Hb, thereby inducing sickling. In a study of cultured human red cells and mice, the induction of adenosine A(2B) receptor led to increased levels of DPG in the cells, consequently inducing more sickling.[50] Free heme alters the kinetics of sickling; increasing amounts of free heme added to dialyzed Hb S solutions enhance polymerization.[51]

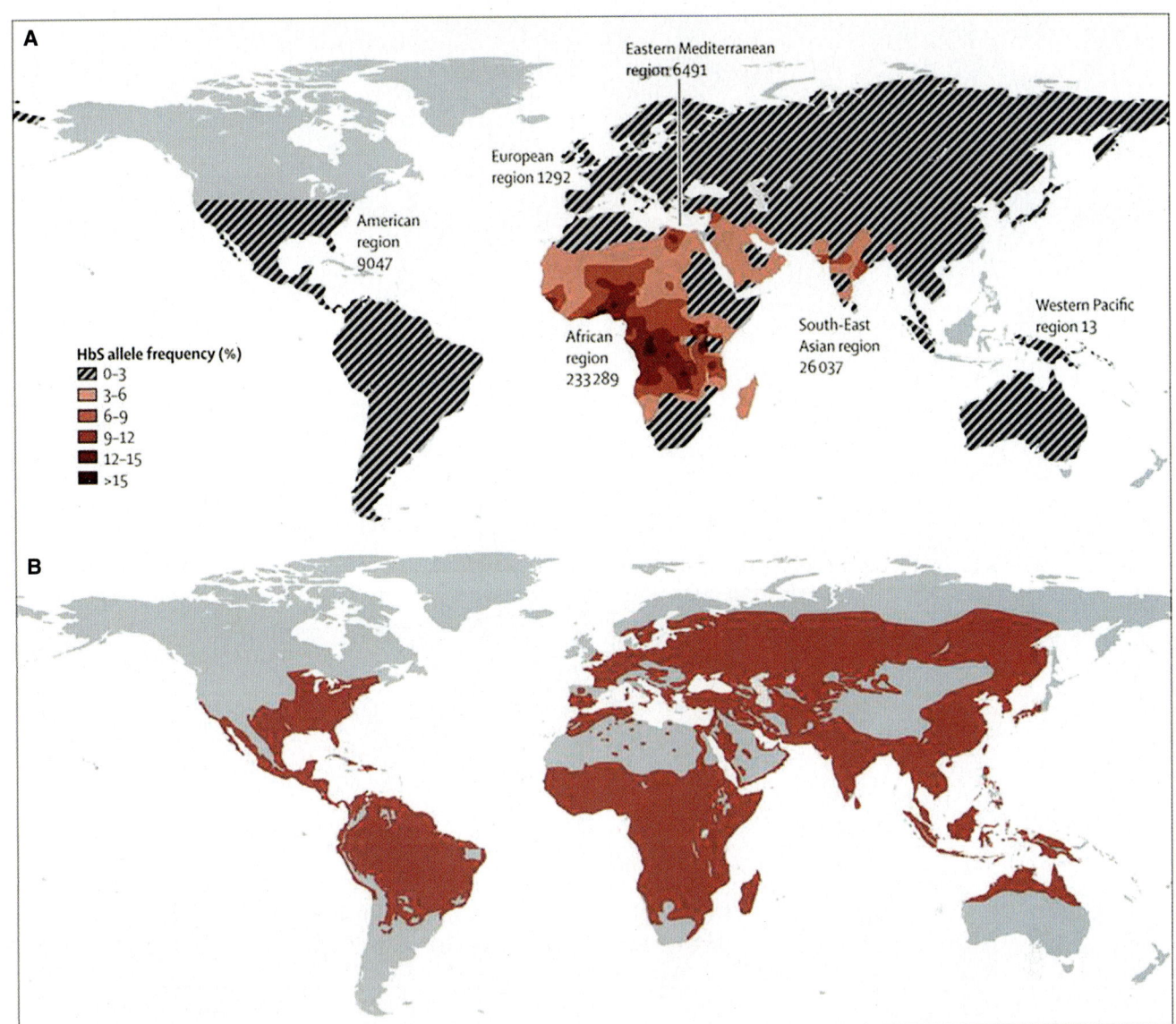

FIGURE 34.1 Global distributions of Hb S and malaria. This map shows the distribution of the Hb S allele. A, Estimates for the combined yearly total number of individuals affected by Hb SS, Hb SC, and Hb Sβ-thalassemia by World Health Organization region. B, The global distribution of malaria (red) before intervention to control malaria. (Reprinted from Rees DC, Williams TN, Gladwin MT. Sickle-cell disease. *Lancet.* 2010;376(9757):2018-2031. Copyright © 2010 Elsevier. With permission.)

(Vertical sidebar text:) Disorders of Red Blood Cells

Red Cell Sickling

The sickling of erythrocytes containing Hb S is induced by the same physicochemical perturbations as those responsible for the gelation of Hb S solutions. Arterial blood, having a high oxygen saturation, contains fewer sickle cells than blood collected from various sites in the venous circulation. The oxygen affinity is abnormally sensitive to pH fluctuations in the physiologic range; a decrease in pH from 7.4 to 7.2 results in twice the normal decrement in oxygen affinity. Sickling is greatly potentiated by increasing the intracellular concentration of Hb S. Predictably, red cells containing relatively more Hb F sickle less readily and survive longer than cells containing little Hb F.[43]

Membrane Alterations

Red cell sickling is associated with reversible membrane changes. With repeated cycles of sickling and unsickling, aberrations in membrane function and structure become increasingly pronounced, culminating in fixation of the membrane in the sickled configuration. From 5% to 50% of cells from individuals with SCA are irreversible sickle cells (ISCs), permanently stabilized in their abnormal crescent or oval shape.[52] ISCs contain substantially less Hb F than reversibly sickled cells, and their endowment of Hb F appears to be the primary determinant of irreversible sickling. In the ISC, the quantity of membrane lipids is decreased consistent with membrane loss, probably as a result of vesiculation. The normal phospholipid organization of the red cell membrane (phosphatidyl choline and sphingomyelin in the outer monolayer and phosphatidyl ethanolamine and phosphatidyl serine [PS] in the inner monolayer) is altered by deoxygenation, resulting in negatively charged PS on the red cell surface. This phospholipid may initiate blood clotting by enhancing the conversion of prothrombin to thrombin, as suggested by the findings of increased plasma levels of fragment 1.2 in the circulation.[53]

Dehydration

Two pathways play a major role in the formation of dense cells: the Ca^{2+}-activated K^+ channel (Gardos pathway) and the K-Cl cotransport channel (KCC). The transient increase in free Ca^{2+} induced by red cell deoxygenation and sickling leads to activation of the Gardos pathway and subsequent activation of KCC with further K^+ loss. In ISCs, unlike reversibly sickled cells, K^+ loss exceeds Na^+ gain, and there is overall loss of cell water and increased concentration of intracellular Hb S.

The rate of dehydration of sickle cells is uneven, and those destined to become ISCs dehydrate by a fast-track process. Reversible

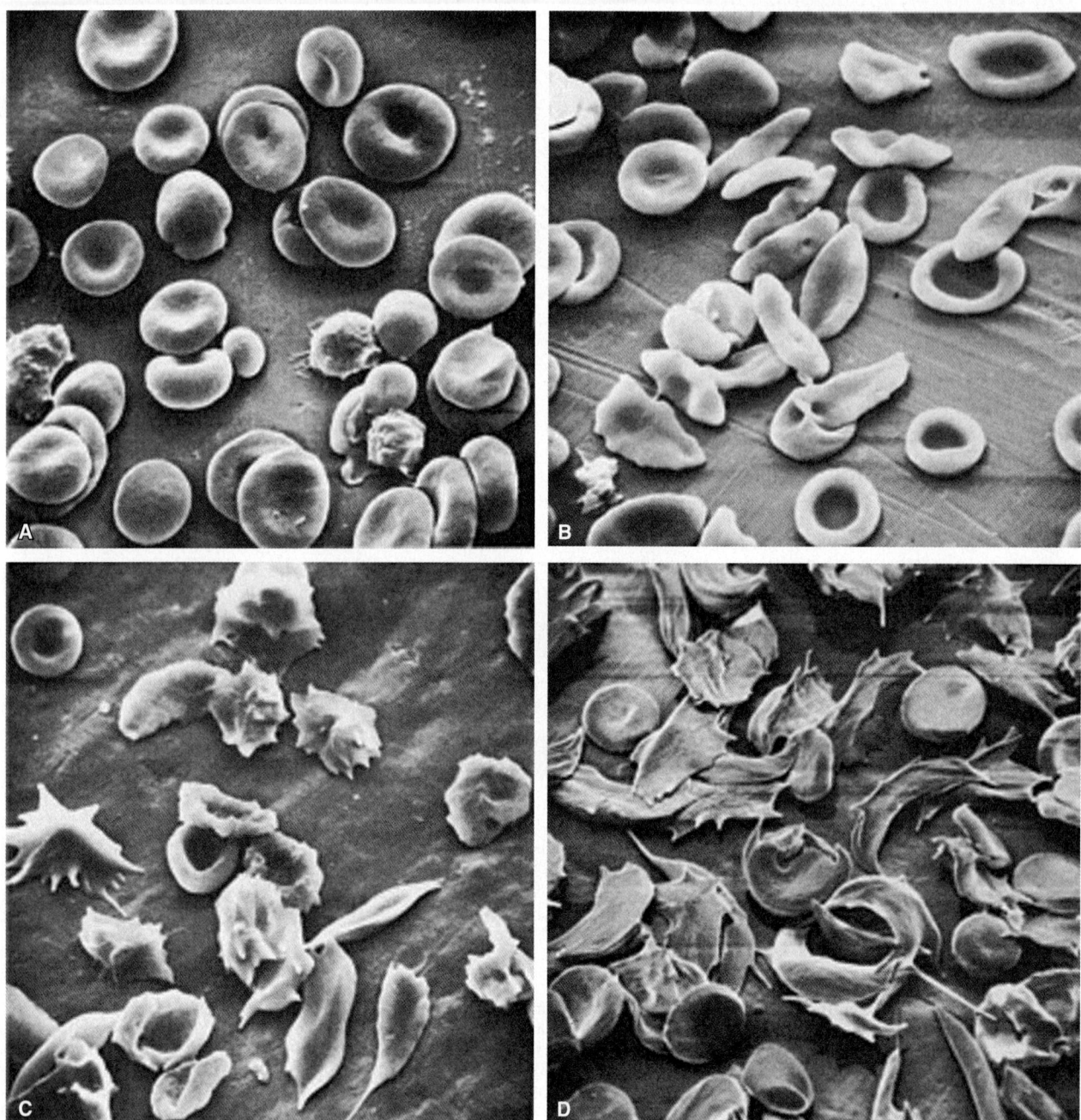

FIGURE 34.2 Erythrocytes from a patient with sickle cell anemia examined with scanning electron microscopy. A, Oxygenated blood. Red cells appear normal except for one microspherocyte. Three leukocytes are evident in the field. B, Oxygenated irreversibly sickled cells are smooth in texture and outline but are ovoid or boatlike in shape. C, Partial deoxygenation causes the cells to assume bizarre shapes with spikes, spicules, and filaments that protrude from the cells. D, More complete deoxygenation causes the cells to assume sickled shapes with longitudinal surface striations.

permeability pathways for Na^+, K^+, Mg^{2+}, and Ca^{2+}, sometimes referred to as the *sickling-induced pathway*, are the result of ionic shifts affecting cell hydration. The combined activity of the Gardos channel and K-Cl cotransport leads to rapid dehydration of a relatively young subpopulation of sickle cells, many with the characteristics of ISCs. The antimycotic agent clotrimazole is an inhibitor of the Gardos channel and prevents dehydration of sickle cells in vitro and in vivo.[54,55]

In vitro, KCC is activated by cell swelling, low pH, or urea. When activated, K^+ and Cl^- leave the cell via facilitated diffusion down their concentration gradients. Water follows their efflux, leading to cell dehydration. The activity of the KCC is abnormally increased in SCA.[56,57] Regulation of its activity involves phosphorylation and dephosphorylation reactions in membrane-bound serine/threonine

kinases and phosphatases. Magnesium is abnormally reduced in sickle erythrocytes and increasing cell magnesium produces a marked decrease in the activity of K-Cl cotransport.[54]

Adhesion
Sickle red cells demonstrate abnormal adherence to vascular endothelium, monocytes, macrophages, and model lipid membranes. Compared with normal red cells, sickle cells are 2 to 10 times more adherent to bovine and human endothelial cells.[58] This property of sickle blood is imparted by deformable sickle cells rather than by ISCs,[59,60] perhaps because rigid cells are unable to form multiple surface contacts with endothelial cells. Furthermore, red cell deformability has a strong positive correlation with the frequency and severity of pain crises.[59]

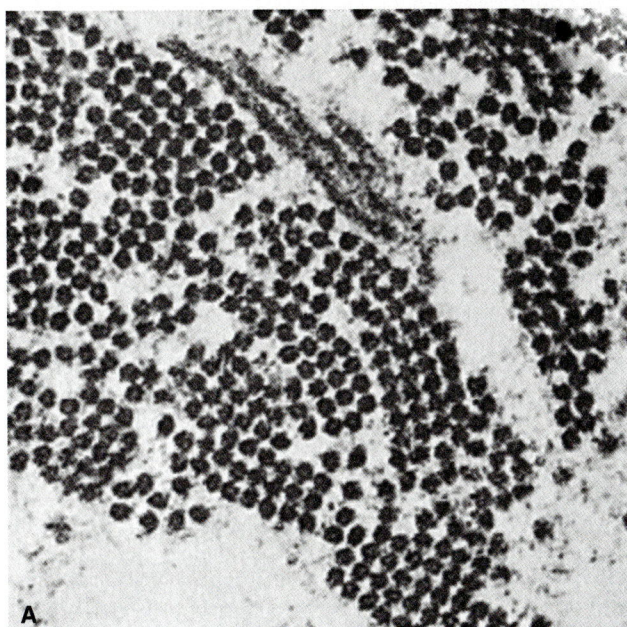

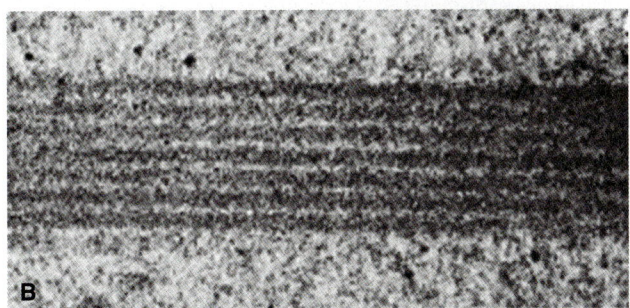

FIGURE 34.3 Electron photomicrographs of cell-free pellets of deoxyhemoglobin (Hb) S. A, Transverse section through fibers of polymerized Hb S (×97 000). B, Longitudinal section through same (×102 000). (From Finch JT, Perutz MF, Bertles JF, et al. Structure of sickled erythrocytes and of sickle cell hemoglobin fibers. *Proc Natl Acad Sci U S A.* 1973;70:718, with permission.)

When examined under dynamic conditions, red cell adherence is noted primarily at sites of turbulence rather than where flow is laminar. Several mechanisms for increased adherence have been proposed. Overexpression of adhesion molecules, such as basal cell adhesion molecule-1 and Lutheran, is involved in the process of RBC adhesion.[61] P-selectin may also mediate SS red cell adhesion to endothelial cells in vitro.[62] Sickle erythrocytes utilize multiple adhesive pathways, potentially first binding to the endothelium and later to other cells, such as leukocytes and platelets. The repellent force of the red cell is thought to reside in negatively charged sialic acid residues that are homogeneously distributed over the surface of the membrane. The distribution of negative charges on membranes of sickle red cells is patchy and interrupted, creating surface areas that may have an electrostatic attraction for other cells. Induction of excessive free radical generation in normal red cells is associated with increased adherence under conditions that allow the influx of calcium.

Conditions and factors that promote the expression of adhesion receptors by endothelial cells include hypoxia, thrombin, tissue necrosis factor, platelet-activated factor, and interleukin (IL)-1.[63] These conditions/factors also cause increased adhesion of sickle cells to endothelium in vitro. Thrombospondin may be an important plasma adhesogen because of its ability to bridge CD36 expressed on sickle reticulocytes.[64] Erythrocyte membrane sulfatide, a sulfated glycosphingolipid, may also play an important role in adhesion and its blockage with specific antibodies significantly prevents endothelial adhesion.[65] Different mechanisms may predominate under various circumstances or in different parts of the circulation. Coagulopathy

might cause thrombospondin release and precipitate vaso-occlusion in microvessels, and dehydration-induced vasopressin elevation might stimulate von Willebrand factor release and precipitate vaso-occlusion in large postcapillary venules.

Circulating activated endothelial cells have been assayed using immunohistochemical examination of buffy coat smears with antiendothelial cell antibodies.[66] In one study, patients with SCA with acute painful episodes had higher levels of circulating endothelial cells than patients with no recent events, who, in turn, had higher levels than controls. Circulating endothelial cells were predominantly microvascular (CD36+) and expressed markers of endothelial cell activation (intercellular adhesion molecule-1, vascular cell adhesion molecule [VCAM]-1, E-selectin, and P-selectin). This suggested that vascular endothelium is activated in patients with SCA and that adhesion proteins on the cells may have a role in the vascular pathology.

Rheology of Sickle Cells

The clinical features of SCA are directly or indirectly related to increased blood viscosity. The viscosity of plasma in sickle cell subjects is slightly higher than that of plasma from normal subjects because of higher total protein concentration. However, at all shear rates, the viscosity of oxygenated sickle blood is lower than that of normal blood, mainly due to lower hematocrit values. The viscosity of a sickle blood sample increases with decreased oxygen saturation, primarily because of reduced cellular deformability. When the cell concentration of sickle blood is raised in vitro to 45%, viscosity becomes higher than that of normal blood. The extent to which membrane rigidity, Hb polymerization, and increased intracellular Hb concentration contribute to altered blood flow depends in part on the method used to study the properties of sickle red cells. Cellular dehydration, as well as the resulting increase in cytoplasmic viscosity, is a major determinant of abnormal rheologic behavior of oxygenated sickled red cells. Sickled red cell membranes demonstrate extensional rigidity and persistent deformation, as documented by videomicrographs of micropipette aspiration. The rheologic properties of oxygenated sickle cells are strongly influenced by the state of cell hydration and the increased propensity for oxidative damage to the membrane. The already compromised deformability of oxygenated sickle cells is dramatically reduced further after deoxygenation. Under physiologic conditions, increased viscosity results primarily from cellular dehydration. The poor deformability of ISCs, as measured by ektacytometry, can be rectified by osmotically hydrating them to a normal mean corpuscular hemoglobin concentration (MCHC). The membrane rigidity of oxygenated sickle cells can also be returned to a normal level by replacing Hb S with Hb A, suggesting that the interaction of Hb S with the cell membrane is an important determinant of cellular rigidity.[67] Peripheral vascular resistance is increased in proportion to ISC numbers, the extent of ISC deoxygenation, and ISC density. The functional significance of the impaired flow properties of sickle red cells has been demonstrated by measuring exercise tolerance before and after partial exchange transfusion. By increasing the relative number of cells containing Hb A without increasing the total Hb concentration, exercise capacity improved significantly.[68]

Pathogenetic Role of Hemolysis

Extravascular hemolysis is the primary hemolytic mechanism in sickle cell disease and may occur by two mechanisms: monocyte and macrophage recognition and phagocytosis of red cells that have undergone sickling- or oxidation-induced membrane changes and physical entrapment of rheologically compromised red cells. Intravascular hemolysis results from the lysis of complement-sensitive red cells[69] and Hb lost during sickling- or shear-induced membrane fragmentation. The multiple mechanisms for intra- and extravascular hemolysis in SCA result in complex interactions involving red cell dehydration, sickling, increased sensitivity to complement-mediated lysis, and clustering of membrane protein band 3 leading to accumulation of immunoglobulin G and complement on the cell surface, collectively leading to red cell trapping and fragmentation, osmotic lysis, and erythrophagocytosis.

Hemolysis can be quantitated utilizing different biomarkers (e.g., lactate dehydrogenase [LDH], reticulocyte count), but the accepted measures of hemolytic rate are the direct red cell survival (red cell lifespan) assessment or the amount of plasma Hb. Traditional red cell survival measurement involves exposure to radioactive chromium 51; however, other methods utilizing erythrocyte labeling with different biotin densities may be safer.[70]

Cell-free Hb, a direct result of hemolysis, is a known cause of consumption of nitric oxide (NO), although other mechanisms may also result in low NO levels, such as increased plasma arginase levels, and increased levels of an NO inhibitor, asymmetric dimethylarginine.[71,72] Individuals with SCA are recognized to be NO deficient, but the role of NO deficiency in the development of vasculopathy and endothelial dysfunction is incompletely understood. Because of the multitude of mechanisms involved in the pathophysiology of SCA (e.g., inflammation, adhesion, hemolysis, hypoxia-reperfusion injury), the contribution of NO consumption in the genesis of vascular dysfunction in SCA is not completely defined.

Two distinct clinical phenotypes have been proposed to classify patients based on the type of disease complications and the pathophysiologic role of hemolysis. The first includes clinical manifestations of sickle cell disease linked to hyperviscosity: vaso-occlusive pain crises and acute chest syndrome (ACS), which are associated with high white blood cell (WBC) counts and relatively elevated steady-state Hb levels.[73] The second encompasses clinical complications attributed to hemolysis-induced "dysregulation of NO metabolism" leading to endothelial dysfunction (vasculopathy) and includes pulmonary hypertension (PHT), leg ulceration, priapism, and possibly stroke. This classification has recently been called

into question, as classic biomarkers of intravascular hemolysis, such as LDH and reticulocyte count, are not consistently elevated in all cases of "hyperhemolysis." Additional mechanisms other than hemolysis-induced low NO levels may be involved in the promotion of endothelial dysfunction. For instance, the pathophysiology of renal dysfunction may be related to induction of heme oxygenase-1, release of heme, and Hb S instability.[74]

Pathogenesis of Vaso-Occlusion

Vaso-occlusion occurs following a series of steps beginning with endothelial activation, recruitment of adherent leukocytes, interactions of sickle RBCs with adherent neutrophils, and vascular clogging by heterotypic cell-cell aggregates[75] (*Figure 34.4*). Consistent alterations in platelet number and function have suggested the involvement of platelets in vaso-occlusive events. Platelet activation is profoundly inhibited by NO, and this inhibition is blocked by plasma Hb-mediated NO scavenging.[76] These processes and events are highly interconnected, leading to clinically significant outcomes, and often reinforcing or producing a "vicious cycle" of vaso-occlusion.

In sickle cell transgenic mice, induction of hypoxia followed by reoxygenation enhances peroxide production and increases leukocyte recruitment.[77] In addition, ischemia-reperfusion injury causes inhibition of oxygen-sensing prolyl hydroxylase enzymes, leading to activation of hypoxia and inflammatory signaling cascades, altering the stability of transcriptional factors hypoxia-inducible factor and nuclear factor-κB.[78] Examples of biomarkers of inflammation that are elevated in sickle cell disease are C-reactive protein (CRP), erythrocyte sedimentation rate, ILs, and secretory phospholipase A_2 (sPLA$_2$; linked to the development of ACS), among others.

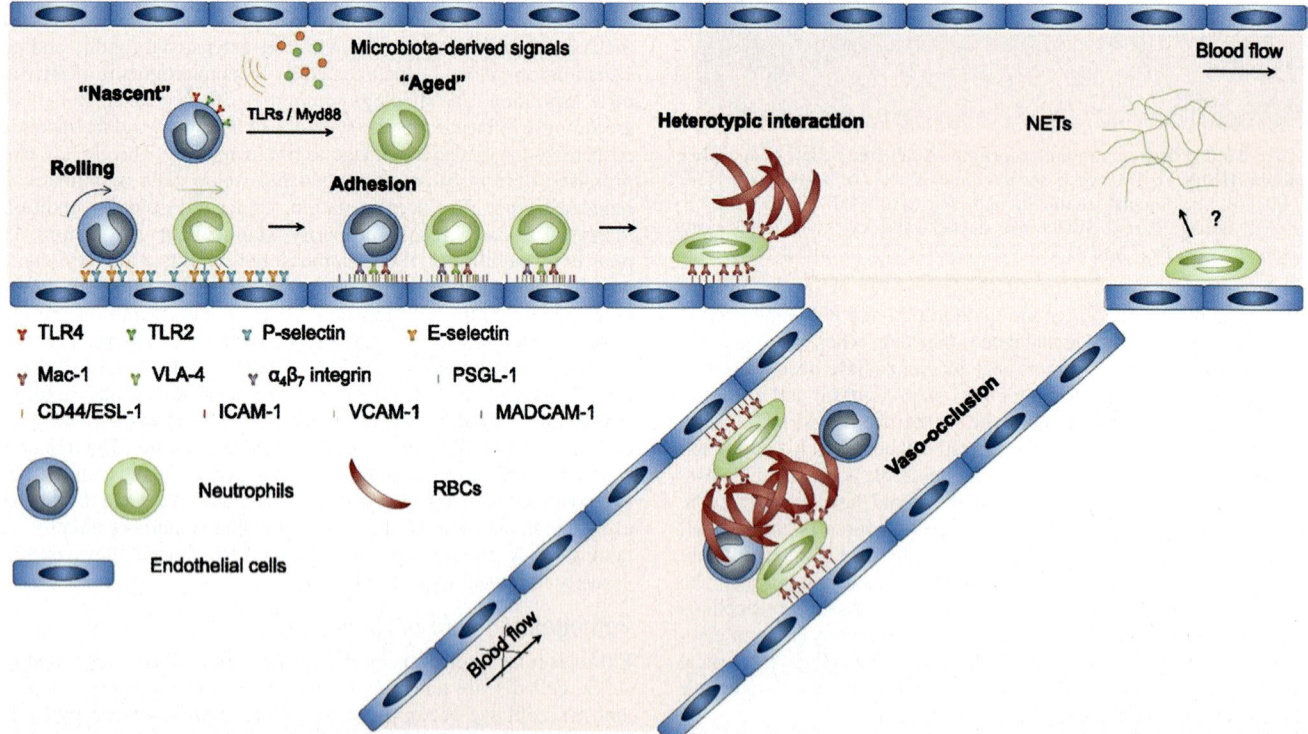

FIGURE 34.4 Multicellular and multistep model of sickle cell vaso-occlusion. Sickle cell vaso-occlusion arises from a cascade of interactions among RBCs, neutrophils, and endothelial cells. Activation of endothelial cells leads to the recruitment of neutrophils, which is initiated by rolling of neutrophils on endothelial selectins, followed by adhesion mediated by integrins. Adherent neutrophils receive a secondary wave of signals transduced through E-selectin, leading to the activation of $\alpha_M\beta_2$ (Mac-1) integrin on the leading edge. Activated Mac-1 on adherent neutrophils mediates the capture of circulating sickle RBCs, producing a temporary or prolonged obstruction of venular blood flow. Circulating neutrophils exhibit considerable heterogeneity in their proinflammatory properties. Signals derived from the microbiota drive the neutrophil aging in the circulation, generating an overly active aged subset that exhibits enhanced Mac-1 activation and NETs formation. Aged neutrophils play an important role in promoting sickle cell vaso-occlusion. Currently, whether NET formation plays a role in the vaso-occlusive process remains unclear. ESL-1, E-selectin ligand-1; ICAM-1, intercellular adhesion molecule-4; MADCAM-1, mucosal vascular addressin cell adhesion molecule-1; NET, neutrophil extracellular trap; PSGL-1, P-selectin glycoprotein ligand-1; VCAM-1, vascular cell adhesion molecule-1; VLA-4, very late antigen-4. (Reprinted from Zhang D, Xu C, Manwani D, et al. Neutrophils, platelets, and inflammatory pathways at the nexus of sickle cell disease pathophysiology. *Blood.* 2016;127(7):801-809. Copyright © 2016 American Society of Hematology. With permission.)

SICKLE CELL ANEMIA (HEMOGLOBIN SS)

Clinical Features

The clinical features of SCA may be divided into those that are acute and episodic and those that are chronic and often progressive. Although signs and symptoms attributed to Hb S have been observed in early infancy, affected individuals characteristically are asymptomatic until the second half of the first year of life. The lack of clinical expression of the Hb SS genotype during fetal and early postnatal life is explained by the production of a sufficient quantity of Hb F to limit clinically important sickling. Because erythrocytes contain proportionally increasing amounts of Hb S and decreasing amounts of Hb F over the first several months of life, the conditions for sickling under physiologic conditions are gradually met. Prospective studies of affected infants followed from birth indicate a close temporal relationship between the postnatal decline in Hb F and evolution of anemia.[79,80] Mild anemia is apparent by 10 to 12 weeks of age (*Figure 34.5*).

Clinical features change with age. In the first year of life, splenomegaly (usually noted after 6 months of age), dactylitis, and ACS are commonly seen. Loss of function of the spleen has been documented as early as 5 months of age, and death from overwhelming infection is an increased risk before 12 months of age. Majority of patients experience their first vaso-occlusive episode before 4 years of age, and some not until late childhood or adulthood. During adolescent and especially young adult years, organ dysfunction (e.g., renal, pulmonary, cardiac, and hepatic dysfunction) becomes more prevalent and, in older adults, frequently causes mortality.[81,82]

The Cooperative Study of Sickle Cell Disease (CSSCD) and the Jamaican Cohort Study, the two largest prospective sickle cell cohorts to date, have generated information regarding the "natural history" of sickle cell disease in thousands of pediatric and adult patients. The Dallas Cohort, Belgium Registry, and, more recently, the Sickle Cell Clinical Research and Intervention Program (SCCRIP), a lifespan cohort study, have offered important data about survival and risk factors in sickle cell disease discussed in the next sections.[83-85]

Acute Events: Characteristics, Management, Prevention

Vaso-Occlusive Events: Dactylitis and Pain

The term *sickle cell crisis* was introduced to describe a recurring attack of pain involving the skeleton, chest, abdomen, or all three. Using the term in a broader sense, vaso-occlusive "crises," preferably called acute sickle cell pain, comprise a variety of syndromes that are typically recurrent and potentially catastrophic. Clinical manifestations are sudden in onset and are directly attributable to obstruction of the microcirculation by intravascular sickling. Modest exacerbation of anemia and increased leukocytosis are common. Infections often precede vaso-occlusive episodes in children, suggesting that fever, dehydration, and acidosis may be contributing factors. In adults, a triggering event is not often identified, however.

Often, the initial vaso-occlusive episode in infants involves the small bones of the hands and feet, referred to as hand-foot syndrome or dactylitis. By 2 years of age, nearly 50% of Jamaican children and 25% of American children with SCA have experienced at least one episode of dactylitis.[79,86] Typically, the dorsa of the hands and/or feet are swollen, nonerythematous, and exquisitely painful. Fever and leukocytosis are common. Radiographic changes are limited initially to soft tissue swelling; cortical thinning and destruction of metacarpals, metatarsals, and phalanges appear 2 to 3 weeks after the onset of symptoms. Dactylitis is sudden in onset and may last 1 or 2 weeks. It may recur until the patient is about 3 years of age.

After the first year of life, interruption of blood flow typically occurs in the larger bones of the extremities, spine, rib cage, and periarticular structures, producing painful crises of the bones and joints. The sinusoidal circulation of the bone marrow provides an ideal vascular bed for the sickling phenomenon.

In the CSSCD, epidemiologic features of pain crises were analyzed in a large group of patients with sickle cell disease and showed that the frequency of pain crisis increased with age.[87]

Pain resulting from ischemia of the bone marrow is gnawing and progressive in severity. Although pain can affect any bone in the body, the most frequent sites are the long bones (humerus, tibia, and femur). Involvement of facial bones is less common but is well documented. The swelling associated with infarction of the orbital bone may be sufficient to produce proptosis and ophthalmoplegia (*Figure 34.6*). Swelling of the elbows or knees may mimic rheumatic fever or septic arthritis.

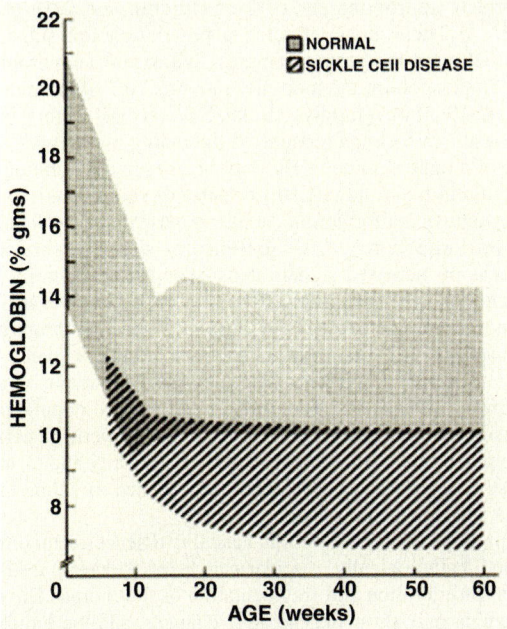

FIGURE 34.5 Hemoglobin concentration as a function of age in infants with sickle cell anemia. (Reprinted from O'Brien RT, McIntosh S, Aspnes GT, et al. Prospective study of sickle cell anemia in infancy. *J Pediatr.* 1976;89(2):205-210. Copyright © 1976 Elsevier. With permission.)

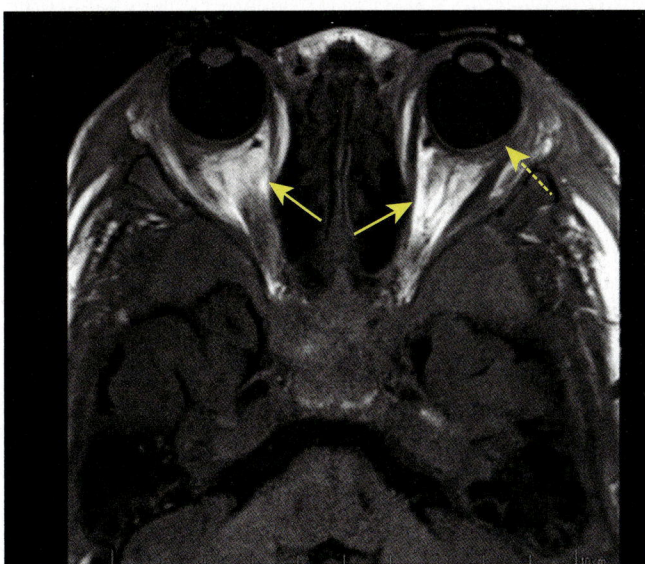

FIGURE 34.6 MRI of the orbits showing orbitopathy from vaso-occlusion. Within orbits, voluminous subperiosteal hemorrhagic masses are seen bilaterally under the orbital roofs (solid arrows), causing grade 2 proptosis bilaterally, especially the left globe that is elongated (dashed arrow). Patient underwent decompressive orbitotomy and fully recovered with normal vision. (Courtesy of Dr. Zoltan Patay.)

Disorders of Red Blood Cells

Infarcts involving deep bones are usually not associated with detectable swelling, erythema, or surface temperature change. Laboratory findings, too, are inconstant and nonspecific. The radiographic features of bone infarction and periostitis usually do not appear until after the resolution of symptoms. Increased signal with T2-weighted images is seen by magnetic resonance imaging (MRI) in approximately one-third of pain crises, posing a challenge to differentiate between osteomyelitis and a vaso-occlusive event.[88] Although radionuclide bone and bone marrow scans theoretically enable differentiation of bone infarcts from osteomyelitis, in practice they are of limited value. Unlike osteomyelitis, bone infarcts are associated with no more than a low-grade fever, little or no left shift in the leukocyte differential, and only occasional edema. As a cause of bone pain, infarction is >50 times as common as osteomyelitis.

An abdominal pain crisis, a diagnosis of exclusion, is attributed to small infarcts of the mesentery and abdominal viscera. Severe abdominal pain and signs of peritoneal irritation characterize this condition; however, other causes of abdominal pain (e.g., cholecystitis, pancreatitis, constipation, urinary tract infection, ACS) should always be considered. Diagnosis is facilitated by prior experience with the patient because the pattern of pain tends to repeat itself from crisis to crisis. Atypical clinical or laboratory features should suggest one of several complications to which patients with SCA are especially susceptible.

In general, painful crises last for 4 or 5 days in children and tend to last longer (sometimes weeks) as patients age. Data from the CSSCD indicate that an increased frequency of painful events is associated with a high hematocrit and a low Hb F level.[87] Adults with high rates of pain episodes tend to die earlier than those with low rates.[87] Of therapeutic significance, it was noted in the CSSCD that even when the Hb F level was low, a small increase was associated with an ameliorating effect on the pain rate and potentially improved survival.

Besides acute pain crisis episodes, chronic and neuropathic forms of pain are also seen, especially in adults.[89] Chronic pain is described as pain present in single or multiple sites, on at least 50% of days, for over 3 or 6 months.[90,91] This pain can persist between acute pain episodes (crisis), the so called chronic on acute pain.[92] Neuropathic pain is initiated by dysfunction of the somatosensory nervous system. It has an estimated prevalence of 25% to 40% in adolescents and adults with SCA.[93] Risk factors found to positively correlate with neuropathic pain include older age, female sex, and hydroxyurea use.[94]

The cornerstones of present-day therapy are fluids and analgesics. The volume of fluids administered should be sufficient to abolish any deficit, correct hypertonicity, and fully compensate for ongoing losses imposed by fever, hyposthenuria, vomiting, or diarrhea. Typically, a normal saline (NS) bolus followed by intravenous (IV) hypotonic fluids is used in the first 12 to 24 hours of the pain event, and subsequently reduced gradually. However, the use of NS, a hyperosmolar fluid during treatment of pain crisis, is controversial. Exposure to NS was associated with reduced sickle RBC deformability, prolonged transit time in capillary-sized microchannels, and increased sickle RBC adhesion in in vitro microfluidic model.[95,96] In a recent retrospective chart review for 60 SCD patients 3 to 21 years old treated for uncomplicated pain crisis with or without NS bolus, use of NS bolus was shown to negatively affect the final pain scores ($P = .05$).[97] On the other hand, preliminary studies report reduced frequency of vaso-occlusive events and improvement in pain with administration of hypotonic fluids.[98,99] Due to the paucity of clinical evidence,[100] the American Society of Hematology has not made any recommendations on the use of IV fluids in the management of pain crisis,[101] and prospective studies to assess the safety and efficacy of different types of fluids administered during pain crisis need to be conducted, Additionally, precipitants of the crisis should be sought and eliminated. Infection, a common precipitating cause in children, may require antibiotic therapy. Oxygen therapy in the absence of documented hypoxemia is without benefit and triggers an increase in the number of ISCs when discontinued.[102] RBC transfusions *are not indicated in the treatment of the acute pain crisis*, unless there is associated accentuated anemia (e.g., parvovirus B19-induced "aplastic crisis"). Furthermore, because fever and back pain are common features of pain crises, transfusion reactions may escape early recognition.

While control of pain requires the use of analgesics, opioid addiction is unlikely as long as analgesics are used for pain control and monitored. However, education on limitations and harms of opioid therapy are recommended by national guidelines.[101,103] Nonsteroidal inflammatory drugs (NSAIDs) used in association with opioids offer benefit but should be used with caution in patients with renal dysfunction. Regardless of the use of opioids and/or NSAIDs, pain should be treated promptly (within 60 minutes of emergency department arrival) and reevaluated within 30 to 60 minutes after the first analgesic dose, according to published quality of care indicators and national guidelines.[104] The use of patient-controlled analgesia enables patients to administer opioids to themselves as needed and provides an element of self-control in pain management. Patient-to-patient variability in the response to pain treatment is common; therefore, the use of individualized pain plans is preferable and shown to reduce hospital admissions[105,106] and improves patient satisfaction.[107] Some of this individual variation may be explained by polymorphic cytochrome P450 (CYP) 2D6 variant alleles that are commonly observed among African Americans and may lead to impaired codeine conversion to morphine.[108] In fact, ultrarapid or poor metabolizer CYP2D6 genotypes are found in 7.1% and 1.4% of children with sickle cell disease, respectively, causing individuals to be over sedated or not respond adequately to codeine, respectively.[109] Use of adjunct medications like subanesthetic dose of NMDA receptor agonist ketamine (starts at 0.1-0.3 mg/kg/h with a maximum of 1 mg/kg/h) and lidocaine infusions has also been shown to be both opioid-sparring and effective in reducing pain.[110-112] A randomized controlled study showed that IV ketamine at 1 mg/kg dose had comparable analgesic effectiveness as IV morphine 0.1 mg/kg in the treatment of acute pain crisis.[113] Neuropathic pain-specific medications are highly underutilized in SCA patients, and while their efficacy has not been systematically studied, some preliminary studies suggest benefit in reducing frequency of pain crisis.[114,115] Nonpharmacologic management of pain, such as with self-hypnosis, transcutaneous electrical nerve stimulation, massage, and virtual reality, has been used successfully for pain control in selected subjects.[116] Local use of warm packs may be beneficial in some. Prophylactic approaches to pain management are discussed later in this chapter.

Central Nervous System Events

Stroke is a catastrophic complication of SCA. Data from <4000 patients followed for an average of 5 years indicated that infarctive stroke affects approximately 10% of children and 24% of young adults.[117,118] These data reflected a population not substantially exposed to disease-modifying therapies (hydroxyurea or chronic transfusions). In this cohort, the mortality rate was 26% after hemorrhagic stroke, but 0% after infarctive stroke. Several risk factors for acute cerebral insults have been recognized, including low oxygen delivery (because of a rapid decline in Hb level or oxygen desaturation),[119,120] altered cerebral blood flow (CBF) because of vasculopathy (e.g., stenosis, moyamoya malformation), acute increase in metabolic demands (e.g., severe infection),[121] the presence of silent cerebral infarcts (SCIs, areas of increased signal intensity on MRI, primarily in deep white matter or watershed areas of the cerebral cortex, not attributable to an overt neurologic event or finding),[122,123] and an abrupt increase in Hb concentration (e.g., a transfusion raising the Hb level to >11 g/dL).[124,125] The risk of stroke is also increased in patients with Hb F levels <8%.[126] Risk factors for stroke in the general population (e.g., hypertension, smoking, obstructive sleep apnea, hypertriglyceridemia) may also place sickle cell disease patients, especially adults, at higher risk for stroke, but further investigation is needed to define the additional risk in sickle cell disease.

The pathogenesis of cerebral vascular disease is incompletely understood. Pathologically, vascular narrowing (stenosis) results from segmental proliferation and fragmentation of the intima. The internal elastic lamina may show degenerative changes, and the tunica media may be disrupted by fibrosis and hemorrhage (*Figure 34.7*). Occlusion is the result of progressive proliferation of vascular smooth muscle, superimposed thrombosis, or embolus. Increased adherence of sickle red cells to the endothelium of vessel walls and decreased cerebral

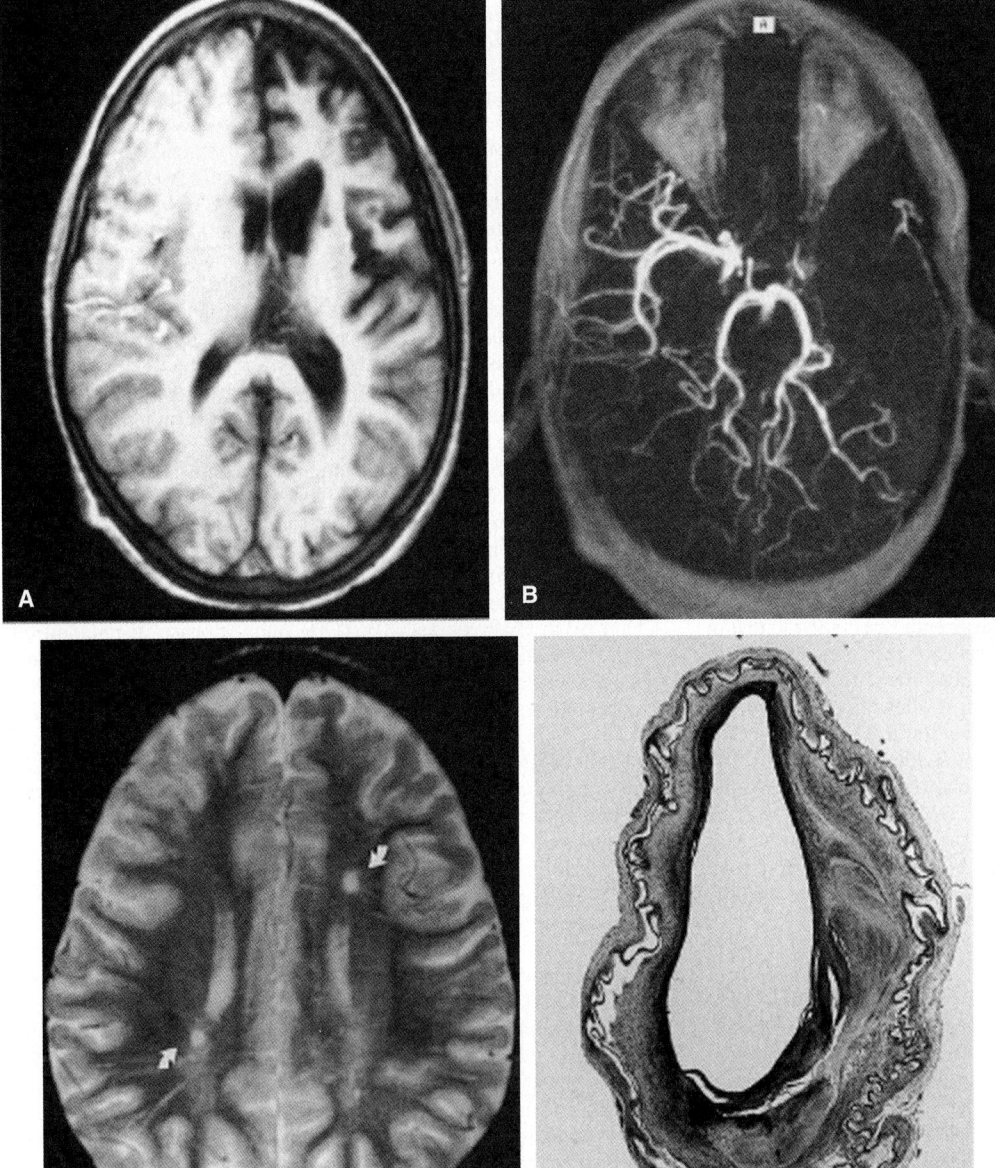

FIGURE 34.7 Vaso-occlusive effects in the central nervous system. A, T1-weighted magnetic resonance imaging (MRI) in a 6-year-old girl with hemoglobin (Hb) SS and a history of stroke. There is extensive atrophy involving the distributions of the left anterior and middle cerebral arteries with compensatory enlargement of the left lateral ventricle. B, Magnetic resonance angiography in the same patient showing occlusion of left middle cerebral artery and diminished flow through both anterior cerebral arteries. C, T2-weighted sagittal MRI in a 4-year-old boy with "silent infarcts." Small areas of leukomalacia are seen in deep white matter in frontal and parietal areas (arrows). D, Pathologic section of internal carotid artery showing fibrinous thrombus with parallel layers of fibrin deposited on intimal surfaces and atrophic media. (Courtesy of Dr J. J. Jenkins, St Jude Children's Research Hospital.)

Disorders of Red Blood Cells

vessel CO_2 responsiveness (reflecting diminished reserve capacity for vasodilatation) may be additional mechanisms.[127,128] Aneurysms can be demonstrated in some patients who have sustained intracranial hemorrhage, but may also be observed as an incidental finding, which may or may not be associated with the presence of moyamoya vascular malformation.[129,130]

In response to chronic anemia and hypoxemia, CBF is markedly increased in SCA.[131] Cerebral flow velocities in the major cerebral arteries (measured by transcranial Doppler ultrasound, TCD) are influenced by both stenosis and anemia and are abnormally elevated in patients at high risk for stroke.[132,133] Several factors modulate cerebral flow velocities and stroke risk. Hb oxygen desaturation, glucose 6-phosphate dehydrogenase (G6PD) deficiency, and higher hemolysis markers are all associated with elevated cerebral flow velocities and stroke.[120,134,135] The most common sites of ischemic stroke are the parenchymal areas supplied by the anterior and middle cerebral arteries and the border zones between their distal circulations. To compensate for the anemia, SCA patients have elevated CBF and oxygen extraction

fraction (OEF) compared to healthy controls.[136,137] When acute or chronic conditions leading to diminished oxygen availability (e.g., an episode of ACS, an aplastic crisis, nocturnal hypoxemia) arise, the increased hypoxic stress coupled with the inability of the cerebrovasculature to undergo further dilatation (limited cerebral reserve) leads to ischemia.[119] MRI sequence with voxel-wise measurement of OEF and CBF showed that the regions with elevated OEF fall within the border zone where CBF nadirs and aligned with the regions with high infarct density. This suggests that elevated OEF could be an indicator of cerebral metabolic stress.[138]

Increasing evidence for genetic modifiers of stroke has accumulated. The risk of stroke appears to be reduced among individuals with SCA who coinherited α-thalassemia (silent carrier or trait).[135,139,140] Association studies have identified two gene polymorphisms, GOLGB1 (Y1212C) and ENPP1 (K173Q), significantly associated with decreased risk for stroke[141]; however, validation studies have not yet confirmed these findings. Associations between several other genes, such as VCAM-1, adenylate cyclase 9 (ADCY9), and tumor necrosis factor-α (TNF-α),[140,142,143] and stroke (both increasing and decreasing risk) have been reported, but in replication studies, only five polymorphisms had significant influence ($P < .05$): single nucleotide polymorphisms (SNPs) in the *ANXA2*, *TGFBR3*, and *TEK* genes were associated with increased stroke risk, whereas α-thalassemia and an SNP in the ADCY9 gene were linked with decreased stroke risk.[144]

Clinically, strokes are characterized by the abrupt onset of hemiparesis, aphasia, seizures, sensory deficits, and altered consciousness, occurring singly or together. The patient may make a full recovery, or there may be incomplete resolution of neurologic deficits. Diffusion-weighted MRI imaging permits noninvasive early visualization of focal ischemia. Emergent treatment TCD stroke includes vigorous hydration, simple transfusion, and patient stabilization, followed by exchange transfusion once the Hb concentration is at least 7 or 8 g/dL.

Strokes tend to be repetitive because of the progressive nature of cerebral vascular disease. Patients with vasculopathy (intracranial stenosis or moyamoya) are more than twice as likely to incur subsequent stroke or transient ischemic attack despite transfusion treatment.[145,146] In general, unless patients begin a long-term transfusion program, they are at high risk for recurrent cerebral infarctions with progressive neurologic deterioration. Chronic transfusion therapy designed to maintain the level of Hb S at <30% reduces the risk of recurrent strokes (within 36 months) from approximately 70% to 90% to 10% to 20%.[127] Interruption or termination of treatment, even after 8 years of chronic transfusion, is associated with a stroke recurrence rate similar to that of untransfused patients, suggesting that transfusion therapy for secondary stroke prophylaxis should be continued indefinitely. However, reduction of the intensity of chronic transfusion to allow pretransfusion Hb S levels to reach 50% appears safe after the first few years of prophylaxis[147,148] and is routinely utilized by many sickle cell centers.[149]

An abnormal TCD ultrasound examination (defined by a time-averaged mean maximum velocity ≥200 cm/s in the distal internal carotid or proximal middle cerebral artery) predicts a 40% stroke risk in Hb SS patients.[132] In the STOP trial, 130 patients with abnormal TCD velocities were prospectively randomized to receive chronic transfusion or standard observation.[150] A 92% reduction in the risk of stroke occurred in the patients receiving chronic transfusion. Subsequently, the STOP II study investigated if discontinuation of transfusion was safe. After 30 months of transfusions, patients were randomly assigned to continue or stop transfusion; among the 41 children enrolled in the discontinuation-of-transfusion group, abnormal TCD results developed in 14 and stroke in 2 others within a mean of 4.5 months (range 2.1-10.1 months) of the last transfusion. None of these endpoint events occurred in the 38 children who continued to receive transfusions. Extrapolation of the STOP I and II data has led to recommendations for the frequency of TCD screening in children with Hb SS/Sβ⁰ thalassemia between the ages of 2 and 16 years (*Table 34.2*) and are endorsed by national guidelines.[151] Information regarding the utility of TCD examination in adults is extremely limited, although velocities are probably intermediate between those found in children with sickle cell disease and normal adult controls.[152]

Participants of the STOP II trial demonstrated that among children who discontinued transfusion there was significant progression of SCI (*Figure 34.7C*) in comparison with those who continued transfusion.[153] In a separate cohort of children who were receiving chronic transfusion therapy for primary stroke prevention after having had abnormal TCD velocities, transfusions were successful in preventing progression of vasculopathy.[154] The same protection does not seem to be conferred by transfusions to children with prior overt strokes.[146,155]

Following publication of the results of the STOP trials, TCD programs have led to a dramatic reduction of stroke incidence in some centers.[151,156,157] However, despite the well-publicized results, only half of children with SCA in the United States receive TCD exams as recommended by national guidelines.[158] The main barriers to TCD implementation included logistical difficulties in scheduling and scheduling coordination, while facilitators included reminders, education, provider investment, and patient positive experience and convenient location.[159] Post STOP study, a long-term follow-up study (median duration 10.3, range 0-15.4 years) of patients that participated in STOP and/or STOP 2 trials, demonstrated an ischemic stroke incidence rate of 2.1%.[160] Majority (63%) of these events occurred due to improper implementation of STOP protocol including lack of appropriate TCD screening or treatment of abnormal TCD.[161]

Alternatives to long-term transfusions for preventing recurrence of stroke have been intensively investigated. The Stroke with Transfusions Changing to Hydroxyurea (SWiTCH) study, a phase III randomized, multicenter clinical trial, compared standard treatment (transfusions with iron chelation) to alternative treatment (hydroxyurea with phlebotomy) for stroke prophylaxis in children who had experienced prior stroke. SWiTCH was a noninferiority trial with a composite primary endpoint of stroke and hepatic iron overload.[162] This study was interrupted early because more strokes were observed in the hydroxyurea/phlebotomy arm and only equivalence in liver iron content was seen in the two arms. Chronic transfusion therapy and iron chelation remains the standard treatment for secondary prevention of stroke in children with SCA (*Figure 34.8*). However, the protection offered by transfusions is not absolute especially in patients with progressive vasculopathy (stenosis or moyamoya).[145,146,155] Revascularization surgery as adjunct therapy to chronic transfusions may be beneficial in patients with underlying vasculopathy,[166] while hematopoietic stem cell (HSC) transplant offers a more definitive option for secondary stroke prevention.[167,168]

The phase III multicenter randomized TCD with Transfusions Changing to Hydroxyurea (TWiTCH) trial investigated the role of hydroxyurea for primary stroke prevention. It enrolled children who had received blood transfusions for at least 12 months (because of having had abnormal TCD velocities) and did not have severe cerebral vasculopathy. In the TWiTCH trial, these children were randomized to continue transfusion, or to discontinue transfusion and begin hydroxyurea after a period of overlap between the two treatment arms.[164] TCD velocities were 143 cm/s (95% confidence interval [CI] 140-146) in children who received standard transfusions and 138 cm/s (95% Confidence Interval [95%CI] 135-142) in those who received hydroxyurea. Criteria for noninferiority and posthoc superiority were met. Therefore, children with SCA and abnormal TCD, who have received at least 1 year of transfusion, and have no magnetic resonance angiography–defined severe vasculopathy, can substitute hydroxyurea treatment for chronic transfusion to maintain lower TCD velocities and prevent primary stroke (*Figure 34.8*). Outside of high resource setting, monthly transfusions present a difficult option. Observational studies conducted in low- and middle income countries using hydroxyurea upfront for primary stroke prevention in children with abnormal TCD measurements showed hydroxyurea to be safe and effective in decreasing TCD velocities when given in either fixed or escalating dose.[169-171]

Although the relative risk of primary stroke is lower among patients with conditional TCD velocities (time-averaged mean maximum velocity 170-199 cm/s) than those with abnormal velocities (risk 2%-5% vs 9% per year), more children have conditional TCD velocities (17% vs 9% prevalence), so the absolute number at risk for

Table 34.2. Recommended TCD Screening Schedule in Children With Sickle Cell Disease

Initial TCD Result[a]	Frequency of Testing		
	Age (y)		
	2-5	6-11	12-16
Normal	Yearly	Yearly × 3	Yearly × 2
Low conditional	Every 6 mo	Every 6 mo	Every 6 mo
High conditional	Every 3 mo	Every 3 mo	Every 3 mo
Abnormal	Within 1 mo	Within 1 mo	Within 1 mo

[a]TCD result: normal, <170 cm/s; low conditional, 170 to 184 cm/s; high conditional, 185 to 199 cm/s; abnormal, ≥200 cm/s.
Abbreviation: TCD, transcranial Doppler.

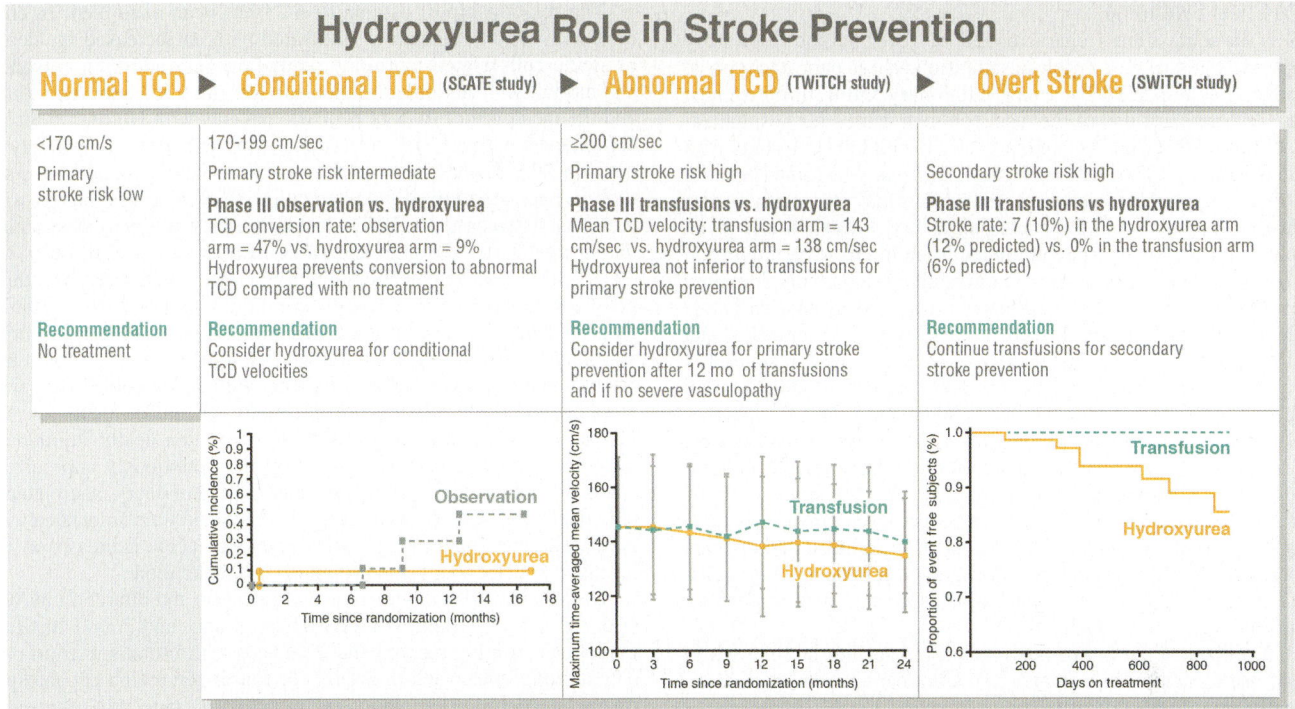

FIGURE 34.8 **Summary of studies investigating the role of hydroxyurea in primary and secondary stroke prevention in sickle cell anemia.** In phase III randomized trials, hydroxyurea was shown to reduce the risk of conversion from conditional to abnormal velocity (SCATE study)[154,163] and was at least equivalent to transfusions in reducing TCD velocities in patients with abnormal TCD (after progressive change from transfusions to hydroxyurea, TWiTCH study),[151,164] but not equivalent to transfusions for secondary stroke prevention (SWiTCH study).[150,165] Prepared by Brandon Stelter, Biomedical Communications, St Jude Children's Research Hospital.

stroke without therapy is comparable. The risk of conversion from a conditional to abnormal TCD velocity is highest in children under 10 years of age.[172,173] The phase III multicenter Sparing Conversion to Abnormal TCD Elevation (SCATE) study investigated whether hydroxyurea therapy in children under age 11 years with conditional TCD was less likely to develop abnormal TCD velocities than those who were observed.[163] Although the SCATE trial was terminated early, in intention-to-treat analysis, the cumulative incidence of abnormal conversion was 9% (95%CI = 0%-35%) in the hydroxyurea arm and 47% (95%CI = 6%-81%) in the observation arm at 15 months. Thus, hydroxyurea reduced TCD velocities in children with SCA and conditional velocities and can be considered for prevention of TCD conversion into the abnormal range requiring transfusion treatment (*Figure 34.8*).

SCI occurs in 27% of children with SCA under 6 years of age[174] and 37% by their 14th birthday.[175] Prevalence of SCI can be as high as 50% by 30 years of age.[176] Data from the CSSCD and other cohorts have shown that children with SCI had an increased incidence of new stroke and new or more extensive SCI[122] and that SCIs were the strongest independent predictor of stroke.[123,177] Data from the STOP trial indicated that those who had SCI (in addition to abnormal TCD velocities) were at higher risk for developing a new SCI or stroke compared with those whose MRI showed no abnormality.[178] Low Hb, acute anemic events, elevated systolic blood pressure, and cerebral vasculopathy are other well-established risk factors for SCI.[179-181] While presence of intracranial vasculopathy is predictive of SCI recurrence in children with abnormal TCD or prior stroke,[146] it is rarely seen in children with normal TCD and SCI, and is not likely a major risk factor for future SCI.[182] The majority of the SCIs have been shown to be symmetrically located in the deep white matter of the internal border zone, where resting CBF is at the lowest.[183,184]

Data from the CSSCD gathered over a 10-year period of follow-up of school-aged children with Hb SS indicated that those with SCI had significantly lower scores for math and reading achievement, full-scale

IQ (FSIQ), verbal IQ, and performance IQ, when compared with individuals with normal MRI of the brain.[185]

A comparison of patients who were in both the CSSCD and STOP studies indicated that those who had abnormal TCDs did not have an unusually high frequency of MRI abnormality; conversely, those who had SCI did not have an unusually high frequency of abnormal TCD velocities, suggesting that those findings are independent events and represent different aspects of the pathophysiology of the brain in children with sickle cell disease.[186]

The Silent Cerebral Infarct Transfusion trial was a phase III multicenter randomized study that enrolled children with SCA and SCI identified by MRI screening to determine whether transfusion therapy could prevent overt clinical stroke or new or progressive SCI in comparison with children randomized to observation.[187] A total of 196 children were randomly assigned to the observation or transfusion group and were followed for a median of 3 years. Fewer children in the transfusion arm had a stroke or a new or enlarged SCI. Regular blood-transfusion therapy significantly reduced the incidence of recurrent cerebral infarct in children with SCA and can be considered as a therapy option for this disease complication. However, analysis in subset of 157 SIT Trial participants showed that transfusion therapy did not prevent brain volume percent loss.[188] On the other hand, hydroxyurea has not been extensively studied as a therapy for SCI prevention. While in a single-site prospective pediatric study, children treated with hydroxyurea at the maximum tolerated dose when compared to baseline (38%) had no significant increase in incidence of SCI at 3 (41%) or 6 years (41%).[189] Another study showed that in individuals treated with hydroxyurea, high fetal Hb measured in childhood was associated with lower hazard of SCI progression on MRI.[190] On the other hand, there are other small observational studies that suggest that hydroxyurea alone may not be sufficient to decrease infarct recurrence in individuals with prior SCI.[191,192] Transfusion and hydroxyurea have not yet been directly compared for the prevention of SCI (new or progressive lesions).

Acute Chest Syndrome

ACS is an acute illness characterized by fever and/or respiratory symptoms/signs (e.g., oxygen desaturation, chest pain, tachypnea, dyspnea), accompanied by a new pulmonary infiltrate on a chest X-ray. ACS remains one of the most common causes for hospitalization, critical care utilization, and mortality in children and adults with sickle cell disease. The term *acute chest syndrome* was coined because it is often not possible to determine the relative importance of vascular occlusion vs infection in the acute pulmonary process in any given patient. Infection tends to predominate in children, while infarction and fat embolism are more common in adults. Additionally, impaired access of oxygen to infected segments of the lung likely enhances local sickling, with resulting focal microvascular thrombotic disease. Data from the CSSCD indicate that the rate of ACS is highest in children 2 to 4 years of age (25/100 patient-years) and decreases gradually with increasing age to that seen in adults (9/100 patient-years).[193] A higher ACS rate is associated with a higher rate of mortality from all causes. The risk of ACS is associated with a lower fetal Hb level and a higher steady-state hematocrit and leukocyte count. A more severe form of ACS characterized by rapid and progressive development of symptoms ("rapidly progressive ACS") has been recognized and appears to represent a distinct phenotype. It occurs more frequently in adults, is preceded by thrombocytopenia, and is associated with multiorgan failure and high risk of death.[194]

Before the availability of pneumococcal vaccines and the widespread use of penicillin prophylaxis, pulmonary events in children typically were the result of bacterial infection.[195,196] *Streptococcus pneumoniae* was the most common causative organism. Infiltrates often affected multiple lobes, and resolution was slower than in the general population. Identified infectious agents have included *Mycoplasma pneumoniae*,[197] *Chlamydia pneumoniae*,[198] parvovirus B19,[199] and respiratory viruses. The National Acute Chest Syndrome Study Group reported causes and outcomes based on an analysis of 671 episodes of ACS.[199] Patients who were 20 years of age or older had a more severe course. A specific cause of ACS was identified in 38% of all episodes and in 70% of episodes with complete data (*Table 34.3*).[199] The most common specific causes were pulmonary fat embolism, chlamydia, mycoplasma, miscellaneous viruses, and bacterial infections resulting from coagulase-positive *Staphylococcus aureus* and *S. pneumoniae*. Influenza, especially H1N1, was shown to be associated with increased risk and severity of ACS, and therefore should be prevented with yearly immunization.[200] While severe pain crisis episodes appear to precede ACS events,[199,201,202] the incidence of neurological complications including SCI or overt stroke is higher after ACS events.[203,204] An association between smoking (and second-hand smoke exposure) and increased rate of ACS and pain events has been observed among adults and children with sickle cell disease.[205,206]

The relationship of asthma to ACS has been examined. In children with Hb SS, asthma is associated with an increased incidence of sickle cell–related morbidity, including ACS and pain episodes, and mortality.[207] A similar relationship was observed between asthma and the incidence of ACS in pediatric patients with Hb SC.[208] Sickle cell patients with a history of asthma were four times more likely to develop ACS during a hospital admission for pain and had a substantially longer duration of hospitalization.[209] Similarly, children with pulmonary function test (PFT)–documented lower airway obstruction had a greater risk for pain and ACS hospitalization (risk ratio 2.0, CI 1.3-3.3).[210] In Jamaican children with sickle cell disease, asthma and bronchiolar hyperreactivity were more common than in ethnic-matched controls and were associated with recurrent ACS.[211] Incentive spirometry with the use of maximal inspirations every 2 hours has been shown to prevent ACS in patients with sickle cell disease who were hospitalized with chest or back pain. Occlusion of major pulmonary vessels is a recognized cause of sudden death. Pulmonary fat emboli are found more commonly than previously appreciated when a diagnosis is sought by fat staining of pulmonary macrophages obtained by bronchoalveolar lavage.[212] Fat emboli are associated with bone pain, chest pain, neurologic symptoms, acute decreases in Hb level and platelet count, and prolonged hospitalization.

Because the relative importance of infection and infarction in ACS is difficult to ascertain, National Heart, Lung, and Blood Institute guidelines strongly recommend treatment with broad-spectrum parenteral antibiotics, such as a third- or fourth-generation cephalosporin, and a macrolide antibiotic (to cover *Mycoplasma* and *Chlamydia*), despite the paucity of evidence and lack of clinical trials on antibiotic treatment for ACS.[213] A recent retrospective data analysis using a large nationwide database Children's Hospital Association's Pediatric Health Information System showed that children receiving guideline-adherent antibiotics had a lower 30- day all-cause readmission rate when compared to those who received non-guideline adherent antibiotic regimens.[214] Of utmost importance is the correction of hypoxemia. If the arterial Po_2 value is <75 mm Hg or the O_2 saturation by pulse oximetry is significantly below baseline, the clinician should consider prompt simple transfusion, or partial exchange transfusion for more severe cases. IV dexamethasone was shown to result in a shorter hospital stay and reduced need for blood transfusion and oxygen when compared with placebo in children with ACS.[215] Because there appeared to be a high risk of recurrent symptoms and readmission to the hospital after dexamethasone was abruptly discontinued, a randomized study investigated the use of tapered oral dexamethasone for ACS treatment.[216] Despite a very small number of participants, this trial showed a reduction in hospitalization duration in the dexamethasone arm, but higher rates of rebound pain. sL-selectin was found elevated among patients with rebound pain and could be a useful

Table 34.3. Causes of Acute Chest Syndrome

Cause	(N = 670)	Number of Episodes Percentage	Age at Episode of Acute Chest Syndrome 0-9 y (N = 329)	10-19 y (N = 188)	≥20 y (N = 153)
Fat embolism, with or without infection	59	8.8	24	16	19
Chlamydia	48	7.2	19	15	14
Mycoplasma	44	6.6	29	7	8
Virus	43	6.4	36	5	2
Bacteria	30	4.5	13	5	12
Mixed infections	25	3.7	16	6	3
Legionella	4	0.6	3	0	1
Miscellaneous infections	3	0.4	0	3	0
Infarction	108	16.1	50	43	15
Unknown	306	45.7	139	88	79

From Vichinsky EP, Neumayr LD, Earles AN, et al. Causes and outcomes of the acute chest syndrome in sickle cell disease. National Acute Chest Syndrome Study Group. *N Engl J Med.* 2000;342(25):1855-1865. Copyright © 2000 Massachusetts Medical Society. Reprinted with permission from Massachusetts Medical Society.

biomarker during ACS. NO inhalation has been utilized in the regulation of hypoxic pulmonary vasoconstriction,[217] but definitive trials have not yet substantiated its therapeutic role. Monthly bolus dosing of vitamin D3 (100,000 or 12,000 IU/mo) for 2 years in a randomized phase 2 study showed a >50% reduction in respiratory events (respiratory illnesses, asthma exacerbation, or ACS) during the second year of vitamin D3 supplementation.[218,219]

Priapism

Priapism is an unwanted, painful, and persistent erection of the penis. The incidence of priapism in patients with sickle cell disease has been reported to be between 3% and 60% and rises steeply with age.[220,221] Most priapism episodes begin during sleep or early in the morning; they may be associated with physiologic dehydration and hypoventilation, which results in metabolic acidosis followed by increases in sickling and stagnation of blood within the penile sinusoids or the corpora cavernosa. In data from the CSSCD and French cohorts, subjects with priapism had significantly lower levels of Hb and higher levels of bilirubin, reticulocytes, LDH, WBCs, and platelets, suggesting an association of priapism with increased hemolysis, perhaps related to a diminished availability of circulating NO, which plays an important role in erectile function.[222,223] Although priapism is usually self-limited and of relatively short duration, it is often recurrent and may become chronic. "Stuttering" priapism refers to multiple episodes, each <4 hours in duration, which may occur several times a week and may herald a prolonged event. Usually, these do not require medical intervention. Typically, priapism results from engorgement of the paired cavernosal bodies with sparing of the glans and corpus spongiosum and is maintained by the partial obstruction of venous drainage. However, tricorporal priapism may occur, especially in postpubertal patients, and is associated with a poor prognosis. The repetitive trapping of cells in the corpora cavernosa, with or without surgical intervention, may lead to fibrosis of the septa and impotence. Of particular concern is an increased rate of impotence reported in sickle cell patients whose attacks lasted >24 hours.

As with other complications resulting from the sludging of sickled erythrocytes, aggressive hydration and adequate analgesia are of primary importance and should be pursued within the first few hours of symptoms. If no response is seen within 12 to 24 hours, partial exchange transfusion to lower the Hb S level to <30% may be performed; this is occasionally sufficient. An association of sickle cell disease, priapism, exchange transfusion, and neurologic events, including seizures and obtundation, referred to as ASPEN syndrome, is of concern if a rapid rise in the hematocrit is promoted.[125,224] An examination of the long-term safety and efficacy of blood exchange transfusions in adults with severe recurrent priapism has shown no neurologic complications and resolution or partial resolution in 80% of men.[225] Additionally, response of recurrent severe stuttering priapism episodes to transfusion therapy is immediate with significant clinical improvement seen after the first transfusion.[226] If no resolution occurs within another 12 to 24 hours, corporal aspiration and irrigation with saline may be indicated through such means as a Winter procedure,[227] in which a fistula between the glans penis and the corpora cavernosa is created using a biopsy needle. Rapid complete detumescence during episodes of prolonged priapism can be achieved with aspiration and irrigation with a dilute epinephrine solution.[228] If penile aspiration is unsuccessful, creation of a cavernosa spongiosum shunt or a venous bypass may be considered.

Prevention of recurrent priapism has been accomplished in some patients with chronic transfusion, particularly through exchange transfusion.[229] The role of hydroxyurea for priapism prevention is unclear. α-Adrenergic agonists increase contraction of the smooth muscle of the trabecular arteries of the cavernosa and facilitate venous outflow from the corpora, promoting detumescence. α-Adrenergic agents including etilefrine, pseudoephedrine, and phenylephrine may be administered either orally or by intracavernous injection.[230,231] Other approaches have been the administration of diethylstilbestrol, the gonadotropin-releasing hormone analog leuprolide acetate, and low-dose antiandrogens, finasteride; however, none of them have shown definitive results.

Sildenafil, a phosphodiesterase type 5 inhibitor, is reported to improve priapism in nonrandomized trials,[232,233] but can trigger pain as a side effect.[233] In a small case series, inhaled nitrous oxide was shown to result in complete resolution of acute priapism event, but this needs to be evaluated further.[234] Recently, studies using microfluidic adhesion assay demonstrated that RBCs from SCA patients with history of priapism when compared to those with no prior priapic episodes had significantly higher hypoxia-enhanced adhesion to the sub-endothelial protein laminin.[235,236] The safety and efficacy of antiadhesion agent like crizanlizumab in priapism is currently being evaluated.[237] Despite either conservative or aggressive treatment, >25% of patients have some degree of impotence[238] and may be candidates for a penile prosthesis after 6 to 12 months.

Exacerbation of Anemia

Hematologic "crises," characterized by sudden exaggeration of anemia, are pathogenetically and temporally unrelated to vaso-occlusive crises. If they are unrecognized or untreated, the decrease in Hb concentration may be so precipitous and severe as to cause heart failure and death within hours.

Transient Aplastic Crises

Epidemiologic studies clearly implicate human parvovirus B19 as the cause for almost all transient aplastic crises. Aplasia is the result of direct cytotoxicity of the parvovirus B19 to erythroid precursors, especially colony-forming units, erythroid.[239] However, not all parvovirus infections result in problems; serologic evidence of previous infection was found in 71% of subjects with SCA who reached adulthood, but only 27% had a previous clinically recognized aplastic crisis.[240]

In the early phase of a transient aplastic crisis, peripheral blood reticulocytes and bone marrow normoblasts disappear or are greatly reduced in number. Because red cell survival in Hb SS is no more than 10 to 20 days, cessation of erythropoiesis is followed by a rapid decrease in Hb concentration. The process is self-limited, however; within 10 days, red cell production resumes spontaneously, and large numbers of reticulocytes and nucleated erythrocytes appear in the peripheral blood. Thereafter, the Hb concentration returns to its pre-crisis level. Often, the patient is first seen early in the recovery phase, when differentiation from a hemolytic crisis may be difficult. Although leukocytes and platelets are usually normal, all marrow elements may be affected. Treatment consists of supportive care with red cell transfusion when necessary. Of note, for patients with sickle cell disease treated with hydroxyurea, the need for transfusion may be reduced,[241] as RBC survival is increased under this therapy.

Susceptible hospital workers exposed to patients with aplastic crises are at high risk of contracting nosocomial erythema infectiosum. Because infection during the mid-trimester of pregnancy may result in hydrops fetalis and stillbirth, respiratory isolation precautions are a necessity if an aplastic crisis is suspected.

In addition to causing an aplastic crisis, an acute parvovirus infection not infrequently will lead to a prolonged vaso-occlusive pain crisis or may trigger acute splenic sequestration.[242,243] Less frequently, it is associated with long-term problems, such as glomerulonephritis, which may cause end-stage renal failure, cardiac dysfunction, and stroke.[244,245] Currently, there are no vaccines clinically available to prevent parvovirus B19 infection in humans. Given the lifelong protection conferred by this infection, vaccine development is warranted for individuals with sickle cell disease to prevent the development of transient aplastic crisis.

Acute Splenic Sequestration

Acute splenic sequestration is characterized by sudden trapping of blood in the spleen. Splenic sequestration is characterized by a decrease in the steady-state Hb concentration of at least 2 g/dL from baseline, thrombocytopenia, evidence of compensatory marrow erythropoiesis (reticulocytosis), and an acutely enlarging spleen. This complication occurs in infants and young children whose spleens are chronically enlarged before autoinfarction and fibrosis. Although splenic sequestration has been documented in infants as young as 3 to 4 months of age,[246] it is observed most commonly during the second 6 months of life and is a less frequent finding after 2 years of age; however, it can be observed in adults.[247] In a large pediatric French cohort study, the risk of recurrence decreased with age: when the first episode occurred after 2 years, the risk was lower than when it occurred before 1 year of age (hazard ratio [HR] 0.60).[248]

There has been wide variability in the long-term management of patients with splenic sequestration, and currently, no consensus exists. Chronic transfusion and surgical splenectomy have both been used to avoid recurrence. Because of concerns about invasive encapsulated organisms in the asplenic child, monthly erythrocyte transfusions are often used under 12 months of age and total splenectomy is delayed until an age after which the risk of sepsis is lower. This practice has been less utilized recently given the decline in infection by invasive encapsulated organism with adequate pneumococcal and meningococcal immunization and prophylactic penicillin use. Partial splenectomy has also been used in an attempt to preserve immunologic function in children with SCA and recurrent splenic sequestration.[249] Long-term outcomes of partial splenectomy have been compared with total splenectomy and found comparable, including the risk of post splenectomy sepsis.[250] Although it is encountered much less frequently, sudden trapping of blood in the liver (hepatic sequestration crisis) also occurs.[251]

Hemolytic Crises (Hyperhemolytic Crises)

Hemolytic (hyperhemolytic) crises result from a sudden acceleration of the hemolytic process. They have been described in association with coinherited hereditary spherocytosis[252] and concurrent mycoplasma infection.[197] They occur in all sickle genotypes and are most commonly associated with acute or delayed hemolytic transfusion reactions (usually Coombs test positive) and more rarely with drug-induced hemolysis.[253] Although about 10% of black male patients with SCA have the unstable A variant of G6PD deficiency,[254] they have no more severe anemia and no greater frequency of acute hemolytic episodes than those with normal levels of G6PD, even when challenged with oxidant drugs and infections, because of the young mean age of sickle RBCs.[255]

Megaloblastic Crises

Megaloblastic crises result from the sudden arrest of erythropoiesis by folate depletion. Chronic erythroid hyperplasia imposes a drain on folate reserves, and biochemical evidence of mild folate deficiency has been demonstrated with high frequency in subjects with SCA.[256] Megaloblastic crises likely occur when food consumption is interrupted by illness or alcoholism or when the folate requirement is augmented by rapid growth or pregnancy. Currently, folic acid deficiency, as a cause of exaggerated anemia in sickle cell disease, appears to be extremely rare in the United States. Nevertheless, it is common practice to prescribe prophylactic folic acid (1 mg/d) to patients with sickle cell disease in areas of the world where folate is not routinely added to grain-derived products.

Infections

Overwhelming infection may be the presenting manifestation of SCA in early childhood. The pathophysiologic basis for increased susceptibility to aggressive infection relates in large part to the loss of spleen function. During the first few years of life, recurrent perivascular hemorrhage and infarction reduce the spleen to a small siderofibrotic vestige. Despite the frequent occurrence of splenomegaly in the first few years, spleen function often is impaired by 6 to 12 months of age.[257] Howell-Jolly bodies and "pits" (depressions in the RBC membrane) are seen in peripheral blood erythrocytes of asplenic patient. Spleen function is necessary for effective host response to *S. pneumoniae* in the absence of preformed antibodies; in the presence of antibody, organisms are trapped effectively at extrasplenic sites. Because the acquisition of pneumococcal antibodies occurs with advancing age, young children without spleen function fare less well than older children and adults. Other mechanisms may contribute to the vulnerability of children with sickle cell disease to infections: serum

immunoglobulin M levels are decreased,[258] the alternative pathway for complement activation may be defective,[259] and chronic vascular inflammation promoting upregulation of the ligand for pneumococcal invasion occur.[260,261]

Acute infection has been one of the most common causes of hospitalization and previously was the most frequent cause of death, particularly during the first 3 years of life. *S. pneumoniae* is the usual infecting organism; the blood and spinal fluid are the major sites of infection. Previously, the incidence of invasive infection with *S. pneumoniae* was about 7 per 100 patient-years in children with SCA who were <5 years of age; this rate was 30 to 100 times than which would be expected in a healthy population of this age.[262,263] More than 70% of meningitis in children with SCA also resulted from *S. pneumoniae*.[264] The mortality rate of pneumococcal sepsis was as high as 35%, but widespread improvement in parental education and aggressive management of the febrile child has greatly improved the likelihood of surviving a septic event. Furthermore, penicillin prophylaxis and pneumococcal vaccines have dramatically lowered the risk of invasive pneumococcal infection. Despite the dramatic decline in the rate of pneumococcal sepsis in recent decades (secondary to widespread use of pneumococcal immunization and penicillin prophylaxis), invasive pneumococcal infection still exists and may be life threatening. A major threat to continued success in prevention and management of *S. pneumoniae* invasive infection has been the emergence of antibiotic-resistant pneumococcal organisms over the past 2 decades.[265,266] In addition, selective pressure from penicillin prophylaxis, pneumococcal vaccines, and the sickle cell host environment promotes changes in the pneumococcal genome, allowing the pathogen to adapt, despite exposure to conjugate vaccine coverage by capsule switching and also through retaining invasive capacity.[267]

Beyond 5 years of age, gram-negative bacteria replace *S. pneumoniae* as the major infectious agents. In contrast to infections in young children, those in older children and adults generally have an identifiable source or focus (e.g., *Escherichia coli* associated with urinary tract infection). Osteomyelitis, sometimes involving multiple sites, occurs with increased frequency at all ages. The increased risk of osteomyelitis may stem from tissue ischemia and infarction associated with pain crises; these provide a potential nidus for infection in the long bones. Although >80% of hematogenous osteomyelitis in the general population is caused by *Staphylococcus*, most cases of osteomyelitis occurring in individuals with SCA are caused by *Salmonella*. A positive blood culture for *Salmonella* in a patient with SCA strongly suggests the diagnosis of osteomyelitis.[268] Staphylococcal bone infection, clinically indistinguishable from *Salmonella* infection, also occurs with increased frequency in sickle cell disease.

Bloodstream infections in hospitalized adults with sickle cell disease have been increasingly recognized. In one series,[269] 28% were caused by *S. aureus*, the majority of which were methicillin resistant. Gram-negative organisms, anaerobes, and yeast were also found and >80% of the infections were considered to be catheter related. Bloodstream infections frequently are associated with bone and joint infection.[270]

Prevention of Infection. The use of penicillin prophylaxis has been a major advance in the management of sickle cell disease. Two controlled trials, one in Jamaica and one in the United States, led to the widespread acceptance of penicillin prophylaxis as standard therapy.[271,272] In the latter trial (prophylactic penicillin study), twice-daily oral penicillin V resulted in an 84% reduction in the incidence of pneumococcal bacteremia in infants <36 months of age. Current recommendations are to initiate penicillin prophylaxis by 2 months of age and to continue it at least until 5 years of age in children with Hb SS or Hb Sβ[0]-thalassemia (or longer if there was a history of surgical splenectomy, incomplete pneumococcal immunization, or invasive pneumococcal infection).[273] A multi–institutional controlled trial found no further advantage of penicillin in the prevention of invasive pneumococcal infection in children >5 years of age.[274] The use of prophylaxis in young children with Hb SC disease or Hb Sβ[+]-thalassemia is debated, but most centers maintain all children with sickle cell disease on penicillin until 5 years of age.

Unfortunately, the pneumococcal serotypes that are most prevalent in the community and most highly virulent (types 6A, 14, 19, and 23F) are least immunogenic. Although the immunologic response of children 2 years of age and older to polysaccharide-conjugated pneumococcal vaccine is comparable to that of the general population,[275] antibody titers fall more rapidly than in adults. Children with sickle cell disease should receive a primary immunization with the 23-valent polysaccharide vaccine (PPSV23) at 2 years of age and a booster immunization 5 years later[276]; the vaccine is ineffective in children <2 years of age. A booster of PPSV23 should be administered in the young adulthood years, and many centers advocate for a booster once every 5 to 10 years thereafter.

In contrast, the 13-valent protein-conjugated pneumococcal vaccine is immunogenic in the first few months of life and is routinely administered to infants in the United States. This vaccine (which includes serotypes 1, 3, 4, 5, 6A, 6B, 7F, 9V, 14, 18C, 19A, 19F, and 23F) is administered at 2, 4, 6, and 12 months of age (same immunization schedule as in the general pediatric population) and produces adequate antibody concentrations even if administered after PPSV23 immunization.[277] The protein-conjugated vaccine has been reported to lower the incidence of invasive pneumococcal disease between 65% and >90% in children with sickle cell disease,[278,279] but it has not completely eliminated invasive pneumococcal infection.[265]

The conjugated *Haemophilus influenzae* type B vaccine induces protective antibody levels in young infants with SCA and has virtually eliminated invasive *H. influenzae* infection in this population. Yearly influenza virus vaccine (including H1N1 strains) and the complete series with three doses of hepatitis B vaccine offer further protection. Meningococcal polysaccharide diphtheria toxoid–conjugated vaccine offers protection against serogroups A, C, Y, and W-135 meningococcus and is recommended in children with sickle cell disease at ages 2, 4, 6, and 12 months. A booster every 5 years is recommended. Meningococcal serogroup B vaccine series are also recommended in addition to ACYW vaccines and are given as two-dose series (30 days-6 months apart) for patients >10 years of age.[280] For updated information regarding the recommended schedule of immunization in children and adults in the United States, the CDC website (www.CDC.gov) should be consulted. The high frequency of parvovirus B19 infections in children with sickle cell disease, their life-threatening nature, and the associated risk of complications indicate the need for a vaccine that would confer lifelong immunity. A vaccine for parvovirus B19 (viral particles 1 and 2 proteins expressed in a baculovirus system with adjuvant MF59) has been developed and tested in phase I studies, but side effects stalled further studies.[281] More recently, a yeast-based virus-like particle was shown to be immunogenic in wild type mice and also in sickle mice when coadministered with the adjuvant MF59.[282,283] Clinical trials of this new parvovirus B19 vaccine have not yet been initiated.

Management of Fever. Any fever ≥38.5 °C in a child with SCA must be considered a medical emergency because of the potential risk of overwhelming pneumococcal sepsis, especially during the high-risk period between 6 months and 3 years of age.[273] The majority of febrile patients can be managed in the emergency department and the outpatient setting if they do not have high-risk characteristics (e.g., toxic appearance, very high fever, serious localized infection, exceptionally high or low WBC count, a history of invasive infection, or inadequate capacity for close follow-up). These children may be managed with prompt assessment, rapid administration of ceftriaxone, observation for at least 2 hours, and close outpatient follow-up.

Chronic Organ Damage
Growth and Development
The sickling syndromes profoundly affect growth and development. Although normal at birth, the height and weights of children with SCA were significantly delayed by 2 years of age.[284-286] Increases in velocity of adolescent height and weight growth occur later, and the magnitude of the growth spurt is substantially less than in healthy children. This was also seen in the SCCRIP cohort where approximately 58% of the study cohort fell below the 50th percentile (z score = 0) curve for stature of age $(P = .007)$[287](*Figure 34.9A* and *B*). Owing to the greater exposure to disease-modifying therapies for sickle cell disease, recent cohort studies have shown a growing number of children with normal or above normal weight for height and age.[288] Puberty also is delayed. Menarche occurs 2 to 3 years later than in the general population (median age 14.0-15.5 years), and Tanner stage V is not achieved until the median ages of 17.3 and 17.6 years for girls and boys, respectively. As in normal subjects, progression through Tanner stages is orderly and appropriate for bone age, and the age of menarche correlates closely with age and weight. By adulthood, both men and women with sickle cell disease appear to acquire normal or near-normal heights, but their mean weights are still lower than those of controls.[284] The normal relationship of puberty and growth pattern seen in most patients suggests that the delay in skeletal maturation represents constitutional delay rather than gonadal or pituitary failure.

The basis for delay in weight gain is not fully understood, although it has been hypothesized that chronic hemolysis leads to a state of high protein turnover and increased basal metabolic requirements.[289] Studies have shown that decreased growth velocity in children with SCA was independently associated with decreased Hb concentration and increased total resting energy expenditure.[290,291] In fact, recent data have shown an association between higher Hb and overweight.[288]

Other studies have suggested increased requirements for zinc, folate, riboflavin, vitamin B_6, ascorbate, and the fat-soluble vitamins A and E, but consistent correlations between deficiencies and growth retardation have not been established.[292,293] Defective growth hormone secretion, decreased insulin-like growth factor-1, and partial resistance to growth hormone in short children with sickle cell disease were reported.[294,295]

Bones and Joints
In addition to the acute episodes of skeletal pain, chronic and progressive destruction of the bones and joints may take place in the absence of clearly defined episodes of pain. The most prominent changes evolve slowly from the cumulative effect of recurrent small episodes of ischemia or infarction within the spongiosa of bone. Radiographs of the long bones of adults show a mottled strand-like increase in density randomly distributed within the medullary region (*Figure 34.10*). These irregular areas of increased density are produced by new bone laid down on devitalized trabeculae. Because the bone is weakened during the early stages of repair, weight bearing may collapse the femoral head, producing the clinical and radiologic features of osteonecrosis (also known as avascular necrosis of the femoral head), which affects patients with all the genotypes of sickle cell disease, but occurs most often in those with Hb SS and α-thalassemia (4.5 cases/100 patient-years).[296] Osteonecrosis is associated with decreased bone mineral density, which should be corrected by height in children with SCD (*Figure 34.9C* and *D*).[287] The overall prevalence of symptomatic osteonecrosis of the hip in persons with sickle cell disease is approximately 10%, but it occurs in 50% in those >35 years of age.[296] The prevalence of symptomatic osteonecrosis of the humeral head is approximately one-half as much.[297] Typically, the pain from osteonecrosis of the hip begins insidiously, is brought on by walking or quick movements, and is localized to the groin or buttock. In the early phases, plain radiographic films usually cannot identify bone damage; therefore, MRI is a more sensitive method for the early phases of osteonecrosis.[298] With progressive bone damage, radiographs may show areas of increased density mixed with areas of increased lucency, followed by the appearance of a "crescent sign," segmental collapse, molding of the femoral head, loss of joint space, involvement of the acetabulum, and complete degeneration of the joint. When osteonecrosis occurs in the femoral capital epiphysis before closure, healing with minimal destruction may occur. However, long-term follow-up showed, in the majority of cases, the hip is painful and permanently damaged and can affect quality of life by predisposing to chronic pain[287] and resulting in high health care utilization.[299] Because weight bearing is not required for the shoulder joint, the prognosis of osteonecrosis of the humeral head is substantially better. Only about 20% of patients have pain or limited range of movement at the time of diagnosis,[297] but

Disorders of Red Blood Cells

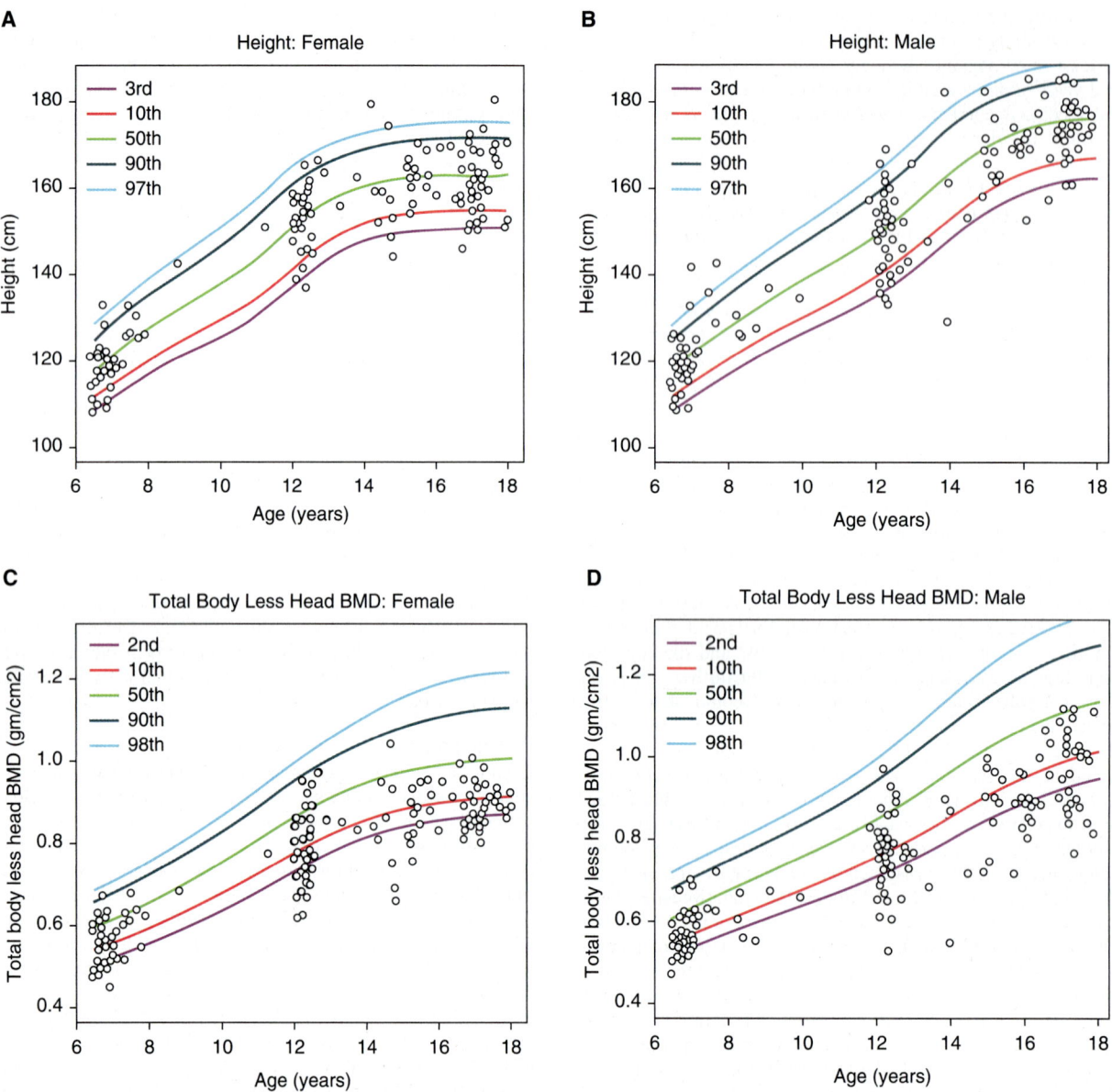

FIGURE 34.9 Sex differences in height-for-age and total body less head (TBLH) areal bone mineral density (aBMD)-for-age curves in the Sickle Cell Clinical Research and Intervention Program (SCCRIP) pediatric cohort. Stature-for-age curves for female subjects (A) and male subjects (B) in the SCCRIP pediatric cohort, compared with reference data from healthy children and adolescents from the US National Center for Health Statistics. TBLH aBMD vs chronological age for female subjects (C) and male subjects (D) in the SCCRIP pediatric cohort. The TBLH aBMD reference curves were obtained from healthy African American control subjects, ages 6 to 18 years, enrolled in the BMDCS. The 50th percentile (green line) represents the mean value-for-age (z score = 0) of the reference populations. (Reprinted from Adesina OO, Gurney JG, Kang G, et al. Height-corrected low bone density associates with severe outcomes in sickle cell disease: SCCRIP cohort study results. *Blood Adv.* 2019;3(9):1476-1488. Copyright © 2019 American Society of Hematology. With permission.)

functional abnormalities of the shoulder may be a long-term consequence in adults. Although screening for asymptomatic osteonecrosis with MRI of the femoral head is not recommended,[273] many asymptomatic cases may go undiagnosed until symptoms occur at a very late stage (collapse of the femoral head). Simpler screening methods could be employed, with careful joint exam and questions related to physical function.

Avoidance of weight bearing in the early phases of bone necrosis may permit sufficient repair to preserve reasonable joint function. More often, however, the deformity is progressively crippling. Total hip replacement is usually recommended for the painful hip in stage III or IV or for restoration of joint movement if this is desired. However, hip replacement is not definitive and may require revision. However, durable long-term results were recently reported with noncemented total hip arthroplasty with almost 97% implant survivorship at 10 years and 94% at 15 years.[300] For stage I and II osteonecrosis,

core decompression, in which a core of cancellous bone <8 mm in diameter is removed from the neck and head of the femur through an incision in the lateral cortex, has been of benefit.[301,302] However, in a prospective randomized trial, physical therapy alone appeared to be as effective as hip core decompression followed by physical therapy, improving hip function and postponing the need for additional surgical intervention at a mean of 3 years after treatment.[303] Grafting with autologous bone marrow–derived mononuclear cells obtained from the iliac crest is a possible new option for osteonecrosis of the hip.[304,305] This technique, which is currently investigational, appears most effective in the early stages of osteonecrosis, before subchondral collapse has occurred, and provides progenitor cells to the proximal femur which stimulate bone remodeling. The effect of hydroxyurea on the natural history of osteonecrosis is still unclear. While hydroxyurea therapy may slow down the progression of osteonecrosis in children and adolescents,[306,307] spontaneous regression without surgical

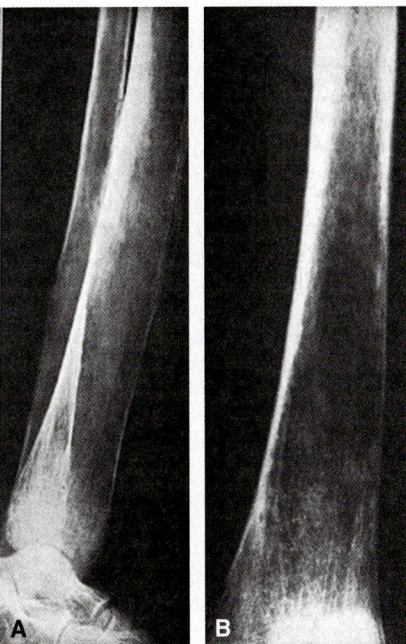

FIGURE 34.10 Long bones in sickle cell anemia. A, Femur. The cortex is thinned, and the normal bony architecture is disturbed. Adjoining small areas of translucency are areas of sclerosis. B, Tibia and fibula. Marked thinning of the cortex of the bones as well as periosteal reaction and disarrangement of the trabeculae. The latter changes and the extensive coarseness of the cortical layers suggest the bone is involved from within.

or significant physical therapy interventions has been reported particularly in younger children (9.9 ± 2.5 years vs 14.6 ± 2.2 years, $P = .002$) and seems to be independent of hydroxyurea exposure.[308] Hospital discharge data from California's Office of Statewide Health Planning and Development (1991-2013) that spanned the decades before and after the Food and Drug Administration (FDA) approval of hydroxyurea for SCA patients showed a decrease in incidence of osteonecrosis in the posthydroxyurea era when compared to the prehydroxyurea (1.52 per 100 person years; 95%CI: 1.41, 1.63 vs 2.37 per 100 person years; 95%CI: 2.18, 2.56). The authors speculated that this was most likely due to decreased opportunity to diagnose osteonecrosis secondary to reduced emergency room utilization and hospitalization for vaso-occlusive events.[309]

Another characteristic bone change develops in the vertebral column of some individuals during the second decade of life. Recurrent infarcts of the main vertebral arteries lead to ischemic damage of the central portion of the vertebral body growth plates. Because the outer portion of the plates is supplied by numerous apophyseal arteries, vertebral growth is irregular, producing a "fish-mouth" deformity, in which symmetric cuplike depressions are confined to the central three-fifths of the vertebral plates. Other skeletal changes result from expansion of medullary cavities owing to long-standing erythroid hyperplasia. Radiographs of the skull show a thickening of the diplöe and thinning of the outer table of the calvaria in the frontal and parietal regions. Gnathopathy (prominent maxillary overbite) may result from overgrowth of maxillary bone and frequently leads to significant malocclusion.

Low bone mass density (osteopenia and osteoporosis) has been recognized in adults and even in children,[310,311] despite correcting for short stature.[287] It has been associated with severity of hemolysis,[312] and chronic pain.[287] Vitamin D levels are low in sickle cell disease. With vitamin D deficiency as a level <20 ng/mL, prevalence estimates in sickle cell disease populations range from 56% to 96.4%.[313] Vitamin D replacement in those cases of vitamin D deficiency has been reported to improve bone density,[314] but its efficacy in reducing osteonecrosis or other bone abnormalities is yet to be determined.

Joints may be affected by avascular necrosis of adjacent bone. The joint effusion, pain, fever, and leukocytosis accompanying such infarcts make differentiation from septic arthritis difficult. Numerous neutrophils and sickled erythrocytes are found in the joint fluid. Less commonly, joint disease is related to infection, gout, or synovial hemosiderosis. Adults may have deformities of the hands and feet with shortening of the digits, the remote sequelae of dactylitis during early childhood.

Cognitive Function

Cognitive function refers to cerebral activities that lead to knowledge and the means and mechanisms of acquiring and processing information. Multiple studies have reported deficits in global and specific cognitive functioning in school-aged children with sickle cell disease when compared with their siblings or healthy children.[185,315,316] Children with sickle cell disease underperform relative to controls in FSIQ and on measures of verbal ability, as well as domain-specific areas such as memory, language, and executive function.[317,318] A recent meta-analysis showed significant deficits in FSIQ, verbal reasoning, and executive function even in infants and preschool aged children.[319] Data show a slow but steady decline in cognitive function over time.[320-322] Although cognitive deficits are found even in the absence of apparent abnormalities on brain MRI overall, these deficits are proportional to the degree of injury to the brain.[319,320,323,324] Children with SCA who have experienced an overt stroke have significant cognitive impairment, reduced language function, and problems in adjustment.[325] Children with SCI had twice the rate of school difficulties as those without SCI, including poor educational attainment.[326] Additionally, in the United States, compared with children without sickle cell diseases, grade retention is 10 times more likely in sickle cell disease.[327]

Similar to children, adults with SCA have poorer cognitive performance when compared with healthy controls, even without a history of prior stroke.[328] Cognitive deficits occur in all sickle genotypes, but are more prevalent in those with SCA.[327] Significant areas of deficit in adults with SCA were in working memory, processing speed, and other measures of executive function.[329] Lower FSIQ in the adult SCA population is associated with higher unemployment rates, low instrumental activities of daily living, and poor engagement with the adult care system.[330-332]

Risk factors for impaired cognitive function in sickle cell disease are multifactorial, including biologic and environmental factors. Brain ischemic lesions (SCI presence, SCI volume,[333] overt stroke) are among the most recognizable risk factors for cognitive dysfunction in sickle cell disease; however, although necessary, they are not sufficient, because decreased cognitive function occurs in patients with normal brain MRI exams (by conventional techniques). A meta-analysis of 17 reports of cognitive functioning in children concluded that sickle cell disease is associated with detrimental effects, even in the absence of cerebral infarction on MRI.[320] Compared with matched healthy controls, adults with sickle cell disease with reduced basal ganglia and thalamus volumes on brain MRI had lower IQ and performed worse on measures of executive function (perceptual organization and working memory).[334] The occurrence of an SCI at an early age places children with sickle cell disease at a particular risk for future cognitive impairments. SCI before age 5 is associated with greater subsequent progressive MRI abnormalities, concurrent brain vessel stenosis, decreased cognitive ability, including attention, and executive function deficits, with consequential hindered academic attainment.[177]

Other recognized risk factors for decreased cognitive function are hypoxemia and lower Hb concentration. Lower Hb concentration is a reported risk factor for both the development of SCI and neurocognitive impairments.[179,335] Decreases in Hb oxygen saturation and/or increased sleep arousals are associated with lower neuropsychological measures of executive function.[336] In addition, elevated blood flow velocity by TCD in children with SCA was associated with decreased language function (syntactical skills), even when controlling for the degree of anemia.[337,338] Elevated cytokine levels, including IL-4, IL-5, IL-8, and IL-13, were also shown to be associated with lower standardized test measurements of executive function, pointing to a potential role for inflammatory processes in cognitive outcomes in these children.[339]

Finally, whereas ischemic brain injury and other biologic factors account for impairment in FSIQ, socioenvironmental factors, including parental educational level, maternal depression, household income, and financial stress, all play significant role in cognitive impairment.[318,340,341]

New MRI modalities that examine CBF perfusion (e.g., arterial spin-labeling), neuroconnectivity (e.g., default mode network), and the effect of oxygenation on the magnetic properties of blood Hb (e.g., blood oxygenation level dependent) deserve further investigation and may prove useful in diagnosing and monitoring brain microvasculature damage and its relationship with neurocognition in sickle cell disease.[342,343]

Interventions for improving neurocognitive performance in patients with sickle cell disease are lacking. Studies evaluating the neuroprotective effect of hydroxyurea have shown an association of oral hydroxyurea therapy with better performance in verbal comprehension, fluid reasoning, general cognitive ability, verbal IQ, reaction speed, and sustained attention.[344-346] In a recent prospective study, children with Hb SS or Hb S/β0 thalassemia were evaluated 1 year after hydroxyurea initiation and saw a significant improvement in mean FSIQ (82.8 (±12.6) to 83.6 (±13.7); $P = 0.059$) and reading comprehension (79.4 (±17.2) to 81.6 (±17.3); $P = .033$).[347] Early initiation of hydroxyurea and longer duration of therapy positively correlated with cognitive performance.[322,346] While this impact on cognition by hydroxyurea can be explained by the improvement in anemia[346] and oxygen delivery to the brain,[344,348] an alternative mechanism through increased fetal Hb production without affecting the degree of anemia has also been proposed.[322,346] Additionally, the decreased TCD velocity with hydroxyurea treatment has been associated with increased performance on math fluency.[347] Neuropsychologic performance in patients who have undergone successful bone marrow transplants has been measured, and it appears that FSIQ levels have at least stabilized.[349,350] Central nervous system stimulants used for the treatment of attention deficit hyperactivity disorders (e.g., methylphenidate) have not been tested systematically in children with sickle cell disease, but have improved measures of memory and inhibitory control in a small group of children.[351] A pilot interventional study using home visitation (Parent as Teachers program) for a small number of preschool children with sickle cell disease showed improvements in the cognitive and expressive language domains of the Bayley Scales of Infant/Toddler Development-III,[352] addressing the socioenvironmental component of cognitive dysfunction in this population. However, effective interventions that improve preschool readiness are lacking.

Heart

Relative to other organs, cardiac complications in sickle cell disease are insufficiently studied or understood, despite, along with pulmonary complications, accounting for 30% of deaths among adults with sickle cell disease.[353,354] Cardiac enlargement has been known to occur in sickle cell disease for many years. It is observed from childhood onward, particularly an increase in left ventricular (LV) dimensions and mass, although systolic function is preserved.[355,356] The typical physical examination reveals a hyperdynamic precordium and a grade II–III (out of VI) systolic ejection murmur with wide radiation.

The mechanism for progression of myocardial dysfunction that leads to sudden death is not fully understood. LV hypertrophy is an adaptive mechanism to the anemia-related volume overload. Findings from a sickle cell mouse model point toward an additional mechanism causing LV hypertrophy-chronic inflammation induced by hypercoagulability. In the BERK sickle cell mouse, a reduction in tissue factor level was associated with less cardiac hypertrophy, which was corroborated by a decline in IL-6 levels and heart hypertrophy after treatment with rivaroxaban (factor Xa inhibitor).[357] Right ventricular (RV) preload and systolic function typically do not worsen during childhood; however, RV mass index, RV myocardial strain, and the prevalence of PHT increase, consistent

with rising pulmonary vascular resistance.[358,359] Myocardial ischemia, on the other hand, is observed in sickle cell disease, but, in general, in the absence of atherosclerotic coronary heart disease. Adults may present with clinical signs of acute myocardial infarction in the absence of atherosclerosis or coronary occlusion.[360,361] In children, rare cases of myocardial infarction and transient ventricular dysfunction have been reported.[362,363] Myocardial perfusion abnormality, measured by thallium-201 myocardial scintigraphy or single-photon emission computed tomography, may be relatively frequent, especially after inducing stress with exercise or dipyridamole.[364,365] Early findings of microvasculature perfusion deficits, coupled with recent information from new cardiac MRI techniques using gadolinium-diethylenetriamine pentaacetic acid (DTPA), have indicated myocardial perfusion deficits and reduced perfusion reserve.[366,367] The same MRI-DTPA technique has disclosed diffuse myocardial fibrosis in individuals with sickle cell disease.[368] These findings are revamping our current understanding of cardiac disease progression in sickle cell disease.

Systolic dysfunction is rare and is seen in adults. Myocardial strain is more sensitive than the conventional echocardiographic measure left ventricular ejection fraction in identifying subclinical systolic dysfunction. A recent meta-analysis reported that RV and LV global longitudinal strain are abnormal and mostly decreased in SCA.[369] Diastolic dysfunction is common, begins early in life, and easily diagnosed and monitored using tissue Doppler and speckle tracking echocardiography techniques.[370,371] LV diastolic dysfunction is associated with Hb concentration, but not with iron deposition in the myocardium.[372] Diastolic dysfunction, as reflected by a low E/A ratio in the tissue Doppler, was associated with mortality with a risk ratio of 3.5, even after adjustment for elevated tricuspid regurgitant jet velocity (TRV). The presence of both diastolic dysfunction and elevated TRV conferred a risk ratio for death of 12.0.[373] Other markers of abnormal diastolic function including lower diastolic myocardial tissue velocity (lateral e′) were also predictive of increased mortality.[374] Diastolic dysfunction has also been shown to be associated with exercise intolerance (decreased 6-minute walk distance) in both adults and children.[375,376]

Varying degrees of myocardial fibrosis including focal or diffuse have been reported in autopsy studies in SCA patients.[367,377] Diffuse myocardial fibrosis as determined by an increased extracellular volume on cardiac MRI was found in SCA patients and was associated with diastolic dysfunction.[368] The etiology of myocardial fibrosis remains to be determined and is thought to be secondary to microvascular vaso-occlusion, wall stress, or effects of hemolysis on myocardium. Electrophysiology changes have also been noted in patients with sickle cell disease. In a screening study of sickle cell subjects between the ages of 10 and 24 years, prolongation of the QTc interval was observed in 29 of 76 (38%) subjects, and was not associated with the presence of LV hypertrophy.[378] Myocardial fibrosis and ongoing myocardial injury from compromised microvascular perfusion predispose to dysrhythmias and sudden death in sickle cell disease.[379] Recently, a higher expression of the profibrotic cytokine IL18 was reported in SCA patients with myocardial fibrosis or QTc prolongation, indicating a possible role of IL-18 in mediating sickle cardiomyopathy and being a potential therapeutic target for patients at risk of sudden cardiac death.[380]

A unifying mechanism for the progression of myocardial dysfunction, including diastolic dysfunction and PHT, has been proposed. This model purports an intrinsic cardiomyopathy with features of both restrictive physiology and anemia-induced hyperdynamic physiology.[381,382] A unique aspect of the proposed restrictive physiology model is that the decreased ventricular compliance occurs in the setting of LV dilation and LV eccentric hypertrophy, differing from the classic myocardial restrictive physiology, in which the LV is not dilated. The proposed sequence of events begins with restrictive LV filling, which leads to subsequent left atrium enlargement and increased left atrial pressure, which in turn leads to backpressure within the pulmonary venous circulation, pulmonary venous hypertension (PVH), and increased TRV.

In summary, the progression of cardiac disease in sickle cell disease is complex and not completely understood. Recent data support a model that likely involves the downstream effects of anemia-induced LV hypertrophy and ongoing myocardial ischemic injury, causing decreased ventricular compliance, cardiomyocyte loss, fibrosis, arrhythmia, diastolic dysfunction, elevated pulmonary pressure, and eventually sudden death (*Figure 34.11*).

Lungs

Chronic pulmonary disease is common in both children and adults with sickle cell disease and includes pulmonary function abnormalities (i.e., restrictive and obstructive patterns), recurrent wheezing, asthma, sleep-disordered breathing, and PHT (pre- and postcapillary).

Pulmonary function abnormalities have been thought to be primarily restrictive, especially among adults[383,384] and in those with history of ACS.[383,385] Typically, the total lung capacity and gas mixing and exchange (diffusion capacity of the lung for carbon monoxide) are compromised.[386] Recent data have pointed to substantial obstructive pathology, accounting for a significant proportion of abnormal pulmonary function in sickle cell disease, especially among children.[387,388] The underlying pathophysiology for abnormal lung function is not fully understood, but recurrent vaso-occlusion in the lungs (especially recurrent ACS events) causes acute and chronic inflammation. Furthermore, lung vaso-occlusion causes blood to be shunted through poorly aerated or collapsed segments of the lung, creating a disparity between ventilation and perfusion. The resulting reduction in the functional pulmonary vascular tree is responsible for a decrease in arterial oxygen tension to 70 to 90 mm Hg and desaturation of arterial blood. Hb oxygen saturation is lower in children with Hb SS/Sβ⁰ thalassemia compared with those with Hb SC/Sβ⁺ thalassemia.[389,390] Although pulse oximetry may underestimate true arterial saturation (because of the right shift of the Hb dissociation curve), pulse oximetry values correlate positively with Hb and fetal Hb levels in patients with Hb SS.[391,392]

There is a high prevalence of asthma and increased airway responsiveness among pediatric patients with sickle cell disease.[211,393,394] Up to 70% of children with sickle cell disease have airway hyperresponsiveness.[395] The presence of both asthma and airway hyperresponsiveness is linked to a higher incidence of pain, ACS events, and early death in children.[396,397] Wheezing is common in SCA and is seen even in the absence of an asthma diagnosis.[387,398] In children, history of wheezing (recent or remote) was the strongest predictor of decline in PFT (FEV$_1$/FVC) in children,[399] while adults with recurrent episodes of wheezing had higher pain and ACS events, decreased lung function, and increased risk of death.[400] Additionally, among adults with sickle cell disease, a forced expiratory volume in 1 second less than 70% of predicted was associated with early mortality.[401] Hemolysis has recently been linked to the pathophysiology of increased airway responsiveness. A cross-sectional study of children with sickle cell disease found an association of LDH levels and airway responsiveness following methacholine test.[402]

The pathophysiology of asthma in sickle cell disease does not seem to follow the same biology as in the general population, as supported by the lack of increased NO flux in the presence of obstruction in the PFT.[403] Because of the high prevalence of asthma and airway hyperresponsiveness in sickle cell disease, the overlap of symptoms of asthma exacerbation and ACS, and the inheritance pattern of asthma within families of patients with sickle cell disease, it is hypothesized that asthma, or perhaps even airway hyperresponsiveness, is in fact part of the pathophysiology of sickle cell disease, rather than being two separate comorbid conditions.[404] Further investigation is needed to elucidate asthma biology in sickle cell disease.

PHT is a major cause of morbidity and mortality among adults with sickle cell disease.[405,406] PHT is defined by a mean pulmonary artery pressure (mPAP) ≥20 mm Hg. PHT in SCA can have features of precapillary or pulmonary arterial hypertension (mPAP >20 mm Hg, pulmonary vascular resistance ≥3 Wood units), postcapillary hypertension (PVH secondary to LV dysfunction), or both. PHT as diagnosed by right heart catherization is present in 6% to 10% of adults with sickle cell disease.[407,408] Although not corresponding to cardiac catheterization documented PHT in all cases, the elevation of TRV on the echocardiogram has been used to estimate PHT. In validation studies against cardiac catheterization, however, a TRV of ≥2.5 m/s had a sensitivity of 78% and specificity of 19%, whereas a higher TRV cutoff of >2.9 m/s had a higher specificity of 81%, but lower sensitivity of 67%.[407,408] Nevertheless, a TRV ≥2.5 m/s is associated with increased mortality among adults with sickle cell disease.[405,409,410] More recently, data from the Pulmonary Hypertension and the Hypoxic Response study, which prospectively followed a cohort of children, adolescents, and young adults with SCD, showed that 20% of patient who died had a TRV ≥2.7 m/s compared to 4.6% of those who survived (*P* = .012).[411] TRV ≥2.5 m/s is present in approximately 30% of adults and children with sickle cell disease.[412-414] Although not fully understood, this prognostic role of TRV elevation appears to point toward disease severity, as demonstrated by studies linking TRV elevation and increased frequency of vaso-occlusive pain, ACS episodes, and proteinuria.[409,415,416] TRV was found to be inversely associated with flow-mediated dilation, a measure of endothelial function, suggesting that endothelial dysfunction and TRV elevation share a common pathophysiology.[417,418]

A potential diagnostic approach and risk stratification for PHT in adults (but not in children) with sickle cell disease has been proposed by the American Thoracic Society utilizing a combination of TRV, N-terminal-proBNP (NT-proBNP), and 6-minute walk tests results.[419] In these guidelines, increased mortality risk was defined as a TRV ≥2.5 m/s, an NT-proBNP level ≥160 pg/mL, or PHT confirmed by right heart catheterization.

Disorders of Red Blood Cells

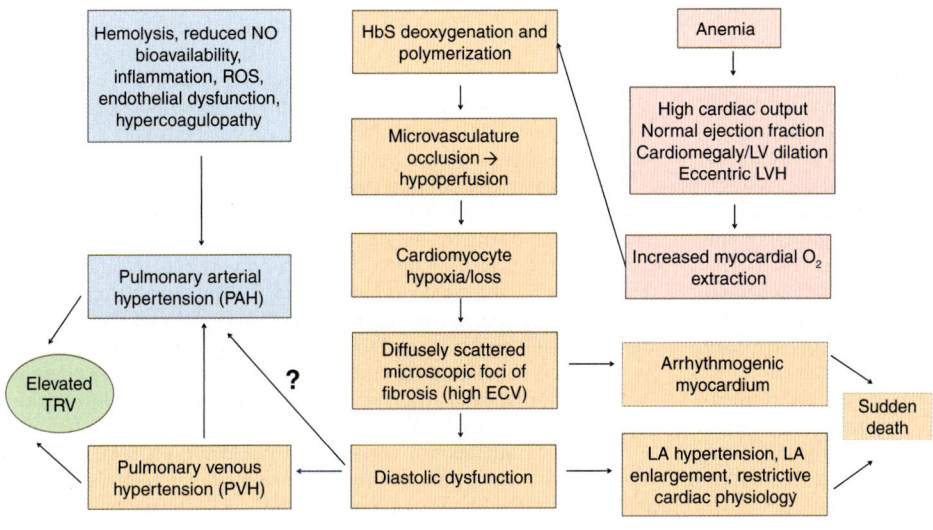

FIGURE 34.11 Proposed mechanism for the development of the cardiomyopathy of sickle cell disease. ECV, extracellular volume fraction; LA, left atrium; LV, left ventricle; LVH, left ventricular hypertrophy; NO, nitric oxide; TRV, tricuspid regurgitation jet velocity. (From Rai P, Niss O, Malik P. A reappraisal of the mechanisms underlying the cardiac complications of sickle cell anemia. *Pediatr Blood Cancer.* 2017;64(11):e26607. Copyright © 2017 Wiley Periodicals, Inc. Reprinted by permission of John Wiley & Sons, Inc.)

Therapeutic intervention for PHT has been limited. Data regarding the effect of disease-modifying therapy like hydroxyurea and monthly blood transfusions have been conflicting.[123,417,420-427] A recent large singe center prospective longitudinal study reported hydroxyurea use to be associated with a 5% decrease in mean TRV over a 2-year period.[428] Sildenafil, a phosphodiesterase 5-inhibitor, was tested in a large multicenter placebo-controlled double-blinded trial of adults with sickle cell disease with elevated TRV and low exercise capacity by the 6-minute walk distance test (walk-PHaSST study); however, the trial was stopped early because of a higher percentage of subjects experiencing serious adverse events (pain) in the sildenafil arm.[429] There was no evidence of a treatment effect on the 6-minute walk, TRV, or NT-proBNP. It is unclear why sildenafil increased the incidence of painful events, but lowering of the pain threshold has been postulated as a possible explanation. Other management considerations include other pulmonary vasodilators, such as endothelin receptor agonists (ambrisentan and bosentan), and various forms of prostaglandin therapy.[430] Endothelin receptor agonists were tested in two clinical trials (ASSET studies), but because of low accrual rate, the studies were interrupted early and were underpowered to show any benefit.[431] Intrapulmonary thromboembolism has been postulated as a modulator of PHT by promoting decreased perfusion on radionuclide lung scans.[432] Although this has not been confirmed by subsequent studies,[433,434] investigation of the role of anticoagulation in patients with sickle cell disease and PHT is warranted.

At present, treatment of PHT includes intensification of antisickling therapies (hydroxyurea and chronic transfusions) and referral to specialists for confirmation of diagnosis and possibly use of pulmonary vasodilators.[419]

Sleep Disorders

Sleep-disordered breathing (e.g., obstructive sleep apnea, snoring, insomnia, restless leg syndrome) is increased among patients with sickle cell disease, although most studies have been retrospective and did not utilize polysomnography to confirm findings, but rather relied on validated sleep disorder questionnaires.[435] In children with SCA, the prevalence of obstructive sleep apnea by polysomnography in a large pediatric cohort was 41% for apnea-hypopnea index (AHI) ≥1 and 10% for AHI ≥5.[436] The prevalence of sleep-disordered breathing appears to increase with age, exemplified by a small adult sample with an overall prevalence of AHI ≥5 of 44%.[437] Although sparse, there is some linkage between nightly oxygen Hb desaturation and central nervous system insults, nocturnal enuresis, painful vaso-occlusive crisis events, and priapism.[119,438,439] Further investigation in this area might establish supportive therapeutic options to reduce nightly oxygen desaturation.

Hepatobiliary and Gastrointestinal Systems

Liver enlargement is present by 1 year of age and persists to a moderate degree throughout life. Analysis of histologic sections reveals distention of sinusoids with sickled cells, Kupffer cell erythrophagocytosis, and varying degrees of periportal fibrosis and hemosiderin pigment.[440] It is not unusual for hyperbilirubinemia (with increases in both direct and indirect bilirubin) to punctuate the course of SCA. These episodes may result from hemolysis, intercurrent infectious hepatitis, intrahepatic sickling (hepatic crisis, "sickle hepatopathy"), or choledocholithiasis. Coexistent G6PD deficiency may be a contributing factor.[441]

Hepatitis A virus may be a frequent cause of acute icteric hepatitis in endemic areas and may result in fulminant hepatic failure and death.[442] Sickle cell patients respond normally to hepatitis B vaccine,[443] although surface antibody titers after immunization should be measured to identify those who do not convert and require booster injections.[444] Evidence of prior hepatitis C virus infection has been found in 10% to 21% of SCA patients,[445,446] but since the advent of screening of transfused blood for hepatitis C, new cases of this infection have become extremely rare. Liver biopsies may show progression to chronic active hepatitis and cirrhosis. The use of liver transplantation for end-stage liver disease has been reported in 22 cases worldwide with slowly improving results.[447]

Acute enlargement of the liver may occur with sequestration of sickle cells, subcapsular infarction, or hepatic vein thrombosis[448,449] and is associated with right upper quadrant tenderness or pain. The histologic consequences of intrahepatic sickling include impaction of hepatic sinusoids with sickled erythrocytes, patchy areas of hepatocellular necrosis, engorgement of Kupffer cells, and bile stasis.[440,450] Sickle hepatopathy, referring to intrahepatic cholestasis, may be defined by a total serum bilirubin concentration >13 mg/dL, not explained by severe acute hemolysis, viral hepatitis, extrahepatic obstruction, or hepatic sequestration.[451] In children, manifestations of sickle hepatopathy are relatively mild and transient. These include right upper quadrant pain, hepatomegaly, fever and leukocytosis, mild elevation of serum transaminase levels, and moderate to marked elevation of serum bilirubin and alkaline phosphatase levels.[452] Although the course in children is benign and symptoms usually resolve in 1 to 3 weeks, progression to fulminant hepatic failure, generalized bleeding, and death are much more frequent in adults[451] and are occasionally seen in adolescents.[453] Total serum bilirubin level of >13.0 mg/dL has been reported to be predictive of end organ injury and associated with an increased need for blood products.[454] Prompt exchange transfusion and, occasionally, chronic transfusion have been effective therapies in these patients.

Because of a sustained increase in heme catabolism, the frequency of pigmentary gallstones in sickle cell disease is high. The incidence of gallstones increases with age, from 12% in the 2- to 4-year-old age group to 42% in the 15- to 18-year-old age group and 60% in adults.[455] When ultrasonography is used routinely, the finding of gallbladder sludge with or without concurrent stones is common[456]; even if it is not present initially, patients with sludge eventually develop stones. Genetic variations in the uridine diphosphate-glucuronosyltransferase 1α promoter significantly influence serum bilirubin levels and the development of symptomatic cholelithiasis in children with SCA.[457] Chronic transfusion, even if used for prolonged periods, does not seem to prevent the development of gallstones.[458] Laparoscopic cholecystectomy has replaced open cholecystectomy in most centers because it results in shorter hospitalization and decreased postoperative pain and other complications.[459,460] While a shorter postoperative hospitalization stay was seen with elective or symptomatic cholecystectomy when compared to emergent cholecystectomy,[461] the use of elective cholecystectomy for asymptomatic cholelithiasis is still controversial.[462]

The chronic use of blood transfusions eventually leads to significant accumulation of iron in the liver (hemosiderosis). Although iron initially accumulates in reticuloendothelial cells of the liver (sinusoids), with continued transfusions, it is incorporated in parenchymal cells (hepatocytes), increasing the risk of liver injury with hepatocyte damage, synthetic dysfunction, fibrosis, and eventually cirrhosis.[463]

Kidneys

A variety of defects in renal function have been described,[464] and a number of histologic alterations noted.[465] Even in the absence of clinically apparent renal disease, small cortical infarcts of varying ages are evident,[466] hemosiderin is deposited in the epithelium of proximal convoluted tubules, glomerular arterioles are dilated and congested, glomerular surface area relative to kidney size is increased,[465] and varying degrees of juxtamedullary glomerular hypertrophy and sclerosis are seen. Symmetric enlargement of the kidneys is a regular feature.

Hyposthenuria[467,468] is a result of tubular damage and is present after 6 to 12 months of age. Disruption of the countercurrent multiplication system owing to sludging of sickle cells in the more hypertonic portions of the renal medulla has been proposed as the mechanism responsible for the concentrating defect.[467] The demonstrated obliteration of a portion of the vasa rectae is in keeping with this hypothesis.[466] Presumably because of the large fluid consumption necessitated by the renal-concentrating defect, most patients experience enuresis.[469] Nocturnal enuresis is prevalent and associated with low health-related quality of life.[470,471]

Urinary acidification is abnormal in sickle cell patients, probably resulting from an incomplete form of distal tubular acidosis attributable to diminished ability of the collecting duct to maintain hydrogen ion gradient.[472,473] Impaired potassium excretion by the kidney and subsequent hyperkalemia, increased phosphate reabsorption, and increased uric acid clearance have also been described.[474,475]

Hematuria is common and may be both brisk and prolonged. Bleeding may originate in one kidney or both. The most common lesion is an ulcer in the renal pelvis at the site of a papillary infarct (acute papillary necrosis).[476,477] The possibility that painless hematuria may be the result of poststreptococcal glomerulonephritis,[478] renal medullary carcinoma,[479] or other disorders unrelated to the hemoglobinopathy should not be overlooked. Idiopathic hematuria rarely requires more than symptomatic treatment. The risk of clotting within the collecting system is best minimized with a high fluid intake. Although there is no controlled study of its use, ε-aminocaproic acid is said to shorten the duration of hematuria in both SCA and sickle trait subjects.[480,481] Its use, however, is attended by a risk of ureteral obstruction resulting from blood clots.

The nephrotic syndrome is an infrequent but well-documented complication of SCA that occurs in adolescents and adults. The syndrome may be associated with hypertension, hematuria, parvovirus B19 infection,[245] and progressive renal insufficiency culminating in renal failure. Pathologic lesions include glomerular enlargement and focal segmental glomerulosclerosis.[450,482] Glomerular enlargement is secondary to the increased glomerular filtration rate and effective renal plasma flow that are found in children but that decline to subnormal levels with increasing age or from adverse effects of nonsteroidal anti-inflammatory agents.[483,484] In addition, the increased cardiac output and vasodilation from increased production of prostacyclins contributes to the glomerular hyperfiltration. Glomerular damage in adults is very common and associated with albuminuria and progressive renal failure.[485] Glomerular hyperfiltration occurs in children with higher levels of hemolysis, has a prevalence of 76% in one pediatric cohort, progressively decreases with age, and has an inverse association with cystatin-C levels and systolic blood pressure.[486] In a recent longitudinal study, participants who developed albuminuria had a significant increase in their mean estimated glomerular filtration rate (eGFR) during early childhood ($P = .003$) as compared to those who had not yet developed albuminuria ($P = .26$), suggesting that hyperfiltration may precede the development of albuminuria in children.[487] Close monitoring of eGFR is recommended; however, equations for estimation of GFR have not shown good precision in patients with sickle cell disease. Equations using cystatin C seem to perform better,[488] but development of sickle cell–specific equations to estimate GFR is needed.

While albuminuria occurs commonly in adults (up to 26%-68%), in children its prevalence is lower at 26%.[489] Multiple studies have shown that short-term treatment (6 months) with angiotensin-converting enzyme inhibitors (ACEis) or angiotensin receptor blockers (ARBs) significantly decreased urinary albumin excretion from baseline (>25%-30% reduction).[490,491] The long-term benefit of these agents was evaluated in a single-center retrospective study (median treatment duration 2.28 years) and showed a slower rate of decline in eGFR (rate of eGFR decline 2.78 mL/min/1.73 m^2 vs 4.70 mL/min/1.73 m^2, $P <.0001$) and progression to chronic kidney disease (CKD) in those treated with ACEi or ARBs.[492] Hydroxyurea, used in conjunction with ACEi or alone, might offer additional benefit in reducing proteinuria and improving renal urine concentrating ability in both children and adults, although a randomized prospective trial has not been reported.[493,494] Endothelin receptor (ET_A) antagonists improved proteinuria in mouse models and are being explored as a potential therapeutic agents.[495] Chronic red cell transfusion begun at an early age may be protective against microalbuminuria.[496]

The overall incidence of hypertension in patients with Hb SS is low (2%-6%), compared with a published incidence of 28% for the black population in the United States.[497] Data from the CSSCD confirmed that individuals with sickle cell disease have a significantly lower blood pressure than the general population, but hypertension is still a risk factor for stroke and increased mortality.[498] Intermittent hypertension occurring during sickle cell crises and associated with transient elevation of plasma renin activity has been attributed to the reversible sludging of red cells in the small vessels of the kidney.

Incidence of acute kidney injury (AKI) in children was found to be higher in the setting of hospitalization for ACS or pain crisis.[499,500] While older age, acute drop in Hb, volume depletion, and frequent NSAID use have been identified as risk factors for developing AKI, hydroxyurea had a protective effect.[500] Hospitalizations complicated with AKI were associated with increased morbidity and resource utilization (prolonged hospitalization, escalation of care),[501] and recurrent episodes potentially increased long-term risk of developing CKD.[502] CKD, which occurs in 12% of patients with SCA, has a median age of onset of 37 years,[82] and is a significant cause of mortality in adults.[81] The preazotemic manifestations of hypertension, proteinuria, and increasingly severe anemia predict end-stage renal failure with an average survival (despite dialysis) of 4 years after diagnosis.[503] Recently, nocturnal hypertension and hyperuricemia have been found to be risk factors for CKD in children, whereas increased Hb and Hb F levels have been protective.[504,505] Newer measures of declining renal function include serum cystatin-C, LDH (as an indicator of hemolysis), and markers of tubular damage (e.g., increased serum β_2 microglobulin, urinary N-acetylglucosaminidase, urinary kidney injury molecule-1, and urinary transforming growth factor-β1, plasma endothelin-1).[506,507] In addition, two genes (MYH9 and APOL1 G1 and G2 variants) have been identified as having SNPs associated with proteinuria and end-stage renal disease (ESRD).[508-510]

Both hemodialysis[511] and peritoneal dialysis, when used in conjunction with a transfusion program, are efficacious in transiently correcting uremic complications. Renal transplantation has been performed, but in a limited numbers of patients.[512] A report from the North American Pediatric Transplant Cooperative Society described nine patients with end-stage sickle cell nephropathy for whom graft survival was 71% at 2 years after transplant.[513] In another report, 82 patients with end-stage sickle cell nephropathy received renal allografts.[514] The short-term result was similar to that seen with other causes of ESRD, and this approach seemed to improve survival in comparison with those patients managed with chronic dialysis.[515] Pharmacologic doses of exogenous erythropoietin have been effective in correcting anemia,[516] but higher hematocrits have been associated with increased pain events.[517]

Eyes

A variety of ocular lesions result from occlusion of the small vessels of the eye by sickled erythrocytes (*Figure 34.12*). The prominence of end arterioles within the retina renders this tissue especially vulnerable to irreversible injury after vascular occlusion.

Vaso-occlusive disease of the retina is responsible for both nonproliferative and proliferative (neovascular) changes. The former consists of "salmon patches," produced by small intraretinal hemorrhages; iridescent spots, representing collections of iron-loaded retinal macrophages; and schisis cavities, left after resorption of blood. Hemorrhages that break into the potential space between the sensory retina and pigment epithelium stimulate pigment production and migration, giving rise to black, disc-shaped scars known as "black sunbursts." Proliferative changes begin with the formation of arteriovenous anastomoses, followed by the development of vascular fronds resembling sea fans.[518] Vessels grow anteriorly toward the pre-equatorial, ischemic portion of the retina. Inspection of sea fans with ultraviolet light after the IV injection of fluorescein usually reveals small leaks into the vitreous. Major hemorrhages from sea fans that extend into the visual axis can generate visual symptoms. More often, however, they are confined to the peripheral portions of the retina and go undetected except by ophthalmoscopy. With time, repeated vitreous hemorrhages cause vitreous degeneration and vitreoretinal traction, which in turn produces retinal holes, tears, and detachment.

The prevalence of sickle retinopathy (both proliferative and nonproliferative) increases with age and is more common among patients with Hb SC than those with Hb SS. In a large study of sickle cell patients, the prevalence of sickle retinopathy was 54.6% and 18.1% in patients with Hb SC and Hb SS, respectively, and was more common among men than women.[519] No correlation has been found between retinopathy and various hematologic parameters except Hb F level,

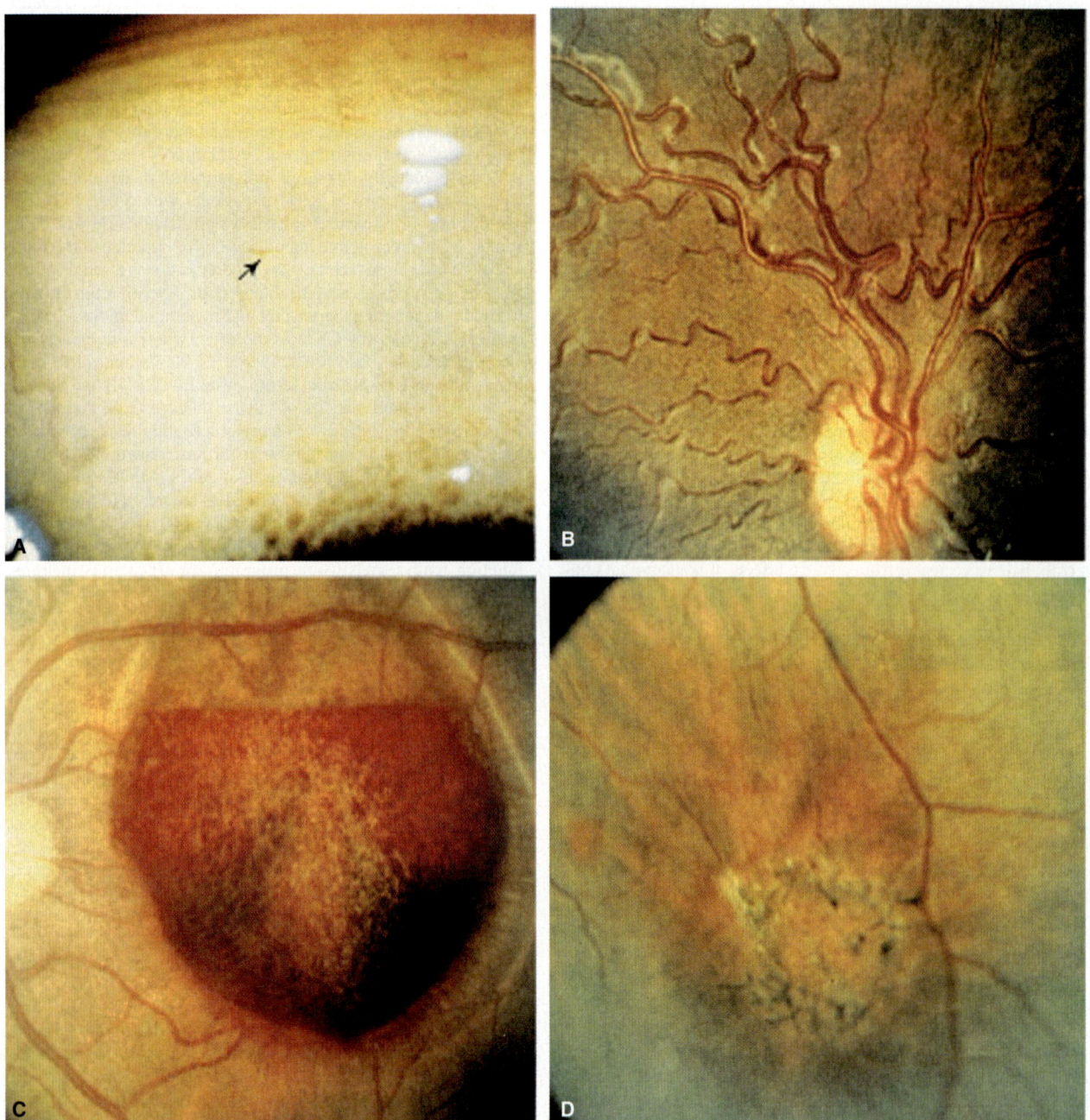

FIGURE 34.12 Ocular abnormalities in sickle cell anemia. A, "Comma" vascular sign: superficial conjunctival vessel that contains densely packed sickled cells (arrow). B, Widened veins and tortuous large vessels of the retina. C, Large preretinal hemorrhage of approximately 2 weeks' duration. There is partial resorption and exposure of a darkened area that was the probable site of intraretinal hemorrhage. D, Old pigmented chorioretinal scar. (Photographs courtesy of Professor Mansour Armaly, The George Washington University Medical Center.)

which is higher in less-affected patients.[520] Screening for sickle retinopathy is recommended beginning at 10 years of age and should be done annually for Hb SC and biannually for other genotypes.

Proliferative retinal disease may be arrested by laser photocoagulation or cryocoagulation to seal off the feeder vessels of neovascular patches and coagulate vascular leaks. A recent Cochrane review of laser therapy for retinopathy in sickle cell disease[521] identified only two randomized trials comparing laser photocoagulation to no treatment. The studies involved 341 eyes in 238 subjects, aged 13 to 67 years. Data from these studies suggested that laser photocoagulation prevented visual loss at a mean follow-up of over 1 year and that it had a protective effect for the occurrence of vitreous hemorrhage. However, because the long-term complication rate is relatively high, most retinal specialists have abandoned feeder vessel treatment in

favor of sectoral scatter photocoagulation, except in recalcitrant cases with repetitive bleeding.[522] Expression of proangiogenic cytokines (HIF-1α and VEGF) by the ischemic retina not adjacent to the neovascular seafans might explain the ineffectiveness of sectoral photocoagulation in some patients, and support the use of broad sectoral and circumferential scatter laser for treatment of proliferative retinal disease.[523] Anti-VEGF therapy has been shown to be safe and beneficial in small case series but needs to be studied further.[524]

An additional ocular complication of sickle cell disease is hyphema. Bleeding into the anterior chamber leads to trapping of sickled red cells, mechanical obstruction of the outflow apparatus, compromised circulation of the aqueous humor, and increased intraocular pressure, which may result in sudden blindness. This complication, which can also occur with sickle cell trait red cells, may be managed effectively by lowering intraocular pressure through anterior-chamber paracentesis.

Mild edema of the eyelids is frequently seen in association with vaso-occlusive pain crises, but more significant sickle "orbitopathy" has been described in approximately 20 patients.[525] A vaso-occlusive process in the marrow space around the orbit may result in frontal headache, fever, eyelid edema, and orbital compression. Subperiosteal hematomas are common and appear to result from bone marrow infarction. Although supportive care is usually adequate, the presence of optic nerve dysfunction or unusually large hematomas may require surgical evacuation to prevent loss of vision.

Skin Ulcers

Breakdown of the skin over the malleoli and distal portions of the legs is a recurring problem during adult life. Less commonly it may happen in other locations, such as the feet (*Figure 34.13*). Stasis of blood in the small vessels supplying these areas may interfere with the healing of minor traumatic abrasions. Ulcers were observed in 2.5% of sickle cell patients >10 years of age in North America,[526] but they affect as many as 75% of adults with SCA who live in tropical areas.[527] Numerous other risk factors have been identified. Ulcers are common in patients with Hb SS but quite rare in those with Hb SC disease or Hb Sβ[+]-thalassemia.[526] They are more common in men than in women and in those >20 years of age. There is a positive correlation with a low steady-state Hb concentration and with a low level of Hb F.[526] Recently, associations with severity of hemolysis and with SNPs in the *Klotho* gene and transforming growth factor-β pathway genes have been reported.[528]

The ulcers typically form a shallow depression with a smooth and slightly elevated margin; often, they have a surrounding area of edema. There may be exudation, crusting, and granulation at the base. Secondary infection of the ulcer with undermining of the edges and progressive extension are common. Single or multiple bacterial organisms may be cultured from the lesions and may contribute to their refractoriness. Healing leaves a thinned depigmented epithelium that is often surrounded by areas of hyperpigmentation and hyperkeratosis. This fragile epithelium is likely to break down with minimal trauma or edema, leading to recurrence rates >70%.

Healing of leg and ankle ulcerations is facilitated by bed rest, elevation of the affected extremities, wet-to-dry dressings, and eradication of documented wound infections with systemically administered antibiotics. When acute inflammation has subsided, occlusive zinc oxide–impregnated gel boots (Unna boots) are applied, and partial ambulation is permitted. In refractory or progressive cases, the healing process may be enhanced if the level of Hb S is maintained at <40% with transfusions. Split-thickness skin grafting may be necessary. Many alternative approaches have also been described in recent years. Zinc deficiency has been invoked to explain slow tissue healing,[529] and oral zinc therapy may hasten healing in some patients.[530] Hydroxyurea has been linked to the development of leg ulcers anecdotally, but larger studies have not found this association. The use of collagen-matrix dressings (arginylglycylaspartic acid [RGD] peptide matrix) resulted in greater ulcer closure in a controlled collaborative trial.[531] A topical Na nitrite cream may also be of value.[532] Newer therapies like the oxygen affinity-enhancing voxelotor are promising. A posthoc data analysis from the phase 3 randomized placebo-controlled HOPE study showed that >70% and >90% participants receiving voxelotor (1500 and 900 mg) had an improvement or resolution of their leg ulcers by week 24 and 72, respectively. This improvement was associated with an improvement in anemia and decrease in markers of hemolysis.[533]

Pregnancy

Pregnancy poses potentially serious problems for the woman with SCA, as well as for the fetus and neonate. Women with sickle cell disease have increased risk of maternal mortality and pre-eclampsia/eclampsia compared with women who do not have sickle cell disease.[534] The jeopardy imposed by pregnancy is explained in part by marginal health status before conception and in part by the sinusoidal circulation of the placenta, whereby a high degree of oxygen extraction provides an excellent milieu for sickling, stasis, and infarction. Although life-threatening complications generally are not encountered until the third trimester, an increased incidence of pyelonephritis, hematuria, and thrombophlebitis is noted throughout pregnancy. Anemia is more severe and may be compounded by folate deficiency. ACS events occur more frequently during late pregnancy and the early postpartum period and are one of the leading causes of death.[535] A majority of these ACS events are preceded by pain crisis episodes requiring hospitalization.[536] However, there is a significant reduction in the incidence of pain (1.8-0.3 events/patient-years; *P* < .001) and ACS (0.4-0 events/patient-years; *P* = .001) events during the postpartum period.[536] With optimal multidisciplinary care, however, mortality and morbidity are reduced substantially, even in difficult settings in Africa.[537]

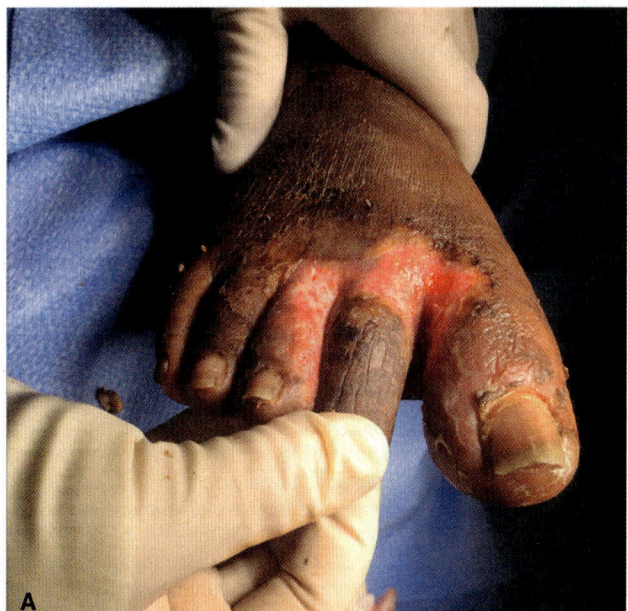 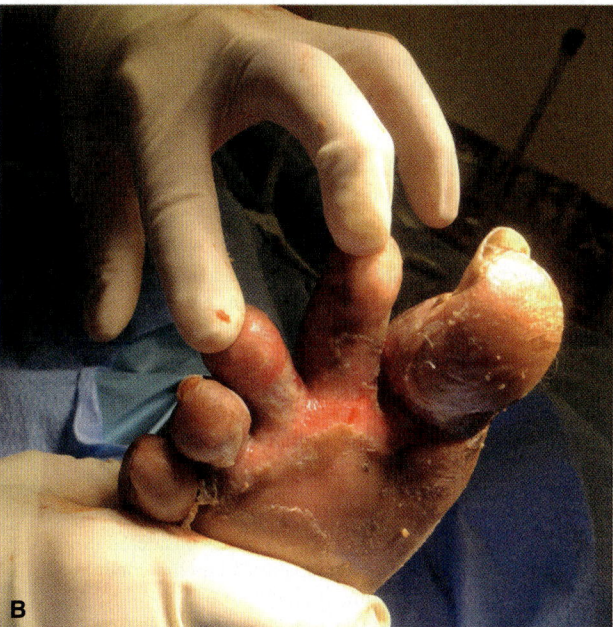

FIGURE 34.13 Chronic foot ulcers in an adolescent patient with Hb SS. (Courtesy of Heather Havens, PNP, and Paul Lavoie, PA-C, St Jude Children's Research Hospital.)

Disorders of Red Blood Cells

The incidence of congenital malformations or susceptibility to complications is comparable to that shared by all preterm infants.[538] Opiates are not associated with teratogenicity or congenital malformations, but higher maternal doses have been linked to greater severity of neonatal abstinence syndrome.[539] Hydroxyurea, even when used throughout pregnancy, has not been associated with teratogenic changes, either in individual pregnancies or among adults who participated in the Multicenter Study of Hydroxyurea (MSH) trial, and was followed for up to 17 years. Nevertheless, it is a teratogen in animals and should be stopped once pregnancy is recognized.

Infants born to women with SCA are at greater risk of preterm birth, low birth weight, being small for gestational age, and neonatal jaundice. According to a CSSCD report, 21% of infants were small for their gestational age.[540] Possible etiologic factors for small birth weight and preterm labor are severe maternal anemia, frequent episodes of vaso-occlusion leading to hypoperfusion and hypoxia of the placenta, increased risks of abruptio placentae, placenta previa, and toxemia of pregnancy, diminished maternal nutrition, and increased narcotic use in the mother. Additional risk factors for preterm labor and prematurity include increased urinary tract infection and chorioamnionitis. The final weeks of pregnancy are often complicated by vaso-occlusive events that may have devastating consequences for both mother and fetus. In an attempt to prevent progressive placental infarction and premature delivery, some clinicians advocate the use of transfusion therapy during pregnancy. A systematic review of retrospective cohort studies concluded that prophylactic transfusion during pregnancy was associated with a reduction in maternal mortality, pain episodes, pulmonary complications, pyelonephritis, perinatal mortality, neonatal death, and preterm birth.[541] A recent retrospective cross-sectional study showed that women treated with prophylactic erythrocytapheresis did not have severe vaso-occlusive crisis, sepsis/severe infection, or preeclampsia/eclampsia.[542]

The reproductive life span is reduced in women with sickle cell disease, as indicated by an accelerated decline in ovarian reserve starting in 25- to 30-year-olds.[543] While hydroxyurea use has been linked to decline of ovarian reserve in some individuals, the data are limited.[544-546] This potential concern on the future fertility has to be addressed with parents and patients in the context of the strong evidence of its benefits in preventing organ injury.[547,548] There is also a lack of studies systematically investigating the efficacy and safety of various methods of contraception in women with sickle cell disease. Despite a theoretical possibility of enhancing thrombotic risk, low-estrogen–dose birth control pills are sometimes recommended. Studies in Nigeria and Brazil found no adverse effects from the progestational contraceptive implant and a possible improvement in Hb F level.[549,550] A review of progesterone-only contraceptive use suggested that they are safe and result in less frequent and severe painful crises.[551]

Prognosis

The prognosis for persons with SCD has undergone dramatic change in the past 4 decades in high-income countries. In the United States today, greater than 95% of children with SCD live beyond the age of 18 years.[39,354,552] This increase in survival from prior decades is due to universal newborn screening for the disease and advances in comprehensive supportive care, including infection prevention (penicillin prophylaxis and immunization)[83] and greater use of disease-modifying therapies (hydroxyurea and erythrocyte transfusions).[39,552,553] Despite major improvements in the outcomes of pediatric SCD patients in high-income countries, the median life expectancy of affected individuals remains low at approximately 48 years, and is strongly associated with SCD-related onset and progression of end organ damage[554] that frequently initially manifests during childhood.[85,190,287,510,555-561] The increased survival, albeit with significant end organ damage, represents a paradigm shift for SCD that was once considered primarily an acute disease, but today is predominantly a chronic condition with cumulative organ damage and high morbidity.

Globally, approximately 300,000 babies a year are born with SCD with the largest burden being in sub-Saharan Africa.[1] The dramatic improvements in outcomes for children with SCD in high-income countries have not been widely reproduced in low-income countries where the greatest burden of the disease is manifest. As an example, Nigeria has highest SCD burden in the world with 3% of all newborns affected,[562] accounting for ~100,000 newborns each year being born with the disease.[1] Nevertheless, there is no universal newborn screening program in Nigeria and poor utilization of standard-of-care treatment practices for infants with SCD throughout the country.[563] Without early diagnosis and treatment, most affected children die during the first few years of life, with reported excess mortality reaching up to 92%.[564] Importantly, in low-income countries where newborn screening programs have been implemented, these programs reduce infant and under-5 mortality rates to levels approximating those of the general population.[565,566]

Determinants of Severity

A large degree of phenotypic variability is observed in SCD-related acute manifestations, end-organ onset and progression, and in individual therapeutic responses observed. Some of this variability is influenced by genetic modifiers, a concept first supported by observations of varying degrees of disease severity in selected geographic regions and in ethnic lines. In the eastern oases of Saudi Arabia, for example, SCA is clinically benign,[567,568] whereas in western Saudi Arabia, it is comparable in severity to that seen in African Americans.[569]

Recent advances in genomics have identified multiple genetic modifiers that influence the pathophysiology of SCD at many levels. Many common and rare variants influence Hb S polymerization directly by altering erythrocyte traits. These include alpha thalassemia,[570] beta thalassemia,[570,571] and variants that regulate HbF expression.[572-574] These erythrocyte-specific genetic modifiers are expected to influence SCD phenotypes broadly, while other non–erythrocyte-specific variants act downstream of Hb S polymerization, independent of the erythrocyte, and influence SCD phenotypes selectively. For example, APOL1 risk alleles accelerate SCD-related kidney injury,[510,558,575-577] UGT1A1 variants are associated with hyperbilirubinemia and cholelithiasis,[578,579] and multiple variants influence pain sensitivity.[580]

Fetal hemoglobin (Hb F, $\alpha_2\gamma_2$) predominates in the human fetus, but postnatally it declines during the first 5 years of life in children with SCD[581] and is restricted to a subpopulation of erythrocytes, termed F-cells.[582] Endogenous Hb F levels, which vary widely,[87,583,584] ameliorate SCD severity because neither homo-($\alpha_2\gamma_2$) nor heterotetramers ($\alpha_2\gamma\beta^S$) participate in polymerization,[585] which results in reductions in acute clinical manifestations,[87,586-588] organ damage,[561,588] and mortality.[81] Endogenous Hb F levels in patients with SCA are determined by the distribution of F cells (pancellular vs a fractional distribution), the Hb F concentration within each F cells, and the survival of F cells.[589] The proportion of reticulocytes containing Hb F is relatively constant over time, but it varies greatly among affected individuals (2%-50%) and is under genomic influence.[590]

In the eastern province of Saudi Arabia[567,591] and in Kuwait,[592] Iran,[593] India,[594] and the West Indies,[595] mild disease is associated with Hb F levels of 15% to 30%. Evidence from the CSSCD indicates that even when the fetal Hb level is low, small increments in the level may have an ameliorating effect on the pain rate and may ultimately improve survival.[87] The limited capacity of Hb F levels to predict disease severity, however, does not negate the importance of Hb F production. Hb F levels are determined not only by synthetic rates but also by the extent to which F cells are enriched by differential cell survival. Thus, high levels of Hb F may reflect increased synthesis, resulting in mild disease, or greater amplification through accelerated destruction of cells containing no Hb F, a manifestation of more severe disease.[589] Coinheritance of SCA and α-thalassemia is common. Nearly 30% of black Americans have a single α-gene deletion, and in about 2% deletion of two of the four α-globin genes is found.[570,580] Hematologic studies provide support for the clinical relevance of α-thalassemia. Subjects with SCA and α-thalassemia have a higher Hb concentration, lower mean corpuscular volume (MCV) and MCHC, fewer ISCs, a lower reticulocyte count, lower serum bilirubin concentration, and relatively more Hb A$_2$ than subjects without concurrent α-thalassemia. The α-gene deletion is also associated with improved cell deformability,[596] a decreased fraction of dense cells,[596,597] protection against cation leak,[598] and improved red cell survival.[599] There is relatively little effect of α-thalassemia on Hb F levels,[600,601] although in patients with the Senegal haplotype, Hb F levels are higher.[602]

Data from the CSSCD demonstrated that coexistent α-thalassemia is associated with a diminished mortality risk in patients >20 years of age.[81] In addition, stroke risk is decreased in the presence of α-thalassemia.[135,141] The rheologic benefits of more deformable α-thalassemic sickle cells are offset by rheologic impairment associated with the greater viscosity of a higher hematocrit induced by α-thalassemia. Thus, α-thalassemia is associated with more frequent vaso-occlusive pain crises by virtue of its effect on hematocrit.[87] Osteonecrosis and perhaps sickle retinopathy occur more often in sickle cell subjects with coexistent α-thalassemia.[603,604]

A cohort of 392 infants with Hb SS or Hb Sβ⁰-thalassemia from the CSSCD were followed for an average of 10 years beginning at <6 months of age. Eighteen percent had an adverse outcome, defined as death, stroke, frequent pain, or recurrent ACS.[605] Three statistically significant predictors of an adverse outcome could be identified at 2 years of age: Hb level <7 g/dL, leukocytosis in the absence of infection, and an episode of dactylitis before 1 year of age. However, in a report from the Dallas newborn cohort, hospitalizations in the first 3 years of life for pain (other than dactylitis), ACS, and dactylitis did not predict death or stroke.[606] Nevertheless, early pain and ACS both predicted a modest increase in later pain episodes, and early ACS strongly increased the odds of more frequent ACS throughout childhood.

Sickle cell disease should no longer be considered a single-gene disorder. No current single genetic marker, clinical feature, or biomarkers can predict disease severity or early mortality. Following the sequencing of the human genome in 2003, genome-wide association studies (GWAS) allowed for examination of common SNPs and correlation of this variation with clinical traits. Potential candidate genes associated with ACS, leg ulcers, osteonecrosis, pain crises, priapism, and stroke have been identified through GWAS, but most of these findings have not been validated in follow-up studies on separate cohorts. Fetal Hb modifier genes have been an exception; elevated levels of Hb F have been correlated with improved clinical outcome in sickle cell disease, and GWAS have identified several genes (*BCL11 A*, *MYB*, *HBB*) that regulate Hb F levels.[273,607,608] *KLF1*, another gene that regulates Hb F levels, was identified by direct DNA sequencing. However, only about 30% to 50% of the heritability of Hb F levels is known.[574,608] In the Sickle Cell Clinical Research and Intervention Cohort (SCCRIP), 567 individuals with SCD underwent whole genome sequencing and previously identified genomic modifiers of globin expression (*BCL11A*, *MYB*, *KLF1*, and *HBB*) were validated as being associated with Hb F levels but no other loci were identified. Thus, the currently unexplained fraction of Hb F heritability is likely regulated by combinations of many genetic variants with low-frequency and/or low-magnitude effect size.[580] Understanding how rare variants in a specific gene can modify SCD now may require interrogation of relatively large cohorts of well-phenotyped cohorts. Nevertheless, understanding the role of *BCL11A* and other loci, and their relationship with the globin switch that occurs early in life, has facilitated to the development of treatment compounds and gene therapy strategies that reactivate Hb F production.[609]

Laboratory Features
Red Blood Cells

In SCA, a moderately severe normocytic, normochromic anemia manifests by 3 months of age and persists throughout life.[257] The average Hb concentration is 8 g/dL, with a range from <6 to 11 g/dL. Mean Hb levels vary with gender and with age; they are higher in adult men compared with women and higher in males between the ages of 20 and 39 years. In adults with Hb SS, the mean MCV is <90 fL, and the mean MCHC is <34.0 g/dL. The MCV and MCHC are substantially lower (means 72 fL and 32.5 g/dL, respectively) in patients with concurrent α-thalassemia minor (−α/−α genotype) and in children with incidental iron deficiency.

Blood smears contain variable numbers of sickled forms, target cells, and ovalocytes (*Figure 34.14*). The morphologic features of accelerated erythropoiesis, which include polychromatophilia (because of reticulocytosis) and nucleated RBCs, are prominent. The mean reticulocyte count is about 10%, with a range of 4% to 24%. Howell-Jolly bodies reflect functional asplenia. Numerous pits in red cell membranes, also a feature of the asplenic state, require phase-interference contrast microscopy for visualization.

Erythrokinetic studies performed in the steady state indicate a fourfold to fivefold increase in red cell production and erythron iron turnover and a comparable shortening of red cell survival. Chronic hemolysis, most of which is extravascular, is responsible for an increase in endogenous carbon monoxide generation and for elevated serum levels of unconjugated bilirubin and heme proteins.

White Blood Cells

The WBC count is consistently elevated owing to an increase in the number of mature granulocytes. The mean leukocyte count under steady-state conditions is 12 to 15 × 10⁹/L, with a range of 6 to 20 × 10⁹/L. This increase is explained to a large extent by a shift of granulocytes from the marginated to the circulating compartments. Both total and segmented leukocyte numbers increase during vaso-occlusive crises and infections, but only with bacterial infections does a consistent increase occur in bands (nonsegmented neutrophils), often to levels >1 × 10⁹/L.

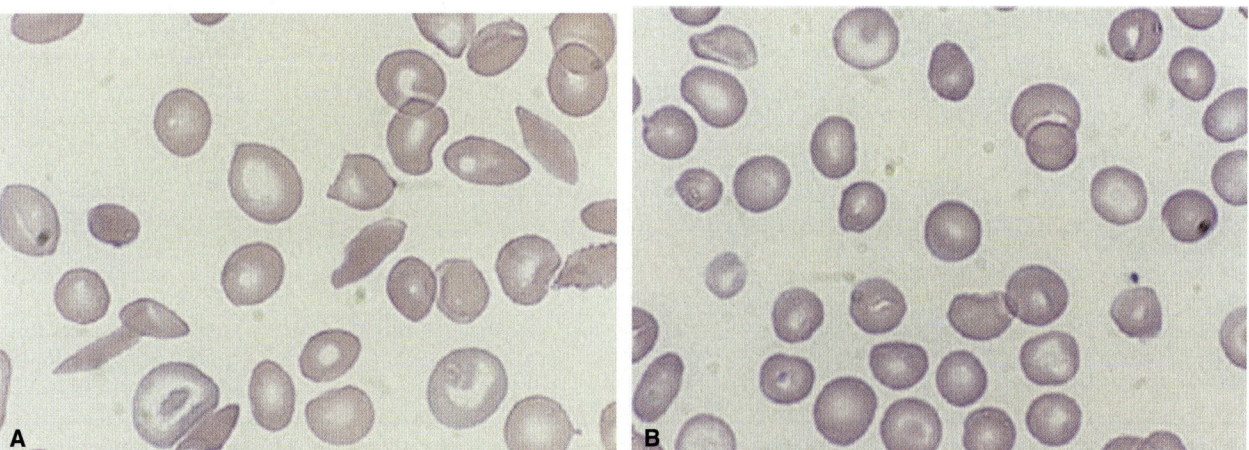

FIGURE 34.14 Blood smears of patients with hemoglobin Hb SS and Hb SC disease. A, Red blood cell morphology in sickle cell anemia is characterized by sickled forms (dense elongated cells with pointed ends), target cells, ovalocytes, and polychromatophilia. B, Hb SC disease is characterized by target cells, relatively few sickled forms, and a small proportion of cells that contain dark blunt protuberances (hemoglobin "crystals").

Platelets and Coagulation

The platelet count is increased (mean ~440 × 10^9/L), reflecting reduced or absent splenic trapping and a hyperinflammatory effect. During vaso-occlusive crises, the plasma β-thromboglobulin level is elevated.[610] Contact factors are decreased,[611] whereas factor VIII activity, fibrinogen concentration, and fibrinolytic activity are increased.

Other Laboratory Tests

Sickle cell disease may be considered a "heightened inflammatory state." Inflammatory markers, such as CRP, sPLA$_2$, fibrinogen, von Willebrand factor, ILs, serum ferritin, and TNF-α, are all elevated, in addition to elevation of WBC. The sedimentation rate is difficult to interpret because of the presence of anemia, hyperfibrinogenemia, and the failure of sickle cells to undergo rouleaux formation.

Diagnosis

The diagnosis of SCA rests on the electrophoretic or chromatographic separation of Hbs in hemolysates prepared from peripheral blood. The predominant Hb is S; Hb F is present in varying concentrations; and Hb A$_2$ is normal. There is no Hb A. Electrophoresis using cellulose acetate and an alkaline buffer is rapid, inexpensive, and effective in the separation of normal Hbs from common variants. Whole blood, blood specimens dried on filter paper, or Hb solutions may be used. Only a few of the doubly heterozygous states involving Hb S and a relatively rare β-globin variant are associated with the clinical and hematologic features of sickling. The interaction of Hb S with β^0-thalassemia gives an electrophoretic pattern that is indistinguishable from that of homozygous SCA, except for an increase in Hb A$_2$. In general, the appropriate diagnosis can be made by taking into consideration associated hematologic data and family studies (*Table 34.4*). Hb separation

Table 34.4. Newborn and Adult Hemoglobin Fractionation Patterns of Sickle Hemoglobinopathies

Diagnosis	Birth Hb Fractionation	Hb Pattern	Adulthood Hb Fractionation	Hb Genotype	Blood Count
Sickle cell trait	HbF 80%-90%, HbA ~6%, HbS ~4%, HbA$_2$ 0	FAS	HbA 55%-60%, HbS 35%-40%, HbA$_2$ <3.5%, HbF 1%-2%	AS	Normal for age and sex
Sickle cell trait with alpha thalassemia trait**	HbF 80%-90%, HbA ~7%, HbS ~3%, HbA$_2$ 0, Hb Bart 5%-10%	FAS + Fast Band	HbA 60%-70%, HbS 20%-30%, HbA2 <3.5%, HbF 1%-2%	AS	Mild anemia (Hb 10-12 g/dL and microcytosis (MCV 70-75 fL). Target cells seen on the peripheral blood smear
Sickle cell anemia (homozygous β^s)	HbF 80%-90%, HbS 10%-20%, HbA 0, HbA$_2$ 0	FS	HbS 80%-90%, HbF 1%-30%***, HbA$_2$ <3.5%, HbA 0	SS	Mild to severe anemia (Hb 6-10 g/dL) and normal MCV (80-90 fL)
Sickle cell anemia (homozygous β^s) with alpha thalassemia trait**	HbF 80%-90%, HbS 10%-20%, HbA 0, HbA$_2$ 0, Hb Barts 5%-10%	FS + Fast Band	HbS 80%-90%, HbF 5%-10%***, HbA$_2$ <3.5% (but may be higher), HbA 0	SS	Mild to moderate anemia (Hb 8-11 g/dL) and microcytosis (MCV 70-75 fL). Target cells seen on the peripheral blood smear
Sickle beta zero thalassemia	HbF 80%-90%, HbS 10%-20%, HbA 0, HbA$_2$ 0	FS	HbS 80%-95%, HbF 5%-10%***, HbA$_2$ 4%-6%, HbA 0	Sβ^0 thalassemia	Mild to severe anemia (Hb 7-9 g/dL) and microcytosis (MCV 60-80 fL). Target cells seen on the peripheral blood smear
Sickle beta plus thalassemia	HbF 80%-90%, HbS ~7%, HbA ~3%, HbA2 0	FSA	HbS 50%-80%, HbA 5%-30% (occasionally higher, but always lower than HbS), HbF 1%-20%***, HbA$_2$ 4%-6%	Sβ$^+$ thalassemia	Moderate anemia (Hb 9-12 g/dL) and microcytosis (MCV 60-80 fL). Target cells seen on the peripheral blood smear
Sickle hemoglobin C disease	HbF 80%-90%, HbS ~4.5%, HbC ~4.5%, HbA 0, HbA$_2$ 0	FSC	HbS 45%-50%, HbC 45%-50%, HbF 1%-6%***, HbA$_2$ <3.5%, HbA 0	HbSC	Mild anemia (Hb 9-14 g/dL) and microcytosis (MCV 70-75). Target cells seen on the peripheral blood smear
Sickle hemoglobin E disease	HbF 80%-90%, HbS 6%, HbE 4%****, HbA 0	FSE	HbS 55%-60% HbE ~30%-35%****, HbF 1%-5%***, HbA 0	HbSE	Mild anemia (Hb 8-14 g/dL) and microcytosis (MCV 71-97 fL). Target cells seen on the peripheral blood smear
Sickle hemoglobin D-Punjab/D-Los Angeles disease	HbF 80%-90%, HbS 6%, HbD 4%****, HbA 0	FS	Hb S ~ 45%, Hb D ~ 45%, Hb A$_2$ <3.5%, and Hb F = 5%-7%. Hb S and D separable on citrate agar at acid pH	HbSD	MIld-moderate anemia (5-10 g/dL), reticulocytosis (5%-20%), macrocytosis (MCV 110-120 fL). Target cells, seen on peripheral blood smear
Sickle cell with δβ^0 thalassemia	HF 80%-90%, HbS 10%-20%, HbA 0, HbA$_2$ 0	FS	HbS 60%-80%, HbF 15%-20% ***(heterocellular pattern), HbA$_2$ <3.5, HbA 0	HbS/δβ^0 thalassemia	Mild anemia (Hb 10-12 g/dL) and microcytosis (MCV 76-85 fL)
Sickle cell with hereditary persistence of fetal hemoglobin (HPFH)	HbF 80%-90%, HbS 10%-20%, HbA 0, HbA$_2$ 0	FS	HbS 60%-70%, HbF 25%-35% ***(pancellular pattern), HbA$_2$ <3.5, HbA 0 (deletion-HPFH)	Hb S/HPFH	Mild or no anemia (Hb 10-15 g/dL) and microcytosis (MCV 68-88 fL)

Notes: Hemoglobin quantification results as measured by High Performance Liquid Chromatography (HPLC). Hb denotes hemoglobin. β^s denotes the sickle mutation in the beta globin gene. β^c denotes the C mutation in the beta globin gene. β^E denotes the E mutation in the beta globin gene. β^0 denotes absence of beta globin gene function. β$^+$ denotes decreased beta globin production. *HbA is lower is premature babies. ** Alpha thalassemia trait can be a deletion either in cis (--/αα) or in trans (α-/α-). *** HbF varies by β^S haplotype (e.g., higher in Arab-Indian haplotype) and variants in other locus (e.g., BCL11a) and may be as high as 30% even in the absence of exposure to hydroxyurea. ****HbE coelutes with HbA2 on HPLC, hence not distinguishable from each other.

by isoelectric focusing or high-performance liquid chromatography (HPLC) has replaced Hb electrophoresis in most labs. Structural analysis of Hb (by protein chemistry, mass spectrometry, or sequencing of polymerase chain reaction–amplified DNA) may be required to characterize accurately the genotypic basis for a sickling disorder.

A variety of simple tests permit detection of Hb S. The sickling phenomenon can be induced by sealing a drop of blood under a coverslip to exclude oxygen or by adding agents that induce chemical deoxygenation, such as 2% sodium metabisulfite or sodium dithionite. The decreased solubility of deoxy Hb S forms the basis for tests in which blood is added to a buffered solution of a reducing agent. Hb S is insoluble and precipitates in solution, rendering it turbid, whereas solutions containing Hbs other than Hb S remain clear. Hyperglobulinemia and other sickling Hbs may cause false positive results; false negatives may result from the addition of an inadequate number of red cells. Neither the sickle cell preparation nor solubility tests differentiate SCA from sickle cell trait or detect Hb variants that interact with Hb S. Thus, they should never be used as a primary screening test. Their principal value has been as an adjunct to electrophoretic identification of Hb S. Recent development of quantitative point-of-care testing devices and single-molecule long-read DNA sequencing appears to be particularly useful in limited resource settings and may allow large-scale screening of local populations.[612,613]

Although the diagnosis of Hb SC disease is straightforward, that of Hb Sβ-thalassemia may sometimes be problematic. In Hb Sβ+-thalassemia, there is a preponderance of Hb S, with Hb A comprising 5% to 30% of the total, and elevation of Hb A_2. This must be distinguished from sickle cell trait, in which Hb A exceeds Hb S, and from the presence of Hb A resulting from RBC transfusions within the previous 3 to 4 months. Hb Sβ⁰-thalassemia produces an electrophoretic pattern that is visually indistinguishable from that of SCA, but a diagnosis can be suggested by the presence of an elevated Hb A_2 level and a decreased MCV. In addition, upon examination of the peripheral blood, both Hb Sβ+-thalassemia and Hb Sβ⁰-thalassemia display large numbers of target cells, as well as hypochromia. However, because SCA with coincident α-thalassemia also has a phenotype with reduced MCV and mildly elevated Hb A_2, family- or DNA-based studies may be necessary to make this distinction.[580]

Neonatal Diagnosis

The first statewide newborn hemoglobinopathy screening program was initiated in New York in 1975, but the impetus for universal screening came from the demonstration that early diagnosis and comprehensive care could reduce morbidity and mortality in infants with SCA through the prevention of pneumococcal sepsis with penicillin prophylaxis. Universal rather than targeted newborn screening is necessary to ensure that all with disease are identified and none are discriminated against or stigmatized.

It is estimated that between 2000 and 3000 children are born yearly with sickle cell disease in the United States,[39] and approximately 280,000 worldwide.[614] A review of newborn screening in the United States during the past 2 decades found that the highest incidence of sickle cell disease (and of sickle cell trait) was in the District of Columbia, followed by Mississippi and South Carolina.[615] Most newborn screening programs use dried blood spots on filter paper, because Hb testing can easily be integrated into existing metabolic programs with established methods of sample collection, specimen processing, data management, and quality control. Isoelectric focusing and HPLC have replaced cellulose acetate electrophoresis in most screening programs. Using these techniques, it was found that compared to term newborns, preterm newborns (<28 weeks) with trait were more often misidentified as having SCA or Hb C disease on newborn screening especially if the abnormal Hb (HbS or Hb C) level is higher than Hb A level.[616] Additionally, newborn screening is unable to distinguish between certain mild and severe disease states where the Hb pattern is similar at birth like in HbS/HPFH and Hb SS or HbS/β⁰thalassemia where the Hb pattern is FS.

The primary goal of newborn screening for sickle syndromes is reduction of morbidity and mortality by identifying affected infants at birth, referring them to treating centers, initiating prophylactic penicillin early, and providing ongoing care by knowledgeable health professionals (*Figure 34.15*). The number of early deaths avoided has been estimated at 0.6 to 1.2 per 100 births.[617] All cases of suspected disease still must be confirmed with a separate sample from the infant, because clerical errors may be encountered (*Figure 34.15*). Using public health

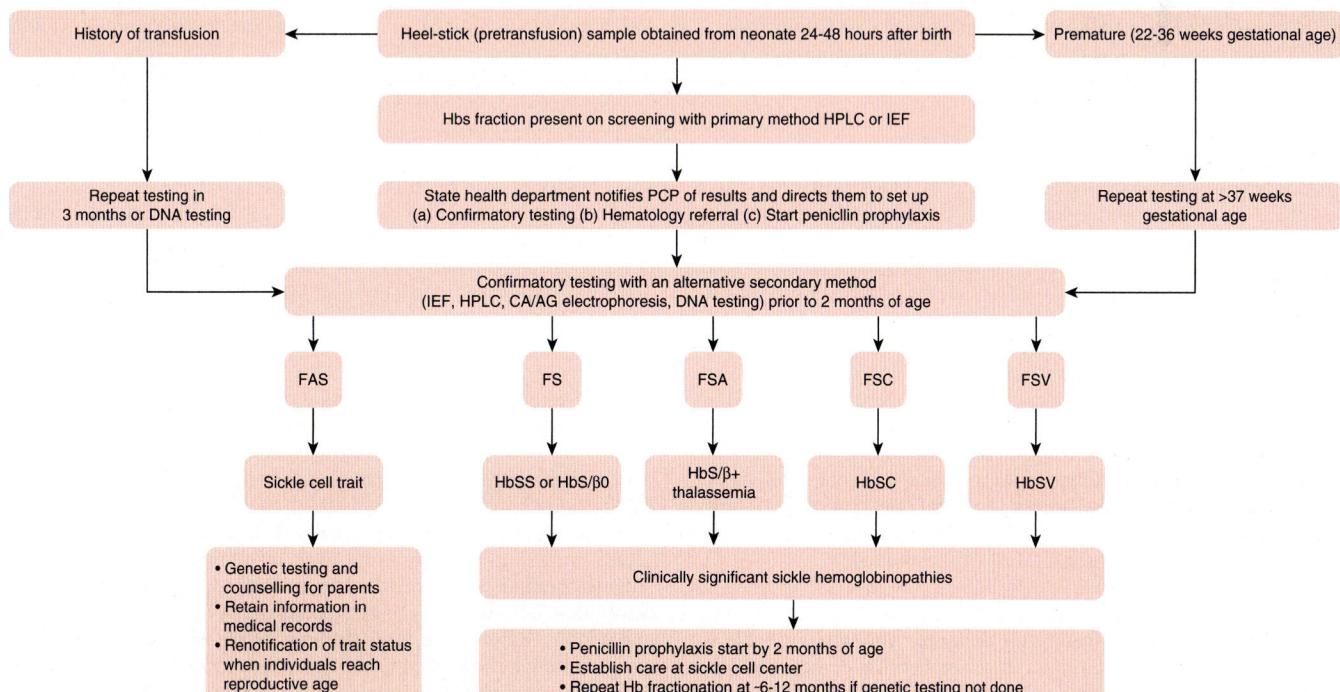

FIGURE 34.15 **Approach to screening and follow-up of sickle hemoglobinopathies in newborns.** Flowchart illustrating how to interpret newborn screening hemoglobinopathy results and the follow-up steps to confirm diagnosis and establish early care. CA/AG electrophoresis, cellulose acetate/agarose gel electrophoresis; Hb A, adult hemoglobin A; Hb F, fetal hemoglobin; Hb S, sickle hemoglobin; Hb V, variant hemoglobin; HPFH, hereditary persistence of fetal hemoglobin; HPLC, high-performance liquid chromatography; IEF, isoelectric focusing; PCP, primary care provider.

Disorders of Red Blood Cells

and state genetic program resources, it is possible to provide parents with individual counseling, education, and extended family testing.[618] Prenatal education for expectant mothers, which includes information about newborn sickle cell screening, significantly increases the follow-up rate for infants with sickle cell trait and contributes to a greater retention of information. Newborn screening programs in sub-Saharan Africa and India are in their infancy,[619,620] but they have been estimated to be cost-effective in most countries based on Disability Adjusted Life Years averted.[621] A recent study of 10 years of newborn screening in Rio de Janeiro, Brazil, found that 912 (out of 1.2 million screened) had sickle cell disease and all were referred to the sickle cell center in that city. Although 3.7% of these children died, early diagnosis and treatment was associated with improved survival and quality of life.[553]

Prenatal Diagnosis

The clinical application of recombinant DNA techniques to the prenatal diagnosis of SCA permits a high level of diagnostic accuracy with relatively little risk to the fetus. Prenatal diagnosis provides earlier diagnostic information, thereby permitting termination of pregnancy in the first trimester when desired, when it is safer for the mother. The least invasive method of prenatal diagnosis uses fetal cells from the maternal circulation isolated by a variety of techniques such as flow cytometry.[622] Preimplantation genetic diagnosis (PGD) allows couples who are sickle cell carriers to select unaffected embryos prior to in vitro fertilization. In some cases, PGD has been performed in combination with human leukocyte antigen (HLA) typing, allowing the delivery of an unaffected child who is also HLA identical to an affected sibling, therefore providing an ideal stem cell donor for the affected child.[623] However, PGD is expensive and has a pregnancy success rate of only 13% to 30%.[623,624] Reduction in the rate of affected births has not been observed in the United States, despite genetic counseling efforts by sickle cell programs. Greece has observed a decline in the number of new births with sickle cell disease and thalassemia, which has been attributed to aggressive education and early pregnancy termination.[625]

Treatment

In addition to prophylactic measures aimed at preventing specific complications of sickle cell disease, three treatment options have been used increasingly for overall management: chronic blood transfusion, hydroxyurea, and HSC transplantation. Gene therapy approaches are just beginning to be utilized.

Preventive Measures

Until a safe and widely applicable mechanism for the prevention of intravascular sickling is found, a high priority must be placed on the prevention of complications. Because vaso-occlusive crises are precipitated by infection, fever, dehydration, acidosis, hypoxemia, and cold exposure, measures to prevent or remedy these conditions assume importance. Optimal hydration is essential, especially during febrile illnesses. In estimating fluid requirements, the hyposthenuria of SCA, as well as increased insensible losses, must be considered. Because the liberal use of salicylates imposes an acid load, acetaminophen is the preferred antipyretic. Sudden transition to high altitude and exposure to situations likely to cause chilling should be avoided.

The high risk of overwhelming pneumococcal disease in children mandates the use of penicillin prophylaxis and pneumococcal vaccination. Preventive measures and early medical intervention for febrile illnesses substantially reduce mortality. Effective primary prevention of stroke using TCD screening has been discussed earlier.

Blood Transfusion

One of the most effective therapeutic measures presently available is the transfusion of normal red cells. However, because of the complications of transfusion therapy, it is reserved for selected indications, such as severe anemia, stroke prevention, pregnancy, progressive or recurrent organ damage, preparation for surgery, and certain severe acute vaso-occlusive events. Transfusion therapy facilitates improved blood and tissue oxygenation, reduces the propensity for vaso-occlusion by diluting host cells, and temporarily suppresses the production of red cells containing Hb S. The viscosity of deoxygenated sickle cell blood is disproportionately reduced by the addition of normal red cells. A mixture of one-fourth Hb A cells and three-fourths Hb S cells reduces the viscosity of deoxygenated blood by 50%.[626] Repeated partial exchange transfusion, which can be performed through erythrocytapheresis, greatly reduces the net gain of iron.[627,628] However, the long-term central venous access, which is often required, may be associated with an unusually high rate of catheter infection, thrombosis, and premature removal of the central line. Repeated simple transfusions are probably equally effective in terminating the consequences of in vivo sickling. Packed red cell transfusions at 3- to 4-week intervals generally are sufficient to maintain the relative number of donor cells in the circulation at >70%, but Hb S is more easily suppressed in some patients than others.

Although it is effective in circumventing the numerous complications of SCA, chronic transfusion therapy is limited by logistic and toxicity considerations. The requisite commitment of personnel and blood resources is considerable, and the risks of alloimmunization and hemosiderosis are cumulative and potentially life-limiting. Among individuals with SCA, 18% to 36% become alloimmunized, considerably more than with other forms of anemia.[629,630] The greater risk of alloimmunization in SCA is primarily a result of racial differences between the blood donor and recipient populations. The development of multiple antibodies is a relatively common problem; antibodies against C, E, and Kell (K) antigens account for most of the alloantibodies. The use of racially matched and selected minor blood group antigen-matched blood for chronically transfused patients with sickle cell disease has been recommended to prevent alloimmunization. However, despite the use of extended cross-matching (for C, E, and K) and, in some programs, African American donors, RBC alloimmunization is still a frequent occurrence,[631,632] because of RBC variants that are not detected on routine screening and transfusions at institutions where extended RBC typing is not done. DNA-based assay using SNPs associated with blood group antigen expression leads to improved accuracy of RBC antigens and is the primary method for RBC typing in at least one institution.[633]

Delayed hemolytic transfusion reactions are associated with as many as 3% of transfusions. Most occur several days after the transfusion and are accompanied by a falling hematocrit, hemoglobinuria, increased jaundice, and, frequently, a pain episode. In some cases, a delayed hemolytic transfusion reaction may lead to a fall in Hb level to a level lower than before transfusion, with a life-threatening or fatal outcome resulting from attempts to provide further transfusions.

Iron overload has been an inevitable result of chronic transfusion. The severity of iron overload has traditionally been monitored with serum ferritin concentration, and there is a strong intrapatient correlation between ferritin levels and volumes transfused. However, there is wide interpatient variability, indicating a need to assess iron stores more directly, such as by quantitative MRI or liver biopsy, to determine the necessity for iron chelation. As little as 10 units of packed RBCs per year will increase the liver iron concentration (LIC) obtained by biopsy above 3 mg Fe/g of dry weight liver, the normal upper limit of LIC.[634] Calibration studies have shown excellent correlation between LIC and quantitative MRI (both R2* and R2) at low and moderate LIC values.[635,636] These noninvasive MR methods to measure iron levels have improved the clinical management of iron overload in the liver and the heart.

With repeated transfusions, iron will accumulate progressively in several organs in addition to the liver, including the heart, pancreas, kidneys, pituitary, and gonads. Iron endocrinopathy and myocardial hemosiderosis have not been as problematic in SCA as in thalassemia major.[372,637] Reasons for these differences are not completely understood, but might be related to the age when transfusions are initiated, total cumulative volume of transfusion, differences in iron metabolism (e.g., lower nontransferrin bound iron levels in sickle cell disease), and the chronic inflammatory state of sickle cell disease, which may confer hepcidin-mediated protection against the toxic effects of iron on the tissues.[638,639]

The availability of iron chelation beginning with deferoxamine (Desferal) in the 1970s has dramatically improved the management of transfusion-dependent iron overload. Vision and hearing need to be monitored yearly during deferoxamine use because of the potential of the drug for ototoxicity and retinal damage. The tridentate chelator deferasirox (Exjade) is given as a single daily oral dose because of its long half-life. The dissolvable powder has a recommended daily dose ranging from 20 to 40 mg/kg/d. Several clinical trials have shown the efficacy of deferasirox in reducing LIC, and recent evidence points toward use of higher doses of deferasirox (30-40 mg/kg/d) to produce adequate liver iron clearance. In addition, there is some evidence to support the efficacy of deferasirox in reducing myocardial iron and improving function.[640,641] However, a comparison in a prospective randomized trial of deferasirox and deferiprone for removing cardiac iron has not been performed. Common side effects of deferasirox included rash (11%) and transient gastrointestinal symptoms (10%-15%); in addition, many patients complained of unpleasant drug taste and texture, prompting the development of a capsule form of the drug (Jadenu). The drug combination of an oral chelator and deferoxamine has been used in patients with thalassemia major and provided improved negative iron balance,[642] but no large trials have been conducted in patients with sickle cell disease.

Deferiprone (L1; Ferriprox), an oral chelator licensed in the United States in 2011, is a small molecule with a short half-life that is believed to have better access to intracellular iron. It is administered three times a day and its side effects are well recognized: agranulocytosis occurring in 0.6 per 100 patients per year, and, more commonly, transient neutropenia, arthropathy, zinc deficiency, increased transaminase levels, and gastrointestinal symptoms. Encouraging preliminary reports suggestive of effective penetration into cardiac cells prompted a large retrospective study, which showed a significantly lower rate of cardiac death and cardiac events in patients treated by deferiprone (75 mg/kg/d) compared to those treated by standard subcutaneous deferoxamine.[643] Randomized prospective trials have shown an advantage of deferiprone over deferoxamine in decreasing myocardial iron as measured by T2* MRI and in improving LV function in thalassemia patients.[644,645]

Although oral chelators have the potential to improve therapy for iron overload by improving compliance and therefore clinical response, suboptimal adherence is the dominant barrier to successful chelation.[646] Current recommendations for the management of iron overload in sickle cell disease are to monitor serum ferritin and LIC (preferably by MRI) longitudinally and to initiate iron chelation when LIC becomes >3.5 mg Fe/g dry weight or ferritin >1000 μg/L.[646]

Indications for Transfusions

Anemia. During hematologic crises, the Hb concentration may fall precipitously, requiring rapid correction. Transient aplastic crisis caused by parvovirus B19 infection often requires a single packed red cell transfusion before erythropoiesis eventually returns. A severe splenic sequestration crisis may require an immediate transfusion to restore blood volume and oxygen-carrying capacity. In children with recurrent acute splenic sequestration, chronic transfusion therapy to maintain splenic function has been used as an alternative to splenectomy. However, recurrences of sequestration have occurred despite transfusion. Transfusions are not indicated during acute vaso-occlusive painful events. Transfusions may be used in ESRD when Hb is not maintained at adequate levels.

Surgery. Anesthesia, surgery, and postsurgical convalescence expose patients to the formidable consequences of hypoventilation, hypotension, cooling, dehydration, acidosis, and immobilization. Although recommendations regarding the preparation of patients for surgery are varied, simple transfusions before elective procedures and partial exchange transfusions before emergency surgery have been used. A large multicenter prospective trial compared the rates of perioperative complications among patients randomly assigned to receive either an aggressive transfusion regimen (to decrease the Hb S level to <30%) or a conservative regimen (to increase the Hb level to 10 g/dL).[647] Perioperative complications, including ACS, were similar in the two

groups except for transfusion-associated complications, which were more common in the aggressively treated group. It was concluded that with good perioperative management, it is unnecessary to markedly reduce the Hb S level before surgery.[647] In the multicenter Transfusion Alternatives Preoperatively in Sickle Cell Disease study of patients undergoing mild-to-moderate risk surgery, subjects were randomized to receive no transfusion or transfusion to an Hb level of 10 g/dL.[648] Significantly more patients in the no-transfusion group had perioperative complications compared with those transfused (39% vs 15%), with most of the events being ACS.

Pharmacotherapy

Antisickling agents can be roughly divided into those that affect "upstream" targets and ones that act on "downstream" targets (*Figure 34.16*). A recent review of therapies approved by the US FDA for SCD has been published[649] and a summary of these therapeutic options is provided in *Table 34.5.*

Hemoglobin F Inducers

Reversal of ontogeny with reinstitution of Hb F synthesis is a long-standing objective that appears increasingly attainable. This therapeutic strategy is based on the observation that clinical expression of the sickle gene is prevented by Hb F synthesis in the perinatal period, as well as throughout life in individuals with HPFH.

Initial attempts to augment γ-globin synthesis were based on the observation that DNA in the vicinity of a wide variety of expressed genes is undermethylated relative to the DNA flanking inactive genes. 5-Azacytidine, a cytidine analog that blocks DNA methylation, reactivated dormant genes in cultured cells and increased Hb F synthesis in anemic baboons. When given to patients with severe SCA, 5-azacytidine caused a fourfold to sixfold increase in net γ-globin synthesis, a marked increase in the proportion of reticulocytes containing Hb F (F reticulocytes), and a precipitous decrease in the number of ISCs and dense red cells.[650]

Because of the known carcinogenic potential of 5-azacytidine, alternative stimulants of fetal Hb were sought. Hydroxyurea, a cytotoxic drug that has no known effect on DNA methylation, also increases Hb F production in anemic primates and in patients with severe disease. Hydroxyurea preferentially arrests the development of the more mature erythroid precursors, perhaps resulting in the recruitment of earlier erythroid progenitors with a greater capacity for Hb F synthesis.[651] Alternatively, hydroxyurea may have a direct effect on "reprogramming" globin synthesis by early erythroid progenitors, a suggestion that is supported by the fact that the increase in F-reticulocyte numbers that follows hydroxyurea administration occurs sooner (within 2-3 days) than would be expected if the effect represented recovery from bone marrow suppression.[652,653] Alterations in the physical properties of red cells produced under the influence of 5-azacytidine and hydroxyurea appear to be out of proportion to modest changes in the level of Hb F.

Patients taking hydroxyurea consistently develop macrocytosis, which may occur before any change in Hb F takes place (*Figure 34.17*). They also show a rapid correction toward normal red cell density distribution and improved whole-blood viscosity. Hydroxyurea therapy is associated with the intravascular and intraerythrocytic generation of NO, which may have a role in the clinical response that precedes the improvement in fetal Hb level.

In 1995, a double-blind multiinstitutional trial of hydroxyurea vs placebo (MSH) in about 300 adults with moderate to severe SCA was concluded with convincing evidence of clinical benefit from the drug.[654] Patients treated with hydroxyurea had approximately 40% to 50% lower rates of pain crises, ACS, hospitalization, and transfusion. There was wide variability in drug tolerance and clinical response, but the primary toxicity and dose-limiting factor was mild neutropenia. In addition to reducing acute events, hydroxyurea therapy has been reported to reduce mortality among adult patients with SCA.[655] Retrospective data from a large pediatric population have also shown substantial reduction in mortality in those receiving hydroxyurea.[553] Because of the favorable outcome in the majority of treated patients,

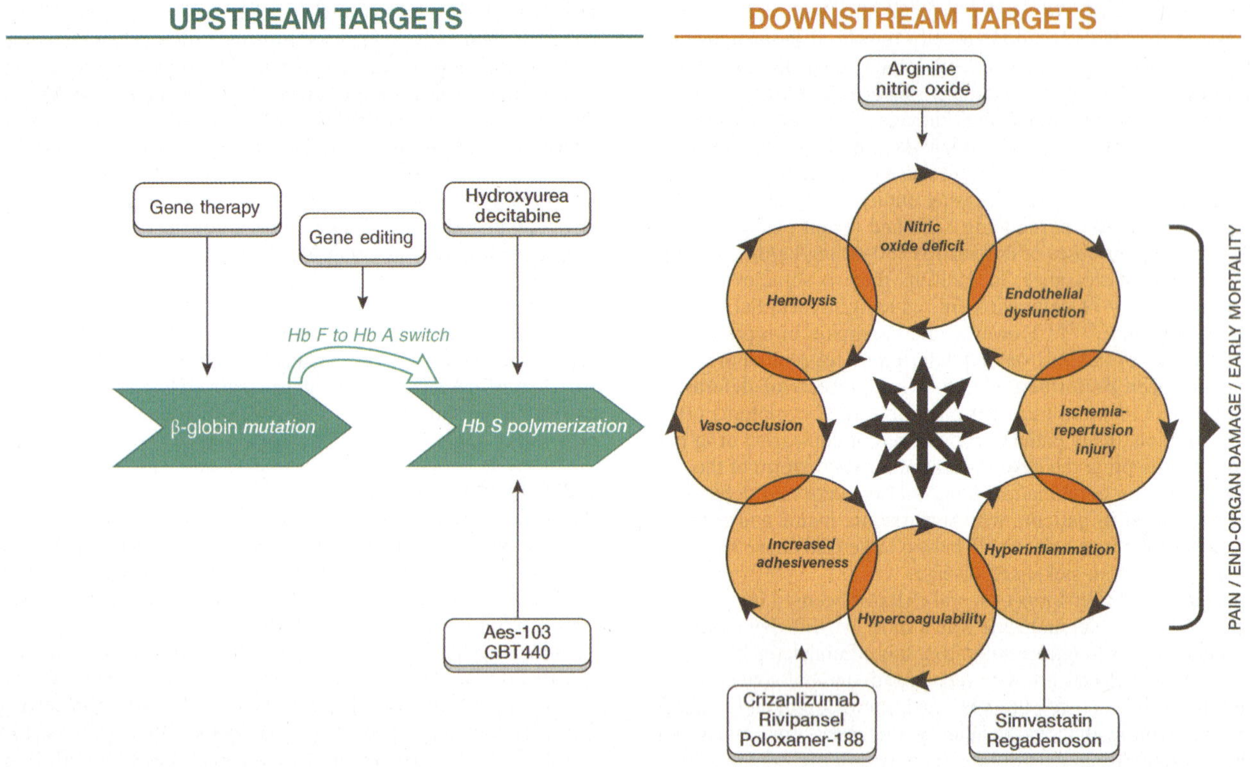

FIGURE 34.16 Therapeutic targets in sickle cell disease. Arrows point to primary sites in the pathophysiologic process targeted by the interventions. (Modified from Nottage KA, Estepp J, Hankins J. Future perspectives for the treatment of sickle cell anemia. In: Costa FF, Conran N. *Sickle Cell Anemia: From Basic Science to Clinical Practice.* 1st ed. Springer International Publishing; 2016. Prepared by Brandon Stelter, Biomedical Communications, St Jude Children's Research Hospital.)

Table 34.5. Summary Characteristics of FDA-Approved Disease-Modifying Therapies for SCD

	Hydroxyurea	L-Glutamine	Crizanlizumab	Voxelotor
Age (years)	**≥2**	**≥5**	**≥16**	**≥4**
Genotypes	HbSS and HbSβ⁰-thalassemia	All Genotypes (only studied in HbSS and HbSβ⁰-thalassemia)	All Genotypes	All Genotypes
Mechanism	Multiple, but primarily by reducing Hb S polymerization by increasing Hb F production	Uncertain, but increases NAD redox potential, possible decrease in cell adhesion	P-selectin inhibitor (decreases adhesion of WBCs and RBCs to vascular endothelium)	Decreases Hb S polymerization by increasing Hb—oxygen affinity
Route and frequency of administration	Oral; Once Daily (capsules/tablets/suspension)	Oral; Twice Daily (powder)	Intravenous; Monthly	Oral; Once Daily (tablets/tablets for oral suspension)
Initial daily dose	15 mg/kg (adults) 20 mg/kg (children)	<30 kg: 10 g 30-65 kg: 20 g >65 kg: 30 g	5 mg/kg	1500 mg$^{\&}$
Dose escalation	Yes (to MTD)	No	No	No
Safety Monitoring	Yes*	None	None	None
Clinical effects	Reduces VOC, ACS, hospitalization, transfusion, decreases stroke risk	Decreases VOC, ACS, and hospitalization	Decreases VOC	Improves hemoglobin and markers of hemolysis
Effect size for primary endpoint	44% reduction in acute pain per year (median from 4.5 to 2.5), IRR = 0.56	45% reduction in pain crises per year (median from 4.30 to 2.37)	45% reduction in pain crises per year (median from 3 to 1.6), IRR = 0.55	5.5-fold increase in Hb responders (9%-59%) at 24 wk, incidence proportion ratio = 6.6
Common toxicities	Myelosuppression# , nail and skin hyperpigmentation, nausea and emesis	Constipation, nausea, diarrhea, headaches, abdominal pain	Nausea, arthralgia	Headache, diarrhea, nausea
Long-term toxicities	Possible infertility in males	Unknown	Unknown Possible development of Antibodies against crizanlizumab	Unknown
Cost	$	$$$	$$$$$	$$$$$

Notes: *CBCs should be done at least once every 2 to 3 months. #Reversible side-effect. ^hydroxyurea is used in non-Hb SS and HbSβ⁰-thalassemia genotypes on an individual basis. $^{\&}$Voxelotor needs dose adjustment for patients with strong CYP3A4 inducers/inhibitors and pregnancy test and premedication with acetaminophen and diphenhydramine is recommended before each dose.
Abbreviations: ACS, acute chest syndrome; Hb, hemoglobin; HbF, fetal hemoglobin; HbS, sickle hemoglobin; MTD, maximum tolerated dose; NAD, nicotinamide adenine dinucleotide; PRBCs, packed red blood cells; RBC, red blood cell; VOC, vaso-occlusion.

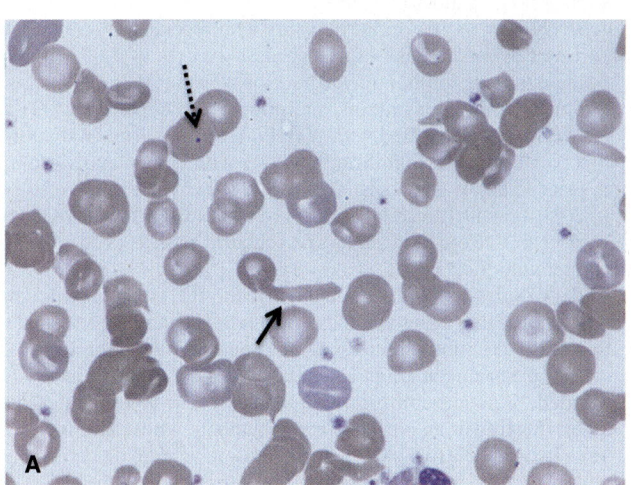 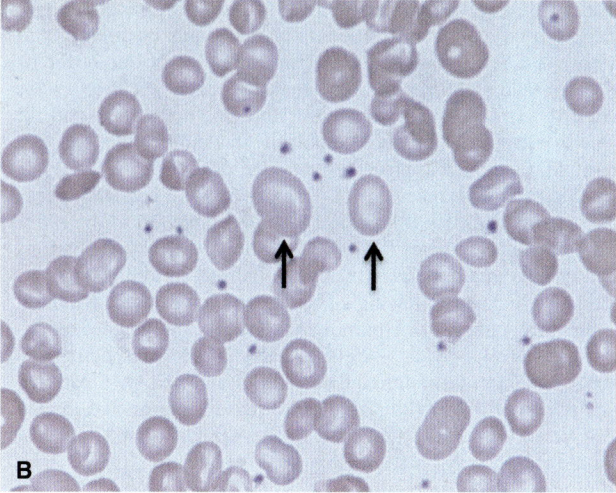

FIGURE 34.17 Effect of hydroxyurea on red blood cells. A, Peripheral blood smear of patient with Hb SS prior to treatment with hydroxyurea showing sickle forms (solid arrow), polychromasia, Howell-Jolly body (dashed arrow), and anisocytosis. B, Peripheral blood smear of same patient after 12 months of hydroxyurea therapy shows significant decrease in number of sickle forms, macrocytosis (solid arrows), and decreased polychromasia. (Courtesy of Hematology Department, St Jude Children's Research Hospital.)

hydroxyurea has become widely used in the treatment of adult patients who experience frequent vaso-occlusive crises and was approved by the FDA in the United States for this indication.

The phase III randomized placebo-controlled trial for infants (ages 9-18 months) with SCA (BABY HUG study) assessed the effect of hydroxyurea therapy on organ dysfunction and clinical complications and examined laboratory findings and toxic effects.[656] Ninety-six patients received hydroxyurea and 97 placebo. Hydroxyurea significantly decreased pain, dactylitis, ACS, hospitalization rates, and transfusion requirement. Spleen and renal functions were not improved when assessed by[140] Tc-spleen scan and[140] Tc-DTPA clearance, respectively. Analysis of secondary endpoints of the BABY HUG study, however, did show reduction of pitted cell and Howell-Jolly body counts, suggesting improvement of splenic function in the hydroxyurea-treated arm. In addition, urine-specific gravity improved, and total kidney volume decreased at study exit, suggesting preservation of renal function. Toxicity was limited to mild-to-moderate neutropenia. The results of the BABY HUG study contributed to the strong recommendation of the National Heart, Lung, and Blood Institute's Expert Panel Report on Evidence-Based Management of Sickle Cell Disease in 2014 that "in infants 9 months of age and older, children, and adolescents with SCA, treatment with hydroxyurea should be offered regardless of clinical severity to reduce sickle cell disease–related complications."[273] In 2017, hydroxyurea was approved by the US FDA based on results from an open-label, single-arm trial of 405 children aged 2 to 18 years who had improved hematologic parameters and reductions in vaso-occlusive episodes, ACS, SCD-related hospitalizations, and transfusion requirements.[10]

Hydroxyurea can be utilized as an oral solution (100 mg/mL) which has been shown to be bioequivalent to capsule formulations[11] and is especially convenient for young children. A modified dose based on hydroxyurea pharmacokinetics in patients with renal dysfunction has been recommended.[12] Erythropoietin therapy may allow more aggressive hydroxyurea dosing in high-risk sickle cell patients and in the setting of mild renal insufficiency, common to the older sickle cell population.[13] Furthermore, erythropoietin appears to be safe when used in conjunction with hydroxyurea.

Cross-sectional and prospective studies of hydroxyurea treatment have examined potential acquisition of genotoxicity with chromosomal karyotype, illegitimate variable-diversity-joining gene segments recombination events, white cell cytostasis and cytotoxicity development, and micronucleated reticulocyte formation. These have not shown significant increases in genotoxicity compared with

the measurements prior to initiation of therapy or those performed on placebo-controlled sickle cell disease subjects.[14,15] Although caution about the long-term carcinogenic and teratogenic potential of hydroxyurea is needed, to date there is no evidence that the drug leads to an increased cancer risk or to congenital anomalies in offspring of women who became pregnant while taking hydroxyurea (or whose partners were taking hydroxyurea). An unanswered question is whether hydroxyurea has a negative impact on male fertility. Males have conceived healthy babies while taking hydroxyurea, including during the original MSH trial[654]; however, some studies suggest that hydroxyurea therapy is associated with transient reduction in sperm counts in adult males.[16] More recently, hydroxyurea therapy initiated prior to the onset of puberty was not associated with semen volume, sperm concentration, total sperm count, or spermatozoa motility, morphology, and vitality compared to individuals who were not given hydroxyurea therapy.[17]

Decitabine, an azacytidine analog (5-aza-2′-deoxycytidine), causes induction of Hb F through DNA hypomethylation.[18] In recent small-scale clinical trials in patients with SCD, treatment with decitabine resulted in significant increases in mean γ-globin synthesis, Hb F levels, and the number of F cells (RBCs that contain Hb F).[18,19] A current clinical trial is testing decitabine in adults with sickle cell disease who do not tolerate hydroxyurea because of hematologic or other toxicities[20] (*Figure 34.16*).

Cyclic guanosine monophosphate (cGMP) depended on signaling pathways are theorized to be therapeutic target for induction of Hb F synthesis in patients with SCD. The cGMP-specific phosphodiesterase 9 (PDE9) enzyme degrades cGMP, and inhibition of PDE9 increases cGMP resulting in elevation of Hb F.[21] A novel and selective PDE9 inhibitor (IMR-687) is being evaluated in SCD.[22,23]

Improved understanding of the physiologic "switch" from fetal-to-adult Hb in humans and silencing factors for the γ-globin genes[24-26] has resulted in the development of multiple genetic therapeutic approaches aimed at curing individuals with SCD.[27]

Other Antisickling Agents Targeting Hb S Polymerization

Increasing Hb F interferes with polymerization of Hb S molecules, a process considered to be "upstream" of the pathophysiologic mechanisms. Other approaches to inhibiting polymerization might include blocking intermolecular contacts in the sickle fiber, reducing the concentration of DPG, increasing oxygen affinity, and reducing red cell density (intracellular Hb concentration).[45] The latter three approaches have led to recent clinical trials and FDA approvals for novel therapeutic approaches to SCD.

Voxelotor (Oxbryta, previously GBT440) is a first-in-class, small molecule, Hb oxygen affinity modulator that binds covalently and reversibly via a Schiff-base to the N-terminal valine of one of the α-chains of Hb and stabilizes the oxygenated R state.[28,29] It is a once daily oral therapy, designed to inhibit HbS polymerization and, in turn, improve anemia and reduce hemolysis. In a multicenter, phase 3, double-blind, randomized, placebo-controlled trial, 51% (95% CI 41-61) of participants who received 1500 mg of voxelotor had an increase of at least 1.0 g/dL in Hb following 24 weeks compared to 7% (95% CI 1-12) in the placebo arm ($P < .001$). Additional efficacy evaluations included change in Hb, percent change in indirect bilirubin, and percent reticulocyte count following 24 weeks. In the voxelotor 1500 mg group, the mean change for Hb, indirect bilirubin, and percent reticulocyte count were 1.14 g/dL, −29.08%, and −19.93%, respectively.[30] In 2019, voxelotor was approved for adults and pediatric patients 12 years of age or older with sickle cell disease under an accelerated approval based on the improvements in anemia. Continued approval for this indication may be contingent upon verification and description of clinical benefit in confirmatory trials. In 2021, voxelotor was granted a supplemental New Drug Application to expand the previous approval to include children aged 4 to 12 years.

Activation of erythrocyte pyruvate kinase (PKR) is being targeted as a novel therapeutic mechanism for SCD. Hypothetically, activation of PKR would result in a reduction of 2,3DPG concentration and increase adenosine triphosphate. Mitapivat, a novel, first-in-class oral small molecule allosteric activator of PKR, has been shown to be safe and effective in adults with pyruvate kinase deficiency[31] and is being evaluated in patients with SCD.[32,33] Etavopivat, a second oral, small molecule activator or PKR, is also being evaluated in patients with SCD.[34,35]

Reduction of Red Cell Density

The therapy designed to reduce the MCHC is based on the fact that small decrements in the MCHC significantly delay the rate of deoxy Hb S polymerization and inhibit red cell sickling. The delay time of gelation of deoxy Hb S is inversely proportional to the 30th power of Hb S concentration. The analog Senicapoc (ICA-17043) was shown to decrease the RBC membrane cation permeability by decreasing the Gardos channel activity and K^+ efflux. In a phase II clinical trial in adult patients treated for 12 weeks, hematologic efficacy was demonstrated in the higher dose treatment arm and the activity of the Gardos channel decreased significantly.[36] However, in a phase III multicenter clinical trial, despite improvements in anemia and hemolysis, Senicapoc failed to reduce the frequency of painful events, leading to an early closure of the study.[657]

In another randomized phase II study, the combination approach of oral hydroxyurea and magnesium in children and adults with Hb SC disease failed to demonstrate effects from magnesium on hyperdense RBCs or vaso-occlusive events.[658] In addition, a recent multicenter randomized trial of IV magnesium for sickle cell pain crisis in children did not shorten the length of hospitalization, decrease opioid use, or improve quality of life.[659]

Reduction of Adhesion

After the formation of sickle cells, tissue injury results in inflammation and increased adhesion among sickle cells, WBCs, and vascular endothelium. Selectins decelerate sickle red cells and leukocytes in the circulation to facilitate adhesion among blood cells and endothelium and platelets also mediate intercellular adhesion, therefore, these processes have been targets of recent therapeutic approaches.[660]

Because platelets also mediate intercellular adhesion during vaso-occlusion in sickle cell disease, therapy with antiplatelet agents has been explored. In a large placebo-controlled international trial involving 13 countries, the rate of vaso-occlusive events was not significantly different in children receiving the antiplatelet agent prasugrel and those receiving placebo.[661] However, recent studies of agents directed against adhesion-promoting selectin molecules have yielded more promising results. In a randomized, placebo-controlled multicenter phase II trial, two different doses of crizanlizumab, (Adakveo),

a monoclonal antibody against P-selectin, were compared against placebo (*Figure 34.16*).[662] Participants who received IV crizanlizumab 14 times over 52 weeks experienced an average of 1.63 crises (composite endpoint combining vaso-occlusive pain, ACS, hepatic sequestration, spenic sequestration, and priapism) compared to 2.98 crises per year in those treated with placebo ($P = .01$). The median time to first pain crises was significantly longer with crizanlizumab compared to placebo and was associated with a low incidence of adverse events. In 2019, crizanlizumab was approved by the FDA for the reduction of vaso-occlusive crises in adults and pediatric patients aged 16 years and greater with SCD.

Poloxamer-188, also known as RheothRx, is a nonionic copolymer emulsifying agent that may counteract the tendency of sickle cells to adhere to endothelium by decreasing the interaction between red cells and fibrinogen (*Figure 34.16*). A phase 3, randomized, double-blinded, placebo-controlled, multicenter, trial evaluated poloxamer-188 infusions on its effect in patients with acute moderate or severe vaso-occlusive pain requiring hospitalization on parental opioid administration, but did not significantly shorten the time to last opioid administration during vaso-occlusive pain episodes.[663]

Oxidative Stress

Nicotinamide adenine dinucleotide (NAD^+) is a cofactor required for oxidation-reduction reactions in erythrocytes, and NAD^+ (and NADH, in reduced form) is required for maintained erythrocyte health and individuals with SCD have reduced redox potential in erythrocytes compared to health controls.[664,665] Oral administration of L-glutamine improved redox potential in patients with SCD by increasing erythrocyte NAD levels and was associated with improved patient-reported outcomes in seven adults with SCD.[666] A subsequent multicenter, randomized, placebo-controlled, double-blinded, phase 3 trial enrolled 230 patients (aged 5-58 years) to receive L-glutamine twice a day for 48 weeks. Patients treated with L-glutamine had fewer pain episodes and hospitalizations.[667,668] Endari (L-glutamine) was approved by the FDA in 2017, for individuals aged 5 years and older with SCD to reduce severe SCD-related complications.

Anti-inflammatory Agents

Sickle cell disease patients live in a state of "baseline heightened inflammation," which contributes to and sustains the pathophysiologic cycle of vaso-occlusion and tissue damage. Attenuation of the inflammatory response in sickle cell disease could potentially ameliorate symptoms of the disease.

Statins are cholesterol-lowering agents that provide protection from vascular injury by suppressing inflammation. In a recent trial in adults with SCA, a daily dose of simvastatin for 3 months resulted in a significant reduction in the frequency of pain, oral analgesic use, and a number of circulating biomarkers of inflammation (*Figure 34.16*).[669] Results were greatest in subjects receiving concurrent hydroxyurea, suggesting a possible synergistic effect.

Adenosine is a purine nucleoside that modulates many intracellular processes, such as signal transduction and energy transfer. The concentration of adenosine rises rapidly in response to cellular damage, such as tissue ischemia. Excessive adenosine signaling occurs in sickle cell disease, as both adenosine and DPG concentrations are elevated in individuals with sickle cell disease and induce sickling in vitro.[50] Adenosine A_{2A} receptor agonists reduced iNKT cell activation and decreased inflammation in sickle cell mice.[660] In a phase I trial, a 24-hour infusion of the A_{2A} receptor agonist regadenoson during pain crises decreased iNKT cell activation without toxicity (*Figure 34.16*).[670]

Modification of Nitric Oxide Metabolism

Intravascular hemolysis is thought to impair NO bioavailability and cause oxidative stress, leading to regional vasoconstriction and clinical complications including PHT, leg ulcers, priapism, CKD, and ischemic stroke. A multicenter placebo-controlled trial of up to 72 hours of inhaled NO gas was given to adult patients presenting with vaso-occlusive pain crises (*Figure 34.16*).[671] Although significant increases in plasma nitrate occurred in the treatment group, the use of inhaled NO did not improve time to crises resolution. Arginine is a semi essential amino acid that is the precursor to NO and a number of other metabolites, and low arginine bioavailability has been associated with pain severity in both adults and children with sickle cell disease (*Figure 34.16*).[672] In a single-center randomized placebo-controlled trial of arginine therapy in children with sickle cell disease and pain requiring hospitalization, a significant reduction in opioid use was seen in those receiving arginine, leading to ongoing larger trials.[673]

Bone Marrow (Hematopoietic Stem Cell) Transplantation

Excellent outcomes in HSC from HLA-identical siblings, improvements in preconditioning regimens, advances in graft-vs-host disease (GVHD) prophylaxis, and alternative donor approaches have all increased availability and acceptability of HSC transplant for individuals with SCD. HSC has the potential to normalize Hb synthesis and is currently the only curative treatment for SCD. The first transplant was performed in a child with both SCA and acute myeloblastic leukemia in 1984; bone marrow from an HLA-identical sibling abolished both diseases.[674] Since then, approximately 1200 patients with SCA have been transplanted, primarily using HLA-identical sibling donors. Analysis of the largest registry experience, which came from France (1986-2013), found that event-free survival was lower with increasing age at transplant and higher for treatment after 2006.[675,676] HLA-matched sibling donor transplant series collectively have shown excellent results, with overall survival of 95% and event-free survival of 92%.[675] In general, treatment-related mortality has ranged from 2% to 7%, and the most common causes of death have been complications of GVHD, sepsis, and stroke (primarily hemorrhagic). The incidence of GVHD has varied from 10% to 20%. Most transplants have used myeloablative conditioning with pretransplant regimens of busulfan, methotrexate, cyclophosphamide, and antithymocyte globulin. A nonmyeloablative regimen in adults[677] and reduced intensity conditioning regimen in children[678] have yielded event-free survivals of 87% and 91%, respectively.

In a retrospective cohort study composed from data submitted to the Center for International Blood and Marrow Transplant Research, 910 patients with SCD underwent transplantation between 2008 and 2017 and were available for analysis. 558 (61%) had HLA-matched sibling donors, 137 (15%) haploidentical-related donors, 111 (12%) matched unrelated donors, and 104 (11%) had mismatched unrelated donors. In this cohort, event-free survival was worse in older (>13 years) participants (HR 1.74, 95%CI: 1.24-2.45; *P* = .004) and in participants who had a haploidentical donor (HR 5.0, 95%CI: 3.17-8.86; *P* < .0001), matched unrelated donors (HR3.71, 95%CI: 2.39-5.75; *P* < .0001) and mismatched unrelated donors (HR 4.34, 95%CI: 2.58-7.32; *P* < .0001) compared to matched sibling donors. There was no significant difference in event-free survival between recipients who received transplants from non–sibling donor sources. Data suggestive that event-free survival remains higher in individuals who undergo transplant prior to 12 years of age and with an HLA-matched sibling donor, but in patients without access to an HLA-matched sibling, no alternative donor source is favored over others.[679] Recent guidelines were developed to provide evidence-based recommendations for HSC transplant in SCD.[680] The evidence utilized to support the recommendations was low to very low in certainty due to lack of randomized controlled trials for transplant in SCD. However, the recommendations were as follows: HLA-matched sibling donors should be considered for all individuals at risk of neurologic injury (abnormal TCD or previous overt stroke), with recurrent vaso-occlusive pain crises or ACS. Additionally, when feasible, transplantation should be pursued at the earliest age possible. All patients, even those with an HLA-matched donor, with severe SCD-related complications should be counseled on transplant options with non–HLA-matched donor options. In adults with an HLA-matched donor, nonmyeloablative conditioning therapies are recommended. Alternative donor options and newer myeloablative condition regimens should be undertaken in the context of a clinical trial.

A recent review discusses current understanding of the indications, condition strategies, donor options, timing, outcomes, and decisions making for transplant in SCD.[681] A consensus statement has addressed the need to carefully evaluate the late effects of HSC transplant in children.[675] Resolution of chronic pain, pulmonary, cardiac and gonadal function, growth, and effects of iron overload all warrant systematic long-term assessment. The impact of transplant on central nervous system function is particularly pertinent; most patients have had stabilization of preexisting cerebrovascular disease, although acute strokes were not entirely eliminated following transplant.[682,683] It is conceivable that transplant may ameliorate the cognitive decline known to occur with increasing age in sickle cell disease, but only a small study of longitudinal cognitive outcomes has been published.[684] Among 15 children transplanted at a mean age of 8.9 years, the median FSIQ increased from 87 to 94 at 3 and 5 years posttransplant.

The possibility of infertility is a concern among patients undergoing myeloablative conditioning regimens for stem cell transplant. Recently, ovarian stimulation followed by oocyte retrieval and cryopreservation provided fertility preservation in an adolescent girl with severe sickle cell disease scheduled to undergo a HSC transplant.[685] This approach, along with sperm banking in men, can be alternatives for young sickle cell patients who undergo stem cell transplant and aspire to have families in the future.

The availability and the relative success of bone marrow transplantation worldwide have raised a number of social and ethical questions about its use. For example, how severe must sickle cell disease be to justify a transplant-associated mortality rate of 5% to 10%? In the United States, only 6% of patients with SCA met the criteria for transplantation specified in a study protocol; furthermore, a survey estimated that only 18% would have sibling donors.[686] Although these criteria would result in approximately 1% of American children with SCA being eligible for transplantation, criteria used in Belgium were based on the poor prognosis of children with sickle cell disease who were returning to a setting of limited medical care in central Africa.[687] Another point of view has been that transplantation is warranted in virtually all patients for whom a suitable donor is available,[688] particularly before organ dysfunction and transfusion exposure occur. It has been noted that the transplant enrollment criteria parallel those of studies using hydroxyurea treatment.[689] When these two modalities are compared, transplantation offers a definitive cure for SCA but a significant risk of mortality, whereas hydroxyurea offers amelioration of the clinical symptoms with short-term complications that appear to be reversible and small.

Other approaches to transplantation have been developed outside of sickle cell disease. Cord blood stem cells harvested from HLA-identical newborn sibs, as well as unrelated donors, have been successfully transplanted.[690,691] Directed donor banking of cord blood from a sibling of a child with a disorder treatable by stem cell transplantation provided a cord blood allograft that was successful in 16 of 17 cases.[692] A trial of unrelated donor marrow transplantation for children with severe sickle cell disease was conducted by the BMT Clinical Trials Network, but the 2-year event-free survival rate was only 69% and the acute and chronic GVH rates were high, indicating that the reduced intensity conditioning regimen used was unsatisfactory.[693] A reduced intensity haploidentical transplant trial also in children with severe sickle cell disease resulted in an overall survival of 97%, but a disease-free survival of only 57% because of graft rejection.[694] However, a modified multicenter haploidentical transplant protocol is in progress.

When stable mixed chimerism is established after stem cell transplant, even a minority of donor cells with a selective advantage may overcome a genetic defect. In an analysis of 50 patients with successful allografts, 5 had chimerism with a relatively low proportion of donor cells (range 11%-74%). These five patients had normal Hb levels and much lower Hb S fractions than the proportion of donor chimerism, suggesting that donor erythroid progenitors or erythrocytes had a survival advantage over their recipient sickle cell counterparts.[695] Because these patients were also clinically asymptomatic, it appears that full-donor chimerism is not necessary to cure nonmalignant disorders, and reduced intensity regimens that allow mixed chimerism may be effective.[695,696] In fact, reduced intensity stem cell transplantation from matched donors has been described in 10 adults with sickle cell disease, and sustainable marrow engraftment with stable mixed chimerism was achieved in 9 out of the 10 subjects. This regimen utilized low-dose total body irradiation, alemtuzumab, and sirolimus, and appears to be a viable option for patients who would otherwise not be able to tolerate an aggressive conditioning regimen.[697]

Worldwide, HSC transplant is underutilized in patients with SCD, a multifactorial phenomenon resulting from high costs, lack of expertise, lack of available HLA-matched donors, insufficient referral to transplant centers, and increased use of disease-modifying therapies (hydroxyurea, erythrocyte transfusions) among other reasons. In one study, when transplantation, periodic prophylactic blood transfusion, and hydroxyurea were compared in a decision analysis study for children with severe sickle cell disease, bone marrow transplant was the strategy treatment of choice.[698] However, in another study, therapy preference and decision-making among patients with severe SCA and their families were analyzed after they received standardized nondirective presentations and educational materials. Ten percent expressed preference for stem cell transplant, 17% for chronic transfusion, and 70% for hydroxyurea.[699] Many patients and families still perceive transplant to be dangerous in comparison with other therapies, such as hydroxyurea and chronic transfusions, and choose not to pursue transplant even when a matched HLA sibling donor is available.[699,700]

Gene Therapy

Major limitations hinder widespread applicability of HSC transplant as a curative option for SCD, such as lack of matched donor availability, high cost, acute mortality rates of 5% to 10%, and the risk of late effects (i.e., GVHD, decreased fertility, immunosuppression, risk of secondary malignancies, graft rejection). Gene therapy aims to insert a gene that codes a desired RNA product or protein into a patient's own HSCs and has expression levels sufficient to halt polymerization of Hb S.

The development of a variety of approaches to gene therapy over the past decades has now led to the initiation of clinical trials in persons with hemoglobinopathies. Previously, low efficiency of gene transfer to stem cells and suboptimal globin gene expression, as well as safety concerns, have limited progress, but recent use of lentiviral vectors derived from the human immunodeficiency virus genome has allowed more efficient transduction of human cells. Two transgenic mouse strains with human SS disease were transduced using lentiviral vectors using globin genes linked to regulatory elements of the locus control region, resulting in reduced sickling, improved renal-concentrating capacity, and human β-globin synthesis at 10% to 50% of the level of endogenous β-globin production.[701] This led to initial treatment of an adult with thalassemia (Hb E/β⁰-thalassemia) who has remained transfusion-independent for several years after lentiviral β-globin gene transfer.[702] A 13-year-old boy with Hb SS and frequent vaso-occlusive events despite previous treatment with hydroxyurea and chronic transfusion received lentiviral vector–mediated addition of an antisickling β-globin gene inserted into autologous HSCs.[703] Fifteen months after treatment, the level of therapeutic antisickling β-globin remained high and the patient had no recurrence of sickle crises and correction of the biologic hallmarks of the disease. More recently, 35 patients with SCD have received a LentiGlobin infusion with a median follow-up of 17.3 months (range, 3.7-37.6). All 35 patients engrafted following autologous transplant and showed robust hematologic responses, with improvements in total Hb levels to an average of 11 g/dL and reduction in markers of hemolysis.[703]

New genetic manipulation approaches, that is, gene editing, have been made possible by increased molecular understanding of Hb F inheritance. BCL11A was identified as a critical fetal Hb silencer and numerous interacting factors have been elucidated.[704] In a meta-analysis of 2040 patients with SCA from 7 cohorts, examination of SNPs from GWAS confirmed that *BCL11A* and *HBS1L-MYB* were the major modifiers of Hb F in African Americans (although together they accounted for only about 15% of the variability in Hb F).[705] Gene editing enables modification of the genome which typically ensues from site-specific double-strand breaks in DNA followed by

nonhomologous end joining or homology-directed repair.[706] The finding that disruption of erythroid-specific *BCL11A* enhancers through gene editing nucleases resulted in marked Hb F induction in primary human erythroid precursors has led to the development of current gene editing trials.[707] As a proof of concept, a gene editing strategy in SCD was based on the clinical knowledge that coinheritance of the Hb S and HPFH genes alleviates clinical manifestations. CRISPR-Cas9–mediated genome editing of human blood progenitors to mutate a 13-nucleotide sequence present in the promoters of the two γ-globin genes (and found in one form of HPFH) yielded RBCs with markedly increased Hb F.[708] In a recent proof of principle, two adult patients (one with transfusion-dependent thalassemia and one with SCD) underwent autologous CD34⁺ HSC transplantation following clustered regularly interspaced short palindromic repeats (CRISPER)-Cas9 targeting of the *BCL11A* enhancer, which resulted in pancellular distribution of Hb F, transfusion independence, and elimination of vaso-occlusive pain in the patient with SCD, 12 months after therapy.[709] In a second therapeutic approach aimed at downregulating *BCL11A*, six patients with SCD received a lentiviral vector that mediates potent erythroid-specific knockdown of *BCL11A* through RNA interference (RNAi), using a microRNA-adapted short hairpin RNA,[710,711] and all six patients had full engraftment following autologous transplant and stable Hb F production following at least 6 months of therapy.[712]

These encouraging and exciting revelations with gene therapy and gene editing provide long-awaited hope from the SCD community that new avenues for curative approach for SCD are on the horizon. In 2021, clinical trials utilizing gene therapy were placed on transient suspension after participants developed acute myelogenous leukemia/myelodysplastic syndrome.[713] Some authors theorized after gene therapy for SCD, the stress of switching from homeostatic to regenerative hematopoiesis by transplanted cells drove clonal expansion and leukemogenic transformation of pre-existing premalignant clones, eventually resulting in AML/MDS.[714] The long-term risk of acquired malignancy following curative intent gene therapy either from exposure from alkylating agents during conditioning, insertional mutagenesis, expansion of preexisting premalignant clones, some combination of all or none of these reasons will need to be addressed moving forward.

SICKLE CELL TRAIT

Sickle cell trait, the heterozygous state for the Hb S gene, is present in about 8% of black Americans and in as many as 20% of some African populations (*Table 34.1*).

Clinical Features

Sickle cell trait is known to confer a better prognosis from malarial infection. It rarely is associated with clinical or hematologic manifestations of significance. Individuals have no anemia, and red cell morphology is normal. Growth and development proceed normally, and no increased frequency of bone and joint disease is observed. A prospective study of pregnant women with sickle cell trait documented an overall incidence of complications and a distribution of birth weights similar to those of a control group.[715] Life expectancy and overall mortality rate for persons with sickle cell trait are the same as for the general population. The prevalence of the trait among professional football players is the same as that in the black population, suggesting that it imposes no limitation in physical capabilities. Nevertheless, most of the complications associated with SCA have been described in individuals with sickle cell trait. In such reports, the presence of Hb S was likely an incidental finding, unrelated to the observed deficit. For example, studies of sudden death in soldiers and athletes undergoing strenuous physical conditioning lack pertinent information concerning the relative amounts of Hb A and Hb S and the presence of potential but undetected underlying illness.[716,717] Nevertheless, a comprehensive analysis of sudden unexplained deaths among more than 2 million recruits undergoing basic training in the United States Armed Forces demonstrated a small increase in such deaths, especially those related to exertional heat illness, in association with sickle cell trait.[718]

Following this finding, an interventional trial examined the hypothesis that preventing exertional heat illness would reduce mortality for all recruits, including those with sickle cell trait.[719,720] The intervention consisted of monitoring core temperature, minimizing efforts in hot weather, increasing water consumption, and using light clothing, among other measures. *No deaths among individuals with or without sickle cell trait were observed when precautionary measures were undertaken*, which was significantly less than the predicted 13 deaths. Currently, sickle cell trait is not a disqualifying condition for entry into the United States Armed Forces, and universal precautions against exertional heat illness have been fully implemented.

A study of almost 2 million National Collegiate Athletic Association (NCAA) athletes found 273 deaths between 2004 and 2008, with 5 (2%) of these deaths occurring in athletes with sickle cell trait, all in association with exertional heat illness.[721] The study concluded that the risk of exertional death was 37 times greater in athletes with sickle cell trait than that among those without it. This study, however, did not have information on the sickle cell trait status of the entire cohort, and estimated trait prevalence based on prior epidemiologic studies. Nevertheless, this report prompted the NCAA to adopt a policy requiring Division I institutions in the United States to perform testing for sickle cell trait in all incoming athletes. However, the risk under even the most adverse circumstances is low (1 in 3200 in the Armed Forces study), and concerns were raised that millions of black individuals, including aspiring athletes, with sickle cell trait should not be stigmatized or labeled as sick. A retrospective analysis of approximately 48,000 black soldiers on active duty in the United States Army between 2011 and 2014 was conducted to test whether the risks of exertional rhabdomyolysis and mortality varied according to sickle cell trait status.[722] There was no significant difference in the risk of death, although there was a higher risk of exertional rhabdomyolysis, similar in magnitude to that associated with tobacco use.

Other complications of the trait are well documented but relatively rare: hematuria, urinary tract infection, and splenic infarction. Hematuria is generally transient and is probably related to poor perfusion of the renal papillae; frank renal papillary necrosis has been described.[477] Of note, although renal medullary carcinoma is a rare malignancy, most of the reported cases have occurred in individuals with sickle cell trait and sickle cell disease. Urine concentrating ability is also impaired in trait, although renal acidification is normal. A Jamaican study of older adult women showed an increased frequency of bacteriuria in those with sickle cell trait. In Reasons for Geographic and Racial Differences in Stroke, a population-based cohort study, individuals with SCT had an HR for ESRD of 2.03 (95%CI, 1.44-2.84) when compared to noncarriers. In fact, the degree of risk for ESRD conferred by SCT status was similar to that conferred by APOL1 high-risk genotypes.[723] During pregnancy, women with sickle cell trait have increase in bacteriuria and pyelonephritis. There are numerous reports of splenic infarction in individuals with sickle cell trait who were exposed to altitudes of 10,000 ft or more in unpressurized aircraft, but this has not been reported in commercial flights, in which cabin pressure is equivalent to about 8000 ft. Recent studies have noted a twofold increased risk of pulmonary embolism but not an elevated deep vein thrombosis risk,[724,725] as well as an increased D-dimer level.[726] However, in recent studies, in African American adults, sickle cell trait was not associated with reduced fitness[727] or with an increased risk of heart failure or abnormalities of cardiac structure and function,[728] or with an increased incidence of ischemic stroke,[729] or cognitive decline/dementia.[730]

Diagnosis

Sickle cell trait is characterized by an electrophoretic pattern containing both Hb A and Hb S, but there is more Hb A than Hb S. The interaction of α-thalassemia with sickle cell trait is responsible for a trimodal distribution of Hb S with means of about 41%, 35%, and 28%, corresponding to the $\alpha\alpha/\alpha\alpha$, $-\alpha/\alpha\alpha$, and $-\alpha/-\alpha$ genotypes, respectively. The positive correlation between the proportion of Hb S and the output of α genes indicates the greater affinity of β^A chains than of β^S chains for α chains in the formation of Hb tetramers. Excess β^S chains

presumably are destroyed by proteolysis. The relative amount of Hb S is also decreased by iron and folate deficiencies.

Screening Programs

There are two possible reasons to screen groups for the presence of sickle cell trait: (1) to inform affected persons of health risks and (2) to provide information that might affect an individual's reproductive decisions. Most hemoglobinopathy screening is now done to identify sickle cell disease in neonates. Therefore, identification of sickle cell trait occurs at a time when counseling of the affected individual is impossible. Counseling of family members of newborns with sickle cell trait may be of value but is only performed sporadically in most states. The technique chosen for screening should be genetically diagnostic and should clearly differentiate between sickle cell trait and those disorders of Hb that have implications for health.

OTHER SICKLING SYNDROMES

Several of the doubly heterozygous states for Hb S and a second disorder of Hb synthesis are characterized by clinical and hematologic aberrations that to some extent mimic the features of SCA. The clinically significant disorders resulting from double heterozygosity for Hb S and a second Hb variant are considered to be forms of sickle cell disease.

Hemoglobin SC Disease

Hb SC disease results from the inheritance of an Hb S gene from one parent and an Hb C gene from the other. Red cells contain approximately equal amounts of the two Hbs. Hb A is absent, and Hb F is normal or slightly increased. The disorder occurs with an approximate frequency of 1 in 1100 births among black Americans and 1 in 1400 births in Jamaica. In Ghana, the presumed site of origin of the Hb C mutation, Hb SC disease is as prevalent as SCA, and in some regions it affects as many as 25% of the population.

The clinical and laboratory features of Hb SC disease cannot be explained by copolymerization of Hb C with Hb S. The solubility of mixtures of deoxy Hb S and Hb C is no different from that of mixtures of Hb S and Hb A. Differences in the sickling properties of sickle trait cells and Hb SC cells are related to two factors: a higher proportion of Hb S and a higher concentration of Hb in Hb SC cells compared with Hb AS cells. The 10% to 15% greater proportion of Hb S in Hb SC cells is the result of differences in rates of subunit assembly, which, in turn, are determined by the net surface charges of β^A, β^S, and β^C.[731] The higher MCHC of Hb SC cells is the result of Hb C inducing, by mechanisms not fully understood, an increase in the activity of K-Cl cotransport, which causes loss of K^+ and consequently of intracellular water.

Clinical Features

The clinical manifestations of Hb SC disease are similar to, but on average less frequent than, those of SCA. Growth and sexual development are delayed compared with normal children, but less so than in children with SCA.[732] The most common symptom is episodic abdominal or skeletal pain, qualitatively similar to that caused by vaso-occlusive events in SCA. The average number of painful episodes per year for Hb SC patients is approximately one-half that for persons with SCA (0.4 vs 0.8 episodes per year).[87] Hb (*P* = .02) and MCHC (*P* = .003) were independently associated with pain crisis episodes in Hb SC patients.[733] Moderate enlargement of the spleen is present in approximately two-thirds of children and often persists into adult life. Spleen perfusion is intact, however, and as a result, symptomatic splenic infarction and acute splenic sequestration may occur in adults as well as in children. Loss of spleen function is more gradual and occurs at a later age than occurs in SCA.[734] The frequency of infections of patients with Hb SC disease is increased, but fatal pneumococcal septicemia, although well documented, is less of a risk than is noted in SCA. The incidence of bacteremia drops abruptly after 2 years of age, a contrasting pattern to SCA, in which the incidence declines gradually between 2 and 6 years of age.[262] Because bacteremia rarely progresses to septicemia and a fatal outcome in young children with Hb SC disease, some investigators believe that prophylactic penicillin is not necessary. However, fatal pneumococcal septicemia was reported in a series of seven children with Hb SC, six of whom were >3 years of age.[735] Central nervous system deficits, asymptomatic hematuria, ankle ulceration, priapism, and other complications of sickling occur with Hb SC disease but are infrequent events. TCD velocities are substantially lower in Hb SC disease,[736] but a higher-than-expected prevalence of SCI has been reported.[737] In the United States, the median lifespan for male and female Hb SC patients is 60 and 68 years of age, respectively.

Because of the frequency with which they occur, certain complications of Hb SC disease deserve special comment. Proliferative retinopathy is more common and more severe than in SCA. Progressive loss of vision may have its onset early in the second decade, and patients should be encouraged to have an annual ophthalmologic examination starting at 10 years of age. Aseptic necrosis of the femoral head has been reported to have a greater frequency in Hb SC disease than in Hb SS, but the age-adjusted prevalence is lower.[296,534] The exaggerated vulnerability of individuals with Hb SC disease to certain complications is thought to be a function of the higher viscosity of the blood relative to that in SCA.

Moderately severe complications of in vivo sickling occur in Hb SC-Harlem disease[738] and in the Hb SC/α-thalassemia syndrome.[739] Combined Hb SC disease and hereditary spherocytosis was documented as the cause of recurrent splenic sequestration crises.[740]

Laboratory Features

Anemia is mild or may be nonexistent; 75% of children 2 to 15 years of age have a hematocrit between 28% and 38%, and 75% of adults have a hematocrit between 28 and 42 (with males having higher levels than females). Compared with Hb SS, the MCV may be decreased (10-15 fL lower), and the MCHC may be increased owing to cellular dehydration. Reticulocytes are modestly increased in number. Blood films contain as many as 50% target cells. Although sickled cells are relatively rare, cells containing Hb "crystals" are noted regularly.[741] These hyperchromic shrunken cells are distorted into pyramidal or elongated contours by condensed aggregates of Hb (*Figure 34.14*). The WBC count and leukocyte differential are normal. Additionally, laboratory investigations of Hb SC patients also revealed increased lipid determinations including total cholesterol, HDL, and LDL.[733,742]

Treatment

Unlike the extensive investigations of the use of hydroxyurea in adults and children with Hb SS, data in patients with Hb SC disease are sparse, as are studies regarding management in general. The first randomized clinical trial specifically targeting individuals with Hb SC was a phase II multicenter double-blinded trial comparing the effects of hydroxyurea and magnesium (pidolate).[658] Subjects were randomized to hydroxyurea + placebo, magnesium + placebo, hydroxyurea + magnesium, or placebo + placebo. The primary endpoint was the proportion of hyperdense RBCs after 8 weeks of treatment, but the study was terminated early. In the combined hydroxyurea groups, MCV and Hb F were increased, but differences were not seen in hyperdense red cells or vaso-occlusive events. Recently, a retrospective multicenter study has described a cohort of 133 adult and pediatric patients with Hb SC disease who received hydroxyurea.[743] As in previous reports, treatment was associated with a stable Hb level, increased Hb F (but much less than that in SCA patients), increased MCV, and decreased absolute neutrophil and reticulocyte counts, as well as reduced pain events in patients older than 15 years. Elevation of hematocrit from hydroxyurea is a concern related to increased blood viscosity. However, none of the 133 patients treated with hydroxyurea required phlebotomy to reduce blood viscosity,[743] and it is unclear if phlebotomy is needed during hydroxyurea therapy in Hb SC patients.

Hemoglobin Sβ-Thalassemia

The doubly heterozygous condition of Hb S and β-thalassemia is designated as Sβ⁰-thalassemia if there is no β-globin synthesis from the affected allele and Sβ⁺-thalassemia if β-globin synthesis is present but reduced. The clinical manifestations are quite variable, and patients may be nearly asymptomatic or have problems similar to those occurring in the worst cases of SCA. In general, Hb Sβ⁰-thalassemia resembles Hb SS in severity (and therefore is often included under the designation "sickle cell anemia"), and Hb Sβ⁺-thalassemia is somewhat milder than Hb SC disease. Patients with Hb Sβ⁰-thalassemia have a slightly higher Hb level, a greater Hb A_2 level (4%-6%), and a smaller MCV (65-75 fL) than those with Hb SS. Hb Sβ⁺-thalassemia patients have a higher Hb level and lower reticulocyte count than those with Hb Sβ⁰-thalassemia. In children with Hb Sβ⁰-thalassemia, splenic dysfunction measured by pit cell counts occurs within the first year of life, but only 20% of those with Hb Sβ⁺-thalassemia have elevated pit counts by 20 years of age. Patients with Hb Sβ⁺-thalassemia, unlike those with SCA, often have splenomegaly beyond the first few years of childhood. However, hydroxyurea has been found to decrease hospitalizations in pediatric patients with Hb Sβ⁺-thalassemia.[744]

Hemoglobin S/Hereditary Persistence of Fetal Hemoglobin

In HPFH, Hb F levels are elevated relative to the patient's age. Deletional mutations typically involve large segments of DNA and result in a pancellular distribution of Hb F. Approximately 1 in 1000 African Americans carry a deletion HPFH gene. Nondeletion mutations result in more variable levels of Hb F (4%-30%) and heterocellular or pancellular distribution. The doubly heterozygous condition for Hb S and HPFH results in a heterogeneous disorder that is generally extremely mild and associated with a pancellular distribution of Hb F, normal blood counts, microcytosis, target cells, and 20% to 30% Hb F.[745,746] Overall, there is <1 case of Hb S/HPFH for every 100 cases of Hb SS, but it is important to identify this condition because of its extremely good prognosis. Hb S/Black (ᴬγδβ)⁰-thalassemia is a very rare sickle cell disease variant previously thought to behave clinically as Hb S/HPFH. Recent data have demonstrated that its clinical course is more similar to that of Hb Sβ⁺-thalassemia, likely because of a less than pancellular distribution of Hb F, despite Hb F levels of >20%.[747]

Hemoglobin SE Disease

Hb E is characterized by the substitution of lysine for glutamic acid at position 26 of the β chain and results in a mild β-thalassemia phenotype. Because of the increase in the Asian population in the United States, the doubly heterozygous condition of Hb SE is now occasionally seen. Patients with Hb SE may have mild anemia and microcytosis along with <30% Hb E, but blood smears look relatively normal (except for target cells), and patients are usually asymptomatic.

Hemoglobin SD Disease

Of the 16 variants fulfilling the electrophoretic and solubility criteria for Hb D or Hb G, at least 9 have been recognized in association with Hb S. With one exception, the doubly heterozygous states for Hb S and Hb D or Hb G are clinically silent. Hb D-Punjab (Hb D-Los Angeles) interacts with Hb S to produce mild to moderate hemolytic anemia and symptoms that mimic those of mild to moderate sickle cell disease. The Hb SD-Punjab syndrome was first detected in a Caucasian man whose case had been previously reported as an instance of SCA in the white race. Subsequently, Hb SD-Punjab disease was recognized in a number of subjects, most of African origin. In each of these subjects, the clinical and hematologic features were those of mild to moderate sickle cell disease. Persisting splenomegaly is more common than in Hb SS. Although in Middle Eastern Kuwaiti sickle cell patients, elevated Hb F level was not protective against pain events in patients with Hb SD,[748] elevation of HbF with hydroxyurea has been shown to be protective in other populations with HbSD.[749]

Hemoglobin SO-Arab Disease

Hb O-Arab interacts strongly with Hb S in vitro. As Hb S fraction forms a higher proportion of the total Hb than Hb O-Arab, as expected the doubly heterozygous state is clinically and hematologically as severe as SCA.[750] Functional asplenia occurs at an early age and is followed by progressive splenic infarction. The disorder is differentiated readily from Hb SC disease, with which it is confused on electrophoretic grounds, by the greater prominence of symptoms, the severity of the anemia, and the presence of numerous ISCs on blood smears.

Hemoglobin C Disorders

In Hb C, lysine replaces glutamic acid in the sixth position of the β-chain. The positive charge resulting from this substitution gives the variant a slow electrophoretic mobility at both an acid and an alkaline pH. This variant appears to have originated on the west coast of Africa, where the carrier rate is as high as 25%. Although less convincing than for Hb S, the distribution of Hb C in Africa suggests that it may also have conferred a survival advantage in areas endemic for malaria. Among the Dogon of West Africa, where the gene frequency of Hb C is high and that of Hb S is low, cerebral malaria and other forms of severe malaria are uncommon in those having Hb C. Although not providing full protection against malaria, Hb C appears to minimize the risk of severe infection. These clinical observations are supported by in vitro studies that demonstrate the inability of Hb CC red cells to release merozoites by cell lysis at the appropriate stage of parasite development.[751] The heterozygous state is noted in 2% to 3% of blacks, and homozygous Hb C disease affects <1 in 5000. As with Hb S, Hb C has been identified in individuals with no known African ancestry. The β^C gene can be identified in fetal DNA by using restriction fragment length polymorphisms and by sequence-specific oligonucleotide probes.

Hemoglobin C Trait

The heterozygous state for Hb C (Hb AC) is clinically silent. Although the Hb concentration is within the broad range of normal, the mean for groups of subjects is low. The red cell mass and red cell survival may also be decreased. Reticulocyte numbers, however, are not increased. The physiologic basis for the apparent failure of appropriate erythropoietic response to shortened cell survival is probably similar to that operative in Hb CC disease. The peripheral blood smear contains moderate numbers (5%-30%) of target cells. By electrophoretic analysis, 30% to 40% of the Hb is Hb C, and 50% to 60% is Hb A; Hb A_2 (separated chromatographically) is increased slightly. The relative amount of Hb C with coexistent α-thalassemia is less, reflecting the higher affinity of β^A-compared with β^C-globin for limited amounts of α-globin during Hb assembly.

Hemoglobin C Disease

Hemoglobin C disease (Hb CC) is a mild disorder that is characteristically detected through newborn hemoglobinopathy screening programs or during the investigation of an unrelated medical problem. Growth and development are appropriate, and pregnancy and surgery are well tolerated. Mild intermittent abdominal discomfort, arthralgia, and headaches are noted in some reports, but their relationship to the hemoglobinopathy, if any, is unclear. The spleen is enlarged in many affected individuals, and spontaneous rupture of the organ has been reported. Spleen function is unaffected, however, and unusual infectious problems are not observed. As with other hemolytic disorders, cholelithiasis occurs with increased frequency.

Anemia is mild to moderate in severity.[752] The mean packed cell volume is 33%; individual values often fall within the normal range. Reticulocyte counts are elevated only slightly (2%-6%). Erythrocyte morphology is strikingly abnormal, with microcytosis, target cells (≥90%), occasional spherocytes, and cells distorted by what appear to be crystals of Hb. Target cells appear more plump and smaller in diameter than those seen in individuals with liver disease, although their resistance to osmotic lysis is similar to that of other target cells. RBC survival is shortened with evidence of splenic sequestration. Considering the relative indolence of the hemolytic process, it is surprising that anemia is not fully compensated by a greater erythropoietic effort. This apparent inconsistency is explained by a decrease in the oxygen affinity of Hb of Hb CC erythrocytes, which have an intracellular pH lower than that of normal cells. The right-shifted oxygen dissociation curve of whole blood permits normal tissue oxygenation despite a smaller than normal RBC mass. Shortened red cell survival is probably related to the decreased solubility of deoxy Hb C, a consequence of electrostatic interactions between positively charged β-6 amino groups and negatively charged groups on adjacent molecules. When suspended in hypertonic medium, Hb CC cells form intracellular crystals, a process that begins along the membrane and is enhanced by deoxygenation. Intracellular aggregates of Hb limit cell deformability by increasing internal viscosity, thereby predisposing to fragmentation, spherocyte formation, and splenic sequestration. Diagnosis rests on the electrophoretic or chromatographic analysis of Hb. The major fraction is Hb C, Hb A is absent, and Hb F is slightly increased. Therapy is neither available nor needed; however, genetic counseling and clinical monitoring are advised.

KEY POINTS

1. Sickle cell disease is a common worldwide genetic disorder with an autosomal recessive pattern.
2. Sickle cell disease is a chronic condition with intermittent and unpredictable acute vaso-occlusive episodes (e.g., pain, ACS, splenic sequestration, priapism).
3. The most common and also the most severe genotype is Hb SS. Hb Sβ⁰-thalassemia is frequently classified with Hb SS because of its similar phenotype. Together they are called SCA.
4. Pathophysiology involves a complex intertwined array of processes including vaso-occlusion in the microcirculation, hypoxia-reperfusion injury, chronic hemolysis, increased endothelial adhesion, hypercoagulability, and enhanced inflammatory response.
5. All tissues can be affected, causing progressive organ dysfunction and eventually organ failure.
6. The overall survival in sickle cell disease has improved in the last few decades because of early diagnosis, prophylaxis against infection, and use of disease-modifying therapies.
7. Effective therapies include hydroxyurea, chronic blood transfusion, and stem cell transplantation.
8. New therapies are being successfully translated to clinical trials and clinical use, targeting the genetic lesion (e.g., gene therapy and gene editing), sickling (e.g., Hb O_2 affinity modulators and PK activators), or the downstream effects of sickling (e.g., anti-inflammatories and antioxidants).

Websites of Interest

The following websites offer useful information about sickle cell disease, both for patients and for medical providers:

- www.NHLBI.nhi.gov
- www.CDC.gov
- www.SCDAA.org

The website http://www.clinicaltrials.gov offers information about prospective clinical trials. Using the search option, trials investigating sickle cell disease can be retrieved.

References

1. Piel FB, Hay SI, Gupta S, Weatherall DJ, Williams TN. Global burden of sickle cell anaemia in children under five, 2010-2050: modelling based on demographics, excess mortality, and interventions. *PLoS Med.* 2013;10(7):e1001484. doi:10.1371/journal.pmed.1001484
2. Konotey-Ahulu FI. The sickle cell diseases. Clinical manifestations including the "sickle crisis." *Arch Intern Med.* 1974;133(4):611-619.
3. Herrick JB. Peculiar elongated and sickle-shaped red blood corpuscles in a case of severe anemia. 1910. *Yale JBiolMed.* 2001;74(3):179-184.
4. Mason V. Sickle cell anemia. *J Am Med Assoc.* 1922;79:1318-1320.
5. Piel FB. The present and future global burden of the inherited disorders of hemoglobin. *Hematol Oncol Clin North Am.* 2016;30(2):327-341. doi:10.1016/j.hoc.2015.11.004
6. Pagnier J, Mears JG, Dunda-Belkhodja O, et al. Evidence for the multicentric origin of the sickle cell hemoglobin gene in Africa. *Proc Natl Acad Sci U S A.* 1984;81(6):1771-1773.
7. Serjeant GR. The geography of sickle cell disease: opportunities for understanding its diversity. *Ann Saudi Med.* 1994;1994(14):237-246.

Disorders of Red Blood Cells

8. Antonarakis SE, Boehm CD, Serjeant GR, Theisen CE, Dover GJ, Kazazian HH Jr. Origin of the beta S-globin gene in blacks: the contribution of recurrent mutation or gene conversion or both. *Proc Natl Acad Sci U S A.* 1984;81(3):853-856.

9. Mears JG, Beldjord C, Benabadji M, et al. The sickle gene polymorphism in North Africa. *Blood.* 1981;58(3):599-601.

10. de Montalembert M, Voskaridou E, Oevermann L, et al. Real-life experience with hydroxyurea in patients with sickle cell disease: results from the prospective ESCORT-HU cohort study. *Am J Hematol.* 2021;96(10):1223-1231. doi:10.1002/ajh.26286

11. Estepp JH, Melloni C, Thornburg CD, et al. Pharmacokinetics and bioequivalence of a liquid formulation of hydroxyurea in children with sickle cell anemia. *J Clin Pharmacol.* 2016;56(3):298-306. doi:10.1002/jcph.598

12. Yan JH, Ataga K, Kaul S, et al. The influence of renal function on hydroxyurea pharmacokinetics in adults with sickle cell disease. *J Clin Pharmacol.* 2005;45(4):434-445.

13. Little JA, McGowan VR, Kato GJ, et al. Combination erythropoietin-hydroxyurea therapy in sickle cell disease: experience from the National Institutes of Health and a Literature Review. *Haematologica.* 2006;91(8):1076-1083.

14. McGann PT, Flanagan JM, Howard TA, et al. Genotoxicity associated with hydroxyurea exposure in infants with sickle cell anemia: results from the BABY-HUG Phase III Clinical Trial. *Pediatr Blood Cancer.* 2012;59(2):254-257. doi:10.1002/pbc.23365

15. Maluf S, Pra D, Friedrisch JR, et al. Length of treatment and dose as determinants of mutagenicity in sickle cell disease patients treated with hydroxyurea. *Environ Toxicol Pharmacol.* 2009;27(1):26-29. doi:10.1016/j.etap.2008.04.004

16. Berthaut I, Bachir D, Kotti S, et al. Adverse effect of hydroxyurea on spermatogenesis in patients with sickle cell anemia after 6 months of treatment. *Blood.* 2017;130(21):2354-2356. doi:10.1182/blood-2017-03-771857

17. Joseph L, Jean C, Manceau S, et al. Effect of hydroxyurea exposure before puberty on sperm parameters in males with sickle cell disease. *Blood.* 2021;137(6):826-829. doi:10.1182/blood.2020006270

18. DeSimone J, Koshy M, Dorn L, et al. Maintenance of elevated fetal hemoglobin levels by decitabine during dose interval treatment of sickle cell anemia. *Blood.* 2002;99(11):3905-3908.

19. Saunthararajah Y, Hillery CA, Lavelle D, et al. Effects of 5-aza-2'-deoxycytidine on fetal hemoglobin levels, red cell adhesion, and hematopoietic differentiation in patients with sickle cell disease. *Blood.* 2003;102(12):3865-3870. doi:10.1182/blood-2003-05-1738

20. Hsieh M. *Decitabine for High-Risk Sickle Cell Disease.* 2011. ClinicalTrials.gov Identifier: NCT01375608. https://clinicaltrials.gov/ct2/show/NCT01375608?term=NCT01375608&draw=1&rank=1

21. McArthur JG, Svenstrup N, Chen C, et al. A novel, highly potent and selective phosphodiesterase-9 inhibitor for the treatment of sickle cell disease. *Haematologica.* 2020;105(3):623-631. doi:10.3324/haematol.2018.213462

22. Attie K. *A Study of IMR-687 in Subjects With Sickle Cell Disease.* 2020. ClinicalTrials.gov Identifier: NCT04474314. https://clinicaltrials.gov/ct2/show/NCT04474314?term=NCT04474314&draw=2&rank=1

23. Mant T. *A Study of IMR-687 in Adult Patients with Sickle Cell Anaemia (Homozygous HbSS or Sickle-B0 Thalassemia).* 2018. ClinicalTrials.gov Identifier: NCT03401112. https://clinicaltrials.gov/ct2/show/NCT03401112?term=NCT03401112&draw=2&rank=1

24. Sankaran VG, Xu J, Ragoczy T, et al. Developmental and species-divergent globin switching are driven by BCL11A. *Nature.* 2009;460(7259):1093-1097. doi:10.1038/nature08243

25. Sankaran VG, Menne TF, Xu J, et al. Human fetal hemoglobin expression is regulated by the developmental stage-specific repressor BCL11A. *Science.* 2008;322(5909):1839-1842. doi:10.1126/science.1165409

26. Sankaran VG, Nathan DG. Reversing the hemoglobin switch. *N Engl J Med.* 2010;363(23):2258-2260. doi:10.1056/NEJMcibr1010767

27. Doerfler PA, Sharma A, Porter JS, Zheng Y, Tisdale JF, Weiss MJ. Genetic therapies for the first molecular disease. *J Clin Invest.* 2021;131(8). doi:10.1172/JCI146394

28. Metcalf B, Chuang C, Dufu K, et al. Discovery of GBT440, an orally bioavailable R-state stabilizer of sickle cell hemoglobin. *ACS Med Chem Lett.* 2017;8(3):321-326. doi:10.1021/acsmedchemlett.6b00491

29. Oksenberg D, Dufu K, Patel MP, et al. GBT440 increases haemoglobin oxygen affinity, reduces sickling and prolongs RBC half-life in a murine model of sickle cell disease. *Br J Haematol.* 2016;175(1):141-153. doi:10.1111/bjh.14214

30. Vichinsky E, Hoppe CC, Ataga KI, et al. A phase 3 randomized trial of voxelotor in sickle cell disease. *N Engl J Med.* 2019;381(6):509-519. doi:10.1056/NEJMoa1903212

31. Grace RF, Rose C, Layton DM, et al. Safety and efficacy of mitapivat in pyruvate kinase deficiency. *N Engl J Med.* 2019;381(10):933-944. doi:10.1056/NEJMoa1902678

32. Thein SL. *Safety, Tolerability, Pharmacokinetics, and Pharmacodynamics of Long-Term Mitapivat Dosing in Subjects with Stable Sickle Cell Disease: An Extension of a Phase 1 Pilot Study of Mitapivat.* 2020. ClinicalTrials.gov Identifier: NCT04610866. https://clinicaltrials.gov/ct2/show/NCT04610866?term=NCT04610866&draw=2&rank=1

33. Agios Pharmaceuticals, Inc. *A Study Evaluating the Efficacy and Safety of Mitapivat (AG-348) in Participants with Sickle Cell Disease.* 2021. ClinicalTrials.gov Identifier: NCT05031780. https://clinicaltrials.gov/ct2/show/NCT05031780?term=NCT05031780&draw=2&rank=1

34. Kelly P. *A Study of FT-4202 in Patients with Thalassemia or Sickle Cell Disease.* 2021. ClinicalTrials.gov Identifier: NCT04987489. https://clinicaltrials.gov/ct2/show/NCT04987489?term=NCT04987489&draw=2&rank=1

35. Black V. *A Study of Etavopivat in Adults and Adolescents with Sickle Cell Disease (HIBISCUS).* 2020. ClinicalTrials.gov Identifier: NCT04624659. https://clinicaltrials.gov/ct2/show/NCT04624659?term=NCT04624659&draw=2&rank=1

36. Ataga KI, Smith WR, De Castro LM, et al. Efficacy and safety of the Gardos channel blocker, senicapoc (ICA-17043), in patients with sickle cell anemia. *Blood.* 2008;111(8):3991-3997. doi:10.1182/blood-2007-08-110098

37. Smeltzer MP, Nolan VG, Yu X, et al. Birth prevalence of sickle cell trait and sickle cell disease in shelby county, TN. *Pediatr Blood Cancer.* 2016;63(6):1054-1059. doi:10.1002/pbc.25936

38. Prevention CfDCa. *The Registry and Surveillance System for Hemoglobinopathies (New York).* Accessed April 14, 2014. http://www.cdc.gov/ncbddd/sicklecell/documents/scd_in_ny_prov.pdf

39. Hassell KL. Population estimates of sickle cell disease in the U.S. *Am J Prev Med.* 2010;38(4 suppl):S512-S521. doi:10.1016/j.amepre.2009.12.022

40. Rees DC, Williams TN, Gladwin MT. Sickle-cell disease. *Lancet.* 2010;376(9757):2018-2031. doi:10.1016/s0140-6736(10)61029-x

41. Piel FB, Patil AP, Howes RE, et al. Global distribution of the sickle cell gene and geographical confirmation of the malaria hypothesis. *Nat Commun.* 2010;1:104. doi:10.1038/ncomms1104

42. Schechter AN, Noguchi CT. Sickle hemoglobin polymer: structure-function correlates. In: Embury SH, Hebbel RP, Mohandas N, Steinberg MH, eds. *Sickle Cell Disease: Basic Principles and Clinical Practice.* Raven Press; 1994:33-51.

43. Franco RS, Yasin Z, Palascak MB, Ciraolo P, Joiner CH, Rucknagel DL. The effect of fetal hemoglobin on the survival characteristics of sickle cells. *Blood.* 2006;108(3):1073-1076. doi:10.1182/blood-2005-09-008318

44. Bunn HF. The triumph of good over evil: protection by the sickle gene against malaria. *Blood.* 2013;121(1):20-25. doi:10.1182/blood-2012-08-449397

45. Eaton WA, Bunn HF. Treating sickle cell disease by targeting HbS polymerization. *Blood.* 2017;129(20):2719-2726. doi:10.1182/blood-2017-02-765891

46. Eaton WA, Henry ER, Hofrichter J, Mozzarelli A. Is cooperative oxygen binding by hemoglobin really understood? *Nat Struct Biol.* 1999;6(4):351-358. doi:10.1038/7586

47. Hofrichter J, Ross PD, Eaton WA. Kinetics and mechanism of deoxyhemoglobin S gelation: a new approach to understanding sickle cell disease. *Proc Natl Acad Sci U S A.* 1974;71(12):4864-4868. doi:10.1073/pnas.71.12.4864

48. Ware RE, de Montalembert M, Tshilolo L, Abboud MR. Sickle cell disease. *Lancet.* 2017;390(10091):311-323. doi:10.1016/S0140-6736(17)30193-9

49. Steinberg MH, Chui DH, Dover GJ, Sebastiani P, Alsultan A. Fetal hemoglobin in sickle cell anemia: a glass half full? *Blood.* 2014;123(4):481-485. doi:10.1182/blood-2013-09-528067

50. Zhang Y, Dai Y, Wen J, et al. Detrimental effects of adenosine signaling in sickle cell disease. *Nat Med.* 2011;17(1):79-86. doi:10.1038/nm.2280

51. Uzunova VV, Pan W, Galkin O, Vekilov PG. Free heme and the polymerization of sickle cell hemoglobin. *Biophys J.* 2010;99(6):1976-1985. doi:10.1016/j.bpj.2010.07.024

52. Smith CM, Krivit W, White JG. The irreversibly sickled cell. *Am J Pediatr Hematol Oncol.* 1982;4(3):307-315.

53. Kuypers FA, Yee M, Vichinsky E, Lubin BH. Activation of the prothrombinase complex in sickle cell anemia. *Blood.* 1992;80:75.

54. Brugnara C. Therapeutic strategies for prevention of sickle cell dehydration. *Blood Cells Mol Dis.* 2001;27(1):71-80.

55. Stocker JW, De Franceschi L, McNaughton-Smith G, et al. A novel Gardos channel inhibitor, ICA-17043, prevents red blood cell dehydration in vitro and in a mouse model (SAD) of sickle cell disease. *Blood.* 2000;96:486a.

56. Bennekou P, De Franceschi L, Pedersen O, et al. Treatment with NS3623, a novel Cl-conductance blocker, ameliorates erythrocyte dehydration in transgenic SAD mice: a possible new therapeutic approach for sickle cell disease. *Blood.* 2001;97(5):1451-1457.

57. Joiner CH, Jiang M, Claussen WJ, Roszell NJ, Yasin Z, Franco RS. Dipyridamole inhibits sickling-induced cation fluxes in sickle red blood cells. *Blood.* 2001;97(12):3976-3983.

58. Hebbel RP, Yamada O, Moldow CF, Jacob HS, White JG, Eaton JW. Abnormal adherence of sickle erythrocytes to cultured vascular endothelium: possible mechanism for microvascular occlusion in sickle cell disease. *J Clin Invest.* 1980;65(1):154-160.

59. Ballas SK, Larner J, Smith ED, Surrey S, Schwartz E, Rappaport EF. Rheologic predictors of the severity of the painful sickle cell crisis. *Blood.* 1988;72(4):1216-1223.

60. Barabino GA, McIntire LV, Eskin SG, Sears DA, Udden M. Endothelial cell interactions with sickle cell, sickle trait, mechanically injured, and normal erythrocytes under controlled flow. *Blood.* 1987;70(1):152-157.

61. Maciaszek JL, Andemariam B, Abiraman K, Lykotrafitis G. AKAP-dependent modulation of BCAM/Lu adhesion on normal and sickle cell disease RBCs revealed by force nanoscopy. *Biophys J.* 2014;106(6):1258-1267. doi:10.1016/j.bpj.2014.02.001

62. Matsui NM, Borsig L, Rosen SD, Yaghmai M, Varki A, Embury SH. P-selectin mediates the adhesion of sickle erythrocytes to the endothelium. *Blood.* 2001;98(6):1955-1962.

63. Hebbel RP. Blockade of adhesion of sickle cells to endothelium by monoclonal antibodies. *N Engl J Med.* 2000;342(25):1910-1912. doi:10.1056/NEJM200006223422512

64. Sugihara K, Sugihara T, Mohandas N, Hebbel RP. Thrombospondin mediates adherence of CD36+ sickle reticulocytes to endothelial cells. *Blood.* 1992;80(10):2634-2642.

65. Zhou Z, Thiagarajan P, Udden M, Lopez JA, Guchhait P. Erythrocyte membrane sulfatide plays a crucial role in the adhesion of sickle erythrocytes to endothelium. *Thromb Haemost.* 2011;105(6):1046-1052. doi:10.1160/TH10-11-0716

66. Solovey A, Lin Y, Browne P, Choong S, Wayner E, Hebbel RP. Circulating activated endothelial cells in sickle cell anemia. *N Engl J Med.* 1997;337(22):1584-1590.

67. Evans EA, Mohandas N. Membrane-associated sickle hemoglobin: a major determinant of sickle erythrocyte rigidity. *Blood.* 1987;70(5):1443-1449.

68. Miller DM, Winslow RM, Klein HG, Wilson KC, Brown FL, Statham NJ. Improved exercise performance after exchange transfusion in subjects with sickle cell anemia. *Blood.* 1980;56(6):1127-1131.

69. Test ST, Kleman K, Lubin B. Characterization of the complement sensitivity of density-fractionated sickle cells. *Blood.* 1991;(78 suppl):202a.

70. Mock DM, Matthews NI, Zhu S, et al. Red blood cell (RBC) survival determined in humans using RBCs labeled at multiple biotin densities. *Transfusion.* 2011;51(5):1047-1057. doi:10.1111/j.1537-2995.2010.02926.x

71. Morris CR, Kato GJ, Poljakovic M, et al. Dysregulated arginine metabolism, hemolysis-associated pulmonary hypertension, and mortality in sickle cell disease. *J Am Med Assoc.* 2005;294(1):81-90.

72. Schnog JB, Teerlink T, van der Dijs FP, Duits AJ, Muskiet FA, Group CS. Plasma levels of asymmetric dimethylarginine (ADMA), an endogenous nitric oxide synthase inhibitor, are elevated in sickle cell disease. *Ann Hematol.* 2005;84(5):282-286. doi:10.1007/s00277-004-0983-3

73. Kato GJ, Gladwin MT, Steinberg MH. Deconstructing sickle cell disease: reappraisal of the role of hemolysis in the development of clinical subphenotypes. *Blood Rev.* 2007;21(1):37-47. doi:10.1016/j.blre.2006.07.001

74. Nath KA, Katusic ZS. Vasculature and kidney complications in sickle cell disease. *J Am Soc Nephrol.* 2012;23(5):781-784. doi:10.1681/ASN.2011101019

75. Zhang D, Xu C, Manwani D, Frenette PS. Neutrophils, platelets, and inflammatory pathways at the nexus of sickle cell disease pathophysiology. *Blood.* 2016;127(7):801-809. doi:10.1182/blood-2015-09-618538

76. Radomski MW, Palmer RM, Moncada S. Endogenous nitric oxide inhibits human platelet adhesion to vascular endothelium. *Lancet.* 1987;2(8567):1057-1058.

77. Kaul DK, Hebbel RP. Hypoxia/reoxygenation causes inflammatory response in transgenic sickle mice but not in normal mice. *J Clin Invest.* 2000;106(3):411-420.

78. Eltzschig HK, Carmeliet P. Hypoxia and inflammation. *N Engl J Med.* 2011;364(7):656-665. doi:10.1056/NEJMra0910283

79. Gill FM, Sleeper LA, Weiner SJ, et al. Clinical events in the first decade in a cohort of infants with sickle cell disease. Cooperative Study of Sickle Cell Disease. *Blood.* 1995;86(2):776-783.

80. Powars DR. Natural history of sickle cell disease–the first ten years. *Semin Hematol.* 1975;12(3):267-285.

81. Platt OS, Brambilla DJ, Rosse WF, et al. Mortality in sickle cell disease. Life expectancy and risk factors for early death. *N Engl J Med.* 1994;330(23):1639-1644. doi:10.1056/NEJM199406093302303

82. Powars DR, Chan LS, Hiti A, Ramicone E, Johnson C. Outcome of sickle cell anemia: a 4-decade observational study of 1056 patients. *Medicine (Baltimore).* 2005;84(6):363-376. doi:10.1097/01.md.0000189089.45003.52

83. Quinn CT, Rogers ZR, McCavit TL, Buchanan GR. Improved survival of children and adolescents with sickle cell disease. *Blood.* 2010;115(17):3447-3452. doi:10.1182/blood-2009-07-233700

84. Le PQ, Gulbis B, Dedeken L, et al. Survival among children and adults with sickle cell disease in Belgium: benefit from hydroxyurea treatment. *Pediatr Blood Cancer.* 2015;62(11):1956-1961. doi:10.1002/pbc.25608

85. Hankins JS, Estepp JH, Hodges JR, et al. Sickle Cell Clinical Research and Intervention Program (SCCRIP): a lifespan cohort study for sickle cell disease progression from the pediatric stage into adulthood. *Pediatr Blood Cancer.* 2018;65(9):e27228. doi:10.1002/pbc.27228

86. Stevens MC, Padwick M, Serjeant GR. Observations on the natural history of dactylitis in homozygous sickle cell disease. *Clin Pediatr (Phila).* 1981;20(5):311-317.

87. Platt OS, Thorington BD, Brambilla DJ, et al. Pain in sickle cell disease. Rates and risk factors. *N Engl J Med.* 1991;325(1):11-16. doi:10.1056/NEJM199107043250103

88. Mankad VN, Williams JP, Harpen MD, et al. Magnetic resonance imaging of bone marrow in sickle cell disease: clinical, hematologic, and pathologic correlations. *Blood.* 1990;75(1):274-283.

89. Boogaard S, De Vet HC, Faber CG, Zuurmond WW, Perez RS. An overview of predictors for persistent neuropathic pain. *Expert Rev Neurother.* 2013;13(5):505-513. doi:10.1586/ern.13.44

90. Dampier C, Palermo TM, Darbari DS, Hassell K, Smith W, Zempsky W. AAPT diagnostic criteria for chronic sickle cell disease pain. *J Pain.* 2017;18(5):490-498. doi:10.1016/j.jpain.2016.12.016

91. Dampier C, Ely E, Brodecki D, O'Neal P. Home management of pain in sickle cell disease: a daily diary study in children and adolescents. *J Pediatr Hematol Oncol.* 2002;24(8):643-647. doi:10.1097/00043426-200211000-00008

92. Kent ML, Tighe PJ, Belfer I, et al. The ACTTION-APS-AAPM pain taxonomy (AAAPT) multidimensional approach to classifying acute pain conditions. *J Pain.* 2017;18(5):479-489. doi:10.1016/j.jpain.2017.02.421

93. Sharma D, Brandow AM. Neuropathic pain in individuals with sickle cell disease. *Neurosci Lett.* 2020;714:134445. doi:10.1016/j.neulet.2019.134445

94. Brandow AM, Farley RA, Panepinto JA. Neuropathic pain in patients with sickle cell disease. *Pediatr Blood Cancer.* 2014;61(3):512-517. doi:10.1002/pbc.24838

95. Carden MA, Fay M, Sakurai Y, et al. Normal saline is associated with increased sickle red cell stiffness and prolonged transit times in a microfluidic model of the capillary system. *Microcirculation.* 2017;24(5):1-5. doi:10.1111/micc.12353

96. Carden MA, Fay ME, Lu X, et al. Extracellular fluid tonicity impacts sickle red blood cell deformability and adhesion. *Blood.* 2017;130(24):2654-2663. doi:10.1182/blood-2017-04-780635

97. Carden MA, Patil P, Ahmad ME, Lam WA, Joiner CH, Morris CR. Variations in pediatric emergency medicine physician practices for intravenous fluid management in children with sickle cell disease and vaso-occlusive pain: a single institution experience. *Pediatr Blood Cancer.* 2018;65(1). doi:10.1002/pbc.26742

98. Rosa RM, Bierer BE, Thomas R, et al. A study of induced hyponatremia in the prevention and treatment of sickle-cell crisis. *N Engl J Med.* 1980;303(20):1138-1143.

99. Guy RB, Gavrilis PK, Rothenberg SP. In vitro and in vivo effect of hypotonic saline on the sickling phenomenon. *Am J Med Sci.* 1973;266(4):267-277. doi:10.1097/00000441-197310000-00005

100. Okomo U, Meremikwu MM. Fluid replacement therapy for acute episodes of pain in people with sickle cell disease. *Cochrane Database Syst Rev.* 2017;7:CD005406. doi:10.1002/14651858.CD005406.pub5

101. Brandow AM, Carroll CP, Creary S, et al. American Society of Hematology 2020 guidelines for sickle cell disease: management of acute and chronic pain. *Blood Adv.* 2020;4(12):2656-2701. doi:10.1182/bloodadvances.2020001851

102. Embury SH, Garcia JF, Mohandas N, Pennathur-Das R, Clark MR. Effects of oxygen inhalation on endogenous erythropoietin kinetics, erythropoiesis, and properties of blood cells in sickle-cell anemia. *N Engl J Med.* 1984;311(5):291-295.

103. Ballas SK. Update on pain management in sickle cell disease. *Hemoglobin.* 2011;35(5-6):520-529. doi:10.3109/03630269.2011.610478

104. Yawn BP, John-Sowah J. Management of sickle cell disease: recommendations from the 2014 expert panel report. *Am Fam Physician.* 2015;92(12):1069-1076.

105. Schefft MR, Swaffar C, Newlin J, Noda C, Sisler I. A novel approach to reducing admissions for children with sickle cell disease in pain crisis through individualization and standardization in the emergency department. *Pediatr Blood Cancer.* 2018;65(10):e27274. doi:10.1002/pbc.27274

106. Mager A, Pelot K, Koch K, et al. Opioid management strategy decreases admissions in high-utilizing adults with sickle cell disease. *J Opioid Manag.* 2017;13(3):143-156. doi:10.5055/jom.2017.0382

107. Krishnamurti L, Smith-Packard B, Gupta A, Campbell M, Gunawardena S, Saladino R. Impact of individualized pain plan on the emergency management of children with sickle cell disease. *Pediatr Blood Cancer.* 2014;61(10):1747-1753. doi:10.1002/pbc.25024

108. Kirchheiner J, Schmidt H, Tzvetkov M, et al. Pharmacokinetics of codeine and its metabolite morphine in ultra-rapid metabolizers due to CYP2D6 duplication. *Pharmacogenomics J.* 2007;7(4):257-265. doi:10.1038/sj.tpj.6500406

109. Gammal RS, Crews KR, Haidar CE, et al. Pharmacogenetics for safe codeine use in sickle cell disease. *Pediatrics.* 2016;138(1). doi:10.1542/peds.2015-3479

110. Tawfic QA, Faris AS, Kausalya R. The role of a low-dose ketamine-midazolam regimen in the management of severe painful crisis in patients with sickle cell disease. *J Pain Symptom Manage.* 2014;47(2):334-340. doi:10.1016/j.jpainsymman.2013.03.012

111. Hagedorn JM, Monico EC. Ketamine infusion for pain control in acute pediatric sickle cell painful crises. *Pediatr Emerg Care.* 2019;35(1):78-79. doi:10.1097/PEC.0000000000000978

112. Puri L, Morgan KJ, Anghelescu DL. Ketamine and lidocaine infusions decrease opioid consumption during vaso-occlusive crisis in adolescents with sickle cell disease. *Curr Opin Support Palliat Care.* 2019;13(4):402-407. doi:10.1097/SPC.0000000000000437

113. Lubega FA, DeSilva MS, Munube D, et al. Low dose ketamine versus morphine for acute severe vaso occlusive pain in children: a randomized controlled trial. *Scand J Pain.* 2018;18(1):19-27. doi:10.1515/sjpain-2017-0140

114. Schlaeger JM, Molokie RE, Yao Y, et al. Management of sickle cell pain using pregabalin: a pilot study. *Pain Manag Nurs.* 2017;18(6):391-400. doi:10.1016/j.pmn.2017.07.003

115. Correia CR, Soares AT, Azurara L, Palare MJ. Use of gabapentin in the treatment of chronic pain in an adolescent with sickle cell disease. *BMJ Case Rep.* 2017;2017:bcr2016218614. doi:10.1136/bcr-2016-218614

116. Zeltzer L, Dash J, Holland JP. Hypnotically induced pain control in sickle cell anemia. *Pediatrics.* 1979;64(4):533-536.

117. Ohene-Frempong K, Weiner SJ, Sleeper LA, et al. Cerebrovascular accidents in sickle cell disease: rates and risk factors. *Blood.* 1998;91(1):288-294.

118. Powars D, Wilson B, Imbus C, Pegelow C, Allen J. The natural history of stroke in sickle cell disease. *Am J Med.* 1978;65(3):461-471.

119. Kirkham FJ, Hewes DK, Prengler M, Wade A, Lane R, Evans JP. Nocturnal hypoxaemia and central-nervous-system events in sickle-cell disease. *Lancet.* 2001;357(9269):1656-1659.

120. Quinn CT, Sargent JW. Daytime steady-state haemoglobin desaturation is a risk factor for overt stroke in children with sickle cell anaemia. *Br J Haematol.* 2008;140(3):336-339. doi:10.1111/j.1365-2141.2007.06927.x

121. Dowling MM, Quinn CT, Plumb P, et al. Acute silent cerebral ischemia and infarction during acute anemia in children with and without sickle cell disease. *Blood.* 2012;120(19):3891-3897. doi:10.1182/blood-2012-01-406314

122. Pegelow CH, Macklin EA, Moser FG, et al. Longitudinal changes in brain magnetic resonance imaging findings in children with sickle cell disease. *Blood.* 2002;99(8):3014-3018.

123. Miller ST, Macklin EA, Pegelow CH, et al. Silent infarction as a risk factor for overt stroke in children with sickle cell anemia: a report from the Cooperative Study of Sickle Cell Disease. *J Pediatr.* 2001;139(3):385-390. doi:10.1067/mpd.2001.117580

124. Serjeant G. Blood transfusion in sickle cell disease: a cautionary tale. *Lancet.* 2003;361(9369):1659-1660. doi:10.1016/S0140-6736(03)13293-X

125. Rackoff WR, Ohene-Frempong K, Month S, Scott JP, Neahring B, Cohen AR. Neurologic events after partial exchange transfusion for priapism in sickle cell disease. *J Pediatr.* 1992;120(6):882-885.

126. Powars DR, Schroeder WA, Weiss JN, Chan LS, Azen SP. Lack of influence of fetal hemoglobin levels or erythrocyte indices on the severity of sickle cell anemia. *J Clin Invest.* 1980;65(3):732-740.

127. Russell MO, Goldberg HI, Hodson A, et al. Effect of transfusion therapy on arteriographic abnormalities and on recurrence of stroke in sickle cell disease. *Blood.* 1984;63(1):162-169.

128. Nur E, Kim YS, Truijen J, et al. Cerebrovascular reserve capacity is impaired in patients with sickle cell disease. *Blood.* 2009;114(16):3473-3478. doi:10.1182/blood-2009-05-223859
129. Birkeland P, Gardner K, Kesse-Adu R, et al. Intracranial aneurysms in sickle-cell disease are associated with the hemoglobin SS genotype but not with moyamoya syndrome. *Stroke.* 2016;47(7):1710-1713. doi:10.1161/STROKEAHA.116.012664
130. Dmytriw AA, Martinez JL, Marotta T, Montanera W, Cusimano M, Bharatha A. Use of a flow-diverting stent for ruptured dissecting aneurysm treatment in a patient with sickle cell disease. *Interv Neuroradiol.* 2016;22(2):143-147. doi:10.1177/1591019915617323
131. Prohovnik I, Pavlakis SG, Piomelli S, et al. Cerebral hyperemia, stroke, and transfusion in sickle cell disease. *Neurology.* 1989;39(3):344-348.
132. Adams R, McKie V, Nichols F, et al. The use of transcranial ultrasonography to predict stroke in sickle cell disease. *N Engl J Med.* 1992;326(9):605-610.
133. Adams RJ, Nichols FT III, Aaslid R, et al. Cerebral vessel stenosis in sickle cell disease: criteria for detection by transcranial Doppler. *Am J Pediatr Hematol Oncol.* 1990;12(3):277-282.
134. Quinn CT, Variste J, Dowling MM. Haemoglobin oxygen saturation is a determinant of cerebral artery blood flow velocity in children with sickle cell anaemia. *Br J Haematol.* 2009;145(4):500-505. doi:10.1111/j.1365-2141.2009.07652.x
135. Bernaudin F, Verlhac S, Chevret S, et al. G6PD deficiency, absence of alpha-thalassemia, and hemolytic rate at baseline are significant independent risk factors for abnormally high cerebral velocities in patients with sickle cell anemia. *Blood.* 2008;112(10):4314-4317. doi:10.1182/blood-2008-03-143891
136. Gevers S, Nederveen AJ, Fijnvandraat K, et al. Arterial spin labeling measurement of cerebral perfusion in children with sickle cell disease. *J Magn Reson Imaging.* 2012;35(4):779-787. doi:10.1002/jmri.23505
137. Jordan LC, Gindville MC, Scott AO, et al. Non-invasive imaging of oxygen extraction fraction in adults with sickle cell anaemia. *Brain.* 2016;139(pt 3):738-750. doi:10.1093/brain/awv397
138. Fields ME, Guilliams KP, Ragan DK, et al. Regional oxygen extraction predicts border zone vulnerability to stroke in sickle cell disease. *Neurology.* 2018;90(13):e1134-e1142. doi:10.1212/WNL.0000000000005194
139. Joly P, Garnier N, Kebaili K, et al. G6PD deficiency and absence of alpha-thalassemia increase the risk for cerebral vasculopathy in children with sickle cell anemia. *Eur J Haematol.* 2016;96(4):404-408. doi:10.1111/ejh.12607
140. Belisario AR, Nogueira FL, Rodrigues RS, et al. Association of alpha-thalassemia, TNF-alpha (-308G>A) and VCAM-1 (c.1238G>C) gene polymorphisms with cerebrovascular disease in a newborn cohort of 411 children with sickle cell anemia. *Blood Cells Mol Dis.* 2015;54(1):44-50. doi:10.1016/j.bcmd.2014.08.001
141. Flanagan JM, Sheehan V, Linder H, et al. Genetic mapping and exome sequencing identify 2 mutations associated with stroke protection in pediatric patients with sickle cell anemia. *Blood.* 2013;121(16):3237-3245. doi:10.1182/blood-2012-10-464156
142. Hoppe C, Klitz W, Cheng S, et al. Gene interactions and stroke risk in children with sickle cell anemia1. *Blood.* 2004;103(6):2391-2396.
143. Hoppe C, Klitz W, D'Harlingue K, et al. Confirmation of an association between the TNF(-308) promoter polymorphism and stroke risk in children with sickle cell anemia. *Stroke.* 2007;38(8):2241-2246. doi:10.1161/STROKEAHA.107.483115
144. Flanagan JM, Frohlich DM, Howard TA, et al. Genetic predictors for stroke in children with sickle cell anemia. *Blood.* 2011;117(24):6681-6684. doi:10.1182/blood-2011-01-332205
145. Dobson SR, Holden KR, Nietert PJ, et al. Moyamoya syndrome in childhood sickle cell disease: a predictive factor for recurrent cerebrovascular events. *Blood.* 2002;99(9):3144-3150.
146. Hulbert ML, McKinstry RC, Lacey JL, et al. Silent cerebral infarcts occur despite regular blood transfusion therapy after first strokes in children with sickle cell disease. *Blood.* 2011;117(3):772-779. doi:10.1182/blood-2010-01-261123
147. Cohen AR, Martin MB, Silber JH, Kim HC, Ohene-Frempong K, Schwartz E. A modified transfusion program for prevention of stroke in sickle cell disease. *Blood.* 1992;79(7):1657-1661.
148. Miller ST, Jensen D, Rao SP. Less intensive long-term transfusion therapy for sickle cell anemia and cerebrovascular accident. *J Pediatr.* 1992;120(1):54-57.
149. Aygun B, McMurray MA, Schultz WH, et al. Chronic transfusion practice for children with sickle cell anaemia and stroke. *Br J Haematol.* 2009;145(4):524-528. doi:10.1111/j.1365-2141.2009.07630.x
150. Adams RJ, McKie VC, Hsu L, et al. Prevention of a first stroke by transfusions in children with sickle cell anemia and abnormal results on transcranial Doppler ultrasonography. *N Engl J Med.* 1998;339(1):5-11.
151. McCarville MB, Goodin GS, Fortner G, et al. Evaluation of a comprehensive transcranial Doppler screening program for children with sickle cell anemia. *Pediatr Blood Cancer.* 2008;50(4):818-821. doi:10.1002/pbc.21430
152. Valadi N, Silva GS, Bowman LS, et al. Transcranial Doppler ultrasonography in adults with sickle cell disease. *Neurology.* 2006;67(4):572-574. doi:10.1212/01.wnl.0000230150.39429.8e
153. Abboud MR, Yim E, Musallam KM, Adams RJ, Investigators SIS. Discontinuing prophylactic transfusions increases the risk of silent brain infarction in children with sickle cell disease: data from STOP II. *Blood.* 2011;118(4):894-898. doi:10.1182/blood-2010-12-326298
154. Bishop S, Matheus MG, Abboud MR, et al. Effect of chronic transfusion therapy on progression of neurovascular pathology in pediatric patients with sickle cell anemia. *Blood Cells Mol Dis.* 2011;47(2):125-128. doi:10.1016/j.bcmd.2011.06.002
155. Brousse V, Hertz-Pannier L, Consigny Y, et al. Does regular blood transfusion prevent progression of cerebrovascular lesions in children with sickle cell disease?. *Ann Hematol.* 2009;88(8):785-788. doi:10.1007/s00277-008-0670-x
156. Fullerton HJ, Adams RJ, Zhao S, Johnston SC. Declining stroke rates in Californian children with sickle cell disease. *Blood.* 2004;104(2):336-339.
157. Enninful-Eghan H, Moore RH, Ichord R, Smith-Whitley K, Kwiatkowski JL. Transcranial Doppler ultrasonography and prophylactic transfusion program is effective in preventing overt stroke in children with sickle cell disease. *J Pediatr.* 2010;157(3):479-484. doi:10.1016/j.jpeds.2010.03.007
158. Kanter J, Phillips S, Schlenz AM, et al. Transcranial Doppler screening in a current cohort of children with sickle cell anemia: results from the DISPLACE study. *J Pediatr Hematol Oncol.* 2021;43(8):e1062-e1068. doi:10.1097/MPH.0000000000002103
159. Phillips SM, Schlenz AM, Mueller M, Melvin CL, Adams RJ, Kanter J. Identified barriers and facilitators to stroke risk screening in children with sickle cell anemia: results from the DISPLACE consortium. *Implement Sci Commun.* 2021;2(1):87. doi:10.1186/s43058-021-00192-z
160. Adams RJ, Lackland DT, Brown L, et al. Transcranial Doppler re-screening of subjects who participated in STOP and STOP II. *Am J Hematol.* 2016;91(12):1191-1194. doi:10.1002/ajh.24551
161. Kwiatkowski JL, Voeks JH, Kanter J, et al. Ischemic stroke in children and young adults with sickle cell disease in the post-STOP era. *Am J Hematol.* 2019;94(12):1335-1343. doi:10.1002/ajh.25635
162. Ware RE, Helms RW, Investigators SW. Stroke with transfusions changing to hydroxyurea (SWiTCH). *Blood.* 2012;119(17):3925-3932. doi:10.1182/blood-2011-11-392340
163. Hankins JS, McCarville MB, Rankine-Mullings A, et al. Prevention of conversion to abnormal transcranial Doppler with hydroxyurea in sickle cell anemia: a Phase III international randomized clinical trial. *Am J Hematol.* 2015;90(12):1099-1105. doi:10.1002/ajh.24198
164. Ware RE, Davis BR, Schultz WH, et al. Hydroxycarbamide versus chronic transfusion for maintenance of transcranial Doppler flow velocities in children with sickle cell anaemia-TCD With Transfusions Changing to Hydroxyurea (TWiTCH): a multicentre, open-label, phase 3, non-inferiority trial. *Lancet.* 2016;387(10019):661-670. doi:10.1016/S0140-6736(15)01041-7
165. Helton KJ, Adams RJ, Kesler KL, et al. Magnetic resonance imaging/angiography and transcranial Doppler velocities in sickle cell anemia: results from the SWITCH trial. *Blood.* 2014;124(6):891-898.
166. Hall EM, Leonard J, Smith JL, et al. Reduction in overt and silent stroke recurrence rate following cerebral revascularization surgery in children with sickle cell disease and severe cerebral vasculopathy. *Pediatr Blood Cancer.* 2016;63(8):1431-1437. doi:10.1002/pbc.26022
167. Bernaudin F, Dalle JH, Bories D, et al. Long-term event-free survival, chimerism and fertility outcomes in 234 patients with sickle-cell anemia younger than 30 years after myeloablative conditioning and matched-sibling transplantation in France. *Haematologica.* 2020;105(1):91-101. doi:10.3324/haematol.2018.213207
168. Fitzhugh CD, Cordes S, Taylor T, et al. At least 20% donor myeloid chimerism is necessary to reverse the sickle phenotype after allogeneic HSCT. *Blood.* 2017;130(17):1946-1948. doi:10.1182/blood-2017-03-772392
169. Galadanci NA, Umar Abdullahi S, Vance LD, et al. Feasibility trial for primary stroke prevention in children with sickle cell anemia in Nigeria (SPIN trial). *Am J Hematol.* 2017;92(8):780-788. doi:10.1002/ajh.24770
170. Lagunju I, Brown BJ, Oyinlade AO, et al. Annual stroke incidence in Nigerian children with sickle cell disease and elevated TCD velocities treated with hydroxyurea. *Pediatr Blood Cancer.* 2019;66(3):e27252. doi:10.1002/pbc.27252
171. Tshilolo L, Tomlinson G, Williams TN, et al. Hydroxyurea for children with sickle cell anemia in sub-Saharan Africa. *N Engl J Med.* 2019;380(2):121-131. doi:10.1056/NEJMoa1813598
172. Adams RJ, Brambilla DJ, Granger S, et al. Stroke and conversion to high risk in children screened with transcranial Doppler ultrasound during the STOP study. *Blood.* 2004;103(10):3689-3694.
173. Hankins JS, Fortner GL, McCarville MB, et al. The natural history of conditional transcranial Doppler flow velocities in children with sickle cell anaemia. *Br J Haematol.* 2008;142(1):94-99. doi:10.1111/j.1365-2141.2008.07167.x
174. Kwiatkowski JL, Zimmerman RA, Pollock AN, et al. Silent infarcts in young children with sickle cell disease. *Br J Haematol.* 2009;146(3):300-305. doi:10.1111/j.1365-2141.2009.07753.x
175. Bernaudin F, Verlhac S, Arnaud C, et al. Impact of early transcranial Doppler screening and intensive therapy on cerebral vasculopathy outcome in a newborn sickle cell anemia cohort. *Blood.* 2011;117(4):1130-1140, quiz 1436. doi:10.1182/blood-2010-06-293514
176. Kassim AA, Pruthi S, Day M, et al. Silent cerebral infarcts and cerebral aneurysms are prevalent in adults with sickle cell anemia. *Blood.* 2016;127(16):2038-2040. doi:10.1182/blood-2016-01-694562
177. Cancio MI, Helton KJ, Schreiber JE, Smeltzer MP, Kang G, Wang WC. Silent cerebral infarcts in very young children with sickle cell anaemia are associated with a higher risk of stroke. *Br J Haematol.* 2015;171(1):120-129. doi:10.1111/bjh.13525
178. Pegelow CH, Wang W, Granger S, et al. Silent infarcts in children with sickle cell anemia and abnormal cerebral artery velocity. *Arch Neurol.* 2001;58(12):2017-2021.
179. DeBaun MR, Sarnaik SA, Rodeghier MJ, et al. Associated risk factors for silent cerebral infarcts in sickle cell anemia: low baseline hemoglobin, sex, and relative high systolic blood pressure. *Blood.* 2012;119(16):3684-3690. doi:10.1182/blood-2011-05-349621
180. Thangarajh M, Yang G, Fuchs D, et al. Magnetic resonance angiography-defined intracranial vasculopathy is associated with silent cerebral infarcts and glucose-6-phosphate dehydrogenase mutation in children with sickle cell anaemia. *Br J Haematol.* 2012;159(3):352-359. doi:10.1111/bjh.12034
181. Houwing ME, Grohssteiner RL, Dremmen MHG, et al. Silent cerebral infarcts in patients with sickle cell disease: a systematic review and meta-analysis. *BMC Med.* 2020;18(1):393. doi:10.1186/s12916-020-01864-8

182. Choudhury NA, DeBaun MR, Ponisio MR, et al. Intracranial vasculopathy and infarct recurrence in children with sickle cell anaemia, silent cerebral infarcts and normal transcranial Doppler velocities. *Br J Haematol*. 2018;183(2):324-326. doi:10.1111/bjh.14979

183. Ford AL, Ragan DK, Fellah S, et al. Silent infarcts in sickle cell disease occur in the border zone region and are associated with low cerebral blood flow. *Blood*. 2018;132(16):1714-1723. doi:10.1182/blood-2018-04-841247

184. Chai Y, Bush AM, Coloigner J, et al. White matter has impaired resting oxygen delivery in sickle cell patients. *Am J Hematol*. 2019;94(4):467-474. doi:10.1002/ajh.25423

185. Armstrong FD, Thompson RJ Jr, Wang W, et al. Cognitive functioning and brain magnetic resonance imaging in children with sickle cell disease. Neuropsychology Committee of the Cooperative Study of Sickle Cell Disease. *Pediatrics*. 1996;97(6 pt 1):864-870.

186. Wang WC, Gallagher DM, Pegelow CH, et al. Multicenter comparison of magnetic resonance imaging and transcranial Doppler ultrasonography in the evaluation of the central nervous system in children with sickle cell disease. *J Pediatr Hematol Oncol*. 2000;22(4):335-339.

187. DeBaun MR, Gordon M, McKinstry RC, et al. Controlled trial of transfusions for silent cerebral infarcts in sickle cell anemia. *N Engl J Med*. 2014;371(8):699-710. doi:10.1056/NEJMoa1401731

188. Darbari DS, Eigbire-Molen O, Ponisio MR, et al. Progressive loss of brain volume in children with sickle cell anemia and silent cerebral infarct: a report from the silent cerebral infarct transfusion trial. *Am J Hematol*. 2018;93(12):E406-E408. doi:10.1002/ajh.25297

189. Nottage KA, Ware RE, Aygun B, et al. Hydroxycarbamide treatment and brain MRI/MRA findings in children with sickle cell anaemia. *Br J Haematol*. 2016;175(2):331-338. doi:10.1111/bjh.14235

190. Champlin G, Hwang SN, Heitzer A, et al. Progression of central nervous system disease from pediatric to young adulthood in sickle cell anemia. *Exp Biol Med (Maywood)*. 2021;246(23):2473-2479. doi:10.1177/15353702211035778

191. Rigano P, De Franceschi L, Sainati L, et al. Real-life experience with hydroxyurea in sickle cell disease: a multicenter study in a cohort of patients with heterogeneous descent. *Blood Cells Mol Dis*. 2018;69:82-89. doi:10.1016/j.bcmd.2017.08.017

192. Jordan LC, Kassim AA, Donahue MJ, et al. Silent infarct is a risk factor for infarct recurrence in adults with sickle cell anemia. *Neurology*. 2018;91(8):e781-e784. doi:10.1212/WNL.0000000000006047

193. Castro O, Brambilla DJ, Thorington B, et al. The acute chest syndrome in sickle cell disease: incidence and risk factors. The Cooperative Study of Sickle Cell Disease. *Blood*. 1994;84(2):643-649.

194. Chaturvedi S, Ghafuri DL, Glassberg J, Kassim AA, Rodeghier M, DeBaun MR. Rapidly progressive acute chest syndrome in individuals with sickle cell anemia: a distinct acute chest syndrome phenotype. *Am J Hematol*. 2016;91(12):1185-1190. doi:10.1002/ajh.24539

195. Fullerton HJ, Gardner M, Adams RJ, Lo LC, Johnston SC. Obstacles to primary stroke prevention in children with sickle cell disease. *Neurology*. 2006;67(6):1098-1099.

196. Cappellini MD, Cohen A, Piga A, et al. A phase 3 study of deferasirox (ICL670), a once-daily oral iron chelator, in patients with beta-thalassemia. *Blood*. 2006;107(9):3455-3462.

197. Miller ST, Hammerschlag MR, Chirgwin K, et al. Role of Chlamydia pneumoniae in acute chest syndrome of sickle cell disease. *J Pediatr*. 1991;118(1):30-33.

198. Lowenthal EA, Wells A, Emanuel PD, Player R, Prchal JT. Sickle cell acute chest syndrome associated with parvovirus B19 infection: case series and review. *Am J Hematol*. 1996;51(3):207-213. doi:10.1002/(SICI)1096-8652(199603)51:3<207::AID-AJH5>3.0.CO;2-0

199. Vichinsky EP, Neumayr LD, Earles AN, et al. Causes and outcomes of the acute chest syndrome in sickle cell disease. National Acute Chest Syndrome Study Group. *N Engl J Med*. 2000;342(25):1855-1865. doi:10.1056/NEJM200006223422502

200. Strouse JJ, Reller ME, Bundy DG, et al. Severe pandemic H1N1 and seasonal influenza in children and young adults with sickle cell disease. *Blood*. 2010;116(18):3431-3434. doi:10.1182/blood-2010-05-282194

201. Creary SE, Krishnamurti L. Prodromal illness before acute chest syndrome in pediatric patients with sickle cell disease. *J Pediatr Hematol Oncol*. 2014;36(6):480-483. doi:10.1097/MPH.0000000000000146

202. Takahashi T, Okubo Y, Handa A. Acute chest syndrome among children hospitalized with vaso-occlusive crisis: a nationwide study in the United States. *Pediatr Blood Cancer*. 2018;65(3). doi:10.1002/pbc.26885

203. Henderson JN, Noetzel MJ, McKinstry RC, White DA, Armstrong M, DeBaun MR. Reversible posterior leukoencephalopathy syndrome and silent cerebral infarcts are associated with severe acute chest syndrome in children with sickle cell disease. *Blood*. 2003;101(2):415-419. doi:10.1182/blood-2002-04-1183

204. Quinn CT, McKinstry RC, Dowling MM, et al. Acute silent cerebral ischemic events in children with sickle cell anemia. *JAMA Neurol*. 2013;70(1):58-65. doi:10.1001/jamaneurol.2013.576

205. Sadreameli SC, Eakin MN, Robinson KT, Alade RO, Strouse JJ. Secondhand smoke is associated with more frequent hospitalizations in children with sickle cell disease. *Am J Hematol*. 2016;91(3):313-317. doi:10.1002/ajh.24281

206. Cohen RT, DeBaun MR, Blinder MA, Strunk RC, Field JJ. Smoking is associated with an increased risk of acute chest syndrome and pain among adults with sickle cell disease. *Blood*. 2010;115(18):3852-3854. doi:10.1182/blood-2010-01-265819

207. Boyd JH, Macklin EA, Strunk RC, DeBaun MR. Asthma is associated with acute chest syndrome and pain in children with sickle cell anemia. *Blood*. 2006;108(9):2923-2927.

208. Poulter EY, Truszkowski P, Thompson AA, Liem RI. Acute chest syndrome is associated with history of asthma in hemoglobin SC disease. *Pediatr Blood Cancer*. 2011;57(2):289-293. doi:10.1002/pbc.22900

209. Boyd JH, Moinuddin A, Strunk RC, DeBaun MR. Asthma and acute chest in sickle-cell disease. *Pediatr Pulmonol*. 2004;38(3):229-232.

210. Boyd JH, DeBaun MR, Morgan WJ, Mao J, Strunk RC. Lower airway obstruction is associated with increased morbidity in children with sickle cell disease. *Pediatr Pulmonol*. 2009;44(3):290-296. doi:10.1002/ppul.20998

211. Knight-Madden JM, Forrester TS, Lewis NA, Greenough A. Asthma in children with sickle cell disease and its association with acute chest syndrome. *Thorax*. 2005;60(3):206-210.

212. Vichinsky E, Williams R, Das M, et al. Pulmonary fat embolism: a distinct cause of severe acute chest syndrome in sickle cell anemia. *Blood*. 1994;83(11):3107-3112.

213. Marti-Carvajal AJ, Conterno LO, Knight-Madden JM. Antibiotics for treating acute chest syndrome in people with sickle cell disease. *Cochrane Database Syst Rev*. 2015;(3):CD006110. doi:10.1002/14651858.CD006110.pub4

214. Bundy DG, Richardson TE, Hall M, et al. Association of guideline-adherent antibiotic treatment with readmission of children with sickle cell disease hospitalized with acute chest syndrome. *JAMA Pediatr*. 2017;171(11):1090-1099. doi:10.1001/jamapediatrics.2017.2526

215. Bernini JC, Rogers ZR, Sandler ES, Reisch JS, Quinn CT, Buchanan GR. Beneficial effect of intravenous dexamethasone in children with mild to moderately severe acute chest syndrome complicating sickle cell disease. *Blood*. 1998;92(9):3082-3089.

216. Quinn CT, Stuart MJ, Kesler K, et al. Tapered oral dexamethasone for the acute chest syndrome of sickle cell disease. *Br J Haematol*. 2011;155(2):263-267. doi:10.1111/j.1365-2141.2011.08827.x

217. Gladwin MT, Schechter AN, Shelhamer JH, Ognibene FP. The acute chest syndrome in sickle cell disease. Possible role of nitric oxide in its pathophysiology and treatment. *Am J Respir Crit Care Med*. 1999;159(5 pt 1):1368-1376.

218. Brittenham GM. *Vitamin D for Sickle-Cell Respiratory Complications*. 2011. ClinicalTrials.gov Identifier: NCT01443728. https://clinicaltrials.gov/ct2/show/NCT01443728?term=NCT01443728&draw=2&rank=1

219. Lee L, Draper B, Chaplin N, et al. An APRIL-based chimeric antigen receptor for dual targeting of BCMA and TACI in multiple myeloma. *Blood*. 2018;131(7):746-758. doi:10.1182/blood-2017-05-781351

220. Serjeant G, Hambleton I. Priapism in homozygous sickle cell disease: a 40-year study of the natural history. *West Indian Med J*. 2015;64(3):175-180. doi:10.7727/wimj.2014.119

221. Furtado PS, Costa MP, Ribeiro do Prado Valladares F, et al. The prevalence of priapism in children and adolescents with sickle cell disease in Brazil. *Int J Hematol*. 2012;95(6):648-651. doi:10.1007/s12185-012-1083-0

222. Nolan VG, Wyszynski DF, Farrer LA, Steinberg MH. Hemolysis-associated priapism in sickle cell disease. *Blood*. 2005;106(9):3264-3267.

223. Cita KC, Brureau L, Lemonne N, et al. Men with sickle cell anemia and priapism exhibit increased hemolytic rate, decreased red blood cell deformability and increased red blood cell aggregate strength. *PLoS One*. 2016;11(5):e0154866. doi:10.1371/journal.pone.0154866

224. Siegel JF, Rich MA, Brock WA. Association of sickle cell disease, priapism, exchange transfusion and neurological events: ASPEN syndrome. *J Urol*. 1993;150(5 pt 1):1480-1482.

225. Ballas SK, Lyon D. Safety and efficacy of blood exchange transfusion for priapism complicating sickle cell disease. *J Clin Apher*. 2016;31(1):5-10. doi:10.1002/jca.21394

226. Tsitsikas DA, Orebayo F, Agapidou A, Amos RJ. Distinct patterns of response to transfusion therapy for different chronic complications of sickle cell disease: a useful insight. *Transfus Apher Sci*. 2017;56(5):713-716. doi:10.1016/j.transci.2017.08.001

227. Winter CC. Priapism cured by creation of fistulas between glans penis and corpora cavernosa. *J Urol*. 1978;119(2):227-228.

228. Mantadakis E, Ewalt DH, Cavender JD, Rogers ZR, Buchanan GR. Outpatient penile aspiration and epinephrine irrigation for young patients with sickle cell anemia and prolonged priapism. *Blood*. 2000;95(1):78-82.

229. Ekong A, Berg L, Amos RJ, Tsitsikas DA. Regular automated red cell exchange transfusion in the management of stuttering priapism complicating sickle cell disease. *Br J Haematol*. 2018;180(4):585-588. doi:10.1111/bjh.14393

230. Okpala I, Westerdale N, Jegede T, Cheung B. Etilefrine for the prevention of priapism in adult sickle cell disease. *Br J Haematol*. 2002;118(3):918-921.

231. Gbadoe AD, Atakouma Y, Kusiaku K, Assimadi JK. Management of sickle cell priapism with etilefrine. *Arch Dis Child*. 2001;85(1):52-53.

232. Burnett AL, Anele UA, Trueheart IN, Strouse JJ, Casella JF. Randomized controlled trial of sildenafil for preventing recurrent ischemic priapism in sickle cell disease. *Am J Med*. 2014;127(7):664-668. doi:10.1016/j.amjmed.2014.03.019

233. Lane A, Deveras R. Potential risks of chronic sildenafil use for priapism in sickle cell disease. *J Sex Med*. 2011;8(11):3193-3195. doi:10.1111/j.1743-6109.2011.02440.x

234. Greenwald MH, Gutman CK, Morris CR. Resolution of acute priapism in two children with sickle cell disease who received nitrous oxide. *Acad Emerg Med*. 2019;26(9):1102-1105. doi:10.1111/acem.13822

235. Kim M, Alapan Y, Adhikari A, Little JA, Gurkan UA. Hypoxia-enhanced adhesion of red blood cells in microscale flow. *Microcirculation*. 2017;24(5). doi:10.1111/micc.12374

236. Yuan C, Quinn E, Kucukal E, Kapoor S, Gurkan UA, Little JA. Priapism, hemoglobin desaturation, and red blood cell adhesion in men with sickle cell anemia. *Blood Cells Mol Dis*. 2019;79:102350. doi:10.1016/j.bcmd.2019.102350

237. Novartis Pharmaceuticals. *A Study to Evaluate the Safety and Efficacy of Crizanlizumab in sickle Cell Disease Related Priapism (SPARTAN)*. ClinicalTrials.gov:NCT03938454. 2019.

Disorders of Red Blood Cells

238. Fowler JE Jr, Koshy M, Strub M, Chinn SK. Priapism associated with the sickle cell hemoglobinopathies: prevalence, natural history and sequelae. *J Urol.* 1991;145(1):65-68.

239. Young N. Hematologic and hematopoietic consequences of B19 parvovirus infection. *Semin Hematol.* 1988;25(2):159-172.

240. Zimmerman SA, Davis JS, Schultz WH, Ware RE. Subclinical parvovirus B19 infection in children with sickle cell anemia. *J Pediatr Hematol Oncol.* 2003;25(5):387-389.

241. Hankins JS, Penkert RR, Lavoie P, Tang L, Sun Y, Hurwitz JL. Original Research: parvovirus B19 infection in children with sickle cell disease in the hydroxyurea era. *Exp Biol Med (Maywood).* 2016;241(7):749-754. doi:10.1177/1535370216636723

242. Krishnamurti L, Lanford L, Munoz R. Life threatening parvovirus B19 and herpes simplex virus associated acute myocardial dysfunction in a child with homozygous sickle cell disease. *Pediatr Blood Cancer.* 2007;49(7):1019-1021. doi:10.1002/pbc.20855

243. Yates AM, Hankins JS, Mortier NA, Aygun B, Ware RE. Simultaneous acute splenic sequestration and transient aplastic crisis in children with sickle cell disease. *Pediatr Blood Cancer.* 2009;53(3):479-481. doi:10.1002/pbc.22035

244. Balkaran B, Char G, Morris JS, Thomas PW, Serjeant BE, Serjeant GR. Stroke in a cohort of patients with homozygous sickle cell disease. *J Pediatr.* 1992;120(3):360-366.

245. Quek L, Sharpe C, Dutt N, et al. Acute human parvovirus B19 infection and nephrotic syndrome in patients with sickle cell disease. *Br J Haematol.* 2010;149(2):289-291. doi:10.1111/j.1365-2141.2009.08062.x

246. Walterspiel JN, Rutledge JC, Bartlett BL. Fatal acute splenic sequestration at 4 months of age. *Pediatrics.* 1984;73(4):507-508.

247. Naymagon L, Pendurti G, Billett HH. Acute splenic sequestration crisis in adult sickle cell disease: a report of 16 cases. *Hemoglobin.* 2015;39(6):375-379. doi:10.3109/03630269.2015.1072550

248. Brousse V, Elie C, Benkerrou M, et al. Acute splenic sequestration crisis in sickle cell disease: cohort study of 190 paediatric patients. *Br J Haematol.* 2012;156(5):643-648. doi:10.1111/j.1365-2141.2011.08999.x

249. Mouttalib S, Rice HE, Snyder D, et al. Evaluation of partial and total splenectomy in children with sickle cell disease using an Internet-based registry. *Pediatr Blood Cancer.* 2012;59(1):100-104. doi:10.1002/pbc.24057

250. Englum BR, Rothman J, Leonard S, et al. Hematologic outcomes after total splenectomy and partial splenectomy for congenital hemolytic anemia. *J Pediatr Surg.* 2016;51(1):122-127. doi:10.1016/j.jpedsurg.2015.10.028

251. Hatton CS, Bunch C, Weatherall DJ. Hepatic sequestration in sickle cell anaemia. *Br Med J(Clin Res Ed).* 1985;290(6470):744-745.

252. Maurer HS, Vida LN, Honig GR. Homozygous sickle cell disease with coexistent hereditary spherocytosis in three siblings. *J Pediatr.* 1972;80(2):235-242.

253. Goyal M, Donoghue A, Schwab S, Hasbrouck N, Khojasteh S, Osterhoudt K. Severe hemolytic crisis after ceftriaxone administration. *Pediatr Emerg Care.* 2011;27(4):322-323. doi:10.1097/PEC.0b013e3182131fa8

254. Bienzle U, Sodeinde O, Effiong CE, Luzzatto L. Glucose 6-phosphate dehydrogenase deficiency and sickle cell anemia: frequency and features of the association in an African community. *Blood.* 1975;46(4):591-597.

255. Steinberg MH, West MS, Gallagher D, Mentzer W. Effects of glucose-6-phosphate dehydrogenase deficiency upon sickle cell anemia. *Blood.* 1988;71(3):748-752.

256. Pearson HA. Folic acid studies in sickle cell anemia. *J Lab Clin Med.* 1964;64:913.

257. O'Brien RT, McIntosh S, Aspnes GT, Pearson HA. Prospective study of sickle cell anemia in infancy. *J Pediatr.* 1976;89(2):205-210.

258. Gavrilis P, Rothenberg SP, Guy R. Correlation of low serum IgM levels with absence of functional splenic tissue in sickle cell disease syndromes. *Am J Med.* 1974;57(4):542-545.

259. Bjornson AB, Lobel JS. Direct evidence that decreased serum opsonization of Streptococcus pneumoniae via the alternative complement pathway in sickle cell disease is related to antibody deficiency. *J Clin Invest.* 1987;79(2):388-398.

260. Miller ML, Gao G, Pestina T, Persons D, Tuomanen E. Hypersusceptibility to invasive pneumococcal infection in experimental sickle cell disease involves platelet-activating factor receptor. *J Infect Dis.* 2007;195(4):581-584. doi:10.1086/510626

261. Rosch JW, Boyd AR, Hinojosa E, et al. Statins protect against fulminant pneumococcal infection and cytolysin toxicity in a mouse model of sickle cell disease. *J Clin Invest.* 2010;120(2):627-635. doi:10.1172/jci39843

262. Zarkowsky HS, Gallagher D, Gill FM, et al. Bacteremia in sickle hemoglobinopathies. *J Pediatr.* 1986;109(4):579-585.

263. Wong WY, Overturf GD, Powars DR. Infection caused by Streptococcus pneumoniae in children with sickle cell disease: epidemiology, immunologic mechanisms, prophylaxis, and vaccination. *Clin Infect Dis.* 1992;14(5):1124-1136.

264. Overturf GD, Powars D, Baraff LJ. Bacterial meningitis and septicemia in sickle cell disease. *Am J Dis Child.* 1977;131(7):784-787.

265. McCavit TL, Quinn CT, Techasaensiri C, Rogers ZR. Increase in invasive Streptococcus pneumoniae infections in children with sickle cell disease since pneumococcal conjugate vaccine licensure. *J Pediatr.* 2011;158(3):505-507. doi:10.1016/j.jpeds.2010.11.025

266. Hsu KK, Shea KM, Stevenson AE, Pelton SI. Changing serotypes causing childhood invasive pneumococcal disease: Massachusetts, 2001-2007. *Pediatr Infect Dis J.* 2010;29(4):289-293. doi:10.1097/INF.0b013e3181c15471

267. Carter R, Wolf J, van Opijnen T, et al. Genomic analyses of pneumococci from children with sickle cell disease expose host-specific bacterial adaptations and deficits in current interventions. *Cell Host Microbe.* 2014;15(5):587-599. doi:10.1016/j.chom.2014.04.005

268. Givner LB, Luddy RE, Schwartz AD. Etiology of osteomyelitis in patients with major sickle hemoglobinopathies. *J Pediatr.* 1981;99(3):411-413.

269. Chulamokha L, Scholand SJ, Riggio JM, Ballas SK, Horn D, DeSimone JA. Bloodstream infections in hospitalized adults with sickle cell disease: a retrospective analysis. *Am J Hematol.* 2006;81(10):723-728.

270. Zarrouk V, Habibi A, Zahar JR, et al. Bloodstream infection in adults with sickle cell disease: association with venous catheters, *Staphylococcus aureus*, and bone-joint infections. *Medicine (Baltimore).* 2006;85(1):43-48.

271. John AB, Ramlal A, Jackson H, Maude GH, Sharma AW, Serjeant GR. Prevention of pneumococcal infection in children with homozygous sickle cell disease. *Br Med J.* 1984;288(6430):1567-1570.

272. Gaston MH, Verter JI, Woods G, et al. Prophylaxis with oral penicillin in children with sickle cell anemia. A randomized trial. *N Engl J Med.* 1986;314(25):1593-1599.

273. Yawn BP, Buchanan GR, Afenyi-Annan AN, et al. Management of sickle cell disease: summary of the 2014 evidence-based report by expert panel members. *J Am Med Assoc.* 2014;312(10):1033-1048. doi:10.1001/jama.2014.10517

274. Falletta JM, Woods GM, Verter JI, et al. Discontinuing penicillin prophylaxis in children with sickle cell anemia. Prophylactic Penicillin Study II. *J Pediatr.* 1995;127(5):685-690.

275. Overturf GD, Rigau-Perez JG, Selzer J, et al. Pneumococcal polysaccharide immunization of children with sickle cell disease. I. Clinical reactions to immunization and relationship to preimmunization antibody. *Am J Pediatr Hematol Oncol.* 1982;4(1):19-23.

276. Weintrub PS, Schiffman G, Addiego JE Jr, et al. Long-term follow-up and booster immunization with polyvalent pneumococcal polysaccharide in patients with sickle cell anemia. *J Pediatr.* 1984;105(2):261-263.

277. De Montalembert M, Abboud MR, Fiquet A, et al. 13-valent pneumococcal conjugate vaccine (PCV13) is immunogenic and safe in children 6-17 years of age with sickle cell disease previously vaccinated with 23-valent pneumococcal polysaccharide vaccine (PPSV23): results of a phase 3 study. *Pediatr Blood Cancer.* 2015;62(8):1427-1436. doi:10.1002/pbc.25502

278. Halasa NB, Shankar SM, Talbot TR, et al. Incidence of invasive pneumococcal disease among individuals with sickle cell disease before and after the introduction of the pneumococcal conjugate vaccine. *Clin Infect Dis.* 2007;44(11):1428-1433. doi:10.1086/516781

279. McCavit TL, Xuan L, Zhang S, Flores G, Quinn CT. Hospitalization for invasive pneumococcal disease in a national sample of children with sickle cell disease before and after PCV7 licensure. *Pediatr Blood Cancer.* 2012;58(6):945-949. doi:10.1002/pbc.23259

280. Folaranmi T, Rubin L, Martin SW, Patel M, MacNeil JR. Use of serogroup B meningococcal vaccines in persons aged >/=10 Years at increased risk for serogroup B meningococcal disease: recommendations of the advisory committee on immunization practices, 2015. *MMWR Morb Mortal Wkly Rep.* 2015;64(22):608-612.

281. Bernstein DI, El Sahly HM, Keitel WA, et al. Safety and immunogenicity of a candidate parvovirus B19 vaccine. *Vaccine.* 2011;29(43):7357-7363. doi:10.1016/j.vaccine.2011.07.080

282. Chandramouli S, Medina-Selby A, Coit D, et al. Generation of a parvovirus B19 vaccine candidate. *Vaccine.* 2013;31(37):3872-3878. doi:10.1016/j.vaccine.2013.06.062

283. Penkert RR, Young NS, Surman SL, et al. Saccharomyces cerevisiae-derived virus-like particle parvovirus B19 vaccine elicits binding and neutralizing antibodies in a mouse model for sickle cell disease. *Vaccine.* 2017;35(29):3615-3620. doi:10.1016/j.vaccine.2017.05.022

284. Platt OS, Rosenstock W, Espeland MA. Influence of sickle hemoglobinopathies on growth and development. *N Engl J Med.* 1984;311(1):7-12.

285. Phebus CK, Gloninger MF, Maciak BJ. Growth patterns by age and sex in children with sickle cell disease. *J Pediatr.* 1984;105(1):28-33.

286. Stevens MC, Maude GH, Cupidore L, Jackson H, Hayes RJ, Serjeant GR. Prepubertal growth and skeletal maturation in children with sickle cell disease. *Pediatrics.* 1986;78(1):124-132.

287. Adesina OO, Gurney JG, Kang G, et al. Height-corrected low bone density associates with severe outcomes in sickle cell disease: SCCRIP cohort study results. *Blood Adv.* 2019;3(9):1476-1488. doi:10.1182/bloodadvances.2018026047

288. Galadanci NA, Sohail M, Akinyelure OP, Kanter J, Ojesina AI. Treatment-related correlates of growth in children with sickle cell disease in the DISPLACE cohort. *J Pediatr Hematol Oncol.* 2022;44(5):249-254. doi:10.1097/MPH.0000000000002296

289. Borel MJ, Buchowski MS, Turner EA, Peeler BB, Goldstein RE, Flakoll PJ. Alterations in basal nutrient metabolism increase resting energy expenditure in sickle cell disease. *Am J Physiol.* 1998;274(2 pt 1):E357–E364.

290. Rhodes M, Akohoue SA, Shankar SM, et al. Growth patterns in children with sickle cell anemia during puberty. *Pediatr Blood Cancer.* 2009;53(4):635-641. doi:10.1002/pbc.22137

291. Wolf RB, Saville BR, Roberts DO, et al. Factors associated with growth and blood pressure patterns in children with sickle cell anemia: silent Cerebral Infarct Multi-Center Clinical Trial cohort. *Am J Hematol.* 2015;90(1):2-7. doi:10.1002/ajh.23854

292. Barden EM, Zemel BS, Kawchak DA, Goran MI, Ohene-Frempong K, Stallings VA. Total and resting energy expenditure in children with sickle cell disease. *J Pediatr.* 2000;136(1):73-79.

293. Westerman MP, Zhang Y, McConnell JP, et al. Ascorbate levels in red blood cells and urine in patients with sickle cell anemia. *Am J Hematol.* 2000;65(2):174-175.

294. Luporini SM, Bendit I, Manhani R, Bracco OL, Manzella L, Giannella-Neto D. Growth hormone and insulin-like growth factor I axis and growth of children with different sickle cell anemia haplotypes. *J Pediatr Hematol Oncol.* 2001;23(6):357-363.

295. Soliman AT, el Banna N, alSalmi I, De SV, Craig A, Asfour M. Growth hormone secretion and circulating insulin-like growth factor-I (IGF-I) and IGF binding protein-3 concentrations in children with sickle cell disease. *Metabolism.* 1997;46(11):1241-1245.

296. Milner PF, Kraus AP, Sebes JI, et al. Sickle cell disease as a cause of osteonecrosis of the femoral head. *N Engl J Med.* 1991;325(21):1476-1481.
297. Milner PF, Kraus AP, Sebes JI, et al. Osteonecrosis of the humeral head in sickle cell disease. *Clin Orthop.* 1993;(289):136-143.
298. Sachan AA, Lakhkar BN, Lakhkar BB, Sachan S. Is MRI necessary for skeletal evaluation in sickle cell disease. *J Clin Diagn Res.* 2015;9(6):Tc08-12. doi:10.7860/jcdr/2015/12747.6095
299. Yu T, Campbell T, Ciuffetelli I, et al. Symptomatic avascular necrosis: an understudied risk factor for acute care utilization by patients with SCD. *South Med J.* 2016;109(9):519-524. doi:10.14423/SMJ.0000000000000512
300. Ilyas I, Alrumaih HA, Rabbani S. Noncemented total hip arthroplasty in sickle-cell disease: long-term results. *J Arthroplasty.* 2018;33(2):477-481. doi:10.1016/j.arth.2017.09.010
301. Styles LA, Vichinsky EP. Core decompression in avascular necrosis of the hip in sickle-cell disease. *Am J Hematol.* 1996;52(2):103-107.
302. Mukisi-Mukaza M, Manicom O, Alexis C, Bashoun K, Donkerwolcke M, Burny F. Treatment of sickle cell disease's hip necrosis by core decompression: a prospective case-control study. *Orthop Traumatol Surg Res.* 2009;95(7):498-504. doi:10.1016/j.otsr.2009.07.009
303. Neumayr LD, Aguilar C, Earles AN, et al. Physical therapy alone compared with core decompression and physical therapy for femoral head osteonecrosis in sickle cell disease. Results of a multicenter study at a mean of three years after treatment. *J Bone Joint Surg.* 2006;88(12):2573-2582.
304. Daltro GC, Fortuna V, de Souza ES, et al. Efficacy of autologous stem cell-based therapy for osteonecrosis of the femoral head in sickle cell disease: a five-year follow-up study. *Stem Cell Res Ther.* 2015;6:110. doi:10.1186/s13287-015-0105-2
305. Lebouvier A, Poignard A, Coquelin-Salsac L, et al. Autologous bone marrow stromal cells are promising candidates for cell therapy approaches to treat bone degeneration in sickle cell disease. *Stem Cell Res.* 2015;15(3):584-594. doi:10.1016/j.scr.2015.09.016
306. Gupta R, Adekile AD. MRI follow-up and natural history of avascular necrosis of the femoral head in Kuwaiti children with sickle cell disease. *J Pediatr Hematol Oncol.* 2004;26(6):351-353. doi:10.1097/00043426-200406000-00004
307. Adekile AD, Gupta R, Al-Khayat A, Mohammed A, Atyani S, Thomas D. Risk of avascular necrosis of the femoral head in children with sickle cell disease on hydroxyurea: MRI evaluation. *Pediatr Blood Cancer.* 2019;66(2):e27503. doi:10.1002/pbc.27503
308. Itzep NP, Jadhav SP, Kanne CK, Sheehan VA. Spontaneous healing of avascular necrosis of the femoral head in sickle cell disease. *Am J Hematol.* 2019;94(6):E160-E162. doi:10.1002/ajh.25453
309. Adesina O, Brunson A, Keegan THM, Wun T. Osteonecrosis of the femoral head in sickle cell disease: prevalence, comorbidities, and surgical outcomes in California. *Blood Adv.* 2017;1(16):1287-1295. doi:10.1182/bloodadvances.2017005256
310. Chapelon E, Garabedian M, Brousse V, Souberbielle JC, Bresson JL, de Montalembert M. Osteopenia and vitamin D deficiency in children with sickle cell disease. *Eur J Haematol.* 2009;83(6):572-578. doi:10.1111/j.1600-0609.2009.01333.x
311. Sarrai M, Duroseau H, D'Augustine J, Moktan S, Bellevue R. Bone mass density in adults with sickle cell disease. *Br J Haematol.* 2007;136(4):666-672. doi:10.1111/j.1365-2141.2006.06487.x
312. Adegoke SA, Braga JA, Adekile AD, Figueiredo MS. The association of serum 25-hydroxyvitamin D with biomarkers of hemolysis in pediatric patients with sickle cell disease. *J Pediatr Hematol Oncol.* 2017;40(2):159-162. doi:10.1097/mph.0000000000000783
313. Nolan VG, Nottage KA, Cole EW, Hankins JS, Gurney JG. Prevalence of vitamin D deficiency in sickle cell disease: a systematic review. *PLoS One.* 2015;10(3):e0119908. doi:10.1371/journal.pone.0119908
314. Adewoye AH, Chen TC, Ma Q, et al. Sickle cell bone disease: response to vitamin D and calcium. *Am J Hematol.* 2008;83(4):271-274. doi:10.1002/ajh.21085
315. Fowler MG, Whitt JK, Lallinger RR, et al. Neuropsychologic and academic functioning of children with sickle cell anemia. *JDevBehavPediatr.* 1988;9(4):213-220.
316. Swift AV, Cohen MJ, Hynd GW, et al. Neuropsychologic impairment in children with sickle cell anemia. *Pediatrics.* 1989;84(6):1077-1085.
317. Hijmans CT, Fijnvandraat K, Grootenhuis MA, et al. Neurocognitive deficits in children with sickle cell disease: a comprehensive profile. *Pediatr Blood Cancer.* 2011;56(5):783-788. doi:10.1002/pbc.22879
318. Yarboi J, Compas BE, Brody GH, et al. Association of social-environmental factors with cognitive function in children with sickle cell disease. *Child Neuropsychol.* 2017;23(3):343-360. doi:10.1080/09297049.2015.1111318
319. Prussien KV, Jordan LC, DeBaun MR, Compas BE. Cognitive function in sickle cell disease across domains, cerebral infarct status, and the lifespan: a meta-analysis. *J Pediatr Psychol.* 2019;44(8):948-958. doi:10.1093/jpepsy/jsz031
320. Schatz J, Finke RL, Kellett JM, Kramer JH. Cognitive functioning in children with sickle cell disease: a meta- analysis. *J Pediatr Psychol.* 2002;27(8):739-748.
321. Wang W, Enos L, Gallagher D, et al. Neuropsychologic performance in school-aged children with sickle cell disease: a report from the Cooperative Study of Sickle Cell Disease. *J Pediatr.* 2001;139(3):391-397.
322. Heitzer AM, Longoria J, Okhomina V, et al. Hydroxyurea treatment and neurocognitive functioning in sickle cell disease from school age to young adulthood. *Br J Haematol.* 2021;195(2):256-266. doi:10.1111/bjh.17687
323. Hogan AM, Pit-ten Cate IM, Vargha-Khadem F, Prengler M, Kirkham FJ. Physiological correlates of intellectual function in children with sickle cell disease: hypoxaemia, hyperaemia and brain infarction. *Dev Sci.* 2006;9(4):379-387. doi:10.1111/j.1467-7687.2006.00503.x
324. Kawadler JM, Clayden JD, Clark CA, Kirkham FJ. Intelligence quotient in paediatric sickle cell disease: a systematic review and meta-analysis. *Dev Med Child Neurol.* 2016;58(7):672-679. doi:10.1111/dmcn.13113
325. Hariman LM, Griffith ER, Hurtig AL, Keehn MT. Functional outcomes of children with sickle-cell disease affected by stroke. *Arch Phys Med Rehabil.* 1991;72(7):498-502.
326. King AA, Rodeghier MJ, Panepinto JA, et al. Silent cerebral infarction, income, and grade retention among students with sickle cell anemia. *Am J Hematol.* 2014;89(10):E188-E192. doi:10.1002/ajh.23805
327. Jorgensen DR, Metti A, Butters MA, Mettenburg JM, Rosano C, Novelli EM. Disease severity and slower psychomotor speed in adults with sickle cell disease. *Blood Adv.* 2017;1(21):1790-1795. doi:10.1182/bloodadvances.2017008219
328. Vichinsky EP, Neumayr LD, Gold JI, et al. Neuropsychological dysfunction and neuroimaging abnormalities in neurologically intact adults with sickle cell anemia. *J Am Med Assoc.* 2010;303(18):1823-1831. doi:10.1001/jama.2010.562
329. Crawford RD, Jonassaint CR. Adults with sickle cell disease may perform cognitive tests as well as controls when processing speed is taken into account: a preliminary case-control study. *J Adv Nurs.* 2016;72(6):1409-1416. doi:10.1111/jan.12755
330. Sanger M, Jordan L, Pruthi S, et al. Cognitive deficits are associated with unemployment in adults with sickle cell anemia. *J Clin Exp Neuropsychol.* 2016;38(6):661-671. doi:10.1080/13803395.2016.1149153
331. Longoria JN, Pugh NL, Gordeuk V, et al. Patient-reported neurocognitive symptoms influence instrumental activities of daily living in sickle cell disease. *Am J Hematol.* 2021;96(11):1396-1406. doi:10.1002/ajh.26315
332. Saulsberry-Abate AC, Partanen M, Porter JS, et al. Cognitive performance as a predictor of healthcare transition in sickle cell disease. *Br J Haematol.* 2021;192(6):1082-1091. doi:10.1111/bjh.17351
333. van der Land V, Hijmans CT, de Ruiter M, et al. Volume of white matter hyperintensities is an independent predictor of intelligence quotient and processing speed in children with sickle cell disease. *Br J Haematol.* 2015;168(4):553-556. doi:10.1111/bjh.13179
334. Mackin RS, Insel P, Truran D, et al. Neuroimaging abnormalities in adults with sickle cell anemia: associations with cognition. *Neurology.* 2014;82(10):835-841. doi:10.1212/wnl.0000000000000188
335. Lebensburger JD, Hilliard LM, McGrath TM, Fineberg NS, Howard TH. Laboratory and clinical correlates for magnetic resonance imaging (MRI) abnormalities in pediatric sickle cell anemia. *J Child Neurol.* 2011;26(10):1260-1264. doi:10.1177/0883073811405054
336. Hollocks MJ, Kok TB, Kirkham FJ, et al. Nocturnal oxygen desaturation and disordered sleep as a potential factor in executive dysfunction in sickle cell anemia. *J Int Neuropsychol Soc.* 2012;18(1):168-173. doi:10.1017/s1355617711001469
337. Sanchez CE, Schatz J, Roberts CW. Cerebral blood flow velocity and language functioning in pediatric sickle cell disease. *J Int Neuropsychol Soc.* 2010;16(2):326-334. doi:10.1017/s1355617709991366
338. Bakker MJ, Hofmann J, Churches OF, Badcock NA, Kohler M, Keage HA. Cerebrovascular function and cognition in childhood: a systematic review of transcranial Doppler studies. *BMC Neurol.* 2014;14:43. doi:10.1186/1471-2377-14-43
339. Andreotti C, King AA, Macy E, Compas BE, DeBaun MR. The association of cytokine levels with cognitive function in children with sickle cell disease and normal MRI studies of the brain. *J Child Neurol.* 2015;30(10):1349-1353. doi:10.1177/0883073814563140
340. Drazen CH, Abel R, Gabir M, Farmer G, King AA. Prevalence of developmental delay and contributing factors among children with sickle cell disease. *Pediatr Blood Cancer.* 2016;63(3):504-510. doi:10.1002/pbc.25838
341. King AA, Strouse JJ, Rodeghier MJ, et al. Parent education and biologic factors influence on cognition in sickle cell anemia. *Am J Hematol.* 2014;89(2):162-167. doi:10.1002/ajh.23604
342. Helton KJ, Paydar A, Glass J, et al. Arterial spin-labeled perfusion combined with segmentation techniques to evaluate cerebral blood flow in white and gray matter of children with sickle cell anemia. *Pediatr Blood Cancer.* 2009;52(1):85-91. doi:10.1002/pbc.21745
343. Colombatti R, Lucchetta M, Montanaro M, et al. Cognition and the default mode network in children with sickle cell disease: a resting state functional MRI study. *PLoS One.* 2016;11(6):e0157090. doi:10.1371/journal.pone.0157090
344. Puffer E, Schatz J, Roberts CW. The association of oral hydroxyurea therapy with improved cognitive functioning in sickle cell disease. *Child Neuropsychol.* 2007;13(2):142-154.
345. Apollonsky N, Lerner NB, Zhang F, Raybagkar D, Eng J, Tarazi R. Laboratory biomarkers, cerebral blood flow velocity, and intellectual function in children with sickle cell disease. *Adv Hematol.* 2020;2020:8181425. doi:10.1155/2020/8181425
346. Partanen M, Kang G, Wang WC, et al. Association between hydroxycarbamide exposure and neurocognitive function in adolescents with sickle cell disease. *Br J Haematol.* 2020;189(6):1192-1203. doi:10.1111/bjh.16519
347. Wang WC, Zou P, Hwang SN, et al. Effects of hydroxyurea on brain function in children with sickle cell anemia. *Pediatr Blood Cancer.* 2021;68(10):e29254. doi:10.1002/pbc.29254
348. Fields ME, Guilliams KP, Ragan D, et al. Hydroxyurea reduces cerebral metabolic stress in patients with sickle cell anemia. *Blood.* 2019;133(22):2436-2444. doi:10.1182/blood-2018-09-876318
349. Walters MC, Storb R, Patience M, et al. Impact of bone marrow transplantation for symptomatic sickle cell disease: an interim report. Multicenter investigation of bone marrow transplantation for sickle cell disease. *Blood.* 2000;95(6):1918-1924.
350. Dallas MH, Triplett B, Shook DR, et al. Long-term outcome and evaluation of organ function in pediatric patients undergoing haploidentical and matched related hematopoietic cell transplantation for sickle cell disease. *Biol Blood Marrow Transplant.* 2013;19(5):820-830. doi:10.1016/j.bbmt.2013.02.010
351. Daly B, Kral MC, Brown RT, et al. Ameliorating attention problems in children with sickle cell disease: a pilot study of methylphenidate. *J Dev Behav Pediatr.* 2012;33(3):244-251. doi:10.1097/DBP.0b013e31824ba1b5

352. Fields ME, Hoyt-Drazen C, Abel R, et al. A pilot study of parent education intervention improves early childhood development among toddlers with sickle cell disease. *Pediatr Blood Cancer.* 2016;63(12):2131-2138. doi:10.1002/pbc.26164

353. Fitzhugh CD, Lauder N, Jonassaint JC, et al. Cardiopulmonary complications leading to premature deaths in adult patients with sickle cell disease. *Am J Hematol.* 2010;85(1):36-40. doi:10.1002/ajh.21569

354. Hamideh D, Alvarez O. Sickle cell disease related mortality in the United States (1999-2009). *Pediatr Blood Cancer.* 2013;60(9):1482-1486. doi:10.1002/pbc.24557

355. Lindsay J Jr, Meshel JC, Patterson RH. The cardiovascular manifestations of sickle cell disease. *Arch Intern Med.* 1974;133(4):643-651.

356. Lamers L, Ensing G, Pignatelli R, et al. Evaluation of left ventricular systolic function in pediatric sickle cell anemia patients using the end-systolic wall stress-velocity of circumferential fiber shortening relationship. *J Am Coll Cardiol.* 2006;47(11):2283-2288.

357. Sparkenbaugh EM, Chantrathammachart P, Chandarajoti K, Mackman N, Key NS, Pawlinski R. Thrombin-independent contribution of tissue factor to inflammation and cardiac hypertrophy in a mouse model of sickle cell disease. *Blood.* 2016;127(10):1371-1373. doi:10.1182/blood-2015-11-681114

358. Qureshi N, Joyce JJ, Qi N, Chang RK. Right ventricular abnormalities in sickle cell anemia: evidence of a progressive increase in pulmonary vascular resistance. *J Pediatr.* 2006;149(1):23-27.

359. Whipple NS, Naik RJ, Kang G, et al. Ventricular global longitudinal strain is altered in children with sickle cell disease. *Br J Haematol.* 2018;183(5):796-806. doi:10.1111/bjh.15607

360. Sherman SC, Sule HP. Acute myocardial infarction in a young man with sickle cell disease. *J Emerg Med.* 2004;27(1):31-35. doi:10.1016/j.jemermed.2004.02.007

361. Robard I, Mansencal N, Soulat G, Deblaise J, El Mahmoud R, Dubourg O. Myocardial infarction with normal coronary arteries in double heterozygous sickle-cell disease. *Int J Cardiol.* 2015;180:120-121. doi:10.1016/j.ijcard.2014.11.165

362. Deymann AJ, Goertz KK. Myocardial infarction and transient ventricular dysfunction in an adolescent with sickle cell disease. *Pediatrics.* 2003;111(2):E183–E187.

363. Johnson WH Jr, McCrary RB, Mankad VN. Transient left ventricular dysfunction in childhood sickle cell disease. *Pediatr Cardiol.* 1999;20(3):221-223.

364. Acar P, Maunoury C, de Montalembert M, Dulac Y. Abnormalities of myocardial perfusion in sickle cell disease in childhood: a study of myocardial scintigraphy. Article in French. *Arch Mal Coeur Vaiss.* 2003;96(5):507-510.

365. Acar P, Sebahoun S, de Pontual L, Maunoury C. Myocardial perfusion in children with sickle cell anaemia. *Pediatr Radiol.* 2000;30(5):352-354.

366. Bratis K, Kattamis A, Athanasiou K, et al. Abnormal myocardial perfusion-fibrosis pattern in sickle cell disease assessed by cardiac magnetic resonance imaging. *Int J Cardiol.* 2013;166(3):e75-e76. doi:10.1016/j.ijcard.2013.01.055

367. Desai AA, Patel AR, Ahmad H, et al. Mechanistic insights and characterization of sickle cell disease-associated cardiomyopathy. *Circ Cardiovasc Imaging.* 2014;7(3):430-437. doi:10.1161/CIRCIMAGING.113.001420

368. Niss O, Fleck R, Makue F, et al. Association between diffuse myocardial fibrosis and diastolic dysfunction in sickle cell anemia. *Blood.* 2017;130(2):205-213. doi:10.1182/blood-2017-02-767624

369. Whipple NS, Joshi VM, Naik RJ, et al. Sickle cell disease and ventricular myocardial strain: a systematic review. *Pediatr Blood Cancer.* 2021;68(6):e28973. doi:10.1002/pbc.28973

370. Eddine AC, Alvarez O, Lipshultz SE, Kardon R, Arheart K, Swaminathan S. Ventricular structure and function in children with sickle cell disease using conventional and tissue Doppler echocardiography. *Am J Cardiol.* 2012;109(9):1358-1364. doi:10.1016/j.amjcard.2012.01.001

371. Ahmad H, Gayat E, Yodwut C, et al. Evaluation of myocardial deformation in patients with sickle cell disease and preserved ejection fraction using three-dimensional speckle tracking echocardiography. *Echocardiography.* 2012;29(8):962-969. doi:10.1111/j.1540-8175.2012.01710.x

372. Hankins JS, McCarville MB, Hillenbrand CM, et al. Ventricular diastolic dysfunction in sickle cell anemia is common but not associated with myocardial iron deposition. *Pediatr Blood Cancer.* 2010;55(3):495-500. doi:10.1002/pbc.22587

373. Sachdev V, Machado RF, Shizukuda Y, et al. Diastolic dysfunction is an independent risk factor for death in patients with sickle cell disease. *J Am Coll Cardiol.* 2007;49(4):472-479.

374. Shah P, Suriany S, Kato R, et al. Tricuspid regurgitant jet velocity and myocardial tissue Doppler parameters predict mortality in a cohort of patients with sickle cell disease spanning from pediatric to adult age groups - revisiting this controversial concept after 16 years of additional evidence. *Am J Hematol.* 2021;96(1):31-39. doi:10.1002/ajh.26003

375. Sachdev V, Kato GJ, Gibbs JS, et al. Echocardiographic markers of elevated pulmonary pressure and left ventricular diastolic dysfunction are associated with exercise intolerance in adults and adolescents with homozygous sickle cell anemia in the United States and United Kingdom. *Circulation.* 2011;124(13):1452-1460. doi:10.1161/CIRCULATIONAHA.111.032920

376. Alsaied T, Niss O, Powell AW, et al. Diastolic dysfunction is associated with exercise impairment in patients with sickle cell anemia. *Pediatr Blood Cancer.* 2018;65(8):e27113. doi:10.1002/pbc.27113

377. Junqueira FP, Fernandes JL, Cunha GM, et al. Right and left ventricular function and myocardial scarring in adult patients with sickle cell disease: a comprehensive magnetic resonance assessment of hepatic and myocardial iron overload. *J Cardiovasc Magn Reson.* 2013;15:83. doi:10.1186/1532-429X-15-83

378. Liem RI, Young LT, Thompson AA. Prolonged QTc interval in children and young adults with sickle cell disease at steady state. *Pediatr Blood Cancer.* 2009;52(7):842-846. doi:10.1002/pbc.21973

379. Rai P, Niss O, Malik P. A reappraisal of the mechanisms underlying the cardiac complications of sickle cell anemia. *Pediatr Blood Cancer.* 2017;64(17):e26607. doi:10.1002/pbc.26607

380. Gupta A, Fei YD, Kim TY, et al. IL-18 mediates sickle cell cardiomyopathy and ventricular arrhythmias. *Blood.* 2021;137(9):1208-1218. doi:10.1182/blood.2020005944

381. Bakeer N, James J, Roy S, et al. Sickle cell anemia mice develop a unique cardiomyopathy with restrictive physiology. *Proc Natl Acad Sci U S A.* 2016;113(35):E5182-E5191. doi:10.1073/pnas.1600311113

382. Niss O, Quinn CT, Lane A, et al. Cardiomyopathy with restrictive physiology in sickle cell disease. *JACC Cardiovasc Imaging.* 2016;9(3):243-252. doi:10.1016/j.jcmg.2015.05.013

383. Knight-Madden JM, Forrester TS, Lewis NA, Greenough A. The impact of recurrent acute chest syndrome on the lung function of young adults with sickle cell disease. *Lung.* 2010;188(6):499-504. doi:10.1007/s00408-010-9255-2

384. Miller AC, Gladwin MT. Pulmonary complications of sickle cell disease. *Am J Respir Crit Care Med.* 2012;185(11):1154-1165. doi:10.1164/rccm.201111-2082CI

385. Al Biltagi M, Bediwy AS, Toema O, Al-Asy HM, Saeed NK. Pulmonary functions in children and adolescents with sickle cell disease. *Pediatr Pulmonol.* 2020;55(8):2055-2063. doi:10.1002/ppul.24871

386. Klings ES, Wyszynski DF, Nolan VG, Steinberg MH. Abnormal pulmonary function in adults with sickle cell anemia. *Am J Respir Crit Care Med.* 2006;173(11):1264-1269. doi:10.1164/rccm.200601-125OC

387. Galadanci NA, Liang WH, Galadanci AA, et al. Wheezing is common in children with sickle cell disease when compared with controls. *J Pediatr Hematol Oncol.* 2015;37(1):16-19. doi:10.1097/MPH.0000000000000239

388. Koumbourlis AC. Lung function in sickle cell disease. *Paediatr Respir Rev.* 2014;15(1):33-37. doi:10.1016/j.prrv.2013.10.002

389. Homi J, Levee L, Higgs D, Thomas P, Serjeant G. Pulse oximetry in a cohort study of sickle cell disease. *Clin Lab Haematol.* 1997;19(1):17-22.

390. Quinn CT, Ahmad N. Clinical correlates of steady-state oxyhaemoglobin desaturation in children who have sickle cell disease. *Br J Haematol.* 2005;131(1):129-134.

391. Blaisdell CJ, Goodman S, Clark K, Casella JF, Loughlin GM. Pulse oximetry is a poor predictor of hypoxemia in stable children with sickle cell disease. *Arch Pediatr Adolesc Med.* 2000;154(9):900-903.

392. Fitzgerald RK, Johnson A. Pulse oximetry in sickle cell anemia. *Crit Care Med.* 2001;29(9):1803-1806.

393. Field JJ, Stocks J, Kirkham FJ, et al. Airway hyperresponsiveness in children with sickle cell anemia. *Chest.* 2011;139(3):563-568. doi:10.1378/chest.10-1243

394. Ozbek OY, Malbora B, Sen N, Yazici AC, Ozyurek E, Ozbek N. Airway hyperreactivity detected by methacholine challenge in children with sickle cell disease. *Pediatr Pulmonol.* 2007;42(12):1187-1192. doi:10.1002/ppul.20716

395. Leong MA, Dampier C, Varlotta L, Allen JL. Airway hyperreactivity in children with sickle cell disease. *J Pediatr.* 1997;131(2):278-283.

396. Boyd JH, Macklin EA, Strunk RC, DeBaun MR. Asthma is associated with increased mortality in individuals with sickle cell anemia. *Haematologica.* 2007;92(8):1115-1118.

397. Glassberg JA, Chow A, Wisnivesky J, Hoffman R, Debaun MR, Richardson LD. Wheezing and asthma are independent risk factors for increased sickle cell disease morbidity. *Br J Haematol.* 2012;159(4):472-479. doi:10.1111/bjh.12049

398. Musa BM, Galadanci NA, Rodeghier M, Debaun MR. Higher prevalence of wheezing and lower FEV1 and FVC percent predicted in adults with sickle cell anaemia: a cross-sectional study. *Respirology.* 2017;22(2):284-288. doi:10.1111/resp.12895

399. Bendiak GN, Mateos-Corral D, Sallam A, et al. Association of wheeze with lung function decline in children with sickle cell disease. *Eur Respir J.* 2017;50(5):1602433. doi:10.1183/13993003.02433-2016

400. Cohen RT, Madadi A, Blinder MA, DeBaun MR, Strunk RC, Field JJ. Recurrent, severe wheezing is associated with morbidity and mortality in adults with sickle cell disease. *Am J Hematol.* 2011;86(9):756-761. doi:10.1002/ajh.22098

401. Kassim AA, Payne AB, Rodeghier M, Macklin EA, Strunk RC, DeBaun MR. Low forced expiratory volume is associated with earlier death in sickle cell anemia. *Blood.* 2015;126(13):1544-1550. doi:10.1182/blood-2015-05-644435

402. Field JJ, Horst J, Strunk RC, White FV, DeBaun MR. Death due to asthma in two adolescents with sickle cell disease. *Pediatr Blood Cancer.* 2011;56(3):454-457. doi:10.1002/pbc.22891

403. Lunt A, Ahmed N, Rafferty GF, et al. Airway and alveolar nitric oxide production, lung function, and pulmonary blood flow in sickle cell disease. *Pediatr Res.* 2016;79(2):313-317. doi:10.1038/pr.2015.217

404. Field JJ, DeBaun MR. Asthma and sickle cell disease: two distinct diseases or part of the same process? *Hematology Am Soc Hematol Educ Program.* 2009;(1):45-53. doi:10.1182/asheducation-2009.1.45

405. Castro O, Hoque M, Brown BD. Pulmonary hypertension in sickle cell disease: cardiac catheterization results and survival. *Blood.* 2003;101(4):1257-1261.

406. Sutton LL, Castro O, Cross DJ, Spencer JE, Lewis JF. Pulmonary hypertension in sickle cell disease. *Am J Cardiol.* 1994;74(6):626-628.

407. Fitzgerald M, Fagan K, Herbert DE, Al-Ali M, Mugal M, Haynes J Jr. Misclassification of pulmonary hypertension in adults with sickle hemoglobinopathies using Doppler echocardiography. *South Med J.* 2012;105(6):300-305. doi:10.1097/SMJ.0b013e318256b55b

408. Parent F, Bachir D, Inamo J, et al. A hemodynamic study of pulmonary hypertension in sickle cell disease. *N Engl J Med.* 2011;365(1):44-53. doi:10.1056/NEJMoa1005565

409. Forrest S, Kim A, Carbonella J, Pashankar F. Proteinuria is associated with elevated tricuspid regurgitant jet velocity in children with sickle cell disease. *Pediatr Blood Cancer.* 2012;58(6):937-940. doi:10.1002/pbc.23338

410. Lee MT, Small T, Khan MA, Rosenzweig EB, Barst RJ, Brittenham GM. Doppler-defined pulmonary hypertension and the risk of death in children with sickle cell disease followed for a mean of three years. *Br J Haematol.* 2009;146(4):437-441. doi:10.1111/j.1365-2141.2009.07779.x

411. Nouraie M, Darbari DS, Rana S, et al. Tricuspid regurgitation velocity and other biomarkers of mortality in children, adolescents and young adults with sickle cell disease in the United States: the PUSH study. *Am J Hematol.* 2020;95(7):766-774. doi:10.1002/ajh.25799

412. Gladwin MT, Sachdev V, Jison ML, et al. Pulmonary hypertension as a risk factor for death in patients with sickle cell disease. *N Engl J Med.* 2004;350(9):886-895. doi:10.1056/NEJMoa035477

413. Ataga KI, Sood N, De Gent G, et al. Pulmonary hypertension in sickle cell disease. *Am J Med.* 2004;117(9):665-669. doi:10.1016/j.amjmed.2004.03.034

414. Kato GJ, Onyekwere OC, Gladwin MT. Pulmonary hypertension in sickle cell disease: relevance to children. *Pediatr Hematol Oncol.* 2007;24(3):159-170. doi:10.1080/08880010601185892

415. Darbari DS, Onyekwere O, Nouraie M, et al. Markers of severe vaso-occlusive painful episode frequency in children and adolescents with sickle cell anemia. *J Pediatr.* 2012;160(2):286-290. doi:10.1016/j.jpeds.2011.07.018

416. Minniti CP, Sable C, Campbell A, et al. Elevated tricuspid regurgitant jet velocity in children and adolescents with sickle cell disease: association with hemolysis and hemoglobin oxygen desaturation. *Haematologica.* 2009;94(3):340-347. doi:10.3324/haematol.13812

417. Detterich JA, Kato RM, Rabai M, Meiselman HJ, Coates TD, Wood JC. Chronic transfusion therapy improves but does not normalize systemic and pulmonary vasculopathy in sickle cell disease. *Blood.* 2015;126(6):703-710. doi:10.1182/blood-2014-12-614370

418. Friedman D, Szmuszkovicz J, Rabai M, Detterich JA, Menteer J, Wood JC. Systemic endothelial dysfunction in children with idiopathic pulmonary arterial hypertension correlates with disease severity. *J Heart Lung Transplant.* 2012;31(6):642-647. doi:10.1016/j.healun.2012.02.020

419. Klings ES, Machado RF, Barst RJ, et al. An official American Thoracic Society clinical practice guideline: diagnosis, risk stratification, and management of pulmonary hypertension of sickle cell disease. *Am J Respir Crit Care Med.* 2014;189(6):727-740. doi:10.1164/rccm.201401-0065ST

420. De Castro LM, Jonassaint JC, Graham FL, Ashley-Koch A, Telen MJ. Pulmonary hypertension associated with sickle cell disease: clinical and laboratory endpoints and disease outcomes. *Am J Hematol.* 2008;83(1):19-25. doi:10.1002/ajh.21058

421. Colombatti R, Maschietto N, Varotto E, et al. Pulmonary hypertension in sickle cell disease children under 10 years of age. *Br J Haematol.* 2010;150(5):601-609. doi:10.1111/j.1365-2141.2010.08269.x

422. Ataga KI, Moore CG, Jones S, et al. Pulmonary hypertension in patients with sickle cell disease: a longitudinal study. *Br J Haematol.* 2006;134(1):109-115. doi:10.1111/j.1365-2141.2006.06110.x

423. Gordeuk VR, Minniti CP, Nouraie M, et al. Elevated tricuspid regurgitation velocity and decline in exercise capacity over 22 months of follow up in children and adolescents with sickle cell anemia. *Haematologica.* 2011;96(1):33-40. doi:10.3324/haematol.2010.030767

424. Ambrusko SJ, Gunawardena S, Sakara A, et al. Elevation of tricuspid regurgitant jet velocity, a marker for pulmonary hypertension in children with sickle cell disease. *Pediatr Blood Cancer.* 2006;47(7):907-913.

425. Pashankar FD, Carbonella J, Bazzy-Asaad A, Friedman A. Longitudinal follow up of elevated pulmonary artery pressures in children with sickle cell disease. *Br J Haematol.* 2009;144(5):736-741. doi:10.1111/j.1365-2141.2008.07501.x

426. Tsitsikas DA, Seligman H, Sirigireddy B, Odeh L, Nzouakou R, Amos RJ. Regular automated red cell exchange transfusion in the management of pulmonary hypertension in sickle cell disease. *Br J Haematol.* 2014;167(5):707-710. doi:10.1111/bjh.13031

427. Liem RI, Nevin MA, Prestridge A, Young LT, Thompson AA. Tricuspid regurgitant jet velocity elevation and its relationship to lung function in pediatric sickle cell disease. *Pediatr Pulmonol.* 2009;44(3):281-289. doi:10.1002/ppul.20996

428. Rai P, Joshi VM, Goldberg JF, et al. Longitudinal effect of disease-modifying therapy on tricuspid regurgitant velocity in children with sickle cell anemia. *Blood Adv.* 2021;5(1):89-98. doi:10.1182/bloodadvances.2020003197

429. Machado RF, Barst RJ, Yovetich NA, et al. Hospitalization for pain in patients with sickle cell disease treated with sildenafil for elevated TRV and low exercise capacity. *Blood.* 2011;118(4):855-864. doi:10.1182/blood-2010-09-306167

430. Gladwin MT, Kato GJ. Cardiopulmonary complications of sickle cell disease: role of nitric oxide and hemolytic anemia. *Hematology Am Soc Hematol EducProgram.* 2005;2005:51-57.

431. Barst RJ, Mubarak KK, Machado RF, et al. Exercise capacity and haemodynamics in patients with sickle cell disease with pulmonary hypertension treated with bosentan: results of the ASSET studies. *Br J Haematol.* 2010;149(3):426-435. doi:10.1111/j.1365-2141.2010.08097.x

432. Anthi A, Machado RF, Jison ML, et al. Hemodynamic and functional assessment of patients with sickle cell disease and pulmonary hypertension. *Am J Respir Crit Care Med.* 2007;175(12):1272-1279. doi:10.1164/rccm.200610-1498OC

433. van Beers EJ, Spronk HM, Ten Cate H, et al. No association of the hypercoagulable state with sickle cell disease related pulmonary hypertension. *Haematologica.* 2008;93(5):e42-e44. doi:10.3324/haematol.12632

434. van Beers EJ, van Eck-Smit BL, Mac Gillavry MR, et al. Large and medium-sized pulmonary artery obstruction does not play a role of primary importance in the etiology of sickle-cell disease-associated pulmonary hypertension. *Chest.* 2008;133(3):646-652. doi:10.1378/chest.07-1694

435. Hankins JS, Verevkina NI, Smeltzer MP, Wu S, Aygun B, Clarke DF. Assessment of sleep-related disorders in children with sickle cell disease. *Hemoglobin.* 2014;38(4):244-251. doi:10.3109/03630269.2014.919941

436. Rosen CL, Debaun MR, Strunk RC, et al. Obstructive sleep apnea and sickle cell anemia. *Pediatrics.* 2014;134(2):273-281. doi:10.1542/peds.2013-4223

437. Sharma S, Efird JT, Knupp C, et al. Sleep disorders in adult sickle cell patients. *J Clin Sleep Med.* 2015;11(3):219-223. doi:10.5664/jcsm.4530

438. Lehmann GC, Bell TR, Kirkham FJ, et al. Enuresis associated with sleep disordered breathing in children with sickle cell anemia. *J Urol.* 2012;188(4 suppl):1572-1576. doi:10.1016/j.juro.2012.02.021

439. Roizenblatt M, Figueiredo MS, Cancado RD, et al. Priapism is associated with sleep hypoxemia in sickle cell disease. *J Urol.* 2012;188(4):1245-1251. doi:10.1016/j.juro.2012.06.015

440. Johnson CS, Omata M, Tong MJ, Simmons JF Jr, Weiner J, Tatter D. Liver involvement in sickle cell disease. *Medicine (Baltimore).* 1985;64(5):349-356.

441. Smits HL, Oski FA, Brody JI. The hemolytic crisis of sickle cell disease: the role of glucose-6-phosphate dehydrogenase deficiency. *J Pediatr.* 1969;74(4):544-551.

442. Yohannan MD, Arif M, Ramia S. Aetiology of icteric hepatitis and fulminant hepatic failure in children and the possible predisposition to hepatic failure by sickle cell disease. *Acta Paediatr Scand.* 1990;79(2):201-205.

443. Sarnaik SA, Merline JR, Bond S. Immunogenicity of hepatitis B vaccine in children with sickle cell anemia. *J Pediatr.* 1988;112(3):429-430.

444. Hord J, Windsor B, Koehler M, Blatt J, Janosky J, Mirro J. Diminished antibody response to hepatitis B immunization in children with sickle cell disease. *J Pediatr Hematol Oncol.* 2002;24(7):548-549.

445. DeVault KR, Friedman LS, Westerberg S, Martin P, Hosein B, Ballas SK. Hepatitis C in sickle cell anemia. *J Clin Gastroenterol.* 1994;18(3):206-209.

446. Hasan MF, Marsh F, Posner G, et al. Chronic hepatitis C in patients with sickle cell disease. *Am J Gastroenterol.* 1996;91(6):1204-1206.

447. Gardner K, Suddle A, Kane P, et al. How we treat sickle hepatopathy and liver transplantation in adults. *Blood.* 2014;123(15):2302-2307. doi:10.1182/blood-2013-12-542076

448. Jeng MR, Rieman MD, Naidu PE, et al. Resolution of chronic hepatic sequestration in a patient with homozygous sickle cell disease receiving hydroxyurea. *J Pediatr Hematol Oncol.* 2003;25(3):257-260.

449. Sty JR. Ultrasonography: hepatic vein thrombosis in sickle cell anemia. *Am J Pediatr Hematol Oncol.* Summer1982;4(2):213-215.

450. Rosenblate HJ, Eisenstein R, Holmes AW. The liver in sickle cell anemia. A clinical-pathologic study. *ArchPathol.* 1970;90(3):235-245.

451. Ahn H, Li CS, Wang W. Sickle cell hepatopathy: clinical presentation, treatment, and outcome in pediatric and adult patients. *Pediatr Blood Cancer.* 2005;45(2):184-190.

452. Buchanan GR, Glader BE. Benign course of extreme hyperbilirubinemia in sickle cell anemia: analysis of six cases. *J Pediatr.* 1977;91(1):21-24.

453. Stephan JL, Merpit-Gonon E, Richard O, Raynaud-Ravni C, Freycon F. Fulminant liver failure in a 12-year-old girl with sickle cell anaemia: favourable outcome after exchange transfusions. *Eur J Pediatr.* 1995;154(6):469-471. doi:10.1007/BF02029357

454. Haydek JP, Taborda C, Shah R, et al. Extreme hyperbilirubinemia: an indicator of morbidity and mortality in sickle cell disease. *World J Hepatol.* 2019;11(3):287-293. doi:10.4254/wjh.v11.i3.287

455. Sarnaik S, Slovis TL, Corbett DP, Emami A, Whitten CF. Incidence of cholelithiasis in sickle cell anemia using the ultrasonic gray-scale technique. *J Pediatr.* 1980;96(6):1005-1008.

456. Winter SS, Kinney TR, Ware RE. Gallbladder sludge in children with sickle cell disease. *J Pediatr.* 1994;125(5 pt 1):747-749.

457. Passon RG, Howard TA, Zimmerman SA, Schultz WH, Ware RE. Influence of bilirubin uridine diphosphate-glucuronosyltransferase 1A promoter polymorphisms on serum bilirubin levels and cholelithiasis in children with sickle cell anemia. *J Pediatr Hematol Oncol.* 2001;23(7):448-451.

458. McCarville MB, Rogers ZR, Sarnaik S, et al. Effects of chronic transfusions on abdominal sonographic abnormalities in children with sickle cell anemia. *J Pediatr.* 2012;160(2):281.e1-285.e1. doi:10.1016/j.jpeds.2011.07.050

459. Al Mulhim AS, Al Mulhim FM, Al Suwaiygh AA. The role of laparoscopic cholecystectomy in the management of acute cholecystitis in patients with sickle cell disease. *Am J Surg.* 2002;183(6):668-672.

460. Ware RE, Kinney TR, Casey JR, Pappas TN, Meyers WC. Laparoscopic cholecystectomy in young patients with sickle hemoglobinopathies. *J Pediatr.* 1992;120(1):58-61.

461. Goodwin EF, Partain PI, Lebensburger JD, Fineberg NS, Howard TH. Elective cholecystectomy reduces morbidity of cholelithiasis in pediatric sickle cell disease. *Pediatr Blood Cancer.* 2017;64(1):113-120. doi:10.1002/pbc.26179

462. Curro G, Meo A, Ippolito D, Pusiol A, Cucinotta E. Asymptomatic cholelithiasis in children with sickle cell disease: early or delayed cholecystectomy? *Ann Surg.* 2007;245(1):126-129. doi:10.1097/01.sla.0000242716.66878.23

463. Hankins JS, Smeltzer MP, McCarville MB, et al. Patterns of liver iron accumulation in patients with sickle cell disease and thalassemia with iron overload. *Eur J Haematol.* 2010;85(1):51-57. doi:10.1111/j.1600-0609.2010.01449.x

464. Buckalew VM Jr, Someren A. Renal manifestations of sickle cell disease. *Arch Intern Med.* 1974;133(4):660-669.

465. Elfenbein IB, Patchefsky A, Schwartz W, Weinstein AG. Pathology of the glomerulus in sickle cell anemia with and without nephrotic syndrome. *Am J Pathol.* 1974;77(3):357-374.

466. Khademi M, Marquis JR. Renal angiography in sickle-cell disease. A preliminary report correlating the angiographic and urographic changes in sickle-cell nephropathy. *Radiology.* 1973;107(1):41-46.

467. Keitel HG. Hyposthenuria in sickle cell anemia. A reversible renal defect. *J Clin Invest*. 1956;35:998.
468. Perillie P, Epstein FH. Sickling phenomenon produced by hypertonic solutions: a possible explanation for the hyposthenuria of sicklemia. *J Clin Invest*. 1963;42:570.
469. Suster G, Oski FA. Enuresis in sickle cell anemia. *Am J Dis Child*. 1967;113(3):311.
470. Nelli AM, Mrad FCC, Alvaia MA, et al. Prevalence of enuresis and its impact in quality of life of patients with sickle cell disease. *Int Braz J Urol*. 2019;45(5):974-980. doi:10.1590/S1677-5538.IBJU.2019.0026
471. Porter JS, Paladino AJ, Russell K, et al. Nocturnal enuresis in sickle cell: sociodemographic, medical, and quality of life factors. *J Pediatr Psychol*. 2022;47(1):75-85. doi:10.1093/jpepsy/jsab079
472. Goossens JP, Statius van Eps LW, Schouten H, Giterson AL. Incomplete renal tubular acidosis in sickle cell disease. *Clin Chim Acta*. 1972;41:149-156.
473. Ho PK, Alleyne GA. Defect in urinary acidification in adults with sickle-cell anaemia. *Lancet*. 1968;2(7575):954-955. doi:10.1016/s0140-6736(68)91175-6
474. de Jong PE, dJ-van Den Berg LT, Statius van Eps LW. The tubular reabsorption of phosphate in sickle-cell nephropathy. *Clin Sci Mol Med*. 1978;55(5):429-434.
475. Diamond HS, Meisel A, Sharon E, Holden D, Cacatian A. Hyperuricosuria and increased tubular secretion of urate in sickle cell anemia. *Am J Med*. 1975;59(6):796-802.
476. Allen TD. Sickle cell disease and hematuria: a report of 29 cases. *J Urol*. 1964;91:177.
477. Harrow BR, Sloane JA, Liebman NC. Roentgenologic demonstration of renal papillary necrosis in sickle-cell trait. *N Engl J Med*. 1963;268(18):969-976.
478. Susmano S, Lewy JE. Sickle cell disease and acute glomerulonephritis. *Am J Dis Child*. 1969;118(4):615-618.
479. Davis CJ Jr, Mostofi FK, Sesterhenn IA. Renal medullary carcinoma. The seventh sickle cell nephropathy. *Am J Surg Pathol*. 1995;19(1):1-11.
480. Bennett MA, Heslop RW, Meynell MJ. Massive haematuria associated with sickle-cell trait. *Br Med J*. 1967;1(541):677-679.
481. Black WD, Hatch FE, Acchiardo S. Aminocaproic acid in prolonged hematuria of patients with sicklemia. *Arch Intern Med*. 1976;136(6):678-681.
482. Bhathena DB, Sondheimer JH. The glomerulopathy of homozygous sickle hemoglobin (SS) disease: morphology and pathogenesis. *J Am Soc Nephrol*. 1991;1(11):1241-1252.
483. Allon M, Lawson L, Eckman JR, Delaney V, Bourke E. Effects of nonsteroidal antiinflammatory drugs on renal function in sickle cell anemia. *Kidney Int*. 1988;34(4):500-506.
484. Hatch FE Jr, Azar SH, Ainsworth TE, Nardo JM, Culbertson JW. Renal circulatory studies in young adults with sickle cell anemia. *J Lab Clin Med*. 1970;76(4):632-640.
485. Guasch A, Navarrete J, Nass K, Zayas CF. Glomerular involvement in adults with sickle cell hemoglobinopathies: prevalence and clinical correlates of progressive renal failure. *J Am Soc Nephrol*. 2006;17(8):2228-2235.
486. Aygun B, Mortier NA, Smeltzer MP, Hankins JS, Ware RE. Glomerular hyperfiltration and albuminuria in children with sickle cell anemia. *Pediatr Nephrol*. 2011;26(8):1285-1290. doi:10.1007/s00467-011-1857-2
487. Lebensburger JD, Aban I, Pernell B, et al. Hyperfiltration during early childhood precedes albuminuria in pediatric sickle cell nephropathy. *Am J Hematol*. 2019;94(4):417-423. doi:10.1002/ajh.25390
488. Lebensburger JD, Gossett J, Zahr R, et al. High bias and low precision for estimated versus measured glomerular filtration rate in pediatric sickle cell anemia. *Haematologica*. 2021;106(1):295-298. doi:10.3324/haematol.2019.242156
489. Ataga KI, Derebail VK, Archer DR. The glomerulopathy of sickle cell disease. *Am J Hematol*. 2014;89(9):907-914. doi:10.1002/ajh.23762
490. Haymann JP, Hammoudi N, Stankovic Stojanovic K, et al. Renin-angiotensin system blockade promotes a cardio-renal protection in albuminuric homozygous sickle cell patients. *Br J Haematol*. 2017;179(5):820-828. doi:10.1111/bjh.14969
491. Quinn CT, Saraf SL, Gordeuk VR, et al. Losartan for the nephropathy of sickle cell anemia: a phase-2, multicenter trial. *Am J Hematol*. 2017;92(9):E520-E528. doi:10.1002/ajh.24810
492. Thrower A, Ciccone EJ, Maitra P, Derebail VK, Cai J, Ataga KI. Effect of renin-angiotensin-aldosterone system blocking agents on progression of glomerulopathy in sickle cell disease. *Br J Haematol*. 2019;184(2):246-252. doi:10.1111/bjh.15651
493. Alvarez O, Miller ST, Wang WC, et al. Effect of hydroxyurea treatment on renal function parameters: results from the multi-center placebo-controlled BABY HUG clinical trial for infants with sickle cell anemia. *Pediatr Blood Cancer*. 2012;59(4):668-674. doi:10.1002/pbc.24100
494. Fitzhugh CD, Wigfall DR, Ware RE. Enalapril and hydroxyurea therapy for children with sickle nephropathy. *Pediatr Blood Cancer*. 2005;45(7):982-985.
495. Kasztan M, Fox BM, Speed JS, et al. Long-term endothelin-A receptor antagonism provides robust renal protection in humanized sickle cell disease mice. *J Am Soc Nephrol*. 2017;28(8):2443-2458. doi:10.1681/ASN.2016070711
496. Alvarez O, Montane B, Lopez G, Wilkinson J, Miller T. Early blood transfusions protect against microalbuminuria in children with sickle cell disease. *Pediatr Blood Cancer*. 2006;47(1):71-76.
497. van Eps LW, De Long P. Sickle cell disease. In: Schrier R, Gottschalk C, eds. *Diseases of the Kidney*. 6th ed. Little Brown & Co; 1997:561.
498. Pegelow CH, Colangelo L, Steinberg M, et al. Natural history of blood pressure in sickle cell disease: risks for stroke and death associated with relative hypertension in sickle cell anemia. *Am J Med*. 1997;102(2):171-177.
499. Lebensburger JD, Palabindela P, Howard TH, Feig DI, Aban I, Askenazi DJ. Prevalence of acute kidney injury during pediatric admissions for acute chest syndrome. *Pediatr Nephrol*. 2016;31(8):1363-1368. doi:10.1007/s00467-016-3370-0
500. Baddam S, Aban I, Hilliard L, Howard T, Askenazi D, Lebensburger JD. Acute kidney injury during a pediatric sickle cell vaso-occlusive pain crisis. *Pediatr Nephrol*. 2017;32(8):1451-1456. doi:10.1007/s00467-017-3623-6
501. McCormick M, Richardson T, Warady BA, Novelli EM, Kalpatthi R. Acute kidney injury in paediatric patients with sickle cell disease is associated with increased morbidity and resource utilization. *Br J Haematol*. 2020;189(3):559-565. doi:10.1111/bjh.16384
502. Hsu CY. Yes, AKI truly leads to CKD. *J Am Soc Nephrol*. 2012;23(6):967-969. doi:10.1681/ASN.2012030222
503. Powars DR, Elliott-Mills DD, Chan L, et al. Chronic renal failure in sickle cell disease: risk factors, clinical course, and mortality. *Ann Intern Med*. 1991;115(8):614-620.
504. Lebensburger J, Johnson SM, Askenazi DJ, Rozario NL, Howard TH, Hilliard LM. Protective role of hemoglobin and fetal hemoglobin in early kidney disease for children with sickle cell anemia. *Am J Hematol*. 2011;86(5):430-432. doi:10.1002/ajh.21994
505. Lebensburger JD, Cutter GR, Howard TH, Muntner P, Feig DI. Evaluating risk factors for chronic kidney disease in pediatric patients with sickle cell anemia. *Pediatr Nephrol*. 2017;32(9):1565-1573. doi:10.1007/s00467-017-3658-8
506. Scheinman JI. Tools to detect and modify sickle cell nephropathy. *Kidney Int*. 2006;69(11):1927-1930.
507. Gurkan S, Scarponi KJ, Hotchkiss H, Savage B, Drachtman R. Lactate dehydrogenase as a predictor of kidney involvement in patients with sickle cell anemia. *Pediatr Nephrol*. 2010;25(10):2123-2127. doi:10.1007/s00467-010-1560-8
508. Ashley-Koch AE, Okocha EC, Garrett ME, et al. MYH9 and APOL1 are both associated with sickle cell disease nephropathy. *Br J Haematol*. 2011;155(3):386-394. doi:10.1111/j.1365-2141.2011.08832.x
509. Freedman BI, Kopp JB, Langefeld CD, et al. The apolipoprotein L1 (APOL1) gene and nondiabetic nephropathy in African Americans. *J Am Soc Nephrol*. 2010;21(9):1422-1426. doi:10.1681/asn.2010070730
510. Zahr RS, Rampersaud E, Kang G, et al. Children with sickle cell anemia and APOL1 genetic variants develop albuminuria early in life. *Haematologica*. 2019;104(9):e385-e387. doi:10.3324/haematol.2018.212779
511. Friedman EA, Rao TK, Sprung CL, et al. Uremia in sickle-cell anemia treated by maintenance hemodialysis. *N Engl J Med*. 1974;291(9):431-435.
512. Montgomery R, Zibari G, Hill GS, Ratner LE. Renal transplantation in patients with sickle cell nephropathy. *Transplantation*. 1994;58(5):618-620.
513. Warady BA, Sullivan EK. Renal transplantation in children with sickle cell disease: a report of the North American pediatric renal transplant cooperative study (NAPRTCS). *Pediatr Transplant*. 1998;2(2):130-133.
514. Ojo AO, Govaerts TC, Schmouder RL, et al. Renal transplantation in end-stage sickle cell nephropathy. *Transplantation*. 1999;67(2):291-295.
515. Sharpe CC, Thein SL. Sickle cell nephropathy - a practical approach. *Br J Haematol*. 2011;155(3):287-297. doi:10.1111/j.1365-2141.2011.08853.x
516. Steinberg MH. Erythropoietin for anemia of renal failure in sickle cell disease. *N Engl J Med*. 1991;324(19):1369-1370.
517. Breen CP, Macdougall IC. Improvement of erythropoietin-resistant anaemia after renal transplantation in patients with homozygous sickle-cell disease. *Nephrol Dial Transplant*. 1998;13(11):2949-2952.
518. Goldberg MF. Natural history of untreated proliferative sickle retinopathy. *Arch Ophthalmol*. 1971;85(4):428-437.
519. Leveziel N, Lalloum F, Bastuji-Garin S, et al. Sickle-cell retinopathy: retrospective study of 730 patients followed in a referral center. *J Fr Ophtalmol*. 2012;35(5):343-347. doi:10.1016/j.jfo.2011.10.007
520. Kent D, Arya R, Aclimandos WA, Bellingham AJ, Bird AC. Screening for ophthalmic manifestations of sickle cell disease in the United Kingdom. *Eye*. 1994;8(pt 6):618-622.
521. Myint KT, Sahoo S, Thein AW, Moe S, Ni H. Laser therapy for retinopathy in sickle cell disease. *Cochrane Database Syst Rev*. 2015;(10):Cd010790. doi:10.1002/14651858.CD010790.pub2
522. Emerson GG, Lutty GA. Effects of sickle cell disease on the eye: clinical features and treatment. *Hematol Oncol Clin North Am*. 2005;19(5):957-973, ix.
523. Rodrigues M, Kashiwabuchi F, Deshpande M, et al. Expression pattern of HIF-1alpha and VEGF supports circumferential application of scatter laser for proliferative sickle retinopathy. *Invest Ophthalmol Vis Sci*. 2016;57(15):6739-6746. doi:10.1167/iovs.16-19513
524. Cai C, Linz M, Scott A. Intravitreal bevacizumab for proliferative sickle retinopathy: a case series. *J Vitreoretin Dis*. 2018;2:32-38. doi:10.1177/2474126417738627
525. Curran EL, Fleming JC, Rice K, Wang WC. Orbital compression syndrome in sickle cell disease. *Ophthalmology*. 1997;104(10):1610-1615.
526. Koshy M, Entsuah R, Koranda A, et al. Leg ulcers in patients with sickle cell disease. *Blood*. 1989;74(4):1403-1408.
527. Serjeant GR. Leg ulceration in sickle cell anemia. *Arch Intern Med*. 1974;133(4):690-694.
528. Nolan VG, Adewoye A, Baldwin C, et al. Sickle cell leg ulcers: associations with haemolysis and SNPs in Klotho, TEK and genes of the TGF-beta/BMP pathway. *Br J Haematol*. 2006;133(5):570-578.
529. Hallbook T, Lanner E. Serum-zinc and healing of venous leg ulcers. *Lancet*. 1972;2(7781):780-782.
530. Serjeant GR, Galloway RE, Gueri MC. Oral zinc sulphate in sickle-cell ulcers. *Lancet*. 1970;2(7679):891-892.
531. Wethers DL, Ramirez GM, Koshy M, et al. Accelerated healing of chronic sickle-cell leg ulcers treated with RGD peptide matrix. RGD Study Group. *Blood*. 1994;84(6):1775-1779.
532. Minniti CP, Gorbach AM, Xu D, et al. Topical sodium nitrite for chronic leg ulcers in patients with sickle cell anaemia: a phase 1 dose-finding safety and tolerability trial. *Lancet Haematol*. 2014;1(3):e95-e103.
533. Minniti CP, Knight-Madden J, Tonda M, Gray S, Lehrer-Graiwer J, Biemond BJ. The impact of voxelotor treatment on leg ulcers in patients with sickle cell disease. *Am J Hematol*. 2021;96(4):E126-E128. doi:10.1002/ajh.26101

534. Oakley LL, Mitchell S, von Rege I, et al. Perinatal outcomes in women with sickle cell disease: a matched cohort study from London, UK. *Br J Haematol.* 2021;196(4):1069-1075. doi:10.1111/bjh.17983

535. Asare EV, Olayemi E, Boafor T, et al. A case series describing causes of death in pregnant women with sickle cell disease in a low-resource setting. *Am J Hematol.* 2018;93(7):E167-E170. doi:10.1002/ajh.25115

536. Asare EV, Olayemi E, Boafor T, et al. Third trimester and early postpartum period of pregnancy have the greatest risk for ACS in women with SCD. *Am J Hematol.* 2019;94(12):E328-E331. doi:10.1002/ajh.25643

537. Asare EV, Olayemi E, Boafor T, et al. Implementation of multi-disciplinary care reduces maternal mortality in women with sickle cell disease living in low-resource setting. *Am J Hematol.* 2017;92(9):872-878. doi:10.1002/ajh.24790

538. Perkins RP. Inherited disorders of hemoglobin synthesis and pregnancy. *Am J Obstet Gynecol.* 1971;111(1):120-159.

539. Shirel T, Hubler CP, Shah R, et al. Maternal opioid dose is associated with neonatal abstinence syndrome in children born to women with sickle cell disease. *Am J Hematol.* 2016;91(4):416-419. doi:10.1002/ajh.24307

540. Smith JA, Espeland M, Bellevue R, Bonds D, Brown AK, Koshy M. Pregnancy in sickle cell disease: experience of the cooperative study of sickle cell disease. *Obstet Gynecol.* 1996;87(2):199-204.

541. Malinowski AK, Shehata N, D'Souza R, et al. Prophylactic transfusion for pregnant women with sickle cell disease: a systematic review and meta-analysis. *Blood.* 2015;126(21):2424-2435, quiz 2437. doi:10.1182/blood-2015-06-649319

542. Vianello A, Vencato E, Cantini M, et al. Improvement of maternal and fetal outcomes in women with sickle cell disease treated with early prophylactic erythrocytapheresis. *Transfusion.* 2018;58(9):2192-2201. doi:10.1111/trf.14767

543. Pecker L, Hussain S, Mahesh J, Varadhan R, Christianson MS, Lanzkron S. Diminished ovarian reserve in young women with sickle cell anemia. *Blood.* 2022;139(7):1111-1115. doi:10.1182/blood.2021012756

544. Queiroz AM, Lobo CLC, Ballas SK. Menopause in Brazilian women with sickle cell anemia with and without hydroxyurea therapy. *Hematol Transfus Cell Ther.* 2021;43(3):386-388. doi:10.1016/j.htct.2020.06.009

545. Pecker LH, Hussain S, Christianson MS, Lanzkron S. Hydroxycarbamide exposure and ovarian reserve in women with sickle cell disease in the Multicenter Study of Hydroxycarbamide. *Br J Haematol.* 2020;191(5):880-887. doi:10.1111/bjh.16976

546. Elchuri SV, Williamson RS, Clark Brown R, et al. The effects of hydroxyurea and bone marrow transplant on Anti-Mullerian hormone (AMH) levels in females with sickle cell anemia. *Blood Cells Mol Dis.* 2015;55(1):56-61. doi:10.1016/j.bcmd.2015.03.012

547. Thornburg CD, Files BA, Luo Z, et al. Impact of hydroxyurea on clinical events in the BABY HUG trial. *Blood.* 2012;120(22):4304-4310. doi:10.1182/blood-2016-10-748764

548. Pecker LH, Sharma D, Nero A, et al. Knowledge gaps in reproductive and sexual health in girls and women with sickle cell disease. *Br J Haematol.* 2021;194(6):970-979. doi:10.1111/bjh.17658

549. Ladipo OA, Falusi AG, Feldblum PJ, Osotimehin BO, Otolorin EO, Ojengbede OA. Norplant use by women with sickle cell disease. *Int J Gynaecol Obstet.* 1993;41(1):85-87.

550. Nascimento ML, Ladipo OA, Coutinho EM. Nomegestrol acetate contraceptive implant use by women with sickle cell disease. *Clin Pharmacol Ther.* 1998;64(4):433-438.

551. Legardy JK, Curtis KM. Progestogen-only contraceptive use among women with sickle cell anemia: a systematic review. *Contraception.* 2006;73(2):195-204.

552. Lanzkron S, Carroll CP, Haywood C Jr. Mortality rates and age at death from sickle cell disease: U.S., 1979-2005. *Public Health Rep.* 2013;128(2):110-116.

553. Lobo CL, Pinto JF, Nascimento EM, Moura PG, Cardoso GP, Hankins JS. The effect of hydroxcarbamide therapy on survival of children with sickle cell disease. *Br J Haematol.* 2013;161(6):852-860. doi:10.1111/bjh.12323

554. Chaturvedi S, Ghafuri DL, Jordan N, Kassim A, Rodeghier M, DeBaun MR. Clustering of end-organ disease and earlier mortality in adults with sickle cell disease: a retrospective-prospective cohort study. *Am J Hematol.* 2018;93(9):1153-1160. doi:10.1002/ajh.25202

555. DeBaun MR, Ghafuri DL, Rodeghier M, et al. Decreased median survival of adults with sickle cell disease after adjusting for left truncation bias: a pooled analysis. *Blood.* 2019;133(6):615-617. doi:10.1182/blood-2018-10-880575

556. Chaturvedi S, Labib Ghafuri D, Kassim A, Rodeghier M, DeBaun MR. Elevated tricuspid regurgitant jet velocity, reduced forced expiratory volume in 1 second, and mortality in adults with sickle cell disease. *Am J Hematol.* 2017;92(2):125-130. doi:10.1002/ajh.24598

557. Zahr RS, Hankins JS, Kang G, et al. Hydroxyurea prevents onset and progression of albuminuria in children with sickle cell anemia. *Am J Hematol.* 2019;94(1):E27-E29. doi:10.1002/ajh.25329

558. Rashkin SR, Rampersaud E, Kang G, et al. Generalization of a genetic risk score for time to first albuminuria in children with sickle cell anaemia: SCCRIP cohort study results. *Br J Haematol.* 2021;194(2):469-473. doi:10.1111/bjh.17647

559. Estepp JH, Cong Z, Agodoa I, et al. What drives transcranial Doppler velocity improvement in paediatric sickle cell anaemia: analysis from the Sickle Cell Clinical Research and Intervention Program (SCCRIP) longitudinal cohort study. *Br J Haematol.* 2021;194(2):463-468. doi:10.1111/bjh.17620

560. Maroda AJ, Spence MN, Larson SR, et al. Screening for obstructive sleep apnea in children with sickle cell disease: a pilot study. *Laryngoscope.* 2021;131(3):E1022-E1028. doi:10.1002/lary.29036

561. Estepp JH, Smeltzer MP, Wang WC, Hoehn ME, Hankins JS, Aygun B. Protection from sickle cell retinopathy is associated with elevated HbF levels and hydroxycarbamide use in children. *Br J Haematol.* 2013;161(3):402-405. doi:10.1111/bjh.12238

562. Odunubun ME, Okolo AA, Rahimy CM. Newborn screening for sickle cell disease in a Nigerian hospital. *Publ Health.* 2008;122(10):1111-1116. doi:10.1016/j.puhe.2008.01.008

563. Galadanci N, Wudil BJ, Balogun TM, et al. Current sickle cell disease management practices in Nigeria. *Int Health.* 2014;6(1):23-28. doi:10.1093/inthealth/iht022

564. Grosse SD, Odame I, Atrash HK, Amendah DD, Piel FB, Williams TN. Sickle cell disease in Africa: a neglected cause of early childhood mortality. *Am J Prev Med.* 2011;41(6 suppl 4):S398-S405. doi:10.1016/j.amepre.2011.09.013

565. McGann PT, Ferris MG, Ramamurthy U, et al. A prospective newborn screening and treatment program for sickle cell anemia in Luanda, Angola. *Am J Hematol.* 2013;88(12):984-989. doi:10.1002/ajh.23578

566. Rahimy MC, Gangbo A, Ahouignan G, Alihonou E. Newborn screening for sickle cell disease in the Republic of Benin. *J Clin Pathol.* 2009;62(1):46-48. doi:10.1136/jcp.2008.059113

567. Pembrey ME, Wood WG, Weatherall DJ, Perrine RP. Fetal haemoglobin production and the sickle gene in the oases of Eastern Saudi Arabia. *Br J Haematol.* 1978;40(3):415-429.

568. Perrine RP, Pembrey ME, John P, Perrine S, Shoup F. Natural history of sickle cell anemia in Saudi Arabs. A study of 270 subjects. *Ann Intern Med.* 1978;88(1):1-6.

569. Acquaye JK, Omer A, Ganeshaguru K, Sejeny SA, Hoffbrand AV. Non-benign sickle cell anaemia in Western Saudi Arabia. *Br J Haematol.* 1985;60(1):99-108.

570. Serjeant GR, Vichinsky E. Variability of homozygous sickle cell disease: the role of alpha and beta globin chain variation and other factors. *Blood Cells Mol Dis.* 2018;70:66-77. doi:10.1016/j.bcmd.2017.06.004

571. Day ME, Rodeghier M, DeBaun MR. Children with HbSbeta(0) thalassemia have higher hemoglobin levels and lower incidence rate of acute chest syndrome compared to children with HbSS. *Pediatr Blood Cancer.* 2018;65(11):e27352. doi:10.1002/pbc.27352

572. Lettre G, Bauer DE. Fetal haemoglobin in sickle-cell disease: from genetic epidemiology to new therapeutic strategies. *Lancet.* 2016;387(10037):2554-2564. doi:10.1016/S0140-6736(15)01341-0

573. Akinsheye I, Alsultan A, Solovieff N, et al. Fetal hemoglobin in sickle cell anemia. *Blood.* 2011;118(1):19-27. doi:10.1182/blood-2011-03-325258

574. Galarneau G, Palmer CD, Sankaran VG, Orkin SH, Hirschhorn JN, Lettre G. Fine-mapping at three loci known to affect fetal hemoglobin levels explains additional genetic variation. *Nat Genet.* 2010;42(12):1049-1051. doi:10.1038/ng.707

575. Kormann R, Jannot AS, Narjoz C, et al. Roles of APOL1 G1 and G2 variants in sickle cell disease patients: kidney is the main target. *Br J Haematol.* 2017;179(2):323-335. doi:10.1111/bjh.14842

576. Saraf SL, Zhang X, Shah B, et al. Genetic variants and cell-free hemoglobin processing in sickle cell nephropathy. *Haematologica.* 2015;100(10):1275-1284. doi:10.3324/haematol.2015.124875

577. Schaefer BA, Flanagan JM, Alvarez OA, et al. Genetic modifiers of white blood cell count, albuminuria and glomerular filtration rate in children with sickle cell anemia. *PLoS One.* 2016;11(10):e0164364. doi:10.1371/journal.pone.0164364

578. Haverfield EV, McKenzie CA, Forrester T, et al. UGT1A1 variation and gallstone formation in sickle cell disease. *Blood.* 2005;105(3):968-972. doi:10.1182/blood-2004-02-0521

579. Milton JN, Sebastiani P, Solovieff N, et al. A genome-wide association study of total bilirubin and cholelithiasis risk in sickle cell anemia. *PLoS One.* 2012;7(4):e34741. doi:10.1371/journal.pone.0034741

580. Rampersaud E, Kang G, Palmer LE, et al. A polygenic score for acute vaso-occlusive pain in pediatric sickle cell disease. *Blood Adv.* 2021;5(14):2839-2851. doi:10.1182/bloodadvances.2021004634

581. Brown AK, Sleeper LA, Miller ST, Pegelow CH, Gill FM, Waclawiw MA. Reference values and hematologic changes from birth to 5 years in patients with sickle cell disease. Cooperative Study of Sickle Cell Disease. *Arch Pediatr Adolesc Med.* 1994;148(8):796-804. doi:10.1001/archpedi.1994.02170080026005

582. Boyer SH, Belding TK, Margolet L, Noyes AN. Fetal hemoglobin restriction to a few erythrocytes (F cells) in normal human adults. *Science.* 1975;188(4186):361-363. doi:10.1126/science.804182

583. Steinberg MH, Hsu H, Nagel RL, et al. Gender and haplotype effects upon hematological manifestations of adult sickle cell anemia. *Am J Hematol.* 1995;48(3):175-181. doi:10.1002/ajh.2830480307

584. Serjeant GR. Natural history and determinants of clinical severity of sickle cell disease. *Curr Opin Hematol.* 1995;2(2):103-108. doi:10.1097/00062752-199502020-00001

585. Sunshine HR, Hofrichter J, Eaton WA. Gelation of sickle cell hemoglobin in mixtures with normal adult and fetal hemoglobins. *J Mol Biol.* 1979;133(4):435-467. doi:10.1016/0022-2836(79)90402-9

586. Wood WG. Increased HbF in adult life. *Baillieres Clin Haematol.* 1993;6(1):177-213. doi:10.1016/s0950-3536(05)80070-8

587. Powars DR, Chan L, Schroeder WA. The influence of fetal hemoglobin on the clinical expression of sickle cell anemia. *Ann N Y Acad Sci.* 1989;565:262-278. doi:10.1111/j.1749-6632.1989.tb24174.x

588. Powars DR, Weiss JN, Chan LS, Schroeder WA. Is there a threshold level of fetal hemoglobin that ameliorates morbidity in sickle cell anemia? *Blood.* 1984;63(4):921-926.

589. Dover GJ, Boyer SH, Charache S, Heintzelman K. Individual variation in the production and survival of F cells in sickle-cell disease. *N Engl J Med.* 1978;299(26):1428-1435.

590. Bhatnagar P, Purvis S, Barron-Casella E, et al. Genome-wide association study identifies genetic variants influencing F-cell levels in sickle-cell patients. *J Hum Genet.* 2011;56(4):316-323. doi:10.1038/jhg.2011.12

591. Miller BA, Salameh M, Ahmed M, et al. Analysis of hemoglobin F production in Saudi Arabian families with sickle cell anemia. *Blood.* 1987;70(3):716-720.

Disorders of Red Blood Cells

592. Ali SA. Milder variant of sickle-cell disease in Arabs in Kuwait associated with unusually high level of foetal haemoglobin. *Br J Haematol*. 1970;19(5):613-619.

593. Haghshenass M, Ismail-Beigi F, Clegg JB, Weatherall DJ. Mild sickle-cell anaemia in Iran associated with high levels of fetal haemoglobin. *J Med Genet*. 1977;14(3):168-171.

594. Kar BC, Satapathy RK, Kulozik AE, et al. Sickle cell disease in Orissa State, India. *Lancet*. 1986;2(8517):1198-1201.

595. Serjeant GR. Fetal haemoglobin in homozygous sickle cell disease. *Clin Haematol*. 1975;4(1):109-122.

596. Embury SH, Clark MR, Monroy G, Mohandas N. Concurrent sickle cell anemia and alpha-thalassemia. Effect on pathological properties of sickle erythrocytes. *J Clin Invest*. 1984;73(1):116-123.

597. Fabry ME, Mears JG, Patel P, et al. Dense cells in sickle cell anemia: the effects of gene interaction. *Blood*. 1984;64(5):1042-1046.

598. Embury SH, Backer K, Glader BE. Monovalent cation changes in sickle erythrocytes: a direct reflection of alpha-globin gene number. *J Lab Clin Med*. 1985;106(1):75-79.

599. De Ceulaer K, Higgs DR, Weatherall DJ, Hayes RJ, Serjeant BE, Serjeant GR. alpha-Thalassemia reduces the hemolytic rate in homozygous sickle-cell disease. *N Engl J Med*. 1983;309(3):189-190.

600. Higgs DR, Aldridge BE, Lamb J, et al. The interaction of alpha-thalassemia and homozygous sickle-cell disease. *N Engl J Med*. 1982;306(24):1441-1446.

601. Steinberg MH, Rosenstock W, Coleman MB, et al. Effects of thalassemia and microcytosis on the hematologic and vasoocclusive severity of sickle cell anemia. *Blood*. 1984;63(6):1353-1360.

602. Schroeder WA, Powars DR, Kay LM, et al. Beta-cluster haplotypes, alpha-gene status, and hematological data from SS, SC, and S-beta-thalassemia patients in southern California. *Hemoglobin*. 1989;13(4):325-353.

603. Fox PD, Higgs DR, Serjeant GR. Influence of alpha thalassaemia on the retinopathy of homozygous sickle cell disease. *Br J Ophthalmol*. 1993;77(2):89-90.

604. Hayes RJ, Condon PI, Serjeant GR. Haematological factors associated with proliferative retinopathy in homozygous sickle cell disease. *Br J Ophthalmol*. 1981;65(1):29-35.

605. Miller ST, Sleeper LA, Pegelow CH, et al. Prediction of adverse outcomes in children with sickle cell disease. *N Engl J Med*. 2000;342(2):83-89.

606. Quinn CT, Shull EP, Ahmad N, Lee NJ, Rogers ZR, Buchanan GR. Prognostic significance of early vaso-occlusive complications in children with sickle cell anemia. *Blood*. 2007;109(1):40-45. doi:10.1182/blood-2006-02-005082

607. Menzel S, Garner C, Gut I, et al. A QTL influencing F cell production maps to a gene encoding a zinc-finger protein on chromosome 2p15. *Nat Genet*. 2007;39(10):1197-1199. doi:10.1038/ng2108

608. Orkin SH, HiggsMedicine DR. Sickle cell disease at 100 years. *Science*. 2010;329(5989):291-292. doi:10.1126/science.1194035

609. Williams DA, Esrick E. Investigational curative gene therapy approaches to sickle cell disease. *Blood Adv*. 2021;5(23):5452. doi:10.1182/bloodadvances.2021005567

610. Mehta P. Significance of plasma beta-thromboglobulin values in patients with sickle cell disease. *J Pediatr*. 1980;97(6):941-944.

611. Gordon EM, Klein BL, Berman BW, Strandjord SE, Simon JE, Coccia PF. Reduction of contact factors in sickle cell disease. *J Pediatr*. 1985;106(3):427-430.

612. Christopher H, Burns A, Josephat E, Makani J, Schuh A, Nkya S. Using DNA testing for the precise, definite, and low-cost diagnosis of sickle cell disease and other Haemoglobinopathies: findings from Tanzania. *BMC Genom*. 2021;22(1):902. doi:10.1186/s12864-021-08220-x

613. Dexter D, McGann PT. Saving lives through early diagnosis: the promise and role of point of care testing for sickle cell disease. *Br J Haematol*. 2022;196(1):63-69. doi:10.1111/bjh.17678

614. Modell B, Darlison M. Global epidemiology of haemoglobin disorders and derived service indicators. *Bull World Health Organ*. 2008;86(6):480-487.

615. Therrell BL Jr, Lloyd-Puryear MA, Eckman JR, Mann MY. Newborn screening for sickle cell diseases in the United States: a review of data spanning 2 decades. *Semin Perinatol*. 2015;39(3):238-251. doi:10.1053/j.semperi.2015.03.008

616. Hustace T, Fleisher JM, Sanchez Varela AM, Podda A, Alvarez O. Increased prevalence of false positive hemoglobinopathy newborn screening in premature infants. *Pediatr Blood Cancer*. 2011;57(6):1039-1043. doi:10.1002/pbc.23173

617. Karnon J, Zeuner D, Ades AE, Efimba W, Brown J, Yardumian A. The effects of neonatal screening for sickle cell disorders on lifetime treatment costs and early deaths avoided: a modelling approach. *J Public Health Med*. 2000;22(4):500-511.

618. Day SW, Brunson GE, Wang WC. Successful newborn sickle cell trait counseling program using health department nurses. *Pediatr Nurs*. 1997;23(6):557-561.

619. Piety NZ, George A, Serrano S, et al. A paper-based test for screening newborns for sickle cell disease. *Sci Rep*. 2017;7:45488. doi:10.1038/srep45488

620. Tubman VN, Marshall R, Jallah W, et al. Newborn screening for sickle cell disease in Liberia: a pilot study. *Pediatr Blood Cancer*. 2016;63(4):671-676. doi:10.1002/pbc.25875

621. Kuznik A, Habib AG, Munube D, Lamorde M. Newborn screening and prophylactic interventions for sickle cell disease in 47 countries in sub-Saharan Africa: a cost-effectiveness analysis. *BMC Health Serv Res*. 2016;16:304. doi:10.1186/s12913-016-1572-6

622. Price JO, Elias S, Wachtel SS, et al. Prenatal diagnosis with fetal cells isolated from maternal blood by multiparameter flow cytometry. *Am J Obstet Gynecol*. 1991;165(6 pt 1):1731-1737.

623. Rechitsky S, Kuliev A, Tur-Kaspa I, Morris R, Verlinsky Y. Preimplantation genetic diagnosis with HLA matching. *Reprod Biomed Online*. 2004;9(2):210-221.

624. Oyewo A, Salubi-Udu J, Khalaf Y, et al. Preimplantation genetic diagnosis for the prevention of sickle cell disease: current trends and barriers to uptake

in a London teaching hospital. *Hum Fertil (Camb)*. 2009;12(3):153-159. doi:10.1080/14647270903037751

625. Voskaridou E, Ladis V, Kattamis A, et al. A national registry of haemoglobinopathies in Greece: deducted demographics, trends in mortality and affected births. *Ann Hematol*. 2012;91(9):1451-1458. doi:10.1007/s00277-012-1465-7

626. Murphy JR, Wengard M, Brereton W. Rheological studies of Hb SS blood: influence of hematocrit, hypertonicity, separation of cells, deoxygenation, and mixture with normal cells. *J Lab Clin Med*. 1976;87(3):475-486.

627. Adams DM, Schultz WH, Ware RE, Kinney TR. Erythrocytapheresis can reduce iron overload and prevent the need for chelation therapy in chronically transfused pediatric patients. *J PediatrHematolOncol*. 1996;18(1):46-50.

628. Kim HC, Dugan NP, Silber JH, et al. Erythrocytapheresis therapy to reduce iron overload in chronically transfused patients with sickle cell disease. *Blood*. 1994;83(4):1136-1142.

629. Rosse WF, Gallagher D, Kinney TR, et al. Transfusion and alloimmunization in sickle cell disease. The cooperative study of sickle cell disease. *Blood*. 1990;76(7):1431-1437.

630. Vichinsky EP, Earles A, Johnson RA, Hoag MS, Williams A, Lubin B. Alloimmunization in sickle cell anemia and transfusion of racially unmatched blood. *N Engl J Med*. 1990;322(23):1617-1621.

631. O'Suoji C, Liem RI, Mack AK, Kingsberry P, Ramsey G, Thompson AA. Alloimmunization in sickle cell anemia in the era of extended red cell typing. *Pediatr Blood Cancer*. 2013;60(9):1487-1491. doi:10.1002/pbc.24530

632. Chou ST, Jackson T, Vege S, Smith-Whitley K, Friedman DF, Westhoff CM. High prevalence of red blood cell alloimmunization in sickle cell disease despite transfusion from Rh-matched minority donors. *Blood*. 2013;122(6):1062-1071. doi:10.1182/blood-2013-03-490623

633. Casas J, Friedman DF, Jackson T, Vege S, Westhoff CM, Chou ST. Changing practice: red blood cell typing by molecular methods for patients with sickle cell disease. *Transfusion*. 2015;55(6 pt 2):1388-1393. doi:10.1111/trf.12987

634. Inati A, Musallam KM, Wood JC, Taher AT. Iron overload indices rise linearly with transfusion rate in patients with sickle cell disease. *Blood*. 2010;115(14):2980-2981. doi:10.1182/blood-2009-09-243568

635. Hankins JS, McCarville MB, Loeffler RB, et al. R2* magnetic resonance imaging of the liver in patients with iron overload. *Blood*. 2009;113(20):4853-4855. doi:10.1182/blood-2008-12-191643

636. Wood JC, Enriquez C, Ghugre N, et al. MRI R2 and R2* mapping accurately estimates hepatic iron concentration in transfusion-dependent thalassemia and sickle cell disease patients. *Blood*. 2005;106(4):1460-1465. doi:10.1182/blood-2004-10-3982

637. Noetzli LJ, Coates TD, Wood JC. Pancreatic iron loading in chronically transfused sickle cell disease is lower than in thalassaemia major. *Br J Haematol*. 2011;152(2):229-233. doi:10.1111/j.1365-2141.2010.08476.x

638. Inati A, Musallam KM, Cappellini MD, Duca L, Taher AT. Nontransferrinbound iron in transfused patients with sickle cell disease. *Int J Lab Hematol*. 2011;33(2):133-137. doi:10.1111/j.1751-553X.2010.01224.x

639. Walter PB, Fung EB, Killilea DW, et al. Oxidative stress and inflammation in ironoverloaded patients with beta-thalassaemia or sickle cell disease. *Br J Haematol*. 2006;135(2):254-263. doi:10.1111/j.1365-2141.2006.06277.x

640. Wood JC, Kang BP, Thompson A, et al. The effect of deferasirox on cardiac iron in thalassemia major: impact of total body iron stores. *Blood*. 2010;116(4):537-543. doi:10.1182/blood-2009-11-250308

641. Pennell DJ, Porter JB, Cappellini MD, et al. Deferasirox for up to 3 years leads to continued improvement of myocardial T2* in patients with beta-thalassemia major. *Haematologica*. 2012;97(6):842-848. doi:10.3324/haematol.2011.049957

642. Kwiatkowski JL. Real-world use of iron chelators. *Hematology Am Soc Hematol Educ Program*. 2011;2011:451-458. doi:10.1182/asheducation-2011.1.451

643. Borgna-Pignatti C, Cappellini MD, De Stefano P, et al. Cardiac morbidity and mortality in deferoxamine- or deferiprone-treated patients with thalassemia major. *Blood*. 2006;107(9):3733-3737. doi:10.1182/blood-2005-07-2933

644. Pennell DJ, Berdoukas V, Karagiorga M, et al. Randomized controlled trial of deferiprone or deferoxamine in beta-thalassemia major patients with asymptomatic myocardial siderosis. *Blood*. 2006;107(9):3738-3744. doi:10.1182/blood-2005-07-2948

645. Maggio A, Vitrano A, Lucania G, et al. Long-term use of deferiprone significantly enhances left-ventricular ejection function in thalassemia major patients. *Am J Hematol*. 2012;87(7):732-733. doi:10.1002/ajh.23219

646. Coates TD, Wood JC. How we manage iron overload in sickle cell patients. *Br J Haematol*. 2017;177(5):703-716. doi:10.1111/bjh.14575

647. Vichinsky EP, Haberkern CM, Neumayr L, et al. A comparison of conservative and aggressive transfusion regimens in the perioperative management of sickle cell disease. The Preoperative Transfusion in Sickle Cell Disease Study Group. *N Engl J Med*. 1995;333(4):206-213.

648. Howard J, Malfroy M, Llewelyn C, et al. The Transfusion Alternatives Preoperatively in Sickle Cell Disease (TAPS) study: a randomised, controlled, multicentre clinical trial. *Lancet*. 2013;381(9870):930-938. doi:10.1016/s0140-6736(12)61726-7

649. Rai P, Ataga KI. Drug therapies for the management of sickle cell disease. *F1000Res*. 2020;9:F1000. doi:10.12688/f1000research.22433.1

650. Charache S, Dover G, Smith K, Talbot CC Jr, Moyer M, Boyer S. Treatment of sickle cell anemia with 5-azacytidine results in increased fetal hemoglobin production and is associated with nonrandom hypomethylation of DNA around the gamma-delta-beta-globin gene complex. *Proc Natl Acad Sci U S A*. 1983;80(15):4842-4846.

651. Torrealba-de Ron A, Papayannopoulou T, Knapp MS, Fu MF, Knitter G, Stamatoyannopoulos G. Perturbations in the erythroid marrow progenitor cell pools may play a role in the augmentation of Hb F by 5-azacytidine. *N Engl J Med*. 1984;63:201.

652. Humphries RK, Dover G, Young NS, et al. 5-Azacytidine acts directly on both erythroid precursors and progenitors to increase production of fetal hemoglobin. *J Clin Invest*. 1985;75(2):547-557.
653. Veith R, Galanello R, Papayannopoulou T, Stamatoyannopoulos G. Stimulation of F-cell production in patients with sickle-cell anemia treated with cytarabine or hydroxyurea. *N Engl J Med*. 1985;313(25):1571-1575.
654. Charache S, Terrin ML, Moore RD, et al. Effect of hydroxyurea on the frequency of painful crises in sickle cell anemia. Investigators of the Multicenter Study of Hydroxyurea in Sickle Cell Anemia. *N Engl J Med*. 1995;332(20):1317-1322. doi:10.1056/NEJM199505183322001
655. Steinberg MH, Barton F, Castro O, et al. Effect of hydroxyurea on mortality and morbidity in adult sickle cell anemia: risks and benefits up to 9 years of treatment. *J Am Med Assoc*. 2003;289(13):1645-1651.
656. Wang WC, Ware RE, Miller ST, et al. Hydroxycarbamide in very young children with sickle-cell anaemia: a multicentre, randomised, controlled trial (BABY HUG). *Lancet*. 2011;377(9778):1663-1672. doi:10.1016/s0140-6736(11)60355-3
657. Ataga KI, Reid M, Ballas SK, et al. Improvements in haemolysis and indicators of erythrocyte survival do not correlate with acute vaso-occlusive crises in patients with sickle cell disease: a phase III randomized, placebo-controlled, double-blind study of the Gardos channel blocker senicapoc (ICA-17043). *Br J Haematol*. 2011;153(1):92-104. doi:10.1111/j.1365-2141.2010.08520.x
658. Wang W, Brugnara C, Snyder C, et al. The effects of hydroxycarbamide and magnesium on haemoglobin SC disease: results of the multi-centre CHAMPS trial. *Br J Haematol*. 2011;152(6):771-776. doi:10.1111/j.1365-2141.2010.08523.x
659. Brousseau DC, Scott JP, Badaki-Makun O, et al. A multicenter randomized controlled trial of intravenous magnesium for sickle cell pain crisis in children. *Blood*. 2015;126(14):1651-1657. doi:10.1182/blood-2015-05-647107
660. Field JJ. Can selectin and iNKT cell therapies meet the needs of people with sickle cell disease? *Hematology Am Soc Hematol Educ Program*. 2015;2015:426-432. doi:10.1182/asheducation-2015.1.426
661. Heeney MM, Hoppe CC, Abboud MR, et al. A multinational trial of prasugrel for sickle cell vaso-occlusive events. *N Engl J Med*. 2016;374(7):625-635. doi:10.1056/NEJMoa1512021
662. Ataga KI, Kutlar A, Kanter J, et al. Crizanlizumab for the prevention of pain crises in sickle cell disease. *N Engl J Med*. 2017;376(5):429-439. doi:10.1056/NEJMoa1611770
663. Casella JF, Barton BA, Kanter J, et al. Effect of poloxamer 188 vs placebo on painful vaso-occlusive episodes in children and adults with sickle cell disease: a randomized clinical trial. *JAMA*. 2021;325(15):1513-1523. doi:10.1001/jama.2021.3414
664. Zerez CR, Lachant NA, Lee SJ, Tanaka KR. Decreased erythrocyte nicotinamide adenine dinucleotide redox potential and abnormal pyridine nucleotide content in sickle cell disease. *Blood*. 1988;71(2):512-515.
665. Al-Ali AK. Pyridine nucleotide redox potential in erythrocytes of saudi subjects with sickle cell disease. *Acta haematologica*. 2002;108(1):19-22. doi:10.1159/000063062
666. Niihara Y, Zerez CR, Akiyama DS, Tanaka KR. Oral L-glutamine therapy for sickle cell anemia: I. Subjective clinical improvement and favorable change in red cell NAD redox potential. *Am J Hematol*. 1998;58(2):117-121. doi:10.1002/(sici)1096-8652(199806)58:2<117::aid-ajh5>3.0.co;2-v
667. Niihara Y, Miller ST, Kanter J, et al. A phase 3 trial of l-glutamine in sickle cell disease. *N Engl J Med*. 2018;379(3):226-235. doi:10.1056/NEJMoa1715971
668. Zaidi AU, Estepp J, Shah N, et al. A reanalysis of pain crises data from the pivotal l-glutamine in sickle cell disease trial. *Contemp Clin Trials*. 2021;110:106546. doi:10.1016/j.cct.2021.106546
669. Hoppe C, Jacob E, Styles L, Kuypers F, Larkin S, Vichinsky E. Simvastatin reduces vaso-occlusive pain in sickle cell anaemia: a pilot efficacy trial. *Br J Haematol*. 2017;177(4):620-629. doi:10.1111/bjh.14580
670. Field JJ, Lin G, Okam MM, et al. Sickle cell vaso-occlusion causes activation of iNKT cells that is decreased by the adenosine A2A receptor agonist regadenoson. *Blood*. 2013;121(17):3329-3334. doi:10.1182/blood-2012-11-465963
671. Gladwin MT, Kato GJ, Weiner D, et al. Nitric oxide for inhalation in the acute treatment of sickle cell pain crisis: a randomized controlled trial. *J Am Med Assoc*. 2011;305(9):893-902. doi:10.1001/jama.2011.235
672. Bakshi N, Morris CR. The role of the arginine metabolome in pain: implications for sickle cell disease. *J Pain Res*. 2016;9:167-175. doi:10.2147/jpr.s55571
673. Morris CR, Kuypers FA, Lavrisha L, et al. A randomized, placebo-controlled trial of arginine therapy for the treatment of children with sickle cell disease hospitalized with vaso-occlusive pain episodes. *Haematologica*. 2013;98(9):1375-1382. doi:10.3324/haematol.2013.086637
674. Johnson FL, Look AT, Gockerman J, Ruggiero MR, Dalla-Pozza L, Billings FT III. Bone-marrow transplantation in a patient with sickle-cell anemia. *N Engl J Med*. 1984;311(12):780-783.
675. Shenoy S, Angelucci E, Arnold SD, et al. Current results and future research priorities in late effects after hematopoietic stem cell transplantation for children with sickle cell disease and thalassemia: a consensus statement from the second pediatric blood and marrow transplant consortium international conference on late effects after pediatric hematopoietic stem cell transplantation. *Biol Blood Marrow Transplant*. 2017;23(4):552-561. doi:10.1016/j.bbmt.2017.01.009
676. Gluckman E, Cappelli B, Bernaudin F, et al. Sickle cell disease: an international survey of results of HLA-identical sibling hematopoietic stem cell transplantation. *Blood*. 2017;129(11):1548-1556. doi:10.1182/blood-2016-10-745711
677. Hsieh MM, Fitzhugh CD, Weitzel RP, et al. Nonmyeloablative HLA-matched sibling allogeneic hematopoietic stem cell transplantation for severe sickle cell phenotype. *J Am Med Assoc*. 2014;312(1):48-56. doi:10.1001/jama.2014.7192
678. King AA, Kamani N, Bunin N, et al. Successful matched sibling donor marrow transplantation following reduced intensity conditioning in children with hemoglobinopathies. *Am J Hematol*. 2015;90(12):1093-1098. doi:10.1002/ajh.24183
679. Eapen M, Brazauskas R, Walters MC, et al. Effect of donor type and conditioning regimen intensity on allogeneic transplantation outcomes in patients with sickle cell disease: a retrospective multicentre, cohort study. *Lancet Haematol*. 2019;6(11):e585-e596. doi:10.1016/S2352-3026(19)30154-1
680. Kanter J, Liem RI, Bernaudin F, et al. American Society of Hematologyguidelines for sickle cell disease: stem cell transplantation. *Blood Adv*. 20212021;5(18):3668-3689. doi:10.1182/bloodadvances.2021004394C
681. Krishnamurti L. Hematopoietic cell transplantation for sickle cell disease: updates and future directions. *Hematology Am Soc Hematol Educ Program*. 2021;2021(1):181-189. doi:10.1182/hematology.2021000251
682. Bernaudin F, Socie G, Kuentz M, et al. Long-term results of related myeloablative stem-cell transplantation to cure sickle cell disease. *Blood*. 2007;110(7):2749-2756. doi:10.1182/blood-2007-03-079665
683. Walters MC, Hardy K, Edwards S, et al. Pulmonary, gonadal, and central nervous system status after bone marrow transplantation for sickle cell disease. *Biol Blood Marrow Transplant*. 2010;16(2):263-272. doi:10.1016/j.bbmt.2009.10.005
684. Bockenmeyer J, Chamboredon E, Missud F, et al. Development of psychological and intellectual performance in transplanted sickle cell disease patients: a prospective study from pretransplant period to 5 years after HSCT. Article in French. *Arch Pediatr*. 2013;20(7):723-730. doi:10.1016/j.arcped.2013.04.012
685. Dovey S, Krishnamurti L, Sanfilippo J, et al. Oocyte cryopreservation in a patient with sickle cell disease prior to hematopoietic stem cell transplantation: first report. *J Assist Reprod Genet*. 2012;29(3):265-269. doi:10.1007/s10815-011-9698-2
686. Mentzer WC, Heller S, Pearle PR, Hackney E, Vichinsky E. Availability of related donors for bone marrow transplantation in sickle cell anemia. *Am J Pediatr Hematol Oncol*. 1994;16(1):27-29.
687. Hayes RJ, Beckford M, Grandison Y, Mason K, Serjeant BE, Serjeant GR. The haematology of steady state homozygous sickle cell disease: frequency distributions, variation with age and sex, longitudinal observations. *Br J Haematol*. 1985;59(2):369-382.
688. Piomelli S. Bone marrow transplantation in sickle cell diseases: a plea for a rational approach. *Bone Marrow Transplant*. 1992;10(suppl 1):58-61.
689. Platt OS, Guinan EC. Bone marrow transplantation in sickle cell anemia–the dilemma of choice. *N Engl J Med*. 1996;335(6):426-428.
690. Brichard B, Vermylen C, Ninane J, Cornu G. Persistence of fetal hemoglobin production after successful transplantation of cord blood stem cells in a patient with sickle cell anemia. *J Pediatr*. 1996;128(2):241-243.
691. Gore L, Lane PA, Quinones RR, Giller RH. Successful cord blood transplantation for sickle cell anemia from a sibling who is human leukocyte antigen-identical: implications for comprehensive care. *J PediatrHematolOncol*. 2000;22(5):437-440.
692. Reed W, Smith R, Dekovic F, et al. Comprehensive banking of sibling donor cord blood for children with malignant and nonmalignant disease. *Blood*. 2003;101(1):351-357.
693. Shenoy S, Eapen M, Panepinto JA, et al. A trial of unrelated donor marrow transplantation for children with severe sickle cell disease. *Blood*. 2016;128(21):2561-2567. doi:10.1182/blood-2016-05-715870
694. Bolanos-Meade J, Fuchs EJ, Luznik L, et al. HLA-haploidentical bone marrow transplantation with posttransplant cyclophosphamide expands the donor pool for patients with sickle cell disease. *Blood*. 2012;120(22):4285-4291. doi:10.1182/blood-2012-07-438408
695. Walters MC, Patience M, Leisenring W, et al. Stable mixed hematopoietic chimerism after bone marrow transplantation for sickle cell anemia. *Biol Blood Marrow Transplant*. 2001;7(12):665-673.
696. Gaziev J, Lucarelli G. Stem cell transplantation for hemoglobinopathies. *Curr Opin Pediatr*. 2003;15(1):24-31.
697. Hsieh MM, Kang EM, Fitzhugh CD, et al. Allogeneic hematopoietic stem-cell transplantation for sickle cell disease. *N Engl J Med*. 2009;361(24):2309-2317. doi:10.1056/NEJMoa0904971
698. O'Brien SH, Hankins JS. Decision analysis of treatment strategies in children with severe sickle cell disease. *J Pediatr Hematol Oncol*. 2009;31(11):873-878. doi:10.1097/MPH.0b013e3181b83cab
699. Hankins J, Hinds P, Day S, et al. Therapy preference and decision-making among patients with severe sickle cell anemia and their families. *Pediatr Blood Cancer*. 2007;48(7):705-710. doi:10.1002/pbc.20903
700. Hansbury EN, Schultz WH, Ware RE, Aygun B. Bone marrow transplant options and preferences in a sickle cell anemia cohort on chronic transfusions. *Pediatr Blood Cancer*. 2012;58(4):611-615.
701. Pawliuk R, Westerman KA, Fabry ME, et al. Correction of sickle cell disease in transgenic mouse models by gene therapy. *Science*. 2001;294(5550):2368-2371. doi:10.1126/science.1065806
702. Cavazzana-Calvo M, Payen E, Negre O, et al. Transfusion independence and HMGA2 activation after gene therapy of human beta-thalassaemia. *Nature*. 2010;467(7313):318-322. doi:10.1038/nature09328
703. Ribeil JA, Hacein-Bey-Abina S, Payen E, et al. Gene therapy in a patient with sickle cell disease. *N Engl J Med*. 2017;376(9):848-855. doi:10.1056/NEJMoa1609677
704. Sankaran VG, Xu J, Byron R, et al. A functional element necessary for fetal hemoglobin silencing. *N Engl J Med*. 2011;365(9):807-814. doi:10.1056/NEJMoa1103070
705. Bae HT, Baldwin CT, Sebastiani P, et al. Meta-analysis of 2040 sickle cell anemia patients: BCL11A and HBS1L-MYB are the major modifiers of HbF in African Americans. *Blood*. 2012;120(9):1961-1962. doi:10.1182/blood-2012-06-432849
706. Hoban MD, Bauer DE. A genome editing primer for the hematologist. *Blood*. 2016;127(21):2525-2535. doi:10.1182/blood-2016-01-678151
707. Hoban MD, Orkin SH, Bauer DE. Genetic treatment of a molecular disorder: gene therapy approaches to sickle cell disease. *Blood*. 2016;127(7):839-848. doi:10.1182/blood-2015-09-618587

708. Traxler EA, Yao Y, Wang YD, et al. A genome-editing strategy to treat beta-hemoglobinopathies that recapitulates a mutation associated with a benign genetic condition. *Nat Med.* 2016;22(9):987-990. doi:10.1038/nm.4170

709. Frangoul H, Altshuler D, Cappellini MD, et al. CRISPR-Cas9 gene editing for sickle cell disease and beta-thalassemia. *N Engl J Med.* 2021;384(3):252-260. doi:10.1056/NEJMoa2031054

710. Brendel C, Guda S, Renella R, et al. Lineage-specific BCL11A knockdown circumvents toxicities and reverses sickle phenotype. *J Clin Invest.* 2016;126(10):3868-3878. doi:10.1172/JCI87885

711. Guda S, Brendel C, Renella R, et al. miRNA-embedded shRNAs for lineage-specific BCL11A knockdown and hemoglobin F induction. *Mol Ther.* 2015;23(9):1465-1474. doi:10.1038/mt.2015.113

712. Esrick EB, Lehmann LE, Biffi A, et al. Post-transcriptional genetic silencing of BCL11A to treat sickle cell disease. *N Engl J Med.* 2021;384(3):205-215. doi:10.1056/NEJMoa2029392

713. Goyal S, Tisdale J, Schmidt M, et al. Acute myeloid leukemia case after gene therapy for sickle cell disease. *N Engl J Med.* 2022;386(2):138-147. doi:10.1056/NEJMoa2109167

714. Jones RJ, DeBaun MR. Leukemia after gene therapy for sickle cell disease: insertional mutagenesis, busulfan, both, or neither. *Blood.* 2021;138(11):942-947. doi:10.1182/blood.2021011488

715. Blattner P, Dar H, Nitowsky HM. Pregnancy outcome in women with sickle cell trait. *J Am Med Assoc.* 1977;238(13):1392-1394.

716. Cooper MR, Toole JF. Sickle-cell trait: benign or malignant? *Ann Intern Med.* 1972;77(6):997-998.

717. Jones SR, Binder RA, Donowho EM Jr. Sudden death in sickle-cell trait. *N Engl J Med.* 1970;282(6):323-325.

718. Kark JA, Posey DM, Schumacher HR, Ruehle CJ. Sickle-cell trait as a risk factor for sudden death in physical training. *N Engl J Med.* 1987;317(13):781-787.

719. Goldsmith JC, Bonham VL, Joiner CH, Kato GJ, Noonan AS, Steinberg MH. Framing the research agenda for sickle cell trait: building on the current understanding of clinical events and their potential implications. *Am J Hematol.* 2012;87(3):340-346. doi:10.1002/ajh.22271

720. Grant AM, Parker CS, Jordan LB, et al. Public health implications of sickle cell trait: a report of the CDC meeting. *Am J Prev Med.* 2011;41(6 suppl 4):S435-S439. doi:10.1016/j.amepre.2011.09.012

721. Harmon KG, Drezner JA, Klossner D, Asif IM. Sickle cell trait associated with a RR of death of 37 times in National Collegiate Athletic Association football athletes: a database with 2 million athlete-years as the denominator. *Br J Sports Med.* 2012;46(5):325-330. doi:10.1136/bjsports-2011-090896

722. Nelson DA, Deuster PA, Carter R III, Hill OT, Wolcott VL, Kurina LM. Sickle cell trait, rhabdomyolysis, and mortality among U.S. Army soldiers. *N Engl J Med.* 2016;375(5):435-442. doi:10.1056/NEJMoa1516257

723. Naik RP, Irvin MR, Judd S, et al. Sickle cell trait and the risk of ESRD in blacks. *J Am Soc Nephrol.* 2017;28(7):2180-2187. doi:10.1681/ASN.2016101086

724. Folsom AR, Tang W, Roetker NS, et al. Prospective study of sickle cell trait and venous thromboembolism incidence. *J Thromb Haemost.* 2015;13(1):2-9. doi:10.1111/jth.12787

725. Noubiap JJ, Temgoua MN, Tankeu R, Tochie JN, Wonkam A, Bigna JJ. Sickle cell disease, sickle trait and the risk for venous thromboembolism: a systematic review and meta-analysis. *Thromb J.* 2018;16:27. doi:10.1186/s12959-018-0179-z

726. Naik RP, Wilson JG, Ekunwe L, et al. Elevated D-dimer levels in African Americans with sickle cell trait. *Blood.* 2016;127(18):2261-2263. doi:10.1182/blood-2016-01-694422

727. Liem RI, Chan C, Vu TT, et al. Association among sickle cell trait, fitness, and cardiovascular risk factors in CARDIA. *Blood.* 2017;129(6):723-728. doi:10.1182/blood-2016-07-727719

728. Bello NA, Hyacinth HI, Roetker NS, et al. Sickle cell trait is not associated with an increased risk of heart failure or abnormalities of cardiac structure and function. *Blood.* 2017;129(6):799-801. doi:10.1182/blood-2016-08-705541

729. Hyacinth HI, Carty CL, Seals SR, et al. Association of sickle cell trait with ischemic stroke among african Americans: a meta-analysis. *JAMA Neurol.* 2018;75(7):802-807. doi:10.1001/jamaneurol.2018.0571

730. Chen N, Caruso C, Alonso A, et al. Association of sickle cell trait with measures of cognitive function and dementia in African Americans. *eNeurologicalSci.* 2019;16:100201. doi:10.1016/j.ensci.2019.100201

731. Bunn HF. Subunit assembly of hemoglobin: an important determinant of hematologic phenotype. *Blood.* 1987;69(1):1-6.

732. Landefeld CS, Schambelan M, Kaplan SL, Embury SH. Clomiphene-responsive hypogonadism in sickle cell anemia. *Ann Intern Med.* 1983;99(4):480-483.

733. da Guarda CC, Yahouedehou S, Santiago RP, et al. Sickle cell disease: a distinction of two most frequent genotypes (HbSS and HbSC). *PLoS One.* 2020;15(1):e0228399. doi:10.1371/journal.pone.0228399

734. Pearson HA, McIntosh S, Ritchey AK, Lobel JS, Rooks Y, Johnston D. Developmental aspects of splenic function in sickle cell diseases. *Blood.* 1979;53(3):358-365.

735. Lane PA, Rogers ZR, Woods GM, et al. Fatal pneumococcal septicemia in hemoglobin SC disease. *J Pediatr.* 1994;124(6):859-862.

736. Vieira C, de Oliveira CN, de Figueiredo LA, et al. Transcranial Doppler in hemoglobin SC disease. *Pediatr Blood Cancer.* 2017;64(5). doi:10.1002/pbc.26342

737. Guilliams KP, Fields ME, Hulbert ML. Higher-than-expected prevalence of silent cerebral infarcts in children with hemoglobin SC disease. *Blood.* 2015;125(2):416-417. doi:10.1182/blood-2014-10-605964

738. Moo-Penn W, Bechtel K, Jue D, et al. The presence of hemoglobin S and C Harlem in an individual in the United States. *Blood.* 1975;46(3):363-367.

739. Honig GR, Gunay U, Mason RG, Vida LN, Ferenc C. Sickle cell syndromes. I. Hemoglobin SC-alpha-thalassemia. *Pediatr Res.* 1976;10(6):613-620.

740. Warkentin TE, Barr RD, Ali MA, Mohandas N. Recurrent acute splenic sequestration crisis due to interacting genetic defects: hemoglobin SC disease and hereditary spherocytosis. *Blood.* 1990;75(1):266-270.

741. Diggs LW, Bell A. Intraerythrocytic hemoglobin crystals in sickle cell hemoglobin C disease. *Blood.* 1965;25:218.

742. Aleluia MM, Fonseca TCC, Souza RQ, et al. Comparative study of sickle cell anemia and hemoglobin SC disease: clinical characterization, laboratory biomarkers and genetic profiles. *BMC Hematol.* 2017;17:15. doi:10.1186/s12878-017-0087-7

743. Luchtman-Jones L, Pressel S, Hilliard L, et al. Effects of hydroxyurea treatment for patients with hemoglobin SC disease. *Am J Hematol.* 2016;91(2):238-242. doi:10.1002/ajh.24255

744. Lebensburger JD, Patel RJ, Palabindela P, Bemrich-Stolz CJ, Howard TH, Hilliard LM. Hydroxyurea decreases hospitalizations in pediatric patients with Hb SC and Hb SB+ thalassemia. *Hematol Res Rev.* 2015;6:285-290. doi:10.2147/jbm.s97405

745. Kinney TR, Ware RE. Compound heterozygous states. In: Embury SH, Hebbel RP, Mohandas N, Steinberg MH, eds. *Sickle Cell Disease: Basic Principles and Clinical Practice.* Raven Press; 1994:437-451.

746. Serjeant GR. *Sickle Cell Disease.* 2nd ed. Oxford University Press; 1992.

747. Cancio MI, Aygun B, Chui DHK, et al. The clinical severity of hemoglobin S/Black (A gammadeltabeta)0 -thalassemia. *Pediatr Blood Cancer.* 2017;64(11):10.1002/pbc.26596. doi:10.1002/pbc.26596

748. Adekile A, Mullah-Ali A, Akar NA. Does elevated hemoglobin F modulate the phenotype in Hb SD-Los Angeles? *Acta Haematol.* 2010;123(3):135-139. doi:10.1159/000276998

749. Patel S, Purohit P, Mashon RS, et al. The effect of hydroxyurea on compound heterozygotes for sickle cell-hemoglobin D-Punjab–a single centre experience in eastern India. *Pediatr Blood Cancer.* 2014;61(8):1341-1346. doi:10.1002/pbc.25004

750. Huisman TH. Combinations of beta chain abnormal hemoglobins with each other or with beta-thalassemia determinants with known mutations: influence on phenotype. *Clin Chem.* 1997;43(10):1850-1856.

751. Olson JA, Nagel RL. Synchronized cultures of P falciparum in abnormal red cells: the mechanism of the inhibition of growth in HbCC cells. *Blood.* 1986;67(4):997-1001.

752. Cook CM, Smeltzer MP, Mortier NA, et al. The clinical and laboratory spectrum of Hb C [beta6(A3)Glu–>Lys, GAG>AAG] disease. *Hemoglobin.* 2013;37(1):16-25. doi:10.3109/03630269.2012.753547

Chapter 35 ■ Thalassemia Syndromes: Quantitative Disorders of Globin Chain Synthesis

EUGENE KHANDROS • JANET L. KWIATKOWSKI

INTRODUCTION

The thalassemia syndromes are a group of disorders that result from decreased or absent synthesis of one or more of the globin subunits that form the normal human hemoglobins (Hbs). The majority are caused by the effect of different genetic molecular defects. The most common thalassemias are referred to as α-, β-, γ-, or $\delta\beta$-thalassemia, depending on which globin chain synthesis is impaired. The resulting imbalance in globin synthesis is responsible for the ineffective erythropoiesis (intramedullary destruction of erythroid precursors) and hemolysis (peripheral destruction of red cells) typically observed in the thalassemia syndromes. Mutations resulting in structural variants produced at reduced rates (e.g., HbE, Hb Lepore) or leading to unstable Hb variants (thalassemic hemoglobinopathies) also cause a thalassemia phenotype, and strict differentiation from the hemoglobinopathies (qualitative changes in Hb structure) may not be clinically helpful. In the past few years, the advances of DNA analysis have permitted a better understanding of the basic aspects of gene structure and function and have allowed for the characterization of the molecular basis for deficient globin synthesis. The combination of recent medical and scientific advances has resulted in an improvement in the lives of people with thalassemic syndromes.

PREVALENCE, GEOGRAPHIC DISTRIBUTION, AND THE ROLE OF MALARIA

According to the most current *Bulletin of the World Health Organization*, inheritance of thalassemic mutations represents a significant public health problem in a majority of nations (71% of 229 countries). It is estimated that up to 1.5% of the entire population may carry a genetic mutation affecting Hb production or about 270 million persons[1] and approximately 1% of couples worldwide are at risk for having children with an Hb disorder.[2]

Thalassemia gene mutations occur most frequently in a broad geographic belt extending from the Mediterranean basin through the Middle East, Indian subcontinent, Burma, Southeast Asia, Melanesia, and the islands of the Pacific Ocean.[3] Many different mutations in either the α- or β-globin genes have developed, and each has different frequencies in different countries. Even within countries, because of the low migration and resultant consanguinity, there may be differences in prevalence and frequency of thalassemic mutations. In addition, with increased migration and travel, thalassemic mutations are found worldwide. The estimated annual worldwide number of births is 22,989 for β-thalassemia major, 5183 for Hb Barts hydrops fetalis syndrome, 9568 for HbH disease (the intermediate form of α-thalassemia), and 19,128 for HbE/β-thalassemia.[2,3]

Disorders caused by α-thalassemia are more common in Southeast Asia and China, with up to 40% of the regional population being carriers, and less commonly in India, Kuwait, the Middle East, Greece, Italy, and Northern Europe. The frequency of these mutations varies widely between nations and even within individual countries.[1] In a random population sample, the gene frequency of deletion-type α-thalassemia-2 ($-\alpha$) was 0.18 in Sardinians and 0.07 in Greek Cypriots; the occurrence of nondeletion α-thalassemia is estimated to be one-third that of the deletion type.[4] In African Americans, α-thalassemia is relatively common but rarely is of clinical significance as a result of most patients carrying the trans-type configuration.[5]

About 3% of the world's population (150 million people) carry β-thalassemia genes. They are particularly prevalent in inhabitants of Italy and Greece. In Italy, the highest prevalence of the carrier state,

in descending order, has been found in Sardinia (10.3%), the Delta region of the Po River near Ferrara (8%), and Sicily (5.9% with an almost equal distribution over the entire island).[6] In Greece, the prevalence varies considerably, ranging from <5% to nearly 15% in the southern and central areas.[7] In Cyprus, 1 individual in 7 is a carrier of β-thalassemia and 1 individual in 1000 is currently homozygous, whereas in Sardinia, the incidence of homozygous β-thalassemia is 1 in 250 live births.[8] The epidemiologic changes in the prevalence of Hb disorders have important implications for public health programs, including new laboratory strategies, newborn screening, counseling, patient management, and political and family planning.[9] Detailed information on the frequency of thalassemia in different world regions is available and updated by the World Health Organization.[2]

The Role of Malaria

The hypothesis that malaria had an influence in promoting the high prevalence of mutations in the globin genes in the world was first proposed in 1949 by Haldane, who hypothesized that the small red cells of the carriers of thalassemia were more resistant to infection by malaria parasites.[10] A few years earlier, Neel and Valentine had calculated that, in the absence of some kind of selective pressure, the mutation rate for thalassemia had to be in the order of 1 in 2500.[11] Molecular studies have shown that a very high number of β-thalassemia mutations are regionally specific and that an association with specific β-globin gene haplotypes exists. The regional specificity of mutations suggests that local processes have played a role in the generation of high mutation frequencies, while the close association with specific haplotypes suggests a recent cause. These observations point to the conclusion that the selective pressure of malaria has amplified the β-thalassemia genes to high frequency so recently that neither migration, recombination, nor genetic drift could have had sufficient time to bring them into spatial or genetic equilibrium with their background.[3]

The mechanism by which the thalassemia heterozygote state protects from malaria is still not established. Immunologic mechanisms protecting carriers of thalassemia from malaria and possibly from other diseases as well are hypothesized. However, recent in vitro studies using red blood cells (RBCs) with common hemoglobinopathies (e.g., α- and β-thalassemias, HbS, HbC, HbE) and enzyme (glucose-6-phosphate dehydrogenase) defects have shown a reduced parasite invasion/growth and an increased susceptibility to phagocytosis of the infected RBC as a malaria-protective effect.[12] A recent systematic review and meta-analysis of studies that estimated the risk of malaria in patients with and without hemoglobinopathies showed a decreased risk of severe *Plasmodium falciparum* malaria in sickle cell carriers, homozygous and heterozygous HbC, and homozygous and heterozygous α-thalassemia. These hemoglobinopathies differ substantially in the degree of protection provided and confer mild or no protection against uncomplicated malaria and asymptomatic parasitemia.[13]

GENETIC MECHANISMS AND MOLECULAR PATHOLOGY

Synthesis of Hb, the molecule used for oxygen transport, is directed by two gene clusters: (1) the α locus, which contains the embryonic ζ gene and two adult α genes, and (2) the β cluster, which contains the embryonic ε, the fetal Gγ and Aγ, and the adult δ and β genes (*Figure 35.1*). Two globin gene switches take place during development. First, the embryonic switch to fetal globin genes (ε to γ and ζ to α). This starts very early in pregnancy and is completed at 10 weeks of gestation. Second, the fetal switch to adult globin genes (γ to β), which

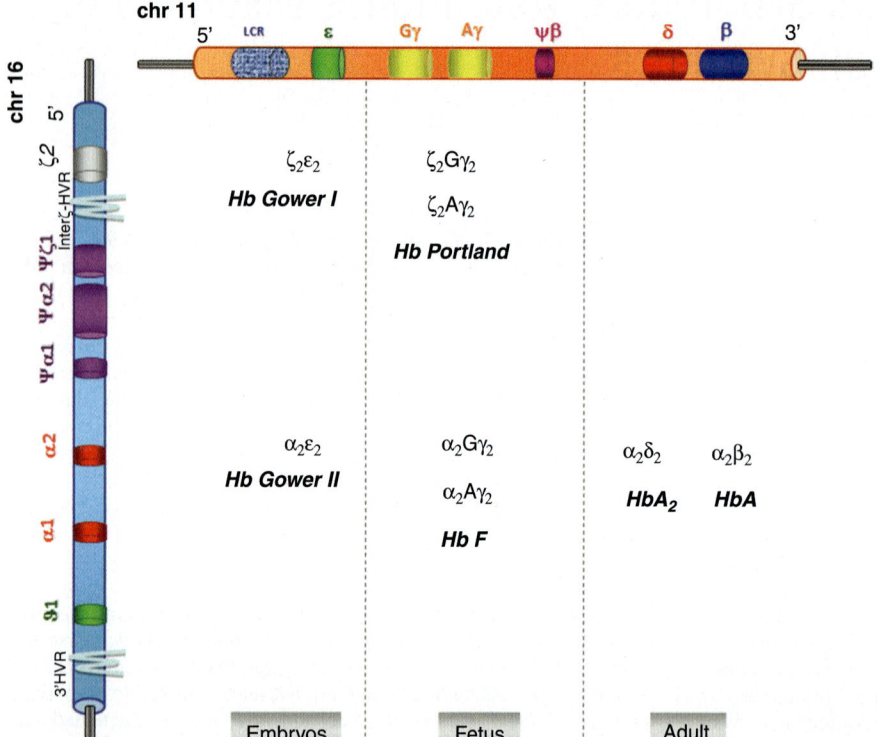

FIGURE 35.1 *α*- and *β*-globin gene clusters and hemoglobins (Hbs) produced during development. LCR, locus control region.

occurs during the perinatal period.[14] These globin gene switches result in changes in Hb composition, which parallel morphologic and biochemical characteristics of the erythropoietic cell line, including the shift from the nucleated megaloblast to macrocyte and to the definitive normocyte; the shift in the site of erythropoiesis from the yolk sac to the liver, spleen, and bone marrow; and changes in the membrane antigenic profile and in the red cell glycolytic activity.

The individual genes of the β-globin gene cluster are regulated through developmental stage-specific chromatin interactions with the locus control region (LCR) (*Figure 35.2*). The globin genes are relatively small and composed of three exons, coding for functional domains of Hb, and two intervening sequences (introns).[15] The differential globin gene expression observed during development is controlled through the action of transcription factors and regulatory elements (promoters, enhancers, and silencers) that flank each globin gene and more remote sequences important for the regulation of the cluster (see below). The promoter of each globin gene contains sequences that act as binding sites for erythroid-restricted or ubiquitously expressed transcription factors responsible for tissue- and developmental-specific regulation of the globin genes. Relevant promoter sequences are the TATA box, situated 30 bp upstream of the initiation site, and the CAAT and CACCC boxes at approximately −70 and −110 bp from the initiation site, respectively.[15] GATA-1 is the first of a family of DNA-binding proteins, whose binding sites are present in one or more copies in almost all regulatory elements of the globin gene. Nuclear factor-erythroid 2, KLF1, FOG-1, and SP1 are other transcription factors involved in the expression of the β-globin gene. Recent work has identified BCL11A and ZBTB7A (LRF) as major repressors of γ-globin expression in adults.[16-24] BCL11A is a zinc finger transcription factor that directly binds to elements in the HBG1 and HBG2 promoters and recruits the NuRD repressor complex to block γ-globin gene expression.[19] ZBTB7A/LRF likewise also directly represses transcription of the fetal globin genes.[24,25] KLF1 is a zinc-finger erythroid-specific transcriptional regulator, which also activates the β-globin gene through direct binding to the critical CACCC box promoter element, which activates *BCL11A* expression by associating with the *BCL11A* promoter.[26] Therefore, KLF1 has a dual role in globin gene regulation, functioning as a direct activator of the β-globin

gene and an indirect repressor of the γ-globin gene. These discoveries have provided novel therapeutic targets for the β-hemoglobinopathies.

The process of globin gene expression consists of the following steps: transcription of DNA into a primary messenger RNA (mRNA) transcript; processing of the primary mRNA, involving modifications at both its 5′ (capping) and 3′ (polyadenylation) ends together with removal of the introns and joining of the exons (splicing) to produce mature mRNA, the final template for protein synthesis; and translation

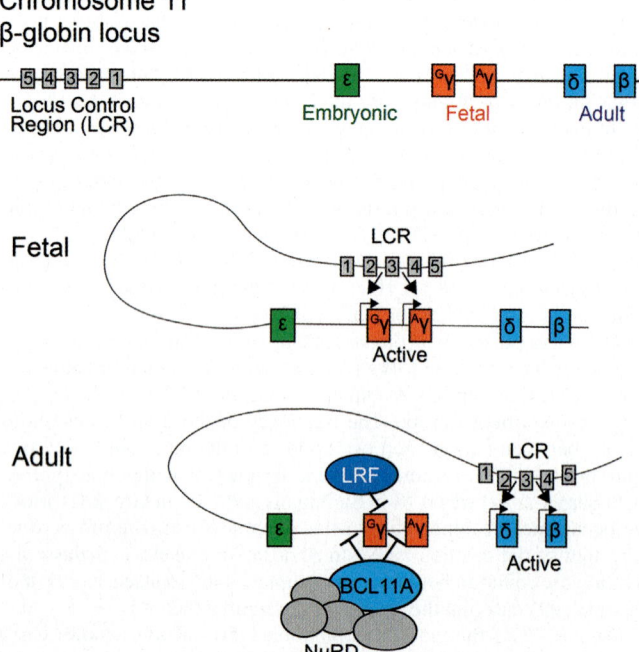

FIGURE 35.2 Current hemoglobin switching model. LCR, locus control region. NuRD, nucleosome remodeling and deacetylase complex.

of mRNA in the globin protein. Transcription and RNA processing occur in the nucleus, whereas translation occurs in the cytoplasm. Thalassemia syndromes result from a large series of molecular defects, which alter the expression of one or more globin genes. Like other genes, globin genes possess a series of motifs critical for their expression: the CAP site, which indicates the start of transcription; the ATG initiation codon, which is the signal for starting translation in mRNA; the donor and acceptor splice sites, which are involved in the processing (splicing) of mRNA; the termination codon, which interrupts translation; and the polyadenylation signal, which is crucial for the addition of a poly (A) tail to the mRNA. The importance of these critical sequences is underscored by the fact that nucleotide substitutions that either alter or create new similar regulatory sequences in a globin gene result in abnormal mRNA processing and constitute the molecular basis for most types of thalassemia. Detailed information on positions, genotypes, and phenotypes for the known globin gene variants are available at the websites listed at the end of this chapter.[15,27,28]

α-Thalassemia

Two α-globin genes are located in the telomeric region of chromosome 16 (16p13.3) in a cluster containing an embryonic α-like gene (ζ_2) and three pseudogenes (pseudo ζ_1, pseudo α_1, and pseudo α_2) (*Figure 35.1*).[15] Thus, wild-type individuals carry 4 α-globin genes. A gene (θ) with unknown function, but whose mRNA can be found through all stages of development, is part of the α cluster. Several regions of the cluster contain tandem arrays of short GC-rich sequences (minisatellites), identified as hypervariable regions, and many Alu family repeats. The α cluster is surrounded by several widely expressed genes. Upstream of the α cluster, four highly conserved noncoding sequences or multispecies conserved sequences (MCSs), called MCS-R1-R4, serve as transcriptional regulators of the α-like globin genes, with MCS-R2/HS-40 having the most significant effect.[15] When the multipotent hemopoietic progenitors committed to the erythroid lineage begin differentiation, several specific erythroid transcription factors, including GATA-1, GATA-2, and SCL, NF-E2, and cofactors such as FOG, pCAF, and p300, bind to the MCS-R elements and the α-like globin gene promoters, causing extended modifications associated with chromatin activation. Then, RNA polymerase II is engaged both at the upstream regulatory regions and at the globin gene promoters beginning transcription in erythroid progenitors.[29] Rare deletions in the *MCS* gene produce α-thalassemia, demonstrating their importance in regulation.[30] The human α-globin gene cluster of normal individuals contains a series of DNA sequence variations; for example, single nucleotide polymorphism (SNP), variations in the number of tandem repeats, and copy number variants have helped in analysis of evolutionary aspects of the gene cluster, in defining the origin of α-thalassemia mutations, and in identifying functionally important areas of the cluster.[29]

The α complex is arranged in the order of expression during development: $5'\zeta_2 \ldots \alpha_2$-$\alpha_1$. There is a high homology between α_2 and α_1 genes; they differ only in the IVS-2 (two base substitutions and a 7-bp insertion/deletion) and in the 3' noncoding region (18 base substitutions and a single-base deletion in the 3'-untranslated region [UTR]).[29,31] The embryonic ζ gene shows 58% homology with the α gene coding region. The level of transcription of the two α genes differs: the α_2 gene expresses two to three times more α-globin than α_1.[32-34] This would imply that Hb is made up of approximately 35% α_2 gene and 15% α_1 globin structural variants. This is not universally accepted, and it is proposed that the differential expression of the α genes is important not only for the α-globin structural variants but also for the pathophysiology of the deletional and nondeletional forms of α-thalassemia.[32] Individuals most often have four α-globin genes, but as a result of unequal genetic exchange, some people may exhibit five or six α genes, while being phenotypically normal.[35] Multiple arrangements with three to six ζ-like embryonic genes have also been reported.[36] The α-thalassemias are classified by mutations; those that result in a complete absence of globin production are designated α^0 and those that lead to a reduced production of α-chains are designated α^+ thalassemia.

Deletional α-Thalassemia

α-Thalassemia is most frequently caused by deletional mutations that involve one or both α-globin genes. The α-globin genes are embedded within two highly homologous regions extending for about 4 kb, whose homology has been maintained by gene conversion and unequal crossover events. Three homologous subsegments (X, Y, and Z), separated by nonhomologous elements, have been defined. Reciprocal recombination between Z boxes (3.7 kb apart) and between X boxes (4.2 kb apart) gives rise to chromosomes with only one α-gene. These common α-thalassemia determinants are referred to as $-\alpha$ 3.7-kb rightward deletion or $-\alpha$ 4.2-kb leftward deletions, respectively (*Figure 35.3*).[37] Based on the exact location within the Z box where the crossover took place, the $-\alpha$ 3.7-kb deletion is further subdivided into $-\alpha$ 3.7 I, $-\alpha$ 3.7 II, and $-\alpha$ 3.7 III. Besides the deletion α-thalassemia determinants, the nonreciprocal crossover produces chromosomes with three α-globin genes: $\alpha\alpha\alpha$ anti-3.7 and $\alpha\alpha\alpha$ anti-4.2.[29] More complex recombination events result in chromosomes with four or five α genes. The result of a single α-globin gene deletion is the reduced production of α-chains from the affected chromosome (α^+-thalassemia). Measurements of α-globin mRNA in patients with $-\alpha$ 4.2 determinants suggest that there is a compensatory increase in expression of the remaining α_1 gene, whereas in the chromosome with $-\alpha$ 3.7 deletion, the remaining α gene is expressed roughly halfway between a normal α_2 and α_1 gene.[29] These differences in expression may result from several mechanisms: (1) changes in the transcription rate, (2) new combinations of flanking sequences, (3) modification in chromatin structure resulting from the deletion, or (4) variation in the interaction with the HS-40 (MCS-R2) regulatory element.[34] Deletions that remove all or part of the α-globin gene cluster, including both α genes (entirely or in part) and sometimes the embryonic ζ_2 gene, result in α^0-thalassemia. The extent of the deletions, completely removing both α-globin genes, is from 100 to over 250 kb, and sometimes other flanking genes, such as a DNA repair enzyme, a protein disulfide isomerase, and several anonymous housekeeping genes, are removed (*Figure 35.3*).[38] However, in individuals with these large deletions, the only phenotypic manifestation is α-thalassemia. Several molecular mechanisms (illegitimate recombination, reciprocal translocation, and truncation of chromosome 16) are responsible for these large deletions and an α^0-thalassemia phenotype. At present, approximately 50 deletions that completely or partially delete both α-globin genes, resulting in α^0 thalassemia, have been reported.

A series of naturally occurring human deletions that remove MCS regulatory elements have been identified.[39] Despite the presence of intact α-globin genes, these MCS deletions have the α°-thalassemia phenotype. Human and murine studies of the four regulatory elements (MCS-R1 to R4) have demonstrated that the most relevant for α-globin gene expression is MCS-R2, located 40 kb upstream of the ζ globin gene. However, MCS-R2 is not absolutely required for α-globin gene expression.[40] Subsequent studies demonstrated that the deletion juxtaposes the normal α_2 globin gene with a downstream widely expressed gene (*Luc 7L*). Transcription of antisense RNA from *Luc 7L* through the α_2 gene mediates methylation of the associated CpG island, with subsequent silencing of α_2 globin gene expression. These findings indicate another mechanism underlying human genetic disease.[41]

Nondeletional α-Thalassemia

Single nucleotide mutations or oligonucleotide deletions/insertions in regions critical for α-globin gene expression produce α-thalassemia. Nondeletional α^+-thalassemias are relatively common with over 70 described mutations, resulting in mutations affecting RNA splicing, the poly (A) addition signal, the initiation of mRNA translation, chain termination mutations, in-frame deletions, and frameshift mutations. The majority of nondeletional mutants occur in the α_2 gene and, as expected, have a more severe effect on α-globin gene expression; Hb Constant Spring (α 142 TAA→CAA, StopSGln) affects Southeast Asian populations and is the most common of the nine chain termination mutants, which change the stop codon to one amino acid, allowing mRNA translation to continue to the next in-phase stop

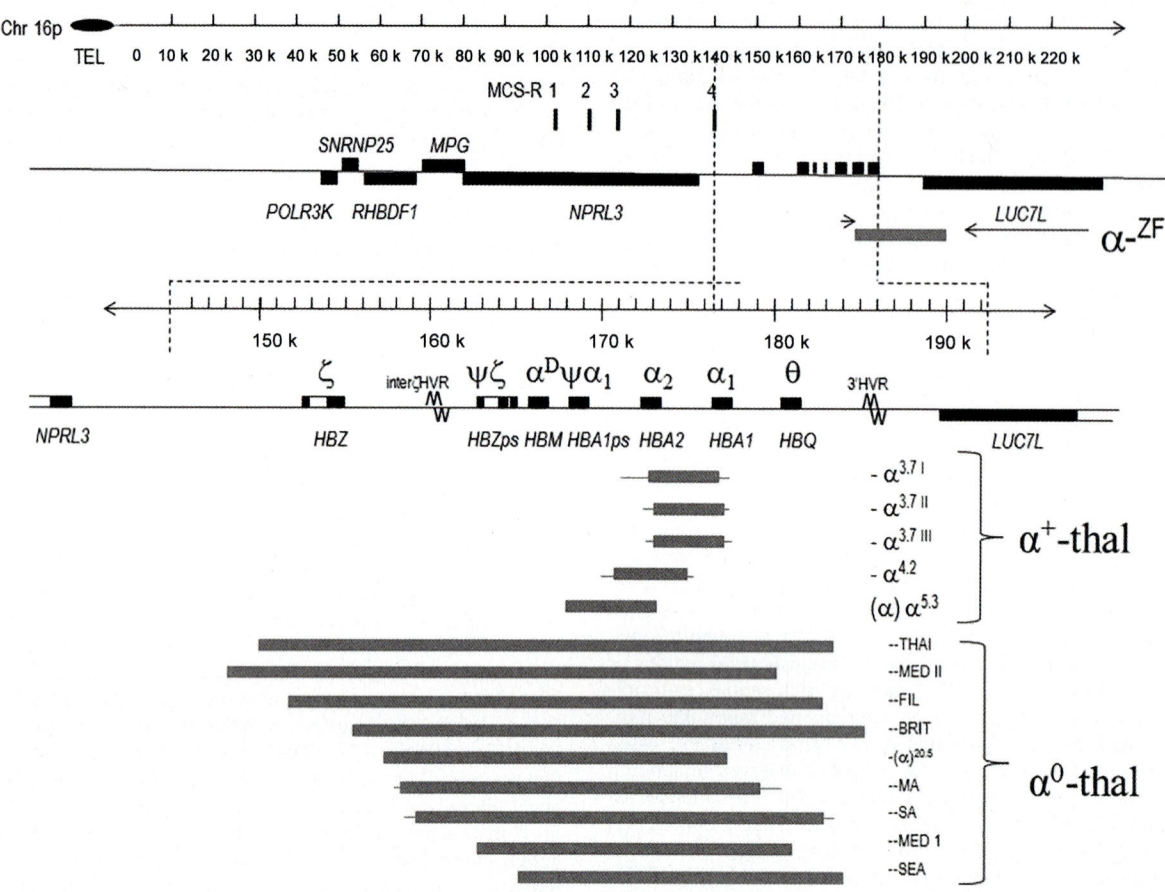

FIGURE 35.3 **Most common deletional α-thalassemia defects.** (Reprinted from Farashi S, Harteveld CL. Molecular basis of α-thalassemia. *Blood Cells Mol Dis.* 2018;70:43-53.)

codon located within the polyadenylation signal.[42] The result of this class of mutation is the production of a very small amount (~1%) of a 31-amino-acid elongated α-chain variant. A proposed reason for the reduced production of the elongated variants is the instability of the mRNA because of disruption of the 3′-UTR. Other extended α-chain variants are Hb Icaria (α 142 Lys), Koya Dora (α 142 Ser), Seal Rock (α 142 Glu), and Paksé (α 142 Tyr).[43] Heterozygotes for α-globin elongated chains, besides the presence of a very small amount of the Hb variant, have the phenotype of α-thalassemia. Mutations of α-globin genes that result in the production of highly unstable globin variants, such as Hb Quong Sze (α 125 Leu→Pro), Hb Heraklion (α 37 Pro→0), and Hb Agrinio (α 29 Leu→Pro), which rapidly degrade, exhibit an α-thalassemia phenotype.[44] A novel mechanism proposed for the nondeletional α-thalassemia phenotype observed in some Melanesian patients who have intact α genes is the creation of a GATA-1–binding site with increased affinity for transcription factors over the α-globin promoters, thereby causing α-thalassemia.[45] A regularly updated overview of these variants can be found at the Hb Var website.

β-Thalassemia

The β-globin gene is located on the short arm of chromosome 11 in a cluster region containing the δ gene, the embryonic ε gene, the fetal Gγ and Aγ genes, the long non-coding RNA BGLT3, and the pseudogene HBBP1 (*Figure 35.1*).[46] The five functional globin genes are arranged in the order of their developmental expression. The complete sequencing of the β-globin gene complex has shown interspersed repetitive sequences, which may play a role in the generation of deletions of the β cluster. The region also contains many polymorphic base substitutions, which produce restriction fragment length polymorphisms, combined in a restricted number of haplotypes in linkage disequilibrium with β-thalassemia mutations.[47] Variations in the number of β cluster genes, mostly involving the γ genes (which may be present in

one to five copies), have been reported. Like the α genes, β-globin genes are subject to a complex regulatory mechanism, acting at the level of single genes or the entire β cluster. The appropriate expression of the different β-like globin genes in erythroid tissues during development depends on a highly conserved mammalian major regulatory region, named the LCR, that is located 5 to 25 kb upstream from the ε-globin gene.[48,49] Five DNAase hypersensitive sites (HSs) have been described in this region, and each HS contains one or more binding motifs for erythroid-specific transcriptional activator 1 (GATA-1 and NF-E2) and for ubiquitous DNA-binding proteins. The importance of the LCR for the control of β-like globin gene expression has also been suggested by a series of naturally occurring deletions that totally or partially remove the HSs and result in the inactivation of the intact downstream β-globin gene.[50,51] More than 200 different mutations producing β-thalassemia have been so far described; the large majority are point mutations in functionally important sequences of the β-globin gene, whereas, in contrast to α-thalassemia, gene deletion is a rare cause of β-thalassemia (*Table 35.1*). Similar to the nomenclature of α-thalassemia mutations, β-thalassemia mutations resulting in complete absence of β-globin chains are designated β⁰-thalassemia, whereas those causing a variable reduction of β-globin production are referred to as β⁺-thalassemia. A complete updated list of published β-thalassemia mutations is available through the globin gene server websites (see the end of the chapter).

Nondeletional β-Thalassemia

Point mutations resulting in β-thalassemia are single nucleotide substitutions or oligonucleotide insertions/deletions that affect the β gene expression (*Table 35.1*). Three main categories can be identified: (a) mutations altering β gene transcription (promoter and 5′-UTR mutants); (b) mutations affecting mRNA processing (splice junction and consensus sequence mutants, exon and intron cryptic site mutants,

Table 35.1. Mutations Causing α-Thalassemia

Transcriptional Mutants	Phenotype	Number of Mutations
Promoter	Silent	3
	Mild	6
	β^+	17
5′-UTR	Silent	4
	Mild	1
	β^+	2
RNA Processing		
Splice junction	β^0	27
Consensus splice sites	Silent	2
	β^0	1
	Mild	1
	β^+	8
Cryptic splice sites in introns	β^0/β^+	1
	β^0	1
	β^+	3
Cryptic splice sites in exons	Mild	2
	β^+	3
3′-UTR RNA cleavage: poly (A) signal	Silent	1
	Mild	4
	β^+	5
Others	Silent	1
	Mild	1
	β^+	1
RNA Translation		
Initiation codon	β^0	9
Nonsense codons	β^0	16
Frameshift	β^0	72
Deletions	β^0	15
Dominant α-Thalassemias		
Missense mutations	β^0	12
Deletion or insertion of intact codons	β^0	9
Premature termination	β^0	2
Frameshift or aberrant splicing	β^0	23

Abbreviation: UTR, untranslated region.
Data from Thein SL, Wood WG, Steinberg MH, et al. The molecular basis of β thalassemia, δβ thalassemia, and hereditary persistence of fetal hemoglobin. In: Steinberg MH, Forget BG, Higgs DR, Weatherall DJ, eds. *Disorders of Hemoglobin: Genetics, Pathophysiology, and Clinical Management.* Cambridge University Press; 2009:323-356.

the polyadenylation site, and other 3′-UTR mutants); and (c) mutations resulting in abnormal mRNA translation (nonsense, frameshift, and initiation codon mutants).

Transcription Mutations

Promoter Mutations

Several mutations are described in or around the conserved motifs in the 5′ flanking sequence of β-globin genes (TATA box, proximal and distal CACCC box). They reduce binding of RNA polymerase, thus reducing the rate of mRNA transcription to 20% to 30% of normal and a moderate decrease in β-globin chain output (β⁺-thalassemia),

with a mild phenotype. A C→T mutation at position −101 of the β-globin gene (distal CACCC box) is unusually mild and associated with a silent phenotype in carriers and a mild non-transfusion-dependent thalassemia (NTDT).[52]

5′-UTR Mutations

Several mutations (single-base substitution and minor deletions) are reported in this 50-nucleotide region, all causing mild effects on gene transcription. Heterozygotes have normal or borderline red cell indices and HbA2, and compound heterozygotes, with severe β-thalassemia alleles, usually have a mild phenotype. The only homozygous state for a mutation at the β-globin gene mRNA capsite (Cap +1 A-C) shows hematologic values consistent with the thalassemia trait.[53,54]

Mutations Affecting mRNA Processing

RNA processing consists of the removal of the intervening sequences and the splicing of the coding regions to produce functional mRNA. The precision of this process relies on critical sequences present at intron/exon boundaries: the invariant dinucleotides—GT—at the 5′ (donor) and—AG—at the 3′ (acceptor) splice junctions and the flanking sequences (consensus sequences).[55]

Splice Junction and Consensus Sequence Mutants

The efficiency of normal splicing may be decreased by mutations within the consensus sequences immediately adjacent to the splice junctions. The reduction of β-globin production is quite variable, and the resulting phenotypes range from mild to severe. Mutations of the invariants 5′—GT—and 3′—AG—dinucleotides completely abolish normal splicing and result in β⁰-thalassemia. Twenty-seven base substitutions or short deletions involving the invariant dinucleotides have been identified. Other cryptic splice sites present elsewhere in precursor mRNA are used for alternative splicing, but miss-spliced mRNA cannot be translated into functional β-globin.[55] Mutations at position five of IVS-1 (G→C, G→T, G→A) produce a consistent reduction of β-globin synthesis and hence a severe β⁺-thalassemia phenotype, whereas the IVS-1–6 T→C mutation (Portuguese mutation), quite common in Mediterraneans, only mildly affects normal splicing and results in a mild (NTDT) clinical picture.[56] Even in the consensus sequence mutations, abnormal alternative splicing using neighboring cryptic sites may occur.

Cryptic Site Mutants in Introns and Exons

Along introns and exons, there are sequences similar to those found at the intron/exon boundaries, which normally are not used for splicing ("cryptic" splice sites). A number of nucleotide substitutions involving these sequences transform a cryptic site into a legitimate one. This new splice signal competes with the normal consensus sequence for splicing and, if is preferentially spliced (up to 90% in the IVS-1–110 G→A substitution and almost 100% in the IVS-1–116 T→G substitution) leads to a severe β⁺- or β⁰-thalassemia phenotype.[55] Two cryptic splice site mutations in IVS-1 and three in IVS-2 have been described. In the exons, three cryptic splice sites can be activated by nucleotide substitution: one at codon (cd) 10 (C→A), a second at codon 19 (A→G), and a third by mutations at codons 24 (T→A), 26 (G→A), 26 (A→C), or 27 (G→T). The nucleotide substitutions partially activate the cryptic splice sites, resulting in both normally and abnormally spliced β-mRNA.

Poly (A) and Other 3′-UTR Mutants

Downstream of the mRNA terminal codon, there is a highly conserved AAUAAA sequence, which represents a signal for cleavage and polyadenylation reaction, as a part of the RNA transcript processing. Because polyadenylation is important in determining the stability of mRNA, mutations at the AAUAAA sequence affect the efficiency of translation, resulting in β⁺-thalassemia of variable severity.[57] Seven nucleotide substitutions at different positions, two oligonucleotide deletions (of two and five bases), and one deletion of the total AATAAA sequence have been described. Mutations in the 3′-UTR (+1480 C→G) also produce β⁺-thalassemia.[58]

Mutations Affecting mRNA Translation

A large group of mutations that alter the different steps of mRNA translation can be grouped into three categories: initiation codon mutations, nonsense mutations, and frameshift mutations.

Initiation Codon Mutations

The initiator codon ATG, which encodes for methionine, is a critical signal for starting translation. Nine different point mutations of the initiation codon have been reported as a cause of β^0-thalassemia.[59]

Nonsense Mutations

Single nucleotide substitutions may change a codon for a given amino acid to one of the three possible chain termination codons: TAA, TAG, or TGA. The result is a premature interruption of mRNA translation, with the absence of β-globin production (β^0-thalassemia). A very low level of β-mRNA has been detected in erythroid cells affected by mutations in exons 1 and 2 as a consequence of rapid degradation of the mutant β-mRNA.[60] This process is referred to as nonsense-mediated decay and may be a mechanism to eliminate mRNAs encoding truncated polypeptides, with potential harmful effects for the erythroid cell. Nonsense mutations in exon 3 are associated with β-mRNA levels comparable with normal levels. The protective process does not occur, and mutant β-mRNA is probably translated to produce the abnormal globin (see "Hyperunstable Globins"). The most common nonsense mutation in the Mediterranean population is the C→T base substitution at codon 39.[61] This mutation likely accounts for 95% of β-thalassemia cases in Sardinia. In the Chinese and Thai populations, the nonsense mutation at codon 17 A→T has a high frequency.[62]

Frameshift Mutations

Insertion or deletion of nucleotides (other than in multiples of three) alters the reading frame of the encoded mRNA starting at the site of the mutation. The new reading frame usually results in an abnormal amino acid sequence and in a premature termination further downstream. The mutant globin chain is rapidly degraded with a β^0-thalassemia phenotype.[63] The frameshift resulting from a single-base deletion at codon 6 (−A) is relatively common in the Mediterranean population, whereas the −4 nucleotides deletion at codons 41 and 42 is common in Chinese and Asian Indian populations. The position of the premature termination (in exon 1, 2, or 3) caused by the frameshift mutation affects the mutant mRNA level and processing, similar to the nonsense mutations.

β-Globin Gene Deletions

Deletions involving only the β-globin gene, from 290 bp to 67 kb, have been reported.[64] A 619-bp deletion, removing the 3′ end of the β-globin gene, is relatively common in the Sind and Punjab populations of India and Pakistan. All others are rare and have in common the deletion of the promoter region and at least part of the β-globin gene. The phenotype is that of β^0-thalassemia with high levels of HbA2 and HbF in heterozygotes. This is probably the result of the removal of competition for the upstream LCR, thus allowing increased interaction between the LCR and the γ and δ genes in cis, resulting in a more efficient expression of these genes. Total deletions of the β cluster result in the lack of any β-like globin production and hence $\epsilon\gamma\delta\beta^0$-thalassemia.[65] Deletions of the β-LCR that leave the β gene intact inactivate the β-globin gene.[50] Approximately 15 deletions removing the whole β-globin cluster and several that remove the upstream LCR have been reported.[59] These deletions confirm, in vivo, the critical importance of the LCR for the control of expression of the β-globin genes.

β-Thalassemic Hemoglobinopathies

This group includes some structurally abnormal Hbs associated with a thalassemia phenotype. They are classified according to the molecular mechanism:

a. $\delta\beta$ hybrid genes
b. Activation of cryptic splice sites
c. Hyperunstable β-globins
d. Unknown mechanisms

δβ Hybrid Genes

Unequal crossing over between the homologous δ- and β-globin genes results in the formation of hybrid $\delta\beta$ (Lepore) and $\beta\delta$ (anti-Lepore) genes. The Lepore Hbs contain the N-terminal amino acid sequence of the normal δ-chain and the C-terminal sequence of the normal β-chain, and depending on the point of transition from δ to β sequence, three different variants of Hb Lepore have been described: Boston or Washington ($\delta87/\beta$IVS-2–8), Baltimore ($\delta68/\beta84$), and Hollandia ($\delta22/\beta$IVS-1–16).[66] The rate of production of the Lepore Hbs (about 10% in the carriers) likely depends on the structure of the hybrid gene, which has the promoter of the δ gene (this would explain the lower Hb Lepore amount as compared with normal HbA), and the IVS-2 of the β gene, which probably contains an enhancer (explaining the higher level of Hb Lepore as compared with HbA2). Moreover, the relative instability of Lepore mRNA may be responsible for the low level of synthesis. Nonhomologous crossover between the β and δ genes also results in the production of a hybrid $\beta\delta$ gene in a chromosome also containing the normal β and δ genes. These anti-Lepore genes produce about 15% to 20% of the abnormal Hb. Based on the position of the fusion point, several anti-Lepore Hbs have been identified (Hb Miyada, P Congo, P Nilotic, and Hb Lincoln Park, which has in addition a valine residue deleted at position 137). Carriers have normal Hb levels and normal red cell indices.

Activation of Cryptic Splice Sites

This group, which includes HbE, Hb Malay, and Hb Knossos, has been previously described.

Hyperunstable Globins

A singular group of β-globin gene mutants are characterized by amino acid substitutions, additions, or deletions in the β-globin chain associated with a clinically detectable thalassemic phenotype in the heterozygous state. For this reason, they are referred to as dominantly inherited β-thalassemia. The molecular lesions include 12 missense mutations, 9 small deletions or insertions of intact codons resulting in severe β-globin destabilization, 2 premature terminations, and 23 frameshift or aberrant splicing producing elongated or truncated β-globin chains. Most of these mutations are located in exon 3.[67]

In contrast with the typical recessively inherited forms of β-thalassemia, which lead to a reduced synthesis of normal β-globin chains, this group of mutations results in the production of β-globin variants, which are extremely unstable. These hyperunstable globins fail to form functional tetramers and precipitate in the erythroid precursors, leading to ineffective erythropoiesis, which is exacerbated by the concomitant relative excess of α-chains. Most of the patients exhibit an NTDT phenotype, a few patients have thalassemia trait, and some may even have a severe anemia requiring RBC transfusions. Laboratory findings consist of varying degrees of hypochromic microcytic anemia, increased HbA2, and an imbalanced α- to β-globin synthesis ratio. In most of the cases, the Hb variant cannot be detected in the peripheral blood.

Unknown Mechanisms

Adams et al reported a patient with 8% of an abnormal hemoglobin (Hb Vicksburg $\beta75$ Leu→0) and the phenotype of NTDT.[68] The reason for the NTDT phenotype associated with Hb Vicksburg has not yet been defined. The original patient has been reexamined, and despite the use of the new technologies of DNA analysis, the predicted Hb Vicksburg deletion was not present. Moreover, the Hb variant was not detected on two occasions, whereas HbA, absent at the beginning, has now been detected. DNA analysis showed that the patient was a compound heterozygote for the −88 C→T β^+ allele and IVS-2–849 A→G mutation that causes β^0-thalassemia.[69] It has been proposed that Hb Vicksburg arose as a stem cell mutation on the β^+-thalassemia chromosome. The variable Hb composition at different ages suggests that, over time, there were at least two clones of erythroid progenitors contributing to erythropoiesis. A phenotype of mild heterozygous β-thalassemia with microcytosis and increased levels of HbA2 has been reported in patients with two Hb variants: Hb North Shore (β134 Val→Glu) and Hb Woolwich (β132 Lys→Glu).[4] In both cases, a mild deficit of β-globin chain synthesis has been reported. DNA analysis of these patients has not been performed, and the mechanism responsible for the thalassemic phenotype remains unknown.

δ-Thalassemia

Several mutations of the δ-globin gene, which result in reduced (δ^+-thalassemia) or absent (δ^0-thalassemia) production of δ-globin chains, have been described. These conditions do not have clinical relevance, but the coinheritance with β-thalassemia mutations may create problems in β-carrier identification because the HbA2 may be normal or borderline. The classes of mutations are similar to those responsible for β-thalassemia. Some δ-thalassemia mutations have been described in cis to β-thalassemia. The δ^+27 C→T, fairly common in the Mediterranean population, has been reported in cis to β^+IVS-2–745 C→G, $\beta^0$39 C→T, and β^+27 G→T (Hb Knossos).[70] Also, the Corfu deletion (−7.2 kb) has been reported in isolation or association with the β^+IVS-1–5 G→A mutation.[71]

$\delta\beta$-Thalassemia

$\delta\beta$-Thalassemia includes a group of disorders characterized by reduced or absent production of both δ- and β-globin chains and by a variable increase in γ-chain synthesis, which is only partially able to balance the δ- and β-chain deficiency.[72] The most common molecular mechanism consists of a deletion of variable extent of the β-like globin cluster, which involves the δ- and β-globin genes. Based on the presence of one (Gγ) or both (Gγ and Aγ) globin genes, and hence on the residual synthesis of only Gγ- or both Gγ- and Aγ-globin chains, two groups of $\delta\beta^0$-thalassemia have been identified: Gγ Aγ($\delta\beta$)^0-thalassemia and Gγ Aγ($\delta\beta^0$)-thalassemia. The different deletions with their sizes are summarized in *Table 35.2*.

Aγ($\delta\beta^0$) and the Black Gγ Aγ($\delta\beta$)^0 are described in large populations, with homozygotes reported as well. For some deletions, the 3′ breakpoint has not been defined. The majority of the deletions that result in $\delta\beta$-thalassemia are caused by illegitimate recombination. Similar but more complex mechanisms have been invoked to explain other $\delta\beta^0$-thalassemias, such as Macedonian/Turkish Gγ Aγ($\delta\beta$)^0 thalassemia, which is characterized by a double deletion/inversion rearrangement.[73] The reasons for the increased expression of the γ genes in $\delta\beta^0$-thalassemia and for the differences between $\delta\beta^0$-thalassemia and hereditary persistence of fetal hemoglobin (HPFH; see later) have not been defined. Juxtaposition to the globin genes of new sequences as a result of the deletion, removal of intergene sequences critical for control of γ-globin gene expression, and altered spatial relationships between the LCR and the genes of the β cluster (with changes in LCR/globin gene promoter interaction and competition) have been postulated to explain the upregulation of the γ-globin genes and the phenotypic differences between $\delta\beta$-thalassemia and deletion HPFH. It is possible that a combination of the above mechanisms plays a role and that a balance between regulatory sequences, with positive or negative effects on the γ gene expression, may determine the amount of HbF in the red cells. A study of three families with elevated HbF identified using comparative genomic hybridization, breakpoint DNA sequencing, and chromatin immunoprecipitation identified a 3.5-kb intergenic region near the 5′ end of the β-globin gene, which is necessary for γ-globin gene silencing.[17] This region binds the fetal Hb silencing factor BCL11A and its partners in the chromatin of adult erythroid cells. The Corfu $\delta\beta$-thalassemia is characterized by a deletion of 7.2 kb, which removes the δ gene associated with the β-IVS-1–5 G→A mutation. Carriers of this mutation have the unusual hematologic phenotype of heterozygous β-thalassemia with normal levels of HbA2, whereas homozygotes have relatively high levels of HbF and a mild clinical phenotype.

Hereditary Persistence of Fetal Hemoglobin

HPFH is characterized by the presence of increased levels of HbF in adult life in the absence of relevant hematologic abnormalities,

Table 35.2. Mutations Responsible for Deletional and Nondeletional $\delta\beta$-Thalassemia

	Deletion Size (kb) Deletion Sizes From[72]
Deletional	
Gγ Aγ($\delta\beta$)^0-thalassemia	
Mediterranean	13.378
Southeast Asian	12.584
Eastern European	9.124
Black	11.767
Macedonian/Turkish	11.465
Macedonian/Turkish	1.593
Indian	32.621
Spanish	~95
Japanese	113.629
Turkish	~30
Gγ Aγ($\delta\beta$)^0-thalassemia	
Black	35.811
Chinese	78.847
Indian	0.834
Indian	7.460
Italian	~52
Belgian	~50
Yunnanese	~88
German	~52
Turkish	36.211
Southeast Asian	79.208
Malaysian 2	~42
Nondeletional	
Sardinian	Aγ-196 C→ T/$\beta^0$39
Chinese	Not defined

with a variable range of HbF in carriers from 2.0% to 30%, reflecting a marked molecular heterogeneity. Both deletion and nondeletion defects have been described. The deletions resulting in HPFH, listed in *Table 35.3*, extend from 13 kb (HPFH-5 or Sicilian HPFH) to about 106 kb (HPFH-1 or black HPFH).[72] They remove δ- and β-globin genes but spare both Gγ and Aγ genes. As in $\delta\beta^0$-thalassemia, the most common mechanism producing deletions is an illegitimate recombination followed by unequal crossing over. Nondeletion HPFH is usually the result of mutations in the promoter regions of Gγ and Aγ genes (*Table 35.3*). Most of these mutations are single nucleotide substitutions in or very close to the conserved sequences that bind various regulatory transcription factors.[74-77] As a consequence, there are changes in the binding of repressor or activator proteins that may modify the balance of the competition between the promoter and the LCR, resulting in increased HbF synthesis in adult life. Several patterns of inheritance for HPFH have been identified: autosomal or X-linked dominant and autosomal recessive. Candidate-gene association studies and genome-wide association studies identified a common SNP in the HBS1L-MYB intergenic region on chromosome 6p23 and in the IVS2 of BCL11A gene in chromosome 2p16.1, associated with increased HbF levels in healthy subjects, in β-thalassemia, and in sickle cell anemia.[16,78,79]

These SNPs explain a significant proportion of the interindividual variation of HbF levels and of the thalassemia severity and represent potential therapeutic targets for HbF induction.

Table 35.3. Mutations Responsible for Hereditary Persistence of Fetal Hemoglobin (HPFH)

	Deletion Size (kb) Deletion Sizes From[72]
Deletional	
$\gamma\beta$ Fusion	
Hb Kenya	22.675
$G\gamma\ A\gamma(\delta\beta)^0$-thalassemia	
Black	84.918
Ghanaian	83.679
Indian	47.733
Italian	~40
Sicilian	12.910
Southeast Asian	~28
Nondeletional	
$G\gamma$ mutations	
Black	−202 C→G
Tunisian	−200+ C
Black/Sardinian/British	−175 T→C
Japanese	−114 C→T
Australian	−114 C→G
$A\gamma$ mutations	
Black	−202 C→T
British	−198 T→C
Italian/Chinese	−196 C→T
Brazilian	−195 C→G
Black	−175 T→C
Greek/Black	−117 G→A
Black	−114 to −102 del
Georgia	−114 C→T

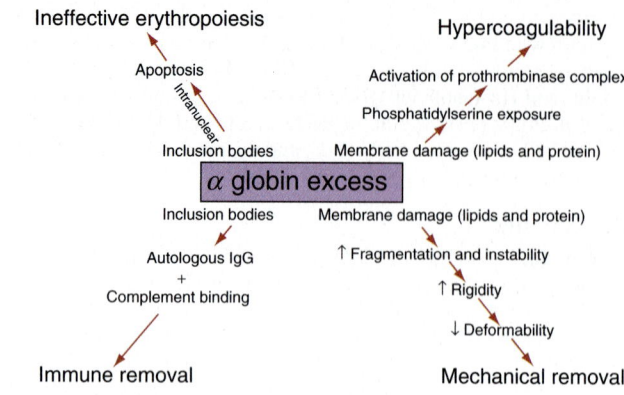

FIGURE 35.4 **Pathophysiology of β-thalassemia.** Ig, immunoglobulin.

Unusual Causes of β-Thalassemia

Insertion of a transposable element into IVS2 of the β-globin gene results in the expression of approximately 15% of normal β-globin mRNA and was reported with the phenotype of β-thalassemia.[80] Mutations in the general transcription factor TFIIH, involved in basal transcription and DNA repair, cause trichothiodystrophy and are frequently associated with the phenotype of β-thalassemia trait.[81] Some mutations in the erythroid transcription factor GATA have been reported as a cause of β-thalassemia associated with thrombocytopenia.[82] Large somatic deletions at chromosome 11 p15.5, including the β-globin cluster and leading to NTDT, have been reported in patients with heterozygous β-thalassemia.[83] The deletion in a subpopulation of erythroid cells resulted in a somatic mosaic with 10% to 20% of erythroid cells heterozygous with one normal copy of the β-globin gene and the rest homozygous without any normal β-globin gene.

PATHOPHYSIOLOGY

The pathophysiology of the thalassemia syndromes is complex. Understanding of both the intracellular processes as well as organism-wide effects is essential to explain the variable clinical phenotypes of the α- and β-thalassemias as well as to target potential interventions.

β-Thalassemia

The basic defect in β-thalassemia is a reduced or absent production of β-globin chains, resulting in a relative excess of α-chains. The direct consequences are a net decrease in Hb production and an imbalance of the globin chain synthesis. The former is more evident in carriers, leading to a reduction of mean cell hemoglobin (MCH) and mean cell volume (MCV), and has a minor clinical significance. The latter has dramatic effects on the red cell precursors, ultimately resulting in their extensive premature destruction in the bone marrow and extramedullary sites. This process is referred to as ineffective erythropoiesis and is the hallmark of β-thalassemia. Using ferrokinetic analysis, it has been shown that, in patients with β-thalassemia, only 15% of ^{59}Fe was incorporated in circulating erythrocytes, indicating that ineffective erythropoiesis could account for as much as 60% to 75% of total erythropoiesis.[84] Hemolysis of the erythrocytes that reach peripheral blood is a minor cause of anemia, particularly in transfusion-dependent thalassemia (TDT) (*Figure 35.4*).

The excess α-chains may, in minor amounts, combine with residual β- (in β^+-thalassemia) and γ-chains (whose synthesis persists usually in small quantity after birth), undergo proteolysis, or become associated with the erythroid precursors and red cell membrane, causing deleterious effects on erythroid maturation and survival. Therefore, the main determinant of the clinical severity is the extent of the relative excess of α-chains in red cell precursors and the degree of α/non-α imbalance. In 1966, Fessas et al described the presence of inclusion bodies in erythroblasts of thalassemic patients, suggesting that they were precipitated by α-chains.[85] The composition of inclusion bodies in β-thalassemia, completely consisting of precipitated α-chains, has been confirmed by immunoelectron microscopy. Oxidation of excess α-chains results in the formation of hemichromes, whose basic structure consists of the covalent binding of distal histidine E7 to the sixth coordination site of the heme iron. Irreversible hemichromes and denatured α-chains precipitate as inclusion bodies early during differentiation and throughout erythroid maturation.[86] α-Chain precipitation in the red cell membrane causes structural and functional alterations with changes in deformability, stability, and red cell hydration. Isolated red cell membranes from β-thalassemia intermedia, particularly from splenectomized patients, are rigid and unstable. Protein 4.1, a major component of the cytoskeleton, undergoes partial oxidation in β-thalassemia, resulting in its defective capability to mediate the formation of the spectrin–protein 4.1–actin complex, which is critical to maintain cytoskeleton stability.[87] In vitro experiments, using purified α-chains released within normal RBCs, support the role of aggregated α-chains in causing red cell membrane rigidity. A further consequence of the membrane-bound hemichromes is their association with the cytoplasmic domain of protein band 3, creating a neoantigen, which is subjected to opsonization with autologous immunoglobulin G (IgG) and complement and immune removal of the cell by macrophages.[88] RBCs in β-thalassemia lose K^+, store Ca_2^+, and are dehydrated, resulting in altered deformability. Finally, free α-chains are subjected to degradation and the formation of denatured α-globin protein, heme, and free iron, which play a role in damaging erythroid precursors and red cell membranes.

Free iron, via the Fenton reaction, generates reactive oxygen species, which cause lipid and protein peroxidation with consequent damage to red cell membranes and intracellular organelles.[89] High levels of iron, closely associated with denatured Hb, have been found in the membrane of β-thalassemic red cells and are thought to decrease red cell survival.[90] Recently, a new protein relevant for α-globin stabilization has been discovered. This protein, named α-hemoglobin–stabilizing protein (AHSP), is an abundant erythroid protein that specifically binds free α-globin chains, stabilizes their structure, and limits their ability to participate in chemical reactions that generate reactive oxygen species, although its significance in modifying the β-thalassemia phenotype in humans is unclear.[91,92] Finally, there is evidence that RBC precursors can degrade and detoxify α-globin thorough the ubiquitin proteasome system as well as autophagy but that these processes can become overwhelmed and limiting.[93-95] Ultimately α-globin-mediated damage leads to apoptosis of erythroid precursors in the bone marrow, significantly contributing to ineffective erythropoiesis. Of the two major pathways of apoptosis, the mitochondrial pathway and the cell surface death domain pathway, the death domain pathway seems to be primarily involved.[96]

Ineffective erythropoiesis and anemia result in several clinical sequelae. The first response to anemia is an increased production of erythropoietin, causing a marked erythroid hyperplasia, which may range between 10 and 30 times normal.[97] Anemia may produce cardiac enlargement and sometimes severe cardiac failure. Erythroid expansion produces skeletal deformities, osteoporosis, and, occasionally, extramedullary masses and contributes to splenomegaly. Untreated or undertreated patients with TDT have poor growth as a result of anemia and the excessive metabolic burden imposed by erythroid expansion. Environmental factors, such as poor nutrition and infections, may also contribute to growth failure. The high vascularization of expanded marrow results in an increase in plasma volume, which, associated with splenomegaly, aggravates the anemia.

Ineffective erythropoiesis is associated with increased iron absorption due to several interacting mechanisms, which converge either on liver hepcidin production or on ferroportin expression on intestinal epithelial cells.[98,99] Erythroferrone was recently identified as a hormone secreted by erythroblasts downstream of the erythropoietin-JAK2-STAT5 pathway activation. Erythroferrone functions to suppress hepcidin production and therefore increase intestinal iron absorption.[100,101] In addition, ferroportin is upregulated in intestinal epithelial cells directly by HIF2α in response to hypoxia. The net result is increased iron absorption and retention. In transfusion-dependent patients, iron overload is largely caused by repeated blood transfusions (see "Complications of Transfusions"). Iron overload damages several organs (heart, liver, and endocrine glands), leading to severe complications. Removal of the abnormal RBCs by the reticuloendothelial elements of the spleen results in splenomegaly and hypersplenism, which, when severe, may exacerbate anemia and cause thrombocytopenia and leukopenia. This may result in the need for increased frequency of erythrocyte transfusions.

Patients with β-thalassemia have been reported to be thrombophilic.[102,103] This is attributed to RBC membrane damage from loss of the normal asymmetric distribution and increased surface exposure of the procoagulant, negatively charged phospholipids phosphatidylserine and phosphatidylethanolamine.[104] Perturbation of the cell membrane causes thalassemic RBCs to become rigid and deformed, increasing their cohesiveness and tendency to aggregate.[105] The anionic phospholipids increase thrombin generation, which leads to activation of platelets and endothelial cells. Further evidence of the chronic platelet activation has been documented in patients with thalassemia, as evidenced by increased platelet aggregation and expression of CD62P (P-selectin) and CD63, shorter platelet survival, and elevated levels of urinary metabolites of prostacyclin (PGI2) and thromboxane A2, two markers of hemostasis.[106]

Moreover, thrombocytosis and increased platelet aggregation associated with splenectomy contribute to the higher risk of thromboembolic events. Decreased levels of naturally occurring anticoagulants, such as protein C and protein S, and elevated plasma levels of the thrombin-antithrombin III complex, have been reported.[107] It has also been shown that adherence of thalassemic red cells to endothelial cells is markedly enhanced as compared with that of normal red cells and that elevated levels of endothelial adhesion proteins (intracellular adhesion molecule-1, E-selectin, vascular cell adhesion molecule-1, and von Willebrand factor) in the serum and plasma of thalassemic patients have been described.[105] Finally, thrombogenic microparticles are enriched in samples from splenectomized thalassemic patients and may enhance adhesion to endothelium.[108]

α-Thalassemia

As in the case of β-thalassemia, the primary defect in α-thalassemia is the imbalance of globin biosynthesis, which leads to an excess of β- and/or γ-globin chains. Unlike α-chains, which are highly unstable and unable to form soluble tetramers, excess γ-chains in fetal life and β-chains in extrauterine life associate to form relatively soluble γ_4 tetramers (Hb Barts) and β_4 tetramers (HbH), respectively. These excess non-α-chains damage mature RBCs and erythroid precursors, leading to hemolysis and, to a lesser degree, ineffective erythropoiesis. The different characteristics of the excess chains in α-thalassemia are of great importance in determining its pathophysiology; in addition, the functional properties of HbH and Hb Barts and the number of α genes contribute to the difference in severity of α-thalassemia as compared with β-thalassemia syndromes. RBCs in α-thalassemia are rigid, as in β-thalassemia, but unlike in β-thalassemia, they are hyperhydrated and have red cell membranes that are hyperstable. The pathophysiology leading to hyperhydration is hypothesized to be a consequence of the effect of excess β-chains on the KCl cotransporter system. Membrane skeleton-bound β-globins become partially oxidized, with consequent membrane damage. In vitro studies have shown that entrapment of β-chains in normal red cells does not result in any significant change in membrane protein function or thiol concentrations, but rather produces changes in red cell deformability, as reported in vivo in patients with HbH disease.[109] Interaction of excess β-globin with the cytoplasmic domain of protein band 3 is abnormal in HbH disease because β_4 tetramers tend to adhere tightly to protein band 3. β-Globin tetramers precipitate as the red cell ages, forming inclusions. These inclusions can be microscopically visualized by staining of peripheral blood with vital stains, such as brilliant cresyl blue or new methylene blue, and are more common in splenectomized patients. Membrane-bound inclusion bodies perturb the flow velocity during transit through the spleen capillaries, ultimately resulting in mechanical trapping and macrophagic phagocytosis. β_4 Inclusion bodies alter the normal membrane phospholipid bilayer, exposing phosphatidylserine, which represents a signal for the development of apoptosis and red cell removal by the macrophages in the spleen and other reticuloendothelial organs.[110]

Red cell membrane deformability and stability is even more affected in patients with HbH/HbCS.[111] As compared with patients with HbH disease, patients with HbH/HbCS have a higher amount of HbH and a higher percentage of erythrocytes with inclusion bodies and with translocated phosphatidylserine. All these characteristics may account for the increased hematologic severity of HbH/HbCS disease. γ-Globin tetramers (Hb Barts) are much less prone than β-globin tetramers to precipitate and form inclusions.[110] Besides the characteristics of excess β- and γ-globin chains discussed earlier, other functionally abnormal properties are important in determining the pathophysiology of α-thalassemia. HbH and, even more, Hb Barts have a very high oxygen affinity and show no heme/heme interaction or Bohr effect, hence severely reducing their oxygen-carrying capacity.[112] Some α-globin chain variants barely symptomatic in the heterozygous state are either unstable because of folding defects and/or defective in binding to AHSP and are associated with the α-thalassemia phenotype.[113]

Genotype-Phenotype Correlation in Thalassemia

Understanding of the mechanisms of globin gene regulation and expression has helped elucidate the relationship between genotype and phenotype. This knowledge is helpful in clinical practice for planning the management of the patients and in genetic counseling for the prediction of phenotype from genotype in couples at risk. However, there is significant variation in phenotype for patients with identical mutations,[114] and while the genotype data are helpful, ultimately the hematological and clinical manifestations guide the need for transfusions. In β-thalassemia, the globin chain imbalance is the main determinant of clinical severity. The presence of factors that reduce the globin chain imbalance results in a milder form of thalassemia. These factors include the coinheritance of α-thalassemia or of genetic determinants that increase γ-chain production and the presence of silent or mild β-thalassemia alleles, associated with a high residual output of β-globin. Examples of these alleles are the silent -101 C→T and the mild IVS-1-6 T→C mutation in the Mediterranean population and the -29 A→G in Africans. Deletional and nondeletional HPFH mutations, associated with a high HbF level in carriers, when in genetic compounds with severe β-thalassemia alleles, result in mild NTDT. A mild phenotype may also be caused by coinheritance of genetic determinants associated with γ-chain production, mapping outside the β-globin cluster. Several SNPs at the BCL11A gene on 2 p16.1 and HBS1L-MYB intergenic region on 6q23.3 have been associated with variable HbF levels in patients with thalassemia and sickle cell disease.[78,79] The effect of α-thalassemia determinants in ameliorating the disease severity is less consistent, but the coinheritance of the deletion of two α-globin genes with homozygous β^+-thalassemia, and sometimes even with β^0-thalassemia, produces the clinical picture of NTDT. Variants at the three main quantitative trait loci regulating HbF levels (i.e., BCL11A, HBS1L-MYB intergenic region, Xmn1 CG $-\gamma$ gene) and α-thalassemia have been associated with an NTDT phenotype and a delayed need for transfusions in patients with homozygous β^0-thalassemia.[72]

The precise definition of the phenotype from the genotype is helpful in genetic counseling and prenatal diagnosis in at-risk couples, where coinheritance of the β-globin -101 C→T mutation or the triple α-gene arrangement can worsen the phenotype while a coinherited HPFH mutation associated with high levels of HbF should exhibit a milder phenotype. The ameliorating effect that results from the presence of mild β-thalassemia alleles is less constant. The mild β-thalassemia allele IVS-1-6 T→C, common in the Mediterranean population, shows remarkable phenotypic diversity in some populations, such as the Jewish population.[2] Despite the progress in better defining genetic determinants able to influence the clinical severity of β-thalassemia, phenotype prediction from genotype is not always accurate. However, the information obtained from extended genetic analysis may be used for planning appropriate management and for providing adequate genetic counseling and may also reveal potential new targets for therapeutic intervention. As reported earlier, the wide range of phenotypic manifestations of thalassemia results from the heterogeneity of the primary mutation and from the coinheritance of other globin gene–associated determinants, which may ameliorate or worsen the disease severity.[115] However, other known or unknown genetic determinants may modify the clinical expression of the thalassemia syndromes. Several secondary genetic modifiers have been identified in the recent years. The presence of (TA)7 polymorphism in the promoter region of the uridine diphosphoglucuronosyltransferase gene, which, in the homozygous state, is associated with Gilbert syndrome, is a risk factor for the development of cholelithiasis in TDT and NTDT and in patients with HbE/β-thalassemia.[116] Other candidate genes for modification of the thalassemia phenotype are the apolipoprotein E4 allele, which seems to be a genetic risk factor for left ventricular failure in homozygous β-thalassemia.[117]

In α-thalassemia, the symptomatic form of HbH disease shows a wide phenotypic diversity. The phenotype varies depending on the number of α genes affected and on the type of mutation present.[118] Studies that have correlated hematologic and clinical findings with α-globin genotypes indicate that HbH patients with nondeletion

α-thalassemia defects have a more severe clinical expression. Unlike with β-thalassemia, limited progress has been made in the search for genetic modifiers of HbH.

CLINICAL AND LABORATORY FEATURES

α-Thalassemia: Clinical Forms

Despite the large number of different α-thalassemia alleles (overall more than 100), only four hematologic phenotypes with clinical conditions of increasing severity are observed: silent carrier, α-thalassemia trait, HbH disease, and Hb Barts hydrops fetalis.[118]

Silent Carrier

This condition results from the presence of a single α-globin gene defect associated with the 3.7- or 4.2-kb deletion ($-\alpha/aa$) and from nondeletional defects. This genotype is characterized in the newborn period by a very mild increased percentage (1%-2%) of Hb Barts, a tetramer of four γ-globin chains (γ_4), which is produced when there is an excess of γ-chains in relation to α-chains. However, failure to demonstrate Hb Barts in cord blood does not exclude the silent carrier state.[119] Among black Americans, the incidence of the silent carrier state determined by gene mapping is about 27%, yet Hb Barts is detected in only 12% of cord samples. Similar trends have been found in Mediterranean and Saudi Arabian populations.

Adult individuals with three functional α genes may have a completely silent phenotype (normal RBC indices) or exhibit a minimal thalassemia-like phenotype (reduced MCV and MCH, minimal anemia) with normal HbA2 and HbF.[118] Analysis of globin chain synthesis in vitro in peripheral blood reticulocytes displays a reduced α:β ratio in the range of 0.8 to 0.9. At birth, children with the $-\alpha$4.2 deletion, which affects the α_2 gene, have a more severe phenotype than children with the $-\alpha$3.7 deletion, which deletes most of the less productive α_1 gene, resulting in a hybrid gene consisting of the 5′ part of the α_2 gene linked to the 3′ part of the α_1 gene.[110] However, with increasing age, the two genotypic forms become phenotypically indistinguishable, presumably because of upregulation of α-globin production by the α_1-gene in subjects with the $-\alpha$4.2 deletion.

α-Thalassemia Trait

This condition is characterized in the newborn by more pronounced increased levels of Hb Barts (5%-6%) and in the adult by thalassemia-like red cell indices, normal HbA2 and HbF, and a reduced α:β-globin chain synthesis ratio in the range of 0.7 to 0.8.[118] Subjects with two residual functional α genes, either in the cis configuration, both mutations affecting genes on the same chromosome ($-/aa$ or α^0-thalassemia carriers), or in trans configuration, with mutations in opposite chromosomes ($-\alpha/-\alpha$, homozygous α^+-thalassemia), both have the α-thalassemia carrier state. Carriers of nondeletion defects have variable hematologic phenotypes ranging from the α-thalassemia trait to the silent carrier state (see above). Double heterozygotes for $-\alpha/$and nondeletion α-thalassemia ($-\alpha/[aa]$T) and homozygotes for nondeletion defects ([aa]T/[aa]T) have the typical phenotype of the α-thalassemia carrier state. However, homozygotes with nondeletional forms of α-thalassemia may have a mild HbH disease.[118] It should be noted that homozygotes for the Hb Constant Spring mutation, the most common nondeletion defect in the Asian population, have a clinical syndrome that is similar to HbH disease (see below). The α-thalassemia carrier state must be differentiated from iron deficiency and from δ- and β-thalassemia interaction (see "Carrier Detection"). This differentiation has important practical consequences.

HbH Disease

HbH disease is common in Southeast Asia and relatively frequent in Mediterranean countries and parts of the Middle East, while occurring rarely in populations of African descent. This clinical condition results from the presence of one functional α gene, usually as a consequence of the compound heterozygous state for α^0-thalassemia/α^+-thalassemia ($-/-\alpha$ or $-/\alpha$Tα). As a consequence of the relative excess of β-chains, individuals with HbH disease produce a variable amount of this abnormal Hb, a tetramer of β-globin chains (β4). The HbH is unstable and precipitates inside the red cells and to some extent in erythroid precursors, causing membrane damage and premature erythrocyte destruction. As reported earlier, the predominant mechanism for anemia in HbH disease is hemolysis. HbH has a higher oxygen affinity than HbA, and this may worsen the severity of anemia in patients with HbH disease.[112] In the neonatal period, subjects with the HbH disease genotype have a consistently elevated Hb Barts (~25%), which may still be detected in small amounts in some adults with HbH disease. The syndrome of HbH disease shows a considerable variability in clinical and hematologic severity. The majority of patients have few clinical manifestations. The most salient features are microcytosis, hypochromia, hemolytic anemia, hepatosplenomegaly, jaundice, and moderate thalassemia-like skeletal modifications.[120] The Hb concentration is usually in the range of 7 to 10 g/dL, and the MCV is low and varies with age (being around 58 fL in childhood and around 64 fL in adulthood), whereas the MCH is around 18 pg irrespective of age. Reticulocytes range between 5% and 10%, and the α:β-globin chain synthesis ratio is markedly reduced, in the order of 0.20 to 0.60. Hb electrophoresis at alkaline pH shows a fast-moving band (HbH) in amounts ranging from 1% to 40%. Sometimes, because of the low quantity and the possible loss owing to instability in the preparation of the hemolysate, HbH may escape detection. The most sensitive method to detect HbH consists of the incubation of peripheral blood cells for 1 to 2 hours at 37 °C in the presence of supravital dyes (brilliant cresyl blue or methyl violet), which induce precipitation of the abnormal Hb as inclusion bodies, easily recognizable at the microscope (*Figure 35.5*).[115] Determination of the α-globin genotype may be useful for prognosis of HbH disease because the nondeletional forms are more severe than the deletion forms. Anemia is accentuated during pregnancy and may worsen quite dramatically with infections, fever, ingestion of oxidant drugs, pure red cell aplasia associated with Parvovirus B19, and hypersplenism. Splenomegaly is almost always present, whereas liver enlargement is less common. A mild phenotype of HbH disease may result from the homozygous state for nondeletional α-thalassemia. Although the phenotype in some cases is closer to that of the homozygous state for $α^+$-thalassemia, the degree of anemia and hypochromia may be more severe. In particular, homozygotes for the elongated α-chain variant Hb Constant Spring are asymptomatic but show mild pallor and jaundice with liver and spleen enlargement in about 50% of the cases. The Hb level ranges from 9 to 11 g/dL, and the MCV tends to be normal (88 ± 6 fL), whereas the MCH is slightly reduced (26 ± 3 pg). The peripheral blood contains HbA2, HbA, Hb Constant Spring, and traces of Hb Barts rather than HbH. The severity of HbH disease shows a good correlation with the degree of α-chain deficiency. Thus, the more severe and variable phenotypes are associated with interactions involving nondeletion α-thalassemia defects that affect the dominant $α_2$ gene, including (−/αConstant Springα), (−/αNcoIα), and (−/αHphIα). Patients with nondeletional genotypes

present younger, with more severe hemolytic anemia, significant growth delay, dysmorphic facial features, and more marked hepatosplenomegaly, and require more transfusions. Patients with HbH disease resulting from the interaction of $α^+$-thalassemia (−α) with the deletion of the MCS regulatory region have been reported.[121] A severe HbH phenotype resulting from deletions of both upstream MCS-Rs, with four intact α-globin genes, has been recently described.[39,122]

A few cases of HbH disease associated with hydrops fetalis caused by coinheritance of $α^0$- and $α^+$-thalassemia have been described.[123] In four cases, the $α^+$-thalassemia alleles were mutations of the $α_2$ gene associated with hyperunstable α-globin variants. The interaction between two relatively common forms of α-thalassemia ($−^{Med}/α^{TSaudi}α$) can present with HbH hydrops fetalis.[124] In these families, prenatal diagnosis is indicated. Patients with HbH disease may develop complications including hypersplenism, leg ulcers, gallstones, and abnormal left ventricular dysfunction.[115] Hypersplenism has been reported in 10% of Thai patients with HbH disease, but it seems to be rare elsewhere. Iron overload as assessed by serum ferritin is increased in a large proportion (50%-75%) of patients and is correlated with age.

In general, patients with deletional HbH disease do not require ongoing treatment to raise the hemoglobin level. Clinicians often recommend folic acid supplementation, similar to other hemolytic anemias. Patients should avoid oxidant drugs because of the risk of hemolytic crisis. Occasional blood transfusions may be required as a consequence of hemolytic or aplastic crisis. Transfusions are more frequently needed with nondeletional HbH disease, and occasionally regular red cell transfusions are used to improve anemia or manage clinical complications in this subpopulation. Pregnant women with HbH disease need careful monitoring of Hb levels. Splenectomy may be indicated in the presence of hypersplenism or severe anemia, but the potential complication of venous thrombosis, reported in some patients with HbH disease following splenectomy, should be considered.[125] Chelation therapy should be initiated in patients with elevated serum ferritin and/or increased liver iron stores.

Hb Barts Hydrops Fetalis Syndrome

Hb Barts hydrops fetalis syndrome is the most severe α-thalassemia clinical condition, often associated with the absent function of all four α-globin genes (homozygous $α^0$-thalassemia or −/−). A few cases of hydrops fetalis have been reported in infants with very low levels of α-chain synthesis.[126] Hb Barts hydrops fetalis syndrome is most common in Southeast Asian populations, whereas in Mediterranean populations, it is relatively rare owing to the low frequency of $α^0$-thalassemia. Because of the extreme rarity of the cis conformation (−/aa genotype) in people of African descent, this disorder also rarely affects infants of African background. A fetus homozygous for $α^0$-thalassemia produces mainly Hb Bart's (γ4), which is functionally useless for oxygen transport, and survival to late pregnancy is because of the presence of small amounts of embryonic Hbs Portland 1 ($ζ_2γ_2$) and Portland 2 ($ζ_2β_2$). There is a marked variability in the intrauterine clinical course of fetuses with Hb Barts hydrops fetalis. Many pregnancies terminate unnoticed or early in gestation. In some cases, pregnancy proceeds to term but the fetus is stillborn or severely ill; in others, the fetus does not become hydropic and is born normally.[81,127,128] The clinical features of this syndrome are those of a very severe anemia (Hb level range, 3-8 g/dL), with marked hepatosplenomegaly, generalized edema, signs of cardiac failure, and extensive extramedullary erythropoiesis.[110] Maternal complications during pregnancy are common and include preeclampsia (hypertension, fluid retention with or without proteinuria), polyhydramnios or oligohydramnios (increased or reduced accumulation of amniotic fluid, respectively), and antepartum hemorrhage. Postpartum complications include placenta retention, eclampsia (seizures and coma), hemorrhage, anemia, and sepsis. Given the severity of this syndrome and of the maternal obstetric complications, early termination of affected pregnancies often is pursued and several regions have initiated universal prenatal screening programs to address homozygous α-thalassemia. More recently, administration of intrauterine erythrocyte transfusions after noninvasive monitoring by Doppler ultrasonography has been utilized to rescue affected fetuses

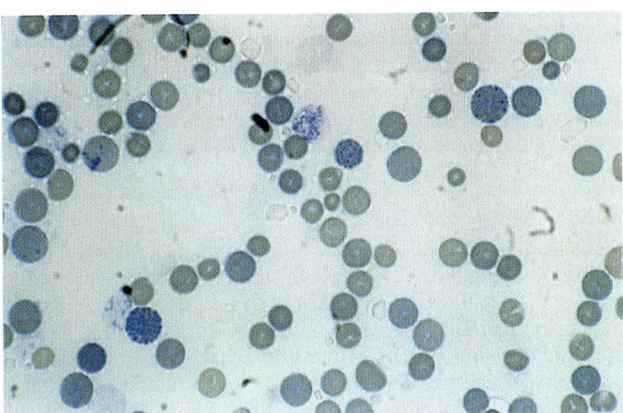

FIGURE 35.5 Hemoglobin H inclusion bodies.

to reduce the risk of hydrops and improve birth outcomes.[127] Postnatal continuation of regular transfusions or curative hematopoietic stem cell transplantation (HSCT) is necessary. Data from an international registry of 69 patients with Hb Barts hydrops fetalis syndrome found that 39 (58%) survived beyond age 5 years.[127] However, congenital abnormalities are common in survivors, including urogenital abnormalities (48%), limb abnormalities (16%), and atrial septal defect (10%), and growth delay was reported in 40% to 50%. Although most patients had either normal development or mild delay, 20% had unfavorable long-term neurodevelopmental outcomes. Intrauterine HSCT before 25 weeks' gestation, typically utilizing a haploidentical parent donor, is under study with the possibility of inducing fetal immunological tolerance that could allow a postnatal stem cell boost.

Unusual Forms of α-Thalassemia

There are two unusual forms of α-thalassemia: acquired HbH disease associated with myelodysplasia and α-thalassemia associated with mental retardation syndrome.

α-Thalassemia/Myelodysplasia Syndrome (OMIM Catalog #300448)

Patients with myelodysplasia may rarely develop an unusual form of HbH disease characterized by the presence of classic HbH inclusion bodies in RBCs, often detectable levels of HbH (1%-57%), and a severe microcytic hypochromic anemia with anisopoikilocytosis. Both α- to β-globin mRNA and synthesis ratios are markedly reduced (0.06-0.50 and 0.28, respectively).[123] Structural analysis of the α-globin genes and their flanking regions has revealed no abnormalities. Recent studies have shown that some patients with α-thalassemia/myelodysplasia syndrome have point mutations and/or splicing abnormalities in the *ATRX* gene.[129] In one patient a large deletion of the telomeric region on the short arm of one allele of chromosome 16, including both α-globin genes, was reported.[130]

α-Thalassemia and Intellectual Disability Syndromes

There are two different syndromes in which α-thalassemia is associated with intellectual disability. The first is characterized by a relatively mild intellectual disability and a variety of facial and skeletal abnormalities. These subjects have extended (1-2 megabases) deletions resulting from rearrangements of the short arm of chromosome 16. The deletions remove both α-globin genes and up to 52 other genes.[131] This condition is called ATR-16 syndrome (OMIM catalog #141750).

The second group of patients has a complex phenotype characterized by severe intellectual disability, hypertelorism, flat nasal bridge, triangular upturned nose, wide mouth, urogenital abnormalities, developmental abnormalities, and defective α-globin synthesis, resulting in a relatively mild form of HbH disease. No structural changes of the α cluster or 16p chromosome have been found in these patients, and the transmission is X linked.[132] This syndrome is associated with mutations in an X-encoded gene, the *ATRX* gene, a member of the DNA helicase family.[133] To date, 128 acquired and/or inherited mutations predominantly lying in two highly conserved domains of the ATRX protein have been identified. ATRX, a large protein with 2492 residues, is a member of the SNF2 family of adenosine triphosphate–dependent remodeling proteins and a key regulatory component of nucleosomal dynamics and higher-order chromatin conformation. ATRX protein plays a prominent role in the control of gene transcription and in the maintenance of chromosome stability. Mutations in this gene downregulate the expression of the α-globin genes and of other unidentified genes, thus producing the complex phenotype.[133] This condition is referred to as ATRX syndrome (OMIM catalog #301040). Detailed information about the forms of α-thalassemia associated with intellectual disability or myelodysplasia and about the role of ATRX are reported in published reviews.[134]

α-Thalassemia in Association With Structural Variants

A number of syndromes result from the interaction of α-thalassemia genes with those producing structurally abnormal Hbs. In some

disorders, thalassemia mutations, which are normally clinically silent, are relevant in the presence of a variant Hb. The relative amount of the variant Hb is altered by the thalassemia gene in these cases. Features common to these syndromes are red cell hypochromia and microcytosis and the presence of a Hb variant. Some mutations causing α-chain structural variants appear to have occurred in chromosomes with only a single α-globin gene. Thus, Q/α^0-thalassemia has a clinical phenotype similar to that of HbH disease and synthesized no HbA.[135] This disorder has been described in individuals from Thailand, China, Iran, and India.[136] The mutation responsible for HbG-Philadelphia sometimes occurs on a chromosome with a single α-globin gene and other times on a chromosome containing both α genes and is encountered primarily in black individuals.[137] In persons with a normal α-globin gene on the same chromosome containing the HbG mutation, HbG-Philadelphia/α^0-thalassemia ($\alpha^G\alpha/-$) is characterized clinically by α-thalassemia minor, whereas in individuals with no normal α-gene cis to the α^G-gene ($-\alpha^{G/-}$), the doubly heterozygous state resembles clinically HbH disease. The variant Hb constitutes approximately 40% of the total concentration of Hb in the former situation and more than 90% in the latter. HbI/α-thalassemia has been reported in a black patient.[138] That the gene for HbI is not linked in cis with an α-thalassemia gene is indicated by the presence of 30% HbA. The combination of α-thalassemia with β-chain variants, such as HbS and HbE, is associated with a decrease in the relative amount of the variant Hb and a clinical picture similar to that of the heterozygous state for the structural variant. The lower-than-usual percentage of the variant Hb is attributed to the preferential binding of α-chains with βA-chains. The interaction of α-thalassemia and the HbS trait produces a trimodal distribution in the relative amount of HbS. Individuals with a full complement of α-globin genes have more than 35% HbS compared with 28% to 35% in those with the ($-\alpha/aa$) genotype, 25% to 30% in those with the ($-\alpha/-\alpha$) genotype, and no more than 20% in those with the rare ($-/-\alpha$) genotype.[139] Reductions in MCV and MCH are also observed. α-Thalassemia modifies some of the hematologic consequences of homozygous sickle cell anemia. Subjects with the ($-\alpha/-\alpha$) genotype have a higher Hb concentration, lower red cell indices, fewer irreversibly sickled cells, a lower reticulocyte count, and lower serum bilirubin levels than subjects without concurrent α-thalassemia.[140,141] The ameliorating effect of α-thalassemia is probably mediated by a decreased red cell concentration of HbS. This also reduces the risk of certain clinical complications such as stroke[142] but coinheritance of α-thalassemia does not completely overcome the clinical expression of sickle cell anemia. For the interaction of α-thalassemia and HbE, see "HbE Syndromes" in this chapter.

Transfusion-Dependent Thalassemia (β-Thalassemia Major)

The β-thalassemia syndromes represent the most clinically relevant forms of thalassemia. The designation commonly used to describe the β-thalassemia syndromes is based on severity of clinical phenotype. Historically, the most severe form was known as *β-thalassemia major* characterized by transfusion-dependent anemia (more than eight red cell transfusions per year). *Thalassemia intermedia* designates a form of anemia that, independent from the genotype, does not require regular transfusion but may be treated with sporadic or intermittent transfusions. *Thalassemia minor, or thalassemia trait*, refers to the heterozygous state, which is usually completely asymptomatic. Newer categorization focuses on transfusion need and divides the phenotype into TDT and NTDT.

History

Originally, a disease called *anemia splenic infantum* included several conditions, characterized by growth failure, pallor, splenomegaly, and bone deformities leading to distinct appearance after 6 months of age. The disease was often present in siblings. The first systematic descriptions came from Cooley and Lee from Michigan, who observed the disease in Italian and Greek children,[143] and from Maccanti, a pediatrician from Ferrara, Italy, who noted that the children were coming from malarial areas near the Po river.[144] Anemia, leukocytosis, and normoblastemia were always present. Both groups tried unsuccessfully to identify effective therapies (arsenium, fresh veal bone marrow, sunshine, the quartz lamp, cod liver oil, and, of course, iron) and even blood transfusions, which were helpful but temporary in one patient and caused increased hemolysis in another. Splenectomy and Roentgen irradiation of the spleen were also performed without benefit. All children died shortly after presentation. Detailed information from autopsies demonstrated peculiar abnormalities in the bones and spleen fibrosis. Simultaneously, Rietti, also from Ferrara, had reported three adult patients, two of whom were father and son, who presented with "primitive hemolytic jaundice" associated with decreased osmotic fragility. Anemia, microcytosis, anisocytosis, and basophilic stippling were noted. This clinical entity was probably a form of NTDT and, for many years, referred to as *Rietti-Greppi-Micheli* in Italy. In 1932, Whipple and Bradford proposed the name of *thalassemia*, from the Greek word *thalassa*, meaning sea, in reference to the Mediterranean origin of patients with Cooley anemia.[145] Subsequently, severe and mild phenotypes of thalassemia were termed *thalassemia major* and *thalassemia minor*, respectively.

The lack of communication between the two sides of the Atlantic made research in this field, as in others, proceed slowly in parallel. In 1940, Wintrobe reported the presence of a familial hemopoietic disorder in adolescents and adults of Italian origin, whereas in Italy, between 1943 and 1947, Silvestroni and Bianco defined the hematologic, clinical, and epidemiologic characteristics of thalassemia minor and its relationship with thalassemia major.[146,147] Further clarification occurred with the identification of HbA2 and its increase in the parents of patients affected by thalassemia major. The patients, on the other hand, were found to be completely devoid of HbA and to have, in addition to elevated HbA2, an alkali-resistant variant usually found in the newborn, HbF.[148] The idea of thalassemia resulting from a defect in production of adult Hb is as a result of the contribution of many investigators. The understanding of globin chain synthesis was able to support this hypothesis. Recent developments in molecular biology continue to clarify more aspects of the disease.

Clinical Features

The clinical picture of TDT includes features that are a result of the disease itself and others that represent the consequences of therapy.

Anemia

The initial symptoms of the disease appear in the latter half of the first year of life, when the synthesis of γ-chains is not replaced by the synthesis of β-chains. In one study from Sardinia, TDT presented most commonly at around 8 months, whereas NTDT presented around 2 years of age.[149] The age at diagnosis is influenced by the molecular defect and by the degree of suspicion of the treating physician. Pallor is usually the first sign, accompanied by splenomegaly of various severity, fever, and failure to thrive.

Bone Deformities

Inadequate red cell transfusions lead to the development of typical bone abnormalities, which were described in the first reports of the disease and are caused by increased erythropoiesis, and consequent expansion of the bone marrow (up to 15-30 times normal). The skull is large and deformed by frontal and posterior bossing with the diploe increased in thickness. The outer and inner tables are thin and the trabeculae arranged in vertical striations, resulting in a "hair-on-end" appearance on x-ray (*Figure 35.6*).[150] The zygomatic bones are prominent, the base of the nose is depressed, pneumatization of the sinuses is delayed, and overgrowth of the maxilla produces severe malocclusion. Metatarsal and metacarpal bones expand as a consequence of increased erythropoiesis (*Figure 35.7*). The ribs are broad, often with a "rib-within-rib" appearance, and the vertebral bodies are square. The trabeculation of the medullary space gives the bones a mosaic pattern. Shortening of long bones is common, resulting from premature fusion of the humeral and femoral epiphyseal lines.[151] Extramedullary erythropoiesis gives rise to masses that protrude from bones where red marrow persists.[152]

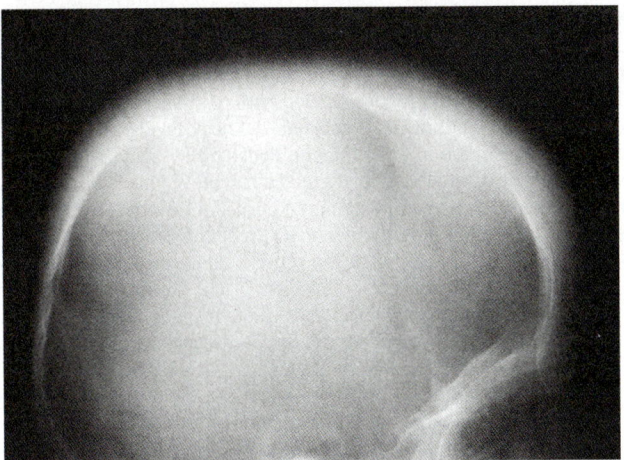

FIGURE 35.6 Radiograph of the skull. In the frontal area, the bone has a lamellated structure, parallel to the inner table of the diploe. In the parietal area, erythroid hyperplasia has perforated the outer table, producing a characteristic "hair-on-end" appearance. (Courtesy of Dr. C. Orzincolo.)

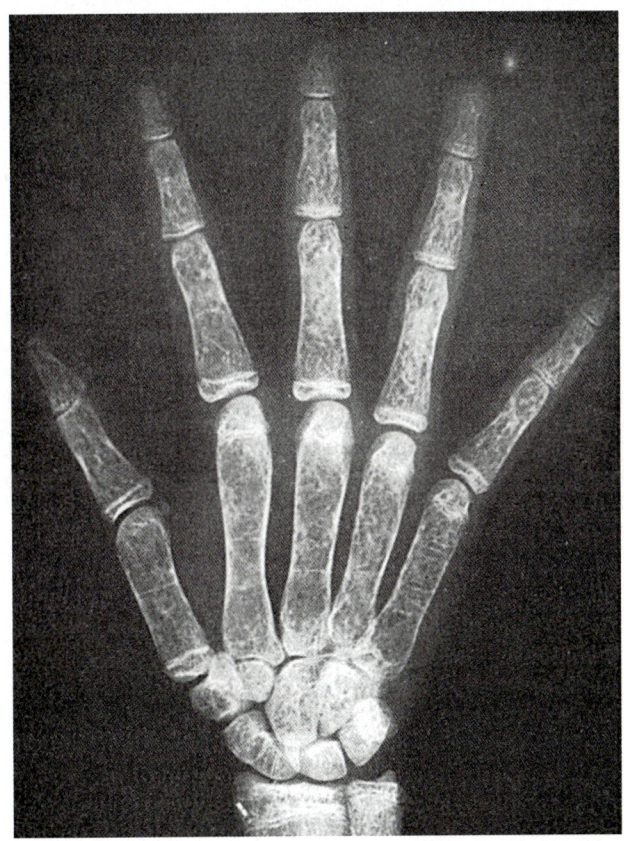

FIGURE 35.7 Mosaic pattern produced by trabeculation in the bones of the hand of a patient with thalassemia major. Note the rectangular contour of the metacarpals.

Overgrowth of vertebral bodies can cause cord compression and paraparesis. Audiologic impairment as a result of extramedullary marrow growing in the middle ear and progressive visual loss caused by compressive optic neuropathy can occur.[153] This kind of picture is more often present in patients with NTDT, in whom transfusions are avoided at the price of intense autologous marrow hyperactivity. Improvement in skeletal complications with optimized regular transfusions can be avoided if begun at an early age. However, skeletal abnormalities of a different nature, such as short truncal height, can occur as a consequence of excessive deferoxamine (DFO) therapy.

Osteoporosis

Reduced bone mineral density and consequent susceptibility to fractures in thalassemic patients have been the subject of intense research. Mineral density is usually investigated with dual-energy x-ray absorptiometry at the spinal (L1-L4) and femoral neck levels. Osteoporosis, defined as a decrease in bone mineral density ≥2.5 standard deviation (SD) below the normative data corrected for age,[154] has been found to affect 48% of the patients, with an additional 44% affected by osteopenia (–1 to >2.5 SD). Although more frequent and severe in males than in females, this complication represents an important cause of morbidity in adult patients of both sexes.[155] The pathogenesis of osteoporosis in TDT is multifactorial and results from a variety of genetic and acquired factors. The polymorphism at the Sp1 site of the collagen type I gene (*COLIA1*) has been associated with severe osteoporosis and pathologic fractures of the spine and the hip.[156] Moreover, the vitamin D receptor Bsm1 and Fok1 polymorphisms were found to be risk factors for bone mineral damage, low bone mineral density, and short stature in prepubertal and pubertal patients.[157] However, different studies of genetic polymorphisms have given contradictory results. Other contributing factors include the primary disease itself, causing ineffective hematopoiesis with progressive bone marrow expansion, and exogenous factors such as endocrine dysfunction, iron overload and chelation therapy, vitamin deficiencies, and decreased physical activity may contribute. In particular, vitamin D deficiency is frequent among adolescents.[158] Male sex, lack of spontaneous puberty, and diabetes represent significant risk factors for osteoporosis, whereas transfusional history, chelation, and erythropoietic activity do not.[159,160]

Defective osteoblastic activity is a major pathogenetic mechanism for osteoporosis. In addition, there is evidence of increased osteoclast activation. Elevated markers of bone resorption, such as urinary N-terminal peptides of collagen type I and serum tartrate–resistant acid phosphatase isoform 5b, have been demonstrated.[161] The increased osteoclast activity seems to result from an overproduction of cytokines, which affect osteoclast differentiation and function.[162] Evidence suggests that the receptor activator of nuclear factor κB ligand (RANKL)/osteoprotegerin (OPG) pathway mediates osteoclast proliferation in thalassemia and contributes to osteoporosis.[163] The hypothesis that the RANKL/OPG system is involved in mediating the action of sex steroids on bone has not been confirmed. Fractures, often secondary to mild or moderate trauma, are more frequent in thalassemic patients than the general population. In a retrospective study, 12% of patients with TDT had suffered from fractures, with an equal distribution between males and females, and prevalence increased with age.[164] The presence of other endocrinopathies, anthropometric parameters, heart disease, or hepatitis C were not significant independent predictors of fractures.[165] Bone pain of varying severity is a common complaint among adult patients and has been attributed to expanded bone marrow with consequent pressure on the cortical bone. Magnetic resonance imaging (MRI) in these cases show the reappearance of hypercellular areas in bones previously replaced by fatty marrow. Reduced and irregular mineralization of the bone has been found using microradiography and x-rays.[166] Back pain is sometimes associated with compression fractures and intervertebral disc degeneration.

In a recent study, pain was found to be associated with low vitamin D, lower bone density, and bisphosphonate use.[167] Osteoporosis is a progressive disease; thus, early detection, prevention, and treatment are essential for effective control of this potentially debilitating condition.[168] Annual evaluation for bone health should be started during adolescence. Interventions include sex hormone replacement therapy, regular exercise, and a diet rich in calcium and vitamin D. Low zinc levels have been found in patients with thalassemia,[169] which can contribute to osteopenia; zinc supplementation was shown to improve bone density.[170] Because the medical literature has shown reduced osteoblastic activity in thalassemic patients and a greater rate of bone resorption, antiresorptive drugs such as bisphosphonates are being increasingly used. To date, alendronate, pamidronate, and zoledronate have been reported to be effective in improving bone mineral density and normalizing bone turnover.[171] Neridronate has improved bone mineral density and reduced back pain in a cohort of thalassemic patients with osteoporosis.[172] One study evaluating the effect of calcitonin on bone mass showed that it prevented bone pain, improved radiologic findings, and decreased the number of fractures.[173]

Cholelithiasis

Gallstones may occur in thalassemia (*Figure 35.8*)[174]; the frequency is variable, depending on the transfusion regimens and amount of ineffective erythropoiesis and hemolysis, timing of splenectomy, and, more importantly, on the associated presence of the (TA)7 promoter mutation of uridine diphosphoglucuronosyltransferase gene.[175] A recent cooperative study of 858 transfusion-dependent thalassemic patients found a cholelithiasis prevalence of 30%. The Gilbert genotype (homozygosity for the [TA]7 motif) influenced both the prevalence of cholelithiasis and the age at clinical presentation. Ultrasonography of the gallbladder should be performed if symptoms of cholelithiasis are present. In addition, if gallstones are present at the time of splenectomy, cholecystectomy should be performed.

Thromboembolic Complications

Thalassemic patients have an increased risk of thromboembolic events. In a multicenter study, the frequency of thromboembolic events was found to be 4% in patients with TDT and 10% in patients with NTDT.[176] Other groups have reported similar prevalences.[177] In a large study of 8860 patients from different countries, female sex, history of splenectomy, and degree of anemia were thrombophilic risk factors.[178] Among patients with NTDT, older age, splenectomy, and higher ferritin levels were associated with an increased thrombosis risk and transfusions were

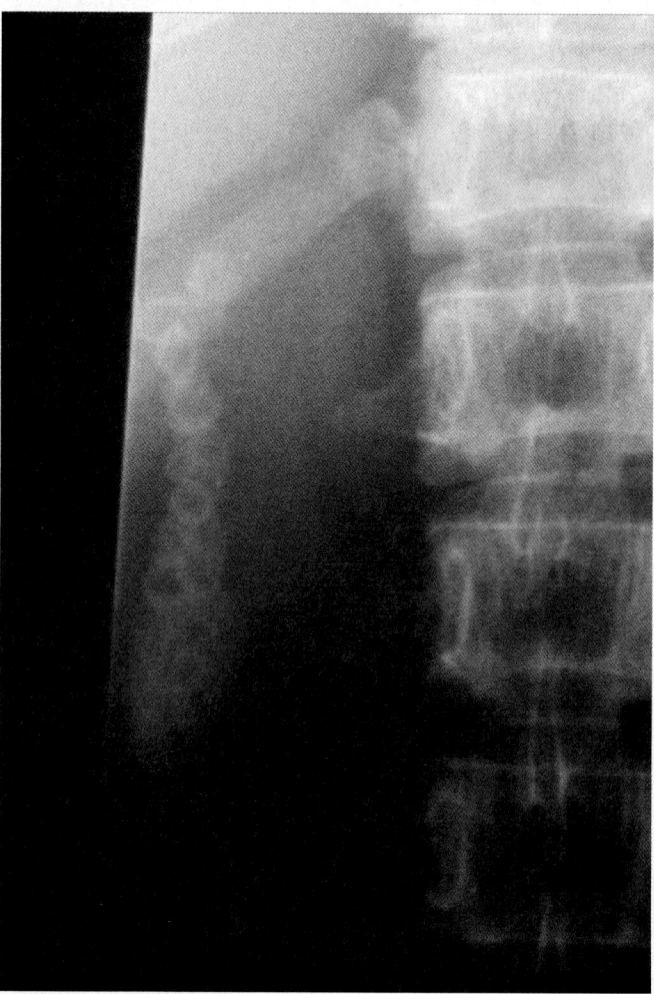

FIGURE 35.8 Spine of a 35-year-old patient with thalassemia major. Reduced mineral bone density is evident, in addition to a gallstone-filled gallbladder.

associated with a reduced risk.[179] Although the mechanisms underlying hypercoagulability in thalassemia are still unclear, it is hypothesized that the presence of a chronic hypercoagulable state could be because of the procoagulant effect of the anionic phospholipids exposed on the surface of damaged circulating red cells and to endothelial derangement in the inflammatory state associated with thalassemia. In addition, vascular endothelial cell injury and the peroxidative status because of iron overload are possible pathogenic mechanisms.[102,180] Concomitant prothrombotic conditions in thalassemic patients after the first decade of life frequently include insulin-dependent diabetes, estrogen therapy, atrial fibrillation, and postsplenectomy thrombocytosis. Prophylactic measures may be indicated for some clinical events (e.g., surgery, parturition, immobilization)[177] (see also "Non-Transfusion-Dependent Thalassemia [Thalassemia Intermedia]").

Pseudoxanthoma Elasticum

An acquired pseudoxanthoma elasticum (PXE)-like syndrome has been described in several hemolytic disorders including thalassemia.[181-183] The condition affects multiple elastic tissues and characteristically presents with lesions of the skin (small yellowish papules or larger coalescent plaques), eyes (breaks of the elastic lamina of Bruch membrane called angioid streaks), and arteries (degeneration of the elastic lamina of the arterial wall often accompanied by arterial calcification).[184] The PXE-like syndrome appears to be age dependent and more common in NTDT and is associated with thrombotic events as well as gastrointestinal and intracranial bleeding.

Laboratory Findings and Diagnosis

Laboratory data at presentation are characterized by HbF levels ranging from 10% to 100%; HbA2 may be normal or increased to 5% to 7%; the remaining percentage constitute HbA and HbF, which are heterogeneously distributed among red cells. The reticulocyte count is low, usually below 1%; the MCV is decreased, typically 60 to 70 fL; and the MCH is 12 to 18 pg/cell. In the peripheral blood smear, a large variation in size and shape of the erythrocytes is always present. Microcytes, tear drop cells, and nucleated red cells may be seen, together with large and pale target cells (*Figure 35.9*). The Hb

composition varies according to the patient's genotype. Homozygotes for β^0-thalassemia mutations have only HbF (93%-97%) and HbA2 (3%-7%) and a complete absence of HbA, whereas homozygotes for β^+-thalassemia mutations and β^0/β^+ genetic compounds have HbA, HbA2, and a variable, but elevated amount of HbF (10%-90%). HbA2 in homozygous β-thalassemia may be normal or increased and thus nondiagnostic. Hb separation to determine the Hb pattern can be performed with different methods (electrophoresis at alkaline or acidic pH, isoelectric focusing, and high-performance liquid chromatography [HPLC]).[185] In the case of transfused patients, diagnosis can be made by globin chain synthesis analysis from peripheral blood reticulocytes, which shows a severe α/non-α imbalance (usually higher than 2), or by β-globin gene analysis to identify the various DNA mutations.

Medical Interventions

Blood Transfusion

The decision to start erythrocyte transfusions in a child with thalassemia is not easy and should be based on the level of Hb and the presence of clinical complications. Initiation of transfusion is recommended if the hemoglobin level when not ill is consistently below 7 g/dL. In addition, evidence of growth delay, increasing splenomegaly, bony expansion with modification of facial features, even in the setting of hemoglobin levels above 7 g/dL, should prompt initiation of a transfusion program.[186,187] The target pretransfusion hemoglobin level is based on adequate suppression of erythropoiesis to limit clinical complications and, to a lesser extent, limiting iron loading. In patients kept at a pretransfusion Hb level between 9 and 10 g/dL, the erythroid marrow activity, evaluated through the measurement of serum transferrin receptor, was between one and four times normal levels, indicating adequate marrow suppression.[188] Transfusion requirements and serum ferritin levels also were lower with this target Hb compared with higher trough levels of 10 to 12 g/dL.[189]

On the basis of these studies, the standard transfusion regimen maintains an Hb level trough of 9 to 10.5 g/dL and posttransfusion Hb is 14 to 15 g/dL. Leukoreduced red cells are recommended for minimizing adverse reactions attributed to contaminating white cells and preventing platelet alloimmunization.

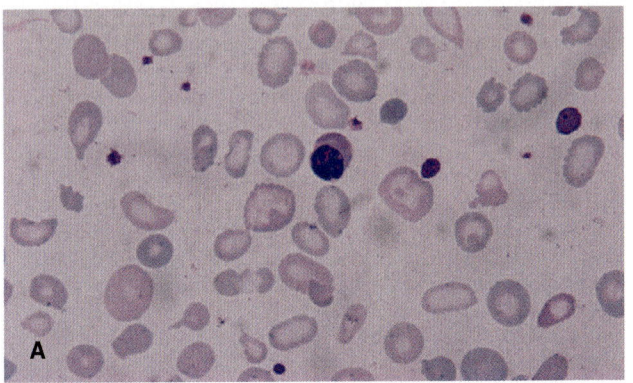

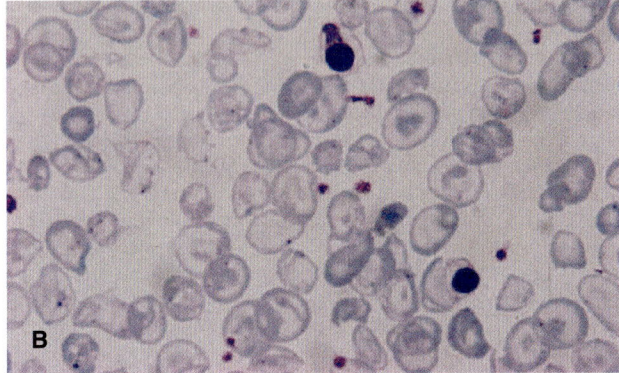

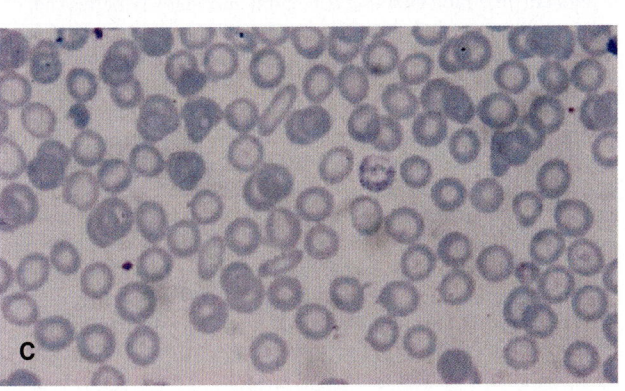

FIGURE 35.9 Peripheral blood smears in β-thalassemia major (A) and intermedia (B) and in heterozygous β-thalassemia (C).

Disorders of Red Blood Cells

In general, the transfusion rate is 5 to 6 mL/kg/h. In patients with cardiac failure, blood should be infused at a slower rate (no more than 3-4 mL/kg/h) and the administration of diuretics before transfusion is advised. The recommended interval between transfusions should take into account the patient's clinical needs and schedule considerations, but it typically begins with every 4 weeks and ranges every 2 to 6 weeks. It is helpful for the center to be able to provide after-hours transfusions, especially for children going to school and for working patients. Extended red cell antigen typing, including at least the Rh antigens, Duffy, Kidd, and Kell, is recommended to prevent alloimmunization. Prior to red cell transfusion, this can be done by traditional antigen typing. If a patient is already on a red cell transfusion regimen, then DNA typing may be performed. It is recommended that matching for Rh antigens and Kell be performed for all transfusions in thalassemia, when possible. Extended antigen matching may be employed, especially in the setting of known alloimmunization or when the racial profile of thalassemic patients does not match the blood donor population. Donor *RH* variant alleles may be an underappreciated risk factor for alloimmunization in thalassemic patients, and provision of *RH* genotype-matched red cells may be a future strategy to mitigate this risk.[190]

The red cell additive, which contains nutrients to prolong the red cell shelf life, affects the concentration of red cells in a unit. Typically, a red cell unit has a hematocrit of 80%, whereas with an additive, this may decrease to 60%. An additional observation to note is that the hematocrit of the unit may be lower during the warm months than in cold months. Possible mechanisms include expansion of plasma volume with resultant hemodilution in the patient and a lower Hb content in donor blood.[191] Thus, when there is difficulty achieving the goal Hb, these possible factors are taken into consideration because the red cell mass delivered will differ at a similar volume. In addition, this may affect the calculation of total iron received.

An accurate record of the total amount of blood transfused should be maintained in order to calculate the iron intake of the patient.[192] The annual intake is expressed in mL/kg/y of pure red cells, assuming that 1 mL of pure red cells contains 1.08 mg of iron in units without additives, or hematocrit of 80%.[193] Transfusion of young red cells (neocytes) obtained by centrifugation has been proposed in the attempt to reduce the total blood requirement, but the results obtained were not sufficient to justify the increased cost and the exposure to a larger number of donors.[194]

Complications of Transfusions

Although blood transfusions are life-saving for thalassemic patients, who no longer die of anemia, they can be complicated by transfusion reactions, alloimmunization, infections, and hemosiderosis.

Febrile Nonhemolytic Transfusion Reactions. A cooperative effort conducted 30 years ago, which reviewed more than one hundred thousand red cell transfusions in Italy and Greece, found that transfusion reactions occurred with 1% of all transfusions and in 16% of patients.[195] About 90% of the red cell units infused were leukocyte poor. Chills, fever, urticaria, headache, and chest pain accounted for more than 80% of symptoms reported, and in two-thirds of cases, reactions were reported during transfusion. Alloimmunization to human leukocyte antigens on leukocytes is the most common cause of febrile reaction in multiply transfused thalassemic patients. If blood is not filtered prestorage, cytokines may develop during storage and cause a reaction. Treatment includes acetaminophen or hydrocortisone. Allergic reactions, caused by plasma proteins and manifesting as hives, pruritus, and more rarely edema, are treated with antihistamines.

Alloimmunization. Alloimmunization and autoimmunization are complications of transfusion therapy. The frequency of alloimmunization against red cell antigens varies, with the lower percentages found in patients who received blood matched for the ABO, Rhesus, and Kell systems from their first transfusion. In a multicenter study, alloantibodies and autoantibodies were reported in 16.5% and 4.9% of patients, respectively. Splenectomized patients were 2.5 times more likely to have developed alloantibodies.[196] Another study from a single large center found that 19.5% of the thalassemic patients developed

alloantibodies, 94% of them being against the Rhesus or Kell antigens. Older age, higher transfusion frequency, and splenectomy were risk factors for alloimmunization.[197]

The risk of developing alloantibodies is not uniform and is probably genetically determined. Transfusion in infancy seems to induce immune tolerance.[198] Asians appear to be at a higher risk of developing alloantibodies and autoantibodies.[199] In addition, the risk of alloimmunization is higher in individuals from ethnic minorities because they are less represented in the donor pool compared with the general population.[200]

This phenomenon is present also in Europe, where the immigrant population, potentially at risk for hemoglobinopathies, is increasing in recent years. Donation by ethnic minorities should be encouraged to prevent the formation of RBC alloantibodies, which can result in hemolytic transfusion reactions and difficulty in finding appropriate RBCs for future transfusions. In addition, expanded crossmatching of the RBCs should decrease this risk substantially.

Infections. The risk of transfusion-transmitted viral infections is well known. Among the most frequent and clinically relevant are hepatitis B and hepatitis C viruses (HBV and HCV). The prevalence of infection of these viruses in chronically transfused patients is different in different parts of the world and is directly related to the frequency in that population. Worldwide, from 0.3% to 5.7% of thalassemic patients are hepatitis B surface antigen positive[201] and from 4.4% to 85% are positive for anti-hepatitis C antibodies.[202] The prevalence of HBV chronic infection is higher in countries in Asia and Southeast Asia, whereas HCV chronic infection is widespread throughout the world. Nucleic acid amplification technology (NAT) screening has greatly reduced the risk of transmission of these viruses from blood products. The DNA-recombinant vaccine against HBV, safe and effective, is available and should be administered to all patients who have not yet been infected. HGV and GB virus C are RNA viruses that were independently identified in 1995 and were subsequently found to be isolates of the same virus. They are common among thalassemic patients but have not been found to contribute to chronic hepatocellular damage.[203] West Nile virus infection has become a concern in recent years. Epidemics have been reported, and the virus can be transmitted through blood transfusion. In the United States, testing for West Nile virus antibodies has been implemented in 2003, and NAT is widely used in Europe in endemic areas.

Cytomegalovirus (CMV) is widespread in most populations. A European collaborative study revealed a positive CMV IgG test in two-thirds of the thalassemic patients.[204] HIV infection has dramatically decreased with the implementation of systematic screening including NAT of blood donations. In 1987, the prevalence of HIV in thalassemic patients from 13 European or Mediterranean countries was found to be 1.56%. Two years later, no HIV seroconversion was observed in the same areas when a total of 2972 patients affected by thalassemia who had received 96,518 blood units were examined.[205] Since 2004, several cases of transfusion-associated variant Creutzfeldt-Jakob disease have been reported and linked to blood collected from preclinically affected donors. Animal data suggest that all blood components are vectors for prion disease transmission.[206] Malaria can be transmitted by transfusion in endemic areas.[207] Screening programs for *Trypanosoma cruzi*, a parasitic infection endemic in Central and South America that causes Chagas disease, and is becoming increasingly diagnosed in other countries owing to travel and immigration, were implemented in 1998 in the United Kingdom[208] and in 2007 in the United States. Although significant improvements have been made to further decrease the incidence of transfusion-transmitted infections, risks remain for infectious disease agents specific to RBC concentrates. Emerging viruses, bacteria, protozoa, and residual contaminating leukocytes continue to be of risk.[209-211] Thus, development of pathogen and leukocyte inactivation methods that do not affect RBC viability continues to be of interest. Pathogen inactivation systems have been approved for platelets and plasma and are actively being studied for RBCs.[212,213]

Predisposing factors for bacterial infections include prior splenectomy, iron overload, and use of the iron chelator DFO. Despite the availability of immunizations against encapsulated organisms, the risk of infections is still high in splenectomized patients.[214] Iron overload and DFO favor the growth of organisms such as *Yersinia enterocolitica* and *Klebsiella pneumoniae*, *Yersinia* being more prevalent in temperate regions and *Klebsiella* in tropical and subtropical areas. *Yersinia* infection should be suspected in the presence of fever, diarrhea, right-lower quadrant abdominal pain, and a palpable abdominal mass because abdominal suppurative complications have been reported.[215] DFO, but not deferiprone (DFP) or deferasirox (DFX), enhances the growth of *Yersinia*, which can use the drug as a siderophore and as a source of iron. Growth of *Klebsiella*, on the contrary, is only moderately enhanced by DFO and unaffected by DFP or DFX. Several reports have described infection with *Aeromonas hydrophila* in Asia, although growth is not affected by the three chelators.[216]

Hemosiderosis

Without iron chelation, the accumulation of iron is an inevitable adverse side effect of chronic, regular red cell transfusions, which causes considerable morbidity and ultimately leads to death. A unit of blood contains approximately 200 mg of iron; thus, a patient who receives 25 to 30 U of blood a year by the third decade of life accumulates over 70 g of iron.[217] In addition to the iron administered through blood transfusions, the increased bone marrow activity leads to increased iron absorption that will contribute, although marginally, to the total body iron load. Ineffective erythropoiesis leads to suppression of hepcidin, a 25-amino-acid peptide, synthesized in the hepatocytes, that controls the concentration of ferroportin on the intestinal epithelium.[218] Ferroportin is the primary means of cellular iron efflux and a key component of iron metabolism. Hepcidin regulates ferroportin activity by inducing its internalization and degradation. Low levels of hepcidin correlate with higher levels of ferroportin, resulting in increased intestinal iron absorption. Duodenal iron absorption is regulated by the hepcidin-ferroportin axis, and hepcidin, in turn, is regulated by plasma iron concentration and iron stores. In addition, hepcidin is homeostatically regulated by the iron requirements of erythroid precursors for Hb synthesis. As a consequence, in β-thalassemia, whenever the bone marrow is not completely suppressed by blood transfusions, iron absorption is increased, even in the presence of iron overload.[219]

Excessive iron damages cells by several mechanisms. In patients who have fully saturated transferrin, a significant fraction of the total iron in plasma circulates in the form of low-molecular-weight complexes not bound to transferrin, referred to as non-transferrin-bound iron (NTBI).[220] Although the exact mechanism of tissue damage remains unclear, the most important pathogenetic factor appears to be NTBI-induced peroxidative injury to the phospholipids of lysosomes and mitochondria. The redox active component of NTBI is referred to as the labile plasma iron, and it can be identified with oxidant-sensitive fluorescent methods.[221] Control of circulating labile plasma iron is crucial to prevent oxidative damage and to decrease the risk of organ dysfunction. At present, an easy method for serial NTBI/labile plasma iron measurements is not available.

Excessive iron stores and NTBI lead to depletion of substances that defend against free radical attack, for example, among others, ascorbic acid, which is oxidized to oxalate, and vitamin E.[222] This, in turn, causes sequestration of the iron in the reticuloendothelial system, somehow protecting tissues from siderosis. At suboptimal concentration, ascorbic acid is a pro-oxidant and enhances the catalytic effect of iron in free radical formation.[223] The presence of the genetic hemochromatosis mutations does not seem to influence the degree of iron overload and its consequences in regularly transfused and chelated patients with TDT.

Assessment of Iron Stores. The ability to measure the total body iron stores in patients with thalassemia is crucial to their medical management. After a few years of transfusion, transferrin is completely saturated in the majority of patients. In TDT, serial serum ferritin has been found to correlate with iron stores, as measured by phlebotomy, and with liver iron, measured directly either by liver biopsy or by MRI.[224] Significantly higher ferritin levels are present in patients with endocrinopathies,[225] cardiac failure, and arrhythmias than in patients

without these complications. Levels above 2500 ng/dL are reported to be associated with an increased risk of death.[226]

Several variables can interfere with the reliability of ferritin as a marker of iron overload. Ferritin is an acute-phase reactant and is increased in infections, chronic disease, malignancy, and inflammatory disorders. A ferritin concentration of 4000 µg/L is the maximum level of physiologic synthesis, whereas higher values would represent the release of intracellular ferritin from damaged cells.[227] Ascorbic acid deficiency can lead to decreased synthesis and release of ferritin, which can lead to ferritin levels that are only mildly elevated in the presence of massive iron stores. A low level of hepcidin also results in iron depletion of macrophages, decreasing secretion of ferritin resulting in lower serum ferritin levels. This phenomenon is particularly evident in NTDT. Conversely, patients with active liver disease or inflammation may have high levels of serum ferritin that do not accurately reflect body iron load.[228] Despite these potential confounding factors, serial measurements of serum ferritin are widely used to evaluate iron overload and efficacy of chelation therapy. It remains the most practical assessment of total iron burden owing to the wide availability, is a noninvasive test, and is less costly than other methods. By reviewing trends in the ferritin levels over time, some of factors affecting accuracy in reflecting total body iron are minimized.

The total iron burden is estimated by measurement of iron concentration in the liver. Needle biopsy specimens of 1 mg dry weight are adequate. The measurement is done by atomic absorption spectrometry on washed or lyophilized samples and correlates well with the total amount of blood transfused and the extent of hepatic fibrosis.[229] Removal of body iron by phlebotomy after bone marrow transplantation has demonstrated that total body iron stores (in mg/kg of body weight) are equivalent to 10.6 times the hepatic iron concentration. The correlation's standard error is <7.9. In the absence of cirrhosis, the correlation is linear up to a body iron burden of 250 mg/kg. The variation in iron concentration throughout the liver, however, increases with the iron loading and the presence of cirrhosis. The coefficient of variation for multiple needle biopsy measurements ranges from an average of 19% for disease-free liver to more than 40% for end-stage cirrhosis.[230] Magnetic susceptometry is another noninvasive method for measuring liver iron content and is based on the magnetic response of ferritin and hemosiderin iron contained in the liver.[231] This method requires specialized equipment, which is referred to as SQUID, superconducting quantum interference device. It has a very limited availability and is available at only four sites (the United States [two], Germany, and Italy). Currently, the standard method to measure iron stores relies on MRI, and spin echo (R2) or gradient echo (R2*) MRI are widely used for the evaluation of iron stores.

A validated, noninvasive method of measuring and imaging liver iron concentration (LIC) in vivo using R2 MRI was reported by St. Pierre et al.[229] High degrees of sensitivity and specificity of mean liver proton transverse relaxation rates (R2) were found at clinically significant LICs. Although most 1.5-T magnets are able to perform iron estimation measurements, specialized software and local expertise are required for accurate assessment. Thus, some centers have chosen to purchase commercial software and outsource image analysis to a central facility where the data are interpreted remotely.

The T2*, the reciprocal of R2*, technique for the measurement of tissue iron was developed in 2001 and validated by chemical estimation of iron in patients undergoing liver biopsy.[232]

T2* is a magnetic relaxation property of any tissue and is inversely related to intracellular iron stores. Iron deposits shorten T1, T2, and T2*. T2* has become widely used because it is the most sensitive to iron deposition. Measurement is simple and robust and has high reproducibility. An additional advantage of the technique is that, during acquisition of the cardiac iron data, ventricular function can also be assessed. Cardiac T2* MRI predicts the risk of developing iron-related cardiac failure or arrhythmias (see below). Iron calibration in humans for cardiovascular magnetic resonance T2* against myocardial iron concentration has been reported.[233] An MRI multislice multiecho T2* technique for global and segmental measurement of iron overload in the heart has been validated and shown to be reproducible.[234] More recently, MRI T2* is used for assessing iron in the pancreas,[235] hypophysis,[236] brain, and kidneys.

Clinical Manifestations of Iron Overload

Heart

Cardiac complications are the most worrisome complication of iron overload, resulting in heart failure and arrhythmias, which are responsible for 70% of the deaths of patients treated with DFO.[224] An Italian cooperative study demonstrated that, of 776 patients with TDT, 22% carried the diagnosis of one or more cardiac problems, including heart dysfunction (66%), arrhythmias (14%), and both (19%).[237] The prevalence of heart dysfunction and/or arrhythmias is significantly higher in males than in females. Heart disease caused by iron overload is mediated through the labile iron-induced peroxidative injury to the phospholipids of lysosomes and mitochondria. This has been demonstrated both in vitro and in animal models.[238] In the absence of chelation, subclinical dysfunction appears in the second decade of life, or when approximately 20 g of iron has been accumulated. Subsequently, cardiomegaly and left ventricular deterioration progress to congestive heart failure, and sudden death from arrhythmias can occur. In asymptomatic thalassemic patients with normal myocardial mass, diastolic dysfunction appears to be an early event, even when the systolic function is mildly impaired. The classic picture of end-stage iron-induced cardiomyopathy is a combination of left ventricular diastolic dysfunction, pulmonary hypertension, and right ventricular dilatation.[239]

The measurement of cardiac iron, until recently, was difficult to obtain. Endomyocardial biopsies are not always accurate, and traditional diagnostic tools (electrocardiography, 24-hour tracings, echocardiography, and nuclear studies), which are routinely performed in monitoring, are not predictive of subsequent cardiac dysfunction.[240] When positive, the myocardiopathy is often advanced. As previously mentioned, the cardiovascular magnetic resonance relaxation parameter R2* (or cardiac T2* MRI) measured in the ventricular septum has greatly increased the amount of information on heart iron content and function. A fast spin-echo sequence permits acquisition of multiple images in one breathhold.[241] The technique has recently been validated against 12 human hearts from transfusion-dependent patients.[233]

The predictive value of cardiac T2* for heart failure and arrhythmia in thalassemia has been assessed on 652 patients with TDT from 21 UK centers. The relative risk of developing heart failure within 1 year was 160 with cardiac T2* values <10 ms (compared with >10 ms) and 270 with a T2* < 6 ms. Cardiac T2* was <10 ms in 98% of patients who developed heart failure and had a greater predictive value than serum ferritin and LIC[242] (*Figure 35.10*). Hepatic iron levels do not predict cardiac iron levels accurately, indicating the importance of proper monitoring and management of cardiac iron loading in chelated patients. A

study of a cohort of patients on long-term DFO therapy showed a prevalence of myocardial iron loading (T2* < 20 ms) of 65% and severe iron overload (T2* < 8 ms) of 13%. There was no correlation between myocardial and hepatic iron loading, and of the five individuals with the lowest myocardial T2* and left ventricular ejection fraction <45%, only one had severe hepatic iron loading (liver T2* < 1.4 ms) (*Figure 35.11*).[243] Regular assessment of cardiac T2* with adjustments in iron chelation has been associated with a lower risk of heart failure.[244]

Right ventricular dysfunction, which mirrors the decrease in left ventricular function, is demonstrated with worsening of cardiac iron loading.[245] Finally, the correlation between myocardial and liver iron is inconsistent, underscoring the importance of regular MRI monitoring of both the liver and heart (*Figure 35.12*).

In the past, the prognosis for thalassemic patients with heart failure was considered to be poor.[246] More recently, the availability of intensive chelation regimens, often incorporating combined chelation agents, with particular efficacy on the reduction of cardiac iron load, has modified the course of the disease, making cardiac failure and arrhythmia now considered reversible complications. Improvements of 2% to 3% in ejection fraction as measured by MRI significantly reduce the risk of cardiac failure over a year if maintained. DFO has been crucial in improving survival and decreasing iron-induced heart disease. However, with the introduction of MRI T2*, myocardial siderosis was found in two-thirds of patients with TDT on DFO treatment and associated with a high prevalence of left ventricular dysfunction.[247] DFO given at high doses of 50 to 60 mg/kg/d as a continuous infusion removes cardiac iron and improves heart function.[248]

Data support that DFP is more effective than DFO in chelating iron from the heart. In a highly influential study, 52 cardiac events, including 10 cardiac deaths, in patients treated with DFO, only, was observed over a 9-year period, whereas no cardiac events developed in patients who were switched to DFP.[249] In a randomized controlled trial in patients with moderate cardiac siderosis, DFP also was superior to DFO for improvement in both cardiac T2* and left ventricular ejection fraction.[250]

High-dose DFX also has been shown to be effective at removing iron from the heart[251,252] and was noninferior to DFO at cardiac iron removal in the setting of moderate cardiac siderosis (T2* 6-20 ms) without left ventricular dysfunction.[253] Some studies have suggested that DFX may be less effective with severe cardiac siderosis[254] or severe hepatic iron loading.[255] At present, for patients with severe myocardial siderosis and impaired left ventricular function, combined chelation therapy with subcutaneous DFO and oral DFP is indicated. This combination of therapy appears to reduce myocardial iron and improves cardiac function.[246]

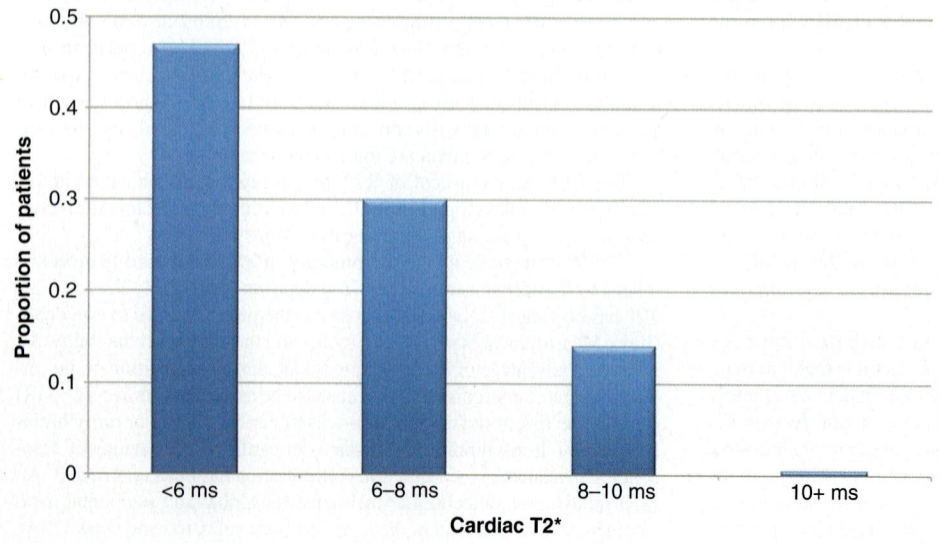

FIGURE 35.10 Proportion of patients developing heart failure after 1 year, according to different baseline cardiac T2* values. (Adapted from Kirk P, Roughton M, Porter JB, et al. Cardiac T2* magnetic resonance for prediction of cardiac complications in thalassemia major. *Circulation.* 2009;120:1961-1968.)

In one long-term study, combined therapy with DFO and DFP was shown to prevent deaths related to iron overload. Results of multivariable analysis demonstrated a 7.4-fold improved survival for each year on combined therapy.[246] Similarly, one study showed a lower risk of cardiac death with the oral chelators, which are smaller molecules and have better myocardial iron removal: 9.5 cardiac deaths per 1000 patient-years for DFO, 2.5 for DFP, and 1.4 for combined therapy. In the DFX group, no cardiac deaths were recorded. The risk for a de novo cardiac event for patients on DFO was 9.1 times greater than for patients on DFP and 23.6 times greater than for those on the combination of DFP and DFO. For DFX, there was one cardiac event over 269 patient-years.[256] Addition of amlodipine to standard chelation can help further reduce cardiac iron through blocking iron entry via myocardial calcium channels; a small effect was demonstrated in a recent small phase 3 trial.[257]

In addition, a striking reduction in cardiac deaths was observed in the United Kingdom in the past decade and has been attributed to the combined benefits of T2*, which identifies myocardial siderosis, and individualized intensification of chelation therapy based on the response.[258] Prior to effective iron chelation, acute episodes of sterile pericarditis were seen in about half of patients with massive iron overload, but these are now uncommon in regularly transfused patients. Diabetes represents an independent risk for cardiac complications, even when other variables have been taken into account. The presence of iron overload in the pancreas predicts heart siderosis.[235] Pulmonary hypertension is a possible concomitant cause that contributes to cardiac dysfunction.[244] An elevated tricuspid regurgitant jet velocity has been described in one-third of transfusion-dependent thalassemic patients, in both adults and children, but this has been a variable finding in TDT.[259] Age, splenectomy, hepatitis C, and smoking were significant univariate risk factors. However, the use of tricuspid regurgitant jet velocity as a surrogate marker of pulmonary hypertension could be inadequate in patients with chronic anemia and hyperdynamic cardiac activity.

An analysis of a database of Italian thalassemic patients reported approximately 19% of regularly transfused and chelated patients with TDT needed cardiovascular drug therapy. This subgroup was characterized by a dilated and mildly hypokinetic left ventricle when compared with the majority of patients with TDT who did not need cardioactive drugs.[260] Management of cardiac complications in patients with TDT has been described.[261] In asymptomatic or minimally symptomatic patients with left ventricular dysfunction, the angiotensin-converting enzyme inhibitor enalapril produced significant improvement in systolic and diastolic function, as demonstrated by echocardiography. The treatment of arrhythmias is difficult, and the risk of proarrhythmic effects of antiarrhythmic drugs is high. The help of a cardiac electrophysiologist is often necessary. Heart transplantation has led to variable outcomes. However, with the advent of effective chelation and supportive therapy, cardiac transplantation should be rarely indicated.[262]

Liver

Liver disease is a major complication of TDT and is caused by the damage produced by iron overload and the effects of transfusion-transmitted viral infections. Liver iron assessment includes a variety of methods. The current standard method to assess iron content is the MRI R2, or its reciprocal T2*. A correlation between T2* and LIC, as measured by biopsy, has been observed with a good sensitivity and specificity for levels above 3.2 mg Fe/g dry tissue. Sensitivity and specificity for higher LICs are less satisfactory (e.g., at 7 mg Fe/g, dry tissue sensitivity and specificity are 70% and 88%, respectively). The R2 (1/T2) technique (Ferriscan) has been registered in the European Union and is US Food and Drug Administration (FDA) approved in the United States and can be done on a standard MRI scanner, with data sent electronically to a commercial organization for analysis.[263]

Hepatic siderosis in the absence of chelation is present from the very early stages of iron loading and progresses to fibrosis and

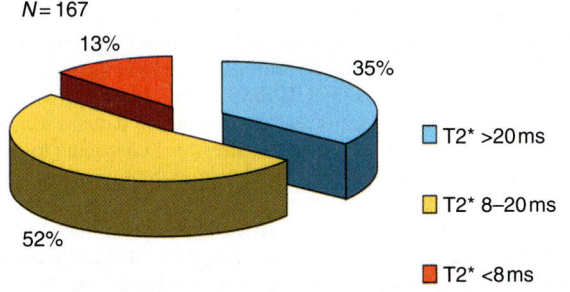

FIGURE 35.11 Myocardial iron loading in patients on long-term deferoxamine treatment.

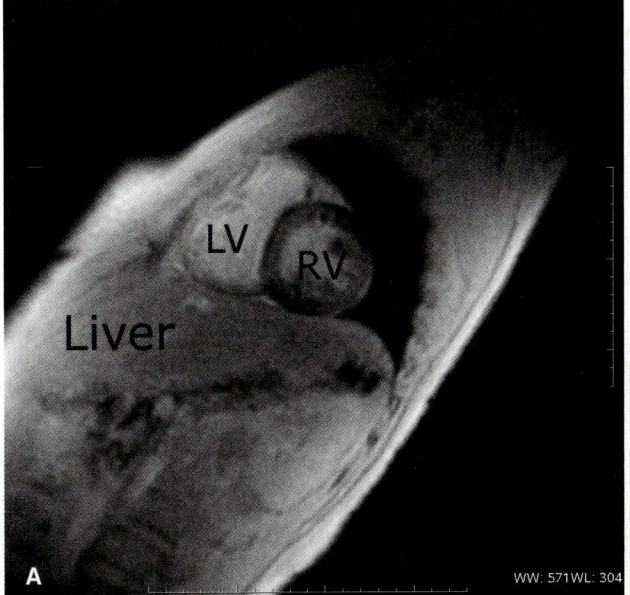
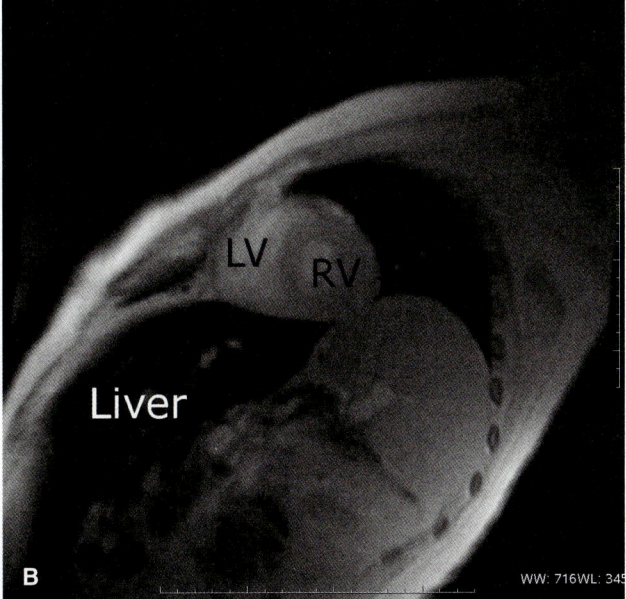

FIGURE 35.12 Heart multislice multiecho MRI T2* obtained with a 1.5-T scanner. The short-axis plane shows discordance of liver and heart iron deposition. A, Heart iron deposition, in contrast with minimal liver iron load. B, Severe hepatic iron overload and normal heart iron. MRI, magnetic resonance imaging. (Courtesy of Alessia Pepe, Magnetic Resonance Unit Fondazione G. Monasterio CNR, Tuscany Region, Italy.)

Disorders of Red Blood Cells

cirrhosis.[264,265] The mechanisms responsible for the effects of iron are not completely clear. Animal model data suggest that peroxidation of intracellular organelles (lysosomes and mitochondria) and membrane components by reactive oxygen species is the major cause of tissue toxicity and organ damage.[266] Liver biopsy remains the standard to assess liver inflammation and fibrosis.[267] The degree of liver fibrosis is best documented histologically by the Ishak score. However, liver biopsy is an invasive procedure associated with some discomfort, and its accuracy for the evaluation of liver fibrosis is questionable in relation to inadequate tissue sampling and intraobserver/interobserver variability. Transient elastography, a technique that uses both ultrasound and low-frequency elastic waves whose propagation velocity is directly related to the elasticity of the liver tissue, is increasingly used to measure liver stiffness in chronic hepatitis C and appears to be a reasonably accurate method for detection of cirrhosis in thalassemic patients, regardless of the degree of iron overload.[268] Fibrosis of the liver directly correlates with age, number of units of blood transfused, and LIC.

HCV infection is common in thalassemic patients who were transfused before 1989, when the virus was identified, and before a systematic screening of blood units was mandated.[269] The residual risk of transfusion-transmitted infections associated with the window-period donations is extremely low in industrialized countries, especially after the introduction of NAT technology, which practically eliminates window periods, but remains significant where the prevalence of infection in the population is high.[270] In the past, treatment with interferon and ribavirin was challenging due to the risk of increased hemolysis. Newer regimens using direct antivirals have been shown to be safe and efficacious in thalassemia.[271,272]

Other hepatotropic viruses, such as GB virus C and transfusion-transmitted virus, are also common among thalassemic patients but have not been found to contribute to chronic hepatocellular damage.

Hepatocellular carcinoma represents the most frequent cause of death in patients with both genetic hemochromatosis and liver cirrhosis, and this frequently complicates the course of cirrhosis due to chronic HCV and HBV. As a consequence of the numerous risk factors present in chronically transfused patients, there is an increased risk with advanced age, requiring surveillance to enable early diagnosis and treatment.[273] Because α-fetoprotein determination lacks adequate sensitivity and specificity for effective surveillance or diagnosis, all patients with chronic HBV and patients with HCV and cirrhosis should undergo liver ultrasound every 6 months. Diagnosis of hepatocellular carcinoma should then be based on imaging techniques and/or biopsy.[274]

Kidney

Renal failure caused by very high doses of DFO has been described.[275] In a small series, 40% of the patients on subcutaneous DFO developed a clinically significant decrease in glomerular filtration rate.[276] DFX also may cause nephrotoxicity that is dose related (see below). Novel measures of renal function allowing the early detection of kidney disease and the introduction of a chelator, which can cause nephrotoxicity, have produced a flurry of interest in assessing renal function in thalassemia. In one study from the US Thalassemia Clinical Research Network, regular transfusions were associated with a decrease in creatinine clearance, and almost one-third of the patients had hypercalciuria. Albuminuria was found in over half of patients but was not consistently associated with transfusion therapy.[277] Other studies have shown impaired renal function with elevated cystatin C levels, glomerular dysfunction with proteinuria, and tubulopathy with hypercalciuria increasing with age and duration of blood transfusion.[278,279] Most adults with TDT followed for 10 years maintained the estimated glomerular filtration rate within the normal range. However, patients with evidence of tubular dysfunction developed an abnormal estimated glomerular filtration rate. Renal tubular dysfunction may be related to the disease itself, the effects of iron overload, or to chelation. Some patients with thalassemia have demonstrated an increased creatinine clearance, leading to hyperfiltration. Iron can be found in the kidneys;

however, kidney MRI T2* does not correlate well with the liver and cardiac T2*.[280]

Endocrine Glands

Iron deposition is the main cause of damage to the endocrine glands, directly or through the hypothalamic-pituitary axis.[281,282] Direct damage to almost all endocrine glands has been demonstrated histologically and by MRI. High ferritin levels, poor compliance with chelation, and splenectomy increase the risk of endocrinopathies. Intensive iron chelation can normalize the iron load and, thereby, prevent or even reverse endocrine dysfunction.[283]

Growth Impairment

Growth impairment is common in thalassemia and is characterized by normal growth during childhood, decreased growth velocity at the end of the first decade of life, and growth failure at the expected age of puberty in patients who lack sexual maturation. Poor pubertal growth, however, was found to be present in a group of thalassemic patients regardless of hypogonadism.[284]

Sitting height may be reduced as a consequence of spinal growth abnormalities. A recent survey from the United States found that approximately 25% of patients with a thalassemia syndrome had short stature.[158] In children, however, growth was mildly affected and final height was close to midparental height. A report from India concluded that the majority of adult patients with thalassemia were less than 150 cm in height, highlighting the importance of adequate Hb levels for normal growth,[285] confirming observations made in the United States and Europe before the introduction of hypertransfusion regimens.[286]

The decrease in height in a subset of children with thalassemia (between 12% and 54%) may be attributed to growth hormone (GH) deficiency. Dysfunction of the GH–IGF-1 axis, hypothyroidism and hypogonadism, chronic liver disease, and in some patients zinc deficiency, malnutrition, and psychosocial stress can contribute to growth disturbance. In clinical practice, regular growth assessment in both standing and sitting positions every 4 to 6 months, annual determination of bone age, and annual pubertal staging should be performed from the age of 11 years. Treatment with recombinant human GH improves height velocity, but most patients remain below their target height.[287] Adults with GH deficiency have a decreased life expectancy. Therefore, the role of treatment with GH in selected deficient adults who present with cardiomyopathy or severe bone disease needs to be evaluated.[288]

DFO toxicity is responsible, in some cases, for reduced or absent growth velocity, platyspondyly with short trunk, metaphyseal irregularity of long bones, and widened growth plates, in particular of the wrist and knee.[289] These abnormalities were first reported in patients on high-dose subcutaneous DFO before the age of 3 years, but they were later also observed in patients on a standard dose of DFO.[290] A negative correlation between the maximum dose of DFO and height was later described in a group of adolescent patients.[291]

Hypogonadism

Hypogonadism is very common, affecting more than 50% of thalassemic patients.[292] It ranges from complete lack of sexual maturation to arrested or delayed puberty. Secondary amenorrhea affects 65% of females who experienced spontaneous menarche.[293] Significant improvement in spontaneous sexual maturation has been observed in patients born after 1975, suggesting a crucial role for adequate chelation. Hypogonadism is likely caused by free radical oxidative damage from iron deposition in the anterior pituitary and/or in the hypothalamus. Clinical evaluation of the diagnosis of pubertal hypogonadism includes bone age measured by x-ray of the wrist and hand, study of the hypothalamic-pituitary-gonadal axis (gonadotropin-releasing hormone [GnRH] test), dosage of sex steroids, and pelvic ultrasound in females.

Hormonal replacement therapy with small doses of oral conjugated estrogens or transdermal 17β-estradiol and progesterone for female and testosterone enanthate in males may be administered to stimulate puberty. An initial trial of 3 to 6 months is prescribed, and if puberty does not develop spontaneously within 6 months after the end of treatment, sex steroids are reintroduced at increasing doses. Hormone replacement, in addition to inducing the secondary sexual characteristics, enhances height velocity, contributes to the prevention of osteoporosis, improves mood and energy, and has enormous psychological benefits. Fertility is normal in female patients with normal menstrual function, or it can be induced with human menopausal gonadotropin or follicle-stimulating hormone (FSH).[294] Decreased fertility in men with TDT is attributed to lower sperm count and sperm motility, and the proportion of sperm with normal morphology is significantly lower than in control individuals.[295]

Gonadotropin treatment, using human chorionic gonadotropin plus human FSH or GnRH, is given to stimulate spermatogenesis and induce fertility.[296]

Pregnancy

In women with hypogonadotropic hypogonadism, gonadal function is usually intact and fertility is often restorable. Hundreds of pregnancies have taken place, and severe obstetric complications have been quite rare.[297] Ninety-one percent of the pregnancies recently reported by an Italian cooperative group resulted in successful delivery, and no secondary complications of iron overload developed or worsened during pregnancy.[298] Anemia should be avoided to protect the fetus from hypoxia (suggested Hb levels of 10 g/dL), and chelation therapy should be discontinued owing to potential teratogenicity. Over 80 cases reported normal outcomes from pregnancies involving a wide range of DFO exposure and it may be used, especially in the last trimester, in the setting of severe iron overload.[299]

Preexisting cardiomyopathy, expanded plasma volume, increased cardiac output, continuous iron accumulation in the absence of chelation, and reduced glucose tolerance can deteriorate maternal health during pregnancy. Cardiac failure, with some leading to fatalities, have been reported. However, many successful outcomes of pregnancy in mothers with thalassemia are described. Delivery has been performed by elective cesarean delivery in approximately half of the cases. As a consequence of gonadotropin-induced ovulation, multiple pregnancies and preterm births are not rare.[297] To decrease the risk of thromboembolic events, the use of low-molecular-weight heparin is recommended peripartum, especially in splenectomized women with thrombocytosis. Low-dose aspirin during the entire pregnancy for women with high platelet counts is indicated. At present, a healthy and uncomplicated delivery can be expected in a pregnant woman with thalassemia but must involve the care by an expert multidisciplinary team to prevent serious complications. This is best ensured with early referral to a high-risk obstetrics center. Genetic counseling should be offered to all patients considering pregnancy, and even postconception, to ensure the understanding of maternal risks.

Hypothyroidism

Hypothyroidism is the second most common endocrine disorder after hypogonadism, having been reported in 5.6% to 17% of patients.[300] The majority of patients have subclinical or mild forms, whereas approximately one-third develop overt clinical symptoms. Central hypothyroidism is less frequently encountered. Regular assessment of free thyroxine and thyroid-stimulating hormone is recommended after the first decade of life. Thyroid ultrasonography may show an irregular echogenic pattern with thickening of the capsule. Abnormal thyroid function has been reversed with intensive chelation therapy with DFO, or in combination with DFP.[283]

Hypoparathyroidism

Hypoparathyroidism affects 3% to 10% of thalassemic patients and is attributed to iron deposition in the parathyroid glands.[301] Males seem to be affected more often than females.

Early detection requires periodic estimation of calcium homeostasis. Serum calcium levels below 8 mg/dL (2 mmol/L), phosphorus levels above 7 mg/dL (2.6 mmol/L), and low 1,25-dihydroxy vitamin D are suggestive of hypoparathyroidism. Symptoms are usually mild and include paresthesias, muscle pain, and, when severe, tetany and even convulsions. Extreme hypocalcemia is a late event. Intracranial calcifications have been reported in 40% of patients with hypoparathyroidism in the absence of symptoms and independently from the severity of the hormonal deficit.[302] In mild cases, normalization of calcium and phosphate with calcitriol, at a dosage of 0.25 to 1 μg twice daily, and careful monitoring of the serum calcium are warranted.

Adrenal

Clinically symptomatic adrenal insufficiency is uncommon but has been reported in older thalassemic patients.[303] However, abnormalities in the integrity of the pituitary-adrenal axis and adrenal insufficiency with provocative testing were identified in 61% of patients in one study.[304] Monitoring for adrenal insufficiency should be performed, as hypoadrenalism may become clinically relevant in major stressful events.[305]

Diabetes

Diabetes mellitus with varying frequency, between 4.9% and 14%, with a mean age at diagnosis of 18 to 22 years, has been reported.[306] The observed prevalence of insulin-dependent diabetes and of impaired glucose tolerance is significantly lower in patients born after 1975, probably as a result of chelation therapy. The peak incidence of diabetes was observed in 1986 (3.9%), decreasing to 0.8% in 2007 in parallel with improved chelation and the progressive decrease in the annual mean serum ferritin levels. Patients with a serum ferritin level >2500 μg/L were 3.5 times more likely to have diabetes mellitus.[225] Iron deposition in the pancreas resulting in excess collagen deposition, fibrosis, and fatty degeneration results in progressive β cell.[307] Pancreatic iron, as evaluated by MRI, is the strongest predictor of β-cell toxicity, but total body iron burden, age, and body habitus also influence glucose regulation.[308]

It has been suggested that liver damage contributes to the impairment of islet cell function.[309] HCV infection may induce insulin resistance by causing aberrations of the insulin-signaling pathways and direct cytopathic effect at the islet cell level, reducing insulin release.[310] Approximately one-third of HCV-positive patients are diagnosed with diabetes or have an abnormal fasting blood glucose, which is significantly higher than in HCV-negative patients.[311] Impaired glucose tolerance characterized by insulin resistance can precede the appearance of symptoms by a few months to several years and can be followed by progressive insulin deficiency, leading to overt diabetes. Impaired β-cell function, as reflected by a reduction in the insulin secretion index, can be found in normoglycemic patients.[312]

Asymptomatic hyperglycemia is the presenting sign in the overwhelming majority of patients. Ketoacidosis is uncommon, and retinopathy develops in one-quarter of patients, a percentage that is approximately half that of age- and sex-matched diabetic controls without thalassemia.[313] Intensive chelation may reverse glucose intolerance and postpone the onset of insulin-dependent diabetes, but once diabetes develops, it is not reversible.[283] Impaired glucose tolerance is often responsive to oral hypoglycemic drugs. In the insulin-dependent form, therapy needs to be closely monitored because glucose control is often difficult.

Exocrine Glands

Low serum levels of chymotrypsin and lipase have been described in patients with thalassemia and have been attributed to hemosiderosis of the pancreatic acinar tissue.[314,315] An ultrasonographic study demonstrated hyperechogenicity of the pancreas, and a decrease in size on ultrasound is observed when compared with controls, and these are significantly correlated with patient's age and duration of transfusion therapy.

Eye

Ocular involvement may be encountered in patients with thalassemia and is usually of moderate severity. In a recent report from India, more than half of the patients had some eye problems. Lenticular opacities were the most common ocular finding (44%).[316] It has been known for a long time that retinal pigmentary changes may complicate hemochromatosis. Accordingly, retinal hyperpigmentation detected in a group of thalassemic patients was attributed to iron overload. Also reported were abnormal electroretinographic potentials, similar to those observed in experimental siderosis bulbi,[317] and severity was directly correlated with iron overload. The presence of retinal angioid streaks should raise the suspicion of PXE.[318] Nevertheless, most eye problems in patients with TDT are a consequence of DFO toxicity, particularly when the dose of DFO is high relative to the iron burden.

Pulmonary Problems

Pulmonary problems, primarily ventilatory-restrictive impairment, have been reported in patients with TDT.[319] Iron deposition in the respiratory system has been proposed as a potential cause. However, no correlation was found between restrictive impairment and iron deposition in the respiratory system evaluated by MRI.[320]

Chelation

Because iron is recycled in the body, and there is little ability to excrete iron, thalassemic patients who require regular transfusions of red cells invariably develop transfusion-related iron overload. To prevent this transfusional hemosiderosis, pharmacologic chelation of iron that allows for iron excretion is crucial. The goal of a neutral or negative iron balance is achieved when the daily excretion is sufficient to eliminate the iron introduced by transfusion. This amount approximates, in most patients, 0.3 to 0.5 mg/kg. The two main sources of chelatable iron are (1) the intracellular labile pool, derived from lysosomal catabolism of ferritin and from transferrin-bound iron and NTBI, and (2) the iron derived from red cell catabolism in macrophages.[321] The first contributes chiefly to the hepatocellular load and is excreted as fecal iron, whereas the second is the major source of urinary iron. Ferric iron has six coordination sites, which need to be chelated completely, for the generation of harmful free radicals to be prevented. Three chelators are currently available: DFO, DFP, and DFX (*Figure 35.13*). DFO is hexadentate and forms stable iron-chelate complexes using a single molecule. The molecules of DFP and DFX are bidentate and tridentate, respectively, and, in theory, could dissociate from iron at suboptimal concentrations and promote, rather than prevent, iron toxicity.[322]

Adherence to chelation therapy is particularly challenging for several reasons: (1) transfusion-related iron overload is asymptomatic until end-organ damage has occurred, (2) the benefits of therapy require long-term adherence and are not perceived immediately, and (3) side effects from chelation can occur. Children are in general the most adherent (parents are responsible for drug administration), followed by adolescents and adults. Compliance appears to be better with oral chelation compared with subcutaneous or intravenous delivery, although switching from one chelator to another has been shown to be beneficial for overall adherence. The relationship between the patient and the health team is an important factor in promoting and supporting adherence with iron chelation in thalassemic patients.[323,324]

The rate of transfusional iron intake strongly influences the effectiveness of the iron chelators.[192] Doses at the higher end of therapeutic typically are needed for patients with high transfusional iron intake, especially above 0.5 mg/kg/d.

Regular monitoring and assessment of the total cumulative volume of packed RBCs received, the trend in ferritin levels, and the iron content of the liver, heart, and pancreas are important to determine an adequate chelation dose.

Deferoxamine

DFO, a trihydroxamic acid produced by *Streptomyces pilosus*, was first used for the treatment of transfusional hemosiderosis in 1962.[325] Because of its large molecular weight, it is not efficiently absorbed from the gut and cannot be administered orally. Initially, the drug was given by intramuscular injection, and because of its short half-life and the finite chelatable iron pool available at any given time, a negative iron balance was not achievable. A seminal study performed in the United Kingdom demonstrated that patients treated with DFO for 7 years had lower ferritin levels and lower LIC than those not chelated.[326] It was only with the administration of prolonged parenteral infusions, intravenous or subcutaneous, that negative iron balance was achieved, preventing complications of iron overload.[327] Today, DFO is most frequently administered subcutaneously, by means of a portable battery-operated pump, at a dose ranging between 20 and 60 mg/kg/d over 8 to 12 hours at night.

Pharmacokinetic studies have shown that a plateau is reached 4 to 8 hours after starting a DFO infusion and that, at the end of it, the plasma levels fall rapidly.[328] NTBI is efficiently bound by DFO so that the effects of free radical formation and lipid peroxidation are prevented. However, due to the short half-life, when administered as an infusion over 8 to 12 hours, NTBI will not be effectively bound for part of the day.[329] This is most relevant in the setting of iron-associated cardiac dysfunction, so 24-hour continuous infusion is recommended in that setting. The efficacy of DFO in reducing the iron burden, in improving organ function, and in improving survival has been repeatedly demonstrated.[224,226,330]

In order to avoid severe effects on growth and bone metabolism, DFO should be started when ferritin levels reach 1000 ng/mL, when the LIC reaches 5 to 7 mg/g dw, or after 10 to 15 units of blood have been given.[193,331] A decrease in growth velocity is an indication to lower the dose of DFO. The adequacy of therapy is monitored by repeated measurements of serum ferritin and by direct quantification of heart and liver iron concentrations, usually by MRI techniques.

In the case of cardiac dysfunction or symptoms of cardiac failure from gross iron overload, continuous 24-hour DFO infusion delivered via an intravenous catheter implanted in a large vein has been used with positive outcomes, although the drug is more efficient on the liver than on the heart.[332] Improvement of cardiac function can usually be demonstrated even before the total iron load is significantly reduced, probably as an effect of the binding of the toxic labile plasma iron.[248] Frequent catheter-related complications have been observed and include infection and thromboembolism, at rates of 1.15 and 0.48 per 1000 catheter days, respectively.[332] In heart cell cultures, studies have demonstrated that DFO removes the iron directly from iron-loaded heart cells, inhibits lipid peroxidation, and reverses the abnormalities in cellular contractility and rhythmicity induced by iron.

The administration of DFO by twice-daily subcutaneous bolus injection has been demonstrated to induce the same urinary iron excretion as the slow, pump-mediated infusion and is well tolerated, especially by older patients.[333,334] The primary limitation of DFO is the inconvenience of parenteral administration. Patient adherence, therefore, is often poor, especially during the teenage years.[335,336]

Deferoxamine Toxicity

The most common side effects of DFO are usually noted around the time of administration and include local redness and soreness at the

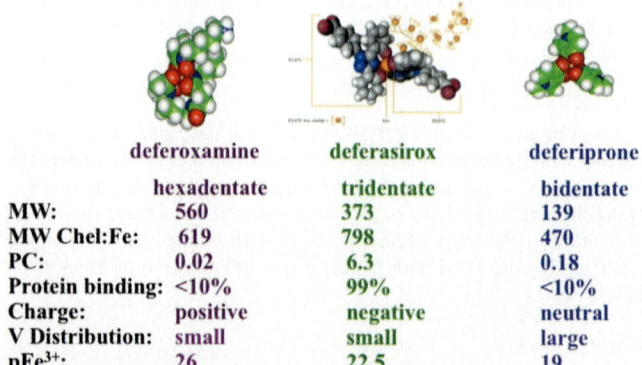

	deferoxamine	deferasirox	deferiprone
	hexadentate	tridentate	bidentate
MW:	560	373	139
MW Chel:Fe:	619	798	470
PC:	0.02	6.3	0.18
Protein binding:	<10%	99%	<10%
Charge:	positive	negative	neutral
V Distribution:	small	small	large
pFe³⁺:	26	22.5	19

FIGURE 35.13 Molecular structure and chemical properties of the three chelators presently available.

site of infusion. Inflammation, necrosis, and even ulceration can occur from the intradermal insertion of the needle. If the reaction persists after appropriate needle placement in the subcutaneous tissue, hydrocortisone (5-10 mg) can be added in the syringe. The direct and rapid injection of DFO in a vessel can cause brief episodes of nausea, hypotension, and collapse. Systemic allergic reactions and anaphylaxis require desensitization or changing chelator.[337]

Less commonly reported and associated with dosing of DFO are ocular, auditory, and skeletal side effects. Retinal and optic nerve disturbances, manifesting as loss of central vision, night blindness, and finally amaurosis, were reported in patients treated with high-dose intravenous or subcutaneous DFO.[338] All cases reported were reversible upon discontinuation of therapy, and the resumption of chelation with DFO was well tolerated. High-frequency sensorineural hearing loss was observed in a large percentage of patients during intensive DFO therapy. The defect was correlated with the total monthly dose of DFO received, and it was more frequent in younger patients with low serum ferritin levels.[339] Auditory toxicity can often be prevented by keeping a therapeutic index devised for that purpose (mean daily dose of DFO [mg/kg] divided by the serum ferritin [ng/L]) below 0.025. The hearing defect should be detected early, by performing an audiogram at least yearly, or whenever symptoms, even subtle, are reported. In fact, significant improvement has been observed after reduction of the DFO dose in patients with a mild defect, whereas only a small benefit has been gained by those severely affected.[340]

Stunted growth and rickets-like bone abnormalities have been described when treatment was initiated early, at a dosage higher than 40 mg/kg, or when the iron burden was not severe.[341] Sitting height is more often affected than standing height, as a consequence of vertebral growth impairment or flatness of vertebral bodies. Cupping of the ulnar, radial, and tibial metaphyses, which are poorly ossified and with irregular sclerotic margins, can be demonstrated radiographically and, when more advanced, can produce severe deformity of the knees and elbows (*Figure 35.14*). Reduction of the DFO dose is sufficient to reestablish normal growth velocity, but orthopedic surgery has sometimes been required for correction of advanced varus and valgus deformities of the knees. An acute, often lethal, pulmonary infiltration syndrome has been observed in patients treated intensively with very high doses of DFO (10-20 mg/kg/h).[342] Renal failure has also been reported in this context.[275] Infection with *Y. enterocolitica* is a well-known complication of hemosiderosis.[215] The presence of DFO in plasma and tissues facilitates the growth of the organism, which uses the drug as a siderophore. Fever and gastrointestinal symptoms are an indication to temporarily discontinue DFO. Antibiotic therapy is indicated as *Yersinia* infection can be severe and even life-threatening. *Klebsiella*, whose growth is only moderately favored by DFO, is becoming more frequent in thalassemia, especially in tropical and subtropical countries.

Deferiprone

DFP (L1) is a member of the family of the hydroxypyridin-4-one chelators.[343] DFP has the advantage in that it is an orally active alternative to DFO for the treatment of transfusional iron overload. Because each molecule provides two coordination sites, three molecules of DFP are required to fully bind the six coordination sites of an iron atom. The iron-chelate complex that is formed has a lower stability than the one formed by DFO. Another advantage is that DFP is a much smaller sized molecule and thus can enter cells and can theoretically chelate intracellular iron.[344] The sources of chelatable iron are, therefore, both parenchymal and in reticuloendothelial cells. In addition, iron is mobilized from transferrin, lactoferrin, and hemosiderin. The drug is excreted in the urine within 3 to 4 hours after having been glucuronidated in the liver.[345,346] The recommended dosage is 75 to 99 mg/kg/d in two to three divided doses, depending on formulation. DFP is easily absorbed from the gut, and a peak concentration is reached in the plasma 45 minutes after ingestion.[346] Food reduces the rate of absorption but not the total amount absorbed. DFP is available as film-coated, immediate-release tablets containing either 500 or 1000 mg of the active agent and as a liquid formulation containing 100 mg/mL. A newer twice-daily formulation of 1000 mg tablet is also available. The majority of iron is excreted in the urine, whereas fecal excretion ranges between 5% and 20%. The dose of 75 mg/kg/d has been shown to induce a urinary iron excretion equivalent to that achieved with 40 mg/kg/d of DFO.[347] Greater excretion can be obtained with a dose of 100 mg/kg/d, without an increase in side effects. Ascorbic acid does not enhance iron excretion with DFP chelation. DFP, as well as the other oral chelator, DFX, were also both found to be efficient scavengers of the labile iron pools of cardiomyocytes and to restore contractility impaired by iron overload.[344]

DFP was licensed for clinical use in India in 1995 and in Europe in 1999. The FDA approved the drug in the United States as a second-line agent in 2011 and as a first-line agent in 2021. DFP is particularly efficacious in removing iron from the heart. In a randomized trial comparing the efficacy over 1 year of DFP and DFO, the former was found to be significantly more effective than DFO in improving asymptomatic myocardial siderosis. Left ventricular ejection fraction also increased significantly more with DFP than with DFO.[250]

Numerous publications have reported the increased chelation effectiveness of combining DFP and DFO. Results have usually demonstrated an additive effect of combination therapy because the two drugs access different pools of iron. It has been suggested that DFP being able to pass through membranes, could "shuttle" tissue iron to DFO in the bloodstream and then be reused.[348] Combination therapy

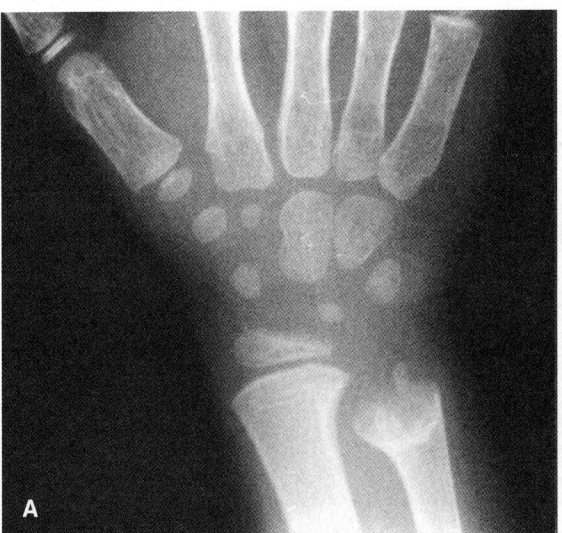
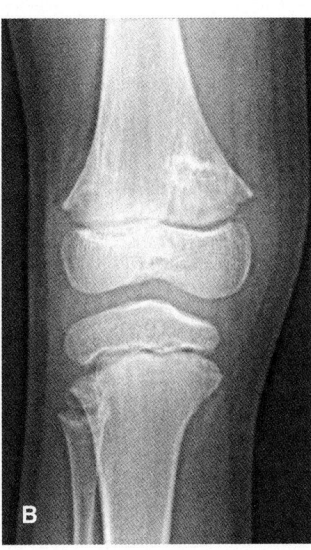

FIGURE 35.14 A, Deferoxamine toxicity. The growth plate of the distal ulna is wide, and the metaphysis exhibits a cuplike deformity with sclerotic and irregular borders. B, A similar picture is present in the metaphyses of the femur and fibula. (Courtesy of Dr. C. Orzincolo.)

Disorders of Red Blood Cells

is now widely used. A randomized, placebo-controlled clinical trial demonstrated that, in comparison with the standard chelation monotherapy of DFO, combination treatment with additional DFP reduced myocardial iron and improved ejection fraction and endothelial function in patients with TDT with mild to moderate cardiac iron load.[349] A small nonrandomized study and several case reports have confirmed the efficacy of combined therapy in the context of severe cardiac iron overload, showing a rapid decrease in both ferritin levels and cardiac iron, as measured by T2*, while at the same time improving cardiac function in severely iron-overloaded patients.[350] In addition, the reversal of some endocrinopathies was observed after normalization of iron stores with intensive combined iron chelation.[351] Alternating DFP and DFO can improve adherence and, in a long-term prospective study, decreased mortality compared with DFO alone.[352,353]

A growing body of literature supports that DFP is effective in pediatric patients with iron overload with a similar safety profile to adults. In a randomized controlled trial of 393 pediatric patients, 91% of whom had thalassemia, improvement in ferritin and control of cardiac T2* over 12 months with DFP was noninferior to DFX.[354] In addition, DFP given to infants with transfusion-dependent thalassemia prior to the development of significant iron overload (ferritin >400 and <1000 ng/mL) had an acceptable safety profile, slowed the time to reach ferritin levels above 1000 ng/mL, and better controlled labile plasma iron levels compared with children who did not receive iron chelation.[355]

DFP Toxicity

The most frequent adverse effects are gastrointestinal discomfort or nausea, reported by 33% of the patients in the first year and decreasing to 3% thereafter. The intensity is usually mild to moderate, with only a small percent of patients abandoning treatment with DFP, and may be reduced by taking the drug with food. The new liquid formulation seems to cause a lower incidence of gastrointestinal side effects. The most severe adverse effects observed with DFP are agranulocytosis and neutropenia. In a prospective multicenter study, the overall frequency of agranulocytosis was 0.5%, and the incidence was 0.2 per 100 patient-years. Milder neutropenia occurred in 8.5% of patients.[356] Neutropenia occurred more frequently in nonsplenectomized patients.[357] Agranulocytosis usually appears within the first 6 months after starting therapy but has been reported as long as 9 years after beginning DFP. Rechallenge with the drug can produce relapse of the agranulocytosis and is not recommended. The concomitant administration of drugs that can induce neutropenia (e.g., interferon and hydroxyurea [HU]) should be avoided.

Arthropathy, particularly of the knees, occurs in 6% to 39% of patients and appears to be more frequent in patients who have more severe iron overload.[358] It has been hypothesized that the formation of 1:1 or 1:2 DFP iron complexes can induce inflammatory changes, possibly mediated by free radicals. Other unwanted effects include excessive appetite, zinc deficiency, and fluctuation in liver enzymes. Reversible neurologic symptoms occurred in two patients when a dose three times higher than suggested was mistakenly given for over 2 years.

Deferasirox

This compound is a member of a class of tridentate iron-selective synthetic chelators, the bis-hydroxyphenyl-triazoles. As a tridentate chelator, two molecules of DFX bind one molecule of iron. The plasma half-life is 8 to 16 hours.[359] DFX is orally administered. It was first available as a dispersible tablet to drink as an oral suspension, with dosing for TDT ranging from 20 to 40 mg/kg/d. The newer, ingestible film-coated tablet or pediatric granule formulation are easier to take and may have fewer gastrointestinal side effects; these formulations are dosed at 14 to 28 mg/kg/d. DFX is administered orally once daily on an empty stomach or with a light, low-fat meal. Aluminum-containing antacid preparations may interfere with the absorption of DFX and should be avoided. In a large randomized trial comparing DFX and DFO, DFX was found to be noninferior in reducing liver iron when administered at doses of 20 and 30 mg/kg.[360]

The ability to reduce cardiac iron stores is critical for reducing the morbidity and mortality in thalassemia. Clinical data suggest that DFX is able to remove cardiac iron. Myocardial iron, assessed by cardiovascular T2* magnetic resonance, was measured in patients on a mean DFX dose of 33.6 ± 9.8 mg/kg/d. After 3 years, over half of patients demonstrated a decrease in cardiac iron content as measured by cardiac T2*. Left ventricular ejection fraction did not vary significantly.[361] In a randomized study comparing DFX with DFO in patients with myocardial iron loading but without cardiac dysfunction, cardiac T2* increased from a mean of 11.2 ms at baseline to 12.6 ms at 1 year, which was noninferior to DFO.[253]

The safety and efficacy of DFX in pediatric patients is similar to adults, and younger pediatric patients responded similarly to older pediatric patients.[362] The recommended starting dose and dosing modifications are also the same for children and adults. One study reporting on 111 children concluded that DFX is at least as effective as DFO in maintaining safe serum ferritin levels and normal growth progression.[363] The height and weight SD scores in children treated with DFX did not differ from those of patients treated with DFO. Fluctuations in liver enzymes and nonprogressive increases in serum creatinine were the most common adverse events.[362] DFX was approved in 2005 by the FDA in the United States, and in 2006 in Europe, for use in patients aged over 2 years.

DFX Toxicity

The most common adverse effects are related to gastrointestinal discomfort, including nausea, vomiting, and abdominal pain.[362] Because lactose monohydrate is among the inactive ingredients of the dispersible tablet, some cases of diarrhea can be attributed to lactose intolerance. The possibility of this side effect should be considered because lactose intolerance occurs more commonly in the same ethnicities that are affected by thalassemia. The film-coated tablet and granule formulations do not contain lactose, which may reduce the gastrointestinal adverse effects.

A skin rash can develop, usually within the first month of treatment (*Figure 35.15*). For rashes of mild to moderate severity, the drug may be continued without dose adjustment because the rash often resolves spontaneously. In severe cases, DFX may be interrupted and reintroduced at a lower dose with gradual escalation, in combination with a short course of oral steroids.

Approximately one-third of patients develop increases in serum creatinine >33% above baseline, but only about 2% reach the abnormal range.[360] Acute renal failure with DFX also has been reported in postmarketing experience. Therapy should not be started in patients with a creatinine clearance below 40 mL/min or with a serum creatinine >2 times the age-appropriate upper limit of normal.

Several cases of Fanconi syndrome have been reported with the use of DFX.[364] Fanconi syndrome is secondary to generalized dysfunction of the renal proximal tubule and results in renal losses of phosphate,

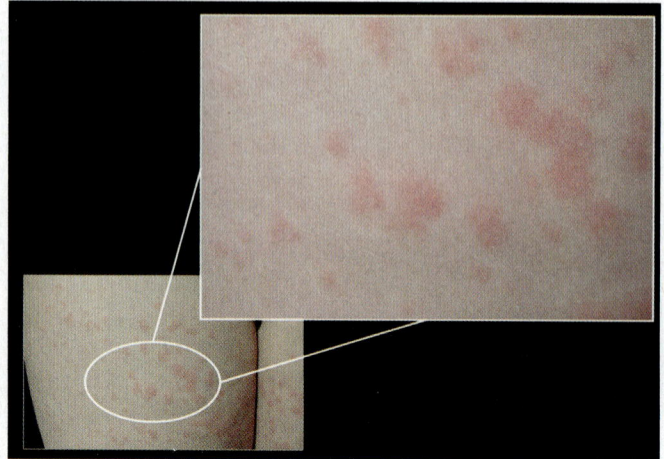

FIGURE 35.15 Typical rash appearing in patients on deferasirox therapy.

amino acids, bicarbonate, glucose, urate, and other molecules. Close monitoring of renal function and serum ferritin levels, with appropriate dose adjustment, in patients receiving DFX is indicated. Regarding hepatic toxicity, in the original phase 3 study, 6% of patients treated with DFX developed elevations in alanine transaminase (ALT) levels >5 times the upper limit of normal. Of these, two patients had drug-induced hepatitis, proven by liver biopsy.[360] Increased ALT levels >10 times above the upper limits of normal were reported in 1.0% of patients. Fulminant hepatic failure has been reported in postmarketing experience, and regular monitoring of hepatic function is required.

There have been postmarketing reports (both spontaneous and from clinical trials) of cytopenias, including agranulocytosis, neutropenia, and thrombocytopenia. The relationship of these episodes to treatment with DFX is uncertain. Interruption of treatment should be considered in patients who develop unexplained cytopenia. Reintroduction of therapy with DFX may be considered once the cause of the cytopenia has been elucidated. Nonfatal upper gastrointestinal tract irritation, ulceration, and gastrointestinal bleeding have been reported in patients, including children and adolescents receiving DFX. Thus, particular caution should be used when DFX is taken concomitantly with nonsteroidal anti-inflammatory drugs, corticosteroids, oral bisphosphonates, or anticoagulants. Many of the adverse effects of DFX, such as increases in serum creatinine, are dose related, and may improve with dose reduction. Alternating DFX with DFP has been used successfully to overcome intolerance to both drugs.[365]

Vitamin Supplementation

Vitamins and trace minerals are buffers against the oxidative stress owing to iron overload. Chronic demands on oxidative buffering capacity may produce deficiencies in key amino acids and enzymatic cofactors.[366] Siderosis of the exocrine pancreas sometimes causes a decrease in circulating pancreatic trypsin and stool elastase levels that results in vitamin malabsorption. In addition, liver damage may play a role in the depletion of lipid-soluble antioxidants, such as vitamins E and A. Surveys reveal inadequate diet intake in thalassemic patients, which is worse with increasing age, in particular for vitamin A, vitamin C, vitamin B_6, folate, thiamine, calcium, magnesium, and zinc.

Circulating levels of serum 25-OH vitamin D remained insufficient in the majority of subjects despite daily supplementation.[367] Vitamin D is essential for intestinal calcium absorption. Vitamin D receptors are found in nearly all tissues and is believed to play a systemic role. Cardiac iron loading was found to be more common in thalassemic patients with vitamin D deficiency and secondary parathyroid hormone elevation, but the association of this deficit with left ventricular dysfunction is unproven. Vitamin D deficiency is also inversely related to hepatic iron concentration and ferritin, as previously described in hereditary hemochromatosis, because of inhibition of hepatic 25-hydroxylation by excess iron.[368]

DFO-induced iron excretion is enhanced by ascorbic acid supplementation because of the expansion of the chelatable iron pool that DFO can access.[369] However, ascorbate, a natural reducing agent, accelerates iron-induced lipid peroxidation in biologic systems at low concentrations and has been shown to alter the function of rat myocardial cells in culture. In addition, anecdotal echocardiographic observations have suggested cardiotoxicity.[370] Vitamin C supplementation is, therefore, recommended for patients not affected by myocardiopathy, with unsatisfactory iron excretion, and demonstrated ascorbate deficiency. When necessary, 50 mg/d of ascorbate in children up to 10 years of age and 100 mg/d thereafter should be sufficient. Vitamin C should be given when DFO infusion is already under way.

α-Tocopherol, a lipid-soluble antioxidant, is able to interrupt the membrane lipid peroxidation process. Supplementation with vitamin E is, therefore, frequently suggested, but data demonstrating its efficacy are lacking. Folic acid deficiency was reported in early studies from Thailand.[371] Folate supplementation is advised for patients with a hyperactive bone marrow, like those with NTDT, and during pregnancy. Zinc has been found to be low in patients with TDT.[372] Nevertheless, these patients have a normal zinc-binding capacity,

which is generally increased in nutritional zinc deficiency.[373] Zinc supplementation can become necessary when DFO and DFP are given in combination. In conclusion, chronically transfused patients with TDT have broad-spectrum nutritional deficiencies of both water- and fat-soluble nutrients.

Splenectomy

Splenectomy was an intervention commonly used in the clinical management of thalassemic patients. It was often performed shortly after diagnosis because the spleen quickly reached an enormous size and caused severe hypersplenism, frequently leading to profound neutropenia and thrombocytopenia. More recently, splenectomy is less frequently utilized owing to an increased awareness of the long-term complications post splenectomy including thromboembolic events and pulmonary hypertension. A cooperative observational study involving 872 regularly transfused thalassemic patients born between 1960 and 1999 found that, overall, 67% of the patients had not been splenectomized, but the probability of having undergone the procedure was strongly influenced by the date of birth (*Figure 35.16*).[374] For patients born in 1960 and in 1980, the probability of being splenectomized was 57% and 7%, respectively. No patient younger than 5 years was splenectomized after 1987. Nonetheless, splenectomy may still be useful, particularly when transfusion requirements are very high. Clinical criteria for splenectomy were first proposed by Modell,[375] who suggested splenectomy when blood consumption increased over 50% above the average consumption of the splenectomized population—or when more than 200 to 250 mL/kg/y of pure red cells are required to maintain a pretransfusional Hb of 9 to 9.5 g/dL. Splenectomy can reduce the transfusion requirement to approximately 150 mL/kg/y and maybe long-lasting.

Cytopenias and symptoms remain primary indications for intervention. Risks associated with splenectomy include an increased susceptibility to encapsulated bacterial infections and an increase in thromboembolic events. Laparoscopic splenectomy, when possible, avoids the disfiguring scar created by laparotomy, reduces the hospital stay, and does not increase overall cost.[376] However, the large size of the spleen, when splenectomy is considered necessary, may make laparoscopic surgery difficult. In addition, the risk of thrombosis of the portal vein seems to be increased.[377]

Postsplenectomy sepsis with encapsulated organisms has been recognized as a risk for many years.[378] These infections are often abrupt in onset and rapidly fatal. The clinical spectrum of serious bacterial

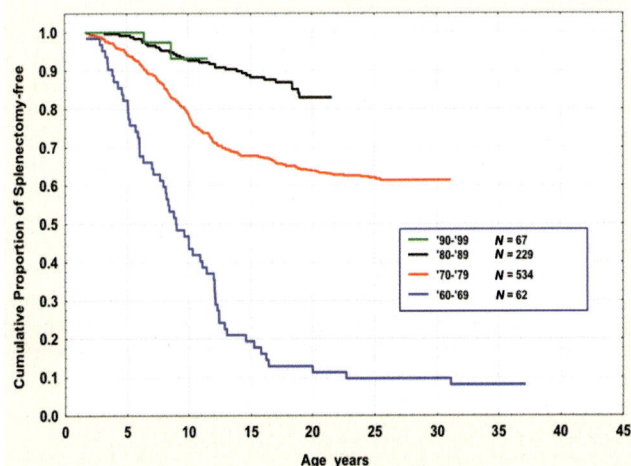

FIGURE 35.16 Cumulative proportion of splenectomy-free survival in different birth cohorts (1960-1969, 1970-1979, 1980-1989, and 1990-1999). During the period of observation, 284 patients (32.6%) were splenectomized, whereas 588 patients (67.4%) still had their spleen in at the end of the study ($P < .0001$). (Reprinted from Piga A, Serra M, Longo F, et al. Changing patterns of splenectomy in transfusion-dependent thalassemia patients. *Am J Hematol.* 2011;86(9):808-810.)

postsplenectomy infections among patients with hemoglobinopathies includes sepsis (the most common and severe complication), bacteremia, pneumonia, skin and liver abscesses, and urinary tract infections. Overwhelming postsplenectomy sepsis results from the removal of a major site of antibody production (in particular the splenic marginal zone) and, possibly, the long-term decrease in T-cell subsets of functional relevance for primary immune responses.[379] Splenic macrophages are critical in clearing opsonized encapsulated bacteria and intraerythrocytic parasites, such as those causing malaria and babesiosis, which explains the fulminant nature of these infections in persons with anatomic or functional asplenia.[380]

The most frequently responsible bacteria are *Streptococcus pneumoniae, Haemophilus influenzae,* and *Neisseria meningitidis.* A study from Israel reported that 35% of splenectomized patients with hemoglobinopathies, despite being vaccinated against *S. pneumoniae* and on prophylactic penicillin, developed serious infections, two of which were fatal. The most common bacteria involved was *Escherichia coli,* followed by *S. pneumoniae* and *Campylobacter.*[214] *Klebsiella* appears to be an increasingly common cause of infection, particularly in Asia. Although the risk for severe infection is greatest in younger children and in the first immediate postoperative year after splenectomy, the risk remains lifelong after the procedure.

Guidelines for the prevention of postsplenectomy infections are published by the British Committee for Standards in Haematology.[381] The guidelines recommend antibiotic prophylaxis with penicillin, amoxicillin, or erythromycin, lifelong for patients with the highest ongoing risk (under 16 or over 50 years old, prior history of pneumococcal infection, inadequate vaccination response). Patients should be immunized against pneumococcus, optimally at least 2 weeks prior to splenectomy, with guidance available for the PPSV23 polysaccharide immunization as well as the pneumococcal conjugate vaccine. The American Academy of Pediatrics likewise recommends immunization for pneumococcus, *H. influenzae,* and meningococcus, as well as antibiotic prophylaxis without a defined duration outside of sickle cell disease.[382]

Thrombocytosis, owing in part to the presence in the circulation of platelets previously marginated in the spleen, develops in 75% of the splenectomized patients, and in 15%, it reaches 1,000,000/mm^3 or more, peaking between 8 days and 4 months after surgery.[383,384] A correlation between splenectomy and pulmonary hypertension has been suggested on the basis of the high prevalence of asplenia found among patients with unexplained pulmonary hypertension. Recurrent pulmonary thromboembolism could be responsible for the phenomenon.[385]

Several alternatives to splenectomy have been proposed, with mixed results. Partial splenectomy and partial dearterialization of the spleen have an immediate beneficial effect, but of short duration.[386] Partial embolization of the spleen has been successfully performed with long-lasting results, but it has sometimes led to other complications. It has the advantage of not requiring general anesthesia and not leaving a scar. The procedure is followed by severe pain lasting several days and requires spinal anesthesia. The hypothesis that a residual portion of spleen protects the patient from infections and thrombotic events is still unproven. It has been theorized that the spleen could represent a reservoir for the transfused iron and that splenectomy would expose the patient to the risk of more massive siderosis of the liver. However, the iron content of the spleen at splenectomy is low, amounting to no more than one-fifth to one-tenth of the liver iron content.[387] As demonstrated by modern MRI techniques, splenic iron content plateaus at 1 to 1.5 g, even as hepatic content continues to grow.[388]

PROGNOSIS WITH CONVENTIONAL THERAPY

The improved survival of patients with TDT has been attributed to improvement in transfusion therapy, better understanding of mechanisms of organ damage from iron, more effective iron chelation, the availability of magnetic resonance for the evaluation of cardiac iron overload, and the referral of patients to centers of excellence. Between 1949 and 1957, in Ferrara, only 9% of the patients reached 6 years of age, and at the end of the 1970s, half of the Italian patients had already

died at age 12 years. A review of patients followed between 1960 and 1976 at Cornell Medical Center (New York City, USA) reported a median survival of 17.1 years for patients transfused with low Hb level goals and no chelation, whereas for hypertransfused and well-chelated patients, the median survival was 31 years. Currently, in developed countries, the majority of thalassemic patients are expected to reach adulthood.[389]

A large cooperative Italian study demonstrated better survival for patients born in more recent years and for females (*Figure 35.17*),[390] but mortality remains increased compared with the general population. In 2010, 68% of the patients were alive at the age of 35 years, with 67% of the deaths being due to heart disease. Infections represented the second cause of death, being responsible for 15% of the deaths, followed by liver disease and thromboembolic events, both at 4%. Similar data are reported from most world centers. In a report of over 1000 Greek thalassemic patients, the overall survival at 50 years was 65%.[391] The standardized mortality ratio compared with the general population improved significantly from 28.9 in 1990 to 1999, to 13.5 in 2000 to 2008, whereas the standardized cardiac mortality ratio decreased from 323 to 107, respectively.

The importance of good chelation in improving life expectancy has been well demonstrated. In fact, lower ferritin levels are associated with a lower probability of heart failure and with prolonged survival, using a cutoff of 1000 ng/mL.[224] Both in the Italian and the Greek series, birth cohort had a significant effect on survival ($P < .001$). In Cyprus, where mortality of thalassemic patients had been high, a marked improvement in survival was noted for patients of all ages since 2000.[392] This observation was also made in the United Kingdom[258] and in Italy (*Figure 35.18*).[224] The use of MRI and the introduction of oral iron chelation have produced significant improvement in terms of reduction of iron overload among US patients.[393]

Complications remain frequent and are primarily because of the oxidative damage mediated by labile iron. With extended survival, new complications are appearing that will change the classic picture of thalassemia and will require new therapeutic interventions. Several studies investigating the effects of thalassemia on psychosocial adjustment have different conclusions. According to a survey from Greece, 42% of patients had psychiatric problems, whereas other authors demonstrated that thalassemic adults have normal psychological development, with better social adjustment and self-esteem than their nonthalassemic peers.[394] A study from the Thalassemia Clinical Research Network comparing health-related quality of life in 264 thalassemic patients over age 14 years to US healthy controls found that patients reported a statistically significant worse quality of life on five of the eight subscales (physical functioning, role-physical, general health, social functioning, and role-emotional).[395] Women, older

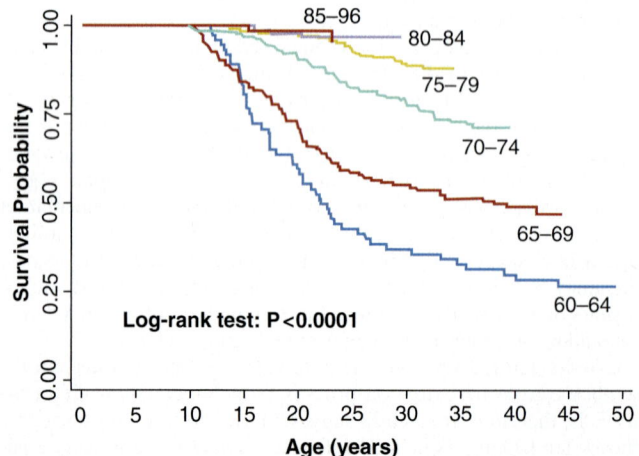

FIGURE 35.17 Kaplan-Meier survival curve after the first decade of life, subdivided by cohort of birth of patients from an Italian cooperative study. The survival data were collected in 2009. The role of the cohort of birth is evident.

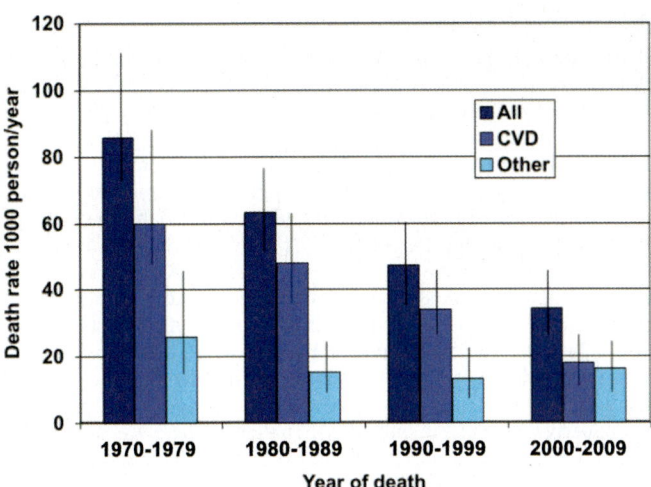

FIGURE 35.18 Decrease in death rate in a multitransfused population of Italian patients with thalassemia by year at death. Death constantly decreased because of the decrease in cardiac causes. (Data collected in 2009 as part of the 7 Centers Study.)

patients, and those with more disease complications and side effects from chelation fared worse.

A survey of the education and employment status of patients with thalassemia in the United States and Canada revealed that 70% of adults were employed. Sixty percent had a college degree, and 14% had achieved some post-college education.[396] Eighty-two percent of school-aged children were at expected grade level. Neither transfusion nor chelation was associated with lower employment or educational achievement.

In countries with lower economic resources, where sanitary problems are an issue and the health care systems do not have the resources to support the optimal management of thalassemia, the clinical picture and outcomes are different. In developing nations, many thalassemic patients are not regularly transfused or chelated. Their survival is limited, and their quality of life poor.

Some countries have adopted aggressive family planning measures, according to the World Health Organization recommendations. However, very few of the poorest and least developed countries have begun to address the public health issue of thalassemia.

Hematopoietic Stem Cell Transplantation

HSCT is a well-established intervention in the treatment of TDT and thus far the only curative measure. Thousands of thalassemic patients have received stem cell transplants worldwide. The vast majority had TDT, whereas a few had NTDT, HbE/β-thalassemia, or HbH disease. The largest experience has been recorded in Italy by Lucarelli et al, who suggested that patients be classified into three levels of transplantation risk based on the presence or absence of portal fibrosis, hepatomegaly, and regular chelation.[397,398] The lowest risk are patients regularly chelated and without liver fibrosis or hepatomegaly. Patients poorly chelated, with hepatomegaly and portal fibrosis, have the highest risk, whereas the intermediate-risk group includes patients with one or two risk factors. The ideal donor is an HLA-identical donor. At present, the prognosis for HSCT from an HLA-matched sibling donor is excellent. A recent review by the European Bone Marrow Transplantation Group of 1061 thalassemic patients of a median age of 7 years, from 28 countries, reported overall survival and thalassemia-free survival of 91% and 83%, respectively.[399] The age threshold for better results was 14 years. In a smaller multicenter study reporting on 179 young patients with TDT, 7 years was found to be the age above which mortality risk was higher.[400] A recent analysis of data from 50 transplant centers in the United States, China, and India showed outcomes using myeloablative conditioning with matched related donor were best for children 6 years and younger, with a 5-year event-free survival of 86%.[401] In contrast, event-free survival was only 63% for

patients 16 to <25 years old and intermediate at 80% for children 7 to 15 years. In adult patients, transplant-related mortality remains high. Lucarelli et al transplanted 107 adult patients with a probability of survival, event-free survival, nonrejection mortality, and rejection of 66%, 62%, 37%, and 4%, respectively, with a median follow-up of 12 years.[402] A second group of 15 patients with a median age of 21 years was treated with a reduced-dose intensity-conditioning regimen that produced some improvement in thalassemia-free survival (67%). Transplant-related mortality (27%) and risk of developing chronic graft-vs-host disease (cGVHD) remained high.

Alternative Donors

Alternative donors have been used as a source of hematopoietic cells because only one-third of thalassemic patients will have HLA-compatible siblings. HLA-identical relatives can be found in families from small ethnic communities or where consanguinity is accepted. A higher risk of rejection mortality, infection, and GVHD was reported in eight patients transplanted from an HLA-identical parent.[403] Matched unrelated donors can be considered a viable alternative when a matched sibling is unavailable. A suitable donor can be found for approximately 40% to 50% of Caucasian patients with TDT. Initially, these HSCTs were aggravated by high risk of death and GVHD, but more precise characterization of HLA alleles using stringent criteria of compatibility with the recipient (ie, identity or single allelic disparity for HLA-A, HLA-B, HLA-C, DRB1, and DQB1 loci) and high-resolution molecular typing for both class I and class II loci can reduce the risk of immune-mediated complications and fatal events.[404] The probability of cure after HSCT was about 85% for children belonging to both class I and class II of the Pesaro classification and 65% for children belonging to class III and for adults.[405] In a more recent series of 48 patients age 2 to 11 years, thalassemia-free survival was reported to be 100% with a modified conditioning regimen.[406]

Additional genetic characteristics have been reported to be of prognostic value in choosing the potential donor more accurately.[407]

Conditioning Regimen

The bone marrow of thalassemic patients is hypercellular, and the conditioning regimen must be able to empty the marrow space and be sufficiently immunosuppressive to permit sustained engraftment. For many years, the standard preparatory regimen for thalassemia consisted of busulfan (intravenous dimethyl busulfan or oral busulfan at 14 mg/kg) and cyclophosphamide (120-200 mg/kg). More recently, a conditioning regimen combining treosulfan with thiotepa and fludarabine was demonstrated in 60 thalassemic patients (median age 7 years, range 1-37 years) to be safe and effective. Neither the class of risk nor the donor source influenced outcome.[408] Reduced-intensity preparative regimens have been investigated in matched unrelated donors[409] and in matched sibling donors,[410] with some promising results, although some regimens have shown high rates of mixed chimerism and graft loss.

GVHD prophylaxis with cyclosporine and a short course of methotrexate is effective in preventing acute GVHD and cGVHD. Antithymocyte globulin is often given to maintain immunosuppression, in particular for transplants from unrelated donors or when an HLA disparity is present. Patterns of graft rejection are variable.[411] Patients may fail initial engraftment, develop aplasia, or, more often, have autologous reconstitution of the thalassemic marrow after engraftment. The most common transplant-related cause of death is infection, especially in patients who remain aplastic after graft rejection. A few splenectomized patients have died after transplant of overwhelming sepsis.

Persistent mixed chimerism has been observed, over a period of time varying between 2 and 11 years after bone marrow transplant, in 11% of posttransplant thalassemic patients.[412-414] Despite the presence of large numbers of residual host cells, these patients no longer required RBC transfusions, producing levels of HbA ranging from 8.3 to 14.7 g/dL. The mechanisms underlying this apparent state of immunologic tolerance or education are not clear. However, these observations may be useful in defining optimal strategies for gene therapy and in utero HSCT.

Related Alternative Sources

Umbilical cord blood has rapidly become a valuable alternative stem cell source for allogeneic HSCT. In thalassemic patients, related cord blood transplantation appears to have a probability of success comparable with that offered by bone marrow transplantation, and, in addition to avoiding general anesthesia to the donor, it is associated with lower risks of transplant-related mortality, cGVHD, and transmission of viral infections. A large study comparing HLA-matched sibling bone marrow with cord blood transplants showed overall survival and thalassemia-free survival to be very similar in the two groups, in the order of 95% to 97% and 80% to 88%, respectively.[415] Acute GVHD and cGVHD were almost double in bone marrow recipients (20% and 12% vs 10% and 5% for cord blood recipients). The mean age in the two groups were similar, 8 vs 6 years, and almost all patients belonged to good-risk classes. The main disadvantage of cord blood is represented by the longer time necessary to reach safe platelet and neutrophil counts. Studies have shown that the number of nucleated cells infused is the most significant predictor of success.[416] These results support targeted efforts to bank family cord blood units that can be used for a sibling diagnosed with thalassemia or other diseases that can be cured by allogeneic HSCT.

Haploidentical related donor HSCT expands the donor pool but is associated with a higher risk of graft rejection, GVHD, and death. More recently, improved immunosuppression and use of T-cell depletion techniques with either ex vivo CD34+ selection or depletion of TCRα/β+/CD19+ lymphocytes or in vivo posttransplant cyclophosphamide have reduced these risks and improved survival. A recent report of haploidentical transplantation utilizing pretransplant hypertransfusion and immunosuppression; reduced-intensity conditioning with ATG, busulfan, and fludarabine; and posttransplant immunosuppression with cyclophosphamide, mycophenolate mofetil, and a calcineurin inhibitor showed excellent outcomes with overall and event-free survival of 96%.[417] However, cGVHD developed in 40% of patients but extensive GVHD was less common, occurring in only 4%. Currently, haploidentical transplantation should be performed in the setting of a research trial in centers with appropriate experience.

Unrelated Alternative Sources

Umbilical cord blood is less restricted with regard to HLA matching, so that a mismatch at 1 or 2 loci is usually tolerated without a significant increase in GVHD or impaired survival.

The use of unrelated cord blood as a source of stem cells for thalassemic patients has not been explored in well-designed clinical trials. In a recent report of 35 unrelated transplants, the 5-year overall survival and thalassemia-free survival were 88% and 74%, respectively. However, 40% of the patients developed skin cGVHD.[418]

Peripheral blood stem cell transplantation has been tried in patients with thalassemia.[419] The results showed that major outcomes obtained with this source of hematopoietic cells are not statistically different from those obtained with bone marrow in terms of rejection and disease-free survival. However, an increased risk of cGVHD was observed.

Side Effects of Stem Cell Transplantation

Chronic Graft-vs-Host Disease

cGVHD, a multiorgan disorder with features of an autoimmune disease, is a risk to consider when transplanting patients, such as those with thalassemia, a nonmalignant disease, who undergo transplantation more to improve quality of life. In an historic series, the incidence of cGVHD was 27%.[420] The risk of GVHD is lower after cord blood transplantation.

Grafts from unrelated donors chosen using strict criteria for HLA compatibility have comparable risks of GVHD. T-cell depletion techniques also can reduce the risk of GVHD.

Growth, Development, and Fertility

Short stature is present in a significant percentage of children transplanted for thalassemia. There appears to be a strict correlation between age at the time of transplant and final adult height. In one study, the patients whose age at transplant was <7 years reached their genetic target for height, whereas those who were >7 years did not.[421] This is in contrast with most studies in children transplanted for hematologic malignancies that have demonstrated that the younger the patient was at the time of HSCT, the greater the loss in height. The deleterious effects on growth of iron and DFO at an early age are likely more profound than the effects of pretransplant conditioning.[422] Results on pubertal maturation remain unsatisfactory after HSCT. In a series of 50 prepubertal patients with TDT, who had been transplanted during childhood or in the peripubertal period, clinical and hormonal evidence of gonadal dysfunction was found, and normal puberty developed in only 40% of patients. There was no correlation between pubertal maturation and age at HSCT or serum ferritin levels.[423] Sterility from pretransplant conditioning is also considered a possible side effect of the procedure. In fact, the myeloablative-conditioning regimen including busulfan and cyclophosphamide may induce gonadal dysfunction in males and females, especially when high doses of busulfan are used. Nevertheless, a few successful cases of spontaneous pregnancy and paternity have been reported in patients transplanted for thalassemia.[424]

Pretransplant sperm banking should be offered to postpubertal males, and cryopreservation of testicular tissue is being studied for younger boys.[425] Cryopreservation of ovarian tissue collected before transplantation is feasible and can maintain fertility even after a long period of time. Several pregnancies have been recorded following autologous reimplantation of frozen ovarian tissue harvested after puberty.[426]

Malignancies

A few solid tumors and several cases of early and late non-Hodgkin lymphoma have been observed in patients transplanted for thalassemia. In one large cohort of transplanted thalassemic patients, a 30-year cumulative incidence of secondary solid cancers was 13.24%, significantly higher than in controls.[427]

Normalization of Iron Status

The iron overload present at the time of grafting will not disappear after transplantation without intervention. After HSCT, ferritin increases, reaching a peak around the third month after the procedure, probably as a consequence of bone marrow aplasia and shifting of iron to the storage compartment.

The conditioning regimen can contribute to the increase in NTBI levels. In one study, NTBI peaked as early as 4 days prior to transplantation and was detectable for 6 to 18 days in all patients.[428] Normally, endogenous antioxidants play a role in scavenging toxic free radicals and preventing cell damage. However, in patients undergoing HSCT, chemotherapy-based conditioning regimens can result in a pro-oxidant status, as indicated by a reduced total radical antioxidant parameter of plasma. After transplant, ferritin usually returns to pretransplant levels. In the absence of therapy, the iron content of the body remains stable, potentially for many years. One study demonstrated that ferritin levels normalized only in moderately to severely iron-overloaded pediatric patients as a result of the use of storage iron for growth.[429]

The effects of persistent iron overload on the long-term morbidity of HSCT recipients (particularly as it relates to late-organ dysfunction) have not been investigated.

Considering the damage that iron induces in nontransplanted thalassemic patients, iron reduction therapy is indicated for patients with high ferritin levels and/or high parenchymal iron concentration measured before transplant. Iron reduction therapy often is not initiated until a year after transplant, due to concerns for interference with engraftment and exacerbation of transplant-related organ toxicity. In a study of 30 patients, early initiation of iron reduction therapy with DFO or phlebotomy at 3 months after HSCT was found to be safe and effective.[430] Early initiation or iron reduction therapy thus can be considered, especially in the setting of severe iron overload or iron-related organ dysfunction.[431,432] Serial phlebotomy typically is utilized if the hemoglobin level is above 10.5 g/dL and there is adequate peripheral venous access. Venesection may be performed every 2 weeks to 3 months depending on the severity of iron overload and is usually continued until the ferritin level falls below 300 ng/mL and/or the LIC is below 3 mg/g dw. Iron chelation therapy may be used in lieu of phlebotomy if the hemoglobin level is low or venous access is difficult, and it has also been used in combination with phlebotomy to increase iron removal. DFX or DFO may be utilized while DFP is not usually given in the early post-HSCT setting due to its potential toxicity on the myeloid cell line. In one report, DFX was used in seven patients transplanted for thalassemia without negative effects on donor chimerism or liver function. Serum ferritin levels decreased, whereas serum creatinine significantly increased, but it remained within normal limits in all patients.[431,432] In a recent randomized study in pediatric patients after HSCT, treatment with DFX at 10 to 20 mg/kg/d or phlebotomy of 15 mL/kg every 2 weeks both led to an improvement in LIC and serum ferritin levels with an acceptable safety profile.[433] Among patients with high ferritin levels above 1000 ng/mL at baseline, the reduction in LIC with DFX was significantly better than with phlebotomy. Regardless of whether phlebotomy or chelation therapy is utilized, it may take several years before iron stores are normalized especially in the setting of high pretransfusion iron burden.[434]

Quality of Life After HSCT

The long-term prognosis of thalassemic patients who are treated according to modern practice is satisfactory and continuously improving. Therefore, the choice to undergo HCST must be carefully considered. On one hand, the freedom from transfusion and chelation and, if the transplant is done early enough, from the consequences of iron overload, and on the other, the immediate risks of death and of acute GVHD and cGVHD and, possibly, of the long-term effects of toxic conditioning regimens need to be considered.

Not many data are available in this regard. In a report of 28 children with β-thalassemia from Middle Eastern countries who underwent allogeneic HSCT in Italy, child self-reports and parent proxy-reports were collected to prospectively evaluate health-related quality of life. The study demonstrated that physical functioning declined significantly from the time of transplant to 3 months after it but then increased significantly up to 18 months after the procedure. As expected, cGVHD was significantly associated with lower scores.[435]

Novel Therapeutic Approaches
Modulators of Ineffective Erythropoiesis

Transforming growth factor beta (TGF-β) family ligands via signaling through the SMAD 2/3 pathway are involved in the ineffective erythropoiesis that characterizes severe β-thalassemia. Luspatercept is a recombinant fusion protein containing the human activin receptor type IIb fused to immunoglobulin that competes for TGF-β family molecules.[436] The drug is administered as a subcutaneous injection every 3 weeks. In the phase 3 randomized placebo controlled BELIEVE trial in TDT, significantly more patients treated with luspatercept (70.5%) achieved at least a 33% reduction in RBC transfusion requirements compared with placebo (29.5%) during any 12-week period on the trial.[437] In addition, with luspatercept, 11% of the patients achieved transfusion independence. Luspatercept was approved for the treatment of transfusion-dependent β-thalassemia by the FDA and the EMA in 2019 and 2020, respectively. Another molecule in this class, sotatercept, has been studied but is not currently in development for thalassemia.[438]

Pharmacologic HbF Reactivation

For patients with homozygous β-thalassemia, an increased γ-globin chain production would result in a more balanced α/non-α ratio with amelioration of the severity of the anemia. In fact, γ-chains can neutralize the harmful excess of α-chains and allow a better survival of erythroid precursors in the bone marrow and of the red cells in the peripheral blood. Many efforts in the past decades have focused on the pharmacologic induction of fetal Hb in patients with hemoglobinopathies, and while most studies have focused on sickle cell disease, they are applicable to β-thalassemia.[439–442] Different therapeutic classes of γ-globin inducers have been investigated, including cytostatic-hypomethylating agents (e.g., HU, 5-azacytidine, decitabine); short-chain fatty acid derivatives, some of which are histone deacetylase inhibitors (e.g., sodium phenylbutyrate, arginine butyrate, isobutyrate); other epigenetic modifiers; and recombinant erythropoietin. The mechanisms for the majority of these are still not completely elucidated. Several promising compounds have been trialed in patients. Cytostatic-hypomethylating compounds, preferentially killing dividing cells, alter the kinetics of erythropoiesis and induce γ-globin gene hypomethylation. Accelerated erythropoiesis is associated with the emergence of stress erythroid progenitors, which are more committed to HbF synthesis. 5-Azacytidine,[443,444] decitabine,[445,446] and butyrate[447,448] have shown some modest effects in clinical trials, but their use has been limited by toxicity concerns. Erythropoietin has been trialed with some success in raising fetal hemoglobin.[449,450] HU has a well-established track record for HbF induction in sickle cell disease, but there have not been high-quality trials of its use in β-thalassemia. A small number of studies have demonstrated a reduction in transfusion burden in patients with TDT and NTDT.[451,452] Dosing of HU is typically lower than in sickle cell disease (starting at 10 mg/kg/d) and may be limited by thrombocytopenia and neutropenia especially in patients who have an intact spleen. IMR-687 is a newer fetal hemoglobin stimulating agent under study in thalassemia. This oral drug selectively inhibits phosphodiesterase 9, which increases fetal hemoglobin expression by raising intracellular cGMP.[453] Preliminary data from a phase 2a trial in sickle cell disease showed only modest mean absolute increase in HbF of 1.7% with an 18.1% increase in F cells[454]; it remains to be seen whether levels high enough to ameliorate ineffective erythropoiesis in thalassemia can be achieved.

Gene Therapy

The β-thalassemias affect the hematopoietic system and have defined molecular lesions in a genetic locus that was among the first characterized; they are therefore an ideal candidate for curative gene therapy approaches.[455] All currently used approaches utilize the ex vivo modification of autologous hematopoietic stem cells and their reinfusion following myeloablative therapy. The two most successful approaches so far are either gene addition of a β-like hemoglobin or reactivation of fetal hemoglobin. Gene addition strategies typically utilize integrating lentiviral vectors capable of infecting hematopoietic stem and progenitor cells (HSPCs) with a high efficiency; these vectors in addition to the β-globin or β-globin like coding sequence must include regulatory elements that ensure high-level expression of the transgene specifically in erythroid cells. Significant work has been done to define the necessary regulatory elements from the β-globin LCR to allow efficient and specific expression within the packaging size constraints of the lentivirus. There are several different approaches to fetal hemoglobin reactivation. The γ-globin repressor BCL11A provides an attractive target.[16,19,20,456] Current studies have used either CRISPR-Cas9 technology or other targeted nucleases to ablate an erythroid-specific enhancer of BCL11A and disrupt its expression specifically in erythroid cells. Another group has used a short hairpin RNA that blocks translation and causes degradation of the BCL11A mRNA[457]; this is expressed from a lentivirus using erythroid-specific regulatory elements and currently is being studied in sickle cell disease. Finally, fetal hemoglobin activation can be achieved by CRISPR-mediated deletion of genetic sequences within the β-globin locus that are typically bound by repressors such as BCL11A.[77,458,459] This method essentially recreates HPFH mutations in HSPCs.

There are several significant obstacles to all these strategies. First, all current approaches require myeloablation for autologous transplantation, although studies are ongoing for reduced-toxicity nonmyeloablative approaches. Lentiviral approaches for gene addition or HbF activation require expertise with making high-titer replication-deficient lentivirus while ensuring lineage-appropriate expression of the transgene. Because lentiviruses integrate throughout the genome, there is the potential for insertional mutagenesis through inactivation of a tumor suppressor or activation of an oncogene. Early experience from treating X-linked severe combined immunodeficiency with retroviral vectors showed that several patients, cured of their disease, developed leukemia as a result of insertional mutagenesis.[460] In the first gene therapy trial for hemoglobinopathies, two patients with thalassemia were treated. In the first patient, the gene-corrected bone marrow failed to reconstitute and the patient required a rescue with untransduced backup bone marrow. The second patient had recently been reported to be free of transfusion for more than 3 years of post–gene therapy follow-up, maintaining an Hb level between 9 and 10 g/dL.[461] However, further analysis of the patient discovered a dominant cell clone with an integration site into the *HMGA2* gene, a potential oncogene, and a possible risk for evolution into a leukemic state. Gene targeting using either synthetic zinc finger nucleases or Cas9/Cas12 nuclease guided by a targeting guide RNA rely on double-stranded DNA cuts followed by repair that creates insertions and deletions. This method relies on optimizing the technology for high-level transduction of HSCs with the nuclease protein, as well as ensuring the specificity of cleavage to avoid double-stranded DNA cuts at off-target sites.

Several gene therapy trials for β-thalassemia have been completed or are ongoing, and one product has received conditional approval for use in Europe. The most complete studies have been done using the BB305 lentiviral vector expressing β-globin with a T87Q mutation that provides anti-sickling effect for sickle cell disease therapy as well as allows tracking of transgene-specific production. A phase 1/2 study in patients with TDT showed that, at median 26 months of follow-up, 12 of 13 patients with non-β^0/β^0 genotypes achieved transfusion independence with hemoglobin levels of 8.2 to 13.7 g/dL. In contrast, only three of nine patients with β^0/β^0 genotypes became transfusion independent but the annual transfusion volume was reduced by 73% in the remaining patients.[462] Importantly, the safety profile was similar to that expected for myeloablative conditioning and no evidence of clonal integration has been found in the patients with β-thalassemia treated with this therapy. Phase 3 studies are ongoing with this product using an improved transduction protocol for patients with β^0/β^0 and non-β^0/β^0 TDT. A second gene addition approach utilizes the GLOBE lentiviral vector expressing the human ß globin gene and intraosseous infusion of the modified hematopoietic stem cells.[463] Among seven patients, most with severe ß-globin genotypes, treated in a phase 1/2 trial, three of four pediatric patients achieved transfusion independence while the fourth pediatric patient and all three adult patients had a reduction in transfusion requirements. Early data have also been published for a trial using CRISPR-Cas9 targeting of the BCL11A erythroid enhancer; one patient with TDT with the β^0/β^+ (IVS-I-110) genotype has been treated and achieved transfusion independence with hemoglobin levels at 18 months of ~14 g/dL composed predominantly of HbF.[464] There are additional trials using different gene addition approaches and gene editing, and overall there is a significant promise of curative therapy. All of these approaches require long-term follow-up to ensure durability of response and to monitor for late adverse effects.

THALASSEMIA MINOR

Classic Form: Clinical Picture

The classic heterozygous carrier of β-thalassemia is usually asymptomatic, and the diagnosis is made by chance, because of positive family history or during population screening. Several series have been published on the clinical and hematologic features of people with thalassemia minor.[465] Anemia is mild or absent. In pregnancy, anemia can be more severe than in unaffected women, and folate supplementation, at the dose of 5 mg daily, is recommended; red cell transfusion occasionally is needed. Iron absorption is increased, and frank iron

overload has been reported.[466] Inappropriate administration of iron has been proposed as a possible cause in some of the patients. The β-thalassemia trait aggravates the clinical picture of hemochromatosis in individuals homozygous for the mutations C282Y and H63D, favoring higher rates of iron accumulation and the possible development of iron-related complications.[467] Serum bilirubin levels are variable. Homozygosity for the mutation typical of Gilbert syndrome is one of the factors determining hyperbilirubinemia in these individuals but an increase in gallstone risk is associated with β-thalassemia trait alone.[175] Men have a lower risk of myocardial infarction than the general population.[468] A partially improved cardiovascular risk profile has been observed in terms of low hematocrit, low-density lipoprotein (LDL) cholesterol, and apo-B in carriers of β-thalassemia. The LDL lowering effect of the thalassemia trait is evident even in patients with familial hypercholesterolemia.[469]

Laboratory Features

The reported mean Hb concentration in affected Italian men and women was 12.7 and 10.9 g/dL, respectively; in Greek men, 13.9 g/dL[470]; and in East Asian men and women, 12.1 and 10.8 g/dL, respectively.[471] A slightly lower Hb concentration was noted in Jamaicans with heterozygous β^0-thalassemia (11.3 g/dL) compared with those having heterozygous β^+-thalassemia (12.5 g/dL). Hb is less markedly decreased in Africans than in Mediterraneans. The red cell count is elevated, and the MCV and MCH values are reduced. The mean cell hemoglobin concentration (MCHC) is normal or only slightly decreased. In one series of 244 cases of β^0-thalassemia carriers, the MCV was 67 ± 4.6 fL (mean ± 1 SD), the MCH was 22.4 ± 1.6 pg, and the MCHC was 32.9 ± 0.8 g/dL RBCs.[472] The degree of reduction in the MCV is directly related to the degree of reduction in β-globin production. The MCVs produced by β^0 mutations are lower than those produced by β^+ mutations. Reticulocytes are generally increased to twice the normal numbers and have been found to correlate with the Hb level. In children, the MCV is lower than in adults and normally increases with age; this correlation with age is less evident with the thalassemia trait. The evolution of hematologic parameters in children at various ages is reported in *Table 35.4*.[473] Free erythrocyte protoporphyrin is normal or slightly increased. Osmotic fragility is decreased. Studies of red cell survival, measured by 51Cr, shows mild ineffective erythropoiesis, rather than peripheral hemolysis.[474] HbA2 is constantly elevated in heterozygous carriers of β-thalassemia in all the ethnic groups studied. The values range from 3.5% to 7% with a mean of 5%.[475] This increase appears to be determined by an increased output of δ-chains from both loci, in cis and in trans, to the thalassemia gene. HbF is increased in half of the patients, but the values observed are generally in the range of 1% to 3%. A minority of carriers show unusually high levels of HbA2 (>6.5%) associated with a variable increase in HbF. The molecular basis of these forms is large deletions

Table 35.4. Main Hematologic Parameters of β-Thalassemia Carriers According to Age

Age	Hb (g/dL)	MCV (fl)	HbA₂ (%)	HbF (%)
At birth	18.3 ± 2.3	99 ± 8	0.5 ± 0.2	73.8 ± 10.1
4 mo	10.1 ± 1.1	70 ± 6	3.2 ± 0.7	27.0 ± 10.5
7 mo	10.5 ± 0.8	59 ± 4	4.8 ± 0.7	8.2 ± 4.0
9-10 mo	11.1 ± 0.9	59 ± 2	5.1 ± 0.5	4.4 ± 2.1
2 y	11.2 ± 0.9	58 ± 2	4.8 ± 0.4	4.1 ± 2.1
2-6 y	10.7 ± 1.0	61 ± 4	5.3 ± 0.6	Nd
6-12 y	11.0 ± 1.0	62 ± 5	5.2 ± 0.6	Nd
Adult male	13.3 ± 0.8	67 ± 6	5.0 ± 0.5	1.0 ± 0.5
Adult female	11.8 ± 0.9	66 ± 4	5.0 ± 0.5	0.9 ± 0.6

Abbreviations: Hb, hemoglobin; MCV, mean corpuscular volume; nd, not determined.

of the β-globin gene, which remove its 5′ promoter region.[476] Globin chain synthesis analysis in heterozygous β-thalassemia shows variable imbalance correlated to the severity of the β-globin chain defect. The physiologic decrease in HbF in the first weeks of life is slower in β-thalassemia heterozygotes (*Table 35.4*).

Atypical Carriers

The typical phenotype of the β-thalassemia trait, essentially characterized by reduced MCV and MCH, and increased HbA2, may be modified by several genetic and acquired factors, causing problems in carrier identification. The coinheritance of heterozygous β-thalassemia with homozygous α⁺-thalassemia (−α/−α) or heterozygous α⁰-thalassemia (−/αα) has a substantial effect on MCV and MCH, which increase sometimes up to normal values (*Figure 35.19*).[477] However, the HbA2 in these double heterozygotes remains in the carrier range, thus allowing their identification. Atypical carriers with reduced MCV and MCH and normal or borderline HbA2 include double heterozygotes for δ- and β-thalassemia and carriers of some mild mutation, such as the −87 C→G, the −29 A→G, and IVS-1 –6 T→C (*Table 35.5*). The differential diagnosis includes iron deficiency and the α-thalassemia trait. Specific tests and sometimes family studies allow correct identification (see below).[478] A third group of atypical β-thalassemia carriers is represented by heterozygotes for very mild or silent β-thalassemia mutations (*Table 35.5*). As a result of minimal deficiency of β-globin production, these carriers have normal MCV and MCH and normal or borderline HbA2.[479] The α- to β-globin chain synthesis ratio is normal or slightly higher than 1, confirming that these mutations cause only a very mild reduction in the expression of the β-globin gene. The carrier state of the triple α-globin gene arrangement (*aaa/aa*) also may be considered a very mild β-thalassemia allele due to the excess of α-globin chain produced.[480] An extreme, although rare, instance of complex thalassemia gene combination that may lead to an almost silent phenotype is the coinheritance of α-, δ-, and β-thalassemia. Acquired factors able to modify the typical phenotype of β-thalassemia trait are iron deficiency anemia and folate deficiency. Iron deficiency anemia, when severe, may decrease the high HbA2 levels typical of heterozygous β-thalassemia, reducing its reliability for β-thalassemia carrier identification.[481] Folate deficiency may increase the MCV up to normal values. When these deficiency anemias are present, other tests, such as DNA analysis to identify the β-globin gene mutation or retesting after correction of the deficiency, are warranted to make a correct diagnosis.

δβ and Hereditary Persistence of Fetal Hb Carriers

δβ⁰-Thalassemia carriers show RBC changes milder than those observed in the β-thalassemia trait. Overall, MCV and MCH are around 70 fL and 24 pg, respectively. HbA2 is normal or reduced, and HbF is increased (5%-20%) and heterogeneously distributed among red cells. The degree of globin chain imbalance is mild (α to non-α ratio around 1.5). Heterozygotes for deletional HPFH are characterized mostly by normal MCV, MCH, and HbA2. Only in some cases is there a mild reduction of red cell indices and HbA2. HbF ranges from 15% to 30% with pancellular distribution. α-/Non-α–globin synthesis is normal or mildly unbalanced.[482] Nondeletional HPFH heterozygotes have red cell indices, HbA2, and α- to non-α ratios similar to those of deletional HPFH carriers, whereas mean HbF levels vary from 1.5% to 27%.

Carrier Detection

β-Thalassemia and δβ-Thalassemia

Carrier detection methods should be able to identify typical and atypical heterozygous β-thalassemia as well as δβ-thalassemia and the Hb variants, such as HbS and HbE, which, by interacting with β-thalassemia, may result in the production of clinically significant syndromes. As compared with most genetic diseases, carrier detection in hemoglobinopathies is relatively easy because it may be achieved through hematologic examination rather than DNA analysis. However, DNA analysis is needed for the identification of globin gene mutation, which is essential for prenatal diagnosis. Basic hematology methods for carrier detection consist of RBC indices determination and Hb pattern analysis. More specialized tests (including iron status determination and globin chain synthesis analysis) and eventually DNA analysis are required in some cases for definitive diagnosis.[483]

The recommended method for blood count is the electronic measurement of red cell indices. All red cell indices are important in the evaluation, but the most useful for thalassemia carrier identification are MCV and MCH, with cutoff values of <80 fl and 27 pg, respectively. Hb pattern analysis can be obtained in a single step by HPLC. This method gives an accurate quantitation of HbA2 and HbF and

Table 35.5. Genotype and Phenotype of Atypical β-Thalassemia Carriers

Phenotype	Genotype
Normal MCV and MCH, high HbA₂	Coinheritance of α-thalassemia
Reduced MCV and MCH, borderline/normal HbA₂	Some mild β-thalassemia alleles Coinheritance of δ-thalassemia εγδβ-thalassemia Corfu δβ-thalassemia
Normal MCV-MCH, and borderline/normal HbA₂	Very mild/silent alleles Triplicated α-globin gene KLF1 mutations
Significant clinical phenotype	Coinheritance of α-globin gene defects: triple alpha locus and HbH disease genotype (−/−α) Hyperunstable globins

Abbreviations: Hb, Hemoglobin; MCH, mean cell hemoglobin; MCV, mean cell volume.

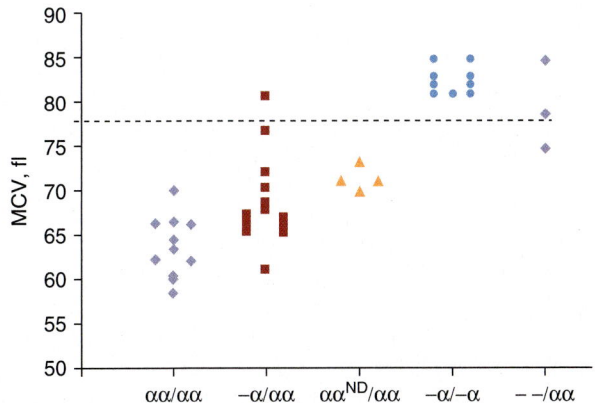

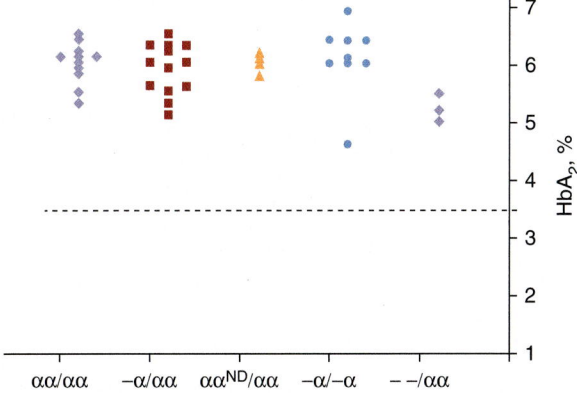

FIGURE 35.19 **Effect of coinheritance of different α-thalassemia alleles in β-thalassemia carriers.** Hb, hemoglobin; MCV, mean cell volume.

detects the large majority of Hb variants. Several automatic devices for Hb separation and quantitation are available, and a comparative study has shown that all provide reliable detection of Hb variants and good HbA2 quantification.[484] Alternatively, cellulose acetate electrophoresis or isoelectric focusing can be used for detecting Hb variants, but quantitation of HbA2 and HbF should be performed, respectively, by microchromatography and alkali denaturation. Elution of HbA2 and HbF bands after electrophoresis is an accurate but time-consuming method. Iron studies, including ferritin, are useful supplementary methods. Family studies may be helpful in some atypical cases, particularly in genetic compounds for two different alleles. The carrier detection procedure should be designed in order not to miss any carrier or couple at risk. Based on the frequency and heterogeneity of thalassemia types present in a population, appropriate screening programs are set out. A sample diagnostic flowchart is shown in *Figure 35.20*.[485] Several mathematical indices derived from red cell parameters, measured using electronic counters, have been proposed to identify β-thalassemia carriers, discriminating thalassemia trait from iron deficiency (Mentzer, England and Fraser, Shine and Lal). However, these indices turned out to be inaccurate, particularly in pregnant women, in children, and in α-thalassemia–β-thalassemia interaction, predicting the correct diagnosis in 80% to 90% of the patients.[486]

Two common problems in screening for β-thalassemia are the presence of borderline HbA2 values (ie, HbA2 = 3.2%-3.8%) and the differential diagnosis of microcytosis with normal to borderline HbA2.[487] Borderline HbA2 may be associated with low or normal MCV and MCH. Several β-thalassemia genotypes have been associated with borderline HbA2, including mild $β^+$-thalassemia mutations (i.e., HBB c.92+6 TC), coinherited δ- and β-thalassemia, and β promoter mutations (i.e., HBB c.-142 CT).[487] However, all these determinants explain only a limited proportion of borderline HbA2 levels, and the unexplained cases pose relevant screening and genetic counseling problems. Recently, mutations of the *KLF1* gene have been described in a consistent proportion of subjects with borderline HbA2, and this facilitates carrier detection and genetic counseling.[488] A phenotype characterized by microcytosis, hypochromia, normal or borderline HbA2, and normal HbF may result from iron deficiency, α-thalassemia, δ-+ β-thalassemia interaction, mild β-thalassemia, or, very rarely, εγδβ-thalassemia. After exclusion of iron deficiency by erythrocyte zinc protoporphyrin determination, serum ferritin level, and/or evaluation of transferrin saturation, the different thalassemia determinants leading to this phenotype are discriminated by globin chain synthesis analysis and eventually by α-, δ-, and β-globin gene analysis.

$δβ^0$-Thalassemia carriers and HPFH heterozygotes, both characterized by increased HbF levels, can be clearly differentiated by globin chain synthesis analysis, showing an α/non-α imbalance in the former. Identification of the molecular defect by globin gene DNA analysis may be requested to confirm the diagnosis.

The presence of the Hb Lepore can be suspected in the presence of an abnormally slow Hb band on the electrophoretic pattern associated with reduced MCV, MCH, and HbA2 and usually a mild increase (~2%-5%) of HbF. The diagnosis is confirmed by DNA analysis of the β-globin gene cluster. In couples at risk identified by the carrier detection procedures described earlier, the specific mutation is defined by globin gene DNA analysis using polymerase chain reaction (PCR)-based methods. There are now many different PCR-based techniques that can be used to detect globin gene mutations, including dot blot analysis, reverse dot blot analysis, the amplification refractory mutation system, denaturing gradient gel electrophoresis (DGGE), mutagenically separated PCR, gap-PCR, restriction endonuclease analysis, real-time PCR, Sanger sequencing, pyrosequencing, multiplex ligation-dependent probe amplification, and gene array systems.

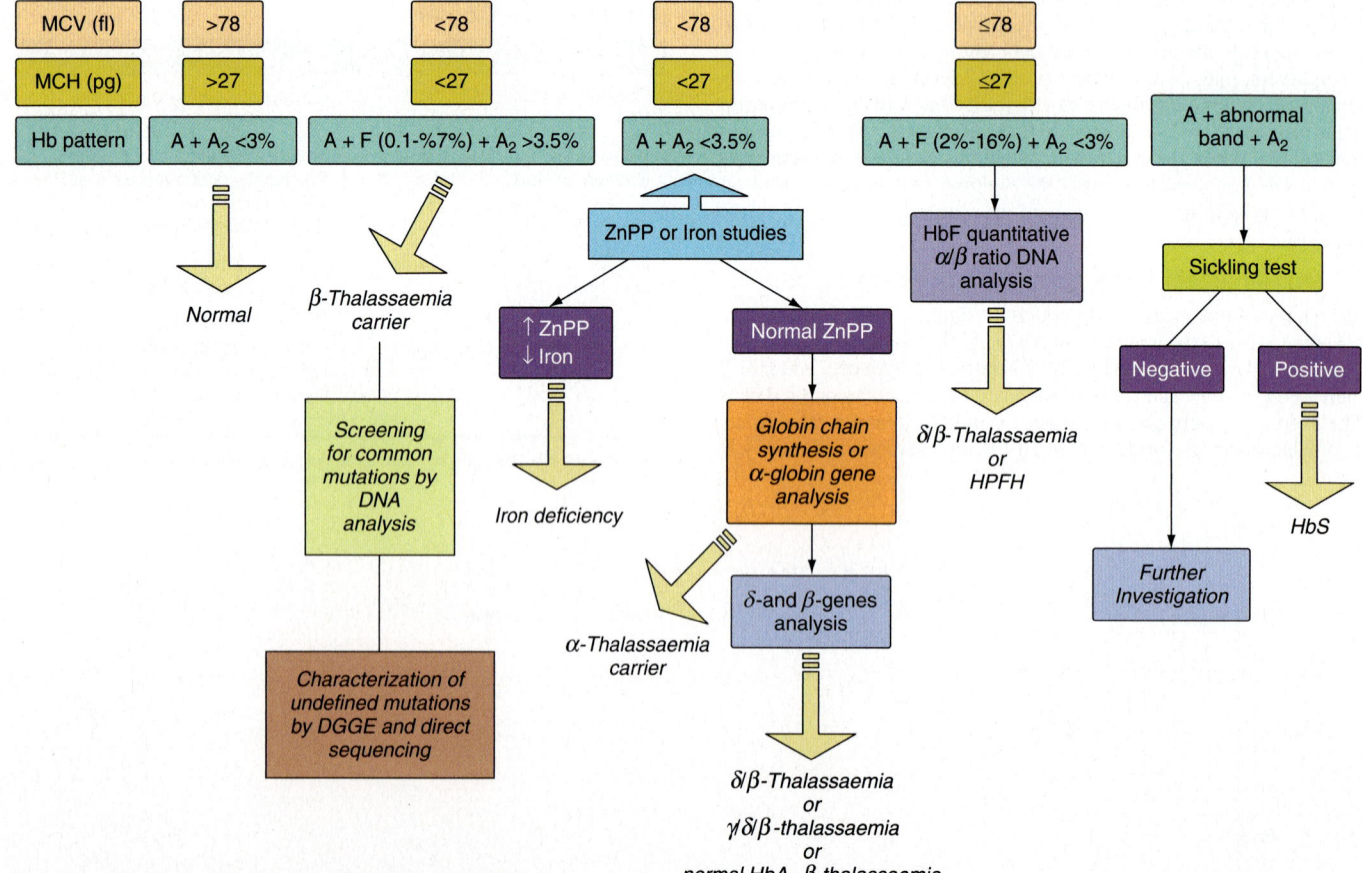

FIGURE 35.20 **Flowchart for the diagnosis of thalassemia syndromes.** DGGE, denaturing gradient gel electrophoresis; Hb, hemoglobin; MCH, mean cell hemoglobin; MCV, mean cell volume. (Adapted from Brancaleoni V, Di Pierro E, Motta I, Cappellini MD. Laboratory diagnosis of thalassemia. *Int J Lab Hematol.* 2016;38(S1):32-40. Copyright © 2016 John Wiley & Sons Ltd. Reprinted by permission of John Wiley & Sons, Inc.)

Each method has advantages and disadvantages, and the choice depends not only on the technical expertise of the laboratory but also on the type and variety of the mutations likely to be encountered in the populations being tested.[489] In fact, despite the marked heterogeneity of thalassemia mutations, a limited number of molecular defects are prevalent in each population (*Table 35.6*). This information is very useful in practice because the most appropriate probes or primers can be selected according to the carriers' ethnic origin. It is advisable for any diagnostic laboratory to have at least two alternative methods for detecting mutations (*Table 35.7*).

α-Thalassemia

α-Thalassemia carriers are more difficult to identify than β- or δβ-thalassemia carriers because they do not have typical changes in HbA2 or HbF levels. MCV and MCH are always reduced in carriers of $-\alpha/-\alpha$ and $-/\alpha\alpha$ genotypes, whereas $-\alpha/\alpha\alpha$ carriers often have normal or sometimes a mild reduction of MCV and MCH values. The Hb pattern in adult α-thalassemia carriers is normal, although as a group, they have slightly lower levels of HbA2. In the newborn, the electrophoretic detection of Hb Barts (γ^4), a fast-moving band, is useful for diagnosis of the α-thalassemia trait. α^+-Thalassemia carriers usually show up to 3% of Hb Barts, and α^0-thalassemia carriers ($-/\alpha\alpha$) and α^+-thalassemia homozygotes ($-\alpha/-\alpha$) may have 3% to 8%. However, in some carriers, Hb Barts may be undetectable.[119]

A simple test for detecting α-thalassemia carriers is the incubation of the peripheral blood with brilliant cresyl blue; the smear examination may show rare RBCs with HbH inclusion bodies, although their absence does not exclude α-thalassemia carrier status.[490] While measurement of $\alpha{:}\beta$ globin chain ratios using radioisotope labeling is helpful for identifying α-thalassemia trait in some situations, this test is not routinely available outside of research settings and molecular testing

should be used. Definitive diagnosis of α-thalassemia carriers can be achieved with DNA analysis of the α-globin genes. The methods used depend upon the type of mutations expected in each population and are divided into those that detect deletions (gap-PCR and Multiplex Ligation-Dependent Probe Amplification) and those that detect point mutations, that is, nondeletion α-thalassemia (direct detection by restriction enzyme analysis, allele-specific oligonucleotide hybridization, DGGE, and DNA sequencing).[491] The α^0-thalassemia phenotype can be detected with an anti-ζ globin monoclonal antibody because small amounts of embryonic ζ globin are produced in adult life by chromosomes lacking both α-globin genes.[492,493] Detection of α^0-thalassemia carriers is important for prevention of Hb Barts hydrops fetalis syndrome, for which prenatal diagnosis is always indicated, also to avoid the severe toxemic maternal complications during pregnancy.

Hemoglobin E

The diagnosis of heterozygous HbE is based on the Hb pattern analysis by electrophoresis or HPLC separation. At alkaline pH (8.4), HbE moves at the same position as HbA2 and can be distinguished by its

Table 35.6. Most Common Silent and Mild β-Thalassemia Mutations

Silent
−101 C→T
−92 C→T
IVS-2-2–844 C→G
6′-UTR mutants
3′-UTR mutants

Mild
Transcriptional Mutants
Proximal CACCC box
−88 C→T
−87 C→G
TATA box
−30 T→A
−29 A→G
Alternative splicing site
cd 19 A→C
cd 24 T→A
cd 27 G→T
Consensus splicing sequence
IVS-1–6 T→C
Poly (A) site
AACCCC
AATGAA

Abbreviations: cd, codon; UTR, untranslated region.

Table 35.7. β-Thalassemia Mutations Occurring in Specific Populations With High Frequency

Population	Alleles
African American	−88 C→T
	−29 A→G
Italians	IVS-1–1 G→A
	IVS-1–6 T→C
	IVS-1–110 G→A
	cd 39 C→T
	IVS-2–745 C→G
Greek	IVS-1–1 G→A
	IVS-1–6 T→C
	IVS-1–110 G→A
	cd 39 C→T
	IVS-2–745 C→G
Indian	cd 8/9 +G
	IVS-1–1 G→T
	IVS-1–5 G→C
	cd 41/42-TTCT
	619-bp deletion
Thai	−28 A→G
	cd 17 A→T
	cd 19 A→G
	IVS-1–1 G→T
	IVS-1–5 G→C
	cd 41/42-TTCT
	IVS-2–645 C→T
Chinese	−28 A→G
	cd 17 A→T
	cd 41/42-TTCT
	IVS-2–645 C→T
Middle East	cd 8-AA
	cd 8/9 +G
	IVS-1–5 G→C
	cd 39 C→T
	cd 44 C
	IVS-2–1 G→A
Israeli	−28 A→G
	IVS-1–110 G→A
	cd 39 C→T
	cd 44 C
	IVS-2–1 G→A
North African	Cd 6-A
	IVS-1–1 G→A
	IVS-1–110 G→A
	cd 39 C→T

Abbreviation: cd, codon.

high concentration; usually 25% to 30% HbE has the same elution time of HbA2 at HPLC.[494] Lower proportions of HbE in carriers indicate the presence of coinheritance α-thalassemia or of iron deficiency anemia. The blue dye dichlorophenolindophenol can be used as a screening test for HbE, which will dissociate and precipitate at the bottom of the tube upon incubation with this dye at 37 °C.[495]

PRENATAL DIAGNOSIS

The availability of prenatal diagnosis added a new option to couples at risk for a major hemoglobinopathy, leading to a significant change in the effectiveness of screening and counseling in hemoglobinopathy prevention. Prenatal diagnosis of both α- and β-thalassemia was carried out for the first time in the 1970s using globin chain synthesis analysis in fetal blood, obtained by fetoscopy or placental aspiration around the 19th week of gestation.[496] The advent of DNA analysis and the introduction of chorionic villus sampling resulted in a notable improvement in prenatal diagnosis that can now be performed within the first trimester of pregnancy, generally at 10 to 12 weeks of gestation. Fetal DNA can also be obtained from amniocytes at 15 to 17 weeks of pregnancy. Chorionic villus sampling is carried out transcervically or transabdominally, and the risk of fetal loss with this procedure has given contrasting results, ranging from 0.5% to 4.5%. However, in experienced hands, the fetal loss rate appears to be 0.5% to 1%, similar to natural wastage for pregnancies of this duration.[497] After sampling, fetal DNA analysis is performed by the PCR-based methods. Methods aimed at identifying the mutations are traditionally separated into direct (those designed to interrogate samples for the presence/absence of specific candidate mutations known to be present in the population) or indirect methods (those that screen regions of genes to identify/exclude sequence variation of genes within each gene region. As a consequence of recent immigrations and the admixture of different ethnic groups, the spectrum of mutations, particularly in Western countries, has increased, making more generic methods such as DNA sequencing indicated. The results of DNA analysis are very accurate, but misdiagnosis may occur for several reasons (e.g., failure to amplify the target DNA fragment, mispaternity, maternal contamination, sample exchange). Recently, noninvasive prenatal testing using cell-free DNA from maternal blood has become a viable alternative to these invasive techniques.[498-500]

The advent of DNA amplification has made it possible to define the genotype of a single cell biopsied from cleaving embryos (preimplantation diagnosis) and to analyze the polar body obtained during the maturation of the oocyte (preconception diagnosis), which allows identification and transfer only of healthy embryos established from in vitro fertilization.[501] Successful experiences in many couples with this approach have been reported in hemoglobinopathies. However, preimplantation genetic diagnosis (PGD) is technically challenging and requires the close collaboration of a team of specialists. PGD is now an established reproductive alternative to prenatal diagnosis, offered in several specialized centers (http://www.eshre.com). PGD is also very expensive and may not be feasible for a wider population. β-Thalassemia prevention programs adapted to meet the need of different communities have been implemented in several at-risk countries across the world. These programs are based on education, carrier screening, and genetic counseling and have resulted in decreased incidence of TDT in several countries, including Sardinia, Cyprus, Taiwan, Iran, India, and China (*Figure 35.21*).[502,503]

NON-TRANSFUSION-DEPENDENT THALASSEMIA (THALASSEMIA INTERMEDIA)

Genetic Determinants

The remarkable clinical diversity of NTDT may be produced by a great variety of genotypes. NTDT most commonly is associated with a homozygous or compound heterozygous state for two β-thalassemia alleles.[504] However, several patients with this mild clinical picture have only a single β-globin gene affected and are considered heterozygotes for β-thalassemia. It has been clearly established that the severity of the β-thalassemias is related to the degree of globin chain imbalance. Therefore, in homozygous β-thalassemia, any inherited or acquired factor able to reduce the degree of globin imbalance may produce milder clinical forms (*Figure 35.22*). On the other hand, in simple β-thalassemia heterozygotes, the worsening of globin chain imbalance may turn the asymptomatic carrier state into a significant clinical phenotype (*Table 35.5*).[505]

Homozygotes or compound heterozygotes for mild β-thalassemia mutations, characterized by a residual high β-globin chain production, usually exhibit NTDT. Examples are the homozygous state for −29 A→G in black patients and the IVS-1-6 T→C in Mediterranean patients.[506,507] Compound heterozygotes for a mild and a severe mutation may cover a remarkably broad clinical spectrum of severity. This variability can be related to the presence of α-thalassemia or of genetic determinants able to increase the γ-chain production.[508] Few homozygotes for silent mutations have been reported (e.g., β CAP + 1 ASC, IVS-2–844 C→G); they have the hematologic and clinical characteristics of the β-thalassemia trait.[509] Compound heterozygotes for a silent and a severe mutation usually have a very mild NTDT, but exceptions with a severe phenotype have been reported. Coinheritance of α-thalassemia with homozygous β-thalassemia leads to a reduction in the excess of the α-chain pool and in the imbalance of the globin chain (*Figure 35.22A*). Interacting α-thalassemia has been reported in patients with β-NTDT from the Mediterranean and Southeast

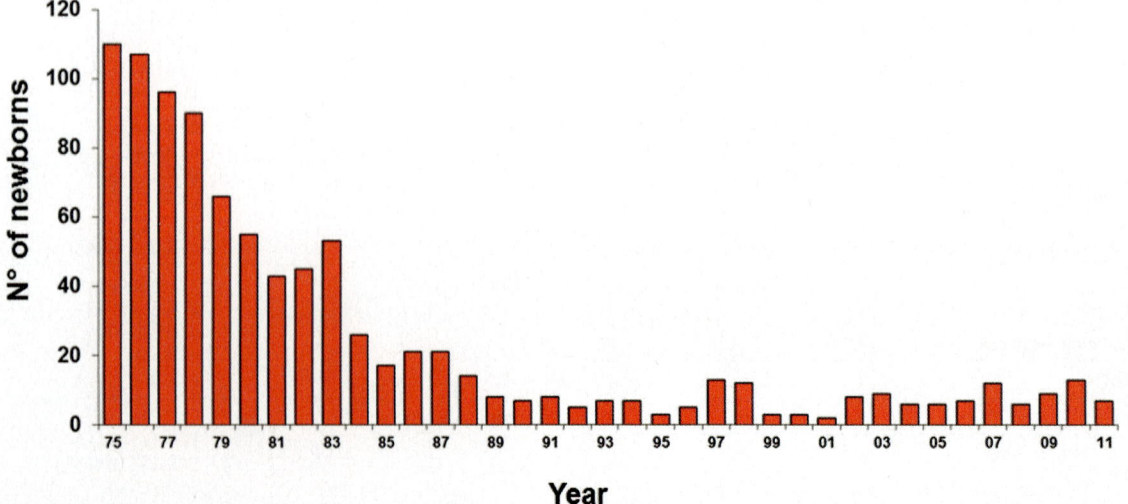

FIGURE 35.21 Fall in the birth rate of infants with homozygous β-thalassemia in Sardinia.

Asia.[510,511] However, the ameliorating effect depends both on the type of coinherited α-thalassemia (the presence of two α genes deleted being more effective) and on the severity of the β-thalassemia allele (α-thalassemia being less effective in ameliorating the homozygous β^0-thalassemia). Genetic determinants maintaining a high γ-chain synthesis after birth result in a reduction of the α/non-α-chain imbalance, thus producing a mild phenotype when coinherited with homozygous severe β-thalassemia. Moreover, high γ-chain synthesis produces a net increase in total Hb synthesis. Rarely, the increase in γ-chain output depends on the type of thalassemia mutations per se because it occurs in $\delta\beta$-thalassemias, caused by deletions of variable extent in the β-globin gene cluster, or in deletions removing the β-globin gene promoter. Most commonly, the persistence of HbF production depends on the cotransmission of specific determinants associated with quantitative trait loci linked or unlinked to the β-globin cluster. The most common of these loci is -158 C$\rightarrow$T Gγ promoter substitution, which is in linkage disequilibrium with several β^0-thalassemia mutations (cd 6 [$-$A], cd 8 [$-$AA], IVS-2–1 G$\rightarrow$A).[512] This mutation leads to enhanced γ-chain production under conditions of erythropoietic stress and partially compensates for the absence of β-chain synthesis with consequent amelioration of the α/non-α imbalance and of the clinical phenotype. The -158 Gγ C$\rightarrow$T substitution has been found occasionally in patients with β^+ IVS-1–6 T$\rightarrow$C and with the severe β^0 39 C$\rightarrow$T mutation.[513] Genetic determinants capable of sustaining a continuous increased production of HbF in adult life and mapping outside the β-globin gene cluster have been identified on chromosome 2p16 (*BCL11A* gene) and on chromosome 6q23 (HBS1L-MYB intergenic region).[78,79,514,515] Several polymorphisms at these loci have been associated with increased HbF levels in patients with different hemoglobinopathies (e.g., β-thalassemia, sickle cell anemia, HbE/β-thalassemia) belonging to different populations (Sardinians, Chinese, Thais, African Americans). Coinheritance of these determinants and α-thalassemia contributes to the amelioration of the phenotype of homozygous β-thalassemia, resulting in an NTDT phenotype. However, in some patients with NTDT homozygous or compound heterozygous for severe β-thalassemia mutations, even of the β^0 type, the inherited modifying factors able to ameliorate the clinical features are still unknown. Less commonly, the phenotype of NTDT has been reported in subjects carrying only one β-globin gene defect. The worsening of the globin chain imbalance, which converts the asymptomatic carrier state into a significant clinical phenotype, depends on several mechanisms (*Figure 35.22B*). Among them, five groups have been defined: (1) the dominantly inherited β-thalassemia mutations (also reported as hyperunstable globins or inclusion body thalassemias)[67,516]; (2) compound heterozygosity for severe β-thalassemia with both deletion and nondeletion pancellular HPFH; (3) compound heterozygosity for β-thalassemia and some structural β-chain variants (HbD-Los Angeles β 121 GluSGln, HbC β 6 Glu$\rightarrow$Lys, HbO-Arab β 121 Glu$\rightarrow$Lys)[517]; (4) coexistence of somatic deletions of a region of chromosome 11p15[518]; and (5) coinheritance of triplicated α-globin gene with excessive α-globin production.[519] This is the most common group. Recently, cases have also been reported of simple β-thalassemia heterozygosity presenting with an intermediate to severe phenotype because of duplication of the complete α-globin gene cluster, including the upstream regulatory element HS-40, resulting in α-globin gene quadruplication. Several patients, heterozygotes for β-thalassemia with the typical NTDT clinical picture, have been reported in whom extensive analysis of β- and α-globin gene cluster and family studies fail to identify any other associated molecular defect. Recently, a novel α-globin chaperone, the α-hemoglobin stabilizing protein (AHSP) has been identified.[92] AHSP stabilizes α-globin chains, and its loss leads to RBC damage and worsens a murine β-thalassemia intermedia phenotype.[91] Although AHSP mutations have been reported, the association with β-thalassemia severity is not yet clear.[520]

Clinical Features

The clinical spectrum of NTDT is heterogeneous and variable in severity, ranging from mild anemia and jaundice to a TDT-like clinical picture. It is usually diagnosed later compared with TDT. About 11% of patients with NTDT presented in the first year of life, 30% in the second year, and 59% later in life.[521] Conventionally, NTDT is considered transfusion independent if Hb is spontaneously maintained at or above 7 to 7.5 g/dL.

However, regular transfusions often become necessary with advancing age, whereas in other cases, they are required only occasionally (infections, hypersplenism, and pregnancy).[522] It is not easy to predict which patients will become transfusion-dependent and at what age. Age at presentation seems to represent an indicator of future transfusion independency. Cao et al, describing a group of 34 patients with NTDT, observed that those who became transfusion dependent were diagnosed at a mean age of 8.5 ± 1.8 months, whereas those who remained transfusion independent were diagnosed at 17.4 ± 11.8 months.[523]

Patients with truly transfusion-independent forms may be completely asymptomatic until adulthood, experiencing anemia of various degrees and mild jaundice, whereas growth and development are not impaired. In severely affected patients, NTDT generally presents between the ages of 2 and 6 years, and although many are able to survive without regular transfusions, growth and development can be delayed. The spleen is palpable in the majority of the patients,

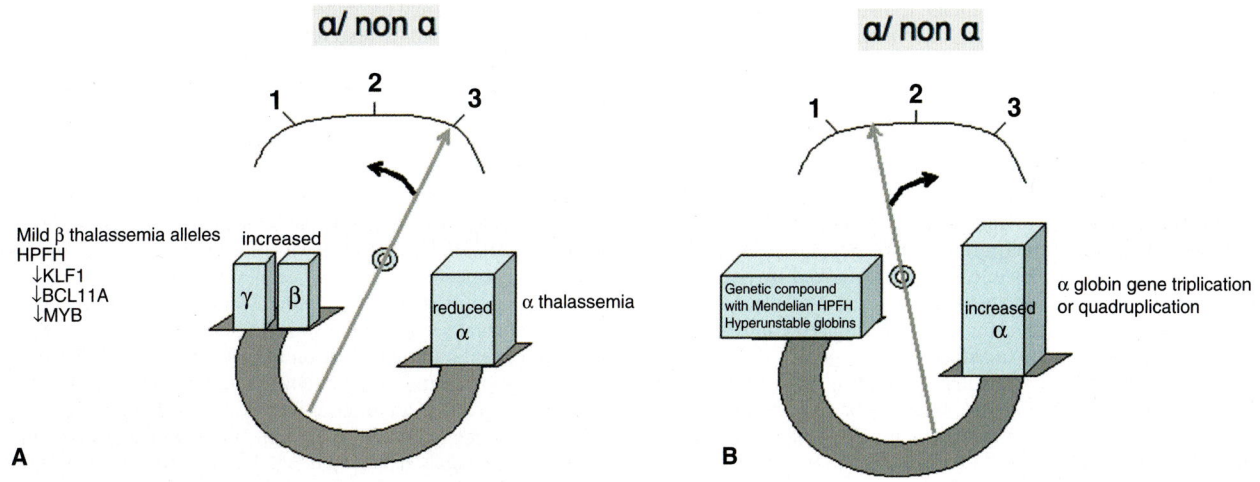

FIGURE 35.22 Mechanisms of β-thalassemia intermedia. A, Reduced globin chain imbalance. B, Increased globin chain imbalance. HPFH, hereditary persistence of fetal hemoglobin.

and its size increases with time. Hypersplenism may develop, causing a decrease in Hb levels and sometimes thrombocytopenia and neutropenia.

Bone and joint pains are also frequently reported and may be a result of different pathophysiology. Bone deformities are common and include frontal bossing, prominence of the zygomatic bones, depression of the base of the nose, shortening of long bones, cortical thinning, and dilatation of the medullary cavities, as described for TDT.[522] The more severe skeletal abnormalities indicate excessive marrow activity secondary to anemia and are an indication to begin transfusions. Extramedullary erythropoiesis is found in up to 65% of patients with NTDT,[524] compared with patients with TDT on regular transfusions, where the prevalence remains below 1%. Symptoms are usually reported during the third and fourth decades of life; however, there have been reports in children.[525]

Ectopic erythropoietic masses may be found in various body sites, including the spleen, liver, lymph nodes, and kidneys, and also in paravertebral, intrathoracic, pelvic, and intracranial locations. Most cases remain asymptomatic and are usually diagnosed incidentally by radiologic techniques, whereas others lead to compression of adjacent structures as tumorlike masses. Paraspinal involvement occurs in 11% to 15% of cases and may present with a variety of neurologic symptoms, including back pain, paraparesis, paraplegia, urinary urgency, and bowel incontinence (*Figure 35.23*).[526] Spinal cord compression causing paraparesis and cauda equina syndrome requires urgent treatment.

The intrathoracic location is often asymptomatic; however, it may present with pleural effusion or mediastinal syndrome[527] (*Figure 35.24*). There is currently no consensus on the best treatment strategy for extramedullary erythropoiesis. HU[528] and transfusions[529] have proven to be effective, but when rapid regression is required, radiotherapy, and, less often, surgical decompression, may be indicated. MRI is considered the method of choice for the diagnosis and follow-up of extramedullary erythropoiesis, especially for paraspinal localizations.

Osteoporosis is frequently found in NTDT and, along with cortical thinning, is responsible for pathologic fractures of long bones and vertebrae. The pathophysiology of bone disease is complex and is caused by bone marrow expansion, endocrine dysfunction, genetic factors, direct iron toxicity to osteoblasts, and increased osteoclast activity.[530] Vitamin D deficiency caused by nutrition or lack of sun exposure may play a role and, in some patients, has been associated with specific polymorphisms in candidate genes (vitamin D receptor, estrogen receptor, calcitonin receptor, and collagen type 1 α_1).[154]

Transfusion Therapy

NTDT is, by definition, transfusion independent. However, at some time during the life of a patient, the decision to initiate transfusion therapy may need to be made. In general, transfusion becomes necessary when the sense of well-being of the patient decreases to a level inadequate to the activities of a normal life. This usually occurs at levels of Hb below 7 g/dL. In children, in addition to the level of Hb, the main indicators are impaired growth, poor general condition, and skeletal deformities.[531]

It is important to consider the consequences of withholding transfusions in terms of medullary and extramedullary hyperplasia. Other circumstances that may require transfusion therapy include infections, hypersplenism, periods of rapid growth, and pregnancy. Parvovirus B19 infections can cause aplastic crises, characterized by peripheral reticulocytopenia and giant and bizarre pronormoblasts in the bone marrow and, sometimes, transient pancytopenia. Anemia is often severe enough to require blood transfusion.

In adult patients who have been transfusion independent for decades, transfusions can become necessary because of reduced marrow activity and development of severe anemia. This phenomenon has been attributed by some authors to a decreased production of erythropoietin, but further research is necessary to confirm this hypothesis. When the decision to transfuse is made, the transfusion regimen should be similar to the one generally adopted for TDT.[532] A level

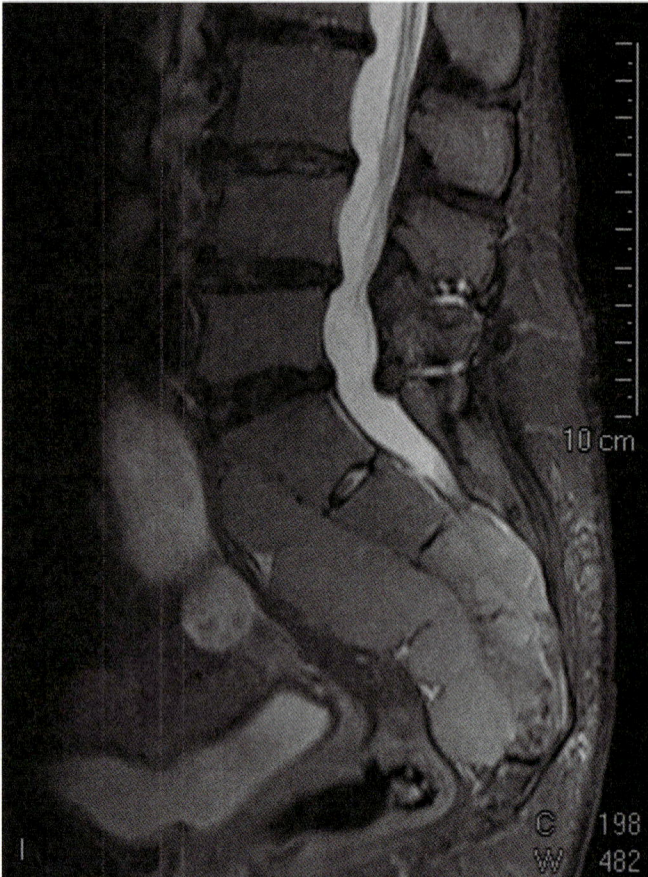

FIGURE 35.23 CT scan of the spine of a 40-year-old patient with thalassemia intermedia showing an extramedullary mass compressing the spinal marrow. CT, computed tomography.

of pretransfusional Hb around 9.5 to 10 mg/dL is usually sufficient to adequately suppress the bone marrow activity, promoting better growth and decreasing iron absorption from the gut. Several authors believe that patients with more severe forms of NTDT, mimicking TDT, should be transfused immediately following diagnosis.

In the OPTIMAL CARE study, a large cooperative effort including heterogeneous patients from the Middle East, Iran, and Italy, and in several observational studies, transfused patients with NTDT experienced fewer complications related to chronic anemia, ineffective erythropoiesis, and hemolysis (extramedullary hematopoiesis, pulmonary hypertension, and thromboembolic events), although with higher rates of iron overload–related endocrinopathy.[179,532] The introduction of transfusions earlier in life will probably increase iron accumulation overload, which can, however, be controlled by effective iron-chelating drugs.

Another reason to start transfusion early is that the risks of alloimmunization and autoimmunization seem to be lower if transfusions are initiated early in life. A Greek study reported a frequency of alloimmunization of 21% vs 47.5% in patients transfused before and after the age of 3 years.[533] The pathogenesis of alloimmunization and autoimmunization is unclear, and it has been attributed to "hidden" antigens from peripheral RBC fragmentation. Transfusion of blood phenotypically matched at least for the ABO, Rh, and Kell systems is necessary and can prevent alloimmunization in many cases.[190,534] Therapy with immune suppressants, intravenous immunoglobulins, HU, and even splenectomy can be attempted. Remission of the hemolytic process has been reported with allogeneic bone marrow transplantation.

Hypersplenism is an almost inevitable complication of NTDT, often leading to transfusion dependency that is usually reversed by splenectomy. An exception is represented by the association of duplication of α genes plus heterozygous β-thalassemia, in which splenectomy

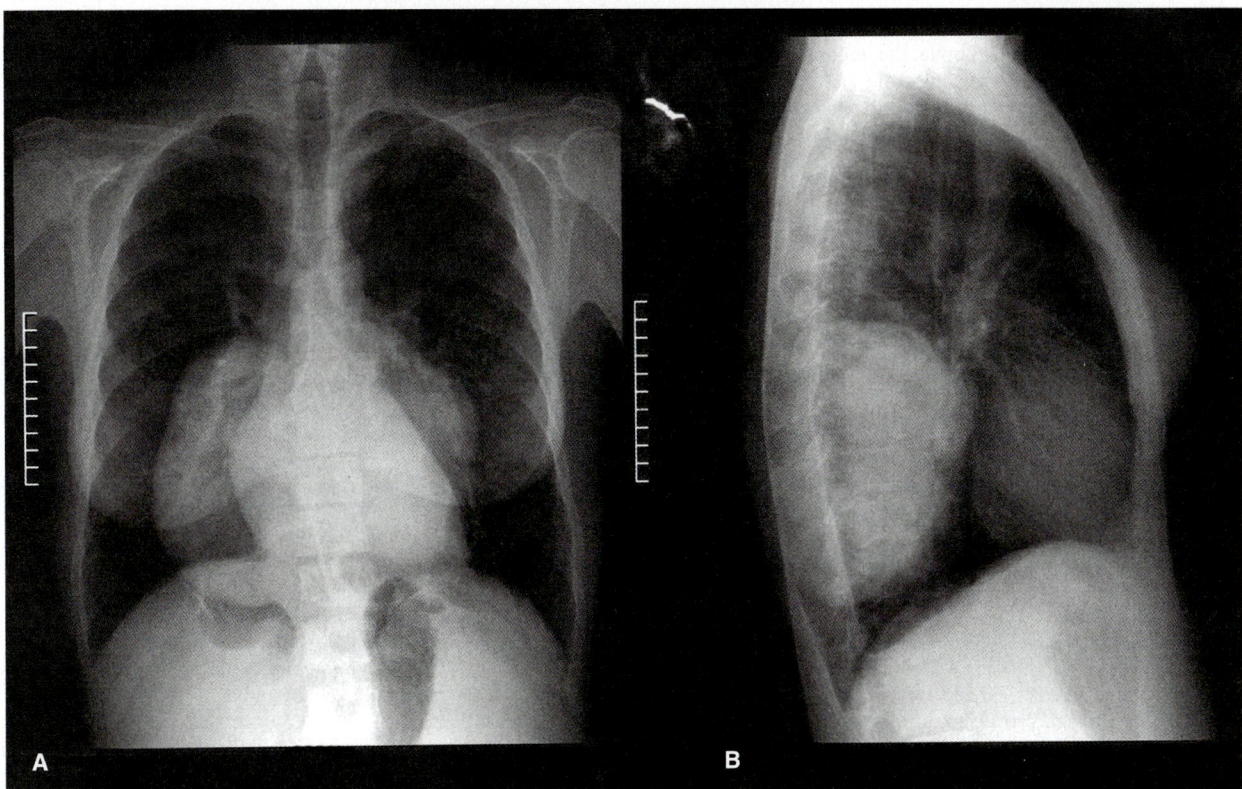

FIGURE 35.24 Extramedullary erythropoiesis manifesting as bulky space-occupying masses in the chest. The patient was a 34-year-old woman, untransfused by her choice. Molecular defect was heterozygous β^0-thalassemia plus α gene duplication. A, Anteroposterior projection. B, Lateral projection.

can aggravate the hemolytic process.[535] The risks of postsplenectomy infection, pulmonary hypertension, and thrombosis should be considered. Given these risks, a course of hypertransfusion often is utilized instead of splenectomy to reduce spleen size.

Iron Overload

Iron overload in NTDT can be caused by two mechanisms: increased intestinal absorption and, from intermittent transfusions. In nontransfused patients, iron overload develops more slowly and accumulates in different sites. There is an inappropriately low hepcidin state and a corresponding increase in ferroportin expression on the intestinal epithelium and hepatic iron accumulation. The lack of hepcidin results not only in hyperabsorption of dietary iron but also in iron depletion of macrophages, lowering their secretion of ferritin, and, consequently, serum ferritin levels. Therefore, reliance on serum ferritin alone may delay adequate treatment.[536]

Iron Chelation

Studies performed by magnetic resonance have shown that, in NTDT, iron tends to accumulate in the liver, whereas the heart is usually spared.[537] Iron assessment in NTDT should include direct LIC by MRI or, if necessary, by biopsy.[538] The decision to start iron chelation in patients with NTDT depends on several factors including degree of iron overload, rate of iron accumulation, duration of exposure to excess iron, and various other factors, including compliance. In one study, elevated LIC was associated with an increased rate of morbidity in patients with phenotypes of any severity. An increase in 1 mg Fe/g dry weight in LIC was independently and significantly associated with higher odds of thrombosis, pulmonary hypertension, hypothyroidism, osteoporosis, and hypogonadism.[539] However, cardiac iron overload is virtually absent in NTDT, and aggressive iron chelation usually is not necessary. Three chelating agents are currently available: DFO, DFP, and DFX. In a randomized, double-blind, placebo-controlled 1-year study that assessed the efficacy and safety of DFX in 166 patients with NTDT, LIC and serum ferritin decreased and the frequency of adverse

events compared favorably with placebo.[540] DFO has demonstrated significant benefits in terms of morbidity and mortality in patients with iron-overloaded TDT. Its use in NTDT was associated with a reduction in LIC and improvement in right ventricular function.[541] Data on the use of the first available oral iron chelator, DFP, in NTDT are also limited. A small clinical trial using DFP in nine intermittently transfused patients with NTDT demonstrated significant reductions in mean serum ferritin, hepatic iron, red cell membrane iron, and serum NTBI levels. Adverse events were mostly mild and included gastrointestinal symptoms and joint pain.[542]

Endocrine Complications and Pregnancy

Endocrine complications are rare in patients with NTDT, but hypogonadism, diabetes, and hypothyroidism have been reported. Although patients generally experience delayed puberty, they have normal sexual development and fertility is usually preserved. Hundreds of children have been born to women and men with NTDT, mostly after spontaneous conception. However, pregnancy may be complicated by miscarriage, preterm delivery, intrauterine growth restriction, and thromboembolic events. In some series, miscarriages seem to be more frequent than in the normal population, especially if severe anemia is present.[543] Anemia becomes more severe during pregnancy, especially during the first and second trimesters, and in order to prevent fetal growth restriction due to hypoxia, blood transfusion is often required.[544] However, transfusions in previously untransfused women may induce alloimmunization, which contributes to worsening of anemia, and alternative approaches, such as erythropoietin administration, have been suggested.[545] Sometimes splenomegaly can interfere with uterus enlargement and splenectomy may become necessary. The risk of thrombosis is high enough to warrant antithrombotic therapy before and after delivery. Folic acid deficiency, a risk factor for neural tube defects, is common in NTDT, and oral folic acid supplementation is recommended during pregnancy for all women with thalassemia. Cesarean delivery is often performed, especially when a fetopelvic disproportion is present.

Leg Ulcers

Trophic leg ulcers developing above the medial malleolus are a common and distressing finding in older patients with NTDT (*Figure 35.25*). The pathophysiology is still unclear, but it seems that the low Hb levels associated with abnormal red cell rheology and increased HbF levels that cause reduced oxygen release determine tissue hypoxia. This promotes thinning of the skin and subcutaneous fragility, which, in turn, increase the risk of lesions both spontaneous and from minimal trauma.[546] Hemolysis-induced low arginine and nitric oxide bioavailability, associated with oxidative stress and hypercoagulability, have been demonstrated in patients with NTDT. These factors contribute to endothelial dysfunction and development of vasculopathy, which have been implicated in the pathogenesis of pulmonary hypertension, stroke, priapism as well as leg ulcers.[547]

Treatment is often unsatisfactory because leg ulcers are difficult to heal and frequently recur. It may include simple measures, like pressure dressing and elevation of legs and feet for a few hours during the day or at night, or, in more complicated cases, skin grafting.[548-550] Regular blood transfusion, associated with HU, may be useful in persistent cases. In one report, a transfusion-independent patient suffering from persistent leg ulcerations responded to 1-year therapy with exchange transfusions, which reduced the percentage of HbF from 70% to 35%.[550] Other reported treatments include topical granulocyte colony stimulating factor, as well as platelet growth factor, zinc supplementation, and local hyperbaric oxygen sessions. More recently, in a phase 2 trial, treatment with luspatercept was associated with improvement in leg ulcers in all six patients with this complication.[551]

Thromboembolic Disease

Hypercoagulability and thromboembolic events have been reported in all thalassemia syndromes. However, they appear to be more common in NTDT compared with a normal age- and sex-matched population and with patients with TDT. In a report on 8860 thalassemic patients from the Mediterranean countries and Iran, thromboembolism occurred in 4% of 2190 patients with NTDT compared with 0.9% of 6670 patients with TDT. In the NTDT group, these events primarily occurred in the venous system and included deep vein thrombosis (40%), portal vein thrombosis (19%), stroke (9%), pulmonary embolism (12%), and others (20%).[178] In an Italian multicenter study, the prevalence of thromboembolic events was found to be 9.6% in patients with NTDT as compared with 4% in patients with TDT.[176] In a large cooperative study, thrombosis was the fifth most common complication, affecting 14% of the patient population. On multivariate analysis, splenectomy, age above 35 years, and a serum ferritin level ≥1000 µg/L were associated with a higher risk for thrombosis. Conversely, a positive history of transfusion and an Hb level ≥9 g/dL were found to be protective against thrombosis.[179] In addition, an MRI study described the presence of silent white matter lesions in the brains of as many as 60% of splenectomized adults. The occurrence and multiplicity of the lesions were associated with older age and transfusion naivety (83% of lesion-positive patients had never had a transfusion vs 25% of lesion-negative patients).[552]

The pathogenesis of the chronic hypercoagulable state is complex. Circulating damaged red cells and erythroid precursors and red cell remnants expose negatively charged phosphatidylserine through the "flip-flop" phenomenon and subsequently activate thrombosis. Splenectomy favors the persistence of these damaged red cells in the circulation, especially in nontransfused patients.[553] Endothelial cells are also activated and damaged by the oxidative stress because of hemolysis and iron overload, leading to increased expression of adhesion molecules and impaired nitric oxide production. Furthermore, increased platelet numbers and aggregation are common in thalassemia. Higher plasma levels of markers of coagulation and of fibrinolysis activation are present in splenectomized patients with NTDT compared with TDT and to healthy individuals.[177]

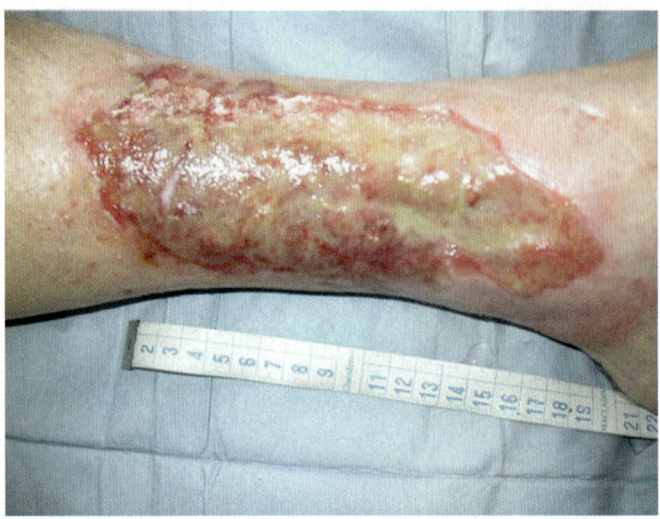

FIGURE 35.25 **Large malleolar ulcer in a patient with thalassemia intermedia.** After numerous unsuccessful attempts, the lesion was cured with compressive bandages.

In a subanalysis of a large cooperative study, platelet counts over 500×10^9/L were an independent and significant predictor of thrombosis in splenectomized patients with NTDT.[554] Therefore, platelet antiaggregants should be given early in the disease, particularly in splenectomized patients. High counts of nucleated RBCs and evidence of pulmonary hypertension were also predictive of the development of thromboembolic events in splenectomized patients with NTDT. Finally, a model for assessing the risk of thrombosis in thalassemia has been proposed to estimate the thrombotic risk as a function of intrinsic (thalassemia type and number of circulating RBCs) and extrinsic (infection, surgery, and splenectomy) factors.[555] Recommended treatment options include platelet antiaggregants, such as aspirin in patients with thrombocytosis, or anticoagulants, such as low-molecular-weight heparin, in patients undergoing surgery and in the peripartum period. Therapeutic anticoagulation with agents such as low-molecular-weight heparin or direct-acting oral anticoagulants, followed by long-term oral anticoagulants or antiplatelet agents, is indicated after thromboembolic events. Although reasonable and widely applied, these recommendations are not supported by compelling evidence from the literature.

Liver Disease

Hepatocellular carcinoma has been reported in adult patients with NTDT as a consequence of iron overload and chronic viral infection.[556] Gallstones are more common in NTDT than in TDT because of greater ineffective erythropoiesis and peripheral hemolysis, in the absence of regular transfusions. Coinheritance of the Gilbert syndrome (mutation of the A[TA]nTAA motif of the promoter of the bilirubin in uridine diphosphoglucuronosyltransferase gene) increases the indirect bilirubin level and the risk of gallstones in thalassemia syndromes.[175,557] The effect is even more evident in patients with NTDT, in whom the prevalence of gallstones seems to be related to allele dosage: 27% in patients with normal (TA)6/(TA)6 genotype, 68% in heterozygous patients for the mutated (TA)7, and 80% in homozygotes (TA)7/(TA)7.[558] Pronounced jaundice is a frequent consequence of hemolysis, especially in patients with coexistent Gilbert syndrome, and may be bothersome to patients for aesthetical reasons.

Cardiac Disease

Although heart disease as a consequence of iron overload is the most common cause of death in TDT, patients with NTDT are usually not affected by severe hemosiderosis and are, therefore, less prone to cardiac problems. MRI data have demonstrated that, in patients with NTDT, cardiac iron overload is virtually absent.[537] Nevertheless, a large multicenter study of 110 Greek patients found that 5.4% had congestive heart failure, 8% acute pericarditis, 34% chronic pericardial changes, and more than half had some kind of valvular defect.[559]

Chronically high cardiac output in nontransfused patients has an important role in left ventricular remodeling, which has been demonstrated to be more pronounced than in regularly transfused patients with TDT.[560] Regular transfusions seem to be protective toward the development of heart failure. However, pulmonary hypertension is known to be the leading cause of cardiac failure in NTDT.

Pulmonary Hypertension

Pulmonary hypertension is defined as systolic pulmonary artery pressure >25 mm Hg at rest and >30 mm Hg during exercise with a normal pulmonary artery wedge pressure <15 mm Hg and an increased pulmonary vascular resistance greater than three Wood units. It is now considered the leading cause of cardiac failure in NTDT.

In the previously mentioned Greek study, pulmonary hypertension was found in 59% of cases, and all the patients with congestive heart failure had severe pulmonary hypertension with normal systolic left ventricular function.[559] Risk factors for pulmonary hypertension have been identified as being splenectomized, having high nucleated RBC counts, not being transfused, and not being treated with HU or iron chelation. In addition, a previous history of thromboembolism is a risk factor.[561]

The mechanisms underlying pulmonary hypertension in NTDT are unclear. There is evidence that chronic hemolysis, through the induction of nitric oxide and arginine depletion, may lead to vasoconstriction, vessel wall hypertrophy, hypercoagulability, local thrombosis, and increase in thromboxane and endothelin, resulting in chronic organ damage and endothelial dysfunction.[562]

Platelet activation has been shown to be significantly higher in NTDT compared with TDT.[561] Complex interactions between platelets, coagulation factors, erythrocytes, and endothelial cells with inflammatory and vascular mediators may also contribute to the endothelial dysfunction and subsequent pulmonary vascular remodeling.

Thus, screening for pulmonary hypertension is an essential part of the diagnostic follow-up in patients with NTDT. Treatment of pulmonary hypertension includes initiation of regular red cell transfusions, if possible. Regular transfusions associated with adequate iron chelation are thought to reduce tissue hypoxia, ineffective erythropoiesis, and circulation of damaged erythrocytes, therefore preventing hemolysis and hypercoagulability that contribute to the development of pulmonary hypertension.[563] However, the preventive role of transfusion is still controversial. Pulmonary hypertension has also been described among patients with TDT, mostly after splenectomy, implying that, in some cases, regular transfusions do not prevent the disease.[564] HU reduces hemolysis and hypercoagulation by increasing HbF synthesis and reducing thrombocytosis. A retrospective study found no pulmonary hypertension in 50 patients with NTDT treated with HU for 7 years.[565]

Specific treatments for pulmonary hypertension are being studied. New agents, such prostacyclin analogues (epoprostenol, iloprost, and oral beraprost), endothelin receptor antagonists (bosentan and sitaxsentan), and phosphodiesterase-5 inhibitors (sildenafil), have been successfully used to treat pulmonary hypertension. Some of these have been used in patients with hemoglobinopathies.[566-568] Further studies including larger groups of patients are necessary to establish the long-term safety and efficacy of these new agents in patients with NTDT.

Pseudoxanthoma Elasticum

As discussed in the section on TDT, an acquired PXE-like syndrome has been reported in thalassemias, more commonly in older patients with NTDT. In a study published in 1998 and including patients affected by NTDT older than 30 years, arterial calcifications were found in 55%, skin lesions in 20%, and ocular alterations in 52%. Eighty-five percent had at least one of the three typical lesions.[569]

The pathophysiology remains unclear and is attributed to iron-induced oxidative tissue damage, caused by hemolysis and iron overload. Although no effective therapy is available, phosphate binders, a group of drugs given in the attempt to limit the intestinal absorption of phosphate and consequently normalizing the serum calcium phosphate product, could offer a means of reducing the calcium/phosphate load in patients with PXE.

Other Complications

Folic acid deficiency can be present because of increased folate utilization by the hyperactive bone marrow.[570] Daily supplementation with 1 mg of folic acid is advised for patients with NTDT.

β-THALASSEMIA IN ASSOCIATION WITH β-CHAIN STRUCTURAL VARIANTS

HbS Thalassemia Syndromes

The term sickle cell disease refers not only to homozygous HbSS but also to all genotypes in which HbS interacts with other globin gene mutations, including β^0-thalassemia, β^+-thalassemia, $\delta\beta$-thalassemia, HPFH, and Hb Lepore. The clinical course of these phenotypes is extremely variable; however, the thalassemia gene is expressed with some degree of microcytosis, hypochromia, and variation in the relative proportions of HbA2 and HbF. Sickling symptoms, if present, are often milder than those noted in patients with homozygous sickle cell anemia.

HbS–β-Thalassemia

The double heterozygous state for HbS and β-thalassemia is the most common variant of sickle cell disease in individuals of Mediterranean ancestry and the second most common sickling disorder. In the United States, it is estimated to affect about 1 in 1667 Americans at birth.[571] HbS/β^0-thalassemia occurs approximately once in every 23,000 African Americans and, in Jamaica, has a frequency of 1 in 6750.

HbS/β-thalassemia is clinically more similar to sickle cell disease than to TDT or NTDT. The severity depends on the type of β-thalassemia mutation. Patients who inherit a β^0 gene are clinically indistinguishable from those with homozygous sickle cell anemia and have absent HbA, whereas patients with β^+ genes present milder phenotypes and may even be asymptomatic because of the higher levels of HbA.[572]

Hematologically, HbS/β-thalassemia presents with higher RBC counts and HbA2 levels and lower MCV and MCH values (mean 68 fL and 20 pg, respectively) compared with HbSS.[573]

The risk of stroke in patients with HbS/β^0-thalassemia is considered high, and therefore, transcranial Doppler screening is recommended, as in homozygous HbSS.[574]

Complications of both diseases are frequently seen, including delayed growth and puberty, vaso-occlusive events, and acute chest syndrome.

Splenomegaly is more common in patients with HbS/β-thalassemia, compared with HbSS, and the spleen tends to remain enlarged and functional in adulthood.[575] As a consequence, several cases of fatal splenic sequestration have been reported in patients with HbS–β^+-thalassemia.

Avascular necrosis of the femoral head is more frequent and appears earlier in sickling disorders with higher hematocrits, like HbS/β^+-thalassemia or HbSC disease.[576]

Proliferative sickle retinopathy also seems to be more common and severe in sickle-thalassemia than in homozygous HbSS.[577]

Various phenotypes of sickle cell disease may have a milder course when associated with a concomitant α-thalassemia trait as a result of a decrease in the MCHC, which lowers HbS polymer formation.

Other genetic modifiers can influence the phenotype, as hypothesized on the basis of the discordance of symptoms in affected members of a single family. In particular, the relative amount of HbF plays an important role in disease severity.[578] Precise diagnosis is important to predict the clinical course and prognosis and to perform correct genetic counseling.

In HbS/β-thalassemia, HbS is the most abundant Hb, HbA2 is increased, and HbF may be normal or variably increased. HbA accounts for less than 30% of the total amount of Hb in patients with β^+ gene mutations, whereas it is virtually absent in HbS–β^0-thalassemia.

The electrophoretic picture of HbS/β^+-thalassemia and sickle cell trait may be similar, but usually the relative proportions of HbS and HbA allow a correct diagnosis. On the other hand, HbS–β^0-thalassemia and homozygous sickle cell anemia may be indistinguishable.

Although consistently elevated by 1 year of age, HbA2 may be difficult to measure accurately with electrophoresis because of its proximity to the HbS band, and with HPLC because of coelution of minor components with HbA2 (secondary to posttranslational modifications of HbS).[484]

HbS–$\delta\beta$-Thalassemia

$\delta\beta$-Thalassemia is a condition characterized by high levels of HbF. The coinheritance with sickle cell disease has been described in African Americans, Indians, and individuals of Mediterranean origin.[579]

Patients are usually asymptomatic and may show signs only of mild anemia or hematologic alterations, including microcytosis, the presence of target cells, and, rarely, sickle cells. The electrophoretic pattern is characterized by the prevalence of HbS and elevated HbF (15%-40%), associated with the absence of HbA and decreased HbA2. Some patients, however, may present with a severe clinical course because of heterogeneous distribution of HbF among peripheral RBCs.

HbS-Hereditary Persistence of Fetal Hb

Compound heterozygosity for HbS and HPFH is characterized by a relatively benign clinical picture. A recent study demonstrated that, in patients with HbS-HPFH, HbF levels are 50% to 90% during infancy and tend to decline steeply within the first few years of life, stabilizing at approximately 30% between the ages of 3 and 5 years. Furthermore, hematologic parameters are nearly normal, with average Hb concentration being 13 ± 1 g/dL and average MCV 75 ± 4 fL.[578]

In adults, the electrophoretic pattern is similar to that of homozygous sickle cell anemia: HbS 70% to 80% of the total Hb, HbF 20% to 30%, decreased HbA2, and absent HbA. In patients with HbS-HPFH, all RBCs contain uniformly distributed HbF in sufficient concentration to dilute HbS and inhibit its polymerization despite the high percentage of HbS.

A correct diagnosis is necessary in order to allow appropriate counseling and alleviate anxiety associated with the diagnosis of sickle cell disease. Therefore, in patients with sickle cell with elevated HbF levels after the age of 1 year, molecular testing should be performed.

HbS-Hb Lepore

The double heterozygosity for sickle Hb with Lepore Hb is a relatively rare condition. The Hb Lepore gene alone or in combination with the HbS gene manifests as microcytosis; therefore, the HbS/Hb Lepore is similar to microdrepanocytosis. This syndrome is usually characterized by a disorder of moderate severity, with chronic hemolytic anemia, splenomegaly, and rare and recurrent painful crises.[580,581]

The electrophoretic mobility of Hb Lepore at an alkaline pH is identical to that of HbS; therefore, the condition can be confused with sickle cell anemia. At an acid pH, however, Hb Lepore migrates with HbA. HbS accounts for 60% to 80% of the Hb, Hb Lepore for approximately 10%, and HbF for 9% to 25%. HbA2 is decreased, and HbA is absent.

HbC Thalassemia

The association of HbC with β-thalassemia, especially with β^+-thalassemia in Africans (more common than β^0-thalassemia in this ethnic group), results in a clinical picture similar to homozygous HbCC, with mild hemolytic anemia, splenomegaly, and a benign clinical course.[582] The MCV is lower in HbC/β-thalassemia than with homozygous HbCC.

In Italian, North African, and Turkish individuals, HbC may be coinherited with β^0-thalassemia, resulting in a more severe clinical course, similar to NTDT.[583] The diagnosis is based on the presence of target cells, specific intraerythrocytic HbC crystals in blood smear, and HbC level at 100%. HbC-Hb Lepore has been described in an African American and an Algerian family.[584]

HbE Syndromes

HbE is the most common abnormal Hb of Southeast Asia and has been reported from other Asian regions, such as Pakistan and India.[585] It is estimated that 30 million people are heterozygous for HbE and that 1 million are homozygous.

As a consequence of migratory fluxes, the epidemiology of thalassemia has changed in most industrialized countries. In North America, HbE–β-thalassemia affects 13% of patients with a hemoglobinopathy and is more common in the Western states.[114]

HbE is a thalassemic hemoglobinopathy because the nucleotide substitution G→A at codon 26 of the β gene changes the encoded amino acid (Lys→Glu) and creates a new alternative splice site in exon 1. This results in the synthesis of structurally abnormal variant hemoglobin HbE by the normally spliced β-mRNA and in a β^+-thalassemia phenotype because of the use of the new splice site. Its molecular and clinical features have been reviewed.[494] When HbE is present, alone or in different combinations with α- and β-thalassemia or with other abnormal Hbs, a range of phenotypes of different HbE syndromes are observed, which can be divided into asymptomatic and symptomatic forms.

Asymptomatic Forms

HbE heterozygotes are clinically normal with only minimal hematologic changes. RBCs are normocytic or slightly microcytic with minor morphologic changes, such as target cell morphology. HbE constitutes 25% to 30% of the total Hb, and this amount is reduced by the coexistence of α-thalassemia.[585]

Patients homozygous for HbE are usually asymptomatic and have normal Hb levels, although in some cases, mild anemia may be present. They show microcytosis and 20% to 80% of target red cells at peripheral blood smear examination. Hb analysis reveals 85% to 95% of HbE with the remainder being HbF. The α/non-α–globin chain synthesis ratio is around 2.0.

Symptomatic Forms

The clinical spectrum of the disease is very heterogeneous, ranging from a mild phenotype to a severe transfusion-dependent anemia.[586] This heterogeneity depends only in part on the different interacting β-thalassemia alleles. HbE–β^0-thalassemia is characterized by HbE and HbF, only while in Hb–β^+-thalassemia, some HbA is detected in addition to HbE and HbF. HbE in association with β-thalassemia is considered to represent one-half of all the severe thalassemia syndromes worldwide.

A large study has been going on since 1997 in Sri Lanka, attempting to define the genetic and environmental factors that modify the severity of HbE thalassemia.[587] Considerable phenotypic heterogeneity occurred within a relatively narrow range of Hb values. Major genetic factors included the type of β-thalassemia mutation, the coinheritance of α-thalassemia, and polymorphisms associated with increased synthesis of fetal Hb. The presence of the Xmn-1 polymorphism in the promoter region of the Gγ gene explains the variation of HbF production. Among the environmental factors, coinfection with the malaria parasite, previous splenectomy, a variable increase in response to erythropoietin, and attenuation of this response with time appear to be important. The remarkable variation and instability of clinical phenotypes requires periodic reassessment of the need for transfusion therapy.

As a consequence of the interaction of HbE with HbH disease and Hb Constant Spring, three symptomatic syndromes have been identified[588,589]:

a. HbAE Barts disease, resulting from the interaction of HbH disease with heterozygous HbE;

b. HbEF Barts disease, which is caused by the interaction of HbH disease with homozygous HbE or HbE-β-thalassemia;

c. Homozygous HbE with homozygous Hb Constant Spring syndrome.

The anemia in these forms is moderate to severe, and the various genotypes can be suspected on the basis of the Hb pattern and/or family studies, but DNA analysis is required for the definition of the exact genotype. Phenotypes similar to TDT can be predicted from the early onset of clinical symptoms and the requirement of regular blood transfusion from infancy.

Clinical Picture

There is significant heterogeneity in the clinical presentation of HbE β-thalassemia, ranging from mild NTDT to transfusion dependence. Patients with HbE β-thalassemia appear to be able to compensate for anemia by a right shift in their oxygen dissociation curves compared with other forms of β-thalassemia and may tolerate hemoglobin levels in the 6- to 7-g/dL range without the need for regular transfusions.[590]

Erythropoiesis is markedly increased, and extramedullary masses are common.[591] As is the case in other forms of sporadically transfused thalassemias, alloimmune and autoimmune hemolytic anemia develops frequently.

Infections, mostly caused by gram-negative bacteria, are a major complication and cause of death in patients with HbE β-thalassemia, especially after splenectomy.[592,593] Prospective studies indicate increased susceptibility to bacterial, fungal, and viral infections. Gallstones are present in 50% of the patients and are strongly associated with the 7/7 genotype of the *UGTA1A* promoter.[594] An increased risk of thrombosis reported in these patients, especially after splenectomy, can be explained by chronic low-grade coagulation and platelet activation, chronic low-grade inflammation, endothelial cell injury, impaired fibrinolysis, and decreased naturally occurring anticoagulants. Hypoxemia is observed in the majority of splenectomized patients.[595] The underlying mechanism is unknown, but it has been attributed to increased aggregation of platelets in the pulmonary vessels, based on the autopsy finding of pulmonary arterial occlusion in a large number of such patients.[596] Accordingly, the administration of aspirin can ameliorate the degree of hypoxemia in the majority of cases.[597] HSCT has proven effective. Some, but not all, patients with β-thalassemia/HbE respond to HU treatment.[598] In an Indian trial, patients who responded showed an increase in Hb, mean corpuscular volume, MCH content, fetal Hb, and F cells. In a study, membrane deformability and cell hydration, whose improvement is important for extending the life span of erythrocytes, did not change significantly, except in splenectomized patients.[599]

Pregnancy in women affected by β-thalassemia/HbE disease is possible, but the cases reported were significantly associated with an increased risk of fetal growth restriction, preterm birth, and low birth weight.[600]

Survival of patients with β-thalassemia/HbE in Thailand has been reported to be 30 years, significantly longer than the 10 years reported for homozygous β-thalassemia.[601]

Websites

http://www.bx.psu.edu
http://phencode.bx.psu.edu

ACKNOWLEDGMENTS

The authors wish to thank Michael Jeng and Ellis Neufeld for their very thorough chapter on Thalassemia Syndromes in the previous edition, which provided an excellent template for our update of this chapter.

References

1. Weatherall DJ. The evolving spectrum of the epidemiology of thalassemia. *Hematol Oncol Clin North Am*. 2018;32(2):165-175.
2. Modell B, Darlison M. Global epidemiology of haemoglobin disorders and derived service indicators. *Bull World Health Organ*. 2008;2008(6):480-487.
3. Williams TN, Weatherall DJ. World distribution, population genetics, and health burden of the hemoglobinopathies. *Cold Spring Harb Perspect Med*. 2012;2(9):a011692.
4. Pirastu M, Lee KY, Dozy AM, et al. Alpha-thalassemia in two Mediterranean populations. *Blood*. 1982;60(2):509-512.
5. Dozy AM, Kan YW, Embury SH, et al. α-Globin gene organisation in blacks precludes the severe form of α-thalassaemia. *Nature*. 1979;280(5723):605-607.
6. Cao A, Congiu R, Sollaino MC, et al. Thalassaemia and glucose-6-phosphate dehydrogenase screening in 13- to 14-year-old students of the Sardinian population: preliminary findings. *Community Genet*. 2008;11(3):121-128.
7. Loukopoulos D. Current status of thalassemia and the sickle cell syndromes in Greece. *Semin Hematol*. 1996;33(1):76-86.
8. Galanello R, Eleftheriou A, Traeger-Synodinos J. *Prevention of Thalassemia and Other Haemoglobin Disorders*. Vol 1. Thalassemia International Federation; 2001.
9. Sayani FA, Kwiatkowski JL. Increasing prevalence of thalassemia in America: implications for primary care. *Ann Med*. 2015;47(7):592-604.
10. Haldane JBS. The rate of mutation of human genes. *Hereditas*. 1949;35(S1):267-273.
11. Neel JV, Valentine WN. Further studies on the genetics of thalassemia. *Genetics*. 1947;32(1):38-63.
12. Daou M, Kituma E, Kavishe R, et al. α-Thalassaemia trait is associated with Antibody prevalence against malaria antigens AMA-1 and MSP-1. *J Trop Pediatr*. 2015;61(2):139-142.
13. Taylor SM, Parobek CM, Fairhurst RM. Haemoglobinopathies and the clinical epidemiology of malaria: a systematic review and meta-analysis. *Lancet Infect Dis*. 2012;12(6):457-468.
14. Stamatoyannopoulos G, Grosveld F. Hemoglobin Switching. In: Stamatoyannopoulos G, Majerus P, Perlmutter R, eds. *The Molecular Basis of Blood Disease*. 3rd ed. W.B.Saunders Publishing Co; 2001:135-182.
15. Forget BG, Hardison RC, Steinberg MH, et al. The normal structure and regulation of human globin gene clusters. In: Steinberg MH, Forget BG, Higgs DR, Weatherall DJ, eds. *Disorders of Hemoglobins: Genetics, Pathophysiology and Clinical Management*. Cambridge University Press; 2009:46-61.
16. Bauer DE, Kamran SC, Lessard S, et al. An erythroid enhancer of BCL11A subject to genetic variation determines fetal hemoglobin level. *Science*. 2013;342(6155):253-257.
17. Sankaran VG, Xu J, Byron R, et al. A functional element necessary for fetal hemoglobin silencing. *N Engl J Med*. 2011;365(9):807-814.
18. Xu J, Bauer DE, Kerenyi MA, et al. Corepressor-dependent silencing of fetal hemoglobin expression by BCL11A. *Proc Natl Acad Sci U S A*. 2013;110(16):6518-6523.
19. Liu N, Hargreaves VV, Zhu Q, et al. Direct promoter repression by BCL11A controls the fetal to adult hemoglobin switch. *Cell*. 2018;173(2):430-442.e17.
20. Sankaran VG, Xu J, Ragoczy T, et al. Developmental and species-divergent globin switching are driven by BCL11A. *Nature*. 2009;460(7259):1093-1097.
21. Lettre G, Sankaran VG, Bezerra MAC, et al. DNA polymorphisms at the BCL11A, HBS1L-MYB, and β-globin loci associate with fetal hemoglobin levels and pain crises in sickle cell disease. *Proc Natl Acad Sci U S A*. 2008;105(33):11869-11874.
22. Uda M, Galanello R, Sanna S, et al. Genome-wide association study shows BCL11A associated with persistent fetal hemoglobin and amelioration of the phenotype of β-thalassemia. *Proc Natl Acad Sci U S A*. 2008;105(5):1620-1625.
23. Sankaran VG, Menne TF, Xu J, et al. Human fetal hemoglobin expression is regulated by the developmental stage-specific repressor BCL11A. *Science*. 2008;322(5909):1839-1842.
24. Masuda T, Wang X, Maeda M, et al. Transcription factors LRF and BCL11A independently repress expression of fetal hemoglobin. *Science*. 2016;351(6270):285-289.
25. Norton LJ, Funnell APW, Burdach J, et al. KLF1 directly activates expression of the novel fetal globin repressor ZBTB7A/LRF in erythroid cells. *Blood Adv*. 2017;1(11):685-692.
26. Zhou D, Liu K, Sun CW, Pawlik KM, Townes TM. KLF1 regulates BCL11A expression and γ- to β-globin gene switching. *Nat Genet*. 2010;42(9):742-744.
27. Giardine BM, Joly P, Pissard S, et al. Clinically relevant updates of the HbVar database of human hemoglobin variants and thalassemia mutations. *Nucleic Acids Res*. 2020;49(D1):D1192-D1196.
28. Hardison RC, Chui DHK, Giardine B, et al. HbVar: a relational database of human hemoglobin variants and thalassemia mutations at the globin gene server. *Hum Mutat*. 2002;19(3):225-233.
29. Higgs DR, Gibbons RJ. The molecular basis of α-thalassemia: a model for understanding human molecular genetics. *Hematol Oncol Clin North Am*. 2010;24(6):1033-1054.
30. Sollaino MC, Paglietti ME, Loi D, et al. Homozygous deletion of the major alpha-globin regulatory element (MCS-R2) responsible for a severe case of hemoglobin H disease. *Blood*. 2010;116(12):2193-2194.
31. Liebhaber SA, Goossens M, Kan YW. Homology and concerted evolution at the α1 and α2 loci of human α-globin. *Nature*. 1981;290(5801):26-29.
32. Orkin SH, Goff SC. The duplicated human α-globin genes: their relative expression as measured by RNA analysis. *Cell*. 1981;24(2):345-351.
33. Liebhaber SA, Cash FE, Ballas SK. Human alpha-globin gene expression. The dominant role of the alpha 2-locus in mRNA and protein synthesis. *J Biol Chem*. 1986;261(32):15327-15333.

34. Proudfoot NJ. Transcriptional interference and termination between duplicated α-globin gene constructs suggests a novel mechanism for gene regulation. *Nature.* 1986;322(6079):562-565.

35. Gu YC, Landman H, Huisman TH. Two different quadruplicated α globin gene arrangements. *Br J Haematol.* 1987;66(2):245-250.

36. Winichagoon P, Higgs DR, Goodbourn SE, et al. Multiple arrangements of the human embryonic zeta globin genes. *Nucleic Acids Res.* 1982;10(19):5853-5868.

37. Bowden DK, Hill AV, Higgs DR, et al. Different hematologic phenotypes are associated with the leftward (-alpha 4.2) and rightward (-alpha 3.7) alpha+− thalassemia deletions. *J Clin Invest.* 1987;79(1):39-43.

38. Farashi S, Harteveld CL. Molecular basis of α-thalassemia. *Blood Cells Mol Dis.* 2018;70:43-53.

39. Ferrão J, Silva M, Gonçalves L, et al. Widening the spectrum of deletions and molecular mechanisms underlying alpha-thalassemia. *Ann Hematol.* 2017;96(11):1921-1929.

40. Mettananda S, Higgs DR. Molecular basis and genetic modifiers of thalassemia. *Hematol Oncol Clin North Am.* 2018;32(2):177-191.

41. Tufarelli C, Stanley JAS, Garrick D, et al. Transcription of antisense RNA leading to gene silencing and methylation as a novel cause of human genetic disease. *Nat Genet.* 2003;34(2):157-165.

42. Hunt DM, Higgs DR, Winichagoon P, Clegg JB, Weatherall DJ. Haemoglobin Constant Spring has an unstable α chain messenger RNA. *Br J Haematol.* 1982;51(3):405-413.

43. Kwaifa IK, Lai MI, Noor SM. Non-deletional alpha thalassaemia: a review. *Orphanet J Rare Dis.* 2020;15(1):166.

44. Wajcman H, Traeger-Synodinos J, Papassotiriou I, et al. Unstable and thalassemic α chain hemoglobin variants: a cause of Hb H disease and thalassemia intermedia. *Hemoglobin.* 2008;32(4):327-349.

45. Gobbi MD, Viprakasit V, Hughes JR, et al. A regulatory SNP causes a human genetic disease by creating a new transcriptional promoter. *Science.* 2006;312(5777):1215-1217.

46. Fritsch EF, Lawn RM, Maniatis T. Molecular cloning and characterization of the human β-like globin gene cluster. *Cell.* 1980;19(4):959-972.

47. Antonarakis SE, Boehm CD, Giardina PJV, Kazazian HH. Nonrandom association of polymorphic restriction sites in the β-globin gene cluster. *Proc Natl Acad Sci U S A.* 1982;79(1):137-141.

48. Talbot D, Collis P, Antoniou M, et al. A dominant control region from the human β-globin locus conferring integration site-independent gene expression. *Nature.* 1989;338(6213):352-355.

49. van Assendelft GB, Hanscombe O, Grosveld F, Greaves DR. The β-globin dominant control region activates homologous and heterologous promoters in a tissue-specific manner. *Cell.* 1989;56(6):969-977.

50. Kioussis D, Vanin E, deLange T, Flavell RA, Grosveld FG. β-Globin gene inactivation by DNA translocation in γβ-thalassaemia. *Nature.* 1983;306(5944):662-666.

51. Rooks H, Clark B, Best S, et al. A novel 506kb deletion causing εγδβ thalassemia. *Blood Cells Mol Dis.* 2012;49(3-4):121-127.

52. Gonzalez-Redondo J, Stoming T, Kutlar A, et al. A C → T substitution at nt − 101 in a conserved DNA sequence of the promotor region of the beta-globin gene is associated with "silent" beta-thalassemia. *Blood.* 1989;73(6):1705-1711.

53. Garewal G, Das R, Awasthi A, Ahluwalia J, Marwaha RK. The clinical significance of the spectrum of interactions of CAP+1 (A→C), a silent β-globin gene mutation, with other β-thalassemia mutations and globin gene modifiers in north Indians. *Eur J Haematol.* 2007;79(5):417-421.

54. Wong C, Dowling CE, Saiki RK, et al. Characterization of β-thalassaemia mutations using direct genomic sequencing of amplified single copy DNA. *Nature.* 1987;330(6146):384-386.

55. Treisman R, Orkin SH, Maniatis T. Specific transcription and RNA splicing defects in five cloned β-thalassaemia genes. *Nature.* 1983;302(5909):591-596.

56. Tamagnini GP, Lopes MC, Castanheira ME, Wainscoat JS, Wood WG. Beta + Thalassaemia—Portuguese type: clinical, haematological and molecular studies of a newly defined form of β thalassaemia. *Br J Haematol.* 1983;54(2):189-200.

57. Orkin SH, Cheng TC, Antonarakis SE, Kazazian HH. Thalassemia due to a mutation in the cleavage-polyadenylation signal of the human beta-globin gene. *EMBO J.* 1985;4(2):453-456.

58. Maragoudaki E, Vrettou C, Kanavakis E, Traeger-Synodinos J, Metaxotou-Mavrommati A, Kattamis C. Molecular, haematological and clinical studies of a silent β-gene C → G mutation at 6 bp 3′ to the termination codon (+1480 C → G) in twelve Greek families. *Br J Haematol.* 1998;103(1):45-51.

59. Thein SL. The molecular basis of β-thalassemia. *Cold Spring Harb Perspect Med.* 2013;3(5):a011700.

60. Baserga SJ, Benz EJ. Nonsense mutations in the human beta-globin gene affect mRNA metabolism. *Proc Natl Acad Sci U S A.* 1988;85(7):2056-2060.

61. Trecartin RF, Liebhaber SA, Chang JC, et al. Beta zero thalassemia in Sardinia is caused by a nonsense mutation. *J Clin Invest.* 1981;68(4):1012-1017.

62. Chang JC, Kan YW. Beta 0 thalassemia, a nonsense mutation in man. *Proc Natl Acad Sci U S A.* 1979;76(6):2886-2889.

63. Thein SL. Dominant β thalassaemia: molecular basis and pathophysiology. *Br J Haematol.* 1992;80(3):273-277.

64. Orkin SH, Old JM, Weatherall DJ, Nathan DG. Partial deletion of beta-globin gene DNA in certain patients with beta 0-thalassemia. *Proc Natl Acad Sci U S A.* 1979;76(5):2400-2404.

65. Game L, Bergounioux J, Close JP, Marzouka BE, Thein SL. A novel deletion causing (εγδβ)° thalassaemia in a Chilean family. *Br J Haematol.* 2003;123(1):154-159.

66. Baglioni C. The fusion of two peptide chains in hemoglobin lepore and its interpretation as a genetic deletion. *Proc Natl Acad Sci U S A.* 1962;48(11):1880-1886.

67. Efremov GD. Dominantly inherited β-thalassemia. *Hemoglobin.* 2009;31(2):193-207.

68. Adams JG, Steinberg MH, Newman MV, et al. beta-Thalassemia present in cis to a new beta-chain structural variant, Hb Vicksburg [beta 75 (E19)Leu leads to 0]. *Proc Natl Acad Sci U S A.* 1981;78(1):469-473.

69. Oggiano L, Guiso L, Frogheri L, et al. A novel mediterranean "δβ-thalassemia" determinant containing the δ+27 and β°39 point mutations in cis. *Am J Hematol.* 1994;45(1):81-84.

70. Loudianos G, Cao A, Pirastu M, et al. Molecular basis of the delta thalassemia in cis to hemoglobin Knossos variant. *Blood.* 1991;77(9):2087-2088.

71. Traeger-Synodinos J, Tzetis M, Kanavakis E, Metaxotou-Mavromati A, Kattamis C. The Corfu δβ thalassaemia mutation in Greece: haematological phenotype and prevalence. *Br J Haematol.* 1991;79(2):302-305.

72. Thein SL, Wood WG, Steinberg MH, et al. The molecular basis of β thalassemia, δβ thalassemia, and hereditary persistence of fetal hemoglobin. In: Steinberg M, Forget B, Higgs D, Weatherall D, eds. *Disorders of Hemoglobin: Genetics, Pathophysiology and Clinical Management.* Cambridge University Press; 2009;323-356.

73. Kulozik A, Bellan-Koch A, Kohne E, Kleihauer E. A deletion/inversion rearrangement of the beta-globin gene cluster in a Turkish family with delta beta zero-thalassemia intermedia. *Blood.* 1992;79(9):2455-2459.

74. Martyn GE, Wienert B, Kurita R, et al. A natural regulatory mutation in the proximal promoter elevates fetal globin expression by creating a de novo GATA1 site. *Blood.* 2019;133(8):852-856.

75. Collins FS, Metherall JE, Yamakawa M, et al. A point mutation in the Aγ-globin gene promoter in Greek hereditary persistence of fetal haemoglobin. *Nature.* 1985;313(6000):325-326.

76. Wienert B, Martyn GE, Kurita R, et al. KLF1 drives the expression of fetal hemoglobin in British HPFH. *Blood.* 2017;130(6):803-807.

77. Martyn GE, Wienert B, Yang L, et al. Natural regulatory mutations elevate the fetal globin gene via disruption of BCL11A or ZBTB7A binding. *Nat Genet.* 2018;50(4):498-503.

78. Thein SL, Menzel S, Peng X, et al. Intergenic variants of HBS1L-MYB are responsible for a major quantitative trait locus on chromosome 6q23 influencing fetal hemoglobin levels in adults. *Proc Natl Acad Sci U S A.* 2007;104(27):11346-11351.

79. Menzel S, Garner C, Gut I, et al. A QTL influencing F cell production maps to a gene encoding a zinc-finger protein on chromosome 2p15. *Nat Genet.* 2007;39(10):1197-1199.

80. Lanikova L, Kucerova J, Indrak K, et al. β-Thalassemia due to intronic LINE-1 insertion in the β-globin gene (HBB): molecular mechanisms underlying reduced transcript levels of the β-GlobinL1 allele. *Hum Mutat.* 2013;34(10):1361-1365.

81. Viprakasit V, Gibbons RJ, Broughton BC, et al. Mutations in the general transcription factor TFIIH result in β-thalassaemia in individuals with trichothiodystrophy. *Hum Mol Genet.* 2001;10(24):2797-2802.

82. Yu C, Niakan KK, Matsushita M, et al. X-linked thrombocytopenia with thalassemia from a mutation in the amino finger of GATA-1 affecting DNA binding rather than FOG-1 interaction. *Blood.* 2002;100(6):2040-2045.

83. Galanello R, Perseu L, Perra C, et al. Somatic deletion of the normal β-globin gene leading to thalassaemia intermedia in heterozygous β-thalassaemic patients. *Br J Haematol.* 2004;127(5):604-606.

84. Finch CA, Deubelbeiss K, Cook JD, et al. Ferrokinetics in man. *Medicine.* 1970;49(1):17-54.

85. Fessas P, Loukopoulos D, Kaltsoya A. Peptide analysis of the inclusions of erythroid cells in β-thalassemia. *Biochim Biophys Acta.* 1966;124(2):430-432.

86. Polliack A, Yataganas X, Rachmilewitz EA. Ultrastructure of the inclusion bodies and nuclear abnormalities in β-thalassemic erythroblasts. *Ann N Y Acad Sci.* 1974;232(1):261-282.

87. Shinar E, Rachmilewitz EA, Lux SE. Differing erythrocyte membrane skeletal protein defects in alpha and beta thalassemia. *J Clin Invest.* 1989;83(2):404-410.

88. Mannu F, Arese P, Cappellini MD, et al. Role of hemichrome binding to erythrocyte membrane in the generation of band-3 alterations in beta-thalassemia intermedia erythrocytes. *Blood.* 1995;86(5):2014-2020.

89. Grinberg LN, Rachmilewitz EA, Kitrossky N, Chevion M. Hydroxyl radical generation in β-thalassemic red blood cells. *Free Radic Biol Med.* 1995;18(3):611-615.

90. Repka T, Shalev O, Reddy R, et al. Nonrandom association of free iron with membranes of sickle and beta- thalassemic erythrocytes. *Blood.* 1993;82(10):3204-3210.

91. Kong Y, Zhou S, Kihm AJ, et al. Loss of α-hemoglobin–stabilizing protein impairs erythropoiesis and exacerbates β-thalassemia. *J Clin Invest.* 2004;114(10):1457-1466.

92. Kihm AJ, Kong Y, Hong W, et al. An abundant erythroid protein that stabilizes free alpha-haemoglobin. *Nature.* 2002;417(6890):758-763.

93. Khandros E, Thom CS, D'Souza J, Weiss MJ. Integrated protein quality-control pathways regulate free α-globin in murine β-thalassemia. *Blood.* 2012;119(22):5265-5275.

94. Khandros E, Weiss MJ. Protein quality control during erythropoiesis and hemoglobin synthesis. *Hematol Oncol Clin North Am.* 2010;24(6):1071-1088.

95. Lechauve C, Keith J, Khandros E, et al. The autophagy-activating kinase ULK1 mediates clearance of free α-globin in β-thalassemia. *Sci Transl Med.* 2019;11(506):eaav4881.

96. Maria RD, Testa U, Luchetti L, et al. Apoptotic role of fas/fas ligand system in the regulation of erythropoiesis. *Blood.* 1999;93(3):796-803.

97. Rivella S. The role of ineffective erythropoiesis in non-transfusion-dependent thalassemia. *Blood Rev.* 2012;26:S12-S15.

98. Rivella S. Iron metabolism under conditions of ineffective erythropoiesis in β-thalassemia. *Blood.* 2019;133(1):51-58.

99. Origa R, Galanello R, Ganz T, et al. Liver iron concentrations and urinary hepcidin in β-thalassemia. *Haematologica.* 2007;92(5):583-588.

100. Kautz L, Jung G, Valore EV, et al. Identification of erythroferrone as an erythroid regulator of iron metabolism. *Nat Genet.* 2014;46(7):678-684.

101. Arezes J, Foy N, McHugh K, et al. Antibodies against the erythroferrone N-terminal domain prevent hepcidin suppression and ameliorate murine thalassemia. *Blood.* 2020;135(8):547-557.

102. Cappellini MD, Motta I, Musallam KM, Taher AT. Redefining thalassemia as a hypercoagulable state. *Ann N Y Acad Sci.* 2010;1202(1):231-236.

103. Eldor A, Rachmilewitz EA. The hypercoagulable state in thalassemia. *Blood.* 2002;99(1):36-43.

104. Kuypers FA, Yuan J, Lewis RA, et al. Membrane phospholipid asymmetry in human thalassemia. *Blood.* 1998;91(8):3044-3051.

105. Butthep P, Bunyaratvej A, Funahara Y, et al. Alterations in vascular endothelial cell-related plasma proteins in thalassaemic patients and their correlation with clinical symptoms. *Thromb Haemost.* 1995;74(04):1045-1049.

106. Ruf A, Pick M, Deutsch V, et al. In-vivo platelet activation correlates with red cell anionic phospholipid exposure in patients with β-thalassaemia major. *Br J Haematol.* 1997;98(1):51-56.

107. Eldor A, Durst R, Hy-Am E, et al. A chronic hypercoagulable state in patients with β-thalassaemia major is already present in childhood. *Br J Haematol.* 1999;107(4):739-746.

108. Kheansaard W, Phongpao K, Paiboonsukwong K, et al. Microparticles from β-thalassaemia/HbE patients induce endothelial cell dysfunction. *Sci Rep.* 2018;8(1):13033.

109. Shalev O, Shinar E, Lux SE. Isolated beta-globin chains reproduce, in normal red cell membranes, the defective binding of spectrin to alpha-thalassaemic membranes. *Br J Haematol.* 1996;94(2):273-278.

110. Higgs DR, Steinberg MH, Forget BG, Higgs DR, Weatherall DJ. The pathophysiology and clinical features of α thalassaemia. In: Steinberg M, Forget B, Higgs D, eds. *Disorders of Hemoglobin: Genetic, Pathophysiology and Clinical Management.* Cambridge University Press; 2009:266-295.

111. Shinar E, Rachmilewitz EA. 2 Haemoglobinopathies and red cell membrane function. *Baillieres Clin Haematol.* 1993;6(2):357-369.

112. Benesch RE, Ranney HM, Benesch R, Smith GM. The chemistry of the Bohr effect II. Some properties of human hemoglobin H. *J Biol Chem.* 1961;236(11):2926-2929.

113. Yu X, Mollan TL, Butler A, et al. Analysis of human α globin gene mutations that impair binding to the α hemoglobin stabilizing protein. *Blood.* 2009;113(23):5961-5969.

114. Vichinsky EP, MacKlin EA, Waye JS, Lorey F, Olivieri NF. Changes in the epidemiology of thalassemia in north America: a new minority disease. *Pediatrics.* 2005;116(6):e818-e825.

115. Fucharoen S, Viprakasit V. Hb H disease: clinical course and disease modifiers. *Hematology Am Soc Hematol Educ Program.* 2009;2009:26-34.

116. Italia KY, Jijina FF, Jain D, et al. The effect of UGT1A1 promoter polymorphism on bilirubin response to hydroxyurea therapy in hemoglobinopathies. *Clin Biochem.* 2010;43(16-17):1329-1332.

117. Dimou NL, Pantavou KG, Bagos PG. Apolipoprotein E polymorphism and left ventricular failure in beta-thalassemia: a multivariate meta-analysis. *Ann Hum Genet.* 2017;81(5):213-223.

118. Lal A, Goldrich ML, Haines DA, et al. Heterogeneity of hemoglobin H disease in childhood. *N Engl J Med.* 2011;364(8):710-718.

119. Higgs DR, Lamb J, Aldridge BE, et al. Inadequacy of Hb Bart's as an indicator of α thalassaemia. *Br J Haematol.* 1982;51(1):177-178.

120. Vichinsky E, Cohen A, Thompson AA, et al. Epidemiologic and clinical characteristics of nontransfusion-dependent thalassemia in the United States. *Pediatr Blood Cancer.* 2018;65(7):e27067-e27068.

121. Huang LY, Yan JM, Zhou JY, et al. A severe case of hemoglobin H disease due to compound heterozygosity for deletion of the major α-globin regulatory element (MCS-R2) and α0-thalassemia. *Acta Haematol.* 2017;138(1):61-64.

122. Coelho A, Picanço I, Seuanes F, Seixas MT, Faustino P. Novel large deletions in the human α-globin gene cluster: clarifying the HS-40 long-range regulatory role in the native chromosome environment. *Blood Cells Mol Dis.* 2010;45(2):147-153.

123. Higgs DR, Buckle VJ, Gibbons R, et al. Unusual types of α thalassaemia. In: Steinberg MH, Forget BG, Higgs DR, Weatherall DJ, eds. *Disorders of Hemoglobin: Genetics, Pathophysiology, and Clinical Management.* Cambridge University Press; 2009:296-320.

124. Traeger-Synodinos J, Papassotiriou I, Karagiorga M, et al. Unusual phenotypic observations associated with a rare HbH disease genotype (–Med/αTSaudiα): implications for clinical management. *Br J Haematol.* 2002;119(1):265-267.

125. Tso SC, Chan TK, Todd D. Venous thrombosis in haemoglobin H disease after splenectomy. *Aust N Z J Med.* 1982;12(6):635-638.

126. Lorey F, Charoenkwan P, Witkowska HE, et al. Hb H hydrops foetalis syndrome: a case report and review of literature. *Br J Haematol.* 2001;115(1):72-78.

127. Songdej D, Babbs C, Higgs DR, Consortium BI. An international registry of survivors with Hb Bart's hydrops fetalis syndrome. *Blood.* 2017;129(10):1251-1259.

128. Beaudry MA, Ferguson DJ, Pearse K, et al. Survival of a hydropic infant with homozygous α-thalassemia-1. *J Pediatr.* 1986;108(5):713-716.

129. Gibbons RJ, Pellagatti A, Garrick D, et al. Identification of acquired somatic mutations in the gene encoding chromatin-remodeling factor ATRX in the α-thalassemia myelodysplasia syndrome (ATMDS). *Nat Genet.* 2003;34(4):446-449.

130. Steensma DP, Viprakasit V, Hendrick A, et al. Deletion of the α-globin gene cluster as a cause of acquired α-thalassemia in myelodysplastic syndrome. *Blood.* 2004;103(4):1518-1520.

131. Lamb J, Harris PC, Lindenbaum RH, et al. Detection of breakpoints in submicroscopic chromosomal translocation, illustrating an important mechanism for genetic disease. *Lancet.* 1989;334(8667):819-824.

132. Wilkie AO, Gibbons RJ, Higgs DR, Pembrey ME. X linked alpha thalassaemia/mental retardation: spectrum of clinical features in three related males. *J Med Genet.* 1991;28(11):738.

133. Gibbons RJ, Picketts DJ, Villard L, Higgs DR. Mutations in a putative global transcriptional regulator cause X-linked mental retardation with α-thalassemia (ATR-X syndrome). *Cell.* 1995;80(6):837-845.

134. León NY, Harley VR. ATR-X syndrome: genetics, clinical spectrum, and management. *Hum Genet.* 2021;140(12):1625-1634.

135. Lie-Injo LE, Dozy AM, Kan YW, Lopes M, Todd D. The alpha-globin gene adjacent to the gene for HbQ-alpha 74 Asp replaced by His is deleted, but not that adjacent to the gene for HbG-alpha 30 Glu replaced by Gln; three-fourths of the alpha-globin genes are deleted in HbQ-alpha-thalassemia. *Blood.* 1979;54(6):1407-1416.

136. Lie-Injo LE, Pillay RP, Thuraisingham V. Further cases of Hb Q-H disease (Hb Q-alpha thalassemia). *Blood.* 1966;28(6):830-839.

137. Rieder RF, Woodbury DH, Rucknagel DL. The interaction of α-thalassemia and haemoglobin G philadelphia. *Br J Haematol.* 1976;32(2):159-166.

138. Atwater J, Schwartz IR, Erslev AJ, Montgomery TL, Tocantins LM. Sickling of erythrocytes in a patient with thalassemia-hemoglobin-I disease. *N Engl J Med.* 1960;263(24):1215-1223.

139. Steinberg MH, Adams JG, Dreiling BJ. Alpha thalassaemia in adults with sickle-cell trait. *Br J Haematol.* 1975;30(1):31-37.

140. Higgs DR, Aldridge BE, Lamb J, et al. The interaction of alpha-thalassemia and homozygous sickle-cell disease. *N Engl J Med.* 1982;306(24):1441-1446.

141. Embury SH, Dozy AM, Miller J, et al. Concurrent sickle-cell anemia and alpha-thalassemia: effect on severity of anemia. *N Engl J Med.* 1982;306(5):270-274.

142. Flanagan JM, Frohlich DM, Howard TA, et al. Genetic predictors for stroke in children with sickle cell anemia. *Blood.* 2011;117(24):6681-6684.

143. Cooley TB, Witwer ER, Lee P. Anemia in children: with splenomegaly and peculiar changes in the bones report of cases. *Am J Dis Child.* 1927;34(3):347-363.

144. Maccanti A. Contributo alla conoscenza dell'anemia splenica infantile a tipo famigliare. *Riv Clin Pediatr.* 1928;26:620-640.

145. Whipple GH, Bradford WL. Racial or familial anemia of children: associated with fundamental disturbances of bone and pigment metabolism. *Am J Dis Child.* 1932;44(2):336-365.

146. Wintrobe MM, Matthews E, Pollack R, Dobyns BM. A familial hemopoietic disorder in Italian adolescents and adults: resembling mediterranean disease (thalassemia). *Am J Med Assoc.* 1940;114(16):1530-1538.

147. Silvestroni E, Bianco I. Some observations on family members of Cooley disease patients and on the frequency of microcythemia carriers in the Ferrara area. Article in Italian. *Ric Sci.* 1947;17(5):655-657.

148. Kunkel HG, Wallenius G. New hemoglobin in normal adult blood. *Science.* 1955;122(3163):288.

149. Cao A, Galanello R, Rosatelli MC, Argiolu F, Virgiliis SD. Clinical experience of management of thalassemia: the Sardinian experience. *Semin Hematol.* 1996;33(1):66-75.

150. Orzincolo C, Castaldi G, Scutellari PN, Franceschini F. The "lamellated" skull in β-thalassemia. *Skeletal Radiol.* 1989;18(5):373-376.

151. Wonke B. Bone disease in β-thalassaemia major. *Br J Haematol.* 1998;103(4):897-901.

152. Colavita N, Orazi C, Danza SM, Falappa PG, Fabbri R. Premature epiphyseal fusion and extramedullary hematopoiesis in thalassemia. *Skeletal Radiol.* 1987;16(7):533-538.

153. Eskazan AE, Ar MC, Baslar Z. Intracranial extramedullary hematopoiesis in patients with thalassemia: a case report and review of the literature. *Transfusion.* 2012;52(8):1715-1720.

154. Origa R, Fiumana E, Gamberini MR, et al. Osteoporosis in β-thalassemia: clinical and genetic aspects. *Ann N Y Acad Sci.* 2005;1054(1):451-456.

155. Perrotta S, Cappellini MD, Bertoldo F, et al. Osteoporosis in β-thalassaemia major patients: analysis of the genetic background. *Br J Haematol.* 2000;111(2):461-466.

156. Khalifa N, Hesham M, Elbaz N, Omran A, AbdElmonem D. Study of relationship between SP1 polymorphism in the collagen type I alpha-1 (COLIA1) gene and osteoporosis in patients with beta-thalassemia. *ZUMJ.* 2017;23(1):1-13.

157. Haidar R, Musallam KM, Taher AT. Bone disease and skeletal complications in patients with β thalassemia major. *Bone.* 2011;48(3):425-432.

158. Vogiatzi MG, Macklin EA, Trachtenberg FL, et al. Differences in the prevalence of growth, endocrine and vitamin D abnormalities among the various thalassemia syndromes in North America. *Br J Haematol.* 2009;146(5):546-556.

159. Sanctis VD, Soliman AT, Elsedfy H, et al. Osteoporosis in thalassemia major: an update and the I-CET 2013 recommendations for surveillance and treatment. *Pediatr Endocrinol Rev.* 2013;11:167-180.

160. Vogiatzi MG, Macklin EA, Fung EB, et al. Bone disease in thalassemia: a frequent and still unresolved problem. *J Bone Miner Res.* 2009;24(3):543-557.

161. Morabito N, Russo GT, Gaudio A, et al. The "lively" cytokines network in beta-Thalassemia Major-related osteoporosis. *Bone.* 2007;40(6):1588-1594.

162. Morabito N, Gaudio A, Lasco A, et al. Osteoprotegerin and RANKL in the pathogenesis of thalassemia-induced osteoporosis: new pieces of the puzzle. *J Bone Miner Res.* 2004;19(5):722-727.

163. Pietrapertosa AC, Minenna G, Colella SM, et al. Osteoprotegerin and RANKL in the pathogenesis of osteoporosis in patients with thalassemia major. *Panminerva Med.* 2009;51(1):17-23.

164. Vogiatzi MG, Macklin EA, Fung EB, et al. Prevalence of fractures among the Thalassemia syndromes in North America. *Bone.* 2006;38(4):571-575.

165. Michelson J, Cohen A. Incidence and treatment of fractures in thalassemia. *J Orthop Trauma.* 1988;2(1):29-32.

Disorders of Red Blood Cells

166. Angastiniotis M, Pavlides N, Aristidou K, et al. Bone pain in thalassaemia: assessment of DEXA and MRI findings. *J Pediatr Endocrinol Metab.* 1998;11(suppl 3):779-784.

167. Trachtenberg F, Foote D, Martin M, et al. Pain as an emergent issue in thalassemia. *Am J Hematol.* 2010;85(5):367-370.

168. Terpos E, Voskaridou E. Treatment options for thalassemia patients with osteoporosis. *Ann N Y Acad Sci.* 2010;1202(1):237-243.

169. Shamshirsaz AA, Bekheirnia MR, Kamgar M, et al. Metabolic and endocrinologic complications in beta-thalassemia major: a multicenter study in Tehran. *BMC Endocr Disord.* 2003;3(1):4.

170. Fung EB, Kwiatkowski JL, Huang JN, et al. Zinc supplementation improves bone density in patients with thalassemia: a double-blind, randomized, placebo-controlled trial. *Am J Clin Nutr.* 2013;98(4):960-971.

171. Tsartsalis AN, Lambrou GI, Tsartsalis D, et al. The role of biphosphonates in the management of thalassemia-induced osteoporosis: a systematic review and meta-analysis. *Hormones (Athens).* 2018;17(2):153-166.

172. Forni GL, Perrotta S, Giusti A, et al. Neridronate improves bone mineral density and reduces back pain in β-thalassaemia patients with osteoporosis: results from a phase 2, randomized, parallel-arm, open-label study. *Br J Haematol.* 2012;158(2):274-282.

173. Canatan D, Akar N, Arcasoy A. Effects of calcitonin therapy on osteoporosis in patients with thalassemia. *Acta Haematol.* 1995;93(1):20-24.

174. Origa R, Galanello R, Perseu L, et al. Cholelithiasis in thalassemia major. *Eur J Haematol.* 2009;82(1):22-25.

175. Borgna-Pignatti C, Rigon F, Merlo L, et al. Thalassemia minor, the Gilbert mutation, and the risk of gallstones. *Haematologica.* 2003;88(10):1106-1109.

176. Pignatti CB, Carnelli V, Caruso V, et al. Thromboembolic events in beta thalassemia major: an Italian multicenter study. *Acta Haematol.* 1998;99(2):76-79.

177. Cappellini MD, Robbiolo L, Bottasso BM, et al. Venous thromboembolism and hypercoagulability in splenectomized patients with thalassaemia intermedia. *Br J Haematol.* 2000;111(2):467-473.

178. Taher A, Isma'eel H, Mehio G, et al. Prevalence of thromboembolic events among 8,860 patients with thalassaemia major and intermedia in the Mediterranean area and Iran. *Thromb Haemost.* 2006;96(4):488-491.

179. Taher AT, Musallam KM, Karimi M, et al. Overview on practices in thalassemia intermedia management aiming for lowering complication rates across a region of endemicity: the OPTIMAL CARE study. *Blood.* 2010;115(10):1886-1892.

180. Sirachainan N. Thalassemia and the hypercoagulable state. *Thromb Res.* 2013;132(6):637-641.

181. Chassaing N, Martin L, Calvas P, Bert ML, Hovnanian A. Pseudoxanthoma elasticum: a clinical, pathophysiological and genetic update including 11 novel ABCC6 mutations. *J Med Genet.* 2005;42(12):881.

182. Hamlin N, Beck K, Bacchelli B, et al. Acquired pseudoxanthoma elasticum-like syndrome in β-thalassaemia patients. *Br J Haematol.* 2003;122(5):852-854.

183. Fabbri E, Forni GL, Guerrini G, Borgna-Pignatti C. Pseudoxanthoma-elasticum-like syndrome and thalassaemia: an update. *Dermatol Online J.* 2009;15(7):7.

184. Cianciulli P, Sorrentino F, Maffei L, et al. Cardiovascular involvement in thalassaemic patients with Pseudoxanthoma elasticum-like skin lesions: a long-term follow-up study. *Eur J Clin Invest.* 2002;32(9):700-706.

185. Munkongdee T, Chen P, Winichagoon P, Fucharoen S, Paiboonsukwong K. Update in laboratory diagnosis of thalassemia. *Front Mol Biosci.* 2020;7:74.

186. Wolman I. Transfusion therapy in cooley's anemia: growth and health as related to long-range hemoglobin levels. A progress report. *Ann N Y Acad Sci.* 1964;119(1):736-747.

187. Piomelli S, Danoff SJ, Becker MH, Lipera MJ, Travis SF. Prevention of bone malformations and cardiomegaly in Cooley's anemia by early hypertransfusion regimen. *Ann N Y Acad Sci.* 1969;165(1):427-436.

188. Cazzola M, Stefano PD, Ponchio L, et al. Relationship between transfusion regimen and suppression of erythropoiesis in beta-thalassaemia major. *Br J Haematol.* 1995;89(3):473-478.

189. Cazzola M, Borgna-Pignatti C, Locatelli F, et al. A moderate transfusion regimen may reduce iron loading in beta-thalassemia major without producing excessive expansion of erythropoiesis. *Transfusion.* 1997;37(2):135-140.

190. Waldis SJ, Uter S, Kavitsky D, et al. Rh alloimmunization in chronically transfused patients with thalassemia receiving RhD, C, E, and K matched transfusions. *Blood Adv.* 2021;5(3):737-744.

191. Borgna-Pignatti C, Ventola M, Friedman D, et al. Seasonal variation of pretransfusion hemoglobin levels in patients with thalassemia major. *Blood.* 2006;107(1):355-357.

192. Cohen AR, Glimm E, Porter JB. Effect of transfusional iron intake on response to chelation therapy in beta-thalassemia major. *Blood.* 2008;111(2):583-587.

193. Cappellini MD, Cohen A, Porter J, Taher A, Viprakasit V. *Guidelines for the Management of Transfusion Dependent Thalassaemia (TDT).* Thalassaemia International Federation; 2014.

194. Marcus RE, Wonke B, Bantock HM, et al. A prospective trial of young red cells in 48 patients with transfusion-dependent thalassaemia. *Br J Haematol.* 1985;60(1):153-159.

195. Rebulla P. Transfusion reactions in thalassemia. A survey from the cooleycare programme. The cooleycare cooperative group. *Haematologica.* 1990;75(suppl 5):122-127.

196. Thompson AA, Cunningham MJ, Singer ST, et al. Red cell alloimmunization in a diverse population of transfused patients with thalassaemia. *Br J Haematol.* 2011;153(1):121-128.

197. el-Danasoury AS, Eissa DG, Abdo RM, Elalfy MS. Red blood cell alloimmunization in transfusion-dependent Egyptian patients with thalassemia in a limited donor exposure program. *Transfusion.* 2012;52(1):43-47.

198. Vichinsky E, Neumayr L, Trimble S, et al. Transfusion complications in thalassemia patients: a report from the centers for disease control and prevention (CME). *Transfusion.* 2014;54(4):972-981, quiz 971.

199. Singer ST, Wu V, Mignacca R, et al. Alloimmunization and erythrocyte autoimmunization in transfusion-dependent thalassemia patients of predominantly asian descent. *Blood.* 2000;96:3369-3373.

200. Shaz BH, Hillyer CD. Minority donation in the United States; challenges and needs. *Curr Opin Hematol.* 2010;17(6):544-549.

201. Mirmomen S, Alavian SM, Hajarizadeh B, et al. Epidemiology of hepatitis B, hepatitis C, and human immunodeficiency virus infecions in patients with beta-thalassemia in Iran: a multicenter study. *Arch Iran Med.* 2006;9(4):319-323.

202. Al-Kubaisy WA, Al-Naib KT, Habib M. Seroprevalence of hepatitis C virus specific antibodies among Iraqi children with thalassaemia. *East Mediterr Health J.* 2006;12(1-2):204-210.

203. Gamberini MR, Fresconi R, Fortini M, et al. HCV and HGV infection, iron overload and liver disease in multitransfused patients with thalassaemia and persistently normal or abnormal transaminase levels. *Pediatr Endocrinol Rev.* 2004;2(suppl 2):259-266.

204. de Montalembert M, Girot R, Mattlinger B, Lefrère JJ. Transfusion-dependent thalassemia: viral complications (epidemiology and follow-up). *Semin Hematol.* 1995;32(4):280-287.

205. Lefrere JJ, Girot R. Haemoglobinopathies O behalf of the study group on H infection in thalassaemia patients of the E and MWWG on. Risk of HIV infection in polytransfused thalassaemia patients. *Lancet.* 1989;334(8666):813.

206. McCutcheon S, Blanco ARA, Houston EF, et al. All clinically-relevant blood components transmit prion disease following a single blood transfusion: a sheep model of vCJD. *PLoS One.* 2011;6(8):e23169.

207. Choudhury NJ, Dubey ML, Jolly JG, et al. Post-transfusion malaria in thalassaemia patients. *Blut.* 1990;61(5):314-316.

208. Kitchen AD, Hewitt PE, Chiodini PL. The early implementation of Trypanosoma cruzi antibody screening of donors and donations within England: preempting a problem. *Transfusion.* 2012;52(9):1931-1939.

209. Leiby DA. Babesiosis and blood transfusion: flying under the radar. *Vox Sang.* 2006;90(3):157-165.

210. Mohammed H, Linnen JM, Muñoz-Jordán JL, et al. Dengue virus in blood donations, Puerto Rico, 2005. *Transfusion.* 2008;48(7):1348-1354.

211. Aubry M, Finke J, Teissier A, et al. Seroprevalence of arboviruses among blood donors in French Polynesia, 2011-2013. *Int J Infect Dis.* 2015;41:11-12.

212. Kleinman S, Stassinopoulos A. Risks associated with red blood cell transfusions: potential benefits from application of pathogen inactivation. *Transfusion.* 2015;55(12):2983-3000.

213. Drew VJ, Barro L, Seghatchian J, Burnouf T. Towards pathogen inactivation of red blood cells and whole blood targeting viral DNA/RNA: design, technologies, and future prospects for developing countries. *Blood Transfus.* 2017;15(6):512-521.

214. Sakran W, Levin C, Kenes Y, Colodner R, Koren A. Clinical spectrum of serious bacterial infections among splenectomized patients with hemoglobinopathies in Israel: a 37-year follow-up study. *Infection.* 2012;40(1):35-39.

215. Adamkiewicz TV, Berkovitch M, Krishnan C, et al. Infection due to Yersinia enterocolitica in a series of patients with β-thalassemia: incidence and predisposing factors. *Clin Infect Dis.* 1998;27(6):1362-1366.

216. Chan GC, Chan S, Ho PL, Ha SY. Effects of chelators (deferoxamine, deferiprone and deferasirox) on the growth of Klebsiella pneumoniae and Aeromonas hydrophila isolated from transfusion-dependent thalassemia patients. *Hemoglobin.* 2009;33(5):352-360.

217. Shah FT, Sayani F, Trompeter S, Drasar E, Piga A. Challenges of blood transfusions in beta-thalassemia. *Blood Rev.* 2019;37:100588.

218. Gupta R, Musallam KM, Taher AT, Rivella S. Ineffective erythropoiesis: anemia and iron overload. *Hematol Oncol Clin North Am.* 2018;32(2):213-221.

219. Gardenghi S, Marongiu MF, Ramos P, et al. Ineffective erythropoiesis in β-thalassemia is characterized by increased iron absorption mediated by down-regulation of hepcidin and up-regulation of ferroportin. *Blood.* 2007;109(11):5027-5035.

220. Hershko C, Graham G, Bates GW, Rachmilewitz EA. Non-specific serum iron in thalassaemia: an abnormal serum iron fraction of potential toxicity. *Br J Haematol.* 1978;40(2):255-263.

221. Esposito BP, Breuer W, Sirankapracha P, et al. Labile plasma iron in iron overload: redox activity and susceptibility to chelation. *Blood.* 2003;102(7):2670-2677.

222. Breuer W, Shvartsman M, Cabantchik ZI. Intracellular labile iron. *Int J Biochem Cell Biol.* 2008;40(3):350-354.

223. Cohen A, Cohen IJ, Schwartz E. Scurvy and altered iron stores in thalassemia major. *N Engl J Med.* 1981;304(3):158-160.

224. Borgna-Pignatti C, Rugolotto S, Stefano PD, et al. Survival and complications in patients with thalassemia major treated with transfusion and deferoxamine. *Haematologica.* 2004;89(10):1187-1193.

225. Belhoul KM, Bakir ML, Saned MS, et al. Serum ferritin levels and endocrinopathy in medically treated patients with beta thalassemia major. *Ann Hematol.* 2012;91(7):1107-1114.

226. Olivieri NF, Nathan DG, MacMillan JH, et al. Survival in medically treated patients with homozygous beta-thalassemia. *N Engl J Med.* 1994;331(9):574-578.

227. Worwoon M, Cragg SJ, Jacobs A, et al. Binding of serum ferritin to concanavalin A: patients with hornozygous β thalassaemia and transfusional iron overload. *Br J Haematol.* 1980;46(3):409-416.

228. Angelucci E, Brittenham GM, McLaren CE, et al. Hepatic iron concentration and total body iron stores in thalassemia major. *N Engl J Med.* 2000;343(5):327-331.

229. Pierre TGS, Clark PR, Chuaanusorn W, et al. Noninvasive measurement and imaging of liver iron concentrations using proton magnetic resonance. *Blood.* 2005;105(2):855-861.

230. Emond MJ, Bronner MP, Carlson TH, et al. Quantitative study of the variability of hepatic iron concentrations. *Clin Chem.* 1999;45(3):340-346.
231. Brittenham GM, Farrell DE, Harris JW, et al. Magnetic-susceptibility measurement of human iron stores. *N Engl J Med.* 1982;307(27):1671-1675.
232. Anderson LJ, Holden S, Davis B, et al. Cardiovascular T2-star (T2*) magnetic resonance for the early diagnosis of myocardial iron overload. *Eur Heart J.* 2001;22(23): 2171-2179.
233. Carpenter J-P, He T, Kirk P, et al. On T2* magnetic resonance and cardiac iron. *Circulation.* 2011;123(14):1519-1528.
234. Kirk P, He T, Anderson LJ, et al. International reproducibility of single breathhold T2* MR for cardiac and liver iron assessment among five thalassemia centers. *J Magn Reson Imaging.* 2010;32(2):315-319.
235. Noetzli LJ, Papudesi J, Coates TD, Wood JC. Pancreatic iron loading predicts cardiac iron loading in thalassemia major. *Blood.* 2009;114(19):4021-4026.
236. Noetzli LJ, Panigrahy A, Mittelman SD, et al. Pituitary iron and volume predict hypogonadism in transfusional iron overload. *Am J Hematol.* 2012;87(2):167-171.
237. Marsella M, Borgna-Pignatti C, Meloni A, et al. Cardiac iron and cardiac disease in males and females with transfusion-dependent thalassemia major: a T2* magnetic resonance imaging study. *Haematologica.* 2011;96(4):515-520.
238. Link G, Athias P, Grynberg A, Pinson A, Hershko C. Effect of iron loading on transmembrane potential, contraction, and automaticity of rat ventricular muscle cells in culture. *J Lab Clin Med.* 1989;113(1):103-111.
239. Ehlers KH, Levin AR, Markenson AL, et al. Longitudinal study of cardiac function in thalassemia major. *Ann N Y Acad Sci.* 1980;344(1):397-404.
240. Barosi G, Arbustini E, Gavazzi A, Grasso M, Pucci A. Myocardial iron grading by endomyocardial biopsy. A clinico-pathologic study on iron overloaded patients. *Eur J Haematol.* 1989;42(4):382-388.
241. Kim D, Jensen JH, Wu EX, Sheth SS, Brittenham GM. Breathhold multiecho fast spin-echo pulse sequence for accurate R2 measurement in the heart and liver. *Magn Reson Med.* 2009;62(2):300-306.
242. Kirk P, Roughton M, Porter JB, et al. Cardiac T2* magnetic resonance for prediction of cardiac complications in thalassemia major. *Circulation.* 2009;120(20):1961-1968.
243. Tanner M, Galanello R, Dessi C, et al. Myocardial iron loading in patients with thalassemia major on deferoxamine chelation. *J Cardiovasc Magn Reson.* 2006;8(3):543-547.
244. Pepe A, Meloni A, Rossi G, et al. Prediction of cardiac complications for thalassemia major in the widespread cardiac magnetic resonance era: a prospective multicentre study by a multi-parametric approach. *Eur Heart J Cardiovasc Imaging.* 2018;19(3):299-309.
245. Kremastinos DT, Tsetsos GA, Tsiapras DP, et al. Heart failure in beta thalassemia: a 5-year follow-up study. *Am J Med.* 2001;111(5):349-354.
246. Telfer PT, Warburton F, Christou S, et al. Improved survival in thalassemia major patients on switching from desferrioxamine to combined chelation therapy with desferrioxamine and deferiprone. *Haematologica.* 2009;94(12):1777-1778.
247. Anderson LJ, Westwood MA, Prescott E, et al. Development of thalassaemic iron overload cardiomyopathy despite low liver iron levels and meticulous compliance to desferrioxamine. *Acta Haematol.* 2006;115(1-2):106-108.
248. Anderson LJ, Westwood MA, Holden S, et al. Myocardial iron clearance during reversal of siderotic cardiomyopathy with intravenous desferrioxamine: a prospective study using T2* cardiovascular magnetic resonance. *Br J Haematol.* 2004;127(3):348-355.
249. Borgna-Pignatti C, Cappellini MD, Stefano PD, et al. Cardiac morbidity and mortality in deferoxamine- or deferiprone-treated patients with thalassemia major. *Blood.* 2006;107(9):3733-3737.
250. Pennell DJ, Berdoukas V, Karagiorga M, et al. Randomized controlled trial of deferiprone or deferoxamine in beta-thalassemia major patients with asymptomatic myocardial siderosis. *Blood.* 2006;107(9):3738-3744.
251. Pennell DJ, Porter JB, Cappellini MD, et al. Continued improvement in myocardial T2* over two years of deferasirox therapy in beta-thalassemia major patients with cardiac iron overload. *Haematologica.* 2011;96(1):48-54.
252. Pennell DJ, Porter JB, Cappellini MD, et al. Efficacy of deferasirox in reducing and preventing cardiac iron overload in beta-thalassemia. *Blood.* 2010;115(12):2364-2371.
253. Pennell DJ, Porter JB, Piga A, et al. A 1-year randomized controlled trial of deferasirox vs deferoxamine for myocardial iron removal in beta-thalassemia major (CORDELIA). *Blood.* 2014;123(10):1447-1454.
254. Ho PJ, Tay L, Teo J, et al. Cardiac iron load and function in transfused patients treated with deferasirox (the MILE study). *Eur J Haematol.* 2017;98(2):97-105.
255. Wood JC, Kang BP, Thompson A, et al. The effect of deferasirox on cardiac iron in thalassemia major: impact of total body iron stores. *Blood.* 2010;116(4):537-543.
256. Ladis V, Chouliaras G, Berdoukas V, et al. Relation of chelation regimes to cardiac mortality and morbidity in patients with thalassaemia major: an observational study from a large Greek Unit. *Eur J Haematol.* 2010;85(4):335-344.
257. Fernandes JL, Loggetto SR, Verissimo MPA, et al. A randomized trial of amlodipine in addition to standard chelation therapy in patients with thalassemia major. *Blood.* 2016;128(12):1555-1561.
258. Modell B, Khan M, Darlison M, et al. Improved survival of thalassaemia major in the UK and relation to T2* cardiovascular magnetic resonance. *J Cardiovasc Magn Reson.* 2008;10(1):42.
259. Morris CR, Kim HY, Trachtenberg F, et al. Risk factors and mortality associated with an elevated tricuspid regurgitant jet velocity measured by Doppler-echocardiography in thalassemia: a Thalassemia Clinical Research Network report. *Blood.* 2011;118(14):3794-3802.
260. Derchi G, Formisano F, Balocco M, et al. Clinical management of cardiovascular complications in patients with thalassaemia major: a large observational multicenter study. *Eur J Echocardiogr.* 2011;12(3):242-246.
261. Pennell DJ, Udelson JE, Arai AE, et al. Cardiovascular function and treatment in beta-thalassemia major: a consensus statement from the American Heart Association. *Circulation.* 2013;128(3):281-308.
262. Caines AE, Kpodonu J, Massad MG, et al. Cardiac transplantation in patients with iron overload cardiomyopathy. *J Heart Lung Transplant.* 2005;24(4):486-488.
263. Anderson LJ. Assessment of iron overload with T2* magnetic resonance imaging. *Prog Cardiovasc Dis.* 2011;54(3):287-294.
264. Maira D, Cassinerio E, Marcon A, et al. Progression of liver fibrosis can be controlled by adequate chelation in transfusion-dependent thalassemia (TDT). *Ann Hematol.* 2017;96(11):1931-1936.
265. Lisboa PE. Experimental hepatic cirrhosis in dogs caused by chronic massive iron overload 1. *Gut.* 1971;12(5):363.
266. Britton RS, Bacon BR, Recknagel RO. Lipid peroxidation and associated hepatic organelle dysfunction in iron overload. *Chem Phys Lipids.* 1987;45(2-4):207-239.
267. Angelucci E, Baronciani D, Lucarelli G, et al. Needle liver biopsy in thalassaemia: analyses of diagnostic accuracy and safety in 1184 consecutive biopsies. *Br J Haematol.* 1995;89(4):757-761.
268. Fraquelli M, Cassinerio E, Roghi A, et al. Transient elastography in the assessment of liver fibrosis in adult thalassemia patients. *Am J Hematol.* 2010;85(8):564-568.
269. Seed CR, Kiely P, Keller AJ. Residual risk of transfusion transmitted human immunodeficiency virus, hepatitis B virus, hepatitis C virus and human T lymphotrophic virus. *Intern Med J.* 2005;35(10):592-598.
270. Velati C, Fomiatti L, Baruffi L, et al. Impact of nucleic acid amplification technology (NAT) in Italy in the three years following implementation (2001-2003). *Euro Surveill.* 2005;10(2):3-4.
271. Ponti ML, Comitini F, Murgia D, et al. Impact of the direct-acting antiviral agents (DAAs) on chronic hepatitis C in Sardinian patients with transfusion-dependent Thalassemia major. *Dig Liver Dis.* 2019;51(4):561-567.
272. Nagral A, Sawant S, Nagral N, et al. Generic direct acting antivirals in treatment of chronic hepatitis C infection in patients of thalassemia major. *J Clin Exp Hepatol.* 2017;7(3):172-178.
273. Sanctis VD, Soliman AT, Daar S, et al. A concise review on the frequency, major risk factors and surveillance of hepatocellular carcinoma (HCC) in beta-thalassemias: past, present and future perspectives and the ICET-A experience. *Mediterr J Hematol Infect Dis.* 2020;12(1):e2020006.
274. Mangia A, Bellini D, Cillo U, et al. Hepatocellular carcinoma in adult thalassemia patients: an expert opinion based on current evidence. *BMC Gastroenterol.* 2020;20(1):251.
275. Koren G, Bentur Y, Strong D, et al. Acute changes in renal function associated with deferoxamine therapy. *Am J Dis Child.* 1989;143(9):1077-1080.
276. Koren G, Kochavi-Atiya Y, Bentur Y, Olivieri NF. The effects of subcutaneous deferoxamine administration on renal function in thalassemia major. *Int J Hematol.* 1991;54(5):371-375.
277. Quinn CT, Johnson VL, Kim HY, et al. Renal dysfunction in patients with thalassaemia. *Br J Haematol.* 2011;153(1):111-117.
278. Ponticelli C, Musallam KM, Cianciulli P, Cappellini MD. Renal complications in transfusion-dependent beta thalassaemia. *Blood Rev.* 2010;24(6):239-244.
279. Bhandari S, Galanello R. Renal aspects of thalassaemia a changing paradigm. *Eur J Haematol.* 2012;89(3):187-197.
280. ElAlfy MS, Elsherif NH, Ebeid FSE, et al. Renal iron deposition by magnetic resonance imaging in pediatric β-thalassemia major patients: relation to renal biomarkers, total body iron and chelation therapy. *Eur J Radiol.* 2018;103:65-70.
281. Toumba M, Sergis A, Kanaris C, Skordis N. Endocrine complications in patients with thalassaemia major. *Pediatr Endocrinol Rev.* 2007;5:642-648.
282. Italian Working Group on Endocrine Complications in Non-Endocrine Diseases. Multicentre study on prevalence of endocrine complications in thalassaemia major. *Clin Endocrinol.* 1995;42(6):581-586.
283. Farmaki K, Tzoumari I, Pappa C, Chouliaras G, Berdoukas V. Normalisation of total body iron load with very intensive combined chelation reverses cardiac and endocrine complications of thalassaemia major. *Br J Haematol.* 2010;148(3):466-475.
284. Caruso-Nicoletti M, Sanctis VD, Raiola G, et al. No difference in pubertal growth and final height between treated hypogonadal and non-hypogonadal thalassemic patients. *Horm Res.* 2004;62(1):17-22.
285. Prakash A, Aggarwal R. Thalassemia major in adults: short stature, hyperpigmentation, inadequate chelation, and transfusion-transmitted infections are key features. *N Am J Med Sci.* 2012;4(3):141-144.
286. Poggi M, Pascucci C, Monti S, et al. Prevalence of growth hormone deficiency in adult polytransfused β-thalassemia patients and correlation with transfusional and chelation parameters. *J Endocrinol Invest.* 2010;33(8):534-538.
287. Cavallo L, Sanctis VD, Cisternino M, et al. Final height in short polytransfused thalassemia major patients treated with recombinant growth hormone. *J Endocrinol Invest.* 2005;28(6):363-366.
288. van Bunderen CC, van Nieuwpoort IC, Arwert LI, et al. Does growth hormone replacement therapy reduce mortality in adults with growth hormone deficiency? Data from the Dutch National Registry of Growth Hormone Treatment in adults. *J Clin Endocrinol Metabolism.* 2011;96(10):3151-3159.
289. Chan YL, Pang LM, Chik KW, Cheng JC, Li CK. Patterns of bone diseases in transfusion-dependent homozygous thalassaemia major: predominance of osteoporosis and desferrioxamine-induced bone dysplasia. *Pediatr Radiol.* 2002;32(7):492-497.
290. Virgilis SD, Congia M, Frau F, et al. Deferoxamine-induced growth retardation in patients with thalassemia major. *J Pediatr.* 1988;113(4):661-669.

Disorders of Red Blood Cells

291. Piga A, Luzzatto L, Capalbo P, et al. High-dose desferrioxamine as a cause of growth failure in thalassemic patients. *Eur J Haematol.* 1988;40(4):380-381.

292. Gamberini MR, Sanctis VD, Gilli G. Hypogonadism, diabetes mellitus, hypothyroidism, hypoparathyroidism: incidence and prevalence related to iron overload and chelation therapy in patients with thalassaemia major followed from 1980 to 2007 in the Ferrara Centre. *Pediatr Endocrinol Rev.* 2008;6(suppl 1):158-169.

293. Singer ST, Sweeters N, Vega O, et al. Fertility potential in thalassemia major women: current findings and future diagnostic tools. *Ann N Y Acad Sci.* 2010;1202(1):226-230.

294. Skordis N, Christou S, Koliou M, Pavlides N, Angastiniotis M. Fertility in female patients with thalassemia. *J Pediatr Endocrinol Metab.* 1998;11(suppl 3):935-943.

295. Safarinejad MR. Evaluation of semen quality, endocrine profile and hypothalamus-pituitary-testis axis in male patients with homozygous β-thalassaemia major. *J Urol.* 2008;179(6):2327-2332.

296. Cisterno M, Manzoni SM, Coslovich E, Autelli M. Hormonal replacement therapy with HCG and HU-FSH in thalassaemic patients affected by hypogonadotropic hypogonadism. *J Pediatr Endocrinol Metab.* 1998;11(suppl 3):885-890.

297. Carlberg KT, Singer ST, Vichinsky EP. Fertility and pregnancy in women with transfusion-dependent thalassemia. *Hematol Oncol Clin North Am.* 2018;32(2):297-315.

298. Origa R, Piga A, Quarta G, et al. Pregnancy and beta-thalassemia: an Italian multicenter experience. *Haematologica.* 2010;95(3):376-381.

299. Singer ST, Vichinsky EP. Deferoxamine treatment during pregnancy: is it harmful? *Am J Hematol.* 1999;60(1):24-26.

300. Chirico V, Valeria C, Lacquaniti A, et al. Thyroid dysfunction in thalassaemic patients: ferritin as a prognostic marker and combined iron chelators as an ideal therapy. *Eur J Endocrinol.* 2013;169(6):785-793.

301. Satictis VD, Vullo C, Bagni B, Chiccoli L. Hypoparathyroidism in beta-thalassemia major. *Acta Haematol.* 1992;88(2-3):105-108.

302. Karimi M, Rasekhi AR, Rasekh M, et al. Hypoparathyroidism and intracerebral calcification in patients with beta-thalassemia major. *Eur J Radiol.* 2009;70(3):481-484.

303. Baldini M, Mancarella M, Cassinerio E, et al. Adrenal insufficiency: an emerging challenge in thalassemia? *Am J Hematol.* 2017;92(6):E119-E121.

304. Huang KE, Mittelman SD, Coates TD, Geffner ME, Wood JC. A significant proportion of thalassemia major patients have adrenal insufficiency detectable on provocative testing. *J Pediatr Hematol Oncol.* 2015;37(1):54-59.

305. Scacchi M, Danesi L, Cattaneo A, et al. The pituitary–adrenal axis in adult thalassaemic patients. *Eur J Endocrinol.* 2010;162(1):43-48.

306. Sanctis V, Soliman A, Yassin M. Iron overload and glucose metabolism in subjects with beta-thalassaemia major: an overview. *Curr Diabetes Rev.* 2013;9(4):332-341.

307. Sanctis VD, Soliman A, Tzoulis P, et al. The Pancreatic changes affecting glucose homeostasis in transfusion dependent beta- thalassaemia (TDT): a short review. *Acta Biomed.* 2021;92(3):e2021232.

308. Noetzli LJ, Mittelman SD, Watanabe RM, Coates TD, Wood JC. Pancreatic iron and glucose dysregulation in thalassemia major. *Am J Hematol.* 2012;87(2):155-160.

309. Sanctis VD, D'Ascola G, Wonke B. The development of diabetes mellitus and chronic liver disease in long term chelated beta thalassaemic patients. *Postgrad Med J.* 1986;62(731):831.

310. Sougleri M, Labropoulou-Karatza C, Paraskevopoulou P, Fragopanagou H, Alexandrides T. Chronic hepatitis C virus infection without cirrhosis induces insulin resistance in patients with β-thalassaemia major. *Eur J Gastroenterol Hepatol.* 2001;13(10):1195-1199.

311. Negro F, Alaei M. Hepatitis C virus and type 2 diabetes. *World J Gastroenterol.* 2009;15(13):1537-1547.

312. Angelopoulos NG, Zervas A, Livadas S, et al. Reduced insulin secretion in normoglycaemic patients with β-thalassaemia major. *Diabet Med.* 2006;23(12):1327-1331.

313. Incorvaia C, Parmeggiani F, Mingrone G, Sebastiani A, Sanctis VD. Prevalence of retinopathy in diabetic thalassaemic patients. *J Pediatr Endocrinol Metab.* 1998;11(suppl 3):879-883.

314. Hussain M, Dandona P, Fedail SS, et al. Serum immunoreactive trypsin in beta-thalassaemia major. *J Clin Pathol.* 1981;34(9):970.

315. Gullo L, Corcioni E, Brancati C, et al. Morphologic and functional evaluation of the exocrine pancreas in β-thalassemia major. *Pancreas.* 1993;8(2):176-180.

316. Taneja R, Malik P, Sharma M, Agarwal MC. Multiple transfused thalassemia major: ocular manifestations in a hospital-based population. *Indian J Ophthalmol.* 2010;58(2):125-130.

317. Gelmi C, Borgna-Pignatti C, Franchin S, Tacchini M, Trimarchi F. Electroretinographic and visual-evoked potential abnormalities in patients with beta-thalassemia major. *Ophthalmologica.* 1988;196(1):29-34.

318. Aessopos A, Farmakis D, Loukopoulos D. Elastic tissue abnormalities resembling pseudoxanthoma elasticum in beta thalassemia and the sickling syndromes. *Blood.* 2002;99(1):30-35.

319. Bourli E, Dimitriadou M, Economou M, et al. Restrictive pulmonary dysfunction and its predictors in young patients with β-thalassaemia major. *Pediatr Pulmonol.* 2012;47(8):801-807.

320. Sohn EY, Noetzli LJ, Gera A, et al. Pulmonary function in thalassaemia major and its correlation with body iron stores. *Br J Haematol.* 2011;155(1):102-105.

321. Kwiatkowski JL. Current recommendations for chelation for transfusion-dependent thalassemia. *Ann N Y Acad Sci.* 2016;1368(1):107-114.

322. Hider RC, Zhou T. The design of orally active iron chelators. *Ann N Y Acad Sci.* 2005;1054(1):141-154.

323. Chong CC, Redzuan AM, Sathar J, Makmor-Bakry M. Patient perspective on iron chelation therapy: barriers and facilitators of medication adherence. *J Patient Exp.* 2021;8:2374373521996958.

324. Fortin PM, Fisher SA, Madgwick KV, et al. Interventions for improving adherence to iron chelation therapy in people with sickle cell disease or thalassaemia. *Cochrane Db Syst Rev.* 2018;2018(5):CD012349.

325. Smith RS. Iron excretion in thalassaemia major after administration of chelating agents. *Br Med J.* 1962;2(5319):1577.

326. Barry M, Flynn DM, Letsky EA, Risdon RA. Long-term chelation therapy in thalassaemia major: effect on liver iron concentration, liver histology, and clinical progress. *Br Med J.* 1974;2(5909):16.

327. Brittenham GM, Griffith PM, Nienhuis AW, et al. Efficacy of deferoxamine in preventing complications of iron overload in patients with thalassemia major. *N Engl J Med.* 1994;331(9):567-573.

328. Porter JB. Deferoxamine pharmacokinetics. *Semin Hematol.* 2001;38(1 suppl):63-68.

329. Porter JB, Abeysinghe RD, Marshall L, Hider RC, Singh S. Kinetics of removal and reappearance of non-transferrin-bound plasma iron with deferoxamine therapy. *Blood.* 1996;88(2):705-713.

330. Wolfe L, Olivieri N, Sallan D, et al. Prevention of cardiac disease by subcutaneous deferoxamine in patients with thalassemia major. *N Engl J Med.* 1985;312(25):1600-1603.

331. Shah FT, Porter JB, Sadasivam N, et al. Guidelines for the monitoring and management of iron overload in patients with haemoglobinopathies and rare anaemias. *Br J Haematol.* 2021;196(2):336-350.

332. Davis BA, Porter JB. Long-term outcome of continuous 24-hour deferoxamine infusion via indwelling intravenous catheters in high-risk beta-thalassemia. *Blood.* 2000;95(4):1229-1236.

333. Borgna-Pignatti C, Cohen A. Evaluation of a new method of administration of the iron chelating agent deferoxamine. *J Pediatr.* 1997;130(1):86-88.

334. Franchini M, Gandini G, de Gironcoli M, et al. Safety and efficacy of subcutaneous bolus injection of deferoxamine in adult patients with iron overload. *Blood.* 2000;95(9):2776-2779.

335. Porter JB, Evangeli M, El-Beshlawy A. The challenges of adherence and persistence with iron chelation therapy. *Int J Hematol.* 2011;94(5):453-460.

336. Trachtenberg F, Vichinsky E, Haines D, et al. Iron chelation adherence to deferoxamine and deferasirox in thalassemia. *Am J Hematol.* 2011;86(5):433-436.

337. Miller KB, Rosenwasser LJ, Bessette JA, Beer DJ, Rocklin RE. Rapid desensitization for desferrioxamine anaphylactic reaction. *Lancet.* 1981;317(8228):1059.

338. Olivieri NF, Buncic JR, Chew E, et al. Visual and auditory neurotoxicity in patients receiving subcutaneous deferoxamine infusions. *N Engl J Med.* 1986;314(14):869-873.

339. Porter JB, Jaswon MS, Huehns ER, East CA, Hazell JW. Desferrioxamine ototoxicity: evaluation of risk factors in thalassaemic patients and guidelines for safe dosage. *Br J Haematol.* 1989;73(3):403-409.

340. Gallant T, Boyden MH, Gallant LA, Carley H, Freedman MH. Serial studies of auditory neurotoxicity in patients receiving deferoxamine therapy. *Am J Med.* 1987;83(6):1085-1090.

341. Olivieri NF, Koren G, Harris J, et al. Growth failure and bony changes induced by deferoxamine. *Am J Pediatr Hematol Oncol.* 1992;14(1):48-56.

342. Freedman MH, Grisaru D, Olivieri N, MacLusky I, Thorner PS. Pulmonary syndrome in patients with thalassemia major receiving intravenous deferoxamine infusions. *Am J Dis Child.* 1990;144(5):565-569.

343. Hider RC, Hoffbrand AV. The role of deferiprone in iron chelation. *N Engl J Med.* 2018;379(22):2140-2150.

344. Glickstein H, El RB, Link G, et al. Action of chelators in iron-loaded cardiac cells: accessibility to intracellular labile iron and functional consequences. *Blood.* 2006;108(9):3195-3203.

345. Kontoghiorghes GJ, Goddard JG, Bartlett AN, Sheppard L. Pharmacokinetic studies in humans with the oral iron chelator 1,2-dimethyl-3-hydroxypyrid-4-one. *Clin Pharmacol Ther.* 1990;48(3):255-261.

346. al-Refaie FN, Sheppard LN, Nortey P, Wonke B, Hoffbrand AV. Pharmacokinetics of the oral iron chelator deferiprone (L1) in patients with iron overload. *Br J Haematol.* 1995;89(2):403-408.

347. Olivieri NF, Freedman MH, Koren G, et al. Comparison of oral iron chelator L1 and desferrioxamine in iron-loaded patients. *Lancet.* 1990;336(8726):1275-1279.

348. Link G, Konijn AM, Breuer W, Cabantchik ZI, Hershko C. Exploring the "iron shuttle" hypothesis in chelation therapy: effects of combined deferoxamine and deferiprone treatment in hypertransfused rats with labeled iron stores and in iron-loaded rat heart cells in culture. *J Lab Clin Med.* 2001;138(2):130-138.

349. Tanner MA, Galanello R, Dessi C, et al. A randomized, placebo-controlled, double-blind trial of the effect of combined therapy with deferoxamine and deferiprone on myocardial iron in thalassemia major using cardiovascular magnetic resonance. *Circulation.* 2007;115(14):1876-1884.

350. Origa R, Bina P, Agus A, et al. Combined therapy with deferiprone and desferrioxamine in thalassemia major. *Haematologica.* 2005;90(10):1309-1314.

351. Farmaki K, Angelopoulos N, Anagnostopoulos G, et al. Effect of enhanced iron chelation therapy on glucose metabolism in patients with β-thalassaemia major. *Br J Haematol.* 2006;134(4):438-444.

352. Galanello R, Kattamis A, Piga A, et al. A prospective randomized controlled trial on the safety and efficacy of alternating deferoxamine and deferiprone in the treatment of iron overload in patients with thalassemia. *Haematologica.* 2006;91(9):1241-1243.

353. Pantalone GR, Maggio A, Vitrano A, et al. Sequential alternating deferiprone and deferoxamine treatment compared to deferiprone monotherapy: main findings and clinical follow-up of a large multicenter randomized clinical trial in -thalassemia major patients. *Hemoglobin.* 2011;35(3):206-216.

354. Maggio A, Kattamis A, Felisi M, et al. Evaluation of the efficacy and safety of deferiprone compared with deferasirox in paediatric patients with transfusion-dependent haemoglobinopathies (DEEP-2): a multicentre, randomised, open-label, non-inferiority, phase 3 trial. *Lancet Haematol.* 2020;7(6):e469-e478.

355. Elalfy MS, Adly A, Awad H, et al. Safety and efficacy of early start of iron chelation therapy with deferiprone in young children newly diagnosed with transfusion-dependent thalassemia: a randomized controlled trial. *Am J Hematol.* 2018;93(2):262-268.

356. Cohen AR, Galanello R, Piga A, Sanctis VD, Tricta F. Safety and effectiveness of long-term therapy with the oral iron chelator deferiprone. *Blood.* 2003;102(5):1583-1587.

357. Cohen, Galanello, Piga, et al. Safety profile of the oral iron chelator deferiprone: a multicentre study. *Br J Haematol.* 2000;108(2):305-312.

358. Agarwal MB, Gupte SS, Viswanathan C, et al. Long-term assessment of efficacy and safety of L1, an oral iron chelator, in transfusion dependent thalassaemia: Indian trial. *Br J Haematol.* 1992;82(2):460-466.

359. Tanaka C. Clinical pharmacology of deferasirox. *Clin Pharmacokinet.* 2014;53(8):679-694.

360. Cappellini MD, Cohen A, Piga A, et al. A phase 3 study of deferasirox (ICL670), a once-daily oral iron chelator, in patients with beta-thalassemia. *Blood.* 2006;107(9):3455-3462.

361. Pennell DJ, Porter JB, Cappellini MD, et al. Deferasirox for up to 3 years leads to continued improvement of myocardial T2* in patients with beta-thalassemia major. *Haematologica.* 2012;97(6):842-848.

362. Cappellini MD, Bejaoui M, Agaoglu L, et al. Iron chelation with deferasirox in adult and pediatric patients with thalassemia major: efficacy and safety during 5 years' follow-up. *Blood.* 2011;118(4):884-893.

363. Aydinok Y, Unal S, Oymak Y, et al. Observational study comparing long-term safety and efficacy of Deferasirox with Desferrioxamine therapy in chelation-naïve children with transfusional iron overload. *Eur J Haematol.* 2012;88(5):431-438.

364. Rafat C, Fakhouri F, Ribeil JA, Delarue R, Quintrec ML. Fanconi syndrome due to deferasirox. *Am J Kidney Dis.* 2009;54(5):931-934.

365. Balocco M, Carrara P, Pinto V, Forni GL. Daily alternating deferasirox and deferiprone therapy for "hard-to-chelate" β-thalassemia major patients. *Am J Hematol.* 2010;85(6):460-461.

366. Claster S, Wood JC, Noetzli L, et al. Nutritional deficiencies in iron overloaded patients with hemoglobinopathies. *Am J Hematol.* 2009;84(6):344-348.

367. Soliman A, Sanctis VD, Yassin M. Vitamin D status in thalassemia major: an update. *Mediterr J Hematol Infect Dis.* 2013;5(1):e2013057.

368. Noetzli LJ, Carson S, Coates TD, Wood JC. Revisiting the relationship between vitamin D deficiency, cardiac iron and cardiac function in thalassemia major. *Eur J Haematol.* 2011;86(2):176-177.

369. Hussain MA, Green N, Flynn DM, Hoffbrand AV. Effect of dose, time, and ascorbate on iron excretion after subcutaneous desferrioxamine. *Lancet.* 1977;309(8019):977-979.

370. Nienhuis AW. Vitamin C and iron. *N Engl J Med.* 1981;304(3):170-171.

371. Vatanavicharn S, Anuvatanakulchai M, Na-Nakorn S, Wasi P. Serum erythrocyte folate levels in thalassaemic patients in Thailand. *Scand J Haematol.* 1979;22(3):241-245.

372. Silprasert A, Laokuldilok T, Kulapongs P. Zinc deficiency in beta-thalassemic children. *Birth Defects Orig Artic Ser.* 1987;23(5A):473-476.

373. Arcasoy A, Canatan D, Sinav B, et al. Serum zinc levels and zinc binding capacity in thalassemia. *J Trace Elem Med Biol.* 2001;15(2-3):85-87.

374. Piga A, Serra M, Longo F, et al. Changing patterns of splenectomy in transfusion-dependent thalassemia patients. *Am J Hematol.* 2011;86(9):808-810.

375. Modell B. Total management of thalassaemia major. *Arch Dis Child.* 1977;52(6):489.

376. Luks FI, Logan J, Breuer CK, et al. Cost-effectiveness of laparoscopy in children. *Arch Pediatr Adolesc Med.* 1999;153(9):965-968.

377. Winslow ER, Brunt LM, Drebin JA, Soper NJ, Klingensmith ME. Portal vein thrombosis after splenectomy. *Am J Surg.* 2002;184(6):631-635.

378. Tahir F, Ahmed J, Malik F. Post-splenectomy sepsis: a review of the literature. *Cureus.* 2020;12(2):e6898.

379. Wolf HM, Eibl MM, Georgi E, et al. Long-term decrease of CD4+CD45RA+ T cells and impaired primary immune response after post-traumatic splenectomy. *Br J Haematol.* 1999;107(1):55-68.

380. Smith CH, Erlandson ME, Stern G, Hilgartner MW. Postsplenectomy infection in cooley's anemia — an appraisal of the problem in this and other blood disorders, with a consideration of prophylaxis. *N Engl J Med.* 1962;266(15):737-743.

381. Davies JM, Lewis MPN, Wimperis J, et al. Review of guidelines for the prevention and treatment of infection in patients with an absent or dysfunctional spleen: prepared on behalf of the British committee for standards in haematology by a working party of the haemato-oncology task force. *Br J Haematol.* 2011;155(3):308-317.

382. American Academy of Pediatrics. Asplenia and functional asplenia. In: Kimberlin DW, Brady MT, Jackson MA, Long SS, eds. *Red Book: 2018 Report of the Committee on Infectious Diseases.* American Academy of Pediatrics; 2018.

383. Hathirat P, Mahaphan W, Chuansumrit A, et al. Platelet counts in thalassemic children before and after splenectomy. *Southeast Asian J Trop Med Public Health.* 1993;24(suppl 1):213-215.

384. Salter PP, Sherlock EC. Splenectomy, thrombocytosis, and venous thrombosis. *Am Surg.* 1957;23(6):549-554.

385. Palkar AV, Agrawal A, Verma S, et al. Post splenectomy related pulmonary hypertension. *World J Respirol.* 2015;5(2):69-77.

386. de Montalembert M, Girot R, Revillon Y, et al. Partial splenectomy in homozygous beta thalassaemia. *Arch Dis Child.* 1990;65(3):304.

387. Borgna-Pignatti C, Stefano PD, Bongo IG, Avato F, Cazzola M. Spleen iron content is low in thalassemia. *Am J Pediatr Hematol Oncol.* 1984;6(3):340-342.

388. Brewer CJ, Coates TD, Wood JC. Spleen R2 and R2* in iron-overloaded patients with sickle cell disease and thalassemia major. *J Magn Reson Imaging.* 2009;29(2):357-364.

389. Telfer P. Update on survival in thalassemia major. *Hemoglobin.* 2009;33(suppl 1):S76-S80.

390. Borgna-Pignatti C. The life of patients with thalassemia major. *Haematologica.* 2010;95(3):345-348.

391. Ladis V, Chouliaras G, Berdoukas V, et al. Survival in a large cohort of Greek patients with transfusion-dependent beta thalassaemia and mortality ratios compared to the general population. *Eur J Haematol.* 2011;86(4):332-338.

392. Telfer P, Coen PG, Christou S, et al. Survival of medically treated thalassemia patients in Cyprus. Trends and risk factors over the period 1980-2004. *Haematologica.* 2006;91:1187-1192.

393. Ballas SK, Zeidan AM, Duong VH, DeVeaux M, Heeney MM. The effect of iron chelation therapy on overall survival in sickle cell disease and β-thalassemia: a systematic review. *Am J Hematol.* 2018;93(7):943-952.

394. Politis C, Palma AD, Fisfis M, et al. Social integration of the older thalassaemic patient. *Arch Dis Child.* 1990;65(9):984.

395. Sobota A, Yamashita R, Xu Y, et al. Quality of life in thalassemia: a comparison of SF-36 results from the thalassemia longitudinal cohort to reported literature and the US norms. *Am J Hematol.* 2011;86(1):92-95.

396. Pakbaz Z, Treadwell M, Kim HY, et al. Education and employment status of children and adults with thalassemia in North America. *Pediatr Blood Cancer.* 2010;55(4):678-683.

397. Lucarelli G, Galimberti M, Polchi P, et al. Bone marrow transplantation in patients with thalassemia. *N Engl J Med.* 1990;322(7):417-421.

398. Lucarelli G, Clift RA, Galimberti M, et al. Marrow transplantation for patients with thalassemia: results in class 3 patients. *Blood.* 1996;87(5):2082-2088.

399. Baronciani D, Angelucci E, Potschger U, et al. Hemopoietic stem cell transplantation in thalassemia: a report from the European society for blood and bone marrow transplantation hemoglobinopathy registry, 2000-2010. *Bone Marrow Transplant.* 2016;51(4):536-541.

400. Sabloff M, Chandy M, Wang Z, et al. HLA-matched sibling bone marrow transplantation for beta-thalassemia major. *Blood.* 2011;117(5):1745-1750.

401. Li C, Mathews V, Kim S, et al. Related and unrelated donor transplantation for β-thalassemia major: results of an international survey. *Blood Adv.* 2019;3(17):2562-2570.

402. Gaziev J, Sodani P, Polchi P, Andreani M, Lucarelli G. Bone marrow transplantation in adults with thalassemia: treatment and long-term follow-up. *Ann N Y Acad Sci.* 2005;1054(1):196-205.

403. Gaziev D, Galimberti M, Lucarelli G, et al. Bone marrow transplantation from alternative donors for thalassemia: HLA-phenotypically identical relative and HLA-nonidentical sibling or parent transplants. *Bone Marrow Transplant.* 2000;25(8):815-821.

404. Nasa GL, Littera R, Locatelli F, et al. Status of donor-recipient HLA class I ligands and not the KIR genotype is predictive for the outcome of unrelated hematopoietic stem cell transplantation in beta-thalassemia patients. *Biol Blood Marrow Transplant.* 2007;13(11):1358-1368.

405. Locatelli F, Littera R, Pagliara D, et al. Outcome of unrelated donor bone marrow transplantation for thalassemia major patients. *Blood.* 2011;118(21):149.

406. Sun L, Wang N, Chen Y, et al. Unrelated donor peripheral blood stem cell transplantation for patients with β-thalassemia major based on a novel conditioning regimen. *Biol Blood Marrow Transplant.* 2019;25(8):1592-1596.

407. Orrù S, Orrù N, Manolakos E, et al. Recipient CTLA-4*CT60-AA genotype is a prognostic factor for acute graft-versus-host disease in hematopoietic stem cell transplantation for thalassemia. *Hum Immunol.* 2012;73(3-2):282-286.

408. Bernardo ME, Piras E, Vacca A, et al. Allogeneic hematopoietic stem cell transplantation in thalassemia major: results of a reduced-toxicity conditioning regimen based on the use of treosulfan. *Blood.* 2012;120(2):473-476.

409. Shenoy S, Walters MC, Ngwube A, et al. Unrelated donor transplantation in children with thalassemia using reduced-intensity conditioning: the URTH trial. *Biol Blood Marrow Transplant.* 2018;24(6):1216-1222.

410. King AA, Kamani N, Bunin N, et al. Successful matched sibling donor marrow transplantation following reduced intensity conditioning in children with hemoglobinopathies. *Am J Hematol.* 2015;90(12):1093-1098.

411. Galimberti M, Andreani M, Lucarelli G, et al. Patterns of graft rejection after bone marrow transplant in thalassemia. *Prog Clin Biol Res.* 1989;309:223-229.

412. Andreani M, Nesci S, Lucarelli G, et al. Long-term survival of ex-thalassemic patients with persistent mixed chimerism after bone marrow transplantation. *Bone Marrow Transplant.* 2000;25(4):401-404.

413. Andreani M, Manna M, Lucarelli G, et al. Persistence of mixed chimerism in patients transplanted for the treatment of thalassemia. *Blood.* 1996;87(8):3494-3499.

414. Fouzia NA, Edison ES, Lakshmi KM, et al. Long-term outcome of mixed chimerism after stem cell transplantation for thalassemia major conditioned with busulfan and cyclophosphamide. *Bone Marrow Transplant.* 2018;53(2):169-174.

415. Locatelli F, Kabbara N, Ruggeri A, et al. Outcome of patients with hemoglobinopathies given either cord blood or bone marrow transplantation from an HLA-identical sibling. *Blood.* 2013;122(6):1072-1078.

416. Wagner JE, Barker JN, DeFor TE, et al. Transplantation of unrelated donor umbilical cord blood in 102 patients with malignant and nonmalignant diseases: influence of CD34 cell dose and HLA disparity on treatment-related mortality and survival. *Blood.* 2002;100(5):1611-1618.

417. Anurathapan U, Hongeng S, Pakakasama S, et al. Hematopoietic stem cell transplantation for severe thalassemia patients from haploidentical donors using a novel conditioning regimen. *Biol Blood Marrow Transplant.* 2020;26(6):1106-1112.

Disorders of Red Blood Cells

418. Jaing TH, Hung IJ, Yang CP, et al. Unrelated cord blood transplantation for thalassaemia: a single-institution experience of 35 patients. *Bone Marrow Transplant.* 2012;47(1):33-39.

419. Ghavamzadeh A, Iravani M, Ashouri A, et al. Peripheral blood versus bone marrow as a source of hematopoietic stem cells for allogeneic transplantation in children with class I and II beta thalassemia major. *Biol Blood Marrow Transplant.* 2008;14(3):301-308.

420. Djavid G, Paola P, Maria G, et al. Graft-versus-host disease after bone marrow transplantation for thalassemia. *Transplantation.* 1997;63(6):854-860.

421. Simone MD, Verrotti A, Iughetti L, et al. Final height of thalassemic patients who underwent bone marrow transplantation during childhood. *Bone Marrow Transplant.* 2001;28(2):201-205.

422. Cohen A, Rovelli A, Bakker B, et al. Final height of patients who underwent bone marrow transplantation for hematological disorders during childhood: a study by the Working Party for Late Effects-EBMT. *Blood.* 1999;93(12):4109-4115.

423. Sanctis VD, Galimberti M, Lucarelli G, et al. Pubertal development in thalassaemic patients after allogeneic bone marrow transplantation. *Eur J Pediatr.* 1993;152(12):993-997.

424. Borgna-Pignatti C, Marradi P, Rugolotto S, Marcolongo A. Successful pregnancy after bone marrow transplantation for thalassaemia. *Bone Marrow Transplant.* 1996;18(1):235-236.

425. Balduzzi A, Dalle JH, Jahnukainen K, et al. Fertility preservation issues in pediatric hematopoietic stem cell transplantation: practical approaches from the consensus of the Pediatric Diseases Working Party of the EBMT and the International BFM Study Group. *Bone Marrow Transplant.* 2017;52(10):1406-1415.

426. Leonel ECR, Lucci CM, Amorim CA. Cryopreservation of human ovarian tissue: a review. *Transfus Med Hemother.* 2019;46(3):173-181.

427. Santarone S, Pepe A, Meloni A, et al. Secondary solid cancer following hematopoietic cell transplantation in patients with thalassemia major. *Bone Marrow Transplant.* 2018;53(1):39-43.

428. Sahlstedt L, Ebeling F, Bonsdorff LV, Parkkinen J, Ruutu T. Non-transferrin-bound iron during allogeneic stem cell transplantation. *Br J Haematol.* 2001;113(3):836-838.

429. Lucarelli G, Angelucci E, Giardini C, et al. Fate of iron stores in thalassaemia after bone-marrow transplantation. *Lancet.* 1993;342(8884):1388-1391.

430. Li C, Lai D, Shing M, et al. Early iron reduction programme for thalassaemia patients after bone marrow transplantation. *Bone Marrow Transplant.* 2000;25(6):653-656.

431. Giardini C, Galimbbrti M, Lucarelli G, et al. Desferrioxamine therapy accelerates clearance of iron deposits after bone marrow transplantation for thalassaemia. *Br J Haematol.* 1995;89(4):868-873.

432. Yesilipek MA, Karasu G, Kazik M, Uygun V, Ozturk Z. Posttransplant oral iron-chelating therapy in patients with beta-thalassemia major. *Pediatr Hematol Oncol.* 2010;27(5):374-379.

433. Inati A, Kahale M, Sbeiti N, et al. One-year results from a prospective randomized trial comparing phlebotomy with deferasirox for the treatment of iron overload in pediatric patients with thalassemia major following curative stem cell transplantation. *Pediatr Blood Cancer.* 2017;64(1):188-196.

434. Aboobacker FN, Dixit G, Lakshmi KM, et al. Outcome of iron reduction therapy in ex-thalassemics. *PLoS One.* 2021;16(1):e0238793.

435. Caocci G, Efficace F, Ciotti F, et al. Prospective assessment of health-related quality of life in pediatric patients with beta-thalassemia following hematopoietic stem cell transplantation. *Biol Blood Marrow Transplant.* 2011;17(6):861-866.

436. Suragani RN, Cadena SM, Cawley SM, et al. Transforming growth factor-β superfamily ligand trap ACE-536 corrects anemia by promoting late-stage erythropoiesis. *Nat Med.* 2014;20(4):408-414.

437. Cappellini MD, Viprakasit V, Taher AT, et al. A phase 3 trial of luspatercept in patients with transfusion-dependent β-thalassemia. *N Engl J Med.* 2020;382(13):1219-1231.

438. Cappellini MD, Porter J, Origa R, et al. Sotatercept, a novel transforming growth factor beta ligand trap, improves anemia in beta-thalassemia: a phase 2, open-label, dose-finding study. *Haematologica.* 2019;104(3):477-484.

439. Steinberg MH. Fetal hemoglobin in sickle cell anemia. *Blood.* 2020;136(21):2392-2400.

440. Pace BS, Liu L, Li B, Makala LH. Cell signaling pathways involved in drug-mediated fetal hemoglobin induction: strategies to treat sickle cell disease. *Exp Biol Med.* 2015;240(8):1050-1064.

441. Musallam KM, Taher AT, Cappellini MD, Sankaran VG. Clinical experience with fetal hemoglobin induction therapy in patients with beta-thalassemia. *Blood.* 2013;121(12):2199-2212, quiz 2372.

442. Lavelle D, Engel JD, Saunthararajah Y. Fetal hemoglobin induction by epigenetic drugs. *Semin Hematol.* 2018;55(2):60-67.

443. Ley TJ, DeSimone J, Anagnou NP, et al. 5-Azacytidine selectively increases γ-globin synthesis in a patient with β+ thalassemia. *N Engl J Med.* 1982;307(24):1469-1475.

444. Dunbar C, Travis W, Kan YW, Nienhuis A. 5-Azacytidine treatment in a βo-thalassaemic patient unable to be transfused due to multiple alloantibodies. *Br J Haematol.* 1989;72(3):467.

445. Olivieri NF, Saunthararajah Y, Thayalasuthan V, et al. A pilot study of subcutaneous decitabine in beta-thalassemia intermedia. *Blood.* 2011;118(10):2708-2711.

446. Kalantri SA, Ray R, Chattopadhyay A, et al. Efficacy of decitabine as hemoglobin F inducer in HbE/β-thalassemia. *Ann Hematol.* 2018;97(9):1689-1694.

447. Collins AF, Pearson HA, Giardina P, et al. Oral sodium phenylbutyrate therapy in homozygous beta thalassemia: a clinical trial. *Blood.* 1995;85(1):43-49.

448. Sher GD, Ginder GD, Little J, et al. Extended therapy with intravenous arginine butyrate in patients with β-hemoglobinopathies. *N Engl J Med.* 1995;332(24):1606-1610.

449. Rachmilewitz EA, Aker M, Perry D, Dover G. Sustained increase in haemoglobin and RBC following long-term administration of recombinant human erythropoietin to patients with homozygous beta-thalassaemia. *Br J Haematol.* 1995;90(2):341-545.

450. Singer ST, Vichinsky EP, Sweeters N, Rachmilewitz E. Darbepoetin alfa for the treatment of anaemia in alpha- or beta- thalassaemia intermedia syndromes. *Br J Haematol.* 2011;154(2):281-284.

451. Algiraigri AH, Wright NAM, Paolucci EO, Kassam A. Hydroxyurea for lifelong transfusion-dependent β-thalassemia: a meta-analysis. *Pediatr Hematol Oncol.* 2017;34(8):1-14.

452. Algiraigri AH, Wright NAM, Paolucci EO, Kassam A. Hydroxyurea for nontransfusion-dependent β-thalassemia: a systematic review and meta-analysis. *Hematol Oncol Stem Cell Ther.* 2017;10(3):116-125.

453. McArthur JG, Svenstrup N, Chen C, et al. A novel, highly potent and selective phosphodiesterase-9 inhibitor for the treatment of sickle cell disease. *Haematologica.* 2020;105(3):623-631.

454. Andemariam B, Bronte L,Gordeuk V, et al. The safety, pharmacokinetics & pharmacodynamic effects of IMR-687, a highly-selective PDE9 inhibitor, in adults with sickle cell disease: phase-2A placebo-controlled & open-label extension studies. Abstract S263. Presented at the EHA 2021 Virtual Congress, June 9-17, 2021. Accessed June 27, 2021. https://imaratx.com/wp-content/uploads/2021/06/Imara-EHA-2021-Presentation.pdf

455. Walters MC. Induction of fetal hemoglobin by gene therapy. *N Engl J Med.* 2021;384(3):284-285.

456. Canver MC, Smith EC, Sher F, et al. BCL11A enhancer dissection by Cas9-mediated in situ saturating mutagenesis. *Nature.* 2015;527(7577):192-197.

457. Brendel C, Guda S, Renella R, et al. Lineage-specific BCL11A knock-down circumvents toxicities and reverses sickle phenotype. *J Clin Invest.* 2016;126(10):3868-3878.

458. Traxler EA, Yao Y, Wang YD, et al. A genome-editing strategy to treat β-hemoglobinopathies that recapitulates a mutation associated with a benign genetic condition. *Nat Med.* 2016;22(9):987-990.

459. Wienert B, Funnell APW, Norton LJ, et al. Editing the genome to introduce a beneficial naturally occurring mutation associated with increased fetal globin. *Nat Commun.* 2015;6(1):7085.

460. Kohn DB, Sadelain M, Glorioso JC. Occurrence of leukaemia following gene therapy of X-linked SCID. *Nat Rev Cancer.* 2003;3(7):477-488.

461. Cavazzana-Calvo M, Payen E, Negre O, et al. Transfusion independence and HMGA2 activation after gene therapy of human β-thalassaemia. *Nature.* 2010;467(7313):318-322.

462. Thompson AA, Walters MC, Kwiatkowski J, et al. Gene therapy in patients with transfusion-dependent β-thalassemia. *N Engl J Med.* 2018;378(16):1479-1493.

463. Marktel S, Scaramuzza S, Cicalese MP, et al. Intrabone hematopoietic stem cell gene therapy for adult and pediatric patients affected by transfusion-dependent ß-thalassemia. *Nat Med.* 2019;25(2):234-241.

464. Frangoul H, Altshuler D, Cappellini MD, et al. CRISPR-Cas9 gene editing for sickle cell disease and beta-thalassemia. *N Engl J Med.* 2021;384(3):252-260.

465. Luo H, Chui DHK. Diverse hematological phenotypes of β-thalassemia carriers. *Ann N Y Acad Sci.* 2016;1368(1):49-55.

466. van der Weyden MB, Fong H, Hallam LJ, Harrison C. Red cell ferritin and iron overload in heterozygous beta-thalassemia. *Am J Hematol.* 1989;30(4):201-205.

467. Martins R, Picanço I, Fonseca A, et al. The role of HFE mutations on iron metabolism in beta-thalassemia carriers. *J Hum Genet.* 2004;49(12):651-655.

468. Gallerani M, Scapoli C, Cicognani I, et al. Thalassaemia trait and myocardial infarction: low infarction incidence in male subjects confirmed. *J Intern Med.* 1991;230(2):109-111.

469. Maioli M, Vigna GB, Tonolo G, et al. Plasma lipoprotein composition, apolipoprotein(a) concentration and isoforms in β-thalassemia. *Atherosclerosis.* 1997;131(1):127-133.

470. Rosatelli C, Leoni GB, Tuveri T, et al. Heterozygous β-thalassemia: relationship between the hematological phenotype and the type of β-thalassemia mutation. *Am J Hematol.* 1992;39(1):1-4.

471. Mazza U, Saglio G, Cappio FC, et al. Clinical and haematological data in 254 cases of beta-thalassaemia trait in Italy. *Br J Haematol.* 1976;33(1):91-99.

472. Millard DP, Mason K, Serjeant BE, Serjeant GR. Comparison of haematological features of the β0 and β+ thalassaemia traits in Jamaican negroes. *Br J Haematol.* 1977;36(2):161-170.

473. Borgna-Pignatti C, Zonta L, Bongo I, Stefano PD. Red blood cell indices in adults and children with heterozygous beta-thalassemia. *Haematologica.* 1983;68(2):149-156.

474. Bernini L, Latte B, Siniscalco M, et al. Survival of 51Cr-labelled red cells in subjects with thalassaemia-trait or G6PD deficiency or both abnormalities. *Br J Haematol.* 1964;10(2):171-180.

475. Galanello R, Melis MA, Ruggeri R, Cao A. Prospective study of red blood cell indices, hemoglobin A2, and hemoglobin F in infants heterozygous for β-thalassemia. *J Pediatr.* 1981;99(1):105-108.

476. Shepard MK, Weatherall DJ, Conley CL. Semi-quantitative estimation of the distribution of fetal hemoglobin in red cell populations. *B Johns Hopkins Hosp.* 1962;110:293-310.

477. Melis MA, Pirastu M, Galanello R, et al. Phenotypic effect of heterozygous alpha and beta 0-thalassemia interaction. *Blood.* 1983;62(1):226-229.

478. Galanello R, Barella S, Ideo A, et al. Genotype of subjects with borderline hemoglobin A2 levels: implication for, β-thalassemia carrier screening. *Am J Hematol.* 1994;46(2):79-81.

479. Bianco I, Cappabianca MP, Foglietta E, et al. Silent thalassemias: genotypes and phenotypes. *Haematologica.* 1997;82(3):269-280.

480. Galanello R, Paglietti ME, Addis M, et al. Pitfalls in genetic counselling for β-thalassemia: an individual with 4 different thalassemia mutations. *Clin Genet.* 1988;33(3):151-155.

481. Verhovsek M, So C, O'Shea T, et al. Is HbA2 level a reliable diagnostic measurement for β-thalassemia trait in people with iron deficiency? *Am J Hematol.* 2012;87(1):114-116.

482. Gianni AM, Bregni M, Cappellini MD, et al. A gene controlling fetal hemoglobin expression in adults is not linked to the non-alpha globin cluster. *EMBO J.* 1983;2(6):921-925.

483. Traeger-Synodinos J, Harteveld CL, Old JM, et al. EMQN Best Practice Guidelines for molecular and haematology methods for carrier identification and prenatal diagnosis of the haemoglobinopathies. *Eur J Hum Genet.* 2015;23(4):426-437.

484. Galanello R, Barella S, Gasperini D, et al. Evaluation of an automatic HPLC analyser for thalassemia and haemoglobin variants screening. *J Automatic Chem.* 1995;17(2):73-76.

485. Brancaleoni V, Pierro ED, Motta I, Cappellini MD. Laboratory diagnosis of thalassemia. *Int J Lab Hematol.* 2016;38(S1):32-40.

486. Vehapoglu A, Ozgurhan G, Demir AD, et al. Hematological indices for differential diagnosis of beta thalassemia trait and iron deficiency anemia. *Anemia.* 2014;2014:576738.

487. Mosca A, Paleari R, Galanello R, et al. New analytical tools and epidemiological data for the identification of HbA2 borderline subjects in the screening for beta-thalassemia. *Bioelectrochemistry.* 2008;73(2):137-140.

488. Perseu L, Satta S, Moi P, et al. KLF1 gene mutations cause borderline HbA2. *Blood.* 2011;118(16):4454-4458.

489. Old J, Henderson S. Molecular diagnostics for haemoglobinopathies. *Expert Opin Med Diagn.* 2010;4(3):225-240.

490. Fucharoen G, Yooyen K, Chaibunruang A, Fucharoen S. A newly modified hemoglobin H inclusion test as a secondary screening for α⁰-thalassemia in Southeast asian populations. *Acta Haematol.* 2014;132(1):10-14.

491. Galanello R, Sollaino C, Paglietti E, et al. α-thalassemia carrier identification by DNA analysis in the screening for thalassemia. *Am J Hematol.* 1998;59(4):273-278.

492. Lafferty JD, Crowther MA, Waye JS, Chui DHK. A reliable screening test to identify adult carriers of the (−SEA) alpha0-thalassemia deletion. Detection of embryonic zeta-globin chains by enzyme-linked immunosorbent assay. *Am J Clin Pathol.* 2000;114(6):927-931.

493. Luo HY, Clarke BJ, Gauldie J, et al. A novel monoclonal antibody based diagnostic test for alpha-thalassemia-1 carriers due to the (-SEA/) deletion. *Blood.* 1988;72(5):1589-1594.

494. Vichinsky E. Hemoglobin E syndromes. *Hematology.* 2007;2007(1):79-83.

495. Frischer H, Bowman J. Hemoglobin E, an oxidatively unstable mutation. *J Lab Clin Med.* 1975;85(4):531-539.

496. Rosatelli MC, Saba L. Prenatal diagnosis of β-thalassemias and hemoglobinopathies. *Mediterr J Hematol Infect Dis.* 2009;1(1):e2009011.

497. Salomon LJ, Sotiriadis A, Wulff CB, Odibo A, Akolekar R. Risk of miscarriage following amniocentesis or chorionic villus sampling: systematic review of literature and updated meta-analysis. *Ultrasound Obstet Gynecol.* 2019;54(4):442-451.

498. Ge H, Huang X, Li X, et al. Noninvasive prenatal detection for pathogenic CNVs: the application in alpha-thalassemia. *PLoS One.* 2013;8(6):e67464.

499. Jiang F, Liu W, Zhang L, et al. Noninvasive prenatal testing for beta-thalassemia by targeted nanopore sequencing combined with relative haplotype dosage (RHDO): a feasibility study. *Sci Rep.* 2021;11(1):5714.

500. Chen C, Li R, Sun J, et al. Noninvasive prenatal testing of alpha-thalassemia and beta-thalassemia through population-based parental haplotyping. *Genome Med.* 2021;13(1):18.

501. Vrettou C, Kakourou G, Mamas T, Traeger-Synodinos J. Prenatal and preimplantation diagnosis of hemoglobinopathies. *Int J Lab Hematol.* 2018;40:74-82.

502. Monni G, Peddes C, Iuculano A, Ibba RM. From prenatal to preimplantation genetic diagnosis of β-thalassemia. Prevention model in 8748 cases: 40 Years of single center experience. *J Clin Med.* 2018;7(2):35.

503. Angastiniotis M, Petrou M, Loukopoulos D, et al. The prevention of thalassemia revisited: a historical and ethical perspective by the thalassemia international federation. *Hemoglobin.* 2021;45(1):5-12.

504. Ho PJ, Hall GW, Luo LY, Weatherall DJ, Thein SL. Beta-thalassaemia intermedia: is it possible consistently to predict phenotype from genotype? *Br J Haematol.* 1998;100(1):70-78.

505. Panigrahi I, Marwaha RK, Kulkarni K. The expanding spectrum of thalassemia intermedia. *Hematology.* 2013;14(6):311-314.

506. Gonzalez-Redondo JM, Stoming TA, Lanclos KD, et al. Clinical and genetic heterogeneity in black patients with homozygous beta-thalassemia from the southeastern United States. *Blood.* 1988;72(3):1007-1014.

507. Cao A, Galanello R. Beta-thalassemia. *Genet Med.* 2010;12(2):61-76.

508. Safaya S, Rieder RF, Dowling CE, Kazazian HH, Adams JG. Homozygous beta-thalassemia without anemia. *Blood.* 1989;73(1):324-328.

509. Rosatelli MC, Pischedda A, Meloni A, et al. Homozygous β-thalassaemia resulting in the β-thalassaemia carrier state phenotype. *Br J Haematol.* 1994;88(3):562-565.

510. Wainscoat JS, Kanavakis E, Wood WG, et al. Thalassaemia intermedia in Cyprus: the interaction of α and β thalassaemia. *Br J Haematol.* 1983;53(3):411-416.

511. Winichagoon P, Fucharoen S, Weatherall D, Wasi P. Concomitant inheritance of alpha-thalassemia in beta 0- thalassemia/Hb E disease. *Am J Hematol.* 1985;20(3):217-222.

512. Efremov DG, Dimovski AJ, Huisman TH. The -158 (C→T) promoter mutation is responsible for the increased transcription of the 3' gamma gene in the Atlanta type of hereditary persistence of fetal hemoglobin. *Blood.* 1994;83(11):3350-3355.

513. Efremov DG, Dimovski AJ, Baysal E, et al. Possible factors influencing the haemoglobin and fetal haemoglobin levels in patients with β-thalassaemia due to a homozygosity for the IVS-I-6 (T→C) mutation. *Br J Haematol.* 1994;86(4):824-830.

514. Garner C, Mitchell J, Hatzis T, et al. Haplotype mapping of a major quantitative-trait locus for fetal hemoglobin production, on chromosome 6q23. *Am J Hum Genet.* 1998;62(6):1468-1474.

515. Sedgewick AE, Timofeev N, Sebastiani P, et al. BCL11A is a major HbF quantitative trait locus in three different populations with β-hemoglobinopathies. *Blood Cells Mol Dis.* 2008;41(3):255-258.

516. Thein SL, Hesketh C, Taylor P, et al. Molecular basis for dominantly inherited inclusion body beta-thalassemia. *Proc Natl Acad Sci U S A.* 1990;87(10):3924-3928.

517. Thein SL. Structural variants with a beta thalassaemia phenotype. In: Steinberg MH, Forget BG, Higgs DR, Nagel RL. eds. *Disorders of Hemoglobin: Genetics, Pathophysiology, and Clinical Management.* Cambridge University Press; 2001:342-355.

518. Badens C, Mattei M, Imbert A, et al. A novel mechanism for thalassaemia intermedia. *Lancet.* 2002;359(9301):132-133.

519. Camaschella C, Kattamis AC, Petroni D, et al. Different hematological phenotypes caused by the interaction of triplicated alpha-globin genes and heterozygous beta-thalassemia. *Am J Hematol.* 1997;55(2):83-88.

520. Ray R, Kalantri SA, Bhattacharjee S, et al. Association of alpha hemoglobin-stabilizing protein (AHSP) gene mutation and disease severity among HbE-beta thalassemia patients. *Ann Hematol.* 2019;98(8):1827-1834.

521. Modell B, Berdoukas V. *The Clinical Approach to Thalassaemia.* Grune and Stratton; 1983.

522. Borgna-Pignatti C, Marsella M, Zanforlin N. The natural history of thalassemia intermedia. *Ann N Y Acad Sci.* 2010;1202(1):214-220.

523. Cao A. Diagnosis of beta-thalassemia intermedia at presentation. *Birth Defects Orig Artic Ser.* 1988;23(5B):219-226.

524. Dore F, Cianciulli P, Rovasio S, et al. Incidence and clinical study of ectopic erythropoiesis in adult patients with thalassemia intermedia. *Ann Ital Med Int.* 1992;7(3):137-140.

525. Ieri T, Azk F, Ertem M, Uysal Z, Gozdasoglu S. Extramedullary hematopoiesis with spinal cord compression in a child with thalassemia intermedia. *J Pediatr Hematol Oncol.* 2009;31(9):681-683.

526. Haidar R, Mhaidli H, Taher AT. Paraspinal extramedullary hematopoiesis in patients with thalassemia intermedia. *Eur Spine J.* 2010;19(6):871-878.

527. Taher A, Skouri H, Jaber W, Kanj N. Extramedullary hematopoiesis in a patient with beta-thalassemia intermedia manifesting as symptomatic pleural effusion. *Hemoglobin.* 2001;25(4):363-368.

528. Meo A, Cassinerio E, Castelli R, et al. Effect of hydroxyurea on extramedullary haematopoiesis in thalassemia intermedia: case reports and literature review. *Int J Lab Hematol.* 2008;30(5):425-431.

529. Chehal A, Aoun E, Koussa S, et al. Hypertransfusion: a successful method of treatment in thalassemia intermedia patients with spinal cord compression secondary to extramedullary hematopoiesis. *Spine.* 2003;28(13):E245-E249.

530. Sanctis VD, Soliman AT, Elsefdy H, et al. Bone disease in beta thalassemia patients: past, present and future perspectives. *Metabolis.* 2018;80:66-79.

531. Salah NB, Bou-Fakhredin R, Mellouli F, Taher AT. Revisiting beta thalassemia intermedia: past, present, and future prospects. *Hematology.* 2017;22(10):607-616.

532. Taher AT, Musallam KM, Cappellini MD, Weatherall DJ. Optimal management of β thalassaemia intermedia. *Br J Haematol.* 2011;152(5):512-523.

533. Spanos T., Karageorga M, Ladis V, et al. Red cell alloantibodies in patients with thalassemia. *Vox Sang.* 1990;58(1):50-55.

534. Compernolle V, Chou ST, Tanael S, et al. Red blood cell specifications for patients with hemoglobinopathies: a systematic review and guideline. *Transfusion.* 2018;58(6):1555-1566.

535. Graziadei G, Refaldi C, Barcellini W, et al. Does absolute excess of alpha chains compromise the benefit of splenectomy in patients with thalassemia intermedia? *Haematologica.* 2012;97(1):151-153.

536. Pakbaz Z, Fischer R, Fung E, et al. Serum ferritin underestimates liver iron concentration in transfusion independent thalassemia patients as compared to regularly transfused thalassemia and sickle cell patients. *Pediatr Blood Cancer.* 2007;49(3):329-332.

537. Origa R, Barella S, Argiolas GM, et al. No evidence of cardiac iron in 20 never- or minimally-transfused patients with thalassemia intermedia. *Haematologica.* 2008;93(7):1095-1096.

538. Taher AT, Musallam KM, Wood JC, Cappellini MD. Magnetic resonance evaluation of hepatic and myocardial iron deposition in transfusion-independent thalassemia intermedia compared to regularly transfused thalassemia major patients. *Am J Hematol.* 2010;85(4):288-290.

539. Musallam KM, Cappellini MD, Wood JC, et al. Elevated liver iron concentration is a marker of increased morbidity in patients with beta thalassemia intermedia. *Haematologica.* 2011;96(11):1605-1612.

540. Taher AT, Porter JB, Viprakasit V, et al. Deferasirox demonstrates a dose-dependent reduction in liver iron concentration and consistent efficacy across subgroups of non-transfusion-dependent thalassemia patients. *Am J Hematol.* 2013;88(6):503-506.

541. Ricchi P, Meloni A, Pistoia L, et al. The effect of desferrioxamine chelation versus no therapy in patients with non transfusion-dependent thalassaemia: a multicenter prospective comparison from the MIOT network. *Ann Hematol.* 2018;97(10):1925-1932.

542. Pootrakul P, Sirankapracha P, Sankote J, et al. Clinical trial of deferiprone iron chelation therapy in β-thalassaemia/haemoglobin E patients in Thailand. *Br J Haematol.* 2017;122(2):305-310.

Disorders of Red Blood Cells

543. Nassar AH, Naja M, Cesaretti C, et al. Pregnancy outcome in patients with beta-thalassemia intermedia at two tertiary care centers, in Beirut and Milan. *Haematologica.* 2008;93(10):1586-1587.

544. Petrakos G, Andriopoulos P, Tsironi M. Pregnancy in women with thalassemia: challenges and solutions. *Int J Womens Health.* 2016;8:441-451.

545. Bennett M, Macri CJ, Bathgate SL. Erythropoietin use in a pregnant Jehovah's witness with anemia and beta-thalassemia: a case report. *J Reprod Med.* 2005;50(2):135-137.

546. (Goldschmidt) ZG, Wexler MR, Rachmilewitz EA. Juvenile leg ulceration in β-thalassemia major and intermedia. *Plast Reconstr Surg.* 1982;69(2):320-323.

547. Morris CR. Mechanisms of vasculopathy in sickle cell disease and thalassemia. *Hematology.* 2008;2008(1):177-185.

548. Fracchia E, Elkababri M, Cantello C, Gori A, Partsch H, Forni GL. Venous-like leg ulcers without venous insufficiency in congenital anemia: successful treatment using compression bandages. *Dermatol Surg.* 2010;36(8):1336-1340.

549. Levin C, Koren A. Healing of refractory leg ulcer in a patient with thalassemia intermedia and hypercoagulability after 14 years of unresponsive therapy. *Isr Med Assoc J.* 2011;13(5):316-318.

550. Aessopos A, Kati M, Tsironi M, Polonifi E, Farmakis D. Exchange blood transfusions for the treatment of leg ulcerations in thalassemia intermedia. *Haematologica.* 2006;91(5 suppl):ECR11.

551. Piga A, Perrotta S, Gamberini MR, et al. Luspatercept improves hemoglobin levels and blood transfusion requirements in a study of patients with β-thalassemia. *Blood.* 2019;133(12):1279-1289.

552. Taher AT, Musallam KM, Nasreddine W, et al. Asymptomatic brain magnetic resonance imaging abnormalities in splenectomized adults with thalassemia intermedia. *J Thromb Haemost.* 2010;8(1):54-59.

553. Cappellini MD, Grespi E, Cassinerio E, Bignamini D, Fiorelli G. Coagulation and splenectomy: an overview. *Ann N Y Acad Sci.* 2005;1054(1):317-324.

554. Taher AT, Musallam KM, Karimi M, et al. Splenectomy and thrombosis: the case of thalassemia intermedia. *J Thromb Haemost.* 2010;8(10):2152-2158.

555. Cappellini MD, Musallam KM, Marcon A, Taher AT. Coagulopathy in Beta-thalassemia: current understanding and future perspectives. *Mediterr J Hematol Infect Dis.* 2009;1(1):e2009029.

556. Borgna-Pignatti C, Vergine G, Lombardo T, et al. Hepatocellular carcinoma in the thalassaemia syndromes. *Br J Haematol.* 2017;124(1):114-117.

557. Galanello R, Piras S, Barella S, et al. Cholelithiasis and Gilbert's syndrome in homozygous β-thalassaemia. *Br J Haematol.* 2001;115(4):926-928.

558. Galanello R, Perseu L, Melis MA, et al. Hyperbilirubinaemia in heterozygous β-thalassaemia is related to co-inherited Gilbert's syndrome. *Br J Haematol.* 1997;99(2):433-436.

559. Aessopos A, Farmakis D, Karagiorga M, et al. Cardiac involvement in thalassemia intermedia: a multicenter study. *Blood.* 2001;97(11):3411-3416.

560. Vaccari M, Crepaz R, Fortini M, et al. Left ventricular remodeling, systolic function, and diastolic function in young adults with β-thalassemia intermedia A Doppler echocardiography study. *Chest.* 2002;121(2):506-512.

561. Singer ST, Kuypers FA, Styles L, et al. Pulmonary hypertension in thalassemia: association with platelet activation and hypercoagulable state. *Am J Hematol.* 2006;81(9):670-675.

562. Atichartakarn V, Likittanasombat K, Chuncharunee S, et al. Pulmonary arterial hypertension in previously splenectomized patients with β-thalassemic disorders. *Int J Hematol.* 2003;78(2):139-145.

563. Fraidenburg DR, Machado RF. Pulmonary hypertension associated with thalassemia syndromes. *Ann N Y Acad Sci.* 2017;1368(1):127-139.

564. Phrommintikul A, Sukonthasarn A, Kanjanavanit R, Nawarawong W. Splenectomy: a strong risk factor for pulmonary hypertension in patients with thalassaemia. *Heart.* 2006;92(10):1467.

565. Karimi M, Borzouee M, Mehrabani A, Cohan N. Echocardiographic finding in beta-thalassemia intermedia and major: absence of pulmonary hypertension following hydroxyurea treatment in beta-thalassemia intermedia. *Eur J Haematol.* 2009;82(3):213-218.

566. Littera R, Nasa GL, Derchi G, et al. Long-term treatment with oral sildenafil in a thalassemic patient with pulmonary hypertension. *Blood.* 2002;100(4):1516-1517.

567. Derchi G, Balocco M, Bina P, et al. Efficacy and safety of sildenafil for the treatment of severe pulmonary hypertension in patients with hemoglobinopathies: results from a long-term follow up. *Haematologica.* 2014;99(2):e17-e18.

568. Barst RJ, Mubarak KK, Machado RF, et al. Exercise capacity and haemodynamics in patients with sickle cell disease with pulmonary hypertension treated with bosentan: results of the ASSET studies. *Br J Haematol.* 2010;149(3):426-435.

569. Aessopos A, Samarkos M, Voskaridou E, et al. Arterial calcifications in β-thalassemia. *Angiology.* 1998;49(2):137-143.

570. Mojtahedzadeh F, Kosaryan M, Mahdavi MR, Akbari J. The effect of folic acid supplementation in beta-thalassemia major: a randomized placebo-controlled clinical trial. *Arch Iran Med.* 2006;9(3):266-268.

571. Motulsky AG. Frequency of sickling disorders in U.S. Blacks. *N Engl J Med.* 1973;288(1):31-33.

572. Tyagi S, Choudhry VP, Saxena R. Subclassification of HbS syndrome: is it necessary? *Clin Lab Haematol.* 2003;25(6):377-381.

573. Stevens MCG, Maude GH, Beckford M, et al. Haematological change in sickle cell–haemoglobin C disease and in sickle cell-beta thalassaemia: a cohort study from birth. *Br J Haematol.* 1985;60(2):279-292.

574. Goldstein LB, Adams R, Becker K, et al. Primary prevention of ischemic stroke. *Circulation.* 2001;103(1):163-182.

575. Koduri PR, Kovarik P. Acute splenic sequestration crisis in an adult with sickle beta-thalassemia. *Ann Hematol.* 2006;85(9):633-635.

576. Milner PF, Kraus AP, Sebes JI, et al. Sickle cell disease as a cause of osteonecrosis of the femoral head. *N Engl J Med.* 1991;325(21):1476-1481.

577. Clarkson JG. The ocular manifestations of sickle-cell disease: a prevalence and natural history study. *Trans Am Ophthalmol Soc.* 1992;90:481-504.

578. Ngo DA, Aygun B, Akinsheye I, et al. Fetal haemoglobin levels and haematological characteristics of compound heterozygotes for haemoglobin S and deletional hereditary persistence of fetal haemoglobin. *Br J Haematol.* 2012;156(2):259-264.

579. Onimoe G, Smarzo C. HbS-Sicilian (δβ)0-Thalassemia: a rare variant of sickle cell. *Case Rep Hematol.* 2017;2017:9265396.

580. Seward DP, Ware RE, Kinney TR. Hemoglobin sickle-Lepore: report of two siblings and review of the literature. *Am J Hematol.* 1993;44(3):192-195.

581. Fairbanks VF, McCormick DJ, Kubik KS, et al. Hb S/Hb Lepore with mild sickling symptoms: a hemoglobin variant with mostly δ-chain sequences ameliorates sickle-cell disease. *Am J Hematol.* 1997;54(2):164-165.

582. Konotey-Ahulu FID, Ringelhann B. Sickle-cell anaemia, sickle-cell thalassaemia, sickle-cell haemoglobin C disease, and asymptomatic haemoglobin C thalassaemia in one Ghanaian family. *Br Med J.* 1969;1(5644):607.

583. Fattoum S, Guemira F, Abdennebi M, Abdeladhim AB. HbC/beta-thalassemia association. Eleven cases observed in Tunisia. Article in French. *Ann Pediatr (Paris).* 1993;40(1):45-48.

584. Sangare A, Sanogo I, Meite M, et al. Clinical and hematological profile of lepore hemoglobin in ivory coast. Article in French. *Med Trop (Mars).* 1994;54(1):43-46.

585. Fucharoen S, Weatherall DJ. The hemoglobin E thalassemias. *Cold Spring Harb Perspect Med.* 2012;2(8):a011734.

586. Olivieri NF, Pakbaz Z, Vichinsky E. HbE/beta-thalassemia: basis of marked clinical diversity. *Hematol Oncol Clin North Am.* 2010;24(6):1055-1070.

587. Premawardhena A, Fisher C, Olivieri N, et al. Haemoglobin E β thalassaemia in Sri Lanka. *Lancet.* 2005;366(9495):1467-1470.

588. Rees DC, Styles L, Vichinsky EP, Clegg JB, Weatherall DJ. The hemoglobin E syndromes. *Ann N Y Acad Sci.* 1998;850(1):334-343.

589. Fucharoen S, Winichagoon P, Thonglairuam V, Wasi P. EF Bart's disease: interaction of the abnormal α- and β-globin genes. *Eur J Haematol.* 1988;40(1):75-78.

590. Allen A, Fisher C, Premawardhena A, et al. Adaptation to anemia in hemoglobin E-ss thalassemia. *Blood.* 2010;116(24):5368-5370.

591. Suriyun T, Kaewsakulthong W, Khamphikham P, et al. Association of the degree of erythroid expansion and maturation arrest with the clinical severity of β0-thalassemia/hemoglobin E patients. *Acta Haematol.* 2021:1-12.

592. Fucharoen S, Piankijagum A, Wasi P. Deaths in beta-thalassemia/Hb E patients secondary to infections. *Birth Defects Orig Artic Ser.* 1987;23(5A):495-500.

593. Aswapokee N, Aswapokee P, Fucharoen S, Wasi P. A study of infective episodes in patients with beta-thalassemia/Hb E disease in Thailand. *Birth Defects Orig Artic Ser.* 1987;23(5A):513-520.

594. Chandrcharoensin-Wilde C, Chairoongruang S, Jitnuson P, Fucharoen S, Vathanopas V. Gallstones in thalassemia. *Birth Defects Orig Artic Ser.* 1988;23(5B):263-267.

595. Wasi P, Fucharoen S, Youngchaiyud P, Sonakul D. Hypoxemia in thalassemia. *Birth Defects Orig Artic Ser.* 1982;18(7):213-217.

596. Sonakul D, Fucharoen S. Pulmonary thromboembolism in thalassemic patients. *Southeast Asian J Trop Med Public Health.* 1992;23(suppl 2):25-28.

597. Fucharoen S, Youngchaiyud P, Wasi P. Hypoxaemia and the effect of aspirin in thalassaemia. *Southeast Asian J Trop Med Public Health.* 1981;12(1):90-93.

598. Italia KY, Jijina FF, Merchant R, et al. Effect of hydroxyurea on the transfusion requirements in patients with severe HbE-β-thalassaemia: a genotypic and phenotypic study. *J Clin Pathol.* 2010;63(2):147.

599. Singer ST, Vichinsky EP, Larkin S, et al. Hydroxycarbamide-induced changes in E/beta thalassemia red blood cells. *Am J Hematol.* 2008;83(11):842-845.

600. Luewan S, Srisupundit K, Tongsong T. Outcomes of pregnancies complicated by beta-thalassemia/hemoglobin E disease. *Int J Gynecol Obstet.* 2009;104(3):203-205.

601. Riewpaiboon A, Nuchprayoon I, Torcharus K, et al. Economic burden of beta-thalassemia/Hb E and beta-thalassemia major in Thai children. *BMC Res Notes.* 2010;3(1):29.

Chapter 36 ■ Hemoglobins With Altered Oxygen Affinity, Unstable Hemoglobins, M-Hemoglobins, and Dyshemoglobinemias

MADELEINE VERHOVSEK • MARTIN H. STEINBERG

Almost 1400 mutations affecting the globin subunits of hemoglobin have been described (http://globin.cse.psu.edu/). Among them, sickle cell disease along with hemoglobinopathies associated with HbE, HbC, and the β- and α-thalassemias are the most common single-gene disorders worldwide (see Chapters 34 and 35). Far less common are hemoglobin mutations discussed in this chapter that affect the ability of the molecule to bind and release oxygen (149 variants); reduce hemoglobin stability (153 variants); allow heme iron to be oxidized (13 variants). Exogenous agents can also oxidize normal hemoglobin, interfering with oxygen transport. Hemoglobin can also oxidize as a result of rare nonglobin gene–associated mutations. Most hematologists never encounter a patient with any of these rare genetic diseases. Anemia, hemolysis, erythrocytosis, abnormal pulse oximetry and/or cyanosis, not readily explained by more common causes, should bring these disorders to mind.

HEMOGLOBINS WITH ALTERED OXYGEN AFFINITY

Hemoglobin oxygen affinity is characterized by the amount of oxygen bound to hemoglobin at any given oxygen tension. P_{50}, the partial pressure of oxygen at which hemoglobin is 50% saturated, is a common measure of hemoglobin oxygen affinity. Oxygen affinity is modified by pH, temperature, and organic phosphates. The normal cooperativity of hemoglobin, or heme-heme interactions in the hemoglobin tetramer, determines the sigmoidal shape of the hemoglobin-oxygen dissociation curve. This is a result of the fact that the deoxygenated T (tense) form of hemoglobin has a lower affinity for oxygen than the oxygenated R (relaxed) form (see Chapter 6). Consequently, globin gene mutations that alter areas of the molecule involved with T-R interactions can lead to alterations in oxygen affinity. Both high- and low-oxygen-affinity hemoglobin variants are encountered, and any globin gene can be affected.

High-Oxygen-Affinity Hemoglobins

Globin gene mutations that increase the affinity of hemoglobin for oxygen usually cause erythrocytosis. One hundred one high-oxygen-affinity variants have been cataloged in the Hb Var database (https://globin.bx.psu.edu/hbvar/menu.html).[1] Familial erythrocytosis is a valuable clue to their presence; isolated cases are caused by new mutations. These mutations are dominant disorders, expressed clinically in the heterozygote. Homozygotes for α-globin variants will already have polycythemia in utero and at birth due to increased oxygen affinity of both fetal hemoglobin (HbF; $\alpha 2\gamma 2$) and the adult hemoglobin variant. One γ-globin variant (HbF-Monserrato-Sassari, HBG2 cys93arg) in a normal newborn and a possible δ-globin variant (Hb Noah Mehmet Oesteurk, HBD his143tyr) have also been described. Homozygotes for β-globin high-oxygen-affinity variants have been described, and these individuals can have more severe disease.[2-5] Compound heterozygotes with a high-oxygen-affinity β-globin variant and β^0-thalassemia can mimic homozygosity for the variant as normal adult hemoglobin A (HbA) is not present.

Pathophysiology

Hemoglobin is a tetrameric molecule with two α- and two non-α-globin chains. Stabilization of the R state of the hemoglobin tetramer, with its high affinity for oxygen, or destabilization of the low-oxygen-affinity T state is caused by globin gene mutations in critical areas that can effect R → T transitions (Table 36.1).[6] The increased avidity for oxygen (low P_{50}) of these variants reduces oxygen delivery to tissues, thereby stimulating erythropoietin production and increasing red cell mass. Patients with high-oxygen-affinity hemoglobins with erythrocytosis will have normal erythropoietin levels at steady state. However,

erythropoietin levels increase when they are phlebotomized to a normal red cell mass.[7,8] Individuals with these hemoglobin variants appear to be reasonably compensated for the low P_{50} by the increased red cell mass. Oxygen consumption and arterial pO_2 are normal, but in some cases there is reduced mixed venous pO_2 and decreased resting cardiac output.

Not unexpectedly, the JAK2 V617F mutation found in individuals with polycythemia vera is absent in patients with high-oxygen-affinity hemoglobin variant-induced erythropoiesis.[9]

Diagnosis

The diagnosis of high-oxygen-affinity hemoglobins is suspected by finding isolated erythrocytosis without accompanying leukocytosis, thrombocytosis, or splenomegaly, as seen in polycythemia vera. A family history of erythrocytosis is also suggestive of a high-oxygen-affinity hemoglobin variant. The differential diagnosis of increased red cell mass and other disorders expressed in the erythrocyte that cause isolated erythrocytosis are discussed in Chapter 45.

In a review of a 42-year reference laboratory experience, 762 patients were found to have 81 high-O_2-affinity variants. Up to half of the variants could not be isolated from HbA by a single hemoglobin protein-based diagnostic-like high-performance liquid chromatography (HPLC). This extensive experience employing many different diagnostic tests suggested the need for an algorithmic approach to diagnosis.[10] Determination of the red cell oxygen equilibrium curve and P_{50} is the benchmark for the diagnosis of erythrocytosis due to high-oxygen-affinity hemoglobins. The oxygen-binding characteristics of hybrid tetramers ($\alpha_2 \beta^A \beta^{var}$) are likely to be intermediate between purified HbA and purified variant, and the shape of the hemoglobin-oxygen dissociation curve can at times be biphasic. Measurement of blood P_{50} confirms the shift in the hemoglobin-oxygen dissociation curve. Rarely, the P_{50} of intact erythrocytes is normal, requiring study of dialyzed purified hemoglobin. An accurate P_{50} value is difficult to "calculate" from pO_2 data, and it is best to measure the pO_2 and hemoglobin saturation directly. P_{50} measurements are not widely available but can be done with several instruments.

High oxygen affinity is observed in both erythrocytes and purified dialyzed hemoglobin. The concentration of 2,3-bisphosphoglyceric acid (BPG) is normal, indicating that altered oxygen affinity is not caused by reduced levels of this modulator of hemoglobin function. This is in contrast to what is seen in the rare instance of red cell 2,3-BPG mutase deficiency, where both erythrocytes and whole blood have high oxygen affinity, while the oxygen affinity of the purified hemolysate stripped of 2,3-BPG is normal.[11]

HPLC may reveal an abnormal hemoglobin, but a normal study does not exclude the possibility of a high-affinity hemoglobin whose migration overlaps that of HbA. Testing with other hemoglobin separation methods, such as capillary zone electrophoresis or mass spectroscopy, may at times enable separation of the variant from HbA. As with most evaluations for rare abnormal hemoglobins, protein-based methods of variant detection are not often conclusive. Determining the DNA sequence of the globin genes provides the definitive information; it is also a prerequisite before genetic counseling.

Examples of high-oxygen-affinity hemoglobins that illustrate their varying mechanisms and heterogeneous phenotypes are discussed next. Understanding the structure of hemoglobin and the role of each residue in determining function allows a molecular explanation of most of their clinical abnormalities.

α-Globin Chain Variants

Because there are four α-globin genes, most stable α-globin variants form 25% or less of the total hemoglobin, compared with 40% to 50%

Table 36.1. Sites of Globin Mutation Associated With Increased Oxygen Affinity[a]

α1β2 Interface contacts (sliding contact) connecting α1β1 and α2β2 dimers
α1β1, α2β2 Interface
Mutations that reduce 2,3-BPG binding
Heme pocket mutations
Miscellaneous

[a]In addition to single amino acid substitutions, these mutations can include small deletions and insertions of amino acids, reading frameshifts, fusion globins, and elongated globin chains.

for stable β-globin variants. As a result, the clinical effects of α-globin variants are less striking than those of β-globin variants. However, the coinheritance of a β-thalassemia mutation can modulate the concentration of high-affinity α-variant hemoglobins and homozygosity for a high-oxygen-affinity variant affecting α-globin chains has been described.

Hb Chesapeake (*HBA* arg92leu) was the first reported high-affinity hemoglobin variant.[12] It was discovered in an 81-year-old patient with erythrocytosis, an abnormal hemoglobin detected by hemoglobin electrophoresis, and erythrocytes with increased oxygen affinity. Fifteen members of the proband's family were similarly affected. Hb Chesapeake represented ~20% of the total hemoglobin. With a P_{50} of 19 mm Hg (normal ~26 mm Hg), Hb Chesapeake produced moderate erythrocytosis. The mutation affected a residue that is invariant in all hemoglobins, which stabilizes the R state at the α1β2 area of contact, making the T state less favored.

Hb Nunobiki (*HBA1* arg141cys) is one of four mutations of this invariant residue, all of which exhibit high oxygen affinity and moderate to mild erythrocytosis.[13] This group of mutations represents an interesting cluster of variants that illustrates the effects of different mutations at the same amino acid position. As a mutant of the 3′-*HBA1* gene that is expressed to a lesser extent than the 5′-*HBA2* gene, Hb Nunobiki makes up ~13% of the hemolysate and is accompanied by only mild erythrocytosis. High oxygen affinity is a result of the breaking of the C terminal–to–C terminal salt bridge that is indispensable for the stabilization of the T state, favoring the R state.

β-Globin Chain Variants

All possible single-base mutations of the β99 site disturbing the α1β2 area of contact have been described and include Hb Kempsey (*HBB* asp99asn), Hb Yakima (asp99his), Hb Radcliffe (asp99ala), Hb Ypsilanti (asp99tyr), Hb Hotel-Dieu (asp99gly), Hb Chemilly (asp99val), and Hb Coimbra (asp99glu). As expected for stable β-globin chain variants, all are present at 40% to 50% of the hemolysate, exhibit moderately high oxygen affinity, and are characterized clinically by erythrocytosis. Hbs Kempsey, Radcliffe, and Hotel Dieu have a decreased response to 2,3-BPG. Hbs Ypsilanti and Radcliffe form stable hybrid tetramers in the hemolysates in which the abnormal β chains coexist with normal β chains.

Six of the possible seven mutations of the C-terminal CAC (his) codon have also been described. One of them, Hb Cochin-Port Royal (his146arg), has nearly normal oxygen affinity but decreased 2,3-BPG interaction and Bohr effect.[14]

Six mutations of β82 lys have been described: Hb Gàmbara (lys-82glu), Hb Tsurumai (lys82gln), Hb Taradale (lys82arg), Hb Rahere (lys82thr), Hb Helsinki (lys82met), and Hb Providence (lys82asn). All have moderately high oxygen affinity and mild to moderate erythrocytosis. These mutants have drastically reduced 2,3-BPG binding as a result of the elimination of one of the normal binding sites for this allosteric effector. Hb Pôrto Alegre (*HBB* ser9cys) has high oxygen affinity and a tendency to aggregate, but erythrocytosis is not present.[15] Polymerization of Hb Pôrto Alegre is based on the formation of disulfide bonds in oxygenated samples and is different from HbS polymerization. Polymerization of this mutant diminishes heme-heme interaction and increases the oxygen affinity.

Hb Tak (*HBB* 147(+AC)) is elongated by 11 amino acid residues because of a modified C-terminal sequence: 147thr-lys-leu-ala-phe-leu-leu-ser-asn-phe-157tyr-COOH).[16,17] It forms 40% of the hemolysate, has a very high oxygen affinity with no cooperativity, and has no allosteric interaction with pH or 2,3-BPG. The C terminus of the β-globin chain is actively involved in the conformational changes of the hemoglobin molecule by stabilizing the T state. By having these stabilizing interactions disrupted, Hb Tak is totally frozen in the R state. The extreme biphasic nature of the hemoglobin-oxygen affinity curve observed in mixtures of Hb Tak and HbA suggests that hybrid tetramer ($α_2β^Aβ^{Tak}$) formation is absent. The top portion of the oxygen equilibrium curve is normal, and it begins to be abnormal only at <40% saturation. Because physiologic oxygen exchange occurs most commonly above that level of saturation, the tissues may not be hypoxic, removing the stimulus for increased erythropoiesis.

Clinical Features

Patients with high-affinity hemoglobins and erythrocytosis may be asymptomatic without complications. Other patients may have symptoms of hyperviscosity (e.g., headaches) or history of unprovoked venous thromboembolism. Ruddy complexion is a common physical finding. Splenomegaly is typically absent. Hemoglobin concentration and hematocrit are increased variably, and usually only moderately, suggesting that modulation by variations in other genes might affect the physiologic response to hypoxia. Some patients with Hb Malmö (*HBB* his97gln) and Hb Potomac[18] have been symptomatic and have benefited from phlebotomy.[19] Long-term follow-up of larger numbers of patients in a rare disease registry would facilitate better understanding of the spectrum of severity and natural history of individuals with high-affinity variants.

Many cases of high-oxygen-affinity hemoglobins are first suspected during a routine hematologic examination or when the family of a proband known to have erythrocytosis is examined. In very limited studies, exercise capacity in the laboratory and the indices of working capacity and cardiac tolerance were similar in patients with high-oxygen-affinity hemoglobins and in controls.[20] It is postulated, however, that patients with high-affinity variants who have undergone phlebotomy therapy would have physiologic reduction in tissue oxygen delivery.

In a population-based study of erythrocytosis, high-oxygen-affinity variants accounted for 3% of all cases.[21] By promptly diagnosing high-affinity hemoglobins, unnecessary invasive diagnostic procedures and inappropriate therapeutic interventions, such as cardiac catheterization or cytotoxic medications, can be avoided. Patients have received ^{32}P treatment based on a mistaken diagnosis of polycythemia vera.

Increased morbidity or mortality in mothers with high-oxygen-affinity hemoglobins or their offspring has not been observed.[20] Low ambient pO_2, as in unpressurized airplanes and ascent to altitude, do not represent a risk, because high-affinity hemoglobins are avid for oxygen. Hypothetically, carriers should be less prone to "the bends" during deep sea diving, because of slower oxygen release during ascension.

Treatment

Patients with high-oxygen-affinity hemoglobins have physiologic compensation for their abnormality via increased baseline hemoglobin concentration, resulting in adequate tissue oxygen delivery despite increases in blood viscosity. Intervention is therefore rarely required. Exercise studies before and after phlebotomy in patients with Hb Osler (*HBB* tyr145asn), a variant with a P_{50} of 10 to 11 mm Hg and a hemoglobin concentration of ~22 g/dL, did not show an impairment after phlebotomy.[20] Limited studies have suggested that phlebotomy generally does not improve exercise performance. However, rare individuals appear to have benefited from phlebotomy, and thus other unknown factors may be interfering with their normal compensation for high hemoglobin oxygen affinity, and increased blood viscosity may have become a burden.[22] Prudence dictates that, before embarking on a regimen of chronic phlebotomy, one should be conservative and review the hematologic and physiologic findings at frequent intervals during the first few years after diagnosis. In older patients, special attention should be directed to blood flow and oxygen delivery to the heart and central nervous system. Thrombosis has been reported in individuals with high-oxygen-affinity variants but a causal relationship has not been established. In an example of a patient with a high-oxygen-affinity hemoglobin with concurrent β-thalassemia, treatment with hydroxyurea reduced the packed cell volume from 61% to 39% and increased HbF from 3.6% to 30% and P_{50} from 6 to 10 mm Hg.[23] This case should not be a recommendation for routine treatment of erythrocytosis due to high-oxygen-affinity hemoglobins with cytostatic agents.

Low-Oxygen-Affinity Hemoglobins

Hemoglobin variants with reduced affinity for oxygen are in many respects the converse of high-oxygen-affinity variants. Forty-eight low-oxygen-affinity variants have been described. They are expressed in the heterozygote, with homozygosity likely to be lethal. A frequent clinical feature is anemia that, in some cases, is accompanied by cyanosis.

Pathophysiology

Alterations of critical molecular regions involved directly in the R-T transition result in the stabilization of the deoxy T state or destabilization of the oxy R state. Low-oxygen-affinity hemoglobins deliver more O_2 to the tissues per gram of hemoglobin, and this is reflected by an oxygen-hemoglobin dissociation curve shifted toward the right of normal and an increase in P_{50}. When hemoglobin has a right-shifted or low-affinity curve, the difference between oxygen binding in the lungs at PO_2 levels of 100 mm Hg and unloading in the tissues at 40 mm Hg can be twice as great as the differences in a hemoglobin with a normal oxygen equilibrium curve. Patients with a moderately right-shifted oxygen equilibrium curve (P_{50} between 35 and 55 mm Hg) may be mildly anemic, but some individuals with P_{50} ~80 are not anemic, perhaps because of the peculiar shape of their oxygen equilibrium curve.[24] A right-shifted oxygen equilibrium curve leads to an increase in the synthesis of 2,3-BPG and a decrease in its destruction.

Diagnosis

The first report of a low-oxygen-affinity hemoglobin was Hb Kansas (*HBB* asn102thr), which presented with asymptomatic cyanosis without anemia.[25] Detection of a low-oxygen-affinity hemoglobin is part of the differential diagnosis of patients with central cyanosis (see later). Before undertaking extensive diagnostic procedures in cases of cyanosis that are not clearly the result of cardiovascular or pulmonary disease, fractionating hemoglobin by HPLC and measuring blood P_{50} is advisable. In individuals with low-oxygen-affinity variants, arterial blood gas typically reveals low arterial oxygen saturation (SaO_2) with normal partial pressure of oxygen (pO_2). A search for low-affinity hemoglobins as an explanation for anemia without cyanosis is less compelling, but if other investigations prove fruitless, unexplained normocytic anemia without reticulocytosis might be evaluated by measuring P_{50}.

A simple bedside test can distinguish cyanosis resulting from low-oxygen-affinity hemoglobins or cardiopulmonary cyanosis from that occurring with methemoglobinemia, M hemoglobins, or sulfhemoglobinemia. When blood from carriers of low-oxygen-affinity hemoglobins or patients with cardiopulmonary disease is exposed to ambient oxygen, it will turn from purple-greenish to bright red. In contrast, blood of patients with methemoglobinemia, sulfhemoglobinemia, or M hemoglobins will remain abnormally colored.

Clinically apparent cyanosis is observed only in carriers of low-oxygen-affinity variants with greatly right-shifted curves and where the variant comprises a substantial portion of the hemolysate. Cyanosis is present from birth in some low-oxygen-affinity hemoglobins due to α-globin chain mutants that affect all hemoglobins. In carriers of β-globin chain mutants, cyanosis may appear from the middle to the end of the first year of life as γ-globin gene expression and HbF synthesis wanes and is replaced by β-globin gene expression and HbA. Neonatal cyanosis has been associated with γ-globin variants that have low oxygen affinity.[26] Globin gene sequencing is the best means of definitive diagnosis.

Clinical Features

Four low-oxygen-affinity variants have been described at β102. Hb Kansas, the best-studied variant, has a whole-blood P_{50} of ~70 mm Hg, decreased cooperativity, and a normal Bohr effect.[25] The β102 asn residue is invariant among β-globin chains and participates in the only hydrogen bond between asn 102 and asp 94 across the α1β2 interface in oxyhemoglobin. This bond is broken when the molecule assumes the T state. The new thr residue is incapable of forming this bond, and low oxygen affinity results from destabilization of the R conformer. The changes induced by this substitution at the α1β2 interface allow Hb Kansas to dissociate into αβ dimers, the near opposite of the high-oxygen-affinity Hb Chesapeake.

Hb Beth Israel (*HBB* asn102ser) was found in a patient with asymptomatic cyanosis.[24] The P_{50} was 88 mm Hg, and SaO_2 was only 63% with a normal pO_2. The hemolysate also had a low oxygen affinity and a normal Bohr effect. Erythrocyte 2,3-BPG was mildly elevated. The molecular mechanism of reduced oxygen affinity is the same as for Hb Kansas, although the defect may be more disruptive locally, because the serine side chain is shorter than that of threonine.

Hb Bologna (*HBB* lys61met) is informative because it was present as a compound heterozygote with β0-thalassemia and comprised 90% of the hemolysate.[27] Adults were neither cyanotic nor anemic despite having a P_{50} of 37.6 mm Hg. During gestation, the high concentration of HbF makes it doubtful that this mutation would have an effect on fetal development.

Hb Bruxelles (*HBB* phe42del) is a low-oxygen-affinity, unstable variant hemoglobin resulting from deletion of the most conserved amino acid residue of hemoglobin.[28,29] Phenylalanine residues at β41 and β42 are conserved in all normal mammalian non-α-globin chains and are indispensable for the structural integrity and oxygen-binding functions of the molecule. From age 4 years, the index case of Hb Bruxelles had severe hemolytic anemia and cyanosis, requiring blood transfusion once. Later in life, her hemoglobin concentration stabilized at 10 g/dL. Reasons for this "switch" of phenotype are unknown. Other mutations of β41 and β42, which are predominately unstable hemoglobins, are discussed later.

Treatment

Treatment is not needed for these variants. The importance of early diagnosis is to avoid unnecessary workup and to alleviate concern for the patient and family.

UNSTABLE HEMOGLOBINS

The unstable hemoglobins result from globin chain mutations that cause hemoglobin tetramer instability and intracellular precipitation of its globin subunits. These intraerythrocytic precipitates are detectable by supravital staining and appear as globular aggregates called Heinz bodies. These inclusions reduce the life of the erythrocyte by binding to the membrane, decreasing cell deformability and increasing membrane permeability. The resultant hemolytic disorder is sometimes called congenital Heinz body hemolytic anemia. Heinz bodies and hemolysis also occurs with certain hereditary erythrocyte enzyme deficiencies (see Chapter 30). One hundred fifty-three unstable variants of both the β- and α-globin chains with widely varying clinical severity have been reported, almost always as heterozygotes for the mutation, although some homozygous cases have been reported. The major clinical features are anemia, reticulocytosis, pigmenturia, and splenomegaly.

Pathophysiology

The pathophysiology of unstable hemoglobins relates to the specific mutations leading to altered heme-globin interaction, the process of Heinz body formation, and destruction of red cells containing denatured hemoglobin.

Mutations That Alter Heme-Globin Interaction

Mutations that change the primary structure (amino acid sequence) of globin, depending on the substitution and its location, can alter the secondary structure (α-helical), the tertiary structure (folding of the globin chain), or the quaternary structure (interactions within the hemoglobin tetramer). The mechanisms that can lead to this hemoglobin instability are listed in *Table 36.2*.

Heme-globin interactions are vital for oxygen delivery and also contribute to molecular stability and intracellular solubility. For example, introduction of a charged amino acid residue into the heme pocket, a site normally formed by residues with nonpolar side chains, results in hemoglobin instability (e.g., Hb Bristol-Alesha *HBB* val67met). Mutations involving residues that interact directly with heme, such as those near the (F8) proximal histidine that reacts with heme-iron (e.g., Hb Köln *HBB* val98met), are associated with hemoglobin instability. Also, mutations associated with nontyrosine substitutions of the (E7) distal histidine (e.g., Hb Zürich *HBB* his63arg) cause molecular instability. An interesting effect of this is that the ligand-binding properties of iron are changed and Hb Zürich has a much higher affinity for CO.[30,31]

Disruption of the secondary structure reduces subunit solubility and is often a result of the introduction of proline residue than cannot be accommodated into the α-helix except in its first two positions. α-Helices comprise ~70% of a globin subunit and must be folded into a globin motif. Introduction of water into the molecule destroys its stability, and this can be caused by substitution of a charged residue, for example, alanine, for a nonpolar residue, such as proline (e.g., Hb Brockton *HBB* ala138pro).[32]

Loss of intersubunit contact hydrogen bonds or salt bridges in the α1β1 contact area will interfere with hemoglobin quaternary structure and also reduce stability. Dissociation of α1β1 contacts normally does not occur in red cells, whereas dissociation of α1β2 contact does take place. Dissociation of α1β1 dimers into monomers is normally minimal, as it generates methemoglobin and consequent instability. Dissociation of chains along the α1β1 contact generates α- and β-globin chains that uncoil, loosening their heme-globin interaction and favoring methemoglobin formation. Mutations affecting the α1β1 interface tend to be more unstable than those affecting the *α1β2* contact. Examples of unstable hemoglobin mutations that are due to decreased α1β1 contact include Hb Philly (*HBB* tyr35pro),[33] Hb Peterborough (*HBB* val111phe),[34] and Hb Stanmore (*HBB* val111ala).[35]

α-Hemoglobin-stabilizing protein (AHSP) binds free *α*-globin chains, protecting them from precipitation (see Chapter 6). In vitro studies suggest that the impaired interaction of AHSP with *α*-globin variants when the mutation lies in the molecular sites where ASHP binds *α*-globin might affect the stability of the variant. In these studies, recombinant Hb Groen Hart (*HBA* pro119ser), Hb Diamant (*HBA* pro-119leu), and *α*-globin termination mutants had impaired interactions with AHSP. These observations suggest an additional mechanism for unstable *α*-globin variants.[36,37]

Heinz Body Formation

Heme loss is inhibited by maintaining heme iron in the reduced ferrous (Fe^{2+}) state by the action of methemoglobin reductases and detoxification of oxygen radicals. Therefore, dimerization and the dispersion and precipitation of free heme is minimized. Hemoglobin dimers autoxidize and lose heme more readily than tetramers. Generation of methemoglobin increases the thermoinstability of hemoglobin, suggesting that the pathways and events accompanying the conversion of ferrous to ferric heme are important for hemoglobin stability.

Heinz bodies are the product of hemoglobin denaturation. First suggested to be heme-depleted globin chains, these inclusions were subsequently identified as hemichromes, derivatives of ferric hemoglobin that have the sixth coordination position occupied by a ligand provided by the globin. Hemichromes are generated when heme is dissociated from the heme pocket and rebinds elsewhere in the globin after the α- or β-chains have denatured. Irreversible hemichromes are a stage in the formation of Heinz bodies (also see Chapter 6). Membranes prepared from the red cells of patients with Hb Köln who have had splenectomies contain aggregates composed of disulfide-linked spectrin, Band 3, globin, and high-molecular-weight complexes composed in part of denatured spectrin.

Red Cell Destruction

Red blood cells containing Heinz bodies have a shortened lifespan. Hemichrome can bind to Band 3 of the erythrocyte membrane. Decreased deformability of the erythrocyte leads to preferential trapping in the spleen, where Heinz bodies are removed. The classic morphologic findings on blood smear are bite cells and blister cells. The coincident loss of small amounts of membrane can convert discoid cells into spherocytes that are eventually removed from circulation. Membrane damage might also result from lipid peroxidation and protein cross-linking because of free-radical formation that is a result of Fenton chemistry.

Hyperunstable hemoglobin variants are an uncommon class of variants in which the mutation, usually in the third exon of the globin gene, leads often to a truncated globin that is barely detectable or is undetectable.[38,39] These hemoglobins, presumably synthesized normally, are rapidly destroyed, creating the phenotype of dominantly inherited thalassemia.

Diagnosis

Patients with unstable hemoglobins may have characteristically dark urine or pigmenturia. This is a result of the presence of dipyrroles that are also present in Heinz bodies. The absence of pigmenturia does not exclude the diagnosis of unstable hemoglobin, and the severity of the hemolysis is unrelated to pigmenturia. For example, carriers of Hb Köln and Hb Zürich both can have pigmenturia, but hemolysis with Hb Köln can be severe, whereas it is usually very mild with Hb Zürich. The P_{50} of unstable hemoglobins is variable and can be normal, low, or high. This is a result of different mutations variously affecting heme-globin interaction and the tertiary and quaternary structures of the molecule.

Blood Smear

Abnormalities of the blood smear are nonspecific. They can include anisocytosis, basophilic stippling, Howell-Jolly bodies, nucleated red blood cells, and microspherocytes. Fragmented cells appear to have had a "bite" taken from them and are thought to result from the phagocytosis of Heinz bodies during passage of the cell through the spleen. The mean corpuscular hemoglobin concentration may be as low as 25 g/dL because of heme loss or Heinz body formation. Some reported values for reticulocytes may be factitiously high, as inclusion bodies are mistaken for reticulocytes.

Heinz Body Preparation

Heinz bodies in circulating red cells are usually seen only after splenectomy or during an acute hemolytic episode. Under such circumstances, >50% of the cells typically contain one or more large, spherical inclusions. Heinz body detection requires the incubation of erythrocytes with a supravital stain such as new methylene blue or crystal violet. The Heinz bodies appear as single or multiple inclusions of 2 μm in diameter or less and often appear attached to the membrane. Heinz bodies may be found in fresh blood, but usually, incubation for 24 hours without glucose is required for their formation. A normal control should always be run simultaneously.

Table 36.2. Sites of Globin Mutation Associated With Unstable Hemoglobins[a]

Weakening or modification of heme-globin interactions
Interference with the secondary structure of a globin subunit
Interference with the tertiary structure of the subunit
Altered subunit interactions interfering with the quaternary structure

[a]In addition to single amino acid substitutions, these mutations can include small deletions and insertions of amino acids, reading frameshifts, fusion globins, and elongated globin chains.

Hemoglobin Stability Tests

The isopropanol test is a good screening test for unstable hemoglobins, but it can give false-positive results when the sample contains >5% HbF.[40] In the heat denaturation test, a hemolysate is incubated for 1 or 2 hours at 50 °C, and hemoglobin instability is suggested by the development of a visible precipitate.[41] Although the test is simple, the results can vary because of different concentrations of the abnormal variant and different temperatures needed for denaturation. Controls with a normal, stable hemolysate must be run simultaneously.

Hemoglobin HPLC

When the mutation is such that heme dissociates from the abnormal globin chain, as in the example of Hb Köln, the partially heme-deficient molecule is susceptible to reversible and irreversible hemichrome formation with subsequent denaturation. Precipitates tend to be pale, and the pattern found during hemoglobin separation is characterized by lack of discrete peaks and multiple diffuse bands when electrophoresis is used, unless stabilized by the addition of hemin. Dipyrroluria is present, suggesting that free heme was converted to dipyrroles rather than bilirubin.

About a quarter of unstable hemoglobins are not detectable by commonly used methods of hemoglobin separation. On HPLC, some unstable hemoglobins such as Hb Köln, Hb Zurich, and Hb Hasharon (*HBA2* asp47his) demonstrate characteristic elution times.

Detection of the Variant Hemoglobin and Mutation Analysis

If clinical and hematologic studies suggest an unstable variant, the determination of the molecular defect becomes the final step in diagnosis. DNA analysis is the ultimate approach to defining the globin mutation. New mutations are common, so a family history of anemia need not be present.

Clinical Features

The presence of an unstable hemoglobin should always be considered when hemolytic anemia is present and its cause is not clearly defined. Chronic hemolysis as a result of unstable hemoglobins can be associated with all of the known complications of hemolysis, including aplastic crisis, jaundice with cholelithiasis, leg ulcers, splenomegaly, and hypersplenism and pulmonary hypertension.[42] A special feature of unstable hemoglobins is pigmenturia. Similar to glucose-6-phosphate dehydrogenase (G6PD) deficiency, increased hemolytic rate can occur with fever, infection, or ingestion of oxidant drugs (see Chapter 30). Dusky cyanosis has been described in some patients with unstable hemoglobins predisposed to methemoglobin formation. In one case in which the γ-globin chain of HbF was affected (HbF-Poole; HBG2 trp130gly), hemolytic anemia was present in the newborn but disappeared as the γ- to β-globin switch was completed.[43] Sometimes the disease is seen in early childhood; it can be found in adults incidentally or when fever or drug treatment induces hemolysis.

Many unstable hemoglobin variants produce mild hemolytic disease with minimal or no anemia. In the steady state, reticulocyte counts range between 4% and 10%. Splenomegaly may be present. Most patients with mild disease are first seen during a hemolytic crisis induced by drugs or infection. More than half of the unstable variants are associated with no hematologic abnormality and are detected through screening programs.

Just as in all other chronic hemolytic anemias, B19 parvovirus infection can temporarily shut down erythropoiesis, rapidly worsening the anemia and resulting in an aplastic crisis. Anemia may also increase during infection and after treatment with oxidant drugs such as sulfonamides. The intensity of hemolysis is variable and is dependent on the mutation and fraction of abnormal hemoglobin present.

Hb Köln, described in multiple kindreds, is the most common unstable hemoglobin and is characterized by anemia, reticulocytosis, splenomegaly, and 10% to 25% Hb Köln.[44] It is not associated with oxidant drug–induced hemolysis. The independent occurrence of this variant in so many apparently unrelated individuals suggests that the Hb Köln mutation, located at a methylated CpG dinucleotide sequence

of the β-globin gene, can act as a "hotspot" for mutation through the deamination of the methylcytosine nucleotide to form thymine.

Hb Zürich has also been reported on multiple occasions.[45] This variant, forming ~25% of the hemolysate, is accompanied by mild anemia exacerbated by oxidant drugs, pigmenturia, and, as discussed previously, an increased affinity for CO. The latter protects the β-globin heme group from oxidation and increased instability. Carriers have a special susceptibility to sulfonamide-induced hemolytic crisis. Investigation of the basis for variation in drug-related hemolysis of family members with Hb Zürich disease suggested that tobacco smoking ameliorated hemolysis, probably because the high affinity of Hb Zürich for CO stabilized the hemoglobin tetramer.[46,47]

Hb Hasharon is another more common variant affecting the α-globin chain, causes hemolysis in newborns but not in most adults.[48,49] This variant comprises 15% to 20% of the hemolysate, and inclusion bodies are not found.

Some unstable hemoglobins are linked to α- or β-thalassemia genes: the α-chain mutants Hb Suan-Dok (*HBA2* leu109arg) and Hb Petah Tikva (*HBA* ala110asp) coexist in cis with α-thalassemia. Compound heterozygosity for a nondeletion α-thalassemia and the unstable Hb Adana (*HBA* gly139asp) caused a severe phenotype. Some β-chain mutants such as Hb Leiden (*HBB* glu6 or 7del), Hb Duarte (*HBB* ala62pro), HbG-Ferrara (*HBB* asn57lys), and Hb Durham-NC (*HBB* leu114pro), for example, coexist with a β[0]-thalassemia mutation in trans and also have a severe phenotype.

Pulmonary Hypertension

Altered nitric oxide (NO) bioavailability has become recognized as a common occurrence in hemolytic anemia and might account for a commonality of clinical findings in what are very different pathophysiologic entities.[50,51] Because a variable fraction of hemolysis occurs within the vasculature, heme and arginase released from the erythrocyte into blood consume NO and deplete supplies of arginine, the substrate of the NO synthases. Pulmonary hypertension and priapism, common complications of hemolytic anemia, have been described in patients with unstable hemoglobins.[52,53]

Miscellaneous

In a case of hemolytic anemia resulting from Hb Bristol-Alesha, moyamoya and transient ischemic attacks occurred in a 10-year-old girl.[54] The authors suggested that chronic hypoxemia may be the cause of occlusive moyamoya in unstable hemoglobinopathies or in hemoglobins with altered oxygen affinity.

Hyperunstable Hemoglobin

Some uncommon globin mutations are hyperunstable. Although these mutants can be synthesized in normal amounts, they are unable to form stable tetramers or even dimers and are rapidly catabolized. These variants therefore have features of both unstable hemoglobins and thalassemias, and they have been called thalassemic hemoglobinopathies. The phenotype is that of severe, dominantly inherited β-thalassemia rather than unstable hemoglobin disease, because the affected globin chain fails to accumulate and participate in tetramer formation. In the first recognized example of this phenotype, three generations of a family had a dominantly transmitted hemolytic anemia with splenomegaly, gross abnormalities of the erythrocytes, dyserythropoiesis, and large inclusion bodies in bone marrow erythroblasts and in nucleated red cells of the peripheral blood.[38,39]

Dominantly inherited β-thalassemias have been identified in many ethnic groups and are caused by missense mutations, deletions or insertions of intact codons, single-base substitutions leading to premature termination of translation (nonsense mutations), and mutations causing frameshifts or aberrant splicing. Most of the mutations are in exon 3 of the affected gene, and this location might permit globin mRNA to escape nonsense-mediated decay and allow enough denatured protein, along with the uninvolved globin chain, to accumulate and damage the developing erythroblast.

Hyperunstable α-globin variants like Hb Charlieu (*HBA1* leu-106pro) also can cause a severe phenotype.

Treatment

Typical unstable hemoglobinopathies are generally mild disorders and do not require therapy except supportive and preventive measures. Administration of folic acid to prevent megaloblastic arrest of erythropoiesis might be warranted, although access to a nutritious diet is probably sufficient. The possibility of fever-associated hemolysis should be recognized, and avoidance of oxidant drugs, including acetaminophen and sulfonamides, are other management considerations. Chronic hemolysis is associated with a high incidence of cholelithiasis.

Severe hemolysis raises the question of therapeutic splenectomy because the spleen plays an important pathophysiologic role in the destruction of Heinz body–containing red cells. As in other chronic hemolytic anemias, the decision to perform a splenectomy must be balanced with the role of the spleen as a defense against pneumococcal infections early in life and the need for antipneumococcal vaccines and prophylactic penicillin in cases where splenectomy is performed in childhood. On balance, splenectomy might be beneficial for individuals with severe unstable hemoglobinopathies, and partial correction of the anemia is sometimes achieved. Nevertheless, predicting the response to splenectomy is difficult. Hydroxyurea has been used to stimulate HbF production and helped repair anemia in two cases of unstable hemoglobin disease due to β-globin gene mutations, but additional reports have noted inconsistent effects.[55,56]

M HEMOGLOBINS

The 13 M (met) hemoglobin variants are characterized by heme-iron oxidation. Heme iron is more stable in the ferric than in the ferrous state. Erythrocyte methemoglobin reductive capacity cannot effectively compensate for this instability of ferrous heme. The major clinical feature of these disorders is cyanosis. They are not noted for clinical severity. The misdiagnosis of other causes of cyanosis and unneeded treatment are the major hazards of these rare variants.

Pathophysiology

In the M hemoglobins, the mutant globin chain creates an abnormal microenvironment for the heme iron, displacing the equilibrium toward the oxidized or ferric (Fe^{3+}) state. A combination of Fe^{3+} and its abnormal coordination with the substituted amino acid generates a visible spectrum that resembles, but is clearly different from, methemoglobin that is not due to a globin gene mutation, in which the heme iron is oxidized but there is no associated amino acid substitution.

In the Iwate prefecture of Japan, "black children" had been observed for more than 160 years, and this was associated with a brownish-colored hemoglobin in the hemolysate of a patient that was eventually characterized as HbM Iwate (*HBA* his87tyr).[57] Four β-, three α-, and two γ-globin HbM variants have been reported. Often the mutation involves the substitution of the distal (E7) or proximal (F8) histidine interacting with the heme iron via tyrosine.

HbM Milwaukee (*HBB* val67glu) is an example of an M hemoglobin that is not caused by mutation of the proximal or distal his residues, but by the nearby β67 (E11) val. In this variant the longer side chain of the glutamic acid residue can reach and perturb the heme iron. Other mutations of val67, such as in Hb Bristol or Hb Sidney

(val67ala), are unstable or have low affinity but do not lead to heme-iron oxidation. X-ray crystallography shows that the carboxylic group of the new glutaminyl residue in Hb Milwaukee occupies the sixth coordination position of the iron and that the proximal his maintains its role as the tenant of the fifth coordinating position, stabilizing the abnormal ferric state of HbM Milwaukee.

In two novel variants that form methemoglobin, an amino acid deletion was suspected to alter the orientations of the distal and proximal his residues.[58] Properties of some M hemoglobins are shown in *Table 36.3*. The strength of attachment of ferric heme to globins differs among M hemoglobins.

Oxygen-Binding Properties and the R → T Transition of M Hemoglobins

HbM Milwaukee, HbM Hyde Park (*HBB* his92tyr), and HbM Boston (*HBA* his58tyr) all adopt deoxy or deoxy-like conformation upon the deoxygenation of the two normal chains, although the abnormal chains cannot off-load oxygen. This, and crystallographic, electron paramagnetic resonance, and nuclear magnetic resonance (NMR) spectroscopy, and 2,3-BPG–binding studies affirm that, after two heme groups become deoxygenated, the entire molecule adopts the deoxy T conformation.

With HbM Milwaukee, HbM Saskatoon (*HBB* his63tyr), and HbM Hyde Park, a normal Bohr effect and P_{50} strongly suggest that the hemoglobin adopts the R state when the two normal chains are oxygenated. NMR studies of HbM Milwaukee support the notion that the conformational changes take place when the normal heme groups are oxygenated. In contrast, HbM Iwate is in the crystallographic T configuration when its normal heme groups are in the ferric state, explaining its decreased oxygen affinity; the molecule does not shift to the R state when the normal heme groups are liganded and remains in the low-affinity T state. A similar situation probably exists in HbM Boston, as the habit of the deoxy crystal remains intact after oxygenation, suggesting that no conformational change has occurred that would require a different crystal structure.

HbM Saskatoon and HbM Boston have different properties despite the common substitution of the distal histidine. This occurs because HbM Saskatoon does not change its conformation when oxygenated, whereas the latter variant does. Why properties of the β-globin chains differ from that of the α-globin chain when their distal histidine is substituted is unresolved.

Iron Oxidation and Spectral Characteristics

In M hemoglobins, the affected heme groups are stabilized in the ferric state and have an abnormal microenvironment. They exhibit an abnormal visible absorption spectrum that is easily distinguished from methemoglobin. This characteristic separates these variants from some unstable hemoglobin mutants that also have a tendency to form methemoglobin.

Heme iron in the abnormal subunits of the M hemoglobin exhibit abnormally low redox potential. They are oxidized more rapidly by molecular oxygen and are resistant, to a variable degree, to reduction by dithionite. Differences also exist in the rate of reduction of the five M hemoglobins with NADH-cytochrome b_5 reductase (*CYB5R3*);

Table 36.3. Hematologic Features of Some HbM Variants of the α- and β-Globin Genes

Variant	Percent	Hb (g/dL)	Reticulocytes (%)	P50	Bohr Effect
HbM Hyde Park (Milwaukee-2) (β)	23–32	10–13	4–6	Normal	Present
HbM Iwate (α)	19	17	—	Decreased	Decreased
HbM Boston (α)	20–30	—	—	Decreased	Decreased
HbM Milwaukee (β)	50	14–15	1–2	Decreased	Present
HbM Saskatoon (β)	35	13–16	0.8–3.2	Normal	Present
HbM Chile (β)	17	13.2	1.2	—	—

HbM Iwate, HbM Hyde Park, and HbM Boston are not reduced at all, whereas HbM Milwaukee is reduced slowly and HbM Saskatoon is reduced normally. These last two variants might be less oxidized in vivo than expected. Full ferric conversion might occur only in vitro, because of the high autoxidation rate of these abnormal hemoglobins. Older red cells might, nevertheless, have fully oxidized abnormal chains consistent with the presence of clinically apparent cyanosis.

Clinical Features and Diagnosis

Clinically, the skin and mucous membranes of HbM carriers have an appearance similar to, but not identical with, cyanosis, sometimes called pseudocyanosis. Pseudocyanosis is not associated with dyspnea or clubbing. In fair-skinned individuals, skin and mucosal surfaces are brownish/slate colored, more like methemoglobinemia, but not as slate blue-purple as true cyanosis. This distinction is subtle and might not be apparent without comparing the two conditions at the same time. Skin tone reflects hemoglobin molecules with an abnormal ferric heme and abnormal spectrum, whereas cyanosis is caused by the presence of more than 5 g/dL of deoxyhemoglobin. Pseudocyanosis is present from birth in α-globin-chain abnormalities and from the middle of the first year of life in the β-chain mutants. The γ-globin gene HbM variants, HbF-M Osaka (*HBG2* his63tyr) and HbF-M Fort Ripley (*HBG2* his92tyr), have been associated with neonatal "cyanosis" that disappears as γ-globin-chain synthesis wanes.[59,60] A mixture of the abnormal pigment and true cyanosis, resulting from hemoglobin desaturation of the normal chains, is observed in the low-oxygen-affinity HbM Boston and HbM Hb Iwate.

A mild hemolytic anemia and reticulocytosis have been observed in HbM Hyde Park and can be explained by the instability of the hemoglobin induced by partial heme loss.

HbM should be considered in all patients with abnormal homogenous coloration of the skin and mucosa, particularly if pulmonary and cardiac functions are normal. The diagnosis can be suspected by observing an abnormal brown coloration of the blood in a tube. To distinguish this coloration from methemoglobin, the addition of KCN to the hemolysate is useful. KCN will turn blood containing methemoglobin red but has little if any effect on HbM-containing hemolysates. Lack of color conversion with KCN is diagnostic of HbM.

A spectrophotometric recording of the visible spectrum of the hemolysate is critical for the diagnosis, and the mutation is confirmed by DNA analysis. M hemoglobins do not have an absorbance peak at 630 to 635 nm that is typical of methemoglobin. In the presence of HbM, accurate measurement of oxygen saturation and CO hemoglobin is difficult with most instruments. Absorption maxima at different wavelengths of all HbM variants have been reported.

Treatment

Treatment for individuals with HbM is neither necessary nor possible. A correct diagnosis is most important, because this will forestall therapeutic and diagnostic misadventures.

METHEMOGLOBINEMIA UNRELATED TO GLOBIN GENE MUTATIONS

Normally, small amounts of hemoglobin are continually being oxidized by endogenous agents, including oxygen itself (auto-oxidation). When oxygen reacts with deoxygenated hemoglobin to produce oxyhemoglobin, one electron from heme iron (Fe^{2+}) is transferred to the bound oxygen, thereby forming a ferric–superoxide anion complex (Fe^{3+}-O_2^{-}). Subsequently, when hemoglobin is deoxygenated, most oxygen is released as O_2, but a small amount leaves as superoxide anion (O_2^{-}). The partially transferred electron is not returned to iron, leaving the heme iron as Fe^{3+} (methemoglobin).[6] Increased temperature and low pH promote auto-oxidation. Usually, methemoglobin levels are <1% of the total hemoglobin, because erythrocytes contain cytochrome b5 reductase that catalyzes its reduction (see Chapter 6). Genetically determined methemoglobinemia, unrelated to globin gene mutations, occurs in individuals with hereditary deficiency of

cytochrome b5 reductase. Acquired methemoglobinemia occurs in normal individuals exposed to drugs and chemicals that oxidize hemoglobin iron at a rate that exceeds the capacity for enzymatic reduction.

Cyanosis

Cyanosis most often is due to cardiac or pulmonary disease, but genetic and acquired disorders of hemoglobin can result in significant arterial desaturation. In the M hemoglobins and with sulfhemoglobin and methemoglobin, the altered visible spectrum of the abnormal pigments is responsible for the brownish/slate skin color. The spectral properties of sulfhemoglobin versus methemoglobin are such that patients can be markedly "cyanotic," with 0.5 g/dL of sulfhemoglobin while 1.5 g/dL of methemoglobin is required to produce "cyanosis"; true cyanosis requires 5.0 g/dL of deoxyhemoglobin.

Although dyspnea is not a feature of M hemoglobins, it can be present even with relatively low levels of methemoglobinemia. Because the altered hemes in HbM, sulfhemoglobin, and methemoglobin do not transport oxygen, affected individuals with all three conditions may have normal hemoglobin concentrations but are functionally anemic, simply because of insufficient operational heme groups. This effect is clinically significant only in extreme cases of methemoglobinemia and sulfhemoglobinemia or when the overall hemoglobin level is low. With HbM, the proportion of normal to abnormal heme is genetically determined and fixed, so that decreased oxygen delivery is problematic only when superimposed on underlying anemia.

The clinical effects of nonfunctional heme groups are not limited to an inability to transport oxygen. Small amounts of nonfunctional heme can have clinical significance if their presence produces a physiologically dysfunctional shift in the oxygenation of neighboring unmodified subunits. This is the molecular basis of the left-shifted oxygenation curve, the impaired oxygen delivery to the tissues, and the resulting respiratory distress seen in relatively mild degrees of methemoglobinemia. This phenomenon, called the Darling-Roughton effect, occurs as oxidized subunits in partially oxidized tetramers are held in an R-like conformation, increasing the oxygen affinity of the remaining subunits. Although mixed venous blood is unusually saturated, the abnormal spectrum of the methemoglobin dominates this effect, causing cyanosis. An analogous left shift in the oxygenation curve, but to a more pronounced degree, is present with CO poisoning, and impaired oxygen delivery exacerbates dyspnea.

Cytochrome b5 Reductase Deficiency

About 50 mutations of the cytochrome b5 reductase 3 gene (*CYB5R3*; 22q13) have been described.[61,62] This gene has two isoforms, a soluble truncated version expressed only in erythrocytes and a membrane bound version present in all cells, especially adipocytes. Only the erythrocyte is affected in type I cytochrome b5 reductase deficiency. Seventeen exon mutations were associated with type 1 disease, 15 with type II, and 1 with both types of disease. Missense, nonsense, deletions, and other classes of mutation have been described. Decreased activity of the soluble form of the erythrocyte enzyme, which is usually a result of missense mutations, results in hereditary methemoglobinemia; *CYB5R3* is a transferase that facilitates electron transfer from NADH to cytochrome b5, which then directly reduces methemoglobin. A second erythrocyte enzyme is NADPH-methemoglobin reductase, which by itself is unable to reduce methemoglobin effectively. Individuals lacking this enzyme do not have methemoglobinemia. However, in the presence of redox compounds such as methylene blue, NADPH methemoglobin reductase rapidly reduces methemoglobin. Thus, this agent is useful in treating methemoglobinemia.

Cytochrome b5 reductase enzyme deficiency is a recessive trait, and only homozygotes or individuals who are compound heterozygotes for two different gene mutations express the disease. Of interest, however, heterozygotes can be at risk for acquired methemoglobinemia when exposed to oxidant drugs.[63,64]

Patients with type I deficiency manifested by only methemoglobinemia are more cyanotic than sick, in the worst cases complaining of fatigue with strenuous exercise. They survive normally, and women have normal pregnancies. Methemoglobin levels vary from 20% to

Disorders of Red Blood Cells

40%. When exposed to methemoglobin-inducing drugs or chemicals, these patients are at risk for developing further methemoglobinemia symptoms. Enzymatic activity of the NADH-dependent methemoglobin reductase system is reduced in the erythrocyte.

Type II deficiency is a generalized form of cytochrome b5 reductase deficiency, affecting 10% to 15% of patients. It is caused by both truncating and missense mutations and is a severe and lethal disease, with strong neurologic components. Although the methemoglobinemia in type II deficiency can be treated, the neurologic syndrome is refractory. Syndromes intermediate between type I and type II disease have been described.

A high incidence of hereditary methemoglobinemia is found among Inuit populations, and among several indigenous communities including in Northwest United States, Navajo, and Yakusk, Siberia, groups that might have common ancestry. In one report from Alaska, the gene frequency was 0.07, but these results were based on enzyme assay and not detection of the abnormal gene. Cytochrome b5 reductase deficiency has also been observed sporadically among populations in Puerto Rico and the Mediterranean.

Acquired (Toxic) Methemoglobinemia

Many chemical agents and drugs can induce methemoglobinemia in normal people (*Table 36.4*). Dapsone- and primaquine-induced methemoglobinemia, at levels of 15% to 33%, have been reported in human immunodeficiency virus–infected patients. Nitrites also are common offenders, and recreational use of amyl, butyl, or isobutyl nitrites is a cause of acquired methemoglobinemia. Infections that release toxins (including nitrites) can produce methemoglobin. Aniline dyes and aniline reduce molecular oxygen and generate methemoglobin. Phenylhydroxylamine, after reducing oxyhemoglobin, can generate nitrosobenzene, which is reduced again to phenylhydroxylamine by red cell enzymes. The cycle can then, in turn, generate more methemoglobin. Henna, a natural product used worldwide as a hair dye and to stain skin and nails, contains a chemical, 2-hydroxy-1,4-naphthoquinone, that can increase methemoglobin production, especially in G6PD-deficient individuals. Use of benzocaine as a topical anesthetic is often associated with methemoglobinemia. Certain medications used to treat diaper rash that contain benzocaine and resorcinol have been reported to produce methemoglobin levels as high as 35%.[62-69]

Newborn infants are at increased risk for methemoglobinemia because of a transient decrease in NADH cytochrome reductase activity during the neonatal period; normal adult enzyme activity is present by 3 to 4 months of age. Infantile methemoglobinemia has occurred in

association with nitrate contamination of the water supply.[66] Children with septic shock also can have methemoglobinemia, presumably because of increased circulating nitrite/nitrate levels. In children with *Plasmodium falciparum* malaria, mean methemoglobin levels are increased, and this is related to disease and anemia severity.[67] Because malaria itself produces hypoxia, the additional reduction in oxygen-carrying capacity because of the presence of methemoglobinemia might be particularly critical for the subgroup of patients who are anemic or acidotic.

Diagnosis

The possibility of acquired methemoglobinemia should be considered in anyone with recent or sudden apparent cyanosis who is unresponsive to 100% oxygen and without cardiopulmonary pathology. Sulfhemoglobinemia (see later) should also be considered in these cases. Acquired methemoglobinemia is not rare; it is much more common than any of the genetic causes of methemoglobinemia. In a retrospective study of acquired methemoglobinemia (methemoglobin level >2%), 138 cases were encountered over a period of 28 months.[69] Patients' ages ranged from 4 days to 86 years, and there was one fatality and three near-fatalities. Dapsone was the most common etiology of acquired methemoglobinemia, accounting for 42% of all cases. The mean peak methemoglobin level among these individuals was 7.6%. In five of the patients with the most severely elevated levels, 20% benzocaine spray was the causative agent and was associated with a mean peak methemoglobin level of 44%. Eleven pediatric patients developed methemoglobinemia either from exogenous exposure, such as drugs, or because of serious illness, such as gastrointestinal infections with dehydration. Ninety-four percent of patients with methemoglobinemia were anemic.

Long-standing symptoms, or symptoms in siblings, is suggestive of a hereditary methemoglobinemia. Because the enzyme deficiency is inherited as a recessive trait, clinical disease is not expected in the parents. The differential diagnosis includes the HbM variants and low-oxygen-affinity hemoglobins. Because of the "dominance" of the HbM genes, one parent often has the same symptoms.

The diagnosis of cytochrome b5 reductase deficiency is made by direct assay of the enzyme. Genetic ascertainment is available for the known mutations. Prenatal diagnosis is available for type II congenital methemoglobinemia.

Treatment

Acquired methemoglobin is treated by stopping the offending agent once it is identified. Direct drug intervention with intravenous methylene blue is indicated in patients with 40% to 60% methemoglobin, particularly when symptoms are present. Methemoglobin levels of 70% can be fatal. The usual dose of methylene blue is 1 to 2 mg/kg, and the maximum dose is 7 mg/kg. It can be given intravenously in acute methemoglobinemia. For intravenous administration, it should be given slowly over 35 minutes to avoid high concentrations and paradoxical methemoglobin production. Rapid improvement in cyanosis and normalization of methemoglobin level usually occurs 30 to 60 minutes after methylene blue injection. If there is coexistent G6PD deficiency, methylene blue is not effective, because of the lack of NADPH production, and its use may result in hemolysis. A transient drop of pulse oximeter arterial oxygen saturation can be seen following methylene blue injection, a result of interference by methylene blue with the light-wave emission of the pulse oximeter. Methemoglobin levels can increase again following successful treatment.[70] In type I cytochrome b5 reductase deficiency, treatment is mainly for cosmetic purposes. Oral methylene blue, 100 to 300 mg daily, can maintain methemoglobin levels of 5% to 10%. Ascorbic acid, 200 to 500 mg daily, also can reverse cyanosis in patients with type I methemoglobinemia.

In aniline-induced methemoglobinemia, methylene blue can couple with oxyhemoglobin to generate free radicals and has sometimes produced hemolysis. In these cases, dosing should be limited.

Automated red blood cell exchange has been used successfully when methylene blue is ineffective and may be superior to manual exchange transfusion.[71]

Table 36.4. Drugs and Agents That Can Cause Methemoglobinemia

Local anesthetics
    Benzocaine
    Lidocaine
    Procaine
    Prilocaine
Analine dyes
Chlorates
Dapsone
Diarylsulfonylureas (sulofenur)
Primaquine
Rasburicase
Nitrates and nitrites
Nitroglycerine
Cerium nitrate
Amynitrate
Isobutyl
Nitrobenzines
Nitrofurans
Pyridium
Primaquine
Sulfonamides
Acetaminophen/phenacetin

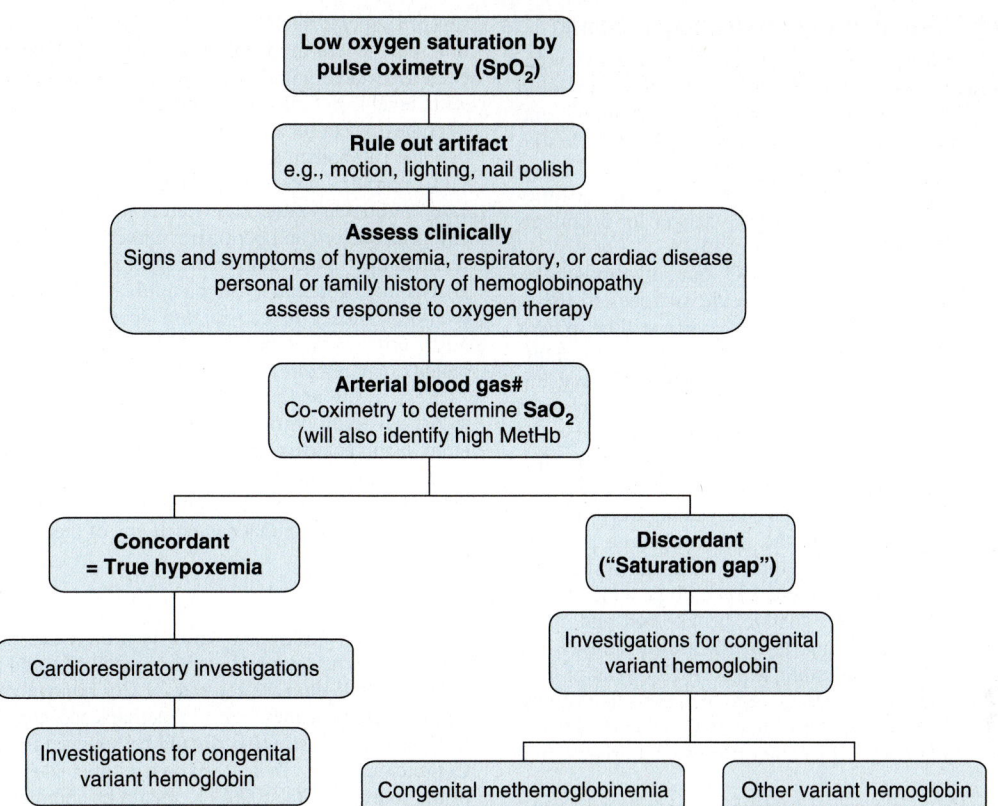

FIGURE 36.1 **An algorithm for evaluation of low SPO₂.** Arterial blood gas should be done on room air and with simultaneous SPO₂ measurement. (From Verhovsek M, Henderson MP, Cox G, et al. Unexpectedly low pulse oximetry measurements associated with variant hemoglobins: a systematic review. *Am J Hematol.* 2011;86:722-725. Copyright © 2011 Wiley-Liss, Inc. Reprinted by permission of John Wiley & Sons, Inc.)

PULSE OXIMETRY

Virtually all of the classes of hemoglobin variants and methemoglobinemia discussed above have examples of variants that have been associated with unexpected low oxygen saturations when this is measured by most pulse oximeters. Some instruments measure met- and carboxyhemoglobins in addition to oxygen saturation, but the reliability of these measurements is yet to be widely accepted. Many low-oxygen-affinity variants had concordantly low pulse oximeter–measured oxygen saturation and low arterial oxygen saturation, although the arterial partial pressure of oxygen was normal.[72-75] Discordant anomalies (i.e., low pulse oximeter–measured oxygen saturation with normal oxygen saturation on arterial blood gas) are due to the altered absorption spectrum of the hemoglobin variant that confound the settings of the pulse oximeter that uses set wavelengths of light to calculate oxygen saturation. Attention should be paid to measurement of blood oxygen saturation when any hemoglobin variant is present. Blood oxygen saturation can be measured using an arterial blood gas analyzer, by pulse oximetry, or by using a CO-oximeter. The first method measures blood partial pressure of dissolved oxygen and provides the PaO_2 and SaO_2. The convenient pulse oximeter provides a transcutaneous measure of absorbance at two wavelengths (660 and 940 nm) but is inaccurate when dyshemoglobins such as methemoglobin, carboxyhemoglobin, and sulfhemoglobin are present. CO-oximetry, the most accurate of all the methods, can be inaccurate in cases of M hemoglobins.

Oxygen saturation calculated from pH and PO_2 should be interpreted with caution, because the algorithms used assume normal hemoglobin oxygen affinity, normal 2,3-BPG concentrations, and no dyshemoglobins such as methemoglobin or hemoglobinopathies. CO-oximeter reports should include the dyshemoglobin fractions in addition to the oxyhemoglobin fraction. In cases of increased methemoglobin fraction, pulse oximeter values trend toward 85%, underestimating the actual oxygen saturation. Hemoglobin M variants may yield normal methemoglobin levels and increased carboxyhemoglobin or sulfhemoglobin fractions measured by CO-oximetry.

In a systematic review, 25 publications and 4 unpublished ones representing 45 patients with low SpO₂ and a confirmed variant hemoglobin were identified.[75] Fifty-seven family members of patients had a confirmed or suspected variant hemoglobin. Three low-oxygen-affinity variant hemoglobins had concordantly low SpO₂ and SaO₂. Eleven variant hemoglobins were associated with unexpectedly low SpO₂ measurements but normal SaO₂. Most variant hemoglobins were associated with spuriously low SpO₂. The differential diagnosis of possible variant hemoglobin should be considered in asymptomatic patients found to have unexpectedly low SpO₂. Otherwise, these patients might be subjected to unneeded extensive cardiopulmonary investigations in search of the cause of their "hypoxemia." An approach to the evaluation of low oxygen saturation is shown in *Figure 36.1*.

DYSHEMOGLOBINEMIAS: CARBOXY-, SULF-, AND NITROSOHEMOGLOBINS

CO and NO are present in normal red cells in very low concentrations, and both can bind to hemoglobin to form carboxyhemoglobin (CO hemoglobin) and nitrosohemoglobin (NO hemoglobin), respectively. Carboxyhemoglobin avidly binds oxygen and cannot release it to the tissues. Nitrosohemoglobin may have critical physiologic functions. In addition to these normally occurring liganded hemoglobins, sulfur compounds can bind to the pyrrole ring of heme, forming a thiochlorin, referred to as sulfhemoglobin (see Chapter 6). Mutations or environmental conditions can increase the concentrations of all these liganded or oxidized hemoglobins, thereby producing dyshemoglobinemias. Sometimes, increased levels of dyshemoglobins are life-threatening, and because effective treatments are available, their presence should be identified promptly.

Carbon Monoxide Poisoning: Carboxyhemoglobinemia

CO, a toxic gas, is odorless, colorless, and tasteless; has a low solubility in water; and is relatively inert. It combines with hemoglobin heme with high affinity and with lesser affinities to myoglobin and cytochrome heme. Under physiologic conditions, its affinity for hemoglobin is ~240 times greater than that of oxygen. Once CO is bound to heme, its "off" rate is very slow, producing a very high affinity constant of CO for heme and a life-threatening danger for organisms exposed to high levels of CO.

Further endangering those exposed to CO, once two molecules of CO are bound to hemoglobin, the molecule switches to the R state, and the two globin chains that can bind oxygen will be in their high-affinity conformation. This high ligand affinity makes more difficult the delivery of oxygen to the tissues by the remaining oxygen-binding sites (Darling-Roughton effect). Consequently, the oxygen equilibrium curve of blood is shifted to the left with increasing CO levels.

In the absence of increased environmental CO, the blood of adults contains ~1% to 2% CO hemoglobin. This endogenous CO is derived from heme catabolism—specifically, the first enzymatic reaction catalyzed by heme oxygenase (see Chapter 6). Caloric restriction, dehydration, and Japanese and Amerindians seem to generate higher endogenous levels of CO. Hemolytic anemia, hematomas, and infection tend to increase CO production up to threefold. Fetuses and newborns have double the normal adult levels of CO hemoglobin, and this increases further in the presence of neonatal hemolysis. Exogenous sources of CO include atmospheric CO, which is a product of incomplete combustion and oxidation of hydrocarbons, and natural sources.

The most commonly used instrument for the detection and quantification of carboxyhemoglobins is the CO-oximeter, which also provides the levels of oxy-, deoxy-, and methemoglobin.

Chronic CO Intoxication

It has been estimated that CO intoxication is responsible for upward of 50,000 Emergency Department visits yearly.[76] Symptoms of CO hemoglobinemia can include irritability, nausea, lethargy, headache, and sometimes a flulike condition. A study of more than 1000 CO-poisoned patients suggested that symptoms might not correlate well with blood levels of CO hemoglobin.[77] Higher CO hemoglobin levels produce somnolence, palpitations, cardiomegaly, and hypertension and might contribute to atherosclerosis. Long-term neuropsychological symptoms can persist and even be permanent.[76] Chronic CO poisoning can produce erythrocytosis, the magnitude of which varies with the level of CO hemoglobin. By increasing red cell production, chronic CO poisoning can mask the mild anemia of thalassemia trait or other acquired or genetic hemolytic disorders.

The most frequent exogenous source of CO is cigarette smoking, which can increase carboxyhemoglobin to 15%. Water pipes have also been associated with CO hemoglobinemia. Pregnant women, fetuses, neonates, and infants are particularly susceptible to CO poisoning from smoking. Because CO hemoglobin increases hemoglobin-O_2 affinity, this may cause erythrocytosis, especially in smokers. The second most common cause of chronic CO exposure is defective heating exhaust systems and vehicles that leak CO into the passenger compartment. Occupational exposure is seen in garage workers, toll booth attendants, tunnel workers and other situations and occupations with poor ventilation, firefighters, and workers with industrial exposure.

Acute CO Intoxication

Carboxyhemoglobin levels >20% are usually required before acute symptoms appear. Accidental exposures to high environmental levels of CO or suicide attempts by deliberate exposure to a CO source are the most frequent causes of acute poisoning in the United States, responsible for over 1000 deaths a year.[78] Unintentional acute CO poisoning is responsible for at least 400 deaths a year,[79] is more severe, and sometimes has unique symptomatology. Children are more likely to have severe sequelae such as leukoencephalopathy, white-matter destruction, and severe myocardial ischemia. Carboxyhemoglobinemia has been associated with high doses of sodium nitroprusside in children, with levels of 5.5% to 7.7%.[80] The mechanism is unclear but is hypothesized to be the induction of heme oxygenase, the first enzyme in heme catabolism that generates CO.[81]

CO rapidly affects the central and peripheral nervous system and cardiopulmonary functions. Cerebral edema is common, as are alterations of sensory and peripheral nerve function. CO induces increased permeability in the lung, resulting in acute pulmonary edema. Cardiac arrhythmia, generalized hypoxemia, and respiratory failure are the common causes of CO-related death. Carboxyhemoglobin levels >40% are present in these cases. In survivors, considerable neurologic deficits may remain.

Less severe acute cases present with the same types of symptoms as patients with chronic intoxication. Arrhythmias, myocardial ischemia, lactic acidosis, convulsions, and coma also can occur. An interesting complication observed several days after the exposure to CO are patches of necrotic skin induced by localized hypoxia. The levels of carboxyhemoglobin that can elicit any of these symptoms vary widely among patients.

Treatment

Treatment of chronic exposure is principally rapid removal of the patient from the source of environmental CO, and if needed, breathing 100% O_2 will increase the rate of CO removal. Hyperbaric oxygen, whose efficacy is unproven,[76,81] perhaps because of the almost inevitable delay in its institution, should be reserved for exceptional cases of CO intoxication.[81] In acute exposure, after identification and removal of the source of CO, 100% O_2 should be administered.

SARS-CoV2 and Dyshemoglobinemia

Both methemoglobin and carboxyhemoglobin levels can be increased in people infected with SARS-CoV2. Most patients hospitalized with severe disease have increased levels of both dyshemoglobins, which can become dangerously high. These increases might be related to disease severity, coincident G6PD deficiency, and exposure to many different therapeutics.

Sulfhemoglobinemia

Sulfhemoglobin is a green-pigmented protein with a sulfur atom incorporated into the heme ring. It is first suspected in a cyanotic patient with near-normal oxygen tension who is felt to have methemoglobinemia but does not respond to therapy with methylene blue. Although it shares a similar absorption peak with methemoglobin, the absorption peak of methemoglobin, unlike that of sulfhemoglobin, is abolished by cyanide. At low concentrations, sulfurated tetramers are shifted toward the deoxy or T form, producing a right shift of the oxygen equilibrium curve. This shift in the hemoglobin-oxygen dissociation curve reduces the likelihood of dyspnea unless the concentrations of sulfhemoglobin are exceptionally high.

Sulfhemoglobin has been associated with the use of certain "oxidant" medications, although mostly when used in doses higher than recommended, during drug abuse, with occupational exposure to sulfur compounds, and with exposure to polluted air.[82] Sulfhemoglobin and methemoglobin have been reported to coexist in some cases of drug-induced hemoglobinopathy, and chemicals and drugs reported to produce these syndromes are similar. Congenital sulfhemoglobinemia is rare and has been described with an unstable hemoglobin. It is likely that, because of drug-related and industrial exposure to sulfur, this condition is underdiagnosed. For equivalent amounts of abnormal pigment, the patient with sulfhemoglobinemia appears bluer than the patient with methemoglobinemia. However, these individuals are less symptomatic than those with methemoglobinemia, as cyanosis occurs at a sulfhemoglobin concentration much lower than the methemoglobin level needed to cause cyanosis. Treatment is rarely required besides withdrawal from the putative offending agent. Exchange transfusion is the sole therapeutic option for symptomatic cases.

Nitrosohemoglobins

NO is generated from L-arginine by nitric oxide synthases (see Chapter 7). NO diffuses out of the originating cells and into nearby target cells, where it binds the heme groups of enzymes and hemoglobin. The reaction of free NO with erythrocytes is diffusion limited. It has been proposed that S-nitrosylhemoglobin is formed in the lungs, while in tissues NO is liberated from hemoglobin leading to vasodilation. It is hypothesized that, by sensing the physiologic oxygen gradient in tissues, hemoglobin exploits conformation-associated changes in the position of β93 cys to bring local blood flow into line with oxygen requirements.[83-88] This hypothesis is controversial, however, and there is little direct evidence that NO is liberated from the β93 cys site as hemoglobin assumes the T state.

References

1. Wajcman H, Galacteros F. Hemoglobins with high oxygen affinity leading to erythrocytosis. New variants and new concepts. *Hemoglobin.* 2005;29:91-106.
2. Papassotiriou I, Traeger-Synodinos J, Marden MC, et al. The homozygous state for Hb Crete [beta129 (H7) Ala → Pro] is associated with a complex phenotype including erythrocytosis and functional anemia. *Blood Cells Mol Dis.* 2005;34:229-234.
3. Tanphaichitr VS, Viprakasit V, Veerakul G, et al. Homozygous hemoglobin Tak causes symptomatic secondary polycythemia in a Thai boy. *J Pediatr Hematol Oncol.* 2003;25:261-265.
4. Venkateswaran L, Swanson KC, Hoyer JD. Homozygous hemoglobin Abruzzo in a North American child. *J Pediatr Hematol Oncol.* 2005;27:618-620.
5. Williamson D, Beresford CH, Langdown JV, et al. Polycythaemia associated with homozygosity for the abnormal haemoglobin Sherwood Forest (beta 104 (G6)Arg → Thr). *Br J Haematol.* 1994;86:890-892.
6. Bunn H, ed. *Hemoglobin: Molecular, Genetic and Clinical Aspects.* WB Saunders; 1986.
7. Adamson JW, Hayashi A, Stamatoyannopoulos G, et al. Erythrocyte function and marrow regulation in hemoglobin Bethesda (β 145 histidine). *J Clin Invest.* 1972;51:2883.
8. Adamson JW, Finch CA. Erythroprotein and the polycythemias. *Ann N Y Acad Sci.* 1968;149:560.
9. McClure RF, Hoyer JD, Mai M. The JAK2 V617F mutation is absent in patients with erythrocytosis due to high oxygen affinity hemoglobin variants. *Hemoglobin.* 2006;30:487-489.
10. Oliveira JL, Coon LM, Frederick LA. Genotype-phenotype correlation of hereditary erythrocytosis mutations, a single center experience. *Am J Hematol* 2018 93:1029-1041.
11. Rosa R, Prehu MO, Beuzard Y, et al. The first case of a complete deficiency of diphosphoglycerate mutase in human erythrocytes. *J Clin Invest.* 1978;62:907.
12. Charache S, Weatherall DJ, Clegg JB. Polycythemia associated with a hemoglobinopathy. *J Clin Invest.* 1966;45:813-822.
13. Shimasaki S. A new hemoglobin variant, hemoglobin Nunobiki [alpha 141 (HC3) Arg—Cys]. Notable influence of the carboxy-terminal cysteine upon various physico-chemical characteristics of hemoglobin. *J Clin Invest.* 1985;75:695-701.
14. Wajcman H, Kilmartin JV, Najman A, et al. Hemoglobin Cochin-Port-Royal: consequences of the replacement of the beta chain C-terminal by an arginine. *Biochim Biophys Acta.* 1975;400:354-364.
15. Tondo C, Bonaventura J, Bonaventura J, et al. Functional properties of hemoglobin Porto Alegre (alpha2A beta2 9Ser leads to Cys) and the reactivity of its extra cysteinyl residue. *Biochim Biophys Acta.* 1974;342:15-20.
16. Flatz G, Kinderlerer JL, Kilmartin JV, et al. Haemoglobin Tak: a variant with additional residues at the end of the beta-chains. *Lancet.* 1971;1(7702):732-733.
17. Imai K, Lehmann H. The oxygen affinity of haemoglobin Tak, a variant with an elongated beta chain. *Biochim Biophys Acta.* 1975;412:288-294.
18. Yudin J, Verhovsek M. How we diagnose and manage altered oxygen affinity hemoglobin variants. *Am J Hematol.* 2019;94:597-603.
19. Giordano PC, Harteveld CL, Brand A, et al. Hb Malmo [beta-97(FG-4)His → Gln] leading to polycythemia in a Dutch family. *Ann Hematol.* 1996;73:183-188.
20. Charache S, Achuff S, Winslow R, et al. Variability of the homeostatic response to altered p50. *Blood.* 1978;52:1156-1162.
21. Percy MJ, Butt NM, Crotty GM, et al. Identification of high oxygen affinity hemoglobin variants in the investigation of patients with erythrocytosis. *Haematologica.* 2009;94:1312-1322.
22. Oliveira A, Warcel D, Huntley N, Eleftheriou P, Porter JB. Symptomatic erythrocytosis due to homozygosity for Hb Luton [HBA2: c.269A>T (or HBA1)] and α-thalassemia—a clinical update. *Hemoglobin.* 2016;40(2):127-129.
23. Gaudreau P-O, Weng X, Cournoyer G, et al. Treatment with hydroxyurea in a patient compound heterozygote for a high oxygen affinity hemoglobin and β-thalassemia minor. *Am J Hematol.* 2009;84:766-768.
24. Nagel RL, Lynfield J, Johnson J, et al. Hemoglobin Beth Israel. A mutant causing clinically apparent cyanosis. *N Engl J Med.* 1976;295:125-130.
25. Bonaventura J, Riggs A. Hemoglobin Kansas, a human hemoglobin with a neutral amino acid substitution and an abnormal oxygen equilibrium. *J Biol Chem.* 1968;243:980-991.
26. Crowley MA, Mollan TL, Abdulmalik OY, et al. A hemoglobin variant associated with neonatal cyanosis and anemia. *N Engl J Med.* 2011;364:1837-1843.
27. Marinucci M, Giuliani A, Maffi D, et al. Hemoglobin bologna (alpha 2 beta 2 61 (E5) lys replaced by met). An abnormal human hemoglobin with low oxygen affinity. *Biochim Biophys Acta.* 1981;668:209-215.
28. Blouquit Y, Bardakdjian J, Lena-Russo D, et al. Hb Bruxelles: alpha 2A beta (2)41 or 42(C7 or CD1)Phe deleted. *Hemoglobin.* 1989;13:465-474.
29. Griffon N, Badens C, Lena-Russo D, et al. Hb Bruxelles, deletion of Phebeta42, shows a low oxygen affinity and low cooperativity of ligand binding. *J Biol Chem.* 1996;271:25916-25920.
30. Williamson D. The unstable haemoglobins. *Blood Rev.* 1993;7:146-163.
31. Ohba Y. Unstable hemoglobins. *Hemoglobin.* 1990;14:353-388.
32. Moo-Penn WF, Jue DL, Johnson MH, et al. Hemoglobin Brockton (beta 138 (H16) Ala—Pro): an unstable variant near the C-terminus of the beta-subunits with normal oxygen-binding properties. *Biochemistry.* 1988;27:7614-7619.
33. Rieder RF, Oski FA, Clegg JB. Hemoglobin Philly (beta 35 tyrosine phenylalanine): studies in the molecular pathology of hemoglobin. *J Clin Invest.* 1969;48:1627-1642.
34. King MA, Wiltshire BG, Lehmann H, et al. An unstable haemoglobin with reduced oxygen affinity: haemoglobin Peterborough, 3 (GI3) Valine lead to Phenylalanine, its interaction with normal haemoglobin and with haemoglobin Lepore. *Br J Haematol.* 1972;22:125-134.
35. Como PF, Wylie BR, Trent RJ, et al. A new unstable and low oxygen affinity hemoglobin variant: Hb Stanmore [beta 111(G13)Val—Ala]. *Hemoglobin.* 1991;15:53-65.
36. Vasseur-Godbillon C, Marden MC, Giordano P, et al. Impaired binding of AHSP to alpha chain variants: Hb Groene Hart illustrates a mechanism leading to unstable hemoglobins with alpha thalassemic like syndrome. *Blood Cells Mol Dis.* 2006;37:173-179.
37. Turbpaiboon C, Limjindaporn T, Wongwiwat W, et al. Impaired interaction of alpha-haemoglobin-stabilising protein with alpha-globin termination mutant in a yeast two-hybrid system. *Br J Haematol.* 2006;132:370-373.
38. Stamatoyannopoulos G, Woodson R, Papayannopoulou T, et al. Inclusion-body beta-thalassemia trait. A form of beta thalassemia producing clinical manifestations in simple heterozygotes. *N Engl J Med.* 1974;290:939-943.
39. Steinberg MH, Adams JG. Thalassemic hemoglobinopathies. *Am J Pathol.* 1983;113:396.
40. Carrell RW, Kay R. A simple method for the detection of unstable haemoglobins. *Br J Haematol.* 1972;23:615-619.
41. Grimes AJ, Meisler A, Dacie JV. Congenital Heinz-body anaemia, further evidence on the cause of Heinz-body production in red cells. *Br J Haematol.* 1964;10:281-290.
42. Kato GJ, Taylor JG6. Pleiotropic effects of intravascular haemolysis on vascular homeostasis. *Br J Haematol.* 2010;148:690-701.
43. Lee-Potter JP, Deacon-Smith RA, Simpkiss MJ, et al. A new cause of haemolytic anaemia in the newborn. A description of an unstable fetal haemoglobin: F Poole, alpha2-G-gamma2 130 trptophan yields glycine. *J Clin Pathol.* 1975;28:317-320.
44. Miller DR, Weed RI, Stamatoyannopoulos G, et al. Hemoglobin Koln disease occurring as a fresh mutation: erythrocyte metabolism and survival. *Blood.* 1971;38:715-729.
45. Tucker PW, Phillips SE, Perutz MF, et al. Structure of hemoglobins Zurich [His E7(63)beta replaced by Arg] and Sydney [Val E11(67)beta replaced by Ala] and role of the distal residues in ligand binding. *Proc Natl Acad Sci U S A.* 1978;75:1076-1080.
46. Zinkham WH, Houtchens RA, Caughey WS. Carboxyhemoglobin levels in an unstable hemoglobin disorder (Hb Zurich): effect on phenotypic expression. *Science.* 1980;209:406-408.
47. Zinkham WH, Houtchens RA, Caughey WS. Relation between variations in the phenotypic expression of an unstable hemoglobin disorder (hemoglobin Zurich) and carboxyhemoglobin levels. *Am J Med.* 1983;74:23-29.
48. Levine RL, Lincoln DR, Buchholz WM, et al. Hemoglobin Hasharon in a premature infant with hemolytic anemia. *Pediatr Res.* 1975;9:7.
49. Tatsis B, Dosik H, Rieder R, et al. Hemoglobin Hasharon: severe hemolytic anemia and hypersplenism associated with a mildly unstable hemoglobin. *Birth Defects.* 1972;8:25.
50. Dejam A, Hunter CJ, Schechter AN, et al. Emerging role of nitrite in human biology. *Blood Cells Mol Dis.* 2004;32:423-429.
51. Gladwin MT, Crawford JH, Patel RP. The biochemistry of nitric oxide, nitrite, and hemoglobin: role in blood flow regulation. *Free Radic Biol Med.* 2004;36:707-717.
52. Andrieu V, Dumonceau O, Grange MJ. Priapism in a patient with unstable hemoglobin: hemoglobin Koln. *Am J Hematol.* 2003;74:73-74.
53. Lode HN, Krings G, Schulze-Neick I, et al. Pulmonary hypertension in a case of Hb-Mainz hemolytic anemia. *J Pediatr Hematol Oncol.* 2007;29:173-177.
54. Brockmann K, Stolpe S, Fels C, et al. Moyamoya syndrome associated with hemolytic anemia due to Hb Alesha. *J Pediatr Hematol Oncol.* 2005;27:436-440.
55. Rose C, Bauters F, Galacteros F. Hydroxyurea therapy in highly unstable hemoglobin carriers. *Blood.* 1996;88:2807-2808.
56. Loovers HM, Tamminga N, Mulder AB, Tamminga RY. Clinical course of two children with unstable hemoglobins: the effect of hydroxyurea therapy. *Hemoglobin.* 2016;40(5):341-344.
57. Percy MJ, McFerran NV, Lappin TR. Disorders of oxidised haemoglobin. *Blood Rev.* 2005;19:61-68.
58. Kutlar F, Hilliard LM, Zhuang L, et al. Hb M Dothan [β 25/26 (B7/B8)/(GGT/GAG→GAG//Gly/Glu→Glu]; a new mechanism of unstable methemoglobin variant and molecular characteristics. *Blood Cells Mol Dis.* 2009;43:235-238.
59. Glader BE, Zwerdling D, Kutlar F, et al. Hb F-M-Osaka or alpha 2G gamma 2(63) (E7)His—Tyr in a Caucasian male infant. *Hemoglobin.* 1989;13:769-773.
60. Priest JR, Watterson J, Jones RT, et al. Mutant fetal hemoglobin causing cyanosis in a newborn. *Pediatrics.* 1989;83:734-736.

61. Siendones E, Ballesteros M, Navas P. Cellular and molecular mechanisms of recessive hereditary methaemoglobinaemia type II. *J Clin Med*. 2018;7(10):341.

62. Coleman MD, Coleman NA. Drug-induced methaemoglobinaemia. Treatment issues. *Drug Saf*. 1996;14:394-405.

63. Cohen RJ, Sachs JF, Wicker DJ, et al. Methemoglobinemia provoked by malarial chemoprophylaxis in Vietnam. *N Engl J Med*. 1968;279:1127-1131.

64. Umbreit J. Methemoglobin—it's not just blue: a concise review. *Am J Hematol*. 2007;82:134-144.

65. Linz AJ, Greenham RK, Fallon LF, Jr. Methemoglobinemia: an industrial outbreak among rubber molding workers. *J Occup Environ Med*. 2006;48:523-528.

66. Greer FR, Shannon M. Infant methemoglobinemia: the role of dietary nitrate in food and water. *Pediatrics*. 2005;116:784-786.

67. Uko EK, Udoh AE, Etukudoh MH. Methaemoglobin profile in malaria infected children in Calabar. *Niger J Med*. 2003;12:94-97.

68. Mansouri A, Lurie AA. Concise review: methemoglobinemia. *Am J Hematol*. 1993;42:7-12.

69. Ash-Bernal R, Wise R, Wright SM. Acquired methemoglobinemia: a retrospective series of 138 cases at 2 teaching hospitals. *Medicine (Balt)*. 2004;83:265-273.

70. Fitzsimons MG, Gaudette RR, Hurford WE. Critical rebound methemoglobinemia after methylene blue treatment: case report. *Pharmacotherapy*. 2004;24:538-540.

71. Golden PJ, Weinstein R. Treatment of high-risk, refractory acquired methemoglobinemia with automated red blood cell exchange. *J Clin Apher*. 1998;13:28-31.

72. Bruns CM, Thet LA, Woodson RD, et al. Hemoglobinopathy case finding by pulse oximetry. *Am J Hematol*. 2003;74:142-143.

73. Deyell R, Jackson S, Spier S, et al. Low oxygen saturation by pulse oximetry may be associated with a low oxygen affinity hemoglobin variant, hemoglobin Titusville. *J Pediatr Hematol Oncol*. 2006;28:100-102.

74. Haymond S, Cariappa R, Eby CS, et al. Laboratory assessment of oxygenation in methemoglobinemia. *Clin Chem*. 2005;51:434-444.

75. Verhovsek M, Henderson MP, Cox G, et al. Unexpectedly low pulse oximetry measurements associated with variant hemoglobins: a systematic review. *Am J Hematol*. 2011;86:722-725.

76. Weaver LK. Carbon monoxide poisoning. *N Engl J Med*. 2009;360:1217-1225.

77. Hampson NB, Dunn SL. Symptoms of carbon monoxide poisoning do not correlate with the initial carboxyhemoglobin level. *Undersea Hyerb Med*. 2012;39:657-685.

78. Hampson NB. U.S. mortality due to carbon monoxide poisoning, 1999-2014. Accidental and intentional deaths. *Ann Am Thorac Soc*. 2016;13:1768-1774.

79. Sircar K, Clower J, Shin MK, et al. Carbon monoxide poisoning deaths in the United States, 1999 to 2012. *Am J Emerg Med*. 2015;33:1140-1145.

80. Lopez-Herce J, Borrego R, Bustinza A, et al. Elevated carboxyhemoglobin associated with sodium nitroprusside treatment. *Intensive Care Med*. 2005;31:1235-1238.

81. Fisher JA, Iscoe S, Fedorko L, Duffin J. Rapid elimination of CO through the lungs: coming full circle 100 years on. *Exp Physiol*. 2011;96:1262-1269.

82. Gopalachar AS, Bowie VL, Bharadwaj P. Phenazopyridine-induced sulfhemoglobinemia. *Ann Pharmacother*. 2005;39:1128-1130.

83. Gow AJ. The biological chemistry of nitric oxide as it pertains to the extrapulmonary effects of inhaled nitric oxide. *Proc Am Thorac Soc*. 2006;3:150-152.

84. Gow AJ, Singel D. NO, SNO, and hemoglobin: lessons in complexity. *Blood*. 2006;108:3224-3225. author reply 3226-3227.

85. Gow AJ, Stamler JS. Reactions between nitric oxide and haemoglobin under physiological conditions. *Nature*. 1998;391:169-173.

86. Jia L, Bonaventura C, Bonaventura J, et al. S-nitrosohaemoglobin: a dynamic activity of blood involved in vascular control. *Nature*. 1996;380:221-226.

87. Kim-Shapiro DB, Schechter AN, Gladwin MT. Unraveling the reactions of nitric oxide, nitrite, and hemoglobin in physiology and therapeutics. *Arterioscler Thromb Vasc Biol*. 2006;26:697-705.

88. Stamler JS, Jia L, Eu JP, et al. Blood flow regulation by S-nitrosohemoglobin in the physiological oxygen gradient. *Science*. 1997;276:2034-2037.

Chapter 37 ■ Megaloblastic Anemias: Disorders of Impaired DNA Synthesis

SALLY P. STABLER

HISTORY OF MEGALOBLASTIC ANEMIA

An anemia which was presumed related to the digestive system was recognized in the first half of the 19th century and then described in detail by Addison in 1849 in a patient who likely had severe pernicious anemia.[1] It was associated with atrophic gastritis by Fenwick in 1870 and Remier described the clinical presentation as progressive pernicious anemia in 1872. It was recognized early that some of the patients had neurological abnormalities also.[2,3] This disease was invariably fatal until Minot and Murphy described treatment with an oral liver diet in 1926.[4] Many attempts over 2 decades eventually resulted in the discovery of the active principal in the liver with contributions from Karl Folkers, Thomas Wood, Norman Brink, Edward Rieckes, and Frank Koniuszy.[2] The crystallized cobalamin (Cbl), vitamin B_{12}, achieved in 1947 was a red compound, which contributed to the success of the chromatography attempts. This discovery was possible because of the collaboration with a clinician, Randolph West, MD, who was able to find patients with pernicious anemia who could be used as a bioassay for the chromatographic fractions, demonstrating reticulocytosis after ingesting an active fraction. The crystalline structure was reported by Dorothy Hodgkin in 1965.[5] Eventually, work by Dr. Mary Shorb led to a microbiologic assay using *Lactobacillus lactis Dorner*, an organism dependent on Cbl for growth.[6] Later, the chemical structure was determined and methods of fermentation for large-scale production were developed obviating the need for large quantities of liver as a starting material. Pernicious anemia is a unique nutritional model because of the specific malabsorption of Cbl in an otherwise healthy individual, unlike many other nutritional deficiencies, so the study of these patients has led to much of the knowledge of the role of Cbl in normal physiology.

Meanwhile, Dr. Lucy Wills was studying macrocytic anemia in pregnancy and reported improvement with yeast extracts in 1931,[7] which led to the discovery of the folates, which were isolated in 1948 by Robert Stokstad and colleagues.[8] It is likely that oral liver therapy may have cured folate as well as Cbl deficiency. But once the active purified vitamins were available, it became necessary to distinguish between the specific etiologies of megaloblastic anemia.

Because treatment is so simple and inexpensive, it is surprising that clinicians still encounter life-threatening, undiagnosed megaloblastic anemia often in its near terminal stages. In addition, there are very few demyelinating diseases of the central nervous system that can be cured or at least greatly ameliorated with a simple treatment. Therefore, Cbl deficiency should be investigated in any compatible clinical situation.

NORMAL PHYSIOLOGY AND PATHOPHYSIOLOGY

Megaloblastic anemia is usually due to either Cbl or folate deficiency, both causing an identical pancytopenia due to impaired DNA synthesis.[9,10] The two cofactors intersect at the conversion of homocysteine to methionine by methionine synthase, a reaction that requires N^5-methyl-tetrahydrofolate and methylcobalamin.[11] Although they contribute to this reaction equally, other aspects of the clinical syndromes and physiology are different between the two vitamins. There are also a number of drugs and enzymatic defects that cause megaloblastic anemias largely unrelated to either Cbl or folate metabolism.

Cobalamin

Cbl is a structurally complex macromolecule (see *Figure 37.1*) with a molecular weight of 1355 Da, in which a central cobalt is coordinated to four nitrogen atoms in pyrrole residues, which form a tetrapyrrolic corrin ring. The cobalt also binds a lower axial ligand, 5, 6-dimethylbenzimidazole linked by a ribose-phosphate group. An upper axial ligand is also coordinated to the cobalt and can be a methyl or 5′-deoxyadenosyl group present in the two active cofactors or glutathionyl, aquo (hydroxyl), or cyano group. The different forms can be interchanged enzymatically.[9-13] The most stable form is cyanoCbl that is most frequently used in treatment. A decyanase activity has been reported.[14] The hydroxoCbl form is readily converted to the active coenzymes. The central cobalt exists in three reduction states cob (III), cob (II), and cob (I). There is a family of corrinoids in which the 5, 6-dimethylbenzimidazole residue is replaced by another nucleotide such as adenine or methyladenine, which are active cofactors for many microorganisms. Although these Cbl analogues are present in large quantities in human feces and in the environment, they do not satisfy

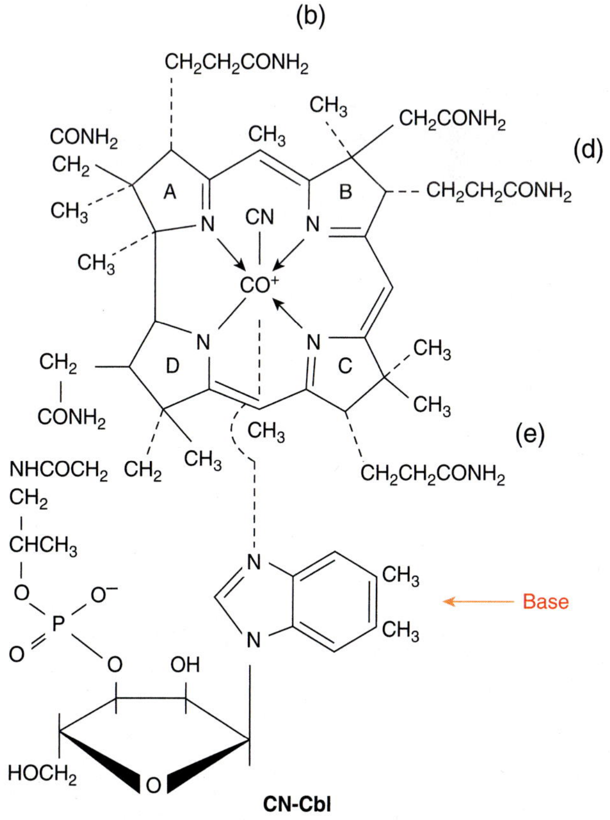

FIGURE 37.1 **Structure of cobalamin.** CN is shown bound to the central cobalt in the tetrapyrrole corrin ring. 5,6-dimethylbenzimidazole is the nucleotide base shown. CN can be substituted by methyl, adenosyl, hydroxo (aquo), or glutathionyl groups. The e chain off of the C ring can be modified to make inhibitory analogues such as C-lactam Cbl.

the requirement for Cbl.[15] Intracellular processing of the Cbl is necessary to form the two active cofactors, methylCbl and adenosylCbl.[13] The study of individuals with inborn errors has elucidated the many reactions and genes necessary for trafficking of Cbl and synthesizing these active cofactors.

Propionyl-CoA Metabolism

Propionyl-CoA and methylmalonyl-CoA metabolism are shown in *Figure 37.2*. Thymine, valine, isoleucine, methionine, odd chain fatty acids, and the other compounds shown are converted to propionyl-CoA, which is carboxylase by propionyl-CoA carboxylate to form the D-isomer of methylmalonyl-CoA. After racemization by methylmalonyl-CoA epimerase (MCE, MCEE gene), L-methylmalonyl-CoA is converted by L-methylmalonyl-CoA mutase to succinyl-CoA utilizing adenosylCbl as a cofactor. The D isomer of methylmalonyl-CoA can be cleaved by a hydrolase (D-methylmalonyl-CoA hydrolase, 3-hydroxyisobutyryl-CoA hydrolase)[16,17] to form methylmalonic acid (MMA), a compound which has a largely unknown metabolic role but is a sensitive indicator of a block in L-methylmalonyl-CoA mutase activity.[11,18-20] When this pathway is inhibited by Cbl deficiency, concentrations of propionyl-CoA increase so that citrate synthase utilizes it instead of acetyl-CoA to form 2-methylcitric acid instead of citric acid.[21,22] Although the propionyl-CoA pathway is not a major energy source in humans (unlike ruminants), a severe deficiency of the mutase or of adenosylCbl causes a devastating buildup of MMA and methylcitric acid with resulting severe acidosis and many secondary metabolic abnormalities in some inborn errors of Cbl metabolism.[23,24] The mutase is not fully saturated with Cbl *in vivo* (25% in liver) and withdrawal of Cbl quickly increases MMA concentrations in animal models,[25] cell cultures,[26] and human patients.[18,27,28] The buildup of methylmalonyl-CoA has consequences on the total CoA pool and increases propionyl-carnitine in urine and

short-chain acylcarnitines in plasma and liver.[23,29,30] It also appears to contribute to increases in odd chain and branched chain fatty acids in tissues.[31-33] Some metabolic abnormalities due to deficiency of Cbl are shown in *Table 37.1*.

Cobalamin and Methionine Metabolism

Methionine metabolism is shown in *Figure 37.3*, which features interrelationships between Cbl and folate metabolism and the second Cbl-dependent enzyme, methionine synthase (MTR).[9,11] Cbl bound to MTR is reduced to cob (I), which can bind the methyl in N^5-methylTHF and transfer it to homocysteine with tetrahydrofolate (THF) and methionine as resulting products. Occasionally, the cob (I) is oxidized to cob (II) and another enzyme methionine synthase reductase (MTRR) transfers a methyl group from S-adenosylmethionine (SAM) and reduces it back to cob (I).[34] The THF produced in this reaction is necessary for the production of substrates for DNA synthesis after the conversion to other folate forms and will be described below in the section on Folate Metabolism. This intersection between the two vitamins underlies the indistinguishable megaloblastic anemia caused by deficiency of either one.[10,11,19,35]

N^5-methylTHF must be demethylated to THF in order to undergo all of the other folate-dependent reactions and is thus metabolically inactive. This has led to a concept of a "methyl trap" such that severe Cbl deficiency results in an accumulation of methylTHF, which since it is a poor substrate for folylpoly-x-glutamate synthetase, is released from cells and lost in the urine causing a secondary folate deficiency.[35,36] THF has another role as the inhibitor of N-glycine methyltransferase, an enzyme that controls the quantity of intracellular SAM, thereby regulating the balance of methylation of many critical compounds.[37,38] This inhibition may have a sparing effect on the availability of SAM in Cbl deficiency when methylTHF is trapped.[38]

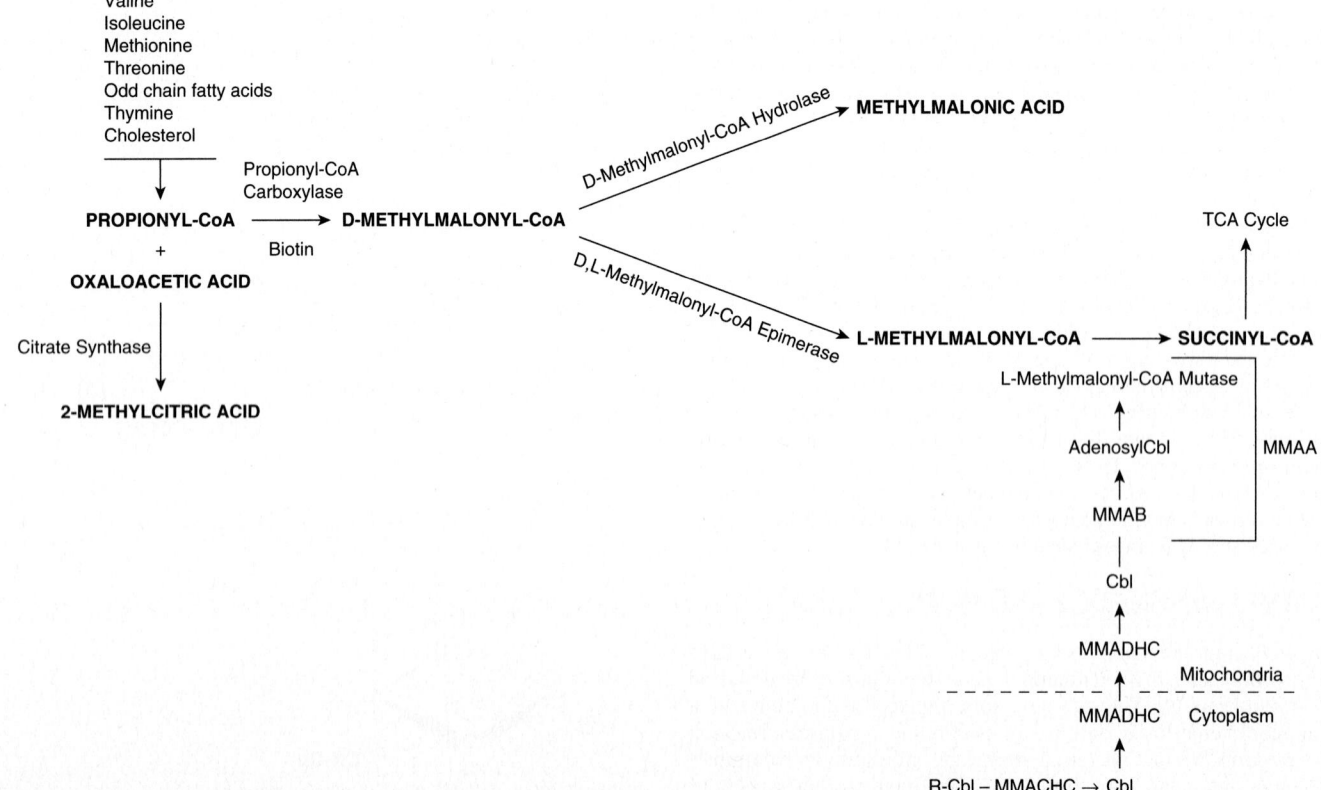

FIGURE 37.2 The mitochondrial reactions of propionyl and methylmalonyl-CoA metabolism are shown with the intracellular steps of processing of Cbl to the adenosylCbl cofactor for L-methylmalonyl-CoA mutase activity. CoA, coenzyme A; MMAA methylmalonic aciduria type A; MMAB, methylmalonic aciduria type B; MMACHC, methylmalonic aciduria cbl C with homocystinuria; MMADHC, methylmalonic aciduria cbl D type with homocystinuria; R-Cbl, cobalamin with an unspecified ligand coordinated to the central cobalt.

Table 37.1. Accumulation of Metabolites Due to Clinical Cobalamin and/or Folate Deficiency

	Cbl	Folate
Methylmalonic acid – serum, CSF, urine	High (>95%)[a]	Normal
2-methylcitric acid – serum, urine	High (95%)	Normal
Total homocysteine - serum, CSF	High (>95%)	High (>95%)
Cystathionine – serum	High (80%)	High (84%)
N-methylglycine – serum	Normal	High (40%)
N, N-dimethylglycine – serum	Normal	High (72%)
S-adenosylmethionine (SAM) – serum	Low (13%)	Unknown
S-adenosylhomocysteine (SAH) – serum	High (86%)	Unknown
SAM/SAH ratio – serum	Low (87%)	Unknown

[a]The percentage shown refers to the fraction of affected patients with abnormality. CSF, cerebrospinal fluid

Folate

Folates are a group of compounds containing a pteridine ring bound to p-aminobenzoate with a polyglutamate tail of varying length as shown in *Figure 37.4*. Two of the nitrogen atoms, N^5 and N^{10}, can bind one-carbon units or hydrogens. The reaction of MTR has been described above because of its role in megaloblastic anemia, wherein the N^5-methylTHF is reduced to THF. THF is thus available after formation of the various cofactors shown in the pathways (*Figure 37.3*)

to participate in reactions important in production of purines and pyrimidines, which are necessary for DNA synthesis and thus hematopoiesis.[11,39] Other reactions are important in formate metabolism.[40] The folates are compartmentalized in the cytoplasm, mitochondria, and nucleus. The one-carbon reactions in the cytoplasm result in the production of purines, thymidylate, and methylation of homocysteine. Formate is generated in the mitochondria from serine and glycine and transferred back to the cytoplasm. Thymidylate is synthesized in the

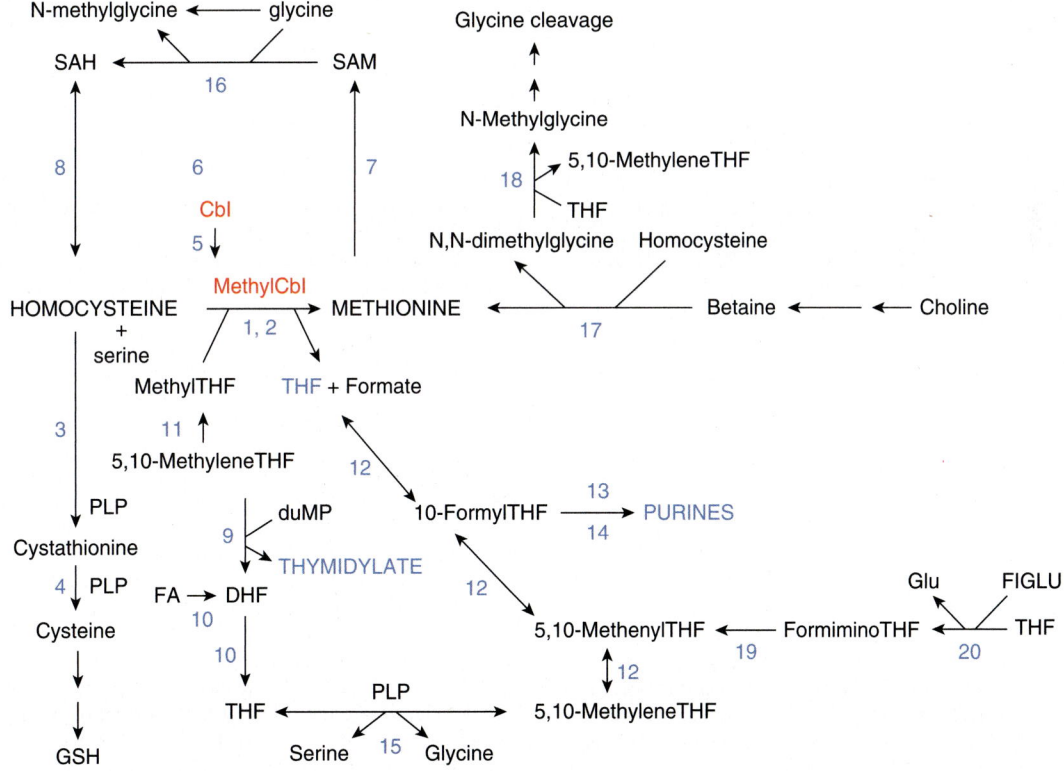

FIGURE 37.3 Reactions and interrelationships between cobalamin (Cbl), folate, and methionine metabolism are shown. The central reaction of methylation of homocysteine to methionine with MethylCbl as a cofactor demethylates N5-methyltetrahdrofolate (THF) to THF, which can be converted to the forms needed for thymidylate and purine synthesis required for DNA synthesis. The enzymes in the pathway are numbered. 1. Methionine synthase, 2. Methionine synthase reductase, 3. Cystathionine beta-synthase, 4. Gamma-cystathionase, 5. Methylmalonic aciduria cbl D type with homocystinuria, 6. Methylmalonic aciduria cbl C with homocystinuria, 7. Methionine adenosyltransferase I/III, II, 8. S-adenosylhomocysteine hydrolase, 9. Thymidylate synthase, 10. Dihydrofolate reductase, 11. 5,10-MethyleneTHF reductase, 12. MTHFD1, methyleneTHF dehydrogenase 1, cyclohydrolase, and formylTHF synthetase, 13. Glycinamide ribonucleotide transformylase, 14. 5(4)amino-imidazole-4-(5)-carboxamide ribonucleotide transformylase, 15. Serine hydroxymethyltransferase, 16. Glycine N-methyltransferase, 17. Betaine homocysteine methyltransferase, 18. Dimethylglycine dehydrogenase, 19. FormiminoTHF cyclodeaminase, 20. Glutamate formiminotransferase. Cbl, cobalamin; DHF, dihydrofolate; dUMP, deoxyuridine monophosphate; FA, folic acid; FIGLU, formiminoglutamic acid; Glu, glutamic acid; GSH, glutathione; MethylCbl, Methylcobalamin; PLP, pyridoxal 5''phosphate; SAH, S-adenosylhomocysteine; SAM, S-adenosylmethionine; THF, tetrahydrofolate.

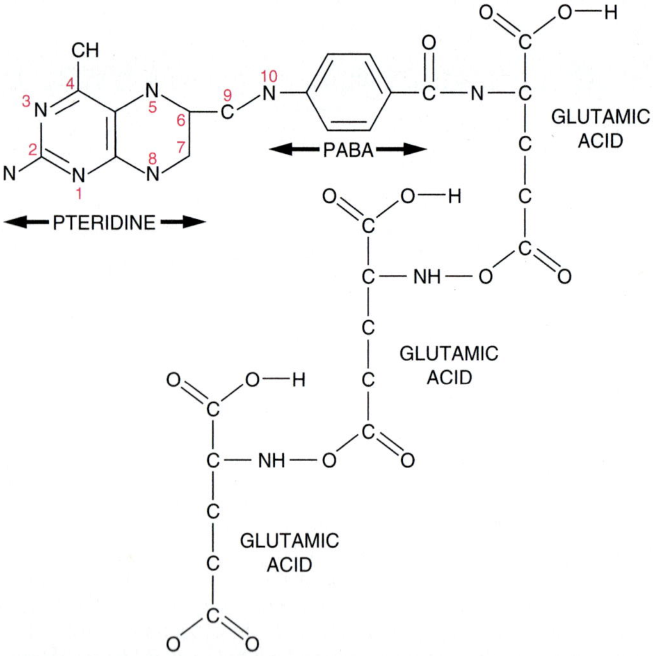

FIGURE 37.4 Structure of folate. Folates contain a pteridine ring bound to *p*-aminobenzoic acid (PABA) and one or more glutamic acid residues bound by a gamma-carboxyl linkage. The nitrogen atoms are numbered. Reduction of positions 5, 6, 7, and 8 are necessary to form tetrahydrofolate. Various one-carbon moieties are attached to position 5 or 10 or bridging 5 and 10 for the cofactor activity specific to the enzymes shown in *Figure 37.3*.

nucleus from uridylate and serine after sumoylation and import of SHMT, thymidylate synthase (TYMS), and dihydrofolate reductase (DHFR).[39,40] The different forms of folates have varying length of polyglutamate tails from 3 to 8, which helps for cellular retention and for specific enzymatic reactions. The primary circulating folate, N^5-methylTHF is not a good substrate for polyglutamation.[35] Folic acid is a fully oxidized stable form and is widely used as a food additive, in multivitamin supplements, and as a therapeutic for folate deficiency. Folic acid can be reduced to dihydrofolate and THF by DHFR and then is available to accept one-carbon units.

The folates participate in many reactions including one-carbon transfer, cellular methylation reactions, amino acid reactions, and nucleotide biosynthesis. Enzymatic pathways and reactions involving folates are shown in *Figure 37.3*.

Transmethylation and Transsulfuration

Homocysteine is at a branchpoint between conversion to methionine or to cystathionine.[11,41,42] Methionine is converted to SAM—the major physiologic methyl donor.[43] Clearance of homocysteine by cystathionine beta-synthase to form cystathionine and hence cleavage to cysteine is necessary for the production of glutathione—the most important physiologic reducing agent. When methionine and, thus, SAM are abundant, cystathionine beta-synthase is activated and homocysteine is shunted toward transsulfuration.[41] SAM also inhibits $N,^{5-10}$ methylenetetrahydrofolate reductase (MTHFR) thus, decreasing the quantity of N^5-methylTHF formed. In conditions of low methionine, homocysteine is shunted toward methionine production instead and MTHFR produces more N^5-methylTHF. SAM is a crucial methyl donor for most cellular methylation reactions. The bulk of the methylation reactions are for the production of creatine and phosphatidylcholine but also used for methylating proteins, histones, neurotransmitters, and nucleic acids.[41,43]

Cobalamin Physiology

Nutrition

Cbl and the related corrinoids are synthesized by micro-organisms and all higher animals obtain Cbl directly or indirectly by ingesting these products. Ruminants have bacteria in the digestive tract that synthesize Cbl. Other animals including humans obtain Cbl from eating animal source food, which include dairy products, meats and shellfish, invertebrates,[44-46] or fermented foods, the latter which contain both true Cbl and its analogues.[47] Although there is Cbl synthesized by bacteria in the human colon, it is not available for absorption and is less than 2% of the total corrinoids, the remainder being the naturally occurring analogues containing different bases.[15] AdenosylCbl and hydroxo-Cbl are found in natural food bound to the enzymes. Many foods are also fortified with cyanoCbl in the western world, especially true of meat and dairy vegetarian alternative foods, energy bars, and drink supplements used to promote athletic performance. Certain algae[48-50] and fermented plant food such as tempe[51,52] and enset[53] have been shown to contain true Cbl as well as analogues. Shellfish such as clams and oysters have the highest concentrations of Cbl followed by organ meats, particularly liver, kidney, and heart. Bovine meat is higher is Cbl content than pork, and fowl is considerably lower.[44,45]

Cobalamin intake varies widely throughout the world. Those consuming an omnivorous diet with large amounts of animal products average 4 to 6 µg/d but populations for whom such food is too scarce or expensive consume much less and mild to severe Cbl deficiency is common.[44] The bioavailability of food Cbl is approximately 50%.[54] In the United States, the dietary reference intake has been set at 2.4 µg/d with higher intakes recommended for pregnancy and lactation—2.6 and 2.8 µg/d, respectively. Intakes for infants range from 0.4 µg/d to 1.8 for prepubescent children.[55] Total body content of Cbl is estimated between 1 and 5 mg, which has implications for replacement therapy in deficient individuals.[56] Most clinical Cbl deficiency results from malabsorption of Cbl and can be overcome by large doses of oral Cbl in which 1% is absorbed by passive diffusion.[57-59] Otherwise, Cbl absorption is limited by the availability of intrinsic factor (IF), so a lower fraction is absorbed from a meal high in Cbl content.[54]

Cobalamin Absorption

There are only trace quantities of Cbl in food and it is bound to proteins. Thus, elaborate processes have evolved to deliver it to cells.[9,13,19,44,60] The proteins important in assimilation and transport of Cbl are shown in *Table 37.2*. As food is ingested, it is mixed with saliva containing haptocorrin (HC), a non–specific glycoprotein binder of Cbl and other corrinoids and then delivered to the stomach[61] as shown in *Figure 37.5*. The gastric parietal cells secrete IF, a glycoprotein that has high affinity and high specificity for true Cbl[62] with much less for the naturally occurring analogues.[63] Digestion of food in the stomach releases Cbl from proteins, and after binding to HC, it is passed to the duodenum where HC is released in the alkaline environment containing pancreatic enzymes freeing Cbl for binding to IF.[64] The IF-Cbl complex is carried to the distal ileum, the site of the cubam receptor for uptake of the IF-Cbl complex. Cubam exists of two proteins: cubulin, the ligand-binding component, and amnionless (ANM), a type 1 transmembrane protein to which it is attached. Both are needed for endocytosis of IF-Cbl.[64,65] After IF is removed, Cbl exits the ileal cell by the multidrug resistance protein 1 and then binds to transcobalamin (TC) or HC in the portal bloodstream. The uptake in the ileum is limited by the amount of cubam receptor to about 1.5 to 2.5 µg. Thus, a lower fraction of Cbl is absorbed from a Cbl rich meal. It takes about 4 to 6 hours after a meal for the receptors to recycle.

Inborn errors of IF,[64,66] the cubam receptor,[64,65] and TC[67] all cause Cbl deficiency, but the role of HC in normal physiology is much less known.[68,69] The Cbl bound to HC (holo-HC) likely has a slower turnover than that bound to TC.[62] HC is cleared by hepatic asialoglycoprotein receptors and the internalized Cbl is secreted into bile where it can be reabsorbed through IF mediated uptake. This enterohepatic circulation of Cbl prevents loss from the body to about only 1 µg/d.[19,70] HC is present in high concentrations in many secretions such as saliva, gastric juice, amniotic fluid, tears, and breast milk.[68] Since HC binds to naturally occurring Cbl analogues, it is thought that it may have a role in removing these from the body. Granulocytes contain HC and it is intriguing to speculate that this is from ingested bacteria containing analogues or has some protective scavenging role in infection.

Table 37.2. Cobalamin Binding Proteins

Protein	Intrinsic Factor (IF)	Transcobalamin (TC)	Haptocorrin (HC)
Gene	*GIF (chr. 11q13)*	*TCN2 (chr. 22q12.2)*	*TCN1 (chr. 11q11-q12.3)*
Role	Binds Cbl in upper intestinal tract and delivers to ileal IF receptor	Carries Cbl in circulation and delivers to all cells	Binds Cbl in mouth and stomach then releases in upper small intestine Binds Cbl in milk Sequesters analogues from IF and TC
Cbl and analogue binding characteristics	High affinity for Cbl Kd < 1pM, low affinity for analogues	High affinity for Cbl, variable affinity for analogues	High affinity for all corrinoids at neutral and high pH
Origin	Gastric parietal cells	Endothelial cells and others	Saliva, gastric juice, secretions, granulocytes
Distribution	Gastric juice	Plasma, CSF, amniotic fluid, semen, 20% of total Cbl in plasma	Plasma, secretions, CSF, semen 80% of total Cbl in plasma
Receptors	Cubilin-amnionless (Cubam) complex in distal ileum	TC receptor (CD320) on all cells and megalin in proximal renal tubule	None for intact HC, but taken up by hepatic asialoglycoprotein receptor after processing
Protein Structure	48 kDa glycoprotein	43 kDa polypeptide	66 kDa glycoprotein
Turnover	4-6 h	90 mi	9 d

COBALAMIN ABSORPTION AND DEFECTS

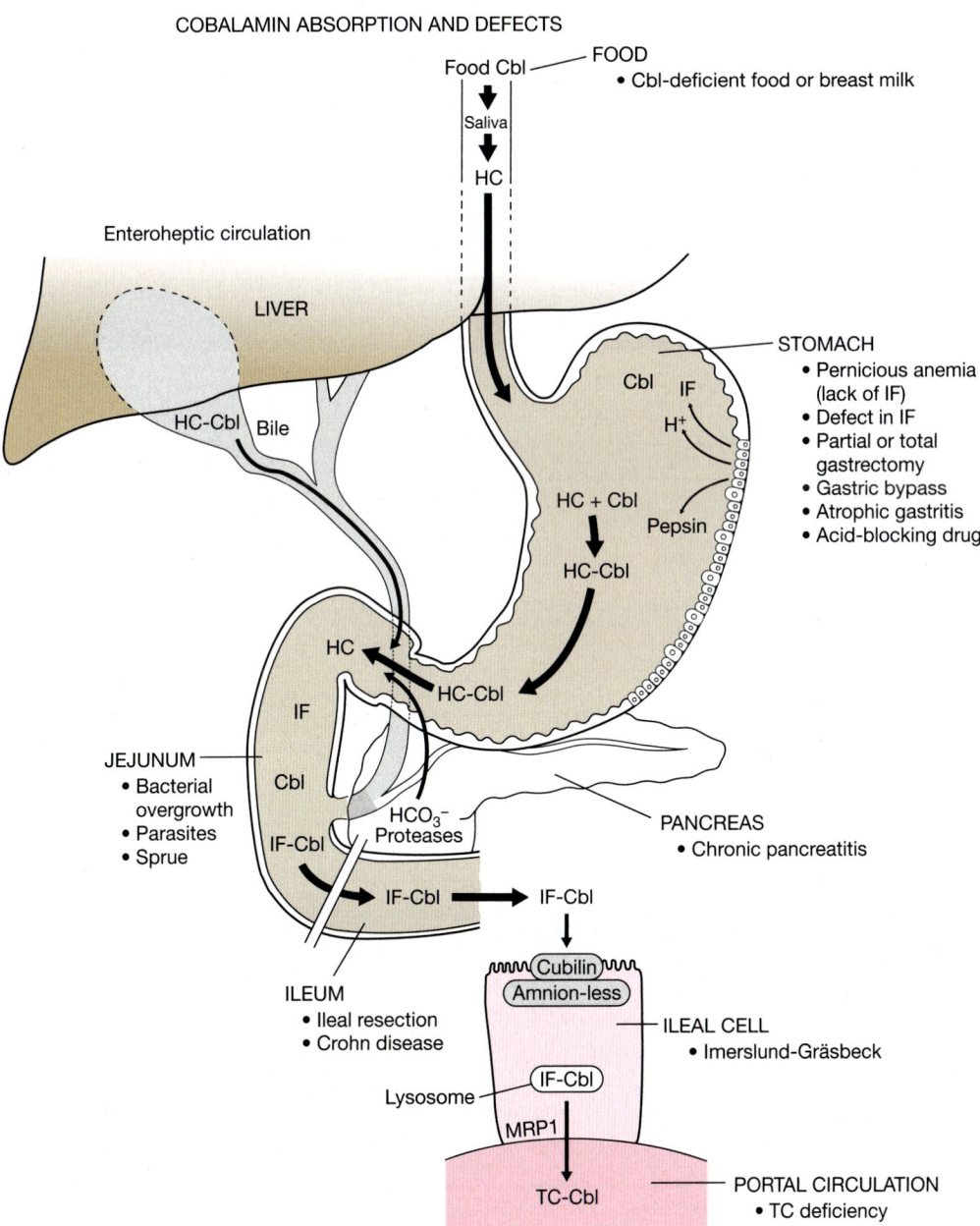

FIGURE 37.5 Processes of absorption of cobalamin (Cbl) by the gastrointestinal tract are shown. Food is mixed with saliva containing haptocorrin (HC) and processed by acid and pepsin in the stomach. Parietal cells release intrinsic factor (IF) and after release of Cbl from HC in the duodenum in the presence of pancreatic secreted bicarb and proteases, the IF-Cbl travels to the distal ileum to be bound to the CUBAM receptor (Cubilin and Amnionless complex) and internalized. HC-Cbl is present in bile and available to bind to IF thus recycled by the enterohepatic circulation.

Measurements of serum/plasma Cbl largely reflect the HC binding of Cbl rather than TC, 80% vs 20% leading to difficulties with the specificity and sensitivity of Cbl assays for defining tissue deficiency.

Intracellular Metabolism

Holo-transcobalamin (holo-TC) is delivered to the liver and to all cells through the vascular system and is taken up by the CD320 receptor by cellular endocytosis.[71,72] The TC is degraded in lysosomes and Cbl release is dependent on the lysosomal membrane proteins LMBRD1[73] and ABCD4[74] and then processed to form the cofactors for cytoplasmic MTR and adenosylCbl for mitochondrial L-methylmalonyl-CoA mutase. Methylmalonic aciduria Cbl C type with homocystinuria (MMACHC) protein binds and removes the upper axial ligand by decyanation or dealkylation[75] and chaperons the cob I to another protein methylmalonic aciduria CbD type with homocystinuria (MMADHC),[76] which can deliver Cbl to MTR in the cytosol or to the mitochondria for the mutase. ABCG, an ATP-binding cassette transporter, may play a role in transporting Cbl into the mitochondria.[13] The mitochondrial methylmalonic aciduria type B protein[77] sequesters the Cbl and synthesizes the adenosylCbl cofactor. The next step is the transfer of the cofactor to the mutase by methylmalonic aciduria type A protein[78] in complex with the mutase. This intracellular metabolism described above and in *Table 37.3* was discovered by examining patients with inborn errors of metabolism causing methylmalonic aciduria and/or homocystinuria.

Cobalamin Issues of Nutrition

There is no storage form of Cbl analogous to ferritin for iron with the body store of Cbl bound to the two enzymes and carriers. The total body content ranges from 1 to 5 mg depending on body size. The efficient enterohepatic uptake of biliary Cbl salvages much of the bile Cbl.[19] TC-Cbl is reabsorbed by megalin in the kidney proximal tubules. Human and animal feces contain large quantities of corrinoids but only a small percent is true Cbl as most intestinal bacteria use analogues with bases other than 5,6-dimethylbenzimidazole.[15] These bacteria remove the corrin ring from high doses of oral Cbl and synthesize analogues.[15] Dietary deficiency takes 5 to 10 years to develop because the loss of Cbl is so low compared to the total body content. However, if depletion starts in utero with the Cbl deficient mother feeding low content breast milk, then consequences for the infant can develop in months.[79,80] Long-standing dietary deficiency cannot be cured quickly with the small amounts of Cbl in food or in most multivitamin preparations because of the IF-mediated limited absorption and will take many months absorbing only 4 µg/d to replace 1 to 4 mg.[81] Trials of Cbl replacement in pregnancy and childhood have often failed to recognize this.

Folate Physiology

Nutrition

Folates are found in almost all fruits and leafy green vegetables. Orange juice, nuts, legumes, organ meats, and yeast preparations are rich in content.[82] Dairy foods and muscle meats are lower. Food folates are soluble and can be lost if cooking water is discarded. In order to prevent some neural tube defects, folic acid was added to enriched grain products in the United States in 1998 and soon after Canada.[83,84] At least 80 countries around the world now fortify enriched grain products[85] with recent inclusion of the United Kingdom[86] and most EU countries. The US target concentration was 140 µg of folic acid

Table 37.3. Inborn Errors of Cobalamin Assimilation and Metabolism

	Disorder					
	Defect (Gene)	Low Cbl	High MMA	High Hcys	MA	Neuro
IF deficiency	IF (*GIF*)	Yes	Yes	Yes	Yes	Yes
Imerslund-Gräsbeck syndrome	CUBAM Ileal IF-Cbl receptor (*AMN* or *CUB*)	Yes	Yes	Yes	Yes	Yes
TC deficiency	TC synthesis (*TCN2*)	No	Yes	Yes	Yes	Yes
TC Receptor deficiency	TC receptor synthesis (*TCblR/CD320*)	No	Yes	No	No	No
HC deficiency	HC Synthesis	Yes	No	No	No	No
Disorders of Intracellular Processing						
Cbl-A defect	Mitochondrial reduction of Cbl (*MMAA*)	No	Yes	No	No	Related to acidosis, FTT
Cbl-B defect	Cob(1)alamin transferase (*MMAB*)	No	Yes	No	No	Related to acidosis, FTT
Cbl-C defect	Cbl reduction and chaperone (*MMACHC*)	No	Yes	Yes	Yes	Yes
Cbl-X defect	Regulates MMACHC transcription (*HCFC1*)	No	Yes	Yes	?	Yes
(Not named)	Regulation of MMACHC (*ZNF143*) (*THAPII*)	No	Yes	Yes	?	Epilepsy, multiple defects
Cbl-D defect	(*MMADHD*)	No				Yes
Combined	Both	No	Yes	Yes	Yes	Yes
Variant 1	Affects methylCbl	No	No	Yes	Yes	Yes
Variant 2	Affects adenosylCbl	No	Yes	No	No	Yes
Cbl-E defect	Methionine synthase reductase (*MTRR*)	No	No	Yes	Yes	Yes
Cbl-F defect	Cbl release from lysosome (*LMBRD1*)	No	Yes	Yes	Yes	Yes
Cbl-G defect	Methionine synthase (*MTR*)	No	No	Yes	Yes	Yes
Cbl-J defect	Cbl release from lysosome (*ABCD4*)	No	Yes	Yes	Yes	Yes
Mut defect	Absent or defective mutase	No	Yes	No	No	Related to acidosis, FTT
MMA-CoA epimerase deficiency	MMA-CoA racemase (*MCEE*)	No	Yes	No	No	No

Abbreviations: AMN, amionless; Cbl, cobalamin; CUB, cubilin; FTT, failure to thrive; GIF, gastric intrinsic factor; HC, haptocorrin; Hcys, homocysteine; IF, intrinsic factor; MA, megaloblastic anemia; neuro demyelination, myeloneuropathy; MMA, methylmalonic acid; MUT, L-methylmalonyl-CoA mutase; TC, transcobalamin.

per 100 g flour, although there was overage initially by food manufacturers. Serum and red cell folate concentrations increased markedly in fortified populations virtually eliminating clinical folate deficiency.[84,85,87-89] Folate deficiency remains a problem in nonfortified countries.[87] The Institute of Medicine has published Dietary Reference Intakes,[55] with reference intakes through the lifespan ranging from 65 μg for young infants, 150 to 200 for school-aged children, 300 to 400 for adolescent females, and 400 μg for adults. The recommended intake is increased to 600 μg for pregnancy and 500 μg for lactation. Other countries often recommend lower values such as 225 μg in the Netherlands. An upper level of intake has been set at 1000 μg for supplements and fortified food together.[55]

Folate Absorption and Intracellular Metabolism

Food folates are a mixture of reduced folates with a predominance of N_5-methylTHF and are often polyglutamated.[82,83] Many prepared foods are supplemented with folic acid, which is an oxidized monoglutamate of folate. Folic acid has a higher bioavailability than the natural food folates and a dietary folate equivalent has been devised such that it equals the natural food folate plus 1.7 times the quantity of folic acid.[83]

Polyglutamated folate in food must be converted to the monoglutamate by folylpoly-gamma-glutamate carboxypeptidase (glutamate carboxypeptidase II), found in the jejunal brush border membrane with a pH optimum of 6.5.[90-92] The deconjugated folates are transported by the proton coupled folate transporter (PCFT, $SLC46A1$) with a pH optimum of about 5.5[91] (*Table 37.4*). This is a saturable system in the brush border of the upper small intestinal membranes. Inborn errors of this carrier cause hereditary folate malabsorption.[93] Both reduced and oxidized folates are transported. PCFT also transports folates into the choroid plexus in the central nervous system. There is another unsaturable pathway for high luminal concentrations of folates. Absorbed folates are converted to N_5-methylTHF. However, folic acid can appear in the blood stream after large doses are ingested. The absorbed monoglutamate is polyglutamated in tissues by folylpolyglutamate synthetase, which increases retention of folate in the cell. The glutamate tail can also be removed by gamma-glutamyl hydrolase a lysosomal protein. Transporters such as PCFT, multidrug resistance proteins, and breast cancer resistance protein release folates from cells. It is estimated there is about 15 to 30 mg total body content of folate in the liver. Folate is filtered by the glomerulus in the kidney and then reabsorbed in the proximal renal tubules. Some folates are subject to the enterohepatic circulation mediated by *MRP2, BCRP,*

OATP1B1, and *OATP1B3*. Enteric bacteria synthesize folates that may be absorbed.[94] It is not known how much folate is lost in feces. There appear to be both fast turnover pools of folates 0.5 to 2 days and larger slow turnover pools of about 200 days.[95] It is estimated that 0.5% to 1% of total body content of 30 to 100 mg is lost per day and must be replaced.[95,96]

The large daily loss of folates is why dietary folate deficiency occurs much faster than dietary Cbl deficiency. Experimental folate deficiency caused megaloblastic anemia after about 2 to 3 months[82] and plasma homocysteine elevation may occur much more rapidly as folates are depleted.

The tissue uptake and release of folates is mediated by the reduced folate carrier (RFC, SCL19A1),[97] which is a member of the SLC19 family or by three glycosylphosphatidylinositol anchored receptors, termed folate receptors (FR and FRB). There is also a mitochondrial folate transporter SLC25A32.[97] RFC transports reduced folates including the antifolate drugs, thus, is important in oncology. The FRs are expressed in the renal tubules and many other epithelial tissues and in some tumors and mediate folate uptake by an endocytic pathway.[97]

Folates in cells are compartmentalized into cytosolic, mitochondrial, and nuclear pools. The cytosolic and mitochondrial pools support one carbon metabolism with the enzymes SHMT, CH2-THF dehydrogenase/CH+-THF cyclohydrolase, and 10 formyl-THF synthase activities in parallel.[11,39,40] The products, serine, glycine, and formate, traverse the mitochondrial membrane and connect such that mitochondrial formate is used in the cytoplasmic reactions for purine, thymidine, and methionine biosynthesis as shown in *Figure 37.3*. The most important reactions for prevention of megaloblastic anemia are the MTR reaction, thymidylate synthesis, and the donation of two formate groups for the synthesis of purines.[98,99]

CLINICAL AND LABORATORY FEATURES OF MEGALOBLASTIC ANEMIA

Severe deficiency of either Cbl or folate results in impairments in the rapidly dividing tissues of the body, especially the bone marrow causing megaloblastic anemia and gastrointestinal malabsorption and glossitis.[9,10,19,20,100,101] In addition, Cbl deficiency specifically causes demyelination in the central and peripheral nervous system.[102] Both deficiencies result in accumulation of plasma homocysteine,[103,104] sometimes to extreme values[105] and resulting vascular pathology such as thrombosis.[106,107] Both vitamins are important in normal neural

Table 37.4. Inborn Errors of Folate Assimilation and Metabolism

Disorders	Defect (Gene)	Low Plasma Folate	High Hcys	MA	Cerebral Folate Def	Other
Hereditary folate malabsorption	PCFT (*SLC46A1*)	Yes	Yes	Yes	Seizures, developmental delay	Immunodeficiency
Dihydrofolate reductase deficiency	DHFR (*DHFR*)	No	No	Yes	Seizures, developmental delay	
5, 10-MethyleneTHF dehydrogenase deficiency	Trifunctional enzyme (*MTHFD1*)	No	Yes	Yes	Seizures, developmental delay	Immunodeficiency, aHUS
5, 10-MethyleneTHF reductase deficiency	MTHFR (*MTHFR*)	No	Yes	No	Developmental delay	
Glutamate formiminotransferase deficiency	Histidine catabolism (*FTCD*)	No	No or mild	Yes, no	Benign to severe	High FIGLU
Cerebral folate deficiency	FRα (*FOLR1*)	No	No	No	Seizures, developmental delay	
5, 10-MethenylTHF synthetase deficiency	MTHFS (*MTHFS*)	No	No	Yes, no	Seizures, developmental delay	

Abbreviations: aHUS, atypical hemolytic uremic syndrome; DHFR, dihydrofolate reductase deficiency; FIGLU, formimino glutamic acid; FRα, folate receptor α; FTCD, formiminotransferase-cyclodeaminase; Hcys, homocysteine; MA, megaloblastic anemia; MTHFD, methylene tetrahydrofolate dehydrogenase; MTHFR, methylene tetrahydrofolate reductase; MTHFS, methenyltetrahydrofolate synthetase deficiency; PCFT, proton coupled folate transporter.

Disorders of Red Blood Cells

tube development. Deficiencies cause pregnancy complications and failure to thrive in infants and children. There may also be roles in preventing cognitive and psychiatric conditions although such data remain controversial.[107]

Pathophysiology of Megaloblastic Anemia

Because folate and Cbl deficiency cause identical megaloblastic anemia, it has been assumed that the most important biochemical defect is impairment in MTR activity with accumulation of N^5-methylTHF and thus starvation of the other folate-dependent enzymatic reactions. TYMS utilizes 5, 10-methylene-THF for the production of dTMP from deoxyuridine monophosphate. Uracil can be misincorporated in DNA that during repair leads to DNA strand breaks.[98,108,109] 10-Formyl-THF donates two carbon groups to the purine ring through the reactions of phosphoribosylglycinamide formyltransferase and 5-aminoimidazole-4-carboxamide ribonucleotide formyltransferase/IMP cyclohydrolase. The abnormal erythroblasts in culture can be rescued with a combination of thymidine and purines.[98,108-111] Megaloblastic red cell precursors are arrested late in development and many undergo apoptosis, causing ineffective erythropoiesis and intramedullary hemolysis.[98] Those surviving have slowed differentiation, increased time in S phase, and increase in cell size since RNA is affected less than DNA synthesis. This has been described as nuclear-cytoplasmic dissociation. A murine model of folate deficiency suggested that apoptosis was independent of p53.[98] However, recent data show high expression of p53 in megaloblastic human bone marrow cells.[112-115] Oxidant stress has been shown in fibroblast cultures of MMAHC cells with increased levels of reactive oxidant species (ROS) produced. Cbl incubation of the fibroblasts improved ROS levels and decreased apoptosis.[116] The cell lines with elevated homocysteine were more affected than those from isolated methylmalonicaciduria patients. Medications such as azidothymidine and azathioprine cause megaloblastic anemia by impairing thymidine and purine synthesis, respectively, which gives credence to these theories of megaloblastosis. Cyclin D3 is reported to regulate cell size and number but links to megaloblastic anemia are largely unexplored.[117]

Macrocytosis

Macrocytosis is simply an elevated mean red cell volume (MCV), whereas megaloblastosis implies an impairment in DNA synthesis.[118] Many causes of macrocytosis are shown in *Table 37.5*. Textbooks and reviews have often defined it as a red cell MCV value of greater than 100 fL. Reference and hospital labs often have different values such as greater than 97 or 99 fL as a cut point to define macrocytosis. However, the best definition of macrocytosis in the specific patient is a value higher than the historic values that were associated with a normal hemoglobin. The previously cited ranges for the definition of macrocytosis have not taken into consideration the lower MCV in persons who may have thalassemias.[119,120] One report from Louisiana found mean MCV of 87.5 vs 90.1 for black and white men, respectively.[119] Another report found that 30% of African Americans had an alpha 3.7 gene deletion with median MCV of 84 fL as compared to the African Americans with no deletion whose MCV was 90 fL.[120] Beta-thalassemia trait is also common in many populations and MCV will be less than 80 fL. Hemoglobin-E occurs in up to 40% of southeast Asians. Thus, it is apparent that a large rise in MCV would still place the aforementioned individuals in the "normal" range. The red cell distribution width (RDW) may be increased without an abnormal MCV and provides a clue that macrocytic cells are being produced.[121] Macro-ovalocytes may be apparent on the blood smear also providing a clue to a macrocytic condition.

An investigation of consecutive patients with macrocytosis in a large hospital revealed that drugs are the most common cause followed by alcohol, liver disease, and reticulocytosis. Megaloblastic anemia was diagnosed in 6%.[118] Some of the implicated drugs cause impairments in DNA synthesis or in folate metabolism as noted in *Table 37.5*. Reticulocytosis is a prominent cause of an increased MCV[118,122] and can be associated with secondary folate deficiency. Macrocytosis due to liver disease, especially due to alcohol use

Table 37.5. Causes of Macrocytosis[a]

Megaloblastic Anemia	MCV > 110 fL[b]
Cobalamin deficiency	++
Nitrous oxide abuse	++
Folate deficiency	
Antifols - Methotrexate, pemetrexed, anticonvulsants, trimethoprim, sulfas	
Thiamine responsive megaloblastic anemia	
Lesch-Nyhan disease	
Hereditary orotic acidemia	+
Drugs affecting DNA synthesis	++
Azathioprine, hydroxyurea, alkylating, and anti-metabolite chemotherapy agents	++
Antiretroviral agents - zidovudine, lamivudine, stavudine	+
Marrow Disorders	
Acquired	
Myelodysplastic syndromes, leukemias, multiple myeloma	++
Aplastic anemia, pure red cell aplasia	++
Sideroblastic anemia	+
Copper deficiency	+
Hereditary	
Fanconi anemia	+
Diamond-Blackfan anemia	+
Congenital dyserythropoietic anemia	+
Macrocytosis	
Reticulocytosis	++
Alcohol use	+
Chronic liver disease ± alcohol abuse	+
Pulmonary hypertension, hypoxia	+
Cold agglutinins and paraproteinemias	
Hyperglycemia, hyponatremia	
Hypothyroidism	
Tyrosine kinase inhibitors - imatinib, sunitinib	
Postsplenectomy	

[a]Macrocytosis may be defined as >97 or 100 fL but is best defined as greater than the historical normal for a particular patient.
[b]++ = common; + = occasional; MCV, mean red cell volume.

disorder, may be exacerbated by folate deficiency; however, severe liver disease causes macrocytosis due to red cell membrane abnormalities independently.[122]

Pathology of Megaloblastic Anemia

Examples of peripheral blood smears and a bone marrow aspirate and biopsy are shown in *Figure 37.6*. Inspection of the peripheral blood smear will show a wide range in red cell size with obvious macro-ovalocytes. Anisocytosis is often prominent with teardrop cells and misshapen, fragmented cells resembling schistocytes. This can cause confusion with microangiopathic hemolytic anemia.[122-127] In one series, teardrop cells were more prominent and mean lactate dehydrogenase (LDH) was higher in Cbl deficiency than thrombocytopenic thrombotic microangiopathy. Occasionally, a megaloblastic nucleated red blood cell or myelocyte is present. There will be progressive thrombocytopenia and neutropenia as the anemia becomes more severe.[122,124] Hypersegmented granulocytes are present and may be an

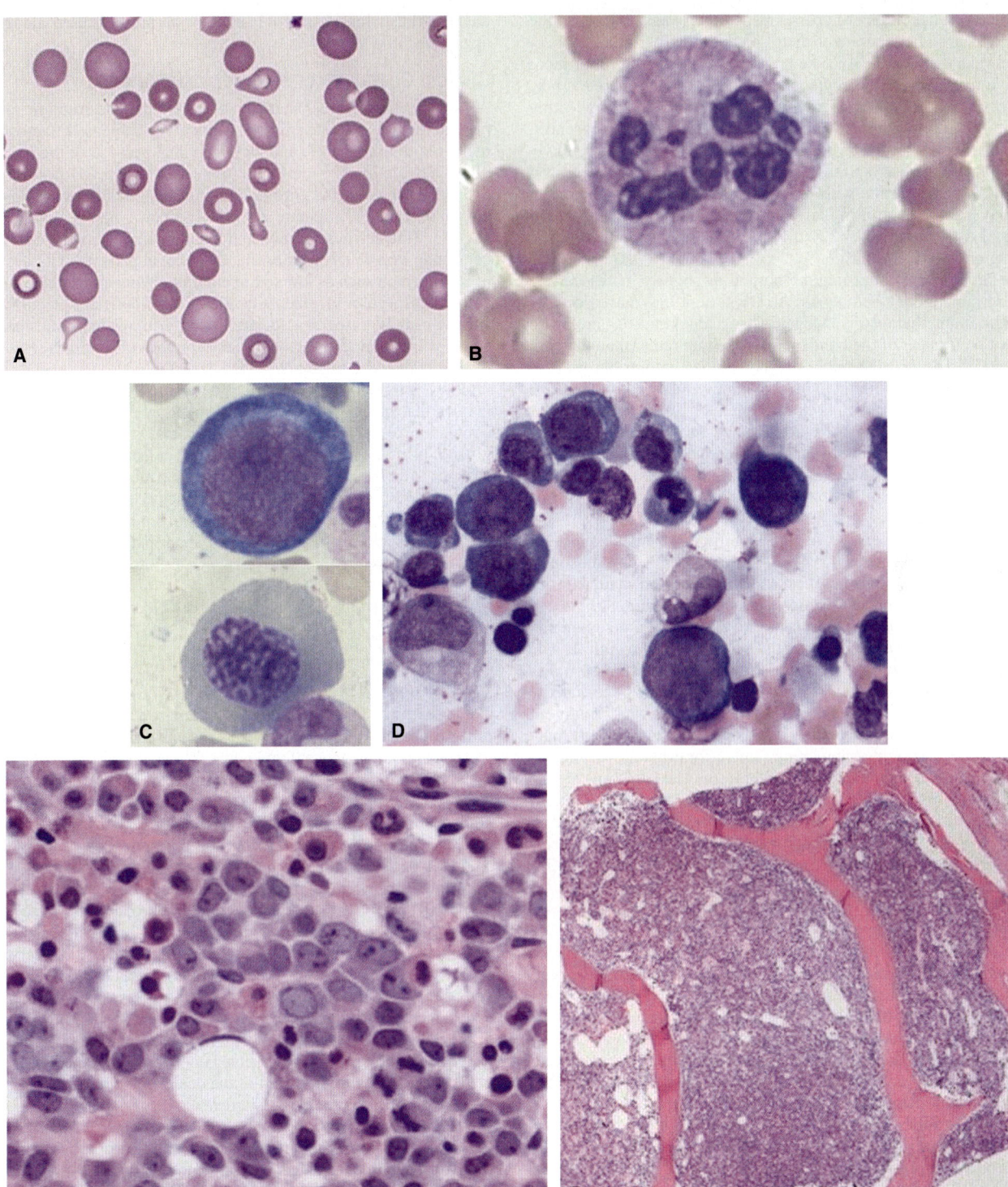

FIGURE 37.6 Photomicrographs from patients with severe cobalamin–deficient megaloblastic anemia. Panel A: anisocytosis and poikilocytosis in a peripheral blood smear from a patient with thalassemia and cobalamin deficiency. Macrocytes, teardrop cells, fragmented cells and background hyperchromic, microcytic cells are present. Panel B: hypersegmented neutrophil. Panel C: Bone marrow aspirate–stained megaloblastic orthochromatophilic normoblast. There is appearance of hemoglobin in the cytoplasm, whereas the nucleus is still large with open lacy chromatin. Top, and erythroblast, Bottom. Panel D: Cluster of differentiating megaloblastic erythroid precursors with poorly condensed chromatin and dysplastic features. One red cell nucleus has a dumbbell shape. A giant band and a metamyelocyte with open chromatin are also shown. Panel E: Bone marrow biopsy with near 100% cellularity. Panel F: High power view of the biopsy shown in E demonstrating the clusters of large megaloblastic erythroblasts which have been mistaken for leukemic blasts as reported in numerous case reports. (Panel B, Adapted from Stabler SP, Megaloblastic anemias: Pernicious anemia and folate deficiency. In: Young NS, Gerson SL, High KA, eds. *Clinical Hematology*. Mosby Elsevier; 2006:242-251. Copyright © 2006 Elsevier. With permission. Panel D and E, Adapted from Stabler SP, Megaloblastic anemias. In: Goldman L, Schafer AI, eds. *Goldman-Cecil Medicine*. 26th ed. Elsevier; 2020:1069-1077. Copyright © 2020 Elsevier. With permission.)

Disorders of Red Blood Cells

early sign. The definition of hypersegmentation is vague but each lobe should appear to be separate or there should be only a small connection between the lobes.[128,129] The presence of one six-lobed, or more than five five-lobed granulocytes per 100 cells, is considered abnormal. Sepsis or other acute illness may cause a bandemia complicating the interpretation of hypersegmentation. The presence of pseudo-Pelger-Huet cells or other hyposegmented neutrophils are more likely indicative of a myelodysplastic process.[130] Signs of underlying iron deficiency or thalassemia with microcytic, hyperchromic, and target cells may also be helpful in diagnosing megaloblastic anemia in the setting of a normal MCV.[126] Red blood cells may show basophilic stippling or other inclusions.[126]

The reticulocyte count may be normal or slightly increased due to the intramedullary hemolysis. A rare patient may have coexisting autoimmune hemolysis. Megaloblastic abnormalities are more apparent on a smear of the bone marrow aspirate rather than the core biopsy.[10,100] The marrow may be hypercellular with erythroid predominance and many mitotic figures, pyknotic and dysplastic red cell precursors. The erythroid cells show large nuclei with open reticular or lacey chromatin despite differentiation of the cytoplasm. The differences between the open blastic nuclei and the maturing cytoplasm have been referred to as nuclear-cytoplasmic dissociation. The maturation of white blood cell precursors is also delayed with open chromatin of the nuclei and giant metamyelocytes and bands.[101] Case reports abound about persons diagnosed initially as leukemia instead of megaloblastic anemia.[131-139] There are reports of chromosomal fragility, cytogenetic abnormalities, and abnormal flow cytometry all suggestive of an erroneous diagnosis of acute leukemia.[134,137,138] A review on the differential diagnosis of myelodysplasia recommends an MMA assay for every patient with Cbl value <400 pg/mL. It was also stated that a few patients had even undergone stem cell transplantation for Cbl deficiency.[130] Megaloblastosis of the bone marrow corrects in 1 to 3 days after a parenteral dose of Cbl; thus, treatment should be delayed until after the biopsy is performed. The bone marrow biopsy and aspirate is not a requirement for evaluation of megaloblastic anemia but should be reserved for unusual situations highly suggestive of hematologic malignancy or metastatic involvement of the bone marrow. Empiric therapy with Cbl can be considered in patients without circulating blasts who may show a response prior to receiving send-out bone marrow pathology results from smaller hospitals or rural areas.

Laboratory Evaluation of Megaloblastic Anemia

Evaluation for megaloblastic anemia begins with routine testing such as a complete blood count with red cell indices, a reticulocyte count, and clinical chemistries with markers of hemolysis.[9,10,19,100,101,124,131] Pernicious anemia is often slowly progressive, with decrease in hemoglobin or increase in MCV that can be apparent over several years in the medical record. The MCV will rise above the patient's setpoint and is accompanied by an increase in the mean corpuscular hemoglobin and reticulocyte hemoglobin. The RDW will increase, and in some cases, extreme values are seen when the smear shows a wide range of size including macro-ovalocytes as well as small, fragmented cells.[121] The blood smear abnormalities have been described in the section on pathology. The red blood cell count and hemoglobin may be normal with only a subtle rise of MCV in mild megaloblastic anemia, yet the patient may have severe biochemical abnormalities of Cbl deficiency and disabling myeloneuronopathy. The incompletely treated patient with pernicious anemia may have steady increase in MCV as the first sign of treatment failure.

The progression of anemia may be so gradual that with hemoglobin values less than 5 g/dL volume overload with hypokalemia, metabolic alkalosis, and resulting high output heart failure may be present.

The megaloblastic anemia of folate deficiency is as described above. However, as folate deficiency is often accompanied by alcohol use disorder, there may be specific changes due to alcohol toxicity combined with megaloblastic anemia.[104,140] For instance, alcohol can cause vacuolation of both bone marrow erythroid and especially myeloid precursors. Alcohol is a common cause of sideroblastic

anemia; thus, ringed sideroblasts may be present often along with aggregated iron.[140]

Clinical Chemistry of Megaloblastic Anemia

All of the biochemical markers of blood cell destruction may be present such as elevated indirect bilirubin, decreased haptoglobin, increased transaminases, and elevated LDH because of the intramedullary destruction.[10,82,100,141] Extreme values of LDH occur, higher even than seen in the thrombotic microangiopathies and aggressive malignancies, a feature not widely known among general clinicians.[123] Transferrin saturation and ferritin will increase unless there is coexisting iron deficiency anemia. Occasional patients will have signs of malnutrition such as low serum albumin, hypogammaglobulinemia, and malabsorption of other vitamins. Folate-deficient megaloblastic anemia usually arises in association with alcoholism or intestinal diseases, which may cause global malabsorption of nutrients, especially other vitamins and minerals.[82,140]

Flow cytometry that is routinely used to identify cell populations in bone marrow aspirates may show a marked expansion of the CD34 population of hematopoietic precursors and CD235A cells marking glycophorin-A in erythroblasts and other early erythroids. These changes from the normal patterns have been misinterpreted as indicating myelodysplastic syndromes or even acute leukemias as published frequently in case reports.[136] Cytogenetics may show a fragmented pattern but occasionally also a clonal abnormality, which will correct with Cbl therapy.[133]

NEUROLOGIC ABNORMALITIES IN COBALAMIN DEFICIENCY

Pathophysiology

Cbl is necessary for the initial development and maintenance of myelin in the central and peripheral nervous systems although the biochemical mechanisms are largely still unknown.[100] The dorsal lateral columns of the spinal cord are particularly vulnerable to demyelination.[102,142,143] Areas of hyperintensity in T2-weighted images can be seen on magnetic resonance imaging (MRI) in the spinal cord, particularly in the cervical regions but extending into the thoracic area also (*Figure 37.7*). Cross-sectional views may show an inverted "V" sign.[142,144-149] Periventricular changes in white matter have also been described in brain MRI due to Cbl deficiency. Optic neuropathy has rarely been described.[150] Electrophysiology studies show abnormal visual evoked potentials, motor and somatosensory evoked potentials, and nerve conduction.[142,149-152] The signs and symptoms of Cbl deficiency in the nervous system are listed in *Table 37.6*. Both experimental animal models and human pathologic studies have demonstrated spongy vacuolation in the involved areas of white matter with swelling of myelin sheaths, destruction and splitting of myelin lamellae, and formation of vacuoles. The lesions appear to start in the dorsal columns and spread laterally.[153,154] Infants with severe Cbl deficiency may show global delay in myelination on imaging and brain choline deficiency.[155]

The underlying biochemical abnormalities and pathophysiology have been studied in animal models such as nitrous oxide (N_2O) exposed fruit bats and pigs and dietary deprived primates but still remain to be elucidated.[153,156] Increases in branched chain and odd chain fatty acids and lipids have been found and attributed to the block in methylmalonyl-CoA mutase with resulting build up in propionyl-CoA and L-methylmalonyl-CoA.[31-33] However, patients with congenital methylmalonicaciduria do not present the same demyelinating disease of the nervous system despite having extreme values of MMA. Other theories have pointed toward impaired SAM-dependent methylation of myelin proteins or neurotransmitters, yet folate deficient–impaired MTR alone is not associated with this demyelinating syndrome. Alcohol abuse (usual cause of folate deficiency) causes peripheral neuropathy and related nutritional defects such as thiamine deficiency and other neurologic toxicities, which differ from Cbl deficiency. It appears that either the combined biochemical lesions of impaired mutase and MTR or an unknown pathway that

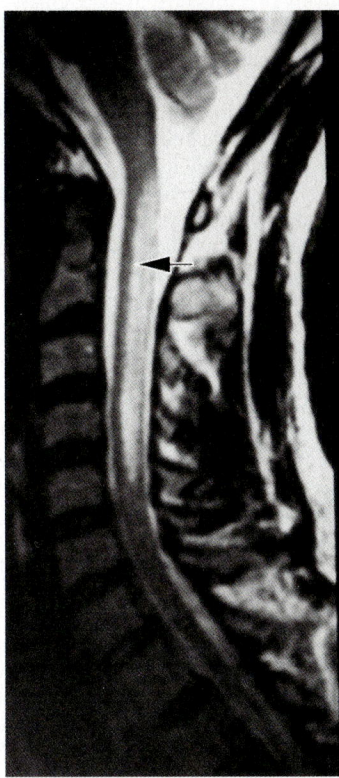

FIGURE 37.7 Magnetic resonance imaging (T2 weighted) of a sagittal section of the cervical spine of a patient with pernicious anemia and severe myelopathy. The arrow points to the posterior area of the high-signal intensity lesion. (Reproduced from Larner AJ, Zeman AZ, Allen CM, et al. MRI appearances in subacute combined degeneration of the spinal cord due to vitamin B12 deficiency. *J Neurol Neurosurg Psychiatry.* 1997;62(1):99-101, with permission from BMJ Publishing Group Ltd.)

Table 37.6. Neurological Abnormalities Due to Cobalamin Deficiency

Spinal Cord

Paresthesias
Proprioceptic loss
    Vibration, position, positive Romberg sign, ataxic gait
Spasticity – hyperreflexia
Lhermitte sign
Limb weakness
Segmental cutaneous sensory level
Paraplegia

Peripheral Nerve

Cutaneous sensory loss
Hyporeflexia
Weakness
Paresthesias

Brain

Cognitive defects
Optic atrophy, anosmia
"Megaloblastic madness"
    Mania, paranoia, irritability, delusions, emotional lability, depression
Autonomic nervous system

Infants

Coma, movement disorders, developmental regression, delayed myelination, permanent disability

is Cbl-dependent in the brain are necessary for the development of this specific lesion. Inborn errors involving MTR alone or some of the folate-dependent enzymes and cerebral folate deficiency do cause

neurologic dysfunction, particularly seizures, mental retardation, and developmental disabilities but likely have a different pathophysiology. No difference in metabolic abnormalities in MMA, homocysteine, 2-methylcitric acid, cystathionine, N-methylglycine, N, N-dimethylglycine, or methionine were seen in a cohort of patients with proven Cbl-deficient neurologic disease vs those with just megaloblastic anemia.[22] Some investigations have shown an increase in neurotoxic molecules such as nerve growth factor, tumor necrosis factor (TNF), and soluble CD40: CD40 ligand in a gastrectomized rat model that develops massive increases in MMA.[157] There were also decreased neurotropic molecules such as epidermal growth factor and Il6. A few Cbl-deficient subjects were found to have similar elevations in serum TNF-α and decreases in serum epidermal growth factor as compared to controls and iron deficient subjects.[158] The cerebrospinal fluid (CSF) level of TNF was increased in 14 subjects with Cbl deficiency associated with a decrease in epidermal growth factor, similar to the animal model.[159] Another study reported that glial migration and synapse formation in Cbl-deficient *Caenorhabditis elegans* is regulated through control of an isoform-specific expression of leukocyte-common antigen-related receptor type tyrosine protein phosphatase.[160] Cell culture studies have shown that an inhibitory Cbl analogue, c-lactam, could change astrocytes from a quiescent to reactive state, which included an increase in cell size with giant cells containing multiple nuclei and reorganization of their actin cytoskeletons. There was increased expression of the glial fibrillary acidic protein and vimentin, changes that are seen in other neurodegenerative diseases.[161] The cells were also shown to express various caspases but without causing apoptotic death. Reactive astrogliosis could be a result of deficient Cbl-induced endoplasmic reticulum stress in another model of Cbl-deficient dopaminergic cells.[162] One of the barriers to investigating depleted Cbl in the central nervous system is the lack of good animal models. Rodents, dogs, and other small mammals have been resistant to development of neurological damage with prolonged N_2O exposure, dietary, or analogue manipulations. Primates, pigs, and fruit bats have shown neurologic defects but are cumbersome or unavailable models. Zebra fish may prove to be a convenient model although it may be difficult to apply the findings to human physiology. Another promising animal model is that of a CD320 knockout mouse, which has a normal circulating Cbl value but brain Cbl depletion.[163] This model has shown spinal cord demyelination with increased expression of myelin basic and glial fibrillary acidic protein and increases in TNF-α. The changes were associated with increased latency to a thermal challenge, which documents a sensory defect.[163]

Central Nervous System: Clinical Manifestations

One of the most interesting and largely unexplained manifestations of the central nervous system disease is its inverse correlation of severity with that of megaloblastic anemia, which has been noted for over 100 years.[102,142,143] The hematologist must be aware that only subtle hematologic megaloblastic anemia may be present in subjects with severe demyelinating myeloneuropathy; yet, the metabolic abnormalities of elevated MMA and homocysteine are seen in those with or without anemia.[22] Hematologists and neurologists in two New York hospitals reported the details in all cases of proven Cbl-deficient neurologic patients over a 17-year period.[102] Paraesthesia or numbness were the most common initial complaints in more than 70% of the patients usually in the feet although about 20% started in the hands. This was accompanied by gait ataxia, leg weakness, and impaired manual dexterity in some patients. Gait ataxia occurred alone in about 15%; impairment in senses, memory loss, psychosis, and decreased visual acuity were seen in a few other patients. The neurological exam was normal in 20% even though the patients complained of paresthesias and ataxia. The most common exam sign was a diminished vibratory sense in the feet or legs up to the knees and in severe cases to the ileal crest, lower thoracic area, and hands to elbows. Proprioception was diminished or absent in the toes or ankles in many and always accompanied by abnormal vibratory sensation. Positive Romberg signs and Lhermitte phenomenon were also seen. Cutaneous touch and pain sensation was reduced in a stocking distribution, occasionally accompanied by a weakness of the lower limbs in about 30%. Some patients had hyperreflexia, extensor planter responses, and spasticity. Bilateral optic atrophy rarely manifests as a progressive bilateral loss of vision. Prompt treatment can improve or in some cases resolve the impairment. Mental impairment was seen in approximately 15 patients with global dementia, recent memory loss, depression, agitation, hypomania, paranoid psychosis, or personality change. However, virtually all of these patients had other neurologic abnormalities also. Severity of the neurologic dysfunction was related to the duration of the symptoms before recognition and was more severe with increasing hematocrit. Treatment resulted in complete response in 47% but was less complete in those who had severe pretreatment severity score and had the longest duration of neurologic symptoms before treatment.

Electrophysiology studies have shown abnormal sural and peroneal nerve conduction, abnormal tibial somatosensory potentials, and visually evoked potentials.[151,152] Nerve conduction abnormalities were found in half of a cohort of patients with severe symptomatic Cbl-deficient neuropathy, which was consistent with mixed demyelinating and axonal damage in the majority. Sural nerve biopsy has shown acute axonal degeneration with formation of myelin ovoids and focal depletion of myelinated fiber loss.[152] In some with prolonged duration of illness, there was endoneurial fibrosis and some axonal regeneration. It is recognized that Cbl-deficient neurologic disease involves both the central and peripheral nervous system and occasionally the brain with the underlying pathology appearing to be loss of myelin. The many case reports and small case series in the literature describe symptoms, signs, and radiologic studies with consistent findings.

Neurological Aspects of Cobalamin Deficiency in Infants

The breastfed infant[80,164] of a Cbl-deficient mother is at risk for severe complications during the first year of life because of the rapid brain growth and myelination that occurs during this period.[79,165-167] The reported symptoms include failure to thrive, hypotonia, movement disorders with tremor and myoclonus, extreme irritability, and either developmental delay or regression in developmental milestones. Hematologic abnormalities may or may not be severe as in the adult patient with Cbl-related neurologic disease.[168,169] The most extreme cases will have microcephaly and MRI imaging can show cortical atrophy with ventriculomegaly and myelination delay.[167,169,170] Treatment induces rapid responses usually first in hypotonia, responsiveness, irritability, and movement disorders.[167,169,170] Unfortunately, prolonged depletion along with failure of brain growth may lead to permanent disabilities. Newborn screening is improving early detection and outcome.[79,171,172]

OTHER CLINICAL MANIFESTATIONS OF COBALAMIN OR FOLATE DEFICIENCY

Glossitis of the tongue, which is due to atrophy of tongue papillae may occur in severe Cbl or folate deficiency.[173,174] Tissues with rapid turnover may also show megaloblastic changes such as intestinal villi resulting in malabsorption and the uterine cervix cells. Weight loss may be prominent. There may be decreased spermatogenesis or other fertility defects. Areas of skin hyperpigmentation may appear, especially in those with darker skin.[121,126,175] Both folate and Cbl deficiency are implicated in increased risk for neural tube defects and other poor reproductive outcomes such as low birth weight, preeclampsia, and maternal hypertension.[176-179] There are controversial data regarding the risk of osteoporosis and bone remodeling in Cbl deficiency, but serum alkaline phosphatase may be low.[180,181] Both acquired folate and Cbl deficiency raise serum/plasma total homocysteine sometimes to values that overlap with the inborn errors of methionine metabolism and other homocystinurias.[105] Thrombotic risk is increased in the deficient patients with high homocysteine.[105,106,182-186] The medical literature is replete with the thrombotic presentation of pernicious anemia with hyperhomocysteinemia.

Hyperhomocysteinemia and Vascular Disease

Soon after classical homocystinuria, a defect in cystathionine beta-synthase, was discovered, it was recognized that hyperhomocysteinemia was also present in inborn errors of Cbl and folate and that these conditions all had greatly increased risk of both thrombotic disease and arteriosclerotic vascular lesions. This was widely publicized as the homocysteine theory of increased vascular disease risk[187] and led to thousands of investigations studying what role elevated homocysteine plays in the etiology of these common disorders (Reviewed in Reference 107). Early literature was compromised by the lack of recognition that poor renal function is a cause of moderate elevations of homocysteine and vascular disease.[188,189] Elevated homocysteine has consistently been shown to be a risk factor for cardiovascular disease and stroke.[190-192] Large trials of single or combinations of B-vitamins were employed in either primary or secondary prevention of cardiac and vascular disease, once it was realized that the homocysteine values could be lowered, but in general, provided little proof of efficacy.[193,194] Signals for benefit were stronger for cerebral vascular disease and stroke than for ischemic cardiac disease.[195] The treatment trials in the United States and Canada were compromised by the implementation of folate food fortification in 1998, which lowered population homocysteine values and virtually eliminated folate deficiency. Newer data from a massive study of combined folic acid (0.8 mg) and antihypertensive treatment in China showed a decrease in incident stroke rate,[196] and combination vitamins halved the incidence of high altitude–related venous thrombosis in a cohort of Indian soldiers.[197] It seems likely that there is a role for homocysteine-lowering in populations with low folate and Cbl intake.

There has also been intensive investigation of the role of homocysteine, folate, and Cbl status in neurocognitive disorders, especially the treatment of cognitive decline and Alzheimer disease and in autism and related disorders.[107]

DIAGNOSTIC TESTING FOR MEGALOBLASTIC ANEMIA

Serum Cobalamin Measurement

The serum Cbl measurement is usually the first test and often combined with a serum/plasma folate value for diagnosis of vitamin-deficient megaloblastic anemia. Unfortunately, neither vitamin assay has impressive sensitivity or specificity for diagnosis unless extremely low values result. It is not surprising that serum values might not reflect body content since Cbl has no intravascular biochemical role. It circulates bound to HC 80% and only 10% to 20% on transcobalamin, (holo-TC) and clinical laboratory assays measure total Cbl, that bound to HC and holo-TC together.[68] There are individuals with low HCs (15% with unexplained low Cbl)[69,198] and, thus, low total Cbl but normal tissue delivery. In addition to the above biochemical variables, there are multiple clinical chemistry issues with the current widely used chemiluminescence immunoassays.[199-207]

Microbiological assays were the first serum Cbl assays and much of the older literature about sensitivity and specificity of a cutoff value for normal was based on these assays. In general, lower values were obtained than with the current tests. The next assays were competitive protein binding radioassays usually in kits with cobalt-57 labeled Cbl and I-25 labeled folic acid that measured both simultaneously. Initial problems were with nonspecificity of the Cbl binding protein but replacement with pure hog IF made these assays very useful. However, in the mid-1990s, many laboratories turned to competitive binding luminescence assays (CBLAs), which were performed on multianalyte analyzers and avoided radioisotopes. The Cbl binding protein used is IF, and anti-IF antibodies can bind the reagent. Most of the instruments require a fresh supply of reducing agent to denature these anti-IF antibodies common in serum from patients with pernicious anemia. Case reports of patients and series of patients with false-positive normal or actual high values of Cbl began to proliferate after the introduction of these assays.[199-207] A very detailed description of patient samples was reported in 2012,[200] in which aliquots were sent to three hospital-based clinical laboratories in New York using different CBLA systems. The labs reported 22% to 35% false normal values as compared to the previously performed radiodilution assay. This was a major problem in subjects who had positive anti-IF antibodies. The literature has since emphasized that hematologists be aware of this clinical problem. Other methodologic problems must exist as shown by a recent survey of the laboratory performance of serum Cbl in the United Kingdom.[202] It showed that Cbl values ranged from 86 to 258 pg/mL on an aliquoted sample with a target of 173 pg/mL as performed by 350 laboratories using eight different analyzers. The lab interpretations ranged from low and indeterminant to normal also on the same sample aliquot. The clinician should not depend on any particular cut-off of "normal" of Cbl as the determinant for further testing, but should be guided by the clinical picture.

A traditional lower cut point for normal serum Cbl has often been defined at around 200 pg/mL.[10,100] Studies correlating the Cbl value with elevated MMA in population series suggest that the Cbl cutpoint should be higher often at about 300 to 350 pg/mL, which will increase sensitivity[208-210] at the great expense of specificity.[208,210-213] If Cbl is measured in persons with common nonspecific symptoms such as fatigue, malaise, and poor concentration, then virtually no patients with values less than 200 to 300 pg/mL will have associated elevated MMA or a clinical, hematologic, or exam documented neurologic response after treatment. A definition of response should include normalization of complete blood counts, fall in MCV, or correction of neurologic symptoms such as paresthesias, vibration sense, and ataxic gait. In general, the lower the measured serum Cbl, the more likely the patient will have elevated MMA and/or homocysteine and a documented response to replacement. Most patients with serum Cbl less than 100 pg/mL are genuinely deficient. However, subjects with Cbl as high as 300 pg/mL[209] may have documented responses even with the older assays before the current problems with the CBLA assays. Before prescribing a lifetime of Cbl treatment, clinicians should pursue other testing such as pretreatment MMA and/or homocysteine. Positive anti-IF antibodies or antiparietal cell antibodies may help but are not positive in all pernicious anemia patients. Alternatively, if megaloblastic anemia is corrected with solely Cbl treatment (no folic acid or iron), then deficiency has been proven and lifelong treatment should be instituted.

Methylmalonic Acid Testing in Cobalamin Deficiency

MMA increases in tissues and body fluids[213,214] when L-methylmalonyl-CoA mutase activity is blocked by Cbl deficiency.[18,27,28,208,209] Mutase is extremely sensitive to the withdrawal of Cbl. Patients with dietary or malabsorption-associated Cbl deficiency[18,27,28,104,212,215] and animal[25] or cellular[26] models of deficiency all develop elevated MMA. MMA was elevated greater than 376 nmol/L in 434 episodes of Cbl deficiency, vigorously defined by response to therapy in virtually every patient and documentation of pernicious anemia or other well-known cause of Cbl deficiency.[104] *Figure 37.8* shows results from these and other subjects[104,215] where the MMA was plotted against the simultaneous serum homocysteine. Inspection of the graph shows only a small number of these clinically symptomatic patients with MMA values between 500 and 1000 nmol/L, and in many, values overlap those seen in the inborn errors of Cbl metabolism. MMA was greater than 2000 nmol/L in 12/19 and greater than 800 nmol/L in all 19 patients with megaloblastic anemia due to Cbl deficiency in a prospective evaluation of macrocytosis.[118]

Another cohort from the same authors show that MMA was elevated in 38 Cbl-deficient patients with normal hemoglobin and or MCV and neurologic deficiency who had a clinical response to therapy as well as a fall or normalization of serum MMA after treatment.[143] The MMA was elevated in 13 prospectively followed patients with low serum Cbl and neurologic symptoms who had clear cut subjective and objective neurologic responses to therapy accompanied by hematologic responses in 10. In the same cohort, there was no response in 25 patients with comparable low Cbl levels and normal MMA. Another report demonstrated a rigorous response to Cbl treatment in

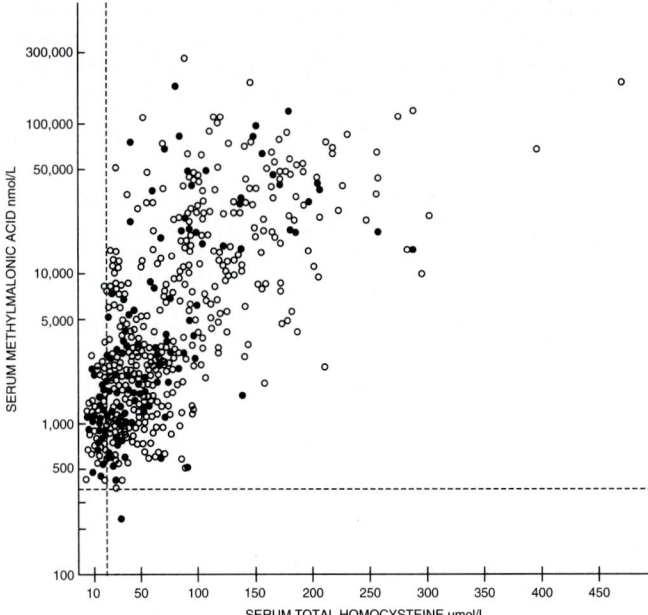

FIGURE 37.8 Serum methylmalonic acid vs serum homocysteine concentrations from 491 episodes of clinical cobalamin deficiency. Most of the patients had confirmed pernicious anemia or other known cause of deficiency as well as a documented response to therapy. The open circles represent patients with anemia and the closed circles represent those with hematocrit of 38% or higher. The dashed lines represent a methylmalonic acid value of 376 nmol/L (y axis) and homocysteine of 21.3 µmol/L (x axis). (From Stabler SP. Clinical practice. Vitamin B12 deficiency. *N Engl J Med.* 2013;368(2):149-160. Copyright © 2013 Massachusetts Medical Society. Reprinted with permission from Massachusetts Medical Society.)

86 prospectively followed patients who had Cbl less than 200 pg/mL and elevated MMA (86%) as compared to 59 subjects with low Cbl who had no response to treatment and in which MMA was elevated in 20% although half of the latter subjects had serologic evidence of pernicious anemia.[216]

Another report detailed laboratory and neurologic exams in 48 consecutive patients with low-normal serum Cbl values between 135 and 237 pg/mL as defined by the authors.[212] MMA was elevated greater than 370 nmol/L in only 21% of these subjects but did fall to low levels (120-210 nmol/L) in all 10 after treatment proving metabolic deficiency. Only one of those with elevated MMA had anemia with MCV of 77 fL suggesting iron deficiency. Neurologic symptoms or signs were present in 5 of the 10 with elevated MMA but also in 15 of 38 with normal MMA leading the authors to conclude that such symptoms were too commonly caused by comorbidities to be specific for Cbl deficiency with most low to low-normal serum Cbl false positive low.

Pernicious anemia patients with interruption of Cbl treatment have increases in serum MMA before hematologic abnormalities or low Cbl values.[209] Low meat eaters or those following a vegan diet have higher MMA than their omnivorous peers.[217]

MMA normalizes following Cbl treatments whether parenteral or high dose oral, and thus, must be measured prior to any treatment.[143,208,213,216] A common clinical error is to measure MMA after weeks of therapy because the patient has had no clinical response and likely initially had a false-positive low Cbl value. Inspection of *Figure 37.8* shows that few clinically ascertained Cbl-deficient patients have MMA less than 500 and most are over 1000 nmol/L. Small increases in serum MMA do reflect metabolic vitamin depletion in many cases (since they fall with therapy)[211,212] yet rarely can be correlated with anemias or myeloneuropathy.[218]

The major influence on serum MMA besides Cbl is renal status.[21,218-221] Serum MMA increases in renal insufficiency although usually under 1000 nmol/L, even in dialysis patients, thus unlikely to overlap with megaloblastic anemia. 2-methylcitric acid is formed when propionyl-CoA accumulates (see *Figure 37.2*), and the concentration is usually about 25% to 40% of that of the concurrent MMA value in Cbl deficiency or the inborn errors.[21] However, 2-methylcitric acid is more dependent on renal excretion than MMA; thus, when 2-methylcitric acid is higher or equal to the MMA value, it is most likely that renal failure is the cause of the elevated MMA.[21]

A common polymorphism in HIBCH, an enzyme in valine catabolism, caused a modest increase in MMA in a population study but that would rarely overlap with the values seen in clinical Cbl deficiency. It is not known yet whether treatment would lower the values in those with the polymorphism.[222] Intestinal bacterial overgrowth in tropical sprue patients was shown to cause elevated MMA which fell after antibiotics.[223]

All major reference laboratories in the United States offer MMA testing, often in panels including 2-methylcitric acid, homocysteine, and cystathionine. Stable isotope dilution, gas chromatography/mass spectrometry (MS), and liquid chromatography (LC)-MS are the most widely used methodologies. CSF and urine (with urine creatinine to normalize values) can also be measured. Unfortunately, review articles continue to decry MMA testing as expensive and unavailable, which is only true in countries that elected to not provide it through national health programs.[224] MS is commonly used for drug assay worldwide and can be adapted to MMA testing.

Homocysteine Testing in Cobalamin and/or Folate Deficiency

Figure 37.3 shows that a block in MTR or cystathionine beta-synthase activity can cause a buildup of homocysteine. This was shown in the early studies of hereditary homocystinurias where only the disulfide, homocystine, was detected in urine.[225] Newer methods were developed in the 1980s, which could quantitate total homocysteine,[226] the sum of homocysteine bound to protein, homocystine, and mixed disulfide with cysteine.[227] Cohorts of patients with Cbl or folate deficiency were analyzed using the new methods.[103,228] Serum or plasma total homocysteine was elevated in greater than 95% of patients with clinically diagnosed Cbl or folate deficiency with megaloblastic anemia, in the large cohorts previously analyzed for MMA.[104] Values in Cbl-deficient vs folate-deficient patients are indistinguishable[22] and both overlap those seen in classical homocystinuria and other inborn errors of Cbl and folate metabolism.[105] Folate-deficient subjects did not have elevated MMA except for minor elevations in patients with hypovolemia or renal insufficiency.[104] Because elevated homocysteine is present in either vitamin deficiency, or in combined deficiency, it is necessary to assay MMA or perform other testing to determine that the patient with pernicious anemia is not treated with high-dose folic acid alone. Large reference laboratories in the United States offer panels that combine MMA and total homocysteine testing often also including cystathionine and 2-methylcitric acid, which can pinpoint which vitamin is deficient. Unfortunately, the health services in some countries have elected to offer the less specific homocysteine assay rather than MMA as a secondary test for Cbl deficiency. Serum homocysteine falls within hours after replacement with the proper vitamin,[103] normalizing in hours to days. If the Cbl-deficient patient is treated with folic acid, then homocysteine does not normalize and vice versa.[223] The elevation in serum total homocysteine correlates with the severity of hematologic abnormalities.[104]

Homocysteine is exquisitely sensitive to folate status in subjects with normal Cbl and renal status. The serum folate concentrations more than doubled in NHANES III (1999-2000) as compared to NHANES (1991-1994) accompanied by a drop in homocysteine of 1 to 2 µmol/L after food folate fortification started in the United States in 1998.[84,229,230] A more recent update evaluating NHANES (2003-2006) showed a geometric mean homocysteine of 8.8 µmol/L with corresponding serum folate 9.4 ng/mL and RBC folate 234 ng/mL, in the entire cohort of 3337 who were not taking supplements.[231] The age group over 60 years had homocysteine of 11.1 µmol/L and serum folate of 10.6 and red cell folate of 256 ng/mL. Homocysteine was highest in non-Hispanic whites followed by non-Hispanic blacks and Mexican Americans. The serum Cbl in non-Hispanic whites was lower (393 pg/mL) and MMA slightly higher (152 nmol/L), which might complicate

interpretation of the slightly higher serum homocysteine found in the non-Hispanic whites as compared to non-Hispanic blacks.[231] Users of supplements containing folic acid had lower homocysteine by about 1 umol/L in every cohort. A study from Israel, without mandatory fortification, shows that with a mean serum folate of 8 to 10 ng/mL plasma homocysteine values were 12.6 for men and 9.6 µmol/L for women, respectively. In male patients selected to have serum folate less than 5.3 ng/mL, homocysteine rose to 15 µmol/L and if folate less than 3 ng/mL, rose to 32.4 µmol/L.[232] These data show the strong inverse relationship between serum folate and homocysteine.

A result of the improved folate status in the fortified countries is that most patients with elevated homocysteine likely have Cbl rather than folate deficiency, notable exceptions being those with alcohol use disorder and users of antifolate medications. Pernicious anemia should be considered in all patients with elevated homocysteine that do not have the previously mentioned risk factors.

Reference labs offer commercial assays for other amino acids in the methionine pathway (*Figure 37.3*). Serum methionine has not been found to be low in Cbl or folate-deficient patients unlike in severely affected infants and children with inborn errors of folate or Cbl metabolism.[22] Serum cystathionine is elevated in the majority of patients with either Cbl or folate deficiency despite expectation that cystathionine beta-synthase activity should be impaired in the methylation disorders.[22,105,233] Cystathionine normalizes in both vitamin disorders after treatment. Serum total cysteine is usually normal in Cbl and folate-deficient patients.[22] N-methylglycine (sarcosine) and N, N-dimethylglycine values are elevated in folate deficient but not often in Cbl-deficient patients.[38] These secondary metabolites are mainly of research interest since homocysteine is also elevated in these same patients.

S-adenosylhomocysteine is an immediate precursor of homocysteine as shown in *Figure 37.3*. It is generated after a SAM-dependent methylation transfers a methyl group to a variety of substrates in transmethylation reactions. Impaired methylation has long been postulated to play a role in the pathophysiology of megaloblastic anemias. Serum SAM was found to be elevated approximately 2 to threefold without a low SAM value and with a 10-fold elevation in total homocysteine in 15 Cbl-deficient subjects with megaloblastic anemia.[234] Total homocysteine fell by more than 90%, S-adenosylhomocysteine by 50%, and SAM decreased slightly as hemoglobin and MCV both normalized after treatment. The small difference in S-adenosylhomocysteine as compared to simultaneous homocysteine values in megaloblastic anemia means it is unlikely that this will be a useful diagnostic test. In addition, post vivo changes in collected specimens lead to false elevations in S-adenosylhomocysteine unless samples are prepared promptly, which would not be possible in the clinical laboratory setting.[235]

Holo-Transcobalamin vs Total Cobalamin Testing; Specificity and Sensitivity

The serum Cbl has low specificity for associated elevated MMA or homocysteine unless highly selected patients with probable megaloblastic anemia are tested. A report of results from four different analyzers in the same laboratory showed that approximately the same percentage of samples resulting below the manufacturers' reference range had elevated MMA, 55% to 65%.[201] Thus, about 40% of samples likely had a false-positive low value in this population of patients chosen to include those with low serum Cbl. An NHANES survey showed that 1% of a cohort of 12,000 adult participants had both elevated MMA (mean 813 nmol/L) and Cbl < 200 pg/mL, likely representing true deficiency.[236] However, twice as many, (2%), of the same cohort had low Cbl, but MMA was less than 271 nmol/L. Also, MMA was elevated in 5% of the entire cohort, when Cbl was greater than 200 pg/mL. Another report from NHANES on the same population showed that with an even lower cut off value for normal Cbl of 170 pg/mL only 2.5% of the group had MMA > 366 nmol/L with a median for this group with low Cbl of only 281 nmol/L.[237] It is clear that a low serum Cbl is a poor predictor for metabolic deficiency in unselected groups; thus, most low values obtained for nonspecific clinical indications will be false-positive low values.

holo-TC is the protein-bound Cbl which is delivered to the TC receptor (CD320) on all cells so is theoretically a better measure for detecting deficiency than total Cbl.[238] Commercial assays for holo-TC are available in Europe and often referred to as "active B12."[239] There are inverse correlations between MMA and holo-TC similar to that with Cbl but again the specificity is low. In one report, the samples with the lowest 10% percentile of holo-TC (<25.7 pg/mL) had a median MMA of 269 nmol/L with only 42% over 300 nmol/L.[240]

Another group reported that only 20% with holo-TC between 34 and 41 pg/mL had MMA > 500 and samples > 1000 nmol/L were spread throughout the range from 34 to 68 pg/mL in subjects with normal renal function.[241] There is little consensus in the literature as to the definition of a low value, ranging from approximately 27 to 50 pg/mL in different publications.[240-246] There is only a slight improvement in sensitivity and specificity when tested against total serum Cbl as defined by identifying elevated MMA or homocysteine.[242,246] Sensitivities ranged from 46% to 87% and specificities from 28% to 94% as reviewed in Reference 242. The cutpoints for holo-TC and MMA were also different between the different studies. The sensitivity for detecting elevated MMA and total homocysteine in a population of seniors was 59.5% for holo-TC vs 48.6% for total Cbl and the specificity was slightly lower for holo-TC at 93.7% vs 95.3%, respectively.[247] The mean serum MMA was 2 to 3 times higher when both values were low than if only one indicator was abnormal. The positive predictive values for holo-TC and Cbl were low, 14.7 vs 21%, in a cohort of patients with neurologic disease compatible with Cbl deficiency.[248] Holo-TC has yet to be tested in a population of pernicious anemia patients with megaloblastic anemia and/or myeloneuropathy. Another issue is that there is a common single nucleotide polymorphism (776C > G) in high prevalence which has been associated with lower values of serum holo-TC.[249] Also, holo-TC increases in renal insufficiency, thus, confounding interpretation.[238] Holo-TC is a marker of absorption of Cbl and remains lower posttreatment in pernicious anemia patients.[238] In addition, a point mutation has been associated with a false low–holo-TC in a patient with apparent normal Cbl status and the population prevalence of this mutation is unknown.[250]

Combined Indicator of Vitamin B12 Status (cB12)

A mathematically derived calculated indicator using between two and four of the biomarkers including Cbl, holo-TC, MMA, and total homocysteine has been devised.[251] This combined indicator may not be useful in clinical practice, as it has been developed mostly in populations that do not have clearly defined megaloblastic anemia or myeloneuropathy due to pernicious anemia or other severely Cbl-deficient subjects. In one report, serum MMA between 350 and 1700 nmol/L is listed under "transitional B12 status," (cB12 of -0.5-2.5)[251] and another (3cB12 of <1.2-0.5) with the 50th to 97.5th percentile for MMA of 440 to 1950 nmol/L also defined as "transitional vitamin B12 status."[252] Inspection of *Figure 37.8* shows that a large number of patients found to have megaloblastic anemia or neurologic abnormalities that corrected with Cbl and otherwise rigorously defined as deficient have MMA values between 500 and 1950 nmol/L and would be poorly served by such a definition. This indicator should be studied in patients with proven responses to Cbl therapy prior to applying it to screening healthy populations who likely have a high prevalence of false positive low Cbl and holo-TC.

Folate Assays

Serum folate should be measured in patients suspected of having megaloblastic anemia. It is now performed, often in tandem with Cbl, by the automated chemiluminescent assays utilizing folate-binding protein on multianalyte instruments. The first folate assays were microbiological assays with *Lactobacillus casei*, followed by radio dilution assays that have largely been phased out also.[82,253-255] The serum/plasma folate reflects fairly recent intake over weeks to a few months and can be low due to an acute illness rather than a chronic condition. New assays utilizing stable isotope dilution tandem MS can distinguish between folate vitamers and were shown to give values similar to the radioassays but less than the microbiologic assay in one report.[256]

Measuring the red cell folate should theoretically give a measure of longer-term folate status although it can be low in severe Cbl–deficient megaloblastic anemia making it less useful to distinguish between the two disorders.[255] Most of the circulating serum folate is N5-methylTHF,[256,257] which can be trapped in severe Cbl deficiency, and thus, lost in the urine so that some Cbl-deficient patients will have a low serum folate despite normal intake and absorption. Methodologic issues hamper the use of the red cell folate as shown by large variations between laboratories.[258] The blood cell folylpolyglutamates must be converted to monoglutamates with difficulties in extraction of the folate and instability of the different forms. Hemolysis of samples may increase the serum folate concentrations.[258]

The food folic acid fortification program has had a profound effect on US population serum folate and red cell folate values.[229-231] It has also been shown that there is circulating, unmetabolized folic acid in a significant proportion of the American population, for example, 38% of older NHANES participants.[259] Investigations are ongoing as to whether this is a public health problem.[260,261] Because previously defined low folate values are rare in fortified countries, many US laboratories have raised the lower limit of the reference range to 5 to 6 ng/mL, which actually overlaps with the median values in unfortified populations. Previous cutpoints for deficiency were usually about <3 ng/mL.[104] Such a low value in a patient from a folate-fortified population indicates severe drug or alcohol-induced deficiency or intestinal malabsorption. Extreme serum homocysteine values despite modest decreases in serum folate are seen in alcoholism.[104] Some hospitals in folate-fortified countries have advised against measuring serum or red cell folates.[262] Isotope dilution methods such as LC-MS/MS are useful to determine the proportions of other folate forms in addition to N5-methylTHF.[256] There are different patterns of folates in individuals with the MTHFR 677TT genotype.[263] Folates can be measured in CSF, which is important for management of the cerebral folate deficiencies.

5, 10-Methylenetetrahydrofolate Reductase Enzyme Polymorphism: Effect on Folate

There is a common ancient polymorphism (C677T) in MTHFR found worldwide except in Africa in which the substitution confers thermolability on the enzyme activity. This instability leads to lower serum folate and higher homocysteine values in non–folate-fortified populations. Because of its association with hyperhomocysteinemia, many investigations have explored the relationship of the polymorphism to cardiovascular disease, neural tube defects, pregnancy complications, and other health risks that have been associated with elevated homocysteine.[264] Many older studies were flawed by a lack of recognition that the prevalence is variable ranging from about 2% in the African American population increasing to 20% to 30% in Italians and Mexicans as found in a study of newborns.[265] There were even striking differences in comparing southern China at about 8% vs northern China at 15%. Hematologists working with unfortified populations will need to consider this polymorphism as a possible explanation for elevated homocysteine but not as a risk for megaloblastic anemia. Patients with severe 5, 10-MTHFR deficiency (not the polymorphism) have brain abnormalities, developmental delay, and thrombotic disease but not megaloblastic anemia, since reduced folates are available for thymidine and purine synthesis.[266]

CAUSES OF MEGALOBLASTIC ANEMIA

Cobalamin Deficiency

Pernicious Anemia and Atrophic Gastritis

The most common cause of severe Cbl deficiency is pernicious anemia,[9,10,19,20,44,100,101,124,131,141,224,267-271] which is a misnomer since it is actually a gastric disease in which an autoimmune attack on the parietal cells prevents the secretion of acid and IF. The parietal cells are a target of CD4+ T lymphocytes causing eventual atrophy of the oxyntic mucosa with achlorhydria in the corpus of the stomach with antral sparing. Because the parietal cells produce acid and IF, both are lost in the autoimmune induced atrophy.[267-270] The lack of acid causes G cells in the antrum to continuously produce gastrin. The mucosal H+K+ATPase is the primary target of the T cells and patients with pernicious anemia usually have antiparietal cell antibodies. The enterochromaffin-like cells assist with acid production by producing histamine. Chief cells in the mucosa produce pepsinogen and are also lost in the autoimmune attack. In 50% to 70% of the patients, antibodies to IF also appear and are more specific for pernicious anemia than the antibodies directed against the parietal cells. *Helicobacter pylori* infects the stomach, causes antral gastritis, and may play a role in causing atrophic gastritis also, although controversial. Atrophic gastritis increases the risk of gastric adenocarcinoma and carcinoid tumors. Historically, autoimmune gastritis was diagnosed at endoscopy with biopsy and by demonstrating histamine-fast achlorhydria, but such testing is rarely done currently. The loss of gastric acid leads to malabsorption of iron in the small intestine and there may be a history of poorly explained, recurrent iron deficiency in patients that subsequently are proven to have pernicious anemia.[272] The prevalence of autoimmune gastritis based on biopsies varies from 0.3% to 2.7% with usually a female predominance.[267] Not all patients with atrophic gastritis will present with anemia, either megaloblastic or iron deficiency anemia.[272] The prevalence of pernicious anemia rises with age and may be as high as 2% to 3% in those over 60 years.[267] It affects all races and ethnic groups but is particularly prevalent in those of European and African ancestry. Although, the incidence is lower in Asia, the clinical features have been reported to be similar.[271] There is a female predominance.[268] The age at onset appears to be younger in nonwhite populations. It is common that patients with pernicious anemia have associated autoimmune disease such as autoimmune thyroid disease, type 1 diabetes mellitus, vitiligo and rarely Addison disease, myasthenia gravis, and others.[267,273] There may be a family history of autoimmune disorders.[274] A genome-wide association study study found five risk loci for pernicious anemia with candidate genes with known roles in other autoimmune conditions identified.[275]

The lack of IF leads to a failure of reabsorption of Cbl from the bile secreted into the duodenum, and thus, fairly rapid depletion of total body Cbl. Cessation of Cbl treatment in patients with pernicious anemia usually leads to relapse within 1 to 2 years. If anti-IF antibodies are positive or atrophic gastritis with achlorhydria were diagnosed on endoscopy, then a diagnosis of pernicious anemia would be proven, although these findings may predate the actual development of megaloblastic anemia by several years. Antiparietal cell antibodies are reported to be more common and less specific for pernicious anemia but when positive also support the diagnosis.[276] Elevated fasting serum gastrin and low pepsinogen-I may also help confirm the diagnosis of autoimmune gastritis. Proving malabsorption of Cbl is difficult since the classic Schilling test, which utilized radiolabeled Cbl, is no longer available in most centers. Some investigators have demonstrated that a test showing an increase in plasma holo-TC after unlabeled oral Cbl dosing is a good substitute. This is known as the CobaSorb test wherein an untreated deficient patient ingests 3.9 µg doses of Cbl in 24 hours and the increase in Holo-TC documents absorption.[277] Absorption of cyano-Cbl resulted in a two-fold increase over hydroxoCbl in a modified test.[278] This test will not be practical if holo-TC assays are not available. Other tests have been reported ingesting C-14–labeled dimethylbenzimidazole moiety in Cbl with analysis by an accelerator mass spectrometer,[279] or a carbon-13 corrin ring label, utilizing ultra HPLC-MS.[54] Hopefully, these methodologies will be developed and tested in patients with pernicious anemia. An egg yolk Cbl absorption test has also been used to define food-bound Cbl malabsorption in the past mainly as a research tool.[280]

Gastric Surgery

Total gastrectomy leads to complete absence of IF and inevitable Cbl deficiency in 1 to 5 years depending on the criteria used to diagnose deficiency. Less complete resections such as partial gastrectomy and gastroduodenostomy or gastrojejunostomy (Billroth 1 and 2) operations are done less frequently, but older patients may have undergone the surgery (now forgotten) and have malabsorption of Cbl.[281]

The most frequent surgical causes of malabsorption are the bariatric surgeries including the Roux-en-Y gastric bypass and sleeve gastrectomy, which can lead to Cbl, iron, folate, and copper deficiencies.[282,283] Bariatric surgery causes a decrease in gastric acid and IF release in the remaining gastric pouch as well as separation of the food bolus from the IF secretion. In addition, the bile and pancreatic secretions are no longer present in the duodenum, to recycle Cbl. Changes are likely less with sleeve gastrectomy.[284] However, a recent study showed that the Cbl status decreased following both Roux-en-Y gastric bypass and sleeve gastrectomy with decreased plasma Cbl.[285] However, more importantly, holo-TC and MMA changes were seen within in 2 months. Cbl absorption was tested by an increase in holo-TC after 2 days of three 9 µg doses and was markedly lower 2 months postoperatively decreasing from 20 pmol/L to 5 pmol/L.[285] Thus, high-dose oral Cbl therapy should start soon after bariatric surgery.

Age-Related Chronic Gastritis

Screening studies of senior populations with serum Cbl best accompanied by serum MMA and/or homocysteine have shown an age-related increase in the prevalence of apparent Cbl deficiency rising to as high as 30%.[208,210,211,218,220,286-291] Most of these subjects did not have anti-IF antibodies specific for pernicious anemia, many have atrophic gastritis,[290] and presumed malabsorption of food Cbl. These populations also have the highest prevalence of pernicious anemia, which would be difficult to distinguish in the 50% of pernicious anemia patients who do not have anti-IF blocking antibody. There are controversies as to the significance of the generally milder and potentially nonprogressive nature of the chronic, incomplete malabsorption of Cbl in these populations also termed subclinical Cbl deficiency. It is clear that the small quantities of Cbl in standard multivitamin preparations (approximately 6-30 µg) are not enough to correct MMA[208,210,220] as at least 500 to 1000 µg of Cbl orally daily may be necessary.[292,293] This condition is more common in white seniors as compared to those of African or Asian ancestry.[220,289,294] The metabolite abnormalities in these seniors readily respond to high-dose Cbl alone[208,291,292] or combined with other vitamins[211,286,295] showing that it is actual vitamin malabsorption, but it is difficult to correlate any clinical benefits with treatment.[211] Anemia in particular usually fails to respond, unless it has features of classic megaloblastic anemia.[211,296] The high prevalence of chronic renal insufficiency, iron deficiency, and anemia of inflammation all contribute to anemia in this elderly population. Many seniors in the United States take multivitamins and other supplemented foods and, thus, are exposed to higher intakes of folic acid than might be appropriate if the patient has an underlying severe Cbl deficiency. This situation can cause high serum folate and low Cbl simultaneously, which is a subject of active investigation.[261] Some studies suggest impaired cognition and other poor outcomes in this situation.[297] It may be prudent to utilize high-dose oral Cbl in all seniors with low Cbl values or elevated MMA rather than trying to distinguish milder forms of malabsorption from true pernicious anemia, since most seniors are already taking supplements in the United States.[298]

Small Intestinal Bacterial Overgrowth and Parasites

Bacterial overgrowth may occur in patients with anatomic abnormalities in the upper small intestine such as jejunal diverticula, fistulas, or strictures and also in motility disorders, particularly long-standing diabetes.[299] The bacteria compete with IF for Cbl and deficiency may ensue. *Diphyllobothrium latum*, a parasite which develops in freshwater fish may cause rare cases of Cbl deficiency.[300]

Ileal Resections and Reconstruction Surgery

The distal ileum is the site of cubam, the IF-Cbl receptor; thus, diseases or resection of the ileum will cause Cbl malabsorption. Necrotizing enterocolitis in premature infants with ileal resection may not manifest as Cbl deficiency for many years.[301] Crohn disease and ulcerative colitis may affect the distal ileum, leading to deficiency. Distal ileum is used in surgeries to form conduits, pouches, or neobladders postradical cystectomy. The various procedures use differing lengths of ileum from short segments up to 60 cm. Therefore, the risk of Cbl malabsorption varies with the amount of ileum removed and the duration of life postsurgery. One study reported a 29% incidence of elevated MMA within 5 years after cystectomy, which was increased in elderly patients, thus, may have been complicated by the age-related increasing incidence of Cbl deficiency.[302]

Tropical sprue causes diarrhea and malabsorption likely due to gastrointestinal infections, which lead to villus damage, throughout the entire small intestine and particularly the terminal ileum. Cbl deficiency often with folate deficiency is seen in 50% to 90% of the patients.[104,303] Although seen mainly in tropical areas of the world, visitors and immigrants from such regions may have undiagnosed tropical sprue. It is often confused with gluten enteropathy, although the latter does not usually cause Cbl deficiency.[304] The treatment includes antibiotics, high-dose folic acid, and Cbl substitution.

Drug-Induced Cobalamin Deficiency

Abuse of N_2O can cause severe myeloneuropathy occasionally with permanent disability and macrocytic anemia.[305,306] The users are either associated with dental offices or anesthesia services or users of pressurized N_2O canisters used for whipping cream. Serum Cbl values are normal to low, but MMA and homocysteine are invariably elevated. Treatment regimens vary greatly but should include rapid replacement with parenteral Cbl until at least MMA and homocysteine have normalized. There are also cases of anesthesia-induced acceleration of probable underlying Cbl deficiency since patients develop symptoms rapidly postexposure and may have undiagnosed pernicious anemia.[307]

Proton pump inhibitors and H2 receptor antagonists are acid-blocking drugs in wide usage. Theoretically, they could decrease absorption of Cbl due to the lack of stomach acid, which leads to impaired release of Cbl from food proteins.[290,308] It has been difficult to prove whether long-term use of these medications leads to clinical Cbl deficiency. They are often used in seniors with already increased risk of Cbl deficiency.

Metformin, a diabetes drug, impairs calcium-dependent binding of IF-Cbl complex to cubam in the distal ilium. Many studies show a dose-dependent decrease in serum Cbl with long-term metformin use,[308] but the clinical significance is unknown.

Cobalamin Deficiency in Infants and Children

Many countries have instituted newborn screening programs for treatable hereditary illnesses.[79,171,172] Acquired Cbl deficiency can be detected by elevations of propionyl-carnitine (C3), which had been implemented to screen for the methylmalonic and propionic acidurias utilizing tandem MS.[172] Second tier testing of MMA and in some cases homocysteine can confirm diagnosis. A recent study from Heidelberg, Germany, showed that 1 in 5300 newborns had Cbl deficiency ranging from mild to severe.[79] The prevalence in newborns depends on the Cbl status of the women in a country but also by criteria for detection. A study from Barcelona found an acquired Cbl deficiency incidence of 1 in 1989, which is much higher than those with genetic disorders.[172] Acquired Cbl deficiency had a higher percentage of elevated homocysteine than those with the genetic disorders. The detection of infants with Cbl deficiency and early treatment should prevent the tragic later development of potentially permanent neurologic disability in the exclusively breast-fed infant of a deficient mother.[171] There are a wide range of causes of Cbl deficiency in these mothers with many having undiagnosed pernicious anemia, usually asymptomatic but also including mothers following vegan or other diets limiting animal-source foods, women with short-gut syndromes, and postbariatric surgery.[165] Human milk has a much lower concentration of Cbl than cow's milk and exclusively breast-fed normal infants usually have lower serum Cbl and some even higher MMA concentrations as compared to their formula fed counterparts. Very low levels of milk Cbl have been documented in vegans, 68 ng/L, as compared to nutritionally adequate mother's milk being almost five-times higher (420 ng/L).[80] Milk Cbl is bound to HC.

Symptoms of Cbl deficiency in infants not detected at newborn screening are usually delayed to about 6 months but can range up to 2 years old. Cbl-deficient infants often refuse to take complimentary feeding, which exacerbates their deficiency. The neurologic symptoms include hypotonia, apathy, lethargy, and movement disorders with tremor, myoclonus, and loss of developmental milestones. The presence of megaloblastic anemia is variable noting that MCV values are lower in infants than adults. Homocysteine and MMA may be greatly elevated. Serum MMA is somewhat higher in infants than older children but usually less than 1000 nmol/L.

Pernicious anemia is rare in children and adolescents but has been reported with the same associations with anti-IF antibodies and other autoimmune disorders. The inborn errors of Cbl absorption also are seen in early to late childhood and are described in another section. Infants with necrotizing colitis may have surgery removing distal ilium which will result in Cbl deficiency if not empirically treated.[301] Children with short-gut syndrome or inflammatory bowel diseases are also subject to Cbl deficiency.

Dietary intake of Cbl varies widely throughout the world depending on the availability of animal source food. There is also increased interest in plant-based diets, which can subject children to deficiencies in Cbl as well as other nutrients. One study from Poland showed that unsupplemented vegan children had higher homocysteine and inadequate Cbl status as compared to their omnivorous counterparts.[309]

Vegetarianism

Dietary deficiency of Cbl results from the avoidance of animal source foods in the diet, which may be based on the practice of veganism or due to the lack of access to expensive animal foods in many parts of the world.[44,45,138,217,309-311] In addition, religious practices may limit animal food intake. Shellfish, organ meats, fish, and beef are good sources of Cbl.[44] Chicken and other fowl are approximately only 10% of Cbl in beef and pork is about 1/3 the content of beef. Goat milk Cbl is much lower than cow milk Cbl. These variations in animal product content could have effects on the total content of an omnivorous diet.[44,45,217] In addition, the definition of a portion of animal food (meat) varies considerably. Some fermented plant foods[51,52] such as tempeh and fermented fish sauce contain Cbl. Dried algae may also have Cbl along with Cbl analogues.[50] Cbl-supplemented foods are widely available in the United States and elsewhere,[309] particularly in milk and meat substitutes, and can prevent deficiency. Dietary Cbl deficiency is common in the Indian subcontinent, Mexico, Central and South America and areas of Africa and the Middle East, and is less common in Asia, except in those following vegetarian diets.[44] A review of vegetarians vs omnivores from many parts of the world showed that plasma Cbl was lower and homocysteine generally higher despite presumed higher intake of folates in those on a plant-based diet.[45]

Causes of Folate Deficiency

Dietary

Dietary folate deficiency can occur in 3 to 4 months of a severely inadequate diet or in the setting of anorexia or cancer cachexia. A widely quoted self-experiment by Victor Herbert in 1962 revealed that a definite increase in the neutrophil lobe average and increase in MCV occurred after 18 weeks of consuming a triple boiled diet. This was accompanied by megaloblastic bone marrow and a marked decrease in red cell folate.[82] Dietary deficiency has become rare in the countries that have fortified grain products with folic acid.[85] Folate deficiency is prevalent worldwide in populations that do not have access to fruits, fresh vegetables, or organ meats. Cooking practices that discard water used to cook vegetables for prolonged periods markedly decrease food folate content. The food folic acid fortification program in the United States was so successful in raising population intake that now there is concern that folate intake may be excessive, particularly true in children and in seniors. The use of folic acid supplements is widespread in the United States with extra folic acid added to sports drinks, energy bars, etc. It would be very rare to attribute megaloblastic anemia to dietary folate deficiency in a folic acid–fortified population.

Malabsorption

Folates are absorbed in the upper intestinal tract. Folate deficiency with elevated homocysteine occurs in inflammatory bowel disease, gluten enteropathy (celiac sprue) with villus atrophy of the upper small intestine, and in tropical sprue.[299,303,304] These disorders usually also cause iron malabsorption and deficiency, which can mask macrocytosis. Intestinal infections occurring in patients with bone marrow or solid organ transplants or HIV and other immunodeficiency syndromes will cause folate deficiency. The folic acid added to grain products has been beneficial in these conditions.

Increased Cellular Folate Requirements

The rapid red cell turnover in the hemolytic anemias, both acquired, and the hemoglobinopathies or other hereditary hemolytic syndromes have been shown to cause folate depletion and hyperhomocysteinemia.[312] In general, the practice is to prevent these complications by treating with folic acid in the United States. Severe exfoliative skin diseases and highly proliferative cancers such as leukemia may also cause depletion of folates.[313]

Renal Dialysis

Water-soluble vitamins are lost during dialysis; thus, patients are usually treated with combination vitamin therapeutics including folic acid and Cbl. Homocysteine is usually elevated in these patients despite vitamin treatment and it is only partially responsive to high-dose combinations of folic acid, vitamin B6, and Cbl.[314] The hyperhomocysteinemia is likely due to a combination of factors including low methionine status in renal failure and elevated cysteine.

Drug Interference With Folate Metabolism

There are many drugs in common usage that either cause folate deficiency or interfere with folate metabolism and some have been shown to cause megaloblastic anemia in individuals without a high folate intake.[315] Methotrexate[316] is the most common antifol used followed by pemetrexate and antibiotics such as trimethoprim, sulfasalazine, and others as listed in *Table 37.7*. The older anticonvulsants including carbamazepine, phenytoin, valproic acid, lamotrigine, and phenobarbital cause folate depletion.[315,317] The newer anticonvulsants such as levetiracetam and lacosamide do not seem to deplete folate or raise homocysteine. Some drugs such as high-dose niacin, levodopa,[318] and the over-the-counter supplement, alpha-lipoic acid,[319] are methylated and have been shown to deplete methyl-groups, raise homocysteine, and in the case of L-dopa cause poor health outcomes. Most of the drugs cited in *Table 37.7* are given with supplemental folic acid without a loss of efficacy.

Alcohol

Many clinicians hoped that the folic acid added to grain products would eliminate alcohol-induced folate-deficient megaloblastic anemia.[89] It is likely that this has benefitted moderate and heavy social drinkers; however, severe folate–deficient megaloblastic anemia is still seen in emergency rooms and hospitals. A recent study of a safety net hospital showed that 5.5% of tested serum folates were <4 ng/mL associated with anemia in 87%, macrocytosis in 25%, and macrocytic anemia in 17%. The demographics showed that about 12% of the patients were homeless, 25% were born outside of the United States, and 33% had active substance use disorder.[89] This report shows that it is still worthwhile to test for folate deficiency post food folic acid fortification.

In addition, moderate to severe hyperhomocysteinemia with only modest decrease in serum folate is also encountered in patients with macrocytic anemia[118] and alcohol use in hematology clinics.[104] Suspected alcoholics often are treated with glucose containing intravenous fluids with folic acid, thiamine, and other multivitamins in order to prevent thiamine–deficient neurologic disease immediately on admission. The unwary clinician will assume the resulting normal folate value precludes a diagnosis of folate–deficient megaloblastic anemia. Homocysteine may still be elevated in the early hours post-vitamin administration. Megaloblastic anemia in alcohol use disorder

Table 37.7. Causes of Cobalamin and Folate Deficiency

Cobalamin Deficiency
Lack of intrinsic factor
Pernicious Anemia (Type A gastritis, autoimmune gastritis)
Gastrectomy, Roux-en-Y gastric bypass or sleeve gastrectomy
Hereditary gastric intrinsic factor deficiency
Food cobalamin malabsorption
Atrophic gastritis (Type B gastritis, *Helicobacter pylori* associated)
Gastric hypo or achlorhydria
Exocrine pancreatic dysfunction
Disorders of the distal ileum
Surgical resection of distal 1-2 ft.
Inflammatory bowel disease
Surgical reconstruction – ileal conduit or cystoplasty
Imerslund-Gräsbeck syndrome, hereditary defects of CUBAM
Usurption of intestinal cobalamin
Tropical sprue, bacterial overgrowth, blind intestinal loops
Parasitic infection – Diphyllobothrium latum and Giardia lamblia
Nutritional cobalamin deficiency
Breast-fed infant of a deficient mother
Diet lacking animal source food, vegan, lacto-ovo vegetarian or impoverished low meat diet
Drug induced cobalamin deficiency
Nitrous oxide abuse or anesthesia in a cobalamin deficient patient
Metformin, gastric acid blockers, proton pump inhibitors or histamine blockers
Inborn errors of cobalamin metabolism
Transport – transcobalamin deficiency
Cellular metabolism – mutations that cause combined methylmalonic acidemia and/or just homocystinuria (CblC-J, X)
Folate Deficiency
Nutritional folate deficiency
Lack of fresh fruit, green leafy vegetables, legumes, organ meats
Anorexia nervosa and other eating disorders
Alcohol abuse combined with poor nutrition
Folate malabsorption
Celiac or tropical sprue
Crohn disease and other small intestinal diseases
Atrophic gastritis and bariatric surgery
Increased demand or loss
Pregnancy
Hemolytic anemias
Proliferative skin disorders
Leukemias
Hemodialysis
Drug-caused folate deficiency
Antifolates – methotrexate, pemetrexed, pralatrexate, pyrimethamine, sulfasalazine, trimethoprim
Anticonvulsants – phenytoin, carbamazepine, valproic acid
Methylation-requiring drugs – L-Dopa, high-dose niacin, α-lipoic acid
Inborn Errors of Folate Metabolism
MTHFD1 deficiency
PCFT (SLC46A1) mutation
DHFR mutation
MTHFR mutation

Abbreviations: CblC-J,X, complementation groups of mutations in cobalamin metabolism; CUBAM, cubilin-amnionless complex; DHFR, dihydrofolate reductase; MTHFD1, 5,10-methyleneTHF dehydrogenase; MTHFR, 5,10-methylenetetrahydrofolate reductase; PCFT, proton-coupled folate transporter.

is often complicated by sideroblastic anemia due to iron utilization defects and overload and vitamin B6 deficiency.[140,320,321] However, many others have iron deficiency from variceal or gastritis–related blood loss.

Alcohol interferes with folate metabolism in multiple ways.[322,323] Because of the high caloric content of alcohol, there is usually decreased food intake including the fortified grain products. Alcohol induces intestinal folate malabsorption by causing megaloblastic changes in enterocytes and by impairing the hydrolysis of dietary N-pteroylpolyglutamyl.[323] A study of humans ingesting tritium labeled folic acid showed decreased jejunal uptake. There is also evidence that the hepatic folate storage is decreased, the acetaldehyde metabolite of alcohol impairs MTR activity,[322,323] and the renal excretion of folates is increased as shown in humans and in animal models. The multiple effects on folate metabolism may explain why homocysteine is elevated out of proportion to the apparent drop in serum folate. In fact, elevated homocysteine can be used as a marker of alcohol use disorder.

Inborn Errors of Cobalamin Absorption and Metabolism

The inborn errors that cause megaloblastic anemia due to either inadequate Cbl status or folate status will be discussed. Methylmalonic aciduria without homocystinuria does not cause megaloblastic anemia, although there may be anemia and neutropenia due to acidosis or other metabolic abnormalities. Likewise, severe MTHFR deficiency does not cause megaloblastic anemia.

Inherited Disorders of Absorption

The inherited disorders of Cbl absorption cause symptoms months to even years after birth when the fetal supply of Cbl is exhausted.[64,324] The symptoms are similar to acquired Cbl deficiency in babies, toddlers, and children with impaired growth, developmental delays, neurodegeneration of brain and spinal cord, immunodeficiencies,[325] and megaloblastic anemia. Serum Cbl values are low and both homocysteine and MMA are elevated in serum or urine. The malabsorption can be detected by the Schilling test, although this is no longer available; thus, genetic testing is needed to pinpoint the disorder.[324]

Imerslund-Gräsbeck syndrome, megaloblastic anemia I (OMIM261100), is caused by a deficiency of either the cubulin gene (CUBN) or ANM, which both cause selective malabsorption of Cbl and proteinuria. They form the cubam dimer, which is the ileal receptor for the gastric IF (GIF)-Cbl complex.[65] Deficiency of GIF (IFD, OMIM261000) also causes impaired Cbl absorption.[66] Many different mutations in these three genes have been described and there are founder effects in some consanguineous populations. One large study of 154 families revealed mutations in 126, 42% had mutations in CUBN, 36% in AMN and 22% in GIF. There was a common Finnish mutation in CUBN. An ancient founder mutation in AMN was found causing 15% of the cases worldwide and more than 50% among Middle Eastern patients. Several founder mutations were also found in GIF[326] and are discussed in detail elsewhere.[324] Details are found in reference 324. The presence of proteinuria can help localize the defect to the cubam receptor. One striking finding in case reports is the lack of continuous treatment in the patients with many episodes of relapse, possibly because a nutritional cause was suspected rather than malabsorption.[327] Many treatment regimens have been reported with both parenteral and high-dose oral dosing on a daily or weekly basis. Family members should be investigated in consanguineous kinships since the clinical presentation is quite variable.

Disorders of Cobalamin Transport

TC transports Cbl and presents it to cells where it is taken up by the TC receptor (CD320). TC deficiency (OMIM275350) causes combined methylmalonic aciduria, homocystinuria, and patients present usually within the first few months of life.[67] They have megaloblastic anemia and pancytopenia as well as failure to thrive and occasionally immunodeficiency.[325] The serum Cbl level will not be low due to the intact HC. The best treatment results have been with at least weekly intramuscular injection of hydroxo- or cyanoCbl with hydroxoCbl preferred. Deficiency of HC causes low Cbl levels and is generally benign since TC is the important delivery protein.[68,69] It may be as common as 15% of patients with low Cbl levels. MMA and homocysteine will not be elevated and there is an absence of megaloblastic anemia.

Inborn Errors of Intracellular Cobalamin Metabolism With Megaloblastic Anemia

The disorders of Cbl metabolism have been placed in complementation groups A-J.[11,42,328] CblA and cblB only cause methylmalonic aciduria and not megaloblastic anemia. CblC is the most common with a defect in MMACHC, methylmalonic aciduria Cbl C type with homocystinuria, which acts as a chaperone and processes Cbl to a cob(II)alamin form. Patients with cblC deficiency may be identified by newborn screening, family history, or by symptoms. There is a common mutation c.394C > T (p.Arg132*). Neurologic symptoms, developmental delays, seizures, and psychiatric disorders are prominent. Some patients may have hemolytic uremic syndrome and thrombotic microangiopathy. The MMA and homocysteine values are markedly elevated and methionine may be below the normal range. Large daily doses of parenteral hydroxoCbl 1 to 7.5 mg have been employed with the addition of betaine and folic acid. It appears that early and aggressive treatment will improve the clinical outcome. An occasional patient may not be diagnosed until early adulthood with the onset of neurologic symptoms. Mutations have also been found in another chaperone enzyme, MMADHC that targets Cbl to either MTR or mutase. The site of the mutation determines whether there is methylmalonic aciduria, homocystinuria, or combined.[328] The clinical presentation varies as to where the mutation is such that the cblD patients with combined methylmalonic aciduria-homocystinuria may have megaloblastic anemia as do the cblD homocystinuric alone patients but not those who only have methylmalonic aciduria. Megaloblastic anemia occurs in the cblG defect, loss of MTR function, with accumulation of homocysteine and a related defect, cblE, loss of the enzyme MTRR, which reduces MTR when it has been oxidized from cob(I)alamin to cob(II)alamin. Megaloblastic anemia also occurs also in cblF due to defective LMBDI and cblJ ABCD4 gene, which are proteins involved in lysosomal release of Cbl.

Megaloblastic Anemia Due to Disorders of Folate Uptake and Metabolism

Hereditary folate malabsorption is caused by defects in the PCFT so that there is impaired folate transport in both the intestines and the choroid plexus of the central nervous system.[93] Mutations are found in SLC46A1.[329] The patients present with megaloblastic anemia, immunodeficiency,[325] and neurologic defects including seizures and developmental delay. Despite treatment with leucovorin, the CSF N^5-methyl-THF levels remain low although megaloblastic anemia can resolve.

A patient has been reported with recurrent, severe megaloblastic anemia due to a defect in the RFC, which is encoded by SLC19A1G.[329] The patient presented with severe macrocytic anemia with hemolysis and hyperhomocysteinemia at age 15 years and had normal serum folate, low Cbl, but normal MMA, and did not respond to parenteral Cbl injections until after high-dose folic acid was added to the treatment regimen. Defects in methylenetetrahydrofolate dehydrogenase (MTHFD1),[93,330] a trifunctional enzyme that catalyzes synthesis of 10-formyltetrahydrofolate and subsequent conversion to 5,10-methylenetetrahydrofolate, have been reported in patients from three families who have megaloblastic anemia, immunologic dysfunction, and atypical hemolytic uremic syndrome.[331] Treatment with folinic acid has improved the anemia and metabolic abnormality.

A homozygous mutation in DHFR was found in several children who presented with megaloblastic anemia responsive to folate treatment and cerebral folate deficiency with severe developmental delay.[332-334] 5,10-methenyltetrahydrofolate synthetase deficiency has also been reported to cause megaloblastic anemia and cerebral folate deficiency.[335,336]

Megaloblastic Anemias Not Related to Folate or Cobalamin Metabolism

Thiamine Responsive Megaloblastic Anemia

Thiamine responsive megaloblastic anemia (SLC19A2 dysfunction) is a defect in thiamine transport that presents with diabetes mellitus, megaloblastic anemia, and hearing loss.[337] About 100 cases have been described, many from consanguineous families. High-dose thiamine may improve or normalize hemoglobin. Patients usually present in childhood.

Lesch-Nyhan Disease

Lesch-Nyhan disease is caused by deficiency of hypoxanthine-guanine phosphoribosyltransferase, which has a role in recycling hypoxanthine and guanine into purine nucleotides. The major manifestations are neurological and behavioral abnormalities with overproduction of uric acid. However, macrocytic red blood cells, with or without anemia, are present in most patients and may even be a clue to the diagnosis in young children with undiagnosed neurologic problems.[338]

Hereditary Orotic Acidemia

The inborn error of pyrimidine metabolism caused by mutations in uridine-5-monophosphate synthase causes orotic aciduria and immunodeficiency with megaloblastic anemia that does not respond to vitamin administration. It can be diagnosed by measuring urinary excretion of orotic acid and treated with uridine.[339]

Drugs Inducing Macrocytosis

Sunitinib and imatinib cause reversible macrocytosis that was not accompanied by anemia or pancytopenia.[340] It has been suggested that this is an effect of inhibition of the c-KIT pathway.

The antiretroviral agents, zidovudine, lamivudine, and stavudine, have all been associated with macrocytosis. Stavudine and lamivudine appear to cause less anemia than higher dose[341,342] zidovudine.

A practical approach to megaloblastic anemia is outlined in Table 37.8.

TREATMENT OF COBALAMIN DEFICIENCY

Megaloblastic Anemia and Myeloneuropathy

The goal of treatment is to quickly restore normal tissue Cbl content, which ranges from 2 to 5 mg depending on size of the individual. The time-honored approach to treatment has been to use parenteral cyano-Cbl or hydroxoCbl intramuscular[9,224,343] or subcutaneous injections of 1000 μg. About 150 μg will be retained from each injection; thus, up to 20 injections might be required to fully replete the severely deficient patient. The frequency of injections often relies on the convenience of access such that hospitalized patients with severe megaloblastic anemia are well served by daily injections until discharge. Others should have twice a week or at least weekly injections for about 8 doses, followed by at least monthly injections with cyanoCbl. It may also be convenient to combine daily high-dose oral tablets with the parenteral treatment. There is some evidence that hydroxoCbl is retained better than the cyano form and some practioners (especially in Europe) decrease frequency of injections to every 2 to 3 months in the former.[224] Reticulocytosis will increase within 4 to 7 days and can reach high levels of approximately 20%. Some patients will gain several grams of hemoglobin in a week. Hypersegmentation will take longer to resolve in the peripheral blood.[129] Elevated MMA and homocysteine values immediately decrease with homocysteine normalizing in days to a week.[18,59,100,103,143,213,216,234] Extreme values of MMA may take several weeks to a month to normalize. Megaloblastic changes in the bone marrow are corrected quickly; thus, if indicated, bone marrow biopsy or aspirate should be performed prior to treatment with Cbl. The biochemical markers of red cell destruction will also clear. Thrombocytopenia and neutropenia are often corrected within a week. Transferrin saturation will fall as iron is utilized in erythropoiesis. If the patient is also iron deficient, then ferritin may decrease to low values, often laboratory signs of iron deficiency will ensue, and

Table 37.8. Practical Approach to Megaloblastic Anemia

Is there macrocytic anemia/pancytopenia?
• Increasing MCV, macrocytes, high RDW, neutropenia, thrombocytopenia
• High LDH, low haptoglobin, high indirect bilirubin
Is there low serum cobalamin or low folate?
Serum Cobalamin
<300 pg/mL Sensitive but not specific
<100 pg/mL Not sensitive but more specific
Serum Holo-TC[a] < 30 pg/mL sensitivity and specificity poorly defined
Serum Folate < 3-4 ng/mL
Is there metabolic evidence of deficiency?
Serum methylmalonic acid > 500 nmol/L
or
Serum homocysteine > 14 μmol/L
Is there a causative disorder?
Pernicious anemia (Type A gastritis, autoimmune gastritis)   • Anti-intrinsic factor antibodies (50% positive, very specific)   • Antiparietal cell antibodies (80% positive but less specific)   • Low serum pepsinogen I < 30 μg/L or I/II ratio < 3   • High fasting serum gastrin > 100 pmol/L
Chronic atrophic gastritis (Type B gastritis, *Helicobacter pylori* associated)
History of gastric or ileal surgery or intestinal diseases
Vegan unsupplemented diet
Alcohol use disorder (Folate deficiency only)
Is there a prompt response to therapy?
Reticulocytosis in 4-7 d
Correction of neutropenia and thrombocytopenia in a week
Correction of hemoglobin in 2 mo
Normalization of methylmalonic acid and/or homocysteine

[a]Holo-TC not available in USA or worldwide.
Abbreviations: LDH, lactate dehydrogenase; MCV, mean red cell volume; RDW, red cell distribution width.

hemoglobin may not reach normal levels. Previous concerns about hypokalemia occurring with Cbl therapy[344] seem to be overemphasized, but patients with volume overload should be monitored. Red blood cell transfusion should not be delayed in the severely anemic patient as it may be lifesaving and will not affect the diagnosis except to decrease the MCV by dilution with normal red blood cells. Folic acid supplementation can be given if the serum folate is unexpectedly low but is usually not needed and may lead to the patient taking folic acid without Cbl supplementation in the future.

A report from Mexico showed that an IM dose of 10,000 μg of hydroxoCbl corrected severe megaloblastic anemia for at least 3 months with continuing normalization of the anemia for 6 months, although MMA and homocysteine increased in some of the subjects.[345] The authors finally recommended repeating at 3-month intervals. Concentrated preparations of hydroxoCbl are not widely available however, but this could be a convenient alternative to monthly injections.

Cbl can be absorbed by mass action in the small intestine although studies with radiolabeled Cbl showed that it was limited to 0.5% to 2% of the dose.[57,58] High doses of oral Cbl (at least 1000 μg/d) are effective in treating PA, total gastrectomy patients, and other causes of Cbl deficiency.[59,346-349]

Intranasal preparations of Cbl are available as an alternative to parenteral treatment but likely are swallowed and similar to oral preparations.[349] A 2 mg puff of a Cbl nasal spray increased Cbl to high levels in children.[350] One study compared daily 50 µg sublingual dosing and 2000 µg sublingual weekly dosing for 90 days in a group of vegans/vegetarians showing increase in Cbl and holo-TC values but not a correction in mean serum MMA in the weekly group as the value remained approximately 500 nmol/L although homocysteine was corrected to 10 µmol/L in both groups.[351] The high-dose once weekly group could have been expected to absorb on average 24 µg vs the daily group at 31 µg since the daily preparation would also be absorbed more frequently by IF-mediated uptake. Both doses were likely low as compared to studies using daily treatment of 500 µg or 2000 µg sublingual dosing.[352,353] Sublingual dosing is likely swallowed and should be as effective as oral Cbl so long as the expected absorbed dose matches the enterohepatic circulation loss of Cbl of 2 to 9 µg/d. Proponents of oral dosing cite convenience and low cost. Opponents say the lack of oversight since the patient is not being directly observed may lead to noncompliance. There is availability of high dose oral Cbl in grocery stores and pharmacies in the United States without prescription, but this is limited in some countries.

The form of Cbl used for treatment is less important than the actual appropriate utilization of treatment and life-long persistence in those with malabsorption; however, cyano-, hydroxo-, and methylCbl are all available for administration. MethylCbl has been widely touted as treatment for neurologic disorders and in general is more expensive than cyanocobalamin.[354] MethylCbl and adenosylCbl (rarely used) must be protected from light, which is not true for the stable, cyano-Cbl form. When the former are exposed to light, they are converted to aquocobalamin, which is also effective for treatment. Concerns that the cyano-group will cause poisoning are unfounded as the extremely small quantity in the preparations is much less than the allowable amount of cyanide in drinking water.[355] All of the forms of Cbl are bound tightly by the transporters and eventually delivered to the cells. The upper axial ligand of Cbl is removed by MMACHC and then Cbl can be methylated or adenosylated as the cell requires.[356] Hydroxocobalamin is generally used for treatment of patients with the inborn errors of intracellular trafficking and processing of Cbl. So far there is no proof that one form is more effective than the others in acquired Cbl deficiency.[356]

A specific diagnosis of Cbl deficiency is important since the symptoms of Cbl deficient neurologic dysfunction overlap with many common diseases, including diabetic neuropathy, spinal stenosis, paraproteinemias, hereditary neurodegenerative syndromes, and especially multiple sclerosis. Myelopathy may take months to respond but should not worsen after the first few weeks of treatment. Longer pretreatment interval and higher severity score pretreatment are correlated with incomplete responses.[102]

Cobalamin Replacement in Infants and Children

It should be determined whether an infant or child with proven Cbl deficiency has an inborn error of absorption or metabolism vs dietary deficiency due to deficient breast milk or vegetarian diet. Initial treatment should be aggressive in all patients in order to provide catch up brain growth and development and fully replace tissue content. One successful treatment regimen is to give cyanoCbl 0.5 mg liquid orally for 3 days and then 0.1 mg day until correction of all abnormal laboratory tests. Oral 5 µg/d can then be given in dietary deficiency. Cbl injections of 1 mg for 4 days to rapidly replete stores have also been recommended. Oral supplementation or formula feeding should follow.[165] School-aged and especially adolescent children should receive adult doses of 1000 µg/d if parenteral treatment is chosen followed by weekly and monthly doses as per in adults. Sublingual or nasal preparations are particularly attractive to avoid parenteral therapy in children but should be monitored by serum MMA and/or Cbl values to make sure frequency of dosing is adequate.

Treatment Considerations in Seniors

Senior populations have both an increased incidence of pernicious anemia but also age-related atrophic gastritis, which may cause a milder malabsorption of Cbl.

It has been assumed that smaller doses of oral Cbl would suffice for treatment in food Cbl malabsorption; however, reports show that MMA is not corrected in most with standard multivitamin doses.[210,220] Sequential oral doses of 25 µg followed by 100 µg did not correct MMA in most of the subjects who when changed to a dose of 1000 µg normalized[292] in one study. Another report found that oral doses between 647 and 1000 µg were required for a maximum reduction in MMA.[293] Because elevated MMA and homocysteine are prevalent in senior populations, it has been tempting to assume that there is an age-related increase which is nonvitamin related in these metabolic markers and that the reference ranges should be shifted upwards, especially since MMA and homocysteine are affected by renal function. However, mean MMA fell from 434 to 240 nmol/L and mean homocysteine from 12.7 to 9.6 µmol/L in 39 senior subjects (mean age 79) after 3 months of 1000 µg daily oral treatment.[291] Those with creatinine > 109 µmol/L had posttreatment MMA of 256 vs 227 nmol/L in those with lower serum creatinine and homocysteine was 11.4 vs 8.3 µmol/L, respectively. S-adenosylhomocysteine remained elevated at 46 compared to 29 nmol/L posttreatment in the same groups. These posttreatment values of MMA and homocysteine are well within the reference ranges seen in younger persons. It has been difficult to prove benefit in cognition, anemias, or other measures of health posttreatment, however, despite the responses in metabolites. Higher doses of Cbl that actually improve metabolite status should be recommended for seniors instead of the low doses in most multivitamin since their use is widespread.

Cobalamin Replacement in Vegetarians

There are many issues to consider when recommending Cbl replacement in persons who avoid animal source food. About 50% of ingested food Cbl is absorbed with limited IF-mediated absorption so that increasing dietary Cbl results in a lower fraction of the dose being absorbed. A study of vegetarians and low meat eaters showed that serum Cbl, holo-TC, MMA, and homocysteine were optimum with intakes between 4 and 7 µg/d,[217] similar to amounts reported from omnivorous diets. This amount is not obtainable in populations with poor access to expensive animal source food or those who choose to avoid such foods. The other important consideration for replacement is the duration of low intake. Multigenerational deficiency will impact the current status of some of the subjects. It will take many months to replace tissue stores (2-5 mg) with small doses, since IF-related absorption is limited to at most 5 µg/d. The Cbl-deficient pregnant woman is in an emergency situation and should be loaded with high-dose oral or parenteral Cbl. A recent report of adults with nutritional Cbl deficiency taking 3 µg cyano- or hydroxoCbl showed that the biochemical markers of MMA and homocysteine did not normalize after 8 weeks of the supplement.[81] Clearly this approach would not be satisfactory unless high-dose therapy was employed first. Processed milk and meat alternative foods are frequently supplemented with Cbl in the United States for informed consumers. For populations without access to such foods, there is interest in finding enriched plant foods or even fortified salt[357] or tea.[358] Micro-organisms have long been harnessed for the vitamins produced when they are used to ferment plant foods such as tempeh[52] or enset[53] and thus are a source of Cbl as well as other vitamins. Algae products, such as dried sea weeds,[49] dried nori, and blue green algae, also contain Cbl, but the naturally occurring Cbl analogues are the dominant form of corrinoids in these foods.

TREATMENT OF FOLATE DEFICIENCY

Folic acid, folinic acid (leucovorin, 5-formylTHF), and L-methylfolate are available over the counter in the United States, by prescription and in combination therapies with other B-vitamins, especially Cbl and pyridoxine. Folic acid is available in doses up to 1 mg tablets over the counter although the usual amount in most multivitamins is 400 µg. This dose is recommended by the Centers for Disease Control for all women of child-bearing age to prevent neural tube defects. All three forms of folate can be used to treat dietary folate deficiency, which is rare in the countries that have fortified food with folic acid. Folic acid 1 mg daily is widely prescribed for alcohol use disorder, inflammatory bowel diseases, celiac disease, postgastric bypass, and other malabsorption syndromes and for persons with hemolytic anemias. Many of these conditions have associated Cbl malabsorption; thus, high-dose oral Cbl should also be instituted or pretreatment serum MMA should be assayed. High doses of methylfolate have been recommended as being effective adjunctives to the treatment of depression and neurocognitive disorders such as mild cognitive decline and autism, but treatment effects appear to be slight. There is much misinformation in the lay literature about the requirement for L-methylfolate rather than folic acid for persons with thermolabile MTHFR polymorphism. Folic acid will cure hyperhomocysteinemia in such individuals. Folinic acid is used in cancer treatments in two opposing ways; high-dose methotrexate is routinely rescued with leucovorin IV in order to ameliorate the expected mucositis and pancytopenia, and conversely used with 5-flurouracil to augment the chemotherapeutic toxicity in some regimens.

TREATMENT OF HYPERHOMOCYSTEINEMIA

Moderate (>50 μmol/L) and severe (>100 μmol/L) hyperhomocysteinemia is associated with increased risk of thrombotic and arteriosclerotic disease, no matter the underlying etiology.[105,106,359] Clinicians may discover elevated homocysteine values in persons with otherwise unexplained deep vein thrombosis, particularly in younger patients where it will be more likely to be tested as part of a thrombophilia work-up.[182-185,360] It is necessary to make a specific diagnosis in these patients since treatment and follow-up varies widely and includes family studies in those with inborn errors of metabolism. MMA should be assayed in addition to homocysteine in those with any indication of megaloblastic anemia or demyelinating CNS symptoms in order to avoid treating a patient with pernicious anemia with folic acid alone. There are many case reports of a thrombotic presentation of severe Cbl deficiency some treated with only folic acid.[182,184-186]

Hyperhomocysteinemia without megaloblastic anemia may be due to one of the disorders of methionine metabolism such as cystathionine beta-synthase, classical homocystinemia. Severely affected individuals are discovered with newborn screening[359] or in childhood. Some affected individuals present as adults with thrombotic disease and a lack of other symptoms.[105,359,360] It is treated with combinations of high-dose pyridoxine, folate, Cbl, and betaine with methionine restriction in the nonresponsive patients, which has been shown to greatly reduce the risk of thrombosis. The common polymorphism of MTHFR (C677T) may cause moderate to severe hyperhomocysteinemia in folate deficient patients (usually from nonfortified countries) not associated with megaloblastic anemia and can be treated with folic acid. Gamma cystathionase deficiency causes extremely high serum cystathionine with mild to moderate hyperhomocysteinemia, is not a cause of megaloblastic anemia, and appears to usually be a benign disorder.[361]

Patients with malabsorption syndromes or chronic renal insufficiency with hyperhomocysteinemia may be treated conveniently with a high-dose combination preparation of cyanoCbl, folic acid, or methylfolate and pyridoxine as long as adequate Cbl dosage is included (at least 1000 μg).

Lowering Homocysteine for Prevention or Treatment of Vascular Disease

Despite the almost universal finding that persons with vascular disease have higher homocysteine than their healthy counterparts,[107] the large trials of B-vitamin therapy have largely been negative for many reasons that are outside the scope of this chapter.[193] There are indications from some trials that prevention of stroke may be a beneficial outcome as was seen in a massive trial from China which added folic acid to a blood pressure medication.[196] Potential benefits are more likely in a folate deficient population.

MANAGEMENT OF THE NONRESPONDING PATIENT

The differential diagnosis of macrocytic pancytopenia anemia includes myelodysplastic syndrome and other heme malignancies but most commonly the macrocytic pancytopenia of chronic liver disease with

hypersplenism. Cardiac-associated mechanical anemias with reticulocytosis and platelet consumption are often confused with megaloblastic anemia also. Needless to say these other entities will not respond to Cbl or folate treatment unless there is an accompanying vitamin deficiency. Mild elevations of MMA (<500 nmol/L) and homocysteine are common in seniors as are the myelodysplastic syndromes and the latter will not improve with Cbl although MMA will decrease. Pancytopenia in chronic liver disease associated with alcohol use disorder may respond only partially to folic acid. Erythropoietin (EPO) deficiency due to chronic kidney disease is very common in the senior population and EPO injections may be needed in addition to vitamin replacement for maximum results. Iron deficiency may become unmasked during the treatment of Cbl deficiency and full response will require iron replacement.

Serum Cbl is frequently measured in patients with nonspecific symptoms of fatigue, difficulty concentrating, transient paresthesias, depression, and other vague complaints without macrocytic anemia. The care of the patient will be greatly enhanced by measuring MMA and/or homocysteine (MMA more sensitive) prior to embarking on a course of Cbl therapy. Parenteral Cbl with its red color has great placebo potential, which eventually wears off. This commonly leads to an increased frequency of injections and disappointment. It will be impossible to determine whether the patient actually had Cbl deficiency, realizing that almost all low Cbl values in younger persons are false positive low if there are no hematologic abnormalities or documented physical exam signs. If there are genuine neurologic signs and no response to Cbl, then an alternative diagnosis such as multiple sclerosis should be pursued. The lay literature and websites abound with recommendations for self-treating with methylCbl or methylfolate for these symptoms. A patient can be weaned off Cbl therapy by testing for MMA every 3 months for about 2 years to see if values rise. MMA values will remain normal but Cbl will likely fall back to the false low value that the patient had initially so should not be measured.

MANAGEMENT OF THE CAUSES OF DEFICIENCY

Pernicious anemia cannot be cured and requires lifelong Cbl treatment. It is associated with other autoimmune illnesses that could possibly require treatment especially autoimmune thyroid disease such as Graves disease. Conversely, women with autoimmune thyroid disease must be informed of the risks of Cbl deficiency in pregnancy and breast feeding. Patients should be informed that the risk of pernicious anemia in their siblings and other family members is increased also.[274] Coexisting or the later development of iron deficiency should be evaluated with gastrointestinal endoscopy. There is a small increased risk of gastric adenocarcinoma and carcinoid tumors in patients with pernicious anemia.[268,270] There may also be celiac disease in patients with combined Cbl and iron deficiency, which requires specific treatment. Folate-deficient megaloblastic anemia is a marker for occult alcohol use disorder or intestinal malabsorption syndromes in folate fortified populations. Referral to the appropriate specialist is indicated on diagnosis.

PREVENTION OF COBALAMIN AND FOLATE DEFICIENCY WORLDWIDE

There is much interest in improving vitamin nutrition in the populations with poor access to animal source foods in the case of Cbl[44,45,357,358,362,363] and fresh fruits and vegetables in the case of folate. A large number of countries have already fortified grain products with folic acid and it is clear that this decreases the risk of neural tube defects up to 50%,[87] depending on the previous folate status of the population.[364] It has been more difficult to discover inexpensive sources for Cbl fortification although bread and rice can be fortified similar to folic acid.[365-367] Many areas in the world rely on local processing of grains and are poorly impacted by such fortification programs. A recent report showed that tea bags can be fortified with folic acid 1 mg and 100 or 500 μg of Cbl, which raised serum folate and Cbl into the normal range in most of the subjects after 2 months consumption of only 1 cup of tea daily.[357] Sources of plant-derived Cbl are also being explored although these often contain more Cbl analogues than true Cbl.[49,50] Another recent report studied *Wolffia globosa* or mankai, a form of duck weed, which is high in essential amino acids, iron, folates, and Cbl. The corrinoid present was proven to be Cbl by LC-MS/MS.[48] Serum Cbl values increased after 18 months of a diet changed to include a shake made of the mankai. There is also interest in developing insects as food. The Cbl content has been studied using ultra performance LC and with MS to confirm the identity of the corrinoids. MS showed that only about 5% of the corrinoids in cricket powders were true Cbl with the remainder being pseudo Cbl.[46] The content was about 3 μg/100 g dry weight.

The content of food Cbl can be overestimated with the commonly employed microbiologic method of quantitation with *Lactobacillus delbrueckii* because this organism can grow on deoxyribosides or deoxynucleotides instead so the assay must correct for an alkaline resistance factor.[47] This organism also grows in the presence of pseudoCbl, thus, will overestimate the Cbl content in edible cyanobacteria and some edible shellfish. Cbl-dependent *Escherichia coli* mutants can also be used in the microbiologic assay, which distinguish between Cbl and pseudocobalamin. Whether ingesting the analogues found in these plant materials is harmful is not known. The reader should determine whether specific methods were used in the older literature.

Edible purple laver porphyra species, known as "nori" is widely eaten in the Far East but now also worldwide, because of the popularity of sushi. It contains Cbl but also pseudoCbl.[49] A number of clinical studies of dietary nori in vegans demonstrate that there likely is absorption of Cbl but also reports that MMA remained elevated, suggesting impaired bioavailability. Tempeh is a vegetarian product made from beans inoculated with fungus spores and incubated for several days. This traditional food has been shown to contain Cbl due to the bacterial fermentation that also occurs.[52] It will be difficult for the consumer to know whether a particular product contains Cbl in adequate amounts to satisfy a daily requirement unless specifically labeled. *Chlorella pyrenoidosa* is a unicellular green algae that contains Cbl. One study showed that a group of vegans taking 9 g of chlorella daily had decreased mean serum MMA levels, decreased serum homocysteine, and increased serum Cbl by 60 days.[50]

CONTROVERSIES AND KNOWLEDGE GAPS IN FOLATE AND COBALAMIN DEFICIENCY

Improved folate status has reached all members of society in food folate–fortified countries, which has raised concern about the subgroups with Cbl deficiency and high folate status. This concern stems from the early days when folates had just been discovered and very high doses of folic acid, 10 to 40 and even 400 mg/day, both orally and by parenteral administration, were given to patients with pernicious anemia resulting in some remissions of anemia. After the early enthusiasm, it was noted that there were suboptimal remissions and relapses and that myeloneuropathy was not responding without additional injections of liver extract. These results[368] have led to the medical dogma of not treating Cbl-deficient patients with only folic acid, and explain why there is a limit to over-the-counter folic acid content in vitamin preparations. It is difficult to extrapolate from these ultrahigh doses to the present.[369-371] A number of reports have suggested or disputed that low Cbl status combined with high folate status or presence of unmetabolized folic acid increased the risk for cognitive impairment in seniors. The recent data are reviewed in Reference 369, which outlines the issues in interpreting the data since the definition of deficiency and cognitive testing varied widely.[369] Those with high MMA and high folate in folate-fortified countries are the individuals with probable Cbl malabsorption and more likely to have true deficiency.

Older studies have shown that elevated homocysteine with Cbl deficiency in some was a risk factor for decreased cognitive function or decline. These studies led to trials of vitamin replacement in different cohorts. A meta-analysis in 2014[372] evaluated 11 trials of homocysteine-lowering on cognitive decline and found that, although vitamin nutrition was improved in these trials, there was no significant effect on the various measures of cognition. Another meta-analysis[373] and a large cohort study concluded the same in 2021.[374] A consensus statement in 2018 suggested that more trials needed to be done since treatment with B-vitamins is safe and inexpensive.[375]

The role of high-dose vitamin therapy for reducing homocysteine in chronic kidney disease also remains controversial with some studies showing potential harm.[314]

Patients with major depressive disorders have often been found to have elevated homocysteine, which can be improved with B-vitamin therapy easily. A recent meta-analysis suggests that adjunct therapy with L-methylfolate or folic acid improved treatment response,[376] although others did not.[373,377] The studies evaluated had variations in treatment periods and doses. In general, the doses were high, especially with L-methylfolate (up to 15 mg/d).

MethylCbl has been recommended widely as a treatment for symptoms of peripheral neuropathy, particularly diabetic neuropathy. A recent meta-analysis suggests that high doses either oral or parenteral as single treatment or with many different combinations of treatments may be effective in diabetic neuropathy.[354] However, pain scores were not improved with the treatment. Another review suggested that there was level II evidence of methylCbl in postherpetic neuralgia and for painful peripheral neuropathy.[378]

The effectiveness of Cbl therapy with or without folates in autism has been reviewed recently.[379] Few studies were double-blind placebo controlled. Gastrointestinal disorders and limited diet choices are frequent in autism spectrum disorder and could result in nutrient deficiency which should be treated.[379]

A diet high in fruits and vegetables, thus high in natural folates, has been promoted as part of a cancer-reducing lifestyle. There has been intense interest in determining whether the high folic acid intake in North America has decreased the incidence of colorectal or other cancers, after folic acid food fortification. Several large studies have shown that high intake of both natural food folates and folic acid supplements show a modest decrease in colorectal cancer.[380,381] A meta-analysis of folate treatment trials showed no effect on cancer incidence.[382] More data and years of follow-up are needed before the effect of high folate status on cancer will be known.[383]

ACKNOWLEDGMENTS

Figures 37.4 and *37.7* were previously published as *Figures 37.1* and *37.6* in the previous edition of this chapter authored by Ralph Carmel in Megaloblastic Anemias: Disorders of Impaired Synthesis.

References

1. Addison T. Anemia disease of the supra-renal capsules. *London Med Gaz.* 1849;43:517-518.
2. Folkers K. History of vitamin B12: pernicious anemia to crystalline cyanocobalamin. In: Dolphin D, ed. *B12*. 1st ed. Wiley-Interscience; 1975:1-15.
3. Castle WB. The history of corrinoids. In: Babior BM, ed. *Cobalamin: Biochemistry and Pathophysiology*. Wiley-Interscience; 1975:1-17.
4. Minot GR, Murphy WP. Treatment of pernicious anemia by a special diet. *JAMA.* 1926;87:470-474.
5. Hodgkin DC, Kamper J, Mackay M, et al. Structure of vitamin B12. *Nature.* 1956;178:64-66.
6. Shorb MS. Unidentified growth factors for Lactobacillus lactis in refined liver extracts. *J Biol Chem.* 1947;169:455.
7. Wills L. Treatment of "Pernicious anaemia of pregnancy" and "Tropical anaemia". *Br Med J.* 1931;1:1059-1064.
8. Jukes TH, Stokstad EL. Pteroylglutamic acid and related compounds. *Physiol Rev.* 1948;28:51-106.
9. Green R, Allen LH, Bjørke-Monsen AL, et al. Vitamin B12 deficiency. *Nat Rev Dis Prim.* 2017;3:17040.
10. Stabler SP. Megaloblastic anemias. In: Goldman LS, Schafer AI, eds. *Goldman-Cecil Medicine*. 26th ed.. Elsevier; 2019:1069-1077.
11. Froese DS, Fowler B, Baumgartner MR. Vitamin B12, folate, and the methionine remethylation cycle-biochemistry, pathways, and regulation. *J Inherit Metab Dis.* 2019;42:673-685.
12. Banerjee R, Gouda H, Pillay S. Redox-linked coordination chemistry directs vitamin B12 trafficking. *Acc Chem Res.* 2021;54:2003-2013.

Disorders of Red Blood Cells

13. Gherasim C, Lofgren M, Banerjee R. Navigating the B(12) road: assimilation, delivery, and disorders of cobalamin. *J Biol Chem.* 2013;288:13186-13193.

14. Kim J, Gherasim C, Banerjee R. Decyanation of vitamin B12 by a trafficking chaperone. *Proc Natl Acad Sci USA.* 2008;105:14551-14554.

15. Allen RH, Stabler SP. Identification and quantitation of cobalamin and cobalamin analogues in human feces. *Am J Clin Nutr.* 2008;87:1324-1335.

16. Kovachy RJ, Copley SD, Allen RH. Recognition, isolation, and characterization of rat liver D-methylmalonyl coenzyme A hydrolase. *J Biol Chem.* 1983;258:11415-11421.

17. Shimomura Y, Murakami T, Nakai N, et al. 3-hydroxyisobutyryl-CoA hydrolase. *Methods Enzymol.* 2000;324:229-240.

18. Stabler SP, Marcell PD, Podell ER, Allen RH, Lindenbaum J. Assay of methylmalonic acid in the serum of patients with cobalamin deficiency using capillary gas chromatography-mass spectrometry. *J Clin Invest.* 1986;77:1606-1612.

19. Sobczyńska-Malefora A, Delvin E, McCaddon A, Ahmadi KR, Harrington DJ. Vitamin B12 status in health and disease: a critical review. Diagnosis of deficiency and insufficiency—clinical and laboratory pitfalls. *Crit Rev Clin Lab Sci.* 2021;58:399-429.

20. Hannibal L, Lysne V, Bjørke-Monsen AL, et al. Biomarkers and algorithms for the diagnosis of vitamin B12 deficiency. *Front Mol Biosci.* 2016;3:27.

21. Allen RH, Stabler SP, Savage DG, Lindenbaum J. Elevation of 2-methylcitric acid I and II levels in serum, urine, and cerebrospinal fluid of patients with cobalamin deficiency. *Metabolism.* 1993;42:978-988.

22. Allen RH, Stabler SP, Savage DG, Lindenbaum J. Metabolic abnormalities in cobalamin (vitamin B12) and folate deficiency. *FASEB J.* 1993;7:1344-1353.

23. Haijes HA, Jans JJM, Tas SY, Verhoeven-Duif NM, van Hasselt PM. Pathophysiology of propionic and methylmalonic acidemias. Part 1: complications. *J Inherit Metab Dis.* 2019;42:730-744.

24. Luciani A, Denley MCS, Govers LP, Sorrentino V, Froese DS. Mitochondrial disease, mitophagy, and cellular distress in methylmalonic acidemia. *Cell Mol Life Sci.* 2021;78(21-22):6851-6867.

25. Stabler SP, Brass EP, Marcell PD, Allen RH. Inhibition of cobalamin-dependent enzymes by cobalamin analogues in rats. *J Clin Invest.* 1991;87:1422-1430.

26. Kolhouse JF, Stabler SP, Allen RH. Identification and perturbation of mutant human fibroblasts based on measurements of methylmalonic acid and total homocysteine in the culture media. *Arch Biochem Biophys.* 1993;303:355-360.

27. Cox EY, White AM. Methylmalonic acid excretion: an index of vitamin-B12 deficiency. *Lancet.* 1962;2:853-856.

28. Norman EJ, Martelo OJ, Denton MD. Cobalamin (vitamin B12) deficiency detection by urinary methylmalonic acid quantitation. *Blood.* 1982;59:1128-1131.

29. Brass EP, Tahiliani AG, Allen RH, Stabler SP. Coenzyme A metabolism in vitamin B-12-deficient rats. *J Nutr.* 1990;120:290-297.

30. Brass EP, Allen RH, Ruff LJ, Stabler SP. Effect of hydroxycobalamin[c-lactam] on propionate and carnitine metabolism in the rat. *Biochem J.* 1990;266:809-815.

31. Garton GA, Scaife JR, Smith A, Siddons RC. Effect of vitamin B12 status on the occurrence of branched-chain and odd-numbered fatty acids in the liver lipids of the baboon. *Lipids.* 1975;10:855-857.

32. Ramsey RB, Scott T, Banik NL. Fatty acid composition of myelin isolated from the brain of a patient with cellular deficiency of co-enzyme forms of vitamin B12. *J Neurol Sci.* 1977;34:221-232.

33. Frenkel EP. Abnormal fatty acid metabolism in peripheral nerves of patients with pernicious anemia. *J Clin Invest.* 1973;52:1237-1245.

34. Koutmos M, Datta S, Pattridge KA, Smith JL, Matthews RG. Insights into the reactivation of cobalamin-dependent methionine synthase. *Proc Natl Acad Sci USA.* 2009;106:18527-18532.

35. Shane B, Stokstad EL. Vitamin B12-folate interrelationships. *Annu Rev Nutr.* 1985;5:115-141.

36. Smulders YM, Smith DE, Kok RM, et al. Cellular folate vitamer distribution during and after correction of vitamin B12 deficiency: a case for the methylfolate trap. *Br J Haematol.* 2006;132:623-629.

37. Luka Z, Mudd SH, Wagner C. Glycine N-methyltransferase and regulation of S-adenosylmethionine levels. *J Biol Chem.* 2009;284:22507-22511.

38. Allen RH, Stabler SP, Lindenbaum J. Serum betaine, N,N-dimethylglycine and N-methylglycine levels in patients with cobalamin and folate deficiency and related inborn errors of metabolism. *Metabolism.* 1993;42:1448-1460.

39. Stover PJ, Field MS. Trafficking of intracellular folates. *Adv Nutr.* 2011;2:325-331.

40. Misselbeck K, Marchetti L, Priami C, Stover PJ, Field MS. The 5-formyltetrahydrofolate futile cycle reduces pathway stochasticity in an extended hybrid-stochastic model of folate-mediated one-carbon metabolism. *Sci Rep.* 2019;9:4322.

41. Mudd SH, Brosnan JT, Brosnan ME, et al. Methyl balance and transmethylation fluxes in humans. *Am J Clin Nutr.* 2007;85:19-25.

42. Watkins D, Rosenblatt DS. Inherited disorders of folate and cobalamin transport and metabolism. In: Valle D, Beaudet AL, Vogelstein B, et al, eds. *The Online and Molecular Basis of Inherited Disease.* McGraw-Hill Medical; 2017.

43. Clarke S, Banfield K. S-adenosylmethionine dependent methyltransferases. In: Carmel R, Jacobsen DW, eds. *Homocysteine in Health and Disease.* Cambridge University Press; 2001:63-78.

44. Stabler SP, Allen RH. Vitamin B12 deficiency as a worldwide problem. *Annu Rev Nutr.* 2004;24:299-326.

45. Obeid R, Heil SG, Verhoeven MMA, et al. Vitamin B12 intake from animal foods, biomarkers, and health aspects. *Front Nutr.* 2019;6:93.

46. Okamoto N, Nagao F, Umebayashi Y, et al. Pseudovitamin B12 and factor S are the predominant corrinoid compounds in edible cricket products. *Food Chem.* 2021;347:129048.

47. Watanabe F, Bito T. Determination of cobalamin and related compounds in foods. *J AOAC Int.* 2018;101:1308-1313.

48. Sela I, Yaskolka Meir A, Brandis A, et al. *Wolffia globosa-Mankai* plant-based protein contains bioactive vitamin B12 and is well absorbed in humans. *Nutrients.* 2020;12:3067.

49. Bito T, Teng F, Watanabe F. Bioactive compounds of edible purple laver porphyra sp. (Nori). *J Agric Food Chem.* 2017;65:10685-10692.

50. Merchant RE, Phillips TW, Udani J. Nutritional supplementation with chlorella pyrenoidosa lowers serum methylmalonic acid in vegans and vegetarians with a suspected vitamin B12 deficiency. *J Med Food.* 2015;18:1357-1362.

51. Bisping B, Hering L, Baumann U, et al. Tempe fermentation: some aspects of formation of gamma-linolenic acid, proteases and vitamins. *Biotechnol Adv.* 1993;11:481-493.

52. Mo H, Kariluoto S, Piironen V, et al. Effect of soybean processing on content and bioaccessibility of folate, vitamin B12 and isoflavones in tofu and tempe. *Food Chem.* 2013;141:2418-2425.

53. Gibson RS, Abebe Y, Stabler S, et al. Zinc, gravida, infection, and iron, but not vitamin B12 or folate status, predict hemoglobin during pregnancy in Southern Ethiopia. *J Nutr.* 2008;138:581-586.

54. Devi S, Pasanna RM, Shamshuddin Z, et al. Measuring vitamin B12 bioavailability with [13C]-cyanocobalamin in humans. *Am J Clin Nutr.* 2020;112:1504-1515.

55. Institute of Medicine (US) Standing Committee on the Scientific Evaluation of Dietary Reference Intakes and its Panel on Folate, Other B-Vitamins, and Choline. *Dietary Reference Intakes for Thiamin, Riboflavin, Niacin, Vitamin B6, Folate, Vitamin B12, Pantothenic Acid, Biotin, and Choline.* National Academies Press (US); 1998:306-356.

56. Adams JF, Tankel HI, MacEwan F. Estimation of the total body vitamin B12 in the live subject. *Clin Sci.* 1970;39:107-113.

57. Doscherholmen A, Hagen PS. A dual mechanism of vitamin B12 plasma absorption. *J Clin Invest.* 1957;36:1551-1557.

58. Gaffney GW, Watkin DM, Chow BF. Vitamin B12 absorption: relationship between oral administration and urinary excretion of cobalt 60-labeled cyanocobalamin following a parenteral dose; study of doses of 2 to 250 mu g in 148 apparently health men 20 to 92 years old. *J Lab Clin Med.* 1959;53:525-534.

59. Kuzminski AM, Del Giacco EJ, Allen RH, Stabler SP, Lindenbaum J. Effective treatment of cobalamin deficiency with oral cobalamin. *Blood.* 1998;92:1191-1198.

60. Nielsen MJ, Rasmussen MR, Andersen CB, Nexø E, Moestrup SK. Vitamin B12 transport from food to the body's cells: a sophisticated, multistep pathway. *Nat Rev Gastroenterol Hepatol.* 2012;9:345-354.

61. Blakeley M, Sobczyńska-Malefora A, Carpenter G. The origins of salivary vitamin A, vitamin B12 and vitamin D-binding proteins. *Nutrients.* 2020;12:3838.

62. Alpers DH, Russell-Jones G. Gastric intrinsic factor: the gastric and small intestinal stages of cobalamin absorption. a personal journey. *Biochimie.* 2013;95:989-994.

63. Kolhouse JF, Allen RH. Absorption, plasma transport, and cellular retention of cobalamin analogues in the rabbit. Evidence for the existence of multiple mechanisms that prevent the absorption and tissue dissemination of naturally occurring cobalamin analogues. *J Clin Invest.* 1977;60:1381-1392.

64. Kozyraki R, Cases O. Vitamin B12 absorption: mammalian physiology and acquired and inherited disorders. *Biochimie.* 2013;95:1002-1007.

65. He Q, Madsen M, Kilkenney A, et al. Amnionless function is required for cubilin brush-border expression and intrinsic factor-cobalamin (vitamin B12) absorption in vivo. *Blood.* 2005;106:1447-1453.

66. Tanner SM, Li Z, Perko JD, et al. Hereditary juvenile cobalamin deficiency caused by mutations in the intrinsic factor gene. *Proc Natl Acad Sci USA.* 2005;102:4130-4133.

67. Trakadis YJ, Alfares A, Bodamer OA, et al. Update on transcobalamin deficiency: clinical presentation, treatment and outcome. *J Inherit Metab Dis.* 2014;37:461-473.

68. Morkbak AL, Poulsen SS, Nexo E. Haptocorrin in humans. *Clin Chem Lab Med.* 2007;45:1751-1759.

69. Carmel R, Parker J, Kelman Z. Genomic mutations associated with mild and severe deficiencies of transcobalamin I (haptocorrin) that cause mildly and severely low serum cobalamin levels. *Br J Haematol.* 2009;147:386-391.

70. Doets EL, In 't Veld PH, Szczecińska A, et al. Systematic review on daily vitamin B12 losses and bioavailability for deriving recommendations on vitamin B12 intake with the factorial approach. *Ann Nutr Metab.* 2013;62:311-322.

71. Gick GG, Arora K, Sequeira JM, et al. Cellular uptake of vitamin B12: role and fate of TCblR/CD320, the transcobalamin receptor. *Exp Cell Res.* 2020;396:112256.

72. Boachie J, Adaikalakoteswari A, Goljan I, et al. Intracellular and tissue levels of vitamin B12 in hepatocytes are modulated by CD320 receptor and TCN2 transporter. *Int J Mol Sci.* 2021;22:3089.

73. Rutsch F, Gailus S, Suormala T, Fowler B. LMBRD1: the gene for the cblF defect of vitamin B12 metabolism. *J Inherit Metab Dis.* 2011;34:121-126.

74. Kitai K, Kawaguchi K, Tomohiro T, et al. The lysosomal protein ABCD4 can transport vitamin B12 across liposomal membranes in vitro. *J Biol Chem.* 2021;296:100654.

75. Lerner-Ellis JP, Tirone JC, Pawelek PD, et al. Identification of the gene responsible for methylmalonic aciduria and homocystinuria, cblC type. *Nat Genet.* 2006;38:93-100.

76. Coelho D, Suormala T, Stucki M, et al. Gene identification for the cblD defect of vitamin B12 metabolism. *N Engl J Med.* 2008;358:1454-1464.

77. Lerner-Ellis JP, Gradinger AB, Watkins D, et al. Mutation and biochemical analysis of patients belonging to the cblB complementation class of vitamin B12-dependent methylmalonic aciduria. *Mol Genet Metab.* 2006;87:219-225.

78. Dobson CM, Wai T, Leclerc D, et al. Identification of the gene responsible for the cblA complementation group of vitamin B12-responsive methylmalonic acidemia based on analysis of prokaryotic gene arrangements. *Proc Natl Acad Sci USA.* 2002;99:15554-15559.

79. Gramer G, Hoffmann GF. Vitamin B12 deficiency in newborns and their mothers-novel approaches to early detection, treatment and prevention of a global health issue. *Curr Med Sci.* 2020;40:801-809.

80. Dubascoux S, Richoz Payot J, Sylvain P, Nicolas M, Campos Gimenez E. Vitamin B12 quantification in human milk: beyond current limitations using liquid chromatography and inductively coupled plasma—mass spectrometry. *Food Chem.* 2021;362:130197.

81. Greibe E, Mahalle N, Bhide V, et al. Effect of 8-week oral supplementation with 3-μg cyano-B12 or hydroxo-B12 in a vitamin B12-deficient population. *Eur J Nutr.* 2019;58:261-270.

82. Stabler SP. Clinical folate deficiency. In: Bailey L, ed. *Folate in Health and Disease.* 2nd ed. Taylor and Francis Group, LLC; 2009:409-428.

83. Bailey LB, Stover PJ, McNulty H, et al. Biomarkers of nutrition for development-folate review. *J Nutr.* 2015;145:1636S-1680S.

84. Pfeiffer CM, Hughes JP, Lacher DA, et al. Estimation of trends in serum and RBC folate in the U.S. population from pre- to postfortification using assay-adjusted data from the NHANES 1988-2010. *J Nutr.* 2012;142:886-893.

85. Bailey RL, McDowell MA, Dodd K, et al. Total folate and folic acid intakes from foods and dietary supplements of US children aged 1-13 y. *Am J Clin Nutr.* 2010;92:353-358.

86. Haggarty P. UK introduces folic acid fortification of flour to prevent neural tube defects. *Lancet.* 2021;398(10307):1199-1201.

87. Martinez H, Pachón H, Kancherla V, Oakley GP. Food fortification with folic acid for prevention of spina bifida and anencephaly: the need for a paradigm shift in evidence evaluation for policy-making. *Am J Epidemiol.* 2021;190:1972-1976.

88. Pfeiffer CM, Sternberg MR, Zhang M, et al. Folate status in the US population 20 y after the introduction of folic acid fortification. *Am J Clin Nutr.* 2019;110:1088-1097.

89. Hildebrand LA, Dumas B, Milrod CJ, Hudspeth JC. Folate deficiency in an urban safety net population. *Am J Med.* 2021;134(10):1265-1269. S0002-9343/00322-00323.

90. Galivan J, Ryan TJ, Chave K, et al. Glutamyl hydrolase. pharmacological role and enzymatic characterization. *Pharmacol Ther.* 2000;85:207-215.

91. Visentin M, Diop-Bove N, Zhao R, Goldman ID. The intestinal absorption of folates. *Annu Rev Physiol.* 2014;76:251-274.

92. Ohrvik VE, Witthoft CM. Human folate bioavailability. *Nutrients.* 2011;3:475-490.

93. Watkins D, Rosenblatt DS. Update and new concepts in vitamin responsive disorders of folate transport and metabolism. *J Inherit Metab Dis.* 2012;35:665-670.

94. Lakoff A, Fazili Z, Aufreiter S, et al. Folate is absorbed across the human colon: evidence by using enteric-coated caplets containing 13C-labeled [6S]-5-formyltetrahydrofolate. *Am J Clin Nutr.* 2014;100:1278-1286.

95. Bailey LB, Gregory JF, III. Folate. In: Bowman BA, Russell RM, eds. *Present Knowledge in Nutrition.* 9th ed. International Life Science Institute; 2006:278.

96. Lin Y, Dueker SR, Follett JR, et al. Quantitation of in vivo human folate metabolism. *Am J Clin Nutr.* 2004;80:680-691.

97. Hou Z, Matherly LH. Biology of the major facilitative folate transporters SLC19A1 and SLC46A1. *Curr Top Membr.* 2014;73:175-204.

98. Koury MJ, Price JO, Hicks GG. Apoptosis in megaloblastic anemia occurs during DNA synthesis by a p53-independent, nucleoside-reversible mechanism. *Blood.* 2000;96:3249-3255.

99. Koury MJ. Abnormal erythropoiesis and the pathophysiology of chronic anemia. *Blood Rev.* 2014;28:49-66.

100. Stabler SP. Clinical practice. Vitamin B12 deficiency. *N Engl J Med.* 2013;368:149-160.

101. Socha DS, DeSouza SI, Flagg A, Sekeres M, Rogers HJ. Severe megaloblastic anemia: vitamin deficiency and other causes. *Cleve Clin J Med.* 2020;87:153-164.

102. Healton EB, Savage DG, Brust JC, Garrett TJ, Lindenbaum J. Neurologic aspects of cobalamin deficiency. *Medicine (Baltimore).* 1991;70:229-245.

103. Stabler SP, Marcell PD, Podell ER, et al. Elevation of total homocysteine in the serum of patients with cobalamin or folate deficiency detected by capillary gas chromatography-mass spectrometry. *J Clin Invest.* 1988;81:466-474.

104. Savage DG, Lindenbaum J, Stabler SP, Allen RH. Sensitivity of serum methylmalonic acid and total homocysteine determinations for diagnosing cobalamin and folate deficiencies. *Am J Med.* 1994;96:239-246.

105. Stabler SP, Korson M, Jethva R, et al. Metabolic profiling of total homocysteine and related compounds in hyperhomocysteinemia: utility and limitations in diagnosing the cause of puzzling thrombophilia in a family. *JIMD Rep.* 2013;11:149-163.

106. Levy J, Rodriguez-Guéant RM, Oussalah A, et al. Cardiovascular manifestations of intermediate and major hyperhomocysteinemia due to vitamin B12 and folate deficiency and/or inherited disorders of one-carbon metabolism: a 3.5-year cross-sectional study of consecutive patients. *Am J Clin Nutr.* 2021;113:1157-1167.

107. Smith AD, Refsum H. Homocysteine—from disease biomarker to disease prevention. *J Intern Med.* 2021;290:826-854.

108. Chakraborty J, Stover PJ. Deoxyuracil in DNA in health and disease. *Curr Opin Clin Nutr Metab Care.* 2020;23:247-252.

109. Palmer AM, Kamynina E, Field MS, Stover PJ. Folate rescues vitamin B12 depletion-induced inhibition of nuclear thymidylate biosynthesis and genome instability. *Proc Natl Acad Sci USA.* 2017;114:E4095-E4102.

110. Koury MJ, Horne DW. Apoptosis mediates and thymidine prevents erythroblast destruction in folate deficiency anemia. *Proc Natl Acad Sci USA.* 1994;91:4067-4071.

111. Koury MJ, Horne DW, Brown ZA, et al. Apoptosis of late-stage erythroblasts in megaloblastic anemia: association with DNA damage and macrocyte production. *Blood.* 1997;89:4617-4623.

112. Schulz E, Arruda VR, Costa FF, Saad ST. Cytoplasmic overexpression of p53 and p21(ras) in megaloblastic anemia. *Haematologica.* 2000;85:874-875.

113. Yadav MK, Manoli NM, Madhunapantula SV. Comparative assessment of vitamin-B12, folic acid and homocysteine levels in relation to p53 expression in megaloblastic anemia. *PLoS One.* 2016;11:e0164559.

114. Yadav MK, Manoli NM, Vimalraj S, Madhunapantula SV. Unmethylated promoter DNA correlates with p53 expression and apoptotic levels only in vitamin B9 and B12 deficient megaloblastic anemia but not in non-megaloblastic anemia controls. *Int J Biol Macromol.* 2018;109:76-84.

115. Kwan DN, Rocha JTQ, Niero-Melo L, Domingues MAC, Oliveira CC. p53 and p21 expression in bone marrow clots of megaloblastic anemia patients. *Int J Clin Exp Pathol.* 2020;13:1829-1833.

116. Richard E, Jorge-Finnigan A, Garcia-Villoria J, et al. Genetic and cellular studies of oxidative stress in methylmalonic aciduria (MMA) cobalamin deficiency type C (cblC) with homocystinuria (MMACHC). *Hum Mutat.* 2009;30:1558-1566.

117. Sankaran VG, Ludwig LS, Sicinska E, et al. Cyclin D3 coordinates the cell cycle during differentiation to regulate erythrocyte size and number. *Genes Dev.* 2012;26:2075-2087.

118. Savage DG, Ogundipe A, Allen RH, Stabler SP, Lindenbaum J. Etiology and diagnostic evaluation of macrocytosis. *Am J Med Sci.* 2000;319:343-352.

119. Williams DM. Racial differences of hemoglobin concentration: measurements of iron, copper, and zinc. *Am J Clin Nutr.* 1981;34:1694-1700.

120. Beutler E, West C. Hematologic differences between African-Americans and whites: the roles of iron deficiency and alpha-thalassemia on hemoglobin levels and mean corpuscular volume. *Blood.* 2005;106:740-745.

121. Sekhar J, Stabler SP. Life-threatening megaloblastic pancytopenia with normal mean cell volume: case series. *Eur J Intern Med.* 2007;18:548-550.

122. Takahashi N, Kameoka J, Takahashi N, et al. Causes of macrocytic anemia among 628 patients: mean corpuscular volumes of 114 and 130 fL as critical markers for categorization. *Int J Hematol.* 2016;104:344-357.

123. Koshy AG, Freed JA. Clinical features of vitamin B12 deficiency mimicking thrombotic microangiopathy. *Br J Haematol.* 2020;191:938-941.

124. Andrès E, Affenberger S, Zimmer J, et al. Current hematological findings in cobalamin deficiency. A study of 201 consecutive patients with documented cobalamin deficiency. *Clin Lab Haematol.* 2006;28:50-56.

125. Tran PN, Tran MH. Cobalamin deficiency presenting with thrombotic microangiopathy (TMA) features: a systematic review. *Transfus Apher Sci.* 2018;57:102-106.

126. Gurung K, Bain BJ. A normal mean cell volume does not exclude a diagnosis of megaloblastic anemia. *Am J Hematol.* 2021;96(12):1706-1707.

127. Oo TH. Diagnostic difficulties in pernicious anemia. *Discov Med.* 2019;28:247-253.

128. Lindenbaum J, Nath BJ. Megaloblastic anaemia and neutrophil hypersegmentation. *Br J Haematol.* 1980;44:511-513.

129. Nath BJ, Lindenbaum J. Persistence of neutrophil hypersegmentation during recovery from megaloblastic granulopoiesis. *Ann Intern Med.* 1979;90:757-760.

130. Htut TW, Thein KZ, Oo TH. Pernicious anemia: pathophysiology and diagnostic difficulties. *J Evid Based Med.* 2021;14:161-169.

131. Kim M, Lee SE, Park J, et al. Vitamin B(12)-responsive pancytopenia mimicking myelodysplastic syndrome. *Acta Haematol.* 2011;125:198-201.

132. Belen B, Hismi BO, Kocak U. Severe vitamin B12 deficiency with pancytopenia, hepatosplenomegaly and leukoerythroblastosis in two Syrian refugee infants: a challenge to differentiate from acute leukaemia. *BMJ Case Rep.* 2014;2014:bcr2014203742.

133. Parmentier S, Meinel J, Oelschlaegel U, et al. Severe pernicious anemia with distinct cytogenetic and flow cytometric aberrations mimicking myelodysplastic syndrome. *Ann Hematol.* 2012;91:1979-1981.

134. Konda M, Godbole A, Pandey S, Sasapu A. Vitamin B12 deficiency mimicking acute leukemia. *Proc (Bayl Univ Med Cent).* 2019;32:589-592.

135. Singh N, Qayyum S, Wasik MA, Luger SM. Combined B12 and folate deficiency presenting as an aggressive hematologic malignancy. *Am J Hematol.* 2015;90:964-965.

136. Steensma DP. Dysplasia has A differential diagnosis: distinguishing genuine myelodysplastic syndromes (MDS) from mimics, imitators, copycats and impostors. *Curr Hematol Malig Rep.* 2012;7:310-320.

137. Chintagumpala MM, Dreyer ZA, Steuber CP, Cooley LD. Pancytopenia with chromosomal fragility: vitamin B12 deficiency. *J Pediatr Hematol Oncol.* 1996;18:166-170.

138. Sutton L, Mba N. Hematogones detected by flow cytometry in a child with vitamin B12 deficiency. *Pediatr Dev Pathol.* 2017;20:172-175.

139. Narang NC, Kotru M, Rao K, Sikka SM. Megaloblastic anemia with ring sideroblasts is not always myelodysplastic syndrome. Halka sideroblastlı megaloblastik anemi her zaman Miyelodisplastik Sendrom Olmayabilir. *Turk J Haematol.* 2016;33:358-359.

140. Savage D, Lindenbaum J. Anemia in alcoholics. *Medicine (Baltimore).* 1986;65:322-338.

141. Wickramasinghe SN. Diagnosis of megaloblastic anaemias. *Blood Rev.* 2006;20:299-318.

142. Briani C, Dalla Torre C, Citton V, et al. Cobalamin deficiency: clinical picture and radiological findings. *Nutrients.* 2013;5:4521-4539.

143. Lindenbaum J, Healton EB, Savage DG, et al. Neuropsychiatric disorders caused by cobalamin deficiency in the absence of anemia or macrocytosis. *N Engl J Med.* 1988;318:1720-1728.

144. Van Berkel B, Vandevenne J, Vangheluwe R, Van Cauter S. Subacute combined degeneration of the cervical and dorsal spinal cord in a 40-year-old male patient: a case report. *Radiol Case Rep.* 2020;16:13-17.

145. Lee WJ, Poon YC, Chuah JH, So SC. Subacute combined degeneration of the spinal cord. *Am J Med.* 2020;133:1421-1423.

146. Bi Z, Cao J, Shang K, et al. Correlation between anemia and clinical severity in subacute combined degeneration patients. *J Clin Neurosci.* 2020;80:11-15.

Disorders of Red Blood Cells

147. Feldman S, Aljarallah S, Saidha S. Primary progressive multiple sclerosis to be treated with ocrelizumab: a mistaken case of cobalamin deficiency. *BMJ Case Rep.* 2019;12:e229080.

148. Rabhi S, Maaroufi M, Khibri H, et al. Magnetic resonance imaging findings within the posterior and lateral columns of the spinal cord extended from the medulla oblongata to the thoracic spine in a woman with subacute combined degeneration without hematologic disorders: a case report and review of the literature. *J Med Case Rep.* 2011;5:166.

149. Misra UK, Kalita J, Das A. Vitamin B12 deficiency neurological syndromes: a clinical, MRI and electrodiagnostic study. *Electromyogr Clin Neurophysiol.* 2003;43:57-64.

150. Gökçe Çokal B, Güneş HN, Güler SK, Yoldaş TK. Visual and somotosensory evoked potentials in asymptomatic patients with vitamin B12 deficiency. *Eur Rev Med Pharmacol Sci.* 2016;20:4525-4529.

151. Ata F, Bint I Bilal A, Javed S, et al. Optic neuropathy as a presenting feature of vitamin B12 deficiency: a systematic review of literature and a case report. *Ann Med Surg (Lond).* 2020;60:316-322.

152. Kalita J, Chandra S, Bhoi SK, et al. Clinical, nerve conduction and nerve biopsy study in vitamin B12 deficiency neurological syndrome with a short-term follow-up. *Nutr Neurosci.* 2014;17:156-163.

153. Agamanolis DP, Victor M, Harris JW, et al. An ultrastructural study of subacute combined degeneration of the spinal cord in vitamin B12-deficient rhesus monkeys. *J Neuropathol Exp Neurol.* 1978;37:273-299.

154. Arora K, Sequeira JM, Alarcon JM, et al. Neuropathology of vitamin B$_{12}$ deficiency in the Cd320$^{-/-}$ mouse. *FASEB J.* 2019;33:2563-2573.

155. Horstmann M, Neumaier-Probst E, Lukacs Z, et al. Infantile cobalamin deficiency with cerebral lactate accumulation and sustained choline depletion. *Neuropediatrics.* 2003;34:261-264.

156. Scott JM, Dinn JJ, Wilson P, Weir DG. Pathogenesis of subacute combined degeneration: a result of methyl group deficiency. *Lancet.* 1981;2:334-337.

157. Scalabrino G. The multi-faceted basis of vitamin B12 (cobalamin) neurotrophism in adult central nervous system: lessons learned from its deficiency. *Prog Neurobiol.* 2009;88:203-220.

158. Peracchi M, Bamonti Catena F, Pomati M, De Franceschi M, Scalabrino G. Human cobalamin deficiency: alterations in serum tumour necrosis factor-alpha and epidermal growth factor. *Eur J Haematol.* 2001;67:123-127.

159. Scalabrino G, Carpo M, Bamonti F, et al. High tumor necrosis factor-alpha [corrected] levels in cerebrospinal fluid of cobalamin-deficient patients. [published correction appears in Ann Neurol 2005;57:304]. *Ann Neurol.* 2004;56:886-890.

160. Zhang A, Ackley BD, Yan D. Vitamin B12 regulates glial migration and synapse formation through isoform-specific control of PTP-3/LAR PRTP expression. *Cell Rep.* 2020;30:3981-3988.e3.

161. Rzepka Z, Rok J, Kowalska J, et al. Astrogliosis in an Experimental model of hypovitaminosis B12: a cellular basis of neurological disorders due to cobalamin deficiency. *Cells.* 2020;9:2261.

162. Ghemrawi R, Pooya S, Lorentz S, et al. Decreased vitamin B12 availability induces ER stress through impaired SIRT1-deacetylation of HSF1. *Cell Death Dis.* 2013;4:e553.

163. Dreumont N, Mimoun K, Pourié C, et al. Glucocorticoid receptor activation restores learning memory by modulating hippocampal plasticity in a mouse model of brain vitamin B12 deficiency. *Mol Neurobiol.* 2021;58:1024-1035.

164. Dror DK, Allen LH. Vitamin B12 in human milk: a systematic review. *Adv Nutr.* 2018;9(suppl 1):358S-366S.

165. Dror DK, Allen LH. Effect of vitamin B12 deficiency on neurodevelopment in infants: current knowledge and possible mechanisms. *Nutr Rev.* 2008;66:250-255.

166. Hasbaoui BE, Mebrouk N, Saghir S, et al. Vitamin B12 deficiency: case report and review of literature. *Pan Afr Med J.* 2021;38:237.

167. Yaramis A. A variety of abnormal movements in 13 cases with nutritional cobalamin deficiency in infants. *Med Hypotheses.* 2020;142:109796.

168. Keskin M. Hematological findings associated with neurodevelopmental delay in infants with vitamin B12 deficiency. *Acta Neurol Belg.* 2020;120:921-926.

169. Okamura J, Miyake Y, Kamei M, Ito Y, Matsubayashi T. Three infants with megaloblastic anemia caused by maternal vitamin B12 deficiency. *Pediatr Int.* 2020;62:864-865.

170. Acıpayam C, Güneş H, Güngör O, et al. Cerebral atrophy in 21 hypotonic infants with severe vitamin B12 deficiency. *J Paediatr Child Health.* 2020;56:751-756.

171. Mütze U, Walter M, Keller M, et al. Health outcomes of infants with vitamin B12 deficiency identified by newborn screening and early treated. *J Pediatr.* 2021;235:42-48.

172. Pajares S, Arranz JA, Ormazabal A, et al. Implementation of second-tier tests in newborn screening for the detection of vitamin B12 related acquired and genetic disorders: results on 258,637 newborns. *Orphanet J Rare Dis.* 2021;16:195.

173. Mizumoto J. Hunter's glossitis. *Intern Med.* 2021;60:1139.

174. Jin YT, Wu YH, Wu YC, et al. Anemia, hematinic deficiencies, hyperhomocysteinemia, and gastric parietal cell antibody positivity in burning mouth syndrome patients with macrocytosis. *J Dent Sci.* 2021;16:1133-1139.

175. Padhi S, Sarangi R, Ramdas A, et al. Cutaneous hyperpigmentation in megaloblastic anemia: a five-year retrospective review. *Mediterr J Hematol Infect Dis.* 2016;8:e2016021.

176. Douglas Wilson R, Van Mieghem T, Langlois S, Church P. Guideline No. 410: prevention, screening, diagnosis, and pregnancy management for fetal neural tube defects. *J Obstet Gynaecol Can.* 2021;43:124-139.e8.

177. Munger RG, Kuppuswamy R, Murthy J, et al. Maternal vitamin B12 status and risk of cleft lip and cleft palate birth defects in Tamil Nadu state, India. *Cleft Palate Craniofac J.* 2021;58:567-576.

178. Finkelstein JL, Fothergill A, Johnson CB, et al. Anemia and vitamin B12 and folate status in women of reproductive age in southern India: estimating population-based risk of neural tube defects. *Curr Dev Nutr.* 2021;5:nzab069.

179. Morris JK, Addor MC, Ballardini E, et al. Prevention of neural tube defects in Europe: a public health failure. *Front Pediatr.* 2021;9:647038.

180. Liu CT, Karasik D, Xu H, et al. Genetic variants modify the associations of concentrations of methylmalonic acid, vitamin B-12, vitamin B-6, and folate with bone mineral density. *Am J Clin Nutr.* 2021;114:578-587.

181. Oliai Araghi S, Kiefte-de Jong JC, van Dijk SC, et al. Long-term effects of folic acid and vitamin-B12 supplementation on fracture risk and cardiovascular disease: extended follow-up of the B-PROOF trial. *Clin Nutr.* 2021;40:1199-1206.

182. Prajapati K, Sailor V, Patel S, Rathod M. Pernicious anaemia: cause of recurrent cerebral venous thrombosis. *BMJ Case Rep.* 2021;14:e239833.

183. Kalita J, Singh VK, Misra UK. A study of hyperhomocysteinemia in cerebral venous sinus thrombosis. *Indian J Med Res.* 2020;152:584-594.

184. Barrios M, Alliot C. Venous thrombosis associated with pernicious anaemia. A report of two cases and review. *Hematology.* 2006;11:135-138.

185. Raymundo-Martínez GI, Gopar-Nieto R, Carazo-Vargas G, et al. Pulmonary embolism and megaloblastic anemia: is there a link? A case report an literature review. *Radiol Case Rep.* 2018;13:1212-1215.

186. Pang X, Hao Y, Ma L, et al. Subacute combined degeneration of the spinal cord concurrent with acute pulmonary embolism: a case report. *J Int Med Res.* 2021;49:3000605211016815.

187. McCully KS. Vascular pathology of homocysteinemia: implications for the pathogenesis of arteriosclerosis. *Am J Pathol.* 1969;56(1):111-128.

188. Friedman AN, Bostom AG, Selhub J, Levey AS, Rosenberg IH. The kidney and homocysteine metabolism. *J Am Soc Nephrol.* 2001;12:2181-2189.

189. Nygård O, Nordrehaug JE, Refsum H, et al. Plasma homocysteine levels and mortality in patients with coronary artery disease. *N Engl J Med.* 1997;337:230-236.

190. Fan R, Zhang A, Zhong F. Association between homocysteine levels and all-cause mortality: a dose-response meta-analysis of prospective studies. *Sci Rep.* 2017;7:4769.

191. Pusceddu I, Herrmann W, Kleber ME, et al. Subclinical inflammation, telomere shortening, homocysteine, vitamin B6, and mortality: the Ludwigshafen Risk and Cardiovascular Health Study. *Eur J Nutr.* 2020;59:1399-1411.

192. Sacco RL, Anand K, Lee HS, et al. Homocysteine and the risk of ischemic stroke in a triethnic cohort: the NOrthern MAnhattan Study. *Stroke.* 2004;35:2263-2269.

193. Clarke R, Halsey J, Bennett D, Lewington S. Homocysteine and vascular disease: review of published results of the homocysteine-lowering trials. *J Inherit Metab Dis.* 2011;34:83-91.

194. Martí-Carvajal AJ, Solà I, Lathyris D, Dayer M. Homocysteine-lowering interventions for preventing cardiovascular events. *Cochrane Database Syst Rev.* 2017;8:CD006612.

195. Saposnik G, Ray JG, Sheridan P, et al. Homocysteine-lowering therapy and stroke risk, severity, and disability: additional findings from the HOPE 2 trial. *Stroke.* 2009;40:1365-1372.

196. Huo Y, Li J, Qin X, et al. Efficacy of folic acid therapy in primary prevention of stroke among adults with hypertension in China: the CSPPT randomized clinical trial. *JAMA.* 2015;313:1325-1335.

197. Kotwal J, Kotwal A, Bhalla S, Singh PK, Nair V. Effectiveness of homocysteine lowering vitamins in prevention of thrombotic tendency at high altitude area: a randomized field trial. *Thromb Res.* 2015;136:758-762.

198. Carmel R. Mild transcobalamin I (haptocorrin) deficiency and low serum cobalamin concentrations. *Clin Chem.* 2003;49:1367-1374.

199. Carmel R, Brar S, Agrawal A, Penha PD. Failure of assay to identify low cobalamin concentrations. *Clin Chem.* 2000;46:2017-2018.

200. Carmel R, Agrawal YP. Failures of cobalamin assays in pernicious anemia. *N Engl J Med.* 2012;367:385-386.

201. İspir E, Serdar MA, Ozgurtas T, et al. Comparison of four automated serum vitamin B12 assays. *Clin Chem Lab Med.* 2015;53:1205-1213.

202. Mackenzie F, Devalia V. Laboratory performance of serum B12 assay in the United Kingdom (UK) as assessed by the UK national external quality assessment scheme for haematinics: implications for clinical interpretation. *Blood.* 2018;132(suppl 1):2230.

203. Tavares J, Baptista B, Gonçalves B, Horta AB. Pernicious anaemia with normal vitamin B12. *Eur J Case Rep Intern Med.* 2019;6:001045.

204. Iltar U, Göçer M, Kurtoğlu E. False elevations of vitamin B12 levels due to assay errors in a patient with pernicious anemia. *Blood Res.* 2019;54:149-151.

205. Ma Y, Chen C, Guo Y. Letter to the editor regarding megaloblastic anemia with elevated vitamin B12. *Clin Biochem.* 2021;97:85-86. S0009-9120(21)00201-0.

206. Burlock B, Williams JP. Recognizing subacute combined degeneration in patients with normal vitamin B12 levels. *Cureus.* 2021;13:e15429.

207. Thong EWS, Tan SS, Sethi SK, Chee YL, Jen WY. Falsely elevated serum vitamin B12 levels in a case of pernicious anemia. *Ann Hematol.* 2021;101(4):889-892. doi:10.1007/s00277-021-04612-x.

208. Pennypacker LC, Allen RH, Kelly JP, et al. High prevalence of cobalamin deficiency in elderly outpatients. *J Am Geriatr Soc.* 1992;40:1197-1204.

209. Lindenbaum J, Savage DG, Stabler SP, Allen RH. Diagnosis of cobalamin deficiency: II. Relative sensitivities of serum cobalamin, methylmalonic acid, and total homocysteine concentrations. *Am J Hematol.* 1990;34:99-107.

210. Lindenbaum J, Rosenberg IH, Wilson PW, Stabler SP, Allen RH. Prevalence of cobalamin deficiency in the Framingham elderly population. *Am J Clin Nutr.* 1994;60:2-11.

211. Johnson MA, Hawthorne N, Brackett W, et al. Hyperhomocysteinemia and vitamin B12 deficiency in elderly using Title IIIc nutrition services. *Am J Clin Nutr.* 2003;77:211-220.

212. Moelby L, Nielsen G, Rasmussen K, Jensen M, Pedersen K. Metabolic cobalamin deficiency in patients with low to low-normal plasma cobalamins. *Scand J Clin Lab Invest.* 1997;57:209-215.

213. Bolann BJ, Solli JD, Schneede J, et al. Evaluation of indicators of cobalamin deficiency defined as cobalamin-induced reduction in increased serum methylmalonic acid. *Clin Chem.* 2000;46:1744-1750.

214. Stabler SP, Allen RH, Barrett RE, Savage DG, Lindenbaum J. Cerebrospinal fluid methylmalonic acid levels in normal subjects and patients with cobalamin deficiency. *Neurology.* 1991;41:1627-1632.

215. Savage D, Gangaidzo I, Lindenbaum J, et al. Vitamin B12 deficiency is the primary cause of megaloblastic anaemia in Zimbabwe. *Br J Haematol.* 1994;86:844-850.

216. Stabler SP, Allen RH, Savage DG, Lindenbaum J. Clinical spectrum and diagnosis of cobalamin deficiency. *Blood.* 1990;76:871-881.

217. Bor MV, von Castel-Roberts KM, Kauwell GP, et al. Daily intake of 4 to 7 microg dietary vitamin B12 is associated with steady concentrations of vitamin B12-related biomarkers in a healthy young population. *Am J Clin Nutr.* 2010;91:571-577.

218. Johnson MA, Hausman DB, Davey A, et al. Vitamin B12 deficiency in African American and white octogenarians and centenarians in Georgia. *J Nutr Health Aging.* 2010;14:339-345.

219. Moelby L, Rasmussen K, Rasmussen HH. Serum methylmalonic acid in uraemia. *Scand J Clin Lab Invest.* 1992;52:351-354.

220. Stabler SP, Allen RH, Fried LP, et al. Racial differences in prevalence of cobalamin and folate deficiencies in disabled elderly women. *Am J Clin Nutr.* 1999;70:911-919.

221. Vogiatzoglou A, Oulhaj A, Smith AD, et al. Determinants of plasma methylmalonic acid in a large population: implications for assessment of vitamin B12 status. *Clin Chem.* 2009;55:2198-2206.

222. Molloy AM, Pangilinan F, Mills JL, et al. A common polymorphism in HIBCH influences methylmalonic acid concentrations in blood independently of cobalamin. *Am J Hum Genet.* 2016;98:869-882.

223. Allen RH, Stabler SP, Savage DG, Lindenbaum J. Diagnosis of cobalamin deficiency I: usefulness of serum methylmalonic acid and total homocysteine concentrations. *Am J Hematol.* 1990;34:90-98.

224. Devalia V, Hamilton MS, Molloy AM; British Committee for Standards in Haematology. Guidelines for the diagnosis and treatment of cobalamin and folate disorders. *Br J Haematol.* 2014;166:496-513.

225. Mudd SH, Finkelstein JD, Irreverre F, Laster L. Homocystinuria: an enzymatic defect. *Science.* 1964;143:1443-1445.

226. Stabler SP, Marcell PD, Podell ER, Allen RH. Quantitation of total homocysteine, total cysteine, and methionine in normal serum and urine using capillary gas chromatography-mass spectrometry. *Anal Biochem.* 1987;162:185-196.

227. Mudd SH, Finkelstein JD, Refsum H, et al. Homocysteine and its disulfide derivatives: a suggested consensus terminology. *Arterioscler Thromb Vasc Biol.* 2000;20:1704-1706.

228. Kang SS, Wong PW, Norusis M. Homocysteinemia due to folate deficiency. *Metabolism.* 1987;36:458-462.

229. Pfeiffer CM, Johnson CL, Jain RB, et al. Trends in blood folate and vitamin B12 concentrations in the United States, 1988 2004. *Am J Clin Nutr.* 2007;86:718-727.

230. Pfeiffer CM, Osterloh JD, Kennedy-Stephenson J, et al. Trends in circulating concentrations of total homocysteine among US adolescents and adults: findings from the 1991-1994 and 1999-2004 National Health and Nutrition Examination Surveys. *Clin Chem.* 2008;54:801-813.

231. Yang Q, Cogswell ME, Hamner HC, et al. Folic acid source, usual intake, and folate and vitamin B12 status in US adults: National Health and Nutrition Examination Survey (NHANES) 2003-2006. *Am J Clin Nutr.* 2010;91:64-72.

232. Cohen E, Margalit I, Shochat T, Goldberg E, Krause I. Sex differences in folate levels: a cross sectional study of a large cohort from Israel. *Isr Med Assoc J.* 2021;23:17-22.

233. Stabler SP, Lindenbaum J, Savage DG, Allen RH. Elevation of serum cystathionine levels in patients with cobalamin and folate deficiency. *Blood.* 1993;81:3404-3413.

234. Guerra-Shinohara EM, Morita OE, Pagliusi RA, et al. Elevated serum S-adenosylhomocysteine in cobalamin-deficient megaloblastic anemia. *Metabolism.* 2007;56:339-347.

235. Stabler SP, Allen RH. Quantification of serum and urinary S-adenosylmethionine and S-adenosylhomocysteine by stable-isotope-dilution liquid chromatography-mass spectrometry. *Clin Chem.* 2004;50:365-372.

236. Bailey RL, Carmel R, Green R, et al. Monitoring of vitamin B-12 nutritional status in the United States by using plasma methylmalonic acid and serum vitamin B-12. *Am J Clin Nutr.* 2011;94:552-561.

237. Bailey RL, Durazo-Arvizu RA, Carmel R, et al. Modeling a methylmalonic acid-derived change point for serum vitamin B-12 for adults in NHANES. *Am J Clin Nutr.* 2013;98:460-467.

238. Hvas AM, Nexo E. Holotranscobalamin: a first choice assay for diagnosing early vitamin B deficiency? *J Intern Med.* 2005;257:289-298.

239. Heil SG, Bodenburg P, Findeisen P, Luebcke S, Sun Y, de Rijke YB. Multicentre evaluation of the Roche Elecsys® Active B12 (holotranscobalamin) electrochemiluminescence immunoassay. *Ann Clin Biochem.* 2019;56:662-667.

240. Herrmann W, Obeid R. Utility and limitations of biochemical markers of vitamin B12 deficiency. *Eur J Clin Invest.* 2013;43:231-237.

241. Sobczyńska-Malefora A, Gorska R, Pelisser M, et al. An audit of holotranscobalamin ("Active" B12) and methylmalonic acid assays for the assessment of vitamin B12 status: application in a mixed patient population. *Clin Biochem.* 2014;47:82-86.

242. Heil SG, de Jonge R, de Rotte MC, et al. Screening for metabolic vitamin B12 deficiency by holotranscobalamin in patients suspected of vitamin B12 deficiency: a multicentre study. *Ann Clin Biochem.* 2012;49:184-189.

243. Rothen JP, Walter PN, Tsakiris DA, et al. Identification of patients with cobalamin deficiency crucially depends on the diagnostic strategy. *Clin Lab.* 2021;67. doi:10.7754/Clin.Lab.2020.200912

244. Campos AJ, Risch L, Nydegger U, et al. Diagnostic characteristics of 3-parameter and 2-parameter equations for the calculation of a combined indicator of vitamin B12 status to predict cobalamin deficiency in a large mixed patient population. *Clin Lab.* 2020;66(10).

245. Nexo E, Hoffmann-Lücke E. Holotranscobalamin, a marker of vitamin B-12 status: analytical aspects and clinical utility. *Am J Clin Nutr.* 2011;94:359S-365S.

246. Valente E, Scott JM, Ueland PM, et al. Diagnostic accuracy of holotranscobalamin, methylmalonic acid, serum cobalamin, and other indicators of tissue vitamin B12 status in the elderly. *Clin Chem.* 2011;57:856-863.

247. Miller JW, Garrod MG, Rockwood AL, et al. Measurement of total vitamin B12 and holotranscobalamin, singly and in combination, in screening for metabolic vitamin B12 deficiency. *Clin Chem.* 2006;52:278-285.

248. Schrempf W, Eulitz M, Neumeister V, et al. Utility of measuring vitamin B12 and its active fraction, holotranscobalamin, in neurological vitamin B12 deficiency syndromes. *J Neurol.* 2011;258:393-401.

249. Refsum H, Johnston C, Guttormsen AB, Nexo E. Holotranscobalamin and total transcobalamin in human plasma: determination, determinants, and reference values in healthy adults. *Clin Chem.* 2006;52:129-137.

250. Keller P, Rufener J, Schild C, et al. False low holotranscobalamin levels in a patient with a novel TCN2 mutation. *Clin Chem Lab Med.* 2016;54:1739-1743.

251. Fedosov SN, Brito A, Miller JW, Green R, Allen LH. Combined indicator of vitamin B12 status: modification for missing biomarkers and folate status and recommendations for revised cut-points. *Clin Chem Lab Med.* 2015;53:1215-1225.

252. Mineva EM, Sternberg MR, Bailey RL, Storandt RJ, Pfeiffer CM. Fewer US adults had low or transitional vitamin B12 status based on the novel combined indicator of vitamin B12 status compared with individual, conventional markers, NHANES 1999-2004. *Am J Clin Nutr.* 2021;114:1070-1079.

253. Sobczyńska-Malefora A, Harrington DJ. Laboratory assessment of folate (vitamin B$_9$) status. *J Clin Pathol.* 2018;71:949-956.

254. Baril L, Carmel R. Comparison of radioassay and microbiological assay for serum folate, with clinical assessment of discrepant results. *Clin Chem.* 1978;24:2192-2196.

255. Hoffbrand AV, Newcombe FA, Mollin DL. Method of assay of red cell folate activity and the value of the assay as a test for folate deficiency. *J Clin Pathol.* 1966;19:17-28.

256. Pfeiffer CM, Fazili Z, McCoy L, Zhang M, Gunter EW. Determination of folate vitamers in human serum by stable-isotope-dilution tandem mass spectrometry and comparison with radioassay and microbiologic assay. *Clin Chem.* 2004;50:423-432.

257. Sobczyńska-Malefora A, Harrington DJ, Voong K, Shearer MJ. Plasma and red cell reference intervals of 5-methyltetrahydrofolate of healthy adults in whom biochemical functional deficiencies of folate and vitamin B 12 had been excluded. *Adv Hematol.* 2014;2014:465623.

258. Farrell CJ, Kirsch SH, Herrmann M. Red cell or serum folate: what to do in clinical practice? *Clin Chem Lab Med.* 2013;51:555-569.

259. Bailey RL, Mills JL, Yetley EA, et al. Unmetabolized serum folic acid and its relation to folic acid intake from diet and supplements in a nationally representative sample of adults aged > or =60 y in the United States. *Am J Clin Nutr.* 2010;92:383-389.

260. Williams BA, Mayer C, McCartney H, et al. Detectable unmetabolized folic acid and elevated folate concentrations in folic acid-supplemented Canadian children with sickle cell disease. *Front Nutr.* 2021;8:642306.

261. Bailey RL, Jun S, Murphy L, et al. High folic acid or folate combined with low vitamin B12 status: potential but inconsistent association with cognitive function in a nationally representative cross-sectional sample of US older adults participating in the NHANES. *Am J Clin Nutr.* 2020;112:1547-1557.

262. Gilfix BM. Utility of measuring serum or red blood cell folate in the era of folate fortification of flour. *Clin Biochem.* 2014;47:533-538.

263. Smulders YM, Smith DE, Kok RM, et al. Red blood cell folate vitamer distribution in healthy subjects is determined by the methylenetetrahydrofolate reductase C677T polymorphism and by the total folate status. *J Nutr Biochem.* 2007;18:693-699.

264. Liew SC, Gupta ED. Methylenetetrahydrofolate reductase (MTHFR) C677T polymorphism: epidemiology, metabolism and the associated diseases. *Eur J Med Genet.* 2015;58:1-10.

265. Wilcken B, Bamforth F, Li Z, et al. Geographical and ethnic variation of the 677C>T allele of 5,10 methylenetetrahydrofolate reductase (MTHFR): findings from over 7000 newborns from 16 areas worldwide. *J Med Genet.* 2003;40:619-625.

266. Froese DS, Huemer M, Suormala T, et al. Mutation update and review of severe methylenetetrahydrofolate reductase deficiency. *Hum Mutat.* 2016;37:427-438.

267. Rustgi SD, Bijlani P, Shah SC. Autoimmune gastritis, with or without pernicious anemia: epidemiology, risk factors, and clinical management. *Therap Adv Gastroenterol.* 2021;14:17562848211038771.

268. Lenti MV, Rugge M, Lahner E, et al. Autoimmune gastritis. *Nat Rev Dis Prim.* 2020;6:56.

269. Harmandar FA, Dolu S, Çekin AH. Role of pernicious anemia in patients admitted to internal medicine with vitamin B12 deficiency and oral replacement therapy as a treatment option. *Clin Lab.* 2020;66.

270. Hall SN, Appelman HD. Autoimmune gastritis. *Arch Pathol Lab Med.* 2019;143:1327-1331.

271. Song IC, Lee HJ, Kim HJ, et al. A multicenter retrospective analysis of the clinical features of pernicious anemia in a Korean population. *J Korean Med Sci.* 2013;28:200-204.

272. Lenti MV, Lahner E, Bergamaschi G, et al. Cell blood count alterations and patterns of anaemia in autoimmune atrophic gastritis at diagnosis: a multicentre study. *J Clin Med.* 2019;8:1992.

273. Souto Filho JTD, Beiral ES, Azevedo FS, et al. Predictive risk factors for autoimmune thyroid diseases in patients with pernicious anemia. *Med Clin.* 2020;154:344-347.

274. Li X, Thomsen H, Sundquist K, et al. Familial risks between pernicious anemia and other autoimmune diseases in the population of Sweden. *Autoimmune Dis.* 2021;2021:8815297.

275. Laisk T, Lepamets M, Koel M, et al. Genome-wide association study identifies five risk loci for pernicious anemia. *Nat Commun.* 2021;12:3761.

276. Salinas M, Flores E, López-Garrigós M, Leiva-Salinas C. High frequency of anti-parietal cell antibody (APCA) and intrinsic factor blocking antibody (IFBA) in individuals with severe vitamin B12 deficiency: an observational study in primary care patients. *Clin Chem Lab Med.* 2020;58:424-429.

277. Hvas AM, Morkbak AL, Hardlei TF, Nexo E. The vitamin B12 absorption test, CobaSorb, identifies patients not requiring vitamin B12 injection therapy. *Scand J Clin Lab Invest.* 2011;71:432-438.

278. Greibe E, Mahalle N, Bhide V, et al. Increase in circulating holotranscobalamin after oral administration of cyanocobalamin or hydroxocobalamin in healthy adults with low and normal cobalamin status. *Eur J Nutr.* 2018;57:2847-2855.

279. Carkeet C, Dueker SR, Lango J, et al. Human vitamin B12 absorption measurement by accelerator mass spectrometry using specifically labeled (14)C-cobalamin. *Proc Natl Acad Sci USA.* 2006;103:5694-5699.

280. Brito A, Habeych E, Silva-Zolezzi I, Galaffu N, Allen LH. Methods to assess vitamin B12 bioavailability and technologies to enhance its absorption. *Nutr Rev.* 2018;76:778-792.

281. Sumner AE, Chin MM, Abrahm JL, et al. Elevated methylmalonic acid and total homocysteine levels show high prevalence of vitamin B12 deficiency after gastric surgery. *Ann Intern Med.* 1996;124:469-476.

282. Lewis CA, de Jersey S, Seymour M, et al. Iron, Vitamin B12, folate and copper deficiency after bariatric surgery and the impact on anaemia: a systematic review. *Obes Surg.* 2020;30:4542-4591.

283. Lombardo M, Franchi A, Biolcati Rinaldi R, et al. Long-term iron and vitamin B12 deficiency are present after bariatric surgery, despite the widespread use of supplements. *Int J Environ Res Public Health.* 2021;18:4541.

284. Jamil O, Gonzalez-Heredia R, Quadri P, et al. Micronutrient deficiencies in laparoscopic sleeve gastrectomy. *Nutrients.* 2020;12:2896.

285. Kornerup LS, Hvas CL, Abild CB, Richelsen B, Nexo E. Early changes in vitamin B12 uptake and biomarker status following Roux-en-Y gastric bypass and sleeve gastrectomy. *Clin Nutr.* 2019;38:906-911.

286. Joosten E, van den Berg A, Riezler R, et al. Metabolic evidence that deficiencies of vitamin B12 (cobalamin), folate, and vitamin B6 occur commonly in elderly people. *Am J Clin Nutr.* 1993;58:468-476.

287. Björkegren K, Svärdsudd K. Serum cobalamin, folate, methylmalonic acid and total homocysteine as vitamin B12 and folate tissue deficiency markers amongst elderly Swedes: a population-based study. *J Intern Med.* 2001;249:423-432.

288. Morris MS, Jacques PF, Rosenberg IH, Selhub J. Elevated serum methylmalonic acid concentrations are common among elderly Americans. *J Nutr.* 2002;132:2799-2803.

289. Carmel R, Green R, Jacobsen DW, et al. Serum cobalamin, homocysteine, and methylmalonic acid concentrations in a multiethnic elderly population: ethnic and sex differences in cobalamin and metabolite abnormalities. *Am J Clin Nutr.* 1999;70:904-910.

290. Porter KM, Hoey L, Hughes CF, et al. Associations of atrophic gastritis and proton-pump inhibitor drug use with vitamin B-12 status, and the impact of fortified foods, in older adults. *Am J Clin Nutr.* 2021;114(4):1286-1294. nqab193

291. Stabler SP, Allen RH, Dolce ET, Johnson MA. Elevated serum S-adenosylhomocysteine in cobalamin-deficient elderly and response to treatment. *Am J Clin Nutr.* 2006;84:1422-1429.

292. Rajan S, Wallace JI, Brodkin KI, et al. Response of elevated methylmalonic acid to three dose levels of oral cobalamin in older adults. *J Am Geriatr Soc.* 2002;50:1789-1795.

293. Eussen SJ, de Groot LC, Clarke R, et al. Oral cyanocobalamin supplementation in older people with vitamin B12 deficiency: a dose-finding trial. *Arch Intern Med.* 2005;165:1167-1172.

294. O'Logbon J, Crook M, Steed D, Harrington DJ, Sobczyńska-Malefora A. Ethnicity influences total serum vitamin B12 concentration: a study of Black, Asian and White patients in a primary care setting. *J Clin Pathol.* 2021;75(9):598-604. jclinpath-2021-207519

295. Naurath HJ, Joosten E, Riezler R, et al. Effects of vitamin B12, folate, and vitamin B6 supplements in elderly people with normal serum vitamin concentrations. *Lancet.* 1995;346:85-89.

296. Smelt AF, Gussekloo J, Bermingham LW, et al. The effect of vitamin B12 and folic acid supplementation on routine haematological parameters in older people: an individual participant data meta-analysis. *Eur J Clin Nutr.* 2018;72:785-795.

297. Selhub J, Morris MS, Jacques PF. In vitamin B12 deficiency, higher serum folate is associated with increased total homocysteine and methylmalonic acid concentrations. *Proc Natl Acad Sci USA.* 2007;104:19995-20000.

298. Gahche JJ, Bailey RL, Potischman N, Dwyer JT. Dietary supplement use was very high among older adults in the United States in 2011-2014. *J Nutr.* 2017;147:1968-1976.

299. Bures J, Cyrany J, Kohoutova D, et al. Small intestinal bacterial overgrowth syndrome. *World J Gastroenterol.* 2010;16:2978-2990.

300. Nyberg W, Grasbeck R, Saarni M, von Bonsdorff. Serum vitamin B12 levels and incidence of tapeworm anemia in a population heavily infected with Diphyllobothrium latum. *Am J Clin Nutr.* 1961;9:606-612.

301. Valman HB, Roberts PD. Vitamin B12 absorption after resection of ileum in childhood. *Arch Dis Child.* 1974;49:932-935.

302. Knap MM, Lundbeck F, Overgaard J. Early and late treatment-related morbidity following radical cystectomy. *Scand J Urol Nephrol.* 2004;38:153-160.

303. Brown IS, Bettington A, Bettington M, Rosty C. Tropical sprue: revisiting an under-recognized disease. *Am J Surg Pathol.* 2014;38:666-672.

304. Sharma P, Baloda V, Gahlot GP, et al. Clinical, endoscopic, and histological differentiation between celiac disease and tropical sprue: a systematic review. *J Gastroenterol Hepatol.* 2019;34:74-83.

305. Noh T, Osman G, Chedid M, Hefzy H. Nitrous oxide-induced demyelination: clinical presentation, diagnosis and treatment recommendations. *J Neurol Sci.* 2020;414:116817.

306. Zheng R, Wang Q, Li M, et al. Reversible Neuropsychiatric disturbances caused by nitrous oxide toxicity: clinical, imaging and electrophysiological profiles of 21 patients with 6-12 months follow-up. *Neuropsychiatric Dis Treat.* 2020;16:2817-2825.

307. Patel KK, Mejia Munne JC, Gunness VRN, et al. Subacute combined degeneration of the spinal cord following nitrous oxide anesthesia: a systematic review of cases. *Clin Neurol Neurosurg.* 2018;173:163-168.

308. Miller JW. Proton pump inhibitors, H2-receptor antagonists, metformin, and vitamin B12 deficiency: clinical implications. *Adv Nutr.* 2018;9:511S-518S.

309. Desmond MA, Sobiecki JG, Jaworski M, et al. Growth, body composition, and cardiovascular and nutritional risk of 5- to 10-y-old children consuming vegetarian, vegan, or omnivore diets. *Am J Clin Nutr.* 2021;113:1565-1577.

310. Caswell BL, Arnold CD, Lutter CK, et al. Impacts of an egg intervention on nutrient adequacy among young Malawian children. *Matern Child Nutr.* 2021;17:e13196.

311. Benham AJ, Gallegos D, Hanna KL, Hannan-Jones MT. Intake of vitamin B12 and other characteristics of women of reproductive age on a vegan diet in Australia. *Publ Health Nutr.* 2021;24(14):4397-4407.

312. Samarron SL, Miller JW, Cheung AT, et al. Homocysteine is associated with severity of microvasculopathy in sickle cell disease patients. *Br J Haematol.* 2020;190:450-457.

313. Refsum H, Wesenberg F, Ueland PM. Plasma homocysteine in children with acute lymphoblastic leukemia: changes during a chemotherapeutic regimen including methotrexate. *Cancer Res.* 1991;51:828-835.

314. Angelini A, Cappuccilli ML, Magnoni G, et al. The link between homocysteine, folic acid and vitamin B12 in chronic kidney disease. *G Ital Nefrol.* 2021;38:2021.

315. Hesdorffer CS, Longo DL. Drug-induced megaloblastic anemia. *N Engl J Med.* 2015;373:1649-1658.

316. Broxson EH, Jr, Stork LC, Allen RH, Stabler SP, Kolhouse JF. Changes in plasma methionine and total homocysteine levels in patients receiving methotrexate infusions. *Cancer Res.* 1989;49:5879-5883.

317. Chuang YC, Chuang HY, Lin TK, et al. Effects of long-term antiepileptic drug monotherapy on vascular risk factors and atherosclerosis. *Epilepsia.* 2012;53:120-128.

318. Boelens Keun JT, Arnoldussen IA, Vriend C, van de Rest O. Dietary approaches to improve efficacy and control side effects of levodopa therapy in Parkinson's disease: a systematic review. *Adv Nutr.* 2021;12(6):2265-2287.

319. Stabler SP, Sekhar J, Allen RH, O'Neill HC, White CW. Alpha-lipoic acid induces elevated S-adenosylhomocysteine and depletes S-adenosylmethionine. *Free Radic Biol Med.* 2009;47:1147-1153.

320. Mangla G, Garg N, Bansal D, Kotru M, Sikka M. Peripheral Blood and bone marrow findings in chronic alcoholics with special reference to acquired sideroblastic anemia. *Indian J Hematol Blood Transfus.* 2020;36:559-564.

321. Medici V, Peerson JM, Stabler SP, et al. Impaired homocysteine transsulfuration is an indicator of alcoholic liver disease. *J Hepatol.* 2010;53:551-557.

322. Medici V, Halsted CH. Folate, alcohol, and liver disease. *Mol Nutr Food Res.* 2013;57:596-606.

323. Halsted CH, Villanueva J, Chandler CJ, et al. Ethanol feeding of micropigs alters methionine metabolism and increases hepatocellular apoptosis and proliferation. *Hepatology.* 1996;23:497-505.

324. Tanner SM, Sturm AC, Baack EC, Liyanarachchi S, de la Chapelle A. Inherited cobalamin malabsorption. Mutations in three genes reveal functional and ethnic patterns. *Orphanet J Rare Dis.* 2012;7:56.

325. Watkins D, Rosenblatt DS. Immunodeficiency and inborn disorders of vitamin B12 and folate metabolism. *Curr Opin Clin Nutr Metab Care.* 2020;23:241-246.

326. Sturm AC, Baack EC, Armstrong MB, et al. Hereditary intrinsic factor deficiency in chaldeans. *JIMD Rep.* 2013;7:13-18.

327. Ruan J, Han B, Zhuang J, et al. Hereditary intrinsic factor deficiency in China caused by a novel mutation in the intrinsic factor gene—a case report. *BMC Med Genet.* 2020;21:221.

328. Huemer M, Diodato D, Schwahn B, et al. Guidelines for diagnosis and management of the cobalamin-related remethylation disorders cblC, cblD, cblE, cblF, cblG, cblJ and MTHFR deficiency. *J Inherit Metab Dis.* 2017;40:21-48.

329. Svaton M, Skvarova Kramarzova K, Kanderova V, et al. A homozygous deletion in the SLC19A1 gene as a cause of folate-dependent recurrent megaloblastic anemia. *Blood.* 2020;135:2427-2431.

330. Bidla G, Watkins D, Chéry C, et al. Biochemical analysis of patients with mutations in MTHFD1 and a diagnosis of methylenetetrahydrofolate dehydrogenase 1 deficiency. *Mol Genet Metab.* 2020;130:179-182.

331. Burda P, Kuster A, Hjalmarson O, et al. Characterization and review of MTHFD1 deficiency: four new patients, cellular delineation and response to folic and folinic acid treatment. *J Inherit Metab Dis.* 2015;38:863-872.

332. Pope S, Artuch R, Heales S, Rahman S. Cerebral folate deficiency: analytical tests and differential diagnosis. *J Inherit Metab Dis.* 2019;42:655-672.

333. Cario H, Smith DE, Blom H, et al. Dihydrofolate reductase deficiency due to a homozygous DHFR mutation causes megaloblastic anemia and cerebral folate deficiency leading to severe neurologic disease. *Am J Hum Genet.* 2011;88:226-231.

334. Banka S, Blom HJ, Walter J, et al. Identification and characterization of an inborn error of metabolism caused by dihydrofolate reductase deficiency. *Am J Hum Genet.* 2011;88:216-225.

335. Rodan LH, Qi W, Ducker GS, et al. 5,10-methenyltetrahydrofolate synthetase deficiency causes a neurometabolic disorder associated with microcephaly, epilepsy, and cerebral hypomyelination. *Mol Genet Metab.* 2018;125:118-126.

336. Romero JA, Abdelmoumen I, Hasbani D, Khurana DS, Schneider MC. A case of 5,10-methenyltetrahydrofolate synthetase deficiency due to biallelic null mutations

with novel findings of elevated neopterin and macrocytic anemia. *Mol Genet Metab Rep.* 2019;21:100545.

337. Warncke K, Prinz N, Iotova V, et al. Thiamine-responsive megaloblastic anemia-related diabetes: long-term clinical outcomes in 23 pediatric patients from the DPV and SWEET registries. *Can J Diabetes.* 2021;45:539-545.

338. Cakmakli HF, Torres RJ, Menendez A, et al. Macrocytic anemia in Lesch-Nyhan disease and its variants. *Genet Med.* 2019;21:353-360.

339. Al Absi HS, Sacharow S, Al Zein N, Al Shamsi A, Al Teneiji A. Hereditary orotic aciduria (HOA): a novel uridine-5-monophosphate synthase (UMPS) mutation. *Mol Genet Metab Rep.* 2021;26:100703.

340. Schallier D, Trullemans F, Fontaine C, Decoster L, De Greve J. Tyrosine kinase inhibitor-induced macrocytosis. *Anticancer Res.* 2009;29:5225-5228.

341. Khawcharoenporn T, Shikuma CM, Williams AE, Chow DC. Lamivudine-associated macrocytosis in HIV-infected patients. *Int J STD AIDS.* 2007;18:39-40.

342. Geené D, Sudre P, Anwar D, et al. Causes of macrocytosis in HIV-infected patients not treated with zidovudine. Swiss HIV Cohort Study. *J Infect.* 2000;40:160-163.

343. Carmel R. How I treat cobalamin (vitamin B12) deficiency. *Blood.* 2008;112:2214-2221.

344. Lawson DH, Murray RM, Parker JL, Hay G. Hypokalaemia in megaloblastic anaemias. *Lancet.* 1970;2:588-590.

345. Pezina-Cantú C, Gómez-De León A, Jaime-Perez JC, et al. Pernicious anaemia can be treated effectively with a single high dose of cobalamin. *Br J Haematol.* 2020;191:e97-e100.

346. Andrès E, Zulfiqar AA, Serraj K, Vogel T, Kaltenbach G. Systematic review and pragmatic clinical approach to oral and nasal vitamin B12 (cobalamin) treatment in patients with vitamin B12 deficiency related to gastrointestinal disorders. *J Clin Med.* 2018;7:304.

347. Sanz-Cuesta T, Escortell-Mayor E, Cura-Gonzalez I, et al. Oral versus intramuscular administration of vitamin B12 for vitamin B12 deficiency in primary care: a pragmatic, randomised, non-inferiority clinical trial (OB12). *BMJ Open.* 2020;10:e033687.

348. Moleiro J, Mão de Ferro S, Ferreira S, et al. Efficacy of long-term oral vitamin B12 supplementation after total gastrectomy: results from a prospective study. *GE Port J Gastroenterol.* 2018;25:117-122.

349. Andrès E, Zulfiqar AA, Vogel T. State of the art review: oral and nasal vitamin B12 therapy in the elderly. *QJM.* 2020;113:5-15.

350. Estourgie-van Burk GF, van der Kuy PHM, de Meij TG, Benninga MA, Kneepkens CMF. Intranasal treatment of vitamin B12 deficiency in children. *Eur J Pediatr.* 2020;179:349-352.

351. Del Bo' C, Riso P, Gardana C, et al. Effect of two different sublingual dosages of vitamin B12 on cobalamin nutritional status in vegans and vegetarians with a marginal deficiency: a randomized controlled trial. *Clin Nutr.* 2019;38:575-583.

352. Delpre G, Stark P, Niv Y. Sublingual therapy for cobalamin deficiency as an alternative to oral and parenteral cobalamin supplementation. *Lancet.* 1999;354:740-741.

353. Sharabi A, Cohen E, Sulkes J, Garty M. Replacement therapy for vitamin B12 deficiency: comparison between the sublingual and oral route. *Br J Clin Pharmacol.* 2003;56:635-638.

354. Sawangjit R, Thongphui S, Chaichompu W, Phumart P. Efficacy and safety of mecobalamin on peripheral neuropathy: a systematic review and meta-analysis of randomized controlled trials. *J Altern Complement Med.* 2020;26:1117-1129.

355. Stabler SP. Vitamin B12 deficiency. *N Engl J Med.* 2013;368:2041-2042.

356. Obeid R, Fedosov SN, Nexo E. Cobalamin coenzyme forms are not likely to be superior to cyano- and hydroxyl-cobalamin in prevention or treatment of cobalamin deficiency. *Mol Nutr Food Res.* 2015;59:1364-1372.

357. Modupe O, Diosady LL. Quadruple fortification of salt for the delivery of iron, iodine, folic acid, and vitamin B12 to vulnerable populations. *J Food Eng.* 2021;300:110525.

358. Vora RM, Alappattu MJ, Zarkar AD, et al. Potential for elimination of folate and vitamin B12 deficiency in India using vitamin-fortified tea: a preliminary study. *BMJ Nutr Prev Health.* 2021;4:293-306.

359. Keller R, Chrastina P, Pavlíková M, et al. Newborn screening for homocystinurias: recent recommendations versus current practice. *J Inherit Metab Dis.* 2019;42:128-139.

360. Sørensen JT, Gaustadnes M, Stabler SP, et al. Molecular and biochemical investigations of patients with intermediate or severe hyperhomocysteinemia. *Mol Genet Metab.* 2016;117:344-350.

361. Kraus JP, Hasek J, Kozich V, et al. Cystathionine gamma-lyase: clinical, metabolic, genetic, and structural studies. *Mol Genet Metab.* 2009;97:250-259.

362. Elmadfa I, Singer I. Vitamin B12 and homocysteine status among vegetarians: a global perspective. *Am J Clin Nutr.* 2009;89:1693S-1698S.

363. Oh S, Cave G, Lu C. Vitamin B12 (cobalamin) and micronutrient fortification in food crops using nanoparticle technology. *Front Plant Sci.* 2021;12:668819.

364. Rogers LM, Cordero AM, Pfeiffer CM, et al. Global folate status in women of reproductive age: a systematic review with emphasis on methodological issues. *Ann N Y Acad Sci.* 2018;1431:35-57.

365. Garrod MG, Buchholz BA, Miller JW, et al. Vitamin B12 added as a fortificant to flour retains high bioavailability when baked in bread. *Nucl Instrum Methods Phys Res B.* 2019;438:136-140.

366. Chamlagain B, Peltonen L, Edelmann M, et al. Bioaccessibility of vitamin B12 synthesized by *Propionibacterium freudenreichii* and from products made with fermented wheat bran extract. *Curr Res Food Sci.* 2021;4:499-502.

367. Jyrwa YW, Palika R, Boddula S, et al. Retention, stability, iron bioavailability and sensory evaluation of extruded rice fortified with iron, folic acid and vitamin B12. *Matern Child Nutr.* 2020;16(suppl 3):e12932.

368. Savage D, Lindenbaum J. Folate-cobalamin interactions. In: Bailey LB, ed. *Folate in Health and Disease.* Marcel Dekker; 1995:237-285.

369. Molloy AM. Adverse effects on cognition caused by combined low vitamin B12 and high folate status-we must do better than a definite maybe. *Am J Clin Nutr.* 2020;112:1422-1423.

370. Berry RJ. Lack of historical evidence to support folic acid exacerbation of the neuropathy caused by vitamin B12 deficiency. *Am J Clin Nutr.* 2019;110:554-561.

371. Maruvada P, Stover PJ, Mason JB, et al. Knowledge gaps in understanding the metabolic and clinical effects of excess folates/folic acid: a summary, and perspectives, from an NIH workshop. *Am J Clin Nutr.* 2020;112:1390-1403.

372. Clarke R, Bennett D, Parish S, et al. Effects of homocysteine lowering with B vitamins on cognitive aging: meta-analysis of 11 trials with cognitive data on 22,000 individuals. *Am J Clin Nutr.* 2014;100:657-666.

373. Markun S, Gravestock I, Jäger L, et al. Effects of Vitamin B12 supplementation on cognitive function, depressive symptoms, and fatigue: a systematic review, meta-analysis, and meta-regression. *Nutrients.* 2021;13:923.

374. Arendt JFH, Horváth-Puhó E, Sørensen HT, et al. Plasma vitamin B12 levels, high-dose vitamin B12 treatment, and risk of dementia. *J Alzheimers Dis.* 2021;79:1601-1612.

375. Smith AD, Refsum H, Bottiglieri T, et al. Homocysteine and dementia: an international consensus statement. *J Alzheimers Dis.* 2018;62:561-570.

376. Altaf R, Gonzalez I, Rubino K, Nemec EC, IInd. Folate as adjunct therapy to SSRI/SNRI for major depressive disorder: systematic review & meta-analysis. *Complement Ther Med.* 2021;61:102770.

377. Almeida OP, Ford AH, Flicker L. Systematic review and meta-analysis of randomized placebo-controlled trials of folate and vitamin B12 for depression. *Int Psychogeriatr.* 2015;27:727-737.

378. Julian T, Syeed R, Glascow N, Angelopoulou E, Zis P. B12 as a treatment for peripheral neuropathic pain: a systematic review. *Nutrients.* 2020;12:2221.

379. Frye RE, Rossignol DA, Scahill L, et al. Treatment of folate metabolism abnormalities in autism spectrum disorder. *Semin Pediatr Neurol.* 2020;35:100835.

380. Stevens VL, McCullough ML, Sun J, et al. High levels of folate from supplements and fortification are not associated with increased risk of colorectal cancer. *Gastroenterology.* 2011;141:98-105.e1.

381. Gibson TM, Weinstein SJ, Pfeiffer RM, et al. Pre- and postfortification intake of folate and risk of colorectal cancer in a large prospective cohort study in the United States. *Am J Clin Nutr.* 2011;94:1053-1062.

382. Vollset SE, Clarke R, Lewington S, et al. Effects of folic acid supplementation on overall and site-specific cancer incidence during the randomised trials: meta-analyses of data on 50,000 individuals. *Lancet.* 2013;381:1029-1036.

383. Kim YI. Folate and cancer: a tale of Dr. Jekyll and Mr. Hyde? *Am J Clin Nutr.* 2018;107:139-142.

Disorders of Red Blood Cells

Chapter 38 ■ Inherited Aplastic Anemia Syndromes Germline

NINA WEICHERT-LEAHEY • AKIKO SHIMAMURA

INTRODUCTION

The inherited bone marrow failure (BMF) syndromes are a diverse group of disorders that may either primarily affect a single hematopoietic lineage or may affect multiple hematopoietic lineages.[1] Five inherited BMF syndromes associated with aplastic anemia (AA) will be discussed in this chapter: Fanconi anemia (FA), telomere biology disorders (TBDs), Shwachman-Diamond syndrome (SDS), congenital amegakaryocytic thrombocytopenia (CAMT), and GATA2 syndromes. Diamond-Blackfan anemia is discussed in Chapter 40, and the inherited neutropenia syndromes are reviewed in Chapter 58. The thrombocytopenia syndromes with mutations in RUNX1,[2] ETV6,[3,4] and ANKRD26,[5] which are associated with leukemia predisposition, will not be covered in this chapter. These will be reviewed in Chapter 50.

Although individual inherited marrow failure syndromes are rare, as a group they constitute a significant subset of marrow failure.[6,7] Early diagnosis is important for treatment decisions, identification and management of associated comorbidities, optimal cancer surveillance, genetic counseling, family planning, and to inform a hematopoietic stem cell donor search if needed. Careful consideration of these underlying diagnoses must be taken to optimize medical management, and a multidisciplinary treatment plan is often required. Some of the disorders are associated with sensitivity to chemotherapy and radiation, and thus diagnosis of those underlying disorders prior to initiation of treatment of AA or associated malignancies is critical. Although the mechanisms by which marrow failure develops in each of the inherited marrow failure syndromes are unique, it has been proposed that the various pathways center on increases in cellular stress leading to apoptosis of hematopoietic stem/progenitor cells. Studying the inherited marrow failure syndromes has advanced our understanding of hematopoiesis and malignant transformation.[8,9]

Diagnostic Approach

A careful medical and family history together with a thorough physical examination may provide important clues to distinguish acquired from inherited BMF.[10] Poor growth or short stature is a characteristic feature of many inherited bone marrow disorders. The family history can often provide additional clues. A family history suggestive of cancer predisposition, such as malignancies at an unusually young age or preceding cytopenias, may be obtained. A history of excessive toxicity following treatment with genotoxic agents may be present. A personal or family history of congenital anomalies or stigmata characteristic of the inherited BMF syndromes, elevated fetal hemoglobin (HgbF), or a macrocytic anemia with elevated mean corpuscular volume may provide important clues.[11] As part of a comprehensive workup, other potential etiologies for cytopenias should also be considered. Thus, a family history, physical examination, and history are critical to identifying potential inherited BMF syndromes.[12] Laboratory diagnostic tests are focused on determining the severity of marrow failure, ruling out treatable causes of BMF such as infection, assessing for abnormalities suggestive of an inherited condition, and assessing baseline organ function to guide management. Testing includes a complete blood count with differentiation of leukocytes, B and T subsets; electrolytes; kidney, liver, and pancreatic function testing; as well as chromosomal breakage tests with diepoxybutane (DEB) or mitomycin C (MMC), or telomere length testing, which are described further in the following sections.[13] Genetic testing is a critical part of the diagnostic evaluation. Gene panels or whole exome sequencing are available to evaluate germline mutations known to cause BMF or hematologic malignancies.[7,14] For recessively inherited disorders, care must be taken to confirm that mutations are biallelic. Distinction between germline

versus somatic mutations is essential because the clinical implications are vastly different.[6] Somatic mosaicism can confound test results for some disorders. Finally, an understanding of the characteristics and methodologies of the specific genetic tests, including which genes are included in the analysis and which regions of each gene is covered, is essential. It is important to utilize genetic testing panels designed for analysis of germline mutations since these are not interchangeable with somatic mutations panels. Somatic panels may exclude genes important for germline analysis, may not cover important regions essential for evaluation of germline mutations in a given gene, may utilize different analytic pipelines, and may not evaluate copy number variants. It is also important to recognize that mutations identified on somatic panels may be of germline origin. New genes causing BMF continue to be reported, and additional genes likely still remain to be identified.[15] Genetic test results must be interpreted critically and within the clinical context of the patient.

Once the diagnosis of an inherited BMF syndrome is made, it is important to test all family members at risk of the disease regardless of clinical symptoms, as manifestations may vary widely among family members, and some may have no physical stigmata despite carrying the same mutation. This is an especially pertinent issue when family members are being evaluated as donors for hematopoietic stem cell transplant (HSCT). Indeed, the inherited BMF syndromes are increasingly being recognized in adults, who often manifest milder clinical phenotypes or whose first manifestation of an underlying inherited BMF syndrome may be AA or malignancy.[16,17] With the advent of genetic and laboratory diagnostic testing, the diseases are also increasingly recognized in patients who lack the characteristic physical stigmata conventionally associated with the disease. Recent genomic studies have shown that germline mutations in patients with either inherited marrow failure syndrome may be more frequent than previously recognized, underscoring the importance of vigilance for these disorders in the diagnostic evaluation of patients with cytopenias and hematologic malignancies.[6,7,18-20]

Approach to Clinical Management

Timely and accurate diagnosis of inherited marrow failure syndromes is critical for optimizing medical care. Expert consensus recommendations for care are published and serve as references in guiding surveillance and medical decision-making for FA, SDS, and Dyskeratosis Congenita (DC).[21-23] Although the specific details vary with each of the inherited marrow failure syndromes, the general approach involves genetic counseling, baseline screening for associated anomalies or comorbidities, counseling for particular risk factors, surveillance strategies for cytopenias and malignancies, and tailoring of medical treatment, oncologic care, or surveillance, and disease-specific HSCT including evaluation of potential related donors.

Appropriate surveillance of blood counts and bone marrow examinations not only is important for clinical care and decision-making regarding bone marrow transplantation but is also critical to identifying early signs of myelodysplastic syndrome (MDS) or abnormal cytogenetic clones prior to the development of overt leukemia. Leukemia can be especially challenging to treat for some of the marrow failure syndrome because of elevated risks of treatment-related toxicities and/or high relapse risk. Although bone marrow transplantation can be curative, many of the inherited BMF disorders require tailored conditioning regimens for bone marrow transplantation and consideration of late effects after transplant.[24] Some of these syndromes are associated with a high risk of solid tumor development, and early diagnosis when tumors are small and localized is critical, as it allows for an increased chance of curative surgical resection.[25]

Patients may develop marrow failure, which can initially manifest as cytopenias in one or more lineages. Fevers in the setting of neutropenia warrant prompt medical evaluation for appropriate cultures and treatment with broad-spectrum antibiotics. Hematopoietic growth factors (such as recombinant human granulocyte colony-stimulating factor [G-CSF]) may stabilize or improve the neutropenia, and patients should be started at low intermittent doses and titrated to effect. The main indication for G-CSF therapy is serious bacterial or fungal infection related to neutropenia, although some centers opt to initiate treatment based on the neutrophil counts. Patients with a history of recurrent or severe bacterial infections may benefit from prophylactic G-CSF. Although there is a theoretical risk that G-CSF might stimulate the growth or progression of leukemic clones, there is no direct evidence to address this.[26,27] Transfusion support with red cells or platelets should be provided as clinically indicated for severe or symptomatic anemia and thrombocytopenia. Tranexamic acid or aminocaproic acid can be helpful adjunct therapies for bleeding symptoms. There are no published reports to support the use of erythropoietin therapy unless erythropoietin levels are low. As described in the following sections, hematopoietic SCT can be a definitive treatment for marrow failure in these five inherited syndromes, although it carries its own risks and complications.

Finally, many of these syndromes are also associated with congenital anomalies, comorbidities, or specific complications such as pulmonary alveolar proteinosis in GATA2 deficiency or liver cirrhosis in DC. Identifying the appropriate members of a multidisciplinary team, whether they include nephrologists, immunologists, pulmonologists, cardiologists, or other subspecialists for each individual patient, is important in optimizing medical care.

FANCONI ANEMIA

FA is an inherited chromosomal instability syndrome with a variable clinical presentation that includes congenital anomalies, progressive pancytopenia, and cancer susceptibility. Guido Fanconi first reported a familial syndrome of pancytopenia and congenital physical abnormalities in 1927.[28,29] The diagnostic hallmark of FA is increased chromosomal breakage in response to DNA-damaging agents such as MMC or DEB. Remarkable advances in the last decade have elucidated the molecular pathways disrupted in FA cells, with several new FA genes described in the past few years.[30]

FA is found with similar frequencies in both genders and has no known ethnic restriction. The mean age at diagnosis is generally reported to be between 7 and 9 years, with 75% of cases diagnosed between the ages of 4 and 14 years; however, FA has been diagnosed in neonates as well as in adults in their 40s. The heterozygote carrier frequency has been estimated at 1 in 300 in the United States and in Europe,[31] and may be higher than previously anticipated, as many of these studies were performed when fewer causative genes had been identified. Indeed, a study using data from the Exome Sequencing Project and the 1000 Genomes Project identified 10.7% of clinically significant FA disease-associated variants within the cohort, and 78.5% of subjects carried a known FA disease-associated variant that is a much higher carrier frequency than previously estimated.[32]

Diagnostic Testing

The diagnosis of FA is based on the demonstration of increased chromosomal breakage in the presence of DNA cross-linking agents, such as DEB or MMC (*Figure 38.1*).[33,34] The chromosomal breakage test is usually performed on metaphase spreads of peripheral blood lymphocytes treated with MMC or DEB. DEB is preferred in some centers as it is associated with less variability in chromosomal breakage among normal controls. A total of 50 cells in metaphase is typically analyzed for chromosomal breakage, including the formation of radials—a hallmark of this disease. Results are generally reported as aberrations per cell and the number of cells with breaks or radial forms. Increased spontaneous chromosomal breakage may be observed in some patients with FA, particularly with subtype FANCD1, but nonetheless the rate of breakage is markedly enhanced by exposure to MMC or DEB regardless of patient phenotype or severity of disease.[35] Chromosomal breakage in response to MMC/DEB can also be assessed in fetal cells obtained for prenatal diagnosis by amniocentesis or chorionic villus sampling.[36] If the disease-causing mutations are known for a given family, DNA sequencing can be used for prenatal diagnosis or preimplantation genetic diagnosis.[37] Clonal somatic reversion to wild type has been observed in a subset of lymphocytes from some patients with FA. The reversion to normal cellular phenotype has been attributed to recombination or gene conversion or reversion-mutation events leading to selective advantage of the reverted lymphocytes.[38-40] Somatic reversion has also been reported in earlier hematopoietic lineages.[41] In such patients, increased levels of chromosomal breakage may be limited to a subpopulation of lymphocytes, but patients with a high degree of wild-type lymphocyte mosaicism may be difficult to diagnose. In cases with a high degree of suspicion for FA and normal blood breakage analysis, the MMC/DEB test should be performed on skin fibroblasts.

FA patient cells also exhibit cell cycle abnormalities with G_2 phase prolongation and arrest by flow cytometry.[42,43] While some studies have documented an increase of serum α-fetoprotein in patients with FA, it is not found to be consistently elevated in all patients with FA, and the lack of its specificity has limited its diagnostic utility.[44,45]

FA heterozygous carriers cannot be reliably detected by testing for chromosomal breakage. Genetic testing is available for some of the FA genes.

Clinical Features

FA should be considered in patients with congenital anomalies, AA, or a family history of BMF or cancer susceptibility. The International

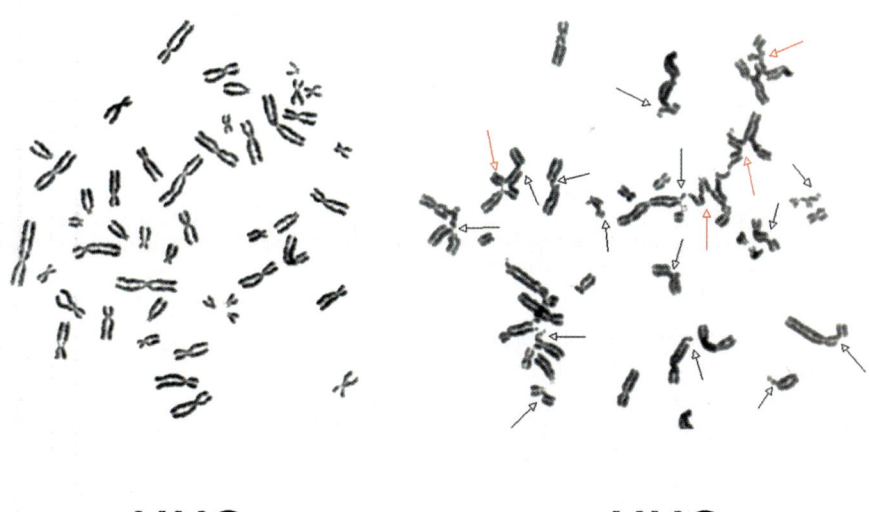

FIGURE 38.1 Chromosomal breakage in Fanconi anemia (FA). Peripheral blood lymphocytes from a patient with FA were cultured without (left panel) or with (right panel) mitomycin C (MMC). The black arrows indicate chromosomal breaks. The red arrows indicate radial chromosomal fusions characteristic of FA. (Courtesy of Lisa Moreau, Dana Farber Cancer Institute, Boston, MA.)

−MMC   +MMC

Disorders of Red Blood Cells

Fanconi Anemia Registry analysis of 370 patients found that nearly 40% of patients had no reported physical findings, and a 20-year follow-up of clinical information on 754 patients with FA highlights the heterogeneity of presentations and has collected information with the goal of improving the understanding of the relationship between genotype and phenotype.[46,47] The manifestations of FA can also vary between affected members of the same family, suggesting that additional factors, possibly genetic, epigenetic, or environmental, likely influence the disease course.

AA or malignancy may be the presenting sign of the underlying diagnosis of FA in the absence of physical anomalies or prior family history. The hematologic complications of FA typically present within the first decade of life. Early manifestations include moderate single or bilineage cytopenias with red cell macrocytosis.[11] Marrow failure may range in severity from mild, asymptomatic cytopenias to severe AA. The cumulative incidence of marrow failure was estimated in one study to be as high as 90% by 40 years of age.[47]

A wide range of congenital anomalies has been reported in patients with FA (*Table 38.1*).[48] A recent meta-analysis of phenotypical abnormalities in patients with FA found that 79% of patients had at least one or more abnormalities: the most common manifestations associated with FA were short stature (43%), upper limb (radial ray) abnormalities (40%), skin pigmentation changes including café au lait macules (37%), renal malformations (27%), and microcephaly (27%).[48] Other classical abnormalities of the skeletal, ocular, renal, genital, aural, gastrointestinal (GI), cardiac, and central nervous systems include those described in the VACTERL-H association (*v*ertebral anomalies, *a*nal atresia, *c*ardiovascular malformations, *t*racheoesophageal fistula, *r*enal and *l*imb anomalies, plus *h*ydrocephalus), and 5% to 30% of patients with FA are reported to meet these criteria.[49] However, a subset of patients with FA lack any apparent physical findings and may present with BMF, MDS, or malignancy as their sole manifestation. Immunologic abnormalities have been variably reported in some patients with FA but are not a common finding. These include lower numbers of total lymphocytes and CD4 T cells and decreased levels of immunoglobulins including IgG, IgA, and IgM in adults with FA. Many, but not all, patients with FA have short stature that may be intrinsic or may be exacerbated by endocrine abnormalities such as growth hormone deficiency.[50] Additional endocrine disorders associated with FA include hypothyroidism with or without thyroid hormone–binding globulin deficiency, abnormal glucose or insulin metabolism, diabetes mellitus, dyslipidemia, hypogonadism, pubertal delay, and impaired fertility.[50] Patients with FA are also at risk of endocrine abnormalities secondary to their medical therapies, including exposure to androgens, treatment with corticosteroids for graft-versus-host disease (GVHD), and/or total-body irradiation and chemotherapy exposure for conditioning with bone marrow transplant.

Patients with FA are at increased risk of developing myelodysplasia (MDS) or acute myeloid leukemia (AML).[51,52] In a cohort study of 145 patients with FA, the cumulative incidence of AML reached 10% by age 24 years and plateaued thereafter,[53] and a similar estimate was found in the National Cancer Institute cohort with a cumulative AML incidence of 10% by age 50 years.[54] Patients with FA are also at increased risk of developing solid tumors, particularly squamous cell carcinomas of the head and neck, skin, GI tract, and genital tract.[55] The cumulative incidence of solid tumors was low in younger patients but increases dramatically for patients 20 years or older and can reach 28% by age 40 to 49 years.[53,56] Patients with the D1 FA subtype manifest an especially high rate of early-onset AML and specific solid tumors (brain tumors and Wilms).[35,57] Patients with FA, particularly those who have received androgen treatment, are also at increased risk of liver tumors and peliosis hepatis.

Differential Diagnosis

Other inherited and acquired causes of BMF should be considered. FA may be considered in patients with characteristic congenital anomalies and may be the underlying diagnosis in some patients with VACTERL-H.[49,58] Screening patients with VACTERL-H for features of FA with the acronym PHENOS (*p*igmentation, small *h*ead, small *e*yes, central *n*ervous system, *o*tology, and *s*hort stature) or assessment for concomitant cytopenia or unexplained red cell macrocytosis may help identify patients who should undergo a diagnostic workup with FA.[49]

Cells derived from patients with other chromosomal breakage syndromes or syndromes with similar constitutional findings, such as Bloom syndrome or ataxia telangiectasia, may exhibit high rates of spontaneous chromosomal breakage; however, they do not show increased chromosomal breakage in response to DNA cross-linking agents such as MMC or DEB. Most other chromosomal breakage syndromes are not typically associated with marrow failure. The exception is Nijmegen breakage syndrome, which may be associated with increased chromosomal breakage with MMC/DEB and may be confused with FA.[59] FA may also be considered in patients with a family history suggestive of cancer predisposition, patients presenting with cancers at an unusually young age, or patients who experience severe toxicity with chemotherapy or radiation. A negative family history does not rule out the diagnosis of FA.

Laboratory Features

Cell morphology on peripheral blood smear is typically unremarkable except for red cell macrocytosis, although this is variably

Table 38.1. Physical Findings Associated With Fanconi Anemia

Skeletal
  Microsomia: Short stature
  Radii: absent or hypoplastic
  Ulnae: short or dysplastic
  Thumb: absent or hypoplastic, bifid, duplicated, attached by a thread, triphalangeal, long, low set
  Hand anomalies: flat thenar eminence, absent first metacarpal, clinodactyly, polydactyly
  Hip and spine anomalies: hip dislocation, spina bifida, scoliosis, hemivertebrae, abnormal ribs, coccygeal aplasia
  Feet: congenital vertical talus ("rocker bottom foot"), club feet, abnormal toes, toe syndactyly

Skin
  Hyperpigmentation: Café au lait spots
  Hypopigmentation

Gastrointestinal malformations
  Esophageal atresia or tracheoesophageal fistula
  Imperforate anus
  Annular pancreas
  Malrotation
  Low birth weight

Genitourinary
  Renal anomalies: horseshoe, ectopic or pelvic, abnormal or dysplastic, absent, hydronephrosis or hydroureter
  Hypogonadism, undescended testes, hypospadias, micropenis, absent testes, bicornuate uterus, uterus malposition, small ovaries

Craniofacial
  Microcephaly
  Hydrocephaly
  Face: triangular, birdlike, dysmorphic, micrognathia, mid-face hypoplasia
  Ophthalmic anomalies: microphthalmia, epicanthal folds, strabismus, hypotelorism, hypertelorism, cataracts, astigmatism, ptosis
  Otic anomalies: external ear anomalies (abnormal shape, dysplastic, atretic, narrow ear canal), abnormal middle ear anomalies, deafness

Cardiac malformations
  Congenital heart disease: patent ductus arteriosus, atrial septal defect, ventricular septal defect, coarctation, situs inversus, truncus arteriosus

Central Nervous System
  Small pituitary, pituitary stalk interruption syndrome, absent corpus callosum, cerebellar hypoplasia, hydrocephalus, dilated ventricles
  Mental retardation, developmental delay

present. Thrombocytopenia or leukopenia typically precede anemia. Pancytopenia may be progressive over time. Erythrocyte macrocytosis and increased hemoglobin F levels may be present even in the absence of cytopenias.

Bone marrow biopsy findings vary from normal cellularity to frank aplasia. Morphologic examination of the bone marrow aspirate may show dysplastic features, with nuclear-cytoplasmic maturation dyssynchrony. Hyposegmented nuclei may be noted in the neutrophil lineage. Dyserythropoiesis with multinucleate forms or nuclear fragmentation may be seen. Bone marrow aspirates should be sent for cytogenetic analysis, as patients with FA are at high risk for malignant transformation. Frequent chromosomal aberrations in patients with FA include gains of the chromosomal regions 1q and 3q and partial or complete loss of chromosome 7.[60] Of these, 7/del7q or amplification or gains of chromosome 3q26q29 or complex cytogenetic abnormalities have been associated with elevated risk of transformation into MDS or AML.[61] The appearance of cytogenetic clones of unclear clinical significance in the absence of morphologic evidence of MDS must be considered carefully, as cases of persistent or transient clonal abnormalities without imminent progression to leukemia have been reported

and were found to predict worse 5-year survival for patients with FA.[62] At a minimum, patients with persistent unexplained changes in blood counts or new cytogenetic marrow abnormalities should be monitored closely with serial blood counts and a follow-up bone marrow examination to assess for possible malignant evolution.

Pathophysiology

Models of the FA biochemical pathway have emerged from molecular studies of the cloned FA gene products. For space reasons, an abbreviated overview is provided here. The reader is referred to recent excellent reviews of this rapidly evolving field for additional information.[63-65] At the time of writing this chapter, at least 23 different FA complementation groups (A, B, C, D1 [*BRCA2*], D2, E, F, G, I, J [*BRIP1/BACH1*], L, M, N [*PALB2*], O [*RAD51C*], P [*SLX4*], Q [*ERCC4*], R [*RAD51*], S [*BRCA1*], T [*UBE2T*], U [*XRCC2*], V [*MAD2L2/REV7*], and W [*RFWD3*]) and their corresponding genes have been identified (*Table 38.2*).[66,67] Other potential genes are being currently investigated, and there are emerging data for *FAAP100* as a potential FA subtype Y.[68-70] With the exception of subtype B, which is X-linked recessive, and subtype R, which is autosomal dominant, all

Table 38.2. Fanconi Anemia Genes

Subtype	Gene	Proportion of Patients with FA (%)	Inheritance Pattern	Chromosome Location	Function
A	*FANCA*	60	Autosomal recessive	16q24.3	FA core complex
B	*FANCB*	2	X-linked recessive	Xp22.31	FA core complex
C	*FANCC*	14	Autosomal recessive	9q22.3	FA core complex
D1	*FANCD1/BRCA2*	3	Autosomal recessive	13q12-13	Homologous recombination, fork stabilization
D2	*FANCD2*	3	Autosomal recessive	3p25.3	Binds to FANCI, localizes to chromatin and recruits DNA repair proteins
E	*FANCE*	3	Autosomal recessive	6p21-22	FA core complex
F	*FANCF*	2	Autosomal recessive	11p15	FA core complex
G	*FANCG*	10	Autosomal recessive	9p13	FA core complex
I	*FANCI*	1	Autosomal recessive	15q25-q26	Binds to D2, localizes to chromatin and recruits DNA repair proteins
J	*FANCJ/BACH1/BRIP1*	2	Autosomal recessive	17q22-q24	Homologous recombination, TLS
L	*FANCL/PHF9/POG*	<1	Autosomal recessive	2p16.1	FA core complex, E3 ubiquitin ligase function
M	*FANCM/Hef*	<1	Autosomal recessive	14q21.3	FAMCM anchor complex, binds to stalled replication forks
N	*FANCN/PALB2*	<1	Autosomal recessive	16p12	Homologous recombination
O	*FANCO/RAD51C*	<1	Autosomal recessive	17q22	Homologous recombination
P	*FANCP/SLX4*	<1	Autosomal recessive	16p13.3	Unhooks ICLs, nuclease scaffold
Q	*FANCQ/ERCC4*	<1	Autosomal recessive	16p13.12	Unhooks ICLs, DNA incision, nucleotide excision repair
R	*FANCR/RAD51*	<1	Autosomal dominant	15q15.1	Homologous recombination, fork stabilization
S	*FANCS/BRCA1*	<1	Autosomal recessive	17q21.31	Homologous recombination, fork stabilization
T	*FANCT/UBE2T*	<1	Autosomal recessive	1q32.1	Associates with FA core complex and FANCM, E2 ubiquitin-conjugating enzyme function
U	*FANCU/XRCC2*	<1	Autosomal recessive	7q36.1	Homologous recombination
V	*FANCV/REV7*	<1	Autosomal recessive	1p36.22	Subunit of TLS polymerase
W	*FANCW/RFWD3*	<1	Autosomal recessive	16q23.1	WD40-containing E3 ubiquitin ligase, accumulates at the replication forks as part of the DNA damage response

Abbreviations: FA, Fanconi anemia; ICLs, interstrand cross-links; TLS, translesion synthesis.

the other FA subtypes follow an autosomal recessive pattern of inheritance. The most common FA subtype is FA-A (66%), followed by FA-C (10%) and FA-G (10%); the other FA subtypes are rare.[71] The mutations associated with FA are highly variable.[72]

The FA genes function in a common molecular pathway to regulate DNA repair.[30] Loss of function of any FA gene results in impaired DNA repair, resulting in sensitivity to DNA interstrand cross-links (ICLs), which can block the progression of DNA replication. Stimuli such as S-phase entry, DNA cross-links induced by agents such as DEB/MMC, or ionizing radiation can lead to activation of the FA core complex. The FA complex consists of three modules, E3 monoubiquitinating ligase FANCB-FANCL-FAAP100, and two other subcomplexes FANCA-FANCG-FAAP20 and FANCC-FANCE-FANCF.[69,73] The FA core complex associates with FANCT (UBE2T), an E2 ubiquitin-conjugating enzyme.[74] This interaction is aided by the FANCM anchor complex (composed of FANCM, FAAP24, FAAP16, and MHF1), which binds to stalled replication forks at sites of unresolved ICLs.[75-78] An intact FA core complex together with FANCT is required for the monoubiquitination of FANCD2 and FANCI, which is required for the assembly of the DNA repair machinery and MMC resistance.[79-81] Of note, FANCD2 monoubiquitination remains intact in BMF syndromes other than FA.[82] The ID2 complex (FANCI and FANCD2) subsequently localizes to chromatin and recruits DNA repair proteins together with FANCS, FANCD1, and FANCR.[64,73] SLX4/FANCP and ERCC4/FANCQ allow unhooking of ICLs and subsequent translesion DNA synthesis.[83] FANCV is one of the subunits within translesion synthesis polymerase Polζ involved in DNA synthesis and was recently described as a new FA gene.[84]

The remaining FA proteins promote homologous recombination (HR) to repair DNA during ICLs repair and include RAD51/FANCR, BRCA2/FANCD1, PALB2/FANCN, RAD51C/FANCO, BRCA1/FANCS, and XRCC2/FANCU.[30,85] Without these FA proteins, ICLs are unable to be resolved, HR cannot occur effectively, and alternative repair pathways such as nonhomologous end joining (NHEJ) are utilized. However, NHEJ leads to a higher incidence of errors with DNA repair as compared with HR,[86] which may contribute to the higher rates of cancer in patients with FA. However, recent studies suggest that repair mechanisms independent of classic NHEJ may contribute to chromosomal aberrations in FA deficient cells.[87]

Elucidation of the FA biochemical pathway in turn led to the identification of interactions between the FA proteins and other known tumor suppressor pathways. These findings provide biochemical support for a role of the FA pathway in tumorigenesis. While FA is caused by biallelic mutations in the FA genes, monoallelic mutations in six of these genes including BRCA1 (also known as FANCS), BRCA2 (also known as FANCD1), FANCJ (also known as BRIP1), FANCM, PALB2 (also known as FANCN), and RAD51C (also known as FANCO) are associated with a higher risk of breast/ovarian cancer or other solid tumors such as head and neck cancers.[88,89] The gene for FA complementation group D1 (FA-D1) is the previously identified tumor suppressor gene BRCA2.[90] Interestingly, the spectrum of tumors observed for patients with FA-D1 include T-ALL, medulloblastoma, and Wilms tumor, which differs markedly from that of BRCA2 mutation carriers and other FA complementation groups.[35,57,71]

Given the compelling biochemical data linking the FA pathway to other known DNA repair pathways functioning in tumor suppression, the question of whether asymptomatic FA heterozygotes carry an increased risk of developing malignancies is a subject of active investigation. Heterozygous BRCA1 and BRCA2 mutations are associated with breast and ovarian cancer risk.[91] The reason why breast and ovarian cancer is uncommon in the FA population is not known, but it may be related to decreased estrogen levels in these patients[92] or to competing risks as patients with FA may have a shorter life expectancy below the typical age of onset of breast and ovarian cancers. Currently, not all FANCD1/BRCA2 mutations reported in patients with FA have been associated with increased cancer risk in heterozygous carriers in the general population, and it is currently unclear whether all the FANCD1/BRCA2 variants leading to FA (when both alleles are mutated) will also confer cancer predisposition in family members in

whom only one of these FA-variant BRCA2 alleles may be present.[57] Therefore, counseling of FA-carrier family members of patients with FA requires expertise in cancer genetics.

Another example of interactions between the FA proteins and other known tumor suppressor pathways is FANCD2, which is phosphorylated by the ATM kinase and this step is required for the cell cycle S-phase checkpoint in response to ionizing radiation.[93] Thus, FANCD2 links two DNA repair pathways associated with increased cancer susceptibility, the FA pathway and the ataxia telangiectasia pathway.[93] The FA pathway also intersects with other DNA damage response proteins including ATR, CHK1, and γ-H2AX.

In addition to a nuclear role in DNA repair, numerous studies suggest additional functions for the FA proteins. FA cells are sensitive to many different extracellular apoptotic signals, such as γ-interferon, tumor necrosis factor-α (TNF-α), and double-stranded RNA.[94,95] FA proteins may have additional roles in other signaling pathways, including autophagy, mitophagy, virophagy, mitochondrial quality control, and response to oxidative stress.[96-101] These new findings might explain how the environment influences FA disease progression and perhaps account at least in part for some of the observed heterogeneity between patients with FA. Whether antioxidants can change DNA damage parameters or improve hematopoiesis in patients with FA continues to be studied.[102]

The FA pathway has also been linked to tumor suppressor p53. FA-deficient hematopoietic stem/progenitor cells show activation of the p53/p21 axis and subsequently undergo cell cycle arrest and accelerated terminal differentiation.[103,104] One recent study identified growth arrest specific 6 (GAS6) as a novel target of activated p53 in FA-deficient HPCs, and when targeted, it can rescue hematopoiesis in these cells.[104] These findings are further supported by the demonstration that knockdown of p53 expression in a zebrafish model of FA rescues developmental abnormalities.[105] Because p53 knockdown rescues hematopoietic abnormalities in other marrow failure syndromes, p53 may represent a final common pathway for cellular stress or DNA damage in marrow failure syndromes. Abrogation of DNA damage checkpoints has been associated with a milder marrow failure phenotype; however, these patients with FA remained at risk for malignant transformation to leukemia.[106] A potential role for toxins in the severity of the FA phenotype has been demonstrated in murine models in which disruption of the FA pathway resulted in increased sensitivity to reactive aldehydes associated with an increased risk of developmental anomalies and a propensity to develop leukemias.[107] The understanding of the interaction between FA proteins and the aldehyde pathway has expanded in the past several years after the initial studies demonstrated that Aldh2$^{-/-}$ Fancd2$^{-/-}$ as well as Adh5$^{-/-}$ Fancd2$^{-/-}$ mice develop marrow failure at an accelerated rate compared with Fancd2$^{-/-}$ mice with intact Aldh2 or Adh5 function.[108,109] ALDH2 and ADH5 are enzymes responsible for detoxification of acetaldehydes and formaldehyde, respectively. Aldehydes are natural products of cellular metabolism. ICLs induced by acetaldehyde have been shown to activate the FA pathway through colocalization of Rad51/Fancr in animal models,[110] as well as increase FANCD2 monoubiquitination and BRCA1/FANCS phosphorylation in human cell lines.[111,112]

Human studies performed in Japan, where aldehyde dehydrogenase 2 (ALDH2) mutations are common, demonstrate that concurrent ALDH2 deficiency (from an ALDH2*2 variant E540K polymorphism) and FA correlate with a more severe phenotype including accelerated marrow failure and increased incidence of developmental defects.[113] However, another study could not find any difference in patients with FA regarding their MDS/AML-free survival depending on their ALDH2 genotype.[114] It has been shown that endogenous aldehydes alter the development of particularly susceptible stem cell populations, while damaging their DNA and leading to irreversible mutations.[115,116] Interestingly, aldehyde metabolism may also play a role in idiopathic AA, as the ALDH2*2/ALDH2*2 homozygous genotype was associated with younger age at diagnosis of BMF and these patients had a lower rate of failure-free survival after immunosuppressive therapy.[117] Aldehydes, in part through mutations in ALDH2 and ADH5, may modify the phenotype of patients with FA.[115]

TGF-β had been shown previously to be an important regulator of hematopoiesis but had not been linked to FA until recently.[118] Recent studies implicate that BMF in FA is at least partially caused by a hyperactive growth-suppressive TGF-β pathway and likely also by high expression of *MYC*, which promotes cell differentiation and egress of the FA hematopoietic stem cells (HSCs) from bone marrow to peripheral blood, which may contribute to the BMF with FA.[119] In recent experiments, inhibition of the TGF-β pathway using a potent TGF-β1- and TGF-β3-specific inhibitor led to increased survival of murine FA HSCs and in a human preclinical models of human HPCs from patients with FA.[120] TGF-β pathway inhibition has been shown to tip the balance of DNA repair pathways toward HR and away from the more deleterious NHEJ pathway. Although TGF-β inhibition has not been tested in patients with FA in vivo, pharmacologic inhibition of TGF-β may be a promising way to target the DNA repair defects and decrease apoptosis of HSCs in FA.

Supportive Care

Cancer surveillance and education plays an important role in the management of patients with FA. Physicians should counsel patients regarding established behavioral and environmental factors associated with increased cancer risk such as tobacco or alcohol exposure. Because patients with FA have a defect in DNA repair, imaging studies should minimize exposure to ionizing radiation.

Because of the increased risk of MDS and leukemia in patients with BMF syndromes, frequent complete blood counts (CBCs) and annual bone marrow aspirates and biopsies with cytogenetic analysis have been recommended by an expert panel, particularly as HSCT outcomes are superior for patients transplanted prior to the emergence of leukemia.[121] Patients with FA are at risk for clonal cytogenetic abnormalities.[122] Assessment of the clinical significance of a cytogenetic clonal abnormality requires consideration of the specific clone, the number of chromosomal abnormalities, the presence of significant marrow dysplasia (some baseline mild dysplasia is common in FA), and whether there are concomitant progressive peripheral cytopenias.[60,123] Chromosomal abnormalities common in AML, such as t(8;21), inv(16), or trisomy 8, have not been reported in FA.[124] Amplifications of 3q are common in FA as a clonal abnormality but are rarely seen in other patients with AML. Patients with FA AML have a higher frequency of 1q amplification, loss of part or all of chromosome 7, gain of 13q, and del 20q.[124,125]

Annual examination by an otolaryngologist for leukoplakia or other signs of squamous cell carcinoma of the oral cavity and oropharynx is important for patients with FA, DC, and those patients with FA previously treated with bone marrow transplantation. Annual endoscopy can be considered in older patients with FA. Regular dental examinations are important both for maintenance of oral hygiene and for detecting leukoplakia. Patients should be evaluated immediately for symptoms of pain in the mouth or throat, difficulty swallowing, changes in voice, anorexia, or weight loss. Suspicious lesions should be biopsied, because early surgical excision is the mainstay of cancer therapy in patients with FA.

GI symptoms are common in patients with FA, but attention should be paid to the possibility of GI tumors or liver tumors. Regular liver ultrasound evaluations are recommended, particularly for patients receiving androgen therapy.

Annual gynecologic examinations, including Pap smears and human papilloma virus (HPV) examinations, are recommended at puberty or after the age of 16 years due to the increased risk of vulvar and genital tract tumors. Vaccination against HPV should be offered to patients with FA. Counseling regarding sexual activity should be provided as this poses an increased risk for neutropenic and thrombocytopenic patients. Barrier methods of contraception may be particularly pertinent for the patients with FA who are already at risk of cervical and vulvar malignancies. HPV, which has been associated with an increased risk of squamous cell carcinoma of the head and neck, expresses the high-risk HPV E6/E7 oncoproteins, which disrupt cross-link repair by causing accumulation of FANCD2 at the sites away from DNA damage and delayed FANCD2 deubiquitination, critically important for effective repair of ICLs.[126]

Regular breast examinations are also recommended, although it is not clear what role mammography should play in cancer screening of these patients given the increased sensitivity to radiation. Regular endocrinology evaluations are important, particularly in the pediatric population if the patient exhibits poor growth or delayed puberty. A recent study reported one or more endocrine abnormalities in 79% of patients with FA.[127] Current guidelines recommend assessing thyroid function, growth hormone, glucose and lipid, fertility, and bone health.[50]

Treatment

HSCT is the only curative therapy for the hematologic manifestations of FA. However, conditioning regimens require careful tailoring for patients with FA, as these patients are exquisitely sensitive to the toxicity of the usual chemotherapy and radiation regimens used in preparation for BMT.[128] Conditioning regimens may confer an increased risk of subsequent malignancies, and dose adjustments were necessary to improve the overall survival of patients with FA undergoing HSCT.[129-131] Reduced dose conditioning regimens and low-dose irradiation have been the standard conditioning regimen over the last few decades, often using a matched sibling donor, and have resulted in survivorship of up to 80% for patients with FA with BMF.[132-134] Post-HSCT malignancies, especially squamous cell carcinomas of the head and neck are a long-term risk, especially for patients experiencing chronic GVHD, and are as frequent as 8% and 14% at 10 and 15 years after transplantation in a recent study.[135] Clinical trials replacing radiation with fludarabine, a potent immunosuppressive agent with less cytotoxicity, have reported successful engraftment using either HLA-matched family member donors or alternative donors.[136-138]

Medical therapies are available for patients who lack a suitable HSCT donor or for whom the risk of HSCT is high. Androgens may improve the blood counts in approximately 50% of patients with FA. Experience is greatest with oxymetholone, but widespread use is limited by its associated virilizing side effects, which are particularly problematic for female patients or very young patients. Fewer virilizing side effects are reported with danazol or oxandrolone.[139,140]

Suggested treatment guidelines have been proposed by a consensus committee of the Fanconi Anemia Research Foundation, although these guidelines must be individualized for each patient and undergo continuous modification as new data emerge. The suggestion of the committee is to consider an allogeneic stem cell transplant or androgen therapy for symptomatic or severe BMF defined as hemoglobin below 8 g/dL, platelet count below 30,000/mm^3, or neutrophil count below 500/mm^3. The earliest and most frequent response to androgens is seen in red cells, with reticulocytosis and increase in hemoglobin generally occurring within the first 1 to 2 months of treatment. Responses in the white cell count and platelet count are variable and may not be seen until 6 to 12 months of therapy. Resistance to therapy often develops over time (generally years). A common androgen regimen consists of oxymetholone 2 to 5 mg/kg/d or danazol 5 mg/kg and tapered to 2.6 mg/kg, but the goal of androgen therapy is to taper to the minimal effective dose while carefully monitoring blood counts.[23,140]

Side effects of androgen administration include liver toxicity such as elevated liver enzymes, cholestasis, peliosis hepatis, and increased propensity to develop hepatic tumors (adenomas and hepatomas). Other side effects of androgens include acne, oily skin, enlarged penis/clitoris, hoarseness/voice deepening, hair growth or hair loss, behavioral changes, hot flashes, breast enlargement or tenderness, amenorrhea, hypertension, premature closure of epiphyses, fluid retention, and secondary hypertension. For patients on androgen therapy, regular physical examinations for liver size, liver ultrasound for masses or abnormalities every 6 to 12 months, and frequent liver enzyme tests are recommended given the risk of transaminitis, cholestatic jaundice, hepatic adenomas, hepatocellular carcinomas, and Peliosis hepatis while on androgen therapy. Given the risk of premature epiphyseal closure, bone ages studies are recommended every 6 to 12 months.[23]

Disorders of Red Blood Cells

Hematopoietic growth factors such as G-CSF or GM-CSF have been shown to improve the neutrophil count in the majority of treated patients.[141,142] In a few patients, platelet or red cell counts have also improved following treatment with G-CSF.[142] Growth factor treatment is generally not recommended for patients with MDS and is generally avoided for those with a clonal cytogenetic abnormality of the bone marrow, although there are no available data that directly address whether G-CSF increases leukemia risk. It is reasonable to perform a bone marrow aspirate and biopsy as well as cytogenetic studies prior to the initiation of growth factor therapy and monitor regularly throughout therapy. Alternative medical therapies to improve hematopoiesis are urgently needed, especially for patients who are not candidates for HSCT or who lack a suitable donor.

Results of a gene therapy trial have been first reported in patients with *FANCC*.[143] Three patients with FA-C underwent three to four cycles of retroviral transduction of G-CSF-mobilized peripheral blood CD34+ mononuclear cells (MNCs), whereas a fourth patient received a single infusion of transduced cells. The transduced wild-type *FANCC* gene was detected in peripheral blood and bone marrow MNC in association with increased hematopoietic colony growth in vitro. Transient improvement in bone marrow cellularity accompanied these findings and two patients experienced a transient improvement in blood counts. Using a lentiviral approach, CD34+ cells from four pediatric patients with FA subtype A were mobilized with G-CSF and plerixafor and transduced with corrected *FANCA* lentiviral vector, and the gene-corrected CD34+ cells were infused to the retrospective patients once BMF was evident without receiving any conditioning prior to the infusion.[144] All patients showed robust and progressive engraftment of the gene-corrected infused HSCs with increasing number of corrected leukocytes and presence of corrected CD34+ HSC in the bone marrow, as well as increases in MMC resistance. Of note, using cytogenetic studies and array analysis of myeloid cancer genes have not detected leukemogenic events in any of the treated patients. Further work will need to be done to overcome potential limitations including low CD34+ cell numbers,[145] poor ex vivo expansion of hematopoietic stem/progenitor cells,[146,147] and the residual risk of leukemia associated with the remaining noncorrected hematopoietic cells.[41] The development of leukemia in a few patients receiving gene therapy for X-linked severe combined immunodeficiency raises concerns about the potential growth advantage theoretically conferred by gene correction of a preleukemic hematopoietic stem/progenitor cell in patients with FA.[148] Additional studies to optimize ex vivo expansion of HSCs are ongoing. Gene therapy attempts and approaches in FA are summarized in recent articles.[149,150]

Published data to guide management of cancer in FA are scarce. Treatment of malignancies is limited by the increased sensitivity of patients with FA to the effects of chemotherapy and radiation. Myeloid malignancies in eligible patients with FA have been successfully treated with HSCT.[121,151] However, its treatment is challenging, and although transplant can be effective in the treatment of MDS or AML, the long-term overall survival rate with this therapy is still only around 30% to 40%.[121]

Patients with FA transplanted in complete remission showed better overall survival in a retrospective analysis of the EBMT group.[152] In a recent analysis in Japan, the outcome was significantly better in patients with FA with BMF than in patients with FA with MDS or acute leukemia with a 5-year overall survival of 89%, 71%, and 44%, respectively, after undergoing HSCT,[153] similarly to previous studies.[154] The role of pretransplant cytoreductive chemotherapy remains unclear at this time as patients are susceptible to organ toxicities and prolonged or intractable cytopenias with chemotherapy. Patients also have a better outcome if they undergo transplant at a younger age and have an HLA-matched sibling donor.[121,154,155] Successful treatment of solid tumors is typically best attained with surgical excision of localized tumors. Treatment with chemotherapy or radiation is limited by the high rates of toxic side effects such as mucositis or prolonged or intractable marrow suppression.

Regular and frequent surveillance for cancers is particularly important in this population and is discussed above.

TELOMERE BIOLOGY DISORDERS/DYSKERATOSIS CONGENITA

TBDs are a group of inherited disorders classically characterized by lacey reticular skin pigmentation, nail dystrophy, and leukoplakia (the diagnostic triad). TBD was first described in 1906 and was initially called Zinsser-Cole-Engman syndrome.[156,157] The advent of genetic testing and telomere length analysis revealed a broad spectrum of clinical phenotype; indeed, the classical clinical triad is absent in a subset of patients. X-linked recessive, autosomal dominant, and autosomal recessive inheritance patterns have been reported. Patients exhibit a predisposition to BMF, malignancy, and pulmonary dysfunction. See excellent recent reviews for additional details.[158,159]

Diagnostic Testing

Telomere length analysis is a useful diagnostic screen for TBD as patients with TBD typically exhibit very short (less than first percentile of age-matched controls) telomeres in lymphocytes measured by multicolor flow cytometric fluorescent in situ hybridization (Flow-FISH). Shortened telomere length in granulocytes is a nonspecific finding frequently observed in BMF without a primary telomere disorder. Shortened telomere length below the 1st percentile for age in at least three lymphocyte subsets is highly suspicious for a telomere biology disorder.[160,161] Telomere length can be assessed by multiple methods of analysis including Flow-FISH, which is the clinically validated diagnostic test for TBD; quantitative polymerase chain reaction (qPCR), which provides a relative estimate of telomere length; and Southern blot analysis to estimate the median telomere length of total leukocytes.[162-164] Results of telomere length testing must be interpreted within the clinical context of the patient and by providers experienced in interpreting these results. Caution is warranted in the interpretation of results for patients with conditions with high HSC turnover or primary immunodeficiency, which may show very low lymphocyte telomere length without a constitutional telomere defect. Telomere length may also fall above the 1st percentile for age in a subset of adults with telomere biology disorders. Genetic testing together with telomere length testing, careful assessment for clinical features of TBD, and family history should be integrated in the diagnostic evaluation of TBD. However, given the incomplete genetic characterization of TBD, a subset of patients diagnosed clinically with TBD may not have evidence of a pathogenic mutation in the TBD genes known to date, and measurement of telomere lengths provides a useful diagnostic screen.

It is increasingly apparent that the classical clinical syndrome of TBD represents only one spectrum of the disease. Previously unrecognized milder forms exhibiting only isolated findings or marrow failure alone may now be identified through astute testing. As revertant somatic mosaicism can occur in TBD (similar to FA), if patients have manifestations of TBD such as pulmonary fibrosis or the diagnostic triad with normal telomere length testing of leukocytes, DNA from skin fibroblasts can be used for testing.[165]

Clinical Features

TBD can be inherited in an X-linked recessive, autosomal dominant, or autosomal recessive pattern or mutations in the associated genes can arise de novo. A variety of clinical features have been described in patients with TBD, but its classic triad consists of reticular skin pigmentation, oral leukoplakia, and nail dystrophy. The range of physical findings in female patients is similar to those reported in male patients.[166] Most of the somatic abnormalities are not present early in life but develop progressively with age. Both the tempo of symptom progression and symptom severity are highly variable between patients, and the classic triad of skin, nail, and oral findings is lacking in most patients. These symptoms generally appear between the ages of 5 and 10 years, with a median age of onset between 6 and 8 years (range 0.5-26 years).[166] Nail dystrophy can range from minimal nail irregularities to progressive atrophy and even complete nail loss. TBD may be mistaken for chronic GVHD in patients transplanted for AA, and care must be taken to diagnose these patients prior to transplant.[167,168] Other clinical characteristics include skin pigmentation changes beyond the upper chest and neck, as well as ophthalmic, dental, skeletal, pulmonary, gastrointestinal, liver, hematological, vascular, and immunological abnormalities (*Table 38.3*). The main mortality reasons in patients with TBD are BMF, lung disease, and malignancy such as squamous cell carcinoma of the head/neck or anogenital cancer, MDS, or AML. Peripheral cytopenias of two or more peripheral lineages were affected in most of the Dyskeratosis Congenita Registry patients, although single-lineage cytopenias, most commonly thrombocytopenia, were also reported.[166] The median age

Table 38.3. Summary of Major Physical Findings Associated With Telomere Biology Disorders

Skeletal
Osteoporosis
Aseptic necrosis
Scoliosis
Dental caries/tooth loss
Integumentary
Skin pigmentary abnormalities
Nail dystrophy
Leukoplakia
Hair loss/gray hair/sparse eyelashes
Hyperhidrosis
Gastrointestinal and growth
Esophageal stricture
Liver disease
Enteropathy
Short stature
Intrauterine growth retardation
Genitourinary
Hypogonadism
Urethral stricture
Phimosis
Craniofacial
Microcephaly
Epiphora
Blepharitis
Cognitive/developmental delay
Deafness
Ataxia
Pulmonary Fibrosis
With reduced diffusion capacity
and/or restrictive pulmonary disease
Abnormal vasculature and telangiectasias
Abnormalities in the pulmonary microvasculature
Pulmonary arteriovenous malformations
Gastrointestinal vascular ectasias
Immune dysregulation
Cytopenia
Reduced numbers of B, NK, or T cells
Reduced stimulation by phytohemagglutinin

of onset of pancytopenia was 8 years, with 50% developing pancytopenia below the age of 10 years.[166] BMF or its associated complications accounted for the majority of deaths (67%). The National Cancer Institute Inherited Bone Marrow Failure Syndrome study reported the cumulative incidence of marrow failure as 50% by age 50 years.[54] Approximately 20% of patients develop pulmonary disease with reduced diffusion capacity and/or restrictive pulmonary disease or pulmonary arteriovenous malformations, which may also be the first presenting symptoms of TBD in adults.[166,169-172] Pulmonary complications account for nearly 10% of deaths.[166,173] In addition, patients can also have vascular ectasias in the GI tract similar to the vascular abnormalities that are found in the lung, leading to recurrent GI bleeding.[174]

Patients with TBD have an increased incidence of cancer, for both solid tumors and leukemia. The risk for cancer increases with age and is more likely to affect patients after their third decade of life if they have not undergone HSCT, whereas the risk may increase at an earlier age if they received an HSCT.[175] The cumulative incidence of solid tumors is 20% by age 65 years without HSCT, and it dramatically increases to more than 60% in the third decade of life for patients who undergo HSCT.[175] The actuarial risk of cancer absent of any competing risks is approximately 40% by age 50 years and 60% by age 68 years.[176] An increased incidence of MDS and AML has also been observed, with 20% incidence of MDS and less than 10% incidence of AML by age 50 years.[175]

There are two severe variants of TBD, which typically present at a very early age. The Hoyeraal-Hreidarsson syndrome is associated with poor intrauterine growth, microcephaly with cerebellar hypoplasia, and immunodeficiency.[177] Revesz syndrome is associated with ocular findings of bilateral exudative retinopathy and intracranial calcifications.[178] Coats plus syndrome has findings of Revesz syndrome and telangiectasias, poor bony healing and fractures, and recurrent GI hemorrhages, and intracranial calcifications and leukoencephalopathy.[179]

Differential Diagnosis

TBD must be distinguished from other inherited BMF syndromes that also present with AA, congenital anomalies, and cancer predisposition, such as FA. In contrast to FA, cells from patients with TBD do not manifest increased chromosomal breakage in response to MMC or DEB.[180] Literature reports differ over whether cells from TBD patient cells exhibit increased chromosomal breakage in response to other agents.[181,182] Because patients with TBD may develop AA in the first decade of life prior to the manifestation of skin or nail abnormalities, their underlying diagnosis may be missed.

Laboratory Findings

In addition to peripheral cytopenias, red cell macrocytosis and elevated HgbF may be seen in patients with TBD.[183] However, these signs of stress erythropoiesis are nonspecific, as they are seen in many patients with any of the inherited BMF syndromes. The bone marrow is typically hypocellular, although cellularity may be normal or even increased early in the disease.

Immunologic abnormalities, including low or high immunoglobulins; reduced numbers of B, NK, or T cells; and reduced stimulation by phytohemagglutinin, have been described in some patients with TBD.[166,184,185] These immunologic findings tended to be more prominent in children with TBD as compared with adults with TBD.[184] There may be liver dysfunction with elevation in transaminases and bilirubin and abnormal liver synthetic function including abnormal coagulation factors and albumin.[22]

X chromosome inactivation patterns in female obligate carriers showed complete skewing, consistent with a growth or survival disadvantage for cells expressing only the defective X chromosome allele.[186-189] Spontaneous unbalanced chromosomal translocations have been observed.[190,191]

Pathophysiology

Telomeres are structures that protect chromosome ends and progressively shorten with sequential cell division. Telomeres are bound and protected by a shelterin protein complex. Telomerase is a ribonucleo-protein enzyme complex that prevents loss of terminal repeats at the chromosome ends (telomeres) during DNA replication and consists of TERT, RNA component hTR, and additional complexed proteins including dyskerin, NOP10, NHP2, NAF1, and GAR1.[192,193] Thus telomeres, the telomerase complex, and shelterin complex are integral to prevent chromosomal fusions, rearrangements, and premature shortening of the chromosomal ends.

Telomere loss has also been implicated in contributing to the process of aging and cancer, and TBD may represent a form of premature aging of tissues with a high replicative requirement.[194,195] Cells from patients with TBD manifest abnormally shortened telomeres and reduced telomerase activity.[161,196]

Although telomerase activity is abundant early in development, expression remains robust only in a subset of tissues, including the progenitor cells of the hematopoietic system, expanding lymphocytes, stem cells, and germ cells.[197] Other cells also include the basal layer of the epidermis, intestinal cells, and hair follicles. These tissues mirror those most severely affected in patients with TBD. The type II alveolar epithelial stem cells in the lung are also affected and may contribute to the mechanism behind pulmonary fibrosis.[198] Bone marrow cells from patients with TBD show poor growth in long-term bone marrow culture assays, and the defect is intrinsic to the HSCs.[199] Reduced hematopoietic progenitor cell (HPC) colonies have been described for all three hematopoietic lineages compared with controls.[200-202]

Since the initial observations that patients with TBD have abnormal telomeres, the understanding of the molecular genetics of TBD and telomere disorders has continued to improve as new genes are discovered.[197] The types of mechanisms leading to TBD can be classified into those that lead to (1) decreased telomerase activity, (2) impaired telomerase recruitment to telomeres, (3) impaired telomere duplication, and (4) impaired regulation of the telomere biology–related gene transcripts. Currently, there are 14 known genes that have been mutated in telomere biology disorders (see Table 38.4). DKC1 is X-linked,[203] whereas the other known TBD genes are autosomal recessive (NHP2, NOP10, WRAP53, CTC1, STN1), autosomal dominant (TERC, TINF2, NAF1, ZCCHC8) in inheritance, or both (PARN, TERT, RTEL1, ACD). For several genes, de novo mutations are common, specifically for TINF2 and DKC1. These are discussed in recent reviews.[158,193,197,204] TBD and Hoyeraal-Heidarsson syndrome (HHS) can be caused by mutations in multiple different genes, but only mutations in TINF2 have been associated with Revesz syndrome[178] and mutations in CTC1 or STN1 with Coats plus, although this may expand as additional genes are discovered.[197,205-207]

The most common mechanism of telomere shortening is due to a decrease in telomerase activity. TERT, TERC, DKC1, NHP2, NOP10, and NAF1 mutations have been shown to lead to decreased telomerase levels or activity.[203,208-213] Telomerase must effectively be recruited to telomeres in order to perform their function, and mutations affecting this process can also cause TBD. The shelterin complex is composed of TRF2, RAP1, TRF1, TIN2, TPP1, and POT1 in mammals, and these proteins are required for telomere maintenance. TIN2 (coded by TINF2) of the shelterin complex is recruited to telomeres,[214-216] and TINF2 disease-causing mutations can lead to severe manifestations of TBD such as HHS[217] and Revesz syndromes.[218] A patient with biallelic missense mutations in NHP2 has been reported with HHS manifestation.[219]

Similarly, mutations in the WRAP53 gene, which encodes TCAB1, and ACD, which encodes TPP1, cause defects in telomerase recruitment. Patients with mutations in the TEL patch of TPP1 have reported with manifestations of TBD and HHS.[220] Recently, a sibling pair with homozygous variants in POT1 was described with Coats plus syndrome.[221]

The CTC1-STN1-TEN1 complex is conserved and is integral to C-strand synthesis and recovery from replicative stress. The hallmark of CTC1 defects is the finding of internal gaps of single-stranded telomeric DNA. Many patients with Coats plus syndrome have biallelic mutations in CTC1, although other patients with CTC1 mutations can have other manifestations along the spectrum of TBD.[222-224] Recently,

homozygous mutations in STN1 in two unrelated patients with Coats plus were described.[205] RTEL1 is also critical in DNA repair, DNA replication, and telomere replication. It acts as a DNA helicase that is recruited to telomeres by TRF2 and functions similar to CTC1 in duplex telomeric replication and also acts to counter the formation of telomere circles by SLX1/4 nuclease.[225,226] However, patients with RTEL1 mutations, unlike those with CTC1 mutations, do not develop Coats plus but instead develop HHS.[227,228]

Mutations in other genes not associated with telomerase, the shelterin complex, or telomerase replication can also cause TBD. PARN encodes a poly(A)-specific 3′ exoribonuclease, and disease-causing mutations in PARN can impair mRNA function and ribosomal RNA biogenesis.[229,230]

Patients with heterozygous mutations in PARN have been described with familial pulmonary fibrosis, whereas those with biallelic mutations have been reported to have TBD or HHS.[197,231-233] A subset of patients with TBD remains genetically undefined, suggesting that additional genes or variants are likely yet to be identified.

Supportive Care

Supportive care for patients with TBD is similar to that outlined for patients with AA and FA, including transfusion of red blood cells and platelets as needed for patients with cytopenias. Surveillance for development of marrow failure, clonal abnormalities, MDS, and leukemia is recommended with CBCs and bone marrow studies. Clonal abnormalities can be common in patients with TBD, with skewed X-inactivation and acquired copy neutral loss of heterozygosity identified on single-nucleotide polymorphism analysis.[234]

Multiorgan surveillance is important for optimizing long-term health for patients with TBD, similar to FA. Annual pulmonary function testing is recommended given their risk of developing pulmonary fibrosis.[170] Exposure to pulmonary toxins, such as cigarettes, should be reduced or eliminated as much as possible. Avoiding sun exposure is important in this population because of the increased risk of skin cancer, and patients benefit from dermatologic evaluations. Screening patients for signs and symptoms of GI and hepatic complications is an important part of surveillance and supportive care. In addition, because of patients' increased risk of osteoporosis, their diet, vitamin D, and parathyroid hormone levels and calcium status should be monitored.

Patients with significant immunologic dysfunction resulting in reduced immunoglobulin levels or with frequent infections may benefit from intravenous immunoglobulin replacement therapy; those with severe T-cell lymphopenia may benefit from prophylaxis against *Pneumocystis jirovecii*.[235,236] Patients should be up to date on their immunizations, including influenza and HPV, as clinically indicated.

Given the increased risk of cancer for patients with TBD, these patients are counseled to minimize exposure to ionizing radiation. Solid tumors include head and neck squamous cell carcinomas, hepatocellular carcinomas, lung cancer, and oropharyngeal cancers.[175,176] Screening involves routine dental, nasolaryngoscopic, gynecologic, and dermatologic examinations and bloodwork surveillance with CBCs and liver function tests.[175,176]

Treatment

The only curative treatment for severe hematologic and immunologic complications in TBD remains allogeneic HSCT. However, HSCT does not cure the nonhematologic manifestations of TBD. The current indications for transplant include severe or symptomatic cytopenias, MDS, and leukemia, although careful consideration is needed to assess an individual patient's organ function and potential donors.

Improving the outcome for patients with TBD undergoing HSCT has been a major goal for clinicians in the last 20 years given the high morbidity and mortality in this patient population. Using conventional conditioning, a retrospective analysis of the data from the Center for International Blood and Marrow Transplantation Research (CIBMTR) found that more than 50% of patients with TBD who underwent HSCT died within the first 4 months after the procedure due to infection, graft failure of GVHD.[237] The 5-year overall survival in this analysis was only 46% at 5 years for patients transplanted prior to 2000.[237]

Table 38.4. Clinical Features of the Inherited Aplastic Anemia Syndromes

	Clinical Features	Inheritance Pattern	Gene	Additional Laboratory Testing	Associated Malignancies
Fanconi anemia	Short stature, hyper/hypopigmentation, skeletal abnormalities, genitourinary abnormalities, gastrointestinal abnormalities, cardiopulmonary abnormalities	Autosomal recessive	*FANCA* *FANCC FANCD1* *FANCD2 FANCE* *FANCF* *FANCG* *FANCI* *FANCJ* *FANCL* *FANCM* *FANCN* *FANCO* *FANCP* *FANCQ* *FANCS* *FANCT* *FANCU* *FANCV* *FANCW*	Chromosome breakage	AML, carcinomas (head and neck, gynecologic); brain and Wilms in *D1/BRCA2*
		X-linked recessive	*FANCB*		
		Autosomal dominant	*FANCR*		
Telomere biology disorder	Abnormal nails, reticular rash, leukoplakia, pulmonary fibrosis, liver and GI disease	X-linked recessive or de novo	*DKC1*	Telomere length	AML, carcinomas (head and neck, anogenital)
		Autosomal dominant	*TERC* *TINF2* *NAF1* *PARN* *TERT* *RTEL1* *ACD* *ZCCHC8*		
		Autosomal recessive	*NHP2* *NOP10* *WRAP53* *CTC1* *STN1* *PARN* *TERT* *RTEL1* *ACD*		
Shwachman-Diamond syndrome and SDS-like disorders	Short stature, exocrine pancreatic dysfunction, skeletal dysplasias, marrow failure	Autosomal recessive Autosomal dominant	*SBDS* *DNAJC21* *ELF1* *SRP 54*	Serum trypsinogen, pancreatic isoamylase	AML
Congenital amegakaryocytic thrombocytopenia	Thrombocytopenia, marrow failure MECOM: skeletal abnormalities, cardiac and renal malformations, B-cell deficiency, hearing loss	Autosomal recessive	*C-MPL* *THPO* *MECOM*		AML
GATA2 deficiency syndrome	MonoMac syndrome, DCML deficiency, Emberger syndrome, familial AML	Autosomal dominant	*GATA2*		AML, CMML

Abbreviations: AML, acute myeloid leukemia; ANL, acute nonlymphocytic leukemia; CMML, chronic myelomonocytic leukemia; DCML, dendritic cell, monocyte, B and NK lymphocyte deficiency; GI, gastrointestinal; MDS, myelodysplastic syndrome.

Early and late fatal pulmonary and vascular complications after SCT have been a significant and often fatal complication for patients undergoing HSCT. Alternate donor sources, age > 20 years at the time of transplant, and long interval between diagnosis of BMF and SCT were identified as markers of poor prognosis.[238] The replacement of DNA alkylating agents (cyclophosphamide, busulfan, melphalan, thiotepa) and total body radiation by the use of fludarabine and antibody-based immunosuppressive conditioning regimens have improved patient outcome.[239-242] The goal of these reduced-intensity conditioning regimens is to decrease transplant-related toxicities while still achieving engraftment. With using such a reduced-intensity conditioning regimen for a small cohort of patients with TBD, these investigators had encouraging results with two-thirds of patients alive with a median follow-up for 16 months, while three of these four patients had received an unrelated donor.[240] While a retrospective analysis of 109 patients with TBD showed that the 5- and 10-year survival for patients who underwent HSCT before 2000 was only 57% and 23%, respectively, but improved for patients with an HSCT after 2000 to a 5-year survival of about of 70%, it also showed that the long-term survival in this group was similar to the years before 2000 and only about 28%.[238]

Disorders of Red Blood Cells

Consistent with these results, a more recent analysis of 94 patients with TBD, who received a nonmyeloablative conditioning regimen, also found that the overall survival and event-free survival at 3 years after HSCT were 66% and 62%, respectively.[243] Prospective trials are underway to understand if various reduced-intensity conditioning regimens omitting radiation and alkylators can lead to successful engraftment and minimize both peritransplant and long-term toxicities.[244]

Treatment with the immunosuppressive regimen of ATG and cyclosporine is generally not effective for the treatment of BMF in patients with TBD.[245] Eltrombopag has not been widely used in these patients and failed to improve severe thrombocytopenia in a case report of two affected siblings.[246]

Improvement in peripheral blood counts has been described in some patients following treatment with the androgen therapy; however, there are no clear benefits for extrahematopoietic disease manifestations. A recent phase I/II study using danazol in adults with TBD demonstrated improvement in hematologic parameters in ~80% of patients and has generated renewed interest in using androgens for TBD.[247,248] At least two studies show controversial data if treatment with androgens indeed lead to telomere elongation, and the biological mechanisms are not yet completely understood.[247,249] Side effects included transaminitis and muscle cramps, which occurred in 41% and 33% of patients, respectively.[247] While some patients have a long-lasting effect of androgens on their hematopoiesis and may become transfusion independent for months, androgens are not considered curative. Therefore, there are no uniform recommendations whether androgens should be trialed before patients with TBD undergo HSCT or not. There have been two cases reported in the literature of patients with splenic rupture while on concurrent G-CSF and androgen therapy, and therefore it is recommended that simultaneous therapy with these two agents be avoided if possible.[250]

SHWACHMAN-DIAMOND SYNDROME

SDS is an autosomal recessive disorder characterized clinically by the combination of exocrine pancreatic dysfunction and BMF with an increased risk of MDS and leukemia. SDS can variably be associated with congenital anomalies, skeletal anomalies, short stature, and neurocognitive, hepatic, cardiac, immunologic, and endocrine abnormalities.[21,251] SDS was first characterized in 1964 with increasing understanding of the molecular and genetic pathogenesis of the disorder since then.[252]

Diagnostic Testing

Prior to identifying the underlying genetic cause of most patients with SDS, the diagnosis of SDS was made based on the clinical criteria including neutropenia (detected over two separate occasions over at least a 3-month time) and exocrine pancreatic dysfunction with reduced levels of serum trypsinogen (age < 3 years) or serum pancreatic isoamylase (age > 3 years).[21] However, normal fecal elastase levels and a normal pancreatic appearance on imaging do not rule out a diagnosis of SDS, and further genetic testing should be pursued if clinically indicated.[251] The genetic diagnosis of SDS can be made by testing for biallelic mutations in the Shwachman-Bodian-Diamond syndrome (SBDS) gene, which is located on chromosome 7q11.[253] Over 90% of patients who meet clinical criteria for SDS harbor autosomal recessive mutations in the *SBDS* gene. Although the presence of biallelic pathogenic *SBDS* mutations is helpful in confirming the diagnosis, currently the absence of mutations does not rule out the diagnosis of SDS if the patient meets diagnostic criteria on clinical grounds.[21] Mutations in additional genes (*DNAJC21, ELF1, and SRP54*) have been recently identified in patients with SDS-like phenotypes.[254-256]

Clinical Features

The hallmark of SDS is BMF, which typically presents with neutropenia, along with exocrine pancreatic dysfunction and leukemia predisposition. However, more recently it has become clear that there is a wide range of clinical presentations in SDS by studying patients enrolled in the North American SDS registry.[251]

Exocrine pancreatic insufficiency typically presents in infancy with failure to thrive and loose, foul-smelling stools consistent with steatorrhea. Fecal fat measurements may be helpful, but a normal test does not rule out the diagnosis of SDS as exocrine pancreatic function may improve in a subset of patients. Exocrine pancreatic insufficiency may improve with age to become clinically asymptomatic in a subset of patients. The pancreas in patients with SDS often shows fatty replacement of the pancreatic acini, with sparing of the ducts and islets, and fecal elastase levels, serum trypsinogen, or pancreatic isoamylase can be low. Fat-soluble vitamin deficiencies (vitamins A, D, E, and K) may be seen.

Neutropenia is the most common feature of marrow failure in SDS. Neutropenia may be either intermittent or persistent, and 81% of patients had absolute neutrophil counts of <1500/μL in one series, although 14% had no history of cytopenias at the time of diagnosis.[251,257] Patients are predisposed to infections, particularly bacterial and fungal infections. Abnormalities of T or B cells have also been reported and may contribute to infectious complications.[258] Anemia and/or thrombocytopenia may also be seen, and a subset of patients with SDS develop AA. The red blood cells may be macrocytic.

There is no pathognomonic feature of the bone marrow in patients with SDS; nonetheless, a bone marrow examination with aspirate, biopsy, and cytogenetics is important to rule out other causes of cytopenias. Marrow cellularity may be normal, low, or high. Marrow cytogenetic abnormalities may be seen, such as abnormalities of chromosome 7 (monosomy 7, deletions/translations of 7q, isochromosome 7, as well as del20q).[259] In the absence of morphologic evidence for MDS, the clinical significance of most cytogenetic abnormalities is unclear. Although monosomy 7/del7q is often associated with a high risk of progression to leukemia, other cytogenetic clonal abnormalities such as del20q or isochromosome 7q may wax and wane over time or even disappear.[260] As with other inherited BMF syndromes, mild dysplastic features may be seen in the myeloid and megakaryocytic lineages. There is a risk for progression to pancytopenia and AA (20%-25%) or MDS/AML (5%-33%).[257,261] SDS may even go unrecognized in some patients until myeloid malignancy occurs and the diagnosis may be made while undergoing further diagnostic workup in preparation of HSCT.[262] In a cohort of 36 patients with SDS with MDS or AML, the prognosis was worse than expected from data from individuals without underlying SDS. The 3-year overall survival for individuals with leukemia was 11% with a median survival of 0.99 years and 51% with median survival of 7.7 years for individuals with MDS.[261] Close bone marrow surveillance may allow earlier disease detection. In this retrospective analysis, patients who underwent routine marrow surveillance had improved 3-year overall survival of 62% compared with 28% for patients without surveillance.[261] However, the use of CBCs and monitoring patient's MCV did not indicate evolving MDS or leukemia in patients with SDS and the authors advise caution in relying on the MCV for monitoring of early disease detection.[261]

Additional features that may be variably associated with SDS include skeletal abnormalities, including metaphyseal dysostosis and osteopenia; failure to thrive despite early institution of pancreatic enzyme supplementation (see below); elevated hepatic transaminases (which typically improve over time); and abnormal dentition.[251,263,264]

Differential Diagnosis

The differential diagnosis of SDS includes other inherited and acquired causes of marrow failure as well as other causes of exocrine pancreatic insufficiency, such as cystic fibrosis, Pearson syndrome, and cartilage hair hypoplasia.[21] SDS is the second most common cause of inherited pancreatic insufficiency, after cystic fibrosis.[265] Sweat chloride is normal and serves to distinguish these patients from those with cystic fibrosis.

Laboratory Findings

Similar to other patients with inherited BMF syndromes, patients with SDS may have isolated cytopenias or have multilineage involvement, but neutropenia is the most common type of hematologic abnormality seen. However, only 51% of patients in the North American

Shwachman-Diamond Syndrome Registry presented with the classic combination of neutropenia and steatorrhea.[251] Patients may have macrocytosis on CBCs, and up to 80% of patients show elevated HgbF, both of which can be a marker of stress hematopoiesis.[257]

Serum trypsinogen is generally depressed in patients with SDS before the age of 3 years but may rise to normal levels thereafter.[266] Pancreatic isoamylase levels remain low after the age of 3 years and is the preferred test in this older age group.[266] Other tests for exocrine pancreatic function include pancreatic stimulation or elevated fecal fat measurement, although the latter test is not specific for pancreatic dysfunction. Imaging studies may reveal a fatty, atretic pancreas, although pancreatic imaging may appear normal early in life. Fecal elastase may be decreased, but the sensitivity of this test as a screen for SDS remains to be ascertained.[267] Fat-soluble vitamin levels (vitamins A, D, E, and K) may be low secondary to malabsorption. Skeletal imaging studies may reveal a wide variety of abnormalities, which are often asymptomatic.[268]

Pathophysiology

SDS is an autosomal recessive disorder with an estimated incidence of 1 in 75,000.[269] In the majority (90%) of affected patients reported, mutations have been detected in the *SBDS* gene located on chromosome 7q11.[253,270] The human SBDS protein is found in both the nucleus and the cytoplasm and shuttles in and out of the nucleolus in a cell cycle–associated fashion,[271] playing a key role in ribosome biogenesis.[272] Human SBDS associates with the 60S ribosomal precursor but not with the mature 80S ribosome.[273] Deletion of murine *Sbds* results in early embryonic lethality.[274] Sbds was shown to function in coupling GTP hydrolysis by EFL1 to the release of eIF6 from the nascent 60S ribosomal subunit, which occurs through a conformational switch in EFL1 and competition for an overlapping binding site on the 60S ribosomal subunit.[275,276] As eIF6 sterically hinders the association of the 60S ribosomal subunit to the 40S subunit,[277,278] eIF6 release is required for final assembly of a translationally active 80S ribosomal subunit. SBDS has also been implicated in additional molecular pathways, including mitotic spindle stabilization,[279] cellular stress response,[280] actin dynamics,[281] and signaling downstream of RANK for osteoclast differentiation.[282]

Mutations in *DNAJC21*, *ELF1*, and *SRP54* have been recently identified in patients with SDS-like phenotypes.[254-256] Biallelic mutations in *DNAJC21* have been described in patients with clinical features of SDS or with isolated neutropenia, often complicated by BMF and rarely by the development of AML.[283] *DNAJC21* is ubiquitously expressed and is required for ribosome biogenesis, similar to *SBDS*. Indeed, both are required in the release of maturation factors from the pre60S ribosomal subunit, suggesting that both *DNAJC21* mutations and *SBDS* mutations may result in similar defects in ribosome maturation.[256]

Autosomal recessive alterations in *EFL1* have also been reported in patients sharing clinical features of SDS. Mutated *EFL1* impairs 80S ribosome assembly and causes an SDS-associated ribosomopathy in cell line and animal models.[284] At the time of this writing, no cases of MDS or AML have been reported in patients with *EFL1* mutations.

Other patients with SDS-like features were found to carry autosomal dominant mutations in *SRP54*, which encodes for a component of the ribonucleoprotein complex and mediates the transport of secretory proteins to the endoplasmic reticulum.[285] These patients may have severe neutropenia or exocrine pancreatic insufficiency, but MDS/AML have not yet been reported.[254,286]

The exact mechanisms of how neutropenia and marrow failure develop as a result of *SBDS* mutations or mutations in *DNAJC21*, *ELF1*, and *SRP54* continue to be under investigation. One hypothesis is that altering the ribosome biogenesis and function increases nuclear stress and activates apoptosis.[8] However, a more recent mechanistic study of clonal hematopoiesis in SDS investigated the development and landscape of acquired somatic mutations in patients with SDS longitudinally.[287] The authors found that hematopoietic clones harboring which acquired heterozygous mutations in either *EIF6* or *TP53* established two contrary fitness constraints with different clinical

consequences. EIF6 was associated with limited leukemic potential by ameliorating the underlying SDS ribosome defect and promoting clone fitness. Acquired *EIF6* mutations were shown to rescue the fitness defect caused by *SBDS* deficiency and suppress the defects in ribosome assembly and protein synthesis, either by reducing the eIF6 expression dosage itself or by disrupting its affinity with the 60S subunit, providing evidence for the possibility of indirect somatic genetic reversion in SDS. Acquisition of biallelic *TP53* mutations lead to inactivation of important tumor suppressor checkpoints without correcting the ribosome defect, which subsequently led to the development of leukemia.[287,288]

Supportive Care

Regular monitoring of peripheral blood counts, mean corpuscular volume, peripheral blood smears, and HgbF level and periodic bone marrow examination are recommended to assess for development of cytogenetic abnormalities and MDS.[21,261] However, as with the other inherited BMF syndromes, surveillance for the development of MDS in this population can be difficult as cytogenetic abnormalities of unclear clinical significance and mild dysplastic features may be present in some patients with SDS without portending a poor prognosis.

Patients with SDS are at risk of secondary infections not only due to neutropenia and absolute neutrophil number but also because some studies suggest that neutrophil function might be impaired. Decreased NK-cell, T-cell, B-cell, and complement activation have also been reported.[289] In a comprehensive review of infectious complications in 153 patients with SDS, 33% developed pneumonia, 29% had recurrent otitis media, and 15% had developed skin infections and/or abscesses.[289] Patients with a history of recurrent or severe bacterial infections may benefit from prophylactic G-CSF.

Endocrinology evaluation is useful in these patients to rule out treatable comorbid conditions that could further exacerbate short stature or osteopenia. About 26% of patients with SDS have endocrinologic abnormalities.[290] Dietary counseling may be helpful to ensure adequate intake of calcium and vitamin D, and patients may have poor nutritional status and micronutrient deficiencies, such as of vitamin A and selenium.[290] Because of the fat malabsorption from pancreatic insufficiency, patients may develop vitamin K deficiency and subsequent deficiency of vitamin K–dependent coagulation factors. Fat malabsorption is treated with the administration of oral pancreatic enzymes. Exocrine pancreatic functions may vary over time, and thus regular assessment by a gastroenterologist is recommended.[291] Patients benefit from supplementation with vitamins A, D, E, and K. Fecal fat measurements, vitamin levels, and prothrombin time provide useful measures of exocrine pancreatic function. In addition, annual dental examinations and monitoring of bone health and neurodevelopment are both recommended.[21]

Treatment

Therapy in SDS is initiated based on the patients' clinical manifestations. Bone marrow transplantation can cure the hematologic aspects of SDS and has been evaluated as a potential therapy in patients with SDS with marrow failure and severe or symptomatic cytopenias, MDS, or AML.[292-294] Patients who undergo transplant for BMF have superior outcomes as compared with patients who undergo transplant for MDS or leukemia: In a retrospective analysis of 39 patients with SDS-associated BMF and 13 patients with MDS or AML undergoing HSCT, patients with BMF had a 5-year overall survival of 72%, whereas only 15% of patients in the MDS/AML group survived.[295] In another retrospective analysis of 36 patients with MDS/AML, the 3-year survival for patients who developed AML was only 11%, but 51% in those with MDS. Most deaths were caused by disease relapse/resistance or treatment-related toxicities.[261] Others have reported similar numbers: Data from the European Society for Blood and Marrow Transplant showed a 5-year overall survival of 70% for patients with BMF and 28.8% for patients with MDS/AML.[296] There was no significant difference of overall survival between patients who received reduced intensity versus a myeloablative conditioning, nor did outcome depend on the source of transplant donor.[296] Given the poor survival rates of patients with leukemia, regular surveillance of blood counts and consideration of bone marrow examinations have been recommended to monitor for early signs of malignant transformation.

CONGENITAL AMEGAKARYOCYTIC THROMBOCYTOPENIA

CAMT is a rare autosomal recessive and genetically heterogenous disorder, which often presents already in the neonatal period with thrombocytopenia and bleeding symptoms and progresses to AA in the majority of patients in childhood. Alterations in the *c-Mpl* gene, encoding for the receptor of thrombopoietin (TPO), were the first known genetic cause of CAMT.[297,298] More recently, mutations in the thrombopoietin gene *(THPO)* itself and *MECOM* (MDS1 and EVI1 complex locus) were found in patients with CAMT-like phenotypes.[299-303]

Clinical Features

Patients with CAMT typically present in the neonatal period with thrombocytopenia, which may manifest with petechiae, purpura, or bleeding typically involving the skin, mucous membranes, or GI tract.[11,304,305] In a recent analysis of a large cohort of 56 patients with CAMT, intracranial bleedings occurred in 23% of patients either during pregnancy or in the perinatal period.[305] Thrombocytopenia was detected at birth in 38 of 52 patients with a median platelet count of 15,000. A family history of miscarriages has been reported.[304] Two clinical phenotypes of CAMT have been described.[306] Patients in CAMT group I are characterized by severe, persistent thrombocytopenia and early onset of pancytopenia, whereas patients in CAMT group II are characterized by transient increase in platelet counts to over 50,000/µL early in life and either a delayed onset of pancytopenia or lack of pancytopenia to date.[306] Patients are at risk of subsequently developing cytopenias in all three hematopoietic lineages as a sign of developing bone marrow exhaustion, which may progress to severe AA and often develops in childhood. More than two-thirds of patients were younger than 4 years, when they developed aplasia, and half of them were not even 2 years of age in a recent study.[305] The development of AML or MDS has been reported in only a few cases of CAMT.[304,305]

Cerebral malformations have been detected and likely represent sequelae of prior intracranial hemorrhage. Patients with germline mutations in MECOM present with a variable phenotype pattern, varying from radioulnar synostosis alone to severe, early-onset BMF with or without multiple organ manifestations, including skeletal abnormalities, cardiac and renal malformations, B-cell deficiency, and presenile hearing loss.[15,302,303,307-313]

Differential Diagnosis

Thrombocytopenia in the neonate may be secondary to other causes such as infections (e.g., TORCH: toxoplasmosis, rubella, cytomegalovirus, herpes simplex, other viruses), sepsis, Kasabach-Merritt syndrome, thrombosis, or medications. Infants may exhibit transient thrombocytopenia in the setting of maternal HELLP syndrome. Immune-mediated thrombocytopenia from transplacentally acquired maternal alloantibodies or autoantibodies is also common in the neonatal period. Other rare causes of thrombocytopenia include the giant platelet syndromes: Bernard-Soulier syndrome, Glanzmann thromboasthenia, and May-Hegglin disease.

The presence of congenital anomalies together with thrombocytopenia should prompt diagnostic workup for other disorders such as FA, thrombocytopenia-absent radii (TAR) syndrome, amegakaryocytic thrombocytopenia with radioulnar synostosis (ATRUS), Paris-Trousseau syndrome, or the Hoyeraal-Hreidarsson variant of DC. While patients with TAR exhibit thrombocytopenia at an early age, platelet counts generally improve with age, although counts may fluctuate. In contrast to CAMT, AA has not been reported in patients with TAR, although cases have been reported of patients with TAR who developed AML or MDS.[314-316] Additional inherited syndromes associated with thrombocytopenia, such as GATA-1 mutations[317] or other inherited BMF syndromes, must also be considered.

Laboratory Findings

Unlike other inherited platelet disorders with micro- or macrothrombocytopenia, the platelet size and morphology in CAMT is usually normal. The platelet count ranges around 20,000/µL, but higher platelet counts do not rule out the diagnosis. Laboratory tests for platelet function are also normal. Mean platelet volume is typically normal. The red cells may be normocytic or macrocytic. TPO levels are typically elevated (see below) in *Mpl*-deficient patients, but not in *THPO*-deficient patients. In a recent study of patients with mutations in *MECOM* with plasma samples available, TPO levels were elevated.[302] When examining the bone marrow of patients with CAMT, there are decreased megakaryocytes, lacking Mpl expression on the cell surface. *Mpl* gene mutations can be identified by sequencing the *Mpl* gene at the coding regions and the splice sites of exons 1 and 2.[306,318] However, the lack of an *Mpl* gene mutation does not exclude the diagnosis of CAMT, and there is new evidence that biallelic mutations of the *THPO* gene itself can result in CAMT as well.[299-301] MECOM patients with mutations affecting the eighth zinc finger have low B-lymphocyte counts, recurrent bacterial and fungal infections, and in some cases hypogammaglobulinemia.[302] The bone marrow of these patients is hypocellular, pointing to advanced exhaustion of hematopoiesis and progression to AA.[15]

Pathophysiology

Mutations in the *c-Mpl* gene, which encode the receptor for TPO, were the first known genetic cause for CAMT, which is an autosomal recessively inherited disorder.[298,318] However, alterations in genes up- or downstream of the receptor for TPO, such as mutations in the *THPO* gene itself or *MECOM,* have been found in patients with CAMT-like phenotype but with normal *Mpl*.[299-301] Mpl is a transmembrane protein that is expressed on cells of the megakaryocytic lineage, and binding of TPO to Mpl leads to activation of signaling pathways necessary for megakaryopoiesis.

Mutations in *c-Mpl* may be located throughout the gene and include nonsense, missense, and splicing mutations. A correlation between clinical severity and mutation classification has been observed.[305,306,319] Patients with a complete loss of function (CAMT I) as a result of *c-Mpl* mutations with defective presentation of the TPO receptor to the cell surface, decreased TPO binding and receptor activation present with persistent thrombocytopenia and rapid progression to AA.[306,320-323] *c-Mpl* missense mutations generally allow for a residual function of the TPO receptor resulting in the milder clinical phenotype (CAMT II).[306,324]

Patients with CAMT with biallelic missense alterations in *THPO* show impaired TPO secretion, which is synthesized in the liver, and have extremely low TPO plasma levels,[300] while patients with *c-Mpl* mutations exhibit high TPO serum levels[325] and their endogenous serum TPO appears functional.[326]

The TPO/Mpl axis is important not only for megakaryocyte development but also for HSC survival. Mice deficient in either *THPO* or *c-Mpl* exhibit both thrombocytopenia as well as reduced numbers of HSCs and progenitors.[327] Interestingly, *c-MPL*-deficient mice also show a neonatal maturation defect of megakaryocytes and shorter platelet survival, increasing the bleeding risk in neonates.[328]

Study of the effect of TPO on embryonic stem cells in mice showed that treatment of ES cells with TPO and simultaneous activation of BMP4 signaling activity may provide a new method for stem cell expansion.[329] Stem cell dependency on TPO likely contributes to the development of AA in patients with CAMT.

The *MECOM* locus encodes the differentially spliced transcripts of *MDS1-EVI1, MDS1,* and *EVI1* resulting in their respective protein isoform. The protein encoded by this locus is a transcription factor, important for normal embryonic development, hematopoiesis, and oncogenesis. In mice, complete *Evi1* knockout is embryonic lethal and causes pancytopenia with reduced HSCs and defective self-renewing capacity, whereas *Evi1* haploinsufficiency presents with an intermediate phenotype and a reduced ability for hematopoietic reconstitution.[330,331] In contrast to patients described with *MECOM* haploinsufficiency and their pronounced BMF early on in life independent of which isoform is impacted, *Mecom* haploinsufficiency in mice does not alter hematopoiesis.[332]

Supportive Care

Indications for platelet transfusion vary, but generally they are reserved for patients who experience bleeding symptoms. Prophylactic platelet transfusions may be considered for patients posing a high bleeding risk (e.g., neonates, prior to surgery). Antifibrinolytic medications such as aminocaproic acid or tranexamic acid may be helpful in stabilizing clots, particularly for mucous membrane bleeding such as oral or nasal bleeding. Agents that inhibit platelet function, such as aspirin or nonsteroidal anti-inflammatory agents, should be avoided. Desmopressin acetate (DDAVP) has been used in some patients with thrombocytopenia, although side effects such as the Syndrome of inappropriate secretion of antidiuretic hormone (SIADH) must be monitored.

Treatment

Treatment options for patients with CAMT depend on the underlying genetic cause and mechanism contributing to the phenotype. Although TPO mimetics have been used in other types of inherited thrombocytopenias, they are not efficacious in *Mpl*-deficient CAMT patients, unless the mutation leads to decreased binding of TPO to MPL.[320,333] In contrast, patients with *THPO* deficiency have been successfully treated with TPO mimetics, resulting in sustained trilineage response.[300,301] While HSCT is the only curative treatment for patients with *MPL* or *MECOM* mutations, it would not be successful in *THPO*-deficient patients, since thrombopoietin is synthesized in nonhematologic tissues such as the liver, so the defective megakaryopoiesis and marrow failure are not corrected by HSCT.[302,334]

HLA typing can be sent at the time of diagnosis for both the patient and the siblings. Transplantation with sibling donors is preferred if an HLA-matched sibling donor is available,[304,335-339] and testing potential sibling donors for biallelic *c-Mpl* mutations is recommended.[297,304] Whether *c-Mpl* carrier status affects transplant outcomes is unclear, but such donors should be carefully evaluated for possible phenotypic abnormalities concerning for CAMT as single mutated *c-Mpl* alleles have been reported in patients with CAMT phenotype.[305]

Alternative donor transplants have also been explored in recent years, including haploidentical transplants, umbilical cord blood transplants, matched unrelated donor transplants, and T cell–depleted transplants.[340-345] However, for those without HLA-matched family donors, transplant-related mortality and graft failure are high.[304,305,346] Considerations for timing of transplant include minimizing the risk of allosensitization from donor blood products or infectious complications secondary to neutropenia. Gene editing strategies to rescue mutant *Mpl* loss of function are under current investigation.[347]

GATA2 SYNDROMES

The phenotypic spectrum of patients with *GATA2* alterations is broad and not only includes MonoMAC syndrome (characterized by recurrent mycobacterial infections secondary to monocytopenia)[348] and dendritic cell, monocyte, B and NK lymphoid (DCML) deficiency,[349] as well as the Emberger syndrome (characterized by lymphedema and MDS),[350] but importantly may also present with isolated neutropenia, BMF, or myeloid malignancy.[351]

Clinical Features

Patients with germline *GATA2* mutations present with variable pleiotropic clinical manifestations, including the hematopoietic, immune, lymphatic, vascular, urogenital, and pulmonary abnormalities (*Figure 38.2*). The overall penetrance of such is high, and it has been estimated that up to 75% of carriers may develop myeloid neoplasms.[352-354] Immunodeficiency is a common manifestation of *GATA2* deficiency, but many patients lack a history of infections.[355] Some patients are identified as having familial MDS/AML, whereas others show manifestations consistent with MonoMAC syndrome characterized by recurrent infections, mostly mycobacterial infections secondary to monocytopenia, and DCML deficiency, leading to increased frequency of viral (HPV, herpes simplex virus, varicella-zoster virus, Epstein-Barr virus, and cytomegalovirus) and bacterial infections.[348] The predisposition to MDS/AML in association with lymphedema and congenital deafness was first described by Emberger et al (Emberger syndrome).[350] Patients can also develop pulmonary complications including pulmonary alveolar proteinosis, diffusion and ventilatory defects, and pulmonary hypertension. In addition, patients can have problems with their vasculature including increased risk of thromboses, and patients have been reported to have hypothyroidism, miscarriages, and sensorineural hearing loss.[356]

Patients with germline *GATA2* mutations, regardless of their clinical manifestations, are at increased risk of marrow failure, MDS, AML, and MDS/MPN. Pediatric MDS in GATA2 patients is characterized by a hypocellular marrow, dysplasia predominantly in the megakaryocytic lineage, and increased fibrosis.[357] Of 426 cases in the European Working Group of MDS in Childhood (EWOG-MDS), constitutional *GATA2* mutations were found in 15% of patients with previously undiagnosed advanced MDS and represented 7% of all primary MDS cases, but they were notably absent in cohorts with secondary MDS or acquired AA.[358] These 57 patients with germline *GATA2*

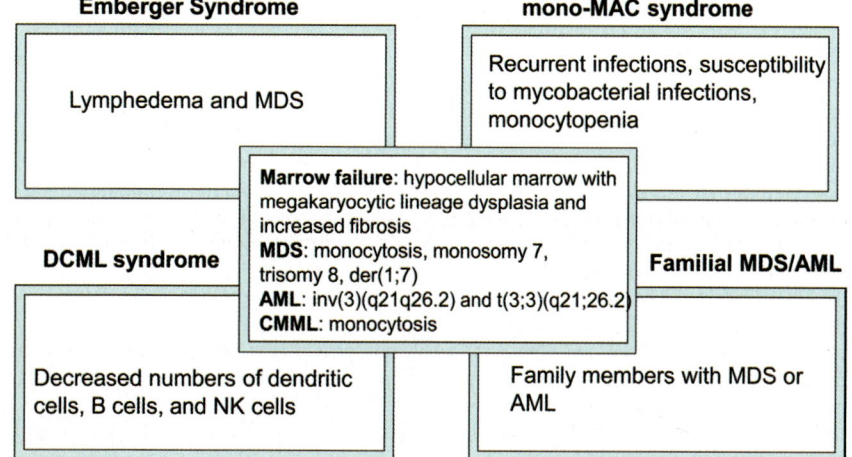

FIGURE 38.2 Clinical features of patients with GATA2 deficiency. Patients can present with familial myelodysplastic syndrome (MDS)/acute myeloid leukemia (AML), Emberger syndrome, DCML syndrome, or MonoMAC syndrome, or can present with isolated MDS, AML, or marrow failure. All patients with GATA2 deficiency are at risk of marrow failure, MDS, AML, and chronic myelomonocytic leukemia. Other clinical extrahematopoietic features of patients with GATA2 deficiency are pulmonary alveolar proteinosis, lymphatic abnormalities, vascular abnormalities, sensorineural hearing loss, and hypothyroidism.

Emberger Syndrome

Lymphedema and MDS

mono-MAC syndrome

Recurrent infections, susceptibility to mycobacterial infections, monocytopenia

Marrow failure: hypocellular marrow with megakaryocytic lineage dysplasia and increased fibrosis
MDS: monocytosis, monosomy 7, trisomy 8, der(1;7)
AML: inv(3)(q21q26.2) and t(3;3)(q21;26.2)
CMML: monocytosis

DCML syndrome

Decreased numbers of dendritic cells, B cells, and NK cells

Familial MDS/AML

Family members with MDS or AML

*Other clinical features of patients with GATA2 deficiency: pulmonary alveolar proteinosis, lymphatic abnormalities, vascular abnormalities, sensorineural hearing loss, hypothyroidism

mutations in the EWOG-MDS cohort were more likely to have monocytosis and monosomy 7 or trisomy 8, with 72% of adolescents with monosomy 7 found to have a *GATA2* mutation. Patients with *GATA2* mutations and MDS also had other characteristic cytogenetic abnormalities including trisomy 8 and der(1;7) in addition to monosomy 7, but their transplant outcome was not influenced by their *GATA2* mutational status.[358] AML in these patients can be associated with recurring inv(3)(q21q26.2) and t(3;3)(q21; 26.2), which may raise suspicion for *GATA2* deficiency. These have been demonstrated to be associated with decreased *GATA2* expression.[359,360]

Differential Diagnosis

The other inherited marrow failure syndromes should be considered in the differential for a patient presenting with marrow failure. For patients who present with AML and have a family history of AML, consideration should be given to testing for other familial cancer predisposition syndromes including familial platelet disorder with propensity to myeloid malignancy (RUNX1), or thrombocytopenia 5 (ETV6), familial AML with mutated DDX41 or ANKRD26, or familial AML (mutations in CEBPA). If patients have a preceding history of neutropenia or family history of neutropenia, the inherited neutropenia syndromes can also be considered. Readers are referred to excellent reviews on the workup of familial myeloid leukemia and hereditary predispositions to MDS.[361-364]

Laboratory Findings

Patients diagnosed with *GATA2* deficiency may have normal blood counts initially but eventually develop trilineage cytopenias over time. This was shown in one report, where 50% of affected patients had normal hemoglobin levels, 61% had normal neutrophil numbers, and 39% had normal platelet numbers, underscoring that patients do not always have abnormal hematologic parameters.[365] Patients with MonoMAC syndrome and other *GATA2* deficiency patients can also present with decreased NK and B cell numbers, as well as monocytopenia. GATA2 patients often show relative T-cell lymphocytosis with inverted CD4:CD8 T-cell ratio, differentiating GATA2 patients from patients with idiopathic AA.[351,365]

It has been demonstrated that patients with GATA2 syndrome have increasing levels of FLT3 ligand as well as circulating CD34$^+$ progenitors over time until the development of MDS.[349,365] These may be markers of stress erythropoiesis. In addition, patients have increased reticulin fibrosis on their bone marrow as well as multilineage dysplasia, which is most striking in the megakaryocytes.[357]

Diagnostic workup for patients with suspected *GATA2* deficiency should include DNA sequencing of the coding sequence, copy number analysis to identify *GATA2* gene deletion, and sequencing of the intron 4 enhancer region.[366,367] For the confirmation of germline status, skin fibroblast testing is recommended for patients presenting with MDS or AML since GATA2 may also be mutated somatically.

Pathophysiology

The *GATA2* gene is located on chromosome 3q21 and encodes a hematopoietic transcription factor with two zinc finger domains, occupying GATA motifs in thousands of target genes through a DNA-binding domain. The *GATA* gene family encodes a group of transcription factors that are evolutionarily conserved and are important in development and differentiation. *GATA2* is important in early erythroid development; thrombopoiesis; maturation of the myeloid, monocytic, and dendritic cell lineages; and in both vascular and lymphatic development.[357] *GATA2* mutations result in loss of function through decreased levels of GATA2 protein, haploinsufficiency, or impairment of DNA binding.[356] Mutations include missense, nonsense, frameshift, duplication, regulatory region alterations, deletions, and substitutions and partial or whole gene deletions.[359,360,366,368] Interestingly, noncoding *GATA2* variants were found in 10.5% of patients with pediatric MDS, in particular in intron 4.[354,368]

In mice studies, *Gata2* knockout embryos cannot survive past day 10 to day 11 of gestation and have decreased self-renewal and proliferation of HPCs.[369,370] Mouse models of *Gata2* heterozygote adult mice

demonstrate that the self-renewal potential of the stem cell compartment remains intact but hematopoietic cells have a disadvantage with competitive transplantation and have a higher fraction of quiescent primitive cells with decreased cell cycling and increased apoptosis.[371]

GATA2 is not only critical in hematopoiesis but also crucial in lymphatic development and is localized in lymphatic vessels. Patients with Emberger syndrome and lymphedema tend to have mutations, which lead to haploinsufficiency through gene deletions or frameshift mutations. Knockdown of *Gata2* in primary lymphatic endothelial cells leads to decreased expression of *Prox1*, *Foxc2*, *Angpt2*, and *Itga9*, which are involved in the development of lymphatic valves.[372]

Supportive Care

Currently, no uniform consensus guidelines exist for monitoring patients with germline *GATA2* mutations. Given the increased incidence of AA, MDS, and leukemia, screening with serial CBCs is advised, and monitoring with bone marrow biopsy and cytogenetics may be considered.[373]

Because of the immunodeficiency associated with *GATA2* mutations, it has been suggested that patients should be vaccinated against HPV and prophylaxis against mycobacterial or bacterial infections can be considered as clinically indicated.[373] Care coordination should be considered with an immunologist for patients with immunodeficiency and with a pulmonologist for patients with pulmonary manifestations.

Treatment

Treatment for these patients includes treatment for marrow failure, MDS, or AML, as well as infections or immunodeficiency. Gaining control over concurrent infections prior to transplantation is an important piece of the pretransplant workup for these patients.

To date, the only curative approach for the immunodeficiency, AA, and MDS has been an HSCT. Severe or symptomatic cytopenias, high-risk clonal abnormalities, MDS, leukemia, or severe symptomatic immunodeficiency are indications for HSCT. However, the optimum timing for transplant and the type of transplant (both conditioning and donor source) have yet to be determined. Nonmyeloablative HSCT has been reported in patients with *GATA2* deficiency with successful immune reconstitution and eradication of the pretransplant malignant clone, although certain groups have recommended myeloablative conditioning with busulfan and fludarabine without prior cytoreductive chemotherapy depending on the clinical context.[374,375] A variety of donor sources have been reported, including umbilical cord blood, bone marrow, and peripheral blood stem cells from HLA-matched unrelated or related donors, or haploidentical donors.

CONCLUSION

The inherited AA syndromes are a heterogeneous group of disorders with germline genetic mutations that lead to variable presentations of AA. Several of these syndromes are also associated with congenital anomalies, cancer predisposition, and variable sensitivity to chemotherapy and/or radiation. Although these disorders are rare individually, they are not as rare as previously suspected when considered as a group of inherited marrow failure syndromes. As described above, maintaining a high level of clinical suspicion for inherited AA syndromes is important in the workup of patients with cytopenias, with hematologic malignancies or congenital anomalies. Thoughtful incorporation of functional and genetic testing along with a comprehensive history and physical examination as part of the diagnostic workup of patients is critical as early diagnosis is important for optimizing surveillance and cancer screening, genetic counseling, and treatment considerations.

ACKNOWLEDGMENTS

The authors regret any omissions of literature citations due to space limitations. This research was supported in part by the National Institutes of Health NIDDK R24 DK099808 (A.S.).

References

1. Sieff CA. Introduction to acquired and inherited bone marrow failure. *Hematol Oncol Clin North Am*. 2018;32:569-580.

2. Mangan JK, Speck NA. RUNX1 mutations in clonal myeloid disorders: from conventional cytogenetics to next generation sequencing, a story 40 years in the making. *Crit Rev Oncog*. 2011;16:77-91.

3. Zhang MY, Churpek JE, Keel SB, et al. Germline ETV6 mutations in familial thrombocytopenia and hematologic malignancy. *Nat Genet*. 2015;47:180-185.

4. Melazzini F, Palombo F, Balduini A, et al. Clinical and pathogenic features of ETV6-related thrombocytopenia with predisposition to acute lymphoblastic leukemia. *Haematologica*. 2016;101:1333-1342.

5. Noris P, Favier R, Alessi MC, et al. ANKRD26-related thrombocytopenia and myeloid malignancies. *Blood*. 2013;122:1987-1989.

6. Keel SB, Scott A, Sanchez-Bonilla M, et al. Genetic features of myelodysplastic syndrome and aplastic anemia in pediatric and young adult patients. *Haematologica*. 2016;101:1343-1350.

7. Muramatsu H, Okuno Y, Yoshida K, et al. Clinical utility of next-generation sequencing for inherited bone marrow failure syndromes. *Genet Med Off J Am Coll Med Genet*. 2017;19:796-802.

8. Glaubach T, Minella AC, Corey SJ. Cellular stress pathways in pediatric bone marrow failure syndromes: many roads lead to neutropenia. *Pediatr Res*. 2014;75:189-195.

9. Tsai FD, Lindsley RC. Clonal hematopoiesis in the inherited bone marrow failure syndromes. *Blood*. 2020;136:1615-1622.

10. Shimamura A, Alter BP. Pathophysiology and management of inherited bone marrow failure syndromes. *Blood Rev*. 2010;24:101-122.

11. Khincha PP, Savage SA. Neonatal manifestations of inherited bone marrow failure syndromes. *Semin Fetal Neonatal Med*. 2016;21:57-65.

12. Elghetany MT, Punia JN, Marcogliese AN. Inherited bone marrow failure syndromes: biology and diagnostic clues. *Clin Lab Med*. 2021;41:417-431.

13. Shimano KA, Narla A, Rose MJ, et al. Diagnostic work-up for severe aplastic anemia in children: consensus of the North American pediatric aplastic anemia consortium. *Am J Hematol*. 2021;96(11):1491-1504. doi:10.1002/ajh.26310

14. Blombery P, Fox L, Ryland GL, et al. Utility of clinical comprehensive genomic characterization for diagnostic categorization in patients presenting with hypocellular bone marrow failure syndromes. *Haematologica*. 2021;106:64-73.

15. Bluteau O, Sebert M, Leblanc T, et al. A landscape of germ line mutations in a cohort of inherited bone marrow failure patients. *Blood*. 2018;131:717-732.

16. Crysandt M, Brings K, Beier F, Thiede C, Brümmendorf TH, Jost E. Germ line predisposition to myeloid malignancies appearing in adulthood. *Expet Rev Hematol*. 2018;11:625-636.

17. Wilson DB, Link DC, Mason PJ, Bessler M. Inherited bone marrow failure syndromes in adolescents and young adults. *Ann Med*. 2014;46:353-363.

18. Zhang MY, Keel SB, Walsh T, et al. Genomic analysis of bone marrow failure and myelodysplastic syndromes reveals phenotypic and diagnostic complexity. *Haematologica*. 2015;100:42-48.

19. Ghemlas I, Li H, Zlateska B, et al. Improving diagnostic precision, care and syndrome definitions using comprehensive next-generation sequencing for the inherited bone marrow failure syndromes. *J Med Genet*. 2015;52:575-584.

20. Alabbas F, Weitzman S, Grant R, et al. Underlying undiagnosed inherited marrow failure syndromes among children with cancer. *Pediatr Blood Cancer*. 2017;64:302-305.

21. Dror Y, Donadieu J, Koglmeier J, et al. Draft consensus guidelines for diagnosis and treatment of Shwachman-Diamond syndrome. *Ann N Y Acad Sci*. 2011;1242:40-55.

22. Savage SA, Cook EF. *Dyskeratosis Congenita and Telomere Biology Disorders: Diagnosis and Management Guidelines*. Dyskeratosis Congenita Outreach, Inc; 2015.

23. Hays L, Frohnmayer D, Frohnmayer L, et al. *Fanconi Anemia: Guidelines for Diagnosis and Management*. 4 edn. Vol 4. Fanconi Anemia Research Fund; 2014.

24. Dietz AC, Duncan CN, Alter BP, et al. The second pediatric blood and marrow transplant consortium international consensus conference on late effects after pediatric hematopoietic cell transplantation: defining the unique late effects of children undergoing hematopoietic cell transplantation for immune deficiencies, inherited marrow failure disorders, and hemoglobinopathies. *Biol Blood Marrow Transplant J Am Soc*. 2017;23:24-29.

25. Yu QH, Wang SY, Wu Z. Advances in genetic studies of inherited bone marrow failure syndromes and their associated malignancies. *Transl Pediatr*. 2014;3:305-309.

26. Donadieu J, Leblanc T, Meunier BB, et al. Analysis of risk factors for myelodysplasias, leukemias and death from infection among patients with congenital neutropenia. Experience of the French Severe Chronic Neutropenia Study Group. *Haematologica*. 2005;90:45-53.

27. Rosenberg PS, Alter BP, Bolyard AA, et al. The incidence of leukemia and mortality from sepsis in patients with severe congenital neutropenia receiving long-term G-CSF therapy. *Blood*. 2006;107:4628-4635.

28. Fanconi G. Familiare infantile perniziosaartige Anamie (pernizioses Blutbild und Konstitution). *Z Kinderheilkunde*. 1927;117:257.

29. Fanconi G. Familial constitutional panmyelocytopathy, Fanconi's anemia (F.A.). I. Clinical aspects. *Semin Hematol*. 1967;4:233-240.

30. Mamrak NE, Shimamura A, Howlett NG. Recent discoveries in the molecular pathogenesis of the inherited bone marrow failure syndrome Fanconi anemia. *Blood Rev*. 2017;31:93-99.

31. Swift M. Fanconi's anaemia in the genetics of neoplasia. *Nature*. 1971;230:370-373.

32. Rogers KJ, Fu W, Akey JM, Monnat RJ. Global and disease-associated genetic variation in the human Fanconi anemia gene family. *Hum Mol Genet*. 2014;23:6815-6825.

33. Sasaki MS, Tonomura A. A high susceptibility of Fanconi's anemia to chromosome breakage by DNA cross-linking agents. *Cancer Res*. 1973;33:1829-1836.

34. Auerbach AD, Wolman SR. Susceptibility of Fanconi's anaemia fibroblasts to chromosome damage by carcinogens. *Nature*. 1976;261:494-496.

35. Hirsch B, Shimamura A, Moreau L, et al. Association of biallelic BRCA2/FANCD1 mutations with spontaneous chromosomal instability and solid tumors of childhood. *Blood*. 2004;103:2554-2559.

36. Auerbach AD, Adler B, Chaganti RS. Prenatal and postnatal diagnosis and carrier detection of Fanconi anemia by a cytogenetic method. *Pediatrics*. 1981;67:128-135.

37. Verlinsky Y, Rechitsky S, Schoolcraft W, Strom C, Kuliev A. Preimplantation diagnosis for Fanconi anemia combined with HLA matching. *JAMA*. 2001;285:3130-3133.

38. Lo Ten Foe JR, Kwee MLB, Rooimans MA, et al. Somatic mosaicism in Fanconi anemia: molecular basis and clinical significance. *Eur J Hum Genet EJHG*. 1997;5:137-148.

39. Waisfisz Q, Morgan NV, Savino M, et al. Spontaneous functional correction of homozygous fanconi anaemia alleles reveals novel mechanistic basis for reverse mosaicism. *Nat Genet*. 1999;22:379-383.

40. Gross M, Hanenberg H, Lobitz S, et al. Reverse mosaicism in Fanconi anemia: natural gene therapy via molecular self-correction. *Cytogenet Genome Res*. 2002;98:126-135.

41. Gregory JJ, Wagner JE, Verlander PC, et al. Somatic mosaicism in Fanconi anemia: evidence of genotypic reversion in lymphohematopoietic stem cells. *Proc Natl Acad Sci USA*. 2001;98:2532-2537.

42. Kubbies M, Schindler D, Hoehn H, Schinzel A, Rabinovitch PS. Endogenous blockage and delay of the chromosome cycle despite normal recruitment and growth phase explain poor proliferation and frequent edomitosis in Fanconi anemia cells. *Am J Hum Genet*. 1985;37:1022-1030.

43. Dutrillaux B, Aurias A, Dutrillaux AM, Buriot D, Prieur M. The cell cycle of lymphocytes in Fanconi anemia. *Hum Genet*. 1982;62:327-332.

44. Alter BP, Giri N. Serum alpha fetoprotein levels in Fanconi anaemia. *Br J Haematol*. 2019;184:1074-1076.

45. Cassinat B, Darsin D, Guardiola P, et al. Intermethod discordance for alpha-fetoprotein measurements in Fanconi anemia. *Clin Chem*. 2001;47:1405-1409.

46. Giampietro PF, Davis JG, Adler-Brecher B, Verlander PC, Auerbach AD, Pavlakis SG. The need for more accurate and timely diagnosis in Fanconi anemia: a report from the International Fanconi Anemia Registry. *Pediatrics*. 1993;91:1116-1120.

47. Kutler DI, Singh B, Satagopan J, et al. A 20-year perspective on the international fanconi anemia registry (IFAR). *Blood*. 2003;101:1249-1256.

48. Fiesco-Roa MO, Giri N, McReynolds LJ, Best AF, Alter BP. Genotype-phenotype associations in Fanconi anemia: a literature review. *Blood Rev*. 2019;37:100589.

49. Faivre L, Portnoï MF, Pals G, et al. Should chromosome breakage studies be performed in patients with VACTERL association? *Am J Med Genet A*. 2005;137:55-58.

50. Petryk A, Kanakatti Shankar R, Giri N, et al. Endocrine disorders in Fanconi anemia: recommendations for screening and treatment. *J Clin Endocrinol Metab*. 2015;100:803-811.

51. Savage SA, Dufour C. Classical inherited bone marrow failure syndromes with high risk for myelodysplastic syndrome and acute myelogenous leukemia. *Semin Hematol*. 2017;54:105-114.

52. Butturini A, Gale R, Verlander P, Adler-Brecher B, Gillio A, Auerbach A. Hematologic abnormalities in fanconi anemia: an international fanconi anemia registry study. *Blood*. 1994;84:1650-1655.

53. Rosenberg PS, Greene MH, Alter BP. Cancer incidence in persons with Fanconi anemia. *Blood*. 2003;101:822-826.

54. Alter BP, Giri N, Savage SA, et al. Malignancies and survival patterns in the National Cancer Institute inherited bone marrow failure syndromes cohort study. *Br J Haematol*. 2010;150:179-188.

55. Alter BP. Fanconi's anemia and malignancies. *Am J Hematol*. 1996;53:99-110.

56. Rosenberg PS, Alter BP, Ebell W. Cancer risks in fanconi anemia: findings from the German fanconi anemia registry. *Haematologica*. 2008;93:511-517.

57. Alter BP, Rosenberg PS, Brody LC. Clinical and molecular features associated with biallelic mutations in FANCD1/BRCA2. *J Med Genet*. 2007;44:1-9.

58. Alter BP, Giri N. Thinking of VACTERL-H? Rule out fanconi anemia according to PHENOS. *Am J Med Genet A*. 2016;170:1520-1524.

59. Nakanishi K, Taniguchi T, Ranganathan V, et al. Interaction of FANCD2 and NBS1 in the DNA damage response. *Nat Cell Biol*. 2002;4:913-920.

60. Cioc AM, Wagner JE, MacMillan ML, DeFor T, Hirsch B. Diagnosis of myelodysplastic syndrome among a cohort of 119 patients with fanconi anemia: morphologic and cytogenetic characteristics. *Am J Clin Pathol*. 2010;133:92-100.

61. Tönnies H, Huber S, Kuhl JS, Gerlach A, Ebell W, Neitzel H. Clonal chromosomal aberrations in bone marrow cells of Fanconi anemia patients: gains of the chromosomal segment 3q26q29 as an adverse risk factor. *Blood*. 2003;101:3872-3874.

62. Alter BP, Caruso JP, Drachtman RA, Uchida T, Velagaleti GVN, Elghetany MT. Fanconi anemia: myelodysplasia as a predictor of outcome. *Cancer Genet Cytogenet*. 2000;117:125-131.

63. Walden H, Deans AJ. The Fanconi anemia DNA repair pathway: structural and functional insights into a complex disorder. *Annu Rev Biophys*. 2014;43:257-278.

64. Lemonidis K, Arkinson C, Rennie ML, Walden H. Mechanism, specificity, and function of FANCD2-FANCI ubiquitination and deubiquitination. *FEBS J*. 2021;289(16):4811-4829. doi:10.1111/febs.16077

65. García-de-Teresa B, Rodríguez A, Frias S. Chromosome instability in fanconi anemia: from breaks to phenotypic consequences. *Genes*. 2020;11:E1528.

66. Taniguchi T, D'Andrea AD. Molecular pathogenesis of Fanconi anemia: recent progress. *Blood*. 2006;107:4223-4233.

67. Ceccaldi R, Sarangi P, D'Andrea AD. The Fanconi anaemia pathway: new players and new functions. *Nat Rev Mol Cell Biol*. 2016;17:337-349.

68. Ling C, Ishiai M, Ali AM, et al. FAAP100 is essential for activation of the Fanconi anemia-associated DNA damage response pathway. *EMBO J*. 2007;26:2104-2114.

69. Huang Y, Leung JWC, Lowery M, et al. Modularized functions of the Fanconi anemia core complex. *Cell Rep*. 2014;7:1849-1857.

70. Shakeel S, Rajendra E, Alcón P, et al. Structure of the Fanconi anaemia monoubiquitin ligase complex. *Nature.* 2019;575:234-237.

71. Levitus M, Rooimans MA, Steltenpool J, et al. Heterogeneity in Fanconi anemia: evidence for 2 new genetic subtypes. *Blood.* 2004;103:2498-2503.

72. Faivre L, Guardiola P, Lewis C, et al. Association of complementation group and mutation type with clinical outcome in fanconi anemia. European Fanconi Anemia Research Group. *Blood.* 2000;96:4064-4070.

73. Swuec P, Renault L, Borg A, et al. The FA core complex contains a homo-dimeric catalytic module for the symmetric mono-ubiquitination of FANCI-FANCD2. *Cell Rep.* 2017;18:611-623.

74. Machida YJ, Machida Y, Chen Y, et al. UBE2T is the E2 in the Fanconi anemia pathway and undergoes negative autoregulation. *Mol Cell.* 2006;23:589-596.

75. Coulthard R, Deans AJ, Swuec P, et al. Architecture and DNA recognition elements of the Fanconi anemia FANCM-FAAP24 complex. *Struct Lond Engl.* 2013;21:1648-1658.

76. Kim JM, Kee Y, Gurtan A, D'Andrea AD. Cell cycle-dependent chromatin loading of the Fanconi anemia core complex by FANCM/FAAP24. *Blood.* 2008;111:5215-5222.

77. Singh TR, Saro D, Ali AM, et al. MHF1-MHF2, a histone-fold-containing protein complex, participates in the Fanconi anemia pathway via FANCM. *Mol Cell.* 2010;37:879-886.

78. Panday A, Willis NA, Elango R, et al. FANCM regulates repair pathway choice at stalled replication forks. *Mol Cell.* 2021;81:2428-2444.e6.

79. Sims AE, Spiteri E, Sims RJ, et al. FANCI is a second monoubiquitinated member of the Fanconi anemia pathway. *Nat Struct Mol Biol.* 2007;14:564-567.

80. Smogorzewska A, Matsuoka S, Vinciguerra P, et al. Identification of the FANCI protein, a monoubiquitinated FANCD2 paralog required for DNA repair. *Cell.* 2007;129:289-301.

81. Rennie ML, Lemonidis K, Arkinson C, et al. Differential functions of FANCI and FANCD2 ubiquitination stabilize ID2 complex on DNA. *EMBO Rep.* 2020;21:e50133.

82. Shimamura A, de Oca RM, Svenson JL, et al. A novel diagnostic screen for defects in the Fanconi anemia pathway. *Blood.* 2002;100:4649-4654.

83. Zhang J, Walter JC. Mechanism and regulation of incisions during DNA interstrand cross-link repair. *DNA Repair.* 2014;19:135-142.

84. Bluteau D, Masliah-Planchon J, Clairmont C, et al. Biallelic inactivation of REV7 is associated with Fanconi anemia. *J Clin Invest.* 2016;126:3580-3584.

85. Zhao W, Steinfeld JB, Liang F, et al. BRCA1-BARD1 promotes RAD51-mediated homologous DNA pairing. *Nature.* 2017;550:360-365.

86. Adamo A, Collis SJ, Adelman CA, et al. Preventing nonhomologous end joining suppresses DNA repair defects of Fanconi anemia. *Mol Cell.* 2010;39:25-35.

87. Thongthip S, Conti BA, Lach FP, Smogorzewska A. Suppression of non-homologous end joining does not rescue DNA repair defects in Fanconi anemia patient cells. *Cell Cycle Georget. Tex.* 2020;19:2553-2561.

88. Cancer Genome Atlas Research Network. Integrated genomic analyses of ovarian carcinoma. *Nature.* 2011;474:609-615.

89. Fang CB, Wu HT, Zhang ML, Liu J, Zhang GJ. Fanconi anemia pathway: mechanisms of breast cancer predisposition development and potential therapeutic targets. *Front Cell Dev Biol.* 2020;8:160.

90. Howlett NG, Taniguchi T, Olson S, et al. Biallelic inactivation of BRCA2 in Fanconi anemia. *Science.* 2002;297:606-609.

91. King MC, Marks JH, Mandell JB. New York Breast Cancer Study Group. Breast and ovarian cancer risks due to inherited mutations in BRCA1 and BRCA2. *Science.* 2003;302:643-646.

92. D'Andrea AD. Susceptibility pathways in Fanconi's anemia and breast cancer. *N Engl J Med.* 2010;362:1909-1919.

93. Taniguchi T, Garcia-Higuera I, Xu B, et al. Convergence of the fanconi anemia and ataxia telangiectasia signaling pathways. *Cell.* 2002;109:459-472.

94. Rathbun RK, Christianson TA, Faulkner GR, et al. Interferon-gamma-induced apoptotic responses of Fanconi anemia group C hematopoietic progenitor cells involve caspase 8-dependent activation of caspase 3 family members. *Blood.* 2000;96:4204-4211.

95. Río P, Bueren JA. TGF-β: a master regulator of the bone marrow failure puzzle in Fanconi anemia. *Stem Cell Invest.* 2016;3:75.

96. Pang Q, Christianson TA, Keeble W, et al. The Fanconi anemia complementation group C gene product: structural evidence of multifunctionality. *Blood.* 2001;98:1392-1401.

97. Sumpter R, Levine B. Novel functions of Fanconi anemia proteins in selective autophagy and inflammation. *Oncotarget.* 2016;7:50820-50821.

98. Sumpter R, Sirasanagandla S, Fernández ÁF, et al. Fanconi anemia proteins function in mitophagy and immunity. *Cell.* 2016;165:867-881.

99. Orvedahl A, Sumpter R, Xiao G, et al. Image-based genome-wide siRNA screen identifies selective autophagy factors. *Nature.* 2011;480:113-117.

100. Pagano G. Mitomycin C and diepoxybutane action mechanisms and FANCC protein functions: further insights into the role for oxidative stress in Fanconi's anaemia phenotype. *Carcinogenesis.* 2000;21:1067-1068.

101. Cumming RC, Lightfoot J, Beard K, Youssoufian H, O'Brien PJ, Buchwald M. Fanconi anemia group C protein prevents apoptosis in hematopoietic cells through redox regulation of GSTP1. *Nat Med.* 2001;7:814-820.

102. El-Bassyouni HT, Afifi H, Eid M, et al. Oxidative stress -a phenotypic hallmark of fanconi anemia and down syndrome: the effect of antioxidants. *Ann Med Health Sci Res.* 2015;5:205-212.

103. Ceccaldi R, Parmar K, Mouly E, et al. Bone marrow failure in Fanconi anemia is triggered by an exacerbated p53/p21 DNA damage response that impairs hematopoietic stem and progenitor cells. *Cell Stem Cell.* 2012;11:36-49.

104. Marion W, Boettcher S, Ruiz-Torres S, et al. An induced pluripotent stem cell model of Fanconi anemia reveals mechanisms of p53-driven progenitor cell differentiation. *Blood Adv.* 2020;4:4679-4692.

105. Liu TX, Howlett NG, Deng M, et al. Knockdown of zebrafish Fancd2 causes developmental abnormalities via p53-dependent apoptosis. *Dev Cell.* 2003;5:903-914.

106. Ceccaldi R, Briot D, Larghero J, et al. Spontaneous abrogation of the G2DNA damage checkpoint has clinical benefits but promotes leukemogenesis in Fanconi anemia patients. *J Clin Invest.* 2011;121:184-194.

107. Langevin F, Crossan GP, Rosado IV, Arends MJ, Patel KJ. Fancd2 counteracts the toxic effects of naturally produced aldehydes in mice. *Nature.* 2011;475:53-58.

108. Garaycoechea JI, Crossan GP, Langevin F, Daly M, Arends MJ, Patel KJ. Genotoxic consequences of endogenous aldehydes on mouse haematopoietic stem cell function. *Nature.* 2012;489:571-575.

109. Pontel LB, Rosado IV, Burgos-Barragan G, et al. Endogenous formaldehyde is a hematopoietic stem cell genotoxin and metabolic carcinogen. *Mol Cell.* 2015;60:177-188.

110. Kotova N, Vare D, Schultz N, et al. Genotoxicity of alcohol is linked to DNA replication-associated damage and homologous recombination repair. *Carcinogenesis.* 2013;34:325-330.

111. Marietta C, Thompson LH, Lamerdin JE, Brooks PJ. Acetaldehyde stimulates FANCD2 monoubiquitination, H2AX phosphorylation, and BRCA1 phosphorylation in human cells in vitro: implications for alcohol-related carcinogenesis. *Mutat Res.* 2009;664:77-83.

112. Abraham J, Balbo S, Crabb D, Brooks PJ. Alcohol metabolism in human cells causes DNA damage and activates the Fanconi anemia-breast cancer susceptibility (FA-BRCA) DNA damage response network. *Alcohol Clin Exp Res.* 2011;35:2113-2120.

113. Hira A, Yabe H, Yoshida K, et al. Variant ALDH2 is associated with accelerated progression of bone marrow failure in Japanese Fanconi anemia patients. *Blood.* 2013;122:3206-3209.

114. Yabe M, Koike T, Ohtsubo K, et al. Associations of complementation group, ALDH2 genotype, and clonal abnormalities with hematological outcome in Japanese patients with Fanconi anemia. *Ann Hematol.* 2019;98:271-280.

115. Van Wassenhove LD, Mochly-Rosen D, Weinberg KI. Aldehyde dehydrogenase 2 in aplastic anemia, Fanconi anemia and hematopoietic stem cells. *Mol Genet Metabol.* 2016;119:28-36.

116. Garaycoechea JI, Crossan GP, Langevin F, et al. Alcohol and endogenous aldehydes damage chromosomes and mutate stem cells. *Nature.* 2018;553:171-177.

117. Kawashima N, Narita A, Wang X, et al. Aldehyde dehydrogenase-2 polymorphism contributes to the progression of bone marrow failure in children with idiopathic aplastic anaemia. *Br J Haematol.* 2015;168:460-463.

118. Blank U, Karlsson S. TGF-β signaling in the control of hematopoietic stem cells. *Blood.* 2015;125:3542-3550.

119. Rodríguez A, Zhang K, Färkkilä A, et al. MYC promotes bone marrow stem cell dysfunction in fanconi anemia. *Cell Stem Cell.* 2021;28:33-47.e8.

120. Rodríguez A, Yang C, Furutani E, et al. Inhibition of TGFβ1 and TGFβ3 promotes hematopoiesis in Fanconi anemia. *Exp Hematol.* 2021;93:70-84.e4.

121. Peffault de Latour R, Soulier J. How I treat MDS and AML in Fanconi anemia. *Blood.* 2016;127:2971-2979.

122. Meyer S, Neitzel H, Tönnies H. Chromosomal aberrations associated with clonal evolution and leukemic transformation in fanconi anemia: clinical and biological implications. *Anemia.* 2012;2012:349837.

123. Schaefer EJ, Lindsley RC. Significance of clonal mutations in bone marrow failure and inherited myelodysplastic syndrome/acute myeloid leukemia predisposition syndromes. *Hematol Oncol Clin North Am.* 2018;32:643-655.

124. Rochowski A, Olson SB, Alonzo TA, Gerbing RB, Lange BJ, Alter BP. Patients with Fanconi anemia and AML have different cytogenetic clones than de novo cases of AML. *Pediatr Blood Cancer.* 2012;59:922-924.

125. Quentin S, Cuccuini W, Ceccaldi R, et al. Myelodysplasia and leukemia of Fanconi anemia are associated with a specific pattern of genomic abnormalities that includes cryptic RUNX1/AML1 lesions. *Blood.* 2011;117:e161-e170.

126. Khanal S, Galloway DA. High-risk human papillomavirus oncogenes disrupt the Fanconi anemia DNA repair pathway by impairing localization and de-ubiquitination of FancD2. *PLoS Pathog.* 2019;15:e1007442.

127. Rose SR, Myers KC, Rutter MM, et al. Endocrine phenotype of children and adults with Fanconi anemia. *Pediatr Blood Cancer.* 2012;59:690-696.

128. Ebens CL, MacMillan ML, Wagner JE. Hematopoietic cell transplantation in Fanconi anemia: current evidence, challenges and recommendations. *Expet Rev Hematol.* 2017;10:81-97.

129. Anur P, Friedman DN, Sklar C, et al. Late effects in patients with Fanconi anemia following allogeneic hematopoietic stem cell transplantation from alternative donors. *Bone Marrow Transplant.* 2016;51:938-944.

130. Rosenberg PS, Socié G, Alter BP, Gluckman E. Risk of head and neck squamous cell cancer and death in patients with Fanconi anemia who did and did not receive transplants. *Blood.* 2005;105:67-73.

131. Guardiola P, Socié G, Li X, et al. Acute graft-versus-host disease in patients with Fanconi anemia or acquired aplastic anemia undergoing bone marrow transplantation from HLA-identical sibling donors: risk factors and influence on outcome. *Blood.* 2004;103:73-77.

132. Dufour C, Rondelli R, Locatelli F, et al. Stem cell transplantation from HLA-matched related donor for Fanconi's anaemia: a retrospective review of the multicentric Italian experience on behalf of AIEOP-GITMO. *Br J Haematol.* 2001;112:796-805.

133. Farzin A, Davies SM, Smith FO, et al. Matched sibling donor haematopoietic stem cell transplantation in Fanconi anaemia: an update of the Cincinnati Children's experience. *Br J Haematol.* 2007;136:633-640.

134. Torjemane L, Ladeb S, Ben Othman T, Abdelkefi A, Lakhal A, Ben Abdeladhim A. Bone marrow transplantation from matched related donors for patients with Fanconi anemia using low-dose busulfan and cyclophosphamide as conditioning. *Pediatr Blood Cancer.* 2006;46:496-500.

135. Bonfim C, Ribeiro L, Nichele S, et al. Long-term survival, organ function, and malignancy after hematopoietic stem cell transplantation for fanconi anemia. *Biol. Blood Marrow Transplant J Am Soc Blood Marrow Transplant*. 2016;22:1257-1263.

136. de la Fuente J, Reiss S, McCloy M, et al. Non-TBI stem cell transplantation protocol for Fanconi anaemia using HLA-compatible sibling and unrelated donors. *Bone Marrow Transplant*. 2003;32:653-656.

137. Tan PL, Wagner JE, Auerbach AD, DeFor TE, Slungaard A, MacMillan ML. Successful engraftment without radiation after fludarabine-based regimen in Fanconi anemia patients undergoing genotypically identical donor hematopoietic cell transplantation. *Pediatr Blood Cancer*. 2006;46:630-636.

138. Bitan M, Or R, Shapira MY, et al. Fludarabine-based reduced intensity conditioning for stem cell transplantation of Fanconi anemia patients from fully matched related and unrelated donors. *Biol Blood Marrow Transplant*. 2006;12:712-718.

139. Rose SR, Kim MO, Korbee L, et al. Oxandrolone for the treatment of bone marrow failure in Fanconi anemia. *Pediatr Blood Cancer*. 2014;61:11-19.

140. Scheckenbach K, Morgan M, Filger-Brillinger J, et al. Treatment of the bone marrow failure in Fanconi anemia patients with danazol. *Blood Cells Mol Dis*. 2012;48:128-131.

141. Guinan EC, Lopez KD, Huhn RD, Felser JM, Nathan DG. Evaluation of granulocyte-macrophage colony-stimulating factor for treatment of pancytopenia in children with fanconi anemia. *J Pediatr*. 1994;124:144-150.

142. Rackoff WR, Orazi A, Robinson C, et al. Prolonged administration of granulocyte colony-stimulating factor (filgrastim) to patients with Fanconi anemia: a pilot study. *Blood*. 1996;88:1588-1593.

143. Liu JM, Kim S, Read EJ, et al. Engraftment of hematopoietic progenitor cells transduced with the Fanconi anemia group C gene (FANCC). *Hum Gene Ther*. 1999;10:2337-2346.

144. Río P, Navarro S, Wang W, et al. Successful engraftment of gene-corrected hematopoietic stem cells in non-conditioned patients with Fanconi anemia. *Nat Med*. 2019;25:1396-1401.

145. Croop JM, Cooper R, Fernandez C, et al. Mobilization and collection of peripheral blood CD34+ cells from patients with Fanconi anemia. *Blood*. 2001;98:2917-2921.

146. Habi O, Delisle M-C, Messier N, Carreau M. Lack of self-renewal capacity in Fancc-/- stem cells after ex vivo expansion. *Stem Cells*. 2005;23:1135-1141.

147. Haworth KG, Ironside C, Ramirez MA, et al. Minimal conditioning in Fanconi anemia promotes multi-lineage marrow engraftment at 10-fold lower cell doses. *J Gene Med*. 2018;20:e3050.

148. Hacein-Bey-Abina S, von Kalle C, Schmidt M, et al. A serious adverse event after successful gene therapy for X-linked severe combined immunodeficiency. *N Engl J Med*. 2003;348:255-256.

149. Adair JE, Sevilla J, Heredia C, Becker P, Kiem HP, Bueren J. Lessons learned from two decades of clinical trial experience in gene therapy for fanconi anemia. *Curr Gene Ther*. 2017;16:338-348.

150. Verhoeyen E, Roman-Rodriguez FJ, Cosset FL, Levy C, Rio P. Gene therapy in fanconi anemia: a matter of time, safety and gene transfer tool efficiency. *Curr Gene Ther*. 2017;16:297-308.

151. Mehta PA, Ileri T, Harris RE, et al. Chemotherapy for myeloid malignancy in children with Fanconi anemia. *Pediatr Blood Cancer*. 2007;48:668-672.

152. Giardino S, Latour RP, Aljurf M, et al. Outcome of patients with Fanconi anemia developing myelodysplasia and acute leukemia who received allogeneic hematopoietic stem cell transplantation: a retrospective analysis on behalf of EBMT group. *Am J Hematol*. 2020;95:809-816.

153. Yabe M, Morio T, Tabuchi K, et al. Long-term outcome in patients with Fanconi anemia who received hematopoietic stem cell transplantation: a retrospective nationwide analysis. *Int J Hematol*. 2021;113:134-144.

154. Peffault de Latour R, Porcher R, Dalle JH, et al. Allogeneic hematopoietic stem cell transplantation in Fanconi anemia: the European Group for Blood and Marrow Transplantation experience. *Blood*. 2013;122:4279-4286.

155. Ayas M, Saber W, Davies SM, et al. Allogeneic hematopoietic cell transplantation for fanconi anemia in patients with pretransplantation cytogenetic abnormalities, myelodysplastic syndrome, or acute leukemia. *J Clin Oncol*. 2013;31:1669-1676.

156. Cole HN, Rauschkolb J, Toomey J. Dyskeratosis congenita with pigmentation, dystrophia unguium and leucokeratosis oris; review of the known cases reported to date and discussion of the disease from various aspects. *AMA Arch Dermatol*. 1955;71:451-456.

157. Zinsser F. Atrophia cutis reticularis cum pigmentione, dystrophia unguium et leukokeratosis oris. *Ikonogr Dermatol*. 1906;5:219-223.

158. Niewisch MR, Savage SA. An update on the biology and management of dyskeratosis congenita and related telomere biology disorders. *Expet Rev Hematol*. 2019;12:1037-1052.

159. Agarwal S. Evaluation and management of hematopoietic failure in dyskeratosis congenita. *Hematol Oncol Clin North Am*. 2018;32:669-685.

160. Alter BP, Rosenberg PS, Giri N, Baerlocher GM, Lansdorp PM, Savage SA. Telomere length is associated with disease severity and declines with age in dyskeratosis congenita. *Haematologica*. 2012;97:353-359.

161. Alter BP, Giri N, Savage SA, Rosenberg PS. Telomere length in inherited bone marrow failure syndromes. *Haematologica*. 2015;100:49-54.

162. Aubert G, Hills M, Lansdorp PM. Telomere length measurement-caveats and a critical assessment of the available technologies and tools. *Mutat Res*. 2012;730:59-67.

163. Alter BP, Baerlocher GM, Savage SA, et al. Very short telomere length by flow fluorescence in situ hybridization identifies patients with dyskeratosis congenita. *Blood*. 2007;110:1439-1447.

164. Ferreira MSV, Kirschner M, Halfmeyer I, et al. Comparison of flow-FISH and MM-qPCR telomere length assessment techniques for the screening of telomeropathies. *Ann N Y Acad Sci*. 2020;1466:93-103.

165. Jongmans MCJ, Verwiel ETP, Heijdra Y, et al. Revertant somatic mosaicism by mitotic recombination in dyskeratosis congenita. *Am J Hum Genet*. 2012;90:426-433.

166. Dokal I. Dyskeratosis congenita in all its forms. *Br J Haematol*. 2000;110:768-779.

167. Ling NS, Fenske NA, Julius RL, Espinoza CG, Drake LA. Dyskeratosis congenita in a girl simulating chronic graft-vs-host disease. *Arch Dermatol*. 1985;121:1424-1428.

168. Ivker RA, Woosley J, Resnick SD. Dyskeratosis congenita or chronic graft-versus-host disease? A diagnostic dilemma in a child eight years after bone marrow transplantation for aplastic anemia. *Pediatr Dermatol*. 1993;10:362-365.

169. Paul SR, Perez-Atayde A, Williams DA. Interstitial pulmonary disease associated with dyskeratosis congenita. *Am J Pediatr Hematol Oncol*. 1992;14:89-92.

170. Giri N, Ravichandran S, Wang Y, et al. Prognostic significance of pulmonary function tests in dyskeratosis congenita, a telomere biology disorder. *ERJ Open Res*. 2019;5:00209-02019.

171. Shomali W, Brar R. Late presentation of dyskeratosis congenita. *Br J Haematol*. 2019;187:273.

172. Armanios M. Syndromes of telomere shortening. *Annu Rev Genom Hum Genet*. 2009;10:45-61.

173. Khincha PP, Bertuch AA, Agarwal S, et al. Pulmonary arteriovenous malformations: an uncharacterised phenotype of dyskeratosis congenita and related telomere biology disorders. *Eur Respir J*. 2017;49:1601640.

174. Higgs C, Crow YJ, Adams DM, et al. Understanding the evolving phenotype of vascular complications in telomere biology disorders. *Angiogenesis*. 2019;22:95-102.

175. Alter BP, Giri N, Savage SA, Rosenberg PS. Cancer in the National Cancer Institute inherited bone marrow failure syndrome cohort after fifteen years of follow-up. *Haematologica*. 2018;103:30-39.

176. Alter BP, Giri N, Savage SA, Rosenberg PS. Cancer in dyskeratosis congenita. *Blood*. 2009;113:6549-6557.

177. Glousker G, Touzot F, Revy P, Tzfati Y, Savage SA. Unraveling the pathogenesis of Hoyeraal-Hreidarsson syndrome, a complex telomere biology disorder. *Br J Haematol*. 2015;170:457-471.

178. Karremann M, Neumaier-Probst E, Schlichtenbrede F, et al. Revesz syndrome revisited. *Orphanet J Rare Dis*. 2020;15:299.

179. Crow YJ, McMenamin J, Haenggeli C, et al. Coats' plus: a progressive familial syndrome of bilateral Coats' disease, characteristic cerebral calcification, leukoencephalopathy, slow pre- and post-natal linear growth and defects of bone marrow and integument. *Neuropediatrics*. 2004;35:10-19.

180. Coulthard S, Chase A, Pickard J, Goldman J, Dokal I. Chromosomal breakage analysis in dyskeratosis congenita peripheral blood lymphocytes. *Br J Haematol*. 1998;102:1162-1164.

181. Pai GS, Yan Y, DeBauche DM, Stanley WS, Paul SR. Bleomycin hypersensitivity in dyskeratosis congenita fibroblasts, lymphocytes, and transformed lymphoblasts. *Cytogenet Cell Genet*. 1989;52:186-189.

182. DeBauche DM, Pai GS, Stanley WS. Enhanced G2 chromatid radiosensitivity in dyskeratosis congenita fibroblasts. *Am J Hum Genet*. 1990;46:350-357.

183. Reichel M, Grix AC, Isseroff RR. Dyskeratosis congenita associated with elevated fetal hemoglobin, X-linked ocular albinism, and juvenile-onset diabetes mellitus. *Pediatr Dermatol*. 1992;9:103-106.

184. Giri N, Alter BP, Penrose K, et al. Immune status of patients with inherited bone marrow failure syndromes. *Am J Hematol*. 2015;90:702-708.

185. Sölder B, Weiss M, Jäger A, Belohradsky BH. Dyskeratosis congenita: multisystemic disorder with special consideration of immunologic aspects. A review of the literature. *Clin Pediatr (Phila)*. 1998;37:521-530.

186. Devriendt K, Matthijs G, Legius E, et al. Skewed X-chromosome inactivation in female carriers of dyskeratosis congenita. *Am J Hum Genet*. 1997;60:581-587.

187. Ferraris AM, Forni GL, Mangerini R, Gaetani GF. Nonrandom X-chromosome inactivation in hemopoietic cells from carriers of dyskeratosis congenita. *Am J Hum Genet*. 1997;61:458-461.

188. Vulliamy TJ, Knight SW, Dokal I, Mason PJ. Skewed X-inactivation in carriers of X-linked dyskeratosis congenita. *Blood*. 1997;90:2213-2216.

189. Xu J, Khincha PP, Giri N, Alter BP, Savage SA, Wong JMY. Investigation of chromosome X inactivation and clinical phenotypes in female carriers of DKC1 mutations. *Am J Hematol*. 2016;91:1215-1220.

190. Scappaticci S, Fraccaro M, Cerimele D. Chromosome abnormalities in dyskeratosis congenita. *Am J Med Genet*. 1989;34:609-610.

191. Dokal I, Bungey J, Williamson P, Oscier D, Hows J, Luzzatto L. Dyskeratosis congenita fibroblasts are abnormal and have unbalanced chromosomal rearrangements. *Blood*. 1992;80:3090-3096.

192. Shay JW, Wright WE. Telomeres and telomerase: three decades of progress. *Nat Rev Genet*. 2019;20:299-309.

193. Grill S, Nandakumar J. Molecular mechanisms of telomere biology disorders. *J Biol Chem*. 2021;296:100064.

194. Marciniak RA, Johnson FB, Guarente L. Dyskeratosis congenita, telomeres and human ageing. *Trends Genet TIG*. 2000;16:193-195.

195. Shay JW. Role of telomeres and telomerase in aging and cancer. *Cancer Discov*. 2016;6:584-593.

196. Mitchell JR, Wood E, Collins K. A telomerase component is defective in the human disease dyskeratosis congenita. *Nature*. 1999;402:551-555.

197. Bertuch AA. The molecular genetics of the telomere biology disorders. *RNA Biol*. 2016;13:696-706.

198. Alder JK, Barkauskas CE, Limjunyawong N, et al. Telomere dysfunction causes alveolar stem cell failure. *Proc Natl Acad Sci USA*. 2015;112:5099-5104.

199. Marsh JC, Will A, Hows J, et al. "Stem cell" origin of the hematopoietic defect in dyskeratosis congenita. *Blood*. 1992;79:3138-3144.

200. Friedland M, Lutton JD, Spitzer R, Levere RD. Dyskeratosis congenita with hypoplastic anemia: a stem cell defect. *Am J Hematol*. 1985;20:85-87.

Disorders of Red Blood Cells

201. Alter BP, Knobloch M, He L, et al. Effect of stem cell factor on in vitro erythropoiesis in patients with bone marrow failure syndromes. *Blood*. 1992;80:3000-3008.

202. Colvin BT, Baker H, Hibbin JA, Gordon-Smith EC, Gordon MY. Haemopoietic progenitor cells in dyskeratosis congenita. *Br J Haematol*. 1984;56:513-515.

203. Heiss NS, Knight SW, Vulliamy TJ, et al. X-linked dyskeratosis congenita is caused by mutations in a highly conserved gene with putative nucleolar functions. *Nat Genet*. 1998;19:32-38.

204. Kam MLW, Nguyen TTT, Ngeow JYY. Telomere biology disorders. *NPJ Genomic Med*. 2021;6:36.

205. Simon AJ, Lev A, Zhang Y, et al. Mutations in STN1 cause Coats plus syndrome and are associated with genomic and telomere defects. *J Exp Med*. 2016;213:1429-1440.

206. Lin H, Gong L, Zhan S, Wang Y, Liu A. Novel biallelic missense mutations in CTC1 gene identified in a Chinese family with Coats plus syndrome. *J Neurol Sci*. 2017;382:142-145.

207. Acharya T, Firth HV, Dugar S, et al. Novel compound heterozygous STN1 variants are associated with coats plus syndrome. *Mol Genet Genomic Med*. 2021;9(12):e1708. doi:10.1002/mgg3.1708

208. Armanios M, Chen JL, Chang YPC, et al. Haploinsufficiency of telomerase reverse transcriptase leads to anticipation in autosomal dominant dyskeratosis congenita. *Proc Natl Acad Sci USA*. 2005;102:15960-15964.

209. Vulliamy T, Beswick R, Kirwan M, et al. Mutations in the telomerase component NHP2 cause the premature ageing syndrome dyskeratosis congenita. *Proc Natl Acad Sci USA*. 2008;105:8073-8078.

210. Walne AJ, Vulliamy T, Beswick R, Kirwan M, Dokal I. TINF2 mutations result in very short telomeres: analysis of a large cohort of patients with dyskeratosis congenita and related bone marrow failure syndromes. *Blood*. 2008;112:3594-3600.

211. Stanley SE, Gable DL, Wagner CL, et al. Loss-of-function mutations in the RNA biogenesis factor NAF1 predispose to pulmonary fibrosis-emphysema. *Sci Transl Med*. 2016;8:351ra107.

212. Savage SA, Stewart BJ, Weksler BB, et al. Mutations in the reverse transcriptase component of telomerase (TERT) in patients with bone marrow failure. *Blood Cells Mol Dis*. 2006;37:134-136.

213. Terada K, Miyake K, Yamaguchi H, et al. TERT and TERC mutations detected in cryptic dyskeratosis congenita suppress telomerase activity. *Int J Lab Hematol*. 2020;42:316-321.

214. Kalathiya U, Padariya M, Baginski M. Molecular basis and quantitative assessment of TRF1 and TRF2 protein interactions with TIN2 and Apollo peptides. *Eur Biophys J EBJ*. 2017;46:171-187.

215. Frescas D, de Lange T. TRF2-tethered TIN2 can mediate telomere protection by TPP1/POT1. *Mol Cell Biol*. 2014;34:1349-1362.

216. Pike AM, Strong MA, Ouyang JPT, Greider CW. TIN2 functions with TPP1/POT1 to stimulate telomerase processivity. *Mol Cell Biol*. 2019;39:e005933-18.

217. Zhang MJ, Cao YX, Wu HY, Li HH. Brain imaging features of children with Hoyeraal-Heidarsson syndrome. *Brain Behav*. 2021;11:e02079.

218. Savage SA, Giri N, Baerlocher GM, Orr N, Lansdorp PM, Alter BP. TINF2, a component of the shelterin telomere protection complex, is mutated in dyskeratosis congenita. *Am J Hum Genet*. 2008;82:501-509.

219. Benyelles M, O'Donohue MF, Kermasson L, et al. NHP2 deficiency impairs rRNA biogenesis and causes pulmonary fibrosis and Høyeraal-Hreidarsson syndrome. *Hum Mol Genet*. 2020;29:907-922.

220. Guo Y, Kartawinata M, Li J, et al. Inherited bone marrow failure associated with germline mutation of ACD, the gene encoding telomere protein TPP1. *Blood*. 2014;124:2767-2774.

221. Takai H, Jenkinson E, Kabir S, et al. A POT1 mutation implicates defective telomere end fill-in and telomere truncations in Coats plus. *Genes Dev*. 2016;30:812-826.

222. Anderson BH, Kasher PR, Mayer J, et al. Mutations in CTC1, encoding conserved telomere maintenance component 1, cause Coats plus. *Nat Genet*. 2012;44:338-342.

223. Walne AJ, Bhagat T, Kirwan M, et al. Mutations in the telomere capping complex in bone marrow failure and related syndromes. *Haematologica*. 2013;98:334-338.

224. Keller RB, Gagne KE, Usmani GN, et al. CTC1 Mutations in a patient with dyskeratosis congenita. *Pediatr Blood Cancer*. 2012;59:311-314.

225. Sarek G, Vannier J-B, Panier S, Petrini JHJ, Boulton SJ. TRF2 recruits RTEL1 to telomeres in S phase to promote t-loop unwinding. *Mol Cell*. 2015;57:622-635.

226. Le Guen T, Jullien L, Touzot F, et al. Human RTEL1 deficiency causes Hoyeraal-Hreidarsson syndrome with short telomeres and genome instability. *Hum Mol Genet*. 2013;22:3239-3249.

227. Ballew BJ, Yeager M, Jacobs K, et al. Germline mutations of regulator of telomere elongation helicase 1, RTEL1, in Dyskeratosis congenita. *Hum Genet*. 2013;132:473-480.

228. Touzot F, Kermasson L, Jullien L, et al. Extended clinical and genetic spectrum associated with biallelic RTEL1 mutations. *Blood Adv*. 2016;1:36-46.

229. Montellese C, Montel-Lehry N, Henras AK, Kutay U, Gleizes PE, O'Donohue MF. Poly(A)-specific ribonuclease is a nuclear ribosome biogenesis factor involved in human 18S rRNA maturation. *Nucleic Acids Res*. 2017;45:6822-6836.

230. Benyelles M, Episkopou H, O'Donohue MF, et al. Impaired telomere integrity and rRNA biogenesis in PARN-deficient patients and knock-out models. *EMBO Mol Med*. 2019;11:e10201.

231. Tummala H, Walne A, Collopy L, et al. Poly(A)-specific ribonuclease deficiency impacts telomere biology and causes dyskeratosis congenita. *J Clin Invest*. 2015;125:2151-2160.

232. Stuart BD, Choi J, Zaidi S, et al. Exome sequencing links mutations in PARN and RTEL1 with familial pulmonary fibrosis and telomere shortening. *Nat Genet*. 2015;47:512-517.

233. Moon DH, Segal M, Boyraz B, et al. Poly(A)-specific ribonuclease (PARN) mediates 3'-end maturation of the telomerase RNA component. *Nat Genet*. 2015;47:1482-1488.

234. Perdigones N, Perin JC, Schiano I, et al. Clonal hematopoiesis in patients with dyskeratosis congenita. *Am J Hematol*. 2016;91:1227-1233.

235. Wiedemann HP, McGuire J, Dwyer JM, et al. Progressive immune failure in dyskeratosis congenita. Report of an adult in whom Pneumocystis carinii and fatal disseminated candidiasis developed. *Arch Intern Med*. 1984;144:397-399.

236. Rose C, Kern WV. Another case of Pneumocystis carinii pneumonia in a patient with dyskeratosis congenita (Zinsser-Cole-Engman syndrome). *Clin Infect Dis*. 1992;15:1056-1057.

237. Gadalla SM, Sales-Bonfim C, Carreras J, et al. Outcomes of allogeneic hematopoietic cell transplantation in patients with dyskeratosis congenita. *Biol Blood Marrow Transplant*. 2013;19:1238-1243.

238. Barbaro P, Vedi A. Survival after hematopoietic stem cell transplant in patients with dyskeratosis congenita: systematic review of the literature. *Biol Blood Marrow Transplant*. 2016;22:1152-1158.

239. Nelson AS, Marsh RA, Myers KC, et al. A reduced-intensity conditioning regimen for patients with dyskeratosis congenita undergoing hematopoietic stem cell transplantation. *Biol Blood Marrow Transplant*. 2016;22:884-888.

240. Dietz AC, Orchard PJ, Baker KS, et al. Disease-specific hematopoietic cell transplantation: nonmyeloablative conditioning regimen for dyskeratosis congenita. *Bone Marrow Transplant*. 2011;46:98-104.

241. Brown M, Myers D, Shreve N, Rahmetullah R, Radhi M. Reduced intensity conditioning regimen with fludarabine, cyclophosphamide, low dose TBI and alemtuzumab leading to successful unrelated umbilical cord stem cell engraftment and survival in two children with dyskeratosis congenita. *Bone Marrow Transplant*. 2016;51:744-746.

242. Bhoopalan SV, Wlodarski M, Reiss U, Triplett B, Sharma A. Reduced-intensity conditioning-based hematopoietic cell transplantation for dyskeratosis congenita: single-center experience and literature review. *Pediatr Blood Cancer*. 2021;68(10):e29177. doi:10.1002/pbc.29177

243. Fioredda F, Iacobelli S, Korthof ET, et al. Outcome of haematopoietic stem cell transplantation in dyskeratosis congenita. *Br J Haematol*. 2018;183:110-118.

244. Agarwal S, Williams DA, London WB, et al. Full donor myeloid engraftment with minimal toxicity in dyskeratosis congenita patients undergoing allogeneic bone marrow transplantation without radiation or alkylating agents. *Blood*. 2014;124(21):2941.

245. Al-Rahawan MM, Giri N, Alter BP. Intensive immunosuppression therapy for aplastic anemia associated with dyskeratosis congenita. *Int J Hematol*. 2006;83:275-276.

246. Trautmann K, Jakob C, von Grünhagen U, et al. Eltrombopag fails to improve severe thrombocytopenia in late-stage dyskeratosis congenita and diamond-blackfan-anaemia. *Thromb Haemostasis*. 2012;108:397-398.

247. Townsley DM, Dumitriu B, Liu D, et al. Danazol treatment for telomere diseases. *N Engl J Med*. 2016;374:1922-1931.

248. Vieri M, Kirschner M, Tometten M, et al. Comparable effects of the androgen derivatives danazol, oxymetholone and nandrolone on telomerase activity in human primary hematopoietic cells from patients with dyskeratosis congenita. *Int J Mol Sci*. 2020;21:E7196.

249. Khincha PP, Bertuch AA, Gadalla SM, Giri N, Alter BP, Savage SA. Similar telomere attrition rates in androgen-treated and untreated patients with dyskeratosis congenita. *Blood Adv*. 2018;2:1243-1249.

250. Giri N, Pitel PA, Green D, Alter BP. Splenic peliosis and rupture in patients with dyskeratosis congenita on androgens and granulocyte colony-stimulating factor. *Br J Haematol*. 2007;138:815-817.

251. Myers KC, Bolyard AA, Otto B, et al. Variable clinical presentation of shwachman-diamond syndrome: update from the North American shwachman-diamond syndrome registry. *J Pediatr*. 2014;164:866-870.

252. Shwachman H, Diamond LK, Oski FA, Khaw KT. The syndrome of pancreatic insufficiency and bone marrow dysfunction. *J Pediatr*. 1964;65:645-663.

253. Boocock GRB, Morrison JA, Popovic M, et al. Mutations in SBDS are associated with Shwachman-Diamond syndrome. *Nat Genet*. 2003;33:97-101.

254. Carapito R, Konantz M, Paillard C, et al. Mutations in signal recognition particle SRP54 cause syndromic neutropenia with Shwachman-Diamond-like features. *J Clin Invest*. 2017;127:4090-4103.

255. Stepensky P, Chacón-Flores M, Kim KH, et al. Mutations in EFL1, an SBDS partner, are associated with infantile pancytopenia, exocrine pancreatic insufficiency and skeletal anomalies in aShwachman-Diamond like syndrome. *J Med Genet*. 2017;54:558-566.

256. Dhanraj S, Matveev A, Li H, et al. Biallelic mutations in DNAJC21 cause Shwachman-Diamond syndrome. *Blood*. 2017;129:1557-1562.

257. Smith OP, Hann IM, Chessells JM, Reeves BR, Milla P. Haematological abnormalities in Shwachman-Diamond syndrome. *Br J Haematol*. 1996;94:279-284.

258. Dror Y, Ginzberg H, Dalal I, et al. Immune function in patients with Shwachman-Diamond syndrome. *Br J Haematol*. 2001;114:712-717.

259. Valli R, De Paoli E, Nacci L, Frattini A, Pasquali F, Maserati E. Novel recurrent chromosome anomalies in Shwachman-Diamond syndrome. *Pediatr Blood Cancer*. 2017;64(8).

260. Dror Y, Durie P, Ginzberg H, et al. Clonal evolution in marrows of patients with Shwachman-Diamond syndrome: a prospective 5-year follow-up study. *Exp Hematol*. 2002;30:659-669.

261. Myers KC, Furutani E, Weller E, et al. Clinical features and outcomes of patients with Shwachman-Diamond syndrome and myelodysplastic syndrome or acute myeloid leukaemia: a multicentre, retrospective, cohort study. *Lancet Haematol*. 2020;7:e238-e246.

262. Lindsley RC, Saber W, Mar BG, et al. Prognostic mutations in myelodysplastic syndrome after stem-cell transplantation. *N Engl J Med*. 2017;376:536-547.

263. Burroughs L, Woolfrey A, Shimamura A. Shwachman-Diamond syndrome: a review of the clinical presentation, molecular pathogenesis, diagnosis, and treatment. *Hematol Oncol Clin N Am*. 2009;23:233-248.

264. Toiviainen-Salo S, Durie PR, Numminen K, et al. The natural history of Shwachman-Diamond syndrome-associated liver disease from childhood to adulthood. *J Pediatr.* 2009;155:807-811.e2.

265. Cipolli M. Shwachman-Diamond syndrome: clinical phenotypes. *Pancreatology.* 2001;1:543-548.

266. Ip WF, Dupuis A, Ellis L, et al. Serum pancreatic enzymes define the pancreatic phenotype in patients with Shwachman-Diamond syndrome. *J Pediatr.* 2002;141:259-265.

267. Myers KC, Rose SR, Rutter MM, et al. Endocrine evaluation of children with and without Shwachman-Bodian-Diamond syndrome gene mutations and Shwachman-Diamond syndrome. *J Pediatr.* 2013;162:1235-1240, 1240.e1.

268. Mäkitie O, Ellis L, Durie P, et al. Skeletal phenotype in patients with Shwachman-Diamond syndrome and mutations in SBDS. *Clin Genet.* 2004;65:101-112.

269. Goobie S, Popovic M, Morrison J, et al. Shwachman-Diamond syndrome with exocrine pancreatic dysfunction and bone marrow failure maps to the centromeric region of chromosome 7. *Am J Hum Genet.* 2001;68:1048-1054.

270. Woloszynek JR, Rothbaum RJ, Rawls AS, et al. Mutations of the SBDS gene are present in most patients with Shwachman-Diamond syndrome. *Blood.* 2004;104:3588-3590.

271. Austin KM, Leary RJ, Shimamura A. The Shwachman-Diamond SBDS protein localizes to the nucleolus. *Blood.* 2005;106:1253-1258.

272. Warren AJ. Molecular basis of the human ribosomopathy Shwachman-Diamond syndrome. *Adv Biol Regul.* 2018;67:109-127.

273. Ganapathi KA, Austin KM, Lee CS, et al. The human Shwachman-Diamond syndrome protein, SBDS, associates with ribosomal RNA. *Blood.* 2007;110:1458-1465.

274. Zhang S, Shi M, Hui CC, Rommens JM. Loss of the mouse ortholog of the shwachman-diamond syndrome gene (Sbds) results in early embryonic lethality. *Mol Cell Biol.* 2006;26:6656-6663.

275. Weis F, Giudice E, Churcher M, et al. Mechanism of eIF6 release from the nascent 60S ribosomal subunit. *Nat Struct Mol Biol.* 2015;22:914-919.

276. Finch AJ, Hilcenko C, Basse N, et al. Uncoupling of GTP hydrolysis from eIF6 release on the ribosome causes Shwachman-Diamond syndrome. *Genes Dev.* 2011;25:917-929.

277. Ceci M, Gaviraghi C, Gorrini C, et al. Release of eIF6 (p27BBP) from the 60S subunit allows 80S ribosome assembly. *Nature.* 2003;426:579-584.

278. Gartmann M, Blau M, Armache JP, Mielke T, Topf M, Beckmann R. Mechanism of eIF6-mediated inhibition of ribosomal subunit joining. *J Biol Chem.* 2010;285:14848-14851.

279. Austin KM, Gupta ML, Coats SA, et al. Mitotic spindle destabilization and genomic instability in Shwachman-Diamond syndrome. *J Clin Invest.* 2008;118:1511-1518.

280. Ball HL, Zhang B, Riches JJ, Gandhi R, Li J, Rommens JM, Myers JS. Shwachman-Bodian Diamond syndrome is a multi-functional protein implicated in cellular stress responses. *Hum Mol Genet.* 2009;18:3684-3695.

281. Orelio C, Kuijpers TW. Shwachman-Diamond syndrome neutrophils have altered chemoattractant-induced F-actin polymerization and polarization characteristics. *Haematologica.* 2009;94:409-413.

282. Leung R, Cuddy K, Wang Y, Rommens J, Glogauer M. Sbds is required for Rac2-mediated monocyte migration and signaling downstream of RANK during osteoclastogenesis. *Blood.* 2011;117:2044-2053.

283. Tummala H, Walne AJ, Williams M, et al. DNAJC21 mutations link a cancer-prone bone marrow failure syndrome to corruption in 60S ribosome subunit maturation. *Am J Hum Genet.* 2016;99:115-124.

284. Tan S, Kermasson L, Hoslin A, et al. EFL1 mutations impair eIF6 release to cause Shwachman-Diamond syndrome. *Blood.* 2019;134:277-290.

285. Juaire KD, Lapouge K, Becker MMM, et al. Structural and functional impact of SRP54 mutations causing severe congenital neutropenia. *Structure.* 2021;29:15-28.e7.

286. Bellanné-Chantelot C, Schmaltz-Panneau B, Marty C, et al. Mutations in the SRP54 gene cause severe congenital neutropenia as well as Shwachman-Diamond-like syndrome. *Blood.* 2018;132:1318-1331.

287. Kennedy AL, Myers KC, Bowman J, et al. Distinct genetic pathways define premalignant versus compensatory clonal hematopoiesis in Shwachman-Diamond syndrome. *Nat Commun.* 2021;12:1334.

288. Tan S, Kermasson L, Hilcenko C, et al. Somatic genetic rescue of a germline ribosome assembly defect. *Nat Commun.* 2021;12:5044.

289. Grinspan ZM, Pikora CA. Infections in patients with Shwachman-Diamond syndrome. *Pediatr Infect Dis J.* 2005;24:179-181.

290. Pichler J, Meyer R, Köglmeier J, Ancliff P, Shah N. Nutritional status in children with Shwachman-diamond syndrome. *Pancreas.* 2015;44:590-595.

291. Cipolli M, D'Orazio C, Delmarco A, Marchesini C, Miano A, Mastella G. Shwachman's syndrome: pathomorphosis and long-term outcome. *J Pediatr Gastroenterol Nutr.* 1999;29:265-272.

292. Hsu JW, Vogelsang G, Jones RJ, Brodsky RA. Bone marrow transplantation in Shwachman-Diamond syndrome. *Bone Marrow Transplant.* 2002;30:255-258.

293. Cesaro S, Oneto R, Messina C, et al. Haematopoietic stem cell transplantation for Shwachman-Diamond disease: a study from the European Group for blood and marrow transplantation. *Br J Haematol.* 2005;131:231-236.

294. Bhatla D, Davies SM, Shenoy S, et al. Reduced-intensity conditioning is effective and safe for transplantation of patients with Shwachman-Diamond syndrome. *Bone Marrow Transplant.* 2008;42:159-165.

295. Myers K, Hebert K, Antin J, et al. Hematopoietic stem cell transplantation for shwachman-diamond syndrome. *Biol Blood Marrow Transplant.* 2020;26:1446-1451.

296. Cesaro S, Pillon M, Sauer M, et al. Long-term outcome after allogeneic hematopoietic stem cell transplantation for Shwachman-Diamond syndrome: a retrospective analysis and a review of the literature by the Severe Aplastic Anemia Working Party

297. of the European Society for Blood and Marrow Transplantation (SAAWP-EBMT). *Bone Marrow Transplant.* 2020;55:1796-1809.

297. Geddis AE. Congenital amegakaryocytic thrombocytopenia. *Pediatr Blood Cancer.* 2011;57:199-203.

298. Ballmaier M, Germeshausen M. Congenital amegakaryocytic thrombocytopenia: clinical presentation, diagnosis, and treatment. *Semin Thromb Hemost.* 2011;37:673-681.

299. Dasouki MJ, Rafi SK, Olm-Shipman AJ, et al. Exome sequencing reveals a thrombopoietin ligand mutation in a Micronesian family with autosomal recessive aplastic anemia. *Blood.* 2013;122:3440-3449.

300. Pecci A, Ragab I, Bozzi V, et al. Thrombopoietin mutation in congenital amegakaryocytic thrombocytopenia treatable with romiplostim. *EMBO Mol Med.* 2018;10:63-75.

301. Seo A, Ben-Harosh M, Sirin M, et al. Bone marrow failure unresponsive to bone marrow transplant is caused by mutations in thrombopoietin. *Blood.* 2017;130:875-880.

302. Germeshausen M, Ancliff P, Estrada J, et al. MECOM-associated syndrome: a heterogeneous inherited bone marrow failure syndrome with amegakaryocytic thrombocytopenia. *Blood Adv.* 2018;2:586-596.

303. Kjeldsen E, Veigaard C, Aggerholm A, Hasle H. Congenital hypoplastic bone marrow failure associated with a de novo partial deletion of the MECOM gene at 3q26.2. *Gene.* 2018;656:86-94.

304. King S, Germeshausen M, Strauss G, Welte K, Ballmaier M. Congenital amegakaryocytic thrombocytopenia: a retrospective clinical analysis of 20 patients. *Br J Haematol.* 2005;131:636-644.

305. Germeshausen M, Ballmaier M. CAMT-MPL: congenital Amegakaryocytic Thrombocytopenia caused by MPL mutations - heterogeneity of a monogenic disorder - comprehensive analysis of 56 patients. *Haematologica.* 2020;106(9):2439-2448. doi:10.3324/haematol.2020.257972

306. Germeshausen M, Ballmaier M, Welte K. MPL mutations in 23 patients suffering from congenital amegakaryocytic thrombocytopenia: the type of mutation predicts the course of the disease. *Hum Mutat.* 2006;27:296.

307. van der Veken LT, Maiburg MC, Groenendaal F, et al. Lethal neonatal bone marrow failure syndrome with multiple congenital abnormalities, including limb defects, due to a constitutional deletion of 3' MECOM. *Haematologica.* 2018;103:e173-e176.

308. Weizmann D, Pincez T, Roussy M, Vaillancourt N, Champagne J, LaverdièreC. New MECOM variant in a child with severe neonatal cytopenias spontaneously resolving. *Pediatr Blood Cancer.* 2020;67:e28215.

309. Niihori T, Ouchi-Uchiyama M, Sasahara Y, et al. Mutations in MECOM, encoding oncoprotein EVI1, cause radioulnar synostosis with amegakaryocytic thrombocytopenia. *Am J Hum Genet.* 2015;97:848-854.

310. Lord SV, Jimenez JE, Kroeger ZA, et al. A MECOM variant in an African American child with radioulnar synostosis and thrombocytopenia. *Clin Dysmorphol.* 2018;27:9-11.

311. Loganathan A, Munirathnam D, Ravikumar T. A novel mutation in the MECOM gene causing radioulnar synostosis with amegakaryocytic thrombocytopenia (RUSAT-2) in an infant. *Pediatr Blood Cancer.* 2019;66:e27574.

312. Bouman A, Knegt L, Gröschel S, et al. Congenital thrombocytopenia in a neonate with an interstitial microdeletion of 3q26.2q26.31. *Am J Med Genet A.* 2016;170A:504-509.

313. Nielsen M, Vermont CL, Aten E, et al. Deletion of the 3q26 region including the EVI1 and MDS1 genes in a neonate with congenital thrombocytopenia and subsequent aplastic anaemia. *J Med Genet.* 2012;49:598-600.

314. Camitta BM, Rock A. Acute lymphoidic leukemia in a patient with thrombocytopenia/absent radii (Tar) syndrome. *Am J Pediatr Hematol Oncol.* 1993;15:335-337.

315. Fadoo Z, Naqvi SMA. Acute myeloid leukemia in a patient with thrombocytopenia with absent radii syndrome. *J Pediatr Hematol Oncol.* 2002;24:134-135.

316. Go RS, Johnston KL. Acute myelogenous leukemia in an adult with thrombocytopenia with absent radii syndrome. *Eur J Haematol.* 2003;70:246-248.

317. Nichols KE, Crispino JD, Poncz M, et al. Familial dyserythropoietic anaemia and thrombocytopenia due to an inherited mutation in GATA1. *Nat Genet.* 2000;24:266-270.

318. Ihara K, Ishii E, Eguchi M, et al. Identification of mutations in the c-mpl gene in congenital amegakaryocytic thrombocytopenia. *Proc Natl Acad Sci USA.* 1999;96:3132-3136.

319. Ballmaier M, Germeshausen M. Advances in the understanding of congenital amegakaryocytic thrombocytopenia. *Br J Haematol.* 2009;146:3-16.

320. Varghese LN, Zhang JG, Young SN, et al. Functional characterization of c-Mpl ectodomain mutations that underlie congenital amegakaryocytic thrombocytopenia. *Growth Factors Chur Switz.* 2014;32:18-26.

321. Gandhi MJ, Pendergrass TW, Cummings CC, Ihara K, Blau CA, Drachman JG. Congenital amegakaryocytic thrombocytopenia in three siblings: molecular analysis of atypical clinical presentation. *Exp Hematol.* 2005;33:1215-1221.

322. Gurney AL, Wong SC, Henzel WJ, de Sauvage FJ. Distinct regions of c-Mpl cytoplasmic domain are coupled to the JAK-STAT signal transduction pathway and Shc phosphorylation. *Proc Natl Acad Sci USA.* 1995;92:5292-5296.

323. Basso-Valentina F, Levy G, Varghese LN, et al. CALR mutant protein rescues the response of MPL p.R464G variant associated with CAMT to eltrombopag. *Blood.* 2021;138(6):480-485. blood.2020010567, doi:10.1182/blood.2020010567

324. Tijssen MR, di Summa F, van den Oudenrijn S, et al. Functional analysis of single amino-acid mutations in the thrombopoietin-receptor Mpl underlying congenital amegakaryocytic thrombocytopenia. *Br J Haematol.* 2008;141:808-813.

325. Mukai HY, Kojima H, Todokoro K, et al. Serum thrombopoietin (TPO) levels in patients with amegakaryocytic thrombocytopenia are much higher than those with immune thrombocytopenic purpura. *Thromb Haemostasis.* 1996;76:675-678.

326. Cremer M, Schulze H, Linthorst G, et al. Serum levels of thrombopoietin, IL-11, and IL-6 in pediatric thrombocytopenias. *Ann Hematol.* 1999;78:401-407.

Disorders of Red Blood Cells

327. Murone M, Carpenter DA, de Sauvage FJ. Hematopoietic deficiencies in c-mpl and TPO knockout mice. *Stem Cells Dayt. Ohio.* 1998;16:1-6.

328. Lorenz V, Ramsey H, Liu ZJ, et al. Developmental stage-specific manifestations of absent TPO/c-MPL signalling in newborn mice. *Thromb Haemostasis.* 2017;117:2322-2333.

329. Pramono A, Zahabi A, Morishima T, Lan D, Welte K, Skokowa J. Thrombopoietin induces hematopoiesis from mouse ES cells via HIF-1α-dependent activation of a BMP4 autoregulatory loop. *Ann N Y Acad Sci.* 2016;1375:38-51.

330. Yuasa H, Oike Y, Iwama A, et al. Oncogenic transcription factor Evi1 regulates hematopoietic stem cell proliferation through GATA-2 expression. *EMBO J.* 2005;24:1976-1987.

331. Goyama S, Yamamoto G, Shimabe M, et al. Evi-1 is a critical regulator for hematopoietic stem cells and transformed leukemic cells. *Cell Stem Cell.* 2008;3:207-220.

332. Christodoulou C, Spencer JA, Yeh SCA, et al. Live-animal imaging of native haematopoietic stem and progenitor cells. *Nature.* 2020;578:278-283.

333. Fox NE, Lim J, Chen R, Geddis AE. F104S c-Mpl responds to a transmembrane domain-binding thrombopoietin receptor agonist: proof of concept that selected receptor mutations in congenital amegakaryocytic thrombocytopenia can be stimulated with alternative thrombopoietic agents. *Exp Hematol.* 2010;38:384-391.

334. Germeshausen M, Ballmaier M. Congenital amegakaryocytic thrombocytopenia - not a single disease. *Best Pract Res Clin Haematol.* 2021;34:101286.

335. Lonial S, Bilodeau P, Langston A, et al. Acquired amegakaryocytic thrombocytopenia treated with allogeneic BMT: a case report and review of the literature. *Bone Marrow Transplant.* 1999;24:1337-1341.

336. Muraoka K, Ishii E, Ihara K, et al. Successful bone marrow transplantation in a patient with c-mpl-mutated congenital amegakaryocytic thrombocytopenia from a carrier donor. *Pediatr Transplant.* 2005;9:101-103.

337. Steele M, Hitzler J, Doyle JJ, et al. Reduced intensity hematopoietic stem-cell transplantation across human leukocyte antigen barriers in a patient with congenital amegakaryocytic thrombocytopenia and monosomy 7. *Pediatr Blood Cancer.* 2005;45:212-216.

338. Al-Ahmari A, Ayas M, Al-Jefri A, Al-Mahr M, Rifai S, Solh HE. Allogeneic stem cell transplantation for patients with congenital amegakaryocytic thrombocytopenia (CAT). *Bone Marrow Transplant.* 2004;33:829-831.

339. Yeşilipek, Hazar V, Küpesiz A, Yegin O. Peripheral stem cell transplantation in a child with amegakaryocytic thrombocytopenia. *Bone Marrow Transplant.* 2000;26:571-572.

340. Mahadeo KM, Tewari P, Parikh SH, et al. Durable engraftment and correction of hematological abnormalities in children with congenital amegakaryocytic thrombocytopenia following myeloablative umbilical cord blood transplantation. *Pediatr Transplant.* 2015;19:753-757.

341. Dalle JH, Peffault de Latour R. Allogeneic hematopoietic stem cell transplantation for inherited bone marrow failure syndromes. *Int J Hematol.* 2016;103:373-379.

342. Tarek N, Kernan NA, Prockop SE, et al. T-cell-depleted hematopoietic SCT from unrelated donors for the treatment of congenital amegakaryocytic thrombocytopenia. *Bone Marrow Transplant.* 2012;47:744-746.

343. Rao AAN, Gourde JA, Marri P, Galardy PJ, Khan SP, Rodriguez V. Congenital amegakaryocytic thrombocytopenia: a case report of pediatric twins undergoing matched unrelated bone marrow transplantation. *J Pediatr Hematol Oncol.* 2015;37:304-306.

344. Even-Or E, NaserEddin A, Dinur Schejter Y, Shadur B, Zaidman I, Stepensky P. Haploidentical stem cell transplantation with post-transplant cyclophosphamide for osteopetrosis and other nonmalignant diseases. *Bone Marrow Transplant.* 2021;56:434-441.

345. Gasior Kabat M, Bueno D, Sisinni L, et al. Selective T-cell depletion targeting CD45RA as a novel approach for HLA-mismatched hematopoietic stem cell transplantation in pediatric nonmalignant hematological diseases. *Int J Hematol.* 2021;114:116-123.

346. MacMillan ML, Davies SM, Wagner JE, Ramsay NK. Engraftment of unrelated donor stem cells in children with familial amegakaryocytic thrombocytopenia. *Bone Marrow Transplant.* 1998;21:735-737.

347. Cleyrat C, Girard R, Choi EH, et al. Gene editing rescue of a novel MPL mutant associated with congenital amegakaryocytic thrombocytopenia. *Blood Adv.* 2017;1:1815-1826.

348. Hsu AP, Sampaio EP, Khan J, et al. Mutations in GATA2 are associated with the autosomal dominant and sporadic monocytopenia and mycobacterial infection (MonoMAC) syndrome. *Blood.* 2011;118:2653-2655.

349. Bigley V, Haniffa M, Doulatov S, et al. The human syndrome of dendritic cell, monocyte, B and NK lymphoid deficiency. *J Exp Med.* 2011;208:227-234.

350. Ostergaard P, Simpson MA, Connell FC, et al. Mutations in GATA2 cause primary lymphedema associated with a predisposition to acute myeloid leukemia (Emberger syndrome). *Nat Genet.* 2011;43:929-931.

351. McReynolds LJ, Calvo KR, Holland SM. Germline GATA2 mutation and bone marrow failure. *Hematol Oncol Clin North Am.* 2018;32:713-728.

352. Wlodarski MW, Collin M, Horwitz MS. GATA2 deficiency and related myeloid neoplasms. *Semin Hematol.* 2017;54:81-86.

353. Bruzzese A, Leardini D, Masetti R, et al. GATA2 related conditions and predisposition to pediatric myelodysplastic syndromes. *Cancers.* 2020;12:E2962.

354. Hirabayashi S, Wlodarski MW, Kozyra E, Niemeyer CM. Heterogeneity of GATA2-related myeloid neoplasms. *Int J Hematol.* 2017;106:175-182.

355. Dickinson RE, Griffin H, Bigley V, et al. Exome sequencing identifies GATA-2 mutation as the cause of dendritic cell, monocyte, B and NK lymphoid deficiency. *Blood.* 2011;118:2656-2658.

356. Spinner MA, Sanchez LA, Hsu AP, et al. GATA2 deficiency: a protean disorder of hematopoiesis, lymphatics, and immunity. *Blood.* 2014;123:809-821.

357. Ganapathi KA, Townsley DM, Hsu AP, et al. GATA2 deficiency-associated bone marrow disorder differs from idiopathic aplastic anemia. *Blood.* 2015;125:56-70.

358. Wlodarski MW, Hirabayashi S, Pastor V, et al. Prevalence, clinical characteristics, and prognosis of GATA2-related myelodysplastic syndromes in children and adolescents. *Blood.* 2016;127:1387-1397. quiz 1518.

359. Yamazaki H, Suzuki M, Otsuki A, et al. A remote GATA2 hematopoietic enhancer drives leukemogenesis in inv(3)(q21;q26) by activating EVI1 expression. *Cancer Cell.* 2014;25:415-427.

360. Gröschel S, Sanders MA, Hoogenboezem R, et al. A single oncogenic enhancer rearrangement causes concomitant EVI1 and GATA2 deregulation in leukemia. *Cell.* 2014;157:369-381.

361. Bannon SA, DiNardo CD. Hereditary predispositions to myelodysplastic syndrome. *Int J Mol Sci.* 2016;17:E838.

362. DiNardo CD, Bannon SA, Routbort M, et al. Evaluation of patients and families with concern for predispositions to hematologic malignancies within the hereditary hematologic malignancy clinic (HHMC). *Clin Lymphoma, Myeloma & Leukemia.* 2016;16:417-428.e2.

363. Rafei H, DiNardo CD. Hereditary myeloid malignancies. *Best Pract Res Clin Haematol.* 2019;32:163-176.

364. Klco JM, Mullighan CG. Advances in germline predisposition to acute leukaemias and myeloid neoplasms. *Nat Rev Cancer.* 2021;21:122-137.

365. Dickinson RE, Milne P, Jardine L, et al. The evolution of cellular deficiency in GATA2 mutation. *Blood.* 2014;123:863-874.

366. Callier P, Faivre L, Marle N, et al. Detection of an interstitial 3q21.1-q21.3 deletion in a child with multiple congenital abnormalities, mental retardation, pancytopenia, and myelodysplasia. *Am J Med Genet A.* 2009;149A:1323-1326.

367. Hsu AP, Johnson KD, Falcone EL, et al. GATA2 haploinsufficiency caused by mutations in a conserved intronic element leads to MonoMAC syndrome. *Blood.* 2013;121:3830-3837, S1-7.

368. McReynolds LJ, Yang Y, Yuen Wong H, et al. MDS-associated mutations in germline GATA2 mutated patients with hematologic manifestations. *Leuk Res.* 2019;76:70-75.

369. Tsai FY, Keller G, Kuo FC, et al. An early haematopoietic defect in mice lacking the transcription factor GATA-2. *Nature.* 1994;371:221-226.

370. Tsai FY, Orkin SH. Transcription factor GATA-2 is required for proliferation/survival of early hematopoietic cells and mast cell formation, but not for erythroid and myeloid terminal differentiation. *Blood.* 1997;89:3636-3643.

371. Rodrigues NP, Janzen V, Forkert R, et al. Haploinsufficiency of GATA-2 perturbs adult hematopoietic stem-cell homeostasis. *Blood.* 2005;106:477-484.

372. Kazenwadel J, Secker GA, Liu YJ, et al. Loss-of-function germline GATA2 mutations in patients with MDS/AML or MonoMAC syndrome and primary lymphedema reveal a key role for GATA2 in the lymphatic vasculature. *Blood.* 2012;119:1283-1291.

373. Hsu AP, McReynolds LJ, Holland SM. GATA2 deficiency. *Curr Opin Allergy Clin Immunol.* 2015;15:104-109.

374. Cuellar-Rodriguez J, Gea-Banacloche J, Freeman AF, et al. Successful allogeneic hematopoietic stem cell transplantation for GATA2 deficiency. *Blood.* 2011;118:3715-3720.

375. Grossman J, Cuellar-Rodriguez J, Gea-Banacloche J, et al. Nonmyeloablative allogeneic hematopoietic stem cell transplantation for GATA2 deficiency. *Biol Blood Marrow Transplant.* 2014;20:1940-1948.

Chapter 39 ■ Acquired Aplastic Anemia

AMY E. DEZERN • ROBERT A. BRODSKY

HISTORICAL BACKGROUND

The earliest case description of aplastic anemia was by Dr. Paul Ehrlich in 1888.[1] He described a young woman who succumbed with a severe presentation including anemia, bleeding, hyperpyrexia, and a markedly hypocellular bone marrow. In 1904, Dr. Chauffard lent the name "aplastic anemia" for this disorder. In 1972, a patient with aplastic anemia was the first recipient of a successful allogeneic bone marrow transplantation (BMT).[2] The advancement of BMT and enhancement of potent immunosuppressive therapy (IST) in the 1970s greatly improved the prognosis for patients with aplastic anemia. The illness was previously almost uniformly fatal within a few years of diagnosis, whereas now remissions are possible. While aplastic anemia remains a potentially overwhelming disease due to complications of delayed diagnosis and appropriate treatment, innovations in therapeutics and supportive care now allow most patients to survive the disease and many can be cured with BMT.

ACQUIRED VS CONSTITUTIONAL APLASTIC ANEMIA

Acquired aplastic anemia can occur in any age and is most often the consequence of an autoimmune attack by T cells against hematopoietic stem cells. There is no distinction in the pathophysiology of acquired disease in pediatrics compared with adults. However, awareness of the less common inherited forms of bone marrow failure is critical in the assessment of any younger patient with aplastic anemia (Chapter 38) and even in older patients as they may present into adulthood. Inherited disorders can masquerade as acquired aplastic anemia but rarely respond to immunosuppressive therapies given their separate pathophysiology; management usually consists of supportive care, or in appropriate cases, BMT.[3-5] Many inherited forms of bone marrow failure commonly present in the first decade of life and are often associated with physical anomalies (e.g., short stature, upper-limb anomalies, hypogonadism, café-au-lait spots). Some patients have a positive family history of cytopenias, highlighting the importance of taking a careful family history when evaluating patients with aplastic anemia.[6] Some patients may have overt manifestations (e.g., short stature, hyperpigmentation, triphalangeal thumbs) that had been overlooked previously, whereas the findings in some disorders (e.g., hair graying and reticulate pigmentation in dyskeratosis congenita (DKC), premature menopause in Fanconi anemia) can become more obvious with age.

The most common inherited mimickers of acquired aplastic anemia include Fanconi anemia, short telomere syndromes (STSs) (also called DKC), amegakaryocytic thrombocytopenia, and Shwachman-Diamond syndrome. Previous reports have suggested that a significant number of patients present with Fanconi anemia (9%) or STS (46%) over the age of 16 years.[6] With improved testing and a higher index of suspicion, it is becoming evident that these numbers are likely an underestimate. Fanconi anemia is usually an autosomal recessive disorder that is characterized by defects in DNA repair and a predisposition to leukemia and solid tumors.[7] STSs are inherited bone marrow failure syndromes that may be autosomal dominant, autosomal recessive, or X-linked, and some patients also have de novo germline mutations. The median age at diagnosis is around 15 years (range 0-75). Males are disproportionately affected, with a male:female ratio of approximately 3:1.[8] Although STS (previously DKC) classically presents with the triad of abnormal skin pigmentation, nail dystrophy, and mucosal leukoplakia, these findings can be subtle and the syndrome is now know to include multiple other manifestations.[9] X-linked recessive, autosomal dominant, and autosomal recessive forms of STS are recognized.[10] Telomerase reverse transcriptase (TERT) and the RNA component of telomerase (TERC) form the core of the active telomerase complex. Autosomal dominant STS can result from mutations of TERC[11] or TERT.[12] The X-linked recessive STS results from mutations in the gene STS1, whose gene product, dyskerin, is important for stabilizing the telomerase RNA-protein complex.[13] Mutations of the TINF2 gene can also lead to STS. TINF2 mutations result in dysfunction of the shelterin complex, interfering with its protection of telomeres and leading to reduced telomere length. Accelerated telomere shortening leads to bone marrow failure, genetic instability, and premature aging.[14] An extreme phenotype of a disorder in the telomere maintenance is the Hoyeraal-Hreidarsson syndrome.[15,16] These individuals have progressive bone marrow failure with an association of intrauterine growth retardation, cerebellar hypoplasia, and immunodeficiency. The mutations reported in this severe syndrome include STS1, TERC, TERT, TPP1 encoded by SCD, TINF2, RTEL1, and PARN.[17-21] Inherited amegakaryocytic thrombocytopenia is characterized by severe thrombocytopenia and megakaryocyte absence at birth. Missense or nonsense mutations in the c-mpl gene are present in most patients. A high percentage of these patients subsequently develop multilineage bone marrow failure in the second decade of life.[22] Shwachman-Diamond syndrome is an autosomal recessive disorder characterized by pancreatic exocrine dysfunction, metaphyseal dysostosis, and bone marrow failure.[23] Similar to Fanconi anemia, there is an increased risk of developing myelodysplasia or leukemia at an early age. The SBDS gene is important for ribosome biogenesis, but how this leads to bone marrow failure is unclear. These inherited forms of aplastic anemia are described in more detail in Chapter 38. The remainder of this chapter focuses on acquired aplastic anemia, hereafter referred to as aplastic anemia.

EPIDEMIOLOGY

Incidence, Age, and Geographic Distribution

Exact estimates of the incidence of aplastic anemia are confounded by the imprecision in establishing the diagnosis. Aplastic anemia is primarily a disease of children and younger adults. There is another peak in incidence in patients 60 years and older, although in these older patients some reported cases of aplastic anemia may represent cases of hypoplastic myelodysplastic syndrome (MDS). Aplastic anemia is rare in Western Europe and the United States (less than 2 cases per million population per year). Aplastic anemia is more common in Asia than in Western countries, and several epidemiological studies have determined an incidence of 3.9 cases per million in Bangkok, 6 cases per million in rural areas of Thailand, and 14 cases per million in Japan.[24,25] The higher incidence in Asian countries has been linked to environmental factors, such as exposure to chemicals like insecticides, more than genetic factors. Both males and females are equally affected for acquired disease. The initial evaluations of a patient with concern for aplastic anemia can be seen in *Table 39.1.*[26]

Drugs and Chemicals

A plethora of case reports and small series have implicated drugs as the cause of bone marrow failure; however, proving a causal association in these rare idiosyncratic reactions is difficult. The more common substances implicated in causing aplastic anemia are listed in *Table 39.2.* Nevertheless, drugs were not found to be a common cause of aplastic anemia in two large, controlled, population-based studies.[24]

Table 39.1. Standard Workup in the Evaluation of a Patient With Suspected Aplastic Anemia to Encompass Risk of Inherited Disorders

Test	Purpose
Heme: Long-standing cytopenia(s) or macrocytosis? Unexplained cytopenia(s) or macrocytosis, AA, MDS, AML in 1 or more close relative(s)?	Could suggest IBMFD due to identification of cytopenias at early age
Developmental: Short stature, physical anomalies (especially thumb/radial ray, cardiac, or renal)?	FA or DKC or thrombocytopenia-absent radius
Immunologic/Infectious Disease: Severe, recurrent, or atypical infections (e.g., mycobacterial, viral, fungal)?	Could suggest GATA2
Dermatologic: Gray hair prior to 25 y? Leukoplakia or nail dysplasia? Reticulated skin pigmentation, café au lait macules?	Could suggest DKC or another STS
Pulmonary: Pulmonary fibrosis and/or early-onset emphysema, pulmonary alveolar proteinosis, fungal or mycobacterial infection?	Could suggest DKC or another STS or GATA2
Abdominal: Pancreatic insufficiency, liver fibrosis, renal anomaly or malplacement?	
Neurologic: Ataxia, nystagmus? Cognitive dysfunction?	
Cardiac/Lymphatic: Cardiac anomaly, lymphedema?	
Oncologic: H&N or anogenital SCC, early-onset GI cancers or multiple cancers in patient or close relatives?	Could suggest STS
Complete blood count with differential and blood smear review	Assess severity of cytopenias and for alternative etiologies
Reticulocyte count	Assess marrow response to anemia and use in AA severity assessment
Hemoglobin F%	Elevated levels can indicate an IBMFD may be present
Vitamin B12, folate, copper, zinc, ferritin	Rule out vitamin or mineral deficiencies as cause or contributor to cytopenias
Hepatitis A/B/C, HIV, EBV, parvovirus, and CMV serologies	Rule out infectious disease contributors to cytopenias and identify comanagement needs during treatment and transplant
LDH, haptoglobin	Rule out a hemolysis component to anemia
PNH clone	Assess presence or absence of GPI anchored protein expression; presence suggests acquired over inherited disease
ANA with reflex to anti-double-stranded DNA if positive	Assess for systemic lupus erythematosus
Immunoglobulins A, G, M quantification	Assess for additional immune deficits
Flow cytometry to assess B, T, NK cell numbers	Assess for additional immune deficits
Telomere length measurement of peripheral blood lymphocytes by Flow FISH	Determine lymphocyte telomere length by Flow FISH; if <1st percentile, patient may have an STS and be at risk of increased transplant-related toxicity with standard preparative regimens and an STS-specific regimen should be considered.
Chromosome breakage analysis on peripheral blood	Evaluate for FA; if test is positive and consistent with a diagnosis of FA, patient is at increased risk of transplant-related toxicity and an FA-specific regimen should be utilized.
Bone marrow aspirate and biopsy	Assess cellularity, iron stores, and reticulin fibrosis and rule out other marrow pathologies
Conventional karyotyping	
HLA typing	Determine HLA profile for stem cell donor search
Myeloid malignancy gene sequencing from peripheral blood or bone marrow	Evaluate for mutations in genes recurrently mutated in AA (e.g., *PIGA*, *BCOR*, *BCORL1*) and/or MDS (e.g., epigenetic mutations, *TP53*)
Inherited bone marrow failure gene panel sequencing	Evaluate for multiple IBMFD at once. Overlapping phenotypes and lack of physical features and family history in a substantial subset of those with IBMFD make universal testing of young patients warranted. Tissue source for this testing should ideally be cultured skin fibroblasts (see text for discussion).
Erythrocyte adenosine deaminase	Screen for Diamond Blackfan anemia
Serum pancreatic isoamylase (age >3 y)	Screen for pancreatic insufficiency suggestive of Schwachman Diamond syndrome
Fecal elastase	Screen for pancreatic insufficiency suggestive of Schwachman Diamond syndrome

Abbreviations: AA, aplastic anemia; AML, acute myeloid leukemia; ANA, antinuclear antibodies; CMV, cytomegalovirus; EBV, Epstein-Barr virus; FA, Fanconi anemia; FISH, fluorescence in situ hybridization; GI, gastrointestinal; H&N, head and neck; HIV, human immunodeficiency virus; IBMFD, inherited none marrow failure disorder; LDH, lactate dehydrogenase; MDS, myelodysplastic syndrome; NK, natural killer; SCC, squamous cell cancer; STS, short telomere syndrome.

Table 39.2. Drugs and Chemicals Associated With Aplastic Anemia

Drugs and Toxins
Nonsteroidal Analgesics
• Phenylbutazone
• Indomethacin
• Sulindac
• Diclofenac
• Piroxicam
Anticonvulsants
• Hydantoins
• Carbamazepine
• Phenacemide
Antibiotics
• Sulfonamides
• Chloramphenicol
• Antiprotozoals
• Quinacrine
• Chloroquine
Antithyroid Drugs
• Methimazole
• Propylthiouracil
• Gold
Benzenes
Solvents
Glues

Interestingly, no increased risk was associated with chloramphenicol, which is often a drug implicated in case reports; however, chloramphenicol use in this study was infrequent.[24]

When drugs are implicated in causing aplastic anemia, it is important to recognize that, unlike agranulocytosis and drug-induced thrombocytopenia, stopping the putative drug does *not* usually lead to hematopoietic recovery. Most cases of drug-induced aplastic anemia lead to an idiosyncratic immune response directed against hematopoietic progenitor cells and are managed similarly to all patients with idiopathic aplastic anemia with the addition of stopping the offending agent. Notable exceptions include patients who receive high doses of cytotoxic chemotherapy drugs (e.g., alkylating agents, antimetabolites, antimitotics) or rare individuals who have thiopurine methyltransferase deficiency (TPMT). TPMT catalyzes the *S*-methylation of 6-mercaptopurine, 6-thioguanine, and azathioprine. Most individuals have high or intermediate activity of TPMT; however, there are rare individuals (0.1% of the population) with undetectable levels of TPMT. Exposure to even low dosages of 6-thioguanine, azathioprine, or 6-mercaptopurine, as used in inflammatory bowel disease and lupus, can result in severe bone marrow failure within weeks of starting the drug. Withdrawal of the drug usually leads to hematopoietic recovery in 2 to 4 weeks. Reliable polymerase chain reaction–based methods are now available for detecting the major inactivating mutations at the human TPMT locus.[27]

Viruses

Viruses are often implicated but seldom proven to cause aplastic anemia. Viral infections, especially in chronically ill patients, often lead to transient cytopenias, but frank aplastic anemia is uncommon. These transient cytopenias can be due directly to infection and cytolysis of hematopoietic cells or indirectly through the elaboration of inhibitory cytokines. True aplastic anemia following an infection with a virus also appears to result usually from an idiosyncratic immune response directed against hematopoietic stem cells. Acute infection with Epstein-Barr virus (EBV) is often associated with peripheral blood cytopenias. Rarely, acute EBV infection can be complicated by the development of aplastic anemia.[28] There are no convincing data that B19 parvovirus causes aplastic anemia, but this virus is often linked with aplastic anemia due to the unfortunate term "aplastic crisis," used to describe the transient red cell aplasia and severe anemia that occurs

in patients with sickle cell anemia (or others with chronic hemolytic anemia) who are acutely infected with B19 parvovirus. The only known natural host cell of parvovirus B19 is the human erythroid progenitor.[29] The receptor for the virus is a neutral glycolipid, globoside, also known as the erythrocyte P antigen.[30] Globoside is expressed on erythroid progenitors, erythrocytes, fetal myocardium, placenta, some megakaryocytes, and endothelial cells; it is not present on hematopoietic stem cells. Other viruses, including a variety of herpes viruses and the human immunodeficiency virus, have been implicated in triggering aplastic anemia, but convincing causal data are lacking. Spontaneous recovery, response to immunosuppression, and response to antiviral therapy have all been described; however, for those with severe disease, conventional therapy (immunosuppression or BMT) should be initiated early.

Seronegative (non-A through non-G) hepatitis precedes the diagnosis of aplastic anemia in 3% to 5% of cases and is recognized as hepatitis-associated aplastic anemia.[31] In most cases, the hepatitis resolves spontaneously; however, when severe aplastic anemia (SAA) follows, it often presents within a few months after the onset of hepatitis.[31] After orthotopic liver transplantation for fulminant seronegative hepatitis, up to 30% of patients will develop aplastic anemia (HAA).[32] The pathophysiology of HAA is unknown but is thought to be immune mediated because it responds to IST. Furthermore, patients with HAA have a skewed T-cell repertoire, and liver biopsies from these patients show lymphocytic infiltration.[33]

Benzene and Environmental Toxins

The medical literature is replete with case reports of aplastic anemia associated with environmental exposures, most notably benzene or radiation exposure. However, rigorous epidemiologic studies supporting an association between environmental toxins and aplastic anemia are lacking. A major confounder is that benzene and other toxins predispose people to MDS and leukemia. Older literature was unlikely to distinguish different types of marrow failure, such as aplastic anemia or MDS, leading to an overestimation of the association between benzene and aplastic anemia. Although the magnitude of the risk remains uncertain, benzene is probably not a major risk factor for aplastic anemia in countries with modern standards of industrial hygiene. A large case-controlled study in Thailand employing modern diagnostic and epidemiologic methods found that individuals of lower economic status and younger age are at greater risk for developing aplastic anemia than their counterparts in other countries following exposure to solvents, glues, and hepatitis A. Grain farmers were also found to have a higher risk of developing aplastic anemia (relative risk = 2.7) regardless of whether they used insecticides. These same investigators noted marked differences in incidence between northern and southern rural regions of Thailand and among Bangkok suburbs, implicating potential environmental factors in causing the disease.[34]

Radiation

Ionizing radiation is directly toxic to bone marrow stem/progenitor cells, and high doses (>1.5 Gy to the whole body) can lead to severe pancytopenia within 2 to 4 weeks after exposure; the LD_{50} has been estimated at about 4.5 Gy, and a dose of 10 Gy or greater is thought to have 100% mortality.[35] Although pancytopenia is common after a single high dose of radiation, an increased risk of aplastic anemia is not well documented as a delayed event from atomic bomb survivors.[36] Although the principles of managing pancytopenia following radiation exposure are similar to those of aplastic anemia, it is important to recognize that the mechanism of bone marrow failure is different. Bone marrow failure in most cases of community-acquired aplastic anemia is due to autoimmune destruction of bone marrow stem/progenitor cells; however, radiation-induced bone marrow failure is dose dependent and is a consequence of direct toxicity to stem and progenitor cells. Supportive care with blood transfusions, granulocyte colony-stimulating factor, and antibiotics is the mainstay of therapy for radiation-induced bone marrow failure, inasmuch as autologous reconstitution will occur in most patients who survive the immediate consequences of radiation exposure.

Disorders of Red Blood Cells

Pregnancy

Pregnancy-associated aplastic anemia is a rare entity, and despite numerous case reports, the association is not well understood.[37,38] The onset of aplastic anemia can occur during pregnancy or shortly after delivery.[39] Moreover, in women with a history of aplastic anemia who had been treated into remission with IST, there is an increased risk for relapse of aplastic anemia during pregnancy. The European Group for Blood and Marrow Transplantation performed a retrospective study on the outcome of pregnancy in 36 women who had received IST to treat aplastic anemia.[38] Seven of the pregnancies (19%) were complicated by relapse of aplastic anemia. In contrast to idiopathic aplastic anemia, pregnancy-associated aplastic anemia is often associated with spontaneous remissions. However, in patients with severe disease, therapy should be initiated promptly, because maternal and fetal mortality are not uncommon.[40]

PATHOPHYSIOLOGY

Autoimmunity

Aplastic anemia was originally thought to result from a direct toxic effect on hematopoietic stem cells. In the late 1960s, Mathé and colleagues were among the first to postulate an autoimmune basis for aplastic anemia.[41] After administering antilymphocyte globulin for conditioning, they performed BMT in patients with aplastic anemia using partially mismatched donors. Although the transplanted marrow failed to engraft, some patients experienced autologous recovery of hematopoiesis, suggesting that growth and differentiation of the patient's hematopoietic stem cells were being suppressed by the immune system. An analysis by the International Bone Marrow Transplant Registry of identical twin bone marrow transplants in patients with aplastic anemia also suggests an autoimmune etiology for the majority of patients. Attempts to treat aplastic anemia by simple transfusion of bone marrow from an identical twin fails to reconstitute hematopoiesis in about 70% of patients.[42] However, repeating the procedure following a high-dose cyclophosphamide conditioning regimen is successful in most patients.[43]

The first laboratory evidence of autoimmunity in aplastic anemia was provided by experiments showing that lymphocytes from patients with aplastic anemia inhibit allogeneic and autologous hematopoietic colony formation in vitro.[44] Subsequently, cytotoxic T lymphocytes were found to mediate the destruction of hematopoietic stem cells in aplastic anemia.[45,46] These cytotoxic T cells are more conspicuous in the bone marrow of patients with aplastic anemia than in the peripheral blood[47-49] and they overproduce interferon-γ and tumor necrosis factor (TNF).[50] TNF and interferon-γ are direct inhibitors of hematopoiesis and appear to upregulate Fas expression on CD34$^+$ cells.[51] Immortalized CD4$^+$ and CD8$^+$ T-cell clones from patients with aplastic anemia also secrete Th1 cytokines and are directly toxic to autologous CD34 cells.[45,46] There is also evidence for a humoral autoimmune response in aplastic anemia; autoantibodies against kinectin, a 1300-amino-acid molecule expressed on human hematopoietic cells, liver, ovary, testis, and brain cells have been found in approximately 40% of patients with aplastic anemia.[52] Studies in patients with aplastic anemia examining T-cell diversity using complementarity-determining region (CDR3) spectratyping further implicate an autoimmune pathophysiology in aplastic anemia. T cells from patients with aplastic anemia have limited T-cell receptor β-chain heterogeneity, suggesting oligoclonal T-cell expansion in response to a specific, but as yet unrecognized, antigen[46,53] (*Figure 39.1*).

Stem Cells

A reduction in the number of hematopoietic stem/progenitor cells is a universal laboratory finding in aplastic anemia. CD34$^+$ cells, assayable hematopoietic progenitors, and long-term culture-initiating cells are strikingly reduced in aplastic anemia.[54,55] However, some healthy hematopoietic stem cells persist in most patients with aplastic anemia as demonstrated by the fact that complete recovery of normal hematopoiesis can occur post effective IST.[56,57] T cells from patients with

aplastic anemia kill hematopoietic stem cells in an HLA-DR restricted manner[45,46] via Fas ligand.[51] Hematopoietic stem cells represent several classes of cells with varying capacity for long-term production of the different hematopoietic lineages and variable expression of Fas ligand and HLA-DR.[58] The most primitive hematopoietic stem cells express little or no HLA-DR[58,59] or Fas,[60,61] and the expression of both HLA-DR and Fas increases as the stem cells mature. Thus, the primitive hematopoietic stem cells, which normally represent less than 10% of the total CD34$^+$ cells, may be relatively invisible to the autoreactive T cells; conversely, the more mature hematopoietic stem cells may be the principal targets of the immune attack in aplastic anemia.[62] The primitive hematopoietic stem cells eluding the autoimmune attack may be responsible for the slow hematopoietic recovery that occurs in patients with aplastic anemia following the administration of high-dose IST.

Clonality and Aplastic Anemia

At the time of diagnosis, 60% to 70% of patients with aplastic anemia are suspected to demonstrate clonality, and many of these patients will develop aggressive MDSs 5 to 10 years after IST.[63] Unfortunately, this clonality is not eliminated post IST alone and often is the source of relapse and/or progression.[63,64] This suggests that the increase in MDS and paroxysmal nocturnal hemoglobinuria (PNH) following IST is not a direct consequence of treatment. Rather, the increased survival following IST allows time for these underlying clones to develop and expand.[65]

MDS is a clonal hematopoietic stem cell disorder that produces multilineage hematologic cytopenias (Chapter 80). It is associated with heterogeneous karyotypic abnormalities, often involving chromosomes 5, 7, or 8. Up to 15% of children and adults with aplastic anemia will develop MDS following IST, with monosomy 7 being the most common chromosomal abnormality to emerge.[66,67]

PNH results from the expansion of an abnormal hematopoietic stem cell that harbors a somatic mutation of the X-linked gene, *PIGA*.[68-70] The *PIGA* gene product is required for glycosylphosphatidylinositol (GPI) anchor biosynthesis; consequently, PNH cells are deficient in all GPI-anchored proteins (GPI-AP). The GPI-APs (CD59 and CD55) protect cells from complement-mediated destruction; their absence explains the complement-mediated intravascular hemolysis associated with PNH.

Small to moderate PNH clones are found in up to 70% of patients with aplastic anemia.[71] Typically, less than 20% GPI-AP-deficient granulocytes are detected in patients with aplastic anemia at diagnosis, but occasional patients may have larger clones. DNA sequencing of the GPI-AP-deficient cells from patients with aplastic anemia reveals clonal *PIGA* gene mutations.[72] Moreover, many of these patients exhibit expansion of the *PIGA* mutant clone and progress to clinical PNH. Although it was once thought that PNH evolving from aplastic anemia is more benign than classical PNH, this observation may be a consequence of lead time bias, as many of these patients eventually develop classical PNH symptoms after the *PIGA* mutant clone expands. Interestingly, the PNH clone can regress, remain stable, or expand in patients with aplastic anemia treated with IST; however, expansion of the PNH clone is commonly associated with relapse.[73,74]

The mechanism whereby PNH clones expand is not entirely clear; however, a preponderance of data suggests that the PNH stem cell has a conditional growth advantage in the setting of aplastic anemia. Specifically, it has be suggested that PNH cells may be relatively resistant to an autoimmune attack on the bone marrow, possibly because they are deficient in GPI-anchored UL binding proteins (ULBP) that serve as receptors for NKG2D, a ligand that is important for natural killer cells and T cells.[75,76] Alternatively, it has been proposed that "second hit" mutations may also give the PNH clone a growth advantage.[77] These hypotheses are not mutually exclusive.

Newer methodology for sequencing of somatic molecular mutations also show higher demonstration of clonal hematopoiesis in aplastic anemia.[63,64,78-80] The clinical utility of these mutations has yet to be fully elucidated, but in-depth molecular testing is an area of current research[26] and is performed on a research rather than a clinical basis.

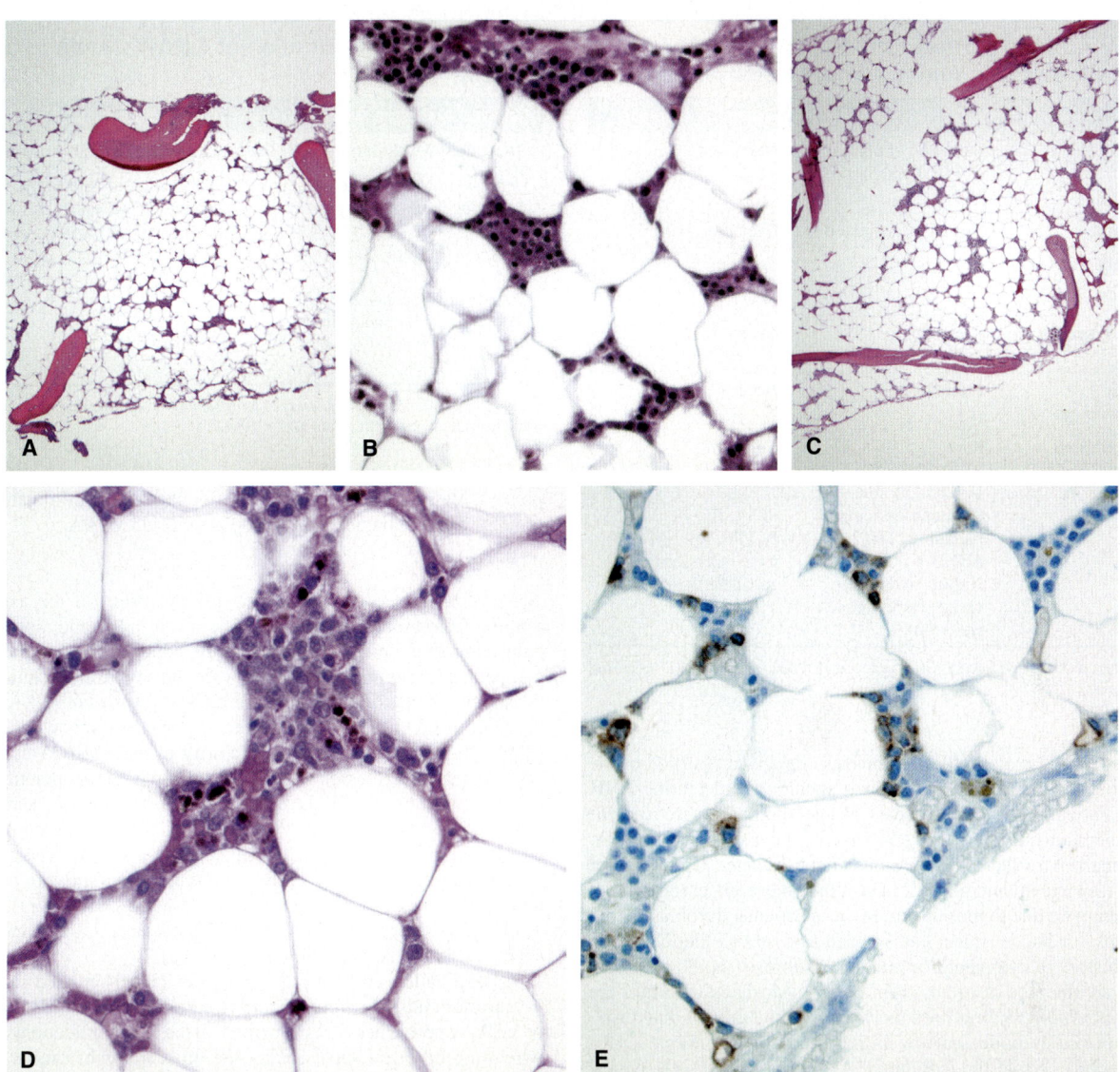

FIGURE 39.1 Aplastic anemia vs hypoplastic myelodysplastic syndrome (hMDS). A, Bone marrow biopsy from a patient with aplastic anemia. B, Higher power of biopsy from (A) showing cluster of nucleated red cells. C, Low-power view of biopsy from a patient with hMDS. D, High-power view of bone marrow from patient in (C) showing small blast population. Brown pigment represents iron. E, CD34 immunoperoxidase stain (brown) of marrow from patient with hMDS.

Presently, 60% to 70% of idiopathic AA patients are now known to demonstrate acquired clonality at the time of diagnosis using sensitive next-generation sequencing and array-based karyotyping (CGH).[63] Unfortunately, these clones are often not eliminated post nontransplant therapy and are frequently the source of relapse and/or progression.[63,64] The presence of clonal hematopoiesis at AA diagnosis or evolution post therapy is not truly uncommon.

CLINICAL FEATURES AND DIAGNOSIS

Aplastic anemia can present abruptly over days, or more gradually over weeks to months. AA is a diagnosis of exclusion, and no single test that can be used to consistently diagnose AA vs other causes of marrow failure. Clinical manifestations are proportional to the peripheral blood cytopenias and may include dyspnea on exertion, fatigue, easy bruising, petechia, epistaxis, gingival bleeding, heavy menses, headache, and fever. The differential diagnosis can be found in *Table 39.3*.

A complete blood count, leukocyte differential, reticulocyte count, and a bone marrow aspirate and biopsy can establish the diagnosis. Peripheral blood flow cytometry to rule out PNH[81,82] and bone marrow karyotyping to help exclude hypoplastic myelodysplastic syndromes

Table 39.3. Differential Diagnosis of Pancytopenia With a Hypocellular Bone Marrow

Acquired aplastic anemia
Inherited aplastic anemia
Fanconi anemia
Dyskeratosis congenita
Shwachman-Diamond syndrome
Amegakaryocytic thrombocytopenia
Reticular dysgenesis
Hypoplastic myelodysplastic syndromes
Large granular lymphocytic leukemia (rare)
Hypoplastic paroxysmal nocturnal hemoglobinuria (aplastic anemia)

(hMDS) should be performed on all patients. Flow cytometric assays to detect PNH cells can be performed with either monoclonal antibodies[82] or a fluorescein-conjugated proaerolysin variant known as FLAER.[81] Unlike monoclonal antibodies that bind the protein portion

Table 39.4. Bone Marrow Findings That Help to Discriminate Aplastic Anemia From Myelodysplasia

	MDS	Aplastic Anemia
Cellularity	Increased or normal* (* 15% hypoplastic MDS)	Decreased
CD34 count	Normal or increased	Decreased (<0.1%)
Dyserythropoiesis	Common	Common
Ringed sideroblasts	Common	Never
Myeloid dysplasia or blasts	Common	Never
Dysplastic megakaryocytes	Common	Never
PNH population	Rare	Common
Abnormal karyotype	Common	Rare
NGS profile	Common: splicing mutations, TET2, ASXL1; Higher mutational variant allele frequencies seen	PIGA, BCOR/BCORL1; DNMT3A more often seen; variant allele frequencies <10%

Abbreviations: MDS, myelodysplastic syndrome; PNH, paroxysmal nocturnal hemoglobinuria.

of a GPI-anchored protein, FLAER binds to the glycan portion of the GPI anchor and is highly sensitive and specific for detecting PNH cells.[65,81] Patients less than 40 years of age should be screened for Fanconi anemia using the clastogenic agents diepoxybutane or mitomycin C that test for increased chromosomal breakage.[7] Up to 10% of patients with Fanconi anemia will have a false-negative chromosomal breakage analysis due to mosaicism. In these patients, fibroblasts from a skin biopsy or buccal smear can be used to establish the diagnosis. A family history of cytopenias or pulmonary fibrosis should raise suspicion for an inherited disorder, even when physical abnormalities are not present.[80] *Table 39.1* outlines the workup at the time of diagnosis.

A hypocellular bone marrow is required for the diagnosis of aplastic anemia. While the cellularity is often profoundly decreased (<10%), small islands of hematopoiesis can be seen. The criteria for the diagnosis of AA require either bone marrow with <25% of the normal cellularity or bone marrow with <50% normal cellularity in which less than 30% of the cells are hematopoietic. The marrow aspirates in AA do not show overt dysplastic changes nor are blasts increased. Mild dyserythropoiesis is not uncommon in aplastic anemia, especially in cases with simultaneous small to moderate-sized PNH populations; however, the presence of a small percentage of myeloid blasts or dysplastic features in the myeloid or megakaryocyte lineages favors a diagnosis of hMDS (*Table 39.4*).

Distinguishing between aplastic anemia and hMDS is often challenging, especially in older patients where hMDS is more common. The percentage of CD34+ cells in the bone marrow is often helpful.[83,84] CD34 is expressed on hematopoietic progenitors and is fundamental to the pathophysiology of both diseases; in MDS clonal expansion emanates from a CD34+ stem cell, and in aplastic anemia the CD34+ stem cells are the target of an autoimmune attack. Accordingly, the percentage of CD34+ cells is usually ≤0.3% in aplastic anemia, whereas the CD34 percentage is either normal (0.5%-1.0 %) or elevated in hMDS.[83] Furthermore, next-generation sequencing is increasingly performed in this setting. There is considerable overlap between the mutational spectrum in AA and MDS with mutations in *BCOR/BCORL1*, *DNMT3A*, and *ASXL1* common to both disease states[63] at similar VAFs. The reported frequencies of somatic mutations in AA range from 5% to over 70% in some series.[63,64,85-88] For example, the prevalence of BCOR and BCORL1 mutations is estimated at 5% in MDS[89] vs 4%[64] or 7% to 10% in AA.[63] It should be noted that, at

Table 39.5. Classification of Aplastic Anemia by Severity

Severe Aplastic Anemia[a]	Moderate Aplastic Anemia
Bone marrow cellularity <30%	Decreased bone marrow cellularity
Depression of at least two of the following three hematopoietic lineages: Absolute neutrophil count <0.5 × 10⁹/L Transfusion dependence, with absolute reticulocyte count, <60 × 10⁹/L Platelet count <20 × 10⁹/L	Depression of at least two of three hematopoietic lineages not fulfilling the severity criteria as specified in the left column

[a]Very severe aplastic anemia is reserved for patients who fulfill criteria for severe AA but with an absolute neutrophil count <0.2 × 10⁹/L.

present, mutations in these genes do not have the discriminating power to help with the diagnosis of hypoplastic MDS vs AA.

Classification

Aplastic anemia encompasses a wide spectrum of disease activity ranging from mild to severe. The risk of morbidity and mortality from aplastic anemia correlates best with the depth of the peripheral blood cytopenias rather than bone marrow cellularity. Thus, acquired aplastic anemia is classified as nonsevere (NSAA), severe (SAA), or very severe (VSAA) based on the degree of peripheral blood pancytopenia (*Table 39.5*). A bone marrow cellularity of less than 25% and markedly decreased values of at least two of three hematopoietic lineages (neutrophil count <500/μL, platelet count <20,000/μL, and absolute reticulocyte count of <60,000/μL) define SAA. VSAA satisfies the above criteria except the neutrophil count is <200/μL, whereas NSAA is characterized by a hypocellular bone marrow, but with cytopenias that do not meet the criteria for severe disease. *Moderate* AA is characterized by depression of blood counts not fulfilling the definition of severe disease (Camitta criteria *Table 39.5*).

Classification and natural history are closely related in AA. The 2-year mortality rate with supportive care alone for patients with SAA or VSAA approaches 80%,[90] with invasive fungal infections and overwhelming bacterial sepsis being the most frequent causes of death. Nonsevere disease is seldom life-threatening and in many instances requires no therapy when comfort is developed with stable mild count depression.

SUPPORTIVE CARE

Transfusions

Patients with symptomatic anemia and/or thrombocytopenia associated with wet purpura or bleeding require immediate blood transfusions. All transfusions in patients with suspected aplastic anemia should be irradiated to prevent transfusion-associated graft-vs-host disease (GVHD). If the patient is a potential BMT candidate and is cytomegalovirus (CMV) negative or the CMV status is unknown, CMV transmission should be avoided by either leukoreduction or the use of CMV-negative products. Blood donation from family members should be avoided to prevent alloimmunization that could also complicate future BMT. After stabilization of the patient, blood products should be used judiciously to prevent cardiopulmonary compromise and to reduce the risk of hemorrhage; a platelet goal of 10,000/μL will suffice for most patients, although some patients will tolerate even lower platelet goals without bleeding or petechiae.[91] Granulocyte transfusions have not been shown to be of benefit to patients with aplastic anemia.[92]

Antibiotics

Fungal and bacterial infections are a major cause of death in patients with SAA.[93] However, an active fungal infection should not delay more definitive therapy such as IST or BMT.[94] However, for patients with absolute neutrophil counts that are consistently <200 μL, prophylaxis with oral antibiotics, such as a quinolone and a triazole antifungal, is reasonable. Patients with febrile neutropenia should be treated promptly with broad-spectrum antibiotics; in patients with persistent fever after the initiation of antibacterial antibiotics, aspergillus coverage should be added. Prophylaxis for *Pneumocystis carinii pneumonia* should be given to all patients for at least 6 months after IST, BMT, or high-dose cyclophosphamide therapy.[95]

Growth Factors

Hematopoietic growth factor deficiency (such as erythropoietin, granulocyte colony-stimulating factor, thrombopoietin, or granulocyte-monocyte colony-stimulating factor) is not responsible for the bone marrow failure in aplastic anemia; levels of measurable hematopoietic growth factors are markedly elevated in patients with aplastic anemia in a compensatory attempt to increase blood production. Hence, these factors should not be used in lieu of definitive therapy. Hematopoietic growth factors are often used after IST or high-dose cyclophosphamide therapy to accelerate hematopoietic recovery, but their use has not been shown to improve survival.[96] Eltrombopag, a thrombopoietic mimetic, will be discussed separately.

DEFINITIVE TREATMENT

The decision to treat patients with AA is based on disease severity (*Table 39.5*). Definitive treatment with either IST or allogeneic hematopoietic stem cell transplantation (BMT) is necessary for patients with *severe* AA, while no standard of care exists for moderate AA. Once severity criteria are fulfilled, the type of treatment used is mainly influenced by the patient's age and the availability of a matched sibling donor (MSD). A younger age (typically <40 years) and the presence of an MSD favor the use of allogeneic HSCT, while older age (>40 years) and absence of an MSD favor the use of IST (IST), which typically uses a combination of antithymocyte globulin (ATG), cyclosporine (CsA), and eltrombopag in adults.[97-99] However, BMT from alternative donors is increasingly being used as front line therapy for children and adults.

Nonsevere (Moderate) Aplastic Anemia

There are limited data on the long-term prognosis of patients with moderate aplastic anemia. Although moderate aplastic anemia can progress, many patients will remain stable for years, and some may spontaneously improve, even in the absence of specific treatment.[100] Treatment should be based on the depths of the cytopenia, not bone marrow cellularity. Patients with asymptomatic cytopenias require no therapy. Patients with more significant cytopenias, such as symptomatic anemia, may benefit from a trial of IST with antithymocyte globulin and cyclosporine (ATG/CsA)[101] or CsA alone.[102] It is not clear that treatment of moderate aplastic anemia will effect survival or the natural history and evolution of the marrow failure.[103]

Definitive Therapy for Severe Aplastic Anemia
Bone Marrow Transplantation

Adolescents and young adults (age of <40-50 years) meeting criteria for severe disease who have an HLA-matched sibling donor should proceed directly to BMT. *Table 39.6* lists large trials that have allowed this approach to be the standard for appropriate patients for the last several decades. Several conditioning regimens can be used after HLA-matched sibling and unrelated donor BMT. Various reviews and retrospective studies have shown essentially no differences in survival between regimens.[111,112] Rabbit-derived ATG compared with equine-derived ATG has been associated with a lower risk of acute GVHD but not chronic GVHD, which makes this more common in preparation regimens.[111]

Results of BMT for SAA have improved over the last few decades, particularly in regards to use of donors other than matched family members. A report from the European Group for Blood and Marrow Transplantation (EBMT) of over 1500 patients transplanted from 1991 to 2002 confirmed that predictors of survival following BMT included matched sibling donor, recipient age of less than 16 years, early BMT (time from diagnosis to BMT of less than 83 days) and a nonradiation conditioning regimen.[113] An advantage of BMT over standard IST is a marked reduction in the risk of relapse and mitigation of the risk for the development of secondary clone disorders. The risks of acute and chronic GVHD remain a challenge after BMT in historical series. Improving BMT outcomes in adolescents and young adults is an area of active research, including choice of donor as well as source of stem cells.

Alternative Donor Bone Marrow Transplantation

Unrelated donors and mismatched transplants have previously had reports almost twice the transplant-related mortality and risk of GVHD as matched sibling donor transplants (*Table 39.7*).[120] Less than 30% of patients will have an HLA-matched sibling donor. Further development of alternative donor options has recently shown very promising results in haploidentical[119,121-123] as well as unrelated donor BMT.[124] Increasingly, the field is moving more toward BMT up front and less concern is given to historical lower survival rates as the results are so promising. Historically, the more favorable results with unrelated and mismatched transplants are seen in patients under 21 years with disease duration of less than 1 year.[115,125] The International Bone Marrow Transplant Registry reported on the results of 318 alternative donor transplants between 1988 and 1998.[114] Most patients in this series were young, heavily transfused, and of poor performance status. The probability of graft failure was 20% and the survival probability at 5 years was less than 40%. The Fred Hutchinson Cancer Research Center reported on the results of unrelated allogeneic BMT in aplastic

Table 39.6. Representative Results From Large Mature Studies of Bone Marrow Transplantation for Severe Aplastic Anemia Using Matched Sibling Donors

Institution	Years	N	Median Age (Range)	Engraftment (%)	Survival (%)	Median Follow-Up (Years)	Acute GVHD (%)	Chronic GVHD (%)
IBMTR[104]	1988-1992	471	20 (1-51)	84	66	3	19	32
EBMT[105]	1991-1998	71	19 (4-46)	97	86	5	30	35
Seattle[106]	1988-2004	81	25 (2-63)	96	88	9	24	26
Seoul[107]	1995-2001	113	28 (16-50)	85	89	6	11	12
Taipei[108]	1985-2001	79	22 (4-43)	92	74	5	7	35
Sao Paulo[109]	1993-2001	81	24 (3-53)	82	56	6	37	39
EBMT[110]	1998-2007	239	42 (30-67)	86	61	4	20	25

Abbreviations: EBMT, European Group for Blood and Marrow Transplantation; IBMTR, International Bone Marrow Transplant Registry.

Disorders of Red Blood Cells

Table 39.7. Representative Results From Mature Studies of Bone Marrow Transplantation From Alternative Donors

Institution	Years	N	Median Age (Range)	Donor Source	Survival	Median Follow-Up (Years)	Acute GVHD	Chronic GVHD
IBMTR[114]	1988-1998	318	16 (1-55)	MUD 181: MMRD 86; MMUD 51	39% for MUD	5	48% for MUD	29% for MUD
Seattle[115]	1988-2004	87	19 (1-53)	MUD 62; MMUD 25	55%	5	70%	52%
Japan Marrow Donor Program[116]	1993-2000	154	17 (1-46)	MUD 79; MMUD75	56%	5	29%	30%
EBMT[117]	1998-2007	100	20 (3-53)	MUD 87; MMRD 13	77%	3.5	10%	43%
China[118]	2012-2015	101	19 (2-45)	Haplo	89%	1.3 mo (3-43.6)	33.7% grade II-IV	10% extensive
Baltimore[119]	2014-2018	37	25 (4-69)	Haplo	94%	~3 y (32 mo)	11%	8%

Abbreviations: EBMT, European Group for Blood and Marrow Transplantation; GVHD, graft-vs-host disease; IBMTR, International Bone Marrow Transplant Registry; MMRD, mismatched-related donor; MMUD, mismatched unrelated donor; MUD, matched unrelated donor.

anemia after conditioning with low-dose total body irradiation, high-dose cyclophosphamide, and ATG.[115] The median age was 19 years, and with a median follow-up of 7 years, 61% of HLA-identical and 40% of HLA-nonidentical transplant recipients survived the procedure; however, more than 70% of patients acquired acute GVHD, and over 50% developed chronic GVHD. However, improved typing, newer conditioning regimens, and better GVHD prophylaxis are leading to better survival, higher engraftment rates, and less GVHD. There has been a recent interest in pediatrics for upfront unrelated donor transplant, which has shown similar results to matched sibling transplants.[124]

Multiple efforts have been ongoing to improve results with BMT in patients with refractory SAA. In the recently published multicenter BMTCTN 0301 trial of fludarabine, ATG, and total body irradiation (2 Gy)-based conditioning for use with unrelated donors in refractory severe aplastic anemia,[126] the investigators explored dose de-escalations of cyclophosphamide (100, 50, and 0 mg/kg) in the conditioning regimen with the goal of allowing sustained hematopoietic engraftment and survival while decreasing the treatment-related mortality. Nearly all patients had been treated previously with ATG. In 96 patients, 8% had graft failure with cyclophosphamide 50 mg/kg and 15% with cyclophosphamide 100 mg/kg. The 0301 cohort treated without cyclophosphamide was closed after accrual of three patients because of secondary graft failure. Four (11%) patients had major regimen-related toxicity with cyclophosphamide 50 mg/kg and 22% with cyclophosphamide 100 mg/kg. The 1-year incidence of chronic GVHD was 22.5% (95% confidence interval [CI] 10.3-37.5) at 50 mg/kg and 31.7% (18.1-46.2) at 100 mg/kg. Overall survival was >95% in both cohorts.

There have been several more recent experiences with haploidentical BMT in severe aplastic anemia with heterogeneous results depending on the patient population and also limited by small sample size.[118,119,123,127-132] In small case series, rejection has been between 6% and 25%, acute GVHD between 12% and 30%, chronic GVHD between 20% and 40%, and overall survival between 62.5% and 84.6%.[131-133] In a large cohort from China,[118] 101 patients prospectively received haplo BMT from June 2012 through October 2015. The median time for myeloid engraftment in this group was 12 days (range, 9-25) and 15 days (range, 7-101). With a median follow-up of 18.3 (3.0-43.6) months, there was a cumulative incidence of grade II-IV acute GVHD (aGVHD) of 33.7% and chronic GVHD of 22.4% at 1 year. In the United Kingdom, there was a pilot study performed in eight patients with refractory SAA or patients who rejected a prior URD or cord blood transplant using as similar reduced intensity conditioning with posttransplant cyclophosphamide. Six of the eight patients engrafted and only one patient had grade II skin GVHD.[132] Another

promising approach to facilitate engraftment and to mitigate the risk of GVHD is the use of posttransplant cyclophosphamide for GVHD prophylaxis.[134,135] The Baltimore group has shown outcomes of haplo donors after reduced-intensity conditioning with intensive GVHD prophylaxis including posttransplantation cyclophosphamide in relapsed/refractory and treatment-naïve patients with SAA. The results in pediatric and adult patients with SAA using a variety of related haplo donors showed an overall survival for all patients of 94% (90% CI: 88,100%) at 1 and 2 years.[119] The cumulative incidence of grade II-IV aGVHD at day 100 is 11%. The cumulative incidence of chronic GVHD at 2 years is 8%. Given that BMT performed in this fashion associated with durable engraftment without greater early toxicity, increasingly upfront BMT from the best available donor is a discussion with many patients. Further study into quality-of-life metrics and fertility outcomes is ongoing.

Immunosuppressive Therapy

IST has combined ATG and cyclosporine (CsA) for years, with more recent standard of care containing eltrombopag,[99] and is often first-line therapy for adolescent and young adult patients with SAA who lack matched sibling donors as well as older adults.[37] As above, alternative donor transplants are increasingly common, though. Two ATG preparations are commonly used in clinical practice: horse (hATG) and rabbit ATG (rATG). Some data support that hATG is superior to rATG in the frontline treatment of severe AA.[98] The standard protocol uses a dose of 40 mg/kg/day of hATG for 4 days, while CsA is given at 12 to 15 mg/kg in divided doses twice daily. Corticosteroids are also administered during the first 2 weeks to prevent serum sickness. The early results of a phase 2 study with the addition of eltrombopag to the hATG and CsA backbone were promising in older patients, but this augmented response was not demonstrated in children.[136] However, longer-term data show that eltrombopag is not a substantial improvement over the hATG/CsA platform, especially considering the added cost (>100,000 US dollars). Recently, a 4-year follow-up report revealed a cumulative relapse rate of 39% in responding patients who received CsA maintenance as well as clonal evolution of 15% in all treated patients at 4 years. Relapse occurred at distinct timepoints: after CsA dose reduction and eltrombopag discontinuation at 6 months, and after 2 years when CsA was discontinued.[137] (*Table 39.8* reviews immunosuppressive therapies.)

Further strengthening the argument for BMT over IST was a separate long-term follow-up paper published in 2020 of patients treated with hATG + CsA from Europe. The median follow-up was 11.7 years (95% CI, 10.9-12.5) and demonstrated an overall survival at 15 years of 60%. Unfortunately, the event-free survival over the same time was

Table 39.8. Representative Results of Trials of Immunosuppressive Therapy for Severe Aplastic Anemia

Study	Regimen	Years	N	Median Age (Range)	Survival (%)	Response (%)	Relapse (%)	Median Follow-Up	MDS or Leukemia (%)
German[138]	ATG with or without CsA	1986-1989	84	32 (7-80)	58	70	38	11 y	8
EGBMT[56]	ALG, CsA, pred, G-CSF	1991-1999	100	16 (1-72)	87	77	12	3 y	3
NIH[139,140]	ATG, CsA, pred	1991-1998	122	35	55	61	35	7 y	11
NIH[141]	ATG, CsA, MMF, pred	1995-2001	103	30 (3-76)	80	62	37	2 y	9
Japan[142]	ATG, CsA, danazol	1992-1997	119	9 (1-16)	84	68	30	4 y	3
Baltimore[143]	High-dose CY, G-CSF	1996-2008	44	32 (2-68)	88	71	7	5 y	5

Abbreviations: ATG, antithymocyte globulin; CsA, cyclosporine; CY, cyclophosphamide; EGBMT, European Group for Blood and Marrow Transplantation; G-CSF, granulocyte colony-stimulating factor; MMF, mycophenolic acid; NIH, National Institutes of Health; pred, prednisone.

only 23%. Events included relapse, nonresponse at day 120, subsequent BMT, myeloid cancers, solid cancer, PNH, or death.[144]

High-Dose Cyclophosphamide

High-dose cyclophosphamide remains (often in conjunction with ATG) the most commonly used BMT conditioning regimen for aplastic anemia.[145] Interestingly, complete reconstitution of autologous hematopoiesis occurs in 10% to 15% of patients undergoing allogeneic BMT for aplastic anemia.[146-148] Most of these patients have maintained long-term remissions despite autologous reconstitution. The EMBT reported that 10% of patients with SAA experience autologous reconstitution following BMT using a cyclophosphamide + ATG conditioning regimen. Interestingly, 10-year survival (84%) in patients with autologous recovery was equivalent or better than in patients who engrafted (74%).[149]

High-dose cyclophosphamide without BMT has been used to treat patients with aplastic anemia who lack a suitable donor.[143,150-153] Despite the high response rate and low risk of relapse and secondary clonal disease, many investigators are unwilling to accept the relatively long period of aplasia associated with this therapy. This approach is used far less often now, given favorable outcome with BMT and posttransplant cyclophosphamide.

Relapsed and Refractory Severe Aplastic Anemia

There is no standard algorithm for managing patients with SAA who fail to respond, or relapse, after treatment with ATG/CsA; however, inasmuch as 30% to 40% of patients do not respond to initial therapy and another 20% to 40% of responding patients relapse, these patients pose a common treatment dilemma. Therapeutic options include allogeneic BMT (usually from an unrelated or mismatched donor), retreatment with ATG/CsA, alemtuzumab, eltrombopag, or high-dose cyclophosphamide. Alternative donor allogeneic BMT probably offers the best chance for cure and is increasingly well tolerated in pediatric and older patients. Patients with relapsed aplastic anemia are more likely to respond to a second course of ATG/CsA or to high-dose cyclophosphamide than patients with primary refractory disease. Clonal evolution post repeated treatment with IST is increasingly a reason to pursue BMT at the time of relapse. However, response rates to a second course of horse or rabbit ATG/CsA ranges from 20% to 70% with the weighted average closer to 30%.[154-158] High-dose cyclophosphamide or alemtuzumab may also salvage up to 30% of patients with refractory SAA.[159,160]

There has been a single new drug approved for SAA in the past 30 years: eltrombopag, which has a 20% response rate (using traditional response criteria). In responders, the association with relapse and secondary clonal disease[161-163] is similar to IST. Eltrombopag may be used in an attempt to improve the cytopenias in patients at the refractory state.[164] More recently there is increasing experience with the use of alternative donor transplants in the refractory setting that show very promising results. Previous reports with haploidentical BMT in SAA have produced heterogeneous results depending on the population and are also limited by small sample size.[118,127-133,165] In these series, graft rejection has been between 0% and 25%, acute GVHD between 12% and 30%, chronic GVHD between 20% and 40%, and overall survival between 60% and 85%.[131-133] In a cohort from China,[118] 101 patients prospectively received haploidentical BMT with cumulative incidence of grade II-IV aGVHD of 33.7% and chronic GVHD of 22.4% at 1 year. In the United Kingdom, a pilot study performed in eight refractory patients who failed a prior transplant used reduced-intensity conditioning with posttransplant cyclophosphamide. Six of the eight patients engrafted and only one patient had grade II skin GVHD.[132] The US experience using nonmyeloablative conditioning and posttransplant cyclophosphamide has shown early success with 100% engraftment, no chronic GVHD, and no transplant-related mortalities nor significant transplant-related complications,[119,165] and many offer BMT much earlier in a patient's course now to avoid prolonged cytopenias.

All of these potential options should be discussed with patients; however, patient age, performance status, timing and availability of a bone marrow donor, insurance coverage, and institutional expertise are factors in the decision process.[162]

Treatment of Hepatitis-Associated Severe Aplastic Anemia

There are no large prospective series to determine the best treatment for HAA, in part due to the rarity of the disease. Most reports consist of registry data, case series, or single case reports. Because HAA predominantly occurs in children, allogeneic BMT from an HLA-identical sibling is usually considered as first-line therapy. In patients without an HLA-identical sibling, ATG/CsA and high-dose cyclophosphamide have produced durable remissions.[166,167] The EBMT performed a retrospective cohort study from 257 centers to assess the epidemiology and treatment out of HAA.[168] They identified 214 patients managed between 1990 and 2007. The incidence of HAA was 5%, and the response rate and outcome did not appear to differ from that of idiopathic SAA. Similar results were reported by the Japan Childhood Aplastic Anemia Study Group who analyzed the outcome of 44 children with HAA. They reported a 70% response rate with IST and an 88% overall survival at 10 years.[169]

Other Therapies

Numerous reports suggest that anabolic steroids are effective in treating aplastic anemia[170-173]; however, for SAA, controlled clinical trials have shown no benefit in terms of hematopoietic improvement[174] or survival.[90] Although it is clear that androgens should not be used as first-line therapy in SAA, a 3- to 6-month trial is not unreasonable in patients with refractory disease. Danazol, oxymetholone, and decanoate are often tried in such cases. Careful monitoring of liver function tests and vigilance for other hepatic complications (adenomas, tumors, etc.) are required. Eculizumab and ravulizumab are humanized monoclonal antibodies that block terminal complement activity and prevent intravascular hemolysis in PNH.[175-177] These drugs are US Food and Drug Administration approved for the treatment of PNH (see Chapter 32) but do not improve bone marrow function; thus it should not be used to treat aplastic anemia.

CONCLUSION

Aplastic anemia is the prototypical disorder of marrow failure characterized by markedly reduced marrow cellularity and markedly decreased hematopoiesis.[178] Patients suffer significant risk of morbidity and death due to its progressive natural history and/or to complications of suboptimal therapy.[6,178] In the current era, overall survival is around 70% in patients over 16 years of age from historical series, including with use of BMT.[113] The hematopoietic response rate after this IST is about 70%-80%, and the probability of survival at 5 years ranges from 60% to 85%.[99,179] The effect of IST can be durable, but only if medications like cyclosporine are continued for months to years.[99] Failure-free survival (survival without relapse or secondary clonal disease beyond 10 years) after IST is less than 50%.[98,180-183] Survival outcomes continue to improve for alternative donor BMT, including URD and haploidentical.[119,124,184] Alternative donor, especially haplo, BMT shows favorable rates of engraftment and survival in relapsed and treatment-naïve patients as well as limited to no GVHD without greater early toxicity, compared with IST.[119]

References

1. Ehrlich P. Ueber einem Fall von Anamie mit Bemer-kungen uber regenerative Veranderungen des Knochenmarks. *Charite-Annalen.* 1888;13:301-309.
2. Thomas ED, Storb R, Fefer A, et al. Aplastic anaemia treated by marrow transplantation. *Lancet.* 1972;1(7745):284-289.
3. Khan NE, Rosenberg PS, Alter BP. Preemptive bone marrow transplantation and event-free survival in Fanconi anemia. *Biol Blood Marrow Transplant.* 2016;22(10):1888-1892.
4. Hsu JW, Vogelsang G, Jones RJ, Brodsky RA. Bone marrow transplantation in Shwachman-Diamond syndrome. *Bone Marrow Transplant.* 2002;30(4):255-258.
5. Dalle JH, Peffault de Latour R. Allogeneic hematopoietic stem cell transplantation for inherited bone marrow failure syndromes. *Int J Hematol.* 2016;103(4):373-379.
6. Shimamura A, Alter BP. Pathophysiology and management of inherited bone marrow failure syndromes. *Blood Rev.* 2010;24(3):101-122.
7. Bagby GC, Jr. Genetic basis of Fanconi anemia. *Curr Opin Hematol.* 2003;10(1):68-76.
8. Armanios M. Syndromes of telomere shortening. *Annu Rev Genom Hum Genet.* 2009;10:45-61.
9. Vulliamy TJ, Dokal I. Dyskeratosis congenita: the diverse clinical presentation of mutations in the telomerase complex. *Biochimie.* 2008;90(1):122-130.
10. Walne AJ, Dokal I. Dyskeratosis Congenita: a historical perspective. *Mech Ageing Dev.* 2008;129(1-2):48-59.
11. Ly H, Schertzer M, Jastaniah W, et al. Identification and functional characterization of 2 variant alleles of the telomerase RNA template gene (TERC) in a patient with dyskeratosis congenita. *Blood.* 2005;106(4):1246-1252.
12. Armanios M, Chen JL, Chang YP, et al. Haploinsufficiency of telomerase reverse transcriptase leads to anticipation in autosomal dominant dyskeratosis congenita. *Proc Natl Acad Sci U S A.* 2005;102(44):15960-15964.
13. Heiss NS, Knight SW, Vulliamy TJ, et al. X-linked dyskeratosis congenita is caused by mutations in a highly conserved gene with putative nucleolar functions. *Nat Genet.* 1998;19(1):32-38.
14. Mason PJ, Bessler M. The genetics of dyskeratosis congenita. *Cancer Genet.* 2011;204(12):635-645.
15. Hoyeraal HM, Lamvik J, Moe PJ. Congenital hypoplastic thrombocytopenia and cerebral malformations in two brothers. *Acta Paediatr Scand.* 1970;59(2):185-191.
16. Hreidarsson S, Kristjansson K, Johannesson G, Johannsson JH. A syndrome of progressive pancytopenia with microcephaly, cerebellar hypoplasia and growth failure. *Acta Paediatr Scand.* 1988;77(5):773-775.
17. Glousker G, Touzot F, Revy P, Tzfati Y, Savage SA. Unraveling the pathogenesis of Hoyeraal-Heidarsson syndrome, a complex telomere biology disorder. *Br J Haematol.* 2015;170(4):457-471.
18. Dhanraj S, Gunja SM, Deveau AP, et al. Bone marrow failure and developmental delay caused by mutations in poly(A)-specific ribonuclease (PARN). *J Med Genet.* 2015;52(11):738-748.
19. Moon DH, Segal M, Boyraz B, et al. Poly(A)-specific ribonuclease (PARN) mediates 3′-end maturation of the telomerase RNA component. *Nat Genet.* 2015;47(12):1482-1488.
20. Jullien L, Kannengiesser C, Kermasson L, et al. Mutations of the RTEL1 helicase in a Hoyeraal-Heidarsson syndrome patient highlight the importance of the ARCH domain. *Hum Mutat.* 2016;37(5):469-472.
21. Walne AJ, Vulliamy T, Kirwan M, Plagnol V, Dokal I. Constitutional mutations in RTEL1 cause severe dyskeratosis congenita. *Am J Hum Genet.* 2013;92(3):448-453.
22. Ballmaier M, Germeshausen M. Congenital amegakaryocytic thrombocytopenia: clinical presentation, diagnosis, and treatment. *Semin Thromb Hemost.* 2011;37(6):673-681.
23. Ellis SR, Gleizes PE. Diamond Blackfan anemia: ribosomal proteins going rogue. *Semin Hematol.* 2011;48(2):89-96.
24. Issaragrisil S, Kaufman DW, Anderson T, et al. The epidemiology of aplastic anemia in Thailand. *Blood.* 2006;107(4):1299-1307.
25. Young NS, Kaufman DW. The epidemiology of acquired aplastic anemia. *Haematologica.* 2008;93(4):489-492.
26. DeZern AE, Churpek JE. Approach to the diagnosis of aplastic anemia. *Blood Adv.* 2021;5(12):2660-2671.
27. Yates CR, Krynetski EY, Loennechen T, et al. Molecular diagnosis of thiopurine S-methyltransferase deficiency: genetic basis for azathioprine and mercaptopurine intolerance. *Ann Intern Med.* 1997;126(8):608-614.
28. Lazarus KH, Baehner RL. Aplastic anemia complicating infectious mononucleosis: a case report and review of the literature. *Pediatrics.* 1981;67(6):907-910.
29. Young NS, Brown KE. Parvovirus B19. *N Engl J Med* 2004;350(6):586-597.
30. Brown KE, Anderson SM, Young NS. Erythrocyte P antigen: cellular receptor for B19 parvovirus. *Science.* 1993;262(5130):114-117.
31. Kiem HP, Storb R, McDonald GB. Hepatitis-associated aplastic anemia. *N Engl J Med.* 1997;337(6):424-425.
32. Tzakis AG, Arditi M, Whittington PF, et al. Aplastic anemia complicating orthotopic liver transplantation for non-A, non-B hepatitis. *N Engl J Med.* 1988;319(7):393-396.
33. Lu J, Basu A, Melenhorst JJ, Young NS, Brown KE. Analysis of T-cell repertoire in hepatitis-associated aplastic anemia. *Blood.* 2004;103(12):4588-4593.
34. Issaragrisil S, Leaverton PE, Chansung K, et al. Regional patterns in the incidence of aplastic anemia in Thailand. The aplastic anemia study group. *Am J Hematol.* 1999;61(3):164-168.
35. Baverstock KF, Ash PJ. A review of radiation accidents involving whole body exposure and the relevance to the LD50/60 for man. *Br J Radiol.* 1983;56(671):837-844.
36. Ichimaru M, Ishimaru T, Tsuchimoto T, Kirshbaum JD. Incidence of aplastic anemia in A-bomb survivors. Hiroshima and Nagasaki 1946-1967. *Radiat Res.* 1972;49(2):461-472.
37. Marsh JC, Ball SE, Cavenagh J, et al. Guidelines for the diagnosis and management of aplastic anaemia. *Br J Haematol.* 2009;147(1):43-70.
38. Tichelli A, Socie G, Marsh J, et al. Outcome of pregnancy and disease course among women with aplastic anemia treated with immunosuppression. *Ann Intern Med.* 2002;137(3):164-172.
39. Killick SB, Bown N, Cavenagh J, et al. Guidelines for the diagnosis and management of adult aplastic anaemia. *Br J Haematol.* 2016;172(2):187-207.
40. Deka D, Malhotra N, Sinha A, Banerjee N, Kashyap R, Roy KK. Pregnancy associated aplastic anemia: maternal and fetal outcome. *J Obstet Gynaecol Res.* 2003;29(2):67-72.
41. Mathe G, Amiel JL, Schwarzenberg L, et al. Bone marrow graft in man after conditioning by antilymphocytic serum. *Br Med J.* 1970;2:131-136.
42. Hinterberger W, Rowlings PA, Hinterberger-Fischer M, et al. Results of transplanting bone marrow from genetically identical twins into patients with aplastic anemia [see comments]. *Ann Intern Med.* 1997;126(2):116-122.
43. Champlin RE, Perez WS, Passweg JR, et al. Bone marrow transplantation for severe aplastic anemia: a randomized controlled study of conditioning regimens. *Blood.* 2007;109(10):4582-4585.
44. Hoffman R, Zanjani ED, Lutton JD, Zalusky R, Wasserman LR. Suppression of erythroid-colony formation by lymphocytes from patients with aplastic anemia. *N Engl J Med.* 1977;296(1):10-13.
45. Nakao S, Takami A, Takamatsu H, et al. Isolation of a T-cell clone showing HLA-DRB1*0405-restricted cytotoxicity for hematopoietic cells in a patient with aplastic anemia. *Blood.* 1997;89(10):3691-3699.
46. Zeng W, Maciejewski JP, Chen G, Young NS. Limited heterogeneity of T cell receptor BV usage in aplastic anemia. *J Clin Invest.* 2001;108(5):765-773.
47. Zoumbos NC, Gascon P, Djeu JY, Trost SR, Young NS. Circulating activated suppressor T lymphocytes in aplastic anemia. *N Engl J Med.* 1985;312:257-265.
48. Maciejewski JP, Hibbs JR, Anderson S, Katevas P, Young NS. Bone marrow and peripheral blood lymphocyte phenotype in patients with bone marrow failure. *Exp Hematol.* 1994;22(11):1102-1110.
49. Melenhorst JJ, van Krieken JHJM, Dreef E, Landegent JE, Willemze R, Fibbe WE. T cells selectively infiltrate bone marrow areas with residual haemopoiesis of patients with acquired aplastic anaemia. *Br J Haematol.* 1997;99:517-519.
50. Nakao S, Yamaguchi M, Shiobara S, et al. Interferon-gamma gene expression in unstimulated bone marrow mononuclear cells predicts a good response to cyclosporine therapy in aplastic anemia. *Blood.* 1992;79(10):2532-2535.
51. Maciejewski JP, Selleri C, Sato T, Anderson S, Young NS. Increased expression of Fas antigen on bone marrow CD34+ cells of patients with aplastic anaemia. *Br J Haematol.* 1995;91(1):245-252.

52. Hirano N, Butler MO, Bergwelt-Baildon MS, et al. Autoantibodies frequently detected in patients with aplastic anemia. *Blood.* 2003;102(13):4567-4575.
53. Melenhorst JJ, Fibbe WE, Struyk L, van der Elsen PJ, Willemze R, Landegent JE. Analysis of T-cell clonality in bone marrow of patients with acquired aplastic anaemia. *Br J Haematol.* 1997;96(1):85-91.
54. Bacigalupo A, Figari O, Tong J, et al. Long-term marrow culture in patients with aplastic anemia compared with marrow transplant recipients and normal controls. *ExpHematol.* 1992;20:425-430.
55. Schrezenmeier H, Jenal M, Herrmann F, Heimpel H, Raghavachar A. Quantitative analysis of cobblestone area-forming cells in bone marrow of patients with aplastic anemia by limiting dilution assay. *Blood.* 1996;88(12):4474-4480.
56. Bacigalupo A, Bruno B, Saracco P, et al. Antilymphocyte globulin, cyclosporine, prednisolone, and granulocyte colony-stimulating factor for severe aplastic anemia: an update of the GITMO/EBMT study on 100 patients. European group for blood and marrow transplantation (EBMT) working party on severe aplastic anemia and the Gruppo Italiano Trapianti di Midolio Osseo (GITMO). *Blood.* 2000;95(6):1931-1934.
57. Brodsky RA, Sensenbrenner LL, Jones RJ. Complete remission in severe aplastic anemia after high-dose cyclophosphamide without bone marrow transplantation. *Blood.* 1996;87(2):491-494.
58. Van Zant G, de Haan G, Rich IN. Alternatives to stem cell renewal from a developmental viewpoint. *Exp Hematol.* 1997;25(3):187-192.
59. Rusten LS, Jacobsen SE, Kaalhus O, Veiby OP, Funderud S, Smeland EB. Functional differences between CD34- and DR- subfractions of CD34+ bone marrow cells. *Blood.* 1994;84(5):1473-1481.
60. Nagafuji K, Shibuya T, Harada M, et al. Functional expression of Fas antigen (CD95) on hematopoietic progenitor cells. *Blood.* 1995;86(3):883-889.
61. Kim H, Whartenby KA, Georgantas RW,III, Wingard J, Civin CI. Human CD34+ hematopoietic stem/progenitor cells express high levels of FLIP and are resistant to Fas-mediated apoptosis. *Stem Cell.* 2002;20(2):174-182.
62. Brodsky RA, Jones RJ. Aplastic anaemia. *Lancet.* 2005;365(9471):1647-1656.
63. Yoshizato T, Dumitriu B, Hosokawa K, et al. Somatic mutations and clonal hematopoiesis in aplastic anemia. *N Engl J Med.* 2015;373(1):35-47.
64. Kulasekararaj AG, Jiang J, Smith AE, et al. Somatic mutations identify a subgroup of aplastic anemia patients who progress to myelodysplastic syndrome. *Blood.* 2014;124(17):2698-2704.
65. Mukhina GL, Buckley JT, Barber JP, Jones RJ, Brodsky RA. Multilineage glycosylphosphatidylinositol anchor-deficient haematopoiesis in untreated aplastic anaemia. *Br J Haematol.* 2001;115(2):476-482.
66. DeZern AE. Nine years without a new FDA-approved therapy for MDS: how can we break through the impasse? *Hematology Am Soc Hematol Educ Program.* 2015;2015(1):308-316.
67. Garcia-Manero G. Myelodysplastic syndromes: 2015 update on diagnosis, risk-stratification and management. *Am J Hematol.* 2015;90(9):831-841.
68. DeZern AE, Brodsky RA. Paroxysmal nocturnal hemoglobinuria: a complement-mediated hemolytic anemia. *Hematol Oncol Clin North Am.* 2015;29(3):479-494.
69. Nakao S, Sugimori C, Yamazaki H. Clinical significance of a small population of paroxysmal nocturnal hemoglobinuria-type cells in the management of bone marrow failure. *Int J Hematol.* 2006;84(2):118-122.
70. Sugimori C, Chuhjo T, Feng X, et al. Minor population of CD55-CD59- blood cells predicts response to immunosuppressive therapy and prognosis in patients with aplastic anemia. *Blood.* 2006;107(4):1308-1314.
71. Wang H, Chuhjo T, Yasue S, Omine M, Nakao S. Clinical significance of a minor population of paroxysmal nocturnal hemoglobinuria-type cells in bone marrow failure syndrome. *Blood.* 2002;100(12):3897-3902.
72. Nagarajan S, Brodsky R, Young NS, Medof ME. Genetic defects underlying paroxysmal nocturnal hemoglobinuria that arises out of aplastic anemia. *Blood.* 1995;86:4656-4661.
73. Scheinberg P, Marte M, Nunez O, Young NS. Paroxysmal nocturnal hemoglobinuria clones in severe aplastic anemia patients treated with horse anti-thymocyte globulin plus cyclosporine. *Haematologica.* 2010;95(7):1075-1080.
74. Pu JJ, Mukhina G, Wang H, Savage WJ, Brodsky RA. Natural history of paroxysmal nocturnal hemoglobinuria clones in patients presenting as aplastic anemia. *Eur J Haematol.* 2011;87(1):37-45.
75. Hanaoka N, Kawaguchi T, Horikawa K, Nagakura S, Mitsuya H, Nakakuma H. Immunoselection by natural killer cells of PIGA mutant cells missing stress-inducible ULBP. *Blood.* 2006;107(3):1184-1191.
76. Savage WJ, Barber JP, Mukhina GL, et al. Glycosylphosphatidylinositol-anchored protein deficiency confers resistance to apoptosis in PNH. *Exp Hematol.* 2009;37(1):42-51.
77. Inoue N, Izui-Sarumaru T, Murakami Y, et al. Molecular basis of clonal expansion of hematopoiesis in 2 patients with paroxysmal nocturnal hemoglobinuria (PNH). *Blood.* 2006;108(13):4232-4236.
78. Mufti GJ, Kulasekararaj AG, Marsh JC. Somatic mutations and clonal hematopoiesis in aplastic anemia. *N Engl J Med.* 2015;373(17):1674-1675.
79. Ogawa S. Clonal hematopoiesis in acquired aplastic anemia. *Blood.* 2016;128(3):337-347.
80. Keel SB, Scott A, Sanchez-Bonilla M, et al. Genetic features of myelodysplastic syndrome and aplastic anemia in pediatric and young adult patients. *Haematologica.* 2016;101(11):1343-1350.
81. Brodsky RA, Mukhina GL, Li S, et al. Improved detection and characterization of paroxysmal nocturnal hemoglobinuria using fluorescent aerolysin. *Am J Clin Pathol.* 2000;114(3):459-466.
82. Hall SE, Rosse WF. The use of monoclonal antibodies and flow cytometry in the diagnosis of paroxysmal nocturnal hemoglobinuria. *Blood.* 1996;87(12):5332-5340.
83. Matsui WH, Brodsky RA, Smith BD, Borowitz MJ, Jones RJ. Quantitative analysis of bone marrow CD34 cells in aplastic anemia and hypoplastic myelodysplastic syndromes. *Leukemia.* 2006;20(3):458-462.
84. Orazi A, Albitar M, Heerema NA, Haskins S, Neiman RS. Hypoplastic myelodysplastic syndromes can be distinguished from acquired aplastic anemia by CD34 and PCNA immunostaining of bone marrow biopsy specimens. *Am J Clin Pathol.* 1997;107(3):268-274.
85. Lane AA, Odejide O, Kopp N, et al. Low frequency clonal mutations recoverable by deep sequencing in patients with aplastic anemia. *Leukemia.* 2013;27(4):968-971.
86. Babushok DV, Perdigones N, Perin JC, et al. Emergence of clonal hematopoiesis in the majority of patients with acquired aplastic anemia. *Cancer Genet.* 2015;208(4):115-128.
87. Huang J, Ge M, Lu S, et al. Mutations of ASXL1 and TET2 in aplastic anemia. *Haematologica.* 2015;100(5):e172-e175.
88. Heuser M, Schlarmann C, Dobbernack V, et al. Genetic characterization of acquired aplastic anemia by targeted sequencing. *Haematologica.* 2014;99(9):e165-e167.
89. Damm F, Chesnais V, Nagata Y, et al. BCOR and BCORL1 mutations in myelodysplastic syndromes and related disorders. *Blood.* 2013;122(18):3169-3177.
90. Camitta BM, Thomas ED, Nathan DG, et al. A prospective study of androgens and bone marrow transplantation for treatment of severe aplastic anemia. *Blood.* 1979;53:504-514.
91. Killick SB, Bown N, Cavenagh J, et al. Guidelines for the diagnosis and management of adult aplastic anaemia. *Br J Haematol.* 2015.
92. Quillen K, Wong E, Scheinberg P, et al. Granulocyte transfusions in severe aplastic anemia: an eleven-year experience. *Haematologica.* 2009;94(12):1661-1668.
93. Aytac S, Yildirim I, Ceyhan M, et al. Risks and outcome of fungal infection in neutropenic children with hematologic diseases. *Turk J Pediatr.* 2010;52(2):121-125.
94. Aki ZS, Sucak GT, Yegin ZA, Guzel O, Erbas G, Senol E. Hematopoietic stem cell transplantation in patients with active fungal infection: not a contraindication for transplantation. *Transplant Proc.* 2008;40(5):1579-1585.
95. Dezern AE, Brodsky RA. Clinical management of aplastic anemia. *Expet Rev Hematol.* 2011;4(2):221-230.
96. Marsh JC, Ganser A, Stadler M. Hematopoietic growth factors in the treatment of acquired bone marrow failure states. *Semin Hematol.* 2007;44(3):138-147.
97. Afable MG,IInd, Shaik M, Sugimoto Y, et al. Efficacy of rabbit anti-thymocyte globulin in severe aplastic anemia. *Haematologica.* 2011;96(9):1269-1275.
98. Scheinberg P, Nunez O, Weinstein B, Biancotto A, Wu CO, Young NS. Horse versus rabbit antithymocyte globulin in acquired aplastic anemia. *N Engl J Med.* 2011;365(5):430-438.
99. Townsley DM, Scheinberg P, Winkler T, et al. Eltrombopag added to standard immunosuppression for aplastic anemia. *N Engl J Med.* 2017;376(16):1540-1550.
100. Howard SC, Naidu PE, Hu XJ, et al. Natural history of moderate aplastic anemia in children. *Pediatr Blood Cancer.* 2004;43(5):545-551.
101. Frickhofen N, Kaltwasser JP, Schrezenmeier H, et al. Treatment of aplastic anemia with antilymphocyte globulin and methylprednisolone with or without cyclosporine. *N Engl J Med.* 1991;324:1297-1304.
102. Maschan A, Bogatcheva N, Kryjanovskii O, et al. Results at a single centre of immunosuppression with cyclosporine A in 66 children with aplastic anaemia. *Br J Haematol.* 1999;106(4):967-970.
103. Nakao S, Gale RP. Are mild/moderate acquired idiopathic aplastic anaemia and low-risk myelodysplastic syndrome one or two diseases or both and how should it/they be treated? *Leukemia.* 2016;30(11):2127-2130.
104. Horowitz MM. Current status of allogeneic bone marrow transplantation in acquired aplastic anemia. *Semin Hematol.* 2000;37(1):30-42.
105. Locatelli F, Bruno B, Zecca M, et al. Cyclosporin A and short-term methotrexate versus cyclosporin A as graft versus host disease prophylaxis in patients with severe aplastic anemia given allogeneic bone marrow transplantation from an HLA-identical sibling: results of a GITMO/EBMT randomized trial. *Blood.* 2000;96(5):1690-1697.
106. Kahl C, Leisenring W, Deeg HJ, et al. Cyclophosphamide and antithymocyte globulin as a conditioning regimen for allogeneic marrow transplantation in patients with aplastic anaemia: a long-term follow-up. *Br J Haematol.* 2005;130(5):747-751.
107. Ahn MJ, Choi JH, Lee YY, et al. Outcome of adult severe or very severe aplastic anemia treated with immunosuppressive therapy compared with bone marrow transplantation: multicenter trial. *Int J Hematol.* 2003;78(2):133-138.
108. Bai LY, Chiou TJ, Liu JH, et al. Hematopoietic stem cell transplantation for severe aplastic anemia--experience of an institute in Taiwan. *Ann Hematol.* 2004;83(1):38-43.
109. Dulley FL, Vigorito AC, Aranha FJ, et al. Addition of low-dose busulfan to cyclophosphamide in aplastic anemia patients prior to allogeneic bone marrow transplantation to reduce rejection. *Bone Marrow Transplant.* 2004;33(1):9-13.
110. Maury S, Bacigalupo A, Anderlini P, et al. Improved outcome of patients older than 30 years receiving HLA-identical sibling hematopoietic stem cell transplantation for severe acquired aplastic anemia using fludarabine-based conditioning: a comparison with conventional conditioning regimen. *Haematologica.* 2009;94(9):1312-1315.
111. Kekre N, Zhang Y, Zhang MJ, et al. Effect of antithymocyte globulin source on outcomes of bone marrow transplantation for severe aplastic anemia. *Haematologica.* 2017;102(7):1291-1298.
112. Bejanyan N, Kim S, Hebert KM, et al. Choice of conditioning regimens for bone marrow transplantation in severe aplastic anemia. *Blood Adv.* 2019;3(20):3123-3131.
113. Locasciulli A, Oneto R, Bacigalupo A, et al. Outcome of patients with acquired aplastic anemia given first line bone marrow transplantation or immunosuppressive treatment in the last decade: a report from the European Group for Blood and Marrow Transplantation (EBMT). *Haematologica.* 2007;92(1):11-18.
114. Passweg JR, Perez WS, Eapen M, et al. Bone marrow transplants from mismatched related and unrelated donors for severe aplastic anemia. *Bone Marrow Transplant.* 2006;37(7):641-649.

115. Deeg HJ, O'Donnell M, Tolar J, et al. Optimization of conditioning for marrow transplantation from unrelated donors for patients with aplastic anemia after failure of immunosuppressive therapy. *Blood.* 2006;108(5):1485-1491.

116. Kojima S, Matsuyama T, Kato S, et al. Outcome of 154 patients with severe aplastic anemia who received transplants from unrelated donors: the Japan Marrow Donor Program. *Blood.* 2002;100(3):799-803.

117. Bacigalupo A, Socie G, Lanino E, et al. Fludarabine, cyclophosphamide, antithymocyte globulin, with or without low dose total body irradiation, for alternative donor transplants, in acquired severe aplastic anemia: a retrospective study from the EBMT-SAA Working Party. *Haematologica.* 2010;95(6):976-982.

118. Xu LP, Wang SQ, Wu DP, et al. Haplo-identical transplantation for acquired severe aplastic anaemia in a multicentre prospective study. *Br J Haematol.* 2016;175(2):265-274.

119. DeZern AE, Zahurak ML, Symons HJ, et al. Haploidentical BMT for severe aplastic anemia with intensive GVHD prophylaxis including posttransplant cyclophosphamide. *Blood Adv.* 2020;4(8):1770-1779.

120. Bacigalupo A, Oneto R, Bruno B, et al. Current results of bone marrow transplantation in patients with acquired severe aplastic anemia. Report of the European group for blood and marrow transplantation. On behalf of the working party on severe aplastic anemia of the European group for blood and marrow transplantation. *Acta Haematol.* 2000;103(1):19-25.

121. Im HJ, Koh KN, Choi ES, et al. Excellent outcome of haploidentical hematopoietic stem cell transplantation in children and adolescents with acquired severe aplastic anemia. *Biol Blood Marrow Transplant.* 2013;19(5):754-759.

122. Xu LP, Liu KY, Liu DH, et al. A novel protocol for haploidentical hematopoietic SCT without in vitro T-cell depletion in the treatment of severe acquired aplastic anemia. *Bone Marrow Transplant.* 2012;47(12):1507-1512.

123. DeZern AE, Zahurak M, Symons H, Cooke K, Jones RJ, Brodsky RA. Alternative donor transplantation with high-dose post-transplantation cyclophosphamide for refractory severe aplastic anemia. *Biol Blood Marrow Transplant.* 2017;23(3):498-504.

124. Dufour C, Veys P, Carraro E, et al. Similar outcome of upfront-unrelated and matched sibling stem cell transplantation in idiopathic paediatric aplastic anaemia. A study on behalf of the UK Paediatric BMT Working Party, Paediatric Diseases Working Party and Severe Aplastic Anaemia Working Party of EBMT. *Br J Haematol.* 2015;171(4):585-594.

125. Deeg HJ, Amylon ID, Harris RE, et al. Marrow transplants from unrelated donors for patients with aplastic anemia: minimum effective dose of total body irradiation. *Biol Blood Marrow Transplant.* 2001;7(4):208-215.

126. Anderlini P, Wu J, Gersten I, et al. Cyclophosphamide conditioning in patients with severe aplastic anaemia given unrelated marrow transplantation: a phase 1-2 dose de-escalation study. *Lancet Haematol.* 2015;2(9):e367-375.

127. Zhu H, Luo RM, Luan Z, et al. Unmanipulated haploidentical haematopoietic stem cell transplantation for children with severe aplastic anaemia. *Br J Haematol.* 2016;174(5):799-805.

128. Zhang Y, Guo Z, Liu XD, et al. Comparison of haploidentical hematopoietic stem cell transplantation and immunosuppressive therapy for the treatment of acquired severe aplastic anemia in pediatric patients. *Am J Therapeut.* 2017;24(2):e196-e201.

129. Sarmiento M, Ramirez PA. Unmanipulated haploidentical hematopoietic cell transplantation with post-transplant cyclophosphamide in a patient with paroxysmal nocturnal hemoglobinuria and secondary aplastic anemia. *Bone Marrow Transplant.* 2016;51(2):316-318.

130. Esteves I, Bonfim C, Pasquini R, et al. Haploidentical BMT and post-transplant Cy for severe aplastic anemia: a multicenter retrospective study. *Bone Marrow Transplant.* 2015;50(5):685-689.

131. Wang Z, Zheng X, Yan H, Li D, Wang H. Good outcome of haploidentical hematopoietic SCT as a salvage therapy in children and adolescents with acquired severe aplastic anemia. *Bone Marrow Transplant.* 2014;49(12):1481-1485.

132. Clay J, Kulasekararaj AG, Potter V, et al. Nonmyeloablative peripheral blood haploidentical stem cell transplantation for refractory severe aplastic anemia. *Biol Blood Marrow Transplant.* 2014;20(11):1711-1716.

133. Gao L, Li Y, Zhang Y, et al. Long-term outcome of HLA-haploidentical hematopoietic SCT without in vitro T-cell depletion for adult severe aplastic anemia after modified conditioning and supportive therapy. *Bone Marrow Transplant.* 2014;49(4):519-524.

134. Luznik L, Fuchs EJ. High-dose, post-transplantation cyclophosphamide to promote graft-host tolerance after allogeneic hematopoietic stem cell transplantation. *Immunol Res.* 2010;47(1-3):65-77.

135. Dezern AE, Luznik L, Fuchs EJ, Jones RJ, Brodsky RA. Post-transplantation cyclophosphamide for GVHD prophylaxis in severe aplastic anemia. *Bone Marrow Transplant.* 2011;46(7):1012-1013.

136. Groarke EM, Patel BA, Gutierrez-Rodrigues F, et al. Eltrombopag added to immunosuppression for children with treatment-naive severe aplastic anaemia. *Br J Haematol.* 2021;192(3):605-614.

137. Patel BA, Groarke EM, Lotter J, et al. Long-term outcomes in severe aplastic anemia patients treated with immunosuppression and eltrombopag: a phase 2 study. *Blood.* 2022;139(1):34-43.

138. Frickhofen N, Heimpel H, Kaltwasser JP, Schrezenmeier H. Antithymocyte globulin with or without cyclosporin A: 11-year follow-up of a randomized trial comparing treatments of aplastic anemia. *Blood.* 2003;101(4):1236-1242.

139. Rosenfeld SJ, Kimball J, Vining D, Young NS. Intensive immunosuppression with antithymocyte globulin and cyclosporin as treatment for severe aplastic anemia. *Blood.* 1995;85:3058-3065.

140. Rosenfeld S, Follmann D, Nunez O, Young NS. Antithymocyte globulin and cyclosporine for severe aplastic anemia: association between hematologic response and long-term outcome. *JAMA.* 2003;289(9):1130-1135.

141. Scheinberg P, Nunez O, Wu C, Young NS. Treatment of severe aplastic anaemia with combined immunosuppression: anti-thymocyte globulin, ciclosporin and mycophenolate mofetil. *Br J Haematol.* 2006;133(6):606-611.

142. Kojima S, Horibe K, Inaba J, et al. Long-term outcome of acquired aplastic anaemia in children: comparison between immunosuppressive therapy and bone marrow transplantation. *Br J Haematol.* 2000;111(1):321-328.

143. Brodsky RA, Chen AR, Dorr D, et al. High-dose cyclophosphamide for severe aplastic anemia: long-term follow-up. *Blood.* 2010;115(11):2136-2141.

144. Tichelli A, Peffault de Latour R, Passweg J, et al. Long-term outcome of a randomized controlled study in patients with newly diagnosed severe aplastic anemia treated with antithymocyte globuline, cyclosporine, with or without G-CSF: a Severe Aplastic Anemia Working Party Trial from the European Group of Blood and Marrow Transplantation. *Haematologica.* 2020;105(5):1223-1231.

145. Storb R, Etzioni R, Anasetti C, et al. Cyclophosphamide combined with antithymocyte globulin in preparation for allogeneic marrow transplants in patients with aplastic anemia. *Blood.* 1994;84:941-949.

146. Thomas ED, Storb R, Giblett ER, et al. Recovery from aplastic anemia following attempted marrow transplantation. *Exp Hematol.* 1976;4:97-102.

147. Sensenbrenner LL, Steele AA, Santos GW. Recovery of hematologic competence without engraftment following attempted bone marrow transplantation for aplastic anemia: report of a case with diffusion chamber studies. *Exp Hematol.* 1977;77(1):51-58.

148. Gmur J, von Felten A, Phyner K, Frick PG. Autologous hematologic recovery from aplastic anemia following high dose cyclophosphamide and HLA-matched allogeneic bone marrow transplantation. *Acta Haematol.* 1979;62:20-24.

149. Piccin A, McCann S, Socie G, et al. Survival of patients with documented autologous recovery after SCT for severe aplastic anemia: a study by the WPSAA of the EBMT. *Bone Marrow Transplant.* 2010;45(6):1008-1013.

150. Baran DT, Griner PF, Klemperer MR. Recovery from aplastic anemia after treatment with cyclophosphamide. *N Engl J Med.* 1976;295:1522-1523.

151. Brodsky RA, Sensenbrenner LL, Smith BD, et al. Durable treatment-free remission after high-dose cyclophosphamide therapy for previously untreated severe aplastic anemia. *Ann Intern Med.* 2001;135(7):477-483.

152. Jaime-Perez JC, Gonzalez-Llano O, Gomez-Almaguer D. High-dose cyclophosphamide in the treatment of severe aplastic anemia in children. *Am J Hematol.* 2001;66(1):71.

153. Gamper CJ, Takemoto CM, Chen AR, et al. High-dose cyclophosphamide is effective therapy for pediatric severe aplastic anemia. *J Pediatr Hematol/Oncol.* 2016;38(8):627-635.

154. Tichelli A, Passweg J, Nissen C, et al. Repeated treatment with horse antilymphocyte globulin for severe aplastic anaemia. *Br J Haematol.* 1998;100(2):393-400.

155. Marsh JC, Hows JM, Bryett KA, Al-Hashimi S, Fairhead SM, Gordon-Smith EC. Survival after antilymphocyte globulin therapy for aplastic anemia depends on disease severity. *Blood.* 1987;70(4):1046-1052.

156. Means RT, Jr, Krantz SB, Dessypris EN, et al. Re-treatment of aplastic anemia with antithymocyte globulin or antilymphocyte serum. *Am J Med.* 1988;84(4):678-682.

157. Stein RS, Means RT, Jr, Krantz SB, Flexner JM, Greer JP. Treatment of aplastic anemia with an investigational antilymphocyte serum prepared in rabbits. *Am J Med Sci.* 1994;308(6):338-343.

158. Di Bona E, Rodeghiero F, Bruno B, et al. Rabbit antithymocyte globulin (r-ATG) plus cyclosporine and granulocyte colony stimulating factor is an effective treatment for aplastic anaemia patients unresponsive to a first course of intensive immunosuppressive therapy. Gruppo Italiano Trapianto di Midollo Osseo (GITMO). *Br J Haematol.* 1999;107(2):330-334.

159. Audino AN, Blatt J, Carcamo B, et al. High-dose cyclophosphamide treatment for refractory severe aplastic anemia in children. *Pediatr Blood Cancer.* 2010;54(2):269-272.

160. Brodsky RA, Chen AR, Brodsky I, Jones RJ. High-dose cyclophosphamide as salvage therapy for severe aplastic anemia. *Exp Hematol.* 2004;32(5):435-440.

161. Desmond R, Townsley DM, Dumitriu B, et al. Eltrombopag restores trilineage hematopoiesis in refractory severe aplastic anemia that can be sustained on discontinuation of drug. *Blood.* 2014;123(12):1818-1825.

162. Marsh JC, Kulasekararaj AG. Management of the refractory aplastic anemia patient: what are the options? *Hematology Am Soc Hematol Educ Program.* 2013;2013:87-94.

163. Olnes MJ, Scheinberg P, Calvo KR, et al. Eltrombopag and improved hematopoiesis in refractory aplastic anemia. *N Engl J Med.* 2012;367(1):11-19.

164. Desmond R, Townsley DM, Dunbar C, Young NS. Eltrombopag in aplastic anemia. *Semin Hematol.* 2015;52(1):31-37.

165. Dezern A, Dorr D, Luznik L, et al. Using haploidentical (haplo) donors and high-dose post-transplant cyclophosphamide (PTCy) for refractory severe aplastic anemia (SAA). *Blood.* 2015;126(23):2031.

166. Savage WJ, DeRusso PA, Resar LM, et al. Treatment of hepatitis-associated aplastic anemia with high-dose cyclophosphamide. *Pediatr Blood Cancer.* 2007;49(7):947-951.

167. Brown KE, Tisdale J, Barrett AJ, Dunbar CE, Young NS. Hepatitis-associated aplastic anemia [see comments]. *N Engl J Med.* 1997;336(15):1059-1064.

168. Locasciulli A, Bacigalupo A, Bruno B, et al. Hepatitis-associated aplastic anaemia: epidemiology and treatment results obtained in Europe. A report of the EBMT aplastic anaemia working party. *Br J Haematol.* 2010;149(6):890-895.

169. Osugi Y, Yagasaki H, Sako M, et al. Antithymocyte globulin and cyclosporine for treatment of 44 children with hepatitis associated aplastic anemia. *Haematologica.* 2007;92(12):1687-1690.

170. Shahidi NT, Diamond LK. Testosterone-induced remission in aplastic anemia. *Am J Dis Child.* 1959;98:293-302.

171. Shahidi NT, Diamond LK. Testosterone-induced remission in aplastic anemia of both acquired and congenital types. Further observations in 24 cases. *N Engl J Med.* 1961;264:953-967.

172. Gardner FH, Juneja HS. Androstane therapy to treat aplastic anaemia in adults: an uncontrolled pilot study. *Br J Haematol.* 1987;65(3):295-300.

173. Townsley DM, Dumitriu B, Liu D, et al. Danazol treatment for telomere diseases. *N Engl J Med.* 2016;374(20):1922-1931.

174. Young N, Griffith P, Brittain E, et al. A multicenter trial of antithymocyte globulin in aplastic anemia and related diseases. *Blood.* 1988;72:1861-1869.

175. Brodsky RA. How I treat paroxysmal nocturnal hemoglobinuria. *Blood.* 2009;113(26):6522-6527.

176. Brodsky RA. How I treat paroxysmal nocturnal hemoglobinuria. *Blood.* 2021;137(10):1304-1309.

177. Kulasekararaj AG, Hill A, Rottinghaus ST, et al. Ravulizumab (ALXN1210) vs eculizumab in C5-inhibitor-experienced adult patients with PNH: the 302 study. *Blood.* 2019;133(6):540-549.

178. Bacigalupo A. How I treat acquired aplastic anemia. *Blood.* 2017;129(11): 1428-1436.

179. Scheinberg P, Young NS. How I treat acquired aplastic anemia. *Blood.* 2012;120(6):1185-1196.

180. de Fontebrune FS, Socie G. Long-term issues after immunosuppressive therapy for aplastic anemia. *Curr Drug Targets.* 2016.

181. Chuncharunee S, Wong R, Rojnuckarin P, et al. Efficacy of rabbit antithymocyte globulin as first-line treatment of severe aplastic anemia: an Asian multicenter retrospective study. *Int J Hematol.* 2016;104(4):454-461.

182. Marsh JC, Bacigalupo A, Schrezenmeier H, et al. Prospective study of rabbit antithymocyte globulin and cyclosporine for aplastic anemia from the EBMT Severe Aplastic Anaemia Working Party. *Blood.* 2012;119(23):5391-5396.

183. Tichelli A, Schrezenmeier H, Socie G, et al. A randomized controlled study in patients with newly diagnosed severe aplastic anemia receiving antithymocyte globulin (ATG), cyclosporine, with or without G-CSF: a study of the SAA Working Party of the European Group for Blood and Marrow Transplantation. *Blood.* 2011;117(17):4434-4441.

184. Dufour C, Pillon M, Passweg J, et al. Outcome of aplastic anemia in adolescence: a survey of the severe aplastic anemia working party of the European group for blood and marrow transplantation. *Haematologica.* 2014;99(10):1574-1581.

Disorders of Red Blood Cells

Chapter 40 ■ Red Cell Aplasia: Acquired and Congenital Disorders

ANUPAMA NARLA • JEFFREY M. LIPTON • ROBERT T. MEANS JR

INTRODUCTION

Red cell aplasia is characterized by anemia, severe reticulocytopenia (reticulocyte count <1%), and an almost complete absence of erythroblasts from the bone marrow (erythroblasts <0.5%). In contrast to aplastic anemia, in which the aplasia involves all three cell lines, pure red cell aplasia (PRCA) is selective for the erythroid cell lineage so that patients often, but not always, have normal leukocyte and platelet counts.[1] Red cell aplasia may occur as a primary disorder or may develop as a hematologic complication in the course of a variety of diseases. In this chapter, differing etiologies of red cell aplasia and their associated pathogenic mechanisms are described. Secondary etiologies are arranged in approximate order of clinical significance or frequency. Finally, Diamond-Blackfan anemia (DBA), a genetic/congenital cause of PRCA also will be reviewed.

ACQUIRED PURE RED CELL APLASIA

PRCA, which was first described in 1922, is a rare disorder that affects any age group and both males and females equally. Today, the term PRCA is used primarily to describe this disorder in adults, although some of the causes of red blood cell (RBC) aplasia in adults are seen in children also. PRCA may be primary or secondary to a variety of autoimmune or infectious diseases (*Table 40.1*). Primary acquired PRCA can occur in individuals of any age in the absence of any underlying disorder. It may run an acute and usually self-limited course or may persist chronically. In adults, the acute form of primary PRCA is very rarely identified except in patients with congenital hemolytic anemia and the chronic form of PRCA predominates. Acute PRCA in otherwise healthy adults may escape diagnosis because acute arrest of erythropoiesis of short duration may not produce significant anemia as a result of the long life span of the red cells and the ability of marrow to increase red cell production rapidly during the recovery process.

Primary Acquired (Autoimmune) Pure Red Cell Aplasia

In primary acquired PRCA, many studies have indicated that the arrest of erythropoiesis is caused by the presence in the patient's plasma of an erythropoietic inhibitor. Early studies in mice showed that injection of patients' plasma led to a significant suppression of in vivo erythropoiesis, as measured by radioactive iron incorporation into newly formed red cells.[2] Evaluation of the response of patients' marrow cells to erythropoietin (Epo) by measuring heme synthesis in vitro showed that, in the presence of normal plasma, PRCA marrow responds normally to Epo, but in the presence of a patient's autologous plasma, a significant decline in heme synthesis is observed, suggesting the presence in the patient's plasma of an inhibitor acting on erythroid cells.[3] In about 60% of cases, patients' marrow cells respond to Epo in a normal way by increasing the rate of heme synthesis by 2- to 9-fold, and in about 40% of patients an inhibitor of erythropoiesis can be detected in their plasma. This inhibitor was localized to the immunoglobulin G (IgG) fraction, and it disappears from the plasma after remission of PRCA.[3,4]

The stage of erythropoiesis at which the arrest occurs has been studied by assaying PRCA marrow cells in semisolid media for erythroid progenitors. Despite a conspicuous absence of erythroblasts from the PRCA marrow, in at least 60% of patients normal numbers of early burst-forming unit erythroid (BFU-E) and late colony-forming unit erythroid (CFU-E) progenitors can be detected, indicating that the arrest occurs at some level between CFU-E and basophilic erythroblasts. In the remainder of patients the erythroid cell compartment is affected at a stage earlier than the CFU-E, so that the CFU-E or BFU-E marrow pools are significantly reduced.[5,6] The presence of normal numbers of erythroid progenitors has been associated with a favorable outcome following immunosuppressive therapy.[6] The patient's serum IgG inhibits maturation and differentiation of erythroid progenitors into erythroblasts in vitro. The inhibition is dose dependent and is no longer present in the IgG fraction of the patient's plasma collected in remission.[4] The inhibitory effect of the IgG is specific for erythroid cells, and no effect on myeloid progenitor cell growth is detected.[6]

The target antigen and mode of action of the IgG inhibitor of erythropoiesis has been investigated in many cases of primary autoimmune PRCA but appears to be variable. As already discussed, it may target erythroid CFU-E or BFU-E progenitors, or it may be directed against morphologically recognizable erythroblasts.[7] The molecule(s) on the erythroid cell membrane with which the PRCA IgG inhibitor interacts has not yet been defined. In rare cases, endogenous Epo itself appears to be the target antigen.[8] In some cases of autoimmune hemolytic anemia concurrent with PRCA, the antibody causing hemolysis can also suppress erythroid progenitor colony formation, whereas in other cases the two processes result from two different antibodies.[9,10]

In addition to antibody-mediated PRCA, cases of PRCA have been reported in which the immunologic mechanism is T cell mediated. These cases appear to be particularly associated with thymoma.[11] Somatic mutations in *STAT3* are found in CD8-expressing T lymphocytes of 43% of patients with PRCA overall. These mutations may be seen in more than 70% of patients with PRCA associated with T-cell large granular lymphocyte leukemia, and also in 20% to 30% of patients with other types of PRCA.[12] There are also cases of PRCA in which no immune pathogenic mechanism or other known mechanism can be established by in vitro assays. These cases can be classified as idiopathic PRCA. However, failure to demonstrate an immune mechanism does not necessarily exclude an immune pathogenesis because the outcome of treatment with immunosuppressive agents seems to be the same for both cases demonstrated to be autoimmune and idiopathic cases. It is important to keep in mind that a patient with no demonstrable autoimmunity who fails to respond to immunosuppressive therapy, and who has birth defects or a family history of red cell failure may, in fact, have DBA presenting in adulthood (see section on "Diamond-Blackfan Anemia").

Transient Erythroblastopenia of Childhood

This rare disorder is a cause of acquired red cell aplasia in young children because of a transient antibody-mediated suppression of normal erythropoiesis. It is characterized by the gradual (over weeks) development of normocytic anemia (hemoglobin level of 2-8 g/dL), reticulocytopenia, and a pronounced reduction of bone marrow erythroblasts. The platelet count is usually normal to increased, and the leukocyte count is usually normal, although 20% of children may have significant neutropenia. The disorder uniquely occurs in previously healthy young children from 6 months to 4 years of age and is seen with equal frequency in boys and girls. The natural history of transient erythroblastopenia of childhood (TEC) is that all patients recover spontaneously in a few weeks and there are no long-term sequelae. No specific therapy other than careful observation is necessary.[13] RBC transfusions are indicated only if a child is symptomatic from anemia, and rarely is more than one transfusion needed. Neither iron nor steroid therapy has any role in the management of this disorder. The diagnosis is often confused with that of iron deficiency anemia, although the erythrocytes in patients with TEC are normocytic. TEC had historically been confused with DBA, although the latter most often, but not always, presents before 6 months of age, is associated with congenital abnormalities in about half the cases, and is characterized

Table 40.1. Classification of PRCA

Congenital PRCA
Diamond-Blackfan Anemia
Acquired PRCA
Primary
  Primary autoimmune PRCA (includes transient erythroblastopenia of childhood)
  Primary myelodysplastic PRCA
Secondary, associated with:
Immunologic disorders
  Autoimmune/collagen vascular disorders
  Other immunologic processes
Neoplasia
  Lymphoproliferative disorders
  Nonlymphoproliferative hematologic malignancies
  Thymoma
  Nonthymoma solid tumors
Infectious diseases
  B19 parvovirus
  Viral infections other than parvovirus
  Bacterial infections
Drugs and chemicals (see *Table 40.2*)
Miscellaneous
  Pregnancy
  Renal failure
  Severe malnutrition
  Vitamin deficiency (B$_{12}$, folate, riboflavin)

Abbreviation: PRCA, pure red cell aplasia.
Modified from Means RT. Pure red cell aplasia. *Blood.* 2016;128(21):2504-2509. Copyright © 2016 American Society of Hematology. With permission.

by macrocytic erythrocytes with many features of fetal erythropoiesis and an elevated erythrocyte adenosine deaminase (eADA) activity. The ability to confirm a clinical diagnosis of DBA genetically in the majority of cases is helpful in rare instances when there is confusion regarding the diagnosis (see section "Diamond-Blackfan Anemia").

Myelodysplastic Primary Pure Red Cell Aplasia

A small percentage of cases of idiopathic PRCA, usually refractory to treatment, may evolve into acute leukemia, and these cases are classified as myelodysplastic PRCA. In a sense, such cases should be regarded not as part of a PRCA syndrome but rather as a myelodysplastic syndrome (MDS) morphologically resembling PRCA.[1,5] These patients may also have molecular or cytogenetic abnormalities characteristic of MDS.

Parvovirus-Induced Pure Red Cell Aplasia

It has been known for many years that human B19 parvovirus is responsible for the aplastic crisis seen in patients with chronic hemolytic anemia. It was subsequently demonstrated that B19 parvovirus can produce chronic PRCA in immunocompromised patients, including those with human immunodeficiency virus (HIV) or on immunosuppressive drugs.[14] Parvovirus B19 directly infects human erythroid progenitors by a process requiring the red cell surface P antigen. Individuals who do not express P antigen are not susceptible to parvovirus infection.[15] Parvovirus B19 induces apoptosis in erythroid progenitors.[16] The precise mechanism by which this occurs is unclear but appears to involve the N terminus of viral nonstructural protein 1. Hypoxia appears to upregulate expression of viral messages in infected cells; the specific role of the HIF-1 pathway, STAT5, and MEK in this effect is being explored.[17] In patients with a functioning spleen, the decreased production can be compounded by sequestration in an enlarged spleen.

Recombinant Epo-Induced Immune Pure Red Cell Aplasia

As noted earlier, autoimmune PRCA caused by antibodies against endogenous Epo has been described infrequently. Beginning in the mid- to late 1990s, cases of PRCA associated with antibodies against recombinant human (rh) Epo began to appear.[18] These cases occurred in patients with end-stage renal disease receiving rhEpo for anemia management. These cases were unusual in that more than 90% involved a particular rhEpo product and were primarily associated with subcutaneous treatment, the vast majority occurred outside the United States, and there was wide nation-to-nation variation, even allowing for use of specific rhEpo products. Eventually, the process was attributed to features of the rhEpo product administration system (such as adjuvant effects of the material used in prefilled syringes). In response to changed packaging, the problem has largely resolved.[19,20]

Thymoma

The association between thymic neoplasms and PRCA has been known for many years. PRCA may precede the development of thymoma, coexist with thymoma, or even develop years after the surgical removal of a thymoma. Although at one time the presence of thymoma in patients with PRCA was reported to be as high as 50%, more recent series suggest the actual percentage is 7% to 10%. The pathogenic mechanism involved is uncertain but presumably related to an immune T cell–mediated process.[21,22]

Lymphoproliferative Disorders

Various lymphoproliferative syndromes have been associated with severe erythroid aplasia (see *Table 40.1*), including chronic lymphocytic leukemia (CLL) of B- or T-cell type and large granular lymphocyte (LGL) syndrome, or with clonal T-cell disorders that are not otherwise clinically apparent but detectable only by molecular studies.[23,24] The incidence of severe erythroid aplasia among patients with CLL may be as high as 6%, with many cases missed because severe normochromic anemia and reticulocytopenia are frequent manifestations of advanced-stage CLL and are often attributed to the primary disease process.[25] The development of erythroid aplasia does not affect the prognosis of CLL and in the majority of cases does not seem to be related to previous cytotoxic chemotherapy. PRCA has also been described in association with Hodgkin and non-Hodgkin lymphomas, multiple myeloma, Waldenström macroglobulinemia, angioimmunoblastic lymphadenopathy, and Castleman disease.[26]

In CLL, PRCA appears to derive from immune suppression, but not typically through inhibitory antibodies. Various studies have demonstrated that in T-cell CLL and LGL syndrome, the T lymphocytes are responsible for the suppression of erythropoiesis. The suppression is mediated by direct cell-to-cell interaction, mainly between a subset of T cells expressing receptors for the γ chain of IgG (Tγ cells) and erythroid progenitors, and is human leukocyte antigen-antigen D related (HLA-DR) restricted. The suppression is selective for the erythroid cells and is not detectable after remission of the PRCA.[27] Similar findings have been reported in B-cell CLL, in which there seems to be a progressive increase in the marrow of Tγ cells, which, when they reach a critical concentration, suppress erythropoiesis and cause red cell aplasia.[28] In LGL lymphocytosis, clonal expansion of LGLs of the γ/δ type expressing killer-cell inhibitory receptors for class I HLA antigens has been shown to be responsible for lysis of erythroblasts, most likely related to the declining density, with eventual disappearance, of HLA-I antigens in late marrow erythroid cells. However, the role of killer-cell inhibitory receptors in the pathogenesis of PRCA in LGL lymphocytosis remains unclear because such receptors are also detectable in patients with large granular lymphocytosis without PRCA.[29] Expansion of the marrow population of CD8$^+$/perforin$^+$ memory T cells has also been noted in patients with thymoma-associated PRCA.[30] As noted earlier, *STAT3* mutations are common in patients with PRCA with clonal T-cell populations.[12]

Other Hematologic Malignancies

PRCA has been reported in association with chronic myelogenous leukemia, chronic myelomonocytic leukemia, chronic eosinophilic leukemia, primary myelofibrosis, essential thrombocythemia, and acute lymphoblastic leukemia. Few cases have been studied in detail, but in general the course of PRCA appears to run independently of the associated disease and may reflect a coincident autoimmune disorder.[1]

Nonthymic Solid Tumors

There have been many reports of PRCA observed in patients with nonthymic, nonhematologic malignancies (*Table 40.1*). Given that these reports are rare and that the primary malignancy and PRCA typically run independent courses, it is likely that the association is coincidental.[1,5]

Autoimmune Disorders/Collagen Vascular Disease

It should not be surprising that PRCA is a hematologic complication of various autoimmune diseases, including collagen vascular diseases, such as systemic lupus erythematosus, rheumatoid arthritis, mixed connective tissue disease, Sjögren syndrome, autoimmune hemolytic anemia, multiple endocrine gland insufficiency, autoimmune hypothyroidism, inflammatory bowel disease, autoimmune liver disease, pyoderma gangrenosum, and pernicious anemia.[1] PRCA may occur prior to, during, or after the onset of these disorders. When investigated in detail, cases of PRCA associated with autoimmune or collagen vascular diseases are typically found to be mediated by antibodies that inhibit erythropoiesis.[31]

ABO-Incompatible Stem Cell Transplantation

PRCA may occur as a consequence of ABO-incompatible bone marrow or stem cell transplantation. In one recent series and review, this complication occurred in 7.5% of ABO-incompatible transplants and was most common in circumstances where a blood group O recipient was transplanted from a blood group A donor. Erythroid precursors express surface blood group antibodies, and anti-A or anti-B isoagglutinins from recipient plasma cells are the etiologic agents. There is a 60% to 70% frequency of spontaneous recovery, but the remainder may develop sustained PRCA requiring treatment.[32]

Pure Red Cell Aplasia With Infections Other Than Parvovirus

Acute, self-limited PRCA may develop in the course of various infections. Viral hepatitis and infectious mononucleosis, in particular, have been reported many times in association with PRCA. In general, PRCA remits with treatment or resolution of the underlying infection.[1,33] Studies on the pathogenesis of PRCA in the course of viral hepatitis, infectious mononucleosis, and human T-lymphotropic virus type 1 (HTLV-1) infection have suggested that the suppression of erythropoiesis is mediated by cytotoxic T lymphocytes.

Drugs and Chemicals

Many drugs and chemicals have been reported as causes of PRCA (*Table 40.2*). Drug-induced PRCA is usually an acute disorder that resolves soon after discontinuation of the drug or cessation of exposure to the chemical. PRCA may appear after the first exposure to the drug or a significant time after the drug's initiation. In most instances, the association of a drug with PRCA is circumstantial and is based on the evidence that PRCA remits after discontinuation of the drug. The mechanisms by which implicated drugs cause erythroid aplasia have been studied infrequently and appear to differ between agents.[1,5] IgG inhibitors of erythropoiesis have been reported with diphenylhydantoin and rifampicin but not with other drugs studied.[34-36]

Pregnancy

Pregnancy also has been associated with PRCA that usually, but not always, remits after delivery. Development of PRCA during one pregnancy does not necessarily predict recurrence of the disease in subsequent pregnancies, although recurrence has been reported.[37]

Miscellaneous Disorders

In rare cases, PRCA has been associated with renal failure, with severe malnutrition producing marasmus or kwashiorkor, and with riboflavin, vitamin B_{12}, or folic acid deficiencies.[5]

Table 40.2. Drugs and Chemicals Associated With Pure Red Cell Aplasia

Antiviral/Antimicrobial
Ampicillin
Cepalothin
Chloramphenicol
Chloroquine
Dapsone/pyrimethamine
Isoniazid
Lamuvidine
Linezolid
Mepacrine
Micafungin
Penicillin
Ribavirin
Sulfathiazole
Thiamphenicol
Trimethoprim/sulfamethoxasole
Zidovudine
Anticonvulsants
Carbamazepine
Diphenylhydantoin
Phenobarbital
Valproic acid
Immunomodulatory/Chemotherapy/Growth Factors
Alemtuzumab
Azathioprine
Cladribine
Erythropoietin (recombinant)
Fludarabine
Gold (colloidal)
Interferon
Mycophenylate
Nivolumab
Pembrolizumab
Sulfasalazine
Tacrolimus
Analgesics/Anesthetics
Fenoprofen
Halothane
Sulindac
Cardiovascular
Clopidogrel
Methyldopa
Procainamide
Metabolic
Allopurinol
Chlorpropamide
Estrogen
Penicillamine
Miscellaneous
Benzene
Bromsulphthalein

Clinical Presentation

There are no clinical features or physical findings characteristic of PRCA other than the signs and symptoms of anemia. Because a complete arrest of erythropoiesis would cause a decline of red cell mass of roughly 1% a day, the development of anemia in PRCA is gradual, allowing for physiologic compensation that would mitigate symptomatology for any given degree of anemia. In secondary cases, physical findings related to the underlying disease may be present.

Laboratory Evaluation

Peripheral Blood Counts

In acquired PRCA, the erythrocytes are normochromic and normocytic, and the reticulocyte percentage is inappropriately low (<1%), with absolute reticulocyte count typically less than 10,000/μL. An uncorrected reticulocyte percentage >1% should raise a serious doubt about the diagnosis of PRCA, although in TEC a reticulocyte percentage greater than 1% may indicate early spontaneous recovery. The white cell count and differential and platelet count are usually normal. Occasionally, mild leukopenia, lymphocytosis, eosinophilia, and either thrombocytosis or mild thrombocytopenia may be present. When present, these abnormalities typically reflect a state of immune activation or marrow suppression caused by the associated disorder.

Bone Marrow

The hallmark of PRCA is the absence of erythroblasts from an otherwise normal marrow. The overall cellularity of the marrow is normal to slightly increased. Markedly increased cellularity with elimination of fat spaces should suggest an alternative diagnosis. In typical cases, the erythroblasts are either totally absent or constitute <1% on the marrow differential count (*Figure 40.1*). In a small number of cases, a few proerythroblasts or basophilic erythroblasts may be seen, not exceeding 5% of the differential count.[5] The presence of large proerythroblasts

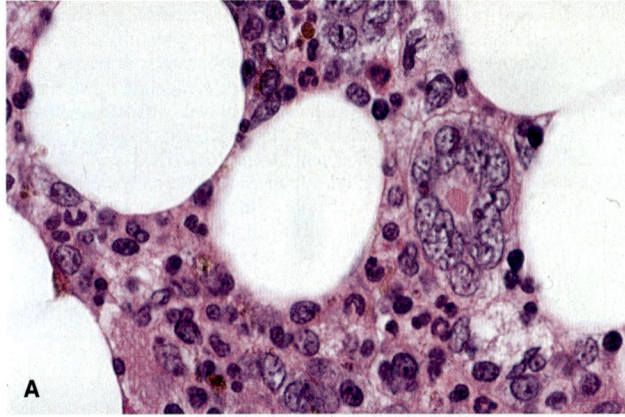

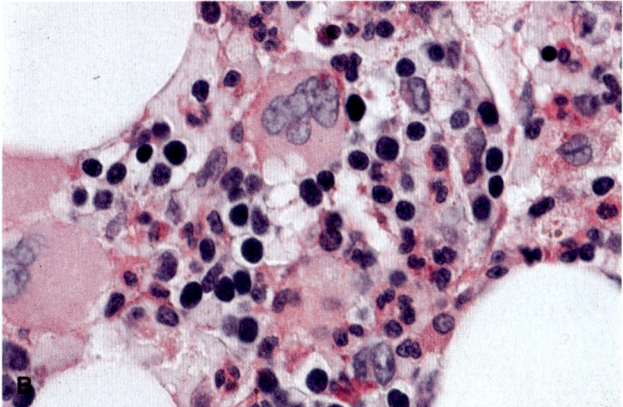

FIGURE 40.1 A. Characteristic bone marrow biopsy from a patient with pure red cell aplasia. B. Bone marrow biopsy from the same patient after successful response to immunosuppression. Note easily identifiable erythroblasts.

("giant pronormoblasts") with vacuolated cytoplasm and pseudopodia formation may raise the suspicion of an active B19 parvovirus infection but is not diagnostic.[38]

In some cases, a phase of ineffective erythropoiesis characterized by erythroid hyperplasia with maturation arrest at the stage of proerythroblasts or basophilic erythroblasts in the marrow and reticulocytopenia in the blood may precede the development of PRCA, develop during the course of PRCA, or appear after partial response to treatment and before the return of erythropoiesis to normal.[39] Although this morphologic picture in the absence of dysplastic changes in other lineages or cytogenetic abnormalities should raise suspicion of PRCA, bone marrow examination would need to be repeated at a later time to confirm the diagnosis.

Cytogenetics/Molecular Diagnostics

The myeloid cells and the megakaryocytes in the marrow are normal and exhibit full maturation. An increased number of lymphocytes on marrow smear; an increased number of polyclonal lymphoid aggregates in marrow biopsy; or a mild increase in plasma cells, eosinophils, or mast cells may be seen. These findings are presumed to reflect inflammatory/immune activation. Iron stores are normal or increased and normally distributed, but during recovery or the phase of ineffective erythropoiesis, a few ring sideroblasts may be seen.

Cytogenetic studies on marrow cells in PRCA are normal. An abnormal karyotype indicates MDS with the morphologic appearance of erythroid hypoplasia.[5,40] Such patients typically do not respond well to immunosuppression,[41] although exceptions have been reported.[42-44] In a number of patients, the presence of lymphocytes with γ or δ T-cell receptor gene rearrangement has been described. These findings demonstrate PRCA secondary to a T-cell lymphoproliferative disorder and frequently respond to immunosuppression, although patients with STAT3 mutations are less likely to have a good response.[12,23]

Other Laboratory Abnormalities

Vitamin B_{12}, folic acid, ferritin, serum iron, and transferrin saturation are normal or elevated. Patients extensively transfused prior to diagnosis may have evidence of iron overload. Serum Epo levels are increased in proportion to the severity of the anemia.[45] A range of immunologic abnormalities have been reported in patients with chronic PRCA, including hypogammaglobulinemia, monoclonal gammopathies, cryoproteins, decreased complement, antinuclear antibodies, decreased or increased B cells, and impaired phytohemagglutinin-induced lymphocyte cytotoxicity.[5] Patients who are refractory to treatment and who are supported by regular red cell transfusions may develop a significant hemolytic component after alloimmunization or development of hypersplenism.[5]

Evaluation and Treatment

PRCA, MDS, and other primary marrow failure disorders are suspected in similar clinical circumstances, and the initial diagnostic approach is bone marrow examination. Specimens should be sent for cytogenetics, T-cell receptor gene rearrangement, and flow cytometry as well as routine pathology, including iron stain. In PRCA, a normocellular marrow in which there is almost a complete absence of erythroblasts but with normal myeloid cells and megakaryocytes is expected. A hypocellular marrow with trilineage hypoplasia suggests aplastic anemia; dyspoietic marrow morphology, hypercellularity, or ringed sideroblasts suggests MDS.

In all patients with PRCA, polymerase chain reaction (PCR) testing for parvovirus DNA should be performed. Parvovirus serology is misleading in the immunocompromised, and PCR on peripheral blood is the test of choice.[46] If parvovirus testing is negative, computerized tomography should be performed on all adult patients to rule out thymoma. Flow cytometry studies performed on the diagnostic bone marrow will identify a lymphoproliferative disorder as the possible etiology of PRCA. Abnormal cytogenetics would indicate an MDS. In particular 5q⁻ MDS can appear, in adults as well as children, as a pure red cell failure mimicking

PRCA or DBA.[40] Although it is uncommon at present, patients with renal failure who develop PRCA while being treated with rhEpo should be evaluated for anti-Epo antibodies. Testing for underlying autoimmune disorders can be performed if otherwise clinically indicated but typically would not alter therapy. In patients with PRCA who do not respond well to immunosuppression and do not have abnormal cytogenetics or clonal T-cell mutations, a next-generation sequencing panel for mutations associated with myeloid malignancies should be considered.

Immunosuppressive/Immunomodulatory Therapy

Drugs should be reviewed as possible contributors to PRCA, and any active infection should be treated. Underlying lymphoproliferative disorders, MDS, or other malignancies should be treated as would otherwise be indicated by disease stage and clinical features.[1] Otherwise, in the absence of documented parvovirus infection or thymoma, the initial approach to PRCA is immunosuppression or immunomodulation (*Table 40.3*). *Figure 40.1A* and *B* display bone marrow biopsy results from a patient before and after immunosuppression. Approximately two-thirds of patients with PRCA will respond to an immunosuppression approach.[1,5,6,41,47]

Cyclosporine

Of the drugs with which there is substantial experience in PRCA, cyclosporine appears to be the single most effective immunosuppressive used for PRCA (*Table 40.3*) and should be considered the immunosuppressive drug of choice for this disorder.[47] *Figure 40.2* shows the response of a patient refractory to several other agents prior to cyclosporine therapy.[4] Cyclosporine is substantially more expensive than prednisone and requires monitoring of drug levels and of renal function.

Cyclosporine may be used as a single agent or concurrently with low-dose prednisone (usually 30 mg prednisone/day or less). The usual starting dose of cyclosporine is 6 mg/kg/d, although higher initial doses have been used.[1,4,47] Target trough levels are 150 to 250 ng/mL. When the hematocrit approaches target levels (usually 35%-36%), a slow taper is begun. Some patients may require maintenance therapy. If a patient has not responded in 3 to 4 months, cyclosporine should be tapered off and another agent started.

Although cyclosporine is not leukemogenic, as are some of the cytotoxic drugs used for PRCA, there are reports of lymphoma development in patients with PRCA treated with cyclosporine.[4] Whether these cases represented treatment-induced lymphomas or were cases of lymphoma-associated PRCA is not clear.

Corticosteroids

Corticosteroids were the traditional first-line drugs in PRCA prior to cyclosporine, and in certain circumstances, such as pregnancy-associated PRCA, they may still be the first choice. Prednisone is given orally at a dose of 1 mg/kg/d until a remission is induced. As indicated in *Table 40.3*, approximately 40% of patients will have a remission on steroids. Corticosteroid-induced remission usually occurs within 4 weeks, and continuation of a trial with prednisone longer than 12 weeks is not recommended.[48] Once the hematocrit reaches a level of 35%, the dose of prednisone can be tapered very slowly and the drug can be eventually discontinued, preferably after 3 to 4 months. Rapid tapering of prednisone may lead to recurrence of anemia. As with cyclosporine, a number of responders may be prednisone dependent, requiring small doses of the drug to maintain a normal hematocrit.[48] For patients who do not respond to prednisone within 2 to

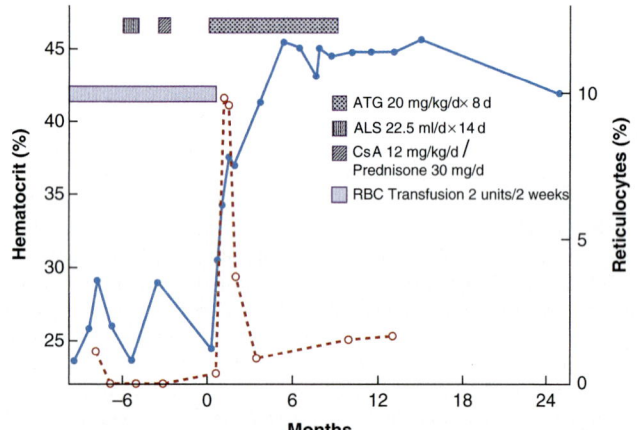

FIGURE 40.2 **Time course of response of patient 9 to cyclosporine A (CsA).** Hematocrit (closed circles) and uncorrected reticulocyte count (open circles) are shown. Treatments administered in the 8 months prior to CsA (equine antithymocyte globulin [ATG] and rabbit antilymphocyte serum [ALS]), and the duration of CsA therapy, are indicated in the figure. Prior to beginning CsA (time 0), the patient had required biweekly transfusion to maintain his hematocrit at the levels indicated. No transfusions have been required subsequently. RBC, red blood cell. (From Means RT Jr, Dessypris EN, Krantz SB. Treatment of refractory pure red cell aplasia with cyclosporine A: disappearance of IgG inhibitor associated with clinical response. Br J Haematol. 1991;78(1):114-119. Copyright © 1991 British Society for Haematology. Reprinted by permission of John Wiley & Sons, Inc.)

Table 40.3. Response of PRCA to Various Immunosuppressive Therapies

Study	Dessypris[5]	Lacy et al[41]	Charles et al[6]	Sawada et al[47]	Total
Number of patients	49	47	37	62	195
Primary PRCA	32	25	18	62	137
Secondary PRCA	17	22	19	0	58
Cyclosporine	3/4	4/5	2/3	28/36	37/48 (77%)
Corticosteroids	18/41[a]	9/29	9/36	14/22	50/128 (39%)
Cytotoxic agents[b]	24/54	14/29	8/27	0/3	46/113 (41%)
Antithymocyte γ-globulin	2/6	0/1	8/12	—	10/19 (53%)
Intravenous immunoglobulin G	—	1/2	2/8	—	3/10 (30%)
Plasmapheresis	—	—	0/2	—	0/2 (0%)
Splenectomy	4/23	0/1	0/1	—	4/25 (16%)
Multiple treatments	35/49	28/47	28/37	—	91/133 (68%)

Abbreviation: PRCA, pure red cell aplasia.
Many patients did not respond to treatment or had relapses, so one patient may be included in more than one treatment modality.
[a]Number of responders/number of patients treated.
[b]Including cyclophosphamide, azathioprine, or methotrexate, each given either alone or in combination with prednisone.

3 months, the dose should be rapidly tapered to approximately 20 to 30 mg daily and the use of a different agent considered.

Cytotoxic Agents

In patients not responding to cyclosporine, prednisone, or both, cyclophosphamide or azathioprine can be given alone, or with small doses of prednisone, which seems to increase the effectiveness of treatment. The overall response rate to cytotoxic agent–based therapy is approximately 40% (*Table 40.3*). The initial dose of either agent is 50 mg orally daily. If the white blood cell and platelet counts allow it, it is increased by 50 mg weekly or biweekly to a maximum of 150 mg daily until remission occurs or bone marrow suppression develops. The mean time to response is about 11 to 12 weeks, with a broad range of 2 to 26 weeks.[5,6,41,48]

If response occurs, prednisone is tapered, and then the dose of cytotoxic agent is progressively decreased and eventually discontinued. If bone marrow toxicity develops, the drug is discontinued, and the marrow is allowed to recover. If, after 3 months of treatment, no response and no marrow toxicity are seen, the dose can be increased progressively (by 50 mg biweekly) to a maximum tolerable dose or 250 mg daily under close monitoring of the blood counts. If reticulocytosis or stabilization of the hematocrit is noticed, the dose is gradually reduced. If the absolute neutrophil count decreases to <1000/μL or the platelet count drops to <100,000/μL, the cytotoxic drug is discontinued. In many patients, with the return of granulocytes and platelets to normal a reticulocytosis is seen, followed by a return of erythropoiesis to normal. If no response occurs, another type of immunosuppressive treatment should be initiated.

Sirolimus

Sirolimus, which is the assigned generic name for the natural product rapamycin, is an immunosuppressive agent most commonly used in the prevention of graft rejection after transplantation. A number of recent small series and case reports have described sirolimus as a highly effective agent in refractory PRCA.[49,50] The limited number of case series reported suggest a response rate at least comparable with cyclosporine, possibly better (*Table 40.3*). In one series, 91.3% of patients had a complete or partial initial response, with 75% of responses persisting at 1 year.[49] The sirolimus dose used for PRCA is most commonly 2 mg/d, although use of 1 mg/d and 3 mg/d have also been reported.[49,50] Median time to onset of response is typically 3 to 4 months, and about half of patients experience adverse events during treatment. As experience with this agent in PRCA treatment increases, its precise role in PRCA treatment will become clearer. It is certainly reasonable to consider it in patients refractory to cyclosporine or who have failed a second line of treatment. The related immunosuppressant tacrolimus has been shown to be effective in refractory PRCA, but the experience is smaller.[51] Tacrolimus has also been implicated as a potential cause of PRCA (*Table 40.2*).

Other Immunosuppressive/Immunomodulatory Modalities

It is reasonable to expect that many, if not most, immunosuppressive or immunomodulatory agents may have some activity in specific cases of PRCA. Rituximab, a humanized monoclonal antibody against CD20, has been reported to be effective in PRCA whether primary/autoimmune or associated with lymphoproliferative disorders.[52] It has also been used effectively in PRCA following ABO-incompatible stem cell transplantation.[53] Other agents that have been reported to be effective include daratumumab,[54] daclizumab,[55] bortezomib,[56] or alemtuzumab.[57] Donor lymphocyte infusion has been reported to be effective in PRCA following ABO-incompatible stem cell transplantation.[58]

There are a number of immunomodulatory modalities used primarily in patients with PRCA who are refractory to other approaches. High-dose intravenous γ-globulin is primarily used for the treatment of parvovirus-induced PRCA. It has also been shown to be effective in patients with immune-mediated PRCA, whether primary or secondary.[59] Plasmapheresis may be considered in patients who have failed other immunosuppressive approaches.[60] Antithymocyte globulin

(ATG), formerly the routine therapy after corticosteroids and cytotoxic agents, is now used uncommonly in refractory patients.[48] The overall response rate to ATG is approximately 50% (*Table 40.3*). ATG is given on the same treatment schedule that is used for aplastic anemia. The European Society for Blood and Marrow Transplantation has reviewed 33 patients who underwent allogenic stem cell transplantation for acquired PRCA. While transplantation was potentially curative, overall survival at 1 year was only 55%, with a high frequency of graft failure and infectious complications.[61]

Splenectomy has also been used as a final therapeutic maneuver in patients who are refractory to all other forms of treatment. Responses to splenectomy have been reported in ~17% of such recalcitrant-to-treatment cases within the first 2 to 3 postoperative months.[5] After splenectomy, patients may become responsive to agents against which they were previously resistant.

Parvovirus-Associated Pure Red Cell Aplasia

As was discussed earlier, in immunocompetent individuals, B19 parvovirus infection produces transient and self-limited erythroid suppression that is generally unnoticed except in patients with chronic hemolytic disorders. In immunocompromised patients, parvovirus infection can lead to chronic PRCA. Patients with PRCA and documented parvovirus infection (demonstrated by PCR on peripheral blood) should be treated with high-dose intravenous γ-globulin 400 mg/kg/d for 5 days, which confers passive immunity.[14] More than 90% of immunocompromised patients will respond to treatment, but approximately a third of these will relapse and require retreatment. The reported mean time to relapse is 16 to 18 weeks.[62] In patients with HIV, relapses of parvovirus-induced PRCA are rare in patients with CD4 lymphocyte count greater than 300/μL.[63]

Thymoma-Associated Pure Red Cell Aplasia

In the presence of a thymoma, thymectomy should be performed. While 30% to 40% of patients with thymoma and PRCA will have recovery of erythropoiesis, this recovery is typically incomplete and immunosuppression is typically required.[64,65] Thymectomy in the absence of thymoma is not recommended. Responses to octreotide and tacrolimus have been reported in thymoma-associated PRCA.[51,66]

Anti-Epo Antibody–Associated Pure Red Cell Aplasia

As noted earlier, many cases of anti-Epo antibody–mediated PRCA induced by rhEpo therapy in patients with renal failure have been reported. Such patients should be managed with immunosuppression, like other patients with immune-mediated PRCA.[67] The overall response rate to immunosuppression has been reported to be 78%, with cyclosporine being the most effective agent and steroids the least effective.[68] Patients who undergo renal transplantation may have remission of PRCA.[69] There are case reports of eventual recovery with no therapy apart from cessation of rhEpo therapy and transfusion support.[70]

The issue of whether or not a patient who has experienced anti-Epo antibody–induced PRCA can ever be retreated with rhEpo or a different rhEpo product remains controversial. The reported antibodies appear to cross-react with all available rhEpo agents.[71] Although there are several case reports of successful rechallenge with epoetin or darbepoetin (in some cases changing to intravenous administration rather than subcutaneous administration), and even of recovery while continuing rhEpo therapy, the practice is not recommended.[72,73]

Refractory Pure Red Cell Aplasia

For patients who respond and relapse, retreatment is often effective.[74] Despite the variety of therapeutic modalities available, there will be some patients with PRCA who do not respond to therapy. These individuals will require transfusion support, with chelation management to minimize complications of iron overload.

Survival After Immunosuppressive Therapy

In the series reported by the Japanese PRCA Consortium, patients with primary autoimmune PRCA had median survival greater than

Disorders of Red Blood Cells

250 months, whereas patients with thymoma and LGL-associated PRCA had median survivals of 148 and 142 months, respectively. Relapse and refractoriness to therapy were predictors of death.[22] Patients with myelodysplastic PRCA have shorter survival, compatible with their underlying disease. The 3% to 5% of patients with PRCA who develop acute myeloid leukemia (AML) typically come from this latter category.[74] Development of subsequent aplastic anemia in patients with PRCA has been reported but is rare.[75]

DIAMOND-BLACKFAN ANEMIA

Background

DBA was originally described by Josephs in 1936[76] and further characterized by Diamond and Blackfan in 1938[77] as congenital hypoplastic anemia. In addition to presenting hypoplastic anemia, the disorder classically presents in children under 1 year of age and is characterized by macrocytosis, reticulocytopenia, and a selective decrease or absence of erythroid precursors in an otherwise normocellular bone marrow. Fetal-like erythropoiesis, fetal membrane antigen "i," and increased fetal hemoglobin (HbF) are often present. A useful, but not well understood, finding is the presence of elevated erythrocyte adenosine deaminase (eADA) activity. In addition, half of patients with DBA also present with physical abnormalities including short stature, thumb abnormalities (classically a triphalangeal thumb as seen in *Figure 40.3*), craniofacial defects, and cleft lip/palate (*Table 40.4*).[78]

DBA was the first disease to be linked to impaired ribosome biogenesis/function and is the founding member of a group of disorders now known as ribosomopathies.[79] Several other inherited bone marrow failure syndromes including Shwachman Diamond syndrome and dyskeratosis congenita have subsequently been linked to mutations in genes encoding proteins required for normal ribosome biogenesis and/or function (Chapter 39). In addition, recent evidence confirms DBA as a cancer predisposition syndrome of moderate penetrance.[80,81] The most common DBA-associated malignancies are colorectal cancer and osteogenic sarcoma. Skin cancer and acute myeloid leukemia follow in incidence. There is also a markedly increased incidence of MDS.[82] More cases of breast cancer are being reported.[83]

Of note, acquired mutations in genes encoding ribosomal proteins have been identified in several cancers, most commonly breast cancer (*RP* gene mutations in 30%-40% of cases), melanoma and multiple myeloma (20%-30% in each), endometrial, uterine cancer, glioblastoma multiforme, and relapsed CLL (10%-20% in each) and less commonly in colorectal and gastric cancer as well as T-cell lymphoblastic leukemia (T-ALL; 10% in each). The mutated *RP* genes are *RPL5* (breast cancer, melanoma, multiple myeloma, and glioblastoma multiforme), *RPL22* (endometrial, colorectal, and gastric cancer and T-ALL), *RPL23A* (uterine cancer), *RPS15* (relapsed CLL), and *RPL10* (T-ALL).[84]

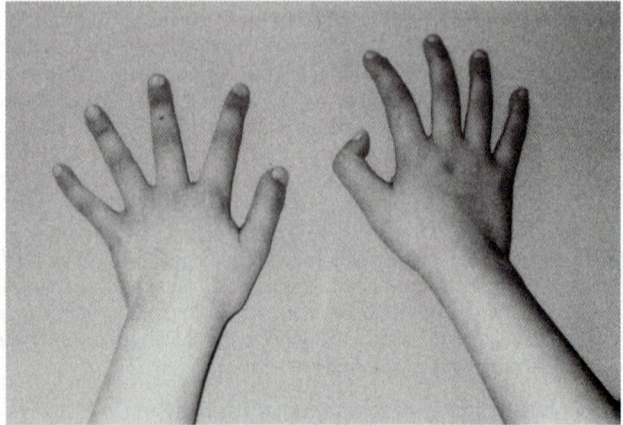

FIGURE 40.3 Typical displaced and "trigger" thumbs in a patient with Diamond-Blackfan anemia. (Image courtesy of A. Narla.)

Clinical Presentation

DBA typically presents in infancy, most commonly with pallor and lethargy, with an estimated incidence of 5 to 10 cases per million live births. There is often a family history of the disease.[78] The Diamond Blackfan Anemia Registry of North America (DBAR), a database of >800 patients, was established in 1991 and provides important information regarding the epidemiology and biology of DBA. DBA is heritable as an autosomal dominant condition with a large proportion of cases being new dominant mutations. The male to female ratio of cases is approximately 1:1 with only very rare cases of X-linked inheritance. The median age at presentation is 8 weeks, with a median age at diagnosis of 12 weeks. More than 90% of the reported cases present **clinically** by 1 year of age. Older patients with no, or only a subtle, phenotype are diagnosed well into adulthood, often as consequence of a family study.

Physical anomalies, not including short stature, are found in nearly 50% of patients (*Table 40.4*). Short stature is clearly a constitutional feature of DBA, but it may also be caused by chronic anemia, iron overload, corticosteroid administration, or a combination of all these. The constellation of physical anomalies includes a high percentage of craniofacial anomalies (50% of patients) as well as anomalies of upper limb and hand, in particular the thumb (38%), as well as genitourinary (39%) and cardiac (30%) abnormalities.

Genetics

Prior to the identification of causative mutations, Alter at al. estimated that there is more than one affected family member in ~10% of cases.[85,86] Early data from the DBAR provided a comparable or higher rate when robust clinical examination, imaging, hematologic, and genetic data were available. Early case reports are worth mentioning as they are representative of the now known genetics of DBA. In these families, there were reports of affected same- and opposite-sex siblings, including identical twins, and maternal or paternal half-siblings. There

Table 40.4. Physical Abnormalities in Patients With Diamond-Blackfan Anemia

General
Low birth weight
Short stature
Head and Neck
Micro- or macrocephaly
Cleft palate and/or lip
Macroglossia
Flat nasal bridge
Abnormal ears
Short, webbed neck
Eyes
Hypertelorism
Epicanthal folds
Ptosis
Strabismus
Congenital cataracts
Glaucoma
Thumb
Triphalangeal
Duplicated or bifid
Subluxed or hypoplastic
Renal
Cardiac

were also instances of parental transmission. Striking evidence of autosomal dominant inheritance is illustrated in one case report of DBA in a male infant who had an affected mother and maternal grandfather.[86]

With the identification of the first DBA gene, *RPS19*, a gene that encodes an RP located at chromosome 19q13.2,[87] and a second gene coding for *RPS24*,[88] it became obvious that other RP genes would be implicated in the fundamental molecular pathogenesis of DBA. Based on the original technique used to describe *RPS19* (cloning of a cytogenetic abnormality from an informative patient), linkage analysis, resequencing of the known ribosome-associated protein genes, or, most recently, a variety of techniques for the detection of copy number variants in the genome as well as whole exome sequencing, many additional *RP* gene mutations/deletions have been identified, accounting for approximately 80% of all cases of DBA. The addition of whole genome sequencing to the armamentarium will unquestionably increase the identification of RP-associated causes of DBA.[89]

Currently, there are over 20 genes encoding RP mutated in DBA.[84,90] DBA results from RP haploinsufficiency with mutations studied so far largely resulting from either complete loss of function or nonexpression of the mutated allele. When a specific gene (*RPS19* most commonly) is knocked down in cellular models, there is resulting failure of erythropoiesis. Furthermore, a number of murine and zebrafish models have been developed confirming the role of RP haploinsufficiency in erythroid failure.[90] In these in vitro models, the erythroid defect can also be corrected when the normal gene is overexpressed.

In addition, mutations in the gene encoding the transcription factor *GATA1* and the *RPS26* chaperone *TSR2*,[91] both with X-linked inheritance, have been described. Owing to the functional relationship of these gene products with ribosomal proteins, the diagnosis of DBA is restricted to disorders resulting mainly from RP haploinsufficiency and rarely mutations of GATA1 and TSR2. *HSP70*, the chaperone of GATA1, and *CERC1*, which encodes the growth factor adenosine deaminase 2 (ADA2) and an erythropoietin mutation, have been identified and are being studied as their phenotypes may mimic DBA. They should be considered in the differential diagnosis of DBA.

Despite our increased understanding of the genetics of DBA, the mechanism of erythroid failure and the other clinical manifestations are only partially explained. Much work needs to be done to connect faulty ribosome biogenesis and function with red cell failure, specific congenital anomalies and cancer predisposition.[92] The disease is also known to have incomplete penetrance, as demonstrated both by the observation of family members who carry the same mutation who are discordant with the proband for the presence of anemia and congenital anomalies as well as by the occurrence of spontaneous remissions and differences in response to treatment in some affected family members. This suggests a role for modifying genes that also need to be explored further.[93]

Pathogenesis

A number of theories have been proposed to account for the pathophysiology of DBA. The fundamental lesion appears to be a faulty translational apparatus created by RP haploinsufficiency leading to nucleolar stress signaling activating downstream cell cycle inhibition and apoptotic pathways. This results from a complex of *RPL5*, *RPL11*, and *5S* rRNA binding to *MDM2* and its human ortholog *HDM2*, leading to a decrease in its ubiquitin ligase activity essential for *p53* degradation, thereby stabilizing *p53*, resulting in accelerated apoptosis.[94] The regulatory pathway utilizing *RPL5* and *RPL11* to bind to *HDM2* seems central to this stress signaling, so much so that even when small ribosome-associated proteins are deficient, offering no excess of *RPL5* and *RPL11*, as is the case for large subunit-associated haploinsufficiency resulting in degraded large subunits, the *RPL5* and *RPL11* TOP (terminal oligopyrimidine tract) messenger RNAs (mRNAs) appear to be translationally upregulated.[95]

The fact that both *RPL5* and *RPL11* are DBA genes and that they represent a more severe congenital anomaly phenotype tells us that there is much more to be learned about how *HDM2* is regulated when their encoding genes are haploinsufficient as well as extraribosomal roles for these proteins. Furthermore, the tissue specificity of defects

manifested by a germ line mutation in a ribosome-associated protein, as opposed to a relatively more erythroid-restricted transcription regulator such as *GATA1*, requires an explanation.

There are several other potential complementary or alternate hypotheses. One is that the synthesis of hemoglobin and metabolic proteins in the erythron results in an extraordinarily high translational requirement that cannot be met by a limited number of ribosomes. Another hypothesis is that the translation of certain canonical proteins is favored over others and that those proteins may be overrepresented in the erythron. Another possibility is that the makeup of ribosomes is tissue specific (i.e., not all 80 RPs are required in every tissue), favoring translation in some tissues and not others as a consequence of any particular RP haploinsufficiency.[96] Another potentially provocative explanation is that delayed globin synthesis caused by faulty translation in DBA leads to the accumulation of unbound heme, toxic to the developing erythron.[97]

There are likely multiple explanations related to the complexity of tissue-specific translation and to the pathogenesis of DBA overall. In particular, upregulating translation with the branched-chain amino acid L-leucine through the mTOR pathway and targeting the knockdown of p53, albeit potentially risky in a cancer predisposition syndrome, have each been successful in ameliorating the DBA phenotype in DBA models[98,99] suggesting scientifically rational clinical trials utilizing each approach. Of note, a clinical trial with L-leucine in transfusion-dependent patients with DBA elicited an erythropoietic response in 7 of 43 patients[100] and a trial modulating p53 with the calmodulin inhibitor trifluoperazine is underway (https://clinicaltrials.gov/ct2/show/NCT03966053) as well as a trial with the thrombopoietin-mimetic Eltrombopag (https://clinicaltrials.gov/ct2/show/NCT04269889). Elucidating all the downstream events leading to accelerated cell death and understanding the interdicting mutations that lead to cancer in DBA are important subjects of inquiry.

Laboratory Evaluation

Classic DBA is characterized by severe anemia, with hemoglobin levels at presentation as low as 2 to 3 g/dL. There is a marked reticulocytopenia and usually no significant abnormalities in other cell lines. Occasionally, there is mild to moderate neutropenia, particularly in patients with *RPL35a* mutations, and infrequently severe neutropenia requiring G-CSF support or thrombocytopenia. However, a normal platelet count or even thrombocytosis in the range of 400,000 to 700,000 is more common. Although originally described as a normochromic, normocytic anemia, macrocytosis was noted at presentation in ~30% of cases reviewed by Alter et al in patients for whom data were available.[85] Indeed, the persistence of "fetal-like" red cells, with macrocytosis, "i" antigen, increased fetal hemoglobin (HbF), and red cell glycolytic and hexose-monophosphate (HMP) shunt enzyme activities characteristic of fetal cells is a consistent finding, although the etiology of the macrocytosis is still not completely understood.

Although glycolytic and HMP shunt enzymes have a fetal pattern, eADA, a purine salvage pathway enzyme, is increased in activity in patients with DBA but not in normal fetal or cord blood erythrocytes. When compared with controls with normal eADA activity obtained from patients with hemolytic anemia, Fanconi anemia, and those with steroid-dependent nephrosis, as well as virtually all patients with TEC, approximately 85% of the patients with typical DBA have elevated eADA activity, which makes it a useful tool to distinguish DBA from TEC.[101] (See *Table 40.4*.) In some patients with DBA with normal eADA activity, there is markedly elevated orotidine decarboxylase activity. Although abnormalities in purine or pyrimidine biosynthesis are consistent findings in most patients with DBA and in some animal models, and serve as a valuable screening tool, this observation has not yet been helpful in understanding the pathophysiology of DBA.

Vitamin B_{12}, folate, serum iron, ferritin, and transferrin saturation can be elevated or normal in patients with DBA and should be part of the initial evaluation of patients. Examination of the bone marrow biopsy and aspirate at diagnosis in childhood usually reveals normal cellularity with a paucity of erythroid precursors. Myeloid and megakaryocyte lineages usually appear normal. Myeloid to erythroid (M:E)

Disorders of Red Blood Cells

ratios at diagnosis are usually around 10:1 and with time may become as high as 100:1. This progression of erythroid failure (with time) seems to parallel the more severe abnormalities in in vitro progenitor differentiation and decreased bone marrow cellularity observed in older chronically affected patients as compared with those newly diagnosed.[102]

Although all patients have a profound reticulocytopenia, the erythroid arrest in DBA has been demonstrated by progenitor assays to occur at all stages of maturation from the multipotent myeloid progenitor to the late normoblast. These and other observations suggest that the defect may become more profound with age and that the arrest in erythropoiesis moves to an earlier stage of differentiation as patients get older. This is, however, somewhat confounding in light of the presence of remissions.

Imaging studies are useful to help delineate congenital abnormalities that may be present in patients with DBA. Skeletal surveys and, in particular, computed tomography scans are not usually warranted in light of the increased risk of cancer in DBA, but selected radiographs may define suspected bony anomalies. Renal and cardiac ultrasonography is warranted and may detect clinically unsuspected and perhaps significant anomalies.

Given our increasing understanding of the genetics of the disease, for patients with a suspicion for DBA, we recommend genetic testing. Furthermore, genetic testing of family members is essential to detect occult disease and to avoid hematopoietic stem cell transplants using a DBA-affected hematopoietic stem cell donor (see Treatment below). With the discovery of genetic mutations, there are many patients who have been identified with no or only subtle hematologic manifestations.

Differential Diagnosis

The differential diagnosis of classical DBA includes the normochromic, normocytic (or macrocytic) anemias that present from birth through the first year of life. These anemias are pathophysiologically distinct from the majority of causes of PRCA seen in adults that are frequently associated with an underlying disorder (*Table 40.1*). However, it is clear that DBA can present in adulthood, and these cases are often undiagnosed. Conversely, a patient presenting with red cell failure at age 5 years and diagnosed with atypical DBA was confirmed to have 5q⁻ MDS some 20 years later.[103] And the association of PRCA with thymoma, as described in adults, has not been described in infancy, although it has been observed in a 5-year-old girl.[104] Thus, an index of suspicion for DBA should be maintained with regard to all cases of PRCA presenting at any age. In contrast, rare genetic disorders with variable clinical phenotypes may mimic DBA. For instance, the autosomal recessive disorders ADA2 deficiency, which is most commonly associated with vasculitis,[105] and a mutation affecting the binding kinetics of erythropoietin[106] may each present with pure red cell aplasia mimicking DBA.

In classical cases, the differential almost always consists of DBA versus TEC (*Table 40.5*). Of note, patients with Pearson syndrome, resulting from large deletions of the mitochondrial genome, may present with pure red cell failure. Clinical suspicion or the presence of vacuolated erythroid precursors in the marrow should prompt a stain for ringed sideroblasts and the evaluation for a mitochondrial DNA deletion. A careful history, physical examination, and examination of the peripheral blood smear can usually rule out hemorrhage, myelosuppression resulting from infection, renal failure, infiltrative disease, severe protein malnutrition, or drug-related red cell failure, as well as the aplastic crisis of a chronic hemolytic anemia (such as sickle cell anemia or hereditary spherocytosis).

Because folate deficiency as a cause of the hypoplastic crises associated with chronic hemolytic anemia is prevented by prophylactic administration of the vitamin, acquired hypoplastic anemia in these patients is now most frequently a consequence of human parvovirus B19 infection. Evidence of human parvovirus B19 infection (see Parvovirus-Induced Pure Red Cell Aplasia) has been found in patients with all congenital hemolytic disorders. Thus, parvovirus infection should be ruled out in all atypical instances of red cell failure in children. This can be best accomplished by PCR analysis, as IgM and IgG

Table 40.5. Differential Diagnosis of DBA versus TEC

	DBA	TEC
Pure red cell aplasia	Present	Present
Age	<1 y	>1 y
Inheritance	Mutation analysis available for known DBA genes	Not inherited
Congenital anomalies	Present	Absent
Mean corpuscular volume	Elevated	Normal
Fetal hemoglobin	Elevated	Normal
i RBC antigen	Present	Absent
Erythrocyte ADA activity	Elevated	Normal

Abbreviations: ADA, adenosine deaminase; DBA, Diamond-Blackfan anemia; RBC, red blood cell; TEC, transient erythroblastopenia of childhood.
All RBC characteristics except ADA activity are helpful only when tested in a reticulocytopenic child. During recovery from TEC, a transient wave of fetal-like erythropoiesis may be detected.

antibody evidence will be lacking in the presence of significant immunodeficiency. Giant pronormoblasts are characteristic.

A bone marrow examination revealing red cell aplasia or severe hypoplasia with no abnormalities in myeloid or megakaryocyte lineages, as well as no evidence of infiltrative disease, congenital dyserythropoietic anemia, vacuolated precursors, giant pronormoblasts, or ringed sideroblasts in an infant or young child, suggests either DBA or TEC. *Table 40.5* outlines the important features that distinguish TEC, a temporary immune-mediated suppression of erythropoiesis that frequently follows a viral infection, from DBA. In all instances a genetic diagnosis is desirable to identify nonpenetrant affected family members and to rule out rare genetic disorders that mimic DBA.

Treatment

The current standard of care for DBA includes corticosteroids or chronic red blood cell transfusions, with the only definitive treatment for the hematologic manifestation of DBA being stem cell transplantation. Approximately 80% of patients respond initially to corticosteroids with an improvement in, or complete remission of, their anemia.[107] However, prolonged corticosteroid treatment has been problematic for many patients such that only about 40% of patients will achieve a tolerable and effective dose of corticosteroids allowing treatment for an appreciable time. With existing treatments, the overall survival of patients, as reported by the Diamond Blackfan Anemia Registry, is 75.1% at 40 years of age; median overall survival is 58 years.[107] As understanding of the pathophysiology of the ribosomopathies increases, the goal will be to be able to translate these findings into novel therapeutic options for patients with DBA.

If the diagnosis of DBA vs TEC is in doubt and the child has symptomatic anemia, the patient should be carefully transfused to a hemoglobin level of 7 to 8 g/dL so that erythropoiesis will not be suppressed, delaying recovery in those patients who have TEC. The use of corticosteroids in TEC is ineffective and should be avoided. In 1951, corticosteroid treatment in the form of adrenocorticotropic hormone was first shown to be effective in DBA.[108] However, the transfusion of packed RBCs is often the initial treatment. Owing to the significant adverse effects of corticosteroids administered to infants and young children transfusions should continue until the patient is older than 1 year if possible. The ability to defer corticosteroid treatment is dependent on the availability of a safe blood supply and the ability to maintain appropriate venous access.

The current approach is to start patients on prednisone, 2 mg/kg/d orally with a maximum dose of 100 mg in two or three divided doses. By delaying the start of corticosteroids, it is anticipated that many of the significant side effects associated with early steroid administration (growth retardation, developmental delay, osteopenia, hyperglycemia, hypertension, etc.) can be avoided.[109] A reticulocyte response usually occurs within 1 to 2 weeks.[110] After an acceptable hemoglobin is reached, a taper to a dose that does not lead to toxicity while maintaining an acceptable hemoglobin is instituted. If there is no response from the initial dose by 4 weeks, corticosteroids should be discontinued. Escalation beyond a dose of 2 mg/kg/d or a duration of 4 weeks, even when there is an erythropoietic response, will not lead to a durable response and an ultimate steroid taper to an acceptable and effective dose. The clinical response to prednisone therapy is variable. Data from the DBAR reveal that 79% of patients were initially responsive to corticosteroids, 17% were nonresponsive, and 4% were never treated with steroids. At the time of the analysis, only 37% of patients were using corticosteroids.[109]

Steroid-related side effects were observed in most patients, at least transiently, with 48%, 22%, and 12% manifesting cushingoid features, pathologic fractures, and cataracts, respectively. Thirty-one percent of the patients were receiving red cell transfusions. Some patients responded rapidly and could be tapered off prednisone, remaining in remission for extended periods of time; others responded but required continued therapy, with erythropoiesis ceasing rapidly if steroids were discontinued. Thus, the ability of responders to achieve an effective every-other-day dose schedule is variable. Of the transfused patients enrolled in the DBAR, 35% were never steroid responsive, 22% became steroid refractory, 33% could not be weaned to an acceptable dose, and 5% were never on steroids. A few were transfused for unspecified reasons.

Some patients may be tapered off steroids even after many years. Indeed, as of the last analysis, the actuarial likelihood of remission is 20% by age 25 years, with 72% entering remission during the first decade of life. Patients appear to remit equally from steroid and transfusion therapy. Almost 75% of these patients have what appears to be a sustained remission. Although high-dose corticosteroid pulses may evoke an erythroid response in some patients, the potential side effects and the need for repeat pulses and the failure of this modality in subsequent studies have limited its utility.

Trials of cyclosporine (CsA), erythropoietin, interleukin-3, metoclopramide, and other agents, despite anecdotal reports of success in patients with DBA, have not been particularly encouraging.[109] The potential toxicity of these agents makes them less preferable to red cell transfusions for those patients who cannot be weaned to an acceptable corticosteroid dose. Anecdotal reports suggest the effectiveness of androgen therapy. However, experienced clinicians do not advocate the use of androgens in DBA because of their limited effectiveness and considerable side effects. If there is no response within a month, prednisone is discontinued in favor of transfusion and iron chelation. These patients may receive periodic trials of prednisone in the hopes that they may respond at a later date.

In patients for whom there is a response to prednisone, the hemoglobin is followed until a level of 10 g/dL is achieved. The steroid dose is then tapered until the patient is on the smallest possible alternate-day dose. A Monday-Wednesday-Friday dose schedule is usually effective and easier to comply with than a strict every-other-day regimen. The dosage in a Monday-Wednesday-Friday schedule may range from a few milligrams even in adolescents to as much as 40 to 50 mg. The target dose is 0.5 mg/kg/d or 1 mg/kg every other day. Arbitrary discontinuation of therapy should be discouraged, because reestablishment of erythropoiesis after discontinuation of an effective every-other-day course of prednisone will likely require reinstitution of the original daily dose.

For patients who are steroid refractory or for whom the dose cannot be tapered to an alternate-day regimen and thus require high daily doses that cause toxicity, chronic transfusion is instituted. Data from the DBAR and accumulated international experience demonstrate that more patients than originally anticipated have significant steroid-related side effects even on a low-dose, every-other-day schedule. These include pathologic fractures and cataracts as well as poor growth, osteoporosis, and osteonecrosis, which may require the discontinuation of corticosteroids in favor of chronic transfusion therapy. Patients must be carefully monitored and steroid therapy should be

discontinued when significant side effects ensue, even if the dose is within the "accepted" range.

In recent years, hematopoietic stem-cell transplantation (HSCT) has been used in DBA patients with good results. The first successful transplant for DBA was performed by August and colleagues in 1976.[111] In a 1998 review of stem cell transplantation in DBA by Alter et al that analyzed 35 of the 37 cases reported to that date in the literature, the actuarial survival for predominantly allogeneic HLA-matched donor transplants was 66%.[112] Two more recent studies suggest that the actuarial survival is in the range of 90% for matched related HSCT in young, otherwise healthy patients. The most recent analysis from the DBAR reports an overall HLA-matched related-donor transplant survival of 76.9% ± 8.4 %, with a 93.8% ± 6.1% survival for patients equal to or less than 9 years of age. For unrelated donor transplants, the overall survival has improved from 32.1% ± 11.7% (1994-1999) to 85.7% ± 13.2% (2000-present).[113,114] The historical substantial risks associated with alternative-donor bone marrow transplantation favor transfusion and chelation in those patients unable to achieve an every-other-day steroid schedule; however, the hesitancy to use unrelated donors is changing, as evidenced by dramatically better results from patients transplanted since 2000, likely as the result of more precise high-resolution HLA typing, an expanded donor pool, and better pretransplant management of iron overload.

Modern chelation regimens seem to be very effective in reducing the consequences of iron overload in chronically transfused patients, but the long-term results of these programs are currently not known. The recent availability of oral chelating agents promises to improve compliance with better-tolerated chelation regimens than the traditional nightly continuous subcutaneous infusions. This uncertainty and the other risks of transfusion (i.e. sensitization and infection) make the decision regarding bone marrow transplantation (when a suitable alternative donor exists) versus chelation therapy for patients with DBA who are steroid refractory or steroid intolerant one that must be individualized and constantly reevaluated. In particular, poor compliance with chelation regimens has resulted in significant morbidity and mortality in young adult patients with transfusion-dependent DBA. Two articles[107,109] provide a detailed approach to the treatment of DBA including iron chelation approaches. There are also several open clinical trials (details available at https://clinicaltrials.gov) for patients with DBA and more in development including gene therapy.

Prognosis

The DBAR describes an overall actuarial survival rate at ~40 years of age as 75.1% ± 4.8%, with 86.7% ± 7.0% for corticosteroid-maintainable patients and 57.2% ± 8.9% for transfusion-dependent patients. There is a statistically significant survival advantage for steroid-maintainable versus transfusion-dependent patients. However, despite modern chelation schemes, transfusion-related hemosiderosis remains a leading cause of death in patients with DBA.

For several years, it has been recognized that DBA is a syndrome predisposing to cancer, both hematopoietic and nonhematopoietic malignancies. A recent analysis from 2016 of the prospective cohort of 702 patients enrolled in the DBAR since 1991 was performed to provide an updated quantitative assessment of cancer incidence in patients with DBA. Among the 702 patients, there were 12,376 person-years of follow-up. There were 39 cancers; 5 in post–hematopoietic stem cell transplant patients. The median age at the first cancer diagnosis was 35 years. AML was observed in 3 and solid tumors in 26 non-HSCT patients. The cancer incidence in DBA is significantly elevated, with an observed-to-expected (O/E) ratio of 4.8 for all cancers and 352 for MDS, 29 for AML, 45 for colon cancer, 43 for osteogenic sarcoma, and 7.1 for cervical and 172 for vaginal squamous cell cancers, respectively.[80,81]

In 2021, an update revealed 51 patients with 60 cancers, 8 post-HSCT, from a cohort of 813 patients. In particular, the high incidence of colorectal cancer in patients with DBA has resulted in a preliminary screening and surveillance strategy for patients 20 years and older.[82] Clearly, in addition to understanding the mechanism of cancer predisposition in DBA, surveillance strategies for other cancers must be carefully considered for this at-risk population. Indeed, although transplant-related mortality appears to be declining, there is a recognition that death from DBA-associated cancers is rising as the DBAR matures.

Future Directions

Advances in cellular and molecular biology have dramatically increased our understanding of the pathophysiology of DBA. In the majority of cases, DBA has been shown to be caused by abnormal ribosome assembly and function. Greater than 20 *RP* genes as well as the transcription regulator GATA1 and the RP 26 chaperone TSR2 have been implicated. Careful clinical investigation has helped to define the syndrome and the study of the cellular biology of the disorder has borrowed from and contributed to the understanding of the mechanism of hematopoietic progenitor cell differentiation. Using the DBAR and other international databases, important epidemiologic, clinical, and laboratory observations have been made with regard to the clinical presentation and inheritance of DBA. These databases have yielded other important observations on the genetics of the congenital malformations in DBA, the therapeutic outcomes including the efficacy of HSCT, and the recognition of DBA as a cancer-predisposition syndrome. In particular, the patients, families, and registries have provided the essential substrate necessary for gene discovery and future therapies.

ACKNOWLEDGMENTS

Dr Louis Diamond, who over a career spanning more than 60 years, had been a teacher to many and an inspiration to the rest, would be pleased to know that his description of an esoteric and rare disease has led to extraordinary insights into the regulation of hematopoiesis and the mechanisms of oncogenesis.

The authors would also like to acknowledge the contributions of Dr. Emmanuel Dessypris and Dr. Bertil Glader, whose excellent work on previous editions of this chapter continues to serve as the template for the subsequent versions.

References

1. Means RT. Pure red cell aplasia. *Blood*. 2016;128(21):2504. doi: 10.1182/blood-2016-05-717140
2. Zalusky R, Zanjani ED, Gidari AS, Ross J. Site of action of a serum inhibitor of erythropoiesis. *J Lab Clin Med*. 1973;81(6):867-875.
3. Krantz SB, Kao V. Studies on red cell aplasia. I. Demonstration of a plasma inhibitor to heme synthesis and an antibody to erythroblast nuclei. *Proc Natl Acad Sci U S A*. 1967;58(2):493-500.
4. Means RT, Dessypris EN, Krantz SB. Treatment of refractory pure red cell aplasia with cyclosporine A: in vitro correlation of clinical response. *Br J Haematol*. 1991;78:114-119.
5. Dessypris EN. *Pure Red Cell Aplasia*. Johns Hopkins University Press; 1988:1-156.
6. Charles RJ, Sabo KM, Kidd PG, Abkowitz JL. The pathophysiology of pure red cell aplasia: implications for therapy. *Blood*. 1996;87(11):4831-4838.
7. Zaentz SD, Luna JA, Baker AS, Krantz SB. Detection of cytotoxic antibody to erythroblasts. *J Lab Clin Med*. 1977;89:851-860.
8. Peschle C, Marmont AM, Marone G, Genovese A, Sasso GF, Condorelli M. Pure red cell aplasia: studies on an IgG serum inhibitor neutralizing erythropoietin. *Br J Haematol*. 1975;30(4):411-417.
9. Meyer RJ, Hoffman R, Zanjani ED. Autoimmune hemolytic anemia and periodic pure red cell aplasia in systemic lupus erythematosus. *Am J Med*. 1978;65(2):342-345.
10. Taniguchi S, Shibuya T, Morioka E, et al. Demonstration of three distinct immunological disorders on erythropoiesis in a patient with pure red cell aplasia and autoimmune haemolytic anaemia associated with thymoma. *Br J Haematol*. 1988;68(4):473-477.
11. Masuda M, Arai Y, Okamura T, Mizoguchi H. Pure red cell aplasia with thymona: evidence of T-cell clonal disorder. Case Reports. *Am J Hematol*. 1997;54(4):324-328.
12. Kawakami T, Sekiguchi N, Kobayashi J, et al. Frequent STAT3 mutations in CD8+ T cells from patients with pure red cell aplasia. *Blood Adv*. 2018;2(20):2704-2712.
13. van den Akker M, Dror Y, Odame I. Transient erythroblastopenia of childhood is an underdiagnosed and self-limiting disease. *Acta Paediatr*. 2014;103(7):e288-e294.
14. Frickhofen N, Chen ZJ, Young NS, Cohen BJ, Heimpel H, Abkowitz JL. Parvovirus B19 as a cause of acquired chronic pure red cell aplasia. *Br J Haematol*. 1994;87(4):818-824.
15. Brown KE, Hibbs JR, Gallinella G, et al. Resistance to parvovirus B19 infection due to lack of virus receptor (erythrocyte P antigen). *N Engl J Med*. 1994;330(17):1192-1196.
16. Yaegashi N, Niinuma T, Chisaka H, et al. Parvovirus B19 infection induces apoptosis of erythroid cells in vitro and in vivo. *J Infect*. 1999;39(1):68-76.
17. Pillet S, Le GN, Hofer T, et al. Hypoxia enhances human B19 erythrovirus gene expression in primary erythroid cells. *Virology*. 2004;327(1):1-7.
18. Casadevall N, Eckardt KU, Rossert J. Epoetin-induced autoimmune pure red cell aplasia. *J Am Soc Nephrol*. 2005;16(suppl 1):S67-S69.
19. Bennett CL, Starko KM, Thomsen HS, et al. Linking drugs to obscure illnesses: lessons from pure red cell aplasia, nephrogenic systemic fibrosis, and Reye's syndrome. a report from the Southern Network on Adverse Reactions (SONAR). *J Gen Intern Med*. 2012;27(12):1697-1703.
20. Macdougall IC, Casadevall N, Locatelli F, et al. Incidence of erythropoietin antibody-mediated pure red cell aplasia: the Prospective Immunogenicity Surveillance Registry (PRIMS). *Nephrol Dial Transplant*. 2015;30(3):451-460.
21. Bernard C, Frih H, Pasquet F, et al. Thymoma associated with autoimmune diseases: 85 cases and literature review. *Autoimmun Rev*. 2016;15(1):82-92.
22. Hirokawa M, Sawada K, Fujishima N, et al. Long-term outcome of patients with acquired chronic pure red cell aplasia (PRCA) following immunosuppressive therapy: a final report of the nationwide cohort study in 2004/2006 by the Japan PRCA collaborative study group. *Br J Haematol*. 2015;169(6):879-886.
23. Masuda M, Teramura M, Matsuda A, et al. Clonal T cells of pure red-cell aplasia. *Am J Hematol*. 2005;79(4):332-333.
24. Hirokawa M, Sawada K, Fujishima N, et al. Acquired pure red cell aplasia associated with malignant lymphomas: a nationwide cohort study in Japan for the PRCA Collaborative Study Group. *Am J Hematol*. 2009;84(3):144-148.
25. D'Arena G, Vigliotti ML, Dell'Olio M, et al. Rituximab to treat chronic lymphoproliferative disorder-associated pure red cell aplasia. *Eur J Haematol*. 2009;82(3):235-239.
26. Vlachaki E, Diamantidis MD, Klonizakis P, Haralambidou-Vranitsa S, Ioannidou-Papagiannaki E, Klonizakis I. Pure red cell aplasia and lymphoproliferative disorders: an infrequent association. *ScientificWorldJournal*. 2012;2012:475313.
27. Lipton JM, Nadler LM, Canellos GP, Kudisch M, Reiss CS, Nathan DG. Evidence for genetic restriction in the suppression of erythropoiesis by a unique subset of T lymphocytes in man. *J Clin Invest*. 1983;72(2):694-706.
28. Abkowitz JL, Kadin ME, Powell JS, Adamson JW. Pure red cell aplasia: lymphocyte inhibition of erythropoiesis. *Br J Haematol*. 1986;63(1):59-67.
29. Qiu ZY, Fan L, Wang L, et al. STAT3 mutations are frequent in T-cell large granular lymphocytic leukemia with pure red cell aplasia. *J Hematol Oncol*. 2013;6:82.
30. Nitta H, Mihara K, Sakai A, Kimura A. Expansion of CD8+/perforin+ effector memory T cells in the bone marrow of patients with thymoma-associated pure red cell aplasia. *Br J Haematol*. 2010;150(6):712-715.
31. Dessypris EN, Baer MR, Sergent JS, Krantz SB. Rheumatoid arthritis and pure red cell aplasia. *Ann Intern Med*. 1984;100(2):202-206.
32. Aung FM, Lichtiger B, Bassett R, et al. Incidence and natural history of pure red cell aplasia in major ABO-mismatched haematopoietic cell transplantation. *Br J Haematol*. 2013;160(6):798-805.
33. Kumar V, Gupta S, Singh S, Goyal VK, Yadav M. Pure red cell aplasia associated with cytomegalovirus infection. *J Pediatr Hematol Oncol*. 2010;32(4):315-316.
34. Giannone L, Kugler JW, Krantz SB. Pure red cell aplasia associated with administration of sustained-release procainamide. *Arch Intern Med*. 1987;147(6):1179-1180.
35. Mariette X, Mitjavila MT, Moulinie JP, et al. Rifampicin-induced pure red cell aplasia. Case Reports. *Am J Med*. 1989;87(4):459-460.
36. Hoffman R, McPhedran P, Benz EJ, Jr, Duffy TP. Isoniazid-induced pure red cell aplasia. *Am J Med Sci*. 1983;286(1):2-9.
37. Edahiro Y, Yasuda H, Ando K, Komatsu N. Self-limiting pregnancy-associated pure red cell aplasia developing in two consecutive pregnancies: case report and literature review. *Int J Hematol*. 2020;111(4):579-584.
38. Au WY, Cheng VC, Wan TS, Ma SK. Myelodysplasia masquerading as parvovirus-related red cell aplasia with giant pronormoblasts. *Ann Hematol*. 2004;83(10):670-671.
39. Keefer MJ, Solanki DL. Dyserythropoiesis and erythroblast-phagocytosis preceding pure red cell aplasia. Case Reports. *Am J Hematol*. 1988;27(2):132-135.
40. Cerchione C, Catalano L, Cerciello G, et al. Role of lenalidomide in the management of myelodysplastic syndromes with del(5q) associated with pure red cell aplasia (PRCA). *Ann Hematol*. 2015;94(3):531-534.
41. Lacy MQ, Kurtin PJ, Tefferi A. Pure red cell aplasia: association with large granular lymphocyte leukemia and the prognostic value of cytogenetic abnormalities. *Blood*. 1996;87(7):3000-3006.
42. Grigg AP, O'Flaherty E. Cyclosporin A for the treatment of pure red cell aplasia associated with myelodysplasia. *Leuk Lymphoma*. 2001;42(6):1339-1342.
43. Garcia-Suarez J, Pascual T, Munoz MA, Herrero B, Pardo A. Myelodysplastic syndrome with erythroid hypoplasia/aplasia: a case report and review of the literature. *Am J Hematol*. 1998;58(4):319-325.
44. Vo AK, Kollsete Gjelberg H, Hovland R, Lindstad Brattas MK, Bruserud O, Reikvam H. Pure red cell aplasia with del(20q) sensitive for immunosuppressive treatment. *Case Rep Hematol*. 2020;2020:1262038.
45. Krantz SB. Pure red-cell aplasiaReview. *N Engl J Med*. 1974;291(7):345-350.
46. Frickhofen N, Young NS. Polymerase chain reaction for detection of parvovirus B19 in immunodeficient patients with anemia. *Behring Institute Mitteilungen*. 1990(85):46-54.
47. Sawada K, Fujishima N, Hirokawa M. Acquired pure red cell aplasia: updated review of treatment. *Br J Haematol*. 2008;142(4):505-514.
48. Clark DA, Dessypris EN, Krantz SB. Studies on pure red cell aplasia.XI. Results of immunosuppressive therapy of 37 patients. *Blood*. 1984;63:277-286.
49. Chen Z, Liu X, Chen M, Yang C, Han B. Successful sirolimus treatment of patients with pure red cell aplasia complicated with renal insufficiency. *Ann Hematol*. 2020;99(4):737-741.

50. Jiang H, Zhang H, Wang Y, et al. Sirolimus for the treatment of multi-resistant pure red cell aplasia. *Br J Haematol*. 2019;184(6):1055-1058.
51. Yoshida S, Konishi T, Nishizawa T, Yoshida Y. Effect of tacrolimus in a patient with pure red-cell aplasia. Case Reports. *Clin Lab Haematol*. 2005;27(1):67-69.
52. Gupta RK, Ezeonyeji AN, Thomas AS, Scully MA, Ehrenstein MR, Isenberg DA. A case of pure red cell aplasia and immune thrombocytopenia complicating systemic lupus erythematosus: response to rituximab and cyclophosphamide. *Lupus*. 2011;20(14):1547-1550. Case Reports.
53. Zhidong W, Hongmin Y, Hengxiang W. Successful treatment of pure red cell aplasia with a single low dose of rituximab in two patients after major ABO incompatible peripheral blood allogeneic stem cell transplantation. *Transfus Med*. 2012;22(4):302-304.
54. Bathini S, Holtzman NG, Koka R, et al. Refractory postallogeneic stem cell transplant pure red cell aplasia in remission after treatment with daratumumab. *Am J Hematol*. 2019;94(8):E216-E219.
55. Sloand EM, Olnes MJ, Weinstein B, et al. Long-term follow-up of patients with moderate aplastic anemia and pure red cell aplasia treated with daclizumab. *Haematologica*. 2010;95(3):382-387.
56. Khan F, Linden MA, Zantek ND, Vercellotti GM. Subcutaneous bortezomib is highly effective for pure red cell aplasia after ABO-incompatible haematopoietic stem cell transplantation. *Transfus Med*. 2014;24(3):187-188.
57. Risitano AM, Selleri C, Serio B, et al. Alemtuzumab is safe and effective as immunosuppressive treatment for aplastic anaemia and single-lineage marrow failure: a pilot study and a survey from the EBMT WPSAA. *Br J Haematol*. 2010;148(5):791-796.
58. Helbig G, Stella-Holowiecka B, Wojnar J, et al. Pure red-cell aplasia following major and bi-directional ABO-incompatible allogeneic stem-cell transplantation: recovery of donor-derived erythropoiesis after long-term treatment using different therapeutic strategies. *Ann Hematol*. 2007;86(9):677-683.
59. Mouthon L, Guillevin L, Tellier Z. Intravenous immunoglobulins in autoimmune- or parvovirus B19-mediated pure red-cell aplasia. *Autoimmun Rev*. 2005;4(5):264-269. Review.
60. Messner HA, Fauser AA, Curtis JE, Dotten D. Control of antibody-mediated pure red-cell aplasia by plasmapheresis. Case Reports. *N Engl J Med*. 1981;304(22):1334-1338.
61. Halkes C, de Wreede LC, Knol C, et al. Allogeneic stem cell transplantation for acquired pure red cell aplasia. *Am J Hematol*. 2019;94(11):E294-E296.
62. Crabol Y, Terrier B, Rozenberg F, et al. Intravenous immunoglobulin therapy for pure red cell aplasia related to human parvovirus b19 infection: a retrospective study of 10 patients and review of the literature. *Clin Infect Dis*. 2013;56(7):968-977.
63. Koduri PR, Kumapley R, Valladares J, Teter C. Chronic pure red cell aplasia caused by parvovirus B19 in AIDS: use of intravenous immunoglobulin—a report of eight patients. *Am J Hematol*. 1999;61(1):16-20.
64. Thompson CA, Steensma DP. Pure red cell aplasia associated with thymoma: clinical insights from a 50-year single-institution experience. *Br J Haematol*. 2006;135(3):405-407.
65. Hirokawa M, Sawada K, Fujishima N, et al. Long-term response and outcome following immunosuppressive therapy in thymoma-associated pure red cell aplasia: a nationwide cohort study in Japan by the PRCA collaborative study group. *Haematologica*. 2008;93(1):27-33.
66. Zaucha R, Zaucha JM, Jassem J. Resolution of thymoma-related pure red cell aplasia after octreotide treatment. *Acta Oncol*. 2007;46(6):864-865.
67. Macdougall IC. Epoetin-induced pure red cell aplasia: diagnosis and treatment. *Curr Opin Nephrol Hypertens*. 2007;16(6):585-588. Review.
68. Fraer M, Campbell A, Sawaya BP. Response to cyclosporine A in a patient with pure red cell aplasia due to antierythropoietin-alpha antibodies. *Semin Dial*. 2006;19(3):251-254. SDI163 pii. doi:10.1111/j.1525-139X.2006.00163.x
69. Alonso Melgar A, Melgosa Hijosa M, Pardo de la Vega R, Garcia Meseguer C, Navarro Torres M. Antierythropoietin antibody-induced pure red cell aplasia: post-transplant evolution. *Pediatr Nephrol*. 2004;19(9):1059-1061. Case Reports.
70. Katagiri D, Shibata M, Katsuki T, et al. Antiepoetin antibody-related pure red cell aplasia: successful remission with cessation of recombinant erythropoietin alone. *Clin Exp Nephrol*. 2010;14(5):501-505. Case Reports.
71. Casadevall N, Nataf J, Viron B. Pure red-cell aplasia and antierythropoietin antibodies in patients treated with recombinant erythropoietin. *N Engl J Med*. 2002;346:469-475.
72. Praditpornsilpa K, Tiranathanagul K, Kupatawintu P, et al. Biosimilar recombinant human erythropoietin induces the production of neutralizing antibodies. *Kidney Int*. 2011;80(1):88-92.
73. Praditpornsilpa K, Tiranathanakul K, Jootar S, Tungsanga K, Eiam-Ong S. Rechallenge with intravenous recombinant human erythropoietin can be successful following the treatment of anti-recombinant erythropoietin associated pure red cell aplasia. *Clin Nephrol*. 2014;81(5):355-358.
74. Dessypris EN, Fogo A, Russell M, Engel E, Krantz SB. Studies on pure red cell aplasia. X. Association with acute leukemia and significance of bone marrow karyotype abnormalities. *Blood*. 1980;56(3):421-426.
75. McMahon JN, Egan EL. Aplastic anaemia in a patient with pure red cell aplasia. *Ir J Med Sci*. 1980;149(5):212-214. Case Reports.
76. Josephs HW. Anaemia of infancy and early childhood. *Medicine (Baltim)*. 1936;15(3):307-451. doi: 10.1097/00005792-193615030-00001
77. Diamond LK, Blackfan KD. Hypoplastic anemia. *Am J Dis Child*. 1938;56:464-467.
78. Lipton JM, Ellis SR. Diamond-Blackfan anemia: diagnosis, treatment, and molecular pathogenesis. *Hematol Oncol Clin N Am*. 2009;23(2):261-282.
79. Narla A, Ebert BL. Ribosomopathies: human disorders of ribosome dysfunction. *Blood*. 2010;115(16):3196-3205.
80. Vlachos A, Rosenberg PS, Atsidaftos E, Alter BP, Lipton JM. Incidence of neoplasia in Diamond Blackfan anemia: a report from the Diamond Blackfan anemia Registry. *Blood*. 2012;119(16):3815-3819.
81. Vlachos A, Rosenberg PS, Atsidaftos E, et al. Increased risk of colon cancer and osteogenic sarcoma in Diamond-Blackfan anemia. *Blood*. 2018;132(20):2205-2208.
82. Lipton JM, Molmenti CLS Hussain M, et al. Colorectal cancer screening and surveillance strategy for patients with Diamond Blackfan anemia: preliminary recommendations from the Diamond Blackfan anemia Registry. *Pediatr Blood Cancer*. 2021;68(8):e28984. doi:10.1002/pbc28984
83. Narla A, Ruddy KJ, Ebert BL, Mar B. Whole exoome sequencing of a breast tumor in a patient with Diamond Blackfan Anemia. *Blood Cells Mol Dis*. 2021;89:102566.
84. Kampen KR, Sulima SO, Vereecke S, De Keersmaecker K. Hallmarks of ribosomopathies. *Nucleic Acids Res*. 2020;48(3):1013-1028.
85. Alter BP, Nathan DG. Red cell aplasia in children. *Arch Dis Child*. 1979;54(4):263-267.
86. Alter BP. Bone marrow failure syndromes in children. *Pediatr Clin North Am*. 2002;49(5):973-988.
87. Draptchinskaia N, Gustavsson P, Andersson B, et al. The gene encoding ribosomal protein S19 is mutated in Diamond-Blackfan anaemia. *Nat Genet*. 1999;21(2):169-175.
88. Gazda HT, Grabowska A, Merida-Long LB, et al. Ribosomal protein S24 gene is mutated in Diamond-Blackfan anemia. *Am J Hum Genet*. 2006;79(6):1110-1118.
89. Bodine DM, Lipton JM, Vlachos A. Whole genome sequencing identifies small deletions in ribosomal genes causing Diamond Blackfan anemia. *Blood*. 2019;134(suppl_1):2502. (abstract) doi: 10.1182/blood-2019-121710
90. Vlachos A, Blanc L, Lipton JM. Diamond Blackfan anemia: a model for the translational approach to understanding human disease. *Expet Rev Hematol*. 2014;7(3):359-372.
91. Gripp KW, Curry C, Olney AH, et al. Diamond-Blackfan anemia with mandibulofacial dystostosis is heterogeneous, including the novel DBA genes TSR2 and RPS28. *Am J Med Genet*. 2014;164A(9):2240-2249.
92. Ruggero D, Shimamura A. Marrow failure: a window into ribosome biology. *Blood*. 2014;124(18):2784-2792.
93. Ulirsch JC, Verboon JM, Kazerounian S, et al. The genetic landscape of Diamond-Blackfan anemia. *Am J Hum Genet*. 2018;103(6):930-947.
94. Donati G, Peddigari S, Mercer CA, Thomas G. 5S ribosomal RNA is an essential component of a nascent ribosomal precursor complex that regulates the Hdm2-p53 checkpoint. *Cell Rep*. 2013;4(1):87-98.
95. Gazda HT, Sheen MR, Vlachos A, et al. Ribosomal protein L5 and L11 mutations are associated with cleft palate and abnormal thumbs in Diamond-Blackfan anemia patients. *Am J Hum Genet*. 2008;83(6):769-780.
96. Ludwig LS, Gazda HT, Eng JC, et al. Altered translation of GATA1 in Diamond-Blackfan anemia. *Nat Med*. 2014;20(7):748-753.
97. Yang Z, Keel SB, Shimamura A, et al. Delayed globin synthesis leads to excess heme and the macrocytic anemia of Diamond Blackfan anemia and del(5q) myelodysplastic syndrome. *Sci Transl Med*. 2016;8(338):338ra367.
98. Taylor A, Humphries JM, White R, Murphey RD, Burns C, Zon LI. Hematopoietic defects in rps29 mutant zebrafish depend upon p53 activation. *Exp Hematopoiesis*. 2012;40(3):228-237. E5.
99. Jaako P, Debnath S, Olsson K, Bryder D, Flygare J, Karlsson S. Dietary L-leucine improves the anemia in a mouse model for Diamond-Blackfan anemia. *Blood*. 2012;120:2225-2228.
100. Vlachos A, Atsidaftos E, Lababidi ML, et al. L-leucine improves anemia and growth in patients with transfusion-dependent Diamond-Blackfan anemia: results from a multicenter pilot phase I/II study from the Diamond-Blackfan Anemia Registry. *Pediatr Blood Cancer*. 2020;67(12):e28748. doi: 10.1002/pbc.28748
101. Fargo JH, Kratz CP, Giri N, et al. Erythrocyte adenosine deaminase: diagnostic value for Diamond-Blackfan anaemia. *Br J Haematol*. 2013;160(4):547-554.
102. Gri N, Kang E, Tisdale JF, et al. Clinical and laboratory evidence for a trilineage haematopoietic defect in patients with refractory Diamond-Blackfan anaemia. *Br J Haematol*. 2000;108(1):167-175. doi: 10.1046/j.1365-2141.2000.01796.x
103. Vlachos A, Farrar JE, Atsidaftos E, et al. Diminutive somatic deletions in the 5q region lead to a phenotype atypical of classical 5q-syndrome. *Blood*. 2013;122(14):2487-2490.
104. Talerman A, Amigo A. Thymoma associated with aregenerative and aplastic anemia in a five-year-old child. *Cancer*. 1968;21(6):1212-1218.
105. Hashem H, Egler R, Dalal J. Refractory pure red cell aplasia manifesting as deficiency of adenosine deaminase 2. *J Pediatr Hematol Oncol*. 2017;39(5):e293-e2e6.
106. Kim HR, Ulirsch JC, Wilmes S, et al. Functional selectivity in cytokine signaling revealed through a pathogenic EPO mutation. *Cell*. 2017;168(6):1053-1064.e15.
107. Vlachos A, Ball S, Dahl N, et al. Diagnosing and treating Diamond Blackfan anaemia: results of an international clinical consensus conference. *Br J Haematol*. 2008;142(6):859-876.
108. Gasser C. Aplastic anemia (chronic erythroblastophthisis) and cortisone. [Article in Undetermined language]. *Schweiz Med Wochenschr*. 1951;81(50):1241-1242.
109. Vlachos A, Muir E. How I treat Diamond-Blackfan anemia. *Blood*. 2010;116(19):3715-3723.
110. Ashley RJ, Yan H, Wang N, et al. Steroid resistance in Diamond Blackfan anemia associates with p57Kip2 dysregulation in erythroid progenitors. *J Clin Invest*. 2020;130(4):2097-2110. doi: 10.1172/JCI132284
111. August CS, King E, Githens JH, et al. Establishment of erythropoiesis following bone marrow transplantation in a patient with congenital hypoplastic anemia (Diamond-Blackfan syndrome). *Blood*. 1976;48(4):491-498.
112. Alter BP. Bone marrow transplant in Diamond-Blackfan anemia. *Bone Marrow Transplant*. 1998;21(9):965-966.
113. Vlachos A, Federman N, Reyes-Haley C, Abramson J, Lipton JM. Hematopoietic stem cell transplantation for Diamond Blackfan anemia: a report from the Diamond Blackfan anemia Registry. *Bone Marrow Transplant*. 2001;27(4):381-386.
114. Dietz AC, Mehta PA, Vlachos A, et al. Current knowledge and priorities for future research in late effects after hematopoietic cell transplantation for inherited bone marrow failure syndromes: consensus statement from the second pediatric blood and marrow transplant Consortium international conference on late effects after pediatric hematopoietic cell transplantation. *Biol Blood Marrow transplant*. 2017;23(5):726-735.

Chapter 41 ■ Congenital Dyserythropoietic Anemias

THEODOSIA A. KALFA • BERTIL GLADER • GARY KUPFER

INTRODUCTION

The congenital dyserythropoietic anemias (CDAs) are a heterogeneous group of inherited blood disorders characterized by anemia and dyserythropoiesis, as evidenced by morphologic abnormalities of the erythroid precursors in the bone marrow.[1-3] Ineffective erythropoiesis associated with iron overload disproportionate to the history of transfusions is a hallmark of most cases. These disorders principally affect the erythroid lineage, whereas the other hematopoietic lineages seem to be unaffected. The classification of CDAs was based for decades on the morphologic classification of bone marrow pathology proposed by Heimpel and Wendt in 1968, in which CDA types I, II, and III were defined based on structural similarities.[1] After 2000, specific genetic causes of the different types were identified, suggesting a phenotype-genotype correlation. Currently, CDAs are additionally classified by their genetic cause into CDA types I, II, and III, the transcription-factor-related CDA type IV, X-linked thrombocytopenia with or without dyserythropoietic anemia (XLTDA), and several other rare CDA variants.[2,4,5] Less than 1000 patients with CDA have been reported so far in the literature.[2,5,6] The European CDA registry reported 218 patients enrolled in the period 1995 to 2019,[2] while the American CDA registry, initiated in 2016, had enrolled 38 patients up to 2020.[5] CDA II is the most common type in both registries, followed by CDA I.[2] The disease-causing genes for CDA I, II, III, IV, XLTDA, and CDA variants identified so far[7-17] are shown in *Table 41.1*, along with the pattern of inheritance and characteristic bone marrow pathology findings on light and electron microscopy.

CLINICAL PRESENTATION

The clinical presentation is frequently nonspecific, typically including anemia, neonatal and chronic or intermittent jaundice, and splenomegaly, and may overlap with various common hemolytic disorders such as RBC membrane disorders and thalassemias, posing challenges in diagnosis and leading sometimes to misdirected treatments.[18] Suboptimal reticulocytosis and macrocytosis are consistent with ineffective and stress erythropoiesis, which typically leads to accelerated iron overload that is in addition to that due to transfusions.[19,20] Increased erythroblast-derived hormone erythroferrone (ERFE) and/or increased growth differentiation factor 15 (GDF15), a member of the transforming growth factor-β superfamily of cytokines, downregulate the iron-regulatory protein hepcidin, leading to excessive iron absorption and systemic iron overload, as has also been described in thalassemias.[21-23] Dyserythropoiesis results in a variety of dysplastic features of erythroblasts in the bone marrow, which collectively are characteristic for each CDA subtype and the associated causative gene: internuclear chromatin bridges, karyorrhectic nuclei, binuclearity, multinuclearity, vacuolation of the cytoplasm, and duplication of the plasma membrane.[24] Diagnosis of CDA relies on light and electron microscopy analyses to identify the characteristic morphologic abnormalities of the erythroblasts in the bone marrow,[25] although given the identification of numerous causative genes (*Table 41.1*), molecular diagnosis utilizing next-generation sequencing (NGS) panels has become a primary diagnostic tool, eliminating the need for a bone marrow diagnostic procedure in many cases. Of note, severe hemolytic anemias caused by globin, red cell membrane, or enzyme disorders with a brisk erythropoietic response may demonstrate erythroid dysplasia in bone marrow studies, which can be misdiagnosed as CDA. Molecular diagnostic tools, including NGS, has allowed the identification of the correct diagnosis, such as pyruvate kinase deficiency, hereditary xerocytosis, unstable hemoglobins, or hereditary spherocytosis.[2,5]

CDA should be suspected in any individual with chronic anemia and evidence of ineffective erythropoiesis or with unexplained iron overload. The presence of ineffective erythropoiesis is characterized by a low absolute reticulocyte count for the degree of anemia despite erythroid hyperplasia in the marrow. Further suggestive laboratory data include a low serum haptoglobin level and increased serum lactic dehydrogenase activity. Generally, the anemia is mildly or moderately macrocytic in CDA-I, normocytic in CDA-II, mildly macrocytic in CDA-III, and normocytic in CDA-IV.

CDA SUBTYPES

Congenital Dyserythropoietic Anemia Type I

CDA-I is inherited in an autosomal recessive pattern and represents the second most common form of CDA.[20] While the disease was initially described in several members of a large Bedouin tribe in Israel and other areas of Middle East with parental consanguinity, patients with CDA-I have now been identified in a multitude of ethnic backgrounds, including Western Europeans, Indians, Japanese, Latino-Hispanic, and African.[5,26] Biallelic mutations in *CDAN1* and *CDIN1* have been found causative for CDA-Ia and CDA-Ib, respectively.[7,10]

Clinical Features

The anemia in CDA-I can range from mild to severe, with the most severe cases presenting in infancy and the milder during adolescence or later.[27,28] Some degree of anemia is present in about two-thirds of neonates, often requiring transfusion, but less than 10% of cases remain transfusion dependent later in life.[27,29] Severe anemia in the fetus due to CDA-I has been described as a cause of hydrops fetalis with pericardial and pleural effusions and edema, occasionally leading to stillbirth or fetal demise in the third trimester without intrauterine transfusion support.[5,30] Jaundice and splenomegaly are common findings at all ages. Gallstones may develop and require cholecystectomy. Nonhematological features are frequently noted and include distal limb malformations, such as syndactyly, absence of phalanges and/or nails, an additional phalanx, and duplication or hypoplasia of the metatarsals; café-au-lait spots; skin pigmentation; macrocephaly; dolichocephaly; scoliosis; flattened vertebral bodies; hypoplastic rib; Madelung deformity; and short stature.[5,26,31] Deafness[26] and deterioration of vision with retinal angioid streaks and macular degeneration[32-34] have been rarely described. Several patients have been reported to have had persistent pulmonary hypertension of the newborn in early infancy requiring mechanical ventilation.[5,35,36] Ineffective erythropoiesis is the major cause of the iron overload in CDA-I via suppression of hepcidin and resulting increased iron absorption,[37,38] and it has been associated with significantly increased levels of GDF15[39] more than increased erythroferrone.[40] In addition, Shalev et al reported high levels of soluble serum hemojuvelin, a key regulator of iron homeostasis, in patients with CDA-I.[41]

Laboratory Features

Patients with CDA-I usually have macrocytic anemia with mean corpuscular volume values up to 115 fL; patients with CDA-I with normocytic anemia still display macrocytes and thus an increased red cell distribution width. Anisocytosis, poikilocytosis (including teardrop-shaped poikilocytes), and basophilic stippling are other features of the peripheral blood smear (*Figure 41.1A*). Increased hemoglobin A_2 levels and unbalanced globin chain synthesis are found in some cases in the absence of β-thalassemia mutations.[42,43] Bone marrow examination reveals marked erythroid hyperplasia and megaloblastic erythroblasts. About 3% to 10% of the erythroblasts are binucleated,

Table 41.1. Types of Congenital Dyserythropoietic Anemias, Causative Genes, and Bone Marrow Pathology Findings

CDA Type	Gene	Inheritance Pattern	Bone Marrow Pathology Findings	
			Light Microscopy	**Electron Microscopy**
Ia **Ib**	*CDAN1* *CDIN1*	AR AR	3%-10% binucleated erythroblasts, occasional thin chromatin bridges between nuclei of divided erythroblasts	Spongy appearance of heterochromatin in intermediate and late erythroblasts ("Swiss cheese" appearance)
II	*SEC23 B*	AR	10%-30% binucleated, occasional multinucleated erythroblasts ~2% of the cells with karyorrhexis	Erythroblast plasma membrane duplicated at sites Peripheral cisternae loaded with ER protein
IIIa **IIIb**	*KIF23* *RACGAP1*	AD AR	Giant multinucleated erythroblasts with up to 12 nuclei (gigantoblasts)	Intranuclear clefts into heterochromatin Autophagic vacuoles
IV	*KLF1*	AD	Binucleated and multinucleated erythroblasts, karyorrhexis, and nuclear pyknosis	Invagination of nuclear membrane and nuclear blebbing
XLTDA	*GATA1*	XLR	Abundant but dysplastic megakaryocytes with small eccentric nuclei; giant platelets; erythroblasts megaloblastic with bi- and multinucleation and nuclear irregularities	Megakaryocytes with abundance of smooth endoplasmic reticulum; decreased alpha granules in platelets
X-linked macrocytic dyserythropoietic anemia in females	*ALAS2*	XLD	Megaloblasts with nuclear-cytoplasmic asynchrony, occasional binucleation and karyorrhexis, rare erythroblasts with siderotic granules	NR
Chronic recurrent multifocal osteomyelitis and CDA (Majeed syndrome)	*LPIN1*	AR	Binucleate erythroblasts, internuclear bridging	NR
Uridine-responsive CDA-II-like disease with epileptic encephalopathy	*CAD*	AR	5%-10% binucleated late erythroblasts, rare trinucleate forms, and prominent cytoplasmic bridging	NR
CDA variant with severe neurodevelopmental delay	*VPS4A*	AD/AR	Binucleated erythroblasts and erythroblasts with cytoplasmic bridges	NR
Nontypable variants	TBD	TBD	Variable dyserythropoiesis findings including bi- and multinucleated nuclear lobation or fragmentation, cytoplasmic bridges between divided erythroblasts	

Abbreviations: AD, autosomal dominant; AR, autosomal recessive; NR, not reported; TBD, to be determined; XLD, X-linked dominant; XLR, X-linked recessive.

frequently with the two nuclei being in different stages of maturation; occasional cells have three or four nuclei, and irregular nuclear outlines and karyorrhexis are also noted (*Figure 41.1B* and D). One of the defining features of CDA-I is the presence of thin internuclear chromatin bridges between nearly completely separated erythroblasts in 0.6% to 2.8% of cells (*Figure 41.1C*).[20,25,44,45]

A second defining structural feature of CDA I is multiple rounded, electron-lucent areas within the electron-dense heterochromatin seen in up to 60% of erythroblasts, giving the nucleus a spongy or "Swiss cheese" appearance (*Figure 41.2A*).[25,46-48] Widening of the nuclear pores and marked invaginations or evaginations of the nuclear envelope can also be seen (*Figure 41.2B*); the invaginations carry cytoplasm and cytoplasmic organelles such as mitochondria into the nucleus.[49] Bone marrow macrophages may also be seen to have phagocytosed morphologically abnormal erythroblasts (*Figure 41.3*).

Historically, because of its remarkable clinical variability and overlap with other hematologic conditions, delayed or misdiagnosis of CDA-I was common, with a median age of 17.3 years at the time of diagnosis.[29] Molecular diagnosis utilizing NGS panels that include the CDA-I-associated genes *CDAN1* and *CDIN1*, along with the other known genes leading to the phenotype of hereditary hemolytic anemia, has improved and expedited accurate diagnosis for CDA-I to early childhood or infancy for the most severe cases.[2,5]

Management

CDA-I is phenotypically variable, ranging from severe, transfusion-dependent anemia to mild anemia, requiring red cell transfusions in infancy, episodes of infections, and during pregnancy. The presentation in late pregnancy and the neonatal period can be dramatic, and the developing fetus may require intrauterine transfusions for a favorable outcome. Splenectomy has been used in the past and was thought to ameliorate anemia in some patients[26,28]; however, long-term follow-up revealed poor hematologic efficacy and the potential for significant morbidity with pulmonary hypertension in young adulthood, likely due to aggravated intravascular hemolysis post splenectomy.[18,29,50] Erythropoietin administration has no effect on the anemia of CDA-I.[51] Following the fortuitous observation that treatment of hepatitis C in a patient with CDA-I with interferon-α2a led to a substantial hematologic improvement,[52] several additional patients as young as 1 year have been treated with interferon-α2a, interferon-α2b, or their pegylated forms, and these patients also have experienced hematologic improvement.[5,31,53-56] Such treatment may also help reduce iron overload by decreasing ineffective erythropoiesis or by allowing for therapeutic phlebotomy.[38,53] Therefore, interferon-α should be considered in the management of CDA-I with significant anemia. Careful monitoring for secondary hemochromatosis is also important, along with iron chelation therapy as needed.[2,5,57-59] Shalev et al[50] examined retrospectively the clinical and laboratory features of 32 adult patients with CDA-I, demonstrating the significant morbidity and mortality of these patients. Splenectomy was performed in six patients, and three patients died at ages 46 to 56 years, one due to pulmonary hypertension and the other two due to gram-negative sepsis. In addition to monitoring iron overload, the authors suggested stem cell transplantation, chronic transfusion therapy with iron chelation, or interferon-α in patients with significant disease.

Disorders of Red Blood Cells

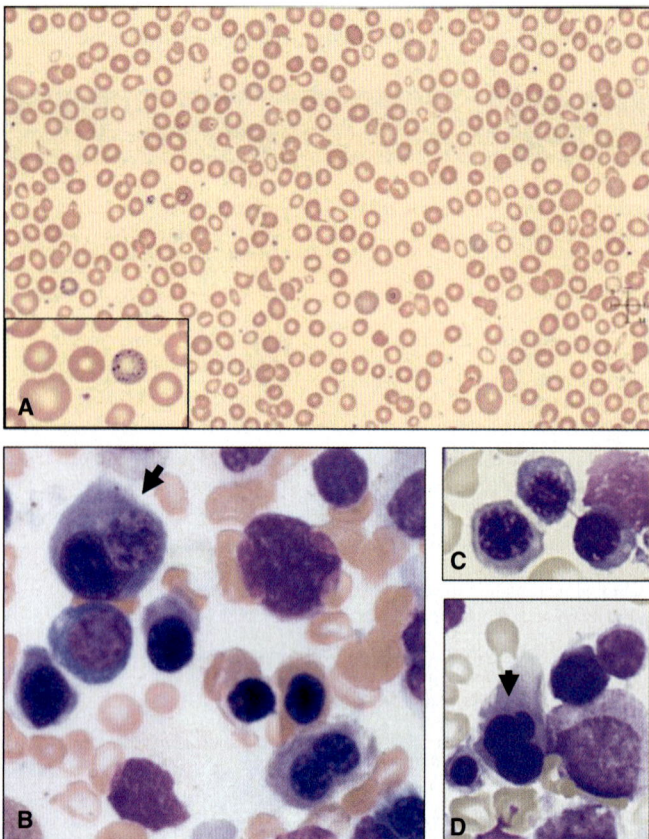

FIGURE 41.1 A, Peripheral blood smear of a patient with CDA-I with profound anisocytosis and poikilocytosis. Several macrocytes, hypochromic cells, and bizarre poikilocytes are seen. The inset shows a cell with intense basophilic stippling and a macrocyte. B, Bone marrow smear of a patient with CDA-I, showing two binucleated erythroblasts, the one showing asynchronous nuclear differentiation (arrow). C, Erythroblasts joined by internuclear chromatin bridge, a pathognomonic morphological characteristic for CDA-I. D, Erythroblast nuclear lobation (arrow).

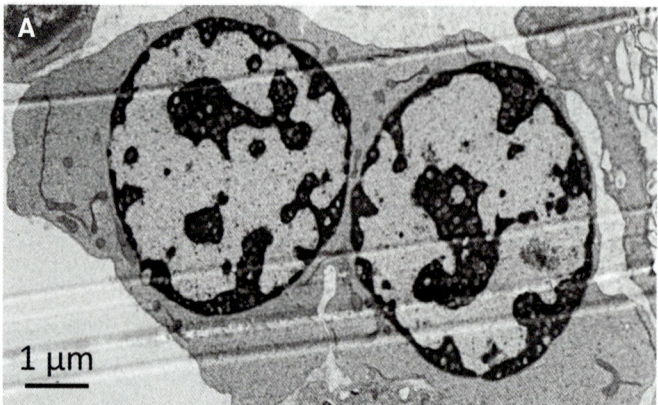

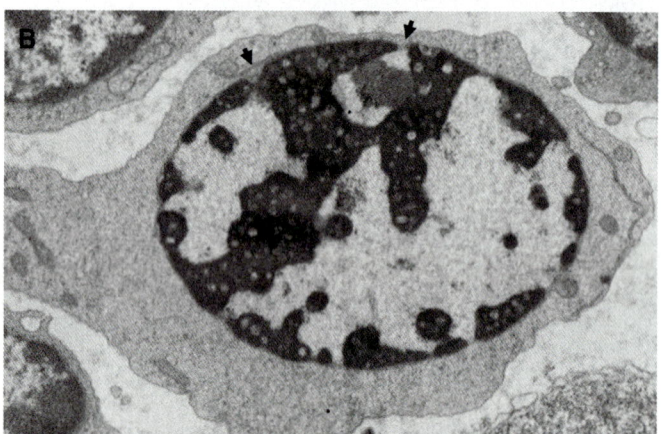

FIGURE 41.2 A, Electron microscopy of a CDA-I binucleated erythroblast. Multiple electron-lucent areas within the electron-dense heterochromatin giving the nucleus a spongy or Swiss cheese appearance. B, Widening of the nuclear pores and invaginations carrying cytoplasm into the nucleus (arrows).

Molecular Biology of CDA-I

In 1998, the gene for CDA-I was localized to chromosome 15q15.1-15.3,[60] and it is now recognized that CDA-I is caused by mutations in the *CDAN1* gene.[7] *CDAN1* has 28 exons spanning 15 kb of genomic DNA and encodes a highly conserved yet poorly understood protein termed codanin-1. Mutations in the *CDAN1* gene are mainly located in the 3' half of the gene, and no homozygote for null type mutations has been identified, suggesting that the complete absence of codanin-1 is likely embryonic lethal,[61] a conclusion supported by studies in knock-out mouse models of CDA-I.[62] One founder missense mutation is observed mainly in Israeli Bedouins with CDA-I, which converts arginine to tryptophan at codon 1042 and generates an *Nco*I restriction site.[7] This same missense mutation was found in 11 individuals with CDA-I of two unrelated Lebanese families. More than 30 additional mutations have been identified, including missense, splicing, frameshift, and deletion/insertion mutations.[2,38,58,63] A single mutation in *CDAN1* has been found in several sporadic cases, and, in one case, no mutations in *CDAN1* were found,[7] implicating either deep intronic mutations in *CDAN1*, promoter or other regulatory mutations, or potentially other genes involved in the same pathogenetic pathway. An additional CDA-I disease gene has been identified, *C15ORF41*, now named *CDIN1* (CDAN1 Interacting Nuclease 1), which encodes for a novel endonuclease member of the Holliday junction resolvase proteins.[10]

Analysis of codanin-1 orthologs revealed that the *Drosophila* homolog, *dlt*, is required for cell survival and cell cycle progression through the S phase.[64] Interestingly, Noy-Lotan et al showed that codanin-1 increases during the S phase in HeLa cells and is phosphorylated and

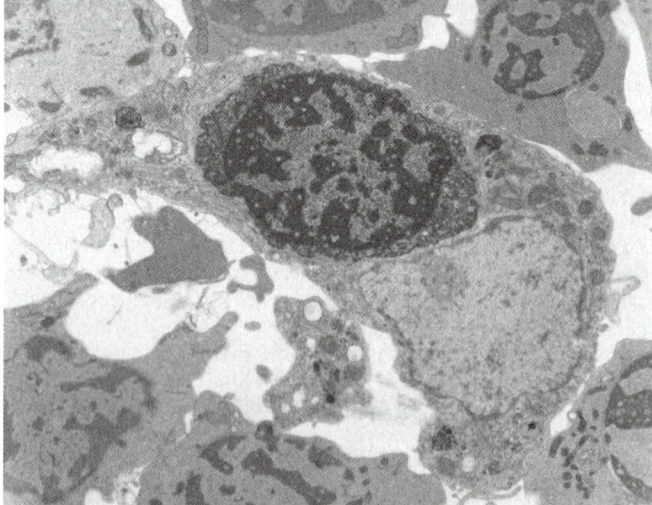

FIGURE 41.3 Macrophage in a bone marrow aspirate from a case with CDA-I containing an ingested erythroblast with a typical abnormal nucleus containing spongy heterochromatin

excluded from condensed chromosomes during mitosis.[65] This study also showed codanin-1 localizes to heterochromatin in the nucleus during interphase and is regulated by the E2F1 transcription factor. Renella et al found that overall chromatin structure as indicated by genome-wide epigenetic marks of several histone modifications is normal in CDA-I erythroblasts.[66] Moreover, they evaluated human erythroblasts by immunofluorescence and confirmed codanin-1 localization to the nucleus, but, in erythroblasts of patients with CDA-I, they found abnormal accumulation of heterochromatin protein 1 (HP1α) and the mutant codanin-1 in the Golgi apparatus.[66] Codanin-1 was also shown to interact with histone chaperone Asf1, histones H3.1–H4, and importin-IV in the cytoplasm to regulate histone supply during DNA replication, thus regulating the import of histones during DNA replication.[67] *CDAN1* knockdown increases the amount of chromatin-bound Asf1, enhancing DNA synthesis. Conversely, forced expression of codanin-1 interferes with Asf1 function due to Asf1 sequestration in the cytoplasm. Thus, codanin-1 may act as a negative regulator of replication.

This close association with heterochromatin suggests that codanin-1 may be involved in mechanisms controlling gene transcription, chromatin structure remodeling, and nuclear condensation necessary for terminal erythroid differentiation. An improved understanding of the biochemical interactions and behavior of codanin-1 is needed to provide us insight into its role in normal erythropoiesis and in CDA-I.

Congenital Dyserythropoietic Anemia Type II

CDA-II was first categorized as such by Heimpel and Wendt in 1968.[1] It is the most common type of CDA, and several hundred patients have been described.[6] The mode of inheritance is autosomal recessive due to *SEC23B* mutations.

Clinical Features

CDA-II is usually a normocytic anemia with evidence of ineffective erythropoiesis and hemolysis, with premature peripheral red cell destruction causing jaundice and splenomegaly. Hepatosplenomegaly may also be present as a sign of significant extramedullary erythropoiesis. In very mild cases, the anemia may be so slight as to remain undiscovered until late in life, although a majority of patients display a hemoglobin <11 g/dL. Overall, a third of affected children require transfusion in the first year of life, but transfusion requirements decrease in subsequent years, and only 5% of patients remain transfusion dependent in adulthood.[68] As in other congenital disorders in which ineffective erythropoiesis is a prominent feature, such as β-thalassemia major, complications of extramedullary hematopoiesis may occur, such as dysmorphic facies, particularly in severely affected individuals.[69,70] Cholelithiasis and secondary hemochromatosis are frequent complications, with iron overload as the presenting manifestation in some cases.[71] Transient red cell aplasia secondary to parvovirus B19 infection has been reported.[72] Mental retardation,[6] fibromuscular dysplasia of the extracranial internal carotid artery with ischemic stroke,[73] hemihypertrophy,[6] piebaldism, and vaginal atresia[74] have all been reported, each in a single case of CDA-II. Since these are rare occurrences and some of the patients with CDA-II are offspring of consanguineous parents, the pathogenesis for these nonhematopoietic manifestations is likely unrelated to the molecular pathogenesis of CDA-II.

Overexpression of GDF15 has been reported in patients with CDA-II,[75] as seen in CDA-I, as well as increased levels of the erythroblast-derived hormone erythroferrone (ERFE),[76] both implicating ineffective erythropoiesis and hepcidin suppression as major contributors to the iron-overload phenotype.

Laboratory Features

Peripheral blood smear features include significant anisocytosis, mild poikilocytosis, and frequent cells with decreased central pallor and spherocytes (*Figure 41.4A*). The combination of hemolysis with jaundice, splenomegaly, and spherocytes in the peripheral smear leads not infrequently to the misdiagnosis of hereditary spherocytosis (HS). The accompanying anisocytosis along with suboptimal reticulocytosis for the degree of anemia may provide a hint to the diagnosis of CDA-II instead.[6] Indications of iron overload disproportionate to the history of transfusions should also raise suspicion for CDA-II rather than HS.

Bone marrow examination reveals marked erythroid hyperplasia without megaloblastosis. The defining erythroblast abnormality is a prominent binuclearity. Proerythroblasts are morphologically normal, but basophilic and mainly polychromatic and orthochromatic erythroblasts are binucleated, with up to 10% to 35% of late erythroblasts being so (*Figure 41.4B*). Multinucleated erythroblasts are also seen

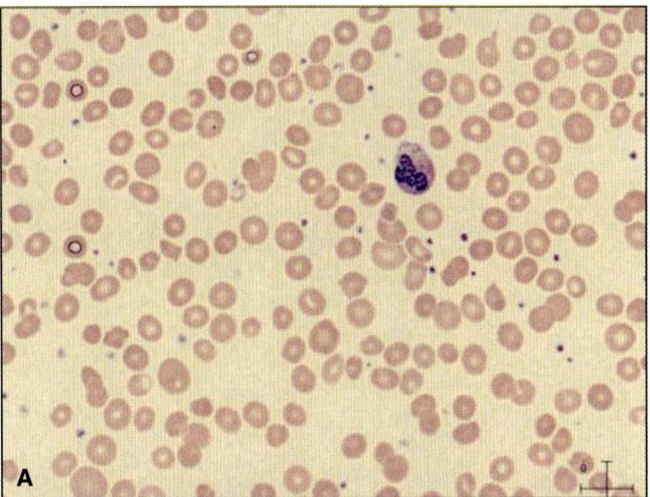

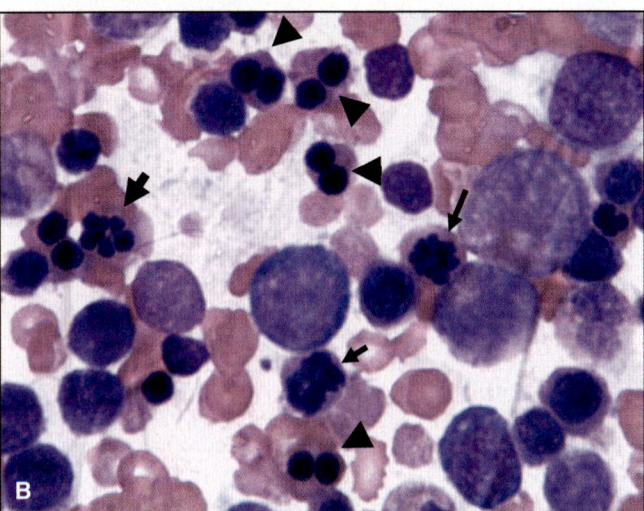

FIGURE 41.4 A, Peripheral blood smear of a patient with CDA-II with significant anisocytosis, mild poikilocytosis, and frequent spherocytic cells. B, Bone marrow smear of a patient with CDA-II, with several binucleated erythroblasts (arrowheads), a multinucleated erythroblast (arrow), and two erythroblasts with karyorrhexis (thin arrows).

as well as erythroblasts with nuclei with irregular contour or demonstrating karyorrhexis. The nuclei in the binucleated erythroblasts are typically equal in size, and each of the two nuclei has diploid DNA content, suggesting that these cells resulted from a failure of cytokinesis following normal mitosis. The phagocytosis of red cells and erythroblasts by bone marrow macrophages may lead to the formation of Gaucher-like macrophages (pseudo-Gaucher cells).[77]

Electron microscopy reveals the characteristic presence of peripheral cisternae in erythroid cells.[78] These are discontinuous double membranes running parallel to and 40 to 60 nm inward from the inner surface of the cell membrane (*Figure 41.5*).[46,79] Peripheral cisternae are found in red cells and a substantial proportion of mononucleate and binucleate late erythroblasts. They appear to represent endoplasmic reticulum (ER), as they contain protein disulfide isomerase and calreticulin, which are known to be present in ER.[80]

When tested against a panel of ABO-compatible acidified sera (pH 6.8) from normal individuals; about 30% of the sera lyses CDA-II red cells (acidified serum lysis test or Ham test). Unlike paroxysmal nocturnal hemoglobinuria (PNH), there is rarely lysis of the patient's red cells by his or her own serum. In addition, CDA-II cells do not lyse in isotonic sucrose as PNH cells do. The lysis in acidified heterologous sera is due to a naturally occurring complement-binding immunoglobulin (Ig) M antibody against an unidentified antigen on CDA-II cells. The combination of the characteristic morphologic abnormalities and the serologic finding led Crookston et al[81] to propose the acronym

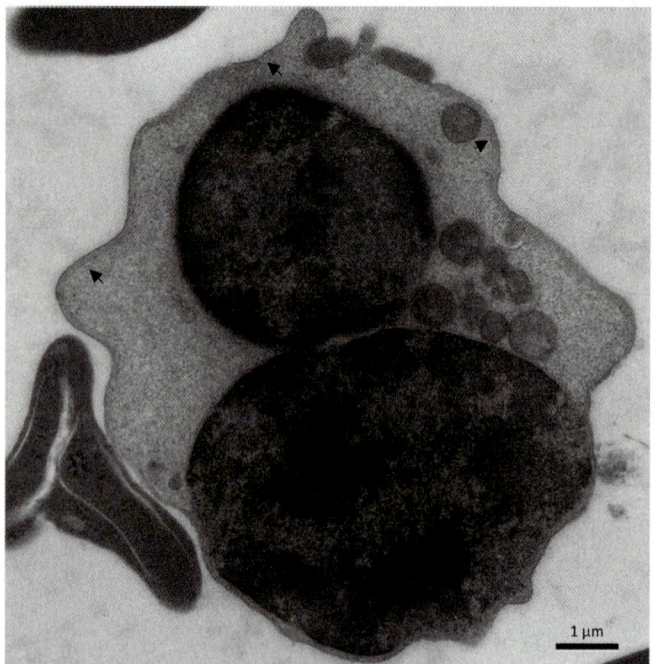

FIGURE 41.5 Electron microscopy of a binucleated erythroblast from a patient with CDA-II with discontinuous double plasma membrane (arrows).

HEMPAS (*h*ereditary *e*rythroblastic *m*ultinuclearity with *p*ositive *a*cidified *s*erum test) for CDA II. While the acidified serum lysis test previously was most informative and useful to diagnose PNH, this test now has been replaced by quantitation of CD55 and CD59 by flow cytometry (see Chapter 32). As a consequence, there is decreased availability of the Ham test in clinical laboratories, and this test is not used commonly to identify CDA II.

Defective *N*-glycosylation of the erythrocyte membrane sialoglycoproteins including band 3 (anion-exchange protein 1) and band 4.5 (glucose transporter 1) was found as a characteristic biochemical feature of CDA-II in the early 1980s.[82-84] This causes band 3 and band 4.5 to migrate at a lower molecular weight on sodium dodecyl sulfate–polyacrylamide gel electrophoresis (SDS-PAGE).[85] During normal maturation of erythroid cells, the erythrocyte membrane proteins are glycosylated with polylactosaminoglycans, and band 3 and band 4.5 proteins normally contain long polylactosamine chains attached to complex *N*-linked oligosaccharides. However, in CDA-II, erythrocyte membrane proteins carry altered *N*-glycans with truncated polylactosamine structures.[86] As a result, glycosylation is shifted to lipid acceptors resulting in the accumulation of polylactosamines as glycolipids. Immunogold electron microscopy analysis using anti-band 3 antibodies reveals irregular clustering of underglycosylated band 3 protein in CDA-II erythrocyte membranes, as compared with normal erythrocytes,[87] likely contributing to loss of membrane and the erythrocyte phenotype of CDA-II resembling HS. SDS-PAGE of red cell membrane proteins was used as a diagnostic criterion in lieu of a positive acidified serum lysis test until *SEC23B* was discovered as the gene causing CDA-II and molecular diagnosis for *SEC23B* mutations became widely available. It is still used in research laboratories as evidence of CDA-II in cases where biallelic pathogenic *SEC23B* variants cannot be identified.

Management

Patients with CDA-II present with a wide spectrum of severity; most have mild anemia, 10% are asymptomatic, and 20% are transfusion dependent.[2,88,89] Splenectomy may modestly improve anemia (by an average of 1.1 to 1.3 g/dL Hgb in two retrospective studies[6,88]) but not the tendency for iron overload, so the current recommendation is to consider splenectomy in CDA-II for severely anemic patients and/or for those with symptomatic splenomegaly.[90]

Patients with CDA-II should be monitored closely for secondary hemochromatosis, which can occur even in the absence of regular transfusion as a result of ineffective erythropoiesis with increased iron absorption.[2,91] The extent of iron overload increases progressively with age,[6,68,88] and about 20% of cases develop cirrhosis, as well as heart failure, diabetes mellitus, and hypergonadotropic hypogonadism without timely intervention with iron chelation treatment.[2,6]

Therefore, close monitoring for iron overload is needed even in transfusion-independent patients. While phlebotomy has been used occasionally in patients with CDA and mild anemia, caution is advised since phlebotomy may aggravate stress erythropoiesis and consequently iron overload. Hematopoietic stem cell transplant (HSCT) has been reported in a few patients in single case reports,[92-94] as well as in a retrospective case series of HSCT for patients with CDA by Miano et al[95] This recent report included 13 patients with CDA-II who received a transplant from sibling (*n* = 5) or from matched unrelated donors (*n* = 8). Overall survival at 36 months was reported as 61%; iron overload was a negative predictive factor, indicating the need for aggressive and early treatment of this complication. Long-term follow-up of patients with CDA who received transplant is needed to evaluate for any unexpected long-term side effects, and care for the identification of donor genotype in related donor transplant is necessary.

Molecular Biology of CDA-II

Abnormalities in two Golgi enzymes had been previously thought to be implicated in the pathogenesis of CDA-II: *N*-acetylglucosaminyltransferase II and α-mannosidase II.[96,97] In fact, an α-mannosidase II knockout mouse reproduces a phenotype similar to CDA-II.[98] However, further familial studies excluded linkage of CDA II to the *N*-acetylglucosaminyltransferase and α-mannosidase II genes.[99]

From studying several families, the causative gene for CDA-II was eventually localized to chromosome 20p11.23-20p12.1. Based on the hypothesis that this gene would likely code for a secretory pathway component since the severe truncation of N-glycans in red cell membrane proteins pointed to a defect in Golgi processing in the erythroblasts, *SEC23B* was identified as the causative gene in 2009 by two different teams.[8,100] *SEC23B* encodes one component of a large group of proteins that assemble to form the coat protein complex II (COPII). COPII-coated vesicles transport secretory proteins from the ER to the Golgi apparatus.[101] The majority of patients with CDA-II harbor biallelic mutations in the *SEC23B* gene, in which more than 100 different mutations have been identified.[2] The most frequent *SEC23B* mutations are the coding-region missense mutations, R14W and E109K, but many more private family missense variants exist.[8,88,100] Several nonsense, frameshift, and splice-site mutations have also been reported.[88,102] Compound heterozygosity for a frameshift or nonsense mutation and a missense mutation result in a more severe CDA II phenotype than does homozygosity or compound heterozygosity for two missense mutations, establishing a genotype-phenotype relationship.[102] In some patients with a CDA-II phenotype, only one *SEC23B* variant has been identified. The existence of deep intronic mutations altering expression, mutations in regulatory elements of *SEC23B*, and digenic inheritance has been hypothesized in these cases.[88] A case of digenic inheritance with a *SEC23B* pathogenic variant and the *GATA1* polymorphism c.-183G>A has been reported.[103] It is notable, as in CDA-I, that patients with CDA II homozygous for nonsense mutations have never been reported, suggesting that some SEC23B expression is necessary for embryonic viability.[8,100]

CDA II cases with *SEC23B* hypomorphic genotypes with low-expression splicing variants have been analyzed for the expression of the SEC23 paralog, *SEC23A*; an upregulation in *SEC23A* expression was reported, suggesting a compensatory mechanism between the SEC23 paralogs.[104] Although *SEC23B* is expressed ubiquitously, *SEC23B* mutations lead to the erythroid-specific phenotype of CDA-II. The expression of its paralog *SEC23A* has been shown to decline significantly during human but not mouse erythroblast differentiation,[105] making SEC23B the critical COPII SEC23 component for human erythroblasts. In contrast, the *SEC23B* knock-out mice do not have an erythropoietic phenotype.[106] Alternatively or in addition to the tissue-specific differential expression of *SEC23B* versus *SEC23A* in terminal human erythropoiesis, SEC23B loss of function may affect the erythroid lineage differentially due to the need for erythroid-specific cargoes (such as band 3), requiring high levels of SEC23B and full function of COPII for the transport from the ER to the Golgi.[2,107] Interestingly, interaction of phosphorylated SEC23B with two other COPII components, SEC24A and SEC24B, was shown to be required for autophagic flux.[108-110] Since autophagy is a process necessary for reticulocyte maturation,[111] further studies are needed to evaluate if *SEC23B* mutations may also affect this final stage of erythropoiesis.

Congenital Dyserythropoietic Anemia Type III

CDA-III was the first CDA to be described in 1951 in an American family by Wolfe and von Hofe under the name familial erythroid multinuclearity. In 1962, Bergström and Jacobsson identified and reported the same as hereditary benign erythroreticulosis in a Swedish family.[112,113] The disease demonstrated an autosomal dominant pattern of inheritance in these families, and it has been found now to be due to a monoallelic *KIF23* mutation (CDA-IIIa). A few sporadic cases, seemingly of an autosomal recessive inheritance or arising de novo, with similar bone marrow morphology of giant multinucleated erythroblasts with up to 12 nuclei (gigantoblasts), were also described.[114-118] Some of these cases were recently shown to be due to biallelic *RACGAP1* mutations (CDA-IIIb).[13,14]

Clinical Features

Affected individuals may experience fatigue, weakness, and episodes of abdominal pain resulting from gallstones. Jaundice exacerbated at times of hemolytic crisis is also reported. Splenomegaly is absent in the dominantly inherited cases, but it is present in most sporadic cases. Marrow hyperplasia with skull erythropoiesis has also been reported in sporadic cases.[117,118] Intravascular hemolysis and consequent hemosiderinuria are reported in both CDA-IIIa and CDA-IIIb. Patients with CDA-IIIa do not appear to have significant stress erythropoiesis, and they have not developed iron overload, possibly because of chronic iron loss due to hemosiderinuria.[119] However, one patient with CDA-IIIb was reported to have significant iron overload, associated with increased medullary and extramedullary stress erythropoiesis.[118] In the Swedish family, the prevalence of monoclonal gammopathy of unknown significance and myeloma is increased,[119] and visual disturbances due to macular degeneration and angioid streaks may be seen in older patients.[120] Interestingly, these additional issues have not been reported in the American family with the same *KIF23* mutation. Single sporadic cases have been reported to develop Hodgkin disease and malignant T-cell lymphoma.[121,122]

Laboratory Features

The macrocytic anemia in patients with CDA-IIIa is generally mild to moderate. Patients with CDA-IIIb have a variable phenotype ranging from mild to transfusion-dependent disease. The peripheral blood smear displays basophilic stippling, irregularly contracted erythrocytes, poikilocytosis, and impressive anisocytosis with "gigantocytes" (*Figure 41.6*).[3] A distinguishing feature of both CDA-IIIa and IIIb is markedly abnormal erythroblast cytokinesis resulting in giant binucleated and multinucleated erythroblasts with up to 16 nuclei (*Figures 41.7* and *41.8*). Electron microscopy

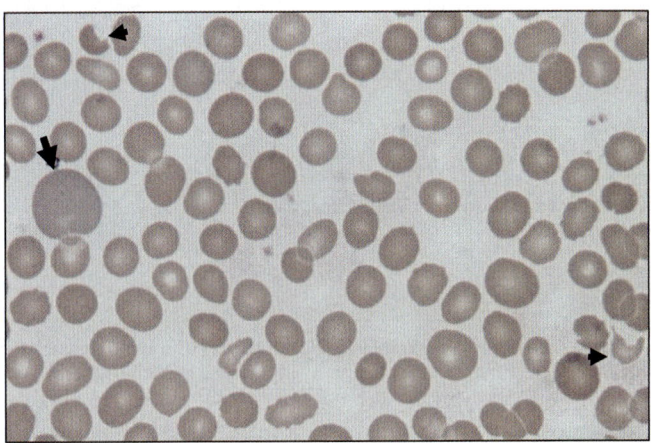

FIGURE 41.6 Peripheral blood smear of a patient with CDA-III due to *KIF23* c.2747C > G (p.P916R) with significant anisocytosis, a giant reticulocyte (arrow), and occasional fragmented cells (arrowheads).

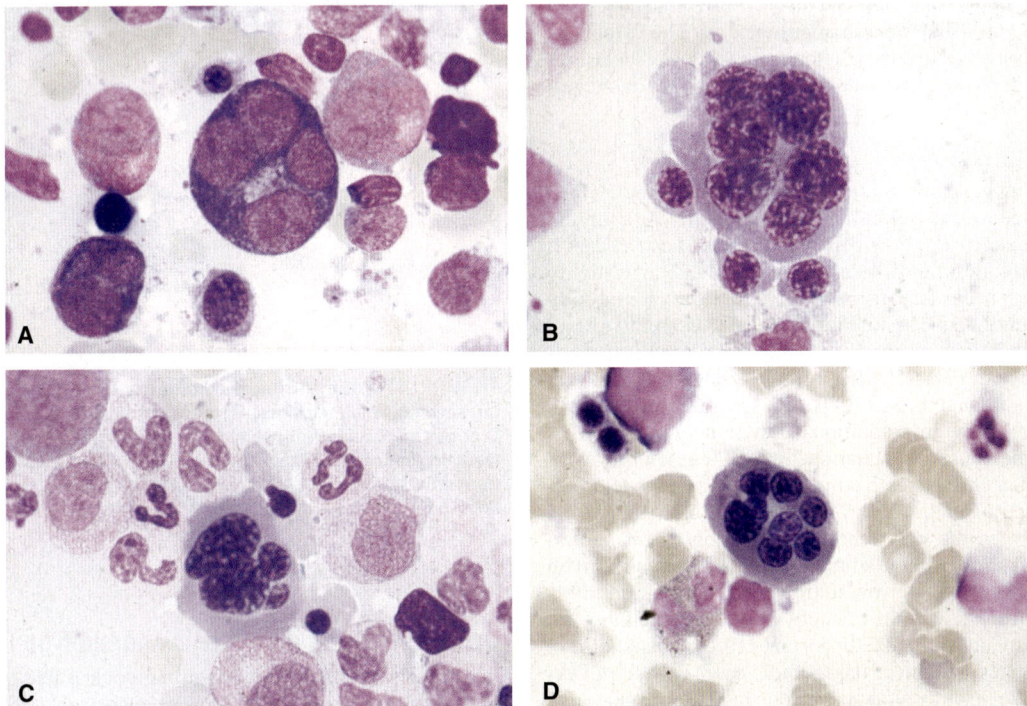

FIGURE 41.7 Multinucleate erythroblasts from the bone marrow of a patient with CDA-IIIa. A, Tetranucleate basophilic erythropoietic cell. B-D, Polychromatic erythroblasts with 6, 4, and 8 nuclei, respectively.

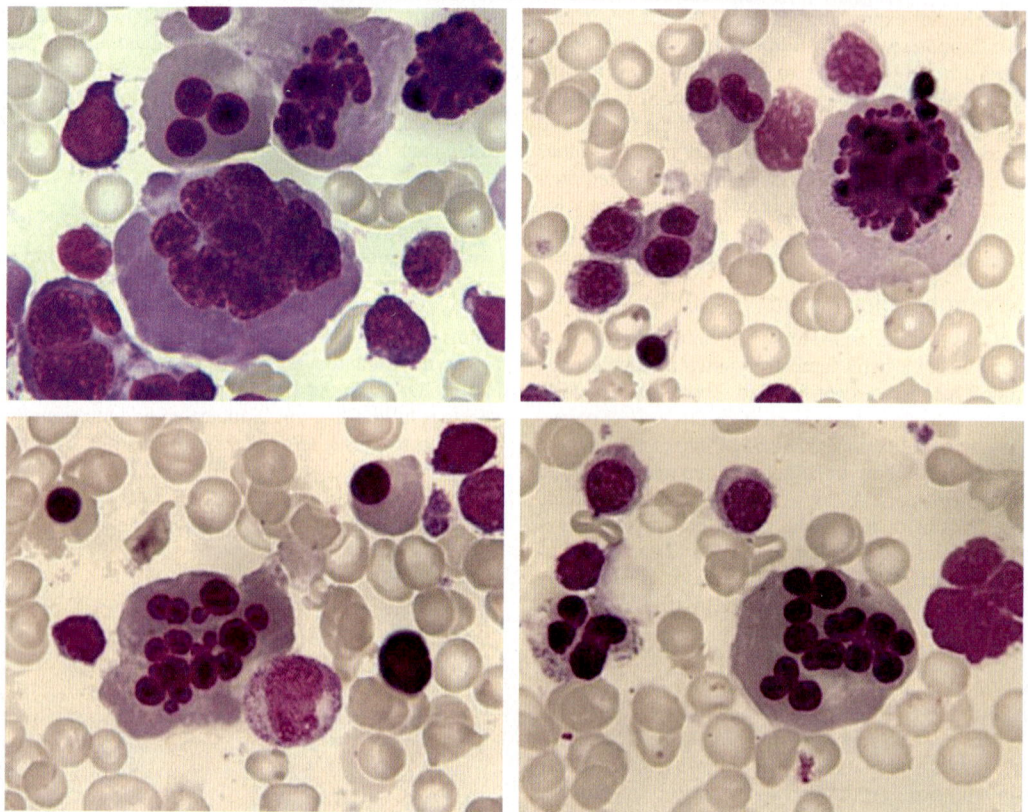

FIGURE 41.8 **Giant erythroblasts (gigantoblasts) with multiple nuclei and additional karyorrhexis from the bone marrow of a patient with CDA-IIIb due to *RACGAP1* mutations.** (Images kindly donated by Dr. Rosario M. Morales-Camacho, Virgen del Rocío, Sevilla, Spain and Dr. Mayka Sanchez, Universitat Internacional de Catalunya (UIC), Sant Cugat del Vallès, Barcelona, Spain.)

shows multinucleated erythroblasts with multiple nuclear clefts in the heterochromatin, which may lead to nuclear lobulation and karyorrhexis (*Figure 41.9*)[123] Individual nuclei within the same multinucleated cells (with up to 16 nuclei) can display different shapes and sizes and abnormal heterochromatin appearance.[123] The cytoplasm of many erythroblasts contains large autophagic vacuoles, inclusions containing β-globin chains, iron-laden mitochondria, and intracytoplasmic myelin figures.[116]

Molecular Biology of CDA III

The disease-causing gene in the autosomal dominant form of CDA-IIIa, which had been localized in the Swedish family to a 4.5-cm interval on chromosome 15q21-q25,[124] was identified as *KIF23*.[9] It encodes for the mitotic kinesin-like protein 1 (MKLP1), a highly conserved protein necessary for central spindle and midbody assembly. The same missense mutation c.2747C.G (p.P916R) in *KIF23* was identified in both the Swedish and the American family as segregating with disease. After MKLP1 knockdown, normal *KIF23* but not the mutant *KIF23* p.P916R was able to rescue the cytokinesis failure, providing additional functional evidence that this was indeed the causative mutation.[9] MKLP1 assembles with RacGAP1/CYK-4, a GTPase-activating protein, to form a heterotetramer, named centralspindlin.[125,126] Centralspindlin organizes the microtubules between the sister chromatids during anaphase into the central spindle, which then stimulates the actomyosin-driven contraction of the cleavage furrow until a microtubule-rich intercellular bridge is formed with the midbody at its center defining the site of absicion.[127] Confirming the importance of centralspindlin in erythroblast cytokinesis, some of the sporadic cases with the CDA-IIIb phenotype were recently shown to be due to biallelic mutations of *RACGAP1*, the gene that encodes the second partner protein in centralspindlin.[13,14]

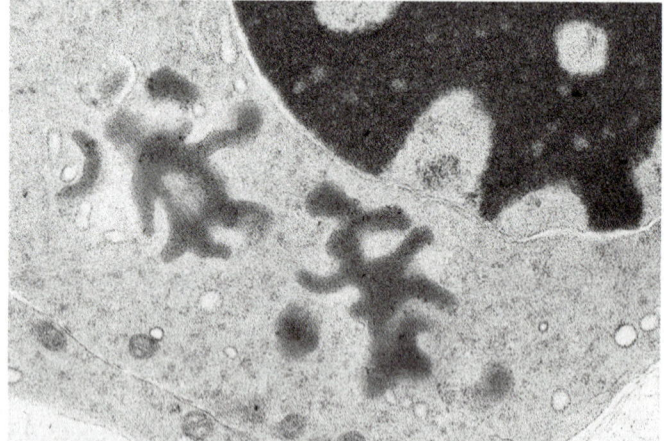

FIGURE 41.9 **Erythroblast from a case of CDA-III showing stellate intracytoplasmic inclusions.** (From Wickramasinghe SN, Wahlin A, Anstee D et al. Observations on two members of the Swedish family with congenital dyserythropoietic anaemia, type III. *Eur J Hematol.* 1993;50(4):213-221. Copyright © 1993 Munksgaard. Reprinted by permission of John Wiley & Sons, Inc.)

Congenital Dyserythropoietic Anemia Type IV

In the early 1990s, a patient with an unclassified type of CDA and high fetal hemoglobin (HbF) was extensively studied.[128-131] In 2010, the erythroid transcription factor *KLF1* was identified as the causative gene,[11] and the disease was classified as CDA-IV. To date, seven additional patients with the similar phenotype have been reported in the literature, all having the dominant (monoallelic) missense variant p.E325K in *KLF1*.[11,128-133]

Clinical Features

The patient with CDA-IV described by Arnaud et al[11] required frequent blood transfusions due to hemolytic anemia, and treatment with erythropoietin or interferon-α was ineffective. Following splenectomy, the patient became transfusion independent. In the small number of patients described so far, there is significant phenotypic variability with increased severity (hydrops fetalis, transfusion dependency until splenectomy, and moderate anemia persisting after splenectomy) in patients with a 46, XY karyotype. Interestingly, there is also a very high possibility of gonadal dysgenesis in patients with 46, XY, with female external genitalia and undescended testicles, which require removal in early childhood to avoid testicular malignancy.[130] Significant iron overload disproportionate to the history of transfusions, as expected with ineffective erythropoiesis, has also been noted.[129]

Laboratory Features

Patients with CDA-IV have hemolytic anemia along with normal or slightly increased reticulocyte count at baseline, pointing to decreased red cell survival along with ineffective erythropoiesis despite significant erythroid hyperplasia in bone marrow evaluation. Patients after splenectomy have reticulocytosis and multiple orthochromatic erythroblasts in the peripheral blood. CDA-IV orthochromatic erythroblasts were shown to have decreased enucleation capacity in comparison with normal control counterparts produced in erythropoiesis cultures in vitro.[11] The circulating erythroblasts and mature erythrocytes in CDA-IV are deficient in the adhesion molecule CD44 and have reduced expression of *AQP1*, which codes for aquaporin 1, a water channel-forming protein (also called Channel-Like Integral Membrane Protein, 28-KD; CHIP28).[134] Since the Indian (In) blood group antigens (In^a and In^b) are located on erythrocyte CD44 glycoprotein and the Colton blood group antigens reside on aquaporin-1, these patients have the unique blood group phenotype being negative for both Indian and Colton blood groups In(a-b-) and Co(a-b-).[135] Increased hemoglobin F (HbF) up to 40% to 50% and small amounts of ζ- and ε-globin chains are also characteristic of CDA-IV, indicating dysregulation of globin gene expression.[11,134-137]

Peripheral blood smear reveals significant anisopoikilocytosis, hypochromia, and multiple nucleated and some binucleated red blood cells (*Figure 41.10*). Light microscopy of the bone marrow aspirate reveals erythroid hyperplasia with binucleate and multinucleate erythroblasts (typically less than 10%), as well as erythroblasts with karyorrhexis and nuclear pyknosis. Rare internuclear bridges may be also seen.[11,129] Electron microscopy analysis demonstrates erythroblasts with invagination of nuclear membrane, abnormally large nuclear pores, and cytoplasmic inclusions.[11,128,129]

Molecular Biology of Congenital Dyserythropoietic Anemia Type IV

Since CDA-IV red cells have multiple molecules altered, including globins and membrane proteins, it was thought that an erythroid transcription factor regulating the expression of multiple genes may be affected. Arnaud et al sequenced first *GATA1* and then *KLF1* and found that two patients with CDA-IV had a de novo variant in exon 3 of the *KLF1* gene, which corresponds to a highly conserved residue in the zinc finger 2 domain, converting glutamate-325 to lysine (E325K).[11] More than 100 *KLF1* variants have been reported, which are classified in four classes: (1) variants with no or minor functional consequences, (2) hypomorphic variants with reduced function, (3) truncating loss-of-function variants, and (4) dominant-negative variants.[138] Compound heterozygosity for null (class 3) *KLF1* mutations was found in a neonate who had kernicterus after presenting with severe nonspherocytic hemolytic anemia (NSHA) with resulting hydrops fetalis, hepatosplenomegaly, and marked erythroblastosis.[139] Such variants in heterozygous status, causing *KLF1* haploinsufficiency as well as the class 1 and 2 variants, are associated with variable benign phenotypes including hereditary persistence of fetal hemoglobin and/or mildly elevated levels of Hb A2 and the rare In(Lu) blood group phenotype (weakly expressed Lutheran antigens).[140] Compound heterozygosity of a class 2 and a class 3 variant is associated with NSHA of variable severity depending on the class 2 variant present.[138,141-144] *KLF1* is a master regulator of erythropoiesis that regulates expression of multiple target genes, including globins, erythrocyte transmembrane and cytoskeletal proteins, RBC enzymes, and those involved in iron metabolism of erythroid precursors, including heme synthetic enzymes and proteins regulating the processing of iron. Mutations in KLF1 thus cause multiple phenotypes other than CDA-IV.[138,144] The only *KLF1* variant of class IV to date is the missense variant p.E325K, which has a strong dominant

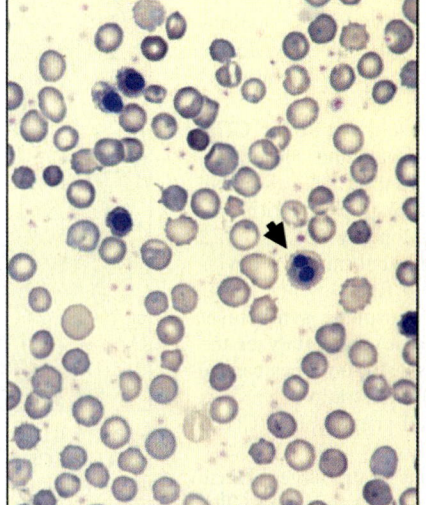
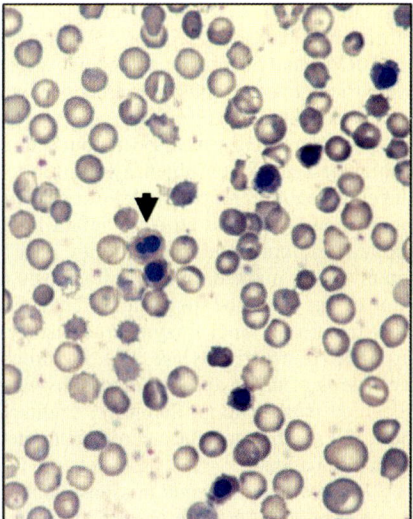

FIGURE 41.10 Peripheral blood smear images of a patient with CDA-IV, with karyotype 46,XY and severe disease, now transfusion independent post splenectomy, with anisocytosis, poikilocytosis, spherocytes, stomatocytes, hypochromic cells, spiculated cells, and multiple nucleated erythrocytes and erythroblasts, some of them binucleated (arrows).

negative effect with ectopic binding across the genome of erythroid progenitor cells and aberrant expression of normal *KLF1*-target and nontarget genes to a "genetic disarray," therefore thought to have a "neomorphic" function for *KLF1*.[145-147]

Congenital Dyserythropoietic Anemia Variants

Certain mutations in *GATA1*, the X-linked critical transcription factor necessary for megakaryopoiesis and erythropoiesis, cause CDA associated with thrombocytopenia.[12,148] The mutation p.V205M was described in two hemizygous boys, half-siblings, born to a mother with mild chronic thrombocytopenia and carrier of this *GATA1* variant. The patients had severe fetal anemia requiring in utero red blood cell transfusions and had anemia and severe thrombocytopenia since birth.[12] Peripheral blood smear was characterized by paucity of platelets and RBC poikilocytosis and anisocytosis. The bone marrow was hypercellular with an abundance of large, multinucleated and binucleated, erythroid precursors and many small and dysplastic megakaryocytes. Interestingly, both boys also had cryptorchidism; normal testicular tissue with germ cells present was identified by biopsy at the time of surgical correction. The variants p.D218G and p. D218Y have been associated with macrothrombocytopenia and mild dyserythropoiesis without anemia,[148] while multiple other mutations of *GATA1* cause different hematologic phenotypes without dyserythropoiesis in an analogous fashion to *KLF1*.[2]

The *ALAS2* variant p.Y365H was reported to cause macrocytic dyserythropoietic anemia in females in a family in an X-linked dominant fashion.[149,150] This missense variant was shown to impair the binding of the enzyme's essential cofactor pyridoxal 5′-phosphate, resulting in loss of function that was not responsive to treatment with pyridoxine. The patients also had iron overload, despite no significant history of transfusions, supporting ineffective erythropoiesis. No male carriers were identified in this family, implying that hemizygosity for this variant may be lethal in utero.[149]

Majeed syndrome is a syndromic form of CDA presenting with chronic recurrent multifocal nonbacterial osteomyelitis (CRMO) and inflammatory neutrophilic dermatosis.[151-154] The disease has significant phenotypic variability even in family members carrying the same mutations.[154,155] Patients frequently present within the first 2 years of life with failure to thrive, bone pain, recurrent fever, evidence of osteitis on MRI, and microcytic anemia of variable severity with high inflammatory markers. Bone marrow evaluation reveals binucleate erythroblasts and internuclear bridging. This syndrome is due to biallelic mutations in *LPIN2*, coding for lipin-2, a magnesium-dependent phosphatidate phosphatase that catalyzes the conversion of phosphatidate to diacylglycerol. Lipin-2 regulates MAPK activation, which mediates synthesis of pro-IL-1β during inflammasome priming.[156] In agreement with these findings the CRMO and microcytic anemia in patients with Majeed syndrome were found to be responsive to treatment with IL1-blockade by anakinra or canakinumab.[153,155]

Two more genes have been found to cause a syndromic CDA characterized by combined dyserythropoietic anemia and neurodevelopmental defects. Biallelic mutations in the *CAD* gene have been shown to cause an early infantile encephalopathy with epilepsy (developmental and epileptic encephalopathy-50) and mild anemia with marked anisopoikilocytosis and abnormal glycosylation of the erythrocyte proteins band-3 and RhAG.[2,17,157] CAD is a multifunctional enzyme (carbamoyl phosphate synthetase, aspartate transcarbamylase, and dihydroorotase) that catalyzes the first steps of de novo pyrimidine biosynthesis. Pyrimidines can be recycled from uridine; therefore, uridine administration improves both the anemia and the neurodevelopmental phenotype of CAD-deficient patients.[17,157]

De novo heterozygous missense mutations in the large ATPase domain of VPS4A were identified as a cause of syndromic CDA with a severe neurodevelopmental disorder,[15,158] while one patient with similar but milder disease had a homozygous variant (p.Ala28Val) in the highly conserved alanine-zipper region of the microtubule-interacting and transport domain of the protein. VPS4A is an ATPase that regulates the ESCRT III machinery in a variety of cellular processes, including cell division and endosomal vesicle trafficking.[159,160] Bone marrow studies showed binucleated erythroblasts and erythroblasts with cytoplasmic bridges (*Figure 41.11*) indicating abnormal cytokinesis and daughter cell separation (abscission), suggesting a critical role of VPS4A in centrosome and spindle assembly.[160,161] Ineffective erythropoiesis is signified by the tendency for significant iron overload, while interestingly this form of CDA has also significant reticulocytosis even before splenectomy. However, there is also significant hemolysis, rendering several patients transfusion dependent. Circulating red blood cells were found to retain transferrin receptor (CD71) in their membrane, demonstrating that VPS4A and the ESCRT III machinery contribute to the process of normal reticulocyte membrane maturation.

Several other cases with anemia and dyserythropoietic features resembling the above described CDAs remain to have their genetic basis identified.[4,5,162-166] These are certainly rare examples, with each affecting only a few families or even a single case, but their study has the potential to offer significant insights on critical molecular pathways for erythropoiesis.

In addition to the congenital dyserythropoietic disorders discussed in this chapter, acquired conditions occasionally can be associated with ineffective erythropoiesis and dyserythropoiesis.[20,24,26] These include nutritional deficiencies such as vitamin B_{12} or folate, severe iron deficiency, the thalassemias, unstable hemoglobins, sideroblastic anemias, myelodysplastic syndromes (MDSs), acute myeloid leukemia, aplastic anemia, malaria, kalaazar, alcohol abuse, and liver disease. It is noteworthy that morphologic features characteristic of CDA-I, -II, and -III may be seen in some acquired dyserythropoietic states. For example, internuclear chromatin bridges such as those seen in CDA-I may be found in MDS, inherited bone marrow failure, in *Plasmodium falciparum* malaria, and during marrow regeneration following transplantation. A high proportion of binucleate late erythroblasts such as those seen in CDA II may be encountered in MDS (*Figure 41.12A*), and marked multinuclearity of erythroblasts as found in CDA III is seen in some cases of erythroleukemia and thiamine-responsive anemia (*Figure 41.12B*).

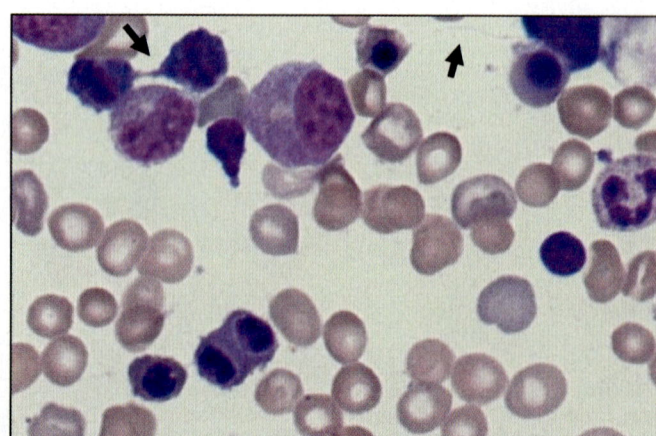

FIGURE 41.11 Bone marrow aspirate smear of a patient with *VPS4A*-associated CDA: binucleated and dysplastic erythroblasts and cytoplasmic rather than chromatin bridges joining erythroblasts post division (arrows).

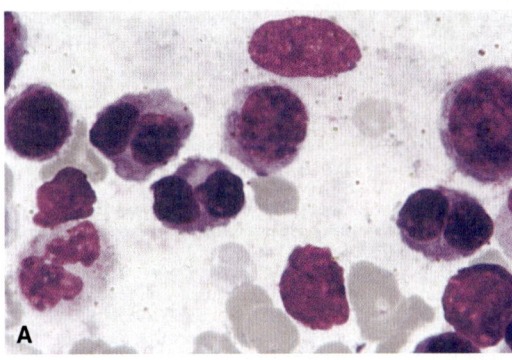
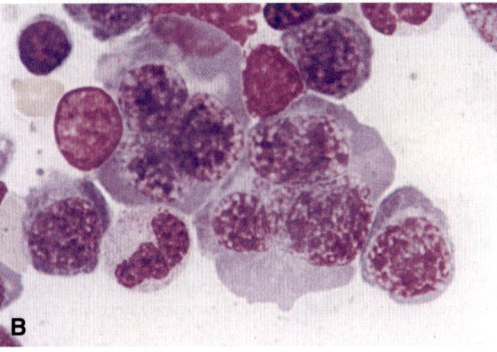

FIGURE 41.12 Bone marrow aspirate smears resembling those of congenital dyserythropoietic anemia. A, Myelodysplastic syndrome with frequent binucleate late polychromatic erythroblasts. B, Thiamine-responsive anemia with multinucleate megaloblasts. (B, Reprinted from Wickramasinghe SN. Macrocytic anemia. In: Wickramasinghe SN, McCullough J, eds. *Blood and Bone Marrow Pathology*. Churchill Livingstone; 2003:229-247. Copyright © 2003 Elsevier. With permission.)

SUMMARY

Although the CDAs are rare, they represent a group of disorders that have progressed from a dusty collection of heterogeneous descriptions to those characterized by their genetic alterations and pathophysiological insights in this modern age of NGS. As a result, our classification scheme can be sorted by virtue of CDA and its molecular biology in a fashion that has true diagnostic power. While disparate biochemical processes are affected, from transcriptional regulation all the way to cytokinesis, and various stages of erythroid development implicated, they are united in the cell biology of erythropoiesis, and in true to form for rare disease, these subtypes have greatly informed our understanding of normal and disease-causing processes. As with any research effort, the increased information that has been uncovered has stimulated entire new areas of investigation, resulting in more questions than answers.

In addition, the heterogeneity overall and within each subtype of CDA demands a healthy respect and humility for the clinician engaged in the diagnosis and management of patients with CDA, also begging the question of whether CDA has been underdiagnosed. Use of modern tools such as NGS in combination with an increased suspicion of CDA suggests a more widespread problem. Thus 21st century hematology practice still demands physicians schooled in both the science and art of clinical care.

References

1. Heimpel H, Wendt F. Congenital dyserythropoietic anemia with karyorrhexis and multinuclearity of erythroblasts. *Helv Med Acta.* 1968;34(2):103-115.
2. Iolascon A, Andolfi I, Russo R. Congenital dyserythropoietic anemias. *Blood.* 2020;136(11):1274-1283.
3. Renella R, Wood WG. The congenital dyserythropoietic anemias. *Hematol Oncol Clin North Am.* 2009;23(2):283-306.
4. Wickramasinghe SN, Vora AJ, Will A, et al. Transfusion-dependent congenital dyserythropoietic anaemia with non-specific dysplastic changes in erythroblasts. *Eur J Haematol.* 1998;60(2):140-142.
5. Niss O, Lorsbach RB, Berger M, et al. Congenital dyserythropoietic anemia type I: first report from the congenital dyserythropoietic anemia registry of North America (CDAR). *Blood Cells Mol Dis.* 2021;87:102534.
6. Heimpel H, Anselstetter V, Chrobak L, et al. Congenital dyserythropoietic anemia type II: epidemiology, clinical appearance, and prognosis based on long-term observation. *Blood.* 2003;102(13):4576-4581.
7. Dgany O, Avidan N, Delaunay J, et al. Congenital dyserythropoietic anemia type I is caused by mutations in codanin-1. *Am J Hum Genet.* 2002;71(6):1467-1474.
8. Schwarz K, Iolascon A, Verissimo F, et al. Mutations affecting the secretory COPII coat component SEC23B cause congenital dyserythropoietic anemia type II. *Nat Genet.* 2009;41(8):936-940.
9. Liljeholm M, Irvine AF, Vikberg AL, et al. Congenital dyserythropoietic anemia type III (CDA III) is caused by a mutation in kinesin family member, KIF23. *Blood.* 2013;121(23):4791-4799.
10. Babbs C, Roberts NA, Sanchez-Pulido L, et al. Homozygous mutations in a predicted endonuclease are a novel cause of congenital dyserythropoietic anemia type I. *Haematologica.* 2013;98(9):1383-1387.
11. Arnaud L, Saison C, Helias V, et al. A dominant mutation in the gene encoding the erythroid transcription factor KLF1 causes a congenital dyserythropoietic anemia. *Am J Hum Genet.* 2010;87(5):721-727.
12. Nichols KE, Crispino JD, Poncz M, et al. Familial dyserythropoietic anaemia and thrombocytopenia due to an inherited mutation in GATA1. *Nat Genet.* 2000;24(3):266-270.
13. Wontakal SN, Britto M, Zhang H, et al. RACGAP1 variants in a sporadic case of CDA III implicates the dysfunction of centralspindlin as the basis of the disease. *Blood.* 2022;139(9):1413-1418.
14. Romero-Cortadellas L, Hernández G, Ferrer-Cortès X, et al. Autosomal recessive congenital dyserythropoietic anemia type III is caused by mutations in the central-spindlin RACGAP1 component. *Blood.* 2021;138(suppl 1):847.
15. Seu KG, Trump LR, Emberesh S, et al. VPS4A mutations in humans cause syndromic congenital dyserythropoietic anemia due to cytokinesis and trafficking defects. *Am J Hum Genet.* 2020.; 107(6):1149-1156.
16. Emberesh M, Giger Seu K, Emberesh S, et al. Peroxiredoxin II (PRDX2) is a novel candidate gene for congenital dyserythropoietic anemia. *Blood.* 2018;132(suppl 1):3605.
17. Russo R, Marra R, Andolfo I, et al. Uridine treatment normalizes the congenital dyserythropoietic anemia type II-like hematological phenotype in a patient with homozygous mutation in the CAD gene. *Am J Hematol.* 2020;95(11):1423-1426.
18. Chonat S, McLemore ML, Bunting ST, Nortman S, Zhang K, Kalfa TA. Congenital dyserythropoietic anaemia type I diagnosed in a young adult with a history of splenectomy in childhood for presumed haemolytic anaemia. *Br J Haematol.* 2018;182(1):10.
19. Kamiya T, Manabe A. Congenital dyserythropoietic anemia. *Int J Hematol.* 2010;92(3):432-438.
20. Wickramasinghe SN. Congenital dyserythropoietic anaemias: clinical features, haematological morphology and new biochemical data. *Blood Rev.* 1998;12(3):178-200.
21. Coffey R, Ganz T. Erythroferrone: an erythroid regulator of hepcidin and iron metabolism. *Hemasphere.* 2018;2(2):e35.
22. Cazzola M, Barosi G, Bergamaschi G, et al. Iron loading in congenital dyserythropoietic anaemias and congenital sideroblastic anaemias. *Br J Haematol.* 1983;54(4):649-654.
23. Tanno T, Bhanu NV, Oneal PA, et al. High levels of GDF15 in thalassemia suppress expression of the iron regulatory protein hepcidin. *Nat Med.* 2007;13(9):1096-1101.
24. Wickramasinghe SN. Dyserythropoiesis and congenital dyserythropoietic anaemias. *Br J Haematol.* 1997;98(4):785-797.
25. Heimpel H, Forteza-Vila J, Queisser W, Spiertz E. Electron and light microscopic study of the erythroblasts of patients with congenital dyserythropoietic anaemia. *Blood.* 1971;37(3):299-310.
26. Wickramasinghe SN, Wood WG. Advances in the understanding of the congenital dyserythropoietic anaemias. *Br J Haematol.* 2005;131(4):431-446.
27. Shalev H, Kapelushnik J, Moser A, Dgany O, Krasnov T, Tamary H. A comprehensive study of the neonatal manifestations of congenital dyserythropoietic anemia type I. *J Pediatr Hematol Oncol.* 2004;26(11):746-748.
28. Shalev H, Kapleushnik Y, Haeskelzon L, et al. Clinical and laboratory manifestations of congenital dyserythropoietic anemia type I in young adults. *Eur J Haematol.* 2002;68(3):170-174.
29. Heimpel H, Schwarz K, Ebnother M, et al. Congenital dyserythropoietic anemia type I (CDA I): molecular genetics, clinical appearance, and prognosis based on long-term observation. *Blood.* 2006;107(1):334-340.
30. Stone P, Zuccollo J. Lethal congenital dyserythropoietic anaemia type I in siblings presenting as pericardial effusions in the second trimester. *Fetal Diagn Ther.* 1999;14(1):11-14.
31. Goede JS, Benz R, Fehr J, Schwarz K, Heimpel H. Congenital dyserythropoietic anemia type I with bone abnormalities, mutations of the CDAN I gene, and significant responsiveness to alpha-interferon therapy. *Ann Hematol.* 2006;85(9):591-595.
32. Tamary H, Offret H, Dgany O, et al. Congenital dyserythropoietic anaemia, type I, in a Caucasian patient with retinal angioid streaks (homozygous Arg1042Trp mutation in codanin-1). *Eur J Haematol.* 2008;80(3):271-274.
33. Roberts E, Madhusudhana KC, Newsom R, Cullis JO. Blindness due to angioid streaks in congenital dyserythropoietic anaemia type I. *Br J Haematol.* 2006;133(5):456.

Disorders of Red Blood Cells

34. Frimmel S, Kniestedt C. Angioid streaks in types I and II Congenital Dyserythropoietic Anaemia (CDA). *Klin Monbl Augenheilkd.* 2016;233(4):482-487.

35. El-Sheikh AA, Hashem H, Holman C, Vyas YM. Congenital dyserythropoietic anemia type I presenting as persistent pulmonary hypertension with pigeon chest deformity. *Pediatr Blood Cancer.* 2014;61(8):1460-1462.

36. Shalev H, Moser A, Kapelushnik J, et al. Congenital dyserythropoietic anemia type I presenting as persistent pulmonary hypertension of the newborn. *J Pediatr.* 2000;136(4):553-555.

37. Kawabata H, Doisaki S, Okamoto A, et al. A case of congenital dyserythropoietic anemia type 1 in a Japanese adult with a CDAN1 gene mutation and an inappropriately low serum hepcidin-25 level. *Intern Med.* 2012;51(8):917-920.

38. Roy NBA, Babbs C. The pathogenesis, diagnosis and management of congenital dyserythropoietic anaemia type I. *Br J Haematol.* 2019;185(3):436-449.

39. Tamary H, Shalev H, Perez-Avraham G, et al. Elevated growth differentiation factor 15 expression in patients with congenital dyserythropoietic anemia type I. *Blood.* 2008;112(13):5241-5244.

40. Meznarich JA, Draper L, Christensen RD, et al. Fetal presentation of congenital dyserythropoietic anemia type 1 with novel compound heterozygous CDAN1 mutations. *Blood Cells Mol Dis.* 2018;71:63-66.

41. Shalev H, Perez-Avraham G, Kapelushnik J, et al. High levels of soluble serum hemojuvelin in patients with congenital dyserythropoietic anemia type I. *Eur J Haematol.* 2013;90(1):31-36.

42. Tamary H, Shalev H, Luria D, et al. Clinical features and studies of erythropoiesis in Israeli Bedouins with congenital dyserythropoietic anemia type I. *Blood.* 1996;87(5):1763-1770.

43. Alloisio N, Jaccoud P, Dorleac E, et al. Alterations of globin chain synthesis and of red cell membrane proteins in congenital dyserythropoietic anemia I and II. *Pediatr Res.* 1982;16(12):1016-1021.

44. Heimpel H, Wendt F, Klemm D, Schubothe H, Heilmeyer L. Congenital dyserythropoietic anemia. [Article in German]. *Arch Klin Med.* 1968;215(2):174-194.

45. Clauvel JP, Cosson A, Breton-Gorius J, et al. Congenital dyserythropoiesis (study of 6 cases). [Article in French]. *Nouv Rev Fr Hematol.* 1972;12(5):653-672.

46. Breton-Gorius J, Daniel MT, Clauvel JP, Dreyfus B. Ultrastructural abnormalities of erythroblasts and erythrocytes in 6 cases of congenital dyserythropoietic anemia. [Article in French]. *Nouv Rev Fr Hematol.* 1973;13(1):23-49.

47. Lewis SM, Nelson DA, Pitcher CS. Clinical and ultrastructural aspects of congenital dyserythropoietic anaemia type I. *Br J Haematol.* 1972;23(1):113-119.

48. Conde E, Mazo E, Baro J, et al. Transmission and scanning electron microscopy study on congenital dyserythropoietic anemia type I. *Acta Haematol.* 1983;70(4):243-249.

49. Hiraoka A, Kanayama Y, Yonezawa T, Kitani T, Tarui S, Hashimoto PH. Congenital dyserythropoietic anemia type I: a freeze-fracture and thin section electron microscopic study. *Blut.* 1983;46(6):329-338.

50. Shalev H, Al-Athamen K, Levi I, Levitas A, Tamary H. Morbidity and mortality of adult patients with congenital dyserythropoietic anemia type I. *Eur J Haematol.* 2017;98(1):13-18.

51. Tamary H, Shalev H, Pinsk V, Zoldan M, Zaizov R. No response to recombinant human erythropoietin therapy in patients with congenital dyserythropoietic anemia type I. *Pediatr Hematol Oncol.* 1999;16(2):165-168.

52. Lavabre-Bertrand T, Blanc P, Navarro R, et al. Alpha-Interferon therapy for congenital dyserythropoiesis type I. *Br J Haematol.* 1995;89(4):929-932.

53. Lavabre-Bertrand T, Ramos J, Delfour C, et al. Long-term alpha interferon treatment is effective on anaemia and significantly reduces iron overload in congenital dyserythropoiesis type I. *Eur J Haematol.* 2004;73(5):380-383.

54. Shamseddine A, Taher A, Jaafar H, et al. Interferon alpha is an effective therapy for congenital dyserythropoietic anaemia type I. *Eur J Haematol.* 2000;65(3):207-209.

55. Parez N, Dommergues M, Zupan V, et al. Severe congenital dyserythropoietic anaemia type I: prenatal management, transfusion support and alpha-interferon therapy. *Br J Haematol.* 2000;110(2):420-423.

56. Abu-Quider A, Asleh M, Shalev H, et al. Treatment of transfusion-dependent congenital dyserythropoietic anemia Type I patients with pegylated interferon alpha-2a. *Eur J Haematol.* 2020;105(2):216-222.

57. Smithson WA, Perrault J. Use of subcutaneous deferoxamine in a child with hemochromatosis associated with congenital dyserythropoietic anemia, type I. *Mayo Clin Proc.* 1982;57(5):322-325.

58. Gambale A, Iolascon A, Andolfo I, Russo R. Diagnosis and management of congenital dyserythropoietic anemias. *Expert Rev Hematol.* 2016;9(3):283-296.

59. Asleh M, Levitas A, Daniel S, Abu-Quider A, Ben-Harosh M, Kapelushnik J. Hepatic and cardiac iron load as determined by MRI T2* in patients with congenital dyserythropoietic anemia type I. *Ann Hematol.* 2020;99(11):2507-2512.

60. Tamary H, Shalmon L, Shalev H, et al. Localization of the gene for congenital dyserythropoietic anemia type I to a <1-cM interval on chromosome 15q15.1-15.3. *Am J Hum Genet.* 1998;62(5):1062-1069.

61. Tamary H, Dgany O, Proust A, et al. Clinical and molecular variability in congenital dyserythropoietic anaemia type I. *Br J Haematol.* 2005;130(4):628-634.

62. Noy-Lotan S, Dgany O, Marcoux N, et al. Cdan1 is essential for primitive erythropoiesis. *Front Physiol.* 2021;12:685242.

63. Tamary H, Dgany O. Congenital dyserythropoietic anemia type I. In: Adam MP, Ardinger HH, Pagon RA, et al., eds. 1993. *GeneReviews((R)).*

64. Pielage J, Stork T, Bunse I, Klambt C. The Drosophila cell survival gene discs lost encodes a cytoplasmic Codanin-1-like protein, not a homolog of tight junction PDZ protein Patj. *Dev Cell.* 2003;5(6):841-851.

65. Noy-Lotan S, Dgany O, Lahmi R, et al. Codanin-1, the protein encoded by the gene mutated in congenital dyserythropoietic anemia type I (CDAN1), is cell cycle-regulated. *Haematologica.* 2009;94(5):629-637.

66. Renella R, Roberts NA, Brown JM, et al. Codanin-1 mutations in congenital dyserythropoietic anemia type 1 affect HP1{alpha} localization in erythroblasts. *Blood.* 2011;117(25):6928-6938.

67. Ask K, Jasencakova Z, Menard P, Feng Y, Almouzni G, Groth A. Codanin-1, mutated in the anaemic disease CDAI, regulates Asf1 function in S-phase histone supply. *EMBO J.* 2012;31(8):2013-2023.

68. Iolascon A, Delaunay J, Wickramasinghe SN, Perrotta S, Gigante M, Camaschella C. Natural history of congenital dyserythropoietic anemia type II. *Blood.* 2001;98(4):1258-1260.

69. Hines GL. Paravertebral extramedullary hematopoiesis (as a posterior mediastinal tumor) associated with congenital dyserythropoietic anemia. *J Thorac Cardiovasc Surg.* 1993;106(4):760-761.

70. Lugassy G, Michaeli J, Harats N, Libson E, Rachmilewitz EA. Paravertebral extramedullary hematopoiesis associated with improvement of anemia in congenital dyserythropoietic anemia type II. *Am J Hematol.* 1986;22(3):295-300.

71. Greiner TC, Burns CP, Dick FR, Henry KM, Mahmood I. Congenital dyserythropoietic anemia type II diagnosed in a 69-year-old patient with iron overload. *Am J Clin Pathol.* 1992;98(5):522-525.

72. Heimpel H, Wilts H, Hirschmann WD, et al. Aplastic crisis as a complication of congenital dyserythropoietic anemia type II. *Acta Haematol.* 2007;117(2):115-118.

73. Ozcan A, Patiroglu T, Acer H, et al. Fibromuscular dysplasia complicated with cerebral stroke in a child with congenital dyserythropoietic anemia type II. *J Pediatr Hematol Oncol.* 2016;38(8):e333-e335.

74. Koklu S, Ertugrul D, Onat AM, et al. Piebaldism associated with congenital dyserythropoietic anemia type II (HEMPAS). *Am J Hematol.* 2002;69(3):210-213.

75. Casanovas G, Swinkels DW, Altamura S, et al. Growth differentiation factor 15 in patients with congenital dyserythropoietic anaemia (CDA) type II. *J Mol Med (Berl).* 2011;89(8):811-816.

76. Russo R, Andolfo I, Manna F, et al. Increased levels of ERFE-encoding FAM132B in patients with congenital dyserythropoietic anemia type II. *Blood.* 2016;128(14):1899-1902.

77. Van Dorpe A, Broeckaert-van O, Desmet V, Verwilghen RL. Gaucher-like cells and congenital dyserythropoietic anaemia, type II (HEMPAS). *Br J Haematol.* 1973;25(2):165-170.

78. Verwilghen RL, Lewis SM, Dacie JV, Crookston JH, Crookston MC. Hempas: congenital dyserythropoietic anaemia (type II). *Q J Med.* 1973;42(166):257-278.

79. Wong KY, Hug G, Lampkin BC. Congenital dyserythropoietic anemia type II: ultrastructural and radioautographic studies of blood and bone marrow. *Blood.* 1972;39(1):23-30.

80. Alloisio N, Texier P, Denoroy L, et al. The cisternae decorating the red blood cell membrane in congenital dyserythropoietic anemia (type II) originate from the endoplasmic reticulum. *Blood.* 1996;87(10):4433-4439.

81. Crookston JH, Crookston MC, Burnie KL, et al. Hereditary erythroblastic multinuclearity associated with a positive acidified-serum test: a type of congenital dyserythropoietic anaemia. *Br J Haematol.* 1969;17(1):11-26.

82. Mawby WJ, Tanner MJ, Anstee DJ, Clamp JR. Incomplete glycosylation of erythrocyte membrane proteins in congenital dyserythropoietic anaemia type II (CDA II). *Br J Haematol.* 1983;55(2):357-368.

83. Fukuda MN, Papayannopoulou T, Gordon-Smith EC, Rochant H, Testa U. Defect in glycosylation of erythrocyte membrane proteins in congenital dyserythropoietic anaemia type II (HEMPAS). *Br J Haematol.* 1984;56(1):55-68.

84. Scartezzini P, Forni GL, Baldi M, Izzo C, Sansone G. Decreased glycosylation of band 3 and band 4.5 glycoproteins of erythrocyte membrane in congenital dyserythropoietic anaemia type II. *Br J Haematol.* 1982;51(4):569-576.

85. Anselstetter V, Horstmann HJ, Heimpel H. Congenital dyserythropoietic anaemia, types I and II: aberrant pattern of erythrocyte membrane proteins in CDA II, as revealed by two-dimensional polyacrylamide gel electrophoresis. *Br J Haematol.* 1977;35(2):209-215.

86. Denecke J, Kranz C, Nimtz M, et al. Characterization of the N-glycosylation phenotype of erythrocyte membrane proteins in congenital dyserythropoietic anemia type II (CDA II/HEMPAS). *Glycoconj J.* 2008;25(4):375-382.

87. Fukuda MN, Klier G, Yu J, Scartezzini P. Anomalous clustering of underglycosylated band 3 in erythrocytes and their precursor cells in congenital dyserythropoietic anemia type II. *Blood.* 1986;68(2):521-529.

88. Russo R, Gambale A, Langella C, Andolfo I, Unal S, Iolascon A. Retrospective cohort study of 205 cases with congenital dyserythropoietic anemia type II: definition of clinical and molecular spectrum and identification of new diagnostic scores. *Am J Hematol.* 2014;89(10):E169-E175.

89. Bianchi P, Schwarz K, Hogel J, et al. Analysis of a cohort of 101 CDAII patients: description of 24 new molecular variants and genotype-phenotype correlations. *Br J Haematol.* 2016;175(4):696-704.

90. Iolascon A, Andolfo I, Barcellini W, et al. Recommendations regarding splenectomy in hereditary hemolytic anemias. *Haematologica.* 2017;102(8):1304-1313.

91. Halpern Z, Rahmani R, Levo Y. Severe hemochromatosis: the predominant clinical manifestation of congenital dyserythropoietic anemia type 2. *Acta Haematol.* 1985;74(3):178-180.

92. Iolascon A, Sabato V, de Mattia D, Locatelli F. Bone marrow transplantation in a case of severe, type II congenital dyserythropoietic anaemia (CDA II). *Bone Marrow Transplant.* 2001;27(2):213-215.

93. Modi G, Shah S, Madabhavi I, et al. Successful allogeneic hematopoietic stem cell transplantation of a patient suffering from type II congenital dyserythropoietic anemia A rare case report from Western India. *Case Rep Hematol.* 2015;2015:792485.

94. Unal S, Russo R, Gumruk F, et al. Successful hematopoietic stem cell transplantation in a patient with congenital dyserythropoietic anemia type II. *Pediatr Transplant.* 2014;18(4):E130-E133.

95. Miano M, Eikema DJ, Aljurf M, et al. Stem cell transplantation for congenital dyserythropoietic anemia: an analysis from the European Society for Blood and Marrow Transplantation. *Haematologica*. 2019;104(8):e335-e339.

96. Fukuda MN, Dell A, Scartezzini P. Primary defect of congenital dyserythropoietic anemia type II. Failure in glycosylation of erythrocyte lactosaminoglycan proteins caused by lowered N-acetylglucosaminyltransferase II. *J Biol Chem*. 1987;262(15):7195-7206.

97. Fukuda MN, Masri KA, Dell A, Luzzatto L, Moremen KW. Incomplete synthesis of N-glycans in congenital dyserythropoietic anemia type II caused by a defect in the gene encoding alpha-mannosidase II. *Proc Natl Acad Sci U S A*. 1990;87(19):7443-7447.

98. Chui D, Oh-Eda M, Liao YF, et al. Alpha-mannosidase-II deficiency results in dyserythropoiesis and unveils an alternate pathway in oligosaccharide biosynthesis. *Cell*. 1997;90(1):157-167.

99. Iolascon A, Miraglia del Giudice E, Perrotta S, Granatiero M, Zelante L, Gasparini P. Exclusion of three candidate genes as determinants of congenital dyserythropoietic anemia type II (CDA-II). *Blood*. 1997;90(10):4197-4200.

100. Bianchi P, Fermo E, Vercellati C, et al. Congenital dyserythropoietic anemia type II (CDAII) is caused by mutations in the SEC23B gene. *Hum Mutat*. 2009;30(9):1292-1298.

101. Gomez-Navarro N, Miller EA. COP-coated vesicles. *Curr Biol*. 2016;26(2):R54-R57.

102. Iolascon A, Russo R, Esposito MR, et al. Molecular analysis of 42 patients with congenital dyserythropoietic anemia type II: new mutations in the SEC23B gene and a search for a genotype-phenotype relationship. *Haematologica*. 2010;95(5):708-715.

103. Russo R, Andolfo I, Gambale A, et al. GATA1 erythroid-specific regulation of SEC23B expression and its implication in the pathogenesis of congenital dyserythropoietic anemia type II. *Haematologica*. 2017;102(9):e371-e374.

104. Russo R, Langella C, Esposito MR, et al. Hypomorphic mutations of SEC23B gene account for mild phenotypes of congenital dyserythropoietic anemia type II. *Blood Cells Mol Dis*. 2013;51(1):17-21.

105. Satchwell TJ, Pellegrin S, Bianchi P, et al. Characteristic phenotypes associated with congenital dyserythropoietic anemia (type II) manifest at different stages of erythropoiesis. *Haematologica*. 2013;98(11):1788-1796.

106. King R, Lin Z, Balbin-Cuesta G, et al.. SEC23A rescues SEC23B-deficient congenital dyserythropoietic anemia type II. *Sci Adv*. 2021;7(48):eabj5293.

107. Russo R, Esposito MR, Iolascon A. Inherited hematological disorders due to defects in coat protein (COP)II complex. *Am J Hematol*. 2013;88(2):135-140.

108. Davis S, Wang J, Ferro-Novick S. Crosstalk between the secretory and autophagy pathways regulates autophagosome formation. *Dev Cell*. 2017;41(1):23-32.

109. Jeong YT, Simoneschi D, Keegan S, et al. The ULK1-FBXW5-SEC23B nexus controls autophagy. *Elife*. 2018;7:e42253.

110. Ishihara N, Hamasaki M, Yokota S, et al. Autophagosome requires specific early Sec proteins for its formation and NSF/SNARE for vacuolar fusion. *Mol Biol Cell*. 2001;12(11):3690-3702.

111. Griffiths RE, Kupzig S, Cogan N, et al. Maturing reticulocytes internalize plasma membrane in glycophorin A-containing vesicles that fuse with autophagosomes before exocytosis. *Blood*. 2012;119(26):6296-6306.

112. Wolff JA, Von Hofe FH. Familial erythroid multinuclearity. *Blood*. 1951;6(12):1274-1283.

113. Bergstrom I, Jacobsson L. Hereditary benign erythroreticulosis. *Blood*. 1962;19:296-303.

114. Sandstrom H, Wahlin A. Congenital dyserythropoietic anemia type III. *Haematologica*. 2000;85(7):753-757.

115. Wickramasinghe SN, Parry TE, Williams C, Bond AN, Hughes M, Crook S. A new case of congenital dyserythropoietic anaemia, type III: studies of the cell cycle distribution and ultrastructure of erythroblasts and of nucleic acid synthesis in marrow cells. *J Clin Pathol*. 1982;35(10):1103-1109.

116. Villegas A, Gonzalez L, Furio V, et al. Congenital dyserythropoietic anemia type III with unbalanced globin chain synthesis. *Eur J Haematol*. 1994;52(4):251-253.

117. Perez-Jacoiste Asin MA, Ruiz Robles G. Skull erythropoiesis in a patient with congenital dyserythropoietic anaemia. *Lancet*. 2016;387(10020):787.

118. Oh A, Patel PR, Aardsma N, et al. Non-myeloablative allogeneic stem cell transplant with post-transplant cyclophosphamide cures the first adult patient with congenital dyserythropoietic anemia. *Bone Marrow Transplant*. 2017;52(6):905-906.

119. Sandstrom H, Wahlin A, Eriksson M, Bergstrom I, Wickramasinghe SN. Intravascular haemolysis and increased prevalence of myeloma and monoclonal gammopathy in congenital dyserythropoietic anaemia, type III. *Eur J Haematol*. 1994;52(1):42-46.

120. Sandstrom H, Wahlin A, Eriksson M, Holmgren G, Lind L, Sandgren O. Angioid streaks are part of a familial syndrome of dyserythropoietic anaemia (CDA III). *Br J Haematol*. 1997;98(4):845-849.

121. Byrnes RK, Dhru R, Brady AM, Galen WP, Hopper B. Congenital dyserythropoietic anemia in treated Hodgkin's disease. *Hum Pathol*. 1980;11(5):485-486.

122. McCluggage WG, Hull D, Mayne E, Bharucha H, Wickramasinghe SN. Malignant lymphoma in congenital dyserythropoietic anaemia type III. *J Clin Pathol*. 1996;49(7):599-602.

123. Bjorksen B, Holmgren G, Roos G, Stenling R. Congenital dyserythropoietic anaemia type III: an electron microscopic study. *Br J Haematol*. 1978;38(1):37-42.

124. Lind L, Sandstrom H, Wahlin A, et al. Localization of the gene for congenital dyserythropoietic anemia type III, CDAN3, to chromosome 15q21-q25. *Hum Mol Genet*. 1995;4(1):109-112.

125. White EA, Glotzer M. Centralspindlin: at the heart of cytokinesis. *Cytoskeleton (Hoboken)*. 2012;69(11):882-892.

126. Traxler E, Weiss MJ. Congenital dyserythropoietic anemias: III's a charm. *Blood*. 2013;121(23):4614-4615.

127. Lekomtsev S, Su KC, Pye VE, et al. Centralspindlin links the mitotic spindle to the plasma membrane during cytokinesis. *Nature*. 2012;492(7428):276-279.

128. de-la-Iglesia-Inigo S, Moreno-Carralero MI, Lemes-Castellano A, Molero-Labarta T, Mendez M, Moran-Jimenez MJ. A case of congenital dyserythropoietic anemia type IV. *Clin Case Rep*. 2017;5(3):248-252.

129. Jaffray JA, Mitchell WB, Gnanapragasam MN, et al. Erythroid transcription factor EKLF/KLF1 mutation causing congenital dyserythropoietic anemia type IV in a patient of Taiwanese origin: review of all reported cases and development of a clinical diagnostic paradigm. *Blood Cells Mol Dis*. 2013;51(2):71-75.

130. Ravindranath Y, Johnson RM, Goyette G, Buck S, Gadgeel M, Gallagher PG. KLF1 E325K-associated congenital dyserythropoietic anemia type IV: insights into the variable clinical severity. *J Pediatr Hematol Oncol*. 2018;40(6):e405-e409.

131. Kohara H, Utsugisawa T, Sakamoto C, et al. KLF1 mutation E325K induces cell cycle arrest in erythroid cells differentiated from congenital dyserythropoietic anemia patient-specific induced pluripotent stem cells. *Exp Hematol*. 2019;73:25-37 e28.

132. Ortolano R, Forouhar M, Warwick A, Harper D. A case of congenital dyserythropoietic anemia type IV caused by E325K mutation in erythroid transcription factor KLF1. *J Pediatr Hematol Oncol*. 2018;40(6):e389-e391.

133. Russo R, Andolfo I, Manna F, et al. Multi-gene panel testing improves diagnosis and management of patients with hereditary anemias. *Am J Hematol*. 2018;93(5):672-682.

134. Agre P, Smith BL, Baumgarten R, et al. Human red cell Aquaporin CHIP. II. Expression during normal fetal development and in a novel form of congenital dyserythropoietic anemia. *J Clin Invest*. 1994;94(3):1050-1058.

135. Parsons SF, Jones J, Anstee DJ, et al. A novel form of congenital dyserythropoietic anemia associated with deficiency of erythroid CD44 and a unique blood group phenotype [In(a-b-), Co(a-b-)]. *Blood*. 1994;83(3):860-868.

136. Tang W, Cai SP, Eng B, et al. Expression of embryonic zeta-globin and epsilon-globin chains in a 10-year-old girl with congenital anemia. *Blood*. 1993;81(6):1636-1640.

137. Wickramasinghe SN, Illum N, Wimberley PD. Congenital dyserythropoietic anaemia with novel intra-erythroblastic and intra-erythrocytic inclusions. *Br J Haematol*. 1991;79(2):322-330.

138. Perkins A, Xu X, Higgs DR, et al. Kruppeling erythropoiesis: an unexpected broad spectrum of human red blood cell disorders due to KLF1 variants. *Blood*. 2016;127(15):1856-1862.

139. Magor GW, Tallack MR, Gillinder KR, et al. KLF1-null neonates display hydrops fetalis and a deranged erythroid transcriptome. *Blood*. 2015;125(15):2405-2417.

140. Waye JS, Eng B. Kruppel-like factor 1: hematologic phenotypes associated with KLF1 gene mutations. *Int J Lab Hematol*. 2015;37(suppl 1):78-84.

141. Huang J, Zhang X, Liu D, et al. Compound heterozygosity for KLF1 mutations is associated with microcytic hypochromic anemia and increased fetal hemoglobin. *Eur J Hum Genet*. 2015;23(10):1341-1348.

142. Viprakasit V, Ekwattanakit S, Riolueang S, et al. Mutations in Kruppel-like factor 1 cause transfusion-dependent hemolytic anemia and persistence of embryonic globin gene expression. *Blood*. 2014;123(10):1586-1595.

143. Belgemen-Ozer T, Gorukmez O. A very rare congenital dyserythropoietic anemia variant-type IV in a patient with a novel mutation in the KLF1 gene: a case report and review of the literature. *J Pediatr Hematol Oncol*. 2020;42(6):e536-e540.

144. Perkins AC, Bieker J. Congenital anemia phenotypes due to KLF1 mutations. *J Pediatr Hematol Oncol*. 2021;43(1):e148-e149.

145. Ilsley MD, Huang S, Magor GW, Landsberg MJ, Gillinder KR, Perkins AC. Corrupted DNA-binding specificity and ectopic transcription underpin dominant neomorphic mutations in KLF/SP transcription factors. *BMC Genom*. 2019;20(1):417.

146. Kulczynska K, Bieker JJ, Siatecka M. A Kruppel-like factor 1 (KLF1) mutation associated with severe congenital dyserythropoietic anemia alters its DNA-binding specificity. *Mol Cell Biol*. 2020;40(5).

147. Varricchio L, Planutis A, Manwani D, et al. Genetic disarray follows mutant KLF1-E325K expression in a congenital dyserythropoietic anemia patient. *Haematologica*. 2019;104(12):2372-2380.

148. Freson K, Thys C, Wittewrongel C, Vermylen J, Hoylaerts MF, Van Geet C. Molecular cloning and characterization of the GATA1 cofactor human FOG1 and assessment of its binding to GATA1 proteins carrying D218 substitutions. *Hum Genet*. 2003;112(1):42-49.

149. Sankaran VG, Ulirsch JC, Tchaikovskii V, et al. X-linked macrocytic dyserythropoietic anemia in females with an ALAS2 mutation. *J Clin Invest*. 2015;125(4):1665-1669.

150. Sankaran VG, Ulirsch JC, Tchaikovskii V, et al. X-linked macrocytic dyserythropoietic anemia in females with an ALAS2 mutation. *J Clin Invest*. 2020;130(1):552.

151. Al-Mosawi ZS, Al-Saad KK, Ijadi-Maghsoodi R, El-Shanti HI, Ferguson PJ. A splice site mutation confirms the role of LPIN2 in Majeed syndrome. *Arthritis Rheum*. 2007;56(3):960-964.

152. Ferguson PJ, Chen S, Tayeh MK, et al. Homozygous mutations in LPIN2 are responsible for the syndrome of chronic recurrent multifocal osteomyelitis and congenital dyserythropoietic anaemia (Majeed syndrome). *J Med Genet*. 2005;42(7):551-557.

153. Herlin T, Fiirgaard B, Bjerre M, et al. Efficacy of anti-IL-1 treatment in Majeed syndrome. *Ann Rheum Dis*. 2013;72(3):410-413.

154. Rao AP, Gopalakrishna DB, Bing X, Ferguson PJ. Phenotypic variability in Majeed syndrome. *J Rheumatol*. 2016;43(6):1258-1259.

155. Roy NBA, Zaal AI, Hall G, et al. Majeed syndrome: description of a novel mutation and therapeutic response to bisphosphonates and IL-1 blockade with anakinra. *Rheumatology (Oxford)*. 2020;59(2):448-451.

156. Lorden G, Sanjuan-Garcia I, de Pablo N, et al. Lipin-2 regulates NLRP3 inflammasome by affecting P2X7 receptor activation. *J Exp Med*. 2017;214(2):511-528.

Disorders of Red Blood Cells

157. Koch J, Mayr JA, Alhaddad B, et al. CAD mutations and uridine-responsive epileptic encephalopathy. *Brain*. 2017;140(2):279-286.

158. Rodger C, Flex E, Allison RJ, et al. De novo VPS4A mutations cause Multisystem disease with abnormal neurodevelopment. *Am J Hum Genet*. 2020;107(6):1129-1148.

159. Scott A, Gaspar J, Stuchell-Brereton MD, Alam SL, Skalicky JJ, Sundquist WI. Structure and ESCRT-III protein interactions of the MIT domain of human VPS4A. *Proc Natl Acad Sci U S A*. 2005;102(39):13813-13818.

160. Morita E, Colf LA, Karren MA, Sandrin V, Rodesch CK, Sundquist WI. Human ESCRT-III and VPS4 proteins are required for centrosome and spindle maintenance. *Proc Natl Acad Sci U S A*. 2010;107(29):12889-12894.

161. Mierzwa BE, Chiaruttini N, Redondo-Morata L, et al. Dynamic subunit turnover in ESCRT-III assemblies is regulated by Vps4 to mediate membrane remodelling during cytokinesis. *Nat Cell Biol*. 2017;19(7):787-798.

162. Carter C, Darbyshire PJ, Wickramasinghe SN. A congenital dyserythropoietic anaemia variant presenting as hydrops fetalis. *Br J Haematol*. 1989;72(2):289-290.

163. Woessner S, Trujillo M, Florensa L, Mesa MC, Wickramasinghe SN. Congenital dyserthropoietic anaemia other than type I to III with a peculiar erythroblastic morphology. *Eur J Haematol*. 2003;71(3):211-214.

164. Heimpel H, Kohne E, Schrod L, Schwarz K, Wickramasinghe S. A new type of transfusion-dependent congenital dyserythropoietic anemia. *Haematologica*. 2007;92(10):1427-1428.

165. Kenny MW, Ibbotson RM, Hand MJ, Tector MJ. Congenital dyserythropoietic anaemia with unusual cytoplasmic inclusions. *J Clin Pathol*. 1978;31(12):1228-1233.

166. Wickramasinghe SN, Spearing RL, Hill GR. Congenital dyserythropoiesis with intererythroblastic chromatin bridges and ultrastructurally-normal erythroblast heterochromatin: a new disorder. *Br J Haematol*. 1998;103(3):831-834.

Chapter 42 ■ Anemia of Inflammation and of Systemic Disorders

ROBERT T. MEANS JR

ANEMIA OF INFLAMMATION

Anemia of Inflammation/Chronic Disease

The anemia that is often observed in patients with infectious, inflammatory, or neoplastic diseases that persists for more than 1 or 2 months was traditionally called *anemia of chronic disease* (ACD). The term was a problematic one, as it usually was not considered to include anemias caused by renal insufficiency, hepatic disease, or endocrinopathy, even when those disorders were chronic. Those other syndromes are discussed in the sections "Anemia of Chronic Kidney Disease," "Anemia in Cirrhosis and Other Liver Diseases," and "Anemias Associated with Endocrine Disorders" in this chapter. More recently, it has become almost universally referred to as the *anemia of inflammation* (AI). Regardless of the name used, the characteristic feature of this syndrome is the occurrence of hypoferremia in the presence of ample reticuloendothelial iron stores.[1-4] The term AI will be used in this chapter, with certain exceptions relating to historical association of specific syndromes with ACD.

Associated Syndromes

AI is extremely common and, overall, is probably more common than any anemia syndrome other than blood loss with consequent iron deficiency. Cash and Sears evaluated all the anemic individuals admitted to the medical service of a busy municipal hospital during two 2-month periods in 1985 and 1986.[5] After patients with active bleeding, hemolysis, or known hematologic malignancy were excluded, 52% of anemic patients met laboratory criteria for "ACD." While 60% of these patients with ACD had one of the infectious, inflammatory, or neoplastic diseases traditionally associated with ACD, an additional 16% had renal insufficiency, with the remaining 24% having an assortment of other disorders. It has been reported that AI is present in 27% of outpatients with rheumatoid arthritis,[6] 15% of patients with ankylosing spondylitis requiring anti–tumor necrosis factor (TNF) agents,[7] and 17% of patients with severe COVID-19 at the time of hospital admission.[8] In a database of anemic patients with rheumatoid arthritis, AI is present in 55%, frequently with concurrent iron deficiency.[9] Clinical disorders commonly associated with AI are listed in *Table 42.1*.

Clinical and Laboratory Description

The clinical manifestations of AI vary widely, reflecting the differing clinical syndromes with which it is associated. The signs and symptoms of the underlying disorder usually overshadow those of the anemia, but on rare occasions, developing anemia provides the first evidence of the primary condition. This situation may be observed particularly in difficult-to-diagnose clinical syndromes, such as temporal arteritis.[10]

Anemia
Development and Severity

Typically, anemia develops during the first 1 to 2 months of illness and thereafter does not progress. The hematocrit usually is maintained above 25%,[2] but significantly lower values are observed in 20% to 30% of patients.[5,6] The hemoglobin concentration and hematocrit generally provide an accurate reflection of the extent to which the circulating red cell mass is reduced, although in certain cases, expansion of the total blood volume would mean that the reduction in red cell mass is less than what the hemoglobin or hematocrit indicates.[11]

A general correlation exists between the degree of anemia and the severity of the underlying disease.[2] For example, patients with rheumatoid arthritis may show a correlation between anemia severity and arthritis activity.[12]

Typically, the percentage of reticulocytes is normal or reduced, although on rare occasions it may be slightly increased.[2] The absolute reticulocyte count and reticulocyte production index are decreased, although not to the same degree seen in primary marrow failure states like aplastic anemia or pure red cell aplasia.

Morphologic Features

The erythrocytes usually are normocytic and normochromic; however, hypochromia and microcytosis may be observed. Microcytosis (mean corpuscular volume [MCV] < 80 fL) can occur in AI but is usually not as striking as that commonly associated with iron deficiency anemia; values for MCV < 75 fL are rare in AI. Hypochromia (mean corpuscular hemoglobin concentration, normal range 26-32 g/dL) is more common than microcytosis. It is observed in almost half

Table 42.1. Conditions Associated With Anemia of Inflammation

Infections
Chronic fungal disease
Chronic urinary tract infections
Human immunodeficiency virus
Meningitis
Osteomyelitis
Pelvic inflammatory disease
Pulmonary infections: abscesses, emphysema, tuberculosis, pneumonia
SARS-CoV-19
Subacute bacterial endocarditis
Noninfectious Inflammation
Ankylosing spondylitis
Rheumatic fever
Rheumatoid arthritis (including juvenile rheumatoid arthritis)
Severe trauma
Systemic lupus erythematosus
Temporal arteritis/polymyalgia rheumatic/giant cell arteritis
Thermal injury
Vasculitis
Malignant Diseases
Carcinoma
Hodgkin disease
Non-Hodgkin lymphoma
Leukemia
Multiple myeloma
Miscellaneous
Alcoholic liver disease
Congestive heart failure
Thrombophlebitis
Ischemic heart disease
Idiopathic

Disorders of Red Blood Cells

of patients with AI[13] and may be observed even though the hematocrit remains within normal limits. Another distinction from iron deficiency is that hypochromia typically precedes microcytosis in AI but typically follows the development of microcytosis in iron deficiency.[2] Slight anisocytosis and poikilocytosis may be detected, but such changes tend to be less prominent than in iron-deficient subjects. Routine examination of the blood smear rarely reveals specific morphologic abnormalities. The width of the erythrocyte size distribution curve (red cell distribution width) is typically elevated to a moderate degree and generally does not help in distinguishing iron deficiency and AI.

Laboratory Markers of Iron Status

Characteristically, serum iron concentration is decreased, total iron-binding capacity (or serum transferrin concentration) is reduced, and transferrin saturation may be below normal, sometimes in the range observed with iron deficiency. In patients with infection, hypoferremia develops early in the course of the illness, often within 24 hours, and is observed even in acute, self-limited febrile diseases, or after experimentally induced fever in humans or animals.[14] When the infection is of short duration, the serum iron returns to normal and anemia does not develop; in prolonged illnesses, the serum iron level remains low as long as the disease is active.

In bone marrow aspirates stained for iron, the number of sideroblasts is reduced to 5% to 20% of the total quantity of normoblasts (normal, 30%-50%). In contrast, the amount of hemosiderin within macrophages usually is increased; exceptions to this probably represent AI cases complicated by concurrent iron deficiency, a fairly common finding.[2,9]

Serum ferritin level is a useful indicator of iron status in patients without underlying inflammatory disorders. In patients with AI, however, the serum ferritin level indicative of adequate reticuloendothelial iron stores requires upward adjustment. Serum ferritin values usually increase in patients with inflammatory diseases,[15] and extreme elevations of serum ferritin may be a nonspecific indicator of significant underlying disease.[16,17] When iron deficiency coexists, the serum ferritin level falls but may not reach values as low as those found in uncomplicated iron deficiency. Values of 60 to 100 ng/mL, previously suggested as the appropriate lower limit of normal for serum ferritin in chronic inflammation, may be too low, and adjustment of the ferritin cutoff may be required.[15,18] At one institution, all hospitalized patients undergoing bone marrow examination with serum ferritin levels <30 ng/mL lacked stainable iron on marrow examination but so did approximately one-third of hospitalized patients with serum ferritin levels between 100 and 200 ng/mL.[19] Adjusting the serum ferritin level indicative of iron deficiency with other parameters, such as erythrocyte sedimentation rate and C-reactive protein, increases its sensitivity for detecting iron deficiency, but there is no consensus on how to make such an adjustment.[15] A patient with chronic inflammatory disease and a serum ferritin <30 ng/mL is certainly iron deficient, and a patient with a serum ferritin >200 ng/mL is certainly not iron deficient; in other circumstances, other studies may be required. The recognition of concurrent iron deficiency in patients with chronic inflammatory states is not a trivial issue: in one study in which iron deficiency was diagnosed by bone marrow examination, it was present in 27% of anemic patients with active rheumatoid arthritis. A more recent study using biochemical parameters reported that 55% of patients had both iron deficiency and AI.[9]

Elevated concentration of soluble transferrin receptors (sTfRs) in serum is another way to identify iron-deficient individuals with normal serum ferritin concentrations.[20] Serum or plasma sTfR concentration is elevated in iron deficiency but is not elevated in uncomplicated AI. It will be elevated in AI cases complicated by iron deficiency.[21] sTfR concentration is most accurately interpreted in the context of the serum ferritin concentration and is often expressed as a ratio to the log of the serum or plasma ferritin concentration (called the transferrin receptor index or transferrin/ferritin index).[9]

Newer parameters calculated by automated hematologic analyzers, such as reticulocyte hemoglobin content (CHr) or reticulocyte

hemoglobin equivalent (RET-He), can distinguish AI from AI with concurrent iron deficiency or iron deficiency alone.[22,23]

As will be discussed later in this chapter, the iron regulatory peptide hepcidin is the driver of the pathogenesis of AI. Circulating hepcidin concentration is expected to be elevated in AI.[4] Well-studied and reproducible assays for hepcidin have been developed, and although none are available for routine clinical use at present, it is probable that they will be available in the near future.[24,25] It has been proposed that the combination of elevated serum hepcidin and normal CHr will distinguish AI from both iron deficiency (normal hepcidin, high CHr) and the combined state of AI and iron deficiency (low CHr, high hepcidin).[26]

Erythrocyte Survival

Erythrocyte survival is modestly but significantly reduced in patients with AI. Depending on the methodology used, red cell survival is 10% to 20% shorter in anemic patients with chronic inflammation.[27] At this low level of hemolysis, changes in bilirubin and lactate dehydrogenase are not apparent.

Pathogenesis

Efforts to clarify the pathogenesis of AI have focused on three principal abnormalities: shortened erythrocyte survival, impaired marrow response, and disturbance in iron metabolism. The modest shortening of the erythrocyte survival creates an increased demand for red cell production on the marrow. Normally, the marrow could easily accommodate this demand, but in the setting of AI, the marrow is unable to respond fully because of a combination of a blunted erythropoietin (Epo) response, an inadequate progenitor response to Epo, and limited iron availability (*Figure 42.1*).

Cytokines

AI is one manifestation of the systemic response to immunologic or inflammatory stress, which results in the production of various cytokines.[28,29] The ability to trigger this cytokine response appears to be the common pathogenetic factor shared by the various conditions associated with this anemia syndrome. The central role of these molecules suggests that AI may be best understood as a cytokine-mediated process.[29] The cytokines most often implicated in the pathogenesis of AI are TNF, interleukin (IL)-1, IL-6, and the interferons, the concentrations of which have been reported to be increased in the serum or plasma of patients with disorders associated with AI and which have been shown to suppress erythroid colony formation in vitro.[30] Therapeutic administration of TNF or interferon may induce anemia.[31,32] The role of IL-6 is complex: IL-6 is a potent inducer of hepcidin, the usual mediator of AI,[33] but can also produce AI by hepcidin-independent processes.[34,35]

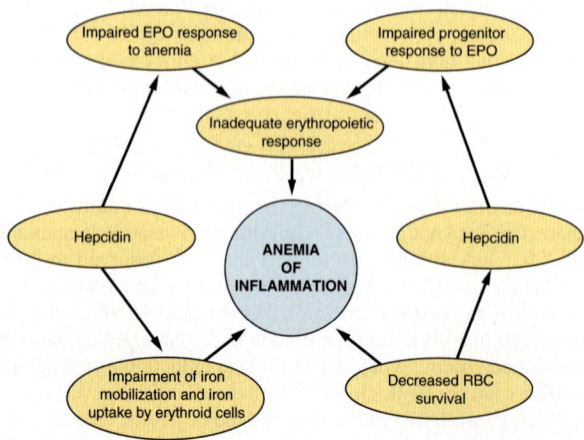

FIGURE 42.1 Schematic diagram representing contributing mechanisms in the pathogenesis of anemia of inflammation. EPO, erythropoietin; RBC, red blood cell.

The Role of Hepcidin

Although inflammation-induced cytokine activation is clearly the initial event in the pathogenesis of AI, the liver-produced antimicrobial peptide hepcidin is the most important mediator through which cytokines exert their effects on the pathogenetic mechanisms of AI. Hepcidin is an acute-phase-reacting peptide, largely regulated by IL-6, but it is also regulated by cytokine pathways not linked to IL-6.[33,36] Hepcidin promotes macrophage iron retention by causing internalization of the iron export protein ferroportin.[37]

Of the pathogenetic mechanisms shown in *Figure 42.1*, hepcidin clearly drives the abnormalities in iron metabolism. However, it may be linked to other elements as well. Under conditions of limited Epo availability, hepcidin is associated with impaired erythroid colony formation in vitro.[38] Increased circulating hepcidin appears to be linked to the degree of resistance to recombinant (rh) Epo therapy in dialysis patients.[39] Hepcidin and Epo production appear to be regulated in an inverse relationship by hypoxia-inducible factor (HIF),[40] which may potentially provide some linkage between hepcidin and the relative Epo deficiency of AI. This latter connection remains to be demonstrated.

Shortened Erythrocyte Survival

Cross-transfusion studies performed in patients with ACD in the 1950s demonstrated that shortened red cell survival in patients with AI reflects the reticuloendothelial/vascular environment rather than an intrinsic red cell defect.[2] IL-1 levels and shortened red cell survival are correlated in anemic patients with rheumatoid arthritis,[41] and mice that become anemic after exposure to TNF in vivo also exhibit a shortened red cell survival.[42] However, red cell survival is normal in hepcidin-expressing transgenic mice.[43] Neocytolysis, a selective hemolysis of newly formed erythrocytes associated with Epo deficiency, has been proposed as a mechanism for shortened red blood cell survival in AI.[44,45]

Impaired Marrow Response

Normal bone marrow, capable of a 6- to 8-fold increase in the red cell production rate, should easily compensate for such a modest reduction in erythrocyte survival. Its failure to do so in AI suggests that impaired production capacity is of fundamental importance in the pathogenesis of this condition. The possible defects in erythropoiesis fall into three categories: inappropriately low Epo secretion, diminished marrow response to Epo, and iron-limited erythropoiesis.

An inverse relationship between serum or plasma Epo levels and hemoglobin normally exists: As the hemoglobin decreases, the Epo level rises. A similar inverse relationship between hemoglobin and Epo level exists in anemic individuals with rheumatoid arthritis, cancer, and human immunodeficiency virus infection[46-49]; however, for any given anemic patient in these disease categories, the Epo level was lower than that found in equally anemic individuals with iron deficiency, indicating that the Epo response to anemia was blunted. This impaired Epo response may be directly cytokine mediated in the case of IL-1, TNF-α, and transforming growth factor-β, with downregulation of Epo occurring at the messenger RNA level.[30] As discussed earlier, there may be cross talk between hepcidin and Epo regulation. It has been proposed that this inadequate Epo secretion is adaptive; that is, it reflects reduced tissue oxygen use so that normal oxygenation is maintained despite reduced hemoglobin levels. Changes that ordinarily signify erythrocyte adaptation to tissue hypoxia, such as increased erythrocyte 2,3-diphosphoglycerate levels and slightly decreased hemoglobin oxygen affinity, are observed in AI.[50]

Although the Epo levels of patients with AI are lower than those observed in equally anemic iron-deficient individuals, they are still higher than are observed in normal individuals who are not anemic. This implies that inhibition of Epo production cannot entirely account for the impaired erythropoiesis associated with AI and that the erythroid progenitors themselves exhibit an abnormal response to Epo. Studies of anemic patients with cancer support this concept.[51,52] Hepcidin-overexpressing transgenic mice also show relative resistance to Epo.[43]

TNF, IL-1, and interferon (α, β, and γ) have all been demonstrated to inhibit erythropoiesis in vivo and in vitro.[30] An important point to consider in reviewing the various models for cytokine inhibition of erythropoiesis is that none of the systems described operates in isolation in vivo. Thus, TNF induces IL-1 production by macrophages, IL-1 induces interferon-γ production by T lymphocytes, and interferon-γ can exhibit positive or negative feedback on production of IL-1 and TNF. A recent study has indicated that interleukin (IL)-33 acts downstream to the Epo receptor to inhibit the response to erythropoietin.[53]

Treatment with recombinant human Epo (rhEpo) can correct AI in many cases; similarly, inhibition of in vitro erythroid colony formation by interferon-γ, but not interferon-α and interferon-β, can be corrected by exposure to high concentrations of Epo.[54,55] Epo-induced erythropoiesis suppresses hepcidin production through induction of the regulatory peptide erythroferrone.[56]

Abnormal Iron Metabolism

The dominant factor in the iron abnormalities of AI is clearly hepcidin, discussed above and at greater length in Chapter 25. A number of other processes of less overarching significance that may contribute under particular circumstances to the iron anomalies observed in AI are listed in *Table 42.2*.

The major contributor to hypoferremia in patients with AI is a shift of iron from a transferrin-bound, available circulating state to an intracellular storage state, creating a functional iron deficiency. Iron absorption appears to be normal, but iron tends to remain in the mucosal cell and in hepatocytes.[62,63] Macrophages, the major site from which iron is obtained for erythropoiesis, also exhibit increased iron storage. This process is mediated by hepcidin, which downregulates the iron egress regulatory ferroportin, thus trapping iron intracellularly.[37]

In addition to decreased availability of iron, erythroid progenitors may also be unable to fully utilize the iron available to them. Erythroblasts from anemic patients with rheumatoid arthritis express fewer surface TfRs than do erythroblasts from normal individuals. These TfRs also exhibit lower binding affinity for transferrin.[64] Furthermore, acute-phase reactants, such as α1-antitrypsin, impair transferrin binding to erythroblasts and also inhibit transferrin internalization.[65] rhEpo appears to induce a greater level of TfR expression on erythroid cells.[66]

Anemia in Patients With Cancer

Much of the anemia commonly observed in patients with cancer can be attributed to the mechanisms involved in AI; however, certain processes unique to malignancy may also contribute. Erythroid precursors may be displaced from marrow by metastatic tumor,[67] tumor-induced fibrosis,[68] or tumor-associated marrow necrosis.[69] The treatment of cancer can also produce or exacerbate anemia by a variety of mechanisms, including impaired Epo production[70] and cytotoxic effects of therapy on erythroid progenitors.[71]

Diagnosis

As described in *Table 42.1*, not all cases are associated with a classic chronic disease,[5] but virtually all cases are associated with states of cytokine or immune activation. This is likely the mechanism

Table 42.2. Alternate Processes That Restrict Iron for Erythropoiesis in Anemia of Inflammation

Process	Mechanism
Increased apoferritin synthesis in response to increased intracellular iron concentration	Excess apoferritin diverts iron to a slow-release pathway[57]
Inflammatory cytokine-induced ferritin synthesis	Increased ferritin acts as a "trap" for iron otherwise available for erythropoiesis[58,59]
Lactoferrin release in inflammation/phagocytosis	Lactoferrin transfers iron from a circulating state to a storage state[60,61]

associated with the many reports of AI in congestive heart failure.[72] The diagnosis is confirmed by demonstrating hypoferremia with adequate reticuloendothelial iron stores in a patient with an appropriate clinical syndrome. Typically, the serum transferrin is either low or low normal, and sTfR concentration is normal in AI. The major differential diagnosis is iron deficiency anemia. This is not a trivial distinction. The diagnosis of iron deficiency mandates identification of a source of blood loss. Incorrectly labeling a patient with AI as iron deficient exposes that patient to intrusive and expensive diagnostic procedures and to ineffective therapy. Mislabeling an iron-deficient patient as having AI may result in failure to diagnose an underlying gastrointestinal malignancy at a curable stage and in failure to offer inexpensive and effective therapy. The diagnosis of iron deficiency is discussed in detail in Chapter 25 and in the section "Abnormal Iron Metabolism." It has been suggested that a marker of inflammation or cytokine activation, such as C-reactive protein or IL-6, should be an element of the diagnosis of AI.[73] This may not be necessary in cases of AI associated with "classic" AI-related disease, like rheumatoid arthritis, but may be helpful in AI that are less typical or perhaps complicated by iron deficiency.

In principle, absence of an elevated serum or plasma hepcidin concentration could rule out AI. As hepcidin assays become available for routine use in a clinical context, it will be important to carry out well-designed studies to determine whether they will contribute more to diagnosis than currently available clinical markers of iron status.[25]

Treatment

The focus of therapy should be on the underlying disorder. The anemia itself is rarely an important clinical problem. Thus, direct approaches to correction of the anemia are rarely necessary. Fewer than 30% of patients have anemia sufficiently severe to consider transfusion, and assessment of the symptomatic state should always be considered before administration of blood products.

rhEpo and its analogs/variants are effective in AI but expensive,[74] and many if not most third-party payers will not reimburse for its use in AI. It is not currently approved for this purpose in the United States. Limitations on the use of rhEpo in anemic patients with cancer for safety reasons (discussed below) also limit the use of rhEpo in AI at present. Because most patients were not symptomatic from their anemia, reports of symptomatic benefit or improved global assessment/performance status results vary in different trials.[75] rhEpo has been used for patients with AI who wish to donate blood for autologous transfusion at elective surgery but are too anemic to do so or to permit autologous blood donation by a patient with AI and multiple alloantibodies.[76,77] It has been proposed that rhEpo administration may be of benefit in anemic patients with congestive heart failure, although results from clinical trials vary.[78]

It is debated whether or not to administer iron routinely to patients receiving therapy with Epo products.[79] It has been this author's practice to do so in the absence of elevated serum ferritin levels. In one study of anemic patients with rheumatoid arthritis, the concurrent use of iron supplementation was a powerful predictor of response to Epo[80]; however, many of the patients in this study may have been iron deficient. Iron therapy by itself is likely to be useful only in patients who have concurrent iron deficiency, and then only for the component of anemia caused by iron deficiency.[81] Anemic patients with cancer treated with concurrent intravenous iron and rhEpo appear to have a better response than those treated with no iron supplementation or with iron supplementation alone.[82]

Studies of the use of rhEpo in patients with cancer have been associated with increased adverse outcomes in certain cases,[83] leading to restrictions on circumstances in which rhEpo can be used in cancer therapy. Although there is debate in the literature as to whether the observed outcomes reflected unique features of particular rhEpo regimens or of specific patient populations, the clinician is encouraged to review current guidelines prior to initiating therapy.[84]

As noted earlier, Epo-driven erythropoiesis downregulates hepcidin production. Given the significant role of hepcidin in the pathogenesis of AI, therapy directed against hepcidin is an attractive concept

under investigation.[74] At present, however, there are no specific anti-hepcidin agents available for clinical use.

ANEMIA OF CHRONIC KIDNEY DISEASE

Anemia is a frequent complication of severe chronic kidney disease (CKD), often contributing substantially to the morbidity of the condition. The prevalence of anemia in CKD ranges from 8.4% at stage 1 (estimated glomerular filtration rate [eGFR] > 90 mL/min/1.73 m^2) to 53.4% in stage 5 (eGFR < 15/mL/min/m^2), when patients are either on or approaching dialysis. *Anemia of chronic kidney disease* refers to that anemia resulting directly from failure of the endocrine and filtering functions of the kidney. The kidney is the major source of Epo, and the ability to secrete this hormone is lost as the kidney fails. In addition, renal failure is associated with other pathologic processes, including some that may inhibit erythropoiesis (such as cytokine activation-induced hepcidin production[85]) and others that may shorten erythrocyte survival. Lack of sufficient Epo is by far the most important of these anemia-causing factors; consequently, the hypoproliferative features of the anemia tend to predominate.[86]

In clinical settings associated with CKD, additional factors may also contribute to the development of anemia, but these should be considered complications rather than fundamental components of the anemia of CKD itself. In the presence of infection or inflammation, additional hepcidin production contributes to the development of a more severe degree of anemia (and may improve with antibiotic therapy, for example).[85] Actual iron deficiency anemia with depletion of iron store, distinct from hepcidin-induced functional iron deficiency (see Chapter 25), may develop because of blood loss from the gastrointestinal tract or (less frequently) hematuria or from retention of blood in the hemodialysis tubing.[87] Folate transport can be abnormal in CKD even when plasma levels are normal and can contribute to anemia.[88] Certain types of renal disease, including the hemolytic-uremic syndrome or thrombotic thrombocytopenic purpura, are associated with microangiopathic hemolytic anemia (see Chapter 49). Although rare in current dialysis practice, aluminum intoxication can cause microcytic anemia in dialysis patients.[89] Zinc deficiency may contribute to anemia in CKD.[90]

Clinical Description

Anemia is less severe in polycystic kidney disease: otherwise, the degree of anemia does not distinguish different etiologies of CKD. In polycystic kidney disease, the Epo-secreting function of the kidney is relatively preserved even as filtering function is lost.[91] Cysts contain erythropoietin, resulting from HIF-2 activation in pericystic interstitial cells.

In most instances, the patient seeks medical attention because of symptoms related to the underlying renal disease, and anemia is an incidental finding. Occasionally, however, the renal symptoms are so subtle and so slowly progressive that the patient cites only symptoms of pallor, exertional dyspnea, or other signs of the cardiovascular adjustment to anemia. The severity of the anemia bears a rough relationship to the degree of renal insufficiency. Anemia is not routinely observed until the creatinine clearance falls to <45 mL/min/1.73 m^2 body surface area, which corresponds roughly to a serum creatinine of 2.0 to 2.5 mg/mL in an average-sized adult. At creatinine clearance rates below that, a statistically significant correlation between creatinine clearance and hematocrit has been reported.[92,93] However, the variation in the results of these studies is so great that the hemoglobin level in an individual patient cannot be predicted on the basis of renal function.

Laboratory Findings

Anemia tends to become more severe as renal failure worsens, but in most patients, the hematocrit ultimately stabilizes around a mean of 25%.[94] Because regulation of body water and electrolyte balance is impaired in renal disease, the apparent degree of anemia may be exaggerated or minimized by alterations in plasma volume.

The erythrocytes usually are normocytic and normochromic. The majority of red cells appear normal on blood smears. Occasionally, however, "burr" cells (*Figure 42.2*) are observed along with some triangular, helmet-shaped, or fragmented cells. Although the reticulocyte count expressed as a percentage often is within normal limits or even moderately increased,[95] the absolute reticulocyte is decreased.

The leukocyte count typically is normal, and the proportion of granulocytes tends to be higher than in healthy individuals. Granulocytosis is not uncommon. The typical platelet count is either normal or slightly increased.[94] Platelet counts may decrease with intravenous iron therapy, suggesting an element of iron deficiency.[96] Platelet function may be severely impaired despite normal numbers, resulting in defective hemostasis (see Chapter 53).

The bone marrow tends to be moderately hypercellular, and slight erythroid hyperplasia may be observed. Erythroid maturation appears morphologically normal in most cases.[94] In some instances, especially when renal failure is relatively acute or severe, hypoplasia of erythroid elements is noted.[97] In a study of 100 predialysis renal failure patients with hemoglobin concentrations less than 11 g/dL and not treated with rhEpo, 48% of patients had no detectable bone marrow iron.[98]

Serum iron may be normal or decreased. Serum ferritin is typically in the usual normal range, but may be elevated out of proportion to iron stores because of inflammation. In one series, patients with early-stage CKD were iron deficient in 17% of cases and had impaired iron utilization in an additional 12%.[99] Iron absorption from the gastrointestinal tract is generally decreased in CKD and appears to be related to disturbances in iron balance and not related to the degree of anemia, the rate of erythropoiesis, or the degree of azotemia.[100] This is consistent with the known role of hepcidin as a regulator of iron absorption.[85] Serum hepcidin levels in dialysis patients appear to track with iron status and to be low in the iron deficient.[101] At any given level of iron stores, higher hepcidin levels appear to predict anemia progression.[102]

Pathogenesis

It has been known for many years that three processes are involved in the pathogenesis of anemia of chronic renal failure—Epo deficiency, suppression of marrow erythropoiesis, and shortened red cell survival.[103] The success of recombinant Epo in the treatment of anemia of renal failure[104,105] has caused the other two contributors to be underemphasized since the late 1980s. More recently, studies on hepcidin metabolism in CKD have emphasized the contribution of iron availability to the anemia of CKD.

As renal function deteriorates, renal Epo secretion decreases.[106] Measured Epo values in renal failure vary widely and are not an effective guide to management. Even normal or "increased" Epo concentrations that may be observed in this syndrome are still strikingly low for the degree of anemia.[107] Overall, the usual relationship between Epo and hemoglobin concentrations is lost, indicating a loss of customary feedback mechanisms.[93] Some capacity to induce Epo secretion is preserved, however, because even the very low levels of Epo secretion in renal disease change in response to hemorrhage or transfusion.[108] Hepatic production of Epo accounts for some of the activity found in serum, especially that found in anephric subjects.[107] This extrarenal Epo secretion does not increase sufficiently in response to anemia to compensate for deficiencies at the renal source.

There is also a significant body of data suggesting that the inadequate marrow response to anemia is not due solely to Epo deficiency, beginning with the observation almost 60 years ago that the rate of erythropoiesis improved in patients treated with dialysis, even though Epo levels were unchanged.[109] Some proposed mechanisms of erythropoietic suppression other than Epo deficiency are listed in *Table 42.3*. As discussed earlier, iron deficiency is fairly frequent in patients with CKD. Cytokine and hepcidin studies both confirm that AI/ACD mechanisms also contribute to the impaired erythropoietic response in CKD.[114,116]

A third pathogenetic factor is hemolysis. Erythrocyte survival, although often within normal limits, may be reduced by 20% to 30%.[117] Key potential contributors to shortened erythrocyte survival are listed in *Table 42.4*. While the shortened erythrocyte survival was traditionally attributed to extracorpuscular factors associated with uremia producing oxidative or metabolic membrane damage, neocytolysis (selective hemolysis of the youngest erythrocytes), which occurs at the endothelium/macrophage interface in the presence of decreased Epo, is a major contributor.[118]

Management and Course
Erythropoiesis-Stimulating Agents

The term erythropoiesis-stimulating agent is the preferred description of the class of drugs required to correct anemia in CKD. This class is largely composed of rhEpo and its analogs such as darbepoetin and rhEpo biosimilars. Since its introduction in the mid-1980s, rhEpo has revolutionized the treatment of anemia of renal disease.[126] Therapy with rhEpo or its analogs has been reported to improve quality of life and cognitive function in small studies, although meta-analyses generally cannot support that conclusion because of design differences between the individual studies.[127] Similarly, meta-analyses do not show that one rhEpo product is clearly superior to another, either in safety or efficacy.[128] rhEpo or its analogs are the treatment of choice

Table 42.3. Mechanisms of Erythropoietic Suppression in Addition to Erythropoietin Deficiency

Suppression of erythropoiesis by polyamines (spermine) and other compounds that accumulated in renal failure and may be removed by dialysis[110,111]
Suppression of erythropoiesis by parathyroid hormone in secondary hyperparathyroidism[112]
Replacement of erythropoietic marrow by fibrosis induced by parathyroid hormone[113]
Suppression of erythropoiesis by inflammatory cytokines (anemia of inflammation-like mechanisms)[114,115]

Table 42.4. Mechanisms Contributing to Shortened Red Cell Survival in Chronic Kidney Disease

Neocytolysis[118]
Increased intracellular oxidative stress
· Pentose phosphate pathway inhibition[119]
· Glutathione reductase inhibition[120]
· Phosphoglyceromutase inhibition[121]
· Oxidant drugs
Abnormal cation transport[122]
Red cell membrane lipid peroxidation[123]
Splenic sequestration[124]
Toxic effects of compounds accumulated in renal failure (guanidine, guanidine metabolites)[125]

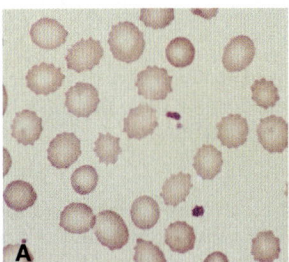
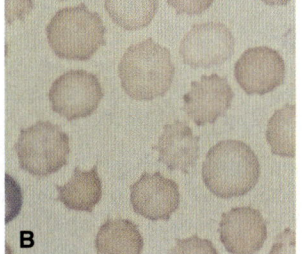

FIGURE 42.2 A, Crenated cells in renal disease (×1500). B, Burr cells in renal disease (×3000).

for anemia in CKD, being effective in patients receiving peritoneal or hemodialysis and in anemia because of renal insufficiency that is not sufficiently advanced to require dialysis, but in which the creatinine clearance is <45 mL/min/1.73 m(2) body surface area or the serum creatinine is >2.5 mg/mL.[129]

rhEpo can be administered intravenously or subcutaneously. Subcutaneous administration typically allows lower doses for comparable effects.[130] Although rhEpo was originally given three times weekly (to coincide with dialysis schedules) and still is frequently given that way, single weekly or less frequent dosing schedules can be similarly efficacious if the dose is increased appropriately.[131] Less frequent dosing can also be achieved with agents that have been modified to prolong rhEpo half-life, whether by increased glycosylation as with darbepoetin or by pegylation as with the continuous erythropoietin activator (CERA) class of rhEpo analogs. A standard starting dose for rhEpo would be 100 to 150 U/kg/wk or its equivalent. Higher doses result in faster correction of anemia but are generally not advised because of concerns of overshooting the target level of correction; target hemoglobin is typically attained within 6 to 8 weeks.[132] Iron supplementation is generally necessary, particularly in patients on hemodialysis. Intravenous iron is generally the modality of choice for iron supplementation or replacement in CKD at stage 3 or higher.[133] Iron should be administered with caution if at all at ferritin concentrations near or above 500 ng/mL and should not be given at all when the ferritin is >800 ng/mL.[129] The target hemoglobin range is to be no higher than 11 to 12 g/dL; higher levels may have an adverse clinical impact and do not convey added benefit.[134] A reasonable starting dose for the long-acting Epo analog darbepoetin (novel erythropoiesis-stimulating protein) is 0.45 µg/kg/wk for patients on dialysis, and 0.45 µg/kg/4 wk for predialysis patients. However, current guidelines should be reviewed prior to initiating rhEpo therapy.[135]

Side Effects/Adverse Reactions

As noted earlier, rhEpo products are generally safe but complications may occur. When used for anemia in renal disease, increased blood pressure is an important complication, experienced by up to 35% of patients. Rarely, the hypertension is abrupt and severe with encephalopathy and seizures.[136]

The occurrence of hypertension appears to be more closely related to the rate of increase in the blood hemoglobin level than the dose of rhEpo. It tends to be a transient phenomenon confined to the first 3 to 6 months of treatment. The pathogenesis is incompletely understood and probably multifactorial.[137] Although initially attributed to the effects of expanded blood volume with increased erythropoiesis, Epo can also contribute to hypertension through vasopressor effects, often mediated by nitric oxide, which appear most active in renal insufficiency.[88,138,139]

In early studies, prolonged or less effective dialysis and increased thrombotic events were thought to be problems associated with Epo treatment, but these concerns were not borne out in a large study.[140] Anaphylaxis in response to Epo has been described but is extremely rare.[141] Pure red cell aplasia due to rhEpo-induced antierythropoietin antibodies is a well-described phenomenon. It appears to have been a result of packaging and delivery characteristics of particular Epo products (especially in Western Europe and Canada), rather than a reaction to Epo itself and is now uncommon. This topic is discussed at length in Chapter 40.

Erythropoietin Resistance

As mentioned earlier, more than one-fourth of hemodialysis patients have a hematocrit < 30%. The failure of patients to respond optimally to rhEpo therapy or a requirement for unusually high doses is referred to as *erythropoietin (Epo) resistance*. Possible causes of Epo resistance are listed in *Table 42.5*.

Iron deficiency is the most common cause of Epo resistance.[142] The 2012 Kidney Disease: Improving Global Outcomes (KDIGO) Guideline set ferritin ≤500 ng/mL and transferrin saturation ≤30% as thresholds of iron parameters for patients with CKD.[135] As noted

Table 42.5. Causes of Erythropoietin Resistance

Iron deficiency
Blood loss (in dialysis apparatus, gastrointestinal, genitourinary)
Insufficient iron supplementation
Concurrent cytokine activation
Infection
Inflammation
Neoplasm
Insufficient dialysis intensity
Vitamin D deficiency
Secondary hyperparathyroidism
Folate deficiency
Angiotensin-converting enzyme inhibitors
Renal allograft failure
Antierythropoietin antibody-mediated resistance
Pure red cell aplasia
Other
Splenomegaly
Aluminum toxicity

above, intravenous iron is the preferred replacement modality and may lead to higher hemoglobin levels with less rhEpo use.[143] In order to avoid iron overload, intravenous iron replacement is reviewed when the ferritin exceeds 500 ng/mL and should be held when the ferritin exceeds 800 ng/mL.[129]

Inadequate hemodialysis is associated with Epo resistance. As a general rule, the intensity of dialysis must be sufficient to reduce the blood urea nitrogen by 65% or more to ensure optimal rhEpo response. Such factors as the frequency and duration of dialysis and characteristics of the dialyzer may need to be adjusted to achieve this goal.[144,145]

As discussed earlier, secondary hyperparathyroidism often accompanies renal failure, and the associated marrow fibrosis may contribute to the anemia and to Epo resistance (*Table 42.3*). Parathyroidectomy has been employed, but treatment with vitamin D_3 can also decrease rhEpo requirements and improve hemoglobin values.[146] However, vitamin D deficiency can cause Epo resistance independently of secondary hyperparathyroidism, through its effects on the hepcidin/cytokine axis.[147] Aluminum toxicity from dialysis water is now an uncommon cause of anemia but responds to chelation therapy.[148]

Elevated homocysteine and folate deficiency or impaired folate availability are common in CKD. Serum folate levels may be less helpful than red cell folate in this situation. If Epo resistance is associated with an increased MCV, empiric folate supplementation is appropriate.[149]

Associated infections or inflammatory states, as in AI, may provoke cytokine-mediated anemia mechanisms. In addition, there are a number of minor etiologies of Epo resistance (*Table 42.5*). Antierythropoietin antibodies can contribute to Epo resistance, although this is uncommon.

Renal Replacement Therapy

Renal replacement approaches (transplantation and dialysis) aim to restore or substitute for lost renal function. As such, they may have some effects on anemia associated with renal failure.

Renal Transplantation

In many ways, renal transplantation is the most complete and satisfactory treatment for severe CKD. With a successful graft, the hematologic response is often striking. Anemia is usually corrected over an 8- to 10-week period.[150] For the most part, the improvement results from Epo secretion by the grafted kidney. Two peaks of Epo secretion have been documented. There is an early peak seen only in patients with delayed graft function and not associated with hematologic improvement, in which serum Epo levels increase approximately 9-fold and then return to baseline after approximately 7 days. The second peak is associated with recovery of renal function from the graft and is presumed to be the important factor in the hematologic response. The increase in Epo levels is smaller but more sustained and begins on approximately day 8, accompanied by reticulocytosis and a gradual increase in hemoglobin levels. Epo values stabilize in the usual normal range when the hematocrit reaches 32%.[150,151]

Approximately 80% of patients experience an increase in blood hemoglobin concentration after renal allograft. Failure to respond usually can be explained on the basis of hemorrhage, vigorous immunosuppression, or graft rejection. Graft rejection often is accompanied transiently by increased Epo levels, but this is followed by a profound reduction in Epo levels and reticulocyte counts.[152-155] In approximately 20% of transplant patients, erythrocytosis follows correction of the anemia.[156] This complication is discussed in Chapter 49.

Dialysis

Most patients with end-stage renal disease are maintained on dialysis. As a modality for managing anemia, dialysis has been essentially eclipsed by the availability of rhEpo and is primarily of interest because the mild increment observed in hemoglobin concentration provides circumstantial evidence for the role of circulating inhibitors. Red cell production increases slightly in patients on hemodialysis, with attendant small increases in hematocrit and decreases in transfusion requirement.[157]

As a general rule, anemia is less severe in patients receiving peritoneal dialysis compared with hemodialysis, with consequently lower rhEpo, intravenous iron, and transfusion requirements, although there is extensive variation in anemia management practices between countries. The reasons for this lesser degree of anemia severity are unclear and have been attributed to better clearance of inhibitors of erythropoiesis or a higher degree of endogenous renal function.[158]

In the Epo era, the importance of other treatments of anemia of renal disease, such as androgens, has become of primarily historical interest. Blood transfusion support may still be required for patients who fail to respond to rhEpo products. The risks of blood-borne infections and of iron overload are significantly increased by the use of transfusion.[159]

HIF Prolyl Hydroxylase Inhibitors

HIF prolyl hydroxylase inhibitors (roxadustat, molidustat, vadadustat, daprodustat, among others) stabilize HIF and contribute to the correction of anemia in CKD both by enhancing Epo levels and by suppressing hepcidin, thus mobilizing iron.[160] These orally administered drugs could be an attractive alternative to rhEpo. They are available in some countries but are not currently approved in the United States.

ANEMIA IN CIRRHOSIS AND OTHER LIVER DISEASES

Some degree of anemia is commonly observed in patients with liver disease. Although it has been studied most extensively in patients with alcohol-induced cirrhosis, changes in red cell morphology and other contributors to anemia have been observed in various other liver diseases, including biliary cirrhosis, hemochromatosis, postnecrotic cirrhosis, and viral hepatitis. When the term *anemia of liver disease* is used, it refers to the mild to moderate anemia associated with liver disease in the absence of any complicating factors such as blood loss, marrow suppression by exogenous agents, or nutritional deficiency. This syndrome apparently results from a combination of intravascular dilution because of blood volume expansion, shortened red cell survival, and impaired ability of the marrow to respond optimally to the anemia. In addition, some patients develop a severe hemolytic anemia associated with morphologically abnormal erythrocytes (spur cells). Hemolytic anemia associated with Wilson disease (hepatolenticular degeneration) is discussed in Chapter 33.

The anemia actually observed in patients with liver disease reflects both the "uncomplicated" anemia discussed above and the consequences of factors extrinsic to the liver itself. Alcohol abusers can develop a characteristic sideroblastic anemia, often accompanied by impaired folate metabolism or overt folate deficiency (see Chapter 37), or may have direct suppression of hematopoiesis by alcohol.[161] Individuals with cirrhosis of any etiology are at increased risk for hemorrhage. Blood loss occurs in 24% to 70% of patients with alcoholic cirrhosis. The upper gastrointestinal tract is the major site of bleeding, but loss of blood from the nose, hemorrhoids, and uterus often occurs in association with coagulopathy of hepatic origins.[162]

Prevalence and Clinical Manifestations

Approximately 75% of patients with chronic liver disease develop anemia.[163] The total blood volume in liver disease (especially cirrhosis) averages 10% to 15% greater than normal but may be as much as 30% to 35% increased; thus, hemodilution tends to exaggerate the prevalence and degree of anemia (*Table 42.6*). For the same reason, the hematocrit may be decreased despite a normal red cell mass. In the absence of bleeding, the hemoglobin/hematocrit in patients with chronic liver disease is more heavily influenced by plasma volume than red cell mass.[164]

In cirrhotic patients, the hemoglobin level average is usually 10 to 12 g/dL.[164] The hemoglobin level rarely falls below 10 g/dL in the absence of bleeding or severe hemolysis. Depending on the population of patients with liver disease studied, 10% to 30% of patients with cirrhosis develop spur cell hemolytic anemia (>5% spur cells) and hemoglobin concentrations <10 g/dL. Spur cell anemia may be seen chronically with cirrhosis, or it may develop rapidly in association with fulminant hepatic failure. Morphologic and hemolytic abnormalities may resolve or diminish if liver function improves. In patients with cirrhosis, more than 5% spur cells in the red cell population carries an adverse prognosis for survival.[165,166] Spur cell anemia can also occur in infants with cholestatic liver disease.[167]

Episodic hemolysis can occur in association with alcoholic liver disease even before cirrhosis. These episodes are typically related to binge drinking, are usually mild to moderate in severity, and tend to resolve in 2 to 4 weeks if the patient abstains. Splenomegaly is not a major finding in these patients. When accompanied by jaundice and hyperlipidemia, episodic hemolysis in liver disease is known as *Zieve syndrome*.[168] It is unclear whether this transient form of hemolysis in liver disease is a syndrome of discrete and characteristic pathogenesis or simply a coincident constellation of independent abnormalities to which patients with liver disease are prone.

Table 42.6. Changes in Blood Volume in Patients With Cirrhosis

Measurement	Normal Subjects	Patients With Cirrhosis (% Change From Normal Subjects)	
		Without Ascites	With Ascites
Hematocrit (%)	42	35 (−17%)	34 (−19%)
Red cell mass (mL/kg)	23	20 (−13%)	19 (−17%)
Plasma volume (mL/kg)	42	57 (+35%)	55 (+31%)
Whole blood volume (mL/kg)	65	74 (+14%)	74 (+14%)

Values are means of 24 normal subjects, 63 patients with cirrhosis and no ascites, and 34 patients with cirrhosis and ascites. All groups included approximately twice as many men as women.
Data modified from Lieberman FL, Reynolds TB. Plasma volume in cirrhosis of the liver. *J Clin Invest.* 1967;46:1297-1308.

Disorders of Red Blood Cells

Hematologic Findings

More often than not, anemia of liver disease is mildly macrocytic. In a characteristic series, mean MCV was 107 fL, with a range of 100 to 139 fL. Alcoholics without established liver disease had a similar mean with a range of 101 to 125 fL. MCV was less than 114 fL in the majority of cases unless megaloblastic features were present, suggesting folate deficiency or (more rarely) pernicious anemia.[169,170] The degree of folate deficiency, when present, does not correlate with the degree of liver disease but is more frequent with higher alcohol consumption and is related to poor nutrition.[170,171] The reported proportion of patients with liver disease who have increased MCV varies from 30% to 76%, depending on the specific liver disease.[171] In a sense, macrocytes in liver disease are the mirror image of the microspherocytes observed in autoimmune hemolysis. The latter result from a decreased membrane pulled more tightly over a constant volume of hemoglobin and enzymes; the former result from a membrane that is expanded and sitting more loosely over a constant volume.

The reticulocyte count expressed as a percentage often is increased, but this depends on the point in the natural history of disease at which it is measured and whether alcohol is involved. After acute alcohol withdrawal, reticulocytosis is common.[161] Sustained reticulocytosis of 15% or more is unusual in the absence of hemorrhage, spur cell anemia, or other complicating conditions.

Target cells and cells with increased diameters are evident on blood smear (*Figure 42.3*). The cells appear hypochromic, but the appearance is related to the thinness of the cell rather than to reduced hemoglobin concentration. When spur cell hemolytic anemia supervenes, characteristic acanthocytes—erythrocytes covered with 5 to 10 spikelike projections—are evident. The acanthocytes are morphologically indistinguishable from the distorted erythrocytes found in patients with abetalipoproteinemia. Stomatocytes have been reported in association with the transient hemolytic episodes associated with acute fatty liver disease, but they are also noted in alcoholics who display no evidence of hemolysis.[172,173]

Approximately 50% of patients with cirrhosis have mild thrombocytopenia, but values <50 × 10(^{9})/L are uncommon. A variety of leukocyte abnormalities may be observed with neutropenia and lymphopenia the most common. Neutrophil mobilization and bactericidal function may be impaired in alcohol abuse.[174]

Older studies (frequently using sternal marrow specimens) tended to report bone marrow cellularity to be increased, whereas more recent studies generally find the cellularity to be normal.[175] Erythroid hyperplasia is common. In alcoholic liver disease, vacuolated erythroblasts and myeloblasts, ring sideroblasts, and plasma cell iron may be seen, with the abnormalities reversible by abstinence. Frank megaloblastosis is seen in <20% of patients.[176]

Pathogenesis

Shortened Erythrocyte Survival/Hemolysis

It has been known for many years that red cell survival is decreased in the majority of patients with liver disease, both alcoholic and nonalcoholic. The precise degree varied depending on the technique used to

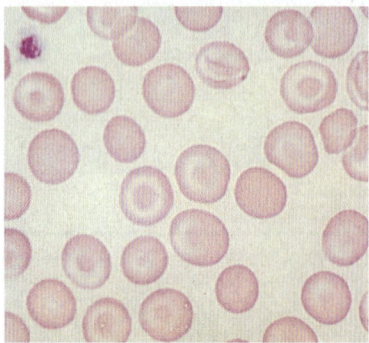

FIGURE 42.3 Macrocytes and target cells in liver disease (×1500).

measure survival, but it was usually of only moderate degree. Shorter survival tends to be observed in more anemic patients.[177-179]

The mechanism for the observed decrease in red cell lifespan is not fully understood; it is most probably multifactorial. Congestive splenomegaly and splenic sequestration may be major contributors, particularly when portal hypertension is presence.[163] In some cases, correction of the hemolytic process may occur after splenectomy. Studies of splenic bypass shunting suggest that the determining factor may be splenic blood flow per unit volume rather than spleen size itself.[180]

Abnormal erythrocyte oxidative metabolism is a possible intracorpuscular factor leading to reduced erythrocyte survival in liver disease. Activity of the pentose phosphate shunt is decreased in chronic liver disease, with consequent glutathione instability and a tendency to form Heinz bodies.[181] This and related metabolic abnormalities render the cell sensitive to oxidant hemolysis.[182] In addition, increased nontransferrin-bound iron associated with iron overload in liver disease (see Chapter 27) may contribute to the generation of free radicals in red cells.[183] Oxidant drugs can produce hemolysis in liver disease, as when patients with hepatitis C are treated with ribavirin.[184] Another metabolic abnormality encountered occasionally in liver disease is hypophosphatemia, with reduced erythrocyte adenosine triphosphate levels and consequent hemolysis. Hypophosphatemia can be exacerbated by antiviral therapy in hepatitis B.[185]

Characteristic alterations in red cell membrane lipids are found in patients with hepatitis, cirrhosis, and obstructive jaundice and may also be another contributor to shortened red cell survival.[186] In the usual uncomplicated case, a 25% to 50% increase in both cholesterol and lecithin is noted in the membrane. These changes result in an increased cell surface area associated with the target cells or macrocytes that are characteristic of liver disease. The loss of sialic acid from the red cell surface may contribute to impaired viability of the cell.[187] In patients with alcoholic liver disease, changes in the red cell membrane saturated/unsaturated fatty acid ratio were most pronounced in patients with severe hemolysis.[188]

Spur cell anemia is the classic example of hemolysis associated with lipid abnormalities in the red cell membrane. In spur cell anemia, the erythrocyte membrane accumulates excess cholesterol without a corresponding increase in lecithin, resulting in the characteristic morphologic abnormality. This change is accompanied by a pronounced reduction in erythrocyte survival, probably because the distorted cells are less deformable than normal and thus become trapped by splenic macrophages. Passage through the spleen causes loss of cell surface with transformation of echinocytes to acanthocytes.[189,190] The mechanism whereby the red cell lipid pattern becomes altered is not well understood. Patients with spur cell anemia have been reported to have plasma lipoprotein abnormalities involving apolipoproteins A-I and A-II, as well as in the high-density lipoprotein-3 and low-density lipoprotein fractions.[165,191] Splenectomy may ameliorate severe hemolysis[189] but may have other complications that offset this benefit. Zieve syndrome (mentioned earlier) is another example of a syndrome where hemolysis has been attributed to plasma lipid abnormalities, although hypertriglyceridemia by itself does not cause hemolysis.[192] Dietary or alcohol-induced vitamin E deficiency with decreased polyunsaturated fatty acids in membrane lipids may cause hemolysis in some patients.[192]

Iron deficiency can also contribute to the anemia observed in liver disease, usually because of gastrointestinal bleeding. Portal hypertensive gastropathy, variceal bleeding, peptic ulcers, and gastric antral vascular ectasia (or "watermelon stomach") account for much of the observed iron deficiency.[162]

Impaired Erythropoiesis

In addition to the shortened erythrocyte survival, the marrow response to the anemia in patients with liver disease may be inadequate. Alcohol, in particular, depresses erythropoiesis, and if the patient is studied before the effects of alcohol ingestion subside, marrow function appears depressed.[193] Serum from cirrhotic patients can suppress hematopoietic colony formation in vitro,[194] and cytokines implicated in the inhibition of erythropoiesis have been found to be increased in patients with liver disease.[195] Dyserythropoiesis with morphologic abnormalities and intramedullary hemolysis has also been reported in severe liver disease.[196] It has been suggested that extrarenal Epo production by the liver is abnormal in patients with liver disease, but in fact, the expected inverse relationship between hemoglobin and Epo production has been found to be preserved in liver disease and to result in levels appropriate for the degree of anemia.[197,198] In hepatitis C, erythropoietin response to anemia has been reported to be suppressed by treatment, which supports a rationale for rhEpo therapy in anemic patients on antiviral therapy.[199]

Hepcidin

Hepcidin is produced in the liver and so abnormalities in hepcidin production would be expected in hepatocellular disease.[200] Decreased hepcidin levels have been reported with cirrhosis and in hepatitis C and may contribute to iron overload in various liver diseases.[201,202] Hepcidin production may increase with antiviral therapy in hepatitis C.[199]

ANEMIAS ASSOCIATED WITH ENDOCRINE DISORDERS

A mild to moderate anemia may be seen in disorders affecting the thyroid, adrenals, parathyroids, gonads, or pituitary. It is usually not associated with symptomatology (other than that associated with the underlying endocrinopathy) and in fact may reflect a physiologically appropriate hemoglobin concentration because the hormone deficiency can be associated with reduced oxygen requirements. The anemia is therefore "adaptive."[203] In consultative hematology practice, these individuals present as referrals for evaluation of moderate anemia with normal iron, B_{12}, and folate studies, frequently with a question from the referring doctor of whether molecular studies or marrow examination are required. The endocrine disorder is frequently undiagnosed at the time of referral.

Hypothyroidism

Anemia is observed in 21% to 60% of hypothyroid patients and is more common in hypothyroid men than in hypothyroid women.[204] The frequency of anemia may be higher in overt hypothyroidism than in subclinical disease, although the difference may be small.[205,206]

Although typically listed as a macrocytic anemia, the uncomplicated anemia of hypothyroidism is either normocytic or only slightly macrocytic.[205] Hypochromic microcytic anemia found in association with hypothyroidism should prompt investigation for concurrent iron deficiency.[207] Iron deficiency in hypothyroidism responds (at least in part) to iron therapy, even if thyroid hormone is not administered, but does not typically respond to thyroid hormone without iron. Both iron and thyroid replacement should be used in hypothyroid patients with iron deficiency.[208] Hypothyroid individuals are more likely to become iron deficient because of predisposition to menorrhagia and autoimmune gastritis.[209,210] Severely macrocytic anemia usually results from complicating deficiency of vitamin B_{12} or folate.

When patients with iron, folate, or vitamin B_{12} deficiency are excluded, the remaining individuals should be considered to have "uncomplicated anemia of hypothyroidism," which is a primary manifestation of the hormone deficiency itself.[204] All or nearly all children with anemia and hypothyroidism have the uncomplicated form of the syndrome.[211] Anemia usually affects children whose height is below the third percentile. The anemia usually is mild, with the hematocrit rarely falling below 35%. The plasma volume often is decreased, which tends to make the reduction in hematocrit less than might be expected for a given decrease in red cell mass.[212]

White cell and platelet counts and red cell morphology are typically normal, although acanthocytes are occasionally seen in severe cases.[213] The bone marrow may show some erythroid hypoplasia but is typically normal otherwise.[214] Hemoglobin A_2 levels are reduced slightly.[215]

Pathogenesis

The anemia of hypothyroidism results from decreased red cell production.[211] As noted earlier, the anemia of hypothyroidism is considered "adaptive"—that is, a physiologic adjustment to the reduced needs of the organism for oxygen. Epo secretion is reduced in hypothyroid patients and 2,3-DPG levels are not increased, which differs from what occurs in most anemic and hypoxic states.[216] Thyroid hormones can enhance erythropoiesis in vitro and presumably in vivo as well.[217]

The response of anemia of hypothyroidism to thyroid hormone is gradual. No striking reticulocytosis occurs, and the hematocrit returns to a normal value only gradually over approximately a 6-month period (range, 3-12 months). The MCV almost always decreases, regardless of its initial value or the presence or degree of anemia, and stabilizes after 4 to 6 months or more.[204,218]

Hyperthyroidism

A mild anemia with no other apparent etiology occurs in 10% to 25% of patients with hyperthyroidism.[219,220] Anemia is primarily observed in individuals with severe or prolonged hyperthyroidism. More typically, the hemoglobin value falls somewhat but remains within normal limits.[219] The anemia of hyperthyroidism is in many ways the mirror image of that observed in hypothyroidism. MCV is either normal or modestly decreased and, consistent with the comparison with hypothyroidism, may be decreased even in the absence of anemia.[219] Hemoglobin A_2 levels are slightly increased but not as much as in thalassemia.[215] Both the anemia and the microcytosis are corrected when the hyperthyroidism is successfully treated.

The pathogenesis of anemia and microcytosis of hyperthyroidism is not well understood. Plasma volume may be increased, suggesting dilution.[221] Erythropoiesis usually is accelerated but ineffective. Increased plasma Epo levels have been reported, the opposite of what is described for hypothyroidism.[214]

Adrenal Insufficiency

Although a decreased red cell mass is common and probably nearly universal in adrenal insufficiency, anemia may be masked by the intravascular volume contraction characteristic of this syndrome.[222,223] In a series of patients with untreated Addison disease, the average blood hemoglobin level was 13.2 g/dL (range, 9.4-18.0 g/dL).[224] The red cells were normocytic and normochromic. After institution of hormone replacement, the average hemoglobin fell to 10.7 g/dL and the hematocrit from 42% to 33%, presumably reflecting the expansion of plasma volume associated with clinical improvement. Later in the course of the disease, reticulocytosis and a return to normal hemoglobin levels occurred.[224] Pernicious anemia is observed in 3% to 16% of cases of nontuberculous adrenal insufficiency and may complicate 13% of adrenal insufficiency cases associated with the polyglandular autoimmune syndrome type I.[225]

Androgen Deficiency

After puberty, values for the hematocrit, blood hemoglobin concentration, and red cell count average ~10% to 13% higher in men than in women.[226] The differences in red cell parameters between the sexes are accounted for chiefly by the stimulating effect of androgens on erythropoiesis. In castrated men, these values fall to within the normal female range.[227] Since androgens act on erythropoiesis by increasing renal synthesis of Epo, this finding is almost certainly because of a difference in Epo production, although the relationship between hemoglobin and Epo concentration does not differ between the sexes.[228] After the sixth decade, male hemoglobin values fall back toward those observed in women.[226]

The anemia of testosterone deficiency is normocytic and normochromic and the hemoglobin concentration rarely falls below 10 to 12 g/dL in the absence of another process. Measuring Epo levels does not help in making a diagnosis. In a study of elderly men with low testosterone and otherwise unexplained anemia, approximately half of the subjects experienced a significant increase in hemoglobin concentration with testosterone therapy.[229] Since a similar proportion of patients did not respond to testosterone replacement, the finding of low testosterone levels by itself does not diagnose anemia of androgen deficiency. Androgens can also stimulate erythropoiesis in normal subjects and may be a cause of secondary polycythemia (see Chapter 45).

Hypopituitarism

Moderately severe anemia is a well-recognized feature of pituitary insufficiency, regardless of cause. In an extensive review of cases of primary panhypopituitarism in the first half of the 20th century, the average blood hemoglobin concentration was ~10 g/dL, with similar values reported in patients with hypopituitarism that arose from neoplasms.[230-232] Anemia is also evident in prepubertal pituitary dwarfs but tends to be underappreciated because of contracted plasma volume.[233] The anemia usually is normocytic and normochromic, and the red cells appear normal morphologically. In some patients, slight hypochromia or macrocytosis has been observed[231,234]; however, complicating deficiencies of iron or folate were not excluded in those reports. Erythrokinetic studies demonstrated reduced red cell production.[235] Marrow hypoplasia and even pancytopenia may be seen.

The anemia of hypopituitarism results chiefly from deficiencies of the hormones of target glands controlled by the pituitary, especially the thyroid and adrenal hormones, and also from deficiency of androgens. In addition, lack of other pituitary factors, such as growth hormone, prolactin, or factors characterized less clearly, may be of importance.[233,235,236]

As suggested for the anemia of hypothyroidism, panhypopituitarism probably produces its effects on erythropoiesis chiefly by reducing tissue oxygen consumption. Treatment with a combination of hormones (such as thyroxine, cortisone, and growth hormone) corrects both the anemia and the marrow hypoplasia and is more effective than any single hormone by itself.[237] In one reported case of panhypopituitarism secondary to craniopharyngioma, anemia persisted and progressed despite replacement hormone therapy. Administration of rhEpo (6000 IU/d) was followed by correction of the anemia, with the blood hemoglobin level rising from 6 g/dL to normal over a 3-month period.[238]

Hyperparathyroidism

Secondary hyperparathyroidism as a contributor to anemia of renal failure has been discussed earlier. Anemia is a known complication of primary hyperparathyroidism. At one institution, 17 of 332 patients (5.1%) with primary hyperparathyroidism were anemic, with hematocrit values ranging from 23% to 37%.[239] At another institution, 14 of 28 patients with primary hyperparathyroidism had anemia attributed to hyperparathyroidism.[112] The anemia was normocytic and normochromic, and no reticulocytosis was reported. The majority of patients undergoing bone marrow examination showed significant marrow replacement by fibrosis. The hematocrit increased in the majority of patients who underwent parathyroidectomy. In one of the series, improvement after surgery occurred in the patients with marrow fibrosis exclusively.[112]

The cause of the anemia in these patients remains obscure. Although renal failure and gastrointestinal bleeding occur in association with hyperparathyroidism, they could not be implicated as an etiologic factor in this group of anemic patients, nor was incidental iron deficiency evident. Some authors conclude that parathyroid hormone decreases the proliferation of erythroid precursors in culture.[240] Marrow fibrosis may also be a result of excess hormone levels.[241,242] Myelofibrosis is a common finding in bone marrow biopsy specimens, but the usual morphologic signs of myelophthisis are lacking in these patients.[243]

When hyperparathyroidism is secondary to renal disease, it is difficult to ascertain the relative importance of the hormone excess versus the Epo deficit characteristic of renal failure as a contributor to the observed anemia. Of note, however, is that medical treatment of hyperparathyroidism with vitamin D_3 can bring about improvement in anemia and decreased requirements for rhEpo in some patients.[146]

Anorexia Nervosa

Anemia is observed in roughly a third of patients with anorexia nervosa overall,[244] with a much higher frequency among hospitalized patients. The anemia is typically normocytic and normochromic. A moderate degree of leukopenia and occasional thrombocytopenia may also be observed. Bone marrow examination shows gelatinous transformation with necrosis, as well as decreased cellularity in most cases. These are essentially the findings observed in starvation, and they return to normal with improved nutrition.[244,245] A small number of cases of hemolytic anemia occurring during refeeding have also been reported in anorexia nervosa.[246,247] These are attributed to transient hypophosphatemia (see Chapter 33).

Diabetes Mellitus

Anemia is fairly common in patients with diabetes, with a prevalence of 40% reported among inpatients and 29% in outpatients. Anemia in diabetes is more common in women than in men. Anemia in diabetes does not appear to be an intrinsic feature of the condition that correlates with the degree of diabetes control but is rather associated with its chronic complications such as renal disease, diabetic foot infections, and other systemic findings, which are themselves associated with anemia.[248,249] Serum hepcidin levels are elevated in diabetic patients with a normal glomerular filtration rate.[250]

References

1. Bentley DP. Anaemia and chronic disease. *Clin Haematol.* 1982;11:465-479.
2. Cartwright GE. The anemia of chronic disease. *Semin Hematol.* 1966;3:351-375.
3. Lee GR. The anemia of chronic disease. *Semin Hematol.* 1983;20:61-80.
4. Weiss G, Ganz T, Goodnough LT. Anemia of inflammation. *Blood.* 2019;133(1):40-50.
5. Cash JM, Sears DA. The anemia of chronic disease: spectrum of associated diseases in a series of unselected hospitalized patients. *Am J Med.* 1989;87(6):638-644.
6. Baer AN, Dessypris EN, Krantz SB. The pathogenesis of anemia in rheumatoid arthritis. A clinical and laboratory analysis. *Semin Arthritis Rheum.* 1990;19:209-223.
7. Niccoli L, Nannini C, Cassarà E, Kaloudi O, Cantini F. Frequency of anemia of inflammation in patients with ankylosing spondylitis requiring anti-TNFα drugs and therapy-induced changes. *Int J Rheum Dis.* 2012;15(1):56-61.
8. Bellmann-Weiler R, Lanser L, Barket R, et al. Prevalence and predictive value of anemia and dysregulated iron homeostasis in patients with COVID-19 infection. *J Clin Med.* 2020;9(8):2429.
9. Scholz GA, Leichtle AB, Scherer A, et al. The links of hepcidin and erythropoietin in the interplay of inflammation and iron deficiency in a large observational study of rheumatoid arthritis. *Br J Haematol.* 2019;186(1):101-112.
10. Healey LA, Wilske KR. Presentation of occult giant cell arteritis. *Arthritis Rheum.* 1980;23:641-643.
11. Atkins MB, Kappler K, Mier JW, Isaacs RE, Berkman EM. Interleukin-6-associated anemia: determination of the underlying mechanism. *Blood.* 1995;86(4):1288-1291.
12. Eastgate JA, Wood NC, DiGiovine FS, Symons JA, Grinlinton FA, Duff GW. Correlation of plasma interleukin1 levels with disease activity in rheumatoid arthritis. *Lancet.* 1988;2:706-709.
13. Chernow B, Wallner SF. Is the anemia of chronic disease normocytic and normochromic? *Mil Med.* 1978;143:345-346.
14. Elin RJ, Wolff SM, Finch CA. Effect of induced fever on serum iron and ferritin concentrations in man. *Blood.* 1977;49:147-153.
15. Namaste SM, Rohner F, Huang J, et al. Adjusting ferritin concentrations for inflammation: Biomarkers Reflecting Inflammation and Nutritional Determinants of Anemia (BRINDA) project. *Am J Clin Nutr.* 2017;106(suppl 1):359s-371s.
16. Lee MH, Means RT. Extremely elevated serum ferritin levels in a university hospital: associated diseases and clinical significance. *Am J Med.* 1995;98:566-571.
17. Moore C, Jr, Ormseth M, Fuchs H. Causes and significance of markedly elevated serum ferritin levels in an academic medical center. *J Clin Rheumatol.* 2013;19(6):324-328.
18. Koulaouzidis A, Cottier R, Bhat S, Said E, Linaker BD, Saeed AA. A ferritin level >50 microg/L is frequently consistent with iron deficiency. *Eur J Intern Med.* 2009;20(2):168-170.
19. North M, Dallalio G, Donath AS, Melink R, Means RT. Serum transferrin receptor levels in patients undergoing evaluation of iron stores:correlation with other parameters, and observed versus predicted results. *Clin Lab Haematol.* 1997;19:93-97.
20. Means RT, Allen J, Sears DA, Schuster SJ. Serum soluble transferrin receptor and the prediction of marrow aspirate results in a heterogeneous group of patients. *Clin Lab Haematol.* 1999;21:161-167.
21. Koulaouzidis A, Said E, Cottier R, Saeed AA. Soluble transferrin receptors and iron deficiency, a step beyond ferritin. A systematic review. *J Gastrointestin Liver Dis.* 2009;18(3):345-352.
22. van Santen S, van Dongen-Lases EC, de Vegt F, et al. Hepcidin and hemoglobin content parameters in the diagnosis of iron deficiency in rheumatoid arthritis patients with anemia. *Arthritis Rheum.* 2011;63(12):3672-3680.
23. Auerbach M, Staffa SJ, Brugnara C. Using reticulocyte hemoglobin equivalent as a marker for iron deficiency and responsiveness to iron therapy. *Mayo Clin Proc.* 2021;96(6):1510-1519.
24. Girelli D, Nemeth E, Swinkels DW. Hepcidin in the diagnosis of iron disorders. *Blood.* 2016;127(23):2809-2813.
25. Means RT, Jr. Hepcidin in differential diagnosis: ready for the clinic? *Eur J Haematol.* 2015;94(1):2-3.
26. Thomas C, Kobold U, Balan S, Roedddiger R, Thomas L. Serum hepcidin-25 may replace the ferritin index in the Thomas plot in assessing iron status in anemic patients. *Int J Lit Humanit.* 2011;33:187-193.

27. Cavill I, Bentley DP. Erythropoiesis in the anaemia of rheumatoid arthritis. *Br J Haematol.* 1982;50(4):583-590.

28. Means RT, Krantz SB. Progress in understanding the pathogenesis of the anemia of chronic disease. *Blood.* 1992;80:1639-1647.

29. Means RT. Pathogenesis of the anemia of chronic disease: a cytokine-mediated anemia. *Stem Cell.* 1995;13:32-37.

30. Means RT, Jr. Recent developments in the anemia of chronic disease. *Curr Hematol Rep.* 2003;2(2):116-121.

31. Blick M, Sherwin SA, Rosenblum M, Gutterman J. Phase I study of recombinant tumor necrosis factor in cancer patients. *Cancer Res.* 1987;47:2986-2989.

32. Vadhan-Raj S, Al-Katib A, Bhulla R, et al. Phase I trial of recombinant interferon gamma in cancer patients. *J Clin Oncol.* 1986;4:137-146.

33. Nemeth E, Valore EV, Territo M, Schiller G, Lichtenstein A, Ganz T. Hepcidin, a putative mediator of anemia of inflammation, is a type II acute phase protein. *Blood.* 2003;101:2461-2463.

34. Langdon JM, Yates SC, Femnou LK, et al. Hepcidin-dependent and hepcidin-independent regulation of erythropoiesis in a mouse model of anemia of chronic inflammation. *Am J Hematol.* 2014;89(5):470-479.

35. McCranor BJ, Kim MJ, Cruz NM, et al. Interleukin-6 directly impairs the erythroid development of human TF-1 erythroleukemic cells. *Blood Cells Mol Dis.* 2014;52(2-3):126-133.

36. Armitage AE, Eddowes LA, Gileadi U, et al. Hepcidin regulation by innate immune and infectious stimuli. *Blood.* 2011;118(15):4129-4139.

37. Nemeth E, Tuttle MS, Powelson J, et al. Hepcidin regulates iron efflux by binding to ferroportin and inducing its internalization. *Science.* 2004;306:2090-2093.

38. Dallalio G, Law E, Means RT, Jr. Hepcidin inhibits in vitro erythroid colony formation at reduced erythropoietin concentrations. *Blood.* 2006;107:2702-2704.

39. Kato A. Increased hepcidin-25 and erythropoietin responsiveness in patients with cardio-renal anemia syndrome. *Future Cardiol.* 2010;6(6):769-771.

40. Mastrogiannaki M, Matak P, Mathieu JRR, et al. Hepatic hypoxia-inducible factor-2 down-regulates hepcidin expression in mice through an erythropoietin-mediated increase in erythropoiesis. *Haematologica.* 2012;97(6):827-834.

41. Rogers J, Durmowicz G, Kasschau K, Lacroix L, Bridges K. A motif within the 5' non-coding regions of acute phase mRNA mediates control of ferritin translation by IL-1[b] and may contribute to the anemia of chronic disease. *Blood.* 1991;78(suppl 1):361a.

42. Moldawer LL, Marano MA, Wei H, et al. Cachectin/tumor necrosis factor alters red blood cell kinetics and induces anemia in vivo. *FASEB J.* 1989;3:1637-1643.

43. Roy CN, Mak HH, Akpan I, Losyev G, Zurakowski D, Andrews NC. Hepcidin antimicrobial peptide transgenic mice exhibit features of the anemia of inflammation. *Blood.* 2007;109(9):4038-4044.

44. Rice L, Alfrey CP, Driscoll T, Whitley CE, Hachey DL, Suki W. Neoctyolysis contributes to the anemia of renal disease. *Am J Kidney Dis.* 1999;33:59-62.

45. Trial J, Rice L, Alfrey CP. Erythropoietin withdrawal alters interactions between young red blood cells, splenic endothelial cells, and macrophages: an in vito model of neocytolysis. *J Invest Med.* 2001;49:335-345.

46. Baer AN, Dessypris EN, Goldwasser E, Krantz SB. Blunted erythropoietin response to anaemia in rheumatoid arthritis. *Br J Haematol.* 1987;66:559-564.

47. Hochberg MC, Arnold CM, Hogans BB, Spivak JL. Serum immunoreactive erythropoietin in rheumatoid arthritis: impaired response to anemia. *Arthritis Rheum.* 1988;31:1318-1321.

48. Miller CB, Jones RJ, Piantadosi S, Abeloff MD, Spivak JL. Decreased erythropoietin response in patients with the anemia of cancer. *N Engl J Med.* 1990;322:1689-1692.

49. Spivak JL, Barnes DC, Fuchs E, Quinn TC. Serum immunoreactive erythropoietin in HIV-infected patients. *JAMA, J Am Med Assoc.* 1989;261:3104-3107.

50. Douglas SW, Adamson JW. The anemia of chronic disorders: studies of marrow regulation and iron metabolism. *Blood.* 1975;45(1):55-65.

51. Dowlati A, RZik S, Fillet G, Beguin Y. Anaemia of lung cancer is due to impaired erythroid marrow response to erythropoietin stimulation as well as relative inadequacy of erythropoietin production. *Br J Haematol.* 1997;97(2):297-299.

52. Corazza GR, Valentini RA, Andreani ML, et al. Subclinical coeliac disease is a frequent cause of iron-deficiency anaemia. *Scand J Gastroenterol.* 1995;30(2):153-156.

53. Swann JW, Koneva LA, Regan-Komito D, Sansom SN, Powrie F, Griseri T. IL-33 promotes anemia during chronic inflammation by inhibiting differentiation of erythroid progenitors. *J Exp Med.* 2020;217(9).

54. Means RT, Krantz SB. Inhibition of human erythroid colony forming units by gamma interferon can be corrected by recombinant human erythropoietin. *Blood.* 1991;78:2564-2567.

55. Means RT, Krantz SB. Inhibition of human erythroid colony-forming units by interferons alpha and beta: differing mechanisms despite shared receptor. *Exp Hematol.* 1996;24:204-208.

56. Ganz T. Erythropoietic regulators of iron metabolism. *Free Radic Biol Med.* 2019;133:69-74.

57. Gelvan D, Fibach E, Meyron-Holtz EG, Konijn AM. Ferritin uptake by human erythroid precursors is a regulated iron uptake pathway. *Blood.* 1996;88(8):3200-3207.

58. Alvarez-Hernandez X, Liceaga J, McKay IC, Brock JH. Induction of hypoferremia and modulation of macrophage iron metabolism by tumor necrosis factor. *Lab Invest.* 1989;61:319-322.

59. Recalcati S, Taramelli D, Conte D, Cairo G. Nitric oxide-mediated induction of ferritin synthesis in J774 macrophages by inflammatory cytokines: role of selective iron regulatory protein-2 downregulation. *Blood.* 1998;91(3):1059-1066.

60. Van Snick JL, Masson PL, Heremans JF. The involvement of lactoferrin in the hyposideremia of acute inflammation. *J Exp Med.* 1974;140(4):1068-1084.

61. Goldblum SE, Cohen DA, Jay M, McClain CJ. Interleukin 1-induced depression of iron and zinc: role of granulocytes and lactoferrin. *Am J Physiol.* 1987;252(1 pt 1):E27-E32.

62. Hershko C, Cook JD, Finch CA. Storage iron kinetics IV. The effect of inflammation on iron exchange in the rat. *Br J Haematol.* 1974;28:67-75.

63. Schade SG. Normal incorporation of oral iron into intestinal ferritin in inflammation. *PSEBM (Proc Soc Exp Biol Med).* 1972;139:620-622.

64. Feelders RA, Vreugdenhil G, van Dijk JP, Swaak AJ, van Eijk HG. Decreased affinity and number of transferrin receptors on erythroblasts in the anemia of rheumatoid arthritis. *Am J Hematol.* 1993;43(3):200-204.

65. Graziadei I, Gaggl S, Kaserbacher R, Braunsteiner H, Vogel W. The acute phase protein-1-antitrypsin inhibits growth and proliferation of human early erythroid progenitor cells (burst-forming units-erythroid) and of human erythroleukemic cells (K562) in vitro by interfering with transferrin iron uptake. *Blood.* 1994;83:260-268.

66. Weiss G, Houston T, Kastner S, Johrer K, Grunewald K, Brock JH. Regulation of cellular iron metabolism by erythropoietin: activation of iron-regulatory protein and upregulation of transferrin receptor expression in erythroid cells. *Blood.* 1997;89(2):680-687.

67. Bezwoda WR, Lewis D, Livini N. Bone marrow involvement in anaplastic small cell lung cancer. Diagnosis, hematologic features, and prognostic implications. *Cancer.* 1986;58:1762-1765.

68. Jacobs SC. Spread of prostate cancer to bone. *Urology.* 1983;21:337-344.

69. Deucher A, Wool GD. How I investigate bone marrow necrosis. *Int J Lab Hematol.* 2019;41(5):585-592.

70. Schapira L, Antin JH, Ransil BJ, et al. Serum erythropoietin levels in patients receiving intensive chemotherapy and radiotherapy. *Blood.* 1990;76:2354-2359.

71. Abdel-Razeq H, Hashem H. Recent update in the pathogenesis and treatment of chemotherapy and cancer induced anemia. *Crit Rev Oncol Hematol.* 2020;145:102837.

72. Okonko DO, Mandal AK, Missouris CG, Poole-Wilson PA. Disordered iron homeostasis in chronic heart failure: prevalence, predictors, and relation to anemia, exercise capacity, and survival. *J Am Coll Cardiol.* 2011;58(12):1241-1251.

73. Weiss G, Goodnough L. Anemia of chronic disease. *N Engl J Med.* 2005;352(10):1011-1023.

74. Weiss G. Anemia of chronic disorders: new diagnostic tools and new treatment strategies. *Semin Hematol.* 2015;52(4):313-320.

75. Marti-Carvajal AJ, Agreda-Perez LH, Sola I, Simancas-Racines D. Erythropoiesis-stimulating agents for anemia in rheumatoid arthritis. *Cochrane Database Syst Rev.* 2013;2013(2):Cd000332.

76. Means RT. Clinical application of recombinant human erythropoietin in the anemia of chronic disease. *Hematol Oncol Clin North Am.* 1994;8:933-944.

77. Thompson FL, Powers JS, Graber SE, Krantz SB. Use of recombinant human erythropoietin to enhance autologous blood donation in a patient with multiple red cell allo-antibodies and the anemia of chronic disease. *Am J Med.* 1991;90:398-400.

78. Lipsic E, van der Meer P, van Veldhuisen DJ. Erythropoiesis-stimulating agents and heart failure. *Cardiovascular therapeutics.* 2011;29(4):e52-e59.

79. Eschbach JW. Iron requirements in erythropoietin therapy. *Best Pract Res Clin Haematol.* 2005;18(2):347-361.

80. Nordstrom D, Lindroth Y, Marsal L, et al. Availability of iron and degree of inflammation modifies the response to recombinant human erythropoietin when treating anemia of chronic disease in patients with rheumatoid arthritis. *Rheumatol Int.* 1997;17:67-73.

81. Amstad Bencaiova G, Krafft A, Zimmermann R, Burkhardt T. Treatment of anemia of chronic disease with true iron deficiency in pregnancy. *Journal of pregnancy.* 2017;2017:4265091.

82. Auerbach M, Ballard H, Trout JR, et al. Intravenous iron optimizes the response to recombinant human erythropoietin in cancer patients with chemotherapy-related anemia: a multicenter, open-label, randomized trial. *J Clin Oncol.* 2004;22:1301-1307.

83. Bohlius J, Schmidlin K, Brillant C, et al. Erythropoietin or Darbepoetin for patients with cancer--meta-analysis based on individual patient data. *Cochrane Database Syst Rev.* 2009;2009(3):Cd007303.

84. Bohlius J, Bohlke K, Castelli R, et al. Management of cancer-associated anemia with erythropoiesis-stimulating agents: ASCO/ASH clinical practice guideline update. *Blood Adv.* 2019;3(8):1197-1210.

85. Ganz T, Nemeth E. Iron balance and the role of hepcidin in chronic kidney disease. *Semin Nephrol.* 2016;36(2):87-93.

86. Adamson JW, Eschbach J, Finch CA. The kidney and erythropoiesis. *Am J Med.* 1968;44(5):725-733.

87. Tanaka S, Tanaka T. How to supplement iron in patients with renal anemia. *Nephron.* 2015;131(2):138-144.

88. Bukhari FJ, Moradi H, Gollapudi P, Ju Kim H, Vaziri ND, Said HM. Effect of chronic kidney disease on the expression of thiamin and folic acid transporters. *Nephrol Dial Transplant.* 2011;26(7):2137-2144.

89. Touam M, Martinez F, Lacour B, et al. Aluminum induced reversible microcytic anemia in chronic renal failure: clinical and experimental studies. *Clin Nephrol.* 1983;19:295-298.

90. Pan CF, Lin CJ, Chen SH, Huang CF, Lee CC. Association between trace element concentrations and anemia in patients with chronic kidney disease: a cross-sectional population-based study. *J Invest Med.* 2019;67(6):995-1001.

91. Hanudel MR, Salusky IB, Pereira RC, et al. Erythropoietin and fibroblast growth factor 23 in autosomal dominant polycystic kidney disease patients. *Kidney Int Rep.* 2019;4(12):1742-1748.

92. de Klerk G, Wilmink JM, Rosengarten PC, Vet RJ, Goudsmit R. Serum erythropoietin (ESF) titers in anemia of chronic renal failure. *J Lab Clin Med.* 1982;100(5):720-734.

93. Pavlovic-Kentera V, Clemons GK, Djukanovic L, Biljanovic-Paunovic L. Erythropoietin and anemia in chronic renal failure. *Exp Hematol.* 1987;15(7):785-789.

94. Weng CH, Lu KY, Hu CC, Huang WH, Wang IK, Yen TH. Bone marrow pathology predicts mortality in chronic hemodialysis patients. *BioMed Res Int*. 2015;2015:160382.

95. Talwar VK, Gupta HL, Shashinarayan. Clinicohaematological profile in chronic renal failure. *J Assoc Phys India*. 2002;50:228-233.

96. Hazara AM, Bhandari S. Intravenous iron administration is associated with reduced platelet counts in patients with chronic kidney disease. *J Clin Pharm Therapeut*. 2015;40(1):20-23.

97. Ahn JH, Yoon KS, Lee WI, et al. Bone marrow findings before and after treatment with recombinant human erythropoietin in chronic hemodialyzed patients. *Clin Nephrol*. 1995;43(3):189-195.

98. Stancu S, Stanciu A, Zugravu A, et al. Bone marrow iron, iron indices, and the response to intravenous iron in patients with non-dialysis-dependent CKD. *Am J Kidney Dis*. 2010;55(4):639-647.

99. Lukaszyk E, Lukaszyk M, Koc-Zorawska E, Tobolczyk J, Bodzenta-Lukaszyk A, Malyszko J. Iron status and inflammation in early stages of chronic kidney disease. *Kidney Blood Press Res*. 2015;40(4):366-373.

100. Eschbach JW, Cook JD, Finch CA. Iron absorption in chronic renal disease. *Clin Sci*. 1970;38(2):191-196.

101. Bratescu L, Barsan L, Munteanu D, Stancu S, Mircescu G. Is hepcidin-25 a clinically relevant parameter for the iron status in hemodialysis patients? *J Ren Nutr*. 2010;20:S77-S83.

102. Niihata K, Tomosugi N, Uehata T, et al. Serum hepcidin-25 levels predict the progression of renal anemia in patients with non-dialysis chronic kidney disease. *Nephrol Dial Transplant*. 2012;27(12):4378-4385.

103. Eschbach JW, Adamson JW. Anemia of end-stage renal disease (ESRD). *Kidney Int*. 1985;28:1-5.

104. Eschbach JW, Kelly MR, Haley NR, Abels RI, Adamson JW. Treatment of the anemia of progressive renal failure with recombinant human erythropoietin. *N Engl J Med*. 1989;321(3):158-163.

105. Winearls CG, Oliver DO, Pippard MJ, Reid C, Downing MR, Cotes PM. Effect of human erythropoietin derived from recombinant DNA on the anaemia of patients maintained by chronic haemodialysis. *Lancet*. 1986;2:1175-1178.

106. McGonigle RJ, Wallin JD, Shadduck RK, Fisher JW. Erythropoietin deficiency and inhibition of erythropoiesis in renal insufficiency. *Kidney Int*. 1984;25(2):437-444.

107. Caro J, Brown S, Miller O, Murray T, Erslev AJ. Erythropoietin levels in uremic nephric and anephric patients. *J Lab Clin Med*. 1979;93(3):449-458.

108. Sexauer CL, Matson JR. Anemia of chronic renal failure. *Ann Clin Lab Sci*. 1981;11(6):484-487.

109. Mann DL, Donati RM, Gallagher NI. Erythropoietin assay and ferrokinetic measurements in anemic uremic patients. *JAMA*. 1965;194(12):1321-1322.

110. Hotta T, Maeda H, Suzuki I, Chung TG, Saito A. Selective inhibition of erythropoiesis by sera from patients with chronic renal failure. *Proc Soc Exp Biol Med*. 1987;186(1):47-51.

111. Radtke HW, Rege AB, LaMarche MB, et al. Identification of spermine as an inhibitor of erythropoiesis in patients with chronic renal failure. *J Clin Invest*. 1981;67(6):1623-1629.

112. Bhadada SK, Bhansali A, Ahluwalia J, Chanukya GV, Behera A, Dutta P. Anaemia and marrow fibrosis in patients with primary hyperparathyroidism before and after curative parathyroidectomy. *Clin Endocrinol*. 2009;70(4):527-532.

113. Zingraff J, Drueke T, Marie P, Man NK, Jungers P, Bordier P. Anemia and secondary hyperparathyroidism. *Arch Intern Med*. 1978;138(11):1650-1652.

114. Means RT. Commentary: an anemia of chronic disease, after all? *J Invest Med*. 1999;47:203.

115. Allen DA, Breen C, Yaqoob MM, Macdougall IC. Inhibition of CFU-E colony formation in uremic patients with inflammatory disease:role of IFN-gamma and TNF-alpha. *J Invest Med*. 1999;47:204-211.

116. Honda H, Hosaka N, Ganz T, Shibata T. Iron metabolism in chronic kidney disease patients. *Contrib Nephrol*. 2019;198:103-111.

117. Korell J, Vos FE, Coulter CV, Schollum JB, Walker RJ, Duffull SB. Modeling red blood cell survival data. *J Pharmacokinet Pharmacodyn*. 2011;38(6):787-801.

118. Trial J, Rice L. Erythropoietin withdrawal leads to the destruction of young red cells at the endothelial-macrophage interface. *CurrPharmDes*. 2004;10(2):183-190.

119. Rosenmund A, Binswanger U, Straub PW. Oxidative injury to erythrocytes, cell rigidity, and splenic hemolysis in hemodialyzed uremic patients. *Ann Intern Med*. 1975;82(4):460-465.

120. Yawata Y, Tanaka KR. Red cell glutathione reductase: mechanism of action of inhibitors. *Biochim Biophys Acta*. 1973;321(1):72-83.

121. Yawata Y, Howe R, Jacob HS. Abnormal red cell metabolism causing hemolysis in uremia. A defect potentiated by tap water hemodialysis. *Ann Intern Med*. 1973;79(3):362-367.

122. Cheng JT, Kahn T, Kaji DM. Mechanism of alteration of sodium potassium pump of erythrocytes from patients with chronic renal failure. *J Clin Invest*. 1984;74(5):1811-1820.

123. Zachee P, Ferrant A, Daelemans R, Goossens W, Boogaerts MA, Lins RL. Reduced glutathione for the treatment of anemia during hemodialysis: a preliminary communication. *Nephron*. 1995;71(3):343-349.

124. Hartley LC, Morgan TO, Innis MD, Clunie GJ. Splenectomy for anaemia in patients on regular haemodialysis. *Lancet*. 1971;2(7738):1343-1345.

125. Giovannetti S, Balestri PL, Barsotti G. Methylguanidine in uremia. *Arch Intern Med*. 1973;131(5):709-713.

126. Eschbach JW, Egrie JC, Downing MR, Browne JK, Adamson JW. Correction of the anemia of end-stage renal disease with recombinant human erythropoietin. Results of a combined phase I and II clinical trial. *N Engl J Med*. 1987;316(2):73-78.

127. Collister D, Komenda P, Hiebert B, et al. The effect of erythropoietin-stimulating agents on health-related quality of life in anemia of chronic kidney disease: a systematic review and meta-analysis. *Ann Intern Med*. 2016;164(7):472-478.

128. Palmer SC, Saglimbene V, Mavridis D, et al. Erythropoiesis-stimulating agents for anaemia in adults with chronic kidney disease: a network meta-analysis. *Cochrane Database Syst Rev*. 2014;12:Cd010590.

129. National Collaborating Centre for Chronic Conditions. *Anaemia Management in Chronic Kidney Disease: National Clinical Guideline for Management in Adults and Children*. Royal College of Physicians of London (UK); 2006.

130. Patel TV, Robinson K, Singh AK. Is it time to reconsider subcutaneous administration of epoetin? *Nephrol News Issues*. 2007;21(11): 57, 59, 63-57, 59, 64.

131. Lago M, Perez-Garcia R, De VMSG, Anaya F, Valderrabano F. Efficiency of once-weekly subcutaneous administration of recombinant human erythropoietin versus three times a week administration in hemodialysis patients. *Nephron*. 1996;72(4):723-724.

132. Locatelli F, Aljama P, Barany P. Revised European best practice guidelines for the management of anaemia in patients with chronic renal failure. *Nephrol Dial Transplant*. 2004;19:ii1-ii47.

133. Shepshelovich D, Rozen-Zvi B, Avni T, Gafter U, Gafter-Gvili A. Intravenous versus oral iron supplementation for the treatment of anemia in CKD: an updated systematic review and meta-analysis. *Am J Kidney Dis*. 2016;68(5):677-690.

134. Besarab A, Bolton WK, Browne JK. The effects of normal as compared with low hematocrit values in patients with cardiac disease who are receiving hemodialysis and epoetin [lsqb]see comment[rsqb]. *N Engl J Med*. 1998;339:584-590.

135. Fishbane S, Spinowitz B. Update on anemia in ESRD and earlier stages of CKD: core curriculum 2018. *Am J Kidney Dis*. 2018;71(3):423-435.

136. Boyle SM, Berns JS. Erythropoietin and resistant hypertension in CKD. *Semin Nephrol*. 2014;34(5):540-549.

137. Kokot F, Wiecek A. Arterial hypertension in uraemic patients treated with erythropoietin. *Nephron*. 1995;71(2):127-132.

138. Vaziri ND, Zhou XJ, Smith J, Oviesi F, Baldwin K, Purdy RE. In vivo and in vitro pressor effects of erythropoietin in rats. *Am J Physiol*. 1995;268:F838-F845.

139. Wang XQ, Vaziri ND. Erythropoietin depresses nitric oxide synthase expression by human endothelial cells. *Hypertension*. 1999;33:894-899.

140. Eschbach JW, Abdulhadi MH, Browne JK, et al. Recombinant human erythropoietin in anemic patients with end-stage renal disease. Results of a phase III multicenter clinical trial. *Ann Intern Med*. 1989;111(12):992-1000.

141. Garcia JE, Senent C, Pascual C, et al. Anaphylactic reaction to recombinant human erythropoietin. *Nephron*. 1993;65:636-637.

142. Tarng DC, Chen TW, Huang TP. Iron metabolism indices for early prediction of the response and resistance to erythropoietin therapy in maintenance hemodialysis patients. *Am J Nephrol*. 1995;15(3):230-237.

143. Pollak VE, Lorch JA, Means RT, Jr. Unanticipated favorable effects of correcting iron deficiency in chronic hemodialysis patients. *J Investig Med*. 2001;49(2):173-183.

144. Ifudu O, Feldman J, Friedman EA. The intensity of hemodialysis and the response to erythropoietin in patients with end-stage renal disease. *N Engl J Med*. 1996;334(7):420-425.

145. Vigano SM, Filippo SD, Milia VL, Pontoriero G, Locatelli F. Prospective randomized pilot study on the effects of two synthetic high-flux dialyzers on dialysis patient anemia. *Int J Artif Organs*. 2012;35(5):346-351.

146. Argiles A, Mourad G, Lorho R, et al. Medical treatment of severe hyperparathyroidism and its influence on anaemia in end-stage renal failure. *Nephrol Dial Transplant*. 1994;9(12):1809-1812.

147. Icardi A, Paoletti E, De Nicola L, Mazzaferro S, Russo R, Cozzolino M. Renal anaemia and EPO hyporesponsiveness associated with vitamin D deficiency: the potential role of inflammation. *Nephrol Dial Transplant*. 2013;28(7):1672-1679.

148. Goch J, Birgegard G, Danielson BG, Wikstroem B. Treatment of erythropoietin-resistant anaemia with desferrioxamine in patients on haemofiltration. *Eur J Haematol*. 1995;55(2):73-77.

149. Teschner M, Kosch M, Schaefer RM. Folate metabolism in renal failure. *Nephrol Dial Transplant*. 2002;17(suppl 5):24-27.

150. Kessler M. Erythropoietin and erythropoiesis in renal transplantation. *Nephrol Dial Transplant*. 1995;10(suppl 6):114-116.

151. Abbrecht PH, Greene JA, Jr. Serum erythropoietin after renal homotransplantation. *Ann Intern Med*. 1966;65(5):908-921.

152. Hoffman GC. Human erythropoiesis following kidney transplantation. *Ann N Y Acad Sci*. 1968;149(1):504-508.

153. Sun CH, Ward HJ, Paul WL, Koyle MA, Yanagawa N, Lee DB. Serum erythropoietin levels after renal transplantation. *N Engl J Med*. 1989;321(3):151-157.

154. Murphy GP, Mirand EA, Grace JT, Jr. Erythropoietin activity in anephric or renal allotransplanted man. *Ann Surg*. 1969;170(4):581-587.

155. Besarab A, Caro J, Jarrell BE, Francos G, Erslev AJ. Dynamics of erythropoiesis following renal transplantation. *Kidney Int*. 1987;32(4):526-536.

156. Alzoubi B, Kharel A, Machhi R, Aziz F, Swanson KJ, Parajuli S. Post-transplant erythrocytosis after kidney transplantation: a review. *World J Transplant*. 2021;11(6):220-230.

157. Eschbach JW, Jr, Funk D, Adamson J, Kuhn I, Scribner BH, Finch CA. Erythropoiesis in patients with renal failure undergoing chronic dialysis. *N Engl J Med*. 1967;276(12):653-658.

158. Perlman RL, Zhao J, Fuller DS, et al. International anemia prevalence and management in peritoneal dialysis patients. *Perit Dial Int*. 2019;39(6):539-546.

159. Brenner N, Kommalapati A, Ahsan M, Ganguli A. Red cell transfusion in chronic kidney disease in the United States in the current era of erythropoiesis stimulating agents. *J Nephrol*. 2020;33(2):267-275.

160. Li ZL, Tu Y, Liu BC. Treatment of renal anemia with roxadustat: advantages and achievement. *Kidney Dis*. 2020;6(2):65-73.

161. Eichner ER. The hematologic disorders of alcoholism. *Am J Med*. 1973;54(5):621-630.

162. Gkamprela E, Deutsch M, Pectasides D. Iron deficiency anemia in chronic liver disease: etiopathogenesis, diagnosis and treatment. *Ann Gastroenterol.* 2017;30(4):405-413.

163. Gonzalez-Casas R, Jones EA, Moreno-Otero R. Spectrum of anemia associated with chronic liver disease. *World J Gastroenterol: WJG.* 2009;15(37):4653-4658.

164. Otto JM, Plumb JOM, Clissold E, et al. Hemoglobin concentration, total hemoglobin mass and plasma volume in patients: implications for anemia. *Haematologica.* 2017;102(9):1477-1485.

165. Privitera G, Meli G. An unusual cause of anemia in cirrhosis: spur cell anemia, a case report with review of literature. *Gastroenterol Hepatol Bed Bench.* 2016;9(4):335-339.

166. Alexopoulou A, Vasilieva L, Kanellopoulou T, Pouriki S, Soultati A, Dourakis SP. Presence of spur cells as a highly prognostic factor of mortality in patients with cirrhosis. *J Gastroenterol Hepatol.* 2014;29(4):830-834.

167. Cynamon HA, Isenberg JN, Gustavson LP, Gourley WK. Erythrocyte lipid alterations in pediatric cholestatic liver disease: spur cell anemia of infancy. *J Pediatr Gastroenterol Nutr.* 1985;4(4):542-549.

168. Liu MX, Wen XY, Leung YK, et al. Hemolytic anemia in alcoholic liver disease: Zieve syndrome – a case report and literature review. *Medicine (Baltim).* 2017;96(47):e8742.

169. Takahashi N, Kameoka J, Takahashi N, et al. Causes of macrocytic anemia among 628 patients: mean corpuscular volumes of 114 and 130 fL as critical markers for categorization. *Int J Hematol.* 2016;104(3):344-357.

170. Sanvisens A, Zuluaga P, Pineda M, et al. Folate deficiency in patients seeking treatment of alcohol use disorder. *Drug Alcohol Depend.* 2017;180:417-422.

171. Maruyama S, Hirayama C, Yamamoto S, et al. Red blood cell status in alcoholic and non-alcoholic liver disease. *J Lab Clin Med.* 2001;138(5):332-337.

172. Davidson RJ, How J, Lessels S. Acquired stomatocytosis: its prevalence of significance in routine haematology. *Scand J Haematol.* 1977;19(1):47-53.

173. Wisloff F, Boman D. Acquired stomatocytosis in alcoholic liver disease. *Scand J Haematol.* 1979;23(1):43-50.

174. Girard DE, Kumar KL, McAfee JH. Hematologic effects of acute and chronic alcohol abuse. *Hematol Oncol Clin North Am.* 1987;1(2):321-334.

175. Batista JN, Santolaria F, Gonzalez-Reimers E, et al. Evaluation of marrow cellularity in alcoholism and hepatic cirrhosis, by aspiration, biopsy and histomorphometric. *Drug Alcohol Depend.* 1988;22(1-2):27-31.

176. Michot F, Gut J. Alcohol-induced bone marrow damage. A bone marrow study in alcohol-dependent individuals. *Acta Haematol.* 1987;78(4):252-257.

177. Sheehy TW, Berman A. The anemia of cirrhosis. *J Lab Clin Med.* 1960;56:72-82.

178. Jackson S, Fleege L, Fridman M, Gregory K, Zelop C, Olsen J. Morbidity following primary cesarean delivery in the Danish National Birth Cohort. *Am J Obstet Gynecol.* 2012;206(2):139 e1-139 e5.

179. Pitcher CS, Williams R. Reduced red cell survival in jaundice and its relation to abnormal glutathione metabolism. *Clin Sci.* 1963;24:239-252.

180. Nishiwaki M, Ashida H, Nishioka A, Utsunomiya J. Red cell survival in patients with nonalcoholic liver cirrhosis before and after distal splenorenal shunt. *J Gastroenterol.* 1997;32(3):318-323.

181. Smith JR, Kay NE, Gottlieb AJ, Oski FA. Abnormal erythrocyte metabolism in hepatic disease. *Blood.* 1975;46(6):955-964.

182. Loguercio C, Taranto D, Vitale LM, Beneduce F, Del Vecchio Blanco C. Effect of liver cirrhosis and age on the glutathione concentration in the plasma, erythrocytes, and gastric mucosa of man. *Free Radic Biol Med.* 1996;20(3):483-488.

183. Fiorelli G, De Feo TM, Duca L, et al. Red blood cell antioxidant and iron status in alcoholic and nonalcoholic cirrhosis. *Eur J Clin Invest.* 2002;32(suppl 1):21-27.

184. Van Vlierbergh H, Delange JR, DeVos M, Leroux-Roel G, Committee BS. Factors influencing ribavirin-induced hemolysis. *J Hepatol.* 2001;34:911-916.

185. Tanaka M, Suzuki F, Seko Y, et al. Renal dysfunction and hypophosphatemia during long-term lamivudine plus adefovir dipivoxil therapy in patients with chronic hepatitis B. *J Gastroenterol.* 2014;49(3):470-480.

186. Cooper RA. Hemolytic syndromes and red cell membrane abnormalities in liver disease. *Semin Hematol.* 1980;17(2):103-112.

187. Powell LW, LaMont JT, Isselbacher KJ. Haemolysis in experimental cholestasis: possible role of erythrocyte sialic acid. *Gut.* 1974;15(10):794-798.

188. Benedetti A, Birarelli AM, Brunelli E, et al. Modification of lipid composition of erythrocyte membranes in chronic alcoholism. *Pharmacol Res Commun.* 1987;19(10):651-662.

189. Cooper RA, Kimball DB, Durocher JR. Role of the spleen in membrane conditioning and hemolysis of spur cells in liver disease. *N Engl J Med.* 1974;290(23):1279-1284.

190. Shohet SB. Acanthocytogenesis—or how the red cell won its spurs. *N Engl J Med.* 1974;290(23):1316-1317.

191. Duhamel G, Forgez P, Nalpas B, Berthelot P, Chapman MJ. Spur cells in patients with alcoholic liver cirrhosis are associated with reduced plasma levels of apoA-II, HDL3, and LDL. *J Lipid Res.* 1983;24(12):1612-1625.

192. Goebel KM, Goebel FD, Schubotz R, Schneider J. Red cell metabolic and membrane features in haemolytic anaemia of alcoholic liver disease (Zieve's syndrome). *Br J Haematol.* 1977;35(4):573-585.

193. Straus DJ. Hematologic aspects of alcoholism. *Semin Hematol.* 1973;10(3):183-194.

194. Ohki I, Dan K, Kuriya S, Nomura T. A study on the mechanism of anemia and leukopenia in liver cirrhosis. *Jpn J Med.* 1988;27:155-159.

195. Tilg H, Wilmer A, Vogel W, et al. Serum levels of cytokines in chronic liver diseases. *Gastroenterology.* 1992;103:264-274.

196. Hadnagy C, Laszlo GA. Acquired dyserythropoiesis in liver disease (letter). *Br J Haematol.* 1991;78:283.

197. Pirisi M, Fabris C, Falleti E, et al. Evidence for a multifactorial control of serum erythropoietin concentration in liver disease. *Clin Chim Acta.* 1993;219:47-55.

198. Means RT, Jr, Mendenhall CL, Worden BD, Moritz TE, Chedid A. Erythropoietin and cytokine levels in the anemia of severe alcoholic liver disease. *Alcohol Clin Exp Res.* 1996;20(2):355-358.

199. van Rijnsoever M, Galhenage S, Mollison L, Gummer J, Trengove R, Olynyk JK. Dysregulated erythropoietin, hepcidin, and bone marrow iron metabolism contribute to interferon-induced anemia in Hepatitis C. *J Interferon Cytokine Res.* 2016;36(11):630-634.

200. Fleming RE, Sly WS. Hepcidin: a putative iron-regulatory hormone relevant to hereditary hemochromatosis and the anemia of chronic disease. *Proc Natl Acad Sci U S A.* 2001;98:8160-8162.

201. Varghese J, Varghese James J, Karthikeyan M, et al. Iron homeostasis is dysregulated, but the iron-hepcidin axis is functional, in chronic liver disease. *J Trace Elem Med Biol.* 2020;58:126442.

202. Means RT, Jr. Hepcidin and iron regulation in health and disease. *Am J Med Sci.* 2013;345(1):57-60.

203. Bomford R. Anaemia in myoedema. *Q J Med.* 1938;7:495-536.

204. Horton L, Coburn RJ, England JM, Himsworth RL. The haematology of hypothyroidism. *Q J Med.* 1976;45(177):101-123.

205. M'Rabet-Bensalah K, Aubert CE, Coslovsky M, et al. Thyroid dysfunction and anaemia in a large population-based study. *Clin Endocrinol.* 2016;84(4):627-631.

206. Erdogan M, Kösenli A, Ganidagli S, Kulaksizoglu M. Characteristics of anemia in subclinical and overt hypothyroid patients. *Endocr J.* 2012;59(3):213-220.

207. Kandhro GA, Kazi TG, Afridi HI, et al. Evaluation of iron in serum and urine and their relation with thyroid function in female goitrous patients. *Biol Trace Elem Res.* 2008;125(3):203-212.

208. Ravanbod M, Asadipooya K, Kalantarhormozi M, Nabipour I, Omrani GR. Treatment of iron-deficiency anemia in patients with subclinical hypothyroidism. *Am J Med.* 2013;126(5):420-424.

209. Sweet MG, Schmidt-Dalton TA, Weiss PM, Madsen KP. Evaluation and management of abnormal uterine bleeding in premenopausal women. *Am Fam Physician.* 2012;85(1):35-43.

210. Castoro C, Le Moli R, Arpi ML, et al. Association of autoimmune thyroid diseases, chronic atrophic gastritis and gastric carcinoid: experience from a single institution. *J Endocrinol Invest.* 2016;39(7):779-784.

211. Chu JY, Monteleone JA, Peden VH, Graviss ER, Vernava AM. Anemia in children and adolescents with hypothyroidism. *Clin Pediatr (Phila).* 1981;20(11):696-699.

212. Park CW, Shin YS, Ahn SJ, et al. Thyroxine treatment induces upregulation of renin-angiotensin-aldosterone system due to decreasing effective plasma volume in patients with primary myxoedema. *Nephrol Dial Transplant.* 2001;16(9):1799-1806.

213. Savage RA, Sipple C. Marrow myxedema. Gelatinous transformation of marrow ground substance in a patient with severe hypothyroidism. *Arch Pathol Lab Med.* 1987;111(4):375-377.

214. Das KC, Mukherjee M, Sarkar TK, Dash RJ, Rastogi GK. Erythropoiesis and erythropoietin in hypo- and hyperthyroidism. *J Clin Endocrinol Metabol.* 1975;40(2):211-220.

215. Kuhn JM, Rieu M, Rochette J, et al. Influence of thyroid status on hemoglobin A2 expression. *J Clin Endocrinol Metabol.* 1983;57(2):344-348.

216. Zaroulis CG, Kourides IA, Valeri CR. Red cell 2,3-diphosphoglycerate and oxygen affinity of hemoglobin in patients with thyroid disorders. *Blood.* 1978;52(1):181-185.

217. Golde DW, Bersch N, Chopra IJ, Cline MJ. Thyroid hormones stimulate erythropoiesis in vitro. *Br J Haematol.* 1977;37:173-177.

218. Tudhope GR, Wilson GM. Anaemia in hypothyroidism: incidence, pathogenesis, and response to treatment. *Q J Med.* 1960;24:513-537.

219. Nightingale S, Vitek PJ, Himsworth RL. The haematology of hyperthyroidism. *Q J Med.* 1978;47(185):35-47.

220. Rivlin RS, Wagner HN, Jr. Anemia in hyperthyroidism. *Ann Intern Med.* 1969;70(3):507-516.

221. Muldowney FP, Crooks J, Wayne EJ. The total red cell mass in thyrotoxicosis and myxoedema. *Clin Sci (Lond).* 1957;16(2):309-314.

222. Franco-Saenz R. Diseases of the adrenal cortex. In: *The Adrenal Gland.* Mulrow PG, ed. Elsevier; 1986.

223. Bethune JE. The diagnosis and treatment of adrenal insufficiency. In: *Endocrinology.* DeGroot LJ, ed. WB Saunders; 1989.

224. Irvine WJ, Stewart AG, Scart L. A clinical and immunological study of adrenocortical insufficiency (Addison's disease). *Clin Exp Immunol.* 1967;1:31.

225. Neufield M, Maclaren NK, Blizzard RM. Two types of autoimmune Addison's disease associated with different polyglandular autoimmune (PGA) syndromes. *Medicine (Baltim).* 1981;60:355.

226. Cheng CK, Chan J, Cembrowski GS, van Assendelft OW. Complete blood count reference interval diagrams derived from NHANES III: stratification by age, sex, and race. *Lab Hematol.* 2004;10(1):42-53.

227. Alexanian R. Erythropoietin and erythropoiesis in anemic man following androgens. *Blood.* 1969;33(4):564-572.

228. Krantz SB, Jacobson LO. *Erythropoietin and the Regulation of Erythropoiesis.* University of Chicago; 1970:1-330.

229. Roy CN, Snyder PJ, Stephens-Shields AJ, et al. Association of testosterone levels with anemia in older men: a controlled clinical trial. *JAMA Intern Med.* 2017;177(4):480-490.

230. Escamilla RF, Lisser H. Simmonds' disease - a clinical study with review of the literature, differentiation from anorexia nervosa by statistical analysis of 595 cases, 101 of which were proved pathologically. *J Clin Endocrin.* 1942;2(2):65-96.

231. Daughaday WH, Williams RH, Daland GA. The effect of endocrinopathies on the blood. *Blood.* 1948;3(12):1342-1366.

232. Greig HB, Metz J, Sunn L. Anaemia in hypopituitarism; treatment with testosterone and cortisone. *S Afr J Lab Clin Med.* 1956;2(1):52-61.

Disorders of Red Blood Cells

233. Jepson JH, McGarry EE. Hemopoiesis in pituitary dwarfs treated with human growth hormone and testosterone. *Blood.* 1972;39(2):229-248.

234. Summers VK. The anaemia of hypopituitarism. *Br Med J.* 1952;1(4762):787-790.

235. Jepson JH, Lowenstein L. Effect of prolactin on erythropoiesis in the mouse. *Blood.* 1964;24:726-738.

236. Lindemann R, Trygstad O, Halvorsen S. Pituitary control of erythropoiesis. *Scand J Haematol.* 1969;6(2):77-86.

237. Nishioka H, Haraoka J. Hypopituitarism and anemia: effect of replacement therapy with hydrocortisone and/or levothyroxine. *J Endocrinol Invest.* 2005;28(6):528-533.

238. Nomiyama J, Shinohara K, Inoue H. Improvement of anemia by recombinant erythropoietin in a patient with postoperative hypopituitarism. *Am J Hematol.* 1994;47(3):249-250.

239. Boxer M, Ellman L, Geller R, Wang CA. Anemia in primary hyperparathyroidism. *Arch Intern Med.* 1977;137(5):588-593.

240. Potasman I, Better OS. The role of secondary hyperparathyroidism in the anemia of chronic renal failure. *Nephron.* 1983;33(4):229-231.

241. Barbour GL. Effect of parathyroidectomy on anemia in chronic renal failure. *Arch Intern Med.* 1979;139(8):889-891.

242. Podiarny E, Rathaus M, Korzets Z, Blum M, Zevin D, Bernheim J. Is anemia of chronic renal failure related to secondary hyperparathyroidism? *Arch Intern Med.* 1981;141(4):453-455.

243. Mallette LE. Anemia in hypercalcemic hyperparathyroidism. Renewed interest in an old observation. *Arch Intern Med.* 1977;137(5):572-573.

244. Hutter G, Ganepola S, Hofmann WK. The hematology of anorexia nervosa. *Int J Eat Disord.* 2009;42(4):293-300.

245. Smith RR, Spivak JL. Marrow cell necrosis in anorexia nervosa and involuntary starvation. *Br J Haematol.* 1985;60(3):525-530.

246. Kaiser U, Barth N. Haemolytic anaemia in a patient with anorexia nervosa. *Acta Haematol.* 2001;106(3):133-135.

247. Van Dissel JT, Gerritsen HJ, Meinders AE. Severe hypophosphatemia in a patient with anorexia nervosa during oral feeding. *Miner Electrol Metabol.* 1992;18(6):365-369.

248. Almoznino-Sarafian D, Shteinshnaider M, Tzur I, et al. Anemia in diabetic patients at an internal medicine ward: clinical correlates and prognostic significance. *Eur J Intern Med.* 2010;21(2):91-96.

249. Alsayegh F, Waheedi M, Bayoud T, Al Hubail A, Al-Refaei F, Sharma P. Anemia in diabetes: experience of a single treatment center in Kuwait. *Prim Care Diabetes.* 2017;11(4):383-388.

250. Hong JH, Choi YK, Min BK, et al. Relationship between hepcidin and GDF15 in anemic patients with type 2 diabetes without overt renal impairment. *Diabetes Res Clin Pract.* 2015;109(1):64-70.

Chapter 43 ■ Anemias During Pregnancy and the Postpartum Period

ROBERT T. MEANS JR

OVERVIEW/EPIDEMIOLOGY

At least a mild reduction in maternal hemoglobin concentration or hematocrit is almost universal by the end of the second trimester of pregnancy.[1] Significant anemia (defined as a hemoglobin concentration <10 g/dL) occurs with a prevalence ranging between 2% and 26%, depending on the population studied.[2-4] Anemia is a major contributor to maternal and fetal morbidity and mortality. While this association is most striking in less developed countries, it has been observed in high resource countries also.[2-7]

Anemia in pregnancy represents a combination of various potential etiologies. The common underlying mechanism is a consequence of the physiology of pregnancy itself (see Physiologic Anemia of Pregnancy). Superimposed on this can be nutrient deficiency (typically in the context of a preexisting deficiency exacerbated by childbearing), hemolysis, or bone marrow failure syndromes. Pregnant women also remain susceptible to etiologies of anemia unrelated to their pregnancy.[8] In some cases, such as sickle cell anemia, the underlying condition has major implications for the management of pregnancy.

PHYSIOLOGIC ANEMIA OF PREGNANCY

Expansion of the plasma volume is the cause of the physiologic anemia of pregnancy (*Table 43.1*). The expanded plasma volume drives a decrease in the volume-dependent indicators of anemia (the hematocrit, the blood hemoglobin concentration, and the circulating erythrocyte count) but does not reduce the absolute amount of hemoglobin or of erythrocytes in the circulation as a whole. It has been speculated that the physiologic anemia of pregnancy serves the purpose of reducing maternal blood viscosity, thereby enhancing placental perfusion and facilitating oxygen and nutrient delivery to the fetus.[9] Beginning approximately in the 6th week of pregnancy, the plasma volume increases disproportionately to the red cell mass. The plasma volume generally reaches a maximum value at approximately 24 weeks' gestation but may continue increasing into the late third trimester. At its peak, the plasma volume is about 40% to 50% higher than at the start of pregnancy.[10] The reduction in the hematocrit, hemoglobin concentration, and circulating erythrocyte count is generally apparent by the 7th to 8th week of pregnancy and continues until a new equilibrium is reached at the 16th to 22nd week.[11] As a result of this new physiologic equilibrium, it has been suggested that a hemoglobin concentration <11 g/dL in the late first trimester and <10.5 g/dL in the second and third trimesters are the lower limits for physiologic anemia:

Table 43.1. Features of the Physiologic Anemia of Pregnancy

Plasma volume begins to increase during the sixth week of pregnancy.
There is no significant increase in erythrocyte production during the first trimester.
Dilutional anemia is first apparent by the seventh to eighth week.
Increase in erythrocyte production is apparent during the second trimester.
Lowest hemoglobin explainable by dilutional effect (the physiologic anemia of pregnancy) is 11 g/dL in the first trimester and 10.5 g/dL in the second and third trimesters.
Physiologic anemia of pregnancy is normochromic, is normocytic, does not worsen during the third trimester, and does not require additional evaluation or specific treatment.

below these a pathologic cause should be sought.[12] In patients with β-thalassemia trait who have only modest anemia at baseline, hemoglobin concentration may drop significantly after the first trimester of pregnancy.[13]

During pregnancy, a 15% to 25% increase in the red cell mass generally occurs but is concealed by the dilutional effect of the increase in plasma volume.[11] This is driven by an increase in serum erythropoietin concentrations during the late second and early third trimesters.[14] A greater increase in the red cell mass occurs if the mother takes iron supplements.[1] Studies of reticulocyte subpopulations and serum transferrin receptor concentration indicate that maternal erythropoiesis increases late in gestation and returns to normal by about 1 month after delivery.[15]

Maternal plasma volume generally decreases during the final weeks of pregnancy, and consequently, the hematocrit, hemoglobin, and circulating erythrocyte count increase.[10] The maternal blood volume generally returns to prepregnancy levels within 1 to 6 weeks after delivery, in part reflecting blood loss at delivery.

IRON DEFICIENCY DURING PREGNANCY

The physiologic anemia of pregnancy is normochromic and normocytic. If a pregnant woman has a microcytic or macrocytic anemia, nonphysiologic causes must be considered. Iron deficiency with or without anemia is common in women of childbearing age and is certainly the most common cause of nonphysiologic anemia during pregnancy.[16] It is particularly common in economically and socially disadvantaged populations but no population group is free of it.[17] The prevalence of iron deficiency ranges from 16% to 55% in pregnant women during the third trimester. This partially reflects utilization of iron by the fetus and partially reflects the high prevalence of preexisting iron deficiency among women of childbearing years.[16,18] In a large review of women of childbearing age, 20% had presumed iron reserves of >500 mg (defined as a serum ferritin concentration >70 µg/L), 40% had iron stores of 100 to 500 mg (serum ferritin 30-70 µg/L), and 40% had undetectable iron stores (serum ferritin <30 µg/L). The latter two categories require supplementation during pregnancy.[19] In a study of healthy nonanemic women in the first trimester, 42% had iron deficiency.[16] The fetus is a privileged recipient of the nutrients required for hemoglobin synthesis: the hemoglobin concentration of infants born to mothers who have severe iron deficiency anemia is normal, and the child's serum iron, transferrin saturation, and serum ferritin levels are unrelated to maternal iron status in most situations.[20,21] The demand for absorbed iron increases from 0.8 mg/d in early pregnancy to 7.5 mg/d in late pregnancy.

There is evidence that the risks of premature delivery, low birth weight, and infant death are increased by severe iron deficiency. However, it is sometimes difficult to distinguish the effects of iron deficiency itself from the effects of the conditions that led to the deficiency. Maternal iron deficiency may also have effects on early neurocognitive development, although that is not clearly established.[22] In a review of published reports, routine iron supplementation decreased the frequency of anemia at term by 73% and the frequency of iron deficiency anemia by 67%.[23] A large case-control study from Venezuela indicated that maternal iron deficiency was associated with increased risk of premature delivery (risk ratio, 1.70; 95% confidence interval, 1.18-2.57).[24] A similar review showed comparable effects on maternal anemia but had no detectable effect on maternal or fetal outcome.[25] It is not clear that maternal iron deficiency reduces the fetal iron supply.[26] It has been reported that iron deficiency anemia in the first trimester is associated with low birth weight but that later development of iron deficiency is not.[27] Iron deficiency leads to placenta hypertrophy, the significance of which is unclear.[28]

In one study of iron supplementation (78 mg/d), 81.5% of women receiving iron (mean hemoglobin 12.4 g/dL) and only 16% of women not supplemented (mean hemoglobin at term 10.9 g/dL) had stainable marrow iron present at term.[1] An iron supplement of 65 mg elemental iron mg per day beginning at or before 20 weeks' gestation generally is adequate to prevent iron deficiency during pregnancy.[19] Oral iron supplementation 2 or 3 days per week appear to give comparable benefits in pregnancy outcomes, although mothers are slightly more anemic at the time of delivery.[29] Some authors recommend that all pregnant women receive iron supplements beginning at 18 to 20 weeks, whereas others recommend that iron supplementation be provided selectively. Routine iron supplementation is considered low risk but is not recommended in the United Kingdom (UK) guidelines; the United States Preventive Services Task Force and the American College of Obstetrics and Gynecology do not take a position on this issue at present (reviewed in[22]).

Approaches to selective supplementation are generally based on risk for iron deficiency or on estimates of iron status. These include treating patients at high risk (based on underlying disorders or prevalence of iron deficiency in the geographic or socioeconomic context) with 80 to 100 mg elemental iron per day and those at low risk with 30 to 40 mg/d.[30] An alternate approach based on serum ferritin provides no iron supplementation for serum ferritin >70 µg/L, low-risk-level iron supplementation for serum ferritin 30 to 70 µg/L, and high-risk-level iron supplementation for lower values.[31] Selective supplementation guided by serum hepcidin concentrations has been studied also.[32]

The usual criteria for diagnosing iron deficiency are valid during pregnancy (see Chapter 25). The most effective indicator of iron status in pregnancy is the serum ferritin. Ferritin cutoff values for iron deficiency from 10 to 30 ng/mL have been reported: a ferritin value of 30 ng/mL is 98% specific and 92% sensitive for iron deficiency (reviewed in[22]). Measurement of serum transferrin receptors may be useful in complicated situations in which inflammatory disease makes the serum ferritin value less reliable.[33] Expression of the iron-regulatory peptide hepcidin appears to be suppressed during pregnancy, consistent with an increased iron demand.[34]

Actual iron deficiency anemia should be treated as in individuals who are not pregnant (see Chapter 25). Once-daily or every-other-day dosing of oral iron appears as effective as more frequent administration.[35] Constipation may be an especially problematic side effect in pregnant women. As a general rule, hematologists are only consulted when pregnant patients are intolerant of, or unresponsive to, oral iron or when patients present for prenatal care late in pregnancy and have significant iron deficiency anemia. The safety and efficacy of intravenous iron in the second and third trimesters is well established.[36]

Recombinant erythropoietin administration, combined with iron replacement, has been reported to be an effective treatment for moderate or severe iron deficiency anemia during pregnancy, although a meta-analysis of this topic suggests that the benefits from erythropoietin are relatively modest.[37]

DEFICIENCY OF FOLATE AND OTHER NUTRIENTS DURING PREGNANCY

Macrocytic anemia of pregnancy is typically megaloblastic and, in most cases, results from deficiency of folic acid. However, folic acid deficiency or B_{12} deficiency in pregnancy may be normocytic if iron deficiency or a thalassemia syndrome is present. Megaloblastic anemia complicates fewer than 5% of pregnancies in the developed world but is much more frequent in less developed countries. Anemia from folate or B_{12} deficiency during pregnancy begins most often in the third trimester or shortly after delivery.[38] Folate requirements increase during pregnancy, and the diets of many pregnant patients are insufficient to meet the increased need.[39] Folate deficiency during pregnancy is relatively common, although its frequency depends on the population studied.[40] Although folate deficiency occurs more frequently in

economically disadvantaged patients, this consequence of inadequate eating habits is not confined to the poor or calorically malnourished: obesity in pregnancy is also associated with folate deficiency.[41] In uncomplicated pregnancies, the gastrointestinal absorption of dietary folate (polyglutamate) and folic acid (monoglutamate) is normal.[42] Not all pregnant patients in whom the serum concentration of folate is low have tissue folate deficiency or develop megaloblastic anemia.[38]

However, the most important consequences of folate deficiency during pregnancy are not hematologic. Folate deficiency is clearly associated with fetal neural tube defects and cleft palate, and these defects are established very early in fetal development, long before maternal megaloblastic anemia is developed. The association between low serum folate during the first trimester of pregnancy and fetal neural tube defects has been known for over 25 years.[43] Preconceptional folate supplementation reduces the incidence of neural tube defects to a relative risk of 0.28 (95% confidence interval, 0.13-0.58). Folate does not increase miscarriage, ectopic pregnancy, or stillbirth. Multivitamins without folate do not prevent neural tube defects, and adding multivitamins to folate supplementation does not further reduce the incidence of neural tube defects.[44]

Megaloblastic anemia during pregnancy, as in the nonpregnant patient, is suggested by an increased mean corpuscular volume with oval macrocytes and hypersegmented granulocytes on blood smear. Folate deficiency must be distinguished from vitamin B_{12} deficiency. The latter is rare in pregnancy, and the distinction can often be made on clinical grounds, especially on the basis of a careful nutritional history. Infants born to mothers with the folate-related megaloblastic anemia of pregnancy have no anemia and no biochemical evidence of folate deficiency.[45]

Recommended levels of folate supplementation for neural tube defect prevention are sufficient to prevent folate-deficiency anemia except in circumstances of excess folate demand (hemolysis, urinary tract infection, or bleeding with sustained reticulocytosis).[46] Current US, Canadian, and UK guidelines recommend 0.4 mg/d folate for pregnant women at standard risk and 4 to 5 mg/d at high risk (history of neural tube defects, circumstances noted earlier).[47] In countries that do not fortify food with folate, 0.8 to 1.0 mg/d is recommended.[48]

Anemia because of vitamin B_{12} deficiency is not common in pregnancy, and when it occurs, typically results from preexisting absorption problems or a vegan-equivalent diet without vitamin supplementation.[49] Vitamin B_{12} levels fluctuate in a healthy normal pregnancy, with 15% of patients at 18 weeks having low plasma concentrations (<200 pg/mL), increasing to 43% at 39 weeks but falling back to 3% by 8 weeks postpartum.[50]

Infants of vitamin B_{12}-deficient mothers are generally protected from vitamin B_{12} deficiency during gestation and at birth,[41] but exclusively breast-fed children of vitamin B_{12}-deficient mothers may develop megaloblastic anemia and neurologic damage unless supplemented.[51]

With the possible exception of homocysteine levels, for which there are conflicting results regarding utility for identifying vitamin B_{12} or folate deficiency in pregnancy,[52] the diagnosis and treatment of folate or vitamin B_{12} deficiency in pregnancy follows the usual guidelines (see Chapter 37). If the possibility of vitamin B_{12} or folate-deficiency anemia cannot be distinguished, concurrent therapy should be used.

Anemia because of zinc deficiency has been associated in some studies with fetal growth restriction, congenital abnormalities, and neurodevelopmental delay.[53] Although supplementation with other micronutrients (magnesium, selenium, copper, calcium, and iodine) has generally been shown to improve pregnancy outcome in less developed countries, associations with maternal anemia are less clear.[54] Vitamin A supplementation in developing countries appears to improve pregnancy outcomes and decrease both maternal and neonatal anemia.[55]

MATERNAL ANEMIA ASSOCIATED WITH PRENATAL INFECTIONS

Most clinically significant infections of the fetus are viral or protozoal, but generally these conditions result in minimal evidence of infection in the mother. Specifically, women carrying a fetus infected with cytomegalovirus, toxoplasmosis, rubella, herpes simplex, or parvovirus B_{19} generally have no anemia related to the infection. However, certain infectious diseases during pregnancy do result in maternal anemia. For example, intestinal helminth infections, common in certain parts of the world, produce or exacerbate iron deficiency during pregnancy, resulting in anemia, and this iron deficiency anemia is improved by anthelmintic therapy.[56]

Malaria can cause both maternal and fetal anemia. Maternal anemia from malaria may be a significant contributor to poor outcomes of pregnancy.[57] It has been estimated that 75,000 to 200,000 annual infant deaths are associated with maternal malaria and that maternal malaria itself carries a 17% to 25% maternal mortality.[58]

HEMOLYTIC ANEMIA IN PREGNANCY

Pregnancy-Induced Hemolytic Anemia

A variety of hemolytic anemia syndromes can occur in pregnant women just as in nonpregnant women. The term "pregnancy-induced hemolytic anemia" refers to a rare disorder presenting as a severe idiopathic hemolytic anemia that occurs during pregnancy, resolves completely after pregnancy, and recurs during subsequent pregnancy (*Table 43.2*). The pathogenesis of this anemia is not known. It is likely that some cases are a variant of autoimmune hemolytic anemia occurring during pregnancy,[59] but some lack any defined autoimmune mechanism.[60] Clinical features are outlined in *Table 43.2*. Corticosteroids and intravenous immunoglobulin (IVIG) have been reported to be successful in some cases, but the mainstay of treatment is transfusion support.

Autoimmune Hemolytic Anemia During Pregnancy

In cases of autoimmune hemolytic anemia during pregnancy, whether idiopathic or of an identified variety, the degree of hemolysis is generally more severe in the mother than that in the fetus.[61] However, the therapy that ameliorates the maternal disease (such as corticosteroids or IVIG) often does not protect the fetus. This is in contrast to autoimmune thrombocytopenia during pregnancy, in which maternal and fetal platelet counts are likely to be concordant.

Hemolysis, Elevated Liver Enzymes, and Low Platelets Syndrome

Preeclampsia is characterized by gestational hypertension and proteinuria or pathologic edema; eclampsia is complicated by the additional occurrence of seizures. Preeclampsia and eclampsia are systemic diseases involving the kidney, liver, heart, and central nervous system. Hematologic complications have been recognized for some time and include microangiopathic hemolytic anemia with characteristic fragmented red blood cells (RBCs) in the peripheral blood, thrombocytopenia, and well-defined abnormalities of the coagulation system. This subset of patients with severe preeclampsia/eclampsia are considered to have HELLP syndrome, characterized

by hemolysis (*H*), elevated liver (*EL*) enzymes, and low platelet (*LP*) counts (*Table 43.3*).[62]

It is considered that RBC fragmentation and thrombocytopenia associated with HELLP are the results of a number of interrelated, largely mechanical factors. These include endothelial damage, vasoconstriction coupled with hypertension, and the deposition of fibrin in injured vessels. Women with preeclampsia have abnormalities in coagulation, including signs of chronic intravascular coagulation, shortened platelet life span, decreased plasma antithrombin III activity, abnormalities in circulating fibrinogen multimers, and increased fibrin deposition within the kidney and the liver. Molecular abnormalities in folate metabolism and factor V Leiden may also be seen.[62-64] Women with preeclampsia also have an increased plasma ratio of the antiangiogenic factor soluble fms-like tyrosine kinase (sFlt)-1 to the proangiogenic placental growth factor (PlGF). An elevated sFlt-1/PlGF ratio suggests preeclampsia/HELLP rather than other pregnancy-associated thrombotic microangiopathies.[65]

HELLP syndrome is reported to occur in 20% of women with severe preeclampsia and 10% of women with eclampsia. Most cases present between 27 and 37 weeks of gestation, with 10% occurring earlier and 20% later in pregnancy. Clinical findings at presentation include malaise, right upper quadrant tenderness, nausea and vomiting, hypertension, and edema.[62] Most women with HELLP syndrome are not anemic at presentation, although the proportion of hemoglobin relative to the volume of blood lost at delivery may drop.[66] Anemia and thrombocytopenia are not actually required for the diagnosis, but rather evidence of hemolysis by microangiopathic changes and elevated lactate dehydrogenase (LDH) or decreased haptoglobin.[65]

Laboratory features include elevated liver enzymes (that is, alanine aminotransferase and aspartate aminotransferase [AST]), thrombocytopenia <100,000/μL in most patients, and evidence of compensated hemolysis. The latter is probably the most specific abnormality associated with HELLP syndrome, but it is sometimes difficult to detect. The peripheral blood smear usually reveals schistocytes and sometimes burr cells and polychromatophilia.[62] In one study, however, schistocytes were seen in only a small fraction of patients, and it was proposed that the fragmented cells may have been removed by the spleen.[67] Hemoglobinemia and hemoglobinuria occur in <10% of cases. The one consistent abnormality noted in women with HELLP syndrome is a decreased serum haptoglobin in virtually all patients, and this may be considered a highly sensitive test to detect this RBC abnormality when only a few schistocytes are present on smear.[67] Patients with HELLP syndrome have been reported to have mild to moderate reduction in the von Willebrand factor–cleaving protease a disintegrin and metalloproteinase with a thrombospondin type 1 motif, member 13 (ADAMTS-13) compared with nonpregnant women or women experiencing an uncomplicated pregnancy. These reduced levels were not due to inactivating antibodies.[68] Severely reduced ADAMTS-13 levels would suggest a diagnosis of thrombotic thrombocytopenic purpura (TTP) rather than HELLP. TTP is also distinguished from HELLP by an increased serum LDH/AST ratio.[69]

The management of preeclampsia with HELLP syndrome is a matter of some obstetric debate and is beyond the scope of this chapter. In general, the issues are related to immediate delivery or close observation, and these in turn are governed by maternal clinical status and fetal gestational age.[65] The most common approach is to deliver the fetus as soon as possible or, if it is likely that there is fetal lung immaturity because of gestational age, steroids are administered to the mother for 2 to 3 days and then the infant is delivered. In contrast to TTP, currently, there are no data indicating a role for plasmapheresis.

One of the most serious (but fortunately very rare) complications is hepatic rupture, with 18% to 86% maternal mortality and up to 80% fetal mortality. Other complications include disseminated intravascular coagulation, renal failure, pulmonary edema, and placental abruption.[62] Overall, maternal mortality is 1% to 2%. Hematologic and chemical abnormalities resolve within a few days of delivery. Neonatal mortality is 7.4% to 34%, and this is more a reflection of fetal age rather than any specific complication of maternal HELLP issues.[62]

Table 43.2. Features of Idiopathic Pregnancy-Induced Hemolytic Anemia

There is no consistently identifiable mechanism.
Anemia becomes apparent in the third trimester.
Anemia remits completely within 2 mo of delivery.
Anemia generally recurs in subsequent pregnancies.
Anemia is usually severe, even life threatening.
Corticosteroids and intravenous immunoglobulin are sometimes helpful.
Red cell transfusions are the mainstay of treatment for severe anemia.
Donor cells have a shortened survival.
Neonates generally have transient, nonsevere hemolysis.

Disorders of Red Blood Cells

Table 43.3. Major Clinical Characteristics of HELLP Syndrome, TTP, and aHUS

Clinical Features	HELLP Syndrome	TTP	aHUS
Target organ/ system involved	Liver	Neurologic	Renal
Gestational age	Second to third trimesters	Second trimester	Postpartum
Platelets	Decreased	Decreased	Decreased
PT/PTT	Normal	Normal	Normal
Hemolysis	Present	Present	Present
Fibrinogen	Normal	Normal	Normal
Creatinine	Normal/increased	Increased	Increased
Liver enzymes	Increased	Normal	Normal
sFlt-1/PlGF ratio	>85 prior to 34 wk; >110 after 34 wk	<38	<38
Decreased ADAMTS-13	Mild to moderate	Severe/ absent	Variable; >10%

Abbreviations: aHUS, atypical hemolytic-uremic syndrome; HELLP, hemolysis (*H*), elevated liver (*EL*) enzymes, and low platelet (*LP*) counts; PT, prothrombin time; PTT, partial thromboplastin time; sFlt-1/PlGF, soluble fms-like tyrosine kinase-1/placental growth factor; TTP, thrombotic thrombocytopenic purpura.

Modified/updated from Saphier CJ, Repke JT. Hemolysis, elevated liver enzymes, and low platelets (HELLP) syndrome: a review of diagnosis and management. *Semin Perinatol.* 1998;22(2):118-133. Copyright © 1998 Elsevier. With permission; and Fakhouri F, Scully M, Provôt F, et al. Management of thrombotic microangiopathy in pregnancy and postpartum: report from an international working group. *Blood.* 2020;136(19):2103-2117. Copyright © 2020 American Society of Hematology. With permission.

Pregnancy-Associated Thrombotic Thrombocytopenic Purpura and Atypical Hemolytic-Uremic Syndrome

In most reported studies of thrombotic microangiopathy with pregnancy, TTP and atypical (complement-mediated) hemolytic-uremic syndrome (aHUS) have been distinguished based on the predominant symptomatology, neurologic or renal. TTP most commonly occurs antepartum, with a significant majority of cases presenting before 24 weeks' gestation. Postpartum TTP is less common but can occur. Pregnancy-associated aHUS, on the other hand, typically (94%) occurs after a normal delivery and a short (48-72 hours) symptom-free interval and is characterized by acute-onset renal failure and microangiopathic hemolytic anemia. It should be noted that pregnancy-associated TTP and aHUS may experience worsening in the first 72 hours after delivery. The majority of cases occur with the first pregnancy. Hypertension is almost always found.[70] A small fraction (10%-15%) of patients with aHUS and TTP have signs of preeclampsia. Sometimes TTP/aHUS is not correctly diagnosed until the patient, thought to have preeclampsia, has an atypical prolonged recovery in the postpartum period.[65,70,71]

Laboratory results show the expected hemolytic anemia with many RBC fragments. Severe thrombocytopenia is usually present. Fibrin breakdown products are often increased, but the findings of coagulation studies are usually normal.[72] In postpartum aHUS, azotemia is the rule, but it is rare in TTP. The PLASMIC score will usually be suggestive of TTP but has not been validated in pregnancy.[71]

While ADAMTS-13 levels normally decline in pregnancy to as low as 25%, ADAMTS-13 activity <10% is diagnostic of TTP. Although congenital ADAMTS-13 deficiency represents only 5% of all cases of TTP, it represents approximately 25% of cases of pregnancy-associated TTP and is diagnosed by the absence of ADAMTS-13 antibodies.[71] In an extensive case review, the overall maternal mortality was 44%. Mortality was reduced or eliminated with plasma therapy, but was 68% if plasma therapy was not instituted.[72-76] The pregnancy should not be terminated because this does not cure the disease, and the fetus may survive with successful therapy. Patients with congenital TTP will require prophylactic plasma infusions throughout pregnancy. Recurrence of

antibody-mediated TTP does not occur in all cases. Patients with a history of antibody-mediated TTP should have monitoring of ADAMTS-13 levels. If levels are persistently above 20%, no special management is required. If levels are between 10% and 20%, corticosteroids are used to suppress antibody production. If ADAMTS-13 activity falls below 10%, prophylactic weekly plasma exchange is started unless there is clinical evidence of overt TTP. If there is clinical TTP, daily plasma exchange is initiated.[71] Although there have been no randomized studies, the anticomplement agent eculizumab appears to be safe and to produce remissions in more than 80% of cases.[70] There is less experience with newer anticomplement agents.

BONE MARROW FAILURE SYNDROMES ASSOCIATED WITH PREGNANCY

Aplastic Anemia/Pure Red Cell Aplasia

Pregnancy may occur in patients with existing bone marrow failure syndromes,[77] although this is uncommon and requires cooperation between a high-risk obstetrics expert and a hematologist experienced with bone marrow failure syndromes. Predictors of a poor outcome include thrombocytopenia and aplastic anemia associated with paroxysmal nocturnal hemoglobinuria.[78] Even more uncommon is aplastic anemia that develops during pregnancy. Whether this is a coincident association in most cases is unclear: the observation that approximately 25% of these individuals experience a spontaneous remission after delivery suggests that it is not a coincidence. Patients are generally managed with supportive care during pregnancy and receive specific immunosuppressive therapy subsequently if necessary.

Pure red cell aplasia may also have its initial onset in pregnancy. These patients should also be managed with supportive care, and the majority will experience a remission after delivery. In some cases, subsequent pregnancies are associated with recurrence.[79,80]

Sideroblastic Anemia

There have been a number of case reports and small series of sideroblastic anemia with onset during pregnancy. Some cases appear to represent a coincident association with idiopathic sideroblastic anemia, whereas others appear to be pregnancy induced and may recur with subsequent pregnancies.[81-83] A pregnancy-associated syndrome with morphologic features of both sideroblastic anemia and amegakaryocytic thrombocytopenia has been described, which responds to immunosuppression, but it may also undergo spontaneous remission after delivery.[84]

POSTPARTUM ANEMIA

Postpartum anemia is common, with a reported overall incidence of 27%. Prenatal anemia was the best predictor of postpartum anemia, and like prepartum anemia, postpartum anemia is associated with lower socioeconomic status and decreased access to care. Anemia during pregnancy, maternal obesity, multiple births, and formula feeding also predict postpartum anemia.[7,17]

Peripartum hemorrhage is an obvious and common cause of postpartum anemia. An estimated blood loss at delivery in excess of 500 mL is reported to be a good predictor of postpartum anemia.[85] Unsuccessful vacuum extraction can cause peripartum hemorrhage and subsequent postpartum maternal anemia.[86]

Secondary postpartum hemorrhage refers to hemorrhage occurring a week or more after delivery and has a high morbidity rate. In one large series,[87] secondary postpartum hemorrhage occurred in approximately 1% of women, with most presenting in the second week after delivery. Previous primary postpartum hemorrhage or manual removal of the placenta was the only significant risk factor identified. In all, 84% of these women were rehospitalized, 63% required surgery, and 17% received blood transfusions. After control of bleeding, patients require treatment of iron deficiency in most cases.

Peripartum hemolysis is another cause of postpartum anemia. Hemolytic reactions have been described in women receiving second- and third-generation cephalosporins, such as cefotetan, administered prophylactically for cesarean delivery.[88]

Recombinant erythropoietin has been used in the treatment of postpartum anemia. A recent meta-analysis was not able to demonstrate superiority of erythropoietin over iron alone.[89] Intravenous iron administration for postpartum anemia is safe and effective in patients intolerant of or unresponsive to oral iron therapy.[90]

References

1. de Leeuw NK, Lowenstein L, Hsieh YS. Iron deficiency and hydremia in normal pregnancy. *Medicine (Baltim)*. 1966;45(4):291-315.
2. Levy A, Fraser D, Katz M, Mazor M, Sheiner E. Maternal anemia during pregnancy is an independent risk factor for low birthweight and preterm delivery. *Eur J Obstet Gynecol Reprod Biol*. 2005;122(2):182-186.
3. Adebisi OY, Strayhorn G. Anemia in pregnancy and race in the United States: blacks at risk. *Fam Med*. 2005;37(9):655-662.
4. Xiong X, Buekens P, Fraser WD, Guo Z. Anemia during pregnancy in a Chinese population. *Int J Gynaecol Obstet*. 2003;83(2):159-164.
5. Kozuki N, Lee AC, Katz J; Child Health Epidemiology Reference G. Moderate to severe, but not mild, maternal anemia is associated with increased risk of small-for-gestational-age outcomes. *J Nutr*. 2012;142(2):358-362.
6. Brabin BJ, Hakimi M, Pelletier D. An analysis of anemia and pregnancy-related maternal mortality. *J Nutr*. 2001;131(2S-2):604S-614S.
7. Harrison RK, Lauhon SR, Colvin ZA, McIntosh JJ. Maternal anemia and severe maternal morbidity in a United States cohort. *Am J Obstet Gynecol MFM*. 2021;3(5):100395.
8. Gangopadhyay R, Karoshi M, Keith L. Anemia and pregnancy: a link to maternal chronic diseases. *Int J Gynaecol Obstet*. 2011;115(suppl 1):S11-S15.
9. Stangret A, Skoda M, Wnuk A, Pyzlak M, Szukiewicz D. Mild anemia during pregnancy upregulates placental vascularity development. *Med Hypotheses*. 2017;102:37-40.
10. de Haas S, Ghossein-Doha C, van Kuijk SM, van Drongelen J, Spaanderman ME. Physiological adaptation of maternal plasma volume during pregnancy: a systematic review and meta-analysis. *Ultrasound Obstet Gynecol*. 2017;49(2):177-187.
11. Horowitz KM, Ingardia CJ, Borgida AF. Anemia in pregnancy. *Clin Lab Med*. 2013;33(2):281-291.
12. Recommendations to prevent and control iron deficiency in the United States. Centers for Disease Control and Prevention. *MMWR Recomm Rep (Morb Mortal Wkly Rep)*. 1998;47(Rr-3):1-29.
13. Lao TT. Obstetric care for women with thalassemia. *Best Pract Res Clin Obstet Gynaecol*. 2017;39:89-100.
14. Milman N, Graudal N, Nielsen OJ, Agger AO. Serum erythropoietin during normal pregnancy: relationship to hemoglobin and iron status markers and impact of iron supplementation in a longitudinal, placebo-controlled study on 118 women. *Int J Hematol*. 1997;66(2):159-168.
15. Choi JW, Pai SH. Change in erythropoiesis with gestational age during pregnancy. *Ann Hematol*. 2001;80(1):26-31.
16. Auerbach M, Abernathy J, Juul S, Short V, Derman R. Prevalence of iron deficiency in first trimester, nonanemic pregnant women. *J Matern Fetal Neonatal Med*. 2019;34(6):1-4.
17. Bodnar LM, Scanlon KS, Freedman DS, Siega-Riz AM, Cogswell ME. High prevalence of postpartum anemia among low-income women in the United States. *Am J Obstet Gynecol*. 2001;185(2):438-443.
18. Berger J, Wieringa FT, Lacroux A, Dijkhuizen MA. Strategies to prevent iron deficiency and improve reproductive health. *Nutr Rev*. 2011;69(suppl 1):S78-S86.
19. Milman N, Graudal N, Agger AO. Iron status markers during pregnancy. No relationship between levels at the beginning of the second trimester, prior to delivery and post partum. *J Intern Med*. 1995;237(3):261-267.
20. El-Farrash RA, Ismail EA, Nada AS. Cord blood iron profile and breast milk micronutrients in maternal iron deficiency anemia. *Pediatr Blood Cancer*. 2012;58(2):233-238.
21. Lee S, Guillet R, Cooper EM, et al. Prevalence of anemia and associations between neonatal iron status, hepcidin, and maternal iron status among neonates born to pregnant adolescents. *Pediatr Res*. 2016;79(1-1):42-48.
22. Means RT. Iron deficiency and iron deficiency anemia: implications and impact in pregnancy, fetal development, and early childhood parameters. *Nutrients*. 2020;12(2):447.
23. Yakoob MY, Bhutta ZA. Effect of routine iron supplementation with or without folic acid on anemia during pregnancy. *BMC Publ Health*. 2011;11(suppl 3):S21.
24. Marti A, Pena-Marti G, Munoz S, Lanas F, Comunian G. Association between prematurity and maternal anemia in Venezuelan pregnant women during third trimester at labor. *Arch Latinoam Nutr*. 2001;51(1):44-48.
25. Mahomed K. Iron and folate supplementation in pregnancy. *Cochrane Database Syst Rev*. 2000;900(2):CD001135.
26. Harthoorn-Lasthuizen EJ, Lindemans J, Langenhuijsen MM. Does iron-deficient erythropoiesis in pregnancy influence fetal iron supply? *Acta Obstet Gynecol Scand*. 2001;80(5):392-396.
27. Turgeon O'Brien H, Santure M, Maziade J. The association of low and high ferritin levels and anemia with pregnancy utcome. *Can J Diet Pract Res*. 2000;61(3):121-127.
28. Huang A, Zhang R, Yang Z. Quantitative (stereological) study of placental structures in women with pregnancy iron-deficiency anemia. *Eur J Obstet Gynecol Reprod Biol*. 2001;97(1):59-64.
29. Pena-Rosas JP, De-Regil LM, Gomez Malave H, Flores-Urrutia MC, Dowswell T. Intermittent oral iron supplementation during pregnancy. *Cochrane Database Syst Rev*. 2015;10:Cd009997.
30. Milman N. Oral iron prophylaxis in pregnancy: not too little and not too much. *J Pregnancy*. 2012;2012:514345.
31. Milman N. Iron prophylaxis in pregnancy—general or individual and in which dose? *Ann Hematol*. 2006;85(12):821-828.
32. Bah A, Muhammad AK, Wegmuller R, et al. Hepcidin-guided screen-and-treat interventions against iron-deficiency anaemia in pregnancy: a randomised controlled trial in the Gambia. *Lancet Global Health*. 2019;7(11):e1564-e1574.
33. Akinsooto V, Ojwang PJ, Govender T, Moodley J, Connolly CA. Soluble transferrin receptors in anaemia of pregnancy. *J ObstetGynaecol*. 2001;21(3):250-252.
34. Koenig MD, Tussing-Humphreys L, Day J, Cadwell B, Nemeth E. Hepcidin and iron homeostasis during pregnancy. *Nutrients*. 2014;6(8):3062-3083.
35. Moretti D, Goede JS, Zeder C, et al. Oral iron supplements increase hepcidin and decrease iron absorption from daily or twice-daily doses in iron-depleted young women. *Blood*. 2015;126(17):1981-1989.
36. Auerbach M, James SE, Nicoletti M, et al. Results of the first American prospective study of intravenous iron in oral iron-intolerant iron-deficient gravidas. *Am J Med*. 2017;130(12):1402-1407.
37. Dodd J, Dare MR, Middleton P. Treatment for women with postpartum iron deficiency anaemia. *Cochrane Database Syst Rev*. 2004;4:CD004222.
38. Achebe MM, Gafter-Gvili A. How I treat anemia in pregnancy: iron, cobalamin, and folate. *Blood*. 2017;129(8):940-949.
39. Lundqvist A, Johansson I, Wennberg A, et al. Reported dietary intake in early pregnant compared to non-pregnant women - a cross-sectional study. *BMC Pregnancy Childbirth*. 2014;14:373.
40. Milman N, Byg KE, Hvas AM, Bergholt T, Eriksen L. Erythrocyte folate, plasma folate and plasma homocysteine during normal pregnancy and postpartum: a longitudinal study comprising 404 Danish women. *Eur J Haematol*. 2006;76(3):200-205.
41. Carter MF, Powell TL, Li C, et al. Fetal serum folate concentrations and placental folate transport in obese women. *Am J Obstet Gynecol*. 2011;205(1):83.e17-83.e25.
42. Iyengar L, Babu S. Folic acid absorption in pregnancy. *Br J Obstet Gynaecol*. 1975;82(1):20-23.
43. Campbell BA. Megaloblastic anemia in pregnancy. *Clin Obstet Gynecol*. 1995;38(3):455-462.
44. Lumley J, Watson L, Watson M, Bower C. Periconceptional supplementation with folate and/or multivitamins for preventing neural tube defects. *Cochrane Database Syst Rev*. 2001;3:CD001056.
45. Grossowicz N, Izak G, Rachmilewitz M. The effect of anemia on the concentration of folate derivatives in paired fetal-maternal blood. *Isr J Med Sci*. 1966;2(4):510-512.
46. Willoughby ML. An investigation of folic acid requirements in pregnancy. II. *Br J Haematol*. 1967;13(4):503-509.
47. Moussa HN, Hosseini Nasab S, Haidar ZA, Blackwell SC, Sibai BM. Folic acid supplementation: what is new? Fetal, obstetric, long-term benefits and risks. *Future science OA*. 2016;2(2):Fso116.
48. Obeid R, Schon C, Wilhelm M, Pietrzik K, Pilz S. The effectiveness of daily supplementation with 400 or 800 microg/day folate in reaching protective red blood folate concentrations in non-pregnant women: a randomized trial. *Eur J Nutr*. 2018;57:1771-1780.
49. Piccoli GB, Clari R, Vigotti FN, et al. Vegan-vegetarian diets in pregnancy: danger or panacea? A systematic narrative review. *BJOG*. 2015;122(5):623-633.
50. Milman N, Byg KE, Bergholt T, Eriksen L, Hvas AM. Cobalamin status during normal pregnancy and postpartum: a longitudinal study comprising 406 Danish women. *Eur J Haematol*. 2006;76(6):521-525.
51. Jain R, Singh A, Mittal M, Talukdar B. Vitamin B12 deficiency in children: a treatable cause of neurodevelopmental delay. *J Child Neurol*. 2015;30(5):641-643.
52. Malinow MR, Duell PB, Williams MA, et al. Short-term folic acid supplementation induces variable and paradoxical changes in plasma homocyst(e)ine concentrations. *Lipids*. 2001;36(suppl):S27-S32.
53. Shamim AA, Kabir A, Merrill RD, et al. Plasma zinc, vitamin B(12) and alpha-tocopherol are positively and plasma gamma-tocopherol is negatively associated with Hb concentration in early pregnancy in north-west Bangladesh. *Publ Health Nutr*. 2013;16(8):1354-1361.
54. Haider BA, Bhutta ZA. Multiple-micronutrient supplementation for women during pregnancy. *Cochrane Database Syst Rev*. 2017;4:Cd004905.
55. McCauley ME, van den Broek N, Dou L, Othman M. Vitamin A supplementation during pregnancy for maternal and newborn outcomes. *Cochrane Database Syst Rev*. 2015;2015(10):Cd008666.
56. Nurdia DS, Sumarni S, Suyoko, Hakim M, Winkvist A. Impact of intestinal helminth infection on anemia and iron status during pregnancy: a community based study in Indonesia. *Southeast Asian J Trop Med Publ Health*. 2001;32(1):14-22.
57. Bardaji A, Martinez-Espinosa FE, Arevalo-Herrera M, et al. Burden and impact of Plasmodium vivax in pregnancy: a multi-centre prospective observational study. *PLoS Neglected Trop Dis*. 2017;11(6):e0005606.
58. Desale M, Thinkhamrop J, Lumbiganon P, Qazi S, Anderson J. Ending preventable maternal and newborn deaths due to infection. *Best Pract Res Clin Obstet Gynaecol*. 2016;36:116-130.
59. Katsuragi S, Sameshima H, Omine M, Ikenoue T. Pregnancy-induced hemolytic anemia with a possible immune-related mechanism. *Obstet Gynecol*. 2008;111 (2 pt 2):528-529.
60. Kumar R, Advani AR, Sharan J, Basharutallah MS, Al-Lumai AS. Pregnancy induced hemolytic anemia: an unexplained entity. *Ann Hematol*. 2001;80(10):623-626.
61. Batalias L, Trakakis E, Loghis C, et al. Autoimmune hemolytic anemia caused by cold agglutinins in a young pregnant woman. *J Matern Fetal Neonatal Med*. 2006;19(4):251-253.
62. Haram K, Svendsen E, Abildgaard U. The HELLP syndrome: clinical issues and management. A Review. *BMC Pregnancy Childbirth*. 2009;9:8.
63. Haram K, Mortensen JH, Nagy B. Genetic aspects of preeclampsia and the HELLP syndrome. *J Pregnancy*. 2014;2014:910751.

64. Gardiner C, Vatish M. Impact of haemostatic mechanisms on pathophysiology of preeclampsia. *Thromb Res.* 2017;151(suppl 1):S48-S52.

65. Fakhouri F, Scully M, Provôt F, et al. Management of thrombotic microangiopathy in pregnancy and postpartum: report from an international working group. *Blood.* 2020;136(19):2103-2117.

66. Curtin WM, Weinstein L. A review of HELLP syndrome. *J Perinatol.* 1999;19(2):138-143.

67. Wilke G, Rath W, Schutz E, Armstrong VW, Kuhn W. Haptoglobin as a sensitive marker of hemolysis in HELLP-syndrome. *Int J Gynaecol Obstet.* 1992;39(1):29-34.

68. Lattuada A, Rossi E, Calzarossa C, Candolfi R, Mannucci PM. Mild to moderate reduction of a von Willebrand factor cleaving protease (ADAMTS-13) in pregnant women with HELLP microangiopathic syndrome. *Haematologica.* 2003;88(9):1029-1034.

69. Keiser SD, Boyd KW, Rehberg JF, et al. A high LDH to AST ratio helps to differentiate pregnancy-associated thrombotic thrombocytopenic purpura (TTP) from HELLP syndrome. *J Matern Fetal Neonatal Med.* 2011;25(7):1059-1063.

70. Gupta M, Govindappagari S, Burwick RM. Pregnancy-associated atypical hemolytic uremic syndrome: a systematic review. *Obstet Gynecol.* 2020;135(1):46-58.

71. Ferrari B, Peyvandi F. How I treat thrombotic thrombocytopenic purpura in pregnancy. *Blood.* 2020;136(19):2125-2132.

72. Weiner CP. Thrombotic microangiopathy in pregnancy and the postpartum period. *Semin Hematol.* 1987;24(2):119-129.

73. Egerman RS, Witlin AG, Friedman SA, Sibai BM. Thrombotic thrombocytopenic purpura and hemolytic uremic syndrome in pregnancy: review of 11 cases. *Am J Obstet Gynecol.* 1996;175(4 pt 1):950-956.

74. Ezra Y, Rose M, Eldor A. Therapy and prevention of thrombotic thrombocytopenic purpura during pregnancy: a clinical study of 16 pregnancies. *Am J Hematol.* 1996;51(1):1-6.

75. Rose M, Rowe JM, Eldor A. The changing course of thrombotic thrombocytopenic purpura and modern therapy. *Blood Rev.* 1993;7(2):94-103.

76. Scully M, Starke R, Lee R, Mackie I, Machin S, Cohen H. Successful management of pregnancy in women with a history of thrombotic thrombocytopaenic purpura. *Blood Coagul Fibrinolysis.* 2006;17(6):459-463.

77. Faivre L, Meerpohl J, Da Costa L, et al. High-risk pregnancies in Diamond-Blackfan anemia: a survey of 64 pregnancies from the French and German registries. *Haematologica.* 2006;91(4):530-533.

78. Tichelli A, Socie G, Marsh J, et al. Outcome of pregnancy and disease course among women with aplastic anemia treated with immunosuppression. *Ann Intern Med.* 2002;137(3):164-172.

79. Choudry MA, Moffett BK, Laber DA. Pure red-cell aplasia secondary to pregnancy, characterization of a syndrome. *Ann Hematol.* 2007;86(4):233-237.

80. Means RT. Pure red cell aplasia. *Blood.* 2016;128(21):2504.

81. Barton JR, Shaver DC, Sibai BM. Successive pregnancies complicated by idiopathic sideroblastic anemia. *Am J Obstet Gynecol.* 1992;166(2):576-577.

82. Jackson N, Hamizah I. Sideroblastic anemia recurring during two pregnancies. *Int J Hematol.* 1996;65(1):85-88.

83. Impey L, Greenwood C, Taylor A, Redman C, Wainscoat J. Recurrent acquired sideroblastic anemia in a twin pregnancy. *J Matern Fetal Med.* 2000;9(4):248-249.

84. Natelson EA. Pregnancy-induced pancytopenia with cellular bone marrow: distinctive hematologic features. *Am J Med Sci.* 2006;332(4):205-207.

85. Swaim LS, Perriatt S, Andres RL, Paradissis J, Watson MN. Clinical utility of routine postpartum hemoglobin determinations. *Am J Perinatol.* 1999;16(7):333-337.

86. Sheiner E, Shoham-Vardi I, Silberstein T, Hallak M, Katz M, Mazor M. Failed vacuum extraction. Maternal risk factors and pregnancy outcome. *J Reprod Med.* 2001;46(9):819-824.

87. Hoveyda F, MacKenzie IZ. Secondary postpartum haemorrhage: incidence, morbidity and current management. *BJOG.* 2001;108(9):927-930.

88. Shariatmadar S, Storry JR, Sausais L, Reid ME. Cefotetan-induced immune hemolytic anemia following prophylaxis for cesarean delivery. *Immunohematol/American Red Cross.* 2004;20(1):63-66.

89. Markova V, Norgaard A, Jorgensen KJ, Langhoff-Roos J. Treatment for women with postpartum iron deficiency anaemia. *Cochrane Database Syst Rev.* 2015;2015(8):Cd010861.

90. Iyoke CA, Emegoakor FC, Ezugwu EC, et al. Effect of treatment with single total-dose intravenous iron versus daily oral iron(III)-hydroxide polymaltose on moderate puerperal iron-deficiency anemia. *Therapeut Clin Risk Manag.* 2017;13:647-653.

Chapter 44 ■ Anemias Unique to the Fetus and Neonate

ROBERT D. CHRISTENSEN • ROBIN K. OHLS

INTRODUCTION

Diagnosing anemia in a fetus or neonate requires the aid of appropriate reference intervals. Erythropoietic development during the fetal period creates constantly increasing hemoglobin and hematocrit values[1,2]; thus, a hemoglobin or hematocrit that is normal (within the reference interval) for a neonate born prematurely at 25 weeks' gestation might very well constitute an anemic value of a neonate born at term. Once anemia is recognized in a fetus or neonate, the differential diagnosis is unique from that at all other ages. In this chapter, we display the pertinent reference intervals and review the underlying differences in erythropoiesis, erythrocyte structure, function, and metabolism that make anemias in the fetus and neonate so unique.

ERYTHROPOIETIN BIOLOGY IN THE FETUS AND NEONATE

During human fetal and neonatal development, erythropoietin has critical erythropoietic and nonerythropoietic actions (*Table 44.1*).[3,4] Although initially described by, and principally known for, its actions on erythroid progenitors, erythropoietin is also an important physiologic growth factor for fetal small intestinal villous enterocytes and neurons.[4-6]

Human amniotic fluid contains erythropoietin in concentrations of 25 to 40 mU/mL. In the third trimester, a fetus swallows 200 to 300 mL of amniotic fluid per kilogram body weight per day, thus ingesting 10 to 15 U of erythropoietin per kg/d.[7] In humans, erythropoietin does not cross the placenta from the maternal to the fetal circulation, and it appears that the source of the erythropoietin in amniotic fluid is not the maternal circulation. In the second and third trimesters, amniotic fluid is largely derived from fetal urine, with minor constituents from fetal tracheal effluent and the placenta and fetal membranes. However, erythropoietin in amniotic fluid does not appear to come from fetal urine. Studies using in situ hybridization and immunohistochemistry indicate that the source of erythropoietin in amniotic fluid is largely placental, from mesenchymal and endothelial cells in the deciduae and from the amnion.[8]

Erythropoietin is present in human colostrum and breast milk in concentrations of 10 to 20 mU/mL.[4-7] Erythropoietin concentrations in mother's milk do not correlate with erythropoietin concentrations in her blood. In fact, over the first weeks of lactation, maternal serum erythropoietin concentrations fall, whereas milk erythropoietin concentrations increase, reaching the highest concentrations in women breast-feeding for a year or more. The source of erythropoietin in breast milk appears to be mammary gland epithelium.[6,7]

Erythropoietin in human amniotic fluid, colostrum, and breast milk is relatively protected from proteolytic digestion in the fetal and neonatal gastrointestinal tract.[8] Rather than being absorbed from the gastrointestinal tract into the blood, the erythropoietin swallowed by the fetus and neonate binds to erythropoietin receptors on the luminal surface of villous enterocytes, where it serves topically as a growth and development factor. Indeed, experimental animals artificially fed formulas devoid of erythropoietin have retarded villous development, a condition that can be remedied by enteral recombinant erythropoietin and blocked by anti-erythropoietin antibody.[4-9]

Erythropoietin is produced by cells in the developing central nervous system and is present in relatively high concentrations in fetal cerebrospinal fluid (CSF).[9-12] Among newborn infants, the highest concentrations of erythropoietin in the CSF are seen in the most premature neonates, and by several years of age CSF erythropoietin concentrations are generally below 1 mU/mL. Erythropoietin receptors are expressed on human fetal neurons, and at least small quantities of recombinant erythropoietin, administered intravenously, cross the blood-brain barrier and appear in the CSF.[13] Erythropoietin in the central nervous system is a neuroprotectant from hypoxia. Erythropoietin production and erythropoietin receptor expression increase rapidly in the brain during hypoxia; when erythropoietin binds to receptors on neurons, antiapoptotic activity is induced. Cell culture systems and whole animal models illustrate a marked neuroprotective effect of erythropoietin.[14] The clinical utility of recombinant erythropoietin as a neuroprotectant is a topic of recent and ongoing studies.[15-17]

The liver is the primary site of erythropoietin production in the fetus. The kidney does not become the primary site until several months after birth. In the human fetus, the kidney produces about 5% of the total erythropoietin during mid-gestation. The developmental mechanisms regulating the switch in erythropoietin production from the liver to the kidney are not completely known but may involve developmental expression of transcription activators such as hypoxia inducible factor and hepatic nuclear factor 4, or developmental methylation of promoter and enhancer regions. The switch might also involve the GATA transcription factors, particularly GATA-2 and GATA-3, which are negative regulators of erythropoietin gene transcription.

Erythropoietin ameliorates experimental damage to the placenta and fetal liver induced by lipopolysaccharide.[18] Elevated concentrations of erythropoietin in fetal blood and/or amniotic fluid may indicate fetal hypoxia. Although erythropoietin may have a protective role for some fetal cells such as neuronal, placental, hepatic, and intestinal villous cells, it might also be a marker for poor neurodevelopmental outcome on the basis of severe or chronic hypoxia.[19,20] The Preterm Epo for Neuroprotection (PENUT) trial indicated that administering recombinant erythropoietin to extremely low-birth-weight neonates significantly reduced blood transfusions[21] but did not result in a lower risk of severe neurodevelopmental impairment or death at 2 years of age.[22] Also, recent studies in lambs indicate that, while recombinant erythropoietin treatment can reduce brain injury after experimental hypoxic ischemic injury, it may not be additive to hypothermia treatment.[23]

Table 44.1. Erythropoietin in the Human Fetus

Site of Erythropoietin Production	Mechanism of Erythropoietin Delivery to Target Cells	Actions at Target Cells
Hepatocyte/hepatic macrophages	Paracrine	Erythropoiesis/angiogenesis
Glia	Paracrine	Neural migration and protection from hypoxia
Decidua and amniotic membranes (amniotic fluid)	Swallowed by fetus	Small bowel villous development
Mammary epithelia (breast milk)	Swallowed by neonate	Small bowel villous development

REFERENCE INTERVALS FOR ERYTHROCYTE VALUES DURING HUMAN FETAL DEVELOPMENT

"Normal ranges" for erythrocyte values of the human fetus and neonate are not available. This is because blood is not drawn on healthy neonates to establish such ranges. Instead, "reference intervals" are used. These consist of the 5th to the 95th percentile values compiled from laboratory tests performed on neonates who were thought to have minimal pathology relevant to the laboratory test or pathology unlikely to significantly affect the test results. The premise on which the reference interval concept is based is that these values approximate normal ranges, although they were admittedly obtained for a clinical reason and not from healthy volunteers.[1,2]

Erythrocytes in the mid- and third-trimester fetus have features reminiscent of what is called "stress erythropoiesis" in adults. These features include marked anisocytosis, poikilocytosis, macrocytosis, and a relatively high percentage of nucleated erythrocytes. Marrow cellularity in the fetus is relatively high, and because the available marrow space is almost fully cellular, the fetus and newborn infant have little marrow reserve on which to call. Erythroid precursors account for 30% to 65% and myeloid cells 45% to 75% of nucleated marrow cells at birth.[24] The myeloid to erythroid ratio at birth is approximately 1.5:1. Marrow cellularity decreases after birth, attaining a normal adult density by 1 to 3 months. Initially, this decrease in cellularity results from a rapid decline in red blood cell precursors. By 1 week of age, erythroid elements account for only 8% to 12% of nucleated cells and the myeloid to erythroid ratio exceeds 6:1. The normal adult proportion of myeloid to erythroid precursors is not established until the third month. Both the percentage and absolute number of lymphocytes increase during the first 2 months, so that by 3 months of age, they constitute nearly 50% of marrow nucleated cells. Differential counts of bone marrow aspirates from preterm infants are the same as those for term infants.[24]

Reference intervals for the hemoglobin concentration on the day of birth, at gestational ages ranging from 22 to 42 weeks, are shown in *Figure 44.1*. The ranges gradually increase during this period in utero, and unlike in adults and older children there are no differences between genders.[25] In newborn infants, the anatomic site of the blood drawn to measure the hemoglobin and hematocrit influences the test result.[26] Perfusion of small vessels in the extremities can be relatively poor, particularly in the hours after birth or during hypotension or skin cooling, and this can result in increased transudation of fluid and capillary hemoconcentration. Consequently, the hemoglobin concentration and packed cell volume of capillary blood are 5% to 10% higher than those of venous blood.[2] The difference between capillary and venous values is greatest at birth but disappears by 3 months of age. The discrepancy is greatest in preterm infants and in those with hypotension, hypovolemia, and acidosis.[27] Differences can be minimized, but not fully resolved, by warming the extremity before sampling, obtaining freely flowing blood, and discarding the first few drops. The interpretation of serial observations necessitates the consistent use of one site of blood sampling.

Hemoglobin concentrations increase during the first hours after birth attributable in part to a shift of fluid from the intravascular compartment and also to the transfusion of fetal red blood cells from the placenta at the time of birth.[1] After the first day, the reference ranges for hemoglobin and hematocrit gradually decrease, as shown in *Figure 44.2* (term and late preterm neonates) and *Figure 44.3* (preterm neonates).

The mean corpuscular volume (MCV) at birth is highly dependent on gestational age, as shown in *Figure 44.4*.[28] MCV values below the 5th percentile are seen in neonates with α-thalassemia trait, hemoglobin H disease or hereditary spherocytosis.[29-31] A low MCV at birth owing to fetal iron deficiency is less common, but this can occur with chronic fetomaternal hemorrhage or twin-to-twin transfusion syndrome. The mean corpuscular hemoglobin (MCH), like the MCV, is high at birth, by adult standards, and is highly dependent on gestational age. In contrast, the MCH concentration (MCHC) does not change with gestational age and should be in the range of 33 to 35 g/dL in all neonates whether born prematurely or at term. An MCHC value >36.5 g/dL can suggest hereditary spherocytosis, particularly if accompanied by an MCV below the reference range for gestational age.[30,31]

The relative reticulocytosis and normoblastosis in fetal and neonatal blood reflect accelerated erythropoiesis. Reticulocyte counts at birth are approximately 5%, with a range of 4% to 7%.[1] Counts in preterm infants are slightly higher, averaging 6% to 10%. Reticulocytes remain

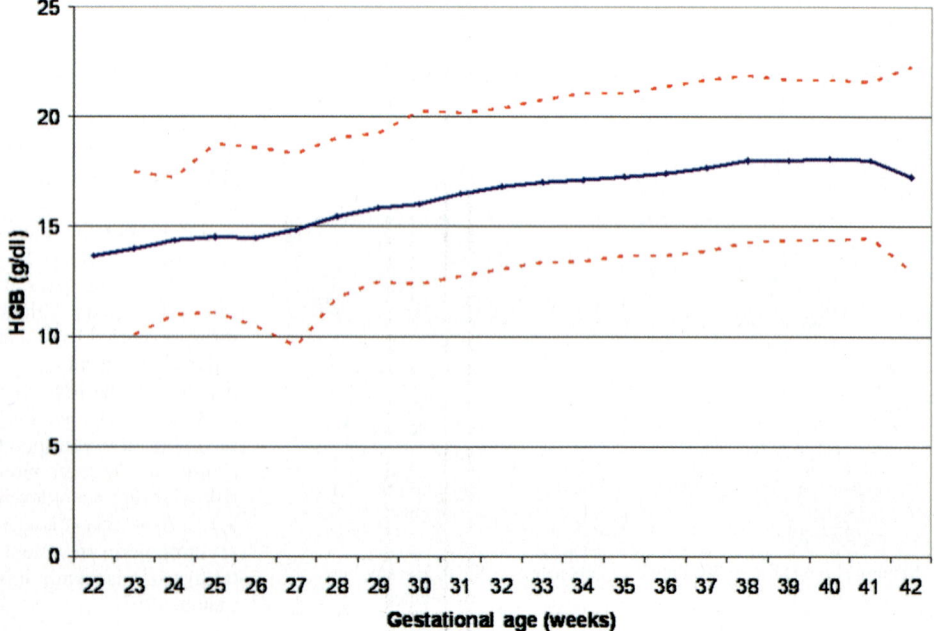

FIGURE 44.1 Reference intervals for blood hemoglobin (HGB) concentration at birth. Values are shown from 24,416 subjects after 22 to 42 weeks' gestation. The solid line shows the mean value, and the dashed lines show the 5% and the 95% reference range. (Reproduced with permission from Jopling J, Henry E, Wiedmeier SE, et al. Reference ranges for hematocrit and blood hemoglobin concentration during the neonatal period: data from a multihospital healthcare system. *Pediatrics.* 2009;123:(2)e333-e337. Copyright © 2009 by the American Academy of Pediatrics.)

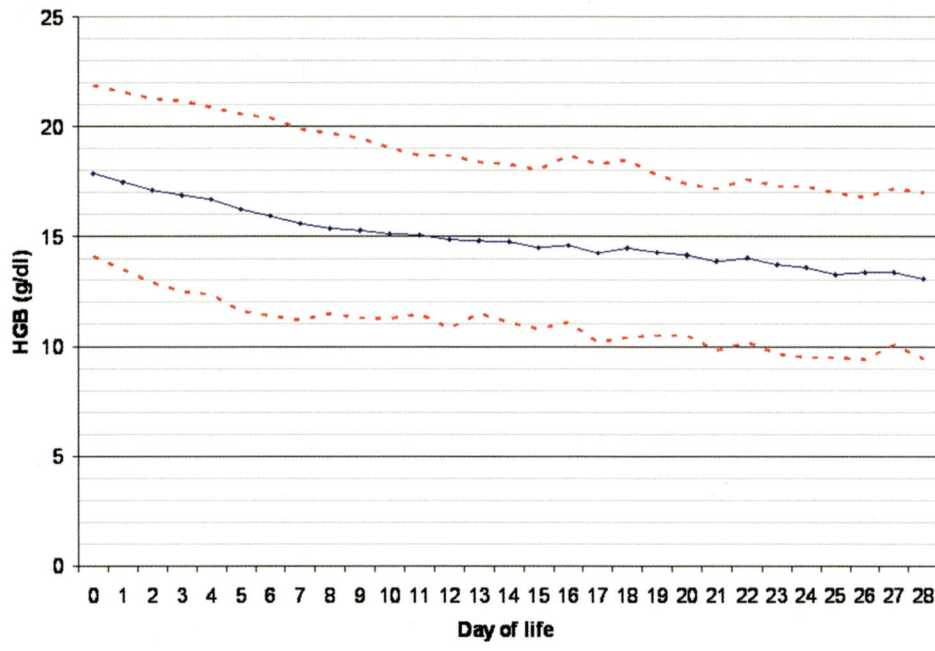

FIGURE 44.2 Reference intervals for blood hemoglobin (HGB) concentration of term and late preterm neonates during the first month after birth. The solid line shows the mean value, and the dashed lines show the 5% and the 95% reference range. (Reproduced with permission from Jopling J, Henry E, Wiedmeier SE, et al. Reference ranges for hematocrit and blood hemoglobin concentration during the neonatal period: data from a multihospital healthcare system. *Pediatrics.* 2009;123(2):e333-e337. Copyright © 2009 by the American Academy of Pediatrics.)

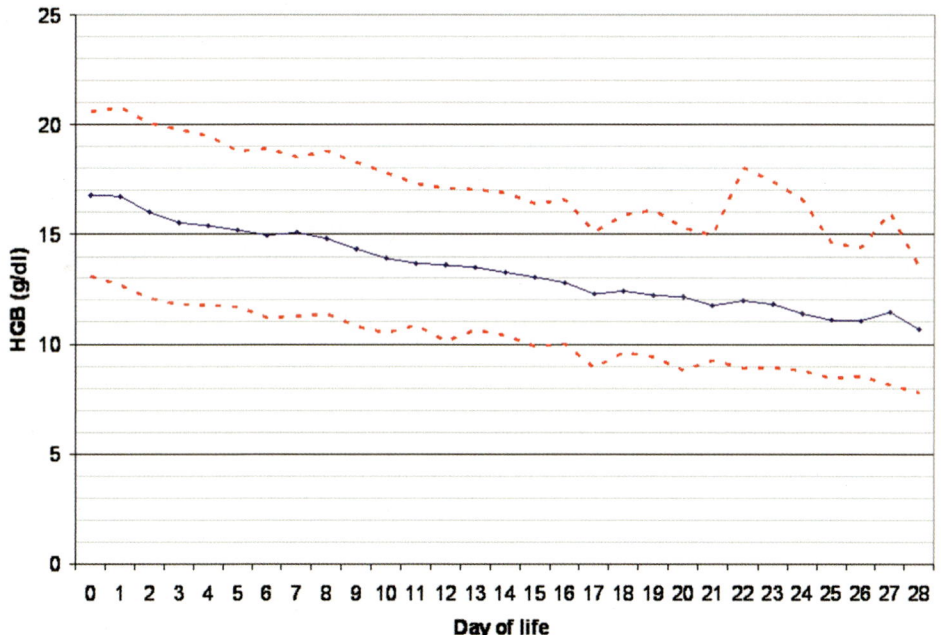

FIGURE 44.3 Reference intervals for blood hemoglobin (HGB) concentration of neonates of 29 to 34 weeks' gestation during the first month after birth. The solid line shows the mean value, and the dashed lines show the 5% and the 95% reference range. (Reproduced with permission from Jopling J, Henry E, Wiedmeier SE, et al. Reference ranges for hematocrit and blood hemoglobin concentration during the neonatal period; data from a multihospital healthcare system. *Pediatrics.* 2009;123(2):e333-e337. Copyright © 2009 by the American Academy of Pediatrics.)

elevated for the first 1 to 2 days of life, then drop abruptly to 0% to 1%. Reference intervals for the reticulocyte parameters, such as reticulocytes per microliter of blood, the immature reticulocyte fraction, and the reticulocyte hemoglobin content, are shown in *Figure 44.5*.[32]

Nucleated red blood cells (NRBCs) are seen regularly on blood smears during the first day of life. The reference ranges for NRBC, according to gestational age at birth, are shown in *Figure 44.6*.[33] Elevations in NRBC in preterm infants correlate with adverse outcomes of intraventricular hemorrhage (IVH) and periventricular leukomalacia, while elevations in NRBC in term infants correlate with hypoxic ischemic encephalopathy and with adverse neurodevelopmental outcomes.

Red blood cell morphology in the newly born preterm or term neonate is characterized by macrocytosis and poikilocytosis. Target cells and irregularly shaped cells are particularly prominent. A high proportion of stomatocytes is noted when viewed by phase contrast microscopy.[34] Similarly, a high proportion of siderocytes (3.16% vs normal male adult mean of 0.09%) is seen.[35] Differential staining of

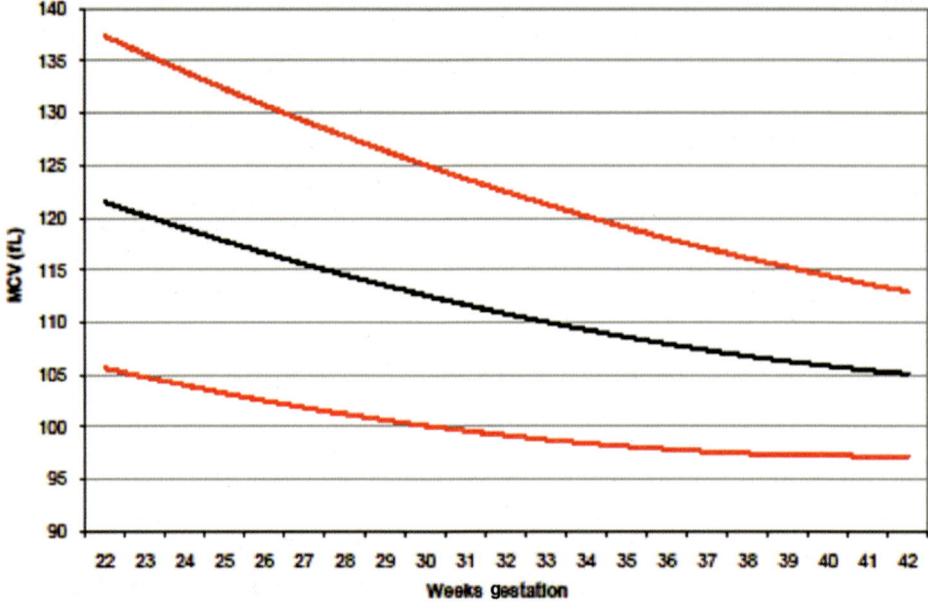

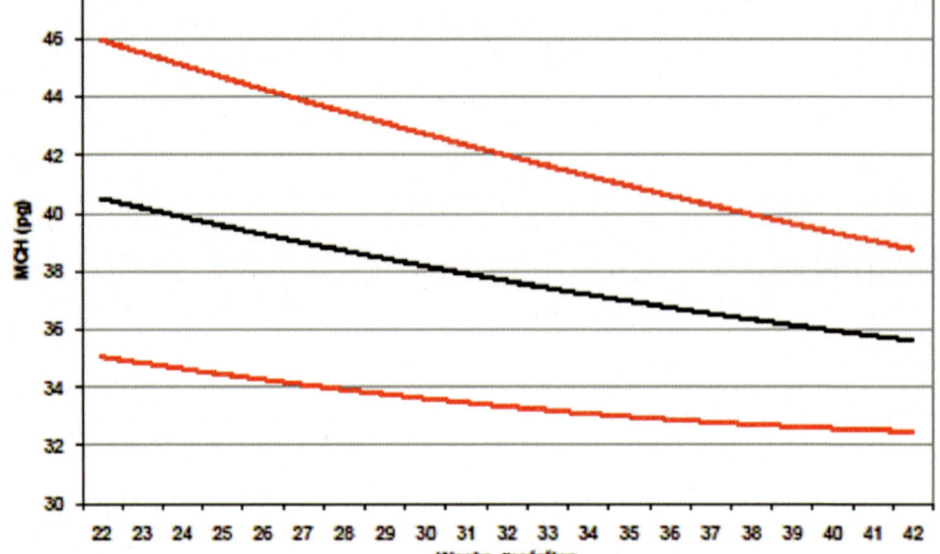

FIGURE 44.4 Reference intervals for mean corpuscular volume (MCV) (top) and mean corpuscular hemoglobin (MCH) (bottom) on the day of birth. Values are shown from subjects after 22 to 42 weeks' gestation. The solid line shows the mean value, and the dashed lines show the 5% and the 95% reference range. (Reprinted by permission from Nature: Christensen RD, Jopling J, Henry E, et al. The erythrocyte indices of neonates, defined using data from over 12,000 patients in a multihospital health care system. *J Perinatol.* 2008;28(1):24-28. Copyright © 2007 Springer Nature.)

red blood cells for fetal hemoglobin (HbF) provides a demonstration of the switch in hemoglobin synthesis that precedes birth: the younger macrocytes contain a minimal amount of HbF, whereas the smaller, older cells are rich in HbF.[36]

Variations in red blood cell size and shape are somewhat greater than those observed in term infants, and cytoplasmic vacuoles are evident in nearly half of all cells when viewed using interference-contrast microscopy. Red blood cell survival is shorter in preterm than in term infants. The capacity of a fetus or neonate to deliver oxygen to tissues is better estimated by the circulating red blood cell volume than by the hematocrit or hemoglobin concentration. However, measuring the circulating red blood cell volume in a fetus or neonate is particularly difficult. Therefore, either the hematocrit or the hemoglobin is often used in making transfusion decisions. Mock et al used a nonradioactive method, based on in vivo dilution

of biotinylated RBC enumerated by flow cytometry, to estimate the correlation between hematocrit and circulating RBC volume in infants below 1300 g, between 7 and 79 days of life. They found that venous hematocrit values correlated highly with the circulating erythrocyte volume (r = 0.907; P < .0001).[37]

Neonates have a shorter red blood cell survival than do children and adults.[38] The life span of red blood cells from term infants is estimated to be 60 to 80 days with use of the ^{51}Cr method and 45 to 70 days using methods involving ^{59}Fe.[38] Fetal studies using [^{14}C] cyanate-labeled red blood cells in sheep revealed an average red blood cell life span of 63.6 ± 5.8 days.[39] The mean red blood cell life span in sheep increased linearly from 35 to 107 days, as the fetal age increased from 97 days (mid-gestation) to 136 days (term).

Neonatal red blood cells transfused into adults have a similarly short survival,[40] indicating that factors *intrinsic* to the newborn red

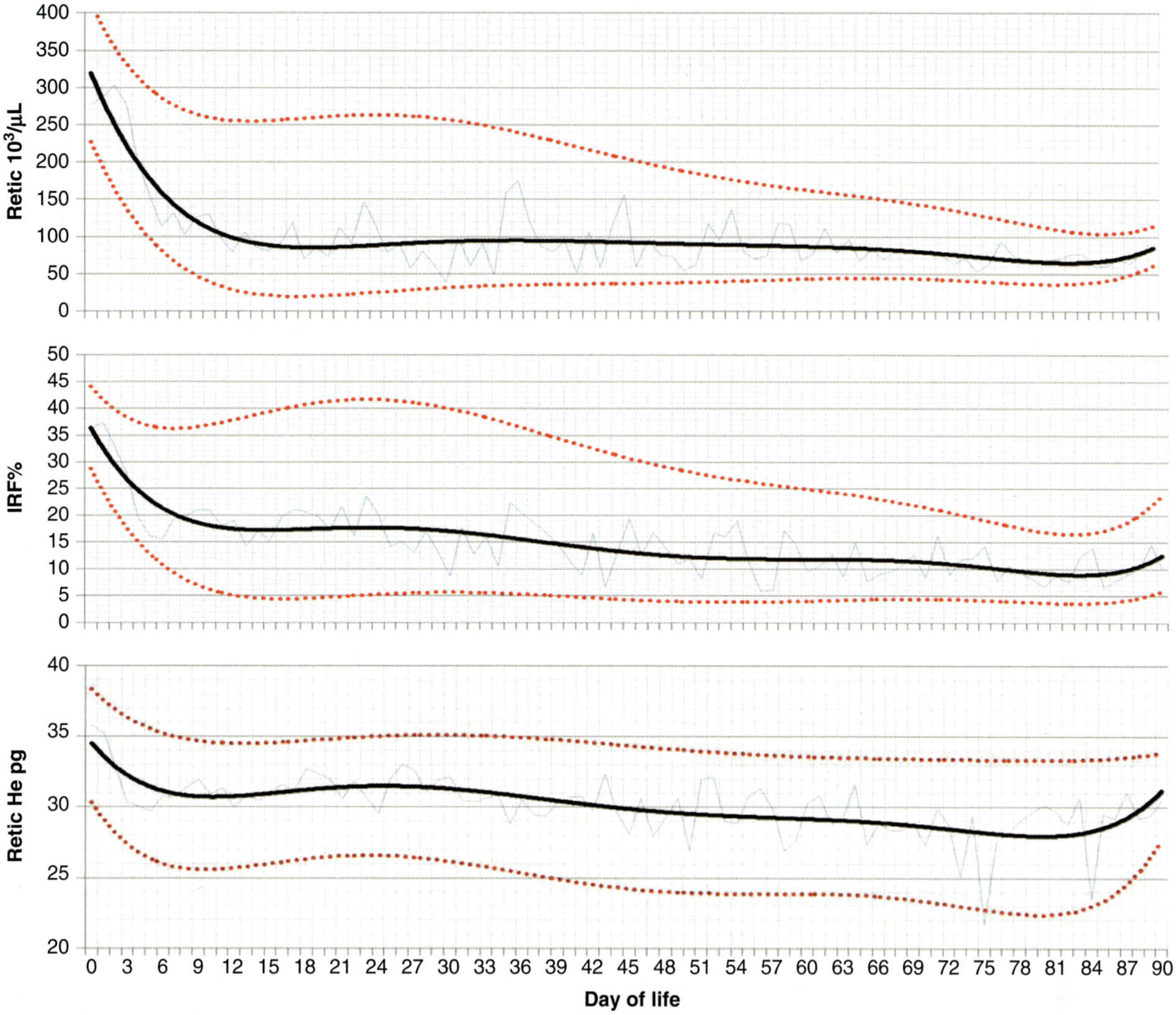

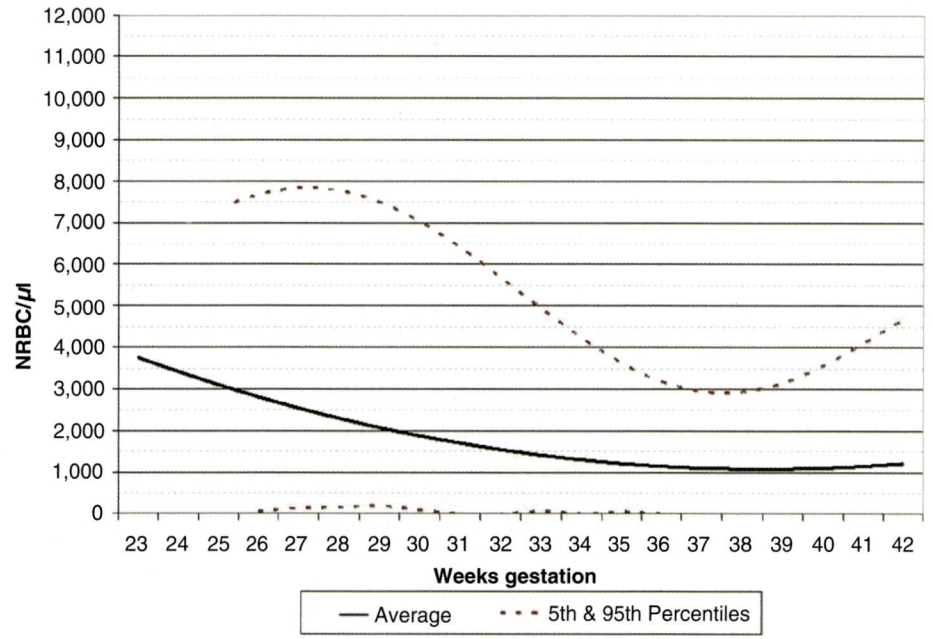

FIGURE 44.5 Reference intervals for reticulocyte parameters during the first 90 days after birth. Top, Reticulocytes (Retic, × 10³/μL blood). Middle, Immature reticulocyte fraction (IRF, %). Bottom, Reticulocyte hemoglobin (Retic He) content (pg). The solid lines show the mean values, and the dashed lines show the 5% and the 95% reference intervals. (Reprinted by permission from Nature: Christensen RD, Henry E, Bennett ST, et al. Reference intervals for reticulocyte parameters of infants during their first 90 days after birth. *J Perinatol*. 2016;36(1):61-66. Copyright © 2015 Springer Nature.)

FIGURE 44.6 Reference ranges for blood concentrations of nucleated erythrocytes on the day of birth. Values are shown from subjects after 23 to 42 weeks' gestation. The solid line shows the mean value, and the dashed lines show the 5% and the 95% reference intervals. NRBC, nucleated red blood cells. (From Christensen RD, Henry E, Andres RL, et al. Reference ranges for blood concentrations of nucleated red blood cells in Neonates. *Neonatology*. 2011;99(4):289-294. Copyright © 2011 Karger Publishers, Basel, Switzerland.)

Disorders of Red Blood Cells

blood cell are responsible. Also, adult red blood cells survive normally in newborn recipients.[41] The life span is not parametrically distributed, in that most cells are destroyed before the mean survival is reached. Shortened red blood cell survival as well as demands imposed by an expanding red blood cell mass accounts for erythropoietic rates at the time of birth that are three to five times higher than those of normal adults.

The transition from the uterus to an oxygen-rich environment triggers responses that have a profound effect on erythropoiesis. During the first 2 months of life, the infant experiences both the highest and the lowest hemoglobin concentrations that occur at any time in development. The highest hemoglobin concentrations are at birth, likely because as a fetus they developed in an environment where oxygen was less available than following birth. Thus, erythropoietin levels at birth usually are well above the normal adult range, as is the hemoglobin concentration, hematocrit, red blood cell count, MCV, and reticulocyte count. Then, erythropoietin levels fall in the immediate postnatal period, with a half-life of 2.6 ± 0.5 hours in infants with polycythemia and 3.7 ± 0.9 hours in infants born to mothers with preeclampsia.[42] By 24 hours, the erythropoietin value is below the normal adult range, where it remains throughout the first month. The decrease in erythropoietin is followed by a decline in the number of bone marrow precursors and a fall in the reticulocyte count, hemoglobin concentration, hematocrit, and MCV.[43]

The combination of shortened cell survival, decreased production, and growth-related expansion of the blood volume is responsible for a progressive fall of the hemoglobin concentration to a mean of approximately 11 g/dL at 2 months of age.[1] The lower range of normal for infants of this age is approximately 9 g/dL. This nadir is called *physiologic anemia*, because it is not associated with apparent distress and is not prevented with nutritional supplements. Stabilization of the hemoglobin concentration is heralded by an increase in reticulocytes at 4 to 8 weeks. Thereafter, the hemoglobin concentration rises to a mean level of 12.5 g/dL, where it remains throughout infancy and early childhood.

At term, the placenta and umbilical cord contain 75 to 125 mL of blood, or approximately one-fourth to one-third of the fetal blood volume. The umbilical arteries constrict shortly after birth but the umbilical vein remains dilated, and blood flows in the direction of gravity. Infants whose umbilical cords remain unclamped can receive half of the placental blood volume (30-mL) in 1 minute. In a randomized trial, 546 infants were randomized at delivery to be held at the introitus ($n = 197$) or to be placed on their mother's abdomen or chest ($n = 192$).[44] Infants were weighted prior to placement and again 2 minutes after, when the umbilical cord was clamped. There was no difference in mean weight change (56 g in the introitus group vs 53 g in the abdomen group) between the two groups. Thus, infant placement on the mother's chest or abdomen during delayed cord clamping results in similar increases in blood volume as maintaining the infant at the level of the introitus.

The blood volume of infants with early cord clamping averages 72 mL/kg, whereas the volume of infants with delayed cord clamping averages 93 mL/kg. Linderkamp et al compared postnatal alterations in blood viscosity, hematocrit, plasma viscosity, red blood cell aggregation, and red blood cell deformability in the first 5 days in full-term neonates with early (less than 10 seconds) and late (3 minutes) cord clamping.[45] The residual placental blood volume decreased from 52 ± 8 mL/kg of neonatal body weight after early cord clamping to 15 ± 4 mL/kg after late cord clamping. The neonatal blood volume was 50% higher in the late cord-clamped infants than in the early cord-clamped infants.

It is possible to promote placental transfer of blood to preterm infants by delaying the clamping of the umbilical cord. In fact, transfer of about 10 mL/kg body weight can be expected using this method.[46] Randomized trials by Mercer et al showed that (1) delayed cord clamping among infants <1500 g birth weight resulted in less IVH and less late-onset sepsis,[47] and (2) generated no greater problem with jaundice.[48]

An alternative approach involves "milking" or "stripping" of the umbilical cord after delivery, while the placenta is still attached to the uterus. This maneuver moves fetal blood toward the fetus before the umbilical cord is clamped. Delayed clamping and cord stripping are roughly equivalent means of providing a small transfusion before birth of a very-low-birth-weight (VLBW) infant, thereby reducing the odds that a donor blood transfusion will be needed during the first days after birth when phlebotomies for laboratory tests commonly result in transfusions to replace the rapidly depleted red blood cell mass.[46,49-51]

An evidence base supporting the practice of delayed cord clamping (and selective cord milking, or "stripping") has expanded in recent years. The differential effect of a 1-, 2-, or 3-minute delay was tested in a randomized study in India among 147 women. Three minutes was superior for reducing subsequent iron deficiency, with no negative effects observed on mothers or babies.[52] Similar outcomes were found in sub-Saharan Africa.[53] Three minutes of delay in cord clamping in term and preterm deliveries has been advocated on the basis of improved neurodevelopmental outcomes.[54] Likewise, 3-year follow-up of 350 Nepalese deliveries indicated more "at-risk" abnormalities in motor development in those randomized to early cord clamping (19% vs 6% with delayed clamping [$P = .02$]). The improved outcomes were exclusively among female neonates.[55] A Canadian study focused on whether delayed cord clamping should be advocated among small for gestational age infants (weight <10th percentile lower reference interval). Using a retrospective cohort of 9722 infants, those who received delayed clamping ≥30 seconds had lower odds of mortality or major morbidity (odds ratio 0.6: 95% confidence interval, 0.42-0.86).[56] An Italian study asked whether delayed cord clamping altered umbilical cord blood gasses, potentially confusing the clinical diagnosis of asphyxia. With 6884 clamped vs unclamped cord gas comparisons, they found slightly lower pH and base excess values with delayed clamped cords, but the authors suggested the differences were so small as to not be of any clinical relevance.[57] An important but unresolved issue is the advisability of performing umbilical cord milking as a potentially more rapid method of accomplishing a cord transfusion. This technique is particularly appealing in cases where time is relevant because a nonvigorous neonate needs resuscitation.[58] In 2020 the American Academy of Pediatrics did not recommend cord milking for neonates <28 weeks' gestation[59]; however, Dani et al expressed lack of confidence in that recommendation, citing benefits in several studies and calling for more and better investigations.[60]

FETAL AND NEONATAL ERYTHROCYTE MEMBRANE AND METABOLISM

Red blood cell membranes of neonates differ slightly from those of adults. The percentage of spectrin dimers and the spectrin tryptic peptide patterns are the same as in adult cells but neonatal cells have more immunoreactive myosin.[61] The quantity and distribution of lipids differ in several respects from adult red blood cells. Total lipid, phospholipid, and cholesterol are increased out of proportion to the surface area of newborn red blood cells.[62] Neonatal cells also exhibit increased endocytosis in response to membrane-active agents, suggesting that the membranes of neonatal cells are less stable and are capable of greater reorganization.[63]

Antigen expression in neonatal red blood cells differs from that of adult cells. The A, B, S, and Lutheran antigens are present in decreased amounts. Replacement of the *i* antigen with its adult counterpart I requires its conversion from a linear polylactosamine to a branched polylactosamine. Reduced A and B antigenicity may result in part from decreased branching and increased stimulation of glycoproteins on neonatal red blood cells.[64] Baseline deformability and viscoelastic properties of RBC of neonates are normal, but they may be more susceptible to endotoxin-induced changes than are those of adults.[65]

Increased concentrations of certain erythrocyte enzymes in neonates can be explained by the young mean age of red blood cells. The increase in glycolytic enzymes is comparable in magnitude to that observed in high-reticulocyte adult blood.[66,67] Increased glycolytic

Table 44.2. Characteristics of Fetal/Neonatal Red Blood Cells

Characteristics Explained by Young Mean Cell Age

- Increased activity of the following enzymes: hexokinase, aldolase, triosephosphate isomerase, phosphoglycerate mutase, pyruvate kinase, lactic dehydrogenase, glucose-6-phosphate dehydrogenase, 6-phosphogluconate dehydrogenase, glutathione reductase, glyoxalase I and II, galactokinase, galactose-1-phosphate uridyl transferase.
- Increased glucose and galactose consumption
- Increased levels of ATP

Characteristics not explained by young cell age and distinctive for neonatal red blood cells

- Embden-Meyerhof pathway: Increased activity of phosphoglycerate kinase, enolase, glucose phosphate isomerase, and glyceraldehyde-3-phosphate dehydrogenase. Decreased activity of phosphofructokinase. 2,3-Diphosphoglycerate instability.
- Pentose phosphate pathway and glutathione metabolism: Decreased glutathione peroxidase and glutathione synthetase. Instability of glutathione and ATP
- Nonglycolytic enzymes: Decreased activity of the following enzymes—carbonic anhydrase, catalase, cholinesterase, adenylate kinase, phosphoribosyl transferase, cytochrome b_5 reductase

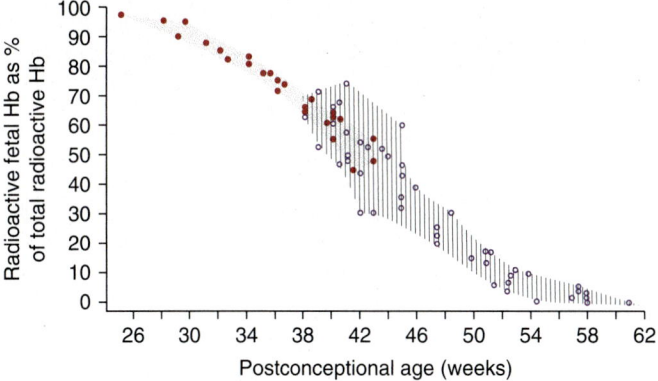

FIGURE 44.7 Decline in fetal hemoglobin (Hb) synthesis as a function of gestational age. Solid dots represent cord blood samples from preterm infants, open circles are samples from term infants. (Used with permission of American Society for Clinical Investigation from Bard H. The postnatal decline of hemoglobin F synthesis in normal full-term infants. *J Clin Invest.* 1975;55(2):395-398; permission conveyed through Copyright Clearance Center, Inc.)

enzyme activity, in turn, is responsible for increased consumption of glucose and galactose and increased levels of adenosine triphosphate (ATP).[68] Unique metabolic characteristics of neonatal erythrocytes are summarized in *Table 44.2.*

In neonates, the activities of four enzymes in the Embden-Meyerhof pathway—phosphoglycerate kinase, enolase, glucose phosphate isomerase, and glyceraldehyde-3-phosphate dehydrogenase—are increased out of proportion to cell age.[69] The activity of phosphofructokinase, a rate-controlling enzyme in glycolysis, is only 40% to 70% of that in adult red blood cells of comparable age.[70] Low levels of phosphofructokinase may produce a block in glycolysis, resulting in the accumulation of glucose-6-phosphate and fructose-6-phosphate and a decrease in the amounts of 2,3-diphosphoglycerate (2,3-DPG) and phosphoenolpyruvate.[71] Decreased activity of phosphofructokinase is probably explained by accelerated decay of a less stable fetal isoenzyme. Neonatal red blood cells contain a homotetramer of liver-type phosphofructokinase subunits rather than the heterotetramer of liver and muscle subunits present in adult cells. Differences in the relative proportions of isoenzymes have also been described for hexokinase and enolase.[72] The concentration of 2,3-DPG falls rapidly during short periods of incubation, apparently because of accelerated breakdown. Preterm infants have lower 2,3-DPG concentrations than term infants. These concentrations gradually increase with gestation.[73] Concentrations can be increased with the use of erythropoietin, thereby shifting the oxygen dissociation curve to the right.[74]

The activities of RBC enzymes are typically increased in neonates, particularly initially after birth, because of a higher reticulocyte count and a young mean red blood cell age. The level of reduced glutathione is equal to or greater than that found in adults, but RBCs of neonates have relative glutathione instability, increased Heinz body formation, and a propensity to increased methemoglobin generation.[75]

Compared with RBCs of adults, ATP levels in neonate's RBCs are elevated, but they fall rapidly during incubation. A disturbance in energy metabolism has been postulated to be responsible for accelerated potassium loss during incubation.[76]

Cord blood contains HbF (α_2, γ_2), HbA (α_2, β_2), and HbA2 (α_2, δ_2), with HbF constituting the major fraction (50%-85%) at term. Because of this, hemoglobinopathies involving β-chain synthesis, such as sickle cell disease and β-thalassemia, do not present in the neonatal period. The G-γ to A-γ ratio at birth is approximately 3:1, in contrast to a ratio of 2:3 in adults.[77] HbA accounts for 15% to 40% of the hemoglobin at term, and HbA2 is present in only trace amounts (mean, 0.3%) but increases slowly after birth, reaching the normal adult level

(2%-3%) by 5 months. The level of HbF at birth is influenced by a number of variables, the most significant of which is gestational age. Premature infants have more HbF and postmature infants less (*Figure 44.7*). Neonates who have survived chronic intrauterine hypoxia, such as occurs with maternal heart and lung disease, have higher levels of HbF. The switch from γ-chain synthesis to β-chain synthesis appears to be developmentally programmed.

HbF has an affinity for oxygen that is greater than that of HbA.[78] The oxygen tension at which the hemoglobin of cord blood is 50% saturated is 19 to 21 mm Hg, 6 to 8 mm Hg lower than that of the hemoglobin of normal adult blood. This shift to the left of the hemoglobin-oxygen dissociation curve results from poor binding of 2,3-DPG by HbF.[79] The position of the oxygen dissociation curve is determined by both the percentage of HbA and the red blood cell content of 2,3-DPG.[80] As the relative proportion of HbA increases, the oxygen dissociation curve shifts by approximately 4 to 6 months of age to a position that is normal for the adult (*Figure 44.8*). The increased oxygen affinity of HbF confers a physiologic advantage to the fetus in facilitating the transfer of oxygen from mother to fetus.

HbF is resistant to alkali denaturation, as determined by the Apt test, and unlike HbA is not eluted from fixed blood smears immersed in an acid buffer, as determined by the Kleihauer-Betke (KB) test.[81] This property permits the differential staining of HbF and HbA, a technique used to detect fetal cells in the maternal circulation.

FETAL AND NEONATAL ANEMIA OWING TO HEMOLYSIS

Hemolytic disease of the fetus and newborn does not typically present with significant jaundice before or at birth, owing to the fact that bilirubin is effectively cleared from fetal blood by the placenta and is metabolized by the maternal liver.[82] However, after birth, bilirubin must be processed by the neonate's liver, which is inherently limited in its ability to metabolize bilirubin efficiently, in part because of a relative deficiency of the cytoplasmic acceptor protein ligandin (encoded by *SLCO1B1*) and in part because of decreased activity of uridine diphosphoglucuronyl transferase (encoded by *UGT1A1*).[82]

Causes of hemolytic disease in the newborn are noted in *Table 44.3.* Worldwide, isoimmunization associated with maternal-fetal blood group incompatibility is the most common cause of neonatal hemolytic anemia. Antigens in the Rh, ABO, MN, Kell, Duffy, and Vel systems are well developed on fetal red blood cells during early intrauterine life.[83] They are present in the fifth to seventh gestational week and remain constant through the remainder of intrauterine development. However, other antigens, such as the Lutheran and XgA systems, develop more slowly but are present at birth, unlike Lewis

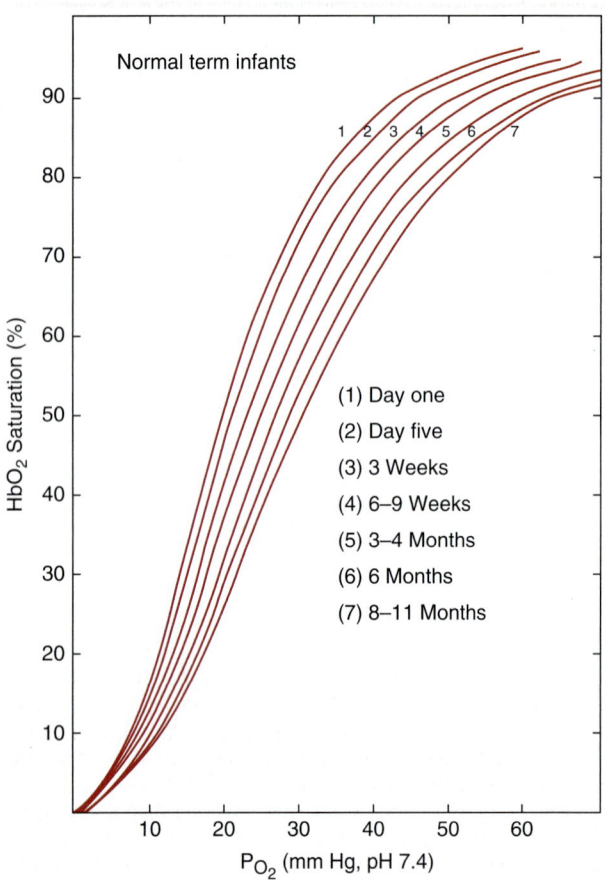

FIGURE 44.8 Oxygen dissociation curves of blood from term infants at different postnatal ages. HbO$_2$, oxygenated hemoglobin; Po$_2$, partial pressure of oxygen. (Reprinted from Oski FA, Delivoria-Papadopoulos M. The red cell 2,3-diphosphoglycerate, and tissue oxygen release. *J Pediatr.* 1970;77(6):941-956. Copyright © 1970 Elsevier. With permission.)

Table 44.3. Causes of Hemolytic Disease in Newborns

Immune-Mediated

Rh incompatibility (anti-D antibody)
ABO, c, C, e, E, G incompatibility
Minor blood group incompatibility such as Fy^a (Duffy), Kell, Jk^a, MNS, Vw
Drug induced (penicillin, methyldopa, cephalosporins)
Maternal autoimmune hemolytic anemia

Non-Immune Mediated

Congenital erythrocyte enzyme defects

Glucose-6-phosphate dehydrogenase deficiency
Pyruvate kinase deficiency
Hexokinase deficiency
Glucose phosphate isomerase deficiency
Pyrimidine 5′ nucleotidase deficiency

Hereditary erythrocyte membrane disorders

Spherocytosis
Elliptocytosis
Stomatocytosis
Pyropoikilocytosis

Infections

Bacterial sepsis (*Escherichia coli*, group B streptococcus)
Parvovirus B19 (typically hyporegenerative, can present with hydrops fetalis)
Congenital syphilis
Congenital malaria
Congenital TORCH infections

Hemoglobin defects

α-Thalassemia syndromes
Gamma or alpha mutations
Macro- and microangiopathic hemolysis
Cavernous hemangiomas or arteriovenous malformations
Renal artery stenosis or thrombosis or other large-vessel thrombi
Severe coarctation of the aorta or valvular stenosis

Other causes

Disseminated intravascular coagulation
Hypothyroidism
Galactosemia
Lysosomal storage diseases
Prolonged metabolic acidosis from metabolic disease

Abbreviation: TORCH, Toxoplasmosis, Other (syphilis, varicella-zoster, parvovirus B19), Rubella, Cytomegalovirus, and Herpes.

antigens, which develop after birth. By 2 years of age, red blood cell and plasma antigens have developed a pattern that is seen throughout the remainder of life.[83]

Rh Hemolytic Disease

Preventing women from developing alloimmunization to the D antigen first became possible in the 1960s and 1970s. Initial investigations showed that Rh-negative men, exposed to the D antigen by transfusing them with Rh-positive red blood cells, could be protected from developing anti-D antibody if, before the transfusion, anti-D immune globulin (RhIG) was administered.[84] Subsequent trials involved Rh-negative pregnant women and demonstrated that administering RhIG within 72 hours following delivery reduced the incidence of D alloimmunization from about 10% to 1% or 2%.[85] Recognizing that fetomaternal hemorrhage in the third trimester contributed to the residual risk of alloimmunization during pregnancy led to the observation that antenatal RhIG prophylaxis, combined with administration after birth, could further reduce the risk of D alloimmunization to <1%.[86]

In the early 1970s, the World Health Organization recommended the practice of administering RhIG to D-negative women after delivery of a D-positive infant and after abortion. Recommendations were introduced in Canada and the United States in 1979 to 1980 and in the United Kingdom in 1998. In the United States, between 1970 and 1986, the incidence of hemolytic disease of the fetus and newborn owing to anti-D fell from 40.5 to 10.6 cases per 10,000 births.[87] Despite these preventive efforts, hemolytic disease of the fetus and newborn owing to anti-D continues to occur in about 6.7 of 1000 live births in the United States.[88] Failure to prevent maternal D alloimmunization is usually owing to failure to administer RhIG or, less commonly, production of anti-D antibodies early in pregnancy.

In countries without RhIG prophylaxis programs, about 15% of affected fetuses are stillborn and half of the affected live born infants have neonatal death or severe brain injury.[89] Even in developed countries, prophylaxis is not 100% effective. Local shortages in RhIG have occurred, failures to follow guidelines are occasionally reported, and a small percentage of women (perhaps 0.1%) become alloimmunized to the D antigen during pregnancy despite full compliance with the prophylaxis protocols.[89,90]

Rh hemolytic disease ranges in severity from intrauterine hydrops fetalis to relatively mild neonatal hyperbilirubinemia and anemia. About half of neonates with detectable maternal anti-D are unaffected or only mildly affected, 30% have moderately severe hemolytic disease, and 20% are severely affected in utero.

Severely affected neonates have cord blood hemoglobin concentrations <12 g/dL and cord bilirubin concentrations >5 mg/dL. If intrauterine transfusions are given, the hemolytic disease may be relatively mild and the blood type at birth may reflect the ABO and D-negative type of the transfused red blood cells. Moderately severe hemolytic disease is predicted by a cord blood hemoglobin of 12 to 14 g/dL and a cord bilirubin of 4 to 5 g/dL. After birth, jaundice may occur within the first 24 hours and bilirubin concentrations typically peak between 3 and 5 days. Mild hemolytic disease is predicted by a cord blood hemoglobin ≥14 g/dL and a cord bilirubin <4 mg/dL.

ABO Hemolytic Disease

ABO hemolytic disease of the newborn is recognized when a mother has blood group O, and a neonate is group A or B, and the neonate has a positive direct antiglobulin test or Coombs test. ABO hemolytic disease of the newborn typically results in an elevated bilirubin level and need for phototherapy. Case reports have described ABO hemolytic disease as causing severe hemolysis and resulting in fetal hydrops with erythroblastosis and significant fetal/neonatal anemia. However, it is possible that such cases had a second, unrecognized cause for the severe hemolytic disease and that it was not the result of ABO incompatibility alone.[91] Similarly, severe neonatal jaundice resulting in kernicterus has been reported to result from ABO hemolytic jaundice, but this remains unproven in large case series.[92] Neonates with ABO hemolytic disease typically have spherocytes on peripheral blood films, whereas those with other varieties of immune-mediated hemolytic disease generally do not.

Hemolytic Disease Owing to Non-Rh, Non-ABO Antigens

Fetuses or newborn infants with hemolytic anemia owing to anti-Kell antibody have lower reticulocyte counts and total serum bilirubin levels than comparable anti-D anemic fetuses.[93] The level of hemolysis caused by anti-Kell antibodies is less than that caused by anti-D antibodies, but fetal erythropoiesis is blunted because Kell sensitization results in both suppression of fetal erythropoiesis and hemolysis. Anti-Kell antibodies cause fetal anemia by suppressing erythropoiesis at the level of erythroid progenitors. Unlike the RhD antigen where a majority of the population are RhD antigen positive, a majority of the population (91% of Caucasians and 98% of African Americans) are Kell antigen negative.[94]

High titers of anti-C antibody have been associated with neonatal hemolytic disease.[95] However, routine screening of anti-C titers during pregnancy is not warranted, because antibody titers do not accurately reflect the severity of hemolytic disease. C(w) is a low-frequency antigen in the Rh blood group system with a prevalence of about 2% among Caucasian populations. Anti-C(w) is not too uncommon in pregnancy (0.1% incidence), but clinically significant hemolytic disease of the newborn is very unusual.[95]

Late Anemia Following Hemolytic Disease of the Fetus and Neonate

Anemia can recur 2 to 10 weeks after treatment of alloimmune-hemolytic disease.[96] This variety can take one of two forms, or it can have elements of both. One form is a continued hemolytic condition on the basis of persistent maternally derived IgG binding to neonatal red blood cells leading to continued destruction. Hemolysis is evident by reticulocytosis, absent serum haptoglobin, presence of free hemoglobin in urine, and elevated end-tidal CO measurements. Maternal IgG can persist in the neonate for 6 weeks or longer, and even after exchange transfusion such antibodies can remain as they may have been extravascular at the time of the exchange.

The second variety of late anemia is a hyporegenerative condition, where the reticulocyte count is low (sometimes 0%) and no evidence of hemolysis is present; serum haptoglobin is measurable, no free hemoglobin is detected in the urine, and end-tidal CO is normal, not elevated. This second variety is likely the result of fetal/early neonatal exposure to large amounts of adult hemoglobin from donor RBC, which markedly increase oxygen delivery to tissues and suppress erythropoietin production.[97,98]

In either variety of late anemia, the hemoglobin concentration can fall sufficiently that signs of anemia are apparent, and problematic, and erythrocyte transfusion can be needed. Late transfusion can, in some instances, be avoided by the administration of recombinant erythropoietin or darbepoetin, thereby increasing erythrocyte production, preventing severe anemia, and obviating the need for a late transfusion.

FETAL AND NEONATAL ANEMIA OWING TO HEMORRHAGE

Hemorrhage can occur at any time during the prenatal, perinatal, and postnatal periods (*Table 44.4*).

Prenatal Hemorrhage

Maternal and fetal erythrocytes cross the placental barrier during pregnancy, generally in small numbers. The volume of fetal blood identified in the maternal circulation at delivery is typically on the order of 0.01 to 0.1 mL. However, approximately 1 in 400 pregnancies are associated with a fetal-to-maternal hemorrhage of 30 mL or more, and approximately 1 in 2000 pregnancies are associated with a potential fetal transplacental hemorrhage of 100 mL or more.[99] To detect and quantify fetal-maternal hemorrhage, flow cytometry–based methods, quantifying red blood cells with fetal hemoglobin in the maternal circulation, are more sensitive than the KB method.[99] Significant fetal-maternal hemorrhage has been described following maternal trauma, and it seems to be more common in preeclampsia, forceps delivery, and manual removal of the placenta,[99] but most cases have no identifiable antecedent.[100]

Term neonates born after a large fetomaternal hemorrhage present with pallor and tachypnea but sometimes have minimal requirements for supplemental oxygen. Hemoglobin concentrations can be extremely low at birth, between 4 and 6 g/dL, and a significant metabolic acidosis is often present as a result of poor perfusion.[101] Quantifying fetomaternal hemorrhage can be relevant to neonatal management, and it can also be important to guide the dose of anti-D IgG that should be administered to a D-negative woman after the birth of a D-positive neonate, where fetomaternal hemorrhage has occurred. Gielezynska et al from Poland tested three flow cytometric methods for quantifying fetomaternal hemorrhage, along with two modifications of the KB test.[102] The flow cytometric tests used antibodies to either fetal hemoglobin, or the D antigen, or to carbonic anhydrase (fetal RBC lack of carbonic anhydrase). They found that the flow cytometric tests outperformed the KB stain unless 10,000 RBCs were enumerated in the KB counting.

Twin-twin transfusion occurs in 5% to 30% of monochorionic twin gestations and involves placental anastomoses that allow net transfer of blood from one twin to the other.[103] The perinatal mortality rate can be as high as 70% to 100%, depending on severity and timing of presentation.

Table 44.4. Causes of Fetal or Neonatal Hemorrhage

Prenatal

Chronic and/or acute twin-to-twin transfusion
Chronic and/or acute fetal-maternal hemorrhage
Hemorrhage after percutaneous umbilical cord blood sampling
Maternal trauma, including trauma after external cephalic version

Perinatal

Placental abruption
Placenta previa
Vasa previa
Trauma to or incision of placenta during cesarean section
Ruptured normal or abnormal (varices, aneurysms, hematoma) umbilical cord
Placental hematoma
Velamentous insertion of the cord
Nuchal cord

Postnatal

Subgaleal hemorrhage
Cephalohematoma
Hemorrhage associated with disseminated intravascular coagulation
Intraventricular/intracranial hemorrhage
Organ trauma (pulmonary, liver, spleen, adrenal, renal, gonadal)
Iatrogenic blood loss

Disorders of Red Blood Cells

Approximately 70% of monozygous twin pregnancies have monochorionic placentas.[103,104] Although vascular anastomoses are present in almost all such cases, not all of those develop twin-twin transfusion.

Acute twin-twin transfusion generally results in twins of similar size but with hemoglobin concentrations that vary by more than 5 g/dL. In chronic twin-twin transfusion, the donor twin becomes progressively anemic and growth retarded, whereas the recipient becomes polycythemic, macrosomic, and sometimes hypertensive. Both can develop hydrops fetalis; the donor twin becomes hydropic from profound anemia, and the recipient from congestive heart failure and hypervolemia. The donor twin often has low amniotic fluid volumes, whereas the recipient twin has increased amniotic fluid.

Chronic twin-twin transfusion can be diagnosed by serial prenatal ultrasounds measuring cardiomegaly, discordant amniotic fluid production, and fetal growth discrepancy of >20%. Percutaneous umbilical blood sampling can determine if hemoglobin concentration differences of greater than 5 g/dL exist between the two fetuses.[105] After birth, the donor twin may require transfusions and can also experience neutropenia, hydrops from severe anemia, growth retardation, congestive heart failure, and hypoglycemia. The recipient twin is often the sicker of the two. Problems include hypertrophic cardiomyopathy, congestive heart failure, pulmonary stenosis/atresia, polycythemia, hyperviscosity, respiratory difficulties, hypocalcemia, and hypoglycemia. Neurologic evaluation and imaging are helpful because the risk of neurologic cerebral lesions is 20% to 30% for both twins.[104]

Conservative prenatal treatment for twin-twin transfusion consists of close monitoring and reduction amniocenteses to decrease uterine stretch and prolong the pregnancy. Staging of twin-twin transfusion syndrome severity as described by Quintero et al[106] has focused on the use of in utero fetoscopic selective laser photocoagulation to ablate bridging vessels. Staging criteria include evaluation of polyhydramnios in the recipient (maximal vertical fluid pocket [MVP] > 8 cm) and oligohydramnios in the donor (MVP < 2 cm), the presence or absence of donor bladder filling, abnormal fetal Doppler values, fetal hydrops, and fetal demise. Initiating laser therapy at stage 2 has resulted in improved survival of both twins (50%-60%) and of at least one twin (70%-80%).[103-106]

Perinatal Hemorrhage

Significant fetal/neonatal blood loss can occur accompanying placenta previa, abruption, incision, or tearing of the placenta during cesarean section, or umbilical cord evulsion. Placental abruption involves premature separation of the placenta from the uterus and occurs in 3 to 6 per 1000 live births.[107] Risk factors for abruption include cigarette smoking, prolonged rupture of the membranes, abdominal trauma, chorioamnionitis, hypertension (before pregnancy and pregnancy induced), and advanced maternal age. The incidence of abruption increases with lower gestational age, and abruption can be a cause of preterm delivery. Mortality ranges from 0.8 to 2.0 per 1000 births or 15% to 20% of the deliveries in which significant abruption occurs.

Placenta previa involves part or all of the placenta overlying the cervical os. Maternal risk factors for developing a placenta previa are essentially the same as those for abruption.[108] Diagnosis of vasa previa (anomalous vessels overlying the internal cervix os) can be made with transvaginal color Doppler, and it should be suspected in any case of antepartum or intrapartum hemorrhage. Although vasa previa is uncommon (1 in 3000 deliveries), the perinatal death rate is high, ranging from 33% to 100% when undetected before delivery.[109]

Infants born after placental abruption or previa can be hypovolemic owing to prenatal hemorrhage. Although the majority of the blood loss with placental abruption is maternal, loss of fetal blood can also occur. Thus, in neonates born after either abruption or previa, it is important to monitor blood pressure, hemoglobin/hematocrit, and tissue perfusion.[109]

Cord rupture can occur during delivery owing to traction on a shortened, weakened, or otherwise abnormal umbilical cord. Cord aneurysms, varices, and cysts can all lead to a weakened cord. Cord infections (funisitis) can also weaken the cord and increase the risk of rupture. Hematomas of the cord occur infrequently (1 in 5000-6000 deliveries) and can be a cause of fetal blood loss and fetal death.

Velamentous insertion of the umbilical cord occurs when the cord enters the membranes distant from the placenta and is present in approximately 0.5% to 2.0% of pregnancies. These vessels are more likely to tear, even in the absence of traction or trauma. The fetal mortality is high in this condition, because rapid detection is difficult.[110]

Postnatal Hemorrhage

Loss of fetal blood during delivery can occur into the placenta. The fetal-placental-umbilical cord unit contains about 120 mL/kg of blood, at term. After delivery, but before the umbilical cord is severed, blood in this unit can flow predominantly toward or away from the neonate. A fetoplacental hemorrhage can occur when the neonate is held significantly higher than the placenta after birth, although studies comparing healthy term neonates held at the introitus with those placed on the mother's abdomen or chest showed no difference in volume gained during delayed cord clamping.[44] It has been suggested that neonates can lose 10% to 20% of their blood volume when born with a tight nuchal cord, which allows blood to be pumped through umbilical arteries toward the placenta, while constricting flow back from the placenta to the baby, through the umbilical vein, which is more easily constricted owing to its thin wall structure. However, in a study of over 200,000 deliveries, those with a tight nuchal cord (6.7%) did not have outcomes different from those with loose nuchal cords or with no nuchal cords.[111] On that basis, it is not clear that tight nuchal cords typically cause clinical problems.

Hemorrhage into the subgaleal space can be a life-threatening neonatal complication.[112,113] It can begin before birth but typically becomes more severe and problematic in the hours after delivery. The spectrum of severity of subgaleal hemorrhage ranges widely, from a small asymptomatic hemorrhage to a massive one causing hypovolemic shock. Associations are well known between vacuum or forceps-assisted delivery and subgaleal hemorrhage, but some cases have occurred when neither vacuum nor forceps were applied. In the Intermountain Healthcare series,[112] all cases were diagnosed within a few hours of birth, and the latest diagnosed were up to 6 or 7 hours after birth. In 38 neonates recently reported with a subgaleal hemorrhage, 21 occurred after vacuum, 2 after forceps, 4 after vacuum followed by forceps, and 11 when neither vacuum nor forceps were used. Thirty-five were admitted to an intensive care unit. Transfusions were given to 13, but no transfusions were given in the group where neither vacuum nor forceps were used, suggesting that their hemorrhages were less severe.

Anemia appearing after the first 24 hours of life in a nonjaundiced infant can be a sign of hemorrhage. Visible hemorrhages, such as a cephalohematoma, as well as internal occult hemorrhages, can occur. Breech deliveries may be associated with renal, adrenal, or splenic hemorrhage into the retroperitoneal space. Delivery of macrosomic infants, such as infants born to diabetic mothers, can result in hemorrhage. Infants with overwhelming sepsis can bleed into soft tissue and organs, such as liver, adrenal glands, and lungs.

The liver in a neonate is prone to iatrogenic rupture, resulting in a high morbidity and mortality.[114] Infants may appear asymptomatic until the liver ruptures and hemoperitoneum occurs. This can occur in term and preterm infants[115] and has been associated with chest compressions during cardiopulmonary resuscitation. Splenic rupture can result from birth trauma or as a result of distention caused by extramedullary hematopoiesis. Abdominal distension and discoloration, scrotal swelling and discoloration, and pallor are clinical signs of splenic rupture; these signs may also be seen with adrenal hemorrhage or hepatic rupture.[116,117] Other rare causes of postnatal hemorrhage include hemangiomas of the gastrointestinal tract, vascular malformations of the skin, and hemorrhage into soft tumors, such as giant sacrococcygeal teratomas or ovarian cysts.

FETAL ANEMIA OWING TO CONGENITAL INFECTION

Neonatal bacterial sepsis can cause anemia on the basis of hemolysis, disseminated intravascular coagulation, and/or hemorrhage. Neonates with sepsis are generally jaundiced and have hepatosplenomegaly. Some bacterial organisms responsible for neonatal sepsis produce hemolytic endotoxins that result in accelerated erythrocyte destruction.[118]

Congenital infections owing to cytomegalovirus, toxoplasmosis, rubella, syphilis, and herpes simplex can also cause hemolytic anemia.[119] Fetal and neonatal infection with parvovirus B19 can cause severe anemia, hydrops, and fetal demise.[120] The fetus or neonate generally presents with a hypoplastic anemia, but hemolysis can occur as well. The virus replicates in erythroid progenitor cells and results in red blood cell aplasia. In utero transfusions for hydropic fetuses can be successful. Intrauterine fetal infusion of B19 IgG-rich titer gammaglobulin has been reported to be successful.[120]

Other fetal infections associated with neonatal anemia include malaria and HIV. Congenital malaria is seen rarely in the United States, generally in large cities where imported cases of malaria are increasing. In certain African countries, congenital malaria has been reported in up to 20% of neonates. Congenital HIV infection in a neonate is generally asymptomatic. However, infants born to mothers on zidovudine can have a hypoplastic anemia owing to suppressive effects of the drug on fetal erythropoiesis.[121]

THE ANEMIA OF PREMATURITY

Infants delivered before 32 completed weeks of gestation typically develop a transient and unique anemia known as the anemia of prematurity.[122] During the first week or two after birth, while in an intensive care unit, anemia secondary to phlebotomy loss is common. However, after this period has passed, a second anemia is often seen, characterized as a normocytic, normochromic, hyporegenerative anemia, with serum erythropoietin concentrations significantly below those found in adults with similar degrees of anemia. This anemia is not responsive to the administration of iron, folate, or vitamin E. Some infants with the anemia of prematurity are asymptomatic, whereas others have clear signs of anemia that are alleviated by erythrocyte transfusion. These signs include tachycardia, rapid tiring with nipple feedings, poor weight gain, increased requirements for supplemental oxygen, episodes of apnea and bradycardia, and elevated serum lactate concentrations.[123-125]

The reason preterm infants do not significantly increase serum erythropoietin concentration during this anemia is not known. Certainly their erythroid progenitors are sensitive to erythropoietin,[126-128] and concentrations of other erythropoietic growth factors appear to be normal.[129]

The molecular and cellular mechanisms involved in the anemia of prematurity are multifactorial and include the transition from fetal to adult hemoglobin, shortened red blood cell survival, and hemodilution associated with a rapidly increasing body mass. Regardless of the mechanism responsible for the anemia of prematurity, exogenous erythropoietin administered to preterm infants accelerates effective erythropoiesis.[130,131] In addition, beneficial neurodevelopmental effects of recombinant erythropoietin administration have been reported in preterm infants.[17,18]

Pharmacokinetic studies of darbepoetin, the long-acting erythropoietic stimulator, have been conducted among neonates with the anemia of prematurity, with the speculation that less frequent dosing and cost savings might render darbepoetin a more attractive alternative than recombinant erythropoietin for treating the anemia of prematurity.[130-133] Following subcutaneous and intravenous dosing, darbepoetin has a considerably shorter terminal half-life in neonates than in adults (*Table 44.5*).

A consistent finding in the largest randomized clinical trials (RCTs) has been an elevation in hematocrit among Epo-treated infants compared with placebo/controls, despite the implementation of strict transfusion guidelines aimed at maintaining hematocrits in a similar range. For those neonatal practitioners electing to maintain hematocrits at higher levels, the use of Epo can gain a "buffer" of 4% to 6% hematocrit points, decreasing the number of transfusions administered.

Table 44.5. Terminal T½ of Darbepoetin in Adults, Children, and Neonates After Subcutaneous or Intravenous Dosing

	After Subcutaneous Dosing (h)	After Intravenous Dosing (h)
Adults	49	25
Children	43	22
Neonates	22	10

IRON DEFICIENCY IN THE FETUS AND NEWBORN INFANT

Although thought to be rare, iron deficiency can definitely exist in a fetus.[134,135] Even if iron is sufficient at birth, deficiency can develop during the neonatal period or during infancy. Central to understanding perinatal iron deficiency is the realization that it is a spectrum, not a dichotomous variable of iron deficiency vs iron sufficiency. Moreover, iron deficiency can exist despite a normal blood hemoglobin concentration, because anemia is a late manifestation of iron deficiency. In fact it is very likely that adverse neurodevelopmental consequences can occur during perinatal biochemical iron deficiency, despite a normal hematocrit and hemoglobin. Consequently, measuring those parameters is a very insensitive method for perinatal iron deficiency screening.

Biochemical iron deficiency exists when metrics indicate the iron supply is low. In a Chinese birth cohort of 854 healthy, normal-birth-weight, term infants, 20% were iron deficient at birth, as diagnosed by a serum ferritin <35 ug/L.[136] When biochemical iron deficiency in a fetus or neonate worsens, iron-deficient erythropoiesis becomes manifest by erythrocyte microcytosis and hypochromia. Perhaps the subtlest evidence of such is an elevation in the Micro-R % and the HYPO-He %,[135] which are evident before a fall in MCV and MCH. In the fetus and newborn, iron is prioritized for red blood cell production at the expense of other tissues, including the brain. Thus, it is critical to optimize iron levels in newborns to support erythropoiesis, growth, and also brain development.

Prematurity, maternal diabetes, maternal smoking, maternal obesity, and small size for gestational age all predispose to congenital iron deficiency.[124,137] The relevance of maternal obesity to fetal/neonatal iron deficiency is an area of current investigation. Maternal obesity increases risks of a variety of fetal and neonatal complications. The underlying pathophysiological mechanisms have been unclear but one contributing factor could be chronic fetal hypoxia. Cord blood erythropoietin was measured among 180 Swedish, healthy full-term singleton pregnancies, half born to women of normal weight and half to women with a body mass index >30 kg/m². A positive association was found between maternal obesity and cord erythropoietin, supporting the hypothesis of chronic fetal hypoxia as a risk factor for complications in the pregnancies of obese women.[137]

The hormonal pathway regulating iron homeostasis in human neonates appears to be intact and similar to that of adults.[138] Following darbepoetin dosing of preterm infants, erythroferrone levels generally increase and hepcidin levels fall, facilitating iron absorption. Some iron-deficient preterm neonates seem to require very high doses of enteral iron in order to increase their serum ferritin or reticulocyte hemoglobin levels.[39] Some of this refractoriness could result from high hepcidin levels accompanying inflammatory conditions.[138,139] Identifying iron-deficient neonates who have high hepcidin levels, or who have other mechanisms causing refractoriness to enteral iron treatment, could permit the use of intravenous iron for those unlikely to respond to high enteral dosing. New oral preparations of iron and also improvements in intravenous iron administration are needed for neonates, as are better noninvasive means of monitoring the efficacy of iron treatment.

Disorders of Red Blood Cells

Studies in infant rhesus monkeys diagnosed as iron deficient on the basis of hematological values show the importance of iron for normal brain development.[140] Neuroimaging studies indicate that a history of iron deficiency is associated with smaller total brain volumes, primarily due to significantly less gray matter. These brain differences were evident even after iron treatment and recovery from the iron-deficiency anemia. These experiments highlight the importance of early detection and preemptive supplementation to limit the neural consequences of neonatal iron deficiency.

ERYTHROCYTE TRANSFUSIONS IN THE NEONATAL PERIOD

Transfusions can be life saving for small and ill neonates with severe anemia or hemorrhage. However, transfusions have risks that should always be weighed against potential benefits. One concern unique to the preterm neonate in the first days after birth is the association between RBC transfusions and the subsequent occurrence of, or extension of, an IVH.[141-144] Another concern is an association between RBC transfusions administered during the third to fourth week and the subsequent occurrence of necrotizing enterocolitis (NEC).[145-148] Much remains to be discovered about these apparent associations with transfusions. Some data suggest that the association between transfusions and NEC is related more to the degree of anemia for which a transfusion is given, rather than with the transfusion itself.[149] Clinically, it is difficult to disentangle the pathogenesis owing to anemia vs owing to transfusion, since severe anemia in a VLBW neonate is almost always treated by transfusion.

Strategies for reducing or avoiding transfusion among VLBW infants are listed in *Table 44.6*. Techniques include the following[147]: (1) delay clamping of the umbilical cord, (2) strip or milk the umbilical cord, (3) draw initial laboratory tests needed from fetal blood in the placenta or umbilical cord (after birth) and thereby draw no blood from the neonate, (4) reduce phlebotomy losses in the first days and weeks, (5) adopt written transfusion guidelines, (6) remove unnecessary indwelling catheters, (7) use early doses of erythropoietin or darbepoetin in neonates likely to qualify for an early transfusion, and (8) optimize nutrition.

The idea of sterilely salvaging anticoagulated fetal blood from the umbilical cord and placenta at the time of birth, for a subsequent autologous transfusion for small or sick neonates, has had limited study.[150-155] A few reports have used a modification of this practice for transfusion immediately after birth, aimed at immediate volume expansion of ill and small neonates. Most such reports describe processing and storing the fetal blood in case a transfusion is needed in the subsequent days or weeks. Reports describe successful cord/placental blood transfusion for neonates with surgical problems.[156-158] As better means are developed for harvesting, storing, and administering autologous fetal blood from extremely preterm deliveries, the benefits of using this blood, rather than donor blood, for early transfusions might be tested.

Table 44.6. Strategies for Reducing Erythrocyte Transfusions Among Very-Low-Birth-Weight Neonates

1. Delay clamping the umbilical cord until 45-60 s after birth.
2. Strip or milk the umbilical cord at birth, moving blood from the placenta and umbilical cord into the neonate, before the umbilical cord is clamped.
3. Draw all initial laboratory blood tests (blood culture, complete blood count, etc.) using fetal blood in the placental side of the umbilical cord, after delayed clamping (or after stripping), thereby initially drawing no blood from the neonate.
4. Develop a consistent approach to minimizing phlebotomy losses.
5. Adopt transfusion guidelines.
6. Remove indwelling catheters once they are not critically needed.
7. Early recombinant erythropoietin or darbepoetin to selected neonates at high risk of requiring transfusion.
8. Optimize nutrition.

In 2016, the Clinical Transfusion Medicine Committee of the American Academy of Blood Banks issued a Committee Report on transfusion-transmitted cytomegalovirus (CMV) infection.[159] Previous recommendations were to use "CMV safe" blood products for infants under 1200 g when mother or infant were CMV seronegative or when their CMV status was unknown. Many blood banks issue CMV-safe red blood cells when any neonate is transfused. CMV safe had been defined as either CMV seronegative (drawn from a donor who test negative for CMV antibody) or leukoreduced. The 2016 report concluded that it is unclear whether leukoreduction is sufficient to reduce transfusion-transmitted CMV or whether CMV serologic testing adds additional benefit to leukoreduction. The committee speculated that it is unlikely that future large-scale clinical trials will be performed to determine whether leukoreduction, CMV serology, or a combination of both is superior. The 2016 report did not issue clinical practice guidelines and concluded that alternative strategies, including pragmatic randomized controlled trials, registries, and collaborations for electronic data merging; nontraditional approaches to inform evidence; or development of a systematic approach to inform expert opinion, may eventually help to address the issue of CMV-safe blood components.

The recent use of bi- or multiprobe near-infrared spectroscopic (NIRS) monitoring in the neonatal intensive care unit (NICU) has provided new evidence of a benefit of RBC transfusions in selected patients.[160-166] Tissue oxygenation is estimated by NIRS on the basis of different near-infrared light absorbance by oxyhemoglobin versus deoxyhemoglobin. Unlike pulse oximetry, NIRS evaluates hemoglobin oxygen saturations deeper in the tissue, about 2 cm below the skin surface, thus reflecting values from mixed arteriolar, venous, and capillary sources. When oxygen delivery to tissues becomes limited by anemia, oxygen extraction increases and venous oxygen saturation falls.

van Hoften et al used NIRS monitoring to evaluate 33 preterm neonates before, during, and after a clinically ordered transfusion of 15 mL/kg RBC infused over a period of 3 hours.[163] They found that regional cerebral tissue oxygen saturation and the fractional tissue oxygen extraction correlated with the pretransfusion hemoglobin level, with lower hemoglobin levels predicting a lower cerebral oxygen tension. Their data supported the conclusion that a blood hemoglobin concentration <9.7 g/dL in a preterm infant corresponds with diminished cerebral oxygenation and that a red blood cell transfusion improves this parameter. Dani et al from Florence, Italy, reported on 15 preterm infants using similar methodology and came to a similar conclusion that, in neonates with a hemoglobin below approximately 6 g/dL, transfusion can often increase cerebral, splanchnic, and renal oxygenation.[164] Bailey et al applied biprobe NIRS monitoring during a 20-minute period just before a clinically ordered packed red blood cell transfusion; 40 such measurements (each integrated over 30 seconds) were made.[165,166] One probe on the forehead assessed cerebral changes, and one on the abdomen assessed splanchnic changes. The measurements from each site were averaged into a ratio of oxygen saturations measured from the cerebral and splanchnic sites. The ratios were expressed as a splanchnic-cerebral oxygenation ratio (SCOR). Ratios were correlated with independent means of judging whether or not the transfusion actually provided a benefit. A SCOR at or below 73% (meaning the average oxygenation in the splanchnic circulation was ≤73% of the cerebral circulation) performed well in identifying the neonates who were likely to benefit from a transfusion.

Using a single NIRS sensor placed on the right lower quadrant of the abdomen, White et al found no differences in fractional tissue oxygen extraction after packed red blood cell transfusions to 23 neonates, running tracings up to 36 hours after transfusions.[136] Mintzer et al used NIRS in a before-versus-after analysis of "booster" transfusions, defined as administering 15 mL/kg RBC after 10 mL/kg phlebotomy loss. They studied 10 neonates 500 to 1250 g at birth and found no change in pH, base deficit, lactate, or cardiopulmonary parameters but an increase in cerebral, renal, and splanchnic tissue oxygenation.[161] Sandal et al found no difference in NIRS measurements among preterm neonates receiving packed red blood cell transfusion over 2 hours versus over 4 hours.[162] With recent technological and other creative advances, it is becoming clear that NICU transfusions should not be ordered simply on the basis of the hemoglobin/hematocrit values.

It can be a challenge determining which neonate with a low hematocrit will benefit from a red cell transfusion. Many preterm infants can adapt to a slowly decreasing hematocrit and can be treated conservatively with supplemental iron and red cell growth factors such as erythropoietin or darbepoetin to avoid the associated risks of transfusion.[16,18] Target hemoglobin and hematocrit have been used as clinical indicators for RBC transfusion; however, it remains uncertain what target hematocrit or hemoglobin will optimally balance the risks and benefits of this intervention.

Better practice guidelines will likely consider NIRS and other measures of oxygen delivery to determine transfusion need. As more mechanistic markers for transfusion need are being evaluated, evidence for benefit or harm of transfusions through randomized controlled trials has provided strong evidence that restrictive transfusion guidelines (similar to those used in pediatric and adult intensive care patients) result in similar neurodevelopmental outcomes as those found in neonates transfused using liberal transfusion guidelines. Two such trials, the Transfusion of Prematures (TOP) trial[167] and the Effects of Liberal vs Restrictive Transfusion Thresholds on Survival and Neurocognitive Outcomes (ETTNO) study,[168] were designed to determine if lower or higher hematocrit thresholds for transfusing preterm infants resulted in better neurodevelopmental outcomes. Both RCTs hypothesized that infants randomized to the higher hematocrit threshold would have better neurodevelopmental outcomes. This hypothesis proved to be incorrect.

Infants in the ETTNO study were 400 to 999 g birth weight and randomized at less than 72 hours of age to the high or low hematocrit threshold. Transfusions of 20 mL/kg were mandated within 72 hours of identifying a threshold hematocrit. In TOP, infants 22 0/7 to 28 6/7 weeks gestation were enrolled within 48 hours of birth and randomized to the high or low group, stratified by gestation. Transfusions of 15 mL/kg were mandated within 12 hours of identifying a threshold hematocrit. Infants enrolled in ETTNO and TOP could not receive red cell growth factors.

The primary outcome for both trials was the combined outcome of death or neurodevelopmental impairment (NDI). NDI was defined similarly in both trials: cognitive score less than 85 on the Bayley Scales of Infant Development (BSID III composite cognitive score for TOP; BSID II mental developmental index for ETTNO); moderate or severe cerebral palsy (gross motor function classification system 2 or greater in TOP; Surveillance of Cerebral Palsy in Europe network definition for ETTNO); severe vision impairment; or severe hearing impairment.

In both trials, outcomes were identical between high and low groups in the primary outcome (*Table 44.7*). Of 1824 extremely low-birth-weight (ELBW) infants enrolled in TOP, the primary outcome (death or NDI) was present in 49.8% in the low group and 50.1% in the high group. There were no differences between groups in the individual components (death or NDI) of the primary outcome. Cognitive delay was the primary factor determining NDI and was identified in 97% of the infants in the high groups and 91% of the infants in the low group who were designated as neurodevelopmentally impaired. No differences between groups were identified in common neonatal hospital morbidities (bronchopulmonary dysplasia, retinopathy of prematurity, grade 3-4 interventricular hemorrhage or periventricular leukomalacia, or necrotizing enterocolitis; *Table 44.8*). Metrics associated with severity of illness such as length of stay (*Table 44.8*), time to full feeds, length of time on a ventilator, and duration of caffeine treatment were similar between low and high groups.

Of 1013 ELBW infants enrolled in ETTNO, the primary outcome was present in 42.9% in the low group and 44.4% in the high group. Similar to TOP, there were no differences between groups in the individual components (death or NDI) of the primary outcome. Cognitive delay (BSID II < 85) was the primary factor determining NDI and was identified in 88% of the infants in the high group and 86% of the infants in the low group who were designated as neurodevelopmentally impaired.

For both studies, the number of transfusions were significantly lower in the low group compared with the high group: 4.4 ± 4.0 versus 6.2 ± 4.3 transfusions in TOP; 1.7 versus 2.6 transfusions in ETTNO (*Table 44.8*). A greater number of infants in the low threshold groups remained untransfused. For both studies, infants randomized to the low threshold groups received more transfusions outside of study protocols (7% vs 0.8% in TOP, 15% vs 5% in ETTNO). These transfusions did not change the primary outcome of either trial, as analyses evaluating infants transfused per protocol yielded similar results as the main trials.

Disorders of Red Blood Cells

Table 44.7. RCTs Comparing Liberal and Restrictive Neonatal Transfusion Guidelines

	TOP High	TOP Low	ETTNO High	ETTNO Low
Number randomized	911	913	492	521
Number evaluated for primary outcome	845	847	450	478
Gestation (wk)	25.9	25.9	26.1	26.4
Birthweight (g)	755	757	745	750
% female	54	51	50	50
Death/NDI	50.1% (423/845)	49.8% (422/847)	44.4% (200/450)	42.9% (205/478)
Death by 24 months	16.2% (146/903)	15.0% (135/901)	8.3% (38/460)	9.0% (44/491)
NDI	39.6% (277/699)	40.3% (287/712)	36% (162/450)	33.7% (161/478)
Cognitive score[a] mean	85.5 ± 15	85.3 ± 14.8	92.6 ± 16.5	92.4 ± 17.5
Cognitive score[a] <85	38.7% (269/695)	37.9% (270/712)	37.6% (154/410)	34.4% (148/430)
Cognitive score[a] <70	12.7% (88/695)	13.5% (96/712)		
Cerebral palsy[b]	6.8% (48/711)	7.6% (55/720)	4.3% (18//419)	5.6% (25/443)

Abbreviations: NDI, neurodevelopmental impairment; NEC, necrotizing enterocolitis; ROP, retinopathy of prematurity.
No differences between high and low groups in each study were identified in any of the measures listed above (analyses not performed *between* ETTNO and TOP studies).
Data from Kirpalani H, Bell EF, Hintz SR, et al. Higher or lower hemoglobin transfusion thresholds for preterm infants. *N Engl J Med*. 2020;383:2639-2651; and Franz AR, Engel C, Bassler D, et al. Effects of liberal vs restrictive transfusion thresholds on survival and neurocognitive outcomes in extremely low-birth-weight infants: the ETTNO randomized clinical trial. *JAMA*. 2020;324:560-570.
[a]Bayley Scales of Infant Development III composite cognitive score for TOP; Bayley Scales of Infant Development II mental developmental index for ETTNO.
[b]Gross motor function classification system 2 or greater for TOP; Surveillance of Cerebral Palsy in Europe network definition for ETTNO.

Table 44.8. Hospital Outcomes of Infants Enrolled in ETTNO and TOP

	TOP High	TOP Low	ETTNO High	ETTNO Low
Hospital days[a]	96 (72-129)	97 (75-127)	93 ± 41	92 ± 38
Untransfused (%)	3	12[c]	21	41[a]
Transfusions (mean)	6.2 ± 4.3	4.4 ± 4.0[c]	2.6	1.7
Volume			40 (16-73)	19 (0-46)
NEC	10.0%	10.5%	5.3%	6.2%
ROP > grade 2	19.7%	17.2%	15.9%	13.0%
Intraventricular hemorrhage grade 3-4[b]	17.1% (146/855)	17.9% (154/859)	8.1% (40/492)	6.7% (35/521)
Periventricular leukomalacia			23/492	30/521
Bronchopulmonary dysplasia	59.0	56.3	28.4	26.0

Data from Kirpalani H, Bell EF, Hintz SR, et al.Higher or lower hemoglobin transfusion thresholds for preterm infants. *N Engl J Med*. 2020;383:2639-2651; and Franz AR, Engel C, Bassler D, et al. Effects of liberal versus restrictive transfusion thresholds on survival and neurocognitive outcomes in extremely low-birth-weight infants: the ETTNO randomized clinical trial. *JAMA*. 2020;324:560-570.

[a]Values are mean and interquartile range for TOP; mean and standard deviation for ETTNO.
[b]Numbers are combined for intraventricular hemorrhage and periventricular leukomalacia for TOP.
[c]*P* < .05, low versus high groups for each study.

The results from these combined transfusion studies encompassing over 2800 ELBW infants provide conclusive evidence that transfusing critically ill ELBW infants at lower hematocrits does not result in adverse outcomes. Infants transfused at higher hematocrits did not do worse. Aside from change in hematocrit, data were not collected on the efficacy of the treatment studied. Because both studies relied on consensus in determining hematocrit thresholds, both studies reported what infants *received*, rather than what they required. Documenting evidence of benefit should be a part of future studies, in order to support ongoing efforts to use blood products judiciously, termed "transfusion stewardship."

Evaluating transfusion guidelines have focused on decreasing administration and led to evaluating the relationship between the number and volume of transfusion and outcomes in ELBW infants. This analysis was performed in preterm infants enrolled in a previous erythropoiesis stimulating agent (ESA) study.[16,17] In that trial, preterm infants were randomized to subcutaneous erythropoietin (400 U/kg three times weekly), darbepoetin (10 µg/kg once weekly), or placebo (sham injections) during their initial hospitalization, and the number and volume of red cell transfusions recorded. Children were evaluated at 18 to 22 months. *Post hoc* analysis[169] revealed that cognitive scores on the Bayley Scales of Infant Development III (BSID-III) at 18 to 22 months were inversely correlated with transfusion volume (*P* = .02). Infants receiving ≥1 transfusion in the placebo group had significantly lower cognitive scores than those that remained untransfused. In the ESA group, cognitive scores were similar between nontransfused and transfused subjects, suggesting ESAs provided neuroprotection from the effects of transfusions.

Transfusions and outcomes were analyzed in similar fashion in the PENUT trial.[170] In that study, erythropoietin 1000 U/kg or placebo was given every 48 hours for a total of 6 doses, followed by 400 U/kg or sham injections 3 times a week through 32 weeks postmenstrual age. A total of 628 infants (315 placebo, 313 erythropoietin) survived and were assessed at 2 years of age. Associations between BSID-III scores and the number and volume of pRBC transfusions were evaluated in a *post hoc* analysis. Each transfusion was associated with a decrease in composite cognitive score of 0.96 (95% confidence interval: −1.34, −0.57), a decrease in composite motor score of 1.51 (−1.91, −1.12), and a decrease in composite language score of 1.10 (−1.54, −0.66). Significant negative associations between transfusion volumes and BSID-III scores were observed in the placebo group but not in the erythropoietin group.

In summary, instituting red cell sparing/enhancing strategies (*Table 44.6*) and implementing restrictive transfusion guidelines similar to those in ETTNO and TOP are reasonable approaches that will decrease transfusions and support judicious use of blood products in the NICU. The goal of limiting red cell donor exposure to zero or one donor for each ELBW infant is achievable and may lead to improved developmental outcomes in the smallest and most critically ill infants.

References

1. Christensen RD. Reference ranges in neonatal hematology. In: de Alarcon P, Werner E, Christensen RD, Sola-Visner MC eds. *Neonatal Hematology*. 3rd ed. Cambridge University Press; 2021;440-469.
2. Henry E, Christensen RD. Reference intervals in neonatal hematology. *Clin Perinatol*. 2015;42:483-497.
3. McPherson RJ, Juul SE. Erythropoietin for infants with hypoxic-ischemic encephalopathy. *Curr Opin Pediatr*. 2010;22:139-145.
4. Shiou SR, Yu Y, Chen S, et al. Erythropoietin protects intestinal epithelial barrier function and lowers the incidence of experimental neonatal necrotizing enterocolitis. *J Biol Chem*. 2011;286:12123-12132.
5. Arsenault JE, Webb AL, Koulinska IN, Aboud S, Fawzi WW, Villamor E. Association between breast milk erythropoietin and reduced risk of mother-to-child transmission of HIV. *J Infect Dis*. 2010;202:370-373.
6. Kling PJ. Roles of erythropoietin in human milk. *Acta Paediatr Suppl*. 2002;91(438):31-35.
7. Juul SE. Nonerythropoietic roles of erythropoietin in the fetus and neonate. *Clin Perinatol*. 2000;27:527-541.
8. Brace RA, Cheung CY, Davis LE, Gagnon R, Harding R, Widness JA. Sources of amniotic fluid erythropoietin during normoxia and hypoxia in fetal sheep. *Am J Obstet Gynecol*. 2006;195:246-254.
9. Juul SE, Yachnis AT, Christensen RD. Tissue distribution of erythropoietin and erythropoietin receptor in the developing human fetus. *Early Hum Dev*. 1998;52:235-249.
10. Dame C, Juul SE, Christensen RD. The biology of erythropoietin in the central nervous system and its neurotrophic and neuroprotective potential. *Biol Neonate*. 2001;79:228-235.
11. Juul SJ, Harcum J, Li Y, Christensen RD. Erythropoietin is present in the cerebrospinal fluid of neonates. *J Pediatr*. 1997;130:428-430.
12. Juul SE, Stallings SA, Christensen RD. Erythropoietin in the cerebrospinal fluid of neonates who sustained CNS injury. *Pediatr Res*. 1999;46:543-547.
13. Juul SE, McPherson RJ, Farrell F, Jolliffe L, Ness DJ, Gleason CA. Erythropoietin concentrations in cerebrospinal fluid of nonhuman primates and fetal sheep following high-dose recombinant erythropoietin. *Biol Neonate*. 2004;85(2):138-144.
14. Statler PA, McPherson RJ, Bauer LA, Kellert BA, Juul SE. Pharmacokinetics of high-dose recombinant erythropoietin in plasma and brain of neonatal rats. *Pediatr Res*. 2007;61(6):671-675.
15. McPherson RJ, Juul SE. Recent trends in erythropoietin-mediated neuroprotection. *Int J Dev Neurosci*. 2008;26(1):103-111.
16. Ohls RK, Christensen RD, Kamath-Rayne BD, et al. A randomized, masked, placebo controlled study of darbepoetin administered to preterm infants. *Pediatrics*. 2013;132:e119-e127.
17. Ohls RK, Kamath-Rayne BD, Christensen RD, et al. Cognitive outcomes of preterm infants randomized to darbepoetin, erythropoietin or placebo. *Pediatrics*. 2014;133:1023-1030.
18. Ohls RK, Cannon DC, Phillips J, et al. Preschool assessment of preterm infants treated with darbepoetin and erythropoietin. *Pediatrics*. 2016;137:1-9.
19. Dijkstra F, Jozwiak M, De Matteo R, et al. Erythropoietin ameliorates damage to the placenta and fetal liver induced by exposure to lipopolysaccharide. *Placenta*. 2010;31(4):282-288.

20. Bhandari V, Buhimschi CS, Han CS, et al. Cord blood erythropoietin and interleukin-6 for prediction of intraventricular hemorrhage in the preterm neonate. *J Matern Fetal Neonatal Med.* 2011;24(5):673-679.

21. Juul SE, Vu PT, Comstock BA, et al. Effect of high-dose erythropoietin on blood transfusions in extremely low gestational age neonates: post hoc analysis of a randomized clinical trial. *JAMA Pediatr.* 2020;174(10):933-943.

22. Juul SE, Comstock BA, Wadhawan R, et al. A Randomized trial of erythropoietin for neuroprotection in preterm infants. *N Engl J Med.* 2020;382(3):233-243.

23. Wassink G, Davidson JO, Fraser M, et al. Non-additive effects of adjunct erythropoietin therapy with therapeutic hypothermia after global cerebral ischaemia in near-term fetal sheep. *J Physiol.* 2020;598(5):999-1015.

24. Gairdner D, Marks J, Roscoe JD. Blood formation in infancy. I. The normal bone marrow. II. Normal erythropoiesis. *Arch Dis Child.* 1952;27:128-133.

25. Jopling J, Henry E, Wiedmeier SE, Christensen RD. Reference ranges for hematocrit and blood hemoglobin concentration during the neonatal period: data from a multihospital health care system. *Pediatrics.* 2009;123(2):e333-e337.

26. Gaitti RA. Hematocrit values of capillary blood in the newborn. *J Pediatr.* 1967;70:117-119.

27. Linderkamp O, Versmold HT, Strohhacker I, Messow-Zahn K, Riegel KP, Betke K. Capillary-venous hematocrit differences in newborn infants. *Eur J Pediatr.* 1977;127(1):9-14.

28. Christensen RD, Jopling J, Henry E, Wiedmeier SE. The erythrocyte indices of neonates, defined using data from over 12,000 patients in a multihospital health care system. *J Perinatol.* 2008;28(1):24-28.

29. Schmairer AH, Mauer HM. Alpha-thalassemia screening in neonates by mean corpuscular volume and mean corpuscular hemoglobin concentration. *J Pediatr.* 1973;83:794.

30. Christensen RD, Henry E. Hereditary spherocytosis in neonates with hyperbilirubinemia. *Pediatrics.* 2010;125(1):120-125.

31. Christensen RD, Yaish HM, Gallagher PG. A pediatrician's practical guide to diagnosing and treating hereditary spherocytosis in neonates. *Pediatrics.* 2015;135(6):1107-1114.

32. Christensen RD, Henry E, Bennett ST, Yaish HM. Reference intervals for reticulocyte parameters of infants during their first 90 days after birth. *J Perinatol.* 2016;36:61-66.

33. Christensen RD, Henry E, Andres RL, Bennett ST. Reference ranges for blood concentrations of nucleated red blood cells in neonates. *Neonatology.* 2011;99:289-294.

34. Zipursky A, Brown E, Palko J, Brown EJ. The erythrocyte differential count in newborn infants. *Am J Pediatr Hematol Oncol.* 1983;5:45-51.

35. Kurth D, Deiss A, Cartwright GE. Circulating siderocytes in human subjects. *Blood.* 1969;34:754-764.

36. Komazawa M, Garcia AM, Oski FA. The relation of red cell size to fetal hemoglobin concentration in the term infant. *J Pediatr.* 1974;85:114-116.

37. Mock DM, Bell EF, Lankford GL, Widness JA. Hematocrit correlates well with circulating red blood cell volume in very low birth weight infants. *Pediatr Res.* 2001;50(4):525-531.

38. Pearson HA. Life-span of the fetal red blood cell. *J Pediatr.* 1967;70:166-171.

39. Brace RA, Langendorfer C, Song TB, Mock DM. Red blood cell life span in the ovine fetus. *Am J Physiol Regul Integr Comp Physiol.* 2000;279(4):R1196-R1204.

40. Bratteby LE, Garby L, Groth T, Schneider W, Wadman B. Studies on erythrokinetics in infancy. XII. Survival in adult recipients of cord blood red cells labeled in vitro with diisopropyl fluorophosphate (DF32P). *Acta Paediatr Scand.* 1968;57:311-320.

41. Mollison PL. The survival of transfused erythrocytes in hemolytic disease of the newborn. *Arch Dis Child.* 1943;18:161-171.

42. Ruth V, Widness JA, Clemons G, Raivio JO. Postnatal changes in serum immunoreactive erythropoietin in relation to hypoxia before and after birth. *J Pediatr.* 1990;116(6):950-954.

43. Kling PJ, Schmidt RL, Roberts RA, Widness JA. Serum erythropoietin levels during infancy: associations with erythropoiesis. *J Pediatr.* 1996;128(6):791-796.

44. Vain NE, Satragno DS, Gorenstein AN, et al. Effect of gravity on volume of placental transfusion: a multicenter, randomized, non-inferiority trial. *Lancet.* 2014;384:235-240.

45. Linderkamp O, Nelle M, Kraus M, Zilow EP. The effect of early and late cord-clamping on blood viscosity and other hemorheological parameters in full-term neonates. *Acta Paediatr.* 1992;81:745-750.

46. Carroll PD, Christensen RD. New and underutilized uses of umbilical cord blood in neonatal care. *Matern Health Neonatol Perinatol.* 2015;1:16.

47. Mercer JS, Vohr BR, McGrath MM, Padbury JF, Wallach M, Oh W. Delayed cord clamping in very preterm infants reduces the incidence of intraventricular hemorrhage and late-onset sepsis: a randomized, controlled trial. *Pediatrics.* 2006;117(4):1235-1242.

48. Mercer JS, Erickson-Owens DA, Collins J, Barcelos MO, Parker AB, Padbury JF. Effects of delayed cord clamping on residual placental blood volume, hemoglobin and bilirubin levels in term infants: a randomized controlled trial. *J Perinatol.* 2016;37(3):260-264.

49. Hosono S, Mugishima H, Fujita H, et al. Umbilical cord milking reduces the need for red cell transfusions and improves neonatal adaptation in infants born at less than 29 weeks' gestation: a randomised controlled trial. *Arch Dis Child Fetal Neonatal Ed.* 2008;93:F14-F19.

50. Rabe H, Jewison A, Alvarez RF, et al. Milking compared with delayed cord clamping to increase placental transfusion in preterm neonates: a randomized controlled trial. *Obstet Gynecol.* 2011;117:205-211.

51. Katheria AC, Lakshminrusimha S, Rabe H, McAdams R, Mercer JS. Placental transfusion: a review. *J Perinatol.* 2016;37(2):105-111.

52. Katariya D, Swain D, Singh S, Satapathy A. The effect of different timings of delayed cord clamping of term infants on maternal and newborn outcomes in normal vaginal deliveries. *Cureus.* 2021;13(8):e17169.

53. Mwangi MN, Mzembe G, Moya E, Verhoef H. Iron deficiency anaemia in sub-Saharan Africa: a review of current evidence and primary care recommendations for high-risk groups. *Lancet Haematol.* 2021;8(10):e732-e743.

54. Andersson O, Mercer JS. Cord management of the term newborn. *Clin Perinatol.* 2021;48(3):447-470.

55. Berg JHM, Isacson M, Basnet O, et al. Effect of delayed cord clamping on neurodevelopment at 3 Years: a randomized controlled trial. *Neonatology.* 2021;118(3):282-288.

56. Brown BE, Shah PS, Afifi JK, et al. Delayed cord clamping in small for gestational age preterm infants. *Am J Obstet Gynecol.* 2022;226(2):247e1-e10.

57. Colciago E, Fumagalli S, Ciarmoli E, et al. The effect of clamped and unclamped umbilical cord samples on blood gas analysis. *Arch Gynecol Obstet.* 2021;304(6):1493-1499. doi: 10.1007/s00404-021-06076-w

58. Katheria AC, Szychowski JM, Essers J, et al. Early cardiac and cerebral hemodynamics with umbilical cord milking compared with delayed cord clamping in infants born preterm. *J Pediatr.* 2020;223:51-56.e1.

59. Aziz K, Lee CHC, Escobedo MB, et al. Part 5: neonatal resuscitation 2020 American heart association guidelines for cardiopulmonary resuscitation and emergency cardiovascular care. *Pediatrics.* 2021;147(suppl 1):e2020038505E.

60. Dani C, Sandri F, Pratesi S. Considering an update on umbilical cord milking for the new guidelines for neonatal resuscitation. *JAMA Pediatr.* 2021;175(9):894-895.

61. Matovcik LM, Gröschel-Stewart U, Schrier SL. Myosin in adult and neonatal human erythrocyte membranes. *Blood.* 1986;67:1668-1674.

62. Fukuda M, Fukuda MN. Changes in cell surface glycoproteins and carbohydrate structures during development and differentiation of human erythroid cells. *J Supramol Struct Cell Biochem.* 1981;17(4):313-324.

63. Linderkamp O, Nash GB, Wu PY, Meiselman HJ. Deformability and intrinsic material properties of neonatal red blood cells. *Blood.* 1986;67:1244-1250.

64. Christensen RD, Yaish HM. Hemolysis in preterm neonates. *Clin Perinatol.* 2016;43(2):233-240.

65. Ito H, Kuss N, Rapp BE, et al. Quantification of the influence of endotoxins on the mechanics of adult and neonatal red blood cells. *J Phys Chem B.* 2015;119:7837-7845.

66. Travis SF, Kumar SP, Paez PC, Delivoria-Papadopoulos M. Red cell metabolic alterations in postnatal life in term infants: glycolytic enzymes and glucose-6-phosphate dehydrogenase. *Pediatr Res.* 1980;14:1349-1352.

67. Gahr M, Meves H, Schröter W. Fetal properties in red blood cells of newborn infants. *Pediatr Res.* 1979;13:1231-1236.

68. Travis SF, Kumar SP, Delivoria-Papadopoulos M. Red cell metabolic alterations in intermediates and adenosine triphosphate. *Pediatr Res.* 1981;15:34-37.

69. Travis SF, Garvin JH. In vivo lability of red cell phosphofructokinase in term infants. The possible molecular basis of the relative PFK deficiency in neonatal red cells. *Pediatr Res.* 1977;11:1159-1161.

70. Vora S, Poimelli S. Fetal isozyme of phosphofructokinase in newborn erythrocytes. *Pediatr Res.* 1977;11:483.

71. Gahr M. Isoelectric focusing of hexokinase and glucose-6-phosphate dehydrogenase isoenzymes in erythrocytes of newborn infants and adults. *Br J Haematol.* 1980;4:529.

72. Scopesi F, Canini S, Mazzella M, Arioni C, Lantieri P, Serra G. 2,3 diphosphoglycerate in preterm newborns. *Acta Bio-Med Ateneo Parmense.* 2000;71(suppl 1):621-626.

73. Barretto OC, Nonoyama K, Deutsch AD, Ramos JL. Physiological red cell, 2,3-diphosphoglycerate increase by the sixth hour after birth. *J Perinat Med.* 1995;23(5):365-369.

74. Soubasi V, Kremenopoulos G, Tsantali C, Savopoulou P, Mussafiris C, Dimitriou M. Use of erythropoietin and its effects on blood lactate and 2,3-diphosphoglycerate in premature neonates. *Biol Neonate.* 2000;78(4):281-287.

75. Glader BE, Conrad ME. Decreased glutathione peroxidase in neonatal erythrocytes. Lack of relation to hydrogen peroxide metabolism. *Pediatr Res.* 1972;6:900-904.

76. Schroter W, Bodemann H. Experimentally induced cation leaks of the red cell membrane. *Biol Neonate.* 1970;15:291-299.

77. Jensen M, Attenberger H, Schneider C, Walther JU. The developmental change in the G-γ- and A-γ-globin proportions in hemoglobin F. *Eur J Pediatr.* 1982;138:311-314.

78. Crowley MA, Mollan TL, Abdulmalik OY, et al. A hemoglobin variant associated with neonatal cyanosis and anemia. *N Engl J Med.* 2011;364(19):1837-1843.

79. Bauer C, Ludwig I, Ludwig M. Different effects of 2,3-diphosphoglycerate and adenosine triphosphate on oxygen affinity of adult and fetal human hemoglobin. *Life Sci.* 1968;7:1339-1343.

80. Delivoria-Papadopoulos M, Roncevic NP, Oski FA. Postnatal changes in oxygen transport of term, premature, and sick infants: the role of red cell 2,3-diphosphoglycerate and adult hemoglobin. *Pediatr Res.* 1971;5:235-245.

81. Kleihauer E, Braun H, Betke K. Demonstration of fetal hemoglobin in erythrocytes of a blood smear. [Article in German]. *Klin Wochenschr.* 1957;35(12):637-638.

82. Wong RJ, Stevenson DK. Neonatal hemolysis and risk of bilirubin-induced neurologic dysfunction. *Semin Fetal Neonatal Med.* 2015;20(1):26-30.

83. Fasano RM. Hemolytic disease of the fetus and newborn in the molecular era. *Semin Fetal Neonatal Med.* 2016;21(1):28-34.

84. Freda VL, Gorman JG, Pollack W. Successful prevention of experimental Rh sensitization in man with an anti-Rh gamma2-globulin antibody preparation: a preliminary report. *Transfusion.* 1964;4:26-32.

85. Freda VL, Gorman JD, Pollack W, Bowe E. Prevention of Rh hemolytic disease—ten years' experience with Rh immunization. *N Engl J Med.* 1975;292:1014-1016.

86. Lee D, Rawlinson VI. Multicentre trial of antepartum low dose anti-D immunoglobulin. *Transfus Med.* 1995;5:15-19.

87. Chavez GF, Mulinare J, Edmonds LD. Epidemiology of Rh hemolytic disease of the newborn in the United States. *JAMA.* 1991;265:3270-3274.

Disorders of Red Blood Cells

88. Moise KJ. Red cell alloimmunization in pregnancy. *Semin Hematol.* 2005;42:169-178.

89. Committee on Practice Bulletins-Obstetrics. Practice bulletin no. 181: prevention of Rh D alloimmunization. ACOG practice bulletin. *Obstet Gynecol.* 2017;130(2):e57-e70.

90. Moise KJ. Fetal anemia due to non-Rhesus-D red-cell alloimmunization. *Semin Fetal Neonatal Med.* 2008;13(4):207-214.

91. Christensen RD, Baer VL, MacQueen BC, et al. ABO hemolytic disease of the fetus and newborn: thirteen years of data after implementing a universal bilirubin screening and management program. *J Perinatol.* 2018;38(5):517-525.

92. Baer VL, Hulse W, Bahr TM, Ilstrup SJ, Christensen RD. Absence of severe neonatal ABO hemolytic disease at Intermountain Healthcare. Why? *J Perinatol.* 2020;40(2):352-353.

93. Slootweg YM, Lindenburg IT, Koelewijn JM, et al. Predicting anti-Kell-mediated hemolytic disease of the fetus and newborn: diagnostic accuracy of laboratory management. *Am J Obstet Gynecol.* 2018;219(4):393.e1-393.e8.

94. Ohto H, Denomme GA, Ito S, et al. Three non-classical mechanisms for anemic disease of the fetus and newborn, based on maternal anti-Kell, anti-Ge3, anti-M, and anti-Jrᵃ cases. *Transfus Apher Sci.* 2020;59(5):102949.

95. Macher S, Wagner T, Rosskopf K, et al. Severe case of fetal hemolytic disease caused by anti-C(w) requiring serial intrauterine transfusions complicated by pancytopenia and cholestasis. *Transfusion.* 2016;56:80-83.

96. Koenig JM, Ashton RD, De Vore GR, Christensen RD. Late hyporegenerative anemia in Rh hemolytic disease. *J Pediatr.* 1989;115(2):315-318.

97. Zuppa AA, Alighieri G, Fracchiolla A, et al. Comparison between two treatment protocols with recombinant human erythropoietin (rHuEpo) in the treatment of late anemia in neonates with Rh-isoimmunization. *Pediatr Med e Chir.* 2012;34(4):186-191.

98. Ohls RK, Wirkus PE, Christensen RD. Recombinant erythropoietin as treatment for the late hyporegenerative anemia of Rh hemolytic disease. *Pediatrics.* 1992;90(5):678-680.

99. Stefanovic V. Fetomaternal hemorrhage complicated pregnancy: risks, identification, and management. *Curr Opin Obstet Gynecol.* 2016;28:86-94.

100. Carr NR, Henry E, Bahr TM, et al. Fetomaternal hemorrhage: evidence from a multihospital healthcare system that up to 40% of severe cases are missed. *Transfusion.* 2021;62(1):60-70. doi: 10.1111/trf.16710

101. Christensen RD, Lambert DK, Baer VL, et al. Severe neonatal anemia from fetomaternal hemorrhage: report from a multihospital health-care system. *J Perinatol.* 2013;33(6):429-434.

102. Gielezynska A, Stachurska A, Fabijanska-Mitek J, Debska M, Muzyka K, Kraszewska E. Quantitative fetomaternal hemorrhage assessment with the use of five laboratory tests. *Int J Lab Hematol.* 2016;38:419-425.

103. Slaghekke F, Zhao DP, Middeldorp JM, et al. Antenatal management of twin-twin transfusion syndrome and twin anemia-polycythemia sequence. *Expert Rev Hematol.* 2016;9:815-820.

104. Müllers SM, McAuliffe FM, Kent E, et al. Outcome following selective fetoscopic laser ablation for twin to twin transfusion syndrome: an 8 year national collaborative experience. *Eur J Obstet Gynecol Reprod Biol.* 2015;191:125-129.

105. Kontopoulos E, Chmait RH, Quintero RA. Twin-to-twin transfusion syndrome: definition, staging, and ultrasound assessment. *Twin Res Hum Genet.* 2016;19:175-183.

106. Quintero R, Kontopoulos EV, Barness E, et al. Twin-twin transfusion syndrome in a dichorionic-monozygotic twin pregnancy: the end of a paradigm? *Fetal Pediatr Pathol.* 2010;29(2):81-88.

107. Schmidt P, Skelly CL, Raines DA. *Placental abruption.* In: *StatPearls* [Internet]. StatPearls Publishing; 2021.

108. Anderson-Bagga FM, Sze A. *Placenta previa.* In: *StatPearls* [Internet]. StatPearls Publishing; 2021.

109. Matsuda Y, Hayashi K, Shiozaki A, Satoh S, Saito S. Comparison of risk factors for placental abruption and placenta previa: case-cohort study. *J Obstet Gynaecol Res.* 2011;37(6):538-546.

110. Ebbing C, Johnsen SL, Albrechtsen S, Sunde ID, Vekseth C, Rasmussen S. Velamentous or marginal cord insertion and the risk of spontaneous preterm birth, prelabor rupture of the membranes, and anomalous cord length, a population-based study. *Acta Obstet Gynecol Scand.* 2017;96(1):78-85.

111. Henry E, Andres RL, Christensen RD. Neonatal outcomes following a tight nuchal cord. *J Perinatol.* 2013;33(3):231-234.

112. Christensen RD, Baer VL, Henry E. Neonatal subgaleal hemorrhage in a multihospital healthcare system: prevalence, associations, and outcomes. *J Neonat Res.* 2011;1:4-11.

113. Colditz MJ, Lai MM, Cartwright DW, Colditz PB. Subgaleal haemorrhage in the newborn: a call for early diagnosis and aggressive management. *J Paediatr Child Health.* 2015;51:140-146.

114. Davies MR. Iatrogenic hepatic rupture in the newborn and its management by pack tamponade. *J Pediatr Surg.* 1997;32(10):1414-1419.

115. Emma F, Smith J, Moerman PH. Subcapsular hemorrhage of the liver and hemoperitoneum in premature infants: report of 4 cases. *Eur J Obstet Gynecol Reprod Biol.* 1992;44(2):161-164.

116. Al Inzi S, Mohiyiddeen G, Dalal N, Pratap C, Gilmour K. Spontaneous rupture of the spleen—a fatal complication of pregnancy. *J Obstet Gynaecol.* 2009;29(6):555-556.

117. Abolmakarem H, Tharmaratnum S, Thilaganathan B. Fetal anemia as a consequence of hemorrhage into an ovarian cyst. *Ultrasound Obstet Gynecol.* 2001;17:527-528.

118. Ng PC, Li K, Leung TF, et al. Early prediction of sepsis-induced disseminated intravascular coagulation with interleukin-10, interleukin-6, and RANTES in preterm infants. *Clin Chem.* 2006;52(6):1181-1189.

119. Macé G, Castaigne V, Trabbia A, et al. Fetal anemia as a signal of congenital syphilis. *J Matern Fetal Neonatal Med.* 2014;27:1375-1377.

120. Sanapo L, Wien M, Whitehead MT, et al. Fetal anemia, cerebellar hemorrhage and hypoplasia associated with congenital Parvovirus infection. *J Matern Fetal Neonatal Med.* 2016;30(16):1887-1890.

121. Shah M, Li Y, Christensen RD. Effects of perinatal zidovudine on hematopoiesis: a comparison of effects on progenitors from human fetuses versus mothers. *AIDS.* 1996;10(11):1239-1247.

122. Widness JA. Pathophysiology of anemia during the neonatal period, including anemia of prematurity. *NeoReviews.* 2008;9:e520.

123. Cibulskis CC, Maheshwari A, Rao R, Mathur AM. Anemia of prematurity: how low is too low? *J Perinatol.* 2021;41(6):1244-1257.

124. Kling PJ. Iron nutrition, erythrocytes, and erythropoietin in the NICU: erythropoietic and neuroprotective effects. *NeoReviews.* 2020;21(2):e80-e88.

125. Ross MP, Christensen RD, Rothstein G, et al. A randomized trial to develop criteria for administering erythrocyte transfusions to anemic preterm infants 1 to 3 months of age. *J Perinatol.* 1989;9(3):246-253.

126. Brown MS, Garcia JF, Phibbs RH, Dallman PR. Decreased response of plasma immunoreactive erythropoietin to "available oxygen" in anemia of prematurity. *J Pediatr.* 1984;105:793-798.

127. Shannon KM, Naylor GS, Torkildson JC, et al. Circulating erythroid progenitors in the anemia of prematurity. *N Engl J Med.* 1987;31:728-733.

128. Rhondeau SM, Christensen RD, Ross MP, Rothstein G, Simmons MA. Responsiveness to recombinant human erythropoietin of marrow erythroid progenitors from infants with the "anemia of prematurity". *J Pediatr.* 1988;112:935-940.

129. Ohls RK, Liechty KW, Turner MC, Kimura R, Christensen RD. Erythroid "burst promoting activity" in the serum of patients with the anemia of prematurity. *J Pediatr.* 1990;116:786-789.

130. Warwood TL, Ohls RD, Wiedmeier SE, et al. Single-dose darbepoetin administration to anemic preterm neonates. *J Perinatol.* 2005;25(11):725-730.

131. Warwood TL, Ohls RK, Lambert DK, et al. Intravenous administration of darbepoetin to NICU patients. *J Perinatol.* 2006;26(5):296-300.

132. Warwood TL, Ohls RK, Lambert DK, et al. Urinary excretion of darbepoetin after intravenous *vs.* subcutaneous administration to preterm neonates. *J Perinatol.* 2006;26(10):636-639.

133. Warwood TL, Lambert DK, Henry E, Christensen RD. Very low birth weight infants qualifying for a 'late' erythrocyte transfusion: does giving darbepoetin along with the transfusion counteract the transfusion's erythropoietic suppression? *J Perinatol.* 2011;31(suppl 1):S17-S21.

134. MacQueen BC, Christensen RD, Baer VL, et al. Screening umbilical cord blood for congenital Iron deficiency. *Blood Cells Mol Dis.* 2019;77:95-100.

135. Bahr TM, Christensen TR, Henry E, et al. Neonatal reference intervals for the complete blood count parameters MicroR and HYPO-He: sensitivity beyond the red cell indices for identifying microcytic and hypochromic disorders. *J Pediatr.* 2021;239:95-100.e2. S0022-3476(21)00757-5.

136. Zhang JY, Wang J, Lu Q, et al. Iron stores at birth in a full-term normal birth weight cohort with a low level of inflammation. *Biosci Rep.* 2020;40(12):BSR20202853.

137. Åmark H, Sirotkina M, Westgren M, Papadogiannakis N, Persson M. Is obesity in pregnancy associated with signs of chronic fetal hypoxia?. *Acta Obstet Gynecol Scand.* 2020;99(12):1649-1656.

138. Bahr TM, Ward DM, Jia X, Ohls RK, German KR, Christensen RD. Is the erythropoietin-erythroferrone-hepcidin axis intact in human neonates? *Blood Cells Mol Dis.* 2021;88:102536.

139. German KR, Vu PT, Comstock BA, Ohls RK, et al. Enteral iron supplementation in infants born extremely preterm and its positive correlation with neurodevelopment; post hoc analysis of the preterm erythropoietin neuroprotection trial randomized controlled trial. *J Pediatr.* 2021;238:102-109.e8. S0022-3476(21)00686-7.

140. Vlasova RM, Wang Q, Willette A, et al. Infantile iron deficiency affects brain development in monkeys even after treatment of anemia. *Front Hum Neurosci.* 2021;15:624107.

141. Baer VL, Lambert DK, Henry E, Snow GL, Butler A, Christensen RD. Among very-low-birth-weight neonates is red blood cell transfusion an independent risk factor for subsequently developing a severe intraventricular hemorrhage? *Transfusion.* 2011;51:1170-1179.

142. Baer VL, Lambert DK, Henry E, Snow GL, Christensen RD. Red blood cell transfusion of preterm neonates with a grade 1 intraventricular hemorrhage is associated with extension to a grade 3 or 4 hemorrhage. *Transfusion.* 2011;51(9):1933-1939.

143. Christensen RD, Ilstrup S. Recent advances toward defining the benefits and risks of erythrocyte transfusions in neonates. *Arch Dis Child Fetal Neonatal Ed.* 2012;98(4):F365-F372.

144. Christensen RD. Associations between "early" red blood cell transfusion and severe intraventricular hemorrhage, and between "late" red blood cell transfusion and necrotizing enterocolitis. *Semin Perinatol.* 2012;36(4):283-289.

145. Christensen RD, Lambert DK, Henry E, et al. Is "transfusion-associated necrotizing enterocolitis" an authentic pathogenic entity? *Transfusion.* 2010;50:1106-1112.

146. Josephson CD, Wesolowski A, Bao G, et al. Do red cell transfusions increase the risk of necrotizing enterocolitis in premature infants? *J Pediatr.* 2010;157:972-978.e1-e3.

147. Carroll PD. Umbilical cord blood—an untapped resource: strategies to decrease early red blood cell transfusions and improve neonatal outcomes. *Clin Perinatol.* 2015;42(3):541-556.

148. Christensen RD, Carroll PD, Josephson CD. Evidence-based advances in transfusion practice in neonatal intensive care units. *Neonatology.* 2014;106(3):245-253.

149. MohanKumar K, Namachivayam K, Song T, et al. A murine neonatal model of necrotizing enterocolitis caused by anemia and red blood cell transfusions. *Nat Commun.* 2019;10(1):3494.

150. Rao M, Ahrlund-Richter L, Kaufman DS. Concise review: cord blood banking, transplantation and induced pluripotent stem cell—success and opportunities. *Stem Cell.* 2012;30:55-60.

151. Strauss RG. Autologous transfusions for neonates using placental blood. A cautionary note. *Am J Dis Child.* 1992;146:21-22.

152. Brune T, Garritsen H, Witteler R, et al. Autologous placental blood transfusion for the therapy of anaemic neonates. *Biol Neonate.* 2002;81:236-243.

153. Khodabux CM, von Lindern JS, van Hilten JA, Scherjon S, Walther FJ, Brand A. A clinical study on the feasibility of autologous cord blood transfusion for anemia of prematurity. *Transfusion.* 2008;48:1634-1643.

154. Strauss RG, Mock DM, Johnson KJ, et al. A randomized clinical trial comparing immediate versus delayed clamping of the umbilical cord in preterm infants: short-term clinical and laboratory endpoints. *Transfusion.* 2008;48:658-665.

155. Jansen M, Brand A, von Lindern JS, Scherjon S, Walther FJ. Potential use of autologous umbilical cord blood red blood cells for early transfusion needs of premature infants. *Transfusion.* 2006;46:1049-1056.

156. Taguchi T, Suita S, Nakamura M, et al. The efficacy of autologous cord-blood transfusions in neonatal surgical patients. *J Pediatr Surg.* 2003;38:604-607.

157. Strauss RG, Widness JA. Is there a role for autologous/placental red blood cell transfusions in the anemia of prematurity? *Transfus Med Rev.* 2010;24:125-129.

158. Khodabux CM, van Beckhoven JM, Scharenberg JG, El Barjiji F, Slot MC, Brand A. Processing cord blood from premature infants into autologous red-blood-cell products for transfusion. *Vox Sang.* 2011;100:367-373.

159. Heddle NM, Boeckh M, Grossman B; AABB; Clinical Transfusion Medicine Committee, et al. AABB Committee Report: reducing transfusion-transmitted cytomegalovirus infections. *Transfusion.* 2016;56:1581-1587.

160. White L, Said M, Rais-Bahrami K. Monitoring mesenteric tissue oxygenation with near-infrared spectroscopy during packed red blood cell transfusion in preterm infants. *J Neonatal Perinatal Med.* 2015;8(2):157-163.

161. Mintzer JP, Parvez B, Chelala M, Alpan G, LaGamma EF. Monitoring regional tissue oxygen extraction in neonates <1250 g helps identify transfusion thresholds independent of hematocrit. *J Neonatal Perinatal Med.* 2014;7(2):89-100.

162. Sandal G, Oguz SS, Erdeve O, Akar M, Uras N, Dilmen U. Assessment of red blood cell transfusion and transfusion duration on cerebral and mesenteric oxygenation using near-infrared spectroscopy in preterm infants with symptomatic anemia. *Transfusion.* 2014;54(4):1100-1105.

163. van Hoften JC, Verhagen EA, Keating P, ter Horst HJ, Bos AF. Cerebral tissue oxygen saturation and extraction in preterm infants before and after blood transfusion. *Arch Dis Child Fetal Neonatal Ed.* 2010;95:F352-F358.

164. Dani C, Pratesi S, Fontanelli G, Barp J, Bertini G. Blood transfusions increase cerebral, splanchnic, and renal oxygenation in anemic preterm infants. *Transfusion.* 2010;50:1220-1226.

165. Bailey SM, Hendricks-Muñoz KD, Wells JT, Mally P. Packed red blood cell transfusion increases regional cerebral and splanchnic tissue oxygen saturation in anemic symptomatic preterm infants. *Am J Perinatol.* 2010;27:445-453.

166. Bailey SM, Hendricks-Muñoz KD, Mally P. Splanchnic-cerebral oxygenation ratio as a marker of preterm infant blood transfusion needs. *Transfusion.* 2012;52:252-260.

167. Kirpalani H, Bell EF, Hintz SR, et al. Higher or lower hemoglobin transfusion thresholds for preterm infants. *N Engl J Med.* 2020;383:2639-2651.

168. Franz AR, Engel C, Bassler D, et al. Effects of liberal vs restrictive transfusion thresholds on survival and neurocognitive outcomes in extremely low-birth-weight infants: the ETTNO randomized clinical trial. *JAMA.* 2020;324:560-570.

169. Shah P, Cannon DC, Lowe JR, et al. Effect of blood transfusions on cognitive development in very low birth weight infants. *J Perinatol.* 2021;41:1412-1418.

170. Vu P, Ohls RK, Mayock DE, et al. Transfusions and neurodevelopmental outcomes in extremely low gestation neonates enrolled in the PENUT Trial: a randomized clinical trial. *Pediatr Res.* 2021;90(1):109-116. doi: 10.1038/s41390-020-01273

Chapter 45 ■ Erythrocytosis

ROBERT T. MEANS JR. • BERTIL GLADER

DEFINITIONS AND TERMINOLOGY

In reading the extensive primary and review literature on polycythemia and erythrocytosis, it is important to understand how specific authors define those terms. Traditionally *polycythemia* ("many cells") referred to an increase in the *total quantity or volume (mass)* of red blood cells (RBCs) in the body ("absolute erythrocytosis"), while *erythrocytosis* meant an increased *concentration* of RBCs, usually measured as hemoglobin concentration (Hb), or hematocrit. Erythrocytosis might or might not be associated with increased red cell mass (RCM). Recent changes in diagnostic criteria for the disease polycythemia vera (Chapter 83) have largely eliminated the clinical meaning of the distinction between erythrocytosis and polycythemia. This chapter will follow evolving standard usage[1] and reserve the term polycythemia for the specific disease polycythemia vera.

PATHOLOGIC PHYSIOLOGY

RBC survival in erythrocytosis and polycythemia is typically normal, implying that increased RCM reflects increased erythropoiesis. As RCM rises, the total blood volume typically increases; concurrent variation in plasma volume means that the degree of Hb/hematocrit increase cannot be predicted reliably from RCM changes.

The clinical manifestations of erythrocytosis are related, in part, to the disorder responsible for erythrocytosis (e.g., thrombosis in patients with polycythemia vera, hypertension in relative erythrocytosis). In addition, the increased blood volume and increased blood viscosity that occur in association with erythrocytosis themselves produce certain symptoms and signs; these are related to the degree of the increase and its resulting effects on blood flow and oxygen transport.[2] Thus, the "ruddy cyanosis" seen in patients with polycythemia vera is a consequence of dilatation of cutaneous vessels caused by expanded blood volume and sluggish local circulation caused by increased blood viscosity.[3] Headache, dizziness, tinnitus, a full feeling in the head, and a bleeding tendency may develop in patients with erythrocytosis and expanded blood volume regardless of the underlying etiology.[4] These symptoms are usually relieved by normalization of the hematocrit.

Blood Viscosity and Oxygen Transport

Viscosity is an intrinsic characteristic of a liquid and represents the tendency of that liquid to resist changes in shape. The viscosity of blood is a result of the interaction of several factors, including RBC content, RBC physical characteristics (deformability, aggregability, and size), the plasma volume, plasma proteins, platelet count, and leukocyte count and differential.[5] In this chapter, because of its implications for viscosity, the proportion of blood volume occupied by RBCs will be referred to as the *hematocrit*, reflecting routine clinical usage. (Other terms used for this parameter in the older literature include packed cell volume or volume of packed red cells [VPRC].) Blood viscosity affects oxygen delivery to tissue. This section focuses primarily on the contribution of RBC concentration to viscosity and oxygen transport; more complete discussions are available elsewhere.[5]

At any given pressure gradient, the flow rate of a liquid through a tube varies directly with the tube's radius and inversely with the tube length and viscosity of the liquid (Poiseuille law). The determinations of the effects of erythrocytosis on blood viscosity were largely made by determining the flow rate of venous blood through an 18-gauge needle under known pressure, thus calculating viscosity.[6] The values thus determined are only an approximation to the in vivo situation. The Poiseuille law is strictly applicable only to fluids that maintain constant viscosity under differing flow rates (Newtonian fluids), which

is not the case with blood (*Figure 45.1*).[7] As the velocity of flow (indicated by the shear rate) increases, the viscosity at any given hematocrit decreases.[6] It has been suggested that, at any given hematocrit, decreased erythrocyte mean corpuscular volume (MCV) is associated with increased viscosity, especially at low flow rates.[8] This appears to result from loss of RBC deformability but may be seen in iron deficiency independent of MCV.[9] This is a clinically significant observation because iron deficiency, typically with a low MCV but with a normal Hb or hematocrit, is a desired end point for the treatment of erythrocytosis and polycythemia vera by phlebotomy.

Clinical observations confirm the effects of an elevated hematocrit on in vivo blood flow.[10-12] Cerebral blood flow in patients with erythrocytosis is significantly reduced compared with controls, whether it is because of an elevated RCM, reduced plasma volume, or from an unknown etiology. Alternatively, hematocrit reduction, either by venesection or by volume expansion, improves cerebral blood flow.

The determination of blood viscosity values at different hematocrits allows the estimation of blood flow rates under different conditions. The Poiseuille law predicts that blood flow decreases linearly with increasing viscosity. The rate of oxygen transport can then be calculated from the blood flow rate and oxygen content. At a given vessel size and pressure gradient, the predicted relation of oxygen transport to hematocrit is expressed by an arch-shaped curve (*Figure 45.2A*).[7,14] At low hematocrits, the reduced Hb content of blood translates into reduced oxygen content. At hematocrits above the 50% to 60% range (>0.5-0.6 VPRC

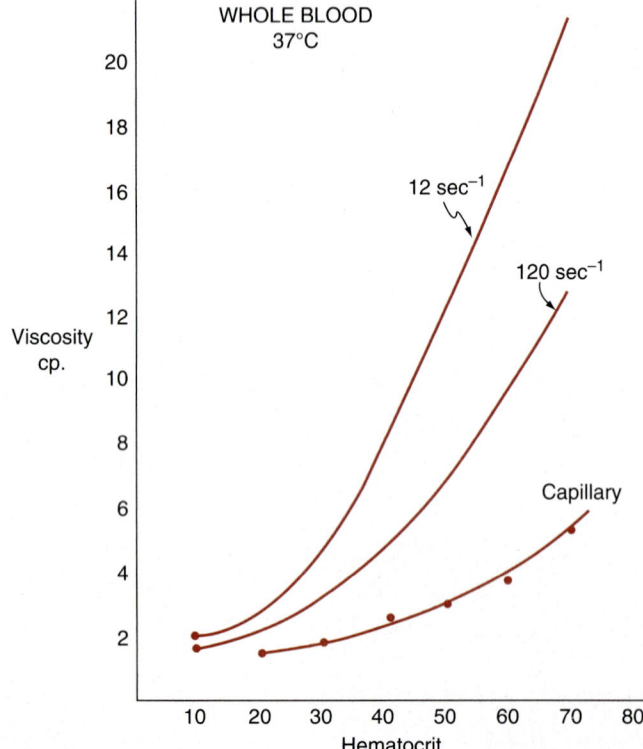

FIGURE 45.1 **Relation of volume of packed red cells (hematocrit) to blood viscosity in centipoise (cp) as measured in a capillary viscosimeter compared with that calculated for shear rates of 120/second (ascending aorta) and 12/second (medium arteriole).** (Reprinted from Wells RE Jr, Merrill EW. The variability of blood viscosity. *Am J Med.* 1961;31:505-509. Copyright © 1961 Elsevier. With permission.)

in *Figure 45.2*), increased viscosity reduces oxygen transport despite increased blood oxygen content. Optimal oxygen transport would be predicted to occur in the normal hematocrit range. Experiments in normovolemic dogs (*Figure 45.2B*, dashed line) support this prediction.[14]

The differences in oxygen transport observed between normovolemic and hypervolemic dogs at different hematocrits reflect the probable situation occurring in patients with erythrocytosis. In erythrocytosis, the associated hypervolemia permits an oxygen transport curve that is similar to that of normovolemic patients but that is elevated and shifted to the right.[14] Therefore, in patients with tissue hypoxia, erythrocytosis is beneficial because it leads to hypervolemia and increases oxygen transport (compare oxygen transport at VPRC of 0.6 on the hypervolemic and normovolemic curves in *Figure 45.2B*). In contrast, in patients who have a normal or decreased total blood volume (called relative or spurious erythrocytosis), erythrocytosis has an adverse effect on oxygen transport.

Relation to Treatment of Erythrocytosis

The physiologic considerations noted above explain not only the consequences of the different etiologies of erythrocytosis but also their treatment. Patients with polycythemia vera have no need for increased tissue oxygen transport. However, in some areas where fixed vessel diameter (from arteriosclerosis) limits increased blood flow, the additional

impeding effect of increased blood viscosity may limit oxygen transport and result in local tissue ischemia. In these latter cases, phlebotomy can bring about a significant clinical benefit (see Chapter 83). When treating by phlebotomy, however, blood volume should not be reduced too greatly at any one time, especially in patients with known symptoms of cardiovascular disease. This is particularly true early in the course of therapy, when hematocrit (and consequently viscosity) is highest.[13] In these instances, time should be allowed for hemodilution to occur between phlebotomies; however, in emergencies, the blood volume should be maintained by infusing saline or some other plasma expander.[3] A concern is that the patient should not suddenly be shifted from the hypervolemic, erythrocytosis-beneficial curve to the normovolemic, erythrocytosis-adverse curve. Another concern is that a sudden fall in blood volume from any cause, such as dehydration or acute hemorrhage, may result in local ischemia because increased cardiac output cannot compensate immediately for the effects of high viscosity. In patients with congestive heart failure, the need for reduction of blood viscosity may be urgent, because the ability to increase cardiac output to compensate for the increased blood viscosity has been compromised. The oxygen-Hb dissociation curve is shifted to the right in such patients.[15]

In contrast to polycythemia vera, patients with erythrocytosis as a result of tissue hypoxia may benefit from an increased hematocrit. Reduced arterial oxygen saturation means that oxygen transport is less efficient at particular Hb or hematocrit levels. Therefore, the curves for oxygen transport would be shifted closer to the origin than those noted in situations in which Hb oxygenation is normal (*Figure 45.2B*). In the presence of decreased arterial oxygen saturation, tissue hypoxia may persist even when erythrocytosis is marked. The main advantage to decreasing blood viscosity and blood volume in hypoxic erythrocytosis is to decrease the cardiac workload. Studies confirm that, in such situations, an increase in tissue oxygen transport and clinical improvement results from phlebotomy.[16] Again, especially early in the course, phlebotomy with preservation of an expanded blood volume may be beneficial.[3,13] To achieve the best balance between increased cardiac work and decreased tissue hypoxia in patients with hypoxemic erythrocytosis, some authors suggest that the hematocrit be maintained between 50% and 55%[3]; however, the subjective symptomatology of the patient is usually the best guide.[17]

CLASSIFICATION AND APPROACH TO THE PATIENT WITH ERYTHROCYTOSIS

The first step in the evaluation of erythrocytosis is to distinguish cases due to decreased plasma volume (*relative* or *spurious erythrocytosis*) from erythrocytosis due to increased red cell production (*Table 45.1*). Patients with relative erythrocytosis will typically have Hb/hematocrit less than 16.5 g/dL/49.5% in women or 18.5 g/dL/55.5% in men and lack clinical features of myeloproliferative disorders like splenomegaly, basophilia, or leukocytosis and thrombocytosis not attributable to an inflammatory process or iron deficiency. Patients with relative erythrocytosis frequently report tobacco or significant alcohol use, hypertension, obesity, renal disease, or use of diuretics.

Actual erythrocytosis (not reflecting decreased plasma volume) can be divided into primary erythrocytosis (*polycythemia vera* and *hereditary* or *familial erythrocytosis*) and erythrocytosis driven by erythropoietin production (*secondary erythrocytosis*). The secondary erythrocytosis syndromes are divided into those that represent a response to tissue hypoxia (physiologically appropriate) and those driven by nonhereditary increases in erythropoietin production not in response to tissue hypoxia (physiologically inappropriate).

An approach to the evaluation of the patient with erythrocytosis is outlined in *Figure 45.3*. Traditionally, relative erythrocytosis and actual erythrocytosis were distinguished by measurement of RCM and blood volume by isotope labeling.[18] Since actual RCM measurement is no longer available for routine clinical use, surrogate measures based on Hb or hematocrit are now the routine basis for separating relative and actual erythrocytosis. In men with a hematocrit >60% or women with a hematocrit >55%, there is reported to be >99% likelihood that

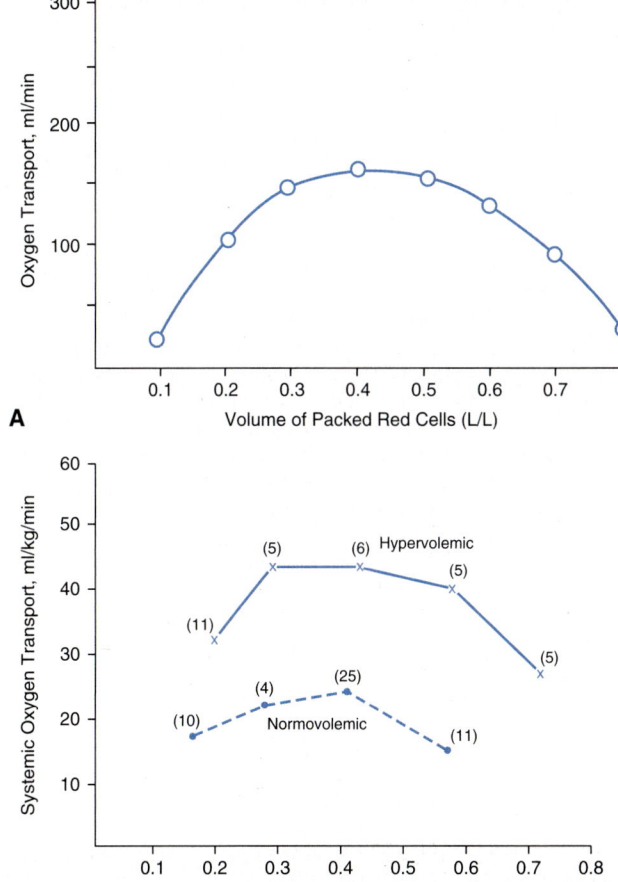

A

B

FIGURE 45.2 Effects of hematocrit on systemic oxygen transport. A, Arterial oxygen transport at different volumes of packed red cells and thus different viscosity values. Values in the curve were calculated from blood viscosity values as measured by Pirofsky,[5] and flow rates were estimated by Castle and Jandl.[13] B, Systemic oxygen transport at different volumes of packed red cells as calculated from cardiac output measured in normovolemic and hypervolemic dogs. (Republished with permission of American Society for Clinical Investigation from Murray JF, Gold P, Johnson BL Jr. The circulatory effects of hematocrit variations in normovolemic and hypervolemic dogs. *J Clin Invest.* 1963;42(7):1150-1159; permission conveyed through Copyright Clearance Center, Inc.)

Table 45.1. Classification of Erythrocytosis

Erythrocytosis With Decreased Plasma Volume

Hemoconcentration

Spurious erythrocytosis (Gaisböck syndrome)

Erythrocytosis With Normal or Increased Plasma Volume (Absolute Erythrocytosis)

Primary erythrocytosis
    Polycythemia vera
    Primary familial erythrocytosis
Secondary erythrocytosis
    Secondary to decreased tissue oxygenation (physiologically appropriate or hypoxic erythrocytosis)
        High-altitude erythrocytosis: acute or chronic (Monge disease)
        Pulmonary disease
            Chronic cor pulmonale
            Pulmonary arterial hypertension (Ayerza syndrome)
        Cyanotic congenital heart disease
        Hypoventilation syndromes
            Primary alveolar hypoventilation
            Pickwickian syndrome, Ondine curse
            Positional desaturation
            Sleep apnea
        Abnormal hemoglobins
            Inherited
            Acquired: drugs and chemicals, carboxyhemoglobin
        Familial erythrocytosis
    Secondary to aberrant erythropoietin production or response (physiologically inappropriate erythrocytosis)
        Tumors, cysts, hemangiomas, etc.
        Androgen abuse
        Erythropoietin/erythropoiesis stimulating agent abuse
        Sodium glucose cotransporter (SGLT-2) use
        Familial erythrocytosis
        Manganese toxicity
        Cobalt toxicity
Idiopathic erythrocytosis

the RCM is elevated.[19] In its 2006 criteria for the diagnosis of polycythemia vera, the World Health Organization (WHO) uses a Hb concentration >18.5 g/dL in men or 16.5 g/dL in women to define an elevated RCM for purposes of identifying erythrocytosis.[20] These criteria generally rule out relative erythrocytosis due to plasma volume contraction, although in certain circumstances of severe hemoconcentration, for example, in the systemic capillary leak syndrome,[21] Hb concentrations or hematocrits in this range may be observed in patients with a normal RCM. Such patients typically exhibit anasarca and other physical findings suggestive of severe intravascular volume depletion and redistribution of intravascular volume. In 2016, the WHO criteria were revised downward to Hb concentration >16.0 g/dL in women/> 16.5 g/dL in men (hematocrit of >48% and >49%, respectively) to allow recognition of prodromal (sometimes called "masked") polycythemia vera before an elevated RBC mass is established[22] (*Table 45.2*). While this represents a clinically significant refinement in the diagnostic approach, it also increases the number of patients who may potentially require screening for possible polycythemia vera. In a review of data from Canada, it has been reported that 4.1% and 0.35% of random blood counts in men and women, respectively, meet the 2016 WHO criteria, increasing the number of patients requiring investigation for polycythemia vera 12- and 3-fold, respectively.[23]

A certain number of patients are not readily classified as having either polycythemia vera or secondary erythrocytosis. These patients fall into a category called *idiopathic erythrocytosis* and appear to represent a heterogeneous group of disorders (see Idiopathic Erythrocytosis).

More than 95% of patients with polycythemia vera express a mutation in the *JAK2* gene in which phenylalanine is substituted for valine at position 617. Patients with *JAK2* V617F mutation-negative polycythemia vera almost invariably have mutations in other exons

of *JAK2*,[24] typically exon 12.[25] The *JAK2* mutation in polycythemia vera is not analogous to the *bcr/abl* mutation in chronic myelogenous leukemia because the *JAK2* V617F mutation is also found in other myeloproliferative disorders.[26] Its implications will be discussed in more detail in Chapter 83, but in terms of differential diagnosis, *JAK2* V617F should be regarded as a marker of a myeloproliferative state. Polymerase chain reaction–based assays for *JAK2* V617F and JAK2 exon 12 mutations are widely available in the United States and Europe at reasonable cost.

A general approach to the evaluation of erythrocytosis based on distinguishing polycythemia vera from other causes of erythrocytosis is outlined in *Figure 45.3*. Prior to beginning an extensive laboratory evaluation, a history should be taken to identify use of medications or supplements associated with erythrocytosis (androgens, sodium glucose transporter-2 inhibitors, cobalt). If these agents are present, discontinuation and observation (possibly accompanied by phlebotomy, depending on the degree of erythrocytosis) should be considered. All patients with erythrocytosis should undergo *JAK2* V617F testing. If negative, *JAK2* exon 12 mutations should be evaluated. Most JAK2-positive patients should undergo bone marrow examination. In a *JAK2* mutation-positive patient with erythrocytosis as defined in the 2016 WHO criteria, a bone marrow with typical features of a myeloproliferative disorder (hypercellularity with trilineage hyperplasia) confirms the diagnosis of polycythemia vera. In a *JAK2* mutation-negative patient, serum erythropoietin should be measured. If the serum erythropoietin is below the assay normal range, a myeloproliferative bone marrow will also confirm a diagnosis of polycythemia vera. If a *JAK2* mutation-positive patient has Hb > 18.5 g/dL men/16.5 g/dL women, the presence of a subnormal serum erythropoietin can confirm the diagnosis without bone marrow examination.[22]

The remainder of this chapter will focus on cause of erythrocytosis other than polycythemia vera or other myeloproliferative diseases. In patients who do not have a *JAK2* mutation, lack myeloproliferative marrow features, but do have low serum erythropoietin, the diagnosis of *primary proliferative erythrocytosis* should be considered (called *primary familial erythrocytosis* if there is a family history). This diagnosis should be confirmed by testing for the associated mutations (*EPOR*, *LNK*). If the clinical features are suggestive of a secondary etiology of erythrocytosis, patients should follow the process outlined in *Figure 45.3*. This involves identifying drivers of increased erythropoietin production: hypoxemia (altitude, cardiopulmonary disease), aberrant erythropoietin production (renal, hepatic, endocrine, or vascular disease, *EPO* mutations), abnormal hemoglobin oxygen release (high-affinity hemoglobins, *BPGM*, *PK*, or *PIEZO*), or modulators of the oxygen sensing pathway that regulate erythropoietin production (*VHL*, *EGLN1*, *EPAS1*), or drugs that induce erythropoietin. These will be discussed in more detail later in the chapter.

RELATIVE ERYTHROCYTOSIS

Lowered fluid intake or marked loss of body fluids or a combination of both causes a decrease in plasma volume and may produce a relative erythrocytosis. The decrease in plasma volume may result from any cause of intravascular fluid loss, insensible fluid loss, persistent vomiting, severe diarrhea, copious sweating, postoperative complications, or shift of fluid into the extravascular space ("third spacing") or may be an effect of high altitude.[27] In severe burns, plasma loss leads to hemoconcentration.

Chronic relative erythrocytosis has been variously referred to as *Gaisböck syndrome*, *"stress" erythrocytosis*, or *spurious erythrocytosis*. Patients with relative erythrocytosis are typically male; the mean age at diagnosis is less than is seen in patients with polycythemia vera.[28] Associated features most commonly include hypertension (the most strongly associated finding) and smoking. Renal disease and alcohol abuse are also common.[29,30] It is probable that this syndrome is not a true clinical entity and includes a significant number of hematologically normal individuals whose values are at the high end of the normal distribution curve.[31] The optimal management of relative erythrocytosis is unknown. As noted previously, phlebotomy

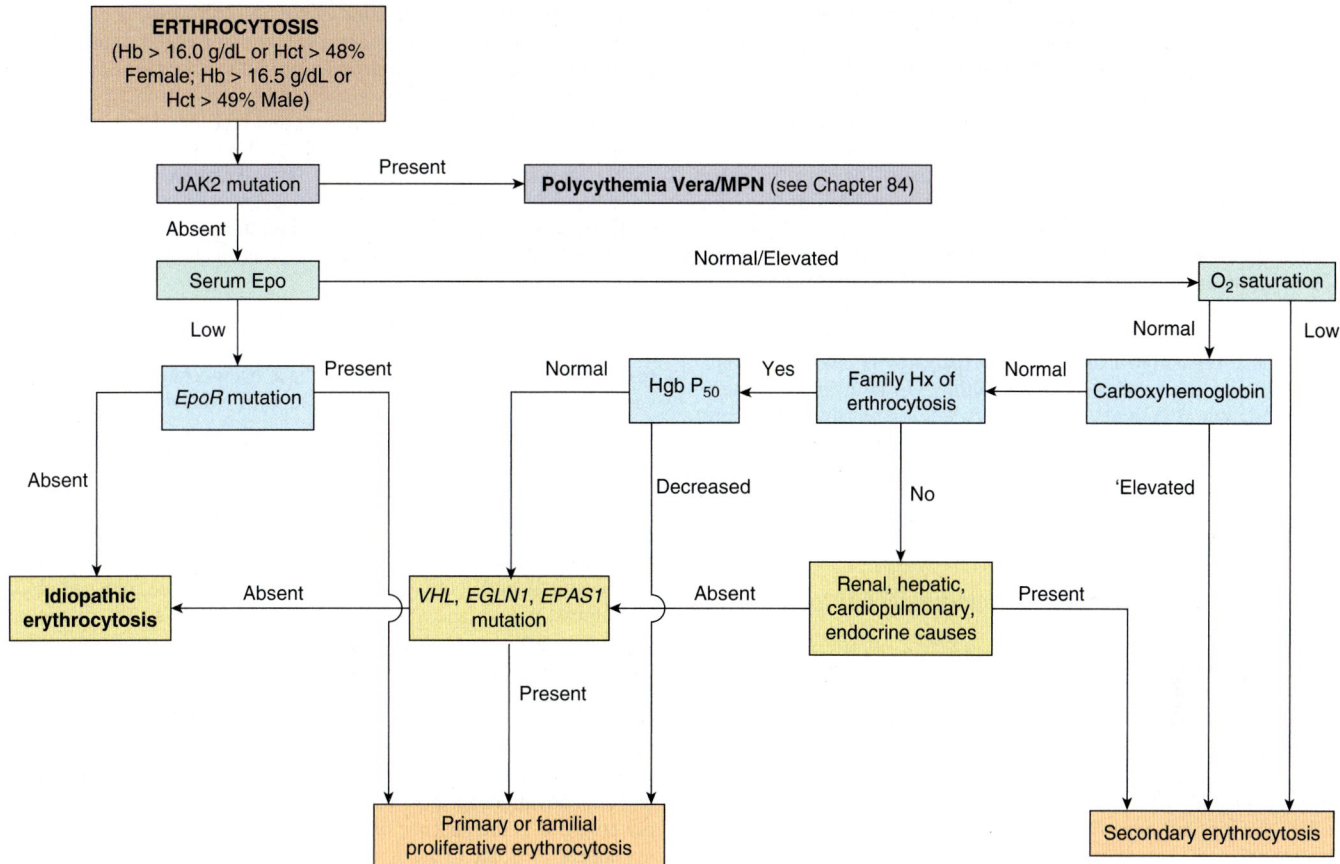

FIGURE 45.3 **Approach to patients with erythrocytosis.** *JAK2* mutation—testing for *JAK2* V617F or other mutations associated with polycythemia vera; low Epo—serum or plasma erythropoietin concentration less than the lower limit of normal; *EGLN1*, prolyl hydroxylase domain-containing protein 2 gene; *EPAS1*, hypoxia-inducible factor 2α gene; Epo, erythropoietin; *EpoR*, Epo receptor gene; Hb, hemoglobin concentration; Hb P$_{50}$, oxygen partial pressure at which Hb is 50% saturated; Hct, hematocrit; *JAK2*, Janus kinase 2 gene; MPN, myeloproliferative neoplasm; *VHL*, von Hippel Lindau protein gene.

Disorders of Red Blood Cells

Table 45.2. World Health Organization Criteria for Diagnosis of Polycythemia Vera

Major Criteria

1. Hb > 16.5 g/dL (or hematocrit > 49%) male; Hb > 16.0 g/dL (or hematocrit > 48%) female
   OR
   Increased RBC mass
2. Bone marrow biopsy showing hypercellularity for age with trilineage hematopoiesis (panmyelosis) including prominent erythroid, granule acidic, and megakaryocytic proliferation with pleomorphic mature megakaryocytes
3. *JAK2* V617F or *JAK2* exon 12 mutation

Minor Criterion

Subnormal serum erythropoietin level

Diagnosis

All three major criteria
   OR
The first two major criteria and the minor criterion[a]

Abbreviation: Hb, hemoglobin.
Adapted from Arber DA, Orazi A, Hasserjian R, et al. The 2016 revision to the World Health Organization classification of myeloid neoplasms and acute leukemia. *Blood.* 2016;127(20):2391-2405. Copyright © 2016 American Society of Hematology. With permission.
[a]If there is sustained erythrocytosis with Hb > 18.5 g/dL (or hematocrit > 55.5%) male; Hb > 16.5 g/dL (or hematocrit > 49.5%) female and both the third major criterion and the minor criterion are also present, then the diagnosis of polycythemia vera can be established without a bone marrow biopsy. However, this would not allow recognition of myelofibrosis at diagnosis, present in 20% of patients with polycythemia vera.

increases cerebral blood flow even in patients with relative erythrocytosis; whether it is of symptomatic benefit is less clear.[12]

Theoretical arguments can be made that contracting the blood volume further in these patients who already are normovolemic or slightly hypovolemic may impair tissue perfusion. Satisfactory control of hematocrit can be obtained in at least two-thirds of patients by reduction of excess weight, improved hypertension control, avoidance of diuretics, and reduction if not cessation of smoking.[28] Cytoreductive therapy is not indicated.

Some types of high-affinity Hbs (Heathrow, Pierre-Benite, and Rahere) may show relative erythrocytosis.[32]

ERYTHROCYTOSIS

Primary Erythrocytosis

Polycythemia Vera

Polycythemia vera is discussed in Chapter 83.

Primary Familial/Primary Proliferative Erythrocytosis

Familial or *hereditary erythrocytosis* is a term used to describe instances in which two or more members of a family have erythrocytosis, do not have polycythemia vera, and have no identifiable "secondary" causes. While responsible mutations have not been identified in the majority of cases studied, when mutations are found they occur in genes regulating the erythropoietin receptor signaling pathway, erythropoietin production, or oxygen-Hb interaction.[33,34]

Familial erythrocytosis is referred to as *primary* when it involves the erythropoietin receptor or the regulation of its signaling pathway. These cases are associated with decreased erythropoietin concentrations. Familial erythrocytosis associated with increased erythropoietin levels is referred to as *secondary familial erythrocytosis*.[35] Most of the molecular abnormalities associated with familial erythrocytosis also have been observed as nonfamilial sporadic cases. The term "*primary proliferative polycythemia (or erythrocytosis)*" has been used in the literature for nonfamilial mutations.

Primary familial erythrocytosis mutations have been reported mostly in the erythropoietin receptor gene (*EPORI*).[36] Mutations in the lymphocyte adaptor protein (LNK) gene have also been associated with primary familial and sporadic erythrocytosis.[37] LNK acts as a negative regulator of the JAK/STAT pathway in cytokine signaling: *LNK* mutations associated with erythrocytosis prevent this negative regulation.[33] Patients with primary familial erythrocytosis are at increased risk of thrombosis and other vascular mortality and are generally managed with phlebotomy. There is a concern that development of iron deficiency from phlebotomy may increase proerythropoietic signaling through the hypoxia-inducible factor (HIF) pathway (described in detail in Chapter 6).[12]

Secondary Erythrocytosis (Physiologically Appropriate [Hypoxic])

The hallmark of secondary erythrocytosis is that it is driven by erythropoietin. Insufficient oxygen supply to the tissues may result from any of the following, alone or in combination: (1) decreased ambient oxygen pressure (e.g., high altitude); (2) pulmonary diffusion or mixing abnormalities; (3) right-to-left cardiopulmonary shunts, as in cyanotic congenital heart disease; (4) hypoventilation; or (5) altered oxygen-carrying affinity of Hb. In all of these disorders, insufficient tissue oxygenation leads to increased erythropoietin production and consequent increase in RCM.

High-Altitude Erythrocytosis

Erythrocytosis develops at high altitudes because of the decreased oxygen tension. Mean Hb concentrations in ethnic Kyrgyz while living at high altitudes is 1.9 g/dL higher than low-altitude dwellers of the same ethnicity and country.[38] A sharp increase in erythropoietin production occurs within the first week of high-altitude exposure and is associated with mobilization of iron stores and evidence of iron-deficient erythropoiesis.[39] Mechanisms of adaptation to living at high altitude apparently are multiple and differ between ethnic groups.[40] Ethnic groups who have relocated to high altitudes comparatively recently (like the Han in Tibet) have more elevated Hb concentration than ethnic groups with a longer history in the region.[41]

The rapid ascent to high altitude is accompanied by symptoms of fatigue, dizziness, pulsating headache, anorexia, nausea and vomiting, insomnia, and irritability—a syndrome referred to as *acute mountain sickness* or *acute altitude disease*.[42] The symptoms first appear 6 to 12 hours after reaching 2500 m or higher but may be delayed for as many as 96 hours, suggesting that the pathogenesis represents more than simple hypoxia. Reported risk factors include previous history of acute mountain sickness, speed of ascent, lack of altitude acclimatization, the actual altitude attained, age less than 46 years, female gender, and history of migraines. Severe acute mountain sickness requires supplemental oxygen or descent to a lower altitude: cerebral edema may require dexamethasone, and pulmonary edema may require nifedipine or phosphodiesterase-5 inhibitors, followed by relocation to a lower altitude when stable.[42]

The pathogenesis of acute mountain sickness may involve hypoxia and subsequent excessive secretion of antidiuretic hormone and adrenal steroids with resulting fluid retention, increased blood volume, and finally cerebral edema or pulmonary congestion or both.[42,43] There is limited evidence supporting a genetic basis for susceptibility to acute mountain sickness.[44]

The events associated with acclimatization after arrival at high altitude are not understood completely but probably include the following:

- An increase in erythrocyte 2,3-diphosphoglycerate (DPG), also referred to as 2,3 bisphosphoglycerate, levels and a shift to the right in the oxygen-Hb dissociation curve, thus allowing better oxygen delivery to tissues despite decreased arterial oxygen saturation.[45]
- Increased erythropoietin production with subsequent increase in iron mobilization, reticulocytosis, and increase in RCM and blood volume.[46] Erythroferrone increases and hepcidin decreases rapidly with ascent to high altitude.[47,48] Since this results in iron-deficient erythropoiesis, administration of intravenous iron prior to ascent may protect against acute mountain sickness.[49]
- Correction of the initial excessive antidiuretic hormone and adrenal steroid secretion and return to the normal diurnal variation of plasma steroid levels.[43]

The final result is a new equilibrium at decreased oxygen saturation and carbon dioxide tension with increases in alveolar ventilation, respiratory frequency, and RCM.[50] These manifestations of acclimatization are quickly lost on descent to sea level, even after many years of residence at high altitude.

In some individuals, however, after a few or many years of good adaptation, arterial oxygen desaturation worsens and erythrocytosis becomes more severe. An incapacitating illness characterized by alveolar hypoventilation and known as *chronic mountain* or *altitude sickness* or *Monge disease*[51] then develops. It is characterized by diminished mental acuity, headaches, dyspnea, fatigue, reduced physical fitness, nausea and vomiting, decreased visual acuity, dizziness, tinnitus, vague or even excruciating pains in the extremities, paresthesias, and cough. If the condition advances, symptoms include incessant dyspnea, aphonia, profound lethargy, and even coma. The face is bluish violet or almost black, the eyelids are edematous and bluish, the sclerae are intensely colored by distended capillaries, the tongue is thick, the hands are enlarged and turgid, the fingers are clubbed, and dependent edema may be observed. The spleen and the liver are not enlarged in the absence of heart failure. Cardiac impairment does not appear until late in the disease course. Autopsies show evidence of pulmonary hypertension and brain and visceral vascular congestion, as well as pulmonary emboli.[52]

Erythrocytosis is more marked than in healthy residents of high altitudes, with hematocrits up to 84% and Hb values as high as 28.0 g/dL. MCV is normal or slightly increased, and the mean corpuscular Hb concentration is normal. Normal reticulocyte and leukocyte counts are usually observed. Hyperbilirubinemia as a result of unconjugated bilirubin may be pronounced. RBC turnover is greater in these individuals than in normal residents of high altitudes or in other patients with other causes of erythrocytosis. Platelet counts are usually normal or high, yet epistaxis is common, and hemoptysis, bleeding of the gums, and purpura may occur. The findings do not appear to be completely explainable by differences in erythropoietin production.[53,54]

It has been suggested that chronic mountain sickness is an exaggeration of the process of acclimatization and aging, because patients with chronic mountain sickness had Hb concentrations within the normally distributed values for large groups of native residents. Support for this suggestion comes from the observation that chronic lung disease increases the likelihood of chronic mountain sickness.[55] Chronic mountain sickness has not been reported to occur in natives of the Himalayas; this observation appears to reflect a common mutation in the hypoxia-sensing pathway prevalent in the population.[56] Investigation of selective gene expression in populations in whom chronic mountain sickness is prevalent may further enhance understanding of this syndrome.[57]

Phlebotomy with concurrent volume replacement may produce rapid symptomatic benefit but is not recommended for long-term management. Descent to sea level produces complete relief of symptoms, together with a pronounced reduction in the blood volume and restoration of normal blood counts. However, return to high elevation leads to recurrence.[52]

Cardiopulmonary Disease

A variety of diseases, such as chronic obstructive pulmonary disease, diffuse pulmonary infiltrates (fibrous or granulomatous), kyphoscoliosis, and multiple pulmonary emboli, lead to erythrocytosis as the result of inadequate oxygenation of the blood circulating through the lungs.

Not all patients with lung disease and decreased arterial oxygen saturation, however, have elevated Hb or hematocrit levels.[58] The reason for this suboptimal response to hypoxia is not clear and may involve defects in the hypoxia-inducible factor oxygen-sensing pathway.[59] If erythrocytosis is present, it is corrected by chronic oxygen administration.[60]

Vascular malformations in the lung may also be associated with erythrocytosis.[61] Pulmonary arteriovenous fistulae should be suspected when a murmur is heard in a lung field in association with erythrocytosis.

Chronic Cor Pulmonale

The clinical picture of chronic cor pulmonale varies, but oxygen deficiency with arterial desaturation and elevated pulmonary artery pressure is of central importance. Erythrocytosis with its associated increase in blood viscosity and volume appears to be the physiologic price of a compensatory mechanism progressively extended to the point at which it is more injurious than beneficial.[62,63]

Cyanotic Heart Disease

Marked degrees of erythrocytosis may be seen in patients with an uncorrected or incompletely corrected partial shunt of the blood from the pulmonary circuit. Hematocrit levels greater than 60% are not uncommon in these cases. The most frequent defects producing such erythrocytosis are pulmonary stenosis (usually with defective ventricular or atrial septum, patent foramen ovale, or patent ductus arteriosus), persistent truncus arteriosus, complete transposition of the great vessels, and the tetralogy of Fallot (pulmonary stenosis, defective ventricular septum, dextroposition of the aorta, and right ventricular hypertrophy). Individuals with such defects exhibit evidence of disturbed cardiorespiratory function, marked cyanosis, clubbing of the fingers and toes, and sometimes stunted growth. In much of the world, modern surgical techniques have substantially reduced the frequency of severe cyanotic heart disease, and severe erythrocytosis in congenital heart disease survivors is now uncommon.

Total plasma volume may be lower than normal, but the increase in RCM is so great that the total blood volume is usually higher than normal. Erythroid hyperplasia is observed in the marrow.[64]

The general consensus is that low oxygen tension resulting from shunting of unoxygenated blood through or around the lungs with consequent desaturation of the arterial blood stimulates erythropoietin production. With successful operative intervention, this value may be significantly corrected, with resolution of erythrocytosis.

Acquired Heart Disease

In 1901, Ayerza described a syndrome characterized clinically by slowly developing asthma, bronchitis, dyspnea, right-sided heart failure, and severe cyanosis with associated erythrocytosis resulting from pulmonary arterial hyperplasia, leading to pulmonary hypertension and right heart failure. In all forms of acquired heart disease, any erythrocytosis that may develop is correlated to some extent with the degree of cardiopulmonary decompensation. It is typically minimal. Erythrocytosis is reportedly accompanied by evidence of intensified erythropoiesis in the bone marrow, an increase in RCM, and some degree of macrocytosis.[65]

Hypoventilation Syndromes

Erythrocytosis is found occasionally in patients who exhibit no evidence of pulmonary disease or cardiovascular shunts. The primary defect in at least some of these patients appears to be an inadequate ventilatory drive from the respiratory center in the brain.[66] A similar defect has been reported in patients with the *Pickwickian syndrome*, so-called because of the description of Joe, the hypersomnolent fat boy, in Dickens's *The Pickwick Papers*.[67] Alveolar hypoventilation and erythrocytosis, however, do not develop in all obese individuals; it appears that only in the presence of an insensitive respiratory center does a massive panniculus limit respiratory function and result in alveolar hypoventilation, hypoxemia, and hypercapnia.[68] In some patients, the decreased ventilatory drive is of unknown cause or is a result of idiopathic disease of the medullary respiratory center (Ondine

curse)[66]; other etiologies include vascular thrombosis and previous encephalitis. In any case, the consequent hypoxemia results in elevated levels of erythropoietin and frequently marked erythrocytosis.

Patients with erythrocytosis and positional arterial oxygen desaturation have also been reported.[69] Obstructive sleep apnea, distinct from alveolar hypoventilation caused by loss of central respiratory drive, is rarely associated with erythrocytosis in the absence of another cause. While patients with obstructive sleep apnea have increased erythropoietin levels (presumably because of episodic erythropoietin secretion during apneic episodes), it has been postulated that inflammatory suppression of erythropoiesis and selective hemolysis of the most recently formed RBCs (neocytolysis; discussed in Chapter 42) prevents erythrocytosis.[70,71]

Abnormal Hemoglobins

Erythrocytosis Due to Inherited Abnormalities of Hemoglobin—Familial Secondary Erythrocytosis (Physiologically Appropriate)

Certain mutant Hbs are characterized by increased oxygen affinity. In this circumstance, oxygen is less readily released to tissues and erythropoietin production is increased (oxygen dissociation curve shifted to the left), leading to erythrocytosis. Since it is driven by erythropoietin, it is categorized as a secondary erythrocytosis. More than 200 high-affinity Hbs have been characterized, of which roughly half produce significant erythrocytosis.[72] Oxygen-Hb dissociation curves are shifted dramatically to the left in individuals carrying these abnormal Hbs. The degree of left shift can be quantified by determining the P_{50} (i.e., the oxygen pressure at which Hb is half saturated). The normal value in whole blood is 23 to 29 mm Hg at standard pH, temperature, CO_2 content, and barometric pressure. The whole-blood P_{50} is almost invariably decreased in patients with a high-affinity Hb; most values fall between 9 and 21 mm Hg. The approach to the diagnosis of high-affinity Hb variants, the characteristics of patients with representative mutations, and the molecular pathology are discussed in Chapter 36.

No treatment is indicated for most patients with high-affinity Hbs.[73] Their erythrocytosis is a compensation for a physiologic state and should be regarded as "normal for them." In the rare patient with high-affinity Hb with erythrocytosis and associated symptoms, phlebotomy may be used, but caution must be used to avoid lowering the hematocrit to a point at which oxygen delivery is impaired. A reasonable approach is to phlebotomize the individual patient to the highest hematocrit at which he/she is no longer symptomatic rather than to a specific number.[74,75] Certainly, reducing blood Hb concentrations to normal levels would be undesirable. Cytoreductive agents should not be used for treatment.

Acquired Abnormalities of Hemoglobin

Moderate elevations of carboxyhemoglobin in erythrocytes shift the oxygen dissociation curve to the left, decreasing the P_{50}. In heavy smokers, carboxyhemoglobin concentration may reach sufficiently high levels (4.0%-6.8%) to produce erythrocytosis.[76]

Familial Secondary Erythrocytosis due to Other Abnormalities of Hb/Oxygen Affinity (Physiologically Appropriate)

Familial defects in 2,3-DPG metabolism, for example, diphosphoglycerate mutase deficiency caused by autosomal recessive loss-of-function mutations in *BPGM*[77] or elevated erythrocyte adenosine triphosphate,[78] which would have the effect of shifting the oxygen dissociation curve to the left, provide other physiologically appropriate reasons for erythrocytosis. A specific pyruvate kinase mutation resulting in higher-than-normal enzyme activity and decreased 2,3-DPG causing erythrocytosis has been described in association with erythrocytosis.[79] Some specific *PIEZO1* mutations in hereditary xerocytosis are associated with erythrocytosis and a left-shifted oxygen dissociation curve.[80]

Secondary Erythrocytosis (Physiologically Inappropriate [Normoxic])

Unlike patients with physiologically appropriate secondary erythrocytosis, individuals with inappropriate erythrocytosis receive no benefit from the higher RBC concentrations. Treatment should be aimed at correcting the underlying disease; phlebotomy can be considered in the symptomatic patient.

Aberrant Erythropoietin Secretion

Erythrocytosis With Inappropriate Increased Erythropoietin Secretion

Erythrocytosis has been described in association with a variety of neoplasms, cysts, vascular abnormalities, and endocrinologic disorders. In the syndromes discussed in the preceding section, erythrocytosis was secondary to increased erythropoietin secretion as an appropriate physiologic response to tissue hypoxia. In this section, disorders in which erythropoietin-driven erythrocytosis bears no relation to physiologic requirements are reviewed.

Most of these disorders (listed in *Table 45.3*) are associated with neoplasms or structural abnormalities or inflammation of organs that normally produce erythropoietin, such as the kidney[109] and liver,[110] or in which erythropoietin production can be activated, such as the cerebellar vasculature,[92] leiomyomas,[95] or uterine fibroid tumors.[94] In many cases, increased erythropoietin levels can be detected in the circulation, in associated fluid as with renal cysts, or in the tissue itself. In the case of tumors or structural abnormalities associated with

erythrocytosis, resection or effective treatment is associated with correction of erythrocytosis. Some cases of cerebellar hemangiomas associated with erythrocytosis are associated with abnormalities of the von Hippel-Lindau signaling pathway.[111] Endocrinologic disorders may be associated with erythrocytosis, particularly Cushing syndrome, primary aldosteronism, and disorders associated with excess androgen secretion.

Erythrocytosis is also observed in patients after renal transplantation. This phenomenon is associated with elevated serum erythropoietin; the source of erythropoietin is presumed to be the transplant recipient's native kidneys. Effective therapeutic modalities include phlebotomy, angiotensin-converting enzyme inhibitors, and theophylline.[88]

There have been a number of reports describing small numbers of patients with human immunodeficiency virus infection and erythrocytosis. It is unclear if there is an actual pathophysiologic association or if this is coincidental.[107]

A syndrome of telangiectasias, elevated erythropoietin with erythrocytosis, monoclonal protein, perinephric fluid collections, and intrapulmonary shunting (TEMPI syndrome) has been described. Patients with this syndrome respond to myeloma therapy, such as bortezomib.[108]

Inherited gain-of-function mutations in the erythropoietin gene (*EPO*) leading to erythropoietin production out of proportion to hypoxia have been reported.[112]

Table 45.3. Disorders Associated With Normoxic Secondary Erythrocytosis

Renal Disease
Renal cell carcinoma[81]
Renal sarcoma[a,82]
Renal adenoma[a,82]
Renal hemangioma[a,82]
Wilms tumor[a,82]
Solitary renal cysts[83]
Polycystic kidney disease[84]
Hydronephrosis[85]
Horseshoe kidney[a,86]
Renal artery stenosis[a,87]
Postrenal transplantation[88]

Hepatic Disease
Hepatocellular carcinoma[89]
Hepatic hamartoma[a,82]
Hepatic metastases[a,82]
Hepatic angiosarcoma[a,90]
Hepatic angioma[a,90]
Viral hepatitis[a,91]

Other Neoplasms
Vascular cerebellar tumors[92]
Uterine leiomyomata[93]
Uterine fibroid tumors[a,94]
Cutaneous leiomyomata[a,95]
Meningioma[a,96]
Placental trophoblastic tumors[a,97]
Chronic lymphocytic leukemia[a,98]
Systemic amyloidosis[a,99]
Atrial myxoma[a,100]

Endocrine Disorders
Cushing syndrome[101]
Primary aldosteronism[102]
Virilizing ovarian tumors[103]
Gonadotropin-secreting pituitary adenoma[104]
Bartter syndrome[a,105]
Pheochromocytoma[a,106]

Other
Human immunodeficiency virus infection[a,107]
Telangiectasias, elevated erythropoietin with erythrocytosis, monoclonal protein, perinephric fluid collections, and intrapulmonary shunting (TEMPI) syndrome[108]

[a]Erythrocytosis infrequently reported.

Secondary Familial Erythrocytosis due to Abnormal Erythropoietin Regulation/Hypoxia Sensing

Mutations in the oxygen sensing pathway are the most common cause of secondary familial erythrocytosis without hypoxia. The most common target for abnormalities involves von Hippel Lindau protein (VHL). VHL stabilizes hypoxia-inducing factor (HIF)1α and HIF2α, inducing Epo production (see Chapter 6). VHL loss of function–driven erythrocytosis was described first among the people of the Chuvashia region of the former Soviet Union, although similar mutations and mechanisms have been described in other populations.[113,114] For that reason, VHL-associated familial erythrocytosis is sometimes referred to as Chuvash erythrocytosis (or polycythemia). *VHL* mutations are generally autosomal recessive. Increased sensitivity to erythropoietin in these patients appears to be mediated by loss of *JAK2* regulation of erythropoiesis.[115] Patients are at increased risk for thrombotic and vascular mortality, including pulmonary hypertension,[114,116] and are generally managed with phlebotomy, although there are data suggesting that phlebotomy in Chuvash erythrocytosis and in patients with the gain-of-function mutations discussed below may not reduce thrombotic risk.[117] Although mechanisms are not fully defined, it has been proposed that phlebotomy-induced iron deficiency, which increases EPO by increasing HIF and inhibiting prolyl hydroxylase domain-containing protein (PHD)-2 production, may contribute to thrombosis.[117] Studies in mouse models of *VHL* mutation-driven erythrocytosis suggest that HIF2α inhibitors may correct erythrocytosis and prevent pulmonary hypertension.[118] Other proteins and genes involved in the oxygen sensing pathway associated with familial erythrocytosis include gain-of-function mutations in the gene encoding HIF2α (*EPAS1*) and a loss-of-function mutation in the gene for PHD-2 (*EGLN1*), which normally downregulates erythropoietin production.[35] These mutations are both autosomal dominant. In a study using next-generation sequencing in 125 patients with otherwise unexplained (idiopathic) erythrocytosis, 45.6% of patients had at least one variant found in pathways regulating erythropoiesis, oxygen sensing, or oxygen transport. Of the 57 variants found,[32] were of either known (10/57) or probable functional significance (22/57), with the remainder being polymorphisms.[119]

Erythrocytosis in families with mutations in the manganese transport protein gene *SLC30A10* exhibit a syndrome of hepatic cirrhosis, dystonia, erythrocytosis, and hypermanganesemia. Erythropoietin production is induced by manganese.[120]

Drug-Induced Erythrocytosis

Anabolic and androgenic steroids may be abused by both recreational and professional athletes for the purposes of improving performance.[121] A consequence of androgen administration, either medicinal or extralegal, may be erythrocytosis.[122] In some cases, the degree of erythrocytosis may be severe.

Recombinant human erythropoietin has also been abused by athletes (particularly those in endurance sports) to increase the RCM and thus oxygen-carrying capacity. Other erythropoiesis-stimulating agents such as HIF regulators could also have the same effects.[123] As indicated earlier in *Figure 45.2*, this may backfire if the athlete becomes hypovolemic as a result of exertion. Stroke, accelerated hypertension, myocardial infarction, and venous thromboembolism can occur as complications. A perceived advantage of erythropoietin over androgens for this purpose is the difficulty of distinguishing natural endogenous erythropoietin from exogenous or induced erythropoietin as well as the lack of hepatic toxicity (compared with androgens). Newer molecular approaches that allow discrimination between exogenous recombinant erythropoietin and endogenous erythropoietin may make this practice less frequent.[123]

Sodium glucose cotransporter-2 (SGLT-2) inhibitors are new agents assuming a large role in the management of diabetes and hyperglycemia. SGLT-2 inhibitors can be associated with erythrocytosis, and higher hematocrit levels may contribute to their favorable cardiovascular effects.[124,125] While hemoconcentration due to increased diuresis contributes in part to the increased hematocrit levels observed, SGLT-2 inhibitors also induce increases in erythropoietin and changes in the hepcidin/erythroferrone axis that support erythrocytosis.[126,127]

Cobalt stabilizes HIF, increasing erythropoietin transcription.[128,129] Exposure to toxic levels of cobalt, either in the environment or ingested, can be associated with erythrocytosis.[130,131] It has also been abused by endurance athletes but has significant side effects that make it an unattractive option.[128]

Idiopathic Erythrocytosis

The term *idiopathic erythrocytosis* refers to patients who have erythrocytosis of unknown etiology after appropriate investigation. It would include most of the patients formerly categorized as "benign erythrocytosis." In reports from the 1990s to the present, this group is estimated consistently to contain 20% to 30% of patients evaluated for erythrocytosis.[69,132] Essentially it represents a failure to characterize all patients with erythrocytosis correctly, which in part reflects the limitations of current knowledge and tools.

Patients remaining in this category after molecular investigation probably represent a mixed bag, including early polycythemia vera, mild secondary erythrocytosis, and normal individuals at the higher end of the bell-shaped curve for RCM,[30] and a cautious approach to management is warranted. Observation may be the most reasonable intervention. As molecular understanding of erythrocytosis increases, it is hoped that this will become an entity of declining frequency.[133]

References

1. Prchal JT, Gordeuk VR. HIF-2 inhibitor, erythrocytosis, and pulmonary hypertension. *Blood.* 2021;137(18):2424-2425.
2. Finch CA, Lenfant C. Oxygen transport in man. *N Engl J Med.* 1972;286(8):407-415.
3. Harrison BD, Stokes TC. Secondary polycythaemia: its causes, effects and treatment. *Br J Dis Chest.* 1982;76(4):313-340.
4. Stanzani Maserati M. Migraine attacks, aura, and polycythemia: a vasculoneural pathogenesis? *J Neural Transm.* 2011;118(4):545-547.
5. Chien S, Gallick S. Rheology in normal individuals and polycythemia vera. In: Wasserman LR, ed. *Polycythemia Vera and the Myeloproliferative Disorders.* WB Saunders; 1995:114-129.
6. Pirofsky B. The determination of blood viscosity in man by a method based on Poiseuille's law. *J Clin Invest.* 1953;32(4):292-298.
7. Wells RE, Jr, Merrill EW. The variability of blood viscosity. *Am J Med.* 1961;31:505-509.
8. Milligan DW, MacNamee R, Roberts BE, Davies JA. The influence of iron-deficient indices on whole blood viscosity in polycythaemia. *Br J Haematol.* 1982;50:467-473.
9. Brandão MM, Castro Mde L, Fontes A, Cesar CL, Costa FF, Saad ST. Impaired red cell deformability in iron deficient subjects. *Clin Hemorheol Microcirc.* 2009;43(3):217-221.
10. Thomas DJ, du Boulay GH, Marshall J, et al. Cerebral blood-flow in polycythaemia. *Lancet.* 1977;2(8030):161-163.
11. Thomas DJ, Marshall J, Ross Russell RW, et al. Effect of haematocrit on cerebral blood-flow in man. *Lancet.* 1977;2:941-943.
12. Humphrey PR, Michael J, Pearson TC. Management of relative polycythaemia: studies of cerebral blood flow and viscosity. *Br J Haematol.* 1980;46(3):427-433.
13. Kiraly JF, Feldmann JE, Wheby MS. Hazards of phlebotmy in polycythemic patients with cardiovascular disease. *J Am Med Assoc.* 1976;236:2080-2081.
14. Murray JF, Gold P, Johnson BL, Jr. The circulatory effects of hematocrit variations in normovolemic and hypervolemic dogs. *J Clin Invest.* 1963;42:1150-1159.
15. Metcalfe J, Dhindsa DS, Edwards MJ, Mourdjinis A. Decreased affinity of blood for oxygen in patients with low-output heart failure. *Circ Res.* 1969;25(1):47-51.
16. Chetty KG, Light RW, Stansbury DW, Milne N. Exercise performance of polycythemic chronic obstructive pulmonary disease patients. Effect of phlebotomies. *Chest.* 1990;98(5):1073-1077.
17. Castle WB, Jandl JH. Blood viscosity and blood volume: opposing influences upon oxygen transport in polycythemia. *Semin Hematol.* 1966;3:193-198.
18. Pearson TC, Messinezy M. The diagnostic criteria of polycythemia rubra vera. *Leuk Lymphoma.* 1996;22(suppl 1):87-93.
19. Djulbegovic B, Hadley T, Joseph G. A new algorithim for the diagnosis of polycythemia. *Am Fam Physician.* 1991;44:113-120.
20. Tefferi A, Thiele J, Orazi A, et al. Proposals and rationale for revision of the World Health Organization diagnostic criteria for polycythemia vera, essential thrombocythemia, and primary myelofibrosis: recommendations from an ad hoc international expert panel. *Blood.* 2007;110:1092-1097.
21. Baloch NU, Bikak M, Rehman A, Rahman O. Recognition and management of idiopathic systemic capillary leak syndrome: an evidence-based review. *Expert Rev Cardiovasc Ther.* 2018;16(5):331-340.
22. Arber DA, Orazi A, Hasserjian R, et al. The 2016 revision to the World Health Organization classification of myeloid neoplasms and acute leukemia. *Blood.* 2016;127(20):2391-2405.
23. Ethier V, Sirhan S, Olney HJ, Busque L. The 2016 WHO criteria for the diagnosis of polycythemia vera: benefits and potential risks (e-letter). *Blood.* 2016;127(20):2391-2405.
24. Stein BL, Oh ST, Berenzon D, et al. Polycythemia vera: an appraisal of the biology and management 10 years after the discovery of JAK2 V617F. *J Clin Oncol.* 2015;33(33):3953-3960.
25. Schnittger S, Bacher U, Haferlach C, et al. Detection of JAK2 exon 12 mutations in 15 patients with JAK2V617F negative polycythemia vera. *Haematologica.* 2009;94(3):414-418.
26. Loscocco GG, Guglielmelli P, Vannucchi AM. Impact of mutational profile on the management of myeloproliferative neoplasms: a short review of the emerging data. *OncoTargets Ther.* 2020;13:12367-12382.
27. Gupta N, Ashraf MZ. Exposure to high altitude: a risk factor for venous thromboembolism? *Semin Thromb Hemost.* 2012;38(2):156-163.
28. Messinezy M, Pearson TC. Apparent polycythaemia: diagnosis, pathogenesis and management. *Eur J Haematol.* 1993;51:125-131.
29. Krishnamoorthy P, Gopalakrishnan A, Mittal V, et al. Gaisböck syndrome (polycythemia and hypertension) revisited: results from the national inpatient sample database. *J Hypertens.* 2018;36(12):2424-2424.
30. Messinezy M, Pearson TC. A retrospective study of apparent and relative polycythaemia: associated factors and early outcome. *Clin Lab Haematol.* 1990;12:121-129.
31. Brown SM, Gilbert HS, Krauss S, Wasserman LR. Spurious (relative) polycythemia: a nonexistent disease. *Am J Med.* 1971;50(2):200-207.
32. Beard ME, Potter HC, Spearing RL, Brennan SO. Haemoglobin Pierre-Benite--a high affinity variant associated with relative polycythaemia. *Clin Lab Haematol.* 2001;23(6):407-409.
33. McMullin MF. Diagnostic workflow for hereditary erythrocytosis and thrombocytosis. *Hematology.* 2019;2019(1):391-396.
34. Bento C, Almeida H, Maia TM, et al. Molecular study of congenital erythrocytosis in 70 unrelated patients revealed a potential causal mutation in less than half of the cases (Where is/are the missing gene(s)?). *Eur J Haematol.* 2013;91(4):361-368.
35. Bento C, Percy MJ, Gardie B, et al. Genetic basis of congenital erythrocytosis: mutation update and online databases. *Hum Mutat.* 2014;35(1):15-26.
36. de la Chapelle A, Sistonen P, Lehaslaiho H, Ikkala E, Juvomen E. Familial erythrocytosis genetically linked to erythropoietin receptor gene. *Lancet.* 1993;1:82-84.
37. McMullin MF, Cario H. LNK mutations and myeloproliferative disorders. *Am J Hematol.* 2016;91(2):248-251.
38. Fiori G, Facchini F, Ismagulov O, Ismagulova A, Tarazona-Santos E, Pettener D. Lung volume, chest size, and hematological variation in low-, medium-, and high-altitude central Asian populations. *Am J Phys Anthropol.* 2000;113(1):47-59.
39. Richalet JP, Souberbielle JC, Antezana AM, et al. Control of erythropoiesis in humans during prolonged exposure to the altitude of 6,542 m. *Am J Physiol.* 1994;266(3 pt 2):R756-R764.
40. Ronen R, Zhou D, Bafna V, Haddad GG. The genetic basis of chronic mountain sickness. *Physiology.* 2014;29(6):403-412.
41. Niermeyer S, Yang P, ShanminaDrolkar, Zhuang J, Moore LG. Arterial oxygen saturation in Tibetan and Han infants born in Lhasa, Tibet. *N Engl J Med.* 1995;333(19):1248-1252.
42. Luks AM, Swenson ER, Bärtsch P. Acute high-altitude sickness. *Eur Respir Rev.* 2017;26(143):160096.
43. Woods DR, Stacey M, Hill N, de Alwis N. Endocrine aspects of high altitude acclimatization and acute mountain sickness. *J Roy Army Med Corps.* 2011;157(1):33-37.

44. MacInnis MJ, Wang P, Koehle MS, Rupert JL. The genetics of altitude tolerance: the evidence for inherited susceptibility to acute mountain sickness. *J Occup Environ Med.* 2011;53(2):159-168.

45. Clench J, Ferrell RE, Schull WJ. Effect of chronic altitude hypoxia on hematologic and glycolytic parameters. *Am J Physiol.* 1982;242(5):R447-R451.

46. Faura J, Ramos J, Reynafarje C, English E, Finne P, Finch CA. Effect of altitude on erythropoiesis. *Blood.* 1969;33(5):668-676.

47. Gassmann M, Muckenthaler MU. Adaptation of iron requirement to hypoxic conditions at high altitude. *J Appl Physiol.* 2015;119(12):1432-1440.

48. Emrich IE, Scheuer A, Wagenpfeil S, Ganz T, Heine GH. Increase of plasma erythroferrone levels during high-altitude exposure: a sub-analysis of the TOP OF HOMe study. *Am J Hematol.* 2021;96(5):E179-E181.

49. Talbot NP, Smith TG, Privat C, et al. Intravenous iron supplementation may protect against acute mountain sickness: a randomized, double-blinded, placebo-controlled trial. *High Alt Med Biol.* 2011;12(3):265-269.

50. Stuber T, Scherrer U. Circulatory adaptation to long-term high altitude exposure in Aymaras and Caucasians. *Prog Cardiovasc Dis.* 2010;52(6):534-539.

51. Monge CC, Whittembury J. Chronic mountain sickness. *Johns Hopkins Med J.* 1976;139(suppl):87-89.

52. Villafuerte FC, Corante N. Chronic mountain sickness: clinical aspects, etiology, management, and treatment. *High Alt Med Biol.* 2016;17(2):61-69.

53. Painschab MS, Malpartida GE, Dávila-Roman VG, et al. Association between serum concentrations of hypoxia inducible factor responsive proteins and excessive erythrocytosis in high altitude Peru. *High Alt Med Biol.* 2015;16(1):26-33.

54. Crawford JE, Amaru R, Song J, et al. Natural selection on genes related to cardiovascular health in high-altitude adapted Andeans. *Am J Hum Genet.* 2017;101(5):752-767.

55. Cogo A, Fischer R, Schoene R. Respiratory diseases and high altitude. *High Alt Med Biol.* 2004;5(4):435-444.

56. Tashi T, Reading NS, Shestakova A, et al. Tibetan gain-of-function variant of prolyl hydroxylase 2 (EGLN1) and selected SNPs of HIF-2-alpha (EPAS1) are associated with lower hemoglobin values in Tibetans. *Blood.* 2015;126(23):3332.

57. Villafuerte FC. New genetic and physiological factors for excessive erythrocytosis and Chronic Mountain Sickness. *J Appl Physiol.* 2015;119(12):1481-1486.

58. Tsantes A, Bonovas S, Tassiopoulos S, et al. A comparative study of the role of erythropoietin in the pathogenesis of deficient erythropoiesis in idiopathic pulmonary fibrosis as opposed to chronic obstructive pulmonary disease. *Med Sci Monit.* 2005;11(4):Cr177-Cr181.

59. Selfridge AC, Cavadas MA, Scholz CC, et al. Hypercapnia suppresses the HIF-dependent adaptive response to hypoxia. *J Biol Chem.* 2016;291(22):11800-11808.

60. Ekström M, Ringbaek T. Which patients with moderate hypoxemia benefit from long-term oxygen therapy? Ways forward. *Int J Chronic Obstr Pulm Dis.* 2018;13:231-235.

61. Pick A, Deschamps C, Stanson AW. Pulmonary arteriovenous fistula: presentation, diagnosis, and treatment. *World J Surg.* 1999;23(11):1118-1122.

62. Wallis PJ, Cunningham J, Few JD, Newland AC, Empey DW. Effects of packed cell volume reduction on renal haemodynamics and the renin-angiotensin-aldosterone system in patients with secondary polycythaemia and hypoxic cor pulmonale. *Clin Sci (Lond).* 1986;70(1):81-90.

63. Wallis PJ, Skehan JD, Newland AC, Wedzicha JA, Mills PG, Empey DW. Effects of erythrapheresis on pulmonary haemodynamics and oxygen transport in patients with secondary polycythaemia and cor pulmonale. *Clin Sci (Lond).* 1986;70(1):91-98.

64. Zabala LM, Guzzetta NA. Cyanotic congenital heart disease (CCHD): focus on hypoxemia, secondary erythrocytosis, and coagulation alterations. *Paediatr Anaesth.* 2015;25(10):981-989.

65. Mazzei JA, Mazzei ME. A tribute: abel Ayerza and pulmonary hypertension. *Eur Respir Rev.* 2011;20(122):220-221.

66. Zaidi S, Gandhi J, Vatsia S, Smith NL, Khan SA. Congenital central hypoventilation syndrome: an overview of etiopathogenesis, associated pathologies, clinical presentation, and management. *Auton Neurosci.* 2018;210:1-9.

67. Bickelmann AG, Burwell CS, Robin ED, Whaley RD. Extreme obesity associated with alveolar hypoventilation; a Pickwickian syndrome. *Am J Med.* 1956;21(5):811-818.

68. Lin CK, Lin CC. Work of breathing and respiratory drive in obesity. *Respirology.* 2012;17(3):402-411.

69. Messinezy M, Sawyer B, Westwood NB, Pearson TC. Idiopathic erythrocytosis - additional new study techniques suggest a heterogenous group. *Eur J Haematol.* 1994;53:163-167.

70. Song J, Sundar KM, Horvathova M, et al. Normal hemoglobin concentrations in obstructive sleep apnea and associated neocytolysis-mediated hemolysis and inflammation mediated suppression of expected elevated hemoglobin. *Blood.* 2019;134(suppl 1):3507.

71. Gangaraju R, Sundar KM, Song J, Prchal JT. Polycythemia is rarely caused by obstructive sleep apnea. *Blood.* 2016;128(22):2444.

72. Wajcman H, Galacteros F. Hemoglobins with high oxygen affinity leading to erythrocytosis. New variants and new concepts. *Hemoglobin.* 2005;29(2):91-106.

73. Gangat N, Oliveira JL, Hoyer JD, Patnaik MM, Pardanani A, Tefferi A. High-oxygen-affinity hemoglobinopathy-associated erythrocytosis: clinical outcomes and impact of therapy in 41 cases. *Am J Hematol.* 2021;96(12):1647-1654.

74. McMullin MF. Congenital erythrocytosis. *Int J Lab Hematol.* 2016;38(suppl 1):59-65.

75. Grace RJ, Gover PA, Treacher DF, Heard SE, Pearson TC. Venesection in haemoglobin Yakima, a high oxygen affinity haemoglobin. *Clin Lab Haematol.* 1992;14(3):195-199.

76. Moore-Gillon J. Smoking—a major cause of polycythemia. *J R Soc Med.* 1988;81(7):431.

77. Cartier P, Labie D, Leroux JP, Najman A, Demaugre F. Familial diphosphoglycerate mutase deficiency: hematological and biochemical study. *Nouv Rev Fr Hematol.* 1972;12(3):269-287.

78. Zurcher C, Loos JA, Prins HK. Hereditary high ATP content of human erythrocytes. *Folia Haematologica Leipzig.* 1965;83:366.

79. Rosa R, Max-Audit I, Izrael V, Beuzard Y, Thillet J, Rosa J. Hereditary pyruvate kinase abnormalities associated with erythrocytosis. *Am J Hematol.* 1981;10(1):47-55.

80. Filser M, Giansily-Blaizot M, Grenier M, et al. Increased incidence of germline PIEZO1 mutations in individuals with idiopathic erythrocytosis. *Blood.* 2021;137(13):1828-1832.

81. Sufrin G, Mirand EA, Moore RH. Hormones in renal cancer. *J Urol.* 1977;117:433-438.

82. Souid AK, Dubansky AS, Richman P, Sadowitz PD. Polcythemia: a review article and case report of erythrocytosis secondary to Wilm's tumor. *Pediatr Hematol Oncol.* 1993;10:215-221.

83. Pejcic T, Hadzi-Djokic J, Markovic B, Naumovic R. Resolving erythrocytosis and hypertension after open surgical extirpation of giant renal cyst measuring 30 cm: case report. *Ren Fail.* 2011;33(2):249-251.

84. Ito K, Asano T, Tominaga S, Yoshii H, Sawazaki H, Asano T. Erythropoietin production in renal cell carcinoma and renal cysts in autosomal dominant polycystic kidney disease in a chronic dialysis patient with polycythemia: a case report. *Oncol Lett.* 2014;8(5):2032-2036.

85. Madeb R, Knopf J, Nicholson C, Rabinowitz R, Erturk E. Secondary polycythemia caused by ureteropelvic junction obstruction successfully treated by laparoscopic nephrectomy. *Urology.* 2006;67(6):1291.e1-1291.e3.

86. Bailey RR, Shand BI, Walker RJ. Reversible erythrocytosis in a patient with a hydronephrotic horseshoe kidney. *Nephron.* 1995;70:104-105.

87. Bhadauria D, Sharma RK, Kaul A, et al. A rare clinical syndrome of refractory secondary hypertension, renal artery stenosis and erythrocytosis. *NDT Plus.* 2011;4(3):175-177.

88. Vlahakos DV, Marathias KP, Agroyannis B, Madias NE. Posttransplant erythrocytosis. *Kidney Int.* 2003;63(4):1187-1194.

89. McFadzean AJ, Todd D, Tso SC. Erythrocytosis associated with hepatocellular carcinoma. *Blood.* 1967;29(5):808-811.

90. Rothman SA, Savage RA, Paul P. Erythropoietin dependent erythrocytosis associated with hepatic angioscarcoma. *J Surg Oncol.* 1982;20:105-108.

91. Bank H, Passwell J. Absolute erythrocytosis in early infectious hepatitis. *Med Chir Dig.* 1974;3:321-323.

92. So CC, Ho LC. Polycythemia secondary to cerebellar hemangioblastoma. *Am J Hematol.* 2002;71(4):346-347.

93. Ossias AL, Zanjani ED, Zalusky R, Estren S, Wasserman LR. Case report: studies on the mechanism of erythrocytosis associated with a uterine fibromyoma. *Br J Haematol.* 1973;25(2):179-185.

94. Takkar D, Kumar A. Polycythemia associated with uterine fibroid. *Indian J Med Sci.* 1994;48:144-146.

95. Venencie PY, Puissant A, Boffa GA, Sohier J, Duperrat B. Multiple cutaneous leiomyomata and erythrocytosis with demonstration of erythropoietic activity in the cutaneous leiomyomata. *Br J Dermatol.* 1982;107(4):483-486.

96. Bruneval P, Sassy C, Mayeux P, et al. Erythropoietin synthesis by tumor cells in a case of menigioma associated with erythrocytosis. *Blood.* 1993;81:1593-1597.

97. Brewer CA, Adelson MD, Elder RC. Erythrocytosis associated with a placental trophoblastic tumor. *Obstet Gynecol.* 1992;79:846-849.

98. Ballard HS, Kouri Y. The association of erythrocytosis and chronic lymphocytic leukemia. *Cancer.* 1992;70:2431-2435.

99. Nagasawa T, Yanagisawa H, Hasegawa Y, Kanma H, Abe T. Polycythemia associated with primary systemic amyloidosis: elevated levels of hemopoietic factors and cytokines. *Am J Hematol.* 1993;43(1):57-60.

100. Siggillino JJ, Crawley CJ, Clauss RH, Reed GE, Tice DA. Myxoma of the right atrium with polycythemia. *Arch Intern Med.* 1963;111:178-183.

101. Gottschalk RG, Furth J. Polycythemia with features of Cushing's syndrome produced by luteomas. *Acta Haematol.* 1951;5(2):100-123.

102. Mann DL, Gallagher NI, Donati RM. Erythrocytosis and primary aldosteronism. *Ann Intern Med.* 1967;66(2):335-340.

103. Kozan P, Chalasani S, Handelsman DJ, Pike AH, Crawford BA. A Leydig cell tumor of the ovary resulting in extreme hyperandrogenism, erythrocytosis, and recurrent pulmonary embolism. *J Clin Endocrinol Metab.* 2014;99(1):12-17.

104. Ceccato F, Occhi G, Regazzo D, et al. Gonadotropin secreting pituitary adenoma associated with erythrocytosis: case report and literature review. *Hormones (Basel).* 2014;13(1):131-139.

105. Erkelens DW, Statius van Eps LW. Bartter's syndrome and erythrocytosis. *Am J Med.* 1973;55(5):711-719.

106. Rezkalla MA, Rizk SN, Ryan JJ. Pheochromocytoma associated with polycythemia: case report. *S D J Med.* 1995;48:349-351.

107. Koduri PR, Sherer R, Teter C. Polycythemia in patients infected with human immunodeficiency virus-1. *Am J Hematol.* 2000;64:80-81.

108. Jasim S, Mahmud G, Bastani B, Fesler M. Subcutaneous bortezomib for treatment of TEMPI syndrome. *Clin Lymphoma Myeloma Leuk.* 2014;14(6):e221-e223.

109. Leung N. Hematologic manifestations of kidney disease. *Semin Hematol.* 2013;50(3):207-215.

110. Muta H, Funakoshi A, Baba T, et al. Gene expression of erythropoietin in hepatocellular carcinoma. *Intern Med.* 1994;33:427-431.

111. Olschwang S, Richard S, Boisson C, Giraud S, Laurent-Puig P. Germline mutation profile of the VHL gene in von Hippel–Lindau disease and in sporadic hemangioblastoma. *Hum Mutat.* 1998;12:424.

112. Zmajkovic J, Lundberg P, Nienhold R, et al. A gain-of-function mutation in *EPO* in familial erythrocytosis. *N Engl J Med.* 2018;378(10):924-930.

113. Sergeyeva A, Gordeuk VR, Tokarev YN, Sokol L, Prchal JF, Prchal JP. Congenital polycythemia in Chuvashia. *Blood.* 1997;89:2148-2154.

114. Sarangi S, Lanikova L, Kapralova K, et al. The homozygous VHL(D126N) missense mutation is associated with dramatically elevated erythropoietin levels, consequent polycythemia, and early onset severe pulmonary hypertension. *Pediatr Blood Cancer.* 2014;61(11):2104-2106.

115. Russell RC, Sufan RI, Zhou B, et al. Loss of JAK2 regulation via a heterodimeric VHL-SOCS1 E3 ubiquitin ligase underlies Chuvash polycythemia. *Nat Med.* 2011;17(7):845-853.

116. Gordeuk VR, Prchal JT. Vascular complications in Chuvash polycythemia. *Semin Thromb Hemost.* 2006;32(3):289-294.

117. Gordeuk VR, Miasnikova GY, Sergueeva AI, et al. Thrombotic risk in congenital erythrocytosis due to up-regulated hypoxia sensing is not associated with elevated hematocrit. *Haematologica.* 2020;105(3):e87-e90.

118. Ghosh MC, Zhang DL, Ollivierre WH, et al. Therapeutic inhibition of HIF-2alpha reverses polycythemia and pulmonary hypertension in murine models of human diseases. *Blood.* 2021;137(18):2509-2519.

119. Camps C, Petousi N, Bento C, et al. Gene panel sequencing improves the diagnostic work-up of patients with idiopathic erythrocytosis and identifies new mutations. *Haematologica.* 2016;101(11):1306-1318.

120. Tuschl K, Clayton PT, Gospe SM, Jr, et al. Syndrome of hepatic cirrhosis, dystonia, polycythemia, and hypermanganesemia caused by mutations in SLC30A10, a manganese transporter in man. *Am J Hum Genet.* 2012;90(3):457-466.

121. Sagoe D, Pallesen S. Androgen abuse epidemiology. *Curr Opin Endocrinol Diabetes Obes.* 2018;25(3):185-194.

122. Anawalt BD. Diagnosis and management of anabolic androgenic steroid use. *J Clin Endocrinol Metab.* 2019;104(7):2490-2500.

123. Salamin O, Kuuranne T, Saugy M, Leuenberger N. Erythropoietin as a performance-enhancing drug: its mechanistic basis, detection, and potential adverse effects. *Mol Cell Endocrinol.* 2018;464:75-87.

124. Gupta R, Gupta A, Shrikhande M, Tyagi K, Ghosh A, Misra A. Marked erythrocytosis during treatment with sodium glucose cotransporter-2 inhibitors-report of two cases. *Diabetes Res Clin Pract.* 2020;162:108127.

125. Packer M. Critical examination of mechanisms underlying the reduction in heart failure events with SGLT2 inhibitors: identification of a molecular link between their actions to stimulate erythrocytosis and to alleviate cellular stress. *Cardiovasc Res.* 2021;117(1):74-84.

126. Ghanim H, Abuaysheh S, Hejna J, et al. Dapagliflozin suppresses hepcidin and increases erythropoiesis. *J Clin Endocrinol Metab.* 2020;105(4):dgaa057.

127. Mazer CD, Hare GMT, Connelly PW, et al. Effect of empagliflozin on erythropoietin levels, iron stores, and red blood cell morphology in patients with Type 2 diabetes mellitus and coronary artery disease. *Circulation.* 2020;141(8):704-707.

128. Ebert B, Jelkmann W. Intolerability of cobalt salt as erythropoietic agent. *Drug Test Anal.* 2014;6(3):185-189.

129. Schuster SJ, Badiavas EV, Costa-Giomi P, Weinmann R, Erslev AJ, Caro J. Stimulation of erythropoietin gene transcription during hypoxia and cobalt exposure. *Blood.* 1989;73(1):13-16.

130. Jefferson JA, Escudero E, Hurtado ME, et al. Excessive erythrocytosis, chronic mountain sickness, and serum cobalt levels. *Lancet.* 2002;359(9304):407-408.

131. Mercier G, Patry G. Quebec beer-drinkers' cardiomyopathy: clinical signs and symptoms. *Can Med Assoc J.* 1967;97(15):884-888.

132. Jalowiec KAA, Vrotniakaite-Bajerciene K, Frey N, et al. JAK2-negative polycythemia: underlying causes, including novel variants of uncertain significance - real life data of 10 years from a tertiary reference center. *Blood.* 2021;138(suppl 1):2003.

133. Blacklock HA, Royle GA. Idiopathic erythrocytosis—a declining entity. *Br J Haematol.* 2001;115(4):774-781.

Index